EMERGENCY MEDICINE

A Comprehensive Review

Third Edition

EMERGENCY MEDICINE
A Comprehensive Review

Third Edition

Editors

Thomas Clarke Kravis, MD
Medical Director
Continental Rehabilitation Hospital
San Diego, California
Associate Medical Director
Emergency Services
CompHealth
Salt Lake City, Utah

Carmen Germaine Warner, MSN, RN, FAAN
Consultant, Community Health Systems,
Emergency Care, and Publishing
Coordinating Editor, Topics in Emergency Medicine
Leucadia, California

Lenworth M. Jacobs, Jr., MD, MPH, FACS
Director, Emergency Medicine
Trauma and LIFE STAR Program
Hartford Hospital
Hartford, Connecticut
Professor of Surgery
University of Connecticut School of Medicine
Farmington, Connecticut

Raven Press ❦ New York

Raven Press, Ltd., 1185 Avenue of the Americas, New York, New York 10036

© 1993 by Raven Press, Ltd. All rights reserved. This book is protected by copyright. No part of it may be reproduced, stored in a retrieval system, or transmitted, in any form or by any means, electronic, mechanical, photocopy, or recording, or otherwise, without the prior written permission of the publisher.

Made in the United States of America

Library of Congress Cataloging-in-Publication Data

Emergency medicine : a comprehensive review / editors, Thomas Clarke
    Kravis, Carmen Germaine Warner, Lenworth M. Jacobs, Jr. — 3rd ed.
       p.   cm.
    Includes bibliographical references and index.
    ISBN 0-7817-0045-0
    1. Emergency medicine.   I. Kravis, Thomas Clarke.   II. Warner,
Carmen Germaine, 1941– . III. Jacobs, Lenworth M.
     [DNLM: 1. Emergency Medical Services.   2. Emergency Medicine.
3. Emergencies.   WB 105 E55 1993]
RC86.7.E585   1993
616.02′5—dc20
DNLM/DLC
for Library of Congress   93-3974
                                                                                                                    CIP

    The material contained in this volume was submitted as previously unpublished material, except in the instances in which credit has been given to the source from which some of the illustrative material was derived.
    Great care has been taken to maintain the accuracy of the information contained in the volume. However, neither Raven Press nor the editors can be held responsible for errors or for any consequences arising from the use of the information contained herein.
    Materials appearing in this book prepared by individuals as part of their official duties as U.S. Government employees are not covered by the above-mentioned copyright.

9 8 7 6 5 4 3 2 1

*To
Mavourneen*

T.C.K.

*To
Dorothy Loreen Warner (1913–1992), my mother,
who taught me the value of completing any task,
not as others would desire it,
but as I would believe in it.*

C.G.W.

*To
Jennifer, a superb human being,
a wonderful flight nurse
who really cared for the patients
and was an inspiration to all of us.*

L.M.J.

Contents

Contributing Authors	xiv
Foreword Richard L. Stennes, MD, FACEP	xxi
Foreword Mildred K. Fincke, RN, BSN	xxiii
Foreword Denis J. Kollar, MD, FACEP	xxiv
Preface to the Second Edition	xxv
Preface	xxvii
Acknowledgments	xxviii

Section I
ORGANIZATION AND DELIVERY OF EMERGENCY MEDICAL CARE

1 Prehospital Emergency Medical Services 1
Barbara Bennett Jacobs, RN, BSN, MPH
Lenworth M. Jacobs, Jr., MD, MPH, FACS

2 Disaster Management 31
Glenn W. Mitchell, MD, MPH, FACEP

3 Emergency Care and the Law 39
Robert W. Heilig, RN, MPA, Esq

4 Hospital Care 45
Eileen Whalen, RN, BSN
Robert W. Heilig, RN, MPA, Esq

5 Quality Assurance/Quality Improvement for the Emergentologist 53
R.S. Venable, MD, FAAFP, FACEP

Section II
SHOCK AND TRAUMA

6 Shock 65
Mark Allen Shaffer, MD, FACEP
Jacek B. Franaszek, MD, FACEP

7 Management of the Multisystem-Injured Patient 93
Lenworth M. Jacobs, Jr., MD, MPH, FACS
Barbara Bennett Jacobs, RN, BSN, MPH
William Kantor, MD

| 8 | Transfusions | 115 |

Frederick B. Epstein, MD, FACEP

| 9 | Emergency Wound Management | 137 |

Davis Cracroft, MD, FACEP

Section III
ORTHOPEDIC EMERGENCIES

| 10 | Musculoskeletal Emergencies: Introduction and Basic Principles | 161 |

Daniel R. Benson, MD

| 11 | Emergencies of the Vertebral Column | 175 |

Daniel R. Benson, MD

| 12 | Upper Extremity Emergency Problems | 195 |

Robert M. Szabo, MD

| 13 | Pelvis and Lower Extremity Fracture Management | 213 |

Timothy J. Bray, MD

Section IV
METABOLIC, ENDOCRINE, AND GENETIC EMERGENCIES

| 14 | Diabetic Emergencies | 233 |

Stephen Hamburger, MD, FACP
David Rush, PharmD

| 15 | Thyroid Disorders | 249 |

Gerald S. Levey, MD

| 16 | Adrenal Insufficiency | 255 |

George L. Higgins III, MD, FACEP

| 17 | Electrolyte Abnormalities | 265 |

Barry E. Brenner, MD, PhD

| 18 | Hypokalemia and Hyperkalemia | 293 |

Paul M. Paris, MD, FACEP

| 19 | Hypomagnesemia, Hypermagnesemia, and Magnesium Therapy | 303 |

Joel Geiderman, MD, FACEP

| 20 | Hypercalcemia | 311 |

Emanuel K. Gordon, MD, FACEP

| 21 | Acid-Base Disturbances | 319 |

Barry E. Brenner, MD, PhD

| 22 | Emergencies in Patients with Connective Tissue Disease | 335 |

Barbara Matteucci, MD
Raphael J. DeHoratius, MD

| 23 | Acute Monoarticular Arthritis | 351 |

Raphael J. DeHoratius, MD
Barbara Matteucci, MD

| 24 | Medical Genetics | 361 |

Joel M. Lamon, MD, FACP

Section V
GENERAL EMERGENCIES

25 Infectious Disease Emergencies 375
    Richard T. Ellison III, MD
    Stephen H. Zinner, MD

26 Burns 417
    G. Richard Braen, MD, FACEP

27 Dermatologic Emergencies 429
    George L. Sternbach, MD, FACEP

28 Gastrointestinal Emergencies 447
    William Linnik, MD

29 Poisoning, Drug Overdose, and Toxic Exposures 469
    John B. Sullivan, Jr., MD

30 Oncology in the Emergency Department 501
    Marc Borenstein, MD, FACEP

Section VI
PEDIATRIC EMERGENCIES

31 Pediatric Cardiopulmonary Resuscitation 513
    James E. Pierog, MD, FACEP

32 Evaluation of Febrile Children Younger Than Two Years of Age 529
    James E. Pierog, MD, FACEP

33 Pediatric Surgical Emergencies 541
    Arthur Cooper, MD, FACS, FAAP, FCCM

34 Upper Airway Obstruction 563
    Michael G. Tunik, MD
    George L. Foltin, MD

35 Lower Respiratory Tract Disorders in Children 573
    Elise W. van der Jagt, MD, MPH

36 Neurologic Emergencies of Infancy and Childhood 589
    Richard M. Cantor, MD, FAAP, FACEP

37 Child Abuse 597
    Celeste M. Madden, MD, FAAP, FACEP

Section VII
ENVIRONMENTAL EMERGENCIES

38 Radiation Emergencies 617
    Charles V. Pollack, Jr., MD

39 Bites and Stings 627
    Robert C. Jorden, MD, FACEP
    Charles V. Pollack, Jr., MD

| 40 | Hyperthermia | 653 |

Eric A. Weiss, MD

| 41 | Hypothermia | 661 |

Jon W. Miller, Jr., MD, FACEP, FACURP

| 42 | Altitude-Related Emergencies | 679 |

Mark A. Selland, MD
Peter H. Hackett, MD

| 43 | Drowning and Near-Drowning | 689 |

Shirley A. Graves, MD
A. Joseph Layon, MD

| 44 | Hyperbaric Emergencies | 701 |

C. Gresham Bayne, MD

| 45 | Dangerous Marine Organisms | 711 |

Kenneth E. Schultz, MD

| 46 | Hazardous Materials | 747 |

Brent T. Burton, MD

| 47 | Occupational Toxicologic Emergencies | 761 |

Robert Harrison, MD, MPH

Section VIII
PSYCHOSOCIAL EMERGENCIES

| 48 | Substance Abuse | 781 |

Carl Klingelberger, MD
Daniel Shine, MD

| 49 | Alcohol Problems | 815 |

William D. Clark, MD

| 50 | Depression and Suicidal Feelings and Behaviors | 829 |

Thomas F. McGee, PhD

| 51 | Domestic Violence | 837 |

Tina M.H. Blair, MD, FACEP
Carmen Germaine Warner, MSN, RN, FAAN

| 52 | Emotional and Spiritual Support | 857 |

Ann R. Schreier, MSN, RN

| 53 | Pain Management | 877 |

*Gary Sparger, RN, MSN, CEN, MICN
K. Sue Hoyt, RN, MSN, CEN
Roland Heidenhofer, MD, FACEP

Section IX
ALTERATIONS OF CENTRAL NERVOUS SYSTEM FUNCTIONS

| 54 | Head Injuries | 891 |

Anthony J. Caputy, MD
Kourosh B. Afshar, MD

---

*Deceased.

| 55 | Cervical Spine Injuries | 903 |

David J. Dula, MD, FACEP

| 56 | Headache | 915 |

James Santiago Grisolía, MD

| 57 | Coma | 927 |

Mark Smith, MD

| 58 | Cerebrovascular Accident | 935 |

Ron M. Walls, MD, FRCPC

| 59 | Seizures | 945 |

Gregg Husk, MD

| 60 | The Confused Patient | 951 |

Gregg Husk, MD

| 61 | Syncope | 959 |

Gregg Husk, MD

Section X
ALTERATIONS OF CIRCULATORY SYSTEM FUNCTIONS

| 62 | Acute Myocardial Infarction | 965 |

Lester B. Jacobson, MD, FACC, FACP

| 63 | Disturbances in Cardiac Rhythm | 997 |

Lester B. Jacobson, MD, FACC, FACP

| 64 | Congestive Heart Failure | 1051 |

Richard G. Friedman, MD, FACC

| 65 | Hypertensive Emergencies | 1059 |

Howard A. Bessen, MD, FACEP

| 66 | Vascular Emergencies | 1069 |

James B. Alexander, MD
Anthony J. DelRossi, MD
Jonathan H. Cilley, Jr., MD

| 67 | Heart and Great Vessel Emergencies | 1077 |

Anthony J. DelRossi, MD
Jonathan H. Cilley, Jr., MD
James B. Alexander, MD

| 68 | Cardiopulmonary Resuscitation | 1083 |

Alan D. Guerci, MD

Section XI
ALTERATIONS OF RESPIRATORY SYSTEM FUNCTIONS

| 69 | Dyspnea and Pulmonary Edema | 1095 |

George L. Sternbach, MD, FACEP

| 70 | Airway Management | 1103 |

Linda Nordeman, MD
Emily J. Lucid, MD, FACEP

71	Croup and Epiglottitis	1113
	Ronald N. Rothenberg, MD, FACEP	
72	Obstructive Airway Disease	1129
	Michael R. Sayre, MD, FACEP	
	Brian W. Carlin, MD, FCCP	
73	Pulmonary Embolism	1141
	Charles M. Shufflebarger, MD	
	D. Kim Zaiser, MD, FACEP	
74	Respiratory Failure	1151
	Rebecca Seip, MD	
	Marcus L. Martin, MD	
75	Miscellaneous Respiratory Emergencies	1159
	Fred Harchelroad, MD, FACEP, ABMT	
	Dietrich Jehle, MD, FACEP	
76	Chest Trauma	1181
	Alan H. Brader, MD	

Section XII
ALTERATIONS IN URINARY AND REPRODUCTIVE FUNCTION

77	Common Genitourinary Emergencies	1195
	Alexander D. Vargas, MD, FACS, FRCPC	
78	Renal Failure	1217
	Jonathan L. White, MD	
	John A. Mitas II, MD, FACP	
	Leonard G. Gomella, MD	
79	Obstetric and Gynecologic Emergencies	1229
	John J. Willems, MD, FRCS, FACOG	
	Dennis E. Sandler, MD, FACOG	
80	Rape and Sexual Assault	1241
	Tina M.H. Blair, MD, FACEP	
	Carmen Germaine Warner, MSN, RN, FAAN	

Section XIII
HEAD AND NECK INJURIES

81	Ocular Emergencies	1259
	James Cabral, MD	
82	Ear, Nose, and Throat Emergencies	1299
	Janice Birney, MD	
	Kenneth Kulig, MD	
	Gordon Genta, MD	
83	Laryngeal Emergencies	1313
	Janice Birney, MD	
	Kenneth Kulig, MD	

| 84 | Maxillofacial Injuries | 1319 |

Stephen V. Cantrill, MD, FACEP

| 85 | Dental Emergencies | 1331 |

John P. Kelly, DMD, MD

Section XIV
PRACTICAL APPLICATIONS OF EMERGENCY CARE

| 86 | Atlas of Emergency Procedures | 1339 |

Thomas Clarke Kravis, MD

| 87 | Emergency Drug Index | 1377 |

Joseph A. Grillo, BS Pharm
Edgar R. Gonzalez, PharmD

Appendix: Temperature Conversion 1455

Subject Index 1463

Contributing Authors

Kourosh B. Afshar, MD
Department of Neurosurgery
Georgetown University Medical Center
3800 Reservoir Road Northwest
Washington, DC 20007

James B. Alexander, MD
Assistant Professor of Surgery
University of Medicine and Dentistry
  of New Jersey
Robert Wood Johnson Medical School
  at Camden
Department of Surgery
Cooper Hospital/University Medical Center
3 Cooper Plaza
Camden, New Jersey 08103

C. Gresham Bayne, MD
Associate Professor
University of California, San Diego
San Diego, California 92106

Daniel R. Benson, MD
Professor
Department of Orthopaedic Surgery
University of California, Davis
2230 Stockton Boulevard
Sacramento, California 95817

Howard A. Bessen, MD, FACEP
Associate Clinical Professor of Medicine
University of California, Los Angeles
Los Angeles, California
Department of Emergency Medicine
Harbor-UCLA Medical Center
1000 West Carson Street
Torrance, California 90509

Janice L. Birney, MD
Swedish Health Park Southwest
6169 South Balsam Way
Littleton, Colorado 80123

Tina M.H. Blair, MD, FACEP
Addison Gilbert Hospital
298 Washington Street
Gloucester, Maine 01930

Marc Borenstein, MD, FACEP
940 High Road
Kensington, Connecticut 06037

Alan H. Brader, MD
Clinical Assistant Professor of Surgery
University of North Carolina
Wake Medical Center
3000 New Bern Avenue
Raleigh, North Carolina 27610

G. Richard Braen, MD, FACEP
Professor and Chairman
Department of Emergency Medicine
Buffalo General Hospital
100 High Street
Buffalo, New York 14203

Timothy J. Bray, MD
Associate
Reno Orthopaedic Clinic
555 North Arlington Avenue
Reno, Nevada 89520
Assistant Clinical Professor
Department of Orthopaedic Surgery
University of California, Davis
Medical Center
Sacramento, California 95817
Assistant Clinical Professor
Orthopaedic Surgery
University of Nevada, Reno
School of Medicine
Reno, Nevada

Barry E. Brenner, MD, PhD
Assistant Clinical Professor of Medicine
University of California, Los Angeles
School of Medicine
Cedars-Sinai Medical Center
8700 Beverly Boulevard
Los Angeles, California 90048

Brent E. Burton, MD
Oregon Poison Center
Oregon Health Sciences University
3181 Southwest Sam Jackson Park Road
Portland, Oregon 97201

James Cabral, MD
Vitreo-Retinal Surgeon
4060 Fourth Avenue
San Diego, California 92103

Richard M. Cantor, MD, FAAP, FACEP
Assistant Professor
Department of Emergency Medicine and
 Pediatrics
State University of New York Health Science
 Center
750 East Adams Street
Syracuse, New York 13210

Stephen V. Cantrill, MD, FACEP
Emergency Medical Services
Denver General Hospital
777 Bannock Street
Denver, Colorado 80204

Anthony J. Caputy, MD
Department of Neurosurgery
Georgetown University Medical Center
3800 Reservoir Road Northwest
Washington, DC 20007
Department of Neurosurgery
Fairfax Hospital
Fairfax, Virginia

Brian W. Carlin, MD, FCCP
Assistant Professor of Medicine and
 Anesthesiology
Medical College of Pennsylvania, Allegheny
 Campus
Pittsburgh, Pennsylvania
Division of Emergency Medicine
Allegheny General Hospital
320 East North Avenue
Pittsburgh, Pennsylvania 15212

Jonathan H. Cilley, Jr., MD
Assistant Professor of Surgery
University of Medicine and Dentistry
 of New Jersey
Robert Wood Johnson Medical School
 at Camden
Division of Cardiothoracic Surgery
Cooper Hospital/University Medical Center
3 Cooper Plaza
Camden, New Jersey 08103

William D. Clark, MD
Bath Memorial Hospital
1356 Washington Street
Bath, Maine 04530

Arthur Cooper, MD, FACS, FAAP, FCCM
Associate Professor and Chief
Pediatric Surgical Critical Care
Division of Pediatric Surgery
College of Physicians and Surgeons of
 Columbia University
Harlem Hospital Center
506 Lenox Avenue
New York, New York 10037

Davis Cracroft, MD, FACEP
Mercy Hospital
4077 Fifth Avenue
San Diego, California 92103

Raphael J. DeHoratius, MD
Professor of Medicine
Division of Rheumatology
Thomas Jefferson Medical College
1015 Walnut Street
Philadelphia, Pennsylvania 19107

Anthony J. DelRossi, MD
Associate Professor of Surgery
University of Medicine and Dentistry
 of New Jersey
Robert Wood Johnson Medical School
 at Camden
Cooper Hospital/University Medical Center
3 Cooper Plaza
Camden, New Jersey 08103

David J. Dula, MD, FACEP
Department of Emergency Medicine
Geisinger Medical Center
Academy Avenue
Danville, Pennsylvania 17822

Richard T. Ellison III, MD
Associate Professor of Medicine
University of Massachusetts School of
 Medicine
Clinical Director of Infectious Disease
University of Massachusetts Medical Center
55 Lake North Avenue
Worcester, Massachusetts 01655

Frederick B. Epstein, MD, FACEP
Director, Emergency Medical Services
Bay Medical Center
615 North Bonita Avenue
Panama City, Florida 32401

George L. Foltin, MD
Assistant Professor of Clinical Pediatrics
New York University School of Medicine
New York, New York
Director, Pediatric Emergency Services
Bellevue Hospital Center
First Avenue and 27th Street
New York, New York 10016

Jacek B. Franaszek, MD, FACEP
P.O. Box 9766
Rancho Santa Fe, California 92067

Richard G. Friedman, MD, FACC
Associate Clinical Professor of Medicine
University of California, San Diego
School of Medicine
San Diego, California
Assistant Director
Cardiac Catheterization Laboratory
Mercy Hospital and Medical Center
4033 Third Avenue
San Diego, California 92103

Joel Geiderman, MD, FACEP
Associate Director
Department of Emergency Medicine
Cedars-Sinai Medical Center
8700 Beverly Boulevard
Los Angeles, California 90048

Gordon Genta, MD
Private Practice
Boise, Idaho

Leonard G. Gomella, MD
Assistant Professor of Urology
Thomas Jefferson University
Philadelphia, Pennsylvania 19107

Edgar R. Gonzalez, PharmD
Associate Professor of Pharmacy and
  Medicine
Department of Pharmacy and Pharmaceutics
Virginia Commonwealth University
Medical College of Virginia
Richmond, Virginia 23298

Emanuel K. Gordon, MD, FACEP
Clinical Assistant Professor of Medicine
University of California, Los Angeles
School of Medicine
Los Angeles, California 90025

Shirley A. Graves, MD
Professor
Departments of Anesthesiology and Pediatrics
Chief, Division of Pediatric Anesthesia
University of Florida College of Medicine
Gainesville, Florida 32610

Joseph A. Grillo, BS Pharm
PharmD Candidate
Department of Pharmacy and Pharmaceutics
Virginia Commonwealth University
Medical College of Virginia
Richmond, Virginia 23298

James Santiago Grisolía, MD
4033 Third Avenue
San Diego, California 92103

Alan D. Guerci, MD
Department of Cardiology
St. Francis Hospital
100 Port Washington Boulevard
Roslyn, New York 11576

Peter H. Hackett, MD
Director, Denali Medical Research Project
Staff Emergency Physician and Air Ambulance
  Director
Humana Hospital, Alaska
2801 Debarr Avenue
Anchorage, Alaska 99508
Affiliate Associate Professor
University of Washington
School of Medicine
Seattle, Washington 98195

Stephen Hamburger, MD, FACP
Associate Professor of Medicine
Department of Medicine
University of Missouri, Kansas City
School of Medicine
Kansas City, Missouri

Fred Harchelroad, MD, FACEP, ABMT
Associate Professor
Department of Emergency Medicine
Medical College of Pennsylvania, Allegheny
  Campus
Pittsburgh, Pennsylvania
Director, Medical Toxicology Treatment
  Center
Allegheny General Hospital
320 East North Avenue
Pittsburgh, Pennsylvania 15212

Robert Harrison, MD, MPH
Associate Clinical Professor of Medicine
Division of Occupational and Environmental
 Medicine
University of California, San Francisco
350 Parnassus Avenue
San Francisco, California 94143

Roland Heidenhofer, MD, FACEP
2440 East Tudor Road
Anchorage, Alaska 99507

Robert W. Heilig, RN, MPA, Esq
Private Practice
4939 Shady Leaf Way
Sacramento, California 95838

George L. Higgins III, MD, FACEP
Clinical Associate Professor of Surgery
University of Vermont
Burlington, Vermont 05401
Chief, Department of Emergency Medicine
Medical Director, Maine Poison Control
 Center
Maine Medical Center
22 Bramhall Street
Portland, Maine 04102

K. Sue Hoyt, RN, MSN, CEN
2040 Capri Court
El Cajon, California 92020

Gregg Husk, MD
Emergency Department
Roosevelt Hospital
428 West 59th Street
New York, New York 10019

Barbara Bennett Jacobs, RN, BSN, MPH
Educational Consultant
Department of Education
Hartford Hospital
Hartford, Connecticut

**Lenworth M. Jacobs, Jr., MD, MPH,
 FACS**
Director, EMS/Trauma/LIFESTAR Program
Hartford Hospital
Hartford, Connecticut
Professor of Surgery
University of Connecticut
Farmington, Connecticut

Lester B. Jacobson, MD, FACC, FACP
Cardiovascular Diseases
California Pacific Medical Center
2340 Clay Street
San Francisco, California 94115

Dietrich Jehle, MD, FACEP
Director of Emergency Services
Erie County Medical Center
462 Grider Street
Buffalo, New York 14215
Associate Professor
Department of Emergency Medicine
State University of New York
 at Buffalo
Buffalo, New York 14222

Robert C. Jorden, MD, FACEP
Chairman, Department of Emergency
 Medicine
Maricopa Medical Center
Phoenix, Arizona 85016

William Kantor, MD
Associate Director
Trauma Program and Critical Care
St. Vincent's Hospital
Worcester, Massachusetts

John P. Kelly, DMD, MD
Department of Oral and Maxillofacial Surgery
Ambulatory Care Center
Massachusetts General Hospital
5 Fruit Street
Boston, Massachusetts 02114

Carl Klingelberger, MD
Chairman, Emergency Medicine Department
Naval Hospital San Diego
San Diego, California 92134

Thomas Clarke Kravis, MD
Medical Director
Continental Rehabilitation Hospital
555 Washington Avenue
San Diego, California 92103
Associate Medical Director
Emergency Services
CompHealth
Salt Lake City, Utah

Kenneth Kulig, MD
University of Colorado Medical School
Rocky Mountain Poison Center
Denver General Hospital
Denver, Colorado

Joel M. Lamon, MD, FACP
Southwest Cancer Care
15524 Pomerado Road
Poway, California 92064

A. Joseph Layon, MD
Associate Professor
Departments of Anesthesiology and Medicine
University of Florida
College of Medicine
Gainesville, Florida 32610

Gerald S. Levey, MD
Senior Vice President
Medical and Scientific Affairs
Merck and Co., Inc.
One Merck Drive
Whitehouse Station, New Jersey 08889

William Linnik, MD
2050 Pacific Beach Drive
San Diego, California 92109

Emily J. Lucid, MD, FACEP
Associate Professor and Chairman of
  Emergency Medicine
Medical College of Pennsylvania, Allegheny
  Campus
Pittsburgh, Pennsylvania
Director, Division of Emergency Medicine
Allegheny General Hospital
320 East North Avenue
Pittsburgh, Pennsylvania 15212

Celeste M. Madden, MD, FAAP, FACEP
Maternal and Child Health Center
516 Prospect Avenue
Syracuse, New York 13208

Marcus L. Martin, MD
Associate Professor
Residency Program Director
Department of Emergency Medicine
Medical College of Pennsylvania, Allegheny
  Campus
Pittsburgh, Pennsylvania
Allegheny General Hospital
320 East North Avenue
Pittsburgh, Pennsylvania 15212

Barbara M. Matteucci, MD
Assistant Professor of Medicine
Division of Rheumatology
Albert Einstein Medical Center
5501 Old York Road
Philadelphia, Pennsylvania 19141

Thomas F. McGee, PhD
Associate Provost and Director
Psychological Services Center
California School of Professional Psychology
6215 Ferris Square
San Diego, California 92121

Jon W. Miller, Jr., MD, FACEP, FACURP
St. Claire Medical Center
222 Medical Circle
Morehead, Kentucky 40351

John A. Mitas II, MD, FACP
Department of Urology
Thomas Jefferson University
1020 Walnut Street
Philadelphia, Pennsylvania 19107

Glenn W. Mitchell, MD, MPH, FACEP
Adjunct Associate Professor of Clinical
  Military and Emergency Medicine
Uniformed Services University of the Health
  Sciences
Bethesda, Maryland
Aeromedical Teaching Faculty
U.S. Air Force School of Aerospace Medicine
Brooks Air Force Base, Texas
Department of Emergency Medicine
Brooks Army Medical Center
San Antonio, Texas 78250

Linda Nordeman, MD
Assistant Professor of Medicine
Medical College of Pennsylvania, Allegheny
  Campus
Pittsburgh, Pennsylvania
Attending Staff
Division of Emergency Medicine
Allegheny General Hospital
320 East North Avenue
Pittsburgh, Pennsylvania 15212

Paul M. Paris, MD, FACEP
Associate Professor and Chief
Division of Emergency Medicine
University of Pittsburgh
School of Medicine
Pittsburgh, Pennsylvania 15213

James E. Pierog, MD, FACEP
Medical Director, Emergency Department
Children's Hospital of Orange County
St. Joseph Hospital, Orange
1100 West Stewart Drive
Orange, California 92668

Charles V. Pollack, Jr., MD
Attending Physician/Associate Research Director
Department of Emergency Medicine
Maricopa Medical Center
Phoenix, Arizona 85016

Ronald N. Rothenberg, MD, FACEP
Associate Clinical Professor
Community and Family Medicine
University of California, San Diego
San Diego, California
Attending Physician
Department of Emergency Medicine
Scripps Memorial Hospital
Encinitas, California

David Rush, PharmD
Professor of Medicine and Clinical Pharmacology
University of Missouri
Truman Medical Center East
7900 Lee's Summit Road
Kansas City, Missouri 64139

Dennis E. Sandler, MD, FACOG
Staff Physician
Division of Obstetrics and Gynecology
Scripps Clinic and Foundation
10666 North Torrey Pines Road
La Jolla, California 92037
Clinical Instructor
University of California, San Diego
225 Dickinson Street
San Diego, California 92103

Michael R. Sayre, MD, FACEP
Assistant Professor
Department of Emergency Medicine
Center for Emergency Care
University of Cincinnati Hospital
231 Bethesda Avenue
Cincinnati, Ohio 45267

Ann R. Schreier, MSN, RN
City of Hope Medical Center
1500 East Duarte Road
Duarte, California 91010

Kenneth E. Schultz, MD
Corporate Medical Director
Risk Management Division
EMSA
1200 South Pine Island Road
Fort Lauderdale, Florida 33324

Rebecca Seip, MD
Assistant Professor
Medical College of Pennsylvania, Allegheny Campus
Pittsburgh, Pennsylvania
Department of Emergency Medicine
Allegheny General Hospital
320 East North Avenue
Pittsburgh, Pennsylvania 15212

Mark A. Selland, MD
Cardiovascular Pulmonary Research Laboratory
University of Colorado Health Sciences Center
781 South High Street
Denver, Colorado 80209

Mark Allen Shaffer, MD, FACEP
Medical Director/President
Centro Medico Latino
San Marcos, California
Attending Physician
Sharp Murrieta Hospital
Murrieta, California 92362
Attending Physician
Sharp Community Hospital
Chula Vista, California

Daniel Shine, MD
Mount Sinai School of Medicine
Beth Israel Hospital
New York, New York

Charles M. Shufflebarger, MD
Department of Emergency Medicine
Methodist Hospital of Indiana
1701 North Senate Boulevard
Indianapolis, Indiana 46206

Mark Smith, MD
Chairman, Department of Emergency Medicine
George Washington University Medical Center
2140 Pennsylvania Avenue Northwest
Washington, DC 20037

Gary Sparger, RN, MSN, CEN, MICN
(Deceased)

George L. Sternbach, MD, FACEP
Clinical Associate Professor of Surgery
Stanford University Medical Center
Stanford, California 94305
Emergency Physician
Seton Medical Center
Daly City, California

John B. Sullivan, Jr., MD
Section of Emergency Medicine
University of Arizona Health Sciences Center
1501 North Campbell
Tucson, Arizona 85724

Robert M. Szabo, MD
Department of Orthopaedics
University of California, Davis
2230 Stockton Boulevard
Sacramento, California 95817

Michael G. Tunik, MD
Assistant Professor of Clinical Pediatrics
New York University School of Medicine
New York, New York
Associate Director, Pediatric Emergency Services
Bellevue Hospital Center
First Avenue and 27th Street
New York, New York 10016

Elise M. van der Jagt, MD, MPH
Strong Children's Critical Care Center
601 Elmwood Avenue
Rochester, New York 14642

Alexander D. Vargas, MD, FACS, FRCPC
3737 Martin Luther King Jr. Boulevard
Lynwood, California 90262

R. S. Venable, MD, FAAFP, FACEP
Chief Medical Officer
Humana Health Care Plans
Clinical Associate Professor
University of South Florida Medical College
Tampa, Florida 33611

Ron M. Walls, MD, FRCPC
Head, Department of Emergency Medicine
Vancouver General Hospital
855 West 12th Avenue
Vancouver, British Columbia, Canada V5Z 1M9

Carmen Germaine Warner, MSN, RN, FAAN
Consultant, Community Health Systems, Emergency Care, and Publishing
Coordinating Editor, Topics in Emergency Medicine
1749 Sky Loft Lane
Leucadia, California 92024

Eric A. Weiss, MD
Assistant Professor
Division of Emergency Medicine
Stanford University Medical Center
300 Pasteur Drive
Stanford, California 94305

Eileen Whalen, RN, BSN
Director of Neonatal Intensive Care Unit
Children's Hospital of Orange County
Orange, California

Jonathan L. White, MD
Department of Urology
Thomas Jefferson University
1020 Walnut Street
Philadelphia, Pennsylvania 19107

John J. Willems, MD, FRCS, FACOG
Staff Physician
Division of Obstetrics and Gynecology
Scripps Clinic and Research Foundation
10666 North Torrey Pines Road
La Jolla, California 92037
Associate Clinical Professor
University of California, San Diego
225 Dickinson Street
San Diego, California 92103

D. Kim Zaiser, MD, FACEP
Assistant Professor
Department of Emergency Medicine
Medical College of Pennsylvania, Allegheny Campus
Pittsburgh, Pennsylvania
Director, Office of Prehospital Care
Division of Emergency Medicine
Allegheny General Hospital
320 East North Avenue
Pittsburgh, Pennsylvania 15212

Stephen H. Zinner, MD
Professor of Medicine
Head, Division of Infectious Diseases
Brown University
Roger Williams Medical Center
Rhode Island Hospital
825 Chalkstone Avenue
Providence, Rhode Island 02908

Foreword

Textbooks represent information which, when transformed, becomes knowledge. Pursuit of knowledge, through academic training, is a prerequisite to the commencement of a professional career. Today, with research and phenomenal acceleration in the development of new information offered through technological advances, the half-life of medical knowledge has grown ever shorter. Thus, the pursuit of new knowledge through continuing medical education, as represented by this textbook, becomes even more important.

Even though I direct my comments specifically to emergency physicians, I hope others will listen in. Innovation and enhanced levels of dialog are in order if administration, managers, and health care specialists, as well as emergency physicians, are to become more effective.

This textbook, especially with its expanded scope represented by chapters on hazardous and toxic materials and occupational health—both areas of rapidly increasing application to the specialty of emergency medicine—will not only help you as an emergency physician stay abreast but also enhance your position as an indispensable professional in your work environment. At no time in history has competition for the health care dollar been more severe or has change been more rampant in the business and practice of medicine than it is today. However, with this competition and change comes opportunity.

The specialty of emergency medicine is officially recognized and accepted within the house of medicine. Gaining widespread respect, however, will require increased participation in medical politics and widely expanded involvement in research and marketing. Tomorrow's emergency physician will need to acquire knowledge and skill in each of the areas presented in this textbook. Coupled with this clinical expertise is the need to participate in the total health care arena by:

- Committing time and dollars to "R & D"
- Developing proficiency in medical economics and politics
- Learning to market yourself and your facility
- Striving to promote and protect quality patient care

Preparing yourself to be unique, with special skills beyond those of general emergency medicine—toxicology, critical care, occupational medicine, emergency medical systems, metabolic/endocrine and genetic emergencies, pediatrics, traumatology, and other areas outlined in this text—is of vital importance. New staffing patterns will emerge as the more highly skilled and trained—and thus the more experienced—will be utilized only for the tasks for which those skills and training are required. The new staffing patterns will include staff reductions. Part of your challenge as the emergency physician member of the administrative team will be to successfully implement these changes and, at the same time, increase quality of patient care.

You will compete in a zero sum game of medical economics. Formerly one could argue for new programs, and additional dollars were authorized by Congress to fund them. Now the amount of dollars available will be relatively fixed, and you will vie with others to retain what you have had, let alone increase the amount; for your gain will be at someone else's expense. Your enthusiasm may be compromised by new stresses of economic problems as emergency departments strain under the demands of socially and legally required, but yet uncompensated, provision of emergency health care. Also we face the continued specter of egregious malpractice suits despite anticipated tort reform and improved patient communications. It is extraordinarily evident that health care professionals can no longer ignore the need to gain optimal knowledge of the scope and impact of local and national economic and political trends.

New attention to health care costs and patient convenience has led to the development of alternative care centers. This, in turn, has provided a catalyst for hospital emergency departments and physicians' offices to develop and promote new marketing programs. The emergency physician of tomorrow must seize these opportunities to act as an important resource to provide needed service to hospital administration and medical staff by actively participating in areas such as long-range planning, hospital promotion, patient relation evaluations, and committee membership.

The challenge of our consumer-oriented health care marketplace demands that we assess the needs and desires of each of our patients and strive whenever possible to incorporate them into our provision of professional services. Our success requires that we confront occasionally-held perceptions of physicians and emergency departments as callous, uncaring entities by offering a heightened degree of sensitivity and demonstrated concern for patients. The ever-increasing options the public has for medical care today also demand that we transmit this same concern and desire for optimal cost-effective service from the perspective of payors such as insurers, health maintenance organizations, preferred provider organizations, or industrial employers.

The emergency physician must be aware of competition, adapt to and take advantage of change, and help shape the transformation to the advantage of our specialty and patient care. I am confident that the authors and content of this textbook have helped point the way. Continuing education will strengthen your foundation and make you better prepared to provide what is, and must remain, your first and foremost goal as an emergency physician—optimally satisfying the emergency patient's health care needs.

Richard L. Stennes, MD, FACEP
Associated Emergency Physician
Medical Group APC
San Diego, California

Foreword

The last decade has seen dramatic changes in the specialty of emergency medicine. Not only has the number of visits to emergency departments shown a continuing increase, but also the changes and complexities of the health care industry have expanded the arena in which emergency care is provided to communities. Emergency services do not, as in the past, encompass the hospital's emergency department alone, but include well-defined prehospital systems, trauma centers, ambulatory care centers, and medical air transportation systems.

The providers of emergency care have become more responsive, working together as a multidisciplinary team to the benefit of those persons who require emergency care. Emergency services encompass a broad scope of practice, and providers have increased and will continue to increase their knowledge, skills, and clinical expertise. Emergency nurses expand their realm of accountability through participation in institutionally based performance verification, independent self-study, and continuing education programs through institutions of higher learning. All these can be precursors to the national examination as a Certified Emergency Nurse (CEN). The challenge and the opportunities awaiting those committed to the practice of emergency services have no limits. Emergency nurses as teachers and leaders, now as ever, must define performance expectations of emergency care for themselves and the emergency department team, for this ultimately provides to the clients receiving care and health education the best possible means for health prevention treatment and survival.

This book is a comprehensive reference on emergency medicine. The up-to-date concepts that it presents challenge the intellect and expand the nurse's knowledge in shaping the emergency health care system.

Mildred K. Fincke, RN, BSN
Clinical Director
Passavant Health Center
Zenienople, Pennsylvania
Past President, ENA
Beaver, Pennsylvania

Foreword

Over the past decade, the cost of health care has grown at rates exceeding the wildest imagination. It consumes 10 percent of the U.S. gross national product, currently surpassing almost every other government expenditure. The federal government's decision to decrease health care expenditures "at whatever price" (e.g., through Medicare's diagnosis-related groups and legislative support of prepaid health care) has created an atmosphere of cost restraint within the private sector. DRGs are just the beginning of the process with capitation as the end result.

As medicine refocuses from "service at any cost" to "the same service for less," the emphasis will be on keeping patients out of the hospital. This will ultimately thrust the specialty of emergency medicine into the role of primary gatekeeper.

Emergency medical services (EMS) mirror the current health care fiscal crisis. Simply infusing the four C's—namely, *c*aring, *c*ompetence, *c*ost-effectiveness, and *c*onvenience—into the practice of emergency medicine may be all that is necessary. Whereas ambulatory care facilities in their myriad forms address convenience and cost, emergency medicine must encourage the delivery of cost-effective medical care within both the hospital and EMS system.

Innovative, low-cost systems that involve paramedics but do not compromise patient care (e.g., firefighter-initiated defibrillator programs) should be planned and implemented. Furthermore, greater priority should be placed on the preventive aspects of illness and injury. The active participation of emergency care personnel in public policymaking pertinent to drunk driving, seat belts, infant car seats, motorcycle helmets, handgun control, and smoking will benefit not only our patients, but also our specialty. Just as important, the individual emergency physician will have to place greater reliance on clinical skills than on diagnostic tests—something our founding fathers did well.

The continued commitment of emergency care physicians to clinical competence through board certification, continuing education, and research; the provision of cost-effective care; and the ongoing support of the multidisciplinary team approach will enhance the delivery of quality emergency care in the latter part of this century. This text's second edition assists the emergency physician in attaining these goals because of its emphasis on clinical medical management and its recognition of the need for all emergency health care professionals, including the emergency physician, emergency nurse, and paramedical personnel, to work together.

In our professional dedication, however, let us not forget caring—probably the most important ingredient to patients. It is the least that patients expect from the specialty that provides 24-hour service. Caring . . . isn't that why we're here?

Denis J. Kollar, MD, FACEP
Past President of the California
   Chapter of the American
   College of Emergency
   Physicians
Member, EMS Commission
   State of California
West Covina, California

Preface to the Second Edition

The second edition of *Emergency Medicine* continues to strive toward enriching and advancing the quality of care afforded all emergency patients. Consequently, the goals and objectives are identical to those envisioned seven years ago when the concept of this text was developed. Specifically, the emphasis is to share with the interested reader the academic and scientific knowledge, rigor, and skills required to provide the optimum level of care to our patients.

The authors' and editors' ultimate intent may in fact have been achieved. This input comes from clinicians, academicians, and reviews, not only in our country, but throughout the world. Continued satisfaction from these comments is derived from the knowledge that this text may have assisted a colleague in salvaging a life or stimulated the emergence of a new prehospital care system in many locations. What has been striking is the heterogenous character of the interest, skill, knowledge, aspirations, and requirements of the many readers who have shared their views regarding this text.

We as editors have taken the liberty of interpreting this positive feedback as confidence in our intuitive decision to include a heterogenous group of contributors from various disciplines in order to meet the diverse expectations of the reader. This includes not only the emergency department physician, but the other integral members of the health care team such as nurses, emergency medical technicians, paramedics, social workers, and spiritual leaders. Each member of this multidisciplinary team offers a valuable piece to the total plan for wholistic, comprehensive patient care. In the same spirit, we sought, directed, and encouraged the efforts of 49 entirely new authors representing not only emergency personnel, but academicians, surgeons, cardiologists, social workers, lawyers, and ministers as well.

The changing dynamics of emergency care has prompted the editors of several new chapters focusing on the emergency needs within these specialty areas. These areas include occupational emergencies, pain management emergencies, oncology, genetic concerns, and hazardous materials emergencies. We believe that the growth, understanding, and acceptance of these new horizons are instrumental in offering a broad based expertise of all emergencies to those in need.

The second edition of *Emergency Medicine* has incorporated the expertise of three section editors. Their talents and careful design have aided in the development of the prehospital care, pediatric, and orthopedic emergencies sections. Each section editor, along with the chapter authors, has included important advances and changes that have emerged during the past three years, making this text a current, up-to-date account of emergency care standards and interventions. An example of this is the use of MRI in the assessment of patients with central nervous system emergencies. Along with these changes and refinements, we have maintained our original organizational strategy and continued our general format: definition of the disease process, etiology, pathophysiology, and clinical correlates including the mechanism of injury, diagnosis, and treatment with an integration of both prehospital and emergency department care.

Finally, with the broad-based acceptance of centigrade conversion for medical use and application, we have included both centigrade and fahrenheit listings throughout. For accuracy and ease of use, a conversion chart has been incorporated in this text and will be found on page 1394.

TCK
CGW

Preface

The third edition of *Emergency Medicine: A Comprehensive Review* continues in the tradition of the previous edition in its goal to provide the knowledge and an outline of the various skills that are required by emergency physicians to provide high-quality, cost-efficient emergency care. Since the first edition was conceived 13 years ago, social, political, and economic pressures have continued to change the character of emergency care. A decade ago emergency medicine was undergoing a revolution that included the development of sophisticated prehospital care systems and high-technology trauma centers. The result of this process was significant increases in the quality of emergency care and access to inpatient care but, at the same time, an enormous increase in health care expenditures. The term *overkill* was increasingly replaced by many with *oversave*.

Two editions later, the character of the evolutionary forces are still in effect as American medicine is poised at the footsteps of major health care reform. There has been an economic depression. Health care costs have been judged by many to be out of control, and the concept of "managed care" has emerged as the panacea. These forces suggest that the American dream of high-quality care for every American at any cost may not be achievable. Indeed, these same pressures have changed many emergency departments into high-volume primary care clinics. This clinic milieu, coupled with an increase in violent multiple trauma victims, has increased the cost per visit: this cost has been borne not only by payors but by the emergency care providers themselves. Concomitantly with these changes, emergency physicians are "burning out" and seeking practice opportunities in new specialties and different practice environments. Just as the volume of patients has erupted, the amount of medical literature in emergency care has exploded in the past several years, and the two original editors are no longer capable of being familiar with all the details and nuances of the many subspecialties now included in the encompassing armamentarium of the emergency physician. Thus, a cadre of respected, knowledgeable, and highly skilled colleagues served as assistant editors to assure that the information provided to the reader of this text would be comprehensive, accurate, and meaningful. Their contributions have been integral to the success of this publication.

With the changing character of emergency medicine, there have been concomitant alterations in this edition that are noteworthy. The earlier editions focused on such topics as systems approaches and roadmaps on how to develop prehospital paramedic systems and advanced trauma life support. Many of these systems have been consolidated and are now often taken for granted. Thus, emergency medicine has empowered talented colleagues such as paramedics, MICNs, nurses, and others to implement these systems while the emergency physician treats emergency patients. Those with administrative inclinations or talents devote more of their time to the supervision and coordination of the individuals and the systems. In the next decade, as care is increasingly "managed," the emergency physician, as one of the last few true 24-hour a day primary care physicians, will continue to participate as an integral part of the "gatekeeper" function in managed competition. As providers "compete" with one another, patients and payors alike will select and pay providers based on patient satisfaction, cost, and clinical outcome. This text is intended to provide the emergency physician with one important tool in this complex process.

Thomas Clarke Kravis, MD
Medical Director

Acknowledgments

With the completion of this, the third edition of *Emergency Medicine*, I am deeply touched by the thousands of voluntary hours that you, the authors, have contributed to this text. For most, this is the second revision of a carefully planned and faithfully written chapter, chapters that signify the intense degree of commitment and determination, making this book an outstanding addition to the field of emergency medical care.

Each of you has put many hours of concentrated effort and enthusiasm into your work. I want to personally thank you and your families and friends for the time you have spent in your desire to share knowledge and expertise with emergency clinicians both nationally and internationally.

I enjoy the long and tedious task of coordinating such a project because of the pleasure I receive in working with each one of you. This is your book, and I thank God for the role you have played in its development and final release.

Even though I may never meet you personally, I shall be indebted to you for your gracious involvement in this project.

In addition I wish to express my gratitude to the editorial and production staffs of Raven Press and Aspen Publishers for all their efforts in the development and production of this volume.

I offer my sincere appreciation.

Carmen Germaine Warner, MSN, RN, FAAN
Coordinating Editor

EMERGENCY MEDICINE

A Comprehensive Review

Third Edition

1. Prehospital Emergency Medical Services

BARBARA BENNETT JACOBS, RN, BSN, MPH
LENWORTH M. JACOBS, JR., MD, MPH, FACS

The federal mandate to improve the response to those with a perceived or actual medical emergency outside a medical facility was initiated with the passage of a federal emergency medical services (EMS) act and allocation of funds beginning in 1974. Although the impetus to improve prehospital care was a concern over the treatment of patients with trauma, the improvements have encompassed the care of trauma patients as well as those who are experiencing an acute medical crisis such as a myocardial infarction or an acute asthma attack. The term *EMS* is recognizable to all providers of emergency medical care, whether they are based in the prehospital or hospital arena. EMS is a multicomponent system designed to respond to a perceived or actual medical emergency. The manner in which EMS systems are delivered across the country has undergone dramatic changes over the last three decades.

HISTORY

Historically, the problem of an ineffectively, inefficiently, and often insufficiently coordinated response system was unveiled in 1966. Since 1963, the National Research Council (NRC) of the National Academy of Sciences (NAS) has been the pivotal group involved in preparing and publishing reports related to injuries and EMS.[1-3] The NAS, located in Washington, DC, was mandated by Congress in 1863 to "advise the federal government on scientific and technical matters."[4(pii)] The NRC was established by the NAS in 1916 and is considered "the principal operating agency of both the National Academy of Sciences and the National Academy of Engineering in providing services to the government, the public, and the scientific and engineering communities."[4(pii)]

The first report to focus on the problems associated with the delivery of prehospital emergency medical care was *Accidental Death and Disability: The Neglected Disease of Modern Society*, which was published in 1966.[5] This report has been referred to as a white paper,[6] a landmark,[7] and a classic.[8] It can be found in the introduction to many books and papers published during the 1970s and early to middle 1980s that deal with subjects related to EMS.[6-9] Although the injured patient was the focus of this report, the disclosure of the dearth of any form of organized, systemic approach to prehospital care was applicable to all persons with a variety of clinical abnormalities. The report made recommendations in the following nine areas: accident prevention; emergency first aid and medical care; development of trauma registries; hospital trauma committees; convalescence, disability, and rehabilitation; medical-legal problems; autopsy of trauma victims; care of casualties under conditions of natural disaster; and trauma research.

Also in 1966, highway safety became an important issue for the federal government. The Governor's Highway Safety Act was signed by President Lyndon Johnson. Authority for promulgating this legislation was bestowed upon the Department of Transportation's (DOT's) Federal Highway Administration through its National Traffic Safety Agency. Standard 11 of the Act addressed EMS and made funds available through the DOT for purchase of ambulances, communications equipment, development of statewide EMS plans, organization and administration of state programs, and support of basic emergency medical technician (EMT) training.[10]

As a result of recommendations made to the Department of Health, Education and Welfare (DHEW) by its Advisory Committee on Traffic Safety, chaired by Dr Daniel Moynihan of the Massachusetts Institute of Technology in 1968, five EMS demonstration projects were funded with $16 million from the Health Services and Mental Health Administration of DHEW. In 1972, these funded areas (the state of Arkansas, a three-county area of southern California, a seven-county area of northeast Florida, the state of Illinois, and a seven-county area of Ohio) were designated to develop various approaches to EMS systems and to serve as models for other communities and states.

Between 1966 and the awarding of funds for pilot EMS projects, two national EMS conferences were held, one in 1969 and the other in 1972. As a result of these conferences, a number of advances occurred: The National Registry of Emergency Medical Technicians was established, the American Trauma Society was founded, ambulance design criteria were developed, and a plea to the President of the United States was made to support the improvement of EMS.

In 1972, which was a year of congressional hearings, a number of EMS-related bills were introduced, and there was some opposition. In 1973, however, Senate bill 2410 passed both the House and Senate and was signed into law by President Richard Nixon. This EMS Act of 1973 was amended in 1976 and again in 1979.[11-13] Administration of these federal monies for EMS development was the responsibility of the Division of Emergency Medical Services of DHEW. This agency divided the states geographically into approximately 300 EMS regions for the purpose of EMS planning and funding. The funding of EMS projects from 1974 through 1981 was founded on some specific principles of EMS[14]:

- EMS is organized on a regional plan
- EMS is a system of care
- EMS is a system of components
- EMS is a system with subsystems for special clinical problems
- EMS is a two-level system of basic life support (BLS) and advanced life support (ALS)

More than $244 million was spent between 1974 and 1981 to establish, expand, and improve EMS across this country. Dr David Boyd, the federal EMS director, reported in 1981 that 98.4% of the nation's EMS regions had received some form of federal support related to EMS.[15] Between 1967 and 1981, more than $532 million was expended on EMS development through a number of agencies. Besides the $244 million from DHEW, additional funds were provided by the National Highway Traffic Safety Administration and the Robert Wood Johnson Foundation (Table 1-1).

EMS systems, although varied in configuration, usually are planned with some reference to the majority of the 15 EMS components originally defined in the 1970s: staffpower, training, communications, transportation, facilities, critical care units, disaster linkages, consumer information, consumer participation, public safety, patient transfers, record keeping, evaluation, mutual aid, and access to care. The specific clinical conditions requiring specialized system planning and organization are trauma, burns, spinal cord injuries, acute cardiac events, poisonings, behavioral emergencies, and high-risk infants and mothers.

Fundamental to the EMS organization is the difference between BLS and ALS. BLS refers to the level of care rendered to patients who use the EMS system and usually refers to noninvasive treatment provided by first responders and basic EMTs. This care may include such interventions as cardiopulmonary resuscitation, splinting, or extrication. ALS is the care rendered to patients that is beyond the basic level and includes such invasive interventions as the administration of medications, definitive airway control (ie, endotracheal intubation), external cardiac defibrillation, or needle chest decompression. ALS response to a scene is provided by either ground ambulance personnel or specialized ALS air medical teams in helicopters and fixed-wing aircraft.

Even though EMS is well into its third decade, and despite the obvious improvements in the delivery of prehospital care, more emphasis is being placed on the treatment and transport of the critically ill or injured patient to decrease morbidity and to prevent mortality. There is little doubt that the sophistication of EMS systems improved the outcome of those patients with acute cardiac events in the field.[16,17] The trauma patient, however, has been the focus of reports since 1966. In 1985, Congress authorized the DOT to investigate the injury issue. The DOT requested that a study be done by the NAS. As a result of this request, the Committee on Trauma Research was established with links to the NRC's

Table 1-1 Grant Funds Allocated for EMS Development, 1974–81

Agency	Year (purpose)	Funds Awarded (dollars)
EMS–DHEW	1974–81 (systems)	244,702,000
EMS–National Center for Health Services Research	1974–80 (research)	31,625,000
EMS–Bureau of Health Manpower–Health Resources Administration	1974–80 (training)	33,099,000
Health Services Mental Health Administration	1972 (EMS projects)	16,000,000
Regional Medical Program	1970–72 (systems)	10,800,000
Robert Wood Johnson	1972–77 (systems)	15,000,000
National Highway Traffic Safety–DOT	1967–81 (Standard 11)	173,709,070
	1967–81 (research)	8,000,000

Commission on Life Sciences and with the NAS's Institute of Medicine. The 16-member committee provided the template for future federal funding in their report *Injury in America*.[18]

Injury in America describes known facts related to injuries and exposes inadequacies and areas with insufficient data, and it makes numerous recommendations to address these issues. All the recommendations are organized into a plan that focuses the injury problem into five categories: epidemiology, prevention, biomechanics, acute care, and rehabilitation. Just as the 1966 report was the forerunner of the establishment of the DHEW's Division of Emergency Medical Services, the 1985 report was the forerunner of an injury control program at the Centers for Disease Control of the Department of Health and Human Services. The Division of Injury Control funds injury research centers and extramural grant programs across the country. With the annual budget increasing since 1985, more funds are available to continue the much-needed research.

COMPONENTS OF AN EMS SYSTEM

As the research continues to develop strategies for injury control, EMS systems are responding to countless calls for medical assistance. The following description of the components of an EMS system highlights the organization and staffpower necessary to meet the medical needs of those persons requesting prehospital emergency medical care. The emphasis on system organization is key to the delivery of prehospital EMS and requires coordination of the following components not only on a planning level but also operationally.

Staffpower and Training

The improvement in the organization and delivery of EMS has strengthened the links between those persons who provide care in the field and the hospital-based health professionals who receive the patient. The most profound advances in the staffpower available for EMS are prehospital providers at both basic and advanced levels. A variety of terms are used to reflect the degree of training, including basic EMT, EMT-intermediate (EMT-I), EMT with additional training in external defibrillation (EMT-D), and the most advanced paramedic (EMT-P).

Basic EMT

DOT funding in the late 1960s led to the development of a standard curriculum for the training of ambulance attendants. Before the development of the DOT curriculum, the Committee on Injuries of the American Academy of Orthopedic Surgeons was the leader in offering training programs beginning in 1964 for emergency care providers.[19] In 1971, *Emergency Care and Transportation of the Sick and Injured*,[19] by the American Academy of Orthopedic Surgeons, was published. Additional texts are now available, but the so-called orange book and its subsequent revisions are classics. The DOT curriculum encompasses the principles of patient assessment; the techniques of patient management (limited to noninvasive management such as splinting, cardiopulmonary resuscitation (CPR), bandaging, oxygen administration, and extrication); and transportation techniques. Table 1-2 outlines the topics of a basic EMT training program. Although the standard curriculum is approximately 81 to 100 hours, there are known EMT training programs that exceed these hours; for example, in Hawaii an EMT training program can be as long as 315 hours.

Table 1-2 Basic EMT Training Course

Introduction to emergency care training
Anatomy and physiology and patient assessment
Airway obstruction and respiratory arrest
Cardiac arrest
Bleeding and shock
Soft tissue injuries
Principles of musculoskeletal care/fractures, upper extremity
Fractures of pelvis, hip, lower extremity
Injuries to head, face, eye, neck, spine
Injuries to chest, abdomen, genitalia
Medical emergencies
Childbirth
Burns and hazardous materials
Environmental emergencies
Psychologic aspects of emergency care
Lifting and moving patients
Principles of extrication
Ambulance operations

The National Association of State Emergency Medical Services Directors, formed in 1980, launched the National EMS Clearinghouse in 1985. The Council of State Governments manages the Clearinghouse in Lexington, Kentucky and offers many research reports and survey results stemming from their biennial survey of state EMS programs. For 1986 to 1987 they report that there were 363,691 EMTs in the 43 states participating in the survey.

The National Registry of Emergency Medical Technicians in Columbus, Ohio conducts testing and certification for basic EMTs and currently has 79,000 registered. Twenty-nine states have reciprocity recognizing national registry certification. In some states, such as California, the certification of EMTs is a county responsibility and therefore may vary across the state. The basic EMT has a well-recognized and standardized role in the provision of prehospital emergency medical care, and the scope of practice is relatively uniform across the nation.

EMT-P

Countries such as England,[20] Ireland,[21] and the former Soviet Union[22] were involved in comprehensive, sophisticated methods of prehospital care utilizing mobile intensive care teams in the 1970s, but the United States was relatively slow in integrating advanced life support into its EMS systems. Although California passed the Wedworth-Townsend Paramedic Act in 1974, other states still do not have ALS capability uniformly throughout their regions. Advanced ambulance services were initiated in the late 1960s and early 1970s, often as a result of a single interested physician leading the effort.[23] The programs that resulted, therefore, were developed and defined at a local level and varied significantly from state to state. Beginning with Dr Eugene Nagel's first advanced EMT training program in 1967, the growing numbers of courses over subsequent years have varied in length, skills taught, depth of academic basis, certification, and testing.

In 1977, the DOT, Department of Labor, and DHEW with consultation from the University of Pittsburgh published the first Emergency Medical Technician–Paramedic National Training Course. Because training in some parts of the country preceded the availability of a national training model, there was considerable concern over the effect of this gap on defining the role and scope of practice of an advanced EMT.[23-25] The role of the EMT-P is predominantly one of providing ALS to patients who require such interventions as the administration of medications, definitive airway control, defibrillation, intravenous fluid resuscitation, and/or electrocardiographic (ECG) monitoring and interpretation.

The National Training Course has been updated over its 14-year history and now contains the modules listed in Table 1-3. The National Registry also administers an examination for the EMT-P and now has approximately 14,200 certified across the United States. The National Clearinghouse reports 41,259 EMT-Ps in its 1986–87 survey, but the number is greater because nine states that do recognize paramedics were not included in this figure. The city of Boston[26] cites the following reasons for the success of its first two paramedic training programs as measured by successful completion of the National Registry certification examination by 28 of 29 students: close adherence to the objectives and curriculum content of the National Training Course; an in-depth academic basis in anatomy and physiology; dedicated course faculty instead of multiple lecturers; comprehensive selection process for students including a written examination, personal interview, previous field experience, and job performance review; comprehensive clinical resources at a major teaching hospital for clinical rotations; a 500-hour field internship including EMS physician or emergency nurse supervision conducted with a service with a large call volume; full-time training schedule; and medical director availability.

Research in the field of prehospital emergency medical care has predominantly been related to those patients treated by some form of advanced EMT. Researchers attempted to prove the usefulness of ALS and its impact on reducing mortality. The controversy regarding the need, expense, and organization of ALS systems has been long-standing, yet it has been the strongest when the care of the injured or traumatized patient is discussed.

Eisenberg et al[17] compared the survival of patients defibrillated in the field by EMTs trained in the recognition of ventricular fibrillation and countershock techniques with that of patients receiving care by standard basic EMTs and found an increased survival with treatment by the more advanced EMTs. Other such studies have reinforced the positive impact that the provision of ALS has on patients with cardiac disease.[27,28]

The controversy, however, persists for patients with trauma. Jacobs et al[29] documented an improvement in survival of trauma patients if they were managed by prehospital ALS providers, yet another group as late as 1985 called the prehospital stabilization of critically injured patients a failed concept.[30] The controversy stems from the influence of scene time and the use of ALS skills. The differences in response time to urban compared to rural areas was documented by Alexander et al,[31] with urban response times being less than 5 minutes in 61% of the calls.

Table 1-3 EMT-P Training Course

Prehospital environment
  Roles and responsibilities
  EMS systems
  Medical-legal aspects
  EMS communications
  Rescue
  Major incident response
  Stress management

Preparatory
  Medical terminology
  General patient assessment
  Airway and ventilation
  Pathophysiology of shock
  General pharmacology

Trauma
  Trauma
  Burns

Medical
  Acute abdomen
  Anaphylaxis
  Toxicology
  Alcohol/drugs
  Infectious diseases
  Geriatrics
  Respiratory system
  Cardiovascular system
  Endocrine system
  Nervous system
  Environmental hazards
  Pediatrics

Obstetrics and gynecology
  Obstetrics and gynecology
  Neonatal care

Behavioral
  Behavioral emergencies

The use of various ALS skills to stabilize patients who have sustained trauma has been researched, but not conclusively. One area in particular that continues to be the subject of investigations is the need for the pneumatic antishock garment (PASG) as part of the ALS treatment of hypotensive patients. Mattox et al[32] in a prospective, randomized study of 911 patients concluded that the PASG was not indicated in patients transported within an urban environment. Others continue to pursue the physiology behind and the use of the PASG. Bivins et al[33] disputed the old thought that the PASG provides the patient with autotransfusion. A study by Gaffney et al[34] supports the theory that the PASG acts as a vasoconstrictor by increasing systemic vascular resistance. The use of the PASG in patients with pelvic fractures to assist in the control of hemorrhage has also been documented.[35] Because the definitive diagnosis of such an injury is impossible in the field, the prehospital provider must rely on sharp assessment techniques and prescribed guidelines for PASG use as developed by local medical authorities. The issue of PASG use also encompasses whether the transport time to a hospital capable of managing the patient is prolonged or short.

The official journal of the National Association of EMS Physicians and the World Association for Emergency and Disaster Medicine in association with the Acute Care Foundation is *Pre-hospital and Disaster Medicine*. This journal features a controversy section in each issue. The PASG controversy was addressed on the pro side by Dr Norman McSwain[36] and on the con side by Dr Kenneth Mattox.[37] McSwain's final argument states:

> In the final analysis, the PASG is a device useful over the short-term for the control of abdominal and pelvic hemorrhage and for improvement of blood flow to the heart and brain. Like any medical device or technique, it has limitations and should be used by medical personnel who understand its use, indications, contraindications, and complications.[36(p44)]

Mattox's final argument states:

> It is time for physicians involved in pre-hospital treatment to lift their heads out of the sand of blind bias and admit to the mistake of imposing on society an untested and potentially dangerous device. They must either mandate removal of such devices from ambulances or produce scientific data documenting the efficacy and safety of the costly [PASG].[37(p40)]

Another controversy in the prehospital phase of emergency medical care is whether time should be taken in the field to stabilize an injured patient and the degree to which the stabilization should extend. There is almost no controversy regarding the cardiac patient who is in cardiopulmonary arrest; most EMS systems with ALS capability mandate full airway control, antidysrhythmic and other medication use, and ECG interpretation with subsequent defibrillation if indicated.

The trauma patient again poses the dilemma of whether the benefits of definitive stabilization compared to quick transport can be determined. The issues of the length of the response time to the scene, the amount of scene time needed to perform such ALS interventions, and whether extrication time automatically prolongs scene time to allow for such interventions need to be in the analysis. It has been reported that the scene times for patients being managed by ALS units are, on average, 7 minutes longer than those for patients managed by BLS units. This study suggested that ALS teams take more time to assess and administer care to patients than BLS teams.[38] Reines and Duffy,[39] in a study related to the survival of patients with injuries from motor vehicle crashes, concluded that the mean time for ALS units to care for patients was 5.9 minutes longer than for BLS units. The issue that ALS units take a longer time in the field is a valid one, but whether the interventions performed during this extra time contribute to better survival is still questionable.

Whether advanced prehospital personnel should be starting intravenous fluid therapy in the field for those patients with trauma is another EMS controversy. Lewis[40] used a computer model to determine the difference, if any, between fluid administration and fluid loss. He concluded that there is no statistically significant benefit to initiating fluid resuscitation in the field if the scene and transport time is less than 30 minutes. Smith et al,[30] who are well known for not totally supporting the use of definitive ALS treatment in the field by ground ALS personnel, concluded that if the scene and transport time is less than 10 to 15 minutes the time it takes to start intravenous infusions is not worth the effort. The complication rate was studied by Lawrence and Lauro,[41] who determined that intravenous therapy initiated in the field had more significant complications compared to therapy initiated in the emergency department. The issue related to prehospital intravenous resuscitation is again one of time and effort expended when transport to a hospital may be delayed as a result.

In the controversy section of *Pre-hospital and Disaster Medicine*, the issue of fluid resuscitation in the field was addressed by Rottman[42] and Lewis.[43] Rottman connects the two points that seem to form the basis of the prehospital fluid resuscitation problem in his concluding argument[42(p128)]: ". . . immediate fluid resuscitation, in tandem with attendant extrication and splinting for blunt trauma, or en route for penetrating injuries, is the sensible pre-hospital practice." Lewis, on the other hand, focuses his argument on the time that it takes to initiate intravenous cannulation and states "There are no convincing data in the literature to support the efficacy for the administration of [intravenous] fluids in the pre-hospital setting."[43(p129)]

Endotracheal intubation in the field by EMS ground personnel has been studied by a number of researchers. Jacobs et al[44] reported an endotracheal intubation success rate of 96.6% in the early 1980s, the group of patients studied being predominantly nontrauma patients (83.7%). The initial training and number of experiences in performing the skill are significant in final successful intubation rates. Stewart et al[45] demonstrated a 90% success rate for intubation over a 27-month period that improved to 94.5% for noninjured comatose or cardiac-arrested patients during the last quarter of the study interval.

Other skills that make use of different types of devices are employed by some ALS and EMT-I providers. One such device, the esophageal obturator airway, was introduced in 1968; since then other similar devices with adaptations such as the esophageal gastric tube airway and the pharyngeal-tracheal lumen airway have been introduced. A more detailed description of these devices and the research resulting from their use is provided in Chapter 7, *Management of the Multisystem-Injured Patient*.

EMT-I

The National Registry of Emergency Medical Technicians in 1980 developed an examination to test at the EMT-I level. It was not until 1982 that the DOT conducted a study through the National Council of State Emergency Medical Services Training Coordinators. The study was designed to collect data from multiple states to define the knowledge needed to train a new level of EMT between the basic EMT and the paramedic. In 1985, the Emergency Medical Technician–Intermediate National Standard Curriculum was published. The introduction to this curriculum mentions that the cost, length, and degree of difficulty of paramedic programs, along with problems associated with skills maintenance and the actual need to learn certain techniques, were all considered when new levels of advanced training were being developed.

The authors of the curriculum caution readers to think of the EMT-I as a person who is trained beyond the basic EMT level with additional cognitive knowledge and manipulative skills. The EMT-I should not necessarily be considered a step toward the EMT-P, however, and therefore should not be thought of as an incomplete paramedic but more appropriately as a provider on his or her own right at a level beyond the basic EMT. The National EMS Clearinghouse for 1986–87 reported that there were 17,733 EMT-Is, but 11 of the states that recognize EMT-Is did not report their totals, so that the actual number is higher. Table 1-4 lists the topics suggested for an EMT-I training program.

EMT-D

EMT-Ds are those persons who have received additional training in the recognition of ventricular fibrillation and the indications for external cardiac defibrillation. Although 28 states do not recognize this level of EMT certification according to the 1986–87 survey done by the National EMS Clearinghouse, there were 5254 reported EMT-Ds in the states of Iowa, Massachusetts, Montana, New Hampshire, North Carolina, North Dakota, Oklahoma, Oregon, Rhode Island, Utah, Vermont, Washington, Wisconsin, and Wyoming.

First Responders

First responders are those persons who, because of their occupation, may be the first persons responding to the scene of a medical emergency. The majority of these persons are police and fire department personnel. The definition is often extended to include lifeguards and persons from other public safety elements, however, such as special police forces (eg, state police). As a group, first responders have been identified as needing specific emergency care training. Such training would focus on the initial management required to meet the needs of emergency patients as well as specific details pertaining to how to gain access to the local EMS system. A National Training Curriculum for First Responders has been published. The average time to train such a person is approximately 40 hours.

Access to Care

A component of any health care system is the availability of the system to all persons. Whether health care is a right of all society or a privilege for those who can afford it, EMS should be available whenever and wherever needed and to whomever needs it. Synonymous with access to care is the provision of such care regardless of the recipient's ability to pay. This availability should extend from the prehospital care scene, through transport to the initial receiving hospital, and on through transport to a tertiary facility and/or a rehabilitation facility.

The majority of EMS systems should have methods to evaluate all portions of the EMS system that may be prohibiting access to any person or group of persons for any reason, be it political, social, or financial. Access to EMS prehospital care depends on the degree of availability of resources in a particular community and may be governed by

---

Table 1-4 EMT-I Training Course

Roles and responsibilities
EMS systems
Medical-legal considerations
Medical terminology
EMS communications
General patient assessment and initial management
Airway management and ventilation
Assessment and management of shock
Defibrillation

local, municipal, or state governments together with local EMS entities such as regional EMS councils. The level of authority held by each of these agencies varies and may be dictated by a state EMS law. Uncompensated care and the numbers of persons who are uninsured and underinsured will greatly affect the reimbursement for EMS yet should not affect access to care.

The federal government, in an attempt to reduce and control government spending, enacted Public Law 96-499, the Omnibus Budget Reconciliation Act, in 1980. A subsequent act, the Consolidated Omnibus Budget Reconciliation Act (COBRA), was passed in 1985. This act addressed the issue of hospitals transferring or "dumping" patients to other facilities because of patients' inability to pay. Such practice was and is a dilemma for EMS prehospital personnel, who are often called to transfer such patients or who may initially bring emergency patients to certain hospitals known to care for indigent or "charity" patients.

The fundamental concern underlying COBRA is that patients must not be denied access to care, especially emergency medical care. The majority of the emphasis of COBRA legislation is on emergency departments. Marasco et al[46] summarized the areas of emergency medical care addressed by the provisions to this legislation and their impact on EMS:

- *Medical screening:* Medical screening must be provided by the hospital and based on its capabilities to determine the presence of an emergency medical condition.
- *Stabilization:* The hospital must stabilize patients by means of its available resources.
- *Patient transfer after stabilization*: Hospitals must ensure that a patient has been stabilized before transfer. If the patient has not been stabilized, then a transfer requires that the patient be informed of the risks of transfer and that a physician sign a transfer certificate indicating that the patient would benefit from being transferred to another facility.

As these authors suggest, the definitional dilemmas are substantial. If the prehospital EMS provider is requested to transfer an unstable patient from one emergency department to another, he or she must face the intent of the COBRA legislation first-hand and deal with the definition of *stable*. This issue is even more profound for air-transport teams, who often transfer the most sick and injured.

Consumer Participation

Although patients are often referred to as consumers of EMS, this particular EMS component does not address the general public as patients but more as planners, supporters, and communicators. A growing management method for public and private planning groups is to involve the general consumer of the service in the planning and organization of the service to be delivered. The DHEW also supports and recommends this method of consumer participation in its original program guidelines.[14] Reasons cited for involvement of consumers in EMS planning are linking health system agencies through consumers with EMS planning entities; providing consumer access to EMS policy planners to promote communications regarding general public needs, to promote involvement in planning, and to promote an exchange forum for policy implementation; and providing consumers an avenue to register and discuss complaints regarding the general system or specific facts of the system. It is imperative that consumers be aware of problems related to financing EMS systems.

Injury preventionists can also participate in activities related to an EMS system. Often those services that provide EMS care are affiliated with local protective agencies such as police and fire departments. Collaboration with these agencies to control injuries and to implement injury prevention strategies often requires the coordination of public groups, civic groups, and special interest groups (eg, Mothers Against Drunk Driving). The scope of EMS systems goes beyond the actual provision of direct emergency medical care and is often linked to many community-based activities designed to improve health and to reduce the need for EMS.

Communications

Telecommunications is an essential component of any EMS system, yet the sophistication of these systems differs geographically, with some states having excellent technical systems and other states still not having universal 911 access. Communications in a variety of forms serve as a coordinating mechanism to link the many other EMS components with patients. Elements of the communications framework include the following:

- telephone access, or the telephone link for the patient, family member, or bystander to notify and gain access to EMS
- triage and ambulance dispatch, where trained EMS communicators receive and prioritize calls for medical assistance by obtaining information about the presenting problem, other pertinent medical information, and, most important, the location of the incident; once the patient is triaged, the closest ambulance is dispatched (after ALS or BLS response is determined)
- hospital-to-ambulance communications, by which trained basic and advanced EMTs are able to transmit clinical information and patient status to the physician and/or nurses in the receiving hospital; they can also

obtain orders for medical intervention from the hospital providing medical direction
- telemetry, which is used to transmit an ECG signal from the patient to the hospital base station that can be monitored by the physician and/or nurse in the emergency department
- record-keeping, which is a function of a communications system that tape-records phone communications and provides an authoritative record for evaluation purposes
- hospital-to-hospital communication links, which can be initiated by an EMS communication command for use during disaster operations
- medical direction, which is the communication between providers in the field and hospital-based staff

The Federal Communications Commission (FCC) plays a central role in EMS communications. Two federal legislative acts, the Governor's Highway Safety Act of 1966 and the EMS Act of 1973, supported the concept of regional EMS systems. Both acts stressed the importance of a comprehensive communications system as the foundation of a multidisciplinary approach to EMS development. In 1974, the FCC decided on the operational channels for EMS. There are 10 UHF radio channels for BLS and ALS; channels 1 through 8 are designated for medical voice and ECG telemetry communications between hospitals and prehospital services (Table 1-5). Channels 9 and 10 are designated for intersystem dispatching and administrative radio traffic.

The communication systems that evolved for EMS activities were predominantly three: the command and control system (CCS), the radio-telephone switch station (RTSS), and the mobile relay system (MRS).

CCS

The CCS utilizes a central, multifaceted communications center with a control console that can interconnect ambulances, hospital physicians and nurses, and ambulance supervisory personnel on a routine minute-to-minute basis. It can also coordinate public safety agencies, such as police, fire, Coast Guard, and air medical systems, during a disaster.

Table 1-5 FCC-Designated EMS UHF Frequencies

Channel	Frequency (MHz)
1	463.000/468.000
2	463.025/468.025
3	463.050/468.050
4	463.075/468.075
5	463.100/468.100
6	463.125/468.125
7	463.150/468.150
8	463.175/468.175

A staff of trained communicators with additional medical triage training is usually essential. A CCS can assign different frequencies to each user and can also coordinate telemetry from the advanced EMTs in the field to the hospital receiving monitor. The system uses radio frequencies, microwave channels, and telephone lines and relies on remote radios and base stations to link ambulances and hospitals.

Kulp[47] described the functions of a CCS as follows:

- telephone screening of medical emergency calls through the public access system
- dispatching of ambulances and rescue units
- coordination of interagency EMS response in mutual aid
- as-needed assignment of medical control radio frequencies, particularly the UHF channels
- manual patching of radio to telephone and VHF to UHF to overcome any incompatibilities in equipment
- coordination of implementing prehospital point-of-entry plans for appropriate patient transportation destination
- direction and routing assistance for ambulance and rescue vehicles, including aircraft and marine medevac units
- technical monitoring for ensuring quality of ECG telemetry signals
- monitoring of the status of hospital bed availability
- multicasualty or disaster coordination
- radio system testing

RTSS

The FCC allowed dedicated UHF frequencies to be connected automatically to the public telephone network; this is the RTSS. This system is particularly useful to cover a large geographic area. An EMS user can gain access to the system by using a multifrequency UHF radio, and then the signal is connected to the telephone network. The RTSS has the ability to locate and select a free channel by means of an internal scanner. The EMS user must have a dual-tone radio. Each hospital in the system has a special dedicated telephone line to a simple telephone in the emergency department. The EMS user can dial the hospital directly by means of the RTSS. The system has conference call capability so that two hospitals or a hospital and a physician in a remote location can monitor the calls and medical direction.

The advantage of the RTSS is that it does not require trained communications personnel and is less expensive to operate than the CCS. The disadvantage is that there is no call prioritization; thus the first user has sole operation of that frequency until termination of the call. This makes it difficult to deal with simultaneous ALS calls. Also, the RTSS cannot interconnect UHF and VHF and cannot be integrated easily into an area that has elements of both. The increased use of mobile cellular phones, however, has contributed to making the RTSS a more attractive system for some areas.

MRS

The MRS is designed to cover large geographic areas. It comprises a UHF base station that receives a transmission from a mobile radio in an ambulance or other transmitting location, enhances and amplifies the signal, and transmits it automatically and simultaneously on a second frequency. The initial signal is about 30 W of output power, and the amplified signal is 60 W or more. The system can therefore dramatically increase the range of radio communications.

The best location for the relay system is the highest natural or constructed point in the given area. This system is simple and effective but subject to the vagaries of the personnel using the system. There is no controlling authority to coordinate, assign, or prioritize frequencies for calls. The field EMS user is at liberty to select any hospital for medical direction. A second EMS user can then begin to transmit, however, disrupting the previous radio traffic. The system is most useful where there are limited EMS radio traffic needs and large geographic areas to cover.

Central EMS Access

To benefit from EMS care, the patient must be able to gain access to the system as swiftly as possible. The concept of a universal simple access number for emergencies originated in Europe. In 1937, cities in Great Britain implemented a single, three-digit number; Moscow and Stockholm followed with the same.

The incentive in the United States was provided by the President's Commission on Law Enforcement in 1967.[48] By 1979, 800 911 systems had been developed across the country.[49] The three-digit access number has the advantage of being universal, simple to remember, easy to dial, and, in a number of locations, toll-free. Decreasing the time needed to gain access to emergency service agencies was the primary reason that 911 was implemented. Another advantage was that emergency medical, police, and fire services would be contacted by a single number. Trained communicators would be dealing with the public, and interservice cooperation such as needed for a burned victim at a fire or an injured person at the scene of a crime could be more easily facilitated.

Telephone 911 access is not universal across the nation. Cline[50] reports, for example, that only half the counties in North Carolina have 911 access and that those that do not may not even have a universal seven-digit number to use. At first 911 was implemented sluggishly because of the overlap of municipal boundaries and 911 catchment areas. The shunting of requests to appropriate towns was time consuming and inefficient. Technologic advances such as selective routing of 911 calls by an automatic system are available to reduce the mismatch dilemma. Automatic location identification, whereby the caller's address and phone number are automatically displayed on the 911 operator's terminal, facilitates operator callback if needed. This is useful if the EMS personnel arrive at the scene and are unable to locate the victim; they can initiate a callback via the 911 operator.

Summary

In general, the communications component of any EMS system is the operational link that holds the EMS system together. Preplanning of the communications network is essential and requires coordination with EMS planners and agencies providing EMS care as well as integration of the providers once they are trained and certified. Central medical emergency direction denotes the communications center at a local, regional, or state level. It is in these centers that the coordination of EMS systems is carried out.

Patient Transfer

The original intent of early EMS planning in the area of patient transfer was to ensure the effective, efficient, appropriate, and timely transfer of patients from one hospital to another if more comprehensive or definitive care was needed. The usual method to initiate such a transfer was, and remains in some locations, physician-to-physician contact. An organized, sustained approach or a definition of the manner in which a transfer can be efficiently executed is a component that can be implemented for an individual patient or for situations involving multiple patients. Patient transfer protocols can be formalized by having hospitals represented on regional EMS committees or councils and collaborate on the development of transfer agreements among each other or with hospitals from neighboring regions.

Transfer agreements should contain the following elements: identification by name of the transferring facility and the receiving facility, identification of the clinical categories of patients whom the receiving hospital is agreeing to accept, identification of the person at the receiving hospital to contact to initiate the transfer, signatures of both hospitals' chief executive officers as well as of the physician chiefs of the particular clinical services, identification of stabilization procedures to be performed before transport, and identification of the particular ambulance service to contact to transport the patient.

Specialized interhospital transport teams are best known in the area of neonatology, where neonatal physicians and nurses are assigned to ground transport teams by means of specially equipped transport vehicles. With the increased number of helicopter EMS, the transfer of critical patients from one hospital to another is frequently done by these services. Stohler and Jacobs[51] describe the components of a transport program as follows: dedicated transport vehicle, dedicated operators, communication system, medical director, medical transport team, specialized equipment, routine equipment, medical control, documentation, and quality assurance. Table 1-6 describes the requirements to fulfill these components in more detail.

The American College of Surgeons[52] has suggested the following criteria for interhospital transfer of trauma patients:

- central nervous system injury that is penetrating or has resulted in a depressed skull fracture, an open injury with or without leakage of cerebrospinal fluid, a patient with a Glasgow coma score (GLS) less than 13 or one with a deteriorating GCS and/or lateralizing signs, and any patient with a spinal cord injury
- chest-injured patients who demonstrate a wide mediastinum, major chest wall injury, or cardiac injury or those who are in need of ventilation assistance
- pelvic-injured patients with unstable pelvic ring disruption, open pelvic injury, or shock and/or continuous hemorrhage with pelvic ring disruption
- patients who have multiple system injury with severe face and head injuries, chest injuries accompanied by head injury, abdominal or pelvic injury with head injury, burns with associated injuries, or multiple fractures
- patients who have injuries indicating high-energy impact (such as a motor vehicle crash or pedestrian injury where the velocity is estimated at greater than 25 mile/hour or where there is displacement of the front axle or front of the car), patients who have been ejected or involved in a roll-over, or accidents where another occupant of the car had fatal injuries
- patients who are younger than 5 or older than 55 years of age and/or those with cardiac, respiratory, or metabolic diseases as cofactors of their injury
- patients who have secondary sequelae of their injuries (such as sepsis, multiple or single organ failure, or major tissue necrosis) or who have a need for mechanical ventilation

The American College of Surgeons also recommends that burn patients with the following characteristics be transported to a burn center:

- second- and third-degree burns of greater than 10% total body surface area (TBSA), younger than 10 or older than 50 years of age
- second- and third-degree burns of greater than 20% TBSA in other age groups
- second- and third-degree burns of the face, hands, feet, genitalia, or perineum or involving the skin over joints
- third-degree burns of greater than 5% TBSA, any age group

Table 1-6 Components of a Transport Program

Components	Requirements
Dedicated transport vehicle (ground ambulance, fixed-wing or rotor-wing aircraft)	Maintenance contract to ensure safety, oxygen supply, 110-V AC inverter, lighting and climate control, two personnel seats with belts, communications system to contact hospital and medical director, medical equipment and storage
Dedicated operators	Individuals who meet or exceed established minimum training and experience, safety training in emergency procedures, adherence to regulations
Communication systems to receive requests	Trained dispatchers, protocols for dispatching, familiarity with geography, FCC adherence, flight following if air transport is used
Medical director	Licensed physician; emergency, surgical, and/or critical care experience; responsibility for quality assurance; knowledge of protocols and system configuration
Medical transport team	Minimum of two crew members; registered nurse preferred, especially for critical patient transfer; second crew member based on need (ie, physician or respiratory therapist, paramedic); specialized training for air transport crew
Equipment	Based on local regulations, standard routine checking protocol/procedure, routine maintenance schedule and battery recharging
Medical control	Designated medical control physician available by telephone or radio, written treatment protocols, knowledge of EMS system configuration
Documentation	Patient written run form, identification of crew members and medical control physician, run form part of in-hospital record
Quality assurance	Quality assurance written guidelines for all phases of patient transfer, routine meetings, written minutes of meetings, procedures for correction of deficiencies

- significant electrical or chemical burns
- inhalation burns
- preexisting medical conditions that could influence treatment or recovery
- other trauma
- pediatric patients who will need specialized resources
- any patient needing specialized social, emotional, or rehabilitative care or those suffering abuse or neglect

Public Education

Public education and information as components of EMS systems span a number of approaches and differ within certain geographic areas. The most predominant indication for public education, however, is to ensure that the public knows how to gain access to the EMS system when the need arises. The public may also desire to know the type of services that are available within their community.

Other communities may expand the role that EMS personnel have in educating the public regarding the initial approach to an injured family member or an individual's role as a bystander to a medical emergency. The teaching of basic CPR, trauma prevention programs, and information regarding what to do in the event of an accidental exposure to a poison have all been programs where EMS personnel have routinely been key participants.

Mutual Aid

Mutual aid, traditionally a public safety phrase, refers to the ability of a certain community to call upon a neighboring community in times of stress, overextension, and other predefined circumstances (eg, if the need for heavy-duty rescue equipment arises). Because many of the EMS prehospital teams are based in fire departments, mutual aid is a well-known activity used when a fire requires the services of many towns or municipalities to control.

The problem of ambulances not being able to cross jurisdictional lines has been and probably will continue to be a stumbling block for EMS planners to hurdle in order to implement mutual aid agreements. Involvement of local political officials and ambulance service chiefs in EMS planning activities will help publicize this issue and perhaps make a solution possible. Local, regional, and state disaster plans, disaster drills, and actual disaster operations usually transcend jurisdictional boundaries and require multiple EMS to cope with a disaster or multiple casualty circumstances.

Public Safety Agencies

Members of such public safety agencies as police departments, fire departments, and special police forces are often involved with the delivery of EMS whether they are the agency responsible for the initial EMS response to a scene or whether they are collaborative responders. Some are first responders to the scene of accidents and/or sudden illnesses, some are trained and certified as EMTs, and some are performing dual functions as operators of ambulance services along with their primary professional role.

Three specific roles of the public safety agencies as they relate to EMS are involvement in the planning and implementation of local and regional EMS systems; integration of their services into day-to-day EMS operations as well as disaster operations; and continuous concentration on initial training and refresher training of public safety agency members as first responders, basic or advanced EMTs, or rescue personnel depending upon the design of the individual system.

Record Keeping

The importance of adequate records related to patient assessment and treatment has long been known to professionals working in health care facilities. The use of written documentation by ambulance professionals is not yet universal, however. The intent of this component, when defined by the Federal Division of Emergency Medical Services, was to standardize data collection and to ensure the documentation of patient management on the basis of management information, process evaluation, and clinical impact studies.

Record obviously refers to a form that is completed by the EMS provider for each individual patient. Achieving a system of data collection within an EMS system necessitates collecting data from the time of the patient's initial contact with the system (eg, the call to 911) through the patient's last contact (eg, hospital emergency department). A specific handbook, published by the Bureau of Medical Services–Division of EMS, outlines the areas where data are collected:

- general data (eg, name, address, age, and gender)
- communications data
- transportation/intervention data
- ambulance and personnel identification
- times: dispatch time, arrival on scene time, scene time, and transport time to hospital
- name of emergency facility receiving the patient

The prehospital run report or patient record is traditionally completed by the EMS team upon arrival at the receiving hospital. The report should become part of the patient's in-hospital record. The use of the above data elements, when known, emphasizes the necessity of their recording.

General data are used for patient identification and for cross-referencing various patient-generated records in the hospitals. They also serve to define the EMS system's needs in terms of numbers of patients who use the system. EMS planners can use these data to evaluate the system's utilization and to redesign the ambulance deployment system to correspond with geographic areas with high demand.

Communications data are used to plot each patient on a time chart so that future time intervals can be used to compare efficiency of the system's response. These data are often used as a quality assurance indicator (eg, scene times can be evaluated when they are prolonged).

Transportation/intervention, ambulance identification, and time data provide the measure to determine the frequency of use of particular ambulances as well as the number of times each EMS provider has responded to a scene. This information can be used to tabulate numbers of transports per provider to correlate skills performed in the field with identification of geographic areas with a high incidence of calls and with individual providers. It can also be used to categorize clinical conditions and to document the intervention in the field in comparison with hospital-based interventions. The efficacy and appropriateness of care rendered by providers can be monitored and used as a basis for refresher or in-service training as well as individual counseling.

Emergency facility data can be cross-referenced with prehospital data to identify individual patients or certain patient tracer groups; to provide data to compare prehospital and hospital-based patient conditions, assessment, and management; to provide statistics related to frequency of ambulance transports, types of patients received, and incidence of patients received by geographic proximity to hospital; and incidence of various grades of seriousness of patient conditions. They can further be used to identify resources that require allocation to meet patient needs, to evaluate intervention by various members of the health care team, to identify delays in treatment, and to facilitate teaching and research projects. Computerized databases are useful to maintain the operational records of many EMS systems.

Although a more detailed description of helicopter EMS systems appears at the end of this chapter, the use of a database system for such operations is discussed here. An example of such a database is the one used in Connecticut by the operator of the state's only air medical EMS system. The LIFE STAR registry is a computer-based data management system utilized to record, analyze, and graphically depict data. The following elements make up the data recording system: flight run number, day of the week, type of call, pilot, physician, lead flight nurse, flight nurse, flight respiratory therapist, injury time, dispatch time, lift-off time, response time, arrival time, departure time, scene time, distance with patient aboard, total flight distance, referring unit, medical classification of the patient, location of injury, mechanism of injury, town of origin of the call, state, transfer hospital, receiving hospital, receiving unit, age, gender, medical procedures performed, laboratory results, trauma score on the scene, trauma score in the receiving emergency department, injury severity score, outcome, length of stay, intensive care unit length of stay, and indications for the call.

The speed and ease of analyzing and graphically representing data enables the LIFE STAR system to evaluate various components in an efficient and effective manner. By the establishment of this database registry, the operator of the services has ensured the careful recording of air medical data and the quick retrieval and analysis of data. The registry contributes to the assurance that system changes and decisions will be guided by objective realities rather than by subjective opinion or intuition. An important aspect of maintaining such a computerized database is the validity and completeness of information provided by the air medical crew who cared for the patient. It is the responsibility of the crew to complete the run report (Fig. 1-1) and to enter the data into the user-friendly data system.

Disaster Linkages

An EMS system may be stressed to its maximum potential during a time of disaster, whether a multicasualty plane crash or a natural disaster. To respond to a disaster situation that has generated multiple injuries and/or casualties, the EMS system as it operates on a day-to-day basis is usually not sufficient. Therefore, a predefined plan for disaster situations is recommended. Such a plan would be designed for incidents resulting from natural disasters (ie, hurricanes, blizzards, or tornadoes), national emergencies (ie, nuclear accidents, bombings, or terrorist attacks), or mass casualties (ie, aviation accidents, extensive fires, mining accidents, or building collapses).

An effective disaster plan cannot be constructed in isolation. A number of agencies have a role in a regional disaster operation, including public safety agencies, civil defense operations, public health agencies, ambulance services, hospitals and specialty care centers, the Red Cross, public government officials and departments, disaster relief groups, specialized groups, the Coast Guard and National Guard, nuclear power plant safety personnel, and volunteer groups.

A written disaster plan may include, but is not limited to, the following components:

- the definition of a disaster for a specific area, which is usually dependent upon the number of victims or the type of incident and may be represented by degree or stages of disaster alert
- the notification or identification of who can activate the disaster plan and the manner in which a disaster situation is confirmed
- the personnel and the method of notifying off-duty personnel to assist in field operations
- any specialized equipment and its location, inventory of supplies and methods for checking the equipment on a routine periodic basis, and methods for getting equipment to the scene of a disaster if needed
- the identification of proceed-out teams who may need to be brought to the scene and their method of transportation
- a communications plan and the use of certain frequencies for radio transmissions as well as location of the disaster communications coordinating center
- the triage system used to identify levels of injury severity, persons authorized to conduct triage, the location of the triage staging areas, and equipment

Figure 1-1 LIFE STAR run report form.

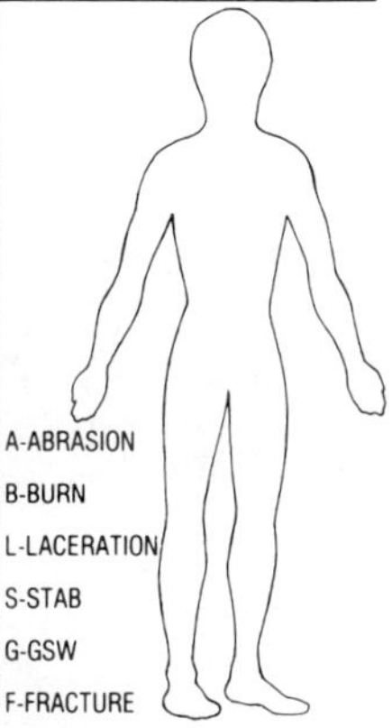

Figure 1-1 continued

- the method for patient identification and the manner in which levels of severity will be determined and the manner in which the patient will be so labeled
- personnel identification and the methods used to designate key personnel necessary for coordination, organization, and security (eg, uniforms, badges, and special headgear)
- the designation of the authority/leadership in charge in the different staging areas
- a point-of-entry plan for the identification of those medical facilities capable of accepting disaster victims for definitive treatment as well as for determining the method of hospital notification and the number of available beds
- identification of decontamination facilities and protocols for securing the incident scene, on-scene management, transport, and in-hospital management of contaminated patients and/or personnel
- transportation plans for air, ground, and sea rescue
- a method for media operations and specific plans for media communications with disaster officials

Although most hospitals have their own internal disaster plans, the integration of EMS systems into a regional disaster plan is optimal. Morris[53] has described the organizational basis for implementing an incident command system (ICS) as part of a regional disaster plan. On the site of a disaster an ICS can organize the disaster scene and the subsequent triage, treatment, and transportation of victims. The designation of one person as the incident commander is key to the operation of an ICS, and it is this person's responsibility to evaluate the disaster and its ramifications, to determine a management scheme, and to communicate with central communications as to the necessity and type of resources needed at the scene.

The ICS utilizes areas divided into sectors, where different roles are executed by sector leaders in such areas as extrication, treatment, support (equipment), and transportation. A staging sector may also be necessary, where transport vehicles and other vehicular apparatus report so as not to congest the actual disaster site. One of the benefits of the ICS is that each sector commander verbally communicates with those assigned to that particular sector. Also, each sector commander is responsible for maintaining communications with the one incident command officer, thereby reducing the need for elaborate radio communications hardware.

Goodwin[54] has described a system for managing mass casualties that was developed by the New England EMS Council and demonstrates the type of planning and organization needed to organize such a system on a six-state basis. In this system there is a strong emphasis on the role of EMS. The command structure identifies one person as the EMS scene control officer, with triage command officers being assigned to head each of four stages of triage. They are the primary triage officer, who identifies those patients with critical, life-threatening conditions; a secondary triage officer, who supervises the tagging of patients; the treatment officer, who identifies and marks the best location for the patient treatment area; and the loading officer, who establishes the transportation sector and organizes the dispatch of vehicles (Fig. 1-2).

Many of the models for disaster and mass casualty operations have been adapted from fire and rescue theories of operation. It is apparent that, regardless of the system used, such operations require organization and planning well in advance of the event, so that the system can be implemented swiftly and each provider, especially EMS personnel, will know his or her role and function.

Transportation

The actual transportation in vehicles was the primary concern of the original investigators who outlined the inadequacies in the delivery of prehospital emergency medical care. Ambulances were largely station wagon or hearse-type vehicles in which patient management and CPR were difficult to perform. The changes in transportation were probably the most visible alterations that have occurred in the last two and a half decades.

The original federal EMS plan suggested the following for BLS units: They should have radio equipment suitable for dispatch and medical consultation, they should meet the DOT General Services Administration (GSA) KKK-1822 specifications, they should be staffed by at least two basic EMTs, they should be located in a place conducive to a response time of no more than 30 minutes in rural areas 95% of the time, and they should utilize a tiered response of vehicles. ALS units should meet all six BLS elements, should be staffed by at least two EMTs trained at ALS levels, and should have communications ability for telemetry.

The federal GSA KKK-1822 specifications were adopted on January 2, 1974 and were revised in 1975 and 1980. The standards expressed a new thinking relative to design and technology and, more important, allowed for a large patient compartment with adequate room for the cot, providers of care, supplies, oxygen, suction, and communications equipment. Although these federal guidelines were available, some states decided to develop their own standards and the degree to which the standards were to be upheld. One state, Massachusetts, developed an ambulance regulation program that licensed ambulance services, inspected vehicles and records, and would withhold a license if certain deficiencies were noted. In 1988, the National EMS Clearinghouse (a service of the National Association of State Emergency Medical Services Directors) estimated that the United States had 35,000 ground ambulance vehicles as part of 12,000 ambulance services. The exact number of vehicles to handle

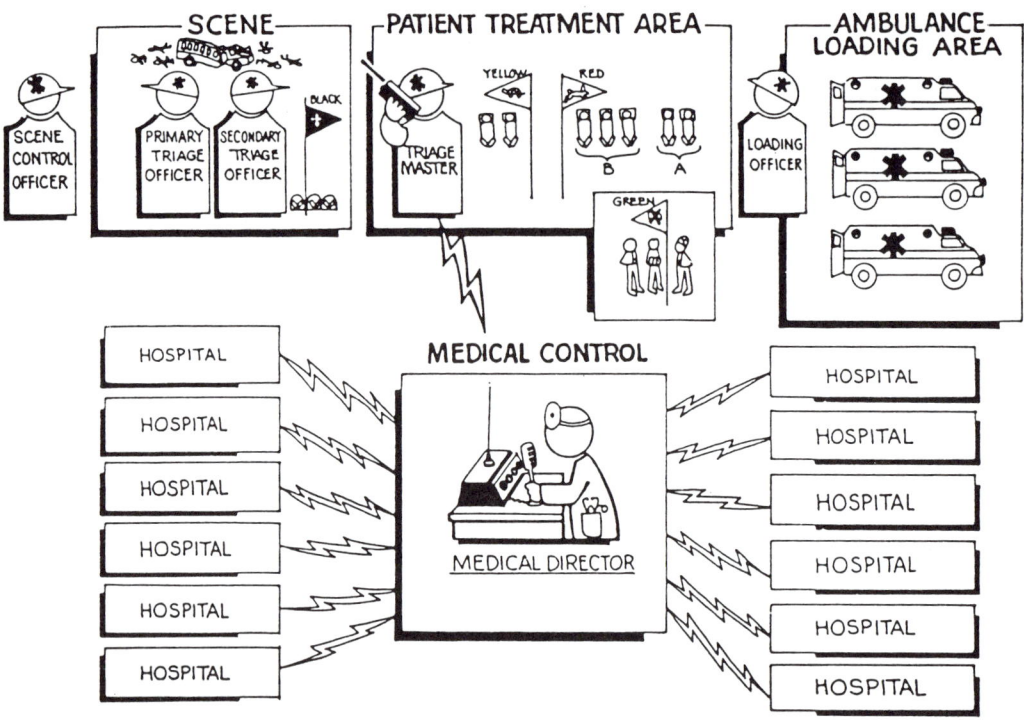

Figure 1-2 System for managing mass casualties.

a certain population is unknown and may depend on the terrain, population densities, and barriers to travel within a certain geographic area (discussed later).

Deployment of vehicles is as important to response times as the equipment and personnel are to the safe management of the patient. A deployment plan usually includes a plan to determine the appropriate number of ambulances needed for a particular area and the most appropriate geographic satellite locations for the ambulances to achieve a given response time and a balanced workload for each unit.

Each city, town, and region has its own financial, political, and geographic restraints that determine the absolute number of ambulances available. The challenge to the EMS operator is how to use these resources to achieve an acceptable short response time and how to maintain skill proficiency by EMTs at all levels of training. Interagency cooperation among police, firefighters, and first responders is usually indicated. Frequently the first responders may be employed by a service different from the one that will actually transport the patient. Fire and police services traditionally have more personnel and equipment geographically interspersed throughout a community. Therefore, if EMS prehospital providers are other than police or firefighters, these two agencies may participate in the system as first-tier responders. Copass[55] reported in 1981 that in Seattle there was a response time of 1.9 minutes for the neighborhood engine company; the district car had a 3.5-minute response time, and the medic unit averaged 7.5 minutes.

Deployment plans may be constrained by a number of factors, some of which are permanently constraining and others that can be alleviated, such as jurisdictional boundaries, inadequate garaging facilities, financial limitations, difficult geographic access, barriers to travel, uneven distribution of workload, and the need for an adequate maintenance and supply system that can respond to multiple satellite locations of vehicles. Larson and Brandeau[56] developed a Hypercube Queueing Model to help the Department of Health and Hospitals of the city of Boston deploy its vehicles. The model is a computer program that inputs historical ambulance data. These data include the number and time of the call, travel time to the scene, average ambulance speed, time spent on the scene, travel time to the hospital, time spent at the hospital, and time taken to return to the satellite location. The EMS provider then locates a given number of ambulances at strategic locations throughout the city, and the program indicates the predicted response time and the percentage of work that each ambulance will perform. A special barriers program was developed to compensate for any geographic barriers such as mountains, rivers, or cemeteries.

For field use, the American College of Surgeons has an algorithm (Fig. 1-3) for deciding when to transport a patient directly to a trauma center.

Facilities

Facilities or hospitals are an EMS component because they are the eventual location where patients are received from prehospital EMS personnel. Organizing hospitals into a coordinated system to respond to changing prehospital prac-

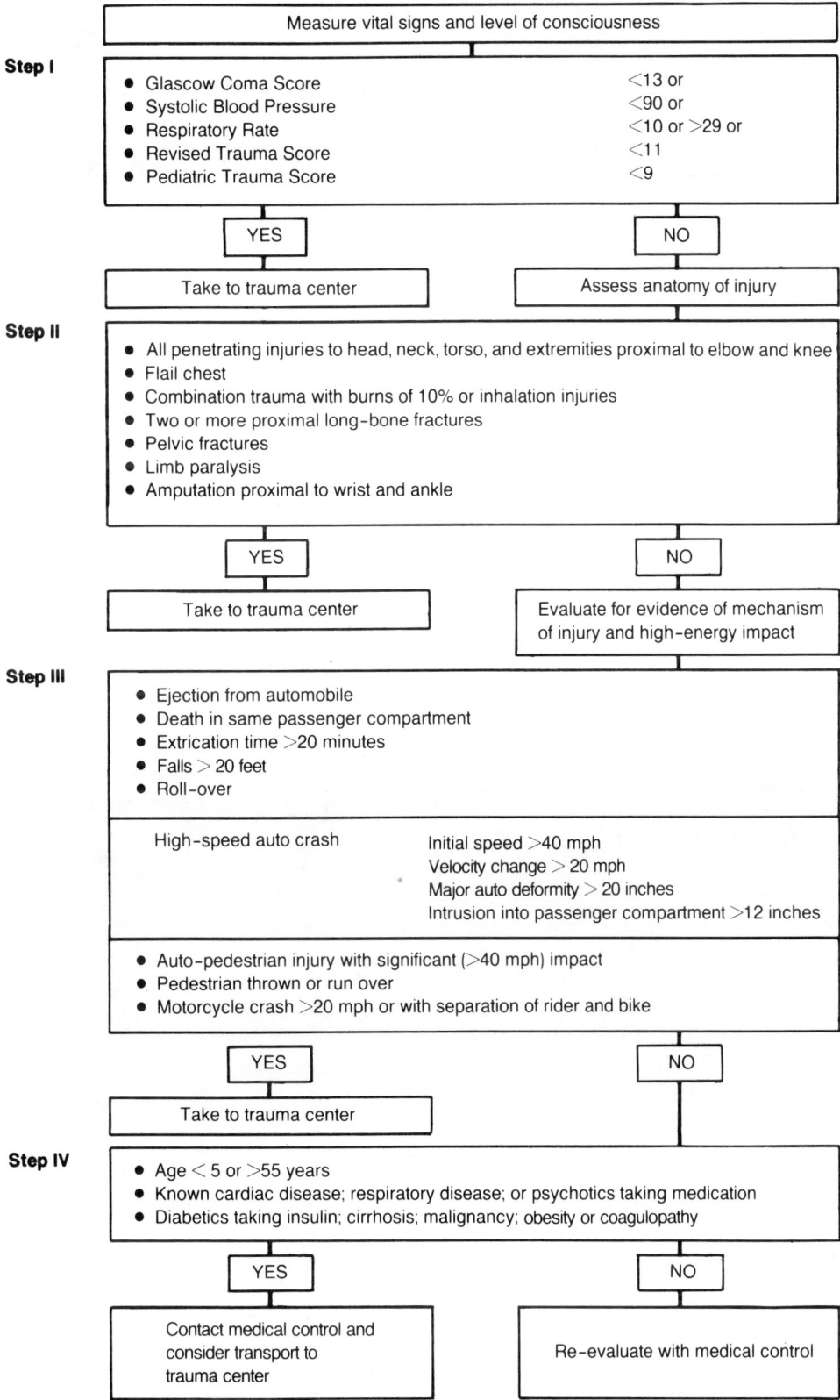

When in Doubt, Take to a Trauma Center

Figure 1-3 Triage decision scheme. *Source:* Reprinted with permission from American College of Surgeons, *Resources for the Optimal Care of the Injured Patient*, p 17, © 1990.

tices was a challenging portion of most EMS grant applications during the 1970s. With little or no funding for communications hardware or any other capital expenses, hospitals were asked to expand and improve services, to participate in provision of medical care outside the hospital setting, and generally to respond to an increase in patient visits. Three specific areas highlight the involvement of hospitals in the sculpturing of EMS systems:

1. categorization of facilities based on resources
2. configuration of the EMS system
3. designation of responsibilities within the system

During the 1970s even the word *categorization* spurred confusion, dispute, criticism, and fear among medical and administrative groups.[57,58] Categorization is a process that utilizes certain criteria to measure the capability of a hospital to manage emergency patients. The point that the hospital closest to the incident should be the receiving hospital for all patients regardless of their level of injury severity is rendered moot. Once this process is achieved, it may be determined that the closest hospital is the most appropriate receiving hospital, but this determination is based on capability and not on geographic proximity.

The first criteria used to categorize emergency facilities were published in 1971 by the American Medical Association (AMA) under the title *Provisional Guidelines for the Optimal Categorization of Hospital Emergency Capabilities*.[59] The term *horizontal categorization*[60] refers to the use of these and similar criteria to determine the general, overall capability of a hospital to manage emergency patients. Once evaluated, each categorizing facility could be labeled comprehensive, major, general, or basic.[59]

The AMA and its Commission on EMS revised the guidelines to meet a different need in the categorization scheme. This need was to determine the capability of a hospital to manage specific emergent conditions. Vertical categorization results in the definition of capability based on particular resources for various types of patients (ie, burns, trauma, spinal cord injury, neonates, etc). The categories resulting from vertical categorization are level 1, or capability to manage all severities of the particular condition with in-house resources; level 2, or capability to manage in the emergency department and intensive care unit but possibly lacking specialized services; and level 3, or capability for rendering initial care to emergency patients with certain physicians on call but probably transferring certain patients to specialty centers.

The discussion of hospital categorization as it relates to prehospital EMS care is essential to the development of a point-of-entry plan that identifies which hospitals should be used for various kinds of patient conditions. Such a plan is ultimately shared with EMS personnel and monitored by the system to be sure that the right patient is getting to the right hospital at the right time. The manner in which patient flow through an EMS system from the original onset of the emergency through rehabilitation is dependent upon how the system is configured and the resources that are available within the EMS region or state.[8]

The categorization and designation of certain hospitals as trauma centers was initiated with the first EMS efforts of the 1970s and continues three decades later. The American College of Surgeons Committee on Trauma has pioneered the efforts to have states plan a system of trauma care that would include the categorization of hospitals as level I, II, or III trauma facilities. Once so designated, the prehospital EMS personnel could utilize a triage decision tree to decide which hospital should receive the patient. In its document *Resources for Optimal Care of the Injured Patient*,[52] the American College of Surgeons has defined the capabilities of the levels of care as follows:

- *level I:* regional resource for trauma care; meets all the requirements to provide total care for all trauma patients at each level of severity; also must have a major commitment toward research and education
- *level II:* a community trauma facility with the resources to resuscitate trauma patients but may need to transfer to a level I center for definitive care
- *level III:* a trauma hospital, perhaps in a rural area where there is no available level I or level II center; does not have the resources definitively to manage trauma patients

It has been reported that only two states, Maryland and Virginia, have a full system of trauma care statewide.[61] Although trauma center designation makes deciding on a receiving hospital for the severe trauma patient an easier task for EMS personnel, the financial implications for those hospitals admitting these patients have resulted in what has been called an American crisis in trauma care reimbursement.[62] Trauma centers in Los Angeles, Chicago, and Miami have abandoned their trauma center designation because of financial problems related to being able to support the care of these patients, many of whom are uninsured or underinsured. Another dilemma for EMS personnel is the diversion status that some hospitals place on incoming ambulances. This means that a particular hospital notifies EMS personnel and tells them not to bring patients there, usually because of the unavailability of an open bed or because of a nursing shortage.

Fischer et al[63] described the effects that a diversion policy used by one of two trauma centers in Houston, Texas had on both the one hospital that diverted and the other that had to receive all the major trauma patients. Although the reasons for diversion, the political precursors, and the subsequent effects are not in the hands of EMS personnel, clearly the diversion policy raises significant concern among these personnel, who have to make difficult decisions regarding their patients' safety.

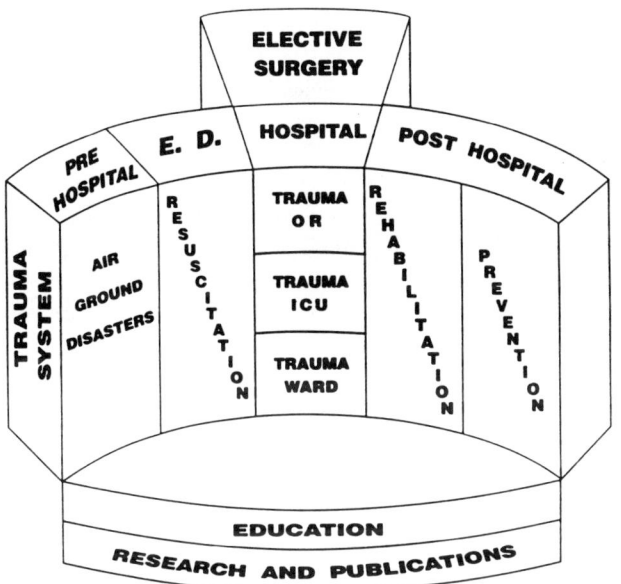

Figure 1-4 Components of a hospital-based trauma program.

Other special conditions such as burns and poisons have received considerable attention in the same way that trauma has. The American Burn Association (ABA) has defined levels of burn care to assist EMS systems to devise a plan for where burn patients should be transported: a burn center or hospital-based burn unit, a hospital with special expertise and a burn program, and a hospital emergency department.[64] The ABA guidelines outline the necessary resources of personnel, equipment, service specialists, and back-up capabilities that all three settings should consider essential or desirable for management of the burn patient. The National Burn Information Exchange, a large database garnering data on burn admissions from a large percentage of the designated burn beds in the United States, has been able to document the increased survival rates of patients treated in facilities where burn care was more organized and utilized a burn team approach to patient care.[65]

Numerous studies have supported the role of trauma centers in improving survival of major trauma patients. Perhaps the most frequently referenced study is the one done in California, where trauma deaths occurring at San Francisco General Hospital were compared to those occurring at smaller nondesignated hospitals in Orange County. The investigators concluded that the number of preventable deaths occurring in Orange County was greater than the number at the trauma center.[66] Certo et al[67] reported on a 5-year study of trauma patients and concluded that bypassing the closest hospital and bringing the patient to a trauma center would have saved more lives.

Cales[68] also reported the effect that the implementation of a regional trauma system had on reducing the numbers of preventable deaths in both trauma centers and nontrauma centers. He concluded that the preventable death rate decreased in trauma centers and remained high in nontrauma centers. The research in the area of the effect of trauma centers on survival and mortality is ongoing, and many defects in research design have been noted, but it is clear that the severely injured trauma patient requires immediate stabilization and early recognition of severe injuries that may require immediate operative intervention. The designation of certain hospitals as trauma centers or burn hospitals is intended to assist EMS personnel in collaborating with their local, regional, or state EMS entities in developing transport protocols that identify the most appropriate hospital for a particular patient.

The current interest in trauma care along with the need for hospitals (aiming to be trauma centers) to formalize their approach to trauma patient care has led to the formation of trauma programs within certain facilities. Jacobs[69] has described the components of the hospital-based trauma program shown in Fig. 1-4.

Evaluation

There are a number of methods to evaluate EMS systems. The individual EMS system itself may decide to develop quality assurance criteria and to measure agreement with those criteria. A management information system that maintains the data discussed in the record-keeping section above would be useful to measure process and outcome objectives. The regional or state EMS council may also participate in evaluation to adjust the EMS system as patient needs dictate. Mortality and morbidity conferences with hospital personnel and EMS personnel are also used by many EMS systems to evaluate the care rendered to patients and to provide a teaching forum for new practices and refinements of on-scene treatment protocols.[70]

Some hospitals employ EMS coordinators to act as liaisons with prehospital personnel; these coordinators may be responsible for monitoring the performance of EMS personnel in terms of patient care and are able to relate to such personnel as a teacher, evaluator, and mediator for smooth transition of the patient from prehospital to hospital-based care.

Subsystems within EMS systems may also develop evaluation strategies. The use of trauma registries in many states has a number of purposes, one of which is EMS system evaluation. Although the first known computerized trauma registry was begun in 1969 at Cook County Hospital in Chicago, a recent survey indicated that hospitals in 35 states have trauma registries.[71] The Center for Environmental Health and Injury Control of the Centers for Disease Control states that "trauma registries can serve as the principal tool for the systematic audit of the quality of patient care provided by a hospital or a trauma system and as a potential source of part of the data needed for injury surveillance."[71(p2280)] Although hospitals are cited as the primary location for evaluation of care, it is clear from the Centers for Disease

Control's recommended core data control for hospital trauma registries that prehospital information is essential. Such data elements from the field include systolic blood pressure, respiratory rate, GCS, mode of transportation, and ambulance response times.[71]

SPECIAL ISSUES IN PREHOSPITAL CARE

Medical Control

Medical control describes the method whereby physicians manage, directly or indirectly, the performance of prehospital ALS personnel. The basic component of medical control is the physician who communicates with advanced EMTs in the field and who provides the actual voice medical direction. The other elements of medical control relate to the manner in which the EMS system is configured to respond to prehospital medical emergencies. These include an identifiable medical director, who is a physician responsible for the medical accountability of the entire prehospital ALS practice; treatment protocols, which are the medically acceptable standards of medical practice in a particular geographic or service area; point-of-entry protocols, which define particular hospitals where patients are taken; and the communications systems, which are used to link the hospital personnel to the advanced EMTs in the field. All these elements are important to build a foundation for a physician-directed prehospital ALS system that permits the practice of medicine by nonphysician field personnel.

The legislative process relative to the practice of medicine in the prehospital setting by ALS paramedic personnel, who are performing tasks as physician surrogates, has not been clearly delineated by statute in many states. Although the physician may have the right to delegate certain aspects of the practice of medicine to his or her surrogates, the physician does remain medically and legally accountable for the actions of the surrogate in the event of inadvertent errors. This clear line of accountability leads to the need for total clarity in operational instructions for prehospital personnel and also the need for careful and accurate recording of all prehospital management ordered by the physician and executed by prehospital personnel.

Because there are various methods for physicians (who are not seeing the patient) to delegate responsibilities, especially to those who are with the patient, Boyd et al[72] described two forms of medical control: on-line and off-line. The on-line medical director is the physician at the resource or base hospital who is directly giving medical direction to the advanced EMT in the field over some form of communications equipment. The forms of medical on-line direction vary; they include a two-tiered medical model involving senior medical/surgical residents in an emergency department providing direction via a base console with attending faculty physicians monitoring these transmissions with a portable radio, emergency physicians in emergency departments who provide total medical direction, and nurses in coronary care units or emergency departments who provide medical direction based on previously determined medical protocols or standing orders.

The administrative off-line medical director is that physician who is responsible for the clinical operation of the prehospital ALS system and therefore is responsible for the appropriateness of the ALS practiced by the on-line physician and the advanced EMTs in the field. This administrative off-line medical director may also be one of the physicians who gives medical on-line direction. In an organized medical control system, the hospitals participating in ALS operations must be categorized, configured, and designated in such a way that the advanced EMTs know exactly who to contact for their medical orders. Treatment protocols are essential. Determination of these protocols clarifies for both the physicians and the advanced EMTs the methods and sequential management plan for any patient. That the physician still has the opportunity to individualize the management of a particular patient is important, but all operating personnel who have an understanding of the general medical approach to clinical problems, including the use of available drugs, will increase their confidence in the system by increasing their familiarity with its management philosophies.

The protocols developed by medical specialists in the community can then be widely disseminated to all the receiving hospitals. This allows any physician whose patient may be treated in the prehospital phase to have input into, and a sound understanding of, the manner in which his or her patient will be managed in the event that the system is used. Although written protocols stand as the most desirable form of medical direction, they still are tools for physicians who are actually communicating with the paramedics or advanced EMTs via radio or telephone.

Another type of medical direction that may be used is the performance of prehospital ALS by standing orders. These standing orders, developed by the physicians, guide advanced EMTs when they perform medical interventions based on whatever management is outlined for a particular medical or surgical problem. One concern with this system is that it is often difficult to record every task performed during a difficult resuscitation effort in an uncontrolled prehospital setting and with minimal assistance. Therefore, the actual intervention can be performed easily yet not recorded or even sometimes not communicated to the awaiting hospital.

A responsibility of the system's medical director is to establish a mechanism whereby regular and systemic review of all ALS transports can be conducted. This evaluation serves a management information purpose as well as a research purpose. Either physicians or specially trained ALS nurse coordinators can review each transport on a daily basis for adherence to protocols, completeness of charting, and accuracy of information. Various record-keeping practices are available to keep track of the utilization of ALS units, frequency of clinical problems, and frequency of specific ALS interventions.

An additional evaluation tool, other than monitoring run reports and tracking patients through the various management phases, is to conduct case review sessions with the physicians and advanced EMTs. In 1981, the Subcommittee on Medical Control[73] agreed on the three basic functions of any medical control design:

1. to ensure that field personnel have immediately available expert direction for emergency care at whatever level they are capable of providing
2. to ensure a continuing high quality of field performance
3. to provide the means for ongoing medical audit of both field performance and the medical control itself

The American College of Emergency Physicians issued a position paper in 1986 entitled *Medical Control of Prehospital Emergency Medical Services* and stated "All prehospital care may be considered to have been provided by one or more of the agents of the physician who controls the pre-hospital system, for this physician has assumed the responsibility for such care." The physician or EMS medical director was the subject of a research survey conducted by Swor and Krome.[74] Although some significant research constraints, such as small sample size, limit the applicability of this research, it does shed some light on the issues of reimbursement and legal risk associated with being an EMS medical director. The surveys were completed by 69 EMS medical directors from 21 states and 2 Canadian provinces who were attending a conference of the National Association of EMS Physicians in 1986 or 1987 along with 55 other physician members of the same association and an additional 14 Michigan-based EMS medical directors (total surveyed, 138).

Interestingly, 22% of the respondents admitted that they had been involved in legal action as a result of their being an EMS program medical director. Six of the legal actions were related to paramedic malpractice, three to system failure, two each to inappropriate destination and dispatch error, and one each to equipment failure, union grievance, withdrawal of medical control, and trauma center designation. Eighteen states have legislation that deals with physician protection from civil liability related to EMS medical control responsibilities.[75]

Others have tried to focus the issue of medical control and the relationship of physicians to the practice of medicine in the field by nonphysicians. Pepe et al,[76] who are physicians with a tendency to gaze at EMS systems with a critical eye, state "When medical supervision is provided properly, paramedic practice no longer is an issue." The reason for such a statement appears to be that, although advanced EMTs are actually rendering medical care to patients in the field, the responsibility and success of such practice rests with those physicians directing such care. These investigators also relate the evolution of EMS medical directors from the early years, when most personally knew the paramedics whom they were supervising, to more comprehensive systems frequently guided by committees of physicians. The crux of their discussion is that, because of the complexities of the EMS systems of today, full-time physician involvement by physicians who have had education and experience in EMS training and operations is essential if the system is to operate safely and in the best interest of the patient.

Medical control and/or direction has been and will continue to be an important issue in prehospital emergency care, especially in those areas where ALS is provided.

Staffing

How many ambulances and personnel are needed to service a community is largely computed from the need and response times that can be achieved. The factors that influence staffing patterns can be so diverse in different communities, however, that actual staffing ratios should be carefully analyzed. Geographic density, age of the population, number of hospitals, and volunteer and public or private paid ambulance services are all important characteristics that determine staffing patterns.

As far back as 1976, Washington state physicians reported that EMS ambulance services respond to 1 true emergency per 10,000 persons.[77] The American College of Surgeons[78] reported the EMS response to patients at a ratio of 50 to 60 injuries and 3 to 4 cardiac arrests per 1,000,000 population/day.

More recent research done by Braun et al[79] at the Northern California Center for Pre-hospital Research and Training provides an excellent picture of the configuration of EMS systems in the 25 cities in the United States with populations between 400,000 and 900,000. Cities interviewed were Atlanta, Baltimore, Boston, Cleveland, Columbus, Dallas, Denver, El Paso, Honolulu, Indianapolis, Jacksonville, Kansas City, Memphis, Milwaukee, Nashville, New Orleans, Phoenix, Pittsburgh, San Antonio, San Diego, San Francisco, San Jose, Seattle, St Louis, and Washington, DC. The following definitions of one- and two-tiered system configurations were used in this study:

- *one-tiered system:* ALS units respond to and transport all patients
- *two-tiered system A:* ALS units respond to all requests; after evaluation, the case can be referred to a BLS unit for transport
- *two-tiered system B:* dispatch decides whether to send a BLS or ALS unit; the ALS unit may be canceled by a first responder or BLS unit, or the ALS unit may refer the patient transport to a BLS unit
- *two-tiered system C:* ALS personnel aboard a non-transport unit and a BLS unit are both dispatched; ALS

personnel, if needed, transport the patient with and in the BLS unit or, if not needed, return to service, and the BLS unit transports patient

Of interest are the following findings. Eighty percent of the cities utilized 911. In 44% of the cities the fire department was the primary ambulance provider, and in 28% of the cities it was the health department; only two of the cities utilized a private ambulance company. Dispatch was the responsibility of personnel minimally trained as an EMT in 58% of the cities; in 16% of the cities paramedics handled dispatch, in 44% of cities basic EMTs did, in 24% it was a combination of civilians and firefighters, in 8% it was a combination of civilians and EMTs, and in 8% dispatch was achieved by a combination of EMTs and paramedics. Thirty-two percent of the cities had computer-aided dispatch. In 16% of the cities, less than 50% of the requests received a code 3 (lights and sirens) priority. In the 96% of the cities that utilized first responder or coresponder programs, they were the responsibility of the fire department, but in 36% of the cities the first responder training level was equivalent to the DOT first responder guidelines, with some cities training to a lesser degree and others to a greater degree. The average first responder response time was 3.2 minutes. Sixty percent of the cities had the one-tiered system and 40% the two-tiered system; of the cities with two-tiered systems, only one (11%) had system A, seven (77%) had system B, and one (11%) had system C.

Of interest in this study in terms of staffing patterns is that the average number of calls per 10,000 population was 2.3, with the range being 0.9 (Honolulu) to 5.2 (Washington, DC). This figure is tempered by the fact that this ratio represented actual calls to dispatch and not patients transported. In other research done in Boston, it was found that of 69,449 calls for medical assistance only 33,196 patients (47.8%) were transported. Calls for assistance are often received for the same incident from a number of callers, or some callers call 911 for the same request more than once.

Also interesting is a comparison of numbers of units and response times in cities with the same population. For example, Boston has a resident population of 665,000 (but swells to 1,000,000 during peak working hours), is 47 square miles, and has three ALS units and twelve BLS units with an average response time of 8.5 minutes (code 3 calls only, which represented 33% of all calls). On the other hand, Jacksonville has a similar population of 625,000 but is 523 square miles and operates 15.5 ALS units and 15.5 BLS units with an average response of 5.2 minutes (all calls are dispatched as code 3). San Antonio, the largest city in the study in terms of area (1,249 square miles) and with a population of 1,000,000, operates 17 ALS units and achieves a response time of 6.7 minutes with all calls dispatched as code 3.

The National EMS Clearinghouse has published a report entitled *Training and Certification of EMS Personnel*.[80] This report found that in general all states recognize EMTs, 11 states do not recognize EMT-Is, 2 states do not recognize paramedics, and 28 states do not recognize EMT-Ds. Although 7 states did not contribute to the survey as it related to numbers of EMTs per 10,000 population, the range for those that reported was from 0.16 EMTs per 10,000 population in Delaware to 5.15 EMTs per 10,000 in West Virginia.

The determination of staffing patterns has to be achieved with a number of factors known to EMS planners, including population both day and night, determination of type of response (ie, one- or two-tiered), funding, medical control configuration, levels and availability of training, local/regional/state EMS plan, budget considerations, and designation of responsibilities and authority within the system.

Rural Emergency Medical Services

The Senate Rural Health Caucus requested that the Office of Technology report on health issues related to rural America. In 1989 a special report concerning those health issues as they relate to EMS was published.[81] The concerns to generate such a report stemmed from perceived inadequacies in EMS systems to meet the needs of those citizens residing in rural areas. Although only 25% of the US population lives in areas considered rural, the actual geographic area represents four-fifths of the US land mass. For example, Johnson[82] has reported that Alaska's EMS systems must cope with a state of 586,000 square miles and a population density of fewer than 1 person per square mile; the total population is 530,000.

Not only has population density been an issue in rural America, but the economic forces facing hospitals and health care facilities have led to the closure of approximately 550 rural hospitals since 1981.[83] The *Rural Emergency Medical Services Special Report*[81] highlights a number of facts and figures previously published; for example, the death rate from unintentional injuries is twice as high in rural areas as in those cities with a population of 1,000,000 or more. If one is severely injured in a rural area, the chance of dying is three to four times greater than in an urban area. Although the frequency of motor vehicle fatalities is less in rural areas, the death rates are higher. In 1986 there was a total of 47,865 motor vehicle–related deaths in the United States. Of these, 31,867 (66%) were in metropolitan areas and 15,998 (34%) in nonmetropolitan areas. The overall death rate was 19.9 per 100,000, but in the metropolitan areas it was 17.3 compared to 28.4 in the nonmetropolitan (rural) areas. In 1988, it was reported that 31 states had rural areas that were not covered by EMS radio communications systems.[84]

Some of the problems specific to rural areas cited in the report[81] are as follows. Rural hospital may be unstable because of the economic problems facing health care facilities. Shortages of health care personnel occur because of recruiting and retaining problems. Because of the closing of some rural hospitals, there may be an increased burden on EMS for even primary care problems. Barriers to detection of an emergency exist (ie, small populations, inaccessible or remote areas, poor road conditions, and limited communications equipment). There is a low level of prehospital provider training programs. Maintaining skills may be difficult because of low patient volumes. Standardized curricula do not meet the educational needs of rural EMS providers. Finally, not enough physician supervision is available.

The report[81] also analyzed data from the American Hospital Association Survey of Hospitals and concluded that of the 1771 metropolitan hospitals 96% had an emergency department, 17% had a trauma center, and 76% had a blood bank. In comparison, of the 2425 nonmetropolitan hospitals 98% had an emergency department, only 8.4% had a trauma center, and 63% had a blood bank.

Some of the solutions (considered options) to rural EMS problems as outlined by the Office of Technology[81] are the following:

- federal funding to improve the supply and level of skills of EMS providers
- congressional requirements that the DOT reevaluate the standardized curricula for EMS providers
- federal legislation to facilitate a national consensus for standards for EMS providers
- federal legislation to facilitate a national consensus for standards for facilities (ie, trauma centers)
- federally mandated technical assistance for states
- federal funding of research through the DOT and DHEW
- increased federal funding through the DHEW's Preventive Health Block Grant Program
- new federal funding through an EMS categorical grant program
- implementation of state plans that particularly address rural EMS problems in programs that provide federal EMS resources to states

Scattered throughout the report[81] are other solutions to specific problems, such as the installation of emergency call boxes along major rural highways to improve EMS access capability, utilization of a mobile EMT training program model that would provide training for volunteers, assigning EMTs who need refresher training to local hospitals, and installing a telephone lecture program whereby learners can use the telephone to attend lectures.

The cost of EMS is an important component of any system analysis. Although state EMS offices are receiving less money since the days of federal EMS funding, this does not mean that EMS are not operating in financially stable conditions. The intent of the original EMS federal initiative was to have states and even EMS regions become self-sustaining. The National EMS Clearinghouse, in a report entitled *The EMS Office: Its Structure and Functions*,[85] concluded that 64% of the 1988 state EMS program funding was from state funds, 10% was from federal Prevention Block Grants, 4% was from other federal funds, and 18% was from local funds. The amount of funds spent on EMS varies not only from state to state but also by the type of service provided by the funds. For example, the five states with the highest expenditures of just state funds toward their total EMS funding are Hawaii ($15.1 million), Florida ($11.3 million), Pennsylvania ($7.7 million), Maryland ($5.5 million), and New York ($5.4 million).[81] California devotes $1.7 million from its Prevention Block Grant to EMS, which, when added to other funding sources, makes California the sixth state to expend the most on EMS at the state level. Per capita spending is the greatest in Hawaii, where state EMS spending is $13.90 per capita. The two states with the lowest per capita EMS spending are Ohio, at $0.02 per capita, and Indiana, at $0.04 per capita.

It does not require state EMS spending, however, to provide EMS services to a community. Maryland, with a large fleet of EMS helicopters operated by the State Police and a dedicated Shock Trauma Unit at the Maryland Institute of Emergency Medical Services, has obviously declared EMS a significant health priority for the state.

Air Medical Systems for Emergency Medical Services

History

Air medical transport of critically ill and injured patients in the United States is a relatively new and innovative method to contribute to the reduction in both morbidity and mortality. Although helicopter transportation was a well-known military activity during both the Korean and Vietnam wars, it was not until the early 1970s that the civilian air medical industry began to flourish.

Early attempts at medical rescue with helicopters was initiated in the 1960s as part of the fire rescue unit in Los Angeles. The Hover Jumpers, when terrain prohibited landing, would jump approximately 20 feet from a hovering helicopter to render medical care to patients.[86] Also during this time, medical helicopters were operated out of the fire and police departments in Chicago and would transfer patients to Cook County Hospital.[87] The National Highway Traffic Safety Administration funded other demonstration projects to test the use of helicopters in civilian EMS and concluded that such a service was expensive, required integration into the ground EMS system, may not have a role in urban settings, and required a medical configuration.[88] The state of Maryland began an air rescue system with State Police helicopters and paramedics in 1969.

Loma Linda Hospital in California initiated a helicopter service in 1972 that was operated by the hospital but was not based at the hospital; this program subsequently was discontinued. The title of *first* actually goes to St Anthony's Hospital in Denver, for it was there that the first hospital-based

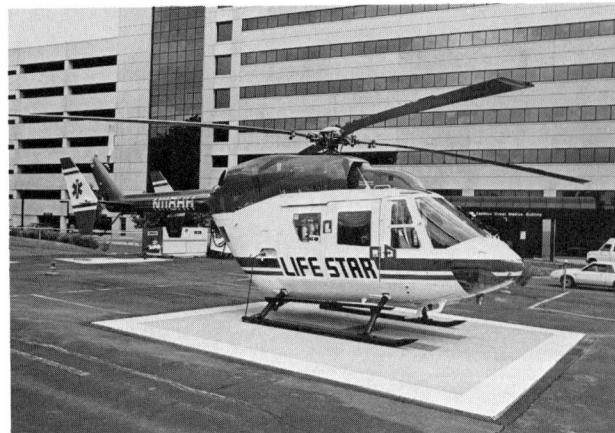 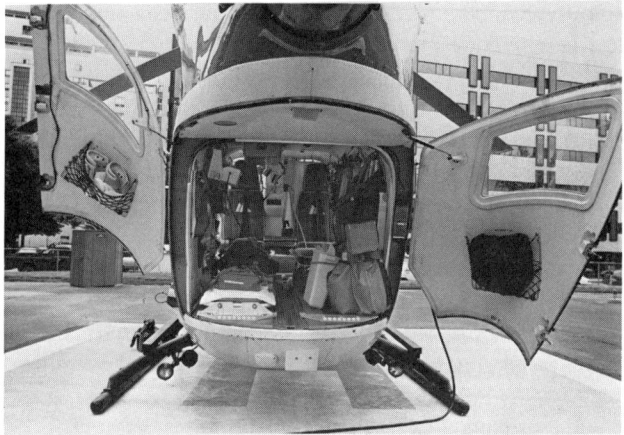

Figure 1-5 Exterior (**A**) and interior (**B**) views of the BK117 helicopter, a third-generation EMS helicopter.

helicopter EMS began that is still operational today.[89] Hospital-based helicopter EMS has been categorized as first-, second-, or third-generation services. First-generation services such as the St Anthony's program have the following characteristics:

- use of a single-engine helicopter
- medical direction and supervision of the service
- ALS-educated flight crews led by nurses
- integration into the existing EMS system of the region
- service provided primarily to the sponsor hospital
- low charges for transport

The light, single-engine helicopters used in first-generation services are readily available and inexpensive and require small landing areas to respond to scene requests. The single-engine Aerospaciale Allouette helicopter has been used frequently in areas such as Colorado, where evacuation capability from high elevations is essential.

The second-generation helicopter EMS are those that became operational during the late 1970s and early 1980s, when a surge of programs flourished. The following characteristics define them:

- a Certificate of Need is required to begin a helicopter EMS
- research reporting effectiveness of the service is necessary to support the Certificate of Need
- expansion of the service beyond caring for trauma patients is expected (ie, transport of neonates and critical medical patients)

Third-generation helicopter EMS, which are now operational, began as the concern for health care costs became a leading issue. The characteristics of third-generation helicopter are as follows:

- use of twin-engine helicopters
- strict adherence to Federal Aviation Administration (FAA) regulations and industry-supported safety guidelines
- involvement of state regulatory agencies
- systems that use multiple hospitals as both transferring and receiving facilities
- refinement of use
- quality assurance standards

Figure 1-5 shows the Messerschmidt Bolkow Blohm BK117 twin-engine helicopter; this is an example of a third-generation EMS helicopter.

Research

Considerable research throughout the development of these generations has been done. Rhee et al[90] reported specific rates for trauma, burns, spinal cord injuries, and neonatal crises as a way to predict prospectively the utilization of a helicopter. MacKenzie et al[91] reported on 760 patients transported from the scene of motor vehicle crashes and concluded that mortality in 49.7% of the patients was due to a head injury with hemorrhage, massive trauma being the second highest cause of death. Baxt and Moody[92] used the Trauma Score and Injury Severity Score to calculate the probability of survival of patients with certain injuries with the Trauma Score/Injury Severity Score (TRISS) methodology described in the American College of Surgeons' major trauma outcome study.[93] This method was used to compare 150 ground transported patients with 150 air transported patients, all of whom ultimately were treated at the same hospital. The investigators concluded that there was a statistically significant difference in the predicted mortality of both groups, with the air transported patients having a 52% reduction in predicted mortality. Other studies supporting the increased survival of patients who are transported by air have been done.[94–96]

The use of air medical transport in rural areas is well accepted. Johnson[82] reports that in Alaska there are nine certified air medical services with one additional service operated out of Seattle, Washington that responds to needs in southeast Alaska. The goal of the Alaskan state EMS program is to add six additional services to meet the needs of its remote rural locations. Advantages of helicopter transport in the rural communities are obvious: Because there are fewer densely populated areas in a larger space, the length and duration of EMS transport gives a significant advantage to air transport. Boyd et al[97] reported on rural interhospital transfer of trauma patients, comparing ground to rotorcraft transport. With two similar cohorts that differed only in the mode of transport, they calculated the probability of survival with the TRISS methodology. The patients transported by ground had the same mortality as predicted by TRISS, but the air transported patients had a 25% reduction from the predicted mortality.

Helicopter EMS in Mass Casualties and Disasters

The benefits of air medical services during disasters and incidents where mass casualties may be sustained are the rapid response time over large geographic areas, the ability to manage the most critically injured, and the ability to facilitate multiple patient transports to trauma receiving hospitals. Five roles of helicopter EMS have been established: an augmented disaster response, triage, medical treatment, air surveillance, and evacuation.

Indications for Air EMS

The Association of Air Medical Services released a position paper on the *appropriate use of emergency air medical services*.[98] The paper is designed to provide boundaries for the use of air medical services in emergencies so that they can be used as a foundation for systems to build individual guidelines. The paper cites the role of such services as a means to transport drugs, equipment, and well-educated personnel to the patient as well as a means of transporting donor organs and/or organ transport teams. The document outlines criteria that can be used to guide medical decisions regarding the mobilization of an air medical team. In general terms, the criteria for utilizing air medical transport based on the needs of patients are as follows:

- General patient population
  1. Critical care requirements (eg, monitoring during transport)
  2. Need for short transport time
  3. Need to avoid potential delays in transport (eg, traffic)
  4. Patient is inaccessible by ground vehicles
  5. Patient requires interventions not available in a particular facility
  6. Patient requires a particular physician's care at another facility
  7. Using a ground transport vehicle would leave the area without sufficient coverage
- Trauma patients
  1. Critical scene patient with extended extrication pending
  2. Motor vehicle mechanism of injury indicators (ie, structural intrusion into occupant compartment of vehicle, patient ejected from vehicle, death of another occupant in same vehicle, pedestrian struck at speed greater than 20 mile/hour, overturned vehicle with occupant unbelted, motorcycle occupant thrown from vehicle traveling at speed greater than 20 mile/hour, more than 30-inch displacement of front bumper to the rear or front axle displaced to the rear)
  3. Fall from more than 20 feet
  4. Penetrating injury between midthigh and head
  5. Near or total amputation
  6. Scalping or degloving injury
  7. Severe hemorrhage (ie, systolic blood pressure < 90 mmHg after resuscitation or need for blood transfusions)
  8. TBSA burn greater than 15%; burns of face, hands, feet, perineum; inhalation burn
  9. Actual or potential spinal cord injury or neurologic deficit
  10. Unstable airway resulting from injuries to face or neck that may require invasive intervention
  11. Severe injury computed by a scoring system (ie, Trauma Score, GCS)
  12. Patient younger than 5 or older than 65 years of age with multiple trauma
  13. Adult with respiratory rate less than 10 or more than 30 per minute or heart rate less than 60 or more than 120 beat/min
- Adult medical/surgical patients
  1. Respiratory or cardiac arrest within 12 hours or respiratory failure
  2. Cardiac output being maintained by vasoactive drugs or mechanical ventricular assistance
  3. Cardiac rhythm being maintained by medications or pacemaker
  4. Unstable airway or patient in need of mechanical ventilation
  5. Deteriorating mental status
  6. Hypothermia requiring invasive treatment
  7. Pulmonary artery catheter, intraaortic balloon pump, intracranial pressure catheter, or arterial line
  8. Respiratory rate less than 10 or more than 30 per minute; heart rate less than 50 or more than

150 beat/min; systolic blood pressure less than 90 or more than 120 mmHg
9. Acidosis (eg, pH < 7.2)
10. Organ transplant or procurement
11. Myocardial infarction, dissecting or leaking aneurysm, cerebrovascular accident requiring diagnostic and therapeutic intervention not available at referring hospital
12. Uncontrollable seizures
13. High-risk pregnancy
- Pediatric patients
  1. Presence or risk for cardiac dysrhythmias or pump failure
  2. Presence or risk of respiratory failure or arrest
  3. Invasive airway procedures needed
  4. Unstable vital signs (ie, respiratory rate less than 10 or more than 60 per minute; systolic blood pressure less than 60 mmHg in neonate, less than 65 mmHg in infant younger than 2 years, less than 70 mmHg in child 2 to 5 years, or less than 80 mmHg in child 6 to 12 years)
  5. Near drowning with hypoxia or altered mental status
  6. Status epilepticus
  7. Acute bacterial meningitis
  8. Acute renal failure
  9. Unstable toxic syndrome
  10. Reye's syndrome
  11. Hypothermia
  12. Multiple trauma

Air Helicopter Safety

In 1982, the number of air medical helicopter accidents reached a record high. Eight accidents that year converted to a rate of 25 per 100,000 patient transports.[99] The Aviation Safety Institute analyzed 84 medical helicopter accidents that occurred from 1975 to 1986.[100] The investigation was initiated because the accident rate for medical helicopters was more than twice the rate for the rest of the helicopter industry (ie, passenger transport, petroleum operations, journalist functions, and forestry operations).

Because of the increased rate, safety issues are a priority for all those involved in air medical transports. Pilot error was cited as a significant cause of helicopter accidents. The FAA strengthened regulations to require certain types of safety equipment on board. The FAA also restricts the number of consecutive hours of a pilot's work shift as well as the number of flying hours per shift.[101] Two other conditions contributing to pilot error were poor weather conditions and night flying. Forty percent of medical helicopter flying occurs at night.[102] Visual flight rules have been improved and refined in regard to weather minimums that depend on the time of day and the expected duration of the flight. These changes were heralded by the Association of Air Medical

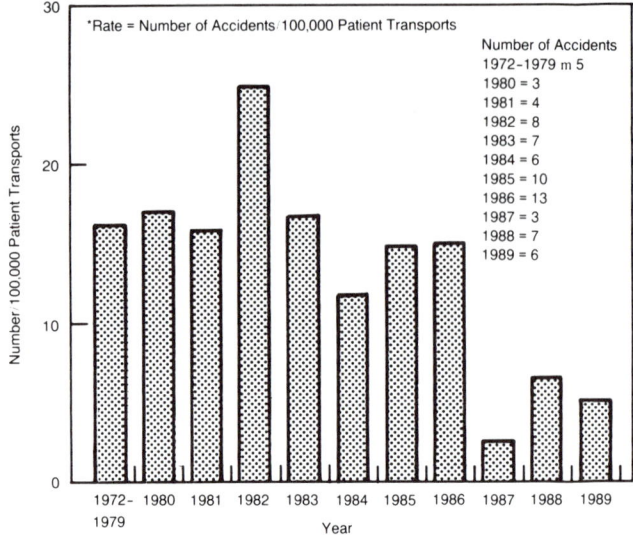

Figure 1-6 Air medical helicopter accident rates,* 1972–89.

Services, the Helicopter Association International EMS Safety Committee, and the National Emergency Service Pilots' Association. The commitment to safety was the primary concern of all in the industry. The number of accidents per 100,000 patient transports declined, with 1987 being the safest year with a rate of three accidents per 100,000 patient transports, a rate that represented only three accidents (Fig. 1-6).

The air medical industry responded to the increased demand of these services and has developed into a mature profession with sustained growth. A standardized curriculum was published in 1988 through a DOT/National Highway Traffic Safety Administration grant and was developed by Samaritan Air Evac of Phoenix, Arizona and the Association of Air Medical Services.[103] The three-volume curriculum identifies five levels of flight crew members: flight physician, flight nurse, flight paramedic, flight EMT-I, and flight EMT. Both basic and advanced texts are available along with an instructor's manual.

Professional associations have been formed to represent the various persons involved in helicopter EMS. The American Society for Hospital-Based Emergency Air Medical Services, now the Association for Air Medical Services (a name that more completely reflects all the members of this group), was founded in 1980, the National Flight Nurses Association in 1981, the National EMS Pilots Association in 1985, and the National Flight Paramedics Association in 1986.[103] There are other groups, such as the Airborne Law Enforcement Association, the Professional Aeromedical Transport Association, and the Helicopter Association International, that have special interest in various aspects of air medical service. The 1990 program listing for air medical services lists 245 programs across the United States, with California (17) and Florida (16) having the most.[104]

CONCLUSION

The three decades of EMS have formed a firm foundation for improved prehospital emergency medical care. During the next few years there will be new concerns for EMS to face. The issue of resuscitating terminally ill patients in the field is a concern that spans ethical, legal, and clinical disciplines. Whether a protocol can be developed that would allow prehospital providers to withhold CPR in certain circumstances is being discussed.[105–108] More involvement of physicians in prehospital EMS at both the planning and the operational levels is necessary.[76]

Standards have been and continue to be a major concern of EMS planners, operators, manufacturers, and providers of care. The American Society for Testing and Materials (ASTM), first founded in 1898, develops voluntary standards for materials, products, systems, and services. ASTM utilizes a consensus model, whereby the representatives of multiple facets meet to agree on standards. Formulating standards in EMS first began in 1984, when the DOT/National Highway Traffic Safety Administration, the DHEW, the Federal Emergency Management Agency, and the National Institute of Standards and Technology met. After that meeting, ASTM formed Committee F-30 on EMS. Support for the development of EMS standards has varied, with some in the EMS industry heralding the diversity of those involved in the standard making as a major step toward better patient care.[109] Other groups, such as the American College of Surgeons Committee on Trauma, have declined to participate in the F-30 process because of such diversity.

As air transport statistics show increasing numbers of patients being transported (125,200 patients were transported by medical helicopters in 1989[110]), the number of programs acquiring more than one helicopter has increased to 46, or 26% of all programs.[111] Whether too many programs exist in a competitive market has been raised as a concern.[81] The uneven distribution of EMS continues to be a concern along with whether such services can survive in some areas that totally rely on volunteerism.

Accreditation is another issue confronting EMS planners and providers. Those programs planning paramedic educational programs can have their program accredited by the Joint Review Committee for EMT-P Training Programs. The Association for Air Medical Services has formed a Commission on Accreditation of Air Medical Services to begin the process of voluntary accreditation of air medical programs.[112]

The passage of Public Law 101-590, the Trauma Care Systems Planning and Development Act, signed by President George Bush on November 16, 1990, is a major step toward renewed federal funding to complete the trauma systems development begun in the 1970s. A state must submit a trauma system plan to qualify for grant funds. The plan must be one that utilizes standards developed by the American College of Emergency Physicians, the American Academy of Pediatrics, and the American College of Surgeons. States that have a trauma system already in place will be able to apply for a waiver that will allow them to use grant funds to reimburse designated trauma centers for the care rendered to patients who do not have any ability to pay for it. This new law establishes an Advisory Council on Trauma Care Systems to the DHEW, establishes a National Clearinghouse on Emergency Medical Services and Trauma Care that will provide technical assistance and be a repository for information, and will provide grants to public and not-for-profit entities to do research and demonstration projects to improve EMS in rural areas. States will be allocated funds, with 80% of the funds depending on population and 20% on geographic size.[113]

As federal funding is renewed, it is incumbent upon the professional providers to be knowledgeable of all the factors that influence prehospital EMS systems. It is through this knowledge that a new shape and new dimensions will ultimately improve the quality of care rendered to the sick and injured.

REFERENCES

1. National Academy of Sciences. *Emergency Medical Services at Midpassage: A Report of the Committee on Emergency Medical Services.* Washington, DC: Assembly of Life Sciences, National Research Council; 1978.
2. National Academy of Sciences. *Medical Control in Emergency Medical Services Systems. Report of the Subcommittee on Medical Control, Committee on Emergency Medical Services.* Washington, DC: National Academy Press; 1981.
3. National Academy of Sciences. *The Emergency Department as a Medical Resource. Report of the Committee on Emergency Medical Services.* Washington, DC: National Academy Press; 1980.
4. National Academy of Sciences, National Research Council, Committee To Review the Status and Progress of the Injury Control Program. *Injury Control: A Review of the Status and Progress of the Injury Control Program of the Centers for Disease Control.* Washington, DC: National Academy Press; 1988.
5. National Academy of Sciences, Division of Medical Sciences. *Accidental Death and Disability: The Neglected Disease of Modern Society.* Rockville, MD: US Dept of Health, Education and Welfare; 1966. DHEW Public Health Service publication 1071-A-13.
6. Cleveland H. Trauma center design. In: Mattox KL, Moore EE, Feliciano DV, eds. *Trauma.* Norwalk, CT: Appleton & Lange; 1988.
7. Flint LM, Richardson JD. Organization for trauma care. In: Richardson JD, Polk HC, Flint LM, eds. *Trauma: Clinical Care and Pathophysiology.* Chicago: Year Book Medical; 1987.
8. Boyd DR. Trauma: a controllable disease in the 1980s. *J Trauma.* 1980;20:14–23.
9. Boyd DR, Edlich RF, Micik SH. *Systems Approach to Emergency Medical Care.* Norwalk, CT: Appleton-Century-Crofts; 1983.
10. Public Law 89-564; *Highway Safety Act of 1966.* 89th Congress, Washington, DC, 1966.
11. Public Law 93-154: *Emergency Medical Services System Act of 1973.* 93rd Congress, Washington, DC, 1973.
12. Public Law 94-573: *Emergency Medical Services Amendments of 1976,* 94th Congress, Washington, DC, 1976.
13. Public Law 96-142: *Emergency Medical Services Amendments of 1979.* 96th Congress, Washington, DC, 1979.

14. Department of Health, Education and Welfare. *Emergency Medical Services Program Guidelines*. Washington, DC: Public Health Service, Health Services Administration, Bureau of Medical Services, Division of Emergency Medical Services; 1975. DHEW publication HSA 75-2013.
15. Boyd D. The conceptual development of emergency medical services systems in the United States. *Emerg Med Serv*. 1982;11:26–35.
16. Eisenberg MD, Copass MK, Hallstrom AP, et al. Treatment of out of hospital cardiac arrests with rapid defibrillation by emergency medical technicians. *N Engl J Med*. 1980;302:1379–1382.
17. Eisenberg MD, Bergner L, Hearne T. Out of hospital cardiac arrest: a review of major studies and a proposed uniform reporting system. *Am J Public Health*. 1980;70:236–240.
18. National Academy of Sciences, Committee on Trauma Research, Commission on Life Sciences, Institute of Medicine. *Injury in America: A Continuing Public Health Problem*. Washington, DC: National Academy Press; 1985.
19. Committee on Allied Health. *Emergency Care and Transportation of the Sick and Injured*. Chicago: American Academy of Orthopedic Surgeons; 1971.
20. Briggs RS, Brown PM, Crabb ME, et al. The Brighton resuscitation ambulances: a continuing experiment in pre-hospital care by ambulance staff. *Br J Med*. 1976;2:1161–1165.
21. Pantridge JF. The effect of early therapy on the hospital mortality from acute myocardial infarction. *Q J Med*. 1970;39:621–622.
22. Scribner R, Raithaus L, Ivanov P. Emergency medical service in the Soviet Union. *J Trauma*. 1974;14:447–452.
23. Page J. *Paramedics: An Illustrated History of Paramedics in Their First Decade in the USA*. NJ: Backdraft; 1979.
24. Romano T, Eisenberg S, Fernandez-Caballero C, et al. Paramedic services: nationwide distribution and management structure. *J Am Coll Emerg Physicians*. 1978;7:99–102.
25. Lambrew C. The paramedic: the problem of defining a role. *J Emerg Nurs*. 1975;1:15–16.
26. Jacobs L, Bennett BR. Emergency medical services. In: *The MGH Textbook of Emergency Medicine*. 2nd ed. Baltimore: Williams & Wilkins; 1983.
27. Eisenberg M, Bergner L, Hallstrom A. Paramedic programs and out of hospital cardiac arrest: factors associated with successful resuscitation. *Am J Public Health*. 1979;69:39–42.
28. Eisenberg MS, Copass MK, Hallstrom A. Management of out of hospital cardiac arrests: failure of basic emergency medical technician services. *JAMA*. 1980;243:1049–1051.
29. Jacobs LM, Sinclair A, Beiser A, et al. Pre-hospital advanced life support: benefits in trauma. *J Trauma*. 1984;24:8–13.
30. Smith P, Bodai BI, Hill AS, et al. Pre-hospital stabilization of critically injured patients: a failed concept. *J Trauma*. 1985;25:65–70.
31. Alexander RH, Pons PT, Krischer J, et al. The effect of advanced life support and sophisticated hospital systems on motor vehicle mortality. *J Trauma*. 1984;24:486–490.
32. Mattox KL, Pepe PE, Bickell WH, et al. The MAST controversy—analysis of 911 hypotensive patients prospectively randomized. *J Trauma*. 1988;28:1091.
33. Bivins HG, Knopp R, Tiernan C, et al. Blood volume replacement with inflation of anti-shock trousers. *Ann Emerg Med*. 1982;11:409–419.
34. Gaffney FA, Thal ER, Taylor WF, et al. Hemodynamic effects of medical anti-shock trousers (MAST garments). *J Trauma*. 1981;21:932.
35. Moreno C, Moore EE, Rosenberger A, et al. Hemorrhage associated with major pelvic fracture: a multispecialty challenge. *J Trauma*. 1986;26:987–994.
36. McSwain NE. Pneumatic anti-shock garment: does it work? *Pre-hosp Disaster Med*. 1987;4:42–44.
37. Mattox K. Blind faith poor judgement. *Pre-hosp Disaster Med*. 1987;4:39–41.
38. Cayten CG, Longmore W, Keuhl A, et al. BLS versus ALS for trauma in an urban setting. *Ann Emerg Med*. 1986;15:23. Abstract.
39. Reines HD, Duffy KH. Survivability of victims of traumatic injuries in eastern South Carolina. *Am Surg*. 1983;49:203–206.
40. Lewis FR. Pre-hospital intravenous fluid therapy: physiologic computer modeling. *J Trauma*. 1986;26:804–811.
41. Lawrence DW, Lauro AJ. Complications from IV therapy: results from field-started and emergency department–started IVs compared. *Ann Emerg Med*. 1988;17:314–317.
42. Rottman SJ. Pre-hospital fluid administration in trauma. *Pre-hosp Disaster Med*. 1989;4:127–128.
43. Lewis FR. Ineffective therapy and delayed treatment. *Pre-hosp Disaster Med*. 1989;4:129–130.
44. Jacobs L, Berrizbeitia L, Bennett B. Endotracheal intubation in the pre-hospital phase of emergency medical care. *JAMA*. 1983;250:2175–2177.
45. Stewart RD, Paris PM, Pelton GH, et al. Effect of varied training techniques on field endotracheal intubation success rates. *Ann Emerg Med*. 1984;13:1032–1036.
46. Marasco ER, DePaola J, Kyes FN. COBRA: impact on EMS. *Emerg Care Q*. 1990;6:62–68.
47. Kulp R. Radio system design considerations affecting medical control and EMS resource coordination. *Emerg Med Serv Q*. 1982;1:14–26.
48. Executive Office of the President of Telecommunications Policy. *The Emergency Telephone Number: A Handbook for Community Planning*. Washington, DC: Publisher; 1973.
49. Dayharsh TI, Yung TJ, Hunter DK, et al. Update on the national emergency number 911. *Trans Veh Technol VT*. 1979;28:292–297.
50. Cline KA. Rural trauma and EMS: where we were, where we are, and where we need to be. *Emerg Care Q*. 1990;6:11–17.
51. Stohler S, Jacobs B. Interhospital transfer of the critical patient. *Emerg Care Q*. 1989;4:66–78.
52. American College of Surgeons. *Resources for the Optimal Care of the Injured Patient*. Chicago: American College of Surgeons; 1990.
53. Morris GP. Applying the incident command system to mass casualty incidents. *Emerg Care Q*. 1986;2:15–27.
54. Goodwin C. Mass casualty care planning, training, and evaluation as organized in the New England states. *Emerg Care Q*. 1986;2:33–50.
55. Copass M. The urban experience in medical control: medical control in Seattle. In: *Medical Control in Emergency Medical Services*. Washington, DC: National Academy Press; 1981.
56. Larson R, Brandeau M. *Implementing the Hypercube Queueing Model To Plan Ambulance Districts in Boston*. Cambridge, MA: Publisher; 1978.
57. Tell R. Categorization: a community based approach. *JACEP*. 1975;4:152–155.
58. Collins J. Categorization of emergency capabilities. *Hosp JAHA*. 1973;47:69–72.
59. American Medical Association. *Provisional Guidelines for the Optimal Categorization of Hospital Emergency Capabilities*. Washington, DC: American Medical Association; 1981.
60. Boyd D, Pizzano W, Murchie P. Categorizing hospital capabilities. *Emerg Med Serv*. 1975;4:24–29.
61. West JG, Williams MJ, Trunkey DD, et al. Trauma systems current status—future challenges. *JAMA*. 1988;259:3597–3600.
62. Champion HR, Mabee MS. *An American Crisis in Trauma Care Reimbursement*. Washington, DC: Washington Hospital Center; 1990. Washington Hospital Center publication 3.90.

63. Fischer RP, Pepe PE, Reed RL, et al. Academic consequences of a trauma system failure. *JAMA*. 1990;30:784–791.
64. American Burn Association. *Specific Optimal Criteria for Hospital Resources for Care of Patients with Burn Injury*. American Burn Association; 1976.
65. Feller I, Jones C. The National Burn Information Exchange: the use of a national burn registry to evaluate and address the burn problem. *Surg Clin North Am*. 1987;67:167–189.
66. West JG, Trunkey DD, Lim RC. Systems of trauma care: a study of two counties. *Arch Surg*. 1979;114:455–459.
67. Certo TF, Rogers RB, Pilcher DB. Review of care of fatally injured patients in a rural state: five-year follow-up. *J Trauma*. 1983;23:559–565.
68. Cales RH. Trauma mortality in Orange County: the effect of implementation of a regional trauma system. *Ann Emerg Med*. 1984;13:1–10.
69. Jacobs L. Forces influencing trauma. Presented at the 1990 meeting of the Eastern Association for the Surgery of Trauma; Month 1990; Sarasota, FL.
70. Bennett BR. Mortality and morbidity conferences: an approach to effective continuing education for the EMT. *EMT J*. 1977;1:68–69.
71. Pollock DA, McClain PW. Trauma registries current status and future prospects. *JAMA*. 1989;262:2280–2283.
72. Boyd DR, Micik S, Lambrew C, et al. Medical control and accountability of emergency medical services (EMS) systems. *Trans Veh Technol VI*. 1979;28:249–261.
73. Committee on Emergency Medical Services, Assembly of Life Sciences. *The Emergency Department: A Regional Medical Resource*. Washington, DC: National Academy Press; 1980.
74. Swor RA, Krome RL. Administrative support of emergency medical services medical directors: a profile. *Pre-hosp Disaster Med*. 1990;5:25–30.
75. National EMS Clearinghouse. *Protection from Liability for EMS Personnel*. Lexington, KY: National EMS Clearinghouse; 1988.
76. Pepe PE, Bonnin MJ, Mattox KL. Regulating the scope of EMS services. *Pre-hosp Disaster Med*. 1990;5:59–63.
77. Cobb LA, Alvarez H, Copass MK. A rapid response system for out of hospital cardiac emergencies. *Med Clin North Am*. 1976;60: 283–290.
78. Pepe PE, Copass MK. Pre-hospital care. In: Moore EE, ed. *Early Care of the Injured*. Philadelphia: Decker; 1990.
79. Braun O, McCallion R, Fazackerley J. Characteristics of midsized urban EMS systems. *Ann Emerg Med*. 1990;19:536–546.
80. National EMS Clearinghouse. *Training and Certification of EMS Personnel*. Lexington, KY: National EMS Clearinghouse; 1989.
81. US Congress, Office of Technology Assessment. *Rural Emergency Medical Services Special Report*. Washington, DC: Government Printing Office; Office of Technology Assessment publication OTA-H-445.
82. Johnson MS. Alaska's EMS system. *Emerg Care Q*. 1990;6:1–9.
83. Merlis M. *Rural Hospitals*. Washington, DC: Congressional Research Service; 1989.
84. Reeder L. Seeding clouds of change: the drought in rural EMS. *J EMS*. 1988;14:42–49.
85. National EMS Clearinghouse. *The EMS Office: Its Structure and Function*. Lexington, KY: Council of State Governors; 1988.
86. Stapleton K. The hover jumpers. *Rotoways*. 1970;2:11.
87. Felix WR. Metropolitan aeromedical service: state-of-the-art. *J Trauma*. 1976;16:873–881.
88. National Highway Traffic Safety Administration. *Helicopters in Emergency Medical Service, NHTSA Experience to Date*. Washington, DC: Government Printing Office; 1972. Dept of Transportation publication DOT HS82-231.
89. Thomas F. The development of the nation's oldest operating civilian hospital—sponsored by the aeromedical helicopter service. *Aviat Space Environ Med*. 1988;59:567–570.
90. Rhee KJ, Burney RE, MacKenzie JR, et al. Predicting the utilization of helicopter emergency medical services: an approach based on need. *Ann Emerg Med*. 1984;13:916–923.
91. MacKenzie CF, Shin B, Fisher R, et al. Two year mortality in 760 patients transported by helicopter direct from the road accident scene. *Am Surg*. 1979;45:101–108.
92. Baxt WG, Moody P. The impact of a rotorcraft aeromedical emergency care service on trauma mortality. *JAMA*. 1983;249: 3047–3051.
93. Champion HR, Sacco WJ, Carnazzo AJ, et al. Trauma score. *Crit Care Med*. 1981;9:672.
94. Anderson TE, Rose WD, Leicht MJ. Physician-staffed helicopter scene response from a rural trauma center. *Ann Emerg Med*. 1987; 16:85–88.
95. Urdaneta LF, Miller BK, Ringenberg BJ, et al. Role of an emergency helicopter transport service in rural trauma. *Arch Surg*. 1987;122: 992–996.
96. Fischer RP, Flynn TC, Miller PW, et al. Urban helicopter response to the scene of injury. *J Trauma*. 1984;24:946–951.
97. Boyd CR, Corse KM, Campbell RC. Interhospital transport: air vs ground. Presented at the second Annual Eastern Association for the Surgery of Trauma Scientific Meeting; Month 1989; Longboat Key, FL.
98. Association of Air Medical Services. Position paper on appropriate use of air medical services. *J Air Med Transp*. 1990;9:29–33.
99. Collett H. Accident trends for air medical helicopters. *Hosp Aviat*. 1989;8:6.
100. Aviation Safety Institute. *Analysis of 84 Aeromedical Helicopter Accidents for the Period 1975–1986*. Washington, DC: Aviation Safety Institute; 1986.
101. Office of the Federal Register. Washington, DC: National Archives and Records Administration; 1989.
102. Collett H. Risk management and the aeromedical helicopter. *Emerg Care Q*. 1986;2:31–39.
103. ASHBEAMS, Samaritan Air Evac. *Air Medical Crew National Standard Curriculum, Instructor Manual*. Pasadena, CA: Publisher; 1988.
104. Program listings of aircraft operators and type. *J Air Med Transp*. 1990;9:36–41.
105. Stratton SJ. Withholding CPR in the prehospital setting. *Pre-hosp Disaster Med*. 1990;5:45–46.
106. Crimmins TJ. The need for a prehospital DNR system. *Pre-hosp Disaster Med*. 1990;5:47–48.
107. Ayres RJ. Current controversies in prehospital resuscitation of the terminally ill patient. Pre-hosp Disaster Med. 1990;5:49–57.
108. McClung JA, Kamer RS. Legislating ethics: implications of New York's do-not-resuscitate law. *N Engl J Med*. 1990;323:270–272.
109. Page JO. In my opinion: a national forum for EMS. *Standardization News*. 1990;18:4–5.
110. Annual transport statistics. *J Air Med Transp*. 1990;9:6.
111. Gabram SGA, Goodwin C, Jacobs LM. Expansion of an established hospital based helicopter emergency medical service. *Emerg Care Q*. 1991;6:69–81.
112. Collett HM. AAMS conference report. *J Air Med Transp*. 1990;9:13.
113. American College of Surgeons. Congress passes trauma bill. *Am Coll Surg Bull*. 1990;7:5.

2. Disaster Management*

GLENN W. MITCHELL, MD, MPH, FACEP

Like cardiac, pediatric, and trauma care, disaster management is an emergency care subsystem that utilizes many of the existing components of a larger emergency medical services (EMS) system.[1,2] Disaster management differs from other subsystems, however, in that it is designed to distribute limited resources among the many, while the others are designed to make sophisticated resources available to the few. Therefore, four aspects of EMS must be modified to meet the special requirements of disaster management:

1. definitions
2. levels
3. components
4. phases

There is no universally accepted definition for a disaster or its management. Because consistency is central to optimal planning and operation, however, standardization is assuming increasing importance. Thus, the American College of Emergency Physicians has offered a definition, describing a disaster as an event in which

> the destructive effects of natural or manmade forces overwhelm the ability of a given area or community to meet the demand for health care.[3]

The Federal Emergency Management Agency also recognized three response levels to facilitate planning for persons injured in mass casualty incidents (MCI).[4] Describing the relationship between resource requirements and availability, these levels define need in terms of local, regional, and state or national mobilization (Table 2-1).

Disaster management systems entail numerous EMS components (see Chapter 1). Because these components were initially designed to meet day-to-day EMS requirements, they must be modified to meet the special needs of disaster management systems.

Finally, the Federal Emergency Management Agency has described four phases of disaster management: (1) mitigation, (2) preparedness, (3) response, and (4) recovery (Table 2-2).[4]

This chapter describes the relationships between definitions, levels, components, and phases in planning, implementing, operating, and evaluating disaster management systems. In addition, the National Disaster Management System is briefly discussed.

Numerous components enter into the medical management of disasters: planning, medical direction, communications, personnel, training, triage, prehospital care, transportation, hospital care, public participation, and medical evaluation.

PLANNING

Although planning has historically received inadequate emphasis, it remains the primary component of disaster

---

*The views, opinions, and/or findings contained in this chapter are those of the author and should not be construed as an official Department of the Army position, policy, or decision.

Table 2-1 Levels for Mass Casualty Incidents

Level I —A localized mass casualty incident wherein local medical resources are available and adequate to provide for field medical treatment and stabilization, including triage. The patients will be transported to the appropriate medical facility for further diagnosis and treatment.

Level II —A mass casualty incident wherein the number of victims or lack of local medical resources require multijurisdictional or regional medical mutual aid.

Level III—A mass casualty incident wherein local and regional medical resource capabilities are exceeded or overwhelmed. Deficiencies in medical supplies and personnel are such as to require assistance from state or federal agencies.

Source: American College of Emergency Physicians Disaster Committee: *Instructor's Manual for Disaster Management and Planning for Emergency Physicians.* Emmitsburg, Md, Federal Emergency Management Agency, chap 1, 1983.

Table 2-2 Phases for Disaster Management

Mitigation	—Activities that actually eliminate or reduce the likelihood of disaster occurrence, including those that reduce the effects of unavoidable disasters.
Preparedness	—Activities necessary to the extent that mitigation measures have not, or cannot, prevent disasters. In this phase governments, organizations, and individuals test plans to save lives and minimize disaster damage. The activities also attempt to enhance disaster response operations.
Response	—Activities that directly follow a disaster that attempt to provide emergency assistance for victims, to reduce the probability of secondary damage, and to speed recovery operations.
Recovery	—Activities that continue until operations return to normal. Short-term recovery addresses vital life support systems while long-term recovery addresses community life.

Source: American College of Emergency Physicians Disaster Committee: *Instructor's Manual for Disaster Management and Planning for Emergency Physicians.* Emmitsburg, Md, Federal Emergency Management Agency, chap 1, 1983.

management. Without planning—the cornerstone of rational management—disasters must be handled by providing "the best possible care under the circumstances," a phrase that suggests inefficiency, delay, and confusion in employing and coordinating the remaining system components. In many situations, such failure contributes to unnecessary morbidity and mortality.

Mitigation. Planning must address each system component in clear, concise language that is easily understood by all responsible persons. Complex, overly specific plans are seldom helpful, especially when read by flashlight on a cold night. Inadequate, confusing, uncoordinated, or obsolete plans are inexcusable, as they may lead to unacceptable outcomes and general chaos.

Central to effective planning are mutual aid agreements to provide the additional personnel and equipment required to handle situations that would otherwise overwhelm available resources. Neighboring communities can thus minimize the duplication of seldom required personnel and equipment. Mutual aid planning for prehospital care for Level II MCIs is relatively simple, because it follows the established practices of the fire and police departments. The problems that do arise generally center around regional and state mismatches in regulations regarding emergency medical technicians (EMTs) and ambulance personnel. Such problems are less likely to occur in Level III MCIs because of preexisting legislation that removes licensing restrictions for prehospital providers in the event of an MCI. Mutual aid agreements between health care facilities are less common, although not necessarily less important. Unfortunately, although sharing key hospital personnel and equipment might optimize medical care, long-standing competition generally results in the transfer of patients instead.

Preparedness. In order to facilitate coordination of activities and minimize disruption of authority, copies of the disaster management plan should be continually available to all affected parties, including those at dispatch and hospital sites and those who operate the command, communications, and response vehicles. Because out-of-date plans can be worse than none, each edition should carry the date and the names of the individuals responsible for receiving, inserting, and verifying periodic updates.

Response. Even the best conceived disaster plan cannot adequately anticipate all possible situations, therefore, each plan should have enough flexibility to allow improvisation when appropriate.[5]

Recovery. Critique and revision based on experience gleaned from drills and incidents are essential parts of disaster management planning.

MEDICAL DIRECTION

Although medical direction in disaster management is similar in philosophy to that exercised in day-to-day EMS operations, it is different in mechanism. At the EMS operational level, day-to-day medical direction focuses on individualizing field medical care for the full array of EMS resources. In practice, such customizing is often based as much on the skills of individual EMTs as on system equipment, medications, and facilities. At the planning and supervisory levels, records are used to evaluate performance retrospectively, often at a remote time and place.

In contrast, medical direction in an MCI allows free use of basic skills and, commonly, of advanced procedures (e.g., those involving airway adjuncts, pneumatic antishock garments, intravenous lines, and medications). In most systems, however, special permission is still required for the performance of such procedures as cricothyrotomy or thoracostomy. Often, individual EMTs are not known to the medical control physicians, and there may be no mechanism for a thorough retrospective evaluation.

Physician availability poses additional problems for medical direction during MCIs. Most on-scene physicians and medical passersby are neither knowledgeable nor skilled in field treatment, while hospital-based teams are usually overwhelmed with their responsibilities for inpatient care. As a result, on-scene physician care can be recommended only for difficult extrications that require field surgery or for other procedures that exceed EMT capabilities. Even then, in order to be most effective, such physicians should be familiar with local plans, policies, and procedures.

Mitigation. Planning for medical direction during MCIs entails the construction and promulgation of training protocols for disaster communications, medical command, and field treatment. Local medical societies and specialty groups should be approached to educate members and obtain their endorsement of the plan.

Preparedness. Realistic disaster drills should be conducted regularly, with written protocols used for medical direction and evaluation. Based on such experience, protocols can be updated as required.

Response. Radio communications should be recorded and transcripts prepared for review. In addition, written records of field and hospital treatment should be reviewed for medical appropriateness.

Recovery. In the critique, all medical aspects of system performance are evaluated, with the system protocols used as standards.

COMMUNICATIONS

The diversity that makes EMS systems useful and flexible renders communications one of the most commonly identified problems in disaster management. Because EMS systems routinely involve high message traffic volumes, numerous prehospital units, and diverse geographical conditions, communication devices and frequencies have proliferated.

Despite the availability of such resources and, in some instances, because of their multiplicity, communicating with neighboring providers is often a challenge. Even when members of established mutual aid networks communicate via radio links instead of vulnerable telephone lines, only rarely is there a way to contact units outside the parent agency. Furthermore, because they use different frequencies, most civilian and military radio links cannot be easily patched. As a result, on-line control ceases, and field units must function independently.

Because such problems go beyond equipment type and availability, additional funding will not solve them. Radio protocols and discipline are required to keep communications channels from becoming overloaded with unnecessary and irrelevant information.

Mitigation. Communications interfaces for all probable frequencies should be installed by the responsible disaster agency. Equipment that is dependent on the physical integrity of lines or cables must have emergency backup systems that are not. Interhospital systems should be completed and regularly tested.

Preparedness. There is no substitute for periodic communications drills, which can be conducted inexpensively from stationary radios and vehicles. Information exchange and joint exercises facilitate coordination with outside agencies. Centralized field command is basic to such exercises.

Response. Alternative and supplementary communications devices, such as low-power citizens band headsets, have proved useful in coordinating search-and-rescue operations. Equipment that covers various frequencies should be centralized at one location, preferably in a vehicle that can also serve as a mobile shelter for rescue coordinators. If commanders are not present, runners can provide rapid links.

Recovery. Communications, such as recordings of radio transmissions, that are used in a critique must include the names of the agencies involved, the frequencies used, the locations of the transmitters and receivers, and the exact times of the communications. The plan must then be revised to resolve any identified problems.

PERSONNEL

Medical personnel qualified for disaster management present a study in contrasts. Individuals willing to help are seldom in short supply, while those willing to follow an efficient relief plan are rarely available.

Several public service agencies participate in disaster management, including the police department, the fire department, transportation agencies, emergency management (formerly Civil Defense), and EMS systems. Some jurisdictions include government agencies, such as the National Guard, the Federal Emergency Management Agency, and the executive branches of state and local governments. Some states have established preparedness committees to formalize planning and administration.

Although the emotional drain involved in routine EMS operations is well recognized, disaster management exceeds normal stress limits for many individuals.[6] Because there are few resources to provide follow-up emotional support, some rescuers are left irrevocably damaged. Effects range from anxiety disorders to marital discord and severe depression. Few rescuers escape unscathed, but most try to hide their psychological wounds. Enlightened systems include routine debriefing sessions in which rescuers can obtain professional psychological help and ventilate emotions, with additional assistance for those who need it.[7,8]

Mitigation. Planning for contingencies and overall coordination remains vital. Agency leaders should be personally acquainted, preferably through periodic meetings and drills. Plans for managing large-scale disasters should detail methods for facilitating interagency communications.

Regional disaster plans that incorporate outside or reserve medical personnel should provide statutory immunity and specify methods for mobilization and transport. In disaster-prone or remote areas, the public should be trained to provide first aid and assist EMS personnel. Psychological intervention should be anticipated and implemented before it is needed.

Preparedness. It is essential to conduct periodic exercises that involve all participating agencies at all response levels. In practice, this requires public recognition and budgetary support. The public should also take part in the drills so that they become familiar with the system. In addition, such exercises should determine the availability of prehospital and hospital personnel, as well as the facilities that require priority in supplementary physician coverage. Personnel should be informed of stress disorders so that they can be prepared as much as possible for the psychological impact of real disasters.

The involved public service agencies and EMS providers should meet annually to review contingency plans for seasonal disasters; for example, hurricane preparedness conferences should be scheduled at the end of each summer.

Response. When several public service agencies provide assistance, each must regularly report to the central field command post; each must be easily and accurately identified. Currently, EMTs provide the bulk of prehospital care, including search and rescue, extrication, stabilization, and transportation. In major disasters, immobilization methods, extrication equipment, and transportation routes should follow predetermined guidelines.

In the hospital setting, personnel must be familiar with institutional policies and procedures, including those that relate to incoming medical personnel. Hospital personnel are not usually transported to the site of a disaster unless prolonged field stabilization or surgical extrication of entrapped victims is required.

Recovery. Officials of the public service agencies remain essential participants in disaster management during the recovery phase because they often facilitate the acquisition and distribution of state and federal relief funds.

It has become increasingly clear that emotional recovery is not routine for disaster management personnel, and prophylactic psychological intervention is desirable to minimize their mood swings and sleep disturbances.[6] Psychologists not only should be present in the field as soon as possible but also should conduct group sessions and debriefings later. Personnel who require more intensive intervention should be referred for additional treatment. Helping disaster management personnel to recover from present disasters mitigates future needs by preserving the abilities of these people to help in a subsequent disaster.

TRAINING

In order to preserve life, improve efficiency, and reduce confusion, training is obviously essential for all medical personnel.[9]

Mitigation. For prehospital and hospital personnel alike, training entails participation in realistic drills and honest critiques to increase their understanding of the goals and objectives of the disaster management system. In this setting, basic medical procedures do not change, although some may be simplified or omitted in large-scale disasters.

Preparedness. Realistic drills that focus on common problems must be conducted periodically at all training levels. Drills that emphasize unlikely events, such as nuclear accidents, should be postponed until more basic system responses have been adequately tested.

Response. At this juncture, it is too late to begin training professionals in disaster management. Preprinted self-help health and safety materials remain useful for the general public, however.

Recovery. Methods must be developed and implemented for rapidly incorporating the lessons learned in a disaster into future training.

TRIAGE

Whenever field teams encounter multiple patients, triage becomes necessary to determine whom the EMTs will attend and in what order. During MCIs, some EMTs perform primary triage at the accident scene, while others perform secondary triage at the treatment area. Patients receive treatment and transportation in an order determined by their needs. Because triage skills in a disaster differ substantially from routine EMS skills, they mandate additional training and experience.[10]

Triage often depends on the injury mechanism. In practice, however, many incidents, such as the Kansas City hotel skyway collapse[11] and the Las Vegas hotel fire,[12] result in unique medical injuries and treatment needs. Although advocates have promulgated various marking systems,[13] few such systems have been adequately evaluated under actual disaster conditions, and no single system has been demonstrated to be superior.

Because there are few opportunities to optimize triage skills for MCIs, there are few learned instructors in this area. Military experience, although extensive, cannot be directly extrapolated to civilian conditions.[14,15] Furthermore, leisurely triage of moulaged victims on clear spring days poorly simulates real events played out in rain and darkness.

Mitigation. Field triage criteria should be developed, evaluated, modified by qualified individuals, and endorsed by the medical community. Likewise, triage marking systems should be adopted and practiced.

Preparedness. Realistic triage drills require properly moulaged victims and evaluation. Exercises should become increasingly complex, with an emphasis on learning rather than competition. All disaster vehicles should have triage and tagging materials on board.

Response. In the event of an actual incident, previously agreed on criteria and tagging techniques should be implemented for triage.

Recovery. The incident critique should address the appropriateness of triage protocols, and system protocols must be appropriately modified, if necessary. Finally, expended tagging materials must be replaced.

PREHOSPITAL CARE

The prehospital component of an EMS system is tested under fire during an MCI.[16] Although the care rendered involves the same skills used in everyday prehospital care, the delivery is radically changed by the circumstances. Much of the care is determined by protocol. Some care, however, requires extraordinary measures that are not commonly used by the EMS system. Under disaster conditions, equipment and supplies may be totally depleted or in such short supply that patients with minor injuries are forced to wait for care, while patients with major, but treatable, injuries may expire.

Mitigation. Well-conceived, properly functioning EMS systems provide EMTs with the wide range of skills necessary to provide disaster treatment. Necessary modifications should be developed and distributed, including appropriate in-service training.

Preparedness. In order to establish a basis for the evaluation of subsequent disaster management, treatment protocols should be used during initial training and disaster drills.

Response. During actual disasters, treatment protocols should be followed whenever possible; extraordinary interventions should be reserved for injuries that threaten life or limb. It may be necessary to improvise equipment for resuscitation and stabilization in large-scale incidents.

Recovery. Critiques, in which care rendered in an actual disaster is compared with treatment protocols, should be made as soon as feasible after the incident.

TRANSPORTATION

Disasters drastically alter patient transportation to and between facilities. Ambulances designed for day-to-day EMS activities are rendered useless in many Level II and all Level III MCIs. In addition, protocols must be developed to accommodate the disruption of normal travel routes and evacuation of remote victims.[17]

Mitigation. Access to alternate vehicles, such as those with four-wheel drive, boats, and rotorcraft, should be predetermined and prearranged. Routes to all involved facilities, both generally traveled and alternate roads, should be reinforced in the minds of all safety, prehospital, and hospital personnel. Protocols for the allocation of patients to system facilities, including interfacility transfer agreements, should also be prepared and tested.

Preparedness. Disaster drills are unique opportunities to develop transportation protocols specific to individual regions, especially if alternate vehicles and access routes require testing. Hospitals without permanent rotorcraft landing zones should designate emergency zones, using system participants to provide ground signals during flight exercises. Air and water transportation safety measures should be incorporated into such exercises.

Response. Although most Level II MCIs can be serviced adequately by routine EMS vehicles, Level III MCIs often require the use of additional vehicles, such as buses, trains, aircraft, and boats. Drivers must be skilled and familiar with all available routes; each driver should be accompanied by at least one individual trained in first aid. The police can sometimes reduce problems caused by private vehicles whose owners are transporting victims to the nearest facility without prior authorization. Interfacility transfers should be attempted only when the care needed cannot be obtained at the original facility.

Recovery. Mechanisms for reimbursing the owners of commandeered vehicles should be developed in advance. If the region is declared a disaster area, federal funds may be available for this purpose. Finally, victim allocation must be evaluated.

HOSPITAL CARE

Although most hospitals have individual plans for handling unusual numbers of disaster victims, few are properly integrated into the disaster management system. To address this problem, methods must be developed to determine and verify the availability of physicians, beds, and operating rooms at each participating facility.[18]

Mitigation. Hospitals should be constructed to withstand likely environmental disasters. For example, electrical power and emergency care facilities should be located above high water marks to ensure that hospitals can continue to function during flooding. In addition, plans must be made to ensure that hospitals have potable water, even if community supplies become contaminated. Finally, to facilitate the allocation of victims among hospitals, protocols must be devised for determining the availability of physician specialists, such as orthopedists and neurosurgeons, and of general and critical care beds.

Preparedness. All hospitals should regularly participate in both small- and large-scale disaster drills. Hospital representatives should attend critiques to receive feedback and gain insight into a regional approach to disaster management.

Response. During an actual disaster, hospitals should closely monitor the interhospital communications network to coordinate the use of resources. Ineffective patient allocation at this juncture results in unnecessary interhospital transfers. Maintenance and housekeeping departments must also be adequately staffed.

Recovery. Once the acute situation stabilizes, interhospital transfer may be required to distribute critical patients more equitably. The attendance of physicians and administrators at hospital and regional critiques remains crucial.

PUBLIC PARTICIPATION

An essential component of all phases of disaster management, including planning, operation, and evaluation, is public participation.

Mitigation. Unlike most other social services, disaster management generally involves limited consumer participation. Unknowledgeable bystanders are at best hindrances and at worst casualties. Therefore, those members of the public who are interested and qualified should have access to planning and critique, especially at a policy level.

Preparedness. Disaster management systems should include programs to educate the public in self-help and public health measures. At a minimum, the populace should be informed of the existence and capabilities of the system, thereby reducing interference by well-meaning bystanders.

Response. In an actual incident, the most important public participation issue revolves around information regarding the incident scene and individual patients. One official at the scene and one at each hospital should be authorized to speak officially; all others should be aware of their responsibility to remain silent.[19]

Recovery. Public participation in critique and revision remains crucial if disaster planning and updating is to accommodate consumer perspectives.

MEDICAL EVALUATION

Commonly called a critique, the medical evaluation of disaster management is a central element in improving performance. Without a critique that includes an assessment of medical direction, recordkeeping, and evaluation, outdated and ineffective plans gather dust while mistakes persist. An open, candid approach that avoids assigning blame for performance shortfalls facilitates the process of identifying problems, suggesting solutions, updating plans, and disseminating changes.[20]

Because prehospital recordkeeping is often inadequate, it is not possible to conduct a proper medical audit in many Level II and Level III MCIs. Even hospital records are often sketchy in a disaster, with census information lagging several hours behind arrivals. As a result, medical evaluation suffers and legal exposure increases.

Mitigation. Field records should be simple, specifying injuries and care. Prenumbered, multipart tags, which should be simple, readily visible, and waterproof, allow victim identification at each checkpoint. Additional information, such as names and addresses, are optional.

Hospital records should likewise remain attached to the patient. They should contain only essential information, although multiple copies may be required to facilitate feedback at control points, such as the radiology department. Each copy should have space for treatment notes, including checkoffs for common interventions. After the situation stabilizes, this temporary record can be incorporated into the conventional inpatient chart.

Preparedness. Leaders must be prepared to monitor the activities of both victims and providers, using observers as necessary for both simulated and real events. Audit trails include tags and records.

Each response vehicle should carry an adequate number of victim tags, prehospital records, and writing instruments. Supplies must also be available at each hospital intake point, both for the hospital's immediate use and for replenishment of field supplies. An attempt should be made to find trained personnel for each triage station; this is difficult, however, since many disasters occur outside the normal 9-to-5 workday.

Response. The orchestration of medical care under adverse circumstances remains the ultimate test of disaster management system effectiveness.[21-23] Proper tag use (e.g., setting priorities for evacuation by means of color coding and controlling patient flow by means of multipart tags) should be verified early. Recordings of on-line communications provide an additional source of information on patient flow.

Both providers and observers should record deviations from established plans and the reasons for them.

Recovery. The critique of victim flow and prehospital care, which may be based on written and taped records, should occur promptly and include all involved parties. Such a debriefing provides an opportunity not only to identify problems and suggest solutions but also to ventilate feelings about stress. The proceedings should be recorded by a secretary and interim reports circulated. Following the final critique, plans should be revised, if necessary, and redistributed.

THE NATIONAL DISASTER MEDICAL SYSTEM

The National Disaster Medical System (NDMS) is a multiplayer partnership designed to coordinate the medical care of victims of large-scale disasters in the United States or of an overseas conventional conflict. Involved are the Department of Health and Human Services, the Department of Defense, the Veterans Administration, the Federal Emergency Management Agency, other federal departments with state agencies, major national professional societies, voluntary agencies, and the private sector. The NDMS has three stated objectives:

1. to assist a disaster-affected area by mobilizing medical assistance teams and medical supplies and equipment
2. to evacuate victims who cannot be cared for in the affected area to designated centers in unaffected areas
3. to provide hospital care in a network of participating hospitals throughout the nation[24]

The NDMS is activated after a request for assistance from a state governor. Both federal and voluntary private sector quick-response medical teams with federal logistic support respond to the scene as required. Appropriate transportation and distribution of victims to unaffected areas of the country is coordinated by NDMS, and both private and Veterans Administration hospitals may receive patients. Liability and payment issues are being addressed by NDMS. A system of recruitment, training, and drills is already in place and has functioned well to date.

The NDMS has taken the systems approach to disaster management defined in this chapter and applied it to potential large-scale events nationwide.[25] It remains for smaller jurisdictions to organize and train at least as well.

REFERENCES

1. Boyd DR, Edlich RD, Micik S, eds. *Systems Approach to Emergency Medical Care*. Norwalk, CT: Appleton-Century-Crofts; 1983.
2. Feldstein BD, Gallery ME, Sanner PH, et al. Disaster training for emergency physicians in the United States: a systems approach. *Ann Emerg Med*. 1985;14:36–40.
3. Disaster Committee. Disaster medical services. *Ann Emerg Med*. 1985;14:1026.
4. American College of Emergency Physicians Disaster Committee. *Instructor's Manual for Disaster Management and Planning for Emergency Physicians*. Emmitsburg, MD: Federal Emergency Management Agency; 1983.
5. Barbash GI, Yoeli N, Ruskin SM, Moeller DW. Airport preparedness for mass disaster: a proposed schematic plan. *Aviat Space Environ Med*. 1986;57:77–81.
6. Durham TW, McCammon SL, Allison EJ Jr. The psychological impact of disaster on rescue personnel. *Ann Emerg Med*. 1985;14:664–668.
7. Sanner PH, Wolcott BW. Stress reactions among participants in mass casualty simulations. *Ann Emerg Med*. 1983;12:426–428.
8. McDaniel EG. Psychological response to disasters. In: Baskett PJF, Weller RM, eds. *Medicine for Disasters*. London: Butterworth; 1988:230–245.
9. Goodwin C. Disaster drills. *Top Emerg Med*. 1986;7:20–33.
10. Champion HR, Moreau MM, Gainer PS. Assessment and triage. In: Baskett PJF, Weller RM, eds. *Medicine for Disasters*. London: Butterworth; 1988:19–35.
11. Orr SM, Robinson WA. The Hyatt Regency skywalk collapse: an EMS-based disaster response. *Ann Emerg Med*. 1983;12:601–605.
12. D'Amore R. The high-rise fire disaster: a plea for a new disaster response. In: *Mass Casualties: A Lessons Learned Approach*. Washington, DC: National Highway Traffic Safety Administration; 1982:257–261. NHTSA report DOT-HS-806 302.
13. Cohen E. A better mousetrap. *J Emerg Med Serv*. 1983;8:30–36.
14. Mitchell GW. The triage process. *Top Emerg Med*. 1986;7:34–45.
15. Vayer JS, Ten Eyck RP, Cowan ML. New concepts in triage. *Ann Emerg Med*. 1986;15:927–930.
16. Cowley RA, Myers RA, Gretes AJ. EMS response to mass casualties. *Emerg Med Clin North Am*. 1984;3:687–693.
17. Leonard R. Mass evacuation in disasters. *J Emerg Med*. 1985;2:279–286.
18. Aghababian RV. Hospital disaster planning. *Top Emerg Med*. 1986;7:46–54.
19. Savage PEA. Public relations and the media. In: Baskett PJF, Weller RM, eds. *Medicine for Disasters*. London: Butterworth; 1988:191–200.
20. Byrd TR. Disaster medicine: toward a more rational approach. *Mil Med*. 1980;144:270–273.
21. Sheng ZY. Medical support in the Tangshan earthquake: a review of the management of mass casualties and certain major injuries. *J Trauma*. 1987;27:1130–1135.
22. Linneman RE. Soviet medical response to the Chernobyl nuclear accident. *JAMA*. 1987;258:637–643.
23. Klausner JM, Rozin RR. The evacuation hospital in civilian disasters. *Isr J Med Sci*. 1986;22:365–369.
24. Mahoney LE, Brinley FJ. The National Disaster Medical System. *Top Emerg Med*. 1986;7:75–86.
25. Mahoney LE, Reutershan TP. Catastrophic disasters and the design of disaster medical care. *Ann Emerg Med*. 1987;16:1085–1091.

3. Emergency Care and the Law

ROBERT W. HEILIG, RN, MPA, Esq

Law serves two broad purposes. First, it is the mechanism by which society translates its values and goals into substantive rules, and second, it provides the procedures by which disputes are resolved and rules enforced. The answer to the question "What is the law?" on a particular subject involves consideration of the four sources of our law: the constitution, statutes, regulations, and judge-made law.

The US Constitution is the supreme law of the land and the foundation for our legal and political system.[1] The most common situation in which health care workers encounter constitutional law is in the area of an individual not having been given adequate due process. The other area of constitutional law involving healthcare workers usually arises out of the denial of a constitutionally guaranteed individual right, such as the right to privacy. All statutes and regulations, whether federal, state, or municipal, must be consistent with the constitution.

STATUTES

Statutes are laws that are passed by a state legislature or Congress and are signed by a governor or president. Most people think of statutes as the law. Statutes may only be changed through the legislative process. Local statutes are usually referred to as ordinances.

REGULATIONS

Regulations are similar to statutes but are promulgated by administrative agencies and generally amplify or implement statutes. A regulation may be changed or modified by the regulatory body that promulgated it.

JUDGE-MADE LAW

Judge-made law is usually called common law and in legal parlance is stare decisis. The bulk of the law we see handed down is based on common law. Stare decisis lends the consistency and predictability of results that are critical to the functioning of our common law system. Despite logic, common law is constantly evolving. Judges rarely explicitly overturn prior decisions; instead, they distinguish the facts in the case before them from those previously decided and make only slight changes. Common law is particularly important to the health care worker in that most actions for malpractice are decided entirely on common law decisions.

THE CONCEPT OF CIVIL REMEDIES FOR CIVIL WRONGS

Of the numerous areas of law (ie, contracts, criminal, real property, etc), the area of tort law most concerns emergency care providers. Tort law addresses private or civil wrongs or injuries. The purpose of tort law is to adjust losses and to afford compensation for injuries sustained by one person as the result of the conduct of another.[2]

A tort is not the same thing as a crime, although the two have many features in common. The distinction lies in the interests affected and the remedy afforded. A crime is an offense against the public at large, and the state or local jurisdiction brings proceedings on behalf of the public. Criminal prosecution is not concerned with compensation to the injured individual. A civil action, on the other hand, is brought by the injured person and is intended to compensate him or her for the harm he or she has suffered. As a general rule, the state may not bring a civil suit against a person.

In some circumstances, the same act may be both a crime against the state and a tort against an individual. The cases, one brought by the state and the other by the harmed individual, are tried in separate courts, and the results, as a general rule, of one case are not admissible in the other. That is, if an individual is convicted of a crime, the results of that trial are not admissible in the civil trial for the same act.

SOCIAL ENGINEERING

Perhaps more than any other branch of the law, the law of torts is a battleground of social theory.[3] The notion of public policy involved in private cases is not new to tort law, but it is only in recent decades that it has played a predominant role.[4] Generally, social engineering involves balancing the interests of society or the public at large. It is rather simple to say that the interests of individuals are to be balanced against one another in the light of those of the general public, but it is far more difficult to say where the public interests may lie.

It is this aspect of the law that provides the most difficulty for the lay public to comprehend. It is easy to state that the law requires that every individual conduct himself or herself in a reasonable manner, not unduly harmful to his or her neighbor; but what is reasonable, and what is undue harm?

NEGLIGENCE

Many writers suggest that the concept of negligence as a separate tort was not recognized before the 19th century.[5] The following passage, however, can be found in the Code of Hannurabi: "Everyone is responsible, not only for the result of his willful acts, but also for an injury occasioned to another by his want of ordinary care or skill in the management of his person or property."[6] Not only did the Code address "reasonable conduct" for the ordinary person, it specifically addressed the medical profession: "If a doctor has treated a man with a metal knife for a severe wound, and has caused the man to die, or has opened a man's tumor with a metal knife and destroyed the man's eye, his hand shall be cut off."[6]

One of the earliest cases that addressed the issue of reasonable care was Weaver v Ward.[7] This 17th century case held that a defendant who accidentally wounded another could be held liable unless he or she could establish that the accident was inevitable, "judged utterly without his fault."[7]

Under modern law, the burden of proof has shifted to the plaintiff, that is, the party alleging the harm. In addition, the plaintiff must now show more than mere conduct. He or she must prove that:

1. the defendant (actor) owed a duty to the plaintiff
2. the defendant breached that duty
3. some form of damage or harm occurred to the plaintiff
4. there is a reasonably close connection between the conduct (or lack thereof) and the damage

Each of these four elements must be proved by the plaintiff before there can be a finding of fault upon which damages may be awarded.

DUTY

One of the more complex of the elements is duty. Duty may be defined as an obligation recognized by the law requiring the actor to conform to a certain standard of conduct for the protection of others against unreasonable risks. This element actually requires the answering of two questions: Does a duty exist, and, if so, what is the extent of that duty?

Medical-legal folklore is full of anecdotal stories regarding the physician who failed to stop and render medical care to an injured person and was sued. Although it may be contrary to someone's moral senses, it appears that there were no actual cases, and the courts have been loath to demand affirmative action by individuals on behalf of stricken strangers. Early Mesopotamian law did require that citizens stop and aid strangers:

> They have no physicians, but when a man is ill they lay him in the public square, and the passersby come up to him, and if they have ever lived his disease themselves or have known anyone who has suffered from it, they give him advice . . . and no one is allowed to pass the sick man in silence without asking him what his ailment is.[6]

Duty then is an obligation to act or refrain from acting in some uniform standard of behavior. From this has risen the so-called reasonable person of ordinary prudence standard.[8]

For emergency health care workers, the duty becomes greater. The standard is elevated to one having superior knowledge, skill, and intelligence. Duty then becomes an issue of how a reasonable and prudent person with similar training and experience would act in the same or similar circumstances. To establish a level of duty or standard, the court allows the use of expert witnesses in circumstances where the average lay juror is not expected to know the standard. That is, medical personnel who are generally considered experts in their fields are called upon to describe to the jury the standards that should be adhered to in similar circumstances to the situation that is the focus of the trial.

BREACH

Once the standard that the defendant is to be measured against is established, the jury must then determine whether the defendant has breached that duty. In other words, did the defendant's actions fall below the accepted standard of care? It is the plaintiff's burden to prove that the defendant's action or lack of action fell below the accepted standard of care.

Although on the surface this may sound relatively simple, it can be a difficult task. Undoubtedly, both parties will have presented expert witnesses to describe what that duty is. The jurors will be left to decide which witness was more credible and whose standard they will accept.

DAMAGES

The plaintiff also has the obligation to show that there was an actual loss or damage. The mere fact that the plaintiff has proven a duty and a breach of that duty is insufficient. The element of damages is one frequently focused upon by the various tort reforms that are taking place across the country.

Most everyone has heard of the multimillion dollar awards in malpractice cases. Damages are broadly divided into three categories: actual damages, emotional damages, and punitive damages. Actual damages are those damages or losses that can be accurately described (eg, medical expenses or lost wages). Emotional damages are frequently referred to as pain and suffering damages. There are no guidelines for a jury to follow in determining how much to award a person who has suffered the loss of a loved one, for instance. Thus it is in this area that juries frequently award large sums of money to compensate a person for his or her emotional suffering. Punitive damages are rarely seen in medical malpractice cases. Punitive damages were designed as a means of punishing the plaintiff for some egregious action or gross negligence. This situation rarely surfaces in medical negligence cases, but when punitive damages are awarded they tend to be very large sums of money. In most cases, punitive damages are not covered by insurance.

CAUSATION

The last of the four elements, and perhaps the most difficult from the attorney's point of view, is causation. The plaintiff must prove that the defendant's breach of duty has a reasonably close relationship to the actual loss or damages. The term frequently used is the *but for* standard. That is, but for the plaintiff's actions or inactions, the defendant would not have suffered the damages as shown. One area of frequent debate is paralysis after a major injury. Did the paralysis occur as the result of the defendant's ineptness or from the actual incident? It would be the plaintiff's burden to prove that the transected cervical spinal cord was the direct result of improper immobilization and not of the actual incident itself. Failure to make this proof destroys the plaintiff's case.

The plaintiff must prove each of the above elements by a preponderance of the evidence for a jury to return a verdict in favor of the plaintiff. Failure to meet this burden must result in a verdict for the defendant.

DEFENSES

As noted above, the plaintiff must prove the four basic elements of negligence to win his or her case. The defense strategy usually centers around one or more of these elements as being inadequately proven. As a general rule, the one element of most controversy is the standard of care. The defendant will present his or her own experts to describe the actions as within the accepted standard of practice given the circumstances of the situation. Other defenses may center on technical issues or certain statutory immunities. Among these immunities are the so-called Good Samaritan laws.

For public policy reasons, over the years certain immunities from civil liability have been granted to various groups including charities, governments, and churches. Although more recently we have seen the erosion of these immunities, we have seen an increase in immunities for certain health care workers. Virtually all states have enacted at least one statute that is designed to provide some protection to health care workers. Recent crises in emergency medical care have seen this protection extended to include certain on-call specialists in a number of states.

Although the Good Samaritan protections may provide an absolute defense to a lawsuit, relying on these protections is a tenuous defense. The Good Samaritan protections are no substitute for good medical care.

CONSENT

It has long been held that every competent adult person has the fundamental right of self-determination over his or her person and property.[3] Even those individuals, such as incompetent adults and minors, who are unable to exercise this right have the right to be represented by another to protect their interests. A person does not necessarily give up this right when he or she seeks medical care. In fact, over the years the area of consent for medical care has expanded to include what is called informed consent.[9] In the absence of consent from a patient before treatment or care, an emergency medical care provider may be liable for battery and/or negligence.

There are two broad categories of consent: express consent and implied consent. Express consent is given by way of actions, words, or written authorization. Express consent may be given by the patient himself or herself or by another individual who is authorized to consent for the patient, as in the case of a minor. In fact, a minor may not legally consent to treatment except under certain special circumstances.

The second major category of consent is implied consent. This level of consent arises when a patient, such as an unconscious or incompetent patient, is unable to consent to treatment. The law implies consent in situations such as emergencies on the theory that if the patient were able, or a qualified legal representative were present, such consent would be given.

There is a third, limited category of consent broadly classified as involuntary consent. In these special circumstances, the courts provide consent or provide the legal authority to consent to another. These circumstances usually arise in the situation where a person is in custody or a child is under the care of a welfare worker.

The area of consent for a child can be difficult at times. The law allows certain circumstances where a child younger than 18 years of age may consent for himself or herself. Some of these conditions are:

- an emancipated minor (usually a child between 15 and 18 years of age who is living away from his or her parents and is not dependent on the parents for financial support)
- a child who is pregnant, and the complaint relates to the pregnancy
- a child whose complaint relates to venereal disease or other serious contagious disease (most states require reporting of certain venereal diseases)
- a child whose complaint involves abuse, either physical or mental/emotional (most states require reporting of suspected child abuse)

Implied consent is applied in the case of a child in a somewhat different manner. In the case of a child suffering from what appears to be a life-threatening illness or injury and there is no specific parental refusal of treatment, consent is implied. There is no requirement as with adults that the child be unconscious or unable to communicate because the child's verbal consent would not be effective.

REFUSAL OF CONSENT

The courts have long held that a patient has the right to control his or her own destiny. Patients who are competent have the right to refuse treatment, either totally or in part. This situation most frequently arises where religious beliefs preclude the use of certain drugs or blood.

Competency is sometimes difficult to define, but generally it may be assumed that a patient presenting himself or herself for treatment is competent unless there is evidence to the contrary. As a general rule, a patient's spouse does not have the legal capacity to consent for the patient simply because the two are married; there may be circumstances, however, where the spouse may give consent on the basis of another legal relationship (eg, the spouse is the patient's attorney-in-fact) or when the patient is incompetent and the spouse is the closest available relative.

A number of states have enacted legislation that allows a person to execute a durable power of attorney authorizing an attorney-in-fact to make health care decisions on his or her behalf. Frequently this legislation allows the attorney-in-fact to authorize withholding of treatment as well as to consent to treatment.

Generally, a competent patient's decision to refuse blood, drugs, treatment, or other procedures should be respected. If the refusal may result in the patient's death or severe disability, however, or if the patient is incompetent, a minor, or pregnant, or if a parent or another person legally authorized to give consent refuses to consent to the recommended medical procedure, it may be advisable to seek court-authorized consent or the establishment of a guardianship. Hospitals should have established policies and protocols to address these circumstances.

The emergency care provider is faced with an ever-changing, complex set of laws relating to consent. It is the exceptions that are difficult and best dealt with in advance. In conjunction with legal counsel, hospitals should develop protocols to deal with the complex consent issues. Health care workers should not have to be reminded that there is no substitution for good documentation.

TRANSFER AND PATIENT ANTIDUMPING LAWS

On August 1, 1986, a new section of the Social Security Act titled *Examination and Treatment for Emergency Medical Conditions and Women in Active Labor* became effective.[10] More commonly known as the COBRA (Consolidated Omnibus Budget Reconciliation Act) antidumping statute, the Act was specifically designed to stop patient dumping through federal legislation. The original Act was amended in 1989, and these amendments became effective on July 1, 1990. Several states, including New York and California, have enacted similar state laws.

The law has the following broad requirements:

- A hospital cannot delay the screening examination to determine a patient's payment status. The screening examination is to determine whether the patient has an emergency medical condition.
- Within the capability of its facilities and staff, a hospital must provide treatment to stabilize a patient with an emergency medical condition.
- Where necessary, the examination and evaluation shall include consultation with specialty physicians qualified to give an opinion or to render treatment necessary to

stabilize the individual. Such consultation may be obtained by telephone; where the emergency and specialty physicians jointly determine it medically necessary, however, the consultation shall include examination and treatment of the individual in person by the specialty physician.
- Physicians who serve in an on-call capacity to the hospital's emergency department cannot refuse to respond to a call on the basis of the individual's race, ethnicity, religion, national origin, citizenship, age, sex, preexisting medical condition, physical or mental handicap, insurance status, economic status, or ability to pay for medical services.

The Act basically precludes the transfer or discharge of patients with an unstabilized emergency medical condition for any reason. There are two exceptions, however:

1. After being fully informed of the risks and consequences involved, of the alternatives, if any, to the transfer or discharge, and of the hospital's obligation to provide such further examination and treatment within its available staff and facilities, the individual or the individual's legal representative requests in writing the transfer or discharge.
2. A physician has signed a certification that, based upon the information available, the medical benefits reasonably expected from the provision of emergency medical treatment at another facility outweigh the increased risks to the individual from effecting the transfer. The receiving hospital must agree to accept and treat the individual being transferred.

Although state and federal antidumping laws regarding emergency transfers apply only to transfers of unstabilized patients or transfers for nonmedical reasons, state licensing regulations and Joint Commission standards apply virtually the same requirements to all transfers.[11]

The emergency department physician is not in violation of the law for a transfer that takes place because an on-call physician either refused to respond or failed to appear in a reasonable period of time. In these situations, the emergency physician is required to include the name and address of the on-call physician in the record.

Violation of the Act can result in severe penalties even when good medical care is being provided. Hospitals and responsible physicians may be subject to termination of Medicare participation and fines of up to $50,000 for a COBRA violation.

The Act also allows for private civil action by anyone who suffers harm, including anxiety, personal injury, and increased medical expenses. Additionally, a facility suffering financial loss because of another facility's violation can sue for damages.

Furthermore, under New York law, patient dumping may be a criminal offense. In November 1989, a nursing supervisor at a local hospital in Queens was convicted of violating New York patient antidumping regulations and was sentenced to 200 hours of community service.

ORGAN TRANSPLANTATION

From donation to transplantation, this is the only medical therapy that is entirely regulated by law. The federal government and, to some extent, the state government monitor and regulate the administrative and financial aspects of this process. The laws controlling organ transplantation are generally viewed as positive by health care professionals. In addition to ensuring that organs are shared on a fair and equitable basis, these laws provide protection for health care professionals so that they may carry out their medical, legal, and ethical responsibilities with assurance and protection.

THE UNIFORM ANATOMICAL GIFT ACT

This Act was passed in 1968 and has been adopted by all 50 states. The Act specifically protects health care professionals from legal liability resulting from organ procurement. In 1987, an amendment to the law was added that eliminated the need for next of kin consent if an organ donor card had been signed. The amendment also required hospitals to establish agreements with other regional hospitals and organ procurement organizations and prohibited the sale or purchase of organs or tissues.

As part of the Budget Reconciliation Act of 1986, all hospitals receiving Medicare and Medicaid reimbursement are required to establish programs encouraging organ and tissue donation. The law also requires that families of potential organ donors be made aware of the option of organ or tissue donation and their option to decline. Thus there is a requirement that health care professionals make this option known to families of potential donors. Frequently emergency medical services workers are the first professionals exposed to patients' families and must consider this issue.

CONCLUSION

During the past decade, we have seen tremendous advances in emergency medicine. Coincident with these advances has been the significant intrusion of the legal system into emergency medicine. There was a time when it was unheard of for someone to sue a paramedic or emergency physician. That time is no longer.

Emergency health care professionals must be cognizant of current laws and regulations. Although this may seem onerous, one can meet the bulk of the requirements of the laws and of the negligence standard by practicing in a common sense manner.

REFERENCES

1. U.S. Constitution.
2. Wright, *Introduction to the Law of Torts,* 1944.8 Camb. L. J. 238.
3. *See generally,* Law of Torts, W.L. Prosser, Ch 1. § 3, 1971.
4. Winfield, *Public Policy and the English Common Law,* 1928, 42 Harv. L. Rev. 76.
5. Winfield, *The History of Negligence in the Law of Torts,* 1926, 42 L.Q. Rev. 184; Prosser, Law of Torts, 1971.
6. Lyons AS. *Medicine: An Illustrated History.* New York: Abrams; 1978.
7. 1616, Hob. 134, 80 Eng. Rep. 284.
8. Vaughn v. Menlove, 1738, 3 Bing. N.C. 468, 132 Eng. Rep. 490.
9. Cobbs v. Grant, 8 Cal. 3d 229 (1972).
10. 42 USC-1395dd.
11. Joint Commission on Accreditation of Healthcare Organizations, *Accreditation Manual for Hospitals: 1990,* Chicago: JCAHO; 1990: E.R. 1.6.

4. Hospital Care

EILEEN WHALEN, RN, BSN
ROBERT W. HEILIG, RN, MPA, Esq

Over the last 10 years, emergency department (ED) visits have increased markedly (Fig. 4-1). As of January 1990, 83.1% of all hospitals in the United States maintain licensed EDs, representing a total of 5133 EDs.[1]

Because the ED is the entrance point for many hospitalized patients, classification schemes for EDs have been used since 1971.[2] These classification schemes provide assurance to the consumer and medical community that a facility meets recognized standards for optimal care delivery.

In systems of regionalized hospital care, horizontal and vertical classifications of institutional capabilities are used to determine categorization and designation.[3] A hospital's horizontal classification indicates its overall capability to respond to a wide variety of emergency conditions. Its vertical classification, in contrast, indicates its capability to provide definitive care for specific medical conditions (ie, trauma, burns, cardiac events, etc).

Hospital categorization is intended to inform the medical community and the public about the capabilities of the individual facility to receive and treat acutely ill and injured patients appropriately. Accordingly, categorization should provide sufficient information to allow patients and providers to choose a hospital wisely and to use its resources efficiently and effectively.

Partly because of the inadequacies of categorization, designation has emerged as a method for directing patient flow. Designation is based on some basic tenets of horizontal and vertical classification used for categorizations, and it facilitates a systems approach by establishing authority and developing standards to verify hospital capability, commitment, and performance.[4]

CLASSIFICATION

Medical care classification is not new, having been used by the military to identify the treatment capabilities of its various facilities (eg, first aid stations, battalion aid stations, and mobile army surgical hospitals). Civilian hospital classification has emerged more recently, however, to provide the basis for categorizing,[3] designating,[4] and accrediting hospital services.

In early classification schemes, broad perspectives were used to evaluate hospital capabilities that ranged from first aid to comprehensive care for general medical problems. This horizontal classification approach proved inadequate for determining a hospital's capability to provide definitive care for certain groups of critically ill and injured patients. To meet this need, a system of vertical classification was developed; this system provides specific information regarding a hospital's critical care capabilities, thus facilitating the admission and transfer of patients who require acute care to qualified facilities.

Horizontal

In 1971, the American Medical Association (AMA) published the first guidelines for the horizontal classification of hospital emergency capabilities,[2] providing the basis for

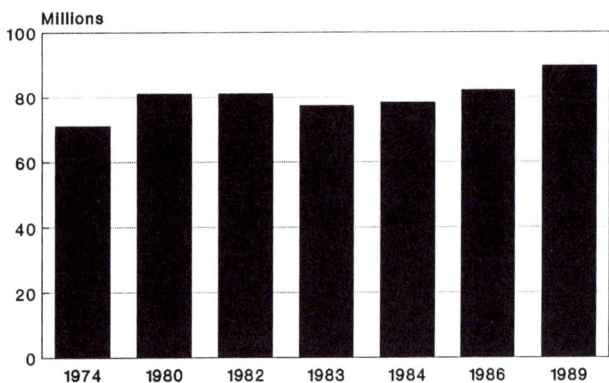

Figure 4-1 Emergency department visits.

numerous regionalization schemes (Fig. 4-2). Two years later, the American Hospital Association recommended a similar approach.[5] Currently the standards developed by the Joint Commission on Accreditation of Healthcare Organizations (JCAHO) are the basis for the accreditation of most hospital emergency services.[6] The JCAHO system is voluntary, but it is the industry standard for validating most hospital emergency services. In evaluating institutional capabilities to respond to general medical emergencies, the JCAHO recognizes four levels of care. The JCAHO considers these levels of care key factors central to the accreditation decision of a facility. The levels of care consist of the following:

- *level I:* 24-hour emergency care with a physician experienced in emergency care on duty in the emergency care area. In-hospital specialty consultation by medical staff members or senior residents is available for at least medical, surgical, orthopedic, obstetric/gynecologic, pediatric, and anesthesia services.
- *level II:* basic 24-hour emergency care with a physician experienced in emergency care on duty in the emergency care area. On-call specialty consultation by members of the medical staff or senior residents is available within approximately 30 minutes.
- *level III:* limited 24-hour emergency care with a physician from a medical staff call roster available to the emergency care area within approximately 30 minutes. Specialty consultation or interhospital transfer is required.
- *level IV:* reasonable standby care for determining whether an emergency exists and for rendering lifesaving first aid. Appropriate referral to the nearest facility capable of providing needed services is available.

These four levels of emergency care are noted as key factors, and compliance is compulsory for accreditation.[6]

Horizontal classification provides health care personnel and the public with important utilization information. For example, emergency medical technicians (EMTs) generally transport patients to hospitals that provide level I or level II services; the staff and resources at such facilities are adequate for 95% of emergency conditions. Some jurisdictions have pursued this concept further, developing minimum standards for receiving hospitals that exceed even these basic requirements and precluding some hospitals and most ambulatory care facilities from receiving advanced life support ambulances. Horizontal classification thus serves notice that, with rare exceptions, level III and IV facilities do not offer the care necessary for most acute medical emergencies.

Vertical

Although horizontal classification of emergency care meets the needs of the overwhelming majority of emergency patients, a small subset remains that requires tertiary care. To meet the needs of these patients, many emergency medical services (EMS) systems have also implemented vertical classification (Fig. 4-2).

In 1973, Congress passed the Emergency Medical Services Systems Act, recognizing seven classified areas for critical care: behavior, burn, cardiac, pediatric, perinatal, toxicologic, and trauma.[7] More recently, the AMA has described nine areas.[3] These classifications recognize that critical care services vary from region to region, depending on a variety of factors (eg, population densities, referral patterns, and facility locations). Accordingly, they are intended to be adapted to meet specific needs.

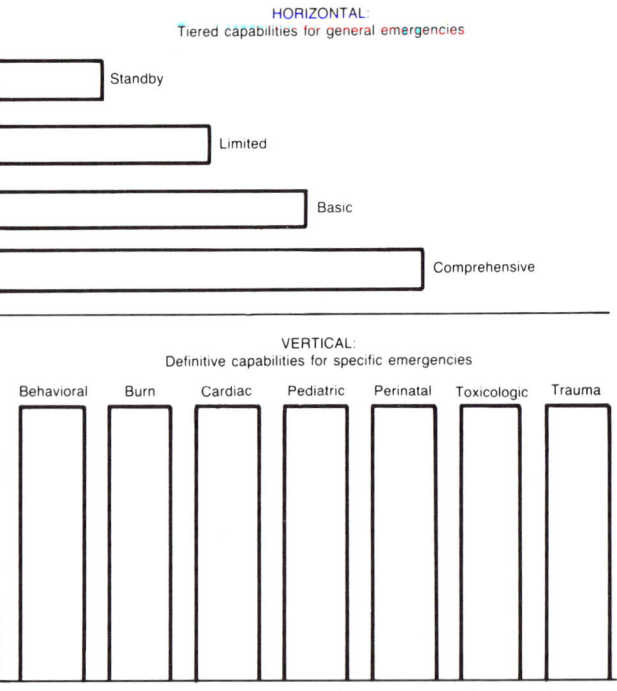

Figure 4-2 Care classifications for emergency medical care systems.

The examples in Fig. 4-2 illustrate horizontal and vertical classification schemes that meet most EMS system needs. Acute, general medical emergencies, recognized by the vertical AMA scheme, do not appear separately because the need is met by systems that classify emergency services horizontally and direct such patients to level I or II services.[3]

Vertical classification schemes that entail three care levels are based on several assumptions regarding hospital capability and responsibility. For example, level I facilities are assumed to have special roles, such as providing system leadership; participating in medical, nursing, and all paraprofessional education; engaging in medical research; and promoting community awareness and prevention programs. Level II hospitals provide an intermediate care level, definitively treating the majority of emergency patients who require special care. Level III facilities, in contrast, have limited resources and offer basic services, expeditiously transferring patients to facilities that provide a higher care level when indicated.

BEHAVIORAL DISORDERS

The AMA guidelines delineate three levels of care for hospitals that receive patients with behavioral emergencies[3]:

- *level I:* 24-hour psychiatric care with an emergency physician on duty in the emergency care area; on-call consultation by a psychiatrist and a psychiatric social worker who are promptly available; secure area for violent or dangerous patients
- *level II:* 24-hour psychiatric care with an emergency physician on duty in the emergency call area; on-call consultation by a psychiatrist who is promptly available
- *level III:* 24-hour psychiatric care with an emergency physician on duty in the emergency care area; on-call consultation by a psychiatrist who is promptly available but who may have courtesy rather than active medical staff privileges

Similarly, the guidelines describe three classifications of behavioral disorders:

1. *major:* life-threatening behavioral disorders in which patients are self-mutilating, intoxicated, psychotic, assaultive, suicidal, or otherwise gravely disabled or a threat to themselves or others
2. *moderate:* intermediate behavioral disorders in which patients are intoxicated, mildly psychotic, or hysterical; are withdrawing from sedatives, narcotics, or alcohol; or are threatening suicide
3. *minor:* mild behavioral disorders in which patients are grieving, anxious, intoxicated, threatening suicide, or requesting medication refills

Optimally, patients with major, moderate, or minor behavioral disorders should be triaged to level I, II, or III hospitals.

BURN INJURIES

The AMA, the American Burn Association, and the American College of Surgeons have published guidelines for hospitals that wish to be considered burn centers.[3,8,9]

Each year in the United States, burn injuries result in more than 500,000 hospital ED visits and approximately 70,000 acute inpatient admissions. Most burn injuries are relatively minor, and patients are discharged after outpatient treatment at the facility where they are originally treated. Approximately 20,000 are directly referred or admitted to burn centers.[9]

The American Burn Association recognizes a burn center as a service system based in a hospital that has made the institutional commitment to meet the criteria specified in its *Guidelines for Development and Operation of Burn Centers*.[8] Likewise, a burn unit is a specific area within a hospital that has committed itself to meeting the criteria of a burn center.[8]

The American Burn Association and the American College of Surgeons have developed criteria for referral to a burn center in an attempt to clarify and quantify for the medical team at referring institutions the difference between major, moderate, and minor burn injuries. The criteria are as follows[8,9]:

1. second- and third-degree burns greater than 10% total body surface area (TBSA) in patients younger than 10 or older than 50 years of age
2. second- and third-degree burns greater than 20% TBSA in other age groups
3. second- and third-degree burns that involve the face, hands, feet, genitalia, perineum, and major joints
4. third-degree burns greater than 5% TBSA in any age group
5. electrical burns, including lightning injuries
6. chemical burns
7. burn injury with inhalation injury
8. burn injury in patients with preexisting medical disorders that could complicate management, prolong recovery, or affect mortality
9. any patient with burns and concomitant trauma in which the burn injury poses the greatest risk of morbidity and mortality; in such cases, if the trauma poses the greater immediate risk, the patient may be treated initially in a trauma center until stable before being transferred to a burn center
10. pediatric burn cases (hospitals without qualified personnel or equipment for the care of children should

transfer children with burns to a burn center with these capabilities)
11. burn injury in patients who will require special social/emotional and/or long-term rehabilitative support, including cases involving suspected child abuse, substance abuse, or elderly abuse

Patients meeting the criteria as stated above are recommended for referral to a burn center. Patients with lesser injuries are usually managed as inpatients at the hospital where they were initially taken; those with minor injuries are treated and discharged from the ED.

CARDIAC EMERGENCIES

Both the AMA[3] and the American Heart Association[10] have developed guidelines for facilities that receive patients with cardiac emergencies. Although the American Heart Association guidelines focus primarily on ED care, they also provide a useful indicator of overall hospital capabilities in the management of cardiac emergencies.

The AMA guidelines delineate three care levels for hospitals that receive cardiac emergency patients[3]:

- *level I:* 24-hour cardiac care with an emergency physician on duty in the emergency care area, consultation by an in-hospital internist or a cardiologist, and on-call consultation by a cardiovascular surgeon who is promptly available; also, promptly available surgical capabilities, including a cardiovascular surgical team, operating room, and coronary care unit
- *level II:* 24-hour cardiac care with an emergency physician on duty in the emergency care area and consultation by an on-call internist or cardiologist who is promptly available; a cardiac care unit
- *level III:* 24-hour cardiac care with an emergency physician on duty in the emergency care area and consultation by an on-call internist who is promptly available

Although cardiac emergency patients would benefit from prehospital triage criteria that identify patients who require tertiary care, there are no generally accepted guidelines for such field determinations because of the complexities involved. Accordingly, most urban and suburban EMS systems transport cardiac patients to the nearest level I or II emergency service, providing interhospital transfer when required for invasive diagnostic or therapeutic procedures.

PEDIATRIC/PERINATAL EMERGENCIES

The AMA has formulated a single set of guidelines for pediatric and perinatal emergencies.[3] The guidelines delineate three care levels for hospitals that receive these patients:

- *level I:* 24-hour pediatric/perinatal care with an emergency physician on duty in the emergency care area; consultation by an in-house pediatrician, a neonatologist, and a pediatric surgeon with on-call consultation by an obstetrician/gynecologist who is promptly available; a separate pediatric/perinatal emergency care area; a pediatric intensive care unit; a neonatal intensive care unit
- *level II:* 24-hour pediatric/perinatal care with an emergency physician on duty in the emergency care area; consultation by an on-call pediatrician and a neonatologist who are promptly available
- *level III:* 24-hour pediatric/perinatal care with an emergency physician on duty in the emergency care area

Currently, there are no generally accepted prehospital triage guidelines that can be used to assess the severity of a patient's condition (with the exception of trauma) in a pediatric/perinatal emergency. Certain jurisdictions have attempted to develop minimum standards for EDs approved for pediatrics, which exceed these basic requirements. This is done on a voluntary basis in a given EMS region, however.

TOXICOLOGIC EMERGENCIES

Classification guidelines for toxicologic emergencies generally focus on a systems approach to poison control, including prevention, referral, treatment, and follow-up. Two organizations have developed standards for hospitals that receive patients with toxicologic emergencies. Presently the American Association of Poison Control Centers describes only tertiary care capabilities.[11] The AMA, however, describes three levels of care[3]:

- *level I:* 24-hour toxicologic care with an emergency physician with special toxicologic competence on duty in the emergency care area; consultation by an in-hospital internist and a pediatrician with on-call consultation by a toxicologist and a pathologist who are promptly available; a comprehensive toxicologic laboratory and a dialysis unit
- *level II:* 24-hour toxicologic care with an emergency physician with special toxicologic competence on duty in the emergency care area; on-call consultation by an internist, a pediatrician, and a pathologist who are promptly available; a toxicologic screening laboratory
- *level III:* 24-hour toxicologic care with an emergency physician on duty in the emergency care area

Currently there are no generally accepted prehospital triage guidelines that can be used to assess the severity of toxicologic emergencies.

TRAUMA

One of the earliest attempts to develop hospital guidelines centered on trauma care. In 1976, the American College of Surgeons developed trauma hospital guidelines,[12] which were updated in 1979,[13] 1983,[14] 1986–87,[15] and most recently in 1990.[9] The AMA has published its own guidelines.[3]

In the 1990 revision of the American College of Surgeons, *Resources for Optimal Care of the Injured Patient*,[9] the Committee on Trauma recognized the individual needs of the pediatric trauma patient and describes two levels of care:

1. *pediatric trauma regional resource hospital:* a children's hospital or general hospital with pediatric surgical service; a pediatric surgeon available promptly 24 hours a day; a pediatric ED fully staffed and equipped; a pediatric intensive care unit fully staffed and equipped; a pediatric trauma service directed by a pediatric surgeon; all appropriate pediatric subspecialists; a pediatric trauma coordinator; and a commitment to research, injury prevention, and quality assurance
2. *adult trauma center with pediatric commitment:* a general hospital with an organized trauma service and pediatric service; a pediatric surgeon available to the general surgeon; a general surgeon with special interest and commitment to the pediatric victim; a designated area in the ED with appropriately trained staff and equipment; a pediatric intensive care unit with appropriately trained personnel and equipment; all appropriate surgical and medical subspecialty physicians; a trauma coordinator; and a commitment to research, injury prevention, and quality assurance

The American College of Surgeons guidelines describe three care levels for hospitals that receive trauma patients[9]:

- *level I:* 24-hour trauma care with an emergency physician on duty in the emergency care area; a trauma team headed by a trauma surgeon who is in the ED on patient arrival and an anesthesiologist who is in-hospital and immediately available; a neurosurgeon who is on call and promptly available; immediately available radiographic capabilities for angiography and computed tomography; and surgical capabilities, including an operating room, a surgical team, and a surgical intensive care unit. Additionally, the level I hospital must maintain a leadership role in the community and should serve as both an acute care and a tertiary referral center. Educational programs must be conducted for physicians, nurses, paramedics, and other trauma personnel. Major outreach programs, public awareness campaigns regarding injury prevention, and a commitment to research at either the clinical or basic sciences level is essential.
- *level II:* 24-hour trauma care with an emergency physician on duty in the emergency care area; a trauma team, headed by a surgeon and an anesthesiologist who may be involved or on call but who are in the ED on patient arrival; on-call consultation by surgical and medical specialists who are promptly available; and immediately available surgical capabilities, including an operating room, a surgical team, and a surgical intensive care unit. A level II facility may find it necessary to transfer patients to a level I center. Appropriate transfer agreements should be written.
- *level III:* 24-hour trauma care with an emergency physician on duty in the emergency care area; on-call consultation by a surgeon and an anesthesiologist who are promptly available; and promptly available surgical capabilities or an interhospital transfer agreement. The intent of a level III facility is to provide the best possible care even in the remote regions, thereby allowing for some flexibility in the guidelines for such a facility.

Field triage guidelines for trauma patients are currently more detailed than those for any other emergency condition. Because there are currently no prehospital methods to differentiate between trauma patients who require level I care and those who require level II care, most urban and suburban trauma care systems transport patients to the nearest level I or level II trauma hospital, providing interhospital transfer when required for special diagnostic or therapeutic procedures.

REGIONALIZATION

Categorization and designation, both used to regionalize hospital care, entail similar horizontal and vertical classifications, but they involve different implementation methods and produce different medical outcomes.[16] As a voluntary, unverified process, categorization is not binding on system providers. Designation, on the opposite end of the regionalization continuum, is a validated process that includes both contractual rights and responsibilities (Table 4-1). Regardless of approach, the success of regionalization in improving the quality of hospital care ultimately depends on the effectiveness of medical direction in determining system standards and directing patients to qualified hospitals.

CATEGORIZATION

Although categorization is a well-established method for regionalizing emergency care services, it has been less effective than designation for improving quality of trauma care.[17] As a voluntary process that requires neither independent

Table 4-1 Regionalization Methods: Comparison of Categorization and Designation

	Categorization	Designation
Binding on prehospital providers	No	Yes
Verified by independent experts	No	Yes
Indicative of hospital commitment	No	Yes
Provides necessary patient volume	No	Yes
Establishes contractual obligation	No	Yes
Standard of care in EMS systems	No	Yes

Source: Adapted from the Oregon State Trauma Plan.

validation nor contractual obligations, categorization involves fewer political hurdles. Furthermore, because categorization requires self-limitation of services and allows all potentially qualified hospitals to provide care, it faces fewer legal challenges from dissatisfied facilities. It yields few medical guarantees, however, and does not provide accountability for capability or commitment.

DESIGNATION

A regionalization method that originated with trauma care systems, hospital designation can be likened to the Certificate of Need process.[4] Because it limits hospital participation, confers a patient monopoly, and entails contractual obligations, designation requires appropriate statutory authority and verification by independent experts. The responsiblities of hospitals designated to provide high levels of care include maintaining a higher state of readiness, sustaining an increased level of medical and administrative staff commitment, contracting with the designating authority, assuming liability for a higher standard of care, and, in some systems, paying user fees to support the emergency medical care system. In return, designated hospitals may expect to receive a larger number of patients because designation is also binding on prehospital providers. Despite the theoretical and proven advantages of designation over categorization, however, there remain only a few EMS systems that have fully implemented a designation system. In 1987, a study was undertaken by West et al[18] to define the current national status of statewide trauma systems in the hope that they could provide a strategy for the development, management, and analysis of such systems. Eight basic components were deemed essential to a statewide system:

1. legal authority to designate trauma centers
2. a formal process in place for designation
3. use of the American College of Surgeons standards for trauma centers
4. use of independent experts for trauma center site review
5. patient volume and population figures available for consideration in determining the number of trauma centers
6. the presence of written triage criteria
7. ongoing monitoring systems
8. a significant percentage of the state population covered by trauma centers

The results of the study indicated that only two states, Maryland and Virginia, have all eight essential components of a regional trauma system. Twenty-nine states have yet to initiate the process of designation. It is clear that in the 22 years since the National Research Council issued a white paper labeling trauma the neglected disease of modern society progress in implementing regional trauma systems has been slow.

REFERENCES

1. American Hospital Association. *Hospital Statistics 1990–1991*. Chicago: American Hospital Association; 1990.
2. Commission on Emergency Medical Services. *Categorization of Hospital Emergency Capabilities*. Chicago: American Medical Association; 1971.
3. Commission on Emergency Medical Services. *Provisional Guidelines for the Optimal Categorization of Hospital Emergency Capabilities*. Chicago: American Medical Association; 1982.
4. Boyd DR, Cowley RA. Systems approach to the care of the trauma patient. In: Boyd DR, Edlich RF, Micek S, eds. *Systems Approach to Emergency Medical Care*. Norwalk, CT: Appleton-Century-Crofts; 1983:ch. 19.
5. American Hospital Association. *Categorization of Hospital Emergency Services: Report of a Conference*. Chicago: American Hospital Association; 1973.
6. Joint Commission on Accreditation of Healthcare Organizations. *Accreditation Manual for Hospitals*. Chicago: Joint Commission on Accreditation of Healthcare Organizations; 1989.
7. Public Law 93-154: Emergency Medical Services Act of 1973; 93rd US Congress; 1973.
8. American Burn Association. Hospital and prehospital resources for the optimal care of patients with burn injury: guidelines for development and operation of burn centers. *J Burn Care Rehabil*. 1990;110:97–104.
9. Committee on Trauma, American College of Surgeons. *Resources for Optimal Care of the Injured Patient*. Chicago: American College of Surgeons; 1990.
10. American Heart Association, Los Angeles Affiliate. *Emergency Heart Care Program*. Los Angeles: American Heart Association; 1985.
11. American Association of Poison Control Centers. *Criteria for Designation as a Regional Poison Control Center*. Washington, DC: American Association of Poison Control Centers; 1982.
12. Committee on Trauma. Optimal hospital resources for care of the seriously injured. *Bull Am Coll Surg*. 1976;61:15–22.
13. Committee on Trauma. Hospital resources for optimal care of the injured patient. *Bull Am Coll Surg*. 1970;64:43–48.
14. Committee on Trauma. Hospital and prehospital resources for optimal care of the injured patient. *Bull Am Coll Surg*. 1983;68:11–18.

15. Committee on Trauma. Hospital and prehospital resources for optimal care of the injured patient. *Bull Am Coll Surg*. 1986;71:4–12.
16. Heilig RW Jr, Cales RH. Development. In: Cales RH, Heilig RW Jr, eds. *Trauma Care Systems*. Gaithersburg, MD: Aspen Publishers; 1986:243–293.
17. Tortella BJ, Trunkey DD. Hospital care. In: Cales RH, Heilig RW Jr, eds. *Trauma Care Systems*. Gaithersburg, MD: Aspen Publishers; 1986:143–162.
18. West JG, Williams MJ, Trunkey DD, et al. Trauma systems: current status, future challenges. *JAMA*. 1988;259:3598–3600.

5. Quality Assurance/Quality Improvement for the Emergentologist

R.S. VENABLE, MD, FAAFP, FACEP

Blendon and Altman[1] report that the public embraces a national contradiction. National polls have indicated that the public wants to have high quality while maintaining the status quo. The medicalization of daily life has brought unrealistic expectations of cure, and at the same time the commercialization of care has led to a decline in the public's trust in health professionals. The public would like the freedom to choose an individual provider but at the lowest common denominator of cost. Managed care may offer one of these lowest common denominators of cost. The public trusts government to explore other potential options for them as well.[2]

It is interesting to note the difference in perceptions that the public and physicians have concerning health care. Physicians disagree with the public sentiment that all costs should be taken to save one life by a margin of 3 to 1. Less than a third of the public believes that it gets good to excellent value for the health care dollar. More than three quarters of physicians believe that we get excellent value. Although the public feels that it should have the best possible health care (by a margin of 91%), it also feels that health insurance should pay for any treatment that will save lives, regardless of the cost to save one life (by a margin of 71%).[3]

With contradictions arising from the public's perception of health care and the physician's perception of its delivery, it is no surprise that there is a great deal of turmoil when federalization of quality measures in health care is consumer based. As the largest purchaser of medical care, the government is intimately involved in establishing its requirements. The consumer guide from the Office of Technology Assessment recommends that the public consider several quality indicators when purchasing health services:[4(p8)]

- hospital mortality rates
- adverse events (including hospital-acquired infections)
- formal disciplinary actions by state boards against physicians
- peer review organization (PRO)/Health and Human Services (HHS) sanctions
- malpractice compensations
- evaluation of physicians' performance based on specific conditions (by process or outcome measures)
- volume of services in hospitals or performed by physicians
- external standards and guidelines for the scope of hospital services (including emergency, cancer, and neonatal care)
- physician specialization as measured by specialty board certification or practicing in one's area of training
- patient assessment of care

The Office of Technology Assessment cautions purchasers that current quality assessment techniques are not adjusted adequately for all patients in all environments, which may influence access to quality health care. Specifically, each individual quality of care indicator should be evaluated based upon the environment in which it is provided. There is an imperfect market access presently based on both consumer knowledge and consumer economic viability. Furthermore, a consumer's impression of overall health care may be influenced by his or her relationship with the family physician.[4] In emergency medicine this relationship is difficult to develop, and rarely does it endow a positive bias in favor of the emergentologist. As a result, consumer advocacy for the emergentologist is usually less than that for the family physician.

McClure[5] emphasizes three components of quality: patient satisfaction, effectiveness, and innovation. These components are best measured by comparing provider performance against an expert quality assessment system. Because these expert systems are idealized, however, the physician must be careful in how the information is presented to the public. Providers who receive quality and efficiency scores compared with expert systems may find that they are sometimes depicted as more inefficient and of lower quality than their fellow physicians whose behavior is closer to that of the expert systems. McClure[5] feels that this is part of the incentive for physicians to improve when they are compared with other physicians in like specialties based on the expert criteria. Hospitals may tend competitively to compare one group against another because of the marketing character of these approaches. Utilizing expert criteria can be a somewhat demanding and perhaps unrealistic approach to comparative evaluation.[5] Therefore, emergentologists should be wary when they are evaluated under these circumstances and be ready to point out that the comparison criteria document deviation from an idealized norm rather than a direct comparison with other physicians.

QUALITY AND OUTCOMES

Since the late 1960s, when Donabedian[6] first promulgated some of the standards of quality assessment and quality measurement in medicine, there has been a continual quest for determining a definition of quality. The emphasis on quality has been more recently brought back into the spotlight with the Health Care Financing Administration's (HCFA) implementation of the standards of the 1986 Health Care Quality Improvement Act.[7] With the HCFA's 1989 establishment of a separate quality improvement division and its 1993 first-released practice guidelines,[7a] emergency physicians can expect to see increasingly more regulation imposed upon practice patterns as determined by outcome measurements. These outcome measurements are, in fact, a reflection of the quality of care and are intimately involved with both quality assessment (a measurement criterion)[8] and quality improvement.[9]

Because it has been federally mandated that there will be an improvement in overall outcome for Medicare patients and, by implication, other third party payor patients, it is imperative that the emergency medicine provider be especially astute as to what quality meter is being used to determine independent management steps that could lead to unexpected outcomes. It is extremely important that a clear distinction be drawn between determining the efficacy of care (appropriate under the circumstances) and the quality of care. To clarify this distinction, the American Medical Association (AMA), in conjunction with the Joint Commission on Accreditation of Healthcare Organizations (Joint Commission), has considered seven elements essential to quality care.[10] Quality care should:

1. optimize a patient's improvement and health
2. emphasize both health promotion and disease prevention
3. be timely in its provision
4. include informed consent
5. be based on accepted medical precepts
6. be empathetic and use technology with the best efficiency available
7. be documented to allow for peer review and improvement

It is significant that this overall definition does not state how these quality elements should be interconnected. Quality must include an assessment of patient goals and values in addition to intended outcomes.

The US government, on the other hand, was quite clear that it planned to regulate quality with implementation of the 1986 Health Care Quality Improvement Act (HCQIA). As noted earlier, the government has delineated its own criteria for quality as well. From the consumer information publication of the Office of Technology Assessment, it is stated that "the quality of medical care is a degree to which the process of care increases the probability of outcomes desired by patients and decreases the probability of undesired outcomes, given the state of medical knowledge."[4(p9)]

In a more global sense, however, quality measurement is not as much an approach to a statistical model as it is a means toward improving patient outcomes. Quality is ultimately the organization and management of a health care system such that appropriate resources are provided within a cost-conscious environment that is relevant, effective, and as free of adverse outcome as possible.[10]

What will be further discussed in this chapter is a current survey of the literature in quality assurance and quality improvement for the emergentologist. Furthermore, the chapter explores how this rapidly changing area can significantly affect practice life in the emergency department.

TRADITIONAL QUALITY ASSURANCE MODALITIES

From Donabedian's[11] initial analysis, quality can be characterized as being based on structure, process, and outcome.

In the early 1980s it was considered that structure and process were much more important than actual outcome measurement. A great deal of literature exists concerning the appropriate measurement techniques necessary statistically to provide a quality of care measurement.[8] Because quality is so difficult to define, being elusive as to its link with eventual outcome in certain cases, it has been increasingly difficult to determine what structures or processes might lead to a positive impact on quality.[12]

Structure refers to the nature of the facility, supplies, managers, and the overall responsiveness of the work environment as it pertains to the provider of health care. Clinically, we have all experienced how inadequate supplies can make it difficult to see patients efficiently. Inadequate staffing can make it difficult to see patients in a timely manner. Lack of certain diagnostic equipment can make it nearly impossible to diagnose a patient's case appropriately. The structure in which the medical care is provided, therefore, is extremely important as a starting point. Facilities management, however, is usually not a problem in the emergency department because of government regulations (Joint Commission, state agencies, and PROs). It has rarely been a problem for the emergentologist to find appropriate equipment or diagnostic tools.[6]

Since there are few facilities problems in most emergency departments, the process of care, therefore, has been the concentration of quality assurance over the last decade.[8,13] In an effort to meet government regulatory concerns about quality assessment, hospitals and clinics have set up quality assurance committees.[12] The quality assurance committee, not always knowing exactly what it is to study and often being necessarily unpopular as a committee, has sometimes become an adversarial committee dedicated to the witch hunt. For that reason, physicians do not have fond memories of quality assurance committees in those circumstances.

By the committee pointing the finger at other physicians who appear to deviate from a standard of care (albeit an artificial one imposed by the committee members at the time), it was felt that the patient would be protected. Little was done as far as educational process, action plan, or intervention to prevent further problems outside of attempting to embarrass the physician being investigated by the quality assurance committee.[13,14]

Although this might not be a desirable approach, it was not necessarily one that physicians resisted unless they were the object of the investigation. Far from being objectionable as an investigatory method, however, this approach is not constructive for improving patient care, especially in view of the new regulatory standards that will certainly affect all practitioners.[7,15] Outcome measures, the third portion of the Donabedian framework[6] for assessing quality, include measures that go beyond simple mortality/morbidity measures. Also included are iatrogenic complications, hospital-acquired infections, and unexpected results of care.[4,8,11]

Another view of quality is that it has two principal dimensions, technical and interpersonal.[15] From this particular reference has emerged concerns over "high-tech" and "high-touch" care. Technical quality will depend on the presence of advancing science and the technology of medicine as applied to treating the patient. Interpersonal skills, however, cannot be supplanted by a physician's technical proficiency. Furthermore, success of interpersonal skills depends on how well a patient's needs are met.[15]

Increasingly, therefore, outcome is the emphasis for many of today's quality assessment and quality assurance studies.[16] This is certainly not new, although the conceptualization of it may be new to many. In 1910, Dr. Ernest A. Codman,[17] a surgeon at Massachusetts General Hospital in Boston, promulgated a quality assurance idea known as the end-result system. He stated that "to affect improvement, the first step is to admit and record the lack of perfection."[17(pxx)] His case by case reviews of surgical outcomes did not engender much goodwill with his fellow professionals. In fact, peers forced him to leave his position. Eventually his work influenced the organization of the American College of Surgeons in 1913, and the hospital standardization program of that college carried on until it evolved into the Joint Commission on Accreditation of Hospitals in 1952 (now known as the Joint Commission on Accreditation of Healthcare Organizations).[17,18]

From the time of the formation of the Joint Commission in 1952, other physicians have sought to link hospital statistics with quality of care. Dr. Paul Lembcke[19] noted wide variations in appendectomy rates in New York state. Much of Dr. Lembcke's work was used as a basis for approaches adopted by future studies.[20–22a]

Early studies emphasized the process of measuring the quality of care. The process of examining the quality of care has become extremely complex from the standpoint of statistical measurement. It has not been determined, however, whether statistical measurement is pertinent to the efficacy and appropriateness of care.[23] Despite this, the US government mandated that a measurable quality improvement plan be in place by 1990 in all hospitals. The Joint Commission implemented a study of quality indicators at multiple medical centers over the period 1988 through 1991. The second cycle of these studies is presently underway and will be helpful in determining what practice patterns indicate a consistent and low adverse outcome approach to care.[16,24]

Results of these indicator surveys will ultimately affect how physicians are allowed to care for patients.[7,22] Even though there will not be a cookbook for physicians, there will be federal regulatory control for failure to meet certain standards.[7,22,25–27] This regulatory control will initially take the form of peer review organization informational investigations. Normally this would not be a problem except for the interface with the new National Practitioner Data Bank. An adverse investigatory outcome from a quality assurance examination will be stored in the National Practitioner Data Bank.[28-30]

POTENTIAL QUALITY PATROL: NATIONAL PRACTITIONER DATA BANK

Before the HCQIA of 1986, hospitals and employers were largely beholden to medical staff members to supply information concerning adverse actions at other places of employment. With the advent of the HCQIA, a new querying databank was mandated.[7,28] It has been sidelined from time to time because of technical difficulties involving everything from information format to problems with UNISYS, the data company awarded this federal contract.

Title IV of the HCQIA set up a databank for malpractice data, disciplinary licensure data, adverse clinical privilege data, and membership data.[30] The National Practitioner Data Bank has been on line since September 1990, but hospitals are just now (1993) able routinely to query and receive a timely response. All hospitals must query the databank every 2 years regarding applicants and present staff members holding clinical privileges. They must also query the databank when negotiating to bring individuals on to their staff or to grant privileges. Hospitals may query at other times, however, regarding questions about practitioners, dentists, and (in the future) nurses.

When checking for malpractice data, any entity (including insurance companies) that makes a malpractice payment on behalf of any licensed health care provider as a result of any judgment or settlement must report this to the National Practitioner Data Bank. Settlements, even as small as $1, must be reported.[31] When a due process examination of clinical performance (usually through peer review) has decided an action that adversely affects clinical privileges, a report must be sent to the databank. All lawsuits filed against a hospital or one of its practitioners (including health maintenance organizations (HMOs) or other organized medical groups within which physicians may work) are reported to the databank. When these lawsuits are filed, a plaintiff or a plaintiff's attorney may access the databank regarding a specific practitioner if the plaintiff's attorney or the plaintiff can prove that the hospital failed to query the databank as required by law.[31]

Individuals may query regarding their own records in the databank, but the data entered may not necessarily relate to their source. Although practitioners may obtain their records at no cost, it is difficult for them to consider any change in the databank because it is treated as analogous to a "write once, read many" computer memory. A practitioner may request changes, however, if this request is made before expiration of the 30-day grace period that starts from notification that there is a matter for potential databank entry.[32]

Further guidelines under the 1986 HCQIA set up a research program through which aggregate data (stripped of all identifiers) will be available to interested parties for study.

Therefore, quality assessments and outside review can be performed. The federal contractor (ie, Medicare and, to some extent, Medicaid) must develop and provide a communication and educational program such that all those involved in the National Practitioner Data Bank will know in advance what their rights are. Efforts are planned to provide educational materials and multiple conferences as a result of these studies.[33]

Under section 5 of Title IV in the HCQIA, state boards of all licensed health practitioner fields must submit data concerning disciplinary licensure actions against practitioners. In addition, state or political subdivisions thereof taking disciplinary action against licensure of health care entities must report to the National Practitioner Data Bank. Therefore, state licensing boards, hospitals, and health care entities are the only ones that can receive data under this section of Title IV.[33] Because of regulations for section 5 currently under development, details pertaining to what other entities may ultimately get data from this section are not clear.

THE HCQIA IN PRACTICE

A review of the HCQIA by any practitioner will immediately reveal that physician leaders of today will be held accountable to provide guidance to their colleagues and to encourage and foster further processes in an ongoing relationship to ensure professional approaches to credentialing, privileging, and peer review. It is hoped that this will be accomplished in a positive educational manner and not in a negative adversarial or punitive way. In the past, medical staff bylaws, rules, and regulations have sometimes been used as a club instead of as an endorsement. The intent of the HCQIA of 1986 is to allow a broadening of the base from which these regulations will be implemented in such a way that a fair and equitable hearing will be afforded.[15,34]

Barring that, many practitioners will find their ability to continue in professional medicine as clinicians severely hampered if unfounded negative reporting is placed in their data file. Although performing peer review is an uncomfortable task for many physicians, it is felt that this task will be less burdensome once better and more precise evaluative tools are available.[34]

It is of interest that the HCQIA has been on the books for more than 7 years and that few practitioners are aware of its broad implications. In July 1990, enforcement powers stemming from this particular law were granted not only to the HCFA but also to divisions of the Department of Justice and the Federal Trade Commission. As discussed in this section, concerning further punishing powers of the federal government this is a broad stroke for the federal government and could eventuate the destruction of many professional lives unless physicians are acutely attuned in a technical way to the various intricacies of these laws and the impact that these various federal agencies will have on their professional lives.

Implementing a hospital- or clinic-based quality assurance program (probably more adequately described now as a quality outcomes management program) will be a daunting task at best.[35]

CONTINUOUS QUALITY IMPROVEMENT

Because there are a significant number of variables making up both the definition and the regulation of medical quality, many practitioners have chosen initially to adopt the standards that are being promulgated by the Joint Commission field surveys. Fourteen potential indicators of hospital-wide performance have been studied from 1988 to 1991 with 14 different medical centers ranging from metropolitan to rural areas. From this has emerged the Joint Commission model of continuous quality improvement. Dr. Dennis O'Leary,[24] President of the Joint Commission, states that continuous quality improvement is perhaps the best approach to ensuring quality. He feels that quality assurance may be an unfortunate semantic selection. Over time he feels that quality improvement will be the model. Certainly this has been adopted by many hospitals and certain managed care plans, to their benefit.[11,26,36]

The old model of quality used by many facilities, which concentrates on getting rid of the bad apples, can improve quality. Recent studies by entities such as Clinical Review Strategies, however, reveal that advancing patient service and care depends on continuous efforts to improve.[10,11] It is felt, therefore, that continuous quality improvement will shift the standard distribution curve to the right.

This is distinguished from the traditional approach where there is an effort to eliminate the bad apples. Eliminating the bad apples, however, will do little more than shift the curve adversely to the left by that 5% that is eliminated. To obtain a fairly high degree of treatment quality as well as patient care, the overall intent of continuous quality improvement is to shift the entire curve to the right (by optimizing performance among all the apples). This optimization approach is ultimately more beneficial to the organization and more supportive of the medical provider.

DESIGN OF A QUALITY MONITORING SYSTEM

Whether one is setting up a hospital-based or a clinic-based quality assurance program, it is imperative to establish an effective system for quality referred issues. When there is a quality concern, multiple professionals should examine it immediately and determine whether, in fact, there was a negative outcome as a result of that quality deviation. Not all quality concerns result in negative outcomes, and vice versa. Practitioners should learn to review objectively their own performance and should be dedicated to quality patient outcomes. Certainly with a more altruistic orientation, physicians and other medical practitioners may protect themselves from the consumer observation that physicians represent nothing but an avaricious trade dealing with human lives.[37]

Therefore, it is proposed that a continuous quality evaluation committee be available for periodic monitoring of activities involving peer review, patient complaints, quality referred issues, complaints from outside departments, and any incident reports. Once these areas are discussed and studied, it may be difficult for these committees to know what to do with the data. Any time a practitioner's performance is challenged, there should be a chance for rebuttal. The final determination of quality evaluation committees should be directed by those dedicated to education and intervention rather than punishment.

A practitioner who has an adverse outcome may improve performance much more quickly if he or she is counseled rather than singled out to make the example. This would also minimize punitive approaches that could lead to adverse action reporting to the National Practitioner Data Bank.[26,38,39]

QUALITY IMPROVEMENT SYSTEMS

Continuous quality improvement models were used initially in industrialization in Japan by Dr. W. Edwards Deming.[40,41] Joseph Juran[42] and, somewhat later, Armand V. Feigenbaum[43] adopted Deming's approach and looked at statistical approaches to production processes. Deming's system is based upon 14 points:

1. Create a constancy of purpose.
2. Adopt the new philosophy promulgated from this new purpose.
3. Cease dependence on continuous inspection (and thus further government intervention from our viewpoint).
4. Cease awarding business based on price alone.
5. Improve continuously and forever.
6. Institute training and retraining on the job.
7. Adopt and institute leadership.
8. Drive out fear.
9. Break down barriers among staff members.
10. Eliminate slogans, exhortations, and targets for the workforce.
11. Eliminate numerical quotas for workers and managers.
12. Improve barriers that rob people of pride in workmanship.
13. Institute a vigorous program of education and self-improvement.
14. Put everyone in the organization to work on this transformation.

Hospital Corporation of America (HCA) has utilized such programs in the past with variable success. It was felt by the HCA that the theories promulgated for quality management processes as outlined above were most productive once used as an educational tool. Once the entire management of an institution learns such new techniques and approaches, new ideas seem to flow quickly.[43]

Currently the technology of medical information systems to monitor quality will still be developing because there are many large and tested routine applications. Industrial modeling has been utilized in the past to afford a method of constant examination. Systems such as COSTAR (Computerized Stored Ambulatory Record), which is utilized at Harvard Community Health Plan, illustrate current approaches in clinical medicine.[40] The Preferred Provider Organization (PPO) and HMO industries are probably leaders in this area of improving their overall systems of quality of care.[36]

Federal regulations will be such that all providers will have sophisticated data analysis tools, and the final benefit of such programs has yet to be seen. Ultimately, algorithms for idealized care will emerge. Whether or not total quality management will work for all medical practitioners remains to be seen.[43-45]

PROS AND THE QUALITY INTERVENTION PROCESS

The Omnibus Budget Reconciliation Act (OBRA) of 1990 establishes rules for the fourth scope of work for PROs. The PRO is charged with ensuring that the quality intervention plans growing from the HCQIA of 1986 are implemented. With this latest scope of work, PROs are to continue their review activities but also have expanded authority, by statute, to deny payments for poor-quality care. Because most health care institutions require Medicare certification to remain in business, guidelines established to meet the federal rules will usually apply in caring for non-Medicare patients as well.[46,46a]

IMPLICATIONS FOR THE FUTURE: THE PROCESS AND PENALTIES OF ADMINISTRATIVE REVIEW

Wyszewianski[13] examined the implications for the future from an emphasis on quality measurement. He states that our somewhat overbearing concern for quality measurement may have missed the big picture in that we have been diverting our attention away from methods to improve quality and therefore to minimize adverse outcomes. What has happened in many centers is an attempt to rate quality of care in a hospital as if it was another financial asset. As a result, practitioners who have not had quality assessment investigations have been rated as high-quality providers. Because this is based on only one measurement and thus fails to acknowledge the process involved in quality medical care, it has been difficult for health care providers to concentrate solely upon performance. There is no feedback available to guide them.

With the advent of the Patient Outcome Research Program, which started in 1986 with Public Law 99-509 (Consolidated Omnibus Budget Reconciliation Act, COBRA) and expanded in 1989 with the Forum for Quality and Effectiveness in Health Care, quality imperatives have been established for American medicine. What was initially thought of as an esoteric concern of physicians such as E. A. Codman 75 years ago has been expanded into a series of federal mandates. Congress has mandated implementation of standards initially set up under the COBRA legislation with follow-up standards in OBRA 1987, OBRA 1989, the HCFA Health Quality Assurance Standards of 1988, and the OBRA update 1990.[47]

Even though it was mandated that a complete quality assurance program be implemented by 1990, this will remain somewhat incomplete, awaiting the quality screening standards that will emerge with practice guidelines. The HCFA seems to be awaiting completion of the Joint Commission multicenter practice parameter studies. If this remains true, physicians have a golden opportunity to work with the Joint Commission in devising these eventual controls on our clinical practices. Initial data anlysis was completed late in 1991, and the first practice parameters were available during late 1992.[24]

PROs will be using generic quality screens to determine quality problems. Even thought it is acknowledged that quality is difficult to determine, there are federal mandates that are construed as reasonable quality interventions. Review criteria will be based upon reviews of inpatient care. These criteria will ultimately be extended to outpatient care. When substandard care is suspected, PROs are required to assign a severity level based on determination of risk to the patient. Significant quality problems will result in certain HCFA-mandated interventions.[47]

PROs can impose sanctions based upon these reviews. These adverse actions are reportable to the National Practitioner Data Bank. All hospitals and other health care industries, including HMOs and group medical practices, must report any peer review activity concerning practitioner competency or professional conduct to the databank if it could be construed to affect outcomes of patient management. All adverse actions taken against a physician or dentist as a result of peer review after due process must be reported.

A physician will accumulate points that are reviewed quarterly and biquarterly. Specific interventions will be considered if there are more than three significant occurrences per quarter or more than five occurrences per biquarter. Significance of occurrence is determined by the PRO and the HCFA. The general quality review process involves the following[46,47]:

- problem identification after case review (this includes timing of reviews, reexaminations, and specified deadlines during problem identification)

- determination of problem source (ie, physician or provider, such as hospital or managed care plan/HMO)
- assignment of severity levels
- notification of quality problems to affected parties
- quarterly profiling and computation of weighted severity levels
- implementation of quality interventions

The PRO must inform the physician and/or provider before making a final determination of a confirmed quality problem. The maximum time for a HCFA/PRO review is 135 days. Of this total, 30 days are afforded to allow for discussion with the responsible party.

There are three severity levels identified from this generic quality screening process:

- *level III:* medical mismanagement resulting in significant adverse effect on the patient
- *level II:* medical mismanagement with the potential for significant adverse effect on the patient
- *level I:* medical mismanagement without potential for significant adverse effect on the patient

A significant adverse effect is defined as unnecessarily prolonged treatment, complications, or readmission or patient management that results in anatomic or physiologic impairment, disability, or death.[48] Therefore, the primary distinction between a level II and a level III problem is outcome. To maintain a level III severity, a clinician must fail to monitor appropriately and recognize and treat in a timely manner potentially life-threatening conditions such that significant adverse effects result. Level II severity concerns are those where only this potential problem exists. A weighted score is assigned based on severity level; level III is scored as 25 points, level II as 5 points, and level I as 1 point.

Profiling is done on a rolling quarter basis (ie, one quarter removed and a successive quarter added); generally two quarters are profiled. Quality interventions are then decided based upon a series of weighted triggers (Table 5-1).

Sanctioning may be considered at any level, even without a 25-point score. Behavior will be sanctioned if it meets the test of being either a gross and/or flagrant violation or a substantial violation in a substantial number of cases. As defined by the HCFA, for use by a PRO gross and flagrant violation means a violation of an obligation in one or more cases that endangers the health, safety, or well-being of a Medicare beneficiary or one that unnecessarily places the beneficiary in a high-risk situation. A substantial violation in a substantial number of cases is based upon a pattern of care that is construed as inappropriate or unnecessary, that does not meet recognized professional standards of care, or that is not supported by required care documentation criteria of the PRO.[46–48]

Table 5-1 Quality Interventions Based on Weighted Triggers

Intervention	Trigger (Points Assigned)
Notification	1
Education	10
Intensification	15
Other interventions	20
Coordination with licensing bodies	25
Sanction consideration	25

It is important for medical providers to understand that quality problems identified by these criteria will always trigger a possible sanction process even though a threshold trigger of 25 has not been attained. Conversely, a threshold trigger of 25 always requires the PRO to consider issuing a sanction notice. The PRO may not issue such a notice if the quality problem does not meet the violation categories as defined above. This must be adequately documented, however, to demonstrate that appropriate corrective action is planned to avoid the HCFA pursuing the sanctioning process.

Quality intervention levels, based upon the weighted scores above, may be summarized as follows. Notification of the problem is undertaken if there are three occurrences per quarter or five occurrences per biquarter. This notification must be made in detail to the responsible party (physician/provider) and must describe all commissions and/or omissions as well as any corrective action recommended (notice of final determination). Because these occurrences, amounting to fewer than 5 weighted points, may occur without any bad outcome from medical care, it is essential that these minor interventions be taken seriously and questioned as to their validity to avoid an accumulation of unfounded points.

Quality intervention assessments may be entered into the National Practitioner Data Bank and are never purged. Therefore, even if a physician has not had any negative outcomes, his or her total score could exceed 25 points over time and be viewed negatively by hiring entities.[46]

Education as an intervention is activated at 10 weighted severity points. It is hoped that this intervention will allow the PRO to be more creative and, therefore, more sensitive to the personal needs of physicians. The draconian approach of most of the overall legislation can be softened as a number of avenues are explored, such as telephone and/or personal discussions with the responsible party, suggested literature reading, self-education courses, meetings with the responsible party, continuing medical education courses, and remedial education plans such as "mini-residencies" as specified by the PRO.

Intensified review occurs at 15 weighted severity points. Although this is not yet at the sanction consideration level, physicians should be especially wary at this level because it can involve 100% retrospective review of cases and a focused intensified review. If quality problems continue from the PRO's standpoint, sanction could be considered.[46,50]

If the PRO refers the matter to a clinic or hospital committee (ie, peer review, quality assurance, or credentials review), this investigation could be reportable to local licensing authorities should a negative standard of care be identified. Note that, although the sanctioning process is considered at 25 weighted points, this is a case where fewer than that could have the same effect as a sanction, namely licensing review for perceived poor-quality care. This negative assessment will be reported to the National Practitioner Data Bank after a 30-day rebuttal period for the physician unless the physician can provide information necessary to reverse the determination of the committee.[50]

Other intervention at higher levels of weighted review are similarly worsening variants of the scenario above. Each elevation within the quality tree can only lead to a greater distance to fall once the determinations come to rest.[46]

THE POWER TO PUNISH BEYOND ADMINISTRATIVE SANCTIONS: POTENTIAL CRIMINAL AND CIVIL PENALTIES

The discussion has yet to identify an interesting twist with these new regulations. Evidence of these professional quality interventions from the PRO and the HCFA may be turned over to the Department of Justice or the Federal Trade Commission if it is determined that potential criminal activity exists. Without belaboring the fact that this is an increasingly complex area of the practitioner's daily life, let us consider the present enforcement scheme under Medicare and Medicaid.

There are three separate areas of potential penalties: criminal, civil, and administrative. Many times, these areas overlap and may appear in the same case. The earlier discussions have been concerned mostly with administrative penalties. Civil monetary penalties under the Civil False Claims Act (31 U.S.C. 3729) assess a mandatory minimum civil penalty of $5,000 and a maximum of $10,000 per false claim and up to three times the damages sustained by the government.[51]

Under provisions of the Stark Bill, physicians having a financial relationship with an entity may not make a referral for services to that entity to bill the federal government. There are narrowly defined exceptions, but these relatively safe harbors may be more trouble than they are worth. Civil sanctions (different from the HCFA/PRO sanctions previously discussed) can include denial of payment, penalties of up to $25,000 for each claim for a service, and penalties of up to $100,000 for any arrangement or scheme that a physician or entity knows or should know has the primary purpose of ensuring referrals by the physician in violation of the act. There is a $10,000 per day fine for each day a physician fails to meet a reporting requirement under the Civil False Claims Act.[49,51]

Administrative sanctions can extend further from the HHS than those discussed specifically from the standpoint of quality concerns of the HCFA. Under the Medicare and Medicaid Patient and Program Protection Act of 1987 (42 U.S.C. 1320a-7), violation can result in mandatory exclusion, formal judgment entered into a federal or state court (nondismissible under bankruptcy code), and conviction relating to fraud or failure to disclose required information or to provide timely access to data required for participation.[49]

False claims are also considered here and may be charged as $2,000 per item or service for which a claim is filed, plus twice the amount claimed for each such item or service, plus a limitless punitive penalty for failure to comply (a chiropractor challenged the system by refusing to cooperate and was assessed 22 times the amount of the claims as a penalty; the penalty was upheld on appeal). This particular assessment can result in up to $1.2 million in fines for a single insurance claim if all potential errors were to occur.[52]

Of significance to physicians in managed care plans is a $2,000 per payment fine for any physician incentive plan from a hospital, HMO, or competitive medical plan that pays, or any physician who accepts a payment or an inducement, to reduce or limit services.

Finally, in the criminal arena, under the Medicare and Medicaid Patient and Program Protection Act of 1987 knowing and willful misrepresentation can result in 5 years imprisonment and a $25,000 fine. The fine and the imprisonment have been disallowed jointly on one appeal, so that the government may seek the criminal avenue more and more in an attempt to more weightily state its case. Kickback schemes, joint ventures, limited partnerships, staffing relationships in hospitals or HMOs, and other medical staff that engage in such activity can also activate such a penalty and potential fine. Excessive charges result in similar criminal penalties.[49]

Sending false or misleading literature to patients (violating Mail Fraud provisions under 18 U.S.C. 1961) may result in a $1,000 fine and/or 5 years imprisonment. If interstate activity was involved (such as mailing a letter interstate) Racketeer-Influenced and Corrupt Organizations Act (RICO) may apply, and a $25,000 fine and/or 20 years imprisonment could result. The sum total of these enormous powers of the federal government is dedicated to limiting unnecessary expenditures while ensuring continually improving quality under the Social Security Act (section 1156).

CONSIDERATIONS DURING A QUALITY INTERVENTION REVIEW

Physicians should cautiously evaluate any inquiry from a federal agency or its representative (ie, the PRO or a licensing authority). It behooves us all to realize that cautious, conscientious medicine can still be professionally rewarding. Nevertheless, it will take some time before these federal interventions can be softened by court challenges of their severity and potential abuse of process.

Individual practitioners are responsible for themselves first under such a scheme. No employer can protect one entirely here. Most managed care physicians will only have to deal with the quality assurance issues discussed earlier, however. Because the results of all these actions are potentially reportable to the National Practitioner Data Bank, cautious concern should be the number one priority for all physicians.

NEW DEVELOPMENTS RELATING TO THE QUALITY PROCESS

Now that it is federally mandated that the hospital query the databank, hospitals will certainly do so. More than just the federal perspective changes with new legislation. It has become apparent that the classic role of the independent contractor protection that a hospital had in dealing with an emergentologist is quickly eroding. What used to be characterized as primarily an arm's length relationship with the hospital has now been colored by the vicarious liability and corporate liability of the hospital contractor.

Hospitals have traditionally felt that it was not their responsibility to supervise medical care; therefore, when malpractice suits arose, they did not feel that they were directly liable for the actions of the practitioners. In the areas of quality assurance/improvement, however, there can be direct corporate liability for inadequate quality measures, predominantly those that relate to credentialing and surveillance. Although much of the change that will eventually be apparent to most practitioners is due to changes in trial case law, a brief survey of significant developments in this area may be medically important for practitioners.

Until 1957, hospitals were protected in most cases by charitable immunity. This was based on a New York court decision. *Schloendorff v. Society of New York Hospitals*, 105 N.E. 92 (N.Y. 1914).[53] This decision held that only physicians in hospitals were licensed to practice medicine. In 1957, however, *Bing v. Theunig*, 143 N.E. 2 d 3 (N.Y. 1957)[54] imposed liability on hospitals for negligence of nurses based on an employment theory of vicarious liability (*respondeat superior*). There was not much made of this decision until much later, when hospitals were found to have some exposure for acts of independent contractors, as was found in *Darling v. Charleston Community Memorial Hospital* (211 N.E. 2 d 253) (Ill. 1965), cert. denied, 383 U.S. 946 (1966).[55] In this decision the Supreme Court of Illinois held that hospitals owe an independent duty of care to supervise the overall medical treatment of both hospital employees and independent contractor physicians.

Since this decision, hospital liability has been extended from *Darling* to include a generalized corporate liability. As a result of this case, hospitals were reminded to be more cautious in their selection and retention of medical staff and to exercise standards concerning availability of specialty care.

Even if a hospital were to avoid its liability for supervising physicians under the HCQIA, further quality issues still arise in the courts concerning the doctrine of ostensible agency. Here, it is significant to note that the independent contractor status does not matter if the hospital creates an appearance that the physician is its employee. In most hospitals the physician who sees the patient is there in the emergency department, and it is not for the patient to dictate whom he or she will see. Ostensible agency theory has been applied in a number of cases, even in states with tort caps such as Indiana.[55] Therefore, hospitals must become intimately involved with some type of quality assessment and outcome improvement methodology or face both serious government fines and losses in the courts.[49,55,56]

Emergentologists have an even more tenuous relationship with their hospitals when one considers that, under the new enforcement provisions of the 1986 HCQIA, physicians are charged (under potential felony penalty) to notify a hospital of poor-quality care concerns. Hospitals will be somewhat protective of their own territory because of the legal concerns just discussed. Hospitals will have to be open with their quality assessment plans to empower physicians to make the changes that they are required to implement by law.[49]

Emergentologists will be called upon more and more to set up statistically reliable methods of quality assessment. Therefore, statistical variation cannot always account for the deviation in physician behavior. Physicians should strongly consider establishing an outcomes review management system for their emergency departments. One method that has been discussed to establish this is setting up clinical consensus panels as a method to determine a norm for practitioner behavior. Peer review should form a strong central core of any such program. It is hoped, however, that any adversarial approach to peer review will be avoided as much as possible.

CONCLUSION

Ultimately, purchasers of health care, whether corporations or governments, will have to decide which quality measures they will use to influence their financial savings in purchasing health care. For more uniform data, a purchaser can demand financial and quality of care data in summary form provided that there is a single source for the care.

Medicare, Xerox, and General Electric have adopted a slightly different approach. It is their contention that the private model dedicated to a single health care provider represents a fundamental misunderstanding that health care is a right for everyone. Although General Electric feels that health care is a local phenomenon, not fundamentally a uniform commodity, and therefore cannot be organized in a decent manner on a national basis, Medicare is organizing on a national basis to negotiate with local and regional preferred provider organizations. This will enable Medicare to gain regulatory emphasis and further clout in its position. The approach by Xerox (having in-house review at all levels) may be optimal for most purchasers. None of these methods of utilization control, however, has yet addressed the entire spectrum of problems with quality and cost containment.[40]

Berwick[36,38] has characterized the difficulty in applying any normative standards to quality care measurement. So difficult have these measurement standards been to promulgate that some have emphasized that we should change our perspective entirely to an overall strategy balanced toward quality improvement and control. This less competitive approach to quality assurance makes the quality assessment (measurement) a portion within an equation that also includes quality improvement and control (action).[13] Much of the newer emphasis on quality assurance as a total environmental approach to care emphasizes appropriateness. Appropriateness may vary depending on the situation and may have variable levels of what was in the past interpreted as quality.[39,57,59]

Business leaders are interested in developing standards and publishing a national database against which physicians could be measured.[37] Dr. Paul Ellwood has taken this one step further; he states that, beyond appropriateness, there lies "our inability to measure and understand the effect of the choices of patients, payors, and physicians on the patient's aspirations for a better quality of life."[16(p1550)] This statement emphasizes once again that quality in medical care includes not only medical but also nonmedical goals of care.[16]

Most recent outcomes management has been characterized as "a technology of patient experience designed to help patients, payors, and providers make rational medical care related choices based on better insight into the effect of these choices on the patient's life."[16(p1554)] Outcomes management has four components:

1. a greater reliance on standards and guidelines against which physicians can select interventions
2. a routine and systematic series of measurements concerning the functioning and well-being of patients
3. pooling of clinical and outcome data on a massive scale
4. analysis and dissemination of results from the segment of the database most appropriate to the concerns of each decision maker

As a result of the emphasis in these areas, Ellwood feels that there will be a shift within the chaotic health system. He believes that payers are currently making purchasing decisions with inadequate information about the impact of those decisions on patients' quality of life.[4] The acceptability of care, access to care, and quality of physician-patient relationships are not presently part of the standard record from a medical encounter.[29]

Looking at outcomes alone, such as mortality database information of such studies as the Rand study, may skew assessments of how institutions will do.[21–23] There needs to be more information about the patient's evaluation of an encounter, as discussed by Ellwood, to draw more correct conclusions about the actual quality of care rendered.[4]

Therefore, the highly regulatory approach to measurement of quality may be shifting more to management of the perception of quality in the future. Despite the consumer interest in quality, it is possible that medical purchasers are not yet able to answer the basic question of what is quality. The purchaser of medical care has presently entered into an area previously reserved for clinicians and patients. Clinicians must now deal with large purchasers of health care and must respond to their concerns about inappropriate utilization.[5,9,36,58]

Derivation of standards will be at best difficult to understand even with organizations such as the Joint Commission and the National Leadership Commission on Health Care to assist us. The federal government has tried to set up concensus development conferences at the National Institutes of Health to influence physician behavior. The results, after more than a decade, are certainly inconclusive and mixed.[25–27]

The AMA has tried to work with other organizations to establish clinical efficacy and efficiency assessment projects. These have been aimed at cost effectiveness and improving overall outcomes.[14] Whether or not public and private agencies, business coalitions, and academic researchers establish a consensus that can influence the current status and appropriateness of medical care has yet to be seen. In the final analysis, clinicians must remain at the forefront, constantly evaluating a change in severity of a patient's condition, evaluating measurements to establish the level of illness severity, validating any quality research program, and helping purchasers find the best quality of care at a reasonable cost to everyone.[34,60]

REFERENCES

1. Blendon RJ, Altman DE. Public attitudes about health care cost: a lesson in national schizophrenia. *N Engl J Med.* 1984;311:613–616.
2. Barsky AJ. The paradox of health. *N Engl J Med.* 1988;318: 318–319.
3. Louis Harris and Associates. *Making Difficult Health Care Decisions.* Boston: Harvard Community Health Plan; 1987.
4. Office of Technology Assessment. *The Quality of Medical Care: Information for Consumers.* Washington, DC: Government Printing Office; 1988. Office of Technology Assessment publication OTA-H-386:8–9.
5. McClure W. Competition and the pursuit of quality: a conversation with Walter McClure. *Health Aff (Millbank).* 1988;7:79–90.
6. Donabedian A. Evaluating the quality of medical care. *Millbank Mem Fund Q.* 1966;44(suppl):166–206.
7. 42 USC Sec. 11101.
7a. PRO Round 4.0. Office of Prepaid Health Care of HCFA. 10/92: Version 1.0, pp 3–45.

8. Donabedian A. Quality assessment and assurance: unity of purpose, diversity of means. *Inquiry*. 1988;25:173–192.
9. Gausz A, Beeler XX. Quality management for the medical/dental professional. *Qual Update*. 1991;10:36–38.
10. Steffen GE. Quality medical care: a definition. *JAMA*. 1988;260:56–61.
11. Donabedian A. The epidemiology of quality. *Inquiry*. 1985;22:282–292.
12. AMA Council on Medical Service. Quality of care. *Conn Med*. 1986;50:832–834.
13. Wyszewianski L. The emphasis on measurement and quality assurance: reasons and implications. *Inquiry*. 1988;25:424–436.
14. Roberts JS, Radany MH, Nash DB. Privileged practice and demanding new environment. *Ann Intern Med*. 1988;180:880–886.
15. Ginsburg PB, Hammons GT. Competition and the quality of care: the importance of information. *Inquiry*. 1988;25:108–115.
16. Ellwood PM. Shattuck lecture—outcomes management: a technology of patient experience. *N Engl J Med*. 1988;318:1549–1556.
17. Codman EA. A study on hospital efficiency. *Surg Gynecol Obstet*. 1914 (January):4916.
18. Couch, JB. *Early Times in Medical Quality Assessment. 1989 Lectures in Quality Assurance and Utilization Management*. City: American Board of Quality Assurance and Utilization Review, 1989.
19. Lembcke PA. Measuring the quality of medical care through vital statistics based on hospital service areas: 1. Comparative study of appendectomy rates. *Am J Public Health*. 1952;42.
20. Winslow CM, Kosecoff JB, Chassin MR, Kanouse DE, Brook RH. The appropriateness of performing coronary artery bypass surgery. *JAMA*. 1988;260:50–59.
21. Winslow C, Solomon DH, Chassin MR, Kosecoff J, Marrick NJ, Brook RH. The appropriateness of carotid endarterectomy. *N Engl J Med*. 1988;318:721–727.
22. Kahn KL, Kosecoff J, Chassin M, et al. Measuring the clinical appropriateness of a procedure: can we do it. *Med Care*. 1988;26:415–422.
22a. Graboys TB, Biegelsen B, et al. Results of second-opinion trial among patients recommended for coronary angiography. *JAMA*. 1992;268:2537–2541.
23. Knauss W, Nash DB. Predicting and evaluating patient outcomes. *Ann Intern Med*. 1988;109:521–522. Editorial.
24. O'Leary D. *Joint Comm Perspect*. 1990;10:2–3.
25. Heinen L, Gorski JA, Rowe W. Quality of care, research and projects in progress. *Health Aff (Millbank)*. 1988;7:145–150.
26. Perry S. The NIH consensus development program. *N Engl J Med*. 1987;317:48–58.
27. Kosecoff J, Kanouse DE, Rogers WH, McCloskey L, Winslow CM, Brook RH. Effects of the National Institutes of Health consensus development program of physician practice. *JAMA*. 1987;258:2708–2713.
28. 42 USC Sec. 11101 *et. seq.*
29. Meyer H. National health care outcome data base proposed. *AMA News*. 1988;31(22):15.
30. 42 USC Sec. 11133,11135.
31. 42 USC Sec. 11131 (d).
32. *National Practitioner Data Bank Guidebooks*, p.2; 45 CFR 60.7 (d).
33. 42 USC Sec. 11137 (b).
34. Goldfield N, Nash DB. *Providing Quality Care: The Challenge to Clinicians*. Philadelphia: American College of Physicians; 1989.
35. Holden S, Craig XX. Medicare and Medicaid Fraud Abuse in Physician's Survival Guide. Nat'l. Health Lawyers Assn./AMA. 1991: Washington, 115–132.
36. Berwick DM. Monitoring quality in HMOs. *Bus Health*. 1987;5:9–12.
37. Freudenheim M. Costly procedures under scrutiny. *New York Times*. July 26, 1988.
38. Berwick DM. Peer review and quality management: are they compatible? *Qual Rev Bull*. 1990:246–251.
39. McClure W. How should behavioral health care be purchased and sold? Presented at Behavioral Healthcare Tomorrow, sponsored by the Institutes for Behavioral Healthcare; September 6, 1991; Boston, MA.
40. Wyszewianski L. Technical aspects of care and broad approaches to quality assurance. *Inquiry*. 1988;25:424–436.
41. Deming WE. *Out of the Crisis*. Cambridge, MA: MIT Press; 1986.
42. Juran MM, Gryna FM. *Juran's Quality Control Handbook*. 4th ed. New York: McGraw-Hill; 1988.
43. Feigenbaum AV. *Total Quality Control*. New York: McGraw-Hill; 1988.
44. Pelberg AL. Quality assurance in ambulatory care. In: *1989 Lectures in Quality Assurance and Utilization Management*. City: American Board of Quality Assurance and Utilization Review; 1989:201–220.
45. Benson DS. System measures ambulatory care quality. *Physician Executive*. 1990;16:15–20.
46. Act of Nov. 5 1990, Pub. L. No. 101–508, *1990 U.S. Code Cong. & Admin. News* (104 Stat.) 1388(286).
47. Krebs-Markrich J. The Medicare PRO: de facto repeal of the prohibition against federal interference. *Physician's Survival Guide*. Washington, DC: National Health Lawyers Association/AMA; 1991: 143–169.
48. 42 C.F.R. 466.98, 54 Fed. Reg. 1956 (January 18, 1991).
49. 42 U.S.C. 1320a-7(h).
50. Cain CP. PRO quality interventional plans—HCFA mandates. In: *1989 Lectures in Quality Assurance and Utilization Management*. City: American Board of Quality Assurance and Utilization Review; 1989:103–112.
51. 31 U.S.C. 3729.
52. Conference of National Health Lawyers with AMA in Phoenix, AZ, 1990.
53. *Schloendorff v. Society of New York Hospitals*, 105 N.E. 92 (N.Y. 1914).
54. *Bing v. Theunig*. 143 N.E. 2d 3 (N.Y. 1957).
55. *Health Care Spec Law Dig*. 1987;8:xx–xx.
56. *J Health Hosp Law*. 1989;22:91–93.
57. Slater CH. An analysis of ambulatory care quality assessment research. *Eval Health Prof*. 1989;12:347–378.
58. Luft HS. HMOs and the quality of care. *Inquiry*. 1988;25:147–156.
59. Udvarhelyi S, Colditz GA, Rai A, Epstein AM. Cost-effectiveness and cost-benefit analyses in the medical literature: Are the methods being used correctly? *Ann Intern Med*. 1992;16(3):238–244.
60. Vdvarhelyi IS, Gatsonis AM, et al. Acute myocardial infarction in the Medicare population: Process of care and clinical outcomes. *JAMA*. 1992;268:2530–2537.

6. Shock

MARK ALLEN SHAFFER, MD, FACEP
JACEK B. FRANASZEK, MD, FACEP

"A rude unhinging of the machinery of life" and "a momentary pause in the act of death" are among the earliest definitions of shock, yet these statements seem to encompass the essence and grim connotation that the shock state implies. Crile and Lower, Henderson, Cannon, and Blalock were just some of the early researchers who laid the groundwork for understanding and treating this enigmatic pathophysiologic entity. Today, despite the decades of efforts by physicians to arrive at accurate definitions that could simplify the recognition and management of the various shock states, considerable controversy remains concerning all aspects of shock states.

Shock, in a broad sense, is a syndrome, a myriad complex of symptoms with varying hemodynamic characteristics. Changes in the many systems designed to supply oxygen and nutrients to the cellular structures allow not only clinical but also microbiological definition.

Damage at any level of these systems leads to a series of events that, if left uncorrected, ultimately affect the transport of oxygen and nutrients to the cells. It is incumbent on the paramedic in the field and the emergency physician and nurse to recognize the early signs and symptoms associated with all shock states, since the crippling long-term damage to vital organs increases as time elapses.

If therapy is not instituted promptly to reverse hypoperfusion and hypoxia, the intracellular structures are forced to utilize other metabolic pathways to survive. This decreases their energy production and efficiency.

The persistence of cellular anoxia and starvation disrupts intracellular organelles, interfering with normal molecular and enzymatic processes. If left uncorrected, shock results in progressive deterioration that ultimately reaches the point of irreversibility and cellular death.

In the initial stages of shock, the changes observed are attempts by the body to compensate for and correct the deficiencies brought about by the insult to the system. If the early pattern of insufficient oxygen delivery or utilization at the cellular level persists, an energy crisis develops, and the metabolism is activated in such a way as to generate end products that may aggravate the initial injurious event. Thus, vital structures (eg, brain, heart, kidneys) undergo changes that secondarily affect the cardiocirculatory system, creating a vicious cycle.

Most of the physiologic derangements that accompany shock result from poor tissue perfusion, which causes inadequate transport of oxygen and nutrients at the cellular level. Four functionally dependent entities interact to maintain normal cardiocirculatory function, cellular oxygenation, and nutrition:

1. heart, the "pump" that generates the power necessary to maintain circulation.
2. conductance (ie, the resistance and capacitance systems). These are composed of (a) arteries and arterioles, the primary functions of which are to conduct blood to the capillary bed and to regulate blood pressure by changes in their caliber; and (b) the venous capacitance bed, which consists of veins and venules that act as a reservoir for blood and regulate circulating

---

The authors wish to thank Anita Shaffer for her invaluable help in the preparation of this manuscript.

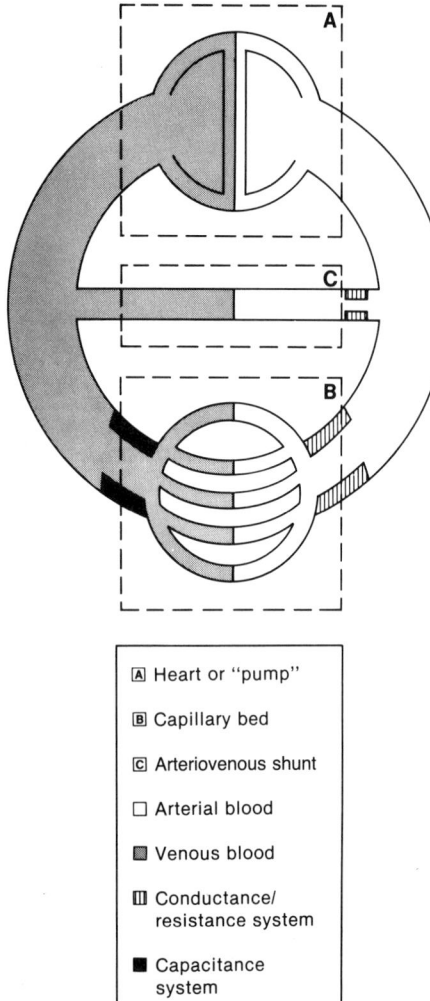

Figure 6-1 Model of normal circulatory system.

Legend:
- A Heart or "pump"
- B Capillary bed
- C Arteriovenous shunt
- ☐ Arterial blood
- ■ Venous blood
- ▥ Conductance/resistance system
- ■ Capacitance system

blood volume by contracting or dilating, directly affecting the capacitance system by means of the precapillaries that bypass the capillary bed.
3. capillary bed, where there is active exchange of oxygen and nutrients. The flow is regulated by precapillary and postcapillary sphincter muscles.
4. blood, which is the "priming" solution of the pump and carrier of oxygen and nutrients.

These four components may be used to construct a diagrammatic representation of the circulatory system (Fig. 6-1).

A number of myocardial factors affect pump function and cardiac output, which is the amount of blood ejected by the heart per unit of time (see Chapter 62, Acute Myocardial Infarction). The cardiac output is the product of stroke volume times the heart rate:

$$\text{Cardiac output} = \text{Stroke volume} \times \text{Heart rate}$$

Stroke volume is the amount of blood ejected by the left ventricle with each contraction; it is determined by the venous return, the myocardial contractility, the length of the myocardial muscle fibers at the beginning of contraction, and the peripheral vascular resistance. Ventricular performance and the stroke volume are thus directly influenced not only by the venous return, increasing with increasing venous return, but also by peripheral vascular resistance, decreasing with increasing resistance. Inadequate stroke volume may result in a narrowed pulse pressure (ie, difference between systolic and diastolic blood pressure), while a large stroke volume is suggested by a widened pulse pressure.

BLOOD PRESSURE

Normal values for systemic blood pressure are variable. One individual may normally have a blood pressure of 90/60 mmHg, yet this blood pressure may be inadequate in another individual who is suffering from acute volume loss. Alternately, a blood pressure of 120/80 mmHg, which is considered well within normal values, may fail to support circulation in an individual who is usually hypertensive.

The size of the blood pressure cuff must be appropriate for the individual in order to ensure valid measurements. Automatic blood pressure monitoring devices facilitate serial blood pressure measurements and are reasonably reliable. Intra-arterial blood pressure recordings are more accurate than are cuff measurements in shock states, however. The placement and maintenance of arterial lines are straightforward, but such lines are underutilized in the emergency setting.

In order to interpret blood pressure measurements correctly, it is very important to obtain an adequate history and to correlate it with clinical findings. Low blood pressure is not considered indicative of shock unless it is accompanied by findings of decreased tissue perfusion. In fact, the interrelationship of all the hemodynamic factors should be considered in the diagnosis of shock (Fig. 6-2):

1. Preload refers to the length of myocardial fiber before contraction. With an increase of the ventricular size at the end of diastole, subsequent myocardial fiber shortening is greater and thus the extent of contraction is greater; this is called Starling's law. Preload is influenced by blood volume, venous tone, intrathoracic pressures, and intrapericardial pressures.
2. Contractility is the force of contraction of myocardial fibers, which is determined by force-generating processes at the contractile sites. The concentration of ionic calcium available to the heart's contractile proteins is one of the factors that determine the extent of myocardial fiber shortening and the velocity of myocardial contraction. Norepinephrine, as well as a

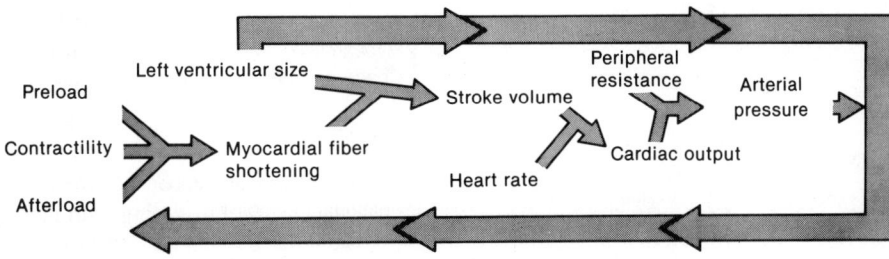

Figure 6-2 Interrelationship of factors supporting hemodynamics.

number of other endogenous and exogenous agents (e.g., digoxin, isoproterenol, and calcium), exert a "positive" inotropic (force or strength of contraction) effect; they increase contractile effectiveness.

3. Afterload is defined as the wall tension that the left ventricle must generate in order to contract and to eject a given blood volume. Chamber size, shape, and wall thickness all contribute to ventricular wall tension. Increases in afterload result in decreases in stroke volume and cardiac output. Peripheral vasoconstriction, which raises arterial pressure and consequently afterload, depresses the extent of myocardial fiber shortening, thus depressing stroke volume. In a "failing" heart, the left ventricular end diastolic volume is increased, and the wall tension required to produce a contraction is greater than normal.

4. Heart rate is a function of the rhythmicity of the pacemaker cells of the heart (see Chapter 63, Disturbances in Cardiac Rhythm). This intrinsic rhythmicity is increased by hyperthermia and hyperthyroidism, and decreased by hypothermia and hypothyroidism. Heart rate and rhythm may be adversely altered by ischemia of the pacemaker cells or surrounding tissues. Rate is also influenced by the extrinsic neural regulation mechanisms, such as β-adrenergic stimulation (increasing heart rate) or parasympathetic stimulation (decreasing heart rate). Extrinsic humoral influences are mediated by circulating catecholamines (Fig. 6-3) and other substances.

Blood pressure is determined by the cardiac output and the peripheral vascular resistance. It is maintained relatively constant by an inverse relationship between the two modalities. Any increase or decrease in peripheral resistance is accompanied by a decrease or increase, respectively, in cardiac output:

Blood pressure = Cardiac output × Peripheral resistance

An excessive increase in afterload, shunting of blood through arteriovenous communications, pooling of blood in the capillary system because of postcapillary sphincter resistance, loss of blood volume, puncture or damage to the

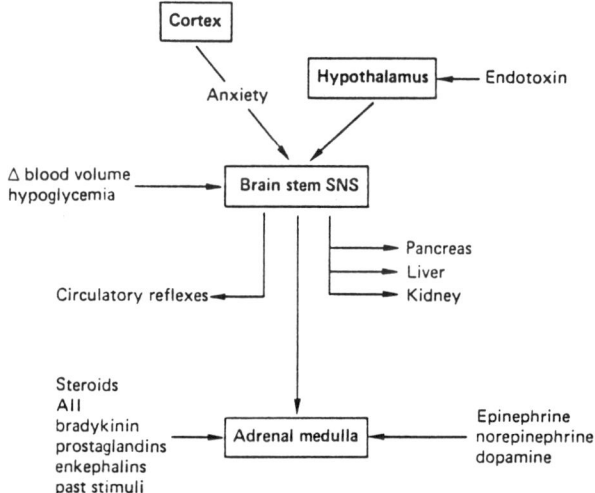

Figure 6-3 Efferent limb leading to catecholamine secretion. *SNS*, sympathetic nervous system; *AII*, angiotensin II. Reprinted with permission from Gann DS, Lilly MP: The endocrine response to injury, in Wilder RJ, McCaffree DR (eds): *Progress in Critical Care Medicine*. Basel, Switzerland, S Karger AG, 1984, vol 1, p 28.

myocardial muscle, or obstruction of the main flow of blood volume accounts for the majority of events that produce acute perfusion failure and clinical signs of shock. In Fig. 6-4, shock states are classified according to the events that precipitate them. This categorization elaborates the abnormal mechanisms that trigger the ultimate damage pattern, disruption of cellular metabolism.

HYPOVOLEMIC SHOCK

Pathophysiology and Compensatory and Decompensatory Mechanisms

Shock caused by a decrease in the intravascular volume relative to the vascular capacity is termed hypovolemic shock (Fig. 6-5). It is generally associated with a circulating blood volume deficit of at least 15% to 25% and is often accompanied by recruitment of large amounts of extra-

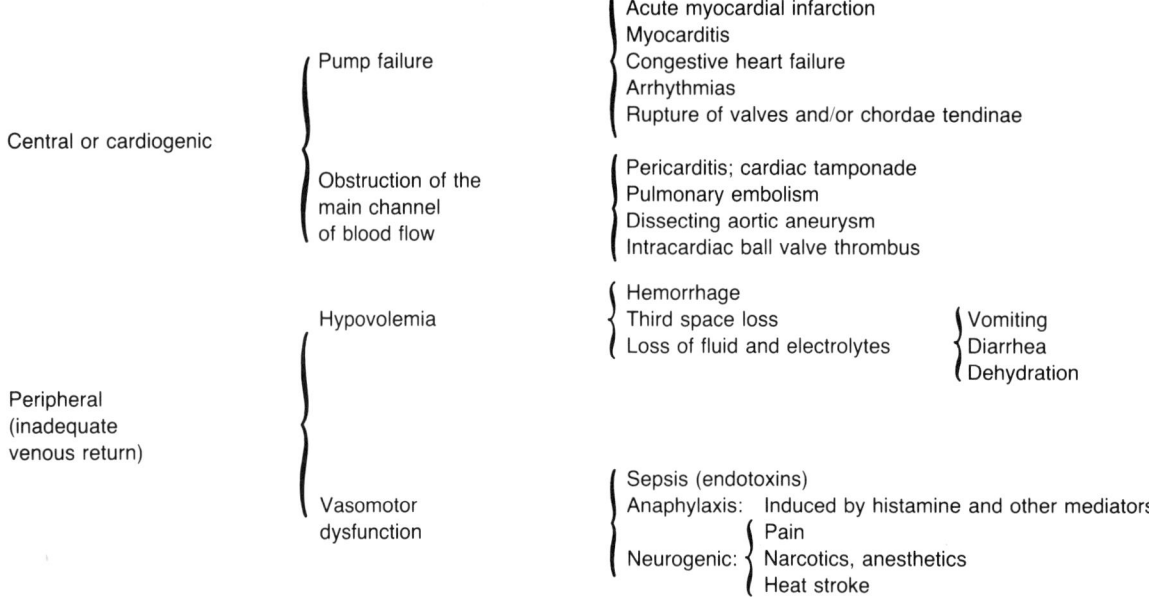

Figure 6-4 Etiologic classification of shock states.

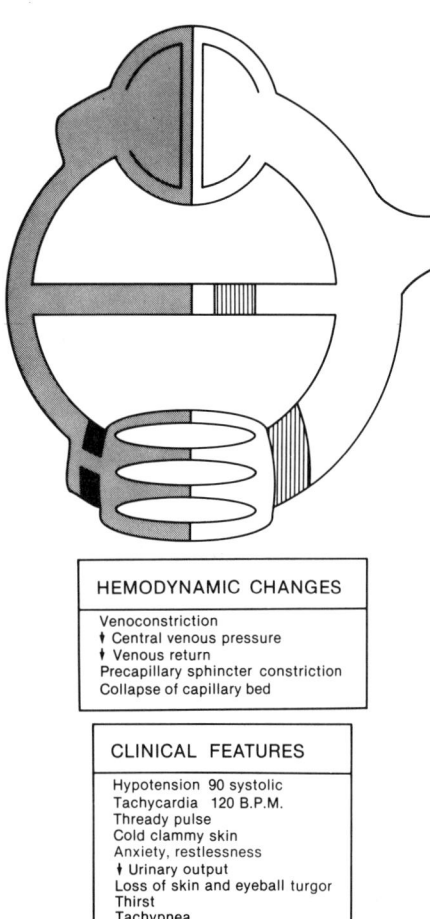

Figure 6-5 Circulatory system in hypovolemic shock (see Fig. 6-1.)

vascular extracellular fluid. The clinical presentation may be characterized by altered mental status, ranging from restlessness and confusion to obtundation and coma; weakness, diaphoresis, tachycardia, hypotension, and tachypnea all reflect poor perfusion at the tissue level. Some of the manifestations may reflect a vigorous catecholamine response to the events that resulted in shock.

The initial response of the body to hypovolemia depends largely on the amount of intravascular volume lost. The rate at which it has been lost, the degree of associated injury, the patient's age, underlying systemic illnesses, and the ability of the cardiovascular system to adjust to the loss determine the clinical presentation (Fig. 6-6). Compensatory mechanisms are initiated in several organ systems in an attempt to maintain adequate perfusion to the peripheral tissues. The interplay of neurohormonal adjustments that occur in shock states is complex (Fig. 6-7); the magnitude of adjustment is variable and temporally dependent.

Contraction of the capacitance system is the initial compensatory response. Intrinsic at first, it is mediated by the release of catecholamines as hypovolemia progresses. This mechanism maintains adequate venous return until 10% to 15% of the volume is lost; metabolic and endocrine responses are minimal with this degree of volume loss. The physical signs and symptoms are transient and nonspecific at this stage. Narrowing of the pulse pressure, reflecting a decrease in stroke volume, is one of the earliest findings in these patients.

As hypovolemia progresses, hypotension and low stroke volume may stimulate baroreceptors and evoke an increase in circulating catecholamines via the vasomotor center's sympathetic discharge. Epinephrine and norepinephrine are

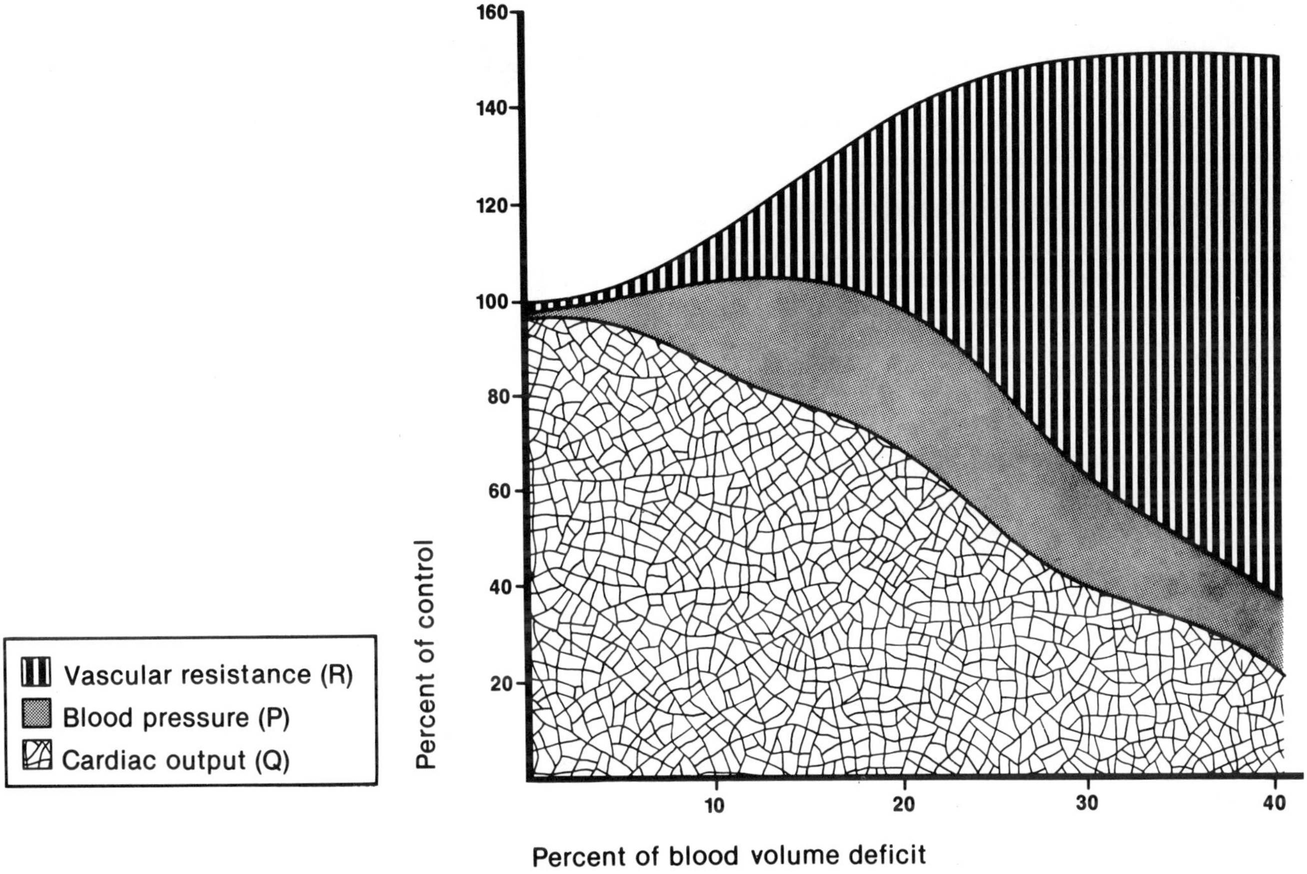

Shock   69

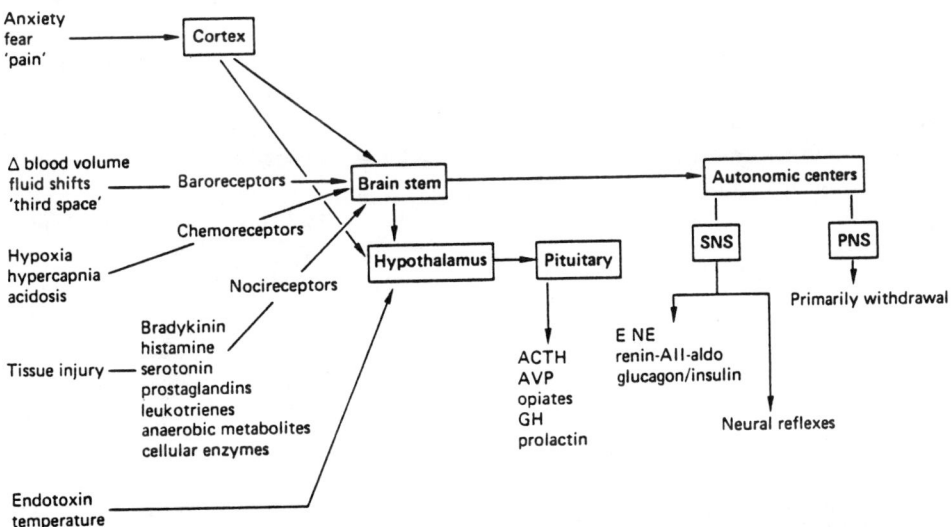

Figure 6-6 Changes in vascular resistance, blood pressure, and cardiac output with increasing blood volume deficits ($P = QR$). *Note:* Because of increasing vascular resistance, the blood pressure is usually maintained until the cardiac output falls approximately 25 to 33 percent.

Figure 6-7 A simplified overview of the reflex response to injury. *SNS*, sympathetic nervous system; *PNS*, parasympathetic nervous system; *ACTH*, adrenocorticotropic hormone; *AVP*, arginine vasopressin; *GH*, growth hormone; *E*, epinephrine; *NE*, norepinephrine; *AII*, angiotensin II; *aldo*, aldosterone. *Source:* Reprinted with permission from Gann DS, Lilly MP: The endocrine response to injury, in Wilder RJ, McCaffree DR (eds): *Progress in Critical Care Medicine.* Basel, Switzerland, S Karger AG, 1984, vol 1, p 17.

Table 6-1 Changes Seen in Acute Hemorrhage

Degree of Volume Loss	Vascular Response	Endocrine Response	Signs and Symptomatology
Mild (0% to 20%)	Contraction of capacitance system	Minimal	Narrowing of pulse pressure Tachycardia Restlessness
	Recruitment of extravascular fluid		Diaphoresis
			Hypotension (90 to 100 mmHg)
Moderate (20% to 30%)	Arteriolar constriction Narrowed pulse pressure Reduced cardiac output	Aldosterone Antidiuretic hormone Catecholamines	Diaphoresis Anxiety Decreased urine output Hypotension (approximately 60 mmHg) Cool, clammy skin Obtundation
Severe (>30%)	Hypotension Drastic reduction of cardiac output	Marked liberation of catecholamines	Dyspnea Coma Death

released, and they act to increase the force and rate of myocardial contraction and to produce vasoconstriction at "nonvital" (eg, renal and mesenteric) structures in an attempt to maintain perfusion pressure to the heart and brain. Concomitantly, the signs and symptoms of adrenergic discharge are seen (ie, tachycardia, restlessness, dry mouth, cool skin, diaphoresis, pallor, and mydriasis, known as the fight or flight response). Orthostatic hypotension, a fall in blood pressure and an increase in heart rate when the patient rises from the supine to the seated position, is a manifestation of hypovolemia. A pulse increase of greater than 30 beats/minute or symptoms of dizziness or syncope upon sitting are significant changes in the orthostatic vital signs of previously healthy patients; lesser changes may be considered significant in patients who have preexisting illnesses. Adrenergic responses are capable of compensating acute volume losses of up to 30%. With a severe volume loss of 45% or more, several vascular, endocrine, and metabolic responses occur in an attempt to correct the underlying pathophysiologic processes. Eventually, however, these responses may change from compensatory to decompensatory, causing a progressive deterioration in metabolic state that, if left uncorrected, leads to death (Table 6-1).

Extracellular Fluid Recruitment

While adrenergic responses are occurring after a moderate volume loss, extracellular fluid is redistributed into the intravascular compartment. Human studies have suggested that, after a loss of 10% to 20% of intravascular volume, plasma is transferred from the extracellular to the intravascular space at a rate of 50 to 90 mL/min during the first 2 hours and averages 40 to 60 mL/hour for 6 to 10 hours. It has been shown that plasma refill rates are considerably brisker in patients with profound volume depletion than in those with mild or moderate volume depletion.

The hematocrit, normally 42% to 52% for a man and 37% to 47% for a woman, is a simple means of estimating red blood cell mass in relation to plasma volume. It may be used in instances of volume loss as a dynamic parameter that aids in determining plasma refill rates. In a healthy 70-kg man, for example, the total blood volume is approximately 5000 mL. Assuming his normal hematocrit is 45%, his red blood cell mass is 2250 mL (45% of 5000 mL) and his plasma volume is 2750 mL. In the first few minutes after an initial depletion of red blood cells, as occurs in acute hemorrhage, these parameters remain constant; with plasma refill, however, the red blood cell mass is diluted, and hematocrit values drop. Plasma refill rates of nearly 1000 mL/hour can follow severe acute blood loss. Thus, the body may compensate by increasing plasma volume. Fluid resuscitation with colloid or crystalloid continues to dilute red blood cell mass. At levels below 30% to 32% of the usual red blood cell mass, the blood's oxygen-carrying capacity is reduced, and hypoxemia may become manifest.

Cellular Metabolism

If the cell is to utilize energy and maintain its structural and functional integrity, it must be supplied with oxygen and nutrients. Most cellular activities are normally accomplished through metabolic pathways that require oxygen (aerobic metabolism). When the cell is forced to produce energy by means of anaerobic metabolic pathways (eg, as a consequence of poor perfusion and hypoxia), it also produces increased amounts of lactic acid, amino acids, fatty acids, and phosphoric acids, resulting in metabolic acidosis.

Acidosis has several deleterious effects. It damages intracellular organelles that contain lytic enzymes, releasing the enzymes and causing death of the cell. Also, when energy production is inadequate, the cell membrane pump does not function, resulting in cellular and mitochondrial edema.

Furthermore, protein synthesis is hampered. In sum, all essential elements of the cell are injured.

Acidosis reduces myocardial contractility, depresses vascular response to catecholamines, and promotes intravascular coagulation. Acidemia promotes hypercoagulability, an effect that may be beneficial, for it tends to inhibit hemorrhage. Blood may stagnate in the face of acidosis, because postcapillary sphincters constrict and precapillary sphincters relax. This facilitates platelet aggregation, which may occlude small vessels, and intravascular coagulation. All these factors can precipitate disseminated intravascular coagulation. The development of microthrombi at the capillary level may contribute greatly to irreversible shock by inhibiting circulation to vital structures.

The serum and tissue lactate levels, which are increased with anaerobic metabolism, may be useful as guidelines in determining whether cellular perfusion is adequate during resuscitation and, to some extent, as prognostic indicators; outcome is likely to be poor when high lactate levels persist. Furthermore, acidosis facilitates release of oxygen and uptake of carbon dioxide at the cellular level (owing to a shift of the oxygen hemoglobin dissociation curve to the right), as well as increases in the respiratory rate and cerebral blood flow. Persistent hypoperfusion of other tissues results in their decompensation.

Myocardial ischemia resulting from hypovolemia may lead to a progressive decrease in coronary blood flow, or it may impair myocardial performance. Adequate cardiac function can be maintained as long as venous return is sufficient; however, in fact, cardiac deterioration has been shown to occur only in very late stages of hypovolemia.

After prolonged ischemia to the kidneys, renal "shutdown" can occur and may become a permanent, devastating complication for long-term survivors (see Chapter 78, Renal Failure). Stress ulceration of the gastric mucosa may occur. The reticuloendothelial system and the intestinal mucosa may be damaged during hypoperfusion of the hepatosplanchnic circulation, destroying barriers against bacterial invasion of the bloodstream. Consequently, sepsis may occur, and close monitoring of the patient for evidence of infection is essential.

Adult respiratory distress syndrome may develop from a variety of causes, including hypovolemia, hypotension-related damage to pulmonary vasculature, and changes in colloid oncotic pressure; it has become a major determinant of the prognosis of patients who survive the initial stages of shock. Appropriate fluid management in the emergency department phase of care to restore volume without inducing fluid overload has a significant bearing on outcome.

Vasoactive Substances

The destruction of intracellular elements that follows prolonged hypotension and hypoperfusion liberates substances that have varied effects on the tone and integrity of the vasculature. Lysosomal enzymes and vasoactive substances are responsible for many of the decompensatory mechanisms found in late shock. Histamine, for example, is a vasodilator that not only affects arteriolar resistance, but also increases capillary permeability; thus, it worsens hypovolemia, especially in the face of persistent venous sphincter tone that allows fluid to be sequestered in the capillary system and exuded into the interstitium. Serotonin, which is abundant in brain cells, intestinal cells, platelets, and mast cells, is felt to have an important role in coagulation and platelet aggregation following trauma. Lysosomal enzymes liberated from damaged cells are capable of converting active kinogens into kinins, which are plasma polypeptides with a potent vasoactive property. Bradykinin, for example, is a potent vasodilator. Another vasoactive polypeptide, myocardial depressant factor, may be produced by an ischemic pancreas; it affects splanchnic vasoconstriction and depresses myocardial contractility.

Hypoxia

In addition to the conditions that arise in the periphery because of hypoperfusion, acid, lysosomal enzymes, and vasoactive substances, hypoxia affects the circulatory system. Tissue hypoxia induces vasodilation at a local level, preferentially in organs that require greater concentrations of oxygen; it stimulates chemoreceptor activity, which induces hyperventilation; it acts on the vasomotor center, which produces peripheral vasoconstriction in an attempt to restore cerebral perfusion; and it also prevents appropriate autonomic circulatory adjustments.

Acid-Base Changes

One of the initial nonspecific responses to trauma, hypotension, or sepsis is alveolar hyperventilation. In the early stages of hypoperfusion, the arterial blood gas and pH measurements are expected to indicate pure respiratory alkalemia. The hypocapnia can further impair hemodynamics by inducing peripheral vasodilation. If hypoperfusion progresses to shock and cellular metabolism is altered, a metabolic acidosis ensues, first within the cell and then in the intravascular blood compartment as hydrogen ions move out of the cell. By the time metabolic acidemia appears, the state of hypoperfusion is very advanced. Care must be taken in the treatment of metabolic acidemia, because excessive intravenous administration of sodium bicarbonate, nasogastric suctioning of gastric acid, excessive diuresis with loss of potassium, and excessive administration of steroids can produce metabolic alkalemia.

In severe shock, a respiratory acidosis due to impairment of gas exchange at the alveolocapillary level, combined with a metabolic acidosis due to acid accumulation resulting from abnormal metabolic processes, is a poor prognostic indicator. The morbidity and mortality are increased even when bicarbonate therapy is instituted (see Chapter 21, Acid-Base Disturbances).

SEPTIC SHOCK

Septic shock is defined as a condition of deranged cellular metabolism and impaired tissue perfusion as a consequence of host invasion by a variety of infectious agents, including bacteria (Gram positive and Gram negative), viruses, fungi, rickettsiae, and toxins produced by microorganisms.

It has been estimated that 70,000 to 300,000 cases of Gram-negative bacteremia occur in the United States annually. Shock, with its attendant spectrum of manifestations, occurs in about 40% of patients with bacteremia; the preponderance of cases is due to Gram-negative organisms. Mixed infections account for 10% to 20% of shock states. Shock develops more commonly in persons older than 60 years of age. Other identified risk factors include immunocompromise, hospitalization, instrumentation, indwelling catheters, drug abuse, and alcoholism.

Gram-negative organisms responsible often have a urinary tract or, less commonly, gastrointestinal tract origin. *Escherichia coli*, followed by *Klebsiella, Enterobacter,* and much less commonly, *Pseudomonas* and *Serratia* species, heads a long list of suspects. *Staphylococcus* and *Streptococcus* organisms top the list of causative Gram-positive species, many from the respiratory tract. Despite modern therapy, mortality remains between 10% and 65%.

An understanding of the range of clinical manifestations is dependent on a knowledge of underlying pathophysiologic events (Fig. 6-8). As bacteria enter the bloodstream, endotoxins (from the cell wall membrane) and exotoxins (intracellular components of some bacteria) are released, activating the coagulation, complement, fibrinolytic, and kinin systems. Although these systems are defensive for the host, their overactivation leads to undesirable consequences, such as disseminated intravascular coagulation and release of a variety of vasoactive substances including bradykinin, histamine, thromboxane, endorphins, and prostacyclin. These initially cause vasodilation and then vasoconstriction and capillary leakage as well as myocardial depression.

Hence, in the early stages of shock (Fig. 6-9), the patient presents in a hyperdynamic state, or so-called arm shock, which is characterized by increased cardiac output, low peripheral vascular resistance, and normal auscultatory blood pressure. This stage, commonly viewed in the emergency department setting, lasts for a matter of hours. There follows the hypodynamic or cold shock state, characterized by decreased cardiac output, hypotension, and lactic acidosis. Thus precise clinical observations are a function of the stage of progression of the disease.

Although fever is usually present, it may be absent, especially in elderly or debilitated patients. Warm, moist skin gives way to cool, clammy skin. Elevated respiratory rate and respiratory alkalosis are seen early in the course;

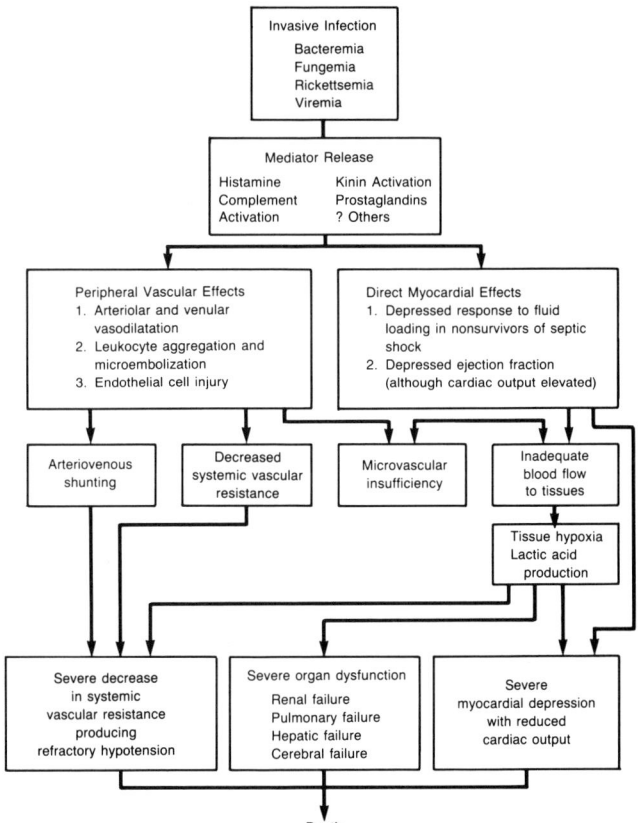

Figure 6-8 Effect of infection on cardiovascular function. Reprinted with permission from Parker MM, Parillo JE: Septic shock: Hemodynamics and pathogenesis. *JAMA* 250(4):3325, December 1983.

alternatively, if the source of infection is pulmonary cough, chest pain, sputum production, and rales may predominate. Nausea and vomiting may be present. Abdominal pain and dysuria will suggest gastrointestinal or genitourinary sources of infection. Altered mental status, from simple lethargy to frank confusion, is a subtle sign of sepsis in the elderly. Chills and prostration are ubiquitous. Advanced hematologic derangements may lead to skin manifestations of thrombocytopenia or overt gastrointestinal bleeding. Adult respiratory distress syndrome, renal failure on the basis of acute tubular necrosis, DIC, and congestive failure are all possible lethal complications.

CARDIOGENIC SHOCK

The simplest definition of cardiogenic shock is a low arterial blood pressure (less than 90 mm Hg systolic) in the setting of acute myocardial infarction (Fig. 6-10). The most common cause of cardiogenic shock after acute myocardial infarction is "pump failure." The hemodynamic abnormalities of pump failure secondary to myocardial infarction are due to paradoxical movement of the infarcted segment of

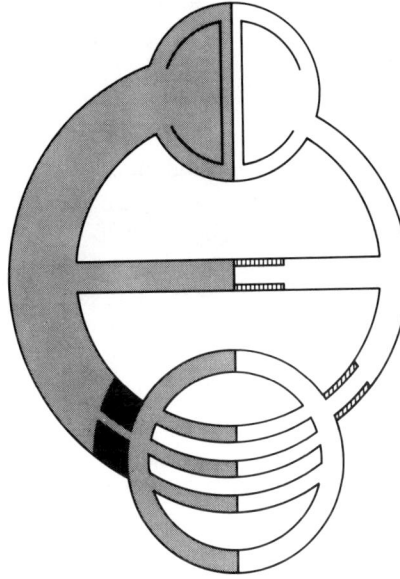

Figure 6-9 Circulatory system in septic shock (see Fig. 6-1).

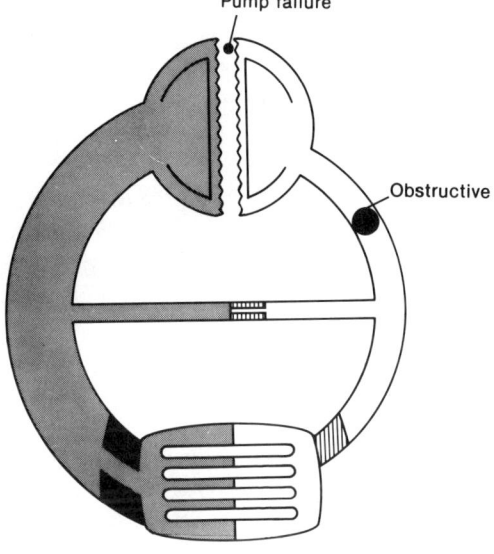

Figure 6-10 Circulatory system in cardiogenic shock (see Fig. 6-1).

myocardium, which leads to a reduction in stroke volume and consequently a fall in cardiac output and elevation of left ventricular pressure. When the reductions in stroke volume and cardiac output are large enough, arterial blood pressure declines, as does coronary blood flow (see Chapters 62, Acute Myocardial Infarction, and 63, Disturbances in Cardiac Rhythm). Cardiogenic shock is an advanced form of pump failure in which low cardiac output causes a functional deficit of tissue perfusion in one or more vital organs.

Because a history of prior myocardial infarction, age of 65 years or greater, and the physical findings of hypertension and congestive heart failure are associated with a poor prognosis, the emergency physician must evaluate all these factors when assessing a patient in cardiogenic shock. The following are the classic features of cardiogenic shock:

1. auscultatory systolic blood pressure less than 90 mm Hg
2. cool, moist skin
3. urine output less than 20 mL/hour
4. impaired state of consciousness
5. lactic acidemia
6. tachypnea

These findings are common to many different varieties of shock with widely varying therapeutic requirements; therefore, it is incumbent on the emergency physician to consider and eliminate noncardiac causes. Of primary importance in this regard is the correction of hypovolemia. Anaphylactic, septic, and neurogenic causes of shock should be revealed by history and physical examination.

Many patients survive an acute myocardial infarction long enough to arrive at a hospital and then develop cardiogenic shock. This ongoing process, or period of deterioration, is termed the preshock syndrome. Pathologic studies have demonstrated damaged cells at the fringes of a zone of infarction, and these damaged cells may or may not survive. Hence, therapeutic interventions should be directed at limiting infarct size. The extent of pump failure is directly proportional to the mass of myocardium disabled by ischemic injury; in cardiogenic shock, more than 40% of the left ventricular myocardium is disabled. Most studies cite the incidence of cardiogenic shock among patients with acute myocardial infarction as 15%. Recently reported lower incidences may reflect a more aggressive approach in the treatment of patients with unstable angina, extending infarcts, and the preshock syndrome, including detection and treatment of congestive heart failure, dysrhythmias, fluid deficits, and metabolic abnormalities. Some therapy of the preshock syndrome may be accomplished in the prehospital care setting. Despite advances in therapy, the mortality rate has remained at 85% to 95%, once the shock syndrome has developed.

Hemodynamic subsets can be used to identify patients with a poor prognosis after myocardial infarction. With normal hemodynamics, the mortality rate is relatively low; however, it reaches 51% to 60% in the presence of pulmonary congestion and clinical evidence of hypoperfusion. Patients with cardiogenic shock associated with gross pulmonary congestion and hypoperfusion have a mortality rate approaching 95%. Survival rates improve with early, aggressive use of intra-aortic balloon counterpulsation, but outcome is still directly linked to left ventricular function. Emergency revascularization surgery and surgery to correct specific mechanical structural abnormalities, such as a post–myocardial infarction ventricular septal defect or mitral regurgitation, are used with varying degrees of success. The intra-aortic balloon pump is useful in stabilizing patients for surgery but is not without complications; for example, arterial occlusion subsequent to this procedure may result in ischemia in an extremity or bowel, local infection, or aortic dissection.

Although acute myocardial infarction is the most common cause of cardiogenic shock, the syndrome may be precipitated by cardiac tamponade, pulmonary embolism, or acute cardiomyopathy. Other less common causes are ventricular septal defects, papillary muscle rupture, myocarditis, cardiomyopathy, valvular disease, myocardial contusion, dysrhythmia, and hypothermia or hyperthermia, all of which produce similar hemodynamic results.

Cardiac Factors

Sympathetic activity is usually enhanced and parasympathetic activity diminished in response to lowered arterial blood pressure. This results in an increased heart rate in an attempt to compensate for reductions in stroke volume and maintain cardiac output. The increase in heart rate may increase the myocardial oxygen demand so that it is out of proportion to supply and exacerbates the ischemia, however.

The endogenous sympathetic discharge may fail to produce adequate changes in myocardial performance because the ischemic myocardium may not respond properly to this stimulus. Lactic acidosis, a consequence of anaerobic metabolism, further impairs contractility. Moreover, cardiac performance may also be compromised by "myocardial depressant factor," a humoral substance that accumulates in the blood in the presence of hypoperfusion.

An important determinant of stroke volume and, therefore, of cardiac output is preload. When volume is depleted, the fiber length decreases, reducing the force and extent of ventricular contraction and thus decreasing stroke volume. In order to increase stroke volume, the heart must be given sufficient volume to increase diastolic fiber length to optimal levels (Starling's law). As diastolic fiber length increases, however, the pressure in the left ventricle increases also. In cardiogenic shock, the left ventricular filling pressure is markedly elevated, and an elevated left ventricular diastolic pressure may inhibit subendocardial perfusion and worsen ischemia, resulting in an even more depressed left ventricular performance.

Another determinant of myocardial oxygen demand is left ventricular wall tension, which is influenced by outflow resistance (impedance), chamber shape, and wall thickness. Increases in left ventricular wall tension during ejection, termed afterload, reduce stroke volume, while decreases in this tension generally increase stroke volume. These observations provide a rationale for vasodilators in therapy for cardiogenic shock with high filling pressures. Increases in left ventricular filling pressure induce elevated pulmonary interstitial pressures; when pulmonary wedge pressure exceeds 25 mm Hg, pulmonary edema develops (see Chapter 69, Dyspnea and Pulmonary Edema).

Peripheral Vascular Factors

When cardiac output falls, arterial pressure falls; systemic vascular resistance reflex increases. While the arterial blood pressure may rise as a consequence, cardiac output may fall as a result of increased afterload. All too often, in cardiogenic shock, blood pressure is raised at the expense of worsening ischemia or regional underperfusion of some vascular beds.

Clinical Findings

Although the clinical picture may vary depending on the etiologic event, in general patients in cardiogenic shock will be tachypneic as a result of hypoxia and acidosis as well as tachycardic as a result of the increased release of catecholamines. If bradycardia is present, inferior wall myocardial infarction should be suspected as a result of stimulation of the vagal nerve.

The blood pressure measurements may be misleading initially because patients may have been chronically hypertensive and present with a normal blood pressure. In time, however, most patients with cardiogenic shock will become truly hypotensive with systolic blood pressures of 70 mmHg and below. Other clinical signs are related to the diversion of blood from the periphery to the central core and include cool skin, cyanosis, pallor, and mydriasis. Frequent presenting signs and symptoms include jugular venous distention, chest pain, shortness of breath, neck pain, cardiovascular findings of failure, murmurs, systolic clicks, and the like. Other more vague findings include generalized weakness, mental status changes ranging from anxiety to coma, focal neurologic signs, and so forth.

ANAPHYLACTIC SHOCK

The hypersensitivity reaction that develops when a previously sensitized individual is exposed to a specific antigen may progress to systemic symptoms and signs; this is termed anaphylaxis. In its more serious form, anaphylaxis may progress to anaphylactic shock. Atopic individuals and persons with asthma are particularly predisposed. Parenteral exposures, particularly via administered drugs, as well as insect stings, foods, and contrast media are commonly responsible for anaphylaxis. Other precipitants include local anesthetics, sulfites, and a variety of other substances (Table 6-2). Anaphylactoid reactions, which mimic anaphylaxis, have similar causes but are not immunologically mediated.

Although 15 to 40 of every 100,000 patients treated with penicillin will experience anaphylaxis, less than 2% of persons given contrast media have such a reaction. Approximately 300 fatalities from penicillin anaphylaxis occur annually as opposed to 60 to 80 deaths from Hymenoptera (bees, wasps, and hornets) stings.

The fundamental pathophysiologic phenomena involve the release of pharmacologic mediators in response to antigenic exposure. These are histamine (a slow-reacting substance of anaphylaxis), bradykinin, and others. The mediators produce airway constriction, peripheral vasodilation, and increased capillary permeability.

Symptoms and signs of anaphylaxis include anxiety, nausea, abdominal cramps, diarrhea, vomiting, rhinorrhea, sneezing, chemosis, angioedema, and, most obviously, urticaria, either singly or in combination. More severe forms of anaphylaxis include laryngeal edema, manifested by stridor; bronchoconstriction, manifested by wheezing if advanced or just cough and dyspnea if less advanced; and hypotension, manifested by low blood pressure and sometimes accompanied by syncope, chest pain, or myocardial infarction if severe enough to produce cerebral or myocardial ischemia. The severity of hypotension may vary from mild (systolic blood pressure, >70 mm Hg and <100 mm Hg) to profound (no blood pressure palpable). Hypotension (anaphylactic shock) is thought to be caused by a relative hypovolemia secondary to capillary leakage.

Table 6-2 Agents Commonly Implicated in Anaphylactic and Anaphylactoid Reactions

Antibiotics	Penicillin and penicillin analogs, cephalosporins, tetracyclines, erythromycin, streptomycin
Nonsteroidal anti-inflammatory agents	Salicylates, aminopyrine
Narcotic analgesics	Morphine, codeine, meprobamate
Other drugs	Protamine, chlorpropamide, parenteral iron, iodides, thiazide diuretics
Local anesthetics	Procaine, lidocaine, cocaine
General anesthetics	Thiopental
Anesthetic adjuncts	Succinylcholine, tubocurarine
Blood products and antisera	Red cell, white cell, and platelet transfusions, gamma globulin, rabies, tetanus, diphtheria antitoxin, snake and spider antivenom
Diagnostic agents	Iodinated radiocontrast agents
Foods	Eggs, milk, nuts, legumes (peanuts, soybeans, kidney beans), fish, shellfish
Venoms	Bees, wasps, hornets, snakes, spiders, jellyfish
Hormones	Insulin, adrenocorticotropic hormone, pituitary extract
Enzymes and other biologicals	Acetylcysteine, pancreatic enzyme supplements
Extracts of potential allergens used in desensitization	Pollen, food, venoms

Source: Reprinted with permission from Shoemaker WC, Thompson WL, Holbrook PR (eds): *Textbook of Critical Care.* Philadelphia, WB Saunders, 1984, p 74.

Clinicians should consider anaphylactic shock in any patient with an appropriate history and classic skin findings accompanied by profound cardiorespiratory compromise or, in a setting in which the airway is compromised, when the blood pressure is low and no obvious explanation exists for findings.

TREATMENT

Early recognition of shock and determination of its possible cause are essential to the appropriate management of patients in shock. Therapy must be individualized to fit the needs of each patient. As there are common pathophysiologic manifestations to all forms of shock, however, certain general principles of therapy may be applied. Cellular anoxia and malnutrition are due to either inadequate circulating blood volume (eg, hypovolemia or pump failure) or loss of tone of the reservoir system (eg, sepsis or anaphylaxis). The goal of therapy is the correction of these derangements.

Management in the first hour after the initial insult directly determines morbidity and mortality; thus, all medical and paramedical personnel should take an aggressive, systematic approach (1) to stabilize and monitor the patient's condition, and (2) to recognize the causative factors in the shock state so that specific and definitive treatment can be instituted with dispatch. The guidelines that should be followed once the diagnosis of shock has been made depend partly on the availability of advanced monitoring systems, regardless of the cause of the shock state.

The first priority is to assess the airway and ensure adequate ventilation. The delivery of high-flow oxygen is essential during the initial resuscitation. Once the airway has been cleared, assisted ventilation, if necessary, can be provided by a bag-valve-mask system. Use of the system is continued until the patient's condition has been stabilized and endotracheal intubation can be performed safely. In cases of traumatic shock, a suction apparatus is invaluable in clearing the airway and preventing aspiration. If the patient is conscious and alert, oxygen at high concentrations can be delivered by nasal prongs or mask; however, the resuscitation team must closely monitor respiratory and mental status and be prepared to assist ventilation in cases of deterioration. The objective is to maintain an arterial P_{O_2} of at least 80 mm Hg.

Once proper oxygenation has been ensured, a quick assessment of the patient's overall condition is important to determine the next step. Under these circumstances, assessment and therapy are almost simultaneous. The initial evaluation includes

- measurement of blood pressure, pulse rate, respiratory rate and depth, and temperature
- inspection of external wounds for signs of hemorrhage
- assessment of mental status
- examination of the skin
- assessment of peripheral perfusion (cyanosis, capillary filling)
- determination of jugular venous pressure

One main concern in the initial stages of resuscitation is the differentiation between pump failure and volume deficiency. This is important largely because the ensuing management depends on the relative contribution of these factors. If the patient is in shock and there is jugular venous distention, a cardiopulmonary cause, such as cardiac tamponade, pulmonary embolus, or myocardial infarction, can be assumed. If the neck veins are flat, hypovolemia should be assumed until proved otherwise.

If hypovolemic shock is evident, a balanced electrolyte solution, such as Ringer's lactate, or a normal saline solution is administered rapidly or over 20 to 40 minutes. This rapid volume administration serves as a therapeutic trial in evaluating pre-existing or continuous blood loss. Markedly hypotensive patients may become normotensive with this regimen if blood loss is minimal. The MAST suit can also function as a quick reversible transfusion and may be very effective in correcting hypotension in both prehospital and hospital settings, although improvement of outcome in multiply traumatized patients is questionable. If the fluid challenge elevates blood pressure and decreases pulse rate only temporarily, the loss of blood volume is assumed to be larger, and other forms of intravascular volume expansion may be considered.

If inadequate cardiac function appears to result from tension pneumothorax, cardiac tamponade, myocardial contusion, or pulmonary embolus, there is little the paramedic can do in the field to treat the underlying cause. In such cases, an initial fluid challenge of lactated Ringer's solution, use of a MAST suit in selected cases, monitoring, and judicious use of inotropic and vasopressor medications are the armamentarium that can be used as temporizing measures until the patient can receive definitive treatment at a medical facility. Other initial measures should include a neurologic assessment (mental status, pupillary response, motor response, and orientation), hemorrhage control by direct pressure or MAST suit, and splinting of fractures. Transport to an emergency facility should not be delayed.

Venous Access

The goal of therapy for hypovolemic shock is the rapid administration of fluid; since the length and diameter of catheters are important factors in the rate of infusion, short, large-bore devices will allow more volume to be infused and should be placed to establish intravenous lines in hypovolemic patients. An optimal flow rate is achieved via a 10-gauge Angiocath or 8F introducer catheter with standard 3.2-mm internal diameter intravenous tubing. The use of 5-mm internal diameter tubing further augments flow, allowing infusion rates of crystalloid and blood in excess of 1,200 mL/min. Fluid may be administered quickly through a central venous catheter if tubing is reduced in length to less than 12 inches and an 8F catheter is used for cannulation. Pressure infusion cuffs also promote fluid delivery. Fluid should be warmed appropriately. At least two large bore intravenous lines should be placed in separate extremities, preferably above and below the diaphragm in the event of a vena cava injury.

Adjuncts to Intravascular Volume Expansion: MAST Suit

The MAST suit, often known as the G-suit or pneumatic suit, was first applied to medical practice by Crile in 1903 for control of hypotension during surgical procedures of the head and neck. In studies conducted in Vietnam, Cutler and Daggett reported the effectiveness of the MAST suit for rapid stabilization of hypotension related to hemorrhage. Kaplan and associates reported successful civilian prehospital use of the MAST suit in hemorrhaging patients. The MAST suit has been used in a variety of prehospital emergencies.

The literature is filled with research that arrives at different conclusions regarding the mechanisms by which the MAST is useful in the clinical setting. At one time, it was thought that a significant component of the beneficial effects of the MAST was due to large amounts of blood being transfused from the lower extremities and pelvic area to the central core, thus diverting blood from nonvital structures into the heart/lung/brain circulation. More current data not only have challenged that notion but in some cases have questioned the justification of the use of the MAST in the treatment of hypotensive trauma patients because of a lack of proper studies.

There seems to be some agreement that the MAST does decrease blood vessel diameter, resulting in decreasing blood flow through injured vessels and diminishing third spacing of fluid. Additionally, there is some consensus that increased peripheral vascular resistance is a mechanism by which the MAST increases blood pressure. Whether this is due to autotransfusion, tamponading of blood vessels and stabilization of fractures, or increased peripheral vascular resistance, there is little doubt that there are clinical situations where the MAST is clearly indicated and where its efficacy far outweighs the possible complications.

The MAST suit is most frequently used in the treatment of hypotension secondary to hemorrhage in the prehospital setting, emergency department, or intensive care unit. It is also commonly used in the management of (a) hemorrhage secondary to severe pelvic fracture and retroperitoneal hematoma, (b) hypotension induced by spinal anesthesia, (c) bleeding arising from hypocoagulation, (d) ruptured atherosclerotic abdominal aortic aneurysms, and (e) cardiogenic shock.

The MAST suit is a polyvinyl three-chambered trouser. It is wrapped around the patient's lower extremities and abdomen, one chamber for each lower extremity and a third chamber for the abdomen. The chambers are secured with Velcro fasteners. Each is independently connected to a foot-activated air pump that can be inflated to an internal pressure of 104 mmHg; each has a pressure relief valve to prevent overinflation. The MAST suit is easy to apply and permits accessibility to the groin area. Its light chambers function both as volume replacers and as air splints.

An important characteristic of the MAST suit is its hemostatic effect. When applied, the external pressure decreases the wall tension of the injured vessel by reducing the difference between internal and external vessel pressure (transmural pressure). Laplace's law states that wall tension (T) varies directly according to the product of transmural pressure (P) and the radius of the lumen (R); ie, $T = P \times R$. Because it is the wall tension that keeps the edges of lacerated vessels apart, reducing the transmural pressure, and thus the wall tension, narrows the separation. The MAST suit also decreases the vessel radius by compressing it, which reduces not only tension, but also flow. The reduction of both tension and flow through the injured vessel probably allows the patient's own clotting mechanism to act and to achieve hemostasis more readily. As a result of MAST application, the blood pressure rises and the heart rate usually decreases, probably as a result of baroreceptor responses to increased aortic pressure and venous return. Carotid blood flow is increased; femoral blood flow, decreased. Vital capacity may be decreased by 5%. Central venous pressure, pulmonary wedge pressure, and stroke volume are all increased.

Contraindications

There is no strong evidence to substantiate the theory that renal or pulmonary disease is a contraindication to MAST suit utilization. The MAST suit should not be used in patients with cardiogenic shock or cerebral edema. The suit has not been demonstrated to raise intracranial pressure in patients who are hypotensive because of hypovolemia. Although its use in patients with injuries or hemorrhage above the diaphragm is controversial, a recent review of patients with a variety of injuries failed to find any detrimental effects when the MAST suit was used in injuries above the diaphragm; indeed, good blood pressure augmentation and outcome were reported. Tension pneumothorax, burns, advanced pregnancy, and evisceration are contraindications.

Complications

Acidosis, both metabolic and respiratory, is a phenomenon of MAST suit use reported in animal and clinical studies. Metabolic acidemia may occur if lactate is produced in ischemic extremities. There are no hard clinical data indicating that this occurs in humans, but respiratory acidemia resulting from restriction of diaphragmatic excursion and thoracic expansion and alveolar hypoventilation is theoretically possible. When this problem was observed in a series of 25 patients on whom a MAST suit had been used for variable periods of time, however, only those patients with head injuries were found to have impaired alveolar ventilation with significant acid-base alterations. In this group of patients, the prognosis was extremely poor.

Acidemia should be corrected as soon as possible, and the acid-base status should be closely monitored by means of arterial blood gas determinations. Alterations in renal and respiratory function occurring with MAST use are difficult to evaluate, because it is not known if they are the consequence of MAST suit application or of hypotension and its attendant complications. Urinary output and pulmonary status must be closely monitored in patients who are treated with the MAST suit for prolonged periods of time. Compartment syndromes have been reported with prolonged use at high pressures.

Recommendations

Potential contraindications and complications of MAST use seem to be related to the magnitude of the inflation pressure. Ideally, pressure should be low enough to avoid problems, yet high enough to maintain hemostasis and permit proper immobilization of patients, especially for transportation. Pressures of 20 to 25 mmHg seem adequate and fulfill these requirements; inflation pressures of 40 mmHg should rarely be exceeded.

Deleterious events all too commonly occur when the MAST suit is removed prematurely. If external pressure is removed without adequate fluid replacement, blood pressure may drop as much as 40 to 60 mmHg. If the MAST suit is to be removed, it should be done cautiously over a 30-minute period; the deflation must be stopped if the blood pressure drops more than 5 mmHg. One compartment at a time, beginning with the abdomen, should be deflated. Should blood pressure drop, fluid must be infused to restore the blood pressure to its initial level before continuing deflation. In some instances, the MAST suit should be removed in the operating room.

In summary, the MAST suit is a valuable adjunct in the prehospital and emergency department management of patients in shock. In the hands of experienced personnel, its use is associated with very low morbidity. The benefits seem to outweigh the potential complications.

Trendelenburg's Position

When a patient is in the recumbent position, more than 50% of blood volume is located in the venous system; when intravascular volume is decreased, pooling occurs in the periphery. Theoretically then, tilting a patient into the head-down position diverts this blood volume into the central circulation, thus increasing cardiac filling and augmenting stroke volume. The efficacy of this maneuver has been debated in the literature, and recent studies do not demonstrate that it results in significant redistribution of blood volume centrally. Some authors hypothesize that not only is it ineffective in improving the hemodynamic status of normotensive and hypotensive patients, but also it may be associated with untoward side-effects in pulmonary ventilation/perfusion, resulting in increased arteriovenous admixture and endotracheal tube displacement. Others support its use with hypotensive patients.

Data suggest that the Trendelenburg position improves hemodynamics in hypotension secondary to loss of vascular tone, but not in hypotension associated with hemorrhage and vasoconstriction. When the effects of the Trendelenburg position on systemic and pulmonary hemodynamics in critically ill, normotensive, and hypotensive patients were studied, all subjects had Swan-Ganz catheters in place, and all important hemodynamic parameters were measured. The results failed to indicate that the Trendelenburg position has any significant beneficial hemodynamic effects. Its failure to increase central blood volume and mean arterial pressure in hypotensive patients is thought to be related to splanchnic pooling of blood. In some instances, a detrimental fall of mean arterial pressure was seen when the patient was in the Trendelenburg position. Considering the potential complications, the augmentation of intravascular volume seems to be better accomplished with the use of intravenous fluid therapy.

Selection of Fluid Therapy

After the initial fluid infusion, the advisability of further fluid replacement must be determined. Again, the basic indicator is the clinical condition of the patient. Once the patient is in the hospital, several monitoring parameters may be used (Table 6-3). Urine output, differences in arterial and venous oxygen levels, colloid osmotic pressure, and measurements of left ventricular function (eg, pulmonary artery wedge pressure) are among the most sensitive and useful parameters to evaluate intravascular volume and cardiac performance, and thus to gauge the necessity of further fluid replacement.

Types of Fluids

In hypoperfusion, the objectives of therapy are to replace lost blood, correct intravascular volume deficits, and identify the reason for the hypoperfusion. The mainstay of therapy for hemorrhagic shock is blood, properly typed and crossmatched, preferably fresh.

The objective of blood therapy is to maintain hemoglobin levels at 12.5 to 14 g/dL or hematocrit at 30% to 32%. This level tends to maintain a better intravascular volume, and

Table 6-3 Cardiopulmonary Monitoring of Critically Ill Patients

All patients	*Patients with incipient respiratory failure*
Vital signs—pulse, blood pressure, temperature, respiratory rate	Monitoring indicated for all patients
Weight	Arterial blood gases
Intake and output	Vital capacity and inspiratory force
Physical examination with special attention to	*Patients on ventilators*
Sensorium	Monitoring indicated for all patients
Respiratory pattern	Ventilator settings
Skin temperature and turgor	Exhaled tidal volume
Neck veins	Inspired oxygen fraction
Peripheral pulses	Inspired gas temperature
Heart	Positive end expiratory pressure
Lungs	Mechanical respiratory rate
Abdomen	Pop-off pressure
Cardiac rate and rhythm	Compliance (dynamic and static)
Chest roentgenography	Sputum Gram's stain and culture
	Ratio of dead space to tidal volume*
	Carbon dioxide production*

*Indicated in certain selected patients only.

Source: Reprinted with permission from Goldenheim PD, Kazemi H: Cardiopulmonary monitoring of critically ill patients. *N Engl J Med* 311:718, 1984.

patients may have a lower risk of respiratory failure. Below these levels, the oxygen-carrying capacity of the blood is reduced significantly, and the ensuing hypoxemia aggravates the clinical state. If the hemoglobin level is adequate, if red blood cell loss has been insignificant, or if whole blood is not readily available, further fluid therapy is carried out with blood substitutes. If multiple transfusions are required, fresh-frozen plasma replacement may be needed to restore clotting factors.

Physiologic Considerations

Starling's famous equation is a key to understanding the controversy surrounding the role of colloid and crystalloid solutions as volume replacements, and their contributing roles in the development of "shock" lung. The formula defines the factors that regulate vascular fluid flux (Fig. 6-11):

$$FH_2O = K_c \times SA (P_c - P_i) + (OP_i - OP_c)$$

All these factors interplay to maintain fluid homeostasis. It can be seen that the extravascular fluid flux (FH_2O) is directly related to the intravascular hydrostatic pressure (P_c) and capillary permeability (K_c) and inversely related to the intravascular colloid oncotic pressure (OP_i). Albumin, a circulating protein that maintains the colloid osmotic pressure, is the major determinant of the flux of fluids at the capillary level. This information can be used to isolate two readily measurable parameters in the clinical setting: the intravascular colloid osmotic pressure and the pulmonary artery wedge pressure. Pulmonary edema can be associated with normal pulmonary artery wedge pressures. Reduction of the colloid osmotic pressure–pulmonary artery wedge pressure gradient, which is normally 10 to 20 mmHg, is associated with the development of pulmonary edema and can be used as a prognostic indicator. In cardiogenic pulmonary edema, the reduction of this gradient is due to an elevation of pulmonary wedge pressure; in noncardiogenic pulmonary edema, it is due to severe reduction of colloid osmotic pressure. This was shown by studies of 17 patients with gradients of 13.6 mmHg who developed noncardiogenic pulmonary edema. Furthermore, severe reduction of colloid osmotic pressure is a reliable prognostic indicator of mortality in 75% of cases.

Early correction of hypovolemia prevents renal and pulmonary complications. Shock lung, congestive atelectasis, and post-traumatic pulmonary insufficiency are some of the terms used to define the pathologic findings associated with the common pulmonary complications of patients in shock. The causes of these complications vary.

Some authors suggest that resuscitation with crystalloid solutions is associated with fewer pulmonary complications, while others feel that resuscitation with colloid solutions results in less morbidity and mortality. Colloid proponents claim that crystalloids alone dilute plasma proteins, thereby reducing plasma colloid osmotic pressures, increasing hydrostatic pressure, and thus facilitating interstitial and intracellular fluid flux. When large amounts of balanced electrolyte solution are given, approximately 25% remains intravascular; the rest distributes itself within the interstitial spaces, promoting edema. Crystalloid proponents claim that albumin enters the interstitial pulmonary compartment, increasing the albumin pool and the interstitial colloid osmotic pressure, thus favoring fluid accumulation. A prospective clinical study, in which crystalloids were used in one group of patients and colloid was added to crystalloids in a second group, showed no significant difference in results; however, the cost of treatment with albumin was much greater.

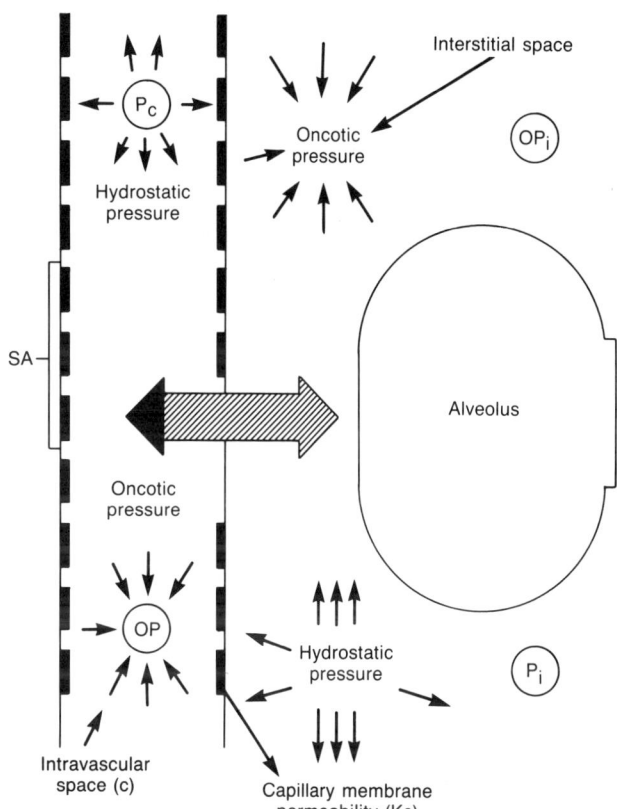

Figure 6-11 Vascular fluid flux.

The role of albumin in the development of interstitial edema during fluid infusion is unclear. In one study, not only was albumin found ineffective in preventing shock lung, but also pulmonary function was worse in patients who received albumin than in those who did not. This is thought to be due to the "secondary effects" of albumin, such as impairment of myocardial performance, which is believed to be caused by a fall in the ratio of ionized to nonionized calcium; impairment of salt and water excretion, which elevates central venous pressure and pulmonary wedge pressure; and interstitial entrapment of albumin within the lungs, which increases interstitial colloid osmotic pressure and extravascular fluid flux.

Table 6-4 Estimated Fluid and Blood Requirements* (Based on Patient's Initial Presentation)

	Class I	Class II	Class III	Class IV
Blood loss (mL)	Up to 750	750–1500	1500–2000	2000 or more
Blood loss (% blood volume)	Up to 15	15–30	30–40	40 or more
Pulse rate	<100	>100	>120	140 or higher
Blood pressure	Normal	Normal	Decreased	Decreased
Pulse pressure (mmHg)	Normal or increased	Decreased	Decreased	Decreased
Capillary blanch test	Normal	Positive	Positive	Positive
Respiratory rate	14–20	20–30	30–40	>35
Urine output (mL/hour)	30 or more	20–30	5–15	Negligible
Mental status	Slightly anxious	Mildly anxious	Anxious and confused	Confused-lethargic
Fluid replacement (3:1 rule)	Crystalloid	Crystalloid	Crystalloid + blood	Crystalloid + blood

*For a 70-kg male.

Source: Adapted with permission from *Advanced Trauma Life Support Course.* Chicago, Committee on Trauma, American College of Surgeons, 1984, p 185.

In the field and in the emergency department, crystalloid resuscitation is sufficient. The quantity and quality of subsequent fluid therapy should be individualized, depending on a set of carefully obtained physiologic data. The causes of shock, shock lung, and pulmonary edema are so varied that no one therapeutic regimen can be recommended; fluid and blood requirements can only be estimated (Table 6-4). Hence, the physician should take into consideration (1) the physiologic actions of each agent, (2) the pathophysiology of the disease entity, and (3) the specific aim of each therapeutic modality. Modern monitoring techniques are helpful in arriving at the proper balance of fluid replacement.

Purified albumin solutions and pasteurized plasma (sold as 5% plasma protein factor) eliminate the risk that infections will be transmitted, but, like albumin, they are costly. Several artificial macromolecular polymers are available as plasma substitutes; they seem partially to correct the problem of rapid interstitial distribution that is seen with crystalloids, and they do not have the described disadvantages of albumin, including cost. They have disadvantages of their own, however. With dextran 70, for example, 70% remains in the circulation initially, and 30% is still present after 24 hours. Complications include a greater tendency for the patient to bleed because the dextran interferes with platelet function and decreases blood viscosity. Furthermore, cross-matching of blood is difficult after dextrans have been used. Dextran 40, although it has a shorter half-life than does dextran 70, carries the same sorts of risks; in addition, it may precipitate renal failure. Both dextrans 70 and 40 are allergenic; severe anaphylactoid reactions with shock and death have occurred.

Hydroxyethyl starch has an intravascular persistence equal to or greater than that of dextran 70. Like the dextrans, it increases bleeding times, but to a lesser degree. The advantage of hydroxyethyl starch is that it does not produce anaphylactoid reactions. It is considered a safe, effective colloidal solution for replacement of lost blood and for augmentation of blood volume. Recently developed fluorochemical blood substitutes need further study, but hold great promise as artificial blood replacements; they are capable not only of expanding blood volume, but also of carrying oxygen. Stroma-free hemoglobin also holds great promise as a synthetic volume-expanding fluid capable of carrying oxygen.

Hypertonic Saline

There have been some studies of the use of hypertonic saline (3.0% to 7.5% sodium chloride). Some of the results demonstrate effectiveness in volume replacement and expansion equal to or greater than those with isotonic saline, affecting not only hemodynamic function but also urine output and other perfusion parameters in hemorrhagic shock. There is a need for further studies before widespread use of hypertonic saline as a volume treatment modality is undertaken.

Blood Transfusion

Whether crystalloids alone or crystalloids in combination with colloids are used in the initial resuscitation of patients in hemorrhagic shock, the patient reaches a critical point beyond which blood replacement is essential. Crystalloids, colloids, and plasma expanders lack oxygen-carrying capacity, and the dilutional effects upon the blood create a drop in the oncotic pressure, which in turn promotes loss of intravascular volume to the interstitial space as a result of the loss of balance between the oncotic and the hydrostatic pressure gradients. Once the hemoglobin level falls to ranges below half normal, the body's compensatory mechanisms start to fail, and tissue perfusion and oxygen-based metabolism become impaired.

When blood transfusions are considered, there are certain guidelines that are appropriate to follow. Any patient suspected of having hemorrhagic shock should be at least typed and cross-matched for 6 U of whole blood. Depending on the urgency of a situation, it may be necessary to replace blood volume with blood products before full type and cross-matching. In such instances, type-specific blood can be used safely, and the turnaround time should be no longer than 5 to 10 minutes. Furthermore, if type-specific blood is unavailable, type O blood can be utilized with little concern regarding side effects.

When large amounts of blood need to be given, the general guidelines are to transfuse 1 U of fresh frozen plasma for every 4 U of blood and 5 U of platelets for every 10 U of blood. Additionally, because of the problems associated with stored blood, it is recommended that 1 g of calcium chloride be given for every 5 U of blood.

Autotransfusion

The safest way of transfusing a patient is with the use of an autotransfuser. Because blood from the chest tubes or other uncontaminated sites from the same patient is used, the risk of immunologic or infectious complications of transfused blood from donors is eliminated.

Whole blood is preferred over packed cells in circumstances where massive transfusions are indicated. Massive blood transfusions are associated with complications such as coagulopathies secondary to platelet abnormalities, deficiencies of factor V or factor VIII, and calcium abnormalities, acid-base disturbances, hypothermia, and transfusion reactions.

Blood Substitutes

The ideal blood substitute would be one that, in addition to transporting oxygen and carbon dioxide effectively, is nontoxic, easily stored, and temperature stable and has a long storage life. To date, no known substance fulfills all these requirements. The two most commonly studied blood substitutes are flousol DA and stroma-free hemoglobin. Both these solutions have been used experimentally in the laboratory and in clinical settings as plasma expanders and solutions that can carry oxygen and carbon dioxide.

The experimental trials with flousol DA have not demonstrated any appreciable benefits over crystalloid therapy for patients with severe anemia. Stroma-free hemoglobin is still in the experimental stages and is currently not available for general use. It is a solution composed of erythrocytes, which results in oxygen transport capabilities and volume expansion properties, but its poor half-life and the tensions at which it unloads oxygen from hemoglobin make clinical and laboratory trials necessary before its widespread clinical use.

Correction of Acid-Base Abnormalities

Most acid-base derangements can be corrected by adequate ventilation, oxygenation, and tissue perfusion. Maintaining the acid-base status as close to normal as possible improves both therapeutic response and physiologic recovery. When the acidemia creates a pH of less than 7.2, the bicarbonate dosage required to correct the deficit should be calculated by multiplying the base deficit by the approximate bicarbonate distribution space (considered to be 30% to 50% of body weight); only one-half the amount should be administered at one time at a rate of 3 to 5 mEq/min. Overcorrection can lead to alkalemia and shift the oxyhemoglobin dissociation curve to the left, increasing hemoglobin affinity for oxygen and decreasing the availability of oxygen at the cellular level (see Chapter 75, Miscellaneous Respiratory Emergencies).

MONITORING THE PATIENT IN SHOCK

Urine Output

If there is no evidence of genitourinary trauma (eg, pelvic fracture or hematuria), a Foley catheter should be inserted in the patient in shock. The flow of urine is a very useful and sensitive parameter of renal perfusion. Through mechanisms such as the aldosterone-renin-angiotensin system and the release of antidiuretic hormone, the kidneys tend to compensate for hypovolemia by reabsorbing water and sodium; consequently, urine output falls. If a critically ill patient has an adequate circulating volume, changes in urine output, milliliter by milliliter and minute to minute, indicate the state of renal perfusion and help to determine the need for volume replacement. The usefulness of this parameter is limited in patients treated with diuretics, however.

Urinary electrolyte levels are used to determine replacement therapy. The urinary sodium concentration is useful in differentiating between a decreased urine output secondary to hypoperfusion (sodium level less than 20 mEq/L) and that secondary to renal insufficiency (sodium level more than 40 mEq/L). In the latter case, sodium is not reabsorbed and is lost in the urine. The urine:plasma creatinine ratio and the urine:plasma osmolality ratio are also used to make this distinction.

Intra-arterial Pressure

Because of discrepancies between central arterial pressures and cuff blood pressures, determination of intra-arterial pressure is required for proper blood pressure monitoring, particularly in those patients with hypotension and peripheral vasoconstriction (ie, with cool upper extremities and thready brachial and radial pulses). This is accomplished by cannulating the radial, brachial, or femoral arteries and connecting the catheter to a pressure transducer and a continuous monitoring device. The catheter also permits frequent blood sampling for determinations of arterial blood gas levels, pH, electrolyte concentrations, glucose levels, and other values.

One therapeutic approach to shock and volume resuscitation, introduced by Jelenko and co-workers, consists of a hypertonic albumin-containing fluid demand (HALFD) regimen. Mean arterial pressure, urine output, weight change, hematocrit, plasma and urinary sodium and potassium levels, and plasma and urinary volume are used as indicators for clinical administration of fluids. The objective is to maintain a normal mean arterial pressure (ie, 60 to 110 mmHg) and a urine volume of 30 to 50 mL/hour. In a prospective, randomized study of 19 burn patients treated with lactated Ringer's solution alone, hypertonic fluid alone, or the HALFD regimen, it was found that the HALFD group made better clinical progress, required the infusion of less fluid, gained less weight, and had less plasma leak.

Acid-Base Determinations

Frequent assessment of oxygenation and saturation of arterial blood as well as pH and Pco_2 is easily accomplished and provides invaluable information for the management of patients in shock.

Central Venous Pressure

There is a wide spectrum of opinion regarding central venous pressure monitoring. Some authors suggest that there is little value in following the relationships between cardiocirculatory function and blood volume, while others find it helpful once certain preexisting factors (eg, myocardial function) have been taken into consideration. In addition to monitoring central pressures, however, large-bore central lines can be used for large volume infusion and are used as ports of entry for pacemaker wires or Swan-Ganz catheters when the appropriate central line sets are used.

It is our opinion that a central venous line should be established as soon as the patient arrives in the emergency department. Several approaches are possible. Physician skill, patient's body habitus, clinical circumstances, age, and any thoracic deformities should be considered in selecting one of the available internal jugular or subclavian techniques (see Chapter 86, Atlas of Emergency Procedures). Common complications of central venous cannulation include pneumothorax, arterial puncture and laceration, air embolus, and sepsis; therefore, the physician must use meticulous aseptic technique. Following insertion, a chest roentgenogram is mandatory to assess placement and detect any immediate complication.

Central venous pressure varies directly with circulating blood volume and inversely with vascular tone or right heart competence. This measurement is of particular value in patients who are in hemorrhagic shock, but are otherwise healthy; in these patients, right atrial and left ventricular end diastolic pressures are closely related, even in the presence of controlled ventilation or positive end expiratory pressure (PEEP). Central venous pressure monitoring is not useful in patients with pre-existing cardiocirculatory disease, since the relationship between the right atrial pressure and the left ventricular end diastolic pressure is variable and clinically misleading in these patients; however, a Swan-Ganz catheter gives accurate information as to left ventricular function by providing pulmonary artery and wedge pressures (see Chapter 86, Atlas of Emergency Procedures).

Trends in central venous pressure measurements in response to the infusion of fluid aliquots are more important than isolated readings. Assuming that right atrial pressure correlates well with left ventricular end diastolic pressure, the central venous pressure can be used to monitor right atrial and left ventricular function in relationship to circulating volume and vascular tone. At 10-minute intervals, 200-mL aliquots of volume-expanding fluids may be infused. If central venous pressure does not increase by more than 2 cmH_2O, the infusion is continued. If it increases by 2 to 5 cmH_2O, the challenge is interrupted briefly, and the patient's needs are reassessed; the challenge is stopped if the increase is more than 10 cmH_2O.

Arterial–Central Venous Oxygen Difference

The measurement of oxygen consumption is a sensitive indicator of cellular metabolism. The oxygen consumption of patients in shock is decreased, owing to (a) limited oxygen transport because of a decrease in blood flow and a reduction of hemoglobin or (b) an inability of the cell to accept or utilize oxygen. Hemorrhagic or cardiogenic shock leads to the former; septic shock, the latter.

The calculation of arterial–central venous oxygen differences is easily performed by drawing arterial and central venous blood samples for Po_2 determination. The arterial–central venous oxygen content difference is calculated in volumes percent. The values may indicate trends in cardiac output,

$$C\,(A\text{-}V\bar{O})\text{ difference} = 1.34 \times Hb\,(aO_2 - V\bar{O}_2) + \frac{0.32}{100}(PaO_2 - P V\bar{O}_2)\,(\text{Vol }\%)$$

where C is oxygen content and Hb is hemoglobin content. If the difference is greater than 6 volumes percent, it can be assumed that cardiac output is depressed. An arterial–central venous oxygen difference of less than 3 volumes percent probably reflects a cardiac output that is abnormally high.

Under normal basal circumstances, oxygen consumption is approximately 145 ± 15 mL/min/m^2 body surface. Oxygen consumption changes when the patient is hyperactive or hypotensive, for example. Yet, changes in the arterial–central venous oxygen difference, regardless of its initial value, provide information on the direction and degree of any change in the cardiac output. If oxygen consumption is assumed to be constant and the arterial–central venous oxy-

Table 6-5 Indications for Pulmonary Artery Lines

1. Myocardial infarctions complicated by
   a. hypotension unresponsive to volume challenge
   b. marked hemodynamic instability requiring intravenous inotropic or vasoactive drugs or mechanical assist devices
   c. hypotension and congestive heart failure
   d. ? cardiac tamponade (equalization of end-diastolic pressures)
   e. ? acute mitral regurgitation (giant V waves)
   f. ? ruptured interventricular septum (step-up in oxygen saturation)
2. Unstable angina requiring intravenous nitroglycerin (most patients)
3. Congestive heart failure unresponsive to conventional therapy, to guide preload and afterload therapy
4. Pulmonary hypertension, for diagnosis and monitoring during acute drug therapy
5. Distinguishing cardiogenic from noncardiogenic pulmonary edema
6. Optimizing PEEP and volume therapy in the adult respiratory distress syndrome
7. Resolving doubts about volume or cardiovascular status if a diuretic or fluid challenge would be unsafe or would yield equivocal results

PEEP: positive end expiratory pressure.

Source: Reprinted with permission from Goldenheim PD, Kazemi H: Cardiopulmonary monitoring of critically ill patients. *N Engl J Med* 311:779, 1984.

gen content difference is known, cardiac output can be calculated by substitution into the Fick principle:

$$Q = \frac{VO_2}{C(a\text{-}V)O_2 \times 10}$$

where Q is cardiac output and VO_2 is oxygen consumption. Cardiac outputs determined in this manner correlate well with measured outputs except at very low and very high ranges. Despite the inaccuracies introduced by the assumptions that oxygen consumption is constant and that right atrial oxygen content is equivalent to central venous oxygen content, the techniques allow an estimate of cardiac output to be made at the patient's bedside.

Pulmonary Artery Pressure

Probably the most sensitive parameter of left ventricular function is pulmonary artery wedge pressure, which can be recorded easily with the Swan-Ganz catheter, a flow-directed, balloon-tipped pulmonary artery catheter that can be used to measure wedge pressure through a continuous electronic pressure monitor. This measurement is of particular value in patients with cardiogenic shock and severe sepsis, because there can be a great difference between central venous pressure and pulmonary artery wedge pressure in these patients.

A pulmonary artery wedge pressure greater than 17 mm Hg is correlated with pulmonary congestion; a pressure greater than 25 mm Hg, with pulmonary edema. With the Swan-Ganz catheter, cardiac output may be measured by the thermodilution method. The prognosis is poor when cardiogenic shock is associated with myocardial infarction and the cardiac output is less than 2.4 L/min/m².

The current trend is toward early placement of the Swan-Ganz catheter, perhaps even in the emergency department, in order to monitor fluid replacement therapy when the central venous pressure is not a clearly reliable indicator of left ventricular function (see Chapter 86, Atlas of Emergency Procedures). Clinical estimates of hemodynamic status correlate poorly with variables measured by means of catheterization; and therapy may be radically altered when more accurate data are available through pulmonary artery catheterization. Indications for pulmonary artery line insertion are given in Table 6-5.

A new monitoring tool useful in emergency practice is the transcutaneous oxygen monitor. This device allows continuous monitoring of oxygen delivery to the peripheral tissues and, thus, makes it possible to determine the efficacy of resuscitation. The transconjunctival oxygen monitor may be even more useful and is suitable for emergency use (Fig. 6-12).

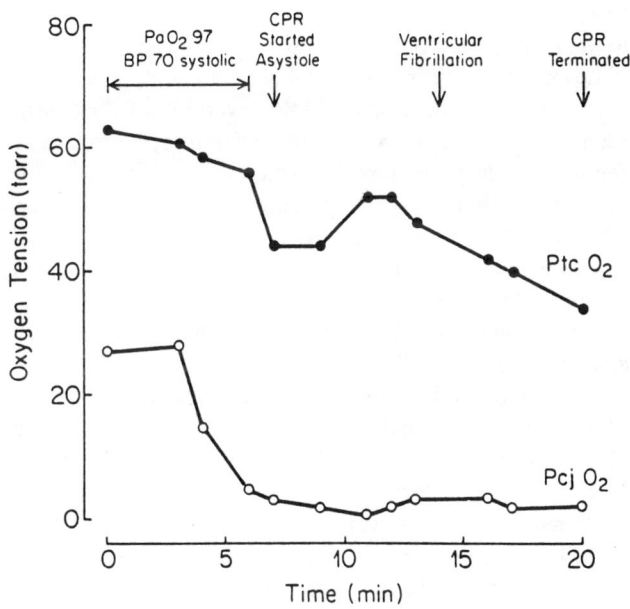

Figure 6-12 $P_{cj}O_2$ and $P_{tc}O_2$ values in a patient with cardiogenic shock. The patient had stable $P_{tc}O_2$ and $P_{cj}O_2$ values with a blood pressure of 70/40 mm Hg for 45 mins before the events shown. Note the decrease in $P_{cj}O_2$ preceding the cardiac arrest: $P_{tc}O_2$ falls at the time of the asystolic arrest. *BP*, blood pressure; *CPR*, cardiopulmonary resuscitation. Reprinted with permission from Abraham E, Smith M, Silver L: Conjunctival and transcutaneous oxygen monitoring during cardiac arrest and cardiopulmonary resuscitation. *Crit Care Med* 12(5):420, 1984.

SPECIFIC THERAPY

Fluid is the keystone to the management of shock, regardless of its cause (unless there are high left ventricular filling pressures). The initial objective is to replace volume, whether it be a few hundred milliliters or several liters. If the cardiocirculatory system cannot function properly when fluid therapy has been adequate (ie, left ventricular filling pressure has been elevated to normal or even moderate levels), shock persists and other therapeutic modalities are necessary (Fig. 6-13).

Inotropic and Vasopressor Agents

If patients remain in shock despite adequate fluid replacement, it may be necessary to administer medications that increase cardiac output, elevate perfusion pressure, or improve tissue perfusion. Most inotropic drugs augment cardiac output by increasing the force and velocity of contraction, which also increases the oxygen demand of the already ischemic myocardium and may be ill-advised when acute myocardial infarction is associated with shock. Vasopressors are useful in raising arterial blood pressure to levels that ensure adequate coronary perfusion, but they may also enhance peripheral vasoconstriction, making tissue perfusion less adequate and increasing the workload of the heart. Therefore, pressors should be used very cautiously and transiently to maintain proper perfusion and vital circulation.

Levarterenol and metaraminol are commonly used vasoconstricting medications. While levarterenol does profoundly increase systemic vascular resistance, it produces a regional underperfusion. Isoproterenol significantly increases cardiac output by increasing contractility and heart rate, but both of these changes increase the myocardial oxygen demand. Clinical trials with isoproterenol have not demonstrated a reduction in the mortality rate for patients with cardiogenic shock, and serious dysrhythmias are often associated with its utilization.

Dopamine, while mimicking the vasoconstrictive effects of levarterenol at high doses, improves renal and mesenteric blood flow at low dosages; it also augments cardiac output. In general, total peripheral vascular resistance remains unaltered when dopamine is administered, and there is little or no increase in heart rate; blood pressure rises because of enhanced output. The drug may precipitate ventricular dysrhythmias, however.

Dobutamine may be superior to dopamine in augmenting cardiac output. It may be used in patients with cardiogenic shock, despite its lack of α-adrenergic effects. Dobutamine acts directly on β-adrenergic receptors in the myocardium to increase cardiac output. Attention to hemodynamic data and appropriate respiratory therapy is important. Ventilatory settings, for example, may alter the volume needs of patients by altering oxygen delivery, venous return, and cardiac output.

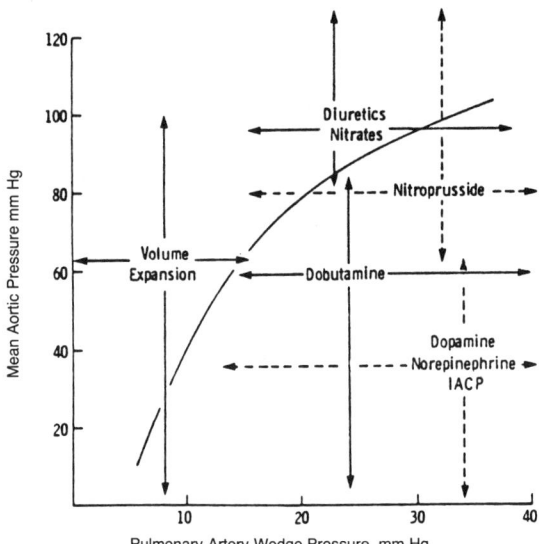

Figure 6-13 The hemodynamic indications for various therapeutic interventions are described by domains or regions in the Frank-Starling diagram. *IACP*, intra-aortic counterpulsation. Reprinted with permission from Ayers SM: Ventricular function, in *Textbook of Critical Care*, W. Shoemaker et al (eds), Philadelphia, WB Saunders, 1984, p 343.

The use of digitalis in patients with congestive heart failure and cardiogenic shock due to acute myocardial infarction is controversial. The drug seems to have beneficial hemodynamic effects in the presence of cardiogenic shock associated with cardiac failure and cardiomegaly, however.

The disadvantage of cardiac glycosides is that they produce a profound splanchnic vasoconstriction, aggravating pre-existing ischemia and enhancing both the release of lysosomal enzyme and the formation of myocardial depressant factor. For this reason, although they improve myocardial performance, they are of questionable benefit in the absence of heart failure and cardiomegaly (see Chapter 64, Congestive Heart Failure).

Amrinone, a recently described inotrope, has been used to increase cardiac output in patients with severe congestive heart failure as a result of cardiomyopathy and in patients with acute myocardial infarction. Because the ensuing increases in cardiac output have been significant, this may be a useful drug in therapy for cardiogenic shock. Consideration should also be given to the administration of nitrates and calcium channel blockers.

Vasodilators in Cardiogenic Shock

A reduction of left ventricular outflow impedance, resistance, and filling pressure may augment cardiac output by decreasing left ventricular workload and myocardial oxygen demand. In patients with acute myocardial infarction, best results are obtained when the left ventricular filling pressure is high and the blood pressure near normal. Among the most commonly used vasodilator drugs are sodium nitroprusside and nitroglycerin. In cardiogenic shock due to myocardial infarction, these medications often improve hemodynamic status, but long-term survival remains poor. Combination therapy (eg, dopamine plus nitroprussides) may have a role in the therapy of cardiogenic shock, but controlled studies of alternative therapeutic regimens, including afterload reduction, are not conclusive.

Dysrhythmia Management

When cardiogenic shock is secondary to dysrhythmia, the underlying cause must be corrected before the shock state can resolve. The first concern is to determine whether the dysrhythmia is the cause of the shock state or a consequence of it. General guidelines for the management of dysrhythmia are extensively reviewed in Chapter 63. Patients with cardiogenic shock also require analgesic therapy, and drugs such as morphine sulfate, hydromorphone, and diazepam are frequently used to relieve anxiety and pain as well as for their positive cardiocirculatory effects.

Anticoagulation

Although the issue of anticoagulation in patients with cardiogenic shock is controversial, it is well accepted in patients who have large infarcts or other medical complications that require extended periods of time of bedrest. Prostaglandins seem to have some effectiveness by increasing cardiac output and decreasing resistance in normal subjects as well as in animals subjected to hemorrhagic shock. There is a need for further experimental research.

Intra-Aortic Balloon Counterpulsation

In intra-aortic balloon counterpulsation, a catheter is threaded through the femoral artery into the thoracic aorta, and a balloon located at the tip is inflated with 30 mL of carbon dioxide; the R wave of the cardiogram is used for timing. The pump activates the balloon; the balloon is deflated before left ventricular systole to lower outflow resistance and then is reinflated at the onset of diastole after aortic valve closure to augment ascending aortic and cerebral arterial pressures and diastolic coronary artery perfusion. With this technique, left ventricular wall tension is reduced, and stroke volume and coronary perfusion are improved. Initial improvements seen in patients with cardiogenic shock may not be supportable in the long term, however.

Intra-aortic balloon counterpulsation allows time for assessment of hemodynamic abnormalities and identification of potentially remediable surgical lesions (eg, aneurysms, mitral regurgitation, rupture, and ventricular septal defects). Still, surgical intervention carries a high mortality rate.

An external counterpulsation device is noninvasive and functions on the same principle, but its usefulness is minimal in profound cardiogenic shock.

Treatment of Septic Shock

Overall treatment principles for septic shock follow those for all critically ill patients, demanding vigorous supportive care, critical care and hemodynamic monitoring, and appropriate life support measures (Fig. 6-14). In addition, pertinent cultures must be obtained before administration of directed but broad spectrum antibiotics. Focal sites of infection must be sought and eradicated. Once the results of bacteriologic tests are available, the clinician should choose the most specific and least toxic antimicrobials available. Side effects, allergic potential, and toxicity are of particular concern because the condition of these patients is already compromised and fragile. Because of vasoconstriction and multiple organ failure, the metabolism of antimicrobials and other drugs may be significantly altered, making the route of administration and organ clearance of antibiotic agents considerations in drug selection.

If the organism is unknown, empiric therapy should endeavor to cover both Gram-positive as well as Gram-negative organisms and should be supplemented with *Bacillus fragilis* coverage if a pelvic or intra-abdominal source is being contemplated. Thus a common initial combination is oxacillin or cephalothin plus aminoglycoside, (eg, gentamicin-tobramycin). Alternatively, oxacillin plus cefotaxime may be used, with vancomycin substituting for the former in penicillin-allergic patients. Chloramphenicol or clindamycin is often added to provide anaerobic coverage. Carbenicillin or ticarcillin is appropriate in leukopenic patients.

Although not completely substantiated, administration of naloxone may be helpful in some patients (Fig. 6-15), having reversed endotoxin shock in some animal models. In addition, vasopressors may be useful to support blood pressure after appropriate volume expansion; dopamine is particularly effective. Dobutamine may be useful in the latter, vasoconstrictive stages of septic shock.

Many effects of corticosteroids make them theoretically attractive for the correction of the severe pathophysiologic derangements so much in evidence in septic shock. Even the anti-inflammatory agent indomethacin has improved endotoxin shock survival in experimental animals. Clinical results with steroids have been disappointing, however. Despite some suggestion that mortality might be ameliorated with early steroid administration, recent large controlled trials failed to demonstrate this benefit or to prevent the development of adult respiratory distress syndrome; moreover, secondary infections were more common in steroid-treated patients. Accordingly, routine use of steroids cannot be recommended.

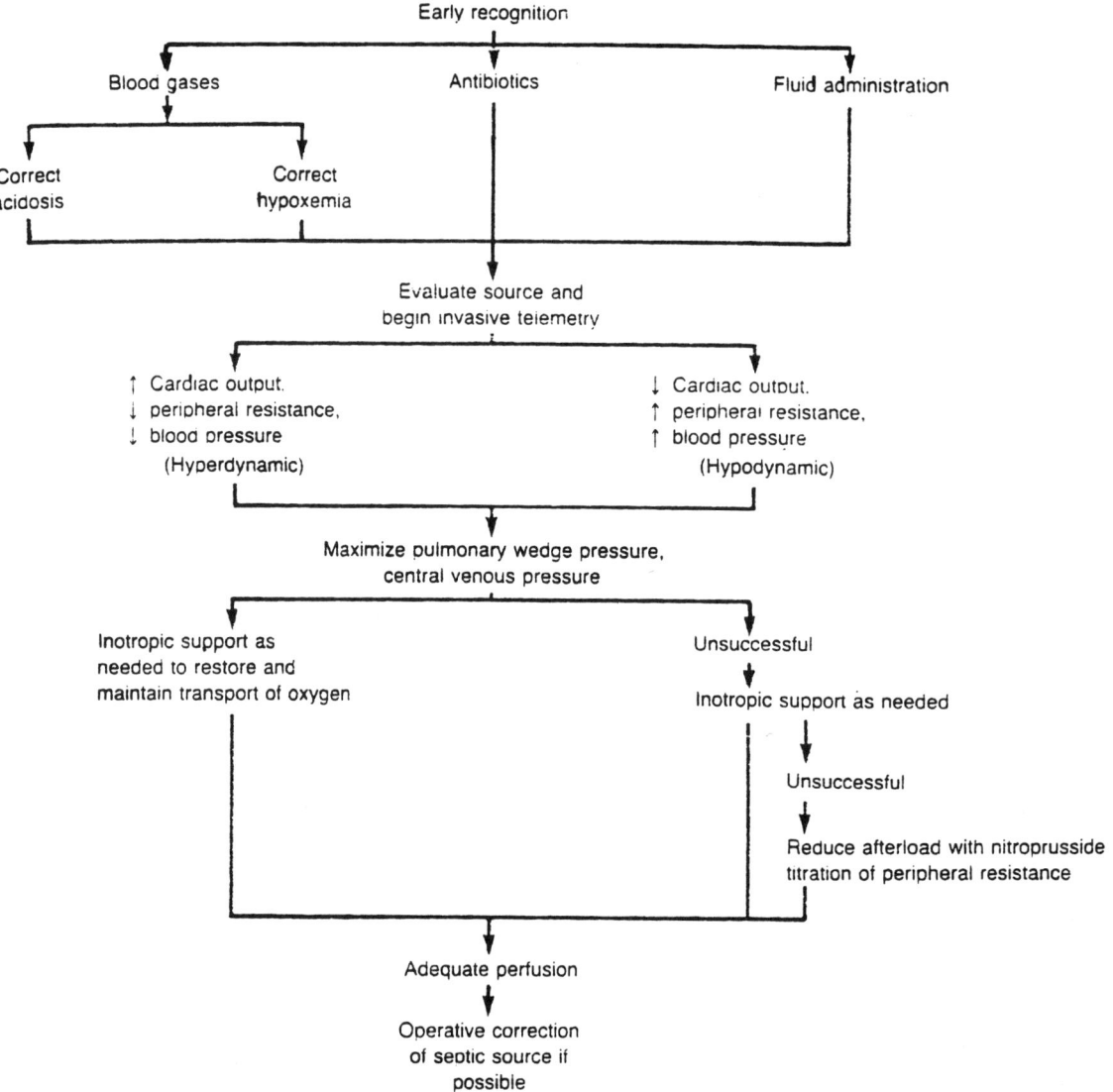

Figure 6-14 Management of septic shock. Reprinted with permission from Schwartz RA, Cerra FB: Shock: A practical approach. *Urol Clin North Am* 10(1):97, 1983.

Therapy for Anaphylaxis

Management depends on the severity of the manifestations. Although mild cases may sometimes be managed with conventional doses of antihistamines (eg, diphenhydramine, 25 mg orally every 4 to 6 hours for 24 hours to 3 days after an initial dose of 50 mg orally or intramuscularly in adults), epinephrine (0.3 to 0.5 mL of a 1:1000 solution subcutaneously) is often required and usually is repeated twice at 20-minute intervals. In refractory cases, the addition of an H2 receptor antagonist (eg, ranitidine) may be helpful.

Patients in anaphylactic shock should be treated similarly to any critically ill person with attention to airway, administration of oxygen, cardiac monitoring, pulse oximetry, securing of intravenous access, serial blood pressure measurements, and close observation, including hemodynamic monitoring in particularly acute cases. Patients with severe airway obstruction should be intubated; failing placement of an airway, a cricothyrotomy should be performed. Parenteral epinephrine and diphenhydramine should be administered concomitantly. Bronchospasm should be treated with these agents as well as with nebulized bronchodilators, typically albuterol (0.5 mL in 3 mL of normal saline), repeatedly if necessary. Aminophylline may be helpful as well.

Hypotension should be treated with volume expansion with normal saline or lactated Ringer's solution. In the hypotensive or life-threatened individual, epinephrine should be given intravenously (3 to 5 mL of a 1:10,000

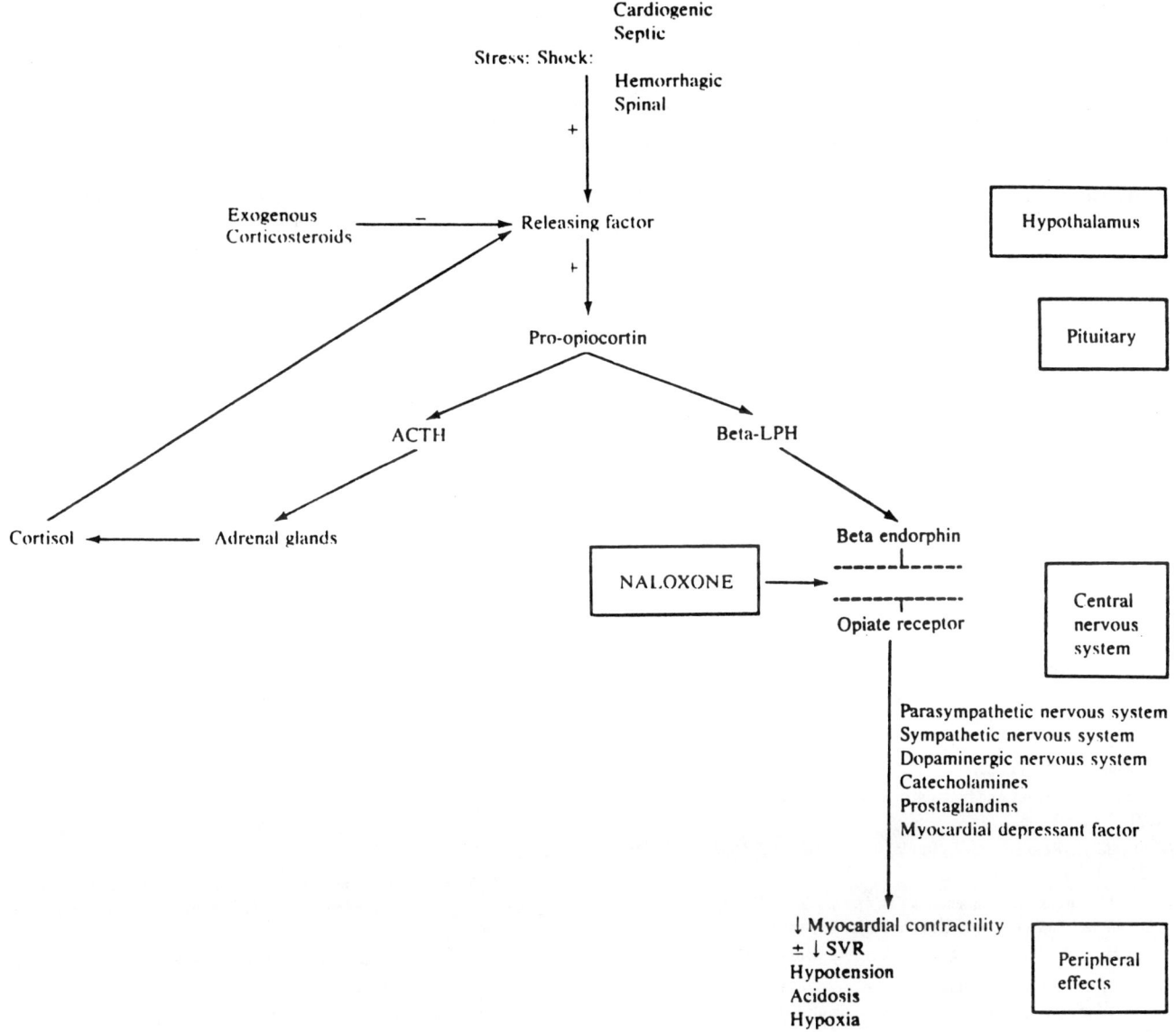

Figure 6-15 Mechanism of naloxone in shock. *ACTH*, adrenocorticotropic hormone; β = *LPH*; *SVR*, systemic vascular resistance. Reprinted with permission from Chen HL: Naloxone in shock. *Am J Emerg Med* 2(5):449, 1984.

solution in the adult or 0.1 mL/kg in the child). An epinephrine drip or additional blood pressure support with pressors such as dopamine may be necessary. Patients with severe or persistent anaphylaxis also should receive steroids (eg, hydrocortisone sodium succinate, 100 mg intravenously). Should outpatient management be chosen subsequently, several days of oral steroid therapy commonly follow.

Some consideration should be given to minimizing the extent of exposure, and, in the case of anaphylaxis provoked by Hymenoptera stings, the provision of a portable epinephrine self-administration kit as well as desensitization therapy. Most patients with severe anaphylaxis will, however, require hospitalization or a protracted period of emergency department observation.

BIBLIOGRAPHY

Abraham E, Smith M, Silver L. Conjunctival and transcutaneous oxygen monitoring during cardiac arrest and cardiopulmonary resuscitation. *Crit Care Med*. 1984;12:419–421.

Alcan KE, Stertzer SH, Walsh E, et al. Current status of intra-aortic balloon counterpulsation in critical care cardiology. *Crit Care Med*. 1984;12: 489–495.

Alexander RS. Venomotor tone in hemorrhage and shock. *Circ Res*. 1955;3:181.

Alonso DR. Pathophysiology of cardiogenic shock: quantification of myocardial necrosis, clinical pathologic and electrocardiographic correlations. *Circulation*. 1973;45:588.

Ayres SM. Mechanisms and consequences of pulmonary edema: cardiac lung, shock lung, and principles of ventilatory therapy in adult respiratory distress syndrome. *Am Heart J*. 1982;103:97–112.

Barach EM, Novak RM, Lee TG, et al. Epinephrine for treatment of anaphylactic shock. *JAMA*. 1984;251:2118–2122.

Bardet J, Masquet C, Kahn J, et al. Clinical and hemodynamic results of intraaortic balloon counterpulsation and surgery for cardiogenic shock. *Am Heart J*. 1977;93:280–288.

Barnard JH. Studies of 400 *Hymenoptera* sting deaths in the United States. *J Allergy Clin Immunol*. 1973;52:259.

Batalden DJ, Wickstrom PH, et al. Valve of the G-suit in patients with severe pelvic fracture. Controlling hemorrhagic shock. *Arch Surg*. 1974;109:326.

Bates RJ, Beutler S, Resnekov L, et al. Cardiac rupture challenge in diagnosis and management. *Am J Cardiol*. 1977;40:429–437.

Bave AE, Chandry IH, Worth MA, et al. Cellular alterations with shock and ischemia. *Angiology*. 1974;25:31–42.

Bergman GE, Reisner FF, Anwar RAH. Orthostatic changes in normovolemic children: An analysis of the tilt test. *J Emerg Med*. 1983;1:137–141.

Bivins HG, Knopp R, dos Santos PAL. Blood volume distribution in the Trendelenburg position. *Ann Emerg Med*. 1985;14:642–643.

Blalock A. Experimental shock: the cause of the low blood pressure produced by muscle injury. *Arch Surg*. 1930;20:959.

Bland JHL, Laver MB, Lowenstein E. Vasodilator effect of commercial 5% plasma protein fraction solution. *JAMA*. 1973;224:1721–1724.

Bounous G, McArdle AH, Hampson LG, et al. The cessation of intestinal mucus production as a pathogenic factor in irreversible shock. *Surg Forum*. 1965;16:11.

Boutros AR, Olson L, et al. Comparison of hemodynamic pulmonary and renal effects of use in three types of fluids after major surgical procedures on the abdominal aorta. *Crit Care Med*. 1979;7:9.

Braunwald E. Control of myocardial oxygen consumption: physiologic and clinical considerations. *Am J Cardiol*. 1970;27:588.

Braunwald E. Structure and function of the normal myocardium. *Br Heart J*. 1971;33(suppl):3–8.

Braunwald E. Regulation of circulation: I. *N Engl J Med*. 1974;290:1124–1129.

Braunwald E, Ross J Jr, Sonnenblick EH. *Mechanisms of Contraction of the Normal and Failing Heart*. Boston: Little, Brown; 1968.

Cannon WB. *Traumatic Shock*. New York: Appleton; 1923.

Carey CL, Lowery BD, Cloutier CT. *Hemorrhagic Shock. Current Problems in Surgery*. Chicago: Year Book Medical; 1971.

Cervera AL, Moss G. Dilutional reexpansion with crystalloid after massive hemorrhage: saline vs balanced electrolyte solutions for maintenance of normal blood volume and arterial pH. *J Trauma*. 1975;15:498.

Chen HL. Naloxone in shock and toxic coma. *Am J Emerg Med*. 1984;2:444–452.

Chisholm CD, Clark DE. Effect of the pneumatic antishock garment on intramuscular pressure. *Ann Emerg Med*. 1984;13:581–583.

Christy JH. Treatment of Gram negative shock. *Am J Med*. 1971;50:77.

Civetta JM, Nussenfeld SR. Prehospital use of military anti-shock trousers (MAST). *JACEP*. 1976;5:581.

Cloutier CT, Lowery BD, Carey LC. The effects of hemodilutional resuscitation on serum protein levels in humans in hemorrhagic shock. *J Trauma*. 1969;9:514.

Cohn JN. Blood pressure measurement in shock: mechanisms of inaccuracy in auscultatory and palpatory methods. *JAMA*. 1967;199:972.

Cohn JN. Shock. In: Hurst JW, ed. *The Heart*. New York: McGraw-Hill; 1978:716–726.

Cook JA, Wise WC, Butler RR, et al. The potential role of thromboxane, and prostacyclin in endotoxic and septic shock. *Am J Emerg Med*. 1984;2:28–37.

Cope O, Litwin SQ. Contribution of the lymphatic system to the replenishment of plasma volume following hemorrhage. *Ann Surg*. 1962;156:655.

Coram AG, Ballantine TV, et al. The effect of crystalloid resuscitation in hemorrhagic shock on acid-base balance: a comparison between normal saline and Ringer's lactate solutions. *Surgery*. 1971;69:874–880.

Craham AJP, Douglas DM. Effect of the head down position on the circulation in hypotensive states. *Lancet*. 1949;2:941.

Crile GW. *Blood Pressure in Surgery in Experimental and Clinical Research*. Philadelphia: JB Lippincott; 1903.

Crile GW, Lower WE. *Anoci-Association*. Philadelphia: Saunders; 1914.

Crowell JW, Houston B. The effect of acidity on blood coagulation. *Am J Physiol*. 1961;201:379.

Crowell JW. Cardiac deterioration as the cause of irreversibility in shock. In: Mills LC, Moyen JH, eds. *Shock and Hypotension. The 12th Hahnemann Symposium*. New York: Grune & Stratton; 1965.

Cutler BS, Daggett WM. Application of the G-suit to the control of hemorrhage in massive trauma. *Ann Surg*. 1971;173:511–514.

Cyres SM. The shock lung. In: *The Organ in Shock. Proceedings of the Second Symposium on Recent Research Developments and Current Clinical Practice in Shock*. 1977:24–32.

Dahn MS, Lucas CE. Negative inotropic effect of albumin resuscitation for shock. *Surgery*. 1979;86:235–241.

Da Luz PL, Weill MH, Shubin H. Current concepts on mechanisms and treatment of cardiogenic shock. *Am Heart J*. 1976;92:103–113.

Darling RC. Ruptured arteriosclerotic abdominal aortic aneurysms. *Am J Surg*. 1976;119:397–401.

Davis SM. Antishock trousers: a collective review. *J Emerg Med*. 1986;4:145–155.

DeMaria EJ, Reichman W, Kenney PR, et al. Septic complications of corticosteroid administration after central nervous system trauma. *Ann Surg*. 1985;202:248–252.

Dranen SC. Proximal saphenous vein cutdown. *Ann Emerg Med*. 1981;10:328–330.

Dronen SC, Maningas PA, Foutch R. Transcutaneous oxygen tension measurements during graded hemorrhage and reperfusion. *Ann Emerg Med*. 1985;14:534–539.

Duncan GW, Sarnoff SJ, Rhode CM. Studies on the effects of posture in shock and injury. *Ann Surg*. 1968;120:24.

Du Point HL, Spink WW. Infections due to Gram negative organisms: an analysis of 860 patients with bacteremia at the University of Minnesota Medical Center, 1958–1966. *Medicine*. 1969;48:307–332.

Eisenberg PR, Jaffe AS, Schuster DP. Clinical evaluation compared to pulmonary artery catheterization in the hemodynamic assessment of critically ill patients. *Crit Care Med*. 1984;12:549–553.

Espinoza MH, Updegrove JH. Clinical experience with the G-suit. *Ann Surg*. 1970;101:36–39.

Fletcher JR, Ramwell PW. *E coli* endotoxin shock in the baboon: treatment with lidocaine or indomethacin. *Adv Prostaglandin Thromboxane Res*. 1978;3:183–192.

Gann DS, Lilly MP. The endocrine response to injury. *Prog Crit Care Med*. 1984;1:15–47.

Geyer RF. Fluorocarbon-polyol artificial blood substitutes. *N Engl J Med*. 1973;289:1077–1082.

Goldenheim PD, Kazemi H. Cardiopulmonary monitoring of critically ill patients: I. *N Engl J Med*. 1984;311:717–720.

Goldenheim PD, Hazemi H. Cardiopulmonary monitoring of critically ill patients: II. *N Engl J Med*. 1984;311:776–780.

Grasswood WD, Pandey N, Jensen CG, et al. Pulmonary changes in treated hemorrhagic shock. *Am J Surg*. 1972;124:738–743.

Gross SD; cited by Mann FC. System of surgery, 1850. *Bull Johns Hopkins Hosp.* 1914;25:205.

Gunnar RM, Loeb HS, Winslow EJ, et al. Hemodynamic measurements in bacteremia and septic shock in man. *J Infect Dis.* 1973;128 (suppl): 5295–5298.

Gunnar, WP, Merlotti GJ, Jonasson O, et al. Resuscitation from hemorrhagic shock: alterations of the intracranial pressure after normal saline, 3% saline and dextran-40. *Ann Surg.* 1986;204:686–692.

Guyton AC, Jones CE, eds. *Physiology Series One: Cardiovascular Physiology.* Baltimore: Butterworth and University Park Press; 1974.

Haller JA, Ward MJ, Cahill JI. Metabolic alterations in shock: the effect of controlled reduction of blood flow on oxidative metabolism and catecholamine response. *J Trauma.* 1967;7:727.

Hansbrough JF, Cain TL, Millikan JS. Placement of a 10-gauge catheter by cutdown for rapid fluid replacement. *J Trauma.* 1983;23:231.

Hardaway RM. *Syndromes of Disseminated Intravascular Coagulation: With Special Reference to Shock and Hemorrhages.* Springfield, IL: Thomas; 1966.

Hardaway RM, James PM, et al. Intensive study of shock in man. *JAMA.* 1967;199:779–790.

Hartong JM, Dixon RS. Monitoring resuscitation of the injured patient. *JAMA.* 1977;237:242–244.

Hayes DF, Weiner MH, Rosenberg IK, et al. Effects of traumatic hypovolemic shock on renal function. *J Surg Res.* 1974;16:490.

Heinonen J, Takki S, Tammisto T. Effect of the Trendelenburg tilt and other procedures on the position of endotracheal tubes. *Lancet.* 1969;1:850.

Heistad DD, Abboud FM. Circulatory adjustments to hypoxia. *Circulation.* 1980;61:463–470.

Henderson Y. Acapnia and shock. *Am J Physiol.* 1909;24:66.

Holaday JW, Faden AI. Naloxone reversal of endotoxin hypotension suggests role of endorphins in shock. *Nature.* 1978;275:450–451.

Holcroft JW, Trunkey DD. Pathophysiology of shock and adult respiratory distress syndrome. *Surg Annu.* 1983;15:1–12.

Iserson KV. Whole blood in trauma resuscitations. *Am J Emerg Med.* 1985;3:358–359.

James PN, Myers RT. Central venous pressure monitoring: misinterpretation, abuses, indications, and a new technique. *Ann Surg.* 1971;175:693–701.

Jelenko C III, Wheeler ML, et al. Shock and resuscitation: II. Volume repletion with minimal edema using the "halfed" method. *JACEP.* 1978;7:326–333.

Jelenko C, Williams JB, et al. Studies in shock and resuscitation: I. Use of a hypertonic albumin containing demand regimen (HALFD) in resuscitation. *Crit Care Med.* 1979;7:157–167.

Kafrouni G. Intraaortic balloon counterpulsation. *Am J Surg.* 1984;147:731–734.

Kaplan BC, Civetta JM, Nagel EL, et al. The military anti-shock trousers in civilian prehospital emergency care. *J Trauma.* 1973;13:843–848.

Knopp R, Dailey R. Central venous cannulation and pressure monitoring. *JACEP.* 1977;6:358–366.

Kuhn LA. Management of shock following acute myocardial infarction: I. Drug therapy. *Am Heart J.* 1978;95:529–534.

Kuhn LA. Management of shock following acute myocardial infarction: II. Mechanical circulatory assistance. *Am Heart J.* 1978;95:789–795.

Lefer AM. Role of a myocardial depressant factor in the pathogenesis of hemorrhagic shock. *Fed Proc.* 1970;29:1836.

Lefer AM, Martin J. Relationship of plasma peptides to the depressant factors in hemorrhage. *Circ Res.* 1970;26:59.

Lefime AA. Results and complications of intra-aortic balloon pumping in surgical and medical patients. *Am J Cardiol.* 1977;40:416.

LeJemtel TH, Keung E, Ribner SH, et al. Sustained beneficial effects of oral amrinone on cardiac and renal function in patients with severe congestive failure. *Am J Cardiol.* 1980;45:123.

Lewis DG, McKenzie A, McNeil LF. The use of the G-suit in the control of bleeding arising from hypocoagulation. *Ann R Coll Surg Engl.* 1973;52:53.

Libby P, Maroko PR, Bloor CM, et al. Reduction of experimental myocardial infarct size by corticosteroids administration. *J Clin Invest.* 1973;52:599–607.

Lister J, McNeill IF, Marshall VC, et al. Transcapillary refilling after hemorrhage in normal man. Basal rates and volumes; effects of norepinephrine. *Ann Surg.* 1963;158:698–712.

Lowe RJ, Moss GS, et al. Crystalloid vs colloid in the etiology of pulmonary failure after trauma—a randomized trial in man. *Crit Care Med.* 1979;7:107–112.

Lucas CE, Ledgerwood AM. The fluid problem in the critically ill. *Surg Clin North Am.* 1983;63:439–454.

Lucas CE, Ledgerwood AM, et al. Impaired pulmonary function after albumin resuscitation from shock. *J Trauma.* 1980;20:446–451.

Lucas CE, Weaver DW, Higgins RP, et al. Effects of albumin versus non albumin resuscitation on plasma volume and renal excretory function. *J Trauma.* 1979;18:564–570.

Luce JM. Pathogenesis and management of septic shock. *Chest.* 1987;91:883–888.

Luz PL, Shubin H, Iveil MH, et al. Pulmonary edema related to changes in colloid osmotic and pulmonary artery wedge pressure in patients after acute myocardial infarction. *Circulation.* 1975;51:350–357.

Mackersie RC, Christensen JM, Lewis FR. The prehospital use of external counter pressure: does MAST make a difference? *J Trauma.* 1984;24:882–888.

Mateer JR, Thompson BM, Aprahamiam C, et al. Rapid fluid resuscitation with central venous catheters. *Ann Emerg Med.* 1983;12:149–152.

Maull KI. Pneumatic anti-shock garment: risks and rewards. *J Arkansas Med Soc.* 1985;82:182–186.

Maull KI, Capehart JE, Cardea JA, et al. Limb loss following military anti-shock trousers (MAST) application. *J Trauma.* 1981;21:60–62.

McCue JD. Gram-negative bacillary bacteremia in the elderly: incidence, ecology, etiology, and mortality. *J Am Geriatr Soc.* 1987;35:213–218.

McSwain NE. Pneumatic trousers and the management of shock. *J Trauma.* 1977;17:719–724.

Miller RD. Complications of massive blood transfusions. *Anesthesiology.* 1973;39:82–92.

Millikan JS, Cain TL, Hansbrough J. Rapid volume replacement for hypovolemic shock: a comparison of techniques and equipment. *J Trauma.* 1984;24:428–431.

Moore FD. *Metabolic Care of the Surgical Patient.* Philadelphia: Saunders; 160.

Moore FD, Daher FD, et al. Hemorrhage in normal man: I. Distribution and dispersal of saline infusion following acute blood loss, clinical kinetics of blood volume support. *Ann Surg.* 1966;163:485–504.

Moran DM, Larsen KR, Russo J, et al. An evaluation of naloxone as a gastric cytoprotective agent during hemorrhagic shock. *J Trauma.* 1984;24:728–730.

Moss GS, Salletta JD. Traumatic shock in man. *N Engl J Med.* 1974;290:724–725.

Mudth ED. Mechanical and surgical interventions for the reduction of myocardial ischaemia. *Circulation.* 1976;53:176.

Mueller H. Effects of isoproterenol, L-norepinephrine and intra-aortic counterpulsation on hemodynamics and myocardial metabolism in shock following acute myocardial infarction. *Circulation.* 1972;45:335.

Mueller U, Ayres SM, Gregory JJ, et al. Hemodynamics of coronary blood flow and myocardial metabolism in coronary shock: response to L-norepinephrine and isoproterenol. *J Clin Invest.* 1970;49:1855–1902.

Nicholson DP. Review of corticosteroid treatment in sepsis and septic shock: pro or con. *Crit Care Clin.* 1989;5:151–155.

Nishijima H, Weil MH, Shubin H, et al. Hemodynamic and metabolic studies on shock associated with gram negative bacteremia. *Medicine.* 1973;52:287–294.

Oettinger W, Berger D, Beger HG. The clinical significance of prostaglandins and thromboxane as mediators of septic shock. *Klin Wochenschr.* 1987;65:61–68.

Oettinger W, Peskar BA, Beger HG. Profiles of endogenous prostaglandin E_2 alpha, thromboxane A_2 and prostacyclin with regard to cardiovascular and organ functions in early septic shock in man. *Eur Surg Res.* 1987;19:65–77.

O'Rourke MF. Acute severe cardiac failure complicating myocardial infarction. *Br Heart J.* 1975;37:169.

Page DL. Myocardial changes associated with cardiogenic shock. *N Engl J Med.* 1971;285:133.

Parker MM, Parillo JE. Septic shock: hemodynamics and pathogenesis. *JAMA.* 1983;250:3325.

Parker MM, Shelhamer JH, Natanson C, et al. Serial cardiovascular variables in survivors and nonsurvivors of human septic shock: heart rate as an early predictor of prognosis. *Crit Care Med.* 1987;15:923–929.

Pelligra R, Sandbeig FC. Control of intractable abdominal bleeding by external counterpressure. *JAMA.* 1979;241:708.

Pepe PE, Bass RR, Mattox KL. Clinical trials of the pneumatic antishock garment in the urban prehospital setting. *Ann Emerg Med.* 1986;15:1407–1410.

Phillips TF, Soulier G, Wilson RF. Outcome of massive transfusion exceeding two blood volumes in trauma and emergency surgery. *J Trauma.* 1987;27:903–909.

Rackow EC, Fein IA, Leppo S. Colloid osmotic pressure as a prognostic indicator of pulmonary edema and mortality in the critically ill. *Chest.* 1977;72:709–713.

Ransom K, McSwain NE. Respiratory function following application of MAST trousers. *JACEP.* 1978;7:15–17.

Ratshin RA. Hemodynamic evaluation of left ventricular function in shock complicating myocardial infarction. *Circulation.* 1972;45:127.

Reed JH Jr, Wood EH. Effect of body position on vertical distribution of pulmonary blood flow. *J Appl Physiol.* 1970;218:303.

Rimailho A, Lampl E, Riou B, et al. Enterococcal bacteremia in a medical intensive care unit. *Crit Care Med.* 1988;16:126–129.

Risk C, Rudo N, et al. Comparison of right atrial and pulmonary capillary wedge pressures. *Crit Care Med.* 1978;6:172–175.

Rock P, Silverman H, Plump D, et al. Efficacy and safety of naloxone in septic shock. *Crit Care Med.* 1985;13:28–33.

Rutherford RB, Buerk CA. *The Pathophysiology of Trauma and Shock in the Management of Trauma.* 3rd ed. Philadelphia: Saunders; 1979:38–79.

Salisbury PF. Acute ischaemia of inner layers of ventricular wall. *Am Heart J.* 1963;66:650.

Sarnoff SJ. Insufficient coronary flow and myocardial failure as a complicating factor in late hemorrhagic shock. *Am J Physiol.* 1954;176:439.

Scheidt S. Intra-aortic balloon counterpulsation in cardiogenic shock. Report of a cooperative clinical trial. *N Engl J Med.* 1973;288:979.

Schein RMH, Bergman R, Marcial EH, et al. Complement activation and corticosteroid therapy in the development of the adult respiration distress syndrome. *Chest.* 1987;91:850–854.

Schwab CW, Shayne JP, Turner J. Immediate trauma resuscitation with type O uncrossmatched blood: a two-year prospective experience. *J Trauma.* 1986;26:897–902.

Schwartz RA, Cerra FB. Shock: a practical approach. *Urol Clin North Am.* 1983;10:89–100.

Shenasky JH, Gillenwater JY. The renal hemodynamic and functional effects of external counterpressure. *Surg Gynecol Obstet.* 1972;134:253–258.

Shine KI. Aspects of the management of shock. *Ann Intern Med.* 1980;93:723–734.

Shires TG. Management of hypovolemic shock. *Bull NY Acad Med.* 1979;55:139–148.

Shoemaker WC. Pathophysiological basis of therapy for shock and trauma syndromes: use of sequential cardiorespiratory measurements to describe natural histories and evaluate possible mechanisms. *Semin Drug Treat.* 1973;3:211–229.

Shoemaker WC, Carl JH. Critique of crystalloid vs colloid therapy in shock and shock lung. *Crit Care Med.* 1979;7:117–124.

Shubin H, Weil WH. Bacterial shock. *JAMA.* 1976;235:421–424.

Shumer W. The microcirculatory and metabolic effects of dibenziline in oligemic shock. *Surg Gynecol Obstet.* 1966;123:787–791.

Shumer W. Pathophysiology and treatment of septic shock. *Am J Emerg Med.* 1984;2:74–77.

Shumer W. Steroids in the treatment of clinical septic shock. *Ann Surg.* 1976;184:333–341.

Shumer W. Septic shock. *JAMA.* 1979;242:1906–1907.

Shumer W, Sperlung R. Shock and its effect on the cell. *JAMA.* 1968;205:75–79.

Sibbald WJ, Patterson NA, Holliday RL, et al. The Trendelenburg position: hemodynamic effects in hypotensive and normotensive patients. *Crit Care Med.* 1979;7:218–224.

Solen J, Muellen HA, Kennedy TJ. Clinical use of the G-suit. *JACEP.* 1976;5:609–611.

Starling EH. On the absorption of fluids from the connective tissue spaces. *J Physiol.* 1896;19:312.

Stein L. Pulmonary edema during volume infusion. *Circulation.* 1975;52:483–489.

Swan HJC. Catheterization of the heart in man with the use of a flow directed balloon tipped catheter. *N Engl J Med.* 1970;283:447.

Swank RL, Hissen W, Bergentz SF. 5-Hydroxytryptamine and aggregation of blood elements after trauma. *Surg Gynecol Obstet.* 1964;119:779.

Taylor J, Weil MH. Failure of the Trendelenburg position to improve circulation during clinical shock. *Ann Surg.* 1941;120:24.

Thompson WL. Rational use of albumin and plasma substitutes. *Johns Hopkins Med J.* 1975;136:220–225.

Timberlake GA, McSwain NE Jr. Autotransfusion of blood contaminated by enteric contents: a potentially life-saving measure in the massively hemorrhaging trauma patient? *J Trauma.* 1988;28:855–857.

Triedman E, Grable E, Fine J. Central venous pressure and direct serial measurements as gauges in blood volume replacement. *Lancet.* 1966;2:609–614.

Trunkey DD, Sheldon GF, Collins JA. The treatment of shock. In: Zuidema GD, Rutherford MD, Ballinger MD, eds. *The Management of Trauma.* Philadelphia: Saunders; 1979.

Valeri CR. Viability and function of preserved red cells. *N Engl J Med.* 1971;284:81.

Van Deventer SJH, Ten Cate JW, Buller HR, et al. Endotoxaemia: an early predictor of septicaemia in febrile patients. *Lancet.* 1988;1:605–608.

Wagensteen SL, De Hall JD, Ludewig RM, et al. The detrimental effects of the G-suit in hemorrhagic shock. *Ann Surg.* 1969;170:187–192.

Walt AJ, Wilson RF. *The Treatment of Shock.* Chicago: Year Book Medical; 1975.

Waxman K, Sadler R, Eisner ME, et al. Transcutaneous oxygen monitoring of emergency department patients. *Am J Surg.* 1983;146:35–37.

Wayne MA. The MAST suit in the treatment of cardiogenic shock. *JACEP*. 1978;7:107.

Wayne MA, Macdonald SC. Clinical evaluation of the antishock trouser: retrospective analysis of five years of experience. *Ann Emerg Med*. 1983;12:342.

Weber KT. Left ventricular dysfunction following acute myocardial infarction. *Am J Med*. 1973;54:697.

Weeden RJ, Cook JH, McElreath RL, et al. Wet lung syndrome after crystalloid and colloid repletion. *Curr Top Surg Res*. 1975;2:335.

Wei JY, Hutchins GM, Bulkley BH. Papillary muscle rupture in fatal acute myocardial infarction. *Ann Intern Med*. 1979;90:149–153.

Weidner MG, Albrecht M, Clowes GH. Relationship of myocardial function to survival after oligemic hypotension. *Surgery*. 1964;55:73.

Weil MH, Shubin H, Carlson R. Treatment of circulatory shock. Use of sympathomimetic vasoactive agents. *JAMA*. 1975;231:1280–1286.

Wilson RF. Acid base abnormalities in clinical shock. In: Schumer W, Nyhus LM, eds. *Treatment of Shock: Principles and Practice*. Philadelphia: Lea & Febiger; 1974:37–52.

Wilson RF, Christensen C, Le Blanc LP. Oxygen consumption in critically ill surgical patients. *Ann Surg*. 1971;174:801–804.

Wilson RF, Gibson D. The use of arterial central venous oxygen differences to calculate cardiac output and oxygen consumption in critically ill surgical patients. *Surgery*. 1978;83:362–369.

Wilson RF, Saruer E, Birks R. Central venous pressure and blood volume determination in clinical shock. *Surg Gynecol Obstet*. 1971;132:631–636.

Young LS, Stevens P, Ingram J. Functional role of antibody against core glycolipid or enterobacteriaceae. *J Clin Invest*. 1975;56:250–261.

Ziegler EJ, McCutchan JA, Brande AL. Clinical trial of core glycolipid antibody in Gram negative bacteremia. *Trans Assoc Am Physicians*. 1978;91:253–258.

7. Management of the Multisystem-Injured Patient

LENWORTH M. JACOBS, JR., MD, MPH, FACS
BARBARA BENNETT JACOBS, RN, BSN, MPH
WILLIAM KANTOR, MD

The first systematic approach to the prehospital management of the multisystem-injured patient arose in early military conflicts. The initial management strategy was essentially to leave the casualties on the battlefield until the end of the hostilities, hours or perhaps days later, and then deal with those who were still alive. Severely injured extremities were generally managed by amputation without anesthesia, followed by cauterization of the stump to control hemorrhage. Infection was a common sequel to any injury, and the outcome of surgical intervention was frequently negative.

Baron Dominique J. Larrey, a surgeon in Napoleon's army, is credited with a major revolutionary change. With the use of horse-drawn wagons as ambulances, he had the injured retrieved during the course of battle and transported to field hospitals close to the battlefield. Although the surgical principles remained rudimentary, the concept of triage, the sorting of injured patients by medically trained personnel into groups of patients with similar medical care needs, was born. Those soldiers who were so severely injured that they were unlikely to survive were made comfortable; those who had sustained only minor injuries were treated and sent back into battle; and those who would benefit most were managed by surgical treatment in the field hospital.

The mortality rate in World War I was 8.2%, and it took many hours for injured soldiers to arrive at a location where they could receive definitive care. In World War II, the mortality rate decreased to 5.8%; the length of time from injury to definitive care also decreased. In Korea, the mortality rate was 2.4%, and the rate in Vietnam was less than 1.7%.[1]

A number of factors contributed to this decrease in the mortality rate: modern surgical techniques, effective anesthesia, a better understanding of the importance of nutrition, and the advent of antibiotics. The most important advance, however, was the recognition that trauma is a time-related disease. The more quickly hemorrhage is controlled and definitive management initiated, the better the outcome. Rapid evacuation by helicopter of severely injured patients and prompt transport—with care provided en route by trained corpsmen—to a definitive surgical hospital where well-trained trauma surgeons were immediately available were standard procedures in Vietnam. The average time from injury to definitive care was 80 minutes.

These principles have been adapted for daily use in civilian prehospital trauma care, as trauma is a national epidemic. In 1989, 150,869 people died from trauma in the United States. Trauma is the fourth leading cause of death for all Americans, with a mortality rate of 61 deaths per 100,000 population. It is the leading cause of death for Americans under the age of 44. It kills more American children than do all other causes combined.[2] The health care system's response to this epidemic was initiated in 1973 when Congress passed the Emergency Medical Services (EMS) Act. Congress appropriated federal monies for EMS regions to plan for and implement systems that, through a central communications network, coordinate prehospital care with designated hospital facilities. As a result, ground and air ambulance personnel (ie, emergency medical technicians [EMTs], paramedics, and nurses) now staff well-equipped ambulances and are uniformly trained in basic and/or advanced life support skills.

Across most of the United States, the standard procedures for prehospital emergency stabilization and resuscitation are based on the curriculum developed for EMTs, the standards for advanced cardiac life support developed by the American Heart Association,[3] and the standards for advanced trauma life support developed by the Committee on Trauma of the American College of Surgeons.[4] Furthermore, ambulance personnel often bypass local hospitals in order to transport patients to fully certified trauma centers that have emergency physicians, trauma surgeons, neurosurgeons, orthopedic surgeons, anesthesiologists, radiologists, computed tomography (CT) scanners, and blood banks immediately available. There is a continuing need for data and well-designed studies to document the impact and effectiveness of these systems on the mortality and morbidity of trauma patients.

A plan for the initial evaluation and emergency management of the trauma patient is essential. The definitive place for the management of major abdominal or thoracic hemorrhage, as well as many neurosurgical or orthopedic problems, is the operating room in a tertiary care hospital. For this reason, the goal of prehospital care is to transport the patient as rapidly as possible to the trauma center. The appropriate prehospital assessment and interventions should be performed on site, but any further interventions should take place while en route to the hospital. In essence, the minimum amount of time that is necessary should be spent in the prehospital setting.

The field management of the trauma patient consists of clearing and controlling the airway, ensuring adequate ventilation, and protecting the cervical spine. Obvious external hemorrhage should be controlled, a pneumatic antishock garment (PASG) placed when indicated, and suspected fractures splinted. If it does not delay transportation, a large-bore intravenous line should be established and volume resuscitation initiated. A study by Pons et al[5] demonstrated that field personnel can initiate an intravenous line as quickly as hospital personnel. It was stated that to be effective large-bore lines should be used and that the bags should be pressurized.[1] There is no indication for prolonged field efforts to stabilize the trauma patient who is in hemorrhagic shock, however. It has been suggested that some prehospital EMTs and paramedics take too long in the field to stabilize patients,[6] although both the Advanced Trauma Life Support course and the Prehospital Trauma Life Support course stress the need for early, rapid transport to a trauma care hospital.

A systematic approach to the prehospital management of the trauma patient hinges on a primary survey and a secondary survey. The primary survey focuses on life-threatening conditions that affect the airway and methods to clear the airway immediately. Once the airway is clear, any anatomical or physiologic compromise that limits ventilation must be identified and corrected. Any external hemorrhage should be controlled with primary pressure. The cervical spine must be assessed and protected during the primary survey. The secondary survey is a comprehensive head-to-toe examination to identify any other injuries.

Providers must have a number of cognitive and manipulative skills for the prehospital management of the trauma victim. Contemporary EMS systems have broadened the scope of advanced life support activities for which prehospital care providers are responsible, and they now use a wide range of noninvasive and invasive techniques (Table 7-1).

Table 7-1 Basic and Advanced Skills and Procedures*

	Basic Skill	Advanced Skill
Airway	Head tilt, neck lift Head tilt, chin lift Jaw thrust maneuver Oropharyngeal airway suction	Endotracheal intubation Nasotracheal intubation Cricothyroidotomy Esophageal obturator airway
Breathing	Artificial ventilation Bag-mask ventilation Manually triggered positive pressure oxygen administration	Bag-tube ventilation Needle decompression for tension pneumothorax
Circulation	Trendelenburg position Hemorrhage control	Pneumatic antishock garment (PASG) Intravenous fluids Cardiotonic drugs
Cervical spine injuries	Rigid cervical collars Short and long spinal boards	Gardner-Wells tongs (recommend to be inserted by trained flight nurses) Intravenous fluids in neurogenic shock
Head injuries	Oropharyngeal airway Oxygen administration	Endotracheal intubation Establishment of intravenous access
Abdominal injuries	Oropharyngeal airway Oxygen administration External hemorrhage control	Intravenous fluids PASG Nasogastric intubation
Skeletal injuries	Appendicular splinting: rigid, inflatable, or soft splints	Intravenous fluids, if necessary
Soft tissue injuries	Hemorrhage control	Intravenous fluids, if necessary

*The basic skills and procedures must be used by both basic and advanced personnel.

PRIMARY SURVEY

Restoring an adequate airway, assisting ventilation, and restoring circulation are the basic goals of all resuscitative efforts.[7] Airway control and prompt initiation of resuscitative efforts have been linked to an improved survival rate for patients who have experienced out-of-hospital cardiac arrests.[8]

Similarly, the survival of trauma patients is dependent on restoration of mechanical ventilation and subsequent diffusion and exchange of oxygen and CO_2 across the alveolar capillary membrane. The key to survival is to maintain perfusion of the tissues by oxygenated, circulating blood. Perfusion cannot occur, however, without restoration of ventilation and diffusion of gases.

Airway

A trauma patient's first need is a clear airway. The oropharynx must be cleared of any foreign materials, such as broken teeth, mucus, or blood. Frequently, the trauma patient is confused or combative because of cerebral hypoxia or ingestion of alcohol. To avoid injury to the examining finger, the examiner should pass it along the lateral aspect of the patient's teeth; the finger should enter the oropharynx at the angle of the mandible and then be swept forward to clear the oropharynx.

The airway is opened with a jaw thrust maneuver that is designed to protect the cervical spine by avoiding hyperextension. Lifting the angle of the mandible forward lifts the posterior tongue and glottis anteriorly. Air then passes freely into the oropharynx through the vocal cords into the tracheobronchial tree. In a patient who is unconscious or whose sensorium is severely compromised, this position must be maintained manually until invasive definitive airway control can be instituted. It may be necessary to insert an oropharyngeal airway and assist ventilation by bag-mask or portable manually triggered oxygen resuscitator. The patient remains at risk for aspiration of gastric contents. If a cervical injury is suspected, the cervical spine must be immobilized with a rigid cervical collar and spinal board in order to protect against aggravating or precipitating a spinal cord injury.

Airway Adjuncts

A number of devices may be used to achieve the vital functions of respiration and ventilation. These devices include the oropharyngeal airway, endotracheal tube, nasotracheal tube, esophageal obturator airway, esophageal gastric tube airway, and pharyngeal-tracheal lumen airway. In the patient who is not breathing or who requires assisted ventilation, none of these devices function without the use of mechanical breathing attachments, such as bag-mask valve units or a manually triggered ventilator. It is desirable for such equipment to be lightweight, easily carried, simple to use, relatively inexpensive, easy to maintain and clean, adaptable to other equipment, and accepted by local or regional medical control protocols.

Bag-Mask Units. Masks that fit over the patient's nose and mouth are essential devices during resuscitation. They must be transparent to permit the detection of any vomitus. In order to prevent air leaks, the mask must fit the contours of the patient's face. Certain criteria are essential for a bag-mask unit:

- The unit should have an inlet for oxygen and a standard 15- to 22-mm coupling size.
- The bag component of the unit should be self-refilling, easy to clean and disinfect, and capable of delivering 95% to 100% oxygen.
- Pediatric-sized bags should have nonrebreathing and pop-off valves.
- The unit should maintain its compliance in varying temperatures and humidity conditions.

A nonaspirating expiratory valve with 360° swivel exhalation port is also a helpful feature to have on these units.

Stewart and his colleagues studied the efficacy of the SEALEASY Mask, the Laerdal Mask, and the Robertshaw Mask.[9] They found that the SEALEASY, which has a balloon fitted over a Guedel modified airway, delivers higher volumes of oxygen than does the Laerdal Mask. It also allows fewer mask leaks than do other types of masks. A major disadvantage of all these units is that they force air into the esophagus, resulting in reflux of gastric contents with the potential for aspiration. Operators must be trained in the use of these units to maintain a tight face seal and to position the patient's head and neck in a way that prevents this complication.

Oropharyngeal and Nasopharyngeal Airways. Designed to support the tongue anteriorly, the oropharyngeal airway alleviates the most common cause of upper airway obstruction—the posterior displacement of the tongue.[10] If the airway is too small or if the distal aspect of the airway does not lie posteriorly in the oropharynx, however, the oropharyngeal airway may displace the tongue posteriorly. Similarly, if the airway is too large, the epiglottis may be maneuvered into a closed position, which obstructs the trachea.

A nasopharyngeal airway is a useful device if the tongue is swollen, the patient's teeth are loose, or it is impossible to open the jaws adequately. The nasopharyngeal airway is usually made of soft rubber. It must be inserted gently, as vigorous and forceful placement through the nares can cause epistaxis. The nasopharyngeal airway allows air to bypass the tongue and is better tolerated by patients who are not totally unresponsive, because it does not generate a gag reflex.

Occasionally, an oropharyngeal airway and a nasopharyngeal airway are used simultaneously to maintain a patent airway. An advantage of both these airways is that

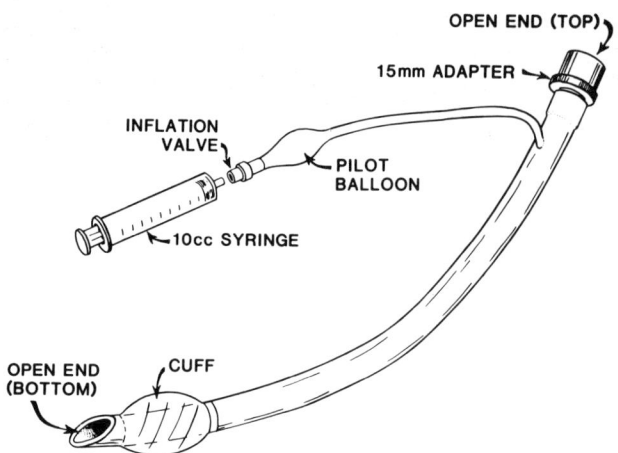

Figure 7-1 Endotracheal tube. *Source:* Reprinted from Lynch J, Bennett B: A review of airway devices. *Emergency Care Quarterly* 1(4):54, 1986.

---

personnel require minimal training to perfect the insertion technique; they can insert the tube without direct radio communication with a medical control physician. Furthermore, once this skill has been mastered, it rarely decays, even if it is not frequently used.

Endotracheal Tube. If the patient does not have a gag reflex or is in actual or imminent respiratory arrest, endotracheal intubation is an effective, definitive way to manage the airway (Fig. 7-1). Personnel require extensive training before they can insert the device, however.[11] Training requires classroom instruction and actual clinical experience with professional supervision in an operating room, but not all EMS systems have the resources to provide this type of training. Exchange programs that allow trainees access to these resources at other facilities (eg, a teaching hospital) help to ensure that prehospital operators develop adequate psychomotor skills to insert invasive airway devices.

Prior to intubation, the patient must be adequately ventilated with a bag-mask valve device, preferably with 100 percent oxygen. A useful technique that can facilitate intubation is Sellick's maneuver. This is a technique designed to reduce the risk of gastric insufflation and gastric acid aspiration into the lungs during intubation or bag-mask ventilation. The method consists of applying pressure on the cricoid cartilage, which compresses the esophagus between the cricoid cartilage and the cervical vertebrae.[12,13] Although this method requires an assistant, it is learned easily and does not require a great deal of specialized skill on the part of the assistant. Sellick demonstrated this method to be efficacious in preventing gastric distension and regurgitation during positive-pressure ventilation applied by face piece or mouth-to-mouth respiration and during induction of anesthesia. A lighted laryngoscope is attached to either a straight or curved blade. The blade determines the method used to pass the endotracheal tube between the vocal cords. The straight blade is designed to lift the epiglottis from beneath, whereas the curved blade is designed to lift the epiglottis by insertion of its tip into the vallecula. It is generally thought that the curved blade technique is less likely to activate pharyngeal reflexes. For infants, the straight blade technique is preferred because of the length and pliability of an infant's epiglottis.

Blades are available in several shapes and sizes. The Wisforreger straight blade has a large flange. The Miller blade has a minimal flange and a slight distal curve. The Phillips straight blade incorporates the flange of the Wisforreger blade with the curve of the Miller blade. The Phillips blade is generally easier to use. All operators should develop manual dexterity with all blades so that they can use the blade most appropriate for each individual patient.

A malleable stylet is a useful adjunct, because it maintains the shape of the endotracheal tube for difficult field intubations. It is also used to displace the tip of the endotracheal tube anteriorly for a more anteriorly placed trachea. A Magill forceps may be used during insertion of a nasotracheal tube to help lift the distal aspect of the tube into the larynx; it may also be used to extract a foreign body from the pharynx.

A lighted stylet within an endotracheal tube has been used for blind intubation.[14] The technique has advantages, especially for patients with a potential cervical spine fracture; a basal skull fracture, or leakage of cerebrospinal fluid from the nares, because it requires neither flexion of the neck nor hyperextension of the head. The stylet is lubricated and inserted through a standard endotracheal tube that has been cut to 25 cm; both are bent at an angle slightly greater than 90°. The tongue or the tongue and jaw are displaced forward after preoxygenation. The tube and stylet are gently guided along the posterior aspect of the tongue in order to elevate the epiglottis and expose the glottic opening. The operator need not stand at the head of the patient. In fact, the operator stands looking at the patient's face and inserts the tube blindly, using the fingers to guide the tube. Every effort must be made to ensure that the tube is not in the esophagus, because the vocal cords are not actually visualized. This particular method is useful in gaining control of the trachea in cramped quarters.

Proper positioning of the tip of a tube blindly inserted in this way is indicated by transillumination; the tip of the lighted stylet should be seen in the midline level of the laryngeal prominence. If the light appears at the right or left of the prominence, it is situated in the piriform sinus. A glow in the submeatal region indicates that the stylet's tip is in the vallecula. Subdued light or no light at all suggests esophageal placement. When transillumination indicates that the endotracheal tube has been correctly placed, the tube is advanced carefully into the trachea. The lighted stylet is then removed. Factors that reduce transillumination and, therefore, may prevent successful intubation are obesity, vomitus, bright daylight, and very pale skin. In some cases, however, stylet transillumination results in prompt intubation when intubation by laryngoscopy has been unsuccessful.

Endotracheal tubes have been modified to aid in difficult intubations. For example, the flex-end or trigger tube has the usual endotracheal shape, but a wire permits anterior flexion of its tip. The wire is incorporated into the wall of the tube, thus eliminating the need for a stylet. The trigger is cut off after intubation to prevent inadvertent flexion and possible dislodging of the tube.[15]

In children under the age of 8 years, a noncuffed endotracheal tube is used. A guideline for the intubation of pediatric patients is that the outside diameter of the appropriately sized endotracheal tube corresponds to the size of the nail bed of the patient's little finger.

At the completion of the intubation, the operator must verify that the tube has passed through the vocal cords into the trachea. The left and right lung fields are auscultated to determine that both lungs are being ventilated. Appropriate anatomical locations for auscultation are the midclavicular line at the third intercostal space and the midaxillary line at the sixth intercostal space. If there are no breath sounds in the left hemithorax and adequate sounds in the right hemithorax, the tip of the endotracheal tube is probably in the right mainstem bronchus. The tube should be pulled back gently until it is located 2 cm above the carina and adequate breath sounds are heard in both the left and right hemithorax.

Next, placing the stethoscope over the patient's stomach, the operator listens for bubbling sounds with ventilation, a sign that the tube is in the esophagus. If so, the tube should be immediately removed and the patient ventilated with 100% oxygen via a bag-mask unit. The vocal cords should then be visualized with a laryngoscope and a second endotracheal tube inserted. The endotracheal tube should not be inserted if the vocal cords cannot be visualized unless specialized equipment is used.

Recent advances for the confirmation of endotracheal tube placement include end-tidal CO_2 detector devices. These have been shown to be effective for confirmation of endotracheal placement. MacCleod et al[16] showed that the device has an 88% sensitivity and an 86% specificity for confirmation of proper placement in all patients. In patients with a palpable pulse, the sensitivity increases to 100%. The intubations in this study were performed in emergency departments, helicopters, and prehospital ground environments. The personnel included emergency medicine physicians, flight nurses, and paramedics. The study concluded that FEF™ colorimetric detectors reliably detect intratracheal placement in the nonarrested patient.

Once the endotracheal tube is in the correct position within the trachea, the cuff is inflated and the tube secured in place. Endotracheal intubation has several major advantages: it affords complete control of the airway, protects the patient from aspiration of gastric contents, and is a conduit for delivery of 100% oxygen.

In a series of 178 patients in Boston, paramedics successfully inserted an endotracheal tube in 172 patients (96.6%).[17] Shea and colleagues reported an 86.7% intubation success rate that improved to 93.4% over 6 months.[18] Other high success rates have been reported.[19,20] Anatomic adversities (eg, a short neck or a fractured mandible) or the presence of vomitus or blood in and about the vocal cords can make endotracheal intubation impossible, however.

Complications occasionally follow endotracheal intubation.[21-23] LoCicero, for example, reported erosion of the trachea and adjacent carotid artery as a result of pressure from the distal end of the endotracheal tube, as well as mucosal damage from the cuff.[24] The patient, who had been intubated for 7 days, subsequently developed hemoptysis and died. Blanc and Tremblay introduced a system for classifying complications from tracheal intubations (Table 7-2).[25]

Table 7-2 Classification for Complications of Endotracheal Intubation

I. Incidents and accidents
   A. First period (during laryngoscopy and insertion of tube)
     1. Traumatic or mechanical complications
       Examples: tooth damage, perforation of esophagus, pyriform sinus
     2. Reflex complications
       a. Laryngovagal: bronchospasm, glottic spasm, bradycardia
       b. Laryngosympathetic: tachycardia, hypertension
       c. Laryngospinal: vomiting
   B. Second period (ETT in position)
     1. Traumatic or mechanical complications
       Examples: respiratory obstruction due to tube kinking, overinflated cuff, or collapsed tube; ruptured cuff; ruptured trachea
     2. Reflex complications (same as above)
     3. Drug-induced complications
       Examples: bronchospasm caused by chemicals in tube
   C. Third period (extubation)
     1. Traumatic or mechanical complications
       Examples: difficult extubations due to nondeflated cuff, large cuff, tube adhesion to tracheal wall
     2. Reflex complications (same as above)
     3. Drug-induced complications
       Examples: glottic edema due to sensitivity to local anesthetics

II. Sequelae to endotracheal intubation
   A. Sore jaw, throat
   B. Dysphagia
   C. Aphonia or dysphonia
   D. Nerve paresis
   E. Lip, mouth, pharynx, larynx ulcerations
   F. Infection
   G. Nasal stricture
   H. Glottic edema
   I. Cord paralysis
   J. Laryngeal granulomas, polyps, fibrosis, webs
   K. Tracheal stenosis

Source: Reprinted from Lynch J, Bennet B: A review of airway devices. *Emergency Care Quarterly* 1(4):61, 1986.

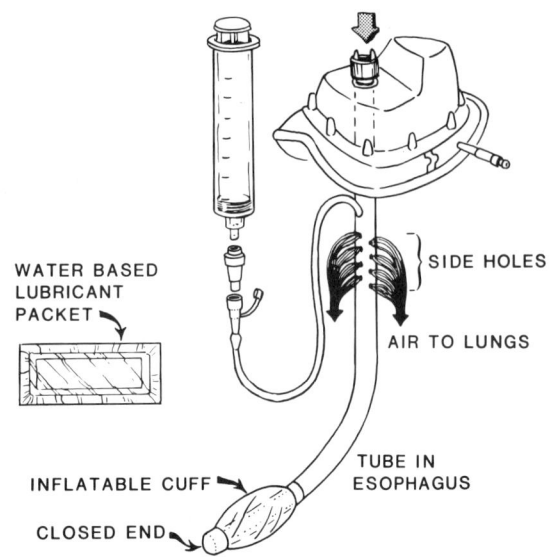

Figure 7-2 Esophageal obturator airway. *Source:* Reprinted from Lynch J, Bennett B: A review of airway devices. *Emergency Care Quarterly* 1(4):56, 1986.

Nasotracheal Tube. When there is a suspected cervical spine injury and immobility of the neck is mandatory, a nasotracheal tube is the definitive airway adjunct. Similarly, a nasotracheal tube is indicated if major trauma to the lower maxilla and mandible has rendered passage of an endotracheal tube technically impossible. It is contraindicated when there is a possible nasal fracture with an associated cerebrospinal fluid leak. Under these circumstances, the tube could be a conduit for ascending infection of the meninges and/or cerebrum, or an inept operator may pass the tube directly into the cranium.

The nasotracheal tube, after it has been lubricated, is inserted through the nares into the posterior oropharynx. The natural curve of the tube carries the tip anteriorly under the epiglottis. The tube should be advanced until it is just proximal to the vocal cords. This point can be identified by the hollow sound that can be heard at the proximal end of the tube as air passes over its distal tip. At the beginning of inspiration, when the vocal cords are maximally abducted, the tube is advanced into the trachea, again following the natural curve of the tube. The patient's head and nares must be aligned in the midline position to ensure that the tip of the tube will pass through the cords. The tube's position in the trachea is confirmed by auscultation over the lung fields.

If the patient is in complete respiratory arrest, it is more effective to use a laryngoscope and a Magill forceps to pass the nasotracheal tube directly between the cords, as there is no respiratory excursion to aid in the positioning of the tube.

Esophageal Obturator Airway. On the assumption that it is easier to pass a tube blindly into the esophagus than into the trachea, the esophageal obturator airway was introduced in 1968.[26] The esophageal obturator airway has been adopted for use in the prehospital arena because it is easy to insert, can be inserted by personnel with minimal training, and allows the patient's head to remain in a neutral position during insertion, thereby preventing manipulation of the cervical spine.

This device has a soft cuffed tube mounted through a face mask and modified with a soft plastic obturator that blocks the distal orifice (Fig. 7-2). The tube is deliberately inserted into the esophagus, and the cuff at the distal end of the obturator is then inflated to prevent pressurized oxygen from reaching the stomach and aspiration from reflux of gastric contents. There are several openings in the upper third of the tube at the level of the pharynx, and oxygen-enriched air administered through the tube passes through these openings into the trachea and lungs.

The esophageal obturator airway has been modified over the years to include a tube that passes down the length of the esophageal obturator into the stomach. The gastric tube, termed the esophageal gastric tube airway (Fig. 7-3), allows for decompression of the stomach.

In order to ensure proper placement of these airways, the operator must use the jaw lift maneuver and insert the tube blindly into the esophagus. Force should never be used; if there is resistance, the tube should not be inserted. Removal of the esophageal obturator airway is frequently followed by immediate regurgitation of stomach contents. For this reason, once the patient arrives in the emergency department, the physician should insert an endotracheal tube before removing the esophageal obturator airway.

A disadvantage of the esophageal obturator airway is that it may require two people to ventilate the patient adequately, one person to secure the mask in place and another to squeeze the bag.[11] Furthermore, numerous complications have been associated with this device: gastric rupture,[27] intubation of

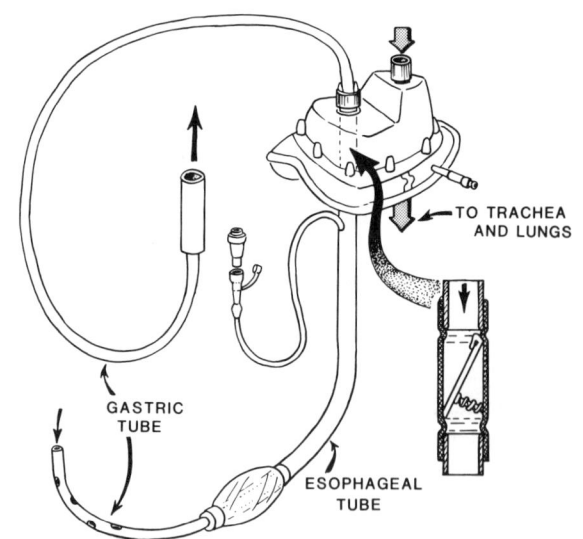

Figure 7-3 Esophageal gastric tube airway. *Source:* Reprinted from Lynch J, Bennett B: A review of airway devices. *Emergency Care Quarterly* 1(4):57, 1986.

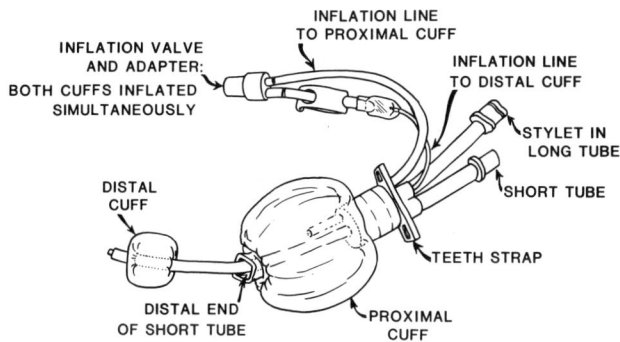

Figure 7-4 Pharyngeal tracheal lumen airway. *Source:* Reprinted from Lynch J, Bennett B: A review of airway devices. *Emergency Care Quarterly* 1(4):58, 1986.

the trachea,[28] kinking of the tube,[29] perforation of the esophagus,[30,31] and other trauma to the esophagus.[32]

Various authors have evaluated the use of the esophageal obturator airway versus the use of the endotracheal tube in the prehospital setting. After comparing the two devices, Meislin concluded that they are equally effective, but that the endotracheal tube is still the mainstay of ventilatory support.[33] These findings were questioned by White,[11] because the mean P_{CO_2} measures were elevated in 50% of Meislin's study sample.[33] Shea and associates[18] concluded that both airway devices could be used in the prehospital setting.

Pharyngeal-Tracheal Lumen Airway. Unlike the other airways, the pharyngeal-tracheal lumen airway has two parallel polyvinyl chloride tubes, each with an internal diameter of 8 mm (Fig. 7-4). One tube is 31 cm long, which prevents it from entering the right mainstem bronchus; the other tube is 21 cm long, which prevents it from occluding the epiglottis. The long tube functions like an endotracheal tube in the trachea. A large balloon cuff on the shorter tube is inflated in the mouth and pharynx to seal the upper airway. An obturator-stylet blocks the larger tube. If the long tube is in the esophagus, ventilation takes place through the short tube. If there are no signs of ventilation, the long tube is in the trachea. In this case, the obturator-stylet is removed, and ventilation takes place through the long tube.

The pharyngeal-tracheal lumen airway has two purported advantages over the esophageal obturator airway. One is that intubation of the trachea is desirable, although not absolutely mandatory; the second is that, if the long tube is in the esophagus, a face mask seal is not required. Although intellectually challenging, this airway is complex. A study by Frass et al[34] demonstrated the esophageal-tracheal combitube (ETC) to be a useful device in cardiopulmonary resuscitation (CPR) routine surgery and in the intensive care unit during mechanical ventilation. Insertion of the ETC was via the esophageal route in all 10 patients, but good to adequate oxygenation, levels of CO_2, and pH in both survivors and nonsurvivors were obtained.[34] It remains to be seen whether this device will be useful in the prehospital setting. Further investigations of this device are needed before it is widely accepted.

Cricothyrotomy

In some patients, it is necessary to perform a cricothyrotomy (ie, surgical incision of the membrane between the thyroid cartilage and the cricoid cartilage) in order to gain access to the airway. This procedure is life-saving in patients who have a fractured larynx with disruption and distortion of the glottis or a completely obstructed glottis secondary to burns or edema. It is a complex and technically difficult procedure in patients with severe facial trauma. It should be performed only by highly trained personnel who have perfected this skill on animals. In the prehospital setting, cricothyrotomy may be performed by physicians and/or nurses involved in emergency transport.

The first step in cricothyrotomy is to identify the thyroid cartilage and palpate the inferior border. The cricoid cartilage is the hard cartilaginous ring inferior to the thyroid cartilage. A horizontal or vertical incision is made over the cricothyroid membrane, which is between the two structures. Care must be taken not to extend the incision too far laterally, as this may lacerate the cricothyroid arteries, compounding respiratory distress with hemorrhage. The membrane is opened sharply, and the handle of the scalpel is inserted into the incision and turned 180°. A 4-mm or 5-mm tube is introduced into the trachea, and the patient is ventilated.

A relatively straightforward procedure for personnel who are accustomed to performing tracheotomies, cricothyrotomy can be an extremely difficult and hazardous procedure in a hypoxic combative patient with trauma to the upper airway. Once the emergency airway has been established and the patient is stable, a tracheotomy should be electively performed and the cricothyrotomy tube removed.

The complications of cricothyrotomy include misplacement of the tube behind the trachea instead of in it, subcutaneous emphysema, mediastinal infections, hemorrhage, and stricture.

Breathing

Once the airway has been opened and controlled, the patient's ventilatory status must be evaluated. The chest is observed for adequate and bilateral expansion. If the patient is failing to ventilate spontaneously, artificial ventilation is initiated. Respiratory compromise may require assisted ventilation with supplemental oxygen. Critical thoracic injuries that can significantly affect breathing are a tension pneumothorax, a flail chest, and open wounds.

Various devices are available for assisting the patient's ventilation in the prehospital setting. The standard anesthesia bag may be connected to the airway via a face mask or attached to an airway device to deliver air or oxygen-enriched air. The Ohio Hope II bag is a manual resuscitator capable of delivering oxygen at high flow rates. It consists of a self-refilling bag with an inlet valve for air or oxygen and a nonrebreathing valve for exhalation. Because most ventilator bags also have a reservoir into which oxygen flows after the bag is filled, the patient may intrain a higher percentage of oxygen on inspiration. The tidal volume is limited by the size of the bag, but it is influenced by the degree of compression exerted. The capacity of an adult bag is approximately 1100 to 1500 mL. The ventilatory rate, which is operator-dependent, may reach 40/min.[35] The operation of a ventilation bag requires two hands.

Thoracic Injuries That Cause Respiratory Compromise

Tension Pneumothorax. A deviated trachea, hyperresonance of the affected hemithorax with absent or diminished breath sounds, and, frequently, distention of the jugular veins suggest tension pneumothorax. This condition occurs when air leaks into the pleural space through an injury to the lung, becoming trapped in the pleural space and increasing intrapleural pressure. As more and more air is forced into this space, the affected lung is compressed and shifted to the unaffected side with subsequent mediastinal shift. As the mediastinum shifts, the inferior and superior vena cavae are kinked, which inhibits venous return to the right side of the heart. A decrease in venous return decreases cardiac output, systemic arterial pressure, and tissue perfusion.

Basic life support consists of maintaining a patent airway and assisting ventilation. Because the condition is an extreme emergency, the affected chest must be decompressed by needle thoracostomy or by closed tube thoracostomy.

A needle thoracostomy not only confirms the diagnosis of tension pneumothorax, but also initiates therapy. Most flight nurses are trained to perform this procedure. A 14-gauge needle is introduced into the affected hemithorax. There are two suitable anatomical locations. The first is the midclavicular line in the second or third intercostal space. This anterior location is safe, as there are no underlying structures that can be penetrated. In well-developed men, however, it may be difficult to pass the needle through the mass of the pectoralis major muscle into the chest. The second suitable location is the midaxillary line in the fifth or sixth intercostal space, 1 to 2 cm below the hairline in the axilla. The ribs are easy to palpate, and the muscle mass that must be penetrated prior to entering the chest is minimal.

Before the needle is introduced into the patient's chest, a finger condom or the fifth finger of a surgical glove is placed over its hub. The needle is then inserted at a 90° angle over the top of the rib to avoid the intercostal vessels underneath the rib. If the patient has a tension pneumothorax, the pressure within the chest is greater than the atmospheric pressure outside the chest and the condom or balloon inflates, confirming the diagnosis. The tension can be relieved by cutting a hole in the condom, allowing air to escape until the pressure inside the chest is equal to the pressure outside. The condom collapses to form a one-way valve. As the lung expands, the air is expelled from the intrapleural space. The needle should be removed before the lung is fully expanded.

The McSwain dart is a 16-French catheter with a central trocar and four expanding wings at its end. The dart is placed directly into the chest after a small skin incision has been made. The same anatomical locations are used. Once the dart is within the chest, the central trocar is removed and the wings allowed to expand within the chest cavity to hold the catheter in place. A one-way valve may be attached to the distal end of the tube, allowing air to escape from the chest cavity, but preventing the entry of air from outside the chest.[36]

The Heimlich valve is a small, plastic, one-way valve that may be attached to one end of the chest tube. Air passes into the plastic container, but is prevented from re-entering the chest cavity by a small rubber flutter valve. The device can be taped to the chest. This valve is light, portable, easy to use, and easy to secure in place; it requires no assembly or underwater seal. If there is an associated hemothorax, however, the blood obstructs the valve and renders it useless. This device is an elegant prehospital adjunct, because it allows the patient to be transported in the supine position without a delay for assembly of a complex underwater sealed system in the prehospital environment.

When the patient requires a closed tube thoracostomy, a large chest tube (32-French) should be prepared, along with a sterile thoracostomy tray and appropriate drainage-collecting apparatus. The lateral chest should be prepared in a sterile fashion and the anatomical entry site selected. An anatomical landmark for locating a site is a point 2 cm inferior to the point at which the axillary hair terminates in the midaxillary line. The skin and periosteum of the rib should be infiltrated with 1 percent lidocaine (Xylocaine). After a 2- to 3-cm incision has been made in the skin, a Kelly clamp is used to dissect bluntly over the top of the preselected rib and to puncture the pleura. A finger should be introduced to confirm that the thoracic cavity has been entered. The clamp is then used to occlude the proximal end of the chest tube, and the tube is inserted superiorly.

If a hemothorax is associated with the tension pneumothorax, extra holes should be cut in the chest tube to permit the free drainage of blood and blood clots. It may even be necessary to place a second chest tube through another incision. A second tube should be directed inferiorly and lie posteriorly on the diaphragm to ensure adequate drainage whether the patient is lying down or standing upright.

The tube should be connected to an underwater seal apparatus or a Pleurovac to confirm that it is correctly placed within the thoracic cavity. If the chest tube is clear plastic, it should fog up with respirations; in addition, the water seal level should fluctuate. If extra holes have been cut in the tube, the distance from the last hole to the tube's proximal end should be measured before the tube is placed in the chest. Once the tube is in place, at least 5 cm beyond the last hole in the tube must be lying within the chest cavity. A simple way to confirm this is to use a second chest tube for comparison. A clamp is placed on the second tube to indicate the position of the last hole in the inserted tube. The exact position of that hole can be gauged by placing the second tube on the chest beside the inserted tube and comparing the two. If no problems are discovered, the first tube should be sutured in place, the wound dressed, and a chest roentgenogram obtained to verify the position of the tube and determine whether the hemopneumothorax has been corrected.

A tension pneumothorax is an unusual occurrence in the prehospital setting. Therefore, it is critical for the medical control physician to be aware of the circumstances and to be involved in the decision-making process. Failure to diagnose tension pneumothorax can be life-threatening. Conversely, incorrectly diagnosing tension pneumothorax when it is not present can result in unnecessary invasive procedures that are also life-threatening.

Flail Chest. The condition in which two or more ribs are broken in two or more places in continuity is termed a flail chest. The involved segment of the chest wall loses continuity with the rest of the thoracic cage, which compromises the mechanics of ventilation. On normal inspiration, the diaphragm contracts and flattens, and the chest increases in diameter, creating a negative intrathoracic pressure and allowing air to flow through the airway into the lungs. The flail segment is pulled inward, however, resulting in paradoxical movement and little or no ventilation of the affected lung. Because the creation of a flail segment requires a great deal of force, a flail chest is usually accompanied by a significant lung contusion. Furthermore, a pneumothorax may occur if a sharp fragment of broken rib lacerates the lung. The intercostal vessels may also be lacerated, resulting in a hemothorax.

The diagnosis is suggested by the inappropriate movement of the flail segment, together with signs of dyspnea, tachypnea, or pain. The diagnosis is confirmed by palpation of the affected hemithorax. Bony crepitus and, usually, pneumocrepitus can be recognized. If pneumocrepitus is present, the patient has an associated pneumothorax.

The flail segment should be splinted with a sandbag or rolled towel. If the segment is in the axillary line, the arm on the affected side should be secured to the chest to prevent the paradoxical movement. The patient requires assisted ventilation with 100% oxygen. If the patient's condition is deteriorating, endotracheal intubation may be necessary so that positive pressure ventilation with 100% oxygen can be used. The patient should be hyperventilated to produce hypocapnia, because this removes the patient's endogenous drive to breathe and allows the patient to tolerate the endotracheal tube more easily. If a hemothorax is present, the patient requires a closed tube thoracostomy in an ED.

Although pain is frequently associated with thoracic injuries, neither analgesia nor muscle relaxants can be administered until full primary and secondary assessments have been performed. No analgesic should be administered in the prehospital setting, unless the surgeon who is to perform the definitive evaluation of the abdomen is present and the patient has no associated head injuries. In general, high tidal volume hyperventilation and verbal assurances are preferable.

If it appears that the flail chest is a minimal one that is not compromising respiratory function, positive pressure ventilation may not be indicated. The patient should be admitted to the intensive care unit for close observation with frequent monitoring of arterial blood gas levels and vital signs, however. There is a risk that respiratory effort may decrease as the patient tires, resulting in insidious hypercapnia and respiratory arrest. For this reason, the patient who has not been intubated requires continuous monitoring.

Open Chest Wounds. Open or sucking chest wounds may lead to a total pneumothorax. The treatment is to seal the wound quickly with a Vaseline gauze. If, after a few minutes, the patient develops signs and symptoms of a tension pneumothorax, the Vaseline seal should be removed and the air in the affected chest allowed to escape. Both venous return to the heart and cardiac output increase. The maneuver may be repeated if there is a recurrence of the tension pneumothorax.[37] A needle with a one-way valve may be inserted not only to relieve the tension, but also to allow for full reexpansion of the lung.

If the patient is hemodynamically stable, a chest roentgenogram should be taken with the patient in the upright position to confirm the presence of a pneumothorax and/or hemothorax. Treatment consists of placing a chest tube in the anatomical location described earlier for needle decompression of tension pneumothorax. The chest tube should not be placed through the open wound, as this procedure contaminates the chest cavity and may create an empyema.

Circulation

Shock

Hemorrhagic shock secondary to blood loss from one or more injuries is the most common form of shock to be seen in the multisystem-injured patient. Blood volume deficits can be staged according to the percent of blood volume lost. In the normal adult, the blood volume accounts for approximately 7% of the total body weight. Stage 1 is a blood loss of 15% or less of the circulating volume; Stage 2, a loss of 15% to 25%; Stage 3, a loss of 25% to 35%; and Stage 4, a loss of more than 35%. The signs and symptoms of the shock syndrome depend on the stage of the volume deficit and the activation of control mechanisms (see Chapter 6, Shock).

Control of Bleeding

Either external or internal bleeding may result from blunt or penetrating trauma. In order to control external bleeding in the field, direct pressure is applied over the site; if an extremity is the site of the bleeding, the extremity should be elevated. Dressings and bandages should not be removed once applied. Firm pressure should be continuous, and additional dressings should be applied if necessary. Pressure applied proximal to the wound on the vessel that is injured can help to control distal bleeding. Pressure points are to be compressed only if bleeding is not controlled by pressure over the wound.

The use of tourniquets originated in the military. It was believed that a tourniquet would occlude arterial inflow and, thus, stop exsanguination from a distal extremity. Tourniquets are rarely indicated in the prehospital setting, however. In the event of a difficult extrication, a prolonged transport time, or the presence of multiple victims, a tourniquet may be inadvertently allowed to remain in place for longer than one hour; this results in tissue ischemia and hypoxia distal to the tourniquet, and it may cause myonecrosis and permanent damage. If the tourniquet occludes venous return, but does not totally occlude arterial inflow, venous oozing may be aggravated. Suffusion of the extremity, leading to compartment syndrome, may also occur. The inappropriate application of a tourniquet may damage accompanying nerves.

If exsanguination is imminent and primary point pressure has failed to control the hemorrhage, a tourniquet may be applied; however, the following precautions must be taken:

- Dress and bandage the wound with a sterile dressing.
- Do not use a thin, narrow device (eg, a rope, wire, or string) as a tourniquet.
- Use a folded cravat proximal to the injury, and adjust it with enough tension to stop the bleeding.
- Apply the tourniquet on the upper arm or upper leg; never apply a tourniquet below the elbow or below the knee, as the ulna and radius, and the tibia and fibula, prevent adequate compression of the intraosseous vessels.
- Record and report the time of application.

Intravenous Management of the Multisystem-Injured Patient

Trauma patients should be given nothing by mouth until all injuries have been assessed and the patients' final disposition determined. The patient who requires surgical intervention continues to have nothing by mouth; thus, an intravenous line must be placed in the severely traumatized patient who is in hypovolemic shock and requires volume resuscitation. The venous catheter used for this should have at least an 18-gauge bore so that blood transfused under pressure can flow rapidly through the needle. Ringer's lactate or normal saline should be rapidly infused until the patient's systolic blood pressure is greater than 100 mmHg. If more than 2000 mL solution is needed to achieve this blood pressure or if blood loss is obviously significant, O-negative or type-specific blood should be administered. Vasopressors are not indicated for hemorrhagic shock that causes hypovolemia.

Several principles are important to the intravenous management of a trauma patient:

- If an abdominal injury may have damaged the vena cava or major hepatic vessels, the intravenous lines should not be placed in the lower extremities; if the vena cava is disrupted, intravenous fluid infused into a lower extremity is transfused into the peritoneum.
- If the patient has a rib fracture or a hemopneumothorax, the central line should be placed on the affected side to ensure that an iatrogenic pneumothorax does not occur on the unaffected side. The subclavian route of intravenous access should be avoided, if possible, as it is associated with an unacceptably high complication rate in the uncooperative, combative trauma patient. The supraclavian approach may be used, however.
- The site of choice for a large-bore intravenous line is a peripheral vein in the upper extremity. If it is technically difficult to establish a line at this site because the patient is in shock, however, another anatomical location should be used.
- When a long intravenous line is introduced, the catheter should not be pulled back through the needle introducer as this may sever the catheter, causing catheter embolization. If the catheter is broken or severed, the vein proximal to the site where the catheter tip was transected should be tamponaded immediately. A surgeon can then retrieve the severed portion of the catheter.
- Intravenous tubing that is used directly for venous access in a saphenous vein cutdown must be extension tubing without a blood filter. A detachable blood filter may then be connected to the extension tube. When the detachable filter is obstructed with debris from multiple blood transfusions, it can be discarded and a new one substituted.

If an intravenous line is to be placed in the external jugular vein, the patient should be placed in the Trendelenburg position to allow jugular venous filling and distention. The external jugular vein can be identified as it passes across the sternomastoid muscle, midway between the angle of the jaw and the midclavicular line. The patient's head is turned to the opposite side and the vein compressed above the clavicle. The needle and catheter are introduced into the vein, with the point aimed at the ipsilateral shoulder. The catheter is threaded into the vein and sutured in place, and the venipuncture site is dressed.

An internal jugular vein approach has the advantage of introducing a large catheter directly into the superior vena cava. The vein passes first medial to and then posterior to the sternocleidomastoid muscle. It lies within the carotid sheath and is 1 to 2 cm in diameter. The vein can be entered by passing a needle posterior to the sternocleidomastoid at the junction of its middle and lower thirds. The needle is aimed toward the suprasternal notch and then advanced slowly until the vein is entered.

For placement of an intravenous line in the subclavian vein, the patient is placed in the head-down position. The needle is introduced under the clavicle at the junction of its medial third, lateral third, and lateral two-thirds. It is then advanced toward the suprasternal notch. The syringe is aspirated until the vein is entered.

Whenever a central line has been placed, a chest roentgenogram should be obtained immediately to verify that the tip of the catheter is located in the superior vena cava and that there is no pneumothorax.

Cardiac Tamponade

Blunt or penetrating trauma may cause blood to accumulate in the pericardial sac. The results of the primary survey should make it possible to differentiate hypotension secondary to hypovolemia from that secondary to tamponade. The accumulation of blood may be sufficient to result in inadequate cardiac filling and poor cardiac output. Beck's triad of (1) a decrease in systolic blood pressure, (2) muffled heart sounds, and (3) distended neck veins may be observed.

The appropriate management in the field is to establish an airway and proceed as quickly as possible to the hospital. If an intravenous line can be established in the moving ambulance, it should be done. No time should be wasted in attempting to establish intravenous access, however.

Cardiac tamponade is a life-threatening condition. Therapy must immediately follow diagnosis, because the patient's cardiac output is severely compromised and cardiac arrest is imminent. The roentgenogram may show widening of the mediastinum, but the patient may be in such critical condition that treatment must be instituted before a roentgenogram can be obtained. Definitive management of cardiac tamponade is to perform a left thoracotomy and open the pericardium. Once the injury to the heart has been sutured, the heart is better able to fill properly; stroke volume is also restored.

A patient with cardiac tamponade who is alert, but borderline hypotensive (ie, a systolic blood pressure of more than 90 mmHg) requires intravenous volume replacement. The patient should be stabilized and rapidly transferred to the operating room, where a surgeon can perform a thoracotomy under aseptic and controlled circumstances, with the assistance of an anesthesiologist and other operating room personnel.

The patient with cardiac tamponade who is in profound shock (ie, a systolic blood pressure of 60 to 90 mmHg) requires intravenous volume resuscitation and, possibly, endotracheal intubation. If the patient's hemodynamic status improves after these procedures, the patient should be immediately transferred to the operating room. If the systolic blood pressure does not respond rapidly, the patient should be given a muscle relaxant and analgesic (morphine), and the left chest should be opened through a fourth or fifth left anterolateral thoracotomy. The tamponade should be relieved and the injury to the myocardium repaired.

When a patient with cardiac tamponade has a pulse, but is atensive or is in electromechanical dissociation, an endotracheal tube should be inserted, large-bore intravenous access established, and an immediate left anterolateral thoracotomy performed. If the physician primarily involved in the immediate assessment is not skilled in open thoracotomy, needle pericardiocentesis can be done as a temporary measure.

Although not the definitive procedure for hemorrhagic cardiac tamponade, a needle pericardiocentesis may allow temporary and/or partial return of cardiac output. The preferred subxiphoid approach avoids both the pleura and the coronary vessels. In the precordial approach, the needle is inserted through the fifth intercostal space, just lateral to the sternal border. Because this anatomical location is not covered by the pleura, the precordial approach eliminates the risk of an iatrogenic pneumothorax; there is a risk of puncture of the left anterior descending coronary artery, however.

A long, large-bore needle attached to a syringe is used for the subxiphoid approach. An alligator clip connected to an electrocardiograph is attached to the needle. The needle is introduced to the left of the xiphoid cartilage and passed superiorly. Aspiration is continuous, and the physician should be able to sense the point at which the needle penetrates the distended pericardium. Contact of the needle with the epicardium produces a large ST segment elevation on the electrocardiogram (ECG). Because the blood aspirated from the pericardium is defibrinated, it does not clot.

The risks of needle pericardiocentesis include ventricular irregularity and fibrillation, myocardial and coronary artery laceration, cardiac air embolism, hemopneumothorax, and the creation of pericardial tamponade if the diagnosis is incorrect. When dealing with tamponade caused by a penetrating injury, it is essential to recognize that pericardiocentesis is only a temporary procedure and that an open thoracotomy is the definitive treatment.

SECONDARY SURVEY

Once the airway has been secured, the patient adequately ventilated, and bleeding controlled, a full examination is performed to assess the extent of the patient's other injuries. The secondary survey includes an assessment of the central and peripheral nervous systems, as well as an examination of the neck, chest, back, abdomen, extremities, and pelvis.

Central Nervous System

Head Injuries

Blunt or penetrating trauma to the head may injure the scalp, skull, and/or cerebral tissue. Rotational forces are most likely to result in injury to the frontal and temporal lobes of the brain. Acceleration or deceleration forces may cause injury to the brain because of the fixed position of the brain stem and the possible rotation of the cerebral hemispheres. The folds of the dura and the bony shelves, such as the petrous temporal ridges, are obstructions against which a decelerating force may thrust the brain, resulting in contusions, lacerations, and/or venous or arterial hemorrhage. Major sequelae of head injury are hypoxia, an increase in Pco_2, acidosis, cerebral edema, and increased intracranial pressure.

Various injuries may occur. A concussion, for example, is a temporary neurologic event induced by trauma. The neurologic manifestations may be a temporary (reversible) loss of consciousness, headache, or visual disturbances. The patient usually recovers within minutes or hours.

Closed head injuries are frequent consequences of energy impacts through mechanical vectors, such as motor vehicles, motorcycles, and falls. Because of its gel-like composition and its flotation within a surrounding layer of cerebrospinal fluid, the brain moves within the cranium on impact. The forces exerted may cause tearing or shearing of nerves and vessels. Hemorrhages that result from torn arteries may lead to intracerebral hematomas. If an artery, such as the middle meningeal artery, is injured, an epidural hematoma may form between the skull and dura mater. Surface veins that tear may lead to a subdural hematoma, a collection of blood below the dura on the brain's surface. The major problems that follow these particular lesions are associated with increases in intracranial volume, diffuse swelling and edema, and an increase in intracranial pressure.

Neck Injuries

Trauma to the neck caused by either penetrating or blunt forces can damage a number of body systems. Seven cervical vertebrae protect the spinal cord, and many large posterior muscles begin at the base of the posterior skull and insert on the scapulae, ribs, and clavicle. The trachea, esophagus, carotid arteries, jugular veins, vagus nerves, and cervical spinal nerves are in the neck area and could be injured by the forces of energy.

Spinal Injuries

Vertebral injuries are associated with fractures, dislocations, or a combination of the two. The more mobile portions of the spine, C4–6 and T11–L2, are common locations of injury. Flexion of the cervical spine can drive the anterior inferior border of a cervical vertebra into the vertebra below it, compressing the spinal cord. In addition, displacement of the posterior portion of a fractured vertebra may compress the spinal cord. In hyperextension of the cervical spine, a spinal cord injury can result from the increased separation between a vertebral disk and vertebral body.

Spinal shock, or complete spinal cord injury that results in loss of both deep tendon and cutaneous reflexes, is accompanied by loss of motor and sensory function. Hypotension may ensue, because the loss of sympathetic innervation leads to subsequent vasodilation of peripheral blood vessels. A complete neurologic examination must be performed; however, it is critical to rule out internal or long bone injuries that add a hemorrhagic component to the neurogenic hypotension. Initial treatment consists of controlling the airway, followed by volume resuscitation with a crystalloid solution. Hemorrhage should be suspected in a patient who requires more than 2000 mL crystalloid to become hemodynamically stable. The use of a vasoconstrictor (eg, phenylephrine hydrochloride [Neo-Synephrine] or levarterenol bitartrate [Levophed]) is controversial, and any vasopressor agent should be given very judiciously. Patients with spinal shock can often tolerate a lower than normal systolic blood pressure. If arterial blood gas levels, urine output, and cerebral mentation are normal, a blood pressure of 90 to 100 mmHg may be tolerable.

The use of steroids in acute spinal cord injuries has been controversial over the years. In a large multicenter, randomized, controlled trial of methylprednisolone given to patients with acute spinal cord injury, Bracken et al[38] concluded that treatment with methylprednisolone in the dose used in the study improves neurologic recovery when given in the first 8 hours of injury. The dose of methylprednisolone, given intravenously, was an initial bolus of 30 mg per kilogram of body weight followed by infusion of 5.4 mg per kilogram per hour for 23 hours. Based on this study, it can be recommended that this protocol be followed in all eligible patients with acute spinal cord injuries. Patients excluded were those who have only cauda equina or root injuries and/or gunshot injuries to the spinal cord.

In a recent prospective, randomized, placebo-controlled, double-blind trial of GM_1 ganglioside, Geisler et al[39] concluded that there was evidence that GM_1 enhances the recovery of neurologic function after 1 year. Although this initial study is encouraging, it was small; a larger study will be needed before the efficacy and safety of GM_1 are proven.

Head and Neck

Assessment of a patient who has had either obvious or obscure injury to the central nervous system (CNS) requires a systematic and organized approach. Environmental circumstances (eg, a fire), the presence of multiple casualties, or the severity of the patient's condition may limit the neurologic examination that is possible in the field, however. Stabilization, assessment, and field diagnosis are essential, but transport to a medical facility is a key objective.

Neurologic assessment includes evaluation of (1) level of consciousness, (2) vital signs, (3) motor function, (4) sensory function, (5) pupillary responses, and (6) primary and secondary surveys. These data are used to set priorities and to formulate a management plan.

An evaluator can judge the severity of injury to the brain by determining (1) the level of consciousness, (2) pupillary function, and (3) the presence of any lateralized weakness of the extremities.[40] Most important, it is necessary in the field to manage the patient in a way that prevents additional injury and preserves maximal neurologic function.

Level of Consciousness

The first step in any assessment of injury is to determine the patient's level of consciousness, as indicated by the patient's wakefulness and mental activity.[41] The actual centers of consciousness are located in the cerebral hemispheres, which are activated by centers in the upper brain stem. Specifically, the reticular system has a significant role in consciousness. Therefore, alteration in a patient's level of consciousness indicates damage or depression of one hemisphere, two hemispheres, the upper brain stem, or a combination of the three.

Field personnel must assess consciousness by eliciting the patient's responses to verbal and painful stimuli. These initial assessment data provide a baseline for subsequent comparisons. The level of consciousness can be grossly tested by asking the patient questions, such as "Are you all right?" or "Can you hear me?" The level of consciousness is best described in terms of the patient's responses to verbal stimulation; if the patient does not respond, various maneuvers can be used to elicit a response to painful stimuli.

The Glasgow Coma Scale is a useful scoring system in the evaluation of the level of consciousness. Unless the examiner is totally familiar with the system, however, it may be advisable to calculate the patient's score after life-saving measures have been started. The examiner determines the patient's verbal responses, motor responses, and eye-opening capabilities, assigning points for each; total points range from 3 to 15. The rating is inaccurate if the patient is under the influence of drugs or alcohol, but it can still be used as a baseline criterion to evaluate subsequent changes in level of consciousness.

It is also helpful to determine the patient's orientation to person, time, and place in establishing the patient's level of wakefulness and mental alertness. At the same time, questions should be asked about the patient's ability to recollect circumstances of the event, about headache, and about other pain. Recordings of blood pressure, pulse, and respirations are important.

Injury to the cervical or upper thoracic cord may so compromise peripheral vascular tone that vasodilation produces hypotension. The accompanying pooling of blood may dissipate heat, leading to hypothermia. Furthermore, the pulse may slow, because the absence of sympathetic tone leaves the parasympathetic or vagal innervation to regulate the heart rate. This bradycardia is often a key diagnostic sign in the differentiation of hypotension caused by hypovolemia from hypotension caused by vasodilation.

Spinal shock may also cause bladder and bowel paralysis, as sympathetic fibers innervate smooth muscle. Sympathetic innervation also regulates the sweat glands; if this innervation is lost, the patient cannot sweat. If spinal shock is not complicated by other shock phenomena, such as blood loss, hypotension and bradycardia are often seen when the patient is alert.

Head-injured patients who develop serious sequelae of cerebral edema and/or elevated intracranial pressure may have an increase in systolic pressure with a subsequent widening of pulse pressure (ie, difference between systolic and diastolic pressures). The mechanism responsible for this systolic rise is Cushing's phenomenon:

1. An increase in cerebrospinal fluid pressure is followed by compression of the brain's arteries.
2. The cerebral ischemia that ensues is followed by a CNS ischemic response, which activates the sympathetic nervous system, leading to vasoconstriction.
3. The vasoconstriction leads to a rise in arterial pressure.

Cushing's phenomenon tends to increase arterial pressure above cerebrospinal fluid pressure to perfuse the brain and correct ischemia.[42]

Vital Signs

Pulse. The pulse is evaluated first for presence, then for rate, rhythm, and quality. A pulse rate in the range of tachycardia may indicate shock, anxiety, and/or stress. A pulse rate in the range of bradycardia strongly suggests the previously mentioned sequelae of head trauma. The mechanism for bradycardia is related to a reflex response to increased intracranial pressure: a slow pulse in combination with a higher blood pressure. The Cushing triad is a slow pulse, increasing systolic pressure with decreasing diastolic pressure, and slow, irregular respiration. The patient's ECG should be continuously monitored if possible.

Respiration. Ventilation involves the mechanics of moving air in and out of the lungs. Respiration is the exchange of oxygen and CO_2 at the alveolar capillary membrane. In the multisystem-injured patient, respiration is evaluated for presence, then rate, depth, exertion, and symmetry.

Particular patterns of respiration reflect the various levels of the brain's influence on the entire respiratory process.

Therefore, the examiner should not only count the number of respirations, but also monitor and record the respiratory pattern. For example, Cheyne-Stokes respiration is a sustained hyperpnea alternating with apnea. The pattern in the head-injured patient may be a sign of impending brain herniation because of a mass above the tentorium. Clearly, the examiner must be able to assess the characteristics of respiratory patterns and to anticipate the need for ventilatory assistance.

Motor Function

The body's motor responses can give information regarding the integrity of the motor system and its consequent ability to produce muscle contraction and internal motor activities. The body, through sensory input, can elicit motor responses that require function at different levels of the nervous system including the spinal cord, the brain stem, and the cerebrum.

Field assessment of the motor function in a neurologically injured patient differs from in-hospital assessment. Certain tests for this component of neurologic function identify the level within the nervous system that may be affected by injury, but such a determination is not relevant for field management and takes valuable time from other important responsibilities for patient care. Simple and quick assessment maneuvers can provide a gross estimate of motor function that is sufficient in the field. The use of these maneuvers depends on the patient's level of consciousness, however.

Motor function can be tested in the more alert patient by examining the muscle groups for abnormalities, assessing muscle tonicity by passive stretching, evaluating the patient's ability to move all four extremities, and determining whether any compromise of muscle strength is lateralized or confined to upper and/or lower extremities. To prevent further injury and to avoid manipulation of extremities that may have local injury, the examiner must not move the patient unnecessarily.

If strength is impaired, but there is no paralysis, the patient has a paresis (weakness). Hemiparesis is a weakness that is limited to one side of the body; hemiplegia is paralysis that is limited to one side of the body. Paraplegia is paralysis in the lower extremities; quadriplegia is paralysis in all four extremities.

Even if the patient is unresponsive, motor function can be tested. The examiner can observe whether there is any purposeful movement away from noxious or painful stimuli and the type of any such movement. The presence or absence of the response, as well as its appropriateness, should be recorded. Positions of body parts in identifiable patterns following stimulation can be classified, and they may alert the examiner to the severity of injury so that management and transport priorities can be set.

Decorticate rigidity is flexion of the arms, wrists, and fingers; abduction and extension of the arms; and internal

Table 7-3 Cranial Nerves and Their Functions

Nerve No.	Name	Function
I	Olfactory	Smell
II	Optic	Vision
III	Oculomotor	Pupil, some extraocular movements
IV	Trochlear	Extraocular movement
V	Trigeminal*	Some movement of jaw; sensation
VI	Abducens	Lateral extraocular movement
VII	Facial	Facial muscle movement Sensation of taste
VIII	Acoustic	Hearing and balance
IX	Glossopharyngeal	Pharynx (motor), ear/pharynx/tongue (sensory)
X	Vagus	Palate, larynx, pharynx, involuntary muscle
XI	Accessory	Sternomastoid/trapezius muscles
XII	Hypoglossal	Tongue

*Sensory divisions (ophthalmic, maxillary, and mandibular).

Source: Reprinted from Bennett B: Assessment of the patient with neurologic injury. *Emergency Care Quarterly* 1(1):16, 1985.

rotation and plantar flexion of the lower extremities. Signs of decerebrate rigidity are adduction, stiff extension, and hyperpronation of the arms; stiff extension of the legs; and plantar flexion of the feet. Decerebrate characteristics in the upper extremities and flaccidity in the lower extremities may indicate severe brain stem injury. For field assessment, the critical concern is not the differentiation among patterns, but rather the observation that stimulation produces such a response.

An examination of the 12 cranial nerves is another component of the neurologic assessment of motion and sensation, but its practicality in the field is questionable (Table 7-3).

Sensory Function and Reflexes

In many tests of function, a sensory stimulus is used to elicit a motor response, such as the muscle stretch reflex (eg, the knee jerk). In general, testing reflexes in the field is unnecessary and does not provide any significant data for decisions regarding field management and transport. There are exceptions, however, and the examiner must exercise judgment in making this determination.

The presence of sensation (eg, pain, temperature, touch, and vibration) can be quickly and accurately tested in the field. Sensation testing can assist the examiner in locating the site of a neurologic injury. The body's dermatomes, skin segments that correspond to the sensory innervation of particular spinal nerve segments, can be used to identify the level at which sensory loss in the spinal cord has occurred.

Pupillary Responses

Pupils are routinely examined for size, shape, equality, and reactivity to light. Any asymmetry in pupillary size must be reported. The autonomic nervous system is a visceral motor system of parasympathetic and sympathetic fibers that are the innervation for smooth muscle, cardiac muscle, and glands. Parasympathetic and sympathetic fibers control constriction and dilation of the pupils, respectively.

If the pupil is nonreactive or sluggish to respond, the brain stem may be involved in the injury. A "blown pupil," a pupil on the same side as the injury that is not reactive to light, is an ominous sign; it is caused by compression of the third oculomotor nerve, which may result from transtentorial herniation. If this condition is bilateral and if the pupils are fixed, midbrain involvement with resulting herniation is likely.

The eyelids should also be examined and observed for the presence of blinking and any involuntary eye movements (in an unresponsive patient). Extraocular eye movements are controlled by six ocular muscles that can be examined in the responsive patient who is asked to move the eyes up, down, to the left, and to the right. Nystagmus is an abnormal oscillation of the eyes that should be noted. Visual acuity should also be determined when a head injury is suspected.

Inspection

The head and neck should be examined for obvious trauma (eg, lacerations, contusions, depressions, asymmetry, facial deformity, or tissue damage). The drainage of fluid that may be cerebrospinal fluid from the ear or nose should be noted, as well as the presence of blood in the ear, raccoon eyes (periorbital ecchymosis) and/or Battle's sign (postauricular ecchymosis), and/or hematoma. Patients with penetrating trauma should be examined for exit and entrance wounds.

History

An injury to the head and/or neck may be considered minor only if critical injuries have been excluded. In order to assist the physician who provides definitive care in making a sound diagnosis, prehospital personnel must gather and record all information. If the mechanism of injury is blunt trauma from a motor vehicle accident, for example, the following information is useful:

- type of vehicle
- speed and circumstances of the accident (eg, struck a tree or hit on the side)
- suspected abuse of alcohol or drugs
- use of a seat belt or helmet
- condition of the vehicle (eg, windshield and steering wheel)
- time of accident, time of extrication, and time to transport
- estimate of blood loss at the scene
- position of the patient in the vehicle
- medications administered
- pre-existing health problems
- condition of other accident victims

Injury to the head and/or neck may also be caused by falls. If the patient's head was struck in a fall to the ground, it is helpful to know the height of the fall. Penetrating injuries may be caused by guns, knives, or other sharp objects. It is important to identify the size, shape, weight, and velocity of the striking object.

The head-injured patient requires continuous monitoring in the field and during transport. Changes in assessment data are extremely significant. Although it may appear that the initial contact with the energy-producing force did not cause injury, appropriate care at the scene and during transport can prevent serious sequelae and permanent disability.

Management of Head and Neck Injuries

The airway of the patient with a head and/or neck injury must be cleared and ventilation assisted, if needed, while cervical immobilization is maintained. The patient with a significant head injury can be hyperventilated in the field. If the patient's airway cannot be controlled or the respiratory rate is inadequate, endotracheal intubation may be necessary. This procedure must be done with increased caution, however, as the intubation could precipitate a rise in intracranial pressure. If the head injury produces respiratory changes that lead to hypercapnia, the cerebral blood vessels dilate, and cerebral blood volume increases. Therefore, hyperventilation causes hypocapnia and cerebral vessel vasoconstriction with a subsequent reduction in cerebral blood volume. The rate of hyperventilation should be 20 to 25 breath/min. Suction and other appropriate measures of protection against vomiting or seizures, such as proper positioning, must be instituted. If the patient is in critical condition, an intravenous access route should be established.

Bleeding from the scalp must be controlled with direct pressure. In the event of an open head injury, a nonadherent type dressing should be applied. The tympanic membranes should be inspected for the presence of hemotympanum. Any impaled objects or protruding bone should be left untouched in the field. An impaled object should be firmly anchored to the skin at the point of entry, however, until definitive treatment can be provided at the trauma center.

Any patient with injury to the neck must be inspected for signs of respiratory distress or subcutaneous emphysema, because air from the trachea or esophagus may leak into the subcutaneous tissue. Immediate transport to a trauma center is essential.

Decerebrate and decorticate posturing are ominous signs of significant cranial injury. Reflexes should also be tested when the patient is in the emergency department. Lateralizing signs, changes in the level of consciousness, bradycardia, and a widening of the pulse pressure are all neurologic signs that necessitate a neurosurgical consultation.

The patient's blood gases and pH should be monitored closely, especially if the patient is being hyperventilated to induce respiratory alkalosis and, thus, decrease cerebral blood volume and intracranial pressure. Computed tomography (CT) should be ordered when intracranial injury is suspected. Most of the injuries that cause intracranial hemorrhage require surgical intervention.

Before any manipulation of the spine, it is critically important to obtain a lateral cervical spine roentgenogram to verify that none of the seven cervical vertebrae is injured. If the patient has a short neck and is very muscular, it may be difficult to see the seventh cervical vertebra. Traction may be placed on the patient's arms to pull the shoulders caudally. If this does not allow a satisfactory roentgenogram, a "swimmer's" view should be obtained. Roentgen rays are directed through the axillae, obliquely across the cervical spine; this gives adequate exposure of the seventh cervical vertebra.

The clinical diagnosis of cervical spine injury is based on the history and on a high index of suspicion, along with paraspinalis muscular spasm and tenderness. Spinal injury may be present even when there are no obvious physical findings, however.

Principles of Spinal Immobilization

The basic principle of spinal immobilization is to immobilize the bony vertebral column sufficiently to prevent any movement that may injure the spinal cord or its nerve pathways. Because injury to the vertebral column can be diagnosed definitively only by a roentgenogram in the hospital, it is accepted practice to immobilize any patient with a suspected injury to the vertebral column. Unnecessary or inappropriate movement of the patient in the field may permanently damage the spinal cord, with subsequent loss of neurologic function and permanent paralysis of the extremities and/or the diaphragm.

Immobilization of the vertebral column requires specialized knowledge and appropriate manipulative skills. The patient's neck should be placed in a neutral position by means of manual cervical traction.[43,44] There are numerous ways to apply cervical traction effectively. The method used should allow both application of any type of cervical collar and maintenance of an open airway by anterior displacement of the lower jaw. One such method can be used when the patient is sitting upright; the provider's hands are placed alongside the patient's head, with the fifth finger placed behind the angle of the jaw. If the patient develops airway problems, the lower jaw can be pushed forward, which displaces the tongue anteriorly and relieves any obstruction. Another method is a modified jaw thrust maneuver in which manual axial traction is applied by the rescuer's thumbs, which are placed on the mandible at the corners of the mouth. The middle fingers, placed behind the angles of the jaw, push the jaw anteriorly.

Placement of the rescuer's hands alongside the patient's head instead of parallel to the line of the mandible and the occiput effectively keeps them out of the way of the cervical column. In this way, a collar can be applied by a second rescuer with minimal manipulation of the first rescuer's hands. The jaw thrust method requires release of traction for the proper application of any of the high-sided extrication type cervical collars, however. Because stiff, opaque collars preclude observation of the neck after they are placed, it is critical to evaluate the neck veins for distention, the trachea for midline position, subcutaneous emphysema or swelling, or hematomas in and around the neck before such a collar is applied.

Soft collars are ineffective and have no place in the prehospital setting for spinal immobilization during extrication or transport of the patient. They do not provide the necessary restriction of flexion, extension, and rotation.[45] Rigid collars are now used for cervical immobilization. The rigid Philadelphia collar, for example, prevents motion of flexion, extension, and rotation. It is also easy to apply because it comes in two premolded pieces. The anterior and the posterior pieces are easily fastened by means of a Velcro strap. A particular advantage of this collar is that the anterior portion can be removed for an inspection of the neck, while the posterior portion maintains immobility.

The Stifneck collar is also a rigid collar made of polyethylene. It has an enlarged opening in its anterior portion that permits examination of the pulse and prevents constriction of the jugular veins. The Cervical Immobilizer Device is a combination of foam and straps that can be used with a long or short board, as well as the scoop type stretcher. This device is lightweight and radiolucent, but can be used only for adults.

The long spinal board with sandbags and 3-inch adhesive tape was found to be superior in immobilization to any collar tested in a series by Podolsky and his colleagues.[46] The backboard used in combination with a Philadelphia collar was found to provide the least amount of motion in all planes, however.

The concept of immobilizing a patient in the sitting position was originated by J.D. Farrington, and the strapping technique used in this procedure is commonly called the Farrington method (Fig. 7-5). This method and all its modifications fix the bottom of the short spine board to a solid bony point to minimize movement (Figs. 7-6 and 7-7). It serves no useful purpose to apply traction to a victim's head and neck, and then secure the head to a splint that is not solidly anchored. The head should be secured last to prevent any movement of the short spine board from causing movement of the patient's head and neck. Once a short spine board

Management of the Multisystem-Injured Patient 109

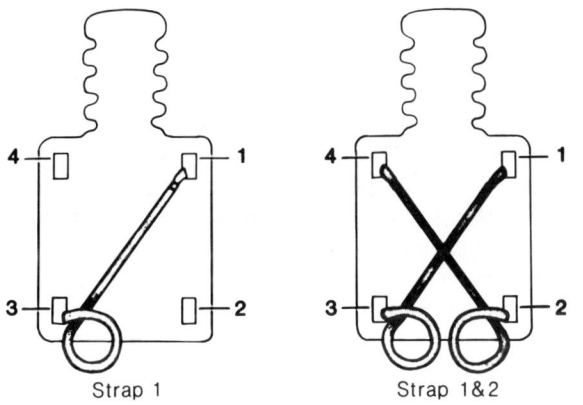

Figure 7-5 Modified Farrington method. *Source:* Reprinted from Weinstein C, Bennett B: Spinal immobilization devices. *Emergency Care Quarterly* 1(4):66, 1986.

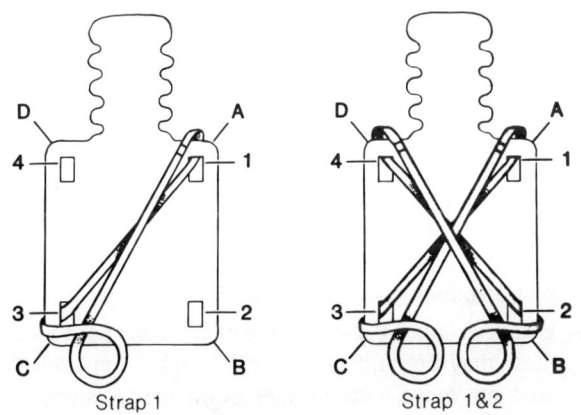

Figure 7-6 W1 modified Farrington method. *Source:* Reprinted from Weinstein C, Bennett B: Spinal immobilization devices. *Emergency Care Quarterly* 1(4):68, 1986.

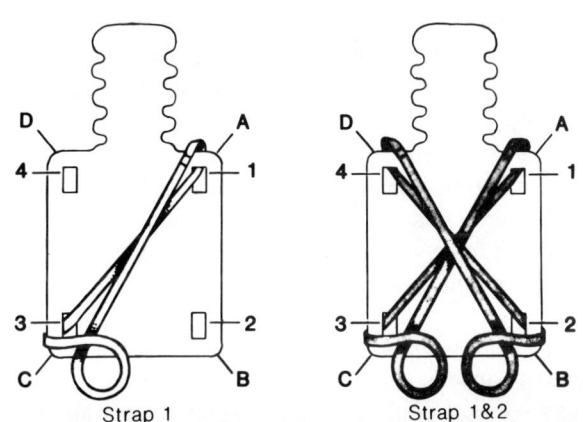

Figure 7-7 W modified Farrington method. *Source:* Reprinted from Weinstein C, Bennett B: Spinal immobilization devices. *Emergency Care Quarterly* 1(4):67, 1986.

has been applied, the victim should be carefully lifted onto a long board and firmly secured to it.

Several other devices are available to immobilize patients. An alternative to the short spine board is the Ferno-KED. Made of a ribbed fabric, the KED is designed to wrap around the patient. Chin and forehead restraints, chest and leg straps, and a neck roll restrict patient movement. The KED is designed for quick application and for use in confined spaces. The Reeves Sleeve is a spinal immobilization device that has an opening for insertion of a rigid board. Once the board has been inserted, the patient is placed onto the sleeve, and the chest and lower extremity vests are wrapped around the patient and fastened with Velcro closures. The Build-a-board is a three-section metal device that consists of a seat section, a back support, and a head board. It is designed for use with a seated patient. A scoop stretcher can be attached to a Build-a-board. Long boards are available in aluminum and plywood.

A vacuum immobilizer, the Coquille, is used for spinal immobilization almost exclusively in France and other European countries. The Coquille is an airtight radiolucent envelope full of tiny plastic balls. After the device is slid around the patient, a small, manually operated vacuum pump is used to withdraw all the air from the envelope. As air is withdrawn, the balls decrease in size, and create a rigid mold around the patient's body, locking the patient into the envelope. The weight of the patient's body is distributed evenly over the envelope, thereby reducing the risk of tissue damage from pressure. The plastic balls also act as thermal insulators to prevent heat loss. This device can be used for a seated or supine patient. The respective costs of some of these devices are found in Table 7-4.

Table 7-4 Current Costs of Immobilization Devices

Device	Cost ($)
Greene body splint	235.00
Ferno-KED	199.00
Extrication back splint	93.00
Reeves Sleeve with case	330.00
Cervical Immobilizer Device	78.00
Sandbags	10.00
Philadelphia cervical collar	19.00
Stifneck cervical collar	20.00
Thomas cervical collar	27.00
Scoop stretcher	265.00
Build-a-board	295.00
Build-a-board/scoop stretcher	425.00
Aluminum spine board, short	100.00
Aluminum spine board, long	120.00
Plywood spine board, short	52.00
Plywood spine board, long	100.00

Source: Reprinted from Weinstein C, Bennett B: Spinal immobilization devices. *Emergency Care Quarterly* 1(1):73, 1986.

Maxillofacial Area

A careful examination of the maxillofacial area for tenderness or crepitation is important. Serosanguineous drainage from the nares should be considered cerebrospinal fluid, the presence of which contraindicates the passage of a nasotracheal or nasogastric tube. Facial fractures may be displaced or undisplaced. Displacement causes further damage, including malalignment of bones. Compression must not be applied to an undisplaced fracture, because it may cause displacement. Field personnel should look for the following signs:

- flatness of a usually rounded cheek
- inability to move the mandible, which may indicate a fracture of the mandible or the zygoma where it articulates
- hemotympanum or blood in the nares (secondary to basilar skull fracture, which results from significant force)
- otorrhea or rhinorrhea (cerebrospinal fluid leaking from the ears or nose)
- unilateral nosebleed, resulting from fracture of the maxillary antrum, which fills the sinus with blood that drains into the nose
- palpable irregularities of the infraorbital rim and the zygomatic arch
- circumorbital or subconjunctival hemorrhage
- postauricular (behind the ear) ecchymosis (Battle's sign)
- altered vision (eye muscle entrapment), enophthalmos (sunken globe), or exophthalmos (protruding globe)

If any of these signs occur, a fracture should be assumed, and the patient should be treated with caution so that the fragments are not displaced. Facial lacerations should be covered with sterile gauze. A light, compressive dressing should be used, but excessive pressure should be avoided.

Injuries around the areas of specialized tissue, such as the parotid gland and its duct, the facial nerve, and the lacrimal apparatus, should be treated with extreme care and finesse to prevent iatrogenic injury. These injuries should be treated by control of bleeding, prevention of contamination and additional trauma, and transport.

Chest

During the secondary survey, the chest is reevaluated to ascertain whether treatment of all the previously identified injuries has been adequate. The heart sounds and neck veins are reevaluated; the breath sounds should also be reevaluated to ensure that any simple or tension pneumothorax has been corrected. Tenderness and bony or pneumocrepitation suggest the possibility of underlying rib fractures and mandate a roentgenogram.

The patient with rib fractures, but without evidence of pneumothorax, who undergoes an abdominal exploration is a candidate for a prophylactic chest tube to prevent the development of a tension pneumothorax under anesthesia. The risk of tension pneumothorax is higher when drug-induced muscle relaxation is part of anesthesia. An unnoticed small pneumothorax can be exacerbated by large tidal volumes of anesthetics and may progress to a tension pneumothorax. Before the induction of anesthesia, this possibility should be discussed with all physicians involved.

Abdomen

By means of percussion, auscultation, inspection, and palpation, the examiner checks the abdomen for contusions, tenderness, signs of peritonitis, organomegaly, distention, and signs of internal hemorrhage. Signs that may be observed are

- Kehr's sign. Free blood in the abdomen irritates the diaphragm and the phrenic nerve. Pain is referred along the phrenic nerve dermatomal distribution to the left shoulder. It is elicited by placing the patient in the Trendelenburg position, which allows the intraperitoneal free blood to bathe the diaphragm. This sign may suggest bleeding from an injured spleen or liver.
- Balance's sign. If there is free blood in the peritoneum, there may be dullness in the left upper quadrant that does not move with changes in the patient's position. This sign also may indicate bleeding from an injured organ.
- Saegesser's sign. Again, free blood in the peritoneal cavity irritates the phrenic nerve. Point pressure, 1 inch above the left clavicle, compresses the phrenic nerve against the transverse process of the cervical vertebrae, causing point tenderness. A similar maneuver on the right side of the neck does not cause discomfort, as the right diaphragm and phrenic nerve are protected by the liver.
- Seat belt sign. Ecchymosis over the lower abdomen results from compression of a lap seat belt against the iliac crest and lower abdomen. The sign indicates that severe force was applied against the abdominal viscera and especially against a distended cecum.

In patients with suspected abdominal trauma, an intravenous peripheral line must be placed for the infusion of Ringer's lactate. Intra-abdominal hemorrhage with subsequent hypotension is an indication for use of the PASG.

Although the use of the PASG remains controversial, its presence is ubiquitous. McSwain,[47] in an excellent review of the literature, made several recommendations on its use and indications. His conclusions, based on extensive review of the literature, were that the PASG should be used to increase blood pressure; to improve brain and heart perfusion; to control intra-abdominal, pelvic, and thigh hemorrhage; and to stabilize pelvic fractures in the prehospital setting. He stated that the PASG also should be used as a stabilizing device for femoral fractures when hypotension coexists.

Mattox et al,[48] however, came to a different conclusion in their large randomized, prospective, and well-controlled study. Their conclusions were that PASG application does not significantly increase the length of total prehospital time; that PASG application does increase the blood pressure; that PASG application does not favorably decrease the length of time in the emergency department, operating room, or hospital; that, when PASG was applied, an overall increased mortality was seen for all patients; that patients with prehospital times longer than 30 minutes and PASG application did not have a better survival rate; that patients with thoracic injury (including cardiac and major thoracic vascular) had a greater chance of dying before arrival at the hospital if PASG was applied; that patients with major abdominal vascular injury did not have a better overall survival rate, nor did they have a better chance of reaching the trauma surgeon alive if PASG was applied; and that a logistic regression model showed that PASG application significantly contributed to chance of dying ($P = 0.003$) and was a greater prognostic indicator of death than mechanism of injury or age.

Peritoneal Lavage

The abdomen of the head-injured or unconscious patient may be difficult to evaluate. In case of blunt abdominal trauma and hypotension, however, intraperitoneal injury is very likely. Peritoneal lavage is a rapid and safe method of evaluating intraperitoneal hemorrhage and injury. The procedure is indicated for patients who have a suspected intra-abdominal pathologic condition, patients who have ingested alcohol or drugs, patients who have head or spinal cord injuries, and patients who will be undergoing prolonged anesthesia for head, orthopedic, or vascular procedures, but whose examination produced equivocal findings. It is contraindicated for patients with previous abdominal surgery, a gravid uterus, or abdominal distention.

The urinary bladder is catheterized before the procedure is started, and the stomach should be decompressed. After the skin on the lower midline abdomen has been prepared, an area one-third the distance from the umbilicus to the symphysis pubis is anesthetized with 1 percent lidocaine (Xylocaine) with epinephrine. The skin, subcutaneous tissues, fascia, and peritoneum are opened with a scalpel under direct vision. The peritoneal dialysis catheter is introduced into the peritoneal cavity and directed into the pelvis. If aspiration produces gross blood, the lavage is considered positive. If no blood is aspirated, Ringer's lactate (10 mL/kg in children or 1 L in adults) is infused into the abdominal cavity. The empty bag is then placed on the floor and the effluent siphoned into it. If it is impossible to read newsprint through the effluent in the bag, the lavage is positive. A positive lavage can be confirmed by laboratory analysis of the effluent that reveals (1) more than 100,000 red blood cells per cubic millimeter, (2) more than 500 white blood cells per cubic millimeter, and (3) the presence of bile or bacteria.

Peritoneal lavage should be performed in consultation with or in the presence of the surgeon responsible for the definitive management of the patient. If the patient is transferred to another hospital, a sample of the effluent and the results of the lavage should accompany the patient. Although a positive lavage indicates an intra-abdominal injury, a negative lavage does not exclude intra-abdominal or retroperitoneal injuries. Therefore, the abdomen should be reexamined frequently.

Nasogastric Intubation

The nares should be rapidly evaluated for a fracture with associated cerebrospinal fluid leakage. If the finding is negative, an 18-French sump nasogastric tube should be inserted to prevent gastric aspiration and treat any gastric dilation that may have occurred during assisted ventilation. The gastric returns should be tested for the presence of blood.

Pelvis and Extremities

If bimanual compression on the iliac crests and downward pressure on the symphysis pubis reveals tenderness, a fractured pelvis is suspected. The vertebrae, clavicles, scapulae, and long bones are digitally examined individually. Bony crepitus, inappropriate movement, loss of function, deformity, or tenderness suggests a fracture, and the involved area should be splinted.

If distal pulses are diminished or absent in the presence of a displaced fracture, in-line traction should be applied to the limb and pulses rechecked. If the pulse does not reappear, arterial injury should be suspected. Depending on the anatomical location, an arteriogram may be indicated. Special attention should be given to the possibility of a compartment syndrome in the affected limb.

Genitourinary System

Injuries to the kidneys, ureters, bladder, or reproductive structures should be suspected in patients who have sustained blunt or penetrating trauma to the lower thorax, abdomen, or pelvis. These areas should be inspected for ecchymoses, contusions, swelling, hematomas, or any masses.

Examination for pelvic fractures should be performed. A kidney, ureter, and bladder roentgenogram of the abdomen should be done.

All multisystem-injured patients should be catheterized. If there is blood at the urethral meatus, the urinary catheter is introduced just far enough to prevent extravasation of dye and a retrograde urethrogram performed. The catheter can be held in place manually or with a Brodsky clamp. If the urethra is intact, the catheter may be inserted into the bladder. If the urethra is lacerated, the catheter is removed, and a cystostomy must be performed by the surgeon or urologist in the operating room. Once the catheter is in the bladder, a filling cystogram, with 350 to 450 mL Renografin is obtained, followed by a voiding cystogram. These radiographs, along with oblique roentgenograms of the bladder, reveal any trauma to the bladder. An intravenous polygram is then obtained. If it shows diminished or absent flow to either kidney, further evaluation by an arteriogram or a CT scan with contrast is required. The complete evaluation of the urinary tract should be performed in consultation with a urologist.

Rectum

All severely traumatized patients must have a rectal examination. If anal tone is absent or diminished, spinal cord injury should be suspected. The position of the prostate gland should be noted. If the area of the prostate gland is boggy, transection of the urethra should be suspected. A stool specimen should be tested for blood.

Tetanus Immunization

Primary surgical debridement of devitalized tissue and cleaning of wounds is most important. If, however, there has been a break in the patient's skin, tetanus prophylaxis should be considered. Full immunization with tetanus toxoid requires three booster injections; once an individual is immunized, however, a booster of tetanus toxoid need be given only every 10 years.

CONCLUSION

The trauma patient presents a dynamic and frequently changing clinical situation. It is critical to reassess the patient frequently so as not to overlook a developing injury or life-threatening situation. Continuous monitoring of the vital signs, urinary output, ECG, and arterial blood gas levels is essential. Management interventions and vital signs must be meticulously recorded as they occur, as it is very difficult to reconstruct them accurately at a later date. A physician asked to appear as an expert witness months or years later finds it nearly impossible to remember the details of a complete resuscitation.

REFERENCES

1. Trunkey DD. Trauma. *Sci Am*. 1983;249:28–35.
2. National Center for Health Statistics. *Advance Report of Final Mortality Statistics*. 1992;40:8.
3. American Heart Association: Standards and guidelines for cardiopulmonary resuscitation (CPR) and emergency cardiac care (ECC). *JAMA*. 1980;244:433–509.
4. Committee on Trauma, American College of Surgeons. *Advanced Trauma Life Support Instructor Manual*. Chicago: American College of Surgeons; 1981.
5. Pons PT, Moore EE, Cusick JM, et al. Prehospital venous access in an urban paramedic system—a prospective on-scene analysis. *J Trauma*. 1985;28:1460–1463.
6. Gervin A, Fischer R. The importance of prompt transport in salvage of patients with penetrating heart wounds. *J Trauma*. 1982;11:6.
7. Criley JM, Niemann JT, Rosborough JP. Cardiopulmonary resuscitation research: 1960–1984. Discoveries and advances. *Ann Emerg Med*. 1984;13:756–758.
8. Thompson RH, Hallstrom AP, Cobb LA. Bystander initiated cardiopulmonary resuscitation in the management of ventricular fibrillation. *Ann Intern Med*. 1970;90:737–740.
9. Stewart RD, Kaplan R, Pennock B, et al. Influence of mask design on bag mask ventilation. *Ann Emerg Med*. 1985;14:403–406.
10. White RD, Goldberg AH, Montgomery WH. *Adjuncts for airway control and ventilation in advanced cardiac life support*. Dallas: American Hospital Association; 1983.
11. White RD. Controversies in out-of-hospital emergency airway control: esophageal obturator or endotracheal intubation? *Ann Emerg Med*. 1984;13:778–781.
12. Sellick BA. Cricoid pressure to control regurgitation of stomach contents during induction of anesthesia. *Lancet*. 1961;2:404–406.
13. Albarran-Sotelo R. Airway control, ventilation, and oxygenation during CPR: part I. *Am Heart Assoc ECC Nat Newsl*. 1985;xx:2–4.
14. Vollmer TP, Stewart RD, Paris PM, et al. Use of a light stylet for guided orotracheal intubation in the prehospital setting. *Ann Emerg Med*. 1985;14:324–328.
15. Isessan KV, Saunders AB, Kaback K, et al. Difficult intubations: aids and alternative. *Am Fam Physician*. 1985;31:99–112.
16. MacCleod B. Verification of endotracheal tube placement with colorimetric end-tidal CO_2 detection. *Ann Emerg Med*. 1991;20:267–270.
17. Jacobs LM, Berrizbeitia LD, Bennett B, et al. Endotracheal intubation in the pre-hospital phase of emergency medical care. *JAMA*. 1983;250:2175–2177.
18. Shea SR, MacDonald JR, Gruzinsky G. Pre-hospital endotracheal tube airway or esophageal gastric tube airway: a clinical comparison. *Ann Emerg Med*. 1985;14:102–112.
19. Stewart RD, Paris PM, Pelton GH, et al. Effect of varied training techniques on field endotracheal intubation success rates. *Ann Emerg Med*. 1984;13:1032–1036.
20. Deleo BC. Endotracheal intubation by rescue squad personnel. *Heart Lung*. 1977;6:851–854.
21. Stauffer JL, Petty TL. Accidental intubation of the piriform sinus: a complication of ''roadside'' resuscitation. *JAMA*. 1977;237:2324–2325.
22. Wolff AP, Kuhn FA, Ogura JH. Pharyngeal esophageal perforations associated with rapid oral endotracheal intubation. *Ann Otolaryngol*. 1971;81:258–261.
23. Myers EM. Hypopharyngeal perforation: a complication of endotracheal intubation. *Laryngoscope*. 1982;92:583–585.
24. LoCicero J. Tracheo-carotid artery erosion following endotracheal intubation. *J Trauma*. 1984;24:907–909.
25. Blanc VF, Tremblay NA. The complications of tracheal intubation: a new classification with a review of the literature. *Anesth Analg*. 1975;53:202–213.

26. Don Michael TA, Labert EH, Mehram A. Mouth to lung airway for cardiac resuscitation. *Lancet*. 1968;2:1329.
27. Adler J, Dykan M. Gastric rupture: an unusual complication of the esophageal obturator airway. *Ann Emerg Med*. 1983;12:224–225.
28. Yancey W, Wears R, Kamajian G, et al. Unrecognized tracheal intubation: a complication of the esophageal obturator airway. *Ann Emerg Med*. 1980;9:18–20.
29. Low RB, Jensen RD, Cavanaugh KJ. Marked anterior displacement of the trachea and larnyx from an esophageal obturator airway. *Ann Emerg Med*. 1982;11:670–672.
30. Pilcher DB. Esophageal perforation following use of esophageal obturator airway. *Chest*. 1976;69:377–380.
31. Carlson WJ, Hunter SW, Bonnabeau RC. Esophageal perforation with obturator airway. *JAMA*. 1979;241:1154–1155.
32. Strate RG, Fisher RP. Medioesophageal perforations by esophageal obturator airway. *J Trauma*. 1976;16:503–511.
33. Meislin H. The esophageal obturator airway: a study of respiratory effectiveness. *Ann Emerg Med*. 1980;9:54–59.
34. Frass M. Esophageal tracheal combitube (ETC) for emergency intubation: anatomical evaluation of ETC placement by radiography. *Resuscitation*. 1989;18:95–102.
35. Carden E, Friedman D. Further studies of manually operated self-inflating resuscitation bags. *Anesth Analg*. 1976;56:202–206.
36. McSwain NE. The McSwain dart: device for relief of tension pneumothorax. *Med Instrum*. 1982;16:249.
37. Lewis FR. Thoracic trauma. *Surg Clin North Am*. 1981;62:97.
38. Bracken M. A randomized, controlled trial of methylprednisolone or naloxone in the treatment of acute spinal-cord injury. *N Engl J Med*. 1990;322:1405–1411.
39. Geisler F. Recovery of motor function after spinal-cord injury—a randomized, placebo-controlled trial with GM_1 ganglioside. *N Engl J Med*. 1991;324:1829–1838.
40. Gennarelli T. Emergency department management of head injuries in emergency medicine. *Clin North Am*. 1984:749–760.
41. Plum F. Disorders of the nervous system and behavior. In: Beeson PB, McDermott W, Wyngaarden JB, eds. *Textbook of Medicine: XI*. Philadelphia: Saunders; 1979:639–930.
42. Guyton AC. *Textbook of Medical Physiology*. Philadelphia: Saunders; 1981.
43. American Academy of Orthopedic Surgeons. *Emergency Care and Transportation of the Sick and Injured*. 3rd ed. Menasha, WA: Banta; 1981.
44. Caroline N. *Emergency Care in the Streets*. 2nd ed. Boston: Little, Brown; 1983.
45. Johnson RM, Hart EL, Simmons EF, et al. Cervical orthoses—a study comparing their effectiveness in restricting cervical motion in normal subjects. *J Bone Joint Surg Am*. 1977;59:332–339.
46. Podolsky SM, Baraff LJ, Simon RR, et al. Efficacy of cervical spine immobilization methods. *J Trauma*. 1983;23:461–465.
47. McSwain Jr N. Pneumatic anti-shock garment: state of the art 1988. *Ann Emerg Med*. 1988;17:506–525.
48. Mattox K, Bickell WH, Pepe PE, et al. Prospective MAST study in 911 patients. *J Trauma*. 1989;29:1104–1112.

8. Transfusions

FREDERICK B. EPSTEIN, MD, FACEP

HISTORY OF TRANSFUSION PRACTICE

Although the modern history of transfusion could not have begun prior to Harvey's description of circulatory anatomy in 1616, the essential property of blood in life sustenance had been recognized since antiquity. Awed by ignorance, ancient physicians ascribed magical properties to its transference. Hopeful young Roman gladiators eagerly drank the blood of their slain mentors; similarly, in 1492, ailing Pope Innocent VIII was persuaded to drink the blood of three sacrificial youths in an attempted rejuvenation.[1] Furthermore, an awareness that blood is composed of functional components is evident in the Hippocratic practice of diagnosis by analysis of blood specimens for the proper proportion of four humors: (1) the "blood" (erythrocytes); (2) the "phlegm" (buffy coat); (3) the "yellow bile" (bilirubin); and (4) the "black bile" (melena).[2] This Hippocratic differentiation between diseases of deranged blood composition and those due to faulty blood containment was precursory to the evolution of physicians and surgeons, respectively, to care for these diseases.

Definition of the essential anatomy by Harvey made intravascular blood transfer feasible. Several concepts had yet to develop scientifically, however, including the medicinal inoculation of the circulation as well as subsequent consideration of the safety and efficacy of donor blood. Christopher Wren, a British naturalist, is credited with founding the practice of intravenous administration of medications in 1657, and fellow countryman Richard Lower concluded a series of animal experiments with the first direct canine transfusion in 1666.[3] Predictably, only 1 year later, transfusion of the first human was recorded by the Frenchman John Baptiste Denys. This first recipient was a 15-year-old boy, who suffered from an obscure fever and who had been made anemic by repeated venesection. The youth reportedly recovered following transfusion of 9 ounces of blood from the carotid artery of a sheep. Buoyed by this apparent success, Denys sought to perform additional heterologous transfusions during the ensuing year.

A series of transfusions that Denys gave to his fourth patient resulted in 150 years of proscribed obsolescence of blood transfusion. This fourth patient was a philanderer whom Denys sought to quiet by transfusion from a docile calf. Noting partial improvement in the patient's behavior, Denys repeated a similar transfusion a few days later; however, this transfusion was attended by development of heat traveling up the arm, dyspnea, flank pain, and subsequent bloody urine. The patient ultimately survived this first recorded transfusion reaction, but two months later became incorrigible, prompting his wife to insist that Denys give her husband another transfusion. The attempted third transfusion was ultimately aborted because of poor patient cooperation. Even so, the patient died the following night, and the widow brought a manslaughter suit against Denys. It was later disclosed that the patient had died of arsenic poisoning at the hands of his wife, who was in collusion with vindictive senior physicians who were bitter about the upstart, celebrated Denys. Nevertheless, the event had not failed in its political impact, and the French Parliament initiated a ban against transfusion that spread throughout Europe.[1]

Transfusion practice was resurrected from interdiction by the careful studies and subsequent practice of the British obstetrician James Blundell.[4] Following a series of animal experiments in which he correctly reasoned that transfusion should be limited to members of the same species, Blundell reported the first homologous human transfusion in 1818. Blood collected from assistants was transfused into a patient hopelessly moribund from inanition caused by pyloric stenosis. Despite brief resurgence, the patient died 3 days later, but an encouraged Blundell pursued the practice. The fifth such patient, a woman dying of uterine hemorrhage, became the first human whose survival was attributable to blood transfusion.

In addition to his interest in the clinical practice, Blundell sought to develop an apparatus by which to facilitate mechanical homologous blood transfer and overcome the difficulties inherent in the indirect transfer of coagulating blood. His most notable product was the "Impellor," the efficacy of which Blundell demonstrated by performing cyclical autotransfusion in a venesected dog. Thus, although widely credited as the founder of autotransfusion, it appears that Blundell never performed human autotransfusion.

Despite the efforts of Blundell and several successors, the problem of anticoagulation was not solved within their century. Not until 1902 did Alexis Carrel develop the surgical technique of direct transfusion by arteriovenous anastomosis; the technique was fraught with complications of volume control and did not survive the development of anticoagulants, but Carrel went on to pioneer the field of vascular surgery.[5,6]

In 1900, Karl Landsteiner made his celebrated description of three erythrocyte antigens A, B, and C (later changed to O to denote zero antigens) and the tendency of incompatible admixed homologous bloods to agglutinate. The codominant expression of AB was inferred by Landsteiner's disciples two years later. By 1907, Jansky[7] had suggested a classification of four blood groups as recognized today. Ottenberg had noted the Mendelian pattern of blood group inheritance by 1908, and was the first active proponent and practitioner of pretransfusion cross-matching for serocompatibility[8]; in 1923, he further speculated on the phenomenon of maternal alloimmunization by placental transfer of fetal blood.[9] In 1940, Landsteiner and Wiener (incorrectly) demonstrated that the agglutinin-causing hemolytic disease of the newborn that reacted with 85% of all human erythrocytes of any group could be produced by immunizing rabbits against red cells obtained from rhesus monkeys (thus, the origin of "Rh").[10] The following year, the true nature of the Rh agglutinin was clarified by Levine.[11]

The remaining significant historical events in the evolution of transfusion therapy involve the development of methods by which blood for transfusion could be stored and preserved. Maintenance of blood fluidity and sterility had confounded physicians since Blundell; solutions to these problems necessitated the search for means to preserve blood viability in storage.

Over 20 years after the demonstration of animal blood anticoagulation by addition of substances such as citrate to form calcium salts, Hustin first reported the human transfusion of citrated blood in 1914.[5] Several other investigators independently reported similar cases within the year, including Lewisohn,[12] who went on to determine scientifically the optimum ratio of citrate additive to blood. Most notable among these initial reports was that of Richard Weil, who exclusively demonstrated not only that such anticoagulated blood facilitated indirect transfusion, but also that such blood could be stored for several days prior to reinfusion without adverse effects.[13] The following year, Rous and Turner reported that the in vitro hemolysis that limited blood storage at that time could be delayed up to 2 weeks by the addition of dextrose.[14] The feasibility and clinical importance of the solutions developed by Rous and Turner were confirmed when the Allied Armies used this blood for treating combat casualties in World War I. In 1918, Canadian medical officer Oswald Robertson reported the successful transfusion of 22 soldiers, noting an additional advance: blood kept on ice could be stored as long as 26 days without adverse effect.[15]

Enthusiasm for the use of stored blood in this era was tempered by the frequent occurrence of febrile reactions. Physicians who collected and administered blood were reconciled to the use of open, glass bottle systems and reusable tubing. Closed, disposable plastic sets did not appear until 30 years later. The problem was further compounded by the fact that the glucose in the anticoagulant solution within the blood collection bottles formed caramel when these bottles were autoclaved. Nevertheless, the practice of transfusion grew exponentially, resulting in the founding of the first true blood bank by Fantus at the Cook County Hospital in 1937.[16] Interestingly, Fantus promoted the concept of patient blood donation for storage 1 or 2 weeks before scheduled surgery in anticipation of (auto)transfusion, a technique that continues to receive controversial endorsement today.[17]

During early World War II, Loutit and his colleagues advanced transfusion therapy by demonstrating that acidification of the sodium citrate-dextrose solutions (acid-citrate dextrose or ACD) by addition of citric acid not only eliminated caramelization of glucose, but also uniformly resulted in acceptable viability of red cells refrigerated for 21 days.[18] In 1957, following the interim clarification of the importance of erythrocyte glycolysis in maintaining viability by preservation of adenosine triphosphate (ATP) stores, Gibson and his co-workers[19] introduced phosphate buffering of the storage solutions (citrate-phosphate dextrose or CPD), improving the 21-day survival of stored cells. CPD was licensed by the Food and Drug Administration (FDA) in 1971, effectively replacing ACD. Continued search by a host of investigators for additives with which to maintain nucleotide levels (especially 2,3-DPG*) led to the study of the effect of direct addition of the precursor adenine. The results led to FDA licensure of CPD-A in 1978 for blood storage as long as 35 days.

Prompted by the increasing use of component therapy, contemporary investigation to improve preservative media has focused on the feasibility of preserving packed cells after virtually all plasma has been removed from the parent unit of whole blood. Historically, the preparation of such ("hard-pack") cells has been prohibited by a regulation requiring that packed cell units not exceed an hematocrit of 80%. This requirement was based on the demonstration that up to 40% of the adenine and glucose was removed during preparation of units of greater hematocrit, resulting in unacceptable 24-hour in vivo red cell survival following transfusion of such units.[20] (Standards require that only storage methods associated with at least 70% post-transfusion red cell survival at 24 hours may be used.)[21]

The anticipated removal of plasma has recently led to revised schemes of blood collection in which the addition of nutrient preservatives, including adenine and extra fuel, is delayed until the hard-packed cells are prepared. Following plasma removal from a unit collected in simple anticoagulant, 100 mL saline containing various commercial proportions of adenine, glucose, and other additives is returned to the packed cells to reconstitute volume and viscosity, as well as enhance viability, of the protein-poor units. Consistent with the pioneering European experience of recent years,[22,23] these units containing additive saline and hence known as AS cells have revolutionized the practice of transfusion therapy in this country. Such units provide the transfusion recipient with a red cell mass and total volume at viscocity-dependent flow rates essentially identical to those of whole blood while limiting much of the inherent risk associated with transfusion of the latter product. This manner of component preparation simultaneously improves the harvest of the nonerythrocytic products derived from the parent donation, thus improving the efficiency of each donation. Further, the FDA currently licenses the storage of AS prepared cells for up to 42 days, in contrast to the 35-day expiration of conventionally prepared products in CPD-A.

REGULATORY STANDARDS AND COLLECTION PRACTICES

Because blood and its components are biological products, they are subject to regulation by the Bureau of Biologics, FDA, Department of Health and Human Services (DHHS) of the federal government. Minimum standards adopted for operation of blood collection and transfusion services must conform to these regulations as written in the *Code of Federal Regulations*.[24] A number of allied organizations are further involved with the regulation and administration of transfusion practice, including the American Red Cross, United Blood Services, the College of American Pathologists, and the Council of Community Blood Centers. Especially notable is the American Association of Blood Banks (AABB), a nonprofit organization founded in 1947 and devoted exclusively to the promotion and advancement of safe transfusion practice. Its official publication, entitled *Standards for Blood Banks and Transfusion Services*,[25] has become the definitive source document in the preparation of the standards and procedural manual required at each blood bank.

The AABB has three types of facilities that collectively administer its volunteer national blood product. The "community blood bank" (also known as a community blood center) is a non–hospital-based facility that collects blood from at least 100 donors annually for subsequent regional distribution. The coordination among these centers is typically supervised by one of the regional offices. A "hospital blood bank" not only must collect blood from at least 100 donors annually, but also must regulate transfusion practice within the facility. A "transfusion service" collects blood from fewer than 100 donors, but must proctor the transfusion of at least 500 U annually. Any of these facilities may perform a variety of allied services, including blood typing and compatibility testing, donor screening for hepatitis and syphilis, preparation of components, HLA screening, and paternity testing. A given unit of blood may have originated from a donor anywhere within the service region and may be days old before it arrives at the source storage facility. Centers that obtain blood from paid donors sell the pooled product to pharmaceutical houses for refinement into various commercial products; these centers must comply with the less stringent regulations that govern the handling of such units.

Volunteer donors must submit to an historical examination certified by affidavit as well as a physical examination in order to qualify for donation. The common factors that influence donor eligibility are summarized in Table 8-1.

Blood is collected into FDA-approved containers that must be pyrogen-free, closed, and sterile. Typically, such collection sets include a series of interconnected closed satellite bags that contain anticoagulant and/or preservative so that subsequent fractionation may be performed within the closed system. The volume of blood drawn from a donor is controlled by balance or vacuum-assisted devices that regulate the additional fluid weight added to the premeasured collection bag and contained anticoagulant. The "ideal" (CPD-A) whole blood unit contains 450 mL whole blood plus 14 mL anticoagulant per 100 mL collected blood, or 513 mL. Regulations permit an added weight of whole blood per each unit ranging from 425 to 520 g (based on blood specific

---

*2,3 Diphosphoglycerate.

Table 8-1 Facts About Being a Blood Donor

Individuals may donate blood if they: Are in good health. Weigh at least 110 pounds.[1] Are at least 17 years of age and have not reached their 66th birthday. Donors over age 66 must have a written statement from their physician dated within 4 weeks of the donation, saying they are in good health. Have not given blood within the past 56 days.		*Blood Disease:*	Must be evaluated by Red Cross nurse.
		Cancer:	Basal cell skin cancer: No deferral. All other forms must be evaluated and approved by written authority of the Blood Services Medical Director.
Medical questions about donating blood:		*Cardiac Condition:*	Donors must have a statement from their cardiologist certifying fitness to donate and exact cardiac condition; charge nurse will evaluate.
AIDS:[2]	Deferral if donor fits in one of the following groups which are considered at increased risk for developing AIDS: • Persons with symptoms and signs suggestive of AIDS. These include severe night sweats, unexplained fevers, unexpected weight loss, lymphadenopathy (swollen glands), or Kaposi's sarcoma (a rare cancer). • Any male engaging in a homosexual contact since 1977. • Recent immigrants or travelers entering the United States from areas identified by the FDA as high risk for endemic HIV transmission. • Present or past abusers of intravenous drugs. • Sexual partners of persons at increased risk of AIDS.	*Chest Pain:*	Must be evaluated by Red Cross nurse.
		Cold:	Deferral if donor does not feel well; no deferral if symptoms are mild and donor feels well.
		Dental:	72-hour deferral for a tooth extraction; there is no deferral for all other dental work unless an infection is involved.
		Diabetes:	No deferral if controlled by diet or oral medications; deferral if insulin controlled.
		Drugs:	Donors must be permanently deferred if they have ever taken self-administered narcotic drugs.
		Epilepsy:	Permanent deferral.
		Exposure to Hepatitis:	6-month deferral after close exposure; should be evaluated through the Blood Services Nursing Department.
Allergies:	No deferral if donor feels comfortable on the day of donation.	*Hepatitis:*[3]	Anyone ever having had hepatitis should not donate blood.
Allergy Shots:	No deferral.		
Antibiotics:	Injections: 2-week deferral for long-acting antibiotics; all others acceptable upon evaluation by Red Cross nurse. Oral: 48-hour deferral if there are no symptoms of infection and donor has been on 5 days or more. Ointments: No deferral. Oral for acne: No deferral for low dosage; 1-month deferral for Accutane.	*HBIG:*	Exposure resulting in hepatitis B immune globulin injection extends deferral to 12 months; regular immune globulin deferral is unchanged (ie, 6 months) after hepatitis exposure.
		Heptavax B:	No waiting.
		Hypertension Treatment:	This must be evaluated by a Red Cross nurse on the day of donation; as long as blood pressure is within Red Cross limits, individual may donate; most anti-hypertensive medications are not reason for deferral.
Artificial Kidney Machine:	Exposure to, or close contact with, a patient on a kidney machine is a 6-month deferral.		
Asthma:	Acceptable upon evaluation by Red Cross nurse.		
Birth Control Pills:	No deferral.	*Immunization Shots:*	Acceptable if symptom-free.

[1] Persons weighting less than 110 pounds may donate proportionately smaller volumes than 1 U whole blood.

[2] Effective March 14, 1985, the FDA mandated serologic screening of all donors for presence of antibodies to HIV-I, formerly known as HLTV-III virus. Effective December 1988 the FDA mandated screening for antibody to HLTV-III virus, a related retrovirus causing leukemia but not AIDS in humans. Effective March 1992 the FDA mandated screening for antibody to HIV-II virus, another retrovirus etiologically identified in a small percentage of current AIDS patients.

[3] In 1986 the FDA mandated "surrogate" donor screening of ALT enzyme levels, as well as HbcAb; in May, 1990 the FDA licensed an assay and mandated screening of donors for antibody to hepatitis-C virus.

Table 8-1 continued

Infectious Mononucleosis:	After 2 months, individual can donate; however, if jaundice occurred during the acute clinical phase of mononucleosis, the donor must be evaluated by a Red Cross nurse at the donation site.	*Shortness of Breath:*	evaluated by a Red Cross nurse; 6-month deferral for C-section. Must be evaluated by a Red Cross nurse.
Malaria:	Must be evaluated by Red Cross nurse.	*Stitches:* *Surgery:*	Deferral until removed. Major: 6-month deferral. Minor: must be evaluated by a Red Cross nurse.
Medications:	Deferral varies with the medication being taken; donors should bring the name of any medication with them to the site, or they can call the Blood Services Nursing Department for clarification.	*Tattoos and Transfusions:* *Travel Outside United States:* *Yellow Jaundice:*	6-month deferral. Must be evaluated by a Red Cross nurse. From causes other than hepatitis, must be evaluated by a Red Cross nurse.
Pregnancy:	A 6-month deferral after a full-term pregnancy, the donor must be		

Source: Courtesy of American Red Cross.

gravity averaging 1.054 g/mL) equivalent to 405 to 495 mL blood. The blood collected is refrigerated at 1° to 6°C (usually 4°C) immediately following collection unless platelets are to be harvested; regardless, the blood must be refrigerated within 4 hours.

Blood issued by the bank may be returned for storage and subsequent reissue, provided that the closed system has not been violated in any fashion and that its temperature has been continuously maintained below 10°C. Once the closed blood container has been entered, the component must be transfused within four hours if stored at room temperature, transfused within 24 hours if immediately returned to 1° to 6°C refrigeration, or discarded.

Whole blood fractionation for component preparation initially involves separation of cells from plasma. The primary separation may result from either active refrigerated centrifuge (5,000g × 5 minutes at 5°C) or from passive sedimentation within the refrigerator. The density of the cell sediment and, thus, the hematocrit of the packed cell unit vary according to the method of sedimentation; conventional centrifuged units typically achieve a higher hematocrit, although not over 80%. In a quality assurance survey conducted by the Red Cross, the average hematocrit of a unit of packed cells was 73%.[26]

The minimum hematocrit of conventional CPD packed cell units is regulated indirectly by prescribed methods for plasma removal. The supernatant plasma is expressed from the unit into a satellite bag by means of a spring-driven press device. Like blood volume taken from a donor, plasma removal is monitored by a weighing technique, with the typical removal of 232 to 258 g, or 225 to 250 mL anticoagulated plasma. The feasibility of physical reconstitution of viscosity for augmentation of flow by addition of crystalloid to packed cells (AS cells) should be evident from this method of primary preparation. Historically, regulation has restricted such additives to normal saline, because there have been no alternate isotonic electrolyte solutions devoid of calcium ions, which neutralize the anticoagulant. There is now available, however, a family of newer, balanced electrolyte solutions devoid of calcium that may be used for hemodilution, as well as volume expansion, which may be preferable in ionic composition to normal saline.

AVAILABLE BLOOD COMPONENTS

A summary chart of the available blood components is presented in Table 8-2.

Red Blood Cells

Packed cells may be further processed by means of special techniques to accomplish specific objectives. Washed and leukocyte-poor red cells, for example, are designed to minimize the antigenic challenge to recipients who have had earlier febrile transfusion reactions or analogous complications resulting from immunization by nonerythrocytic antigens. With the addition of the protective agent glycerol, leukocyte-poor cells may subsequently be cryopreserved, permitting extended storage for up to 3 years. These cryopreserved cells must be thawed and deglycerolized by washing techniques before transfusion, a preparation technique that requires several hours; thus, these cryopreserved cells and the antigen-poor precursor units are rarely used in the common practice of emergency medicine. Further, the recent introduction of simple polyester leukocyte filters, which effectively remove the residual leukocytes from normally prepared components, affords a practical and greatly

Table 8-2 Summary Chart of Blood Components

Component	Contents and Volume	Amount of Active Substance per Transfused Unit	Major Indications	Action	Special Precautions	Hazards[1]	Rate of Infusion
Red cells	Red cells, some plasma, some WBCs and platelets or their degradation products (250–350 mL)	200 mL packed red cell mass	Symptomatic anemia	Restoration of oxygen-carrying capacity, restoration of blood volume	Must be ABO-compatible	Hepatitis allergic reactions, febrile reactions	For massive loss, fast as patient can tolerate
Red cells Leukocytes removed by washing Leukocyte-poor	Red cells, some plasma, few WBCs (200–250 mL)	185 mL red cells	Febrile reactions from leukocyte antibodies, or for which plasma removal is indicated	Restoration of oxygen-carrying capacity, restoration of blood volume	Must be ABO-compatible	Hepatitis	For massive loss, fast as patient can tolerate
FFP	Red cells—no plasma, minimal WBCs and platelets (220–250 mL)	220–250 U factor VIII	Deficit of labile plasma coagulation factors	Source of labile and nonlabile plasma factors	Must be ABO-compatible	Hepatitis, allergic reactions, febrile reactions, circulatory overload	Approximately 10 mL/min
Single donor plasma, frozen or liquid	Plasma, no labile coagulation factors (220–250 mL)		Deficit of stable coagulation factors	Source of nonlabile factors	Must be ABO-compatible	Hepatitis, allergic reactions, febrile reactions, circulatory overload	Approximately 10 mL/min
Cryoprecipitated AHF	Coagulation factors (10–25 mL)	80–100 U factor VIII	Hemophilia and von Willebrand's disease, fibrinogen deficiency	Provides factor VIII, fibrinogen, VWF, factor XIII	Rapid infusion and frequent repeat doses may be necessary	Hepatitis, allergic reactions, febrile reactions	Approximately 10 mL diluted component per minute
Platelets	Platelets, few WBCs, some plasma (30–50 mL)	5.5×10^{10} platelets per pack	Bleeding from thrombocytopenia or platelet function abnormality	Provides platelets as well as trace quantities coagulation factors	Should not use microaggregate filter	Hepatitis, allergic reactions, febrile reactions	Approximately 5 mL/min

[1] All single unit components convey same hepatitis risk as parent unit whole blood; pooled plasma and platelet concentrates or derivatives convey additive hepatitis risk. VWF, von Willebrand factor.

Sources: Blood Component Therapy: A Physician's Handbook, American Association of Blood Banks; and *Circular of Information for the Use of Blood and Blood Components,* a joint publication of the American Association of Blood Banks, American Red Cross, and Council of Community Blood Centers.

simplified means of minimizing the risks (especially simple febrile reactions and cytomegalovirus transmission) associated with these residual cells.

Plasma Components

Single donor plasma (SDP) may be harvested from the parent whole blood unit anytime from collection up to 5 days after the expiration date of the parent unit. Such plasma may be stored liquid at 1° to 6°C in which case it must be used or discarded by 5 days after expiration of the parent unit (ie, up to 40 days from the time of phlebotomy when collected in CPD-A). Alternatively, the plasma may be frozen to at least −18°C (preferably −30°C), after which it may be stored as long as 5 years. SDP is infrequently prepared now, however, in part because of the revised allocation schedules for whole blood and component fractionation attending the evolution of AS cell preparation. Conversely, when plasma is similarly prepared and frozen within 6 hours of collection of the parent unit, the product is designated fresh-frozen plasma (FFP) and may be so stored for up to 1 year. FFP is distinguished from SDP in that the latter is deficient in the labile clotting factors. Following 1 year of frozen storage, FFP is generally also deficient in the labile factors and, therefore, must be redesignated as frozen SDP for the duration of the permissible 5-year storage.

FFP must be thawed briefly at room temperature prior to placement in a thawing bath/agitator apparatus at 37°C before administration. Such units may be prepared for transfusion within approximately 30 minutes when necessary. By contrast, following passive, uninterrupted thawing of FFP to 4°C, there remains an insoluble proteinaceous aggregate rich in antihemophilic factor (AHF), as well as von Willebrand factor, factor XIII, fibrinogen, fibronectin, and other trace constituents. This insoluble cryoprecipitate is recovered by centrifugation and refrozen in less than 15 mL residual plasma, such that 1 "unit" (bag) of factor VIII concentrate (FVIII:C) contains an average of 80 to 100 U of factor VIII. Such bags of cryoprecipitate obtained from multiple donors may also be pooled in saline; the FVIII:C content is assumed to equal or exceed 80 U per contained bag. Similarly, commercially prepared lyophilized factor VIII concentrate may be prepared from pooled units; the assayed potency of the preparation is marked on the vial.

The required AHF dosage for treatment of clinical coagulopathy varies according to the severity of the injury. Various schedules of required Factor VIII activity (in percent) have been suggested; however, a minimum activity of 50% generally renders hemostatic competence to the hemophiliac in any situation. For emergency calculation, assuming that there is no initial activity (but also assuming that antibody to factor VIII does not complicate therapy), the number of bags required may be computed by dividing the product of the patient's weight (in kilograms) and the desired activity level (in percent) by 200. Conversely, in a controlled clinical situation and one in which the precise clotting defect is known with certainty, a heat-treated factor VIII concentrate is the preferred component for treatment of hemophilia A, although cryoprecipitate remains the component of choice for the patient with von Willebrand's disease.

The residual cryoprecipitate-poor plasma remains an effective source of the stable, vitamin K-dependent factors, as well as a colloidal volume expander. Cryoprecipitate-poor whole blood may also be prepared by return of the residual plasma to the parent unit; this has been suggested as a possible solution to the conflict between advocates of the use of whole blood and advocates of the use of blood components in resuscitation of traumatic hypovolemia.[27] The residual plasma may also be pooled for commercial harvesting of plasma protein fraction, albumin, coagulation factor concentrates, immunoglobulins, and related constituents.

Because of concern over the exponential increase in the use of FFP, the National Institutes of Health (NIH) convened a Consensus Development Conference to define the appropriate indications for the administration of FFP and to develop a strategy for improved physician education in order to limit dubious practices.[28] Of interest to practitioners of emergency medicine, it was concluded that the use of FFP is indicated for treatment of "dilutional coagulopathy" as a result of massive blood transfusion (although best evidence indicates that thrombocytopenia is likely to be the cause[27]) and for emergency reversal of warfarin effect in the anticoagulated patient with a hemorrhagic complication.

Platelets

Following removal of platelet-rich supernatant plasma by means of a "light-spin" (centrifugation) of unrefrigerated whole blood within 6 hours of collection, platelets are prepared by extracting the sediment from a subsequent "hard-spin" of the plasma. By regulation, the concentrated platelet "unit" or pack must contain at least 5.5×10^{10} platelets at pH 6 or greater in 30 to 50 mL residual plasma. Platelet concentrates may be stored either at 1° to 6°C for up to 48 hours or, alternatively, at room temperature (20° to 24°C) with continuous gentle agitation for three to five days. The viability of platelets, especially those stored at room temperature, is pH-dependent; the pH tends to vary according to the material construction of the storage bag, which may be either polyolefin or polyvinylchloride.

Platelets bear at least three systems of antigens.[29] In addition to unique antigens, platelets and several other tissues (as well as secretions in persons not homozygous for the recessive secretor allele) bear ABO group antigens; moreover, like all tissues except erythrocytes, platelets bear HLA system antigens. Although it is preferable to transfuse ABO-compatible platelets, it is not essential unless the unit is marked by visible red cell admixture. Recipients of serial platelet transfusions frequently become alloimmunized to HLA antigens, however, necessitating a search for HLA-compatible (two to four antigen match) donors. Such platelets may be obtained by hemapheresis of a single, compatible donor, resulting in production of a "unit" of platelets equivalent in number and volume to six to eight conventional platelet units.

The most common indication for platelet transfusion in emergency medical practice has been dilutional thrombocytopenia attendant to massive blood replacement. Studies have shown that the coagulopathy in these patients usually responds to platelet administration alone;[27,30] such patients frequently have abnormal in vitro coagulation times, but these tend to correlate poorly with clinically evident bleeding and to normalize after successful resuscitation without specific provision of clotting factors.[27] Despite this evidence for efficacy of platelets prophylactically administered to massively transfused patients, the NIH has recently discouraged this or indeed any prophylactic transfusion of blood products, because of the evolving concern for potential transmission of HIV and related pathogens. In choosing to withhold platelets in this circumstance, however, the emergency physician must contrast the benefits and risks associated with intervention into this predictably imminent and almost certainly catastrophic clinical complication of massive transfusion with the relatively minute statistical risk of infectious illness developing remotely.

Occasionally, the physician is confronted by a patient with an oncologic emergency presenting as thrombocytopenic bleeding, particularly when the count falls below 20,000 platelets per microliter blood. Such a patient typically responds to delivery of six to eight regular platelet units, provided that post-transfusion platelet survival is initially normal.[29]

TESTING FOR SEROLOGIC COMPATIBILITY

AABB *Standards* requires that blood banks perform those tests necessary to ensure ABO blood group compatibility between donor and recipient, as well as those tests necessary to identify clinically significant (agglutinating or hemolyzing) recipient antibodies active at 37°C, including but not limited to antiglobulin tests. In practice, these requirements are met by performance of three allied procedures:

1. ABO and D (Rh) blood group typing
2. screening of sera for the presence of unsuspected antibodies
3. cross-matching (in vitro incubation) of intended donor and recipient blood specimens

Early investigators noted the phenomenon of reciprocal isoagglutination, the existence of erythrocyte antigens and the absence of antibodies to those antigens on the cells of the patient. It is now known that these isoagglutinins (antibodies) are not present at birth, but rather are formed early in life in immunologic response to the ubiquitous presence of bacterial polysaccharide antigens closely related to the (absent) red cell antigens.[7] Nevertheless, these predictable antibodies continue to be regarded as naturally occurring in contrast to the unsuspected alloantibodies, which form only in response to occult immunization, including that coincident to pregnancy or prior transfusion. The best known example of the latter is the alloantibody formed by the mother in response to isoimmunization by fetal D (Rh) antigen.

The remaining primary feature by which to distinguish these antibodies is the inherent capacity of each to effect hemolysis or agglutination when mixed with incompatible blood. Unlike the "natural" isoagglutinins that are so named for this activity, many of the alloantibodies that form in response to the minor erythrocyte antigens (eg, Kell, Duffy, Kidd, and Lewis) are incapable of similarly affecting red cells in the normally existing titers. This "incomplete" antibody presence or activity can be demonstrated in vitro, however, either by a variety of enhancement techniques or by antiglobulin (Coombs) testing. Finally, antibody activity may vary according to the ambient temperature; because clinically significant transfusion reactions are usually limited to antibodies with demonstrated in vitro activity at 37°C, detection of antibodies active only at lower temperature is not required in routine compatibility testing.

Typing of donor and recipient blood, thus, refers to the determination and selection of identical ABO and Rh (D) phenotypes to avoid predictable isoagglutinin incompatibility, as well as Rh alloimmunization. Screen refers to the screening of sera, particularly that of the recipient, for the presence of unsuspected alloantibody against Rh, as well as several other minor antigens resulting from prior immunization by any means. Finally, cross-matching refers to the incubated admixture between donor and recipient fractions that has subsequently been treated stepwise with enhancing techniques designed to reveal the presence of incomplete antibodies and to corroborate the compatibility between patient and the intended donor units selected for imminent transfusion.

Blood Typing

Routine ABO group testing is performed by mixing patient cells with commercial anti-A and anti-B sera, known as forward typing or testing, and by mixing commercial A and B cells with patient sera, known as reverse typing. Unlike patient sera used for reverse typing of commercial cells, commercial antisera are cultivated to such high titers that phlebotomized patient cells need not undergo centrifugal separation within the clot tube before being tested for agglutination; similarly, incubation of the reaction to 37°C is unnecessary and, in fact, weakens these reactions. Therefore, forward typing of the patient sample can be completed very expeditiously, which is fortuitous in an emergency.

Forward typing should not be relied on exclusively for typing of specimens, however, unless the patient's blood has been typed in the past, such as occurs with donor blood at the collection facility. The typing of patient (recipient) samples for emergency release of type-specific blood must at least include corroboration of compatibility by the saline immediate spin procedure. Rh grouping is determined by means of commercial antisera in a method analogous to forward ABO typing.

Antibody Screening

AABB *Standards* requires antibody screening of all recipient sera and strongly recommends screening of donor sera obtained from persons with a history of prior transfusion or pregnancy. The regulation in regard to the screening of donor sera is relaxed, because the reaction between donor sera and recipient cells (known as the "minor" transfusion reaction) is expected to be clinically insignificant, owing to the quantitatively limited passive transfer of such sera. This is in contrast to the "major" transfusion reaction that is anticipated when an alloimmunized recipient is challenged with donor cells bearing the corresponding antigen.

Antibody screening is performed by incubating commercial group O cells of defined minor antigenic phenotype with sera to be tested at 37°C and by using enhancing techniques (as well as an antiglobulin phase) to demonstrate any potentially active agglutinin. Group O cells are specifically selected to avoid potentially interfering reactions by naturally occurring ABO isoagglutinins.

Whereas literally hundreds of obscure erythrocyte antigens and corresponding alloantibodies have been identified, the screening procedure is logistically limited to the use of cells bearing not less than the 18 antigens[25] from the Rh, Kell, Duffy, Kidd, Lewis, and similar prevalent systems; typically, fewer than two dozen such antigens are involved. For sensitivity of antibody detection, it is desirable, but not always feasible, to obtain test cells homozygous for various antigens. The problem of distinguishing trace, but potentially dangerous, antibodies from clinically insignificant antibodies necessitates use of techniques such as proteolytic pretreatment[31] of the test cells and suspension of cells in polymerized albumin[32] or low ionic salt solutions,[33] which tend to enhance the activity of incomplete antibodies. In practice, similar enhancement techniques are used during, and antibody screening is typically performed simultaneously with, the cross-matching test for serologic compatibility.

Cross-Matching Test

The cross-matching procedure corroborates the predicted compatibility between recipient blood and donor units selected on the basis of results of the ABO typing and antibody screening procedures. Therefore, it is a confirmatory check of these prior results, as well as a final means to detect unpredictable incompatibility before transfusion of the patient.

Historically, the cross-matching procedure included each of two series of stepwise incubations: that between recipient sera and donor cells, known as the major cross-match, and the reciprocal incubation between donor sera and patient cells, known as the minor cross-match. The results quantitatively indicate the predicted severity of reaction that may be caused by serologic incompatibility following transfusion. The limited passive transfer of donor sera containing antibody to recipient antigens is usually insufficient to effect a clinically significant reaction; thus, AABB *Standards* requires only the major cross-matching test, and the reciprocal test is obsolete in practice.

The complexity of the cross-matching procedure is necessitated by the comprehensive effort to determine whether incompatible alloantibodies are present in recipient sera, particularly those that are inactive in vitro, but may be active in vivo at 37°C. In vivo activity may result from the disproportion in the antibody:donor cell ratio, further augmented by anamnestic immune production of additional alloantibody. Therefore, it is essential to use one or more of a variety of available enhancing techniques designed to disclose the presence of such incomplete, incompatible antibody. It is also essential to perform such steps after incubation to 37°C. Clearly, the time required for the performance of complete cross-matching is in sharp contrast with that required for simple typing procedures, which yield only type-specific blood.

The phenomenon of enhanced cross-matching sensitivity originates in the demonstrated increase in antibody affinity and activity for erythrocyte antigens following incubation in a test medium of reduced ionic strength.[31-34] Such conducive media are most commonly created by addition of low ionic strength solutions (LISS) or solutions that contain hypertonic or polymerized albumin. The minimum acceptable duration of 37°C incubation required for adequate testing is least with the LISS technique, but the difference is only rarely of significance, even in emergency practice.

Several preformed antibodies do not commonly achieve sufficient titer to effect agglutination of incompatible donor cells, despite the presence of offending erythrocyte antigens. Agglutination follows the addition of test sera that contain antibody (antiglobulin) to human immunoglobulin, however, because this increases the concentration of alloantibody-bound erythrocytes (ie, positive indirect Coombs test). The reliability of each negative antiglobulin test result is subsequently confirmed by addition of a commercial Coombs check or control reagent that contains sensitized group O red cells bearing IgG; antiglobulin remaining free after a true negative Coombs test agglutinates the sensitized control cells when they are added.

In a complementary control procedure, one tube that contains only patient cells and sera (autocontrol) is subjected to all steps of the cross-matching procedure in parallel fashion to those tubes that contain patient sera with cells from each donor unit selected (in accord with the number of units requisitioned) for study; agglutination at any step within the autocontrol tube indicates the presence of an autoagglutinin (eg, positive direct Coombs test from autoimmune cold agglutinin), which may not prohibit donor transfusion, but necessitates additional measures to ensure that an alloantibody reactive at the same step in the sequence is not hidden.

Procedurally, cross-matching consists of a stepwise series of reactions between precise volumes of recipient (patient) sera obtained from a centrifuged sample and a 2% to 5% saline suspension of washed donor cells from each selected unit. Historically, the cross-matching procedure was usually initiated with an immediate spin (ie, an immediate centrifugation of a tube containing patient sera and saline) that suspended cells prior to 37°C incubation or addition of any enhancing agents. This optional immediate spin is commonly eliminated in current practice in favor of subsequent, more sensitive steps in the cross-matching procedure. The primary value of the immediate spin is to illuminate ABO incompatibility quickly; cold agglutinins may also be detected, but these are generally considered insignificant unless they are also active after the 37°C incubation. Most blood banks require this quick check of ABO compatibility, however, before the emergency release of units of type-specific blood when complete cross-matching is not temporally feasible.

Typically, after the initial timed incubation of the cell suspension to 37°C, each successive reagent step involves

- decantation of the nonhemolyzed supernatant from the preceding centrifuged step
- resuspension of the sedimented cell button following confirmation of nonagglutination (ie, negative result)
- addition of next test or enhancing reagent
- timed centrifugation
- repeat examination of the (new) supernatant and cell button for positive results: hemolysis and agglutination, respectively

Inspection for agglutination further requires optical assistance, conventionally microscopic examination, before the result can be declared negative. In addition to the test tubes that contain cells from respective potential donor units and the autocontrol, the tubes that contain patient sera and commercial group O cells used for antibody screening are simultaneously subjected to several of the same reagent steps of the cross-matching procedure. There is no precise, preferred cross-matching procedure required by regulation to the exclusion of alternative, equally satisfactory methods, so long as the minimum testing requirements are met. One representative cross-matching procedure is presented in Table 8-3.

Table 8-3 LISS Cross-Matching Procedure

1. Wash donor cells twice with saline.
2. Wash donor cells with LISS.
3. Decant supernatant; resuspend cells to 2% to 5% concentration in LISS.
4. Add equal volumes of patient serum and LISS cells.
5. Centrifuge; examine for hemolysis/agglutination.
6. Incubate 10 minutes at 37°C.
7. Centrifuge; examine for hemolysis/agglutination.
8. Wash resuspended cells repeatedly with saline.
9. Decant completely; add one volume Coombs reagent.
10. Centrifuge; examine for hemolysis/agglutination.
11. If Coombs-negative, add Coombs-sensitized red cells.
12. Centrifuge; examine for hemolysis/agglutination.
13. If no agglutination (step 12), repeat entire procedure.

Source: Compiled from Walker R (Ed): *Technical Manual of the American Association of Blood Banks,* ed 10. Arlington, VA, 1990.

The recent widespread development of challenging surgical practices that demand increased quantities of replacement blood and the proliferation of newer hemotherapies that involve component fractionation have led to the development of schemes designed to conserve the available blood resources, such as consensus surgical blood order schedules and the type-and-screen procedure.[35] The latter is especially appropriate for cases in which the predicted or historical need for actual transfusion is least, as it is an abbreviated testing procedure that spares donor cell units by its use of patient cells and sera exclusively. The appropriate use of the type-and-screen procedure eliminates unnecessary cross-matching, thus containing laboratory costs and, ultimately, conserving blood products.

Criteria for ordering cross-matched blood for patients in the emergency department, conceptually analogous to the development of predetermined surgical blood schedules, have also been devised. Clarke and his associates[36] proposed four independent criteria by which to justify the emergency requisition of cross-matched blood: (1) shock; (2) hematocrit less than 30%; (3) witnessed blood loss exceeding 500 ml or frank gastrointestinal bleeding; and (4) expected emergency surgery with predicted blood loss. These authors demonstrated both prospectively[37] and retrospectively[36] the validity of these critera in reducing unnecessary serologic testing.

FUNCTIONAL CLASSIFICATION AND CLINICAL APPROACH TO COMPONENT USE

Viewed simplistically, the physiologic functions of blood may be classified into three discrete roles: (1) maintenance of energetics, the preservation of normal cellular fuel delivery, metabolism, and excretion; (2) immunocompetence, the capacity to distinguish self from foreign material and to respond to the latter so as to preserve health; and (3) hemostasis, the containment and maintenance of a fluid blood organ. The endogenous constituents of normal blood may be further classified into the cellular and acellular or plasmatic elements that preserve these functions. Erythrocytes, leukocytes, and platelets respectively serve the three functions as delineated; plasma is the fluid admixture of a variety of acellular constituents, each of which is dedicated primarily to one of the three functions (Table 8-4).

Similarly, the available pharmaceutical and banked blood components can be related to these three classes of functions (see Table 8-2). Only rarely does a patient suffer from simultaneous lesions in more than one of the three primary classes. Therefore, salient therapy is devoted exclusively to correction of the specific deficit manifested, with the remaining blood resource conserved as feasible. Advocates of component therapy argue that the use of whole blood for treatment of acute hemorrhage, which typically compromises only energetics, is analogous to the use of pooled simple rather than hyperimmune globulin for delivery of tetanus prophylaxis or use of FFP for treatment of hemophilia B. Furthermore, collection, processing, and distribution must be considered. Banked, refrigerated whole blood, for example, is functionally void of platelets as well as labile clotting factors by the end of 2 to 3 days.

The practicing emergency physician is confronted daily with patients suffering hypovolemia from acute hemorrhage. Data suggest that as many as 25% of patients who die from hemorrhage despite having survived long enough to reach the emergency department may have been salvageable. The most illuminating series of studies demonstrating this phenomenon were initiated by West, Trunkey, and Lim,[38] who reviewed treatment in two populations of 100 consecutive fatal vehicular accident victims who survived to emergency treatment. They contrasted the care provided in San Francisco within a paragon of regionalized trauma care at an academic institution supported by 24-hour in-house traumatologist, anesthesiologist, and intensivist, as well as an active walk-in blood donor program, with care provided in Orange County within an antithetical, nonregionalized community-based practice. Compared with a single preventable death in San Francisco, two-thirds of the nonneurologic Orange County deaths (as well as one-third of the CNS-related deaths) were judged preventable in retrospect. Inadequate management of hemorrhage was responsible for 82% of these preventable, nonneurologic deaths. The publication of this study fueled implementation of a representative system of regionalized trauma care within Orange County, prompting Cales to review 60 vehicular deaths within the renovated system and contrast them with 58 historical controls.[39] Although regionalization decreased preventable deaths from 34% to 15%, inadequate management of hemorrhage remained the cause of more than 80% of these preventable deaths. Inadequate emergency resuscitation from hemorrhage has been similarly implicated in preventable death in other studies.[40,41]

RESUSCITATION FLUIDS

One of the earliest notable investigations into the resuscitation of patients with hemorrhagic shock is perhaps that of Wiggers,[42] who studied the effects of restoration of blood volume in exsanguinated animals following defined periods of hypotension. The basic Wiggers experimental method was later modified by Selkirk, who reasoned that pathologic endpoints (eg, lactic acidemia with systemic pH 7.1) rather than arbitrary time intervals should be observed in order to standardize the severity of the shock lesion prior to

Table 8-4 Comparative Functional Classification of Endogenous and Replacement Blood Components

Function	Component	
	Endogenous	Replacement
Energetics		
Cellular	Erythrocytes (hemoglobin)	Whole blood Packed cells washed leukocyte-poor frozen Stroma-free hemoglobin
Acellular	Serum volume, fuel (crystalloid)	Saline Ringer's lactate Balanced electrolyte solutions Perfluorocarbons
	(colloid)	Albumin Plasma protein fraction Hydroxyethyl starch Dextrans
Immunocompetence		
Cellular	Leukocytes	Granulocyte packs
Acellular	Immunoglobulin (nonspecific)	ISG - Hepatitis Rubella Polio Hypogammaglobulinemia
	(specific)	Tetanus Rabies Hepatitis B Rh antibody Antivenins Antitoxin
Hemostasis		
Cellular	Platelets	Platelet concentrates
Acellular	Coagulation factors	FFP Single donor plasma Cryoprecipitate Commercial concentrates

attempts at comparative resuscitation. The most notable conclusion derived from these early experiments was that isovolemic (shed blood) resuscitation is inadequate, as demonstrated by the 80% mortality in groups of animals subjected to the modified Wiggers preparation. The hypothesis that isovolemic fluid restoration would prove inadequate because of fluid "sequestration" had actually been advanced early in the century by Dale and Crile.[43,44] The inadequacy was grimly corroborated by the military experience coincident to World War II and the Korean conflict, during which time isovolemic resuscitation was practiced.

Prior to the Vietnam era, Moyer advanced his theories regarding the need to replace significant blood losses with quantities of fluids two to three times the volume of the shed blood. By comparing survival rates among groups of animals subjected to an adjusted Wiggers preparation in which 13 different proposed resuscitation fluid compositions and formulae were used, Moyer demonstrated that only blood plus supplemental quantities of crystalloid improved the mortality rate associated with isovolemic blood resuscitation.[45] It remained for Shires, however, to demonstrate the actual transudation of fluid among the various body pools following hemorrhage of graded severity.[46] The corroborated work of Shires and Moyer led to the 3:1 fluid replacement recommendation (see Table 6-4 in Chapter 6, Shock).

There are potentially four classes of fluids that may be considered for specific resuscitation of the hypovolemic patient: two classes of asanguineous plasma expanders (crystalloids and colloids); the class of artificial blood substitutes, distinguished from the conventional plasma expanders by inherent augmented oxygen transport capacity; and the class of proper blood components.

Crystalloids

Early search for an isotonic fluid with which to expand plasma safely led to the development of normal saline as a crystalloid replacement vehicle. Normal saline continues to be widely used in this mode, particularly for replacement of nonhemorrhagic losses. Until recently, saline was the only feasible priming and diluent crystalloid solution accepted by the AABB for use in transfusion. Investigators continued to seek a solution that more closely approximated the actual ionic composition of serum, prompting Ringer to develop a modified saline solution in which the sodium chloride content was "balanced" by the addition of trace quantities of other elemental ions present in serum. Few practical differences could be demonstrated between saline and this original Ringer's solution, however.

The initial advance in crystalloid therapy was the result of attempts by a pediatrician named Hartmann to develop a solution more appropriate for the replacement of gastrointestinal losses caused by dehydration and shock in infants. Hartmann sought in his solution to make the known ionic composition of serum somewhat more hypotonic, consistent with these gastrointestinal losses; he further sought to counter the hyperchloremic acidemia resulting from diarrheal losses and shock by replacing some of the chloride content with bicarbonate.[47] His solution differed from Ringer's solution only in the latter regard.

Commercial attempts to produce the solution Hartmann contrived were initially thwarted by difficulties in preserving the bicarbonate additive in storage; however, the addition of metabolic bicarbonate precursors, such as sodium lactate (or acetate), produced stable solutions of functionally equivalent composition, presuming subsequent normal hepatic metabolism of the infusate. Thus, Ringer's lactate was commercially prepared by comparable modification of the original solution.

Historically, there was a family of lactated Ringer's solutions among which the pH was varied by buffering according to the desired level. In fact, much of Moyer's original work leading to the selection of Ringer's lactate as the crystalloid vehicle of choice derived from experimental use of a solution with a pH of 8.5. Intuitively appropriate for the treatment of acidemic shock states, the potentially adverse effect of such an alkalemic solution on oxyhemoglobin dissociation was not then appreciated. Today, commercial Ringer's lactate is buffered to a pH of 6.5.

The most recent additions to this family of crystalloids comprise the second generation of these balanced electrolyte solutions, in which composition of major ions as well as pH and osmolality have been adjusted to reproduce normal serum values exactly; the notable exception is ionic calcium, which has been deleted entirely. The presence of calcium ions in Ringer's lactate prohibits its use as a blood transfusion vehicle, because the calcium may interfere with the citrate additive and subsequent coagulation. Thus, it is feasible to use one of these newer balanced electrolyte solutions as both the primary crystalloid plasma expander and the priming and diluent solution for associated transfusion of blood products, potentially simplifying the logistic implementation of such therapy. The functional superiority of these solutions remains to be demonstrated, however.[48]

Colloids

There are four colloid fluid preparations commercially available: albumin, plasma protein fraction, dextran, and hydroxyethyl starch. Normal human serum albumin emerged historically as the most widely used colloid solution. It is a plasma derivative that is at least 96% pure albumin. The product is heat-treated for viral inactivation and carries no risk of hepatitis transmission.[49] Albumin is available in 5% and 25% solutions of buffered saline, oncotically equivalent to an equal volume or five times this plasma volume, respectively. Each 20 mL of intravenously administered albumin normally results in a translocation of an additional 70 mL of interstitial fluid, provided hydration is adequate.

Plasma protein fraction is a similar, hepatitis-free derivative of plasma that contains up to 90% albumin, as well as α- and β-globulins, but no ABO agglutinins or clotting factors.[50] The 5% solution is oncotically equivalent to plasma. The utility of plasma protein fraction has been limited by recovery of prekallikrein activator thought to be Hageman factor fragments within the product;[51] the rapid intravenous infusion of this product may thus result in paradoxical hypotension owing to generation of bradykinin.[52]

Dextran is a branched polysaccharide of glucose units available at an average molecular weight of approximately 40,000 (dextran 40, low molecular weight) and 70,000 (dextran 70, clinical dextran).[50] Dextran 40 is available as a 10% solution in either normal saline or dextrose; dextran 70 is available as a 6% solution in saline or glucose. Dextran is known to interfere with coagulation and platelet adhesion, prompting the use of dextran 40 for prophylaxis against thromboembolic disease. Unfortunately, because of prior formation of antibodies directed against dietary bacterial polysaccharides, unpredictable anaphylactic reactions occasionally result in patients who have never previously been exposed to dextran. In early 1983, three deaths as a result of dextran administration were reported to the FDA.[53]

The demonstrated efficacy, but prohibitive cost, of colloid albumin solutions has long impelled a search for alternate solutions. The most promising to date has been hetastarch (HES), which is a commercial derivative of amylopectin, created by ethylene oxidation of this waxy starch to yield hydroxyethyl ether linkages to the integral glucose subunits. The product is a heterogenous solution of molecular chains ranging 100-fold in individual molecular weights. The structural similarity between precursor amylopectin and endogenous glycogen has minimized (but not eliminated) the anaphylactic response that complicates the use of dextran. HES is commercially available as a 6% saline solution.[54]

Studies of volume replacement with HES have demonstrated plasma expansion equivalent to 100% to 170% of the volume of infusate. The approved HES dosage is limited to 20 mL/kg administered over 1 hour for hemorrhagic shock, less rapidly for other shock states. HES promotes in vitro rouleaux formation,[55] which is easily dispersed by saline, but may cause false-positive results in serocompatibility tests performed by an unwary technician. The induction of increased serum amylase levels following HES administration may further confuse diagnosis of pancreatic disorders unless corroborative lipase assays are performed.[55]

The duration of volume expansion following HES administration ranges from 12 to 48 hours, plasma HES residence varying linearly with the dosage. The elimination of HES is biphasic and similar in respects to that of perfluorocarbon; smaller molecules are rapidly excreted in urine, whereas larger molecules persist to phagocytosis by reticuloendothelial cells with an elimination half-life as long as 48 days.[56]

Administration of HES predictably interferes with in vitro coagulation testing; however, a single 20 mL/kg dose does not appear to cause a clinically significant bleeding diathesis.[57] The potential effect of greater doses cannot be stated with certainty. The incidence of anaphylactic reactions is reportedly less than 0.006%.[58]

HES has two indicated extracorporeal uses, each of which is germane to transfusion therapy. The addition of HES to blood within the centrifuge during hemapheresis significantly improves the subsequent yield of both granulocytes and platelets, ensuring the feasibility of adequate collection of these products from a single donor when necessary. A 500-mL dose of HES has also proved to be an effective, safe, and affordable alternative to the administration of albumin as the priming solution for extracorporeal bypass pump units during cardiothoracic surgery.[59]

The controversy regarding the superiority of either colloids or crystalloids for fluid resuscitation has now raged for at least three decades. In the words of one colloid proponent, the "emotional fervor [has been] inversely proportional to the supporting data."[60] Attempts to conduct prospective studies of reliable design have been confounded by the logistical and ethical difficulties in creating controls and comparable treatment regimens, as well as in randomizing patients into groups stratified by injury of comparable severity. It is feasible to propose that, when each is used appropriately, there may be insufficient discrepancy in outcome to reach a conclusion.

Such equivalency in expensive colloid use must be reconciled with the tremendous cost differential, as well as adverse side-effects and an occasional death from use of these pharmaceutical products.[53] The pathophysiology of hemorrhagic shock, involving late failure of oncotic barriers, raises additional questions, at least regarding timing, in colloid administration to such patients. Finally, consideration may be given the colloid properties of FFP;[61] however, questions regarding its indiscriminate use have been raised,[28] and its additive component cost, as well as hepatitis risk, must be remembered when it is used in this fashion.

Artificial Blood Substitutes

Two distinctly different solutions are currently being investigated for possible future use as blood substitutes. Neither is being actively used in current clinical investigation, and neither is likely to revolutionize emergency therapy of hypovolemia in the imminent future, however.

Stroma-Free Hemoglobin

The preservation of function by hemoglobin released from cellular confines has been dramatically demonstrated in isolated case reports of patients who endured prolonged demise despite transfusion-refractory hemocrit levels of zero as a result of clostridial hemolysis.[62] Interest in the development of artificial blood substitutes naturally paralleled development of feasible transfusion practice, and early investigators intuitively considered derivatives of hemoglobin for such a purpose. These attempts were such that, by 1936, Amberson was prompted to review the first 60 years of this investigation.[63]

By the time of Amberson's review, it was already known that the clinical use of these "free hemoglobin" solutions was complicated by the frequent occurrence of coagulopathy and renal failure due to the presence of a lipid substance from the source erythrocytic stroma, which persisted because of technical limitations in the available washing and extraction techniques. The further development of these solutions was arrested for years until the technical sophistication by which to eradicate this contaminant evolved, when interest in these "stroma-free" hemoglobin (SFH) solutions underwent a resurgence.

SFH solutions have several potentially useful features: the oxygen-carrying capacity is excellent; the antigenicity of all extracellular mammalian hemoglobins is such that immunization does not occur, even after heterologous transfusion; and the product may be lyophilized for months or years of shelf storage prior to saline reconstitution.[64]

The problems that limit the feasibility of SFH at present derive primarily from its manner of elimination. The tertiary structure of tetrameric hemoglobin within erythrocytes tends to dissociate following cellular lysis, producing monomeric and dimeric molecules that are sufficiently small to be filtered by the renal glomerulus. The resultant oncotic diuretic effect obviously confounds use of SFH as a volume expander. Furthermore, although the extraordinary affinity of human free hemoglobin for molecular oxygen results in excellent carrying capacity, tissue delivery is so poor that human SFH will actually "steal" oxygen from the ambient erythrocytes, thus aggravating tissue hypoxia. The latter problem may be solved by chemical modification (pyridoxylation) or use of heterologous (particularly bovine) hemoglobin; however, the diuretic limitation persists. Current investigation is directed toward attempts to polymerize or encapsulate SFH artificially to obviate this problem.[65,66]

Perfluorocarbon

The clinical history of perfluorocarbon (PFC) is more contemporary, interest resulting from the 1966 demonstration by Clark and Gollan[67] that mice submerged up to four hours in an oxygenated PFC solution could survive. The PFC solution receiving greatest recent attention has been Fluosol DA-20%, a heterogenous combination of emulsified PFC compounds that has demonstrated favorable elimination kinetics. In addition to oxygen solubility, PFC is characterized by oncotic activity, which makes it an ideal blood substitute (ie, a plasma expander with enhanced oxygen-carrying capacity). Clinical experience to date with PFC solutions is limited, although its efficacy has been demonstrated in severely anemic preoperative patients who refused blood transfusion,[68] and investigational studies of ischemic neuronal[69] and myocardial salvage.[70]

PFC solutions have several features to suggest that their feasibility is superior to that of SFH solutions. As noted, PFC solutions are effective volume expanders; SFH solutions are not. The duration of the volume-expanding effect lasts several hours, following which the PFC solution is cleared from plasma. PFC elimination is biphasic; early renal clearance of smaller molecules is followed by prolonged reticuloendothelial accumulation of larger molecules. Furthermore, oxygen is readily extracted from PFC by tissues. The primary disadvantages of PFC are associated with the limited contribution of plasma-dissolved oxygen to total oxygen delivery, despite PFC augmentation; only when the ambient hematocrit is critically reduced (eg, less than 20%) does PFC-augmented plasma oxygen delivery become significant. Such critical anemia is rarely observed, particularly during the acute phase of hemorrhagic shock. Moreover, the ability of PFC to augment plasma oxygen carriage significantly presumes a P_{O_2} greater than 300 mmHg, which may be impossible to achieve at atmospheric pressure in patients with pulmonary disease, even when tight-fitting, non-rebreathing masks are used.[71]

Following completion of recent clinical investigation under protocol, the FDA disapproved the use of Fluosol DA-20% for use in the United States as a general resuscitation fluid for treatment of shock. Although PFC is a promising agent for ischemic salvage with potential as an adjunct for hypovolemic resuscitation, the inherent problems in the rapid administration of appropriately large doses prohibit its essential role in hemorrhagic shock resuscitation for the foreseeable future.

Blood and Blood Components

The limitations of the "blood substitutes" preserve the essential role of conventional blood products in the fluid resuscitation of critically hypovolemic patients. Whereas crystalloid or colloid plasma expanders suffice in the treatment of less severe losses, more acute reductions in the erythrocyte mass result not only in lesions of intravascular volume, but also lesions in the oxygen-carrying capacity that can be treated only by restoration of the hemoglobin mass.

The traditional controversy in the management of these patients begins with the choice between whole blood or packed cells as the sanguineous replacement fluid. Whole blood advocates argue that this fluid best approximates the shed loss; component advocates propose that the lesion initially manifest is functionally limited to volume and hemoglobin depletion, which may be replaced with expanders and packed cells, respectively (ie, AS cells), conserving the acellular blood reserve to meet the specific needs of other patients. The component advocates continue that, should coagulopathy become clinically evident in the case of massive acute blood loss and replacement, only then need plasma or platelets be transfused.

The potential fallacy in each of these arguments is temporal in origin. First, much of the conventional surgical wisdom in the treatment of massive hemorrhage is a byproduct of the military casualty experience, in which there was a limited capacity for sophisticated blood processing and storage; more importantly, there was an essentially inexhaustible reservoir of fresh, frequently warm, "walking donor" blood. The similarity between such walking donor blood and conventionally banked blood is more apparent than real. As mentioned earlier, banked whole blood that has been stored at 4°C is functionally devoid of viable platelets and progressively deficient in activity of the labile clotting factors. Counts and his associates[27] have demonstrated that the assayed activity of factor V decreases linearly in storage, while the activity of factor VIII decreases exponentially, with an initial half-life of 24 hours.

Because FFP must be harvested within 6 hours in order to preserve activity of these labile factors, component advocates argue that arbitrary allocation schedules that require a retention of whole blood units for a defined time period exhaust the potential for subsequent recovery of the labile plasma factors and derivatives. Whole blood proponents argue reciprocally that the implementation of an aggressive schedule for component fractionation virtually eliminates the availability of fresh, competent whole blood during these initial 1 or 2 days of potency. They further note that subsequent transfusion of component cells plus component plasma subjects the recipient to double the cost of product processing as well as twice the risk of adverse reaction, including hepatitis. This argument must be reconciled against the benefits afforded subsequent recipients of the competent plasma derivatives, as well as the additional hazard presented to recipients of whole blood by the increased transfer of plasma antigens and agglutinins, as well as by the metabolic byproducts (eg, acidemia, hyperkalemia, hyperammonemia, excess citrate) known collectively as the "storage lesion."[72]

Ironically, the best available evidence suggests that the controversy regarding labile factor salvage may be moot. In their study of 27 patients, Counts and his colleagues transfused a mean of 33 whole blood units from which cryoprecipitate had previously been removed; they found that dilutional thrombocytopenia was the exclusive cause of the subsequent bleeding diathesis in 6 of 8 such patients. The remaining two patients required platelets, plus clotting factors, for treatment of disseminated intravascular coagulation. They further demonstrated that no laboratory index except the platelet count correlated with the development of bleeding in these patients.[27] The importance of platelet administration as contrasted with FFP for treatment of bleeding diathesis as a complication of massive transfusion was reiterated at the NIH Consensus Development Conference regarding use of FFP.[28]

Sohmer and Scott reasoned that estimation of formed element dilution by massive transfusion should follow the known mathematics of exchange transfusion.[72] They predicted that transfusion to replace a hemorrhage equivalent to one entire blood volume (approximately 70 mL/kg in an adult) should reduce the original formed elements by 70%, and transfusion of two blood volumes should produce a 90% depletion of these elements. The average patient who receives 2 L crystalloid or equivalent and 5 to 6 U of packed cells (fewer units of whole blood) is thus approaching a one-volume exchange, and significant thrombocytopenia would be predicted. Although platelet counts are essential to guidance of therapy, few physicians willingly permit further dilution of the platelet count below the $100,000/\mu L$ that can be expected following this single volume exchange; once initiated, the efficacy of platelet transfusion may be compromised by continued hemorrhage and transfusion. There is no evidence to support prophylactic administration of FFP,[28] and in view of the poor clinical correlation with laboratory indexes of bleeding,[27] FFP administration is probably best reserved for manifest pathologic bleeding.

Because of the large endogenous reservoir of ionic calcium, toxic reactions to citrate are relatively rare, particularly if packed cells are used to obviate transfusion of much of the anticoagulant that is expressed with supernatant plasma.[30] When the rate of transfused citrate (approximately 20 mL per unit packed cells) exceeds the physiologic capacity of the parathyroid glands to mobilize calcium[73] (ie, when the rate of transfused blood exceeds approximately 70 mL/min)[74]; however, cautious calcium supplementation may be required. Calcium assays and monitoring of electrocardiographic QT interval are recommended to guide such therapy; inadvertent hypercalcemia is otherwise likely to result.[75]

The one and perhaps only indisputable advantage of whole blood for massive transfusion is that its viscosity is less than that of packed cells and, thus, its flow rate is greater. The problem in packed cell administration is easily overcome by the reconstitution of packed units with 100 mL saline, however, and this is one of the benefits of the AS red cell solutions, units of which have been similarly reconstituted following hard-spin harvesting of plasma during processing.

Occasionally, it is necessary to administer blood products incompletely tested for serocompatibility prior to transfusion (ie, transfusion of universal donor and type-specific bloods).

Shortly after the discovery of a blood group lacking A and B antigens, it was hypothesized that this group would become a "universal donor" blood. Indeed, some early investigators were so enthused as to postulate that blood of no other group should be considered for transfusion, thereby eliminating the need for all pretransfusion testing.[76] Such recommendations were not totally heretical, as the sensitivity of cross-matching tests as then practiced was poor and few erythrocyte antigens had been identified at that time. Indeed, Oswald Robertson limited his celebrated World War I transfusions to the use of group O blood.[15] The difficulty in eliminating the cross-matching procedure was initially illuminated by Levine and Mabee,[77] and the hemolytic complications attendant to passive transfer of large quantities of blood that contained anti-A and anti-B agglutinins were soon realized.[78] Therefore, investigators began to search for units of group O blood that contained "low titers" of these agglutinins.

The relative safety and efficacy of universal donor O blood was demonstrated by its extensive use during the Vietnam era. It is recorded that 25% of patients who received five or more units developed minor cross-matching reactions, however, and subsequent transfusion of type- or group-specific blood (unless fortuitously O) could not be initiated for 14 days.[79,80] Use of group O packed cells essentially precludes the passive transfer of these agglutinins, thereby minimizing this risk. The efficacy of universal donor packed group O cells has been demonstrated by Sohmer and Scott at the Maryland Shock-Trauma Unit: only five cases of transfusion reaction resulted in 170 patients transfused an average of 6 U of uncross-matched packed O cells; furthermore, no complications resulted from immediate institution of transfusion with type-specific blood, once it was available.[72] A blood sample must be obtained for typing and antibody testing prior to transfusion of universal donor or other blood to avoid subsequent confusion in the interpretation of these tests.

Because the prevalence of the O-negative phenotype is relatively small (approximately 6% of the population in the United States), the O-negative resource must be used carefully. Conversely, because approximately 85% of the population is Rh-positive, O-positive is an acceptable universal donor for these persons. Barring undiscovered alloimmunization by prior transfusion or pregnancy, the only risk associated with O-positive usage is the possibility of alloimmunization and subsequent maternofetal illness in women of childbearing age; this Rh incompatibility can be conventionally treated by administration of Rh hyperimmune globulin. In summary, consideration may be given to the use of Rh-positive universal donor blood for all men and for women who lack childbearing potential, particularly in resource regions where O-negative blood is scarce.[30,80]

The ultimate safety of type-specific, uncross-matched blood transfusion is evident from the 3-year study of Gervin and Fischer,[81] in which none of the 160 patients who received an average of 5.5 U of type-specific blood subsequently developed a transfusion reaction. The risk involved in the administration of universal donor blood is best managed by judicious selection of appropriate candidates, followed by timely provision of group- (type) specific and, ultimately, cross-matched blood. Appropriate candidates include patients who demonstrate visibly uncontrolled hemorrhage or recent precipitous decline in stability. Type-specific and universal donor transfusion should be curtailed by provision of fully cross-matched blood within approximately 30 minutes, particularly with use of newer, rapid enhancement techniques, such as the LISS technique.

TECHNICAL ADJUNCTS TO TRANSFUSION

The mechanical delivery of cellular blood products requires the use of an administration tubing set with contained or appended filter. The transfusion set may be further subjected to a pressurizing and warming apparatus, particularly when rapid delivery of the blood product is needed.

Tubing

Historically, primarily because of the lack of meaningful differences among commercial products, administration sets were ignored in deference to hospital purchasing agreements governing routine inventory. Despite general agreement regarding the feasibility of improving transfusion flow rates by using greater than conventional gauge (approximately 3.0 to 3.2 mm internal diameter) tubing, only recently have trauma tubing blood administration sets that feature tubing with internal diameters ranging from 3.8 to 6.4 mm become available.

Filters

The current market offers a bewildering array of blood microfilters, yet the significance or necessity of some microfiltration remains uncertain. The tendency of stored blood to form aggregates has been recognized since the inception of blood banking. Indeed, in their description of procedural standards for the first US blood bank, Fantus and Schirmer noted the necessity of filtering blood by first pouring it through "genuine Swiss bolting cloth, No. 150 mesh."[82] Subsequent investigators confirmed the macroscopic and microscopic collection of platelets, leukocytes, and fibrin in stored blood and developed methods by which to quantify their removal.[83]

Available blood filters are each a variant or combination of one of two basic prototypes: (1) screen type filters that use the sieving effect of a broad surface area of mesh of predetermined pore size, and (2) depth type filters that rely on the adsorbent capacity of a wad of permeable material. Most standard administration sets contain a 170-μm mesh filter.

A number of early reports raised concern that, despite 170-μm mesh filtration, massive transfusion of stored blood resulted in pulmonary microembolization, particularly of aggregates in the 10- to 80-μm range, sufficient to result in pulmonary insufficiency evolving days to weeks following transfusion in survivors.[84–87] The relationship between these "microaggregates" and subsequent pulmonary injury has never been conclusively demonstrated to be independent of associated factors attending the massive resuscitation of, physiologic response to, and complications arising during recovery from these injuries, however. Enthusiasm for the proposed "ultrafilters" designed for removal of these smaller particles followed the initial speculative reports, but the consensus at an international symposium[88] was that such correlation was sparse, if real, and that ultrafiltration should be reserved for transfusions exceeding 5 U of blood. Essentially everyone concurs that no ultrafiltration should be performed during the initial resuscitation from critical hypovolemia because of the associated obligate compromise of flow rates.[89,90]

Among available ultrafilters, a number of comparative studies have demonstrated superior flow rates (and acceptable, albeit not necessarily best performance) with use of the Pall 40-μm polyester mesh filter.[90,91] All ultrafilters are contraindicated for granulocyte transfusions,[25] but ultrafilters are neither prohibited[25] nor recommended[29] for transfusion of platelet packs.

A significant improvement in hemotherapy has followed the recent introduction of simple polyester mesh filters specifically designed to entrap residual leukocytes contaminating red cell or platelet component preparations.[92] The effective removal of these residual leukocytes serves to protect the transfusion recipient from complications, including the common allergic and febrile, nonhemolytic reactions resulting from isoantibodies directed against corresponding leukocyte antigens as well as uncommon to rare complications of leukocyte transmission such as cytomegalovirus transmission (primarily of concern only to immunodeficient patients and premature neonates, for whom cytomegalovirus-seronegative products are preferred) and the acute leukoagglutinin reaction characterized by acute pulmonary insufficiency. Multiparous patients and patients previously receiving multiple transfusions are at greatest risk for such leukocyte-dependent reactions and thus especially benefit from the use of such filters. Previously, comparable protection could be provided only by the (relatively inefficient) preparation of either leukocyte-poor or buffy coat–poor packed cells or washed cells, which techniques are considerably more cumbersome, time consuming, and expensive compared to the simple in-line placement of these filters.

Pressure Systems

Although pressurized delivery systems by which to augment transfusion flow rates are commonly used in practice and are frequently included in study protocols that address other integral features of delivery systems, few data are available with which to define or differentiate the contributions of these devices. AABB *Standards* does not address this subject.

A variety of devices have been suggested for use. A manual syringe–driven system (as commonly used for platelet administration) with alternating blood bag aspiration and forced infusion via stopcock is least efficient and effective for rapid blood administration. Dula and his colleagues[93] have shown that either hand-operated bulb-pump systems or pneumatic sleeve systems are far superior to syringe systems; the pneumatic sleeve is probably the superior of the three in terms of absolute flow, as well as operator freedom.

The standard pneumatic sleeve incorporates the blood bag into a semirigid pouch against which a bladder is inflated with air. By common convention, air is typically inflated until the gauge reflects a maximum pressure of 200 to 300 mmHg, although there have been few rigorous studies to determine the survival of transfused red cells subjected to specific pressures. In practice, no adverse clinical results have been reported, whereas other limiting elements in the transfusion apparatus preclude the routine use of higher driving pressures. One potential drawback of the pneumatic sleeve arises from the operator independence; there is a tendency for the driving pressure to wane progressively during transfusion as the blood bag empties. This may be corrected by further serial inflation of the bladder, but attention is often rightfully directed elsewhere during hectic resuscitations. Some recently introduced products address this problem by incorporating the blood bag and bladder within a closed, rigid box that maintains the desired pressure by a stepdown valve connected to a regulated high-pressure gas source.

Blood Warmers

The provision of adequately warmed blood may be the most woefully neglected aspect of transfusion practice today. The temperature dependence of oxyhemoglobin dissociation, as well as the risk of cardiac hypothermia, has long been established,[94,95] yet physicians continue to perform massive transfusions of blood refrigerated at 4°C to unclad shock victims already tending toward hypothermia as if oblivious to the potential detriment. Similarly, a variety of mechanical adjuncts, including special cannulas, tubing sets, and hyperbaric delivery systems specifically designed to augment fluid delivery, have appeared on the market, but the practical utility of these innovations remains compromised by the absence of any independent method to warm blood adequately as it is transfused at these rates.

The first comprehensive review of this problem was performed by Russell,[96] who in 1974 reported the results of comparative trials of the then available products to warm refrigerated blood that was to be transfused at rapid rates. Russell empirically determined that an effective product must be capable of warming blood to at least 32°C while delivering the blood at 150 mL/min. Like others before him,[97] Russell noted that warming coils made of polyethylene performed superiorly.

In recent years, a newer generation of instruments known as "dry heat" blood warmers has supplanted the cumbersome coil and bath units. These instruments provide a broad surface area of electrically warmed aluminum that conducts heat to blood as it flows through an apposed bag placed in series with the administration set. Two such units are marketed in the United States today; each manufacturer reports trial data that exceed the minimum performance criteria of Russell.[98,99] Both units not only are easy to handle, but also feature temperature gauges, alarms, and automatic shut-off controls to simplify safe operation.

There has been recurrent interest in the development of a microwave (or similar electromagnetic) blood-warming apparatus; however, no such device is presently in use in the United States. The greatest potential advantage of such an instrument is the issue of previously warmed blood by the bank, essentially eliminating the step that is currently rate limiting in the rapid transfusion of blood. Preliminary study of the effect of electromagnetic warming on blood indicated that the procedure is safe;[100] furthermore, there was one report of the metabolic superiority of blood so prepared.[101]

The initial studies of Leonard and co-workers[100] culminated in 1970 in the introduction of a commercial microwave warmer in the United States that heats banked blood to 32°C within one minute. There were several subsequent reports of clinical morbidity,[102,103] however, including one death from extracorporeal hemolysis following unit malfunction.[104] These units were withdrawn from the market without subsequent commercial return. The European literature includes a few recent reports that suggest a possible resurgence of the device,[101,105] but no imminent return is apparent.

The primary difficulty encountered with the microwave devices is inhomogenous warming of the various blood fractions, as well as of the plastic containers. Engineering efforts to safeguard against this problem by maintaining cells in suspension and continuously monitoring internal temperature by probe were thwarted by design flaws. Recently, however, attention has been directed to the feasibility of microwaving crystalloid solutions to complement hemotherapy,[106] a practice simplified by the homogeneity of the crystalloid solution. The safety and feasibility of warming blood with a warmed priming and diluent solution remains to be adequately studied.

Integrated Delivery Systems

The newest generation of instruments developed reflects an effort to combine the various adjuncts just described (ie, pressurized and large-bore delivery systems with blood warming capacity) into an integrated apparatus. Several of these devices utilize heat exchanging elements similar to those found in an extracorporeal cardiopulmonary bypass pump. Such instruments thus offer the capacity to warm banked blood to nearly normothermic levels at flow rates capable of sustaining even the most heroic volume resuscitation. Such instrumentation is, however, predictably accompanied by much greater complexity and cost. Further, there are extraordinarily few patients with survivable injuries who cannot otherwise be sustained, particularly during the initial emergency department resuscitation, by the expedient delivery of incompletely cross-matched blood through multiple intravenous lines by means of the more conventional instruments described as indicated.

Autotransfusion

The recorded history of autotransfusion is generally traced to Blundell's "Impellor"[4]; another century transpired, however, before the first extraoperative use of autotransfusion for emergency recycling of hemothorax. The development of homologous transfusion practices early in this century relegated autotransfusion to years of obscurity. Interest was rekindled, however, after the advent of cardiopulmonary bypass procedures, by which the feasibility and occasional need for shed blood reinfusion was demonstrated,[107] and more recently by a recipient patient population concerned with the prospect of transmissible illness.

The AABB recognizes three distinct formats for autologous blood transfusion.[25] Predeposit or scheduled donation, as originally conceived by Fantus, is currently receiving heightened attention because of recent public awareness of transfusion-related AIDS transmission. Significant clinical study of intraoperative autologous blood salvage has also been performed. It is post-traumatic autologous transfusion from hemothorax, however, that is of primary interest to the practicing emergency physician. Conceptually, this form of autotransfusion requires no skills on the part of the practicing emergency physician other than those coincident to the performance of routine thoracostomy drainage. The blood is simply collected into a closed, sterile bag suitable for subsequent reinfusion. Despite the simplicity of the procedure, the technique is infrequently practiced by the emergency physician, perhaps because of a lack of familiarity and training with the equipment.

The emergency transfusion of autologous blood affords several practical advantages under defined circumstances. First, such blood is available immediately, and perfect compatibility is ensured by definition. Second, this blood is thermally and metabolically superior to stored, banked blood; furthermore, it obviates any concern for inherent transmissible disease. Third, no religious prohibitions apply to transfusion of autologous blood. Finally, the cost of autologous transfusion compares favorably with the cost of conventional transfusion of banked products, while sparing the banked products.

The potential complications of autotransfusion may be considered in terms of two broad classes: hematologic aberrations resultant in autotransfused patients and complications attending faulty technique (e.g., microparticulate and air embolism). The in vitro study of hematologic parameters of platelet and clotting factor function following autotransfusion consistently reveals qualitative and quantitative abnormalities,[108] prompting most authorities to recommend at least supplemental platelet transfusion when a substantial volume of blood is autotransfused.[109,110] These indexes normalize by 48 hours with or without treatment, however, and thus such prophylactic platelet administration need be directed only to prevention or treatment of clinical bleeding, rather than attempted normalization of these laboratory indexes.[108–110]

The occasional report of massive air embolism complicating autotransfusion has resulted in repetitive admonitions by all those who discuss the technique. In fact, such massive embolism was due uniquely to use of intraoperative instruments that combined cell washers with an open-air reservoir from which washed blood was returned by a roller-driven pump. Lack of attention to the emptying reservoir resulted in continuous pumping of air into the patient.[111] This design has been eliminated from all instruments in current use and was never descriptive of the apparatus intended for emergency department autotransfusion. Modest air embolism, nevertheless, may complicate use of the latter, because air simultaneously evacuated from hemopneumothorax is also collected by vacuum into the blood bag connected to the chest tube. This air must be expelled from the collection bag by conventional bleeding of the intravenous tubing set prior to reinfusion of blood.

The necessity for filtration of collected autologous blood has been the subject of occasional debate, most authors noting that blood collected from ongoing brisk hemorrhage does not defibrinate despite serosal contact within the pleural cavity.[107–110] These authors therefore recommend conventional CPD anticoagulation of collected blood as well as standard and microparticulate filtration of reinfused blood. The apparatus designed for emergency department use allows either continuous drip or serial titration of CPD into collected blood, as well as in-line screen and depth filtration during reinfusion. Although condemned clinically except when there is no alternative, the reinfusion of even fecally contaminated blood has been shown experimentally to be relatively safe when concomitant broad-spectrum intravenous antibiotic therapy is administered.[112–114]

Published indications for emergency autologous transfusion from hemothorax include the following:

- acute hemothorax of 1000 mL blood or greater
- acute need for blood loss replacement when there is no available compatible blood
- supplementation of banked blood in cases of massive transfusion
- urgent replacement in the patient with religious prohibition to homologous transfusion

Although all are certainly reasonable indications, the first implies an ability to perceive the magnitude of the hemothorax prior to initial chest tube placement if this initial liter of blood is to be reused. These indications must be liberalized or autotransfusion is destined to remain used by only a select group of physicians who staff high-volume, academically oriented trauma centers. Implementation of the autotransfusion apparatus in the collection phase of operation, in lieu of conventional collection systems during thoracostomy, is one means by which the necessary familiarity might be gained; subsequent reinfusion of any blood collected may then be reserved for patients with classic indications. Contraindications to autotransfusion are sepsis and malignancy.

COMPLICATIONS OF TRANSFUSION THERAPY

Estimates suggest that approximately 1% to 3% of all transfusion recipients experience some form of adverse reaction complicating hemotherapy (Table 8-5).[115,116] Febrile or other simple allergic reactions comprise the great majority of these complications, although a life-threatening complication occasionally occurs. Persons at greatest risk are those patients who have received multiple prior transfusions and multiparous women because of the cumulative probability of prior alloimmunization. Similarly, patients transfused with large quantities of products and patients transfused without benefit of completed serocompatibility testing are subject to

Table 8-5 Complications of Transfusion Therapy

Mechanism	Immediate	Delayed
Serologic		
Hemolytic	Intravascular; chills, dyspnea, flank pain, hemoglobinemia, hemoglobinuria	Extravascular; falling hematocrit, jaundice, positive Coombs conversion
Nonhemolytic	Single febrile, allergic reactions	Alloimmunization
Anaphylactic	Typically, reaction of IgA-deficient recipient to IgA in donor sera	
Mechanical	Air or particulate embolism	Adult respiratory distress syndrome Graft-versus-host disease
Physiologic	Hypothermia Hyperkalemia Hypocalcemia Citrate toxicity Dilutional coagulopathy Congestive heart failure	
Infectious	Endotoxemia, bacteremia	Hepatitis AIDS Syphilis

additional risk. By federal regulation, mandatory FDA reporting of selected complications is required of each blood bank medical director. This includes all fatal reactions, which must be communicated to the Director of the Bureau of Biologics within 24 hours and corroborated by written report within 7 days.

Complications may occur during or within hours following blood transfusion. These acute or immediate reactions, of greatest interest to the emergency physician, may or may not result from adverse serologic interaction between donor and recipient bloods; however, the serologic and particularly hemolytic reactions are of greatest probable concern. Thus, by protocol, an investigation into each such reaction especially designed to uncover seroincompatibility must be initiated.[25] Other causes of immediate reactions include the common (allergic, febrile) serologic, nonhemolytic reactions; rare anaphylactic reactions; occasional hemolytic reactions resulting from mechanical rather than serologic causes; complications resulting from technical error (including hypothermia and air embolism); and physiologic or metabolic complications, particularly following massive transfusion.

By contrast, a variety of complications following transfusion may not present for weeks to several months. These include most notably transmitted infectious disease and delayed hemolytic reactions following anamnestic production of incomplete (IgG) alloantibody in previously sensitized individuals. Such delayed hemolytic reactions are characterized by extravascular hemolysis within the reticuloendothelial system, resulting in conversion of the patient's Coombs test to positive associated with an insidiously falling hematocrit and a rising serum bilirubin; this is easily distinguished from the immediate, intravascular hemolytic reaction, which is associated with dramatic symptomatology, hemoglobinemia, hemoglobinuria, and renal failure.

Attention to proper technique and judicious selection of components as clinically feasible minimize the manageable hazards associated with transfusion. A small incidence of unavoidable and potentially emergent complications remains, however. The physician confronted with an acute, adverse transfusion reaction must initially decide whether to stop the transfusion and initiate the protocol for evaluation of such reactions. Stated simply, all but the simplest allergic reactions must be presumptively regarded as hemolytic reactions, requiring cessation of transfusion of the current unit and, circumstance permitting, withholding of subsequent units pending protocol investigation. By contrast, many simple urticarial reactions unaccompanied by other signs of allergy may be managed with intravenous diphenhydramine without interruption of transfusion.

The acute hemolytic reaction typically presents with fever (hence febrile reactions, albeit rarely hemolytic, must be carefully investigated), chills, dyspnea, chest and flank pain, and hemoglobinuria; the reaction may proceed to coagulopathy or DIC and renal failure with a 40% to 60% mortality despite treatment. Following immediate cessation of transfusion, recipient blood and urine specimens must be secured for return, along with the donor blood unit, for laboratory analysis of causation. Most authors recommend vigorous fluid administration accompanied by loop diuresis for prophylaxis from hemoglobinuric renal failure. The incidence of these serologic, hemolytic reactions is approximately 1 per 40,000 transfused units of blood, the great majority of which result from technical or clerical human error rather than from undetectable incompatibility.[117]

A much less common but equally serious complication is the anaphylactic reaction resulting most often from transfusion of plasma containing IgA to previously alloimmunized recipients deficient in IgA. It is estimated that 1 in 500 persons in the population is IgA-deficient and, thus, at risk. These anaphylactic reactions must be vigorously treated with conventional measures, including provision of airway maintenance and administration of intravenous epinephrine, cimetidine, diphenhydramine, and glucocorticoids.[118,119]

Least commonly, fulminating endotoxic shock due to proliferation of cryophilic Gram-negative organisms within refrigerated products may complicate transfusion. Appropriate therapy is that conventionally rendered for Gram-negative bacteremic sepsis; however, mortality in this circumstance is exceedingly high.[117,120]

REFERENCES

1. Maluf NSR. History of blood transfusion. *J Hist Med Allied Sci.* 1954;9:59–107.
2. Todd JK. Non-culture techniques using blood specimens for the diagnosis of infectious disease. *Am J Med.* 1983;75:37–43.
3. Keynes G. The history of blood transfusion. *Br J Surg.* 1943; 31:388–350.
4. Jones HW, Mackmull G. The influence of James Blundell on the development of blood transfusion. *Ann Med Hist.* 1928;10:243–247.
5. Perkins HA. Blood transfusion. *JAMA.* 1983;250:1902–1904.
6. Bing RG. Carrel: a personal reminiscence. *JAMA.* 1983;250: 3297–3298.
7. Bryant NJ. *An Introduction to Immunohematology.* Philadelphia: Saunders; 1976:57–59.
8. Ottenberg R. Transfusion and arterial anastomosis. *Ann Surg.* 1908;47:486.
9. Ottenberg R. Reminiscence on the history of blood transfusion. *J Mt Sinai Hosp.* 1937;4:264.
10. Landsteiner K, Weiner AS. An agglutinable factor in human blood recognized by immune sera for Rhesus blood. *Proc Soc Exp Biol Med.* 1940;43:223.
11. Levine P, Katzin EM, Burnham L. Isoimmunization in pregnancy: its possible bearing on the etiology of erythroblastosis foetalis. *JAMA.* 1941;116:825–827.
12. Lewisohn R. A new and greatly simplified method of blood transfusion. *Med Rec.* 1915;87:141–142.
13. Weil R. Sodium citrate in the transfusion of blood. *JAMA.* 1915;64:425–426.
14. Rous P, Turner JR. The preservation of living red cells in vitro: I. Methods of preservation. *J Exp Med.* 1915;23:219–237.
15. Robertson OH. Transfusion with preserved red blood cells. *Br Med J.* 1918;1:691–695.

16. Fantus B. Blood preservation. *JAMA*. 1937;109:128–131.
17. Kruskall MS, Churchill WH, Brauer M, et al. Designated blood donations. *N Engl J Med*. 1984;310:1194–1195.
18. Loutit JF, Mollison PL, Young IM. Citric acid-sodium citrate-glucose mixtures for blood storage. *Q J Exp Physiol*. 1943;32:183–202.
19. Gibson JG II, Reese B, McManus TJ, et al. A citrate-phosphate-dextrose solution for the preservation of human blood. *Am J Clin Pathol*. 1957;28:569–578.
20. Zuck TF. The in vivo survival of red cells stored in modified CPD with adenine: report of a multi-institutional cooperative effort. *Transfusion*. 1977;17:374.
21. Szymanski IV, Valeri CR. Life span of preserved cells. *Vox Sang*. 1971;21:97.
22. Hogman CF, Hedlund K, Zetterstrom H. Clinical usefulness of red cells preserved in protein-poor mediums. *N Engl J Med*. 1982;299:1377–1382.
23. Herve T. Preservation of human erythrocytes in the liquid state. *Vox Sang*. 1980;39:195.
24. 21 CFR § 640.
25. Schmidt TJ, ed. *Standards for Blood Banks and Transfusion Services*. 11th ed. Arlington, VA: American Association of Blood Banks; 1984.
26. Moroff Dende. *The Additive Solution System Approach to Blood Preservation and Component Preparation. A Background Report*. Cell Preservation Laboratory, American Red Cross Blood Services; 1983.
27. Counts RB, Haisch C, Simon TL, et al. Hemostasis in massively transfused trauma patients. *Ann Surg*. 1979;190:91–99.
28. *Fresh Frozen Plasma: Indications and Risks*. NIH Consensus Development Conference Statement, vol 5, No 5, 1984.
29. Menitove JE, Aster RH. Transfusion of platelets and plasma products. *Clin Hematol*. 1983;xx:238–266.
30. Sohmer PR, Dawson RB. Transfusion therapy in trauma: a review of the principles and techniques used in the MIEMS program. *Am Surg*. 1979;2:109–125.
31. Morton JA, Tickles MM. Use of trypsin in the detection of incomplete Rh antibodies. *Nature*. 1947;159:779.
32. Diamond LK, Denton RL. Rh agglutination in various media with particular reference to the value of albumin. *J Lab Clin Med*. 1945;30:821.
33. Low B, Messeter L. Antiglobulin test in low ionic strength salt solution for rapid antibody screening and crossmatching. *Vox Sang*. 1974;26:53.
34. Beattie K. Control of the antigen-antibody ratio in antibody detection/compatibility tests. *Transfusion*. 1980;20:277.
35. Mintz PD, Henry JB, Boral LI. The type and antibody screen. *Clin Lab Med*. 1982;2:169–179.
36. Clarke JR, Davidson SJ, Bergman GE, et al. Optimal blood ordering for emergency department patients. *Ann Emerg Med*. 1980;9:2.
37. Davidson SJ, Bergman GE, Garbak RC. Optimal blood ordering for emergency department patients: II. Prospective validation. In: Editors? *Proceedings of the University Association for Emergency Medicine Annual Meeting*. 1980.
38. West JG, Trunkey DD, Lim RC. Systems of trauma care: a study of two counties. *Arch Surg*. 1979;114:455–460.
39. Cales RH. Trauma mortality in Orange County: the effect of implementation of a regional trauma system. *Ann Emerg Med*. 1984;13:1.
40. Wright CS, McMurtry RY, Hoyle M, et al. Preventable deaths in multiple trauma: review of deaths at Sunnybrook Medical Centre Trauma Unit. *Can J Surg*. 1983;26:20–23.
41. Certo TF, Rogers FB, Pilcher DB. Review of fatally injured patients in a rural state: 5-year followup. *J Trauma*. 1983;23:559.
42. Wiggers CJ. Present status of shock problem. *Physiol Rev*. 1942;22:74.
43. Crile GW. *Hemorrhage and Transfusion*. New York: Appleton; 1909.
44. Blalock A. *Principles of Surgical Care, Shock and Other Problems*. St Louis: Mosby; 1940.
45. Dillon JL. A bio-assay of treatment of hemorrhagic shock. *Arch Surg*. 1966;93:537.
46. Shires GT. Fluid therapy in hemorrhagic shock. *Arch Surg*. 1964;88:688.
47. Hartmann AF, Senn MJE. Studies in the metabolism of sodium-lactate: I. Response of normal human subjects to intravenous injection of sodium-lactate. *J Clin Invest*. 1932;11:327–335.
48. Traverso LW, Lee WP, Langford MJ, et al. *Fatal Hemorrhagic Shock and Acetate Solutions* (Institute Report no 181). San Francisco: Letterman Army Institute of Research; 1984.
49. Tullis JL. Albumin: background and use. *JAMA*. 1977;237:355–360.
50. Robinson WA. Fluid therapy in hemorrhagic shock. *Crit Care Q*. 1980;24:1–13.
51. Alving BM, Hojima Y, Pisano JJ, et al. Hypotension associated with prekallikrein activator (Hageman factor fragments) in plasma protein fraction. *N Engl J Med*. 1978;299:66–70.
52. Werner PH, Bonchek LI, Olinger GN. Hemodynamic response to rapidly infused protein volume expanders. *Surg Forum*. 1978;29:34–35.
53. *FDA Drug Bull*. 1983;13:23.
54. Hulse JD, Yacobi A. Hetastarch: an overview of the colloid and its metabolism. *Drug Intell Clin Pharm*. 1983;17:334–341.
55. Janes AW, Mishler JM, Lowes B. Serial infusion effects of hydroxyethyl starch on ESR, blood typing and crossmatching and serum amylase levels. *Vox Sang*. 1977;32:131–134.
56. Yacobi A, Stoll RG, Sum CY, et al. Pharmacokinetics of hydroxyethyl starch in normal subjects. *J Clin Pharmacol*. 1982;22:206–212.
57. Stauss RG. Review of the effects of hydroxyethyl starch on the blood coagulation system. *Transfusion*. 1981;21:299–302.
58. Ring J, Messmer K. Incidence and severity of anaphylactoid reactions to colloid volume substitutes. *Lancet*. 1977;1:466–468.
59. Sade RM, Crawford FA, Dearing JP, et al. Hydroxyethyl starch in priming fluid for cardiopulmonary bypass. *J Thorac Cardiovasc Surg*. 1982;84:35–38.
60. Shoemaker WC. Evaluation of colloids, crystalloids, whole blood and red cell therapy in the critically ill patient. *Clin Lab Med*. 1982;2:35–63.
61. Traverso LW, Hollenbach SJ, Deguzman LR, et al. *Fatal Hemorrhagic Shock: The Superiority of Compatible Fresh Frozen Plasma as a Resuscitation Agent* (Institute Report no. 186). San Francisco: Letterman Army Institute of Research; 1984.
62. Terebelo HR. Implications of plasma-free hemoglobin in massive clostridial hemolysis. *JAMA*. 1982;248:20–28.
63. Amberson WR. Blood substitutes. *Biol Rev*. 1937;12:48.
64. Rabiner SF. Further studies with stroma-free hemoglobin solution. *Ann Surg*. 1971;171:615.
65. DeVenuto F. Appraisal of hemoglobin solution as a blood substitute. 1979;149:4–17.
66. Gould SA. Red cells substitutes: hemoglobin solution or fluorocarbon? *J Trauma*. 1982;22:736.
67. Clark LC, Gollan F. Survival of mammals breathing organic liquids equilibrated with oxygen at atmospheric pressure. *Science*. 1966;152:1755.
68. Tremper KK. The pre-operative treatment of severely anemic patients with a perfluorochemical oxygen-transport fluid, Fluosol-DA. *N Engl J Med*. 1982;307:277.

69. Peeress SJ, Ishikawa R, Hunter IG, et al. Protective effect of Fluosol-DA in acute cerebral ischemia. *Stroke*. 1981;12:558–563.
70. Glogard H, Kloner RA, Muller J, et al. Fluorocarbons reduce myocardial ischemic damage after coronary occlusion. *Science*. 1981;211:1439–1441.
71. Geyer RP. Fluorocarbon-polyol artificial blood substitutes. *N Engl J Med*. 1973;289:1077.
72. Sohmer PR, Scott RL. Massive transfusion. *Clin Lab Med*. 1982;2:21–34.
73. Blum JW, Mayer GP, Potts JT. Parathyroid hormone responses during spontaneous hypocalcemia and induced hypercalcemia in cows. *Endocrinology*. 1974;95:84.
74. Committee on Trauma. *Student Manual: Advanced Trauma Life Support Course*. American College of Surgeons; 1981.
75. Wolf PC, McCarthy LJ, Hafleigh B. Extreme hypercalcemia following blood transfusions combined with intravenous calcium. *Vox Sang*. 1970;19:544.
76. Lee RI. A simple and rapid method for the selection of suitable donors for transfusion by the determination of blood groups. *Br Med J*. 1917;2:684.
77. Levine P, Mabee J. A dangerous "universal" donor detected by the direct matching of bloods. *J Immunol*. 1923;8:425.
78. Garner J, Tovey G. Potentially dangerous group O blood. *Lancet*. 1954;1:1001.
79. Barnes A, Allen TE. Transfusions subsequent to administration of universal donor blood in Viet Nam. *JAMA*. 1968;204:695.
80. Barnes A. Transfusion of universal donor and uncrossmatched blood. *Bibl Haematol*. 1980;46:132–142.
81. Gervin AS, Fischer RP. Resuscitation of trauma patients with type-specific uncrossmatched blood. *J Trauma*. 1984;24:327–331.
82. Fantus B, Schirmer EH. The therapy of the Cook County Hospital: blood preservation technique. *JAMA*. 1938;11:317.
83. Swank RL. Alteration of blood on storage: measurement of adhesiveness of "aging" platelets and leucocytes and their removal by filtration. *N Engl J Med*. 1961;265:728.
84. Genevein EP, Weiss DL. Platelet microemboli associated with massive blood transfusion. *Am J Pathol*. 1964;45:313–325.
85. McNamara JJ, Molot MD, Stremple JF. Screen filtration pressure in combat casualties. *Ann Surg*. 1970;172:334–341.
86. Reul GJ, Greenberg SD, Lefrak EA, et al. Prevention of post-traumatic pulmonary insufficiency: fine-screen filtration of blood. *Arch Surg*. 1973;106:386–394.
87. Reul GJ, Beall AC, Greenberg SD. Protection of the pulmonary microvasculature by fine-screen blood filtration. *Chest*. 1974;66:4.
88. Bredenberg CE, Collins JA, Solis RT, et al. International forum: does a relationship exist between massive blood transfusions and the adult respiratory distress syndrome? If so, what are the best preventive measures? *Vox Sang*. 1977;32:311–321.
89. Rosario MD, Rumsey EW, Arakaki G, et al. Blood microaggregates and ultrafilters. *J Trauma*. 1978;18:498–501.
90. Gay P, Thede J, Suehiro G, et al. Filtration of debris from banked blood. *J Trauma*. 1979;19:806–811.
91. Buley R, Lumley J. Some observations on blood microfilters. *Ann R Coll Surg Engl*. 1975;57:262.
92. Sirchia G, Wenz B, Rebulla P, et al. Removal of white cells from red cells by transfusion through a new filter. *Transfusion*. 1990;30:30–33.
93. Dula DJ, Muller HA, Donovan JW. Flow rate variance of commonly used IV infusion techniques. *J Trauma*. 1981;21:480–482.
94. Boyan CP, Howland WS. Blood temperature: a critical factor in massive transfusions. *Anesthesiology*. 1961;22:559.
95. Boyan CP, Howland WS. Cardiac arrest and temperature of banked blood. *JAMA*. 1963;183:58.
96. Russell WJ. A review of blood warmers for massive transfusion. *Anesth Intensive Care*. 1974;2:109–130.
97. Xifaras GP, Healy TEJ. A comparative study of four blood warming coils. *Anaesthesia*. 1971;26:229–234.
98. Thermal dry heat blood warmer 4R4305. Travenol Laboratories, Inc. Deerfield, IL 60015, 1980.
99. DW-1000 Blood/Fluid Warmer. American Hamilton, Two Rivers, WI 54241, 1981.
100. Leonard TF, Restall CJ, Taswell HF, et al. Microwave warming of bank blood. *Anesth Analg*. 1971;50:302–305.
101. Linko K, Hekali R. Influence of the taurus radiowave blood warmer on human red cells. *Acta Anaesthesiol Scand*. 1980;24:46–52.
102. Arens JF, Leonard GL. Danger of over-warming blood by microwave. *JAMA*. 1971;218:1045–1046.
103. McCullough J, Polesky HF, Nelson C, et al. Iatrogenic hemolysis: a complication of blood warmed by a microwave device. *Anesth Analg*. 1972;51:102–106.
104. Staples PJ, Griner PF. Extracorporeal hemolysis of blood in a microwave blood warmer. *N Engl J Med*. 1971;285:317–319.
105. Van der Starre PJA. The Treonic Haemoheater: a new blood warming device. *Anesthesiology*. 1978;33:729–732.
106. Werwath DL, Schwab CW, Robinett WL, et al. Microwave ovens: a safe new method for warming crystalloids. In: *Proceedings of the 14th Annual Meeting of the University Association for Emergency Medicine*. 1984.
107. Jacobs LM, Hsieh JW. A clinical review of autotransfusion and its role in trauma. *JAMA*. 1984;251:3283–3287.
108. Beall W. The hematology of autotransfusion. *Surgery*. 1978;84:695–699.
109. Symbas TN. Autotransfusion in thoracic trauma. In: Hauer JM, Thurere RL, Dawson RB, eds. *Autotransfusion*. New York: Elsevier, 1981:83–92.
110. Davidson SJ. Emergency unit autotransfusion. *Surgery*. 1978;84:703–707.
111. Klebanoff G. Intraoperative autotransfusion with the Bentley ATS-100. *Surgery*. 1978;84:708–712.
112. Klebanoff G, Phillips J, Evans W. Use of a disposable autotransfusion unit under varying conditions of contamination. *Am J Surg*. 1970;120:351–354.
113. Smith RN, Yaw PB, Glover JL. Autotransfusion of contaminated intraperitoneal blood: an experimental study. *J Trauma*. 1978;18:341–344.
114. Boudreaux JP, Bornside GH, Cohn I. Emergency autotransfusion: partial cleansing of bacteria-laden blood by cell washing. *J Trauma*. 1983;23:31–35.
115. Myhre PA. Incidence, symptomatology, and serology of transfusion reactions. *Wis Med J*. 1966;65:247.
116. Wintrobe MM, Lee CR, Boggs DR, et al. *Clinical Hematology*. 8th ed. Philadelphia: Lea & Febiger; 1981.
117. Myhre BA. Fatalities from blood transfusion. *JAMA*. 1980;244:1333–1335.
118. Schmidt AP, Taswell HF, Gleich GJ. Anaphylactic transfusion reactions associated with anti-IgA antibody. *N Engl J Med*. 1969;280:188–193.
119. Vyas GN, Fudenberg HH. Isoimmune IgA causing anaphylactoid transfusion reactions. *N Engl J Med*. 1969;280:1073–1074.
120. Braude AI. Transfusion reactions from contaminated blood. *N Engl J Med*. 1958;258:1289–1293.

9. Emergency Wound Management

DAVIS CRACROFT, MD, FACEP

Essential in the emergency department treatment of any wound is the initial evaluation of the patient's condition. Attention should be directed to the patient's age, allergies, medications being taken (eg, steroids, chemotherapeutic agents), tetanus immunization status, and coexisting illnesses (e.g., diabetes mellitus, coronary artery disease). The establishment of an airway, adequate breathing, and support of the circulation (ABCs) with intravenous (IV) fluid administration, and the treatment of life-threatening medical problems always precede definitive care of any wound. A sterile, dry gauze pad applied with pressure provides adequate hemostasis, prevents further contamination, and allows attention to be directed to more urgent problems. Occasionally, a cavity must be packed firmly to control bleeding; on an extremely rare occasion, a tourniquet is necessary to control the hemorrhage. Under these circumstances, the tourniquet is intended only as a temporary measure to provide a bloodless surgical field, allowing the accurate placement of hemostats and preventing damage to vital structures associated with blind clamping. Once hemostasis is ensured, the tourniquet is removed and some blood flow is restored to the limb until arterial reconstruction can be performed. Only in the case of the severely shattered limb, when amputation is inevitable, should the tourniquet be left in place. It should then be placed as close to the injury as possible in anticipation of amputation proximal to the tourniquet.

WOUND EVALUATION

After the patient has been stabilized and associated injuries or illnesses treated or ruled out, attention can be directed to the wound. Information regarding the history and mechanism of injury is critical to the subsequent management of the patient. The injury may be the consequence of a more serious underlying disease. For example, a scalp laceration may be secondary to a dysrhythmia-induced syncopal episode. Suspicious location or appearance of wounds in children should suggest child abuse and prompt appropriate physical and social investigation. The history given by the patient may be suspect because of drug or alcohol intoxication, head injury, fear of potential legal consequences, senility, toxic or metabolic encephalopathy, and it may be necessary to seek the history of injury from family, friends, paramedics, police, or bystanders at the scene. The clinician should attempt to establish the age of the wound, the nature of any contamination, the causative agent (eg, knife, dog bite, high- or low-velocity missile, blunt object), and the possibility of foreign bodies in the wound or distant sites. This information, combined with the location of the wound and overall physical and mental condition of the patient, allows the physician to plan the treatment of the injury logically.

Age of the Wound

The length of time between injury and treatment and the type and degree of contamination are important considerations in deciding whether to leave a wound open or to proceed with primary closure. Any accidental open wound can be considered contaminated. If left untreated, all but the most superficial wounds become infected. The presence of dead or devitalized tissue, blood clot, foreign bodies, moisture, and warmth enhances and hastens the process. The study of open wounds during World War I revealed that bacterial colony counts doubled at 10 to 12 hours postinjury.[1] It was concluded that wound closure was safe before, but dangerous after, 12 hours had elapsed. Multiple studies have variously placed the safe period for wound closure from less than 6 to more than 24 hours. A recent study from Jamaica showed excellent results with simple, uncontaminated wounds of the trunk and extremity that were closed up to 19 hours postinjury and facial and head wounds closed primarily after more than 24 hours.[2] The number of variables influencing the decision to close a wound should include specifically patient age (with greater risk of infection in the young and elderly), nutritional status, and medical illnesses, with particular attention to diabetes mellitus, congestive heart failure, cirrhosis, peripheral vascular disease, and malignancy. The physician must consider the patient's current medications, especially steroids, immunosuppressants, and anticoagulants. Allergies to local anesthetics, antiseptics, antibiotics, and tape must be determined, and the potential for rabies, tetanus, or other infection from local contamination should be assessed.[3] Certainly the experience and skill of the treating physician play a prominent role in the decision of how to care for any wound. At this time there are no hard and fast rules governing when to close and when to leave a wound open. The "golden period" varies from patient to patient and must be assessed individually.

Contamination and Infection

Infection occurs when the number of organisms at a given site exceeds the ability of local tissue defenses to control them. Most common linear lacerations are usually caused by a shearing force from a sharp object such as a razor, knife, or glass edge. These lacerations require a concentration of 10^6 bacteria per gram of tissue to cause infection with the usual pathogens. With a lower concentration of bacteria, the wound is merely contaminated, and local humoral and cellular defenses prevent infection. Any contaminated wound can be converted to a surgically clean wound by means of mechanical cleansing and meticulous debridement. Infected wounds, however, cannot be converted to clean wounds by any quick, simple procedure. Contamination can be differentiated from infection by the cardinal signs of inflammation—calor, rubor, dolor, and tumor. These signs are associated with infection and are an absolute contraindication to closure, regardless of the length of time the wound has been open.[4]

The wound environment helps determine the likelihood of subsequent infection. The skin microflora vary greatly in both density and diversity in different regions of the body. Moister skin areas such as the perineum, web spaces, intertriginous areas, and axillae provide a rich environment for millions of bacteria per square centimeter. Over most of the dry areas of the body, including the trunk, upper arms, and legs, the bacterial counts are quite low. Wide variability exists in the bacterial counts of exposed body surfaces from the relative sterility of the palms of the hands to an abundance of bacteria on the forehead and scalp. Generally aerobes far outnumber anaerobes, in a ratio of 5:1 to 10:1, but anaerobes are frequently the predominant organism of the upper back, cheeks, and presternum.[5]

The blood supply to the region of injury plays an important role in the natural defense against infection. Facial and scalp lacerations may be closed primarily after 24 hours in many instances, owing to the rich blood supply in these areas. Conversely, as a consequence of diminished venous and lymphatic return and poor arterial supply, there is a high risk that distal lower extremity lacerations will become infected even when treated shortly after injury. The effectiveness of the defense provided by the blood supply to the upper extremity, proximal lower extremity, abdomen, and thorax falls between these two extremes.

Contusional damage to tissue surrounding a traumatic laceration may compromise local defenses and render a relatively clean wound unsuitable for closure. Compressive injuries with shear forces caused by the collision of two bodies are more likely to become infected because the contusion of wound edges and surrounding soft tissue increases damaged tissue and reduces blood flow. A concentration of as little as 10^4 bacteria per gram of tissue may cause infection.[6] Additionally, the size and shape of the wound, the general condition of the patient, and damage to adjacent structures must all be considered by the physician who is deciding whether to close a wound. If there is any doubt, the wound should be left open or surgical consultation should be requested. A primary closure delayed 3 to 5 days does not appreciably alter the time of healing and avoids the discomfort, disability, time, and expense of treating an infected closed wound.

A heavily contaminated or "dirty" wound should under most circumstances be left open. Wounds contaminated with feces or oral secretions from humans or animals contain approximately 10^{11} bacteria per gram of wet weight. Even with mechanical and hydraulic cleansing and antibiotic coverage, many of these wounds become infected with primary closure. The wound should be packed open after debridement and irrigation, and empiric antibiotic therapy should be initiated. If there is no sign of infection after 3 to 4 days, the wound can be closed with a single layer of deep Nylon sutures.

Human hair proves to be a source of potential infection when trapped in the sutures or the wound.[7] Removal of hair around a wound with the standard prep razor, however, significantly increases the incidence of infection.[8] The use of scissors or an electric clipper avoids abrasion of the skin and the potential for bacterial contamination.[9]

Causative Agent

The causative agent of injury may dictate whether the wound should be closed primarily. All partial thickness abrasions, puncture wounds, most animal (including human) bites, and most stab wounds are best treated with cleansing, exploration, debridement, and open drainage. Low-velocity missiles, such as a knife, low-caliber pistol bullet, or blunt object, usually create a relatively weak penetrating force that decelerates along its track. Surrounding injury is usually limited, and the greatest need is to review the anatomy of the region involved and ascertain the damage through the track. The destructive forces radiating from a high-velocity missile produce shock waves that extend several centimeters along its track, shatter bone, disrupt viscera, tear muscles, cause contusions, and usually leave a large, ragged exit wound. Clearly, the emergency treatment of such injuries is centered on resuscitation and prompt transfer to the operating room.

Foreign Body Contamination

If there is any suspicion of foreign body contamination in a wound or distant site, radiographic examination in two planes should precede exploration. Current radiographic techniques allow emergency physicians to localize both metallic and many less opaque foreign bodies. Both leaded and nonleaded glass and various wooden or fibrous spines, thorns, and splinters have been demonstrated with plain radiography or xeroradiography.[10] Radiopaque objects can be located by roentgenogram and removed under fluoroscopy. After the patient has been given local anesthesia, small-gauge (22 to 25) needles are passed through various angles and planes until the object is touched or seen to move. A small cutdown is then performed along the path of the needle in contact with the object, and the foreign body is retrieved. Only the most superficial foreign body (ie, one that is readily seen or palpated after the injection of a local anesthetic) can be retrieved without the aid of fluoroscopy. A search for the proverbial "needle in the haystack" without fluoroscopy usually leads to excessive tissue damage and is often unsuccessful. Multiple shotgun pellets and less radiopaque foreign bodies in soft tissue are best left in place. If the object is not sterile, a localized abscess forms within a few days, allowing accurate removal by simple incision and drainage. Obviously, in the case of deep intraocular, intraarticular, or visceral foreign bodies, appropriate surgical consultation should be sought.

ANESTHESIA

Premedication

In general, premedication is not indicated for procedures performed under local anesthesia in the emergency department; it only adds to the potential complications. Careful explanation and ample reassurance usually allay fear in all but the most recalcitrant patients. When necessary, narcotics provide alleviation of apprehension, analgesia, and often some degree of euphoria. The recommended dose of meperidine hydrochloride (Demerol) is 1.0 to 2.0 mg/kg IV or intramuscularly and of morphine sulfate is 0.1 to 0.2 mg/kg IV or intramuscularly. Naloxone (Narcan, 0.1 mL/kg) readily reverses the respiratory depressant effects of narcotics. The best way to deliver narcotics is by slow titration via the IV route. This avoids the pain of intramuscular injection, the delay in action, and the variability in absorption and consequent unpredictable effect of the drug. Intravenous fentanyl (Sublimaze, 2.0 to 3.0 µg/kg) has been used safely and efficaciously in children requiring repair of facial lacerations.[11] It has a half-life of 20 minutes and can easily be reversed with naloxone. Nitrous oxide (50% mixture) is a useful supplement to local anesthetics. Caution should be used with children under the age of two; a papoose board or other restraint is the safer alternative. For procedures in which the uncooperative patient may jeopardize the outcome, general anesthesia is necessary.

TAC (tetracaine 0.5%, adrenaline 0.05%, and cocaine 11.8%) or TEC (tetracaine, epinephrine, and cocaine) solution is becoming a widely used topical anesthetic for repair of lacerations in the pediatric population. In well-vascularized, nonmucous membrane lacerations of 5.0 cm or less, TAC is equal to infiltrated lidocaine in both anesthetic efficacy and subsequent wound complication rate.[12,13] For wounds smaller than 3 cm in length, 5 mL of the TAC solution on gauze is applied to the wound with firm pressure for 5 to 10 minutes. Up to 10 mL can be used safely in lacerations of from 3 to 6 cm. TAC can be effectively applied by the person accompanying the child to the emergency department, saving nursing time.[14] TAC should not be used in repair of lacerations of the pinna, penis, digits, or nose because of the potent vasoconstriction induced by epinephrine and cocaine. Because of enhanced absorption and the consequent potential for serious side effects, TAC should never be used on mucous membranes, burns, or other areas of partial-thickness skin loss.[15,16] TAC topical anesthetic maximizes patient compliance, avoids the "brutane" approach to pediatric suturing, and prevents the anatomic distortion seen with infiltrative anesthesia.

Local Anesthesia

Most minor soft tissue injuries are best repaired under local infiltrative anesthesia. Lidocaine (Xylocaine), because of its low toxicity, rapid diffusibility, topical activity, and chemical stability, is the drug of choice.[17] Toxic reactions vary from local skin wheals to convulsions, respiratory difficulties, and cardiovascular collapse. Resuscitative drugs and equipment should be readily available whenever local anesthetics are used. True allergic reactions are rare; most adverse reactions are due to overdosage. The maximum safe dose of lidocaine is 5.0 mg/kg in infants and 7.0 mg/kg in older children and adults, up to 500 mg total dose (50 mL of a 1.0% solution). Procaine hydrochloride (Novocain) with a maximal dose of 1000 mg (100 mL of a 1% solution) is a good alternative to lidocaine in allergic patients. Strict limitation of dosages to below toxic levels, combined with aspiration in areas of suspected vascularity, prevents reactions in all but the rare hypersensitive patient.[18]

Most wounds are best infiltrated through the open tissue with fine 25- to 30-gauge needles and systematic injection of the subcutaneous, intradermal, intrafascial, and deeper layers. With the addition of epinephrine (1:200,000), vasoconstriction occurs and absorption is delayed. The clinician should wait about 10 minutes for maximal vasoconstrictive effect. In wounds of the head and neck, the use of lidocaine with epinephrine is standard. Avoid epinephrine-containing solutions where end-arteries are present (digits) or vasoconstriction may further compromise a tenuous blood supply (nasal tip, penis, ear, and skin flaps). Furthermore, avoid unnecessary distention of tissue by injecting small amounts of local anesthetics. High pressure injections only injure tissue, distort anatomy, compromise blood supply, add tension to the wound closure, and increase discomfort. Additionally, neutralizing the pH of the anesthetic solution with bicarbonate greatly lessens the discomfort of injection.[19]

DEBRIDEMENT AND IRRIGATION

Once the decision has been made to close a wound and the area has been properly anesthetized, a technique for converting the contaminated wound to a surgically clean one must be selected. In areas with sufficient tissue, such as the face, trunk, or an extremity, complete excision is by far the simplest and most certain way of eliminating damaged and contaminated tissue. Where excision is not feasible, irrigation and debridement are necessary. Hydraulic cleansing with sterile saline solution under moderate pressure (30 to 40 cmH$_2$O) provides optimal irrigation for the removal of blood clots, loose debris, and foreign bodies.

A commercially available irrigation system (Travenol), consisting of a 12-mL syringe attached via IV tubing to a saline irrigant bottle, makes an ideal irrigation device. With moderate force the irrigation device delivers about 20 psi—the recommended pressure for irrigation of heavily contaminated wounds. For mild to moderate contamination, irrigation with a 19-gauge needle or catheter attached to a 35-mL syringe produces about 7 to 8 psi and is adequate.[20] Irrigation of most wounds with 100 to 200 mL of fluid is optimal. Saline is thought by many to be the best irrigant, although it has no bactericidal properties and mainly works mechanically to remove debris and bacteria. Because povidone-iodine in a 1% solution provides mechanical cleansing and is bactericidal, it is regarded by some to be ideal. The commercially available povidine-iodine solution is 10%, a concentration shown to retard healing. The standard 10% solution must be diluted with 10 times the volume of normal saline to make the 1% irrigation solution. The 10% stock povidine-iodine solution still remains the agent of choice for skin prep around the wound.

Debridement is intended to remove all devitalized tissue and foreign material without doing harm to vital structures. Meticulous and often tedious attention to the removal of all small, often firmly adherent foreign bodies is mandatory if infection and tattooing are to be avoided. Repetitive saline irrigation, sponging with a dry gauze pad, and removal of adherent contaminants with fine-tipped Adson's forceps is recommended. Adequate visualization of the contaminated area may require extension of the wound. Partial thickness abrasions and lacerations should be debrided vigorously by scrubbing under topical, local, or general anesthesia. It must be remembered, however, that overzealous scrubbing can convert a partial thickness abrasion into a full thickness defect that will need skin grafting. Adherent road dirt and other fine particles not removed by scrubbing must be teased or even scraped from the surface of an abrasion with a number 12 scalpel. Scrubbing a full-thickness wound increases the inflammatory response and may destroy otherwise viable tissue. The use of a fine-pore sponge with a detergent to reduce the friction between the sponge and tissue should minimize tissue damage. Scrubbing should be reserved for "dirty" wounds contaminated with large amounts of foreign material.[21]

Excision should be done by sharp dissection, preferably with a scalpel and fine-toothed forceps, although sharp scissors can be used for removal of dead muscle, fat, and fascia. As a general rule, viable tissue bleeds freely and nonviable tissue does not. In skin debridement, only a narrow margin need be excised. On the face and scalp, questionably viable tissue can often be spared debridement; the abundant blood supply increases its chance of survival. Similarly, the facial subcutaneous tissue should be excised sparingly to avoid loss of supporting tissue that would result in a depressed scar. Elsewhere, fat should be excised back to a healthy, yellow plane free of any blood stains. Loose, ragged fragments of fascia should be excised. When ischemic or dead, muscle tissue is ragged and cyanotic; living muscle contracts when cut or pinched, bleeds when cut, and has a glistening, reddish brown color. Excision of muscle must be radical to prevent clostridial or other bacterial growth.

Flap lacerations and avulsions often present a difficult problem in management. Especially with distal-based and contused flaps, viability is not always easy to determine. Color demarcation is one important consideration. A slightly dusky end of a flap without a clear demarcation usually survives; if there is a clear-cut color line between normal tissue and cyanotic tissue, the cyanotic area should be removed. Often a flap has a good arterial supply, blanching and refilling when pressure is applied to its base, but local edema may impair venous return. This may lead to necrosis

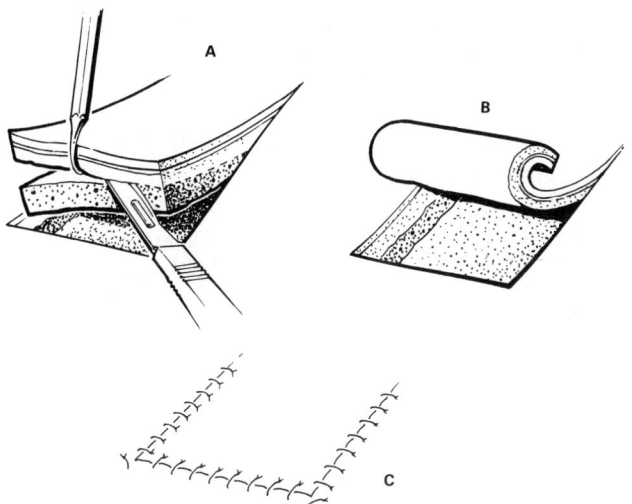

Figure 9-1 Defatting a skin flap. When judged nonviable, a skin flap can be replaced after defatting as a full thickness graft. **(A)** Initially, evert the flap and sharply dissect away all fatty tissues from the overlying dermal layer, using a #15 scalpel, sharp-tipped iris or small Metzenbaum scissors. **(B)** Avoiding penetration of the dermal layer, remove all fat. **(C)** Tack the flap down with fine sutures placed close to the wound edge. As with other full thickness grafts, strict hemostasis, immobilization, and close observation of the wound are recommended.

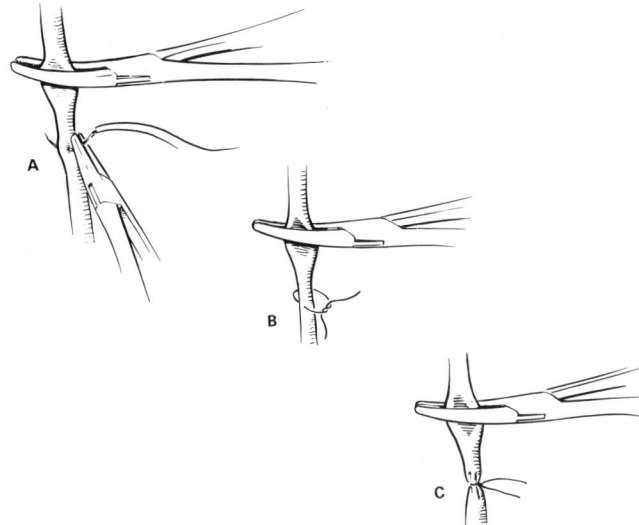

Figure 9-2 Suture ligature technique. **(A)** Suture ligature passed through vessel beneath hemostat. **(B)** Ligature tied with single throw and then passed around vessel and tied again. **(C)** Completed suture ligature. The suture may be tied freehand in a similar fashion or passed with a hemostat when dealing with less accessible vessels.

within the first few days. When doubt exists, the best method is to defat the flap and apply it as a full thickness graft with fine sutures placed close to the wound edges (Fig. 9-1).

HEMOSTASIS

With most routine lacerations, hemostasis can be accomplished initially with a pressure dressing of sterile gauze. Following injection of a local anesthetic and preparation for closure, most wounds resume bleeding as vasodilatation occurs and clots are removed. If bleeding does not follow debridement, the excision was inadequate. In most superficial lacerations hemostasis can be adequately obtained with simple closure of the wound. Should bleeding be evident postclosure, local pressure for 5 minutes or a temporary suture around the bleeding site is normally sufficient. If this does not control hemorrhage, the wound should be reopened and the bleeding vessel ligated. Disposable thermal-loop cautery units can be useful to control hemorrhage from small bleeders. These are ideal for obtaining a bloodless field for skin grafts or closure of thin skin flaps, where the accumulation of a hematoma could cause skin slough. Deeper wounds may require electrocauterization or, most often, suture ligatures of absorbable (4-0 or 5-0) material to effect hemostasis. Care must be taken to ligate only the bleeding vessel and not a large volume of surrounding soft tissue (Fig. 9-2).

The ligature and the necrotic material enclosed in the suture both act as foreign bodies and an inoculum for potential infection.

The physician should not attempt to ligate bleeders in the vascular subcutaneous tissue of the scalp. Most scalp lacerations can be closed primarily with deep, snugly tied skin sutures to control bleeding.[22] In deep scalp lacerations, traction and eversion of the galea with hemostats effectively controls subcutaneous hemorrhage and allows exploration of the wound. In other areas, clamping of larger vessels may be necessary to visualize the wound adequately. The physician should never clamp a vessel blindly; when faced with persistent bleeding, the physician must seek assistance. The assistant can sponge the area frequently, retract the edges of the wound, and apply pressure over the involved feeding artery or vein. Any wound that is too extensive to permit a systematic, thorough approach to its exploration and closure should be closed in the operating room.

SUTURING

Selection of Suture

Suture is used to obliterate spaces, stop hemorrhage, and impart physical strength to a discontinuous surface. The physician should select the best artificial fiber (suture) to maintain the edges in close apposition until a natural fiber (collagen) is synthesized. All suture material invokes a foreign body reaction, but using the most appropriate and finest gauge suture that will do the job lessens the chances of postoperative infection. There are many types of suture available, and the appropriate type can be chosen according to the tissue to be closed, the probable time required for healing, and the potential for infection in the wound.

Absorbable sutures are made of various materials including catgut, collagen, polyglycolic acid (Dexon), and a copolymer of glycolic and lactic acids in a ratio of 90:10 (Vicryl). Catgut sutures are digested by proteolytic enzymes derived from inflammatory cells. Plain catgut incites a greater inflammatory reaction than chromic catgut, and the reaction may persist for a prolonged period if plain catgut is used in or near the skin surface. Polyglycolic acid (Dexon) and polyglactin 910 (Vicryl) are slowly hydrolyzed by water, and the principal reaction occurs with invasion of the interstices of the suture by macrophages. While plain catgut and chromic catgut are digested at a variable rate (2 weeks to 2 years), the synthetic sutures disappear at a more predictable rate. Polyglactin 910 (Vicryl) disappears after approximately 80 days and polyglycolic acid (Dexon) after 100 to 120 days; both suture types are much more rapidly absorbed in the presence of infection. Absorbable sutures lose strength more rapidly than they disappear. At 14 to 21 days, both polyglactin 910 (Vicryl) and polyglycolic acid (Dexon) have lost nearly all their tensile strength. Compared with catgut, however, both synthetic sutures exhibit greater tensile strength and cause less inflammation at all stages of healing in normal, irradiated, and infected tissue.[23] The overall superior qualities of Dexon and Vicryl, combined with their handling ease, make them the logical choice over catgut in emergency department use.

Nonabsorbable sutures are made of silk, cotton, Nylon, polyester (Dacron), polypropylene (Prolene), or steel. They are further classified as monofilament—Nylon, steel, polypropylene—or multifilament (woven)—steel, Nylon, silk, cotton, or polyester. Silk is classified as nonabsorbable, but it has been shown to lose all its tensile strength after 1 year and usually disappears after 2 years. The unfortunate fatalities that have resulted from the failure of silk suture lines used to insert heart valve prostheses during the early years of cardiac surgery bear testimony to the absorbable nature of silk. Nylon may swell and lose some of its strength after 1 year, but this is probably not clinically significant.[24]

All nonabsorbable sutures induce a cellular reaction. Silk and cotton produce the greatest reaction; Nylon, polypropylene, and steel, the least reaction. Polyester is intermediate in its reactivity. Because of their construction, multifilament sutures have a greater potential for infection than do monofilament sutures. Bacteria and tissue fluids can penetrate the interstices of the multifilament suture, but inflammatory cells cannot; the bacteria can multiply and convert a contamination into an infection. Monofilament sutures, on the other hand, provide no place for bacteria to hide and therefore are recommended when the possibility of infection is high.

When other characteristics of suture material are equal, the handling qualities of the suture may dictate the one to choose. Most multifilament sutures are easier to handle than monofilament. Usually, they are more pliable, lie flatter when tied, and do not project stiffly above the skin when cut. The latter is particularly important when suture is used near the eye, as such a projection could be a potentially dangerous corneal irritant. Nylon is notorious for coming untied and requires more knots than silk or cotton to secure. The absolute tensile strength of any suture is insignificant if the knot is weakened. Wire requires two throws to secure; silk, cotton, and other nonabsorbable braided sutures require three. Catgut, polymeric absorbables (Dexon and Vicryl), and the monofilament nonabsorbables—Nylon and polypropylene—require four. All knots should be squared.

Nonabsorbable sutures should be utilized in the closure of skin and fascia, as well as in the approximation of lacerated tendons. Absorbable sutures can be utilized to close the periosteum, muscle, and subcutaneous tissue, and to ligate blood vessels. As a rule, the emergency department physician needs to become familiar with only one or two types of absorbable and nonabsorbable suture. Table 9-1 provides a general guide to suture; Dexon, Vicryl, and Nylon are presented as examples, but personal preferences may be substituted.

Suturing Technique

The various layers of a wound should be placed in close apposition so that a minimal amount of new connective tissue will be required to restore structural integrity. Probably the most important single determinant of the final width of a scar is the tension under which the skin is originally closed. As a rule, the final width of any scar is approximately the size of the defect remaining after the subcutaneous tissue has been approximated. Up until the fifth to sixth day postinjury, the injured tissue has little tensile strength, and the wound edges are held together by the adhesiveness of cells, globular proteins, and fibrin. The deposition of collagen, which gives the tissue strength, is not even demonstrable until the fifth day. Collagen synthesis continues during the first 6 weeks, the proliferative phase of wound healing, but the injured tissue does not gain maximal strength for several months to years. If closed under any tension, the weakened, vulnerable scar will gradually widen for the first few weeks. Ideally, to optimize strength and minimize the tendency for the wound edges to separate, sutures should be left in place for 2 to 3 months. However, any suture left in place for more than 2 weeks produces unsightly railroad track scars or stitch abscesses. To reconcile these two inconsistencies, a subcuticular buried suture should be employed. In wounds that must be closed under tension, the suture material should be nonabsorbable to maintain the tensile strength of the closure until collagen synthesis is complete. In areas where little tension is exerted along the suture line, such as in the closure

Table 9-1 Wound Closure Guide

Site	With Tension	Without Tension	Stitch
Face			
Skin	6-0 Nylon	6-0 Nylon	Simple, running simple
	6-0 silk	6-0 silk	
Subcuticular	4-0 Nylon (running)		Running subcuticular
	5-0, 6-0 Nylon (white or clear)	4-0, 6-0 Dexon, Vicryl	Inverted or horizontal simple
Muscle and fascia	3-0, 4-0 Nylon	3-0, 4-0 Dexon, Vicryl	Simple, horizontal mattress
Fatty tissue	4-0, 5-0 Dexon, Vicryl	None or 5-0, 6-0 Dexon, Vicryl	Simple, inverted simple
Scalp			
Skin	3-0, 4-0 Nylon	3-0, 4-0 Nylon	Simple, running locking
Fascia (galea)	3-0, 4-0 Nylon	3-0, 4-0 Dexon, Vicryl	Simple, horizontal mattress
Trunk	3-0, 4-0 Nylon	3-0, 4-0 Nylon	Simple, vertical mattress, running simple or running vertical mattress
Extremities	4-0, 5-0 Nylon	4-0, 5-0 Nylon	Simple, vertical mattress, running simple or running vertical mattress
Hands, feet	4-0, 5-0 Nylon	4-0, 5-0 Nylon	Simple, vertical or horizontal mattress
Mucous membranes	4-0, 5-0 silk	4-0, 5-0 silk	Simple
	4-0, 5-0 Dexon, Vicryl	4-0, 5-0 Dexon, Vicryl	Inverted or horizontal simple

of facial lacerations parallel to relaxed lines of tension (Fig. 9-3), an absorbable suture combined with external support can be utilized.

Often the face is the only area of the body requiring meticulous closure with subcuticular support. If infection, drainage, or hemorrhage is anticipated, or if local edema and tissue damage are present, loose approximation or open drainage is recommended. A widened scar is an acceptable alternative to devitalization and infection in a wound improperly closed.

There is no hard-and-fast rule dictating the exact number of sutures necessary to close a wound. The physician should use only enough sutures to approximate the wound edges adequately. As a general rule, sutures should be placed as far from the skin edge as they are from each other (Fig. 9-4). The finest gauge suture that is stronger than the tissue to be closed should be used. A wound edge is more effectively controlled when the sutures are placed nearer to that edge, but strangulation and necrosis can occur if the sutures are placed too close or under excessive tension. In general, the suture tension should be just enough to approximate the edges and no more. When tied too tightly, wound edges are inverted, making the suture line appear very fine, but the rolled-under edges heal by secondary intention. To avoid wound edge inversion, a small probe or the tip of a forceps should be inserted along the entire length of the suture line at the end of the procedure. If the skin edges are not abutting, the sutures should be replaced. Excessive suture tension may also herniate subcutaneous tissue to the surface of the wound, producing a scalloped effect.

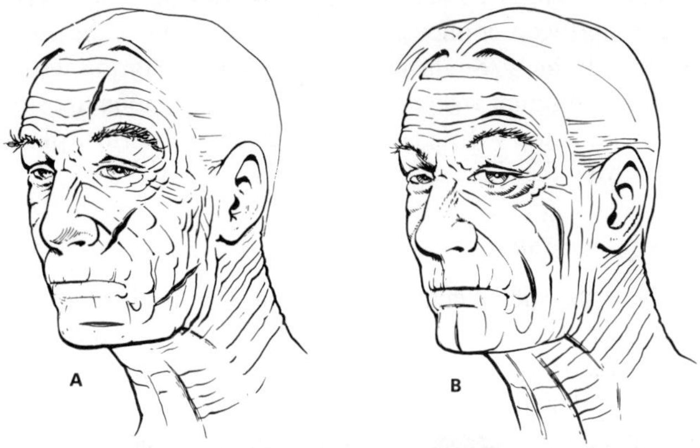

Figure 9-3 Relaxed lines of tension. (**A**) When a laceration runs perpendicular to the relaxed lines of tension, nonabsorbable subcuticular sutures should be used. (**B**) Esthetic results are usually superior when the laceration lies parallel to normal facial tension lines. Absorbable subcuticular sutures can be used.

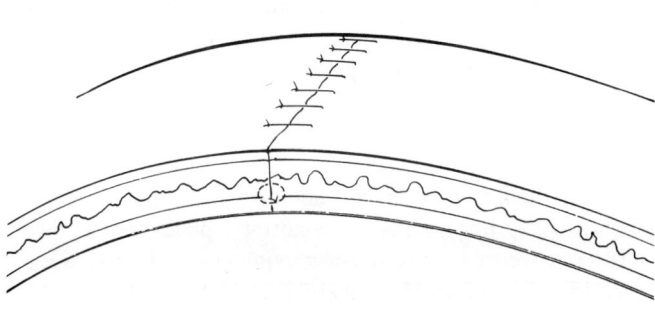

Figure 9-4 Sutures are generally placed as far from the skin edge as they are from each other.

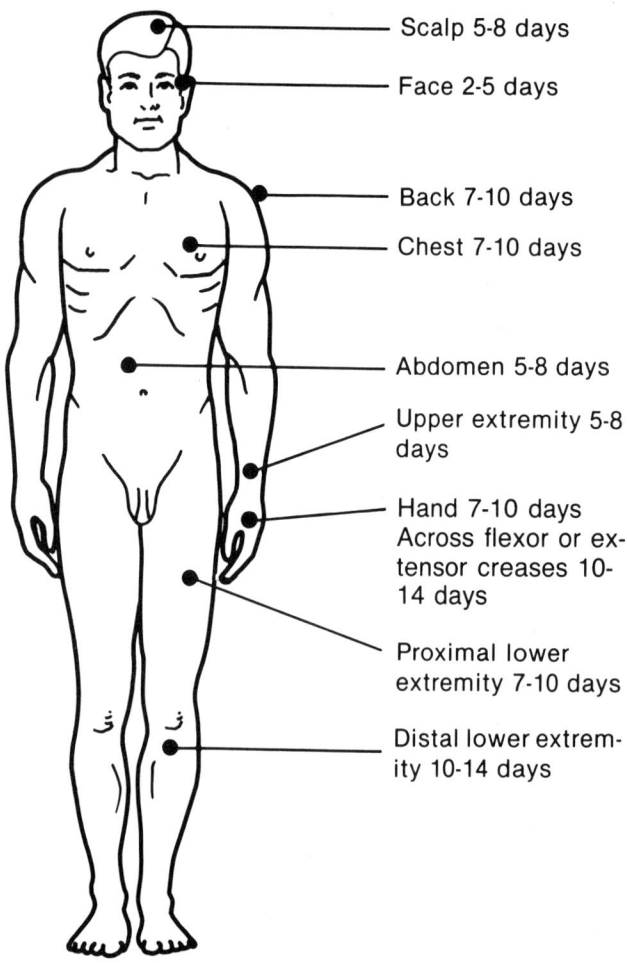

Figure 9-5 Guide to suture removal.

Several hours after closure, a wound should be watertight, unless drainage is excessive. Sutures may be removed from 2 to 14 days after closure if the epithelium has healed adequately. Cross-hatching inevitably occurs at 14 days and may occur sooner if the sutures are tied under excessive tension or infection supervenes. In debilitated patients or in patients with wounds of the distal lower extremity, it may be necessary to leave the stitches in place at least this long, however, in order to ensure wound healing. If there is some question about the removal of a suture, alternate sutures can be removed and the wound rechecked in two days. A general guide to suture removal is provided in Fig. 9-5.

The importance of using sharp, fine instruments in handling tissue should be stressed. An instrument tray for the closure of facial wounds in the emergency department should include diamond-tipped or smooth-tipped needle holders, skin hooks, fine mosquito hemostats, plain and toothed Adson's forceps, curved and straight iris scissors, number 15 and number 11 scalpels, curved Metzenbaum scissors, suture scissors, antiseptic solution, sterile gauze, and saline.

Types of Sutures

The Subcuticular Suture

In the closure of facial lacerations or anywhere where the final cosmetic result is important, subcuticular sutures should be used. They reduce tension on the skin edges and allow epidermal sutures to be removed early. Subcuticular stitches are placed after the underlying muscle fascia and subcutaneous tissue have been closed. Depending on the anticipated tension on the skin, either nonabsorbable (5-0 white silk or Nylon) suture or absorbable (5-0 Vicryl or Dexon) should be used. Care should be taken to place the suture only in the dermis, as any perforation of the epidermis will lead to epithelial migration and the possible formation of an epithelial cyst or abscess. The skin edge is gently grasped and everted with fine-toothed Adson's forceps or skin hooks, and the lowest level of the dermis is approximated. The suture should be inverted with the knot cut close to avoid penetration of the overlying epidermis (Fig. 9-6).

In straight or gently curved lacerations, the running subcuticular stitch may be used instead of interrupted sutures. It prevents the occasional lumpy scar seen with simple interrupted subcuticular sutures and, with practice, can be placed with greater speed. The tensile strength of 4-0 Nylon makes it ideal for a continuous intradermal suture. The needle is placed horizontally through the dermis, and small bites are taken alternatively on each side of the wound. If the laceration is long, it is wise to pass the suture through the skin every 6 to 8 cm to facilitate its removal. The physician should check the suture at the end of the procedure to make sure it slides back and forth easily. The suture can remain in place for 2 to 3 weeks (Fig. 9-6E).

For short or shallow full-thickness lacerations, a useful technique is to orient the simple interrupted subcuticular suture in a horizontal rather than vertical plane. This allows accurate approximation of the dermal layers when the restricted length or depth of the wound would otherwise make it difficult or impossible to pass the needle in the usual vertical fashion. Slight upward angulation with the initial pass of the suture and similar downward angulation to complete the stitch will keep the knot in the subdermal plane away from the skin surface (Fig. 9-7).

The Simple Suture

Once the subcuticular layer has been approximated, the skin edges should be nearly touching. The simple epidermal suture is intended only to adjust the level of the two opposing edges and makes no contribution to the strength of the closure. The suture can be placed shallowly near the skin edge with 6-0 or 7-0 Nylon or silk. In 3 to 4 days it can be cut or, often, lifted off without being cut owing to the normal desquamating process of the skin.

In areas of the body where full thickness single-layer closure of the skin is desirable, the interrupted simple suture

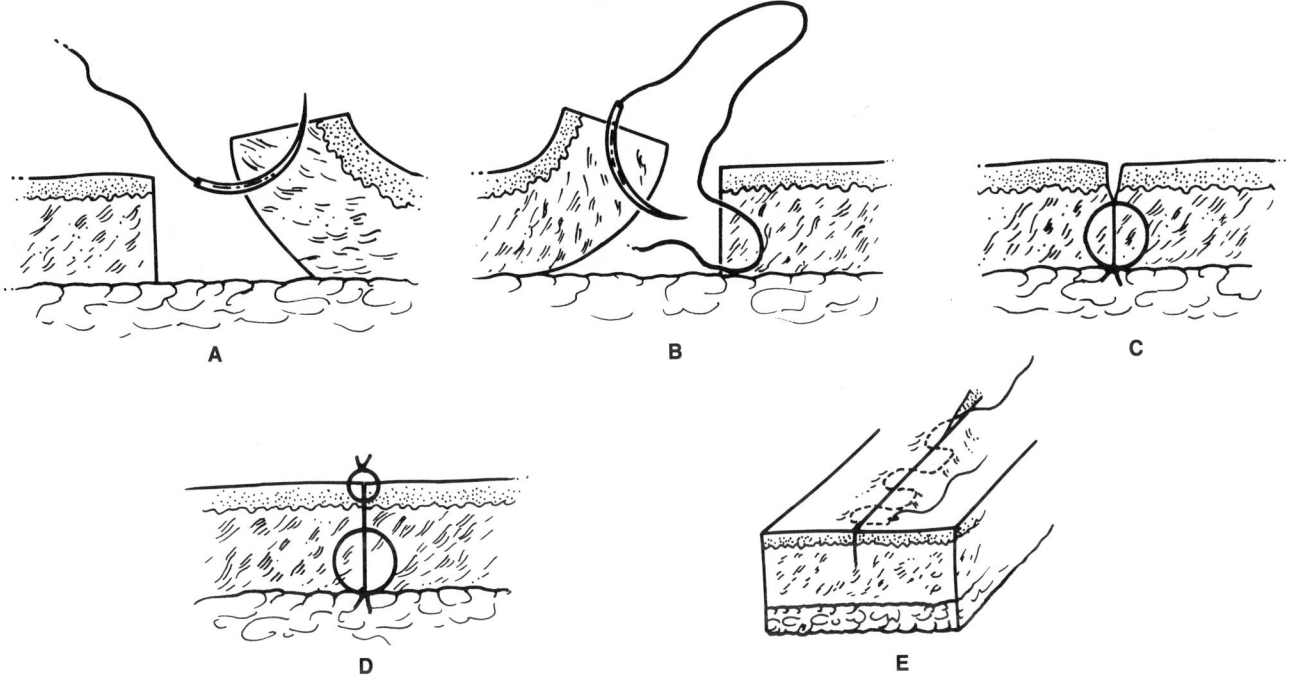

Figure 9-6 (**A** to **C**) Subcuticular (inverted) stitch. (**D**) Subcuticular and cuticular stitch. (**E**) Running subcuticular stitch.

is the mainstay of cuticular sutures. The skin edge is readily everted by enclosing a greater amount of tissue at the bottom of the suture path than near the surface. The curved needle should enter the skin at a 90° angle, at least, with sufficient subcutaneous tissue included in the bite to aid eversion. Similarly, the exit angle of the needle should be at least 90° with an equal amount of subcutaneous tissue taken on the exit side of the wound. Often the needle should be regrasped after the first bite in the center of the wound to allow entry at the same level on the other side. This ensures proper skin edge alignment and obliteration of dead space (Fig. 9-8).

The simple or inverted simple suture is usually used in closure of subcutaneous fat, muscle, and fascia. It is important to take small tissue bites and to use as few sutures as possible in closing the subcutaneous tissue (see Fig. 9-9). The suture should be absorbable (4-0 or 5-0 Vicryl or Dexon) with inverted simple sutures used near the upper levels of the wound. Fascia should be approximated with 4-0 Prolene or Nylon sutures, as sutured fascia attains only 50% of its original strength in 50 days and may take 1 year to reach full strength.

Vertical Mattress Suture

Ideal for everting wound edges, the vertical mattress suture may be used anywhere except the face. It is especially useful in areas where the cut skin naturally inverts, such as on the dorsum of the hand, in web spaces, on the scrotum, at flexion creases, and for any laceration through atrophic skin. The vertical mattress suture is placed initially just like a simple suture, enclosing a larger rectangle of tissue in the base of the wound than near the surface. Instead of tying the knot at this stage, however, the needle is passed through the cuticular layer of skin on both sides of the laceration as near to the edge as possible. The knot is secured, everting and approximating the wound edges. Some physicians alternate vertical mattress and simple interrupted sutures. A running vertical mattress suture may also be utilized (Fig. 9-10).

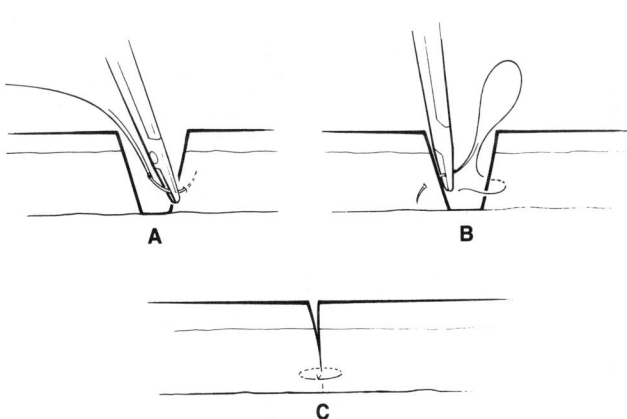

Figure 9-7 Horizontal interrupted subcuticular suture. (**A**) Slight upward angulation with the initial pass and (**B**) downward angulation through the opposite dermal surface keeps the knot away from (**C**), the overlying epidermis. This technique is useful when the wound is either too short or shallow to allow orientation of the needle in the usual vertical plane.

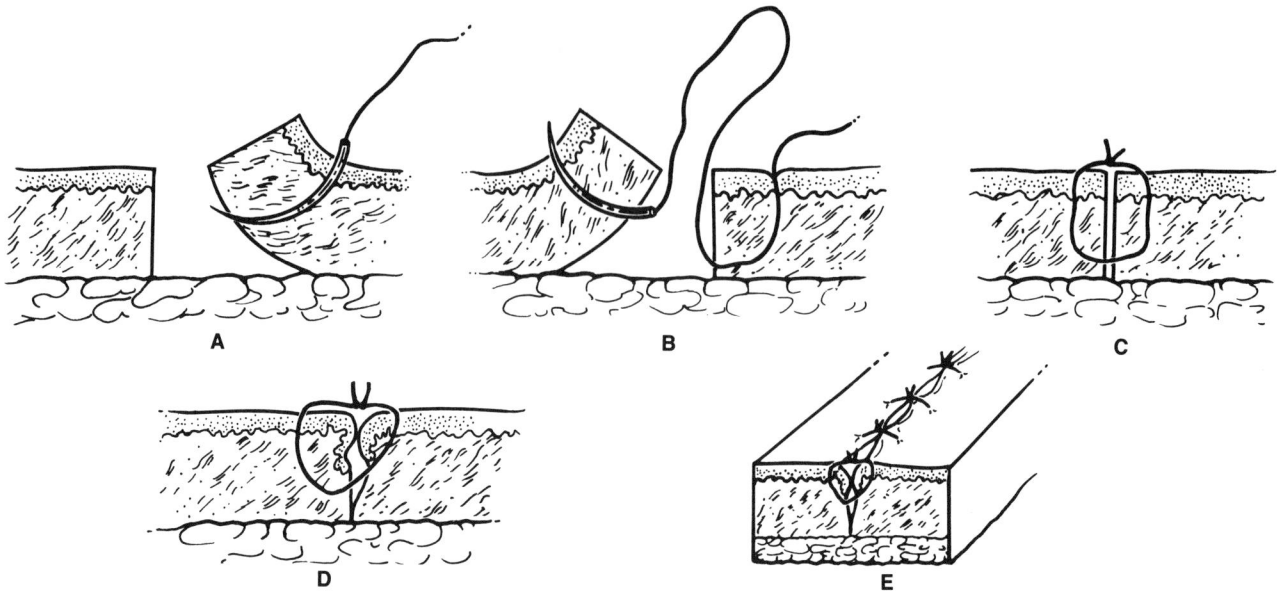

Figure 9-8 (**A** to **C**) Properly placed simple suture. (**D**) Unequal bites produce scars and dead space. (**E**) Bites too shallow and tight produce scalloping.

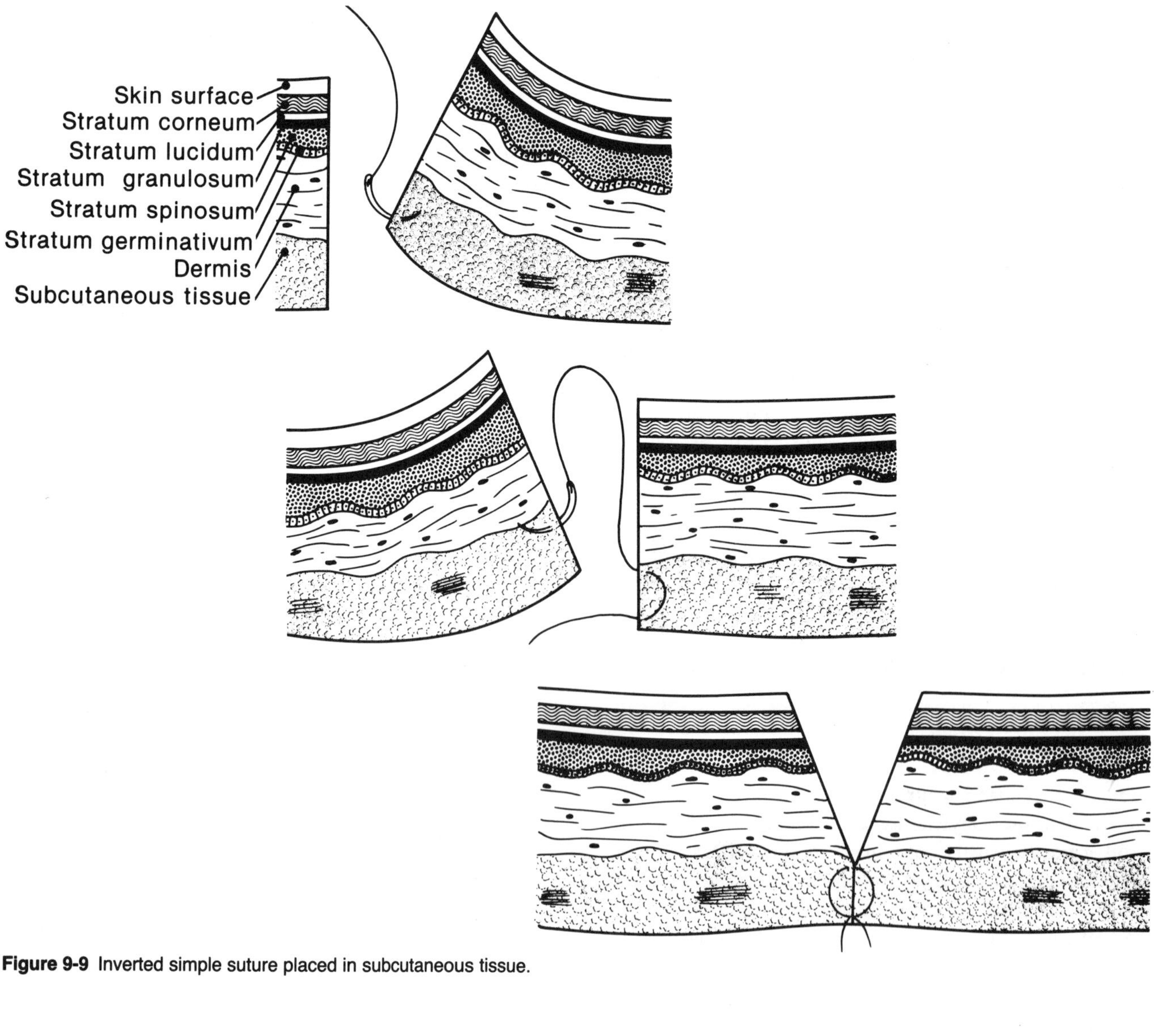

Figure 9-9 Inverted simple suture placed in subcutaneous tissue.

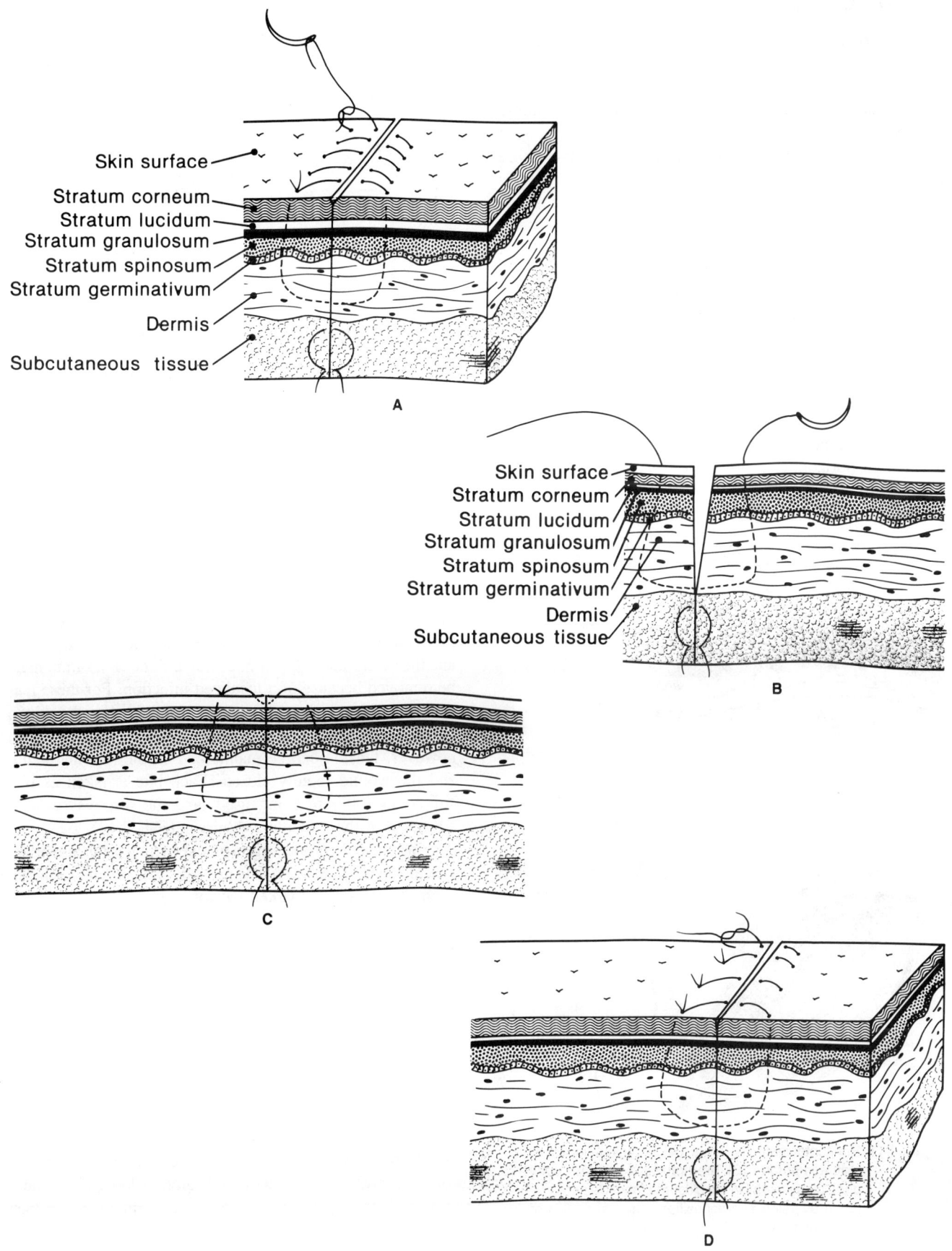

Figure 9-10 (**A**) Running (continuous) vertical mattress. (**B** to **D**) Interrupted vertical mattress.

Horizontal Mattress Suture

The horizontal mattress suture may be used whenever maximal eversion and security of the suture are desired. The horizontal mattress suture is two simple sutures placed parallel with one continuous suture. After the initial simple suture is placed, the needle is regrasped and reenters the skin on the same side as the initial exit wound. The second simple suture is completed, and the knot tied on the same side as the entry wound (Fig. 9–11A). The horizontal mattress suture is particularly useful in the closure of muscle or muscle fascia, where the wider bite aids in securing the suture. Often a simple suture will pull through the loose or stringy fibers of muscle or fascia. Additionally, the horizontal mattress suture aids in the closure of the thick skin of the palms and soles, where optimal eversion cannot be obtained with a simple suture (Fig. 9–11, B and C).

Half-Buried Horizontal Mattress Suture

For approximating the point of a V-shaped laceration, the half-buried horizontal mattress suture is ideal. Passing the buried portion of the suture through the lower portion of the dermis gives the stitch adequate strength and avoids necrosis of the delicate skin tip (Fig. 9-12).

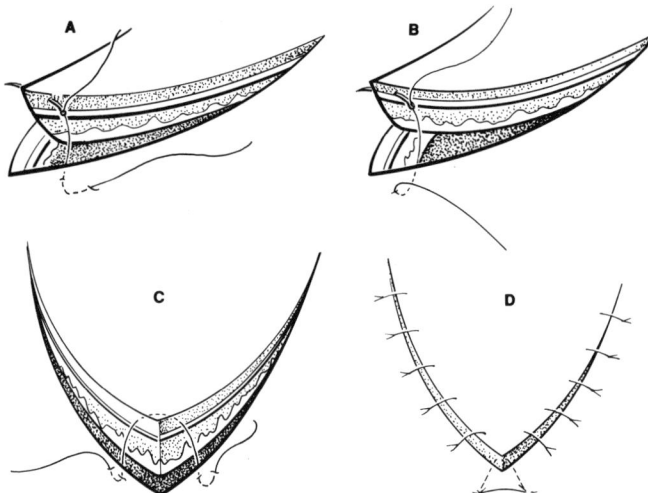

Figure 9-12 Method of tip closure; half-buried horizontal mattress.

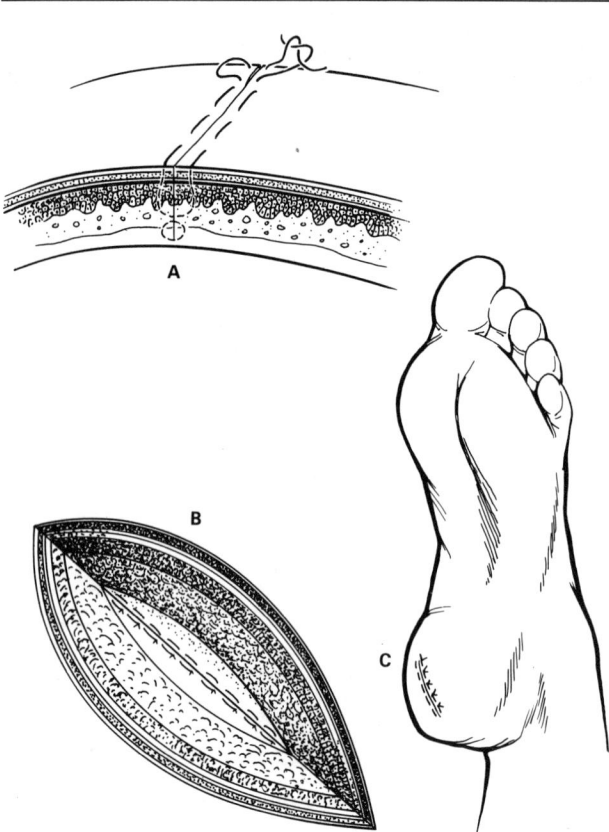

Figure 9-11 Horizontal mattress suture. (**A**) Technique for horizontal mattress suture. (**B**) The horizontal mattress suture is particularly useful in the closure of muscle or fascia and (**C**) in eversion and apposition of the thick skin of the palms or soles.

Running and Running Locking (Blanket) Sutures

Running sutures are generally not used in the emergency department except in the closure of scalp lacerations or very long lacerations when the risk of infection is minimal. The final tension of a running suture is often difficult to adjust, and the suture line is lost if one knot unties or if a suture must be removed because of a localized infection. For these reasons, a running suture should never be used below the skin in wounds treated in the emergency department. In the scalp, however, tension can be maintained on the running suture and the wound rapidly closed. Each bite is taken as if a simple suture were being used, and the suture is usually advanced in the subcutaneous tissue (Fig. 9-13). Each bite may be locked, producing a blanket stitch. The abundant vascularity of the scalp ensures survival, even when the suture is tied under marked tension.

TAPE CLOSURE OF LACERATIONS

Microporous surgical adhesive tape (Steri-strip), easily and quickly applied without anesthesia, can be useful in selected cases. The tape has a backing of viscous rayon fibers that are coated with an adhesive. Although pervious to perspiration, the tape does not permit the passage of blood or purulent material. Tape usually remains in place 1 to 2 weeks; if placed in areas of growing hair, however, it is pushed off in 5 to 7 days. Tape is ineffective over areas in constant motion or over wrinkled, oily, or loose skin. Children and uncooperative patients often remove it, further limiting its usefulness.

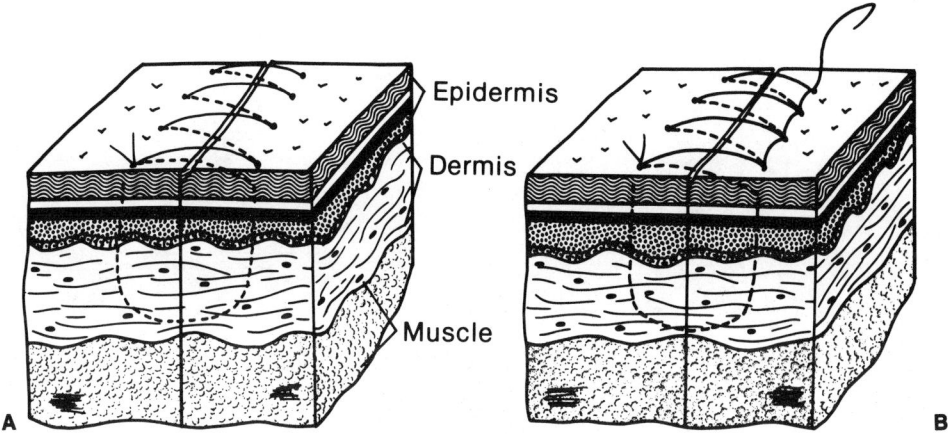

Figure 9-13 (A) Running simple suture. (B) Running locking suture.

Before tape is applied, the skin should be cleansed with soap and water and thoroughly dried; excess oily secretions can be removed with acetone or alcohol. The tape is applied perpendicular to the wound surface, one side first and then the other, bringing the edges together. Adhesives such as benzoin are contraindicated; they strengthen the adhesion initially, but after a few days they actually weaken it.[25]

Unfortunately, Steri-strips do not naturally evert skin edges. A meticulous subcuticular closure must precede their use on the face. Even then, cosmetic results are often inferior to those obtained by suturing. Their particular usefulness comes in the closure of finger burst lacerations and lower leg lacerations where local edema makes standard wound closure risky. In these cases, the use of Steri-strips makes it unnecessary to infiltrate anesthetic into an already edematous area, lessens the risk of marginal necrosis due to tight sutures, and allows prolonged coverage with a splint, cast, or bulky dressing.

All principles of wound closure with sutures apply equally to closure with Steri-strips. The tensile strength of adhesive strips is often greater than that of sutures, but the use of surgical tapes to close an infected or contaminated wound, or to approximate the edges of a puncture wound, is inviting disaster. Used alone or in conjunction with sutures, these tapes can be a valuable tool in delayed primary or secondary wound closure. In addition, by using tapes, the physician can avoid the troublesome bleeding encountered in tacking down skin grafts or approximating the avulsed, thin, atrophic skin frequently seen in steroid-dependent and elderly patients.

STAPLES

Staple closure of lacerations in the emergency department is a useful technique gaining increased popularity among physicians. The staples should be used on linear lacerations with weak tension of the edges in areas of the body where optimal cosmetic results are not required. Stapled skin wounds actually show more resistance to infection than those closed with monofilament Nylon.[26] Staples are particularly useful in the closure of long, linear, nonfacial lacerations in patients who are critically ill. In a busy emergency department where time constraints exist, staples can certainly save time.

TYPES OF LACERATIONS

Scalp Lacerations

Laceration of the scalp is the most common head injury that requires surgical care in the emergency department. Nearly all scalp lacerations can be closed primarily; because of the rich vascularity of the scalp, there is little chance of subsequent infection.

The scalp is the thickest integument and functions as a protective layer for the cranium. It is composed of five distinct layers:

1. the thick (3- to 8-mm) skin
2. the dense and richly vascular subcutaneous layer
3. the epicranium, consisting of the paired occipitalis and frontalis muscles joined by the galea aponeurotica
4. the subepicranial layer (cavum subgalea) of loose areolar tissue that separates the galea from the pericranium
5. the pericranium or periosteum of the skull

There are five paired arteries from the external carotid system with many anastomoses throughout the subcutaneous layer. The veins of the scalp parallel the arterial supply. Unlike the arteries, however, the veins communicate intracranially by way of the diploid and emissary veins to the cavernous, superior sagittal, and lateral sinuses. Any extracranial scalp infection may thus precipitate sinus thrombophlebitis and meningitis.

Scalp lacerations should be thoroughly cleansed and shaved approximately 2 cm around the wound edges. Although shaving the area actually increases the chance of infection, it is necessary to keep hair from becoming entangled in the sutures. Shaving can be avoided in linear lacerations by using a soap solution to part and plaster the hair down along the sides of the laceration. The wound should be explored, thoroughly irrigated, and debrided of devitalized tissue. While an assistant applies local pressure on both sides of the wound, the physician can inspect it for foreign bodies or underlying skull fractures. If pressure fails to control hemorrhage, the galea should be grasped with a series of hemostats and everted over the wound edge to allow adequate visualization. Often, ground-in road dirt or other contaminants may be lodged in the cranium; these should be removed with a rongeur in order to avoid cranial osteomyelitis.

In most scalp lacerations, simple or running sutures of 3-0 or 4-0 Prolene or Nylon effect hemostasis and provide adequate closure. In male patients with frontal or temporal lacerations, careful approximation is paramount as the naturally receding hairline may eventually uncover the scar. When a laceration extends across the galea, muscle pull may result in a gaping wound; separate closure of the galea with 3-0 or 4-0 absorbable suture is recommended in these cases. Irrigation or aspiration of blood clots is necessary to prevent infection. Skull roentgenograms should be obtained to rule out the presence of foreign bodies or associated fractures in all but the most superficial scalp injuries.

Scalp lacerations are often multiple, irregular, stellate, or trapdoor in nature. Simple debridement of only the tissue that is clearly devitalized and careful suturing of scalp flaps and irregular edges usually produce excellent results. In cases of extensive scalp laceration, or partial or total scalping injuries, prompt surgical consultation should be obtained. An avulsed scalp should be placed in a watertight plastic bag on iced saline and accompany the patient to the nearest center where microsurgical anastomosis can be performed.[27]

Facial Lacerations

In the management of a facial laceration, several factors work to the surgeon's advantage. The excellent arterial supply, lymphatic drainage, and venous drainage of the face almost guarantee success with primary closure, even in grossly contaminated wounds. Because of its innate elasticity, the skin can be undermined and mobilized to close lacerations with skin loss. Sutures can be removed early because facial skin heals rapidly. By handling the tissues delicately and accurately approximating the layers with little or no tension on the skin, the surgeon can almost always obtain a pleasing cosmetic result.

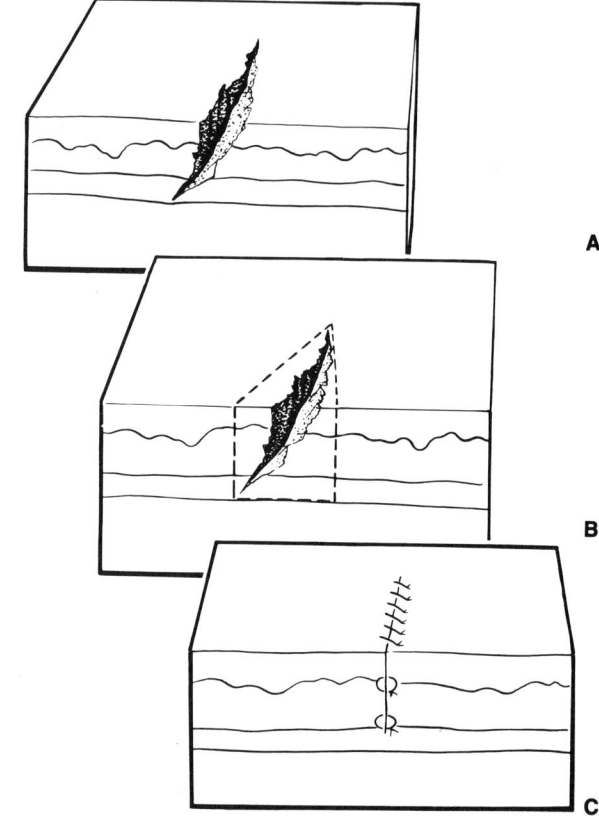

Figure 9-14 Debridement of beveled wound. (**A**) Beveled wound. (**B**) Wound trimmed with a scalpel at sharp right angles. (**C**) Final closure.

Many facial lacerations have a contusional component; the burst type injury damages skin edges, underlying muscle, and subcutaneous tissue. Closure without trimming the beveled skin edge results in a stepped scar. Whenever possible, it is best to trim the wound edges at right angles with a scalpel to ensure accurate everting apposition. Slight inward beveling of the edge also aids in eversion (Fig. 9-14).

The subcutaneous tissue usually requires only minimal debridement; overzealous debridement produces a depressed scar with loss of facial contour. In small, ragged facial lacerations, the best technique includes wound excision, undermining, and closure without tension. Undermining is best accomplished by elevating the skin edge with skin hooks or Adson's forceps and sharply incising along the subdermal plane parallel to the skin surface with a number 15 scalpel. Tension should be tested by grasping the two wound edges and apposing them; more undermining may be necessary if excessive tension is necessary to bring the edges together (Fig. 9-15). A subcuticular supporting suture should be utilized in nearly all facial lacerations. With more complex facial wounds, simplification with trimming to produce straight, gently curved, or sharply angled edges ideal for repair minimizes hypertrophic scar formation (Fig. 9-16).

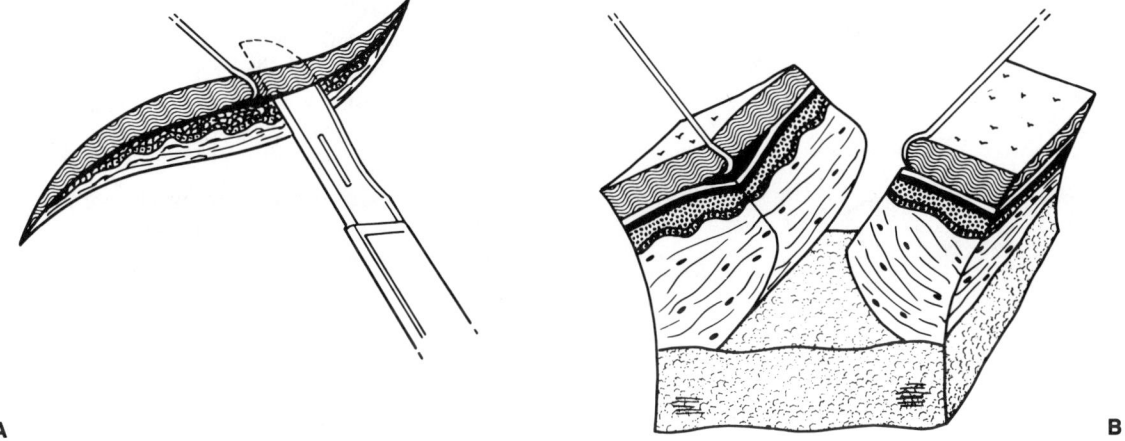

Figure 9-15 (**A**) Method of undermining skin. (**B**) Subdermal plane undermined.

When possible, wounds should be trimmed or mobilized to fit into or parallel to the lines of the patient's facial contour. However, all possible skin should be left in the vicinity of the lower eyelid, the nasal alae, and the angle of the mouth to avoid distortion of the surrounding structures. Similarly, only the nonviable edges of large ragged or stellate lacerations should be trimmed and the pieces of the jigsaw puzzle gently tacked back in place. Often, the results are cosmetically excellent; if not, ample skin remains for revision at a later time. The patient should be informed from the start of the possibility of revision but should be advised to wait at least six months before making any decision.

The Eyebrow

Because eyebrow hair grows very slowly and because it provides an accurate guide to approximation of cut edges, it should never be shaved. By gently grasping the wound edges with fine-tipped forceps and apposing them, the physician can determine the correct placement of sutures to avoid a discontinuity. Most eyebrow lacerations are burst type, and separate closures of muscle, subcuticular tissue, and skin are necessary.

The Eyelid

The location and direction of an eyelid laceration determine the appropriate type of closure. Severe functional and cosmetic deformities can occur if the physician is not aware of a few basic rules in dealing with eyelid lacerations. Unless the emergency physician is experienced with eyelid closure, most vertical through and through lacerations should be handled by a specialist. If the laceration involves the inner one-sixth of the eyelid, the canaliculus may be severed and must be repaired with a stent. Additionally, both lateral and medial lacerations may sever the lateral or medial canthal

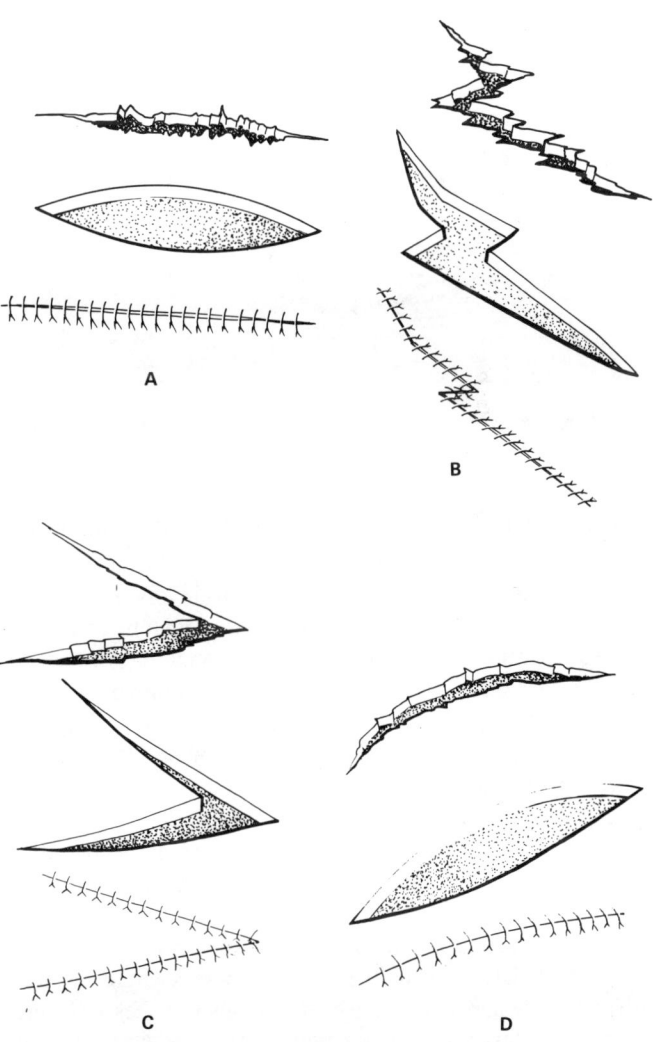

Figure 9-16 Simplification of wounds by excision.

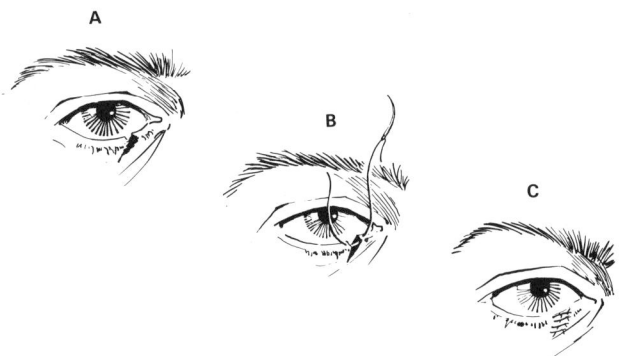

Figure 9-17 (**A**) When faced with a ragged vertical eyelid laceration, wedge resection (**B**) should be performed. The initial suture is placed through the grey line to check alignment of the cilial margin. After closure of the tarsal plate, the grey line suture is secured and the skin approximated with fine silk (**C**).

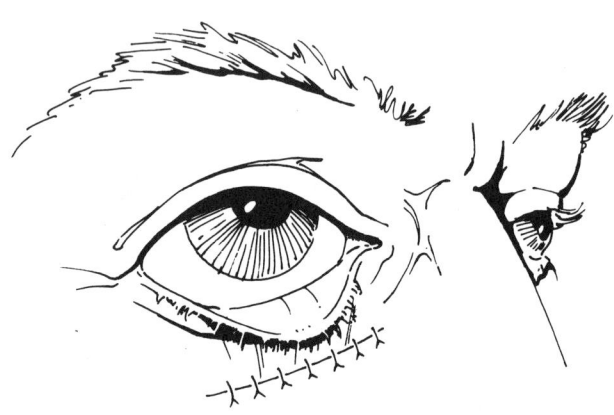

Figure 9-18 Excessive debridement may cause lid ectropian.

ligament. Reapproximation or reimplantation should be done using 4-0 Nylon suture.

When approaching vertical lacerations involving the eyelid, care must be taken to attain proper alignment of the eyelid margin so a step-off deformity or notching is avoided. If the laceration is ragged or uneven, careful pie-shaped wedge resection should be performed (Fig. 9-17). The initial suture is placed at the apex of the cilial margin through the grey line using 6-0 or 7-0 silk. This suture is left untied and used for repeated check of the alignment of the cilial margin throughout the closure. Once proper alignment is obtained, approximation of the tarsal plate should be performed using fine 6-0 or 7-0 Vicryl or Dexon with the knot tied toward the skin to avoid ocular irritation. The conjunctiva is adherent to the tarsal plate and usually does not require separate closure. The muscle and skin of the eyelid are also a cohesive layer, allowing closure of the skin with fine silk as the final step. The initial traction suture through the grey line should be tied prior to closure of the skin to again ensure proper alignment.

Simple lacerations parallel to the lid margin are not subject to the sideways pull of the orbicularis oculi muscle and can be closed as are other facial lacerations. Occasionally, avulsion of the thin eyelid skin creates small flaps of questionable viability. These usually survive if simply tacked back into place using fine silk suture.

With excessive debridement or closure under tension of more complex lacerations, ectropian may occur. Though most often associated with lower eyelid or infraorbital lacerations, ectropian can complicate any wound in the periorbital area (Fig. 9-18). To ensure that sufficient skin exists for debridement of the lower eyelid, pinch the edges of the wound together and have the patient look upward and open his mouth widely. If ectropian does occur with this maneuver, appropriate surgical consultation should be obtained.

The Cheek

When lacerations involve the cheek, injury to the facial nerve, parotid gland, or parotid duct is possible and should be ruled out before closure. Under ordinary circumstances, muscle paralysis on the involved side of the face indicates nerve injury. The parotid duct and buccal branch of the facial nerve course along a line from the tragus to the midportion of the upper lip. Division of the nerve branches medial to the midpupillary line usually does not require nerve repair, as cross innervation and regeneration will reinnervate the appropriate muscle. If the injury is lateral to this point, however, nerve repair should be attempted in order to avoid permanent functional and cosmetic deformity. Severance of the temporal branch of the facial nerve, which is superficial and courses superiorly at a point halfway between the tragus and lateral canthus, causes particular disability (eg, paralysis of the eyelid and potential exposure keratitis). Any suspected proximal nerve injury requires prompt surgical consultation.

Parotid duct injury may accompany injury to the buccal branch of the facial nerve. It is indicated by the leakage of clear fluid from the cut proximal end of the duct or blood at the orifice of Stensen's duct. Reanastomosis over a Silastic catheter or reimplantation of the proximal end into the buccal mucosa requires the skills of a specialist. Simple glandular lacerations need not be repaired; salivary fistulas are common and usually resolve spontaneously in approximately 3 weeks.[28]

The Nose

Because of the structural symmetry of the nose and the absence of excess loose subcutaneous tissue, nasal lacerations should not generally be debrided except in the glabellar and central bridge regions. Nasal alar lacerations should be closed in three layers with absorbable 5-0 suture for the mucosa and cartilage and 6-0 Nylon or silk for the skin. Care must be taken to avoid an alar hematoma by careful hemostasis and packing of the ipsilateral nostril. When full thickness loss occurs or debridement is deemed necessary with any laceration to the lateral nasal bridge, nasal alae, columella or tip of the nose, plastic surgical consultation should be obtained. If surgical consultation is not available, it is often best to simply tack the wound edges and pieces of tissue back together to ensure that adequate tissue remains for later revision. Due to the rich nasal blood supply, the disjointed and apparently devitalized pieces may heal surprisingly well.

Every attempt should be made to close lacerations of the septum or floor of the nostril with direct suturing. Usually 5-0 Vicryl or Dexon is a good choice for closure of cartilage, mucosa, or the skin of the nostril floor. If the laceration is inaccessible to suturing, light packing with vaseline gauze may be used to help approximate the wound edges.

The Lips

Vertical lip lacerations are almost invariably untidy and require some degree of debridement or wedge excision before closure. Defects of up to one-third of the upper or lower lip can be closed by direct suturing after the laceration has been converted to a V or W. The oral commissures, philtrum, and philtral ridges are unique structures, and tissue should not be sacrificed in these areas. Proper alignment of the vermilion border is essential for a good cosmetic result. A traction suture of fine silk initially placed through the white line of the vermilion border allows accurate approximation. The lip is then closed in three layers with inverted 4-0 or 5-0 Vicryl or Dexon for the muscle and subcutaneous tissue and 4-0 or 5-0 silk, Vicryl, or Dexon for the mucosa and skin.

In general, lip debridement should be in a vertical fashion. Horizontal debridement may lead to lip ectropian (Fig. 9-19). As with other facial structures the excellent blood supply to the lips allows healing of apparently nonviable flaps that are simply tacked into place with fine sutures.

Tongue and Mouth

Debridement of any tongue laceration should be limited and, if possible, oriented in a longitudinal direction. Function, not esthetics, dictates the closure of tongue lacerations; every attempt should be made to preserve even marginally viable tissue. Closure of muscle with 4-0 or 5-0 absorbable suture and of the mucosa with 4-0 or 5-0 silk, Vicryl, or Dexon is recommended.

Typical mouth lacerations can be closed as are other mucosal lacerations, with special attention directed to potential injury to underlying structures such as muscle, salivary glands, and ducts.

The Ear

Full thickness ear lacerations should be closed in three layers: absorbable suture in interrupted stitches for the cartilage and 6-0 Nylon or silk simple interrupted stitches for the two skin surfaces. An alternative method that can be used when cartilage must be trimmed to facilitate skin closure is a cutaneous-perichondrial suture. With 5-0 or 6-0 silk or Nylon the skin and perichondrium are closed on both sides of the ear, thus apposing the cartilage without direct suturing. Flap type lacerations of the ear, often with small tenuous pedicles, are common. With careful handling and the use of fine, well-spaced tacking sutures, most of these flaps can be salvaged.

When debridement is deemed necessary, careful wedge resection and approximation of both cartilage and skin produces optimal cosmetic results. Discrepancy of size between the two ears is far less noticeable than deformity of the external structure. Ragged through and through helical lacerations should be debrided in a V-shaped wedge extending into the concha (Fig. 9-20).

Overzealous debridement of the ear lobe should be avoided. Simple closure of even ragged lacerations may often produce excellent results. If excessive tissue loss precludes simple closure, surgical consultation should be sought.

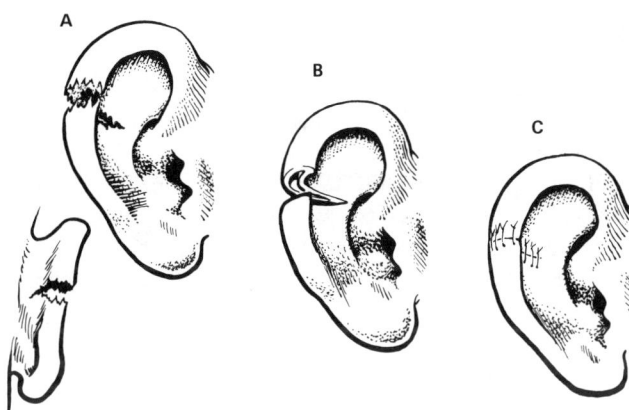

Figure 9-20 (**A**) Ragged through and through lacerations should be debrided (**B**) in a V-shaped wedge extending into the concha. Layered closure (**C**) produces excellent cosmetic results.

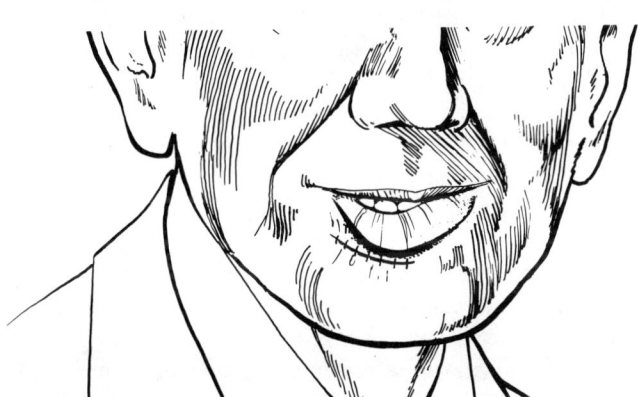

Figure 9-19 Lower lip ectropian caused by excessive debridement in the vertical plane.

Nail Lacerations

Lacerations through the nail and nail beds are a common problem in the emergency department. Lacerations through the nail bed are often seen in association with crush injuries with distal phalangeal tuft fractures. When repairing lacerations of the distal phalanx, one should first approximate the onychal folds on either side of the nail bed laceration and then close the remaining skin. Skin closure with 5-0 Nylon helps align the nail bed for subsequent closure.

If the nail has been completely avulsed, no attempt should be made to replace it. The nail bed laceration can be approximated with 5-0 or 6-0 absorbable suture and a gauze petroleum dressing placed over the nail bed and gently tucked under the proximal cuticle (eponychium). The petroleum gauze serves to keep the cuticle from scarring down to the nail matrix and should be used as a dressing for 3 weeks. The nail bed is friable and thin, and care must be taken to avoid tearing on passage of the needle. If more than one pass is attempted in the same area, usually the suture will not hold. A laceration across an otherwise intact nail can be sutured with simple sutures through the nail to approximate the underlying nail bed. Technical problems encountered with passage of suture through the hard nail and problems with subsequent wound care make nail removal and direct visualization the better alternative. If the germinal nail matrix has been avulsed, it is necessary to reimplant it with a horizontal mattress suture from the base of the nail matrix through the overlying cuticle. Xeroform or plain gauze is placed between the matrix and cuticle to secure the germinal layer.

Distal phalangeal fractures with nail bed lacerations are open fractures. Nail trephination for a subungual hematoma or nail removal for nail bed repair theoretically increase the open nature of the fracture and the consequent chance of tuft osteomyelitis. Most of these heal without problems, but antibiotic therapy is indicated.

Leg and Foot Lacerations

Among the most difficult injuries to deal with in the emergency department are leg and foot lacerations. Without proper initial management, the patient may suffer discomfort and expense for several weeks. The classic example is the elderly or debilitated patient with a triangulated flap laceration over the tibia as a result of a fall against a curb or step. With the full body weight transmitted through the tibia, the injury results in real skin loss through crushing; widespread subcutaneous damage with edema invariably leads to secondary skin loss. The poor arterial supply, decreased venous return, and local edema, together with the patient's compromised ability to heal, render any closure liable to skin necrosis and cellulitis. If the flap is distally based, the blood supply and venous return are even more tenuous, and placing the leg in a dependent position inevitably leads to hematoma formation and flap necrosis.

Puncture wounds of the foot are common, and their innocuous appearance belies the fact that serious complications occur at a significant rate. Cellulitis occurs in 8% of cases and osteomyelitis in 1.8%. The presence of a foreign body in the wound predisposes to the development of osteomyelitis. Conventional X-ray films and xeroradiography should be used to detect any foreign bodies. *Pseudomonas aeruginosa* is the most common pathogen involved in bone infections.

It is recommended that contaminated or dirty puncture wounds, such as those encountered with the ubiquitous rusty nail, be cleansed initially with Poloxamer 188. Antibiotics with *Pseudomonas* organism coverage (eg, cefoperazone, 2 g IV in an adult or 50 mg/kg in a child) are administered to all dirty puncture wounds immediately. The wound is then explored with a blunt probe to determine whether bone or joint cavity is encountered. If the wound is superficial it is dressed with sterile gauze, and the patient is discharged on crutches with foot elevation for 4 days. If the wound is deep, the edges should be excised and the wound thoroughly irrigated and packed with fine-mesh gauze. The wound should be repacked regularly until healing occurs.

Clean wounds such as those caused by a sewing needle or a new (unrusted) nail also require cleansing with Poloxamer 188 and exploration with a blunt probe. For clean wounds that extend to bone or enter the joint, a simple dressing is recommended. The patient should elevate the foot and use crutches for 4 days. If the wound is superficial, then the patient may weight bear as tolerated. Antibiotics are not given for clean wounds.[29] Tetanus prophylaxis should follow the recommendations of the American College of Surgeons, as outlined in Table 9-2.

Simple lacerations without skin loss can be closed primarily, provided the wound edges can be brought together without tension. Fine bites with 4-0 Nylon suture widely placed without tension can be used. The wound should be dressed with sterile gauze and an encircling firm bandage from foot to knee. The lower leg and foot should be immobilized with a posterior plaster padded splint and elevated for the next week. Hospitalization may be required for some patients. If minimal tension is necessary to approximate the wound edges, the laceration should be closed with Steri-strips, combined with a pressure bandage. Immobilization and elevation are also necessary.

Even if there is a residual defect, either from the initial injury or subsequent debridement of nonviable tissue, primary closure under tension should never be considered. The triangulated flap can be tacked without tension to one side of the wound margin and checked for adequate capillary return, bleeding, and color. The remaining defect will require grafting that is best undertaken by a plastic surgeon. Likewise, when bone, tendon, or ligament is exposed or subcutaneous

Table 9-2 Tetanus Prophylaxis of Puncture Wounds

History of Tetanus Immunizations (Doses)	Puncture Wound			
	Non–Tetanus Prone		Tetanus Prone	
	Td*	TIG	Td*	TIG†
Uncertain	Yes	No	Yes	Yes
0–1	Yes	No	Yes	Yes
2	Yes	No	Yes	No‡
3 or more	No§	No	No‖	No

*For children younger than 7 years of age, diphtheria and tetanus toxoids and pertussis vaccine adsorbed (DPT) [or diphtheria and tetanus toxoids adsorbed (DT) if pertussis vaccine is contraindicated] are preferred to tetanus toxoid alone. For persons 7 years and older, Td is preferred to tetanus toxoid alone.
†When TIG and Td are administered concurrently, separate sites and syringes must be used.
‡Yes, if wound is more than 24 hours old.
§Yes, if more than 10 years since last dose.
‖Yes, if more than 5 years since last dose (more frequent boosters are not needed and can accentuate side effects).

damage extends to these structures, hospitalization and plastic surgical care are necessary.

PRESSURE GUN INJURIES

Pressure (paint and grease) gun injuries can lead to profound and permanent disability if inappropriately treated. The small, seemingly innocuous entry wound belies the infiltration of often large amounts of grease or paint throughout the muscles, tendons, and fascial planes. On a rare occasion, the wound is tangential to the skin surface, and roentgenogram examination (if the paint is lead-based) reveals only superficial opacification. The wound can then be debrided or excised and closed. Unfortunately, most wounds are penetrating and require wide debridement in the operating room.[30]

BITES

Dog Bites

With more than 25 million dogs in the United States and 60% of families having at least one dog, it is little wonder that dog bite injuries occur so frequently. In the emergency department dog bite injuries are seen at a rate of 500 to 700 cases per 100,000 population, accounting for 1% to 2% of all surgical cases. They account for more than 90% of animal bites, with cat bites making up most of the remainder. More than 1 million dog bites occur annually, but controlled studies are few and often based on anecdotal information.[31] Controversy still rages around the advisability of closing dog bite wounds primarily and the indications for antibiotic therapy.

Recent studies have shown debridement and irrigation of dog bite wounds to be the most important factors in preventing subsequent infection. Dog bite wounds that are irrigated have shown a 12% infection rate compared to a 69% rate for nonirrigated wounds.[32,33] Debridement of the wound further increases the resistance to infection by a factor of 30.[34] Low-risk wounds include all fascial lacerations and larger lacerations not of the hand, foot, or wrist. In immunocompetent patients younger than 50, these wounds generally can be closed primarily if treated within approximately 6 hours of injury. Facial and scalp lacerations consistently show the lowest infection rates and can be safely closed 12 to 18 hours after injury.[35,36] Most dog bite wounds of the face and scalp are at low risk for infection and probably do not need prophylactic antibiotics. In all children, and especially in infants, a thorough evaluation with skull radiographs to exclude cranial perforation must be performed.

Puncture dog bite wounds are often inflicted with a pressure of more than 400 psi and have a significant contusional component. Adequate local wound care is difficult, and puncture wounds become infected up to 25% of the time. Presently, local debridement with irrigation combined with prophylactic antibiotics appears to be the optimal therapy. Hand, wrist, and foot lacerations from dog bites are considered high-risk injuries and generally should be left open after local wound care. If tendon, bone, joint space, or large vessels are exposed or transected, appropriate consultation should be sought immediately.

Bacteriologic studies of normal canine flora reveal more than 64 species.[37] Infected dog bites reflect this wide array of pathogens, including *Staphylococcus aureus,* hemolytic streptococci, pencillin-resistant Gram-negative rods, and anaerobic strains of *Bacteroides.* Isolation of *Pasteurella multocida* varies, being present 50% of the time, but generally infection of dog bites with *P multocida* is low. Indeed, the overall infection rate of dog bite injuries is only 3.8%. Antibiotic therapy should be reserved for high-risk wounds or for low-risk wounds in older patients and those with immunologic or vascular compromise (see specific recommendations below).

Cat Bites and Scratches

The nature of cat bite injuries is similar to that of dog bite injuries, except that the sharp, slender teeth of the cat often inflict deeper and initially less conspicuous damage. *P multocida* is present in 50% to 80% of normal feline oral flora and accounts for more than 80% of all infections. *Pasteurella multocida* is a small, nonmotile, Gram-negative coccobacillus that grows under both anaerobic and aerobic conditions. It is sensitive to penicillin G, cephalosporins, and tetracycline but is resistant to erythromycin. It is unique in its ability to incite a severe inflammatory reaction within 24 hours of injury; most pathogens require 36 to 72 hours to produce clinical signs of infection. The organism may not be identified on culture unless the laboratory is aware of its possible presence. As with dog bites, *S aureus*, anaerobes, Gram-negative rods, diphtheroids, and streptococci may also be cultured from wounds.[38]

The initial treatment of cat bites and scratches should include cleansing, irrigation, debridement, excision of puncture wounds, dressing, and, when possible, immobilization. Facial lacerations may be closed primarily; in other areas, however, especially the hand, wounds should be left open. A 7- to 10-day course of oral penicillin or erythromycin is indicated. The patient should be seen again in 24 hours. If infection has supervened, hospitalization for intravenous antibiotics is indicated. The wound should be closely examined at both the initial and follow-up visits for tendon, bone, joint, or neurovascular injuries and appropriate consultation obtained.[39]

Human Bites

Inadequate treatment of human bites often leads to serious disabling sequelae. Human bites occur most often during altercations involving young individuals. They are also common in children, the mentally ill, and victims of sexual assault.[40] One of the most discouraging aspects of human bite wounds is the often long delay before the victim seeks treatment. In one study, the average length of time between injury and treatment was 2.5 days; in many cases, it was several weeks.[41]

One of the most common wounds of this type seen in the emergency department is the clenched fist injury, which occurs when the patient's flexed metacarpophalangeal joints are impaled on another person's teeth. The skin stretched over the joint is lacerated, possibly accompanied by damage to the underlying extensor tendon and opening of the joint space. With the fingers extended, tendon and joint injury may go unnoticed. Even with broad spectrum antibiotic coverage the patient with the clenched fist injury stands an almost 50% chance of developing suppurative tenosynovitis, septic arthritis, or osteomyelitis.[42]

The key to reducing the risk of complications associated with a clenched fist injury is prompt and aggressive treatment. The physician should assume that all such wounds enter the joint space until adequate examination proves otherwise. Not only is the risk of infection increased by the shear force involved in the injury, but the resistance to infection of the joint space is tenfold less than that of soft tissue.[43] Radiographs of the hand are crucial to detect foreign bodies (especially tooth fragments), metacarpal or phalangeal fractures, and air in the joints. The wound should be thoroughly inspected under regional block anesthesia after the arm has been elevated for 5 minutes and a blood pressure cuff has been applied at 250 mmHg to ensure a bloodless examination. If the joint capsule has been violated, operating room debridement and hospitalization are indicated. If only a tendon laceration is found, the tendon should be approximated and the wound left open and splinted in extension for 4 weeks. Soft tissue injuries should be debrided and irrigated, a drain should be left in place, and the arm should be immobilized from finger tips to elbow. Movement is allowed at 2 weeks. The dressing and drain should be changed after 48 hours, and dressing changed twice weekly thereafter. This regimen has significantly lessened the permanent disability resulting from such an injury.[44]

All human bite wounds, except those on the face, should be debrided and left open. Antibiotic coverage with a cephalothin is indicated for all but the most trivial of injuries. Group A streptococci, *S aureus*, and *Eikenella corrodens* are the pathogens usually associated with human bite infections. Aerobic Gram-negative rods and anaerobes (*Bacteroides* species) frequently are cultured, but their role in infection remains unclear. Isolated cases in which tetanus, gonorrhea, and syphilis were transmitted by human bites have been noted. *Eikenella corrodens* bacteria are present in a significant number of infected wounds. An anaerobic, Gram-negative bacillus, *E corrodens* is sensitive to penicillin and second- and third-generation cephalosporins. The organism is usually resistant to first generation-cephalosporins and dicloxacillin.[45,46] Hospitalization is required for any patient with a human bite injury showing signs of cellulitis, lymphangitis, abscess formation, or joint penetration. Severe, old, or facial wounds may also require specialized care.

DRESSINGS AND IMMOBILIZATION

All wounds should have a pressure dressing to help prevent local edema and hematoma formation, as well as to immobilize the wound edges and surrounding tissue. Mobility of any wound increases the chance of a cross-hatched scar and may lead to excessive scar formation. Patient comfort and the prevention of contamination are additional benefits of a properly dressed wound.

Facial dressings over convex surfaces, such as the forehead, malar region, or chin, are readily applied with strips of Elastoplast or adhesive tape placed over a fine gauze dressing (cocoon dressing). Where strapping is impossible a collodion and fine mesh gauze dressing is a satisfactory alternative. Elevation of the head lessens edema. The patient should be advised against excessive talking or chewing postoperatively. The dressing can be left in place for 24 to 48 hours. After this time the wound should be swabbed three to four times daily to remove any blood clot and to allow epithelial repair. Abraded skin with sutures does not respond to this therapy, but gentle cleansing and swabbing with an antibiotic ointment keeps the wound from developing a dry eschar. The ear should be gently packed anteriorly and posteriorly with small gauze fluffs to prevent distortion or excessive pressure. Diagonal strips of Elastoplast or an encircling Kerlex bandage is used to exert firm, even pressure to the helix. Following nasal alae repairs, the ipsilateral nostril should be packed with petroleum gauze packing, with an Elastoplast bandage exerting gentle counterpressure externally. After sutures are removed from facial lacerations, external support with strapping or Steri-strips should be continued for 2 weeks.

Scalp lacerations should be dressed with an encircling bandage of Kerlex under moderate pressure. The hemostatic bandage can be left in place for 24 hours, after which a loose, occlusive dressing is applied. Elastic bandages may lead to pressure necrosis and should not be used. Plastic spray dressings should be reserved for only the most superficial lacerations.

Splinting of extremity wounds is an important facet of total wound care; a properly applied splint hastens healing, reduces discomfort, and lessens scar formation. Abrasions, contusions, and lacerations all benefit from splinting. Simple finger lacerations at or near joint lines are best treated with immobilization of the entire digit. A forearm wound should be immobilized from the finger tips to the proximal forearm. The plaster splint should always be applied to the surface of the limb opposite the wound, and the limb should be splinted in the position of function whenever possible. A bulky, well-padded dressing with a splint is an ideal dressing for hand injuries. The finger tips should be left exposed to facilitate neurovascular evaluation. Prolonged immobilization always produces some degree of joint stiffness, and all splints should be removed as soon as the wound is adequately healed. A joint contracture is a poor trade-off for a cosmetically acceptable scar. Splinting and elevation are essential in the treatment of most lower extremity injuries. Slings help decrease dependent edema in upper extremity injuries; when possible, the patient should elevate the arm on pillows.

ANTIBIOTIC THERAPY

Antibiotics are not indicated in the treatment of routine lacerations seen in the emergency department. They will not prevent infection in a wound improperly selected for closure or inadequately irrigated, debrided, or sutured. Antibiotics are costly, have significant side effects (both toxic and allergic), and predispose to the development of superinfection or the emergence of resistant organisms.[47] Emergency department studies have shown an infection rate of about 6% in lacerations not treated with antibiotics.[48,49] When antibiotics are used, most studies indicate a significantly higher infection rate.[50-53]

True antibiotic prophylaxis implies therapy initiated before wounding, a clinical situation only rarely encountered in an emergency department. Antibiotics must be administered within 3 hours of wounding to have any significant effect.[54] They should be given intravenously for the initial dose and started as soon as possible in the emergency department. The American Heart Association provides no formal recommendations for the treatment of wounds in high-risk patients. It is well known that incision and drainage of extremity abscesses result in documented bacteremia up to 40% of the time.[55] It follows that patients with valvular lesions should receive prophylaxis with staphylococcal and streptococcal coverage for most common abscesses. With manipulation of infected wounds of the pelvic or rectal area and intravenous drug abusers' extremity abscesses, Gram-negative and anaerobic coverage should be added. Diabetics and other immunocompromised individuals should receive prophylaxis before any manipulation of infected tissue. Because infection of hip prostheses has been attributed to previous surgical or dental procedures, antibiotic prophylaxis in such patients should also be initiated. Although no study has investigated the problem, it seems logical that patients with cardiac valvular lesions or prosthetic orthopedic devices should probably receive prophylactic antibiotics before manipulation of old or contaminated wounds.

Firm recommendations for antibiotic prophylaxis for wounds seen in the emergency department are surprisingly few. Antibiotic therapy is certainly indicated in open fractures. Initial cultures should be obtained because the culture results are generally predictive of subsequent infection.[56] An intravenous cephalosporin such as cephazolin is a good choice for empiric therapy. Dog bites of the hand and lower leg, puncture wounds including all cat bites, bites in immunologically compromised individuals, crush injuries, and human clenched fist injuries should all receive prophylactic antibiotics. For dog bites dicloxacillin or cephalexin (500 mg orally four times a day; 50 to 100 mg/kg per day in four divided doses in children) is a good regimen when outpatient treatment is deemed adequate. Because of the increased likelihood of *Pasteurella multocida* infection in cat bites, penicillin or dicloxacillin should be started in the same dosages as for dog bites. With human bites of the hand dicloxacillin and penicillin in the same dosages as for dog bites are recommended. If the patient is allergic to penicillin, then erythromycin (500 mg four times a day; 30 to 50 mg/kg per day in four divided doses in children) is a reasonable substitute. Clindamycin therapy for human bites and trimethoprim/sulfamethoxazole for animal bites are recommended alternative regimens in penicillin-allergic patients.

In high-risk mammalian bites parenteral antibiotic therapy within 3 hours of injury is recommended. Ampicillin/sulbactam intravenously or intramuscularly followed by amoxicillin/clavulanate for 3 days offers excellent although expensive coverage in all mammalian bites. Intramuscular ceftriaxone, with its long half-life, is a useful means of sustaining antibiotic levels in the noncompliant patient.[57]

Antibiotic treatment of lacerations is indicated when the probability of infection developing in the wound is deemed high. If there is a delay in treatment of more than 6 hours, if the wound occurs on the distal lower extremities, or if the wound is judged to be dirty, antibiotics may decrease the likelihood of infection. Antibiotic treatment is generally indicated in wounds contaminated by feces, exudate, saliva, or vaginal secretions. Most intraoral lacerations probably do not require routine antibiotic prophylaxis, however. If the degree of contamination is deemed excessive, and if local debridement and irrigation do not create a clean wound, then open wound management is appropriate. In the immunocompromised individual or with soft tissue injury to a lymphedematous extremity, antibiotic therapy should be initiated as soon as possible.

In clearly infected wounds with suppuration, spreading cellulitis, or lymphangitis, a penicillinase-resistant penicillin or first-generation cephalosporin should be given. Sutures, if present, should be removed and local wound care initiated. Occasionally, with early signs of inflammation in a closed wound, prompt antibiotic therapy will eliminate an impending infection. In such cases, close follow-up is mandatory, and sutures must be removed if the inflammation does not subside. In many instances of localized cellulitis and wound abscess formation, suture removal, wound debridement, and frequent dressing changes rapidly bring infection under control. Antibiotics, in such cases, should be held in reserve and used only if local measures fail.

Often the use of prophylactic antibiotic coverage is purely a clinical decision. In crush injuries and other wounds in which the blood supply has been imperiled, antibiotic coverage may prevent a low-grade infection that could lead to loss of valuable flap tips or skin edges. Where skin survival is essential, such as for cosmetic facial repairs or coverage of bone or tendon, many surgeons advocate antibiotic coverage. In every instance, however, proper wound cleansing, handling, and closure provide the optimal conditions for healing; no antibiotic can compensate for poor wound care.

REFERENCES

1. Peacock EE Jr, Van Winkle W Jr. *Wound Repair*. Philadelphia: Saunders; 1976.
2. Berk WA, Osbourne DD, Taylor DD. Evaluation of the "golden period" for wound repair: 204 cases from a Third World emergency department. *Ann Emerg Med*. 1988;17:496.
3. Roberts JR, Hedges JR. *Clinical Procedures in Emergency Medicine*. Philadelphia: Saunders; 1985.
4. Dudley HAF. *Emergency Surgery*. 10th ed. Bristol: Wright; 1977.
5. Pecora DV, Landis RE, Martin E. Location of cutaneous microorganisms. *Surgery*. 1968;64:1114.
6. Simon RR, Brenner BE. *Procedures and Techniques in Emergency Medicine*. Baltimore: Williams & Wilkins; 1982.
7. Dineen P, Drusin L. Epidemics of postoperative infections associated with hair carriers. *Lancet*. 1973;2:1157.
8. Alexander JW, Fischer JE, Boyajian M, et al. The influence of hair removal methods on wound infections. *Arch Surg*. 1983;118:347.
9. Masterson TS, Rodeheaver GT, Morgan RF, et al. Bacterial evaluation of electric clippers for surgical hair removal. *Am J Surg*. 1984;118:301.
10. Pond GD, Lindsey D. Localization of cactus, glass and other foreign bodies in soft tissues. *Ariz Med*. 1977;34:700.
11. Billmire DA, Neale HW, Gregory RO. Use of IV fentanyl in the outpatient treatment of pediatric facial trauma. *J Trauma*. 1985;25:1079–1080.
12. Anderson AB, Colecchi C, et al. Local anesthesia in pediatric patients: topical TAC versus Lidocaine. *Ann Emerg Med*. 1990;19:519–522.
13. Pryor G, Kilpatrick WR, Opp DR. Local anesthesia in minor lacerations: topical TAC versus Lidocaine infiltration. *Ann Emerg Med*. 1980;9:568–571.
14. Lyman JL, McCabe JB. Improving the effectiveness of TAC application. *Ann Emerg Med*. 1984;13:642.
15. Dailey RH. Fatality secondary to misuse of TAC solution. *Ann Emerg Med*. 1988;17:159–169.
16. Fitzmaurice LS, Wasserman GS, Knapp JF, et al. TAC use and absorption of cocaine in a pediatric emergency department. *Ann Emerg Med*. 1990;19:515–518.
17. Goodman LS, Gilman A. *The Pharmacological Basis of Therapeutics*. London: Macmillan; 1970.
18. Moore DC. *Regional Block*. Springfield, IL: Charles C Thomas; 1965.
19. Cristoph RA, Buchanan L, Begalla D, et al. Pain reduction in local anesthetic administration through pH buffering. *Ann Emerg Med*. 1987;480.
20. Stevenson J. Cleansing the traumatic wound by high pressure irrigation. *JACEP*. 1976;5:17.
21. Rodeheaver GT, Smith SL, Thacker JG. Mechanical cleansing of contaminated wounds with a surfactant. *Am J Surg*. 1975;129:241.
22. Thompson RVS. *Primary Repair of Soft Tissue Injuries*. Melbourne: Melbourne University Press; 1969.
23. Barham E, Butz GW, Angell JS. Comparison of wound strength in normal, irradiated and infected tissues closed with polyglycolic acid and chromic catgut sutures. *Surg Gynecol Obstet*. 1978;146:901–907.
24. Mach SD, Krizek TJ. Sutures and suturing: current concepts. *J Oral Surg*. 1978;36:710–712.
25. Grabb WC, Smith JW. *Plastic Surgery*. Boston: Little, Brown; 1979.
26. Johnson A, Rodeheaver GT, Durand LS, et al. Automatic disposable stapling devices for wound closure. *Ann Emerg Med*. 1981;10:631.
27. Dingman RO, Johnson AJ. Surgery of the scalp. *Surg Clin North Am*. 1977;57:1011–1013.
28. Schultz RC, Oldham RJ. An overview of facial injuries. *Surg Clin North Am*. 1977;57:987–994.
29. Edlich RF, Rodeheaver GT, Horowitz JH, et al. Emergency department management of puncture wounds and needlestick exposure. *Emerg Med Clin North Am*. 1986;4:581–582.
30. Gaul JS Jr. Management of hand injuries. *Ann Emerg Med*. 1980;9:140.

31. Kizev KW. Epidemiological and clinical aspects of animal bite injuries. *JACEP*. 1979;8:134–141.
32. Thomson HG, Suitek EV. Small animal bites: the role of primary closure. *J Trauma*. 1973;13:22.
33. Callaham ML. Treatment of common dog bites; infection risk factors. *JACEP*. 1978;7:83.
34. Callaham ML. Emergency medical management—dog bite wounds. *JAMA*. 1980;244:2327.
35. Palmer AE, Rees M. Dog bites of the face: a 15 year review. *J Plast Surg*. 1983;36:315.
36. Callaham ML. Prophylactic antibiotics in common dog bite wounds: a controlled study. *Ann Emerg Med*. 1980;9:410–414.
37. Bailie WE, Stowe EC, Schmitt AM. Aerobic bacterial flora of oral and nasal fluids of canines with reference to bacteria associated with bites. *J Clin Microbiol*. 1978;7:223–231.
38. Goldstein EJC, Citron DM, Wield B, et al. Bacteriology of human and animal bite wounds. *J Clin Microbiol*. 1978;8:667–672.
39. Veitch JM, Omer GE. Case report: treatment of cat bite injuries of the hand. *J Trauma*. 1979;19:201–202.
40. Weinstein RA, Stephen RJ, Morot A, et al. Human bites: review of the literature and report of a case. *J Oral Surg*. 1973;31:792–794.
41. Guba AM, Milliken JB, Hoopes JE. The selection of antibiotics for human bites of the hand. *Plast Reconstr Surg*. 1975;56:538–540.
42. Farmer CB, Mann RJ. Human bite infections of the hand. *South Med J*. 1966;59:515–518.
43. Edlich RF, Spengler BS, Rodeheaver GT, et al. Emergency department management of mammalian bites. *Emerg Clin North Am*. 1986;4:595–604.
44. Chuinard RC, D'Ambrosia RD: Human bite infections of the hand. *J Bone Joint Surg*. 1977;59:416–418.
45. Goldstein EJC. Management of animal and human bites. *Infect Dis*. 1984;14:5.
46. Goldstein EJC, Caffee HH, Price JE, et al. Human bite infections. *Lancet*. 1977;2:90.
47. Guterman JJ. Antibiotic prophylaxis. *Top Emerg Med*. 1989;10:19–21.
48. Gosnold JK. Infection rate of sutured wounds. *Practitioner*. 1977;218:584–585.
49. Hutton PAN, Jones BM, Law DJW. Depot penicillin as prophylaxis in accidental wounds. *Br J Surg*. 1978;65:549–550.
50. Lindsey D, Nava C, Marti M. Effectiveness of penicillin irrigation in control of infection in sutured lacerations. *J Trauma*. 1982;22:186–189.
51. Haughey RE, Lammers FL, Wagner DK. Use of antibiotics in the initial management of soft tissue hand wounds. *Ann Emerg Med*. 1981;10:187–192.
52. Day TK. Controlled trial of prophylactic antibiotics in minor wounds requiring suture. *Lancet*. 1975;2:1174–1176.
53. Worlock P, Boland P, Darrell J, et al. The role of prophylactic antibiotics following hand injuries. *Br J Clin Pract*. 1980;34:290–292.
54. Burke JF. The effective period of preventive antibiotic action in experimental incisions and dermal lesions. *Surgery*. 1961;50:161–168.
55. Fine BC, Sheckman PR, Bartlett JC. Incision and drainage of soft-tissue abscesses and bacteremia. *Ann Intern Med*. 1985;103:645.
56. Patzakis MJ, Harvey JP, Ivler D. The role of antibiotics in the management of open fractures. *J Bone Joint Surg Am*. 1974;56:532–541.
57. Karkal SS, Tandberg D, Talan DA. Minimizing morbidity and mortality from mammalian bites. *Emerg Med Rep*. 1990;11:4–9.

10. Musculoskeletal Emergencies: Introduction and Basic Principles

DANIEL R. BENSON, MD

Musculoskeletal emergencies involve any acute affliction of the extremities or vertebral column, including soft tissue, neural vascular structures, tendons, and bone. If the injury or infection is severe enough, all can be involved simultaneously.

This section is divided into four chapters: Introduction and Basic Principles, Emergencies of the Vertebral Column, Upper Extremity Emergency Problems, and Pelvis and Lower Extremity Fracture Management. Each chapter was written by an orthopedic surgeon who specializes in treating emergencies in the specific area under discussion.

PRINCIPLES OF FRACTURES AND DISLOCATIONS

Understanding the language or description of fractures and dislocations is important. Proper interpretation of roentgenograms will help the emergency physician in deciding treatment or in describing the fracture to a colleague.

A fracture can be described in several different ways:

1. whether the fracture is open (through the skin) or closed
2. its anatomic location (proximal, middle, or distal third of the shaft supracondylar or subtrochanteric)
3. the angle of the fracture line (transverse to the shaft, oblique, or spiral; Figs. 10-1 to 10-3)
4. whether the fracture is one linear crack or is comminuted (a fracture in many fragments; Fig. 10-4)
5. whether or not the fracture is intra-articular (into the joint)

A proper description of a fracture might be as follows: The patient has an open fracture of the proximal right tibia, which is comminuted. This clear description of the fracture provides the treating physician with a great deal of information that can be used in deciding proper treatment. First, the fracture is open and, therefore, contaminated with bacteria and foreign material. This condition automatically requires operating room debridement and irrigation. The comminution indicates that a lot of energy was required to create this fracture, making neurovascular injury or a compartment syndrome a distinct possibility.

Fractures that may not fit into this classification (see the fracture description list at the beginning of this chapter) are impaction or compression fractures and children's fractures. In an impaction fracture, the shaft of long bone is driven into the cancellous bone in the metaphyseal region. This type of injury is most commonly seen in the shoulder. Children's fractures are different because of the relative flexibility of their bones, the thick periosteum, and the growth plate.

One can also classify fractures in terms of the mechanism of injury. By knowing how a fracture is produced, decisions as to the severity of soft tissue trauma and therapeutic management can be made.

Direct trauma is due to the application of force at the fracture site. These can be divided into tapping fractures, crush fractures, and penetrating injuries. A tapping fracture occurs when a relatively small force is applied to a linear

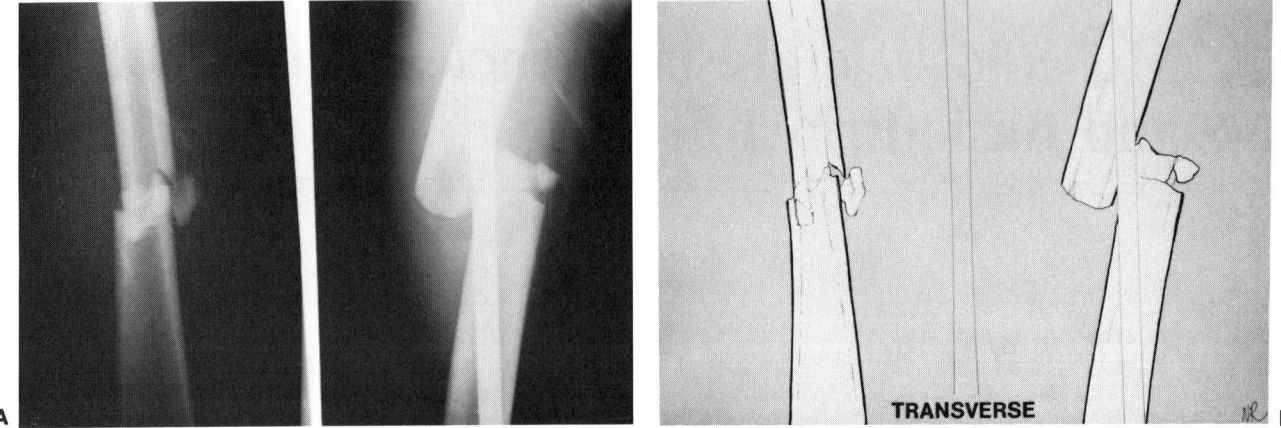

Figure 10-1 (**A**) Roentgenograms of a transverse fracture of a femur. One small fragment is free, but the major fracture elements are transverse. (**B**) A drawing of the roentgenograms demonstrates the anatomy of the fracture even more clearly. Courtesy of George N. Ewing, MD.

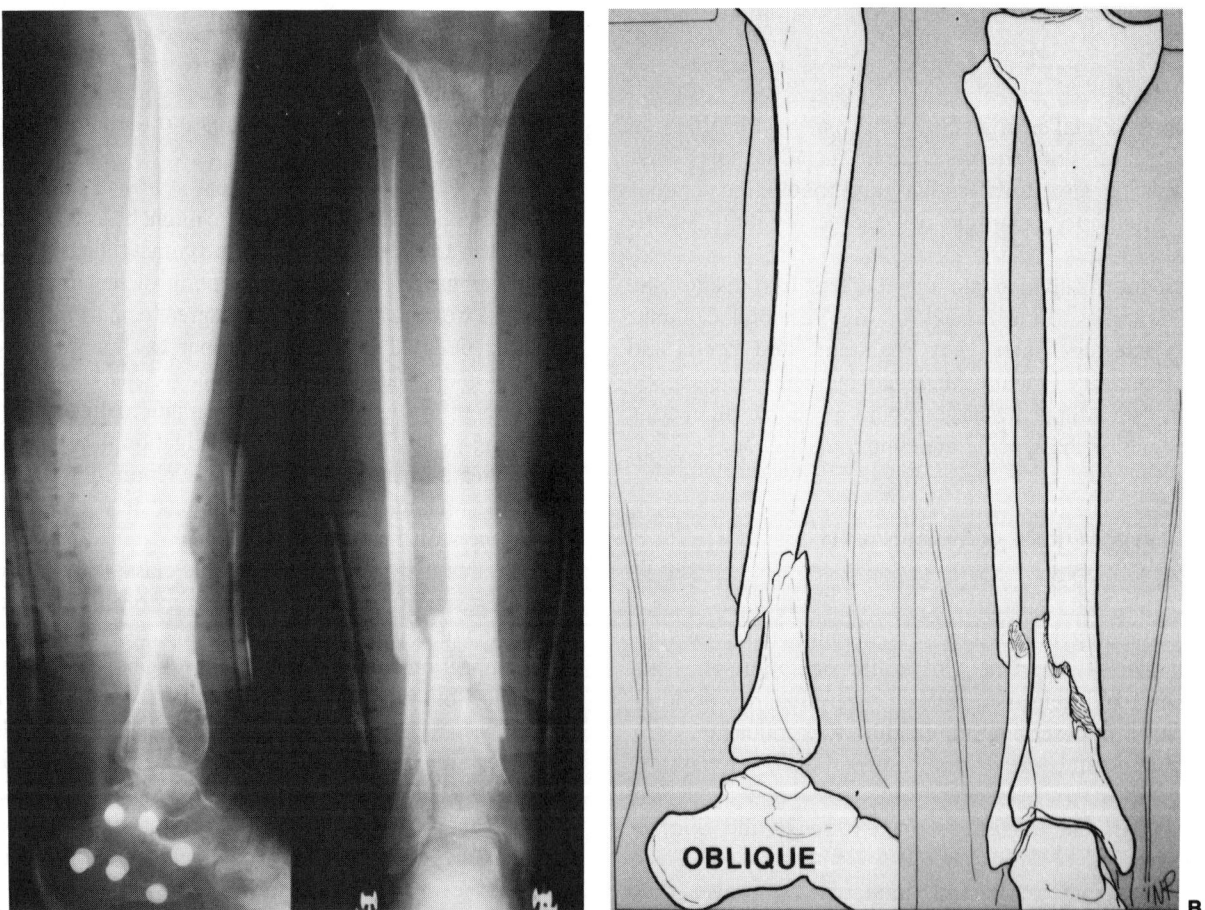

Figure 10-2 (**A**) AP and lateral roentgenograms of an oblique fracture of the distal tibia. The leg is immobilized in a universal splint. (**B**) The roentgenograms have been drawn to demonstrate the oblique nature of the fracture. Courtesy of George N. Ewing, MD.

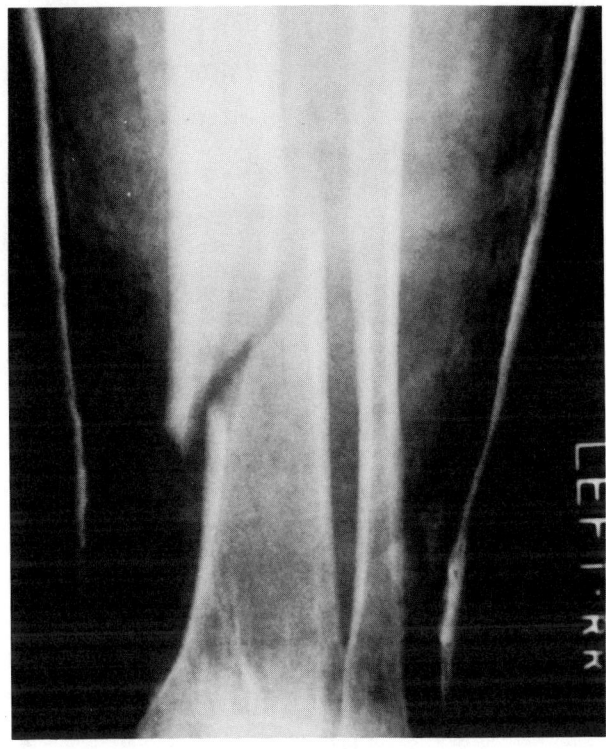
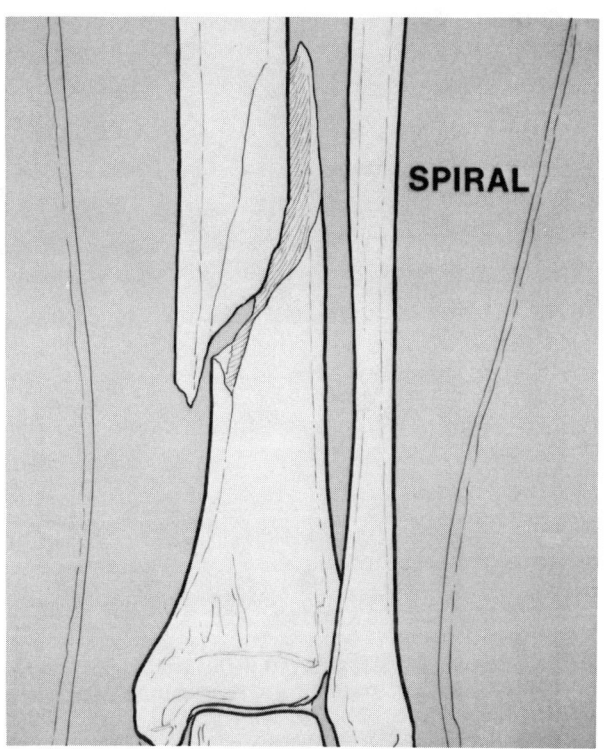

Figure 10-3 **(A)** Roentgenogram of a spiral fracture of a tibia. This was the result of a slow twisting injury to the extremity while patient was learning to ski. **(B)** The spiral fracture is better shown on this artist's interpretation of the fracture. Courtesy of George N. Ewing, MD.

area. This fracture is best represented by a transverse fracture line in a long bone. Since most of the energy is absorbed by the bone, there is little soft tissue damage, although there may be local bruising or a small laceration. A crush fracture is due to a large force applied to the extremity. The bone is usually extensively comminuted or shattered, but may be transversely fractured. Soft tissue injury is extensive and may involve blood vessels and peripheral nerves. Crush fractures are likely to be open and contaminated. A penetrating fracture is caused by a missile. The projectile is most likely to be a bullet of high or low velocity. High-velocity weapons, those with a muzzle velocity greater than 1800 feet per second, inflict severe soft tissue wounds.

Indirect trauma causes fractures at a distance from the applied force. Traction or tension fractures are created by excessive force pulling a portion or piece of bone away. This is represented by avulsion of a patellar tendon by the quadriceps mechanism (Figs. 10-5 and 10-6) or the medial malleolus by the deltoid ligament. Fracture lines in tension fractures are invariably transverse (Fig. 10-1). Excessive angulation of long bones creates fractures that first fail on the convexity in tension, then on the concavity in compression. This mechanism of injury usually produces transverse fractures, but the compression side can shatter into pieces if the force is severe enough. Rotational stress (torque) produces a

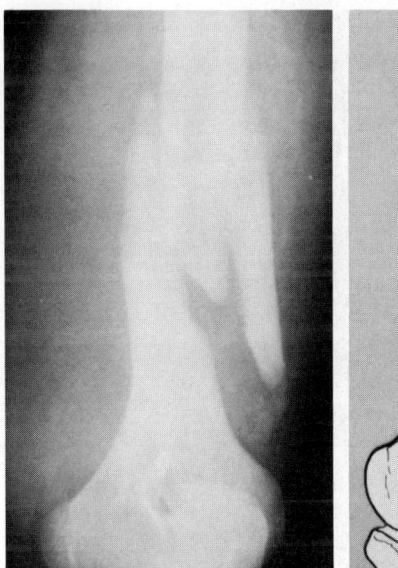
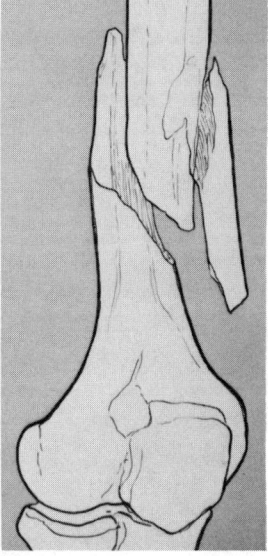

Figure 10-4 **(A)** This humerus has been subjected to a crushing injury with the comminuted fracture representing the amount of energy absorbed by the bone. These high-energy fractures can be shattered into many more pieces than this. **(B)** The artist's drawing of the roentgenogram demonstrates the three major fragments of the fracture. Courtesy of George N. Ewing, MD.

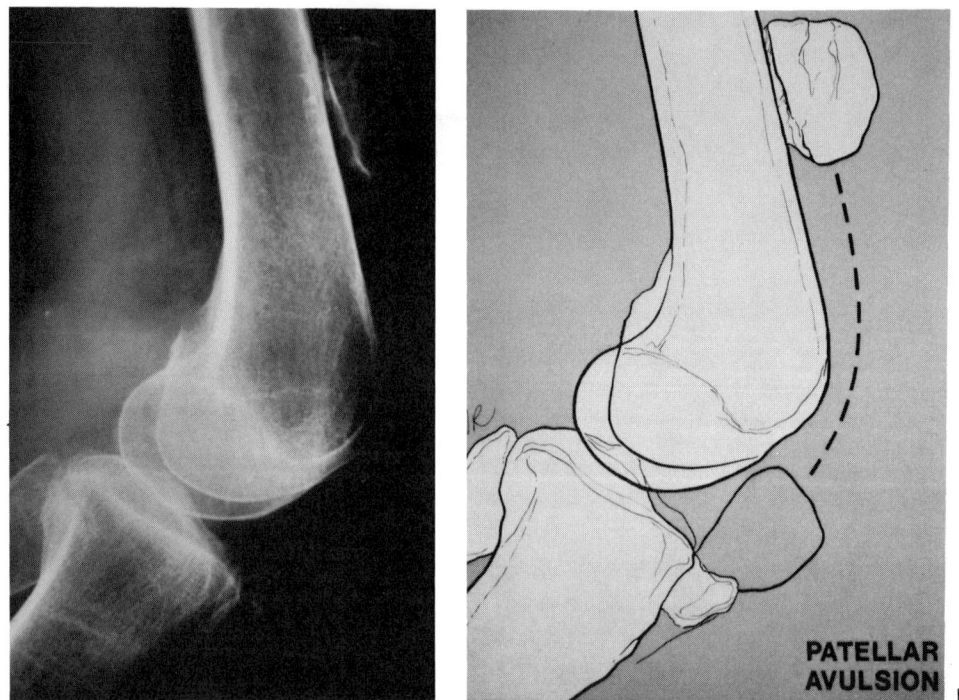

Figure 10-5 (**A**) This roentgenogram demonstrates superior migration of the patella in an athlete. The patient noticed a snap and immediate pain after springing up for a rebound in a basketball game. (**B**) This drawing based on the roentgenogram illustrates both the normal position of the patella and the partial avulsion of the tibial tubercle. Courtesy of George N. Ewing, MD.

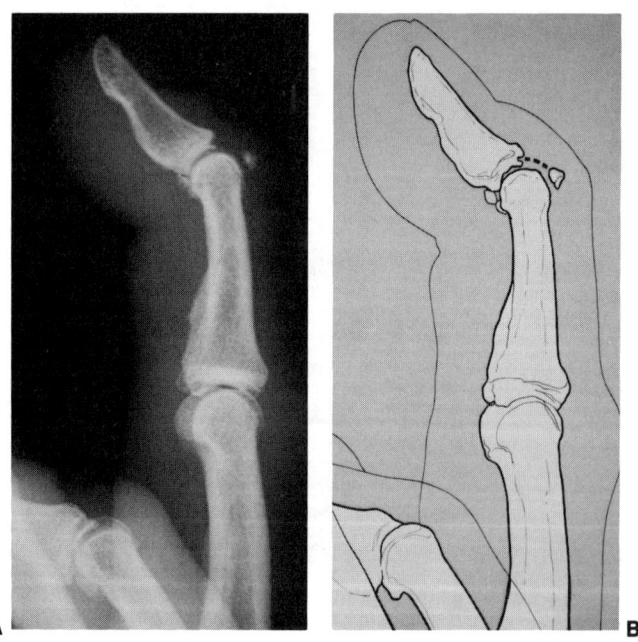

Figure 10-6 (**A**) This mallet finger deformity was the result of excessive stress to the extensor tendon with avulsion of a small piece of the proximal phalanx. (**B**) The illustration based on the roentgenogram nicely defines the avulsion injury. Courtesy of George N. Ewing, MD.

fracture line that falls at 45° to the long axis of the bone. The spiral fracture best demonstrates this abnormal loading (Fig. 10-3). Compression fractures are the result of excessive axial load and are represented by the shaft of long bone being driven into the softer metaphyseal cancellous bone. In children, the force might create a crinkle in the shaft called a torus fracture (Fig. 10-7). Compression fractures are most commonly seen in the spine, where the vertical trabeculae of the vertebral body fail, causing collapse (Fig. 10-8). There can be combinations of these forces, such as in fractures caused by angulation and axial compression or angulation-rotation. Examples of these fractures are the seat-belt fracture and the slice-fracture dislocation in the vertebral column. These are further explained in Chapter 11, Emergencies of the Vertebral Column.

In children, the physeal growth plate, the relative flexibility, and the thick periosteum all play a part in making fractures different. Even the roentgenogram is hard to interpret because the ends of the long bones are composed largely of cartilage (Fig. 10-9). The osseous centers appear at predictable times; these have been charted. An important rule to remember when reading a child's confusing roentgenogram is to take similar views of the opposite extremity. In comparing the injured limb to the uninjured one, subtle differences will be noted. Fractures through the physeal (epiphyseal)

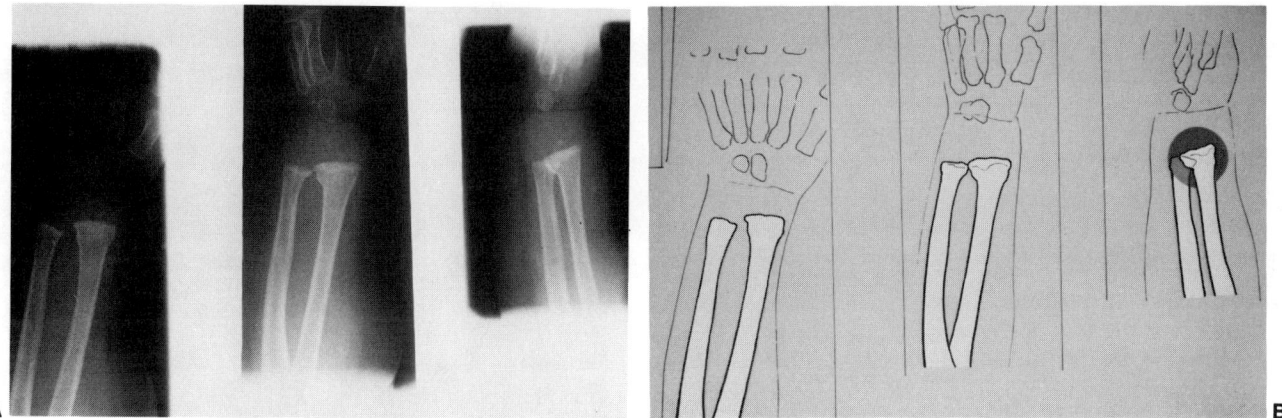

Figure 10-7 (**A**) Three views of this distal radius and ulna in a small child demonstrate a torus fracture of the radius. (**B**) The drawings made point out the area of compression in the radius. Courtesy of George N. Ewing, MD.

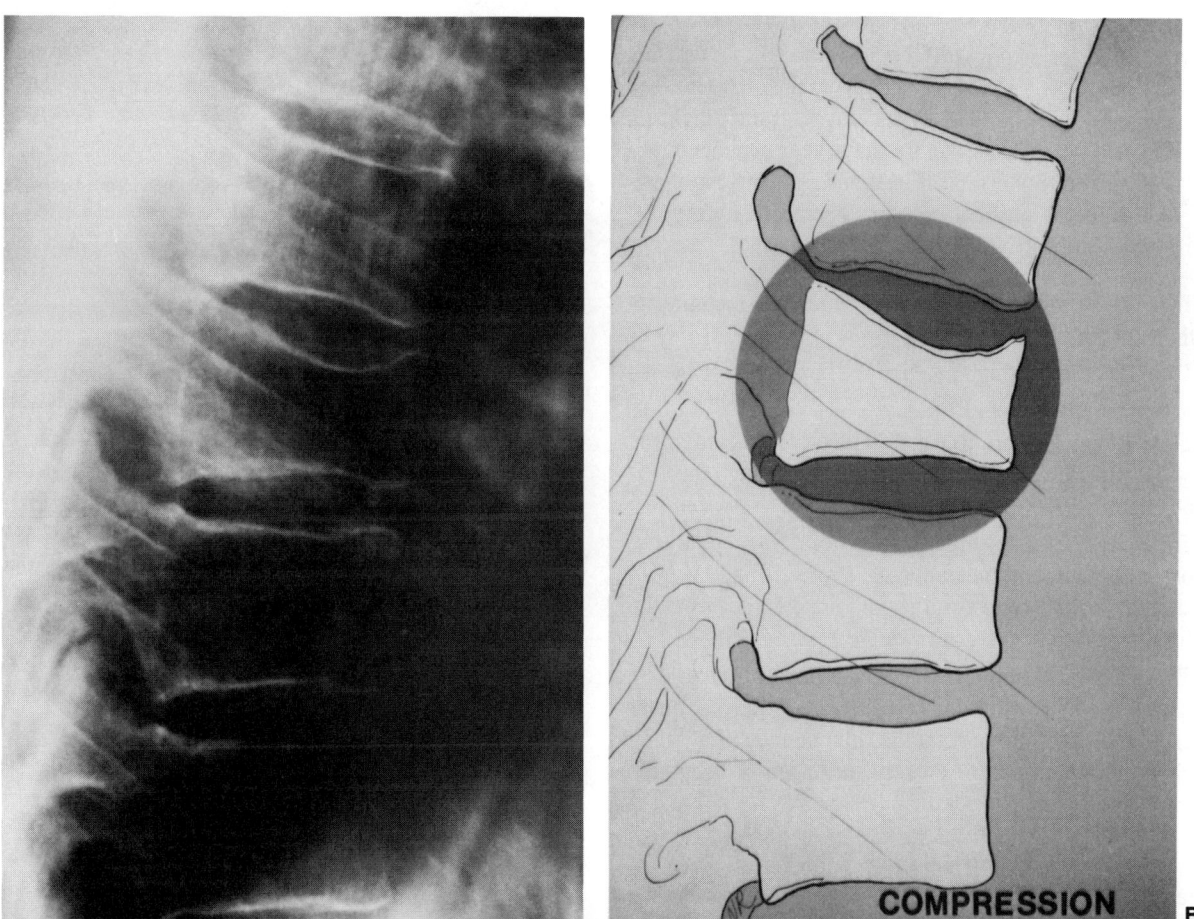

Figure 10-8 (**A**) This roentgenogram of the 12th thoracic vertebra is typical of a mild compression fracture. The disc tissue is pushed through the superior end plate, fracturing the trabeculae of the vertebral body. (**B**) The drawing indicates the area of concern in the 12th thoracic vertebra. Courtesy of George N. Ewing, MD.

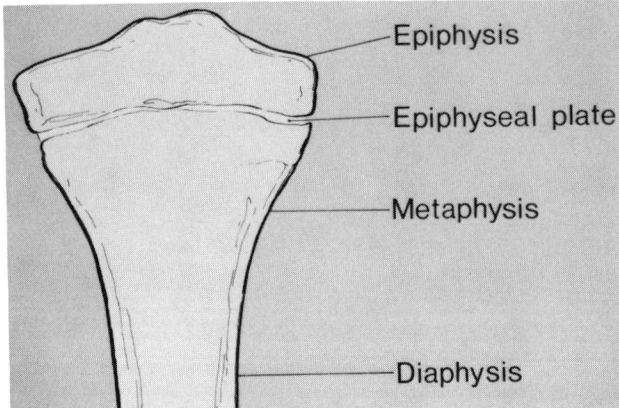

Figure 10-9 The end of a long bone in a child is divided into the epiphysis, epiphyseal plate (physeal plate), metaphysis, and diaphysis. The epiphysis is composed mostly of cartilage at birth and ossifies at a predictable time (each epiphysis has a specific age range of appearance). This leads to difficulties in interpretation of the roentgenograms in young children.

plate are difficult to recognize if there has been a spontaneous reduction. Frequently, a chip of bone from the metaphysis is present (Thurston-Holland sign) and suggests the diagnosis (Fig. 10-10). The physeal fractures have been separated into five categories by Salter and Harris and indicate the prognosis of the future physeal growth. There are five types, Salter-Harris I to V (Fig. 10-11):

- Type I separates the epiphysis from the metaphysis through the physeal plate.
- Type II passes through much of the physis before taking a chip off the metaphysis.
- Type III injuries are a plane of separation through the physeal plate before entering the joint through the epiphysis.
- Type IV injuries occur through the joint line, epiphysis, physeal plate, and metaphysis. (Types III and IV need accurate reduction to ensure both joint congruity and the future growth of the growth plate.)
- Type V is a crushing injury of the physeal plate. The major problem with this type is cessation of linear growth of the long bone at the injured end. In a young child, this can lead to severely shortened or angulated extremities.

The periosteum in the child is very thick and elastic. It frequently will be torn on the tension side of the fracture and intact on the compression side. This can result in a "hinging" effect by the intact side, making reduction or the maintenance of the achieved reduction difficult.

Pathological fractures occur in bones that are weakened by disease. This might be osteoporotic bone or bone thinned by

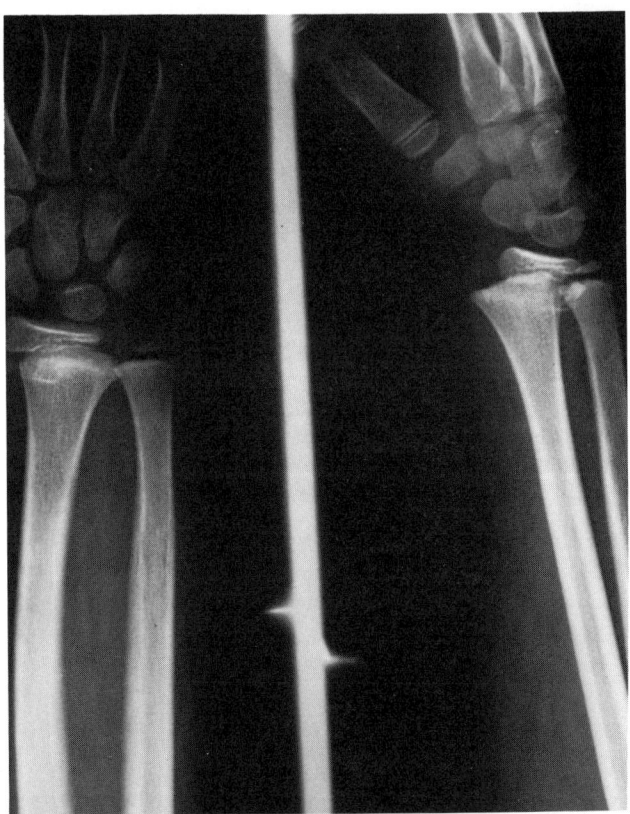

Figure 10-10 This roentgenogram of a distal radius in a child illustrates separation of the epiphysis from the metaphysis with a flake of the metaphysis included in the fracture. This is an example of a Salter-Harris type II physeal fracture.

infection, fibrosis replacement, or tumor. These can occur with very little trauma. Stress fractures are the result of repetitive loading beyond the tolerance of the bone. Cracks develop and may lead to a complete fracture. These are most frequently seen in patients who have had a major change in the amount of activity being performed. Examples might be fractures of the tibia in army recruits marching long distances or metatarsal fractures in ballet dancers with recently increased training schedules (Fig. 10-12).

Open fractures require special attention because of wound contamination at the time of injury. Bacterial contamination is present in 65% of open fractures, and if the organism is present in great enough concentration, it is likely to cause the wound to become infected. It has also been shown that the open fracture type (Gustilo-Anderson I to III), which is based on the amount of tissue destruction, determines the chance of infection. This classification has been modified by a subdivision of the type III fractures.

- Type I: Fractures with a wound less than 1 cm long.
- Type II: Fractures with a wound greater than 1 cm, but without extensive soft tissue damage, flaps, or avulsion.

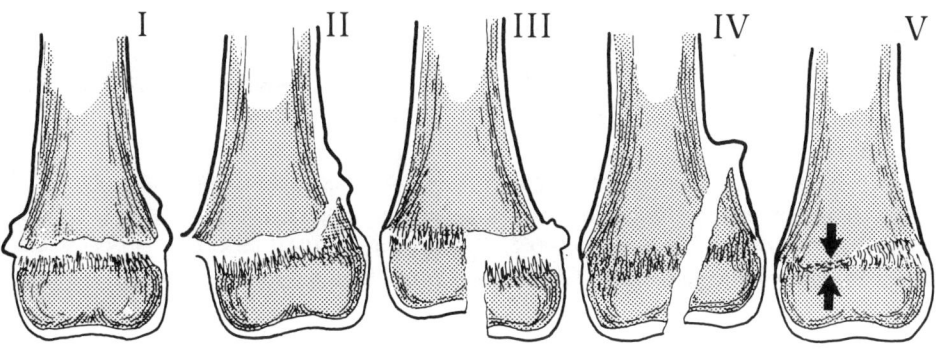

Figure 10-11 Salter-Harris classification. Type I involves a separation of the epiphysis from the metaphysis through the physeal plate. Type II injuries are the most common. The fracture passes through most of the physis before taking a small piece of the metaphysis (Thurston-Holland sign). Type III physeal fractures require the plane of separation to involve a portion of the physeal plate continuing through the epiphysis into the articular joint. Type IV fractures continue through the metaphysis, physeal plate, epiphysis, and into the joint. Types III and IV need accurate reduction to ensure congruity and future longitudinal growth of the growth plate. Type V injuries involve a crushing of the physeal plate. These may be difficult to interpret roentgenographically. They are important because the injury to the growth plate is severe and cessation of linear growth is likely to occur. Modified from M. Rang, *Children's Fractures*, J.B. Lippincott Co, 1974. *Source:* Adapted with permission from *J Bone Joint Surg* 45A: 589, 1963.

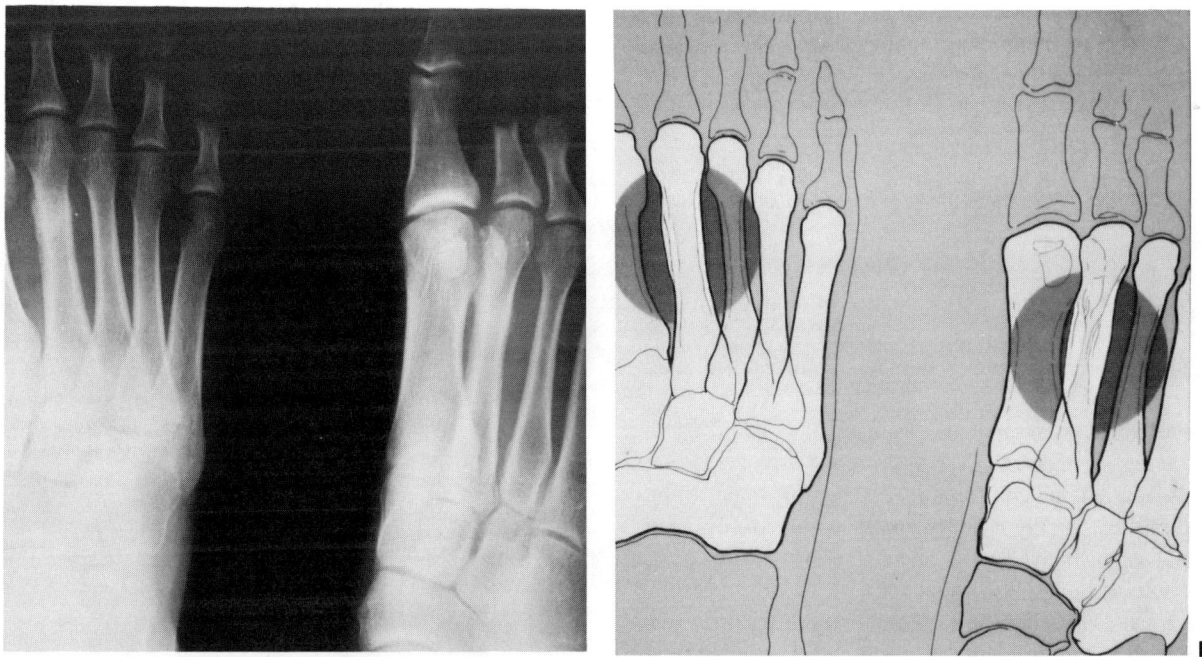

Figure 10-12 (**A**) This roentgenogram was taken after a long-distance runner complained of a fairly severe pain in the forefoot. He had recently increased his daily mileage in preparation for a marathon. An area of callus can be seen in the diaphyseal region of the second metatarsal. (**B**) The mid-shaft of the second metatarsal represents a typical site for the occurrence of a stress fracture. This drawing better demonstrates the pathology.

- Type III: Fractures with a wound longer than 5 cm and with extensive soft tissue damage. Regardless of the amount of wound damage, segmental fractures, fractures with loss of diaphyseal bone, highly contaminated wounds, associated vascular injury, and comminuted fractures are included in this category (if open).

- Type IIIA: Fractures not involving extensive soft tissue stripping of bone.
- Type IIIB: Fractures in which some periosteal stripping of bone has occurred.
- Type IIIC: Fractures in which a major vascular injury has occurred.

The goal in treatment of these injuries is to decrease the incidence of infection and to obtain a united-functional extremity. Debridement and irrigation will significantly decrease the number of bacteria but will not sterilize the wound. The addition of systemic antibiotics to the treatment protocol further decreases the incidence of infection. In one series of open fractures (Patzakis et al), the incidence of infection using no antibiotic (13.9%) was reduced to 9.6% using a penicillin-streptomycin combination, and to 2.3% using cephalothin.

DEFINITIVE TREATMENT OF FRACTURES

When the general condition of the patient is stable, management of the fractures can be considered. The fact that large volumes of blood can be lost from even closed fractures should not be forgotten. Femoral fractures can lose 1 to 2.5 L, tibial fractures 0.5 to 1.5 L, and pelvic fractures can lead to exsanguination. Open fractures can lose even greater volumes, and if the injury is old (more than three hours), it can be difficult to estimate the volume of blood loss.

In the emergency situation, the most important role is to adequately splint the fracture. Adequate splinting is desirable for the following reasons:

1. Further soft tissue damage (particularly to nerves or blood vessels) can be avoided. Closed fractures remain closed.
2. Immobilization lessens the pain.
3. Splinting decreases the incidence of adult respiratory syndromes (from fat embolism) and shock.
4. The obtaining of proper roentgenograms is facilitated.

Conventional splints include cardboard or wooden boards, wire frames, or metal Universal extremity splints. All, if properly applied and comfortable, can be functional. Inflatable splints are widely used by emergency medical technicians and can be both effective and dangerous. These consist of a double-walled polyvinyl jacket with a zip fastener that can be inflated around the injured extremity. They are said to control both bleeding and swelling, but can cause circulatory embarrassment, particularly if the blood flow is already tenuous. Femoral fractures are usually treated with the Thomas splint or one of its modifications (Fig. 10-13). Traction can be applied through a bandage over the boot or shoe to the base of the device. The modern adaptation of this splint has built-in traction capabilities (Fig. 10-14). The vertebral column is treated using a spine board (for thoracolumbar injuries) or "sandbagging" the neck. All of these are discussed in relation to specific fracture types in the text.

Closed treatment consists of some form of manipulation or reduction of the fracture followed by the application of a definitive splint or cast. The earlier the reduction the better, since swelling tends to increase for 6 to 12 hours after the injury. The hemorrhage and edema in the soft tissues may make adequate reduction very difficult after this "golden period." On the other hand, a closed fracture is not a surgical emergency, and the patient's life should not be jeopardized in an overzealous attempt to obtain early reduction.

After adequate roentgenographic evaluation of the fracture is completed, the objectives of the manipulation can be decided. Closed reduction is not necessary or may not be possible in the following circumstances:

1. No significant displacement is present.
2. The displacement present is of little concern (eg, humeral shaft).
3. The reduction, when obtained, cannot be held (eg, compression fracture of a vertebral body).
4. No reduction is possible (eg, comminuted fracture of the head and neck of the humerus).
5. The fracture has been caused by a traction force (eg, patellar fracture with displacement).

In order to achieve reduction, it is necessary to apply traction along the long axis of the limb to reverse the mechanism that caused the fracture and to align the fragment that

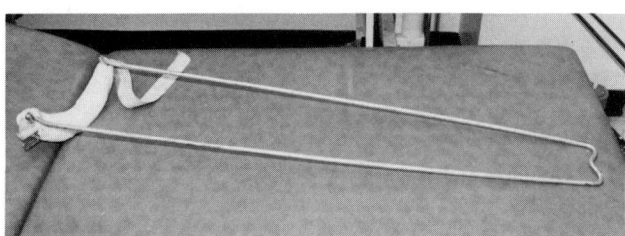

Figure 10-13 The Thomas splint was developed in the latter part of the 19th century by Hugh Owen Thomas. It was popularized by Sir Robert Jones during World War I when it saved many lives. It still remains basically the same and is used for control of the fractured femur. Traction can be applied through a bandage placed over the shoe and attached to the base of the splint.

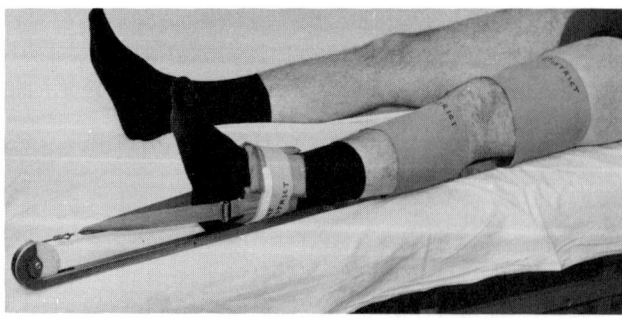

Figure 10-14 This splint is a modern adaptation of the Thomas splint and includes traction capabilities. A pulley and winch near the base provide the traction through a harness placed around the foot.

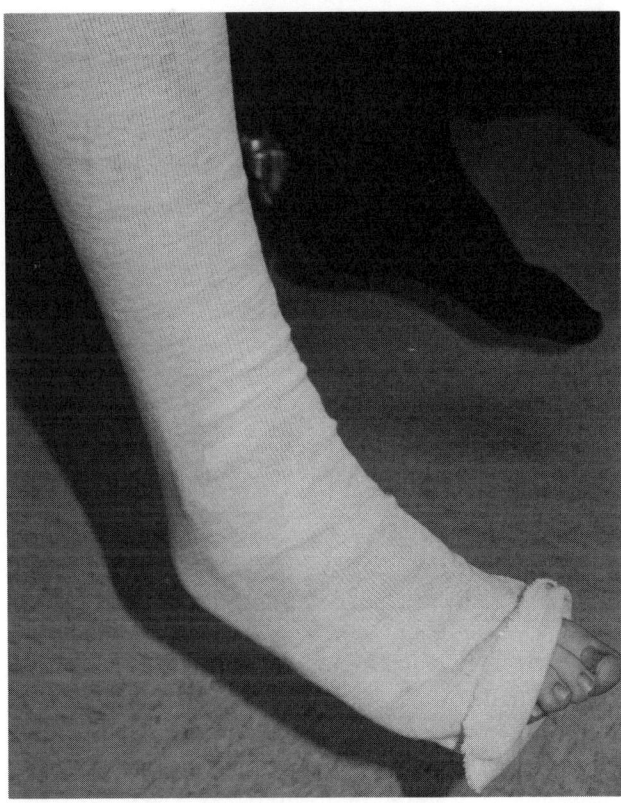

Figure 10-15 The first layer of cast application is the stockinette. It provides a smooth covering for the extremity and can be used to trim the edges of the cast after plaster is applied.

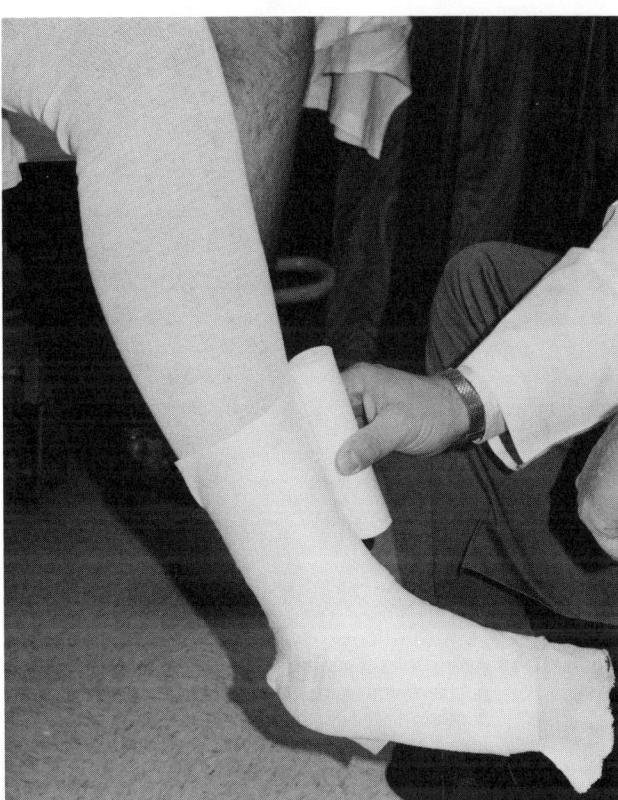

Figure 10-16 Sheet wadding, or "web roll," is used as a padding. It is rolled distally to proximally, making sure that it is applied smoothly. The material can be torn to ensure that the roll is smooth and without unnecessary bulges.

can be controlled (usually the distal one) with the one that cannot be controlled.

Once a fracture is reduced it must be immobilized until primary union takes place. This can be accomplished by means of plaster of Paris casting, continuous traction, or some form of splinting. In using plaster of Paris, certain guidelines should be followed. Stockinette can be applied as a first layer, which can be used to trim the edges of the plaster cast at the end of application (Fig. 10-15). Sheet wadding or "web roll" is then applied distally to proximally, rolling it as smooth as possible (Fig. 10-16). The wadding can be torn so it fits the extremity without any unnecessary bulges. Areas of bony prominence or possible nerve compression (eg, medial malleolus or fibular head) may need extra padding (Fig. 10-17).

The rolled plaster bandages must be thoroughly immersed in water until air bubbles stop rising. The roll can then be gently squeezed to release excess water, being careful to retain the plaster of Paris (Fig. 10-18). The plaster bandage is rolled in the same direction as the wadding. The roll should be in contact with the extremity and is rolled on (Fig. 10-19). Each turn of the bandage should overlap the preceding one by half. The plaster is folded rather than torn to maintain smooth symmetrical rolls (Fig. 10-20). The cast should be two to

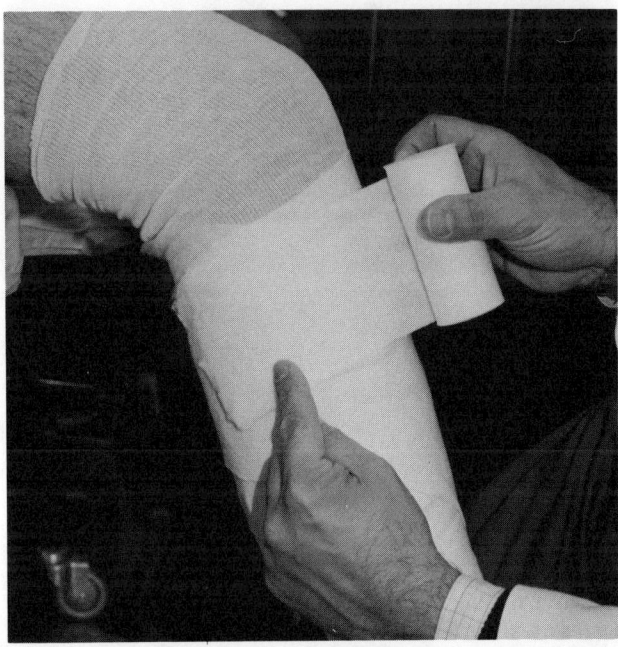

Figure 10-17 Certain areas such as the medial malleolus, proximal fibular head, or humeral condyles will require additional padding to avoid skin breakdown or neural compression. Three layers of web roll are usually enough.

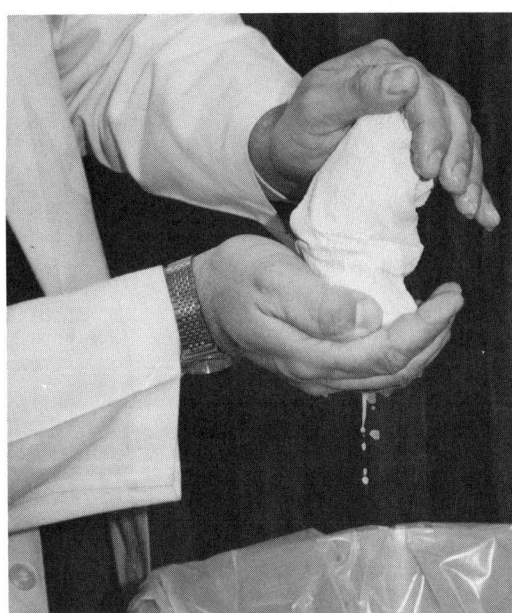

Figure 10-18 After a roll of plaster is immersed in water until the air bubbles stop rising, the roll is removed and gently squeezed. The ends are held to aid in the retention of the plaster of Paris. The roll should be moist but not dripping wet.

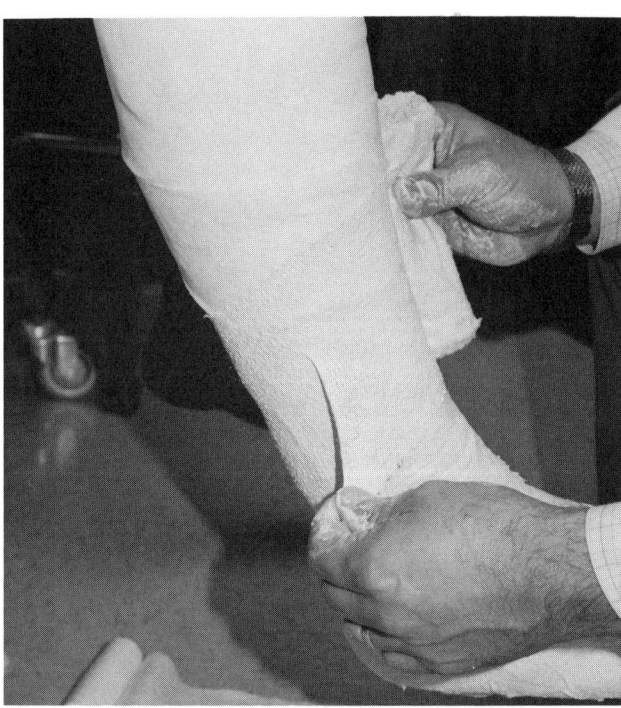

Figure 10-19 The plaster is rolled in the same direction as the wadding. The roll should be in contact with the extremity as it is rolled on. Each turn of the bandage should overlap the preceding one by half. Two to three layers of plaster roll are required for cast strength.

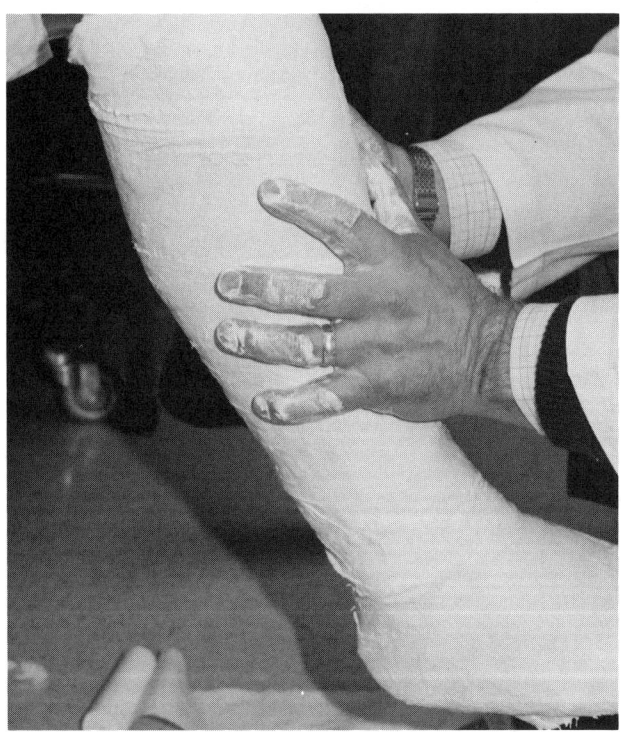

Figure 10-20 To ensure that the plaster rolls are smooth and symmetrical, the plaster is folded rather than torn. After it is applied, the entire cast is smoothed and molded with both hands. This not only makes for pleasing appearance of the cast, but prevents lamination of the layers, which weakens its structure.

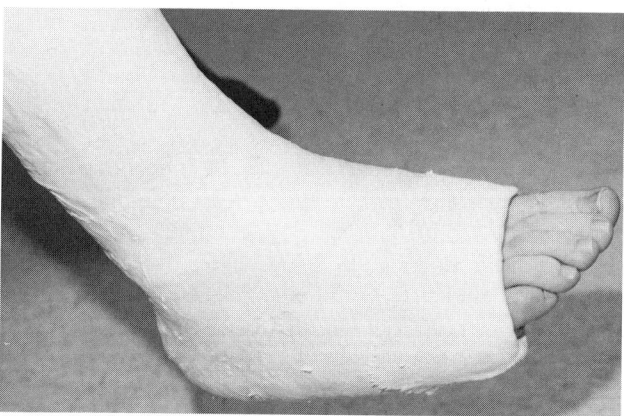

Figure 10-21 After the cast is trimmed, the edges are trimmed along the previously applied stockinette. A few strips of plaster can be used to seal it to the cast and create a good appearance.

three layers thick to provide adequate strength. After it is applied, it is smoothed by using the palms of both hands. This prevents lamination, which weakens the cast. Trimming can be done carefully using a cast saw (when it is dry) or a scalpel. After trimming, the stockinette should overlap the ends of the cast; it is folded down and sealed to the cast with a few strips of plaster to create a good appearance (Fig. 10-21).

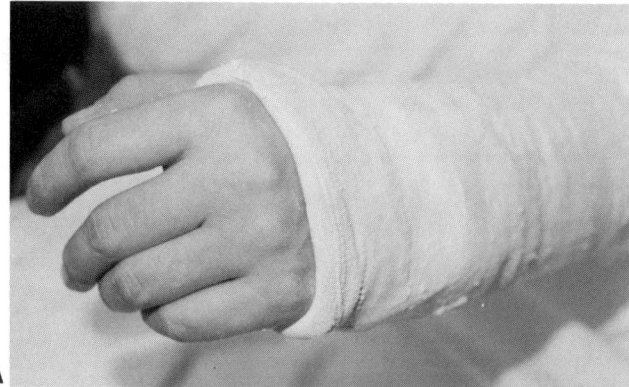
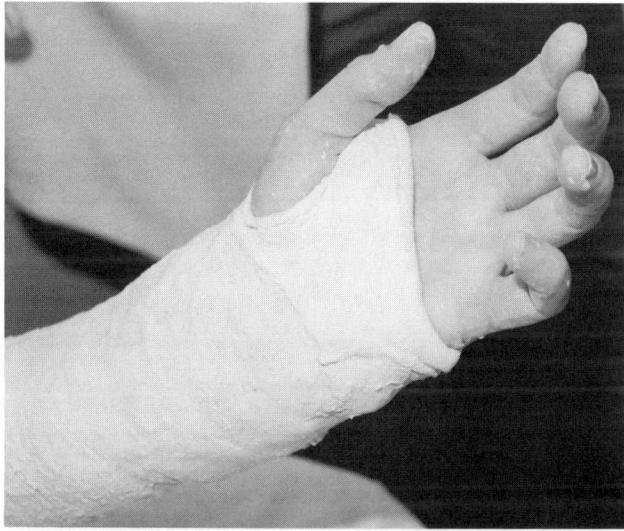

Figure 10-22 (**A**) The upper extremity cast is trimmed distally in line just above the knuckles dorsally and (**B**) across the proximal flexor crease on the palmar side.

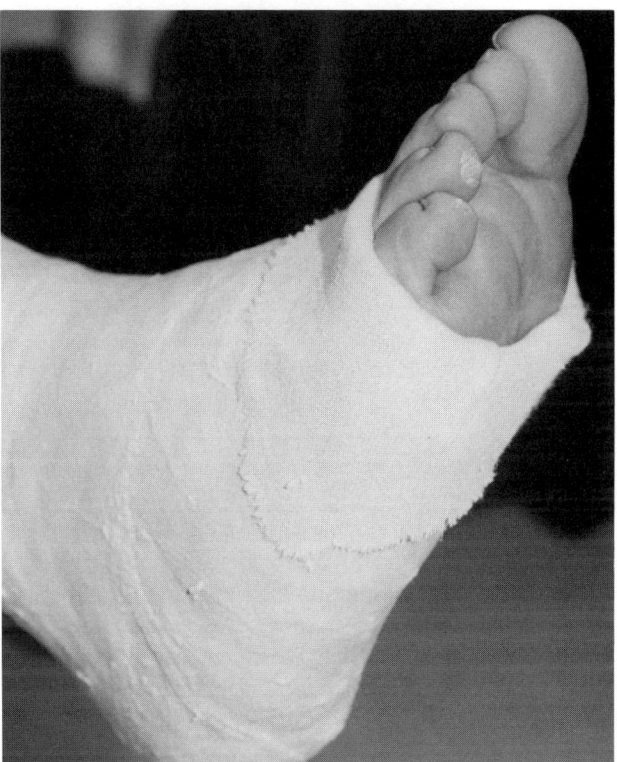

Figure 10-23 Lower extremity casts are usually trimmed in line with the metatarsal heads on the plantar side and at the base of the toes dorsally.

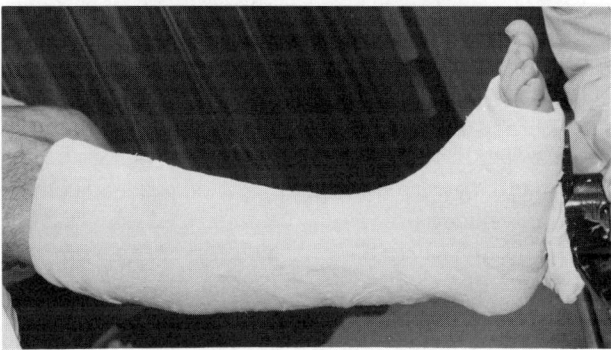

Figure 10-24 If a walking heel is needed, extra layers of plaster are used to accommodate it. It is applied so it is in almost direct line with the tibia rather than more anteriorly.

Upper extremity casts can extend above the elbow or be limited to the forearm. The distal end should be trimmed in line with the knuckles on the dorsum and obliquely across the proximal flexor crease of the palm on the palmar side (Fig. 10-22). This allows unrestricted finger motion. The hole for the thumb should be large and smooth enough to allow it adequate movement. Some fractures (scaphoid) will require that the thumb be included in the cast. This is further described in the specific section devoted to those injuries.

Lower extremity casts such as long leg casts can be applied with the knee flexed or extended. If weight bearing is to be allowed, the knee should be in neutral to 5° of flexion. The cast should be trimmed in line with the metatarsal heads on the plantar side and at the base of the toes dorsally (Fig. 10-23). If a toe plate is used, it should not hyperextend the toes. In most cases, it is best to immobilize the ankle at 90° of dorsiflexion, except when this position displaces the fracture (e.g., distal tibia). If a walking heel is applied, an extra layer of plaster is used to accommodate it to the foot of cast. The heel should be centered almost directly below the line of tibia rather than more anteriorly (Fig. 10-24).

More often than not, splints will be used for acute fractures. The two most common types are the radial slab and sugar tong splints. Both are used in the treatment of Colles' fracture.

The radial slab consists of eight to ten thicknesses of 6-inch plaster with a thumb hole cut in it. Web-roll padding can

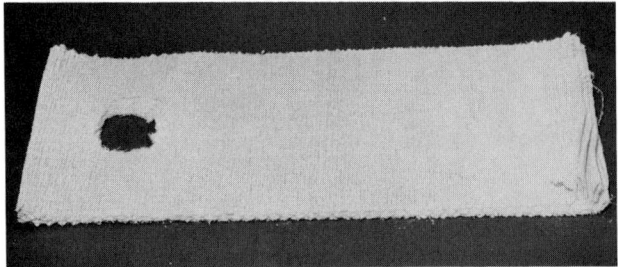

Figure 10-25 A radial slab consists of eight to ten thicknesses of 6-in plaster with a thumb hole cut in it. Web-roll padding can be placed on at least one side of the plaster to protect the skin.

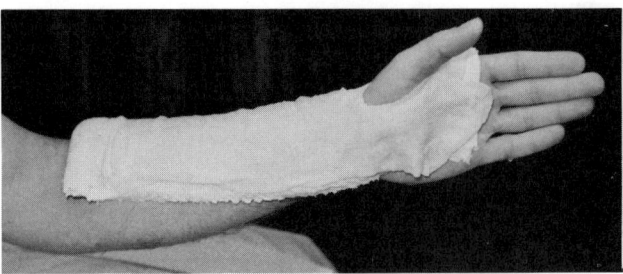

Figure 10-26 After immersion in water, the radial slab is applied over the radial aspect of the forearm, overlapping the dorsal and volar aspects of the wrist.

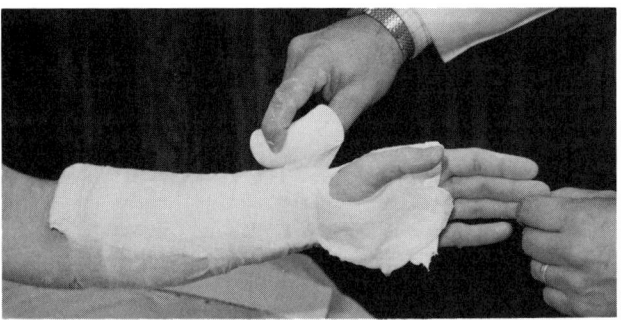

Figure 10-27 The radial slab is bandaged using a wet roll gauze.

be placed on both sides of the laid-out plaster (Fig. 10-25). The splint, after being dunked in water, is applied to the radial aspect of the forearm, overlapping the dorsal and volar aspects of the wrist (Fig. 10-26). When the appropriate position of the extremity is obtained, it is bandaged on with a wet gauze roll (Fig. 10-27). The sugar tong is even more versatile, as it can be used on the upper arm or leg as well as the forearm and wrist. This consists of an 8- to 10-layer sheet of plaster, which is fitted from the dorsum of hand over the forearm, around the flexed elbow, and along the volar aspect of the forearm (Fig. 10-28). It is also wrapped on using a wet gauze bandage.

Another splint, which may be the most valuable of all in the emergency situation, is the Robert Jones dressing. This is an excellent alternative if there is extensive soft tissue injury or swelling, or if the patient needs to be splinted for a hospital transfer. After treatment of the wound, sheet wadding or web-roll padding is applied around the extremity. Then a large roll of cotton padding is rolled on to provide a bulky compression dressing (Fig. 10-29). Slabs of plaster can be used, as in the sugar tong method, for additional immobilization. The cotton is then snugly compressed with bias-cut stockinette rolls (Fig. 10-30). This is a very safe dressing and provides good fracture stabilization. It is not good for maintaining fracture reduction.

The open fracture requires special consideration. An attempt should be made to control the care of open fractures between the place where the accident occurred and the hospital, as this may play a major role in the prevention of infection. Hemorrhage is controlled with a sterile compression dressing before emergency splinting. Unnecessary movement of the fracture site may draw contaminated material into the wound or further damage soft tissue structures. Most long bone fractures can be handled with cardboard or wooden splints. The exception is the femur, which should be traction splinted. These measures should be completed before roentgenographic examination. If the patient will undergo surgery within 1 or 2 hours for formal irrigation and debridement, no further wound care is necessary.

Resuscitation or other organ-system injury may take priority over this "ideal situation." If factors intervene and result in a delay of surgical debridement, the following is recommended: In contaminated type I, type II, and all type III fractures, tetanus toxoid is considered. If previously immunized, the patient should receive 0.5 mL of tetanus toxoid unless it is proven that a booster has been given in the past 6 years. In the absence of immunization, the patient should receive both a minimum of 4500 to 5000 U of heterologous tetanus antitoxin (horse serum) or an equivalent number of units of human serum and three doses of 0.5 mL tetanus toxoid (the first at the time of initial treatment, the second in 3 months, and the third in 6 to 12 months).

A predebridement culture is taken in the emergency department. Gross debris is cleaned from the wound using sterile techniques (gown, gloves, mask). The wound is irrigated with sterile saline (2 or 3 L) and covered with a Betadine-soaked dressing. All patients with type I and II open fractures are given intravenous cefazolin starting with an initial 1-g bolus, which is repeated every 6 hours. Because of the increased risk of Gram-negative contamination, patients with type III fractures also receive an intravenous aminoglycoside, usually gentamicin or tobramycin, in a dosage of 3 to 5 mg/kg every 8 hours. Later, more thorough, meticulous debridement will be done in the operating room.

Musculoskeletal Emergencies 173

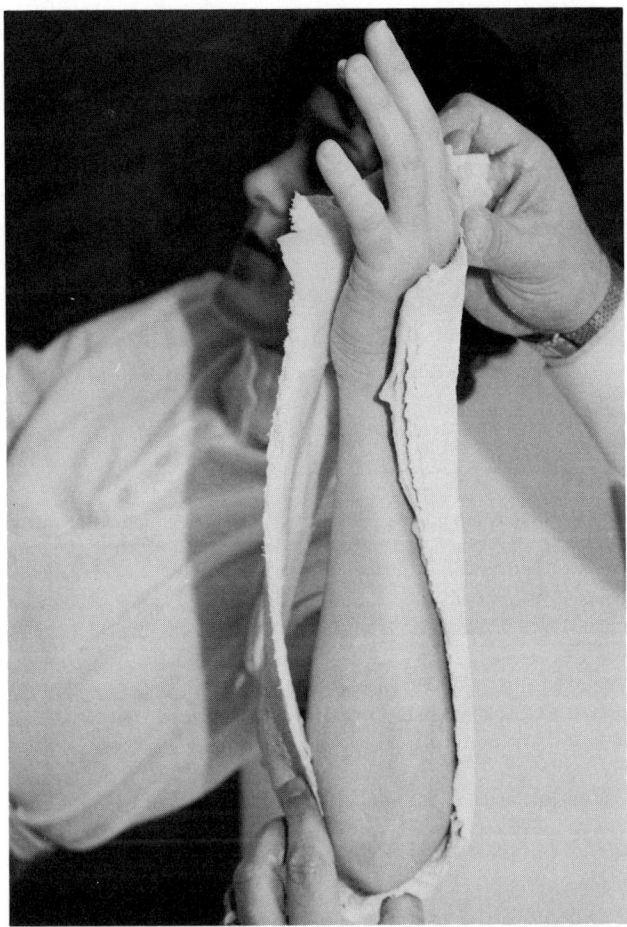

Figure 10-28 The sugar tong is a very adaptable splint that can be used on both the upper and lower extremities. It consists of 8 to 10 layers of 4- to 6-inch plaster, which is fitted over the forearm, around the flexed elbow, and along the volar aspect of the forearm. An additional splint can be used to include the upper arm. It is fitted before water immersion and the distal end is cut to accommodate the thumb. It is wrapped on with a wet gauze bandage.

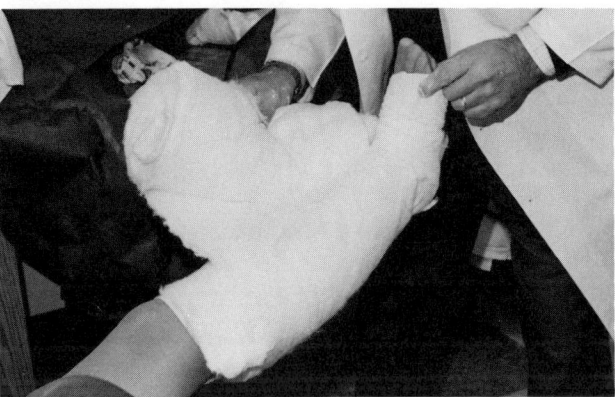

Figure 10-29 The Robert Jones compression dressing consists of large rolls of cotton padding placed over the dressings and web roll. Slabs of plaster in the sugar tong manner can be used to provide additional stabilization.

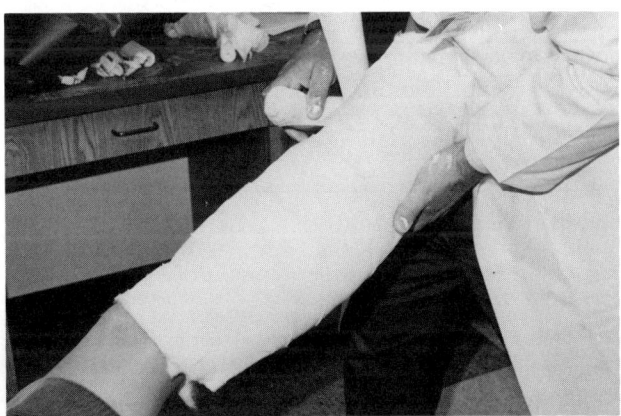

Figure 10-30 The Robert Jones bulky dressing is completed by the application of bias-cut stockinette rolls or Ace wrap to contain the padding and plaster slabs. This is a very safe dressing and provides adequate fracture stabilization; for the crush injury or neurovascularly compromised extremity, it may be the best dressing or splint available.

DISLOCATIONS

A dislocation is a complete disruption of a joint so that the articular surfaces are no longer in contact (Fig. 10-31). A dislocation is properly described in terms of the relationship of the distal segment to the proximal segment. For example, if the tibia is dislocated so that it lies anterior to or in front of the femur, it is identified as an anterior dislocation of the knee. Similarly, the position of the humeral head or femoral head in relation to its respective joint will describe the type of dislocation. Subluxations are less severe disruptions of joints, in which some articular contact remains. Either may be associated with a fracture of a joint surface.

The clinical features of a dislocation consist of pain, loss of normal contours or relationships, and loss of motion. The limb may be held in a diagnostic position (flexed, adducted, internal rotation of the femur in a posterior hip dislocation). Neurovascular complications are particularly apt to occur in some dislocations (eg, knee joint) and are much higher in all dislocations than in fractures.

After careful physical examination, appropriate roentgenograms are obtained to evaluate the dislocation for any associated fractures. The principles of reduction are adequate analgesia, muscle relaxation, and traction. Specific dislocations are discussed in the text. After reduction, splinting of the joint can be accomplished by the same techniques as those applied to fractures. The shoulder usually is treated using a sling-and-swathe, and the hip with some form of traction, until the pain dissipates and motion can be started.

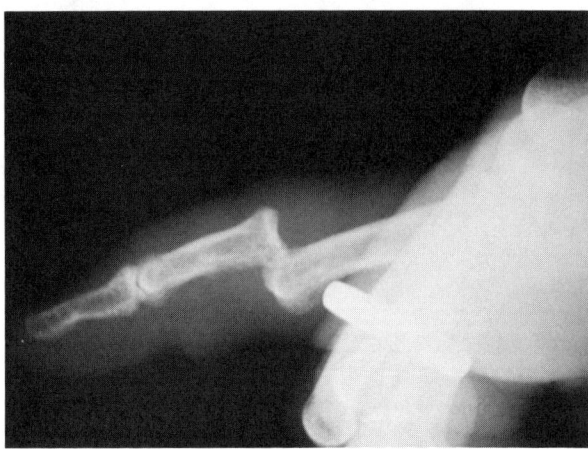 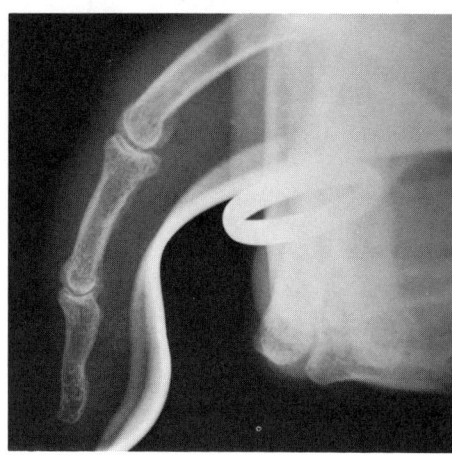

Figure 10-31 (**A**) A dislocation is complete disruption of a joint so that the articular surfaces are no longer in contact. The dislocation is described according to the position of the distal segment involved. Therefore, a tibia which is dislocated anterior to the femur is properly identified as an anterior dislocation of the knee. This roentgenogram illustrates a dorsal dislocation of the proximal interphalangeal joint of the index finger. (**B**) Traction or a combination of traction and some gentle manipulation is required to reverse the mechanism of the dislocation and to reduce it. The finger in this roentgenogram is reduced and in a splint to protect the injured joint and soft tissues. Courtesy of George N. Ewing, MD.

BIBLIOGRAPHY

Benson DR. Management of open fractures. *Contemp Orthop* 1985; 11:113–117.

Blount WP. *Fractures in Children*. Baltimore: Williams and Wilkins; 1955.

Gustillo RB. Management of open fractures. *Minn Med*. 1971;54:185–189.

Gustillo RB, Anderson JT. Prevention of infection in the treatment of 1,025 open fractures of long bones. *J Bone Joint Surg Am*. 1976;58:453–458.

Harkess JW. Principles of fractures and dislocations. In: *Fractures*, Rockwood CA, Green DP, eds. Philadelphia: JB Lippincott; 1975.

Patzakis MJ, Harvey JP Jr, Ivler D. The role of antibiotics in the management of open fractures. *J Bone Joint Surg Am*. 1974;56:532–541.

Rang M. *Children's Fractures*. Philadelphia: Lippincott; 1974.

11. Emergencies of the Vertebral Column

DANIEL R. BENSON, MD

Injury to the vertebral column is generally due to flexion and/or rotational forces placed on the head or torso. The majority are caused by motor vehicle (car) or motorcycle accidents (50%). Falls from a height account for an additional 20%, and sporting accidents cause 15%. The remainder are due to direct blows, penetrating missiles, and miscellaneous trauma. Neurological injury can accompany the associated fractures which occur, or may result from an acutely herniated disc or an epidural hematoma without any fractures.

All of the vertebrae articulate in the same general way. The bodies are joined by the strong anterior longitudinal ligament and the intervertebral disc. The posterior portions of adjacent vertebrae are connected by the articular capsules and the intraspinous ligaments. Direct longitudinal forces stretch these ligamentous tissues, but it is rotational or twisting forces that usually create tearing.

In accidents, the vertebral column is deformed by one (or more) of five mechanisms: pure flexion, flexion and rotation, extension, vertical compression, or a direct shearing force.

This introduction presents the reader with a system for classifying fractures. The individual fractures are discussed in more detail later in the chapter with suggestions as to appropriate emergency treatment.

COMPRESSION FRACTURES

Pure flexion forces create a longitudinal pull on the posterior ligament complex (which usually does not rupture) and compress the anterior position of the vertebral body. The posterior portion of the vertebral body remains intact and acts as a hinge. In severe cases, when the compression is greater than 50% of the vertebral height, the posterior complex can fail. The compression can also be lateral, which is secondary to lateral rather than anterior flexion. The most frequently occurring type of compression fracture is represented by fracture of the superior end plate anteriorly. Occasionally, the inferior end plate is involved or both end plates are involved.

The lateral roentgenogram demonstrates the loss of anterior vertebral height (see Chapter 10, Musculoskeletal Emergencies: Introduction and Basic Principles, Fig. 10-8). The posterior height of the vertebra remains unchanged, as does the posterior vertebral body cortex. There is no subluxation on the vertebral bodies either above or below. The intraspinous distance (posteriorly) can be increased and is related to the amount of compression and angulation. The anterior-posterior roentgenogram will demonstrate lateral compression if present. The computerized tomography (CT) scan will confirm that the vertebral ring (posterior vertebral wall pedicles and lamina) are totally intact. Therefore, the neural canal has not been violated. The anterior vertebral body destruction can be appreciated on the CT scan.

FRACTURE-DISLOCATIONS

When flexion-rotation of the vertebral column occurs, the posterior complex tears and the upper vertebrae twist on the

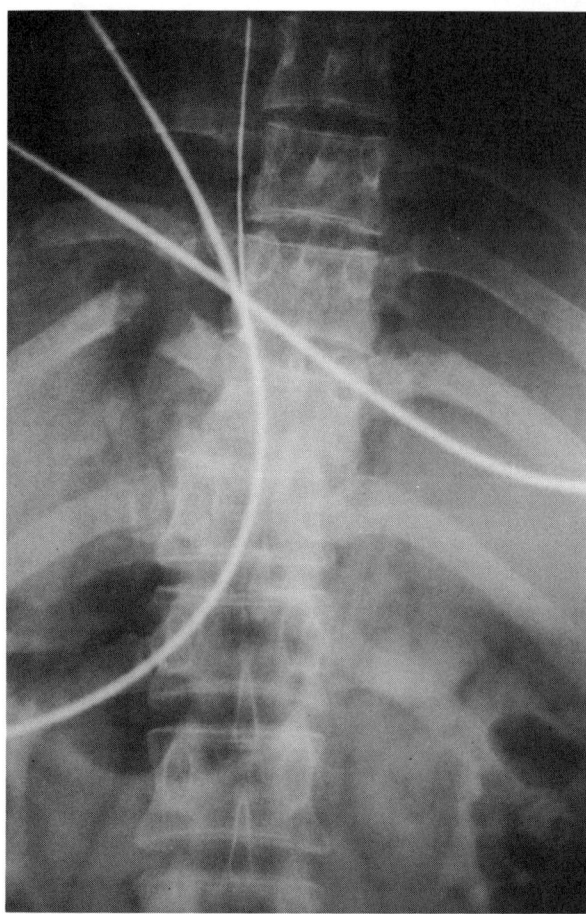

Figure 11-1 This AP roentgenogram demonstrates a fracture dislocation of the thoracic spine. In this case, T-10 is dislocated on T-11. Note the fractured ribs on the right side and the shift of the vertebral body T-10, laterally on T-11. There is preservation of vertebral height and no pedicular widening.

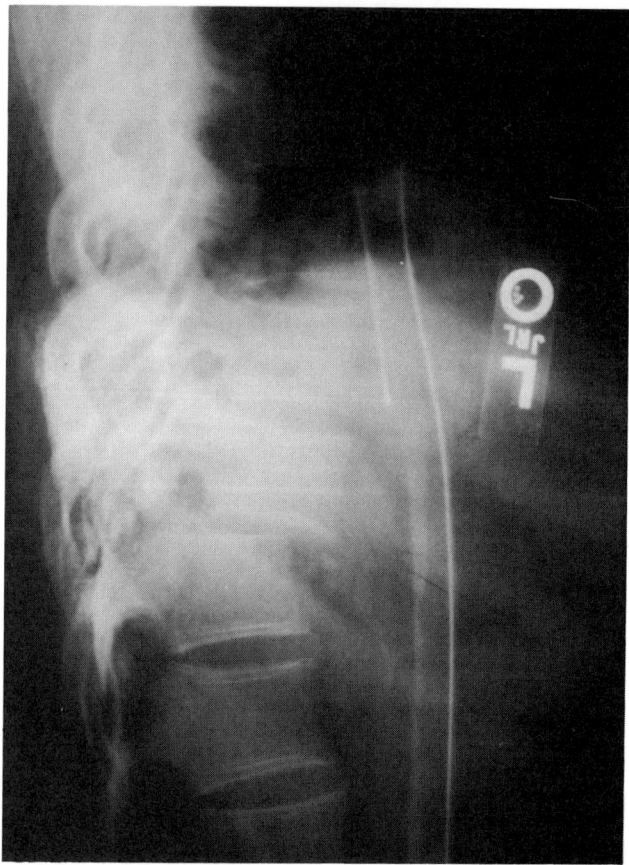

Figure 11-2 The lateral view of the same fracture-dislocation of the spine (Fig. 11-1) demonstrates significant displacement of one vertebra on another. The soft tissue shadows posteriorly cannot be appreciated, but they would demonstrate widening between one spinous process and the next in the area of the dislocation. The patient was felt to have a complete neurologic lesion below the fracture-dislocation. The only possible sign of neurologic sparing was some sensation in the sacral area. This patient had a closed reduction and awoke from anesthesia with complete recovery of both motor and sensory function. This demonstrates that even small amounts of motor or sensory function may indicate that neurologic recovery is possible.

lower ones. The appearance may be different in various parts of the vertebral column, because the anatomy of articular facets varies from being flat and almost horizontal in the cervical region to being larger and having a vertical orientation in the lumbar spine.

In the cervical spine, flexion-rotation ruptures the posterior ligaments and the articular facets are allowed to slide off each other, usually without fracturing. The disc is torn anteriorly, allowing the vertebral bodies to subluxate. In the lumbar spine, the same violence would be likely to fracture one or both articular facets. In addition, rather than the disc tearing, the vertebral body fractures through its upper portion creating the so-called "slice fracture." In both the cervical and lumbar spine, these injuries are considered unstable. Inappropriate handling of the patient could create gross displacement and further jeopardize the spinal cord.

The anterior-posterior (AP) roentgenogram will usually show some evidence of subluxation or dislocation, but spontaneous reduction occasionally occurs. There is good conservation of the posterior wall of the vertebral body and, therefore, preservation of the vertebral height (Fig. 11-1). On the lateral roentgenogram, the displacement can be further appreciated, as well as an increased distance between the spinous processes (Fig. 11-2). Other associated injuries may be seen on the AP view, such as fracture of multiple ribs (thoracic fractures) or transverse processes (lumbar fractures; Fig. 11-1).

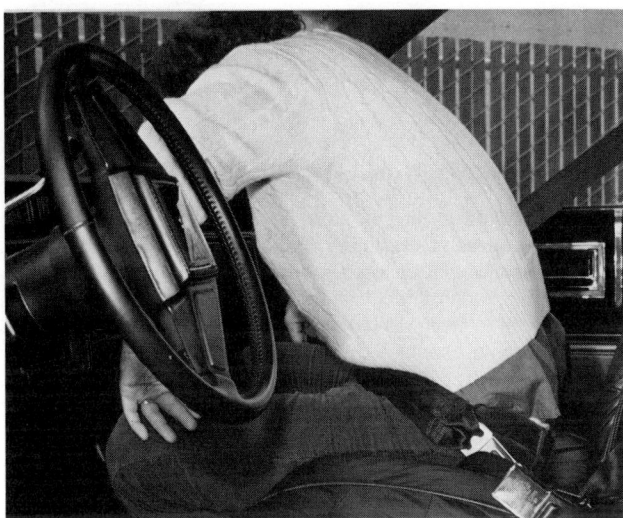

Figure 11-3 The seat-belt injury occurs when the passenger in a car is thrown forward as the car stops abruptly. The lumbar spine fails posteriorly under tension and anteriorly under some flexion. Frequently the seat belt leaves a bruise or mark across the lower abdomen.

SEAT-BELT TYPE INJURIES

Although these fractures do not necessarily occur while the person is wearing a seat belt, the concept of that mechanism is easy to understand. The injury occurs when the lumbar spine fails under tension forces created by a flexion force combined with some distraction (Fig. 11-3). The posterior ligamentous complex and the posterior portion of the disc or vertebral body are pulled apart, while the anterior part of the vertebral body may be compressed but intact.

The AP roentgenogram may demonstrate either widening of two contiguous spinous processes or a split in one of them. The transverse processes and the pedicles can be similarly split, with the fracture continuing into the vertebral body (Chance fracture; Fig. 11-4). In other cases, the injury involves only soft tissue, rupturing the interspinous ligaments, posterior longitudinal ligament, and posterior part of the annulus fibrosis. On the lateral roentgenogram, this will have the appearance of widening of spinous processes and of the disc space. The CT scan does not contribute much, as the neural canal usually is not compromised and the injury is parallel to the plane of the cuts, making the fracture easy to miss.

EXTENSION INJURIES

Extreme extension of the neck can rupture the anterior longitudinal ligament and the disc, dislocating the cervical

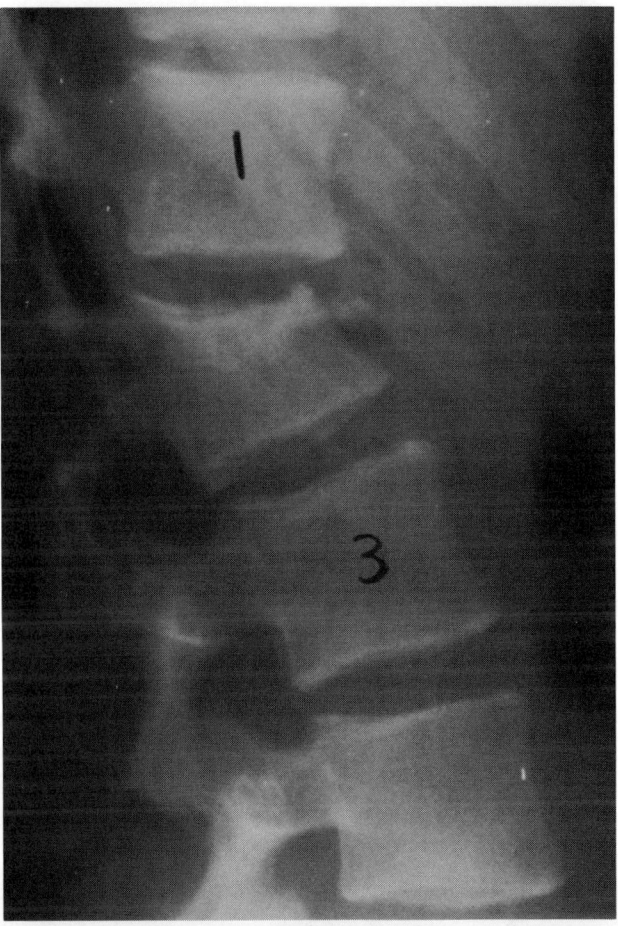

Figure 11-4 The lateral view of this seat-belt injury demonstrates that the spinous process pedicle and a portion of the vertebral body have been split in a tension mode. The anterior portion of the body of L-2 has been compressed slightly. This type of seat-belt injury has been named the Chance fracture. The patient in this case was neurologically intact and remained so after surgical treatment of this lesion.

spine. The anterior longitudinal ligament frequently tears off a flake of bone from one of the vertebral bodies (usually the superior one). This avulsion of bone may aid in diagnosing this injury, since it almost always spontaneously reduces. This dislocation is stable in flexion.

VERTICAL COMPRESSION FRACTURES

Vertical compression or axial load can be applied to those areas of the spine that are mobile enough to be made straight (cervical and lumbar spine). These are also the areas most likely to be axially loaded, the neck from trauma to the head and the lumbar spine due to lower extremity or buttock load-

178 EMERGENCY MEDICINE

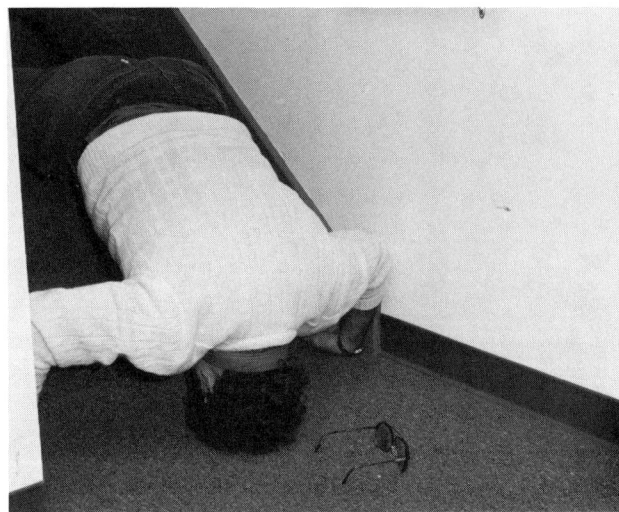

Figure 11-5 Axial loading of the cervical spine can result in an injury to C-1 if the spine is straight, or, if the neck is slightly flexed as in this case, injury to the vertebral body between C-3 and C-7. The sudden load on the cervical spine will cause the vertebra to burst as the disc explodes through the end plate. Frequently, the vertebral body will protrude posteriorly into the area of the spinal canal.

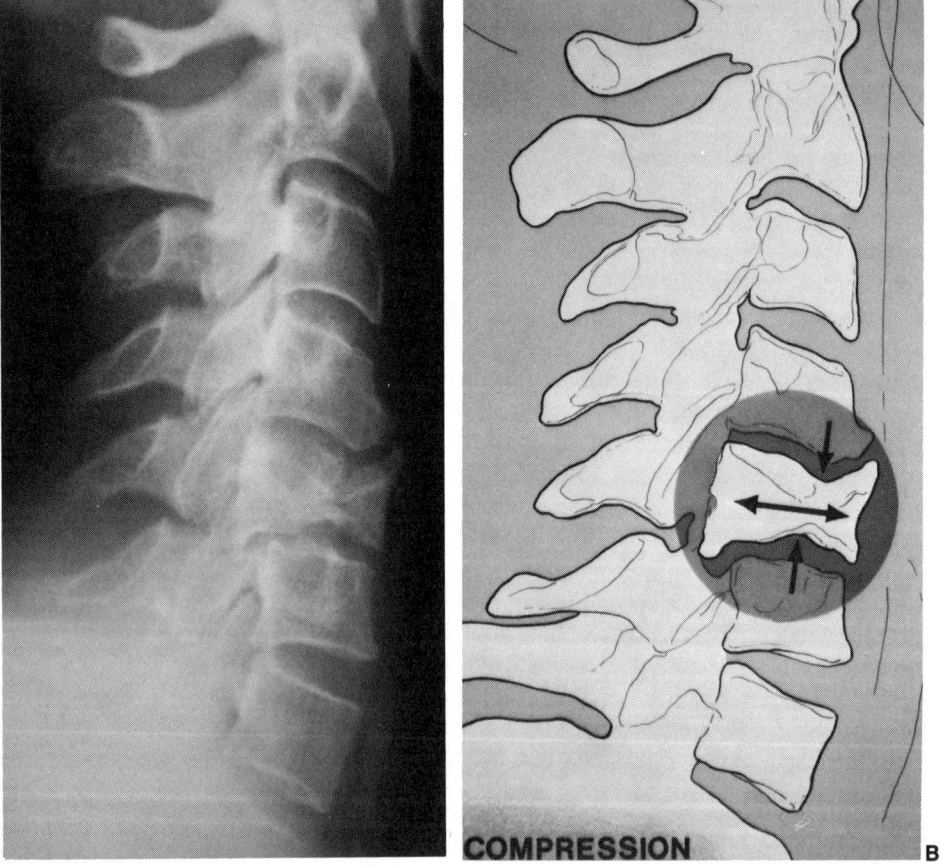

Figure 11-6 (A) The C-5 vertebra in this patient has been burst with some extrusion of the posterior vertebral wall into the spinal canal. Courtesy of George N. Ewing, MD. **(B)** An artist's interpretation of this picture demonstrates the mechanism of loading in the direction in which the portions of the vertebral body are expanded.

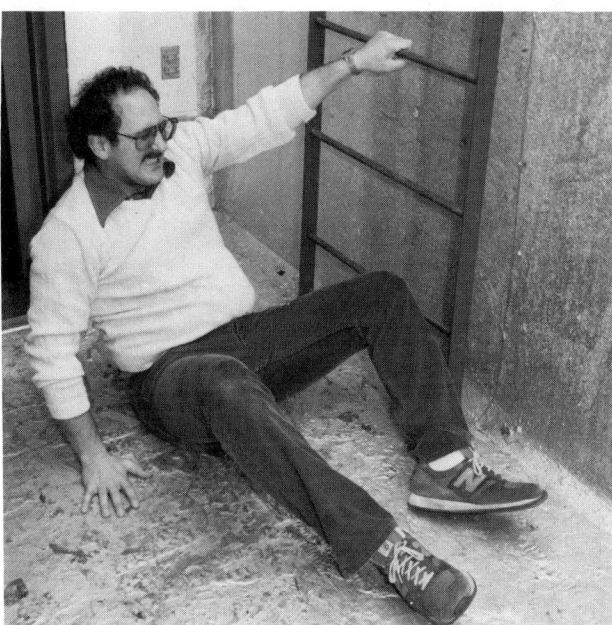

Figure 11-7 The lumbar spine can be axially loaded in a similar manner. In this case, the individual usually falls from a height or is thrown from a vehicle. He may either strike on his buttocks, such as this individual is demonstrating, or fall on his heels, first breaking his calcanei and then fracturing the lumbar spine, as the forces are directed more proximally. The association of fractured calcanei and lumbar spine is very high in the patient who has jumped or fallen from a height.

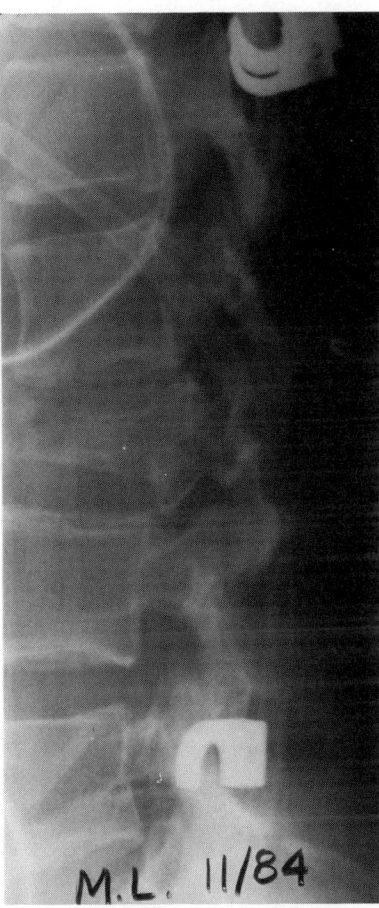

Figure 11-8 This is a lateral view of a young girl who was thrown a distance from her vehicle after it veered off the highway. The L-3 vertebra in this patient has been severely crushed anteriorly and the body exploded posteriorly into the spinal canal. This patient had almost a complete neurologic lesion, but had slight motion in both great toes prior to her treatment.

ing. In the upper cervical spine, the ring of C-1 is disrupted and widened (Jefferson's fracture). If the neck is slightly flexed (Fig. 11-5), the lower vertebral bodies (C-3 to C-7) absorb the sudden load and one of them (usually C-5 or C-6) will burst as the disc explodes through the end plate (Fig. 11-6). The ligaments remain intact, but the body is shattered and frequently driven back into the neural canal.

In the lumbar spine, the vertebral body fails in a similar manner (Fig. 11-7). In the past, these have frequently been confused with compression fractures, but they differ because the posterior portion of the vertebral body is fractured and frequently protrudes into the neural canal. Lateral roentgenograms will reveal the fracture of the posterior vertebral wall cortex, loss of posterior vertebral height, and even the retropulsion of bone into the neural canal (Fig. 11-8). On the AP roentgenogram the classic findings are increase of the interpediculate distance, vertical laminar fractures, and splaying of the posterior articular facet joints (Fig. 11-9). The CT scan is most helpful in these fractures, as it clearly defines the fracture of the posterior vertebral wall and its intrusion into the canal (Fig. 11-10). The laminar fractures and the splaying of the pedicles can also be seen. The degree of neural canal compromise can be determined, aiding in treatment decisions. The burst fractures in the thoracolumbar spine have been categorized by Denis into five types. This classification is not covered in this chapter.

SHEARING FRACTURES

A shearing fracture is specific for the thoracic spine. It occurs when a severe force is applied to the torso (such as being thrown from a motorcycle). It is frequently combined with an element of twist or rotation aiding in the rupture of ligaments and/or bone as one vertebral body is sheared from

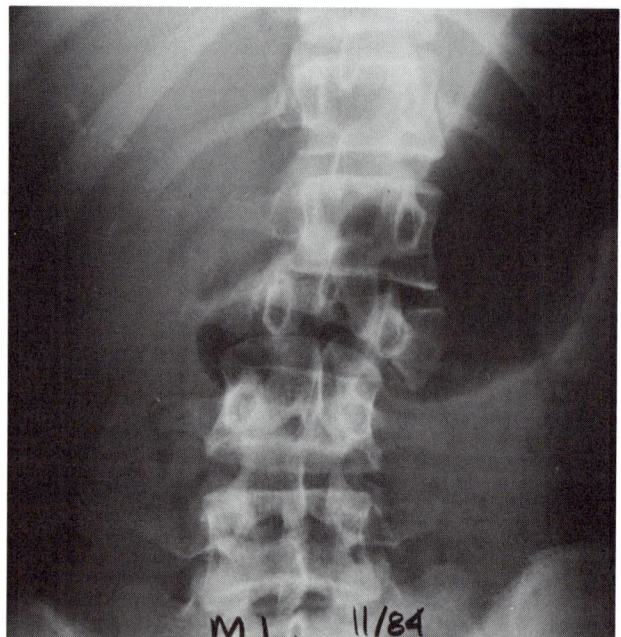

Figure 11-9 The AP radiograph of this same patient (Fig. 11-8) demonstrates the loss of height of the vertebral body, the spreading of the pedicular shadows, and the spreading of the posterior articular facet joints. In this case, the body has also shifted laterally on the vertebra below.

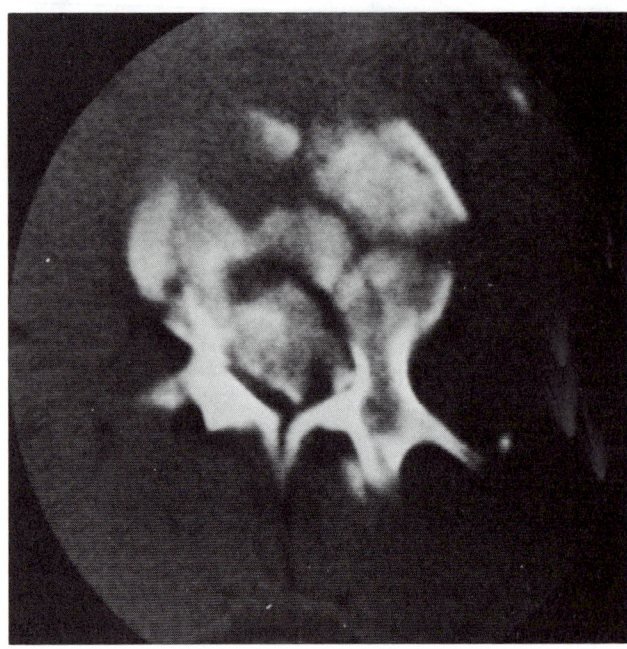

Figure 11-10 A CT scan of this same person (Fig. 11-8) demonstrates the massive amount of vertebral destruction and the amount of bone that has been forced into the spinal canal. In this case, almost the entire spinal canal has been occluded by bone fragments. The cauda equina, which is present at L-3, can be expected to be severely compromised as it was in this young girl. This patient had a posterior stabilization and an anterior vertebrectomy with removal of all bone from the spinal canal and a strut graft from L-2 to L-4. Because of the slight motor sparing in her great toes, which indicated an incomplete lesion, and because of her young age, she was very fortunate and recovered most of her neurologic function. She is now back in high school, ambulating without aids, and beginning to participate in sports.

the one immediately more caudal to it. This fracture-dislocation usually damages the spinal cord, resulting in partial or complete paraplegia. While the thoracic rib cage usually stabilizes these fractures, they may remain considerably displaced.

DIAGNOSIS

Delay in diagnosis of vertebral fractures in the emergency department is not uncommon. The delay in diagnosis ranges from hours to days to even months. The most common causes for missed diagnosis are associated head trauma, alcoholic or drug intoxication, and polytrauma. The patient who is comatose or intoxicated does not complain of vertebral fracture pain. Severe trauma in other areas distracts the examiner from proper examination of the spinal column.

There is a high correlation between head and neck pathology. Therefore, any evidence of head or facial trauma should suggest that cervical spine trauma may also have taken place. Similarly, chest, abdominal, or pelvic trauma might be associated with fractures of the thoracic or lumbar spine.

If conscious, the patient can frequently describe the mechanism of the injury. This provides information on the severity of the accident and the likelihood of fracture to the spinal column. Transient paralysis or even numbness or tingling of the extremities means that the spinal cord or its roots have been injured. Information on earlier conditions is also important, as the weakness or sensory loss discovered on physical examination may be the result of a previous injury or a cerebrovascular accident.

An important point to be considered is the amount of neurologic damage. Usually, the patient who has suffered complete paraplegia or quadriplegia receives intense scrutiny. While this is appropriate, the neurologic status is, in all likelihood, settled and irreversible. On the other hand, the patient with a vertebral fracture and transient or minimal or even normal neurologic findings is occasionally not provided the same careful examination and transport mechanism. The point is that these patients with incomplete neurologic injuries have the potential to either improve or, if injudiciously treated, to deteriorate neurologically. Therefore, if a vertebral injury is suspected, treat it as an unstable situation.

Physical Examination

Observation

The inability to move the neck or refusal to move the lower spine because of pain is a good clue that a fracture may be present. Lacerations or abrasions about the scalp, face, or torso demand that the vertebral column be carefully examined. Any voluntary motion of the arms, legs, feet, fingers, or toes should be recognized and recorded. Sustained penile erection indicates a severe spinal cord injury. The trunk should be examined for contusions, abrasions, or any evidence of trauma. In seat-belt fractures, frequently the belt leaves a band of ecchymosis just superior to the iliac spines.

Palpation

Without moving the patient, careful palpation of the entire cervical and thoracolumbar spine can be done, starting superiorly and working progressively down to the sacrum (Fig. 11-11). The spinous processes should be in a relatively straight line, evenly spaced and not painful. If a gap or offset is felt, rupture of the posterior ligamentous structures or fracture of the vertebral column is likely. If the damage is to the vertebral body, posterior palpation will usually produce some tenderness and may demonstrate paravertebral muscle spasm, with loss of the normal spinal contours. Fractures with severe displacement may have acute angulation (gibbus) at the level of the injury and should be considered highly unstable.

Neurologic Examination

In all cases of suspected injury to the vertebral column, an accurate and complete neurologic examination should be performed and recorded. A good initial neurologic examination is invaluable later in determining any changes and the ultimate neurologic prognosis. This is, without a doubt, the most important single diagnostic procedure that the emergency department physician can perform on the patient with spinal injury. He or she must take time to do it well. A neurologic form, if not available, should be developed to record the findings.

General Principles

The voluntary movement and grade of strength of the trunk and upper and lower extremity muscles are determined. Their strength is graded from zero through five. Zero strength indicates no muscular contraction; grade one (trace) indicates slight contraction without joint motion; grade two (poor), complete range of motion with gravity eliminated; grade three (fair), complete range of motion against gravity only; grade four (good), complete range of motion with some resistance; and grade five (normal), complete range of motion with full resistance.

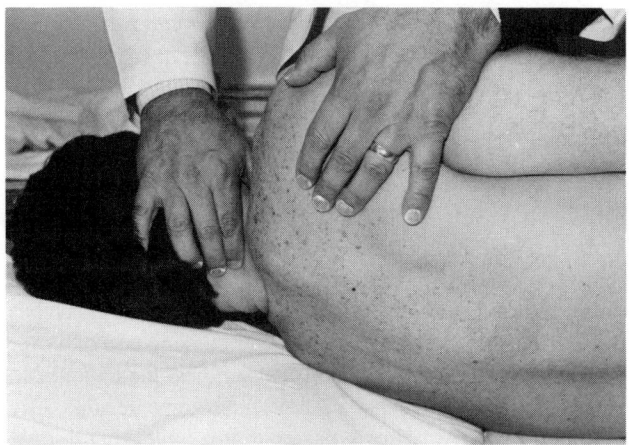

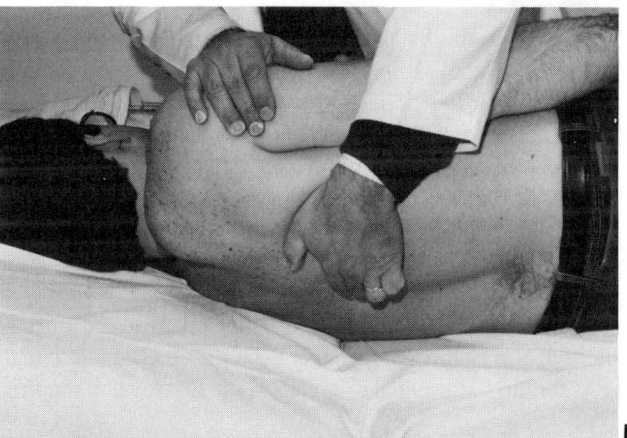

Figure 11-11 (**A**) Examination of the spine when injury is suspected can be done by rolling the patient very carefully from the back to the side. Palpation can then be started superiorly and progressively worked down from the cervical spine to the thoracic spine. (**B**) The entire thoracic and lumbar spine can be palpated for any tenderness, any spreading of the vertebral processes, or angulation of one vertebra on its neighbor. The back should also be inspected for any wounds or ecchymosis.

Elevation or separation of the costal margins with deep inspiration indicates intact intercostal muscles. Abdominal bulging or cephalad migration of the umbilicus when coughing suggests abdominal muscle paralysis. Any voluntary control of finger or toe movement is important to record, as this may be the only clinical sign that the neurologic lesion is incomplete. A digital rectal examination will reveal whether voluntary sphincter tone is intact or if it occurs when testing the bulbocavernosus reflex. This reflex can be tested by pulling on the urethral catheter (if one is present), squeezing the glans penis, or applying pressure to the clitoris. The deep tendon reflexes, abdominal cutaneous reflexes, and the cremasteric reflex should also be tested.

Paralyzed muscles with intact deep tendon reflexes indicate a spinal cord or upper motor neuron injury, while paralyzed muscles with absent deep tendon reflexes suggest cauda equina or nerve root injury. The latter has a much more favorable prognosis.

Initially, the examination of deep tendon reflexes may not be reliable, because post-traumatic spinal shock may create a temporary loss of all spinal reflexes. The absence of spinal reflexes due to spinal shock seldom lasts longer than 24 hours, and during this period the prognosis of neurologic recovery cannot be determined. If the bulbocavernosus reflex returns, this is a reliable sign that spinal shock has passed. If this reflex returns with no documentation of motor or sensory function in the lower extremities, the patient can be predicted to have a complete neurologic lesion. Any motor or sensory sparing indicates an incomplete neurologic lesion with some hope for recovery.

Sensory testing is less reliable because of its subjectivity and inconsistency. It should be done with particular attention being paid to the perianal area, where many spinal cord levels are represented. Presence of cutaneous sensation in this area might be the only evidence that a suspected complete lesion is, in fact, incomplete. The minimal sensory examination should include sharp-dull discrimination with a needle, light touch, deep pain, and proprioception. Any discrepancy between the two sides is important to note.

Thoracolumbar fractures notoriously produce a confusing picture. Holdsworth first clearly described the anatomic reasons for this. The spinal cord ends at the first level of the first

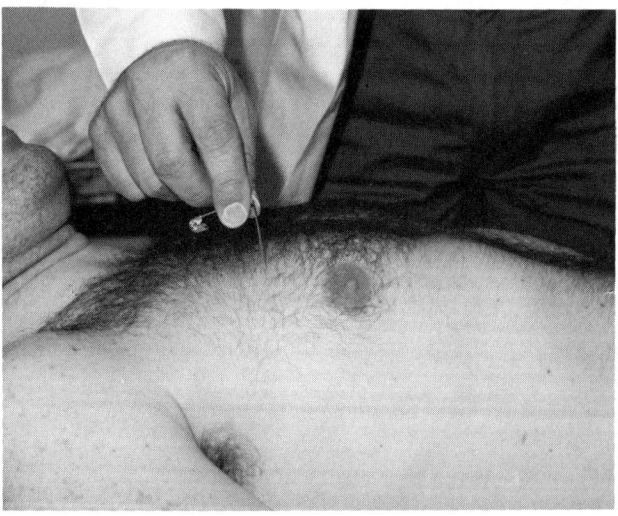

Figure 11-12 The sensory exam can be done using a pin, starting at the occiput and working progressively distal. The nipple line is represented by the level T-4 with T-3 just above it. In this case, the examiner is at the level of T-3. T-2 extends across the chest to the axillae. On the chest, just above T-2, is C-4, the area just beneath the clavicle. This can be confusing if the physician is not familiar with dermatome patterns. C-5 through T-1 are represented in the upper extremity.

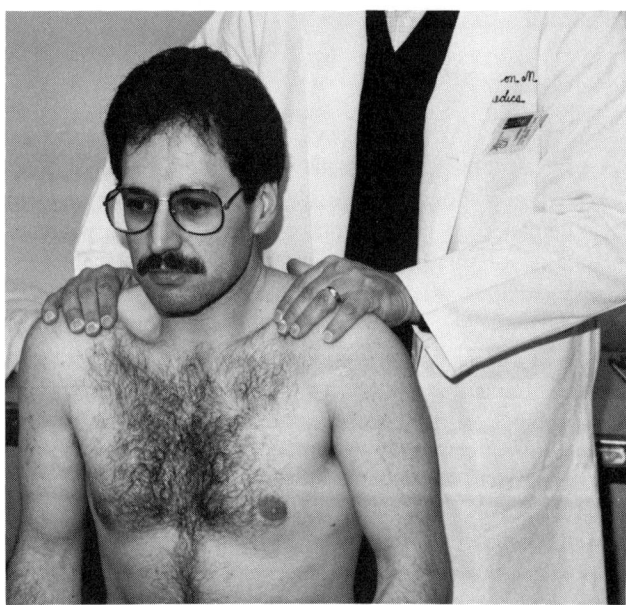

Figure 11-13 Function of the trapezius muscle indicates that the C-4 level is intact.

lumbar vertebra. The first sacral segment lies at the level of the upper part of L-1, and the first lumbar segment lies as high as T-10. Therefore, at the level of T12–L1 lie the spinal cord segments of L-5 and S-1 and all of the nerve roots (cauda equina) of the remaining lumbar levels (L1–L4). Thus, injury at this level could produce cord injury to the sacral segments and root damage to all the lumbar levels. The concept of mixed cord and root lesions explains why seemingly complete lesions at this level recover after a period of weeks or months (the sacral cord lesion remains while the roots recover).

Vital Signs

In the neurologically injured patient, the blood pressure may be low because of the spinal cord shock with its associated decreased vascular tone and absence of reflexes below the cord lesion (sympathectomy effect). Blood pressure may be in the 90/50 range in the traumatic paraplegic. This should not be confused with hemorrhagic shock, as the treatment is entirely different. The pulse rate is usually not elevated.

Sensory Examination

The sensory examination is done using a pin, starting at the occiput and working progressively distally. Dermatome charts are useful in determining the level of spinal cord injury. Sensation may be normal (sharp), oversensitive (hyperesthetic), decreased (hypesthetic), or absent (anesthetic). The nipple line is T-4 with T-3 just above, and T-2 extending across the chest to the axillae (Fig. 11-12). The

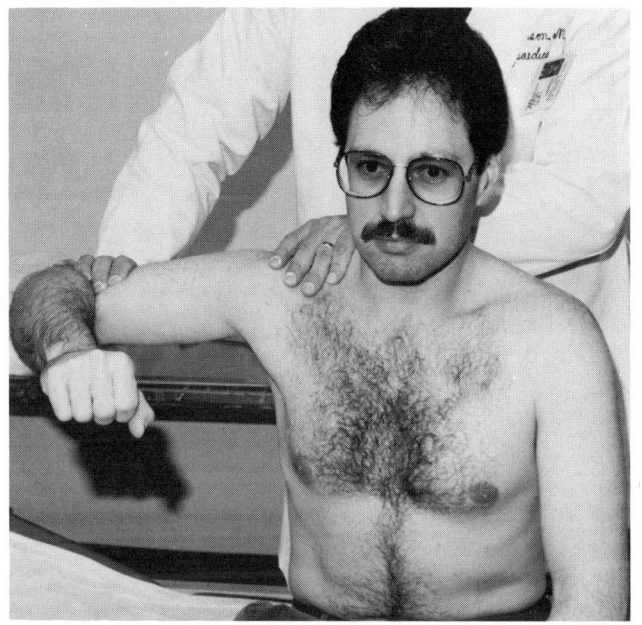
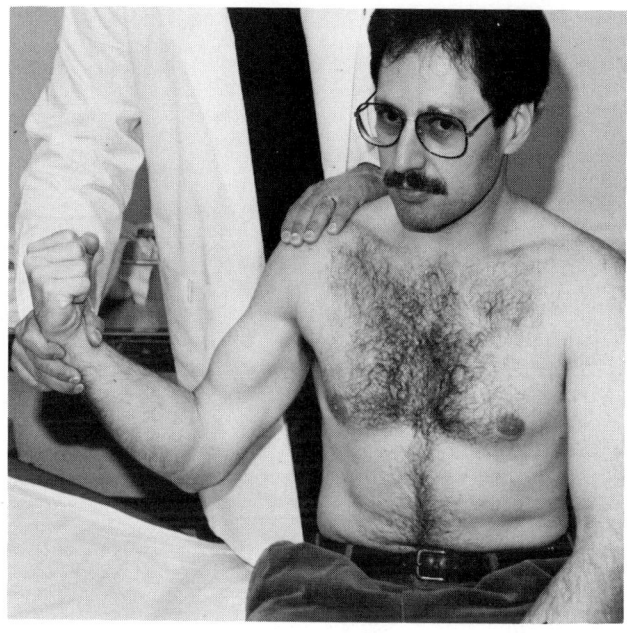

Figure 11-14 (A) Deltoid function can be tested by having the patient abduct his arm and seeing if he can maintain that abduction against resistance. The deltoid is the main muscular force holding this position. The deltoid is innovated by the C-5 nerve root. (B) C-5 is also represented by the biceps muscle and should be similarly tested against resistance.

inner arm and forearm are represented by T-1. On the chest above T-2 is C-4, the area just beneath the clavicle. This can be confusing if the examining physician is not familiar with the normal dermatome distribution. C-5 through T-1 are represented in the upper extremities.

Motor Function Examination

Motor testing is done starting at the shoulder and working into the lower extremities. Quadriplegia of above C-3 is rarely seen, since the diaphragm is paralyzed and the patient cannot breathe independently. An active diaphragm and sternocleidomastoid and trapezius muscles confirm that the C-4 level is intact (Fig. 11-13). Deltoid and biceps functions are present if C-5 is intact (Fig. 11-14); active supination and wrist extension indicate function of C-6 (Fig. 11-15); functioning pronator teres, flexor carpi radialis, triceps, and finger extensors indicate that C-7 is intact (Fig. 11-16); and flexor digitorum sublimi or profundi function activity suggest C-8 activity (Fig. 11-17). The intrinsic function requires that the T-1 root is intact (Fig. 11-18).

In the lower extremities, the hip flexion requires that at least L-1 through L-3 be intact; knee extension, L-3 and L-4 (Fig. 11-19); knee flexion, L-4, L-5 (medial hamstrings) and L-5, S-1 (lateral hamstrings; Fig. 11-20); ankle dorsiflexion (anterior tibial), L-4, L-5 (Fig. 11-21); and plantar flexion, S-1 (Fig. 11-22). The level of spinal cord injury is defined as the first functioning segment.

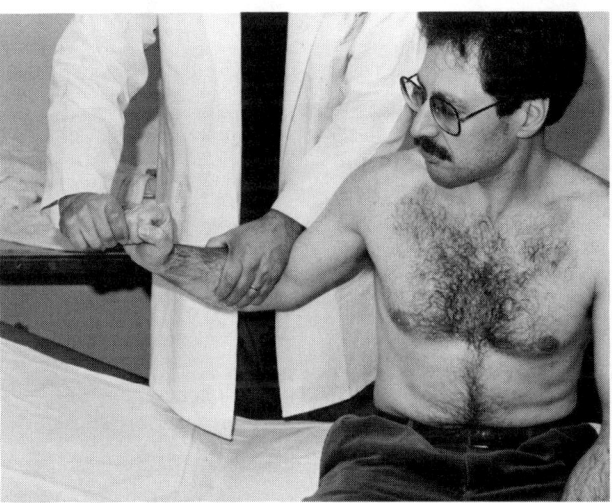

Figure 11-15 The ability to actively extend the wrist and to supinate the forearm indicate that the C-6 level is intact.

INCOMPLETE NEUROLOGIC LESIONS

Injury to the spinal cord can be complete or incomplete. Although most of the incomplete lesions are mixed, there are several well-described syndromes. A sparing distal to the injury constitutes an incomplete lesion, and therefore some recovery is possible.

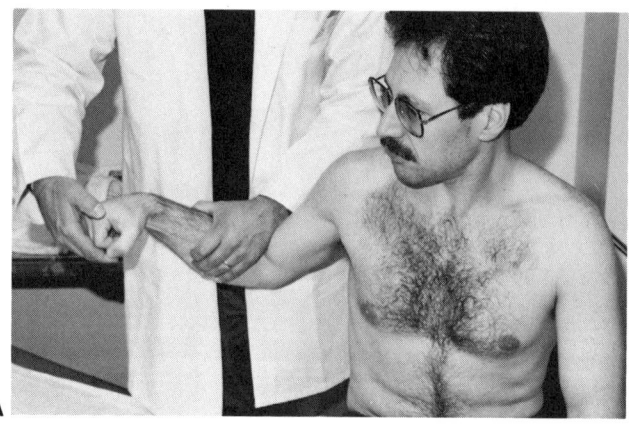
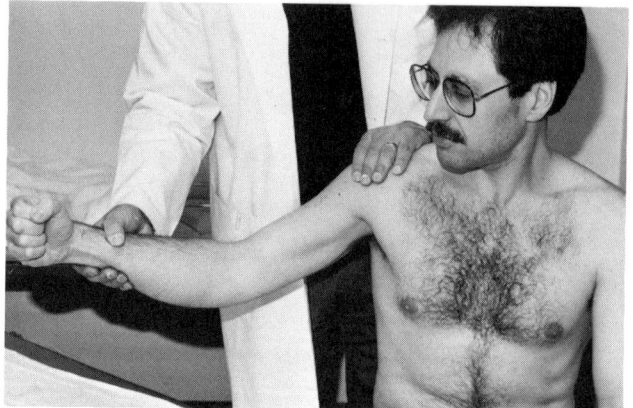

Figure 11-16 (**A**) Activity of the flexor carpi radialis and finger extensors indicates that C-7 is intact. (**B**) The triceps, if active against resistance, indicates that C-7 is intact.

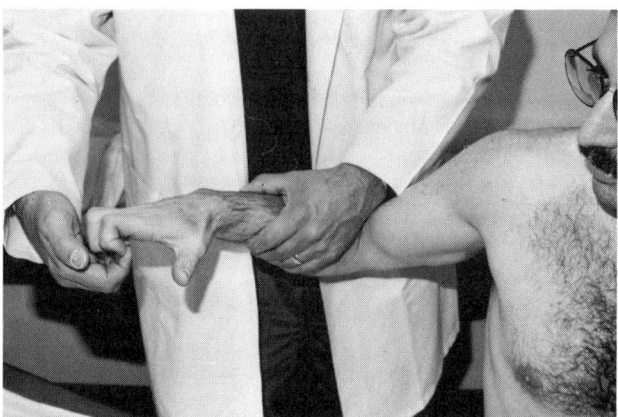

Figure 11-17 The ability to contract the flexor digitorum sublimi or profunda indicates that the C-8 level is intact.

Figure 11-18 Intrinsic function of the hand is best demonstrated by having the patient actively spread the fingers. The interosseous muscle on the radial side of the index finger is being palpated by the examiner's index finger. If this contracts actively, one can assume that the T-1 root is intact.

Root Injury

Individual nerve roots can be damaged at the neural foramen, and because they are peripheral nerves, they are expected to recover. Avulsion can occur in the brachial or lumbosacral plexi but would require fairly severe trauma.

Brown-Sequard Syndrome

An injury to either side of the spinal cord produces ipsilateral muscle paralysis and contralateral hypesthesia to pain and temperature. This syndrome has a good prognosis for recovery, with most patients regaining bowel and bladder control and the ability to walk.

Central Cord Syndrome

This is the most common incomplete spinal cord syndrome and is usually associated with hyperextension injuries in the osteoarthritic spine. The roentgenogram may not demonstrate any fractures or dislocations, but the patient has neurologic damage. The patient presents with spastic paralysis of the lower extremities and the trunk. The sacral tracts, which are located more peripherally in the cord, are usually spared. The prognosis for recovery is only fair in this syndrome. The patients usually recover motor and sensory power to the legs and trunk, but recovery of hand function is poor. The expected result is spastic gait with ambulation and recovery of bowel and bladder control.

Anterior Cord Syndrome

This is an injury to the anterior two-thirds of the spinal cord and is heralded by a quadriplegia that is complete in the lower extremities but incomplete in the upper extremities.

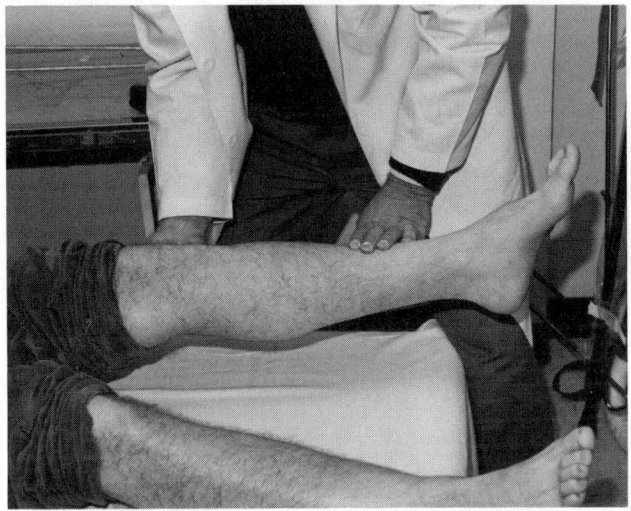

Figure 11-19 Knee extension, which is active, indicates that the L-3 and L-4 roots are intact.

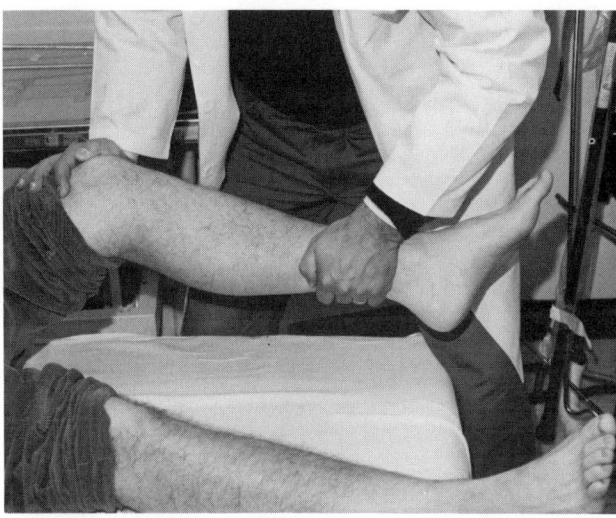

Figure 11-20 Knee flexion is represented by L-4, L-5, which are the medial hamstrings, and L-5, S-1, which are the lateral hamstrings.

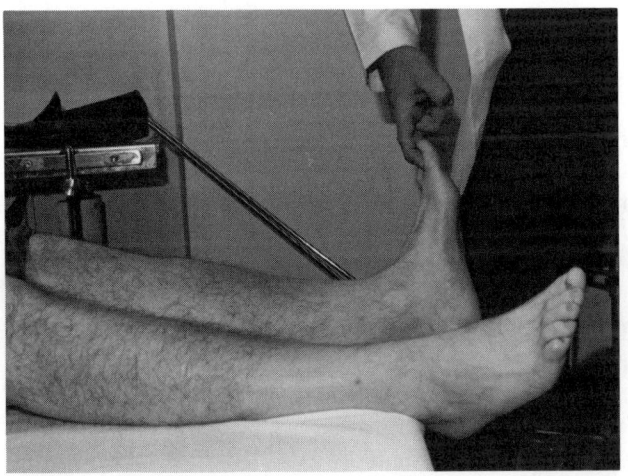

Figure 11-21 Ankle dorsiflexion and dorsiflexion of the great toe indicate function of L-4, L-5.

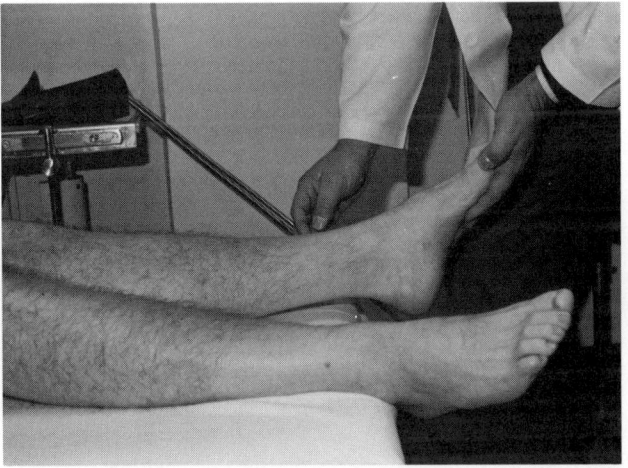

Figure 11-22 Plantar flexion of the foot indicates function of the S-1 root. The level of spinal cord injury is defined as the first functioning segment.

The posterior columns are spared to a degree, enabling the patient to feel deep pressure and retain proprioception in the legs. This injury is common in patients with ankylosing spondylitis resulting from a neck fracture. The prognosis for recovery is poor.

Posterior Cord Syndrome

This syndrome consists of loss of deep pressure, deep pain, and proprioception only. The patient will have fully voluntary involvement, pain, and temperature sensation throughout the body. The gait will be normal except for a slapping of the feet (proprioceptive loss) similar to that seen in tabes dorsalis.

ROENTGENOGRAPHIC DIAGNOSIS

The minimal roentgenographic views of a suspected spinal injury are anterior and lateral views. By careful manipulation of the X-ray equipment or log-rolling the patient as a unit, these views can almost always be safely obtained. The lower cervical spine and the upper levels of the thoracic spine are particularly difficult to visualize and may require tomography for clarification. Oblique or spot views may help to completely evaluate a suspicious area.

The roentgenograms are examined for any evidence of bony comminution, anterior-posterior or lateral displacement, fracture of the neural arch or transverse processes, and

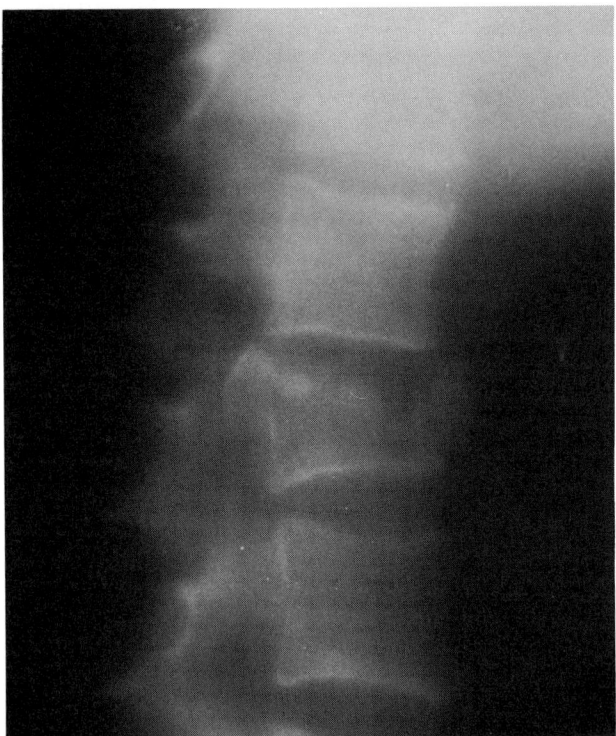

Figure 11-23 The posterior portion of the vertebral wall is scrutinized on the lateral view. In this instance, a tomogram demonstrates that the superior posterior part of this vertebral body has been extruded into the spinal canal.

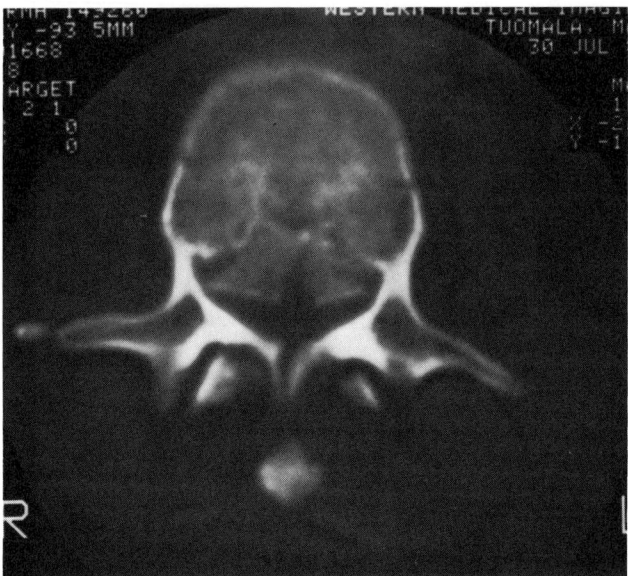

Figure 11-24 CT has been very helpful in evaluating any suspected intrusion of fragments into the spinal canal. This demonstrates bony fragments which have been pushed posteriorly and have occluded almost two-thirds of this spinal canal at L-2.

loss of normal vertebral contours (ie, cervical lordosis, thoracic kyphosis, or lumbar lordosis). The posterior portion of the vertebral body, if fractured, is scrutinized for displacement at the neural canal (Fig. 11-23). CT can assist in the evaluation of the suspected intrusion of fragments into the canal (Fig. 11-24). At times, the addition of metrizamide can help in determining the relationship of the neural elements to the bony and soft tissue compromise of the spinal canal. A myelogram is rarely indicated, unless there is neurologic deficit and no apparent skeletal damage. An unsuspected acute herniated disc may be detected by this study. In the evaluation of the cervical spine, every effort should be made to visualize all seven levels. This may require mild cervical traction, combined with depression of the arms.

The upper cervical spine is best evaluated using an open-mouth or odontoid view to visualize fractures of both the ring of C-1 and the dens. The lateral roentgenogram is also studied for soft tissue injury. Using a bright light, the distance between individual spinous processes can be evaluated. Any abnormal widening between spinous processes indicates tearing of the supraspinous and interspinous ligaments and potential instability of the spine. The prevertebral fascia anterior to C2–3 is thin and should not be greater than 7 mm. Anterior to C-4 and C-5 the soft tissue shadow includes the perilaryngeal muscles and the esophagus. The thickness varies from 9 to 22 mm. Widening suggests bleeding into the prevertebral space, secondary to the injury (Fig. 11-25).

Once a fracture or soft tissue lesion is detected, it can be further evaluated by more specific roentgenographic studies. In 10% of vertebral fractures, more than one level is involved. If all roentgenographic studies are interpreted as normal and yet vertebral injury is suspected, the patient should *not* be discharged from the emergency department until flexion-extension films are obtained. If these show no abnormal motion, it is probably safe to send the patient home to be followed in a clinic situation.

DIFFERENTIAL ROENTGENOGRAPHIC DIAGNOSIS

Old compression fractures, congenital scoliosis or kyphosis, and Scheuermann's disease can all be confused with acute trauma. Congenital scoliosis (hemivertebra) usually will have an extra pedicle or rib. Congenital kyphosis, which is caused by a congenitally absent vertebral body, may be hard to differentiate from an acute fracture. Tomography may help to define the deformity. Scheuermann's disease typically involves more than one, and usually several, vertebral levels with the production of anterior wedging and irregular end plates. An old compression fracture is perhaps the most difficult of differential diagnoses to make. The area of involvement should be nontender unless superimposed

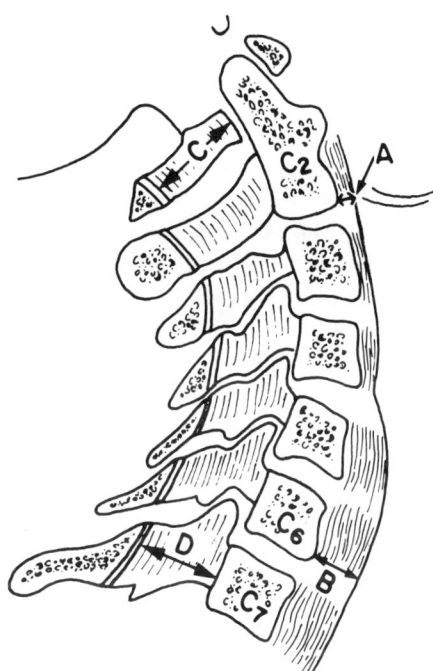

Figure 11-25 The soft tissue spaces anterior to the cervical spine can be determined on the lateral cervical roentgenogram. A fracture or dislocation with bleeding can cause the soft tissue spaces to widen. The retropharyngeal soft tissue space (A) averages 3.5 mm (range, 2 to 7 mm) in children under 15 years of age and 3.4 mm (range, 1 to 7 mm) in adults. This is measured from the anterior-inferior aspect of the second cervical vertebra to the posterior wall of the pharynx. The retrotracheal space (B) measures 7.9 mm (range, 5 to 14 mm) in children and 14.0 mm (range, 9 to 22 mm) in adults. Drawing and information are based on material published by O'Rahilly and Benson in *The Pediatric Spine*, Bradford and Hensinger (eds), New York, Thieme-Stratton, Inc. *Source:* Reprinted with permission from DS Bradford, RM Hensinger (eds): *The Pediatric Spine*. New York, Thieme-Stratton, Inc, 1985, p 13.

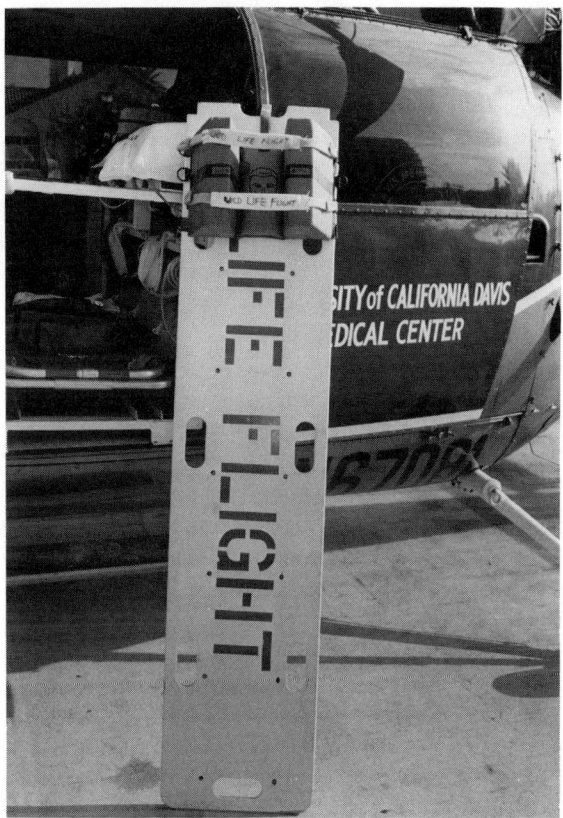

Figure 11-26 A patient with a suspected spinal injury should be lifted as a unit or logrolled onto a hard surface structure or spine board. This spine board is shown standing outside the Life Flight helicopter used by the University of California, Davis, to transport patients from the scene of an accident. The head and neck can be stabilized using the apparatus, shown above, and held in a relatively stable position. The pads come alongside the head bilaterally to keep it from shifting or rolling from side to side.

trauma has occurred. A ^{99m}Tc bone scan will be positive if the fracture is new and negative if it is old.

TREATMENT

Suspected injury to the vertebral column should be treated as an unstable fracture from the scene of the accident until the final roentgenographic analysis is complete and a diagnosis made. An assessment of the circumstances of the injury may be helpful in evaluating the spine. Directly after the injury, the patient may be able to relate transient neurologic symptoms that are later forgotten.

The patient should be lifted as a unit by several persons or logrolled onto a hard stretcher or spineboard (Fig. 11-26). The body, including the head and neck, can be stabilized with straps or tape. When the patient reaches the emergency department, similar methods are used for transfer to the emergency department cart or X-ray table. Acting too hurriedly in retrieving ambulance equipment or obtaining roentgenograms may place the patient's spine in jeopardy.

Other organ systems are frequently injured when the vertebral column is fractured. The head, chest, ribs, abdomen, and genitourinary system should all be examined. Fractures of the thoracolumbar and lumbar spine will create a transient ileus with cessation of bowel sounds. Therefore, the patient should not be given anything by mouth until the gastrointestinal tract is functioning normally.

Medications are given basically to control the pain and anxiety of the patient. Systemic steroids have been proven helpful in spinal cord injury but are potentially harmful. If the fracture is open (penetrating injuries), antibiotics are started after cultures have been taken. These usually consist of a cephalosporin and an aminoglycoside (gentamicin), which are given intravenously. Tetanus toxoid is given if there is no history of the patient having received it in the past 6 years.

In the cervical spine, realignment of the bony fragments or reduction of the dislocated vertebra is important and emergent only if there is progressive neurologic loss. Reduction and maintenance of the obtained reduction are best done with cranial tongs. Gardner-Wells tongs are currently the most widely used because of their effectiveness and ease of application (Fig. 11-27). Traction can be applied through a cranial halo, which later can be connected to a cast or vest as definitive stabilization. Progressive weight, which is applied under roentgenographic control, will reduce most fractures and dislocations in the cervical spine. If reduction does not readily occur, surgical manipulation may be necessary.

Most thoracolumbar fractures can be nursed on a regular hospital bed, although some doctors prefer a turning (Stryker) frame. Turning the patient from side to back to side should be done every 2 hours to prevent pressure areas. This is especially true in the elderly or neurologically impaired patient.

Neurologic examinations are repeated frequently during the first 24 hours to detect any change (for better or worse). The vital signs need to be monitored because spinal injury can affect the blood pressure. If transfer to another facility is necessary, it can be done after the patient is stable. Surgical treatment for any vertebral fracture is usually not an emergency. Total paraplegia or quadriplegia that is unchanged, or a myelographic block, is not an indication to do an immediate laminectomy. The only absolute indication for immediate decompression and/or stabilization is neurologic deterioration or an open fracture.

SPECIFIC INJURIES

Dislocations

Atlanto-occipital dislocation occurs when a violent twisting force tears all the ligaments connecting the occipital to the ring of C-1 (Fig. 11-28). If the patient survives (which is rare), this dislocation should be considered highly unstable. Rigid immobilization, but without traction, is the treatment of choice. The head should be sandbagged for emergency stability until a halo vest can be applied. This injury will ultimately require fusion of the occiput to C-2.

C1–2 dislocation can occur in a variety of ways. Rupture of the transverse ligament can occur with or without fracture of the ring of C-1 (Jefferson's fracture). The atlas–dens interval should not exceed 3.5 mm in the child or 2.5 mm in the adult (Fig. 11-29). An interval greater than 4 mm should alert the examiner to possible rupture of the ligament. Con-

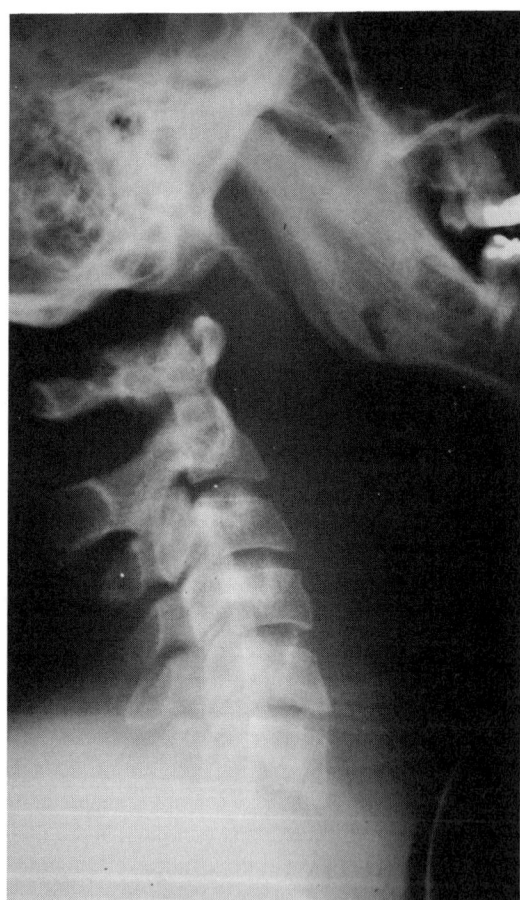

Figure 11-28 Atlanto-occipital dislocations occur when a violent twisting force tears all the ligaments connecting the occiput to the ring of C-1. This injury is noted in the radiograph of this patient, who was having respiratory problems on arrival at the emergency room and subsequently died because of the extent of her injuries.

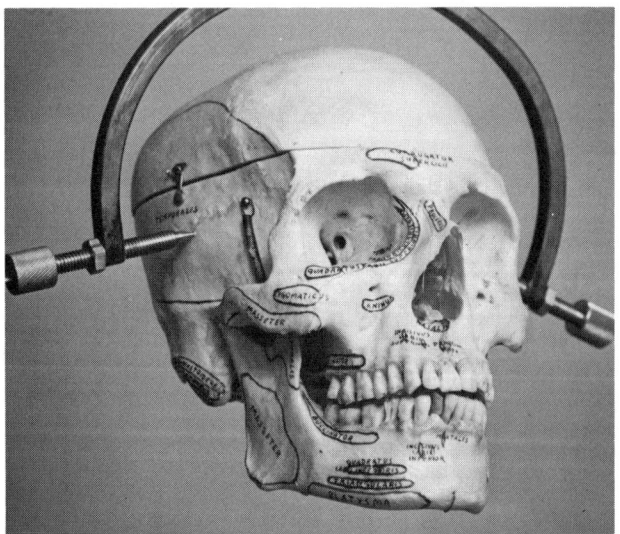

Figure 11-27 Gardner-Wells tongs are currently the most widely used traction device, because they are extremely easy to apply and traction for reduction or stabilization can be applied through the device.

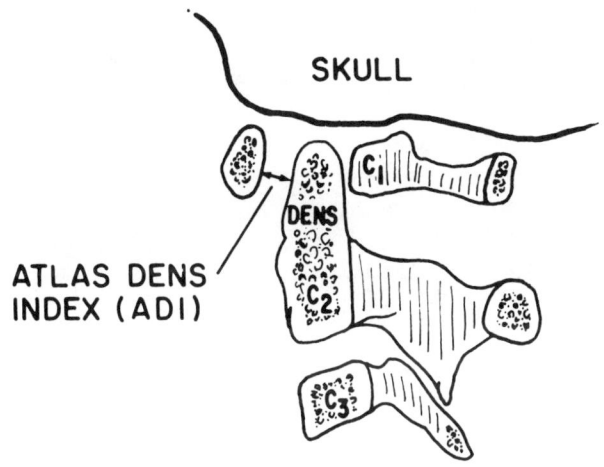

Figure 11-29 The atlas–dens interval should not exceed 4 mm in the child (3 to 15 years) or 2.5 mm in the adult. An interval greater than 4 mm should alert the examiner to the possibility of rupture of the transverse ligament. This suggests an unstable spine. The child's interval is larger than the adult's because a great deal of the dens is made up of cartilage, which makes the measurement apparently larger because the cartilage is not visualized on radiographs. Drawing and information are based on material published by O'Rahilly and Benson in *The Pediatric Spine,* Bradford and Hensinger (eds), New York, Thieme-Stratton, Inc. *Source:* Reprinted with permission from DS Bradford, RM Hensinger, (eds): *The Pediatric Spine.* New York, Thieme-Stratton, Inc, 1985, p 13.

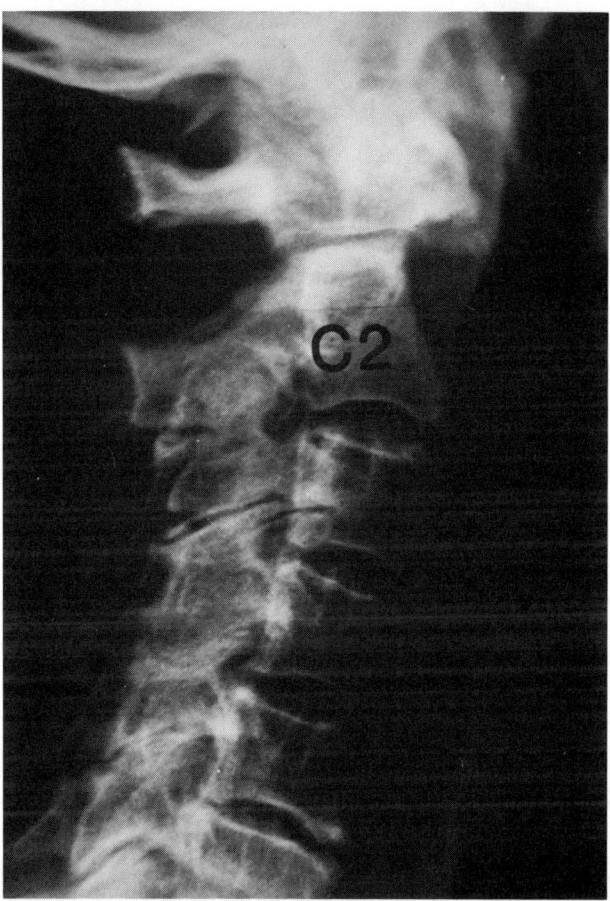

Figure 11-30 Anterior dislocation of C-1 on C-2 can occur with the fracture of the dens. In this case, the dens and the ring of C-1 are shifted anteriorly on the body of C-2.

trolled flexion-extension lateral roentgenograms can be used to confirm the diagnosis. A CT scan may be helpful to determine the extent of the injury. This lesion is dangerous because it allows the dens to migrate posteriorly into the spinal cord. The head and neck should be stabilized with or without traction until a C1–2 fusion can be accomplished. This should be done with the head in extension to effect reduction of the dens against the anterior ring of C-1.

Anterior dislocation secondary to a fracture through the base of the dens can occur (Fig. 11-30). This is basically a bony injury and should heal if immobilized. The fracture is reduced with tongs or halo traction with the neck in extension. This can be maintained for an extended period using a halo cast or vest.

A posterior dislocation of C1–2 can occur due to a blow in the submental area. The anterior ring of the atlas is lifted over the dens and settles posterior to it. The treatment is reduction using longitudinal traction, then extension-flexion manipulation under roentgenographic control. The transverse ligament remains intact; hence prolonged immobilization in a halo body jacket will usually accomplish stability. If not, a C1–2 fusion can be performed later.

Rotary subluxation of C-1 or C-2 occurs when excessive rotary force causes the inferior facet of C-1 to slip anterior to the superior facet of C-2. The facets become fixed, and the patient has marked limitation of motion and pain when attempting to rotate the head. The typical roentgenographic finding is asymmetry of the dens on the open-mouth view. The CT scan is particularly helpful in confirming this dislocation. Traction is usually helpful in both controlling the pain and reducing the facets. All C1–2 dislocations are treated for 12 weeks in a halo jacket. If instability persists, bony fusion is strongly considered.

Dislocations of the lower cervical spine are due to flexion-rotation forces. The posterior ligamentous complex is ruptured, thus allowing the facets and disc to dislocate. The roentgenographic signs of dislocation include loss of alignment of the posterior aspect of the vertebral bodies. Because of overlapping, the facets may be hard to visualize in a unilateral dislocation but can easily be seen in bilateral facet dislocations. On flexion, each vertebral body normally moves 2 to 3 mm forward on the one just inferior to it. However, in neutral there should be no displacement and the posterior edge of each vertebral body should line up. Oblique views, or even oblique tomograms, may offer the best view of the facet dislocation. Usually, a unilateral facet dislocation allows anterior subluxation up to 25% of the width of the inferior vertebral body (Fig. 11-31). Bilateral facet dislocations allow up to 50% displacement (Fig. 11-32). Bilateral dislocations are frequently combined with severe neurologic damage.

Treatment consists of reducing the dislocation as rapidly as possible to allow the spinal cord as much freedom as possible. Skull tongs or a halo ring should be applied with traction in a longitudinal direction. Under roentgenographic control, starting with 20 pounds, more and more weight is applied. Over the course of 1 to 2 hours, up to 45 pounds can be applied. It is usually said that reduction requires 10 pounds for the head and 5 pounds for each cervical vertebra above the dislocation. A C-6 or C-7 dislocation would, thus, require 40 or 45 pounds to reduce. This, of course, varies with the size and age of the patient. This should *not* be done in an unsupervised setting. If reduction cannot be accomplished in the emergency department in a few hours, then open reduction and fusion will probably be required. On occasion, under anesthesia, the spine can be gently manipulated, reducing the dislocation. Closed reductions need to be immobilized for 12 weeks, then checked for stability with flexion-extension films. If stability is in question, it should be accomplished by posterior cervical fusion of the vertebra involved. Sometimes this is done as a primary procedure to avoid the necessity for a long-term halo jacket.

Fractures

A fracture of the ring of C-1 has been named Jefferson's fracture. It is the result of an axial load on the top of the head (eg, diving into a pool). The force of C-1 causes it to fracture anterior and posterior to the facets, widening the ring. Because there is no encroachment on the spinal cord, neurologic injury is usually not a problem. On plain roentgenograms, the diagnosis can be difficult. The AP view may show a lateral shift of the C-1 lateral masses, in relation to the occipital condyles and the C-2 facets. If on this view the overhang of C-1 and C-2 is greater than 7 mm (measured from the outer aspect of C-1 to the outer aspect of C-2 on both sides and the measurements added together), then the transverse ligament is likely to be ruptured. This combination makes it an unstable fracture. A CT scan best shows the extent of the fractures. In most cases, this is a stable situation and is treated with traction until the pain subsides. A halo jacket is then used for 6 to 8 weeks, followed by a cervical brace for an additional 6 weeks. Most cervical fractures are immobilized for a total of 12 weeks.

Odontoid (dens) fractures have been grouped into three types. Type one involves avulsion of the tip by the alar ligaments. Type two are fractures through the isthmus or neck of the dens, superior to the body of C-2. Type three are fractures extending into the body of C-2. Type one is a stable fracture, since the majority of the dens remains intact. Type

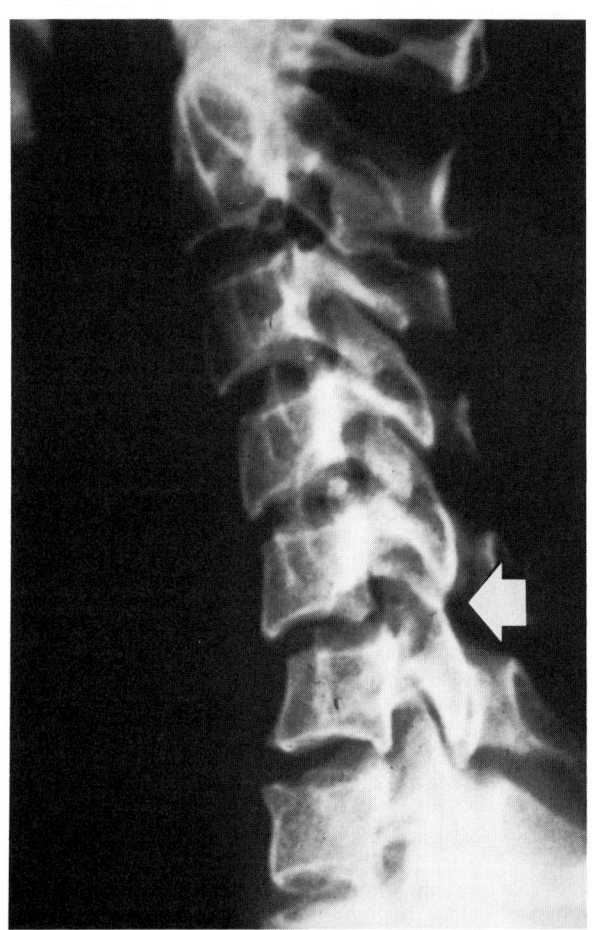

Figure 11-31 A unilateral facet dislocation on routine radiographs is difficult to diagnose because the facet joints tend to overlap and the dislocation can be overlooked. Usually a unilateral facet dislocation will allow the superior vertebra to migrate slightly anterior on the inferior vertebra. This will not exceed 25% of the vertebra width if it is only a unilateral facet dislocation. In this case, C-5 has migrated approximately that amount on C-6. One should also note that the normal cervical lordosis has been lost.

two is unstable and is in some risk of not healing, particularly if it is displaced (more than 4 mm) and if the patient is older than 50 years. Type three fractures heal fairly consistently with immobilization. Diagnosis is made with AP (open-mouth view) and lateral roentgenography. Questionable fractures can be confirmed using tomograms. Treatment is reduction and immobilization for 12 weeks in a halo jacket. Type one fractures need only symptomatic treatment and a soft collar. If the fracture is unhealed at 12 weeks, posterior cervical fusion of C-1 to C-2 is considered. Flexion-extension films will demonstrate abnormal motion of C-1 or C-2. If an unhealed fracture and motion or pain on motion are present at 12 weeks, fusion is probably the treatment of choice.

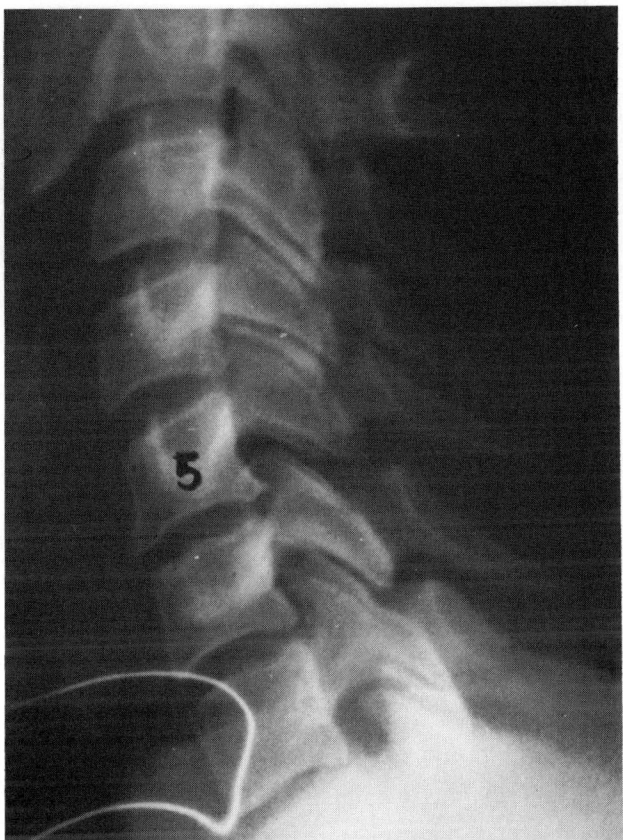
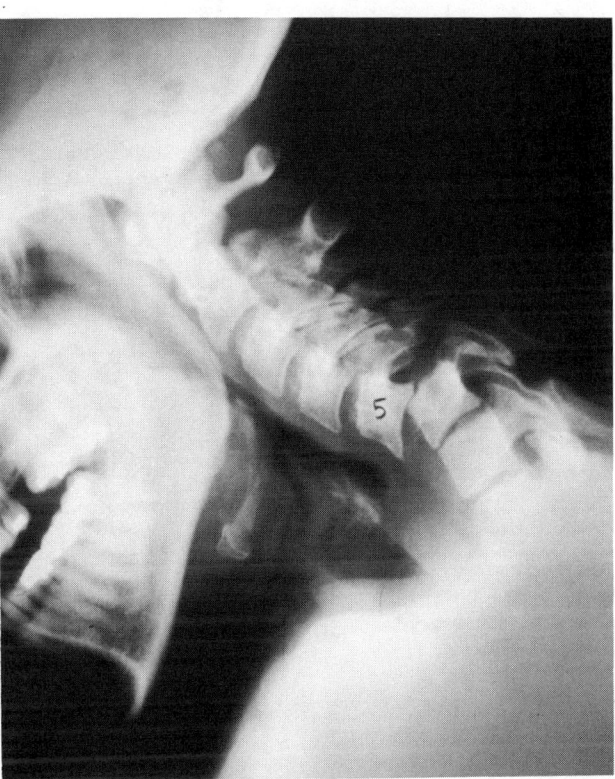

Figure 11-32 (**A**) This view demonstrates the cervical spine in a patient after a rather severe injury to her face and neck. She had a large scalp laceration, which drew attention away from her cervical spine. The apparently normal lateral roentgenogram was not repeated until 6 weeks later, even though the patient complained of severe neck pain. (**B**) Flexion view taken 6 weeks after injury demonstrated the true extent of this patient's injuries, a bilateral facet dislocation. This allowed the superior vertebra to migrate considerably forward. This patient was placed in traction and had surgical fusion with a good result. Fortunately, she had no neurologic damage; most bilateral dislocations are associated with severe neurologic injury.

Fractures through pars interarticularis of C-2 are known as hangman's fractures. These occur when the neck is in extension and a force is placed on the head forcing the occiput into the posterior elements of the atlas and axis, producing a fracture of the pars (head striking a windshield; Fig. 11-33). This fracture allows the body of C-2 to slide anteriorly with the remainder of the cervical spine, giving it the name "traumatic spondylolisthesis." The neural canal is not compromised by this fracture, and it will almost always heal. Roentgenographic diagnosis can be made in the lateral film or with tomograms. Treatment is reduction (if displaced) with traction, followed by halo cast or vest immobilization.

Flexion combined with axial load on the cervical spine produces a comminuted or burst fracture of the lower cervical vertebral bodies. (This injury is sometimes called a "teardrop" fracture, not to be confused with the extension fracture of the cervical spine where a piece of the body is avulsed by the anterior longitudinal ligament.) The burst fracture is a very unstable injury and is likely to be associated with neurologic damage. The most frequent levels are C-5

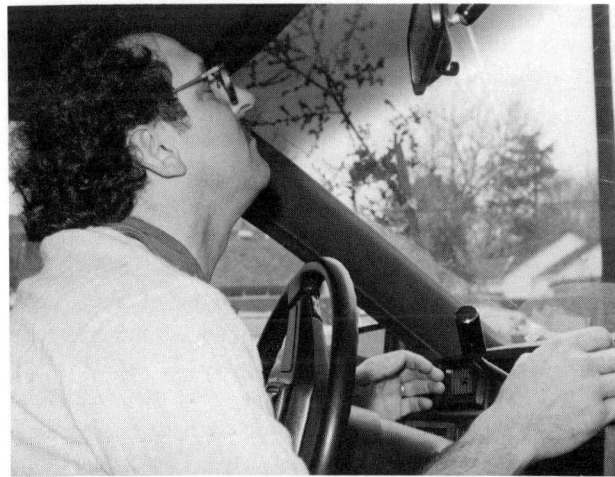

Figure 11-33 The hangman's fracture occurs when the head is axially loaded in extension, such as is demonstrated in this photograph when the head strikes the windshield. This forces the right of C-1 posteriorly into the pars interarticularis of C-2, fracturing it.

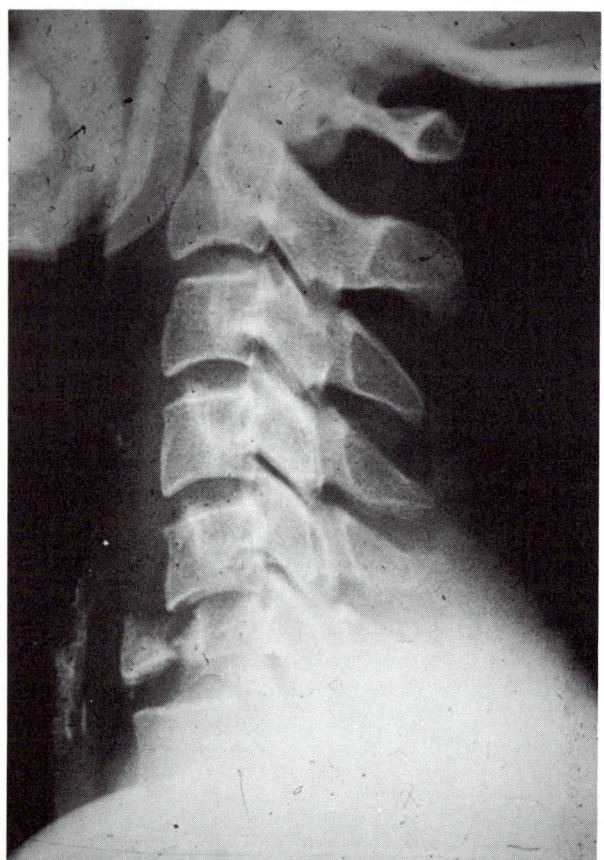

Figure 11-34 A lateral radiograph in the axially loaded cervical spine demonstrates that the vertebral body has been exploded anteriorly and posteriorly with loss of vertebral height.

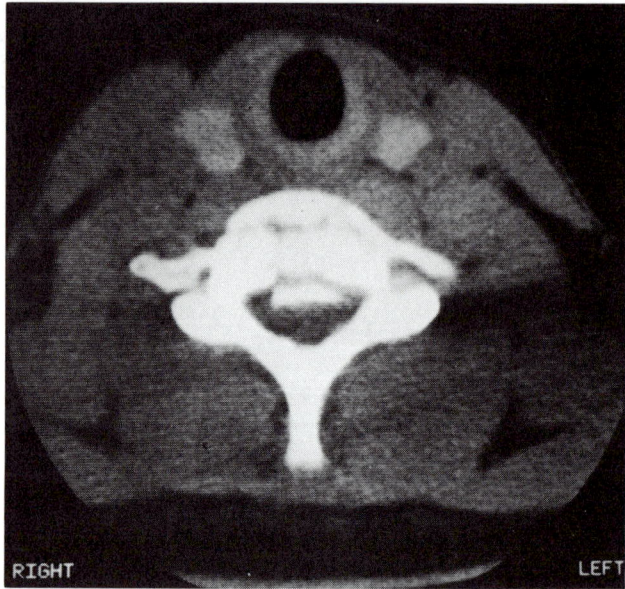

Figure 11-35 The CT scan demonstrates the damage to the vertebral body of C-6, with extrusion of bone into the spinal canal. This patient had a severe neurologic injury.

and C-6, which are the most flexible. These are the fractures seen in the individual who strikes his head diving into shallow water, or in the football linebacker who spears a runner with his helmet. All too frequently the young person is paralyzed, perhaps justifying the "teardrop" designation. The neurologic damage occurs because bone is pushed back into the spinal canal, causing hemorrhage and ischemia of the spinal cord. This fracture is unstable both early and late, as the anterior column has lost structural support. Roentgenograms, particularly the lateral, confirm the diagnosis (Fig. 11-34). CT scans and myelograms better demonstrate the neural canal encroachment but do not aid the prognosis (Fig. 11-35). Treatment is traction followed by immobilization in a fixed traction using the halo jacket. Because of the instability and because most of these fractures occur low in the cervical spine, the halo jacket may not be enough. The position has to be carefully watched. If immobilization fails, anterior strut grafting may be necessary. The only indication for anterior or posterior decompression as an emergency procedure is an incomplete paralysis that has plateaued or is becoming worse, as documented by neurologic examination.

Thoracic and Lumbar Spine

A fracture unique to the thoracic spine is the "slice fracture." Because the chest is rigid, this area of the spine is relatively well protected; hence, fractures occur only with great violence. The thoracic spinal canal is very narrow, making spinal cord injury a likely complication. The slice fracture occurs when a vertebra above slices down in a sagittal plane through the vertebra below, displacing half of the caudal vertebra laterally. Roentgenographically on the AP view, the superior vertebra appears telescoped, overlapping the one below. On the lateral view these appear to be a complete overlap of one vertebra on another. These usually require surgical manipulation and fusion if the deformity is too great to accept.

The seat-belt or Chance fracture occurs in the thoracolumbar spine, damaging the posterior column. It is unstable only if it continues through the anterior column, tearing the anterior longitudinal ligament. The AP roentgenographic features include a split spinous process, transverse processes, and pedicles if the lesion is completely bony (Chance fracture). On the lateral film, the separation posterior can be appreciated, which may be either bony or through the ligaments and disc (Fig. 11-4). Anteriorly the vertebral body may be compressed. These are usually stable injuries and are treated either by extension body casting or by surgical instrumentation and fusion.

Fracture-dislocations of the spine are considered extremely unstable. These should receive gentle care in the emergency department and during roentgenographic diagnosis. The roentgenograms (both AP and lateral; Figs. 11-1 and 11-2) show one vertebra displaced from its partner. Treatment is closed or open reduction followed by either long immobilization or, more likely, surgical instrumentation and fusion.

The burst fracture is the most difficult to understand, because plain roentgenograms do not really demonstrate the pathology. The vertebral body, which is loaded axially, forces the disc through the end plate, shattering the vertebral body. The body, particularly the posterior cortex, is extruded into the neural canal where it compromises the cord or cauda equina. This encroachment of the canal is best demonstrated on the CT scan, which is very helpful in deciding treatment. Although the fracture is basically stable, it is potentially unstable. With time, it can collapse, creating kyphosis and even more neural canal embarrassment. Therefore, the treatment of this fracture is surgical, with attempt being made to free the spinal canal of bone and to reconstruct the vertebral anatomy.

Stable Fractures of the Thoracolumbar Spine

There are several fracture types which, although painful, are not likely to cause any neurologic damage. These include mild compression fractures and fractures of spinous or transverse processes. The compression fracture usually is the result of axial loading of the spine in flexion. The front of the vertebral body will be flattened or decreased in height. The compression, if less than 50% of the expected height, is considered to be stable. Avulsions of the spinous processes and particularly the transverse processes (lumbar spine) can be the result of violent muscle contractions or trauma. They may be combined with other vertebral or rib fractures. Avulsions of spinous and transverse processes have occurred in weight lifters, football linemen, and rugby players, among others.

These lesions, if isolated, can be treated symptomatically. Pain medication and abdominal splinting (lumbosacral corset) may be enough to make the patient comfortable. If bowel sounds are present (an ileus could complicate recovery) and the patient is reliable, he or she could be sent home. However, this should only be done if there is a friend or relative who can bring the patient back if any problems occur. This protocol is only applicable if the physician is absolutely sure of the fracture's stability. Any suspicion of instability would preclude sending the patient home.

THE CAUDA EQUINA SYNDROME

On occasion, a large midline lumbar herniation may compress several roots of the cauda equina. Although it rarely occurs, it can be a catastrophic emergency. The most common level is the L4-5 disc. If the lesion reaches a large size and is slowly progressive, it may mimic a spinal cord tumor. Back and perianal pain predominates and masks the radicular symptoms. The patient experiences difficulty in urination, consisting of frequency or overflow incontinence, and males may have a recent history of impotence. Leg pain may be quickly followed by numbness of the feet and difficulty walking. Perianal numbness and loss of the anal reflex or bulbocavernosus reflex characterize an advanced syndrome.

The significance of this entity is that it is usually progressive, and spontaneous neurologic recovery has not been reported. If incontinence is present, only quick surgical decompression can offer hope of a normal bladder. Similarly, paresis or paraplegia may not recover if surgery is delayed. When the symptoms are severe, a carefully performed myelogram, using a small amount of dye, serves to locate the disc level. A complete block is usually seen.

VERTEBRAL OSTEOMYELITIS

Infection of the vertebral column can present as an emergency but is more likely to be a prolonged diagnostic problem. When it does present quickly, prompt diagnosis and treatment are necessary to avoid bony collapse due to destruction of the vertebral bodies or paralysis. Although most of the reported cases are hematogenous in origin, there are a few associations which should be mentioned. Infection of the lumbar spine with Gram-negative organisms are seen after urinary tract manipulations. *Pseudomonas* and *Serratia* infections of the spine are seen in intravenous drug addicts. Infections occur after surgery to the spine (laminectomy or fusion). Diabetic patients are prone to develop infections anywhere. However, in most cases there is no association, and the diagnosis may be confusing and prolonged.

The patient with a pyogenic infection of the spine will develop severe and unrelenting back pain that is due to both the swelling and bony destruction with instability. If the infection has created collapse of the vertebral body and angular kyphosis, or if an epidural abscess complicates the infection, paralysis may occur.

Roentgenograms will usually show osteoporotic vertebral bodies surrounding a narrowed or even lost disc space. If severe destruction has taken place, the vertebral end plates will appear to be moth-eaten and one vertebra may even collapse into its lower neighbor (Fig. 11-36). There may be paravertebral tissue swelling (particularly in the cervical spine) with soft tissue shadows. CT scans will further demonstrate the loss of vertebral body integrity and the status of the neural canal. A ^{99m}Tc bone scan will help by demonstrating a "hot area" in the involved vertebra.

The white blood count is usually normal to slightly elevated and the differential will show an increase in the percentage of polymorphonuclear leukocytes. The most helpful hematologic test is the sedimentation rate, which is always grossly elevated (usually greater than 100 mm/hour). The blood culture will be positive in a good percentage of patients, the infection being most likely due to *Staphylococcus aureus*.

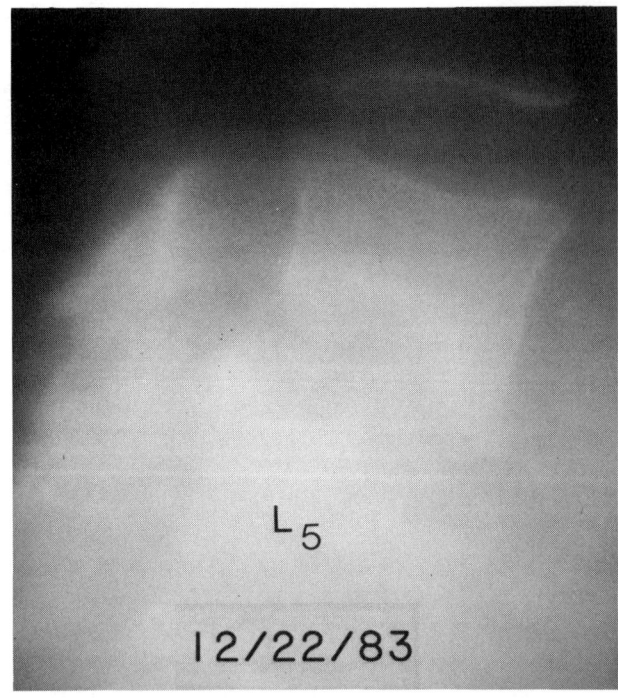

Figure 11-36 This lateral tomogram of the lumbar spine in a 65-year-old woman demonstrates an *Escherichia coli* infection of the L-4, L-5 disc space. Note the extensive destruction of the inferior surface and body of L-4 and of the superior surface and body of L-5. The disc space is all but destroyed. Anterior debridement and fusion plus a 6-week regimen of antibiotics enabled this patient to return to her home in relative comfort and back to full activity. Interestingly, this infection had been misdiagnosed as a carcinoma for over 1 year. Late diagnosis in vertebral infections is not uncommon, and when pain, fever, and an increased sedimentation rate are present, one should think of infection as a possibility.

Once the diagnosis is suspected, it can be verified by needle or open biopsy and then appropriately treated. The emergency physician should be aware of the potential diagnosis and of the implications if left untreated.

BIBLIOGRAPHY

Bohlmann HH, Ducker TB, Lucas JT. Spine and spinal cord injuries. In: Rothman RH, Simeone FA, eds. *The Spine*. Philadelphia: W.B. Saunders; 1982:661–756.

Denis F. The three column spine and its significance in the classification of acute thoracolumbar injuries. *Spine*. 1982;8:817–831.

Holdsworth F. Fractures, dislocations, and fracture-dislocations of the spine. *J Bone Joint Surg Am*. 1970;52:1534–1551.

O'Rahilly R, Benson DR. The development of the vertebral column. In: Bradford DS, Hensinger RM, eds. *The Pediatric Spine*. New York: Thieme-Stratton; 1985:3–17.

Stauffer ES, Kaufer H, Kling TF. Fractures and dislocations of the spine. In: Rockwood CA, Green DP, eds. *Fractures in Adults*. 2nd ed. Philadelphia: Lippincott; 1984.

12. Upper Extremity Emergency Problems

ROBERT M. SZABO, MD

Injuries to the upper extremity are fairly obvious when isolated. The affected part usually exhibits pain, swelling, and deformity. However, in the multiply traumatized individual these same injuries are frequently overlooked; if not treated properly, they can become the main source of that patient's disability. Open fractures, dislocations, vascular injuries, high-voltage electrical burns, and compartment syndromes require precise and early evaluation in order to avoid future disasters.

Circumferential splinting or casting should be avoided in the swollen upper extremity. Instead, a bulky well-padded dressing (Fig. 12-1) with some form of rigid splint can be adapted in most situations to immobilize a fracture or dislocation. Splinting applied at the scene of an accident should be carefully inspected when the patient reaches the emergency department and, in most cases, removed and replaced in order to permit an adequate examination of the extremity. Rings, bracelets, and jewelry of any kind should be removed immediately, before swelling prevents their removal and neurovascular compromise occurs. It is of paramount importance that circulation not be embarrassed and that there be no excessive pressure on any nerve. Gentle manipulation to restore the alignment of an extremity is preferable to applying a splint to an acutely angulated fracture in the position in which it lies. Bleeding in the upper extremity should not be controlled with tourniquets or the use of hemostats plunged into a wound. Rather, a bulky sterile compression dressing should be applied and the extremity elevated. Nerves and tendons have been crushed by injudicious use of hemostats in the emergency department, resulting in unnecessary injuries.

HISTORY

An accurate history, including the patient's age, sex, occupation, and life style, must be considered in relation to the nature of the injury. Previous injury, symptoms, or disability, along with a detailed account of the mechanism of the present injury, can frequently yield a diagnosis even before the physical examination is performed.

PHYSICAL AND RADIOGRAPHIC EXAMINATION

The examiner should avoid focusing on the injury until a careful assessment of the normal extremity and of the extremity proximal and distal to the injury is performed. Any examination of the upper extremity should include a complete neurovascular examination and range of motion of all joints. Most of the time this can be done prior to ordering radiographs, and thus return trips to the radiology department will be avoided. While physicians are criticized for the overuse of radiographs, in upper extremity injuries it is an absolute dictum that the joint above and below the affected part be well visualized on a radiograph. For example, a fracture of the midshaft of the radius cannot be adequately evaluated without an X-ray view that shows both the elbow and wrist joints. All too often, a concomitant dislocation such as the distal radial ulnar joint or proximal radius is missed as a result of a limited X-ray view. Interpretation of the x-ray requires careful thought. A small chip fracture on the palmar aspect of the distal phalanx of a finger may seem

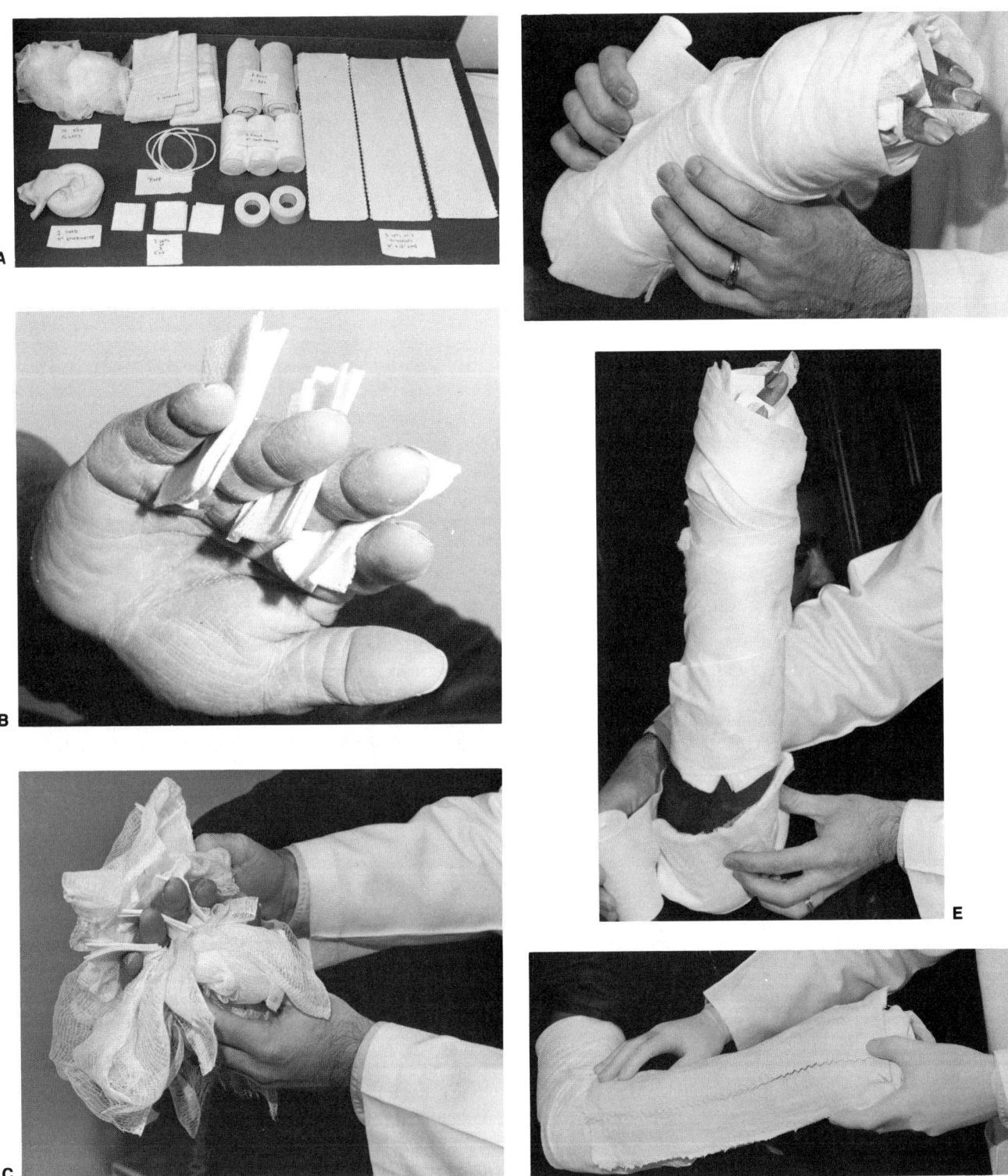

Figure 12-1 Bulky well-padded compression hand dressing. (**A**) The necessary components: 14 4″ x 4″ fluffs; 6 2″ x 2″ gauze; 3 combines; 3 rolls of 4″ cast padding; 2 rolls of 6″ bias stockinette; 1 yard of 4″ stockinette; 21 4″ x 15″ plaster splints; 1½″ tape; rope. (**B**) Three 2″ x 2″ gauze squares are placed between the fingers. (**C**) Fluffs are distributed evenly about the hand. (**D**) A combine is placed dorsally and palmarly around the wrist, and the hand is wrapped with 4″ cast padding. (**E**) An additional combine is placed around the elbow, which is maintained at 90°. (**F**) Plaster slabs (4″ x 15″) are placed dorsally and (**G**) around the elbow. (**H**) Plaster is covered with cast padding. (**I**) The dressing is wrapped with 6″ bias. (**J**) Stockinette (4″) is placed over the dressing. (**K**) The proximal half of the dressing is further secured with 6″ bias. (**L**) Tape is applied and a slot is cut posteriorly. (**M**) Rope is secured into the slot with tape. (**N**) The extremity is elevated with the rope.

Upper Extremity Emergency Problems 197

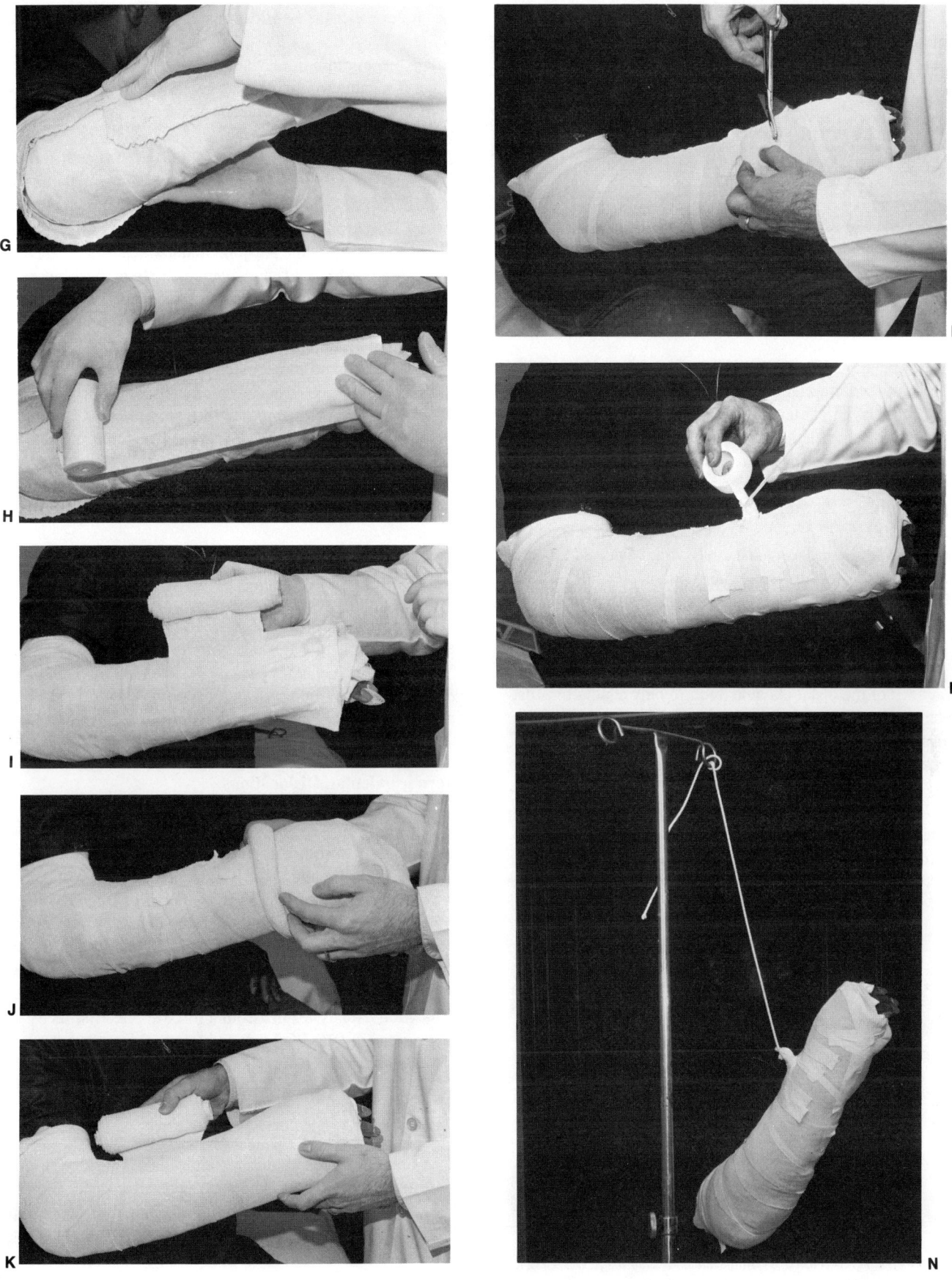

like a trivial injury unless one realizes that the profundus tendon is attached to the small chip, and surgery may be necessary to restore its function.

SPECIFIC UPPER EXTREMITY INJURIES

Clavicle Fractures

The clavicle is one of the bones most frequently fractured during childhood. The majority of clavicle fractures occur in the middle third by a shearing force. Fractures of the distal clavicle result from a direct blow to the shoulder from above. Fractures of the inner third of the clavicle result from direct trauma.

Examination usually reveals tenderness with a clavicle deformity and crepitation at the fracture site. Reduction of midthird clavicle fractures can generally be obtained by drawing the shoulders upward and backward. Maintenance of reduction is not as easy as obtaining the reduction. Most commonly, the proper application of a clavicular figure-8 splint will hold the fragments in adequate position to allow for healing (Fig. 12-2). For the first few days, in addition, an arm sling on the ipsilateral extremity will provide added comfort. While this method works fairly well in children, on occasion the adult will need treatment with a clavicular cast, which is a modified shoulder spica cast, in order to maintain reduction. Healing takes a minimum of 6 weeks in the adult.

Fractures of the inner clavicle, as well as nondisplaced fractures of the distal clavicle, require only a sling for treatment, and the patient may resume activities as pain subsides. Displaced distal clavicle fractures, however, are unstable because of ligamentous disruption and frequently require surgical reduction and fixation.

Careful evaluation for cervical spine or brachial plexus injury should be performed at the time of initial examination. Compression of the brachial plexus or subclavian vessels can also occur during the healing process from exuberant fracture callus and residual deformity.

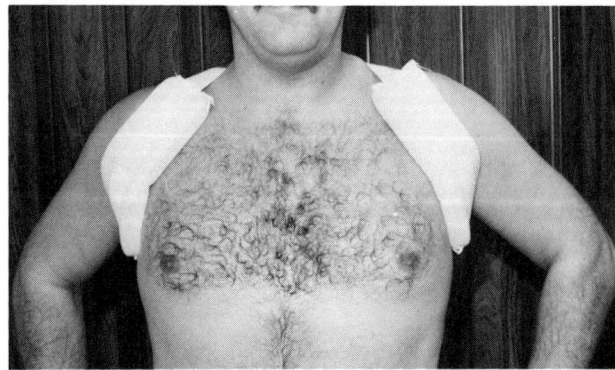

Figure 12-2 Application of a commercially available figure-8 splint for treatment of a midshaft clavicle fracture.

Acromioclavicular Separations

The most common mechanism of injury of this joint is a direct force due to a fall on the shoulder. However, a force from a fall on the outstretched hand may also superiorly displace the acromion from the clavicle. Six types of acromioclavicular injuries are now recognized. Types I, II, and III are classified depending on the type of ligament disruption to the acromioclavicular and the coracoclavicular ligaments. Type I is a sprain of the acromioclavicular (AC) ligament with the integrity of the AC joint maintained. In type II there is disruption of the AC ligament with stretching, but with maintenance of the coracoclavicular ligaments. Type III has complete disruption of the AC and the coracoclavicular ligaments with an upriding clavicle above the AC joint. In type IV the AC and coracoclavicular ligaments are disrupted and the clavicle is grossly displaced posteriorly into or through the trapezius muscle. In type V, the AC and coracoclavicular ligaments are disrupted and the clavicle is grossly displaced superiorly up into the base of the neck. In type VI, the AC and coracoclavicular ligaments are disrupted and the clavicle is dislocated under the coracoid process.

A type I injury may be treated with 7 to 10 days of resting the extremity in a sling until symptoms subside. Treatment of types II and III is more controversial. The spectrum of treatment ranges from "skillful neglect" for the inactive, nonlaboring patient to the use of various adhesive strappings, braces or harnesses, and operative reconstruction. Types IV, V, and VI most often will require some form of operative intervention to restore the grossly displaced clavicle.

Sternoclavicular Dislocations

Ligamentous supporting structure about the sternoclavicular is so strong that this is one of the least commonly dislocated joints in the body. Therefore, a traumatic dislocation usually indicates that a great amount of force has been applied, either directly or indirectly, to the clavicle. A direct force applied to the anterior medial clavicle can push the clavicle posteriorly behind the sternum into the mediastinum. This results in a posterior dislocation. Anterior dislocation usually results from a force applied indirectly to the sternoclavicular joint from a blow to the anterolateral or posterolateral aspect of the shoulder.

Anterior Dislocation

An anterior dislocation is recognized by a visibly prominent medial end of the clavicle. A posterior dislocation is recognized by the absence of the usually palpable medial end of the clavicle. If swelling is present, however, the physical exam can be deceptive. Posterior dislocations can result in venous congestion in the neck or upper extremity, shortness of breath, breathing difficulties, or dysphasia. Special radiographs are frequently required to confirm this diagnosis. These include a true cephalocaudal lateral view of the sternoclavicular joint, conventional tomography, and computed tomography.

Mild sprains and subluxations of the sternoclavicular joint should be treated with the application of ice for 12 hours, followed by moist heat, use of a sling, and 3 to 5 days of rest. With a complete dislocation, reduction should be attempted. Anterior dislocations can be reduced with a combination of downward pressure on the anterior aspect of both shoulders, with another person applying pressure to the medial end of the clavicle. Although the dislocation is frequently unstable, it rarely requires surgical fixation. The patient is instructed to wear a sling for 1 week to 10 days and to begin using the arm as soon as pain subsides. Many of the anterior dislocations in adults under the age of 25 are actually physeal injuries, which heal and remodel in time.

Posterior Dislocation

Treatment of posterior dislocations is more complicated. If any symptoms of mediastinal compression are present, the appropriate specialist should be contacted. A reduction of a posterior dislocation may be attempted with the patient supine and with a sandbag between the scapulae. Gentle traction is applied to the abducted arm in line with the clavicle while countertraction is applied by an assistant. Traction is increased while the arm is brought into extension. Frequently this maneuver is best performed under general anesthesia, and if it is not successful, a towel clip can be used to grasp the medial clavicle. If this is not successful, open reduction will be necessary. Once the posterior dislocation is reduced, the joint is usually stable and is best maintained for a few weeks in a figure-8 dressing.

Scapula Fractures

Fractures of the scapula usually indicate a significant magnitude of trauma and should signal the physician to search for associated injuries. Fractures of the body of the scapula may be treated with a sling for 10 to 14 days. Early exercises should be instituted to regain full range of motion of the shoulder joint. Application of ice within the first 48 hours will minimize bleeding from this bone.

Shoulder Injuries

Anterior Dislocation

The combination of abduction, external rotation, and extension applied to the arm can produce a dislocation of the glenohumeral joint, the most common dislocation of a major joint in the body. The humeral head is levered downward out of the glenoid cavity, until it tears through the inferior portion of joint capsule. The humeral head can then be found beneath the coracoid, a subcoracoid dislocation; inferior to the glenoid, a subglenoid dislocation; or beneath the clavicle, a subclavicular dislocation or intrathoracic dislocation.

The patient with an acute anterior dislocation presents holding the affected extremity in abduction and external rotation. There may be prominence of the anterior shoulder and, on palpation, a cavity may be felt along the lateral border of the acromion. As always, a neurovascular examination should be performed of the extremity. Particular attention should be directed towards the axillary nerve, which can sustain a traction injury during the dislocation. Findings will include decreased sensibility over the lateral aspect of the proximal humerus. Motor function of the deltoid is difficult to evaluate, secondary to pain. Radiographic evaluation should always include an anteriorposterior view in internal and external rotation, and a transaxillary lateral view. If the transaxillary view cannot be obtained, a transthoracic lateral can be useful. To confirm the diagnosis and to learn whether an additional fracture of the greater tuberosity or proximal humerus is present, it is advisable to obtain radiographs before reduction.

Reduction should be accomplished as soon after evaluation as possible, under sedation with an intravenous narcotic. It is preferable to use a narcotic rather than a muscle relaxant in the emergency department, as it may easily be reversed with an opiate blocker. The use of intravenous diazepam can cause profound respiratory depression, particularly in an elderly individual. If reduction cannot be performed gently with the use of intravenous sedation, then general anesthesia is preferable to exerting a large amount of force, which can result in either further fracture or damage to the axillary vessels and brachial plexus.

Straight traction on the arm, in line with the humeral shaft, with gentle rotation may be successful; frequently countertraction needs to be applied by an assistant with a folded sheet underneath the axilla. While maintaining traction the arm is adducted, and if reduction is not immediately obtained, internal and external rotation of the arm with pressure on the humeral head often completes the reduction.

The Kocher maneuver is a technique that should be used with extreme caution. Complications include damage to the axillary vessels and brachial plexus, as well as spiral fractures of the proximal humerus. The Kocher maneuver is performed in the following manner:

1. The elbow is flexed to 90° and traction is applied in line with the humeral shaft.
2. The arm is slowly brought into full external rotation.
3. The arm is bent adducted across the chest to the midline.
4. The arm is internally rotated, placing the hand on the opposite shoulder.

This maneuver causes the humeral head to lever on the anterior glenoid.

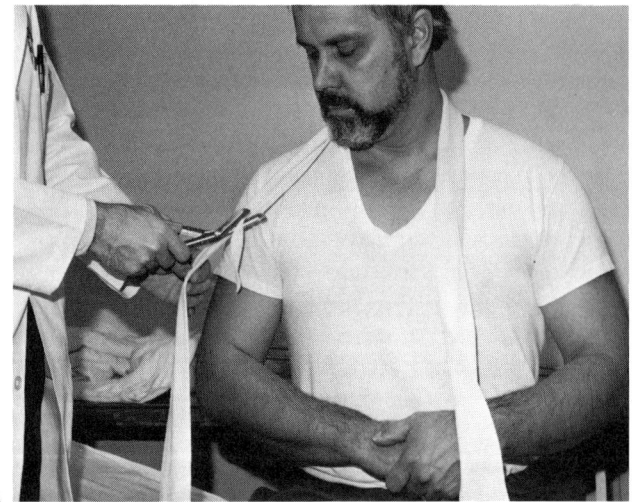
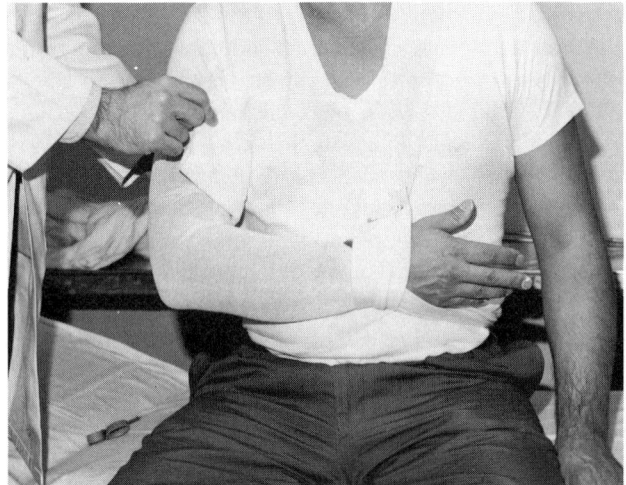

Figure 12-3 Velpeau stockinette shoulder immobilizer. **(A)** A hole is cut in 4" Velpeau stockinette in which to place the affected extremity. **(B)** The extremity is secured to the chest by passing the stockinette around the back and fastening it to the arm. The axilla is then padded.

Another method of reduction is known as the Stimson technique. The patient is placed prone on the table with the injured extremity hanging over the side. Eight to 10 pounds of weight is suspended from the flexed forearm for traction. As spasm of the shoulder muscles subsides, reduction may occur spontaneously.

Postreduction, a Velpeau stockinette dressing (Fig. 12-3) or a commercially available shoulder immobilizer, is applied for 3 to 6 weeks. For patients over the age of 40 years, immobilization can be discontinued after 1 to 3 weeks, and a gentle range-of-motion program should be instituted. In patients who have had a previous dislocation, immobilization is continued for 7 to 10 days for comfort before beginning an exercise program. Vigorous use of the extremity is avoided until normal muscle strength has been achieved.

Posterior Dislocation

Posterior dislocations present a particular problem, as they are frequently misdiagnosed. In fact, the diagnosis is initially missed in nearly 80% of cases. The routine anterior-posterior radiographs of the shoulder often look deceptively normal. The signs and symptoms of a posterior dislocation are as follows:

1. The arm is fixed in adduction and internal rotation.
2. Abduction and external rotation are severely limited.
3. The posterior aspect of the shoulder is rounded, and the anterior aspect of the shoulder is flat compared with the normal shoulder.
4. The coracoid process is more prominent on the dislocated side.

Closed reduction is accomplished with intravenous sedation. The patient is placed in a supine position and traction is applied to the adducted arm. Occasionally, lateral traction on the upper arm is applied by an assistant, using a folded towel. Postreduction, the extremity is placed in a shoulder spica cast, which holds the arm in neutral rotation. Physical therapy is prescribed after 4 weeks of immobilization.

Rotator Cuff Injuries

Fracture of the greater tuberosity with retraction of 1 cm or more is pathognomonic of a tear in the rotator cuff. This injury requires surgical intervention in order to repair the rotator cuff and reposition the greater tuberosity, which will act as a bony impingement in its superiorly displaced position. Minimally displaced fractures of the greater tuberosity are treated with a shoulder immobilizer for 3 to 4 weeks, followed by a progressive, gentle range of motion exercises.

Acute traumatic tear of the rotator cuff can occur with no signs of fracture. Generally the patient is in the fourth decade of life, but all ages can be affected. The presenting symptoms are pain and swelling about the shoulder after a fall on the outstretched hand or a direct blow. Radiographs are generally normal; however, acromioclavicular arthritis with spurring underneath the acromion may indicate previous pathology. On physical examination, the patient is unable to abduct the extremity and demonstrates weakness of shoulder external rotation. Injection of several milliliters of 1% lidocaine under the subacromial space will eliminate much of the pain and allow for a better examination of the shoulder. If weakness persists, an arthrogram or MRI is indicated to confirm the diagnosis.

The treatment is based on the patient's age, functional expectations, and size of tear. Minor tears in older individuals are treated with a short period of immobilization in a sling followed by a progressive physical therapy program. Larger tears, particularly in younger individuals, usually require surgical repair.

Bursitis/Tendonitis

Subacromial bursitis can be distinguished from rotator cuff tear. The underlying pathology in both diseases is in the supraspinatus tendon, but the treatment may be quite different. Presenting features of subacromial bursitis, also known as "impingement syndrome," are similar to those of a rotator cuff tear, that is, pain and weakness of abduction and external rotation. Forced forward flexion with adduction will aggravate symptoms of pain. This test is known as the "impingement test." Anesthetizing the subacromial space with 10 mL of 1% lidocaine will relieve these symptoms and confirm the diagnosis. Once the diagnosis is confirmed, a long-acting steroid may be injected into the subacromial space to relieve the inflammation in the supraspinatus tendon. The patient is placed in a sling for a few days; however, gentle active motion is encouraged early to avoid a resultant stiff shoulder. Aspirin or nonsteroidal anti-inflammatory agents are used for relieving pain and inflammation.

Proximal Humerus Fractures

In proximal humerus fractures, the classical mechanism of injury is a fall on the outstretched arm. Fractures occur between adjacent two or all of four major proximal humeral segments. These are the head (which is the articular segment); the greater tuberosity, to which the external rotators are attached; the lesser tuberosity, to which the subscapularis is attached; and the shaft. When any of the segments are separated by 1 cm or angulated by more than 45°, the fracture is considered to be displaced.

Early signs of pain, swelling, and ecchymosis about the shoulder after injury would direct examination of the proximal humerus radiographically and an exact diagnosis would be made. Integrity of the axillary nerve and vessels, as well as the remainder of the brachial plexus, should be evaluated with this injury.

Minimally displaced fractures are best treated with a commercial shoulder immobilizer, Velpeau stockinette immobilizer, or a sling and swathe. The arm is immobilized for 3 weeks, followed by gradual introduction of functional exercises. Displaced fractures of the head can usually be reduced by traction with the arm in an adducted and flexed position. Displaced greater tuberosity fractures are discussed above.

Three-part and four-part fractures that are displaced require surgical intervention. A shoulder immobilizer or sling and swathe is applied for comfort until proper referral can be made.

Fractures of the Humeral Shaft

The angulation and displacement of fragments of the humeral shaft depend on the nature of the force causing the fracture and the level of the fracture. A bending force will result in a transverse fracture, whereas a torsional force will produce a spiral fracture. Displacement of the fracture fragments depends on the influence of the muscle forces pulling the fragments apart. For instance, a fracture above the level of the pectoralis major insertion will cause abduction and external rotation of the proximal fragment due to the action of the rotator cuff. A fracture below the pectoralis major insertion and above the deltoid insertion will produce adduction of the proximal fragment, and a fracture below the deltoid insertion will cause abduction of the proximal fragment.

Injury to the radial nerve is the most common complication associated with fractures of the shaft of the humerus. The examiner must be alerted to this possible complication and look for the signs of wrist drop and inability to extend the metacarpophalangeal joint of the digits. Examination must be performed before any manipulative reduction and repeated after reduction. Palsy of the radial nerve that is not present initially but is found after reduction must alert the examiner to the possibility that the nerve is caught between the fracture fragments. This situation would dictate exploration of the radial nerve and internal fixation of the fracture. As usual, open fractures necessitate operative irrigation and debridement. All other uncomplicated fractures can be treated by closed methods.

Though there are many methods prescribed for the management of closed humeral shaft fractures, the most frequently employed are (1) hanging cast, (2) coaptation brachial splint, and (3) functional bracing. The hanging cast is a method of applying continuous traction. It is applied with the elbow flexed to 90° and extends from the midpart of the hand to the level of the humeral fracture. The patient must maintain a vertical position for the traction to be effective. A loop is incorporated into the plaster cast at the level of the wrist. A sling is passed through the loop and tied around the neck. The position of the loop will direct the forces to reduce the fracture fragments. Lengthening the sling corrects posterior bowing; shortening the sling corrects anterior bowing. Placing the wrist loop in a more palmar position will correct a valgus deformity, and a more dorsal position will correct a varus deformity.

Radiographs of the fracture are made at weekly intervals, and careful adjustments are made to avoid distraction of the fragments. Circumduction exercises of the shoulder are instituted early, as soon as the patient is comfortable. Transverse fractures are particularly at risk for developing nonunion with this treatment should distraction occur.

The coaptation plaster brachial splint is another acceptable method of treating humeral shaft fractures. A plaster slab extending from the axilla around the elbow and over the deltoid is placed over a few layers of cast padding. The arm is then placed in a sling or collar and cuff.

Functional bracing has increasingly become the method of choice for treating humeral shaft fractures in reliable and cooperative patients. The initial management can be the use of a coaptation splint. When swelling has subsided, a commercial polyethylene functional brace (or one fashioned by an orthotist) is applied to the arm. Active exercises of the shoulder, elbow, wrist, and hand begin immediately. The brace acts to compress the soft tissues surrounding the fracture and thus maintains alignment of the fragments until healing occurs. The use of functional bracing minimizes the stiffness of the adjacent joints. If the patient initially presents with a radial nerve palsy, the physician must not forget to support the wrist in slight dorsiflexion and follow return of function with serial neurologic examinations. If there is no return of function within 3 months of injury, electrodiagnostic studies are ordered and exploration of the radial nerve is considered.

Elbow Injuries

Fractures and Dislocations

Severe complications may be associated with fractures and dislocations about the elbow. Due to the unyielding nature of the fascial envelope surrounding the cubital fossa, bleeding resulting from a displaced fracture or dislocation can lead to increased pressure on the neurovascular structures in this small area. As swelling ensues, a resulting compartment syndrome and subsequent Volkmann's ischemic paralysis can occur.

Circularized plaster only aggravates the situation. The amount of swelling must be considered, and the integrity of the median, ulnar, and radial nerves tested before and after reduction and splinting and at frequent intervals thereafter. Documentation of each examination is imperative.

Elbow radiographs can be difficult to read. Nondisplaced fractures are often missed on routine anterior-posterior and lateral films. The "fat pad" sign is an area of radiolucency found posterior at the level of the distal humerus and indicates distention of the joint capsule by either effusion or hemoarthrosis displacing the fat pad away from the humeral cortex. When there is a high index of suspicion and the fat pad sign is present, further radiographs, such as oblique views, are necessary to identify the pathology.

Supracondylar Fractures

Supracondylar fractures primarily occur in the first decade of life. Because of the potential serious complication of Volkmann's ischemic contracture, all children with displaced supracondylar fractures should be admitted to the hospital for observation. The mechanism of injury is either extension or flexion. The more common extension-type injury occurs from a fall on the extended elbow and is stable only in significant flexion.

Extension-type injuries are further described as being displaced posteromedial or posterolateral, depending on the position of the distal fragment in relation to the proximal fragment. Posteromedial displacement is most commonly found. Making this determination is clinically significant, for the posteromedial fractures have a higher incidence of cubitus varus deformities, whereas the posterolateral fractures tend to develop a valgus deformity. Careful interpretation of the radiograph is important to determine the proper reduction maneuver and position of splinting.

On clinical examination, one finds a very swollen elbow. With a completely displaced fracture one will find an S-shaped deformity created by the prominence of the proximal fragment, flexion of the distal fragment, and prominence of the olecranon. If the proximal spike penetrates into the subcutaneous tissue, one might see dimpling of the skin with subcutaneous hemorrhage in the area of the cubital fossa. This is known as the "dimple" sign. Clinically, a supracondylar fracture may appear similar to a posterior dislocation of the elbow; however, in the latter situation the olecranon is more prominent, as it is displaced posterior to the humeral condyles.

It is desirable to reduce supracondylar fractures in children under adequate anesthesia. Some prefer to do this in the operating room under a general anesthetic; however, it is acceptable to perform a gentle reduction under intravenous sedation in the emergency department. Local infiltration of anesthetic into the fracture area is not advised, because it increases the pressure on the neurovascular structures in the cubital fossa. The method of reduction is to apply traction and countertraction with the elbow in extension. The distal fragment is then lifted anteriorly, while the proximal fragment is pushed posteriorly. At the same time, an assistant maintains traction on the pronated forearm, with the elbow in slight flexion. Lateral displacement is then reduced with direct pressure and the elbow flexed to at least 90°. All the while, the radial pulse is palpated and signs of a neurovascular compromise monitored. The forearm should not be flexed to the point where the radial pulse diminishes. After reduction, a posterior plaster splint with medial and lateral plaster supports is applied, followed by a sling and swathe. Immediate radiographs are taken to confirm the reduction.

A common pitfall is to externally rotate the humerus in order to obtain good radiographs postreduction. This, however, creates rotation at the fracture site with resultant displacement and tilting of the distal fragment into varus position.

Traction, either Dunlop's or overhead skeletal, has been employed in the treatment of supracondylar fractures with a badly swollen elbow, or when closed reduction is unsuccessful. Percutaneous pinning with the use of an image intensifier has recently gained popularity, as it eliminates the need for immobilization in extreme flexion to maintain reduction.

Flexion-type supracondylar fractures are rare and usually occur from a direct force on the posterior elbow. In order to reduce the distal fragment, closed reduction is performed with the forearm flexed. Once the fracture is reduced with traction applied to the flexed forearm, the fracture fragments are locked into place by the anterior periosteal hinge when the elbow is placed into extension.

Lateral Condyle Fractures in Children

A lateral condyle fracture is usually a Salter-Harris type or physeal injury and most commonly is believed to occur when the elbow is forced into varus. The extensor muscles and lateral collateral ligament apply an avulsion force to the lateral condyle.

Immobilization with a plaster cast is all that is necessary for a nondisplaced fracture. A displaced fracture, however, usually requires an accurate open reduction and internal fixation to prevent premature closure of the distal humerus physis. Complications in the treatment of this fracture include nonunion, malunion, angular deformity, avascular necrosis, and neurologic injuries.

Medial Condyle and Epicondyle Fractures

A direct force applied to the posterior aspect of the elbow or a fall on the outstretched arm with the elbow and wrist extended can result in an avulsion of the medial condyle. In younger children where there is only ossification of the medial epicondyle, one may not appreciate that the entire medial condyle is fractured, with intra-articular displacement. Open reduction and internal fixation are required for displaced medial condyle fractures to prevent the development of nonunion and cubitus varus deformities. Cubitus valgus can also occur, secondary to stimulation and overgrowth of the medial condylar fragment.

Medial epicondyle fractures can occur from the same forces that produce condylar fractures; however, only the apophysis will fracture from the pull of the forearm flexors. Nondisplaced or minimally displaced fractures are treated with simple immobilization. Sometimes, however, the epicondylar fragment can become incarcerated in the joint, and I think that this is an indication for operative intervention. This injury is also associated with ulnar nerve symptoms; if such symptoms are present, operative intervention, along with anterior transposition of the ulnar nerve, is indicated.

Intercondylar Fractures of the Distal Humerus in Adults

These fractures result from a direct blow or a fall onto the elbow. Marked displacement is common, and reasonable joint movement cannot be expected unless anatomic reduction is achieved. Therefore, open reduction and stable internal fixation are recommended in order to permit early active exercises and restore elbow motion. In elderly patients or in fractures so badly comminuted that adequate reduction is impossible, either traction or the "bag of bones" technique can be utilized. This technique involves simply placing the arm in a collar and cuff in as much flexion as possible. Hand motion is started immediately and shoulder exercises begun at 7 to 10 days. The patient gradually extends the elbow as swelling and pain diminish. The fracture usually unites in 6 weeks. It should be emphasized, however, that most displaced intra-articular elbow fractures require open reduction and internal fixation.

Radial Head Fractures

Most radial head fractures are caused by a fall on the outstretched hand, resulting in compression of the radial head against the capitellum. Radial head fractures can be classified into four types: (1) nondisplaced fractures, (2) marginally displaced fractures with depression and/or angulation, (3) comminuted fractures, and (4) comminuted fractures associated with dislocation of the elbow.

On physical examination, rotation of the forearm, particularly supination, causes pain in the proximal lateral forearm over the radial head. Nondisplaced fractures may be difficult to see on the initial films; however, a positive fat pad sign is usually present. Nondisplaced fractures are treated with a short period (7 to 10 days) of immobilization using a posterior plaster splint. Early motion is then begun, maintaining the elbow in a sling until pain subsides. Some pain may persist for several weeks until fracture healing is complete.

With displaced fractures, aspiration of the hemarthrosis through a lateral approach is followed by an injection of local anesthetic into the radiocapitellar joint. Examination of passive pronation and supination will then determine if there is a mechanical block due to fracture displacement. If no mechanical block is present, the fracture is treated as if nondisplaced. If, however, a mechanical block is present, there is angulation of the fracture greater than 30°, there is depression greater than 3 mm, or there is involvement of more than one-third of the radial head, surgical intervention should be considered. The surgical management will vary and may consist of either an open reduction and internal fixation or excision of the radial head. Surgery should be performed within the first 24 hours or delayed for several weeks to avoid the complication of myositis ossificans.

Every patient with a radial head fracture needs to be examined for disruption of the distal radial ulnar joint. This pattern of injury, known as the Essex-Lopresti injury, will result in significant wrist pain if it goes unrecognized and untreated.

Olecranon Fractures

Fractures of the olecranon occur from direct violence and indirectly from a strong contraction of the triceps mechanism or a combination of these forces.

Nondisplaced fractures are best treated in a long-arm cast with the elbow at 45° to 90° flexion. Protective range of motion is allowed at 3 weeks, avoiding flexion of the elbow past 90° until 6 to 8 weeks when bone healing is complete.

Displaced fractures require open reduction and internal fixation or, in some cases, excision of the olecranon fragment with repair of the triceps mechanism.

Dislocations of the Elbow

Posterior or posterolateral dislocations account for nearly 90% of all elbow dislocations. The mechanism of injury is usually a fall on the outstretched hand with the arm in extension and abduction. Roentgenograms should include an anterior-posterior view of the forearm, an anterior-posterior view of the humerus, and a lateral of the elbow. Neurovascular function is checked and recorded prior to and after the completion of reduction. Neurovascular function compromised by reduction may indicate a need for operative treatment.

Treatment involves immediate reduction. Reduction can be achieved by gentle traction of the slightly flexed elbow with countertraction on the humerus. Medial and lateral displacement are corrected; pressure is applied over the olecranon as the elbow is brought into further flexion. It is important to flex and extend the elbow through full range of motion immediately after the reduction. This ensures that the joint is stable and that there is no mechanical block of motion within the joint. Reduction can generally be accomplished with intravenous sedation and, at times, can even be accomplished without any anesthesia if the diagnosis is made very early after injury.

The extremity is placed in a long-arm plaster splint with the elbow flexed to at least 90°. The duration of immobilization varies from 3 to 4 days to 3 weeks before the institution of active motion. The choice depends on the stability of the elbow and the preference of the treating physician. If the patient is not hospitalized with an elbow dislocation, strict instructions should be given for observation of the neurologic and vascular status of the extremity.

Subluxation of the Radial Head

This entity, also commonly referred to as "pulled elbow" or "nursemaid's elbow," is found in children 2 to 3 years of age. Probably one to two of these injuries can be found in every emergency department per week. Injury occurs when distal traction is suddenly applied to the pronated forearm if the elbow is extended. Such a mechanism is present when a young child steps from a curb when the parent is holding on to the hand. Familiarity with this entity will avoid confusing the diagnosis, as X-ray findings are usually negative. Following the injury, the child is reluctant to use the involved extremity. Attempts to supinate the forearm or flex the elbow cause pain. Reduction is accomplished by supinating the forearm and hyperflexing the elbow. A snapping sensation of reduction occurs. Within a few minutes, the child will begin to use the affected extremity once again.

Fractures of the proximal radius and septic arthritis of the elbow can be mistaken for the diagnosis of a "nursemaid's" elbow. However, pain will persist after the above manipulation if fracture or infection is present. After reduction, the extremity is placed in a sling or a shirt sleeve pinned to the chest for a short period of time. If the injury has been recurrent, then it is advisable to immobilize the extremity for 3 weeks in plaster. It is important to educate the parent about the mechanism of this injury to avoid repetition.

Septic Arthritis

Three types of infection occur about the elbow: (1) septic arthritis, (2) septic bursitis, and (3) osteomyelitis. As with other joint infections, the clinical setting reveals pain, warmth, erythema, and sometimes fever or frank drainage. While infections usually occur from direct inoculation, hematogenous infection does occur in the elbow joint also. Infection within the joint is heralded by resistance to all motion of that joint. In contrast, a patient with osteomyelitis or septic bursitis will allow gentle passive motion of the elbow joint.

Aspiration of the elbow from a portal between the radial head and the lateral epicondyle will yield fluid for examination. A sympathetic effusion can be differentiated from purulent fluid by simple inspection. However, a Gram stain and culture of the fluid are essential for definitive diagnosis.

The presentation of septic olecranon bursitis varies from an acute onset of cellulitis to a low-grade process present for two or more weeks. Septic arthritis requires immediate operative incision and drainage. Mild cases of septic olecranon bursitis initially may be treated with a single aspiration and a course of oral antibiotics. Surgical drainage is indicated for failure of the above treatment or for a long-standing or chronic infection. With chronic septic olecranon bursitis, excision of the olecranon bursa is advised. Osteomyelitis is treated using the same principles as those used elsewhere in the body.

Tennis Elbow

Elbow tendinitis may be classified as lateral tendinitis or medial tendinitis. The differential diagnosis should include ulnar nerve neurapraxia, carpal tunnel syndrome, radial nerve entrapment, cervical root compression, and intra-articular abnormalities of the elbow. The key to diagnosis is specific point tenderness over either the lateral or medial epicondyles.

First line of treatment includes applying cold, resting the extremity, and using either aspirin or nonsteroidal anti-inflammatory medication. If the patient does not respond to this treatment program, a local steroid injection is appropriate. More than three steroid injections in 1 year may cause harm by weakening the surrounding normal tissues. After the acute stage has passed, some form of counter-force bracing, such as a Froimson strap, should be prescribed along with a graduated exercise and strength training program. Less than 5% of patients with tennis elbow will require surgery.

Forearm Injuries

Fractures

Of all fractures in the upper extremity, the diaphyseal fracture of the radius or ulna exemplifies the need for X-ray examination of the joint above and below the fractured bone. When both bones are fractured, the injury is known as a "both-bones" fracture of the forearm. A fracture of the shaft of the ulna may be associated with a dislocation of the radial head; this injury is known as a "Monteggia" fracture. A single-bone fracture of the ulna without dislocation of the radial head is called a "night-stick" fracture. A single-bone fracture of the distal third of the radius associated with a dislocation of the distal radial ulnar joint is known as a "Galeazzi" fracture.

Children can have an incomplete fracture in the forearm known as a "greenstick" fracture or a compression fracture, particularly in the distal radius, where it is known as a "torus" fracture. In the adult, both-bone fractures and Monteggia and Galeazzi fractures are best treated by open reduction and rigid internal fixation when displaced. Undisplaced diaphyseal fractures of the forearm are rare in adults, with the exception of the ulna. This injury, the night-stick fracture, is initially placed in a long-arm cast with the elbow in 90° of flexion and the forearm in slight supination. After 7 to 10 days the extremity may be placed in an orthoplast sleeve, which allows free motion of the elbow and wrist and pronation and supination. The splint is worn until the fracture is united.

The objective of treatment of forearm injuries is to restore full forearm rotation. This can only be achieved if the rotation and angulation are corrected. Reduction of displaced fractures in the pediatric age group is best achieved under general anesthesia. Multiple attempts at reduction in the emergency department should be avoided because undue swelling results, leading to muscle spasm, further difficulty with reduction, and possible compartment syndromes.

Compartment Syndrome

A compartment syndrome exists when the pressure in a closed osteofascial compartment exceeds the tolerance of those tissues within the compartment. The end result is ischemic necrosis of both muscle and nerve. Closed compartment syndromes are not uncommon following forearm and elbow fractures, as well as crushing injuries to the forearm. Findings include a tense swollen forearm with pain on palpation of the affected compartment. Pain is increased with passive extension of the digits. Next follows decreased sensibility, which can be assessed both by history and careful examination with either Semmes-Weinstein monofilaments, a tuning fork, or two-point discrimination as measured by a paper clip (Fig. 12-4). One should not wait for pulselessness to occur before declaring a compartment syndrome; this is the latest finding and almost always indicates the diagnosis has been missed for a significant time.

Tissue pressure monitoring is useful to confirm the diagnosis and, at times, to establish the diagnosis in a patient who is unresponsive or uncooperative. The differential diagnosis usually includes a neurapraxia or an arterial injury. The treatment of compartment syndrome is wide fasciotomy

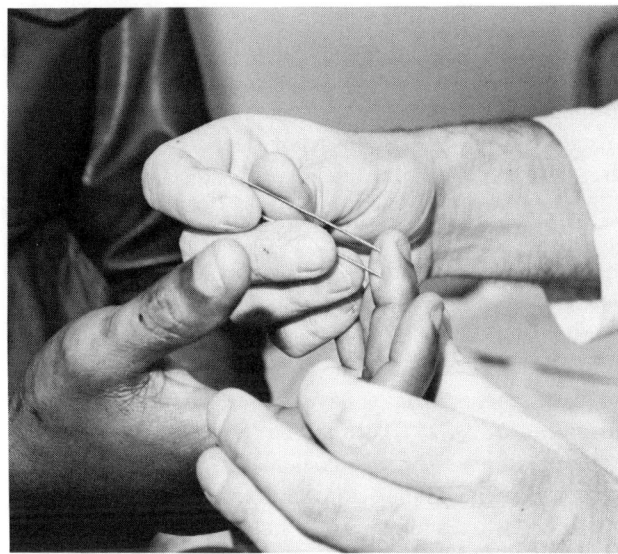

Figure 12-4 Two-point discrimination is measured with a paper clip. Normally one can distinguish the difference between being touched by one or two points separated by 6 mm or less.

from the elbow to the wrist, including decompression of the carpal tunnel. Along with open fractures, compartment syndromes are absolute surgical emergencies, and delay in treatment can result in the loss of a useful limb.

Fractures and Dislocations about the Wrist

The distal radius fracture is the most common fracture of the upper extremity. Three eponyms are commonly used to identify fractures of the distal radius: (1) Colles' fracture denotes dorsal displacement of the distal fragment. (2) Smith's fracture denotes palmar displacement of the distal fragment. (3) Barton's fracture denotes an intra-articular fracture of the dorsal or palmar lip of the distal radius.

Distal radial fractures, in particular Colles' fractures, have been thought to be a fracture of only the osteoporotic individual. While this often is the case, there is a growing population of younger patients with high-velocity type injuries sustained in motor vehicle accidents.

Physical examination reveals a swollen wrist with a "silver-spoon" deformity. Careful neurologic examination might reveal either median or ulnar nerve involvement. The median nerve can be affected by traction from the original injury or from acute pressure within the carpal canal due to swelling and hematoma formation. To differentiate increased pressure from neurapraxia, it may be necessary to measure carpal canal pressures; an acute carpal tunnel syndrome left untreated may create significant consequences for later hand function.

It is essential to take radiographs in the anterior-posterior and lateral projections and to measure dorsal displacement, angulation, proximal displacement, and radial displacement.

Reduction of a Colles' fracture is performed by applying traction to the grasped hand or with Chinese finger-traps and countertraction to the humerus with the elbow flexed. After disimpaction, pressure is applied to the dorsal aspect of the distal fragment and to the palmar aspect of the proximal fragment and in a radial direction to the distal fragment. The wrist is then splinted in no more than 20° of palmar flexion and slight ulnar deviation. Greater flexion may cause dangerously high pressures in the carpal tunnel with resultant median nerve injury.

Maintenance of this reduction can be quite difficult in the face of severe comminution. Therefore, alternative methods to plaster immobilization have become popular in the badly displaced fracture. These include external fixation, percutaneous pinning, and a combination of these two techniques. As with all intra-articular fractures, one principle of treatment is to restore the congruity of the articular surface. Accepting more than 20° to 25° of dorsal angulation can result in late midcarpal instability.

The choice of short-arm or long-arm plaster immobilization is still debated. With a comminuted fracture, a long-arm plaster maintaining the wrist in slight supination may offer a little more protection against displacement. Regardless of the method of treatment, finger motion and shoulder motion should begin immediately, to prevent stiffness. Settling of the fracture can be expected, and frequent X-ray follow-up in the first few weeks of treatment is recommended. Enough healing usually occurs to remove the constant external support within 5 to 7 weeks.

The dorsal fracture, if minimally displaced, is treated by plaster immobilization in a short-arm cast with the wrist in neutral position. Displacement greater than 1 to 2 mm is treated by percutaneous pin fixation or open reduction and fixation.

The palmar fracture dislocation is difficult to reduce, and reduction is even more difficult to maintain. Therefore, this fracture most often requires open reduction and internal fixation with a small plate placed on the palmar aspect of the radius.

Distal radial and ulnar fractures in children are sometimes wrongly referred to as Colles' fractures. Dorsal displacement of the distal radius occurs through an epiphyseal plate fracture. Reduction is accomplished with the same maneuvers as for a Colles' fracture. These injuries, after reduction, are usually stable and can be managed with a below-elbow plaster cast.

Carpal Injuries

Fractures. The most important fracture of the carpus is a fracture of the scaphoid. Limitation of extremes of wrist motion along with point tenderness in the anatomic "snuffbox" will be present. With the presence of the above physical findings, a fracture of the scaphoid cannot be ruled out until roentgenograms repeated ten days after injury are negative. At this point, bony resorption around the nondisplaced fracture will allow for better visualization of the fracture line. If the examination is still suspicious, however, but radiographs are negative, a [^{99m}Tc]phosphate bone scan may help confirm the diagnosis. An undisplaced scaphoid fracture is treated with a short-arm cast, incorporating the thumb into a spica. If pronation and supination are painful, the cast is extended to include the elbow. Immobilization for 12 weeks or more is often necessary; however, radiographs can be repeated at 6-week intervals, and when the fracture is radiographically united and clinically there is no pain or tenderness, immobilization can be discontinued. Displacement of 2 mm or more is indication for open reduction and internal fixation of scaphoid fractures. The rate of nonunion of displaced scaphoid fractures treated by conservative methods is unacceptably high.

Dislocations. There is a spectrum of damage of carpal dislocations that ranges from a partial tear to total disruption of the ligamentous complex of the wrist. Once thought of as distinct injuries, perilunate, lunate, and transscaphoid perilunate dislocations can be considered progressive stages of the same basic injury. The mechanism of injury is usually a fall on the hyperextended wrist. Examination reveals limitation of wrist motion, swelling and tenderness about the wrist, and, with the complete dislocation of the lunate, fullness on the palmar aspect of the wrist. Signs of median nerve compression are frequent.

Confusion exists regarding the various terms used to describe carpal dislocations. Basically there are two major patterns: a dorsiflexion and a palmar flexion instability. Dorsiflexion instability is far more common. Other names used to describe this entity include dorsal intercalary segment instability, scapholunate dissociation, and rotary subluxation of the scaphoid. What is found radiographically, however, is a dorsiflexed lunate, a triangular appearance of the lunate on anterior-posterior films, a "Terry-Thomas" sign (gap between scaphoid and lunate of 2 mm or greater), and a scapholunate angle greater than 70° (30° to 60° is normal, with an average of 47°). The forces may be transmitted in such a manner that the scaphoid fractures but the scapholunate ligament remains intact. The diagnosis is usually apparent due to the noticeable fractured scaphoid on radiographs. In the absence of fracture, however, this injury must be suspected and the radiographic features looked for, lest the diagnosis be missed.

Radial styloid fractures are commonly present with carpal dislocations; therefore, dorsal instability should be specifically looked for when a radial styloid fracture is present.

Initial treatment consists of closed reduction by longitudinal traction, hyperextension of the wrist and, with a completely dislocated lunate, pressure directed dorsally over the palmarly dislocated lunate. While pressure is applied, the wrist is then brought into flexion. Obtaining and maintaining an accurate reduction of this injury is possible, although extremely difficult. For this reason, most physicians have preferred an early open reduction and internal fixation with ligament repair.

Isolated Dislocation of the Distal Radial Ulnar Joint

This injury is frequently missed and diagnosed as a "wrist sprain." Physical examination will reveal pain over the distal radial ulnar joint with a ballotable distal ulna. Radiographs can appear normal. The more common dorsal dislocation is reduced by supination and the palmar dislocation is reduced by pronation. The extremity should be placed into a long-arm cast in the appropriate rotation for 4 to 6 weeks.

A word of caution about wrist sprains is in order. Several entities that cause pain about the wrist are lumped into the category of "sprains" by the uninitiated. These include flexor carpi radialis tendonitis, flexor carpi ulnaris tendonitis, DeQuervain's disease, extensor carpi radialis brevis and longus tendonitis, and extensor carpi ulnaris subluxation. The diagnoses of scaphoid fractures and distal radial ulnar joint disruptions are also sometimes confused as sprains. When a specific diagnosis cannot be made because of either negative radiographs or confusing clinical examinations, it is better to refer this patient early for evaluation than to miss a subtle diagnosis and cause further disability.

Injuries of the Hand

Nowhere else in the body is it so important to recognize the soft tissue injuries that accompany fractures as in the metacarpals and phalanges. The exact area of tenderness will determine what structure is injured and, thus, the appropriate injury treated and position chosen for splinting. Every injured hand must be examined meticulously and systematically to determine the status of the tendons, nerves, intrinsic muscles, and blood vessels. Posterior-anterior, lateral, and oblique views are necessary, and for injuries involving a finger, a true lateral of the individual digit is mandatory.

Fractures of the Distal Phalanx

Most fractures of the distal phalanx are of the crushed "eggshell" type, with severe comminution of the distal tuft. This injury is frequently accompanied by a subungual hematoma. Evacuation of the hematoma can easily be accomplished with a red-hot paper clip or a disposable battery-operated cautery. "Nail-bed" injuries frequently accompany tuft fractures and are more serious than the fracture itself. Careful approximation with fine nonabsorbable sutures is required. The distal phalanx can then be protected with a small aluminum splint, allowing active motion of the proximal interphalangeal joint.

Mallet finger, or baseball finger, is caused by either attenuation or rupture of the extensor tendon at the level of the distal phalanx or by an avulsion of a bony fragment from the distal phalanx. If a fracture fragment involves more than one-third of the dorsal articular surface, there is a tendency for the distal phalanx to sublux palmarly and the fragment to rotate. These injuries require operative treatment. The remainder of acute mallet fingers can be treated with immobilization of the distal phalanx in full extension. This can be accomplished with either a commercial Stack splint (Fig. 12-5) or, preferably, a dorsal padded aluminum splint (Fig. 12-6), which allows for the exposure of the tactile surface of the digit. Immobilization must be continued for at least 8 weeks.

Fractures of the Proximal and Middle Phalanges

Fractures in the fingers can be divided into stable and unstable fractures as well as intra-articular and extra-articular fractures. Generally, all intra-articular fractures should be reduced anatomically. Reduction of a stable frac-

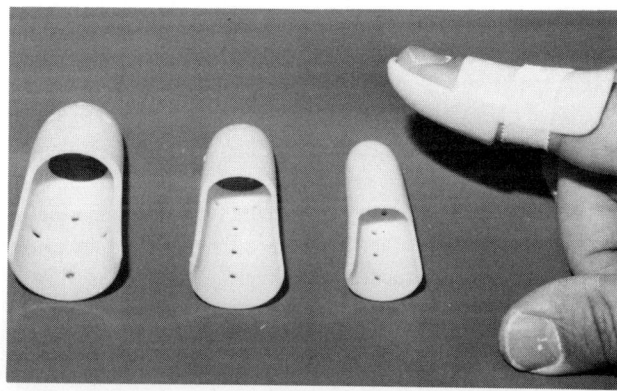

Figure 12-5 Commercially available stick splint used for the treatment of mallet finger deformities.

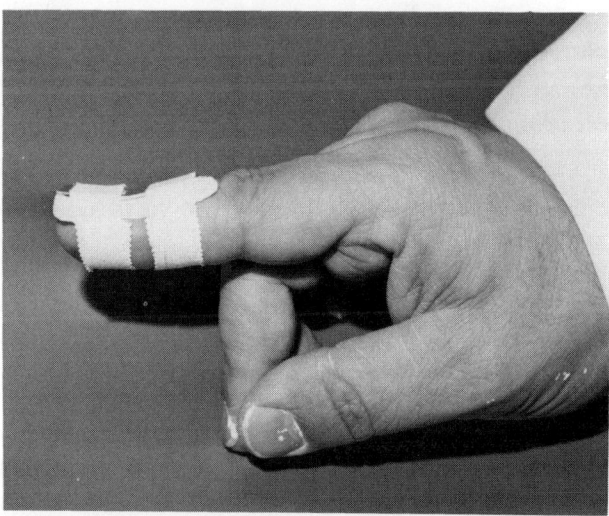

Figure 12-6 Dorsal padded aluminum splint bent to maintain distal phalanx in slight hyperextension (alternative splint for mallet finger deformities).

ture is maintained with a cast or splint. Unstable fractures, however, will lose position after reduction without internal fixation.

Unstable fractures of the proximal phalanx present with the proximal fragment flexed, owing to the forces of the interossei muscles at the base of the proximal phalanx. The extensor mechanism tends to pull the distal portion of the proximal phalanx into hyperextension, creating a fracture with palmar angulation.

The deforming forces acting on a middle phalangeal fracture are mainly the flexor digitorum superficialis, which inserts palmarly, and the central slip of the extensor mechanism, which inserts dorsally.

The most frequent complication of phalangeal fractures is rotational malalignment. The rotation of the fingernail can be compared with that of the opposite hand held in the same position, and rotational alignment can be confirmed if, when the fingers are flexed, they converge to the tuberosity of the scaphoid. Fractures involving the proximal interphalangeal joint tend to result in loss of motion at this joint. Nondisplaced stable fractures of both the proximal and middle phalanges require about 3 weeks of splinting. Alternatively, the injured finger may be taped to an adjacent normal finger and active motion encouraged from the beginning of treatment.

Displaced fractures are unstable but can be divided into those that obtain stability after reduction and those that do not. Those fractures that are stable after reduction are immobilized with the metacarpophalangeal joint in 70° of flexion and the proximal interphalangeal joint in 15° of flexion. A plaster cast incorporating a metal splint for the injured finger and additional "buddy taping" to the adjacent normal finger provide excellent immobilization. Protection continues for 6 weeks after injury; however, active exercises are started after 3 weeks of immobilization.

Fractures that do not obtain stability after reduction require either percutaneous pinning or open reduction and internal fixation for definitive treatment.

Metacarpal Fractures

Metacarpal fractures most commonly result from a direct blow. Frequently, the fourth and fifth metacarpals are involved; fracture of the fifth metacarpal neck is also known as a "fighter's fracture" or "boxer's fracture." The distal fragment always displaces into the palm, therefore resulting in dorsal angulation. There is disagreement in the literature over how many degrees of angulation are acceptable. More angulation can be accepted in the fourth and fifth metacarpals because of the mobility of their carpal-metacarpal joints. In the index and long finger metacarpals, residual angulation over 10° is unacceptable. In the fourth and fifth metacarpals, persistent angulation greater than 30° is an indication for open reduction. Otherwise, the patient may develop pain in the palm during grasp and limitation of metacarpophalangeal motion.

Reduction is performed under local block. Control of the distal fragment is obtained by maximally flexing the metacarpophalangeal joint. The metacarpal head is then pushed dorsally with the flexed proximal phalanx. The metacarpal is immobilized with either an ulnar "gutter" splint (Fig. 12-7) or a palmar plaster splint with an aluminum outrigger (Fig. 12-8), maintaining the metacarpophalangeal joint in 60° of flexion and buddy-taping the injured digit to the adjacent normal digit. If closed reduction is unsuccessful, then open reduction and internal fixation are indicated.

Metacarpal shaft fractures most often can be managed by closed reduction and plaster cast with a splint for immobilization. Plaster should be molded over the apex of angulation and the metacarpophalangeal joint flexed to 60° with free motion of the interphalangeal joints.

Open reduction is indicated for displaced transverse fractures, displaced open fractures, multiple displaced fractures, and oblique or spiral fractures with shortening.

Intra-articular fractures of the base of the metacarpals are important when they involve the fifth metacarpal. This fracture is commonly associated with proximal and dorsal subluxation of the fifth metacarpal created by the pull of the extensor carpi ulnaris tendon. The injury is best delineated on an anterior-posterior view of the hand with the forearm pronated 30° from the full supinated position. Inadequate reduction of this fracture results in weak grip strength and, therefore, open reduction and Kirschner wire fixation are usually indicated.

Fractures of the Thumb Metacarpal

The most significant fracture to recognize at the base of the thumb metacarpal is known as Bennett's fracture and is more properly called a fracture-dislocation. The fracture line is intra-articular and separates the metacarpal from a small palmar lip avulsion fracture. The small fragment is secured to the tubercle of the trapezium by a very strong anterior oblique ligament, while the base of the metacarpal is pulled dorsally and radially by the abductor pollicis longus. Treatment consists of obtaining anatomical reduction, either by closed or open means, followed by Kirschner wire fixation.

Comminuted fractures of the base of the thumb, known as Rolando fractures, are probably best treated by careful molding of the fragments, with the institution of early motion, or skeletal traction followed by early motion. If the comminution is not severe, and major fragments can be assembled to restore articular anatomy, then open reduction and internal fixation can be worthwhile.

Extra-articular fractures of the thumb metacarpal are reduced by closed manipulation and immobilization in a short-arm thumb spica cast for 4 weeks.

Ligamentous Injuries and Dislocations

Collateral ligaments in the hand may rupture with or without dislocation of the joint. Reduction is frequently

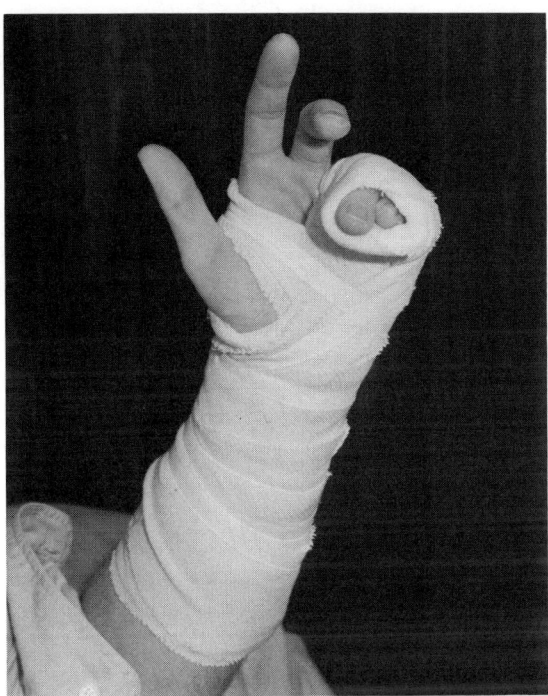

Figure 12-7 Ulnar "gutter" splint.

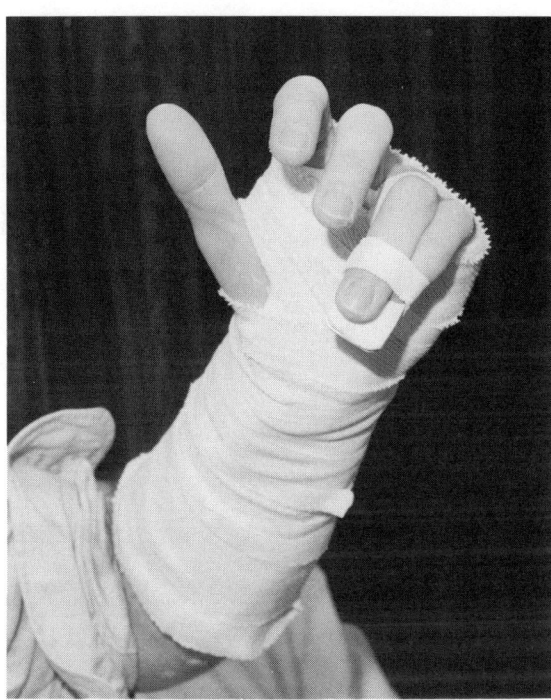

Figure 12-8 Palmar plaster splint with an aluminum outrigger.

performed before the patient is seen by a physician, and thus the dislocation is not appreciated. Swelling and pain in an area of the joint, despite normal-appearing radiographs, demand careful examination for ligamentous stability. Specific point tenderness, whether dorsal, palmar, radial, or ulnar, will direct attention to the injured structure. The structures most commonly injured include the radial and ulnar collateral ligaments, the volar plate, and the central slip over the dorsum of the proximal interphalangeal joint.

A metacarpophalangeal joint dislocation occasionally requires surgical reduction because the metacarpal head becomes trapped between the flexor tendons, the natatory ligament, the lumbricals, and the superficial transverse ligament. Most commonly, the volar plate becomes interposed between the metacarpal head and the proximal phalanx, blocking reduction.

Dislocations of the proximal interphalangeal joint, uncomplicated by fractures, can usually be reduced by manual traction. The joint is immobilized in 30° of flexion for 2 to 3 weeks, followed by buddy-taping and active motion. Complete rupture of the radial collateral ligament of the index finger may be an indication for operative repair. In any case, buddy-taping is continued for a minimum of 6 weeks for protection.

Partial tears (sprains) of the collateral ligaments are treated with buddy-taping for 3 weeks from the onset. The patient is advised to expect prolonged stiffness, tenderness, and some thickening about the joint that may be permanent.

An ulnar collateral rupture of the metacarpophalangeal joint of the thumb is often called a "gamekeeper's" thumb.

The name is derived from a chronic injury sustained by English gamekeepers who would kill a rabbit by holding it between the thumb and index finger and snapping its neck. This repetitive motion would cause a chronic strain of the ulnar collateral ligament of the thumb metacarpophalangeal joint. Today, this injury is most commonly found acutely and has been renamed the "ski pole thumb"; the mechanism of injury is a fall with the ski pole, producing a radial directed force that causes a rupture of the ulnar collateral ligament. It is now recognized that in more than half of the acute ruptures of ulnar collateral ligaments, the adductor aponeurosis becomes interposed between the two ends of the torn ligament, preventing adequate healing. The joint should be examined under adequate anesthesia and, if instability can be demonstrated, primary ligamentous repair is performed. Incomplete tears are immoblized in a thumb spica short-arm cast with the metacarpophalangeal joint in slight flexion for 3 to 6 weeks.

Volar Plate Injuries

Rupture of the volar plate occurs by hyperextension of the proximal interphalangeal joint. The injury is recognized by pain and swelling over the palmar aspect of the proximal interphalangeal joint and frequently is accompanied by a fracture of the volar lip of the middle phalanx. If 20% or more of the articular surface is involved, the middle phalanx subluxates dorsally. This unstable injury is nicely treated with a technique called "extension block splinting." The proximal interphalangeal joint is immobilized in a dorsal

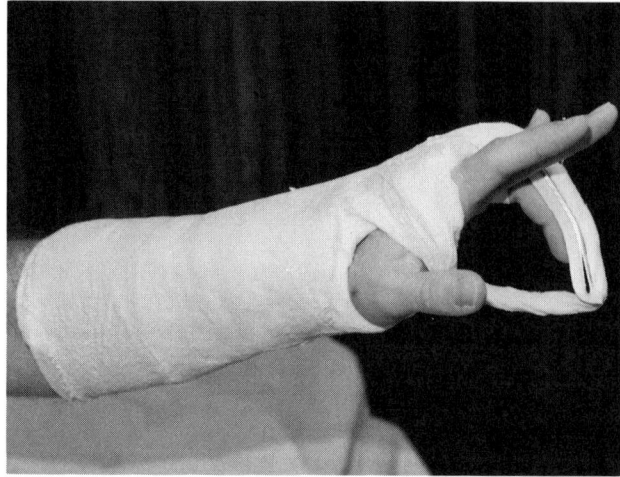

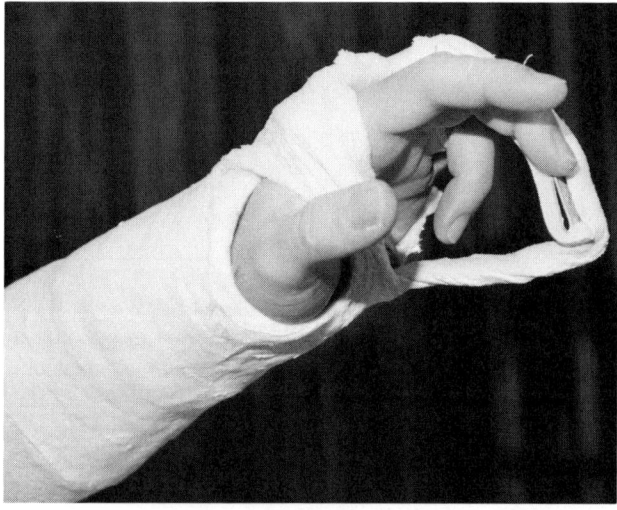

Figure 12-9 Extension block splint. **(A)** A short-arm cast incorporates a 1-inch padded aluminum splint bent to maintain the proximal interphalangeal joint in 50° flexion. **(B)** Active range of motion is performed within the limitations of the splint.

extension block splint as described by McElfresh. First, reduction of the joint is performed. A short-arm cast is applied, incorporating a 1-inch wide padded aluminum splint over the dorsum of the involved finger, which is bent to maintain the proximal interphalangeal joint in about 50° of flexion (Fig. 12-9A). The proximal phalanx is taped to the splint. The tape is removed and active exercises are performed within the limitations of the splint (Fig. 12-9B). A true lateral view is then taken to confirm reduction. Active flexion is encouraged from the onset. The patient is seen weekly and the splint is extended to reduce the amount of flexion in the proximal interphalangeal joint. Usually flexion can be reduced 15° each week so that full extension is achieved by 4 weeks. The splint is then removed and buddy-taped (Fig. 12-10) for 2 to 3 weeks. It must be emphasized that on each weekly examination a true lateral view ray is taken to confirm maintenance of reduction of the proximal interphalangeal joint.

One final word of advice: Do not be satisfied with diagnosing a swollen finger as a "sprain." Be careful to identify the injured structure and direct treatment accordingly.

Infections

Examination begins with careful observation of the hand, noting erythema, edema, tenderness, and the stigmata of intravenous drug abuse. Radiographs are performed to look for foreign bodies and associated fractures or dislocations. The natural history of a hand infection is cellulitis progressing to the formation of an abscess. It is beyond the scope of this chapter to deal with specific organisms and the use of antibiotics; rather, attention will be directed toward general principles and specific infections as defined by their anatomy.

Basic principles of treatment consist of immobilization of the hand in a position of function, elevation of the extremity, the use of appropriate antibiotics, adequate tetanus prophylaxis, and, when pus is present, surgical drainage.

Paronychia. This infection involves the eponychial fold around the fingernail. It is the most common infection in the hand. If untreated, it can progress to an abscess involving the entire perionychium. In the early stages, oral antibiotics and frequent washing of the hands can be curative. Usually, however, a patient presents with frank pus. Treatment consists of elevating the eponychial fold from the nail gently with a blunt instrument or a large sterile needle. Gauze packing is inserted beneath the fold to keep the cavity open for 48 hours. After removal of the gauze, the patient is advised to wash hands several times a day and apply a dry, sterile dressing to the affected digit. Occasionally, an incision will be necessary, or part of the nail will need removal.

Felon. A felon is an abscess in the pulp of the distal phalanx of the finger or thumb. There are multiple fibrous septa that divide the pulp into many small compartments. Treatment consists of surgical drainage with breaking up of the septa.

Herpes simplex infections are frequently confused with paronychia or felons. Since human saliva transmits the disease, physicians, dentists, nurses, and operating room personnel are at high risk. Typically the presentation varies from a single vesicle to multiple vesicles with surrounding erythema. The importance of considering this diagnosis cannot be overemphasized; incising a herpetic vesicle is contraindicated because secondary bacterial infection can ensue.

Web space abscess. Examination reveals a painful web space with swelling most pronounced dorsally where the tissues are loose and can therefore accommodate edema. A "collar button" abscess may be present, consisting of a collection of pus dorsally and palmarly with a thin sinus connection. A common mistake is to only incise the superficial dorsal abscess and leave the deep palmar abscess un-

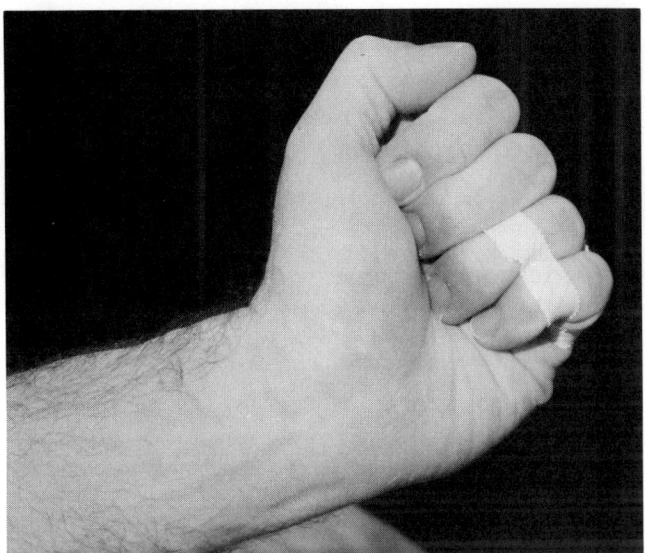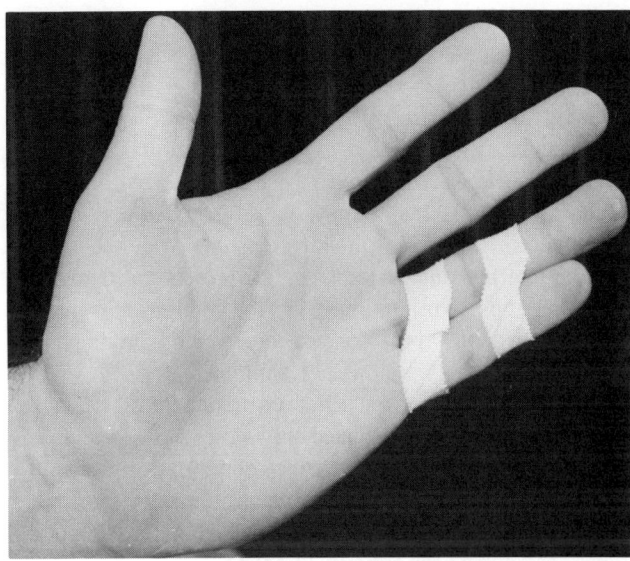

Figure 12-10 Buddy taping. **(A)** Flexion and **(B)** extension exercises are performed with the adjacent finger acting as a splint.

treated. This infection demands careful drainage in the operating room under adequate anesthesia.

Deep palmar space infections. Compartments exist in the hand which are spaces in which infections can occur. There is a potential space deep to the flexor tendons and superficial to the adductor pollicis. This space is divided in half by a thin septum along the midline from the long finger metacarpal. The space radially is known as the "thenar" space, and the space ulnarly is known as the "mid-palmar" space. Another potential space exists deep to the adductor pollicis, known as the "posterior adductor space." More proximally, just superficial to the pronator quadratus muscle, the "Parona's space" is located.

Deep-space infections result either from a direct penetrating wound or from spread of a more distal infection such as a flexor tenosynovitis or finger abscess. The diagnosis is made by tenderness and swelling over the affected space. One must remember that despite infection localizing in a palmar space, the hand will appear more swollen dorsally due to the unyielding nature of the palmar fascia.

All deep space infections require surgical incision and drainage. The surgery should be performed in an operating room under tourniquet control by someone who is knowledgeable about hand anatomy.

Acute pyogenic flexor tenosynovitis. The most important diagnostic consideration in an infected finger is to differentiate cellulitis from a flexor tendon sheath infection. Cellulitis may be treated with antibiotics alone, whereas if a flexor tenosynovitis is not drained, the flexor tendon will necrose and render the finger useless.

There is usually a history of a penetrating wound to the affected digit. Kanavel described four cardinal signs which are pathognomonic of a flexor tenosynovitis: (1) exquisite tenderness over the course of the flexor tendon sheath, (2) semiflexed attitude of the finger, (3) symmetric fusiform swelling of the finger, and (4) marked pain on passive extension of the finger.

If seen very early (within 48 hours of onset of symptoms), the patient may be observed in the hospital on intravenous antibiotics over a period of 24 hours. Unless noticeable resolution of the process can be demonstrated, surgical drainage is imperative. The operative approach most commonly used consists of a through-and-through irrigation of the flexor tendon sheath over a closed catheter system. This method allows for primary wound healing and rapid return of function for the patient.

Clenched fist injury. The "clenched fist" injury is the most commonly mistreated infection of the hand. It is characterized by a small punctate wound over a metacarpophalangeal joint, usually in the ring finger or little finger. It represents a human bite sustained when a clenched fist makes contact with a tooth. Early on, the wound looks quite inocuous and the patient frequently denies the true nature of the injury. As a result, the primary physician will make the error of suturing the wound closed, only to find severe infection a few days later. The danger of this injury is that the metacarpophalangeal joint is usually inoculated with mouth flora. One need not be reminded that the human mouth contains a high concentration of potentially dangerous bacterial organisms. All punctate wounds over the dorsum of the metacarpophalangeal joints, particularly of the ring and little fingers, should be explored in a bloodless field and treated as a clenched fist injury, regardless of the history. Cultures are obtained, the wound is copiously irrigated and left open, and antibiotic therapy is begun immediately.

TENDON LACERATIONS

Extensor tendon lacerations may be repaired primarily in the emergency department if the tendons are easily located without extensive dissection. A simple horizontal mattress suture of 4.0 braided Dacron is used. The wrist and the metacarpophalangeal and proximal interphalangeal joints are splinted in extension to relieve tension. At 4 weeks the proximal interphalangeal joints are set free and at 6 weeks immobilization is discontinued. If the tendon ends have retracted, surgery is best done in the operating room in a bloodless field using atraumatic technique.

Flexor tendon injuries are never repaired in the emergency department and should be treated only by surgeons specializing in hand surgery. In the emergency department the wound is cleansed, not explored, and, if clean, the skin is closed. The extremity is placed in a bulky sterile hand dressing and the patient referred for definitive treatment.

SPECIAL INJURIES

Grease gun injuries result from the introduction of grease under pressure into the digit. The grease dissects through tissue planes and spaces, causing an intense chemical reaction. While the wound can be deceptive and look like a small puncture, severe damage can result if decompression of the involved spaces and debridement is not performed.

High-tension electrical burns frequently involve the upper extremity as contact is first made as a patient grasps the source of current. A thermal injury ensues, producing zones of patchy necrosis. Initial treatment consists of immediate decompression and complete debridement of the necrotic tissue. Repeated exploration and debridements are common and the amputation rate is high.

REPLANTATION

Replantation of amputated parts is best handled at a regional center for replantation. The goal of replantation is to restore greater function to the hand than that which could be provided by a prosthesis. In the emergency department, the general physical status of the patient is assessed. The remaining stump is cleansed and placed in a bulky sterile compression dressing. The amputated part is placed in a container of lactated Ringer's solution, which is then put into a plastic bag filled with crushed ice. To avoid a frostbite wound, the amputated part is never placed directly on ice. The fastest transportation to a replant center is then arranged.

There are several basic indications and contraindications to replantation. Some of these have changed, and others may change as the field evolves; therefore, the final assessment in decision for replantation should be left to the specialist who performs this service. It is important for the emergency department physician to contact the replantation specialist as soon as possible after examining the patient, to discuss and expedite the treatment plan.

BIBLIOGRAPHY

American College of Surgeons. *Early Care of the Injured Patient.* 2nd ed. Philadelphia: Saunders; 1976.

Bohart PG, Gelberman RH, Vandell RF, et al. Complex dislocations of the metacarpophalangeal joint; operative reduction by Farabeuf's dorsal incision. *Clin Orthop.* 1982;164:208–210.

Green DP. *Operative Hand Surgery.* New York: Churchill Livingstone; 1982.

Iversen LD, Clawson DK. *Manual of Acute Orthopaedic Therapeutics.* Boston: Little, Brown; 1977.

Kalisman M, Millendorf JB. Hand infections part I: management of superficial infections. *Infect Surg.* 1982;xx:59–64.

Kanavel AB. *Infections of the Hand.* 7th ed. Philadelphia: Lea & Febiger; 1983.

Luce EA, Dowden WC, Su Chi T, et al. High tension electrical injury in the upper extremity. *Surg Gynecol Obstet.* 1978;147:38–42.

McElfresh EC, Dobyns JH, O'Brien ET. Management of fracture-dislocation of the proximal interphalangeal joints by extension-block splinting. *J Bone Joint Surg Am.* 1972;54:1705–1711.

Neviaser RJ. Closed tendon sheath irrigation for pyogenic flexor tenosynovitis. *J Hand Surg.* 1978;3:462.

Rockwood CA Jr, Green DP. *Fractures in Adults.* 2nd ed. Philadelphia: Lippincott; 1984.

13. Pelvis and Lower Extremity Fracture Management

TIMOTHY J. BRAY, MD

PELVIC FRACTURES

The pelvis is a complex structure that serves a pivotal point in bipedal ambulatory Homo sapiens. The pelvis provides both an osseous support for the spine and a mechanism for the lower extremities to articulate with the hip joint. The pelvic bone is commonly referred to as a "ring structure" in that the two identical hemipelvis structures are connected anteriorly by the pubic symphysis and posteriorly by strong ligamentous structures attached to the sacrum. Therefore, this intact circular bony structure protects vital intra-abdominal organs and provides articular support for the spine and lower extremities.

To completely understand the issue of pelvic stability, one must understand the circular ringed concept and these ligamentous support structures anatomically and radiographically. The anterior and posterior sacroiliac ligaments, the sacrotuberous, and sacrospinous ligaments provide the support structure posteriorly, whereas the pubic symphysis is joined by dense fibrocartilage anteriorly. The magnitude of force required to disrupt this pelvic ring is usually manifested by major motor-vehicle accidents, motorcycle accidents, or falls from great heights.

Classification

The classification of pelvic fractures is based upon the disruption or maintenance of the "pelvic ring." The fractures can be categorized as anterior-posterior (AP) compression injury ("the open book"), lateral compression injury, or vertical shear.

The AP compression injuries usually create a widening of the pubic symphysis. The lateral compression injuries usually result from a laterally directed force resulting in a fracture of the ilium near the sacroiliac joint and fractures of the ipsilateral ramus, or the straddle fracture. These are very difficult to differentiate from the grossly unstable vertical shear injury. The ligamentous disruption associated with the vertical shear causes disruption of the pubic symphysis and the posterior ligamentous structures. The vertical shear injuries are frequently associated with major hemorrhage and genital, urinary, or lower extremity neurologic injury.

Radiographic Assessment

All multiply injured patients should have a lateral C-spine radiograph to include the seven cervical vertebral bodies as well as an AP view of the pelvis. This is extremely important, as many associated pelvic injuries are commonly missed due to the inadequacy of the physical examination in the acute management environment. Pelvic fractures, acetabular fractures, and hip dislocations can frequently be diagnosed with this one simple, cost-effective view. The Pennal views (ie, 45° inlet and 45° outlet views) demonstrate the pelvic brim as well as the anatomy of the pubic symphysis and sacroiliac joints. Therefore, all pelvic fractures should have an AP pelvis, an inlet, and an outlet view.

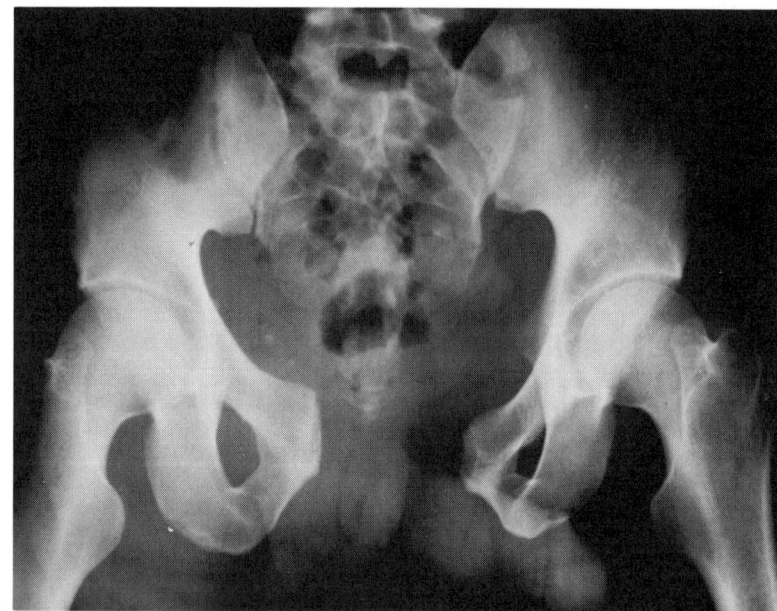
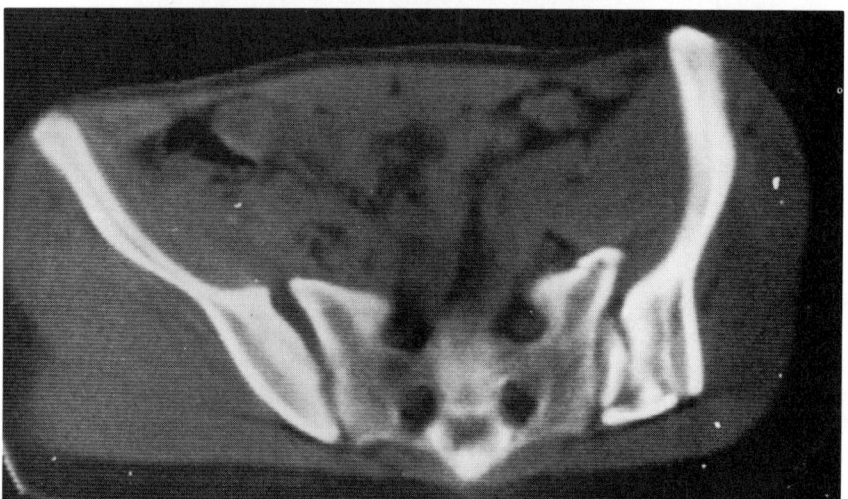
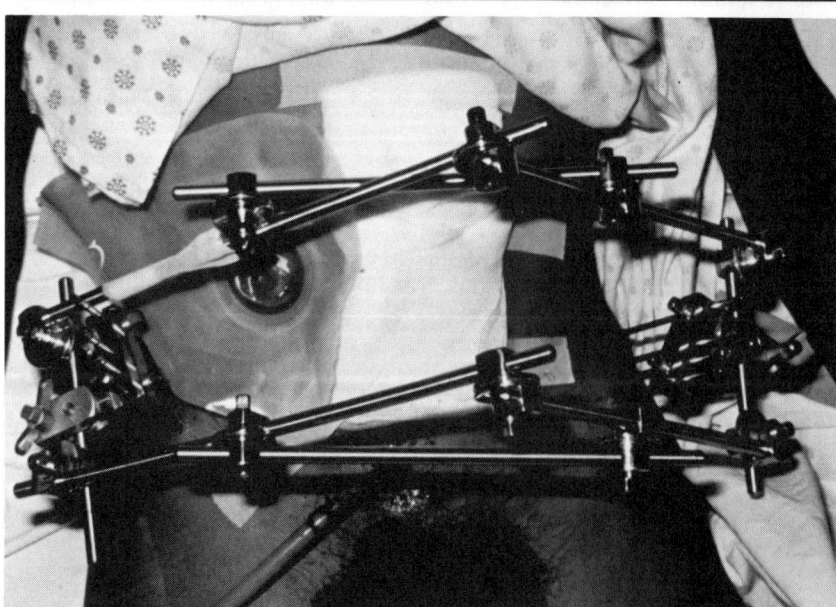

Figure 13-1 (**A**) A 23-year-old male involved in high-speed vehicular trauma with an open, Malgaigne pelvic fracture. On this AP roentgenogram of the pelvis, note the disrupted left sacroiliac joint, the proximal migration of the left hemipelvis, and the wide disrupted pubic symphysis. (**B**) The CT scan of the sacroiliac joints demonstrates a previously unrecognized fracture-dislocation on the left with widening on the right. (**C**) Rigid, stable, external fixation of the pelvis with a diverting colostomy and diverting cystostomy appropriately manages the pelvic instability and open wounds associated with this potentially catastrophic injury.

Associated Injuries

It is extremely important to consider the complications of pelvic fractures in five major areas: (1) hemorrhage; (2) urinary symptoms; (3) open fracture; (4) neurologic complications; and (5) associated trauma.

Acute Management

Most volume problems associated with pelvic fractures should be managed by adequate fluid replacement as monitored by central venous pressure, urine output, and/or balloon catheterization as indicated. External fixation of the unstable pelvis should be performed as soon as possible (Fig. 13-1). Nursing care is facilitated, bleeding is brought under control, and the patients can be mobilized as they are more comfortable when bony stability is achieved. Military antishock trousers, pelvic plaster spicas, and skeletal traction have all been reported as effective but with certain disadvantages. There are no indications for the once-popular pelvic sling.

It must be stressed that fluid management, however, is the keystone to the hypovolemia associated with the acute pelvic fracture. Prior to urinary catheterization to monitor urinary output, a rectal examination should be completed to evaluate the prostate for evidence of a posterior urethral injury, and a retrograde urethrogram should be performed if blood is found on the meatus of the penis. A free-floating prostate and/or blood in the penile meatus are strong clinical findings of a urethral injury. Intravenous pyelography or cystography and a delayed cystometrogram are sometimes required to evaluate the potential bladder injury.

The rectal examination is important to check for both sphincter tone and perirectal sensation that may be indicative of a sacroplexus injury. Occult open pelvic fractures frequently occur with small tears into the vagina as well as the retrosigmoid area. All females with pelvic fractures should have a vaginal examination as well as sigmoidoscopy to rule out the possibility of a puncture wound in the retrosigmoid. The open pelvic fracture is associated with a high incidence of mortality, and strong consideration should be given to laparotomy and diversional colostomy for appropriate wound management.

Open reduction and internal fixation of the pelvis are becoming more popular in treating the displaced pelvic fracture, and in these cases, 12 weeks are generally required prior to full unprotected weight-bearing.

Management of Stable Pelvic Fractures

The AP compression injuries and the stable lateral compression injuries without vertical displacement can be treated without skeletal immobilization. After complete evaluation, these patients will require admission to the hospital for hemodynamic evaluation and bedrest until the pain subsides. When the patient is able to move comfortably in bed, he or she may be progressed to limited weight-bearing with crutches. Prior to discharge, additional weight-bearing radiographic evaluations should be utilized to check for previously unrecognized instability. Anticoagulation should be considered if early mobilization is delayed. Low-dose heparin, sequential pneumatic compression stockings, or low-dose coumadin are all effective protocols. The prognosis is excellent for these injuries, and the patients should be pain-free in a 12-week period. If a neurologic injury occurs, or a major disruption of the sacroiliac joint or a chronic pain syndrome results, additional reconstructive surgery may be required.

ACETABULAR FRACTURES

The hip joint is a diarthrodial joint composed of the cup-shaped acetabulum and the round femoral head. Fractures of the acetabulum that involve intra-articular fragments should be managed as fractures of any lower extremity weight-bearing joint (ie, with anatomic reduction and early mobilization; Fig. 13-2.) There has been hesitancy to apply these principles to internal fixation of acetabular fractures because of the difficulty in surgical approaches and reduction techniques. Clearly, certain displaced intra-articular fractures of the acetabulum are best managed by open reduction and internal fixation.

Classification

Many acetabular fractures are associated with hip dislocation, and there is confusion as to the difference between fracture dislocations of the hip and acetabular fractures. Acetabular fractures are classified as to the fracture patterns of the acetabulum, not necessarily the mechanism of injury. The hemipelvis is divided into an anterior and posterior column as described by Judet, Judet, and Letournel: the anterior column or the iliopubic segment and the posterior column or the ilioischial segment. "Anterior column" fractures predominantly involve the iliopubic segment, and "posterior column" fractures predominantly involve the ilioischial segment. "Both-column" fractures are transverse or complex in nature and involve both anterior and posterior columns (Fig. 13-3).

Physical Examination/Evaluation

Many of the same complications that are associated with pelvic fractures are also of concern when diagnosing and managing acetabular fractures. Associated injuries must be primarily cared for, occult open fractures must be ruled out, and hemorrhagenic complications must be controlled by adequate volume replacement. Neurologic injuries should be suspected with posterior dislocations injuring the sciatic nerve.

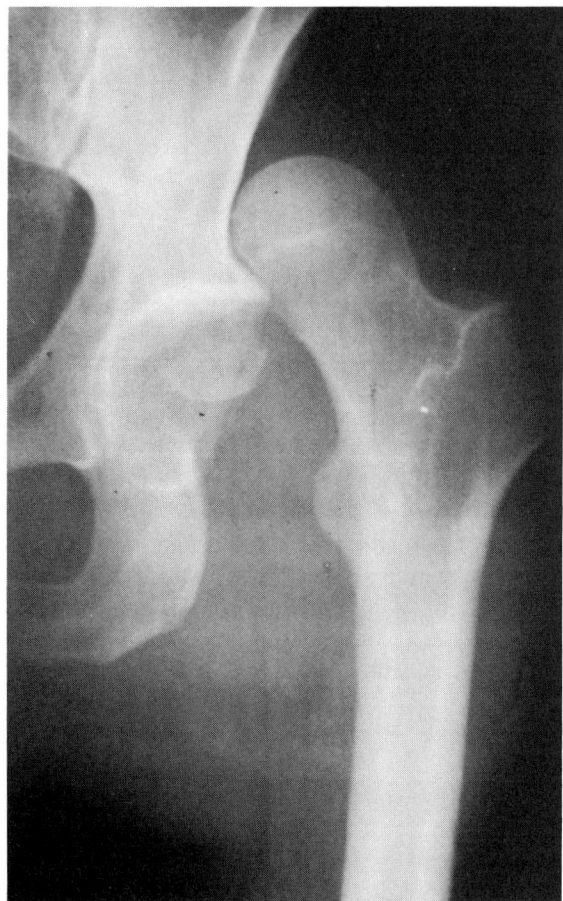

Figure 13-2 Posterior dislocation of the left hip with a small fracture of the femoral head. Note the femoral head fracture fragment contained within the acetabulum. Immediate reduction is mandatory to prevent associated avascular necrosis of the femoral head. The malreduction of the fracture fragment can adequately be reconstructed on an elective basis.

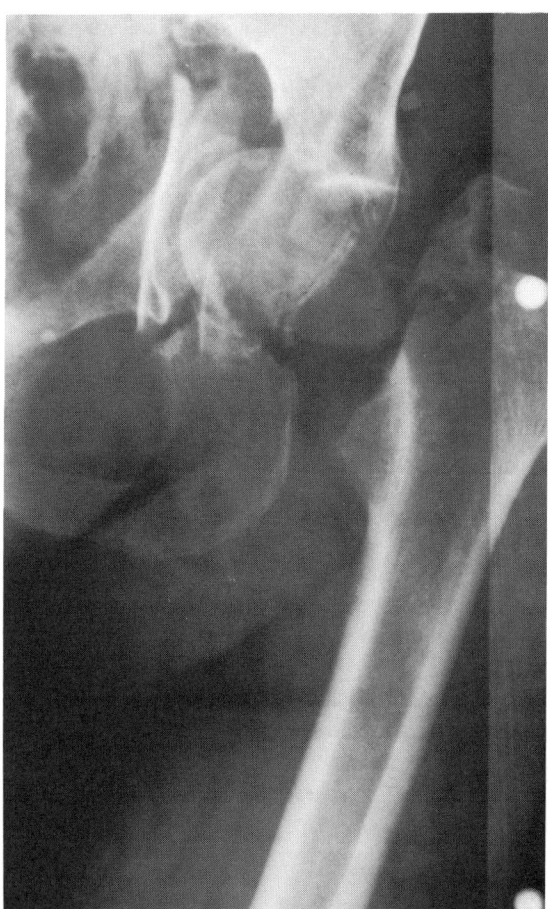

Figure 13-3 A complex fracture of the acetabulum associated with femoral neck fracture in a 65-year-old patient. This high-energy vehicular injury was fatal in this patient.

The principal views of the acetabulum in acute management situations should include an AP of the pelvis as well as two 45° oblique views of the injured acetabulum. These oblique views demonstrate the fracture pattern clearly.

Treatment

If a dislocated hip is present, the hip should be reduced as soon as possible to prevent the complications of avascular necrosis. Ideally, a gentle reduction under general anesthesia may prevent the associated cartilaginous trauma with the reduction maneuver. If a prolonged wait is anticipated, the hip can be gently reduced under adequate analgesia in the emergency department. A "three-man" reduction technique is employed, as described for posterior fracture dislocations. One force is exerted with a perineal sheet in the cephalad direction, a second force is applied by an axial pull on the foot, and a third force is applied by a sheet wrapped around the inside of the thigh and pulled laterally. Therefore, the three forces are applied with resultant controlled, gentle reduction. Once the fracture is reduced, an indication as to its stability should be ascertained by an experienced physician. In general, unstable acetabular fractures will require prolonged skeletal immobilization or open reduction and internal fixation. In the nondisplaced or minimally displaced fracture, tomography or computed tomography (CT) is indicated to rule out previously undiagnosed retained osteochondral fractures, nonconcentric reductions, or previously unrecognized fracture patterns. These fractures usually require prolonged traction to prevent displacement of the fracture fragments.

Prognosis

The prognosis of acetabular fractures depends totally on the mechanism of injury, the magnitude of the injury, and the eventual ability to obtain an anatomic reduction. Fracture patterns without intra-articular displacement have an excellent prognosis, whereas complex fracture patterns with intra-articular loose bodies, a step-off of the articular surface, or nonconcentric reductions have a worse prognosis. Avascular necrosis, post-traumatic arthritis, and myositis ossificans have all been reported as long-term complications. There is a 10% chance of associated sciatic nerve injury, but spontaneous recovery usually occurs. In general, 12 weeks are required for patients to return to full unprotected weight-bearing.

DISLOCATIONS OF THE HIP

Posterior Dislocations

The majority of posterior hip dislocations are so-called "dashboard" injuries. These occur when the patient strikes the dashboard, or vice versa, and a posteriorly directed force pushes the head of the femur out of the acetabular dome. When an associated acetabular fracture occurs, this is usually referred to as a "fracture dislocation." The majority of hip dislocations without fractures occur in the posterior direction, and as with all fractures about the pelvis there is a high association of complex injuries of the head, chest, abdomen, or extremities. All of the prior concerns for pelvic injuries including neurologic injury, hemorrhagic control, and the necessity for early reduction hold true for the hip dislocation.

Radiographic evaluation includes an AP and a lateral view of the hip. The majority of these dislocations can be diagnosed by careful scrutiny of the acetabular dome, femoral head relationships. There are multiple reports of missed posterior dislocations by inappropriate scrutiny or poor lateral roentgenographic evaluations at the time of injury. The physical examination usually reveals a leg that is short, internally rotated, and adducted. The sciatic nerve can be injured in a significant percentage of these injuries, and careful evaluation should include the femoral shaft for possible concomitant fracture, knee instability, and ipsilateral femoral head fracture.

The dislocated hip must be reduced as soon as possible. There is a direct correlation with the prognosis and time to reduction. Under ideal circumstances, a general anesthetic with muscle relaxation and "atraumatic reduction" is indicated. For prolonged waits to obtain a general anesthetic, a reduction should be obtained as soon as possible in the emergency department.

After the reduction is radiographically confirmed in the AP and lateral planes, the patient should be admitted to the hospital and placed in balanced suspension until comfortable. When the patient is able to ambulate with crutches and protected weight-bearing, he or she is then discharged and advanced to full weight-bearing status.

If closed reduction cannot gently be obtained, an open reduction is indicated. Under no circumstance should multiple attempts be made to reduce the posterior dislocation. This may result in severe articular damage to the femoral head. Occasionally, the femoral head is buttonholed through the hip capsule, or the reduction is blocked by the piriformis tendon. Open reduction allows direct visualization of the femoral head and intra-articular debridement of small loose fragments. With single large posterior fragments, open reduction and internal fixation can be obtained with screws and/or buttress-plating as indicated. Depending on the fixation, patients are allowed partial weight-bearing for 8 to 12 weeks and allowed full weight-bearing thereafter.

Anterior Dislocations

The anterior dislocation is usually a forced abduction injury. The motorcyclist who catches his abducted leg on a car or in a severe fall may suffer an anterior dislocation. These are classified as obturator, iliac, or pubic dislocations, depending on the position of the femoral head to the acetabulum at the time of the diagnosis.

The physical examination is quite characteristic. With the obturator dislocation the hip is abducted, externally rotated, and flexed. In the iliac or pubic dislocation, the hip is extended. In all cases careful consideration should be given to the anterior neurovascular structures (ie, the femoral artery and/or femoral nerve).

Reduction is attempted under anesthesia with axial traction and internal rotation. For the iliac or pubic dislocation, the hip is flexed and internally rotated. As with the posterior dislocations, no attempt should be made to multiply reduce these injuries, as severe femoral head injury can occur. Open reduction is indicated when failure of closed reduction occurs. As with the posterior dislocation, post-traumatic arthritis or avascular necrosis can occur, and the prognosis is directly related to timing of the reduction. The rule of thumb: the earlier the reduction, the better the prognosis.

FRACTURES OF THE FEMORAL HEAD

Pipkin's classification of four different fractures of the femoral head is well described and is prognostically important. Most fractures of the femoral head are associated with hip dislocations, and they can be associated with fracture of the acetabulum. Careful neurologic examination, as well as examination of the general condition of the patient, is indicated. These are high-energy injuries, and associated fractures commonly occur.

Special radiographic evaluation is sometimes indicated to make an appropriate diagnosis. CT scans are helpful for identifying loose fragments and undiagnosed fractures, and for evaluating the adequacy of the closed reduction.

Fractures of the femoral head associated with hip dislocations must be reduced as soon as possible. Nevertheless, Pipkin types I, II, and IV are generally treated conservatively. The reductions must be anatomic and proven radiographically. If a minor step-off results, strong consideration should be given to open reduction and internal fixation. Pipkin type III injury is probably best treated with initial open reduction and pinning of the femoral neck fracture. The approach, mechanism of reduction, and trochanteric osteotomy are dependent on the surgeon's experience. Avascular necrosis, degenerative hip disease, and late segmental collapse occurring in the young patient make this fracture particularly worrisome.

HIP FRACTURES

According to the *Orthopaedic Knowledge Update—1 Home Study Syllabus*, 1984, approximately 200,000 hip fractures occur annually in the United States and result in health care costs of $1 billion or more. The most commonly seen patient with hip fracture is an elderly woman in the 6th, 7th, or 8th decade. Mortality rates in the literature are conflicting; however, 30% within the first year is often quoted. Due to the patient's elderly status, many associated medical conditions are found in patients sustaining hip fractures, including cardiac dysrhythmias, severe osteoporosis, metabolic disease, and metastatic disease resulting in pathologic bone conditions.

Classification

Fractures about the hip can be classified as transcervical or femoral neck fractures, intertrochanteric fractures, subtrochanteric fractures, and shaft fractures.

The intracapsular fracture of the femoral neck is often referred to as the "unsolved fracture." There are multiple classifications as to the type of fracture, but the simplest approach is based on the degree of displacement (Fig. 13-4). Nondisplaced fractures of the femoral neck have a much better prognosis than displaced fractures of the femoral neck. This deals exclusively with the anatomy and vascular insult at the time of injury. The femoral head has a very tenuous vascular supply in that the medial and lateral femoral circumflex arteries provide 90% of the vascular blood supply. When the femoral neck is fractured, this blood supply is severely compromised, and avascular necrosis, nonunion, and late collapse frequently occur.

Intracapsular fractures of the hip usually occur in elderly patients sustaining a minor fall. The general medical condition of these elderly patients must be accurately evaluated and cover their neurologic status, cardiopulmonary status, and any evidence of pathologic bony conditions.

In young patients, the femoral neck fracture is usually the result of high-energy, motor vehicular trauma and con-

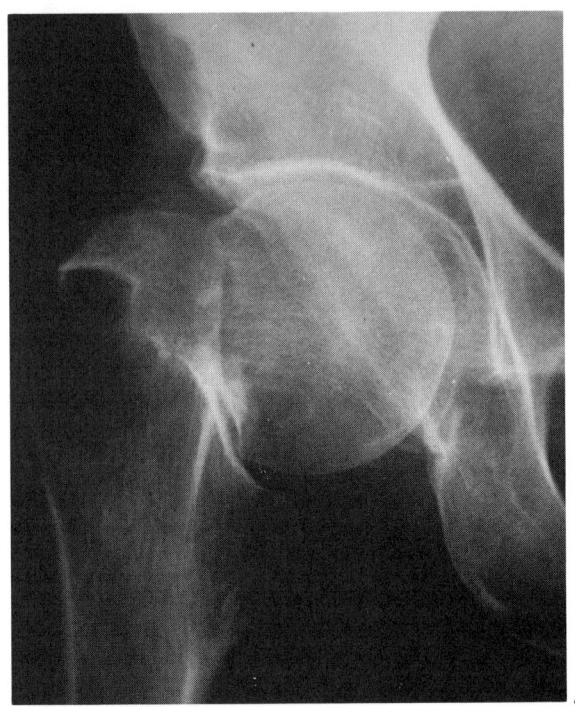

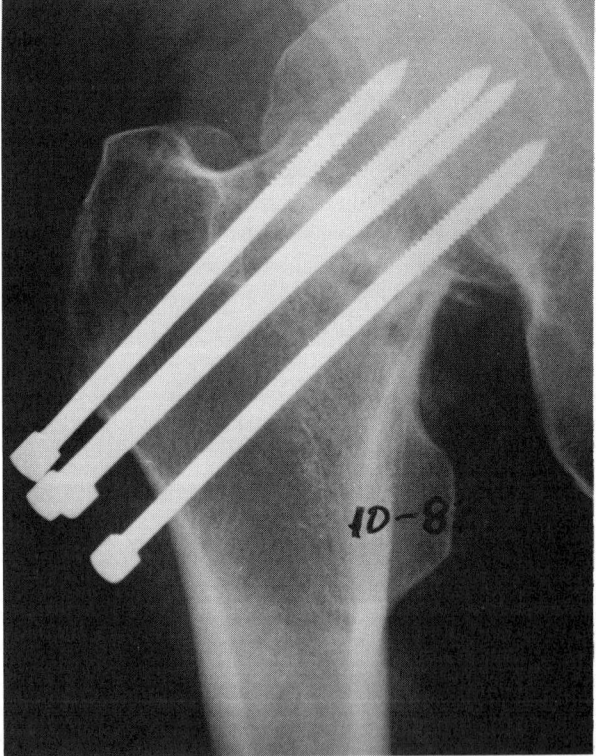

Figure 13-4 **(A)** A 55-year-old man sustained a displaced femoral neck fracture after a fall from a tree. **(B)** This was treated with percutaneous pinning and stabilization with resultant bone union and excellent functional range of motion. Most femoral neck fractures should be pinned in the young patient and hemiarthroplasty reserved for elderly patients with displaced fractures.

stitutes a different category of injury pattern. The general condition of the young, multiply injured patient should also be evaluated for associated head, neck, chest, or abdominal injuries.

Once the patient is stabilized and cleared for surgery, the treatment of choice for most femoral neck fractures is operative. There are relatively few indications for nonoperative therapy in the management of femoral neck fractures.

The nondisplaced femoral neck fracture can be treated with percutaneous pinning. This is usually performed on a fracture table with close radiographic control and adequate pin placement to allow the patient to be up and weight-bearing immediately postoperatively.

The displaced femoral neck fracture can be treated by anatomic closed reduction and percutaneous pinning or prosthetic replacement. Advocates of percutaneous pinning suggest the operation is shorter and quicker with less morbidity as compared to hemiarthroplasty. Hemiarthroplasty advocates state that one operation is generally required with better functional results than the pinned group.

In the young, femoral neck fractures are usually treated with open reduction and internal fixation. Multiple screws and an anatomic reduction appear to be the most recent approach. There is some support in the literature that the earlier the fracture is stabilized, the better the prognosis. Associated fractures of the ipsilateral femoral shaft and neck should be treated by internal, anatomic reduction of the femoral neck and stabilization of the femoral shaft by intramedullary fixation.

Prognosis

Operated, nondisplaced femoral neck fractures have an excellent prognosis, and most patients can be fully weight-bearing immediately postoperatively. The displaced femoral neck fractures treated with open reduction and internal fixation have approximately a 60% chance of good to excellent results. The failures usually result from avascular necrosis, late segmental collapse, and nonunion. Should this occur, a secondary reconstruction is indicated. When hemiarthroplasty is selected as the treatment of choice, barring any complication the result is extremely favorable. However, if the patient develops a dislocation from malposition of the prosthesis or an infection, reconstructive procedures become a major undertaking.

In the young, femoral neck fracture has an extremely poor prognosis. Many studies suggest a 50% incidence of complications including avascular necrosis, nonunion, and late segmental collapse. In passing, it should be mentioned that the occult fracture of the femoral neck, or the undiagnosed stress fracture commonly seen in runners, can pose a diagnostic problem. An elderly patient with a history of a fall or an avid runner with hip pain should be suspect for this injury. Although the physical examination can be benign, most patients will have pain with internal rotation. Tomographic evaluations, CT evaluations, and bone scans may be required to make the diagnosis. These patients should be admitted to the hospital, as displacement of these relatively benign fractures can result in catastrophic complications.

Intertrochanteric Fractures

The intertrochanteric fracture is classified as to the number of free fracture fragments occurring in the intertrochanteric region (Figs. 13-5 and 13-6). The potential free fracture fragments are as follows: femoral head and neck fragment, greater trochanteric fragment, lesser trochanteric fragment, and shaft fragment. The classification therefore depends on the number of free fracture fragments. A two-part intertrochanteric fracture has the femoral head and neck as one fragment and the greater, lesser, and shaft fragment as the other; a three-part intertrochanteric fracture involves the head, neck, and lesser trochanter as one fragment, the greater trochanter as the second fragment, and the shaft as the third fragment; and a four-part intertrochanteric fracture has all four intertrochanteric components free. This anatomic description of the intertrochanteric fracture is quite applicable to radiographic evaluation.

Clinically, these patients are usually elderly and present with a history of a fall. The hip can be swollen, is exquisitely painful to any range of motion, and is usually short and externally rotated. This fracture can usually be diagnosed by observing the patient's lower extremity while the patient is lying supine on the gurney. The extracapsular fracture (ie, the intertrochanteric fracture) should be differentiated from the transcervical or intercapsular fracture, as the hemodynamic stability of the intertrochanteric fracture is far more hazardous. Such a patient can lose up to 3 U of blood in the thigh, as compared to the transcervical fracture where the hematoma is contained within the hip capsule. The elderly patient with the displaced intertrochanteric fracture must not be admitted to a ward sparse on nursing care, because hypovolemia, cardiac dysrhythmia, and death can occur if the patient is not closely observed.

When the patient's medical condition is stabilized and adequate radiographs of the hip reveal the fracture pattern, these patients are treated with open reduction and internal fixation. Generally, these fractures are treated with a standard compression screw and side plate. In patients with metastatic disease or severe pathologic conditions of bone, polymethylmethacrylate has been utilized to provide stability when the fixation device alone does not suffice.

Because of the condition of these elderly debilitated patients, there is a high association of significant mortality and morbidity. Although there is no consensus as to the use of anticoagulation, most surgeons feel that an antithrombotic agent is indicated. Early mobilization is the best prevention for deep vein thrombophlebitis. As soon as these patients are

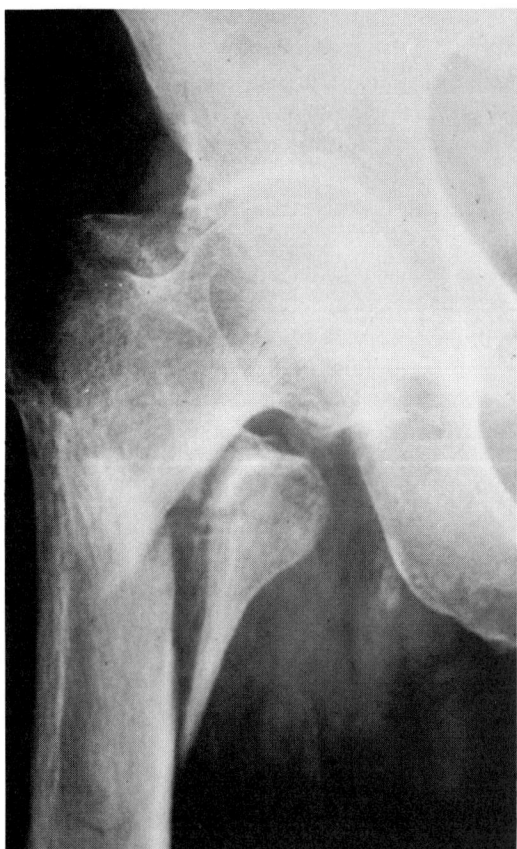

Figure 13-5 A 65-year-old patient with a four-part intertrochanteric hip fracture. Note the fracture of the greater and lesser trochanters with an obvious fracture line through the intertrochanteric area. This fracture is routinely stabilized with a compression screw and side plate to allow patients to be fully ambulatory as soon as possible.

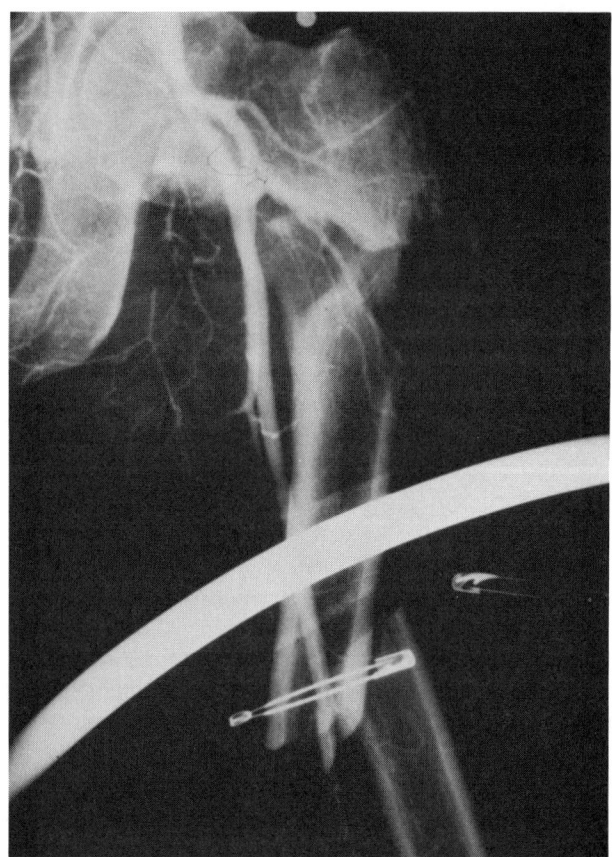

Figure 13-6 Ipsilateral fracture of the femoral shaft and the intertrochanteric zone. This injury is frequently found in young patients subjected to high-energy vehicular trauma. Note the disruption of the femoral artery at the level of the mid-shaft femur fracture. Detailed neurovascular examination is mandatory with femur fractures, especially in the poly-traumatized patient.

stabilized, they are allowed to sit at the bedside for improvement of their pulmonary status, postural urinary stasis, and prevention of pressure sores. The patients are encouraged to begin weight-bearing as tolerated, advancing to the four-posted walker soon thereafter.

Subtrochanteric Fractures

Whereas transcervical and intertrochanteric fractures commonly occur in the elderly patient, the subtrochanteric fracture commonly occurs in the young, healthy patient. There are multiple classifications of this injury; however, the important observation is to differentiate the intertrochanteric fracture and look carefully for extension into the femoral shaft. For these reasons, a radiograph to include the pelvis and complete AP and lateral views of the entire femur, including the knee, are mandatory.

Due to the muscle forces of the subtrochanteric fracture, the proximal segment is usually flexed and is usually palpable in the proximal aspect of the thigh. These patients have severe muscle spasm and are in pain. Femoral nerve, artery, or vein lacerations are reported and a detailed neurovascular examination is indicated. Diagnosis is made radiographically by an AP view of the proximal femur. Careful attention must be paid to the radiographic characteristics of these intertrochanteric fractures. The fixation device is totally dependent on the stability or instability of the fracture pattern.

Open reduction and internal fixation are the mainstays of the management of subtrochanteric fractures. Skeletal traction should be implemented initially, with skeletal traction until operative intervention is possible. Either intramedullary fixation or compression screw is usually selected as the treatment of choice.

Trochanteric Fractures

Isolated fractures of the greater or lesser trochanter are extremely rare and usually benign. If the displacement is less than 1 cm, they can simply be treated with protected weight-bearing until comfortable. If there is displacement of greater than 1 cm, consideration is given to open reduction and internal fixation. The standard radiographic evaluation should be implemented and should include AP and lateral views of the hip.

Hip Fractures in Children

The intertrochanteric and subtrochanteric fracture patterns found in the child are quite different from the adult hip fracture. A traumatic separation of the proximal femoral epiphysis is a particularly dangerous injury in the child, and the parents should be warned against avascular necrosis and proximal femoral growth arrest (Fig. 13-7). Displaced fractures of the femoral neck are treated with open reduction and internal fixation, and undisplaced femoral neck fractures can usually be treated with a 1½ hip spica.

The intertrochanteric fracture found in the child can usually be treated in skeletal traction for approximately 4 to 6 weeks and then converted to a 1½ hip spica. An indication for internal fixation is the association of multiple other injuries or the inability to manage the fracture closed. When treated in traction, subtrochanteric fractures usually pose a problem in maintenance of reduction. In general, these can be reduced in the so-called "90/90" position with a distal femoral traction pin. Although rarely indicated, intramedullary fixation has been selected for the management of certain proximal femur fractures in the multiply injured or head-injured adolescent. This facilitates nursing care and provides anatomic reduction of the fracture; the only objection is the (low) risk of sepsis. The complications associated with proximal fractures in the child are avascular necrosis, leg-length discrepancies, and malrotations.

FRACTURES, LIGAMENTOUS INJURIES, AND DISLOCATIONS ABOUT THE KNEE

The knee is very susceptible to injury in the bipedal human. It is extremely flexible, with great exposure to high-energy trauma, sports injuries, and arthritic disease due to the major weight-bearing forces required of the knee on a daily basis. Fractures about the knee are particularly dangerous in that they frequently involve the articular surface and predispose the knee to early arthritic changes. Neurologic and vascular injuries are commonly associated with traumatic events about the knee because of the close proximity of the common peroneal nerve as well as the arterial trifurcation found distal to the popliteal space of the major arterial blood supply to the leg (Figs. 13-8 and 13-9).

Anatomy

The anatomy of the knee is extremely complex; it requires extensive knowledge to accurately diagnose and recognize pitfalls of the injured knee. The knee is composed of the articular surface of the femur, the medial and lateral femoral condyles, which articulate with the surface of the proximal tibia, commonly referred to as the tibial plateau. The patella is an articular seismoid bone which provides mechanical advantage to the quadriceps extensor mechanism and also serves to protect the anterior articular surface of the femur and tibia. The significant supporting structures include the medial and lateral collateral ligaments, which provide stability to the knee in the varus and valgus planes, as well as the anterior and posterior cruciate ligaments, which prevent anterior and posterior excursion of the femur on the tibia. There are two semicircular menisci found on the medial and lateral aspect of the tibial-femoral joint, which act as shock absorbers and prevent abnormal forces within this major articular complex. The popliteal artery trifurcates into the anterior tibial, posterior tibial, and peroneal arteries at the proximal third of the tibia. This artery is extremely susceptible to injury from fractures and knee dislocations. The com-

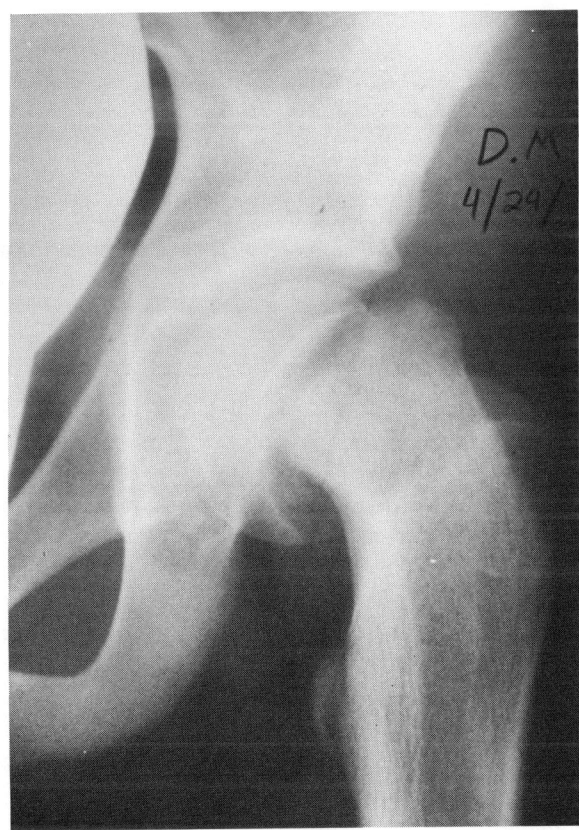

Figure 13-7 This AP view of the left hip of a skeletally immature patient demonstrates a slipped capital femoral epiphysis. This can be confused with a traumatic separation of the proximal femoral epiphysis. Any young patient with a complaint of knee pain should have a mandatory radiographic view of the ipsilateral hip. The differential diagnosis of knee pain in the skeletally immature patient always includes hip pathology.

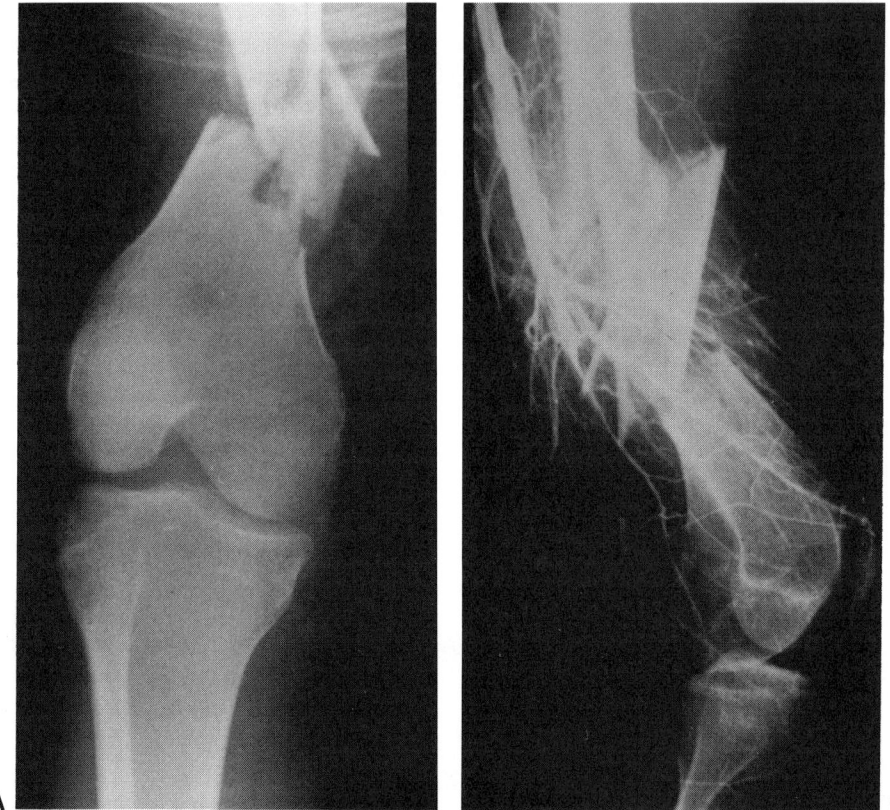

Figure 13-8 (A) This roentgenogram demonstrates an open, comminuted fracture of the distal third of the femur in a young patient. The physical findings were consistent with a femoral arterial lesion. The high-energy nature of these injuries frequently results in concomitant vascular injuries. A detailed neurovascular examination should always be completed. **(B)** A lateral angiographic view of the fracture area illustrates the associated femoral artery disruption. Note the minimal peripheral circulation through the superior geniculate arterial system. This lesion requires both orthopedic and vascular surgical consultation.

mon peroneal nerve is found directly posterior to the fibular head and is susceptible owing to its superficial placement. This can be iatrogenically injured with inappropriate cast placement, tight dressings, and, more commonly, from injury patterns due to lateral stress.

Classification

Fractures of the distal femur and proximal tibia can be characterized as articular or nonarticular fracture patterns. The nonarticular fracture patterns are those that occur in the distal third of the femur, which are usually spiral, short oblique, or transverse. They do not communicate with the knee joint itself. Tomography is often necessary to absolutely rule out intra-articular communication, but the majority of cases can be appropriately diagnosed on routine radiographs. Puncture wounds in the area of distal femur fractures are open fractures until proven otherwise and are orthopedic emergencies requiring surgical debridement and consideration for early fracture stabilization.

Intra-articular fractures of the distal femur are particularly challenging in that anatomic reduction and early mobilization have been found to provide better results than has conservative treatment of those types of fractures. Therefore, the fracture pattern that involves the articular surface will most likely be treated with some form of operative fixation. Conversely, those fractures that do not involve the articular surface can be treated conservatively in a traction apparatus or cast. The emergency evaluation of these fractures includes compulsive attention to the potential of a vascular or neurologic injury; they should be splinted immediately for comfort and to prevent further soft tissue injury from sharp, shearing, bony fragments. The open fracture should be treated with sterile dressings, culture, antibiotics, and preoperative evaluation, including appropriate blood tests, urinalysis, chest radiography, electrocardiography, and nothing by mouth until the operating surgeon has arrived.

Fractures of the patella are usually the result of direct injury. These fractures commonly occur as dashboard injuries and are, quite often, open fractures requiring urgent

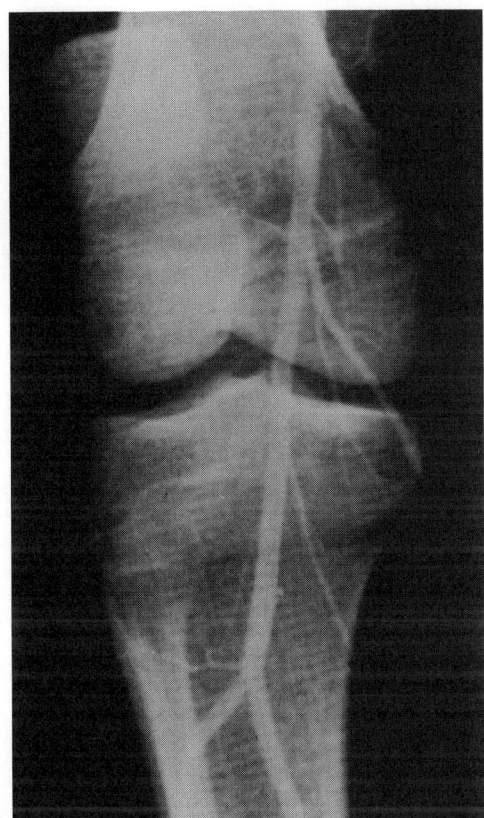 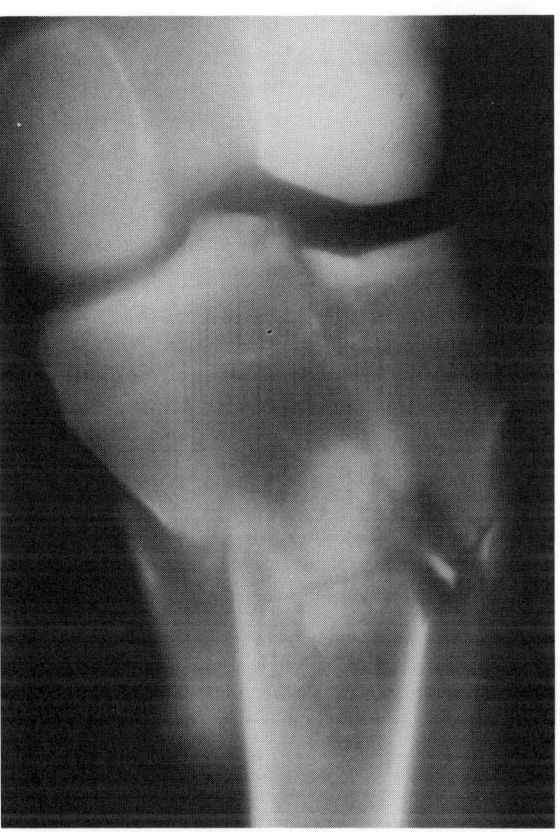

Figure 13-9 (**A**) Routine anterior roentgenogram of a minimally displaced proximal tibia fracture with an angiogram demonstrating normal distal flow through the trifurcation. Proximal tibia fractures are particularly dangerous, as the fracture frequently shears these posterior vascular bundles. (**B**) AP tomogram demonstrating the complex nature of the same fracture as demonstrated on the plain film in **A**. Note the intra-articular extent of the fracture and the transverse proximal third comminution not appreciated on the plain film. Tomography can be a valuable tool in the emergency room evaluation of questionable fracture patterns.

surgery. Most of these fractures are also associated with disruption of the extensor mechanism, medial and lateral to the patella proper. Not only does the patella require stabilization and fixation, but the extensor mechanism must be repaired as well.

Avulsions of the patellar tendon or disruption of the quadriceps mechanism can also occur in the presence of a normal patella. This mechanism is usually the result of the quadriceps muscle contracting against the flexed knee. Careful radiographic evaluation demonstrates an abnormal position of the patella in relation to the femur, as compared to the normal contralateral patella femoral joint. In certain cases, these extensor mechanism injuries must be surgically repaired by a heavy suture attached to the patella. Postoperatively, the knee must be immobilized for 8 to 12 weeks, with a gradual increase in the flexion range of motion. Extensive postoperative rehabilitation is required to return the extremity to normal function.

Patellar dislocations are frequently found in the young patient and are occasionally associated with bony abnormalities of the articular surface of the tibia or femur, angulatory deformities of the knee, and prior histories of dislocation. Arthroscopic evaluation is usually indicated in these injuries, and minor surgery in conjunction with extensive rehabilitation will give most patients an acceptable result. The dislocation is simply reduced with a medially or laterally directed force, after mild analgesic or sedation. A knee immobilizer can be used as a temporizing modality.

Ligamentous Injuries

Due to the popularity of sports in our society, the knee joint is frequently injured. The history is usually that of a valgus-producing stress pattern or a lateral blow to the knee associated with a twisting injury. The patient characteristically complains of pain, swelling, and the inability to obtain a full range of motion. Radiographic evaluation can frequently be normal.

The emergency physician's responsibility includes radiographic evaluation to rule out fractures of the femur, tibia, and patella, or avulsion injuries of the cruciate ligaments.

Next, some indication as to the stability of the knee must be ascertained. In the young patient's knee, with an acute effusion, arthrocentesis is indicated. This procedure must not be done with a cavalier attitude. The knee must be shaved, scrubbed, and prepped in a normal surgical fashion, and the physician should always wear gloves, mask, and drape by strict surgical standards. A 16-gauge needle is then placed in the lateral aspect of the patella/femoral joint through a previously anesthetized area with 0.5% Xylocaine without epinephrine. If blood is obtained, there is a 75% chance of a major ligamentous disruption.

Examination of the knee is then attempted. The cruciate ligaments can be examined by the so-called anterior drawer test, Lackman's, and the pivot shift, which is simply an attempt to sublux the tibia on the femur with the knee flexed at 90°. In the acutely injured knee, this is sometimes extremely difficult and painful, and intra-articular Xylocaine can be helpful. Collateral ligament stability can be examined by a varus or valgus stress applied to the knee flexed at 30°. If a medial or lateral collateral ligament injury is suspected, these ligaments can also be anesthetized with a local anesthetic prior to stress testing. To stress for a right medial collateral ligament, the examiner places the left hand on the lateral aspect of the femur and the right hand on the medial aspect of the tibia, applying a lateral force to the tibia.

To check for a lateral collateral ligament injury, the examiner simply places the hands in the opposite direction and applies an oppositely directed force. Major collateral ligament injuries are sometimes associated with cruciate ligament injuries and meniscal tears ("terrible triad").

The treatment of these injuries has become quite sophisticated in the past few years. MRI provides accurate, noninvasive information to establish an accurate diagnosis and is the mainstay of the evaluation prior to operative intervention. Arthroscopy plays a major role in the treatment of these injuries. An examination of the patient under anesthesia will certainly aid the treating physician in the management of the injury. The arthroscope will provide the physician with the exact nature of the injury. Arthroscopic meniscectomy has favorably changed the treatment of meniscal tears. Partial meniscectomy or meniscal repair is the treatment of choice for meniscal pathology. Ligamentous augmentation for cruciate injuries is usually indicated for the high-demand athlete.

Dislocations and Proximal Tibia Fractures

Both these injuries are usually associated with major vehicular trauma or falls from high positions (Fig. 13-10). With the knee dislocation, most major supporting ligaments of the knee are disrupted. Injuries to the vascular trifurcation and peroneal nerve result in an extremely high incidence of morbidity.

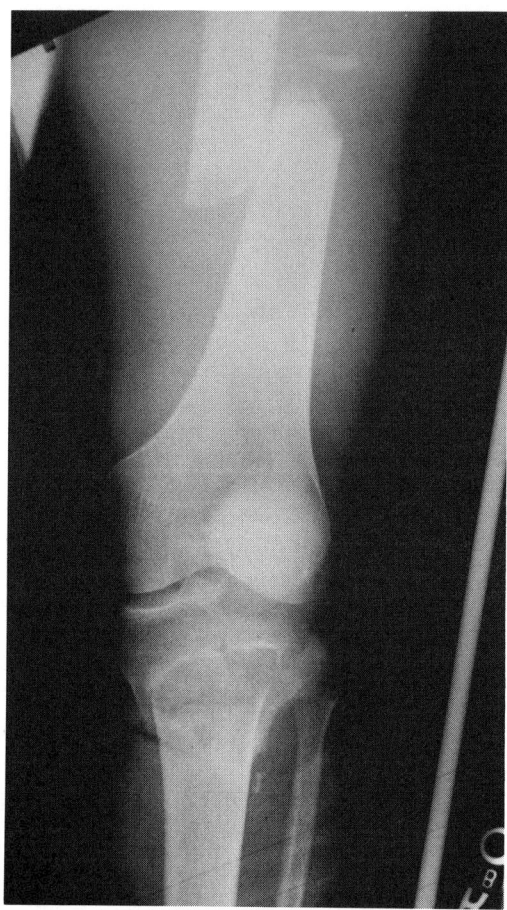

Figure 13-10 This 25-year-old man was involved in high-speed vehicular trauma, sustaining an ipsilateral femoral shaft and comminuted tibial plateau fracture. The so-called "floating knee" requires stabilization of the femur and internal fixation of the intra-articular plateau fracture to achieve an optimum result. Femur fractures are frequently associated with hip dislocations and intra-articular pathology of the knee.

The same holds true for fractures of the proximal tibia. With sharp, shearing bony fragments, the arterial supply and nerve supply to the distal tibia can be acutely injured. The emergency physician's responsibility for both these injuries lies in early recognition of potential problems. If the distal pulse is absent, if the foot demonstrates alteration in its vascularity, or if there is a diminution of palpable pulses, arteriography is recommended. If an arterial injury is found, then vascular surgery should be consulted in addition to orthopedic evaluation for knee or fracture stabilization. Time is of the essence, and these injuries should be given maximum attention. Reduction of the dislocation or proximal tibial fracture is usually not difficult and should be done as soon as possible. In general, a very gentle axial pull at the ankle will realign most fracture fragments or reduce the dislocated knee. A knee immobilizer should immediately be placed loosely, and care should be taken to prevent redislocation while the patient is being evaluated in the emergency department.

Most fractures of the proximal tibia, whether intra-articular or extra-articular, are treated in a similar fashion as those of the distal femur. With intra-articular fractures of the tibial plateau, an anatomic reduction is attempted. If this can be obtained with closed reduction, then closed management is indicated. Frequently, depressed fracture fragments contraindicate closed management, and open reduction with articular surface elevation and bone grafting is required to produce articular congruency. Early motion is indicated to nourish the articular surface and provide early rehabilitation. Fractures of the proximal tibia treated conservatively can usually be managed for 6 weeks in a long-leg walking cast and an additional 6 weeks in a short-leg cast until bone union is obtained.

FRACTURES OF THE TIBIA AND FIBULA

Due to the superficial nature of the tibia and the peripheral placement of this bone in the axial skeleton, the tibia is statistically prone to high rates of injury (Figs. 13-11 and 13-12). The serious complications associated with tibia fractures have been reported in the orthopedic literature for decades. The anatomic relationships of the calf are important when considering compartment syndromes associated with tibial injuries. The anterior compartment, or the compartment that contains the tibialis anterior, the extensor hallucis longus, the extensor digitorum longus, and the peroneus tertius muscles, is responsible for dorsiflexion. If this compartment is violated, dorsiflexion is lost and a foot-drop develops. Conversely, the posterior and lateral compartments are responsible for plantar flexion and eversion. Should these compartments be injured, push-off is altered and smooth gait is altered.

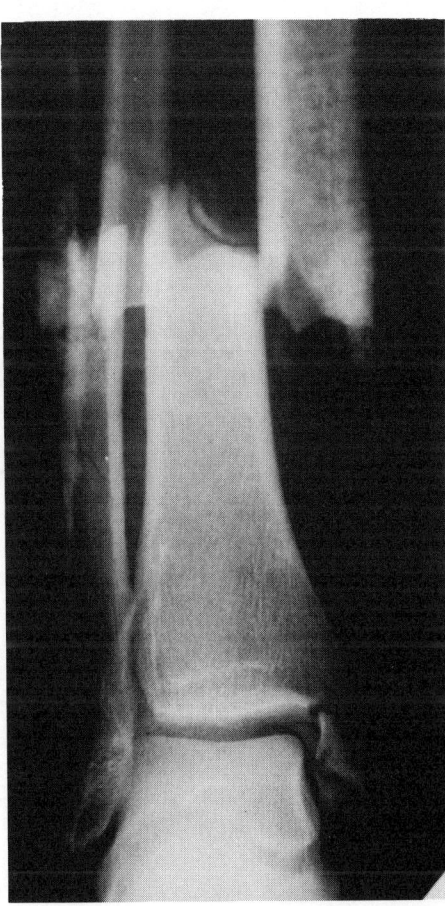

Figure 13-11 This roentgenogram demonstrates a transverse noncomminuted fracture of the tibia and fibula at the level of the junction of the middle and distal thirds. There is also a comminuted, minimally displaced, medial malleolus fracture. Tibia fractures are best described by their anatomic location, fracture characteristic, and whether the fracture is open or closed.

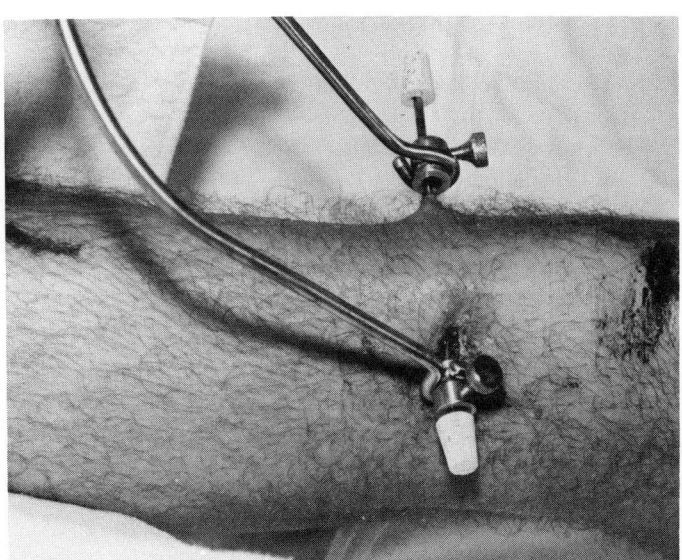

Figure 13-12 A threaded Steinmann pinned placement in the proximal tibia of the left leg in a patient with a femur fracture. Proximal tibial Steinmann pins should be placed from lateral to medial in order to avoid injury to the common peroneal nerve. The landmarks of insertion are one finger-breadth posterior to and one finger-breadth inferior to the tibial tubercle. The skin should be shaved, scrubbed, and prepped. A solution of 0.5% Xylocaine without epinephrine is utilized and the pin placed perpendicular to the long access of the tibia. A sterile dressing should be applied around the pin site.

Most fractures of the tibia occur from high-velocity injuries such as those associated with motorcycles, motor vehicles, and skiing. These fractures are usually described as to their location (ie, proximal, middle, or distal), the characteristic of the fracture (ie, short oblique, transverse, or segmental), and whether or not they are open fractures. The signs and symptoms associated with the tibia fracture are classic in that pain, swelling, and skeletal instability are quite easily identified.

Many tibia fractures can be definitively treated by closed reduction and application of a long-leg cast. However, the open fracture will require immediate irrigation and debridement in the operating suite. The emergency physician's responsibility for managing tibia fractures is the identification of potential complications such as compartment syndromes, nerve or vascular injuries, and associated traumatic injuries above and below the fracture site. Severe swelling and pain are the rule after these fractures are splinted, and it is much safer to have these patients under direct observation in the hospital during the acute stage.

Early consultation with orthopedic surgery is indicated, as few fractures represent so many possible complications. If fracture reduction cannot be maintained by closed manipulation, then operative management is indicated. Several techniques such as pins and plaster, internal fixation, and intramedullary fixation have all been reported to produce good results.

Fractures involving the distal articular joint of the tibia are referred to as "plafond fractures." As with all intra-articular fractures of the lower extremity, these fractures commonly require anatomic reduction and rigid fixation. This allows early mobilization of the joint, which is healthy for cartilaginous regeneration and repair.

The prognosis of tibia fractures is totally dependent on the mechanism of injury, type of fracture, whether the fracture is open, and the patient's age. Young, healthy patients with a relatively benign, minimally displaced fracture will heal within 20 weeks. Conversely, the patient with an open fracture with gross displacement who develops an infected nonunion will require multiple operative procedures and may even require amputation.

The tibia fracture found in the child is generally a midshaft, spiral-type fracture. In the urban trauma center, this can be associated with child abuse. Since this is a most unusual injury in a child, the index of suspicion must be elevated. These fractures can be treated with a long-leg cast for approximately 6 weeks, then cut to a short-leg cast for an additional 6 weeks. Most of these fractures have an excellent result.

The "tibial stress fracture" is a difficult diagnosis and must be differentiated from other entities such as "shin splints" or compartment syndromes. Radiographs taken initially may be normal. However, radiographs taken at follow-up within 2 to 4 weeks will frequently reveal a hypertrophied cortex and even sclerosis transversely in the area of the stress fracture. Stress fractures can be diagnosed early with the use of technetium bone scanning.

Isolated fractures of the fibular shaft 7 cm above the ankle joint and 3 cm below the head of the fibula are usually the result of a direct blow and can be treated with crutches for comfort. Fractures that are found above and below that level can interfere with ankle mechanics and common peroneal nerve function, respectively. The emergency physician must consider stress views of the ankle and specifically check for peroneal nerve function.

FRACTURES OF THE ANKLE

Fractures of the ankle, although anatomically involving the tibia and fibula, are classically differentiated from tibial shaft and tibial plafond fractures (Fig. 13-13). Their mechanism of injury is entirely different. Ankle fractures commonly occur in the athlete and are the result of pronation or supination forces combined with rotational forces.

The anatomy of the ankle is important in order to understand the multiple ligamentous instability problems. The medial side of the ankle is supported by the deltoid ligament, which has a superficial and deep portion (Figs. 13-14 and 13-15). The lateral ligaments of the ankle are referred to as the anterior talofibular ligament, the calcaneofibular ligament, and the posterior tibial-fibular ligament. These ligaments are important to maintain ankle stability and are responsible for chronic ankle sprains, if a disruption occurs.

Ankle fractures can be classified in a number of sophisticated ways. For the emergency physician, the concept of a unimalleolar, bimalleolar, or trimalleolar ankle fracture is easiest to remember.

The most common ankle fracture is the isolated lateral malleolar fracture. This, unfortunately, is the most difficult to manage appropriately, in that the associated deltoid ligament injury can be misdiagnosed or neglected. If either occurs, joint incongruity results. One approach that does not need to be completed emergently is the medial "stress test." By placing a laterally directed force on the foot, the congruity of the deltoid ligament can be checked. If there is a radiographically proven opening on the medial aspect of the ankle, open reduction and internal fixation are indicated. If stress testing is negative, then the isolated distal fibular fracture can be treated with a short-leg walking cast. This concept of stability and maintenance of articular congruency is critical in the appropriate management of ankle fractures.

Isolated medial malleolus fractures must be reduced anatomically. If this cannot be done by closed means, then open reduction and internal fixation are indicated. Displaced bimalleolar ankle fractures, open ankle fractures, or trimalleolar ankle fractures are usually treated with open reduction and internal fixation. The emergency physician's responsi-

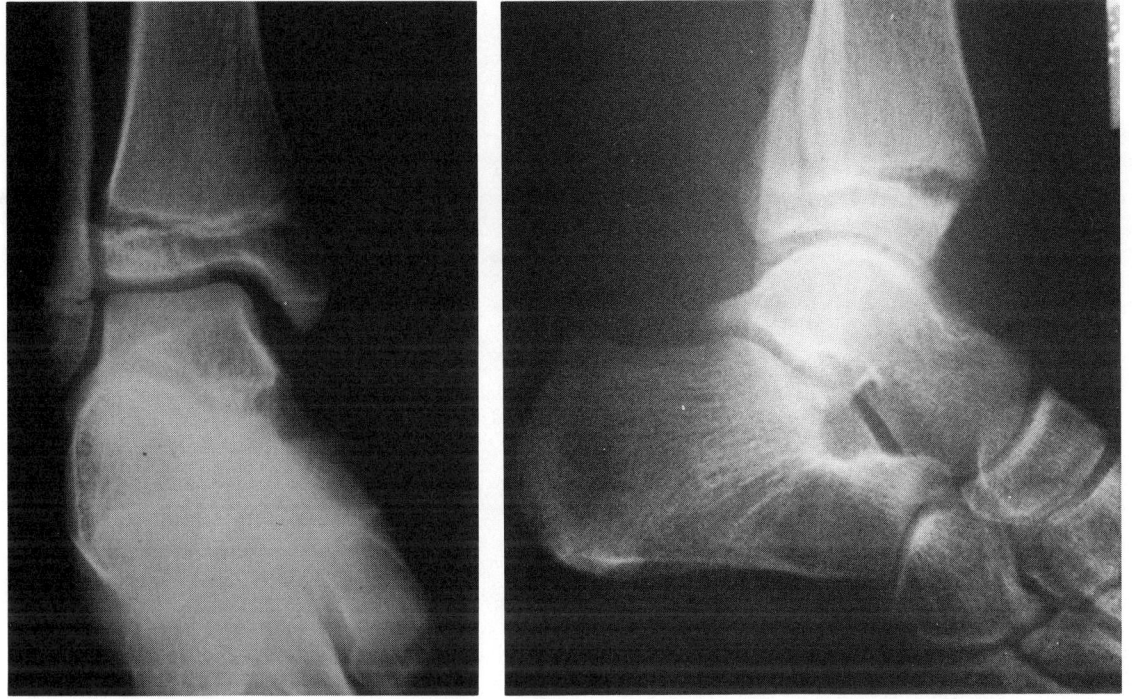

Figure 13-13 Ankle fractures in skeletally immature patients require orthopedic evaluation to assure preservation of the growth plate. The mortise (**A**) and lateral (**B**) views demonstrated here show the classic tri-plane fracture pattern frequently found in the adolescent ankle. There are fracture lines noted in the sagittal, coronal, and horizontal planes. This complex fracture pattern often requires open reduction and internal fixation.

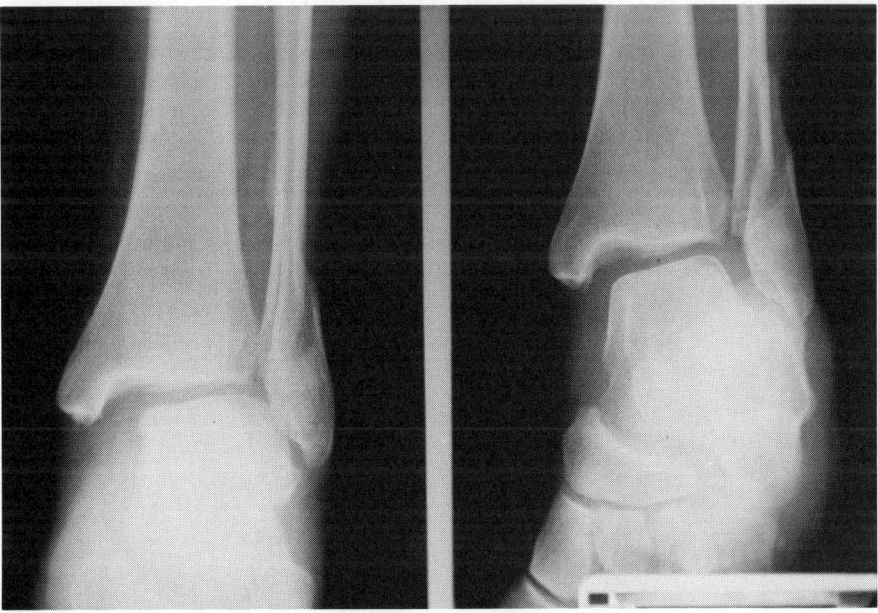

Figure 13-14 Disruption of the medial collateral ligament of the ankle (the deltoid ligament) with lateral displacement of the talus. Note the widened medial clear space. This unstable ankle fracture requires orthopedic attention for anatomic closed reduction or open reduction and internal fixation.

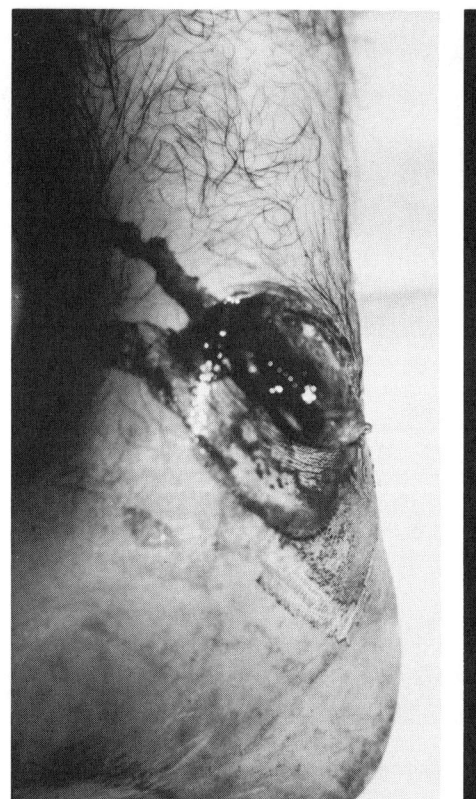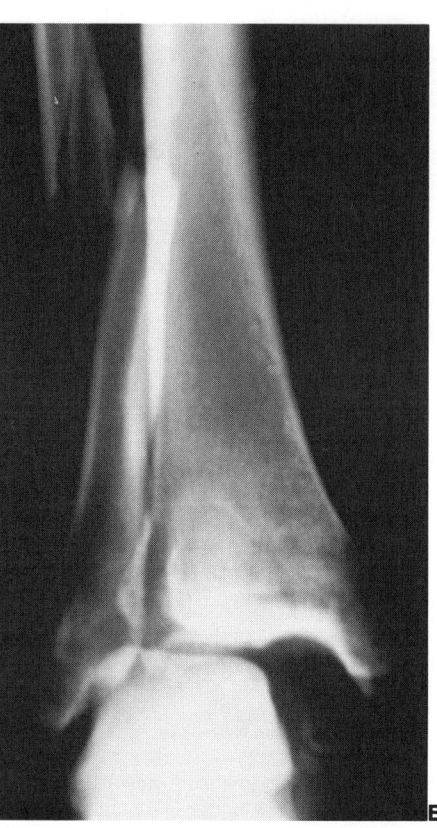

Figure 13-15 (**A**) This open ankle fracture demonstrates protrusion of the medial malleolus with a remnant of the deltoid ligament. The treatment includes culture, a surgical prep, and sterile dressing, plus tetanus and antibiotic prophylaxis. (**B**) This roentgenogram represents a pronation external rotation injury with a wide medial mortise and a high fibular fracture. These open ankle fractures always require urgent operative irrigation, debridement, and surgical stabilization.

---

bility includes reduction and splinting of the dislocation, preoperative evaluation of the patient, and appropriate radiographic evaluation. This includes AP, lateral, and mortise views of the ankle with an AP and a lateral of the entire involved tibia, and a mortise view of the contralateral ankle. These views will help to identify any proximal pathology of the ipsilateral injured tibia and fibula, and the contralateral normal mortise view will help when comparing stress radiography, closed, or open reductions.

Ankle fractures in the child are of particular concern, in that the distal fibula and distal tibial growth plates can potentially be injured. If such injury occurs, leg length discrepancy, malunions, and angulatory deformities may occur. Therefore, any physeal injury in the child should appropriately be evaluated by a fracture surgeon.

SIGNIFICANT FRACTURES OF THE FOOT

Talus

Fractures of the talus are especially worrisome in that they frequently result in avascular necrosis requiring additional reconstructive surgery. Hawkins has described these fractures in relation to the degree of displacement of the neck from the talar body (Fig. 13-16). Fractures of the talar neck with associated subtalar dislocations are of particular concern and are usually treated with open reduction and internal fixation. Post-traumatic arthritis, malunion, nonunion, skin necrosis, infection, and late arthrodesis are associated with these injuries. These fractures should be evaluated early by an orthopedist, as local skin necrosis can interfere with fracture management.

Calcaneus

Fractures of the calcaneus usually result from jumps or falls from heights (Fig. 13-17). They are frequently associated with compression fractures of the lumbar spine. The minimally displaced fracture can usually be treated conservatively with a short-leg cast until comfortable and then advanced in 4 to 6 weeks to a shoe with firm support. The displaced intra-articular comminuted fragment can be treated by closed manipulation and casting, closed manipulation and early motion, or, more recently, with open reduction, internal fixation, and bone grafting. The emergency physician's

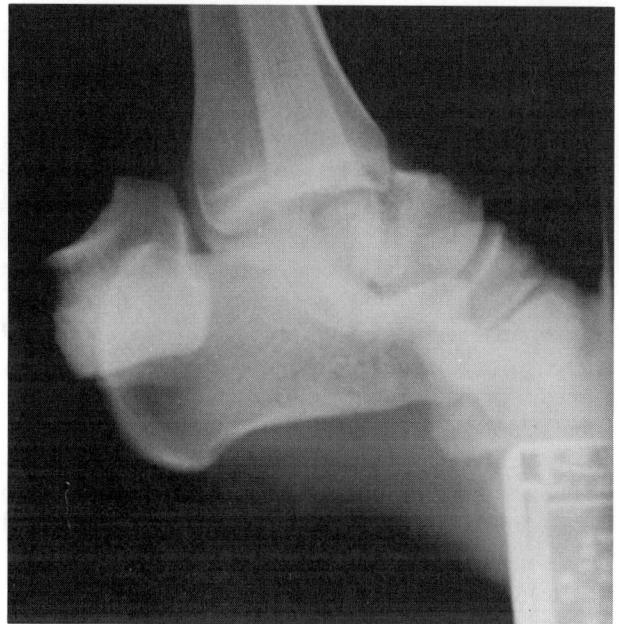
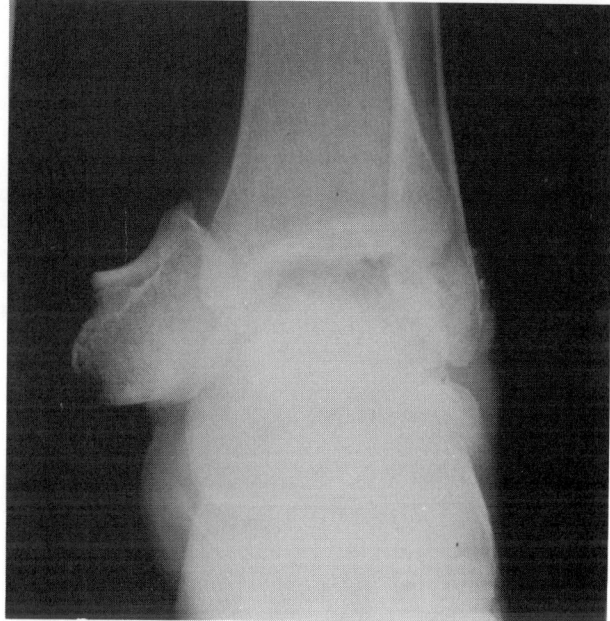
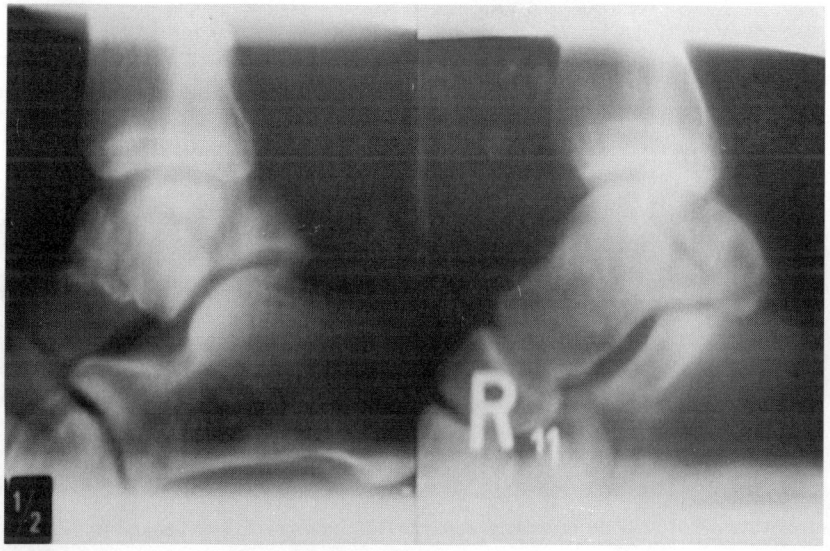

Figure 13-16 (A) This roentgenogram represents a lateral view of the ankle, demonstrating a complete dislocation of the body of the talus with posterior retropulsion. Talus fractures are associated with a high incidence of avascular necrosis and nonunion. This injury frequently requires operative reduction and fixation. (B) The anterior view of the same fracture dislocation of the talus shows the medial extrusion of the fragment. (C) Tomographic evaluation of a comminuted intra-articular fracture of the talus. A single-cut tomographic evaluation is useful in the emergency department to rule out the nondisplaced or undiagnosed talus fracture.

responsibilities for this fracture are appropriate radiographs with a high suspicion of spinal compression fracture, elevation, and admission to the hospital.

Midfoot

Injuries to the tarsometatarsal (Lisfranc's joint) are uncommon. However, early recognition is imperative because the swelling and potential vascular compromise to the skin can significantly affect the long-term result. The metatarsal heads are held together by strong midfoot ligaments that are usually disrupted in this injury pattern. Because of the difficulty in maintaining the reduction, closed manipulation, percutaneous pinning, or more rigid screw fixation constitute the method of choice.

A similar fracture dislocation that occurs at the talonavicular and calcaneocuboid joints (Chopart's joint) also requires early and aggressive anatomic reduction and pinning. Fractures of Chopart's joint pose the same problems as those associated with Lisfranc fractures.

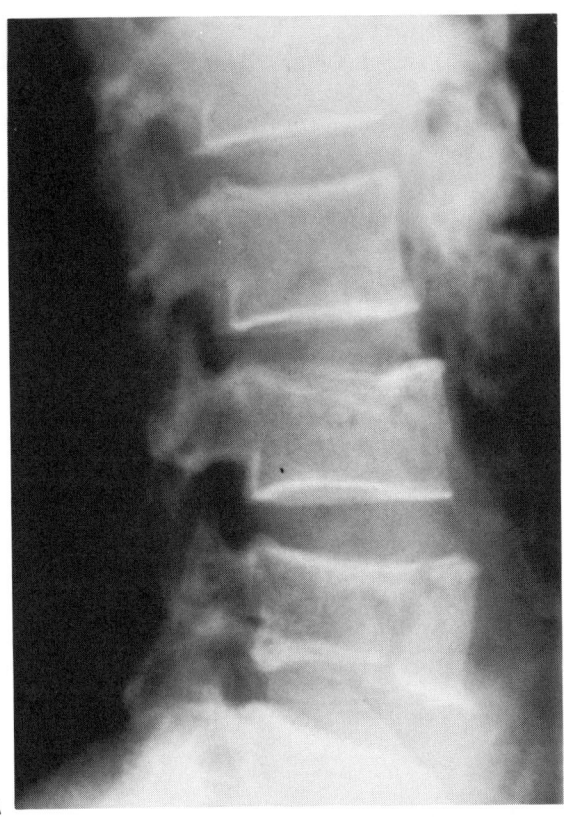

Fractures and Dislocations of the Metatarsals

Most fractures of the metatarsals can be treated with closed manipulation and casting. They can be quite painful and present problems with swelling. Patients should be advised to elevate the extremity. If these fractures are open, appropriate operative irrigation and debridement are indicated.

Dislocations of the interphalangeal joints of the toes can be routinely treated in the emergency department. These are usually reduced atraumatically and "buddy" splinted (ie, taped to the normal medial or lateral toe). If an intra-articular fracture of the great toe results, occasionally open reduction and internal fixation to maintain joint space congruity are indicated. Entrapment of the anterior tibial tendon will inhibit appropriate reduction of the first or second metatarsophalangeal joint, and open reduction with pinning is then necessary.

Sprains

Ankle sprains pose one of the most common problems evaluated by the emergency department. These injuries usually occur in young, healthy individuals and require a thor-

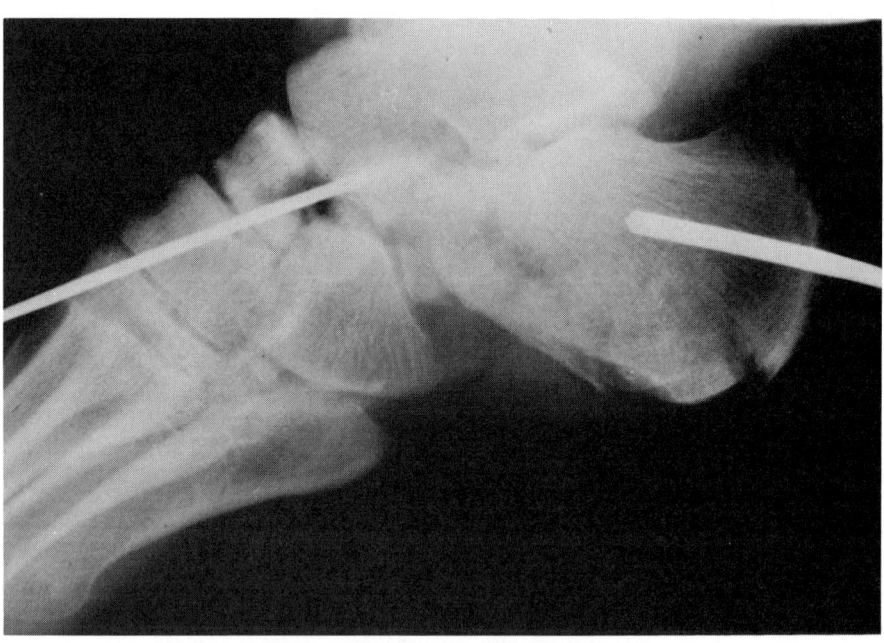

Figure 13-17 (**A**) These compression fractures of L-3 and L-4 were sustained in jumping off an 8-foot brick wall; frequently associated with lumbar compression fractures or calcaneal fractures. (**B**) This comminuted midfoot dislocation and a calcaneal fracture, shown with pins placed for reduction, will require 6 weeks of casting to maintain the reduction. Calcaneal fractures and lumbar compression fractures are injuries that frequently occur concomitantly.

ough evaluation, including radiographs. Several types of therapy have been advocated, including short-leg casting, ice, elevation, and immobilization with a posterior splint. The young, athletic individual may be treated with a more aggressive motion program including contrast baths, tape, and daily therapy. These injuries may require three months to heal appropriately and can be as debilitating as an ankle fracture. Very rarely do severe sprains or complete ligament disruptions about the ankle require emergent surgical reconstruction. These procedures are reserved for chronic instability.

Foot Ulcers

Diabetic foot ulcers can be associated with pyarthrosis or osteomyelitis of the metatarsal head. These usually occur in the insensate foot on the weight-bearing aspect of the metatarsal heads. These will usually require operative debridement, elevation, dressing changes, and intravenous antibiotics. These ulcers often demand some form of amputation and frequently represent the beginning of a long road of hospitalization and lower extremity orthopedic care. Never more clearly is appropriate medical management indicated than in the patient with a diabetic foot. These patients should be advised to wash their feet daily and examine the plantar aspect with a mirror to prevent catastrophic associated amputations.

BIBLIOGRAPHY

Judet R, Judet J, Letournel E. Fractures of the acetabulum: classification and surgical approaches for open reduction. Preliminary report. *J Bone Joint Surg Am*. 1964;46:1615.

14. Diabetic Emergencies

STEPHEN HAMBURGER, MD, FACP
DAVID RUSH, PharmD

DIABETIC KETOACIDOSIS

Diabetic ketoacidosis (DKA) is a medical emergency. Although the introduction of insulin into clinical medicine has lowered the morbidity and mortality rates of DKA tremendously, there is still a 5 to 10% mortality in most medical centers.[1–3] In select subgroups of patients with DKA, such as the elderly, the mortality rate is significantly higher.[4] In recent years, interest in the treatment of DKA has focused mainly on the method of insulin administration.[5–8] Less dramatic, but possibly more important, has been the work involving the various components of fluid and electrolyte therapy: (1) the role of adequate hydration,[9] (2) the potential benefits of early use of phosphate salts,[10] and (3) the role of alkali therapy.[11]

The recent emphasis on the use of insulin in DKA has a potential negative impact; many physicians might assume that the treatment of DKA is standardized. This assumption could not be further from the truth—therapy of DKA must be individualized. As knowledge of the pathogenesis and the effect of the ketotic state on the host has evolved, awareness of the potential risk of DKA and its therapy has increased. There are few other conditions in which careful and continuous vigilance over the clinical and laboratory status of the patient is more important to the eventual outcome.

Pathogenesis

Diabetes mellitus is a complex syndrome. A component of this syndrome is a defect in intermediary metabolism resulting from the relative or absolute deficiency in insulin. DKA is the extreme clinical expression of this deficiency, which might be secondary to endogenous failure of insulin release (eg, in the ketosis-prone diabetic), the exogenous administration of inadequate quantities of insulin in the known diabetic, or the antagonism of insulin by elevated circulating levels of anti-insulin hormones (glucagon, cortisol, growth hormone, and catecholamines) that might occur in numerous stressful conditions (Table 14-1). Whatever the reason, the normal balance between the anabolic hormone insulin and the catabolic anti-insulin hormones (growth hormone has both anabolic and catabolic functions) is shifted to the anti-insulin hormones, resulting in overproduction of glucose and ketone bodies.

The hyperglycemia that is seen in most cases of DKA is a reflection of both overproduction and underutilization.[12] Circulating levels of insulin in these patients are usually quite low; thus, the insulin-dependent tissues, such as liver, muscle, and adipose tissue, which normally assimilate approximately 75% of a glucose load, are unable to use glucose.[13] In fact, the liver, which is normally a glucose-producing organ only during a fasting state, actively contributes to the hyperglycemia in DKA.[14] The increase in hepatic production of glucose is secondary to both glycogenolysis and gluconeogenesis. Both these glucose-producing mechanisms are primed by elevated levels of anti-insulin hormones, especially glucagon, cortisol, and catecholamines. Hyperglycemia results in an osmotic diuresis with loss of sodium, potassium, magnesium, chloride, and phosphorus. The urinary loss is usually hypo-osmolar to plasma. Clini-

Table 14-1 Metabolic Effects of the Anti-Insulin Hormones

	Insulin Release	Muscle Glucose Uptake	Gluconeo-genesis	Lipolysis
Glucagon	↑	↓	↑	↑
Growth hormone	↑	↓		↑
Glucocorticoids	↑	↓	↑	↑

Source: Reprinted from *Family Practice Certification.*

cally, the hyperglycemia is manifested as polydipsia and polyuria, leading to intravascular volume depletion.

Ketoacidosis is the end product of the accumulation of the ketone bodies: β-hydroxybutyric acid and acetoacetate. Another ketone body, acetone, is also formed; unlike β-hydroxybutyric acid and acetoacetate, however, acetone is neither an organic acid nor a hydrogen ion donor.[15] Because of the lack of insulin, there is an excessive lipolysis of triglycerides to free fatty acids and glycerol, as well as an excessive formation of β-hydroxybutyric acid, acetoacetate, and acetone. The free fatty acids are transported to the liver (glycerol is used for gluconeogenesis) where they are either oxidized to carbon dioxide or used in ketogenesis. In DKA, the oxidative capacity of the liver is overwhelmed; thus, ketogenesis is enhanced.

A working definition of DKA may be as follows: DKA is the state of relative or absolute insulin deficiency that results in an excess ketone concentration, a low arterial pH, and a low bicarbonate concentration. Hyperglycemia is *usually* present, and the results of a nitroprusside test are *usually* positive, although neither is a prerequisite to the diagnosis.[16,17] This definition of DKA takes into account the wide spectrum of severity of this illness.

Diagnosis

Clinical Diagnosis

DKA is a common medical disorder that is seen not only in known diabetics but also in previously unrecognized diabetics. Although the symptoms of DKA are variable, most can be explained by the defect in intermediary metabolism and the intravascular volume deficiency that causes poor tissue perfusion (Fig. 14-1). Patients with DKA usually have increased urination and thirst secondary to the osmotic diuresis; increasing weakness and weight loss secondary to the catabolism of body fat and protein stores, anorexia, nausea, and vomiting; and variable mental symptomatology arising from the ketosis and intravascular volume depletion. In a known diabetic, these symptoms in increasing severity strongly suggest DKA; otherwise, the suspicion of DKA is a matter of clinical judgment. DKA should be very uncommon in the known, compliant diabetic, however, because the symptomatology of DKA is usually present for several days prior to severe clinical and metabolic decompensation and should be recognized by the patient. Furthermore, the patient who has had proper training in urinary testing for glucose and ketones will know when the test reflects a poor degree of control and will seek medical attention long before DKA develops.

Initial examination of the patient with DKA must include a meticulous search to determine the precipitating

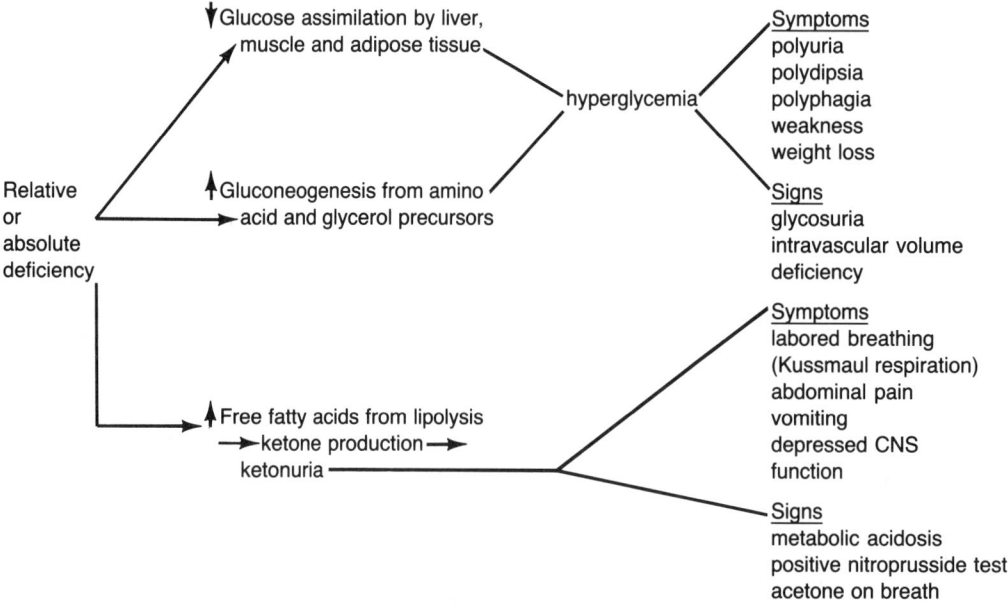

Figure 14-1 Pathophysiology of diabetic ketoacidosis.

event (Table 14-2). Patient noncompliance with the medical regimen or an infection is usually the underlying cause. A skin abscess, especially of the feet, is frequently overlooked. It is particularly important to seek an underlying condition in the elderly patient, since it is not uncommon for a diabetic to have a painless myocardial infarction with DKA.[18,19] The adequacy of the intravascular volume should be evaluated by measurement of blood pressure and pulse in both the supine and erect positions, if possible. Skin turgor and signs of tissue perfusion, such as central nervous system (CNS) symptomatology, urine output, and skin temperature, should be assessed.

The DKA patient with abdominal pain and tenderness presents a problem. Although the diabetic patient is certainly not exempt from surgical problems in the gastrointestinal tract, some DKA patients have a "pseudoappendicitis."[20] The serum amylase level is elevated in a significant percentage of diabetic patients with DKA (as is the amylase-creatinine clearance ratio), but most of these patients do not have clinically significant pancreatitis.[21-23] Leukocytosis is common in uncomplicated DKA; therefore, this finding does not aid in the differential diagnosis. Since the abdominal signs and symptoms subside with treatment of the ketosis, it is of the utmost importance to correct the DKA as rapidly as possible in order to avoid unnecessary surgery. If, in spite of adequate treatment of the DKA, abdominal signs and symptoms persist, the possibility of a surgical condition should be strongly considered. Studies by Campbell and associates suggest that, in any DKA patient over 40 years of age, abdominal pain is very likely to have an underlying precipitating cause. Also, it was found that abdominal pain in patients with a serum bicarbonate level greater than 10 mEq/L is very likely to be caused by an underlying condition. It must be stressed, however, that several of the conditions producing abdominal pain were of medical origin, such as pyelonephritis.[24]

Laboratory Diagnosis

Occasionally there is a significant delay in the laboratory reporting of biochemical determinations; however, any patient with a strongly positive reaction for ketones in undiluted serum, glycosuria, and a low arterial pH may be considered to have DKA and be treated as such. These tests may be done very rapidly in a semiquantitative fashion by means of nitroprusside tablets or reagent strips. Proper interpretation of the nitroprusside test is crucial and requires an understanding of the limitations of the test. It does not measure the level of β-hydroxybutyric acid, but it does reflect the concentration of acetoacetate and acetone.[25] Normally, the ratio of β-hydroxybutyric acid to acetoacetate (acetone is usually quantitatively much less significant) is 3:1. In DKA, the ratio might be greatly elevated, although both compounds are circulating at levels higher than normal.[26] If, as is often the case in DKA, tissue hypoxia leads to an increase in lactic

Table 14-2 Common Precipitating Factors of Diabetic Ketoacidosis

Failure of endogenous insulin
1. Previously undiagnosed diabetic
2. Viral infections of pancreas
3. Pancreatitis
4. Idiopathic/autoimmune

Failure of exogenous insulin
1. Change in diet or exercise
2. Patient noncompliance
    a. inadequate patient education
    b. poor vision
    c. wrong insulin concentration
    d. calibration/injection error
    e. mental deficiency
3. Inadequate dose or type prescribed
4. Insulin antibodies

Hormonal antagonism of insulin
1. Cushing's syndrome
2. Thyrotoxicosis
3. Pheochromocytoma
4. Acromegaly

Stress
1. Infection (eg, pneumonia, abscess, urinary tract infection, gangrene)
2. Pregnancy
3. Myocardial infarction
4. Surgery
5. Trauma
6. Acute psychiatric illness

Source: Modified and reprinted from *Family Practice Certification.*

acid, the β-hydroxybutyric acid–acetoacetate ratio is shifted further to favor β-hydroxybutyric acid. This is secondary to the increased level of NADH that results from tissue hypoxia. Thus, a patient may have a significant degree of ketoacidosis with only a weakly positive ketone test.[17] Then, too, a patient recovering from DKA may continue to have a strongly positive ketone test as the β-hydroxybutyric acid is converted to acetoacetate after the correction of the tissue hypoxia (Fig. 14-2).

The nitroprusside test is a poor indicator of the patient's response to therapy in DKA. This is true not only because the ketone equilibrium shifts as tissue hypoxia is relieved but also because the acetone that might have accumulated in the DKA patient is excreted so slowly. Acetone in high concentration might cause a positive nitroprusside test.[27] Thus, the patient might be fully recovered biochemically from DKA and yet have a positive ketone test if significant acetonemia remains.

Initial laboratory studies include a complete blood cell count; measurements of electrolytes, blood urea nitrogen (BUN), creatinine, magnesium, and blood glucose; urinalysis; and arterial blood gas and pH determinations. Interpretation of the serum sodium value must take into account the "pseudohyponatremia" induced by hyperglycemia.

β-Hydroxybutyric Acid Dehydrogenase

β-Hydroxybutyric Acid (BHB) ⟷ Acetoacetic Acid (AcAc)

NAD ⟷ NADH

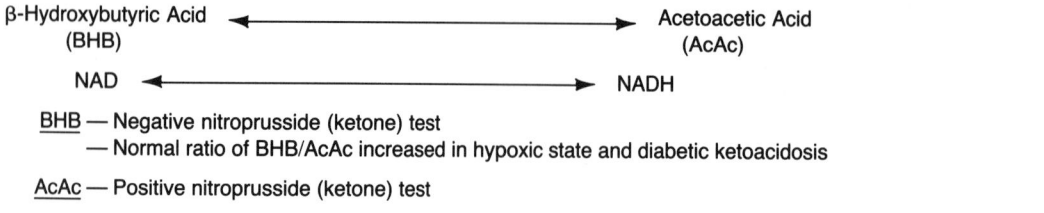

BHB — Negative nitroprusside (ketone) test
— Normal ratio of BHB/AcAc increased in hypoxic state and diabetic ketoacidosis

AcAc — Positive nitroprusside (ketone) test

Acetone — Positive nitroprusside (ketone) test. Color intensity is much less than that of AcAc at equal concentration, but if acetone concentration is greatly increased a positive nitroprusside test will result.

Figure 14-2 Interpretation of the nitroprusside test. NAD, NADH, oxidized and reduced forms of pyridine nucleotide.

Katz demonstrated that for every 100 mg/dL glucose above normal the serum sodium level is reduced by 1.6 mEq/L.[28] Knowledge of this relationship is important in determining the water deficit in such a patient. An elevation in the serum triglyceride level might also result in factitious hyponatremia. A normal or increased serum osmolality, coupled with a low serum sodium level, suggests this possibility.[29] Ultracentrifugation of the serum can remove the triglycerides and result in a correct serum sodium determination, or if this technology is unavailable, the Katz relationship can be used to correct the measured serum sodium value. An elevated uric acid level results primarily from decreased renal perfusion and competitive inhibition of uric acid secretion in the distal tubule of the kidney by the ketone bodies or lactic acid.[30,31] Test of kidney function might be misleading; the BUN, which is almost always high, might have a significant prerenal component in its increase, and the creatinine level might be spuriously elevated by the acetoacetate if the colorimetric method of determination is used.[32] The blood sugar level is invariably elevated, but a small percentage of patients with DKA have a normal glucose level.[16] Arterial blood gas determinations reflect a pure metabolic acidosis with a respiratory alkalosis as compensation in uncomplicated DKA. A superimposed lactic acidosis should be suspected if the nitroprusside test is weakly positive in the presence of significant acidemia and an elevated anion gap.* A baseline electrocardiogram (ECG) should always be obtained to diagnose a painless myocardial infarction. Appropriate Gram stains and cultures should be done to rule out an infection.

---

*Anion gap = $Na^+ - (Cl^- + HCO_3^-)$.
Normal anion gap = 12.4 ± 2 mEq/L.[33]

Treatment

The correction of DKA encompasses the following areas:

- diagnosis and treatment of the precipitating event(s)
- replacement of fluid and electrolyte deficits
- normalization of the intermediary metabolism
- avoidance of complications
- education of the patient to avoid recurrence

All patients with DKA should have a complete and up-to-date flowsheet (Fig. 14-3). This simple monitoring device allows the physician to see at a glance what therapy has previously been rendered and how the patient responded to the various modalities. If possible, central venous pressure lines and urinary catheters should be avoided so as to minimize the risk of a superimposed infection. In the unconscious patient, a patent airway must be established. Supplemental oxygen may be needed. Gastric aspiration benefits the patient with persistent vomiting or gastric atony. In the unconscious patient with an indwelling gastric tube, a cuffed endotracheal tube should be used to prevent an aspiration pneumonia.

Fluid Therapy

In all cases of DKA, it is crucial to replace the significant intravascular volume depletion as soon as possible. The average calculated loss of sodium is 8 mEq/kg; that of water is approximately 75 mL/kg.[34] The average patient with severe DKA requires 4 to 6 L normal and/or half-normal saline during the first 12 to 24 hours of treatment.[35] The choice of normal or half-normal saline is dictated by the

Time	Temp (°F)	BP Sys / Dial	Pulse / Resp	FLUID BALANCE																CONSCIOUSNESS	TREATMENT								
				Intake		Output		Urine	Glucose mg/dL	BUN mg/dL	Na mEq/L	K mEq/L	Cl mEq/L	CO_2 mEq/L	Anion gap		Osmolality	PH	Serum ketone	1. Alert 2. Drowsy 3. Stupor 4. Light Coma 5. Coma	Insulin			Na mEq	K mEq	Bicarb mEq	ECG	Antibiotic	Other
				PO	IV	Urine	Gastric	Glucose / Ketone													Regular IV	Regular SQ / IM	NPH or Lente						

Figure 14-3 Flowsheet for diabetic ketoacidosis.

status of intravascular volume and the serum osmolality. The intravascular volume, which is most easily corrected by normal saline, is measured by following the parameters of volume repletion, such as blood pressure, pulse, mentation, skin temperature, and urine output. During the repletion of the intravascular volume, the physician must continuously evaluate the patient's condition—not only for continued volume depletion but also for the development of signs and symptoms of sodium overload, such as congestive heart failure.

In the initial management of DKA, it is wise to determine the plasma osmolality (either by measurement or estimation*); this helps dictate early therapy and might warn of potential complications as the patient recovers. Most patients with DKA have some increase in plasma osmolality. This abnormality results mainly from loss of urine that is hypotonic to plasma. Studies have shown that the urinary output in DKA resembles half-normal saline with 35 to 63 mEq/L potassium.[35] With repletion of the intravascular volume by saline solutions and the reduction of the blood sugar level by insulin, much of the hyperosmolality is corrected. If the serum osmolality is still elevated, the use of hypotonic fluids such as half-normal saline or free water by mouth lowers the osmolality to within nomal range. It should be emphasized, however, that the rapid correction of the free water deficit has not been shown to be clinically beneficial and might be harmful.[36]

Potassium

Studies that took place in the early 1950s demonstrated that there is a significant loss of total body potassium in DKA.[37,38] Later studies confirmed these observations.[39-41] Additionally, the Helderman studies, which researched the relationship of glucose intolerance and thiazide diuretic use, concluded that the lowering of extracellular potassium is the critical factor in diminishing the insulin response to a glucose load.[42] Causes of potassium depletion include the osmotic diuresis, vomiting, acidemia with resultant intracellular buffering of hydrogen ions by potassium, and the catabolism of intracellular protein. Despite the *average* loss of approximately 6 mEq/kg (some patients may lose as much as 10 mEq/kg),[34] patients with DKA may have hypokalemia, normokalemia, or hyperkalemia. The mean admission concentration of potassium in a study by Beigelman was 5.3 mEq/L (range 2.1 to 8.4), with 4% of the patients having an initial value less than 3.5 mEq/L.[43] Initial hypokalemia signified a larger deficit of potassium, since those patients required a greater amount of parenteral administration of this cation for correction.

Aggressive therapy of DKA decreases the potassium level. This drop in potassium is secondary to rehydration and reuptake of potassium by cells under the influence of insulin therapy. If alkali therapy is begun to correct the acidosis, the decrease in potassium is more significant, owing to the intracellular shift of potassium; hence, additional exogenous potassium must be given to maintain a normal concentration. The study by Hockaday and Alberti showed the rapidity with which potassium is decreased after the start of therapy and the potential for significant hypokalemia without potassium supplementation.[44] Their patients with DKA had an initial mean potassium value of 4.4 mEq/L, which decreased in 1 hour to 3.5 mEq/L with little potassium supplementation. In light of this information, more aggressive potassium therapy was begun in the next group of patients. Five hours after therapy had begun, the mean potassium level was 4 mEq/L (decreased from an initial mean of 4.4 mEq/L), with an average of 87 mEq potassium being given to each patient. This drop in potassium level was inversely related to the amount of exogenous potassium administered. Beigelman's study corroborated the fact that potassium levels drop rapidly with the initiation of treatment and further demonstrated the extreme range of potassium replacement needed to maintain a normal concentration (mean 170, range 0 to 620 mEq).[43]

Extreme hyperkalemia or hypokalemia is potentially lethal. (See Chapter 18, Hypokalemia and Hyperkalemia.) In the absence of known hyperkalemia, ECG changes associated with hyperkalemia, or oliguria, it is recommended that potassium administration be initiated simultaneously with the initiation of other modalities of therapy. If the initial potassium level is found to be elevated, the administration of exogenous potassium should be stopped until the potassium level has decreased to the normal range. Potassium therapy should be individualized to maintain a normal serum concentration. Careful monitoring by frequent blood samples is essential. Serial ECGs to determine the prevailing serum potassium level are not as useful as expected because many changes are nonspecific.[45]

Phosphorus

DKA is associated with total body phosphate depletion.[37,46] As with potassium, the serum level of phosphate can be normal or elevated in the patient with untreated DKA, in spite of the overall deficit.[47] In DKA, the possible deleterious effects of phosphate depletion include decreased oxygenation of peripheral tissues, depressed CNS function, increased risk of infection, and impaired carbohydrate utilization.

Decreased Oxygenation of Peripheral Tissues. Oxygen delivery at the cellular level is partially dependent on cardiac output and the arteriovenous oxygen difference. Phosphate depletion in DKA interferes with both of these mechanisms.

O'Connor and associates demonstrated that, in severely hypophosphatemic patients, the cardiac output (measured by thermodilution and cardiac stroke work) was impaired.[48] After the correction of the phosphate depletion, cardiac output improved significantly—possibly because of the

---

*Estimated serum osmolality = $2(Na^+ + K^+) + \dfrac{glucose}{18} + \dfrac{BUN}{2.8}$

repletion of intracellular adenosine triphosphate (ATP). Since many patients with DKA already have a compromised myocardium and some of the complications in DKA might be related to cellular hypoxia, phosphate repletion seems warranted.

Most of the interest in the treatment of DKA and the oxyhemoglobin dissociation curve (Fig. 14-4) has focused on 2,3-diphosphoglyceric acid (2,3-DPG) and the state of the arterial pH. 2,3-DPG levels are decreased in DKA by several mechanisms. Acidosis impairs the production of 2,3-DPG by inhibiting red cell glycolysis at the phosphofructokinase step.[49,50] Total body phosphate depletion is a factor in the low red cell 2,3-DPG. Travis has suggested that, in the presence of hyperglycemia with an increased conversion of glucose to sorbitol via the polyol pathway, production of 2,3-DPG is reduced.[51] Although the depletion of 2,3-DPG shifts the oxyhemoglobin association curve to the left, most *untreated* patients with DKA have a dissociation curve that approximates normal because the acidosis shifts the curve to the right, compensating for the leftward shift.[52] Clinically significant is the recovery of the 2,3-DPG during the treatment of DKA when phosphate is withheld. Although the pH may return to normal within 24 hours, the return of the 2,3-DPG to adequate levels may take as long as 1 week.[10] Thus, the protective effect of the acidosis on the oxyhemoglobin dissociation curve is lost rapidly, whereas the adverse effect of the depressed level of 2,3-DPG remains. This results in a potentially dangerous situation, that is, the circulating hemoglobin has a high affinity for oxygen, and this may result in cellular hypoxia. The early administration of phosphate would probably help in the recovery phase of 2,3-DPG. Studies in DKA patients who were given phosphate during early therapy have supported this contention.[53] However, although 2,3-DPG concentration does increase with treatment, there appears to be little effect on oxygen saturation of hemoglobin since the P_{50} (50% saturation of hemoglobin at oxygen partial pressure of 26 mmHg) of patients treated and not treated with phosphate does not differ.[54]

In regard to hyperalimentation, another clinical entity associated with hypophosphatemia, Travis has shown that supplemental phosphorus increases the red cell level of 2,3-DPG to the normal range more rapidly.[55]

Depressed CNS Function. CNS symptomatology is quite common in DKA. A depressed sensorium is the most frequent abnormality. Seizures and focal neurologic deficits are unusual in uncomplicated DKA.[56] If these neurologic findings are encountered in a patient with DKA, a secondary precipitating cause is usually present. The reason that seizures are uncommon in DKA may be related to the fact that concentrations of γ-aminobutyric acid (GABA) are normal in the CNS of patients with DKA.[57] Although many causes have been proposed for this depressed sensorium, no one cause is probably at fault in the individual patient. Postulated factors in the pathogenesis of CNS depression in DKA include extracellular hyperosmolality,[58] hyperviscosity of the blood,[59] cellular hypoxia,[60] cerebrospinal fluid and presumably intracellular acidemia in the brain,[61] CNS utilization of the ketones[56] that occur in DKA, and a medical condition, such as a cerebrovascular accident or infection.

The role, if any, of phosphate depletion in the pathogenesis of CNS dysfunction is unclear. Droller and associates have shown that mental obtundation and seizures can occur in severely hypophosphatemic patients during hyperalimentation.[62] Travis and associates are in apparent agreement, but they found that many of the neurologic abnormalities could be prevented by adequate phosphorus supplementation during hyperalimentation.[55] Thus hypophosphatemia, possibly caused by impaired glucose utilization and/or depressed 2,3-DPG with resultant cellular hypoxia, seems to have a potential role in the CNS symptomatology of DKA.

Increased Risk of Infection. Although no defects in humoral antibodies or the complement system have been demonstrated in the diabetic patient, white cell function in patients with DKA or mildly uncontrolled diabetes is impaired.[63] This dysfunction affects not only chemotaxis but also phagocytosis and microbiologic killing of ingested bacteria.[64,65] Therefore, the patient with DKA may be at an increased risk of infection, possibly related to phosphorus depletion. If true, the pathogenesis of this increased risk of infection seems related to a decreased level of intracellular ATP, with a resultant decrease in energy.

Impaired Carbohydrate Utilization. Several studies suggest that glucose utilization is improved following phosphorus administration. In his review of phosphorus depletion, Knochel showed that diabetic patients who received phosphorus had better glucose utilization.[66] In a more

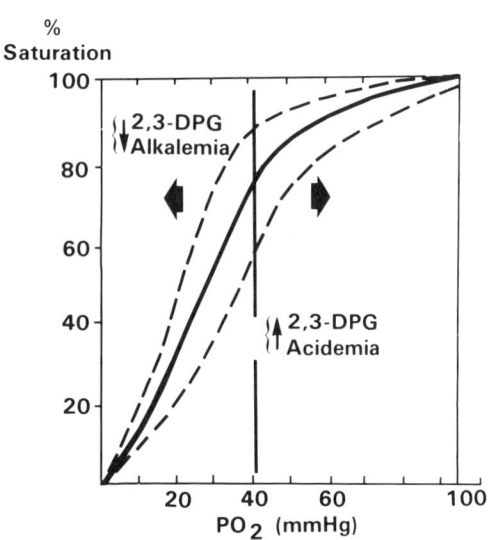

Figure 14-4 Oxyhemoglobin dissociation curve.

recent study, Lichtman and associates showed that phosphorus depletion decreased the utilization of glucose by red blood cells.[67]

Phosphate Therapy. Phosphorus depletion in DKA may be a clinical liability to the patient. Therefore, correction of this deficit in early therapy would seem logical, unless there are known contraindications to phosphate therapy, such as renal failure or a significant increase in the plasma phosphorus value. However, data have shown the major consequences of hypophosphatemia do not develop until the serum phosphorus level approaches or falls below 1.0 mg/dL. In addition, studies have been ambiguous as to the benefits of phosphate therapy in decreasing morbidity or mortality. Thus, phosphate supplementation is suggested only when the phosphate concentration approaches 1.0 mg/dL or there are known complications related to the hypophosphatemia. Intravenous preparations include sodium or potassium phosphate. Therapy must be carefully monitored, especially during intravenous therapy. Complications include hyperphosphatemia with possible metastatic calcifications, hyperkalemia due to the use of potassium phosphate salts, and hypocalcemia.

Magnesium

DKA is associated with a significant urinary excretion of magnesium.[68] As with potassium, the magnesium level might be normal or elevated initially, but it tends to drop with the administration of insulin and fluids. Clinical symptomatology of hypomagnesemia includes tetany, seizures, cardiac dysrhythmias, and CNS depression. It is recommended that the serum magnesium level be determined as soon as possible in all patients with DKA. If low, magnesium should be administered. Intravenous magnesium supplementation is the preferred method of repletion in a severely magnesium-deficient patient. This is particularly true in the early therapy of DKA, as the uptake of magnesium after an intramuscular injection might be less than optimal until adequate hydration has been restored. In the presence of seizures or dysrhythmias of uncertain etiology, magnesium therapy should be considered even if the initial magnesium level is within normal limits. Extreme caution must be used when magnesium is administered to patients with renal insufficiency, since these patients are prone to develop a toxic level. Both the blood level and the deep tendon reflexes, which tend to diminish as the magnesium concentration rises to toxic levels, should be checked frequently in these patients.

Alkali Therapy

The acidemic state in DKA results from the excess production and underutilization of the hydrogen ion–donating ketone bodies β-hydroxybutyric acid and acetoacetate. The consequences of severe acidosis include cardiovascular collapse, respiratory depression, and CNS dysfunction. Although it would seem logical to treat all cases of DKA with alkali, this approach is invalid because insulin can reverse the ketotic state and alkali therapy has detrimental effects.

Lipolysis is inhibited by very low circulating levels of insulin, approximately 40 μU/mL in one study.[69] The metabolism of β-hydroxybutyric acid requires about 100 μU/mL in normal subjects.[70] Therefore, insulin levels readily achieved by current methods of therapy reverse the ketoacidotic state, usually within 24 hours. This fact is clinically documented thousands of times each year as DKA patients are returned to normal without resorting to alkali therapy.

Potential adverse effects of alkali therapy include the following:

- shift of the oxyhemoglobin dissociation curve to the left with resulting cellular hypoxia
- accentuation of the intracellular shift of potassium and phosphate
- accentuation of the "paradoxical" cerebrospinal fluid acidosis to levels associated with coma[71]
- sodium overload
- tetany secondary to hypocalcemia and/or hypomagnesemia
- induction of metabolic alkalosis

Weighing the benefits and risks of alkali therapy, it would appear wise to initiate alkali therapy only in those patients with a pH of approximately 7.0, significant cardiac dysrhythmias in the acidemic state, or a compromised respiratory system. The latter may be suggested by an abnormal elevation of the P_{CO_2} according to the following formula in a primary metabolic acidosis[72]:

$$\text{expected } P_{CO_2} = 1.54(HCO_5) + 8.34 \pm 1.1$$

In any case, the alkali therapy given should be estimated to give a final pH of approximately 7.20.[11]

The alkali therapy of choice is bicarbonate, not lactate, for two reasons:

1. Lactate usually makes a small contribution to the overall acidemic state in DKA.[73]
2. After high-dose insulin therapy, there is a small rise in lactate concentration during the early recovery phase of DKA.[74]

Close surveillance of the result of the bicarbonate therapy by arterial blood gas or venous pH determination is required.

Insulin Therapy

Much has changed in the therapy of DKA in recent years, particularly in regard to the route and amount of insulin administration. Since the highly quoted work by Root, as well as that of Black and Malins, during the 1940s, the supposed benefits of intensive, high-dose insulin therapy have been emphasized.[75,76] The occasional reports of "low"-dose insulin therapy (lower than generally used at the time but nowhere near current standards) during this era were largely ignored by practicing clinicians.[77]

This remarkable decrease in insulin dosage has been derived from elegant studies concerning the physiologic action of insulin in relation to carbohydrate and ketone metabolism in the normal person. It was found that low-dose insulin therapy of DKA results in circulating levels of insulin of approximately 100 µU/mL, which supports the rationale of high physiologic, not pharmacologic, concentrations of insulin for therapy.[78,79] This concentration of insulin has been readily achieved by several routes of administration, including intramuscular and intravenous (Table 14-3).

Intramuscular Administration. Studies by Binder have shown that intramuscularly administered insulin has a half-life of 2 hours.[80] By calculations and in actual practice, Alberti and associates have shown that an initial injection of 20 U insulin, followed by hourly injections of 10 U, results in an insulin concentration of approximately 100 µU/mL in less than 3 hours.[81] The intramuscular method of insulin administration in the treatment of DKA has worked quite well in several studies.[82,83] Advantages include a very predictable fall in the blood glucose level (80 to 100 mg/hour, assuming adequate hydration),[81-83] a decreased incidence of hypokalemia,[81] a decreased incidence of delayed hypoglycemia,[82] and a fall, not a rise, in the blood lactate level.[81] Although not yet documented, a smaller fall in serum phosphorus and magnesium levels, as well as a decreased incidence of cerebral edema, might be a consequence of low-dose insulin therapy of DKA. This regimen is also extremely convenient to administer. The recommended site of insulin injection is the deltoid muscle.[82] In the occasional patient who is adequately hydrated but does not respond to intramuscular insulin therapy (such a patient usually has an infection), a change to continuous infusion of intravenous insulin is recommended. If there is any doubt about the practicality of a continuous insulin infusion, the intramuscular route of insulin administration is the treatment of choice.

Intravenous Administration. Constant infusion of insulin is not new—only the dosage has changed. Since the work by Genuth,[84] who used a loading dose of 50 U regular insulin, followed by 50 U/hour, the dosage has plummeted to only 1 U/hour in one study.[85] The goal of insulin therapy is to normalize the metabolic state of the patient; thus, circulating insulin concentrations of 100 to 200 µU/mL are probably adequate, if not excessive. This level is readily achieved by a constant infusion of regular insulin at a rate of 4 to 8 U/hour.[86,87] A loading dose is not necessary.

Table 14-3 Methods for Low-Dose Insulin Therapy in Diabetic Ketoacidosis

	Subcutaneous	Intramuscular	Intravenous
Dose	1. 0.33 unit regular insulin per kg as initial dose*†	1. 0.22 unit of regular insulin per kg as initial dose	1. 7 units of regular insulin per hour as continuous drip until plasma glucose reaches 250 mg/dL
	2. 7 units of regular insulin per hour thereafter until plasma glucose reaches 250 mg/dL	2. 0.1 unit of regular insulin per kg hourly until plasma glucose reaches 250 mg/dL	2. Priming dose optional
		3. Priming dose optional	
Advantages‡	1. Same as intramuscular	1. Predictable decrease in plasma glucose level (60–100 mg/dL per hour)	1. Same as intramuscular
		2. Possibly lower incidence of hypokalemia	
		3. Possibly lower incidence of hypoglycemia	
		4. Simplification of insulin therapy	
Disadvantages	1. Heavily dependent on intravascular volume replacement	1. Dependent on intravascular volume replacement	1. Dependent on intravascular volume replacement
	2. Occasional nonresponder	2. Occasional nonresponder	2. Occasional nonresponder
			3. Necessary to check infusion set frequently to ascertain that insulin delivery is correct

*If plasma glucose fails to decrease by 10 percent in the first hour, repeat initial dose each hour thereafter until a 10 percent decrease in plasma glucose is obtained.
†If there is no response in the plasma glucose after three doses, switch to intravenous insulin and search for an infection.
‡In a patient with adequate replacement of intravascular volume and careful clinical and biochemical monitoring.

Source: Modified from *Missouri Medicine*.

The advantages of a constant insulin infusion are similar to those of low-dose intramuscular therapy. Treatment should be continuous, since insulin administered intravenously has a half-life of only 5 minutes. Although a great advantage in preventing or in facilitating the recovery from hypoglycemia, the short half-life mandates constant surveillance of the intravenous apparatus. In the rush of the daily hospital routine, an accidental increase or decrease in the intravenous insulin infusion is all too possible.

It is well known that insulin binds with glass and plastic—potentially as much as 30 or 40%.[88,89] Thus, many centers recommend adding human albumin, a gelatin solution, or the patient's own blood to the insulin solution to prevent absorption.[90] The latter is preferred, since there is a risk of hepatitis with albumin and the gelatin solution is not available in the United States. Although of theoretical importance, the clinical significance of this absorption is questionable; several studies have shown excellent results with low-dose insulin therapy when no binding inhibitor was used.[6,91]

Despite the fact that the biologic action of insulin is longer than its immunologic half-life, bolus intravenous therapy is to be discouraged. The insulin levels fluctuate from initial pharmacologic levels to potentially suboptimal concentrations before the next dose is given.[92] Also, bolus therapy has been associated with rapid increases in anti-insulin hormones and lactate levels.[4]

As in other methods of insulin therapy in DKA, constant intravenous infusion is only part of the regimen. Total care of the patient is paramount. If the patient is not responding to the intravenous therapy in spite of adequate hydration, the insulin dosage should be doubled and an insulin-binding inhibitor added, if this has not been done already. As in intramuscular insulin therapy, patients with infections seem to respond more slowly.

Complications. By any method of administration, insulin may induce *hypoglycemia*. With low-dose insulin therapy—because the drop in the blood glucose level is predictable—and with frequent monitoring of the blood sugar level, this complication should be quite infrequent. When the blood sugar level approaches 250 mg/dL, exogenous glucose should be added either intravenously or, preferably, orally. As the exogenous sugar is added, insulin administration must be continued, but the dosage and route of administration should be reviewed. The correction of the acidosis tends to lag behind the normalization of the blood sugar, but this delay should be of little concern as long as the pH continues to improve.[93] In fact, this lag might be beneficial to the patient, because a correction of pH that is too rapid may result in significant complications.

Fortunately, since it is frequently fatal, *cerebral edema* is very uncommon in DKA. This complication should be suspected in any patient whose clinical and biochemical improvement is followed by deterioration in cerebral function. Elevation of the intraocular or cerebrospinal fluid pressures (with or without papilledema) in such a patient strongly suggests cerebral edema. Although no treatment is of proved benefit, free water administration should be stopped and hypertonic saline or mannitol begun in hope of reversing the process.[94] It is hoped that early supplementation of exogenous sugar (at approximately 250 mg/dL) and less reliance on markedly hypotonic solutions to correct the increased serum osmolality will reduce this deadly complication.

Education of the Patient

The often quoted saying "an ounce of prevention is worth a pound of cure" certainly applies to DKA. A second episode of DKA in the same patient should be extremely uncommon. Education begins in the hospital. By the time of discharge, each diabetic patient should be thoroughly versed in proper diet, urine testing, drug therapy, and activity. This education is continued at each follow-up visit and should include the "sick day" management of diabetes mellitus. The following rules should be emphasized:

1. *Do not discontinue daily insulin injections.* Many diabetic patients are under the false impression that, when they have an illness that causes a decrease in the intake of food (eg, the flu or gastroenteritis), insulin is not needed. In reality, the insulin requirement usually increases, because the levels of anti-insulin hormones are elevated during an acute illness.
2. *Check urine fractional for sugar and ketones four times a day.* This should be done by many patients even when their condition is stable, but it is imperative during an acute illness. Double-voided urine specimens are preferred, since they usually reflect the prevailing blood glucose level more accurately.
3. *Know how to use regular insulin.* During an acute illness, a working knowledge of a rapid-acting insulin is essential. Injection of regular insulin at times determined by urine fractionals (approximately every 6 hours) helps prevent the illness from developing into overt DKA.
4. *Initiate a sick day diet.* Frequently, a normal diet cannot be tolerated during an acute illness. Substitution of a liquid or soft diet equal in calories to the food normally consumed is usually adequate. This diet must be adequate in sodium and potassium content as well. Substitutions of this type should be explained as part of the dietary education.
5. *Use common sense.* Close cooperation between patient and physician is essential. If this treatment regimen is not successful, admission to a hospital for more intensive treatment is advisable.

The success of the treatment of any disease must be measured by the decrease of morbidity and mortality that results from therapy versus the risk of treatment. There is no doubt that the treatment of DKA by the various modalities mentioned has considerably brightened the outlook of the patient with DKA. The risk of treatment has been reduced by the introduction of low-dose insulin therapy. Still, there is much to be achieved both in morbidity and mortality in DKA. Low-dose insulin therapy of DKA is not a panacea. Many deaths in DKA are associated with a major precipitating event; only in relation to hypoglycemia, hypokalemia, and possibly cerebral edema does low-dose insulin therapy have any impact. Future research will uncover other avoidable causes of morbidity and mortality in DKA. Until that time, and probably thereafter, the best therapy begins with a diligent physician dedicated to total patient management.

HYPEROSMOLAR HYPERGLYCEMIC NONKETOTIC COMA

In recent years, hyperosmolar hyperglycemic nonketotic coma (HHNK) has become a common complication of diabetes mellitus. Although HHNK was initially described more than a century ago,[95] modern awareness of this syndrome is credited to the work of Sament and Swartz in 1957.[96] Since then, other reports have appeared.[97–99] Despite increased recognition of this syndrome, which is characterized by pronounced hyperglycemia, hyperosmolality, and dehydration in the absence of ketoacidosis, the mortality rate remains significantly higher than that of DKA, even in patients of comparable age.

Pathogenesis

The mechanism of HHNK has not been totally elucidated. Much interest in the pathogenesis of HHNK has focused on the lack of significant ketosis and the depressed sensorium.

Ketone bodies are normally produced by the liver in proportion to the circulating levels of free fatty acids, which act as substrate. Several reports have revealed that the levels of free fatty acids in HHNK are either normal or lower than those found in DKA, implying a defect in lipolysis.[100,101] Although the circulating levels of insulin have been found to be similar in patients with HHNK and DKA, the levels of growth hormone and cortisol, which are lipolytic hormones, have been found to be significantly lower in patients with HHNK than in patients with DKA. This suggests that, in some patients with HHNK, the low levels of free fatty acids and the lack of ketosis reflect a decrease in the activity of lipolytic hormones. Other mechanisms for the lack of ketosis in this syndrome have been postulated. For example, it has been suggested that severe dehydration might be antiketogenic, resulting in low plasma free fatty acid levels and ketone production.[102,103] In addition, in vitro studies have revealed that hyperosmolality inhibits both the release of pancreatic insulin to glucose and the production of free fatty acids from adipose tissue.[104]

Much of the work in the pathogenesis of the depressed sensorium in patients with HHNK has been done by Arieff and Carroll.[105] In a study of 40 patients with HHNK, they found that the depressed sensorium was highly correlated with the plasma osmolality. All stuporous or obtunded patients had a plasma osmolality of at least 350 mOsm/kg, whereas patients with a plasma osmolality of less than 350 mOsm/kg were alert. Sensorium did not correlate with the glucose concentration or the pH of either cerebrospinal fluid or plasma.

Pathophysiology

Fundamental to the pathophysiology of HHNK is a relative lack of insulin and relative excess of anti-insulin hormones, such as growth hormone, cortisol, and glucagon (Fig. 14-5). The net result of the interaction of these hormones is the excessive production and the underutilization of glucose, which lead to a pronounced hyperglycemia. Osmotically active glucose is located only in the extracellular fluid. Total body water generally represents approximately 60% of body weight, with two thirds of the water being intracellular and one third being extracellular. As the plasma glucose level rises, water moves from the intracellular fluid to the extracellular fluid until osmotic equilibrium is achieved. Thus, pronounced hyperglycemia results in the loss of water from the intracellular fluid, producing intracellular dehydration and expanding the extracellular fluid. Both have diagnostic and therapeutic implications. When the plasma glucose level is elevated, the renal threshold for glucose reabsorption may be surpassed, resulting in glycosuria. Generally, the higher the glucose level, the greater the renal excretion of glucose. Glycosuria causes an osmotic diuresis by inhibiting the reabsorption of water, which increases the flow of urine.

In terms of electrolyte loss, the osmotic diuresis in patients with HHNK results in a urinary loss of sodium and potassium of approximately 50 mEq/L each.[106] Thus, the osmotic diuresis produces a greater water loss than sodium loss, resulting in the hyperosmolar state and intracellular loss of water in most patients with HHNK. In addition, the loss of sodium leads to depletion of extracellular fluid volume. Other electrolytes, including magnesium and phosphate, have also been found to be depleted in patients with HHNK.

Much of the hyperglycemia in the HHNK patient probably results from decreased renal excretion of glucose rather than from overproduction or underutilization of glucose. As the extracellular fluid volume is depleted, the glomerular filtration rate decreases, which hampers the normal renal escape mechanism for glucose. Thus, a vicious cycle occurs: (1) the higher the plasma glucose level, the more pronounced the depletion of extracellular volume; (2) the glomerular filtration decreases; (3) less glucose is excreted in the urine; and (4) the plasma glucose level becomes more elevated. A similar circumstance has been shown to occur in patients

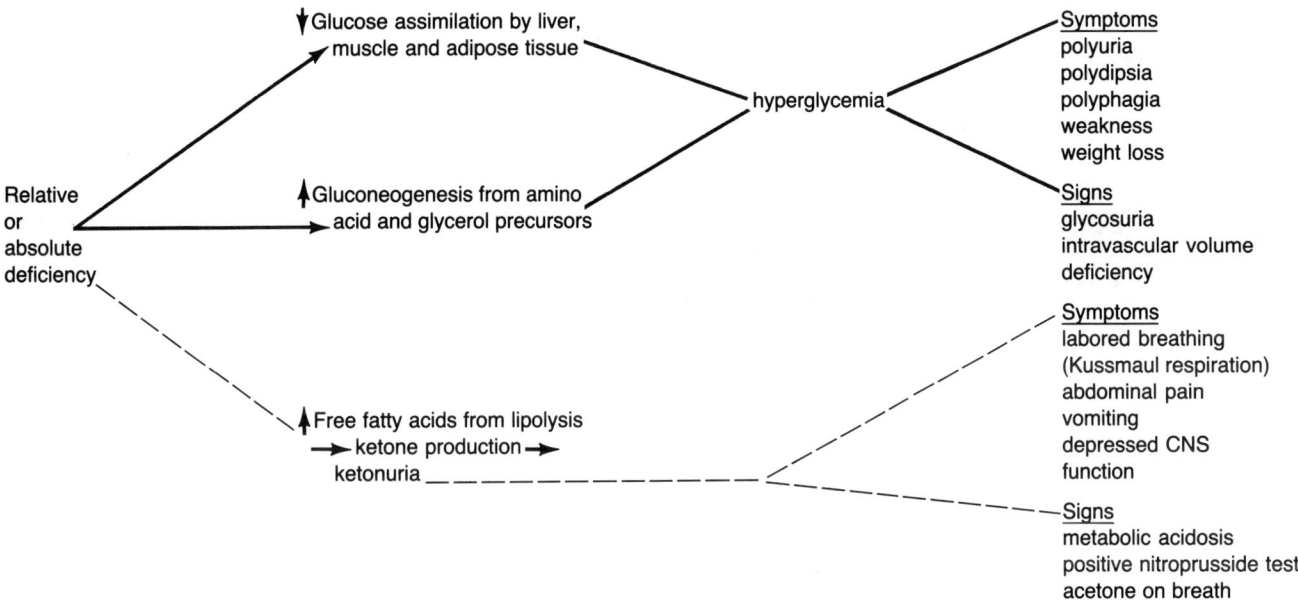

Figure 14-5 Pathophysiology of hyperosmolar hyperglycemic nonketotic coma (HHNK). In HHNK, the actions indicated by broken lines are suppressed.

with DKA; as much as 80% of the hyperglycemia in DKA patients is secondary to impaired excretion of renal glucose.[107] In most instances, patients with HHNK have a more pronounced volume depletion and higher plasma glucose levels than do patients with DKA because of the longer duration of symptoms before therapy is given.

Diagnosis

Clinical Diagnosis

HHNK occurs mainly in the elderly; patients have an average age of 60 years, although one patient recorded was a 9-month-old child. The condition occurs with equal frequency in men and women. Prior to the onset of HHNK, many patients have no history of diabetes mellitus. Even those with diabetes have usually been well controlled with diet or hypoglycemic agents. Although symptoms usually develop over a few days to a week unless there is an acute precipitating cause, HHNK has occurred within several hours after peritoneal dialysis or major surgery. Symptoms (eg, polyuria, polydipsia, and, occasionally, polyphagia) reflect the osmotic diuresis. Probably because ketosis (ketones are anorectic substances) and acidosis are insignificant, patients with HHNK generally have a longer history of illness than do patients with DKA.

Neurologic abnormalities are quite prevalent. As mentioned earlier, seizures are uncommon in uncomplicated DKA, but they are frequent in HHNK and occur in approximately 15% of patients. Localizing signs of a cerebrovascular accident, such as a positive Babinski sign, are also common and often resolve with successful therapy. In many instances, the admitting diagnosis is a cerebrovascular accident, which delays the recognition and management of HHNK. Any comatose patient should have a screening test for glucose in blood and urine in order to prevent such a delay in the diagnosis of HHNK. In pure terms, all patients with HHNK are comatose; in reality, half are either obtunded or stuporous. A distinct minority is alert.

Physical examination usually reveals extensive evidence of extracellular fluid volume depletion. Relative or absolute hypotension and tachycardia are present in the majority of patients. Skin turgor is poor, but this sign is unreliable because most patients are elderly. Many individuals also have a precipitating illness:

- infection, particularly pneumonia
- cardiovascular disease
    myocardial infarction
    cerebrovascular accident
    gastrointestinal bleeding
- miscellaneous
    pancreatitis
    excessive carbohydrate intake
    surgery
    dialysis

In addition, the use of certain drugs has been associated with the onset of HHNK:

- diuretics, particularly thiazides, chlorthalidone, furosemide
- corticosteroids

- propranolol
- immunosuppressive agents
- phenytoin (Dilantin)
- diazoxide

Hospital procedures, such as peritoneal dialysis, hemodialysis, hyperalimentation, and the administration of mannitol have also produced HHNK.

Laboratory Diagnosis

HHNK is easily diagnosed once the syndrome has been considered. No rigid criteria have been set, but a laboratory diagnosis may be defined as follows[107]:

- glycosuria of 3+ or 4+ without ketonuria
- extreme hyperglycemia (ie, glucose usually greater than 600 mg/dL)
- negative or minimally positive nitroprusside test (Acetest)—no greater than 2+ reaction when plasma is diluted 1:1 with water
- serum osmolality greater than 350 mOsm/kg

In addition, the serum sodium level is usually normal to elevated; the serum potassium level is normal to low; and the BUN, creatinine, and BUN-creatinine ratio (which is normally 10:1) are usually elevated.

In the absence of an osmometer, the approximate plasma osmolality may be calculated by using the following formula:

$$\text{Osmolality} = 2\,[\text{serum sodium}] + \frac{\text{blood glucose}}{18} + \frac{\text{BUN}}{2.8}$$

Normal osmolality is 285 to 300 mOsm. A low or low-normal plasma osmolality concomitant with extreme hyperglycemia may alter therapy. In any given series, the individual values for blood glucose and plasma osmolality vary widely. In the report by Arieff and Carroll, the mean blood glucose level was 1166 mg/dL (standard deviation ± 306) and the mean plasma osmolality was 384 mOsm/kg water (standard deviation ± 27).[107]

Initial studies should include a complete blood cell count; determinations of electrolytes, BUN, creatinine, and arterial blood gases; and urinalysis. Interpretation of these studies must take into account many of the same factors that must be considered with laboratory studies on DKA patients, such as "pseudohyponatremia" induced by hyperglycemia and factitious hyponatremia caused by an elevated triglyceride level. Many of the initial studies reflect the marked degree of dehydration. The hemoglobin and hematocrit are commonly elevated, but they return to normal with adequate fluid replacement. Many patients, successfully treated, will have residual impairment of kidney function. Like patients with DKA, those with HHNK have a total body depletion of potassium that is secondary to the osmotic losses in the urine and gastrointestinal tract. Unlike patients with DKA, who are usually acidemic, patients with HHNK are occasionally hyperkalemic. In the series by McCurdy, approximately 12% of patients with HHNK had initial hyperkalemia, whereas almost 30% had initial potassium levels below 4 mEq/L.[98] In the series of patients studied by Arieff and Carroll, the mean initial values for BUN, creatinine, serum sodium, and potassium were 95 mg/dL, 5.6 mg/dL, 144 mEq/L, and 5 mEq/L, respectively.[107] The "normal" serum sodium level in spite of extreme hyperglycemia demonstrates the tremendous loss of body water that occurs in patients with HHNK.

Metabolic acidosis is not infrequent in HHNK. In both the report by McCurdy and that by Arieff and Carroll, metabolic acidosis, as defined by a serum carbon dioxide level of less than 21 mEq/L or an arterial pH of 7.35 or less, occurred in 40 to 60% of the patients.[98,107] Slight lactate elevations were frequent but did not account for the majority of cases of metabolic acidosis. Renal failure accounted for several. In a few patients, even though the nitroprusside test was not impressive, the level of acetoacetic acid (one of the prevalent hydrogen ion-donating ketone bodies in DKA) was slightly elevated, suggesting possible DKA. Interestingly, Sotos and associates have shown that pronounced hyperosmolality per se may cause metabolic acidosis in animals.[108] Thus, the cause for the metabolic acidosis is unknown in the majority of cases in HHNK; in most patients, it is probably multifactorial.

As with DKA, a baseline ECG should always be obtained to identify a painless myocardial infarction, and appropriate bacterial stains and cultures should be done to rule out an infection.

Treatment

The correction of HHNK encompasses four areas: (1) correction of fluid and electrolyte deficits, (2) normalization of the intermediary metabolism, (3) prevention of complications, and (4) diagnosis and treatment of the precipitating event.

All patients with HHNK should have a complete and up-to-date flowsheet like that used in DKA (see Fig. 14-4) to eliminate uncertainty about previous therapy and to indicate how the patient responds to various modalities. Catheters should be avoided if at all possible so as to minimize the risk of a superimposed infection. If required, a Swan-Ganz catheter is preferred to a central venous pressure line.

Fluid and Electrolyte Therapy

Fluid therapy in patients with HHNK is controversial. Some authors suggest fluid replacement with normal saline, whereas others prefer to use half-normal saline provided the patient is not clinically hypotensive or oliguric.[34,109] In actuality, initial therapy is best determined by the clinical presentation of the individual patient. Whatever treatment is chosen, the patient's condition must be carefully monitored to determine progress and changes in fluid requirements.

Total body water loss in patients with HHNK has been estimated to average 24%, with approximately 50 mEq/L each of sodium and potassium lost in the osmotic diuresis. Total body loss of sodium and potassium is similar to that in patients with DKA, that is, an average of 8 mEq/kg and 6 mEq/kg, respectively. Thus, most patients with HHNK initially have marked clinical evidence of sodium depletion (relative or absolute hypotension, tachycardia, oliguria, and poor skin turgor) and require rapid and total correction of the sodium deficit. The amount of normal saline required varies among patients. The criteria mentioned previously indicate the adequacy of sodium repletion. Since most individuals with HHNK are elderly, normal saline may not be innocuous, and hypertension with sodium overload must be carefully avoided.

In the face of clinical intravascular volume depletion, it may be advisable to withhold insulin early in the course of therapy. A few patients have no evidence of sodium depletion on initial presentation, and in these, cautious use of the half-normal saline and insulin may be used. Careful and continuous monitoring of intravascular volume is necessary, however. Replacement with hypotonic fluids with simultaneous lowering of the plasma glucose by insulin has been shown to induce hypotension and oliguria because of the movement of water from the extracellular to the intracellular space.[110] Correction of sodium deficit with normal saline instead of half-normal saline results in a slower drop in the plasma osmolality.

The average loss of water is 75 to 100 mL/kg or, as mentioned previously, 24% of total body water. After the sodium deficit has been corrected, the free water may be replaced. The free water deficit may be calculated by the following formula:

$$\text{Water deficit} = 0.6 \times \text{body weight in kg} \left(1 - \frac{140}{\text{Plasma sodium}}\right)$$

Although this formula is based on several assumptions, it is adequate for the initiation of treatment. It is important to realize that the formula does not take into account the ongoing urinary and nonurinary losses of fluid and electrolytes. Generally, replacement of the water deficit is accomplished by 50% normal saline or 5% dextrose as the plasma glucose level approaches 250 mg/dL. As the patient becomes more alert, water may be taken by mouth. It must be remembered that too rapid correction of the water deficit may result in water intoxication with cerebral edema. Moreover, extreme caution is advisable in those patients with a low plasma osmolality because removal of the osmotic effect of glucose by insulin therapy or use of hypotonic fluids may also cause water intoxication.

Although total body potassium losses are probably higher in HHNK than in DKA, the mean initial potassium level in HHNK is lower. Thus, potassium replacement, with the chloride or phosphate salt, is generally indicated in the initial treatment. Contraindications to early potassium administration include ECG evidence of hyperkalemia, known hyperkalemia, or oliguria. The latter is a relative contraindication, since hydration and insulin-influenced cellular uptake of potassium cause a rapid drop in the potassium level. Careful monitoring of the potassium levels is required, since ECG evidence of hyperkalemia is nonspecific.

Normalization of Intermediary Metabolism

As in DKA, there has been a shift to the use of low-dose insulin therapy in the treatment of HHNK. The main goal of insulin therapy in DKA is to reverse the ketotic state; the goal in HHNK is to return carbohydrate metabolism to normal. Hyperglycemia in HHNK reflects three conditions: (1) underexcretion of glucose by the kidney, (2) hepatic overproduction of glucose, and (3) peripheral underutilization of glucose. Studies have shown that circulating insulin levels of approximately 200 μU/mL are sufficient to inhibit gluconeogenesis and to produce almost maximal glucose uptake by adipose tissue and muscle.[111] This concentration of insulin may be achieved by intramuscular or intravenous administration. Bendezo and associates have shown satisfactory results in the treatment of HHNK with an intravenous loading dose of 5 to 10 U regular insulin, followed by a continuous infusion of 7 to 12 U/hour.[112] It must be emphasized that, no matter how the insulin is given, it is only part of the total management of the patient with HHNK.

For recent reports from the medical literature, see refs. 113–131.

REFERENCES

1. Beigelman PM. Severe diabetic ketoacidosis (diabetic "coma"). *Diabetes*. 1971;20:490–500.
2. Soler NG, Fitzgerald MG, Bennett MA, et al. Intensive care in the management of diabetic ketoacidosis. *Lancet*. 1973;1:951–954.
3. Alberti KGMM. Diabetic ketoacidosis: aspects of management. In: Ledingham JGG, ed. *Tenth Advanced Medicine Symposium*. New York: Pitman Publishing; 1974;68–82.
4. Alberti KGMM. Low-dose insulin in the treatment of diabetic ketoacidosis. *Arch Intern Med*. 1977;137:1367–1376.
5. Felig P. Insulin: rates and route of delivery. *N Engl J Med*. 1974; 291:1031–1032.
6. Page M, Alberti KGMM, Greenwood R, et al. Treatment of diabetic coma with continuous low-dose infusion of insulin. *Br Med J*. 1974;2:687–690.
7. Semple PF, White C, Manderson WG. Continuous intravenous infusion of small doses of insulin in treatment of diabetic ketoacidosis. *Br Med J*. 1974;2:694–698.
8. Kedson W, Casey J, Kraegen E, et al. Treatment of severe diabetes mellitus by insulin infusion. *Br Med J*. 1974;2:691–694.
9. Felig P. Diabetic ketoacidosis. *N Engl J Med*. 1974;290:1360–1363.

10. Ditzel J. Importance of plasma in organic phosphate on tissue oxygenation during recovery from diabetic ketoacidosis. *Horm Metab Res.* 1973;5:471–472.
11. Zimmet PZ, Taft P, Ennis GC, et al. Acid production in diabetic acidosis: a more rational approach to alkali replacement. *Br Med J.* 1970;3:610–612.
12. Felig P. Combating diabetic ketoacidosis and other hyperglycemic ketoacidotic syndromes. *Postgrad Med.* 1976;50:150–153.
13. Felig P, Wahren J, Handler R. Influence of oral glucose ingestion on splanchnic glucose and gluconeogenic substrate metabolism. *Diabetes.* 1975;24:468–475.
14. Nahren J, Felig P, Cerasi E, et al. Splanchnic and peripheral glucose and amino acid metabolism in diabetes mellitus. *J Clin Invest.* 1972;51:1870–1879.
15. McGarry JD, Foster DW. Regulation of ketogenesis and clinical aspects of the ketotic state. *Metabolism.* 1972;21:471–489.
16. Munro JF, Campbell IW, McCuish AC, et al. Euglycaemic diabetic ketoacidosis. *Br Med J.* 1973;2:578–580.
17. Marliss EB, Ohman JL, Aoki TT, et al. Altered redox state obscuring ketoacidosis in diabetic patients with lactic acidosis. *N Engl J Med.* 1970;283:978–980.
18. Faerman I, Faccio E, Milei J, et al. Autonomic neuropathy and painless myocardial infarction in diabetic patients: histologic evidence of their relationship. *Diabetes.* 1977;26:1147–1158.
19. Soler NG, Bennett MA, Peneost BL, et al. Myocardial infarction in diabetes. *Q J Med.* 1975;44:125–132.
20. Beardwood UT Jr. Abdominal symptomatology of diabetic acidosis. *JAMA.* 1935;105:1168–1172.
21. Knight AH, Williams DN, Ellis G. Significance of hyperamylasaemia and abdominal pain in diabetic ketoacidosis. *Br Med J.* 1973;3:128–131.
22. Levine RI, Glauder FI, Berk JE. Enhancement of the amylase-creatinine clearance ratio in disorders other than acute pancreatitis. *N Engl J Med.* 1975;292:329–332.
23. Fridhandler L, Berk JE, Veda M. Isolation and measurement of pancreatic amylase in human serum and urine. *Clin Chem.* 1972;18:1493–1497.
24. Campbell IW, Duncan LJ, Innes JA, et al. Abdominal pain in diabetic metabolic decompensation: clinical significance. *JAMA.* 1975;233:166–168.
25. Page LB, Culver PG, eds. *A Syllabus of Laboratory Examinations in Clinical Diagnosis: Critical Evaluation of Laboratory Procedures in the Study of the Patient*, rev ed. Cambridge, MA: Harvard University Press; 1960.
26. Stephens JM, Sulway MJ, Watkins PJ. Relationship of blood acetoacetate and 3-hydroxybutyrate in diabetes. *Diabetes.* 1971;20:485–489.
27. Sulway MJ, Malins JM. Acetone in diabetic ketoacidosis. *Lancet.* 1970;2:736–740.
28. Katz MA. Hyperglycemia-induced hyponatremia—calculation of expected serum sodium depression. *N Engl J Med.* 1973;289:818–844.
29. Krumlovsky FA. Hyponatremia. *Ration Drug Ther.* 1975;9:1–6.
30. Padova J, Bandersky G. Hyperuricemia in diabetic ketoacidosis. *N Engl J Med.* 1962;267:530–534.
31. Goldfinger S, Klinenberg JR, Seegmiller JE. Renal retention of uric acid induced by infusion of β-hydroxybutyrate and acetoacetate. *N Engl J Med.* 1965;272:351–355.
32. Watkins PJ. The effect of ketone bodies on the determination of creatinine. *Clin Chem Acta.* 1967;18:191–196.
33. Murray T, Long W, Narins RG. Multiple myeloma and the anion gap. *N Engl J Med.* 1975;292:574–575.
34. Kleeman CR, Liberman B. Diabetic acidosis and coma. In: Rand MM, Kleeman CR, eds: *Clinical Disorders of Fluid and Electrolyte Metabolism.* 2nd ed. New York: McGraw-Hill; 1972:971–994.
35. Winegrad AI, Clements RS. Diabetic ketoacidosis. *Med Clin North Am.* 1971;55:899–911, 1971.
36. Martin HH, Smith K, Wilson ML. The fluid and electrolyte therapy of severe diabetic acidosis and ketosis. A study of twenty-nine episodes (twenty-six patients). *Am J Med.* 1958;24:376–389.
37. Nabarro JDH, Spencer AG, Stower JM. Metabolic studies in severe diabetic ketosis. *Q J Med.* 1952;21:225–248.
38. Burnell JH, Villamil MF, Vyeno TB, et al. The effect in humans of extracellular pH changes on the relationship between serum potassium concentration and intracellular potassium. *J Clin Invest.* 1956;35:935–939.
39. Seftel HC, Kew MC. Early and intensive potassium replacement in diabetic acidosis. *Diabetes.* 1966;15:694–696.
40. Beigelman PM, Martin HE, Miller LV, et al. Severe diabetic ketoacidosis. *JAMA.* 1969;219:1082–1086.
41. Clementsen HJ. Potassium therapy: a break with tradition. *Lancet.* 1962;2:175–177.
42. Helderman JH, Elahi D, Andersen DK, et al. Prevention of the glucose intolerance of thiazide diabetics by maintenance of body potassium. *Diabetes.* 1983;32:106–111.
43. Beigelman PM. Potassium in severe diabetic ketoacidosis. *Am J Med.* 1973;54:419–429.
44. Hockaday TDR, Alberti KGMM. Diabetic coma. *Clin Endocrinol Metab.* 1972;1:751–788.
45. Roberts KE, Magida MG. Electrocardiographic alterations produced by a decrease/increase in plasma pH, bicarbonate and sodium as compared with those produced by an increase/decrease in potassium. *Circ Res.* 1953;1:206–213, 214–218.
46. Butler AM. Metabolic studies in diabetic coma. *Trans Assoc Am Physicians.* 1947;60:102–109.
47. Nabarro JDN, Spencer AG, Stowers JM. Metabolic studies in severe ketosis. *Q J Med.* 1952;21:225–243.
48. O'Connor LR, Wheeler WS, Bethune JE. Effect of hypophosphatemia on myocardial performance in man. *N Engl J Med.* 1977;297:901–903.
49. Rorth M. Dependence of oxyhaemoglobin dissociation and introerythrocytic 2,3-DPG on acid-base status of blood: I. In vitro studies on reduced and oxygenated blood. *Adv Exp Med Biol.* 1970;6:57–64.
50. Rapaport S. The regulation of glycolysis in mammalian erythrocyte. *Essays Biochem.* 1968;4:69–103.
51. Travis SF. Metabolic alterations in the human erythrocyte produced by increases in glucose concentration: the role of the polyol pathway. *J Clin Invest.* 1971;50:2104–2112.
52. Bellingham AJ, Detter JC, Lenfant C. Regulatory mechanisms of haemoglobin oxygen affinity in acidosis and alkalosis. *J Clin Invest.* 1971;50:700–706.
53. Stankl E, Ditzel J. The effect of red cell 2,3-DPG changes induced by diabetic ketoacidosis on parameters of the oxygen dissociation curve. *Man Adv Exp Med Biol.* 1976;75:89–95.
54. Gibby DM, Veale KEA, Hayes TM, et al. Oxygen availability from the blood and the effect of phosphate replacement on erythrocyte 2,3-diphosphoglycerate and hemoglobin-oxygen affinity in diabetic ketoacidosis. *Diabetologia.* 1978;15:386.
55. Travis SF, Sugerman AJ, Ruberg RL, et al. Alterations of red cell glycolytic intermediates and oxygen transport as a consequence of

hypophosphatemia in patients receiving intravenous hyperalimentation. *N Engl J Med.* 1971;285:763–768.
56. Guisad OR, Arieff AI. Neurologic manifestations of diabetic comas: correlation with biochemical alterations in the brain. *Metabolism.* 1975;24:665–679.
57. Flock EV, Tyce GM, Owen CA Jr. Glucose metabolism in brains of diabetic rats. *Endocrinology.* 1969;85:428–437.
58. Fulop M, Tannebaum H, Dreyer N. Ketotic hyperosmolar coma. *Lancet.* 1973;2:635–639.
59. Reubi FC. Glomerular filtration rate, renal blood flow and blood viscosity during and after diabetic coma. *Circ Res.* 1953;1:410–413.
60. Ditzel J. Impaired oxygen release caused by alterations of metabolism in the erythrocytes in diabetes. *Lancet.* 1972;1:721–723.
61. Posner JB, Plum F. Spinal fluid pH and neurologic symptoms in systemic acidosis. *N Engl J Med.* 1967;277:605–613.
62. Droller H, Siluis SE, Paragas PB. Paresthesia, weakness, seizures, and hypophosphatemia in patients receiving hyperalimentation. *Gastroenterology.* 1972;62:513–520.
63. Bagdade JD, Rout RK, Bulger RJ. Impaired leucocyte function in patients with poorly controlled diabetes. *Diabetes.* 1974;23:9–15.
64. Molenaar DM, Palumbo PJ, Wilson WR, et al. Leucocyte chemotaxis in diabetic patients and their non-diabetic first degree relative. *Diabetes.* 1976;25(suppl 2):880–883.
65. Bagdade JD. Infection in diabetes—predisposing factors. *Postgrad Med.* 1976;59:160–164.
66. Knochel JP. The pathophysiology and clinical characteristics of severe hypophosphatemia. *Arch Intern Med.* 1977;137:203–220.
67. Lichtman MA, Miller DR, Cohen J, et al. Reduced red cell glycolysis, 2,3-diphosphoglycerate and adenosine triphosphate concentration and increased hemoglobin oxygen affinity caused by hypophosphatemia. *Ann Intern Med.* 1971;74:562–568.
68. Wacker WEC, Vallee BL. Magnesium metabolism. *N Engl J Med.* 1958;259:431–438, 475–482.
69. Zierler KL, Rabiosowitz D. Effect of very small concentrations of insulin on forearm metabolism: persistence of its action on potassium and free fatty acids without its effect on glucose. *J Clin Invest.* 1964;43:950–962.
70. Sherwin RS, Hendler RG, Felig PF. Effect of diabetes mellitus and insulin on the turnover and metabolic response to ketones in man. *Diabetes.* 1976;25:776–784.
71. Ohman JC, Marliss EB, Aoke TT, et al. The cerebral spinal fluid in diabetic ketoacidosis. *N Engl J Med.* 1971;284:283–290.
72. Albert MS, Dell RB, Winters RW. Quantitative displacement of acid-base equilibrium in metabolic acidosis. *Ann Intern Med.* 1967;66:312–322.
73. Watkins PJ, Smith JS, Fitzgerald MG, et al. Lactic acidosis in diabetes. *Br Med J.* 1969;1:744–747.
74. Alberti KGMM, Hockaday TDR. Blood lactate and pyruvic acids in diabetic coma. *Diabetes.* 1972;21:350.
75. Root HF. The use of insulin and abuse of glucose in the treatment of diabetic coma. *JAMA.* 1945;127:557–564.
76. Black AB, Malins JM. Diabetic ketosis: a comparison of results of orthodox and intensive methods of treatment based on 170 consecutive cases. *Lancet.* 1949;1:56–59.
77. Shaw CE, Hurwitz GE, Schmukler M. A clinical and laboratory study of insulin dosage in diabetic acidosis: comparison with small and large doses. *Diabetes.* 1962;11:23–30.
78. Menzel R, Aande E, Jutze E. Treatment of diabetic coma with low-dose injections of insulin. *Endocrinologie.* 1976;67:230–239.
79. Hannan TJ, Stahers GM. Constant low-dose infusion in severe diabetes mellitus. *Med J Aust.* 1976;1:11–13.
80. Binder C. *Absorption of Injected Insulin.* Copenhagen: Ejnar Munksgaaris Forlag; 1969.
81. Alberti KGMM, Hockaday TDR, Turner RC. Small doses of intramuscular insulin in the treatment of diabetic "coma." *Lancet.* 1973;2:515–522.
82. Kitabchi AE, Ayyagari V, Guerra SMO, et al. The efficacy of low-dose versus conventional therapy of insulin for treatment of diabetic ketoacidosis. *Ann Intern Med.* 1976;84:633–638.
83. Moseley J. Diabetic crises in children treated with small doses of intramuscular insulin. *Br Med J.* 1975;1:59–61.
84. Genuth SM. Constant intravenous insulin infusion in diabetic ketoacidosis. *JAMA.* 1973;223:1348–1351.
85. Piters K, Goodman J, Bessman A. Treatment of diabetic ketoacidosis with continuous low-dose intravenous insulin. *Diabetes.* 1975;24:396.
86. Malleson PN. Diabetic ketosis in children treated by adding low-dose insulin to rehydrating fluid. *Arch Dis Child.* 1976;51:373–376.
87. Martin MM, Martin ALD. Continuous low-dose insulin infusion vs. conventional intermittent subcutaneous injections in the treatment of diabetic ketoacidosis in children. *Diabetes.* 1976;25:376.
88. Weisenfeld S, Poldolsky S, Goldsmith L, et al. Absorption of insulin to infusion bottles and tubing. *Diabetes.* 1968;17:766–771.
89. Peterson L, Caldwell J, Hoffman J. Insulin absorbance to polyvinylchloride surfaces with implications for constant infusion therapy. *Diabetes.* 1976;25:72–74.
90. Sonksen PH, Ellis JP, Lowy C, et al. A quantitative evaluation of the relative efficiency of gelatine and albumin in preventing insulin absorption to glass. *Diabetologia.* 1965;1:208–210.
91. Herer D, Molitch M, Sperling M. Low-dose continuous insulin therapy for diabetic ketoacidosis: prospective comparison with "conventional" insulin therapy. *Arch Intern Med.* 1977;137:1377–1380.
92. Clumeck N, DeTruyer A, Naeije R, et al. Treatment of diabetic coma with small intravenous boluses. *Br Med J.* 1976;2:394–396.
93. Soler NG, Fitzgerald MG, Wright AD, et al. Comparative study of different insulin regimens in management of diabetic ketoacidosis. *Lancet.* 1975;2:1221–1224.
94. Feig PV, McCurdy DK. The hypertonic state. *N Engl J Med.* 1977;297:1444–1454.
95. Dreshfeld J. The Bradshawe lecture on diabetic coma. *Br Med J.* 1886;2:358–360.
96. Sament S, Swartz MB. Severe diabetic stupor without ketosis. *S Afr Med J.* 1957;31:893–894.
97. Tyler FH. Hyperosmolar coma. *Am J Med.* 1968;45:485–487.
98. McCurdy DK. Hyperosmolar hyperglycemic non-ketotic diabetic coma. *Med Clin North Am.* 1970;54:683–699.
99. Miller EC. Diabetic emergencies. *Am Fam Physician.* 1978;18:115–121.
100. Gerich JE, Martin MM, Recant L. Clinical and metabolic characteristics of hyperosmolar nonketotic coma. *Diabetes.* 1971;20:228–237.
101. Joffé BI, Krut LH, Goldberg RB, et al. Pathogenesis of nonketotic hyperosmolar diabetic coma. *Lancet.* 1975;1:1069–1071.
102. Passmore R, Johnson RE. The modification of post-exercise ketosis by environmental temperature and water balance. *Q J Exp Physiol.* 1958;43:352–358.
103. Gerich J, Penhos JC, Recant L. Metabolic consequence of hyperosmolarity. *Clin Res.* 1970;18:87.

104. Kuzuya T, Samols E, Williams RH. Stimulation by hyperosmolarity of glucose metabolism in rat adipose tissue and diaphragm in vitro. *J Biol Chem.* 1965;240:2277–2283.
105. Arieff AI, Carroll HJ. Cerebral edema and depression of sensorium in non-ketotic hyperosmolar coma. *Diabetes.* 1974;23:525–531.
106. Clements RS, Vourganti B. Fatal diabetic ketoacidosis: major causes and approaches to their prevention. *Diabetes Care.* 1978;1:314–325.
107. Arieff AI, Carroll HJ. Nonketotic hyperosmolar coma with hyperglycemia: clinical features, pathophysiology, renal function, acid-base balance, plasma-cerebrospinal fluid equilibria and the effects of therapy in 37 cases. *Medicine.* 1972;51:73–94.
108. Sotos JF, Dodge PR, Meara P, et al. Studies in experimental hypertonicity: II. Hypertonicity of body fluids as a cause of acidosis. *Pediatrics.* 1962;30:180–193.
109. Loeb JN. The hyperosmolar state. *N Engl J Med.* 1974;290:1184–1187.
110. Brown RH, Rossini AA, Callaway W, et al. Caveation fluid replacement in hyperglycemic, hyperosmolar, non-ketotic coma. *Diabetes Care.* 1978;1:305–307.
111. Christensen NJ, Orskou J. The relationship between endogenous serum insulin concentration and glucose uptake in the forearm muscle of nondiabetics. *J Clin Invest.* 1968;47:1262–1266.
112. Bendezo R, Wieland RG, Furst BH. Experience with low-dose insulin infusion in diabetic ketoacidosis and diabetic hyperosmolarity. *Arch Intern Med.* 1978;138:60–62.
113. Herlitz J, Karlson BW, Edvardsson N, Emanuelsson H, Hjalmarson A. Prognosis in diabetics with chest pain or other symptoms suggestive of acute myocardial infarction. *Cardiology.* 1992;80:237–245.
114. Muir R. A 15-year-old girl with abdominal pain, vomiting, tachycardia, and tachypnea. *J Emerg Nurs.* 1992;18:357–358.
115. Criado E, De Stefano AA, Keagy BA, Upchurch GR Jr, Johnson G Jr. The course of severe foot infection in patients with diabetes. *Surg Gynecol Obstet.* 1992;175:135–140.
116. Holmwood KI, Williams DR, Roland JM. Use of the accident and emergency department by patients with diabetes. *Diabet Med.* 1992;9:386–388.
117. Mulcahy K. Hypoglycemic emergencies. *Crit Care Nurs.* 1992;3:361–369.
118. Palmer CF. Special issues in the management of the elderly patient with diabetes. *Mt Sinai J Med.* 1991;58:287–292.
119. McCrea DL, McCrea CA. Emergency department care of the patient with an insulin pump. *J Emerg Nurs.* 1991;17:220–224.
120. Quale JM, Lonano F. Salmonella myonecrosis in a patient with diabetes mellitus. *Am J Med Sci.* 1991;301:335–336.
121. Sutherland DE, Gruber SA. Pancreas transplantation. *Crit Care Clin.* 1990;6:947–953.
122. Hirsch IB, McGill JB. Role of insulin in management of surgical patients with diabetes mellitus. *Diabetes Care.* 1990;13:980–991.
123. Hanley RM. Diabetic emergencies. They happen with or without diabetes. *Postgrad Med.* 1990;88:90–96.
124. Patrick AW, Collier A, Hepburn DA, Steedman DJ, Clarke BJ, Robertson C. Comparison of intramuscular glucagon and intravenous dextrose in the treatment of hypoglycaemic coma in an accident and emergency department. *Arch Emerg Med.* 1990;7:73–77.
125. Purnell L. Triage decisions. A 68-year-old unconscious woman with a history of urinary tract infection treated with oral antibiotics. *J Emerg Nurs.* 1990;16:303–304.
126. Akerblom HK, Kaprio EA. Care in diabetic emergencies. *Indian J Pediatr.* 1989;56(suppl 1):871–876.
127. Ankel F, Wolfson AB, Stapczynski JS. Emphysematous cystitis: a complication of urinary tract infection occurring predominantly in diabetic women. *Ann Emerg Med.* 1990;19:404–406.
128. Alberti KG. Diabetic emergencies. *Br Med Bull.* 1989;45:242–263.
129. Ouellet LM, Brook MP. Emphysematous pyelonephritis: an emergency indication for the plain abdominal radiograph. *Ann Emerg Med.* 1988;17:722–724.
130. Bonadio WA, Gutzeit MF, Losek JD, Smith DS. Outpatient management of diabetic ketoacidosis. *Am J Dis Child.* 1988;142:448–450.
131. Kitabchi AE, Rumbak M. The management of diabetic emergencies [see comments]. *Hosp Pract.* 1989;24:129–133.

15. Thyroid Disorders

GERALD S. LEVEY, MD

THYROID STORM

Hyperthyroidism is a readily recognized and treatable endocrine disease that is commonly encountered in the clinical practice of medicine. The clinical syndrome known as thyroid storm or thyroid crisis is one of the most dramatic and feared manifestations of hyperthyroidism. Thyroid storm occurs in a small percentage of patients with hyperthyroidism and accounts for much of the mortality associated with hyperthyroidism. Only prompt institution of appropriate therapy can prevent the dreaded sequelae of this syndrome. A number of excellent reviews have been written on this subject.[1-4]

The pathogenesis of thyroid storm is poorly understood. Such a crisis may occur in patients of either sex and at any age, although it is unusual in children. Thyroid storm almost always occurs in patients with preexistent hyperthyroidism due to diffuse toxic goiter that has been either untreated or inadequately treated before the onset of storm. Although the extent of clinical symptoms is variable, thyroid crisis develops abruptly and is best characterized as a state of unregulated hypermetabolism with fever and tachycardia. Examination of patients with thyroid storm reveals excess sympathetic (adrenergic) activity, as well as evidence of chronically increased levels of thyroid hormone. A number of studies have demonstrated the importance of the interactions of both thyroid hormones and catecholamines as they affect the cardiovascular system, adipose tissue, and the central nervous system.[5-7] It is important to understand the role of both β-adrenergic stimulation and thyroid hormone in thyroid storm in order to institute effective treatment.

Precipitating Factors

Although the pathophysiology of thyroid crisis is poorly understood, the clinical settings in which it arises are well known. In general, there are two classes of precipitating factors in thyroid storm: surgical and medical. Surgical treatment of hyperthyroidism in a patient who has not been rendered euthyroid with antithyroid drugs prior to the operation may induce thyroid storm postoperatively. Operative procedures that do not involve the thyroid but are performed in untreated or inadequately treated hyperthyroid patients may also result in thyroid storm. In this instance, anesthesia per se or the general stress of the procedure may be responsible for the induction of storm.

The medical factors that place patients at risk for thyroid crisis include infection, trauma, diabetic ketoacidosis, pulmonary embolism, toxemia of pregnancy or labor, premature discontinuance of antithyroid drug therapy, and, rarely, radiation thyroiditis secondary to radioactive iodine therapy of hyperthyroidism. The manner in which these physiologic stresses induce thyroid storm is totally unclear. A variety of measurements, including measurements of serum thyroxine (T_4), serum triiodothyronine (T_3), and serum catecholamines, reveal no differences between patients with thyroid storm and those with uncomplicated hyperthyroidism.

Clinical Signs and Symptoms

Frequently thought to represent an exaggerated or decompensated state of ordinary hyperthyroidism, the signs and symptoms of thyroid storm are in some respects similar to those of uncomplicated thyrotoxicosis. The usual signs of hyperthyroidism include goiter; tachycardia; widened pulse pressure; warm, fine, moist skin; tremor; eye signs (eg, lid lag, exophthalmos, ocular muscle palsies, and chemosis); and atrial fibrillation. The more frequent symptoms include nervousness, increased sweating, hypersensitivity to heat, palpitations, fatigue, weight loss, tachycardia, dyspnea, weakness, increased appetite, and frequent bowel movements.

Thyroid storm is characterized by more florid signs of thyrotoxicosis. The additional signs and symptoms include fever, which many consider to be the sine qua non for the diagnosis. The following may also be seen:

- extreme tachycardia
- restlessness, agitation
- emotional lability
- confusion
- psychosis
- diarrhea and vomiting
- jaundice
- hypotension
- coma

The patient may experience cardiovascular collapse and shock. The heart rate is usually increased out of proportion to the extent of the fever. Although the tachycardia is generally sinus in nature, it may be ectopic in origin, most commonly atrial fibrillation; rarely, heart block may be found, and the patient may be in congestive heart failure because of markedly hypertrophied heart muscle and the severity of the tachycardia. These patients are generally profusely diaphoretic; together with severe diarrhea and vomiting, this may produce marked electrolyte disturbances.

Diagnosis

The diagnosis of thyroid storm must be made promptly and is predicated on a careful clinical history and physical examination. Determination of serum T_4 and T_3 levels, and a measure of thyroxine-binding globulin (T_3 resin uptake) are appropriate initial tests, but the results will not be known before therapy is initiated. If possible, a 2-hour radioactive iodine (^{123}I) uptake is useful.

Laboratory tests are useful only in establishing the diagnosis of hyperthyroidism, since there is no specific laboratory test that indicates the presence of thyroid storm. The diagnosis of thyroid storm is considered more frequently than it is actually encountered. Patients with hyperthyroidism and intercurrent infections are particularly difficult to distinguish from patients with thyroid storm because both conditions are associated with fever, tachycardia, and diaphoresis. The treatment under these circumstances is the same, however.

Treatment

When thyroid storm is suspected, therapy should be initiated promptly. It is directed at decreasing the synthesis and release of thyroid hormones, blocking the increased adrenergic activity, treating congestive heart failure and electrolyte abnormalities, and reducing fever. The following treatment is recommended:

1. Give propylthiouracil, 900 to 1200 mg/day, by mouth or by gastric tube in three or four divided doses. Methimazole, 90 to 120 mg/day, may be used instead of propylthiouracil.
2. Administer iodine as 30 drops potassium iodine daily by mouth in three or four divided doses or 1 or 2 g of sodium iodide per day by intravenous drip.
3. Give propranolol, 160 mg/day, by mouth in four divided doses or 1 or 2 mg slowly intravenously every 4 hours under careful monitoring.
4. Order intravenous glucose solutions.
5. Correct dehydration and electrolyte imbalance.
6. Provide cooling blanket for hyperthermia.
7. Order digitalis, if clinically indicated.
8. Diagnose and treat any underlying precipitating diseases (ie, infection, diabetic ketoacidosis, or pulmonary embolism).
9. Give glucocorticoid (eg, hydrocortisone, 100 to 300 mg/day intravenously or intramuscularly).
10. Provide definitive therapy after control of the crisis, which consists of ablation of the thyroid gland with ^{131}I or surgical removal (subtotal thyroidectomy).

If an intercurrent illness is present, it must also be promptly treated.

Iodine

A critical therapeutic intervention involves iodine. In pharmacologic doses, it inhibits the release of T_3 and T_4 from the thyroid within a few hours of administration. Iodine also inhibits the organification of iodine, a transitory effect that lasts from a few days to 1 week. It is administered orally as Lugol's solution, 30 drops per day in three or four divided doses, or is given as sodium iodide, 0.5 to 1 g in 1 L of normal saline every 12 hours. If possible, antithyroid drugs should be administered prior to the initiation of iodine therapy in order to prevent any further incorporation of iodine into thyroid hormone. In practice, however, this is rarely possible in the treatment of thyroid storm.

Propylthiouracil and Methimazole

The standard agents for the treatment of hyperthyroidism are propylthiouracil and methimazole. They decrease organification and impair the coupling of monoiodotyrosines and diiodotyrosines to T_4 and T_3. In addition, large doses of propylthiouracil (in excess of 800 mg/day) block the peripheral conversion of T_4 to T_3 in the liver. Therefore, propylthiouracil should be administered in amounts of 900 to 1200 mg/day. It may be given by mouth, or the tablets may be crushed and administered by nasogastric tube; parenteral preparations are not available. It requires about 24 hours of propylthiouracil therapy to decrease serum T_3 levels significantly; it is approximately 5 to 7 days before serum T_4 levels decline. If methimazole is used, the doses are one-tenth of those of propylthiouracil. Methimazole does not block the peripheral conversion of T_4 to T_3, however.

β-Adrenergic Blocking Drugs

Many of the signs and symptoms of hyperthyroidism are secondary to increased adrenergic activity. β-Adrenergic blocking agents, notably propranolol, have replaced reserpine and guanethidine in the adjunctive treatment of hyperthyroidism. Thyroid storm is one of the major indications for propranolol, since it produces a very rapid decrease in heart rate (within 2 to 3 hours when given orally, in minutes when given intravenously). Propranolol occasionally results in rapid defervescence of fever in thyroid storm. The drug is administered orally in a dosage of 40 to 160 mg daily in four divided doses. If given parenterally, patients should be titrated with 1 to 2 mg intravenously, which may be repeated every 4 hours, not exceeding 6 mg in 24 hours.

Propranolol and other β-adrenergic blocking agents are usually contraindicated in the following instances:

- patients with chronic lung disease, such as asthma, emphysema, and bronchospasm
- patients with second-degree or greater heart block
- hyperthyroid patients with congestive heart failure
- patients with peripheral vascular disease
- diabetics receiving insulin or oral hypoglycemic agents
- patients receiving monoamine oxidase inhibitors
- pregnant women

The presence of any of these conditions should be considered in a plan of therapy. Heart failure is frequently related to the tachycardia. After congestive heart failure has been adequately treated with digitalis, the hyperthyroid patient may be cautiously titrated with propranolol under appropriate conditions of cardiac monitoring.

Plasmapheresis

Patients with thyroid storm sometimes fail to respond to the usual medical measures. Under these circumstances, plasmapheresis has been shown to be a useful adjunct to therapy.[8] The removal of large amounts of protein-bound thyroid hormone abruptly lowers the circulating T_4 and T_3. This measure is generally not used unless the patient's condition is deteriorating under medical management.

Other Measures

Dehydration and hyponatremia due to the fluid and electrolyte losses secondary to diaphoresis, vomiting, and diarrhea must be corrected. Glucose must be administered to prevent or correct hypoglycemia. A cooling blanket and, occasionally, ice packs may be required for the treatment of fever. It has been traditional to administer "stress" doses of adrenal corticosteroids to patients with thyroid storm. Although a convincing rationale for such therapy has not been established, 300 to 400 mg hydrocortisone or its equivalent is generally given by continuous infusion each day.

Prognosis

The mortality of thyroid storm has been estimated at approximately 20%. The statistics are difficult to establish, however, since the incidence of thyroid storm is so low. It should also be noted that the mortality statistics that have been provided were calculated before the advent of β-adrenergic blocking drugs, such as propranolol, and before the development of plasmapheresis. These advances will probably lessen the mortality to some degree. Successful medical therapy generally produces improvement within 24 hours, and recovery occurs within a few days to 1 week. When the patient has recovered and is euthyroid, definitive therapy should be instituted either by ablation of the thyroid gland with ^{131}I or subtotal resection of the thyroid gland.

MYXEDEMA COMA

The end stage of improperly treated, neglected, or undiagnosed primary hypothyroidism is myxedema coma. This is a major medical emergency that requires prompt and effective treatment.[9–12] The underlying cause of the thyroid gland failure may be idiopathic, or it may be associated with autoimmune (Hashimoto's) thyroiditis, therapy (^{131}I) for hyperthyroidism or thyroid cancer, or thyroidectomy.

Precipitating Factors

There are a number of factors that predispose the hypothyroid patient to myxedema coma, including exposure to cold, infection, trauma, and administration of central nervous system depressants, such as morphine, barbiturates, or general anesthetics. Coma is more common in elderly people with advanced coronary and systemic arteriosclerosis.

Clinical Signs

Patients with myxedema coma have many of the signs noted in uncomplicated hypothyroidism: dry skin, puffy appearance, coarse hair, cool skin, slow return of reflexes, carotenemia, periorbital swelling, facial puffiness, glossomegaly, and nonpitting edema. Myxedema coma is characterized by the following additional signs:

- hypothermia
- hypotension
- marked bradycardia
- hypoventilation with respiratory acidosis and carbon dioxide narcosis
- a variety of fluid and electrolyte abnormalities, such as decreased serum sodium level, increased serum lactate level, and inappropriate secretion of antidiuretic hormone
- hypoglycemia
- ileus

Hypothermia is considered by many to be the sine qua non for the diagnosis.

Diagnosis

The diagnosis of myxedema coma is based on the clinical picture; it requires a high index of suspicion and a careful history and physical examination. Uncomplicated hypothyroidism can be diagnosed by measuring the levels of serum T_4 and T_3, which are markedly decreased, and of serum thyroid-stimulating hormone (TSH), which is markedly elevated. These tests require too much time to aid in the early management of myxedema coma, however. Thus, when this life-threatening medical emergency is seriously considered a possibility, therapy is initiated. Treatment can be altered later, depending on the results of the serum T_4, serum T_3, and serum TSH measurements. Serum levels of cortisol should also be determined, since some of these patients may have associated autoimmune adrenal failure.

Treatment

The patient's general medical condition, especially cardiovascular and pulmonary status, must be evaluated promptly and thyroid hormone replaced quickly by the intravenous administration of 500 μg L-thyroxine as a single loading dose, followed by 50 μg L-thyroxine on a daily basis intravenously. The large loading dose is necessary to saturate the unoccupied thyroid-hormone binding sites on thyroxine-binding globulin. Intravenous therapy is required in this life-threatening situation because thyroid hormone is incompletely absorbed after oral administration. Recently, commercial preparation of parenteral triiodothyronine has become available.

Adrenal corticosteroids are routinely administered to patients in myxedema coma; 100 mg hydrocortisone or its equivalent is administered intravenously by direct push, and a total of 300 to 400 mg hydrocortisone is administered in normal saline over the first 24 hours. Corticosteroids, 100 to 300 mg/day, should be continued until the result of the initial plasma cortisol determination is reported and adrenal status established. It is particularly important to administer corticosteroids if there is any suspicion of either adrenal cortical failure or pituitary insufficiency. Carbon dioxide narcosis must be treated promptly with mechanical ventilation, and any airway obstruction must be promptly relieved. Blood gases are monitored frequently. It should be emphasized that patients with hypothyroidism, particularly those in myxedema coma, metabolize drugs very slowly; therefore, narcotics and sedative drugs must be avoided entirely and the dosage of other drugs appropriately reduced. Hypoglycemia must be relieved by the intravenous administration of glucose. Electrolyte and water balance must be carefully monitored to prevent water intoxication because patients with myxedema coma tend to retain water. Pressor amines may be administered cautiously to treat shock, although the effectiveness of pressor agents may be impaired until thyroid hormone is adequately replaced. Hypothermia is best treated by a covering blanket; the patient should not be actively warmed because of the risk of dysrhythmias and peripheral vascular collapse. Other illnesses, such as intercurrent infections, that may have precipitated the myxedema coma must be diagnosed and treated vigorously and promptly.

Prognosis

The mortality rate for patients with inadequately treated myxedema coma is approximately 80%. Promptly treated myxedema is associated with a mortality rate of approximately 30%, one of the highest mortality rates of any medical emergency. Management must be prompt and effective, and all the physician's skills are required. Following recovery, the patient requires lifelong treatment with thyroid hormone.

REFERENCES

1. Rosenberg IN. Thyroid storm. *N Engl J Med*. 1970;283:1052–1053.
2. Mackin JF, Canary JJ, Pittman CS. Thyroid storm and its management. *N Engl J Med*. 1974; 291:1396–1398.
3. Nicoloff JT. Thyroid storm and myxedema coma. *Med Clin North Am*. 1985;69:1005–1017.
4. Bagdade JD. Endocrine emergencies. *Med Clin North Am*. 1986; 70:1111–1128.
5. Levey GS. The heart and hyperthyroidism. *Med Clin North Am*. 1975; 59:1193–1202.

6. Landsberg L. Catecholamines and hyperthyroidism. *Clin Endocrinol Metab.* 1977;3:697–718.
7. Levey GS, Klein I. Catecholamine-thyroid hormone interactions and the cardiovascular manifestations of hyperthyroidism. *Am J Med.* 1990;88:642–647.
8. Ashkar F, Katims RB, Smoak WM III, Gilson AJ. Thyroid storm treatment with blood exchange and plasmapheresis. *JAMA.* 1970;214:1275–1279.
9. Green WL. Guidelines for the treatment of myxedema. *Med Clin North Am.* 1968;52:431–450.
10. Mazzaferri EL. Adult hypothyroidism 1. Manifestations and clinical presentation. *Postgrad Med.* 1986;79:64–72.
11. Mazzaferri EL. Adult hypothyroidism 2. Manifestations and clinical presentation. *Postgrad Med.* 1986;79:75–86.
12. Myers L, Hays J. Myxedema coma. *Crit Care Clin.* 1991;43–46.

16. Adrenal Insufficiency

GEORGE L. HIGGINS III, MD, FACEP

Adrenal insufficiency, in both chronic and acute forms, often manifests itself in ways that bring the patient to the attention of the emergency care provider. Such manifestations range from subtle neuropsychiatric complaints to life-threatening complications. In the busy and hectic atmosphere that exists in many of today's emergency departments, it is difficult at times to follow the superb example of clinical diagnosis set by Thomas Addison when he first described this disorder more than a century ago.[1] The responsibility, then, of the emergency physician is to search for those clues in the history, physical examination, and laboratory data that allow recognition and expeditious management of this gratifyingly treatable disease.

ETIOLOGY

Autoimmune States

Autoimmune destruction of the adrenal glands is emerging as one of the more common causes of gland failure.[2] This recognition has come as developing technology has allowed identification of specific antibodies to specific adrenal gland antigens.[3] Indeed, the detection of adrenal autoantibodies may predate the clinical manifestations of adrenal insufficiency by months or even years.[4] The glandular morphology reveals mononuclear inflammation, fibrosis, and atrophy. Numerous other disease entities that are presumed to have an autoimmune pathogenesis have been associated with this type of hypoadrenalism, such as chronic lymphocytic (Hashimoto's) thyroiditis,[5-7] silent thyrotoxic thyroiditis,[8] Graves' disease,[9] diabetes mellitus,[10-12] hypogonadism,[13-15] pernicious anemia,[16,17] vitiligo,[18] and hypoparathyroidism.[19,20] It is not uncommon for several of these disorders to develop sequentially in the same patient. Therefore, the presence of one of them should raise the possibility of the occult existence of another. Many of the previously so-called idiopathic forms of hypoadrenalism probably have an autoimmune basis. Computed tomography (CT) in patients with autoimmune adrenal insufficiency reveals small and atrophied glands bilaterally.[21-23]

Exogenous Steroid Administration

The frequent use of exogenous steroids in the treatment of various disorders and diseases has brought secondary adrenal insufficiency into prominence. In contrast to the primary type, secondary hypoadrenalism is not associated with hyperpigmentation, aldosterone deficiency,[24] or overproduction of cortisol precursors. Furthermore, the adrenal gland retains the capacity to respond to prolonged treatment with exogenous adrenocorticotropic hormone (ACTH). Most important, secondary hypoadrenalism is potentially a completely reversible disorder, although full recovery of adrenal responsiveness may take nine months or more. Prolonged administration of exogenous steroids is usually required for significant pituitary-adrenal suppression,[25,26] but short-term, high-dose steroid therapy can occasionally suppress adrenal function for a week or more.[27] Dexamethasone appears to have the most potent suppressive effect on ACTH secretion in humans.[28] Even very cautious steroid withdrawal not only can result in adrenal hypofunction but also may exacerbate the underlying disorder being treated.[29] In addition, maintenance doses of steroid occasionally become inadequate when stress is superimposed. It is important, then, to establish the possibility of exogenous steroid ingestion in the medical history.

It should be remembered, however, that the source of exogenous steroid may not always be obvious. Adrenocortical suppression has been found in workers who produce synthetic glucocorticoids, and it is recommended that these workers be screened periodically for adrenal responsiveness.[30] Topical corticosteroids used in the treatment of dermatologic disorders, such as psoriasis, have led to adrenal insufficiency,[31-33] as have inhaled steroids.[34-37a] Switching from oral steroid to inhaled steroid therapy in the asthmatic patient may result in adrenal failure.[38] Maternal steroid therapy has caused adrenal gland suppression in the newborn.[39,40] Both extradural and intrathecal steroid administration have been implicated in secondary adrenal insufficiency.[41,42] Finally, to complicate matters further, there seems to be a true psychologic addiction to steroids. Withdrawing some patients from the drug leads to subjective signs and symptoms of adrenal insufficiency, although biochemically the hypothalamic-pituitary-adrenal axis remains intact and responsive.[43]

Sepsis

Fulminant bacterial infections can lead to or be complicated by absolute or relative hypoadrenalism. Like many other physiologically stressful situations, systemic bacterial infections are usually associated with elevated plasma cortisol levels.[44-47] Not only is adrenal hormonal secretion accelerated with septic stress, but supplemental ACTH administration during systemic infections can also lead to additional hormonal production.

Careful prospective analysis of adrenal response to severe infections has revealed several patterns.[46-48] The highest baseline cortisol levels are usually seen in the most critically ill patients, many of whom succumb to their illness. A larger group of patients demonstrate higher than normal baseline levels and respond to synthetic ACTH administration with increased adrenocortical secretion. However, a significant minority of patients with severe infection have lower than expected baseline cortisol levels and fail to exhibit an appropriate increase in plasma cortisol levels following exogenous ACTH stimulation. Necropsy examination of the adrenal glands in such patients may reveal only cellular hyperplasia without hemorrhage or necrosis.

In the classic syndrome of fulminant meningococcemia, adrenal crisis has been well recognized. Autopsy frequently reveals evidence of bilateral adrenal hemorrhage (the Waterhouse-Friderichsen syndrome).[49] The etiology of this hemorrhage has not yet been fully defined, but it has been ascribed to endotoxin-producing thromboplastic activity as well as direct endothelial damage by the meningococci with subsequent thrombosis. Another postulated cause is that severe stress leads to rapid depletion of lipid hormone from the adrenal cells, causing tubular degeneration and, thus, predisposing the gland to hemorrhage.[50-52] In such cases, early steroid replacement can be life saving.[53]

Hemorrhage

Adrenal gland hemorrhage can rapidly lead to adrenal crisis. Adrenal apoplexy, or idiopathic hemorrhage infarction, is an uncommon but life-threatening development.[54-56] Hemorrhage is usually associated with physiologic stress caused by sepsis, burns, surgery, or trauma.[57] Since it has been demonstrated that marked adrenal stimulation can lead to tubular degeneration and necrosis, as well as increased vascularity, it has been hypothesized that such stress predisposes the adrenal gland to hemorrhagic events.[58] Flank or abdominal pain, a dropping hematocrit, and developing shock may be the initial manifestations of this syndrome. The presumptive diagnosis may erroneously be renal colic or a ruptured abdominal aortic aneurysm. Hemorrhage may be confined to the gland itself or the periadrenal tissues, but it can be massive. Signs and symptoms of adrenal insufficiency may be present. Radiographic procedures, including abdominal CT scanning,[59,60] ultrasound, and angiography, are helpful in localizing the site of hemorrhage and ruling out an aneurysm. Once the diagnosis is established, immediate surgical intervention is indicated.

Anticoagulant-induced adrenal hemorrhage is a well-documented event. A review of over 4000 autopsies revealed 30 cases of adrenal hemorrhage, 10 of which occurred in patients receiving anticoagulants in the treatment of thromboembolism or acute myocardial infarction.[61] In contrast to the fulminant course of adrenal hemorrhage associated with the Waterhouse-Friderichsen syndrome, which usually occurs in younger patients, anticoagulant-associated adrenal hemorrhage more often involves older patients (50 to 70 years of age). The primary medical disorders in these older patients tend to mask the signs and symptoms of hypoadrenalism, thus hindering diagnosis. Both heparin and coumarin compounds may be responsible for adrenal hemorrhage. Even prophylactic subcutaneous heparin therapy has been implicated.[61a] In addition, heparin-induced thrombocytopenia has been associated with acute adrenal insufficiency.[61b,61c] Coagulation parameters are not always excessively prolonged, and there may be no evidence of generalized bleeding in these patients. Development of flank or abdominal pain, hypotension refractory to fluid management, anorexia, vomiting, mental status changes, and fever in patients on anticoagulation therapy should suggest adrenal hemorrhage.[62] Aggressive medical intervention, including corticosteroid replacement, can be life saving.[63-65]

Anticoagulant-associated adrenal hemorrhage is often bilateral, but it may be unilateral. As it does in spontaneous adrenal hemorrhage, stress appears to play a role in this form. In the experimental animal, the administration of ACTH with anticoagulants increases the incidence of hemorrhagic complications significantly,[66] while hypophysectomized animals subjected to stress do not develop hemorrhages.

Neoplastic Disorders

Spontaneous and massive hemorrhage from intrinsic adrenal tumors, such as pheochromocytomas, can lead to adrenal insufficiency.[54] Less well understood is the role played in this syndrome by disease that has metastasized to the adrenal gland. Since the time of Addison, symptoms of terminal metastatic carcinomatosis have occasionally been attributed to adrenal gland replacement with tumor. Empiric treatment of weakness, fatigue, fever, anorexia, and orthostatic reactions with exogenous steroids in the terminally ill cancer patient has led to varying degrees of improvement. Response to this treatment obviously does not imply hypoadrenalism. Indeed, many cancer patients with symptoms resembling those of adrenal insufficiency are found to have elevated plasma cortisol levels and normal pituitary and adrenal glands at the time of autopsy.[67,68] Although some tumors demonstrate corticotropic activity with resultant hypercortisolemia, the stress of terminal carcinomatosis itself appears to be sufficient stimulation for elevated adrenal output.[67,69] Clinical response to administered steroids, then, may be independent of adrenal function, resulting instead from their nonspecific euphoretic effect or anti-inflammatory action. Even when disease that has metastasized to the adrenal glands (usually from lung or breast) leaves less than 20% of apparently normal tissue, adequate adrenal function and reserve remains.[70] Rarely, infiltrative hematologic malignant neoplasms such as lymphoma can lead to clinical adrenal insufficiency.[71] It appears that, although adrenal insufficiency from metastatic disease does indeed occur and may even be the initial manifestation of malignancy,[72] it is a relatively uncommon event. CT can aid in detecting metastatic disease in the adrenal glands,[73-75] with adrenal gland enlargement often being demonstrated.[23]

Surgical Procedures

Adrenal hemorrhage and necrosis may occur during certain abdominal operations that, because of anatomic proximity, result in direct trauma to the gland itself or embarrassment of its blood supply.[76] Operations of the stomach, lower esophagus, spleen, and kidneys appear to be especially prone to produce this complication.[77] In addition to disruption of the arterial supply of the gland, thrombosis or rupture of capsular and intra-adrenal veins can result in hemorrhage and necrosis. Destruction of one adrenal gland during or soon after the severe stress of a major operation may result in acute adrenal insufficiency.

Surgical procedures in areas of the body anatomically remote from the adrenal glands in patients without predisposing factors can also be complicated by postoperative adrenal hypofunction.[78-81] Hyperpigmentation is usually absent. Hypoglycemia, electrolyte abnormalities, and vomiting may be controlled by aggressive routine postoperative care; other manifestations of adrenal insufficiency, such as anorexia, abdominal pain, fever, and confusion, may be attributed to the stress of the operation. Recognition of adrenal insufficiency in these patients depends on a high index of suspicion when the postoperative course is complicated by bizarre, confusing, and apparently inappropriate symptoms. When the diagnosis is entertained, the pretreatment serum cortisol level should be determined and a therapeutic trial of steroid replacement promptly initiated to prevent death.

Abdominal CT scans obtained on victims of blunt abdominal trauma have, on occasion, demonstrated acute adrenal gland hemotomas. Rarely, such hematomas are bilateral, leading to acute adrenal insufficiency.[81a]

Granulomatous Disease

In Addison's time, granulomatous destruction of the gland by tuberculosis was the predominant cause of adrenal insufficiency. Over 70% of Addison's disease could be ascribed to tuberculosis in the early part of this century. The introduction of antitubercular chemotherapy and skin test screening programs has permitted earlier recognition and effective treatment of tuberculosis, dramatically reducing the incidence of adrenal insufficiency caused by this disease. A Danish study that reviewed 108 cases of Addison's disease identified tuberculosis as the primary cause in only 17% of the patients in the series.[82]

In spite of its decreased incidence, tuberculosis adrenal gland destruction in all age groups continues to be reported in the United States.[83-85] The recently recognized increasing prevalence of invasive tuberculosis in AIDS patients is of concern in this regard. Often, active tuberculosis is also apparent in other organs, suggesting hematogenous spread. As might be expected, the symptoms and signs of adrenal insufficiency mimic those of active tuberculosis, making diagnosis difficult.[86] The combination of a suggestive chest roentgenogram, a positive tuberculin skin test result, adrenal gland calcifications (occurring in 5% to 10% of cases), and no serologic evidence of autoimmune adrenal gland destruction should cause the physician to suspect tuberculous involvement of the adrenal glands.[87] CT often reveals gland calcification and enlargement in such cases.[21,23,88,89]

Rifampin is a potent inducer of hepatic enzymes and, therefore, increases the metabolism of glucocorticoids. Its use in the treatment of patients with active tuberculosis who also have marginal adrenal reserve can lead to acute adrenal insufficiency.[90]

There are other, less common causes of granulomatous adrenal gland destruction. Histoplasmosis is a recognized cause of adrenal insufficiency in the Ohio and Tennessee river valleys.[91,92] Disseminated North American blastomycosis frequently involves the adrenal gland and, rarely, can lead to adrenal crisis, suggesting that patients so infected should be screened for adrenal dysfunction.[93,94] Cryptococcosis and coccidioidomycosis have also been implicated in the etiology of adrenal insufficiency. Rarely, paracoccidioidomycosis (South American blastomycosis) can result in hypoadrenalism.[95]

Congenital Idiopathic Adrenal Hypoplasia

A relatively uncommon condition that affects newborns,[96] congenital idiopathic adrenal hypoplasia may not become manifest for several months[97] or even years.[98] There are both sporadic and familial cases,[99] and recessive and sex-linked inheritance occurs.[100–102] The association of anencephaly and adrenal insufficiency was noted as early as 1723 by Morgagni.

Secondary forms of adrenal hypoplasia in the very young have been ascribed to maternal Cushing's syndrome,[103] congenital adrenal cysts,[104] adrenal hemorrhage,[105,106] and steroid therapy during pregnancy.[39,40] The idiopathic type, however, is often associated with maternal pre-eclampsia, very low maternal estriol excretion (the fetal adrenals produce the major portion of maternal urinary estriol precursors),[96,107] and post-term pregnancy. The fetus is alive and radiologically normal. The living newborn may exhibit a salt-losing syndrome with dehydration, hyponatremia, hyperkalemia, acidosis, hypoglycemia, poor eating, failure to thrive, fever, vomiting, diarrhea, vascular collapse, and sudden infant death syndrome.[108] Autopsy findings include a normal pituitary and brain, no evidence of adrenal destruction, and diminished adrenal mass.[109] The mortality rate is high in these infants.

Other Causes

Adrenal insufficiency has been associated with systemic lupus erythematosus,[110] oral contraceptives,[111] methadone,[112] bilateral adrenal venography,[113] hypopituitarism,[87,114] ACTH-releasing factor deficiency,[115] and isolated ACTH deficiency.[116,117] AIDS patients, at risk for developing various infections and neoplasms and exposed to numerous drugs, are also at risk for developing subsequent adrenal insufficiency.

Adrenomyeloneuropathy and adrenoleukodystrophy are rare, recessive sex-linked disorders that can lead to adrenal insufficiency, as well as to central and peripheral neurologic dysfunction (eg, mental deterioration, sphincter disorders, objective sensory deficits, and spastic paraparesis). The neurologic deficits usually precede the endocrine manifestations. Long-chain cholesterol esters accumulate as cytoplasmic inclusions in brain, adrenal, and testes.[118–122]

SYMPTOMATOLOGY

Cutaneous

The diffuse hyperpigmentation of primary adrenal insufficiency, first described by Addison, is common (92% in these patients[82]) and results from melanocyte stimulation by elevated levels of β-lipoprotein. ACTH is a weak melanocyte stimulant,[122] but some patients have a level high enough to produce hyperpigmentation. Diffuse hypermelanosis is by no means unique to primary hypoadrenalism, however; it can be found in association with endocrine and nonendocrine tumors, folate deficiency, cirrhosis, hemochromatosis, pernicious anemia, starvation, and many other disorders.[123] The hyperpigmentation of adrenal insufficiency has a predilection for extensor surfaces, pressure areas, palmar creases, scars from injuries that occurred after the onset of the adrenal disorder, mucous membranes, tongue, gingival margins, breast areola, scrotum, perineum, and the perivaginal and perianal areas.[87] Longitudinal banded pigmentation of fingernails has also been described.[124] An increased ability to tan or a longer lasting tan should raise the possibility of hypoadrenalism.[125] It must be remembered, however, that Addison's disease may exist without hyperpigmentation.[126–128]

An interesting case of Addison's disease associated with excessively salty sweat and ichthyosis has been reported.[129] Steroid replacement brought a dramatic decrease in the sodium and chloride, as well as an increase in the potassium content of the patient's sweat.

Vitiligo, yet another manifestation of autoimmune polyendocrine deficiency, has been associated with autoimmune primary adrenal insufficiency.[18] Cutaneous candidiasis appears to be more common in adrenal insufficient patients,[130] and abnormal calcification of the auricular and costochondral cartilages has been documented.[131,131a]

Cardiovascular

Hypotension occurs in 88% of patients; postural dizziness, in 12%.[82] These findings reflect decreased intravascular volume, as well as diminished inotropy and cardiac output. In addition, glucocorticoid deficiency may enhance the endothelial production of prostacyclin, a potent vasodilator.[132] Syncope may bring the patient to the physician's attention. Patients with severe adrenal insufficiency may develop shock and terminal vascular collapse.[133] The radiographic appearance of a small heart on the chest roentgenogram should raise the possibility of hypoadrenalism.[134] Heart size in untreated, uncomplicated cases of Addison's disease is consistently reduced below normal, probably reflecting the cachectic and hypovolemic states of some of these patients. Steroid administration increases cardiac dimensions. Excessive therapy may lead to cardiomegaly.

Gastrointestinal

Gastrointestinal symptoms occur in 56% of patients.[82] Anorexia, weight loss, nausea, and vomiting are nearly universal.[135] Chronic diarrhea is not uncommon. Abdominal pain, at times severe, can result in "pseudoperitonitis" with signs of intra-abdominal catastrophe and may lead to unfruitful exploratory laparotomies.[136] Nearly all acute abdominal entities, including cholecystitis, pancreatitis, leaking abdominal aneurysm, ischemic or infarcted bowel, retroperitoneal hemorrhage, nephrolithiasis, perforated viscus, and cecal volvulus have been confused with acute adrenal crisis.[80] The exact mechanism of this pain syndrome has not been defined, but improvement with exogenous steroid therapy can be dramatic.

There is a decreased incidence of peptic ulcer disease in patients with adrenal insufficiency, possibly because of diminished gastric acid production.[137]

Neurologic

In addition to the full spectrum of mental status changes that manifest themselves during inadequate adrenal function (eg, confusion, acute psychosis,[138] delirium, and coma), more unusual neurologic disorders have been observed. Adrenal insufficiency has been associated with the polyradiculoneuropathy of Guillain-Barré syndrome, with both disorders responding to steroid administration.[139] Morphologic changes in the adrenal glands, including necrotizing inflammation and inclusion bodies, have been found at autopsy.[140,141]

The abrupt onset of "Addisonian encephalopathy" can be dramatic and confusing[142,143] and must be differentiated from other causes of metabolic encephalopathies. As noted previously, adrenoleukodystrophy and adrenomyeloneuropathy are rare disorders that can lead to adrenal hypofunction and rapidly progressive neurologic deterioration.

Miscellaneous

Adrenal deficiency may be associated with tachydysrhythmia[144]; delayed development of pubic hair[145]; chronic low back pain[146]; sciatica-like back pain[147,148]; flexion contractures,[149] diffuse myalgias and arthralgias[150]; self-mutilation[151]; more acute senses of taste, smell, and hearing[152–154]; and salt craving (in 15% to 20% of patients). One interesting case report describes a woman with undiagnosed adrenal insufficiency who noted that licorice ingestion abolished her lassitude, presumably owing to its mineralocorticoid effect.[155] The recent onset of asthma in a patient with weight loss or other constitutional signs should suggest hypoadrenalism.[156,157]

Laboratory Findings

Hyponatremia is common in adrenal insufficiency, occurring in 88% of patients in one study.[82] The degree of sodium depletion may at times be life threatening. The etiology of this complication appears to be failure of aldosterone-directed renal sodium conservation, as well as poor handling of water loads.[158] Angiotensin-converting enzyme concentrations are increased in untreated adrenal insufficiency but return to normal after corticosteroid replacement therapy.[159]

Hyperkalemia, which occurs in 64% of patients, may become severe enough to produce cardiac dysrhythmias and periodic paralysis.[160,161] Patients are also prone to potassium intoxication when given exogenous potassium. Both mineralocorticoid and glucocorticoid deficiencies play a role in the development of hyperkalemia (see Chapter 18, Hypokalemia and Hyperkalemia).

Hypercalcemia, occurring in 6% of patients, is due to volume depletion with decreased glomerular filtration and increased tubular calcium reabsorption. It can be treated successfully with corticosteroid administration.[162] Hypercalcemic crisis has been reported as the initial manifestation of Addison's disease[163,164] (see Chapter 20, Hypercalcemia).

Hypoglycemia, probably resulting from defective gluconeogenesis and lipolysis, is not uncommon[135] and is unmasked by fasting or excessive exercise. Patients with symptomatic hypoglycemia that has no obvious cause should be screened for adrenal insufficiency. It should be remembered that patients receiving insulin may develop insulin sensitivity as hypoadrenalism develops.

Decreased glomerular filtration rates can lead to elevated serum creatinine and blood urea nitrogen (BUN) determinations.

Eosinophilia has been associated with glucocorticoid deficiency, although it is not invariably present. The eosinopenic effect of steroid administration can be explained by intravenous shift of eosinophils, as well as migration into tissues and diminished bone marrow production of these cells.[165]

Adrenal insufficiency can only be unequivocally diagnosed by biochemically demonstrating an absolute or relative adrenal hormone deficiency with abolished adrenal reserve. The combination of a low plasma cortisol level (less than 5 to 10 µg/dL during stress) and an elevated plasma ACTH level (greater than 200 µg/dL) confirms the diagnosis of primary adrenal deficiency. Both plasma cortisol and

ACTH levels are depressed in exogenous steroid adrenal gland suppression, ACTH deficiency, and ACTH-releasing factor deficiency. However, any of the previously described signs and symptoms may be missing in the patient with hypoadrenalism, and isolated serum and urinary steroid determinations may be in the normal range. It is often necessary, therefore, to establish the status of adrenal gland responsiveness by administering synthetic ACTH and monitoring serial plasma cortisol levels. Normally, 1 hour following the administration of 250 μg cosyntropin, plasma cortisol levels will increase by 15 μg/dL or to an absolute value of 20 to 25 μg/dL. This stimulation test has proved to be a safe, sensitive, and simple screening procedure.[166] It is also very helpful in determining when patients may be safely withdrawn from glucocorticoid therapy following a tapering schedule.[167] To examine the entire hypothalamic-pituitary-adrenal axis, as would be required in secondary adrenal failure, more sophisticated tests, such as metyrapone provocation, are required.[168]

Therapy

The emergency care provider routinely sees physiologically stressed patients. Conditions that can lead to acute adrenal insufficiency, such as systemic sepsis, acute myocardial infarction, trauma, burns, gastroenteritis, and AIDS, are relatively common in most emergency departments. Therefore, it is most important that physicians involved with emergency care consider adrenal crisis in patients who demonstrate the symptoms and signs that have been outlined. Patients being evaluated in the emergency department must be questioned about steroid usage, since augmentation of the daily dose of steroid may be indicated in patients with certain disorders (eg, pneumonia) who are to be managed as outpatients. Conditions that preclude the oral retention of medications (eg, significant vomiting) might require a more liberal attitude toward hospitalization to ensure steroid administration. Obviously, a high index of suspicion is essential.

When the diagnosis of acute adrenal insufficiency is entertained, immediate treatment is mandatory. Blood should be drawn for cortisol, ACTH, electrolyte, glucose, calcium, white blood cell count, hematocrit, BUN, and creatinine determinations. After a secure intravenous line has been established, hydrocortisone phosphate or hemisuccinate (100 mg intravenously over 3 to 5 minutes) is administered. This dose is also sufficient coverage for the patient with known adrenal insufficiency who is to undergo emergent surgery. The onset of action of this steroid is immediate, although it has a relatively short half-life (1½ hours). Over the first 24 hours, the total dosage of exogenous steroid should equal the amount that would be produced by normal adrenal glands subjected to severe stress (eg, up to five times basal levels). Most patients require 100 to 400 mg during the first day, depending on body size. This can be given in the form of an intravenous bolus (eg, 1.5 mg/kg every 6 hours) or, more ideally, as a continuous drip (eg, 100 mg in 1000 mL of 5% dextrose in normal saline to be infused at a rate of 100 to 200 mL/hour). Hydrocortisone in these doses has adequate mineralocorticoid activity; therefore, specific replacement is not usually indicated during the acute management phase. If hypotension or electrolyte abnormalities persist, however, desoxycorticosterone acetate (2 to 3 mg in oil intramuscularly) or fluorohydrocortisone (0.1 to 0.2 mg orally) may be required. Dexamethasone and prednisone lack a mineralocorticoid effect and probably should not be used in the management of adrenal crisis.

Most patients in adrenal crisis exhibit signs of significant dehydration, and an extracellular fluid volume deficit of 20% is not uncommon. Fluid therapy should be aggressive, especially in the presence of hypotension. One liter of 5% dextrose in normal saline should be given over the first 30 minutes to 1 hour, and most patients require 3 to 4 L the first day. Obviously, shock must be even more aggressively treated. Patients with limited cardiac reserve require a more cautious approach. Placement of a central venous pressure or Swan-Ganz catheter can provide valuable monitoring information. If shock is severe, colloid solutions may be required; rarely, vasopressor agents are needed. Persistent shock suggests sepsis or occult blood loss.

Hyponatremia is responsive to the measures that have been discussed. Hypertonic saline should be avoided, if at all possible. Hyperkalemia usually responds to the administration of glucose, steroid, and fluid. Should hyperkalemia be life threatening, the traditional measures for rapidly lowering the serum potassium level should be used. It must be remembered, however, that such patients are sensitive to insulin and may be hypercalcemic. Hypercalcemia usually resolves with the measures described, and an effective calciuresis is established as the glomerular filtration rate improves.

A thorough search for the precipitating cause, especially infection, is mandatory. Appropriate cultures should be obtained and antibiotic therapy administered early when appropriate. Coexisting endocrinopathies, such as hypothyroidism, should also be considered and ruled out when appropriate. Sedatives should be avoided and hypoglycemia corrected. Nonessential procedures should be postponed. If the patient fails to respond to this approach, other complications, such as occult sepsis, gastrointestinal bleeding, and panhypopituitarism, should be considered.

Once the life-threatening manifestations of the acute adrenal insufficiency have been controlled, the steroid dose is gradually tapered and a maintenance oral dose established, typically hydrocortisone (20 mg in the morning and 10 mg in the late afternoon) or the equivalent dose of prednisone (7.5 mg and 5 mg). At this time, the addition of a mineralocorticoid (eg, fluorohydrocortisone, 0.1 to 0.2 mg daily) is often indicated.

REFERENCES

1. Addison T. *On the Constitutional and Local Effects of Disease of the Suprarenal Capsules.* London: Highly; 1855.
2. Nerup J. Addison's disease: Serological studies. *Acta Endocrinol.* 1974;76:142.
3. Nerup J, et al. Antiadrenal cellular hypersensitivy in Addison's disease. *Clin Exp Immunol.* 1969;5:341.
4. Betterle C, et al. Complement-fixing adrenal autoantibodies as a marker for predicting onset of idiopathic Addison's disease. *Lancet.* 1983;1:1238.
5. Faber J, et al. Subclinical hypothyroidism in Addison's disease. *Acta Endocrinol.* 1979;91:674.
6. McHardy-Young S, et al. Serum TSH and thyroid antibody studies in Addison's disease. *Clin Endocrinol.* 1972;1:45.
7. Anderson P, et al. Familial Schmidt's syndrome. *JAMA.* 1980;244:2068.
8. Parker M, et al. Silent thyrotoxic thyroiditis in association with chronic adrenocortical insufficiency. *Arch Intern Med.* 1980;140:1108.
9. Gastineau C, et al. Thyroid disorders in Addison's disease. *Mayo Clin Proc.* 1964;39:939.
10. Riley W, et al. Adrenal autoantibodies and Addison's disease in insulin-dependent diabetes mellitus. *J Pediatr.* 1980;97:191.
11. Nelson R, et al. Schmidt's syndrome in a child with diabetes mellitus. *Diabetes Care.* 1978;1:37.
12. Gharib H, et al. Coexisting Addison's disease and diabetes mellitus: report of 24 cases with review of the literature. *Mayo Clin Proc.* 1969;44:217.
13. Elder M, et al. Gonadal autoantibodies in patients with hypogonadism and/or Addison's disease. *J Clin Endocrinol Metab.* 1981;52:1137.
14. Edmonds M, et al. Autoimmune thyroiditis, adrenalitis, and oophoritis. *Am J Med.* 1973;54:782.
15. Appel G, et al. The syndrome of multiple endocrine insufficiency. *Am J Med.* 1976;61:129.
16. Irvine W, et al. Adrenocortical insufficiency. *Clin Endocrinol Metab.* 1972;1:549.
17. Strickland R. Pernicious anemia and polyendocrine deficiency. *Ann Intern Med.* 1969;70:1001.
18. Betterle C, et al. Vitiligo and autoimmune polyendocrine deficiencies with autoantibodies to melanin-producing cells. *Arch Dermatol.* 1979;115:364.
19. Blizzard R, et al. The incidence of adrenal and other antibodies in the sera of patients with idiopathic adrenal insufficiency. *Clin Exp Immunol.* 1967;2:19.
20. Fisher M, et al. Candidiasis, vitiligo, Addison's disease and hypoparathyroidism. *Arch Dermatol.* 1970;102:110.
21. Doppman J, et al. CT findings in Addison's disease. *J Comput Assist Tomogr.* 1982;6:757.
22. Rzymski K, et al. CT of the adrenal glands in Addison's disease. *ROFO.* 1984;140:48.
23. Vita J, et al. Clinical clues to the cause of Addison's disease. *Am J Med.* 1985;78:461.
24. Liddle G, et al. Dual mechanism regulating adrenocortical function in man. *Am J Med.* 1956;21:380.
25. Graber A, et al. Natural history of pituitary adrenal recovery following long-term suppression with corticosteroids. *J Clin Endocrinol.* 1967;25:11.
26. Meakin J, et al. Pituitary-adrenal function following long-term steroid therapy. *Am J Med.* 1960;29:459.
27. Spiegel R, et al. Adrenal suppression after short-term corticosteroid therapy. *Lancet.* 1979;1:630.
28. Meikle A, et al. Potency and duration of action of glucocorticoids: effects of hydrocortisone, prednisone, and dexamethasone on human pituitary-adrenal function. *Am J Med.* 1977;63:200.
29. Naik R, et al. Serious renal transplant rejection and adrenal hypofunction after gradual withdrawal of prednisolone two years after transplantation. *Br Med J.* 1980;2:1337.
30. Newton RW, et al. Adrenocortical suppression in workers manufacturing synthetic glucocorticoids. *Br Med J.* 1978;1:73.
31. Tan R. Pustular psoriasis with adrenal suppression following topical corticosteroids. *Proc R Soc Med.* 1974;67:719.
32. Carr R, et al. Adrenocortical suppression with topical flumethasone. *Arch Dermatol.* 1967;96:269.
33. Miyachi Y. Adrenal axis suppression caused by a small dose of a potent topical corticosteroid. *Arch Dermatol.* 1982;118:451.
34. Harris D, et al. The effect of intranasal beclomethasone dipropionate on adrenal function. *Clin Allergy.* 1974;4:291.
35. Michels M, et al. Adrenal suppression and intranasally applied steroids. *Ann Allergy.* 1967;25:569.
36. Williams H. Beclomethasone dipropionate. *Ann Intern Med.* 1981;95:464.
37. Smith M, et al. Effects of long-term inhaled high-dose beclomethasone dipropionate on adrenal function. *Thorax.* 1983;38:676.
37a. Wong J, et al. Acute adrenal insufficiency associated with high dose inhaled steroids. *BMJ.* 1992;304:1415.
38. Cayton R, et al. Adrenal failure in bronchial asthma. *Br Med J.* 1973;2:547.
39. Bongiovanni A, et al. Steroids during pregnancy and possible fetal consequences. *Fertil Steril.* 1960;11:181.
40. Grajwer L, et al. Neonatal subclinical adrenal insufficiency: result of maternal steroid therapy. *JAMA.* 1977;238:1279.
41. Chernow B, et al. Secondary adrenal insufficiency after intrathecal steroid administration. *J Neurosurg.* 1982;56:567.
42. Jacobs S. Adrenal suppression following extradural steroids. *Anaesthesia.* 1983;38:953.
43. Dixon R, et al. On the various forms of corticosteroid withdrawal syndrome. *Am J Med.* 1980;68:224.
44. Cornil A, et al. Cortisol secretion during acute bacterial infections in man. *Acta Endocrinol.* 1968;58:1.
45. Melby J, et al. Comparative studies on adrenal cortical function and cortisol metabolism in healthy adults and in patients with shock due to infections. *J Clin Invest.* 1958;37:1971.
46. Migeon C, et al. Study of adrenal function in children with meningitis. *Pediatrics.* 1967;40:163.
47. Sibbald W, et al. Variations in adrenocortical responsiveness during severe bacterial infections. *Am Surg.* 1977;186:29.
48. Sandberg A, et al. Metabolism of adrenal steroids in dying patients. *J Clin Endocrinol.* 1956;16:1001.
49. D'Agati V, et al. The Waterhouse-Friderichsen syndrome. *N Engl J Med.* 1945;232:1.
50. Rick A. A peculiar type of adrenal cortical damage associated with acute infections and its possible relation to circulatory collapse. *Bull Johns Hopkins Hosp.* 1944;74:1.
51. Thomison J, et al. Adrenal lesions in acute meningococcemia. *Arch Pathol.* 1957;63:527.
52. Levin J, et al. Endotoxemia and adrenal hemorrhage. *J Exp Med.* 1965;121:247.

53. Bosworth D. Reversible adrenocortical insufficiency in fulminant meningococcemia. *Arch Intern Med*. 1979;139:823.
54. Lawson D, et al. Massive retroperitoneal adrenal hemorrhage. *Surg Gynecol Obstet*. 1969;128:989.
55. Greendyke R. Adrenal hemorrhage. *Am J Clin Pathol*. 1965;43:210.
56. Batteri A, et al. Adrenal hemorrhage and necrosis in the adult. *Acta Med Scand*. 1964;175:409.
57. Foley F, et al. Adrenal hemorrhage and necrosis in seriously burned patients. *J Trauma*. 1967;7:863.
58. Wilbur O, et al. A study of the role of adrenocorticotrophic hormone (ACTH) in the pathogenesis of tubular degeneration of the adrenals. *Bull Johns Hopkins Hosp*. 1953;93:321.
59. Albert S, et al. Bilateral adrenal hemorrhage in the adult. *JAMA*. 1982;247:1737.
60. Wolverson M, et al. CT of bilateral adrenal gland hemorrhage with acute adrenal gland insufficiency in the adult. *AJR*. 1984;142:311.
61. Amador E. Adrenal hemorrhage during anticoagulant therapy. *Ann Intern Med*. 1965;63:559.
61a. Hardwicke M, et al. Prophylactic subcutaneous heparin therapy as a cause of bilateral adrenal hemorrhage. *Arch Intern Med*. 1992;152:845.
61b. Ernest D, et al. Heparin-induced thrombocytopenia complicated by bilateral adrenal hemorrhage. *Intensive Care Med*. 1991;17:238.
61c. Bleasel J, et al. Acute adrenal insufficiency secondary to heparin-induced thrombocytopenia-thrombosis syndrome. *Med J Aust*. 1992;156:192.
62. Portnay G, et al. Anticoagulant therapy and acute adrenal insufficiency. *Ann Intern Med*. 1974;81:115.
63. Harper J, et al. Bilateral adrenal hemorrhage: a complication of anticoagulant therapy: case report and review of the literature. *Am J Med*. 1962;32:984.
64. Klassen J, et al. Survival after bilateral adrenal hemorrhage during heparin therapy. *Can Med Assoc J*. 1967;97:1162.
65. Danese C, et al. Adrenal hemorrhage during anticoagulant therapy. *Ann Surg*. 1974;179:70.
66. Van Couwenberge G, et al. Effect of ACTH with anticoagulants. *Can Med Assoc J*. 1958;79:536.
67. Cedermark B, et al. Adrenal activity in patients with advanced carcinomas. *Surg Gynecol Obstet*. 1981;152:461.
68. Allot E, et al. Increased adrenocortical activity associated with malignant disease. *Lancet*. 1960;2:278.
69. Bishop M, et al. Adrenocortical activity in relation to prognosis. *Br J Cancer*. 1971;24:719.
70. Cedermark B, et al. The clinical significance of metastases to the adrenal gland. *Surg Gynecol Obstet*. 1981;152:607.
71. Osei K, et al. Primary adrenal insufficiency such as lymphoma can lead to clinical adrenal insufficiency. *Arch Intern Med*. 1983;143:1791.
72. Rosenthal F, et al. Malignant disease presenting as Addison's disease. *Br Med J*. 1978;1:1591.
73. Meyer J, et al. Adrenal insufficiency secondary to metastatic lung carcinoma: CT aided diagnosis. *J Comput Assist Tomogr*. 1983;7:1107.
74. Sheeler L, et al. Adrenal insufficiency secondary to carcinoma metastatic to the adrenal gland. *Cancer*. 1983;52:1312.
75. Gamelin E, et al. Non-Hodgkin's lymphoma presenting with primary adrenal insufficiency. A disease with an underestimated frequency? *Cancer*. 1992;69:2333.
76. Fox B. Adrenal hemorrhage and necrosis resulting from abdominal operations. *Lancet*. 1969;1:600.
77. Henrich W, et al. Adrenal insufficiency after unilateral radical nephrectomy. *Urology*. 1976;8:584.
78. Steer M, et al. Recognition of adrenal insufficiency in the postoperative patient. *Am J Surg*. 1980;139:443.
79. Byyny R. Preventing adrenal insufficiency during surgery. *Postgrad Med*. 1980;67:219.
80. Ting W, et al. Bilateral adrenal hemorrhage after an open heart operation. *Ann Thoracic Surg*. 1992;54:357.
81. Hubay C, et al. Occult adrenal insufficiency in surgical patients. *Ann Surg*. 1975;181:325.
81a. Burks D, et al. Acute adrenal injury after blunt abdominal trauma: CT findings. *Am J Roentgenol*. 1992;158:503.
82. Nerup J. Addison's disease: clinical studies—a report of 108 cases. *Acta Endocrinol*. 1974;76:127.
83. Benini F, et al. Diagnostic and therapeutic problems in a case of adrenal tuberculosis and acute Addison's disease. *J Endocrinol Invest*. 1990;13:597.
84. Morens D. Congenital tuberculosis and associated hypoadrenocorticism. *South Med J*. 1979;72:160.
85. Braedy J. Military tuberculosis presenting as adrenal failure. *Can Med Assoc J*. 1981;124:748.
86. Liddle G. Pathogenesis of glucocorticoid disorders. *Am J Med*. 1972;53:638.
87. Dillon R. *Handbook of Endocrinology*. 2nd ed. Philadelphia: Lea & Febiger; 1980.
88. Sawczuk I, et al. CT findings in Addison's disease caused by tuberculosis. *Urol Radiol*. 1986;8:44.
89. McMurry J, et al. Addison's disease with adrenal enlargement on computed tomographic scanning. *Am J Med*. 1984;77:365.
90. Elansary E, et al. Rifampicin and adrenal crisis. *Br Med J*. 1983;286:1861.
91. Crispell K, et al. Addison's disease associated with histoplasmosis. *Am J Med*. 1956;20:23.
92. Roofen R, et al. Addison's disease due to *Histoplasma capsulatum*. *S Afr Med J*. 1975;47:1953.
93. Eberle D. Disseminated North American blastomycosis occurrence with clinical manifestations of adrenal insufficiency. *JAMA*. 1977;238:2629.
94. Chandler P. Addison's disease secondary to North American blastomycosis. *South Med J*. 1977;70:863.
95. Marsiglea I, et al. Adrenal cortical insufficiency associated with paracoccidioidomycosis: report of four patients. *J Clin Endocrinol Metab*. 1966;26:1109.
96. Colin R. Congenital idiopathic adrenal hypoplasia. *Obstet Gynecol*. 1973;41:655.
97. Tsung S, et al. Sudden infant death and old adrenal hemorrhage. *JAMA*. 1979;241:2507.
98. Sills I, et al. Prolonged survival without therapy in congenital adrenal hypoplasia. *Am J Dis Child*. 1983;137:1186.
99. Mitchell R. Congenital adrenal hypoplasia in siblings. *Lancet*. 1959;1:488.
100. McKusick V. *Mendelian Inheritance in Man*. 3rd ed. Baltimore: Johns Hopkins University Press; 1971.
101. Laverty C, et al. Congenital idiopathic adrenal hypoplasia. *Obstet Gynecol*. 1973;41:655.
102. Wakefield M, et al. X-linked congenital Addison's disease. *Arch Dis Child*. 1981;56:73.
103. Kreines K, et al. Neonatal adrenal insufficiency associated with maternal Cushing's syndrome. *Pediatrics*. 1971;47:516.

104. Moore F, et al. Adrenal cysts and adrenal insufficiency in an infant with fatal termination. *J Pediatr.* 1950;36:91.
105. Dickerman J, et al. Adrenal hemorrhage in the newborn: the phenomenon of "enclosed" hemorrhage as a cause of neonatal jaundice and later adrenal calcifications. *Clin Pediatr.* 1977;16:314.
106. Stevenson J. Calcification of the adrenal glands in young children. *Arch Dis Child.* 1961;36:316.
107. Shackleton C, et al. Deficient 3-beta-hydroxy-5-ene steroid secretion by newborn infants. *J Clin Endocrinol Metab.* 1979;49:247.
108. Russell M, et al. Sudden infant death due to congenital adrenal hypoplasia. *Arch Pathol Lab Med.* 1977;101:168.
109. Favara B, et al. Idiopathic adrenal hypoplasia in children. *Am J Clin Pathol.* 1972;57:287.
110. Eichner H, et al. SLE with adrenal insufficiency. *Am J Med.* 1973;55:700.
111. Das G, et al. Adrenocortical insufficiency related to oral contraceptives. *JAMA.* 1969;207:2438.
112. Pullan P, et al. Methadone induced hypoadrenalism. *Lancet.* 1983;1:714.
113. Eagan R, et al. Adrenal insufficiency following bilateral adrenal venography. *JAMA.* 1971;215:115.
114. Chakurakjian Z, et al. Adrenocortical failure in panhypopituitarism. *J Clin Endocrinol Metab.* 1968;28:25.
115. Fehm H, et al. Adrenal insufficiency secondary to hypothalamic CRF insufficiency with hyperpigmentation: a case report. *Hormone Metab Res.* 1976;8:470.
116. Corrall R, et al. Acute adrenal insufficiency due to isolated corticotrophin deficiency. *J R Soc Med.* 1979;72:530.
117. Stacpoole P, et al. Isolated ACTH deficiency. *Medicine.* 1982;61:13.
118. Toifl K, et al. A combination of spastic paraparesis, polyneuropathy, and adrenocortical insufficiency: a childhood form of adrenomyeloneuropathy. *J Neurol.* 1981;225:47.
119. Davis L, et al. Adrenoleukodystrophy and adrenomyeloneuropathy associated with partial adrenal insufficiency in three generations of a kindred. *Am J Med.* 1979;66:342.
120. Schaumberg H, et al. Adrenomyeloneuropathy: A probable variant of adrenoleukodystrophy. *Neurology.* 1977;27:1114.
121. Menkes J, et al. Adrenoleukodystrophy. *Neurology.* 1977;27:928.
122. Scott A, et al. Adrenocorticotrophic and melanocyte-stimulating peptides in the human pituitary. *Biochem J.* 1974;139:593.
123. Greipp P. Hyperpigmentation syndromes. *Arch Intern Med.* 1978;138:346.
124. Bissell G, et al. Longitudinal banded pigmentation of nails in primary adrenal insufficiency. *JAMA.* 1971;215:1666.
125. Strakosch C, et al. Early diagnosis of Addison's disease: pigmentation as sole symptom. *Aust N Z J Med.* 1978;8:189.
126. Goodwin T, et al. Addison's disease without pigmentation. *Postgrad Med J.* 1973;49:305.
127. Hidden adrenocortical insufficiency. *Br Med J.* 1973;1:5. Editorial.
128. Barrett A, et al. Patients presenting with Addison's disease need not be pigmented. *Postgrad Med J.* 1982;58:690.
129. Chan H, et al. Salty sweat and ichthyosis in Addison's disease. *Br Med J.* 1977;1:145.
130. Blizzard R, et al. Candidiasis studies pertaining to its association with endocrinopathies and pernicious anemia. *Pediatrics.* 1968;42:231.
131. Bedsole A. Calcified auricular cartilages in Addison's disease. *South Med J.* 1966;59:1268.
131a. Talmi Y, et al. Ossified auricle in Addison's disease. *Ann Otol Rhinol Laryngol.* 1990;99:499.
132. Axelrod L. Inhibition of prostacyclin production mediates permissive effect of glucocorticoids on vascular tone: perturbations of this mechanism contribute to pathogenesis of Cushing's syndrome and Addison's disease. *Lancet.* 1983;1:904.
133. Krug J. Cardiac arrest secondary to Addison's disease. *Ann Emerg Med.* 1986;15:735.
134. Jarvis J, et al. Roentgenologic observations in Addison's disease: a review of 120 cases. *Radiology.* 1954;62:16.
135. Cohen E. *Adrenal Cortical Insufficiency, American College of Physicians Course in Clinical Endocrinology, Physiologic Basis for Current Diagnoses and Therapeutic Procedures.* Ann Arbor, MI: American College of Physicians; 1971.
136. Turnipseed W, et al. The acute abdomen in undiagnosed Addison's disease. *Wis Med J.* 1976;75:104.
137. Sparberg M. Addison's disease and peptic ulcer. *Gastroenterology.* 1967;53:450.
138. Harper M, et al. Combined adrenal and thyroid deficiency presenting as an acute psychosis. *Med J Aust.* 1970;1:546.
139. Abbas D, et al. Polyradiculopathy in Addison's disease. *Neurology.* 1977;27:494.
140. Spaar F, et al. Adrenalitis inclusio-necroticans in Landry-Guillain-Barré syndrome. *Z Neurol.* 1968;193:195.
141. Sabin A, et al. Visceral lesions in infectious polyneuritis. *Am J Pathol.* 1941;17:469.
142. Spinnler H, et al. Unusual acute neurologic onset of Addison's disease. *Med J Aust.* 1979;1:280.
143. Kollmannsberger A, et al. Addison's encephalopathy. *Electroencephalogr Clin Neurophysiol.* 1969;26:448.
144. Nora J. Tachyarrhythmia and hyperkalemia in adrenal insufficiency. *Chest.* 1977;71:686.
145. Hochberg Z. Delayed pubarche in adolescents with adrenal insufficiency. *Clin Pediatr.* 1980;19:827.
146. Sheridan P, et al. Addison's disease presenting with chronic low backache. *Br Med J.* 1976;1:77.
147. Zaleske D, et al. Association of sciatica-like pain and Addison's disease. *J Bone Joint Surg Am.* 1984;66:297.
148. Shapiro M, et al. Myalgias and muscle contractures as the presenting signs of Addison's disease. *Postgrad Med J.* 1988;64:222.
149. Susac J, et al. Flexion contracture in adrenal insufficiency. *Arch Phys Med Rehabil.* 1968;49:3.
150. Calabrese L, et al. Musculoskeletal manifestations of Addison's disease. *Arthritis Rheum.* 1979;22:558.
151. Rajathurai A, et al. Self-mutilation as a feature of Addison's disease. *Br Med J.* 1983;287:1027.
152. Henkin R, et al. Studies of olfactory threshold in normal man and in patients with adrenocortical insufficiency. *J Clin Invest.* 1966;45:1631.
153. Henkin R, et al. Studies on auditory threshold in normal man and in patients with adrenocortical insufficiency. *J Clin Invest.* 1967;46:429.
154. Kosowicz J, et al. The "taste" test in adrenal insufficiency. *J Clin Endocrinol Metab.* 1967;27:214.
155. Cotterill J, et al. Self-medication with liquorice in a patient with Addison's disease. *Lancet.* 1973;1:294.
156. Green M, et al. Bronchial asthma with Addison's disease. *Lancet.* 1971;1:1159.
157. Harris P, et al. Bronchial asthma with Addison's disease. *Lancet.* 1971;1:1349.
158. Spital A. Hyponatremia in adrenal insufficiency: review of pathogenetic mechanisms. *South Med J.* 1982;75:581.

159. Falezza G, et al. High serum levels of angiotensin-converting enzyme in untreated Addison's disease. *J Clin Endocrinol Metab*. 1985;61:496.

160. Vilchez J, et al. Hyperkalemic paralysis, neuropathy, and persistent motor neuron discharges at rest in Addison's disease. *J Neurol Neurosurg Psychiatr*. 1980;43:818.

161. Van Dellen R, et al. Hyperkalemic paralysis in Addison's disease. *Mayo Clin Proc*. 1969;44:904.

162. Muls E, et al. Etiology of hypercalcemia in a patient with Addison's disease. *Calcif Tissue Int*. 1982;34:523.

163. Downie W. Hypercalcemic crisis as presentation of Addison's disease. *Br Med J*. 1977;1:145.

164. Siegler D. Idiopathic Addison's disease presenting with hypercalcemia. *Br Med J*. 1970;2:522.

165. Spry C. Eosinophilia in Addison's disease. *Yale J Biol Med*. 1976;49:411.

166. Speckart P, et al. Screening for adrenocortical insufficiency with cosyntropin (synthetic ACTH). *Arch Intern Med*. 1971;128:761.

167. Byyny R. Withdrawal from glucocorticoid therapy. *N Engl J Med*. 1976;295:30.

168. Cunningham S, et al. Normal cortisol response to corticotropin in patients with secondary adrenal failure. *Arch Intern Med*. 1983;143:2276.

17. Electrolyte Abnormalities

BARRY E. BRENNER, MD, PhD

Disorders of electrolytes pervade all areas of emergency medicine: surgery, medicine, pediatrics, and obstetrics and gynecology. Some electrolyte disorders may be life-threatening, even though there may be few symptoms or signs. These disorders may impair the function of critical organs, such as the brain or the heart. Abnormalities of electrolytes may be manifestations of an underlying disease process that is a major threat to the life of the patient; for example, mild lactic acidosis may signify sepsis.

Electrolytic disorders frequently require keen clinical judgment. The emergency physician may diagnose an electrolytic disorder tentatively and await laboratory test results only for confirmation. In an asymptomatic patient with a normal electrocardiogram (ECG), the laboratory may occasionally provide a startlingly abnormal result. It is important, however, to treat the patient, not the laboratory value. The treatment of electrolytic disorders may have serious side-effects, and the treatment must be based on symptoms, signs, and ECG findings rather than on the magnitude of any laboratory abnormality.

The rapidity of treatment should also depend on the clinical or ECG findings. As a general rule, one half of the electrolyte deficit should be corrected over a 6- to 12-hour period; then, the patient's condition should be reevaluated.

HYDRATION

The state of hydration of a given patient is dependent on the total amount of sodium as well as the total amount of fluid in the body.

Fluid Physiology

The human body can be thought of as having two physiologic components: a solid compartment, which makes up 40% of the total body weight, and a fluid compartment, which makes up 60% of the total body weight (Fig. 17-1). The fluid compartment, called the total body water (TBW), in a normal, lean 70-kg man is 42 L. Two thirds of the TBW is intracellular fluid; therefore, in a 70-kg man, the intracellular space contains 28 L fluid. The extracellular space contains both the fluid in the interstitial space and the plasma volume. One third of the TBW consists of extracellular fluid, which is 14 L in a 70-kg man.

The interstitial fluid is the fluid that surrounds each cell and serves as the immediate medium for oxygen and nutrient delivery, as well as for the secretion and excretion of products. The interstitial fluid represents about 75% of the extracellular fluid. In a 70-kg man, interstitial fluid is 11 L.

The plasma volume is the fluid that maintains the intravascular volume and is the fluid portion of blood. It is the supernatant fluid found after the centrifugation of blood in a capillary tube for a "routine" hematocrit. The plasma volume represents about 25% of the extracellular fluid; therefore, in a 70-kg man, it is 3 L.

There is considerable variation in the apportioning of TBW. Variations from this 70-kg model occur because the water content of muscle is greater than that of fat. The more fat, the lower the percentage of TBW. Women have more fat than men; therefore, TBW in a woman is 50% to 55% of weight. Since the newborn has little fat, the TBW is 70% to

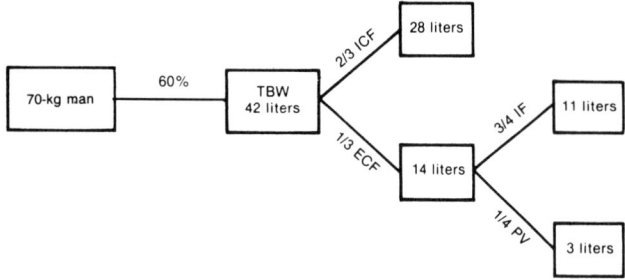

Figure 17-1 Fluid compartments. *TBW*, total body water; *ICF*, intracellular fluid; *ECF*, extracellular fluid; *IF*, interstitial fluid; *PV*, plasma volume.

80% of the newborn's weight; the extracellular fluid is 40% of TBW.

Sodium Physiology

Sodium is a major extracellular cation in the body. Because it maintains extracellular volume by binding hydrogen in water, it plays an important role in metabolism. Sodium metabolism is clearly affected by the daily intake and excretion of sodium. With normal renal function, the daily intake of sodium is equal to the urinary output of sodium; that is, the urinary sodium value is 130 to 260 mEq/day, which is equivalent to the daily sodium intake. Clinically, it is important to remember that urinary electrolytes must be measured when the patient is not taking diuretics because these medications enhance sodium and potassium excretion, making the results difficult to interpret.

Some control mechanisms are involved in the maintenance of normal serum sodium. These mechanisms are thirst, antidiuretic hormone (ADH), and free water excretion.[1]

Thirst

Hypertonicity or an elevation of the plasma osmolarity causes thirst. As independent factors, a decrease in the extracellular fluid or an elevation in the level of plasma angiotensin also induces thirst. Therefore, hypovolemic patients may have increased thirst.

Antidiuretic Hormone

In order to understand the mechanism of action of ADH, it is necessary to understand renal physiology (Fig. 17-2). The plasma is passively filtered into the glomeruli. Sodium, bicarbonate, and small molecules, along with water, are reabsorbed in the proximal tubule, which is located in the renal outer medulla. This filtrate is isotonic. Proceeding from the renal outer medulla, the filtrate descends through the descending limb of the loop of Henle, located in the inner medulla of the kidney. When the urine arrives in the ascending limb of Henle's loop, sodium is actively removed from the filtrate, leaving a hypotonic fluid. The medulla of the kidney is highly hypertonic, owing to the high concentration

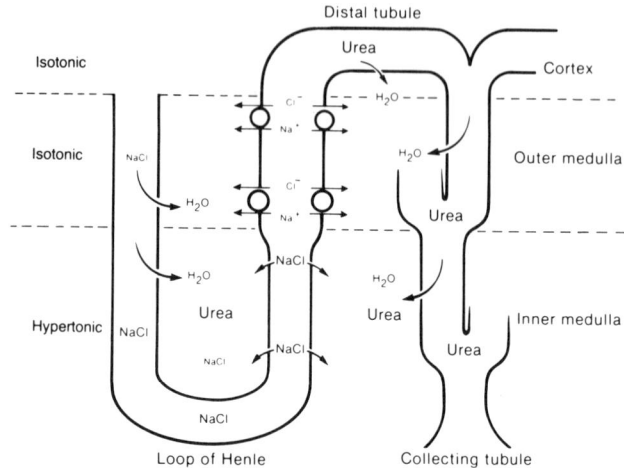

Figure 17-2 Renal physiology.

of urea that is maintained in the medullary interstitium of the kidney. The filtrate next proceeds to the distal tubule, located in the renal cortex. The urine is still hypotonic at this point. In the distal tubule, isotonic sodium and water reabsorption as well as potassium and acid secretion occur. These functions are controlled by the hormone aldosterone (see below). From the distal tubule, the urine enters the collecting tubule, which is located in the hypertonic medullary interstitium. Openings or "pores" in the cells of the collecting tubule permit equilibration between the hypotonic urine and hypertonic medullary interstitium, thereby causing an efflux of water from the hypotonic filtrate into the collecting tubule and the concentration of urine.[2,3] This pore size is regulated by ADH.

The mechanism of ADH action involves the second messenger, cyclic adenosine monophosphate (cAMP). ADH governs the water reabsorption at the collecting tubule and, in healthy individuals, is able to produce a maximum of 800 to 1200 mOsm urine.[2-4] ADH secretion is normally increased during dehydration or hypovolemia.[5]

Free Water Excretion

The last control mechanism involved in the maintenance of a normal serum sodium level is free water excretion. A decrease in free water excretion means that less free water is being presented to the collecting tubule, either because of a decrease in the glomerular filtration rate or because of an increase in the proximal tubular reabsorption of water. Therefore, less free water can be conserved by the ADH mechanism, resulting in a loss of water.

HYPERNATREMIA AND FLUID DEFICIT

Pathophysiology

Since cell membranes are permeable to water, tonicity must be the same on both sides of a cell. Therefore, a decrease in TBW increases serum sodium concentration; conversely, an increase in TBW decreases serum sodium concentration.[6] For example, a 10% increase in the serum sodium level reflects a 10% deficit in TBW. In general, the amount of serum sodium is most highly influenced by TBW; therefore, the serum sodium value is a poor indicator of sodium excess or deficit.[4]

In order to understand hypernatremia, it is necessary to understand the concept of hyperosmolarity or hypertonicity. The tonicity of the extracellular environment is influenced by sodium, glucose, and blood urea nitrogen (BUN). Sodium is maintained almost exclusively in the extracellular environment and is actively transported out of the intracellular space.[7] Owing to its high concentration extracellularly, sodium is the major osmotic agent. Glucose may enter the intracellular space but only at a slow, fixed rate and only when facilitated by a transport mechanism. BUN diffuses freely across cell membranes and is not affected by tonicity in vivo.[4] During in vitro measurements by freezing point depressions, BUN increases serum osmolarity.

The serum osmolarity can be calculated by the following equation[8,9]:

$$\text{Osmolarity} = 2 \times \text{Na} + \frac{\text{Glucose}}{18} + \frac{\text{BUN}}{2.8} \qquad (1)$$

BUN is included in this equation so that the calculated osmolarity will agree with the measured osmolarity obtained from the laboratory; however, BUN does not affect osmolarity in vivo.[4] Hyperosmolarity is defined as a serum osmolarity greater than 350 mOsm.[10,11] Normal serum osmolarity is 270 to 300 mOsm.

Etiology

Hypernatremia and dehydration have many causes.[1,12–14] Patients in nursing homes are highly susceptible to dehydration, for example, because they may not feed themselves adequately and may not be able to communicate with their caretakers when they are thirsty. Likewise, infants cannot communicate when they are thirsty, and the loss of even a small amount of water that is not corrected can rapidly result in dehydration in an infant.

Renal loss of more water than sodium also causes hypernatremia and dehydration. Patients whose renal losses of water are excessive have marked thirst, but, as long as they have access to water, they do not become dehydrated. This process occurs in diabetes insipidus. If patients with diabetes insipidus are not permitted access to water, they dehydrate quite rapidly. An osmotic diuresis, either drug induced or due to the sudden release of urinary tract obstruction, also causes a significant renal loss of more water than sodium.[4] These patients may excrete as much as 1 to 2 L urine every hour with a urine sodium value of more than 10 mEq/L on a "spot" sample. If these patients do not have adequate fluid intake, usually by the intravenous route, severe dehydration rapidly ensues.

Gastrointestinal loss of more water than sodium because of nausea, vomiting, or diarrhea can lead to dehydration. During hot weather or fever, perspiring may cause a patient to lose more water than sodium and thus become dehydrated. Likewise, tachypnea, which may be associated with entities such as asthma, may result in dehydration.

Central neurologic lesions can decrease thirst. The hypothalamus is the area of the brain that controls thirst, and a lesion in the hypothalamus can eliminate thirst and predispose a patient to dehydration. Such lesions are rare, however. In patients with essential hypernatremia,[4,12] the mechanism maintaining a normal serum osmolarity or "osmostat" has been reset to a different level of serum sodium. Therefore, the body may vigorously maintain a serum sodium level of 150 mEq/L in the same fashion that most individuals maintain a serum sodium level of 140 mEq/L. Essential hypernatremia has been associated with the presence of ectopic pinealomas located in the hypothalamus.[12]

Almost all cases of hypernatremia are due to a deficit in TBW, not to sodium excess.[4,12] It is most unusual for sodium excess to cause hypernatremia. Sodium excess, however, may result from excessive sodium bicarbonate administration during cardiopulmonary resuscitation, injection of hypertonic saline into a blood vessel by mistake during a saline abortion, administration of excessive amounts of hypertonic saline in the treatment of hyponatremia, the excessive ingestion of salt tablets or sea water, or, in infants, ingestion of cow's milk with a salt load that exceeds the ability of the infant to excrete sodium.[1,4,12,15]

Central Diabetes Insipidus

ADH is produced by the paraventricular nucleus of the hypothalamus. Central diabetes insipidus results either from damage to the hypothalamus or, in the familial form, a defect in the ADH itself. Other causes of this condition include the following:

- trauma
- primary or metastatic carcinoma, such as carcinoma of the breast
- Hand-Schüller-Christian disease
- granulomas, as seen in tuberculosis, sarcoidosis, and syphilis
- vascular conditions, such as aneurysm, Simmonds' syndrome, and Sheehan's syndrome
- meningitis or encephalitis

The clinical manifestations of central diabetes insipidus include an abrupt onset, usually in patients 10 to 20 years old, with polyuria and polydipsia as major symptoms. The fluid intake and output are both usually 3 to 15 L/day.

Patients maintain a normal serum osmolarity, provided that they have access to water. Even if their intake decreases, however, their obligate production of urine continues because of the ADH deficiency. Therefore, patients with diabetes insipidus tend to develop dehydration. Most of the patients with central diabetes insipidus have only a partial deficit so that oral intake and renal output are only 3 to 5 L/day.

Nephrogenic Diabetes Insipidus

Congenital. The congenital form of nephrogenic diabetes insipidus is rare. The clinical manifestations are fever, vomiting, dehydration, yet the presence of a markedly hypotonic urine.

Acquired. The acquired form of nephrogenic diabetes insipidus is common. In the usual forms of nephrogenic diabetes insipidus, the oral intake balances renal output of 3 to 5 L/day. The etiology of acquired nephrogenic diabetes insipidus includes the following:

- *chronic renal failure.* The diseased kidney may be unresponsive to ADH, but this does not tend to produce dehydration. Since the glomerular filtration rate (GFR) is less than 60 ml/min, less compensatory polydipsia is needed to ensure adequate fluid intake in patients with chronic renal failure.
- *starvation.* When protein intake and urea excretion are diminished, less urea is provided to maintain the hypertonic medullary interstitium of the kidney. Therefore, the urine-concentrating mechanism of the hypertonic medullary interstitium is impaired and the urine cannot be concentrated in the collecting tubule (see above).
- *ethanol.* Not only does ethanol directly inhibit the action of ADH on the collecting tubule, but it also inhibits ADH secretion by the hypothalamus, producing, in part, both a central and a nephrogenic diabetes insipidus.
- *hypercalcemia.* A persistently elevated calcium level may produce nephrocalcinosis, which interferes with the ability of the kidneys to keep the medullary interstitium hypertonic and, therefore, impairs the action of ADH.
- *hypokalemia.* Hypokalemia impairs the renal ability to maintain the hypertonicity of the medullary interstitium. Patients with potassium values persistently less than 3 mEq/L may develop an acquired nephrogenic diabetes insipidus and hypokalemic nephropathy (see below).
- *sickle cell disease and sickle cell trait.* Because they interfere with the vasa recta or the blood supply to the hypertonic renal medullary interstitium, sickle cell disease and sickle cell trait cause edema of the renal papillae.[16] Hence, they impair the urine-concentrating mechanisms of the kidneys.
- *drugs.* Several different drugs have been reported to cause a nephrogenic diabetes insipidus: most commonly lithium, demeclocycline, and amphotericin B.[17] In fact, lithium and demeclocycline have been used successfully in the treatment of excessive and inappropriate levels of ADH (syndrome of inappropriate secretion of ADH).

Clinical Manifestations

The clinical manifestations of dehydration vary with the severity. As the TBW deficit increases, there is a progressive increase in the symptomatology. One of the earliest manifestations of dehydration in children is the absence of tears when they cry; this reflects a 2% to 3% deficit in TBW. Next, sunken fontanelles appear, signifying a 3% to 5% deficit in TBW. Prominent in both adults and children who become dehydrated, dry mucous membranes mean a 4% to 8% deficit in TBW.[18–20] In adults with developed apocrine sweat glands, diminished axillary sweating is a reliable sign of a 4% to 8% TBW deficit. In adults, decreased skin turgor means at least a 6% to 10% deficit in TBW.[21] The most severe sign of dehydration is hypovolemia; orthostatic hypotension may be the earliest sign of hypovolemia, indicating at least a 10% to 15% deficit in TBW and a 20% to 25% deficit in the extracellular fluid.[22]

Mental aberrations, which occur in both adults and children with dehydration, are manifested as lethargy. In children under 2 years of age, hypertonia, irritability, and seizures are seen when the sodium concentration exceeds 160 mEq/L.[1,4,12,15] Also in children, minute cerebral vessels may rupture with dehydration, producing a xanthochromic cerebrospinal fluid with a high protein content. The rupture of these vessels is of no consequence.[23]

In dehydration, oliguria is defined as a urine output less than 10 mL/kg or less than 500 mL/day in adults. This oliguria reflects the physiologic response of ADH and aldosterone secretion to conserve water.[5,24] Adults or their family members may be able to report oliguria. In order to document oliguria it is important to ask parents of infants whether their child's diapers must be changed less often.

Diagnosis

Dehydration

The diagnosis of dehydration is aided by the clinical manifestations. The serum osmolarity should be more than 350 mOsm before it is classified as hyperosmolarity.[10,11] The serum sodium level should be elevated in dehydration to more than 150 mEq/L. If the actual level is more than 170 mEq/L, however, the result of a laboratory determination will be artificially low.[25] This underestimation of the

Table 17-1 Water Deprivation Test

Diagnosis	Initial Serum Osmolarity	Urine Osmolarity After Dehydration	Urine Osmolarity After Vasopressin
Normal	Normal, 275–300	Normal, 1000	No response, 1000
Complete diabetes insipidus	Normal	Dilute, 160	Excellent response, 400
Incomplete diabetes insipidus	Normal	Medium dilute, 440	Good response, 700
Nephrogenic diabetes insipidus	Normal	Dilute or medium dilute	No response
Psychogenic polydipsia	Dilute, 250–275	Isotonic, 300	Slight response, 370

Note: If patients with diabetes insipidus can drink, they have a normal serum osmolarity. Patients with psychogenic polydipsia cannot concentrate their urine secondary to their chronic hypotonicity, which "washes out" the countercurrent dilution mechanism of the interstitium of the medulla of the kidney.

serum sodium value is due to hyperviscosity and hyperosmolarity of the serum, which decreases the amount of serum that can be aspirated into the roller pump diluter. In addition, the standard curves for serum sodium are not linear when sodium values are greater than 170 mEq/L.

To calculate the level of serum sodium, it is necessary only to use Eq. 1. If the serum osmolarity, BUN, and glucose values are known, then the serum sodium level can be calculated. For example, a physician suspects that a patient's serum sodium level of 178 mEq/L may be an underestimation of the serum sodium value. The glucose value is determined to be 180 mg/dL, the BUN is 56 mg/dL, and the serum osmolarity is determined to be 400 mOsm. Using Eq. 1,

$$2 \times Na + \frac{180}{18} + \frac{56}{2.8} = 400 \text{ mOsm}$$

therefore,

$$Na = 185 \text{ mEq/L}$$

In hypernatremia it is helpful to calculate the TBW deficit. In this calculation, it is assumed that the patient's condition is stable and that sodium excess is not the cause of the patient's hypernatremia. The TBW deficit may be used as an estimate of the amount of fluid that the patient will require to be hydrated.[4,6,15] To calculate the TBW in a man, for example, the physician must remember that the TBW represents 60% of total body weight. The total body solute is calculated by multiplying the TBW by the serum osmolarity. For example, a 70-kg man has 42 L TBW. This is multiplied by 400 mOsm in the dehydrated patient, resulting in 16,800 mOsm total body solute. In the calculation of the TBW deficit, a desired osmolarity of approximately 300 mOsm can be used. The total body solute is divided by the desired osmolarity; the expected TBW is subtracted from this result to arrive at the TBW deficit. In the above example, the total body solute, 16,800 mOsm, is divided by 300 mOsm. From this quotient, 56, the expected TBW, 42 L, is subtracted, resulting in a 14-L TBW deficit.

Diabetes Insipidus

If a dehydrated patient has a dilute urine, the physician should suspect diabetes insipidus. It is important to distinguish diabetes insipidus from psychogenic polydipsia. The onset of psychogenic polydipsia is vague rather than abrupt. Frequently, patients with psychogenic polydipsia have a history of psychiatric illness.[4] To distinguish central diabetes insipidus from incomplete diabetes insipidus, nephrogenic diabetes insipidus, and psychogenic polydipsia, a water deprivation test is performed (Table 17-1). In this test, the patient is deprived of water for 12 to 16 hours until there is a decrease in TBW of 3% to 5% or three consecutive urines are unchanged in osmolarity.[26] At this time, serum osmolarity and urine osmolarity are measured. Then, 5 U of aqueous ADH are administered and the serum osmolarity and urine osmolarity are measured over the next hour.

Treatment

Dehydration

The treatment of dehydration depends on the severity of the condition. If a patient is mildly symptomatic and has neither nausea nor vomiting, oral hydration may be possible. The maximum amount of oral hydration that may be considered is 2.5 to 3 L/day.[15]

If the patient is mildly symptomatic and has more than a 5% deficit of TBW, or if the patient cannot tolerate oral hydration, then intravenous hydration is indicated. If hypotension or orthostatic hypotension is present, the TBW deficit is calculated and 1 to 2 L normal saline administered over 48 hours. The baseline rate of fluid administration is equal to the rate of urine output, but the TBW deficit must be replaced by the administration of fluid above and beyond the amount excreted in the urine. The TBW deficit is replaced as 5% dextrose with one-half normal saline in adults.[1,4,15] In children, 5% dextrose with one-fourth normal saline is used.

It is important to treat dehydration over a prolonged period of time, such as 48 hours. The rapid administration of markedly hypotonic fluids, such as 5% dextrose, may cause hemolysis. Furthermore, rapid treatment of dehydration is associated with the development of cerebral edema and the subsequent marked deterioration in the mental status of the patient.[12] This cerebral edema may be due to the development of different osmotic gradients between the blood and the brain. To decrease these osmotic gradients and prevent cerebral edema, some physicians advocate normal saline for rehydration in patients without cardiac or renal disease; if the serum sodium level becomes more than 155 mEq/L, a change to hypotonic fluids is recommended.[27]

During the hydration of children, mild hyperglycemia may develop. This hyperglycemia must not be treated with insulin, because rapid falls in glucose may alter the tonicity between the blood and the brain and predispose children to cerebral edema.[23]

During rehydration, it is important to avoid overhydration. A central venous pressure of 5 mmHg or neck vein distention of 5 cm above the angle of Louis reflects adequate intravascular volume. Urine osmolarity and urine output are also useful determinations in avoiding overhydration. The physician must always be alert to the development of acute tubular necrosis with oliguria, which can develop secondary to the profound hypovolemia and decreased renal blood flow that occurs with severe dehydration. A composition of various solutions may be reviewed in Appendix 17–A.

Sodium Excess

Patients with sodium excess should be treated in the same manner as other patients with dehydration, except that normal saline is contraindicated. These patients should receive only one-fourth or one-half normal saline. Dialysis may be necessary to remove the excess saline in the presence of renal failure.[4]

Central Diabetes Insipidus

The treatment of central diabetes insipidus is beyond the scope of the emergency physician. These patients should be referred to the internist. A convenient and effective therapy for these patients has been developed. Deamino arginine vasopressin, a long-acting nasal spray with a half-life of 20 hours, has been highly effective as a single daily treatment in the patient with central diabetes insipidus.[1,4]

Nephrogenic Diabetes Insipidus

The treatment of congenital nephrogenic diabetes insipidus is the same as the treatment of any dehydration. These patients are treated with 5% dextrose with one-fourth normal saline. Interestingly, however, marked volume contraction with furosemide improves the patient's condition by increasing the proximal reabsorption of sodium and decreasing the delivery of sodium to the distal tubule.[4] Indomethacin has also been effective,[4] although the mechanism is unclear. In children with congenital nephrogenic diabetes insipidus, the combination of indomethacin and diuretics may decrease urine flow from 10 to 12 L/day to 3 to 5 L/day.

Prehospital and Nursing Care

Prehospital and nursing intervention should include the establishment of an intravenous catheter with normal saline or 5% dextrose with one-half normal saline infusion. If the dehydration is perceived to be severe, the nursing team should prepare the patient for admission. Any patient with dehydration so severe that it produces altered mental status, orthostatic hypotension, or hypotension requires prolonged therapy and should be admitted to the hospital.

HYPONATREMIA

Pathophysiology and General Etiology

The causes of hyponatremia may be divided into three categories according to the hydration status of the patient: edema, hypovolemia, and normovolemia.

Edema

Patients with hypervolemia have more water than sodium; the result is hyponatremia. This may occur in patients with nephrotic syndrome or in those with chronic renal failure who ingest excess water. The hypervolemia in congestive heart failure may diminish renal perfusion, causing a diminished sodium and water delivery to collecting ducts and thus decreasing free water excretion.[5,28,29] In addition, ADH secretion increases in an effort to compensate for the renal hypoperfusion, which in turn increases water retention.[5] In patients with chronic congestive heart failure or liver diseases, such as cirrhosis, metabolism of ADH is decreased, which also increases water retention.

Hypovolemia

Patients with hyponatremia and hypovolemia may be divided into two groups; those with renal salt-wasting and those with nonrenal salt losses.[29] Patients with hypovolemia and renal salt-wasting have a urine "spot" sodium of more than 40 mEq/L in association with hypovolemia or orthostatic hypotension.[4] These patients may have hypopituitarism or Addison's disease; their high urine sodium and low serum sodium levels may be due to mineralocorticoid deficiency (see below).[1] In addition, a salt-losing nephropathy would produce severe renal salt losses and hyponatremia. Potent diuretics may produce salt-wasting and hyponatremia.[30]

Nonrenal salt losses occur with increased fluid retention secondary to compensatory and appropriate ADH secretion. In addition, free water excretion is decreased because of hypovolemia.[1,4] These nonrenal losses of fluid can result from gastrointestinal problems, such as diarrhea or vomiting, or retroperitoneal disease, such as pancreatitis.[1] Similarly, salt can be lost by profuse sweating during hot, humid weather; it is lost cutaneously in patients with severe burns.[1] The urine sodium value is less than 10 mEq/L on a spot sample in these patients, owing to the appropriate secretion of mineralocorticoids.[4]

Normovolemia

In the normovolemic patient, hyponatremia may result from several different causes. Hypothyroidism leads to hyponatremia, but the mechanism is unclear.[31] Sickle cell syndrome is a general phrase for a hyponatremia that occurs in patients who have a severe, usually chronic illness.[1,4,32] Both the existence of this disease and its pathophysiologic mechanism are controversial, however. It is postulated that sodium-potassium adenosine triphosphatase is not effective in a severe illness. Therefore, sodium enters the intracellular space and, owing to the ineffective sodium-potassium adenosine triphosphatase, is not actively transported out to the extracellular fluid.[7] Essential hyponatremia is similar to essential hypernatremia in that the pathophysiologic mechanism is that of a reset "osmostat" that maintains a lower serum osmolarity.[1,4] These patients are noted to have an increase in thirst. The existence of this entity is also controversial. Patients with psychogenic polydipsia drink 10 to 40 L water per day. For this volume of fluid ingestion to produce hyponatremia a reset "osmostat" has been demonstrated. In contradistinction to diabetes insipidus, psychogenic polydipsia has a gradual onset.[33]

Pseudohyponatremia may develop secondary to hyperproteinemia or hyperglycemia. Patients with multiple myeloma or hyperlipemia may develop a pseudohyponatremia.[34] In the healthy patient, serum is 93 parts water and 7 parts solute (aqueous plus protein). The sodium is dissolved in the aqueous phase of serum at a concentration of 152 mEq per liter of water. The sodium concentration reported from the laboratory is normally 140 mEq per liter of serum (ie, aqueous plus solid). In patients with hyperproteinemia, the relative proportion of water in serum may be decreased by an elevation of the solid phase (lipid or protein), producing a spurious decrease in the sodium concentration per liter of serum. Although the sodium concentration dissolved in the aqueous phase is unchanged, it shows 152 mEq per liter of water.

In hyperglycemia, the serum sodium level decreases 1.6 mEq/L for each increase in glucose of 100 mg/dL.[35,36] Hyperglycemia produces hypertonicity in the extracellular fluid, and water transfers from the intracellular space to dilute the more hypertonic extracellular fluid. This increase in extracellular water decreases the concentration of sodium, producing hyponatremia. This reflects an actual hyponatremia in the extracellular fluid but does not reflect a total body sodium deficit or TBW excess.

The syndrome of inappropriate secretion of ADH is a diagnosis of exclusion. It is based on the assumption that the patient has normal renal, adrenal, thyroid, and cardiac function. In addition, the patient must not have hypervolemia, which would make the ADH response appropriate and produce hyponatremia by mechanisms that have already been listed. The etiology of this syndrome includes the following[3,4,37]:

- *drugs.* Carbamazepine and chlorpropamide increase ADH secretion. Both chlorpropamide and tolbutamide enhance the effect of ADH on the collecting duct. Amitriptyline hydrocholoride, thioriadazine hydrochloride, narcotics, and barbiturates may also induce this syndrome by unclear mechanisms.
- *ectopic production.* An inappropriate ADH response has been produced by various malignant tumors, ranging from carcinoma of the lung, pancreas, or prostate to lymphomas.
- *pulmonary disease.* Many different pulmonary diseases may cause this syndrome. The most frequent pulmonary causes are pulmonary tuberculosis, pneumonia, and lung abscesses.
- *neurologic conditions.* Since ADH is produced by the hypothalamus, it is not surprising that neurologic aberrations may cause increased secretion of this hormone. Patients with encephalitis, meningitis, brain tumors, cerebral aneurysms, or Guillain-Barré syndrome may develop the syndrome of inappropriate secretion of ADH.
- *miscellaneous factors.* Various stress situations may induce an inappropriate ADH response. Presumably, this increased production of ADH is induced directly by the effect of stress on the hypothalamus. Acute intermittent porphyria, assisted ventilation, or emotional, physical, or surgical stresses are known to produce the syndrome.[38]

Clinical Manifestations

Only patients with a serum sodium level of less than 120 to 125 mEq/L may have symptoms of hyponatremia.[1,4,39] The quicker the fall in the level of serum sodium, however, symptoms occur at higher values of serum sodium.[39] The symptoms of hyponatremia are altered mental status, headache, nausea and vomiting, asterixis, myoclonus, ataxia, and, in the most severe cases, seizures.

Diagnosis

The diagnosis of hyponatremia depends simply on the laboratory values. The presence of edema, congestive heart failure, or chronic renal failure suggests one set of diseases. The presence of hypovolemia with salt wasting suggests a set of diseases different from those suggested by the presence of hypovolemia with nonrenal salt losses. In patients with hyponatremia and normovolemia, the possibility of pseudohyponatremia due to hyperproteinemia or hyperglycemia must be considered. Hypothyroidism, sickle syndrome, and essential hyponatremia are difficult to diagnose confidently in the emergency department. The syndrome of inappropriate secretion of ADH is a diagnosis of exclusion, as noted earlier. If the serum osmolarity is less than 270 mOsm, the urine osmolarity is more than 300 mOsm, and the urine sodium level is more than 40 mEq/L on a spot sample, then the urine is inappropriately concentrated, despite a dilute serum, and the syndrome of inappropriate secretion of ADH is present.

Treatment

Nonsymptomatic Patients

The treatment of the nonsymptomatic patient with hyponatremia should in general be referred to the internist. The patient with hypervolemia or normovolemia requires fluid restriction to an intake of fluid that equals the insensible losses plus only one third of the patient's urine output.[1,4] In patients with the syndrome of inappropriate secretion of ADH, if fluid restriction has been inadequate, the physician must use drugs that interfere with the action of ADH at the renal level. The drugs that have been used with success are lithium and demeclocycline.[40] Patients with hypovolemia and hyponatremia require the infusion of normal saline, which corrects both the volume deficit and the hyponatremia.[4]

Symptomatic Patients

If the patient is symptomatic, then urgent therapy is required. The water excess may be calculated in the same way as the water deficit. Patients with symptomatic hyponatremia should be treated with hypertonic saline.[41,42] Three percent saline may be administered over 3 to 4 hours to a volume of 500 mL if the patient is seizing or if other serious neurologic findings are present. It is important to continue free water restriction. Furosemide, 1 mg/kg, is an important adjunct.[42] The physician must replace urine volume that is lost with an additional 3% saline. The aim of therapy is to remove one half of the calculated water excess over the first 3 to 4 hours of treatment. The physician should check the urine electrolytes every hour, following the serum potassium level and replacing as necessary. With these methods, most patients become asymptomatic in less than 12 hours. This vigorous treatment of hyponatremia is designed to achieve a serum sodium level of 120 mEq/L. Efforts to raise the serum sodium level higher than this are unwarranted, since symptoms are unusual above 120 mEq/L.

Prehospital and Nursing Care

The assessment of hyponatremia by the prehospital or nursing care team is nondiagnostic and nonspecific. The diagnosis is made in the laboratory. Once the diagnosis of hyponatremia has been made, nursing intervention should include establishment of an intravenous line and the preparation for a possible seizure in symptomatic patients.

All patients with symptomatic hyponatremia (eg, altered mental status or seizures) or serum sodium levels lower than 125 mEq/L should be admitted to the hospital.

POTASSIUM

Physiology

Potassium is found in abundance in the body. The normal adult has approximately 160 mEq/L, nearly 98% of which is found inside the cells.[43] Potassium is also found in high concentrations in gastric secretions, bile, and pancreatic secretions. The serum or interstitial compartment contains 3.5 to 5.3 mEq/L. Large fluctuations in intracellular potassium are well tolerated by the body, but even very small fluctuations in serum potassium levels can be life threatening.

An average daily diet contains 40 to 100 mEq potassium. Although some is lost in feces, perspiration, or during vomiting, most is excreted by the kidney. Normal urine potassium is 40 to 80 mEq/day. Potassium excretion in the kidney varies with sodium retention.[43,44] This mechanism is under the influence of aldosterone, a hormone secreted by the adrenal gland.[5] Aldosterone causes reabsorption of sodium and a loss of potassium at the distal tubule. Potassium is lost in spite of a low serum level of potassium because the kidney cannot conserve it effectively. The amount of sodium and potassium exchanged depends on the amount of sodium delivered to the distal tubule and on the serum aldosterone level. A decrease in aldosterone secretion, as might be seen in adrenal insufficiency or Addison's disease, causes a decrease in sodium reabsorption, resulting in an increase in the amount of potassium retained by the tubules. An aldosterone antagonist, such as spironolactone, could increase the risk of hyperkalemia.

Aldosterone is under the influence of many feedback mechanisms (Fig. 17-3). Hypotension, standing, or low renal perfusion stimulate the kidney to secret renin. Renin converts a liver protein, angiotensinogen, to angiotensin I, which is in turn converted to the potent hypertensive agent angiotensin II. Angiotensin II stimulates the zona glomerulosa to release increased amounts of aldosterone. High levels of aldosterone, high renal perfusion, or recumbency inhibits renin secretion by the kidney.[5,45]

The role of potassium parallels that of sodium in extracellular fluids, and its physiologic action is almost solely related to its concentration in extracellular fluids. Potassium plays an important role in muscular contraction, conduction of nerve impulses, enzyme action, cell membrane function, and acid-base balance.

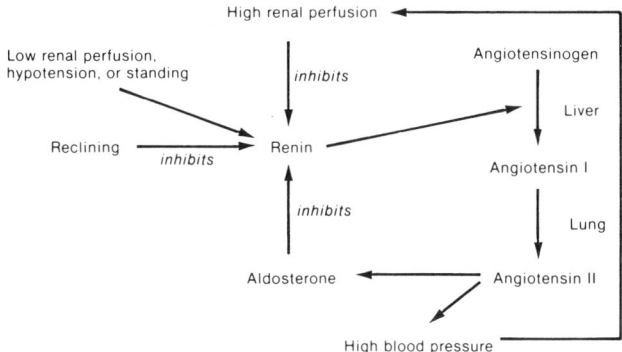

Figure 17-3 Model for aldosterone, renin-angiotensin control mechanisms. *Note:* Pointing arrows signify stimulation unless otherwise noted.

Acid-Base Balance

Body cells contain buffer systems that can either donate or accept hydrogen ions. Both hydrogen ions and potassium ions freely interchange across the cell membrane. In acidosis, the excess hydrogen ions in the serum migrate into the cells, displacing the potassium ions into the serum. Since the level of extracellular potassium is quite low compared with the intracellular levels, even a very small shift in potassium ions across the cell membrane can cause significant changes in the serum level. As a result, acidosis can cause hyperkalemia.[44]

Alkalosis can cause hypokalemia. The intracellular buffers dissociate to release hydrogen ions, which move out of the cell into the serum. To preserve electrical neutrality, potassium ions move into the cell, causing a decrease in the serum level.

An acid-base imbalance can mask a potassium imbalance. For example, a patient with a very low potassium level could appear to have an almost normal serum level if acidosis has caused potassium ions to move out of the cells into the serum.

The kidneys also influence the relationship of acid-base imbalances to potassium imbalances.[44-48] In acidotic states, the kidneys retain sodium ions instead of hydrogen ions,[49] and the excess hydrogen ions in the renal tubules prevent the normal renal excretion of potassium. In alkalotic states, the kidneys retain sodium and hydrogen ions and excrete potassium ions into the renal tubules. By these mechanisms, hyperchloremic metabolic acidosis raises the potassium level 0.6 to 0.9 mEq/L for each 0.1 decrease in serum pH.[50] However, in a metabolic acidosis with an elevated anion gap, a decrease in serum pH of 0.1 may not raise the serum potassium level at all (Fig. 17-4).[51,52]

Nerve Conduction and Muscle Contraction

The resting polarization of neurons and all types of muscle fibers (smooth, cardiac, or striated) is determined by the continual diffusion of potassium ions across the cell membrane. The magnitude or potential of the resting polarization is responsible for the duration and velocity of the subsequent action potentials (depolarization and repolarization).

Resting membrane potential. A nerve cell, to conduct an impulse, or a muscle cell, to contract and relax, must be polarized or "charged." A cell is polarized when ions of opposite charges are arranged on either side of the cell membrane. This ionic imbalance across the cell membrane creates an electrical "tension" or a potential; as long as the membrane remains undisturbed, the cell maintains itself in this state, referred to as the resting membrane potential. No current flows, since current flows only when negative and positive ions are in the same compartment, not separated by a membrane. The strength of the potential depends on the ionic imbalance across the cell membrane. In this resting state, sodium and potassium, both positively charged ions, establish an equilibrium across the cell membrane with more sodium ions outside and more potassium ions inside. Because the cell also contains negatively charged phosphate and protein molecules, the inside of the cell is more negative. Furthermore, in the resting state, the cell membrane is more permeable to potassium than to sodium; since the ratio of potassium ions inside the cell to those outside is 30:1, potassium can slowly leak out of the cell, causing the extracellular fluid to become less negative.[53,54] Normally, a cardiac muscle cell is polarized with an intracellular charge of -90 mV. During the resting potential phase, the cell is ready to receive a stimulus.

Action potentials. A stimulus may be electrical (eg, an impulse from the sinoatrial node), chemical (eg, hypoxia), or mechanical (eg, chamber dilation). This stimulus changes membrane permeability, which allows sodium to enter the cell. The sodium ions rush in, carrying their positive charges, and the inside of the cell becomes rapidly positive. Because polarity has been changed, the cell is said to be

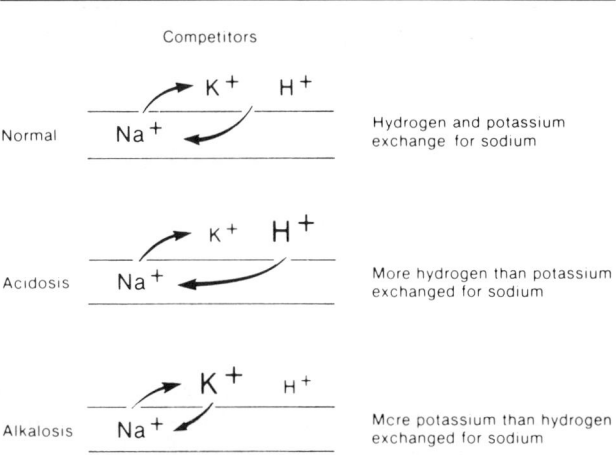

Figure 17-4 Effect of alkalosis and acidosis on potassium–sodium exchange.

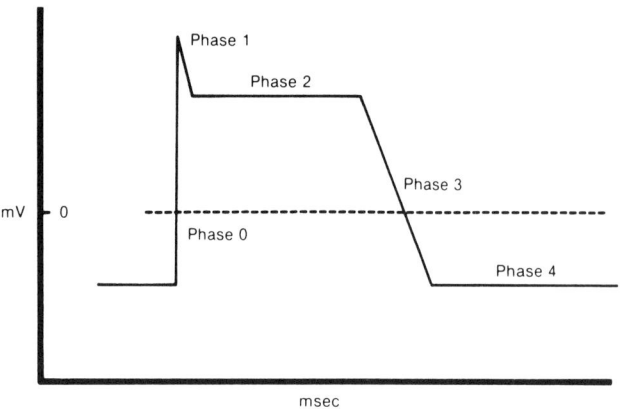

Figure 17-5 Action potential.

depolarized. Depolarization is an electrochemical event that precedes the mechanical event of contraction.

After depolarization, a series of further ionic movements, termed *repolarization*, takes place before the ionic balance is restored to the resting state (Fig. 17-5):

- During phase 4, the cell is in the resting state with an inside negativity of −90 mV. The ionic "pumps" and membrane integrity maintain this resting membrane potential.
- Phase 0 represents the rapid depolarization of the cell. A stimulus causes a sudden change in cellular membrane permeability. Sodium rushes in, changing the polarity and producing the upstroke or first phase of the action potential or depolarization.
- Phase 1 is the initial phase of repolarization.
- During phase 2, the process of repolarization decelerates, causing a plateau in the action potential. This plateau does not occur in skeletal muscles, but it is necessary in cardiac muscle to allow for a sustained contraction to expel all of the stroke volume from the ventricle. During this phase, calcium ions enter the cell.
- Phase 3 represents the last period of repolarization. Potassium ions enter the cell, and the resting membrane potential is restored.[53,54]

Pathophysiology

The magnitude of the resting membrane potential is dependent on the size of the potassium gradient across the membrane. The action potential (in phase 0) is dependent on the strength of the resting membrane potential, its amplitude (the degree of positive charge after depolarization), and the rate at which this amplitude is reached. These factors determine whether the rapid depolarization necessary to ensure adequate conduction velocity is possible. Contiguous muscle fibers are stimulated faster by a strong action potential and a steep rise in phase 0.

If a rubber band were attached to the highest peak, stretched down to the point marked −90 mV, and suddenly released, it would snap upward to a point higher than the peak to which it was attached. Because the position was so high, it would take longer to descend. This analogy approximates events that occur in the presence of hypokalemia, which produces an increased electrical gradient across the membrane. A rubber band stretched only half the distance, however, not only would rise more slowly but also would be unable to rise as high. Because the rubber band did not ascend as high, it would take less time to descend. This analogy approximates the events that occur when levels of potassium ions are elevated in the extracellular fluid and the gradient across the membrane is lessened.

Hypokalemia affects the action potential by increasing the potassium gradient across the cell membrane. The serum deficit facilitates the movement of potassium to the extracellular fluid. This increased negativity increases membrane excitability and interferes with the normal repolarization process. A potassium change from 4 to 2 mEq/L causes the intracellular-extracellular potassium gradient to change from 30:1 to 60:1,[53,54] which increases the negativity of the resting membrane potential and, thus, increases the amplitude of the action potential. Therefore, in hypokalemia, slight to moderate increases in the amplitudes of P and QRS waves are seen on ECGs. The movement of potassium out of the cardiac cell, which occurs during phase 3 of repolarization, involves a lower number of potassium molecules. The T wave of the ECG associated with hypokalemia, which is relatively small, reflects phase 3 of the action potential, or the repolarization process. The fewer potassium molecules moving during phase 3, the smaller the current generated and the smaller the T wave on the ECG. Owing to the increased magnitude of the action potential, phase 3 is prolonged, resulting in a broad T wave.

U waves are positive deflections that are more than 1 mm in height and follow the position of the T waves on the ECG. U waves are characteristic of hypokalemia and are best seen in leads V_2 and V_3. They are secondary to repolarization of Purkinje fibers or to myocardial stretch potentials evoked during myocardial relaxation.

Hyperkalemia with a potassium change from 4 to 8 mEq/liter decreases the intracellular-extracellular potassium gradient from 30:1 to 15:1.[53,54] Such a change decreases both the negativity of the resting membrane potential and the height of the action potential. Hyperkalemia, therefore, decreases the amplitude of the P and QRS waves. Advanced hyperkalemia decreases automaticity, increases atrioventricular conduction abnormalities, and produces asystole.[54] In hyperkalemia, the movement of potassium during phase 3 involves a large number of potassium molecules; therefore, more current is generated and the amplitude of the T-wave height is increased, as is characteristic of hyperkalemia. Owing to the decreased magnitude of the action potential, phase 3 is shortened, resulting in a peaked, short T wave. Hyponatremia and hypocalcemia increase membrane permeability to potassium and enhance the effects of hyperkalemia on the ECG and on the heart.[53]

HYPOKALEMIA

The causes of hypokalemia can be divided into two types: those associated with normotension and those associated with hypertension.

Normotensive Conditions

There are many causes of hypokalemia associated with normotension.

Poor Intake

Hypokalemia is common in cases of starvation. Despite inanition, there is an obligatory potassium loss of 5 to 15 mEq/day in the urine.[55] Ketones produced as a result of starvation serve as organic anions in the distal tubule. Their anionic charge produces an electrical gradient for cations, such as potassium,[56] causing the movement of potassium into the distal tubule and increasing potassium excretion.

Emesis

Another common cause of hypokalemia is emesis. The potassium concentration in gastric secretions is only 10 mEq/L and therefore accounts for only minimal potassium loss during emesis.[43,44] During regurgitation, however, hydrochloric acid is lost from the stomach and a metabolic alkalosis develops. This alkalosis encourages the elimination of potassium by a renal mechanism.[44]

Diarrhea

Potassium concentration is greater than sodium concentration in diarrheal fluid, and diarrhea is a frequent cause of hypokalemia. The potassium loss with diarrhea varies with the volume and frequency of the stool. Villous adenoma in the colon may produce diarrhea and profound potassium depletion, and it should be considered in any patient with diarrhea and marked hypokalemia.[57] Some patients may abuse laxatives, causing diarrhea. Historically, these patients often deny laxative abuse, however. Their condition may simulate Bartter's syndrome, with high renin and low serum aldosterone levels that are unaffected by postural changes (see Fig. 17-3).[58-60]

Bartter's Syndrome

Although there is a familial association with mental retardation, many patients with Bartter's syndrome have normal intelligence. There is an increased incidence in blacks. The histopathology demonstrates a hyperplasia in the cells located between the glomeruli and the macula densa; this is termed *juxtaglomerular hyperplasia*. These juxtaglomerular cells secrete renin.

A model of this syndrome was proposed by Bartter.[61] Although the model does not explain all the more recent findings, such as the role of prostaglandin E_2 in the pathogenesis of this syndrome,[62] it is still quite useful in understanding the different hormonal interactions in these patients. Bartter proposed that the mechanism for this syndrome is a hyporesponsiveness of the vasculature to angiotensin.[61] To compensate and maintain normotension, the juxtaglomerular cells produce excessive amounts of renin. High levels of angiotensin persist, however; these high levels of angiotensin stimulate aldosterone production, which causes hypokalemia. The hypokalemia in Bartter's syndrome impairs the renal ability to form urine (hyposthenuria) and, therefore, produces a nephrogenic diabetes insipidus. The severity of the hypokalemia in Bartter's syndrome usually varies from values of 1.5 to 2.5 mEq/L.

Renal Tubular Acidosis

In type I renal tubular acidosis, hydrogen ions cannot be secreted into the distal tubule. In type II renal tubular acidosis, the kidney is unable to reabsorb bicarbonate in the proximal tubule.[63,64] Hypokalemia occurs because the net effect of renal tubular acidosis is to increase bicarbonate within the lumen of the distal tubule. Bicarbonate, with its negative charge, provides an electrical gradient for the migration of potassium to the lumen as well.[63,64]

Drugs

Carbenicillin and gentamicin both serve as nondiffusible anions within the distal tubule; therefore, they produce an electrical gradient that encourages the positively charged potassium ions to migrate into the distal tubule.[65] In addition, because each gram of carbenicillin contains 4.7 mEq of sodium, carbenicillin increases the delivery of sodium to the distal tubule. This mechanism provides more sodium for exchange with potassium at the distal tubule by the normal physiologic mechanisms of aldosterone.

Amphotericin B may produce hypokalemia by causing a renal tubular acidosis.[66] This is a common finding in patients on amphotericin B.

Acetazolamide is an inhibitor of the enzyme carbonic anhydrase. Because of this inhibition, the urine is alkalinized, which produces an excess of bicarbonate within the renal tubule and an electrical gradient for the migration of potassium within the distal tubule.[67] Therefore, this alkalinization of the urine produces hypokalemia in the same way that renal tubular acidosis does.

Diuretic medications, such as mannitol, glycerol, furosemide, ethacrynic acid, and the thiazides increase delivery of sodium to the distal tubule so that more sodium is available for exchange with potassium.[43,44] This increased availability results in hypokalemia through the normal physiologic mechanisms of aldosterone. Similarly, other causes of diuresis, such as postobstructive diuresis, diabetic ketoacidosis, or the diuretic phase of acute tubular necrosis, may produce hypokalemia.

Acute Leukemia

In patients with acute leukemia, the chronic secretion of lysozyme may cause renal tubular damage.[68] This damage may result in renal potassium wasting and may explain the hypokalemia occasionally seen in these patients.

Transcellular Shifts

The sudden shift of potassium from the extracellular space to the intracellular space may result in hypokalemia on a serum sample. These transcellular shifts occur in several situations.

Alkalosis. Acute respiratory alkalosis, chronic metabolic alkalosis, and acute metabolic alkalosis all induce a renal loss of potassium. For reasons that are still unclear, hypokalemia does not occur in patients with chronic respiratory alkalosis.

Periodic paralysis. The hypokalemic variety of periodic paralysis is inherited as an autosomal dominant trait. In these patients, there is no change in the urinary potassium excretion during periods of hypokalemia; therefore, the hypokalemia must be due to a shift of potassium from the extracellular fluid to the intracellular fluid. Adrenocorticotropic hormone (ACTH) induces attacks, but its effect is blocked by metyrapone, an agent that inhibits glucocorticoid synthesis by the adrenal cortex. The clinical manifestations of the hypokalemic form of periodic paralysis have an abrupt onset, usually within 10 to 20 minutes after various precipitating factors. Such factors include rest following exercise, high carbohydrate intake, infection, trauma, emotional stress, and ethanol ingestion. These manifestations last for approximately 24 hours.[43,44,69]

Insulin. In the therapy of patients with hyperglycemia, insulin encourages transport of glucose into the intracellular space.[70] Along with glucose, potassium is transported into the intracellular space, occasionally resulting in hypokalemia.

Trauma. In patients with marked trauma, hypokalemia seems to correlate with the degree of trauma.[71] The mechanism of this hypokalemia seems to involve a transcellular shift.

Heat Stroke

In patients with heat stroke, an acute respiratory alkalosis that may be due to exercise or to hyperventilation for heat dissipation is prominent. This acute respiratory alkalosis is responsible, in part, for the hypokalemia seen in patients with heat stroke. In addition, mucocutaneous fluid losses and hypovolemia may induce a physiologic aldosteronism that is a contributing factor to this hypokalemia,[72,73] since sweating results in an obligatory potassium loss under the control of aldosterone.[5]

Barium Poisoning

In barium poisoning, which may be induced by the ingestion of certain pesticides or depilatories, the patients have nausea, vomiting, and diarrhea. The severe hypokalemia that occurs is due to gastrointestinal losses.[74] It may be so severe that it produces arrhythmias or flaccid paralysis.

Vitamin B_{12} Therapy

During the therapy of pernicious anemia with vitamin B_{12}, there is a rapid formation of new platelets and erythrocytes. Formation of the new cells involves the formation of an intracellular space for each cell and the rapid uptake of potassium from the extracellular environment.[75] This mechanism is proposed to explain the occurrence of hypokalemia in association with vitamin B_{12} therapy.

Hypertensive Conditions

Hyperaldosteronism or Conn's Syndrome

Patients with inappropriately high levels of aldosterone usually have adrenal adenomas.[76-78] Occasionally, these patients may have adrenal hyperplasia. Patients with adrenal adenoma cannot be distinguished from patients with adrenal hyperplasia by the serum aldosterone level.[77] The striking feature of the high level of aldosterone in these conditions is that it is unresponsive to normal physiologic controls; for example, it persists even when the patient is recumbent (see Fig. 17-3).[77] This hyperaldosteronism continuously and primarily inhibits renin production, resulting in low plasma renin levels. This low renin production is also unresponsive to physiologic controls and persists despite volume contraction with diuretics or prolonged standing.

Cushing's Syndrome

The most common cause of Cushing's syndrome is adenoma of the adrenal cortex. Although unusual, carcinoma of the adrenal gland may also produce Cushing's syndrome. In addition, a pituitary adenoma that secretes excessive amounts of ACTH may induce bilateral adrenal hyperplasia. This cause of Cushing's syndrome is termed *Cushing's disease.*

The clinical manifestations of Cushing's syndrome are truncal obesity, buccal fat pad, purple striae, ecchymosis, acne, hirsutism, and a buffalo hump.

Accelerated Hypertension

Hyperreninemia as a primary cause of accelerated hypertension results in increased serum aldosterone levels (see Fig. 17-3), which, in turn, produces hypokalemia.[79] The clinical manifestations of accelerated hypertension are well described (see Chapter 70, Hypertensive Emergencies).

Renal Artery Stenosis

Renal artery hypoperfusion may induce hyperreninemia and therefore elevate angiotensin levels and serum aldosterone levels, which in turn produces hypokalemia (see Fig. 17-3).[80] The salient clinical manifestations of renal artery stenosis are hypertension with an abdominal bruit.

Hemangiopericytoma or Robertson-Kihara Syndrome

A tumor of the juxtaglomerular cells may cause them to produce an excessive amount of renin.[43,44] The condition, called hemangiopericytoma or Robertson-Kihara syndrome, is characterized by hypertension, hyperreninemia, hyperaldosteronism, and hypokalemia.

Adrenogenital Syndrome

A disease in which there is a defect in the synthesis of adrenocorticoids is referred to as an adrenogenital syndrome. Many of these syndromes result in masculinization. A defect in hydrocortisone synthesis of the zona fasciculata of the adrenal cortex, due to 11-hydroxylase or 17-hydroxylase deficiency, may produce hypertension and hypokalemia in association with the adrenogenital syndrome.[43,44]

Because glucocorticoid levels are diminished in patients with these hydroxylase deficiencies, the pituitary gland secretes more ACTH to maintain adequate glucocorticoid levels. The glucocorticoid that substitutes for hydrocortisone is desoxycorticosterone. The elevated ACTH level also stimulates the zona glomerulosa of the adrenal cortex to synthesize aldosterone, thereby producing hypertension and hypokalemia.

The elevated ACTH levels and the blocked synthesis of hydrocortisone make it necessary for other glucocorticoid synthetic pathways to be used; this results in glucocorticoids with strong androgenic and masculinizing effects. Therefore, this syndrome often is seen in females who have had masculinized features from birth. A masculinized male patient may be less obvious. In addition, childhood hypertension suggests an adrenogenital syndrome.

Licorice Extract (Glycyrrhizic Acid)

Within licorice is a substance called glycyrrhizic acid that is biochemically similar to aldosterone and has many of the same clinical effects as aldosterone.[81] This substance is found in pipe tobacco and extracts for alcoholic beverages.[82] It can cause hypertension, hypokalemia, and laboratory evidence of hyperaldosteronism (ie, a low plasma renin value unresponsive to provocative measures but a low level of serum aldosterone).[81,82]

Clinical Manifestations

A low serum potassium level results in impaired neuromuscular function with profound weakness and cramping of skeletal muscle, leading to impaired ventilation or even rhabdomyolysis, and smooth muscle, producing distention and ileus.[43] In addition, hypokalemia may produce a nephrogenic diabetes insipidus and hyposthenuria (see above), referred to as hypokalemic nephropathy.[44]

The ECG shows decreased amplitude and broadening of T waves, prominent U waves, sagging ST segments, and, at times, T-wave inversion in precordial leads and prolongation of the PR interval. The QT interval often appears prolonged because the T wave is difficult to discern from the U wave; however, it is actually of normal duration. This is referred to as pseudo–QT interval prolongation.[54] The best lead to measure the QT interval is V_L, where the U waves are the smallest.[54]

Hypokalemia potentiates the toxicity of digitalized patients. Atrioventricular conduction defects, ventricular ectopic beats, tachycardias, ventricular fibrillation, or asystole also may occur. Hypokalemia decreases the effectiveness of vasoconstrictive pressors.[72] Myopathy may be severe enough to cause rhabdomyolysis and myoglobulinuria.[43]

Diagnosis

The method by which a potassium value is obtained may strongly affect the result. Hemolysis, which may occur during phlebotomy when the tourniquet remains too long on the arm, may profoundly elevate a serum potassium value. In addition, agitation of a blood sample by passing it through a small-bore needle rapidly or by shaking the sample of blood in a glass tube may cause lysis of erythrocytes.

The serum should be rapidly separated from the cellular elements in the blood sample to obtain an accurate potassium value. If the blood components are not separated for prolonged periods of time, potassium will "leak" from the intracellular space into the serum, artificially raising potassium values. This effect is most prominent in patients with marked thrombocytosis or leukocytosis and produces a pseudohyperkalemia. Some patients have particularly "leaky" cells—a trait that is inherited on an autosomal dominant basis. These "leaky" cells are of no clinical concern, except that they routinely elevate the serum potassium level unless blood samples have the cellular elements rapidly separated from the serum.

Hyperviscosity, as occurs in dehydration or Waldenström's macroglobulinemia, may artificially lower the serum potassium level by decreasing the amount of fluid that can be aspirated by the roller pump diluters of the automated blood analyzers.[25] It is recommended that, if a potassium abnormality is significant and important, a repeat value should be obtained by means of a different technique before intensive therapy for the abnormality is undertaken. The repeat value should be determined from an arterial blood sample that was obtained without a tourniquet on the arm during a phlebotomy.[83] In addition, rapid centrifugation of a plasma sample is preferable.

The ECG changes seen with hypokalemia may raise the index of suspicion for this abnormality even before the potassium value has been determined. The characteristic ECG changes are seen in 75% of patients with a potassium value of less than 3 mEq/L. Occasionally, the characteristic ECG changes of hypokalemia are seen in patients with a normal serum potassium but a depleted total body store of potassium.

Therapy

The following is a useful guide for the estimation of potassium deficits[6]:

- In patients with potassium values of 3 to 3.5 mEq/L, the associated deficit in total body potassium is 150 to 200 mEq.
- Potassium values of 2.5 to 3 mEq/L are associated with a total body potassium deficit of 300 mEq.
- Potassium values of 2 to 2.5 mEq/L are associated with a total body potassium deficit of 500 mEq.

Asymptomatic without Arrhythmias

In patients who are asymptomatic and do not have arrhythmias, one half of the potassium deficit can be replaced over 24 hours and the remainder replaced over the next 48 hours. It is important to account for any urinary losses of potassium that occur during this potassium replacement. In general, the physician should not correct a potassium deficit until an adequate urine output is ensured. In patients who have an asymptomatic hypokalemia without any arrhythmias, the oral route is preferable, provided an ileus is not present and the patient can ingest and absorb oral potassium. The effervescent solution of potassium marketed as Klorvess has been independently evaluated as the best tasting of the oral potassium preparations.[84] In addition, Klorvess is as inexpensive as potassium chloride solution. Potassium chloride salt found in Morton's salt substitute contains 27 mEq of potassium chloride in each one-half teaspoon and is 15-fold less expensive than potassium chloride solution. Morton's salt substitute is an acceptable oral regimen for potassium chloride replacement.[85] If the cause of the hypokalemia is unclear, these patients should be referred to an internist.

Mildly to Moderately Symptomatic without Arrhythmias

The treatment of the patient with mildly to moderately symptomatic hypokalemia without dysrhythmias requires more aggressive potassium replacement than the asymptomatic patient. One half of the deficit of serum potassium should be replaced over the first 12 hours of therapy, with the remainder of the deficit replaced over the next 24 hours. The physician should not replace potassium until adequate urine output is ensured, and all urine potassium lost during replacement must be considered. If possible, the oral route is preferable, and the recommendations for treatment of the asymptomatic hypokalemic patient can be followed. If oral therapy cannot be instituted, then intravenous therapy is indicated. During intravenous therapy ECG monitoring is desirable, since potassium is being administered more rapidly to these patients.

Patients with mildly to moderately symptomatic hypokalemia without dysrhythmias should be admitted to the hospital if the etiology of the hypokalemia is unclear or if oral therapy is not possible, since prolonged therapy over a 36-hour period is indicated.

Severely Symptomatic with Arrhythmias

Patients with severe hypokalemia that causes impaired ventilation, rhabdomyolysis, or dysrhythmias (eg, ventricular tachycardia) require urgent treatment. One half of the potassium deficit should be replaced over the first 6 hours and the remainder replaced over the next 24 hours. For this type of therapy, the intravenous route and ECG monitoring are essential. Potassium chloride at a rate of 40 mEq/hour or in solutions containing more than 40 mEq of potassium should be administered only with ECG monitoring.[6] More than 60 mEq/hour should not be administered except under the most extraordinary circumstances. Potassium should not be administered through a central venous catheter because local hyperkalemia may result in myocardial arrhythmias, heart block, or asystole.[86]

All patients with hypokalemia who are severely symptomatic or manifest arrhythmias due to their hypokalemia should be admitted to the hospital.

Therapy of Specific Causes of Hypokalemia

The therapy of Bartter's syndrome is aided by the use of indomethacin.[62]

The therapy of periodic paralysis involves acetazolamide, which produces a metabolic acidosis and decreases the ability of potassium to enter the intracellular fluid. In addition, these patients are usually placed on spironolactone, which encourages the development of hyperkalemia because it is an aldosterone antagonist.[43,44,69]

Prehospital and Nursing Care

The signs and symptoms of hypokalemia are only suggestive and are highly nonspecific. Only supportive therapy should be instituted before the serum potassium value is known. Clearly, an intravenous catheter should be placed in any patient with significant dysrhythmias.

HYPERKALEMIA

Etiology

Hyperkalemia is one of the most serious electrolytic disturbances and can be immediately life threatening. The emergency physician must be familiar with its etiology.

Pseudohyperkalemia

As mentioned earlier, potassium may "leak" into the serum of patients with thrombocytosis or leukocytosis if the serum is not rapidly removed from the cellular elements.[44] In fact, there is a familial disorder, inherited as an autosomal dominant trait, in which the erythrocytes "leak" potassium in vitro; however, these patients do not have a true elevated serum potassium value,[87] and the condition is of no clinical concern.

Increased Exogenous Potassium Load

Patients with normal renal function can handle large amounts of exogenous potassium, but patients with renal failure may develop hyperkalemia with even small amounts of exogenous potassium. For example, whole blood more than ten days old contains potassium in amounts of 10 to 15 mEq/L and may cause hyperkalemia if administered in large quantities.[88] Both potassium penicillin and oral or intravenous potassium may result in hyperkalemia in patients with any degree of renal failure.[6]

Increased Potassium Production

Tissue destruction may increase the amount of potassium released from the intracellular fluid.[44] This cellular damage occurs in patients with massive crush injury, burns, gangrene, and rhabdomyolysis. Destruction of tumors, such as lymphomas and leukemias, may also damage cells.

The administration of succinylcholine, a depolarizing muscle relaxant, produces muscle contraction and fasciculations that occur before paralysis. These extensive muscular reactions may also induce the release of additional potassium from the muscles and result in hyperkalemia.[89-91] These effects of succinylcholine may be prevented by pretreatment of the patient with diazepam before the administration of succinylcholine.

Transcellular Shifts

Shifting of potassium from the intracellular space to the extracellular space may be responsible for hyperkalemia.

Acute digitalis overdose. Digitalis inhibits the sodium-potassium adenosine triphosphate system, which maintains a normal sodium-potassium gradient in cells.[44] Through this inhibition, excessive amounts of potassium are permitted to remain in the extracellular space, resulting in hyperkalemia.

Periodic paralysis. Patients with periodic paralysis are usually under 10 years of age. The onset of paralysis is abrupt, occurring over a period of 30 minutes; paralysis persists for less than 12 hours. These patients have an increased urinary potassium level but a decreased urinary sodium level. This hyperkalemia is associated with hyponatremia and metabolic acidosis.[44]

Hyperosmolar diuresis. The administration of hypertonic solutions, such as mannitol, may cause a diuresis. Potassium may shift from the intracellular space to the extracellular space,[92] resulting in hyperkalemia.

Acidosis. The mechanism by which acidosis causes hyperkalemia has been discussed (see above). Hyperkalemia in the presence of acidosis is much more prominent in hyperchloremic metabolic acidosis (as with administration of arginine hydrochloride) than in increased anion gap metabolic acidosis.

Decreased renal potassium excretion. Patients with acute or chronic renal failure are unable to excrete potassium. Some patients have a selective renal defect in the excretion of potassium into the distal tubule and, therefore, develop hyperkalemia.

Aldosterone antagonism or deficit. Patients on potassium-sparing diuretics such as triamterene or the aldosterone antagonist, spironolactone, may develop hyperkalemia. Patients with hypoaldosteronism due to Addison's disease or hypopituitarism also may have hyperkalemia.[44]

Juxtaglomerular Hypoplasia

The juxtaglomerular apparatus produces renin (see Fig. 17-3). Some patients have a juxtaglomerular hypoplasia and, therefore, have a hyporeninemic hypoaldosteronism.[93,94] Even when these patients stand or ingest diuretics, the hyporeninemia and the hypoaldosteronism persist. These patients usually have mild to moderate renal disease. This condition is associated with diabetes mellitus, gout, pseudogout, or hyperparathyroidism.[95] Although rare, some patients have a selective deficit in their aldosterone secretion; however, patients with this selective hypoaldosteronism have normal renin levels.[44,96]

Adrenogenital Syndrome

In the form of the adrenogenital syndrome with the 21-hydroxylase deficiency, patients do not synthesize aldosterone.[97] This deficit in the synthesis of aldosterone produces masculinization from birth, hyperkalemia, and salt wasting at the renal level. These patients are normotensive, owing to the effect of other corticosteroids and angiotensin.

Miscellaneous

Heparin and acute barium poisoning may also cause hyperkalemia.

Clinical Manifestations

The ECG provides critical information to the emergency physician. The earliest manifestations of hyperkalemia with potassium values greater than 7 mEq/L are prominent, tall, peaked T waves. Only 20% of patients with potassium values of 7 mEq/L have such T waves.[98]

Potassium values of 8 to 10 mEq/L produce prolonged PR and QRS intervals and decreased P-wave height. At these values, the ST segment may be elevated. Superimposed on the previously mentioned ECG abnormalities, a classic sine wave pattern of hyperkalemia occurs.[53,54] This pattern is frequently accompanied by bradycardia and sudden asystole, without intervening ventricular fibrillation.

Diagnosis

Hyperkalemia should be suspected in the emergency department even before laboratory values have been obtained. In addition, ECG monitoring of any patient with a potassium value of more than 6.5 mEq/L should be initiated at once because hyperkalemia with ECG findings requires immediate therapy.

The differential diagnosis of hyperkalemia is based on the findings on the ECG. Tall, peaked T waves may be found congenitally or may occur early in patients with acute myocardial infarction. The broad QRS complex seen in patients with hyperkalemia must be distinguished from that caused by a left bundle branch block. In hyperkalemia, the left precordial leads show a wide S wave that is not found in patients with left bundle branch block. It is impossible to distinguish a slow, wide complex idioventricular rhythm of an agonal heart from the effects of hyperkalemia.[53]

Therapy

In patients with potassium values less than 7 mEq/L and no ECG changes, it is important to reverse the underlying cause. If this is not possible, the emergency physician should administer sodium polystyrene sulfonate (Kayexalate) to maintain serum potassium values less than 5.5 mEq/L. Kayexalate is a sodium-potassium cation resin that exchanges 2 mEq of sodium for each 1 mEq of potassium. One mEq of the total body potassium store is removed per gram of Kayexalate.[6] The dose of Kayexalate, if administered orally, is 20 g three times a day with 50 mL of 20% mannitol. The mannitol is a cathartic and is added because Kayexalate is highly constipating. This dose of Kayexalate contains 120 mEq sodium per day.[44] These patients should be admitted to the hospital if the cause of the hyperkalemia is unclear or the hyperkalemia proves difficult to reverse. In any case, they should be referred to an internist.

In patients with potassium values more than 7 mEq/L and either no ECG changes or only tall, peaked T waves, it is also important to reverse the underlying cause. These patients should receive Kayexalate to remove potassium from the body. Dosage is the same as that just described.

In patients who are obtunded, Kayexalate can be administered as a 50-g retention enema in 200 mL of mannitol every 1 to 2 hours. Each dose so administered decreases the serum potassium value 0.25 to 0.50 mEq. All patients in this category should be admitted to the hospital.

Severe Hyperkalemia

Patients with hyperkalemia and a broad QRS complex, a prolonged PR interval, or a decreased P-wave height in the appropriate clinical setting, for example, in the presence of renal disease, should receive treatment even before the potassium value returns from the laboratory. The institution of therapy must be immediate—these ECG findings represent a life-threatening emergency.

Calcium gluconate. A first-line drug to be administered to patients with this severe hyperkalemia is calcium gluconate. It increases the permeability of the cell membrane to potassium and immediately reverses electrophysiologic manifestations of hyperkalemia. One to three ampules or 4 to 12 mEq of a 10% solution of calcium gluconate should be administered over 3 to 5 minutes.[44] The patient's ECG should be monitored. The effect of calcium gluconate has its onset within 1 to 5 minutes, but its duration of action is brief, only 30 minutes. More long-lasting therapy is needed.

Glucose-insulin infusion. An important second-line therapy for hyperkalemia is glucose-insulin infusion; it should be administered promptly. The dose is 1 U of insulin per 3 to 4 g of glucose. In a typical solution, 500 mL of 10% dextrose in water is administered with 15 U of regular insulin. This solution should be administered over 30 minutes and the infusion slowed to maintain normokalemia. The onset of action is 30 minutes, and the duration is 4 to 5 hours.[6,44,99]

Sodium bicarbonate. When the acid-base status of the patient is unknown or if the patient is alkalotic, 80 to 120 mEq of sodium bicarbonate in 1 L of 5% dextrose and water should be administered over 1 to 2 hours. This therapy is effective within 20 to 40 minutes, and the duration of its action is 4 to 5 hours. When the acid-base status of the patient, however, shows metabolic acidosis, 80 to 120 mEq of sodium bicarbonate may be administered over 2 to 3 minutes.[44]

Kayexalate. Either orally or by retention enema, Kayexalate should be administered in all patients with severe hyperkalemia. The administration of Kayexalate should not be delayed in the emergency department.

Dialysis. Hemodialysis or peritoneal dialysis is the treatment of choice for hyperkalemia in a patient with moderate to severe renal failure. These patients cannot tolerate the high sodium load that is concomitantly administered with Kayexalate. In addition, any patient who does not respond appropriately to therapy with calcium gluconate, glucose-insulin infusion, sodium bicarbonate, and Kayexalate should be considered for immediate dialysis.

Specific Therapy

Patients with a renal potassium defect should receive diuretics, such as hydrochlorothiazide or furosemide (Lasix), which tend to induce a more normokalemic situation.

Patients with hyporeninemic hypoaldosteronism, selective hypoaldosteronism, or adrenogenital syndrome need mineralocorticoid replacement. The synthetic mineralocorticoid 9α-fluorohydrocortisone (Florinef) may be administered at a dose of 0.1 mg/day.

Prehospital and Nursing Care

If the prehospital care team notes the ECG findings of hyperkalemia in the presence of hypotension, dysrhythmias, electrical mechanical dissociation, or cardiac arrest, immediate therapy is required. Therapy with calcium gluconate, glucose-insulin, and sodium bicarbonate should be instituted as noted. If calcium gluconate is unavailable, calcium chloride may be substituted.

A nurse recognizing ECG manifestations of hyperkalemia should immediately establish an intravenous catheter and obtain a potassium value. The patient should have bedside ECG monitoring. Calcium chloride should be placed at the patient's bedside and the physician notified immediately.

CALCIUM

Physiology

The serum calcium level is affected by several different factors. Parathormone, a hormone secreted by the parathyroid gland, maintains serum calcium by stimulating osteoclastic activity that mobilizes the bony stores of calcium.[100] The renal mechanism involves the conversion of adenosine triphosphate (ATP) to cAMP, a second messenger that affects parathormone action and causes renal tubular excretion of phosphate and reabsorption of calcium and chloride. Parathormone also facilitates transport of calcium across the duodenal mucosa. Parathormone is controlled by feedback inhibition in which hypercalcemia suppresses parathormone secretion.

Vitamin D or calciferol, after absorption, is 25-hydroxylated in the liver and subsequently 1-hydroxylated in the kidney to form the active vitamin D, 1,25-hydroxycalciferol. This active form increases calcium absorption from the gastrointestinal tract.[101]

Calcium is 50% protein bound, mostly to albumin. Calcium values obtained from the laboratory reflect total calcium, that is, free plus protein-bound calcium.[100] This protein-bound calcium is in equilibrium with free calcium, and this balance is affected by the acid-base status of the patient. The free calcium is responsible for symptoms of either hypercalcemia or hypocalcemia. If albumin decreases 0.8 to 1 g/dL, then total calcium diminishes 0.8 to 1 mg/dL, owing to the decrease in protein-bound calcium.[100] The free calcium, however, remains unchanged.

Alkalosis increases the electronegativity of proteins, so that more calcium is bound to the proteins and less calcium is free; therefore, symptoms of hypocalcemia may occur.[100] A respiratory condition such as respiratory alkalosis in association with hyperventilation may reduce the level of free calcium in the serum and produce symptoms identical to those of hypocalcemia. During alkalosis, total calcium (bound plus free) does not change; since the laboratory routinely measures only total calcium, this value is normal in the presence of alkalosis.

Acidosis decreases the electronegativity of proteins; therefore, less calcium is bound to proteins, and more calcium is free. Again, total calcium value remains unchanged.

Pathophysiology

Elevated levels of calcium stimulate the production of gastrin, which increases acid secretion and predisposes to peptic ulcer disease and pancreatitis.[100-104] Patients who have experienced prolonged periods of hypercalcemia may develop renal stones or nephrolithiasis or calcifications throughout the kidney, termed *nephrocalcinosis*, and renal failure.[105]

Hypercalcemia has marked effects on the ECG. It shortens the duration of phase 2 of the action potential and causes a shortening of the ST segment on the ECG (see above).[106] In addition, calcium increases the duration of the ventricular ejection and causes a prolonged inotropic action.

Hypocalcemia has several important pathophysiological effects. A chronically low level of calcium in the serum and a high level of calcium in the lens results in cataracts.[100,107] Low levels of calcium, in addition, prevent troponin from inhibiting actin-myosin interaction; therefore, muscle contraction and even tetany may occur.[100,107]

The cardiac effects of hypocalcemia include a prolongation of the duration of phase 2 of the action potential, thereby causing a prolonged ST segment on the ECG.[106] Hypocalcemia is the only cause of a prolonged ST segment. In addition, hypocalcemia shortens the duration of ventricular ejection.

HYPERCALCEMIA

Etiology

Carcinoma

The most common cause of hypercalcemia is carcinoma; in one series the incidence was 20%.[108-110] There are several mechanisms by which carcinoma produces hypercalcemia. Metastatic disease may induce bony destruction and thereby cause calcium release. Certain tumors may produce a parathormone-like substance that also causes the release of calcium. The mechanism of hypercalcemia in some tumors is unclear, but, in some manner, prostaglandin E_2 seems to be involved.[108,109,111–113] The cancers most often associated with hypercalcemia are those of lung, breast, and kidney, and multiple myeloma. The prognosis of patients with multiple myeloma and hypercalcemia is particularly poor.[114,115]

Hyperparathyroidism

The incidence of hyperparathyroidism is 2 per 100 cases of hypercalcemia. Hyperparathyroidism is frequently diagnosed in asymptomatic patients by means of automated chemistry tests.[116–118] In 80% of cases, the pathogenesis is an adenoma of the parathyroid. In 15 percent of the cases, it is diffuse hyperplasia of the parathyroid glands.[119]

With primary hyperparathyroidism, calcium values may be high or simply high-normal with an inappropriately high value of parathormone. Since parathormone increases the tubular reabsorption of chloride and enhances the secretion of phosphorus, a high chloride to phosphorus ratio, that is, more than 33:1, is maintained in 96% of cases.[120] The serum chloride value is almost invariably more than 102 mEq/L unless the patient has received diuretics; because diuretics enhance chloride secretion, the physician cannot use this criterion in a patient on diuretics.[109] In addition, diuretics such as thiazide may increase the serum calcium level.[100] Since parathormone functions by a cAMP mechanism, the urinary cAMP value also is elevated in cases of primary hyperparathyroidism.

In hyperparathyroidism, there is prominent resorption of subperiosteal bone of the fingers and toes.[119] There is a central resorption of the vertebrae, resulting in alternating radiolucent and radiodense areas of the vertebrae. Owing to excess parathormone secretion, bony cysts may result from resorption of bone; this is called osteitis fibrosa cystica.[119] A late finding in hyperparathyroidism is resorption of the distal one third of the clavicle.

Patients with suspected hyperparathyroidism should be referred to an internist.

Multiple Endocrine Adenopathies

Patients with a type I multiple endocrine adenopathy (eg, Wermer's syndrome) have adenomas in multiple endocrine organs.[100] Hypercalcemia is due to adenomas of the parathyroid. These patients may also have adenomas of the pituitary, adrenal cortex, pancreas, and, less commonly, the adrenal medulla and thyroid gland. Sipple's syndrome, a type II multiple endocrine adenopathy, consists of adenomas of the parathyroid, explaining the hypercalcemia; adenomas of the adrenal medulla with pheochromocytoma; and medullary carcinoma of the thyroid.[100]

Sarcoidosis

Hypercalcemia may occur in association with sarcoidosis. In sarcoidosis there is increased gastrointestinal absorption of calcium and increased reabsorption of bone.[121,122]

Vitamin D

With excessive amounts of exogenous vitamin D (more than 150,000 U/day), gastrointestinal absorption of calcium may be increased.[123,124] These patients are frequently health food faddists. Laboratory examination reveals an elevated serum phosphorus level because the hypercalcemia suppresses parathormone levels.[100] These low parathormone levels, in turn, diminish tubular secretion of phosphorus.

Immobilization

During periods of immobilization, bony stores of calcium are mobilized in children and young adults, and hypercalcemia may occur.[100] Elderly patients with Paget's disease who are immobilized have increased osteoclastic activity that mobilizes their bony calcium stores, and they may also develop hypercalcemia.[100]

Renal Failure

Patients with chronic renal failure are unable to excrete calcium and therefore should be cautioned against excessive calcium intake. An increased calcium load in the presence of acute renal failure may result in hypercalcemia.[125,126] Calcium released during rhabdomyolysis, for example, may produce hypercalcemia because of the diminished ability of the kidney to excrete calcium. Classically, this occurs during the diuretic phase of acute tubular necrosis in patients with rhabdomyolysis.

Milk-Alkali Syndrome (Burnett's Syndrome)

Increased intake of calcium in the form of calcium carbonate antacids and milk in the treatment of peptic ulcer disease has been associated with severe hypercalcemia and nephrocalcinosis.[127] With the use of other treatments for peptic ulcer disease, this syndrome has markedly decreased in frequency.

Miscellaneous

Other conditions, such as hyperthyroidism (20% incidence), acromegaly, pheochromocytoma, and Addison's disease (endocrinopathies), are occasionally associated with hypercalcemia.[100,108,128,129]

Renal Transplant

During the first six months after surgery, renal transplant patients have a mild hypercalcemia.[130]

Thiazide Diuretics

Interference of thiazide diuretics with the renal excretion of calcium may lead to hypercalcemia.[100]

Idiopathic Hypercalcemia of Infancy

Patients with idiopathic hypercalcemia of infancy have enhanced vitamin D synthesis, which produces hypercalcemia. Some cases are associated with supravalvular aortic stenosis.[131]

Clinical Manifestations

The symptoms of mild hypercalcemia are subtle and difficult to discern. These symptoms are quite similar to typical functional complaints: malaise, weakness, anorexia, and arthralgia. In contrast, severe hypercalcemia results in nausea and vomiting, constipation and obstipation, polyuria, polydipsia, altered mental status, and hyporeflexia. In patients with prolonged hypercalcemia, calcium deposits in the lens or brand keratopathy, nephrocalcinosis, or nephrogenic diabetes insipidus may be present.[119,132,133]

Because hypercalcemia shortens phase 2 of the action potential, a short ST segment may be noted on the ECG.[106] The interval, Q-aTc, defined as the time lapse from the beginning of the Q wave to the apex of the T wave measured in seconds divided by the square root of the R-R interval as measured in seconds,[134] is generally less than 0.29 second in hypercalcemia.

$$\text{Q-aTc} = \frac{\text{Q-aT (sec)}}{\sqrt{\text{R-R (sec)}}} \quad (2)$$

Hypercalcemia markedly increases the sensitivity of the heart to digitalis and may induce digitalis toxicity. Therefore, in patients on digitalis, therapy with calcium-containing agents should be avoided.[135]

Diagnosis

Technical artifacts may affect serum calcium values. If the tourniquet is left around a vein for too long (2 to 3 minutes), a transudate may exude from the intravascular space to the interstitial space, leaving a more highly concentrated sample of blood with a high concentration of protein-bound calcium to be assayed for serum calcium level. This may elevate the serum calcium level from 0.5 to 1.5 mg/dL.[136] In addition, erythrocytes may nonspecifically adsorb calcium to their surface and artifactually lower the serum calcium level.[136] Also, the cork stoppers supplied with some tubes of blood may cause a false hypercalcemia.[137]

It is recommended that, if the routine sample shows hypercalcemia, an arterial sample be obtained. An arterial sample is reliable[136] and can be obtained without a tourniquet. It is important not to use anticoagulants, however. For example, edetic acid and oxalates may chelate calcium and falsely lower the serum calcium level. Also, only blood tubes with rubber stoppers should be used.

Treatment

Only patients with symptomatic hypercalcemia should be treated.[6,100,138] The initial treatment of all patients with hypercalcemia is to administer normal saline. A rate of at least 400 mL/hour for 6 hours to induce diuresis is recommended. It is important to try to maintain the urine output at a brisk pace, approximately 300 mL/hour and 5 to 10 L/day.[6] To increase the urine flow, some patients may need a potent diuretic, such as furosemide.[100] It must be recognized that many of these patients are dehydrated. Evaluation of intravascular volume by either neck vein distention or central venous pressure is desirable to maintain the appropriate level of hydration. During this rapid diuresis, it is also important to monitor levels of serum potassium and magnesium, which may be lost in the urine.[138]

If therapy with normal saline has been unsuccessful, the second-line therapy is mithramycin, an antibiotic and antitumor agent that blocks the resorption of bone and inhibits DNA-dependent RNA synthesis.[139,140] This drug is administered in doses of 25 to 50 μg/kg. The effect begins within 1 hour and peaks at 2 to 3 days.[139,140] The notable side effects with this drug are nausea and vomiting.

Calcitonin, secreted by the thyroid gland, mobilizes calcium into bone.[141] In some medical centers it is actively used for the treatment of hypercalcemia, and there have been few side effects. This drug has a rapid onset of action and is given intravenously at 4 U/kg with repeat doses at 12 to 24 hours. Twenty percent to 25% of patients may not respond, and even in those that respond, resistance may develop. However, resistance may be avoidable with concomitant steroid administration.[142]

Edetic acid and phosphate were formerly used in the therapy of hypercalcemia.[143] Normal saline, mithramycin, and calcitonin are less toxic and have replaced these drugs in the treatment of hypercalcemia.

Indomethacin inhibits prostaglandin E_2 and is especially effective in treatment of hypercalcemia associated with metastatic carcinoma. This drug is not effective for the management of acute hypercalcemia, however, because its effect is delayed several days.[144,145]

The mechanism by which corticosteroids inhibit hypercalcemia is not clear. They may inhibit vitamin D, which mediates calcium absorption. Corticosteroids inhibit hypercalcemia associated with vitamin D intoxication, multiple myeloma, sarcoidosis, carcinoma, and, very rarely, hyperparathyroidism.[146-150] Prednisone is given orally 40 mg/day for 7 to 10 days. Corticosteroids do not control acute hypercalcemia, but they are useful for the differential diagnosis and treatment of chronic hypercalcemia.

Prehospital and Nursing Care

Patients with hypercalcemia require no special prehospital or nursing assessment or intervention. Those with newly symptomatic hypercalcemia should be admitted to the hospital. All those with symptomatic hypercalcemia should be under the care of an internist.

HYPOCALCEMIA

Etiology

DiGeorge's Syndrome

Congenital absence of the third and fourth branchial pouches results in an absent thymus and absent T lymphocytes, as well as a congenitally absent parathyroid gland. This is called DiGeorge's syndrome. These patients have profound hypocalcemia.[151]

Hypoparathyroidism

The autosomal dominant form of idiopathic hypoparathyroidism is associated with candidiasis, hypogonadism, hypoadrenocorticism, and pernicious anemia.[152] The sex-linked variety of idiopathic hypoparathyroidism manifests itself early in life as neonatal tetany.[153–155]

Acquired hypoparathyroidism occurs commonly after thyroidectomies or parathyroidectomies.[155] Rarely, tumors of the neck, as in carcinoma, may infiltrate the parathyroid gland. Amyloid may infiltrate the parathyroid, resulting in hypoparathyroidism.[156,157] Medullary carcinoma of the thyroid may produce enough calcitonin to induce hypocalcemia, but this is unusual. Most cases of medullary carcinoma of the thyroid do not secrete enough active calcitonin to lower the serum calcium level.[142]

Hypomagnesemia

A low serum magnesium may cause hypocalcemia by inhibiting parathormone secretion and, thus, its action at the level of the renal tubules.[158–160]

Vitamin D Deficiency

Patients whose vitamin D intake or exposure to sunlight is inadequate may have vitamin D deficiency.[161,162] Since vitamin D is fat soluble, patients with steatorrhea (eg, those with malabsorption syndromes) may have vitamin D deficiency. Malabsorption is a relatively common cause of vitamin D deficiency and hypocalcemia. When vitamin D deficiency and hypocalcemia are prolonged, osteomalacia may result.

Pseudohypoparathyroidism

Patients with pseudohypoparathyroidism, an X-linked dominant trait, demonstrate a marked unresponsiveness to parathormone.[155,163] These patients have characteristic features: round face, short neck; short stature; squat appearance; short, stubby fingers; mental retardation; cataracts; short fourth metacarpal; thick calvaria, and calcifications in the basal ganglia.

Pseudo-pseudohypoparathyroidism is also an X-linked dominant trait. These patients have the somatic features of pseudohypoparathyroidism; however, they have no hypocalcemia.[155,163]

Acute Pancreatitis

In acute pancreatitis, release of parathormone is decreased. It was formerly believed that saponification of calcium by fats released by lipase during pancreatitis caused this hypocalcemia, but this is probably not the mechanism.[164] Serum calcium levels of less than 7 mg/dL correlate with a poor prognosis in hemorrhagic pancreatitis.[165]

Uremia

The mechanism of hypocalcemia in patients with uremia reflects a defect in the conversion of vitamin D into its active form by the kidney (see Chapter 78, Renal Failure).

Diuresis

During diuresis, there is an obligatory calcium loss. Hypocalcemia may accompany the severe diuresis associated with an overdose of a diuretic.

Acute Renal Failure

Hypocalcemia may occasionally accompany acute renal failure.[100]

Massive Transfusion of Blood

During the massive transfusion of blood, citrate, which is used as an anticoagulant in blood, chelates calcium.[161] During massive transfusions, it is important to follow the patient for symptoms of hypocalcemia, prolongation of the QT interval, or low serum calcium values. Some physicians prefer to give 4 to 10 mEq of calcium routinely for each 6 U of whole blood transfused.[100]

Clinical Manifestations

Acute hypocalcemia is manifested by paresthesias; altered mental status, especially surreal feelings; carpal or pedal spasm; irritability; Chvostek's sign (ie, facial spasm, especially at the corner of the lip, caused by tapping along the facial nerve with reflex hammer [this test may be positive in 10% of healthy patients]); and Trousseau's sign (ie, severely painful carpal spasm induced by elevation of blood pressure cuff over the systolic pressure for 3 minutes). In severe cases, opisthotonus, tetany, and general or focal seizures may be seen.[100,161,166]

Patients with chronic hypocalcemia may also have a decrease in hair in the eyebrows, eyelashes, and pubic and axillary regions.[106,155,161] In addition, there is an increased predisposition for these patients to develop cataracts.[161]

Owing to the prolongation of phase 2 of the action potential, there is a prolongation of the ST segment of the QT interval. As mentioned earlier, hypocalcemia is the only cause of QT interval prolongation due to elongation of the ST segment.[106] The QTc is the interval from the beginning of the QRS complex to the terminal part of the T wave measured in seconds divided by the square root of the RR interval as measured in seconds.[167] This calculation is similar to that for the Q-aTC (see Eq. 2).

$$QTc = \frac{QT \text{ (sec)}}{\sqrt{RR \text{ (sec)}}} \quad (3)$$

The QTc calculation takes into account the effect of heart rate on QT interval prolongation (Table 17-2).

Treatment

In the treatment of hypocalcemia,[6,100,165,168] parenteral medication is indicated only for the treatment of symptomatic hypocalcemia. For symptomatic patients, 10 mL of 10% calcium gluconate (4 mEq per 19 mL) should be administered at 2 mEq/min. This drug should be administered at a much slower rate of infusion if the patient is receiving digoxin. The administration of calcium gluconate can be titrated to the patient's symptoms. However, it seems wise not to administer more than 50 mEq of calcium gluconate without checking the serum calcium level, even in a symptomatic patient. In such a patient, the persistent symptomatology may be due more to hypomagnesemia than to hypocalcemia.

Although calcium chloride contains more available calcium (14 mEq per 10 mL), it causes massive tissue necrosis when infiltrated. Therefore, calcium gluconates are preferable in situations other than cardiac arrest, since they do not cause tissue necrosis.[169,170]

Another preparation, calcium gluceptate, is suitable for intramuscular use, although it is irritating to muscle.[170]

A patient with asymptomatic hypocalcemia may be treated with various preparations of calcium. Calcium gluconate (1 g) or calcium lactate (300 mg) may be required in doses up to 8 gm/day orally.

Various vitamin D preparations have been useful in the treatment of hypocalcemia, the most effective of which is 1,25-hydroxycalciferol (calcitriol), which is the active form of vitamin D and is especially useful in the therapy of patients with uremia. The dosage is 0.2 μg/day, with increments of 0.25 μg/day to 4-week intervals, depending on the clinical response.[171] Exposure to sunlight may induce calcitriol production and may be useful in refractory cases.[162]

If 1,25-hydroxycalciferol is unavailable, 50,000 to 100,000 U of dietary supplementation of calciferol per day may be tried.

Prehospital and Nursing Care

Clinical manifestations such as altered mental status, Chvostek's or Trousseau's sign, muscle cramping or carpopedal spasm should lead the prehospital care team or nursing team to suspect hypocalcemia. Patients with suspected hypocalcemia should have an intravenous line, and blood samples should be obtained for calcium, magnesium, electrolytes, albumin, phosphate, and arterial blood gas studies. If an ST segment prolongation is seen on the ECG, calcium chloride should be available at the bedside.

Patients with newly symptomatic hypocalcemia should be admitted to the hospital. The condition of those with asymptomatic hypocalcemia should be evaluated by an internist, provided the albumin level is normal.

MAGNESIUM

Physiology

In a 70-kg man, there is 2000 mEq of magnesium. One half of this magnesium resides in bone; one third in muscle.[172–174] The serum concentration of magnesium remains remarkably constant, ranging from 1.5 to 2 mEq/L. One third of this is protein bound.[172]

Table 17-2 Effect of Heart Rate on QT Interval

Heart Rate	Lower Limit (sec)	Upper Limit (sec)
40	0.40	0.50
50	0.38	0.46
60	0.35	0.43
70	0.33	0.405
80	0.32	0.38
92.5	0.29	0.36
100	0.29	0.35
109	0.27	0.33
120	0.26	0.32
133	0.25	0.30
150	0.23	0.28

Note: These values vary ± 0.02 sec, depending on sex and age of the patient. *Source:* Caty L: *Electrocardiography.* Philadelphia, Lea & Febiger, 1946.

Magnesium plays an important role in many enzyme systems, especially in reactions involving ATP, because it stabilizes the highly negative charges of the triphosphates in such reactions.[173]

Pathophysiology

Although magnesium deprivation causes seizures in rodents, there has been no evidence to show that magnesium deprivation induces seizures in humans. The subject of magnesium-induced seizures is complicated by the fact that magnesium elevates the threshold for seizures.[172] Early investigators believed that hypomagnesemia, which is commonly found in alcoholic patients, was the cause of alcohol withdrawal seizures.[172]

Like potassium, magnesium metabolism is under the influence of aldosterone. Conditions that are frequently associated with hypokalemia are, therefore, frequently associated with hypomagnesemia. Similarly, hypermagnesemia tends to be found in patients with hypoaldosteronism.[172] There is also an obligatory loss of magnesium in the urine, a loss that increases with vigorous diuresis.[172,174]

HYPOMAGNESEMIA

Etiology

Ethanol Abuse

Ethanol inhibits the reabsorption of magnesium at the level of the proximal tubule. In addition, ethanol enhances the effect of aldosterone on the loss of magnesium at the renal level. Ethanol induces a diabetes insipidus, and the ensuing diuresis also increases the loss of magnesium in the urine.[175,176] For these reasons, hypomagnesemia is frequently found in patients who abuse alcohol.

Diabetic Ketoacidosis

Magnesium levels are usually elevated initially in diabetic ketoacidosis. This is due to the effect of acidosis on serum magnesium. During the vigorous diuresis that ensues during the first three to four hours of therapy for diabetic ketoacidosis, the magnesium level may fall precipitously—to dangerously low levels.[177,178]

Diuresis

Hypomagnesemia may occur in patients during periods of vigorous diuresis, such as diuretic overdose, or in patients on normal doses of diuretics but who have a predisposing cause for hypomagnesemia, such as alcohol abuse.[179]

Digitalis Preparations

Digitalis causes an increased renal excretion of magnesium. Hypomagnesemia in patients on digitalis may be responsible for digitalis toxicity, especially in patients refractory to the usual therapies.[180–184]

Malabsorption

In diarrheal fluid there is a large loss of magnesium. Patients with steatorrhea or malabsorptive syndrome may develop hypomagnesemia.[185–187] Hypomagnesemia also may occur in patients who abuse laxatives.

Hyperalimentation

During total parenteral nutrition, it is important for the physician to ensure that the patient is given an adequate supply of all the less common nutrients. Because of the obligatory magnesium loss in the urine, patients receiving hyperalimentation may develop hypomagnesemia without a continuous intravenous supply of magnesium.[188]

Renal Wasting

There are several causes for renal wasting of magnesium.[172–174] Hypercalcemia may cause diuresis and therefore result in an obligatory magnesium loss. Patients with renal tubular acidosis may have an excess of bicarbonate ion within the tubule that serves as a nondiffusible anion and therefore results in excess magnesium loss in the urine to maintain electrical neutrality. Occasionally, patients receiving gentamicin develop hypomagnesemia. Gentamicin within the renal tubule serves as a nondiffusible anion and, to preserve electrical neutrality, magnesium is lost in the kidneys. Patients with hyperthyroidism may have hypomagnesemia due to renal losses. Some patients have an obligatory magnesium loss in the renal tubules for which no reason has been found. In some patients with chronic renal failure, proximal tubular dysfunction may result in renal wasting of magnesium.[172,173]

Acute Pancreatitis

Some patients with acute pancreatitis develop hypomagnesemia. This association may be due to the high frequency of alcohol abuse among patients with acute pancreatitis.[172] The presence of hypomagnesemia, however, seems to correlate with the presence of hypocalcemia.

Multiple Transfusions

The anticoagulants, such as citrate, that are administered during multiple transfusions, may bind magnesium and result in hypomagnesemia.[172]

Clinical Manifestations

The clinical manifestations of hypomagnesemia are anorexia, nausea, vomiting, and diarrhea; in severe cases, carpopedal spasm, tetany, Chvostek's and Trousseau's signs, tremors, hyperreflexia, and altered mental status may be seen.[189,190]

Studies on the ECG manifestations of hypomagnesemia have been complicated by the fact that many of the patients have other electrolytic abnormalities. In one study to evaluate the effect of hypomagnesemia alone on an ECG, it was noted that hypomagnesemia prolonged the QT interval and resulted in a low QRS complex, and a short, fixed PR interval.[191]

Diagnosis

It is not always necessary to determine the magnesium level when serum electrolytes or calcium are measured, but a magnesium level should be obtained in the presence of hypocalcemia or hypokalemia, during clinical manifestations suggestive of hypocalcemia, or in the presence of any of the conditions that may predispose to hypomagnesemia: digitalis intoxication, diabetic ketoacidosis, alcohol abuse, malabsorption, chronic renal failure, or vigorous diuresis. The value of the magnesium level should be used in a qualitative fashion; it should be considered only an indication of the presence or absence of hypomagnesemia. The absolute magnitude of the level of magnesium does not correlate with the severity of the symptoms or the severity of the deficiency. The clinical signs and symptoms determine if a low serum magnesium value reflects mild, moderate, or severe deficiency.

Not uncommonly, the magnesium level is normal, but the clinical manifestations suggest hypomagnesemia. In this instance, the physician should administer 1 g of magnesium sulfate intravenously and collect the urine for 24 hours. The excretion of less than 80% of the administered dose of magnesium sulfate over 24 hours indicates magnesium deficiency.[192,193]

Treatment

Patients who are asymptomatic with hypomagnesemia should receive 10 to 15 mEq/day orally (8.1 mEq of magnesium = 1 g). Oral absorption is erratic, however. The amount of magnesium that is absorbed orally depends on the magnitude of the deficit. In addition, many oral magnesium preparations are poorly tolerated.[6,173]

Several preparations contain magnesium and may be used for magnesium replacement: Maalox (1.2 g per 30 mL), Mylanta II (2.4 g per 30 mL), Milk of Magnesia (2.5 g per 30 mL).[172]

A patient with symptoms secondary to hypomagnesemia needs parenteral administration of magnesium. In these patients, the deficit is expected to be 1.5 mEq/kg or 100 mEq, or approximately 12 g for a 70-kg man.[6,172,173] Even in the presence of an extreme magnesium deficit, the kidneys excrete more than 50% of an administered dose. Therefore, it is necessary to replace double the calculated magnesium deficit. In general, the physician should correct one half of the deficit, or 12 g in a 70-kg man, during the first 24 hours, and the remainder of the deficit should be corrected over the next 48 to 72 hours.[6,172–174] Six grams of magnesium may be given continuously over 4 to 6 hours intravenously, but no more than 12 g should be administered within 12 hours. Alternatively, 2 g magnesium sulfate can be given intramuscularly every 2 to 4 hours.[194,195]

During the initial replacement of magnesium, the physician must monitor the patient's signs, symptoms, and reflexes in order to guide the rate of therapy; magnesium should be replaced at a slower rate once the patient becomes asymptomatic.

All patients with symptomatic hypomagnesemia should be admitted to the hospital.

HYPERMAGNESEMIA

Etiology

Hypermagnesemia is a rare entity that occurs only in certain clinical situations. Most patients with renal failure, for example, have a diminished ability to excrete potassium from the body. Continued intakes of magnesium, as with antacids, in these patients may result in severe hypermagnesemia.[196] In the treatment of eclampsia of pregnancy, magnesium is administered to elevate the seizure threshold. Some physicians may administer magnesium in excessive quantities in the treatment of alcohol withdrawal seizures. In both these instances, hypermagnesemia occasionally may ensue.[172,173]

Clinical Manifestations

If the level of magnesium is less than 3 mEq/L, the patient is asymptomatic. With values of magnesium of 3 to 9 mEq/L, nausea, vomiting, hypotension, bradycardia, and confusion may be seen.[172] At 5 to 6 mEq/L, the deep tendon reflexes are diminished. At values of magnesium exceeding 10 mEq/L, carbon dioxide narcosis, respiratory depression, paralysis, and hypotension may ensue.

On an ECG, hypermagnesemia may prolong the PR interval, increase the duration of the QRS interval, and occasionally cause heart block.[197]

Diagnosis

The diagnosis of hypermagnesemia is made by obtaining a magnesium level.

Therapy

Calcium neutralizes the effect of magnesium on a milliequivalent per milliequivalent basis. When patients are symptomatic with hypermagnesemia and serum levels are either known or suspected to be 5 to 8 mEq/L, or when a patient is asymptomatic but the level is more than 8 mEq/L, then 5 mL of 10% calcium chloride can be administered intravenously over 30 seconds. If the patient is unimproved, calcium chloride may be repeated in 2 minutes. The effect is prompt.[172,198,199] Since calcium is such a rapid antidote of hypermagnesemia, calcium chloride should be at the bedside of all patients receiving parenteral magnesium therapy.

REFERENCES

1. Friedler RM, Koffler A, Kurokawa K. Hyponatremia and hypernatremia. *Clin Nephrol*. 1977;7:163.
2. Stein JH, Reineck HJ. Regulation of the excretion of sodium and other electrolytes by the collecting duct. *Kidney Int*. 1974;6:1.
3. Bartter F. The syndrome of inappropriate secretion of antidiuretic hormone (SIADH). *DM*. 1973;11:1.
4. Berl T, Anderson RJ, McDonald KM, et al. Clinical disorders of water metabolism. *Kidney Int*. 1976;10:117.
5. Robertson G, Athar S. The interaction of blood osmolality and blood volume in regulating plasma vasopression in man. *J Clin Endocrinol Metab*. 1976;42:613.
6. Lindeman RD, Papper S. Therapy of fluid and electrolyte disorders. *Ann Intern Med*. 1975;82:64.
7. Sweadner KJ, Goldin SM. Active transport of sodium and potassium ions: mechanism, function and regulation. *N Engl J Med*. 1980;302:777.
8. Smithline N, Gardner KD Jr. Gaps—anion and osmolal. *JAMA*. 1976;236:1594.
9. Glasser L, Sternglanz PD, Combie J, et al. Serum osmolarity and its applicability to drug overdose. *Am J Clin Pathol*. 1963;60:695.
10. Arieff AI, Carroll HJ. Non-ketotic hyperosmolar coma with hyperglycemia: clinical features, pathophysiology, renal function, acid-base balance, plasma-cerebrospinal fluid equilibria and the effects of therapy in 37 cases. *Medicine*. 1972;51:73.
11. Sotos JR, Dodge PR, Meara P, et al. Studies in experimental hypertonicity: I. Pathogenesis of the clinical syndrome, biochemical abnormalities and cause of death. *Pediatrics*. 1960;26:925.
12. Arieff AI, Guisado R. Effects of the nervous system of hypernatremic and hyponatremic states. *Kidney Int*. 1976;10:104.
13. Zlerler KL. Hyperosmolarity in adults: a critical review. *J Chronic Dis*. 1958;7:1.
14. Harrington JT, Cohen JJ. Measurements of urinary electrolytes: indications and limitations. *N Engl J Med*. 1975;293:1241.
15. Ross EJ, Christie SBM. Hypernatremia. *Medicine*. 1969;48:441.
16. Keitel HG, Thompson D, Itand HA. Hyposthenuria in sickle cell anemia: a reversible renal defect. *J Clin Invest*. 1956;35:998.
17. Singer I, Forrest N Jr. Drug-induced states of nephrogenic diabetes insipidus. *Kidney Int*. 1976;10:82.
18. Bruck E, Abal G, Aceto T. Pathogenesis and pathophysiology of hypertonic dehydration with diarrhea. *Am J Dis Child*. 1968;115:122.
19. Finberg L, Harrison HE. Hypernatremia in infants: an evaluation of the clinical and biochemical findings accompanying this state. *Pediatrics*. 1955;16:1.
20. Skinner AL, Moll FC. Hypernatremia accompanying infant diarrhea. *Am J Dis Child*. 1956;92:562.
21. Dorrington KL. Skin turgor: do we understand the clinical sign? *Lancet*. 1981;1:264.
22. Knopp R, Claypool R, Leonardi D. Use of the tilt test in measuring acute blood loss. *Ann Emerg Med*. 1980;9:72.
23. Finberg L. Hypernatremic (hypertonic) dehydration in infants. *N Engl J Med*. 1973;298:196.
24. Chonko A, Bay W, Stzin J, et al. The role of renin and aldosterone in the salt retention of edema. *Am J Med*. 1977;63:881.
25. Vader HL, Vink CLF. The influence of viscosity on dilution methods: its problems in the determination of serum sodium. *Clin Chim Acta*. 1975;65:379.
26. Miller M, Dalakos T, Moses A, et al. Recognition of partial defects in antidiuretic hormone secretion. *Ann Intern Med*. 1970;73:721.
27. Alberti KGMM, Hockaday TDR. Diabetic coma: a reappraisal after five years. *Clin Endocrinol Metab*. 1977;6:421.
28. McDonald K, Miller P, Anderson R, et al. Hormonal control of renal water excretion. *Kidney Int*. 1976;10:38.
29. Epstein M, Pins D, Schneider N, et al. Determinants of deranged sodium and water homeostasis in decompensated cirrhosis. *J Lab Clin Med*. 1976;87:822.
30. Fichman M, Vorherr H, Kleeman L, et al. Diuretic-induced hyponatremia. *Ann Intern Med*. 1971;75:853.
31. Pettinger W, Talner L, Ferris T. Inappropriate secretion of antidiuretic hormone due to myxedema. *N Engl J Med*. 1965;272:362.
32. Sickle cells and hyponatremia. *Lancet*. 1974;1:342.
33. Hariprasad M, Eisinger RP, Nadler IM, et al. Hyponatremia in psychogenic polydipsia. *Arch Intern Med*. 1980;140:1639.
34. Waugh WH. Utility of expressing serum sodium per unit of water in assessing hyponatremia. *Metabolism*. 1969;18:706.
35. Katz M. Hyperglycemia-induced hyponatremia—calculation of expected serum sodium depression. *N Engl J Med*. 1973;289:843.
36. Moses AM, Miller M. Drug-induced dilutional hyponatremia. *N Engl J Med*. 1974;291:1234.
37. Bartter F, Schwartz W. The syndrome of inappropriate secretion of antidiuretic hormone. *Am J Med*. 1967;42:790.
38. Renzetti AD Jr, Kobayashi T, Bigler A, et al. Regional ventilation and perfusion in silicosis and in the alveolar-capillary block syndrome. *Am J Med*. 1970;49:5.
39. Arieff A, Llach F, Massry S. Neurological manifestations and morbidity of hyponatremia: correlation with brain water and electrolytes. *Medicine*. 1976;55:121.
40. Forrest J, Cox M, Hong C, et al. Superiority of demeclocycline over lithium in the treatment of chronic syndrome of inappropriate secretion of antidiuretic hormone. *N Engl J Med*. 1977;298:173.
41. Tallob L, Needle M. Hyponatremic syndromes. *Med Clin North Am*. 1973;57:1425.
42. Hantman D, Rossier B, Zohlman R, et al. Rapid correction of hyponatremia in the syndrome of inappropriate secretion of antidiuretic hormone: an alternative treatment to hypertonic saline. *Ann Intern Med*. 1973;78:870.
43. Nardone D, McDonald W, Girard D. Mechanisms in hypokalemia: clinical correlation. *Medicine*. 1978;57:435.
44. Kunau RT, Stein JH. Disorders of hypo- and hyperkalemia. *Clin Nephrol*. 1977;7:173.
45. Berliner RW. Renal mechanisms for potassium excretion. *Harvey Lect*. 1960;55:141.
46. Malnic G, DeMello G, Aires M, et al. Potassium transport across renal distal tubules during acid-base disturbances. *Am J Physiol*. 1971;221:1192.
47. Gennari FS, Cohen JJ. Role of the kidney in potassium homeostasis: lessons from acid-base disturbances. *Kidney Int*. 1975;8:1.
48. Schultz R. Recent advances in the physiology and pathophysiology of potassium excretion. *Arch Intern Med*. 1973;131:885.

49. Burnell J, Villamil M, Uyeno B, et al. The effect in humans of extracellular pH change on the relationship between serum potassium concentration and intracellular potassium. *J Clin Invest*. 1956;35:935.
50. Oster JR, Perez GO, Vaamonde CA. Relationship between blood pH and potassium and phosphorus during acute metabolic acidosis. *Am J Physiol*. 1978;235:345.
51. Orringer CE, Eustace JC, Sunsch CD, et al. Natural history of lactic acidosis after grand mal seizures: a model for the study of an anion gap acidosis not associated with hyperkalemia. *N Engl J Med*. 1977;297:746.
52. Fulop M. Serum potassium in lactic acidosis and ketoacidosis. *N Engl J Med*. 1979;300:1087.
53. Surawicz B. Relationship between electrocardiogram and electrolytes. *Am Heart J*. 1967;73:814.
54. Ettinger P, Regan T, Oldewurtel H. Hyperkalemia, cardiac conduction and the electrocardiogram: a review. *Am Heart J*.1974;88:360.
55. Stoa KF, Knutsen KOH. Oestrogen excretion during cortisone therapy. *Acta Endocrinol*. 1957;25:209.
56. Sigler MH. The mechanism of the naturiesis of fasting. *J Clin Invest*. 1975;55:377.
57. Shields R. Absorption and secretion of electrolytes and water by the human colon, with particular reference to benign adenoma and papilloma. *Br J Surg*. 1966;53:893.
58. Gossain VV, Werk EE. Surreptitious laxation and hypokalemia. *Ann Intern Med*. 1972;76:671.
59. Larusso N, McGill D. Surreptitious laxative ingestion: delayed recognition of a serious condition: a case report. *Mayo Clin Proc*. 1975;50:706.
60. Schwartz W, Reuman A. Metabolic and renal studies in chronic potassium depletion resulting from overuse of laxatives. *J Clin Invest*. 1953;32:258.
61. Bartter FC, Pronove P, Gill JR Jr, et al. Hyperplasia of the juxtaglomerular complex with hyperaldosteronism and hypokalemic alkalosis. *Am J Med*. 1962;33:811.
62. Gill J, Frolich J, Bowden R, et al. Bartter's syndrome: a disorder characterized by high urinary prostaglandins and a dependence of hyperreninemia on prostaglandin synthesis. *Am J Med*. 1976;61:43.
63. Morris R Jr. Renal tubular acidosis. Mechanisms classification and implications. *N Engl J Med*. 1969;281:1405.
64. Narins RG, Goldberg M. Renal tubular acidosis: pathophysiology, diagnosis and treatment. *DM*. 1977;23:3.
65. Lipner H, Ruzany F, Dasgupta M, et al. The behavior of carbenicillin as nonreabsorbable anion. *J Lab Clin Med*. 1975;87:183.
66. Douglas J, Healy J. Nephrotoxic effects of amphotericin B, including renal tubular acidosis. *Am J Med*. 1969;46:154.
67. Frazier H, Yager H. Drug therapy. The clinical use of diuretics. *N Engl J Med*. 1973;288:455.
68. Muggia F, Heinemann H, Farhangi M, et al. Lysozymuria and renal tubular dysfunction in monocytic and myelomonocytic leukemia. *Am J Med*. 1969;47:351.
69. Forman BH. Hypokalemic periodic paralysis. *JAMA*. 1971;216:146.
70. Santeusanio F, Faloona G, Knochel JP, et al. Evidence for a role of endogenous insulin and glucagon in the regulation of potassium homeostasis. *J Lab Clin Med*. 1973;81:809.
71. Smith JS Jr. Hypokalemia in resuscitation from multiple trauma. *Surg Gynecol Obstet*. 1978;147:18.
72. Knochel J. Environmental heat illness: an eclectic review. *Arch Intern Med*. 1974;133:841.
73. Sprung CL, Portocarrero CJ, Fernaine AV, et al. The metabolic and respiratory alterations of heat stroke. *Arch Intern Med*. 1980;140:665.
74. Berning J. Hypokalemia of barium poisoning. *Lancet*. 1975;1:110.
75. Lawson DH, Murray RM, Parker JLW. Early mortality in the megaloblastic anemias. *Q J Med*. 1972;41:1.
76. Smithwick RH, Kinsey D, Whitelaw GP. Surgical treatment of hypertension-primary aldosteronism. *N Engl J Med*. 1962;266:160.
77. Vaughan NJA, Slater JDI, Lightman SL, et al. The diagnosis of primary hyperaldosteronism. *Lancet*. 1981;1:120.
78. Primary aldosteronism. *Lancet*. 1980;1:667.
79. Wrong O. Incidence of hypokalemia in severe hypertension. *Br Med J*. 1961;2:419.
80. Simon N, Franklin S, Bleiter K, et al. Clinical characteristics of renovascular hypertension. *JAMA*. 1972;220:1209.
81. Conn JW, Rovner DR, Cohen EL. Licorice-induced pseudoaldosteronism. Hypertension, hypokalemia, aldosteronopenia, and suppressed plasma renin activity. *JAMA*. 1968;205:492.
82. Blachley JD, Knochel JP. Tobacco chewer's hypokalemia: licorice revisited. *N Engl J Med*. 1980;302:784.
83. Ward CF, Arkin DB, Venumof SL, et al. Arterial versus venous potassium: clinical implications. *Crit Care Med*. 1978;6:335.
84. Love DW, Foster TS, Bradley DL. Comparison of the taste and acceptance of three potassium chloride preparations. *Am J Hosp Pharm*. 1978;35:586.
85. Sopko JA, Freeman RM. Salt substitutes as a source of potassium. *JAMA*. 1977;238:608.
86. Surawicz B, Chlebus H, Mazzoleni A. Hemodynamic and electrocardiographic effects of hyperpotassemia: differences in response to slow and rapid increases in concentration of plasma K. *Am Heart J*. 1967;73:647.
87. Stewart GW, Fyffe JA, Corrall RJM. Familial pseudohyperkalemia: a new syndrome. *Lancet*. 1979;2:175.
88. Bostic O, Duvernoy WFC. Hyperkalemic cardiac arrest during transfusion of stored blood. *J Electrocardiol*. 1972;5:407.
89. Roth F, Wuthrick H. The clinical importance of hyperkalemia following suxamethonium administration. *Br J Anaesthesiol*. 1967;41:311.
90. Thomas ET. Circulatory collapse following succinylcholine: report of a case. *Anesth Analg*. 1969;48:333.
91. Mazze R, Escue H, Houston J. Collapse following administration of succinylcholine to the traumatized patient. *Anesthesiology*. 1969;31:540.
92. Maroff DL, daSilva JA, Rosenbaum BJ. On the mechanism of hyperkalemia due to hyperosmotic expansion with saline or mannitol. *Clin Sci Mol Med*. 1971;41:383.
93. deLeiva A, Christlieb AR, Melby JC, et al. Big renin and biosynthetic defect of aldosterone in diabetes mellitus. *N Engl J Med*. 1976;295:639.
94. Szylman P, Better OS, Chaimowitz C, et al. Role of hyperkalemia in the metabolic acidosis of isolated hypoaldosteronism. *N Engl J Med*. 1976;294:361.
95. Tan S, Burton M. Hyporeninemic hypoaldosteronism: an overlooked cause of hyperkalemia. *Arch Intern Med*. 1981;141:30.
96. Spitzer A, Edelmann C Jr, Goldberg L, et al. Short stature, hyperkalemia and acidosis: a defect in renal transport of potassium. *Kidney Int*. 1973;3:251.
97. Iverson T. Congenital adrenocortical hyperplasia with disturbed electrolyte regulations: dysadrenocorticism. *Pediatrics*. 1955;16:875.
98. Braun H, Surawicz B, Beuet S. T waves in hyperpotassemia: their differentiation from simulating T waves in other conditions. *Am J Med Sci*. 1955;230:147.
99. Levinsky NG. Management of emergencies: VI. Hyperkalemia. *N Engl J Med*. 1966;274:1076.
100. Singer FR, Bethune JE, Massry SG. Hypercalcemia and hypocalcemia. *Clin Nephrol*. 1977;7:154.

101. Zerwekh JE. Vitamin D–dependent intestinal calcium absorption. *Gastroenterology.* 1979;76:404.
102. Ostrow JD, Blanchard G, Gray SJ. Peptic ulcer in primary hyperparathyroidism. *Am J Med.* 1960;29:769.
103. Barreras RF, Donaldson RM. Role of calcium in gastric hypersecretion, parathyroid adenoma and peptic ulcer. *N Engl J Med.* 1967;276:1122.
104. Cope O, Culver PS, Mixter CG, et al. Pancreatitis, a diagnostic clue to hyperparathyroidism. *Ann Surg.* 1957;145:857.
105. Parks J, Coe F, Favus M. Hyperparathyroidism in nephrolithiasis. *Arch Intern Med.* 1980;140:1479.
106. Bronsky D, Dubin A, Kushner DS, et al. Calcium and the electrocardiogram: III. The relationship of the intervals of the electrocardiogram to the level of serum calcium. *Am J Cardiol.* 1961;7:840.
107. Juan D. Hypocalcemia: differential diagnosis and mechanisms. *Arch Intern Med.* 1979;139:1166.
108. Muggia FM. Hypercalcemia associated with neoplastic disease. *Ann Intern Med.* 1970;73:281.
109. Lafferty FW. Pseudohyperparathyroidism. *Medicine.* 1966;45:247.
110. Fisken RA, Heath DA, Somers S. Hypercalcaemia in hospital patients: clinical and diagnostic aspects. *Lancet.* 1981;1:202.
111. Stewart AF, Horst R, Deftos LJ, et al. Biochemical evaluation of patients with cancer-associated hypercalcemia: evidence for humoral and non-humoral groups. *N Engl J Med.* 1980;303:1377.
112. Sherwood LM. The multiple causes of hypercalcemia in malignant disease. *N Engl J Med.* 1980;303:1412.
113. Skrabanek P, McPartlin J, Powell D. Tumor hypercalcemia and "ectopic hyperparathyroidism." *Medicine.* 1980;59:262.
114. Kyle RA. Multiple myeloma: a review of 869. *Mayo Clin Proc.* 1975;50:29.
115. Kapadia SB. Multiple myeloma: a clinicopathologic study of 62 consecutively autopsied cases. *Medicine.* 1980;59:323.
116. Boonstra CE, Jackson CE. Hyperparathyroidism detected by routine serum calcium analysis: prevalence in a clinic population. *Ann Intern Med.* 1965;63:468.
117. Mundy GR, Cove DH, Fiskan R, et al. Primary hyperparathyroidism: changes in the pattern of clinical presentation. *Lancet.* 1980;1:1317.
118. Heath H, Hodgson SF, Kennedy MA. Primary hyperparathyroidism: incidence, morbidity, and potential economic impact in a community. *N Engl J Med.* 1980;302:189.
119. Mallette LE, Bilezikian JP, Heath DA, et al. Primary hyperparathyroidism: clinical and biochemical features. *Medicine.* 1974;53:127.
120. Palmer FJ, Nelson JC, Bacchus H. The chloride-phosphate ratio in hypercalcemia. *Ann Intern Med.* 1974;80:200.
121. Winnacker JL, Becker KL, Katz S. Endocrine aspects of sarcoidosis. *N Engl J Med.* 1968;278:427.
122. Cushard WG, Simon AB, Canterbury JM, et al. Parathyroid function in sarcoidosis. *N Engl J Med.* 1972;286:395.
123. Chaplin H Jr, Clark LD, Ropes MW. Vitamin D intoxication. *Am J Med Sci.* 1951;221:369.
124. Paterson CR. Vitamin-D poisoning: survey of causes in 21 patients with hypercalcaemia. *Lancet.* 1980;1:1164.
125. deTorrente A, Berl T, Chon P, et al. Hypercalcemia of acute renal failure, clinical significance and pathogenesis. *Am J Med.* 1976;61:119.
126. Segal AJ, Miller M, Moses A. Hypercalcemia during the diuretic phase of acute renal failure. *Ann Intern Med.* 1968;68:1066.
127. Randall RE, Strauss ME, McNeely WF. The milk-alkali syndrome. *Arch Intern Med.* 1961;107:163.
128. Meier DA, Arnstein AR, Hamburger JI. Symptomatic thyrotoxic hypercalcemia. *Mich Med.* 1974;73:19.
129. Walser M, Robinson BHB, Duckett JW. The hypercalcemia of adrenal insufficiency. *J Clin Invest.* 1963;42:456.
130. Chatterjee SN, Friedler RM, Berne TV, et al. Persistent hypercalcemia after successful renal transplantation. *Nephron.* 1976;17:1.
131. Garcia RE, Friedman WF, Kaback MM, et al. Idiopathic hypercalcemia and supravalvular aortic stenosis: documentation of a new syndrome. *N Engl J Med.* 1964;271:117.
132. David NJ, Verner JV, Engel FL. The diagnostic spectrum of hypercalcemia. *Am J Med.* 1962;33:88.
133. Goldsmith RS. Differential diagnosis of hypercalcemia. *N Engl J Med.* 1966;274:674.
134. Nierenberg DW, Ransil BJ. Q-aTc interval as a clinical indicator of hypercalcemia. *Am J Cardiol.* 1979;44:243.
135. Toda N, West TC. Modification by sodium and calcium of the cardiotoxicity induced by ouabain. *J Pharmacol Exp Ther.* 1965;154:239.
136. Dent CE. Some problems of hyperparathyroidism. *Br Med J.* 1962;2:1419.
137. Smith FE, Reinstein H, Braverman LE. Cork stoppers and hypercalcemia. *N Engl J Med.* 1965;272:787.
138. Aldinger KA, Samaan NA. Hypokalemia with hypercalcemia: prevalence and significance in treatment. *Ann Intern Med.* 1977;87:571.
139. Perlia CP, Gubisch NJ, Walter J, et al. Mithramycin treatment of hypercalcemia. *Cancer.* 1970;25:389.
140. Smith IE, Powles TJ. Mithramycin for hypercalcemia associated with myeloma and other malignancies. *Br Med J.* 1975;1:268.
141. Austin LA, Heath H. Calcitonin: physiology and pathophysiology. *N Engl J Med.* 1981;304:269.
142. Wisneski LA, Croom WP, Silva OL, et al. Salmon calcitonin in hypercalcemia. *Clin Pharmacol Ther.* 1978;24:219.
143. Dudley HR, Ritchie AC, Schilling A, et al. Pathologic changes associated with the use of sodium ethylene diamine tetra-acetate in the treatment of hypercalcemia. *N Engl J Med.* 1953;262:331.
144. Robertson RP, Baylink DJ, Marini JJ, et al. Elevated prostaglandins and suppressed parathyroid hormone associated with hypercalcemia and renal cell carcinoma. *J Clin Endocrinol Metab.* 1975;41:164.
145. Brereton HO, Halushka PV, Alexander RW, et al. Indomethacin-responsive hypercalcemia in a patient with renal-cell adenocarcinoma. *N Engl J Med.* 1974;291:83.
146. Ashkar FS, Miller R, Katims RB. Effect of corticosteroids on hypercalcemia of malignant disease. *Lancet.* 1971;1:41.
147. Deftos LJ. Medical management of the hypercalcemia of malignancy. *Annu Rev Med.* 1974;25:323.
148. Goldsmith RS. Treatment of hypercalcemia. *Med Clin North Am.* 1972;56:951.
149. Watson L, Moxham J, Fraser P. Hydrocortisone suppression test and discriminant analysis in differential diagnosis of hypercalcemia. *Lancet.* 1980;1:1320.
150. Binstock ML, Mundy GR. Effect of calcitonin and glucocorticoids in combination on the hypercalcemia of malignancy. *Ann Intern Med.* 1980;93:269.
151. DiGeorge AM. Congenital absence of the thymus and its immunologic consequences: concurrence with congenital hypoparathyroidism. *Birth Defects.* 1968;4:116.
152. Graham K, Williams BO, Rowe MJ. Idiopathic hypoparathyroidism: a cause of fits in the elderly. *Br Med J.* 1979;1:1460.
153. Peden VH. True idiopathic hypoparathyroidism as a sex-linked recessive trait. *Am J Hum Genet.* 1960;12:323.
154. Richter PI, Chutorian AM. Familial hypoparathyroidism: case reports and a review of the literature. *Neurology.* 1968;18:75.

155. Nusynowitz ML, Frame B, Kolb FO. The spectrum of the hypoparathyroid states: a classification based on physiologic principles. *Medicine*. 1976;55:105.
156. Horwitz C, Myers WP, Foote F Jr. Secondary malignant tumors of the parathyroid glands: report of two cases with associated hypoparathyroidism. *Am J Med*. 1972;52:797.
157. Davis RH, Fourman P, Smith JWG. Prevalence of parathyroid insufficiency after thyroidectomy. *Lancet*. 1961;2:1432.
158. Anast CS, Motts JM, Kaplan SL, et al. Evidence for parathyroid in magnesium deficiency. *Science*. 1972;177:606.
159. Reddy CR, Coburn JW, Hartenbower DL, et al. Studies on mechanism of hypocalcemia of magnesium depletion. *J Clin Invest*. 1973;52:3000.
160. Chase LR, Slatopolsky E. Secretion and metabolic efficacy of parathyroid hormone in patients with severe hypomagnesemia. *J Clin Endocrinol Metab*. 1974;38:363.
161. Juan D. Hypocalcemia: differential diagnosis and mechanisms. *Arch Intern Med*. 1979;139:1166.
162. Holick MF, Vskokovic M, Henley JW. The photoproduction of 1,25-dihydroxyvitamin D_3 in skin: an approach to therapy of vitamin-D–resistant syndromes. *N Engl J Med*. 1980;303:349.
163. Farfel Z, Brickman AS, Kaslow HR, et al. Defect of receptorcyclase coupling protein in pseudohypoparathyroidism. *N Engl J Med*. 1980;303:237.
164. Robertson GM Jr, Moore EW, Switz DM, et al. Inadequate parathyroid response in acute pancreatitis. *N Engl J Med*. 1976;294:512.
165. Edmondson HA, Berne CJ. Calcium changes in acute pancreatic necrosis. *Surg Gynecol Obstet*. 1944;79:240.
166. Blanchard BM. Focal hypocalcemic seizures 33 years after thyroidectomy. *Arch Intern Med*. 1962;110:382.
167. Howard E. Value of the Q-T interval. *Am Heart J*. 1960;59:789.
168. Avioli L. The therapeutic approach to hypoparathyroidism. *Am J Med*. 1974;57:34.
169. Pak CYC, Zisman E, Lotz M. Gluconate carrier in 47 Ca kinetic studies. *J Clin Endocrinol Metab*. 1967;27:433.
170. White RD, Goldsmith RS, Rodriguez R, et al. Plasma ionic calcium levels following injection of chloride, gluconate and gluceptate salts of calcium. *J Thorac Cardiovasc Surg*. 1976;71:609.
171. Calcitriol. *Med Lett Drugs Ther*. 1979;21:50.
172. Graber TW, Yee AS, Baker FJ. Magnesium: physiology, clinical disorders and therapy. *Ann Emerg Med*. 1981;10:49.
173. Massry SG, Seelig MS. Hypomagnesemia and hypermagnesemia. *Clin Nephrol*. 1977;7:147.
174. Geiderman JM, Goodman SL, Cohen DB. Magnesium—the forgotten electrolyte. *J Am Coll Emerg Phys*. 1979;8:204.
175. Kalbfleisch JM, Lindeman RD, Ginn HE, et al. Effects of ethanol administration on urinary excretion of magnesium and other electrolytes in alcoholic and normal subjects. *J Clin Invest*. 1963;42:1471.
176. Mendelson JH, Ogata M, Mello NK. Effects of alcohol ingestion and withdrawal on magnesium states of alcoholics: clinical and experimental findings. *Ann NY Acad Sci*. 1969;162:918.
177. Martin HE, Wertman M. Serum potassium, magnesium and calcium levels in diabetic patients. *J Clin Invest*. 1947;26:217.
178. Martin HE, Smith K, Wilson ML. The fluid and electrolyte therapy of severe diabetic acidosis and ketosis. *Am J Med*. 1958;24:376.
179. Lim P, Jacob E. Magnesium deficiency in patients on long-term diuretic therapy for heart failure. *Br Med J*. 1972;3:620.
180. Iseri LT, Freed J, Bures AR. Magnesium deficiency and cardiac disorders. *Am J Med*. 1975;58:837.
181. Neff MS, Mendelssohn S, Kim KE, et al. Magnesium sulfate in digitalis toxicity. *Am J Cardiol*. 1972;29:377.
182. Seller RH, Cangiano J, Kim KE, et al. Digitalis toxicity and hypomagnesemia. *Am Heart J*. 1970;79:57.
183. Specter M, Schweizer E, Goldman R. Studies on magnesium's mechanism of action in digitalis-induced arrhythmias. *Circulation*. 1975;52:1001.
184. Burch GE, Giles TD. The importance of magnesium deficiency in cardiovascular disease. *Am Heart J*. 1977;94:649.
185. Balint JA, Hirschowitz BI. Hypomagnesemia with tetany in nontropical sprue. *N Engl J Med*. 1961;265:631.
186. Savage DCL, McAdam WAF. Convulsions due to hypomagnesaemia in an infant recovering from diarrhea. *Lancet*. 1967;2:234.
187. Fletcher RF, Henley AA, Sammons HG, et al. A case of magnesium deficiency following massive intestinal resection. *Lancet*. 1960;1:522.
188. Flink EB, Stutzman FL, Anderson AR, et al. Magnesium deficiency after prolonged parenteral fluid administration and after chronic alcoholism complicated by delirium tremens. *J Lab Clin Med*. 1954;43:169.
189. Hanna S, Harrison M, MacIntyre I, et al. The syndrome of magnesium deficiency in man. *Lancet*. 1960;2:172.
190. Shils ME. Experimental human magnesium depletion. *Medicine*. 1969;48:61.
191. Bajpai PC, Hasan M, Gupta AK, et al. Electrocardiographic changes in hypomagnesemia. *Indian Heart J*. 1972;24:271.
192. Fitzgerald MG, Fourman P. An experimental study of magnesium deficiency in man. *Clin Sci Mol Med*. 1956;15:635.
193. Fourman P, Morgan DB. Chronic magnesium deficiency. *Proc Nutr Soc*. 1962;21:34.
194. Pritchard JA. The use of the magnesium ion in the management of eclamptogenic toxemias. *Surg Gynecol Obstet*. 1955;100:131.
195. Flink EB. Therapy of magnesium deficiency. *Ann NY Acad Sci*. 1969;162:901.
196. Randall RE, Cohen MD, Spray CC Jr, et al. Hypermagnesemia in renal failure: etiology of topic manifestations. *Ann Intern Med*. 1964;61:73.
197. Berns AS, Kollmeyer KR. Magnesium-induced bradycardia. *Ann Intern Med*. 1976;85:760.
198. Massry SG. Pharmacology of magnesium. *Annu Rev Pharmacol Toxicol*. 1977;17:67.
199. Wacker WEC, Parisi AF. Magnesium metabolism. *N Engl J Med*. 1968;278:658 (part 1), 712 (part 2), 772 (part 3).

APPENDIX 17-A

Table 17-A1 Solutions

	Glucose (g/L)	Na (mEq/L) NaCl Lactate		KCl (mEq/L)	$CaCl_2$ (mEq/L)	NH_4Cl	PO_4(g/L)
0.9% saline		154					
3% saline		513					
5% saline		856					
5% dextrose in water	50						
2% ammonium chloride						374	
1/6 molar ammonium chloride (0.9%)						167	
Ringer's lactate		103	27	4	4		
Sodium phosphate (pH 5.7)		400					93
Potassium phosphate (pH 6.6)				400			93

Table 17-A2 Common Ampules

	Volume (mL) in Ampule	mEq in Ampule (Not Concentration)
7.5% sodium bicarbonate	50	44
7.5% potassium chloride	20	20
14.9% potassium chloride	20	20
10.0% calcium gluconate	10	4
10.0% calcium chloride	10	14
26.8% ammonium chloride	20	100
25.0% magnesium sulfate	2	4
		Gr in Ampule
25.0% mannitol	50	12.5
50.0% glucose	50	25.0

Table 17-A3 Conversions

	mEq of Anion or Cation/g of Salt	Salt/mEq (mg)
$CaCl_2 \cdot 2H_2O$	14	73
Ca gluconate $\cdot 1H_2O$	4	224
KCl	13	75
$KHCO_3$	10	100
NaCl	17	58
$NaHCO_3$	12	84

18. Hypokalemia and Hyperkalemia

PAUL M. PARIS, MD, FACEP

HYPOKALEMIA

An electrolyte disturbance seen relatively often in emergency medicine, hypokalemia may become life threatening. Therefore, the emergency physician must have a high index of suspicion and search for this condition even when its clinical manifestations are subtle.

Etiology

The causes of hypokalemia can be divided into four general groups, which are outlined below:

I. Dietary
   A. Decreased intake
   B. Clay ingestion
   C. Kayexalate
II. Gastrointestinal Losses
   A. Protracted vomiting
   B. Diarrhea
   C. Gastrointestinal fistulas
   D. Villous adenomas
   E. Laxative abuse
   F. Malabsorption
   G. Ileostomy
III. Renal Losses
   A. Drug induced
      1. Potent saluretic agents
      2. Osmotic diuretics
      3. Carbonic anhydrase inhibitors
      4. Carbenicillin
      5. Nafcillin
      6. Sodium penicillin
      7. Amphotericin B (RTA)
      8. Glycyrrhizic acid (licorice and chewing tobacco)
   B. Mineralocorticoid activity
      1. Cushing's syndrome (adrenal neoplasm, ectopic adrenocorticotropic hormone, steroid therapy)
      2. Primary aldosteronism
      3. Bartter's syndrome
      4. Exogenous steroids
      5. Edematous states (congestive heart failure, cirrhosis, nephrosis)
   C. Acid-base disturbances
      1. Alkali loading
      2. Renal tubular acidosis
      3. Diabetic ketoacidosis
   D. Renal tubular defects
      1. Renal tubular acidosis (types I and II)
      2. Salt-wasting nephropathy
      3. Postobstructive diuresis
   E. Other
      1. Magnesium deficiency
      2. Leukemia
IV. Maldistribution
   A. Alkalosis
   B. Periodic paralysis
   C. Insulin
   D. Excessive exercise
   E. Adrenergic drugs
   F. Barium poisoning

G. Early vitamin B_{12} treatment of megaloblastic anemias
H. Multiple trauma
I. β_2 Agonists

Dietary

It is unusual for clinically significant hypokalemia to result from decreased intake.[1-3] Potassium is present in almost all naturally occurring foods, including meats, vegetables, fruits, and juices.[2] The daily renal, gastrointestinal, and skin obligate losses of potassium are 20 to 30 mEq/day.[3] Few diets contain less than this amount of potassium. In the rare circumstances in which less than 20 mEq of potassium is consumed per day, mild hypokalemia may occur after several weeks, but other manifestations of malnutrition are usually more prominent. Clay ingestion can cause hypokalemia by binding to potassium in the gastrointestinal tract, thus preventing absorption.

Gastrointestinal Losses

All gastrointestinal secretions contain potassium (Table 18-1).[1,4] Any patient with fluid losses from the gastrointestinal tract should be considered a candidate for hypokalemia. Patients with vomiting, diarrhea, tube drainage, gastrointestinal fistulas, and villous adenomas should all be monitored for potassium loss. Hypokalemia may also result from laxative abuse or self-induced vomiting that may not be evident from the patient's history. Much of the hypokalemia that occurs with vomiting is secondary to volume loss, which leads to alkalosis and an increase in aldosterone levels.

Renal Losses

The most common cause of significant hypokalemia is renal loss.[3,5,6] Several mechanisms cause increased urinary losses of potassium (see outline).

Almost all potassium that is filtered in the glomerulus of the kidney is reabsorbed in the proximal tubule and loop of Henle. Any potassium excreted in the urine has been secreted in the distal tubule and collecting duct. Factors that increase such secretions are increased delivery of sodium to the distal tubule, increased delivery of nonreabsorbable anions to the distal tubule, alkalosis, and increased urine flow rate. Loop diuretics, osmotic diuretics, and carbonic anhydrase inhibitors increase both urine flow rates and sodium delivery to the distal tubule, thus causing significant increases in kaliuresis.[1-3,7] Twenty percent to 30% of patients taking 50 mg of hydrochlorothiazide per day and 50% of those taking 50 mg of chlorthalidone per day develop hypokalemia.[8] Most cases of severe hypokalemia are associated with the use of diuretics. Carbenicillin, nafcillin, and sodium penicillin are nonreabsorbable anions that increase potassium secretions in the distal tubule.[9]

Certain chemicals with mineralocorticoid activity, such as licorice, increase distal tubule reabsorption of sodium, which is accompanied by the exchange of either potassium or hydrogen ion.

When an alkalosis is present, the distal tubular cell has a deficiency of intracellular hydrogen; therefore, most of the exchange of sodium is for potassium, which increases losses in the urine. Diabetic ketoacidosis causes significant potassium losses because of several factors. Glycosuria and ketonuria, for example, cause a tremendous osmotic diuresis and increase the delivery of nonreabsorbable anions to the distal tubule. Magnesium deficiency impairs the function of the renal tubular cells with subsequent potassium loss.[2] Edematous states (eg, congestive heart failure, nephrosis, cirrhosis) increase the levels of aldosterone, owing to a decreased effective circulating volume. Aldosterone, like other mineralocorticoids, increases sodium exchange for potassium or hydrogen in the distal tubule. In acute myeloid leukemia, especially monocytic or myelomonocytic, increased loss of potassium in the urine is thought to be due to the effect of lysozymes on the proximal tubule.[1] Bartter's syndrome is a rare, interesting disease in which hyperplasia of the renal juxtaglomerular apparatus results in overproduction of renin. In this syndrome, however, the renin does not cause hypertension but increases aldosterone secretion, thus increasing potassium loss. Renal tubular abnormalities may also cause potassium loss. These tubular abnormalities may be mediated by prostaglandins, since many inhibitors of prostaglandins, such as indomethacin, are helpful in correcting the hypokalemia.[10]

Maldistribution

Normally, 2% of potassium is extracellular. In certain circumstances, potassium is shifted to the intracellular stores, leaving the serum hypokalemic.[1,3,4] With alkalosis, for example, potassium from extracellular stores is transported intracellularly in exchange for hydrogen ion. A rough estimate is that for each 0.1 change in pH there is a 0.6 mEq/L change in the serum potassium level in the opposite direction.[1,3,4]

An unusual disorder caused by hypokalemia due to maldistribution is periodic paralysis. Patients with this disorder are subject to attacks of severe muscle weakness owing to the sudden intracellular shift of potassium. These shifts are frequently precipitated by carbohydrate loads in association with a lack of muscular activity, but the exact etiology is unknown.[11]

Table 18-1 Average Potassium Content of Gastrointestinal Fluids

Fluid	Potassium Content (mEq/L)
Gastric	10 to 15
Pancreatic	5
Biliary	5
Small bowel	5
Diarrheal stool	25 or greater

One action of insulin is to cause potassium to be transported intracellularly. With insulin therapy, therefore, care must always be taken to avoid precipitating hypokalemia. This is especially critical in the treatment of diabetic ketoacidosis, in which several other factors also predispose the patient to hypokalemia.[2,4]

The β_2-adrenergic agents have been shown to shift potassium to the intracellular compartment. This may occur with inhaled β_2 agents or even in states where endogenous catecholamine levels are high.[12–14]

In the early treatment of megaloblastic anemias with vitamin B_{12}, large amounts of potassium are transported into young red blood cells and platelets, which may lead to hypokalemia. Other conditions that may be associated with intracellular transport of potassium include barium poisoning, multiple trauma, and excessive exercise.[15–17]

Clinical Manifestations

Hypokalemia has several manifestations, all of which depend on the severity and the duration of the hypokalemia. Losses greater than 5% to 10% of body potassium are usually symptomatic. The clinical effects of hypokalemia include the following[2,4,18]:

- *skeletal and smooth muscle:* weakness, paralysis, rhabdomyolysis
- *cardiac:* electrocardiogram (ECG) abnormality, increased sensitivity to digoxin, increased premature atrial contractions and premature ventricular contractions
- *neurologic:* mental changes, decreased deep tendons reflexes
- *metabolic:* decreased release and sensitivity to insulin
- *gastrointestinal:* atony of the gastrointestinal tract
- *renal:* decreased concentrating ability, decreased glomerular filtration rate, increased ammonia production, decreased urinary acidification
- *cerebral:* irritability, lethargy, drowsiness, confusion

Neuromuscular Effects

Frequently, the most prominent effect of hypokalemia is that on the neuromuscular system. When potassium is decreased in the extracellular space, the ratio of intracellular potassium to extracellular potassium increases. This change, in turn, increases the transmembrane potential, which widens the difference between the transmembrane potential and the resting potential, thereby impeding impulse conduction and muscular contraction. Skeletal muscle weakness is usually the first sign of this effect. Limb muscles are usually affected before trunk muscles. The classic pattern first involves the lower extremities, especially the quadriceps. The pattern of weakness may resemble ascending paralysis of primary neurologic origin (Guillain-Barré syndrome). Smooth muscle also becomes involved so that nausea, vomiting, constipation, paralytic ileus, and gastric distention are all possible. The muscle weakness may become severe enough to cause respiratory paralysis and death from respiratory failure. Significant neuromuscular symptoms are not usually seen unless the potassium levels are less than 2.5 mEq/L.

When hypokalemia is severe, rhabdomyolysis may be induced by exercise; occasionally, it may occur even without muscular activity. Rhabdomyolysis frequently results in acute tubular necrosis secondary to myoglobinuria. This mechanism has even been implicated in cases of renal failure secondary to licorice ingestion.[19]

Cardiac Effects

Some of the most serious effects of hypokalemia are the cardiac changes (eg, conduction disturbances, rhythm abnormalities, and possible decreases in contractility). The ECG changes that are seen with potassium depletion include the following[2,3,20,21]:

- depression of ST segments
- decreased T-wave voltage and sometimes inversion
- increased U-wave voltage (with more severe changes)
- increased amplitude of P wave
- widening of the QRS complex
- prolongation of PR interval

The ECG changes of hypokalemia do not occur as reliably as those of hyperkalemia. Therefore, significant hypokalemia cannot be ruled out on the basis of an ECG. The most common dysrhythmias seen with hypokalemia are premature atrial and premature ventricular contractions and disturbances in atrioventricular nodal conduction.[22] Severe hypokalemia may lead to the life-threatening ventricular rhythm of torsade de pointes. This rhythm is frequently fatal and is a variant of ventricular tachycardia with unique electrocardiographic features.[23] Digitalis causes a decrease in intracellular potassium and potentiates the cardiac manifestations of hypokalemia. Digitalis toxicity with hypokalemia is a life-threatening emergency. This association must be remembered because many patients taking digitalis preparations are also on diuretics, which predisposes them to hypokalemia. It is essential to monitor potassium levels in these patients. It must also be remembered that patients on diuretics frequently become deficient in magnesium, and correction of the magnesium may be required to correct the ventricular irritability seen with digitalis toxicity. There is some experimental evidence that hypokalemia decreases cardiac contractility and, therefore, may precipitate or exacerbate congestive heart failure.[3]

There is some suggestive evidence that patients with an acute myocardial infarction who are hypokalemic are at a greater risk of ventricular fibrillation. This evidence would suggest that it is wise to check the serum potassium level early in the course of a myocardial infarction and begin potassium replacement if the level is low.[24]

Renal Effects

Hypokalemia affects many aspects of renal function, including glomerular filtration rate, concentrating ability, ammonia production, urinary acidification, and bicarbonate and sodium reabsorption.[4,18,25,26] The renal abnormalities usually take weeks to develop. Because hypokalemia interferes with the kidney's responsiveness to antidiuretic hormone, the kidney's ability to concentrate urine is decreased, leading to polyuria and polydipsia. Hypokalemia induces an increase in the production of ammonia by renal tubular epithelial cells and diminishes the kidney's ability to acidify urine. Reabsorption of bicarbonate is increased, even in the face of alkalosis. Histologic changes associated with hypokalemia are seen in the renal tubular epithelial cells, but all functional and histologic abnormalities can be reversed with potassium replacement.

Metabolic Effects

Hypokalemia causes some interference in the release of insulin, and mild glucose intolerance is one of the signs of hypokalemia.[3] Since potassium is necessary for the synthesis of skeletal muscle and hepatic glycogen, this function is also impaired by hypokalemia.

Diagnosis

The history usually suggests which patients are likely to have hypokalemia. Some patients, however, may have symptomatic hypokalemia without a history to suggest a cause. Patients can become hypokalemic from occult diuretic abuse, self-induced vomiting, or laxative abuse, but these patients frequently deny these practices. Therefore, it is necessary to determine the serum potassium level in patients with symptoms that suggest hypokalemia, even when there is no relevant history. In addition, hypokalemia may result from such entities as villous adenomas or Bartter's syndrome without a history to suggest these causes.

In patients with unexplained hypokalemia, it is frequently helpful to determine the urine potassium level. Patients with hypokalemia due to renal losses usually have a urine potassium level greater than 10 to 20 mEq/L. If the cause is extrarenal, a kidney is usually able to limit its potassium excretion to less than 10 to 20 mEq/L.[2,3] Serum potassium determinations are extremely unreliable in estimating total body potassium deficits, but they are the easiest to obtain.

Treatment

Hypokalemia should be corrected as slowly as the clinical situation will permit. As mentioned previously, serum potassium determinations are very inaccurate, and it is impossible to predict precisely the amount of potassium that must be replaced.[2,3,27] The safest way to correct hypokalemia is via the gastrointestinal tract with oral supplements.[28] In life-threatening situations that involve severe muscle weakness or digitalis toxicity, or when oral preparations are not tolerated, intravenous potassium chloride must be used. When replacing significant quantities of potassium by the intravenous route, ECG monitoring is required to prevent the development of unrecognized transient hyperkalemia with its possible cardiotoxic effects.

Hypokalemia is frequently associated with alkalosis and a chloride deficit. When an alkalosis is present, bicarbonate acts as a nonreabsorbable anion in the distal tubule, leading to continued potassium losses in the urine unless chloride is replaced along with potassium. Therefore, potassium chloride should be used for replacement in this circumstance.[2,3] If no alkalosis is present, many compounds can be used, including potassium chloride, potassium acetate, potassium phosphate, or potassium bicarbonate.

All oral preparations of potassium chloride are irritating to the gastrointestinal tract and may cause ulcerations, especially if gastrointestinal motility is decreased. Even with enteric-coated tablets, ulcerations of the small bowel have been described.

Salt substitutes are a good source of oral potassium supplementation. One gram of most of these preparations contains about 12 mEq of potassium, so that 1 teaspoon will contain 60 mEq.[29]

When intravenous replacement with potassium chloride is used, the rate should be limited to 20 mEq/hour, or a total of 200 to 250 mEq/day, unless losses continue at a rate greater than this.[2,3,29,30] With peripheral intravenous administration, concentration should not exceed 40 mEq/L, owing to the risk of vein irritation. In severe life-threatening situations, 40 mEq of potassium chloride can be administered in 1 hour via a central vein in a concentration of 60 mEq/L, but continuous ECG monitoring is mandatory.

In patients with significant continuous losses of potassium, daily oral administration of potassium chloride may be necessary. The routine use of potassium chloride in all patients on diuretics does not seem to be justified, however. Several studies have shown that only a small minority of patients develop symptomatic hypokalemia on diuretic therapy. The Boston Collaborative Drug Surveillance Program in 1974 studied 4921 patients on potassium chloride and found that 7 had died as a result of hyperkalemia and 21 others had developed life-threatening complications of hyperkalemia.[31] Eighty-six percent of the patients in this study were taking potassium chloride for prophylaxis rather than for any demonstrated hypokalemia. Patients on diuretic therapy should be monitored for the signs and symptoms of hypokalemia, but routine prophylactic potassium supplementation is not necessary in patients with a normal diet. The serum potassium level of patients on digitalis should be monitored more closely. Some patients benefit from the addition of potassium-sparing diuretics, such as spironolactone, triamterene, or amiloride hydrochloride; but, again, patients must be screened carefully for the development of hyperkalemia.[32,33]

Patients with diabetic ketoacidosis are a special group whose serum potassium levels must be extremely carefully monitored. Many of the deaths that occur in this disease are preventable consequences of hypokalemia. In diabetic ketoacidosis, there is a tremendous loss of potassium, owing to the osmotic diuresis and, occasionally, to vomiting. Initial serum potassium levels may be normal or even high. For each 0.1 decrease in pH, there is an approximate serum increase in potassium of 0.6 mEq/L.[1,2,4] As the acidosis is corrected, the serum potassium level may decrease quite rapidly. Also, insulin causes a shift of potassium to the intracellular space. The combination of correcting the acidosis and using insulin therapy causes extremely precipitous drops in potassium levels, and serum levels should be monitored every 1 to 2 hours for the first 12 hours of therapy. Large doses of intravenous potassium supplementation must be anticipated in the treatment of this disease.

When hypokalemia is present, the magnesium level may also be decreased. Serum magnesium levels are notoriously unreliable indicators of body deficits. When hypokalemia is due to malabsorption or diuretic therapy, when losses of magnesium would be expected, it is frequently wise to add magnesium to the potassium supplement, especially if ventricular irritability is a problem. Hypocalcemia may also be associated with hypokalemia, especially in cases of malabsorption. If this is the case, the correction of either deficit without the simultaneous correction of the other will exacerbate the symptoms of the uncorrected deficit.[10,30]

Since serum levels are only a very indirect measure of total body deficits of potassium, treatment should be followed by serial levels but a lag of at least 30 minutes occurs between intravenous administration and intracellular equilibration.[34]

It is difficult to estimate accurately total body potassium deficits from serum levels. If transcellular shifts are not a factor, then a rough estimate of body deficits is 370 mEq for each decrease of 1 mEq/L down to a serum level of 2.0 mEq/L.[35]

HYPERKALEMIA

One of the most serious electrolyte abnormalities seen in emergency medicine is hyperkalemia. This term is usually applied when the plasma potassium level is greater than 5.5 mEq/L. Severe hyperkalemia is life-threatening and represents a true medical emergency. Death due to hyperkalemia has been reported to occur in 1 of every 1000 hospitalized patients.[8]

Etiology

The four main categories of hyperkalemia and differential diagnoses in each category are as follows[4,7,26,31,36-39]:

I. Spurious
  A. Laboratory error
  B. Hemolysis in vitro
  C. Pseudohyperkalemia secondary to thrombocytosis or leukocytosis
  D. Poor venipuncture technique
II. Excessive Intake
  A. Dietary
  B. Intravenous infusions
  C. Potassium salts
III. Transcellular Redistribution
  A. Severe tissue trauma
  B. Intravascular hemolysis
  C. Acidosis
  D. Insulin deficiency
  E. Hyperkalemic periodic paralysis
  F. Massive digitalis overdose
  G. Administration of succinylcholine (especially in burn and trauma victims)
  H. Rapid lysis of malignant cells
  I. Hyperosmolality
IV. Decreased Excretion
  A. Acute renal failure
  B. Chronic renal failure
  C. Adrenal insufficiency
  D. Potassium-sparing diuretics
  E. Hyporeninemic hypoaldosteronism
  F. Renal transplant
  G. Miscellaneous drugs (nonsteroidal anti-inflammatory drugs, angiotensin-converting enzyme inhibitors, cyclosporine)

Spurious

Whenever hemolysis occurs before or after blood sampling, the serum potassium levels are elevated because intracellular potassium, which is present in a concentration of approximately 150 mEq per liter of cell water has been released.[7,38] When markedly elevated platelet counts (greater than 500,000/mm^3) or leukocyte counts (greater than 100,000/mm^3) are present in the serum, potassium may be artificially elevated because potassium has been released in the clotting process.[7,38] When this is suspected, it can be confirmed by comparing simultaneously drawn serum potassium with a heparinized plasma potassium. Spurious hyperkalemia should be suspected when the potassium is elevated without any accompanying changes on ECG.

Excessive Intake

In individuals with normal renal function, the oral intake of potassium is rarely a cause of sustained hyperkalemia. The rapid administration of 50 mEq of potassium can temporarily elevate the potassium level by 0.5 to 1 mEq/L.[26] Individuals with any degree of renal impairment are candidates for significant hyperkalemia from oral and intravenous infusions. The potential sources of potassium include oral and intravenous potassium salts, potassium salts of penicillin (1.7 mEq/10^6 U), salt substitutes, and banked blood. In Lawson's study of 16,048 patients receiving potassium supplements, approximately 4% developed hyperkalemia and 7 died as a result of their hyperkalemia.[29] When patients are being treated for hypokalemia too rapidly, they may develop transient hyperkalemia prior to the intracellular equilibration of the potassium given.

Transcellular Redistribution

Ninety-eight percent of the body's potassium is intracellular. Owing to this high intracellular concentration of potassium, hyperkalemia may be produced by the release of intracellular potassium to the extracellular space. With severe tissue trauma, such as crush injuries or burns, massive amounts of potassium may be released. Hemolysis and the rapid lysis of malignant cells during drug therapy are other mechanisms of potassium release. During acidosis, hydrogen ions enter cells in exchange for potassium or sodium ions, with a resultant increase in the serum potassium level.[26,37–40] Insulin is very important in the intracellular transport of potassium, and hyperkalemia is one stimulus for insulin release.[41] In the presence of an insulin deficiency, the serum potassium level may be elevated because less potassium can be transported intracellularly. Massive digitalis overdoses block the sodium-potassium adenosine triphosphatase pump in cell membranes that are responsible for maintaining the high intracellular concentration of potassium.[26,39] This action greatly elevates the serum potassium level, but it is seen only with massive doses of digitalis, not clinically therapeutic levels.

An increase in osmolality of the extracellular fluids may enhance the outward diffusion of potassium and lead to hyperkalemia. This phenomenon may occur, for example, in diabetics with hyperglycemia.

Succinylcholine is a muscle relaxant that works by allowing potassium to leak out of cells, causing depolarization blockade of impulses.[26,38] Normally, the potassium level increases by only 0.5 mEq/L or less, but significant potassium increases may occur in patients with burns, multiple trauma, or neuromuscular disease if used more than five days after the event. In acute injury or burn, succinylcholine should not increase the potassium level greater than the normal 0.5 mEq/L.[42]

Hyperkalemic periodic paralysis is a hereditary disease characterized by episodes of muscle weakness or paralysis due to sudden increases in serum potassium. Episodes are precipitated by small increases in dietary potassium or by exercise.[26,37,38] These patients have a diminished ability to transfer and maintain potassium intracellularly, but the exact nature of the defect is unknown. Attacks can be prevented by treatment with mineralocorticoids or acetazolamide. Success has also been reported with the use of salbutamol, a β-adrenergic agonist.

Decreased Excretion

Since greater than 90% of potassium excretion is mediated by the kidneys, major changes in the serum potassium level can occur if renal function is decreased.[26,39] The most severe condition is acute oliguric renal failure. In this condition, the potassium level may rise sharply, owing to the inability to excrete potassium. This may be exacerbated both by the acidosis that may develop and by the increased potassium load that results from the catabolic state. In chronic renal failure, the ability to excrete potassium is frequently maintained because the surviving nephrons adapt, excreting four to five times their normal amount of potassium. Maintaining a normal potassium level in the presence of chronic renal failure is highly dependent on urine volumes, however. Patients may be able to maintain potassium at normal levels until the potassium load is increased or potassium-sparing diuretics, such as spironolactone, triamterene, or amiloride, are used. These drugs work by different mechanisms, but all selectively block the aldosterone-mediated distal tubule reabsorption of sodium, thereby limiting the normal mechanism for potassium secretion. Because patients with decreased renal function are very sensitive to these drugs, they should be used with caution in these patients. A case of fatal hyperkalemia due to spironolactone in a patient with entirely normal renal function has been reported.[43]

Other drugs also may cause an increase in potassium levels. Nonsteroidal anti-inflammatory drugs and cyclosporine may suppress renin production, leading to a decrease in aldosterone levels. Angiotensin-converting enzyme inhibitors also inhibit aldosterone production.

Patients with adrenal insufficiency have a decreased production of mineralocorticoid and, therefore, a decreased ability for distal tubular secretion of potassium. In addition, patients with only mild degrees of renal insufficiency may have chronic hyperkalemia. These patients are reported to have decreased levels of renin and, thereby, decreased levels of aldosterone. Patients with this hyporeninemic hypoaldosteronism are frequently also diabetic, and many have a hyperchloremic metabolic acidosis.[26,37,39] Patients with renal transplants frequently have marked difficulty with the tubular mechanisms responsible for potassium excretion.[39,44]

Clinical Manifestations

The major clinical manifestations of hyperkalemia include the following[4,26,37–39]:

- *cardiovascular:* ECG changes, heart block, ventricular arrhythmias
- *neuromuscular:* paresthesias, weakness, flaccid paralysis
- *gastrointestinal:* nausea, vomiting, abdominal pain, ileus

All the manifestations of hyperkalemia can be attributed to the high extracellular potassium level on cell membranes. An increase in the ratio of extracellular to intracellular potassium decreases the resting membrane potential toward threshold levels with resultant delays in depolarization, hastening of repolarization, and decreased conduction velocity. Significant clinical abnormalities are not usually seen until the plasma potassium level exceeds 6.0 to 6.5 mEq/L.

Cardiotoxicity

The most serious medical problem induced by hyperkalemia is cardiotoxicity. Cardiac tissue is very vulnerable to the effects of hyperkalemia. The ECG changes seen with hyperkalemia are relatively reliable; in fact, when hyperkalemia occurs without ECG changes, spurious hyperkalemia should be suspected. With increasing levels of potassium, the following changes are noted[37,38,44–46]:

- peaking of T waves (with normal or slightly decreased QT interval)
- PR lengthening with possible ST segment depression
- disappearing P waves
- increasing degrees of heart block
- widening of the QRS complex
- ventricular arrhythmias with possible sine wave pattern
- ventricular fibrillation or standstill

The most reliable ECG change seen with hyperkalemia is the peaking of T waves, which can sometimes be distinguished from T-wave changes of ischemic heart disease by the lack of U waves and the lack of any T-wave axis changes in the horizontal plane. The presence of any ECG changes of hyperkalemia warrants immediate treatment, since the progression to fatal cardiotoxicity is unpredictable and frequently rapid. Hyponatremia, hypocalcemia, and acidosis all increase the cardiotoxicity of hyperkalemia and should be corrected if they exist.

Neuromuscular Effects

The first neuromuscular sign of hyperkalemia is usually the onset of paresthesias. This may be followed by weakness of several muscle groups in an ascending pattern. If hyperkalemia becomes severe, flaccid quadriplegia may occur. Cerebral and cranial nerve function is usually preserved, and respiratory muscle paralysis is very rare.

Treatment

Hyperkalemia is a life-threatening condition that deserves immediate medical attention. When ECG changes of hyperkalemia are seen, continuous ECG monitoring is mandatory until the hyperkalemia has been corrected. There are four general categories of treatment:

I. Antagonism of membrane effects
   A. Calcium (calcium gluconate or calcium chloride)
   B. Sodium (if hyponatremia exists)
   C. β_2 Agonists
II. Transfer of potassium intracellularly
   A. Sodium bicarbonate
   B. Glucose with or without insulin
III. Removal of potassium from the body
   A. Potassium exchange resins
   B. Hemodialysis
   C. Peritoneal dialysis
   D. Loop diuretics
IV. Correction of underlying defects

The decision as to which modalities should be used in the treatment depends on the degree of potassium elevation and the associated medical conditions.[30,37–39,47,48]

Antagonism of Membrane Effects

When changes of hyperkalemia other than peaked T waves are seen on the ECG, then immediate measures must be taken to prevent ventricular dysrhythmias. The intravenous administration of calcium, either as calcium gluconate or calcium chloride, has the earliest action. Calcium decreases the membrane threshold potentials, counteracting some of the effects of hyperkalemia on cell membranes. These actions are very rapid but temporary; they are to be used only in conjunction with other measures. Calcium chloride or calcium gluconate may be administered intravenously as a 10% solution with 10 to 30 mL given over several minutes. Also, another 10 to 30 mL calcium can be added to a 1-L bottle of a dextrose solution.

Hyponatremia exacerbates the membrane abnormalities induced by hyperkalemia. When a patient has any degree of hyponatremia, the administration of sodium frequently corrects some of the membrane effects of hyperkalemia. Care must be used to avoid fluid overload when sodium is administered as a hypertonic solution, however. The result of sodium use is not as reliable as that of calcium. An excellent way to add sodium is by means of sodium bicarbonate added to a dextrose solution, which combines the beneficial effects of sodium, bicarbonate, and dextrose.

Transfer of Potassium Intracellularly

An extremely useful strategy in the treatment of hyperkalemia is to increase the transfer of extracellular potassium to the intracellular space. When acidosis exists, it should be corrected immediately, since the serum potassium level increases approximately 0.6 mEq/L for each 0.1 decrease in pH.[7,26,37,38] The bicarbonate ion increases the transfer of potassium to the intracellular space even when pH changes do not occur.[43] Fifty to 100 mEq/L sodium bicarbonate can be administered over several minutes.

Insulin also facilitates the transfer of potassium intracellularly. In nondiabetics, administering glucose first as 50 mL of a 50% solution followed by 500 mL of 10% dextrose enhances endogenous insulin secretion. It is frequently helpful to add 5 to 10 U of regular insulin while administering this combination, being careful to avoid hypoglycemia. In patients with diabetes mellitus, insulin should be administered with the dextrose infusion. Approximately 1 U of regular insulin for each 3 g of glucose usually suffices, but serum glucose levels must be monitored.[37]

The use of β_2 agonists such as albuterol causes extracellular potassium to be transported intracellularly. This action may be very prompt and may last for 2 hours.[49]

Removal of Potassium from the Body

Antagonizing the membrane effects of hyperkalemia and increasing the transport of potassium to the intracellular space are both temporary measures. The definitive treatment of hyperkalemia is to remove potassium from the body. The simplest technique to accomplish this is the administration of the cation exchange resin sodium polystyrene sulfonate (Kayexalate). This resin can be administered orally or in a retention enema. For each gram of resin used, approximately 1 mEq of potassium is removed.[26,38] When given orally, 20 to 30 g of Kayexalate can be added to an approximately equal amount of sorbitol. Sorbitol increases the amount of fluid entering the intestinal tract, thereby facilitating ion exchange. Retention enemas can be mixed by adding 50 to 100 g of Kayexalate to 200 mL of water and adding an appropriate amount of sorbitol. The enema must be retained for 30 to 45 minutes.

When extremely large amounts of potassium must be removed, hemodialysis and peritoneal dialysis can be considered. Hemodialysis is extremely effective—it can remove potassium at a rate of 25 to 50 mEq/hour. Peritoneal dialysis is less predictable and may not remove more than 10 to 15 mEq/hour. In patients who are nonoliguric with only minor elevations of serum potassium, the loop diuretics increase the renal excretion of potassium. Patients in cardiac arrest secondary to hyperkalemia should have prolonged resuscitation attempts while correcting the serum potassium. One case report described a 36-year-old man with chronic renal failure who suffered a cardiac arrest due to hyperkalemia. After 145 minutes of external cardiac massage and 75 minutes of hemodialysis the patient was successfully defibrillated and had a totally normal neurologic recovery.[50]

Correction of Underlying Defects

Hyperkalemia is usually a short-term problem, but certain underlying medical conditions require continuing therapy. With hyperkalemia periodic paralysis, mineralocorticoids, acetazolamide, and salbutamol have all been shown to be effective at decreasing episodes of paralysis.[7,26,38] In chronic renal failure, potassium-sparing diuretics and large loads of potassium must be avoided. With adrenal insufficiency and with hyporeninemic hyperaldosteronism, chronic mineralocorticoid therapy is very effective at maintaining potassium within normal levels.

REFERENCES

1. Nardone DA, et al. Mechanisms in hypokalemia: clinical correlation. *Medicine.* 1978;57:435.
2. Rose BD, ed. *Hypokalemia: Clinical Physiology of Acid-Base and Electrolyte Disorders.* New York: McGraw-Hill; 1977.
3. Cohen J Jr, et al. Acid-base disorders of respiratory origin. In: Brenner BM, Stein JH, eds. *Acid-Base and Potassium Homeostasis.* New York: Churchill Livingstone; 1978.
4. Cohen JJ. Disorders of potassium balance. *Hosp Pract.* 1979;1:119.
5. Lowman DH, et al. Severe hypokalemia in hospitalized patients. *Arch Intern Med.* 1979;139:978.
6. Rose DB, ed. *Introduction to Disorders of Potassium Balance: Clinical Physiology of Acid-Base and Electrolyte Disorders.* New York: McGraw-Hill; 1977.
7. Kliger AS, et al. Disorders of potassium balance. In: Brenner BM, Stein JH, eds. *Acid-Base and Potassium Homeostasis.* New York: Churchill Livingstone; 1978.
8. Zull DN. Disorders of potassium metabolism. *Emerg Med Clin North Am.* 1988;7:771.
9. Mohr JA, et al. Nafcillin-associated hypokalemia. *JAMA.* 1979;242:544.
10. Bartter FC. Clinical problems of potassium metabolism. *Contrib Nephrol.* 1980;21:115.
11. Gastel B, Ehrlichman R, eds. Clinical conferences at the Johns Hopkins Hospital—hypokalemic periodic paralysis. *Johns Hopkins Med J.* 1978;143:148.
12. Gelmont DM, et al. Hypokalemia induced by inhaled bronchodilators. *Chest.* 1988;94:763.
13. Brown MJ, et al. Hypokalemia from beta$_2$ receptor simulation by circulating epinephrine. *N Engl J Med.* 1983;309:1414.
14. Rosa RM, et al. Adrenergic modulation of extrarenal potassium disposal. *N Engl J Med.* 1980;302:431.
15. Berning J. Hypokalemia of barium poisoning. *Lancet.* 1975;1:110.
16. Smith JS Jr. Hypokalemia in resuscitation from multiple trauma. *Surg Gynecol Obstet.* 1978;147:18.
17. Carlsson E, et al. B-adrenoceptor blockers; plasma potassium and exercise. *Lancet.* 1978;2:424.
18. Cronin RE, et al. The consequences of potassium deficiency in acid-base and potassium. In: Brenner BM, Stein JH, eds. *Acid-Base and Potassium Homeostasis.* New York: Churchill Livingstone; 1978.

19. Laei F, et al. Licorice, snuff and hypokalemia. *N Engl J Med*. 1980;303:463. Letter.
20. Carlon GC. Drug associations in hypokalemia. *Arch Intern Med*. 1980;140:989. Letter.
21. Schamroth L, et al. A case of prolonged Q-T interval. *Heart Lung*. 1978;7:846.
22. Dychner T, et al. Ventricular extrasystoles and intracellular electrolytes in hypokalemic patients before and after correction of the hypokalemia. *Acta Med Scand*. 1978;204:375.
23. Parrish C, et al. Les torsades des pointes. *Ann Emerg Med*. 1982;3:143.
24. Duke M. Thiazide-induced hypokalemia association with acute myocardial infarction and ventricular fibrillation. *JAMA*. 1978;239:43.
25. Giebisch G, et al. Renal transport and control of potassium excretion. In: Brenner BM, Rector FL, eds. *The Kidney*. 2nd ed. Philadelphia: Saunders; 1981.
26. Cohen JJ, et al. Disorders of potassium balance. In: Brenner BM, Rector FL, eds. *The Kidney*. 2nd ed. Philadelphia: Saunders; 1981.
27. Franklin JE Jr. Long-standing hypokalemia. *Hosp Pract*. 1979;9:153.
28. Ramsay LE, et al. Rational potassium prescribing. *Practitioner*. 1977;219:529.
29. Zeluff GW, et al. Hypokalemia—cause and treatment. *Heart Lung*. 1978;7:854.
30. Levinsky N. Fluid and electrolytes. In: Isselbacher KJ, Adams RD, Braunwald E, et al, eds. *Harrison's Principles of Internal Medicine*. 9th ed. New York: McGraw-Hill; 1980.
31. Lawson DH. Adverse reactions to potassium chloride. *Q J Med*. 1974;171:433.
32. Ramsay LE, et al. Amiloride, spironolactone, and potassium chloride in thiazide-treated hypertensive patients. *Clin Pharmacol Ther*. 1980;4:533.
33. Pearce VR, et al. Total exchangeable potassium in response to amiloride. *Postgrad Med J*. 1978;54:533.
34. Azar I, et al. Rapid correction of chronic hypokalemia in dogs. *Anesth Analg*. 1985;64:192.
35. Elms JJ. Disorders of potassium metabolism. In: Mandal AK, Jeannette JC, eds. *Diagnosis and Management of Renal Disease and Hypertension*. Philadelphia: Lea & Febiger; 1988.
36. Lowenstein J. Hypokalemia and hyperkalemia. *Med Clin North Am*. 1973;57:1435.
37. Daniels GH. Metabolic and endocrine emergencies. In: Wilkins EW Jr, ed. *MGH Textbook of Emergency Medicine*. Baltimore: Williams & Wilkins; 1981.
38. Falls WF. Hyperkalemia: pathophysiology and management. *Va Med*. 1980;107:184.
39. Rose BD, ed. *Hyperkalemia: Clinical Physiology of Acid-Base and Electrolyte Disorders*. New York: McGraw-Hill; 1977.
40. Hassan H, et al. Hypercapnia and hyperkalaemia. *Anaesthesia*. 1979;34:897.
41. Cox M, et al. The defense against hyperkalemia: the roles of insulin and aldosterone. *N Engl J Med*. 1978;299:525.
42. Barnett WM, Paris PM. Hyperkalemia and succinylcholine. *Ann Emerg Med*. 1983;12:654.
43. Welti CV, et al. Fatal hyperkalemia from accidental overdose of potassium chloride. *JAMA*. 1978;240:1339. Letter.
44. Shapiro JB. Bifascicular block produced by hyperkalemia. *Cardiology*. 1979;64:303.
45. Schwartz AB. Potassium-related cardiac arrhythmias and their treatment. *Angiology*. 1978;29:194.
46. Burris AC, et al. Pseudomyocardial infarction associated with acute bifascicular block due to hyperkalemia. *Cardiology*. 1980;65:115.
47. Levinsky NG. Management of emergencies: VI. Hyperkalemia. *N Engl J Med*. 1966;274:1076.
48. Fraley DS, et al. Correction of hyperkalemia by bicarbonate despite constant blood pH. *Kidney Int*. 1977;12:354.
49. Allon M, Dunlay R, Copkney C. Nebulized albuterol for acute hyperkalemia in patients on hemodialysis. *Ann Intern Med*. 1989;110:426.
50. Gomez-Arnau J, et al. Hyperkalemic cardiac arrest: prolonged heart massage and simultaneous hemodialysis. *Crit Care Med*. 1981;9:556.

19. Hypomagnesemia, Hypermagnesemia, and Magnesium Therapy

JOEL GEIDERMAN, MD, FACEP

Disorders of magnesium balance are now being recognized more frequently than they were in the past, owing largely to new techniques that allow rapid and accurate measurement of the cation and to an increased awareness of the manifestations of these disorders. Both hypermagnesemia and hypomagnesemia may be life-threatening emergencies that require prompt medical treatment, or they may be less severe disturbances with subtle symptomatology. Normomagnesemic patients may also benefit from magnesium therapy for some conditions.

MAGNESIUM HOMEOSTASIS

Magnesium is the fourth most abundant cation in the body and the second most plentiful intracellular element. The adult human body contains 21 to 28 g, or about 2000 mEq, of magnesium. Approximately 50% of the total body magnesium is in bone; the other 50% is about equally divided between muscular and nonmuscular soft tissue.[1] Only about 1% of total body magnesium is extracellular. Twenty percent to 30% of serum magnesium is protein bound; the remainder is in diffusible form, mainly as free ionized magnesium.[2] The normal serum magnesium concentration ranges between 1.6 and 2.1 mEq/L.[3]

The level of magnesium in serum does not always accurately reflect total body magnesium stores, since the magnesium in the vascular space is only a fraction of the total body pool of the cation.[4] Serum and intracellular levels vary independently, and deficit or excess in one compartment may not indicate the level in the other.[5] Skeletal muscle biopsy provides the most accurate measurement of total body magnesium stores[6] but is not practical in the emergency setting. Measurement of serum magnesium levels must therefore suffice as the quickest, simplest, and most effective screening tool when magnesium depletion is suspected.[7]

An adult's average daily intake of magnesium is 20 to 40 mEq, much of which is contained in the chlorophyll portion of green vegetables.[1] Other sources include meats, grains, and seafood. The daily requirement of magnesium for the adult is approximately 5 mg/kg, or about 350 mg for a 70-kg person (Table 19-1).[8] This amount is contained in 3.5 g of magnesium sulfate.

Magnesium is absorbed primarily from the proximal small intestine; little is absorbed from the colon. Absorption begins within 1 hour of ingestion, continues at a steady rate for 2 to 6 hours, and has nearly ceased after 12 hours.[4] Under normal circumstances, 30% to 60% of orally ingested magnesium is absorbed. No apparent adaptation in absorption occurs in response to the body's need for the ion.

The kidneys are largely responsible for regulation of the serum magnesium concentration. Approximately 1800 mg of magnesium is filtered at the glomerule each day.[9] Since the diffusible fraction of magnesium is the moiety that is filtered, the filtered load is a function of both the serum concentration of diffusible magnesium and the glomerular filtration rate. Magnesium is actively reabsorbed along the entire nephron but mainly in the proximal tubule. There seems to be a tubular maximum for reabsorption beyond which all magnesium is excreted. Under normal circumstances, 3% to 5% of the filtered load is excreted in the urine.[2]

Table 19-1 Nutritional Requirements for Magnesium

Period of Life	Age (years)	Amount of Magnesium (mg/day)
Infants	0–0.5	50
	0.5–1	70
Children	1–3	150
	4–6	200
	7–10	250
Adults		
Men	11–14	350
	15–18	400
	19 and older	350
Women	11–14	300
	15 and older	300
	During pregnancy	300 + 150
	During lactation	300 + 150

Source: Food and Nutrition Board of National Academy of Sciences and National Research Council, 1980.

Many conditions can affect proximal tubular reabsorption of magnesium and result in variations in urinary excretion.[10] Factors that decrease tubular reabsorption include the following[11]:

- extracellular fluid volume expansion (saline infusions)
- renal vasodilatation
- osmotic diuretics
- diuretics
- hypercalcemia
- alcohol ingestion
- high sodium intake
- growth hormone
- thyroid hormone
- calcitonin
- chronic mineralocorticoid excess
- phosphate depletion
- gentamicin
- tobramycin
- carbenicillin

Renal handling of magnesium is closely associated with that of sodium; in general, those agents that produce natriuresis produce magnesiuria as well.

The major factors that increase tubular reabsorption of magnesium are parathyroid hormone and hypomagnesemia.[2]

BIOCHEMICAL ASPECTS

Magnesium activates an array of enzyme systems that are vital to intracellular metabolism. Most prominent among these enzymes are those that hydrolyze and transfer phosphate groups, which are important in the synthesis of adenosine triphosphate (ATP).[4,12] ATP is necessary for glucose utilization; for synthesis of protein, nucleic acids, nucleoproteins, nucleotides, coenzymes, and carbohydrates; for muscle contraction; and for maintenance of the sodium–potassium pump.[4,8] Magnesium also stabilizes ribosomes and thereby facilitates polypeptide formation. Interference with magnesium balance can therefore affect all of these functions.

HYPOMAGNESEMIA

Clinical Manifestations

The predominant clinical manifestations of hypomagnesemia are gastrointestinal and neurologic, involving both the central and peripheral nervous systems (Fig. 19-1)[1–3,13]:

- anorexia
- nausea, vomiting, diarrhea
- fasciculations
- gross tremor
- athetoid movements
- tetany
- convulsions
- confusion
- stupor, coma
- hallucinations
- supraventricular dysrhythmias
- ventricular dysrhythmias

Magnesium has a curarelike effect at the neuromuscular junction, presumably because it interferes with the release of acetylcholine at the motor neuron terminal.[12] Thus, hypomagnesemia leads to hyperexcitability as a result of the accumulation of acetylcholine at the neuromuscular junction.[14]

Tetany caused by hypomagnesemia is clinically indistinguishable from tetany caused by any other condition.[15] In the past, the existence of tetany in humans as a result of hypomagnesemia alone, in the absence of other measurable serum electrolyte or acid-base disturbances, has been controversial. However, the magnesium-deficiency tetany syndrome is now a recognized clinical entity. The diagnosis of human tetany is based on facial muscle and carpopedal spasm, convulsions, and, occasionally, laryngeal stridor.[15] Latent tetany may be elicited as Chvostek's and Trousseau's signs.

Supraventricular tachycardia, ventricular tachycardia, paroxysmal ventricular fibrillation, and torsades de pointes have all been reported in association with hypomagnesemia.[16–20] Nonspecific changes on the electrocardiogram

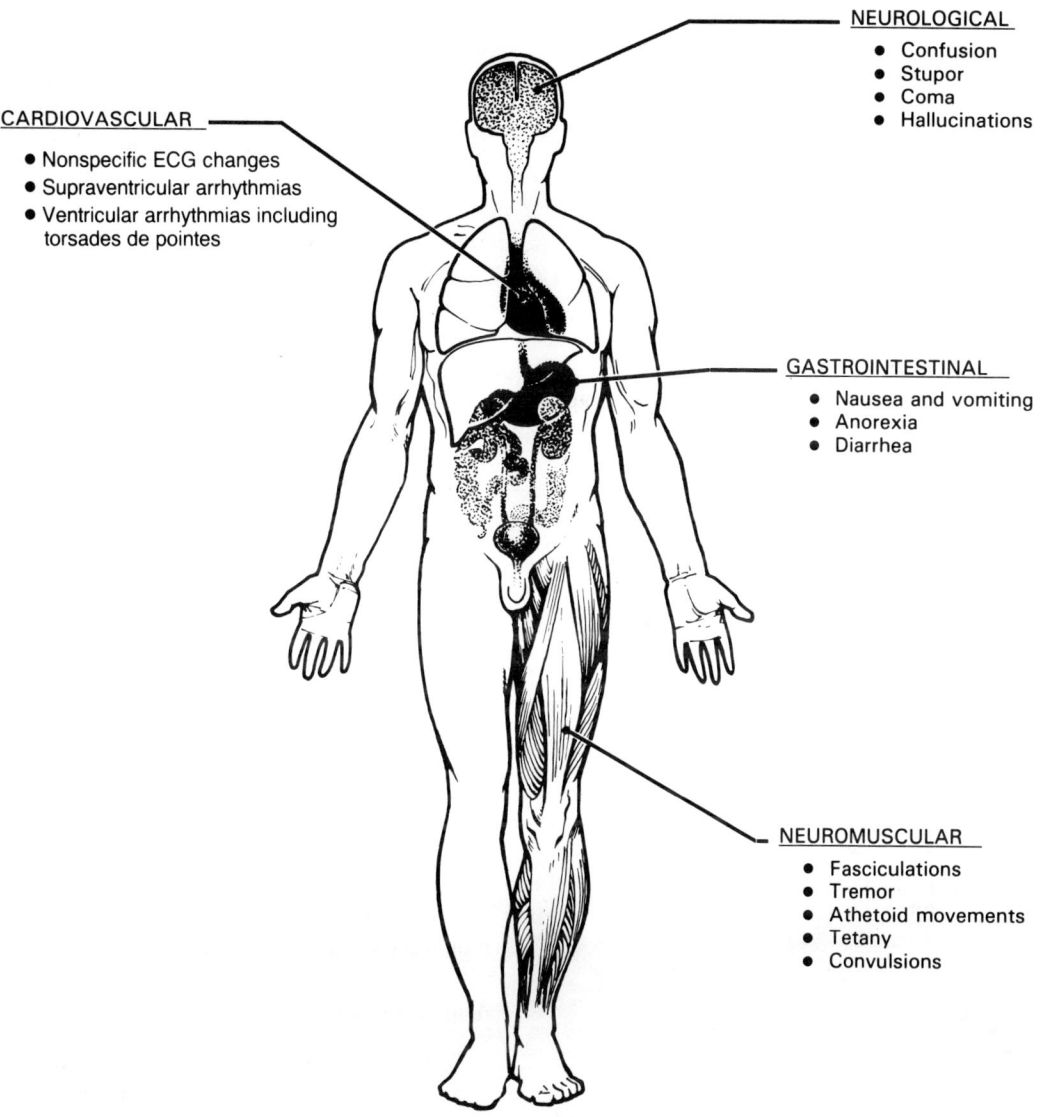

Figure 19-1 Clinical manifestations of hypomagnesemia.

(ECG), such as prolonged PR interval, ST segment depression, and inverted or peaked T waves, also occur.[17] The explanation for the cardiac arrhythmias seen with magnesium deficiency remains speculative.[21,22] Since magnesium deficiency is almost always associated with imbalance of other electrolytes, it is difficult to be certain which electrolyte abnormality is responsible for the ECG changes.

Etiology

Hypomagnesemia may result from poor intake or a defect in absorption or excretion. The following conditions are associated with hypomagnesemia:

- decreased intake
  a. protein-calorie malnutrition
  b. starvation
  c. prolonged intravenous therapy without added magnesium
  d. liquid protein diet
- decreased intestinal absorption
  a. malabsorption syndromes, including nontropical sprue, celiac disease, and tropical sprue
  b. massive surgical resection of small intestine
  c. neonatal hypomagnesemia with selective malabsorption of magnesium
- excessive losses of body fluids
  a. prolonged nasogastric suction
  b. excessive uses of purgatives
  c. intestinal and biliary fistulas
  d. severe diarrhea, as in ulcerative colitis and infantile gastroenteritis
  e. rarely, prolonged lactation
  f. cancer of the colon

- excessive urinary losses
  a. diuretic therapy
  b. diuretic phase of acute renal failure
  c. chronic alcoholism
  d. primary and secondary aldosteronism
  e. hypercalcemic states (eg, malignancy, hyperparathyroidism, and vitamin D excess)
  f. renal tubular acidosis
  g. diabetes, especially during the treatment of acidosis
  h. hyperthyroidism
  i. idiopathic renal magnesium wasting
  j. chronic renal failure with renal magnesium wasting
  k. gentamicin, tobramycin, and carbenicillin therapy
  l. alcoholic cirrhosis
  m. glomerulonephritis
  n. pyelonephritis
  o. familial and sporadic renal magnesium wasting
  p. cisplatin therapy
- miscellaneous
  a. idiopathic hypomagnesemia
  b. acute pancreatitis
  c. porphyria with inappropriate secretion of antidiuretic hormone
  d. multiple transfusions or exchange transfusions with citrated blood
  e. malignant osteolytic disease
  f. cardiopulmonary bypass
  g. infant born of hypomagnesemic mother
  h. hypoparathyroidism

Alcoholism

Alcoholism is the most common cause of hypomagnesemia.[11] A variety of factors, including decreased dietary intake, vomiting, diarrhea, hyperhidrosis, and increased urinary excretion, contribute to the hypomagnesemia.[17,23] Magnesium diuresis results from ethanol's interference with tubular reabsorption of the ion. In patients with alcoholic cirrhosis and ascites, hypomagnesemia may be caused by secondary hyperaldosteronism, which prevents distal tubular reabsorption.[24]

Because magnesium levels fall precipitously soon after the withdrawal of alcohol, the neurologic manifestations of hypomagnesemia may be seen at this time. This must be differentiated from delirium tremens, which may occur simultaneously.[17,23,25] Although hypomagnesemia is common in severe alcoholism and may be symptomatic in some patients, it clearly is not the cause of delirium tremens.[15] The latter may develop and progress, despite vigorous magnesium replacement and normal serum magnesium levels. Each of these closely related symptom complexes must be considered separately.

Malabsorption

Malabsorption syndromes, especially those associated with steatorrhea, may also result in hypomagnesemia.[6] This may be secondary to the excretion of large amounts of magnesium soaps. Steatorrheic hypomagnesemia has been reported in patients with nontropical sprue, following abdominal irradiation, and after extensive small bowel resection. It also may occur after jejunoileal bypass for morbid obesity[16,26,27] and in patients who abuse laxatives.

Severely Decreased Dietary Intake

Patients who are maintained on magnesium-free parenteral fluids for long periods of time are at risk of developing magnesium deficiency.[28] This should be considered in a patient who comes to the emergency department after a recent long hospitalization. Another group of patients predisposed to hypomagnesemia secondary to reduced dietary intake are those on liquid protein diets for obesity.[29]

Diabetic Ketoacidosis

Diabetes is also associated with hypomagnesemia.[28,30] With glycosuria, there is a threefold increase in urinary magnesium excretion, resulting in depletion.[30] In the initial phases of diabetic ketoacidosis, serum magnesium levels may be normal or slightly elevated owing to the acidosis and dehydration.[31] However, fluid and insulin therapy not only lead to large urinary losses of magnesium but also facilitate the movement of the ion intracellularly. This may produce severe hypomagnesemia, resulting in fatal dysrhythmias.[32] It is therefore recommended that magnesium be added to replacement fluids and that serum levels of the ion be monitored during treatment.

Acute Pancreatitis

Patients with acute pancreatitis may develop hypomagnesemia, but this may be associated with the high frequency of alcohol abuse among patients with acute pancreatitis. The presence of hypomagnesemia seems to correlate with the presence of hypocalcemia.

Multiple Transfusions

Anticoagulants such as citrate, administered with transfused blood, may bind magnesium and cause deficiency.

Association with Congestive Heart Failure

A condition commonly seen in the emergency department that may be associated with hypomagnesemia is congestive heart failure[29] (see Chapter 64, Congestive Heart Failure). Several factors may lead to magnesium depletion in these patients. Markedly congested splanchnic vessels may lead to malabsorption of the ion in the gut. Secondary hyperaldosteronism contributes to the hypomagnesemia[33] by preventing reabsorption at the distal convoluted tubule. Cardiac glycosides are known to reduce renal absorption of magnesium also. This can have catastrophic consequences, since hypomagnesemia has been shown to predispose patients

Table 19-2 Suggested Dosage Schedule for Treatment of Magnesium Depletion

Route	Day	Dosage
Intramuscular (50% magnesium sulfate solution)	1	2 g (16.3 mEq) q2h × 3 doses, then 1 g (8.1 mEq) q4h × 4 doses
	2	1 g (8.1 mEq) q4h × 6 doses
	3–5	1 g (8.1 mEq) q6h
Intravenous (<20% magnesium sulfate solution only)	1	6 g (48 mEq) in 1000 mL desired intravenous solution to be infused over 3 hours, then 5 g (41 mEq) in each of two 1-L solutions to be infused over the day
	2–5	6 g (49 mEq) distributed equally in the total fluids of the day

Source: Information from Flink EB: Therapy of magnesium deficiency. Ann NY Acad Sci. 162:901–905, 1969.

taking digitalis to dysrhythmias.[17,34] Serum magnesium and potassium levels should be checked in all patients with suspected digitalis-induced dysrhythmias, and magnesium should be administered if serum concentrations are low. This has been effective in abolishing a number of dysrhythmias.

Finally, thiazide diuretics and furosemide, commonly used in congestive heart failure, both increase renal magnesium clearance.[33,35] Some have suggested routine measurement of serum magnesium in all patients taking diuretics and digitalis.

Treatment

While asymptomatic magnesium-depleted patients may warrant treatment, only symptomatic hypomagnesemia should be treated in the emergency department.[7] Occult magnesium deficiency can be detected in skeletal muscle,[33] but only the magnesium in the intravascular space can be rapidly measured by the emergency physician. Some patients may require treatment on an empiric basis, before magnesium depletion has been demonstrated. This may be especially true in smaller hospitals that do not have the facilities to provide rapid measurements. Renal function must be assessed before therapy is begun, however. Azotemia does not exclude therapy but necessitates modification of dosage.[35]

Convulsive seizures due to magnesium deficiency represent a true medical emergency and require immediate, vigorous treatment. The loading dose for such a patient is 4 g (33 mEq) of magnesium given as a 10% to 20% solution of magnesium sulfate[36] over 5 to 10 minutes, followed by either continuous intravenous or intramuscular administration. Intravenous magnesium sulfate should never be given as the 50% solution. A 20-mL dose of 20% solution (4 g) can be made by mixing 8 mL of 50% magnesium sulfate solution and 12 mL of sterile distilled water. Each magnesium sulfate molecule, with a molecular weight of 246, contains 8.1 mEq/g. Each magnesium chloride molecule, with a molecular weight of 203, contains 9.75 mEq/g.

Serious dysrhythmias occur frequently in the alcohol withdrawal syndrome. They require urgent treatment, since sudden death of patients with the alcohol withdrawal syndrome is probably related to tachydysrhythmias. In case of ventricular tachycardia or ventricular fibrillation in alcohol withdrawal, 2 g (16.3 mEq) of magnesium sulfate as a 10% to 20% solution should be given intravenously over 5 to 10 minutes, followed by continuous intravenous infusion.[36]

Magnesium-depleted patients usually require 1 to 2 mEq/kg for parenteral replacement, and restitution of magnesium stores must take place over a 3- to 4-day period. Thus, magnesium-depleted patients usually require hospitalization, although treatment can be started in the emergency department as outlined in Table 19-2.

It has been shown that plasma levels of magnesium will not exceed 6.5 mEq/L as long as the rate of administration of magnesium salt does not exceed 100 mEq in 12 hours. Furthermore, it has been shown that patients can normally excrete 40 to 60 g of magnesium sulfate every 24 hours.[36] Thus, complications should not occur when the recommended regimen is employed in normal individuals. However, kidney function must be evaluated before treatment is begun. In azotemic patients, therapy must be modified and carefully monitored.[8]

There does not appear to be any therapeutic advantage of the intravenous route over the intramuscular route, except when treating convulsions and dysrhythmias. If any intravenous solution is being given already, magnesium should be added to it; otherwise, the intramuscular route is acceptable.

MAGNESIUM THERAPY IN NORMOMAGNESEMIC PATIENTS

Cardiac

Intractable ventricular tachycardia and ventricular fibrillation have been treated successfully with magnesium in patients with normal serum magnesium levels.[37] These patients, who had failed to respond to standard drug regimens, had their condition successfully controlled with 2 to 3 g of magnesium sulfate given over 1 minute and then with 10 g over 5 hours. Iseri and associates[37] postulate that a high concentration of magnesium may prolong transient inward current, prolong the effective refractory period, and increase the membrane potential, thus controlling ventricular irritability. Torsades de pointes, an unusual type of ventricular tachycardia, has also been shown to respond to infusion of magnesium sulfate, even in the presence of normomagnesemia.[38]

Magnesium sulfate was administered to 100 patients in a double-blind randomized trial of patients admitted after acute myocardial infarction.[39] Compared to 100 placebo-treated patients, those patients receiving magnesium experienced a lower rate of ventricular dysrhythmias and death. This approach merits further study before it can be widely advocated.

Pulmonary

Several small studies showed significant improvement of patients with acute asthma who were treated with magnesium sulfate.[40–43] The dosages used, 1 to 3 g over 20 minutes, are considered safe, and some experts consider magnesium sulfate a safe and effective adjunct to conventional therapy in patients with severe asthma who do not respond to standard therapy.[44]

HYPERMAGNESEMIA

Clinical Manifestations

Hypermagnesemia affects mainly the nervous and cardiovascular systems.[2] Deep tendon reflexes are usually lost when the serum magnesium level reaches 6 mEq/L, and the patient may be sedated. Muscle paralysis, respiratory depression, narcosis, and hypotension may occur as the serum concentration approaches 10 mEq/L. ECG changes include lengthening of the PR interval, progressing to complete heart block, widening of the QRS complex, and transient rise in heart rate followed by bradycardia.[2,11] Asystolic arrest may occur if the level reaches 14 to 15 mEq/L.

Etiology

Hypermagnesemia, less common than hypomagnesemia, may develop in a number of conditions (Table 19-3).[11] The most common cause is severe renal failure,[3] especially when exogenous sources are not restricted. The other major cause is iatrogenic; hypermagnesemia may develop during therapy of the toxemic patient.

Treatment

Symptomatic patients with serum magnesium levels of greater than 5 mEq/L and those with levels of 8 mEq/L, regardless of whether they have symptoms, should be treated.[11] Treatment is 5 mL of 10% calcium chloride solution by slow intravenous push. This may be repeated if symptoms do not subside within 2 minutes, thereafter as dictated by the clinical setting.[11] Peritoneal dialysis or hemodialysis should be considered for persistently high levels.

Table 19-3 Clinical Settings of Hypermagnesemia

Common
- Acute renal failure
- Chronic renal failure with exogenous magnesium intake
- Toxemia therapy

Less Common
- Chronic renal failure without exogenous intake
- Rectal administration of magnesium-containing solutions

Uncommon
- Parasitosis with exogenous magnesium intake
- Lithium therapy
- Hypothyroidism
- Certain neoplasms with skeletal involvement
- Viral hepatitis
- Hyperparathyroidism with renal disease
- Pituitary dwarfism
- Milk-alkali syndrome
- Perforated viscus with exogenous magnesium intake
- Acute diabetic ketoacidosis
- Addison's disease

Source: Modified and reprinted with permission from Graber TW, Yee AS, Baker FJ: Magnesium: Physiology, clinical disorders, and therapy. *Ann Emerg Med.* 10:49–57, 1981.

REFERENCES

1. Wacker WEC, Parisi AF. Magnesium metabolism. *N Engl J Med.* 1968;278:656–661, 712–716.
2. Massry SG, Seelig MS. Hypomagnesemia and hypermagnesemia. *Clin Nephrol.* 1977;7:147–153.
3. Fishman RA. Neurological aspects of magnesium metabolism. *Arch Neurol.* 1965;12:562–569.
4. Swenson SA, Lewis JW, Sebby KR. Magnesium metabolism in man with special reference to jejunoileal bypass for obesity. *Am J Surg.* 1974;127:250–255.
5. Reinhart RA. Magnesium metabolism. *Arch Intern Med.* 1988;148:2415–2420.
6. Booth CC, Babouris N, Hanna S, et al. Incidence of hypomagnesemia in intestinal malabsorption. *Br Med J.* 1963;2:141–144.
7. Geiderman JM, Goodman SL, Cohen DB. Magnesium—the forgotten electrolyte. *JACEP.* 1979;8:204–208.
8. Flink EB. Nutritional aspects of magnesium metabolism (nutrition in medicine). *West J Med.* 1980;133:304–312.
9. Heaton FW. The kidney and magnesium homeostasis. *Ann NY Acad Sci.* 1969;162:901–905.
10. Massry SG. Pharmacology of magnesium. *Ann Rev Pharmacol Toxicol.* 1977;17:67–82.
11. Graber TW, Yee AS, Baker FJ. Magnesium: physiology, clinical disorders, and therapy. *Ann Emerg Med.* 1981;10:49–57.

12. Wacker WEC, Vallee BL. Magnesium metabolism. *N Engl J Med.* 1958;259:431–438.
13. Whang R. Magnesium deficiency: pathogenesis, prevalence, and clinical indications. *Am J Med.* 1987;82(suppl 3A):24–29.
14. Hamed IA, Lindeman RD. Dysphagia and vertical nystagmus in magnesium deficiency. *Ann Emerg Med.* 1978;89:222–223.
15. Vallee BL, Wacker WEC, Ulmer DD. The magnesium-deficiency tetany syndrome in man. *N Engl J Med.* 1960;262:155–160.
16. Iseri LT, Freed J, Bures AR. Magnesium deficiency and cardiac disorders. *Am J Med.* 1975;58:837–844.
17. Burch GE, Giles TD. The importance of magnesium deficiency in cardiovascular disease. *Am Heart J.* 1977;94:649–656.
18. Loeb HS, Petras RJ, Gunnar RM, et al. Paroxysmal ventricular fibrillation in two patients with hypomagnesemia. *Circulation.* 1968;37:210–215.
19. Levine SR, Crawley BA, Hai HA. Hypomagnesemia and ventricular tachycardia. *Chest.* 1982;81:244–247.
20. Topol EJ, Lerman BB. Hypomagnesemic torsades de pointes. *Am J Cardiol.* 1983;52:1367–1368.
21. Dyckner T. Serum magnesium in acute myocardial infarction. *Arch Med Scand.* 1980;207:59–66.
22. Eisenberg MJ. Magnesium deficiency and cardiac arrhythmias. *NY State J Med.* 1986;xx:133–136.
23. Sullivan JF, Wolpert PW, Williams R, et al. Serum magnesium in chronic alcoholism. *Ann NY Acad Sci.* 1969;162:947–962.
24. Kalbfleish JM, Linderman RD, Ginn HE, et al. Effects of ethanol administration on urinary excretion of magnesium and other electrolytes in alcoholic and normal subjects. *J Clin Invest.* 1963;42:1471–1475.
25. Fankushen D, Raskin D, Dimich A, et al. Significance of hypomagnesemia in alcoholic patients. *Am J Med.* 1964;37:802–812.
26. Lipner A. Symptomatic magnesium deficiency after small intestinal bypass for obesity. *Br Med J.* 1977;1:148.
27. Houston BD, Turner T. Severe electrolyte abnormalities in a pregnant patient with a jejunoileal bypass. *Arch Intern Med.* 1978;138:1712–1713.
28. Jackson CE, Meier DW. Routine serum magnesium analysis. *Ann Intern Med.* 1968;69:743–747.
29. Fouty RA. Liquid protein diet, magnesium deficiency, and cardiac arrest. *JAMA.* 1978;240:2632–2633. Letter.
30. Martin HE, Smith K, Wilson ML. The fluid and electrolyte therapy of severe diabetic acidosis and ketosis. *Am J Med.* 1958;24:376–389.
31. Martin HE. Clinical magnesium deficiency. *Ann NY Acad Sci.* 1969;162:891–899.
32. McMullen JK. Asystole and hypomagnesemia during recovery from diabetic ketoacidosis. *Br Med J.* 1977;1:690.
33. Calcium, magnesium and diuretics. *Br Med J.* 1975;1:170–171. Editorial.
34. Ghani MF, Smith JR. The effectiveness of magnesium chloride in the treatment of ventricular tachyarrhythmias due to digitalis intoxication. *Am Heart J.* 1974;88:621–626.
35. Flink EB. Correspondence. *Arch Intern Med.* 1978;138:825.
36. Flink EB. Therapy of magnesium deficiency. *Ann NY Acad Sci.* 1969;162:901–905.
37. Iseri LT, Chung P, Tobis J. Magnesium therapy for intractable ventricular arrhythmias in normomagnesemic patients. *West J Med.* 1983;138:823–828.
38. Tzivoni D, Keren A, Cohen A, et al. Magnesium therapy for torsades de pointes. *Am J Cardiol.* 1984;53:528–530.
39. Smith LF, Heagerty AM, Bing RF, et al. Intravenous infusion of magnesium sulphate after acute myocardial infarction: effects on arrhythmias and mortality. *Int J Cardiol.* 1986;12:175–180.
40. Okayama H, Aikawa T, Okayama NM, et al. Bronchodilating effects of intravenous magnesium sulfate in bronchial asthma. *JAMA.* 1987;257:1076–1078.
41. Rolla G, Bucca C, Caria E, et al. Acute effect of intravenous magnesium sulfate on airway obstruction of asthmatic patients. *Ann Allergy.* 1988;61:338.
42. Skobeloff EM, Spivey WH, McNamara RM, et al. Intravenous magnesium sulfate for treatment of acute asthma in the emergency department. *JAMA.* 1989;262:1210.
43. Noppen M, Vanmade L, Impens N, et al. Bronchodilating effect of intravenous magnesium sulfate in severe bronchial asthma. *Chest.* 1990;97:373.
44. Miller WF. Consider magnesium sulfate when conventional asthma therapy fails? *J Crit Illness.* 1991;6:517–520.

20. Hypercalcemia

EMANUEL K. GORDON, MD, FACEP

Hypercalcemic crisis is a syndrome encountered in a minority of patients with hypercalcemia. A common condition, hypercalcemia occurs in up to 6% of asymptomatic patients who undergo routine screening.[1,2] Only a small proportion of hypercalcemia patients who become symptomatic develop the hypercalcemic crisis syndrome, a true medical emergency. Hypercalcemic crisis may be defined as hypercalcemia that causes the abrupt onset of severe symptoms, most commonly a comatose or semicomatose state, protracted nausea and vomiting accompanied by polyuria that markedly depletes intravascular volume, profound weakness, and deteriorating renal function.

The subgroup of hypercalcemic patients who develop hypercalcemic crisis is not determined simply by the absolute level of the serum calcium concentration. Factors such as the rapidity with which the serum calcium concentration rises, the underlying etiology of hypercalcemia, and variations in individual tolerance to the effects of hypercalcemia all seem to influence the development of hypercalcemic crisis. The syndrome may occur in a patient with an underlying malignancy who has a serum calcium concentration of 12 mg/dL, while an individual with chronic hypercalcemia can be virtually asymptomatic with a serum calcium concentration of 15 mg/dL.

The diagnosis of hypercalcemic crisis is based on the clinical symptoms and the demonstration of an elevated serum calcium concentration. The initial therapy of hypercalcemic crisis should be instituted immediately after the diagnosis is made. Therapy is similar for all patients with hypercalcemic crisis syndrome, no matter what the cause.

DIAGNOSIS OF HYPERCALCEMIC CRISIS

Even though hypercalcemia can produce symptoms referable to nearly every organ system in the body (Fig. 20-1), the diagnosis of hypercalcemic crisis is easily made by determining the serum calcium concentration. It is recommended that a serum calcium level be determined on every patient who comes to the emergency department with a disordered level of consciousness unless the cause is obvious.[3] The symptoms of a delirious or confused patient with a history of renal calculi, cancer, recent immobilization, or a combination of these should alert the physician to check the serum calcium concentration. Seizures are rarely seen in hypercalcemic crisis.[4] Unexplained gastrointestinal symptoms, weakness with hypotonia, and polyuric dehydration may also be initial clues to hypercalcemic crisis. In fact, serum calcium levels should be obtained in all emergency department patients with symptoms of uncertain origin that may be manifestations of hypercalcemic crisis. Once the serum calcium concentration has been determined, the diagnosis of hypercalcemic crisis is usually self-evident.

Interpretation of Serum Calcium Concentration

The normal range of serum calcium concentration is generally stated to be 8.9 to 10.3 mg/dL when determined by the EDTA titration method or 9.1 to 10.5 mg/dL when measured by atomic absorption flame spectrophotometry. This is roughly equivalent to 4.6 to 5.8 mEq/L. Each laboratory

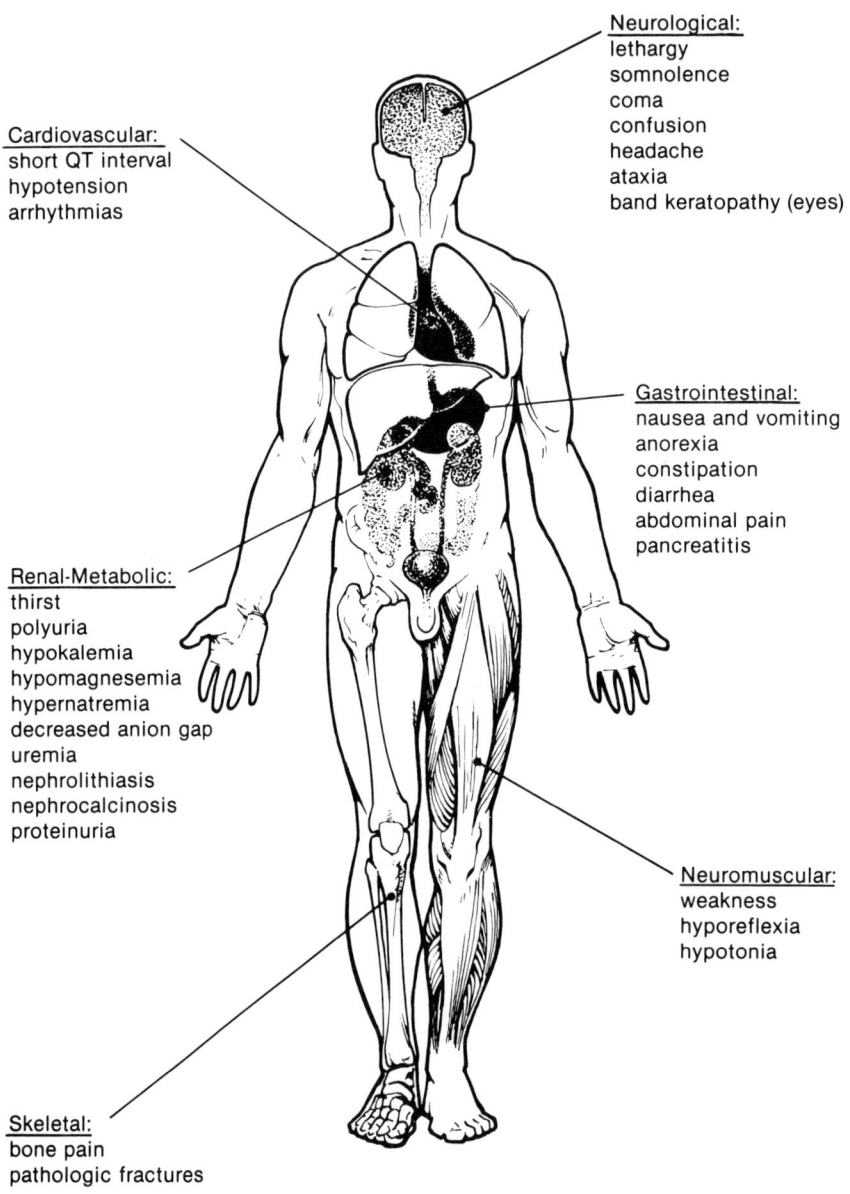

Figure 20-1 Clinical symptoms in hypercalcemia.

should establish its own standard, depending on the technique used.[5]

The total serum calcium concentration measured on routine testing consists of the sum of the ionized and nonionized calcium present in the serum. It is the ionized calcium fraction that is responsible for the clinical disturbances in hypercalcemic crisis. In normal circumstances, the total serum calcium concentration is composed of 47% ionized calcium, 40% protein-bound calcium (primarily bound to albumin), and 13% calcium in a complex with various ions (eg, citrate). A useful approximation is that one half of the measured total serum calcium is ionized under normal circumstances.

Three circumstances may alter the relationship of ionized calcium to calcium that is bound or in a complex:

1. abnormalities in serum protein concentration
2. abnormal serum pH (ie, systemic alkalosis or acidosis)
3. elevations in soluble ligands that form complexes with calcium ions

A change in the serum albumin concentration of 1 g/dL results in a corresponding change in the total serum calcium concentration of 0.8 mg/dL *in the same direction*. Thus, if the serum protein concentration is elevated, the fraction of protein-bound calcium is increased and the proportion of ionized calcium declines. This relationship may be significant when interpreting the total serum calcium concentration. For example, a hypoproteinemic cancer patient may have a low serum albumin concentration that normally leads to an appreciable decrease in total serum calcium concentration. With the decrease in serum albumin concentration, the fraction of ionized calcium increases. Therefore, a normal or slightly elevated total serum calcium level in this patient may actually represent a significantly elevated ionized calcium level. Conversely, a patient with multiple myeloma may have an elevated concentration of abnormal γ-globulin that binds calcium, raising the total serum calcium concentration. This situation may lead to a diagnosis of severe hypercalcemia, which would be in error, since the fraction of ionized calcium is decreased with hypergammaglobulinemia.[6]

It is important to remember that a tourniquet applied for unnecessary lengths of time can raise the concentration of calcium in the venous blood sample taken from that area. This phenomenon is due to the fact that the serum protein concentration of the blood rises as a result of the transudation of protein-free fluid from the capillaries. A tourniquet applied for three minutes has been shown to increase the measured total serum calcium concentration by 10%.[7] Therefore, it is important that the blood drawn for determination of the serum calcium concentration be obtained immediately after the tourniquet is applied.

Alkalosis leads to a decrease in ionized calcium and an increase in protein-bound calcium. Although the total serum calcium concentration may not be changed with alkalosis, the concentration of ionized calcium drops 1.6 mg/dL for each rise of 1.0 in the pH of the blood. This is the reason for symptoms of hypocalcemia (eg, tetany) in cases of severe acute respiratory alkalosis, such as the hyperventilation syndrome. The assumption that 50% of the total serum calcium is ionized should therefore be modified in a patient with severe systemic pH abnormalities.

Abnormal elevations in the concentration of soluble ligands that form complexes with calcium may also make the 50% ionized calcium assumption invalid. This occurs with acute uremia and with elevations of citrate, sulfate, and phosphate levels in the serum.

In the absence of the conditions described, the assumption that the measured total serum calcium concentration reflects the physiologically active ionized serum calcium level is a valid and useful method of evaluating the magnitude of hypercalcemia. Direct measurement of ionized serum calcium is rarely available to the emergency physician on an immediate basis.

An additional rapid diagnostic tool that can indirectly suggest hypercalcemia is the electrocardiogram (ECG). The earliest and most common finding on the ECG associated with hypercalcemia is shortening of the QT interval. This finding is not specific for hypercalcemia, but a rapid rhythm strip demonstrating a short QT interval should increase the suspicion of hypercalcemic crisis in a patient with appropriate symptoms. This information may be obtained while the results of the serum calcium concentration are pending.

CALCIUM HOMEOSTATIC MECHANISMS

Hypercalcemic crisis occurs when homeostatic control of calcium metabolism is severely impaired. Hypercalcemia always results from an increased calcium influx into the circulation, with or without impaired removal of calcium from the circulation; hypercalcemic crisis never results only from impaired removal of calcium from the circulation. Three sources contribute to the influx of calcium into the serum:

1. osteoclastic resorption of mineral from bone stores
2. gastrointestinal absorption of calcium
3. tubular reabsorption of calcium from the glomerular filtrate

The skeletal system contains over 95% of the total body calcium. Most hypercalcemic crises involve a relative increase of bone resorption over bone formation, which releases excess calcium into the blood. Bone resorption may be increased by hormonal agents that stimulate osteoclastic bone resorption or by skeletal osteolytic lesions that liberate calcium into the vascular space. The hormonal agents that increase calcium influx into the blood include parathormone, parathormonelike agents produced by malignancies, and neoplastic production of prostaglandins of the E series (PGE), which have been shown to augment bone resorption in tissue culture.[8]

Increased gastrointestinal absorption of calcium can also be mediated through hormonal mechanisms. The most potent stimulus of gastrointestinal calcium absorption is 1,25-dihydroxyvitamin D. By this means, hypervitaminosis D in faddists who consume enormous quantities of vitamin D is a rare cause of hypercalcemia. Increased gastrointestinal absorption can also result from increased calcium load in the intestine under certain circumstances, such as the milk-alkali syndrome.

Increased tubular reabsorption of calcium in the kidney is stimulated by parathormone, as well as by thiazide diuretics. By itself, increased tubular reabsorption of calcium is rarely a cause of significant hypercalcemia, but it is frequently a factor when combined with increased calcium influx from bone or gastrointestinal absorption.

The essential facts to remember in hormonal control of calcium homeostasis are that parathormone is the major hormone regulating bone resorption and renal reabsorption of calcium, and that vitamin D exerts its major effect on gastrointestinal absorption.

INITIAL THERAPY OF HYPERCALCEMIC CRISIS

It is essential to initiate therapy for hypercalcemic crisis immediately upon diagnosis. The order of priorities in managing hypercalcemic crisis is as follows:

1. Institute general supportive measures to prevent further elevation in serum calcium. Correct life-threatening hypovolemia and associated electrolyte abnormalities.
2. Lower serum calcium concentration by nonspecific methods that decrease calcium influx from bone, renal tubules, and gastrointestinal tract. Initiate therapy to stimulate calcium egress from the vascular space to bone and urine.
3. Determine the cause of the hypercalcemia and initiate specific measures to correct the primary disorder.

General Supportive Measures

A flowsheet, similar to that used in patients with diabetic ketoacidosis, is helpful in the initial therapy of hypercalcemic crisis. A suggested format appears in Table 20-1.

Correcting Hypovolemia

Patients in hypercalcemic crisis have a marked intravascular volume depletion. Nausea, vomiting, and polyuria have usually been present for some time before the patient seeks treatment in the emergency department. Therefore, the most important initial therapeutic measure is to administer intravascular fluids, normal saline in most cases, to restore the markedly depleted extracellular fluid volume to an adequate level. The usual infusion rate is 1 to 2 L of normal saline during the first 2 hours of therapy (Table 20-2). To determine the amount of saline infusion required for volume replacement, insertion of a central line to monitor central venous or pulmonary wedge pressure is recommended; this is mandatory when patients are elderly or when renal function may be inadequate.[9] Urine output should be carefully monitored.

Correcting Electrolyte Abnormalities

Hypokalemia is the electrolyte abnormality most frequently associated with hypercalcemic crisis. Hypomagnesemia is also common in these patients. Correction of hypokalemia and hypomagnesemia should be instituted with the restoration of intravascular volume.

In the case of a patient in hypercalcemic crisis who takes a digitalis preparation, correction of hypokalemia and continuous monitoring are of extreme importance. Because calcium and digitalis are synergistic in their effects on the myocardium, such a patient may exhibit signs of digitalis toxicity as a result of hypercalcemia alone. Hypokalemia introduces an

Table 20-1 Flowsheet for Initial Therapy of Hypercalcemic Crisis

Time	Pulse	Blood Pressure	Central Venous Pressure/ Pulmonary Wedge Pressure	Serum Calcium Level mg/%	Serum Potassium Level mEq/L	Serum Blood Urea Nitrogen/ Creatinine	Intravenous Infusion Rate	Cumulative Total	Urine Output Per Hour	Cumulative Total	Medications	Remarks
00:00	110	90/60	1 cmH$_2$O/ 4 mmHg	16.5	2.5	28/1.2	Normal Saline + 40 mEq/KCl + 10 mg MgSO$_4$ at 1500 mL/hour		40 mL			ECG monitoring: shortened QT interval noted.
01:00	90	110/60	1 cmH$_2$O/ 6 mmHg	16.0	2.9	24/1.1	Normal Saline + 40 mEq/KCl + 10 mg MgSO$_4$ at 1000 mL/hour	1500	90 mL	130 mL		Furosemide is not given until ECF volume has been significantly restored as measured by rise in CVP or PWP.
02:00	90	120/70	3 cmH$_2$O/ 7 mmHg	15.8	3.2	23/1.1	Normal Saline + 30 mEq KCl + 10 mg MgSO$_4$ at 1000 mL/hour	2500	380 mL	510 mL	Furosemide 100 mg IV at 02:00	
03:00	84	120/70	5 cmH$_2$O/ 7 mmHg	15.1	3.4	21/1.0	D$_5$W + 30 mEq KCl + 10 mg MgSO$_4$ at 1000 mL/hour	3500	400 mL	910 mL	Furosemide 100 mg IV at 03:00	Substitute D$_5$W for normal saline every fourth liter of intravenous fluid.
04:00	80	120/74	6 cmH$_2$O/ 7 mmHg	14.4	3.7	19/1.0	Normal Saline + 20 mEq KCl at 1000 mL/hour	4500	580 mL	1490 mL	Furosemide 100 mg IV at 04:00	Goal of maintaining urine output at greater than 500 mL/hour is achieved. Continue saline loading with diuresis until serum calcium falls below 12 mg/%.

Source: Adapted and reprinted with permission from Zwada ET, Lee DL, Kleeman CR: Management of hypercalcemia. *Postgrad Med* 1979;66(4):105.

Table 20-2 Schedule for Initial Therapy in Hypercalcemic Crisis*

Hour	Intravenous Normal Saline	Potassium Chloride (mEq/L)	Magnesium (mEq/L)	Furosemide (mg)
1	500 mL or more†			
2	500 mL or more†	10	5–10	
3	1 L	20	10–20	100–200
4	Equivalent to urinary loss by volume	20	10–20	100–200
5	Equivalent to urinary loss by volume, replacement fluid D_5W	20	10–20	
6	Equivalent to urinary loss by volume	20	10–20	100–200

*In patients with normal renal function and without congestive heart failure.
†Volume of infusion sufficient to restore extracellular fluid volume as monitored by central venous or pulmonary wedge pressure.

Source: Adapted and reprinted with permission from Zawada ET, Lee DL, Kleeman CR: Management of hypercalcemia. Postgrad Med 1979;66:105.

additional risk factor for digitalis toxicity. Any digitalized patient in hypercalcemic crisis should have continuous ECG monitoring until the hypercalcemia and hypokalemia have been corrected. Additional doses of digitalis should be withheld until the hypercalcemic crisis has resolved.

Withholding Medications That May Cause Hypercalcemia

In addition to digitalis, medications that may elevate the serum calcium level should be withheld from the patient in hypercalcemic crisis. The most common drug of this type is a thiazide diuretic. Pharmacologic agents that should also be discontinued during the initial therapy of hypercalcemic crisis include[10,11]:

- androgens and estrogens (especially tamoxifen) in patients with breast cancer
- vitamin D
- vitamin A
- isotretinoin
- lithium
- calcium-containing antacids

Encouraging Mobilization

Immobilization increases the release of calcium into the extracellular fluid from bone. Although it may be impossible to mobilize a patient in hypercalcemic crisis initially, routine turning of the patient and specialized physical therapy regimens are helpful in reducing this source of calcium influx until adequate mobilization is possible.

Reduction of Serum Calcium Concentration

After general supportive measures have been initiated, therapeutic maneuvers to lower the serum calcium level should be begun. The most rapid methods involve urinary calcium excretion.

Increasing Caluresis

Sodium and calcium reabsorption in the kidney are closely correlated. Therefore, therapeutic interventions to increase urinary sodium excretion also increase urinary calcium excretion. The generally accepted method of increasing caluresis in hypercalcemic crisis is a combination of intravenous saline infusion and a loop diuretic, either furosemide (Lasix) or ethacrynic acid (Edecrin). A suggested schedule for the first 6 hours of combined saline and furosemide therapy is shown in Table 20-2. This schedule assumes normal renal function. During the initial 2 hours, saline infusion without furosemide is used to restore the extracellular volume deficit as described earlier. Once this has been accomplished, 1 to 2 L of saline are "loaded" intravenously followed by furosemide (100 to 200 mg) given intravenously. The furosemide doses are repeated at 1- to 2-hour intervals with the goal of maintaining urine output at 500 mL/hour or more. Urine output is replaced on a volume-to-volume basis with intravenous fluid. After each 3 L of normal saline have been infused, 1 L of 5% dextrose in water should be alternated with the saline in replacing urine volume.

Potassium (20 to 40 mEq/L) and magnesium (10 to 20 mEq/L) are added to replace initial losses. Additional replacement therapy of potassium is guided by repeated serum potassium determinations.

Caluresis by combined saline and furosemide administration decreases the serum calcium level rapidly. With careful monitoring to detect fluid overload and oliguria, this method is safe and without side effects. In the patient with renal insufficiency, renal failure, or congestive heart failure, however, it should not be attempted in the aggressive manner described. In these patients, either peritoneal dialysis or hemodialysis is the treatment of choice to remove calcium rapidly from the extracellular fluid.[12]

In the past, chelating or binding agents have been used to increase caluresis. They filter soluble complexes with calcium that are poorly reabsorbed by the renal tubule and thereby increase caluresis. These agents (eg, edetate, sodium sulfate, and sodium citrate) all have serious side effects, including renal tubular damage, renal failure, hypotension, hypernatremia, and potassium and magnesium depletion. They should not be used in the emergency treatment of hypercalcemic crisis unless all safer modalities fail and dialysis is unavailable.

Reducing the Movement of Calcium out of Bone

Three medications can be useful in decreasing the efflux of calcium from bone into the extracellular fluid: mithramycin, calcitonin, and corticosteroids.

Mithramycin is an antibiotic that has been found to be a potent antineoplastic agent. It was observed that serum calcium levels in patients treated with mithramycin for malignancies markedly decreased. This hypocalcemic effect has been used to treat patients in hypercalcemic crisis from both malignant and nonmalignant causes. Mithramycin inhibits RNA synthesis directed by DNA, which is thought to result in osteoclastic refractoriness to parathormone, thus decreasing bone calcium mobilization. The hypocalcemic effect of one dose of mithramycin can be as large as a drop of 7 mg/dL in the serum calcium concentration.[13]

The usual dosage is 25 μg/kg given intravenously over 3 to 8 hours. Reductions in serum calcium levels appear about 12 hours after administration, and the hypocalcemic effect peaks at 36 hours. The hypocalcemic effect of mithramycin may last for 2 weeks after a single administration of the drug. Mithramycin, in the usual dosage, frequently causes nausea and vomiting as side effects. Severe side effects are rare at this dose, although renal impairment, hepatic damage, and hemorrhagic disorders with thrombocytopenia have been reported.

Calcitonin is a polypeptide hormone secreted by the parafollicular cells of the thyroid gland in mammals. Its hypocalcemic action stems from its inhibition of bone resorption by osteoclasts. The calcitonin preparation available to clinicians (Calcimar) is derived from salmon.

Calcitonin is not as potent a hypocalcemic agent as mithramycin, but it has a lower incidence of side effects, the only common ones being nausea and vomiting. The usual decrement in serum calcium concentration with calcitonin therapy is 1 to 2 mg/dL.[13] The onset of action is more rapid than that of mithramycin, occurring within 2 hours. Its hypocalcemic effect may persist up to 24 hours. The potency of calcitonin preparations is assessed by plasma calcium concentration lowering in rats and is measured in British Medical Research Council (MRC) units. The usual dose is 4 MRC units per kilogram given subcutaneously or intramuscularly every 12 hours.

Corticosteroids have also been used in the treatment of hypercalcemic crisis. The efficacy of steroids is ill defined, however, and the mechanism of action remains unclear. Glucocorticoids may lower serum calcium levels by inhibiting osteoclast precursor cells,[7] by inhibiting tumor growth and thus decreasing the efflux of skeletal calcium into the extracellular fluid,[14] or by inhibiting the synthesis of prostaglandins that stimulate bone resorption.[7] Glucocorticoids may also inhibit gastrointestinal calcium absorption and increase urinary calcium excretion. All of the postulated mechanisms are of little net effect in the treatment of hypercalcemic crisis. The hypocalcemic effect of glucocorticoids may take up to 1 week to manifest itself. If given, the recommended dosage is 80 mg of prednisone daily.

Recent studies have demonstrated that PGE inhibitors such as indomethacin and aspirin can cause a decrease in serum calcium levels in hypercalcemic cancer patients who have a clear elevation of circulating PGE.[15,16] These agents are only rarely successful and should not be used in the initial therapy of hypercalcemic crisis.[17]

The diphosphonate 3-amino-1-hydroxypropane-1,1-diphosphonate appears to be useful in treatment of the hypercalcemia of malignancy in recent trials.[16,18]

Stimulating Movement of Calcium from the Extracellular Fluid into Bone

The administration of inorganic phosphates is an effective method of increasing movement of calcium from the extracellular space into bone. Inorganic phosphates stimulate osteoblastic activity, resulting in a shift of calcium and phosphorus into the skeletal system. This phenomenon is associated with

1. a decrease in the serum calcium concentration
2. a reduction in urinary calcium excretion
3. decreased rate of bone resorption

The hypocalcemic effect of inorganic phosphate given intravenously is extremely rapid, beginning within minutes. However, this method of therapy has a high incidence of serious side effects, such as extraskeletal precipitation of calcium, hypotension, renal failure, and hypocalcemia. For this reason, intravenous phosphate is not recommended for therapy of hypercalcemic crisis unless safer methods (eg, saline infusion combined with furosemide) fail to improve the patient's condition and the rapid reduction of serum calcium concentration would clearly be life saving. In these rare circumstances, intravenous phosphorus (In-Phos, Hyper-Phos-K) in a dose of 1.5 g (50 mM) is infused intravenously over 6 to 8 hours. Only one dose should be given.

Oral phosphate therapy is safer but is slow in onset of action (greater than 24 hours) and has no value in the initial therapy of hypercalcemic crisis.

Decreasing Intestinal Calcium Absorption

In the initial therapy of hypercalcemic crisis, very little can be gained by techniques that decrease gastrointestinal calcium absorption. Discontinuance of any calcium-containing foods or medications and vitamin D preparations should be routine, however.

Etiology of Hypercalcemic Crisis

The primary responsibility of the emergency physician is to recognize hypercalcemic crisis and initiate therapy for the syndrome, regardless of its cause. The underlying condition responsible for the hypercalcemic crisis becomes clear in the majority of patients during the initial hours of therapy. Treatment of the underlying disorder does not play a significant part in the initial therapy of hypercalcemic crisis, but it is necessary for prolonged correction of the hypercalcemic state.

The list of causes of hypercalcemia is long:

1. neoplasms
   a. skeletal metastases
   b. increased production of parathormone or parathormonelike factors
   c. PGE production
   d. production of osteoclast-activating factor
2. hyperparathyroidism
   a. primary
   b. secondary
3. pharmacologic agents
   a. thiazides
   b. vitamin D toxicity
   c. vitamin A toxicity (including isotretinoin)
   d. calcium (including massive transfusions)
   e. lithium
   f. androgen and estrogen therapy (especially in breast cancer)
4. hyperthyroidism
5. hypothyroidism
6. acromegaly
7. adrenal insufficiency
8. pheochromocytoma
9. milk-alkali syndrome
10. granulomatous disease
    a. sarcoidosis
    b. tuberculosis
    c. histoplasmosis
    d. coccidioidomycosis
11. renal failure
12. renal transplantation
13. phosphorus-depletion syndrome
14. immobilization
15. idiopathic infantile hypercalcemia

On the basis of the initial history, initial laboratory results, and knowledge of the frequency of various causes of hypercalcemic crisis, however, the underlying disorder responsi-

Table 20-3 Malignancies That Commonly Underlie Hypercalcemia

Type of Malignancy	Incidence of Hypercalcemia (%)	Comments
Breast cancer	25–40	Most common cause: usually due to bone metastases
Lung cancer	10–15	Frequent in epidermoid and anaplastic cell types
Renal cell carcinoma	13	
Multiple myeloma	70	

ble for the development of the syndrome is usually apparent to the emergency physician.

One important axiom should be emphasized in the etiologic diagnosis of hypercalcemic crisis. Conditions leading to hypercalcemia coexist in patients who develop hypercalcemic crisis with a much higher incidence than would be expected by chance. Therefore, the physician should seek multiple causes or coexistent diseases that may combine to precipitate the hypercalcemic crisis syndrome.

The most common underlying disorder in patients with hypercalcemic crisis is malignancy. The overall incidence of hypercalcemia in malignant disease is 10% to 20%. The most common types of cancer underlying the development of hypercalcemic crisis are shown in Table 20-3; they account for over 90% of malignancy-associated cases.[19]

Of interest is the high incidence of hypercalcemia seen in cases of adult T-cell lymphoma. It occurs in over 50% of cases of this tumor and is related to human immunodeficiency virus (HIV) infection.[20,21] Hypercalcemia has been reported in patients with acquired immunodeficiency syndrome (AIDS) and disseminated cytomegalovirus infection. It is unclear whether cytomegalovirus or HIV infection alone was directly responsible, but their occurrence together is a common feature in AIDS. Therefore, the possibility of hypercalcemia should be investigated in AIDS patients exhibiting symptoms compatible with hypercalcemic crisis.[22]

In a patient with known malignancy, initiation of antineoplastic therapy can precipitate hypercalcemic crisis; the most frequent cause in breast cancer patients is tamoxifen. Immobilization, common in patients with malignancies, is a potential precipitating factor.

Primary hyperparathyroidism, although the most common cause of hypercalcemia in the general population, is less likely than malignancy to produce the rapid elevations and high levels of serum calcium concentrations (greater than 14 mg/dL) that usually characterize hypercalcemic crisis. Carcinoma of the parathyroid gland and acute hyperparathyroid crisis can, however, lead to the syndrome. Historical and laboratory evidence suggesting hyperparathyroidism as the cause of hypercalcemic crisis include the following:

- long history of hypercalcemia
- ureteral calculi
- hypophosphatemia
- hypochloremic acidosis
- a ratio of serum chloride to phosphate greater than 33

A serum parathormone level is necessary to confirm the indirect evidence suggesting hyperparathyroidism.

The history obtained on arrival of the patient is important in diagnosing pharmacologic causes of hypercalcemia. The most common agents precipitating hypercalcemic crisis (usually in combination with another hypercalcemic disorder) are thiazide diuretics. Large amounts of vitamin D, vitamin A, or calcium containing antacids can result in hypercalcemia, as can lithium.

A chest roentgenogram, skeletal series, and, once the patient is adequately hydrated, an intravenous pyelogram are helpful in detecting a malignant cause. The chest roentgenogram may also suggest sarcoidosis as an underlying cause. Rouleaux formation seen on the complete blood cell count suggests multiple myeloma.

REFERENCES

1. Prunell DC, Smith LH, Scholtz DA, et al. Primary hyperparathyroidism: a prospective clinical study. *Am J Med*. 1971;50:670–678.
2. Christensson T, Hellström K, Wengle B, et al. Prevalence of hypercalcemia in health screening in Stockholm. *Acta Med Scand*. 1976;200:131–137.
3. Daniels GH. Calcium emergencies. In: Wilkins EW, ed. *MGH Textbook of Emergency Medicine*. Baltimore: Williams & Wilkins; 1978.
4. Plum F, Posner JB. *The Diagnosis of Stupor and Coma*. 3rd ed. Philadelphia: Davis; 1980.
5. Yendt ER, Gagne RJ. Detection of primary hyperparathyroidism with special reference to its occurrence in hypercalcemic females with normal or borderline serum calcium. *Can Med Assoc J*. 1968;98:331–336.
6. Lindgärde F, ZeHervoll O. Hypercalcemia and normal ionized Ca^{++} in a case of myelomatosis. *Ann Intern Med*. 1973;78:396–399.
7. Lee DB, Zwada ET, Kleeman CR. The pathophysiology and clinical aspects of hypercalcemic disorders. *West J Med*. 1978;129:278–320.
8. Robertson RP. Prostaglandins and hypercalcemia of cancer. *Med Clin North Am*. 1981;65:845.
9. Zwada ET, Lee DB, Kleeman CR. Management of hypercalcemia. *Postgrad Med*. 1979;66:105.
10. Stewler GJ, Nissenson RA. Nonparathyroid hypercalcemia. *Adv Intern Med*. 1987;32:235–258.
11. Valentic JP, Elias AN, Weinstein GD. Hypercalcemia associated with oral isotretinoin in the treatment of severe acne. *JAMA*. 1983;250:1899.
12. Strauch BS, Ball MF. Hemodialysis in the treatment of severe hypercalcemia. *JAMA*. 1976;235:1347–1348.
13. Pak CYC. Pathogenesis and management of hypercalcemic states. In: Isselbacher KJ, eds. *Harrison's Principles of Internal Medicine*. 9th ed. New York: McGraw-Hill; 1981.
14. Deftos LJ, Neer R. Medical management of the hypercalcemia of malignancy. *Annu Rev Med*. 1974;25:323–331.
15. Robertson RP. Prostaglandins and hypercalcemia of cancer. *Med Clin North Am*. 1981;65:845–853.
16. Mundy GR, Wilkinson R, Heath DA. Comparative study of available medical therapy for hypercalcemia of malignancy. *Am J Med*. 1983;74:421–432.
17. Insogna KL, Broadus AE. Hypercalcemia of malignancy. *Annu Rev Med*. 1987;38:241–256.
18. O'Dorosio TM, Cataland S. Symptomatic hypercalcemia. *Emerg Med Surv*. 1984;3:123–130.
19. Mundy GR. The hypercalcemia of cancer. *N Engl J Med*. 1984;310:1718–1727.
20. Bunn PA, et al. Clinical course of retrovirus-associated T-cell lymphoma in the United States. *N Engl J Med*. 1983;309:257–264.
21. Odell WD. Paraendocrine syndromes of cancer. *Adv Intern Med*. 1989;34:325–352.
22. Zaloga GP, Chernow B, Eil C. Hypercalcemia and disseminated cytomegalovirus infection in the acquired immunodeficiency syndrome. *Ann Intern Med*. 1985;102:331–333.

21. Acid-Base Disturbances

BARRY E. BRENNER, MD, PhD

In 1923, Bronsted and Lowry independently defined an acid as a chemical that can donate a proton.[1] A base was defined as a chemical that would accept a proton. This concept of an acid and a base has been useful in the understanding of metabolic disturbances.

DISSOCIATION

The acid HA may dissociate into the anion (A^-) and a hydrogen ion (H^+). Henderson demonstrated that the rate of the reaction, K, is directly proportional to the concentration of the reactants (Eqs. 1 and 2).[2]

$$K = \frac{(H^+)(A^-)}{(HA)} \quad (1)$$

$$(H^+) = K \frac{(HA)}{(A^-)} \quad (2)$$

In 1909, Sorenson proposed the concept of pH so that the numbers used to express hydrogen ion concentration would be conveniently small[3]; pH was defined as the negative log of the hydrogen ion concentration (Eq. 3).

$$pH = -\log(H^+) \quad (3)$$

The hydrogen ion concentration in the normal metabolic situation was found to be 40×10^{-9} Eq/L or 40 nEq/L; therefore, the pH in the normal metabolic situation was 7.4. It was found that the normal pH ranged from 7.36 to 7.44.

Another useful formula is the modification of the Henderson equation (Eq. 2) known as the Henderson-Hasselbalch equation.[4] By taking the negative logarithm of Eq. 3, one can derive the following formula:

$$pH = -\log K + \log \frac{(A^-)}{(HA)} \quad (4)$$

The $-\log K$ was defined as the pK. Rewriting this equation results in the formula:

$$pH = pK + \log \frac{(A^-)}{(HA)} \quad (5)$$

From this Henderson-Hasselbalch equation (Eq. 5), it can be seen that, when the salt (A^-) and the acid (HA) are of equal concentration, the pH is equal to the pK.

OTHER METHODS OF EXPRESSING HYDROGEN ION CONCENTRATION

In addition to pH, there are other convenient methods for expressing the hydrogen ion concentration. As noted earlier, the hydrogen ion concentration can be expressed in units of 10^{-9} Eq/L. Another method of expressing hydrogen ion concentration, therefore, is in nanoequivalents per liter. There are three methods for converting pH to hydrogen ion concentration and vice versa.[5]

Method 1

There is a linear relationship between pH and hydrogen ion concentration from pH 7.1 to 7.5. Each 0.01-unit pH change is equivalent to a change of 1 nEq/L in hydrogen ion concentration. Therefore, for each 0.1 unit of pH, there would be a change in hydrogen concentration of 10 nEq/L. For example, a pH of 7.5 is 0.1 pH unit away from normal metabolic pH of 7.4 or 40 nEq/L. Hence, a pH of 7.5 would result in a hydrogen ion concentration of 30 nEq/L. It is important to note that method 1 is only to be used for pH ranging from 7.1 to 7.5.

Method 2

The second method is of value for pH ranging from 6.8 to 7.7. To obtain a hydrogen ion concentration corresponding to each 0.1 pH unit decrement, sequentially multiply nanoequivalents per liter by 1.25. For example, given a pH of 7.2, one would multiply 40 nEq/L by 1.25, resulting in 50 nEq, which corresponds to a pH of 7.3. To arrive at the number of nanoequivalents of hydrogen ions at pH of 7.2, the 50 nEq is again multiplied by 1.25, resulting in 62.5 nEq/L, corresponding to a pH of 7.2. To obtain the hydrogen ion concentration corresponding to each 0.1 pH unit increment, it is necessary to multiply sequentially nanoequivalents per liter by 0.8. For example, to find the hydrogen ion concentration corresponding to a pH of 7.6, one multiplies 40 nEq/L by 0.8, resulting in 32 nEq/L, which corresponds to a pH of 7.5. To find the pH corresponding to 7.6, it is necessary to multiply the 32 nEq/L again by 0.8, resulting in 25.6 nEq/L, which is equivalent to a pH of 7.6.

Method 3

In order to use method 3, it is important to remember that pH is based on a logarithmic scale and that the antilog of 0.3 is 2. Therefore, when the pH changes 0.3 unit, the corresponding hydrogen ion concentration either doubles or halves. For example, when pH rises from 7.4 to 7.7 and then to 8.0, the hydrogen ion concentration falls from 40 to 20 and then to 10 nEq/L, respectively.

HYDROGEN ION CONCENTRATION vs. pH

Commonly pH is used; however, the hydrogen ion concentration may have several advantages over the pH when used with the following equation[6]:

$$(H^+) = 24 \times \frac{P_{CO_2}}{(HCO_3^-)} \qquad (6)$$

This equation is a derivation of the Henderson-Hasselbalch equation (see Eq. 5). The P_{CO_2} and the bicarbonate in this equation are readily obtained by determining blood gas levels. The bicarbonate reflects the metabolic component of acid-base disturbances, and the P_{CO_2} represents the respiratory component of acid-base disturbances. If any two of these three parameters are known, the third parameter can be calculated. Therefore, the physician obtains an arterial blood gas level and can immediately double-check the laboratory results. All that is needed is the interconversion of pH to the hydrogen ion concentration by any of the three methods described. It is important to double-check the results of the laboratory because only the pH and the P_{CO_2} are determined directly. The bicarbonate level is determined from a nomogram, which is occasionally misread in the laboratory. Such an error can be rapidly detected by using this formula.

ACID-BASE PHYSIOLOGY

Acidosis represents processes that cause acid to accumulate; alkalosis reflects processes that cause base to accumulate.[7,8] Neither acidosis nor alkalosis necessarily cause pH to be altered out of the normal range. However, both acidosis and alkalosis cause pH changes to the low side or high side of normal, respectively. For example, alkalosis may increase pH from 7.40 to 7.44, and acidosis may decrease pH from 7.40 to 7.36.

Several terms are important in the understanding of acid-base physiology. The term *acidemia* indicates that the pH is less than 7.35; the term *alkalemia*, that the pH is more than 7.45.[7,8]

The anion gap is pivotal to understanding acid-base disturbances. To maintain electrical neutrality, positive charges (cations) must equal negative charges (anions); if they do not, there is a "gap." Normally, there are unmeasured negative charges within the body, two thirds of which are proteins. Sulfates and phosphates constitute the other one third. The cations and anions normally measured are sodium, chloride, and bicarbonate. The anion gap is calculated according to the following equation[9]:

$$Na - (Cl^- + HCO_3^-) = \text{anion gap} \qquad (7)$$

Normal values for the anion gap are 8 to 16 mEq/L.[10]

METABOLIC ACIDOSIS

Compensation

In an attempt to maintain body pH within the normal range, despite the addition of acid, the respiratory center in the medulla compensates for metabolic acidosis by inducing hyperventilation. This profound hyperventilation decreases P_{CO_2} and causes a more normal pH in the presence of acidosis. This compensatory response is slow to occur, however, and may take 12 to 24 hours to be maximal after the onset of acidosis.[11] The slow response may be due to the

Table 21-1 Effect of Temperature on Blood Gases

Parameter	Increase 1°C	Decrease 1°C
pH	Decrease 0.015	Increase 0.015
P_{CO_2}	Increase 4.4*	Decrease 4.4*
P_{O_2}	Increase 7.2*	Decrease 7.2*

*Percentage change from value at 37°C.

Source: Reprinted with permission from Reuler JB: Hypothermia: Pathophysiology, clinical settings, and management. Ann Intern Med 89:519, 1978.

slow diffusion of hydrogen ions through the blood-brain barrier. In addition, ketoacids that are commonly involved in metabolic acidosis do not cross the blood-brain barrier.

The degree of hyperventilation is directly proportional to the severity of the metabolic acidosis, although lactic acidosis seems to result in more hyperventilation than other acidoses because it directly affects the chemoreceptors of the brain.[5] Provided that the patient is in steady state and has had the metabolic acidosis for 12 to 24 hours, one of the following four methods could be used to calculate the expected response of hyperventilation (ie, expected P_{CO_2}) for a given degree of metabolic acidosis (ie, bicarbonate level).[5]

1. The expected P_{CO_2} can be calculated by the following formula:

$$P_{CO_2} = 1.5 (HCO_3^-) + 8 \pm 2 \quad (8)$$

The P_{CO_2} should be within 2 units of the value calculated by this method. For example, a bicarbonate of 10 should produce a significant respiratory compensation (ie, a P_{CO_2} of 23).
2. The P_{CO_2} is expected to decrease 1.0 to 1.3 mmHg for each 1-mEq fall in bicarbonate. For example, if bicarbonate drops from 25 mEq/L to 10 mEq/L, the P_{CO_2} would be calculated to decrease from 40 mmHg to between 20.5 and 24.0 mmHg.
3. The P_{CO_2} approximates the last two digits of the arterial pH. For example, an arterial pH of 7.19 produces a respiratory compensation that results in a P_{CO_2} of approximately 19 mmHg.
4. For every 10-mEq increase or decrease in bicarbonate level, the pH decreases or increases, respectively, 0.15 unit, provided the P_{CO_2} is unchanged. For example, given a pH of 7.4, a P_{CO_2} of 40 mmHg, and a bicarbonate value of 24 mEq/L, a sudden decrease in the bicarbonate to 14 mEq/L produces a pH of 7.25, provided that the P_{CO_2} has not changed.

Except for the last, these methods for analyzing acid-base disturbances are valid only if the patient is in steady state and the metabolic acidosis has been present for at least 12 to 24 hours. If the degree of compensation is not proportional to the severity of the metabolic acidosis as determined by these methods, then it can be assumed that the patient has a primary respiratory disturbance or the patient's condition is not stable.

In the analysis of acid-base disturbances, the physician must be constantly aware of the possibility of errors in the laboratory values. For example, the patient's temperature has marked effects on pH, P_{CO_2}, and P_{O_2} (Table 21-1).[12] Also, too much heparin in a blood gas syringe lowers P_{CO_2} without affecting pH or P_{O_2}.[13] This causes the calculated bicarbonate level to be low and leads to an interpretation that the patient has a compensated metabolic acidosis.

Normal Anion Gap

The diagnostic approach to metabolic acidosis is greatly simplified when viewed in terms of the anion gap. For example, a normal (hyperchloremic) or high anion gap suggests specific diagnostic possibilities.

The addition of strong acids to body fluids converts bicarbonate to carbonic acid, which is subsequently degraded to water and carbon dioxide. The latter is then lost in the lungs. This loss of bicarbonate not only is acidifying but also represents the loss of anions that were counterbalancing positive charges of sodium.[9] Thus, an anionic moiety is needed to replace the negative charge lost with the bicarbonate. In hyperchloremic metabolic acidosis, each milliequivalent of bicarbonate lost is replaced with chloride, often from the intracellular space. However, if an unmeasured anion replaces bicarbonate, then the anion gap continues to appear increased.[9] Patients who have been vomiting or receiving exogenous bicarbonate have a normal pH and a normal bicarbonate, but the anion gap remains elevated. The normal anion gap is 8 to 16 mEq/L.

The etiology of metabolic acidosis associated with a normal anion gap includes the following[9]:

- *diarrhea.* Hyperchloremic metabolic acidosis is most commonly caused by the loss of bicarbonate in diarrheal fluid.
- *pancreatic fistula.* Bicarbonate is lost from alkalotic pancreatic secretions in the presence of pancreatic fistula.
- *ureteroenterostomy.* A urinary diversion procedure from ureter to sigmoid ileum, a ureteroenterostomy induces urea-splitting organisms to grow and function in the urine, where they produce ammonia and, most important, ammonium ions. The ions are systemically absorbed, causing the metabolic acidosis as well as an increase in the blood urea nitrogen (BUN)/creatinine ratio.
- *acetazolamide (Diamox).* Metabolic acidosis can also be caused by acetazolamide, a carbonic anhydrase inhibitor. The drug causes hydrochloric acid to be reab-

Table 21-2 Distinction Between Proximal and Distal Renal Tubular Acidosis

Parameter	Type I Distal Renal Tubular Acidosis	Type II Proximal Renal Tubular Acidosis
Renal stones or nephrocalcinosis	Common	Rare
Phosphoglycosuria	Rare	Common
Serum bicarbonate	Less than 15	More than 15
Potassium	Low	Low
Urinary pH		
Random	Inappropriately alkaline	Inappropriately alkaline
First morning void	Never less than 6.0	Commonly less than 6.0
Post-acid load	More than 5.3	Less than 5.3
Ease of bicarbonate replacement	2–3 mEq/kg/day (sensitive)	More than 3–5 mEq/kg/day (resistant)

Source: Reproduced with permission from Narins RG, Goldberg M: Renal tubular acidosis: Pathophysiology, diagnosis, and treatment. DM 23:1, 1977.

sorbed and bicarbonate to be excreted in the urine, resulting in alkalinization of the urine.

- *mafenide acetate (Sulfamylon)*. The antibiotic mafenide acetate, useful in burn patients, converts to *p*-carboxybenzene sulfonamide, a carbonic anhydrase inhibitor.[14] The degree of acidosis is highest in the second to fourth hours after its application in the burned patient. Also, the degree of acidosis correlates directly with the amount of partial thickness burn.[14] Acidosis is particularly severe if the patient is in renal failure and cannot excrete this carbonic anhydrase inhibitor.
- *cholestyramine*. Daily oral ingestion of 32 g of cholestyramine, which binds bile salts, causes bicarbonate to decrease by 3 to 4 mEq after 1 to 2 months. The acidosis is secondary to the high chloride content in cholestyramine.[15]

Table 21-3 Causes of Renal Tubular Acidosis

Type I	Type II
Hereditary elliptocytosis	Tyrosinemia or cystinosis
Chronic hydronephrosis	Hereditary fructose intolerance
Hyperthyroidism	Galactosemia
Hyperparathyroidism	Glycogen storage disease (type 1)
Vitamin D intoxication	Myeloma
Hyperglobulinemic states (carcinoma)	Nephrotic syndrome
Amyloid	Amyloid
States associated with edema	Carcinoma
Lithium	Heavy metal poisoning
Amphotericin	Carbonic anhydrase inhibitors
Conn's syndrome	Outdated tetracycline (not a problem unless saved from 1960s)
Wilson's degeneration	
Renal transplantation	Hyperparathyroidism
Medullary sponge kidney	Renal transplantation

Source: Reproduced with permission from Narins RG, Goldberg M: Renal tubular acidosis: Pathophysiology, diagnosis, and treatment. DM 23:1, 1977.

- *excessive acidifying agents*. The use of excessive acidifying agents, such as ammonium chloride, may cause hyperchloremic metabolic acidosis.
- *rapid intravenous hydration*. Sodium and chloride increase during intravenous hydration without a commensurate increase in bicarbonate; hypoaldosteronism is induced by the volume expansion.[16] This may explain why hyperchloremic metabolic acidosis persists approximately 8 hours after treatment of diabetic ketoacidosis, even though the anion gap is decreased. Dilution of the anion gap may also have a role in this situation.[17] The development of a renal tubular acidosis type II, administration of potassium chloride, and the loss of urinary ketones that would have been metabolized to bicarbonate also may explain the decrease in the anion gap and the presence of hyperchloremic metabolic acidosis in the therapy of diabetic ketoacidosis.[5,18]
- *hyperalimentation*. During hyperalimentation of infants, more cationic than anionic amino acids are administered. Metabolism of cationic amino acids causes increased generation of hydrogen ions and metabolic acidosis.[19]
- *post hypocapnia*. Chronic respiratory alkalosis decreases the bicarbonate by no more than 3 to 4 mEq/L.[20] Sudden relief of the respiratory alkalosis, therefore, leaves a mild metabolic acidosis.
- *early renal failure*. In obstructive uropathies or other forms of early renal failure, a renal tubular acidosis may occur.[21]
- *renal tubular acidosis*. In type I renal tubular acidosis, hydrogen ions cannot be secreted at the distal tubule; in type II, bicarbonate cannot be reabsorbed at the proximal tubule (Tables 21-2 and 21-3).[22–25] In patients with a metabolic acidosis and a urine pH greater than 6, the physician should suspect renal tubular acidosis or laboratory error.

Increased Anion Gap

Uremia

Metabolic acidosis is not seen with chronic renal failure unless the glomerular filtration rate is less than 20 mL/minute and the BUN and the serum creatinine exceed 40 and 4, respectively. Fortuitously, the renal excretion of phosphates and sulfates parallels that of acid excretion. The increased anion gap associated with uremia is due to retained sulfates and phosphates, whereas acidosis is due to the inability to excrete acid. It is unusual for the anion gap to be more than 20 to 25 mEq/L in uremia uncomplicated by a second metabolic acidosis.

Lactic Acidosis

The etiology of lactic acidosis includes shock, anemia, hypoxia, metabolic poisons, heat stroke, glycogenoses, malignancies, phenformin, and idiopathic causes.[26-30] An elevated lactate level (more than 5 mEq/L) is the major finding of this covert but serious illness, which may be one of the earliest indications of sepsis. In lactic acidosis, profound degrees of acidosis can develop in a matter of minutes, while most other acidoses, including diabetic ketoacidosis, develop much more slowly. After seizures, pH may be as low as 6.9, but it is rapidly restored to normal, usually in less than 1 hour.[31] During the reparative phase of lactic acidosis, the lactate is fully metabolized to bicarbonate, which returns the anion gap to normal. The physician can minimize the risk of an "alkaline overshoot" by anticipating this conversion and limiting the replacement of bicarbonate to maintain a pH of 7.2.[9] During reasonable respiratory compensation for metabolic acidosis, serum pH may be more than 7.2, but the serum bicarbonate value should be maintained at more than 10 mEq/L. A lower bicarbonate level may induce dysrhythmias and increase the incidence of ventricular fibrillation independent of pH.[32]

Lactic acidosis may be distinguished from ketoacidosis without directly measuring serum lactate. The phosphorus-creatinine ratio varies from 4.4 to 4.7 in lactic acidosis, whereas the ratio ranges from 1.7 to 2.3 in ketoacidosis.[33] These different ratios are due to hyperphosphatemia in lactic acidosis and a spurious elevation in serum creatinine in ketoacidosis.[34]

Ketoacidosis

When the mobilization of free fatty acids from adipose tissue is greatly increased, as it is with insulin deficiency, for example, the oxidative capacity of the liver is overwhelmed, free fatty acids combine, and ketogenesis dominates. Ketones are measured in urine by the nitroprusside reaction (Acetest), which measures *only* acetoacetate; in ketoacidosis, however, the concentration of another ketone, β-hydroxybutyrate, is in equilibrium at a threefold higher concentration with acetoacetate so that the result of the urine Acetest is occasionally only weakly positive. Therefore a patient may have ketoacidosis due to a preponderance of β-hydroxybutyrate but only a weakly positive or negative urine Acetest. Hypoxia may increase the amount of reduced nicotine adenine dinucleotide (NADH) and drive the ratio of these two ketones toward even more β-hydroxybutyrate. When the ketoacidosis begins to resolve, the ratio shifts toward acetoacetate, paradoxically causing increased ketonuria in a patient who is improving.[5]

Isopropyl alcohol also is metabolized to acetone, causing a positive nitroprusside reaction.[35]

Alcoholic ketoacidosis. The pathogenesis of alcoholic ketoacidosis is not fully clear, but it is related to increased lipolysis, an elevation in the plasma cortisol level, and a deficiency in growth hormone and insulin. The patients have a history of abdominal pain, protracted vomiting, and starvation for two to three days.[36,37] They may have low-grade fever (ie, less than 38.3°C), with epigastric tenderness; otherwise, physical examination is normal. The arterial pH may range from 7.0 to 7.6 (alkalosis secondary to severe vomiting), and the anion gap varies from 18 to 25 mEq/L as average values. Hyperglycemia is seen, although it is generally less than 275 mg/dL, and 10% of patients have negative urine and serum nitroprusside reactions. When the urine nitroprusside reaction is negative, an increased β-hydroxybutyrate level is diagnostic. Hyperamylasemia may occasionally occur; hyperuricemia is common.

The treatment of choice is 5% dextrose in water infused at a rate of 125 to 150 mL/hour, which resolves the syndrome in 12 hours. The use of normal saline alone may distort initial laboratory values, and the syndrome may persist even at 24 hours.[38] Glucose infusion restores the ability of the mitochondria to convert NADH to its oxidized form (NAD$^+$) and thereby to oxidize ketones. During therapy, phosphate should be replaced, for the level may fall from 7 to 1 mg/dL during the first 6 hours of therapy.[38] Also, the physician must follow the potassium level. Bicarbonate therapy is rarely needed in this syndrome. Insulin should never be used.

Diabetic ketoacidosis. The therapy of diabetic ketoacidosis involves treatment of hyperglycemia, acidosis, dehydration (usually 10% of body weight), and potassium deficit, once adequate urine output is established. Initially, patients may have hyperkalemia, despite the total body potassium deficit.

Too rapid treatment of dehydration or hyperglycemia may lead to cerebral edema within 4 to 16 hours after the initiation of therapy.[39-42] The exogenous administration of bicarbonate may reduce cerebrospinal fluid pH, even though the serum bicarbonate is rising, because it also reduces the stimulus to hyperventilate.[43] However, this cerebrospinal fluid acidosis has not been a problem and remains more of theoretical interest.[44]

Treatment with insulin usually lowers the glucose level at a rate of 75 mg/dL each hour. The rate is quite constant in a given individual, but this decline occurs only half as fast if an infection is present.[45] Continuous intravenous administration of insulin may be preferred, since absorption by other routes is irregular in the presence of acidosis and dehydration. Furthermore, hypokalemia and hypoglycemia may occur less frequently during the administration of low-dose, intravenous insulin, and the fall in glucose and serum acetone levels during the first 2 hours of therapy may be more rapid.[46,47]

Continuous intravenous infusion of regular insulin (5 to 10 U/hour after 0.33-U/kg priming dose) is an excellent treatment for diabetic ketoacidosis. If 100 mL of solution containing regular insulin (50 U/dL) is first run through the tubing, then there is no loss of insulin during initial infusions because of adherence to the plastic tubing or microscopic cracks in glassware. Once glucose values fall to less than 300 mg/dL, the regular insulin infusion should be stopped and glucose added to the solution used to hydrate the patient.[44] The physician should always check carefully for precipitating causes of diabetic ketoacidosis, such as infection, pancreatitis, or myocardial infarction.[48] During therapy of diabetic ketoacidosis it is important to replace magnesium and phosphorus (2.5 mg/kg over 6 hours) for levels of phosphorus less than 1 mg/dL[49] (see Chapter 14, Diabetic Emergencies).

Paraldehyde Intoxication

There have been few cases of paraldehyde intoxication described in the literature. The typical history is one of abdominal pain and central nervous system depression in an alcoholic.[9] A garlic odor on the breath and leukocytosis of 24,000 to 65,000/μL are characteristic. All patients have survived.

Methanol Intoxication

Methanol is readily available in wood alcohol and paint thinner so that intoxication is inexpensive. The drug is easily absorbed through the skin, respiratory tract, and gastrointestinal tract. Pathologically, the concentration of methyl alcohol is highest per gram of tissue in the eye.[50] Methyl alcohol is oxidized at one fifth of the rate at which ethanol is oxidized; hence, it has a long persistence in the body.[50,51] It is metabolized to formic acid, which is an uncoupling agent and, like aspirin, causes an increase in the concentration of other organic anions and an increase in the anion gap.[52] Variations in individual responses to methyl alcohol are extreme. There is normally a latent period of 24 to 48 hours between ingestion and onset of symptoms, although symptoms may appear in less than 12 hours.

All patients who are frankly acidotic when first seen have visual impairment, and at least 50% with transiently normal bicarbonate have visual difficulties.[50] The most frequent complaint is blurred or indistinct vision. Headache is present in 62%.[50] Patients may have moderate to severe systemic hypertension. Nausea and vomiting are prominent in 52% of patients.[50] The abdominal pain is particularly violent, epigastric, and colicky; the abdomen is strikingly rigid and exquisitely tender, but rebound is not noted. Amylase was over 300 Somogyi units in 66% of patients, and pancreatic necrosis was regularly found at autopsy.[50] Only 25% had true Kussmaul breathing.[50] Patients have dilated pupils and papillitis. It is important to remember that these patients appear intoxicated. Chronic methanol abusers frequently develop an ophthalmic tolerance and do not become blind. The treatment is to keep the pH more than 7.2, maintain ethyl alcohol level at 100 mg/dL, and perform early hemodialysis.[53–55] For treatment protocol with alcohol see ethylene glycol intoxication.

Ethylene Glycol Intoxication

Ethylene glycol, which is contained in antifreeze, is a poor man's alcohol. It has a warm and sweet taste and may be the chosen agent for suicide. Ethylene glycol is nontoxic per se; however, its metabolites are aldehydes that are cytotoxic and oxalates that produce extensive renal damage.[56] High concentrations of oxalic acid, an uncoupling agent, result in the accumulation of organic anions that are responsible for the acidosis and increased anion gap.[9] These patients appear to be drunk, but there is no smell of ethanol on their breath. Central nervous system manifestations occur 30 minutes to 12 hours after ingestion; other symptoms include low-grade fever, nystagmus, ophthalmoplegias, papilledema, and cerebrospinal fluid findings consistent with a meningoencephalitis.[56] Moderate leukocytosis occurs. Hypocalcemia results from chelation of the calcium ion by oxalate. Profuse oxalate and, occasionally, hippurate crystalluria is noted.[56,57] Extreme ethylene glycol poisoning is associated with pulmonary edema, bronchopneumonia, and congestive heart failure. At 24 to 72 hours, the patient develops acute tubular necrosis, although normal renal function usually returns.[56] Early diagnosis and treatment reduce the mortality.[58] The estimated lethal dose is 100 mL, but one patient was saved after a 2-L ingestion.[58]

Treatment includes thiamine and pyridoxine, which are cofactors needed in the degradation of ethylene glycol to less toxic metabolites. Osmotic diuresis increases renal clearance of ethylene glycol and reduces interstitial edema and renal cortical edema. Like methanol, ethylene glycol is a competitive inhibitor of alcohol dehydrogenase, reducing the half-life of ethylene glycol of 3 hours.[56,59] Ethanol should be started if ingestion occurred within 4 to 6 hours, keeping an ethanol level of 100 mg/dL using 0.1 mL/kg/hour of 100% ethanol as a 5% solution in 5% dextrose and water preceded by a 1-mL/kg loading dose administered over 20 minutes.[56,59] Early hemodialysis is life saving and is the procedure of choice. Ethanol infusion is a temporizing measure until hemodialysis can be instituted.

Table 21-4 Toxic Substances Contributing 1 mOsm/kg of Water to the Serum at Their Lethal Levels

Substance	Molecular Weight	Lethal Level (mg/dL)	mOsm/kg Water
Ethanol	46	350	80
Ethyl ether	26	180	70
Isopropanol	60	340 (toxic)	60
Methanol	32	80	27
Acetone	58	55	10
Trichloroethane	133	100	9
Paraldehyde	132	50	4
Ethylene glycol	62	21	4
Chloroform	119	39	3
Salicylate	180	50	3
Chloral hydrate	165	25	2
Ethchlorvynol	144	15	1

Source: Reproduced with permission from Glasser L, Sternglanz PD, Combic J, et al: Serum osmolarity and its applicability to drug overdose. *Am J Clin Pathol* 60:695, 1963.

Osmolar Gap

The final diagnosis of ethylene glycol or methanol intoxication depends on toxicologic analysis, but these tests are difficult to obtain rapidly. Determinations of the serum osmolarity and osmolar gap are rapid screening tests for some circulating toxins, such as methanol and ethylene glycol.[57,60,61] At the concentration present in plasma, the osmotic coefficient of sodium chloride is $1.85 \times (Na^+)$. Doubling the factor (Na^+) in the formula does not overestimate the plasma osmolarity, since other cationic constituents of the plasma (potassium, calcium, and magnesium) are excluded from the calculation.

$$2 \times Na^+ + \frac{Glucose}{18} + \frac{BUN}{2.8} = \text{Calculated serum osmolarity} \quad (9)$$

The limit by which the measured osmolarity may exceed the calculated value is 10 mOsm. If the calculated value exceeds the measured value, either the laboratory made a mistake or there is an arithmetic mistake. If the measured value exceeds the calculated value, there are two possibilities: (1) if the measured serum osmolarity is normal but the calculated value is low, the free water content is decreased, or (2) if the measured and calculated osmolarities are elevated, there is an unmeasured osmole (Table 21-4) and osmolar gap.

Salicylate Intoxication

Aspirin solution is absorbed in less than 30 minutes. Addition of small amounts of antacids to aspirin solution increases the rate of absorption. Peak levels with tablets may take as long as 2 hours. Aspirin inhibits gastric emptying, and plasma salicylate levels may continue to rise for as long as 24 hours.[62]

The pathophysiology of salicylate toxicity involves two basic underlying mechanisms: (1) salicyclic acid directly stimulates the respiratory center of the brain, producing the predominant respiratory alkalosis, and (2) salicylate inhibits oxidative phosphorylation, as does thyroxine.[62,63] Uncoupling of oxidative phosphorylation from electron transport increases heat production, producing fever, tissue glycolysis, and peripheral demand for glucose because adenosine triphosphate is not being generated. This increased peripheral demand for glucose results in the mobilization of fats to free fatty acids and ketones. In addition, glycogen stores are mobilized initially, producing hyperglycemia; the subsequent depletion of the body stores of glucose results in hypoglycemia.[62] Hypoglycemia occurs much more frequently in children than in adults. It is also more commonly reported in chronic salicylate intoxication.

Although metabolic acidosis is commonly associated with salicylate intoxication in children, it is rare in adults; only 10% of patients with a low pH had a metabolic acidosis, 30% had a respiratory alkalosis, and 57% had a combined respiratory alkalosis and a metabolic acidosis with the respiratory alkalosis being the overriding event.[64] Because it is an uncoupling agent, salicylate stimulates net organic acid production and causes a minor elevation in the anion gap.

The signs and symptoms of salicylate intoxication are secondary to all the laboratory value abnormalities that have been described. Other symptoms may be tinnitus, which is common, nausea, vomiting, and sensorineural hearing loss.[65] Anderson and associates studied 73 consecutive cases of adults with salicylate intoxication.[62] Twenty of these patients were older (mean age 53 years), had no psychiatric or suicidal history, and denied aspirin use, although they were taking aspirin for medical conditions. Diagnosis was frequently delayed up to 72 hours. Laboratory evaluation showed a mixed respiratory alkalosis and an anion gap type metabolic acidosis. In this study, the signs and symptoms noted were tachypnea and neurologic abnormalities (eg, confusion, agitation, hyperactivity, slurred speech, hallucinations, generalized seizures, focal seizures [rare], and coma). The severity of the central nervous system manifestations correlated with the brain salicylate level. Cardiac dysfunction occurred as congestive heart failure or sudden death.

Some of the laboratory abnormalities are predictable from the pathogenesis (eg, glucose aberrations, acid-base disturbances, and enhanced ketone formation). The severity of the acidosis varies inversely with age. Severe acidosis may be delayed in onset 12 to 24 hours following ingestion of excessive salicylate. Owing to increased insensible fluid losses from fever, increased renal losses due to a greater solute load, and organic aciduria, dehydration is in the order of 2 to 3 L/m² in moderate intoxications and 4 to 6 L/m² in severe intoxications. Respiratory alkalosis occurs initially and may persist throughout the intoxication. This acute respiratory alkalosis (unlike chronic respiratory alkalosis), together with nausea, vomiting, and dehydration (extracellular fluid contraction), encourages the development of an alkalosis and the renal excretion of potassium. Hypernatremia and hypokalemia are common findings. Occasionally, hyponatremia may occur secondary to inappropriate antidiuretic hormone secretion induced by aspirin. Salicylate intoxication also has hemostatic effects (eg, decreased synthesis of prothrombin, decreased factor VII, and decreased aggregation of platelets).[63] With very high salicylate levels, hepatotoxicity has been described.[66] Neurogenic (ie, noncardiogenic) pulmonary edema has also been described.[67] Owing to inappropriate antidiuretic hormone secretion and/or excessive administration of fluids during forced diuresis, cardiogenic pulmonary edema may ensue in the elderly (see also Chapter 29, Poisoning, Drug Overdose, and Toxic Exposures).

Treatment

In the treatment of metabolic acidosis, it is important to determine the base deficit,[68,69] which can be calculated as follows:

$$\text{Desired plasma HCO}_3^- - \text{Actual plasma HCO}_3^- = \text{Deficit of HCO}_3^-/\text{L}$$

$$\text{Total body water} = 60\% \text{ total body weight} \quad (10)$$

$$\text{Total body HCO}_3^- \text{ deficit} = \text{Total body water} \times \text{Deficit of HCO}_3^-/\text{L}$$

For example, if a bicarbonate level of 18 mEq/L is desired in a 50-kg patient in metabolic acidosis with a bicarbonate level of 12 mEq/L, the bicarbonate deficit is 18 − 12 or 6 mEq/L. Total body water is 0.6 × 50 kg or 30 L. Total body bicarbonate deficit is 30 L × 6 mEq/L or 180 mEq. One half of the initial deficit can be replaced over 5 to 10 minutes and the remainder of the deficit replaced according to the clinical condition of the patient. The proportion of bicarbonate passing into the intracellular space increases with bicarbonate values less than 5 mEq/L. If bicarbonate values are this low, use total body water as 100% of total body weight.[70] To alkalinize urine orally, give 4 g bicarbonate orally and then 1 to 2 g orally every 4 hours.

Vasodilator therapy may help in severe idiopathic lactic acidosis.[71] Some success has been reported with nitroprusside; *tris*-hydroxyaminomethane (THAM) is an interesting buffer and an alternative to bicarbonate. Although THAM regularly depresses ventilation and therefore increases hypoxemia, it has the unusual property of lowering P_{CO_2} at the same time it raises the bicarbonate level. To reduce the P_{CO_2} by 25% for 2 hours, however, requires 500 mM THAM. This drug is useful in a ventilated patient who still has an increased P_{CO_2}, such as a patient in cardiac arrest. In addition, THAM contains no sodium, which may make it the drug of choice in patients with cirrhosis, congestive heart failure, or nephrotic syndrome.[72] THAM is 0.3 M isotonic, with a pH of 10.6 and must be used within 1 hour of reconstitution. It catalyzes the following reaction:

$$(CH_2OH)_3 - C - NH_2 + H^+ \rightleftarrows (CH_2OH)_3 - C - NH_3^+ \quad (11)$$

Seventy-five percent of THAM is in ionized form at pH 7.4. The ionized form penetrates the cell and titrates the intracellular space. Since this removes H^+ without affecting bicarbonate level, P_{CO_2} is decreased because of a shift in equilibrium toward bicarbonate generation by the following reaction:

$$H^+ + HCO_3^- \rightleftarrows H_2CO_3 \rightleftarrows CO_2 + H_2O \quad (12)$$

The decrease in P_{CO_2} may cause hypoventilation. THAM should be given over 1 hour according to the following formula:

$$\text{0.3 M solution THAM (mL)} = \text{kg body weight} \times \text{base deficit (mEq/L)} \quad (13)$$

In cardiac arrest, 100 to 300 mL may be administered via a large-bore intravenous catheter. This solution can occasionally cause hypoglycemia, prolonged prothrombin time, or hyperkalemia. Fifty percent to 75% of THAM is excreted from the body in 24 hours.[73]

All patients with an acute metabolic acidosis should be hospitalized except patients with chronic seizure disorders who have had a seizure within 1 hour.

ELEVATION OF THE ANION GAP WITHOUT ACIDOSIS

If more water is lost than salt, then the concentration of the remaining electrolytes increases.[9] If the loss is 20% of total body water, then electrolytes would be expected to increase by 20% and so would the unmeasured anions; however, a

20% increase in the anion gap (eg, from 10 to to 12 mEq/L) is trivial.

If lactate metabolism is slowed in shock or hypoxia, administration of lactated Ringer's solution has been shown to elevate the anion gap. In addition, each unit of whole blood contains 17 mEq of citrate per liter.[74] This citrate is usually converted to bicarbonate; however, in shock or hypoxia, it is retained, elevating the anion gap.

Carbenicillin at 30 mg/day and penicillin at 50,000 to 100,000 U/day serve as unmeasured anions and elevate the anion gap.[75,76]

The accumulated organic anion in chronic hypocapnia may be lactate, which elevates the anion gap by 3 to 4 mEq/L.[77]

Removal of chloride elevates the anion gap by 3 to 5 mEq/L. It is believed that dehydration increases the concentration of unmeasured anions and alkalosis (pH 7.60), thus increasing the electronegativity of the serum proteins that constitute two thirds of unmeasured anions in the normal anion gap.[78,79]

LOW ANION GAP

In contrast to dehydration, which increases the anion gap, dilution of the extracellular fluid decreases the anion gap.[9]

The replacement of the unmeasured anion albumin with the measured anion chloride in salt-retaining hypoalbuminemic states, such as a cirrhosis or nephrotic syndrome, causes a fall in the anion gap.[9] It is important to remember that albumin is responsible for most of the normal anion gap. The average anion gap in patients with nephrotic syndrome is 2 mEq/L less than expected.

The combination of a spuriously lower than expected serum sodium level plus a high serum chloride level causes a low anion gap in patients with hypernatremia.[9] Hyperviscosity also results in an underestimation of the sodium level and causes a decreased anion gap by the same mechanism as hypernatremia.

The reaction of bromide with the automated analysis reagents is greater than that of chloride, causing a falsely elevated chloride level. A negative anion gap is a clue to this diagnosis. Nervine has bromide in the amount of 25 mEq/L (200 mg/dL) and is the agent usually associated with toxicity. Symptoms and signs involve psychiatric and neurologic aberrations along with an acneiform eruption.[80,81]

The displacement of serum water by protein causes an artifactual decrease in the serum sodium concentration and, therefore, a decrease in the anion gap. In 76 patients with myeloma, the mean anion gap was 9.2 ± 0.4 mEq/L. In fact, one third of the patients had an anion gap less than 6 mEq/L. Other causes of increased globulins (eg, sarcoidosis) did not decrease the anion gap.[82]

The anion gap is affected on milliequivalent by milliequivalent basis with hypercalcemia; therefore, only life-threatening hypercalcemia affects the anion gap.[9] Therapeutic levels of the cation lithium rarely exceed 3 mEq/L, which hardly affects the anion gap. However, suicide attempts with lithium may be quite effective in lowering the anion gap.[9]

METABOLIC ALKALOSIS

Despite a widely diverse collection of clinical situations, hypokalemia or extracellular fluid depletion is nearly always associated with a metabolic alkalosis. For the most part, either acid or potassium is lost in the kidney or the intestinal tract, generating a metabolic alkalosis.[68,83]

Metabolic alkalosis can be rapidly life-threatening. An increase in the serum bicarbonate level of only 15 to 20 mEq/L may cause marked alkalemia, because the compensatory respiratory response is a modest hypoventilation (P_{CO_2} of 50 to 55 mmHg at most).[84,85] The following formula helps to predict the P_{CO_2} for a given value of bicarbonate:

$$P_{CO_2} = 0.9(HCO_3^-) + 9 \qquad (14)$$

A normal or lower than normal P_{CO_2} in the presence of a high bicarbonate level implies a respiratory alkalosis along with a metabolic acidosis.

Metabolic alkalosis can be divided into two groups: (1) that caused by gastric- or diuretic-induced chloride loss with subsequent replacement by the selective proximal reabsorption of bicarbonate in the renal tubules and (2) that caused by direct renal bicarbonate reabsorption without a chloride deficit. In group 1, the "spot" urine chloride is quite low, often less than 10 mEq/L; in group 2, the urine chloride varies with the diet as usual (60 to 100 mEq/L).[86]

Group 1

Gastric Loss

Chloride may be lost secondary to nasogastric suction or vomiting with reabsorption of bicarbonate.[68,83] The alkalosis stimulates a renal loss of potassium. Hypovolemia results in a low urine sodium level (ie, less than 10 mEq/L), whereas normovolemia is associated with a normal value for urine sodium (ie, dependent on intake, but greater than 40 mEq/L).

Contraction Alkalosis and Diuretic-Induced Metabolic Alkalosis

Enhanced excretion of sodium and chloride without the proportional loss of bicarbonate may result in contraction alkalosis and diuretic-induced metabolic alkalosis.[16] Acid excretion is brought on by the potassium depletion, as well as by a volume contraction induced by the physiologic response of aldosterone.

Relief of Chronic Hypercapnia

The abrupt reduction of carbon dioxide levels in patients with chronic hypercapnia may cause a sudden, severe metabolic alkalosis. For example, a patient with chronic obstructive pulmonary disease may have a pH of 7.37, P_{CO_2} of 58 mmHg, and bicarbonate level of 40; when placed on a ventilator, this patient develops a pH of 7.67, P_{CO_2} of 40 mmHg, and bicarbonate level of 40. If the reduction in P_{CO_2} is gradual (over two to three days), the excess bicarbonate is gradually excreted. If these patients are on a low salt diet or are treated with diuretics, however, proximal reabsorption of bicarbonate is enhanced, and the metabolic alkalosis that previously was compensating for a respiratory acidosis becomes primary. This primary metabolic alkalosis may develop even without diuretics; all that is needed is contraction of the arterial volume (eg, congestive heart failure).[87]

Fasting Patients During Initial Feedings

Some patients who have been fasting are initially somewhat hypovolemic. Therefore, excess aldosterone has been secreted. With the addition of glucose, there is an increase in the proximal reabsorption of bicarbonate.

Hypoparathyroidism

Parathormone increases the renal absorption of chloride and enhances the renal loss of bicarbonate. Hypoparathyroidism causes a chloride deficit and a secondary reabsorption of bicarbonate.[68,83]

Hypercalcemia

Suppression of parathormone secretion in association with hypercalcemia causes a chloride deficit and a secondary reabsorption of bicarbonate. Hyperparathyroidism can be distinguished from all other causes of hypercalcemia, therefore, by the serum chloride level. A serum chloride level of greater than 102 mEq/L should occur in hyperparathyroidism, presuming the patient is not on diuretics[68,83] (see Chapter 20, Hypercalcemia).

Excess Bicarbonate Load

The oral intake of 140 g of bicarbonate every day for 3 weeks produces a metabolic alkalosis with bicarbonate levels ranging from 33 to 36 mEq/L.[68,83] In renal failure, smaller doses of bicarbonate may produce a metabolic alkalosis because of the inability of the kidney to excrete this excess bicarbonate.

Congenital Alkalosis with Diarrhea

Although this syndrome is initially seen in infancy, children with congenital alkalosis with diarrhea survive into adulthood.[88] These patients have a defect in the chloride-bicarbonate pump in the ileum and are unable to transport chloride against an electrochemical gradient; this defect causes a loss of chloride and acid in the stool.

Group 2

All the causes of hypokalemia secondary to renal losses are included in group 2 metabolic alkaloses.

Diagnosis

Symptoms of metabolic alkalosis may be tetany secondary to hypocalcemia (low free serum calcium), hyperirritability, convulsions, altered mental status, and respiratory depression.[68,83] Electrocardiographic changes resemble those of hypokalemia. Hepatic failure is worsened by alkalosis secondary to an increase in the ratio of ammoniate ammonium ions in the presence of alkalosis, causing increased ammonia levels in the blood that may cross the blood-brain barrier and worsen hepatic encephalopathy.

The appropriate value to use as the bicarbonate level is controversial and varies among institutions. As an arterial blood gas determination, the calculated bicarbonate level depends on the reliability of the pH and the P_{CO_2}; theoretically, small errors in these measured values could distort the resulting serum bicarbonate level.[89] The venous serum total carbon dioxide should be 2 to 3 mEq/L higher than the calculated bicarbonate obtained from the arterial blood gas determination, since the total carbon dioxide obtained on a venous sample of blood measures the dissolved carbon dioxide, carbonic acid, and bicarbonate. The dissolved carbon dioxide and carbonic acid are usually no more than 2 to 3 mEq/L, a value that must be subtracted when using the total carbon dioxide to calculate the anion gap. Although a measured value, the total carbon dioxide is unreliable and frequently results in two different values on the same sample. It is probably prudent to use the calculated arterial bicarbonate value as the "true" bicarbonate level.

Treatment

When considering therapy for severe metabolic alkalosis, the physician must remember that sodium chloride and potassium chloride infusions can usually correct alkalosis by suppressing renal acid excretion and enhancing the renal excretion of bicarbonate. However, these corrective mechanisms are slow and cannot be relied on for patients with extreme alkalosis, defined as a pH more than 7.6 with symptoms or more than 7.8 without symptoms. Nasogastric drainage should be stopped, if possible, and exogenous bicarbonate therapy discontinued. Patients in group 1 respond to sodium chloride and potassium chloride replacement in 3 to 4 four days, whereas patients in group 2 are chloride resistant but usually respond to spironolactone, an aldosterone antagonist.

In patients who retain sodium chloride (eg, those with congestive heart failure or cirrhosis), arterial hypovolemia causes a secondary hyperaldosteronism with increased bicarbonate reabsorption. Volume expansion would obviously be detrimental in these cases. Spironolactone or acetazolamide (carbonic anhydrase inhibitor) may be given to increase the renal excretion of bicarbonate.

In the presence of extreme alkalosis or hepatic encephalopathy, the use of direct acidifying agents is justified:

1. Arginine hydrochloride supplies hydrochloride during its metabolism. It is the compound that is tolerated best parenterally. If commercial arginine is unavailable, a solution can be prepared from the powder with 50 mEq/dL.
2. Ammonium chloride contains hydrogen ion in a concentration of 167 mEq/L and is well tolerated.
3. Lysine hydrochloride is an alternative to ammonium chloride.
4. Dilute hydrochloric acid can be used. This acid must be given through a central catheter. This method is the best treatment in patients with hepatic encephalopathy because no additional sources of ammonia, such as amino acids, are being supplied. Administration of acid should not prevent therapy with volume expanders and potassium chloride, if needed, since these patients frequently require 4 to 5 L of fluid (isotonic saline) and 500 to 600 mEq of potassium chloride for correction of their metabolic alkalosis. To prepare the solutions, 100 mL of 1N hydrochloric acid is added to 900 mL of normal saline or 5% dextrose in water, resulting in 0.1N hydrochloric acid containing 100 mEq of hydrogen ion per liter and a hypotonic 200 mOsm/L solution. Alternatively, 200 mL of 1N hydrochloric acid can be added to 800 mL of normal saline or 5% dextrose in water, resulting in 0.2N hydrochloric acid with 200 mEq of hydrogen ion per liter and a hypertonic 400 mOsm/L solution.[90–92]
5. Hemodialysis against low chloride and high acetate solution is well suited for uremic patients with severe metabolic alkalosis.

To calculate the amount of acid necessary to treat a metabolic alkalosis, the volume of distribution of bicarbonate must be known. The volume of distribution of bicarbonate is one half of the total body weight.[68,83] This volume is then multiplied by the desired decrement in bicarbonate, resulting in the base excess. In general, the physician should try to obtain a reduction in bicarbonate of 10 mEq/L over 12 to 24 hours. For example, a 70-kg man with a severe metabolic alkalosis has a bicarbonate level of 50 mEq/L, and a decrease in the bicarbonate level to 40 mEq/L is desired. The volume of distribution is one half of 70 kg, or 35 L. Multiplying the volume of distribution (35 L) by the desired decrement (10 L) results in 350 mEq of acid needed to decrease serum bicarbonate by 10 mEq/L. This neutralization could be achieved with 0.2N hydrochloric acid in normal saline administered at a rate of 200 mL/hour. Faster decrements in bicarbonate can be achieved if the clinical situation warrants.

RESPIRATORY ACIDOSIS

Pathophysiology

Carbon dioxide is an end product of metabolism. The level of carbon dioxide reflects the balance between production at the cellular level and excretion by the lungs. Although carbon dioxide is produced at a relatively constant rate, the rate at which it is excreted varies with the efficiency of breathing. If alveolar ventilation is increased, the carbon dioxide level in the blood, or P_{CO_2}, decreases.[93] Conversely, if alveolar ventilation is decreased, arterial P_{CO_2} increases.

Acute respiratory acidosis is uncompensated. There is no renal retention of bicarbonate.[94] For every 10-mmHg increase in P_{CO_2}, the hydrogen ion concentration increases 8 nEq/L or decreases 0.08 pH unit.[5,95] For example, if a patient with a P_{CO_2} of 40 mmHg, a pH of 7.40, and a hydrogen ion concentration of 40 nEq/L develops acute respiratory failure so that the P_{CO_2} becomes 60 mmHg, the hydrogen ion concentration increases by 16 nEq/L or 56 nEq/L and the pH decreases by 0.16 unit to 7.24.

In acute respiratory acidosis, the elevation of P_{CO_2} increases the serum bicarbonate level by a small amount owing to an equilibrium shift in the reaction catalyzed by carbonic anhydrase (see Eq. 12 above).[5] It is not a compensation for respiratory acidosis by the kidneys. Because of the shift in equilibrium, for every 10-mmHg increment in P_{CO_2}, bicarbonate increases 1 mEq/L.

After 6 to 12 hours of acute respiratory acidosis, the renal synthesis and retention of bicarbonate is stimulated, and the patient is in chronic respiratory acidosis.[5,96] With the increased retention of bicarbonate, electrical neutrality is maintained by renal secretion of chloride. The renal compensation for respiratory acidosis is not complete, however. The pH remains in the low normal range from 7.36 to 7.39, provided that the P_{CO_2} is less than 60 mmHg. When the P_{CO_2} is more than 60 mmHg, only 15% of patients are able to compensate and maintain their pH within the normal range. Most of these patients have an arterial pH less than 7.36.[97] If the P_{CO_2} is more than 70 mmHg, only 1% of patients have a pH within the normal range; the remainder have a pH less than 7.35.[97]

The hydrogen ion concentration in chronic respiratory acidosis does not vary as much as it does with acute respiratory acidosis because of the buffering capacity of the elevated bicarbonate values in chronic respiratory acidosis. In chronic respiratory acidosis, for each 10-mmHg increase in P_{CO_2} there is a 3-nEq/L increase in hydrogen ion concentration or a 0.03-unit decrease in pH.[5] For example, if the P_{CO_2} of a patient with a pH of 7.40 and a hydrogen ion concentration of 40 nEq/L is increased from 50 to 60 mmHg, the hydrogen ion concentration is increased from 40 to 43 nEq/L and the pH is decreased from 7.40 to 7.37.

Etiology, Diagnosis, and Treatment

For the etiology, diagnosis, and treatment of respiratory acidosis, see Chapter 74, Respiratory Failure.

RESPIRATORY ALKALOSIS

Mechanism

Respiratory alkalosis develops when ventilation is increased to the point that carbon dioxide excretion exceeds carbon dioxide production.

Acute Respiratory Alkalosis

During acute respiratory alkalosis, a nonrenal compensation occurs secondary to the carbonic anhydrase reaction (see Eq. 12). In this reaction, the decreased level of carbon dioxide shifts the equilibrium so that bicarbonate is consumed, bringing the pH closer to normal and, therefore, functioning as a buffer. To maintain electrical neutrality, lost bicarbonate is replaced by chloride, which results in mild hyperchloremia. For every 10-mmHg decrease of P_{CO_2}, the bicarbonate level decreases 2 mEq,[98] the hydrogen ion concentration decreases 8 nEq/L, and the pH increases by 0.08.[5] For example, if a patient with a pH of 7.4 and a P_{CO_2} of 40 mmHg develops an acute respiratory alkalosis that decreases the P_{CO_2} to 20 mmHg, the hydrogen ion concentration decreases 16 nEq/L to 24 nEq/L and the pH increases by 0.16 to 7.56.

Chronic Respiratory Alkalosis

By definition, chronic respiratory alkalosis is an acute respiratory alkalosis that has persisted for at least 12 to 24 hours and is being compensated for by the renal excretion of bicarbonate. As in all other acid-base abnormalities, the compensated pH is in the high normal range (ie, 7.40 to 7.45). This persistence in a high normal range lasts for 7 to 9 days. After 2 weeks, however, the pH returns to a completely normal value without any superimposed metabolic acidosis.[5] Chronic respiratory alkalosis is unique among the acid-base disturbances in that it is the only one in which a completely normal pH is expected.[5] The serum bicarbonate level can be predicted in a chronic respiratory alkalosis. For every 10-mmHg decrease in P_{CO_2}, the serum bicarbonate level should fall 5 mEq/L.[5,99] For example, if a patient with a pH of 7.4, a P_{CO_2} of 40 mmHg, and a bicarbonate level of 25 mEq/L develops a chronic respiratory alkalosis and a new P_{CO_2} of 20 mmHg, the pH will be 7.4 and the expected serum bicarbonate level is 15 mEq/L after 2 weeks.

Etiology

Hyperventilation Syndrome

Anxiety or stress may cause patients to develop the hyperventilation syndrome. They are usually totally unaware that they are breathing rapidly. Some patients, however, do not have tachypnea but simply increase the depth of inspiration without increasing the rate.

Central Neurogenic Hyperventilation

Massive brain injury may affect the medullary centers that inhibit respiration. Because these centers control the rate and depth of respiration, hyperventilation may follow such an injury. Central neurogenic hyperventilation is seen in patients with brain tumors, massive cerebral vascular accidents, encephalitis, or meningitis.

Respiratory Stimulants

Several entities stimulate the respiratory centers in the medulla. Progesterone secreted during pregnancy is responsible for the chronic respiratory alkalosis seen in pregnancy. During pregnancy, the P_{CO_2} usually is approximately 30 mmHg, and the patient has a normal pH.[100] In fact, progesterone has been successfully used in the treatment of acute respiratory failure in patients with chronic obstructive pulmonary disease as well as in patients with pickwickian syndrome.[101–102] Adrenergic stimulation also may increase the respiratory rate. Excessive catecholamines, as may be seen in pheochromocytoma, may cause respiratory alkalosis. In a similar fashion, patients with analeptic overdose (eg, with amphetamines or cocaine) also develop respiratory alkalosis.

Hepatic Insufficiency

The mechanism is unclear, but patients with marked liver disease frequently have respiratory alkalosis.

Restrictive Pulmonary Disease

Patients whose chest wall motion is restricted may complain of dyspnea. Although not associated with hypoxemia, this dyspnea and hyperventilation results in respiratory alkalosis. It has been postulated that restriction in chest wall motion stimulates the J receptors in the bronchi, which in turn enhance breathing. This mechanism may explain the dyspnea seen in nonhypoxemic patients with tumors of the lung, pneumothorax, pleural effusions, or pneumonia.

Pulmonary Hypoxemia

Chemoreceptors in the carotid body stimulate respiration in response to hypoxemia.[103] In normal individuals, there is a highly varied response to hypoxemia. Some patients develop a profound respiratory alkalosis in response to hypoxemia, while other patients do not hyperventilate at all in response to hypoxemia.[104] It is well known that patients with chronic obstructive pulmonary disease may have a blunted response to hypoxemia[105]; it is less well known that normal patients may also have a blunted response to hypoxemia and hyperventilate less than expected[104] (see Chapter 72, Obstructive Airways Disease).

Tissue Hypoxia

The pathophysiologic mechanisms behind tissue hypoxemia usually involve uncoupling. Uncoupling implies that oxidative phosphorylation has been uncoupled from electron transport in the mitochondria. Therefore, despite an abundant supply of oxygen, adenosine triphosphatase is not being generated. This is perceived by the body as hypoxemia, and hyperventilation ensues. This mechanism explains the respiratory alkalosis found during fever, gram-negative sepsis, hyperthyroidism, and salicylate intoxication (see Chapter 6, Shock).

Another pathophysiologic mechanism of tissue hypoxemia is impaired delivery of oxygen to the tissues. For example, carbon monoxide may occasionally produce respiratory alkalosis in association with a normal Po_2.[106] Carbon monoxide not only shifts the oxygen-hemoglobin dissociation curve to the left, which deprives tissues of oxygen, but also binds strongly to hemoglobin. Both these processes impair the ability of hemoglobin to release oxygen. Therefore, the patient may hyperventilate. Another cause of impaired oxygen delivery is methemoglobinemia, which may be congenital or acquired. The acquired form of methemoglobinemia can result in tissue hypoxia secondary to impaired oxygen delivery and, subsequently, respiratory alkalosis.[107] These patients are quite dyspneic, with a normal Po_2 and a dark brown arterial blood gas sample rather than the normally red arterial blood sample.

Clinical Manifestations

During respiratory alkalosis, the ratio of charges between the cationic and anionic proteins is altered so that more anionic proteins are present. This results simply from the change in pH. The increased anionic proteins bind more free calcium, producing symptoms of hypocalcemia; the serum calcium is unaltered, however, since serum calcium measures both free and bound calcium. Therefore, the symptoms of respiratory alkalosis mimic those of hypocalcemia. Any other manifestations of acute respiratory alkalosis reflect the underlying etiology.

Treatment

The only treatment of respiratory alkalosis is treatment for the underlying condition. Respiratory alkalosis is highly refractory to any other forms of therapy.

REFERENCES

1. Van Slyke DD. Some points of acid-base history in physiology and medicine. *Ann Ny Acad Sci*. 1966;133:5.
2. Henderson LJ. Theory of neutrality regulation in animal organism. *Am J Physiol*. 1908;21:427.
3. Sorenson SPL. Enzymestudien: II. Mitteilung: Uber die Messung und die Bedeutung der Wasserstoffionen-Konzentration bei enzymatischen Prozessen. *Biochem Z*. 1909;21:131.
4. Hasselbalch KA. Die Berechnung der Wasserstoffzahl des Blutes aus der freien und gebundenen Kohlensaure desselben und die Sauerstoffbindung des Blutes als Funktion der Wasserstoffzahl. *Biochem Z*. 1916;78:112.
5. Narins RG, Emmett M. Simple and mixed acid-base disorders: a practical approach. *Medicine*. 1980;59:161.
6. Kassirer JP, Bleich HL. Rapid estimation of plasma carbon dioxide from pH and total carbon dioxide content. *N Engl J Med*. 1965;272:1067.
7. Morgan HG. Acid-base balance in blood. *Br J Anaesthesiol*. 1969;41:196.
8. Kaufman HE, Rosen SW. Clinical acid-base regulation—the Bronsted schema. *Surg Gynecol Obstet*. 1956;103:101.
9. Emmett M, Narins RG. Clinical use of the anion gap. *Medicine*. 1977;56:38.
10. Witte DL, Rodgers JL, Barrett DA. The anion gap: its use in quality control. *Clin Chem*. 1976;22:643.
11. Pierce NF, Fedson DS, Brigham DE, et al. The ventilatory response to acute base deficit in humans: time course during development and correction of metabolic acidosis. *Ann Intern Med*. 1970;72:633.
12. Reuler JB. Hypothermia: pathophysiology, clinical settings and management. *Ann Intern Med*. 1978;89:519.
13. Goodwin NM, Schreiber MT. Effects of anticoagulants on acid-base and blood gas estimations. *Crit Care Med*. 1979;7:473.
14. Asch MJ. Acid-base effects of topical mafenide acetate in the burned patient. *N Engl J Med*. 1971;284:1281.
15. Runeberg L, Miettinen TA, Nikkila EA. Effect of cholestyramine on mineral excretion in man. *Acta Med Scand*. 1972;192:71.
16. Garella S, Chang BS, Kahn SF. Dilution acidosis and contraction alkalosis: review of a concept. *Kidney Int*. 1975;8:279.
17. Oh MS, Carroll HJ, Goldstein DH, et al. Hyperchloremic acidosis during the recovery phase of diabetic ketosis. *Ann Intern Med*. 1978;89:925.
18. Giammarco R, Goldstein M, Halpern M, et al. Renal tubular acidosis during therapy for diabetic ketoacidosis. *Can Med Assoc J*. 1975;112:465.
19. Heird WC, Dell RB, Driscoll JM, et al. Metabolic acidosis resulting from intravenous alimentation mixtures containing synthetic amino acids. *N Engl J Med*. 1972;287:943.
20. Gennari FJ, Goldstein MB, Schwartz WB. The nature of the renal adaptation of chronic hypocapnia. *J Clin Invest*. 1972;51:1722.
21. Batlle DC, Aruda JAL, Kurtzman NA. Hyperkalemic distal renal tubular acidosis associated with obstructive uropathy. *N Engl J Med*. 1981;304:373.

22. Narins RG, Goldberg M. Renal tubular acidosis: pathophysiology, diagnosis and treatment. *DM*. 1977;23:1.
23. Sebastian A, Morris RC Jr. Renal tubular acidosis. *Clin Nephrol*. 1977;7:216.
24. Morris RC Jr. Renal tubular acidosis. *N Engl J Med*. 1981;304:418.
25. Gennari FJ, Cohen JJ. Renal tubular acidosis. *Annu Rev Med*. 1978;29:521.
26. Ritz E, Heidland A. Lactic acidosis. *Clin Nephrol*. 1977;7:231.
27. Kreisberg RA. Lactate, homeostasis and lactic acidosis. *Ann Intern Med*. 1980;92:227.
28. Fraley DS, Adler S, Bruns FJ, et al. Stimulation of lactate production by administration of bicarbonate in a patient with a solid neoplasm and lactic acidosis. *N Engl J Med*. 1980;303:1100.
29. Nadiminti Y, Wang JC, Chou S-Y, et al. Lactic acidosis associated with Hodgkin's disease: response to chemotherapy. *N Engl J Med*. 1980;303:15.
30. Sprung CL, Portocarrero CJ, Fernaine AV, et al. The metabolic and respiratory alterations of heat stroke. *Arch Intern Med*. 1980;140:665.
31. Orringer CE, Eustace JL, Wunsch CD, Gardner LB. Natural history of lactic acidosis after grand-mal seizures: a model for the study of an anion-gap acidosis not associated with hyperkalemia. *N Engl J Med*. 1977;297:796.
32. Gerst PH, Fleming WH, Malm JR. Increased susceptibility of the heart to ventricular fibrillation during metabolic acidosis. *Circ Res*. 1966;19:63.
33. O'Connor LR, Klein KL, Bethune JE. Hyperphosphatemia in lactic acidosis. *N Engl J Med*. 1977;297:707.
34. Molitch ME, Rodman E, Hirsch CA, et al. Spurious serum creatinine elevations in ketoacidosis. *Ann Intern Med*. 1980;93:280.
35. Grant DH. Pharmacology of isopropyl alcohol, a synopsis of available data. *J Lab Clin Med*. 1923;8:382.
36. Cooperman MT, Davidoff F, Spark R, et al. Clinical studies of alcoholic ketoacidosis. *Diabetes*. 1974;23:433.
37. Fulop M, Hoberman HD. Alcoholic ketosis. *Diabetes*. 1975;24:785.
38. Miller PD, Heinig RE, Waterhouse C. Treatment of alcoholic acidosis: the role of dextrose and phosphorus. *Arch Intern Med*. 1978;138:67.
39. Young E, Bradley RF. Cerebral edema with irreversible coma in severe diabetic ketoacidosis. *N Engl J Med*. 1967;276:665.
40. Metzger AL, Rubenstein AH. Reversible cerebral edema complicating diabetic ketoacidosis. *Br Med J*. 1970;3:746.
41. Kitabchi AE, Young R, Sacks H, et al. Diabetic ketoacidosis: reappraisal of therapeutic approach. *Annu Rev Med*. 1979;30:339.
42. Alberti KGMM, Hockaday TDR. Diabetic coma: a reappraisal after five years. *Clin Endocrinol Metab*. 1977;6:421.
43. Ohman JL, Marliss EB, Aoki TT, et al. The cerebrospinal fluid in diabetic ketoacidosis. *N Engl J Med*. 1971;284:283.
44. Kreisberg RA. Diabetic ketoacidosis: new concepts and trends in pathogenesis and treatment. *Ann Intern Med*. 1978;88:681.
45. Soler NG, Fitzgerald MG, Wright AD, et al. Comparative study of different insulin regimens in management of diabetic ketoacidosis. *Lancet*. 1975;2:1221.
46. Kitabchi AE, Ayyagari Y, Guerra SM. The efficacy of low-dose versus conventional therapy of insulin for treatment of diabetic ketoacidosis. *Ann Intern Med*. 1976;84:633.
47. Fisher JN, Shahshahani MN, Kitabchi AE. Diabetic ketoacidosis: low dose insulin therapy by various routes. *N Engl J Med*. 1977;197:238.
48. Knight AH, Williams DN, Ellis G, et al. Significance of hyperamylasemia and abdominal pain in diabetic ketoacidosis. *Br Med J*. 1973;3:128.
49. Lentz RD, Brown DM, Kjellstrand OM. Treatment of severe hypophosphatemia. *Ann Intern Med*. 1978;89:941.
50. Bennett IL Jr, Cary FH, Mitchell GL, et al. Acute methyl alcohol poisoning: a review based on experiences in an outbreak of 323 cases. *Medicine*. 1953;32:431.
51. Erlanson P, Hagstam K-E, Liljenberg B, et al. Severe methanol intoxication. *Acta Med Scand*. 1965;177:393.
52. McMartin KE, Ambre JJ, Tephly TR. Methanol poisoning in human subjects: role for formic acid accumulation in the metabolic acidosis. *Am J Med*. 1980;68:414.
53. Keyvan-Larijarni H, Tannenberg AM. Methanol intoxication: comparison of peritoneal dialysis and hemodialysis treatment. *Arch Intern Med*. 1974;134:293.
54. McCoy HG, Cippole RJ, Ehlers SM, et al. Severe methanol poisoning: application of a pharmacokinetic model for ethanol therapy and hemodialysis. *Am J Med*. 1979;67:804.
55. Gonda A, Gault H, Churchill D, et al. Hemodialysis for methanol intoxication. *Am J Med*. 1978;64:749.
56. Parry MF, Wallach R. Ethylene glycol poisoning. *Am J Med*. 1974;57:143.
57. Cadnapaphornchai P, Taher S, Bhathena D, et al. Ethylene glycol poisoning: diagnosis based on high osmolal and anion gaps and crystalluria. *Ann Emerg Med*. 1981;10:94.
58. Stokes JB, Averon F. Prevention of organ damage in massive ethylene glycol ingestion. *JAMA*. 1980;243:2065.
59. Wacher WEC, Haynes H, Druyan R, et al. Treatment of ethylene glycol poisoning with ethyl alcohol. *JAMA*. 1965;194:173.
60. Smithline N, Gardner KD Jr. Gaps—anion and osmolal. *JAMA*. 1976;236:1594.
61. Glasser L, Sternglanz PD, Combic J, et al. Serum osmolarity and its applicability to drug overdose. *Am J Clin Pathol*. 1963;60:695.
62. Anderson RJ, Potts DE, Gabow PA, et al. Unrecognized adult salicylate intoxication. *Ann Intern Med*. 1976;85:745.
63. Temple AR. Pathophysiology of aspirin overdosage toxicity with implications for management. *Pediatrics*. 1978;62:873.
64. Gabow PA, Potts DE, Schrier RW, et al. The acid-base abnormalities of adult salicylate intoxication. *Clin Res*. 1976;24:126A.
65. Myers EN, Bernstein JM, Fostiropolous G. Salicylate ototoxicity: a clinical study. *N Engl J Med*. 1965;273:587.
66. Zimmerman HJ. Aspirin-induced hepatic injury. *Ann Intern Med*. 1974;80:103.
67. Hrnicek G, Skelton J, Miller WC. Pulmonary edema and salicylate intoxication. *JAMA*. 1974;230:866.
68. Arruda JAL, Kurtzman NA. Metabolic acidosis and alkalosis. *Clin Nephrol*. 1977;7:201.
69. Lindeman RD, Papper S. Therapy of fluid and electrolyte disorders. *Ann Intern Med*. 1975;82:64.
70. Garella GD, Serafino AL, Dana CL, et al. Severity of metabolic acidosis as a determinant of bicarbonate requirements. *N Engl J Med*. 1973;289:121.
71. Taradash MR, Jacobson LB. Vasodilator therapy of idiopathic lactic acidosis. *N Engl J Med*. 1975;293:468.
72. Bleich HL, Schwartz WB. Tris buffer (THAM): an appraisal of its physiologic effects and clinical usefulness. *N Engl J Med*. 1966;274:782.
73. THAM. *American Hospital Formulary Service*. 1979;40:8.
74. Litwin MS, Smith LL, Moore FD. Metabolic alkalosis following massive transfusion. *Surgery*. 1959;45:805.
75. Lipner HI, Ruzany F, Dasgupta M, et al. The behavior of carbenicillin as a nonreabsorbable anion. *J Lab Clin Med*. 1975;86:183.

76. Brunner FD, Frick PG. Hypokalaemia, metabolic acidosis, and hypernatraemia due to "massive" sodium penicillin therapy. *Br Med J.* 1968;4:550.
77. Eldridge F, Salzer J. Effect of respiratory alkalosis on blood lactate and pyruvate in humans. *J Appl Physiol.* 1967;22:461.
78. Kassirer JP, Schwartz WB. The selective depletion of hydrochloric acid: factors in the genesis of persistent gastric alkalosis. *Am J Med.* 1966;40:10.
79. Madias NE, Ayus JC, Adrogue HJ. Increased anion gap in metabolic alkalosis: the role of plasma-protein equivalency. *N Engl J Med.* 1979;300:1421.
80. Blume RS, MacLowry JD, Wolf SM. Limitations of chloride determination in the diagnosis of bromism. *N Engl J Med.* 1968;279:593.
81. Driscoll JL, Martin HF. Detection of brominism by an automated chloride method. *Clin Chem.* 1966;12:314.
82. Murray T, Long W, Narins R. Multiple myeloma and the anion gap. *N Engl J Med.* 1975;292:574.
83. Coe FL. Metabolic alkalosis. *JAMA.* 1977;238:2288.
84. Elkinton JR. Clinical disorders of acid-base regulation. A survey of seventeen years' diagnostic experience. *Med Clin North Am.* 1966;50:1325.
85. Fulop M. Hypercapnia in metabolic alkalosis. *NY State J Med.* 1976;76:19.
86. Harrington JT, Cohen JJ. Measurement of urinary electrolytes—indications and limitations. *N Engl J Med.* 1975;293:1241.
87. Bear R, Goldstein M, Phillipson E, et al. Effect of metabolic alkalosis on respiratory function in patients with chronic obstructive lung disease. *Can Med Assoc J.* 1977;117:900.
88. Bieberdorf FA, Gorden P, Fordtran JS. Pathogenesis of congenital alkalosis with diarrhea: implications for the physiology of normal ileal electrolyte absorption and secretion. *J Clin Invest.* 1972;51:1958.
89. Schwartz WB, Relman AS. A critique of the parameters used in the evaluation of acid-base disorders: "whole-blood buffer base" and "standard bicarbonate" compared with blood pH and plasma bicarbonate concentration. *N Engl J Med.* 1963;268:1382.
90. Wagner CW, Nesbit RR Jr, Mansberger AR. The use of intravenous hydrochloric acid in the treatment of thirty-four patients with metabolic alkalosis. *Am Surg.* 1980;46:140.
91. Frick PG, Senning A. The treatment of severe metabolic alkalosis with intravenous N/10 or N/5 hydrochloric acid. *German Med Monthly.* 1964;9:242.
92. Williams DB, Lyons JH Jr. Treatment of severe metabolic alkalosis with intravenous infusion of hydrochloric acid. *Surg Gynecol Obstet.* 1980;150:315.
93. Pontoppidan H, Geffin B, Lowenstein E. Acute respiratory failure in the adult. *N Engl J Med.* 1972;287:743.
94. Goldring RM, Heinemann HO. Bicarbonate and the regulation of ventilation. *Am J Med.* 1974;57:361.
95. Martinez-Maldonado M, Sanchez-Montserrat R. Respiratory acidosis and alkalosis. *Clin Nephrol.* 1977;7:191.
96. MacDonald FM. Respiratory acidosis. *Arch Intern Med.* 1965;116:689.
97. Van Ypersele de Strihou C, Brasseur CL, DeConnick J. The "carbon dioxide response curve" for chronic hypercapnia in man. *N Engl J Med.* 1966;275:117.
98. Arbus GS, Herbert LA, Levesque PR, et al. Characterization and clinical application of the "significance band" for acute respiratory alkalosis. *N Engl J Med.* 1969;280:117.
99. Gennari FJ, Goldstein MB, Schwartz WB. The nature of the renal adaptation to chronic hypocapnia. *J Clin Invest.* 1972;51:1722.
100. Weinberger SE, Weiss ST, Cohen WR, et al. Pregnancy and the lung. *Am Rev Respir Dis.* 1980;121:559.
101. Sutton FD, Zwillich CW, Creagh E, et al. Progesterone for outpatient treatment of pickwickian syndrome. *Ann Intern Med.* 1975;83:476.
102. Morrison DA, Goldman AL. Oral progesterone therapy in COPD. *Am Rev Respir Dis.* 1978;119:154.
103. Lugliani R, Whipp BJ, Seard C, et al. Effect of bilateral carotid body resection on ventilatory control of rest and during exercise in man. *N Engl J Med.* 1977;285:1105.
104. Hirschman CA, McCullough RE, Weil JV. Normal values for hypoxic and hypercapnic ventilatory drives in man. *J Appl Physiol.* 1975;38:1095.
105. Flenley DC, Franklin DH, Miller JS. The hypoxic drive to breathing in chronic bronchitis and emphysema. *Clin Sci.* 1970;38:503.
106. Myers RAM, Linberg SE, Cowley RA. Carbon monoxide poisoning: the injury and its treatment. *Ann Emerg Med.* 1979;8:479.
107. Green ED, Zimmerman RC, Ghurabi WH, et al. Phenazopyridine hydrochloride toxicity: a cause of drug-induced methemoglobinemia. *Ann Emerg Med.* 1979;8:426.

22. Emergencies in Patients with Connective Tissue Disease

BARBARA MATTEUCCI, MD
RAPHAEL J. DeHORATIUS, MD

There are relatively few rheumatologic emergencies as frequent as acute monoarticular arthritis. These emergencies include various neurologic catastrophes in systemic lupus erythematosus, acute abdominal emergencies due to large vessel vasculitis, acute ocular events, as well as several areas of nonarticular rheumatism. Aside from these particular cases requiring emergency care, there are a number of rheumatologic problems that will undoubtedly present in the emergency department and that should be discussed for several reasons. First, certain symptoms and signs presenting in the setting of an established disease such as systemic lupus erythematosus demand immediate and specific attention, often beyond that given to a patient in good health. Second, connective tissue diseases manifest themselves in all organ systems. Rheumatologic disease should be at least a minor part of the differential diagnosis of a certain percentage of medical cases seen in the emergency department. In this chapter a review of systems will be followed to evaluate the emergencies of the connective tissue diseases that are seen in the emergency department.

FEVER

Significant fever, that is, greater than 38.3°C, especially in a previously healthy person is rarely dismissed without evaluation. The fact, however, that fever is the second most common symptom in systemic lupus erythematosus, occurring in between 80% and 97% of patients during the course of their flares, may lead the examiner away from an infectious cause. Lupus flares are exacerbations of the disease process that become clinically obvious and usually confirmed by laboratory tests. Other symptoms suggestive of infection such as arthritis, pneumonitis, or serositis often accompany flares. Infection in systemic lupus erythematosus remains the major cause of morbidity and mortality and should always be taken seriously. Patients with lupus represent an immunocompromised group, intrinsically from their disease, as well as due to concomitant drug therapy frequently consisting of corticosteroids and/or cytotoxic agents. They are susceptible to unusual organisms such as *Cryptococcus* species and *Pneumocystis carinii* as well as overwhelming bacterial infections. Because of corticosteroid therapy, certain hallmarks of infection may also be masked.

Studies performed to help differentiate flare from infection have yielded few gold standards for diagnosis.[1] These studies have shown that the only symptom found to be significantly present in infection of patients with lupus was chills while lupus flares were not associated with chills. Thus, in patients with systemic lupus erythematosus a history of shaking chills becomes an important differential point.

Historically, certain types of lupus patients are more susceptible to infection (ie, those with active nephritis or recently increased disease activity). In dealing with lupus patients presenting with fever, great care must be taken to rule out infection, reserving the diagnosis of lupus flare as one of exclusion.

CUTANEOUS LESIONS

Several skin lesions are noted to accompany specific types of infectious arthritis (Table 22-1). These include first the papulovesicular lesions of gonococcal arthritis, the distinctive erythema migrans of Lyme arthritis, and the erythema marginatum of rheumatic fever. This section lists other types of rashes that, while not constituting actual emergencies, may be seen by the emergency physician (see Chapter 27, Dermatologic Emergencies).

Systemic Lupus Erythematosus

At least 80% of patients with systemic lupus erythematosus have skin involvement at some point in their illness, and 20% present with some type of rash. The well-demarcated lesions of discoid lupus occur in up to 15% of patients with systemic lupus, but the majority of rashes are more transient and nonspecific. They call to mind a number of diagnoses such as viral exanthem, as well as drug or allergic reactions.

The classic discoid lesion is a well-demarcated annular erythematous plaquelike lesion, with scaling, central atrophy, and telangiectasia. They occur most frequently on the nose, cheeks, forehead, upper back, and chest.

The butterfly rash of lupus is an erythematous blush in the malar area and across the nose, often worsened by sun exposure. At least half of the patients with systemic lupus erythematosus will have this butterfly rash at some point, but many common skin conditions such as rosacea mimic it.

The more diffuse erythematous rashes that are less specific for lupus are generally maculopapular, more common above the waist, often exacerbated by the sun, and sometimes pruritic. Skin lesions may also be bullous, urticarial, or purpuric.

A more foreboding skin presentation of lupus is the spectrum of vasculitic disease. This spectrum includes livedo reticularis (a fine, lacy erythematous pattern of discoloration on the extremities and trunk); tender and often ulcerated lesions of the fingertips, palms, and forearms; and more severe punched-out ulcerations especially of the extremities. These latter lesions may extend deep into muscle and require grafting.

Panniculitis is a collection of subcutaneous tender or nontender nodules occurring more frequently on the extremities and buttocks. This form of skin lesion is fairly rare although it can be quite painful and disabling.

Dermatomyositis

Dermatomyositis is an inflammatory disease of proximal muscles that generally develops gradually over months to years, and so it would be an unusual emergency department case. However, there have been cases of acute myositis, and, in addition, the classic rash may develop prior to muscle involvement and necessitate an emergency department visit.[2] The typical rash is erythematous and patchy and involves the eyelids, cheeks, bridge of the nose, neck, upper chest and back, extensor surfaces of arms and legs, medial malleoli, and knuckles (Gottron's patches). It may be scaly or psoriaform. The eyelids may be edematous with a more lilac hue. The only emergency situation would be the rare case of acute dermatomyositis with severe acute weakness, concomitant rhabdomyolysis, and possible massive myoglobinuria with its associated renal involvement.

Erythema Nodosa

Erythema nodosa represents the common result of various disease processes.[3] It is thought to be a hypersensitivity reaction occurring in subcutaneous tissue to a variety of antigens, most commonly infectious. A rheumatologic process may be suggested erroneously, however, because of the arthralgias often accompanying erythema nodosum.

The clinical presentation is crops of tender, red, painful, at times edematous, warm nodules, predominantly on the anterior lower legs bilaterally. The lesions are small, generally measuring 0.5 to 2 cm. They develop over a day and may last 1 to 3 weeks. They do not ulcerate but eventually darken, may scale, and fade without atrophy. Lesions are present at all stages of development, and the entire process may continue over 1 to 3 months. They are not pruritic. The associated symptoms besides arthralgias may be fever, malaise,

---

Table 22-1 Cutaneous Lesions in Connective Tissue Disease

Specific
  Papulovesicular lesions
    Disseminated gonoccocal infection
  Erythema migrans
    Lyme disease
  Erythema marginatum rheumaticum
    Rheumatic fever
Nonspecific
  Butterfly rash
    Lupus erythematosus
    Erysipelas
    Rosacea
    Jessner's disease
    Granuloma faciale
  Livedo reticularis
    Lupus erythematosus
    Thrombotic thrombocytopenic purpura
    Rheumatoid arthritis
    Rheumatic fever
    Scleroderma
    Cryoglobulinemia
    Polyarteritis nodosa
  Panniculitis
    Erythema nodosum
    Cold-induced panniculitis
    Pancreatitis and pancreatic carcinoma
    Factitial
    Poststeroid panniculitis
    Lupus erythematosus (lupus profundus)
    Weber-Christian disease

and anorexia. The population affected has a 4:1 female to male predominance with peak occurrence in childhood and the third decade.

The most commonly associated illnesses are sarcoid, tuberculosis, and streptococcal infection, although lupus and Behçet's syndrome have also been associated with erythema nodosum. The triad of arthritis, erythema nodosum, and bilateral hilar adenopathy constitute Lofgren's syndrome. Chronic erythema nodosum is more common with sarcoid than the idiopathic variety of erythema nodosum. When associated with Behçet's syndrome the underlying disease is generally complicated by furunculosis, impetigo, and vesicular eruptions.

When a patient with erythema nodosum presents in the emergency department, important initial screening would be complete blood cell count with differential, throat culture, antistreptolysin O titer, chest roentgenogram, and purified protein derivative skin test. Treatment includes bed rest, aspirin or nonsteroidal anti-inflammatory drugs, and elevation of the lower extremities.

Vasculitis

Vasculitis may be a skin manifestation of systemic lupus erythematosus, at times corresponding to a more severe disease process and course. Vasculitic lesions characterized by inflammation and necrosis of various vessels occur in many diseases as well as being systemic diseases in and of themselves. Although the classification of the vasculitides has evolved and been revised again and again over the past 20 years, it still remains complex and overlapping.[4] While it is extremely important diagnostically and therapeutically to distinguish among the various types, the problem at hand in the emergency department is merely to recognize the presence of vasculitis and initiate a work-up.

In the absence of distinguishing systemic symptoms, the vasculitides are all similar in their cutaneous presentations. These include livedo reticularis, purpura, nodules, ulcers, bullae, vesicles, urticaria, and petechiae.[5] Lesions most commonly occur in the lower extremities and dependent areas, especially in the ankles and feet.

With specific entities a specific pattern may be seen. Classic polyarteritis nodosa commonly involves the skin. When it does, lesions consist of subcutaneous nodules and livedo reticularis. Hypersensitivity vasculitis (a primarily small vessel vasculitis type that is acute and has a recognizable precipitating event or exposure) presents predominantly in the skin. The typical lesion is palpable purpura (leukocytoclastic vasculitis), occurring 1 to 10 days after antigenic exposure. All lesions are at the same stage of development.

Wegener's granulomatosis involves the skin in 40% of cases, with purpura and ulcerative lesions being seen. Vasculitis may be a part of many systemic diseases such as serum sickness, systemic lupus erythematosus, rheumatoid arthritis, or malignancies. Additional symptoms should suggest the proper diagnosis, however.

When a patient presents in the emergency department with skin lesions in this descriptive category, especially if involving primarily dependent areas, a thorough history and physical examination must be done to rule out a systemic disease. Routine blood work in the emergency department should be done but most likely will not define the diagnosis. Unless a clear-cut precipitating event or exposure can be elicited, only subsequent follow-up and probably biopsy will yield the answer.

In the case of possible vasculitic lesions, the best therapy is the avoidance of topical preparations or any other specific therapy until the proper diagnosis is made, if necessary by biopsy. Symptomatic relief is best accomplished with aspirin (if no allergy is present) and with antihistamines if pruritus is significant.

OCULAR EMERGENCIES

Ocular manifestations of rheumatologic diseases are fairly common in the group of diseases known as the spondyloarthropathies (eg, Reiter's, reactive arthritis, and ankylosing spondylitis). The ocular findings are generally part of the diagnostic criteria of the disease and so are important to recognize. In terms of emergencies per se, the major diseases to diagnose and treat are temporal arteritis and the neurovascular lesions of systemic lupus erythematosus. These may result in blindness if unrecognized and untreated (see Chapter 81, Ocular Emergencies).

Temporal Arteritis

Temporal arteritis is a granulomatous inflammation of large arteries of unknown etiology.[7,8] The inflammation proceeds insidiously, gradually to occlude arteries by obliterative arteritis. The disease generally remits spontaneously in 2 to 5 years. However, its most serious complication, blindness, occurs in 30% to 50% of patients. A typical patient is older than 50 years of age, and the disease occurs predominantly in women. Headache occurs in 36% to 100% of patients. It is a continuous, boring type of headache with episodic lancinating pain. At times, it radiates to the neck and face and worsens with hair combing and pressure against the temporal arteries. Jaw claudication is present in 4% to 6% of patients. The claudication is described as fatigue of the jaw with talking or chewing, which is relieved with rest. Tender temporal arteries occur frequently. Visual symptoms include transient diplopia, visual field losses, oculomotor ophthalmoplegia, ptosis, and, most seriously, sudden blindness. Most patients with blindness will have had premonitory transient visual symptoms over a period on the average of 3.5 months. Nonspecific systemic symptoms such as malaise, weight loss, fever, and anorexia may be the major presentation. The association of polymyalgia rheumatica and temporal arteritis is between 20% and 40%, so patients may have the typical polymyalgia rheumatic symptom complex of stiffness and achiness in the shoulders and pelvic girdle.

Temporal arteritis may also be occult, presenting as sudden ischemic blindness in one eye with no prodrome. It is extremely important to consider a diagnosis of temporal arteritis, look for the physical findings, and obtain appropriate studies. Involvement of the opposite eye may follow quickly, commonly within 2 weeks. Therefore, rapid diagnosis and treatment are important.

Physical findings classically are tender, nodular temporal arteries with erythematous overlying skin. These classic findings occur infrequently, however, and one may simply note a change in the pulse pressure in the temporal artery on the involved side. There may be ptosis or ocular muscle weakness. The fundoscopic examination, even in acute blindness, is usually normal.

Laboratory values of importance are an elevated erythrocyte sedimentation rate (often greater than 80 mm/hour), anemia, an elevation on the serum protein electrophoresis of α_2- and β-globulins, and mild hepatic dysfunction.

Temporal arteritis should be considered in every patient older than 50 years of age who presents with severe unexplained headache in the temporal artery area; in every patient older than 50 years of age with unexplained visual symptoms, especially with a normal fundic examination; and in the patient with sudden blindness.

Treatment depends on the presentation. If history, physical examination, and laboratory findings point one toward the diagnosis of temporal arteritis, the patient should be treated with high doses of corticosteroids (60 to 80 mg/day) given in divided doses. If a temporal artery biopsy is to be done, the use of corticosteroids for 24 to 48 hours prior to the biopsy will not affect the subsequent specimen.

Systemic Lupus Erythematosus

Ocular manifestations of systemic lupus erythematosus include both inflammatory lesions of the globe itself and lesions in the central nervous system. Retinal disease is present in 9% to 24% of patients, most commonly with cotton wool exudates called cytoid bodies and hemorrhages. Cytoid bodies are exudates near the optic disc identical to diabetic exudates and resulting from ischemia of the retina and microinfarcts. The optic disc may demonstrate mild papilledema, especially with central nervous system disease.

Sudden blindness may occur in systemic lupus erythematosus either secondary to central retinal artery occlusion, ischemic optic neuritis, ocular migraine, or cerebral disease posterior to the optic chiasm.[9] The latter may present as visual field defects, scotomas, unformed or formed hallucinations in the absence of psychosis, or cortical blindness. In a patient with known systemic lupus erythematosus presenting with acute visual deterioration, admission is imperative. If the cause appears to be lupus cerebritis, high doses of corticosteroids would be necessary.

The diagnosis of lupus should be strongly considered in young women presenting with such ocular complaints and a full evaluation instituted.

Rheumatoid Arthritis

Ocular involvement is fairly common in rheumatoid arthritis, with an incidence of scleritis and episcleritis that is greater than in the general population.[10] The danger of ocular pathology in rheumatoid arthritis lies not in blindness per se but in the complications of severe scleritis such as uveitis, cataracts, glaucoma, or globe perforation. Episcleritis is a benign, self-limited inflammation of the subconjunctival vessels. The patient may complain of discomfort but not of severe ocular pain as in scleritis. The inflammation is bright red or salmon pink and commonly involves the temporal and nasal palpebral fissure areas. Treatment is either observation or the topical use of corticosteroid creams.

Scleritis is a much more serious condition since it may result in blindness if not treated properly. The patient complains of severe ocular pain, and the inflammation is of a more purplish hue. The area of the eye most commonly involved is the superior sclera. The scleritis may be of a nodular variety, and thinning of the sclera may be evident by the bluish color imparted by the underlying uveal vessels. Minor trauma may result in uveal prolapse. The topical use of corticosteroids is the initial therapy, but urgent ophthalmologic follow-up is necessary to ensure adequacy of treatment. Subconjunctival steroid injections are contraindicated in rheumatoid arthritis scleritis due to scleral thinning.

Sjögren's Disease

The symptom-complex of Sjögren's disease includes dry mouth plus ocular complaints of burning, photophobia, and a foreign body sensation. Rose bengal staining of the cornea and conjunctiva will be irregular and will lend support to the diagnosis. Definitive diagnosis is made by biopsy of the minor salivary glands in the lip. Therapy is symptomatic with the use of artificial tears.

Seronegative Spondyloarthropathies

Rheumatologic diseases such as Reiter's syndrome, inflammatory bowel disease with arthritis, reactive arthritis, and ankylosing spondylitis will involve the eye as anterior uveitis in up to one third of cases. Iritis may precede the musculoskeletal complaints by months. The features of anterior uveitis are redness, ocular pain, and photophobia. A slit-lamp examination is necessary to view the anterior chamber of the eye for precipitates and cells. The complications of untreated uveitis are anterior and posterior synechiae, glaucoma, and cataracts. Treatment includes the use of topical corticosteroids, cycloplegics, and mild diuretics.

Behçet's Syndrome

Behçet's syndrome is an inflammatory condition of probable immune origin characterized by recurrent oral and genital ulcers plus uveitis. Treatment of the ocular involvement is local corticosteroids.

In terms of incidence of immunologic disorders with anterior uveitis, a study of 896 patients with a presentation of uveitis yielded the following results: in males, 45% were of unknown origin, 28% were secondary to Reiter's syndrome, and 18% were secondary to ankylosing spondylitis. In females, 82% were of unknown origin, 6% were secondary to ankylosing spondylitis, and 4% were secondary to sarcoid.

Finally, iatrogenic ocular problems in rheumatologic disorders need to be kept in mind. The most important drug-related problem for the emergency physician is antimalarial retinopathy. Hydroxychloroquine and chloroquine are antimalarial drugs used in rheumatoid arthritis and systemic lupus erythematosus. They preferentially localize to inner retinal layers, and the degree of injury is dose related. Although patients are required to see an ophthalmologist every 6 months, they do not always do so. Complaints indicative of retinal disease are decreased visual acuity and night blindness. The fundoscopic examination will be normal at this time, and abnormalities will be found on visual field examination using a 1-mm red object or alternatively by fluorescein angiography of the retina.

PULMONARY MANIFESTATIONS

The lung is frequently involved in a connective tissue disease, although the patient may not have specific pulmonary symptoms.[11] Often the routine chest roentgenogram may reveal an otherwise hidden systemic manifestation of the disease. The most common roentgenographic findings in connective tissue diseases are chronic diffuse pneumonitis, pleural effusions and scarring, and nodules. Patients presenting to the emergency department with such pulmonary involvement will be in one of three categories: (1) abnormal routine chest roentgenogram in a patient without known connective tissue disease, (2) abnormal chest roentgenogram in a patient with known connective tissue disease without pulmonary complaints, and (3) acutely symptomatic patient with or without a known connective tissue disease. Obviously, the first two categories necessitate an awareness of the typical pulmonary signs of the diseases to aid in differential diagnosis. The last category of patients requires emergent treatment depending on their particular disease and presentation.

Rheumatoid Arthritis

Pulmonary involvement is very common in rheumatoid arthritis and usually asymptomatic.[12] Involvement takes four different forms: (1) nodules, (2) diffuse interstitial fibrosis, (3) pleural disease, and (4) Caplan's syndrome (a combination of rheumatoid nodules with the interstitial fibrosis found with silicosis).

Half of patients with rheumatoid arthritis will have pleural disease at autopsy. Radiographic findings are effusions (one third are asymptomatic) that may be unilateral or bilateral with pleural thickening. Estimated frequencies are about 8% for men and 1.6% for women. Patients may have pleuritic pain, cough, and dyspnea. Despite a high probability that the effusion is secondary to rheumatoid arthritis, all effusions in rheumatoid arthritis patients should be aspirated at least initially to rule out empyema. Fluids will be exudates with a very low glucose level and high protein and lactic dehydrogenase levels. They should also be Gram stained and cultured.

Diffuse interstitial fibrosis begins as a fine reticulonodular pattern occurring predominantly at the bases. It may progress to a honeycombed appearance with cyst formation. The roentgenographic picture is indistinguishable from idiopathic pulmonary fibrosis. The occurrence of this type of lung involvement is reported to be 1.6% to 40% of patients, and one half are believed to be asymptomatic. Symptoms will be the expected dyspnea on exertion and progressive shortness of breath, with a greater risk of pneumonia and bronchitis. Patients may also have hemoptysis and fever secondary to their lung disease.

In rheumatoid arthritis, as in any of the other connective tissue diseases, it is important to rule out other causes of pulmonary symptoms before attributing them all to the underlying disease. These causes include pulmonary embolism, infection, and bronchogenic carcinoma. Important to keep in mind in evaluating pulmonary changes in patients with rheumatoid arthritis is the fibrosis secondary to drugs used in the treatment of rheumatoid arthritis such as methotrexate.

Cricoarytenoid synovitis is common in rheumatoid arthritis. Infrequently, involvement of these joints may lead to acute airway obstruction with subsequent laryngeal stridor. Respiratory failure may ensue, necessitating a tracheostomy. In the subacute case, systemic corticosteroids may be helpful.

Systemic Lupus Erythematosus

Pulmonary involvement in systemic lupus erythematosus differs from rheumatoid arthritis in that it is generally symptomatic. Pleural involvement, pleuritis, and effusions occur in 50% to 75% of patients at some point and are generally painful and accompanied by fever. It may be a presenting symptom of systemic lupus erythematosus. Patients with drug-induced lupus frequently have pleuropulmonary disease as well as fever and arthralgias. It is important, however, to rule out infection, pulmonary embolism, and congestive heart failure as causes of pleural disease before attributing it to a lupus flare. Pleuritic disease in lupus generally responds well to nonsteroidal anti-inflammatory drugs used for general disease control.

Diffuse interstitial disease of the lung may be present in 3% to 10% of cases of lupus. Most patients have some degree of dyspnea on exertion. Patients may progress to dyspnea at rest and dry cough. The roentgenogram demonstrates reticulonodular infiltrates primarily in the lung bases. In studies of patients with lupus with this symptom-complex, Po_2 was found to be in the range of 53 to 80 mmHg. Pulmonary embolism might be suspected and ventilation-perfusion scans should be done, although they may be difficult to interpret.

Acute lupus pneumonitis is difficult to distinguish from infection. Patients have one or several poorly defined infiltrates on chest roentgenograms. They may be very sick with fever, tachypnea, and hypoxia. The crucial goal is to rule out infection or hemorrhage and later to start corticosteroids.

Acute massive pulmonary hemorrhage is an even more rare complication of lupus but should be kept in mind in the patient with lupus. The symptoms will be acute onset of cough, which is initially dry; dyspnea; high fever; blood-tinged sputum; and then frank hemorrhage. Death occurs in almost all cases. The cause of death is asphyxiation within 12 to 48 hours after admission. The roentgenogram will initially demonstrate diffuse, finely nodular, parahilar infiltrates. This presentation is a medical emergency, and prompt supportive and diagnostic studies are mandatory. Intravenous corticosteroids and perhaps plasmapheresis started promptly within 12 hours of hospitalization may be able to reverse the course.

Scleroderma

Scleroderma involves the lung more frequently than the previously mentioned diseases, with some investigators finding pulmonary disease in nearly all patients at autopsy. Interstitial pulmonary fibrosis is the most common type of lung disease, evolving through a reticulonodular pattern in the lower two thirds of the lung fields to honeycombing and cystic lesions. Spontaneous pneumothorax may occasionally occur and is an entity to consider in the patient with acute shortness of breath. Patients are also prone to aspiration pneumonia secondary to their esophageal dysfunction. The typical pulmonary symptom complex is dyspnea on exertion, cough, and pleuritic chest pain. A search for other etiologies as in rheumatoid arthritis and systemic lupus erythematosus is important in scleroderma before attributing change in symptoms simply to the underlying disease.

Vasculitis

The various vasculitides such as Wegener's granulomatosis may present with patchy, nonspecific pneumonitis similar to infectious and inflammatory disorders. These infiltrates may spontaneously regress. Periarteritis nodosa rarely has pulmonary involvement. Patients with Wegener's granulomatosis, on the other hand, may present with an abnormal chest roentgenogram or may have an explosive onset of fever, chills, arthralgias, cough, and dyspnea.[13] The roentgenograms may show discrete nodules or widespread pneumonitis. The important point to keep in mind is that these diseases are in the differential diagnosis of diffuse infiltrative lung findings. The acute management depends on the clinical status of the patient.

Relapsing Polychondritis

Finally, a rare disease of collagen, relapsing polychondritis, may have important respiratory involvement. This disease is an inflammation of cartilaginous structures. The most common presentation is of bilateral auricular chondritis; in addition, there may be nasal chondritis, ocular inflammation, audiovestibular damage, and respiratory tract chondritis. This latter involvement of the tracheal cartilage may lead to an emergency department presentation for acute airway obstruction.

In general, the lung has a limited number of responses to inflammation. The resultant roentgenographic picture in all these diseases, therefore, is similar. When a patient presents asymptomatically or with mild symptoms with or without a diagnosis of connective tissue disease, the evaluation should include roentgenograms (it is hoped there will be a previous comparison film), complete blood cell count, erythrocyte sedimentation rate, pulmonary function tests, blood chemistries to evaluate for calcium and liver function, skin tests for tuberculosis, and examination of any pleural fluid.

CARDIAC DISEASE

In the emergency department setting a solely cardiac presentation of a rheumatic disease would be unusual. The most common situation would be in systemic lupus erythematosus.

Systemic Lupus Erythematosus

Pericardial involvement in this disease is more commonly symptomatic than in the other rheumatic diseases. Pericarditis occurs in between 25% and 75% of lupus patients as a symptomatic illness and is present in up to 80% of autopsy specimens. Patients more frequently have a rub than have demonstrable fluid on echocardiogram. Pericardial tamponade is a rare complication. Although a patient with systemic lupus erythematosus may present initially as a patient with chest pain, it would be unusual not to have other symptoms and a history to suggest a generalized disease. Treatment of pericarditis is usually with nonsteroidal anti-inflammatory drugs.

Patients with systemic lupus erythematosus may have myocarditis. Coronary disease has been found in a younger population with lupus than in the general population. The etiology of this atherosclerotic coronary artery disease is debatable.[14] Whether corticosteroids promote early coronary disease or the initial arteritis itself is responsible is unclear. The important point is to realize that patients with systemic lupus erythematosus are at greater risk of developing coronary artery disease at a young age, and chest pain should always be thoroughly evaluated. One must also keep in mind the other risk factors that may complicate the lupus cardiac picture, such as renal disease, secondary hypertension, and anemia. Malignant hypertension may occur in up to 22% of lupus patients. Fluid retention, congestive heart failure, and pulmonary edema may result from a precipitous worsening of the patient's renal status. Obviously, these complications are dealt with in the usual manner regardless of the etiology while the evaluation is in progress.

VASCULAR DISEASE

In this section vascular events that may present in the emergency department with or without known connective tissue disease are discussed. The most significant and impressive vascular problem is Raynaud's phenomenon. Other topics to be briefly mentioned are complications secondary to vasculitis in diseases such as rheumatoid arthritis or thrombosis in systemic lupus erythematosus.

Raynaud's phenomenon is a vascular abnormality that may occur as an isolated disorder or in association with connective tissue disease, secondary to hematologic problems, or secondary to environmental problems.[15] It is most frequently found in association with the two connective tissue disorders of scleroderma and systemic lupus erythematosus. The exact cause of vascular spasm is still controversial; the debate involves the vascular versus the neurogenic mechanisms. The clinical picture of Raynaud's phenomenon is a spectrum of color changes in the distal extremities precipitated by such things as cold and anxiety, especially in the hands, toes, nose, and ears. The color changes are associated with paresthesias and pain. The initial vessel spasm causes pallor, then cyanosis of tissue due to stagnant blood in the area, followed by erythema due to reactive vasodilatation.

Patients may present in the emergency department with a complaint of recurrent episodes of this phenomenon, although they would be more likely to consult a general physician or clinic for evaluation. If this presentation should occur, a full work-up would include the following: erythrocyte sedimentation rate, complete blood cell count, rheumatoid factor, antinuclear antibodies, cold agglutinins, cryoglobulins, serum protein electrophoresis, and a chest roentgenogram to rule out thoracic outlet obstruction. A thorough history for associated symptoms of other connective tissue diseases, precipitating events, and drug history (eg, ergot compounds) should be obtained.

The acute presentation of Raynaud's phenomenon with nonremitting cyanosis of a digit over minutes to hours requires immediate attention and probable admission. Such a presentation may be an initial manifestation of the disease or may be occurring within a setting of connective tissue disease. The usual procedure would be a consultation with a vascular surgeon and an immediate arteriogram to determine the etiology of the occlusion.

Treatment of Raynaud's phenomenon other than treatment of the underlying disease depends on the severity or frequency of symptoms. In the acute setting of unremitting occlusion, therapy may include infusion of vasodilating agents, stellate ganglion blockade, or sympathectomy. In the more chronic case simple measures such as avoidance of cold and wearing warm gloves may significantly reduce the attacks. Many medications have been tried, such as reserpine, guanethidine, and, more recently, calcium channel blockers.

Vasculitic lesions were described under skin manifestations of connective tissue disease. As noted, vasculitis may be a significant component of systemic lupus erythematosus and rheumatoid arthritis as well as the primary disorder of periarteritis and allergic angiitis. Vasculitic involvement in these disorders is important to recognize since one may confuse other disease entities with this clinical presentation. For example, small vessel vasculitis can cause focal skin infarctions similar to subacute bacterial endocarditis lesions (ie, splinter hemorrhages, paronychial infarction). Visceral vasculitis may result in major organ pathology such as cerebral infarction, bowel infarction, mononeuritis multiplex, and coronary arteritis.

Finally, there is an increased incidence of thrombophlebitis, both deep and superficial, in patients with systemic lupus erythematosus.[16] Patients may have one of several antibodies to phospholipids, including the lupus anticoagulant responsible for the falsely prolonged partial thromboplastin time (PTT), the antibody to cardiolipin, and the antibody responsible for the false-positive RPR. Despite a prolonged PTT, these patients are actually in a hypercoagulable state.

Behçet's syndrome, an autoimmune disease characterized by the triad of oral ulcers, genital ulcerations, and uveitis, is associated with frequent and recurrent attacks of thrombophlebitis. Treatment for the phlebitis is similar to that for other causes, although it may be more recalcitrant. With a multitude of unusual manifestations of connective tissue disease, it is still important to recognize that common things occur commonly, even to those with connective tissue disease.

GASTROINTESTINAL MANIFESTATIONS

Gastrointestinal manifestations of connective tissue disease will generally not necessitate emergency department presentations but are fairly common.

Scleroderma is the connective tissue disease most commonly associated with esophageal dysfunction, with 90% of patients having some involvement. A decrease in the propulsive force of the lower two thirds of the esophagus represents the major dysfunction, with subsequent complications of peptic esophagitis and strictures. This esophageal dysfunction may be the source of typical or atypical chest pain in an emergency department presentation. A thorough history and examination in the patient with scleroderma should divulge the etiology. These patients may also have duodenal hypomotility with subsequent bacterial overgrowth and malabsorption.

Patients with rheumatoid arthritis who have more severe disease with vasculitis may also have mesenteric vasculitis. Although not as common as in systemic lupus erythematosus, an acute abdomen may ensue from bowel ischemia or perforation. The history of intermittent abdominal pain gradually becoming continuous with a tender, quiet abdomen on examination would suggest this diagnosis among the other causes of acute abdomen (see Chapter 28, Gastrointestinal Emergencies).

Polyarteritis nodosa may present as an acute catastrophic abdominal event, or abdominal symptoms may develop on the background of diffuse disease.[17] Acute mesenteric vasculitis in this disease evolves rapidly. Pain is sharp and intense, may be midepigastric and shifting or more vaguely located, and has usually been present for an average of approximately 11 days. Associated symptoms include fever, tachycardia, abdominal distention, tenderness, and rebound tenderness. The differential diagnosis is much the same as the patient without polyarteritis nodosa, including acute appendicitis, cholecystitis, intra-abdominal hemorrhage, perforation of the stomach or intestine, and ulceration. The diagnosis of polyarteritis nodosa should be considered in any patient in the second to fourth decade presenting with these symptoms in association with signs of low-grade sepsis, and especially polyneuritis. Obviously, acute evaluation of the potential surgical abdomen should proceed as in the case of any other acute abdomen.

Systemic lupus erythematosus involvement in the gastrointestinal tract ranges from the minor esophageal dysfunction to major acute hemorrhagic events. In patients with lupus with even vague symptoms, the results of ischemic vasculitis of intra-abdominal vessels must be strongly considered in the differential diagnosis. Up to 25% of patients with systemic lupus erythematosus may have dilatation of the esophagus and impaired peristalsis. Dysphagia occurs in 5% to 10% of patients. More severe complications such as esophagitis may instigate an emergency department visit for severe retrosternal and epigastric burning. When cardiac causes of epigastric pain have been ruled out, a usual protocol for peptic esophagitis may be begun. Another possible cause of these symptoms in a patient on corticosteroids is esophageal candidiasis.

Catastrophic events such as perforation and hemorrhage are a very real possibility in systemic lupus erythematosus and of course result in high morbidity and mortality.[18] Stomach ulceration and gastritis may be secondary to arteritis or to corticosteroids, as well as nonsteroidal anti-inflammatory drugs. Patients on high-dose corticosteroids have been shown to develop ulcers within weeks of starting therapy. If the patient with typical ulcer pain is stable and not clearly bleeding (negative stool guaiac, stable hematocrit, and vital signs), an ulcer regimen may be started with instructions for early follow-up. The crucial point to be stressed is close follow-up until the etiology is determined as clinical deterioration may occur rapidly (ie, perforation, hemorrhage).

Fulminant, acute pancreatitis occurs not uncommonly in patients with lupus.[19] A more indolent pancreatitis with right upper quadrant pain, anorexia, and increased amylase occurs much more commonly in the outpatient setting. Pancreatitis may be due to a lupus vasculitis or secondary to corticosteroids or azathioprine. The patient with acute pancreatitis presents in a typical manner, with severe abdominal pain, vomiting, fever, and adynamic ileus. When the pancreatitis is secondary to lupus involvement of pancreatic vessels it invariably occurs in the setting of active systemic disease and vasculitis. Pancreatitis of this etiology should respond to an increase in corticosteroids with resolution taking 2 to 3 weeks. The mortality rate is moderate in systemic lupus erythematosus pancreatitis, and the recurrence rate is 25%.

Mesenteric vasculitis represents the most serious abdominal involvement of systemic lupus erythematosus. There is a high mortality rate, especially if treatment is delayed. It has been found at autopsy that up to 50% of patients with lupus have peritoneal involvement. Five percent to 10% of patients have clinical ascites with painful serositis. Patients who develop intestinal complications secondary to small vessel vasculitis generally have active disease elsewhere with peripheral vasculitis, neurologic involvement, and thrombocytopenia. The abdominal pain develops insidiously, usually over 1 month. It typically is dull and cramping and located in the lower quadrants and periumbilically. Patients have anorexia, nausea and vomiting, fever, tachycardia, and abdominal tenderness. More than 75% have abdominal distention, but the classic acute abdominal findings of guarding, rigidity, and absent bowel sounds may be present in only one half of the patients. The acute event of perforation or hemorrhage thus may be atypical in presentation. The differential diagnosis depends on the location of pain to upper (pancreas, ulcer) or lower (intestinal perforation or appendicitis) quadrants. A crucial diagnostic test is paracentesis, and this should be done as part of the evaluation. The presence of bacteria on Gram stain suggests a perforation, while a sterile aspiration suggests serositis, arteritis, or pancreatitis. The highest morbidity and mortality occurred in patients with perforation (as suggested by the finding of bacteria) in whom surgical exploration was delayed. Surgery in systemic lupus erythematosus, especially in the face of active disease, carries a great deal of risk and should not be entered lightly. However, the presence of bacteria is an indication for exploration. If the fluid is initially clear, the situation remains critical but the patient may be admitted, hydrated, cultured, and observed with a greater degree of confidence.

Finally, in discussing the gastrointestinal system in connective tissue disease one should at least mention the complications of drugs used in these diseases. Salicylates and all the nonsteroidal anti-inflammatory drugs as well as corticosteroids and immunosuppressive agents may have adverse effects on the gastrointestinal tract. A careful drug history should always be elicited. With ibuprofen now an over-the-counter drug, specific attention should be paid to its overuse.

NEUROLOGIC MANIFESTATIONS

Although many of the connective tissue diseases may have neurologic involvement, systemic lupus erythematosus is by far the most common and the most serious.[20] Neurologic emergencies in systemic lupus erythematosus represent the other major category of emergencies in rheumatology other than an acute monoarticular arthritis. Before discussing the extensive involvement in systemic lupus erythematosus, the limited neurologic findings in several other diseases will be reviewed.

The cervical spine is a common location for the destructive changes of rheumatoid arthritis, and this involvement may lead to serious neurologic problems. There is destruction of the odontoid process, the lateral atlantoaxial joint, and other intravertebral joints. The rheumatoid pannus infiltrates the ligaments, leading to a laxity of these joints and allowing subluxation. Subluxation can occur at the C1–2 joint or the subaxial areas. The latter area is actually more commonly symptomatic since the spinal canal is more narrow at this point. Erosion of the odontoid allows the skull to sink onto the spine, a process called basal invagination.

Patients with rheumatoid arthritis and cervical spine disease may present in the emergency department with either pain or neurologic symptoms due to this arthritic involvement. The pain would be associated with morning stiffness when acute inflammation is still active. The pain typically is in the occipital area and may spread over the occiput to the temporal and frontal areas and behind the eyes. The pain does not generally correlate with the degree of cervical instability. When a rheumatoid patient presents with this type of pain, cervical spine disease is an important etiology to consider along with other diagnoses such as subarachnoid hemorrhage and trauma. Cervical spine films will help in the diagnosis by demonstrating the rheumatoid arthritis destruction. Patients with pain or symptoms secondary to cervical spine disease will have changes on roentgenography. To assess the degree of subluxation one needs to perform flexion and extension lateral views of the cervical spine. One then measures the space between the front of the odontoid and the inner surface of the anterior arch of the atlas. This space should not exceed 3 mm. The other vertebral bodies are considered subluxed if their posterior surfaces are malaligned by greater than 2 mm. Vertical shift of the odontoid is identified by finding the odontoid tip greater than 4.5 mm above MacGregor's line. This line is drawn from the upper surface of the hard palate to the most caudal point of the occipital curve. Patients who actually have nerve impingement due to these bony changes may be difficult to assess due to severe arthritis in the peripheral joints. Symptoms will vary from paresthesias and numbness usually more distally to acute spastic paraplegia or quadriplegia. Patients may have flexor spasms and long tract signs.

Therapy may be as simple as a cervical collar or as extreme as cervical fusion surgery. The important step is to recognize the problem prior to an unpredictable catastrophic complication. The instability must be assessed prior to intubation to avoid a major neurologic complication.

The various vasculitides may have neurologic associations, most commonly polyarteritis nodosa.[21] Vasculitis should be included in the differential diagnosis of any neurologic event (stroke, encephalopathy, peripheral neuropathy) especially in the younger population without a precipitating etiology (hypertension, diabetes).

The acute presentation of polyarteritis nodosa may be as a diffuse encephalopathy affecting cognitive function. Seizures may be a part of the picture. Patients may have focal lesions as well, such as stroke or spinal cord lesions. Central nervous system disease occurs in 20% to 40% of patients with polyarteritis. The evaluation includes complete blood cell count with differential and urinalysis, with findings usually of an increased erythrocyte sedimentation rate, mild anemia, thrombocytosis, and urinary changes. The diagnosis of vasculitis obviously will not be made in the emergency department, and generally these patients will need admission and full neurologic evaluation.

Meningoencephalitis is one of the components of Behçet's syndrome, with other central nervous system lesions of cerebellar ataxia, corticospinal tract disease, and seizures occurring in 25% of patients. Again, admission and full work-up will delineate the etiology, but consideration of these diseases early will aid in the speed and accuracy of that evaluation.

Central nervous system involvement in patients with systemic lupus erythematosus is believed by some to be present in all patients with lupus. Some may manifest only mild changes in memory while others may present with seizures. Studies cite from 14% to 75% as the frequency of clinically evident central nervous system involvement. The following discussion deals with presentation of lupus neuropsychiatric involvement.

Disturbance of mental function such as psychosis and coma may occur in 35% to 60% of patients with systemic lupus erythematosus. Psychosis may masquerade as a clearly defined process such as acute mania. Coma due to lupus cerebritis is obviously a presentation with a poor prognosis and requires rapid assessment and institution of therapy.[22] In both these cases other possible treatable causes of mental dysfunction must be ruled out prior to attributing the process to lupus per se. These causes include abnormalities of glucose or electrolytes, metabolic derangements, sepsis, uremia, hypertensive encephalopathy, and addisonian crisis in patients on corticosteroids. The immediate evaluation of coma or obtundation is blood work to evaluate these causes, blood cultures, lumbar puncture to rule out infection, and computerized tomography to rule out hemorrhage, mass lesion, or stroke. The evaluation should begin in the emergency department to facilitate early treatment of lupus cerebritis with corticosteroids if all proves negative.

Patients with a psychotic presentation should be evaluated for the above nonsystemic causes of lupus erythematosus. Sedation with haloperidol (Haldol) or other antipsychotics is acceptable as the evaluation proceeds. Clues to the lupus etiology would be other systemic involvement by systemic lupus erythematosus. One should also consider the role of corticosteroids and change in dosage of these agents as causing a psychosis. Although psychosis may be an acute and severe presentation, it rarely causes any residual changes.

Convulsions may occur in 15% to 35% of patients with systemic lupus erythematosus and may be the initial presentation. Anticonvulsants such as phenytoin (Dilantin) may be used to control the seizure while the routine work-up proceeds. An important study done within the first few hours of presentation should be a lumbar puncture. It is essential to rule out infection as an etiology, especially opportunistic infections such as cryptococcosis, aspergillosis, toxoplasmosis, and that due to cytomegalovirus.

Meningitis occurs less commonly but again constitutes an emergency because of possible opportunistic infections. Even in the face of diffuse symptoms of a flare, a diagnosis of aseptic meningitis secondary to lupus is one of exclusion. Aseptic meningitis may also be due to nonsteroidal anti-inflammatory drugs, with cases reported secondary to ibuprofen, indomethacin, naproxen, and sulindac.[23-25] This is an important consideration especially with the new over-the-counter preparation of ibuprofen since patients may take this drug without the knowledge of the physician. Azathioprine may also cause aseptic meningitis. The classic history is that the patient ingested a tablet of the drug and began feeling ill 12 to 18 hours later. Features included chills, fever, headache, abdominal pain, nausea, shortness of breath, cervical adenopathy, and, most notably, nuchal rigidity and lethargy progressing to obtundation.

Cerebrospinal fluid should be examined for organisms, glucose level (which will be decreased), and cells, as well as sent for all cultures. In aseptic meningitis there is often a pleocytosis of lymphocytes, an elevated protein level, and an increased opening pressure. Generally, while results of cultures are pending, broad-spectrum antibiotic therapy will be begun until infection is ruled out. Again, the revelation of a drug ingestion may be extremely diagnostic.

Hemiplegia and transverse myelitis are even more uncommon, but the statistics on recovery versus paralysis underline the importance of awareness of this complication.[26] Patients may present initially with transverse myelitis, which may also occur in the setting of systemic lupus. Symptoms usually evolve over 1 to 2 days. Initial symptoms are vague (ie, numbness, then weakness in the legs in up to 50% of patients). Pain in the lower back, lower abdomen, and midscapular area may develop. Urinary retention and fecal incontinence may evolve as well. Paresthesias and a reduced sensory level will be found. The important point is that full recovery is possible if corticosteroids are begun within 24 hours. If treatment is delayed beyond that time, paraplegia or quadriplegia is almost inevitable. Patients with lupus may at times have bizarre neurologic symptoms as well as an abnormal affect. Because of this, an examiner may at times minimize the vague symptoms of early transverse myelitis. In these cases, an unbiased, complete neurologic evaluation may rescue the patient from paralysis.

SOFT TISSUE RHEUMATISM

Many patients will present in the emergency department with pains and possible neuromuscular symptoms in the extremities that will not actually involve the joint.[27] In some instances, the importance of proper diagnosis is to rule out significant medical problems, such as thrombophlebitis versus a Baker's cyst, a septic joint versus bursitis, and a cardiac etiology in the many chest wall syndromes. The second important reason for the proper recognition of these syndromes of soft tissue rheumatism is to be able to treat these sometimes incapacitating problems (Table 22-2).

Table 22-2 Soft Tissue Rheumatism

Upper extremity
   Bursitis (olecranon, subdeltoid)
   Tendinitis
   Epicondylitis
   Reflex sympathetic dystrophy syndrome
   Trigger points
Lower extremity
   Bursitis (trochanteric, anserine)
   Tendinitis
   Tarsal tunnel syndrome
   Baker's cyst
   Trigger points
Trunk
   Costochondritis
   Tietze's syndrome
   Rib tip syndrome
   Trigger points

Bursitis

Bursae are the sacs lined with synoviallike cells that serve to facilitate the motion between bones and muscles. There are hundreds of bursa in the body as discovered by anatomists centuries ago, lying between muscle, tendons and bone.[28] The more superficial bursae such as the olecranon and prepatellar bursae are believed to have developed after birth secondary to wear and tear to the area. The bursae become inflamed due to acute or chronic trauma (eg, housemaid's knee, miner's elbow), crystal disease, infection, or contiguous joint disease. The most commonly affected bursae are the subdeltoid and subacromial bursae, the olecranon, the greater trochanteric, the anserine bursa, and the prepatellar bursa. The anserine bursa is located on the medial aspect of the proximal tibia.

The most important distinction to make in evaluating a bursitis is whether infection is present.[29] Septic bursitis is not a medical emergency, but early treatment can shorten the disease course and also shorten the treatment. Most bursae become infected locally, for example, by penetration from skin lesions, rather than hematogenously. Patients with diabetes mellitus, a history of an injection, or an alcoholic history are more prone to septic bursitis. The bursae more commonly involved in infection are the prepatellar and olecranon bursa with a ratio of 1:4. It has been found that septic bursitis is more commonly associated with fever, tenderness over the bursa, peribursal cellulitis, and skin involvement over the bursa. Patients with septic bursitis have more intense symptoms and so seek medical attention sooner. A history of trauma is found in both septic and nonseptic bursitis as well as a history of previous bursal disease. Sympathetic effusions may be present in adjacent joints in both cases. The bursal fluid will yield the answer in most cases, being examined for cell count, crystals, Gram stain, and culture. Gram stains are reported to be positive in a majority of patients with an infection. Greater than 90% are due to *Staphylococcus* species. Septic bursae will have an inflammatory fluid, with less than 20,000 polymorphonuclear leukocytes and a lowered glucose level. Nonseptic fluid is usually less inflammatory. Bursal fluid in general will not demonstrate the high cell counts found in septic joints.

In gouty bursitis, the fluid may be yellow, chalky, or bloody.[30] Gouty episodes may be temporally related to trauma with subsequent shedding of monosodium urate crystals into the bursa.

Treatment in the face of infection is the use of the appropriate antibiotics for the organisms found on Gram staining. Antibiotics should be given for 10 days, especially if the infection has been present for more than 1 week. In the case of gout, the use of nonsteroidal anti-inflammatory drugs is recommended along with heat.

The trochanteric bursa of the proximal femur causes a great deal of pain but is amenable to local injections. The area of tenderness can be localized with the patient lying on his unaffected side. The most prominent bony structure of the proximal lateral thigh is the area of the bursa. The patient may be able to localize the spot more easily. The hip joint can be manipulated without pain, which will help to distinguish this condition from arthritis of the hip. Forced abduction of the thigh is painful in trochanteric bursitis. The area should be cleansed and injected with corticosteroids and lidocaine. Heat and mild nonsteroidal anti-inflammatory drugs can be prescribed and a gradual exercise program begun when the pain has diminished.

Up to 3% of the elderly population has calcific bursitis or calcium deposits in the bursa, especially the trochanteric bursa, patella, shoulder, and subacromial bursa. Patients with shoulder involvement by a bursitis have acute pain and limited range of motion. There is point tenderness to palpation and with passive movement. Involvement of the bursa must be distinguished from a bicipital tendinitis or a rotator cuff tear. Distinction from bicipital tendinitis can be found by forced supination of the forearm with the arm held at 90° of flexion. The examiner palpates the intertrochanteric area of the upper humerus or the bicipital groove. In a rotator cuff tear, the patient cannot actively abduct the arm between 45° and 90°.

Tendinitis

Tendinitis is the inflammation of the fibrous tendons that serve to pull and transmit muscle power. Tendinitis more commonly is secondary to chronic wear and tear than to acute trauma. It most often occurs in the shoulder, elbow, hands, and knees. The actual pathology may be rupture, strain of the tendon, stenosis of the sheath, or rupture of the tendon from the sheath.

Shoulder tendinitis is the most common type. The tendons involved are the supraspinatus or others of the rotator cuff. Secondary calcification is often seen on the roentgenogram, although definite trauma may rarely have preceded the inflammation. Usually the injury is secondary to chronic use and is of insidious onset. As noted previously, shoulder tendinitis should be distinguished from bicipital tendinitis. Treatment includes heat, nonsteroidal anti-inflammatory drugs, and maintenance of at least passive range of motion. Later, active range of motion should be performed to prevent adhesive capsulitis. Healing may take 6 months to 1 year.

Lateral epicondylitis (tennis elbow) is secondary to chronic trauma associated with occupation or other activities. Pain is worsened by palpation of the lateral epicondyle and by extending the wrist against resistance with the elbow at 90°. Treatment includes injecting the lateral epicondyle by a method of repeated pricking of the periosteal surface, rest (1 week would be a reasonable period of time), nonsteroidal anti-inflammatory drugs, and the use of an arm band to prevent excessive wrist extension. Patients may require repeated injections if the implicated activity continues, but these should not be done more often than every 3 to 6 months. Medial epicondylitis may also occur, with pain worsened by wrist flexion.

Tendinitis of the abductor pollicis longus and extensor pollicis brevus constitutes a syndrome known as DeQuervain's tenosynovitis. It is caused by chronic stress to the tendons secondary to activity (eg, piano playing). Finkelstein's test is the maneuver that stresses these tendons and should be painful in this syndrome. The patient places the thumb of the affected hand across that palm, curls the fingers over the thumb, and forces the hand into ulnar deviation. Treatment of the tendinitis is local corticosteroid and lidocaine injections, rest, and, if necessary, splinting.

One should consider gonococcus in a patient presenting with tenosynovitis, especially in the susceptible age group. The symptoms of urogenital infection will precede the tendinitis by about 1 week.

In rheumatoid arthritis, nodules may occur on the flexor tendons of the fingers causing locking of the fingers, known as trigger finger. The tendon is able to move through the sheath in flexion, but it may lock when one attempts to return to a neutral position. The point of locking usually occurs at the distal palmar crease where the fascia is tight. Injection of corticosteroids will often improve the situation.

Achilles tendinitis occurs commonly and is most often secondary to trauma, exercise without proper conditioning, or a general connective tissue disease. Heat and nonsteroidal anti-inflammatory drugs are the treatments of choice, with actual immobilization being necessary at times. Injections should not be given into the Achilles tendon since this can predispose to future rupture of the tendon.

Baker's Cyst

Baker's cyst is a swelling in the popliteal fossa caused by the posterior herniation of the synovial membrane through the posterior capsule of the knee joint. It can occur in rheumatoid arthritis, osteoarthritis, and gout, but it is also secondary to meniscal tears and structural joint disease as well as being found in normal individuals. The cyst may dissect into the calf with a subsequent presentation indistinguishable on examination from a thrombophlebitis.[31,32] The patient will have pain, swelling, and stiffness in the calf with engorgement of superficial veins. There will not be cords or specific venous tenderness. One clue to the diagnosis of a ruptured Baker's cyst is the crescent sign. This is a crescent-shaped ecchymotic area that forms beneath the medial malleolus due to pooling of the dissected serosanguineous fluid from the ruptured cyst. It is extremely rare.

Ultrasound will confirm the diagnosis in an asymptomatic Baker's cyst.[33] However, with the symptomatic patient it is important to eliminate thrombophlebitis as the cause of symptoms. This diagnosis would necessitate immediate admission and anticoagulation with heparin. The only definitive diagnostic study to rule out thrombophlebitis is a venogram, and this should be done immediately. An arthrogram is done to confirm a diagnosis in a patient who has a negative ultrasound but a high suspicion clinically of a ruptured Baker's cyst.

Other possible etiologies include a hematoma, ruptured plantaris muscle, acute muscle strain, and rupture of the head of the gastrocnemius muscle.

Treatment of popliteal cysts is local injection of corticosteroids and lidocaine into the knee joint, rest, and nonsteroidal anti-inflammatory drugs.

Shoulder Syndromes

Several soft tissue shoulder syndromes should be discussed because of their frequency and the need for appropriate treatment to prevent permanent disability. Rotator cuff tear and adhesive capsulitis constitute 90% of painful, immobile shoulders.

Rotator cuff tears most frequently involved rupture of the supraspinatus tendon. It is most commonly a partial tear. The patient may give a history of an acute injury with a sensation of a snap in the shoulder and subsequent pain with decreased range of motion. However, a rotator cuff tear may be more insidious in onset as well, indistinguishable from adhesive capsulitis. Abduction between 45° and 90° is painful, and the patient must be assisted with abduction from 90° to 120°.

Routine roentgenograms may show narrowing of the distance between the acromial tip and the head of the humerus, reversal of the acromial convexity, or cyst formation at the acromion process and greater tuberosity. Treatment is with heat, physical therapy, analgesia, and anti-inflammatory drugs. Corticosteroid injections may help in some cases.

Adhesive capsulitis or frozen shoulder is a chronically progressive immobilization of the shoulder with a resultant contracted joint capsule. The etiology is still a mystery. The entity is not specifically related to occupation, injury, or activity. It occurs most frequently in women, is most common in the 40- to 70-year age range, and is progressive over weeks to months. Investigators favor an autonomic dysfunction causing impaired circulation and subsequent fibrosis. Symptomatically, patients have reduced shoulder mobility more marked with internal rotation and abduction.

The differential diagnosis includes rotator cuff tear, hemarthrosis, and anterior capsule tear. Treatment is with intensive physical therapy, local injections, heat, and analgesics. The improvement is very slow, and the patient should be so cautioned. Surgical release may eventually be necessary.

Emergency department treatment of these somewhat chronic conditions should include examination and roentgenograms and possibly corticosteroid injections. The patient should be instructed on the use of heat and simple exercises for the shoulder and given an anti-inflammatory or analgesic drug.

Another etiology of shoulder immobility is the shoulder–hand syndrome, also known as Sudec's atrophy and reflex sympathetic dystrophy or causalgia.[34,35] The shoulder dysfunction is usually of secondary importance, with the patients mostly complaining of redness, swelling, pain, and immobility of the hand. This syndrome is believed to be caused by an overactive sympathetic nervous system, resulting in inappropriate vasomotor activity. It is seen in association with peptic ulcer disease, myocardial infarction, gallbladder disease, cerebral hemorrhage, rheumatoid arthritis, arthritis of the shoulder, and pulmonary neoplasms or may be idiopathic. The mechanism in these varied etiologies seems to be through afferent nerve stimulation.

The syndrome progresses through three stages, and patients may present in any stage. In the first stage, one finds increased blood flow to the hand with pain, swelling, synovitis at the small joints of the hand and wrist, hyperhidrosis, and erythema. The hand symptoms are made worse with excitement or movement and are improved with submersion in cold water or with rest. This phase lasts 3 to 6 months and is the optimum time for treatment to be effective. Treatment includes high doses of corticosteroids, heat, aggressive physical therapy, and, at times, stellate ganglion blockade.

The second stage involves a decrease in swelling but persistence of movement limitation. One finds scant hair distribution and the skin is cool. In the final stage, dystrophic skin changes have evolved, the skin is cool, and there are soft tissue contractures, limited joint motion, adhesive capsulitis, and possible Raynaud's phenomenon. The changes will most likely be irreversible at this point, but physical therapy may improve and maintain mobility.

In the emergency department evaluation it is important to consider the diagnosis in a case of a painful, swollen, erythematous hand with shoulder symptoms without involvement of the intervening elbow. Roentgenograms may show patchy osteoporosis, although early on, the technetium bone scan will be positive.

Paresthesias, pain, and swelling in the arm may be secondary to neurovascular compression producing outlet syndromes. These include cervical rib compression, scalenus anticus hypertrophy, and costoclavicular syndrome. Roentgenograms and vascular maneuvers such as Adson's maneuver will help to distinguish the etiology. Adson's maneuver is performed by locating the radial pulse of the affected side and having the patient extend his neck first forward and then to that side fully while the pulse is being felt. In a positive test, the pulse should diminish with this maneuver. The patient should extend the head in the opposite direction as well.

The carpal tunnel syndrome is the compression of the median nerve as it passes under the transverse carpal ligament of the palm.[36] The syndrome may be bilateral, with initial presentation in the dominant hand. Etiologies of this compression include local wrist derangements, such as a poorly healed fracture, tumor, or callus; excessive wrist flexion secondary to occupation; systemic disease such as diabetes mellitus, rheumatoid arthritis, multiple myeloma, polycythemia vera, myxedema, polymyalgia rheumatica, amyloidosis, acromegaly, and gout; and conditions with tissue edema such as pregnancy.

Initial symptoms are paresthesias and pain of the thumb and second and third digits, later with weakness of these fingers. Poorly localized pain may extend proximally to the elbow or shoulder. The pains are worse at night when involuntary flexion is maintained. Patients find relief by shaking the hands or hanging them over the bed. Activities using wrist motion such as driving, knitting, or carrying packages may worsen the symptoms.

On examination, patients have decreased sensation to pinprick over the median nerve distribution of the thumb and second and third digits. They may have weakness of adduction and opposition of the thumb and thenar wasting. The Tinel test (tapping the wrist at the flexor retinaculum) and Phalen's sign (holding the wrist in forced flexion or extension for 60 seconds) may cause tingling and pain in the median nerve distribution secondary to worsened compression.

Definitive diagnosis requires nerve conduction studies. One is obliged, as well, to determine the presence of any underlying disease such as those noted previously. Routine evaluation includes roentgenograms to rule out local pathology; evaluation of blood sugar level, complete blood cell count, erythrocyte sedimentation rate, and rheumatoid factor; protein electrophoresis; and uric acid and thyroid studies.

If the diagnosis is clear and roentgenograms are negative, an initial corticosteroid injection could be tried in the significantly symptomatic patient while the work-up is pending. One-half milliliter of soluble corticosteroids is injected very superficially at the distal wrist crease on the palmar wrist surface, just lateral to the flexor ulnaris tendon. If the patient experiences tingling of the hand, the needle should be withdrawn slightly. Lidocaine should not be used because of potential nerve infiltration.

Patients may use a wrist splint especially at night along with avoiding aggravating occupations or activities. If several local injections fail, surgery may be necessary.

The final soft tissue rheumatism entity to discuss is the group of conditions that constitutes the chest wall syndrome.[37] All age ranges are affected by these chest wall pains, but the older patients will command more attention and concern owing to potential cardiac etiologies. These syndromes have several common denominators, including the presence of trigger points, the ability of the examiner to reproduce the pain, and the lack of laboratory or roentgenographic abnormalities. A major task in the emergency department is to rule out other more serious causes of chest pain such as diseases of the heart, great vessels, mediastinum, head and neck, and abdomen.

Generally, the pain has been present for weeks to years and may remit spontaneously. The origins of the pain are the muscles, bones, and ligaments of the chest wall.

Costochondritis (costosternal syndrome, anterior chest wall syndrome, parasternal chondrodynia) is the inflammation of one or several costal cartilages. Patients may have dull pain with acute lancinating shocks of pain. They usually have had the pain chronically and relate no precipitating event. The pain may radiate and the patient may complain of tingling in the fingers usually due to hyperventilation from anxiety. The diagnosis is made by palpating the costochondral areas and reproducing the pain.

Tietze's syndrome is the specific involvement of a single costochondral junction (usually the second) or the sternoclavicular junction. It is distinguishable from costochondritis in that the area is swollen and possibly warm and tender. There may be a history of heavy work, coughing, or sudden movement as a precipitant. The pain may be sudden or gradual. It is worsened by bending and recumbency, exertion, lifting, fatigue, sneezing, coughing, and even inspiration. On examination, the patient has a fusiform, nonsuppurative, tender swelling in the area of inflammation. Without the swelling, there is no diagnosis. All laboratory studies and roentgenograms are normal. The major entities to rule out are tumor and infection.

Treatment for these two syndromes is heat, nonsteroidal anti-inflammatory drugs, avoidance of provoking activities, and local corticosteroid and lidocaine injections for severe or intractable pain.

Xiphoidalgia (xiphoid cartilage syndrome) is a similar inflammatory process involving the tip of the xiphoid process. The pain worsens with bending, twisting, lifting, and stooping and also following a large meal. It may radiate deeper within the chest, simulating gastrointestinal or cardiac disease, as well as traveling to the shoulder or back. The time course is the same as the syndromes above. Treatment, again, is with heat, aspirin or nonsteroidal anti-inflammatory drugs, and possibly injection.

Finally, the rib tip syndrome or slipping rib results from hypermobility of the anterior end of the costal cartilage, usually at the tenth rib. There will be pain with pressure, and a clicking sensation may be appreciated with palpation. Pain may be dull and continuous or sharp and stitchlike. Treatment is the same as for the other chest wall syndromes.

All these variations of chest wall syndromes have in common the reproducibility of their pain. Without that component, one should search for another cause. Herpes zoster may present merely with severe chest wall pain prior to the typical rash. Multiple myeloma to a rib is rarely the isolated presentation of this disease but should be a minor consideration in the undiagnosed case. Metastatic disease more commonly affects the posterior rib cage but should be considered. Carcinoma of breast, kidney, thyroid, lung, and prostate most commonly involve the ribs with metastatic disease. Minor trauma may cause rib fracture, and this history should be sought.

In general, the soft tissue rheumatic syndromes are fairly easy to diagnose if attention is paid to pain location, history of precipitating events, and anatomical and functional details of the examination. The major roles of the immediate emergency department evaluation in these cases are to rule out serious illness and to treat the patient symptomatically.

REFERENCES

1. Stohl NL, Klippel JH, Decker JL. Fever in systemic lupus erythematosus. *Am J Med.* 1979;67:935.
2. Bohan A, Peter JB. Polymyositis and dermatomyositis. *N Engl J Med.* 1975;292:344, 403.
3. Blomgren SE. Erythema nodosum. *Semin Arthritis Rheum.* 1974;4:1.
4. Fauci AS, Haynes BF, Katz P. The spectrum of vasculitis. *Ann Intern Med.* 1978;89:660.
5. Diaz-Perez JL, Winkelmann RK. Cutaneous periarteritis nodosa. *Arch Dermatol.* 1974;110:407.
6. Scott DGJ, Bacon PA, Tribe GR. Systemic rheumatoid vasculitis: a clinical and laboratory study of 50 cases. *Medicine.* 1981;60:288.
7. Goodman BW. Temporal arteritis. *Am J Med.* 1979;67:839.
8. Huston KA, Hunder GG, Lie JT, et al. Temporal arteritis, a 25 year epidemiologic, clinical, and pathologic study. *Ann Intern Med.* 1978;88:162.
9. Brandt KD, Lessell S, Cohen AS. Cerebral disorders of vision in systemic lupus erythematosus. *Ann Intern Med.* 1975;83:163.
10. Jayson MIV, Jones DEP. Scleritis and rheumatoid arthritis. *Ann Rheum Dis.* 1971;30:343.
11. Hunninghake GW, Fauci AS. Pulmonary involvement in the collagen vascular diseases. *Am Rev Respir Dis.* 1979;119:471.
12. Walker WC, Wright V. Pulmonary lesions and rheumatoid arthritis. *Medicine.* 1968;47:501.
13. Israel HL, Patchefsky AS. Wegener's granulomatosis of the lung: diagnosis and treatment. *Ann Intern Med.* 1971;74:881.
14. Bulkley BH, Roberts WC. The heart in systemic lupus erythematosus and the changes induced in it by corticosteroid therapy. *Am J Med.* 1975;58:243.
15. Blunt RJ, Porter JM. Raynaud syndrome. *Semin Arthritis Rheum.* 1981;10:282.
16. Mueh JR, Herbst KD, Rapaport SI. Thrombosis in patients with the lupus anticoagulant. *Ann Intern Med.* 1980;92:156.
17. Nightingale EJ. The gastroenterological aspects of periarteritis nodosa. *Am J Gastroenterol.* 1958;152:161.
18. Zizic TM, Shulman LE, Stevens MB. Colonic perforations in systemic lupus erythematosus. *Medicine.* 1973;54:411.
19. Reynolds JC, Immon RD, Kimberly RP, et al. Acute pancreatitis in systemic lupus erythematosus: report of twenty cases and a review of the literature. *Medicine.* 1982;61:25.
20. Bennahum DA, Messner RP. Recent observations on central nervous system lupus erythematosus. *Semin Arthritis Rheum.* 1975;4:253.
21. Moore PM, Cupps TR. Neurological complications of vasculitis. *Ann Neurol.* 1983;14:155.

22. Ellis SG, Verity MA. Central nervous system involvement in systemic lupus erythematosus: a review of neuropathologic findings in 57 cases, 1955–1977. *Semin Arthritis Rheum*. 1979;8:212.
23. Ballas ZK, Donta ST. Sulindac-induced aseptic meningitis. *Arch Intern Med*. 1982;142:165.
24. Ruppert GB, Barth WF. Tolmetin-induced aseptic meningitis. *JAMA*. 1981;245:67.
25. Widener HL, Littman BH. Ibuprofen-induced meningitis in systemic lupus erythematosus. *JAMA*. 1978;239:1062.
26. Andrianakos AA, Duffy JD, Suzuki M, et al. Transverse myelopathy in systemic lupus erythematosus. *Ann Intern Med*. 1975;83:616.
27. Wood PHN, Sturrock AW, Badley EM. Soft tissue rheumatism in the community. *Clin Rheum Dis*. 1979;5:743.
28. Bywaters EGL. Lesions of bursae, tendons and tendon sheaths. *Clin Rheum Dis*. 1979;5:883.
29. Ho G, Tice AD. Comparison of nonseptic and septic bursitis. *Arch Intern Med*. 1979;139:1269.
30. Canuso JJ, Yood RA. Acute gouty bursitis: report of 15 cases. *Ann Rheum Dis*. 1979;38:326.
31. Blumberg S, Kantrowitz FG. The pseudothrombophlebitis syndrome: a reappraisal. *Semin Arthritis Rheum*. 1981;10:278.
32. Katz RS, Zizic TM, Arnold P, Stevens MB. The pseudo-thrombophlebitis syndrome. *Medicine*. 1977;56:151.
33. Lukes PJ, Herberts P, Zochrisson BE. Ultrasound in the diagnosis of popliteal cysts. *Acta Radiol Diagn*. 1979;21:663.
34. Kozin F, Genant HF, Bekerman C, McCarty DJ. The reflex sympathetic dystrophy syndrome. *Am J Med*. 1976;60:332.
35. Kozin F, Ryan LM, Carerra GF, Soin JS. The reflex sympathetic dystrophy syndrome. *Am J Med*. 1981;70:23.
36. Reddy MP. Peripheral nerve entrapment syndromes. *AFP*. 1983;xx:133.
37. Epstein SE, Gerber LH, Borer JS. Chest wall syndrome. *JAMA*. 1979;241:2793.

23. Acute Monoarticular Arthritis

RAPHAEL J. DeHORATIUS, MD
BARBARA MATTEUCCI, MD

The diagnosis and treatment of monoarticular arthritis represent a true medical emergency. Prompt evaluation and treatment of such a joint may mean the difference between normal function and a compromised joint if the cause is infection. The differential diagnosis of such a presentation is quite extensive, and a number of these etiologies will be discussed. The four major disease categories in the differential diagnosis are (1) septic arthritis, (2) crystal-induced arthritis, (3) trauma, and (4) osteomyelitis. Although diagnosis of any of these is important, an untreated septic joint carries a morbidity rate of 50% and a mortality rate as high as 20%. The following discussion describes the proper approach to monoarticular arthritis in general. It is important to recognize that a monoarticular arthritis may be only one manifestation of a generalized systemic disease; additionally, septic arthritis can involve three or fewer joints (pauciarticular) early in the course of infection. For this reason, a thorough history and physical examination are crucial to the appropriate diagnosis and therapy.

HISTORY

Important historical facts include the age and sex of the patient, the joint(s) involved, the type of onset, and precipitating factors. Data from each of these categories can help to focus the differential diagnosis and guide the physician in ordering the most appropriate diagnostic procedures in the individual patient.

Age and Sex of the Patient

Gout rarely affects women prior to menopause or children without an underlying metabolic defect. Gonococcal arthritis, on the other hand, affects primarily women during the second through fourth decades of life. Pseudogout is a disease of later life; patients under 55 years of age are rarely affected.

Joints Involved

As in many arthritic disorders, the knee is the most common joint affected by monoarticular arthritis. However, complacency should not take place with regard to diagnosis. Involvement of the first metatarsophalangeal joint most frequently is gout. Nonetheless, trauma and rarely infection can also involve this joint. Pauciarticular arthritis settling into one joint suggests gonococcal arthritis, especially when associated with a tenosynovitis.[1] Monoarticular arthritis of the shoulder in an elderly woman may represent chronic hydroxyapatite synovitis (Milwaukee shoulder),[2] while monoarthritis of a sternoclavicular joint may suggest infection in a patient with a history of substance abuse.[3]

Type of Onset

Gout frequently has a sudden onset, and a patient may awaken with the symptoms of an acute monoarticular arthritis. A more subtle onset suggests pseudogout or infection.

True synovitis tends to be constant, while periarticular problems, such as bursitis and tendinitis, cause pain with active movement of the adjacent joint.

Precipitating Factors

The patient should be questioned about a history of trauma, either recent or remote, and about alcoholic history both with relationship to gout and to trauma occurring during alcoholic stupor. Recent infection, especially systemic, or dental manipulation would be consistent with septic arthritis. Diuretic usage (especially the thiazides and loop diuretics) is associated with hyperuricemia and the subsequent precipitation of acute gouty arthritis. Both gout and pseudogout can be precipitated by recent surgery. Substance abuse is a cause of septic arthritis in unusual joints caused in part by gram-negative organisms, which need to be sought. Gonococcal arthritis frequently occurs around the time of the menstrual flow. An underlying concurrent arthritis can predispose to septic arthritis, especially in the presence of frequent intra-articular injections of corticosteroids. Septic arthritis also occurs in the immunocompromised host. The patient may be immunocompromised due to endogenous autoimmune disease, to concurrent therapy with high doses of corticosteroids or chemotherapy for malignancy, as well as to the presence of other diseases such as chronic renal failure or diabetes mellitus.

PHYSICAL EXAMINATION

The physical examination may yield an essential clue to the diagnosis and must therefore be thorough. The following areas are particularly important in evaluating monoarticular arthritis. First, vital signs and the presence of fever are important. Fever and chills would be most suggestive of infection, although patients with gout and pseudogout may present with temperatures to 38.9°C on rare occasions. Next, there are several specific skin changes for which to look. Tophi are the nodular collections of monosodium urate crystals found in 20% of patients with gout. They may be only a few millimeters to several centimeters in diameter. They most commonly occur in the ear, olecranon bursa, dorsum of the hands, knees, Achilles tendon, and ulnar surfaces of the forearms. Tophi located over pressure points may be painful in an acute attack of gout. Disseminated gonococcemia causes a characteristic rash that is fairly obscure and must be specifically sought. Lesions are discrete vesicles on extremities that may be pustular, necrotic, or bullous. There may be only one or several in an individual patient. Vasculitic lesions and petechiae are suggestive of autoimmune diseases such as systemic lupus erythematosus. Rheumatoid nodules would be helpful in the diagnosis of rheumatoid arthritis. Erythema marginatum and erythema migrans are the rashes of rheumatic fever and Lyme disease, respectively. Finally, one should be aware of needle tracks on the skin, suggesting substance abuse. Of note also in the general physical examination would be hepatomegaly or liver tenderness to suggest hepatitis with associated arthritis.

Before examining the affected joint, the other joints and periarticular areas should be examined for abnormalities. Previous arthritis such as rheumatoid arthritis, osteoarthritis, or psoriatic arthritis will help in the differential diagnosis. Tenosynovitis involving the hands, wrists, Achilles tendon, and dorsa of the feet occurs in 60% of patients with gonococcal arthritis.

The affected joint should be inspected for the cardinal signs of inflammation: erythema, swelling, and warmth.[4] Erythema may be localized to surrounding soft tissue, and it is important to distinguish joint versus soft tissue inflammation or cellulitis. It is a common error to implicate joint involvement when only cellulitis is present and vice versa. This seems to occur especially in the ankle for some reason. To distinguish between the two, one should first palpate along the joint line to see if this is particularly sensitive. One should then gently evaluate range of motion in the joint, being careful not to grasp the area of inflammation directly. If these two maneuvers do not increase the pain, in all likelihood synovitis is not present. A basic knowledge of joint anatomy should be sufficient to allow one to decide if the inflammation is beyond the limits of the joint capsule. A specific instance of soft tissue inflammation with arthritis occurs in the so-called satellite phenomenon of gout. Here, involvement of a single joint is followed by inflammation of contiguous joints with erythema and warmth of soft tissue in between. Thus an entire foot may appear involved during the course of podagra. Increased heat should be carefully assessed by lightly moving the dorsum of the hand over the joint and adjacent soft tissue. A difference of 1°C can be assessed in this way. This maneuver is particularly important in the patient with rheumatoid arthritis whose deformed, swollen joints make evaluation of a septic joint difficult.

Joints may appear swollen for several reasons. First, the obese patient may appear to have swollen joints when there is excessive subcutaneous fat, for example, in the knees. In all cases, comparison with the opposite limb is crucial. The other two causes of swelling are fluid versus synovial proliferation. The distinction between these two is often difficult even for the rheumatologist. Luckily, the problem should only arise in the setting of a chronic arthritis such as rheumatoid arthritis, an old injured joint, or the rare case of villonodular synovitis. Fluid filling the joint capsule will have fluctuance and feel buoyant, while synovial proliferation has a more gelatinous texture to it or the sensation of a spongy substance beneath the palpating hand. In the knee, a large amount of fluid will be obvious when compared with the opposite side. However, one must look carefully for small effusions of 10 to 15 mL by using the "bulge sign" to demonstrate these effusions. The bulge sign is performed with the leg extended and the quadriceps relaxed. The examiner gently and slowly strokes the medial aspect of the patella from its inferior border to the superior border in an attempt to "milk" the fluid to the other side. After this is done, a gentle tap is delivered to the lateral side of the patella to create a fluid wave to the medial side. The examiner should observe the medial side very closely for a small bulge. When greater than 15 mL of fluid is present, one cannot elicit this sign. Joints may appear swollen, but on palpation the appearance is actually due to bony changes. In osteoarthritis one sees bony swelling at the distal and proximal interphalangeal joints, termed Heberden's and Bouchard's nodes, respectively. The tophi of gout feel more gelatinous than these nodules and can occur in periarticular areas, but again should be distinguished from a possible effusion.

In the elbow, an inflamed olecranon bursa is often mistakenly labeled an arthritis. A bursitis is more common and may be due to infection, trauma, or gout. The bulging, fluid-filled bursa is located over the olecranon tip. Actual involvement of the elbow joint can be ascertained by palpating the groove below the lateral epicondyle, comparing it to the opposite side. A feeling of fluctuance there indicates fluid. Another clue is found in assessing range of motion. If fluid is in the joint, the patient will not be able to fully extend or flex the elbow.

After assessing for inflammation, the joints should be tested for stability or signs of internal derangement with range of motion and various tests of ligamentous pathology. Instability demonstrated on examination will suggest trauma, old or new, or a more chronic process rather than an acute infection.

At times, the symptomatic joint is normal on examination. At these times it is important to examine the more proximal joint. Not infrequently, hip disease is referred to the knee or knee disease is referred to the ankle.[5] It is in these instances that the axiom to examine the joint proximal to the symptomatic one assumes major importance.

DIAGNOSIS

Diagnostic studies include aspiration of joint fluid, roentgenogram studies, and hematologic evaluation of the patient, including blood cultures. The crucial component in the evaluation of monoarticular arthritis is the joint fluid. Whether a patient has classic podagra or a history of trauma, fluid should be examined by Gram stain for signs of infection and crystals examined by polarized light microscopy. It is especially important to look for monosodium urate crystals in a patient with a diagnosis of gout who has never had a joint aspiration performed. As will be discussed, other diseases such as pseudogout may cause a similar clinical picture. However, drugs such as allopurinol will not be helpful in the long-term therapy of pseudogout and may carry a certain degree of risk. Allopurinol has been noted to cause a severe hypersensitivity reaction in patients with compromised renal function leading to vasculitis, dermatitis, hepatitis, and renal toxicity. Corticosteroids are required in many of these cases, and death occurs in some patients.

Aspiration of joints requires sterile technique with hand washing and cleansing with povidone-iodine (Betadine) as well as gloves. Before beginning the aspiration, one should have on hand at least one 20-mL syringe (more if there is a larger effusion), a needle of appropriate gauge for the joint (18 or 19 gauge for the knee and shoulder, 21 gauge for the elbow or wrist, and 23 gauge for small joints of the hands and feet), povidone-iodine, alcohol swabs, and tubes for a complete blood cell count and a glucose level, as well as a tube with a drop or two of sodium heparin for crystal analysis. If gonococcal infection is a consideration, a chocolate agar plate at room temperature for gonococcal culture should be close at hand. Last, 4×4 inch gauze pads, a Band-Aid, and ethyl chloride to anesthetize the skin are helpful. The joint to be aspirated should be kept in a relaxed position and the point of aspiration marked by pressing the skin with a pen top or fingernail (markings will be erased with the cleansing process). The area should initially be cleansed twice with povidone-iodine, ending by swabbing the area with alcohol. Anesthetizing the skin with ethyl chloride will relieve the discomfort of needle insertion to a minor degree. Lidocaine infiltration of the skin is often more painful than the actual skin penetration and is not recommended by some. As much of the fluid as possible should be removed, aided by milking the synovial capsule while the needle is held in place and negative pressure is maintained. Remember that the major pain of aspiration will result from inadvertently pricking the periosteum. Therefore, repeated jabbing of the needle should be avoided in favor of a complete redirection of the needle if no fluid is found.

The aspiration and/or injection techniques for the more commonly involved joints follow. It is important to note here that after any attempt at aspiration even a drop of fluid may have fortuitously been obtained. Always attempt to expel fluid onto a slide even if the syringe appears dry since crystals will have frequently been obtained in the needle barrel. Starting cephalad, the shoulder joint may be aspirated with an anterior or posterior approach, with the anterior approach used almost exclusively (Fig. 23-1). The coracoid process is palpated as the principal landmark, just medial to the humeral head. One can also localize it by finding the midpoint of the convex curve of the clavicle and then palpating just below that point. The joint space to be entered is just lateral to the coracoid process. It can be appreciated by having the patient fix his upper arm against the body while the physician externally and internally rotates the shoulder, palpating the glenohumeral area. The needle should be directed just slightly upward because of the proximity of the lung. It is a good idea to auscultate the lungs after aspiration of the shoulder to ensure that a pneumothorax, a rare complication, has not developed. The elbow joint proper is most easily entered at the radiohumeral joint with the arm flexed at

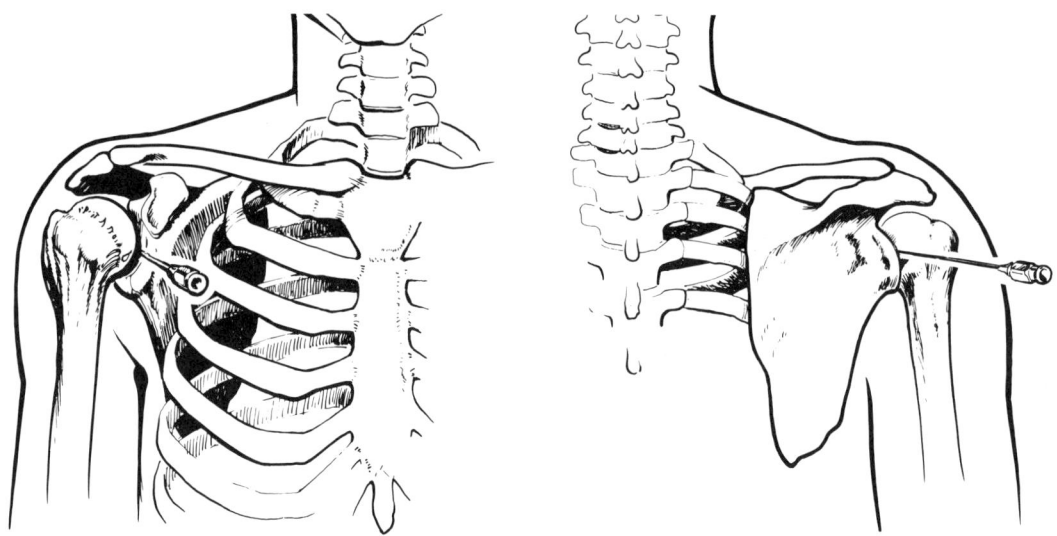

Figure 23-1 Arthrocentesis of the shoulder. (**A**) Anterior approach. (**B**) Posterior approach.

45° to 90° (Fig. 23-2). The lateral epicondyle of the humerus is located, and the needle is inserted just distal to it and proximal to the head of the radius, directed medially and perpendicular to the skin. The space can be appreciated by supinating and pronating the arm while palpating the radial head. The olecranon bursa is entered posteriorly by directing the needle below the skin at the proximal edge of the bursa in a line parallel to the shaft of the forearm. The needle need not be inserted very deeply since the bursa is superficial.

The wrist joint is entered by a dorsal approach with the wrist held in slight passive flexion (Fig. 23-3). The point of insertion is just distal to the bony prominence of the radius and just lateral to the extensor pollicis longus tendon. The needle is properly positioned if one can advance it 1 to 2 cm without resistance.

When a septic arthritis of the hip is suspected, it is best to obtain consultation from orthopedics or rheumatology since this joint is extremely difficult to aspirate. Ideally, the approach would be to aspirate under fluoroscopy to ensure proper needle placement in the joint. With a blind aspiration one does not know if the joint has truly been entered.

The knee is probably the easiest joint to aspirate and is fortuitously the most likely joint to be encountered in monoarticular arthritis (Fig. 23-4). It can be entered either medially or laterally, approaches that, interestingly, are medical and orthopedic styles, respectively. The leg should be extended and relaxed with emphasis to the patient to relax the quadriceps. In the medial approach the midpoint of the posterior surface of the patella is localized and marked. While the examiner gently holds the patella at the inferior

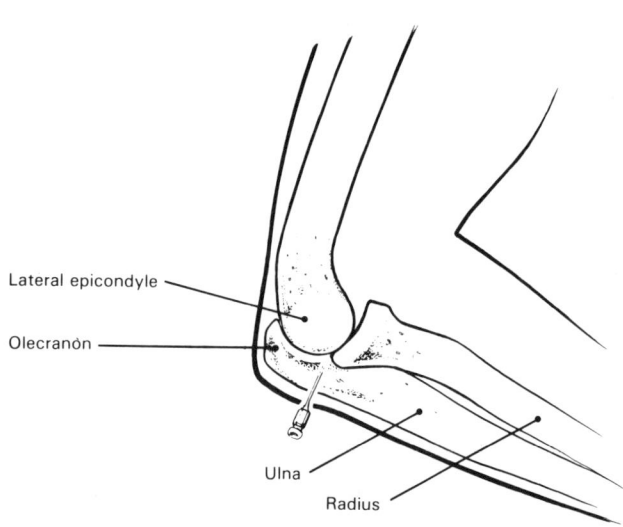

Figure 23-2 Arthrocentesis of the elbow.

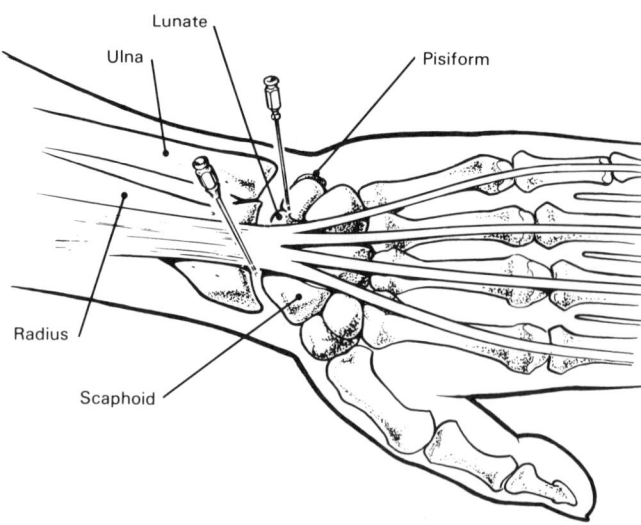

Figure 23-3 Arthrocentesis of the wrist.

and superior surfaces with one hand (for continued localization), the needle is directed through the mark at an angle of 45° to the skin. In other words, one is directing the needle under the patella as the medial patellar surface is beveled. When aspirating from the lateral approach the needle is inserted beneath (ie, posterior to) the upper one third of the lateral patella in a direction perpendicular to the skin. As noted previously, if fluid is not obtained the needle should be partially withdrawn and redirected rather than used in the more painful, jabbing maneuver.

Two sites of aspiration in the ankle are the subtalar joint and the tibiotalar joint (Fig. 23-5). Indications for an aspiration of these sites are pain with eversion and inversion versus pain with flexion and extension, respectively. The subtalar joint is entered at a point just inferior to the tip of the lateral malleolus. One can appreciate the sinus tarsi by first palpating the depression below the malleolus. The tibiotalar joint is entered anteriorly at a point just medial to the extensor halluces tendon and lateral to the medial malleolus. The joint space is several centimeters deep to the surface, and the needle should freely penetrate to this depth without bony resistance if positioned correctly.

Since landmarks may be obscured by extensive soft tissue swelling, the first metatarsophalangeal joint and the needle should be well localized on the uninvolved foot prior to injection. The needle is inserted on the medial side of the joint slightly dorsal to the midline and perpendicular to the skin. Exerting very gentle traction on the toe can help to widen the joint space.

The fluid obtained with aspiration is now analyzed for cell count, glucose, crystals, and bacteria. Appropriate cultures should be sent for and a specimen plated on chocolate agar if gonococcal infection is a possibility. A drop should be placed on a glass slide with a coverslip for crystal examination and a Gram stain done. The fluid is examined grossly for classification into one of four groups. It is examined for clarity (reading print through it), color, and viscosity. Viscosity is tested by placing a drop of fluid between the thumb and index finger and attempting to draw it out in a string by rapidly separating the two fingers. This is the "string test," and a normal fluid should form a strand at least 1 to 2 inches long. An inflammatory fluid is less viscous due to loss of hyaluronic acid. Obviously, if the fluid is grossly purulent, one should not try the string test. Viscosity can also be measured by expressing a drop of fluid from the tip of the needle. Again it should only separate after dropping 1 to 2 inches. The types of fluids as defined by cell count, color, and viscosity are listed in Table 23-1. The cell counts within each group have a degree of overlap, but generally a grossly purulent fluid with more than 50,000/µL indicates infection while a relatively viscous yet cloudy fluid indicates an inflammatory process. Some exceptions include the rare case of gout in which the fluid has an excessively high white cell count in the range of a purulent fluid. Also, in rheumatoid arthritis, the patient may have decreased leukocyte chemo-

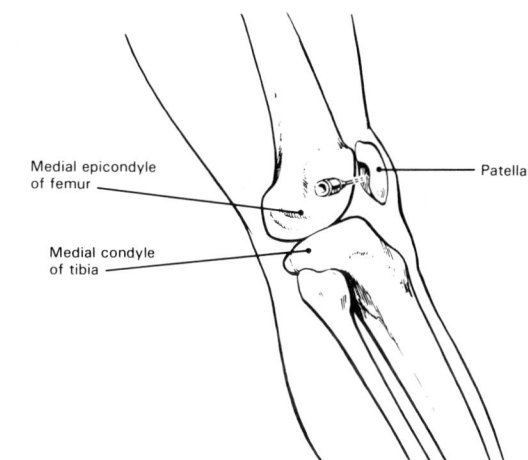

Figure 23-4 Arthrocentesis of the knee.

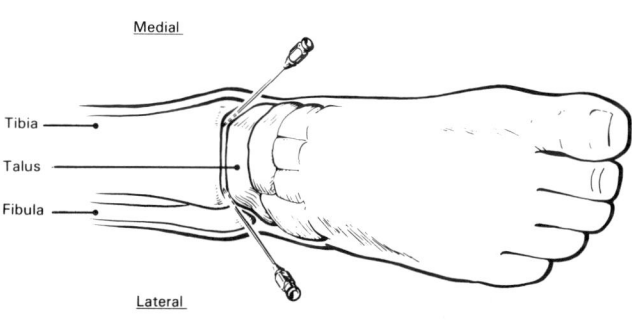

Figure 23-5 Arthrocentesis of the ankle.

taxis and inflammatory response. The cell count in a patient with septic rheumatoid arthritis may only be in the group 2 fluid range. Since these patients are more susceptible to infection due to underlying joint deformity, all fluids obtained in patients with rheumatoid arthritis should be cultured when the possibility of infection is seriously considered. Group 4 fluid is grossly hemorrhagic and can be seen in trauma, blood dyscrasias such as hemophilia, and the rare, pigmented villonodular synovitis.

Gram stains are essential and will be positive in one half to two thirds of cases of septic arthritis, with the greatest yield occurring in joints infected with *Staphylococcus aureus*.

Crystal identification requires the use of a polarizing light microscope. If this is not available, ordinary light microscopy can be used to identify crystal morphology. The prepared slides can then be preserved for later evaluation by someone experienced in crystal identification by sealing the edges of the coverslip with clear nail polish. The major crystals to be identified are monosodium urate (MSU) crystals in gout and calcium pyrophosphate dihydrate (CPPD) crystals in pseudogout. MSU crystals are usually thin and needle shaped, while CPPD crystals are shorter and more rhomboid. Under the polarizing scope MSU crystals demonstrate a bire-

Table 23-1 Joint Fluid Analysis

	Color	Clarity	Viscosity	White Blood Cell Count (cells/μL)	Polymorphonuclear Leukocytes (%)	Diseases
Normal	Yellow	Clear	High	<200	<25	
Group 1: noninflammatory	Yellow	Clear	High	<2000	<25	Osteoarthritis Traumatic arthritis Chronic crystal disease Systemic lupus erythematosus
Group 2: inflammatory	Yellow to white	Slightly cloudy	Low	3000 to 50,000	>70	Rheumatoid arthritis Rheumatic fever Reiter's syndrome Crystal-induced disease Viral arthritis
Group 3: purulent	Yellow to white	Opaque	Very low	50,000 to 300,000	>90	Bacterial infections Severe crystal-induced synovitis
Group 4: hemorrhagic	Bloody	Opaque	Low	Comparable to peripheral blood		Trauma Blood dyscrasias Pigmented villonodular synovitis Sickle cell disease Anticoagulant therapy

fringence, which is labeled "negative birefringence" by convention. When the crystals are aligned parallel to the axis of the polarizing light (which is marked by an arrow on the microscope), they are bright yellow. When the field is rotated 90° and the crystals are perpendicular to the axis, they are bright blue. At a point 45° from the perpendicular, the angle of extinction, MSU crystals disappear completely. CPPD crystals, on the other hand, are positively birefringent. They are yellow when perpendicular to the axis and blue when parallel. In addition, the colors are not as bright, and at the angle of extinction (20° to 30°), the crystals merely fade rather than disappearing completely.

Other crystals can be seen in the fluid, as well as contaminating debris, which may be birefringent. Lithium heparin used in certain Vacutainer tubes appears as rodlike, rhomboid, or rectangular crystals with positive birefringence. Starch from gloves appears as ovoid birefringent forms. Insoluble corticosteroid crystal injections are variable in shape and birefringence. Cholesterol crystals are flat, platelike forms with notched corners. Despite the variety of crystals that one may find, the appearance of MSU or CPPD crystals is distinctive, especially when the crystals are intracellular. One must diligently search the slide, since there may be only a very few crystals. This is especially true if the monoarticular arthritis has been present for several days.

In evaluating the patient with monoarticular arthritis, other laboratory tests include a complete blood cell count, a uric acid study (which may be normal in an acute attack of gout), and evaluation of the erythrocyte sedimentation rate. The white blood cell count will be increased in most cases of septic arthritis and may be mildly increased in crystal-induced synovitis. Cultures of any skin lesions and wounds should be done as well as appropriate examination and culture for *Gonococcus* organisms, if indicated.

Roentgenograms of the affected joint are important, although most likely they will show only soft tissue swelling in early septic arthritis. They may demonstrate injury, fracture, tumor, neuropathic change, or chondrocalcinosis. Chondrocalcinosis is a thin line of calcification typically found in the articular and hyaline cartilage of the knee, symphysis pubis, and the triangular cartilage of the wrist at the ulnocarpal articulation. It is suggestive of pseudogout since CPPD deposits account for the majority of cases of such calcification.

SPECIFIC ETIOLOGIES

Armed with the information gained from a thorough history and physical and laboratory examination, one should be able to reach a definite diagnosis of acute monoarticular arthritis. In the following section, evaluation and treatment of the various entities will be discussed.

Septic Arthritis

The diagnosis of septic arthritis should be made in the presence of purulent synovial fluid, fever, and leukocytosis, with or without a positive Gram stain. If the Gram stain is positive, the patient is admitted and treatment is begun with the appropriate antibiotic. If the Gram stain is negative, one uses the information from the patient's history to decide on the most likely organism, and antibiotics for the infection caused by that organism are begun. This must take into account the epidemiology of organisms in the community. In the general healthy population, the most common organism is *Staphylococcus aureus*, occurring in approximately one half of cases. In the sexually active population, between the ages of 15 and 40, *Gonococcus* is the most common organism. In children under two years of age, the incidence of *Hemophilus influenzae* is increased. Immunocompromised patients such as those with cancer, cirrhosis, or diabetes mellitus, and intravenous drug abusers are more prone to develop infection with Gram-negative organisms. Empiric therapy, then, is with nafcillin, 8 to 12 g/day intravenously for the general population; cefuroxime for those in the age range susceptible to gonococcus; nafcillin plus an aminoglycoside for the immunocompromised patient; and cefuroxime or any third-generation cephalosporin for the pediatric patient. The crucial point in the evaluation of monoarticular arthritis is that one must assume infection is present, admit the patient, and treat the infection while cultures are pending if the diagnosis is not clear from the initial examination. Nonsteroidal anti-inflammatory agents should not be used during the first 48 hours in order that one can observe the temperature curve as well as the response of the joint to antibiotic treatment.

Patients with rheumatoid arthritis represent a distinct subpopulation of patients more prone to pyarthrosis or septic joints. This is due to local factors such as underlying joint deformity and penetration of the joint with corticosteroid injections or to systemic factors such as chronic debility, decreased polymorphonuclear cell numbers and chemotaxis, and concurrent drug therapy for the arthritis. The incidence of septic arthritis is 0.3% to 3.0% of rheumatoid patients. As noted, the leukocyte count in the synovial fluid may be in the group 2 rather than in group 3 range. The major clue that one is dealing with a pyarthrosis rather than rheumatoid arthritis may be inflammation in one joint out of proportion to the other joints. *S aureus* is the etiologic agent in 80% of cases.

Patients on dialysis represent another subgroup of patients prone to septic joints.[6] Important risk factors in these patients include decreased immunocompetency and repeated penetration of the vascular system and presence of a foreign body due to their grafts and dialysis. Diagnosis of an acute monoarticular arthritis may be difficult since patients on dialysis have a high incidence of hydroxyapatite crystal–induced arthritis, especially in the shoulders. Again, one must have an awareness of the possibility of infection, most notably since *S aureus* occurs in 85% of reported cases of septic arthritis in this patient population.

Lyme arthritis is a disease entity, first recognized in 1975.[7] It is part of a disease syndrome including a typical rash following a tick bite, then development of arthritis, neurologic symptoms, carditis, and malaise. It occurs most commonly in late summer or early fall. The causative agent is the spirochete *Borrelia burgdorferi*, which is transmitted by the tick. In a majority of cases, patients give a history of a classic rash of erythema migrans following the tick bite by 3 to 32 days. The rash begins as an expanding area of erythema around the bite with bright red advancing margins. The central area may fade and become vesicular or even necrotic. It may be painful or burn and feels hot to the touch. The patient develops multiple other annular lesions that do not expand and that spare the palms and soles. Patients may have symptoms of malaise, lethargy, meningismus, headache, and neurologic changes such as Bell's palsy and sensory radiculopathy. The rash of erythema migrans generally lasts about 3 weeks. The arthritis follows the rash by days to months, averaging 4 weeks. It is a monoarticular arthritis in 69% of cases, most commonly affecting the knee, and is oligoarticular in 29% of cases. The joint is swollen, with synovial fluid of a group 2 classification. Patients have the same systemic symptoms as described during the rash of erythema migrans. They may give a history of recurrent arthritis since this occurs in 70% of patients. If the diagnosis of Lyme arthritis has been made and the patient treated with penicillin or tetracycline the arthritis will be milder. Established Lyme arthritis can be successfully treated with antibiotics although response is not uniformly successful.[8] Adjunctive therapy with aspirin or occasionally with corticosteroids is also useful.

Crystal Arthritis

The diagnosis of monosodium urate crystal–induced disease is extremely gratifying since the treatment is clear-cut and successful. Treatment for acute gout includes either colchicine, nonsteroidal anti-inflammatory drugs, or injection. The treatment of choice is with any of the nonsteroidal anti-inflammatory drugs. In a patient with peptic ulcer disease, it is best to avoid both drugs orally since either category is a gastric irritant. In patients with congestive heart failure or renal disease, especially if the patient is to be discharged on medication, it is best to avoid nonsteroidal anti-inflammatory drugs due to their effect on the kidney. The dose of colchicine is 0.6 mg orally every hour for six doses or until symptoms resolve or intolerable diarrhea ensues. Diarrhea can be controlled by diphenoxylate (Lomotil) or paregoric. Intravenous colchicine may also be used at a dose of 2 mg in 15 mL of saline given over 15 minutes. The recommended dose of intravenous colchicine is two administrations at 12-hour intervals. It often requires only one dose and so constitutes a legitimate therapy for emergency department use or in the patient with either active gastrointestinal disease or the postsurgical patient who has had nothing by mouth. Care should be taken to avoid soft tissue infiltration since the drug can be irritative. Colchicine will be effective in 90% of patients with gout if given in the first 12 hours of the attack. If the attack is more than 24 hours old, colchicine may not be successful. Another successful mode of therapy for the patient with gastrointestinal disease or the postsurgical patient is with indomethacin suppositories. In pseudogout, colchicine is successful less than 50% of the time. The usual dose of such a nonsteroidal anti-inflammatory drug as indomethacin is 50 mg four times a day for several days, then twice daily subsequently, stopping if the attack has resolved. If neither drug can be used and infection has definitely been ruled out, the joint can be injected with a corticosteroid suspension such as methylprednisolone (Depo-Medrol), 40 mg, and lidocaine. The patient should always be warned about a postinjection flare after intra-articular corticosteroids. This entity is an inflammatory response to the corticosteroid crystals themselves, which occurs in the first 24 hours post injection. Treatment includes patient reassurance and education, aspirin, and ice. All fluids should be cultured, even when crystals are observed, since infection may be present in a joint with crystal arthritis.

Traumatic Arthritis

Trauma as a cause of acute monoarticular arthritis should be evident from history, physical examination, aspiration of bloody fluid, and possible roentgenographic findings. Treatment is dependent on the particular injury sustained.

Osteomyelitis

Children are suspectible to acute osteomyelitis, generally occurring in the metaphysis of long bones such as the tibia, femur, and humerus. The infection may have been due to introduction through a wound but is more commonly secondary to hematogenous spread. The presentation is similar to acute septic arthritis with an extremely tender periarticular area with warm, indurated soft tissue surrounding it, fever, chills, tachycardia, and weakness. It may be difficult to distinguish this from joint involvement, but the evaluation should proceed and antibiotics started for presumed infection (usually due to *S aureus*).

Miscellaneous Arthritis

Any of the rheumatic diseases such as systemic lupus erythematosus, psoriatic arthritis, arthritis associated with inflammatory bowel disease, and Reiter's syndrome can present with a monoarticular arthritis. One may recognize that the arthritis is part of the underlying syndrome by finding other systemic symptoms of that disease. In psoriasis, one should look for the characteristic rash. Reiter's syndrome also has a distinctive rash on the soles, keratodermia blenorrhagica, and involvement of the penis in a scaling rash, balanitis circinata. The important matter to settle in any of these diseases, especially if the patient is on medication such as corticosteroids, is whether or not infection is present.

In most cases of monoarticular arthritis in which no diagnosis can be made on the basis of the initial examination, a diagnostic plan must be used based on the clinical presentation and facts. An immunocompromised or debilitated patient with only group 2 fluid and stable clinical status should be admitted and observed over the next 24 to 48 hours, while cultures are pending and further tests (eg, scans) are done. No medications should be used except analgesics such as codeine, and prompt action must be taken if the patient's condition deteriorates. In a stable, healthy patient without infection, trauma, or crystal disease, a trial with a nonsteroidal anti-inflammatory drug could be started with outpatient follow-up for further rheumatologic evaluation. All patients should be instructed to return for any worsening or change in symptoms.

POLYARTICULAR ARTHRITIS

Patients may present to the emergency department with an acute polyarticular arthritis without a previous history of arthritis. Generally, the decision to admit these patients would depend on their clinical status and the ability of the examiner to rule out a septic process. It would be highly unusual for an adult to have polyarticular involvement in a bacterial septic arthritis, although children may have more than one joint involved. The following discussion lists the more common diseases in the differential diagnosis of acute polyarticular arthritis.

Acute rheumatic fever, although rare, should be a consideration as a cause of migratory polyarticular arthritis in adults, especially if the process is associated with congestive heart failure.[9] The patient may have had recent exposure to *Streptococcus* organisms or had a streptococcal infection, and he or she may have had acute rheumatic fever even up to 20 years prior to this episode. It is believed that recurrent episodes of acute rheumatic fever may occur undiagnosed. The patient will have fever sometimes to 39.4°C and an additive arthritis. Rash and subcutaneous nodules rarely occur in the adult. The patient may have carditis manifested by congestive heart failure with increased cardiac size but generally without murmur. Typically there is marked periarticular tenderness elicited on physical examination of the joints. Treatment is with aspirin and also consideration for prophylactic antibiotics in the future. Involvement of the heart warrants hospitalization.

Rheumatoid arthritis may begin abruptly over 12 to 24 hours as an acute polyarticular arthritis. Generally, the onset is over days to weeks. Fevers may be as high as 39.4°C and a distinguishing factor from acute rheumatic fever is the persistence of the joint pain and stiffness. It is not migratory. Laboratory tests such as antistreptolysin O, antihyaluronidase, and antistreptokinase titers, plus a history of streptococcal infection help differentiate these two diseases. Juvenile rheumatoid arthritis and adult-onset Still's disease demonstrate a characteristic salmon-colored evanescent rash on the face, palms, soles, limbs, and trunk. The rash is generally worse in the late afternoon and may coincide with fever spikes. Joint involvement may be monoarticular, pauciarticular, or polyarticular.

Gonococcal arthritis may present as a migratory arthritis or arthralgia, gradually localizing to one joint. During the polyarticular phase one may see the typical rash and can culture the organism from the primary source, the skin lesions, or the blood. Joint fluid is generally sterile at that time. The patient may have fever, chills, and tenosynovitis.

Many viral illnesses are associated with fever, polyarthralgias, and rash. These include rubella, mononucleosis, hepatitis B, arbovirus, adenovirus, varicella, parvovirus, and smallpox. The arthritis is generally short-lived and causes no residual change in joint structure.

Pseudogout and gout will generally be monoarticular or pauciarticular but could present as an acute polyarticular arthritis with fevers up to 38.3°C and a septic-looking patient. Search for crystals and attempts to rule out infection are the procedures of choice. MSU and CPPD crystals can occur in a septic joint.

Arthritis and arthralgias represent the most frequent symptoms in systemic lupus erythematosus and may be the initial presentation. Other system involvement will aid in the diagnosis.

The spondyloarthropathies and reactive arthritides such as Reiter's syndrome, arthritis associated with inflammatory bowel disease, and psoriasis may present with polyarticular arthritis. In Reiter's syndrome the rash as noted previously may be found along with conjunctivitis.

Finally, sarcoidosis may present with polyarticular arthritis. The triad of arthritis, bilateral hilar adenopathy, and erythema nodosa is termed Lofgren's syndrome. A chest roentgenogram should be included in the initial work-up to rule out this disease.

To summarize, the major thrust of emergency department evaluation in these patients with polyarticular arthritis should be to rule out infection and to admit clinically unstable patients even in the absence of infection. The general work-up includes chest roentgenogram, complete blood cell count, urinalysis, antistreptolysin O titer, erythrocyte sedimentation rate, throat culture, and rheumatoid factor, antinuclear antibody, Venereal Disease Research Laboratory (VDRL), and possibly hepatitis studies. Joint fluid must be examined in all cases.

If the patient is not infected, immunocompromised, or clinically unstable, aspirin may be started in full doses of 5200 mg in divided doses for adults or nonsteroidal anti-inflammatory drugs to tolerance.

REFERENCES

1. Brogadir SP, Schimmer BM, Myers AR. Spectrum of the gonococcal arthritis-dermatitis syndrome. *Semin Arthritis Rheum.* 1979;8:177.
2. McCarty DJ, Halverson PB, Carrera GF, et al. "Milwaukee shoulder"—association of microspheroids containing hydroxyapatite crystals, active collagenase, and neutral protease with rotator cuff defects. *Arthritis Rheum.* 1981;24:464.
3. Yood RA, Goldenberg DL. Sternoclavicular joint arthritis. *Arthritis Rheum.* 1980;23:232.
4. Polley HF, Hunder G. *Physical Examination of the Joints*. Philadelphia: Saunders; 1978.
5. Enis JE. The painful knee. *Hosp Med.* 1980;10–19.
6. Mathews M, Shen FH, Lindner A, et al. Septic arthritis in hemodialized patients. *Nephron.* 1980;25:87.
7. Steere AC, et al. The early clinical manifestations of Lyme disease. *Ann Intern Med.* 1983;99:76.
8. Steere AC, Green J, Schoen RT, et al. Successful parenteral penicillin therapy of established Lyme arthritis. *N Engl J Med.* 1985;321:869.
9. Ben-Dor I, Berry E. Acute rheumatic fever in adults over the age of 45 years: an analysis of 23 patients together with a review of the literature. *Semin Arthritis Rheum.* 1980;10:100.

24. Medical Genetics

JOEL M. LAMON, MD, FACP

Concepts of human genetics are certainly not foreign to medical training. However, the focus of such expertise toward the diagnosis of patients with inherited disease, counseling of patients, evaluation of potentially affected family members, and the management of multisystem problems is rather new in medical practice. This approach has become defined in the past decade as the specialty of medical genetics.

The emergency department is a unique setting for the practice of medicine. The emergency physician spends only a fraction of time in acute life-saving efforts. Immediacy is paramount in the emergency department. Symptom assessment and relief are followed by triage to home, hospital, or specialty services. Among the specialty areas of medicine that are brought to bear by the emergency physician, few would appear less important in the emergency setting than medical genetics.

Recognition of a genetic disease can help the physician provide proper immediate symptom control and referral. There are situations in which this information can prepare the emergency physician to avoid unnecessary and sometimes potentially dangerous procedures. The family history and the physical examination provide the information. The family history may provide the underlying diagnosis and perhaps the cause for these complaints because of previous work-up of a family member. The information is often volunteered by a family member. Inherited diseases may manifest themselves as isolated problems in a single organ system or a single structural defect, but they can also present as a multisystem disorder. The recognition of a positive family history for a specific inherited disease may provide the initial clue that there may be a genetic reason for new and acute symptomatology in the family member being seen. The issue of whether a specific genetic disease exists may require in-depth specialty evaluation.

The second approach to genetic disease in the emergency setting is the physical examination. Recognition that a patient, whether a child or an adult, does not look normal is the first step in using dysmorphology as a clue to an inherited disease. Careful observation may allow the emergency physician to specify the exact nature of the patient's abnormal appearance. Genetic illnesses affect more than one organ system, and the identification of an abnormality affecting the extremities, overall stature, eyes, heart, or the skin, may provide an important clue that abnormalities of other organs may also be present. A patient's acute symptomatology might, therefore, be related to an inherited predisposing condition.

The interaction of medical genetics in the emergency department occurs primarily with the family history and physical examination for identification of possible inherited disease. However, the potential for such a connection must be kept in mind if inherited disease is to be recognized. Since acute symptoms are typically the focus of emergency department visits, certain signs and symptoms will be addressed in this chapter with respect to their differential diagnosis of inherited diseases.

BASIC GENETICS

The basic principles of inheritance as delineated by the Austrian monk Gregor Mendel remain fundamental in our understanding of simple patterns of inheritance. The Mendelian patterns of inherited disease involve abnormalities that we now know are related to specific mutations at distinct loci on chromosomes and are inherited in predictable patterns. These Mendelian patterns of inheritance include dominant, recessive, and X- or sex-linked inheritance. They are also supplemented by concepts of polygenic inheritance, genetic heterogeneity, and genetic epidemiology. Mendelian principles of inheritance are most applicable in the emergency department. They offer simple and straightforward concepts of inheritance and allow one to use specific information regarding family members in order to exclude or maintain a hypothesis of a genetic cause for an individual's symptomatology.

Chromosomes are complex structures of nucleic acid and proteins that can be readily identified using special laboratory studies of cells induced to divide in culture. In humans there are 23 chromosome pairs, which include 22 pairs of autosomes and 1 pair of sex chromosomes. Autosomal dominant diseases are manifested when a single allele or focus of genetic material on only one chromosome of a pair codes for an abnormal protein that defines structure or biochemical function in the body. The significant principle in dominant conditions is that the presence of a normal allele on the other chromosome of the pair cannot compensate for the mutation. The breadth of abnormalities on the cellular and molecular level has become quite complex but involves either deletions or an abnormal sequence of genetic material. Abnormal gene products or a decreased amount of a normal product result from these situations. Other potential regulatory abnormalities will not be considered here. Autosomal recessive genes are expressed only when the identical allele is present on both chromosomes of the pair.

This is a rather simplistic scheme, and it is important to acknowledge that with modern technology of enzymology and other chemical techniques it is frequently possible to measure subtle differences in the products of genes. More recently it has become possible to evaluate genetic information using restriction enzyme technology so that the abnormality may be defined on a molecular level. The sex- or X-linked forms in inheritance manifest variation on the basis of the same mechanisms noted for the autosomal diseases. However, the sex chromosomes are unique in that the X chromosome may be paired with a Y chromosome (male) or with another X chromosome (female). Therefore, recessive disorders that normally require a double genetic "dose" of a mutant allele for expression may be seen only in males when the inheritance is sex chromosome linked. Since the sex is determined by whether the sperm that fertilizes an ovum contains an X or Y chromosome, all males (XY chromosomal pattern) obtain their X chromosome from their mothers and their Y chromosome from their fathers.

With these concepts is mind family pedigrees can be evaluated for insights regarding possible mechanisms of inheritance. In the Mendelian dominant conditions, inheritance is from parent to child and there is no relationship to sex of any affected individual. However, an affected individual's sex may affect manifestation of dominantly inherited conditions if those conditions are affected by hormones or other aspects of environmental differences between the sexes. These are most likely to occur in the post-adolescent years. Dominant diseases are well known for variation in disease expression in various generations, but a basic rule of thumb is that only affected individuals can pass on the abnormal genetic material to their offspring. Therefore, a dominant pattern of inheritance would appear in a pedigree to show affected persons in generations preceding and following the proband. One would expect that each offspring of an affected person would have a 50% likelihood of being affected by a similar condition. Brothers and sisters of the affected individual would have a 50% likelihood of being affected as well. The recessive pattern of inheritance is much more restrictive in presentation. As noted, a "double dose" of the recessive allele must be present. This, of course, requires that both chromosomes of a pair contain the same allelic abnormality. With specific recessive disorders, the possibility that any two unrelated individuals would carry the same genetic disorder is extremely small. The possibility that marriage partners would carry identical recessive alleles would be enhanced if they shared a common ancestry. Therefore, a significant question in evaluating the possibility of a recessive genetic disorder is whether the affected individual's parents are related. Recessive disorders tend to be more severe and manifest themselves at birth or in childhood. Thus, it is more common to see autosomal recessive diseases in the pediatric age group. A pedigree for a recessive disease would likely show only brothers and sisters within the family being affected and neither of the parents manifesting any abnormality. The history of consanguinity would enhance the likelihood of such a condition. In such an instance one would expect the "carrier" state (that is, the heterozygote pattern of one normal and one abnormal chromosome) to be present in other family members. Finally, the sex-linked disorders demonstrate family pedigrees in which only males are affected. By Mendelian genetics, we would expect that mothers of affected males have one normal and one abnormal X chromosome. Their brothers would be at a 50% risk for manifesting the X-linked disease, and, therefore, a pedigree may suggest that the disease is skipping generations rather than the correct interpretation that the disease is being manifested only by males and passed on to future generations via unaffected females. A corollary to this is that female carriers of X-linked diseases may demonstrate mild aspects of the fully expressed disorder. This is based on random inactivation of one of the X chromosomes.

These concepts of Mendelian genetics can be used in the emergency department to ascertain whether a recognized condition or trait may be inherited. The pedigree may also indicate the type of inheritance. It is important to realize that not all genetic diseases manifest a consistent range of abnormalities and that certain aspects of a genetic syndrome may be manifest in some individuals and not in others. These principles, however, can allow the emergency physician to make a more accurate assessment of whether an inherited disease may be present, and whether it may be related to the presenting symptoms.

CLINICAL GENETICS

The evaluation of morphologic features in the individual can often provide significant clues to the etiology of apparent multisystem problems. Frequently it is pertinent to the chronology of embryologic events. Prominent associations of morphological abnormalities either in well-characterized clinical syndromes or developmental anomaly associations are typically recognized in the newborn or young child. Such conditions are frequently diagnosed early in life. When these people are seen in the emergency department, the underlying disease is often well established and the diagnosis is typically provided by parents and family. However, dysmorphic features that may be part of multisystem abnormalities may escape earlier notice if gross structural changes are absent. On occasion, development of observable abnormalities develop with age and may be accentuated during adolescent growth.

Dysmorphology

Dysmorphology is a contemplative diagnostic exercise requiring astute observation and an appreciation of embryologic events. In the emergency department setting, the observation of a single dysmorphic feature may be a clue to an underlying condition. This may lead to an awareness of a condition that may be the predisposing or actual causal factor in the patient's acute symptomatology. Specific aspects of morphology that may lend themselves to the emergency department examination include the patient's stature and within that context the proportionality of abnormal stature—specifically, whether tall or short stature is related to the limbs, the trunk, or is completely proportioned. Ears and eyes are readily examined. They can be assessed with respect to spatial arrangements, functional ability, and for the presence of all normal anatomical features. The thorax and abdomen are frequently examined in the emergency department because of symptoms such as chest pains, breathing difficulties, and abdominal pains. The appearance of the thorax with respect to the sternum, spine, and pigment changes can be easily assessed. The normal morphology of the digits should not be missed since the hands and the feet are frequently available for examination and do not require special efforts to observe morphologic abnormalities there. Unusual curvature of the fingers (clinodactyly), absence of nails, digitalization (triphalangeal) of the thumb (Fig. 24-1), or gross structural defects in the limbs should be readily apparent. Extraordinary changes in the skin might include multiple nevi or evidence of multiple surgeries for skin problems. These observations might prompt one to consider epidermal abnormalities that might be a manifestation of underlying multisystem disease.

These issues of general morphologic abnormalities have been discussed previously in broad general terms, and specific areas of dysmorphologic evaluation have been pointed out. Several physical findings and associated genetic disease are listed in Table 24-1. Multiple associations can be made in genetic diseases, and the table that is presented is intended to provide information with respect to genetic disorders that may be pertinent to the acute symptomatology seen in the emergency department.

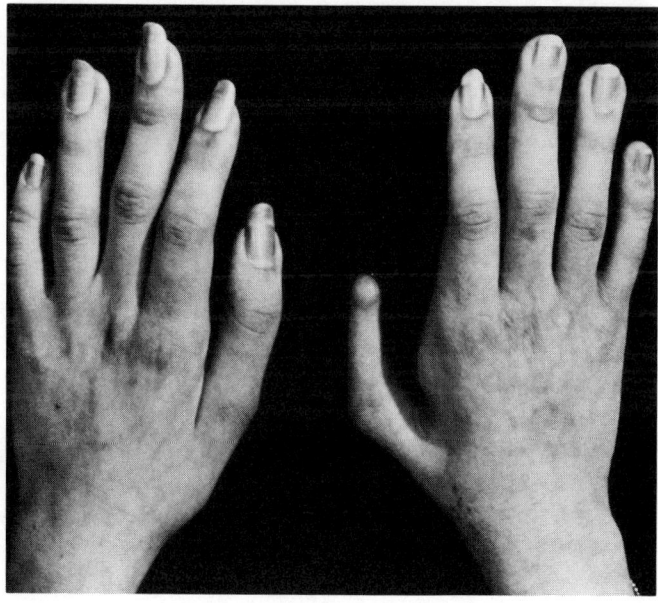

Figure 24-1 Triphalangeal thumb (digitalization). This patient has Holt-Oram syndrome.

Table 24-1 Features of the Physical Examination with Implication for the Presence of Inherited Disease

Name (MIM* number)	Dysmorphology Inheritance	Associated Features
Lens Dislocation		
Homocystinuria (236200)	Recessive	Osteoporosis, arachnodactyly, arterial and venous occlusion
Marfan's syndrome (154700)	Dominant	Aortic dissection, scoliosis, inguinal and femoral hernias, arachnodactyly, mitral valve prolapse, aortic regurgitation
Weil-Marchesani syndrome (277600)	Recessive	Short stature, brachydactyly, carpal tunnel syndrome
Sulfocyteinuria (272300)	Recessive	Unspecified neurologic disease
Pectus excavatum		
Isolated, isolated familial (169300)	Dominant	
Faciogenital dysplasia (305400)	X-linked	Hypertelorism, short stature, shawl scrotum, inguinal hernias, prominent umbilicus
Homocystinuria (236200)	Recessive	
Marfan's syndrome (154700)	Dominant	
Leopard syndrome (151100)	Dominant	Pulmonic stenosis, electrocardiographic abnormalities (prolonged QRS and PR intervals), sensorineural deafness, subaortic stenosis, lentigenes (dark freckling)
Noonan's syndrome (163950)	Dominant	Web neck, short stature, pulmonic stenosis, septal defects, cryptorchidism
Osteogenesis imperfecta (166200–166240, 259400–259450)	Dominant and recessive forms	Blue sclerae, deafness, poorly mineralized bone with multiple fractures, mitral insufficiency
Oto-palatal-digital syndrome (Taybi; 311300)	X-linked	Small stature, fusion of hamate and capitate bones, hip dislocation, clinodactyly, broad thumbs and great toes, conductive hearing loss
Thumb and Radial Defects		
Anemia and triphalangeal thumbs (205600)	Recessive	Leukopenia, hypoplastic anemia, ventricular septal defects
Fanconi's pancytopenia (227650)	Recessive	Small stature, pancytopenia, brown skin pigmentation (groin, anogenital, axillae, trunk), occasional leukemia
Holt-Oram syndrome (142900)	Dominant	Upper limb defects, atrial septal defect
Thrombocytopenia absent radius (TAR; 274000)	Recessive	Megakaryocyte hypoplasia, eosinophilia
Hemangioma and Telangiectasia		
Ataxia telangiectasia (208900)	Recessive	Café au lait pigmentation, ataxia, frequent respiratory infections, bronchiectasis, lymphopenia, lymphoid malignancies
Bloom's syndrome (210900)	Recessive	
Fabry's disease (301500)	X-linked	
Goltz's syndrome (305600)	X-linked	Coloboma of iris, syndactyly, hypoplasia of teeth
Klippel-Trenaunay-Weber syndrome (149000)	Dominant	Asymmetric limb hypertrophy, glaucoma, cataracts
Mafucci's syndrome (166000)	Dominant	Hamartomas, enchondromas with potential malignant change
Osler-Weber-Rendu syndrome (187300)	Dominant	Arteriovenous fistulas (lungs, brain)
Sturge-Weber syndrome (185300)	Dominant	Hemangioma of arachnoid and pia, macrocephaly, coloboma of iris, coarctation of aorta
Tuberous sclerosis (191100)	Dominant	Intracranial calcifications, subungual fibromas, renal cysts, café au lait pigmentation, hamartomas, astrocytoma, cystic changes in lung
Xeroderma pigmentosa (278700–278790)	Recessive	Multiple basal and squamous cell cancers

*Mendelian Inheritance in Man.

Sources: Emery AE, Rimoin DL: *Principles and Practice of Medical Genetics.* New York, Churchill Livingstone, 1990; and McKusick VM: *Mendelian Inheritance in Man,* ed 9. Baltimore, Johns Hopkins University Press, 1990.

A defect in stopping one motor impulse and substituting that impulse or direction for one that is opposite is a phenomenon that can on occasion be observed in the iris and is termed iridodonesis. On rapid horizontal eye motions with a light illuminating the iris from an acute angle a fluttering or wavelike motion of the iris is detected. This physical finding is always abnormal. It demonstrates a lack of posterior support for the iris that is normally provided by the lens. It is most commonly observed in patients who have had cataract surgery. These patients also have coloboma of the iris. However, observing iridodonesis in an individual who has had no previous cataract surgery suggests lens dislocation. Four disorders are listed in Table 24-2 that include lens dislocation as a feature of the disorder. This finding may be a clue to the possibility that a patient's shortness of breath or special foci of pain may be related to thromboembolic disease (homocystinuria). Severe chest pain or abdominal pain with iridodonesis may prompt a careful examination for aortic aneurysm and dissection (Marfan's syndrome).

It is rare that a patient is seen in the emergency department without a cardiopulmonary examination being performed. Deformities of the thorax should be easily observed (Fig. 24-2). Findings could include scoliosis, absence of the clavicles, or deformities of the sternum. This latter area is included in Table 24-1 as pectus excavatum. This is a significant depression of the sternum that has also been termed pectus recurvatum and funnel breast. A severe depression in the sternum can distort the position of the heart, thereby leading to artifactual abnormalities in the electrocardiogram and potential mild changes in the auscultatory findings on cardiac examination. This deformity may be significant in the setting of thromboembolic disease (homocystinuria); with chest or abdominal pains it may herald aortic dissection (Marfan's syndrome; Fig. 24-2); or suggest pulmonic stenosis or cardiac defects (Noonan's syndrome and leopard syndrome).

The hands and arms rarely escape observation in the emergency department and one would not expect defects of the thumb or radial aspect of the upper extremities to be missed (Fig. 24-1 and Table 24-1). However, the observation may not be correlated in the physician's mind with significant underlying pathology. Hypoplastic anemia is a significant feature of the Aase syndrome and Fanconi's pancytopenia. A more specific marrow defect with isolated thrombocytopenia is seen in the TAR syndrome (thrombocytopenia and absent radius). Defects of the thumb, especially those that demonstrate digitalization or a triphalangeal thumb (Fig. 24-1), should immediately bring to mind the potential for cardiac defects (Aase's syndrome and Holt-Oram syndrome).

In observing the skin, hemangiomas and telangiectasias (Table 24-1) may be grossly apparent or quite subtle. The cavernous hemangioma is a very prominent hamartoma that may be present at birth and appears as a red-blue spongy mass that is made up of connective tissue and vascular spaces often filled with blood. This has also been called a strawberry nevus. A more subtle lesion made of capillaries is called a nevus flammeus. Telangiectasias represent a more discrete vascular lesion produced by dilatation of small blood vessels. In the context presented here, telangiectasia connotes dilatation of blood vessels, but telangiectasia of the lymphatics can also occur. Subtle telangiectasia of the conjunctivae may be an important clue when seeing a young child for a respiratory difficulty who may in fact have bronchiectasis, skin pigmentation, or perhaps a history suggestive of ataxia (ataxia telangiectasia; Fig. 24-3). Unusual vascular telangiectasia on the buttocks or abdomen, termed angiokeratoma, may be an important observation in a male experiencing attacks of abdominal pain and may prompt the physician to look for evidence of renal insufficiency (Fabry's disease). Anemia and gastrointestinal bleeding may be a significant issue with the observation of multiple small vascular telangiectasia on the lips or tongue (Osler-Weber-Rendu disease; Fig. 24-4). Hemangioma of the face may provide a clue to underlying similar malformations of the arachnoid and suggest the possibility of coarctation of the aorta (Sturge-Weber syndrome). Adenoma sebaceum is a unique cutaneous abnormality that can be associated with hamartomas, potential seizure disorders with cranial calcifications, and cystic changes in the lungs that may be cause of a spontaneous pneumothorax (tuberous sclerosis; Fig. 24-5).

BLEEDING

Bleeding is a focal issue in the evaluation of many patients. It may be very easy to determine that blood loss is a major issue in a given patient on the basis of acute presentation and observed hematemesis, melena, or a clear history from the patient's family. The complete blood cell count (CBC) provides a white blood cell count, and with newer Coulter counters a platelet count as well as hemoglobin and hematocrit. Thus, a broad hematologic screen is obtained with every CBC. Genetic causes of bleeding are reviewed in Table 24-2. From the standpoint of inherited causes of bleeding, platelet abnormalities delineate an important group of disorders. The ramifications of variable degrees of thrombocytopenia will not be reviewed here, but it will be assumed that all patients with significant thrombocytopenia (less than $100,000/\mu L$) can manifest abnormal hemostasis, which may include easy bruising, epistaxis, and potential mucosal bleeding. Albinism is an unusual and easily appreciated clinical feature and, in association with thrombocytopenia, may suggest the Hermansky-Pudlak syndrome, which may be accompanied as well by pulmonary fibrosis or granulomatous colitis. Thrombocytopenia should prompt an assessment for splenomegaly. Gaucher's disease, one of the most

Table 24-2 Genetic Causes of Blood Loss

Name (MIM number)	Inheritance/Incidence	Associated Features
Thrombocytopenic		
Bernard-Soulier syndrome (231200)	Recessive	Giant platelets
Cyclic thrombocytopenia (188020)	Dominant	
Fanconi's pancytopenia (22765)	Recessive	Usually all marrow elements affected; café au lait spots, thumb deformity; aplasia of radius; malformation of heart, kidney
Gaucher's disease, types I, II, III (230800–231000)	Recessive heterozygote frequency in Ashkenazi Jews of 1 in 13	Splenomegaly; frequent Ashkenazi Jewish background; aseptic necrosis of femoral heads; distal femur deformity (Erlenmeyer flask); organic brain disease (seizure, dysphagia, visual disturbances) in cerebral forms II and III
Gray platelet syndrome (139090)		
Hermansky-Pudlak syndrome (20330)	Recessive	Albinism; pulmonary fibrosis (single report); granulomatous colitis (single report)
Isolated thrombocytopenia (188000)	Recessive	Incomplete penetrance in females
Thrombocytopenia and absent radius (274000)	Recessive	Distinct from Fanconi's pancytopenia without pigment, marrow, chromosomal, or late leukemic problems
Thrombocytopenia, elevated IgA, renal disease (314000)	X-linked	Cow's milk intolerance; occasional congenital heart disease and renal anomalies
Thrombocytopenia (X-linked; 313900)	X-linked	Mild tendency to infection and eczema (uncertain if distinct from Wiskott-Aldrich syndrome)
Thrombocytopenia, platelet dysfunction, hemolysis, imbalanced globin chain synthesis (314050)	X-linked	Moderate thrombocytopenia, petechiae, splenomegaly
Wiskott-Aldrich syndrome (301000)	X-linked/4 per 10^6 live male births in United States	Eczema; small platelets; prone to infection; high risk for lymphoreticular malignancies
Nonthrombocytopenic		
Coagulopathies		
Afibrinogenemia (202400)	Recessive	Occasional mild thrombocytopenic, possible hemorrhagic lesions of liver and bone
Factor VIII deficiency (hemophilia A; 306700)	X-linked	
Factor IX deficiency (hemophilia B, Christmas disease; 306900)	X-linked	
Factor XI deficiency (264900)	Recessive	More frequent in Jewish population; mild bleeding except postoperation when it may be severe and protracted
Glanzmann's thrombasthenia (273800)	Recessive	
Factor XIII deficiency (262800)	Recessive	Umbilical cord stump bleeding
Plasmin inhibitor deficiency (262850)	Recessive	Prolonged bleeding and ecchymosis after minor trauma
Platelet cyclo-oxygenase deficiency (262870)	Recessive	
Von Willebrand disease (193400)	Dominant	Occasional mitral valve prolapse; rare aneurysm and angiodysplasia
Portal Hypertension		
α_1-Antitrypsin deficiency (10740)	Dominant	
Erythropoietic protoporphyria (177000)	Dominant	Severe photosensitivity; cholelithiasis
Idiopathic hemochromatosis (235200)	Recessive	Generalized skin pigmentation; diabetes mellitus; hypogonadism, cardiomyopathy, arthritis
Tyrosinemia (276700)	Recessive	Acute porphyrialike illness
Wilson's disease (277900)	Recessive	Seizures, hemolytic anemia, impaired platelet aggregation, iris abnormality (Kayser-Fleischer rings)

Table 24-2 continued

Name (MIM number)	Inheritance/Incidence	Associated Features
Vascular Abnormalities		
Aortic aneurysm (cystic medial necrosis; 132900)	Dominant	
Ehlers-Danlos type I (gravis; 130000)	Dominant	Aortic dissection, hernia
Ehlers-Danlos type IV (130050)		
Ehlers-Danlos type V (305200)		
Ehlers-Danlos type VI (225400)		
Ehlers-Danlos type VII (130060)		
Pseudoxanthoma elasticum (177850)		

Sources: George JN, et al: Molecular defects in interactions of platelet with the vessel wall. *N Engl J Med* 311:1084–1098, 1984; and McKusick VM: *Mendelian Inheritance in Man*, ed 9. Baltimore, Johns Hopkins University Press, 1990.

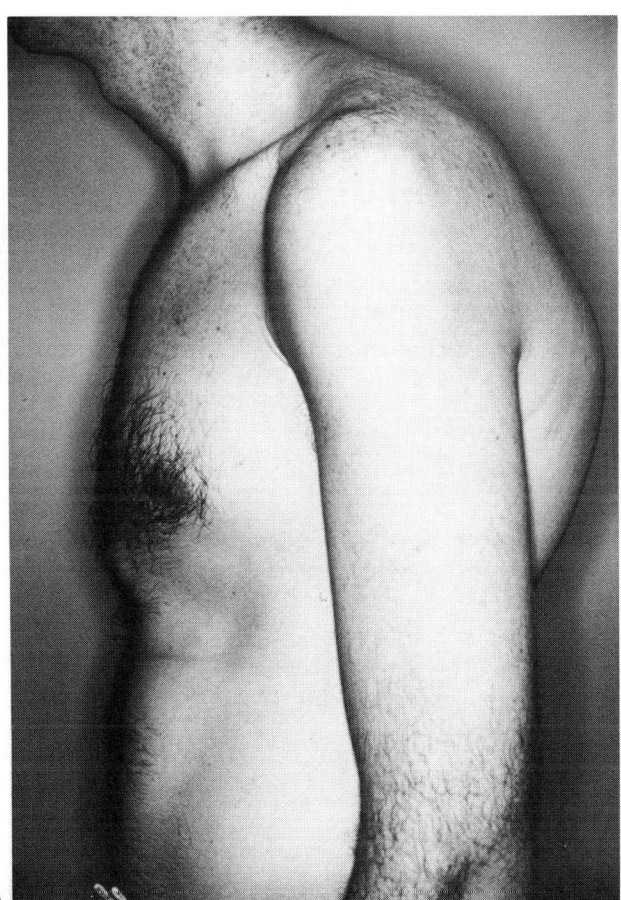
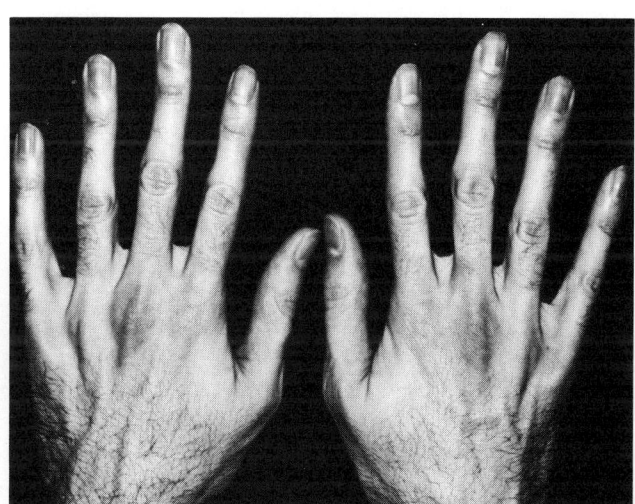
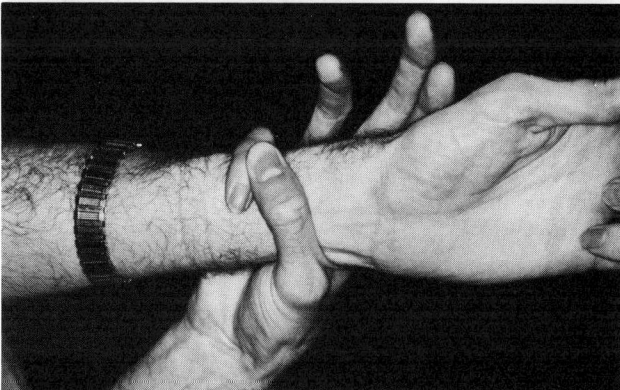

Figure 24-2 Marfan's syndrome. (**A**) Pectus deformity of the chest. (**B**) Arachnodactyly. (**C**) Another method of demonstrating arachnodactyly.

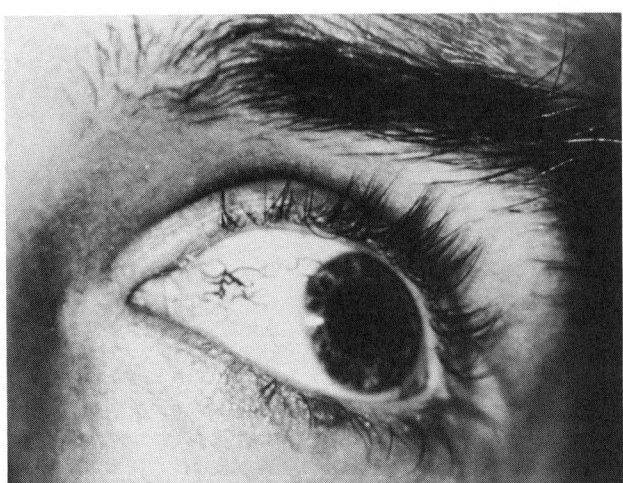

Figure 24-3 Telangiectasia of conjunctival vessels.

prevalent recessive disorders among Ashkenazi Jews, presents with that combination. Gaucher's disease is a multisystem disorder with well-recognized imperatives in genetic counseling. Frequent infections with evidence of eczema in a young male child that are accompanied by thrombocytopenia and petechiae are highly suggestive of Wiskott-Aldrich syndrome. TAR is a recessive disorder, and radial defects should be easily observed on physical examination. Even if previously diagnosed, the recognition of the syndrome allows one to be aware of potential cow's milk allergy and cardiac and renal anomalies that sometimes accompany the syndrome. Café au lait spots and thumb deformities, including aplasia of the radius, may occur in another recessive disorder that is unique for pancytopenia (ie, Fanconi's pancytopenia). There is a high risk of hematologic malignancy in this disorder as well as the possibility of malformations of the heart and kidneys.

ABDOMINAL PAIN

Abdominal pain is a common symptom in the emergency department. The history of similar symptomatology in other family members or a history of recurrence of similar symptoms in the patient, especially if previous diagnostic work has investigated the symptoms and failed to find an answer, might suggest an unusual cause of abdominal pain, such as a genetic illness. The genetic causes of abdominal pain are reviewed in Table 24-3. When one considers the possibility of vascular problems as the cause of abdominal pain, issues of abdominal aneurysm with dissection or abdominal angina are significant. The Marfan syndrome may be suggested by the observation of iridodonesis, striae on the lower back, an aortic valvular murmur, or abnormal stature characterized by a decreased upper segment to lower segment ratio, arachnodactyly (Fig. 24-2, B and C), and/or dolichocephaly.

While taking the blood pressure, one may notice an unusual irregularity of the skin in the antecubital fossa that may resemble the surface of an orange (peau d'orange). This

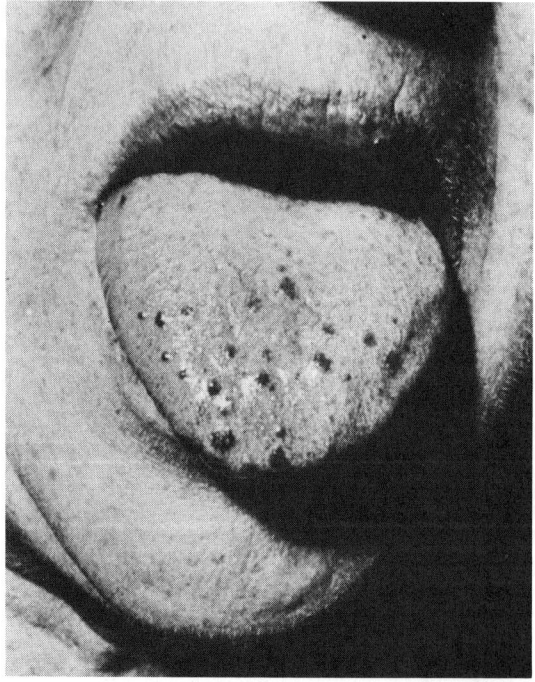
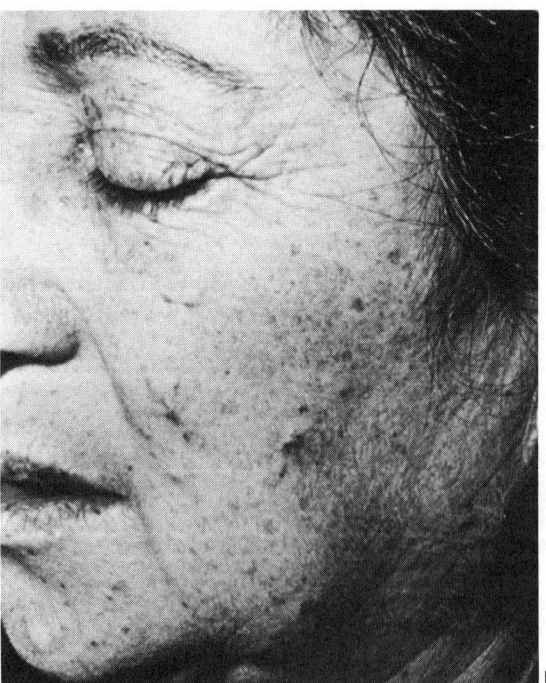

Figure 24-4 Osler-Weber-Rendu disease. (A) Vascular lesions on tongue. (B) Vascular lesions on face.

finding, along with joint laxity and angioid streaks of the retinae might suggest the diagnosis of pseudoxanthoma elasticum (PXE). Celiac artery stenosis has been observed in this condition and may, in fact, lead to symptoms of abdominal angina. This is classically described as abdominal pain occurring sometimes after meals or during any time of increased blood flow to the mesentery. It is important to note that PXE is also associated with vitreous hemorrhage following trauma to the globe and with gastrointestinal hemorrhage.

Inflammatory diseases of the abdomen comprise a wide range of problems, some of which can clearly be attributed to specific organ pathology, such as pancreatitis, peptic ulcer disease, or cholelithiasis. The abdomen is only one of numerous anatomical sites where sickle cell crisis may present with pain. Elevated bilirubin levels, splenomegaly, and a positive family history, which may include cholelithiasis at an unusually young age, may suggest a diagnosis of hereditary spherocytosis. If the hemolytic process is ongoing, the increased bilirubin pigment load may be a cause of gallstones and one should consider the possibility of cholecystitis as a cause of abdominal pain. Studies of pepsinogen deficiency have demonstrated that peptic ulcer disease can be inherited in a Mendelian dominant fashion. As mentioned previously, it is typical for inherited diseases to manifest at unexpected ages and with variable severity. Included in the consideration of premature ulcer disease must be the multiple endocrine adenomatosis syndromes, which may include gastrinomas with excessive secretion of gastric acid. These syndromes are frequently suspected on the basis of other organ system neoplasms or a positive family history for similar disorders. Armenian, Middle Eastern, or Jewish ancestry in the setting of recurrent bouts of abdominal pain and fevers may suggest to the astute observer the possibility of familial Mediterranean fever.

Inherited metabolic disorders may feature abdominal pain, and the etiology of this symptom is often poorly understood. The acute attack or inducible porphyrias may be considered when numerous episodes of abdominal pain have prompted significant evaluation without an established etiology. Many such patients have undergone exploratory laparotomies without success in determining the cause of the abdominal pain. These inducible forms of porphyria are all autosomal dominant. The presentation of a patient with an acute onset of facial or upper airway edema certainly can suggest an acute allergic phenomenon, but careful history may indicate that antecedent trauma and not allergen exposure is the trigger for severe edema. The additional history of abdominal pain in association with multiple episodes of edema may suggest the possibility of hereditary angioedema. Disordered peristalsis and intestinal dilation can occur in myotonic dystrophy. Unlike the sex-linked inheritance of the well-known Duchenne muscular dystrophy, myotonic dystrophy is inherited as a dominant condi-

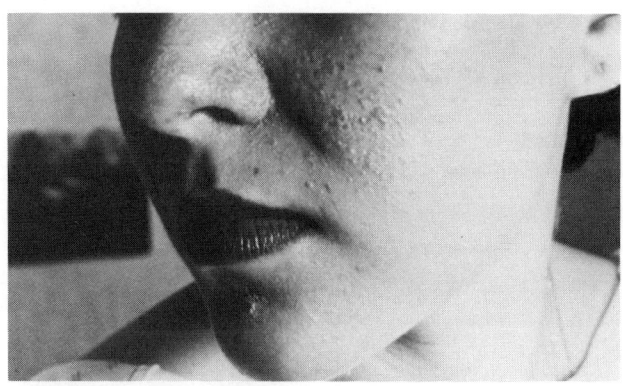

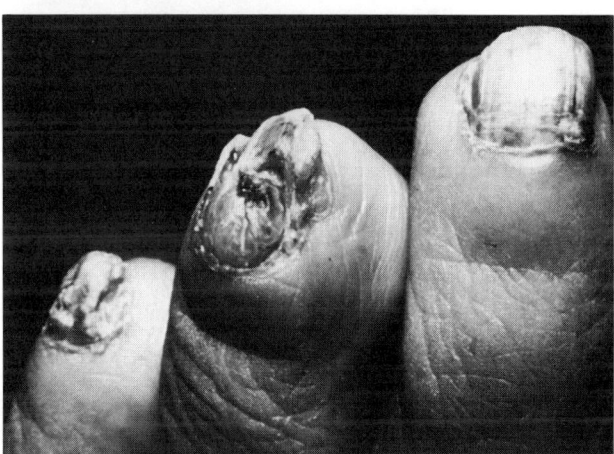

Figure 24-5 Tuberous sclerosis. (**A**) Adenoma sebaceum. (**B**) Subungual fibromas.

tion. Frontal balding and early cataracts accompany the disorder, and typical of dominantly inherited diseases the expression of the illness may be quite variable.

Neoplasms, for purposes of this discussion, should include both malignant and benign or hamartomatous presentations of disease. Colon cancer may present as abdominal pain. This might be the first sign of familial polyposis. This dominant condition is manifested in the preadolescent years, and the risk of colon cancer increases with advancing age. A family history of this condition should prompt significant concern regarding the patient. A hamartoma predisposition in the small bowel with rare risk of malignancy occurs in the Peutz-Jeghers syndrome. Freckling of the lips, buccal mucosa, and digits may be a very useful observation with respect to this disease. Despite the benign nature of the polypoid lesion of the small bowel, intussusception is possible. Multiple cutaneous neurofibromas, prominent café au lait spots with axillary freckling, scoliosis, and hemihypertrophy may all be seen in neurofibromatosis (Von Recklinghausen's disease; Fig. 24-6). These cutaneous neurofibromas are capable of sarcomatous degeneration. The multiple endocrine adenoma syndromes were noted previously and may

Table 24-3 Genetic Causes of Abdominal Pain

Name (MIM number)	Inheritance	Etiology of Pain	Associated Features
Inflammatory			
Sickle cell disease (141900.0243)	Dominant (codominant with other β-hemoglobinopathies)	Splenic infarction, cholecystitis	Black race
Hereditary spherocytosis (182900)	Dominant	Cholecystitis	
Familial Mediterranean fever (249100)	Recessive	Unknown (possible abnormal complement activation)	Elevated sedimentation rate, but a normal white cell count, Armenians and Sephardic Jews; amyloid
Familial lipoprotein lipase deficiency (23860)	Recessive	Pancreatitis	Hepatosplenomegaly, eruptive xanthomas, lactescence of plasma
Hereditary pancreatitis (167800)	Dominant	Pancreatitis	Fever and hyperamylasemia during attacks, occasional reports of thrombosis of portal or splenic vein
Hyperpepsinogen I, duodenal ulcer (126850)	Dominant	Duodenal ulcer	
Tremor, nystagmus, duodenal ulcer (190310)	Dominant	Duodenal ulcer	Essential tremor, often suppressed by alcohol
Metabolic			
Acute attack (inducible) porphyrias			
Acute intermittent porphyria (176000)	Dominant	Unknown	Excess urine porphobilinogen excretion
Hereditary coproporphyria (121300)	Dominant	Unknown	Excess urine porphobilinogen excretion
Variegate porphyria (176200)	Dominant	Unknown	Excess urine porphobilinogen excretion
Fabry's disease (301500)	X-linked	Lipid changes in ganglion cells of the autonomic nervous system	Vascular rash (angiokeratoma), fever, renal failure, characteristic corneal dystrophy seen on slit-lamp examination. Heterozygous females rarely develop renal failure and often show corneal changes
Hereditary angioneurotic edema (106100)	Dominant	Presumed visceral edema	
Myotonic dystrophy (160900)	Dominant	Disordered peristalsis and intestinal dilatation, cholelithiasis	Frontal balding, cataracts, muscle wasting, hypogonadism
Neoplastic			
Familial polyposis (175100)	Dominant	Colon carcinoma with obstruction	
Peutz-Jeghers syndrome (175200)	Dominant	Intussusception	Associated with development of ovarian (granulosa cell) tumor in females; freckles of lips, buccal mucosa, and digits
Pancreatic cancer (260350)	Recessive		
Multiple endocrine adenomatosis			
Type I (131100)	Dominant	Peptic ulcer disease, hyperparathyroidism, and hypergastrinemia	Islet cell tumor with hypoglycemia
Type II (171400)	Dominant	Pheochromocytoma	Medullary carcinoma of thyroid
Type III (162300)	Dominant	Pheochromocytoma	Mucosal neuromas, features resembling Marfan's syndrome (scoliosis, high arched palate, pectus excavation, pes cavus), medullary carcinoma of thyroid
Von Hippel-Lindau disease (193300)	Dominant	Pancreatic carcinoma, pheochromocytoma, renal cell cancer	Angiomata of retina in adults, angiomatous tumors of face

Table 24-3 continued

Name (MIM number)	Inheritance	Etiology of Pain	Associated Features
Von Recklinghausen's disease (162200)	Dominant	Sarcomatous degeneration of hamartomas	Cutaneous neurofibroma, café au lait pigmentation, axillary freckling, scoliosis, homihypertrophy
Vascular			
Marfan's syndrome (154700)	Dominant	Aortic dissection	Characteristic stature, mitral and aortic murmurs, scoliosis, joint laxity
Pseudoxanthoma elasticum (177850, 264800)	Dominant and recessive forms	Celiac artery stenosis (abdominal angina)	Claudication, hypertension, peau d'orange skin changes in flexural areas, choroiditis (angioid streaks)

Sources: McKusick VM: *Mendelian Inheritance in Man*, ed 9. Baltimore, Johns Hopkins University Press, 1990; and Nora JJ, Nora AH: *Genetics and Counseling in Cardiovascular Diseases.* Springfield, Ill, Charles C Thomas, 1978.

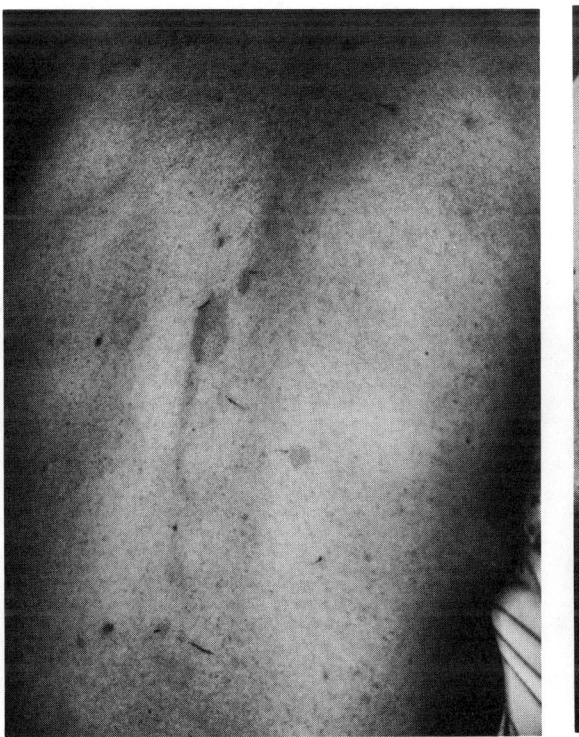 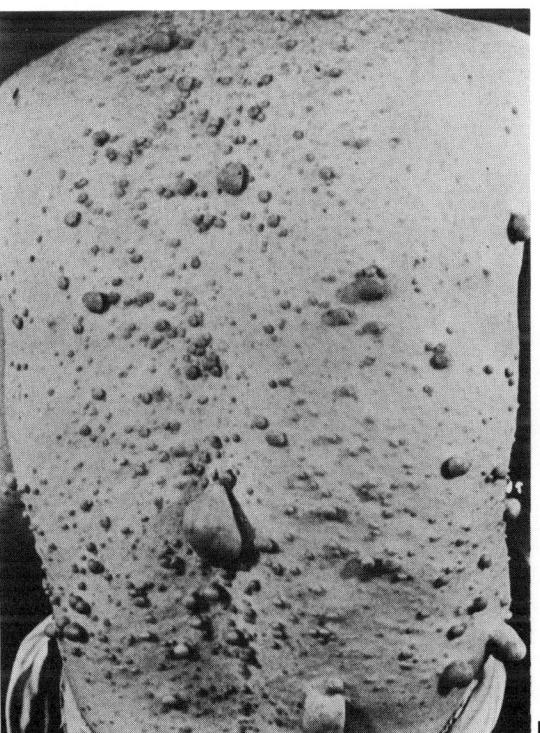

Figure 24-6 Neurofibromatosis (Von Recklinghausen's disease). (**A**) Café au lait spots. (**B**) Multiple hamartomas.

present with endocrine adenomas of the pancreatic islet cells that have metastatic potential in some cases. However, the excess secretion of certain hormones may produce a significant clinical picture with respect to abdominal pain or systemic illness. The excess secretion of gastrin by gastrinoma was mentioned previously. Metastatic islet cell cancer to the liver and multiple lipomas may be other features of an adenomatous process.

GENERAL CONSIDERATIONS

As noted previously in this chapter, dominantly inherited disorders are passed on from parent to child. Only one parent must possess the abnormal allele to pass the trait to the child. It is known that there can be variable expression of the dominant traits and, therefore, one may have the impression that a generation is skipped with respect to the disorder. With

Table 24-4 Ethnic Groups and Genetic Disease

Name (MIM number)	Inheritance	Associated Features
Jews		
Abetalipoproteinemia (Bassen-Kornzweig disease; 200100)	Recessive	Celiac syndrome, ataxia, acanthocytes, hypocholesterolemia
Afibrinogenemia (202400)	Recessive	Variable bleeding tendency; osseous and hepatic lesions of hemorrhagic origin
Bloom's syndrome (210900)	Recessive	Short stature, photosensitivity (facial rash)
Factor XI deficiency (264900)	Recessive	
Familial dysautonomia (Riley-Day syndrome; 223900)	Recessive	Lack of tearing, paroxysmal hypertension, postural hypotension, scoliosis, absent deep tendon reflexes, impaired taste
Familial Mediterranean fever (249100)	Recessive	Often in Armenians, amyloidosis
Gaucher's disease (types I, II, III; 230800)	Recessive	Thrombocytopenia and bleeding, splenomegaly, pathologic fractures
Gilles de la Tourette syndrome (137580)	Dominant	Echolalia, coprolalia, grunting, possible self-mutilation
Mucolipidosis type IV (252650)	Recessive	Corneal clouding, psychomotor retardation
Niemann-Pick disease (257200)	Recessive	Cherry-red macula
Spongy degeneration of central nervous system (271900)	Recessive	Infants only, megalocephaly, blindness, hypotonia
Tay-Sachs disease (272800)	Recessive	Paralysis, dementia, and blindness developing in early childhood
Torsion dystonia (224500)	Recessive	
Finnish		
Congenital nephrosis (Finnish nephrosis; 256300)	Recessive	
Diastrophic dysplasia (222600)	Recessive	Dwarfism, clubbed feet, scoliosis, malformed pinnae, "hitchhiker" thumb
Metaphyseal chondrodyplasia—McKusick type (cartilage-hair hypoplasia; 250250)	Recessive	Dwarfism with fine, sparse, light-colored hair, possible immune defect
Myoclonus epilepsy (25480)	Recessive	Ataxia, eventual dementia
Ornithinemia with gyrate atrophy of the retina (258870)	Recessive	Night blindness
French Canadians (Quebec)		
Agenesis of corpus callosum (218000)	Recessive	Mental retardation
Mucopolysaccharidosis type IVA (Morquio's syndrome; 253000)	Recessive	Corneal clouding, aortic valve defects
Tay-Sachs disease (272800)	Recessive	Paralysis, dementia, and blindness developing in early childhood
Tyrosinemia (276700)	Recessive	Acute porphyrialike illness, juvenile cirrhosis
Amish		
Ellis-van Creveld syndrome (225500)	Recessive	Dwarfism, polydactyly, congenital heart defects
Kaufman's syndrome (236700)	Recessive	Polydactyly, heart defects, transverse vaginal septum
Metaphyseal chondrodysplasia—McKusick type (cartilage-hair hypoplasia; 25025)	Recessive	Dwarfism with fine, sparse, light-colored hair, possible immune defect
Asians		
Alcohol sensitivity (103750)	Dominant	Marked facial flushing and moderate symptoms of intoxication with small amounts of alcohol
α-Thalassemia (141800)	Codominant	

Sources: Goodman RM, Motulsky AG: *Genetic Diseases among Ashkenazi Jews.* New York, Raven Press, 1979; and McKusick VM: *Mendelian Inheritance in Man*, ed 9. Baltimore, Johns Hopkins University Press, 1990.

respect to recessive disorders, the "double dose" phenomenon requires that an identical abnormal allele be inherited from each parent. The chances of such an occurrence in the general population is extremely small, but some recessive disorders, such as cystic fibrosis, have a relatively high heterozygote frequency in the American population. In other recessive disorders, despite a low overall frequency of the heterozygote state, certain groups have an unusually high frequency of this carrier status. Certainly, blood relatives define a unique group that will be more likely than the general population to have similar unique recessive alleles. The Amish of Pennsylvania, Jews of European ancestry, and other ethnic groups have an increased risk for certain recessive disorders. Genetic illnesses that have been observed in specific ethnic groups are compiled in Table 24-4. This is not meant to imply that these diseases are restricted to these ethnic groups. The physician might use information regarding ethnic background to enhance diagnostic considerations.

BIBLIOGRAPHY

Emery AE, Rimoin DL. *Principles and Practice of Medical Genetics*. 9th ed. New York: Churchill Livingstone; 1990.

George JN, Nurden AT, Phillips DR. Molecular defects in interactions of platelet with the vessel wall. *N Engl J Med*. 1984;311:1084.

Goodman RM, Motulsky AG, eds. *Genetic Diseases among Ashkenazi Jews*. New York: Raven; 1979.

McKusick VM. *Mendelian Inheritance in Man*. 9th ed. Baltimore: Johns Hopkins University Press; 1990.

Nora JJ, Nora AH. *Genetics and Counseling in Cardiovascular Diseases*. Springfield, IL: Thomas; 1978.

25. Infectious Disease Emergencies

RICHARD T. ELLISON III, MD
STEPHEN H. ZINNER, MD

Because an increasing number of patients are using the emergency department for walk-in medical care, the emergency physician must have a ready approach to the diagnosis and treatment of common infectious diseases. With the exception of meningitis or septicemia from any source, few of these infections are bona fide emergencies, but prompt recognition and appropriate therapy are required to prevent the spread of infection and the development of potentially life-threatening disease.

Physicians must elicit the history pertinent to the patient's presenting complaint. Certain epidemiologic clues are essential in the evaluation of bites, skin and soft tissue infections, respiratory infections, gastrointestinal infections, and genitourinary illness. The well-informed physician is able to obtain relevant data quickly.

Once the site of the presumed infection has been localized, the etiologic agent must be sought promptly and aggressively. The emergency department should have a simple mechanism to provide for the immediate preparation and reading of diagnostic material, such as Gram stains of sputum, pus, or cerebrospinal fluid; wet mounts of vaginal secretion or urine for the evaluation of trichomoniasis or yeast infection; routine urinalysis; and blood counts. Suitable cultures (eg, of pus, blood, or urine) must be performed, and the emergency physician must have a follow-up system to link the patient with the appropriate culture report. Careful instructions must be given to the patient if therapy is to be based on the results of this culture. A system for data retrieval and patient recall is essential, since emergency physicians may be the patient's only source of medical care. The responsibility of these physicians includes referral for follow-up visits when indicated, such as in the treatment of gonorrhea, urinary tract infections, and other infections that do not necessarily require hospitalization.

In life-threatening infections such as meningitis, the diagnosis must be made and specific appropriate therapy initiated in the emergency department with a minimum of delay. The physician must obtain spinal fluid for diagnostic studies and begin antibiotic therapy immediately. Rapid diagnostic tests such as countercurrent immunoelectrophoresis may be available and can provide rapid feedback to the physician.

Since many infections seen in the emergency department are self-limited, the presence of fever itself does not warrant a therapeutic course of antibiotics. It is imperative, however, that patients whose condition is initially evaluated in an emergency department have access to further medical care if the diagnosis and the proper therapeutic plan is not immediately apparent.

RESPIRATORY TRACT INFECTIONS

Common Cold

Acute upper respiratory infection is the most common illness in the United States. Children under 1 year of age have more than six "colds" each year, and most individuals average more than two per year until the fourth decade.[1] The etiology of upper respiratory infection is almost exclusively viral, although group A β-hemolytic streptococci may cause the illness in very young children. Rhinoviruses are responsible for 25% to 40% of upper respiratory infections; coronaviruses, parainfluenza viruses, adenoviruses, influenza virus, and respiratory syncytial viruses account for the remaining cases in which a pathogen can be identified. No causative agent is found in 30% to 40% of adults and up to 70% of children.[1]

Pathogenesis

More than 100 antigenically distinct viruses circulate among young children, who represent the main reservoir for the respiratory viruses. Although humoral immunity develops after exposure to a given viral strain, exposure to a new strain usually causes clinical illness. Viral infections induce large volumes of protein secretions from the nasal mucosa. In rhinovirus infections, viral particles are shed in the secretions beginning the day after infection; these reach a peak concentration 2 to 4 days into the clinical illness. Shedding may continue through day 7 of illness. It appears that these infections are spread by air-borne particles or by hand-to-hand contact after contamination of hands with nasal secretions.[2,3]

Diagnosis

After a 48- to 72-hour incubation period, a self-limited illness develops with rhinorrhea, nasal obstruction, and a scratchy or sore throat. Nonproductive cough, headache, malaise, myalgias, and loss of smell and taste are less common symptoms. Initially, the rhinorrhea is thin and watery, but over several days it evolves to a mucopurulent discharge. Low-grade fever may occur in children, but this is uncommon in adults. The symptoms are most prominent in the first 2 to 4 days of illness, and usually last for approximately 1 week. Occasionally patients may have persistent symptoms for up to 6 weeks. Examination shows a boggy nasal mucosa and obviously increased nasal secretions. Conjunctivitis and pharyngeal erythema may develop with adenovirus infections.

Differential Diagnosis

The typical syndrome is easily recognized, but a specific etiologic diagnosis usually cannot be made. Although allergic or vasomotor rhinitis can simulate an upper respiratory infection, they can be excluded by a careful history. It is important to rule out associated bacterial infections of the sinuses, the middle ear, or the lower respiratory tree. In patients with an atypical presentation, additional diagnostic studies should be performed (eg, a throat culture), especially in febrile children under 6 years of age.[4]

Treatment

Antibiotics have no role in the treatment of the common cold. Symptomatic therapy consists of oral or intranasal sympathomimetic decongestants, saline gargles, or oral analgesics. If necessary, antitussive therapy can be initiated with agents containing dextromorphan or benzonatate; codeine-containing cough suppressants are rarely required. A petrolatum-based ointment may be effective in preventing irritation of the nares by the nasal secretions. To limit the spread of infection, all patients should be instructed to wash their hands frequently.

Pharyngitis

One of the most frequent complaints brought to the emergency physician is pharyngitis or sore throat. While almost all episodes of pharyngitis are self-limited, the major concern associated with this illness is that rheumatic fever may develop from unrecognized or untreated streptococcal infection. The management of pharyngitis is therefore directed at both treating the acute event and limiting the risk of rheumatic fever.

Etiology

Acute pharyngitis is caused predominantly by viral agents (eg, rhinovirus, coronavirus, and adenovirus), by bacterial agents (eg, group A β-hemolytic *Streptococcus pyogenes*), and by both *Chlamydia pneumoniae* and *Mycoplasma pneumoniae*.[5,6] The following other infectious and noninfectious causes also have been implicated and should be considered:

I. Infection
   A. Localized pharyngitis
      1. Viral
          Herpes simplex virus (types 1 and 2)
          Coxsackievirus A
      2. Bacterial
          Mixed anaerobes
          Neisseria gonorrhoeae
          Corynebacterium diphtheriae
          Corynebacterium hemolyticum
          Treponema pallidum
          Group C streptococci
          *Hemophilus influenzae**
          *Neisseria meningitidis**
      3. Fungal
          Candida species
   B. Contiguous infections
      1. Epiglottitis
      2. Retropharyngeal abscess
      3. Peritonsillar abscess
   C. Systemic infection
      1. Viral
          Rubeola
          Rubella
          Influenza A and B viruses
          Parainfluenza virus

---

*Rare proven cause of pharyngitis.

Epstein-Barr virus
Cytomegalovirus
Poliomyelitis
Varicella zoster
Viral hepatitis
2. Bacterial
Bordetella pertussis
3. Parasitic
Toxoplasma gondii
II. Trauma
A. Heat
B. Chemical injury
C. Endotracheal intubation
III. Inhalation
A. Smoke
B. Industrial exposures
IV. Dehydration
V. Subacute thyroiditis

Unfortunately, a specific etiology will elude definition in 30% to 40% of patients.

Pathogenesis

Adenovirus, coxsackievirus A, and herpes simplex virus directly invade the pharyngeal mucosa and produce local inflammation. Other viruses, such as rhinovirus, induce pharyngeal inflammation secondary to nasopharyngeal infection. Group A β-hemolytic streptococci invade the pharyngeal mucosa and produce inflammation by release of extracellular toxins and proteases including streptolysin, hemolysin, DNAase, and hyaluronidase.

Diagnosis

Acute pharyngitis presents as a sore throat, which may or may not be accompanied by fever and erythema of the pharynx. The erythema, which is related to vascular congestion, may extend to the soft palate and uvula. Frequently, a patchy white or yellow exudate appears on the tonsils, and the anterior cervical lymph nodes may be enlarged and tender. The presentations of viral and bacterial pharyngitis are similar, and no single element or combination of clinical signs reliably indicates the etiologic agent.[4] Occasionally, additional findings may suggest a specific pathogen. A prior history of rheumatic fever is associated with an increased likelihood of both streptococcal pharyngitis and recurrent rheumatic fever. Coryza is occasionally associated with streptococcal infection in children but in adults is indicative of viral infection. A recent history of oral sexual contact increases the likelihood of gonococcal, syphilitic, or herpes simplex type 2 pharyngitis.

Petechiae of the soft palate are associated with viral pharyngitis. Vesicles on the tonsillar pillars and soft palate occur with herpes simplex and coxsackievirus infections (herpangina). The presence of gingivitis and fetid breath suggests a mixed anaerobic infection, usually referred to as Vincent's angina. An ulcer on the soft palate or pharyngeal wall may indicate a syphilitic chancre or a disseminated fungal infection. Any suggestion of stridor should prompt a search for epiglottitis.

Unilateral swelling of the pharyngeal wall is not a feature of uncomplicated pharyngitis and may represent a peritonsillar abscess or peripharyngeal infection. Membrane or pseudomembrane structures may develop in the pharynx in diphtheria, candidiasis, herpes simplex virus infection, Vincent's angina, and paraquat poisoning. Follicular conjunctivitis is present in 30% to 50% of patients with adenoviral pharyngitis. Posterior cervical adenopathy associated with pharyngitis is seen primarily in infectious mononucleosis. A scarlatiniform rash (an erythematous, fine, sandpaper-textured eruption on the trunk and extremities), circumoral pallor, and strawberry tongue are seen predominantly with streptococcal pharyngitis, although this may also occur secondary to localized staphylococcal infection.

Thrush is an infection of the buccal or gingival mucosa with *Candida* species. Although it is usually seen in immunocompromised patients or those on broad-spectrum antibiotics, it can occur in diabetics and, rarely, in completely normal hosts. Recently, an increased incidence of thrush has been seen in individuals infected with the human immunodeficiency virus (HIV), and it is a marker for acquired immunodeficiency syndrome (AIDS)–related complex. It is characterized by grayish-white plaques with an erythematous base on the buccal mucosa, gingivae, and tongue and by budding yeast forms in Gram-stained exudates.

Management

Except for the relatively less common infections with such pathogens as *C diphtheriae*, *Treponema pallidum*, and *Candida* species, pharyngitis is self-limited, and early antibiotic therapy shortens its duration only minimally. The primary concern in the management of pharyngitis is the prevention of acute rheumatic fever. If penicillin therapy is initiated within the first 10 days after the development of streptococcal pharyngitis, the risk of secondary acute rheumatic fever is significantly decreased. Antibiotic treatment also decreases the incidence of other complications of streptococcal pharyngitis and aids in limiting epidemics of streptococcal disease, but these effects are not related to the early timing of therapy. The optimal management of pharyngitis is therefore to treat patients having streptococcal disease with antibiotic therapy and to manage almost all other patients symptomatically.

As there are no diagnostically distinguishing characteristics of streptococcal pharyngitis, a throat culture should be considered in all patients with pharyngitis. However, with the decreasing incidence of rheumatic fever in industrialized nations, it is not economically appropriate to perform throat cultures on all patients with pharyngitis. Several studies have suggested guidelines for performing throat cultures on only selected patients with pharyngitis, and one community health care system has used such guidelines without either a decrease in the number of throat cultures that grew group A β-hemolytic streptococci or the development of a single case of rheumatic fever.[4,7–9]

Throat cultures should be performed at least on all patients over the age of 2 years who have symptoms of pharyngitis without coryza, who have a fever greater than or equal to 38°C (100.4°F) of undetermined cause and upper respiratory tract symptoms; on children aged 2 to 6 years with unexplained fever greater than 38.3°C (101°F) regardless of symptoms; and all symptomatic patients who reside in a community having epidemic disease. Throat cultures should also be performed on currently asymptomatic household contacts of patients who have diagnosed streptococcal pharyngitis and who themselves had pharyngitis without coryza in the previous 2 weeks.[4,7–9]

For optimal throat culture results, a sterile cotton or Dacron swab is used to brush vigorously the mucosa of both tonsillar pillars and the posterior pharyngeal wall. The swabs should be streaked on sheep blood agar or selective streptococcal agar within 15 minutes. Unless special pathogens such as *N gonorrhoeae* or *C diphtheriae* are suspected, the cultures should only be used to identify group A β-hemolytic streptococci. Isolation of other bacteria is neither clinically nor economically useful.

In most patients, it is reasonable to wait for the results of the throat culture before beginning antibiotic therapy. Recent data suggest, however, that severe group A streptococcal pharyngitis with fever and lymphadenitis may respond more rapidly to early therapy.[10] Additionally, reliance on standard culture techniques is dependent on adequate follow-up for all patients with throat cultures positive for group A β-hemolytic streptococci. Therefore, in patients with severe pharyngitis or in those for whom follow-up cannot be ensured, a rapid streptococcal test kit should be used.[11] Patients with a positive result should receive immediate antibiotic treatment, and those with a negative result should have a standard throat culture. Immediate antibiotic therapy is also warranted in patients with a scarlatiniform rash or a history of rheumatic fever.

Penicillin remains the drug of choice for treatment of streptococcal pharyngitis. For adequate therapy significant pharyngeal levels of penicillin must be maintained for 10 days. This can be achieved with either penicillin V potassium (250 mg by mouth four times a day for 10 days) or one intramuscular injection of 1.2×10^6 U of benzathine penicillin. The latter route is preferred for poorly compliant patients. For penicillin-allergic patients, erythromycin (250 mg by mouth four times a day for 10 days) may be used (40 to 50 mg/kg/day of erythromycin ethylsuccinate for a child).

Gonococcal pharyngitis should be treated with ceftriaxone (250 mg intramuscularly). If patients cannot receive ceftriaxone, ciprofloxacin (500 mg orally) as a single dose appears to be the most effective alternative.[12] Oral ampicillin and amoxicillin and intramuscular spectinomycin regimens have unacceptable failure rates for gonococcal disease at this site.

Any patient with suspected diphtheria should be immediately hospitalized. Initial therapy requires antibiotic treatment with either penicillin or erythromycin and the use of diphtheria antitoxin.

The first step in therapy of thrush is to eliminate predisposing factors such as antibiotics when possible. Nystatin may be given as a 4- to 6-mL oral suspension of 100,000 U/mL four times a day to be swished around the oral cavity or as tablets or suppositories. Clotrimazole, given as oral troches (10 mg troche two to five times a day) that are allowed to dissolve in the mouth, is also effective. Oral ketoconzaole (200 mg/day; 5 mg/kg/day for children) may also be used.[13] Because an acid milieu is required for absorption of this agent, however, it should not be given with antacids, cimetidine, or ranitidine. Fluconazole (100 to 200 mg/day orally) can be used to treat thrush in patients with HIV infection or in those in whom other therapy fails.

Follow-up and referral should be arranged for all patients with pharyngitis whose symptoms persist for more than 10 days because uncomplicated pharyngitis usually resolves in this time period.

Epiglottis and Croup

See Chapter 72, Obstructive Airway Disease.

Sinusitis

Acute sinusitis is an inflammation of the accessory nasal sinuses that predominantly develops from bacterial infection. *Hemophilus influenzae* and *Streptococcus pneumoniae* are the most frequent pathogens in adults and children; together they account for more than 60% of documented infections. *Moraxella catarrhalis,* group A β-hemolytic streptococci, and other oral streptococci and anaerobes produce most of the other infections.[14–17] *Staphylococcus aureus* and Gram-negative rods are rarely responsible for community-acquired sinusitis but are the major pathogens in hospital-acquired disease. Additionally, acute fungal sinusitis due to *Aspergillus* or *Mucor* species may occur as fulminant infections in immunocompromised patients. Clinically, chronic sinusitis is considered a persistent or recurrent mucopurulent nasal discharge from a sinus with an associated roentgenographic abnormality. Bacterial pathogens may be present, as they are in acute sinusitis, but this may simply represent colonization of the sinus with nasal flora.

Pathogenesis

The sinuses are lined with a ciliated columnar epithelium covered with mucus produced by goblet cells. This mucus blanket is the primary defense against infection, having an intrinsic antibacterial effect mediated by immunoglobulin A (IgA), lactoferrin, and lysozyme. In addition, a synchronized, rhythmic movement of the epithelial cilia continuously moves mucus out of the sinuses. This mucociliary clearance mechanism removes particulate matter that enters the sinuses and becomes trapped in the mucus (see Chapter 82, Ear, Nose, and Throat Emergencies).

Viral upper respiratory tract infection is the most common factor predisposing patients to acute sinusitis. This infection produces edema of the nasal mucosa and increases the viscosity of the overlying mucus, resulting in obstruction of the sinus ostia and mucus stasis. Inhaled bacteria are not cleared from the sinuses and this leads to infection. Nasal polyps, septal deviation, surgery, or nasal packing can similarly induce sinusitis by ostial obstruction. Acute sinusitis may also develop from contiguous spread of infection from a dental abscess, from infected soft tissues, or from fractures or osteomyelitis of surrounding bone.

Persistent purulent sinusitis, recurrent episodes of acute sinusitis, and/or local trauma may lead to gross and histologic changes in the sinus anatomy that predispose to chronic sinusitis. The epithelium becomes richer in stratified squamous epithelial cells, and the cilia may disappear. Goblet cell hyperplasia can develop with excessive mucus production resulting in chronic mucus stasis. Rarely, congenital abnormalities of the mucociliary clearance mechanism may lead to chronic sinusitis. In cystic fibrosis, mucus is abnormally viscous and is not cleared readily, while in the immotile cilia syndrome there is impaired ciliary activity.

Diagnosis

Clinically acute sinusitis is associated with fever, chills, nasal obstruction, and asymmetric head or facial pain. Purulent nasal discharge may or may not be present depending on the degree of obstruction of the involved sinus. Classically, the pain in frontal sinusitis has been described as localizing to the forehead, in maxillary sinusitis to the face, in ethmoidal sinusitis to the superior lateral nose, and in sphenoidal sinusitis to the base of the skull. Unfortunately, however, it is much more common for the pain to be nonlocalizing.

There may be tenderness over the involved sinus and transillumination can be diagnostic, particularly with maxillary sinusitis. With the room darkened, an intense, well-shielded light source is held against the patient's skin just below the orbital ridge and the hard palate observed through the mouth for the transmission of light. Complete opacity of the sinus is indicative of an abnormal sinus, although partial or dull light transmission is a nonspecific finding.[14,15]

Standard roentgenographic evaluation of the sinuses should be performed to confirm sinusitis when the diagnosis is not clear. Sinusitis is suggested by an air-fluid level, complete opacification, or marked mucosal thickening of the sinus wall to greater than 5 mm.[14] Computed tomography (CT) and magnetic resonance imaging (MRI) are both highly sensitive (and expensive) techniques to define sinusitis.

Precise bacteriologic diagnosis of acute sinusitis can be determined only by direct sinus puncture. Bacteria found by nasal swab cultures do not always correlate with infecting organisms within the sinus. Although lavage via catheter into the sinus ostia often yields infecting organisms, these cultures are usually contaminated with nasal flora. Gram stain and aerobic and anaerobic cultures of material recovered by direct sinus puncture usually will establish the diagnosis, but this technique should be reserved for immunocompromised hosts and patients with persistent acute sinusitis unresponsive to initial therapy.

Differential Diagnosis

The major alternative diagnosis when considering acute sinusitis is a prolonged viral upper respiratory tract infection that may simulate the clinical presentation of sinusitis. Cancer, tuberculosis, mucormycosis, aspergillosis, syphilis, and Wegener's granulomatosis should be considered in the differential diagnosis of chronic sinusitis.

Treatment

Acute sinusitis requires treatment with antibiotics effective against both *Streptococcus pneumoniae* and *H influenzae*. At present, oral ampicillin (500 mg every 6 hours) or amoxicillin (500 mg every 6 to 8 hours) is the best initial agent in most communities. In areas with a high prevalence of ampicillin-resistant *H influenzae* or in the penicillin-allergic patient, trimethoprim-sulfamethoxazole can be used. Cefaclor (500 mg every 6 hours by mouth or 20 mg/kg in three divided doses for children) and amoxicillin-clavulanate (500 mg every 8 hours in adults and 40 mg/kg/day in 3 divided doses for children) are additional alternatives for infection with ampicillin-resistant *H influenzae*. Treatment should be continued for 10 days. Decongestants may promote drainage, and mild analgesics may relieve pain.

Adequate follow-up must be provided to ensure clinical resolution. The complications of poorly treated or untreated sinusitis are severe and include osteomyelitis, meningitis, brain abscess, orbital cellulitis, and cavernous sinus thrombosis.[18] Patients with persistent acute sinusitis not responding to therapy should be referred for direct sinus puncture to precisely define the etiology and guide therapy.

The optimal therapy for chronic sinusitis has not been defined. A complete evaluation by an otolaryngologist is often useful, and surgical drainage might be beneficial.

Otitis

Otitis Externa

Sometimes called "swimmer's ear," otitis externa is an inflammation of the external auditory canal that may be produced by infection, trauma, seborrheic dermatitis, or sensitization to medications. Infection is most commonly caused by *Pseudomonas aeruginosa*, although *Streptococcus pyogenes, Staphylococcus aureus, Proteus* species, and *C albicans* may be isolated. The squamous epithelium of the auditory canal is delicate and may be irritated by the retention of excess moisture. Subsequent inflammation may be exacerbated by scratching with cotton swabs or other objects.

The patient complains of pain and tenderness of the affected ear. The pain may increase with movement of the jaw, and the patient may not be able to sleep on the involved side. Usually, there is no history of an upper respiratory tract infection and no fever. The external canal is tender and erythematous, and it may be completely obstructed by edema and cerumenous exudate. When it can be visualized, the tympanic membrane is found to have normal landmarks and movement.

The initial therapeutic approach is to remove any irritant and to prevent further exposure to irritants. The ear canal should be irrigated carefully. A 5- to 7-day course of a topical antimicrobial agent such as topical 2% acetic acid solution or combined antibiotics and corticosteroids in an acid vehicle may be useful. If such therapy is deemed appropriate, a cotton wick should be inserted down the length of the canal to ensure adequate penetration of the medication and to discourage continued self-trauma. Very prolonged therapy with topical bacitracin, neomycin, polymyxin B, or chloramphenicol should be avoided, because these agents may induce sensitization and contact dermatitis.

Erysipelas and cellulitis are occasional complications of otitis externa. Malignant otitis externa, a deep soft tissue infection, may develop if the infecting organism invades the junction of the cartilaginous and osseous external auditory canals; in such cases *Pseudomonas aeruginosa* is usually found alone or with other pathogens.[19] This complication is seen predominantly in elderly diabetic patients. These patients have persistent pain and may have facial nerve paralysis. They should be hospitalized for intravenous therapy and may require surgical drainage.

Otitis Media

Although otitis media is one of the most common illnesses in the pediatric population, ambiguities in its definition have obscured understanding of the disease. This discussion focuses on the management of acute otitis media, defined as signs and symptoms of acute illness associated with the acute accumulation of a middle ear effusion. Chronic otitis media with persistent symptoms and effusion requires continued evaluation and should be referred to a specialist.

Otitis media may be related to infection, allergy, or anatomical abnormalities. Bacteria are isolated from approximately 90% of specimens obtained by needle aspiration of the middle ear in children with acute otitis media. *Streptococcus pneumoniae* and nontypable *H influenzae* are found in up to 60% of cases. *Moraxella catarrhalis, Staphylococcus aureus*, group A β-hemolytic streptococci, and anaerobic bacteria produce the remaining infections.[20] In infants less than 6 weeks of age, the percentage of infections caused by Gram-negative bacilli and *Staphylococcus aureus* may be higher, but the predominant pathogens remain *H influenzae, Streptococcus pneumoniae*, and *M catarrhalis*.[21] Viruses and *Mycoplasma* play only a minimal role in acute otitis media.

Pathogenesis

The pathogenesis of otitis media is related to abnormalities in the ventilation of the middle ear. If the eustachian tube is obstructed by anatomic changes or edema of the nasal mucosa due to allergy or viral infection, the middle ear is isolated as a closed space. Oxygen and carbon dioxide are absorbed through the middle ear mucosa, and negative pressure subsequently develops in the middle ear chamber. With the negative pressure, fluid crosses the mucosa into the middle ear space, and bacteria migrate up the eustachian tube to infect the effusion.[22] Recent work suggests that intercurrent upper respiratory tract viral infections are major triggering events for this sequence.[23]

Diagnosis

The diagnosis of otitis media should be suspected strongly in any patient with a febrile illness, otalgia, and acute hearing loss; however, only 50% of children may have symptoms relating to the ear. Instead, a child may have gastrointestinal complaints or may show increased irritability. The peak frequency of otitis media occurs between 1 and 2 years of age, and infection recurs in 40% to 50% of patients.

Pneumatic otoscopy is the simplest technique to identify otitis media. It is relatively precise, but not definitive. The full tympanic membrane should be visualized, and its appearance, landmarks, the presence of a light reflex, and motion should be evaluated. With the pneumatic otoscope, gentle pressure changes in the external auditory canal cause the tympanic membrane to move. The normal membrane has a rapid fluttering movement; absent or sluggish movement indicates an effusion. When tympanic membrane motion is normal, the presence of erythema alone is not indicative of otitis media.

Tympanocentesis, aspiration of the middle ear, is the only definitive diagnostic study for otitis media. It is a relatively difficult procedure in an uncooperative patient and should be reserved for those cases in which a pathogen must be isolated as with a critically ill or immunocompromised host, a patient with a suppurative complication, or a patient whose condition deteriorates during antibiotic therapy. Nasopharyngeal cultures have been proposed as a method of determining the etiologic agent in otitis media, but their usefulness is limited by high rates of false-positive and false-negative results. This technique is helpful only in detecting the presence of resistant bacterial strains.

Therapy

Although acute otitis media can resolve without treatment, the decrease in suppurative complications since the advent of antibiotics suggests that therapy of otitis media should be based on the use of antimicrobial agents.[24] The selected antibiotic should be active against both *H influenzae* and *Streptococcus pneumoniae*. Ampicillin (50 to 70 mg/kg/day) and amoxicillin (40 mg/kg/day) have been preferred because they are effective against the predominant pathogens, are inexpensive, and are able to penetrate into the middle ear. With the increasing incidence of *H influenzae* strains resistant to these agents, other antibiotics have been evaluated. Penicillin plus a sulfonamide (100 to 150 mg/kg/day), erythromycin (50 mg/kg/day) plus a sulfonamide, trimethoprim (8 mg/kg/day) with sulfamethoxazole (40 mg/kg/day), cefaclor (40 mg/kg/day), amoxicillin-clavulanate, and cefuroxime axetil or cefixime (slightly more expensive) are all effective alternative regimens for otitis media. Although no clinical studies have been performed to determine the duration of therapy required, otitis media should be treated empirically for 7 to 10 days. Decongestants and antihistamines are used frequently, although controlled clinical trials have not demonstrated efficacy in children.[25] Surgical drainage by myringotomy should be considered in immunocompromised patients and patients who worsen on therapy, but this is not usually necessary in the treatment of the normal host.

In most patients, symptoms resolve within 72 hours, but middle ear effusion may persist for up to 6 months. This may predispose patients to more frequent recurrence and, possibly, to chronic otitis media. Consequently, all patients with otitis media should be seen in follow-up if they remain symptomatic after 3 or 4 days of therapy. If the patient is severely ill, tympanocentesis should be performed. If mild signs persist, then therapy should be adjusted to cover less common pathogens, particularly β-lactamase–producing *H influenzae* and *M catarrhalis*. Patients with persistent effusion beyond 2 weeks should be referred for continued evaluation of their condition.

Oral-Facial Infections

Oral Ulcerative and Vesicular Infections

The most common lesions of the oral mucosa are aphthous ulcers or "canker sores," the etiology of which is unknown. They are recurrent, painful, 1- to 3-mm vesicular lesions that appear singly or in clusters on the buccal mucosa, gingiva, and palate. The vesicles ulcerate, leaving a clean white or gray crater. They occur more frequently in periods of stress and during menses and resolve spontaneously in several days. At present, there is no effective therapy, but saline mouthwashes or topical anesthetic ointments may provide symptomatic relief.

Herpes simplex viruses types 1 and 2 may produce a gingivostomatitis with vesicular ulcerating lesions on the gingiva, buccal mucosa, lips, tongue, and palate.[26] In the initial infection, there is a 2- to 12-day incubation period that is followed by fever, pharyngeal irritation, and diffuse involvement of the oral mucosa with multiple lesions. The typical lesion begins as a vesicle on an erythematous base that rapidly ulcerates. Cervical lymphadenopathy is typical. Infrequently, halitosis and extension of the vesicular lesions onto the lips and cheeks may be seen. Patients normally have a gradual recovery over 7 to 10 days, although their clinical appearance may be unchanged during much of this period. The diagnosis can be confirmed if multinucleated giant cells are found on microscopic examination of material scraped from the base of a fresh ulcer or aspirated from a vesicle. Viral cultures and immunofluorescent antibody slide tests are also available for diagnosis of herpes infections, but they are relatively expensive and should be reserved for situations when a precise diagnosis is essential.

Following the patient's recovery from the initial infection, gingivostomatitis may recur through reactivation of viral organisms that remain in the trigeminal ganglion. Such a recurrence is characterized by a brief syndrome of pain or tingling, followed by the appearance of vesicular lesions that rapidly ulcerate and crust. The mucosal involvement is much less severe than that of the initial infection, and associated adenopathy and systemic toxicity are absent. Lesions may recur as often as several times a month or as infrequently as once or twice a year.

At present, there is no effective therapy for permanently eradicating primary or recurrent gingivostomatitis caused by herpes simplex viruses. Although treatment of an acute episode will not prevent relapse, however, the antiviral agent acyclovir can slightly shorten both the duration of symptoms and viral shedding in immunosuppressed hosts.[27] Comparable data are not available on its use in immunocompetent hosts. Even so, herpes gingivostomatitis is in general a benign illness in the normal host. Considering the cost of therapy, the risks of developing drug-resistant strains of virus, and the limited data available on toxicity of prolonged acyclovir therapy, at present routine therapy with acyclovir does not appear to be warranted. Instead, symptomatic treatment can be offered as for aphthous ulcers. Immunosuppressed or severely ill patients should receive acyclovir treatment intravenously (15 mg/kg/day) or orally (200 mg five times daily) for 7 days.

Several other pathogens may also produce oral lesions. Group A coxsackieviruses cause two syndromes with oral ulcerations, both of which occur primarily but not exclusively in children. Herpangina is a febrile illness that occurs predominantly in summer or autumn epidemics. It is manifested by fever, malaise, pharyngitis, and multiple discrete vesicles on the tonsils, anterior pillars, soft palate, and uvula. It is self-limited and resolves in 5 to 7 days. Hand-foot-mouth disease, a variant of herpangina with a similar seasonal incidence, is associated with tender, painful vesicles on the palms and soles, as well as in the oral cavity. Compared with those in herpangina, the vesicles are small in number, and they may occur anywhere in the oral cavity. This is also a self-limited illness that resolves in approximately 7 days.

Acute necrotizing ulcerative gingivitis is a synergistic anaerobic infection of the periodontal gingiva in patients with poor oral hygiene. It occurs in young adults as an acute febrile illness with bleeding and ulceration of the gingiva, pseudomembrane formation of the interdental papillae, foul breath, and cervical adenopathy. It is mediated by the endogenous fusobacteria and spirochetes of the oral flora and is rare in edentulous patients. The treatment of choice is oral penicillin and hydrogen peroxide mouthwashes.

Oral lesions may be seen as manifestations of several systemic illnesses. Varicella can result in oral vesiculation with its characteristic exanthem. Syphilis not only can involve the mouth with a primary chancre, but also may produce oral lesions during the secondary and tertiary stages. One third of patients with secondary syphilis have nonpainful, symmetric, silvery mucosal ulcerations in the oral cavity. These mucosal lesions occur concurrently with the exanthem of secondary syphilis and are highly infectious. Erythema multiforme and pemphigus vulgaris are two noninfectious processes that must also be considered with oral mucosal ulcerations.

Deep Space Infections

Infections of the oropharynx may extend into the deep fascial spaces of the head and neck, producing maxillary space infections, peripharyngeal abscesses, retropharyngeal abscesses, and submandibular space infections.[28] The natural history of each of these infections is determined by the anatomy of the involved space.

Infection of the canine space anterior to the maxilla can occur secondary to abscesses of the maxillary incisor and canine teeth. As with all infections of dental origin, mixed aerobic and anaerobic bacteria from the mouth predominate, especially *Bacteroides* species, *Peptostreptococcus* species, and *Streptococcus* species. Swelling of the upper lip and soft tissues anterior to the maxilla is dramatic. The infection can spread to the infratemporal space, to the maxillary bone and sinus, and into the orbit.

The peripharyngeal space, or pharyngomaxillary space, is a cone-shaped potential space bordered medially by the pharyngeal wall, laterally by the medial pterygoid muscles of the mandible and the parotid gland, and superiorly by the base of the skull. The carotid sheath passes through this space and may be involved in any infection of this space. Because of its location, the peripharyngeal space can become infected in association with suppurative pharyngitis, a molar tooth abscess, mastoiditis, or suppurative parotitis. The usual pathogens are mixed aerobic and anaerobic bacteria, although suppurative parotitis is usually due to *Staphylococcus aureus*. Clinically, the patient is febrile and may have sore throat, dysphagia, hoarseness, marked facial pain, trismus, medial displacement of the pharyngeal wall, and swelling and induration of the soft tissue below the angle of the jaw. Typically, only a few of these findings are present in an individual patient, and the presentation can be very subtle. Complications from this infection arise either from spread to the retropharyngeal space or from involvement of the carotid sheath, which can cause septic carotid arteritis and septic jugular thrombophlebitis.

The retropharyngeal space lies directly posterior to the posterior pharyngeal wall and anterior to the prevertebral fascia of the cervical and thoracic spine; it extends from the base of the skull to the superior mediastinum. Infection in this space most frequently arises from direct trauma to the posterior pharyngeal wall or contiguous spread of infecting organisms that have caused pharyngitis, peripharyngeal abscess, or vertebral osteomyelitis. The infection is usually caused by the same pathogens as peripharyngeal abscesses. Patients are febrile and complain of dysphagia. Laryngeal edema and bulging of the posterior pharyngeal wall may develop, resulting in upper airway obstruction that resembles epiglottitis. Bilateral cervical adenopathy is common. Upper airway obstruction and secondary suppurative mediastinitis are major complications.

The submandibular space lies below the floor of the mouth and extends posteriorly to the hyoid bone. Direct trauma or erosion of the mandible by a dental abscess permits both aerobic and anaerobic organisms to enter this area and produce an infection termed Ludwig's angina.[29] This space has very loose connective tissue, and once invaded, cellulitis rapidly involves the entire space without typical abscess formation. The patient is febrile and has severe dysphagia. There is submental induration and tenderness, and the entire floor of the mouth is elevated. The upper airway can be rapidly compromised as the tongue is moved superiorly and posteriorly.

Since peripharyngeal, retropharyngeal, and submandibular infections can obstruct the larynx, airway protection is the first priority when such an infection is suspected. With advanced infection (particularly submandibular) this may be difficult, and blind oral or nasotracheal intubation should be avoided when possible. Alternative approaches to airway control are tracheotomy, cricothyroidotomy, or intubation under direct visualization with a fiberoptic laryngoscope. When the situation is not this urgent, a lateral radiograph of the neck with soft tissue technique should be performed to evaluate the airway and to exclude epiglottitis.

With the airway controlled, patients should be hospitalized and kept under supervision with arrangements made for possible rapid surgical intervention. Parenteral antibiotic therapy directed against mixed aerobic-anaerobic flora should be initiated. The best evaluated therapy is penicillin G (8×10^6 to 12×10^6 U/day administered intravenously in 6 divided doses). Because of increasing penicillin resistance in oral *Bacteroides* species, however, in patients with life-threatening infections metronidazole (15 mg/kg loading, then 7.5 mg/kg every 6 hours) should be added. Clindamycin and chloramphenicol are appropriate alternatives in patients with penicillin allergy. Occasionally antibiotic coverage for *Staphylococcus aureus* should be considered when the infection has spread from a parotitis or vertebral osteomyelitis. In these instances, a semisynthetic penicillinase-resistant penicillin, such as nafcillin or oxacillin, should be used in high doses (2 g administered intravenously every 4 hours) in place of penicillin. Because the pathophysiology of these infections is initially more typical of cellulitis than of an abscess, it is possible to treat these deep spaces with antibiotic therapy alone. If there is any indication of airway compromise or progression during antibiotic therapy, however, surgical drainage should be performed emergently (see Chapter 85, Dental Emergencies).

Bronchitis

See Chapter 72, Obstructive Airway Disease.

Pneumonia

Acute pneumonia, "the captain of the men of death," remains a leading cause of morbidity and mortality both as a common community-acquired illness and a major nosocomial infection. Relatively few organisms are responsible for most cases of community-acquired pulmonary infection, but a more complete differential of infectious etiologies includes:

I. Viral
   Children: Respiratory syncytial virus
   Parainfluenza virus
   Influenza A virus
   Adults: Influenza A virus
   Parainfluenza virus
   Adenovirus
   Rhinovirus
   Varicella
   Measles
   Cytomegalovirus
II. Bacterial
   Pneumococcus (*Streptococcus pneumoniae*)
   H influenzae
   Mixed anaerobic species
   Enterobacteriaceae: *Klebsiella pneumoniae*
   Escherichia coli
   Enterobacter species
   Citrobacter species
   Pseudomonas aeruginosa
   Serratia marcescens
   Acinetobacter species
   Staphylococcus aureus
   Legionella pneumophila
   Other *Legionella* species
   Neisseria meningitidis
   Streptococcus pyogenes
   Streptococcus viridans
   Moraxella catarrhalis
   Francisella tularensis
   Yersinia pestis
   Bacillis anthracis
   Nocardia asteroides
   Actinomyces israelii
III. Mycobacterial
   Mycobacterium tuberculosis
   Mycobacterium kansasii
   Mycobacterium avium-intracellulare
IV. Mycoplasmal
   Mycoplasma pneumoniae
V. Chlamydial
   Chlamydia trachomatis
   Chlamydia pneumoniae
   Chlamydia psittaci
VI. Rickettsial
   Coxiella burnetii (Q fever)
VII. Fungal
   Histoplasma capsulatum
   Coccidioides immitis
   Aspergillus species
   Cryptococcus neoformans
   Blastomyces dermatitidis
   Pneumocystis carinii

In young children the predominant pathogens are respiratory syncytial and parainfluenza viruses, with *Mycoplasma pneumoniae, Streptococcus pneumoniae, H influenzae,* and *Chlamydia trachomatis* being implicated somewhat less frequently. In adolescents and adults, *S pneumoniae* and *M pneumoniae* are the most frequent causes of community-acquired pneumonia, with mycoplasmal disease predominating in adolescents and younger adults. *Streptococcus pneumoniae* was traditionally considered the cause of up to 90% of cases of pneumonia requiring hospitalization, but there has been increasing recognition of infections due to *Legionella pneumophila, H influenzae,* mixed oral anaerobes, and *Chlamydia pneumoniae*. Pneumococcal disease now appears to cause at most 60% of severe pneumonias, and there may be regional differences in the relative frequency of the different pathogens.[30,31] Mixed oral aerobic and anaerobic bacteria and Gram-negative bacilli, including *Klebsiella pneumoniae* and *H influenzae,* are more frequent in the elderly and individuals compromised by chronic alcohol consumption. Influenza virus is major worldwide cause of epidemic penumonia in the winter months, and this viral pneumonia can be complicated by superimposed pneumococcal, staphylococcal, and meningococcal bacterial pneumonias.

Immunosuppressed individuals, including those with HIV infection, may present with pneumonias due to a wide spectrum of unusual pathogens.[32] For the HIV-infected patient, *Pneumocystis carinii* is the predominant pathogen, although these patients are also predisposed to pneumonias due to cytomegalovirus, fungi (including *Histoplasma capsulatum, Cryptococcus neoformans,* and *Coccidioides immitis*), and mycobacteria.[33] Additionally, patients with early HIV infection have an increased incidence of bacterial pneumonias, with *Streptococcus pneumoniae* being the predominant pathogen.

Patients who acquire pneumonia while they are in the hospital also may be infected with pneumococci, but infection with staphylococci and Gram-negative rods is more common. In some communities, *Legionella* species are also major nosocomial pathogens.

Pathogenesis

The primary host defenses against pulmonary infection act to prevent infectious agents from reaching the pulmonary parenchyma.[34] The complex airflow past the nasal turbinates and through the nasopharynx and oropharynx aerodynamically filters most inhaled particles larger than 10 μm in diameter as the particles impact on the mucus layer lining the respiratory mucosa. This mucus contains secretory IgA and a variety of proteolytic enzymes and has intrinsic antimicrobial activity. The gag reflex limits the aspiration of oral secretions, and the cough reflex acts to expel large quantities of mucus and particulate material from the lower respiratory tree. Infectious agents that do reach the lower respiratory tree are usually trapped in mucus lining the bronchi and bronchioles. This surface is also covered with a ciliated epithelium that acts to continuously sweep the mucus layer from the peripheral to central airways and then out of the lungs. Those microorganisms that bypass these defenses to reach the pulmonary alveoli may be killed either by alveolar macrophages or by intrinsic antimicrobial activity of the intraalveolar secretions.

Pneumonias due to viral agents, mycoplasmae, chlamydiae, rickettsiae, fungi, mycobacteria, and some unusual bacteria develop as a result of the intrinsic invasiveness of the microorganisms, and even normal hosts may develop infections. However, bacterial pneumonias usually develop because of an impairment in host defenses rather than from contact with particularly virulent organisms. Most individuals aspirate small amounts of pharyngeal secretions during sleep, but the possibility of aspiration is greatly increased when the gag reflexes are blunted by sedatives, ethanol ingestion, heavy smoking, or advanced age. Alcohol, tobacco, and viral infection may impair mucociliary transport, and chronic tobacco use can destroy ciliated epithelia. Congestive heart failure increases intra-alveolar fluid and hinders bacterial clearance by alveolar macrophages.

Although most pulmonary infections are due to inhalation of pathogens or aspiration of oral pharyngeal secretions, pneumonias will occasionally develop from hematogenous seeding of the pulmonary parenchyma. Varicella pneumonia and metastatic staphylococcal pneumonia due to right-sided endocarditis are examples of such infections.

Diagnosis

Community-acquired pneumonia usually presents as one of three patterns: acute lobar pneumonia, atypical generalized pneumonia, or aspiration pneumonia. Acute lobar pneumonia, of which pneumococcal pneumonia is the prototype, usually develops in middle-aged or elderly patients during the winter or early spring, frequently following an upper respiratory tract viral infection. These infections are often associated with underlying illnesses, such as diabetes, chronic obstructive pulmonary disease, or congestive heart failure. The most frequent pathogen in this setting is *Streptococcus pneumoniae,* but *H influenzae, L pneumophila, Staphylococcus aureus, K pneumoniae,* other enteric Gram-negative bacteria, and mixed oral anaerobes can produce this illness.

Lobar pneumonia begins with the abrupt onset of high fever and shaking chills, accompanied by a cough that produces yellow-green to rusty, possibly blood-streaked, sputum. Pleuritic chest pain over the involved lung is common; tachypnea and tachycardia are present. Physical examination typically reveals percussion dullness, increased tactile and vocal fremitus, and bronchovesicular breath sounds with crepitant inspiratory rales over the involved lung segments. The chest roentgenogram usually reveals dense lobar consolidation in one or more lobes, although it may show patchy localized infiltrates. Pleural effusions may occur late in the course of pneumococcal or *Legionella* pneumonia. Significant early effusions are suggestive of empyema. The peripheral white blood cell count is elevated to 15,000/μL to 30,000/μL with a predominance of neutrophils and a shift to immature forms. Arterial blood gas determinations may show significant hypoxemia and an increased alveolar-arterial gradient. Serum levels of hepatic enzymes may be elevated.

Atypical pneumonia is most commonly due to *Mycoplasma pneumoniae*. It is usually seen in young adult or adolescent patients and does not have a particular seasonal predominance. Frequently, there is a prodrome of 3 to 4 days of malaise, myalgias, coryza, headache, low-grade fever less than 39°C (102.2°F), and a cough that is initially nonproductive.[35] Pleuritic chest pain early in the course is less common than in lobar pneumonia. Physical examination may reveal some localized crackles, but other chest findings are not impressive. Chest roentgenogram reveals diffuse, patchy infiltrates often out of proportion to the physical findings. Lower lobe involvement is common and may be unilateral or bilateral. Pleural effusions are unusual, and the white blood cell count is normal or only mildly elevated, often with a relative lymphocytosis.

When atypical pneumonia is due to *Mycoplasma pneumoniae,* it can be associated with bullous or hemorrhagic myringitis, upper respiratory tract symptoms, myalgias, migratory arthralgias, and gastrointestinal symptoms; rarely, it is associated with meningoencephalitis, transverse myelopathy, and ascending paralysis.

A carefully obtained history can aid in evaluating for other possible causes of atypical pneumonia. For example, a recent visit to the San Joaquin Valley in California or other parts of the southwestern United States increases the likelihood of coccidioidomycosis. Histoplasmosis is endemic in the Ohio River Valley and may be associated with exposure to bird or bat guano in this region. Exposure to animals or birds increases the likelihood of psittacosis, tularemia, plague, brucellosis, and Q fever.

Legionnaire's disease may initially resemble atypical pneumonia, but the patient's condition tends to worsen with the development of headache, altered sensorium, and diarrhea—often with laboratory findings of hyponatremia, hypophosphatemia, and liver enzyme elevations. Specific culture or direct fluorescent antibody tests on expectorated sputum or pleural fluid may reveal the presence of *L pneumophila.*

Aspiration pneumonia is associated with an abnormal gag reflex and occurs most commonly in alcoholics or patients who have vomited heavily. The findings depend on the type of material aspirated.[36] Aspiration of toxic secretions, particularly gastric acid, may cause an immediate and intense chemical pneumonitis with acute dyspnea, bronchospasm, and the production of frothy sputum. Patients may be hypotensive, and diffuse inspiratory crackles are present on auscultation. Roentgenograms show mottled densities in the lower lobes that may progress to diffuse infiltrates and possibly pulmonary cavities. Arterial blood gas measurements demonstrate severe hypoxia with normal or low Pco_2. Aspiration of solid particulate matter may cause acute respiratory distress beginning immediately after the aspiration if the particle obstructs the trachea or a major bronchus. Aspiration of particles small enough to reach a peripheral airway produces cough, atelectasis, and recurrent localized infection due to oral anaerobic bacteria.

After the aspiration of oropharyngeal secretions, fever, chills, anorexia, weight loss, and a cough productive of copious, foul-smelling, and foul-tasting sputum develop gradually over an 8- to 14-day period. Physical examination reveals dullness to percussion, increased breath sounds, and bronchovesicular respiration. This process is usually localized to gravitationally dependent lobes. If aspiration took place while the patient was in the supine position, the superior segments of the lower lobes and the posterior segments of the upper lobes are involved; if the patient was in the upright position, the basal segments of the lower lobes are usually involved. Pleural effusions may occur. The peripheral white blood count is usually elevated.

While these clinical syndromes can aid in defining the probable etiology, there is enough overlap in presentation that laboratory studies should aid in diagnosis. Examination of the lower respiratory tract secretions is particularly important. Samples of sputum can be obtained by expectoration, transtracheal aspiration, flexible fiberoptic bronchoscopy, or lung puncture. Examination of expectorated sputum is the simplest, safest, and most economical technique, although it must be recognized that this sample is contaminated with oropharyngeal flora. The sputum specimens should be observed for amount, purulence, color, and odor; and a representative portion of mucopurulent material should be selected for microscopic examination by Gram stain. The presence of columnar epithelial cells and polymorphonuclear leukocytes associated with a predominant bacterial flora intracellularly and extracellularly is indicative of lower respiratory tract infection with these organisms. Alternatively, the presence of large squamous epithelial cells and multiple bacterial forms indicates significant sample contamination with oral secretions. This type of specimen is unreliable for definitive diagnosis.

At best, the Gram-stained sputum smear permits only putative identification of the offending organisms.[37] However, given that contaminating normal mouth flora are always present in expectorated sputum samples, this study is more reliable than sputum culture in defining the etiology of a pneumonia. An expectorated sputum culture can provide etiologic information about a pneumonia only when microscopic examination of the sample indicates that there is relatively little oral contamination *and* there is a good correlation between the culture results and Gram-stain reading. Additional diagnostic studies should be considered when a more definitive diagnosis is required in patients with an uninterpretable expectorated sputum Gram stain or in patients with hospital-acquired pneumonia where the potential pathogens are less predictable.

Transtracheal aspiration by means of a flexible catheter passed through the cricothyroid membrane to the trachea is a technique that avoids specimen contamination with oral secretions.[38] Because of the potential complications of the procedure, it is rarely performed today. In selected situations where a precise diagnosis is necessary, however, it remains useful. In performing a transtracheal aspiration, first a pillow is placed under the patient's shoulders to hyperextend the neck. The cricothyroid membrane, which is between the cricoid and thyroid cartilage, is identified, cleansed with an antibacterial solution, draped, and locally anesthetized. A large-bore indwelling intravenous catheter needle is inserted through the cricothyroid membrane into the trachea. The flexible catheter within the needle is advanced quickly, and the needle is withdrawn, leaving the catheter in place. A sterile syringe is connected to the catheter, and a sputum sample is aspirated. If a sample cannot be obtained in this way, 3 to 5 mL of a nonbacteriostatic sterile saline can be injected into the trachea to induce coughing and produce a suitable specimen. The catheter is removed and firm pressure applied to the puncture site. A Gram stain and aerobic and anaerobic cultures should be performed on the specimen.

Significant complications, including subcutaneous emphysema, local bleeding, and, rarely, death, may follow transtracheal aspiration; consequently, this should not be a routine procedure in the management of pneumonia. It should be reserved for situations when determining the exact etiology is essential. The risk of these complications can be reduced by strict attention to technique and careful patient selection.[38] Minimal morbidity has occurred when (1) the patient is cooperative, (2) the normal cricothyroid membrane is easily identifiable, (3) the results of coagulation studies are normal, (4) arterial P_{O_2} of at least 70 mmHg can be maintained with supplemental oxygen, and (5) the procedure is performed by an experienced physician.

Any pleural effusion associated with a pneumonic process should be aspirated for diagnosis and therapy. In a patient with an undiagnosed pneumonia this procedure is preferred to the other invasive approaches for collecting pulmonary secretions. Blood cultures should be performed on all patients ill enough to be considered for hospitalization, even though the results are positive in only 30% to 40% of patients with bacterial pneumonia.

Additional diagnostic studies can be helpful in selected clinical situations. If tuberculosis is suspected on the basis of patient history or chest roentgenogram, sputum samples should be examined microscopically with an acid-fast smear and sputum sent for mycobacterial culture. In approximately 50% of patients with mycoplasmal pneumonia, cold hemagglutinin titers rise in the first 7 to 10 days of illness and may remain elevated for several weeks. Occasionally, these titers are elevated in infection caused by adenoviruses, Epstein-Barr virus, rubella, influenza, and *Chlamydia psittacii*. Fluorescent antibody techniques may be applied to smears of sputum or pleural fluid for the identification of *L pneumophila* in Legionnaire's disease, and pneumococcal polysaccharides may be detected in the urine or serum by countercurrent immunoelectrophoresis in patients with pneumococcal pneumonia and bacteremia.

Differential Diagnosis of Pneumonia

Pulmonary embolism, atelectasis of a pulmonary segment, congestive heart failure, neoplastic disease, hypersensitivity pneumonitis, collagen vascular diseases, sarcoidosis, and lipoid pneumonia are diagnostic considerations in the evaluation of a pulmonary infiltrate. Although the clinical presentation may indicate an infectious process, the precise diagnosis may be difficult and require additional studies. Pulmonary infarction may be associated with fever and a wedge-shaped pulmonary density on roentgenogram.

Pulmonary angiography, if it is performed early, establishes the diagnosis. In congestive heart failure, a chest roentgenogram may show pleural effusions that change position with properly performed lateral decubitus radiography and an infiltrate that may clear rapidly following diuretic therapy.

Treatment

The management of patients with pneumonia depends on the clinical setting.[39] Young individuals with uncomplicated pneumonia and no underlying disease can be managed outside the hospital, provided that they can be followed closely. Most other patients should be hospitalized. For outpatient therapy, pneumococcal pneumonia can be treated effectively with procaine penicillin (300,000 to 600,000 U intramuscularly twice a day for 7 to 10 days) or phenoxymethyl penicillin V (250 mg orally four times a day). Penicillin-allergic patients or those with an atypical pneumonia presentation can be treated with erythromycin (500 mg orally every 6 to 8 hours). Penicillin is not effective for *Mycoplasma pneumoniae*. Patients with suspected *H influenzae* in communities with a low incidence of β-lactamase–producing *H influenzae* can be treated effectively with oral ampicillin or amoxicillin. Where β-lactamase–producing *H influenzae* strains are prevalent, trimethoprim-sulfamethoxazole, cefuroxime-axetil, or amoxicillin-clavulanate is an effective alternative agent. Psittacosis or Q fever pneumonias can be treated with tetracycline (500 to 750 mg orally four times a day for 10 to 14 days) or doxycycline (100 mg orally twice a day for 10 to 14 days).

For patients requiring hospitalization, the initial antibiotic selection should be based on the clinical presentation and examination of the sputum Gram stain (or other pulmonary secretions if special studies were employed). Patients with presumed pneumococcal disease can be treated with penicillin G intravenously. Because there is an increasing prevalence of relatively resistant *Streptococcus pneumoniae* in the United States, seriously ill patients should receive 6×10^6 to 12×10^6 U intravenously per day (in divided doses given every 4 hours) until results of susceptibility testing for the organism are available. In patients with mixed flora or a predominance of small Gram-negative coccobacillary organisms on Gram stain, ampicillin (1 to 2 g intravenously every 4 to 6 hours) is again appropriate in communities with a low incidence of β-lactamase–producing *H influenzae*. Otherwise, an antimicrobial regimen that is active against both *S pneumoniae* and β-lactamase–producing *H influenzae* should be used. A number of intravenous agents could be used in this situation, including trimethoprim-sulfamethoxazole or a second-generation cephalosporin (cefoxitin, cefuroxime, cefonicid, or cefamandole). When large Gram-negative rod bacteria are the predominant organisms found in appropriate sputum samples, initial therapy should be directed against *K pneumoniae* and *E coli* with either a third-generation cephalosporin or an extended-spectrum penicillin in conjunction with an aminoglycoside agent. If *Legionella* infection is suspected, erythromycin (500 mg intravenously every 6 hours) should be added to the above regimens.[40]

Patients with presumed community-acquired aspiration pneumonia can be managed initially with aqueous penicillin G (8×10^6 to 12×10^6 U intravenously for 7 to 10 days in divided doses given every 4 hours, including at least 5 afebrile days at the end of the course). Clindamycin (600 to 900 mg intravenously every 6 hours) is an alternative for the penicillin-allergic patient.[41]

For individuals presenting with severe atypical pneumonia without a history suggestive of psittacosis, Q fever, influenza, or other unusual pathogens such as acute coccidioidomycosis or histoplasmosis, the possibility of *Pneumocystis carinii* pneumonia should be considered and diagnosis attempted through the use of either an induced sputum specimen stained for the organism or fiberoptic bronchoscopy.[42] Therapy can be initiated with intravenous trimethoprim-sulfamethoxazole (trimethoprim dosage of 15 mg/kg/day given every 6 to 8 hours).[43] For patients with profound sulfonamide allergy, pentamidine (3 to 4 mg/kg/day) is an appropriate alternative, although its use should usually be limited to patients with a confirmed diagnosis of *P carinii* infection.

GASTROINTESTINAL INFECTIONS

Acute Gastroenteritis

The diagnosis of acute gastroenteritis encompasses nausea, vomiting, abdominal cramping, and diarrhea, an increase in the frequency or fluidity of bowel movements in relation to the patient's usual routine. The symptoms may either be predominantly nausea and vomiting or diarrhea, and there may or may not be associated fever and systemic toxicity.

Etiology

Gastroenteritis can be due to a diverse group of infectious and noninfectious agents. Viral agents are the major cause of sporadic diarrhea in children under two years of age and can produce epidemics of explosive nausea, vomiting, and diarrhea in both children and adults.[44,45] Bacterial agents, including *Campylobacter jejuni*, *Shigella* species, *Salmonella* species, *Clostridium* species, *E coli*, *Yersinia enterocolitica*, and *Vibrio cholerae*, produce varied illnesses, ranging from profuse watery diarrhea to severe dysentery with rectal pain and bloody, purulent stools.[45] The protozoans *Giardia lamblia* and *Cryptosporidium* produce watery diarrhea, and *Entamoeba histolytica* may produce a dysenteric syndrome. While the intestinal helminths typically cause asymptomatic infection, they can occasionally produce chronic mild gastroenteritis.

Drug ingestion is a frequent noninfectious cause of acute diarrhea. Many cholinergic agents, antacids, broad-spectrum antibiotics, and antimetabolites produce diarrhea. Acute psychologic stress may be responsible for diarrhea with symptoms usually limited to the morning hours. Toxin or allergen ingestion can cause severe self-limited gastroenteritis. Diverticulitis, fecal impaction, radiation proctitis, ischemic colitis, and inflammatory bowel disease may first present as acute diarrheal illnesses.

Pathophysiology

Acute gastroenteritis due to infectious agents develops from the oral ingestion of microorganisms or their toxins.[45] The defenses against the pathogenic microorganisms include the normal acid environment of the stomach at pH 4, which kills over 99.9% of ingested coliform bacteria (but not *Shigella* species). Normal intestinal motility further helps to clear pathogenic microorganisms, thus decreasing the time available to establish infection. Intraluminal antibodies, either those secreted from plasma cells in the lamina propria of the bowel wall or serum immunoglobulins that migrate through the mucosal capillaries, also block infection. In addition, the pre-existing enteric flora of the normal small and large bowel limit colonization with pathogens.

The effectiveness of these defenses against specific bacteria is quite variable. An inoculum of 10^5 to 10^8 organisms is required to establish enteritis with *E coli*, but the ingestion of only 10 to 50 *Shigella dysenteriae* or *Salmonella* species can produce disease.[45]

If infection is established, gastroenteritis may be produced either by toxin formation or by invasion of the intestinal wall (Table 25-1). Toxin-associated illness can be further subdivided by the type of toxin and by whether the toxin is ingested preformed or is produced within the lumen of the gut. Enterotoxins induce diarrhea by stimulating the small bowel mucosa to produce intestinal secretions at a rate that surpasses the reabsorptive ability of the gut, resulting in profuse watery diarrhea with isotonic fluid loss. Most of the enterotoxin-associated pathogens do not invade the intestinal mucosa. The prototype of the enterotoxin-mediated diarrheas is cholera, in which toxin induces cyclic adenosine monophosphate activity by stimulating adenyl cyclase. Enterotoxigenic *E coli*, one of the major causes of traveler's diarrhea, produces a similar toxin.

Bacterial cytotoxins cause necrosis of the intestinal mucosa and induce an intense polymorphonuclear inflammatory response. The colon is the major site of involvement. The cytotoxin produces a dysenteric syndrome with abdominal cramping and small amounts of bloody or purulent stool. Antibiotic-induced pseudomembranous colitis due to the toxin of *Clostridium difficile* is an example of disease mediated by cytotoxins.

Neurotoxins can induce upper gastrointestinal cramping, nausea, vomiting, and hyperperistalsis. Unlike enterotoxins

Table 25-1 Pathogenic Mechanisms of Infectious Gastroenteritis

Mechanism	Action	Agent
Toxin production	Enterotoxic	Vibrio cholerae Escherichia coli Clostridium perfringens Bacillus cereus Shigella dysenteriae
	Cytotoxic	Clostridium difficile Clostridium perfringens Shigella dysenteriae
	Neurotoxic	Staphylococcus aureus Bacillus cereus Clostridium botulinum Shigella dysenteriae
Invasion of the intestinal wall	Intraepithelial	Shigella dysenteriae Escherichia coli Vibrio parahaemolyticus Campylobacter jejeuni Entamoeba histolytica Neisseria gonorrhoeae
	Submucosal	Salmonella spp Yersinia enterocolitica Campylobacter jejeuni
Undefined		Viral (eg, Norwalk agent, rotavirus) Giardia lamblia Cryptosporidium spp

and cytotoxins, which are produced within the intestinal lumen by ingested bacteria, neurotoxins are ingested preformed; disease develops without an established infection. The most frequent neurotoxin-associated illness is *Staphylococcus aureus* gastroenteritis, with acute gastroenteritis developing 2 to 7 hours after ingestion of toxin-contaminated food.

Bacterial invasion of the intestinal epithelium, which occurs primarily in the colon and distal small bowel, produces an inflammatory response and a dysenteric bloody diarrhea syndrome. *Shigella* species, enteroinvasive *Escherichia coli* strains, and *Entamoeba histolytica* are the major pathogens in this category. The lamina propria of the large and small bowel is invaded by *Salmonella, Y enterocolitica,* and *Campylobacter jejeuni*. Diarrhea produced by these organisms may be watery and bloody and is probably mediated both by enterotoxins and by alteration in the intestinal wall due to bacterial invasion. Bacteremia and systemic febrile illness may accompany these infections.

The pathogenesis of gastroenteritis caused by other well-defined pathogens remains controversial. Viral agents, including rotavirus and the Norwalk agent, appear to infect the mucosa of the proximal small bowel, induce watery diarrhea, and alter the motor function of the upper gastrointestinal tract. *Giardia lamblia* and *Cryptosporidium* colonize the small bowel and produce noninflammatory watery diarrhea by presently undefined mechanisms.

Diagnosis

The acute gastroenteritides can be divided into several distinct clinical syndromes according to the age of the patient, geography, the patient's history, and the characteristics of the stool. For example, children between 4 months and 2 years of age develop watery diarrhea from rotavirus infection, but this agent is unusual in other age groups. Travel provides exposure to exotic pathogens that may cause diarrhea. Recent food ingestion and similar illness in dining companions suggest a food poisoning syndrome. A history of medication use introduces the possibility that the symptoms may be a side effect of therapy. Additionally, current use of either an antibiotic or a chemotherapeutic agent raises concerns about antibiotic-associated colitis due to *Clostridium difficile*. Recent psychologic stress suggests possible psychogenic illness.

The physical examination only occasionally will provide additional diagnostic information, but it is important in assessing the state of the hydration, which is the major criterion of the severity of illness. Examination of the abdomen may indicate severe distention and high-pitched bowel sounds, suggesting intermittent partial bowel obstruction. Severe tenderness and peritoneal irritation may occur from a diffuse process, such as toxic megacolon, or from a localized process, such as diverticulitis.

Stool examination is important and should include testing for both occult blood and fecal leukocytes.[46] The latter test can be performed quickly by mixing two drops of Loeffler's methylene blue with a fleck of mucus or stool on the surface of a glass slide. After a cover slip has been placed, the material is allowed to incubate for 2 to 3 minutes to provide good nuclear staining. The presence of sheets of polymorphonuclear cells indicates an inflammatory diarrhea, while the absence of white blood cells suggests a watery diarrhea syndrome. Occasionally, a small number of mononuclear white blood cells is seen (eg, 10 to 15 white blood cells per high-powered field). This has been associated with a low-grade inflammatory diarrhea caused by *Salmonella* species. The darkfield examination is an additional, inexpensive study that can be performed on watery stools. The presence of comma-shaped bacteria with darting motility is strongly suggestive of *Campylobacter jejeuni* infection.[47]

Following the history, physical examination, and stool examination, most patients can be considered as having one of three syndromes: acute watery diarrhea, dysenteric gastroenteritis, or food poisoning.

Acute Watery Diarrhea

Sporadic, spontaneous, noninflammatory diarrhea is the second leading cause of illness. It occurs most commonly in infants from 6 months to 2 years of age after they have been weaned. Usually, there is a 2- to 3-day illness with frequent watery brown diarrhea, occasional vomiting, and a low-grade fever. The usual etiologic agents are the rotaviruses and, outside the United States, enterotoxigenic *E coli*. While gastroenteritis is so ubiquitous that every child has several episodes in the first 2 years of life, it may also be the first indication of serious systemic infection in patients in this age group.

Both in older children and adults, the watery diarrhea syndrome can be produced by any of the enterotoxigenic bacteria, the invasive or cytotoxin-producing bacteria, *G lamblia*, *Cryptosporidium* species, and viral agents. Typically, there is anorexia, malaise, mild abdominal cramping, and progressive diarrhea. Depending on the volume produced, stool can vary in color and appearance from semiformed to rice-watery. The volume of stool varies with the etiologic agent; the enterotoxin-producing bacteria cause the most profuse diarrhea. If adequate hydration is maintained, these patients usually are not toxic and the disease resolves spontaneously in 3 to 5 days.

Acute, noninflammatory diarrhea is particularly common in individuals who travel. Traveler's diarrhea usually develops as an explosive, watery diarrhea 5 to 15 days after arrival in the new environment. Enterotoxigenic *E coli* is responsible for 75% of the cases worldwide, but other agents should be considered after travel to certain locales. For example, cholera may rarely be acquired after travel to endemic areas, and *G lamblia* has produced water-borne epidemics in Russian and Southeast Asian cities and is endemic in many of the mountain regions throughout the United States.

Recently it has been recognized that *Cryptosporidium* organisms are a cause of watery diarrhea in the normal host and of prolonged fatal disease in immunocompromised patients including those with AIDS. Infrequently, a history of animal exposure can be elicited from affected individuals.[48]

Initial treatment of any patient with gastroenteritis is directed at maintaining adequate hydration. Although fluid loss is not severe in most patients, the loss is so great in some that hospitalization is necessary for parenteral fluid replacement. As diarrheal fluid is isotonic, intravenous therapy should be initiated with normal saline solution. Serum electrolyte levels should be monitored because metabolic acidosis can develop from ongoing bicarbonate loss in the stool; properly diluted sodium bicarbonate is appropriate replacement fluid if acidosis develops. Fluid can be replaced orally in patients who are not severely dehydrated.

In the late 1960s, studies with cholera victims in Bangladesh demonstrated that patients could be effectively rehydrated with oral isotonic glucose-electrolyte solutions containing sodium chloride, potassium, and bicarbonate.[49] The rationale for this therapy is based on the mechanisms for sodium transport in the gut. Normally, sodium is absorbed from the intestinal lumen by several active mechanisms, one that transports sodium alone and others that transport sodium coupled with glucose or neutral amino acids. Once sodium is transported, chloride and water follow passively. In patients with cholera and other enterotoxin-mediated diarrhea, only the transport of sodium is blocked. Coupled sodium transport continues and compensates effectively for the other impaired transport mechanism. Although this approach was designed for treatment of cholera, it is effective for any diarrhea if the small intestinal mucosa is intact.

Several commercial oral rehydration mixtures are available, and a home-prepared oral rehydration regimen has been recommended by the World Health Organization as shown in Table 25-2.[50] While glucose is preferred, sucrose can be substituted if glucose is not available. This therapy does not decrease the stool volume; in fact, the volume will probably increase, as not all the oral fluids will be absorbed. An adequate intravascular volume can be maintained by matching the stool fluid losses with oral therapy.

Several agents have been marketed for the symptomatic treatment of diarrhea, including agents that absorb toxins and water such as kaolin, pectin, and psyllium hydrophilic mucilloid, and agents that decrease intestinal motility such as paregoric, diphenoxylate hydrochloride, and loperamide hydrochloride. While both classes of drugs decrease stool fluidity and frequency, they do not decrease the intestinal fluid loss, and all of them have very limited utility in the management of gastroenteritis. Furthermore, the agents that inhibit intestinal motility are contraindicated in dysenteric syndromes, as they have been demonstrated to prolong the duration of illness with *Campylobacter*, *Salmonella*, and *Shigella* infections and rarely may induce toxic megacolon or perforation. Recent evidence has demonstrated that bismuth

Table 25-2 Oral Therapy of Diarrhea

3.5 g NaCl	(NA+ 90 mEq/L)
2.5 g NaHCO$_3$	(HCO$_3^-$ 30 mEq/L)
1.5 g KCl	(K+ 20 mEq/L)
20 g glucose	(Glucose 110 mM/L)
1 L boiled water	

Source: WHO Weekly Epidemiol Rec 1979;54 (16):121–123.

subsalicylate (30 to 60 mL every 30 minutes for eight doses or two tablets four times daily) will decrease the fluid loss associated with enterotoxin-mediated diarrhea.[51]

Antibiotic therapy is not indicated in patients with enterotoxigenic *E coli* infection. Gastroenteritis caused by *Salmonella* is usually a self-limited illness, and antibiotics prolong the period of bacterial shedding. For selected pathogens, however, antibiotic therapy can be useful. Erythromycin (500 mg orally every 6 hours for 5 days; 40 mg/kg/day orally in four doses for 5 days in children) may be helpful treatment for prolonged *Campylobacter jejeuni* gastroenteritis. *Giardia lamblia* enteritis should be treated with either quinacrine hydrochloride (100 mg orally three times a day for 5 days; 6 to 7 mg/kg/day orally three times a day for 5 days for children) or metronidazole (250 mg orally three times a day for 10 days; 15 mg/kg/day orally three times a day for children).

Patients with very prolonged symptoms should be referred for further work-up. Stool cultures and stool examination for ova and parasites should be performed. If *Campylobacter*, *Yersinia*, or *Cryptosporidium* infection is suspected, the microbiologist should be informed because these pathogens require special growth or examination conditions. When *Salmonella* infection is likely, blood cultures should be obtained as these organisms may cause bacteremia.

Dysenteric Gastroenteritis

Bloody or mucous diarrhea with severe abdominal cramping pain, tenesmus, rectal pain, and systemic toxicity may be seen in infections with the pathogens that invade the mucosal epithelium, such as *Campylobacter jejeuni*, *Shigella* and *Salmonella* species, enteroinvasive and enterohemorrhagic *Escherichia coli*, *Entamoeba histolytica*, *Vibrio parahaemolyticus*, and *Neisseria gonorrhoeae*, and with the cytotoxin-producing pathogens, including *Clostridium difficile*.[52] Further, invasive proctitis due to *Chlamydia trachomatis*, *Treponema pallidum*, or herpesvirus can produce similar symptoms, although these infections are predominantly limited to homosexual men.[53] With the multiplicity of pathogens producing this syndrome, additional studies are required to make a specific diagnosis. All patients should have a stool culture and stool examination for ova and parasites performed, and patients on antibiotics or chemotherapy or those who have had bowel manipulation should undergo an analysis for *Clostridium difficile* cytotoxin as well as having the potential predisposing agent discontinued immediately. In adolescents and adults, a sigmoidoscopic examination should be performed to evaluate the extent of inflammation and to determine whether idiopathic inflammatory bowel disease is present.

Patients with dysenteric syndromes should be hospitalized or followed closely as outpatients for the duration of the illness. Fluid rehydration therapy as outlined above should be initiated. Because of the wide diversity of potential pathogens, unless bowel perforation is suspected antibiotic treatment should usually be withheld until a pathogen is identified. Trimethoprim-sulfamethoxazole (160 mg to 800 mg orally every 12 hours for 5 days; 10 to 50 mg/kg/day orally in two doses for children) is appropriate for known *Shigella* disease, and erthryomycin (500 mg orally every 6 hours for 5 days; 40 mg/kg/day in two doses for children) is appropriate for known *Campylobacter jejeuni*. Alternatively, the quinoline antibiotics norfloxacin and ciprofloxacin each have clinical efficacy against enteroinvasive and enterohemorrhagic *E coli*, *Shigella* species, and *Campylobacter jejeuni*.[54] Ciprofloxacin also may eradicate *Salmonella* carriage and bacteremia. Thus these agents may be used for treating known bacterial dysentery not due to *Clostridium difficile* while culture and susceptibility tests are being performed.[55] Symptomatic intestinal amebiasis should be treated with metronidazole (750 mg orally three times a day for 10 days; 30 to 50 mg/kg/day orally for children) plus diiodohydroxyquin (650 mg orally three times a day for 20 days). Patients with pseudomembranous colitis due to *Clostridium difficile* with severe disease not responsive to discontinuation of the inciting agent can be treated with vancomycin (125 mg orally every 6 hours for 7 to 10 days) or metronidazole (500 mg orally three times a day for 10 days). Both regimens may be associated with relapse, however.

Food Poisoning

Several distinct gastroenteritic syndromes arise after the consumption of contaminated food.[56] These syndromes are most readily distinguished by the duration of the incubation period. Food-related illness is especially likely if two or more individuals develop gastrointestinal or neurologic symptoms within 72 hours of sharing a meal.

Severe nausea, vomiting, abdominal cramping, and watery diarrhea occur within 1 to 6 hours after ingestion of preformed toxin from *Staphylococcus* organisms or *Bacillus cereus* in prepared food that has been stored improperly. Fried rice has been associated with *B cereus* in particular. Disease induced by either bacteria usually resolves in less than 24 hours. The major differential diagnosis is heavy metal poisoning with copper, tin, zinc, or cadmium. Abdominal cramping and watery diarrhea that begin 8 to 16 hours after food ingestion can develop secondary to toxins produced by *Clostridium perfringens* or *B cereus*. Vomiting is unusual, and the illness usually resolves spontaneously in 24 hours. Therapy of these syndromes is symptomatic.

Food-borne gastroenteritis developing 16 to 72 hours after a meal is usually related to *Salmonella*, *Shigella*, *Vibrio parahaemolyticus*, enteroinvasive and enterotoxigenic *E coli*, and *Campylobacter jejeuni*. The norwalk virus also has been identified as a cause of food-borne illness transmitted by contaminated shellfish. Vomiting is a prominent feature, with illness lasting 24 to 48 hours. If a specific bacterial pathogen is defined, therapy should be given as described above.

The development of a dry mouth and weakness or paralysis in association with gastroenteritis strongly suggests *Clostridium botulinum* toxin ingestion. If botulism is suspected, the stomach should be lavaged and the patient hospitalized for observation and supportive care. The Centers for Disease Control should be contacted for consultative assistance and to arrange for the possible use of botulinal antitoxin (telephone weekdays: 404-639-3753; weeknights and weekends: 404-639-2888).

Noninfectious food-borne illnesses include monosodium glutamate intoxication, fish and shellfish poisoning, and mushroom poisoning. The Chinese restaurant syndrome associated with monosodium glutamate ingestion is a self-limited syndrome of headache, paresthesias, flushing, and diaphoresis that develops within minutes of ingestion and lasts for several hours. Scromboid fish poisoning represents acute histamine intoxication and in severe cases may cause urticaria and bronchospasm. Ciguatera fish poisoning is due to a toxin concentrated up the food chain and most commonly occurs after ingestion of contaminated carnivorous reef fish such as sea bass, grouper, or snapper.[57] The illness presents first with gastrointestinal symptoms of cramps, vomiting, and watery diarrhea and then unusual neurologic symptoms that may include nondermatomal numbness and tingling of the lips and limbs, tooth pain, and the sensation of loose teeth. Paralytic shellfish poisoning presents with paresthesias and muscle weakness developing within 30 minutes of ingestion of toxin-containing mussels, clams, scallops, and oysters. With severe cases respiratory failure can occur during the first 12 hours. Depending on the species ingested, toxic mushroom poisoning can present as either delirium, parasympathetic hyperactivity, disulfiramlike reactions, or gastroenteritis with or without hepatorenal failure.

INFECTIONS OF THE URINARY TRACT

Infection of the urinary tract is a frequent cause of emergency department visits. Cystitis and pyelonephritis are primarily infections in women, and the incidence of these infections increases with age. Older men may develop urinary tract infection in association with prostatic hypertrophy and urethral instrumentation.[58] Prostatitis is a disease of men that can be either acute or chronic. The "urethral" syndrome, which consists of symptomatic urethral irritation without evidence of cystitis or vaginitis, has been delineated as a distinct entity in women of childbearing age.[59] While the clinical manifestations of urinary tract infections may be shared, the etiology and pathophysiology vary with the specific site involved.

The terms "cystitis" and "pyelonephritis" are clinical descriptions of acute symptomatic urinary tract infections caused by *Escherichia coli* or other bacteria, such as *Klebsiella* or *Proteus* species, *Pseudomonas aeruginosa*, *Serratia marcescens*, *Enterobacter* species, and enterococci. *Staphylococcus saprophyticus,* a coagulase-negative staphylococcus, is also a cause of lower urinary tract infection and in some clinical series has been the second most common pathogen.[60] Furthermore, *Chlamydia trachomatis* has been recognized as a major pathogen in women with the "urethral" syndrome.[59] The first episodes of bacterial infection of the urinary tract are most frequently due to *Escherichia coli,* which is very sensitive to most antibiotics, but recurrent episodes may be caused by other, more resistant organisms.

Pathophysiology

Bacteria can ascend the urethra and enter the bladder. Urinary tract infection in women results from colonization of the vaginal introitus by organisms that migrate from the fecal reservoir. Intravesical seeding occurs by migration of bacteria up the urethra. Small bacterial inocula may be cleared by normal voiding. Factors that facilitate bacterial migration up the urethra, such as urethral catheterization or sexual intercourse, or those that prevent complete voiding, such as neurogenic bladder, pregnancy, urethral stricture, and benign prostatic hypertrophy, allow bacteria to multiply within the bladder. Failure of local antibacterial defense mechanisms of the bladder mucosa results in the establishment of infection.

Infection may extend to the kidney as a result of reflux of urine from the bladder into the ureter. Bladder infection itself may cause relative incompetence of the ureterovesical valve that permits such reflux to occur. Bacterial infection in the upper urinary tract (kidneys and collecting system) may occur without symptoms, or it may produce the signs and symptoms typical of acute pyelonephritis. Gram-negative bacteria may inhibit normal ureteric peristalsis, and this inhibition facilitates the rapid ascent of bacteria to the renal pelvis and renal parenchyma. Infection usually begins in the renal medullary tubules and spreads cortically, inciting an inflammatory response. Microabscesses may develop in acute bacterial pyelonephritis.

Diagnosis

The clinical manifestations of urinary tract infections are urinary frequency, burning on micturition, pressure sensation over the bladder, urinary urgency, and pyuria and hematuria. However, this clinical constellation alone is not helpful in differentiating between urethral, bladder, and renal parenchymal infection. The additional symptoms of fever greater than 38.5°C (101.3°F), back pain at the costovertebral angles, rigors, nausea, and vomiting are more strongly suggestive of acute pyelonephritis, but there are no reliable, universally available techniques for definitively localizing infection to the upper or lower urinary tract.

The traditional hallmark for acute urinary tract infection has been the presence of a single bacterial species at a concentration equal to or greater than 100,000 colony forming units (ctu) per milliliter urine. However, women may have cystitis with as few as 10^2 coliform bacteria per milliliter of urine.[61] Because of the decreased diagnostic accuracy of the usual midstream urine culture at this bacterial concentration, the high degree of predictability of pathogens producing sporadic episodes of urinary tract infections and the inherent time delay in obtaining culture results, routine culturing of urine in all cases of suspected urinary tract infection is not appropriate. However, it should always be obtained in men, women who are pregnant, and patients who are ill enough to require hospitalization, who have had recurrent infections, or who have recently been hospitalized and may have unusual pathogens.[62]

Particular care must be taken in obtaining a specimen for urine culture. Because the urine sample must not be contaminated with periurethral flora, the urethral orifice and periurethral area should be cleansed carefully with dilute green soap solution, and the patient should collect a urine sample while retracting the foreskin or labia. Although midstream specimens have been recommended, it is very difficult for women to obtain an adequate sample with this technique. Alternatively, an appropriate sample may be obtained by bladder catheterization or by suprapubic bladder aspiration. Either of these techniques can introduce bacteria into the bladder, however. In general, the urine should be obtained with the patient standing over a wide-mouthed collecting jar. The sample should be either refrigerated immediately or transferred to culture media in a quantitative fashion within 30 minutes of collection, as bacteria will continue to multiply in a sample at room temperature. Failure to transport and culture the sample promptly results in artificially high colony counts, usually with multiple bacterial species.

A more useful diagnostic study in the dysuric patient is a microscopic examination of the urine. An examination of unspun urine with a hemocytometer provides a rapid accurate assessment of the number of white blood cells present. The presence of 10 white blood cells or more per microliter is indicative of urinary tract pathology.[63] The finding of one bacterium per high-powered field on examination of at least five fields of unspun urine also correlates well with a urine bacterial colony count of 10^5/mL, which is further strong evidence for cystitis and raises concern about pyelonephritis. If examination of an unspun urine indicates pyuria, a centrifuged urine sample can be examined for white blood cell casts, which is an insensitive but specific marker for renal involvement. In facilities where microscopy is not available, the leukocyte esterase dipstick method is a somewhat less sensitive alternative.[62,64]

A CBC should be performed in the more severely ill patients. The white blood cell count frequently reveals a polymorphonuclear leukocytosis in patients with acute pyelonephritis.

Several rapid screening tests are currently under evaluation as adjuncts or substitutes for the traditional urine culture and microscopic examination. These tests have not yet undergone adequate study to determine their utility.

Differential Diagnosis

The differential diagnosis of acute urinary infection includes vaginitis in women, prostatitis in men, and renal stone disease in both sexes. In some populations, vaginal infections are even more common than urinary tract infections, and they may cause dysuria as well as vaginal discharge or irritation.[64] A pelvic examination should be performed if these symptoms are present. Vaginitis and bacterial urinary tract infection may occur simultaneously in the same patient.

Treatment

Antimicrobial therapy is effective for bacterial and chlamydial infections in the urinary tract and should be instituted based on the clinical signs and symptoms and microscopic examination of the urine. At present there is no clear drug of choice or duration of therapy for these infections. In patients with high fever, hypotension, or shaking chills, Gram-negative rod bacteremia secondary to urinary tract infection should be suspected. These patients should be admitted to the hospital, blood and urine cultures should be obtained, and the patients should be treated with parenteral antibiotic therapy. Therapy with ampicillin (1 g intravenously every 4 hours for an adult) and an aminoglycoside is appropriate pending culture results. In patients where the urine Gram stain suggests that enterococcal infection is unlikely, intravenous therapy with an aminoglycoside alone, trimethoprim-sulfamethoxazole, or a third-generation cephalosporin is a reasonable alternative. The appropriate agent for a given institution should be selected on the basis of local cost and susceptibility considerations.[62]

For patients who can be managed outside the hospital, the optimal selection of antibiotics is also undefined. Clinical studies have suggested that a single dose of one of several antibiotics will cure a "traditionally" defined cystitis in nonpregnant women, but patients with upper urinary tract infections (as defined by antibody-coated bacteria studies) require longer treatment regimens of 10 to 14 days.[65] Also, it appears that nonpregnant women with the "urethral" syndrome having pyuria and less than 10^5 bacteria per milliliter of urine may be best treated with a 7-day course of tetracycline that provides coverage for both *Chlamydia trachomatis* and the usual bacterial pathogens.[66]

Until additional data are available, a reasonable therapeutic approach is to guide antibiotic therapy by the clinical

Table 25-3 Antibacterial Therapy for Urinary Tract Infection

Drug	Dosage Adults	Dosage Children	Drug	Dosage Adults	Dosage Children
10- to 14-day regimens*			Trimethoprim	100 mg orally twice a day	8 mg/kg/day orally given twice a day
Ampicillin or amoxicillin	500 mg to 1 g orally four times a day	100 mg/kg/day orally given in four divided doses in children less than 20 kg	Trimethoprim-sulfamethoxazole	160/800 mg orally twice a day	8 to 40 mg/kg/day orally given twice a day
Cephalexin or cephradine	250 to 500 mg orally four times a day	25 to 50 mg/kg/day orally given in four divided doses	Tetracycline	250 to 500 mg orally four times a day	Not used in children younger than 8 years
Ciprofloxacin	250 mg orally twice a day (not used during pregnancy)	Not used	**Single-dose regimens for nonpregnant, reliable women**		
			Amoxicillin	3.0 g orally	
			Amoxicillin plus clavulanate	500 mg orally	
Norfloxacin	400 mg orally twice a day (not used during pregnancy)	Not used	Ampicillin	3.5 g orally	
			Cephalexin or cefaclor	2 g orally	
			Ciprofloxacin	250 mg orally	
Nitrofurantoin	50 to 100 mg orally three to four times a day	5 to 7 mg/kg/day orally given in four divided doses	Nitrofurantoin	200 mg	
			Norfloxacin	400 mg orally	
			Sulfisoxazole	2 g orally	
			Trimethoprim	400 mg orally	
Sulfisoxazole	500 mg orally four times a day	150 mg/kg/day orally given in four divided doses	Trimethoprim-sulfamethoxazole	320 to 1600 mg orally	

*Three-day regimens also may be effective.

setting and the urinalysis findings. In women without a complicating factor (pregnancy, diabetes, other immunosuppressing conditions, recent antibiotic usage, known urinary tract abnormalities, indwelling foley catheter, history of recurrent urinary tract infections, or hospital-acquired infections) with dysuria and a urinalysis demonstrating white blood cells and no visible bacteria on microscopic examination of urine, a 7-day course of a tetracycline antibiotic (500 mg of tetracycline hydrochloride orally four times a day or 100 mg of doxycycline orally twice daily) appears appropriate. For pregnant women with this presentation, a 10- to 14-day treatment plan with ampicillin or amoxicillin (as in Table 25-3) can be implemented with arrangements for follow-up in 2 to 3 days. Patients who have not improved can then be re-evaluated for a possible resistant bacterial infection or considered for a trial of erythromycin base (500 mg orally four times a day for 7 days) or erythromycin ethylsuccinate (800 mg orally four times a day for 7 days) for chlamydial disease.

Either a single dose or a 3-day course of therapy with any of the agents listed in Table 25-3 could be used for reliable women without a complicating factor who have both white blood cells and bacteria present on microscopic examination of the urine or dipstick analysis. Recent data suggest that higher success rates are noted with trimethoprim or trimethoprim-sulfamethoxazole than with ampicillin or amoxicillin.[62] These patients should be seen in follow-up in 2 to 3 days to ensure resolution of symptoms, and if this cannot be ensured they should receive a 10-day course of therapy. A longer course of therapy should also be given to women with a complicating factor and to men and children. All the agents in Table 25-3 are reasonable alternatives, and selection can be based on possible complications of a given patient as well as on economic considerations.

Patients with recurrent urinary tract infections are frequently infected with organisms that are resistant to many antibiotics. These patients should have a urine culture repeated 24 hours after empiric therapy has been initiated so that the adequacy of treatment can be ascertained. Antibiotics act quickly as they are rapidly excreted into the urine and the bacteriologic response to a treatment regimen is clear within 24 hours. If the antibiotic is appropriate for the infecting organism, the infection should be cleared in this time period. Should this not be the case, the addition of other antibiotics would be appropriate at that time. Patients with a history of recurrent urinary infections usually benefit from long-term suppressive therapy with trimethoprim-sulfamethoxazole or nitrofurantoin. Small doses of these agents can be taken as infrequently as two to three times a week and/or after intercourse in patients whose recurrent infections are related to sexual activity.[67]

Urethritis in Men

Urethritis in men with symptomatic urethral irritation and a urethral discharge is primarily a sexually transmitted disease. Although classically this disease has been associated with *Neisseria gonorrhoeae*, nongonococcal infections account for at least 40% of the cases of urethritis and the prevalence is higher in more affluent socioeconomic classes. Further, 15% to 45% of men with gonococcal urethritis will have a concurrent nongonococcal urethral infection.[68] *Chlamydia trachomatis* is the pathogen in approximately 40% to 50% of cases, and *Ureaplasma urealyticum* has been implicated in another 10% to 20%.[68,69] *Trichomonas vaginalis* and herpes simplex virus also cause nongonococcal urethritis occasionally, but they are responsible for less than 5% of cases. Reiter's syndrome, with uveitis, conjunctivitis, circinate balanitis, oral mucosal ulcerations, and asymmeric arthritis, may be responsible for 1% to 2% of these cases. Unfortunately, an etiology cannot be identified in almost 50% of patients with nongonococcal urethritis.

Pathophysiology

Both gonococcal and chlamydial urethritis are predominantly localized infections. Gonococcal infection is acquired by intimate contact of the organism with a mucosal surface. The bacteria adhere to the epithelial surface and then penetrate to the subepithelial connective tissue where they induce an intense inflammatory response and cause epithelial sloughing. Although untreated infection usually resolves spontaneously within 6 months, periurethral abscesses, urethral strictures, epididymitis, prostatitis, and disseminated gonococcal infection may develop as complications.[70]

Chlamydia trachomatis is an obligate intracellular microorganism that infects columnar epithelial cells. Urethral infection results from contact with another mucosal surface infected with *C trachomatis*. While the infection is localized to the epithelial surface, it may extend along the urethra and produce acute epididymitis.

Diagnosis

The predominant symptom of urethritis is urethral discharge, which may be purulent, mucoid, or watery. Occasionally, this is the only symptom, but dysuria is usually present with frequency, urgency, a sensation of pressure in the groin, or continuous mild urethral pain or pruritus.

Unless the patient is sexually aroused or has just urinated, the presence of any urethral fluid is abnormal and should be considered a discharge. Physical examination should be performed 2 hours or more after the patient has last urinated to permit the accumulation of scant discharges that may have been cleared by the urinary stream. If there is no spontaneous discharge, manual stripping of the penis from the base to the meatus may express fluid from the urethra.

Microscopic examination of the urethral secretions is essential in the diagnosis of urethritis. With careful uniform swabbing of the secretions onto a 2×1 cm^2 area of a glass slide, a Gram stain can provide diagnostic and etiologic information. An average of more than four neutrophils per high-powered field is indicative of urethritis.[69] Gonococcal urethritis is further characterized by the presence of intracellular Gram-negative diplococci in association with the polymorphonuclear exudate. Nongonococcal urethritis is defined by the presence of polymorphonuclear leukocytes without intracellular bacteria, although mixed extracellular coliform and coccobacillary forms may be present. The presence of extracellular Gram-negative diplococcal organisms without intracellular organisms is suggestive but not diagnostic of gonococcal infection. All urethral discharges should be cultured for *N gonorrhoeae*, and rectal and pharyngeal swab cultures should be obtained as indicated by the sexual history.

The urethral culture is taken with a urethral calcium alginate swab and plated immediately on modified Thayer-Martin agar or a specific gonococcal transport medium. At present only a few microbiology laboratories can culture *C trachomatis* and *U urealyticum* routinely. Direct immunofluorescent and enzyme-linked immunosorbent assays are now available to identify chlamydiae in secretions. In symptomatic men their positive predictive value averages between 87% and 93%, and their negative predictive value is between 90% and 98%.[71] Their cost effectiveness is not defined in the asymptomatic individual, however, or in the patient with symptoms who lacks other objective physical or laboratory evidence of chlamydial infection.

Differential Diagnosis

Gonococcal urethritis in men has a short incubation period of 2 to 7 days and is typically associated with significant dysuria and purulent exudate, although it may be asymptomatic. Nongonococcal urethritis has a more prolonged incubation period of 1 to 3 weeks, and frequently a watery or mucoid discharge is the only symptom. When present, dysuria is mild or "itchy." Because of the nonspecificity of these clinical presentations, microscopic examination and culture should be used to confirm the diagnosis in all patients.

The differential diagnosis of urethritis includes prostatitis, cystitis, and epididymitis, but they should be readily distinguished on clinical presentation. Hematuria and hemospermia are not seen with urethritis and suggest disease of the kidneys, bladder, or prostate.

Treatment

The current regimen for treatment of uncomplicated gonococcal infection recommended by the Centers for Disease Control[12] is ceftriaxone (250 mg intramuscularly once) plus doxycycline (100 mg orally two times a day for 7 days). In patients who are allergic to ceftriaxone, the preferred alternative is spectinomycin (2 g intramuscularly in a single dose) followed by the 7-day regimen of doxycycline. Additional potential alternatives for which there is less information about efficacy include ciprofloxacin (500 mg orally once), norfloxacin (800 mg orally once), cefuroxime-axetil (1 g orally once with 1 g of probenecid orally), cefotaxime (1 g intramuscularly once), and ceftizoxime (500 mg intramuscularly once). All these alternative regimens should also be given with the 7-day doxycycline regimen. For patients who cannot take a tetracyline, erythromycin ethylsuccinate (800 mg orally four times a day for 7 days) may be substituted.

The initial therapy of nongonococcal urethritis must be directed at both *Chlamydia trachomatis* and *Ureaplasma urealyticum,* since the precise etiology is not usually established. Although both microorganisms are susceptible to tetracycline and erythromycin, tetracycline (500 mg by mouth four times a day for 7 days) or doxycycline (100 mg orally twice a day for 7 days) may be preferred because these are also effective against gonorrhea and syphilis. If tetracycline therapy has been ineffective or is contraindicated, erythromycin base (500 mg by mouth four times a day for 7 days) is recommended.[12]

The sexual partners of patients with urethritis should be examined and treated also, because both gonococcal and nongonococcal urethritis are sexually transmitted diseases. Failure to eradicate infection in both partners can lead to recurrences.

Serologic studies for syphilis should be done on all patients with urethritis, and the patients should be offered confidential counseling and testing for HIV. Most patients with incubating seronegative syphilis will also be adequately treated by the β-lactam, doxycycline, and tetracycline regimens. Spectinomycin, ciprofloxacin, and norfloxacin are not effective for syphilis.

Follow-up

All patients with gonococcal urethritis should be reexamined in 10 to 14 days, at least 3 days after conclusion of antibiotic therapy. A repeat culture for *Neisseria gonorrhoeae* should be performed and should be negative to confirm cure. Following gonococcal urethritis, a small percentage of patients not treated concurrently for nongonococcal urethritis will develop recurrent urethral symptoms associated with a mucoid discharge. At least 70% of these cases are due to *Chlamydia trachomatis* infection that probably occurred simultaneously with the initial *N gonorrhoeae* infection. These patients usually respond to tetracycline therapy.

It is also reasonable to arrange follow-up for patients with nongonococcal urethritis. Although over 80% of initial chlamydial infections are completely eradicated by tetracycline, patients with nonchlamydial, nongonococcal urethritis have a lower response rate. These patients may have infections with *U urealyticum* strains resistant to tetracycline, or urethritis due to *Trichomonas* organisms or herpes simplex. The first 10 mL of a freshly voided urine sample should be examined by wet mount for *Trichomonas* organisms; if positive, metronidazole (2 g as a single dose or 250 mg three times a day for 7 days) should be given. If *Trichomonas* organisms are not present and if compliance with previous therapy was adequate, a 3-week trial of erythromycin base (500 mg orally four times daily for 3 weeks) can be attempted.[72]

Prostatitis

Acute bacterial prostatitis is caused by *E coli,* other Gram-negative bacteria, or, occasionally, *N gonorrhoeae.*[73] Infection is probably caused by reflux of bacteria from the urethra to the prostate. The normal prostate secretes an antibacterial zinc salt that may be reduced in patients with bacterial prostatitis.

Diagnosis

Acute bacterial prostatitis has an abrupt onset with fever, chills, dysuria, frequency, and perineal and low back pain. Variable degrees of bladder outlet obstruction may occur. The physical examination reveals an enlarged, exquisitely tender prostate. Prostatic massage should be avoided to minimize the risk of bacteremia. Urinalysis reveals pyuria and bacteriuria, and a polymorphonuclear leukocytosis is found in peripheral blood.

Treatment

Hospitalization is required for patients who have severe infections or marked bladder outlet obstruction. Appropriate cultures of urine and blood should be obtained and treatment with parenteral antibiotics begun immediately. An aminoglycoside with or without a broad-spectrum penicillin is reasonable pending culture results. Intravenous trimethoprim-sulfamethoxazole is an alternative agent. Suprapubic bladder drainage and not urethral catheterization should be performed if urinary retention is marked.

Outpatient management is acceptable in less severely ill patients. Few antibiotics other than quinolones, trimethoprim, and erythromycin penetrate well into prostate tissue. Trimethoprim or trimethoprim-sulfamethoxazole (160 mg/800 mg orally twice daily) is adequate therapy for prostatitis caused by sensitive organisms. Ciprofloxacin (250 to 500 mg twice a day) is also effective against susceptible bacteria. Treatment should be continued for up to 30 days and arrangements made for urologic follow-up.

CENTRAL NERVOUS SYSTEM INFECTIONS

The major infectious processes involving the central nervous system (CNS) include meningitis, encephalitis, brain abscess, and very rarely subdural and epidural empyemas. They are caused by a diverse group of pathogens and have differing presentations. However, because of fundamental aspects of CNS, these infections share several pathophysiologic and clinical characteristics. First, the complexity of the nervous system does not allow for the repair of direct damage, and the function of lost nervous tissue either cannot be replaced or must be compensated for by another region of the system. Second, the normal elements of the inflammatory response can further damage the nervous system by compromising the delicate vascular supply or disrupting the function of the cranial nerves or nerve roots. Third, the brain and spinal cord are enclosed in a compartmentalized, rigid, bony and membranous framework. While this protects the CNS, any process that increases the amount of fluid within this framework will cause a rise in overall intracranial pressure and may produce compression injury to nervous tissue.

If a process produces an asymmetric distortion in intracranial anatomy, as happens with a subdural empyema or a localized brain abscess, the risk of compression of vital structures is markedly enhanced because of the compartmentalization of the brain by three septa, the falx cerebri, the falx cerebelli, and the tentorium cerebelli.

Finally, the brain and spinal cord are surrounded by continuously circulating cerebrospinal fluid (CSF). Approximately 85% of this fluid is produced by the choroid plexi within the third, fourth, and lateral ventricles.[74] If there is a blockage in the flow of CSF, the continued production of fluid will produce a localized increase in pressure and consequent compression damage to periventricular nervous tissue.

Purulent Meningitis

Meningitis, inflammation of the subarachnoid space on an infectious or noninfectious basis, has been defined by CSF pleocytosis, characteristically considered to be more than 5 white blood cells per cubic millimeter. Signs and symptoms of meningeal irritation with headache, nuchal rigidity, and Kernig's and Brudzinski's signs are present to varying degrees depending on the etiology of the process. Although there is some overlap, meningitis can be divided into two clinically relevant categories on the basis of the cerebrospinal fluid examination. A positive CSF Gram stain and/or a polymorphonuclear CSF pleocytosis is indicative of purulent meningitis; a negative CSF Gram stain and mononuclear CSF pleocytosis suggests an aseptic meningitis. Purulent meningitis is often an overwhelming infection and is a true medical emergency requiring immediate recognition and the rapid initiation of antibiotic treatment to avoid a tragic outcome.

Etiology

Hemophilus influenzae, *Neisseria meningitidis*, and *Streptococcus pneumoniae* together account for 80% of all cases of purulent meningitis. In about 10% of patients with a classic clinical presentation and CSF findings consistent with bacterial infection, no pathogen will be isolated, often because of prior inadequate antimicrobial therapy.[75] Group B *Streptococcus* and enteric Gram-negative bacilli are important causes of meningitis in the neonate, but are rare in other age groups. *Listeria monocytogenes* is an uncommon pathogen that produces meningitis in the elderly, in immunocompromised hosts, and in neonates. *Staphylococcus aureus* is another infrequent meningeal pathogen causing meningitis secondary to contiguous infected foci or hematogenous seeding during prolonged staphylococcal sepsis.

The relative frequency of microbial pathogens in meningitis varies with the patient's age. Although *H influenzae*, *N meningitidis*, and *S pneumoniae* all produce meningitis in all age groups, *H influenzae* is the predominant pathogen in patients 1 month to 4 years of age and is uncommon after the age of 10 years.[75] *Neisseria meningitidis* is the most frequent cause of meningitis in patients 5 to 30 years of age, and *S pneumoniae* predominates in patients older than 30 years. In patients older than 65 years, enteric Gram-negative bacteria can account for up to 25% of cases, and *L monocytogenes* becomes more frequent.[76]

Pathogenesis

The subarachnoid space is well protected from microbial invasion in that it is surrounded by bone, ligaments, and three distinct membranes. However, CSF lacks intrinsic cellular and humoral immunity and is thus particularly vulnerable to infection when pathogens are introduced. Hematogenous seeding is the predominant route of infection, but the subarachnoid space may be invaded by contiguous spread of infection from otitis or sinusitis, or through CSF leaks due to trauma, surgery, or neuroectodermal defects.

Vascular permeability of the choroid plexus, ependyma, and pia mater is increased by inflammation in the subarachnoid space, contributing to an increased protein content and cellularity of the CSF. With significant inflammation from bacterial meningitis, active transport of glucose into the CSF is decreased and glucose concentration falls. CSF lactate concentration increases with increased anaerobic metabolism. Without prompt therapy, a thick, purulent exudate forms that may obstruct the normal CSF flow and occlude the vascular structures that pass through the subarachnoid space. Inflammation and edema of the underlying brain and cranial nerves may produce cranial nerve palsies, seizures, stupor, coma, and death.

Diagnosis

Most patients with purulent meningitis have fever, severe headache, and nuchal rigidity. Other symptoms that are commonly present include nausea, vomiting, photophobia, and mental aberration. Frequently, patients have had an antecedent upper respiratory tract infection or otitis media. Clinically, the meningeal irritation is reflected in nuchal rigidity, a positive Kernig's sign (pain in the hamstring and paraspinal muscles when the knee is extended with the hip flexed), and a positive Brudzinski's sign (flexion of the knees and hips when the neck is flexed). An abnormal state of consciousness is common with purulent meningitis; only 15% to 20% of patients appear alert on presentation.[75] Approximately 10% of patients present in coma or with convulsions, and these individuals have a significantly worse prognosis. Papilledema is unusual with meningitis alone; if present, a brain abscess or encephalitis should be considered. In infants whose cranial sutures have not fused, the inflammatory response and resultant edema will produce a bulging fontanelle.

The clinical presentation is variable and depends on the patient's age. Very young and very elderly patients may not have the usual signs of meningeal irritation and meningitis may present as lethargy, increased irritability, or gastrointestinal disturbances with or without fever. Occasionally, it is possible to identify an anatomic source predisposing the patient to meningitis and the initial examination should include a thorough evaluation of the sinuses and the middle ears, and a search for the presence of a possible midline dermal sinus or an occult skull fracture.

The major diagnostic test for meningitis is an examination of the CSF. This should be performed in all patients in whom purulent meningitis is a serious diagnostic consideration. The primary means for collection is the lumbar puncture, although when this is not possible an individual highly skilled in the techniques can obtain CSF through cisternal or ventricular punctures. In that lumbar puncture lowers pressure in the spinal canal, individuals with increased intracranial pressure who undergo this procedure are at risk of uncal herniation from the pressure change. Therefore, *individuals with papilledema or focal neurologic deficits (excluding ophthalmoplegias) should not have a lumbar puncture performed until a CT or MRI scan has been performed to exclude the presence of a mass lesion.*

Examination of the CSF should include cell count and differential count, determination of glucose and protein concentrations, and Gram-stained smear of the sediment and culture. As noted above, meningitis is confirmed by the presence of spinal fluid pleocytosis. When purulent meningitis is present, the diagnosis is confirmed in 75% to 85% of cases by a CSF Gram stain demonstrating bacteria.[75,77]

Purulent meningitis has several other characteristic CSF findings: two-thirds of patients have a CSF white blood cell count greater than 1000/μL with a polymorphonuclear leukocytosis, approximately 75% have a CSF glucose concentration less than 50 mg/dL, and 85% have an elevated protein concentration.[77] In patients with a negative CSF Gram stain, a CSF white blood cell count over 1200/μL with either a protein concentration greater than 150 mg/dL or a glucose concentration less than 30 mg/dL strongly suggests purulent meningitis.

It should be recognized that patients with early bacterial meningitis may have normal CSF examinations.[78] If a patient clinically appears to have purulent meningitis but a CSF examination is normal, it is prudent to repeat the study in several hours.

Countercurrent immunoelectrophoresis, Latex agglutination tests, and gas-liquid chromatography are additional rapid techniques to identify bacterial antigens in the CSF. The usefulness of these studies is limited to the management of cases of apparent purulent meningitis with a negative CSF Gram stain.

Differential Diagnosis

The diagnosis is usually clear in overwhelming purulent meningitis. However, aseptic meningitis, partially treated bacterial meningitis, viral encephalitis, brain abscess, epidural or subdural abscess, and vertebral osteomyelitis are alternative diagnostic considerations in patients with a subacute presentation. Elderly patients frequently lose nuchal flexibility as a result of osteoarthritis, and nuchal rigidity may occur in these patients without true meningeal irritation. Localizing neurologic signs are often present with parameningeal abscesses, and vertebral osteomyelitis may produce point tenderness over the infected bone.

The CSF examination is the major discriminating study. Aseptic meningitis, viral encephalitis, and suppurative parameningeal infections are associated with a lymphocytic pleocytosis. The CSF glucose is usually but not always normal in these illnesses, and the CSF protein is only slightly elevated. In parameningeal infections there can be a marked elevation in CSF protein concentration, but it may be an isolated finding not associated with changes in other CSF parameters.

Treatment

The period of highest mortality with bacterial meningitis is the first 24 hours after onset and presentation.[75] Furthermore, the mortality is highest in patients with a rapid onset of disease. Thus it is crucial that diagnostic evaluation be performed immediately if meningitis is suspected and that antibiotic therapy be started as quickly as possible after the diagnosis is established. In patients with possible meningitis who are acutely ill, a brief examination should be performed to exclude focal neurologic deficits or papilledema, blood cultures should be obtained, and a lumbar puncture should be performed immediately. If the CSF is turbid, empiric antibiotic therapy based on the age and condition of the patient should be instituted in the emergency department.[79] In children younger than 4 months, consideration must be given to group B streptococci, E coli, and L monocytogenes; ampicillin (50 mg/kg intravenously every 4 hours) plus a third-generation cephalosporin (eg, cefotaxime 50 mg/kg intravenously every 6 hours) is appropriate. In older children and young adolescents therapy must be directed predominantly at H influenzae with additional consideration for N meningitidis and Streptococcus pneumoniae. A third-generation cephalosporin alone (eg, cefotaxime 50 mg/kg intravenously every 6 hours) should be initiated, although ampicillin (50 mg/kg intravenously every 4 hours) plus chloramphenicol (25 mg/kg intravenously every 6 hours) remains an alternative approach. In the older adolescent and younger adult the major pathogens are N meningitidis and S pneumoniae. In this instance penicillin G (50,000 U/kg intravenously every 4 hours, approximately 20×10^6 to 20×10^6 U/day in adults) still remains highly appropriate therapy. With the prevalence of penicillin-resistant S pneumoniae slowly increasing worldwide, however, a third-generation cephalosporin alone (eg, cefotaxime 2 g intravenously every 6 hours) is an appropriate alternative. In the elderly patient, therapy should comprise ampicillin (2 g intravenously every 4 hours) plus a third-generation cephalosporin (eg, cefotaxime 2 g intravenously every 6 hours) to provide additional coverage for enteric Gram-negative bacteria and L monocytogenes.

In patients who are immunocompromised, who have experienced head trauma or cranial surgery, or who develop meningitis in the hospital, there is an increased risk that infection is due to Staphylococcus aureus or Gram-negative bacilli. Treatment with ampicillin (2 g intravenously every 4 hours) plus a third-generation cephalosporin (eg, cefotaxime 2 g intravenously every 6 hours) should be started in these patients pending culture results unless the CSF Gram stain suggests S aureus, in which case nafcillin should be substituted for ampicillin.

In patients in whom lumbar puncture is contraindicated because of focal findings consistent with a mass lesion, the next considerations are brain abscess, subdural empyema, and viral encephalitis. In patients who are acutely ill, therapy directed at a potential abscess and herpes simplex encephalitis should be initiated pending results of a CT or MR scan. Penicillin G (20×10^6 to 24×10^6 U/day intravenously in an adult) and chloramphenicol (25 to 50 mg/kg intravenously every 6 hours in children, 1 g intravenously every 6 hours in adults) is appropriate for coverage of bacterial infection, and acyclovir (10 mg/kg every 8 hours) is appropriate for herpes infection. Immediate neurosurgical consultation should be obtained in these patients.

With patients whose symptoms are subacute, antibiotic therapy can be withheld until the initial results of lumbar puncture are known. If the studies are consistent with purulent meningitis, antibiotic therapy should be initiated promptly on the basis of either the Gram stain results or the age of the patient when the Gram stain is negative. As noted above, crystalline penicillin G (50,000 U/kg intravenously every 4 hours, approximately 20×10^6 to 24×10^6 U/day in adults) still remains highly appropriate therapy. A third-generation cephalosporin alone (eg, cefotaxime 50 mg/kg intravenously every 6 hours in children, 2 g intravenously every 6 hours in adults) is an appropriate alternative, however. When the Gram stain is suggestive of H influenzae, treatment with a third-generation cephalosporin alone (eg, cefotaxime 50 mg/kg intravenously every 6 hours in children, 2 g intravenously every 6 hours in adults) should be begun until the results of susceptibility testing are known. Ampicillin remains an appropriate alternative for susceptible H influenzae isolates. Staphylococcal meningitis requires high-dose therapy with a semisynthetic penicillinase-resistant penicillin (nafcillin, 2 g intravenously every 4 hours) or vancomycin.

Supportive therapy for purulent meningitis includes maintenance of respiration with mechanical ventilation if necessary, control of seizures, and careful control of fluids to minimize potential cerebral edema. Recent double-blind, placebo-controlled trials have indicated that dexamethosone can decrease the morbidity of H influenzae meningitis in children when given as a regimen of 0.6 mg/kg/day in four intravenous doses for 4 days.[80] There are no available data on its efficacy with other pathogens or in adults, but it should be considered if severe cerebral edema develops and appropriate antibiotic therapy has been instituted.

Prevention

There is an increased incidence of meningococcal disease in household contacts of patients with meningococcal infection and an increased incidence of H influenzae type B disease in children less than 4 years old having household (or day-care) contact with patients with H influenzae type B disease. Consequently, in both of these situations it is desirable to provide some form of prophylaxis for close contacts.

For meningococcal disease both sulfonamide antibiotics and meningococcal vaccine can provide effective prophylaxis in the appropriate setting.[81] Unfortunately, at present sulfonamide resistance is common among strains of meningococci, and there is no effective vaccine available for serogroup B meningococci, the most frequently implicated serogroup in endemic meningococcal disease in the United States. It has been demonstrated that rifampin and minocycline can eradicate nasal carriage of meningococci, although treatment with the latter has been associated with a high incidence of vestibular toxicity. While resistant isolates occasionally develop and chemoprophylactic failures have been reported, therapy with rifampin (600 mg in adults, 5 mg/kg in children under 1 year, and 10 mg/kg for older children given orally every 12 hours in four doses) appears to be the best initial prophylactic option. It is appropriate for close, direct contacts of patients with meningococcal meningitis. Casual contacts, such as fellow workers, schoolmates, or health care workers, do not require prophylaxis.

Rifampin also eradicates carriage of *H influenzae* type B, and the current recommendation of the American Academy of Pediatrics is that rifampin prophylaxis (20 mg/kg/day as a single dose for 4 days) be given to all household contacts where there are other children under the age of 4 years.[82]

Aseptic Meningitis

The finding of a mononuclear CSF pleocytosis and a negative CSF Gram stain in a patient with fever, headache, and signs of meningeal irritation is diagnostic of aseptic meningitis. While this syndrome is most frequently due to viral infection, it must be recognized that it is produced by a wide variety of infectious and noninfectious causes, and that many of the infectious causes may respond to antimicrobial therapy. The critical concern in managing patients with this syndrome is the prompt recognition of those patients who require such therapy.

An etiology is defined in approximately 25% of the 3000 to 4000 cases of aseptic meningitis reported each year, and the most frequently defined pathogens are the enteroviruses. These infections occur predominantly in the summer or early fall, although there may be some rare cases seen throughout the year. Other agents that may cause this syndrome include mumps, herpes simplex types 1 and 2, HIV, varicella zoster, cytomegalovirus, adenovirus, measles, Epstein-Barr virus, hepatitis virus, poliomyelitis, lymphocytic choriomeningitis virus, and the encephalitis viruses. More important, meningeal irritation with mononuclear pleocytosis may be present in partially treated bacterial meningitis, parameningeal bacterial infections, tuberculosis, amebiasis, leptospirosis, Lyme disease, syphilis, and fungal meningitis. Noninfectious causes include systemic lupus erythematosus, sarcoidosis, carcinomatosis, drug reactions, chemical injury from intrathecal medication, Behçet's syndrome, and Mollaret's syndrome.

Diagnosis

Viral aseptic meningitis presents with fever and signs of meningeal irritation (nuchal rigidity, severe headache, Kernig's and Brudzinski's signs) after a short prodromal illness. Unlike purulent meningitis it is uncommon for viral meningitis alone to produce a change in mental status, and the presence of lethargy or confusion indicates either a purulent meningitis or concurrent encephalitis. The presence of sinusitis or otitis media raises the question not only of a purulent meningitis but also of a parameningeal abscess. If there is a history of prior antimicrobial therapy, partially treated bacterial meningitis must be considered. In general, compared with bacterial and viral meningitides, tuberculous and fungal meningitis have a more subacute presentation. Tuberculous infection evolves over a few days to weeks and fungal infections develop over a few weeks to months.

In most patients with viral meningitis the CSF examination reveals a normal glucose concentration, a protein concentration ranging from 50 to 200 mg/dL, and a white blood cell count of $50/\mu L$ to $1000/\mu L$. Very early in the course of the illness neutrophils often predominate, but as the course progresses a shift to more lymphocytic cells occurs within the first 24 hours. A low CSF glucose concentration with a lymphocytic pleocytosis is seen with a few less common viral meningitides including mumps and lymphocytic choriomeningitis virus infections. This CSF profile is more commonly associated with tuberculous or fungal meningitis, with partially treated bacterial meningitis, with parameningeal infections, or with carcinomatous or sarcoid meningitis. A lymphocytic pleocytosis and high CSF protein concentration can occur with viral meningitis, but this profile should increase the concern about a parameningeal pyogenic process.

Other studies may aid in defining the diagnosis. Counterimmunoelectrophoresis or other available rapid studies for bacterial antigens should be obtained if partially treated bacterial meningitis is suspected. An acid-fast smear of concentrated CSF will rarely be positive in tuberculous meningitis; usually the diagnosis must await cultural confirmation. India ink preparations and cryptococcal antigen determinations should be performed on CSF from immunocompromised patients with possible cryptococcosis. In patients with a possible history of exposure to *Coccidioides immitis* and a subacute presentation, a CSF antibody titer against *C immitis* should be determined. Similarly, serologic studies for *Borrelia burgdorferi*, the causative agent for Lyme disease, should be performed in patients from endemic areas developing aseptic meningitis in the late spring or summer months regardless of whether or not there is a history of tick exposure. Counseling and serologic testing for HIV should be considered in patients with a history of high-risk sexual activity or intravenous drug use. If the clinical presentation suggests carcinomatosis, cytocentrifugation of CSF facilitates identification of neoplastic cells.

Management

The appropriate treatment of aseptic meningitis is determined by the clinical setting. For example, during a summer epidemic of viral meningitis, mildly ill alert patients who have a typical CSF examination for an enteroviral meningitis do not necessarily require hospitalization if close follow-up can be arranged.[83] However, if the patient presents during a nonepidemic period for enteroviral or arboviral infections, if there are any unusual features on physical examination or

CSF examination, or if the patient is not alert, then immediate hospitalization is indicated for close observation and additional diagnostic studies.

Patients who clinically have aseptic viral meningitis but whose CSF examination reveals a polymorphonuclear pleocytosis early in the clinical course do not require immediate antimicrobial therapy. If close observation can be assured, these patients can be watched without specific therapy and undergo a repeat CSF examination in 12 to 24 hours. The conversion of the polymorphonuclear pleocytosis to a lymphocytic pleocytosis is consistent with a benign aseptic process.[84] This management approach is appropriate only if repeat CSF examination can be performed immediately if any change in the patient's condition occurs during observation. If this cannot be assured, empiric antimicrobial therapy is indicated as above.

Encephalitis and Brain Abscess

The relative rarity of encephalitis, infection of the brain parenchyma, probably relates to the effectiveness of the host defense system of the CNS. Encephalitis is usually an infrequent complication of a common infection and can be caused by viral, bacterial, rickettsial, or parasitic pathogens. Although an etiologic agent is not defined in many cases of encephalitis, viruses are implicated most frequently. In the United States, epidemic encephalitis may be produced by a variety of arthropod-borne viruses including eastern equine encephalitis, western equine encephalitis, St. Louis encephalitis, and California encephalitis. Colorado tick fever is a tick-borne virus that produces seasonal disease in the Rocky Mountain states, and still other arthropod-borne viruses cause disease outside the United States. Herpes simplex virus is the major cause of sporadic encephalitis. It can cause encephalitis in all age groups at all times of the year. All of the viral agents implicated in aseptic meningitis can also produce encephalitis. Rabies virus and slow viruses are rare causes of encephalitis in the United States.

Rocky Mountain spotted fever and typhus are the major rickettsial diseases associated with encephalitis. The spirochetes of syphilis and Lyme disease can produce encephalitis. Localized bacterial encephalitis, or brain abscess, is predominantly caused by mixed oral anaerobic bacteria and streptococcal species. *Staphylococcus aureus* and enteric Gram-negative bacilli are less frequently implicated. Parasitic brain infections can be due to cysticercosis, malaria, or trypanosomiasis.

Immunocompromised individuals are at risk of encephalitis due to a wider spectrum of agents. The incidence of encephalitis in this group also is higher, particularly in patients with AIDS, among whom up to 30% may develop neurologic disease.[85] Toxoplasmosis is a common cause of encephalitis in patients with AIDS, but encephalitis due to other agents (eg, progressive multifocal leukoencephalopathy) also occurs frequently.

Pathogenesis

The pathogenesis of encephalitis depends on the infectious agent involved. Most arthropod-borne viruses reach the brain hematogenously. Rabies virus and herpes simplex virus reach the brain by retrograde spread along nerve roots, and spread of herpes simplex virus from a silent latent focus in the trigeminal ganglion may contribute to the frequent localization of herpes simplex virus encephalitis to the temporal horn.

Rickettsial and syphilitic encephalitis are vasculitides in which disease develops because of disruption of the vascular supply and not significant direct invasion of the brain parenchyma. Focal bacterial encephalitis does involve invasion of brain parenchyma and develops most frequently as a result of contiguous spread from a chronic sinus or otitic infection. Less commonly noncontiguous bacterial encephalitis can develop from such chronic infections through retrograde flow in the venous system. Hematogenous brain abscesses can occur in patients with sustained bacteremia as in bacterial endocarditis.

Diagnosis

In the normal host, viral encephalitis presents with fever, severe headache, nausea, vomiting, and alterations in state of consciousness ranging from mild lethargy to frank coma. Concurrent signs of meningeal irritation may or may not be present. Although none of these findings is diagnostic of a specific pathogen, herpes simplex virus is the most common cause of encephalitis associated with focal neurologic deficits.[86] Additionally, the occurrence of encephalitis in the summer or early fall and a history of mosquito exposure suggest disease due to an arthropod-borne agent.

Peripheral blood studies are nonspecific. CSF examination is important in the evaluation of these patients, *but individuals with focal neurologic findings should undergo a CT scan to exclude a focal mass lesion prior to having a lumbar puncture.* Findings on CSF examination are similar to those in aseptic meningitis and include mononuclear pleocytosis, normal CSF glucose concentration, and elevated CSF protein concentration. Red blood cells in CSF are seen commonly with herpes simplex virus encephalitis, and approximately 40% of these patients have more than 50 red blood cells per microliter of CSF.[87] Electroencephalography and brain scan may also demonstrate focal deficits in this form of encephalitis.

Brain abscess presents as an expanding intracranial mass lesion with generalized headache, nausea, vomiting, and the development of focal neurologic findings such as seizures and an abnormal state of consciousness.[88] Fever is not universally present and may be seen in only 30% to 40% of these patients.[89] Papilledema is observed occasionally, and 50% of patients with a brain abscess have an apparent extracranial focus of infection.[89,90] The CT scan is the major diagnostic procedure and may demonstrate focal enhancing lesions in most patients with brain abscess. The MR scan may well be more sensitive than the CT scan and should be considered in patients with a normal CT scan in whom an intracranial lesion is strongly suspected.

Historical information and systemic findings are critical to the diagnosis of the other causes of encephalitis such as the rickettsial diseases, Lyme disease, and syphilis.

Management

As with aseptic meningitis, it is critical to identify those patients with encephalitis or brain abscess who may respond to therapy. At present there is no current treatment available for the viral causes of encephalitis with the exception of herpes simplex virus encephalitis. Studies now indicate that vidarabine (15 mg/kg/day for 10 days) and acyclovir (30 mg/kg/day for 10 days) are both effective therapy for herpes simplex virus encephalitis, although the outcome is significantly better in patients treated with acyclovir.[91,92] Brain abscess and systemic bacterial and rickettsial diseases associated with encephalitis will respond to appropriate antibiotic therapy.

Neurosurgical consultation should be arranged for all patients with increased intracranial pressure or focal intracranial lesions. Patients with presumed brain abscess should be initiated on empiric antimicrobial therapy directed against the predominant pathogens. Penicillin G (20×10^6 U/day intravenously in adults) and chloramphenicol (4 g/day intravenously in adults) are effective, although when the bacteriology is defined intravenous metronidazole or a third-generation cephalosporin may be alternative agents.[88]

The usefulness of brain biopsy to confirm the diagnosis of herpes simplex virus encephalitis remains unresolved. In patients who have undergone brain biopsy for presumed herpes simplex virus encephalitis, 50% to 60% have had the diagnosis confirmed, and about 24% have had another potentially treatable illness identified.[93] As the risk of brain biopsy is dependent upon the experience of the neurosurgeon, this decision must be individualized. The complication rate of brain biopsy in the nationwide antiviral treatment studies was less than 2%.[93] This procedure should be considered in all patients with possible herpes simplex virus encephalitis.

Similarly, patients with AIDS or other immunocompromising illnesses who develop encephalitis with focal lesions should also be considered for brain biopsy because of the diversity of possible causes.

Aside from these specific therapies, patients with encephalitis should receive support similar to that of patients with purulent meningitis as described above.

Infectious Mononucleosis Syndrome

The "mono" syndrome is characterized as the clinical constellation of (1) subacute onset of fever, pharyngitis, malaise; (2) lymphadenopathy and/or splenomegaly; and (3) characteristic hematologic abnormalities of an absolute and relative lymphocytosis (greater than 50% of white blood cells) with 10% to 20% atypical lymphocytes.[94,95] In over 90% of cases the causative pathogen has been the Epstein-Barr virus, and the term "infectious mononucleosis" has usually been restricted to cases due to this virus. Cytomegalovirus may cause 5% to 7% of the cases of the syndrome, and *Toxoplasma gondii* is responsible for somewhat less than 1%.

Pathogenesis

Epstein-Barr virus, cytomegalovirus, and *T gondii* produce systemic infection that involves lymph nodes, spleen, and liver. The central nervous system, kidney, bone marrow, and the cardiovascular and respiratory systems are less frequently involved. The hematologic abnormalities associated with Epstein-Barr virus infection are mediated by viral infection of B lymphocytes and secondary proliferation of cytotoxic and suppressor T lymphocytes, which appear as atypical lymphocytes. The spread of this infection is mediated by prolonged low-level excretion of Epstein-Barr virus in salivary secretions. Cytomegalovirus mononucleosis is spread by low-level, close, person-to-person contact and by blood transfusion. Toxoplasmosis primarily follows either the ingestion of uncooked, infected meat or contact with infected cat feces, although water-borne transmission has been recognized.

Diagnosis

The mononucleosis syndrome is most common in patients 15 to 25 years old, although it may occur at any age.[95] The illness begins with a prodrome of fatigue, malaise, headache, and myalgias with the subsequent development of fever (38.3° to 39.5°C, 101° to 103.1°F). A severe exudative pharyngitis is prominent in Epstein-Barr virus disease, but is less common with cytomegalovirus or *Toxoplasma* infections. Tender peripheral lymphadenopathy, involving particularly the anterior or posterior cervical nodes, is present in over 80% of patients infected with Epstein-Barr virus or *T gondii* but is infrequent with cytomegalovirus disease. Splenomegaly may develop with disease from any of the three pathogens.

Other early manifestations of the mononucleosis syndrome include an evanescent erythematous skin rash, periorbital edema, and palatal petechiae.[95] Neurologic complications including encephalitis, cerebellar ataxia, cranial nerve palsies, transverse myelitis, and the Guillain-Barré syndrome may occur, although they are found in less than 1% of cases. Other rare manifestations of mononucleosis include myocarditis, pericarditis, hemolytic anemia, granulocytopenia, thrombocytopenia, interstitial pneumonia, monoarticular arthritis, and splenic rupture. Very rarely Epstein-Barr virus disease can become chronic, progress to malignancy, or result in death.

The atypical lymphocytes seen in the peripheral blood smears are large cells with vacuolated cytoplasm and horseshoe-shaped or oval nuclei that contain dense, irregular chromatin. Initially, mild granulocytopenia may be present, but leukocytosis develops in the second to third week of illness. Uncommonly, a leukemoid reaction is seen. Mild hepatic abnormalities are present in over 80% of patients with the mononucleosis syndrome. While clinical hepatitis is rare, the levels of lactic dehydrogenase (LDH), alkaline phosphatase, bilirubin, and the serum aminotransferases are usually elevated and are useful in confirming the diagnosis.

With Epstein-Barr virus infection, the production of Igs, including IgM heterophil antibodies (reactive against an antigen from another species), is characteristically increased. While several different heterophil antibodies are produced, a distinct elevation of the Paul-Bunnell heterophil antibody (an antibody reactive against sheep erythrocytes that can be absorbed by beef but not guinea pig erythrocytes) is found in infectious mononucleosis, and this has been used as a serologic marker for Epstein-Barr virus disease. Rapid slide tests (eg, Monospot) that utilize formalinized horse or sheep erythrocytes are available to detect the presence of this heterophil antibody.

Antibody titers begin to rise with the onset of clinical illness and may remain elevated for as long as 1 year. The results of a heterophil test are positive in 85% of patients with Epstein-Barr virus mononucleosis, although the titer elevation may not become significant for 6 to 12 weeks in some patients. Serologic studies for Epstein-Barr virus–specific antibodies are available but they are difficult to perform, expensive, and not routinely necessary.

Neither cytomegalovirus nor *T gondii* infection induces heterophil antibodies. Cytomegalovirus mononucleosis is documented by a fourfold rise in serum antibody titers from the time of acute illness to the convalescent period. Either complement-fixing or immunofluorescent IgM assays may be used to determine the presence of antibodies. Toxoplasmosis is documented by specific serology or by lymph node pathology.

Differential Diagnosis

The initial evaluation should include a complete blood count and heterophil antibody study, and these usually establish the diagnosis of mononucleosis in patients with Epstein-Barr virus infection. Patients with the typical hematologic picture and a negative result on a heterophil antibody test during the first 6 weeks of illness may have a cytomegalovirus or *T gondii* infection. Adenovirus, rubella, the hepatitis viruses, Group A streptococci, syphilis, and *Salmonella* species all may produce clinical illnesses that simulate mononucleosis.

Primary infection with HIV, the causative agent of AIDS, also can produce an acute febrile syndrome similar to the "mono" syndrome.[96,97] In the United States this infection is primarily limited to certain high-risk populations, including homosexual and bisexual men, intravenous drug abusers, individuals with hemophilia who received frequent transfusions with coagulation factors in the early 1980s, and the regular sexual partners of individuals in these groups. The relative prevalence of HIV infection in relation to other causes of the "mono" syndrome remains undefined, but it appears to be markedly lower. Still, the diagnosis should be entertained in individuals presenting with symptoms of mononucleosis who are sexually active, use intravenous drugs, or may have been exposed to blood products from an HIV-infected individual.

The frequency of clinical symptoms with initial HIV infection is unclear, with prospective studies reporting symptoms in 55% to 92% of individuals who have seroconverted.[98,99] There appears to be a 3- to 6-week incubation period, and the predominant symptoms are fever, fatigue, lymphadenopathy, and headache. A smaller percentage of patients have had rash and a lymphocytic aseptic meningitis. These symptoms are self-limited, but the patients develop chronic HIV infection, which can be confirmed with serologic studies.

Treatment

There is no specific therapy for Epstein-Barr virus or cytomegalovirus mononucleosis. Both are typically self-limited illnesses that begin to resolve in 2 to 3 weeks, although fatigue may persist for several months. Prolonged bedrest is not indicated. Patients should be advised against vigorous activity or contact sports until splenomegaly recedes. Although short-term oral steroid therapy with 40 to 60 mg of prednisone daily may decrease the duration of fever and symptomatic illness, its use is not necessary in the vast majority of cases.[100] It should be considered if severe pharyngitis threatens the airway or limits nutrition, or if pericarditis, myocarditis, hemolytic anemia, thrombocytopenia, or neurologic complications develop. Because occasional patients have simultaneous streptococcal pharyngitis and infectious mononucleosis, throat cultures should be obtained in patients with pharyngeal disease. The use of ampicillin in patients with Epstein-Barr virus or cytomegalovirus infections is frequently complicated by a prominent erythematous papular rash.

Mild cases of toxoplasmosis do not require therapy. Severe disease, particularly in patients with impaired cell-mediated immunity such as individuals with AIDS, can be treated with pyrimethamine and sulfadiazine, but this therapy requires close supervision.

Although HIV infection remains incurable, treatment with antiviral therapy and prophylaxis for opportunistic infections can prolong life. Patients with primary HIV infection should be advised to avoid sexual activities or needle sharing, which could transmit the infection to others, and should be referred for long-term follow-up with a physician versed in the management of HIV disease.

VIRAL HEPATITIS

The term *viral hepatitis* now refers to disease that is due to at least five distinct viruses: hepatitis A, hepatitis B, hepatitis C, delta agent, and at least one other virus associated with non-A, non-B hepatitis. They all produce an illness characterized by fever, malaise, anorexia, nausea, and jaundice associated with serum biochemical abnormalities from hepatic dysfunction. The infections differ in some clinical and epidemiologic characteristics, but precise diagnosis is dependent on serologic studies.

Hepatitis A virus causes approximately 35% to 40% of the cases of hepatitis in the United States. It is an RNA virus that is primarily spread from person to person through the fecal-oral route.[101] The peak fecal virus excretion occurs just prior to and during the early phase of symptomatic illness. The infection is more common in lower socioeconomic groups, and approximately 50% of the US population will have antibodies to the virus by age 50. There has been recent recognition that transmission often occurs in preschool daycare centers, and sexual transmission through oral-rectal contact has been noted. The severity of illness is associated with patient age; while children under 2 years are commonly asymptomatic, the majority of adults develop symptomatic hepatitis. When associated with symptomatic disease, there is an incubation period of approximately 28 days followed by an abrupt onset of nausea, vomiting, fatigue, aversion to cigarette smoke, jaundice, dark urine, light-colored stools, abdominal pain, and fever. The symptoms typically persist for 3 to 4 weeks; fulminant infection is rare and chronic hepatitis does not occur.

Hepatitis B virus is a DNA virus that is present in the blood and serous fluids of infected individuals.[102] In contrast to the hepatitis A virus, a chronic carrier state can exist and develops in approximately 10% of infected patients. It is transmitted either percutaneously or permucosally, primarily through contaminated needles or sexual contact. Transmission can occur in the setting of continuous, close, interpersonal contact such as that found between mothers and infants or within institutions for the mentally retarded. In these settings viral infection probably develops from inapparent contamination of cutaneous lesions with infective secretions.

The overall prevalence of antibodies to hepatitis B in the general US population has been estimated at between 5% and 20%. However, the distribution of infection is not homogenous and is markedly more prevalent in users of illicit parenteral drugs, homosexually active men, hemodialysis patients, and patients in institutions for the mentally retarded. Furthermore, the disease is highly prevalent in parts of Asia, Africa, and Malaysia, where the chronic carriage rate may exceed 25%.

The majority of hepatitis B infections appear to be asymptomatic. Symptomatic disease is associated with an incubation period of from 60 to 160 days. Occasionally, there are initial manifestations of arthralgias, skin rashes, or arthritis, but usually the symptoms are indistinguishable from hepatitis A. Fulminant hepatitis may develop in up to 1% of patients, and there appears to be a strong epidemiologic link between hepatitis B infection and hepatocellular carcinoma.

The delta agent is a defective RNA virus that produces hepatic infection in chronic carriers of the hepatitis B virus.[103] The agent does not produce its own viral capsid, but instead "hitchhikes" within hepatitis B virus particles. It produces infection only when there is either acute or chronic concurrent infection with the hepatitis B virus. It is transmitted through the same modes as hepatitis B and is common only among populations with a high prevalence of hepatitis B carriage. The infection may be subclinical or parallel the symptoms of the other hepatitides. Both fulminant and chronic infections have occurred.

In addition to these three well-defined viral agents, there are at least two other transmissible agents that have caused the syndrome termed non-A, non-B hepatitis. Two specific viral agents have recently been defined: hepatitis C, which is associated with parenterally transmitted hepatitis in the United States, and hepatitis E, which is associated with enterically transmitted hepatitis in Asia.[104,105] Hepatitis C shares many of the epidemiologic and clinical features of hepatitis B, with infection arising after blood transfusions or parenteral drug abuse.[106] The disease is clinically indistinguishable from the other hepatitides, although the acute illness is usually mild. Between 10% and 60% of patients will go on to develop a chronic hepatitis with abnormal liver function studies persisting for more than 1 year after the onset of symptoms. The epidemiologic and clinical characteristics of hepatitis E are similar to those of hepatitis A, although fulminant disease is more common, particularly in pregnant women. Hepatitis E has been reported in India, Pakistan, Asia, North Africa, and Mexico. Endemic infection in the United States has not been recognized, although imported cases have been seen.

Diagnosis

Confirmation of clinical hepatitis is made by the laboratory finding of significant elevations of serum aminotransferases, serum glutamic-oxaloacetic and glutamic-pyruvic transaminases, and moderate elevations of direct bilirubin and alkaline phosphatase. In severe hepatitis, there may be hypoglycemia, suppression of serum albumin and fibrinogen, and prolongation of the prothrombin time and partial thromboplastin time.

Defining the etiology of viral hepatitis is dependent upon serum serologic studies. Hepatitis A can be diagnosed by the presence of an elevated titer of IgM antibodies against the virus. This may develop as early as 2 days after the onset of symptoms but the peak titer develops approximately 1 month later. The serum IgG antibody titer against hepatitis A remains elevated for years after the infection and cannot be used as a diagnostic study.

Hepatitis B infections can be studied by a variety of serologic studies. Acute infection is associated with positive serum determinations for hepatitis B surface antigen (HBsAg), a surface protein of the virus, and for two internal antigens, the e antigen (HBeAg) and DNA polymerase. The presence of these latter two antigens is highly associated with potential infectivity of the patient for others. Within the first month after the infection, the patient develops antibodies to a core antigen of the virus (anti-HBc) and then later to the surface antigen (anti-HBs). In the usual uncomplicated case of type B hepatitis, HBsAg will persist in the serum for 1 to 6 months and peak at the height of symptomatic illness. Anti-HBc will develop during the symptomatic period, peak in early convalescence, and subsequently wane after several months. Anti-HBs does not develop until resolution of the hepatitis and can be considered a marker for recovery. As noted above, approximately 10% of individuals develop chronic carriage of the virus. They remain persistently positive for HBsAg, HBeAg, and DNA polymerase and do not develop anti-HBs. While all of these studies may rarely be required in the diagnosis of unusual cases, on a routine basis the most cost-effective tests for hepatitis B infection are the HBsAg and anti-HBs determinations.

Delta hepatitis can be diagnosed by the finding of the delta antigen in serum. Serologic assays for hepatitis C and hepatitis E are now available in the United States.

Management

There is no specific therapy for acute viral hepatitis. All five viruses typically cause self-limited disease that resolves over 4 to 6 weeks. In most instances the patient can be managed as an outpatient. Inpatient treatment by a specialist should be considered if the patient cannot maintain adequate hydration, if there is prolongation of the coagulation studies, severe hypoglycemia, or any evidence of hepatic encephalopathy. While prolonged bedrest is not indicated, there should be a restriction from most physical activity until there is resolution of symptoms and vigorous exercise should be avoided until there is normalization of the liver function studies. Consumption of alcohol or other hepatotoxic drugs should be avoided. It should also be recognized that hepatic dysfunction will alter the pharmacokinetics of a wide variety of therapeutic agents.

Recent studies have now shown that prolonged interferon therapy can modify the course of chronic hepatitis due to hepatitis B and C in selected patients.[106a,106b] Patients with these infections should be referred for evaluation for this therapeutic approach.

Prevention

It has now been well established that both hepatitis A and B can be prevented through the appropriate use of Ig preparations and the hepatitis B vaccine.[107] In view of the significant morbidity of both infections and the potential mortality associated with hepatitis B disease, prophylactic measures are warranted for both diseases.

Prophylaxis with Ig provides 80% to 90% protection from clinical illness with hepatitis A if it is given either before or early in the incubation period. Preexposure prophylaxis with this preparation is recommended for travelers to developing countries if they will be eating in settings of poor or uncertain sanitation or if they will have extended contact with the local population. Such individuals should receive a single injection of 0.02 mL/kg of sterile Ig if the intended travel is for less than 3 months. They should receive 0.06 mL/kg every 5 months for prolonged travel.

Postexposure prophylaxis for hepatitis A with Ig should be considered for close personal contacts of infected patients. It should be given as soon as possible after exposure; it is not effective when given more than 2 weeks after the exposure occurred. As the hepatitis A virus is only responsible for 35% to 40% of episodes of viral hepatitis in the United States, serologic confirmation of the diagnosis of hepatitis A in the index case is desirable before the initiation of prophylaxis. The question of who should receive Ig prophylaxis is dependent upon the clinical situation and is summarized in Table 25-4.

Protection from hepatitis B virus infection can now be provided by either Ig preparations or by hepatitis B vaccine. While the current standard Ig preparations contain some anti-HBs, a second Ig preparation produced from plasma preselected for high titers of anti-HBs is available (HBIG) that has an anti-HBs titer of greater than 1:100,000.

The hepatitis B vaccine licensed in the United States is composed of purified HBsAg and is both immunogenic and safe. After a series of three intramuscular injections into the deltoid, over 90% of healthy adults develop protective levels of antibody against HBsAg. Thus, preexposure vaccination with the hepatitis B vaccine should be considered for individuals at high risk for developing hepatitis B infection. This includes individuals who are intravenous drug abusers, homosexually active men, hemodialysis patients, clients and staff of institutions for the mentally retarded, hemophiliacs, sexual contacts of hepatitis B virus carriers, or health care workers who are frequently exposed to blood or blood products.

Postexposure prophylaxis to prevent infection with hepatitis B should be considered for infants born to HBsAg-positive mothers, infants whose primary care provider has acute hepatitis B while they are younger than 12 months of age, individuals who are sexual contacts of an HBsAg-

Table 25-4 Postexposure Prophylaxis for Hepatitis A with Igs

Households	All household and sexual contacts should receive Ig prophylaxis.
Day-care centers	In centers with children in diapers, administer Igs to all staff and attendees if one or more cases are recognized in the day-care center or if cases are recognized in two or more households of center attendees. If three or more households are involved, consider prophylaxis of all members of households whose diapered children attend. In centers without children in diapers, administer Igs to classroom contacts of case.
Schools	Ig prophylaxis is not indicated for classroom contacts of a case in an elementary or secondary school setting.
Institutions for custodial care	Depending upon the epidemiologic situation, Ig prophylaxis should be considered for residents and staff.
Hospitals	Routine Ig prophylaxis is not indicated for hospital personnel.
Offices and factories	Routine Ig prophylaxis is not indicated.
Food handlers	Igs should be administered to other food handlers. Patrons should be considered for Ig prophylaxis if the infected food handler directly worked with food that was not cooked before being eaten, if he or she had had diarrhea or poor hygiene, and if the patrons are identified within 2 weeks of exposure.

Source: MMWR 1990; 39 (No. RR-2)

Table 25-5 Prophylaxis for Hepatitis B After Percutaneous or Permucosal Exposure

Source	Exposed Person	
	Unvaccinated	Vaccinated
Known source, HBsAg positive	1. HBIG prophylaxis immediately (0.06 mL/kg intramuscularly). 2. Initiate hepatitis B vaccine* series.	1. Test exposed person for anti-HBs. 2. If adequate antibody, nothing required. If inadequate antibody,† HBIG prophylaxis immediately plus vaccine booster dose.
Known source, HBsAg negative	Initiate hepatitis B vaccine* series.	Nothing required.
Unknown source or source not tested	Initiate hepatitis B vaccine* series.	Test exposed for anti-HBs. If adequate antibody nothing required. If inadequate antibody,† vaccine booster. If known source was high risk but not tested, may also treat with HBIG prophylaxis.

*The dosage of the Heptavax-B and Engerix-B hepatitis B vaccine preparations is 20 μg intramuscularly for immunocompetent adolescents and adults and 10 μg for infants and children younger than 11 years of age. The dosage of Recombivax HB is 10 μg for adults older than 19 years of age, 5 μg for adolescents 11 to 19 years of age, 5 μg for infants of carrier mothers, and 2.5 μg for other children younger than 11 years of age. The dosage is 40 μg for dialysis and immunocompromised patients for all three preparations. The usual schedule is three doses at 0, 1, and 6 months.

†Less than 10 SRU by radioimmunoassay, negative by enzyme immunoassay.

Source: MMWR 1990; 39 (No. RR-2)

positive person, and individuals who have had accidental needlestick or permucosal exposure to HBsAg-positive blood or secretions. For perinatal exposure, the current recommendations of the Centers for Disease Control are 0.5 mL of hepatitis B Ig intramuscularly within 12 hours of birth and concurrent administration of hepatitis B vaccine at a second site. The dosage of hepatitis B vaccine administered is dependent upon the preparation used (10 μg of Heptavax-B or Engerix-B, 5 μg of Recombivax). A booster dose of vaccine should be administered at 1 and 6 months. Sexual contacts of hepatitis B carriers should receive Ig prophylaxis (0.06 mg/kg) if it can be given within 14 days of sexual contact. In high-risk populations, preprophylaxis serologic screening of the contact should be performed if it will not delay Ig administration beyond 14 days. Regular sexual contacts of chronic hepatitis B carriers should receive the hepatitis B vaccine; this can be initiated concurrently with Ig administration if given at a different site (dosage and vaccine schedule as per Table 25-5). The recommendations for hepatitis B prophylaxis after needlestick or permucosal exposure are dependent upon the status of both the source patient and the exposed person. It is now recommended that when possible the source patient be tested for HBsAg as soon as possible. Table 25-5 is adapted from the current recommendations of the Immunization Practices Advisory Committee of the Centers for Disease Control.[107]

There are no products available that provide protection against infection with the delta antigen. Similarly, there is little information available about prophylactic regimens for hepatitis C or hepatitis E. For persons with percutaneous exposure to blood from a patient with known hepatitis C infection, it is reasonable to consider administering standard Ig (0.06 mL/kg). It is not known whether Ig preparations manufactured in the United States contain any neutralizing antibody to hepatitis E.

COMMUNITY-ACQUIRED SEPSIS

A variety of infections will present as acute sepsis with high fever, toxicity, and possibly shock. Patients with these illnesses will require urgent hospitalization, but initial treatment must be started in the emergency department. The primary focus of therapy is the supportive care necessary for a patient in shock, as discussed in Chapter 6. However, diagnostic studies should be undertaken rapidly to define the etiology of the infection.

The differential diagnosis of an infection presenting as acute sepsis encompasses all classes of infectious agents. Almost any far-advanced local bacterial infection such as pneumonia, cellulitis, or urinary tract infection can potentially advance to a bacteremia. Bacterial infections due to *Neisseria meningitidis*, group A streptococci, *Yersinia pestis*, and *Salmonella typhi* can produce overwhelming primary bacteremias in the normal host, and *Streptococcus pneumoniae* and other encapsulated bacteria can do so in splenectomized patients. Individuals with hepatic cirrhosis are susceptible to all of these as well as spontaneous bacteremia due to a number of "unusual" bacteria that invade through the gastrointestinal system, including *Aeromonas hydrophila*, *Vibrio* species, *Listeria monocytogenes,* and *Campylobacter fetus*. Granulocytopenic patients are quite susceptible to bacterial sepsis arising from inapparent breaks in the skin or gastrointestinal mucosa. Localized colonization of vaginal tampons or superficial cutaneous lesions with toxin-producing strains of *Staphylococcus aureus* can cause a multisystem illness termed "toxic shock syndrome" with skin, mucus membrane, hepatic, renal, and cardiovascular involvement.[108]

Rocky Mountain spotted fever due to *Rickettsia rickettsii* is endemic throughout most of the United States but is particularly common in the southern mid-Atlantic states of the Carolinas, Virginia, and Maryland and in Oklahoma and Missouri.[109] The rickettsiae are introduced into humans by a tick bite and infect cells of the vascular endothelium producing an acute systemic vasculitis. Following an incubation period of approximately 1 week, a febrile illness develops with high fever, myalgias, arthralgias, and headache. A characteristic maculopapular rash typically arises on the third to fifth day of illness. It begins on the distal extremities involving the palms and soles and spreads proximally. Fatal infections have been associated with the late onset of rash as there is usually a delay in consideration of the diagnosis and in the initiation of appropriate therapy.[110]

Although the causative agents are not present in the United States, dengue fever, Lassa fever, and other hemorrhagic fevers due to arena and toga viruses can develop in travelers to the endemic regions of Africa, Asia, and South and Central America. Overwhelming infection due to *Plasmodium falciparum* can occur in travelers to the malarious regions of Africa, Southeast Asia, or South and Central America.

Diagnosis

Most of the information necessary to make a presumptive diagnosis in a patient with sepsis will be obtained from the history and physical examination. A history of prior splenectomy raises concern about sepsis due to encapsulated bacteria, particularly *Streptococcus pneumoniae*. Patients with cirrhosis are also at risk for spontaneous bacteremia with these pathogens along with *Escherichia coli* and the unusual bacteria noted above. Intravenous drug abusers are at risk for both staphylococcal and Gram-negative enteric rod sepsis due to contamination of their drugs or paraphernalia. As noted above, determining a history of travel is extremely important. Animal exposure in the southwestern United States raises concern about plague, and living in or traveling through the endemic areas for Rocky Mountain spotted fever raises concern about this infection (only 60% to 70% of these patients will have a history of a tick bite). Typhoid fever should be considered in any patient who has traveled in underdeveloped countries. It begins with an initial influenzalike prodrome with headache, myalgias, a nonproductive cough, and relative bradycardia, but it can advance to delirium, coma, and septic shock.

The presence of a skin rash can be quite helpful diagnostically. The rash of Rocky Mountain spotted fever has been described above. Meningococcemia is associated with a diffuse palpable purpuric rash. The toxic shock syndrome produces a very erythematous sunburnlike rash and an exanthema with a "strawberry" tongue.

Management

Complete blood counts with differential and blood cultures should be obtained in all patients and should be supplemented by the appropriate studies for possible localized infections as suggested by the initial history and physical examination. Thick and thin smears for malaria should be performed in individuals who have recently traveled to endemic regions. Suspected Rocky Mountain spotted fever can be confirmed by the biopsy of petechial skin lesions and staining the specimen with specific immunofluorescent stains.[111]

Appropriate supportive measures for septic shock should be undertaken as outlined in Chapter 6. Initial empiric antibiotic therapy directed against the suspected pathogen should be started after the appropriate cultures have been obtained. Meningococcemia or group A streptococcal sepsis should be treated with high-dose penicillin G (2×10^6 U every 2 hours for adults, 200,000 U/kg/day for children). Suspected staphylococcal sepsis should be treated with a semisynthetic antistaphylococcal penicillin such as oxacillin or nafcillin unless the epidemiologic setting indicates that there is a high suspicion of a methicillin-resistant strain requiring vancomycin therapy. Possible Gram-negative rod sepsis may be treated with an intravenous aminoglycoside with or without a first-generation cephalosporin or with a third-generation cephalosporin alone. Patients who are presumed to have the toxic shock syndrome should receive an intravenous antistaphylococcal penicillin, and the suspected staphylococcal focus should be drained (eg, removal of tampon if a vaginal site is suspected).

Possible Rocky Mountain spotted fever should be treated with tetracycline (25 to 50 mg/kg/day) or chloramphenicol (50 mg/kg/day). During the peak summer months of tick exposure in areas of high endemicity for Rocky Mountain spotted fever, oral tetracycline or chloramphenicol should be considered for individuals with an otherwise unexplained febrile illness of 2 to 3 days' duration.[112]

Antimicrobial therapy for malaria should be initiated based upon the known drug susceptibility of malaria strains from the country where the infection was acquired, in consultation with a physician well versed in the management of malaria. Up-to-date information on the resistance of strains from different nations can be obtained from the Centers for Disease Control, Atlanta, Georgia. If the infection was acquired in a country where chlorquine-resistant strains of P falciparum have not been recognized, then chlorquine is the drug of choice (chlorquine phosphate, 1 g orally followed by 500 mg in 6 hours, then 500 mg/day for 2 days in adults; 10 mg/kg up to 600 mg maximum followed by half the dose at 6 hours and daily for 2 days in children; for patients unable to take oral medication, chlorquine hydrochloride, 5 mg/kg intramuscularly every 12 hours for 3 days). Patients with possible chlorquine-resistant falciparum malaria require treatment with either combined oral quinine sulfate, pyrimethamine, and sulfadiazine, or intravenous therapy with quinine dihydrochloride obtained through the Centers for Disease Control. Quinidine gluconate given in a dosage of 15 mg/kg intravenously over 4 hours followed by 75 mg/kg every 8 hours for 7 days is an effective alternative to quinine if the latter cannot be obtained promptly.[113]

SKIN AND SOFT TISSUE INFECTIONS

Cutaneous Abscesses

Trauma or obstruction of the eccrine or exocrine glands in the skin can lead to cutaneous abscesses. Rarely, such abscesses may arise from hematogenous spread of infection from a distant focus. They are limited to the dermis, but deeper structures in the hand may be infected owing to the close spatial relations of potential and actual spaces. Infection is usually caused by resident skin flora and varies slightly with the anatomic location. Hand infections are primarily caused by *Staphylococcus aureus*, which is also responsible for most infections of the head, neck, thorax, and extremities; however, some infections in these areas are due to *Streptococcus pyogenes* or mixed anaerobic and aerobic organisms. In perineal abscesses (including inguinal, buttock, pilonidal, and anorectal abscesses), the predominant pathogens are those comprising the anaerobic fecal flora, although *Staphylococcus aureus* is occasionally isolated. The fecal aerobic Gram-negative bacilli are found less commonly.

Diagnosis and Differential Diagnosis

A cutaneous abscess generally occurs as a painful, tender, warm, erythematous mass. Fluctuance is a particularly helpful diagnostic clue, but may be absent. The abscess may be accompanied by spreading cellulitis or lymphangitic streaking. A peripheral leukocytosis with a shift to immature polymorphonuclear leukocytes may be seen with large abscesses, although not with smaller lesions. The aspiration of pus is definitive, and Gram stain and culture of the aspirate determine the etiology.

A few lesions may mimic pyogenic abscesses. Sterile abscesses can develop in parenteral drug abusers owing to talc and other "cutting" materials. Acute relapsing panniculitis is associated with multiple subcutaneous nodules of fat necrosis on the abdomen and extremities. Erythema nodosum may produce similar lesions, primarily on the lower extremities. Herpetic whitlow may resemble staphylococcal paronychial infection. Localized arterial aneurysms may be seen as fluctuant masses, but they should be readily distinguished by the presence of pulsation.

Treatment

Systemic antibiotics do not always reach the center of an abscess cavity in adequate concentration, and the bacterial and phagocytic breakdown products within the abscess inhibit many antimicrobial agents. Consequently, surgical drainage is essential in the treatment of any abscess. The involved site should be scrubbed with organic iodine solution, the area anesthetized, and the abscess cavity incised. Purulent materials should be collected for culture in a syringe, and the cavity should be probed to break up any loculated pus. After irrigation with saline solution, the cavity should be loosely packed with a gauze wick. In most instances, cutaneous abscesses can be treated on an outpatient basis, but infections at several body sites require special attention and, often, hospitalization.

Hand infections are of particular concern. Infections on the palmar surface may be complicated by suppurative tenosynovitis or arthritis. Hospitalization is warranted if exploration of an abscess cavity suggests that infection has penetrated deep into the hand. Infection of the distal phalanges around the nail bed (paronychia) or in the deep pulp (felon) may induce compartmental syndromes. The dense fascial layers within the finger limit swelling, and infection below fascial planes may result in pressure necrosis. If deep space infection is suspected, adequate surgical drainage of the deep compartments must be ensured and careful follow-up maintained.

Anorectal abscesses arise from the anal glands. They are usually limited to the perianal region but extension to the ischiorectal fossa or the supralevator space may occur. All anorectal abscesses should be carefully explored at the time of drainage, and general or spinal anesthesia may be necessary for adequate evaluation.

With uncomplicated cutaneous abscesses, supplemental antibiotics are usually not required after a drainage procedure. They should be used if the patient's defenses are compromised, cellulitis is marked, or infection appears to be systemic. In these instances, presumptive antibiotics should be prescribed, based on Gram-stain results and the anatomic location. When *Staphylococcus aureus* is suspected, treatment should be started with a penicillinase-resistant penicillin (dicloxacillin, 250 to 500 mg orally every 6 hours or oxacillin, 500 to 1000 mg orally or intravenously every 6 hours) or a first-generation cephalosporin (eg, cephalexin 500 mg orally every 6 hours). Vancomycin (500 mg intravenously every 6 hours) is the preferred alternative for the severely ill patient who is allergic to penicillins and cephalosporins. Clindamycin, erythromycin, and trimethoprim-sulfamethoxazole all have variable activity against *S aureus* and could be utilized for mild infections. Hospitalization may be necessary for severely ill patients.

Small, superficial anorectal abscesses may respond to surgical drainage alone. Deeper infections require therapy directed toward anaerobic organisms with agents such as clindamycin, chloramphenicol, cefoxitin, or metronidazole.

Herpetic Whitlow

Herpes simplex viruses types 1 and 2 may produce localized cutaneous infection. Three to 7 days after direct contact with active oral or genital herpetic lesions, painful paresthesias and vesicles develop on the skin, most often on the finger near the nail bed. The vesicles may coalesce and become turbid, mimicking bacterial infection. Regional lymphadenopathy, low-grade fever, and malaise may accompany the initial infection. Complete healing occurs in 14 to 28 days, but, as with oral and genital lesions, frequent recurrences at the infection site can occur (see Chapter 27, Dermatologic Emergencies).

Incision of the lesions should be avoided because it may lead to extension of the herpetic infection or bacterial superinfection. Acyclovir given orally or intravenously (200 mg five times daily for 7 days) can be an effective therapy but in most instances is not necessary. Health care workers should avoid self-infection by wearing gloves during oral and genital examinations.

Occupational Skin Infections

Aside from the typical cutaneous abscesses related to normal skin flora described above and the cellulitides discussed in Chapter 27, unusual skin and wound infections may occasionally develop in individuals exposed to pathogenic microorganisms in an occupational or recreational setting. As would be expected, each setting is associated with a different spectrum of pathogens.

Marine-Associated Infections

Erysipelothrix rhusiopthiae, *Aeromonas* species, *Vibrio* species, and *Mycobacterium marinum* may all produce skin and wound infections in individuals exposed to seafood or the marine environment (including aquariums). *Erysipelothrix rhusiopathiae* is a small Gram-positive pleomorphic rod bacteria that colonizes fish, marine animals, birds, and wild and domestic animals. Inoculation of a wound with organic material colonized with this organism produces erysipeloid, a localized self-limited infection developing at the site of trauma.[114] After a 1- to 4-day incubation period, a slowly progressive, painful, erythematous and violaceous cellulitis develops beginning at the inoculation site. Systemic toxicity is unusual and the patient is typically afebrile and has a normal white blood cell count. Untreated disease will usually resolve spontaneously in several weeks. Rarely, however, there may be systemic involvement with the development of septicemia, arthritis, or endocarditis. Although the diagnosis can be made by Gram stain or culture of the lesion, the organism is fastidious and cultures are often negative. The diagnosis usually rests on the history and the presence of the distinctive rash in a nontoxic patient. Because of the occasional significant complication, antibiotic therapy with penicillin VK (250 mg orally four times a day for 5 to 7 days) is recommended. Erythromycin, a first-generation cephalosporin, or a tetracycline are alternative agents in a penicillin-allergic patient.

Noncholera *Vibrio* species have been associated with severe local and bacteremic infections in individuals exposed to seafood or the coastal environment along the United States southeast and Gulf coasts.[115] Local infections develop in wounds occurring in the marine environment such as those associated with cleaning shellfish or walking on seashells. The infections are frequently severe. Tissue necrosis develops quickly, and surgical debridement is often necessary. The diagnosis is suggested by the clinical setting and should be supported by cultures of the wound and blood. Initial antibiotic therapy could be with either a tetracycline or chloramphenicol, but should be guided by antimicrobial susceptibility testing.

Aeromonas species are Gram-negative bacteria found in fresh water and soil, and traumatic exposure to either has been associated with local infections.[116] Significant muscle involvement can be seen with these infections, but characteristic findings have not been reported and the diagnosis must be based on clinical suspicion and culture results. These organisms are usually susceptible to chloramphenicol, tetracyclines, and the aminoglycosides.

Mycobacterium marinum, an atypical mycobacterium, can be found in both fresh and salt water. Infection develops through the introduction of the organism into the skin after contact with contaminated water. A localized, indolent, nodular lesion develops that occasionally ulcerates. The lesions are usually self-limited and heal slowly. The organism is generally susceptible in vitro to rifampin, ethambutol, and tetracyclines, and combination therapy with these agents can be utilized in nonresolving lesions.

Soil-Associated Infections

Individuals from Asia and Mexico may present with indolent combined bone and soft tissue foot infections due to mixed fungi and higher bacteria. These chronic infections, referred to as mycetoma or "madura foot," arise from repeated trauma to the feet with recurrent contamination of the wounds with soil and water. Although antibiotic therapy should be attempted, surgery is frequently necessary. As both fungal and bacterial pathogens can be involved, antimicrobial treatment cannot be empiric but must be based on the results of properly obtained deep tissue cultures.

The dimorphic fungus *Sporothrix schenckii* can produce indolent infection in individuals exposed to soil, sphagnum moss, or wet or rotting wood or hay. It is commonly associated with rose gardening or working in a forest or nursery setting. Local lymphocutaneous infection developing from inoculation of a wound with the organism is the most frequent presentation, but pulmonary infection can follow inhalation of the fungus. In cutaneous disease, an erythematous, painless, subcutaneous nodule develops from 1 to 12 weeks after inoculation. The nodule slowly enlarges, and secondary nodules and lymphatic cords may develop along the lymphatics draining the primary site. Usually, there is little or no systemic toxicity. The diagnosis is confirmed by culturing the fungus from the lesions. Cutaneous lesions can be treated with a saturated solution of potassium iodide (8 to 12 mL/day of a 1 mg/mL solution in three divided oral doses) continued for 3 weeks after the lesion has healed. Oral ketoconazole may also be effective but only limited data on its use are available. Nonresponsive patients should be referred to a specialist. Amphotericin B may be required for pulmonary or disseminated infection.

Animal-Associated Infections

The most frequent animal-associated cutaneous infections are due to bite wounds and are discussed in detail in Chapter 40, Bites and Stings. A wide variety of other cutaneous infections may develop rarely in farmers, ranch hands, abattoir workers, and other individuals with occupational exposure to animals or animal products.

Localized cutaneous viral infections on the hands and fingers may occur in cattle workers as a result of vaccinia or paravaccinia virus. These lesions develop as localized, painful, erythematous nodules that are similar to herpetic whitlows. They are self-limited in the normal host. Individuals with exposure to sheep and goats may develop a very similar lesion as a result of the Orf virus, which produces a painful nodule that resolves over several weeks.

As noted above, *E rhusiopatiae* is found in domestic animals and may produce erysipeloid in workers exposed to swine and cattle. Tularemia may develop in hunters or trappers after inoculation of a hand or forearm wound with *Francisella tularensis* during the skinning of an infected rabbit, deer, or small carnivore. An ulcerative lesion develops at the site of inoculation in association with regional lymphadenopathy and systemic toxicity. Although now an exceedingly rare disease, anthrax due to *Bacillus anthracis* should be considered in abattoir workers or individuals working with imported hides and furs who develop necrotic skin lesions. If tularemia or anthrax is suspected, the patient should be hospitalized and managed by a specialist.

Tick-Borne Infections

A number of infectious diseases may be transmitted by ticks, including Rocky Mountain spotted fever, Colorado tick fever, and relapsing fever. Two tick-borne diseases that may present as localized dermatologic infections are tularemia and Lyme disease. This latter illness is caused by a spirochete, *Borrelia burgdorferi*, and is endemic in eastern Connecticut, Massachusetts, Long Island, Wisconsin, and some parts of the Pacific Northwest. The geographical distribution appears to be dependent on the distribution of the ticks that carry the spirochete and on the presence of small mammals that may act as intermediate hosts.

Lyme disease is transmitted by tick bite, although it is frequently unrecognized by the patient.[117] After a 4- to 20-day incubation period, an enlarging erythematous lesion develops around the bite, with the gradual development of central pallor. This lesion has been termed erythema chronicum migrans and usually will resolve spontaneously without treatment, although satellite lesions frequently develop. There is often associated lymphadenopathy and constitutional symptoms of low-grade fever, fatigue, malaise, headache, myalgias, and arthralgias. Untreated Lyme disease may be complicated by chronic arthritis, CNS involvement, and myocarditis. Antibiotic treatment with tetracycline (250 mg orally four times a day) for 7 to 10 days can prevent these complications and should be given to patients over age 7 years with the typical rash who have been in endemic areas during the tick season. Penicillin V (250 mg orally four times a day) or amoxicillin is appropriate for younger children or when tetracyclines cannot be used, but they may not be as effective in preventing complications. Individuals with suspected complications from Lyme disease should be referred to a specialist.

Necrotizing Fasciitis and Myositis

Necrotizing infections of deep soft tissue, muscle, and fascia are extremely rare. They are fulminant illnesses that typically develop as complications of wounds due to trauma, peripheral vascular disease, or surgery. Even with optimal modern medical management the mortality rate remains up to 50% depending on the microorganism and site of infection. Clostridial species that produce "gas gangrene" and group A β-hemolytic streptococci are the major pathogens at most sites, but infections involving the pelvic region and the anterior abdominal wall (Fournier's syndrome) may be due to mixed aerobic and anaerobic bacteria of fecal origin.[118–120]

These infections usually arise from direct seeding of the deep soft tissue with bacteria during trauma or surgery. Very rarely, acute "spontaneous" clostridial myonecrosis may develop in previously normal tissue, most often in association with underlying malignancy or intravenous drug abuse. Release of exotoxins from clostridial or streptococcal species causes local cell death and necrosis and allows for the extremely rapid progression of these infections along and through fascial planes. Both group A *Streptococcus pyogenes* and *Clostridium perfringens* elaborate toxins that produce systemic effects including circulatory collapse and disseminated intravascular coagulation. Further, the ongoing rhabdomyolysis can contribute to acute renal failure.

Diagnosis

The clinical presentation of these infections is remarkably similar despite the different pathogens involved. After an incubation period of 8 to 24 hours, severe local pain develops at the wound site associated with marked systemic toxicity. Initially, minimal erythema and a watery nonpurulent discharge are present. As the infection progresses, edema develops around the wound with the formation of hemorrhagic bullae. Bronzing of the skin, cutaneous gangrene, and palpable crepitus due to gas formation may develop over the subsequent 8 to 24 hours in disease due to clostridial species. Nonclostridial infections produce similar local manifestations but the onset may be slightly more prolonged. Streptococcal disease is often associated with significant erythema.

Associated laboratory findings include leukocytosis with a shift to immature forms and elevation of the muscle enzymes LDH and creatine phosphokinase. Soft tissue roentgenograms may demonstrate gas in the involved areas.

Differential Diagnosis

Although fulminant infection is unmistakable, occasionally the early manifestations may appear similar to cellulitis or phlebitis. If there is any question of the possibility of necrotizing fasciitis and myositis, a deep soft tissue incisional biopsy with frozen section analysis should be considered and performed *rapidly* to avoid delay in initiating definite therapy.[121]

The presence of soft tissue gas alone does not indicate necrotizing fasciitis. Isolated anaerobic cellulitis may produce crepitus without involvement of deeper tissues, and gas can be introduced by noninfectious means such as extension from pneumomediastinum, from intravenous catheter sites, and from inadvertent or factitial injection.

Treatment

The necrotizing infections can be managed only within the hospital setting with immediate, aggressive surgical debridement and concurrent high-dose intravenous antibiotic therapy. All necrotic or suspected necrotic material must be excised and, where appropriate, fasciotomies may be required to prevent compartment syndromes. Normal tissue need not be excised, but the extent of involvement may necessitate amputation of an involved extremity. Surgical incisions and explorations should extend well beyond the involved region in all directions because of frequent occult extension of these infections.

Blood and soft tissue cultures must be obtained; early antibiotic therapy should be based on the results of Gram stain of infected material. The presence of large "box-car" shaped Gram-positive bacilli suggests clostridial infection, and treatment can be started with penicillin G (12×10^6 to 24×10^6 U/day intravenously in 4-hour doses) or clindamycin (600 mg intravenously every 6 hours for adults) for penicillin-allergic patients. If Gram-positive cocci are seen alone, high-dose penicillin G is also appropriate; if mixed flora or no bacteria are seen, a mixed aerobic/anaerobic infection should be suspected and therapy should be initiated with penicillin G, clindamycin, and an aminoglycoside.

Once stabilized with antibiotic treatment and supportive measures, almost all patients should undergo repeat surgical exploration within the first 24 to 36 hours to confirm the removal of all necrotic tissue. Antibiotic therapy should be maintained for 10 to 14 days.

Septic Arthritis

A relatively uncommon but serious infection, septic arthritis requires immediate therapy to prevent irreversible joint injury. It is primarily a disease resulting from invasive bacteria and the predominant pathogens vary with the age of the patient.[122,123] In children *Staphylococcus aureus* and *H influenzae* are the most common pathogens. In the sexually active population *Neisseria gonorrhoeae* predominates, followed by *Staphylococcus aureus*. In elderly adults *Staphylococcus aureus* is most common. *Streptococcus pyogenes* and Gram-negative bacilli can produce disease at any age and *Pseudomonas aeruginosa* appears to be particularly frequent in intravenous drug abusers. Other bacteria, such as *Streptococcus pneumoniae*, *Brucella* species, *Neisseria meningitidis*, and anaerobic Gram-negative rods, may also cause septic arthritis. Viruses, fungi, and mycobacteria may produce arthritis, but they are not usually associated with acute, purulent, rapidly destructive disease.

Pathogenesis

Septic arthritis results from invasion of the synovium and joint space by the infecting organism through either direct inoculation or hematogenous or contiguous spread. Parenteral drug use, prior joint disease, chronic illness, joint prostheses, and trauma are predisposing factors for infectious arthritis.

In gonococcal infection, the arthritis is a manifestation of disseminated gonococcal infection occurring as a complication of symptomatic or asymptomatic anogenital or pharyngeal infection.[124] The characteristics of gonococci that produce disseminated disease differ from those of other gonococci in that the former are more resistant to serum bactericidal activity and more sensitive to penicillin. Several cases of gonococcal arthritis due to penicillinase-producing strains of N gonorrhoeae have now been recognized, although at present they are limited to communities where penicillinase-producing N gonorrhoeae have been frequently isolated in uncomplicated infections.

Diagnosis

Patients with septic arthritis develop a painful, tender, swollen, erythematous, and warm joint with fever and systemic toxicity. Concurrent extra-articular infection or sepsis may occur. Synovial effusion is not always obvious, and all the major signs of joint inflammation will be found in only 10% of cases. In infants, the initial complaint is commonly limited to an unwillingness to move the affected joint. Septic arthritis is most common in the knee, wrist, shoulder, elbow, hip, and ankle joints, although parenteral drug abusers have a predilection for sternoclavicular or sacroiliac joint infections. Most cases of nongonococcal arthritis involve a single joint, while gonococcal arthritis may have an asymmetric polyarticular distribution. Peripheral blood leukocytosis and elevated erythrocyte sedimentation rate are usually but not always present.

Arthrocentesis should be performed on any joint believed to be infected (see Chapter 86, Atlas of Emergency Procedures, for the technique of aspirating joints). The synovial fluid should be examined for cell count and differential, glucose determination, Gram stain, culture, and inspection of the mucin clot. In septic arthritis, the synovial fluid leukocyte count is typically 100,000/μL to 150,000/μL with more than 85% polymorphonuclear leukocytes. Glucose concentration is usually less than 40 mg/dL. The mucin clot is characteristically poor, and the Gram stain is positive in approximately 65% of cases. Possible additional diagnostic studies of the synovial fluid include lactic acid determination and countercurrent immunoelectrophoresis for bacterial antigens, but the cost effectiveness of these studies has not been determined. Blood cultures should be obtained in all patients with suspected septic arthritis and are positive in approximately one third to one half of patients with the infection. With gonococcal arthritis, the pathogen may be isolated from a primary urethral, cervical, rectal, or pharyngeal site, and all potential sites should be cultured appropriately for gonococci. Radiologic studies may demonstrate distention of the joint capsule or coexistent osteomyelitis.

Differential Diagnosis

Crystalline-induced synovitis, osteoarthritis, rheumatoid arthritis, Reiter's syndrome, hemophilic hemarthroses, and acute rheumatic fever may resemble suppurative arthritis. Gout and pseudogout may occur simultaneously with septic arthritis. In patients with rheumatoid arthritis, superimposed infection may be seen as a sudden asymmetric flare in joint symptoms. Arthrocentesis is critical to confirm the diagnosis.

Several clinical characteristics may help distinguish gonococcal from nongonococcal septic arthritis. Gonococcal arthritis occurs in healthy, sexually active individuals. It presents three times more frequently in women than in men, and in women it commonly occurs during menstruation, pregnancy, or the postpartum period.[124] Sixty percent of patients have two or more joints involved. The wrists and hands are frequently infected in gonococcal arthritis; in contrast, joints of the lower extremity are more commonly involved in septic arthritis due to other pathogens. Patients with gonococcal arthritis may have concurrent tenosynovitis in the hands, wrists, or ankles. In addition, diffuse, widely scattered skin lesions are present in 30% to 50% of patients. These lesions are painful papules and pustules that are located primarily on the distal extremities.

Nongonococcal septic arthritis is slightly more common in men. Most patients have concurrent extra-articular infection or an underlying predisposing factor. The knee and hip are the most frequently involved joints.

Treatment

Therapy for septic arthritis depends on the pathogen involved, the joint infected, and the presence or absence of prosthetic devices. Gonococcal arthritis is quite responsive to therapy and may be managed with antibiotics alone, although initial hospitalization is suggested for all patients. In patients with Gram-negative diplococci on synovial fluid Gram stain and presumed gonococcal arthritis, the following regimens have been recommended by the Centers for Disease Control as appropriate alternatives: ceftriaxone (1 g intramuscularly or intravenously every 24 hours), or ceftizoxime (1 g intravenously every 8 hours), or cefotaxime (1 g intravenously every 8 hours). Individuals allergic to penicillin or cephalosporin antibiotics may be treated with spectinomycin (2 g intramuscularly every 12 hours). If the infecting organism is proven to be susceptible to penicillin, ampicillin (1 g intravenously every 6 hours) may be used.

Patients with an uncomplicated course can be discharged from the hospital 24 to 48 hours after symptoms resolve to complete 7 days of oral therapy with any of the following agents: oral cefuroxime-axetil (500 mg twice daily), or amoxicillin (500 mg with clavulanic acid three times daily), or ciprofloxacin (500 mg twice daily in nonpregnant patients). Because of possible concurrent chlamydial infection, patients with gonococcal arthritis should also receive 7 days of treatment with tetracycline (500 mg orally four times a day), doxycycline (100 mg orally twice a day), or erythromycin base (500 mg four times daily).

Nongonococcal septic arthritis is more destructive than gonococcal disease, and all patients with this infection should be hospitalized and receive initial parenteral antibiotic therapy. For presumed staphylococcal infection, therapy should include a penicillinase-resistant penicillin (oxacillin or nafcillin) given at a dose of 2 g intravenously every 4 hours. For patients allergic to penicillin, or where methicillin-resistant *Staphylococcus aureus* is suspected, vancomycin (500 mg intravenously every 6 hours) is appropriate. If Gram-negative bacilli are found on Gram stain of synovial fluid, initial therapy should be designed to treat *Pseudomonas aeruginosa*. A combination of an antipseudomonal penicillin (or either cefoperazone or ceftazidime), and an aminoglycoside should be administered. If the Gram stain is negative but the clinical presentation suggests septic arthritis, a healthy, sexually active young adult with no other risk factors for joint infection can be treated initially for gonococcal arthritis. Other adult patients and older children should receive initial therapy directed against *S aureus* and Gram-negative infections pending culture results. Children younger than 2 years of age may be treated for *S aureus* and *H influenzae* with a penicillinase-resistant penicillin (200 mg/kg/day in six doses) and chloramphenicol (100 mg/kg/day in four doses) until results of cultures and susceptibility tests are available. Third-generation cephalosporins such as ceftriaxone can be effective as single agents in this setting, but comparative studies with older agents have not been performed.[125]

In addition to antibiotic therapy, nongonococcal septic arthritis requires drainage of synovial fluid to avoid joint damage. If the synovial fluid is neither loculated nor thick, daily or twice daily needle aspirations may be adequate for infection of joints other than the hip (or shoulder in neonates). Aspirations should be continued until the effusion resolves completely and the response to therapy should be monitored with serial cell counts and cultures. A good therapeutic response can be expected if synovial fluid leukocyte counts progressively decrease and the synovial fluid is sterilized within 4 days.[126] However, if at any time there is an increase in joint symptoms and effusion, a rise in synovial fluid leukocyte counts, or difficulty encountered in effecting complete drainage of the effusion by needle aspiration, then more definitive drainage should be performed surgically. Complete joint immobility is not necessary, but weight bearing should be avoided. The joint should be kept in the functional position as much as possible and passive range of motion exercises should be used to prevent contractures.

Septic Bursitis

One-third of patients with inflammation of the olecranon or prepatellar bursae have septic bursitis.[127] *Staphylococcus aureus* is the causal pathogen in over 90% of the cases, but, rarely, group A β-hemolytic streptococci, *Sporothrix schenckii,* or atypical mycobacteria have been implicated.[128] Infection usually occurs in young or middle-aged men engaged in manual labor who have sustained trauma either directly to or distal to the involved bursa. Previous bursal disease is a predisposing factor. The major clinical features are tenderness, warmth, and distension of the involved bursa associated with erythema and cellulitis of the overlying skin. Fever develops in approximately 40% of patients.

Bursal fluid analysis can distinguish septic from nonseptic bursitis. Gram stain of the fluid demonstrates organisms in 65% to 100% of infected cases, and the white blood cell count is usually greater than $1000/\mu L$, with a predominance of neutrophils. The bursal fluid glucose level is almost always less than 50% of the corresponding serum level. In noninfectious bursitis, the white blood cell count is less than $1000/\mu L$ with predominantly mononuclear cells; the bursal fluid glucose concentration is nearly the same as the serum level in these forms of bursitis.

The major differential diagnoses are traumatic, gouty, or rheumatoid bursitis. Septic bursitis should be suspected if the patient is febrile or has severe bursal tenderness, but as the presentation can be nonspecific, needle aspiration should be performed in all cases of olecranon or prepatellar bursitis. Gouty and septic bursitis can occur simultaneously and all fluid should be examined for crystals as well as for organisms.

Treatment should be initiated with a semisynthetic penicillinase-resistant penicillin pending culture results. Adequate antibiotic levels can be achieved in bursal fluid with oxacillin (500 mg orally four times a day) or a corresponding dosage of cloxacillin or dicloxacillin. The time required to sterilize the bursal space increases with the duration of the untreated bursal infection, and therefore, the length of therapy must be individualized. Repeat needle aspirations of the bursa achieve effective drainage and permit monitoring of the therapeutic response. Therapy for 5 days after the bursa has been sterilized is effective and results in few complications.[129]

REFERENCES

1. Monto AD, Ullman BM. Acute respiratory illness in an American community. The Tecumseh study. *JAMA.* 1974;277:164–169.
2. Gwaltney JM, Moskalski PB, Hendley JO. Hand-to-hand transmission of rhinovirus colds. *Ann Intern Med.* 1978;88:463–467.
3. Dick EC, Jennings LL, Mink KA, Wartgow CD, Inhorn SL. Aerosol transmission of rhinovirus colds. *J Infect Dis.* 1987;156:442–448.
4. Honikman LM, Masser BF. Guidelines for the selective use of throat cultures in the diagnosis of streptococcal respiratory infection. *Pediatrics.* 1971;48:573–581.

5. Glezen WP, Clyde WA, Senior RJ, et al. Group A streptococci, mycoplasmas and viruses associated with pharyngitis. *JAMA*. 1967;202:455–460.
6. Huovinen P, Lahtonen R, Ziegler T, et al. Pharyngitis in adults: the presence and coexistence of viruses and bacterial organisms. *Ann Intern Med*. 1989;110:612–616.
7. Komaroff AL. A management strategy for sore throat. *JAMA*. 1978;239:1429–1432.
8. Bass JW. Treatment of streptococcal pharyngitis revisited. *JAMA*. 1986;256:740–743.
9. Wright RA, Scholes E. Streptococcal disease control in an ambulatory practice. *West J Med*. 1984;140:409–413.
10. Krober MS, Bass JW, Michels GN. Streptococcal pharyngitis. Placebo-controlled double-blind evaluation of clinical response to penicillin therapy. *JAMA*. 1985;253:1271–1274.
11. Radetsky M, Solomon JA, Todd JH. Identification of streptococcal pharyngitis in the office laboratory: reassessment of new technology. *Pediatr Infect Dis*. 1987;6:556–563.
12. Centers for Disease Control. 1989. Sexually transmitted diseases treatment guidelines. *MMWR*.
13. Jones PG, Kauffman CA, McAuliffe LS, et al. Efficacy of ketoconazole v nystatin in prevention of fungal infections in neutropenic patients. *Arch Intern Med*. 1984;144:549–551.
14. Daley CL, Sande M. The runny nose infection of the paranasal sinuses. *Infect Dis Clin North Am*. 1988;2:131–147.
15. Evans FO, Sydnor JS, Moore WEC, et al. Sinusitis of the maxillary antrum. *N Engl J Med*. 1975;293:735–739.
16. Hamory BH, Sande MA, Sydnor A, et al. Etiology and antimicrobial therapy of acute maxillary sinusitis. *J Infect Dis*. 1979;139:197–202.
17. Wald ER, Milmoe GJ, Bowen A, et al. Acute maxillary sinusitis in children. *N Engl J Med*. 1981;304:749–754.
18. Morgan PR, Morrison WV. Complications of frontal and ethmoid sinusitis. *Laryngoscope*. 1980;80:661–666.
19. Rubin J, Yu VL. Malignant external otitis: insights into pathogenesis, clinical manifestations, diagnosis and therapy. *Am J Med*. 1988;85:391–398.
20. Brook I. Otitis media in children: a prospective study of aerobic and anaerobic bacteriology. *Laryngoscope*. 1979;89:992–997.
21. Shurin PA, Howie VM, Pelton SI, et al. Bacterial etiology of otitis media during the first six weeks of life. *J Pediatr*. 1978;92:893–896.
22. Giebink GS, Quie PG. Otitis media: the spectrum of middle ear inflammation. *Annu Rev Med*. 1978;29:285–306.
23. Henderson FW, Collier AM, Sanyal MA, et al. A longitudinal study of respiratory viruses and bacteria in the etiology of acute otitis media with effusion. *N Engl J Med*. 1982;306:1377–1383.
24. Bluestone CD. Otitis media in children: to treat or not to treat? *N Engl J Med*. 1982;306:1399–1404.
25. Cantekim EI, Mandel EM, Bluestone CD. Lack of efficacy of a decongestant-antihistamine combination for otitis media with effusion ("secretory" otitis media) in children. *N Engl J Med*. 1983;308:297–301.
26. Spruance SL, Overall JC, Kern ER, et al. The natural history of recurrent herpes simplex labialis: implications for antiviral therapy. *N Engl J Med*. 1977;297:69–75.
27. Corey L, Spear PG. Infections with herpes simplex viruses. *N Engl J Med*. 1986;314:686–691, 749–757.
28. Chow AW, Roser SM, Brady FA. Orofacial odontogenic infections. *Ann Intern Med*. 1978;88:392–492.
29. Blomquist IK, Bayer AS. Life-threatening deep fascial space infections of the head and neck. *Infect Dis Clin North Am*. 1988;2:237–264.
30. Yu VL, Kroboth FJ, Shonnard J, et al. Legionnaire's disease: new clinical perspective from a prospective study. *Am J Med*. 1982;73:357–361.
31. Woodhead MA, Macfarlane JT, McCracken JS, Rose DH, Finch RG. Prospective study of the aetiology and outcome of pneumonia in the community. *Lancet*. 1987;1:671–674.
32. Williams DM, Krick JA, Remington JS. Pulmonary infection in the compromised host. *Am Rev Respir Dis*. 1976;114:359–394.
33. Cohn DL. Pulmonary infections in the acquired immunodeficiency syndrome. *Semin Respir Med*. 1989;10:1–11.
34. Newhouse M, Sanchis J, Bienenstock J. Lung defense mechanisms. *N Engl J Med*. 1976;295:990–998, 1045–1052.
35. Murray HW, Masur H, Senterfit LB, et al. The protean manifestations of *Mycoplasma pneumoniae* infection in adults. *Am J Med*. 1975;58:229–242.
36. Bartlett JG, Gorbach SL. The triple threat of aspiration pneumonia. *Chest*. 1975;68:560–566.
37. Murray PR, Washington JA II. Microscopic and bacteriologic analysis of expectorated sputum. *Mayo Clin Proc*. 1975;50:339–344.
38. Pratter MR, Irwin RS. Transtracheal aspiration: guidelines for safety. *Chest*. 1979;76:518–520.
39. LaForce FM. Community-acquired lower respiratory tract infections: prevention and cost-control strategies. *Am J Med*. 1985;78(suppl 6B):52–57.
40. Kirby BD, Snyder KM, Meyer RD, et al. Legionnaire's disease: clinical features of 24 cases. *Ann Intern Med*. 1978;89:297–309.
41. Levison ME, Mangura CT, Lorber B, et al. Clindamycin compared with penicillin for the treatment of anaerobic lung abscess. *Ann Intern Med*. 1983;98:466–471.
42. Masur H, Lane C, Kovacs JA, Allegra CJ, Edman JC. Pneumocystis pneumonia: from bench to clinic. *Ann Intern Med*. 1989;111:813–826.
43. Sattler FR, Cowan R, Nielsen DM, Ruskin J. Trimethoprim-sulfamethoxazole compared with pentamidine for treatment of *Pneumocystis carinii* pneumonia in the acquired immunodeficiency syndrome. *Ann Intern Med*. 1988;109:280–287.
44. Blacklow NR, Greenberg HB. Viral gastroenteritis. *N Engl J Med*. 1991;325:252–264.
45. Guerrant RL, Bobak DA. Bacterial and protozoal gastroenteritis. *N Engl J Med*. 1991;325:327–340.
46. Harris JC, Dupont HL, Hornick RB. Fecal leukocytes in diarrheal illness. *Ann Intern Med*. 1972;76:697–703.
47. Paisley JW, Mirrett S, Lauer BA, et al. Darkfield microscopy of human feces for presumptive diagnosis of *Campylobacter fetus* subspecies *jejeuni* enteritis. *J Clin Microbiol*. 1982;15:61–63.
48. Pitlik SD, Fainstein V, Garza D, et al. Human cryptosporidiosis: spectrum of disease. *Arch Intern Med*. 1983;143:2269–2275.
49. Santosham M, Daum RS, Dilman L, et al. Oral rehydration therapy of infantile diarrhea: a controlled study of well nourished children hospitalized in the United States and Panama. *N Engl J Med*. 1982;306:1070–1076.
50. The WHO Diarrheal Diseases Control Programme. *WHO Wkly Epidemiol Rec*. 1979;54:121–123.
51. Dupont HL, Ericsson CD, Johnson PC, et al. Prevention of travelers' diarrhea by the tablet formulation of bismuth subsalicylate. *JAMA*. 1987;257:1347–1350.
52. Blaser MJ, Wells JF, Feldman RA, et al. Campylobacter enteritis in the United States: a multicenter study. *Ann Intern Med*. 1983;98:360–365.

53. Quinn TC, Stamm WE, Goodell SE, et al. The polymicrobial origin of intestinal infections in homosexual men. *N Engl J Med.* 1983; 308:576–582.
54. Wolfson JA, Hooper DC. Fluoroquinolone antimicrobial agents. *Clin Microbiol Rev.* 1989;2:378–424.
55. Goodman LJ, Trenholme GM, Kaplan RL, Segreti J, et al. Empiric antimicrobial therapy of domestically acquired acute diarrhea in urban adults. *Arch Intern Med.* 1990;150:541–546.
56. Horowitz MA. Specific diagnosis of food borne disease. *Gastroenterology.* 1977;73:375–381.
57. Eastaugh J, Shepherd S. Infectious and toxic syndromes from fish and shellfish consumption. *Arch Intern Med.* 1989;149:1735–1740.
58. Lipsky BA. Urinary tract infections in men. *Ann Intern Med.* 1989; 110:138–150.
59. Stamm WE, Wagner KF, Amsel R, et al. Causes of the acute urethral syndrome in women. *N Engl J Med.* 1980;303:409–415.
60. Komaroff AL. Acute dysuria in women. *N Engl J Med.* 1984; 310:368–375.
61. Stamm WE, Counts GW, Running KR, et al. Diagnosis of coliform infection in acutely dysuric women. *N Engl J Med.* 1982;307:463–468.
62. Johnson JR, Stamm WE. Urinary tract infections in women: diagnosis and treatment. *Ann Intern Med.* 1989;111:906–917.
63. Stamm WE. Measurement of pyuria and its relationship to bacteruria. *Am J Med.* 1983:53–58. Infectious disease supplement.
64. Komaroff AL. Urinalysis and urine culture in women with dysuria. *Ann Intern Med.* 1986;104:212–218.
65. Rubin RH, Fang LST, Jones SR, et al. Single-dose amoxicillin therapy for urinary tract infection. *JAMA.* 1980;244:561–564.
66. Stamm WE, Running K, McKevitt M, et al. Treatment of the acute urethral syndrome. *N Engl J Med.* 1981;304:956–958.
67. Stamm WE, McKevitt M, Counts GW, et al. Is antimicrobial prophylaxis of urinary tract infections cost effective? *Ann Intern Med.* 1981;94:251–255.
68. Stamm WE, Guinnan ME, Johnson C, et al. Effect of treatment regimens for *Neisseria gonorrhoeae* on simultaneous infection with *Chlamydia trachomatis. N Engl J Med.* 1984;310:545–549.
69. Felman YM, Nikitas JA. Nongonococcal urethritis: a clinical review. *JAMA.* 1981;245:381–386.
70. Weisner PJ, Thompson SE III. Gonococcal diseases. *DM.* 1980; 20:1–44.
71. Stamm WE. Diagnosis of *Chlamydia trachomatis* genitourinary infections. *Ann Intern Med.* 1988;108:710–717.
72. Hooton TM, Wong ES, Barnes RC, et al. Erythromycin for persistent or recurrent nongonococcal urethritis. A randomized, placebo-controlled trial. *Ann Intern Med.* 1990;43:21–26.
73. Meares EM Jr. Prostatitis and related diseases. *DM.* 1980;26:7–39.
74. Conly JM, Ronald AR. Cerebrospinal fluid as a diagnostic body fluid. *Am J Med.* 1983:102–108. Infectious disease supplement.
75. Geisler PJ, Nelson KW, Levin S, et al. Community acquired purulent meningitis: a review of 1316 cases during the antibiotic era, 1954–1976. *Rev Infect Dis.* 1980;1:725–745.
76. Behrman RE, Meyers BR, Mendelson MH, et al. Central nervous system infections in the elderly. *Arch Intern Med.* 1989;149:1596–1599.
77. Spanos A, Harrell FE, Durack DT. Differential diagnosis of acute meningitis. An analysis of the predictive value initial observations. *JAMA.* 1989;262:2700–2707.
78. Onorato IM, Wormser GP, Nicholas P. "Normal" CSF in bacterial meningitis. *JAMA.* 1980;244:1469–1471.
79. Tunkel AR, Wispelwey B, Scheld WM. Bacterial meningitis: recent advances in pathophysiology and treatment. *Ann Intern Med.* 1990; 112:610–623.
80. Lebel MH, Freij BJ, Syrogiannopoylos GA, et al. Dexamethasone therapy for bacterial meningitis. Results of two double-blind, placebo-controlled trials. *N Engl J Med.* 1988;319:964–971.
81. Lieberman JM, Greenberg DP, Ward JI. Prevention of bacterial meningitis. Vaccines and chemoprophylaxis. *Infect Dis Clin North Am.* 1990;4:703–729.
82. Committee on Infectious Diseases, American Academy of Pediatrics. *The 1988 Red Book.* 21st ed. Elk Grove Village, IL: American Academy of Pediatrics; 1988.
83. Singer JI, Maur PR, Riley JP, et al. Management of central nervous system infections during an epidemic of enteroviral aseptic meningitis. *J Pediatr.* 1980;96:559–563.
84. Varki AP, Puthuran P. Value of second lumbar puncture in confirming a diagnosis of aseptic meningitis: a prospective study. *Arch Neurol.* 1979;36:581–582.
85. Snider WD, Simpson DM, Nielsen S, et al. Neurological complications of acquired immune deficiency syndrome: analysis of 50 patients. *Ann Neurol.* 1983;14:403–418.
86. Whitley RJ. Viral encephalitis. *N Engl J Med.* 1990;323:241–250.
87. Whitley RJ, Soong S, Linneman C Jr, et al. Herpes simplex encephalitis: clinical assessment. *JAMA.* 1982;247:317–320.
88. Mathisen GE, Meyer RD, George WL, et al. Brain abscess and cerebritis. *Rev Infect Dis.* 1984;6:S101–S106.
89. Harrison MJG. The clinical presentation of intracranial abscesses. *Q J Med.* 1982;204:461–468.
90. Brewer NS, MacCarty CS, Wellman WE. Brain abscess: a review of recent experience. *Ann Intern Med.* 1975;82:571–576.
91. Skoldenberg B, Forsgren M, Alestig K, et al. Acyclovir versus vidarabine in herpes simplex encephalitis: randomised multicentre study in consecutive Swedish patients. *Lancet.* 1984;2:707–711.
92. Whitley RJ, Alford CA, Hirsch MS, et al. Vidarabine versus acyclovir therapy in herpes simplex encephalitis. *N Engl J Med.* 1986; 314:144–149.
93. Whitley RJ, Soong S, Hirsch MS, et al. Herpes simplex encephalitis: vidarabine therapy and diagnostic problems. *N Engl J Med.* 1981; 304:313–318.
94. Rapp CE Jr, Hewetson JF. Infectious mononucleosis and the Epstein-Barr virus. *Am J Dis Child.* 1978;132:78–86.
95. Evans AS. Infectious mononucleosis and related syndromes. *Am J Med Sci.* 1978;276:325–339.
96. Cooper DA, Gold J, Maclean P, et al. Acute AIDS retrovirus infection. Definition of a clinical illness associated with seroconversion. *Lancet.* 1985;1:537–540.
97. Ho DD, Sarngadharan MG, Resnick L, et al. Primary human T-lymphotropic virus type III infection. *Ann Intern Med.* 1985; 103:880–883.
98. Fox R, Eldred GJ, Fuchs EJ, et al. Clinical manifestations of acute infection with human immunodeficiency virus in a cohort of gay men. *AIDS.* 1987;1:35–38.
99. Tindall B, Barker S, Donovan B, et al. Characterization of the acute clinical illness associated with human immunodeficiency virus infection. *Arch Intern Med.* 1988;148:945–949.
100. Bender CE. The value of corticosteroids in the treatment of infectious mononucleosis. *JAMA.* 1967;199:529–531.
101. Lemon SM. Type A viral hepatitis. New developments in an old disease. *N Engl J Med.* 1985;313:1059–1068.
102. Hoofnagle JH. Type B viral hepatitis: virology, serology and clinical course. *Semin Liver Dis.* 1982;1:7–14.

103. Rizzetto M, Verme G, Recchia S, et al. Chronic hepatitis in carriers of hepatitis B surface antigen, with intrahepatic expression of the delta antigen. An active and progressive disease unresponsive to immunosuppressive treatment. *Ann Intern Med.* 1983;98:437–441.
104. Alter HJ, Purcell RH, Shih JW, et al. Detection of antibody to hepatitis C virus in prospectively followed transfusion recipients with acute and chronic non-A, non-B hepatitis. *N Engl J Med.* 1989;321:1494–1500.
105. Reyes GR, Purdy MA, Kim JP, et al. Isolation of a cDNA from the virus responsible for enterically transmitted non-A, non-B hepatitis. *Science.* 1990;247:1335–1340.
106. Dienstag JL. Non-A, non-B hepatitis. 1. Recognition, epidemiology, and clinical features. *Gastroenterology.* 1983;85:439–462.
106a. Perrillo RP, Schiff ER, David GL, et al. A randomized, controlled trial of interferon ALFA-2b alone and after prednisone withdrawal for the treatment of chronic hepatitis B. *N Engl J Med.* 1990;323:295–301.
106b. Davis GL, Balart LA, Schiff ER, et al. Treatment of chronic hepatitis C with recombinant interferon ALFA. A multicenter randomized controlled trial. *N Engl J Med.* 1989;321:1501–1506.
107. CDC. Protection against viral hepatitis. Recommendations of the Immunization Practices Advisory Committee (ACIP). *MMWR.* 1990;39(No. RR-2).
108. Chesney PJ, Davis JP, Purdy WK, et al. Clinical manifestations of toxic shock syndrome. *JAMA.* 1981;246:741–748.
109. CDC. Rocky Mountain spotted fever and human ehrlichiosis—United States, 1989. *MMWR.* 1990;39:281–284.
110. Hattwick MAW, et al. Fatal Rocky Mountain spotted fever. *JAMA.* 1978;240:1494–1503.
111. Walker DH, Cain BG, Olmstead PM. Laboratory diagnosis of Rocky Mountain spotted fever by immunofluorescent demonstration of *Rickettsia rickettsii* in cutaneous lesions. *Am J Clin Pathol.* 1978;69:619–623.
112. Vianna NJ, Hinman AR. Rocky Mountain spotted fever on Long Island. *Am J Med.* 1971;51:725–730.
113. Philips RE, Warrell DA, White NJ, et al. Intravenous quinidine for the treatment of severe falciparum malaria. Clinical and pharmacokinetic studies. *N Engl J Med.* 1985;312:1273–1278.
114. Reboli AC, Farrar WE. *Erysipelothrix rhusiopathiae*: an occupational pathogen. *Clin Microbiol Rev.* 1989;2:354–359.
115. Bonner JB, Coker AS, Berryman CR, Pollock HM. Spectrum of *Vibrio* infections in a Gulf coast community. *Ann Intern Med.* 1983;99:464–469.
116. Davis WA, Kane JG, Garagusi VF. Human *Aeromonas* infections: a review of the literature and a case report of endocarditis. *Medicine.* 1978;57:267–277.
117. Steere AC, Hutchinson GJ, Rahn DW, et al. Treatment of the early manifestations of Lyme disease. *Ann Intern Med.* 1983;99:22–26.
118. Dellinger EP. Severe necrotizing soft tissue infections: multiple disease entities requiring a common approach. *JAMA.* 1981;246:1717–1721.
119. Stevens DL. Invasive group A-streptococcus infections. *Clin Infec Dis.* 1192;14:2–13.
120. Kallen PA, Louie JA, Nies KM, et al. Infectious myositis and related syndromes. *Semin Arthritis Rheum.* 1982;11:421–439.
121. Stamenkovic I, Lew PD. Early recognition of potentially fatal necrotizing fasciitis: the use of frozen-section biopsy. *N Engl J Med.* 1984;310:1689–1693.
122. Rosenthal J, Bole GG, Robinson WD. Acute nongonococcal infectious arthritis: evaluation of risk factors, therapy, and outcome. *Semin Arthritis Rheum.* 1980;23:889–897.
123. Goldenberg DL, Reed JI. Bacterial arthritis. *N Engl J Med.* 1985;312:764–772.
124. Masi ASL, Eisenstein BJ. Disseminated gonococcal infection (DGI) and gonococcal arthritis (GCA): II. Clinical manifestations, diagnosis, complications, treatment and prevention. *Semin Arthritis Rheum.* 1981;10:173–197.
125. Frenkel LD. Once-daily administration of ceftriaxone for the treatment of selected serious bacterial infections in children. *Pediatrics.* 1988;82:486–491.
126. Ho G Jr, Su EY. Therapy for septic arthritis. *JAMA.* 1982;247:797–800.
127. Ho G Jr, Tice AD, Kaplan SR. Septic bursitis in the prepatellar and olecranon bursae: an analysis of 25 cases. *Ann Intern Med.* 1978;89:21–27.
128. Ho G Jr, Tice AD. Comparison of nonseptic and septic bursitis: further observations on the treatment of septic bursitis. *Arch Intern Med.* 1979;139:1269–1273.
129. Ho G Jr, Su EY. Antibiotic therapy of septic bursitis. *Arthritis Rheum.* 1981;24:905–911.

26. Burns

G. RICHARD BRAEN, MD, FACEP

In the United States over 2 million people per year suffer thermal burns. A great majority of these burns are minor in nature, while 3% to 5% may be life threatening. Most minor burns heal spontaneously, but inappropriate treatment may delay healing, lead to infection, or cause complications.

Thermal burns include contact with direct flames, superheated gases, steam, hot water, and other agents. Hot tap water is frequently a cause of burns occurring at home. Half of the victims of hot water burns are under 5 years of age and almost 10% are over 65 years of age. Almost all of these hot tap water injuries could have been prevented by lowering the temperature of the water heater to below 54.4° C (130°F) or preferably somewhat lower.[1]

PATHOPHYSIOLOGY OF THERMAL INJURIES

The skin is the largest organ of the body. Its thickness varies from 1 to 3 mm, being thicker on the dorsal and extensor aspects of the body. It not only is a waterproof barrier for the body, but also aids in temperature regulation.

The skin is composed of two layers, the epidermis and the dermis. The epidermis comprises the outer layer of the skin and is further divided into five sublayers. From superficial to deep, these layers include (1) the stratum corneum, (2) the stratum lucidum (present only in thick areas, such as the palms of the hands and soles of the feet), (3) the stratum granulosum, (4) the stratum spinosum, and (5) the stratum germinativum.

The stratum corneum forms the vapor barrier of the body because of its keratin and lipid content. When this layer is damaged, fluid loss may be extensive. The stratum germinativum is the layer from which new epidermal cells are produced. Portions of the stratum germinativum are also found around some of the epidermal appendages that lie in the dermis (eg, hair follicles, sebaceous glands, and sweat glands). If the entire epidermis is damaged, but the epidermal appendages within the dermis remain intact, the stratum germinativum that surrounds these appendages may regenerate a new epidermis.

The dermis contains fibrous connective tissue and blood vessels that support the epidermis and supply it with nutrients. In addition to hair follicles, sebaceous glands, and sweat glands, the dermis contains peripheral nerve fibers that form a plexus near the lipodermal junction. Superficial burns are more painful than deeper burns because these pain-transmitting nerve fibers, which lie deep in the dermis, are irritated in superficial burns rather than being destroyed as they are in a deeper burn.

Beneath the dermis lies a layer of subcutaneous tissue that contains areolar and adipose tissue. The subcutaneous tissue also contains collagen fibers that bind and support the more superficial layers.

The water, lipid content, and vascularity of these various layers influence heat conductivity and subsequent depth of the burn. The greater the water content, the greater the heat conduction, and the more rapidly damage occurs. In highly vascular areas, however, heat can be transferred away from the burn site by blood flow, and this heat dissipation may decrease the depth of burn in such an area.

The water loss from burned skin may be considerable, ranging from 5 to 15 times normal. In conjunction with the evaporation of water, a considerable amount of body heat may be lost, and hypothermia may develop. In order to maintain the body's core temperature, metabolic and caloric demands are increased.[2]

The chance of localized and subsequent systemic infection increases greatly following a burn of the skin. In deeper burns, the skin undergoes coagulation necrosis, which provides an excellent growth medium for bacteria. Since blood vessels within a deeper burn may be destroyed and normal host defense mechanisms, such as white blood cell migration into the wound, may be altered, the natural defense against infection is decreased. Essentially, the immune response of the host decreases in proportion to the extent and depth of the burn.[3]

Almost immediately following a burn injury, the vascularity of the skin in the involved area changes. Three concentric areas of vascular change may be identified on the surface of the skin at the damaged site. The center area, which is called the *zone of coagulation* (seen particularly in deeper burns), is the area of greatest destruction.[4] Within this area, thermal coagulation and irreversible cellular death occur. Also within this area, all blood vessels and capillaries become occluded. As the intensity of the heat or length of exposure increases, this zone of coagulation extends more deeply into the skin, producing a full-thickness destruction.[5]

Surrounding the zone of coagulation is a *zone of stasis* that involves the vasculature of the dermis. Initially, it appears red and blanches on pressure. Within a few minutes, there is an abnormal aggregation of formed blood elements within this area, causing thrombosis. There is also vasoconstriction, which further decreases blood flow to the burned area. Some blood vessels in this zone remain patent, even though the overall blood supply is reduced, and circulation can be restored in these areas with appropriate treatment. Exposure of the wound to drying, further trauma, infection, or improper care may cause irreversible damage to this zone, however, converting it to a zone of coagulation with subsequent necrosis that could result in a full-thickness injury. This is preventable by appropriate treatment.

Surrounding the zone of stasis is a small *zone of hyperemia*, which is the area least affected by the burn. In this area, vascular integrity is maintained, and cellular death is minimal. This zone can be recognized by the bright red color that blanches on pressure. Almost all wounds have this zone of hyperemia at their margins.

Burn Shock

Shock following major thermal injuries is a common but preventable occurrence. Burn shock is due to changes in circulating blood volume and to cardiovascular changes. Circulating blood volume may decrease because of an extravasation of fluid and plasma into the burned area. The interstitial osmotic pressure of burned tissue increases immediately after the burn. This increase of osmotic pressure explains the magnitude of fluid shift into burned tissue, which cannot be explained by increased capillary permeability alone.[6] In addition, there is an initial shunting of water and electrolytes into skeletal muscles throughout the body, even in areas not involved directly by the burn. This shift of sodium and water from the general circulation may play the greatest role in the development of shock during the first 1 to 2 hours following the thermal injury. Within a few more hours of the injury, however, the flow reverses, and sodium and water begin to move back into the intravascular compartment. By 20 to 24 hours following the burn, the fluid shift has largely stabilized.

Along with the fluid shifts, the cardiac output may fall to 30% to 50% of normal when the burn injury is extensive. This may be due in part to a circulating myocardial depressant factor that is created by the burn wound; this factor may directly decrease myocardial contractility, leading to a reduced cardiac output.[7] As the burn wound size and depth increase, the myocardial depression becomes greater, although there is wide variation among patients (see Chapter 6, Shock). The hypothesis that one of the systemic complications of dermal burns is a dysfunction of myocardial contraction has been extensively studied in guinea pigs 24 hours after approximately 47% body surface area full-thickness burns. The hearts of the guinea pigs showed decreased contractility, slowed isovolumic relaxation, and decreased diastolic compliance when compared with controls. These changes would reduce ejection and impede filling of the ventricle.[8]

Other Pathophysiologic Considerations

Immediately following the burn injury, there may be an acute erythrocyte hemolysis because of direct heat damage to the red cells. Up to 15% of the total red blood cell mass may be lost in major burns. In addition to this direct damage to red blood cells, there may be a microangiopathic hemolytic anemia. During this time, both the patient's red blood cells and transfused blood cells have a shortened half-life. Platelets and leukocytes may also have shortened half-lives. This condition may last for up to 2 weeks after the burn episode.[9] The production of immunoglobulins is also altered in burns. Postburn circulating immunoglobulins are initially depressed but return to normal at a variable rate. There is a normal response in these patients to rechallenge with tetanus toxoid.[10]

The kidneys may be damaged indirectly by the burn. Acute tubular necrosis may develop secondary to burn shock. Myoglobinuria may be a cause of renal failure. Fortunately, with adequate fluid resuscitation, acute renal failure due to hypovolemia is uncommon.

An acute adynamic ileus and gastric dilatation may develop after a major burn injury. As burn shock is corrected, the ileus and dilatation diminish. There may be a small amount of coffee ground gastric material aspirated from the stomach of the patient, which is probably due to a self-limited episode of hemorrhagic gastritis. Later, Curling's ulcers, accompanied by massive gastrointestinal bleeding, may develop in the burn patient.

Hypertension has been reported in some burn victims, particularly children. These patients perfuse at an inappropriately high total peripheral resistance and tend to be hypervolemic. There is no difference between hypertensive and normotensive patients in plasma renin activity, aldosterone, catecholamine, or electrolyte levels, suggesting that the combination of hypervolemia along with the vasoconstrictor activity of the plasma renin activity and/or catecholamines must be present for hypertension to develop.[11]

PREHOSPITAL EVALUATION AND CARE

The prehospital care of burn injuries is concerned with (1) home care of a minor burn, possibly supplemented by telephone advice from a nurse or physician, and (2) initial assessment and care of a major burn by an emergency medical technician (EMT), followed by transport of the victim.

Most minor burn injuries occur at home, and it is common for emergency departments to be contacted by a patient or family member for advice on treatment. There are a few rules of general first aid that may be given. First, separate the victim from the cause of the burn; for example, any smoldering clothing should be removed. Next, the burn wound should be covered with a clean cloth (eg, towels, handkerchiefs, sheets) soaked in cool water. This helps to stop the burning process and possibly minimizes the depth of injury by dissipating the heat. It also makes the patient feel more comfortable because it decreases the air currents over the wound.

Chemical burns may also mandate first aid measures. The injury to the skin is directly proportional to the duration of exposure and to the concentration of the offending substance. Any clothing that is soaked by the burning chemical should be immediately removed. (Those helping the victim must themselves avoid coming in contact with the agent.) Dry, powdered chemicals that may cause burning should be brushed off as much as possible. Specific neutralizing antidotes are not recommended, and the treatment of choice is *copious* irrigation with cool tap water. The importance of copious irrigation with water cannot be overemphasized. One study found that the majority of these burns are work related. Among these patients, those that received irrigation at the scene had significantly less full-thickness injury and a more than twofold shorter hospital stay.[12]

Victims who consult emergency departments by telephone should be advised to avoid home remedies, such as butter, grease, or over-the-counter ointments. Some of these home remedies may promote bacterial growth on the burn wound, while others are difficult to remove for later wound evaluation. All patients who report burns should be encouraged to see a physician as soon after the burn as possible, since most burn victims are unable to judge the depth and severity of their own wounds.

EMTs and other ambulance personnel frequently are called to transport a burn victim from the scene of the injury. The EMT must initiate the proper care to decrease the morbidity and mortality of these patients. While the patient is removed from the source of heat, the airway, breathing, and circulation should be evaluated. There are 6000 to 10,000 deaths annually from major burns, and half of these victims die at the scene of the burn, not uncommonly because of a simple problem such as an airway obstruction.[13] Burns that result from motor vehicle accidents are frequently severe and are often associated with other injuries. In motor vehicle accidents associated with burns, the injury associated with death is inhalation injury. Multiple trauma itself has little effect on the overall mortality unless severe, but fractures complicate burn wound care unless surgically stabilized.[14]

After the airway, breathing, and circulation have been ensured and the burning process has been halted, the EMT may proceed to other treatment. The burn should be covered with clean sheets or sterile gauze dressings moistened with normal saline solution. This not only helps to arrest the burning process, but also may relieve some of the pain. Instead of saline moistened dressings, a dry, clean sheet may be used to cover a patient in whom the burning process has been stopped and who feels relatively comfortable.

Some burn victims also require nasal oxygen (5 to 10 L/min). In addition to their burn, these patients may suffer from carbon monoxide–hemoglobin binding. This is particularly common when the patient has lost consciousness or has been burned in an enclosed space.

If the transportation time to the hospital will be short, no further treatment is necessary. However, if the anticipated transportation time is over one-half hour and the EMT or paramedic has the skill, an intravenous line with normal saline or lactated Ringer's solution may be started. During transport, the airway should be frequently reevaluated, particularly in patients with suspected respiratory burns.

EMERGENCY DEPARTMENT CARE OF THERMAL INJURIES

Initial Evaluation and Treatment

In the emergency department, initial evaluation of the burned patient's condition must include another assessment of the airway, breathing, and circulation, as well as an examination for other injuries that may have been sustained during the accident. For example, a patient burned in an automobile accident may have a cervical spine injury.

Since a major contributor to morbidity and mortality is burn wound infection, care should be taken from the onset of treatment to minimize contamination of the burn wound. Important steps include keeping the number of people dealing with the burned patient at a minimum; the use of sterile drapes; the use of surgical caps, masks, gowns, and gloves; and the use of sterile technique when starting intravenous lines.

The most immediate threat to the life of the burned patient is airway damage from an inhalation injury.[15] These injuries occasionally result from direct flame damage, but they more commonly result from superheated gases, steam, smoke, or toxic fumes that produce airway edema, changes in the physiologic properties of pulmonary surfactant, increased exudation in the upper and lower airways, deposition of carbonaceous material in the lungs, atelectasis, traumatic pneumonitis, and other types of damage to the airway and lung tissue.[16]

The diagnosis of an inhalation injury may be based on the history and physical findings. The history is important for the diagnosis, since many of these injuries occur when the victim is burned in an enclosed or confined space, such as an automobile. Physical findings (Fig. 26-1) suggestive of an inhalation injury include burns of the face, lips, tongue, or mucous membranes; singed facial hairs; singed nasal hairs; hoarseness; wheezing; stridor; cough, particularly if it produces a carbonaceous material; or hemoptysis. The finding of stridor is particularly significant because it occurs when there is at least a 70% occlusion of the airway, an ominous sign.

The great majority of patients with inhalation injuries have associated burns of the face or neck, although the presence of head or neck burns does not necessarily indicate an inhalation injury. When these burns are present, a very careful evaluation of the patient's pulmonary status is necessary.

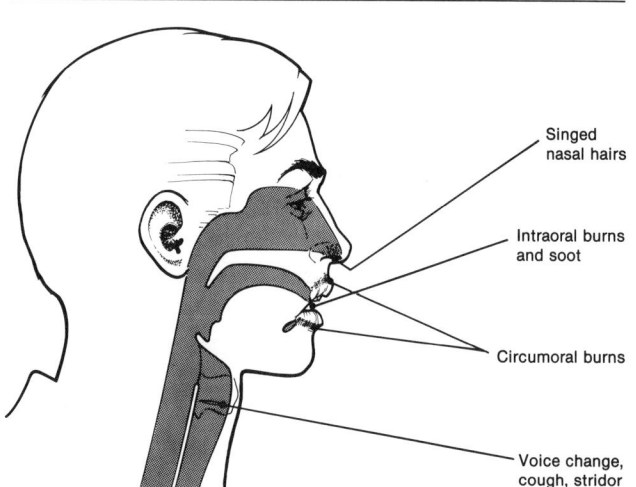

Figure 26-1 Physical findings suggestive of inhalation injury. Source: Adapted with permission from Marion Laboratories, Inc.

Serial chest roentgenograms, arterial blood gases, possibly a diagnostic bronchoscopy, and serial pulmonary function studies are also needed. It is extremely important to consider the possibility of a pulmonary burn because this type of injury may lead to a significant reduction in the oxygen transfer potential of the lung with subsequent respiratory dysfunction and death.[17,18] Because smoke inhalation injury is found in up to 20% of patients admitted to burn centers, some authorities recommend routine fiberoptic bronchoscopy or xenon ventilation, which can result in more frequent and earlier diagnoses.[6]

Circumferential burns of the chest may decrease respiratory excursions if significant edema and a constricting eschar develop. Such circumferential burns of the chest may require incision for release of the bandlike constriction. In addition, respiratory function may be altered by carboxyhemoglobinemia, which decreases the amount of oxygen that can be carried by the hemoglobin molecule, or by methemoglobinemia (due to inhaled chemicals) or a postburn hemolytic anemia, which also decreases the oxygen-carrying capacity of the blood. These factors working in concert may severely limit the transfer of oxygen to the tissues. Once the airway has been ensured, all major burn patients should be started on high-flow oxygen. An exception may occur with some patients having chronic obstructive lung disease, however, because carbon dioxide retention may become a problem in these patients.

If a respiratory burn is suspected, the initial step in treatment is the administration of humidified oxygen at a concentration of 40% to 100% with a flow rate of approximately 10 L/min. The use of humidified oxygen helps to keep the airway moist, inhibiting the inspissation of material that could produce atelectatic areas within the lung. The use of 100% oxygen is also important if carboxyhemoglobinemia is suspected. The half-life of carboxyhemoglobin is approximately 200 minutes in room air, but diminishes to approximately 40 to 50 minutes when 100% oxygen is given. When chronic obstructive lung disease is suspected in a burn patient, oxygen must be used cautiously to prevent the retention of carbon dioxide and subsequent carbon dioxide narcosis with respiratory depression. Initial blood gas determinations should be obtained as soon as possible, and the patient could be started on a 24% or 28% concentration of oxygen via Venturi mask. After 15 minutes, arterial blood gas levels should be measured again. If carbon dioxide has not been retained at that time, a higher concentration of oxygen may be used, followed by another blood gas determination in 15 minutes. When the patient begins to retain carbon dioxide, a lower concentration should be chosen for maintenance oxygen therapy.[17]

Particular attention should be given to the circulatory competence in burned patients. Minor burns generally do *not* require intravenous fluid therapy. If intravenous fluid therapy is necessary, the patient should probably be hospitalized.

With extensive burns, intravenous fluid therapy should be initiated as soon as possible. The solution of choice for the initial resuscitation is Ringer's lactate through a peripheral vein cannulated with a large-bore catheter. Some experts in burn care feel that central venous lines are unnecessary and should be avoided in the management of major burns, except when no other intravenous route can be established. On the other hand, experts in the transport of burn victims feel that a central venous line is easier to maintain in the cramped quarters of a helicopter or ambulance and therefore prefer the use of central venous lines. It has been recognized that infections such as suppurative thrombophlebitis and endocarditis are more common in burn patients when indwelling intravenous catheters are used.[6]

The physician may choose to begin intravenous fluids before the exact fluid requirement has been calculated. In this case, if an adult's burn wound is less than 30% of the body surface, an initial rate of 500 mL/hour may be chosen. Patients with greater than 30% body surface area burn should receive fluids at an initial rate of approximately 1 L/hour.

Following the primary evaluation, the percent of the body surface burned is estimated. This estimation of percentage is used in calculating the amount of fluid to be given. There are several methods of evaluating burn wound size, such as the "rule of nines," the use of a Lund and Browder chart,[19] and the "rule of palms."

Under the rule of nines, the adult body surface is divided into 11 areas, each equal to 9% or multiples thereof (Fig. 26-2). The genitalia are assigned the final 1%. An adult patient with a burn of the entire left arm, the entire right arm, the anterior chest and abdomen, and the genitalia would have a 37% burn (9% + 9% + 18% + 1%), according to the rule of nines. The estimation of the body surface area in children is slightly different; during the first year of life, each leg accounts for 13%, while the head accounts for 18%. Until adolescence, these percentages of body surface in children change by a small amount each year.

The Lund and Browder method is more accurate than the rule of nines. With a Lund and Browder chart (Fig. 26-3), the patient noted in the previous paragraph would have a 9.5% burn (right arm), 9.5% burn (left arm), 13% burn (anterior chest and abdomen), and 1% burn (genitalia), totaling 33% body surface burn.

A very simple method of estimating burns is the rule of palms, by which the examiner compares the palm of the burn victim's hand with the size of the burn wound. Since the palm of the victim's hand approximates 1%, the examiner can compare the size of the burn with the number of "palms" to estimate the size of the burn. This is more useful for small burns than for large burns.

There are many formulas that can be used to calculate the fluid necessary for the resuscitation of burn victims. The lactated Ringer's formula is currently the most popular. According to this formula the only intravenous fluid given

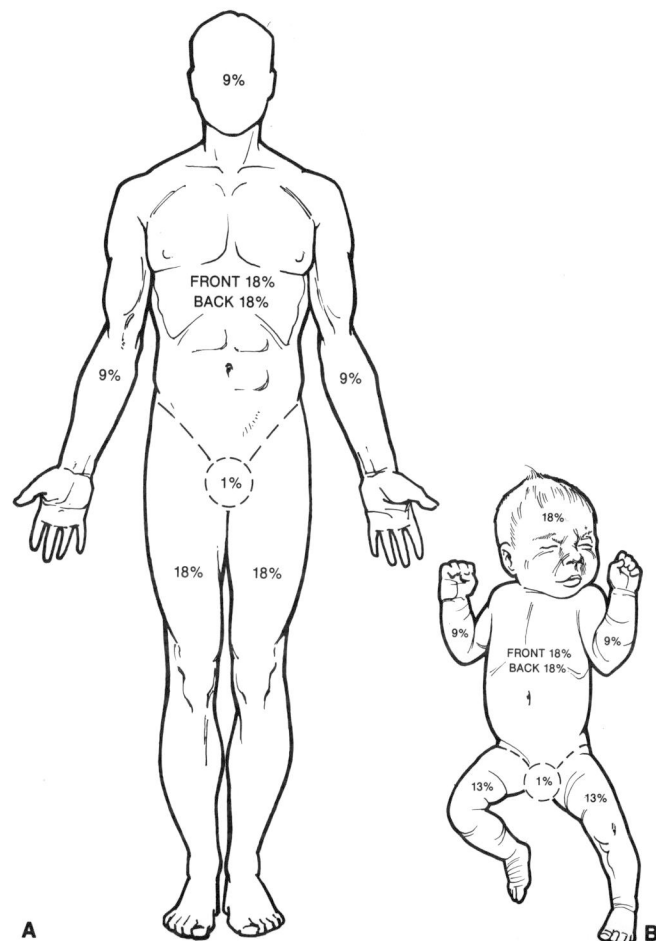

Figure 26-2 Rule of nines. **(A)** Adult. **(B)** Adaptation for children. *Source:* Adapted with permission from Marion Laboratories, Inc.

during the first 24 hours is lactated Ringer's solution. The basic formula is as follows:

$$\text{Percent body surface area burn} \times \text{kg body weight} \times 4 \text{ mL} = \text{Amount for the first 24 hours}$$

One half of this total is given in the first 8 hours *following the burn*, and one quarter of the total is given in the subsequent two 8-hour periods. The first 8 hours after the burn begins with the time of the burn and not with the time that the patient arrives in the emergency department. If 2 hours have elapsed from the time of the burn until the arrival of the patient, then one half of the total 24-hour fluid requirement should be given within the next 6 hours. According to this formula, an 80-kg man with 50% body surface area burn would require 16 L fluid during the first 24 hours of therapy; 8 L would be given during the first 8 hours, 4 L from the 9th through the 16th hours, and 4 L from the 17th through the 24th hours.

To monitor the success of fluid resuscitation, urine output should be monitored in all extensively burned victims. The

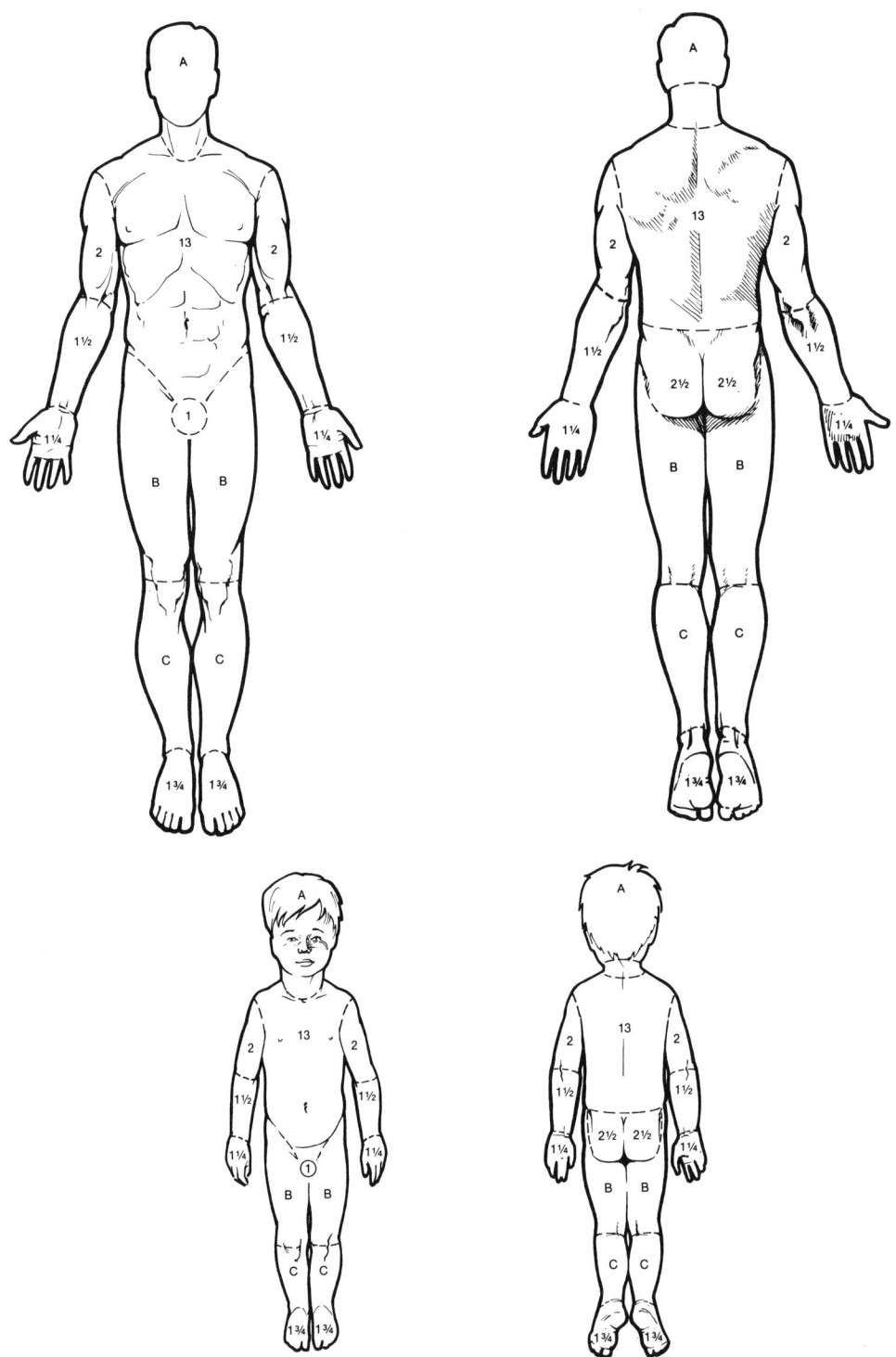

Figure 26-3 Lund and Browder charts. *Source:* Adapted with permission from Marion Laboratories, Inc.

results of adequate fluid resuscitation include a urine production of 50 to 75 mL/hour in the adult, a slowing of the pulse, a stable blood pressure, a return to normal cerebration, and bowel sounds without an ileus. If these parameters neither stabilize nor improve within the first 2 hours of fluid resuscitation, the burn size should be recalculated and fluid administration altered accordingly. In addition, a careful search for hidden injuries that may have altered the fluid requirements should be made.

Two types of patients commonly demonstrate a reduced response to fluid resuscitation: those with massive burns and those with a decreased myocardial reserve, such as the elderly. The circulating myocardial depressant factor of burn shock, which directly depresses myocardial contractility and cardiac output, may be present. The failure of the cardiac output to respond to fluid therapy is manifested by a low blood pressure and elevated central venous pressure (possibly indicated by distended neck veins).

A nasogastric tube should be inserted for seriously burned patients, because it is common for them to develop gastric dilatation, gastric atony, and vomiting. The administration of antacids through the nasogastric tube may help reduce gastric irritation and the development of Curling's ulcers.[20,21] Cimetidine, which inhibits the action of histamine at the histamine receptors of the parietal cells of the stomach, is being used in some centers to reduce the incidence of gastritis and ulcer formation in postburn patients. Cimetidine is rapidly absorbed following oral administration. Its half-life is approximately 2 hours when the patient has normal renal function, but the half-life is prolonged during renal impairment. The drug can also be given intramuscularly or intravenously. In an adult, the oral, intramuscular, and intravenous dosage is 300 mg every 6 hours. Clinical experience with cimetidine in pregnancy, during lactation, and in childhood is limited, and its use is not, therefore, recommended in these situations.

Laboratory Studies

Early in the resuscitation of a major burn victim, emergency care personnel should obtain baseline laboratory determinations on which further treatment can be based. These laboratory studies should include a complete blood count with differential blood cell count; measurements of serum electrolytes, glucose, blood urea nitrogen, creatinine, and arterial carboxyhemoglobin; arterial blood gas determinations, blood typing, and clotting studies. Patients may be under the influence of alcohol or drugs, and blood ethanol and drug screening should be considered. A baseline urinalysis should be obtained; if myoglobinuria is suspected, urinary myoglobin levels should be determined.

Precautions during Early Burn Treatment

There are a few precautions that the emergency personnel should take during the early burn treatment. First, burn victims frequently have associated traumatic injuries that must be treated before the burn wound is treated. For example, patients may have been involved in an automobile accident or an explosion in association with burns, or they may have jumped or fallen from buildings in attempts to flee a fire. Particular attention should be paid to the possibility of skull or cervical spine injuries.

Second, major burn victims should not be cooled excessively. Packing a patient in ice may initially relieve some of the pain of the burn, but this cooling may lead to hypothermia. Core body temperatures below 32.2°C have been reported in burn patients who have been excessively cooled. Hypothermia not only increases the morbidity and mortality of burn patients, but also could freeze tissues, changing partial-thickness burns into full-thickness burns.

Third, narcotics should be avoided during the first few minutes of resuscitation until shock has been corrected and circulation restored. In addition, narcotics should be avoided if surgical consultation for abdominal trauma or neurosurgical consultation for head trauma is to be obtained.

Estimation of the Depth of the Burn

During the emergency phases of the care of major burn victims, it may be impossible to determine the depth of all areas of a burn because the depth of many burns is not clear until debridement has been performed. What may initially appear to be a partial-thickness burn may develop into a full-thickness burn during subsequent days.

First-degree burns, or superficial partial-thickness burns, involve only the most superficial layers of the skin (Fig. 26-4). The key diagnostic feature of the superficial burn is its erythematous, unblistered nature. Second-degree burns, or deeper partial-thickness burns, involve the entire epidermis and parts of the dermis. Blisters form in this type of burn. Third-degree burns, or full-thickness burns, involve the epidermis, dermis, and subcutaneous tissues. Characteristically, the skin appears to be pearly white or charred, and the burn is *insensitive to pin prick*. Recently a "burn depth indicator" has been clinically tested. This apparatus utilizes reflectance ratios of red, green, and infrared light. Results of the testing suggest that use of such an indicator is more accurate than clinical evaluation in determining burn depth and, because it is both portable and noninvasive, it may serve as a triage tool for emergency departments or in combat situations for predicting which wounds should be excised and grafted during the first few days after injury.[22]

The American Burn Association further classifies burns into three categories; (1) major burn injuries, (2) moderate

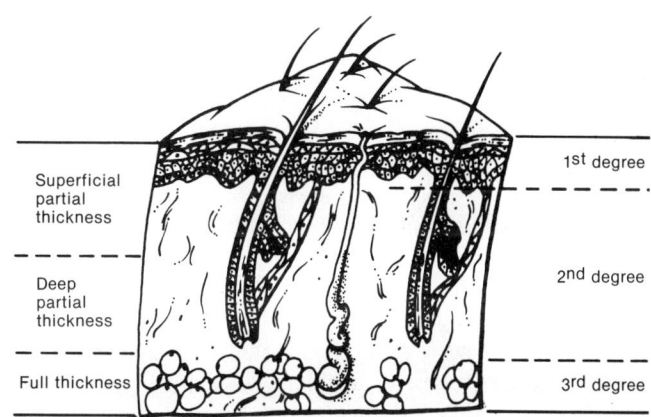

Figure 26-4 Depth of burns. *Source:* Adapted with permission from Marion Laboratories, Inc.

uncomplicated burn injuries, and (3) minor burn injuries. These distinctions have been made because the size and depth are not the only factors in the determination of the magnitude or severity of the injury.

Major burn injuries include

1. second-degree burns over more than 25% of the body surface area in adults and 20% in children
2. all third-degree burns involving 10% or more of body surface area
3. all burns that involve the hand, face, eyes, ears, feet, or perineum
4. all inhalation injuries
5. electrical burns
6. burn injuries complicated by fractures or other major trauma
7. all burns in poor-risk patients, such as those with cardiovascular disease, chronic obstructive pulmonary disease, chronic renal disease, hepatic disease, alcoholism, insulin-dependent diabetes, cerebrovascular accidents with residuals, head injuries associated with a loss of consciousness, severe psychiatric disabilities, and enclosed space injuries.

In addition, patients with sickle cell disease may develop a sickle cell crisis following a major burn. Almost all of these patients should be transferred to a burn center for care.

Moderate uncomplicated burn injuries include (1) second-degree burns of 15% to 20% of the body surface area in adults and 10% to 20% in children, and (2) third-degree burns of 2% to 10% of the body surface area if they do not involve the eyes, ears, face, hands, feet, or perineum. These patients should be cared for by a physician specifically trained in burn management.

Minor burn injuries include second-degree burns of less than 15% of the body surface area in adults and 10% in children, as well as third-degree burns of 2% or less if they do not involve the eyes, ears, face, hands, feet, or genitalia.

FURTHER MANAGEMENT OF THE BURN VICTIM

Drug Administration

The parenteral use of cimetidine and narcotics has been discussed earlier. The administration of penicillin and tetanus toxoid for prophylaxis should also be considered in many major burn victims, even though the use of prophylactic penicillin is controversial. In one study that analyzed the outpatient effectiveness of antibiotics used for burns in an outpatient setting, the infection rates in treated and untreated groups were 3.8% and 3.1%, respectively, arguing against the routine use of systemic antibiotics in the treatment of outpatient burns.[23] The use of prophylactic penicillin in acutely burned, hospitalized patients is also controversial, and it is felt that the routine administration of prophylactic penicillin neither protects against cellulitis and burn wound sepsis nor promotes selection of antibiotic-resistant bacteria in hospitalized patients with acute thermal injury.[24]

All burn patients should have up-to-date tetanus prophylaxis. In the previously unimmunized patient, 250 U of human immunoglobulin should be given intramuscularly in one extremity, and 0.5 mL of tetanus toxoid should be given intramuscularly in another extremity. The patient who has been adequately immunized previously should receive 0.5 mL of tetanus toxoid intramuscularly.

Some anti-inflammatory drugs have been known to stimulate host defense mechanisms. These drugs act as immunomodulators and, experimentally, have shown promise in increasing host resistance to infections if begun shortly after injury.[25]

Management of the Burn Wound

After all pieces of burned clothing, foreign bodies, and loose skin have been removed from the burn and after the initial life-saving resuscitative steps have been taken, care can be directed toward the burn wound itself. The burn wound may be washed gently with an antiseptic solution, with the exception of hexachlorophene-containing solutions in children; it has been reported that hexachlorophene is absorbed and causes an encephalopathy in isolated cases. After the skin has been cleansed with an antiseptic solution, a topical agent may be applied to the burn.

Tar and asphalt burns are unique injuries because the chemical is difficult to remove without inflicting further tissue injury. Principles of management include rapid cooling of tar or asphalt to solidify the agent and to dissipate heat. Removal can then be accomplished with a petroleum-based, surface-active solvent or with an ointment containing Tween-80 (such as neosporin ointment). These burns may require early excision and grafting followed by an early back-to-work philosophy.[26]

Over the past century many agents have been used for the topical therapy of burns. In the 1800s, carbolic oil was the agent most widely used, but early in the 1900s sodium bicarbonate paste was applied, followed by a solution of picric acid. In approximately 1910, the use of ammonium acetate was widespread, but it was replaced in 1918 by the application of warmed paraffin wax. During the Depression, tannic acid was the agent of choice.

Interest in thermal burns increased after World War II, mainly because of a fear of an atomic disaster. During that postwar period, extensive research was devoted to new topical agents and silver nitrate solution was introduced (1965), followed by mafenide acetate (1966), and silver sulfadiazine

(1968). Numerous other compounds have been introduced for the care of major burn wounds, but they have not been as popular as these three.

Silver nitrate is effective on those burns in which an infection is not established. Some disadvantages of silver nitrate, however, have made this agent unpopular. For example, application is painful for the patient, and it leaves a dark stain on almost anything with which it comes in contact.

Mafenide acetate (Sulfamylon) penetrates burn wounds and eschars well, and it has an excellent antibacterial activity in infected wounds. There are, however, several disadvantages to the use of mafenide acetate: pain on application, maceration of the wound when used under a dressing, short duration of antibacterial potency, and the development of metabolic acidosis. Both mafenide acetate and its metabolite are excreted through the kidneys, and impaired renal function increases the risk of metabolic acidosis.

Silver sulfadiazine (Silvadene) is painless on application to burn wounds and does not inhibit carbonic anhydrase. The antibacterial potency of silver sulfadiazine is longer than that of mafenide acetate when used with a dressing. Local and systemic toxicity of silver sulfadiazine is very uncommon. Unlike mafenide acetate, however, silver sulfadiazine does not penetrate well into an eschar and should not be used in extensively infected burn wounds.

Minor burn wounds should be cleansed and debrided; then a number of methods can be used in the treatment of these minor burns. The burn can be treated in an open or closed fashion, with or without topical agents. Factors to be considered include the area of the body to be dressed, the depth and extent of the burn, the age and type of patient, the home or work situation, the patient's ability to care for the wound, and the availability of health care personnel to help in the home.

Some clinicians treat minor burn wounds in selected areas, such as the head and neck, in an open fashion to allow exposure of the burned area to the air. Such exposure theoretically minimizes bacterial growth because moisture is decreased. As an alternative, burns in these areas can be treated with a topical antibacterial agent, but without a dressing. The antibacterial agent would be applied directly to the wound with a sterile tongue blade or a sterile-gloved hand. The dressing should be applied thickly enough to cover the wound completely. The agent is applied twice daily or as necessary if rubbed off. Before each reapplication, dried topical agent and exudate should be removed.

Closed dressings may be used for both outpatient and inpatient treatment. Closed dressings permit ambulatory management of small wounds, allow the patient to wear clothing over the burn, and may be used with or without topical therapy.

Burn dressings consist of a combination of layered materials, the innermost being a nonadherent, porous mesh gauze impregnated with a nonpetroleum-based, water-soluble lubricant. This mesh should be fine enough to prevent the ingrowth of new epithelium, but not so fine that the dressing becomes impermeable to exudation from the wound. Over the fine mesh layer is a layer of bulky, fluffed, coarse mesh gauze that absorbs any exudate and protects the wound from minor trauma. Securing this bulky layer in place is an outer layer of flexible semielastic coarse mesh bandage wrapped to apply a light, even pressure.

Closed, dry dressings are favored by many clinicians who view antibiotic agents as unnecessary for minor burns. Burns that cover less than 1% to 2% of the body surface area generally heal quite satisfactorily if simply enclosed in a dressing such as Xeroform or Adaptic and changed every 3 to 5 days.

Follow-up care for patients with minor burns treated in the emergency department is essential. Timing of the follow-up care depends on the extent and depth of the injury, the frequency with which the dressing must be changed, and the personal preference of the physician. When dressings that incorporate antibacterial agents are used, the first dressing should be changed at the end of 24 hours. When nonadherent, fine-meshed, porous gauze is used, care should be taken to avoid simply pulling off this gauze during the dressing change because the underlying crust may adhere to the gauze. This crust is important because it protects the maturing wound, which is undergoing new epithelial growth.

Patients with newly healed burns should be cautioned against exposing the healed burn to the sun. These tissues are very sensitive to sunburning, and the application of a sun screen agent may be necessary. The patient may also notice itching and irritation of the newly healed burn wound; this can be relieved by the use of a mild lanolin cream (eg, Alpha Keri or Nivea).

Topical antibiotics decrease mortality among burn patients with less than 40% body surface area involvement, but there has been less of an effect with larger burns, particularly those with more than 70% body surface area involvement. Topical antibiotics can also slow burn wound healing.[27] For these reasons, early surgical excision and skin graft closure of deep partial-thickness burns by a technique of tangential excision is becoming a more popular form of inpatient management. Early chemical debridement with sutilains ointment (containing an enzyme derived from *Bacillus subtilis*) is also being used.[6]

Temporary skin substitutes are also being used in both inpatient and outpatient settings. Temporary skin substitutes help reduce the drying of exudate on the wound, which retards reepithelialization. The temporary skin substitute also helps retard the growth of bacteria by promoting normal wound defense mechanisms (eg, phagocytosis). Temporary skin is either biologic (previously living tissue such as amniotic membranes, xenografts, and homografts) or synthetic (silicone polymers, polyurethane polymers, and poly-

Burn transfer checklist

TIME OF _____ AM
DATE_____CALL _____ PM
REFERRING DOCTOR_____
REFERRING HOSPITAL_____
PHONE #_____

CLOSED SPACE	YES	NO
ENDOTRACHEAL TUBE	YES	NO
VENTILATOR	YES	NO
IV LINES	YES	NO

(size & site) _____

CONSCIOUS NOW	YES	NO
DIABETES	YES	NO
HEART DISEASE	YES	NO

Type _____

ALLERGIES?	YES	NO

To what? _____

ASSOCIATED INJURIES: (Fracture, abdominal or chest injury, head trauma, etc) _____
_____

THERAPY GIVEN THUS FAR

IV's	_____	cc Normal Saline
	_____	cc Ringer's
	_____	cc D$_5$W
Foley	_____	cc urine total
	_____	cc urine last hour

IF PATIENT IS ACCEPTED SUGGEST:

1. M.D. accompany (if needed but must come with patient with endotracheal tube)
2. IV Morphine for sedation if needed
3. NG tube for burns over 30% or if drunk or intubated—DON'T CLAMP TUBE.
4. IV fluids—Ringer's fast enough to produce urine output
5. NO topical cream, antibiotics, IM meds of any kind. Debridement of burn wound to be discussed.
6. Escharotomy if needed
7. Does family know about transfer?

Widespread availability of this form for simultaneous use by both referring and receiving physicians will make telephone communication more precise.

PATIENT NAME _____
DATE &
AGE _____ TIME OF BURN _____
TYPE OF BURN: FLAME   SCALD
ELECTRICAL   CHEMICAL   RADIATION

LAB RESULTS: Na____, K____, Cl____,
CO_2____, BUN____, Sugar____,
pH____, PO_2____, PCO_2____
Is there blood in urine? _____
Chest x-ray _____

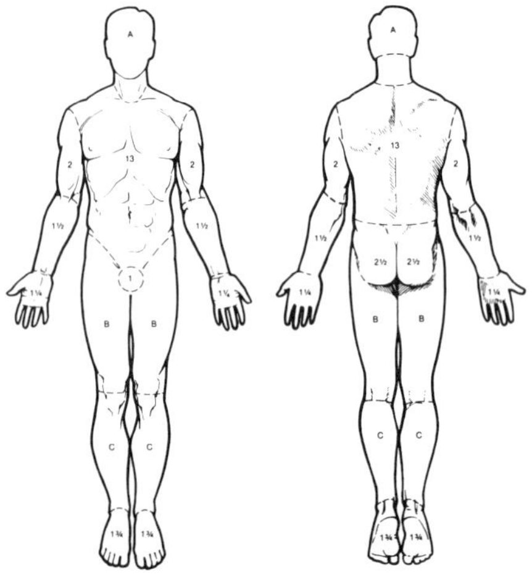

RELATIVE PERCENTAGE OF AREAS AFFECTED BY GROWTH
(age in years)

A: ½ of hand	9½	8½	6½	5½	4½	3½
B: ½ of thigh	2¾	3¼	4	4¼	4½	4¾
C: ½ of leg	2½	2½	2¾	3	3¼	3½

Total Percent Burned _____ 2 + _____ 3 = _____

INSURANCE DATA:
Type: _____
Policy # _____
Workmen's Compensation?   YES   NO
Resident making report _____
Senior resident notified _____
Attending notified _____
Accept patient _____
Refer to _____

Adapted from *JAMA* 238:489–492, 1977.

Figure 26-5 Burn transfer checklist. *Source:* Reprinted with permission from Marion Laboratories, Inc.

---

vinylchloride). Any of these dressings must be permeable to water vapor and oxygen but impermeable to bacteria. These temporary skin substitutes are helpful when even minor burn wound infections are present but will not adhere to the wound if it is grossly infected.

The most exciting advance in major burns is the use of cultured human epidermal cells derived from a small skin biopsy specimen from the patient. After several weeks the culture can produce epithelial sheets capable of covering the entire surface of the body.[6]

SPECIAL SITUATIONS

Myoglobinuria

Electrical and thermal burns occasionally cause myoglobinuria, which may be manifested by a brownish urine. Particularly in a patient who has a decreased urine output, myoglobinuria may damage the renal tubules. Myoglobinuria may be suspected rather than hemoglobinuria when the levels of serum muscle enzymes are greatly increased (especially that of creatine phosphokinase). Myoglobin may be positively identified in the urine by spectrophotometry or electrophoresis on gel or cellulose acetate. Treatment includes diluting the urine by increasing fluid therapy, using an osmotic diuretic such as intravenous mannitol at the rate of 25 g/hour, or alkalizing the urine with intravenous sodium bicarbonate.

Escharotomy

Occasionally, escharotomies are performed in an emergency department. They may be needed in circumferential burns of extremities or chest wall burns when a constricting eschar and edema decrease respiratory excursions. The indications for an escharotomy in a burned extremity include peripheral cyanosis, decreased pulse strength, and a changing neurologic status. The most sensitive of these is a changing neurologic status, for example, the progressive loss of light touch or pin prick sensation of the hand in a burned arm. Early elevation and reglar exercise of a burned extremity may decrease the need for an escharotomy. When edema develops beneath the constricting eschar, the interstitial pressure may rise to a point above that of the venous pressure, which could lead to ischemia and necrosis of otherwise uninjured tissues.

Transfer of Burn Patients

Many hospitals are unable to provide the total care that a patient with a major burn requires. In these cases, transfer may be necessary. The patient should not be transferred, however, until fluid resuscitation is adequate, the airway has been ensured, and there are signs of reversal of burn shock. Even for local transfers, both telephone contact with a receiving physician and the use of a burn transfer checklist are essential.[28] Telephone contact with a receiving physician and hospital should include the following:

- patient's name and age
- extent of burn
- pertinent medical information
- fluid therapy started
- topical burn care initiated
- use of escharotomy
- adequacy of airway
- sedatives and analgesics used
- systemic antibiotics administered
- tetanus immunization given

In addition, the referring physician should outline a precise transfer plan to the receiving hospital, including the expected time of departure and the expected time of arrival, information on all aspects of air and ground transfer (eg, ground ambulance to airplane to ground ambulance), and who will accompany the patient. The burn transfer checklist (Fig. 26-5) should accompany the patient along with any other pertinent medical records from the transferring institution.

CONCLUSION

Burns are not simply injuries to the skin. Many other organ systems can be involved, making this type of injury a challenge to emergency care personnel. In addition, the treatment of a burn brings out almost all of the evaluative skills that are necessary for a practicing emergency care professional. Appropriate emergency care can mean the difference between early recovery or even death.

REFERENCES

1. Katcher M. Scald burns from hot tap water. *JAMA*. 1981;246:1219–1222.
2. Artz CP. What's new in burns. *Med Times*. 1976;104:128–141.
3. Baxter CR. Pathophysiology and treatment of burns and cold injury. In: Hardy JD, ed. *Rhoads Textbook of Surgery, Principles & Practice*. 5th ed. Philadelphia: Lippincott; 1977.
4. Noble HG, Robson MC, Krizek TJ. Dermal ischemia in the burn wound. *J Surg Res*. 1977;23:117–125.
5. Zawacki BE. Reversal of capillary stasis and prevention of necrosis in burns. *Ann Surg*. 1974;180:98–102.
6. Demling RH. Burns. *N Engl J Med*. 1985;313:1389–1398.
7. Baxter CR, Cook WA, Shires GT. Serum myocardial depressant factors of burn shock. *Surg Forum*. 1966;17:1–2.
8. Adams HR, Baxter CR, Izenberg SD. Decreased contractility and compliance of the left ventricle as complications of thermal trauma. *Am Heart J*. 1984;108:1477–1487.
9. Lloyd JA. Thermal trauma: therapeutic achievements and investigative horizons. *Surg Clin North Am*. 1977;57:121–138.
10. Shorr RM, Ershler WB, Gamelli RL. Immunoglobulin production in burned patients. *J Trauma*. 1984;24:319–322.
11. Popp MB, Silberstein EB, Srivastava LS, et al. A pathophysiologic study of hypertension associated with burn injury in children. *Ann Surg*. 1981;193:817–824.
12. Leonard LG, Scheulen JJ, Munster AM. Chemical burns: effect of prompt first aid. *J Trauma*. 1982;22:420–423.
13. Artz CP, Moncrief JA, Pruitt BA. *Burns: A Team Approach*. Philadelphia: Saunders; 1979.
14. Purdue GF, Hunt JL, Layton TR, et al. Burns in motor vehicle accidents. *J Trauma*. 1985;25:216–219.
15. Moylan JA, Chan CK. Inhalation injury—an increasing problem. *Ann Surg*. 1978;188:34–37.

16. Jelenko C, Garrison AF, McKinley JC. Respiratory problems complicating burn injury. *Postgrad Med.* 1975;58:97–102.
17. Boutros AR, Hoyt JL, Boyd WC, et al. Algorithm for management of pulmonary complications in burn patients. *Crit Care Med.* 1977;5:89–92.
18. Diamond AW, Piggott RW, Townsend PLC. Immediate care of burns. *Anesthesia.* 1975;30:791–802.
19. Lund CC, Browder NC. The estimation of areas of burns. *Surg Gynecol Obstet.* 1944;79:352–358.
20. Baxter CR, Marvin JA, Curreri PW. Early management of thermal burns. *Postgrad Med.* 1974;55:131–139.
21. Boswick JA. Burns. *Surg Clin North Am.* 1978;58.
22. Heimbach DM, Afromowitz MA, Engrav LH, et al. Burn depth estimation—man on machine. *J Trauma.* 1984;24:373–378.
23. Boss WK, Brand DA, Acampora D, et al. Effectiveness of prophylactic antibiotics in the outpatient treatment of burns. *J Trauma.* 1985;25:224–227.
24. Durtsch MB, Orgain C, Counts GW, et al. A prospective study of prophylactic penicillin in acutely burned hospitalized patients. *J Trauma.* 1982;22:11–14.
25. Ehrlich HP. Anti-inflammatory drugs in the vascular response to burn injury. *Ann Surg.* 1983;198:53–57.
26. Stratta RJ, Saffle JR, Kravitz M, et al. Management of tar and asphalt injuries. *Am J Surg.* 1983;146:766–769.
27. Feller I, Flora JD Jr, Bawol R. Baseline results of therapy for burned patients. *JAMA.* 1976;236:1943–1947.
28. Stein JM, Stein ED. Safe transfer of civilian burn casualties. *JAMA.* 1977;238:489–492.

27. Dermatologic Emergencies

GEORGE L. STERNBACH, MD, FACEP

Skin conditions frequently induce patients to seek treatment in the emergency department because of the accompanying pruritus or the unaesthetic appearance of the skin lesions. Although common skin lesions are usually not indicative of serious illness, the possibility that a dermatosis may be a marker of infection or systemic illness should always be considered.

ACANTHOSIS NIGRICANS

The association of acanthosis nigricans with internal malignancy is well known, despite the fact that most cases are benign.[1] These benign cases may be familial, or they may be related to endocrine disease or obesity. *Malignant acanthosis nigricans* is the term used to designate that form associated with neoplastic disease. This term may be misleading, since acanthosis nigricans is only a marker of the underlying disease and is never infiltrated with malignant cells.

The lesion appears as a hyperpigmented, verrucous, velvetlike hyperplasia and hypertrophy of the skin, with accompanying accentuation of the skin markings. The chief sites of involvement are the body folds—especially the axillae, antecubital fossae, neck, and groin.

More than 90% of cases of malignant acanthosis nigricans are associated with intra-abdominal malignancies, about two-thirds of which are adenocarcinomas of the stomach.[2] Carcinomas of the breast and lung make up the majority of the remaining cases.[3] Regardless of the tumor type, acanthosis nigricans is associated with tumors that usually are highly malignant and metastasize early.[2] The mechanism by which this dermatosis develops in internal malignant disease is unknown.

ATOPIC DERMATITIS

The cutaneous manifestation of atopy, atopic dermatitis is associated with allergic diseases such as asthma and allergic rhinitis. Patients with atopic dermatitis are known to display both humoral and cell-mediated abnormalities of immunity.[4] Although the skin condition is chronic, patients frequently seek treatment of exacerbation at the emergency department. The pathogenesis is obscure. Although atopic dermatitis is seen with high frequency in some families, its genetic transmission has not been clearly delineated.[5]

Skin lesions appear as inflammatory macules or papules with indefinite borders. The skin is typically dry and scaly, but lesions in the acute phase may be vesicular, weeping, or oozing. The distribution of lesions varies with the age of the patient. Infants may have inflammatory, exudative plaques on the cheeks and in the diaper area. Older children have lesions in the antecubital and popliteal flexion areas. In adults, areas of involvement include the hands, feet, forearms, groin, and scalp.

Intense pruritus is the hallmark of atopic dermatitis, and low itching thresholds have been demonstrated in patients with this disorder.[4] Itching may be focal or generalized. Excoriations may be a prominent part of the clinical picture, and secondary bacterial infection of excoriated lesions is common. Repeated scratching and rubbing produce lichenification, a feature of chronic atopic dermatitis that consists of hyperpigmentation, thickening of the skin, and accentuation of skin furrows. Exacerbation can follow a number of triggering factors. These include exposure to intense heat, cold, or changes in temperature, friction, irritant soaps or detergents, emotional stress, and infection. Patients with atopic dermatitis are very vulnerable to irritant contact dermatitis.[5]

Exudative areas should be treated by application of wet dressings to reduce itching and crusting. Two to three layers of gauze soaked in Burow's solution should be applied for 5 minutes four times a day. Administration of antihistamines not only reduces pruritus, but also has useful sedative and soporific effects. Topical corticosteroids are the cornerstone of therapy, and should be prescribed in ointment form since this form is an effective lubricant for dry skin. Small amounts should be applied to involved areas three to six times daily. One- to 2-week courses of systemic steroids may occasionally be necessary, but should be reserved for severe episodes of exacerbation.

BACTERIAL INFECTIONS

For a discussion of infectious disease emergencies, see Chapter 25.

Erythrasma

An infection caused by *Corynebacterium minutissimum*, erythrasma appears as dry, brown, scaly plaques with sharp margins, frequently localized to the groin. It is more commonly seen in diabetic patients. A coral red fluorescence under Wood's light is characteristic. Erythromycin (250 mg four times a day) is the treatment of choice.[6]

Gonococcal Dermatitis

The most common presentation of disseminated gonococcal disease is the arthritis-dermatitis syndrome.[7] It affects approximately 1% to 2% of patients with gonorrhea and is seen primarily in women.[8] Fever and migratory polyarthralgias frequently precede or accompany skin lesions. The lesions are often multiple and have a predilection for the distal periarticular regions. They begin as erythematous or hemorrhagic papules that may resemble the lesions of meningococcemia. Lesions evolve into pustules and vesicles with an erythematous halo. They are tender and may have a gray necrotic or hemorrhagic center. They usually heal with crust formation within several days, although recurrent crops of lesions may continue to appear for some time.[7,8]

Gram stain occasionally reveals the organisms within the lesions, but culture is usually negative. Immunofluorescent antibody staining of pustular fluid may be a more reliable diagnostic technique.[9] This has been thought to indicate that the lesions are the result of hematogenous dissemination of nonviable gonococci.[7]

Hospitalization of the patient with disseminated gonococcal infection is recommended. The patient should be tested for genital chlamydial infection. Initial antibiotic treatment should be with ceftriaxone (1 g intramuscularly or intravenously every 24 hours), ceftizoxime (1 g intravenously every 8 hours), or cefotaxime (1 g intravenously every 8 hours). Patients allergic to the cephalosporins should be treated with spectinomycin (2 g intramuscularly every 12 hours). The total duration of therapy is 7 days, with oral antibiotics being used to complete the course of treatment after symptoms resolve.[10]

Meningococcemia

The severity of meningococcemia varies from a mild febrile illness to a fulminant infection capable of producing death within hours. The onset is usually sudden, with the development of fever, chills, myalgias, and arthralgias. A rash appears in approximately three-quarters of cases; initially, it consists of nonpruritic, macular, erythematous lesions on the trunk or extremities. The lesions may be 2 to 15 mm in diameter, and they blanch on pressure. Petechiae may be present, and these occasionally coalesce to form large intracutaneous hemorrhages. The latter are seen in the Waterhouse-Friderichsen syndrome, which occurs in 10% of cases. Lesions similar to those of meningococcemia may be encountered in the presence of other infections, such as meningitis due to ECHO virus type 9, acute staphylococcal meningitis, and very rarely in meningitis due to pneumococcus or *Hemophilus influenzae*.[11]

Meningococci can be recovered from blood and cerebrospinal fluid, as well as from fresh skin lesions. Immediate culture and treatment is imperative. Penicillin G is the drug of choice. Adults with meningococcemia or meningococcal meningitis should receive 24×10^6 U daily in divided intravenous boluses. Children require 250,000 U/kg daily. Chloramphenicol can be administered as an alternative drug to patients with penicillin allergy (see Chapter 87, Emergency Drug Index).

Pyoderma

Most bacterial infection of the skin and subcutaneous tissue is caused by streptococci or staphylococci. Patients predisposed to pyoderma are those with various other skin diseases, obesity, diabetes, chronic granulomatous disease, dysglobulinemia, leukemia, and those receiving corticosteroids or immunosuppressive chemotherapeutic agents. Common skin infections include impetigo, the staphylococcal scalded skin syndrome, cutaneous abscess, and cellulitis.

Impetigo

Although impetigo, a pustular eruption, occurs at all ages, it is most commonly seen in preschool-age children. Group A streptococci are the primary pathogens. Poor health and hygiene, malnutrition, and various antecedent dermatoses—scabies, varicella, contact dermatitis, atopic dermatitis—predispose patients to impetigo.

Lesions are found most often on the face and upper extremities. They begin as 1- to 2-mm vesicles with erythematous margins. These break, leaving a red erosion covered with a golden yellow crust. Regional lymphadenopathy is frequently present. Impetigo may be pruritic, but it is not painful as a rule. The infection is very contagious among infants and young children, less so in older children and adults. Postpyodermal acute glomerulonephritis is a recognized complication.

Bullous impetigo, caused by group 2 staphylococci, is less common than the streptococcal form. It is seen primarily in infants and young children. The initial skin lesions are thin-walled, 1- to 2-mm bullae. These persist longer than the vesicles of streptococcal impetigo and leave a thin serous crust when they rupture. Regional lymphadenopathy occurs rarely.

Impetigo should be treated with systemic antibiotics; topical treatment alone is not effective. Although systemic treatment shortens healing time of skin lesions and reduces the number of recurrences, there is no evidence that systemic antibiotics prevent the development of acute glomerulonephritis.[12] Treatment of choice is intramuscular benzathine penicillin: 40,000 U/kg for children under 6 years old, 1.2×10^6 U for older children and adults. Alternatively, phenoxymethyl penicillin (penicillin V) may be given orally, 25 mg/kg daily or 250 to 500 mg four times a day for 10 days. Penicillin-allergic patients may be treated with erythromycin, 250 to 500 mg four times a day.

Bullous impetigo may be treated with cloxacillin, dicloxacillin, or erythromycin. Topical therapy, useful as an adjunct, should consist of soaking in warm water three to four times daily to remove crusts, followed by the application of povidone-iodine (Betadine) or topical antibiotic ointment.

Staphylococcal Scalded Skin Syndrome

Although it generally occurs in children younger than 6 years of age, staphylococcal scalded skin syndrome has infrequently been described in adults.[13] It is also caused by infection with group 2 exotoxin–producing staphylococci. The illness begins with erythema and a crusting lesion around the mouth. The erythema then spreads down the body, and bulla formation and desquamation follow. Mucous membranes are involved to a minor extent, if at all. After desquamation, the lesions tend to dry up quickly; clinical resolution occurs in 3 to 7 days. Although this syndrome resembles toxic epidermal necrolysis in some respects, these two entities can be distinguished both clinically and histologically (see below).

Since most group 2 toxin–producing organisms are penicillin-resistant, treatment has been with penicillinase-resistant penicillins—methicillin or dicloxacillin—although it is recognized that most patients recover completely without any antimicrobial treatment.[14]

Cutaneous Abscess

Folliculitis, furuncles, and carbuncles can be distinguished from each other by their size and the extent of involvement of deeper tissue layers. *Staphylococcus* species are the usual infecting organisms, although other infecting flora may be present simultaneously.[15] Folliculitis is an infection of hair follicles. The skin surrounding the follicle is not involved, and there is little erythema or pain. A furuncle, or boil, may develop from folliculitis as a result of infection of the dermal glands. This lesion begins with swelling and erythema that progresses as the center of the furuncle liquefies. The overlying skin becomes tense and very tender, and there may be significant surrounding induration or cellulitis.

Hidradenitis suppurativa is a disorder of apocrine sweat glands. It is associated with recurrent abscess formation in the axillae and groin. These abscesses should be incised and drained as indicated. The condition tends to be recurrent and may be extremely resistant to therapy. Antistaphylococcal antibiotics are useful if administered early and for a prolonged course.[12] Many cases do not respond, however, and local excision and skin grafting of the involved area may eventually be required. A carbuncle is a large abscess that develops in the thick, inelastic skin of the back of the neck, back, or thighs. Carbuncles produce severe pain and fever. Septicemia may accompany the lesions.

Superficial folliculitis should be treated with local cleansing and application of topical antibiotics. Furuncles and carbuncles should be treated by the local application of heat and they should be incised and drained when they point. Antibiotics need not be administered if incision and drainage are performed unless cellulitis or septicemia is present.

Cellulitis

An infection of subcutaneous tissue, cellulitis is manifested by erythema, swelling, and local tenderness. The margins of the infection are not elevated or sharply defined. Chills and fever may be present. The causative organisms may be *Staphylococcus* or group A *Streptococcus* species. Treatment should include the application of moist heat and administration of antibiotics. If an extremity is involved, it should be immobilized and elevated. Severe or extensive cases may require hospitalization for parenteral administration of penicillin or nafcillin.

Erysipelas is a streptococcal cellulitis that affects the skin and subcutaneous tissue, most frequently on the face. The involved area is red, indurated, and edematous; its borders are elevated and sharply demarcated. Fever, chills, and systemic toxicity may be present. Treatment should consist of daily injections of procaine penicillin G (600,000 U) or oral phenoxymethyl penicillin (250 to 500 mg four times a day for 10 days). Rapid improvement is the rule, but patients who are elderly or suffer from severe chronic illness may require hospitalization.

The appearance of cellulitis in very young children suggests infection with *Hemophilus influenzae*. Patients infected with this organism are usually 6 months to 2 years of age. The infection typically involves the face, causing a bluish or purple-red discoloration, accompanied by marked temperature elevation.[16] Blood cultures are positive for *H influenzae*. Treatment with ampicillin (50 mg/kg/day) or chloramphenicol (50 mg/kg/day) typically results in defervescence and rapid recovery within 24 hours.[17]

Scarlet Fever

Infection with group A hemolytic streptococcal organisms causes scarlet fever. The illness has an abrupt onset with fever, chills, malaise, and sore throat. This is followed within 12 to 48 hours by the appearance of a distinctive rash (ie, a generalized papular eruption overlying a hyperemic base). The eruption begins on the chest and spreads rapidly, occasionally involving the entire body within 24 hours. Classically, it spares the perioral area. The skin has a rough "sandpaper" texture owing to the multitude of pinhead-sized papules. The pharynx is infected, and erythematous or petechial lesions may be seen on the palate. Following resolution of symptoms, desquamation of the involved areas occurs. This desquamation is as characteristic of the disease as is the eruption.

Complications include streptococcal infection of lymph nodes, the middle ear, and the respiratory tract. Rheumatic fever and acute glomerulonephritis may be late complications. Treatment is aimed at providing adequate antistreptococcal blood levels for at least 10 days, and penicillin is the drug of choice. In children younger than 10 years, benzathine penicillin (600,000 U) and aqueous procaine penicillin (600,000 U) should be injected intramuscularly. In older children and adults, the dosage of benzathine penicillin is 900,000 U. In patients allergic to penicillin, erythromycin (250 mg four times a day) may be given orally for 10 days.

Toxic Shock Syndrome

The toxic shock syndrome (TSS) is an acute febrile illness associated with diffuse desquamating erythroderma. Its appearance has frequently been linked to culture of exotoxin-producing *Staphylococcus aureus*. Occurring primarily, though not exclusively, in young women using tampons, TSS is classically characterized by sudden onset of high fever, hypotension, headache, myalgias, vomiting, diarrhea, and skin rash.[18] Criteria for TSS require *fever* (temperature of at least 38.9°C, 102°F), *hypotension* (systolic blood pressure, 90 mmHg or less), *rash*, and involvement of at least three organ systems.[19] Systemic involvement may include mucous membrane hyperemia, clinical abnormalities of the gastrointestinal (vomiting or diarrhea), muscular (myalgias), or central nervous (alteration of consciousness) systems, or laboratory evidence of renal, hepatic, or hematologic dysfunction.

The rash is typically a diffuse, blanching, macular erythroderma. Fading within 3 days of appearance is the rule, as is full-thickness desquamation 5 to 12 days after resolution. Mucous membrane inflammation is common. Pharyngitis, sometimes accompanied by "strawberry tongue," is most frequently seen. Conjunctival or vaginal hyperemia may also be encountered.

Although linked with tampon use in previously healthy young women, TSS has also been associated with various staphylococcal infections, including empyema, septic abortion, osteomyelitis, fasciitis, peritonsillar and subcutaneous abscess, and staphylococcal colonization of mucous membranes.[20]

Initial treatment includes tampon removal, when appropriate, intravenous volume replacement, and initiation of empiric antibiotic therapy. The patient should be hospitalized for definitive treatment and diagnosis.

CONTACT DERMATITIS

Contact dermatitis is an inflammatory reaction of the skin to chemical, physical, or biologic agents that act as irritants or allergic sensitizers. Irritant contact dermatitis is the more common form, with caustics, detergents, and industrial solvents being prominent causes.[21] However, the condition may be seen in settings in which a less strongly irritant substance is repeatedly applied, or where the skin is injured or macerated.[5] Allergic contact dermatitis is a form of delayed hypersensitivity mediated by lymphocytes that have been sensitized by contact of the allergen to the skin. Clothing, jewelry, soaps, cosmetics, plants, and medications contain allergens that frequently cause allergic contact dermatitis. The most common allergens are listed in Table 27-1.[22] However, any chemical is capable of producing allergic contact dermatitis under appropriate circumstances.

The primary lesions of contact dermatitis are papules, vesicles, or bullae on an erythematous bed. Of the allergens, *Rhus* plants are the most likely to cause bullous eruptions. Oozing, crusting, scaling, and fissuring may be found. Lichenification is seen in chronic lesions. The distribution of the eruption depends on the specific contactant, but mucous membranes are usually not involved. A history of exposure and an appropriate distribution of the lesions are the most

Table 27-1 Common Allergens Causing Contact Dermatitis

Source	Sensitizing Agent
Topical medications	Ethylenediamine
Topical antibiotics	Neomycin
Jewelry	Nickel
Hair and fur dyes	Paraphenylenediamine
Leather	Potassium dichromate
Topical and parenteral medications	Thimerosal
Rhus plants: poison ivy, oak, and sumac	Urushiol

Source: Reprinted with permission from Fisher AA. *Contact Dermatitis*, 2nd ed. Philadelphia: Lea & Febiger; 1973.

significant indications of the diagnosis. If there is doubt, the patient should be referred for allergic patch testing.

The first step in treatment is to avoid the irritant or allergen. Oozing or vesiculated lesions should be treated with cool, wet compresses of Burow's solution, applied for 5 minutes three to four times daily. Topical corticosteroid lotions help to reduce inflammation and pruritus. In some instances—such as severe cases of *Rhus* contact dermatitis—a short course of systemic corticosteroids is necessary.[23] Prednisone, 30 to 50 mg daily, may be prescribed initially, with the dosage reduced over a 1- or 2-week period.

DIABETES MELLITUS

A number of skin conditions are associated with diabetes mellitus. The most characteristic is necrobiosis lipoidica diabeticorum, which occurs predominantly in women, usually in the third or fourth decade of life. It precedes the diagnosis of diabetes in about 15% of patients.[24] The typical lesion is an oval or round yellowish plaque with sharply demarcated borders and a shiny atrophic surface, localized to one or both shins. A telangiectatic pattern often develops within the lesions. Control of the diabetic condition has no effect on necrobiosis lipoidica diabeticorum. Its appearance and course are similar in well-controlled and poorly controlled diabetics, as well as in nondiabetics, in whom it also may occur.[25]

Diabetic dermopathy is the most common skin lesion found in diabetics. It is a nonspecific sign, however, since it also appears in nondiabetics. The lesions are oval or round macules located in groups or in a linear pattern, usually on the anterior shins. They are also found on the forearms. They are atrophic and depressed; they may be dull red or hyperpigmented. The lesions of diabetic dermopathy likewise do not fade with control of the hyperglycemia.[26]

Localized pruritus is very common in diabetics. The vulva, perianal area, and legs are frequent sites of involvement. The cause of this itching is often either *Candida* infection or excessive dryness of the skin.[26]

DRUG ERUPTION

Drugs may cause virtually any type of dermatosis, so a rash in a patient taking medication always raises the possibility that the drug is involved. Reactions tend to appear within a week after the drug has been taken, although reactions to the semisynthetic penicillins frequently occur later than this. Skin lesions may appear after a drug has been discontinued if the drug or its metabolites persist in the system.

The most acute and potentially life-threatening allergic reaction is anaphylaxis. Diffuse erythema, pruritus, and urticaria are the skin manifestations of anaphylaxis; they may accompany hypotension, bronchospasm, and laryngeal edema. Any of these manifestations may be seen, isolated or in combination. Although an anaphylactic reaction most frequently follows parenteral drug administration, it may also be triggered by oral ingestion. Symptoms of dyspnea, substernal discomfort, nausea, vomiting, and hyperperistalsis typically develop within 5 to 30 minutes following administration of the drug.

Epinephrine is the drug of choice in treatment. It should be administered subcutaneously (0.3 to 0.5 mL in a 1:1000 solution) unless shock is present. In this case, it may be given intravenously (1 to 2 mL in a 1:10,000 solution). Intravenous fluids should also be administered. Pressor agents such as levarterenol or dopamine should be considered if hypotension cannot be reversed by these measures. Diphenhydramine hydrochloride (Benadryl), 50 mg, may be administered intravenously or orally for treatment of urticaria, but this should be considered of secondary importance in the therapy.

Serum sickness is a systemic allergic reaction comprised of an urticarial or maculopapular rash accompanied by fever, myalgia, arthritis, edema, and lymphadenopathy. Although initially described as a reaction to horse serum, it is now found most frequently associated with drugs. There is a latent period of 5 to 14 days between the administration of the inducing drug and the onset of symptoms. The syndrome is usually self-limited, resolving within 1 week. When a long-acting penicillin or sulfonamide is involved, symptoms may appear as late as 3 weeks after termination of therapy and persist for 1 month.[27] Other medications that cause serum sickness include aspirin, barbiturates, digitalis, insulin, phenylbutazone, and phenytoin.[28] Treatment for serum sickness is far less urgent than that for anaphylaxis. Allergic symptoms may be controlled by discontinuation of the drug and administration of corticosteroids or antihistamines.[29]

Drug eruptions have numerous forms. Skin lesions of urticaria, erythema multiforme, erythema nodosum, and toxic epidermal necrolysis may be drug induced. In addition, drug eruptions may be exanthemic, eczematous, vasculitic, purpuric, photosensitive, and fixed.

Exanthemic drug eruptions are the most common type. Resembling the skin manifestations of various viral infections, they are usually widespread, symmetric maculopapular eruptions. Severe cases may progress to exfoliative dermatitis. Drugs that commonly produce exanthemic reactions include barbiturates, chloral hydrate, insulin, isoniazid, meprobamate, penicillin, phenothiazines, phenylbutazone, quinine, quinidine, salicylates, sulfonamides, tetracycline, and thiazide diuretics.

Eczematous drug rashes resemble contact dermatitis but are generally more extensive. They begin as erythematous or papular eruptions that may become vesicular. Prior sensitization to a topical medication is common. Aminophylline, meprobamate, methyldopa, penicillin, phenothiazines, sulfonamides, and thiazides are common causes of this type of eruption.

Vasculitic lesions begin as erythematous papules or nodules, but they may ulcerate and become gangrenous. Chloramphenicol, quinidine, iodides, guanethidine, quinine, and other antimalarials may cause such lesions. Purpuric drug eruptions may be the result of bone marrow suppression or platelet destruction. In severe cases, inpatient management with systemic corticosteroid administration, platelet transfusion, plasmapheresis, or splenectomy may be necessary. Quinidine is a frequently implicated causative agent.

Photosensitive reactions result from excessive exposure to sunlight. Patients who are subject to photosensitive drug eruptions should utilize sun-screening agents during any prolonged ultraviolet light exposure. Anovulatory drugs and tetracyclines are well-known causes of photosensitive drug eruption.

Fixed drug eruptions are those that appear and recur at the same site following repeated exposures to a drug. The lesions are usually round or oval in shape and sharply marginated. They may be pigmented, erythematous, or violaceous; they may itch.

Treatment of drug eruptions should begin with discontinuation of the inciting agent. Pruritus may be controlled as needed by the application of drying antipruritic lotion (calamine) or lubricant (Eucerin with 0.25% menthol and 1% phenol). Cool compresses or tepid water baths with Aveeno or cornstarch may be useful. Diphenhydramine (Benadryl), 50 mg, or hydroxyzine (Atarax, Vistaril), 25 to 50 mg every 6 hours, is likely to be of benefit. If the condition is severe, systemic corticosteroid therapy—such as prednisone, 25 mg every 6 hours until improvement is noted—should be instituted. This is most likely to be necessary for severe erythema multiforme, drug-induced toxic epidermal necrolysis, or vasculitis.

ERYTHEMA MULTIFORME

An acute disease that is usually self-limiting, erythema multiforme is characterized by skin lesions that are erythematous or violaceous macules, papules, vesicles, or

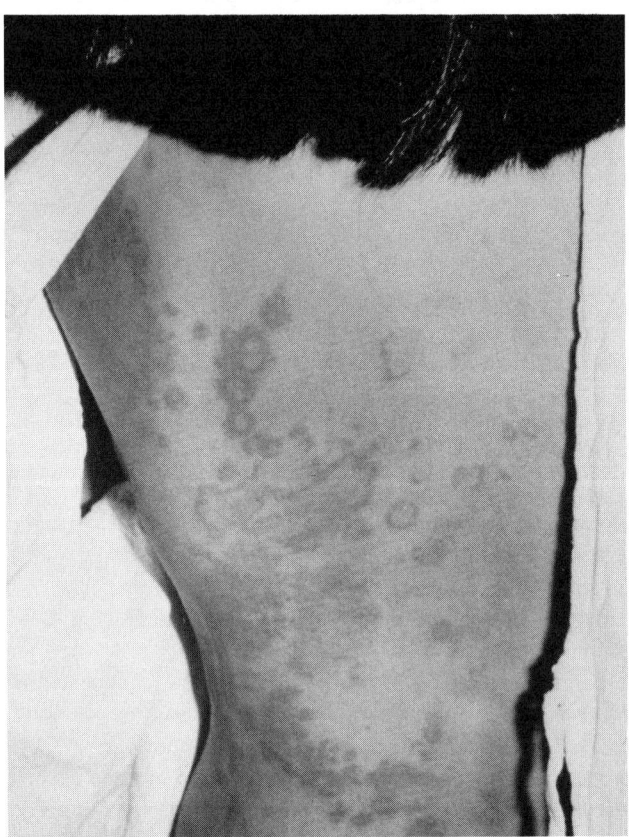

Figure 27-1 Erythema multiforme.

bullae in a symmetric distribution (Fig. 27-1). This involves most frequently the soles and palms, the backs of the hands or feet, and the extensor surfaces of the extremities. Particularly characteristic is the presence of lesions on the soles and palms. The hallmark of erythema multiforme is the target lesion, which may be a papule surrounded by a zone of normal skin or a vesicle surrounded by a halo of erythema. This lesion is frequently found on the hands or wrists.

The Stevens-Johnson syndrome is a severe form of erythema multiforme that is occasionally fatal. It is characterized by bullae, mucous membrane lesions, and multisystem involvement. The patient may be acutely ill, with chills, headache, fever, malaise, tachycardia, and tachypnea, in addition to the skin lesions.

Erythema multiforme has a variety of precipitating causes:

- collagen-vascular disease
    - dermatomyositis
    - periarteritis nodosa
    - rheumatoid arthritis
    - systemic lupus erythematosus
- drugs
- infectious disease

- fungal infection—systemic and dermatologic
- hepatitis
- herpes simplex
- influenza A
- streptococcal infection
- tuberculosis
- malignancy
  - Hodgkin's lymphoma
  - leukemias
- pregnancy

The most common of these are exposure to drugs and herpes simplex infection. Drug-induced erythema multiforme is frequently caused by barbiturates, halogens, penicillin, phenolphthalein, phenothiazines, phenylbutazone, quinine, quinidine, salicylates, and sulfonamides. The long-acting sulfonamides in particular have been linked to the Stevens-Johnson syndrome. In about half of all cases, no provocative factor can be identified.

Treatment should begin with a search for an underlying cause. Severity of the condition varies; mild forms resolve spontaneously over a few weeks, while severe cases may require hospitalization. Treatment for severe cases consists of intravenous hydration and systemic corticosteroid therapy. Bullous lesions should be treated with application of wet compresses soaked in 0.25% silver nitrate solution several times per day.

ERYTHEMA NODOSUM

Patients with erythema nodosum have painful erythematous or violet nodules that represent an inflammatory reaction of the dermis and adipose tissue. The nodules occur most frequently over the anterior tibiae, but may also be seen on the arms or body (Fig. 27-2). Women are affected more frequently than men by a 3:1 ratio.[30]

A number of conditions produce erythema nodosum (eg, tuberculosis, sarcoidosis, coccidioidomycosis, histoplasmosis, ulcerative colitis, regional enteritis, and streptococcal infections). Erythema nodosum has also been found in association with leukemia, Hodgkin's disease, and metastatic carcinoma.[31] As in erythema multiforme, many cases are idiopathic. The relationship of drugs to erythema nodosum has already been noted; oral contraceptive agents are the leading cause of drug-induced cases.[32]

Erythema nodosum is a self-limiting process that usually resolves in 3 to 8 weeks.[32] When an underlying condition can be identified, this should be treated. Bedrest, elastic stockings, and elevation of the legs reduce pain and edema. Aspirin, 600 mg every 4 hours, may also afford some relief. Very symptomatic patients may be treated with potassium iodide, 360 to 900 mg orally daily for 3 to 4 weeks.

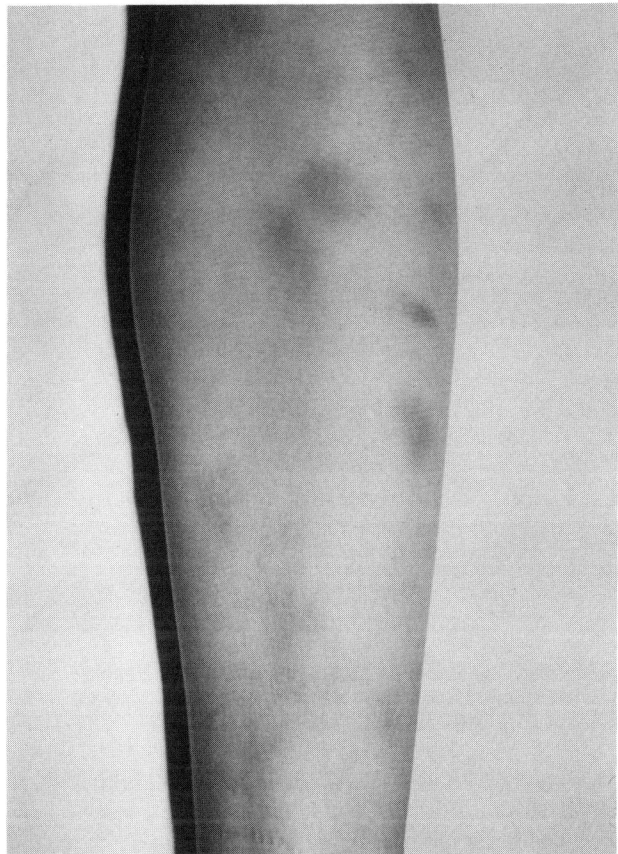

Figure 27-2 Erythema nodosum.

FUNGAL INFECTION

The dermatophytoses are superficial fungal infections of the skin that are characterized by scaling, pruritic lesions. Since dermatophytes generally grow best in hot, moist areas and grow only in the keratin layer of the skin, they are most often found in the areas where keratin tends to accumulate (eg, in the body folds, between the toes, in the groin, and in the axillary and inframammary areas). With the exception of tinea capitis, the dermatophyte infections are not markedly contagious.[33]

Infection of the scalp—tinea capitis—occurs primarily in children. It may cause hair loss, resulting in circular patches of partial baldness. Infected hairs may fluoresce green yellow under long-wave ultraviolet (Wood's) light, although not in all cases. The disease may be transmitted by close child-to-child contact, as well as by contact with household pets, hats, combs, barber's shears, and similar items.

Tinea corporis affects the trunk and extremities. It is classically a sharply marginated, annular lesion with raised or vesicular margins and central clearing (Fig. 27-3). Lesions may be single or multiple. Dermatophytosis of the groin—tinea cruris—is similar in appearance. The perineum, thighs, or buttocks may be involved, but the scrotum

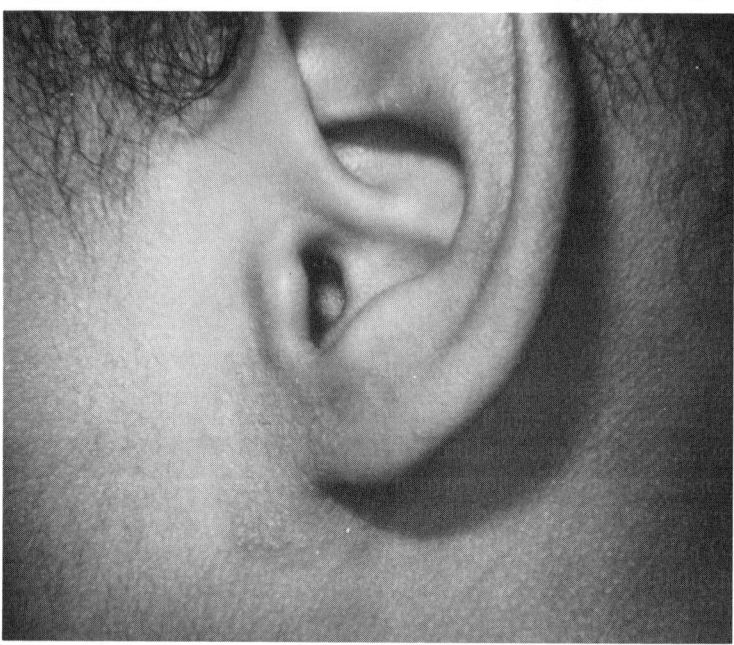

Figure 27-3 Tinea corporis.

is characteristically spared. It is often accompanied by involvement of the feet and toenails.[34]

Tinea pedis, or athlete's foot, is associated with scaling, maceration, vesiculation, and fissuring between the toes and on the plantar surface of the foot. In extensive cases, the entire sole may be involved. Nail involvement—tinea unguium—results in nails that are opaque, thickened, cracked, and crumbled; there are yellowish longitudinal streaks on the nails. The big toe is the digit most frequently involved.

An eruption thought to be a dermatophyte infection should be sampled and examined under the microscope in a potassium hydroxide preparation. The lesion should first be sponged with alcohol and allowed to dry. A specimen from the border of a lesion should be gently scraped onto a glass slide with a scalpel blade. The tops of vesicles or subungual debris can also be examined. A drop of 10% potassium hydroxide solution should then be applied and the specimen covered with a cover slip. The slide is heated over an alcohol lamp flame for a few minutes. The specimen should be examined for the characteristic long, thin, branching hyphae.

Infections of the body, groin, and extremities usually respond to topical measures alone. A number of effective topical antifungal agents are available, including clotrimazole (Lotrimin), haloprogin (Halotex), miconazole (MicaTin), and tolnaftate (Tinactin). The cream or solution of any of these should be applied two to three times a day; most superficial lesions heal in 1 to 3 weeks with this treatment. Acute inflammatory lesions with oozing or blisters should be additionally treated with wet compresses of Burow's solution.

Involvement of hyperkeratotic skin, such as on the palms and soles, may also require the use of a keratolytic agent, such as salicylic acid. Application of the gel form under an occlusive dressing overnight softens hyperkeratotic skin and leads to exfoliation. Keratolytic agents may, however, cause significant skin irritation.

Infections of the scalp and nails require additional treatment. Oral micronized griseofulvin, 5 to 10 mg/kg/day, should be given to patients with tinea capitis until lesions have cleared completely and scrapings are negative. This usually requires 3 to 6 weeks of therapy. There is also some evidence that alternate day or twice-a-week griseofulvin therapy may be as efficacious as daily administration.[35] Shaving or cutting the hair is not a necessary part of treatment.

Tinea unguium often poses a difficult therapeutic problem. Topical therapy of nails alone rarely results in a cure. Administration of griseofulvin (0.5 to 1 g/day for 6 to 12 months) is necessary. Headache, gastrointestinal discomfort, and photosensitization are common side effects.

There are a number of predisposing factors to infection of the skin or mucous membranes by *Candida albicans*. These include infancy, old age, pregnancy, obesity, malnutrition, diabetes and other endocrine imbalances, malignancy, or other debilitating illness. Patients treated with corticosteroids, immunosuppressive agents, and antibiotics are also prone to such infection.

Oral thrush is the most frequent clinical expression of *Candida* infection.[36] It is most frequently due to inoculation of the infant's mouth during the passage through the maternal vaginal canal.[37] It appears as patches of white or grey friable material covering an erythematous base on the buccal mucosa, gingiva, tongue, palate, or tonsils. There may also be fissuring or crusting at the corners of the mouth.

Cutaneous candidiasis favors the moisture and maceration of the intertriginous areas. Lesions appear as moist, bright red plaques with scalloped borders, and small satellite vesicles or pustules are present just peripheral to the main body of the rash. Intertriginous lesions are prone to bacterial superinfection. Potassium hydroxide preparation reveals blastospores—oval budding yeast forms—or pseudohyphae, which have indentations of the septae.

Treatment of thrush involves painting the mouth with oral nystatin suspension—2 mL (100,000 U/mL) for infants, 4 to 6 mL for older children and adults—four times a day. Treatment should be continued for 5 to 7 days after the lesions disappear. Gentian violet (1% to 2% solution) is an alternate treatment.

Treatment of intertriginous lesions requires the removal of excessive moisture and prevention of maceration. Lesions should be exposed to circulating air from a fan several times a day. Inflammatory lesions should be soaked in or covered with compresses of cool water or Burow's solution. Nystatin dusting powder, lotion, cream, or ointment can then be applied. Clotrimazole and miconazole are also effective as topical agents.

PEDICULOSIS

The diagnosis of pediculosis pubis (crabs) is made by identifying louse eggs—nits—in the pubic hair or, occasionally, in other body hair. Nits, which are more commonly found than the adult lice form, appear as white dots attached to the bases of hair shafts. Adult forms look like blue or black grains. Patients complain of intense itching and scratching.

Treatment is the application of gamma benzene hexachloride (GBH—Kwell, Gamene) lotion or cream to the infested and adjacent hairy areas. A thin layer is applied following a warm bath or shower and left in place for 24 hours before being washed off. A second treatment may be administered in 1 week, although it is not usually necessary. GBH should not be applied to the face. Involvement of the eyelashes may be treated with the topical application of 0.5% physostigmine or petrolatum, applied twice a day for 8 days. Itching frequently persists for a short time following treatment.

Sexual partners should also be treated, but other uninfested household members need not be. Underclothing, pajamas, sheets, and pillowcases should be machine-washed and dried (hot cycle), laundered and ironed, or boiled. Pruritus that persists following a course of therapy may be due to irritation of the skin by GBH, sensitization, or anxiety.

Pediculosis capitis (head lice) is seen more frequently in small children than adults. Pruritis is the major symptom, although excoriation frequently results in secondary bacterial infection. Diagnosis is made by identification of nits cemented to hairs at the hair-scalp junction. Treatment consists of shampooing for 4 minutes with 1 tablespoon of GBH shampoo. The shampoo should be applied while the scalp is dry. Shampooing may be repeated in 1 week, if needed. There is no need to cut hair. Household contacts should be examined for involvement, but uninfested persons need not be treated. Clothing and linen should be washed as described earlier. However, the infestation is generally transmitted by direct contact rather than via clothing, and compulsive sterilization of clothing may not be useful.[38]

The organisms that cause pediculosis corporis (body lice) reside in the seams of clothing and bedding materials while they feed on the human host. Except in heavily infested individuals, the parasites are absent from the body itself. Erythematous macules or wheals may be present, along with intense pruritus. Treatment consists of laundering or boiling clothing and bed linen. If nits are found in the body hair, a treatment with GBH lotion may be used, but this is unnecessary in most cases.[39]

PEMPHIGUS VULGARIS

Although pemphigus vulgaris is an uncommon dermatologic disorder, it is an important one because it is potentially fatal. It is a bullous disease that is most common in the 40- to 60-year-old age group and affects men more often than women. The typical lesions are small flaccid bullae that break easily, forming superficial erosions and crusted ulcerations. Any area of the body may be involved, although mucous membrane lesions antedate cutaneous lesions by several months.[40] The most common site of these mucous membrane lesions is in the mouth, especially the gums and vermilion borders of the lips. Blisters may be extended or new bullae formed by firm tangential pressure of a finger on the intact epidermis; this is known as *Nikolsky's sign* and is characteristic of the condition.

The cause of pemphigus is unknown, although studies suggest an autoimmune mechanism.[12] The diagnosis may be confirmed by cytologic testing—Tzanck smear—or serum immunofluorescence. Once the diagnosis is made, treatment with oral glucocorticoids, initial dosage of 100 to 200 mg prednisone daily, should be instituted. Despite the condition's localization to the skin and mucous membranes, mortality in the presteroid era was 95% and continues to be substantial.[40] Most deaths relate to uncontrolled spread of the disease; secondary infection, dehydration, and thromboembolism may also contribute to mortality. Patients may also succumb to the side effects of corticosteroids.

PITYRIASIS ROSEA

A benign skin eruption, pityriasis rosea is seen predominantly in children and young adults. The lesions are multiple oval pink or pigmented papules or plaques, 1 to 2 cm in

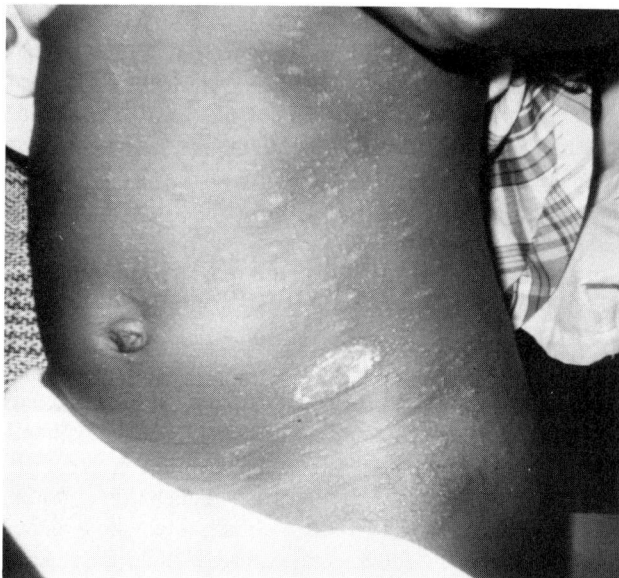

Figure 27-4 Pityriasis rosea.

diameter, appearing on the trunk and proximal extremities. Lesions may be scaly and are arranged parallel to the long axis of the ribs, forming a "Christmas tree" distribution on the trunk. In about one-half of cases, the generalized eruption is preceded by 1 week by a "herald patch." This is a larger lesion—2 to 6 cm in diameter—that resembles the smaller lesions in other respects (Fig. 27-4). The eruption is usually asymptomatic, although pruritus may be present.

Pityriasis rosea is a self-limited condition, usually resolving in 8 to 12 weeks. The etiology is unknown, although a viral etiology is suspected. Recurrences are rare. Treatment is usually unnecessary, except for symptomatic alleviation of pruritus.

ROCKY MOUNTAIN SPOTTED FEVER

Although originally described in the western United States, Rocky Mountain spotted fever occurs in other portions of North, South, and Central America. Most cases are currently reported from the southeastern United States. Rocky Mountain spotted fever is an acute infectious disease caused by *Rickettsia rickettsii*, an organism harbored by certain ticks.

Onset is usually abrupt, with headache, nausea, myalgias, chills, and a fever spiking to 40°C (104°F). Occasionally, the illness begins insidiously, with progressive anorexia, malaise, and fever. The rash usually develops on the second to fourth day of the illness. It consists of erythematous macules that blanch on pressure; they appear first on the wrists and ankles, then spread up the extremities to the trunk and face. This spread is rapid, occasionally occurring in a matter of hours. The presence of lesions on the palms and soles is particularly characteristic. Lesions may become petechial or hemorrhagic, capillary fragility may be increased, and splenomegaly may be present.

The Weil-Felix test is the best known serologic diagnostic test, but Weil-Felix agglutinins are not always present in Rocky Mountain spotted fever, and more specific immunofluorescent procedures have been developed.[41] Treatment should not await the result of such tests, but should begin as soon as the disease is diagnosed on clinical grounds. Diagnosis may be extremely difficult in those patients who do not display a rash. Although less than 10% of patients never develop the rash, the mortality among this group is considered to be very high.[42]

Tetracycline is the antibiotic of choice. It should be given orally, 25 to 30 mg/kg daily in divided doses. If the patient is unable to take oral medications, tetracycline may be administered intravenously, with a 15 mg/kg loading dose followed by a maintenance dose of 15 mg/kg/day. Chloramphenicol may be used in patients allergic to tetracycline. Treatment should be continued until the patient is afebrile for 72 hours.

While deaths can occur in untreated cases, the response to treatment with antibiotics is uniformly favorable. The patient usually shows symptomatic improvement in 24 hours and is afebrile in 3 days. Administration of antibiotics should be continued for 3 days after defervescence.

ROSEOLA INFANTUM

High fever and a rash characterize roseola infantum, but there is a paucity of other physical findings. Ninety-five percent of cases are seen in children 6 months to 3 years old. The fever typically has an abrupt onset and rapid rise to 39.5°C (103°F) to 41°C (106°F). Fever is present consistently or intermittently for 3 to 4 days, then drops precipitously to normal.

The rash appears when the fever subsides. Lesions are discrete pink to rose-colored macules or maculopapules 2 to 3 mm in diameter; they blanch on pressure and rarely coalesce. The trunk is involved initially, with eruption typically spreading to the neck and extremities. The rash clears over 1 to 2 days without desquamation.

Despite the presence of a high fever, the infant may not appear particularly ill. Other physical findings are entirely nonspecific. The etiology of roseola is unknown, and there are no diagnostic tests. The prognosis is uniformly excellent, the most common complication being the occurrence of febrile convulsions.

SCABIES

Epidemics of scabies, a mite infestation characterized by severe itching, have been thought to occur in 15-year cycles, with a 15-year gap between the end of one epidemic and the beginning of the next. The most recent epidemic period began around 1964.[43] For unknown reasons, however, it is extending beyond the usual 15-year period.[44]

Areas of the body most commonly involved are the interdigital web spaces, the flexion areas of the wrists, the axillae, buttocks, lower back, penis, scrotum, and breasts. Infestation tends to be more generalized in infants and children than in adults. Typical lesions are reddish papules or vesicles surrounded by an erythematous border and scratch marks. The pathognomonic lesion of scabies is the burrow, a short, wavy line that often crosses skin lines. It is most commonly seen on the finger web space, elbow, penis, and flexor surface of the wrist.[44] Impetigenization of lesions is common. Close personal contact is involved in transmission of scabies, and multiple family members are likely to become infested. The infestation is also transmitted venereally.

Among effective treatment agents are GBH (Kwell, Gamene) and crotamiton (Eurax) lotion and cream. Patients who do not respond to the former may respond to the latter.[45] Following a warm bath or shower, the scabicide is applied to the entire body, except the face and scalp, even though lesions may be localized. It should be left in place for 12 to 24 hours and then washed off during another bath. Children younger than 5 years should be treated with GBH for 4 hours only; alternatively, crotamiton may be used for these patients. A second treatment course may be applied in 1 week.

All family members and sexual contacts should be treated. In addition, intimate articles of clothing, sheets, and pillowcases should be washed and dried by machine (hot cycle), laundered and ironed, or boiled.[33] It may take several weeks following therapy for signs and symptoms to abate. Hypersensitivity or anxiety may prolong symptoms long after the mites have been destroyed.

Some cases of scabies have been found to be resistant to treatment with lindane. Such cases may be treated with crotamiton or 5% permethrin cream (Nix).[46] Because pruritis may remain for 2 weeks or longer after successful treatment, however, the persistence of itching should not, of itself, indicate treatment failure.

SYPHILIS

The causative organism of syphilis is the spirochete *Treponema pallidum*. The primary lesion appears 10 to 90 days after exposure, remains for 3 to 12 weeks, and heals spontaneously. Six weeks to 6 months following exposure, the disease enters the secondary stage, which may include a variety of mucocutaneous lesions. These lesions also heal spontaneously in 2 to 6 weeks, when the disease enters the latent phase. Either a prolonged latent phase or tertiary syphilis follows. Twenty-five percent of untreated patients have at least one relapse of mucocutaneous lesions during the latent phase.[47] Such lesions are often located in the oral cavity or anogenital region.

The chancre is the principal manifestation of primary syphilis. Although they may be multiple, chancres usually appear as single lesions at the site of spirochete inoculation, generally the mucous membranes of the mouth or genitalia. The chancre begins as a papule and characteristically develops into an indurated ulcer about 1 cm in diameter, with a clean base and raised borders. Painless unless secondarily infected, it may be accompanied by nontender regional lymphadenopathy. This usually develops 7 to 10 days after the appearance of the chancre.

There are a number of cutaneous manifestations of secondary syphilis. Lesions may be erythematous or pink macules or papules, usually with a symmetrical, generalized distribution. Pigmented macules and papules classically appear on the palms and soles. Lesions may be scaly, but are rarely pruritic. Papular, annular, and circinate lesions are more common in nonwhites (Fig. 27-5). Generalized lymphadenopathy and malaise accompany the skin lesions. Symptoms of sore throat, headache, fever, myalgias, hoarseness, and anorexia appear in approximately half of patients. Lymphadenopathy is encountered in 50% to 85% of cases and is usually symmetric.[48] Irregular, patchy alopecia may be seen. Moist, flat, verrucous condylomata lata may appear in the genital area. These lesions are highly contagious.

The diagnosis of primary syphilis is made principally by identification of spirochetes on darkfield microscopy. If darkfield examination is negative, another examination is indicated in 24 hours.[47] The result of the Venereal Disease Research Laboratory (VDRL) test, the most commonly used diagnostic serologic test, is positive in about three-quarters of patients with primary syphilis, but it tends to be negative in the very early stage.[47] The result of the VDRL test is invariably positive in secondary syphilis, usually in titers of 1:16 or greater. Darkfield examination of moist lesions may also be positive.

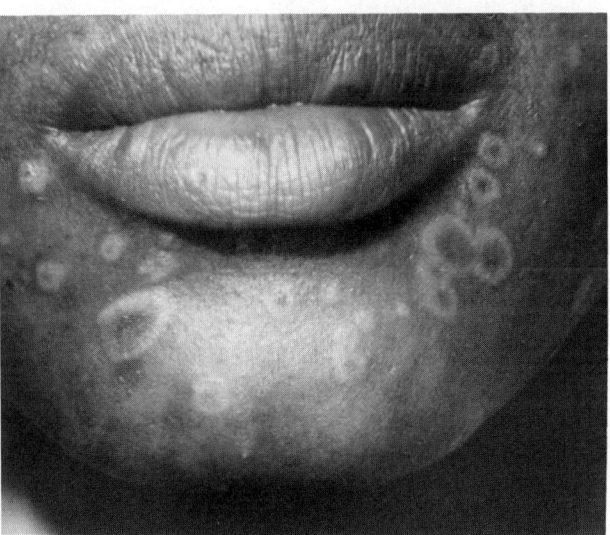

Figure 27-5 Secondary syphilis.

The most specific and sensitive serologic test is the fluorescent treponemal antibody absorption (FTA-ABS) test. A biologic false-positive serologic reaction for syphilis is defined as a positive VDRL test result with a negative FTA-ABS test result. This is seen following vaccination or infections—especially mycoplasmal pneumonia, mononucleosis, hepatitis, measles, varicella, and malaria—and in pregnancy. Chronic biologic false-positive reactions (ie, those lasting longer than 6 months) may occur with systemic lupus erythematosus, thyroiditis, lymphoma, or narcotic addiction; they may also be seen in the elderly. Most false-positive reactions are in low titer ranges of 1:1 to 1:4.[48]

Incubating syphilis—the stage prior to the appearance of primary lesions—may be treated with 4.8×10^6 U of procaine penicillin given intramuscularly along with 1 g of probenecid orally. Primary and secondary syphilis call for treatment with benzathine penicillin G (2.4×10^6 U intramuscularly). Patients allergic to penicillin may be treated with oral tetracycline (500 mg four times a day for 15 days).

TOXIC EPIDERMAL NECROLYSIS

There are two forms of toxic epidermal necrolysis, both of which are characterized by the loosening of large sheets of epidermis from underlying layers of epidermis or dermis. One form is associated with *Staphylococcus aureus* (the staphylococcal scalded skin syndrome; see above) and has an excellent prognosis, regardless of treatment. The other form may be associated with drugs, infection, or medical illness, or it may be idiopathic. This form carries a substantial risk of mortality. The two conditions are histologically distinguishable at skin biopsy.

The main feature of nonstaphylococcal-induced toxic epidermal necrolysis is the separation of large sheets of epidermis from underlying dermis. The full thickness of epidermis is involved. In pigmented skin, the pigment is entirely removed when the skin desquamates. In contrast, substantial pigment remains in staphylococcal scalded skin syndrome. Toxic epidermal necrolysis usually appears first on the face, and mucous membrane involvement is the rule. Erythema usually precedes loosening of the epidermis.

Medications are an important cause of toxic epidermal necrolysis. Among those that have been implicated as inciting agents are the long-acting sulfa drugs, aspirin, penicillin, barbiturates, phenylbutazone, phenytoin, and allopurinol. Toxic epidermal necrolysis has followed vaccination and immunization against poliomyelitis, measles, smallpox, diphtheria, and tetanus. It has also been found in association with lymphoma.

The mechanism that results in toxic epidermal necrolysis is not known. Treatment includes fluid replacement and the administration of systemic corticosteroids. Prednisone, as much as 300 mg daily or its equivalent, has been used, but deaths occur despite high-dose steroid therapy.[49]

URTICARIA

Among the most common skin lesions seen in emergency medicine, urticaria appears as circumscribed, raised wheals that represent localized edema produced by transvascular fluid extravasation (Fig. 27-6). The wheals, or hives, may be slightly erythematous with central clearing. Urticaria is classified as acute or chronic, depending on whether its duration is greater than some arbitrary time limit, usually 4 to 6 weeks. Acute urticaria, which is seen in patients of both sexes, is more likely to have an allergic cause. Chronic urticaria is more common in women in their 40s and 50s, and it may persist for years.

Various mediators, including histamine, bradykinin, kallikrein, and acetylcholine, are thought to play a role in urticaria. Their release may be initiated by immunologic mechanisms, as in anaphylaxis and serum sickness, or by nonimmunologic degranulation of mast cells. The latter may be accomplished by a number of drugs and foods.

Substances that can cause urticaria by contact with the skin include foods, textiles, animal dander and saliva, plants, topical medications, chemicals, and cosmetics.[50] Although virtually any drug can cause urticaria, aspirin and penicillin most frequently produce this eruption.[28,51] Penicillin may be present in trace amounts in dairy products, as well as in medications. Drug-induced urticaria is not invariably allergic. Some drugs—notably the narcotics—may cause urticaria by the direct release of histamine.

A variety of food allergies may result in urticaria, such as sensitivity to fish, eggs, and nuts. In addition, foods such as lobster and strawberries are able to release histamine through a nonimmunologic mechanism. Hereditary forms of urticaria include familial cold urticaria and hereditary angioneurotic edema.

Infections are an uncommon cause of urticaria, although infection with *Candida* organisms, the dermatophytes, bacteria, viruses, and parasites may trigger hives. Bacterial infections usually involve the respiratory or urinary tracts. Viral infections that may produce urticaria include hepatitis, mononucleosis, and coxsackievirus infections.

Inhalation of pollens, mold, animal dander, dust, plant products, and aerosols may produce urticaria. Respiratory symptoms may accompany the dermatosis, and the pattern of occurrence may be seasonal. Stings and bites of insects, arthropods, and various marine animals may produce an urticarial eruption (see Chapter 45, Dangerous Marine Organisms).

Urticaria is uncommonly associated with internal disease and malignancy. It is occasionally found in Hodgkin's disease, more rarely in leukemia and carcinoma. Systemic lupus erythematosus, hyperthyroidism, rheumatic fever, and juvenile rheumatoid arthritis are also occasionally associated with an urticarial eruption.

A number of physical agents produce urticaria. Dermatographia (ie, when firm stroking of the skin produces an

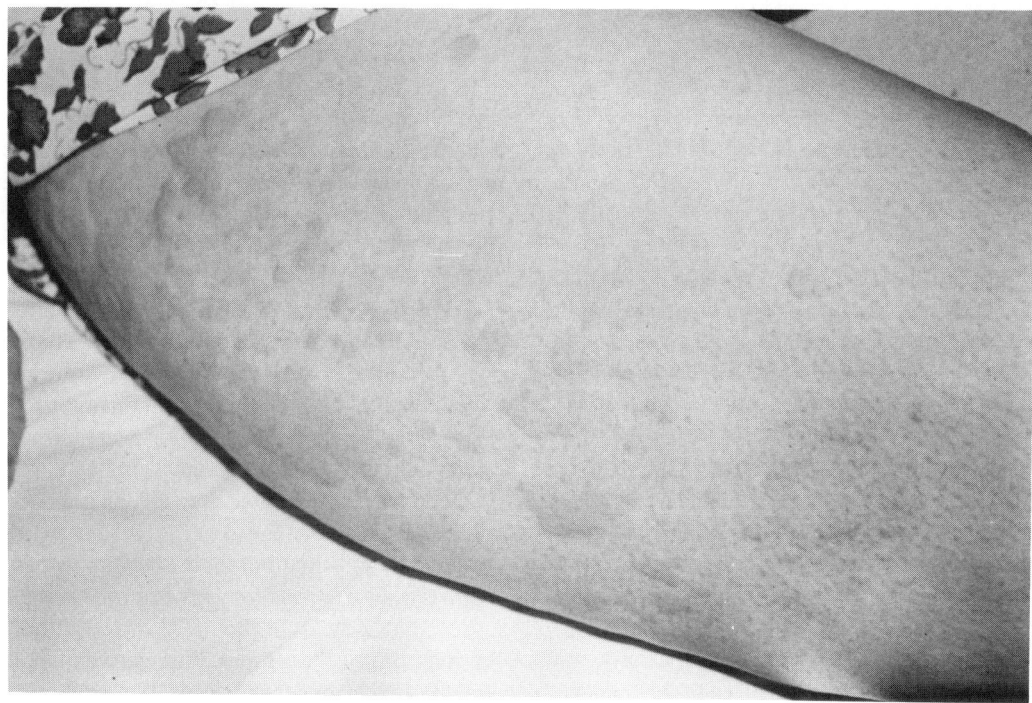

Figure 27-6 Urticaria.

urticarial wheal within 30 minutes), is the most common form of physical urticaria. Pressure urticaria is distinct from dermatographia in that the onset of urticaria is delayed by 4 to 8 hours after the application of physical pressure.

Cold urticaria may be either familial or acquired, although the latter is more common. Cold urticaria may also be associated with underlying illness, such as multiple myeloma, cryoglobulinemia, cryofibrinogenemia, syphilis, and connective tissue disease.[50]

Cholinergic urticaria is induced by exercise, heat, or emotional stress. It may be associated with pruritus, nausea, abdominal pain, and headache.[43] Wheals of cholinergic urticaria are characteristically small, 1 to 3 mm, and surrounded by extensive erythematous flares. Heat rarely induces hives. Solar urticaria, also uncommon, is confined to sun-exposed areas of skin and clears rapidly when light stimulus is removed. Extensive sun exposure may cause wheezing, dizziness, and syncope in the susceptible individual.[52]

Treatment of urticaria involves removal of the inciting factor, where applicable, and administration of antihistamines or other antipruritics. Diphenhydramine (Benadryl, 25 to 50 mg), hydroxyzine (Atarax or Vistaril, 25 to 50 mg), and chlorpheniramine maleate (Chlor-Trimeton, 2 to 8 mg) all provide symptomatic relief. Combined therapy with cimetidine, an H_2 antihistamine, in combination with an H_1 antihistamine has been shown to be effective in treatment of chronic urticaria.[53] However, an H_2 antihistamine should not be used by itself in such treatment.[54] When anaphylaxis accompanies urticaria, treatment of this life-threatening condition obviously takes precedence.

The most important diagnostic steps are a history of inciting factors and a physical examination to investigate the possibility of an underlying illness. An allergic work-up may be in order, especially for acute urticaria. In a significant number of patients with urticaria, however, the cause is not determined.

VIRAL INFECTIONS

Herpes Simplex

Two variants of herpes simplex virus (HSV) are known to cause human infection. These are designated HSV-1, which affects primarily nongenital sites, and HSV-2, which produces lesions in the genital area predominantly. HSV-2 is thought to be transmitted primarily by venereal contact.[55] Lesions found above the waist are usually caused by HSV-1, while those below the waist are generally caused by HSV-2.

The oral region is the most common site of HSV-1 infection, and children are affected more frequently than adults.[56] Initial lesions are small clusters of vesicles, but these are soon broken, leaving irregularly shaped, crusted erosions. Herpetic gingivostomatitis varies in severity from small areas of erosion to extensive ulceration of the mouth, tongue, and gums. Severe cases may be accompanied by fever and cervical lymphadenopathy. Infection may be severe enough to inhibit adequate food and fluid intake. Healing typically takes place in 7 to 14 days, unless the lesions are secondarily infected with streptococci or staphylococci.

The hallmark of HSV infection is the presence of grouped vesicles on an erythematous base. The lesions are usually localized in a nondermatome distribution, although the skin distribution may become more generalized in patients with atopic dermatitis and other skin disease.[56] HSV infection in the immunocompromised host is a potentially fatal infection, owing to its propensity for generalization and dissemination to the internal organs.[57]

HSV-2 infections in the male appear as either a single vesicle or multiple vesicles on the shaft or glans penis. Fever, malaise, and regional lymphadenopathy may also be present. A prodrome of local pain and hyperesthesia may precede the appearance of the cutaneous lesions. Erosion of vesicles after several days to form a crust that heals in 10 to 14 days is the rule. The infection is much more severe in the female. It may involve the introitus, cervix, or vagina; vesicles may be grouped or confluent. Herpetic cervicitis or vaginitis may be the cause of severe pelvic pain, dysuria, or vaginal discharge,[58] and hospitalization may be necessary to control pain. Although recurrences are common, symptoms tend to be less severe in subsequent episodes.

Treatment for a first clinical episode of genital herpes is oral acyclovir (Zovirax, 200 mg 5 times per day for 7 to 10 days or until clinical resolution occurs).[10] Healing is accelerated, the duration of symptoms is diminished, and the period of viral shedding is reduced by treatment with acyclovir. Hospitalization and treatment with intravenous acyclovir should be considered for the immunocompromised patient with HSV infection.[59]

Prevention of recurrent episodes has not been accomplished by treatment with acyclovir. Prophylactic administration may be effective in ameliorating the severity of recurrences, but the effects of long-term acyclovir administration are not known.[60]

Herpes Zoster

Infection with varicella-zoster (V-Z) virus causes herpes zoster, or shingles. Individuals who have previously been infected with chickenpox virus are affected exclusively. The patient typically develops pain in a dermatomal distribution prior to the appearance of the rash. This pain is of variable intensity and is sharp, dull, or burning in quality. It precedes the eruption by 1 to 10 days. The rash consists of grouped vesicles on an erythematous base and involves one or several dermatomes. The thorax or abdomen is involved in the majority of cases. The appearance of herpes zoster in the trigeminal nerve dermatomes is also common.

The vesicles, which are initially clear, become cloudy and then progress to scab and crust formation. This process takes 10 to 12 days, and the crusts heal over the next 2 to 3 weeks. Unusual in children, herpes zoster has a peak incidence in the 50- to 70-year-old age group. The majority of cases occur in healthy individuals.[57] Although the association with Hodgkin's lymphoma and other malignancy is well known, rarely does the appearance of the rash antedate the diagnosis of such disease.[57]

Herpes zoster may be transmitted from patients infected with chickenpox to susceptible individuals. It is generally believed, however, that most herpes zoster is caused by reactivation of V-Z virus present since the initial infection with chickenpox. During the latent period between the two illnesses, the virus is thought to reside in dorsal root ganglion cells.[61]

Herpes zoster has a very low mortality rate, rarely being life threatening even when disseminated to the visceral organs, as occurs occasionally in immunosuppressed patients.[62] Possible complications include central nervous system involvement (eg, meningoencephalitis, myelitis, and peripheral neuropathy). Ocular complications occur in half of the cases that involve the ophthalmic division of the trigeminal nerve.[57] The severity of this varies from mild conjunctivitis to panophthalmitis that threatens the eye. There is a close correlation between eye involvement and the presence of vesicles at the tip of the nose, due to common innervation by the nasociliary nerve. Anterior uveitis, secondary glaucoma, and corneal scarring may result from eye involvement.[63] Ophthalmologic consultation or follow-up should be sought in these cases. Postherpetic neuralgia (ie, pain that persists after lesions have healed) is a troublesome complication. It occurs more frequently in elderly and immunosuppressed patients.[61] The pain may last for months and is often severe and resistant to standard analgesic medications. As much as 5% of patients will have pain that persists indefinitely. Severe pain preceding or accompanying the eruption is associated with a higher incidence of postherpetic neuralgia.[63]

Treatment is rarely necessary. Analgesics may be prescribed as needed. Burow's solution compresses (1:20 to 1:40 diluted in water) may be applied to hasten the drying of lesions. Early systemic corticosteroid therapy may shorten the duration of postherpetic neuralgia, but it does not reduce the severity of pain or accelerate the rate of healing.[56,64]

Although there has been insufficient study of the use of acyclovir in V-Z infection, such treatment should be considered in patients with herpes zoster who are immunocompromised. Because the V-Z virus is less sensitive to acyclovir than HSV, a dose of 400 to 800 mg five times per day for 5 to 10 days has been recommended.[65] The severity of postherpetic neuralgia may be diminished by the administration of acyclovir at the higher dosage.[66]

Measles

A viral illness, measles is highly contagious. Following an incubation period of 10 to 11 days, fever and malaise develop. The fever usually escalates daily until it reaches around 40.5°C (105°F) on the fifth or sixth day of the illness. Cough, coryza, and conjunctivitis begin within 24 hours of the onset of symptoms.

The second day of the illness is marked by the appearance of the pathognomonic Koplik's spots on the buccal mucosa. Although these small, red spots with whitish centers are usually located opposite the molars, they may involve an extensive portion of the oropharynx. The cutaneous eruption begins on the third to fifth day of the illness. Maculopapular erythematous lesions appear on the forehead and upper neck initially, then spread to involve the face, trunk, arms, and finally the legs and feet. The rash begins to fade after 3 days, disappearing from the various sites in the same order. The fever subsides and Koplik's spots begin to disappear during this time.

Otitis media is the most common complication. Other common complications include encephalitis and pneumonitis. Encephalitis occurs in approximately 1 of 1000 cases of measles and carries a 15% mortality. Measles pneumonia may also be life threatening.

If bacterial invasion occurs in the presence of otitis media or pneumonia, antibiotics are indicated. Otherwise, treatment is supportive. Quarantine is of limited value, as others are usually exposed before the appearance of the rash and Koplik's spots render the diagnosis apparent. Measles is not contagious after the rash has been present for 5 days.

The illness can be modified or prevented by the administration of human immune serum globulin, which induces a passive immunity of about 4 weeks' duration. The dosage is 0.22 mL/kg as an intramuscular injection, which is administered within 5 days of exposure.

Rubella

The chief characteristics of rubella, or German measles, are fever, skin eruption, and generalized lymphadenopathy. The incubation period is typically 16 to 18 days. In children, the rash heralds the onset of the illness; in adults, a 1- to 5-day prodrome of headache, malaise, sore throat, coryza, and a low-grade fever antecedes the rash. These prodromal symptoms generally disappear within the first day following the appearance of the skin eruption. Reddish spots on the soft palate may be seen prior to the development of the rash.

The rash first appears on the face, then spreads to the neck, trunk, and extremities. Its appearance is that of pink to red maculopapules. Lesions on the face and trunk may coalesce, but those on the extremities typically do not. Mild pruritus may be present. The rash remains for 1 to 5 days, classically disappearing at the end of 3 days. Clearing is occasionally accompanied by some desquamation.

Lymphadenopathy may be apparent from 1 day to 1 week before the rash appears. In general, the nodes most apparent in their enlargement are the suboccipital, postauricular, and posterior cervical groups. Tender adenopathy may be apparent several weeks after other signs and symptoms subside.

Major complications of rubella (eg, encephalitis, arthritis, and thrombocytopenia) occur more frequently in older children and adults who contract the disease. The most severe complication is fetal damage. Twenty percent of children born to mothers infected during pregnancy have congenital anomalies. Maternal infection may be determined by comparing serum hemagglutination-inhibition antibody during the acute illness with that of 2 weeks later. A fourfold rise in titer is diagnostic of rubella infection.

Varicella

An infection caused by V-Z virus, varicella, or chickenpox, begins with low-grade fever, headache, and malaise, following an incubation period of 14 to 16 days. The exanthem coincides with these symptoms in children, follows them by 1 to 2 days in adults. The skin lesions progress from macules to papules to vesicles to the crusting stage very rapidly, sometimes within hours. The vesicles are usually 2 to 3 mm in diameter and surrounded by an erythematous border. Drying begins centrally, producing umbilication. The dried scabs fall off in 5 to 20 days.

Lesions are most highly concentrated on the trunk. Crops are also common in the scalp, face, and extremities. The hallmark of varicella is the appearance of skin lesions in various stages of development in a single region of the body. Extensive eruptions are often associated with high and prolonged fever.

The illness is self-limited, and treatment should be symptomatic only. Complications include encephalitis, pneumonia, and bacterial cellulitis. As the disease may be transmitted before the diagnosis is clinically evident, isolation of infected patients is futile. The illness is contagious until all vesicles are crusted and dried, so children should be kept at home until this stage is reached.

Other Viral Exanthems

An exanthem is a skin eruption that occurs as a symptom of a systemic disease. Enteroviruses, predominantly the coxsackievirus and ECHO virus groups, and adenoviruses are known to produce exanthems, and other viruses may do so as well. The exanthems of the coxsackievirus and ECHO virus have been the most thoroughly studied. Although most viral exanthems are maculopapular, other forms of rash are occasionally seen (eg, erythematous, vesicular, and petechial eruptions). These are variable in the extent of involvement, are nonpruritic, and do not desquamate. Oropharyngeal lesions, enanthemas, may accompany or precede the skin rash. Fever, meningitis, interstitial pneumonitis, or stomatitis may be part of the viral exanthem syndrome.[67]

DERMATOLOGIC MANIFESTATIONS OF AIDS

The acquired immune deficiency syndrome (AIDS) has become recognized during the past several years as a major public health problem. A number of dermatologic lesions are

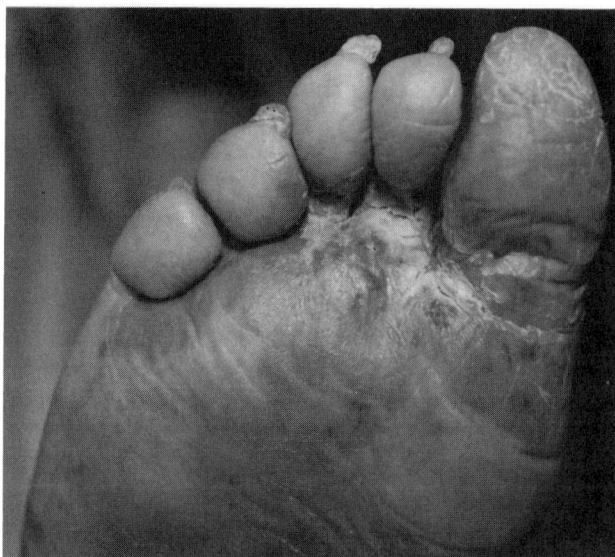

Figure 27-7 Kaposi's sarcoma.

known to be associated with AIDS, most notably Kaposi's sarcoma (KS).

KS, a multifocal neoplasm, is seen in approximately a quarter of AIDS patients. Lesions are macular, papular, nodular, or plaques of reddish-pink, violaceous, or red-brown color (Fig. 27-7). They may be localized, generalized, or present in a pityriasis rosealike pattern following the skin lines. When localized, there is a predilection for the head and neck areas. Mucous membrane involvement is frequent, as is generalized lymphadenopathy.

The course of KS in AIDS is fulminant. There is a 24% mortality reported for KS in these patients and a 63% mortality for those with both KS and *Pneumocystis carinii* pneumonia.[68]

Other dermatologic pathology may be encountered in conjunction with AIDS. Widespread and disseminated herpes simplex infection has been described, as has disseminated herpes zoster and mucocutaneous candidiasis.[69–71] More unusual cutaneous infections, such as cryptococcosis, have also been seen.[72]

There is a high prevalence of syphilis, both active and latent, in patients with human immunodeficiency virus infection.[73] Reactivation of latent syphilis may occur in the AIDS patient.

Several reports have described appearance of widespread lesions of molluscum contagiosum in patients with AIDS.[74,75] These appear as firm, waxy papules 2 to 5 mm in diameter. Molluscum contagiosum, an uncommon viral infection, is otherwise generally encountered in children.

REFERENCES

1. Sibrack LA. Cutaneous signs of internal malignant disease. *Primary Care.* 1978;5:263–280.
2. Safai B, Grant JM, Kurtz R, et al. Cutaneous manifestations of internal malignancies (I). Acanthosis nigricans. *Int J Dermatol.* 1978;17:312–315.
3. Rosenberg FW. Cutaneous manifestations of malignancy. *Cutis.* 1977;20:227–234.
4. Hanifin JM, Lobitz WC. Newer concepts of atopic dermatitis. *Arch Dermatol.* 1977;113:663–670.
5. Galen W. Dermatitis. *Primary Care.* 1983;10:355–367.
6. Robins DN. Cutaneous groin lesions. *Primary Care.* 1978;5:215–232.
7. Bennett RM. Disseminated gonococcal infection: the problems of diagnosis and management. *J Reprod Med.* 1973;11:99–103.
8. Kraus SJ. Complications of gonococcal infection. *Med Clin North Am.* 1972;56:1115–1125.
9. Holmes KK, Weizer PJ, Pederson AHB. The gonococcal arthritis-dermatitis syndrome. *Ann Intern Med.* 1971;75:470–471.
10. Centers for Disease Control. 1989 Sexually transmitted diseases treatment guidelines. *MMWR.* 1989;38:4–43.
11. Swartz MN, Dodge PR. Bacterial meningitis—a review of selected aspects. *N Engl J Med.* 1965;272:725–731.
12. Causey WA. Staphylococcal and streptococcal infections of the skin. *Primary Care.* 1979;6:127–139.
13. Sturman SW, Malkinson FD. Staphyloccocal scalded skin syndrome in an adult and a child. *Arch Dermatol.* 1976;112:1275–1279.
14. Pearson RW. Advances in the diagnosis and treatment of blistering diseases: a selective review. In: Malkinson FD, Pearson RW, eds. *Yearbook of Dermatology.* Chicago: Year Book Medical; 1977;7–52.
15. Meislin HW, Lerner SA, Graves MH, et al. Cutaneous abscesses: anaerobic and aerobic bacteriology and outpatient management. *Ann Intern Med.* 1977;87:145–149.
16. Feingold M, Gellis SS. Cellulitis due to *Haemophilus influenzae* type B. *N Engl J Med.* 1965;272:788–789.
17. Rapkin RH, Bautista G. *Hemophilus influenzae* cellulitis. *Am J Dis Child.* 1972;124:540–542.
18. Tofte RW, Williams DN. Clinical and laboratory manifestations of toxic shock syndrome. *Ann Intern Med.* 1982;96:843–847.
19. Follow-up on toxic shock syndrome. *MMWR.* 1980;29:441–445.
20. Rheingold RL, Hargrett NT, Dan BB, et al. Nonmenstrual toxic shock syndrome. *Ann Intern Med.* 1982;96:871–874.
21. Smith SZ. Contact dermatitis. *Primary Care.* 1978;5:653–659.
22. Farber EM, Abel EA. Contact dermatitis. In: Rubenstein E, Federman DD, eds. *Scientific American Medicine.* New York: Scientific American; 1980;2:1–14.
23. Fisher AA. The notorious poison ivy family of anacardiaceae plants. *Cutis.* 1977;20:570–595.
24. Braverman IM. Cutaneous manifestations of diabetes mellitus. *Med Clin North Am.* 1971;55:1019–1029.
25. Stawiski MA, Voorhees JJ. Cutaneous signs of diabetes mellitus. *Cutis.* 1976;18:415–421.
26. Gouterman IH, Sibrack LA. Cutaneous manifestations of diabetes. *Cutis.* 1980;25:45–54.
27. Parker CW. Drug allergy, part one. *N Engl J Med.* 1975;292:511–514.
28. Fisher AA. Drug eruptions in geriatric patients. *Cutis.* 1976;18:402–409.
29. Parker CW. Drug allergy, part three. *N Engl J Med.* 1975;292:957–960.
30. Soderstrom RM, Krull EA. Erythema nodosum. *Cutis.* 1978;21:806–810.
31. Cormia FE, Domonkos AN. Cutaneous reactions to internal malignancy. *Med Clin North Am.* 1965;47:655–680.
32. Sibulkin D. Drug eruptions. *Primary Care.* 1978;5:233–248.

33. Mescon H, Moretti G. The treatment of cutaneous mycoses. *Med Clin North Am.* 1954;38:1301–1308.
34. Sutton RL Jr, Waisman M. Dermatoses due to fungi. *Cutis.* 1977;19:377–394.
35. Oskui J. Intermittent use of griseofulvin in tinea capitis. *Cutis.* 1978;21:689–692.
36. De Villez RL, Lewis CW. Candidiasis seminar. *Cutis.* 1977;19:69–83.
37. Greenspan JS. Oral mucous membrane disease. *Int J Dermatol.* 1978;17:31–41.
38. Fine BC. Pediculosis capitis. *N Engl J Med.* 1983;309:1461.
39. Orkin M, Epstein E Sr, Maibach HI. Treatment of today's scabies and pediculosis. *JAMA.* 1976;236:1136–1139.
40. Sanders SL, Nelson CT. Pemphigus and pemphigoid. *Med Clin North Am.* 1965;47:681–694.
41. Walker DH, Cain BG, Olmstead PM. Laboratory diagnosis of Rocky Mountain spotted fever by immunofluorescent demonstration of *Rickettsia rickettsii* in cutaneous lesions. *Am J Clin Pathol.* 1978;69:619–623.
42. Westerman EL. Rocky Mountain spotted fever. *Arch Intern Med.* 1982;142:1106–1107.
43. Orkin M, Maibach HI. Scabies in children. *Pediatr Clin North Am.* 1978;25:371–386.
44. Orkin M, Maibach HI. Current views of scabies and pediculosis pubis. *Cutis.* 1984;33:85–116.
45. McRae ME. Scabies. *Cutis.* 1977;20:90–92.
46. Taplin D, Meinking TL, Porcelain SL, et al. Permethrin 5% dermal cream: a new treatment for scabies. *J Am Acad Dermatol.* 1986;15:995–1001.
47. Swartz MN. Syphilis. In: Rubenstein E, Federman DD, eds. *Scientific American Medicine.* New York: Scientific American; 1980;7:1–15.
48. Lee TJ, Sparling PF. Syphilis: an algorithm. *JAMA.* 1979;242:1187–1189.
49. Rosenthal AL, Binnick S, Panber P, et al. Drug induced toxic epidermal necrolysis in children. *Cutis.* 1979;24:437–440.
50. Monroe EW, Jones HE. Urticaria. *Arch Dermatol.* 1977;113:80–90.
51. Fellner MJ, Baer RL. Cutaneous reactions to drugs. *Med Clin North Am.* 1965;49:709–724.
52. Akers WA, Waverson DN. Diagnosis of chronic urticaria. *Int J Dermatol.* 1978;17:616–627.
53. Harvey RP, Wegs J, Schocket AL. A trial of therapy in chronic urticaria. *J Allergy Clin Immunol.* 1981;68:262–266.
54. Monroe EW, Cohen SH, Kalbfleisch J, et al. Combined H_1 and H_2 antihistamine therapy in chronic urticaria. *Arch Dermatol.* 1981;117:404–407.
55. Josey WE, Nahmias AJ, Naib ZM. The epidemiology of type 2 (genital) herpes simplex virus infection. *Obstet Gynecol Surv.* 1972;27:295–302.
56. Olmstead CB. Genital herpes: the newest venereal disease. *Cutis.* 1977;20:113–127.
57. Miller LH. Herpes zoster in the elderly. *Cutis.* 1976;18:427–432.
58. Jarratt M, Smith R, Knox JM. Therapy of herpes simplex infection. *Int J Dermatol.* 1979;18:357–361.
59. Thin RN. Management of genital herpes simplex infections. *Am J Med.* 1988;85(suppl 2A):3–6.
60. Reichman RC, Badger GJ, Mertz GJ, et al. Treatment of recurrent genital herpes simplex infections with oral acyclovir. *JAMA.* 1984;251:2103–2107.
61. Dolin R, Reichman RC, Mazur MH, et al. Herpes zoster-varicella infections in immunosuppressed patients. *Ann Intern Med.* 1978;89:375–388.
62. Gallagher JG, Merigan TC. Prolonged herpes-zoster infection associated with immunosuppressive therapy. *Ann Intern Med.* 1979;91:842–846.
63. Glaser RB. Clinical aspects of herpes zoster. *West J Med.* 1983;139:718–720.
64. Keczkes K, Basheer AM. Do corticosteroids prevent postherpetic neuralgia? *Br J Dermatol.* 1980;102:551–555.
65. Huff JC. Antiviral treatment of chickenpox and herpes zoster. *J Am Acad Dermatol.* 1988;18:204–206.
66. Huff JC, Bean B, Balfour HH, et al. Therapy of herpes zoster with oral acyclovir. *Am J Med.* 1988;85(suppl 2A):84–89.
67. Lerner AM, Klein JO, Cherry JD, et al. New viral exanthems. *N Engl J Med.* 1963;269:678–685, 736–740.
68. Skeen WF. Acquired immunodeficiency syndrome and the emergency physician. *Ann Emerg Med.* 1985;14:267–273.
69. Siegal FP, Lopez C, Hammer GS, et al. Severe acquired immunodeficiency in male homosexuals manifested by chronic perianal ulcerative herpes simplex lesions. *N Engl J Med.* 1981;305:1439–1444.
70. Gottlieb MS, Schroff R, Schanker HM, et al. *Pneumocystis carinii* pneumonia and mucosal candidiasis in previously healthy homosexual men. *N Engl J Med.* 1981;305:1425–1431.
71. Cockerell CC, Friedman-Kien AE. Skin manifestations of HIV infection. *Primary Care.* 1989;16:621–644.
72. Rico MJ, Penneys NS. Cutaneous cryptococcosis resembling molluscum contagiosum in a patient with AIDS. *Arch Dermatol.* 1985;121:901–902.
73. Quinn TC, Glasser D, Cannon RO. Human immunodeficiency virus infection among patients attending clinics for sexually transmitted diseases. *N Engl J Med.* 1988;318:197–203.
74. Lombard PC. Molluscum contagiosum and the acquired immunodeficiency syndrome. *Arch Dermatol.* 1985;121:834–835.
75. Katzman M, Elmets CA, Lederman NM. Molluscum contagiosum and the acquired immunodeficiency syndrome. *Ann Intern Med.* 1985;102:413–414.

28. Gastrointestinal Emergencies

WILLIAM LINNIK, MD

ABDOMEN PAIN: PRESENTATIONS AND CONSIDERATIONS

Patients who present to the emergency department (ED) with classic abdominal pathology are rewarding for the treating physician. This is rarely the case, however; clinicians diagnose acute abdominal pain with inaccuracy in the range of 65%, and the first physician to evaluate a patient with abdominal pain assigns a correct diagnosis in only 40% to 50% of cases. This occurs because in approximately one-third of cases patients with abdominal pain exhibit significantly atypical features. The Staniland investigation of 600 patients showed findings of perforated peptic ulcer in teenagers and cases of diverticulitis in the age group younger than 30 years, and less than 20% of patients with cholecystitis were in their 40s.

The site of pain is only a rough guide. In one study, in 23% of cases of diverticulitis the pain was confined to the left lower quadrant, and in 38% of cases of cholecystitis the pain was limited to the right upper quadrant. In cases of appendicitis, however, 74% of the patients complained of pain confined to the right lower quadrant at the time of admission. The duration of pain was sometimes misleading, most commonly in the young and the aged, where marked delays in presentation occurred. Although the quality of the pain was more significant—that in bile obstruction usually being colicky and that in pancreatitis usually being steady—many patients complaining of colicky or intermittent pain ultimately had appendicitis, and several had perforated peptic ulcers.

In a study of 1000 adult patients with abdominal pain,[3] the two most common final diagnoses of those discharged incorrectly from the ED with surgical disease were acute appendicitis and acute intestinal obstruction. All the patients with obstruction had histories of intra-abdominal surgery and normal initial abdominal radiographs. In those patients who underwent unnecessary laparotomy, the most common postoperative diagnosis was acute salpingitis. The second most common diagnosis was abdominal pain of unknown cause. Approximately 10% of patients older than 50 years who were discharged with this diagnosis ultimately proved to have intra-abdominal cancer.

In summary, the majority of patients who are diagnosed as having abdominal pain of undetermined etiology, even after inpatient work-up, will not have a cause found. Most will remain asymptomatic after the episode has resolved. In those who have a diagnosis made, the predominant problems are appendicitis, gynecologic disorders, and urinary tract problems.[4]

Fried makes five statements regarding the population of patients presenting with acute abdominal pain. (1) Life-threatening illnesses are relatively infrequent; (2) an exact diagnosis will be difficult to make in a large segment of the population; (3) a small percentage of patients sent home will return with significant surgical disease; (4) a large percentage of patients with be admitted with suspected surgical disease that turns out not to be present; and (5) a significant percentage of patients will have abdominal pain of other than gastrointestinal (GI) tract origin.

The priorities in cases of abdominal pain seen in the ED are as follows:

- Does the patient require hemodynamic stabilization?
- Is there a need for immediate or urgent surgical intervention?
- Does the patient's problem warrant admission?
- What is the specific diagnosis?

Diagnosis is least important in most cases, but not in ectopic pregnancy, ischemic bowel, torsion of the testicle, or ruptured abdominal aortic aneurysm.

UPPER GASTROINTESTINAL BLEEDING

Each year, approximately 250,000 patients are admitted to a hospital for upper GI bleeding. This is about 100 admissions per 100,000 population. Mortality as high as 10% exists; it is higher especially in those with bleeding esophageal varices and in those who bleed after being hospitalized. Patients often recognize the symptoms of upper GI bleeding and usually seek evaluation quickly. Patients, however, are not reliable when it comes to estimating the quantity of blood loss.

Patients may describe hemoptysis, coffee-ground emesis, or melanotic stools. One should beware of patients who seek medical care with only fatigue, lightheadedness, or chest pain and syncopy due to blood loss anemia.

Early Management

If the patient is not hypotensive in the supine position, attempt an orthostatic blood pressure check. Upright pulse increase of greater than 15 beat/min or upright blood pressure decrease of greater than 15 mmHg suggests a substantial acute blood loss. If the patient exhibits no alteration in pulse or blood pressure or becomes dizzy upon standing, this is a positive tilt test. In some patients, peripheral arterial constriction can maintain the mean blood pressure at the expense of a markedly decreased cardiac output. β-Blocker medications may affect the pulse changes.

In hypotensive patients, feel the extremity. If it is cool and pale with capillary refill greater than 2 seconds, assume clinical shock. Take a quick look at the neck veins; if flat, consider hypovolemic shock until proven otherwise. Place the patient supine, and prevent unnecessary heat loss by keeping him or her warm. The priorities are to gain access to the circulation, to obtain blood for laboratory tests, to determine the site of blood loss, and to start fluid resuscitation.

For patients in mild shock (up to 20% blood volume loss) showing decreased perfusion of nonvital organs and tissues, who have cool skin, or who feel cold, a 16-gauge peripheral extremity catheter is usually adequate. In moderate shock, where there is 20% to 40% blood volume loss, patients show decreased perfusion of vital organs (liver-gut-kidneys). The manifestation is oliguria or anuria and slight to significant drops in blood pressure on tilt test and sometimes mottling in the extremities (especially the legs). In severe shock, with 40% or more blood volume loss, there will be decreased perfusion of the heart and brain with restlessness, agitation, occasional coma, and electrocardiographic (ECG) irregularities.

Presentations other than mild shock require at least two large-bore (14- to 16-gauge) intravenous lines, one with lactated Ringer's solution and the other with normal saline. Central lines can be used; their complication rate is increased in hypovolemic agitated patients. Once the first line is established, blood should be drawn for type and cross match, complete blood chemistries (CBC), platelet count, prothrombin time (PT), partial thromboplastin time (PTT), electrolytes, blood urea nitrogen (BUN), creatine, and glucose. The patient should have a Foley catheter inserted to monitor urine output. The patient should be placed on a nasal cannula at 3 L of oxygen. A nasogastric tube as large as the patient can comfortably tolerate should be placed. Use of an Ewald tube should be discouraged because it can result in epistaxis and gagging and because the possible complication of varices outweighs the benefits. In resuscitation, lactated Ringer solution is the initial fluid of choice. The liver readily converts lactate to bicarbonate in hypotensive states. Dextrose is not needed in shock because glucose levels are already elevated as a result of circulatory catecholamines.

Whole negative blood typically is immediately available for profound shock. Type-specific blood is usually available within 20 minutes. Fully cross-matched blood typically takes 45 minutes. It is uncommon for a major reaction to occur to type-specific blood. Bank blood is often low in factors V and VIII and in platelets. In whole blood, clotting factors, leukocytes, and platelets are found in reduced amounts also. The patient should receive a fluid challenge of 2 L of crystalloid before a blood transfusion is contemplated.

Only in the most serious, immediately life-threatening situation should the patient be given O-negative blood before crystalloid, colloid, or type-specific blood. In active bleeding associated with vitamin K–dependent factor deficiency, fresh frozen plasma (2 mL/kg) is indicated. Vitamin K alone corrects too slowly. Cirrhotics can easily become citrate intoxicated with whole blood. For them, packed red blood cells reduce citrate load. Platelets will lose 50% of their activity after 24 hours of storage. Actively bleeding patients should have platelet counts above 100,000/mm^3. One unit of platelets raises the count by about 5000/mm^3.

Blood transfusion is generally not necessary if the patient's hematocrit is above 35% and hemoglobin is above 10 and if there are no clinical signs indicating shock. Blood transfusions may aggravate portal hypertension and cause recurrent and prolonged bleeding.

History and Examination

After resuscitation, a history is obtained and a physical examination performed to obtain clues as to the source of the GI bleeding. Seventy-five percent of patients will be found to have peptic ulcer disease or drug-induced gastritis from alcohol or anti-inflammatory medications. Priorities are as follows: (1) Is it varicele or nonvaricele? (2) Is it controlled? Hemoptysis usually means an upper GI bleed. Its absence does not preclude upper GI bleed, and it may be found with small bowel lesions. The most common cause of massive GI hemorrhage is duodenal ulcer. This is followed by erosive gastritis.

Patients with vomiting, coughing, and retching before upper GI bleed may have Mallory-Weiss tears of the gastroesophageal junction. Approximately 40% of these tears are not associated with a history of forceful straining. History of abdominal pain may point to duodenal gastric ulcer disease. Mallory-Weiss tears account for 10% of upper GI bleeds. A history is lacking in 15% of cases. None of the tears is confined to the esophagus. The majority of tears are below the gastroesophageal junction, and only about 9% will extend into the esophagus. Ninety percent stop bleeding spontaneously and 31% require transfusion, and approximately 4% of these patients die because of aspiration, hemorrhage, or liver failure.

Esophageal or gastric varices usually are not associated with abdominal pain unless the patient has gastritis, pancreatitis, or alcohol hepatitis. Twenty percent of patients complaining of intestinal bleeding are in fact not bleeding.

Complaint of melena suggests the digestion of blood, usually from the upper GI tract. A right-sided colonic bleed with stasis may also produce melena. Passage of bright red or maroon blood per rectum occurs in 5% to 10% of all upper GI hemorrhages. Many patients with recurrent episodes of upper GI bleeding often have a different source than that identified in previous episodes. Melanotic stools can be false positive secondary to iron, bismuth, licorice, or charcoal ingestion. The hematocrit test distinguishes this from melena secondary to GI bleeding.

Complaints of fever, chills, and bloody diarrhea suggest typhoid fever, amebiasis, or *Shigella* infection. Complaints of chronic weight loss, anorexia, and malnutrition suggest carcinoma or ischemia. History of salicylate, steroid, anticoagulant, or acute alcohol ingestion suggests gastritis, esophagitis, gastric ulcer, or abnormal clotting profile. Age can be helpful in that usually Meckel's diverticulum occurs in patients younger than 20 years of age and diverticulitis, angiodysplasia, and carcinoma occur usually in patients older than 40 years of age. Angiodysplasia is a venous bleed that is repetitive but usually not profuse. Diverticula are usually arterial bleeds, which are sudden and massive. Meckel's diverticulum from gastric acid erosion has only a 4% incidence of bleeding. Ulcerative colitis bleeds commonly but not massively. Crohn's colitis bleeds less commonly than ulcerative colitis but massively. Aorta and enteric fistulas have a history of aortic graft, ulcer, and bleeding. One hundred percent mortality occurs without surgery, and these patients may require immediate endoscopy. Syncope and presyncope may be the only symptoms.

A history of bleeding from one site is no assurance that bleeding is from the same site. Physical examination of the skin may suggest alcoholism if jaundice, spiderangioma, facial flushing, and palmar erythema are seen. Physical examination is only so helpful. Clinical examination, apart from endoscopy, will only be 40% to 50% accurate in making the diagnosis of the cause of upper GI bleed.

In patients with known varices, endoscopy reveals the source of upper GI bleed to be from another site in one third of cases.[1] Fifteen percent of patients suspected of having a lower GI bleed will be found to have an upper GI bleed.

Laboratory tests may be normal in the acute phase. Blood gases may show metabolic acidosis. Deficient clotting factors often occur in alcoholics. A BUN above 30 is usually seen in a upper GI bleed but not a lower GI bleed. Radiographs help rule out aspiration and associated disease of an aortic graft.

Diagnostic and Therapeutic Modalities

Gastric lavage through the nasogastric tube is time honored. It helps clear the stomach of food and old blood. It is helpful for the endoscopist to determine the activity of bleeding. Adults should get 200-mL aliquots, and then after a minute or two the lavage fluid should be removed. Active bleeding exists if pink or red effluent persists after 1 to 2 L. The best overall choice is probably a room temperature tap water lavage. The dose in children is usually 5 mL/kg per aliquot.

Histamine receptor antagonists, although not arresting acute upper GI bleeding, generally are supportive in treating the underlying peptic ulcer disease. Adults can receive ranitidine (50 mg intravenously every 8 hours) or cimetidine (300 mg intravenously every 8 hours). Endoscopy should be performed on patients suspected of upper GI hemorrhage. The exact diagnosis determines the treatment; today the diagnosis can often be rendered with the endoscope. The diagnosis is made more than 90% of the time. Only about 5% of patients with GI bleed need immediate surgery. Eighty percent to 90% of upper GI hemorrhages stop spontaneously. Lavage is not instrumental in stopping bleeding.

Endoscopic treatment for a bleeding gastric ulcer is photocoagulation. Endoscopy should be performed on an emergency basis if there is active upper GI hemorrhage that is not massive. If the hemorrhage has stopped, the timing of endoscopy is controversial. Endoscopic sclerotherapy for esophageal varices is successful 90% of the time. There is a 20% mortality compared to 80% with emergency portocaval shunt. As with all varices, rebleed is common in the first 4 to 6 weeks (about 25%).

If an endoscopist is not available or if his or her efforts fail to control hemorrhage, three situations can exist. If bleeding is minimal or decreasing and the patient is stable, a conservative approach is appropriate. If the bleeding is significant and/or patient stability cannot be maintained, use intravenous vasopressin, angiography, or surgery. If the bleeding is varicele, add balloon tamponade. The Sengstaken-Blakemore tube or a Minnesota tube has gastric and esophageal balloons that, when inflated, may tamponade actively bleeding varices. They are often accompanied by life-threatening complications. Their use necessitates endoscopic documentation of varicele bleeding before insertion. To use them, check the balloon, partially inflate the gastric balloon, and check the position radiographically. If bleeding stops with the gastric balloon, do not inflate the esophageal balloon. Balloons work 85% to 90% of the time but must be followed by a more definitive procedure. Fifty percent of patients with active bleeding with known esophageal varices will be bleeding from some other source. The most common complication of the Sengstaken-Blakemore tube is pulmonary aspiration. When this tube is used, a nasogastric tube should be taped alongside, ending in the esophagus, to permit suction of the esophagus and decreased aspiration.

Disposition

Patients who are hemodynamically unstable at admission should be admitted to the hospital. If they are older than 40 years, they probably should be in a monitored area. Patients who have bleeding that persists in spite of the previously mentioned measures should be admitted to the intensive care unit, and an endoscopist and general surgeon should be on consult on an emergency basis. Young, reliable patients with inactive and insignificant bleed not requiring fluid resuscitation can be managed as outpatients. In patients who are not having persistent hemorrhage, there is no advantage in terms of mortality, transfusion, or hospitalization with emergent endoscopy. Patients who are admitted to the hospital during their course, however, should have definitive endoscopic verification of the site of hemorrhage.

Endoscopy: Who Needs It?

It is the 10% to 20% of patients who have persistent or recurrent bleeding who would have been endoscoped for diagnosis anyway. Thirty percent of gastric ulcers rebleed during the hospital stay. Duodenal ulcers rebleed slightly less often (about 25%). The most reliable predictor of rebleeding is a visible nonbleeding vessel. If the vessel is elevated, red, and blue and rising from an ulcer base, there is a 50% likelihood of rebleeding. With other stigmata such as an overlying clot without oozing, flat spots, or dark slough, the risk of rebleeding is less than 10%. Oozing is not an indication for endoscopic therapy unless it signals other problems. The chances of finding bleeding points are greatest within 24 hours of the initial hemorrhage. If a patient is bleeding and semistable, immediate action is indicated. Make sure the blood pressure is stable and the patient has proper respiratory support. Pre-endoscopy considerations are as follows: It should be determined whether sedation to be used will compromise respiration and whether the probability of aspiration is enough to require intubation. Before endoscopy has begun, a surgeon should be available in case an emergency operation becomes necessary. Prepping is similar to that for other upper GI endoscopy. Because the patient must be able to swallow an endoscope, the procedure is contraindicated in those who are violent, uncooperative, or psychotic. It probably should not be performed on those who are dying of other causes or on those who cannot tolerate or would not consent to surgery, should that become necessary. Significant derangements of bleeding are also a contraindication, especially if one is unable to correct a significantly abnormal bleeding time by transfusion of platelets. Endoscopy treatment may seal a bleeding artery for a little while, but within 3 days those places often rebleed and usually massively. Currently, lasers are not generally used for emergency hemostasis because of their inconvenience. The bipolar and heater probes are usually cheaper and more portable.

LOWER GASTROINTESTINAL BLEEDING

Rectal bleeding occurs less commonly than upper GI bleeding. At presentation, immediately assess the extent of blood loss, resuscitate, and stabilize the patient's hemodynamic state. As outlined for upper GI bleeding, blood should be drawn at once for laboratory studies, and monitoring is advisable. Large-bore intravenous lines and oxygen should be part of the initial stabilization. A brief history may help if there has been hematochezia, history of cholitis, or change in bowel habits. Painless GI bleeds are seen more commonly in diverticular disease, angiodysplasia, colonic polyps, malignancy, and hemorrhoids. Painful GI bleeding with abdominal cramping often suggests infection, inflammatory bowel disease, or ischemia. A rapid bleed is more likely to be accompanied by syncopy and dizziness. A chronic bleed is more likely to be accompanied by weight loss, change in bowel habits, and anorexia, all pointing to malignancy.

Physical examination in elderly patients with aortic stenosis has shown an association with colonic angiodysplasia. Active bowel sounds suggest an upper GI bleeding source, whereas infrequent bowel sounds suggest a lower GI source. The rectal examination may detect hemorrhoids, fissures, or masses. Black stools suggest a slower or upper GI bleed. Maroon stools suggest possible rapid upper GI bleed. Bloody stools mixed with mucus suggest an inflammatory source for bowel disease or ischemia in the elderly.

The patient should have a 16- or 18-gauge nasogastric tube placed. If the aspirate is negative, this may not rule out upper GI bleeding; 3% of nasogastric aspirates are negative in upper GI bleed. The bleed may be intermittent, and blood may not reflux back through the pylorus. If the patient's history strongly suggests upper GI bleeding, fibroptic endoscopy of the upper GI tract may be considered at this point. If there is no history of recent bowel surgery, especially anastomosis, and if the patient's GI bleeding is not heavy enough to cause unstable vital signs, fibroptic endoscopy of the colon should be carried out. We prefer to start with an anoscope for stable patients. Bleeding beyond the level of the anoscope then requires a full colonoscopy. These patients can be prepared with oral saline lavage with Go-lightly solution. A flat plate of the abdomen may reveal the presence of large or small amounts of stool and allow the endoscopist to proceed without bowel preparation.

Colonoscopy identifies the bleeding site in up to two thirds of patients with active hemorrhage. Bleeding from angiodysplastic or other vascular lesions can be treated by colonoscopic laser or electrocautery at that time. If colonoscopy does not reveal the source of bleeding and if the patient is fairly stable, scanning with ^{99m}Tc-labeled sulfur colloid or [^{99m}Tc]pertechnetate-labeled red blood cells is an option. The sensitivity of labeled red blood cells is 0.1 mL/min. Arteriography requires at least 0.5 mL/min for the site to be seen. The tagged red blood cell requires about 30 to 40 minutes to prepare but displays bleeding from the upper GI tract better than the sulfur colloid, which may miss intermittent bleeding because the half-life is so short. Tagged red cells will remain in the circulation for scanning over the next 24 to 48 hours. A positive radionuclide scan should be followed by arteriography. The first injection is usually in the superior mesenteric artery. If an arterial bleeding site is identified, the catheter may be left in place and attempts made to control the bleeding by embolization or vasopressin infusion, with the dose being tapered over 1 to 2 days. Venous-phase films are mandatory to detect intestinal varices in a patient with portal hypertension. The risk with embolization is infarction.

In summary, lower GI tract bleeding is a surgical disease unless age or medical status dictates otherwise. With massive bleeding, colonoscopy and radionuclide scanning offer little benefit. Surgical decisions in the operating room involve different types of bowel resection.

ESOPHAGUS AND ESOPHAGEAL EMERGENCIES

Chemical Burns

Caustic ingestions occur between 5000 and 10,000 times yearly in children younger than 5 years. In adults, usually this is intentional rather than accidental. The caustics are split into acid substances and alkali substances. Lyes can be solids or liquids, with solid lyes usually producing a deeper tissue injury of the esophagus and less of the stomach. Liquid lye, however, affects the esophagus and stomach equally. The mechanism of injury is liquefaction necrosis. This usually occurs within seconds, limiting the effectiveness of most nonsurgical treatments. Acids tend to cause coagulation necrosis, which produces an eschar that prevents deeper penetration of esophageal and stomach tissues.

There are immediate and delayed injuries that occur with caustic ingestions. The most common of the immediate types are airway edema and compromise. This is due to the hyperthermic injury. Perforation of the esophagus and stomach is the next immediate injury that is encountered. Delayed complications include strictures and an increased incidence of carcinoma decades later.

Presentation

Although the majority of patients present with severe pain, occasionally parents will bring in a child who had bits of lye granules on the mouth and no symptoms. If careful examination of these children reveals intraoral lesions or excessive salivation, this mandates a full work-up including endoscopy and observation in the hospital. The absence of oral lesions does not preclude the possibility of esophageal burns. Many studies have shown that lower GI burns can occur without any oral manifestation. Initial stabilization is similar in both acid and alkali ingestion. Patients in respiratory distress should be intubated. This should be done under direct visualization because blind nasotracheal intubation may perforate edematous soft tissue in the hypopharynx. Laboratory studies include CBC and type and cross-match for 4 U of packed red cells, and the patient should have intravenous lines and oxygen applied if there is any respiratory distress. Radiographs (upright chest and abdomen) may reveal free air in the mediastinum from esophageal perforation or in the abdomen from stomach perforation. Patients should receive nothing by mouth. Emesis and lavage may cause regurgitation of acid contents and reinjury of esophageal structures. In the prehospital area, diluents, preferably milk or water, are probably indicated in solid lye ingestion. In liquid lye, because of the repeated nature of the injury, diluents are of no value. Charcoal is not recommended; it would interfere with endoscopic evaluation of tissue injury. Acute perforation does mandate broad-spectrum antibiotics.

Disposition

Patients with perforations require immediate operative intervention and not endoscopy. Patients without obvious signs of perforation should be referred for endoscopy for evaluation of the extent of burn; most studies show the ideal time of endoscopy intervention to be at 12 to 24 hours, when tissue is less friable and less easily perforated by the endoscope.

Esophagus Obstruction

Obstruction of the esophagus can be mechanical or due to neuromuscular causes. The most common mechanical causes are solid food boluses. These patients often localize the site of their pain and usually give a history that they are unable to pass the bolus despite swallowing liquid. In these patients an upright chest radiograph should be obtained, especially if they vomited against the bolus and were unable to expel it. Glucagon, through its action of relaxing smooth muscle of the esophagus, will often give relief of symptoms within 20 minutes. If the patient is still symptomatic after 20 minutes, an additional 1 mg of glucagon should be given. The patient not responding to glucagon after a brief observation period should probably have endoscopy. Patients who do pass the food bolus should be referred to a gastroenterologist to make sure there was not an occult lesion accounting for the food bolus getting caught.

Suspect mechanical causes of dysphasia especially when solid food sticks and is regurgitated undigested. Suspect neuromuscular causes of dysphasia if the bolus passes after repeated swallowing and drinking of water. Difficulty swallowing liquids is more symptomatic of a motor disorder.

Patients with dysphagia or odynophagia deserve an emergency barium swallow. These results allow disposition for the appropriate diagnosis. Patients with infectious disease causing obstruction, such as herpes or candidiasis, often have oral manifestations. Nystatin swish and swallow can offer relief in candidiasis. Those in the acute phase of herpetic infection may get relief from oral acyclovir (200 mg five times a day for a 7-day course).

Peptic Esophagitis

The esophagus is normally protected from acid by the lower esophageal sphincter, a secondary esophageal peristalsis, and bicarbonate-rich swallowed saliva (1000 to 1500 mL daily). Heartburn is the most common presenting symptom in patients with this esophageal disease. This is due to acid or alkali refluxing onto inflamed esophageal mucosa. Complications of uncontrolled reflux esophagitis are strictures. The mucosa in the injured area may be replaced by columnar epithelium (Barrett's esophagus). Bleeding may also occur but is uncommon. Reflux can occur with or without an associated hiatus hernia. Diagnosis by esophagoscopy with biopsy is considered the most accurate method of determining the presence of esophagitis. In the ED setting, most patients with esophageal reflux are started on nonoperative therapy alone. Treatment is aimed at increasing sphincter tone and diminishing the effects of reflux. Obese patients often get alleviation of symptoms with weight loss. Elevation of the head of the bed and avoidance of tight-fitting garments such as girdles are beneficial. Smoking, alcohol, and caffeine all decrease lower esophageal sphincter tone and increase the incidence of reflux. Anticholinergic agents (metoclopramide) increase lower esophageal sphincter pressure and increase acid clearing from the distal esophagus.

All patients should be referred to a gastroenterologist for follow-up. Heartburn associated with postprandial fullness and occasional vomiting must be looked at closely to make sure there is no paraesophageal diaphragmatic hernia. This can be diagnosed by an upper GI series and requires emergency surgery if incarcerated or obstructed.

Rupture

Pathophysiology of ruptures can be split into anatomic sections of the esophagus. The cervical thoracic area is injured by foreign bodies (eg, laryngoscopes or nasogastric tubes). The midthoracic region is injured by vomiting, as in Boerhaave's syndrome, endoscopy, or biopsy. The abdominal thoracic region is injured by surgery or vomiting, as in Mallory-Weiss syndrome. Perforations can be suspected by history. Anyone who swallows a foreign body that sticks in the esophagus is at risk. Patients who vomit blood or develop chest or abdominal pain after vomiting are suspect. Any unconscious patient with instrumentation should be suspected of having a perforation. Penetrating wounds of the neck or chest or a crushing wound to the chest must be suspected of having a ruptured esophagus. Patients in the ED should have chest radiographic examination for evidence of free air, mediastinal fluid, effusions, or foreign body. If there is evidence of perforation, a water-soluble Gastrograffin study should be done to confirm the diagnosis. Patients who are unconscious after chest trauma may require esophagoscopy management. Survival is inversely proportional to the length of time between perforation and operative repair. Patients with suspected perforation should be given intravenous antibiotics (for adults, 2 g of cefoxitin). The most malignant complication of delay is mediastinitis. In this instance, the fluid from the perforation spreads through the mediastinal tissue, causing a caustic burn to the blood vessels in this region and rapid spread of bacteria. Untreated patients quickly develop shock, septicemia, and death. Although Mallory-Weiss and Boerhaave's syndromes are the most traumatic presentations of esophageal perforation, laceration and perforation have occurred in flexion-hyperextension injuries at the level of the cervical esophagus. Unconscious patients who undergo cardiopulmonary resuscitation and survive should also be suspected of having esophageal perforation, especially if they are instrumented in the prehospital arena.

VARICES

Varices are dilated submucosal veins of the esophagus, usually due to portal hypertension from cirrhosis of the liver. Because of the size and high pressures in the portal system, usually in excess of 180 mmH$_2$O, and because of common coagulopathy in these patients, bleeding from these can be massive and life threatening. These patients present with upper GI bleeding with jaundice, ascites, encephalopathy, and advanced muscle wasting. A history of variceal bleed is no guarantee that a rebleed is from the same cause in these patients. In patients with known varices, endoscopy reveals the source of the upper GI bleed to be from another site in one third of cases. Perform stabilization as outlined above for upper GI bleed. These patients also require a rapid correction of coagulopathies with fresh frozen plasma (2 to 3 mL/kg). Packed red blood cells are preferred over whole blood in these patients because of reduced citrate load and prevention of chelation of calcium with resultant hypocalcemia and seizures. Early manifestations of hypocalcemia will be muscle tremors and a prolonged QT segment, which can be treated immediately with 1 to 10 g of a 10% solution of calcium chloride. Diagnosis of varices is by endoscopic examination. Endoscopic sclerotherapy for varices is 90% successful. There is a 20% mortality. When sclerotherapy is unable to control bleeding esophageal varices, vasopressin can be used. It is a potent vasoconstrictor. It vasoconstricts the prehepatic splenic vessels, resulting in a reduced flow into the portal venous system and a decreased portal venous pressure. As a peripheral venous infusion, start 0.4 U/min and titrate up 0.1 U every 15 minutes until the bleeding ceases. This is followed by a 24-hour infusion of 0.2 U/min and a further 24-hour infusion of 0.1 U/min. The vasopressin causes a significant decrease in coronary blood flow and cardiac output along with bradycardia and hypertension.

Disposition is admission to an intensive care unit and surgical consult for consideration of a shunting procedure. Distal splenorenal shunt appears to be advantageous in that it has a decreased incidence of postoperative encephalopathy. Patients with variceal hemorrhage with easily controllable ascites can be prepared for elective operation. Depending upon patient selection, operative mortality ranges between 10% and 50%.

HICCUPS

Definition

Hiccups are repetitive spasmatic contractions of the diaphragm. If the diaphragm goes into spasm during inhalation, the vocal cords, which stay open to let air through, snap shut, and the characteristic hiccup sound results. The phrenic nerve, which regulates smooth breathing and normally stimulates the diaphragm to contract, often triggers the spasm. The occurrence sometimes has no explanation. Alcohol, gulping food too fast, swallowing cold liquids too quickly, and laughing when the stomach is empty are implicated as causes, as are stress and anxiety. Hiccups seldom last more than a few minutes to a few hours. Intractable hiccups (those lasting longer than 2 days) sometimes signal serious disorders involving the chest, abdomen, or head. Irritation of the phrenic nerve anywhere along its course from the brain to the diaphragm can cause hiccups. Diaphragmatic irritation by an inflamed pancreas can cause hiccups. Diaphragmatic hernias, stomach lesions, brain lesions, and even hardening of the arteries are implicated in the intractable variety of hiccups.

Treatment

There are two methods that have been published in the control of intractable hiccups. Rubbing a cotton swab on the roof of the mouth were the pallet changes from hard to soft can overload the phrenic nerve until it shuts down. The sugar cure calls for swallowing in a sucking fashion a teaspoon of dry granulated white sugar. The granules hitting the back of the throat repeatedly stimulate nerves, interrupting the spasm signals. In one study, this method stopped hiccups in 19 of 20 people, including some who had been hiccupping for several weeks. Hiccups that do not respond to these methods may require antipsychotic medications, including chlorpromazine (25 to 50 mg) or haloperidol. Even anticonvulsants have been used to relieve the muscle spasms. Beyond that, some attempts have been made to anesthetize or surgically crush the phrenic nerve to abolish the repetitive spasms.

LIVER AND BILIARY TRACT DISEASE

Biliary tract disease is thought to affect as many as 15 million people in the United States. Patients often present to the ED with right upper quadrant pain with or without jaundice. Most cases of biliary tract disease are caused by gallstones. Gallstones are found in 20% of women and 8% of men older than 40 years of age, with an incidence of about 1 million new cases of cholecystitis a year. Ten percent of cases of acute cholecystitis occur in the absence of stones (acalculous cholecystitis). Obstruction of the cystic duct by a stone causes ischemia of the gallbladder wall and mucosa with release of bowel components, which attack the mucosa and create an inflammatory response. Bacteria are not present early in the course of the disease but play an important role in most cases that are prolonged. The most common organisms are *Escherichia coli*, group D streptococci, staphylococci, and *Klebsiella* species.

History and Physical Examination

Diagnosis of acute biliary tract disease is often apparent by the history and physical examination. In equivocal cases the physician must use the newer imaging techniques.[1] The differential most commonly includes acute cholecystitis and biliary colic. Additional right upper quadrant pain presentations include pancreatitis, appendicitis (especially in the third trimester of pregnancy), emphysematous cholecystitis, cholangitis, renal stones, pyelonephritis, gonococcal perihepatitis (Fitz-Hugh–Curtis syndrome), liver abscess, and hepatic tumor. More difficult to exclude in the ED are reflux esophagitis, peptic ulcer disease, hepatitis, and diverticulitis. Extra-abdominal causes include right lower lobe pneumonia and cardiac ischemia. Acute cholecystitis is generally a febrile illness with nausea, vomiting, right upper quadrant localized peritoneal irritation, and leukocytosis.

Biliary colic, or transient obstruction of the cystic duct, causes visceral pain without surrounding inflammation. It is generally constant, has a sudden onset, and gradually resolves; it is characterized by maximal pain in the epigastrium and, less commonly, the right upper quadrant.

Acute cholecystitis may be indistinguishable from biliary colic or may induce septic shock. Biliary tract disease with jaundice can sometimes be differentiated by biochemical profiles. Acute viral hepatitis is associated with an enlarged liver, ALT elevated more than the serum glutamic-oxaloacetic acid transaminase (SGOT) level, and a normal alkaline phosphatase level. Alcoholic liver disease closely mimics viral hepatitis, but the SGOT level is usually higher than the ALT level. An elevated alkaline phosphate suggests an obstructive process such as cholecystitis. Chronic active hepatitis produces a picture similar to that of acute hepatitis, often with autoimmune phenomena such as elevated immunoglobulin. Amylase levels greater than 1000 U/dL suggest associated pancreatitis. Charcot's triad (right upper quadrant pain, fever, and jaundice) suggests cholangitis. Reynolds' pentad (Charcot's triad plus shock and mental status changes) suggests suppurative cholangitis or gallbladder perforation, which has a high mortality (30%) and is a true surgical emergency. Perforation is seen more commonly with emphysematous cholecystitis and predominantly affects diabetic men; it has a mortality rate of 10%. The etiology is ischemia resulting in proliferation of anaerobic organisms. Abdominal plain films show gas in the gallbladder. More specific ultrasound findings exist for emphysematous cholecystitis. Surgery and antibiotics with *Clostridium perfringens* coverage must be started immediately.

Diagnostic Imaging

Ultrasonography and gallbladder nuclear scans are the two best tests available to emergency physicians for biliary tract disease. Nuclear scanning involves an intravenous injection and then scanning for approximately 1 hour. It can assess the anatomy of the gallbladder and is the only test for detection of function of the gallbladder. Nonvisualization of the gallbladder with visualization of the liver and common duct is diagnostic of gallbladder disease, acute or chronic. Nuclear scanning is slightly more accurate than ultrasound in diagnosing acute cholecystitis, with 98% sensitivity and specificity greater than 90%. It is more expensive and less readily performed than ultrasound. In patients presenting with right upper quadrant pain who are not jaundiced and do not have an elevated amylase level, many surgeons prefer the hida scan as the first test of choice. In our institution, however, in the ED evaluation of patients with right upper quadrant pain we prefer ultrasound as the first test of choice. Sensitivity is about 90%, and specificity is about 95%. Ultrasound is cheaper and can be performed more readily than nuclear scanning. It identifies most patients with symptomatic stones and proves better at diagnosing other pathology causing right upper quadrant pain. For instance, it can tell whether the pancreatic head is enlarged or, in a young woman on oral contraceptives, whether a ruptured adenoma of the liver or hepatic abscess is present. Ultrasound has less sensitivity for common duct stones but will detect ductal dilation. Ultrasound can give a false sense of security in those patients with intermittent right upper quadrant pain, no jaundice, and no gallstones in the gallbladder. Such patients may still have a common duct stone. Patients with Charcot's triad who present with a suppurative cholangitis often cannot be stabilized for nuclear imaging, and urgent sonograms should be obtained to document the presence or absence of dilated intrahepatic ducts. Medical management alone is associated with nearly 100% mortality in acute suppurative bacterial cholangitis. If the serum bilirubin is greater than 5 mg/dL, suspect common duct stones; if the level is greater than 20 mg/dL, suspect a neoplastic etiology. The differential for fever and right upper quadrant pain with jaundice also includes sclerosing cholangitis, hepatobiliary parasites, and neoplasms, which are difficult to diagnose in the ED.

Emergency Department Management of Acute Biliary Tract Disease

Patients with biliary colic with pain, nausea, and vomiting should receive fluids for hydration and antiemetics and may be discharged from the ED. Follow-up should include outpatient ultrasound and instructions to return if fever, jaundice, increased pain, or vomiting occurs. Elective cholecystectomy is recommended for patients with symptomatic gallstones or calcified gallbladder. The literature is controversial in the management of diabetics with asymptomatic gallstones.

Acute cholecystitis requires hospitalization and surgical consultation. Surgical timing often depends on the surgeon's preference, with hydration, nothing by mouth, and antibiotics often preparing the patient better for surgery. Blood cultures should be obtained in the ED, and antibiotics may be begun. Cefotetan has achieved popularity, providing excellent coverage and being economical and convenient, with dosing at 1 g every 12 hours. Patients with suspected cholangitis and sepsis have traditionally been covered with ampicillin, gentamicin, and metronidazole or clindamycin. The newest drug of choice for this condition is mezlocillin. The serum concentration and therapeutic index, especially bile concentration, of mezlocillin are much higher than those of either ampicillin or gentamicin. Biliary concentration of mezlocillin is 112 times higher than that of ampicillin and 778 times higher than that of gentamicin. In clinical trials 83% of patients treated with mezlocillin were cured compared to 41% of patients treated with ampicillin and gentamicin. Mezlocillin therapy was more effective, less toxic, and less expensive than therapy with ampicillin and gentamicin in patients with cholangitis. Patients presenting from Third World countries, where gallstone disease is unusual, have a wide range of alternative diagnoses, most of which are unusual helminthic diseases. Acute obstruction similar to that in classic biliary colic can occur from *Ascaris* species, *Trichuris* species, and liver flukes, in which worms migrate through the biliary tract via the ampulla of Vater. Conservative management with anthelminthic agents is successful in most cases. Patients infected with the human immunodeficiency virus are more likely to have an acalculous cholecystitis, with etiologies including cytomegalovirus, *Cryptosporidium* infection, and an even higher incidence of sclerosing cholangitis and papillary stenosis. The last two conditions often have resolution of abdominal pain with sphincterotomy.

PANCREAS DISEASE

Pancreatitis is an inflammatory process of the pancreas manifesting as either an acute event or an exacerbation of chronic disease. There are 1.5 cases per 100,000 population in the United States, with an increased frequency occurring at inner city hospitals as a result of increased alcohol abuse in these areas. Biliary tract disease, gallstones, and trauma are the other leading causes of pancreatitis. Alcohol abuse and biliary tract disease account for 90% of cases of acute pancreatitis. Mechanisms involved include precipitation of protein plugs blocking pancreatic ducts, increased sphincter resistance, bowel enzyme release, autodigestion with formation of edema, liquefactive coagulation necrosis, fat necrosis, vascular injury, and hemorrhage.

Estrogens and azathioprine commonly cause pancreatitis. Three percent of cases occur after renal transplant and hyperparathyroidism. Postoperative pancreatitis with surgery on or near the pancreas has a 40% mortality. Parapancreatic edema is prominent in all types of acute pancreatitis. This edema is caused by a protein-rich exudate that escapes into the mesentery, abdominal cavity, and other areas. Additional fluid is found in the stagnant loops of the small bowel. For these reasons, patients on admission often have hemoconcentration with high hematocrit values. This is why these patients tolerate infusion of considerable amounts of colloids and crystalloids without an appreciable increase in their central venous pressure.

Clinical Features

Attacks of pancreatitis often occur after a heavy meal or an episode of acute alcoholism. Acute alcoholic pancreatitis is often seen in male patients 25 to 65 years of age who have been drinking rather heavily for 5 to 10 years. The manifestations vary from vague dyspepsia or slight abdominal pain to an irreversible fulminating collapse with shock and death. The outstanding symptom is steady, severe pain, frequently radiating to the back. It may be intermittent or cramplike. Its location is the midepigastrium; pain in the left or upper right quadrant is not uncommon. Pain is often improved by sitting and aggravated by lying. Persistent vomiting with or without nausea is often present on physical examination. Fever, leukocytosis, and tachycardia are seen in about 90% of cases. Shock occurs from the loss of fluid in the peritoneum and retroperitoneum as well as fluid loss from repeated vomiting. Abdominal tenderness with guarding and distension is usually present. Jaundice may be present in 20% to 30% of cases. Acute renal failure may be present, and carpopedal spasms due to hypocalcemia may be seen. The abdomen is often hypoactive or silent secondary to adynamic ileus.

Diagnosis

Laboratory analysis provides useful but limited information. Serum amylase is the most widely used test but has well-described limitations, not being sensitive enough or specific enough to be the gold standard in diagnosing acute pancreatitis. Ten percent of patients with acute pancreatitis have normal amylase values. Patients with chronic pancreatitis, who present late in the course of an acute episode, or who have hyperlipidemia may have normal amylase levels. There is no correlation between the severity of illness and the degree of serum amylase elevation. The highest values are seen in women with biliary tract disease accompanied by acute pancreatitis. In a series of 154 patients, when the serum amylase was higher than 1000 somogye units there was usually a surgically correctable lesion (usually stones in the biliary tract). When amylase was 200 to 500 somogye units, most patients had idiopathic or alcoholic pancreatitis. In acute pancreatitis amylase rises within 6 to 24 hours, remains high for only a few days, and then returns to normal in 2 to 7 days. The pancreas is virtually the only source of serum lipase, which is secreted into the lumen of the digestive tract. Elevated serum lipase is more specific for pancreatic disease than elevated serum amylase. Serum lipase levels rise with pancreatic inflammation and remain higher longer than amylase levels; they cannot be picked up in the urine.

Table 28-1 Ranson's Criteria for Predicting Severity of Acute Pancreatitis

At admission or on diagnosis:
  Age > 55 years
  Leukocyte count > 16/dL
  Serum glucose > 200 mg/dL
  Serum lactic dehydrogenase > 350 mg/dL
  Serum aspartate aminotransferase > 250 IU/dL

During initial 48 hours:
  Fall in hematocrit > 10%
  BUN rise > 5 mg/dL
  Serum calcium < 8 mg/dL
  Base deficit > 4 mEq/L
  Estimated fluid sequestration > 6 L
  Arterial oxygen tension < 60 mmHg

The goal of ED diagnosis of pancreatitis is to identify patients with serious hemorrhagic pancreatitis and abdominal pain requiring immediate surgery from patients with mild pancreatitis. The criteria suggested by Ranson (Table 28-1) help differentiate severity because clinical criteria alone are inaccurate. Gallstone-induced pancreatitis has slightly different criteria, also suggested by Ranson (Table 28-2). Prognostic signs described by Ranson correlate with increased morbidity and mortality. In a study of 450 patients with acute pancreatitis, those with fewer than three signs had a mortality of 0.9% and morbidity (ie, intensive care monitoring for longer than 1 week) of 2.9%. Those with three to four signs had 16% mortality and 24% morbidity. Patients with five to six signs had 40% mortality and 53% morbidity. Patients with more than six signs had 100% mortality. This classification scheme is far from perfect: Some patients with four to five signs did well and did not require aggressive management. The sensitivity is great in identifying groups of patients at risk. The presence of three or more signs is an indicator of serious disease (sensitivity, 96%).

ED laboratory work should include CBC, BUN, glucose, SGOT, calcium, and lactic dehydrogenase. Abdominal films (flat plate and upright) are often ordered to rule out free air. The KUB may show a sentinel loop (single dilated loop with small bowel in the left upper quadrant). The valvulae are concentric, and the wall of the bowel appears thickened. Colon cut-off sign can be seen (dilatation of the transverse colon with possibility of gas beyond the splenic flexure). The chest radiograph may show diaphragm elevation on the left with a small pleural effusion.

Management

Severe acute pancreatitis with more than three of Ranson's signs requires admission to an intensive care unit. If ileus and abdominal distension is present, a nasogastric tube should be placed and fluid resuscitation performed. A central venous line should be placed if more than 2 L of fluid are needed to maintain a blood pressure greater than 100 mmHg. A Foley catheter should be placed for urine output. Hematocrit, electrolytes, and glucose should be monitored every 4 hours. Patients with mild to acute pancreatitis with fewer than three of Ranson's criteria require intravenous hydration, pain relief with meperidine hydrochloride, and antiemetics such as prochloroperazine (25 mg suppository). After observation in the ED, if the patient is able to take clear fluids by mouth he or she can be discharged to home with oral pain medications for 24 to 48 hours along with rectal suppositories for 24 to 48 hours (prochloroperazine, 25 mg or promethazine, 25 mg every 4 to 6 hours by mouth). Patients should have outpatient follow-up within 24 to 48 hours. Chronic pancreatitis is often managed on an outpatient basis with similar treatment in the ED as for mild acute pancreatitis. Indications for surgery for inpatients include (1) presence of an upper abdominal mass suspected of being a pseudocyst, (2) obstruction of the duodenum or biliary tree, and (3) intra-abdominal leakage. Development of pancreatic abscess with high white blood cell count, fever, and intra-abdominal sepsis requires surgical drainage. If gallstones are found, it is generally safe to remove the gallbladder if the pancreatitis is mild. Cholecystotomy is performed in more severe pancreatic disease with the presence of gallstones.

LIVER DISEASE

Jaundice

Jaundice is a clinical condition in which there is the appearance of yellow bilirubin pigment in skin, sclerae, and mucosal membranes. The condition must be differentiated from carotenemia, which is caused by the accumulation of carotenoid pigments in the skin but not the sclerae. There are few life-threatening processes that require immediate treatment in patients complaining of jaundice.

There are five general mechanisms whereby clinical jaundice may become apparent: (1) increased bilirubin production, (2) decreased hepatic uptake within the liver cell, (3) impaired hepatic conjugation, (4) decreased excretion

Table 28-2 Risk of Death or Major Morbidity: Ranson's Criteria of Severity in Acute Pancreatitis

Criteria number	0–2	3–4	5–6	7–8
Patient number	347	67	30	6
Mortality (%)		1	16	40	100
Patients in intensive care longer than 7 days (%)		3	24	53	

Source: Data from JA Ranson, *Gastroenterology Clinics* (1984;13: 843–863), WB Saunders Company.

into the bile, or (5) obstruction of the bile channels before bilirubin enters the lumen of the intestine. In the first three processes the bilirubin is primarily in unconjugated form, and the conjugated (direct) bilirubin dominates.

Clinical Presentation

Jaundice is usually detected when the sclerae, mucous membranes, skin, or urine turn abnormally yellow as a result of an increased serum concentration of bilirubin (greater than 3 mg/dL). Certain clinical or biochemical features suggest the presence of cholestasis. These include pruritus, dark urine (indicates conjugated hyperbilirubin anemia), and clay-colored stool. Abnormal liver function tests (increased serum transaminase and alkaline phosphatase levels) confirm cholestasis. Determination of direct and indirect reacting bilirubin fractions is of limited diagnostic value. Fever, chills, abdominal pain, or previous biliary tract surgery suggests extrahepatic biliary obstruction. If cholestasis is present, rapid identification of the patient with extrahepatic biliary obstruction is imperative because prompt biliary decompression is required. Even when intrahepatic cholestasis is suspected, noninvasive imaging of the biliary tract is indicated. The abdominal examination may reveal dilated veins consistent with portal hypertension or ascites. A large liver (cancer), normal size liver, or small liver (hepatitis, cirrhosis, or extrahepatic cholestasis) may be seen. Congestive heart failure with an enlarged tender liver, jugular venous distension, rales, and a third heart sound may provide a clue to the jaundice. Examination of serum, urine, and feces often provides confirmatory diagnostic information. A dipstick test of the urine, if positive, may indicate conjugated hyperbilirubinemia. The absence of bile in the urine suggests unconjugated hyperbilirubinemia (ie, impaired hepatic clearance or acquired disorders). The absence of urobilinogen in the urine suggests total bowel obstruction. A rectal examination should be performed in all patients with jaundice. Acholic stools suggest biliary obstruction, and blood implies bleeding from a carcinoma or mucosal lesion in the GI tract. The liver function tests, urine, CBC, and examination of peripheral blood smear should suggest hemolysis, ineffective erythropoiesis (eg, folate or vitamin B_{12} deficiency), or a selective defect in bilirubin transport (eg, Gilbert's syndrome causing unconjugated hyperbilirubinemia or Dubin-Johnson syndrome causing conjugated hyperbilirubinemia). If hepatic obstruction is suspected, ultrasound is the preferred noninvasive imaging technique and is cheaper, exposing the patient to less radiation than computed tomography (CT). Both tests demonstrate duct dilatation in 85% of patients with jaundice due to biliary obstruction. CT is generally more reliable in identifying the level of obstruction. Neither test is reliable in detecting common duct stones, however. In certain situations (eg, recurrent jaundice in a patient who has had a cholecystectomy), it may be appropriate to bypass noninvasive biliary imaging and proceed to direct ductal visualization. False-negative results occur in patients with cirrhosis, sclerosing cholangitis, or choledocholithiasis. If any of these conditions is suspected, or if the index of suspicion for obstruction remains high, obtain direct ductal visualization.

Hepatitis

Viral hepatitis is most commonly caused by hepatitis A virus (HAV) and hepatitis B virus (HBV). Twenty-five percent of sporadic hepatitis and 90% of posttransfusion hepatitis are not related to either HAV or HBV and must be attributed to non-A, non-B hepatitis. Infectious organisms causing infectious hepatitis include Epstein-Barr virus, cytomegalovirus, toxoplasmosis, herpes simplex, leptospira, and yellow fever virus. Etiology of the hepatitis can be gained from a history and physical examination. The most common etiology is viral. A history of travel to a developing country would favor HAV, blood transfusion non-A, non-B, (less likely type B), intravenous drug abuse; B, non-A, non-B, or delta, homosexuality (all types), and work in a daycare center type A. Spiderangiomas, pulmonary edema, gynecomastia, and testicular atrophy are clues to chronic liver disease.

Delta infection occurs exclusively in people are are also infected with HBV; it presents as either an acute, often severe superimposed hepatitis or chronic hepatitis B. It is an acute, often fulminant, hepatitis that represents simultaneous infection with HBV and the delta agent.

Acute alcoholic hepatitis is usually accompanied by jaundice, fever, tender hepatomegaly, leukocytosis, and a serum AST activity less than 300 IU/L but greater than the serum ALT activity. Liver biopsy may be needed to distinguish alcoholic hepatitis from other forms of liver disease. Drugs that are known to produce hepatic injury include halothane, haldomet, isoniazid, diphenylhydantoin, phenothiazines, and acetaminophen.

Non-A, non-B hepatitis, a diagnosis of exclusion, may be caused by the non-A, non-B virus and occasionally by Epstein-Barr virus or cytomegalovirus. Non-A, non-B accounts for most cases of posttransfusion hepatitis and commonly results in chronic liver disease. Uncommonly syphilis, brucellosis, Q fever, Wilson's disease, and *Amanita phalloides* poisoning result in chronic illness. Hepatitis is usually suspected when a patient presents with jaundice or when increased serum transaminase activity (greater than 5 to 10 times normal) is found. If suspected, obtain a CBC with differential, liver function tests, PT and PTT, serum electrolytes, glucose, hepatitis B surface antigen (HBsAg), heterophile antibody, and anti-HAV immunoglobulin M (IgM). SGOT and serum glutamic-pyruvic transaminase increase during the prodrome period and return to normal after jaundice appears. Conjugated hyperbilirubinemia predominates during the icteric stage, and bilirubin levels may be high if there is renal disease or hemolysis. Alkaline phosphate is elevated, but albumin is normal. Leukopenia with atypical lymphocytes may be seen during the prodrome. Clotting abnormalities with prolonged PT (ie, greater than 2 seconds over control) occur in severe disease and are a poor prognostic indicator.

The presence of anti-HAV IgM confirms HAV infection within the preceding 4 weeks. Anti-HAV IgG implies that infection occurred more than 4 weeks before testing. Most common in diagnosing HBV is the surface antigen, HBsAg, which appears in the blood 4 to 6 weeks after exposure and 1 week to 2 months before elevation of transaminase. HBsAg usually disappears 1 to 13 weeks after onset of clinical disease, but if it persists beyond 6 months it defines chronic hepatitis. Antibody against HBsAg (anti-HBs) is protective, lasts indefinitely, and implies recovery from infection in absence of infectivity. It does not appear until clinical hepatitis resolves and cannot be measured until several weeks after the disappearance of HBsAg. This serologic gap occurs when both HBsAg and anti-HBs are absent from the blood. This gap is filled by core antibody (anti-HBc), which is not protective. If all three (HBsAg, anti-HBc, and anti-HBs) are negative, it can be concluded that the patient does not have hepatitis B.

There is no specific therapy for acute viral hepatitis. An attempt to find the etiology should be made because potential hepatotoxins must be removed. Hydrate those patients with severe vomiting. Prophylaxis should be given to those who have infections caused by HAV and HBV.

Patients with anti-HBs have immunity to hepatitis B and do not require prophylaxis after exposure, nor do they require active immunization. Ig is not infective if there is clinical onset of the disease or if it has been greater than 2 weeks since exposure. Because alcoholic hepatitis is directly related to the amount of alcohol consumed, patients who do not stop drinking will progress to cirrhosis 50% of the time. Household contacts and health care personnel attending a patient with HAV only require handwashing and stool precautions and IG prophylaxis. In pediatric patients give 0.02 mL/kg of Ig intramuscularly to all household contacts. Daycare centers require that this dose be given to all children, staff members, and household contacts of non–toilet trained children attending the center. When there is a clear exposure, either percutaneous or mucous membrane contact to blood that is positive for HBsAg, the treatment of choice is both hepatitis B Ig and hepatitis B vaccine; give as soon as possible after exposure but at different sites. The vaccine dose should be repeated at 1 month and 6 months. Patients exposed to high-risk sources with unknown HBsAg status should be vaccinated once, and blood should be sent from the source for HBsAg testing. If that test is positive, give one dose of Ig and then complete the vaccine series at 1 month and 6 months. If the test is negative, complete the vaccination series, but hepatitis B Ig is not necessary. In laboratories that require more than 7 days to run blood for HBsAg, it is best to give the exposed person a dose of Ig pending the result. Nonsexual contacts with HBV infection do not require prophylaxis unless there has been blood exposure or sharing of razors and toothbrushes. Treat this as sexual exposure with one dose of hepatitis B Ig. If, however, the person with HBV infection becomes a chronic carrier, vaccinate all household contacts.

Acute Liver Failure

Acute hepatic failure is uncommon and is due to severe impairment of hepatocytes. Viral infections, inborn errors of metabolism, and glactosemia are the most common etiologies. During childhood and adolescence the etiology is often infectious, toxic, or metabolic, as in Reye's syndrome.

Clinical Presentation

Bleeding manifestations may be present (ecchymosis, prolonged bleeding at the venipuncture site, hematuria, and melena). Progressive neurologic deterioration ensues and is classified in four stages. In stage 1, mild confusion, sleep disorder, and hyperventilation are noted. This is followed by stage 2: irritability, confusion, and inappropriate behavior. Stage 3 is hyperreflexia, liver flap, and electroencephalographic slowing with obtundation. The patient can be aroused. Stage 4 is deep coma, areflexia, seizures, decorticate rigidity, and apnea.

Diagnosis

Look for liver transaminase greater than 3000 U/L, hypoglycemia, prolonged PT, elevated blood ammonia, and hyperbilirubinemia (except in Reye's syndrome). On physical examination, look for jaundice, icteric sclerae, papilledema, hepatomegaly, and right upper quadrant tenderness. Perform a thorough neurologic examination, including assessment of level of consciousness and orientation, pupillary response, extraocular movements, motor response, and reflexes.

Management

Patients require admission to the intensive care unit after intravenous 10% dextrose is started at a maintenance rate. Patients may need fresh frozen plasma (5 mL/kg) intravenously and vitamin K if there are any clotting abnormalities or evidence of bleeding. Blood work with CBC, electrolytes, glucose, BUN, creatinine, SGOT, SGPT, lactic dehydrogenase, alkaline phosphatase, bilirubin, PT, and ammonia is necessary. Once in intensive care, patients should be given enemas and oral neomycin/lactulose to decrease bowel flora and ammonia production. For patients with ascites, paracentesis is a diagnostic procedure needed only if there is evidence of bacterial peritonitis. Transfusion and furosemide may both worsen the encephalitis, increasing the protein on one hand and decreasing the potassium on the other. Increased blood pressure can be associated with encephalopathy that will mimic hepatic encephalopathy, but one does not cause the other. Conditions worsening encephalopathy, if present, include gastrointestinal bleeding, bacterial peritonitis, phenothiazines, and hypokalemia. Those patients with Reye's syndrome may require management for increased intracranial pressure. All patients with hepatic failure, hepatic encephalopathy, and Reye's syndrome should be admitted.

SPLENIC RUPTURE AND INFARCT

Spontaneous, nontraumatic splenic rupture rarely occurs even in classic infectious mononucleosis. In the setting of mononucleosis splenic rupture will occur during the second and third weeks of illness, or patients will complain of left upper quadrant pain and tenderness accompanied by peritoneal irritation and a falling hematocrit. It is also seen in leukemia, lymphoma, amyloidosis, collagen vascular diseases, malaria, and the second half of pregnancy. If the patient is stable, CT scan is preferred to estimate the amount of blood loss to try to preserve the spleen. Splenic thrombosis is more common in patients with sickle cell anemia, in whom splenic infarction usually occurs during childhood. Some myeloproferative disorders and other hematologic disorders can be complicated by vascular thrombosis or functional ischemia. Laboratory studies show anemia and leukocytosis in 50% of the cases. Immediate treatment for symptomatic patients with splenic infarction is bedrest, hydration, and analgesics. Symptoms usually resolve in 7 to 14 days.

ASCITES

Ascites is the accumulation of peritoneal fluid with abdominal distension. Left unchecked, ascites has a high rate of infection; allows high portal hypertension to develop; and decreases renal blood flow, cardiac output, and ventilation. The most common etiology is cirrhosis secondary to alcohol abuse or chronic hepatitis. Initial therapy is bedrest and salt restriction (generally less than 2 g/day). Water restriction is totally unnecessary because ascites is due to the retention of salt, not water. Medications that inhibit prostaglandin synthesis, such as nonsteroidal anti-inflammatory drugs, should be stopped. Patients with low serum sodium levels suggesting high water intake are the only patients who require some water restriction. If these measures are ineffective alone, a diuretic should be given. The newest choice with increased favor among hepatologists is Amiloride, which has a faster onset of action than spironolactone (1 hour compared to 4 days) and is less expensive. It has fewer side effects, such as impotence and painful gynecomastia. This is begun at 10 mg every morning. If no weight reduction occurs, within 24 hours the dose can be increased to 30 to 40 mg/day. If this does not result in adequate diuresis, furosemide (initial dose, 40 mg/day) should be added to the regiment.

When diuretic therapy is unsuccessful, large-volume paracentesis or the creation of a peritovenous shunt is necessary. ED studies have shown that up to a 5-L paracentesis does not cause any change in plasma volume or renal function regardless of whether a patient has peripheral edema. For ED patients with evidence of respiratory distress, renal failure, or diminished cardiac output, paracentesis is a first-line treatment. If there is bowel obstruction or severe coagulopathy, however, this procedure is contraindicated. Patients can have up to 5 L of ascitic fluid removed and should be admitted to the hospital to be monitored for possible hypotension afterward. Clinical manifestations are spontaneous bacterial peritonitis, fever, leukocytosis, and abdominal tenderness; these only appear in 60% of patients. Expect spontaneous peritonitis any time the condition of an ascites patient deteriorates. If more than 250 neutrophils per cubic millimeter are recovered in a small diagnostic tap, antibiotics should be started. The antibiotic most extensively used for that purpose is cefotaxime. It covers the three most common organisms (*Escherichia coli*, *Klebsiella* species, and *Streptococcus pneumoniae*). It is effective with high ascitic fluid levels and is not associated with renal toxicity.

SMALL BOWEL AND COLON DISORDERS

Intestinal Obstruction

Of all patients with abdominal pain, 2.5% have obstruction. Twenty-five percent of patients with abdominal pain of unknown etiology are obstructed; this accounts for 20% of all surgical emergencies. There are 10,000 deaths annually due to intestinal obstruction. There are differences in small and large bowel intestinal obstructions.

The most common causes of small bowel obstruction in the United States are postoperative or posttraumatic adhesions and hernias. In simple mechanical small bowel obstruction, distension of the lumen is a consequence of either gas or fluid accumulation proximal to the anatomic site of the obstruction. Obstruction progresses, intraluminal secretions increase, and there is a shift of intravascular water with resultant fluid electrolyte abnormalities, which are especially worsened by vomiting. Intraluminal pressure decreases in the intravascular supply, causing strangulation, bacterial invasion, and possible gangrene perforation and peritonitis.

Unlike mechanical obstruction, paralytic ileus is intestinal obstruction due to neuromuscular disturbances that cause paralysis and interruption of intestinal motility. Frequently seen after surgery, it manifests with peritonitis, hypokalemia, intestinal ischemia, burns, ureteral calculus, pancreatitis, vertebral or rib fractures, or gastroenteritis. Volume loss can be 9 L in 24 hours.

Presentation

The triad of vomiting, intermittent abdominal pain, and prior surgery or trauma is diagnostic of obstruction until proven otherwise. The pain is colicky and severe and occasionally radiates to the back. Vomiting will occur early with high obstruction and will be copious and light green in color. Low obstruction has delayed vomiting for 24 to 48 hours after pain onset; the vomitus is usually dark green and feculant as a result of bacterial overgrowth. The vomiting is nonprojectile. Bowel sounds are high pitched early and disappear later. They may be normal with very high obstructions. Stool and gas may be passed after complete obstruction. Distension may not be prominent early with high obstruction. Laboratory studies show the white count to be increased in 50% to 60% of cases with strangulation. Studies often reflect hypovolemia and, with vomiting, hypokalemia and hypochloremic alkalosis. Radiographs can show dilated loops of small bowel with air-fluid levels. Five percent of adults show no gas. Significant small bowel gas is uncommon in the adult. Forty percent of patients with obstruction have rectal gas, whereas 50% of normal patients show no rectal gas.

Severely ill patients should have a lateral decubitus view taken. Colon gas differs from small intestine gas in that it is more peripheral and does not transverse the entire colon diameter. If no air is seen in the intestine, look for a sausage-shaped mass and obtain radiographs after nasogastric tube placement. In strangulation obstruction the closed loop rapidly fills up with fluid, giving a normal appearance before any evidence of bowel dilatation occurs. A distended colon and small bowel gas may represent an obstructed colon with an incompetent ileocecal valve. Supine films can be helpful in up to 65% of patients; always look for ectopic gallstones, air in the biliary tree, and free air. Reliance on predetermined criteria for bowel obstruction indicating nonviability of intestine has proven quite misleading. In one series of patients with strangulation obstruction, 70% of the patients had no fever and 42% had no leukocytosis or tachycardia, and radiographs indicated a strangulation obstruction in only 10%.

Management

Any patient with an abdominal scar or an incarcerated external hernia who presents with any signs and symptoms of bowel obstruction should be rapidly volume repleted and treated with nasogastric suction. If any sign of nonviable intestine is present, such as local tenderness, fever, tachycardia, or elevated white blood cell count (greater than 18,000/mm^3), surgical consult should be obtained for prompt operation. If none of these signs is present the patient may have simple obstruction; continued nonoperative management may be successful. In one series of 238 patients it was noted that no patient had dead bowel if all these signs were absent.[19] If one sign was present, some patients had dead bowel; if more than one sign was present, chances were increased. Surgical intervention should be expedient except in cases of partial bowel obstruction, radiation enteritis, postoperative ileus, metastatic malignancy, and selected cases of multiple recurrent adhesive obstruction. All patients should have fluid replacement with lactated Ringer solution and be typed and cross-matched. Potassium should be corrected, and the patient should receive nothing by mouth. A nasogastric tube should be applied and antibiotics begun if strangulation is suspected.

Large Bowel Obstruction

Obstruction of the colon is due to carcinoma, volvulus, and sigmoid diverticulitis in 90% of cases. Obstruction pain is initially crampy or colicky with frequent exacerbations at up to 10-minute intervals coinciding with high-pitched rushes. The pain usually localizes in the lower abdomen for large bowel obstruction. The pain is less intense than that in ischemia, and vomiting is absent or delayed. Later the pain is more constant and diffuse with decreased or absent bowel sounds because abdominal distension usually becomes quite obvious. Without an incompetent ileocecal valve, the risk of distention with perforation is the most significant problem. The cecum is at greatest risk of perforation if a diameter of 8 to 10 cm is present on radiographs. Peritoneal signs are present with perforation. Strangulation is less common and is present in volvulus.

Large bowel volvulus makes up 5% of intestinal obstructions and involves the cecum, transverse colon, and sigmoid. Eighty percent of cases are sigmoid, 20% are cecum, and less than 5% are transverse colon. This is due to rotation of a freely movable segment of bowel about its point of fixation to the mesentery axis. Sigmoid volvulus occurs most often in inactive elderly patients with laxative abuse and medications that exacerbate bowel dysfunction such as psychotropics and narcotics. They usually present late in the course after 1 to 2 days of anorexia, nausea, vomiting, pain, and distension.

Cecal volvulus occurs at any age but is most common in the 25- to 35-year age group without a history of constipation. Presentation is similar to that in mechanical small bowel obstruction. The patient is usually dehydrated and has a tender, diffuse abdominal examination with distension, tympany, and no bowel sounds. The rectum is usually empty.

Plain films are diagnostic in 60% of cases. Sigmoid volvulus shows a dilated single loop of colon bent back on itself in the left half of the abdomen with both ends pointing down to the pelvis. Sigmoid volvulus tends to be vertically oriented on its long axis, whereas cecal volvulus is horizontally oriented. In adynamic ileus, the colon is distended with loss of haustral pattern. The right colon becomes larger than the left. Elderly or mentally deranged patients may have chronic large bowel dilatation. Generalized colonic dilatation in colitis patients can indicate toxic megacolon. Usually the patient presents with extreme illness. Barium enema is usually not necessary for diagnosis of sigmoid volvulus but will reveal the bird's-beak sign. Sigmoid volvulus usually has a double air-fluid level, whereas in cecal volvulus a single air-fluid level is the rule.

The patient should be fluid resuscitated with lactated Ringer solution, and potassium should be corrected. Nasogastric tubes will not relieve large bowel obstruction. Allow the patient nothing by mouth, and begin antibiotics with cefoxitin (1 g) or clindamycin-gentamicin if strangulation is suspected or if pneumoperitoneum is seen on plain films. A high risk of perforation is present when the cecal diameter is greater than 10 cm. Immediate surgical consult is indicated for laparotomy in most instances. Surgeons may be able to decompress and detorse the sigmoid volvulus during sigmoidoscopy by inserting a rectal tube with the resultant passage of a large amount of gas and stool. The success rate is 90% in some series. Barium enemas may reduce the obstruction if rectal tube insertion fails. Because of the high recurrence rate of sigmoid volvulus, elective surgery is often required after successful reduction.

All cecal volvuli should undergo immediate operative repair. Delayed diagnosis results in high morbidity and mortality from mesenteric ischemia. These patients often have no peritoneal findings, nonspecific laboratory studies, and normal radiographs, all of which contribute to the delay of invasive diagnostic tests such as angiography. The superior mesenteric artery lies from the ligament of Treitz to the midtransverse colon. The inferior mesenteric artery supplies the distal colon. The rectum has a large collateral blood supply and seldom infarcts. Older patients with atherosclerosis usually have vascular insufficiency involving the superior mesenteric artery. Aortic dissection, hypercoagulable states, vasculitis, and vascular surgery may result in mesenteric infarct. Mitral stenosis, atrial fibrillation, or ventricular thrombosis from a recent myocardial infarction may be an embolic source to the superior mesenteric artery in younger patients. Of the low-flow states, including shock and anoxia, severe congestive heart failure can cause nonocclusive intestinal infarction. Mesenteric venous thrombosis is most likely to occur in patients with malignancies, sepsis, trauma, renal transplant, or hypercoagulable states.

There is no noninvasive test that is of any use in identifying patients with decreased blood flow to the intestine or in predicting who is at risk for infarction. Initial symptoms of mesenteric ischemia include usually severe but poorly localized midabdominal pain. This is the classic finding of pain out of proportion to symptoms. Patients may have weight loss during the preceding weeks with a history of postprandial abdominal pain. Occult fecal blood is present in the majority of patients; abdominal bruits may be audible.

Peritoneal signs usually are a late finding and suggest a poor prognosis.

Obtain an acute abdominal series to rule out pneumoperitoneum and to exclude intestinal obstruction. Although insensitive signs, thumbprinting of the bowel wall (indicating intramural hematoma formation), separation of bowel loops due to edema, and streaks of gas in the thickened bowel wall or portal vein suggest mesenteric infarction. Abdominal CT achieved 85% sensitivity for bowel infarction in one study. Angiography can often localize the site of mesenteric insufficiency and its etiology. The first flush of the aorta will reveal aneurysm, dissection, or major artery occlusion. Selective superior mesenteric artery injection visualizes the entire intestinal vascular and collateral circulation. The mortality rate for bowel infarction is 70%. Younger patients with embolization in mesenteric venous thrombosis have a better prognosis. Prompt surgical consultation with an exploratory laparotomy is necessary for inspection of bowel and resection of dead bowel.

NONINFECTIOUS INFLAMMATORY BOWEL DISEASE

In the ED setting patients with inflammatory bowel disease may have acute exacerbation of chronic processes such as Crohn's disease and ulcerative proctitis/colitis.

Crohn's Disease

Crohn's disease, a regional enteritis, is an inflammatory disease of the GI tract that is chronic and of uncertain etiology. The disease may involve any part of the GI tract from the mouth to the rectum. The process occurs in young adults and also in those older than 60 years of age. The pathognomonic feature of Crohn's disease is that the inflammatory process extends through all layers of the bowel wall, and there are areas of abnormal mucosa adjacent to areas of normal mucosa.

Clinical Features

Diarrhea, often with urgency, and abdominal pain are the complaints in three fourths of patients. In approximately half, fever is present along with rectal complications such as fistula and abscess. These latter manifestations may be the first clinical clues. Other presenting clinical characteristics include hematochezia, intestinal obstructions, fissures and fistulas, and systemic manifestations including arthralgia, uveitis, liver disease, and skin or oral involvement.

The pain is described as intermittent and often is localized in the right lower quadrant. Increased bowel motility initiated by the eating of food may aggravate the symptoms. The pain may be constant and is often associated with a palpable abdominal mass, which may reflect the presence of thickened bowel, abscess, or fistula. Intestinal obstruction should be considered with associated complaints of nausea and vomiting.

Diarrhea frequently occurs, and the stools are unformed and frequent. Watery diarrhea suggests the presence of partial bowel obstruction (blind loop syndrome), in which an overgrowth of bacteria may lead to diarrhea, steatorrhea, weight loss, anemia, hypoproteinemia, and fat-soluble vitamin deficiencies. Half the patients with Crohn's disease have colon involvement and may have ulcerations of the anus and/or bleeding. The most common lesion is the fissure, which is broad, shallow, and painless.

An emergent complication of Crohn's disease is small bowel obstruction, which may require surgery. Obstruction is often partial and the clinical onset slow, although sudden, complete obstruction can occur, and perforation, although rare, should be considered with the findings of peritonitis. Bleeding, if present, is usually mild and is a cause of accompanying anemia. When the disease is associated with the signs and symptoms of hypovolemia, immediate fluid resuscitation is required.

Patients with Crohn's disease may develop toxic megacolon. This complication may also occur in severe cases of ischemic, ulcerative, amebic, and granulomatous colitis and in *Salmonella* infection. Diagnosis of this life-threatening process, which has a mortality of up to 30%, should be considered. In instances of acute dilatation of all or part of the colon to a diameter greater than 6 cm in association with systemic toxicity, the patient has fever, tachycardia, and profuse diarrhea and may have marked dehydration with severe electrolyte abnormalities. The wall of the colon may show gas and shaggy luminal margins.

Diagnosis

Diagnosis of Crohn's disease is one of exclusion. In patients with fever, acute diarrhea, abdominal pain, and stool that contains mucus, blood, and pus, infectious causes such as *Salmonella, Shigella,* and *Campylobacter* organisms must be excluded. Tuberculosis, lipoma, and ischemic colitis also mimic Crohn's disease.

A peripheral leukocytosis and black positive stools in association with anemia are common. Nonspecific increases in serum alkaline phosphatase levels and other liver enzymes may be observed. Sigmoidoscopic examination of the rectosigmoid may be normal in half the patients, but in others there is the characteristic finding of distinct ulcerations (cobblestone appearance of patches of seemingly normal mucosa). Rectal biopsy may be required for definitive diagnosis.

A plain upright abdominal radiograph may reveal nonspecific dilated loops of bowel, obstruction, or abscess. A contrast barium enema may demonstrate the clinical characteristics of strictures of the lumen, fistula tract, mucosal nodularity, ulceration, skip lesions, eccentric involvement, and a cobblestone or even a normal appearance.

Treatment

A life-threatening emergency may be present in patients with Crohn's disease if bowel obstruction, toxic megacolon, or sepsis is present. A nasogastric tube, intravenous lactated Ringer solution, and correction of electrolyte abnormalities should be instituted. Simple nasogastric suction may clear the bowel and reduce the edema and spasm. Hemoglobin check with correction of blood loss may be necessary. Consult a surgeon if obstruction, megacolon, or abscess is present. Admission for sulfasalazine and steroids is indicated for less severe cases.

Ulcerative Colitis

Ulcerative colitis is an inflammatory process of unknown cause that affects the mucus of the rectum and left colon. The disease is chronic, with acute exacerbations being followed by remission. The diagnosis is one of the exclusion after infectious causes are ruled out. The lesion is limited to the mucosa; deeper layers of the colon are not involved. Crypt abscesses are observed on microscopic examination. In toxic megacolon the disease extends through the deep muscle layers of the colon.

Clinical Features

The major symptoms are bloody diarrhea, abdominal pain, fever, and weight loss. Onset is in the second to fourth decades of life with occasional abrupt acute exacerbations. Mortality is related to the severity of the disease. With ulcerative colitis or toxic megacolon, 10% to 15% mortality is noted during the first attack; 50% mortality is seen in those patients with colonic perforation.

Mild ulcerative colitis involves usually only the sigmoid and rectum. Minimal pain, bleeding, and diarrhea are present. Patients may complain of anorectal or extracolonic manifestations such as arthralgia, uveitis, erythema nodosum, and weight loss.

Diagnosis

Patients with moderate and severe forms of the disease have profuse bloody diarrhea, high fever, massive bleeding, crampy abdominal pain, or progressive dilatation of the colon. The patient may appear acutely ill with fever to 38.9°C, leukocytosis, sepsis, and dehydration. The abdomen is tender and tympanitic with absent bowel sounds and sometimes peritoneal findings. Abdominal films may reveal air in the colon, which can silhouette an irregular colonic mucosa. Tonic megacolon may be noted. Rebound tenderness suggests colonic perforation. In a routine evaluation barium enema may be preferred to colonoscopy, but sigmoidoscopic examination may reveal bleeding with normal mucosa or an irregular, granular-appearing mucosa that is friable and bleeds easily. Rectal biopsy confirms the diagnosis and rules out amebic colitis. Rule out invasive diarrhea due to bacteria by cultures.

Treatment

Except in the most mild cases, inpatient hospital treatment is required. Patients already on steroids need maintenance or alteration of dosage. Patients not previously treated benefit from acute steroids or adrenocortical hormone. Sulfasalazine is useful in the prevention of the recurrence of colitis but not during the acute process. Opioids are ineffective and may predispose to toxic megacolon.

Diverticulitis

Diverticulitis of the colon is a protrusion of the large intestinal mucosa through the muscular coat. Diverticulosis is the presence of diverticula. Inflammation of the structure is diverticulitis. Diverticula penetrate through the circular muscular wall in association with penetrating arteries. They can occur anywhere in the colon but most commonly in the sigmoid.

The incidence of colonic diverticulitis increases with age, but it can be present in young patients. Although up to two thirds of patients older than age 70 are affected by diverticulosis only, a small proportion develop diverticulitis with complications that require hospital admission.

Clinical Features and Diagnosis

Patients have severe, persistent, hypogastric, or left lower abdominal pain with associated tenderness. One fourth of the patients have right lower quadrant pain, which may vary, and occult blood. Distention may be marked; pain in the left lower quadrant with a palpable distal colon is highly suggestive. Dilation may be hazardous and result in perforation. Plain abdominal films are useful to exclude other causes of abdominal pain. CT scan has been helpful in demonstrating the diverticula.

Treatment

Diverticulosis requires no treatment. Daily fiber supplements are advised, as is weight loss in obese patients. Patients without elevated white counts or peritoneal signs and good follow-up can be treated on an outpatient basis with a clear liquid diet, antibiotics, and anticholinergics such as Donnatal. Patients should avoid gassy foods, caffeine, and alcohol. Patients with dehydration, fever, shock, and severe pain require fluid resuscitation, antibiotics, and hospital admission with surgical consult.

IRRITABLE BOWEL SYNDROME

An irritable intestinal tract is a constellation of symptoms including abdominal discomfort, erratic bowel behavior, and alteration between constipation and diarrhea. Certain medications and psychologic stress may trigger the symptoms.

Clinical Features

Patients complain of abdominal stress of variable intensity and location, with erratic bowel behavior alternating between constipation and diarrhea. The stools may be loose, watery, and fragmented but are negative. Gas is often present with excessive bloating.

Diagnosis

Physical findings are nonspecific; patients are anxious and may have a flat or distended abdomen. Rectal examination usually is negative. Laboratory tests are normal. Barium enema often reveals segmental spasm.

Treatment

Reassurance, explanation of normal physiology, and referral to a gastroenterologist are indicated. Symptomatic treatment with dicyclomine (Bentyl) before meals or at bedtime may be used temporarily. Patients should avoid narcotics and add bulk fiber products such as psyllium to their diet.

APPENDICITIS

The appendix is a small organ of lymphoid tissue, the base of which is always located at the posteromedial aspect of the cecum below the ileocecal valve. The free end is in numerous locations; in one third of individuals it is at the brim of the right pelvis, and in two thirds it is retrocecal. It cannot always be located at McBurney's point (5 cm medial to the superior-anterior right iliac spine on a line extending to the umbilicus).

Pathophysiology

Appendicitis occurs when a closed loop obstruction of the lumen (by fecal, lymphoid hypertrophy, barium inspissation, seeds, worms) causes mucus secretions into the lumen with distension, vague midabdominal visceral pain with peristalsis (crampy pain). Multiplication of bacteria (toxins cause fever, tachycardia, and leukocytosis). This distension when it exceeds venous pressure causing nausea and vomiting, vascular congestion, cirrhosal inflammation, (right lower quadrant, parietal pain) and eventual perforation. There is a 7% lifetime incidence of developing appendicitis. The incidents of males to females is roughly 2-1 and the highest incidents in the late teen, twenties and thirties. Ten percent of cases occur in patients younger than 10 years of age and 10% in those older than 50 years of age. The appendix becomes gangrenous and perforates the peritoneal cavity, usually within 36 hours after the onset of symptoms. The classic picture of increasing right lower quadrant pain suddenly relieved at the time of perforation is rarely seen.

Chronic appendicitis are those patients with multiple recurrent right lower quadrant pain with resolution and pathologic evidence for chronic appendicitis does occur. The etiology being spontaneous relief of luminal obstruction as soft fecaliths shift, or lymphoid hypertrophy shrinks slightly.

Clinical Presentation

With the history as outlined above fever is noted uncommonly, and patients often prefer to lie supine with the hips slightly flexed. Peritoneal irritation with voluntary guarding is noted near McBurney's point. Retrocecal appendicitis has more marked right flank tenderness. An appendix lying against the soleus muscle will be more painful if the right hip is extended, stretching the muscle (psoas sign). A pelvic appendix fully localized sometimes in the lower quadrants bilaterally or suprapubic exam is helpful here. A pelvic appendix often lies near the obturator internus muscle, and stretching the obturator by passive internal rotation of the flexed right hip reproduces the pain.

Patients with suspected appendicitis should have at a minimum a white cell count with differential and urinalysis. Ten percent of patients have a normal white cell count; most have a white cell count greater than 10,000/mm^3 with a neutrophil fraction of about 75%. This helps differentiate appendicitis from mesenteric adenitis and gastroenteritis. No significant difference occurs between patients with appendicitis and those with pelvic inflammatory disease. A white cell count with differential, particularly if less than 10,000/mm^3, is helpful. Abdominal radiographs are not indicated for patients with a history and examination typical of appendicitis. Appendicitis with calcified appendocolith was visible on plain films in 1.4% of cases in a series of 570 patients. Urinalysis helps diagnose patients in whom appendicitis is suspected but who actually have urinary tract pathology.

Ultrasound has been used extensively in some centers to diagnose appendicitis. In one study of 76 patients who had abdominal compression ultrasound based on a clinical impression of appendicitis, ultrasound was 80% sensitive, 95% specific, and 92.2% accurate in diagnosing appendicitis. It also provided additional findings leading to alternative diagnoses for abdominal pain. It directly influenced clinical management in 18% of the patients. Its greatest usefulness has been in ovulating women.

Differential Diagnosis of Appendicitis

Mesenteric adenitis, gastroenteritis, and abdominal pain of unknown cause are not distinguishable from appendicitis by duration of pain on admission, anorexia, nausea, vomiting, chills, or fever. The classic history of appendicitis can be consistent with all these and does not distinguish it from this trio of nonoperative diseases (Table 28-3).

Table 28-3 Differentiating Factors in Appendicitis

Patient Population	Differentiating Factors*
Adult men	Localized right lower quadrant tenderness Rebound tenderness Elevated white cell count (>11,500/mm^3) Increase neutrophil fraction (>75%)
Ovulating women	Absence of anorexia, nausea, vomiting Duration of pain > 2 days Onset within 7 days of menstruation History of venereal disease Abdominal tenderness outside right lower quadrant Cervical motion tenderness Bilateral adnexal tenderness

*In men, factors differentiating appendicitis from trio of nonoperative diseases; all favor appendicitis as correct diagnosis. In women, factors differentiating appendicitis from pelvic inflammatory disease; all favor pelvic inflammatory disease as correct diagnosis.

Tenderness is useful in distinguishing appendicitis; it is more often localized to the right lower quadrant, and rebound tenderness is more often present. In addition, in men the white cell count is higher in appendicitis than in this trio of diagnoses. The neutrophil percentage is also useful and is higher in appendicitis than in the nonoperative diseases; thus rebound tenderness and white cell count with differential are the helpful differential points between appendicitis and the trio of mesenteric adenitis, gastroenteritis, and abdominal pain of unknown etiology.

In women appendicitis is usually confused with pelvic inflammatory disease. There are several factors that can differentiate the two and improve on the high negative laparotomy rate for pelvic inflammatory disease.

Complications

Perforation with an associated increase in mortality may occur in up to one third of the patients, particularly in children in whom symptoms have been present for more than 4 days and in whom signs of peritonitis, fever, and leukocytosis are present. Abscess formation may be suggested by peritoneal findings on physical examination; ileus may be suggested by the finding of a palpable mass. Inflammatory irritation of the right hemidiaphragm may be suggested by the radiation of pain to the right shoulder or aggravation of the pain with deep inspiration. Relief of pain after perforation is rare.

Another complication of appendicitis is fistula formation, in which the abscess communicates with an adjacent anatomic structure into the urinary bladder, vagina, or abdominal wall; small bowel obstruction may occur after perforation. Rarely, pyelophlebitis, which is associated with 25% mortality, is suggested by fever, chills, and jaundice. This occurs as a result of suppurative thrombophlebitis of the portal vein.

In mucocele there is an accumulation of appendiceal secretions in the appendix. A tender mass may be felt. Sepsis may occur in 10% of patients with acute appendicitis and perforation.

Treatment

Intravenous fluid resuscitation and nasogastric suctioning in the presence of nausea and vomiting are required. Early surgical care is indicated in patients with peritonitis; in children, the elderly, and pregnant patients; or in patients with abscess formation. Antimicrobial therapy in appendectomy is necessary for perforation in appendicitis. In contrast, patients with normal or inflamed appendices have a low risk of infection after appendectomy and therefore have little need for antimicrobial therapy. In preventing postoperative infections in gangrenous or perforated appendicitis, the combination of clindamycin plus aminoglycoside remains the most effective and established regimen in clinical studies. This combination provides coverage for most anaerobes, including *fragilis* and facultative organisms. The regimen also provides coverage for Gram-negative bacilli including *aeruginosa*, which is isolated in 15% to 20% of cases of perforated appendicitis.[1-5]

INJURIES TO THE RECTUM AND COLON

Injuries to the rectum and colon can occur from externally introduced penetrating materials, such as bullets, knives, or foreign bodies, or from iatrogenic procedures. Foreign bodies may be associated with bleeding or pain, but in some instances the patient offers only a history of a lost foreign body that had been inserted. In some cases, disruption of the anal sphincter may be observed. Acceleration and deceleration injuries, frequently in association with the use of seat belts, may injure the ileum and may cause disruption of the colonic mesentery or injury to the colon itself.

Determining the mechanism of injury is important in the approach to the patient with injury to the rectum or colon. Life-threatening extracolonic injuries should be sought and excluded. If the rectal examination reveals normal findings, proctosigmoidoscopy should ensue. Brunt genographic studies may demonstrate fractures, opaque foreign bodies, intraperitoneal air, and intramural air. Extra-abdominal foreign bodies should be excluded.

Foreign bodies can often be removed in the ED with a tenaculum, ring forceps, snare, or inflated Foley catheter. Removal of the foreign body should be followed by a proctoscopic and physical re-examination with attention to the detection of mucosal lacerations and perforations of the bowel. Perforation of the rectal sigmoid may be asymptomatic or suggested in some cases by peritoneal signs or the observation of free air in the abdomen. In the patient with multiple trauma, establishment of airway, breathing, and circulation takes precedence over treatment of rectal and colon injuries. Nasogastric intubation, placement of a Foley catheter, routine laboratory tests, and fluid resuscitation are indicated. Associated injuries (eg, hematuria) should be followed up with appropriate studies.

In instances in which perforation of the large colon is known, intravenous administration of antibiotics, including an aminoglycoside, clindamycin, or cefoxitin, should be initiated.

Perforation subsequent to barium enema may result from improper technique or from an underlying bowel disease that predisposes to perforation. Intravenous therapy with antibiotics is required, as is surgery. Perforations that occur in association with barium enemas may be serious because both bacterial contents as well as barium may be released into the peritoneum. As in free air perforation, early operation is the treatment of choice.

HEMORRHOIDS

Internal hemorrhoids are submucosal dilated venules that are located in the upper anal canal (ie, above the pectinate and involving the superior hemorrhoidal flexures). They are often found in the right anterior, posterior, or left lateral perianal areas. External hemorrhoids involve dilatation of the external inferior plexus, are located below the pectinate line, and are covered by anal skin. The two types may coexist. The major symptoms include rectal bleeding associated with defecation that is unaccompanied by pain. A history of pain suggests thrombosis of internal hemorrhoids or accompanying fissures or stenoses.

Prolapse of internal hemorrhoids may occur. In first-degree prolapse the anal cushion may merely protrude beyond the dentate line during Valsalva maneuvers. The patient may experience perianal aching and a mucoid rectal discharge. Further degrees of prolapse are suggested by protrusion through the anus, and in severe (fourth-degree) instances the hemorrhoids may become strangulated and irreducible. In acute thrombosis of an internal hemorrhoid the rapid onset of rectal pain may be accompanied by protrusion of a mass covered with reddish mucosa. Thrombosis of an external hemorrhoid is associated with a painful mass at the anal verge. The pectinate line is separate from the mass. Small amounts of blood, which have the appearance of streaks on the outer surface of the stool, may be the first clue of hemorrhoids; this blood loss, if chronic, may lead to iron deficiency anemia. Occasionally bleeding may be brisk, particularly in association with prolapse. The differential diagnosis should include hemorrhoids that occur in the presence of portal hypertension (such as that observed in cirrhosis), those that follow pregnancy, and other causes of rectal bleeding.

Patients with mild symptoms may respond to reassurance and bowel care. Hydrocortisone suppositories after each bowel movement and before sleep have been recommended. Avoidance of straining at the time of defecation and bulk fiber laxatives may be useful. Sitz baths three to four times a day may give local symptomatic relief. Prolapse may be reduced by gentle manual manipulation. External thrombosed hemorrhoids may be decompressed by locally injecting 1% lidocaine with epinephrine, making an elliptic incision over the thrombosed hemorrhoid with a number 11 surgical blade, and subsequently removing all the clots. Local application of gauze or taping the buttocks together may achieve hemostasis. Surgical intervention may be indicated in the presence of severe or persistent bleeding, strangulation, an internal hemorrhoid, or thrombosis that does not respond to the above symptomatic treatment.

ANAL FISSURE

Anal fissure is an interruption of the anal canal involving the area between the pectinate and the anal verge. Fissures are initiated by local trauma due to the passage of stool and are suggested by a burning, gnawing pain after bowel movement. Pruritis, bleeding, or a sentinel pile may be noted. Fissures occur in children and young adults and are most commonly found in the posterior midline. Visual inspection may reveal blood, a sentinel pile at the anus, and the characteristic longitudinal lesion. Rectal examination reveals exquisite tenderness, induration, and spasm. Proctosigmoidoscopic examination is eventually indicated to distinguish other process such as Crohn's disease, syphilis, carcinoma, and tuberculosis. Treatment includes bulk oral agents, warm Sitz baths, and analgesics. Surgical treatment by radical incision may be required for chronic fissures, which are suggested by findings of fissure, atrophied anal papillae, and a sentinel pile.

ANORECTAL DISEASE

An anorectal abscess is an infection of the pelvic, rectal, intersphincteric, or other space around the anal rectum. It may occur in patients with Crohn's disease or in those who are immunocompromised. Patients present with rectal pain that is constant, throbbing, and aggravated by the Valsalva maneuver and defecation. Fever may be present. Rectal examination reveals a soft or indurated mass in the anal canal. The abscess is to be distinguished from tumors, particularly adenocarcinoma. Treatment includes incision and drainage (even if the abscess does not appear fluctuant) and the use of oral antibiotics. Fistula is a common occurrence after incision. Patients who are obese, elderly, toxic, or immunosuppressed require hospitalization.

PROLAPSE OF THE RECTUM

Prolapse of the rectum through the anal wall is easy to identify when the prolapse comes through the anus, but it may be difficult to identify if the prolapse remains in the upper canal. Complete prolapse (procidentia) involves the protrusion of the full thickness of the rectum, including the muscle layer, into the anus. The condition occurs in both the very young and the elderly. Prolapse may occur with defecation and is often associated with incontinence of feces, which may be bloody or mucous. Prolapse may be overlooked unless an examination takes place with the patient in a squatting position. In children the protruding mass may spontaneously reduce or could be manually reduced by the emergency physician. The treatment of procidentia is surgery.

PROCTITIS

Gonococcal proctitis is mainly observed in homosexual men. The patient may be completely asymptomatic or complaining of bleeding, discharge, and pain. Diagnosis is confirmed with the observance of the characteristic diplococci on Gram's stain of the exudate. Treatment is with ceftoriaxone and/or spectinomycin for penicillin-allergic patients.

RECTAL HERPES

Herpes simplex, caused by herpesvirus type II, may be suggested by rectal pain that is aggravated by defecation. The characteristic lesion is observed to be a erythematous area with associated vesicles that may ulcerate. After the appropriate smears and cultures are obtained, symptomatic relief can be provided by frequent Sitz baths, and 5% acyclovir ointment may shorten the clinical duration and impede viral shedding.

BIBLIOGRAPHY

Acute abdomen disorders. *Emerg Med Clin North Am*. August 1989.

Bochanan TG, Zuidema GD. *Reason for delay of the diagnosis of acute appendicitis. SGO* 158:760–766.

Boden TF. Recent advances against ascites. *Emerg Med*. 1989;21(18).

Bressen HA. Evaluation, management and prevention of hepatitis. *Critical Decisions Emerg Med*. (ACEP). 1989; vol. 4, lesson 27.

Brewer RJ, et al. Abdomen pain; analysis of 1000 cases. *Am J Surg*. 1976;131:219.

Cerecht WB, et al. Prospective randomized comparison of mezlocillin therapy alone with combined ampicillin and gentamycin therapy for patients with cholangitis. *Arch Intern Med*. 1989;149:1279–1284 (Prem 14-2[8], Sept. 1989).

Decisions in Critical Care, Aspen, 1984.

Fried PO. Selected topics in abdominal pain. *Written Board Review Course* (ACEP Ill.) 1989.

Harold T, O'Connor R, Hoffman G. *Emergency Medicine Self Assessment and Review*, 2nd ed., 1988.

Hiccup: common remedies work. *Better Health*. Fall 1989.

Iserson KV. Acute abdomen pain, parts I and II. *Prem. 14-6*, 14-7, Jan/Feb 1990.

Jess P, et al. Prognosis of acute non-specific abdominal pain, *Am J Surg*. 1982;144:338–340.

Jordan RC, Marx JA. *Case Studies in Emergency Medicine*, vol. II, no. 8, Aspen.

Kwoon JH, et al. Presentation of intestinal infarction resulting from extensive arterial occlusion disease. *SGO*. 1987;157:321–324.

Mann NS, Mann SK. Upper gastrointestinal bleeding. *Hosp Phys*. 1989;25:15–23.

Matolo NM, Staddnick RC, McGahon JP. Comparison of ultrasonography, computerized tomography, and radionuclide imaging in the diagnosis of acute and chronic cholecystitis. *Am J Surg*. 1982;144:678–681.

Pickelman J. *Problems in General Surgery*, 1982.

Rosen P, et al. Intestinal obstruction: the great masquerader. *ER Rep* 1980;1:21–28.

Sirinekkor, et al. High dose vasopressin for acute variceal hemorrhage. *Arch Surg*. 1988;123.

Sorpure JS. *Pediatric Emergency Trends*, vols. I, II, III, 1987, 1988.

Stellman RM. *General Surgery: Review and Assessment*, 2nd ed. 1983.

Surg Auto Digest. 30(2).

29. Poisoning, Drug Overdose, and Toxic Exposures

JOHN B. SULLIVAN, JR., MD

A patient who has either ingested an overdose of a drug or encounters a toxic exposure should receive special toxicologic and clinical evaluation. Manifestations of such an exposure may range from a paucity of signs and symptoms to coma and complete cardiorespiratory arrest. Not all toxic exposures result in immediate symptomatology. The patient may initially be asymptomatic, but serious morbidity may develop over a period of hours or days. Physiologic antagonists are available for a select number of toxic agents; however, basic and advanced critical care are imperative to the management of the patient with a poisoning or a drug overdose. The emergency physician should understand the clinical toxicology and pharmacology of a drug in overdose, the changing absorptive process, the possible changing kinetic process, and the effect of patient age and disease on drug metabolism.

PREHOSPITAL MANAGEMENT

Basic prehospital care of a poisoned patient does not differ from the care rendered any seriously ill patient. Emergency care personnel should attempt to ascertain what substance was ingested, how much was ingested, and when it was ingested. They should search the area of initial contact with the patient for evidence of an empty container or drug prescription. Supportive prehospital care consists of the following:

- Airway management. Intubation should be considered if the patient is comatose, experiences seizures, or has a depressed gag reflex. The airway should be protected at all times, and the aspiration of vomitus or secretions should be prevented.
- Intravenous lines. Poisoned patients may be hypotensive because of vasodilation, peripheral pooling of intravascular volume, or myocardial depression. Intravenous administration of crystalloid fluids may be indicated to correct hypotension. Administration of other drugs may also be necessary.
- Naloxone, glucose, and oxygen. The intravenous administration of an adequate dose of naloxone with glucose and supplementary oxygen by mask or nasal cannula is not harmful to any comatose patient if the diagnosis is not yet established. Hypoglycemia may be present, or a narcotic may be involved in the overdose.
- Basic and advanced cardiac life support. Cardiopulmonary resuscitation of a poisoned patient is generally the same as that of any other critically ill patient.

EMERGENCY DEPARTMENT MANAGEMENT

The evaluation of the poisoned patient in the emergency department should begin with a baseline history and physical examination. Historical information concerning the poison or drug may be difficult to obtain, however, owing to coma, seizures, cardiopulmonary arrest, or delirium. The history supplied by a friend or family member may not be accurate. A depressed patient who has attempted suicide with a drug may also be reluctant to reveal the substance ingested. The physical examination may provide the only database in a comatose patient when a history is not available. If the patient is not comatose and can supply information, the emergency physician should try to ascertain what was ingested, when it was ingested, and how much was ingested. Also, it is useful to know if any type of first aid treatment was administered by friends or family, for example, an outdated antidote.

The emergency physician must first determine if the patient's life is in immediate danger and if advanced critical care is required. It is also imperative that the physician, in the initial and subsequent evaluations, rule out any associated illness or injury. An acute abdominal, neck, or intracranial injury is easily overlooked in a comatose poisoned patient or in a patient assumed to be poisoned.

Good supportive care is the foundation for proper management of any poisoned patient, and the physician should always provide this basic care instead of hurriedly searching for an antidote.

Airway Management

The poisoned patient who is deeply comatose, is having seizures, or has a depressed gag reflex has an unprotected airway. Endotracheal intubation, either by the oropharyngeal or nasotracheal route, is necessary in these patients. If the patient cannot be intubated, then correct positioning of the head to prevent aspiration or airway occlusion by the tongue is important. Intubation may be required to protect the airway during orogastric lavage, and the endotracheal tube cuff should always be properly inflated. Tracheal intubation may also be necessary to provide ventilatory assistance. Possible complications to tracheal intubation should be anticipated, however.[1] A poisoned patient may be supported on a respirator until a drug is metabolized and eliminated from the body (see Chapter 70, Airway Management).

Fluid Resuscitation of Hypotensive Patients with a Drug Overdose

Hypotension secondary to a drug overdose may result from the following[2,3]:

1. peripheral pooling of vascular volume and vasodilation because of a drug-induced effect on the vascular tone, either directly or through central nervous system action
2. myocardial depression through drug effects on contractility, heart rate, stroke volume, and peripheral resistance
3. direct injury to the vascular endothelium
4. direct caustic effect of the drug on the gastrointestinal tract, producing necrosis and hemorrhage

Fluid resuscitation of shock following a drug overdose should be initiated with a crystalloid. The rapid administration of a crystalloid such as Ringer's lactate or normal saline usually brings about some correction of hypotension, although the administration of large volumes of crystalloid solutions can precipitate noncardiogenic pulmonary edema[4-7] and worsen cerebral edema.[8,9] An adult should be given 500 mL of crystalloid solution rapidly to begin restoration of intravascular volume. A child in shock should be given isotonic saline or Ringer's lactate intravenously (15 to 20 mL/kg) rapidly.[10] If large volumes of fluid are required, the addition of a vasopressor such as dopamine (Intropin) or norepinephrine (Levophed or Levarterenol) should be considered. The pediatric and adult dosage of dopamine is 5 to 10 µg/kg/min by intravenous infusion. The adult dosage of norepinephrine is 0.1 to 0.2 µg/kg/min by intravenous infusion; the pediatric dosage, 0.05 µg/kg/min.[11] The infusion rate can be varied to titrate blood pressure.

Physical Examination and Neurologic Evaluation

Associated illnesses and injuries should be ruled out in the poisoned patient. Neurologic evaluation should include a determination of the level of consciousness, as well as an examination of pupillary reflexes, oculovestibular reflexes, and muscle stretch reflexes. The pattern of respiration should be noted with attention to the rate and depth. Funduscopic examination may provide some information as to the cause of coma. Naloxone, glucose, and oxygen should be administered. The depth of coma should be determined and any changes noted (see Chapter 57, Coma).

Cardiac Monitoring

Many drugs may be associated with cardiac dysrhythmias when taken in overdose. This is especially true with tricyclic antidepressants and phenothiazines. An electrocardiogram (ECG) should be obtained and the PR, QRS, and QT intervals noted.

Electrolyte and Acid-Base Determination

Serum electrolyte and arterial blood gas determinations are helpful in managing a poisoned patient. The presence of metabolic acidosis and electrolyte derangement may help determine the type of toxicity involved.

Advanced Cardiac Life Support

The clinical status of a poisoned patient may deteriorate rapidly. Cardiorespiratory depression, pulmonary edema, deepening coma, seizures, and life-threatening dysrhythmias may occur and must be treated appropriately. The critical care of a poisoned patient is no different from that of any other critically ill patient. Advanced cardiac life support techniques should be applied when necessary.

EMERGENCY TOXICOLOGY DRUG SCREENS

Drug and toxin screens are useful for identifying the unknown and confirming the suspected. The physician ordering the screen, however, frequently does not understand what is being ordered, what specimens to send to the laboratory, and how to interpret the results. This leads to some confusion concerning the utility of drug screening procedures and inappropriate use of these procedures.

The physician should first endeavor to ascertain by examination and history what drugs or toxins could potentially be involved and then decide if toxicologic analysis is really necessary. Common errors made by the ordering physician are: (1) a general screen in blood and urine is requested when only specific analyses are required. This causes the laboratory to waste time and reagents. (2) The proper specimens are not sent to the laboratory. Both urine and blood need to be collected for a complete screen. Most drugs and toxins can be assayed for in urine; however, there is a need for quantitating certain drugs or toxins and this can only be done with blood. (3) A drug screen is sent too soon. Patients may arrive in the emergency department with a history of an ingestion. If urine is sent immediately the drug may not have had time to be metabolized and excreted in the urine. The drug screen should be properly timed. (4) The physician does not communicate with the lab. If the physician suspects that certain toxins or drugs have been ingested, then communicating this to the lab is very helpful. This can speed up the analysis and build better relations with lab personnel. (5) There is generally a lack of understanding by the ordering physician of what the lab can do. The emergency physician should take time to visit the lab and become familiar with what toxicology screens the lab can perform and what drugs and toxins the lab can quantitate. Some labs will be better than others in their capacity to perform analyses.

Techniques and methods for emergency drug and toxin screening have vastly improved over the last few years. Most laboratories will use a combination of thin layer chromatography (TLC), an immunoassay system, gas-liquid chromatography (GLC), and high-pressure liquid chromatography (HPLC). These tools are all useful for drug identification, confirmation, and quantitation. Also, certain well-accepted color tests are employed to rapidly identify some toxins. A general approach to analytical and screening procedures is as follows:

1. Blood and urine are received by the laboratory along with some information about the patient's condition, drugs suspected, and possible time of ingestion.
2. Spot color tests for chloral hydrate and salicylates are performed. If the test is positive for salicylates, then quantitation is performed usually by the Trinder method.
3. A volatile screen is performed on plasma looking for aliphatic alcohols—methanol, ethanol, acetone, and isopropanol. Ethylene glycol is usually not assayed for in the initial volatile screen. If its presence is suspected, special assay procedures are required. If any of these are identified, they are quantitated. At this time also, the lab may perform serum electrolytes, serum glucose, and quantitate any anion gap. This helps confirm the presence of a toxin that could produce a metabolic acidosis. Also, the serum glucose can help detect a possible diabetic ketoacidosis if the screen is positive for acetone. It should also be noted that with isopropanol ingestions the presence of acetone without metabolic acidosis is to be expected. Conversely, if acetone is detected, the presene of isopropanol should be considered.
4. TLC analysis is performed on urine. Many unknown materials are detected by this system. It is rapid, reliable, and has reasonable sensitivity and can distinguish among the variety of drugs or toxins. Acid hydrolysis of the sample is necessary to detect drugs by TLC that have been glucuronated. If this is not done, many drugs will not be detected or confirmed.
5. An immunoassay system is frequently used to detect, confirm, or quantitate drugs along with a TLC system. The immunoassay can screen urine for barbiturates, benzoylecgonine (metabolite of cocaine), benzodiazepines, opiates, propoxyphene, phencyclidine, and methaqualone. The immunoassay system can also be utilized for accurate, reliable quantitation of acetaminophen, theophylline, phenytoin, and other drugs in serum.
6. The presence of drugs detected by TLC and immunoassay systems can be cross-confirmed by these systems or by GLC and HPLC if necessary.

There are certain drugs and toxins whose quantitation is important for patient care. Plasma determination of these compounds will decide treatment and disposition of a patient. These drugs/toxins along with a reliable detection method are listed in Table 29-1. Other drugs and toxins whose quantitation is important are carbon monoxide, methemoglobin, cyanide, lithium, iron, and other heavy metals.

Analysis of gastric contents obtained from emesis or lavage may be of limited value to the emergency physician. However, it can be of forensic value to the laboratory. The emergency physician can have gastric contents analyzed by the same methodologies described. Sometimes, early detection of a nonabsorbed drug can be accomplished. In practical terms, the patient with a drug ingestion already has absorbed, metabolized, and excreted some or all of the drug by the time of arrival in the emergency department. Thus urine is a better matrix for rapid analysis.

Table 29-1 Critical Quantitations

Drug or Toxin	Assay Method
Acetaminophen	HPLC, immunoassay
Salicylate	Spectrophotometry (Trinder), HPLC
Theophylline	HPLC, GLC, immunoassay
Phenytoin	HPLC, GLC, immunoassay
Phenobarbital	HPLC, GLC, immunoassay
Ethanol	GLC, enzyme assay
Methanol	GLC
Ethylene glycol	GLC

Coma, Depressed Reflexes, Hypotension

Many drugs can cause coma when taken in an overdose. Coma of various degrees associated with depressed reflexes is characteristic of the sedative-hypnotic drugs, which include barbiturates, benzodiazepines, ethanol, chloral hydrate, glutethimide, and ethchlorvynol.[12-17] Other drugs associated with coma and flaccidity are narcotics, meprobamate, and valproic acid.[18-21] Many of these drugs can cause coma, respiratory depression, depressed muscle stretch reflexes, loss of oculogyric and oculocephalic reflexes, and hypotension. With the narcotics, however, miosis is generally present. Valproic acid, though, is not known to cause hypotension in overdose. Clonidine hydrochloride overdose has been reported to result in coma, areflexia, and hypotension.[22,23]

Coma, Hyperreflexia, Seizures, Hypertonicity, and Myoclonus

Certain drugs in overdose may be associated with a combination of coma, seizures, increased muscle tone, and myoclonic activity. This toxicologic syndrome is most commonly caused by the anticholinergics such as tricyclic antidepressants and phenothiazines.[24,25] Overdose with methaqualone, a sedative-hypnotic, can result in coma, hyperreflexia, hypertonicity, and seizures.[26,27] Other drugs and toxins associated with this type of symptomatology are phencyclidine hydrochloride, strychnine, amphetamines, cocaine, phenytoin, haloperidol, and fluoroacetate.[28-36] Propoxyphene (Darvon) overdose may be associated with seizure activity, along with coma, miotic pupils, and pulmonary edema.[37] Propranolol and metoprolol overdose has been reported to be associated with seizure and coma, along with the cardiac manifestations of atrioventricular block and hypotension.[38,39]

Overdose with carbamazepine (Tegretol), a drug being employed more frequently as an anticonvulsant for grand mal seizure disorders, may result in coma, hyperreflexia, seizures, and myoclonic activity.[40] Patients with cyanide and carbon monoxide poisoning may manifest seizures, coma, and hypertonicity.[41-44] Isoniazid also produces coma and seizures in overdoses along with metabolic acidosis.

Intense, prolonged seizure activity and myoclonus can result in rhabdomyolysis with possible acute renal failure secondary to myoglobinuria. Rhabdomyolysis has been associated with various drug overdoses[45,46] and is particularly noted with overdose of amphetamine, heroin, phencyclidine hydrochloride, or carbon monoxide.[45,47,48]

Coma, Pulmonary Edema, Hypotension

The syndrome of coma, pulmonary edema, and hypotension may be caused by drug overdoses with sedative-hypnotics, narcotics, or salicylates. Ethchlorvynol (Placidyl) has been reported to be associated with noncardiogenic pulmonary edema.[49,50] Sedative-hypnotic drugs may also be associated with respiratory distress and pulmonary edema secondary to shock and aspiration of gastric contents. Narcotics have long been known to be associated with pulmonary edema, hypotension, and coma.[51,52] An overdose of propoxyphene should be suspected in a comatose patient with pulmonary edema, seizures, and miotic pupils.[37,53] Salicylate toxicity is associated with noncardiogenic pulmonary edema,[54,55] and the mechanism is thought to be increased permeability of alveolar and capillary endothelial cells.[56] Insult to the lungs following shock with development of the respiratory distress syndrome can accompany any drug overdose that produces coma and hypotension.

Narcotic-Opiate Toxicologic Syndrome

All of the opiates and narcotic drugs may produce a similar toxicologic syndrome (ie, a combination of coma, hypotension, areflexia, bradycardia, miosis, pulmonary edema, and seizures). Miosis may not always be present in overdoses with meperidine (Demerol).[57,58] Miosis may not be extreme in some cases, and clinical suspicion is important in making a diagnosis of narcotic toxicity. Bowel sounds may be decreased or absent, and reflexes may be depressed. Lomotil (diphenoxylate and atropine) poisoning may have some anticholinergic symptomatology along with the narcotic syndrome; furthermore, symptomatology may be delayed for 12 or more hours.[59] Treatment with the narcotic antagonist naloxone (Narcan) is warranted if narcotic or opiate toxicity is suspected.

Cardiac Dysrhythmias, Seizures, Coma

Many drugs in overdose are associated with cardiac dysrhythmias, seizures, and coma. The tricyclic antidepressants are probably the most commonly ingested drugs that cause cardiac dysrhythmias in overdose; they are also associated with seizures.[3,24] Other poisons and drugs associated with cardiac dysrhythmias, seizures, and coma in overdose are theophylline, caffeine, arsenic, chloral hydrate, propranolol, cocaine, amphetamine, phencyclidine hydrochloride, fluoroacetate, clonidine, carbamazepine, phenothiazines, lead, digoxin, and lithium. Theophylline and caffeine are known to produce seizures and ventricular dysrhythmias in overdose, as well as gastrointestinal bleeding.[60-62] Arsenic has been associated with ventricular irritability, as has lead, which may also produce a myocarditis.[63,64] Chloral hydrate has produced both supraventricular and ventricular dysrhythmias in overdose.[65] Clonidine overdose can result in coma, seizures, and atrioventricular block of varying degrees.[66,67] Sodium fluoroacetate was previously used in rodenticide preparations, but it is now banned because of its toxic effects on humans. Symptomatology from fluoroacetate may consist of coma, seizures, nystagmus, and cardiac dysrhythmias ranging from ST segment and T wave changes to ventricular premature contractions.[32,68] Propranolol overdose may result in coma, seizures, and atrioventricular block.[69] Carbamazepine overdose has been reported to result in QRS and QT interval prolongation in at least one case, as well as coma and seizures.[40] Cocaine, amphetamines, and phencyclidine hydrochloride are commonly abused drugs that may be associated with cardiac dysrhythmias and hypertension, as well as coma and seizures.[3]

Newer antidepressant drugs have been implicated in producing cardiac dysrhythmias in overdose. This is especially true with the tetracyclic maprotaline (Ludiomil). Amoxapine (Asendin), a new tricyclic antidepressant, can produce seizures, coma, and cardiac dysrhythmias; however, the seizure activity is more commonly seen and can be very difficult to terminate even with aggressive anticonvulsant pharmacotherapy.

Hypothermia and Hyperthermia

A patient who is comatose from a drug ingestion may become hypothermic through exposure to environmental ambient temperature and through loss of heat secondary to peripheral vasodilation and depression of central nervous system thermoregulation. Because hypothermia may add to metabolic acidosis, hypoxemia, central nervous system depression, and cardiac dysrhythmias,[70,71] the temperature of a comatose patient should always be taken rectally to rule out complicating hypothermia. Drugs or poisons frequently associated with hypothermia are ethanol, barbiturates, other sedative-hypnotics, general anesthetics, phenothiazines, tricyclic antidepressants, and carbon monoxide.[72-75]

Hyperthermia may be present with salicylate, phenothiazine, tricyclic antidepressant, phencyclidine hydrochloride, cocaine, and amphetamine overdose.[25,28,73,76] Agents that uncouple oxidative phosphorylation (eg, salicylates, pentachlorophenol, and dinitrophenol) may result in hyperthermia, tachycardia, and coma[76,77] (see Chapter 40, Hyperthermia, and Chapter 41, Hypothermia).

Cyanosis

Many disease processes can produce cyanosis. The differential diagnosis of a cyanotic patient includes acute myocardial infarction, pulmonary thromboembolism, right-to-left arteriovenous shunts, impaired pulmonary function, and abnormal hemoglobins, either hereditary or acquired. Cyanosis is clinically evident when there are more than 5 g of reduced hemoglobin per 100 mL of blood (33% reduced hemoglobin). At this point, the arterial blood is usually less than 80% saturated.[78]

Cyanosis is also clinically evident when there is 1.5 g of methemoglobin per 100 mL of blood (approximately a 10% methemoglobinemia). Many drugs and chemicals can result in methemoglobinemia, and the most common etiologic agents are sulfonamides, nitrates, and nitrites.[79] Aromatic amino and nitro compounds, such as aniline, trinitrotoluene, nitrobenzene, nitrophenol, dinitrobenzene, and nitroaniline, are well absorbed through the skin and can result in methemoglobinemia and hepatotoxicity.[80] Other common causes of methemoglobinemia are azo dye compounds such as those used in urinary analgesics. Most of these products contain phenazopyridine hydrochloride.[81] Benzocaine is present in many proprietary compounds and can cause methemoglobinemia when ingested.[82] The diagnosis of methemoglobinemia should be considered in a patient who is cyanotic, does not respond to oxygen therapy, and has no other historical or cardiac reason for being cyanotic.

Sulfhemoglobinemia is another chemical cause of cyanosis that is again unresponsive to oxygen therapy. This is a rare disorder thought to be due to sulfur-containing drugs or to chronic constipation with absorption of sulfur compounds.[83] Sulfhemoglobinemia is not responsive to methylene blue therapy and lasts the life of red blood cells. As little as 0.5 g of sulfmethemoglobin per 100 mL of blood can result in clinical cyanosis.[84]

Metabolic Acidosis

Anion gap metabolic acidosis may be caused by a toxic ingestion of salicylates, methanol, ethylene glycol, isoniazid, iron, ethanol, or paraldehyde.[76,85-89] Other common causes of metabolic acidosis, such as diabetic ketoacidosis and sepsis, should be ruled out. Phenformin ingestion is associated with a severe lactic acidosis, but it is uncommon now. Renal tubular acidosis without an anion gap has been associated with chronic sniffing abuse of toluene-containing products.[90] Toluene ingestion has also been reported to cause an anion gap metabolic acidosis.[91] Salicylates, methanol, and ethylene glycol are the most commonly ingested substances that cause an anion gap metabolic acidosis and should always be considered in a comatose, acidotic patient. Seizures may also occur with ingestion of these drugs; seizures almost always occur with isoniazid poisoning (see Chapter 21, Acid-Base Disturbances).

DISORDERS OF MOVEMENT

Both nontoxic ingestions and overdoses can cause movement disorders. Phenytoin is known to be associated with movement disorders in both therapeutic and toxic concentrations. Choreoathetosis and orofacial dyskinesias have been reported at therapeutic levels,[92] and choreoathetoid movements have been reported with ingestion of amounts in the toxic range.[93] Phenytoin toxicity is also associated with ataxia and nystagmus.[94] Phenothiazines and the butyrophenone haloperidol (Haldol) are known to cause extrapyramidal reactions. Tricyclic antidepressants in overdose have been associated with choreoathetoid movements.[95] Heavy metals such as lead, mercury, and arsenic can cause movement disorders of ataxia and choreiform motions through chronic toxicity.[63,96,97] Lithium toxicity is associated with ataxia and tremors.[98]

BEHAVIORAL DISORDERS

Drug-induced disorders of behavior include psychoses, delirium, paranoia, hallucinations, excitability, abusive and violent behavior, disorders of perception, extreme agitation, fatigue, and depression. Phencyclidine hydrochloride, cocaine, and amphetamines can produce a toxic psychosis indistinguishable from a true paranoid schizophrenia. Phencyclidine hydrochloride intoxication may be associated with paranoid and violent reactions, as well as agitation and hallucinations.[28,99] Chronic abuse of cocaine and amphetamines can result in depression, paranoia, hallucinations, perceptual difficulties, emotional lability, and irritability as well as a toxic psychosis.[100–102] Anticholinergic drugs such as antihistamines, tricyclic antidepressants, phenothiazines, atropine, scopolamine, and over-the-counter products can produce a syndrome of hallucinations, delirium, and agitation in overdose.[24,25,103,104] Chronic heavy metal poisoning with mercury, lead, or arsenic can produce a toxic psychosis and other behavioral disturbances.[63,96] Caffeine and theophylline toxicity may also produce an acute confusional state with hyperalert behavior. Phenytoin can also produce a confusional state in high therapeutic plasma levels, and in toxic plasma ranges can cause excitation, delirium, nystagmus, myoclonus, and, in rare cases, seizures.

The most common cause of acute confusion in emergency department patients is ethanol. Phenylpropanolamine is found in over-the-counter diet aids and is frequently a cause of acute confusion and excitability when ingested in overdose. The ingestion of a sympathomimetic agent can also cause acute hypokalemia. This is seen also with acute ingestions of theophylline and caffeine.

Abuse of solvents can result in a hyperexcitable state and even seizures. Abuse of gasoline by inhalation can cause confusion, delirium, and result in permanent central nervous system damage due to tetraethyl lead poisoning. Patients with carbon monoxide poisoning can present with symptoms of confusion and disorientation. Those who are started on the β blockers metoprolol or propranolol can develop acute confusion. The drug should be discontinued or changed to atenolol.

GENERAL MANAGEMENT

The general approach to managing a patient with a poisoning or drug overdose can be summarized as (1) prevention of absorption, (2) enhancement of elimination, and (3) use of physiologic antagonists as necessary.

Prevention of Absorption

Skin and Ocular Decontamination

Contamination of the eyes by an alkaline, acidic, or irritating chemical should be managed immediately by flushing the eyes with tap water. A low-pressure continuous stream should be applied to the exposed eye for a minimum of 20 minutes if an alkali is involved, for 10 minutes if an acid or hydrocarbon is involved. The eye should be irrigated for 20 minutes if the substance involved is unknown. Treatment in the emergency department is to continue the irrigation if flushing may have been inadequate and to examine the eyes for corneal injuries.

Gasoline and hydrocarbon solvents not only may cause burns of the skin, but also they may be absorbed dermally.[105] These substances should be removed by means of thorough detergent and water decontamination.

Organophosphate and carbamate insecticides are readily absorbed through clothes and skin. The decontamination procedure for these insecticides should be carried out away from the emergency facility to prevent contamination of medical personnel. The person performing the decontamination should wear a protective apron, gloves, and disposable shoe covers. The patient's clothes should be removed and placed in specially marked plastic bags. Two separate water-detergent washes should be performed. Studies have demonstrated that two separate washes removed up to 94% of skin contamination with an organophosphate 6 hours postexposure.[106,107] It is important to wash all parts of the body, including the hair and under the fingernails.

Induction of Emesis

The clinical condition of the patient and what was ingested determine the appropriateness of inducing emesis. It is contraindicated when the patient:

- has ingested acid or alkali
- is unconscious
- is having seizures
- has a depressed or absent gag reflex

Emesis will remove only up to 30% of the stomach contents and is not indicated in every overdose. Emesis is most beneficial within a short time following an ingestion. Inducing emesis for an ingestion has not been proven more effective than the administration of activated charcoal. Emesis should be induced with syrup of ipecac, which works by both local gastric irritant effects and central nervous system effects.[108] The adult dose is 30 mL; the pediatric dose is 15 mL. After the syrup of ipecac, water should be given to distend the stomach. The dose may be repeated once if vomiting does not occur in 15 to 20 minutes. Stimulation of the pharynx with a tongue blade may also help in inducing emesis.

The use of apomorphine to produce vomiting has no advantage over the use of syrup of ipecac. In fact, because apomorphine may also produce drowsiness and protracted vomiting, it should be avoided. Sodium chloride should not be used as an emetic because of the possibility that it will lead to a serious hypernatremia. Deaths have been reported.

Lavage

If a patient is becoming unconscious, is unconscious, has lost the gag reflex, or is having seizures, endotracheal or nasotracheal intubation followed by the insertion of a large orogastric tube is the preferred method of removing the remainder of the drug. A 28-French Ewald with multihole tip is the smallest bore orogastric tube that should be used. A 36-French Ewald that is about 1 cm in diameter and has large holes is preferable. The usual size nasogastric tube of 16 or 18 French is completely worthless except for liquids. Tablets cannot be aspirated through it. The preferred lavage solution is saline. The patient should be in the left-side, head-down position. Lavage should continue until no solid material returns. Rarely can all the ingested substance be removed at this point, however.

Charcoal

Most drugs are well absorbed by activated charcoal, which can be administered orally or by nasogastric or orogastric tube. The use of activated charcoal as a primary mode to prevent drug or toxin absorption is receiving more attention. Activated charcoal has been demonstrated to be more effective than emesis and catharsis in preventing the absorption of a variety of drugs. Multiple doses of charcoal have been demonstrated to be of benefit in increasing the total body elimination of theophylline and phenobarbital (see below). Multiple doses of activated charcoal have not been shown to increase total body elimination of tricyclic antidepressant overdoses.

There are no known contraindications to the administration of activated charcoal. It should be remembered that activated charcoal also absorbs syrup of ipecac and that these should not be given simultaneously. The dose of activated charcoal is usually 30 to 50 g for an adult and 10 to 15 g for children. The dose of charcoal may be repeated during the clinical course to ensure adequate absorption.

Cathartics

Another method by which drug absorption is prevented is through the use of cathartics to enhance gastric motility. The use of magnesium cathartics is contraindicated in renal failure. Oil-based cathartics should be avoided, owing to the potential for a lipoid pneumonia if aspiration occurs. The cathartic of choice is sorbitol. Sorbitol increases gastrointestinal clearance of charcoal much faster than magnesium-based cathartics. A combination of 70% sorbitol and activated charcoal is available in a single-dose container.

Enhancement of Excretion

Enhancing the removal of a drug includes the techniques of forced diuresis, dialysis, or hemoperfusion.

Forced Diuresis

The excretion of some drugs can be facilitated by a neutral, alkaline, or acid diuresis. Alkaline and acid diureses employ the principle of ion trapping. Drugs with a dissociable group carry a charge at a pH that is distant from the pK_a. At a pH equal to the pK_a, a drug is half-dissociated and half-undissociated. Promoting an alkaline urine to a pH of 7 or greater accelerates the renal elimination of salicylates and phenobarbital, since both of these drugs are weak acids.[109,110] An alkaline urine causes the drugs to remain ionized in the renal tubular lumen and thus not readily able to cross the tubular cell membrane. Forced diuresis is not helpful for drugs with large volumes of distribution, such as tricyclic antidepressants, phenothiazines, and digoxin. Cerebral edema and pulmonary edema may be exacerbated by forced diuresis, and caution is in order in these cases.

Alkaline diuresis is accomplished with bicarbonate administered intravenously in 5% dextrose in water. Since normal saline contains 154 mg of sodium per liter, the addition of $NaHW_3$ to 5% dextrose in water should be limited to two to three ampules per liter. The addition of potassium chloride may be necessary to ensure that the urine becomes alkaline. Alkaline diuresis is useful in the treatment of salicylate and phenobarbital poisoning. The urine pH must be increased to 7.5 to achieve the maximum elimination effect.

Acid diuresis has been accomplished in the past with ammonium chloride (2 to 6 g/day orally in adults and 75 mg/kg orally divided into four doses for children). Acid diuresis has previously been used for amphetamine and strychnine intoxication,[29,111] but its effectiveness is not established.

Also, if rhabdomyolysis has occurred secondary to seizures or myoclonic activity, acid diuresis can precipitate myoglobinuric renal failure. Intense myoclonic activity and seizures can occur with PCP, amphetamines, and strychnine toxicity. Therefore, acid diuresis should be avoided in the vast majority of cases.

Usual urine flow is 0.5 to 2 mL/kg/hour; with forced diuresis, urine flow should be 3 to 6 mL/kg/hour. Alkaline or acid diuresis should be chosen on the basis of the drug's pK_a, protein-binding capacity, and volume of distribution so that ionized drug is trapped in the tubular lumen and not reabsorbed. Osmotic load is also important, and either type of diuretic may be employed. Reabsorption proximally occurs if inadequate osmotic load is not maintained in the tubule.

Dialysis

Hemodialysis or peritoneal dialysis can be useful in some poisonings. Dialysis may be considered if the patient's condition fits any of the following criteria and the drug or toxin is amenable to extracorporeal removal:

1. coma or seizures that are caused by a dialyzable drug and cannot be treated by conservative means
2. acid-base and electrolyte disturbances that cannot be controlled
3. marked hyperosmolality that is not due to easily corrected fluid problems
4. drug-induced hypotension that is uncontrollable and threatens renal or hepatic function
5. renal failure

More specifically, dialysis should be considered if the substance involved is:

- ethylene glycol and acidosis is present
- methanol and acidosis is present
- a heavy metal and chelation is being employed and the patient is in renal failure
- theophylline and seizures and dysrhythmias cannot be controlled or the concentration is extremely high (see below)
- salicylate and pulmonary edema, acidemia, seizures, or cerebral edema is present
- ethanol and the blood level is extremely high and respiratory depression has occurred

The dialyzability of a drug is dependent upon its physiochemical properties and its pharmacokinetic parameters.[112,113] The factors involved in the dialyzability of a drug can be summarized as follows:

1. Molecular weight. Drugs with a lower molecular weight cross the dialyzing membrane more readily than drugs with a higher molecular weight.
2. Solubility. Water-soluble drugs are dialyzed more easily than lipid-soluble drugs in an aqueous dialysate solution.
3. Plasma protein binding. Only free drug is available for removal. Drugs with a high degree of protein binding are poorly dialyzed.
4. Distribution phase. For drugs having a long tissue-to-plasma redistribution phase, extracorporeal methods of removal will be less successful.
5. Apparent volume of distribution. Drugs with large volumes of distribution are highly tissue bound, and very little of the drug is actually present in the vascular compartment. Thus, less is available for removal by dialysis.
6. Elimination half-life. The half-life of a drug in an overdose situation may change as a result of the change in elimination kinetics. A drug's half-life may be shorter or longer in an overdose than in a therapeutic situation.
7. Dialysis clearance relative to total body clearance. The overall clearance must be increased in order to shorten the elimination half-life of the drug. Even if the overall clearance with dialysis is greater than total body clearance, dialysis may not remove a significantly larger fraction of the drug during a reasonable period.
8. Metabolites. The same considerations of dialyzability must be given to metabolites as well as the parent compound. Many metabolites are pharmacologically and toxicologically active.
9. Type of dialysis membrane. A hollow-fiber membrane has been shown to be more effective than other types in theophylline elimination (see below).

Hemoperfusion

The use of hemoperfusion as an extracorporeal technique to remove ingested drugs is increasing in the management of overdoses.[114,115] The technique involves passing the patient's venous blood over a fixed adsorbent bed that consists of either coated activated charcoal or Amberlite resin. The fixed bed provides a solid surface area with a continuous porous phase so that the blood can penetrate the pores and be exposed to a large surface area. Hemoperfusion has a few advantages over hemodialysis. It is particularly useful for drugs with a high degree of protein binding, since both protein-bound and non–protein-bound drug is removed. Charcoal-based hemoperfusion beds can remove both polar and nonpolar drugs, as well as their metabolites. The Amberlite adsorbent, however, removes nonpolar drugs and metabolites better than it removes polar drugs.

The limiting factors of hemoperfusion are the affinity of the drug for the adsorbent material, the rate of blood flow through the adsorbent bed, the volume of distribution of the drug, and the redistribution of the drug back into the vascular compartment following termination of the procedure. A drug with a slow redistribution from tissue to plasma can result in rebound levels after hemoperfusion. Hemoperfusion is best used for drugs that have a low intrinsic clearance and a small volume of distribution. Drugs such as tricyclic antidepressants, phenothiazines, etchlorvynol, and digoxin do not have an effective total body burden clearance. Hemoperfusion can significantly decrease the total body burden of theophylline, salicylates, and phenobarbital. The patient must be heparinized, however, and there is a substantial decrease in platelet count up to one-half the prehemoperfusion value. The platelet count usually returns to normal within 1 to 2 days following the procedure. There may also be a loss of plasma protein and calcium.

Specific Poisons and Their Physiologic Antagonists

Some physiologic antagonists reverse the symptomatology of certain poisons and drug overdoses. It is important to be aware of the pathophysiology of the specific toxic agent involved.

Oxygen

Oxygen is employed in managing carbon monoxide poisoning. Carbon monoxide is produced by incomplete combustion of organic products. Automobile exhaust fumes account for approximately 60% of carbon monoxide emitted per year into the atmosphere. Other causes of carbon monoxide poisoning are fires, industrial processes, gas and water heaters, and methylene chloride exposure. Tobacco smokers may have carboxyhemoglobin levels between 5% and 20%.[116] There is also an endogenous carbon monoxide production that results in a carboxyhemoglobin level of 0.4% secondary to heme catabolism.[117]

Carbon monoxide has an affinity for hemoglobin 200 times that of oxygen. It also has an affinity for other heme-containing proteins, such as cytochrome oxidase, peroxidases, P-450 cytochrome oxidase, and myoglobin. The effect of carbon monoxide on the oxyhemoglobin dissociation curve is a shift to the left, which inhibits the release of oxygen to tissues.[117] The pathophysiology of carbon monoxide is tissue hypoxia and interference with cellular respiration.

Several factors are involved in carbon monoxide poisoning: (1) the concentration of carbon monoxide in the environment, which need not be very high since carbon monoxide has a great affinity for hemoglobin; (2) alveolar ventilation; (3) pre-existing cardiovascular disease and anemia; (4) duration of exposure; (5) cardiac output; (6) physical activity of the person exposed.

The signs and symptoms of carbon monoxide poisoning vary according to carbon monoxide concentration in the environment (Table 29-2). The absolute carboxyhemoglobin concentration may not correlate with the signs and symptoms at all times since the level declines once exposure is terminated. A patient with a low level of carboxyhemoglobin may be comatose and having seizures because the level was very high during primary exposure. The half-life of carboxyhemoglobin is approximately 6 hours in 21% FIO_2 (room air). With 100% oxygen, the half-life is 30 to 60 minutes, and with 2 atm of oxygen (hyperbaric) the half-life is 15 minutes.[118] A person with carbon monoxide poisoning should be given 100% oxygen if a hyperbaric chamber is not available or while preparations are being made for hyperbaric therapy. One hundred percent oxygen therapy should continue until the carboxyhemoglobin concentration is less than 5%. Hyperbaric oxygen is the primary mode of therapy for carbon monoxide poisoning. Any patient symptomatic from carbon monoxide poisoning should be treated by hyperbaric therapy if it is available regardless of the carboxyhemoglobin level. Symptomatic patients with carbon monoxide poisoning should be admitted and observed, post oxygen treatment, for 12 to 24 hours.

Table 29-2 Signs and Symptoms of Acute Carbon Monoxide Poisoning

Level of Carboxy-hemoglobin (%)	Signs and Symptoms
10–20	Headache, fatigue, dizziness
20–30	Headache, fatigue, nausea, vomiting, decreased motor ability
30–40	Syncope, increased respirations, tachycardia, confusion, obtundation
50–60	Coma, convulsions, Cheyne-Stokes respirations
60–70	Cardiorespiratory depression, bradycardia, pulmonary edema
70–80	Cardiovascular failure, death

When a patient is brought to the emergency department following a fire exposure, carbon monoxide poisoning should be considered. However, other toxic gases may also be produced in the combustion process, such as hydrogen cyanide and hydrochloric acid from burning plastic and foam products. Arterial blood gases may be normal in carbon monoxide poisoning except for a decreased oxyhemoglobin saturation. In order to detect a decreased oxyhemoglobin saturation, direct measurement of the concentration by an oximeter is required (see Chapter 47, Occupational Toxicologic Emergencies).

The normal solubility of oxygen in blood is 0.3 mL per 100 mL of blood at a PaO_2 of 100 mmHg (FIO_2 of 21%). With 100% oxygen there is a six- to sevenfold increase in the amount of dissolved oxygen, up to 2 mL per 100 mL of blood. Breathing 100% oxygen should produce a PaO_2 of 673 mmHg at sea level. Hyperbaric (2 atm) oxygen therapy dissolves 4.3 mL per 100 mL of blood. Thus, therapy with oxygen in carbon monoxide poisoning involves increasing the dissolved oxygen in the blood for delivery to tissues.[118] If patients do not improve despite 100% oxygen or hyperbaric oxygen therapy, the possibility of cerebral edema should be considered.

Carbon monoxide poisoning can result in myocardial ischemia and myocardial infarction with increased myocardial oxygen consumption. ST segment and T-wave changes can be seen in acute and chronic carbon monoxide poisoning. Neurologic sequelae can involve cerebral edema, seizures, focal cortical necrosis, cerebellar lesions, focal and disseminated cerebral atrophy, demyelination of white matter, and basal ganglia lesions. Neurologic lesions may thus result in personality changes, dementia, memory impairment, visual loss, and retardation.[119,120] The exposure of a pregnant woman to carbon monoxide may have severe central nervous system effects on the fetus.[121]

Most clinicians are not aware that methylene chloride is a source of carbon monoxide poisoning. Used as an industrial solvent and present in paint remover, methylene chloride can produce carbon monoxide poisoning if used in a poorly ventilated area because it is converted into carbon monoxide. Also, the half-life of carbon monoxide from methylene chloride exposure is twice that from other sources[122] (see Chapter 75, Miscellaneous Respiratory Emergencies).

Cyanide Kit

A cyanide kit is available from Lilly and Company and is presently the only treatment form for cyanide poisoning now available in the United States. The cyanide kit should be in every emergency department and should be checked frequently for expiration. The kit contains an amyl nitrite ampule, a 3% sodium nitrite solution, and a 25% sodium thiosulfate solution. The drugs should be used sequentially. The amyl nitrite ampule should be crushed and the patient made to breathe it for 30 seconds of every 60 seconds until the sodium nitrite can be administered. The sodium nitrite is in an adult dosage form; if a child is being treated, the dose must be adjusted.

The goal of therapy is to produce a state of methemoglobinemia, since the cyanide ion has a great affinity for iron in the ferric (Fe^{3+}) state. The amyl nitrite produces a 5% methemoglobinemia. The 3% sodium nitrite solution is then administered intravenously. The adult dose is 300 mg or 10 mL; the pediatric dose is 10 mg/kg or 0.2 mL/kg, not to exceed 300 mg. If a child is given the adult dose of sodium nitrite, a fatal methemoglobinemia may be produced. The pediatric dosage regimen should be affixed to the kit so it will be readily seen. The 25% sodium thiosulfate solution is then administered intravenously. Packaged as a 50-mL volume (12.5 g), it provides substrate for conversion of cyanide to thiocyanate. Sodium thiosulfate has a low toxicity and is well tolerated. Should symptoms recur, the sodium nitrite and sodium thiosulfate can be repeated but at half the dose previously administered.

There are other agents known to be effective antagonists of cyanide toxicity. Such agents currently being explored are DMAP (4-dimethylaminophenol) and the cobalt-containing compounds hydroxocobalamin and cobalt EDTA.[123–125] These antagonists have actually been around for a number of years and have been intensively investigated. DMAP is a rapid methemoglobin former. Cobalt EDTA is used in Europe and is a direct chelator of cyanide (see below).

Atropine

The cholinergic effects of organophosphate and carbamate insecticides can be reversed by atropine, although the patient's condition will be refractory to the usual doses. An adult may be given 1 to 2 mg intravenously and observed for a reversal of signs and symptoms. The pediatric starting dose is 0.05 mg/kg administered intravenously. Organophosphates and carbamates inhibit acetylcholinesterase enzyme and allow acetylcholine to stimulate the cholinergic receptor sites continually. Atropine blocks the muscarinic effects of increased salivation, pulmonary secretions, bradycardia, bronchospasm, and diarrhea, but it does not block the nicotinic effects of skeletal muscle weakness and paralysis. The amount of atropine required may be tremendously large, sometimes approaching as much as 2 g over a 24-hour period.[126–129]

The end point of treatment with atropine is to dry all secretions. Only when all secretions are dried is the patient fully atropinized. At this point, the patient's heart rate is most likely to be increased and pupils dilated; however, if the pulmonary secretions or oropharyngeal secretions are still present, the patient has not been given enough atropine. A patient who has been fully atropinized may also suffer a respiratory arrest secondary to skeletal muscle paralysis, owing to the fact that the nicotinic receptors have not been blocked. The airway of the patient should be protected at all times, and the physicians should be prepared to intubate the patient and support respiration during the course of the treatment. A patient may even succumb to a respiratory arrest late in the course of treatment. Adjunct therapy, and in some cases a major therapeutic modality, is 2-PAM chloride (pralidoxime).

Pralidoxime (2-PAM, Protopam Chloride)

An acetylcholinesterase regenerator, 2-PAM is useful in organophosphate poisonings in which the red blood cell-cholinesterase level is depressed below 50% of normal. 2-PAM can be a major therapeutic benefit for the patient and should be administered early in the course of the poisoning treatment. It can be beneficial as late as 24 hours or more past the time of the poisoning. In some individual cases, organophosphates may cause a predominance of nicotinic effects and a paucity of muscarinic effects. In these cases 2-PAM is the mainstay of therapy. The dose is 1000 mg for adults intravenously over several minutes. This dose can be repeated every 4 to 6 hours as needed.[130] Both 2-PAM and atropine should be administered to most patients suffering from organophosphate toxicity.

Naloxone (Narcan)

Naloxone, a pure narcotic antagonist with no agonist properties, effectively reverses the central nervous system and cardiorespiratory effects of narcotic overdoses. Naloxone may be administered intravenously, subcutaneously, intramuscularly, or via the endotracheal tube. Because the half-life of naloxone is approximately 60 minutes,[131] the dose may need to be repeated as the antagonistic effect disappears. Naloxone is devoid of respiratory depressant effects. The usual adult dose of naloxone is 0.4 to 0.8 mg, and the usual pediatric dose is 0.01 mg/kg. However, larger doses of naloxone may be required in narcotic overdoses involving methadone, propoxyphene, or pentazocine. Ten times the usually recommended dose may be necessary as an intravenous bolus to reverse the narcotic effects of propoxyphene. Narcotic toxicity may not be reversed until five to ten ampules (2 to 4 mg) are administered as an intravenous bolus. An adequate naloxone trial for any narcotic overdose should be at least 2 mg intravenously.[132-134] Relatively large doses of naloxone have been administered without adverse effects or addictive potential.[135] Some clinicians even administer a constant naloxone infusion following the bolus dose. This can prevent the recurrence of narcotic effects in some cases. Naloxone is available in multidose vials.

Methylene Blue

A nonenzymatic catalyst, methylene blue is used to treat methemoglobinemia caused by nitrates, nitrites, and other nitro compounds. Methemoglobin is the oxidized form of hemoglobin with the iron in the ferric (Fe^{3+}) state. Since methemoglobin is unavailable for oxygen transport and release to tissues, the oxyhemoglobin dissociation curve shifts to the left.[79] An endogenous physiologic methemoglobinemia usually does not exceed 2% because the erythrocyte expends energy to keep hemoglobin in the reduced state. This function is normally performed by methemoglobin reductase enzymes that are NADPH dependent. This system is activated by electron transport carriers such as methylene blue. If the normal methemoglobinemia exists, then the methemoglobin reductase–NADPH system increases its activity about 60-fold. The addition of the nonenzymatic electron carrier methylene blue increases the activity rate of the methemoglobin reductase–NADPH system 10-fold above the rate at which methemoglobin stimulates it.[79]

Methylene blue is oxidized in the enzymatic process as it reduces the methemoglobin to hemoglobin. The secondary methemoglobin reductase system requires an intact pentose phosphate shunt and normal glucose metabolism to provide NADPH as a cofactor. The congenital absence of glucose-6-phosphate dehydrogenase results in an absence of NADPH. Individuals with this condition do not respond to methylene blue and develop a hemolytic process when exposed to oxidant agents. Persons with a deficiency or absence of methemoglobin reductase are also more likely to develop methemoglobinemia from oxidant drugs.

The clinical presentation of a patient with methemoglobinemia depends on the percent of hemoglobin oxidized to the ferric state. Cyanosis, dyspnea, lethargy, coma, seizures, hypotension, bradycardia, and cardiac arrest may occur. At low levels of methemoglobinemia, below 30%, mild symptomatology of headache, cyanosis, and lethargy may occur. As the methemoglobin level increases above 50% to 70%, the symptomatology may progress to coma, hypotension, bradycardia, and seizures with cyanosis. Levels greater than 70% may result in death.[81] Cyanosis develops when the level of methemoglobin is greater than 1.5 g per 100 mL of blood or about 10% methemoglobinemia. The cyanosis is also unresponsive to oxygen therapy. A simple test can be performed at the patient's bedside to determine if a significant methemoglobin level should be investigated. If a drop of the patient's blood on a piece of blotter paper appears darker than a normal control, methemoglobinemia should be suspected.

Treatment of methemoglobinemia is with high-flow oxygen and methylene blue. The dose of methylene blue is 0.1 to 0.2 mL/kg intravenously of a 1% solution.[79-81] Caution is in order since large doses of methylene blue can also cause a methemoglobinemia; therefore, only one repeat dose should be administered if the patient with a severe case of poisoning has not improved. Also, if a patient does not respond to methylene blue therapy, the possibility of a glucose-6-phosphate dehydrogenase deficiency should be considered.

Physostigmine

In order to reverse the severe peripheral and central effects of anticholinergic drug overdose, physostigmine may cautiously be employed. Physostigmine is a reversible inhibitor of acetylcholinesterase and reverses the anticholinergic syndrome of tricyclic antidepressants, antihistamines, atropine, and other drugs with anticholinergic effects in overdose.[136-138] The adverse effects of physostigmine are bradycardia, increased tracheobronchial secretions, decreased atrioventricular conduction, and seizures. Seizures commonly occur following intravenous dosing of 1 to 2 mg of physostigmine. The half-life of physostigmine is estimated to be 20 to 30 minutes. Physostigmine is available as an injectable in 1 mg/mL ampules. The adult dose is 1 to 2 mg slowly administered intravenously. The pediatric dose is 0.5 mg administered intravenously at a slow rate.

The effective dose can be repeated in 20 minutes if needed. However, the dose should be repeated only if the symptomatology is serious enough to warrant continued drug treatment. No maximum dose of physostigmine has been established, but a conservative approach to physostigmine administration is indicated in order to avoid seizures and other adverse effects.

The use of physostigmine for reversal of tricyclic antidepressant toxicity and dysrhythmias is not indicated. The evidence of physostigmine's efficacy in this situation is not established and therefore its use should be avoided.

PHARMACOKINETICS AND DRUG OVERDOSES

A basic understanding of drug pharmacology and pharmacokinetics is helpful in managing and appreciating the clinical condition of the patient with a serious overdose. Pharmacokinetics involves the basic processes of drug absorption, distribution, biotransformation, and elimination from the body. A drug ingested in an overdose may act much differently pharmacokinetically than a drug taken in therapeutic amounts.

Drug Absorption

The various routes of drug administration include intravenous, intramuscular, rectal, subcutaneous, dermal, ocular, sublingual, and inhalation; however, the oral route is the most commonly employed, with the gastrointestinal tract forming the absorptive barrier to entrance into the vascular compartment. After entering the vascular compartment, a drug is distributed to various tissue receptor sites. Various factors affect the absorption of a drug from the gastrointestinal tract and thus the distribution of the drug to the receptor sites in tissues.[139-141]

Absorptive Process

Two barriers affect absorption of a drug through the gastrointestinal tract: the columnar epithelium of intestinal villi and the endothelium of the capillary wall. Because the capillary endothelium is relatively porous, the intestinal villi epithelium is the main biologic barrier to drug absorption. Absorption may be by passive diffusion or by active transport. The integrity of the villi epithelium is very important for drug absorption, and any pathologic state that disrupts this integrity may affect absorption, either increasing it (as in massive iron poisoning), or decreasing it by causing diarrhea and loss of absorptive area.

Fasting State

The absence of food in the stomach increases the absorption of most drugs. Drugs may combine with food particles, which can retard or inhibit absorption.

Gastric Juices and Digestive Enzymes

Some drugs may be destroyed, precipitated, or altered by gastric juices and enzymes present in the stomach.

Drug Dissolution

A drug must be dissolved before it can be absorbed; therefore, the dissolution rate of a drug influences absorption. A drug with a slow dissolution rate has a slow absorptive rate. The dissolution rate of a drug depends on its solubility, the pH of the gastrointestinal juices, food content of the stomach, and the salt or crystalline form of the drug.

Gastrointestinal Surface Area and Motility

The large surface area of the intestinal villi and the rate of emptying of gastric contents are the two most important factors in drug absorption.[140] The absorptive capacity of the small intestines is much greater than that of the stomach; if gastric emptying into the intestines is rapid, drug absorption is not delayed. Any factor that decreases gastric emptying (eg, drugs such as anticholinergics and narcotics) also delays drug absorption.[142] Once the drug is in the small intestines, the large absorptive area compensates for other factors that may affect the absorption.

The motility of the small intestine also influences the absorption of a drug. Decreased intestinal motility increases the contact time with the epithelial surface and, thus, absorption of a drug. Increased intestinal motility decreases surface contact time and delays or decreases absorption. Since the absorptive area of the small intestine is greater in the duodenum and proximal area, absorption would be thought to be expedited here. However, since the motility of the proximal small intestines is greater than that of the distal small intestines, a drug may actually be absorbed in the distal segment because the contact time with the epithelial area there is longer.

pH Influence on Drug Absorption

The influence of gastric pH on the absorption of a drug is not clinically significant. A nonionized drug penetrates a biologic membrane much more rapidly than an ionized drug; however, the large absorptive area of the small intestines more than compensates for pH effect.

First Pass Elimination

The venous blood from the intestinal villi goes directly into the liver via the portal system. A drug may be metabolized to a great extent at this point by the liver before it reaches the general circulation.

Drug Distribution

Following an intravenous dose of a drug, there appears to be an exponential decline in drug concentration over time. The drug is distributed from the vascular compartment into extravascular tissue sites. Some drug in the plasma is bound to plasma proteins at varying extents depending on the drug.

Non-protein-bound drug is free to equilibrate with tissue receptor sites and the plasma proteins. The free drug is the pharmacologically active fraction.

The decline in concentration of many drugs is biexponential when plotted as the log of concentration versus time (Fig. 29-1). This biexponential curve represents a two-compartment model of drug distribution (alpha phase) and drug elimination (beta phase). The two-compartment model is complex and difficult to appreciate at times. The one-compartment model is more useful for the clinician and can easily be used to derive certain clinical pharmacokinetic parameters such as the volume of distribution and half-life of the drug.

The distribution of drug into the vascular space, body water space, and tissue sites is a pharmacologic concept termed the "apparent volume of distribution." This is not a real volume, but a concept that describes the characteristics of the drug (eg, its lipid or water solubility and the extent of its plasma protein binding and tissue binding). A drug that is confined chiefly to the vascular and body water space with relatively low tissue binding has a low volume of distribution; a lipid-soluble drug with a high degree of tissue binding has a large volume of distribution. The volume of distribution is also affected by plasma protein binding. Disease states and other drugs can change the free fraction of a drug by displacing it from protein-binding sites. This would increase the free, pharmacologically active fraction. Increased binding to plasma protein tends to decrease the volume of distribution. Volume of distribution is given in units of liters per kilogram.

A large volume of distribution would be greater than 1 L/kg. The volume of distribution (V_d) is related to the plasma concentration (C_p) and administered drug dose (D) by the following equation (in a simplified one-compartment model):

$$V_d = \frac{D}{C_p}$$

where V_d = L/kg × body weight in kg
D = mg (dose administered intravenously)
C_p = mg/L (μg/mL)

The volume of distribution of a drug can be determined from a one-compartment model or a two-compartment model by extrapolating a straight line from the elimination phase back to what the concentration would have been at C_{p0} (Fig. 29-2). At least three drug concentrations should be obtained once the drug is in the elimination phase in order to more accurately describe this line. The C_{p0} is the assumed drug concentration at time 0 if instantaneous distribution had occurred. C_{p0} can be entered into the above equation along with the administered intravenous dose (D) in milligrams, to obtain the volume of distribution.

The one-compartment model assumes that both distribution and elimination are occurring in only the central

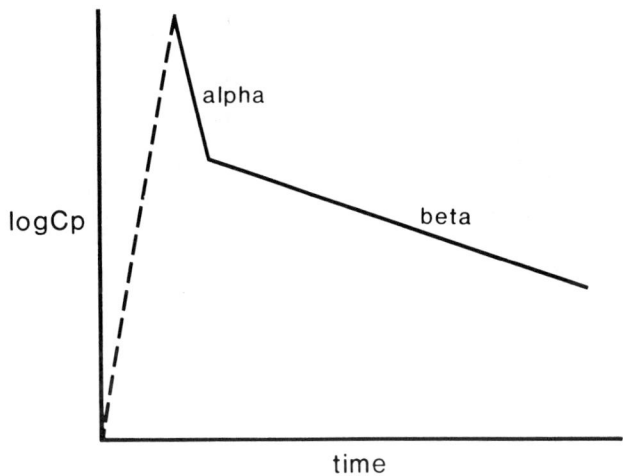

Figure 29-1 Biphasic decline in drug concentration over time following an intravenous drug dose.

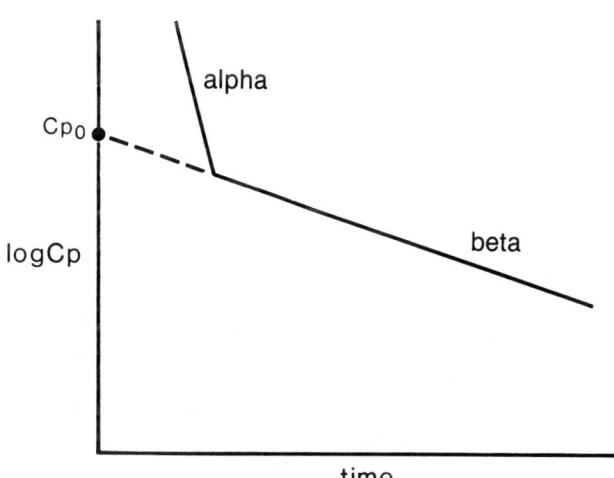

Figure 29-2 The one-compartment model.

(plasma) compartment. In reality, several compartments, representing various tissue areas, are involved. The two-compartment model most closely approximates the real situation since it assumes that the drug is distributed from the central compartment to a peripheral compartment where it must be redistributed back to the central compartment to be metabolized and eliminated. However, the one-compartment model is useful to the clinician.

The volume of distribution can be used to calculate either the amount of certain drugs in the body when plasma concentration is known or to calculate a loading dose needed to obtain a specific plasma concentration (a partial listing of volumes of distribution is given in Table 29-3). For example, using a known volume of distribution (V_d) to calculate the loading dose (D) required (in a one-compartment model),

Table 29-3 Volumes of Distribution (V_d = L/kg)

Drug	Older Children	Adults
Acetaminophen	1–1.2	1–1.2
Digoxin	15	7.5
Furosemide	0.20	0.25
Phenobarbital	0.75	0.75
Phenytoin	0.75	0.60–0.80
Salicylates	0.3–0.6*	0.3–0.6*
Theophylline	0.45	0.45
Ethanol	0.60	0.60

*V_d of salicylate changes in an overdose from 0.30 to 0.60 L/kg.

Source: Modified and reprinted with permission from Kempe CH, Silver HK, O'Brien D (eds): *Current Pediatric Diagnosis and Treatment.* 8th ed. Copyright 1984 by Lange Medical Publications, Los Altos, California.

to obtain a theophylline blood level of 15 μg/mL in a 70-kg adult results in the following calculation:

$$V_d = 450 \text{ mL/kg for theophylline in an adult}$$
$$450 \text{ mL/kg} = \frac{D}{15 \text{ μg/mL}}$$
$$(450 \text{ mL/kg}) \times (70 \text{ kg}) = 31.5 \text{ L}$$
$$15 \text{ μg/mL} = 15 \text{ mg/L}$$
$$31.5 \text{ L} = \frac{D}{15 \text{ mg/L}}$$
$$(31.5 \text{ L})(15 \text{ mg/L}) = 473 \text{ mg}$$
$$D = 473 \text{ mg}$$

Since aminophylline is 80% theophylline, the adjusted dose of aminophylline in a 70-kg adult would be 591 mg administered slowly over 30 minutes intravenously to achieve a 15 μg/mL therapeutic level.

The volume of distribution concept can also be useful when a patient is subtherapeutic on either theophylline or phenytoin and the concentration needs to be increased. In order to increase phenytoin concentration from 5 μg/mL to 15 μg/mL (an increment of 10 μg/mL), the following calculation can be made:

$$V_d = 600 \text{ mL/kg for phenytoin}$$
$$600 \text{ mL/kg} = \frac{D}{10 \text{ μg/mL}}$$
$$(600 \text{ mL/kg})(10 \text{ μg/mL}) = D = 6000 \text{ μg/kg} = 6 \text{ mg/kg}$$

Therefore, to raise a phenytoin blood level 10 μg/mL, 6 mg/kg can be administered intravenously (assuming V_d = 600 mL/kg).

Biotransformation

Elimination of a drug includes biotransformation into pharmacologically active or inactive metabolites. Polar drugs and metabolites are primarily excreted by the kidneys, whereas nonpolar drugs are first metabolized by the liver to more polar compounds. Biotransformation of a drug taken in overdose may be very important clinically. For example, amitriptyline, imipramine, and doxepin are tertiary amines and are metabolized to their respective secondary amines nortriptyline, desipramine, and nordoxepin. Both the parent compounds and metabolites are further hydroxylated. All of these are toxicologically active and influence the clinical course of a tricyclic antidepressant overdose. Amoxapine is metabolized to 7-hydroxy and an 8-hydroxy amoxapine metabolite. The 8-hydroxyamoxapine metabolite has a half-life of 30 hours and may account for prolonged toxicity. Thus drug metabolism and biotransformation may account for prolonged toxicity.

DRUG ELIMINATION, HALF-LIFE, AND CLEARANCE

Following distribution, elimination begins. Elimination is through the central compartment. The elimination phase of drug metabolism may follow one of two pharmacokinetic processes or a combination of two processes: (1) first-order elimination kinetics and (2) zero-order elimination kinetics.

Most drugs are eliminated by a first-order process (ie, the amount of drug metabolized per unit time is a constant fraction of the total drug present and does not vary with the plasma concentration of the drug). Most drugs are eliminated in this manner. In contrast, a constant amount of drug is metabolized per unit time with zero-order elimination. The metabolic mechanism for the drug elimination is saturated and cannot proceed faster than its maximal rate of metabolism.

The time required for one-half of a drug to be eliminated from the body is termed the drug half-life. Since most drugs are eliminated by a first-order process, it can be predicted that 97% of a drug will be removed from the body in five half-lives. Thus, if a patient has a theophylline level of 40 μg/mL with a half-life of 4 hours, then the patient will have a level of 20 μg/mL in 4 hours and 10 μg/mL in 8 hours. Detailed reviews of clinical pharmacokinetics are available elsewhere.[143,144]

Understanding the two processes can be clinically useful in certain overdose instances. For example, phenytoin elimination is normally a first-order process at levels below 20 μg/mL and the drug has a half-life of 22 hours. In an overdose, however, the elimination process changes from first order to zero order as the plasma level rises above 20 μg/mL. Thus, owing to the saturation of the hydroxylation process that is the major metabolic route of phenytoin, the patient with a phenytoin overdose may require several days to eliminate the drug. Knowing this will help the clinician predict the course of a patient with such an overdose.

Clearance is the term applied to the volume of blood or plasma from which drug is eliminated per unit time (mL/min). The sum of individual clearances adds up to a total body clearance. Clearance can be derived from the volume of distribution and the elimination constant (k_{el}). The elimination constant is derived from the (beta) phase of drug elimination and is related to the slope of this phase:

$$\text{slope} = \frac{-k_{el}}{2.303}$$

The product of the k_{el} and the volume of distribution yields the clearance value (Cl) of a drug:

$$k_{el} \times V_d = Cl$$

Once the Cl of a certain drug is known, the maintenance dose for maintaining a steady-state plasma level (C_{pss}) is given by:

$$Cl \times C_{pss} = \text{maintenance dose}$$

Clearance can also be calculated from the rate of administration of an infusion once a steady-state plasma drug concentration is achieved:

$$Cl = \frac{\text{Rate of infusion}}{C_{pss}}$$

Clearance can also be calculated from the area under the curve (AUC) described by the time versus concentration of the drug. After a single intravenous dose, the clearance can be derived from the following equation:

$$Cl = \frac{\text{dose}}{\text{AUC}}$$

Clearance is a more appropriate term than the elimination half-life to describe a drug's total body elimination. The half-life is a pharmacokinetic term that depends on both the clearance and the volume of distribution of a drug:

$$\text{half-life} = 0.693 \, Cl \times V_d$$

The half-life is thus inversely proportional to clearance. The half-life can also be determined from a graphic display of the elimination phase of a drug by noting the time required for the drug concentration to decrease by one half. The half-life is related to the slope of this elimination phase and the constant of elimination by the following equation:

$$\text{half-life} = \frac{0.693}{k_{el}}$$

By plotting out three drug concentration points in the elimination phase the following pharmacokinetic parameters can be estimated: half-life, volume of distribution, constant of elimination, and the clearance.

DRUG DISPOSITIONS AND PHARMACOKINETIC CONSIDERATIONS IN THE NEONATE AND ELDERLY

Patients in the extremes of age groups present special pharmacokinetic problems that must be considered in both therapeutic and overdose situations. The neonate and premature infant generally have a larger volume of distribution because of an increase in the extracellular fluid and the decreased ability of fetal plasma proteins to bind drugs. The premature infant has much less protein-binding ability than the neonate. Adult values for plasma protein may not be attained until the infant is over 1 year of age.[145] Free fatty acids and bilirubin are also increased in neonates, which would tend to displace some drugs from protein-binding sites. Highly protein-bound drugs, such as salicylates and phenytoin, can displace bilirubin from binding sites, leading to possible hyperbilirubinemia. Salicylate plasma protein binding is decreased in the neonate, and the volume of distribution is approximately 600 mL/kg, twice the adult value.[145,146] Premature infants and neonates also have a relative hypoxemia and a lower blood pH that can lead to increased tissue concentrations of salicylates.[145]

The volume of distribution of phenytoin in the neonate is twice that of the adult.[147,148] The level of non–protein-bound phenobarbital is 60% in the neonate versus 50% in the adult.[149] Tricyclic antidepressants are generally greater than 90% protein bound in plasma; however, increased free levels in the neonate can certainly result in increased toxic reactions. In general, the increased volume of distribution of drugs and the decreased plasma protein binding can result in a higher plasma/tissue ratio of the drug than would be expected in an older child or adult, leading to possible toxicity.

The premature infant and neonate also have a decreased ability to biotransform drugs through hydroxylation and a decreased plasma esterase activity.[145] However, the ability to N-demethylate is present.

Renal function is reduced in the newborn; adult functional levels are not reached until 6 to 12 months of age.[150] The renal functions of glomerular filtration and tubular secretion do not mature at the same rate. The development of tubular secretory capacity lags behind the development of glomerular filtration capacity so that the premature infant has difficulty handling some drugs even though glomerular filtration is possible. Furosemide (Lasix), for example, is a drug that depends on both glomerular filtration and active tubular transport.[151] The ability of a premature infant to secrete furosemide actively is much different from that of the full-term infant. Furosemide half-life in the premature infant may be prolonged up to 20 hours, whereas in the full-term infant the half-life may be only 7 hours. In the healthy adult, it is 30 minutes.[152]

The elderly are another group who can have alteration in drug disposition and metabolism. An elderly patient has a decrease in muscle mass with respect to the total body weight. Along with this is a decrease in GFR of around 35%. This decrease in GFR affects drugs like digoxin, procainamide, and lithium.[153] Hepatic blood flow decreases with age 40% to 45% below the normal and as a result drugs whose metabolism depends on hepatic blood flow will be affected.[154] Oxidative metabolism can also be impaired to some extent in the elderly. There is also the suggestion that receptor sensitivity changes. The elderly have increased sensitivity to benzodiazepines and warfarin and reduced sensitivity to β agonists and antagonists.[153] Absorption of drugs from the gastrointestinal tract is not significantly altered in the elderly, although it may be in the neonate because the neonate has irregular peristalsis and prolonged gastric emptying. Also, the premature infant has a relative achlorhydria compared with the full-term infant. The gastric pH of a neonate is 6 to 8, but reaches adult values by 1 year of age.[145] The elderly do not have drastic changes in drug volumes of distribution; however, some decrease in plasma protein binding can occur.

Theophylline is a commonly used drug that has different kinetics in the different age groups. In the premature infant, it has a prolonged elimination half-life, owing to a decreased elimination rate and an increased volume of distribution up to 690 mL/kg.[150] Elderly patients may also have a decreased theophylline elimination; the drug may have a prolonged half-life owing to a decrease in hepatic and renal blood flow secondary to congestive heart failure or decreased cardiac output associated with aging.

The disposition of drugs in the newborn and elderly must be a real concern to the physician in order to manage an intoxication properly or to prevent an iatrogenic complication.

SPECIFIC DRUGS AND TOXINS

Theophylline

The therapeutic range for theophylline is 10 to 20 μg/mL[155] and serum concentrations much above 20 μg/mL can produce toxicity. Overdose of theophylline-containing compounds can cause ventricular dysrhythmias, focal and generalized seizures, hallucinations, tremors, hyperreflexia, hyperpnea, tachypnea, hyperthermia, gastrointestinal hemorrhage, coma, hypotension, tachycardia, and cardiovascular collapse.[60,61,156] Theophylline-induced seizures may be refractory to conventional anticonvulsant therapy; ventricular ectopy may also be difficult to control. Theophylline overdose may result in metabolic derangements that include hypokalemia, hypophosphatemia, hypomagnesemia, hyperglycemia, and mild lactic acidemia. Clinical investigations reveal increased concentrations of circulating epinephrine and norepinephrine[157–159] following overdose. There is increasing evidence that theophylline in high overdose concentrations may be eliminated by mixed first- and zero-order kinetic processes.[160] Prolonged theophylline half-lives with toxic plasma concentrations have been reported.[161]

Theophylline toxicity may also occur secondary to decreased clearance in patients with pulmonary edema, liver disease, and congestive heart failure.[162] These patients require the same theophylline loading dose as other patients, but the maintenance doses should be decreased to avoid toxicity.

Some patients may tolerate very high theophylline levels with a paucity of signs and symptoms.[163] Therefore, if a toxic reaction to theophylline is suspected, the level should be determined as soon as possible. Such a toxic reaction may also be misinterpreted as abdominal pain with gastrointestinal bleeding.

Treatment is mainly supportive. However, if seizures and dysrhythmias occur, conventional antidysrhythmic and anticonvulsive therapy should be employed and hemodialysis should be considered. A patient may be managed conservatively with cardiac monitoring, activated charcoal in multiple doses, and electrolyte replacement as long as the theophylline half-life is not prolonged beyond the normal 6 hours and seizures and dysrhythmias do not occur. Should the half-life be prolonged significantly, then hemodialysis should be considered.

Hemodialysis using hollow-fiber systems has been reported to yield higher theophylline clearance values than coil systems.[164] In fact, this system yields clearance figures comparable to hemoperfusion.[165] Hemodialysis using hollow-fiber systems produced clearance values ranging from 130% to 387% above intrinsic clearance of theophylline.[164] Hemoperfusion or hemodialysis can be life saving in severe theophylline intoxications.

The use of multiple doses of activated charcoal has been shown to increase the elimination of theophylline and reduce the half-life.[166] This effect is more pronounced in patients with prolonged theophylline half-lives below 7 hours with a range of 3.0 to 7.1 hours. The dosing regimen consisted of an initial 40 g followed up with 20 g every 2 hours until the theophylline concentration was below 25 μg/mL.

The clinical use of sustained-release preparations of theophylline has resulted in serious problems following overdose. Prolonged theophylline concentrations result in sustained toxicity. Management consists of a thorough gut cleaning with charcoal and cathartics. Hemoperfusion and hemodialysis have been employed with some success; however, plasma theophylline levels may rebound if the drug is allowed to remain in the gut.

The use of the β blocker propranolol may be beneficial in reducing the systemic effects of increased circulating catecholamines. Small doses given intravenously have resulted in marked clinical improvement in cases of hypotension secondary to tachydysrhythmias. Propranolol may also be of benefit for extreme agitation and tremor.[167,168]

Tricyclic Antidepressants

Commonly ingested in overdose, tricyclic antidepressants may result in a clinical spectrum ranging from lethargy, hyperreflexia, sinus tachycardia, and delirium to coma, seizures, respiratory depression, hypotension, ventricular ectopy, and cardiac arrest. The mechanisms of tricyclic activity are (1) direct anticholinergic effect, (2) direct myocardial depression, and (3) blockade of norepinephrine reuptake. Cardiotoxicity is common, with intraventricular conduction delay, premature ventricular contractions, ventricular tachycardia, and ventricular fibrillation.[169] Neurologic effects include seizures, myoclonus, choreoathetosis, loss of oculovestibular reflexes, loss of muscle stretch reflexes, and pupillary changes.[170] Tricyclics are highly lipophilic, are absorbed rapidly from the small intestines, and have a large volume of distribution, signifying extensive tissue binding. The parent compounds of tricyclic antidepressants have half-lives between 24 and 36 hours. The active metabolites may take much longer to be eliminated.[24] Total plasma levels of tricyclic antidepressants do not correlate with symptomatology and cannot be depended on to predict outcome.

Amitriptyline (Elavil), doxepin (Sinequan), and imipramine (Tofranil) are tertiary amines and are N-demethylated by the liver to the corresponding secondary amines nortriptyline, nordoxepin, and desipramine, which are pharmacologically and toxicologically active. These are further hydroxylated to toxic metabolites.

Treatment is mainly supportive (eg, cardiac monitoring and pulmonary care). Intubation with respiratory support may be required because of respiratory depression. Hypotension can be managed initially with crystalloid fluids and secondarily with a vasopressor. The vasopressor of choice is norepinephrine. Intravenous sodium bicarbonate has been used to reverse ventricular ectopy in tricyclic intoxication. Even though there is speculation as to its mechanism of action, its clinical efficacy is well established. Original investigations using sodium bicarbonate appeared in 1973.[171] The postulated mechanism of action for ectopy reversal was an increase in the plasma binding of toxicologic active-free drug as the plasma pH became more alkaline. This study reported a decrease in the free fraction of amitriptyline from 18% to 2% as the plasma pH was increased from 6.7 to 7.5 in vitro. Other reports since 1973 substantiated the beneficial effects of plasma alkalinization to a pH of 7.4 to 7.5 either with bicarbonate intravenously or by hyperventilation.[172–176]

A recent investigation into the possible mechanism of dysrhythmia reversal with bicarbonate has reconfirmed the original investigation in 1973[177] that there is a significant decrease in the free fraction of drug as the plasma pH becomes more alkaline. This effect of plasma alkalinization on tricyclic antidepressants is similar to that found in studies of basic drugs such as lidocaine, bupivacaine, and propranolol. The plasma protein binding of this class of basic drugs, which are highly bound to α_1–acid glycoproteins in human plasma, all increase their binding as the plasma pH increases and decrease their binding in acidemia. Since tricyclic antidepressants have a high affinity for α_1–acid glycoprotein as the principal binding protein, it makes sense that their binding properties would behave similarly.[178–182]

Another in vivo study[183] reported that normal saline provided antidysrhythmic effects similar to that of sodium bicarbonate. However, the increase in plasma protein binding with an increase in plasma pH appears to be realistic and that in a patient with tricyclic cardiotoxicity and ventricular ectopy, administration of 1 mEq/kg of bicarbonate intravenously is warranted, as is maintaining the plasma pH between 7.4 and 7.5.

The use of physostigmine in reversing tricyclic-induced cardiac toxicity is not indicated. Physostigmine, in the past, had reportedly reversed delirium, agitation, supraventricular tachycardia, coma, and in some cases ventricular ectopy.[184] However, its clinical use in tricyclic antidepressants should be limited and can still be utilized in managing the anticholinergic symptomatology such as delirium and hallucinations if severe. Intravenous physostigmine administration even if given slowly can result in seizures, bradycardia, increased tracheobronchial secretions, and asystole.

Lidocaine and phenytoin have been used with success to reverse ventricular ectopy in tricyclic poisoning.[185] In some circumstances, bretylium has successfully terminated ectopy. Physostigmine, propranolol, and sodium bicarbonate have been shown to counter the effect of amitriptyline on the frequency of extrasystole threshold under experimental design.[185]

Phenytoin has received attention recently with respect to its use therapeutically to reverse dysrhythmias and to narrow a widened QRS interval in serious poisonings. However, there is some disagreement on the prophylactic value of phenytoin. One in vivo study demonstrated the potential efficacy of phenytoin in reversing dysrhythmias and narrowing prolonged QRS intervals.[186] Overall, the antidysrhythmic agents of choice are sodium bicarbonate, lidocaine, phenytoin, and bretylium.[187]

A patient with a history of ingestion of a tricyclic antidepressant should be admitted to the critical care unit for cardiac monitoring and observation if any signs of cardiac complications are present. This includes hypertension, tachycardia, and ECG changes even if the patient is otherwise stable. The tricyclics are absorbed from the gastrointestinal tract and distributed to tissue sites within 6 to 8 hours following ingestion. The maximal symptomatology usually occurs within the first 6 to 12 hours. Cardiac monitoring is necessary until the cardiac complications have abated. The elimination half-life of the parent compound may be 24 hours. Each of the metabolites will have its own elimination half-life. Plasma concentrations of a tricyclic may persist for days and be very high following a large ingestion.

However, plasma concentrations of the tricyclic and/or its metabolite do not correlate with the degree of toxicity. In the case of a symptomatic patient, a qualitative detection of tricyclics in the urine or plasma is sufficient to determine admission to the critical care unit.

The use of extracorporeal procedures such as hemoperfusion has received attention. In most cases where resin hemoperfusion was employed, there was no improvement in the clinical status[188]; however, there have been isolated reports of dramatic clinical improvement upon initiating the procedure.[189] In reviewing these cases of dramatic improvement, the procedure was found to have begun early and may have interrupted the distribution phase of the drug, thus quantitatively decreasing the amount of drug reaching deep tissue sites. At this time, though, hemoperfusion is not a recommended proven modality by which to manage a patient with tricyclic poisoning.

An overall conservative approach of preventing absorption with cleaning out the gut and cardiac monitoring is the nucleus of care. The management of tricyclic-induced cardiotoxicity can be approached as follows:

1. Correct any plasma pH imbalance to 7.4.
2. If ventricular dysrhythmias are occurring, administer 1 mEq/kg sodium bicarbonate intravenously. Raise the arterial pH to between 7.4 and 7.5.
3. If sodium bicarbonate does not reverse the ventricular ectopy, administer a loading dose of lidocaine and start a maintenance infusion to keep the plasma concentration between 2 and 5 μg/mL.
4. Phenytoin can be administered as a loading dose of 15 to 18 mg/kg, or as 1000 mg to an adult, to achieve a plasma concentration between 10 to 20 μg/mL.
5. Hyperventilation can also be employed to raise arterial pH.
6. If the above measures are of no benefit, a loading dose of bretylium may be tried, 5 to 10 mg/kg intravenously.
7. There is no need to give phenytoin prophylactically, even when QRS prolongation is present, if the patient is stable hemodynamically.
8. Stop seizure activity if it is prolonged. Seizure activity will worsen metabolic acidosis and increase risk of cardiac toxicity. General muscular paralysis is indicated in extreme cases for stopping muscular activity in order to control ventricular ectopy.

Other Cyclic Antidepressants

Since the discovery of the more traditional tricyclic antidepressants, newer antidepressants have come on the market for managing depression. Some of these agents are newer tricyclics such as loxapine and amoxapine. Others represent different cyclic structures such as the tetracyclics, maprotiline (Ludiomil) and mianserin (Norval), or bicyclic antidepressants, zimelidine and viloxazine. There is even a new noncyclical class represented by trazodone (Desyrel).

Newer Tricyclics—Loxapine and Amoxapine

Loxapine (Loxitane) and amoxapine (Asendin), newer tricyclic antidepressants, are dibenzoxazepines similar in structure to the tricyclic antidepressant imipramine. Loxapine is actually the parent compound of amoxapine. Pharmacologically these two new drugs share activity similar to antidepressants and antipsychotics. They both inhibit the reuptake of norepinephrine. Loxapine has a half-life of 6 to 8 hours. Its principal metabolite is amoxapine. Amoxapine is hydroxylated by the liver to two primary active metabolites, 8-hydroxyamoxapine and 7-hydroxyamoxapine. The half-life of amoxapine is 8 hours, and the half-lives of the metabolites are 30 hours for the 8-hydroxy metabolite and 4 to 6 hours for the 7-hydroxy metabolite.[190,191] The 8-hydroxyamoxapine, with the prolonged elimination half-life, accumulates in both therapeutic doses and overdoses. Amoxapine and its metabolites also have dopamine receptor blocking properties, which are greater than imipramine but not as great as haloperidol.[190]

Overdose with both loxapine and amoxapine has become more commonplace. Most of the symptomatology is central nervous system depression and seizures. There appears to be little in the way of the severe cardiac complications as seen with the more traditional tricyclics. One small series of cases documented the lack of amoxapine-related cardiotoxicity following overdose.[192] Another larger series pointed out the high incidence of seizure activity associated with overdoses of amoxapine.[193] Management of the overdose situation involving these drugs should include supportive care and aggressive management of seizures.

Tetracyclic Antidepressants

The tetracyclic antidepressants are represented by maprotiline (Ludiomil) and mianserin (Norval). Maprotiline is chemically distinct from the tricyclics because of an ethylene bridge across its central ring giving it a tetracyclic structure. Maprotiline inhibits the reuptake of norepinephrine predominantly and has a weaker effect on inhibiting the reuptake of serotonin. It has strong sedative properties as well as strong anticholinergic effects and α-receptor blocking activities.[194]

Following oral ingestion, maprotiline is completely absorbed and distributed within 9 to 16 hours. The elimination half-life of the parent compound averages 43 hours.[194] Maprotiline is metabolized by N-demethylation, deamination, and hydroxylations of the aromatic and aliphatic rings. The demethylated metabolite appears in appreciable concentrations. The volume of distribution of maprotiline has been estimated to be 231 mL/kg.[194] In overdose, maprotiline can produce lethargy, coma, seizures, cardiac dysrhythmias, cardiac arrest, hypotension, mild hypertension, bradycardia, delirium, and hallucinations.[195-197]

Mianserin (Norval), unlike maprotiline and the tricyclics, does not affect the reuptake of norepinephrine. Instead, it combines presynaptic α-receptor blocking activity with antihistaminic and sedative properties. Mianserin has minimal central nervous system anticholinergic effects. Like maprotiline, it has a large volume of distribution with an elimination half-life of 10 hours. Overdoses with mianserin have been described and symptomatology includes lethargy, coma, hypotension, sinus tachycardia, and mild hypertension.[196]

Overdose management of the tetracyclic antidepressants is concerned mainly with supportive care and seizure management.

Bicyclic Antidepressants

Zimelidine and viloxazine are bicyclic antidepressants currently under investigation. Zimelidine has an elimination half-life of 5 to 8 hours. Its major metabolite, norzimelidine, has an elimination half-life of up to 30 hours and can thus accumulate in therapeutic and overdose situations. The antidepressant action of zimelidine is through its inhibition of serotonin uptake. Norzimelidine is 10 times more potent than the parent drug in this activity. Zimelidine has minimal effects on norepinephrine reuptake.

In overdose, the bicyclics have been associated with coma, seizures, hypotension, miosis, and sinus tachycardia. Management is supportive.

Trazodone

Trazodone (Desyrel) is a new class of antidepressants. Chemically, trazodone is a triazolopyridine derivative with pharmacological properties much different from the other more traditional antidepressants. Trazodone is an inhibitor of serotonin reuptake.[198] In acute overdose, trazodone has shown to be remarkably devoid of major, life-threatening symptomatology.[199-201] Drowsiness, ataxia, nausea, vomiting, dry mouth, and mild hypotension have been reported. The drug appears to be relatively much safer in overdose as compared with other antidepressants. It also appears to lack the significant cardiovascular and respiratory toxic effects associated with the more traditional antidepressants.

Methanol and Ethylene Glycol

These are aliphatic alcohols that cause severe metabolic acidosis with a large anion gap. Both methanol and ethylene glycol are nontoxic as the parent compound, but are metabolized by alcohol dehydrogenase and aldehyde dehydrogenase to their respective acids and aldehydes—which are toxic. Both methanol and ethylene glycol are ingredients of antifreeze and deicers. Ethylene glycol is metabolized to glycoaldehyde by alcohol dehydrogenase and then to glycolic acid by aldehyde dehydrogenase. The glycolic acid is the major metabolite and is most likely responsible for the metabolic acidosis.[202] Other acids are formed in the metabolism of ethylene glycol, but they are rapidly metabolized. Less than 3% of ethylene glycol is actually converted to oxalic acid.[202,203] Ethylene glycol poisoning is diagnosed by findings of a marked anion gap, metabolic acidosis, hyperoxaluria, intoxication similar to ethanol intoxication. Seizures and coma are late sequelae.

Methanol is metabolized by alcohol dehydrogenase to formaldehyde, which is metabolized by aldehyde dehydrogenase to formic acid. Methanol by itself may cause gastrointestinal distress with epigastric pain, but does not seem to produce the intoxication syndrome as ethanol does. Optic nerve damage can occur with methanol poisoning and may result in blindness. The optic nerve damage is possibly due to the accumulation of formate in the choroid plexus and optic nerve tissue, which damages the mitochondria and inhibits cytochrome oxidase activity.[204,205] Another central nervous system aspect of methanol poisoning is putaminal infarction, which can be readily evaluated by computerized tomographic scanning.[206,207]

Treatment of both ethylene glycol poisoning and methanol poisoning includes correction of the metabolic acidosis, prevention of further metabolism of the parent compounds, and consideration of hemodialysis. Ethanol prevents the metabolism of both methanol and ethylene glycol by alcohol dehydrogenase. It has a greater affinity for the alcohol dehydrogenase enzyme and can be given in a loading dose of 1 mL/kg intravenously (diluted in normal saline or dextrose and water) of absolute ethanol to achieve a blood level of approximately 130 mg/dL. Oral loading is also acceptable. An ethanol concentration of 125 mg/dL will almost completely block the metabolism of ethylene glycol and methanol to their respective organic acids.[208] Ethanol loading can also be achieved by giving 10 mL/kg of a 10% ethanol and dextrose solution as an intravenous bolus, to achieve a blood alcohol of 125 mg/dL. Sodium bicarbonate is administered to correct the existing acidosis. After the loading dose of ethanol is given and the blood ethanol level is documented to be over 100 mg/dL, an ethanol maintenance infusion is begun. Ethanol is metabolized at a rate of between 70 and 175 mg/kg/hour.[208] Calculation of the maintenance infusion uses the average metabolic rate of 125 mg/kg/hour as follows:

$$\frac{(125 \text{ mg/kg/hour})(\text{kg wt of patient})}{750 \text{ mg/mL (density of ethanol)}}$$
$$= \text{mL/hour of absolute ethanol to maintain level at 100 mg/dL}$$

The density of 95% ethanol is 750 mg/mL, and dividing by this gives the milliliters per hour of absolute ethanol required to maintain the desired ethanol level. Maintenance dosing is also achieved by a 10% ethanol and dextrose solution (simply multiply the maintenance dose of 95% ethanol by 10). Once the metabolism of ethylene glycol and methanol is blocked, the parent compounds are renally eliminated over a period of days. Hemodialysis should be performed on a patient with ethylene glycol or methanol poisoning. Also, since the renal excretion of methanol and ethylene glycol may require up to 5 days once metabolism is blocked, hemodialysis morbidity can be weighed against the morbidity of ethanol therapy for several days. Ethanol infusions should be maintained during the hemodialysis. The infusion rate will have to be almost doubled because the ethanol is dialyzable also. Hemodialysis is very effective at removing methanol, ethylene glycol, and ethanol.[209] The requirements for intervention by hemodialysis are based on the clinical condition of the patient, the concentration of ethylene glycol or methanol, and the presence of metabolic acidosis.

SALICYLATES

Overdose with aspirin is a common cause of metabolic acidosis with an anion gap. Salicylates have numerous pharmacologic, toxicologic, and metabolic effects in overdose:

- direct stimulation of the central respiratory center with resulting hyperpnea and tachypnea
- uncoupling of oxidative phosphorylation
- interference with glucose metabolism
- interference with the Krebs cycle
- increased lipolysis
- increased plasma amino acids
- fluid and electrolyte loss with total body potassium depletion
- decreased platelet adhesiveness
- decreased prothrombin formation
- decreased level of factor VII
- increased pyruvate and lactic acid with a severe metabolic acidosis.[210,211]

Interference with glucose metabolism most frequently results in hyperglycemia, although hypoglycemia can occur. Salicylates have also been demonstrated to produce a decrease in central nervous system glucose levels with a peripheral normoglycemia.[211,212] Adults usually develop a combined metabolic acidosis and respiratory alkalosis, whereas children and infants develop a profound metabolic acidosis. Hyperpyrexia can also occur as a result of the hypothalamic effect of salicylates and uncoupling of oxidative phosphorylation.

Coma, seizures, and pulmonary edema are signs of serious salicylate intoxication. Morbidity and mortality are related to the central nervous system salicylate concentration, cerebral edema, the severity of the metabolic disorder, and pulmonary edema. Noncardiogenic pulmonary edema as a result of salicylate toxicity is well recognized and is attributed to increased epithelial permeability in the alveolar-capillary membrane.[56] Fluid retention with hyponatremia has been noted in a few cases of salicylate overdose. The central nervous system concentration of salicylates may be the most important factor contributing to morbidity and mortality.[213] The central nervous system and other tissue concentrations of salicylates are directly related to the alkalemia or acidemia of the patient. At a blood pH of 7.4, more than 99% of the salicylate is in an ionized form (pK_a equals 3); as acidemia supervenes, the amount of nonionized salicylate, and thus the amount available to cross biologic membranes, increases. As the pH of blood decreases from 7.4 to 7.2, the amount of nonionized salicylate that is available to enter the central nervous system doubles.[213]

The volume of distribution of salicylates increases with increasing plasma levels. The normal volume of distribution of salicylates ranges from 150 to 300 mL/kg at therapeutic concentrations, but it is increased in overdoses and may be as high as 600 mL/kg.[214] This increase may be attributed to increased tissue binding in an overdose.

The elimination of salicylate is zero order at two metabolic pathways: formation of salicyluric acid and salicyl phenolic glucuronide metabolites. Thus, in an overdose, the elimination kinetics can change from first order to zero order. The metabolites of salicylate are excreted renally when they are formed.[214]

Salicylism can be divided into acute and chronic conditions. Both types are associated with dehydration, potassium depletion, and acidosis, the triad of salicylism. However, in chronic salicylism, the hypokalemia and acidosis are more profound. The salicylate blood level in chronic poisoning can be very low as opposed to a high level seen with an acute overdose. Chronic salicylism results from continued administration of aspirin that saturates the metabolic pathways. Usually, this occurs in a child who is already dehydrated from vomiting and diarrhea and is receiving salicylates for fever therapy. Treatment of salicylate poisoning is often delayed because it is not recognized until late in the clinical course when metabolic acidosis is a prominent feature. The clinical presentation can include lethargy, coma, vomiting, diarrhea, tachypnea, hyperpnea, pulmonary edema, seizures, and hyperthermia, as well as the electrolyte and metabolic derangements. Treatment is aimed at restoring depleted vascular volume and electrolytes, and correcting the metabolic acidosis. Alkaline diuresis has proved effective in increasing renal salicylate elimination by trapping anions in tubular lumen. However, before an alkaline urine can be achieved, total body potassium must be repleted. The patient should be rehydrated with normal saline and receive potassium replacement before alkaline diuresis is begun.

The Done salicylate nomogram is useful in determining the severity of intoxication in acute overdose cases,[215] but the nomogram requires that a salicylate level be obtained no earlier than 6 hours postingestion. Therefore, the nomogram is not helpful with chronic salicylism. Hemodialysis is indicated in salicylate poisoning if the patient is having seizures or severe mental status alteration, has pulmonary edema, or has electrolyte abnormalities and an acid-base imbalance that cannot be controlled (see Chapter 21, Acid-Base Disturbances).

Acetaminophen

Commonly used as an aspirin substitute for analgesia, acetaminophen has become recognized as a cause of hepatotoxicity in overdose. Acetaminophen is a pharmacologically active metabolite of phenacetin. Its metabolism involves sulfate conjugation, glucuronide conjugation, and glutathione conjugation. Although the conjugation with glutathione involves only 3.8% of the metabolic pathway,[216] this is the pathway that determines whether or not hepatotoxicity will occur. Should glutathione reserves be depleted in a massive acute overdose, then a reactive intermediate is formed via this minor metabolic route. This active intermediate covalently binds to protein structures in hepatocytes, causing hepatocellular necrosis. Animal studies indicate that 70% to 80% of the intracellular glutathione stores must be depleted before hepatotoxicity occurs.[216]

The earliest symptoms of an acute overdose are gastrointestinal distress with some epigastric pain. Hepatocellular damage is usually manifested in 48 hours with rising levels of hepatic enzymes. Abnormalities of coagulation and renal failure may also occur. The levels of hepatic enzymes usually peak in 4 to 5 days and then return to normal. A plasma acetaminophen concentration should be obtained, at the earliest, 4 hours following the ingestion. This concentration should be below 150 µg/mL at 4 hours and below 37.5 µg/mL at 12 hours. A nomogram is available to aid in deciding probability of hepatotoxicity as well as the need for treatment with N-acetylcysteine.[217,218]

Treatment involves the administration of N-acetylcysteine (Mucomyst), which acts as a glutathione surrogate to detoxify the active intermediate.[217] N-Acetylcysteine is administered orally as a loading dose of 140 mg/kg and then given as a maintenance dose of 70 mg/kg every 4 hours for 3 days.[217] It should be administered within the first 24 hours following the overdose to be effective. Death from acetaminophen-induced hepatotoxicity is usually due to a combination of hepatic encephalopathy and acute renal failure, but it can be prevented with the administration of N-acetylcysteine within 24 hours of the overdose and with supportive care. If treated prior to 10 hours, the hepatotoxicity can be significantly blunted. Due to the relative lack of symptomatology early in the course following overdose, acetaminophen toxicity can be easily missed.

Intravenous N-acetylcysteine has proven useful in the British experience. This mode of administration is currently being investigated in the United States.

ANTICONVULSANTS

The most common anticonvulsants encountered by the clinician in overdose are phenytoin (Dilantin), phenobarbital, primidone (Mysoline), carbamazepine (Tegretol), and valproic acid (Depakene). Each of these anticonvulsants has its own unique clinical toxicologic spectrum in overdose.

Phenytoin

One drug that changes elimination kinetics from first order to zero order in overdose situations is phenytoin. The therapeutic range for phenytoin is 10 to 20 µg/mL. Below 20 µg/mL, phenytoin is eliminated by first-order process, and the half-life is approximately 22 hours. The half-life may be much shorter in some situations, however. When phenytoin concentrations rise above 20 µg/mL, the enzymatic process that hydroxylates the phenyl ring and forms hydroxylphenyl-phenylhydantoin, the major phenytoin metabolite, becomes saturated and the elimination of phenytoin becomes dependent on a maximal rate of an enzymatic process. Thus, a patient with a phenytoin overdose and high phenytoin plasma levels can be expected to have a prolonged elimination course (ie, over days instead of the usual 22-hour half-life).

The change in phenytoin kinetics also has implications for therapeutic dosage. Because of the saturation process, even small changes in phenytoin doses can lead to large changes in plasma concentrations of the drug.

Phenytoin has a systemic bioavailability of 80% to 95% after oral dosing.[219] It is a weak acid, poorly soluble in water, and slowly absorbed from the small intestines. Being a weak acid, phenytoin precipitates in the acid medium of the stomach. Thus, in an overdose, it would be expected to be slowly absorbed over a period of 6 to 12 hours, and the clinician may see slowly rising plasma levels for hours. Therefore it becomes important to clear the stomach and small intestines of a patient who has overdosed on phenytoin, even if it is 12 hours after ingestion.

Phenytoin has a volume of distribution of approximately 600 mL/kg (body water space) and is about 90% bound to plasma albumin. It is displaced from albumin binding sites by hepatic disease, uremia, valproic acid, and salicylates.[220] Because it also readily crosses placental membranes, neonatal concentrations may be equal to maternal concentrations, a fact to be kept in mind in overdoses involving pregnant women.[220]

The clinical spectrum of phenytoin poisoning may range from nystagmus, slurred speech, and ataxia at lower concentrations to more pronounced cerebellar signs, confusion, choreoathetoid movement disorders, coma, and decerebrate rigidity at higher concentrations.[36,94] Treatment is mainly supportive, with monitoring of vital signs and plasma concentrations. Hemodialysis is of no benefit. The clinician should be aware that plasma phenytoin concentrations in overdose decline slowly over days and that the complete absorption of the drug from the gut may take hours.

Phenobarbital

The volume of distribution of phenobarbital is approximately 600 mL/kg, and the drug is 40% to 50% protein bound. The plasma half-life ranges from 1 to 3 days and is shorter in children than in adults. Metabolism is by hepatic first-order elimination. Therapeutic plasma concentrations range from 20 to 30 μg/mL. Phenobarbital is also a potent inducer of hepatic enzymes. In an overdose, phenobarbital may cause a clinical spectrum ranging from lethargy, nystagmus, and increased muscular activity to deep coma, areflexia, hypotension, hypothermia, and cardiovascular collapse.[221,222] Treatment of phenobarbital intoxication is mainly supportive care and includes the use of alkaline diuresis to increase urinary excretion. There is a fourfold increase in the excretion of phenobarbital when the pH of the urine exceeds 7.5.[223] Alkaline diuresis can result in an increased phenobarbital clearance and a quicker recovery. The effect of an alkaline diuresis is considerably less when a short-acting barbiturate, such as secobarbital or pentobarbital, is ingested. However, because the pK_a of the drug is higher than that of phenobarbital and urine, alkalinization cannot be achieved to that extent.[223] Multiple doses of activated charcoal will also increase phenobarbital clearance. Should pulmonary edema be present, a diuresis would be relatively contraindicated. Hemodialysis can also effectively remove a phenobarbital body burden.

Primidone

An anticonvulsant that is chemically related to phenobarbital, primidone is converted to phenobarbital and phenylethylmalonamide by hepatic metabolism. The anticonvulsant effects of primidone are primarily due to phenobarbital. The parent compound, primidone, and the phenylethylmalonamide metabolite have weak anticonvulsant properties. Therapeutic plasma levels of phenobarbital are obtained with chronic administration of primidone. An overdose of primidone should be managed as if it were a phenobarbital overdose. Primidone itself can result in mild central nervous system depression and over a period of 12 to 24 hours following an acute overdose the phenobarbital concentration should peak.

Carbamazepine

Now being more commonly employed as an anticonvulsant for grand mal seizures, carbamazepine is slowly absorbed from the small bowel over 12 hours.[224] The half-life of carbamazepine in overdose has been reported to range from 10 to 29 hours.[40] Carbamazepine follows first-order elimination, and the major metabolite is carbamazepine-10, 11-epoxide, which has anticonvulsant properties of its own. The clinical spectrum of carbamazepine intoxication may include various degrees of coma, respiratory depression, nystagmus, ataxia, slurred speech, seizures, hyperreflexia, absent bowel sounds, myoclonus, depressed reflexes, atrioventricular conduction delay with prolongation of the QRS interval, and sinus tachycardia.[40] Cyclic coma has been described following acute overdoses.[40,225] Carbamazepine is similar in chemical structure to imipramine hydrochloride and has anticholinergic properties that delay gastric emptying. Supportive care is essential in the management of acute overdoses. The removal of any remaining drug from the gastrointestinal tract is important, since delayed absorption occurs with delayed gastric emptying. Carbamazepine is 75% protein bound and has a volume of distribution ranging from 0.79 to 1.40 L/kg.[226] Data currently available on hemodialysis and hemoperfusion following acute overdoses indicate the efficacy of extracorporeal removal of the drug. Cardiac monitoring is important until the ECG is normal. Therapeutic concentrations of carbamazepine range from 2 to 8 μg/mL, but intoxication is generally evident at concentrations greater than 10 μg/mL.

Valproic Acid

Valproic (dypropylacetic) acid is a fatty acid with a small volume of distribution (100 to 400 mL/kg) and is greater than 90% protein bound. It is absorbed from the gastrointestinal tract within 1 to 4 hours following ingestion and has a plasma elimination half-life of 8 to 15 hours.[227] In neonates and young infants, the elimination half-life may be prolonged to 60 hours. Valproic acid displaces phenytoin from plasma protein binding sites, lowers the total phenytoin plasma level, and increases plasma levels of phenobarbital by interfering with elimination.[227,228] An overdose of valproic acid may cause deep coma. Gastrointestinal irritation with vomiting may also occur. Hepatotoxicity associated with valproic acid has been reported only with therapeutic doses.[229] Therapeutic plasma concentrations range from 50 to 100 μg/mL. Treatment is supportive.

Isoniazid

Isoniazid produces seizures and extreme metabolic acidosis with a large anion gap when ingested in an overdose. It is rapidly absorbed from the gastrointestinal tract; plasma concentrations peak in 1 to 2 hours. The volume of distribution of isoniazid is approximately 600 mL/kg, and the drug is only 15% bound to plasma proteins.[230] Isoniazid is acetylated by the liver to inactive metabolites. One of these metabolites is N-acetylhydrazine, which is thought to be responsible for isoniazid-induced hepatitis. Acetylation of isoniazid may be classified as slow or rapid, based on genetic phenotype; rapid acetylators have an autosomal dominate allele. Ingestion of a single large dose of isoniazid does not result in hepatotoxicity. The hepatitis is a result of chronic therapeutic doses. The half-life for isoniazid varies, depending on whether the patient is a rapid or slow acetylator. In rapid acetylators, the drug has a half-life of approximately 1 hour, in slow acetylators, 2 to 4 hours.[230]

In overdose, isoniazid may cause coma, convulsions, anion gap, metabolic acidosis, and hyperglycemia.[231] Owing to the rapid absorption of isoniazid, symptomatology usually occurs within an hour or less. The metabolic acidosis is due to lactic acidemia. Treatment of acute intoxication is based on controlling seizure activity and correcting the lactic acidosis. Seizures may be difficult to control until the acidosis is also corrected. Isoniazid interferes with the activity of pyridoxine, a cofactor in various important enzymatic reactions. Pyridoxine is a cofactor for central nervous system transaminases that transform glutamate into γ-aminobutyric acid (GABA), decarboxylases that are central to gluconeogenesis, and glycogen phosphorylases. In interfering with pyridoxine activity, various metabolic pathways are disturbed. The resulting decrease in the neuroinhibitor transmitter GABA can produce seizure activity. The other metabolic derangements present following isoniazid overdose are secondary to the various enzymatic systems being interfered with through pyridoxine depletion. Pyridoxine, given intravenously, may help control seizure activity. One gram of pyridoxine for each gram of isoniazid ingested has been recommended and has been clinically beneficial, along with intravenous diazepam, in helping to terminate seizures. Patients who ingest large amounts of isoniazid-pyridoxine combination tablets will also have seizures and acidemia. Once seizures have been terminated and the acidemia corrected, isoniazid is rapidly eliminated, and the coma resolves within 24 hours or less. Isoniazid excretion can be enhanced by a forced neutral diuresis. Also, should the seizures and acidemia be difficult to control, hemodialysis may be beneficial in removing the drug.

OVER-THE-COUNTER DRUGS AND ALERTNESS AGENTS

Nonprescription drugs are commonly ingested in overdoses, sometimes accidentally by small children.[232] Most of these drugs contain various anticholinergic compounds, phenylpropanolamine, caffeine, salicylates, acetaminophen, salicylamide, or phenacetin, and some small volume of ethanol. These drugs are sold as common cold preparations, sleep aids, alertness agents, diet aids, or sedatives. Over-the-counter sleep aids contain methapyrilene hydrochloride or pyrilamine and in overdose may cause seizures, delirium, tachycardia, hypertension, and coma. Children are more susceptible than adults. The anticholinergic syndrome is common with toxic ingestions of the cold preparations and sleep aids. Common cold preparations usually contain a form of antihistamine, such as chlorpheniramine maleate or phenylpropanolamine, together with an antipyretic in many cases. Preparations containing ethanol can result in seriously high blood ethanol levels if ingested by small children.

Management of over-the-counter ingestions is mainly supportive and is directed at controlling the symptomatology that can result from the anticholinergic drugs, such as hypertension, seizures, and tachycardia. The clinician should be aware of other ingredients in these preparations, such as caffeine, which can cause seizures, tachycardia, gastrointestinal bleeding, and cardiac dysrhythmias; acetaminophen, which may result in hepatocellular necrosis; salicylates, which may result in a metabolic acidosis; and ethanol, which can result in coma and hypoglycemia in children. Phenylpropanolamine-containing preparations have been associated with hypertension, headache, and in a few instances cerebral hemorrhage following ingestion of normally recommended doses.[233]

BENZODIAZEPINES, BENZODIAZEPINE ANTAGONIST, AND OTHER SEDATIVE-HYPNOTICS

The benzodiazepines include the commonly used drugs diazepam (Valium), chlordiazepoxide (Librium), oxazepam (Serax), lorazepam (Ativan), flurazepam (Dalmane), chlorazepate (Tranxene), clonazepam (Clonopin), and triazolam (Halcion). The elimination half-lives for diazepam and chlordiazepoxide vary between 20 and 50 hours. Diazepam, chlordiazepoxide, flurazepam, and chlorazepate are long-acting benzodiazepines and have a common pharmacologically active intermediary metabolite—desmethyldiazepam.[234] Chlorazepate undergoes acid hydrolysis in the stomach to desmethyldiazepam, whereas the other long-acting benzodiazepines are demethylated by the liver to desmethyldiazepam. Oxazepam and lorazepam, short-acting benzodiazepines, are both metabolized by hepatic glucuronidation. Oxazepam and lorazepam are metabolites of desmethyldiazepam.

Frequently ingested in overdose, the benzodiazepines have proven to be relatively safe. Large clinical reviews of benzodiazepines and their derivatives substantiate the low order of toxicity following acute oral overdose.[235–237] However, in combination with other central nervous system depressant drugs, the additive depressant effects of benzodiazepines can be very serious. Acute ingestions of ethanol along with a benzodiazepine can result in coma, respiratory depression, and death. Also, the acute ingestion of ethanol will temporarily block oxidative metabolism of drugs that are metabolized by the mixed function oxidase system in the liver, thus resulting in prolonged elimination of the drug as well as a prolongation of symptomatology.[238] Elderly patients with acute ingestions either as an overdose or in therapeutic amounts may have an increased duration of coma or central nervous system depression, especially when the benzodiazepines are combined with β blockers or cimetidine.

Triazolam (Halcion) is a new benzodiazepine with rapid onset after ingestion and a short half-life of both the parent drug (2 to 3 hours) and its metabolite (4 hours). Triazolam has been associated with serious and life-threatening respiratory depression in one overdose situation not involving other drugs.[239] As a result of the frequency of benzodiazepine overdose, research has led to the development of a benzodiazepine antagonist, which appears to be very effective in reversing coma and respiratory depression caused by any member of this category of drugs.[240]

Other sedative-hypnotics encountered in overdose are ethchlorvynol (Placidyl), glutethimide (Doriden), and chloral hydrate. Ethchlorvynol is rapidly absorbed in an overdose. It has a large volume of distribution, signifying a great deal of tissue binding. Clinically, ethchlorvynol overdose produces coma, usually prolonged, and respiratory depression. The half-life for ethchlorvynol is about 70 hours. Supportive care is the mainstay of treatment. Resin hemoperfusion has been advocated to treat serious overdoses,[241] but hemoperfusion techniques are limited by the large tissue distribution of ethchlorvynol plus its very slow redistribution back into plasma from tissue.[242] The benefit of hemoperfusion in ethchlorvynol intoxication remains questionable.

Glutethimide intoxication usually results in coma and respiratory depression. Glutethimide is irregularly absorbed from the gastrointestinal tract, has a large volume of distribution, and a half-life of up to 40 hours in overdose.[243] Conservative management usually results in a good outcome.[244] Chloral hydrate intoxication results in coma, respiratory depression, and sometimes cardiac dysrhythmias. Chloral hydrate is metabolized to trichloroethanol, the active metabolite, by alcohol dehydrogenase. The half-life of trichloroethanol has been calculated to be around 13 hours.[245] Hemodialysis appears to remove the trichloroethanol metabolite and may be beneficial in serious intoxication.[245]

ETHANOL AND ISOPROPANOL

Ethanol is associated with violent acts and dangerous behavior. More than 60% of suicides, homicides, child abuse, and spousal abuse are associated with alcoholism or the abuse of alcohol.[246-248] In the emergency setting, the most common cause of acute delirium and confusion in a patient is alcohol. Patients who are chronic drinkers may have very little in the way of gross motor dysfunction and virtually no obvious impairment at blood ethanol concentrations well above 200 mg/dL. In fact, many of these patients do not appear intoxicated on casual observation. There is a difference between the acute ingestion and chronic ingestion of ethanol in overdose.

The acute ingestion of ethanol in overdose can result in coma, respiratory depression, hyperosmolality, hypoglycemia, gastrointestinal bleeding, and metabolic acidosis.[86] Small children who ingest ethanol-containing products may experience seizures, respiratory depression, and hypoglycemia.[249] The chronic ingestion of ethanol is associated with many problems as a result of interference with carbohydrate, lipid, and protein metabolism.[86] Alcoholic ketoacidosis and lactic acidosis can be seen in the alcoholic population.[250] The management of ethanol ingestion in overdose includes providing respiratory support and correcting electrolyte problems and hypoglycemia. Ethanol can be removed by hemodialysis, if necessary (see Chapter 49, Alcohol Problems).

In acute overdose, ethanol will block the oxidative metabolism of a variety of drugs, including acetaminophen, long-acting benzodiazepines, and other drugs metabolized by the mixed function of oxidase system.[251]

The ingestion of isopropanol can cause gastrointestinal irritation, central nervous system depression, and coma. Approximately 15% to 19% of isopropanol is metabolized to acetone, which can be detected in blood and urine. Treatment is supportive, and hemodialysis is indicated in serious intoxications.

IMMUNOTHERAPEUTICS OF POISONINGS

Employment of antibodies for diagnostics and therapeutics has changed the science and practice of toxicology. Currently, immunotherapy for reversal of poisonings is limited to digoxin F(ab) fragments (Digibind) and antivenins. Development of hybridoma technology has led to large-scale production of monoclonal antibodies that recognize a single antigen only. Research is continuing into the possibility of drug and toxin neutralization by antibodies and antibody fragments.

Reversal of Digoxin Poisoning with Antidigoxin F(ab) Fragments

Digoxin in overdose can result in cardiac dysrhythmias, hyperkalemia, nausea, and vomiting. Cardiac dysrhythmias range from paroxysmal atrial tachycardia with block, premature ventricular contractions, and accelerated atrioventricular junctional rhythm to ventricular tachycardia, ventricular fibrillation, and severe conduction disturbances. Conventional therapy is directed at preventing or reversing dysrhythmias and treating hyperkalemia. Lidocaine, phenytoin, and bretylium have been used to treat ventricular ectopy. Sometimes a pacemaker is essential for high-degree atrioventricular block. Hyperkalemia is managed with insulin-glucose infusions and bicarbonate.

Failure of conventional therapy to reverse a life-threatening, digitalis-induced syndrome is indication for administration of digoxin-specific F(ab) fragments. In 21 of 26 cases initially reported, life-threatening cardiac dysrhythmias and hyperkalemia were reversed immediately.[252] F(ab) fragments are the portion of the whole immunoglobulin G (IgG) antibody retaining affinity for antigen. Digoxin F(ab) fragments were initially produced by papain enzymatic cleavage of sheep antidigoxin IgG antibodies. There are good reasons to use an F(ab) fragment instead of the whole antibody:

1. F(ab) fragments have a molecular weight of 50,000 compared with 150,000 for IgG. This allows for more favorable distribution and elimination kinetics.
2. F(ab) fragments, because of their smaller size, are renally cleared. IgG is cleared by the cells of the immune system and can thus set up future hypersensitivity reactions on re-exposure to the antibody as well as serum sickness reactions.

After antidigoxin F(ab) fragments are administered intravenously in patients with digoxin poisoning, the plasma digoxin level rises quickly. Digoxin redistribution from tissue to plasma is occurring, and binding to the high-affinity F(ab) fragment helps prevent the re-equilibration back into the tissue receptor sites and urinary excretion of bound and free digoxin is increased.[253] Digoxin F(ab) fragments have also been successfully employed in serious digitoxin poisoning; this demonstrates the cross-antigenicity of digoxin and digitoxin.[254]

Ovine source F(ab) fragments (Digibind, Wellcome Laboratories) have recently been approved by the Food and Drug Administration for human use. The cost of this preparation has stimulated research into potential use of hybridomas as a source of large amounts of antidigoxin monoclonal antibodies and F(ab) fragments.

Venom Poisoning and Antivenin

Presently, the only agents available for venom poisoning in the United States are polyvalent Crotalidae antivenin for snake venom poisoning (Wyeth Laboratories), black widow spider antivenin (Merck, Sharp & Dohme), and a scorpion antivenin which is produced in Arizona.

Venoms represent a complex biologic poison, unlike a single drug. There have been numerous proteins isolated from the venom of American poisonous snakes. The immunotherapeutic agent for snake venom poisoning in the United States is produced by hyperimmunization of horses with venom proteins. Hyperimmune serum is processed by ammonium sulfate precipitation and package lyophilized in a vial. Each vial of Wyeth Crotalidae polyvalent antivenin contains approximately 1.5 g of total protein.

Processing of hyperimmune serum with ammonium sulfate does not eliminate all extraneous proteins. Albumin and α and β globulins are still present.[255] Antivenin is given intravenously and a patient may receive as many as 10 to 20 vials for a treatment. Skin testing should always be done according to the package insert before administering any heterologous antivenin. The incidence of serum sickness may be as high as 50% to 75%. The actual IgG component of antivenin is 25% or less with respect to the total protein content of a vial.[255]

Investigations have demonstrated that high-affinity IgG(T), a subclass of equine IgG, can be isolated from hyperimmune serum.[256] This IgG(T) has not produced acute hypersensitivity reactions in animals or human cells in vitro sensitized to horse serum.[256]

Black widow spider antivenin (*Latrodectus mactans*, Merck, Sharp & Dohme) is also equine in source. The use of this antivenin is limited to very few indications, since envenomization by a black widow spider can be managed with conventional analgesics and muscle relaxants. Some authorities believe that small children and the elderly are more susceptible to the venom effects and should be considered for antivenin therapy if severely symptomatic following envenomization. The antivenin is lyophilized and available with 2.5 mL sterile water diluent in the kit. It is usually administered as a one-time dose intravenously. Hypersensitivity reactions and serum sickness can occur following its use. Skin testing can predict IgE-mediated sensitivity and is always recommended before administration of any horse serum product. The majority of black widow spider envenomizations can be safely managed without the antivenin. Black widow spider antivenin is not first-line therapy following envenomization. Patients with sensitivity to horse serum or a history of allergies should not receive black widow spider antivenin; instead they should be managed conservatively.

Scorpion antivenin is available only in Arizona, since this is where the majority of scorpion sting envenomizations occur. The antivenin is produced in goats. The use of this antivenin is restricted and is recommended only after failure of conventional therapy to control symptomatology.

METAL POISONING

Metal poisoning occurs mainly in occupational settings. Children are exposed to metals from contaminated food, soil, and the environment. The most common toxic metal exposures are lead, mercury, and arsenic.

Lead

Occupational exposure occurs in smelting, industrial activities involving paint removal, battery making, and stained glass work. Lead paint remains the major source of exposure in children.[257] Target organ pathophysiology from lead exposure occurs in the nervous system, hematopoietic system, and kidneys. Screening for lead poisoning is best done by measuring a blood lead concentration. In adults, a whole blood lead above 40 μg/dL represents an increased lead absorption. Under OSHA regulations, adults with blood leads above 50 μg/dL must be removed from occupational exposure until the concentration falls below 40 μg/dL.

In children, a blood lead concentration greater than 30 µg/dL reflects increased absorption. In addition to elevated blood lead concentrations, the diagnosis of increased lead exposure is also supported by measuring the erythrocyte protoporphyrin concentration. Elevation of erythrocyte protoporphyrin above 50 µg/dL indicates lead toxicity.

Anemia may be the first objective indication of lead poisoning. It is caused by lead interference with heme biosynthesis. Inhibition of ferrochelatase causes the accumulation of erythrocyte protoporphyrin in red blood cells. The nervous system is very sensitive to lead. High lead concentrations can result in toxic encephalopathy with coma and seizures. Asymptomatic children with lead exposure have been found to have diminished IQ scores. Low levels of lead exposure can produce irreversible changes in intelligence and behavior. Lead induced peripheral neuropathy can be manifested by segmental demyelination.

Lead nephrotoxicity results from damage to proximal tubular cells and glomeruli. Clinically, this can result in decreased glomerular filtration and impairment of renal tubular concentration. Interstitial fibrosis may result in chronic renal failure.

Mercury

Poisoning by mercury can be acute or chronic. Toxicity is caused mainly by inorganic and organic mercurial compounds. In addition, elemental mercury is also extremely poisonous. Mercury poisoning is mainly industrial; however, some acute toxicities occur in suicide attempts with mercury compounds. Methyl and ethyl mercury are used as antifungal agents and pesticides.

Elemental mercury vaporizes at room temperature and may produce acute encephalopathy and pulmonary insult.

Inorganic mercury in the form of mercuric chloride is occasionally ingested in suicide attempts. This results in acute bloody gastroenteritis, hypotension, and renal failure. Chronic inorganic mercury poisoning produces gingivitis, dermatitis, tremor, and central nervous system dysfunction in the form of an organic brain syndrome.

Organic mercury poisoning produces mainly a central nervous system syndrome. Congenital organic mercury poisoning (Minamata disease) can result from pregnant females being exposed to organic mercury compounds.[257]

Exposure is best determined by both blood and urine mercury measurements. Hair analysis is worthless for any metal poisoning determination.

Arsenic

Arsenic occurs in a trivalent (+3) and pentavalent (+5) form. Trivalent arsenic is the more poisonous of the two. Most arsenic poisoning occurs occupationally from mining and agricultural areas. Contaminated water has been a well-recognized source of chronic poisoning from arsenic.[258] Acute poisoning occurs mainly by suicidal ingestion.

Acute poisoning produces a clinical syndrome of gastroenteritis, hematemesis, and bloody diarrhea. Hypotension can result from volume loss due to necrosis of the bowel. Coma and seizures may follow.

Chronic arsenic poisoning targets the skin, nervous system, hematopoietic system, cardiovascular system, and respiratory tract.

Dermatologic lesions include eczematous dermatitis, hyperpigmented areas, and hyperkeratosis of palms and soles. Chronic arsenic exposure is associated with skin cancer. Neurologically, a sensory neuropathy may follow chronic exposure. Angiosarcoma of the liver, as well as cirrhosis, has been described in cases of chronic poisoning. Arsenic is a respiratory tract irritant and produces erosive lesions.[257]

Diagnosis of exposure is made by measuring blood and urinary arsenic concentrations.

COMBUSTION TOXICOLOGY

The combustion process produces a variety of toxic substances of which carbon monoxide is the major human toxin. Depending on the material burning, the toxic byproducts may include hydrogen cyanide, nitrogen dioxide, ammonia, hydrogen chloride, halogen gases, sulfur dioxide, isocyanates, and acrolein.[259]

Hydrogen cyanide, a chemical asphyxiant, is produced from combustion of polyurethane, paper, Nylon, wool, silk, and polyacrylonitrile. Nitrogen dioxide is produced from fabrics and celluloid and is a pulmonary irritant that can produce pulmonary edema and death quickly. Ammonia is produced from burning wool, silk, Nylon, and other inorganic products. Its concentration is generally low in most building fires. Hydrogen chloride is a respiratory irritant which can coat particulate matter inhaled during a fire.[260]

The halogen gases are pulmonary irritants produced by combustion of film and fluorinated resins. Sulfur dioxide is produced from any sulfur-containing compound and is a pulmonary irritant.

Isocyanates, pulmonary irritants, are derived from burning polyurethane and isocyanate polymers.

Acrolein is an aldehyde produced from pyrolysis of celluloids, wood, and polyolefins.[254,250]

Smoke inhalation of complex toxic materials can result in pulmonary injury as well as carbon monoxide and cyanide poisoning (see Chapter 47, Occupational Toxicologic Emergencies).

REFERENCES

1. Applebaum E, Bruce D. Complications of tracheal intubation. In: *Tracheal Intubation*. Philadelphia: Saunders; 1976.
2. Berne R, Levy M. Interplay of central and peripheral factors in the regulation of the circulation. In: *Cardiovascular Physiology*. St Louis, MO: Mosby; 1972.

3. Benowitz N, Rosenberg J, Becker C. Cardiopulmonary catastrophes in drug-overdose patients. *Med Clin North Am.* 1979;63:267–296.
4. Carrico C, Canizaro C, Shires T. Fluid resuscitation following injury: rationale for the use of balanced salt solutions. *Crit Care Med.* 1976;4:46–54.
5. Stein L, Berand J, Morissette M, et al. Pulmonary edema during volume infusion. *Circulation.* 1975;52:483–489.
6. Rackow E, et al. Relationship of colloid osmotic pressure and pulmonary capillary pressure to pulmonary edema. *Cardiovasc Med.* 1978;3:407–412.
7. Rackow E, Fein A. Fulminant noncardiogenic pulmonary edema in the critically ill. *Crit Care Med.* 1978;6:360–363.
8. Shoemaker W. Comparison of the relative effectiveness of whole blood transfusions and various types of fluid therapy in resuscitation. *Crit Care Med.* 1976;4:71–78.
9. Skillman J. The role of albumin and oncotically active fluids in shock. *Crit Care Med.* 1976;4:55–61.
10. Burrington J. Emergencies and accidents. In: Kempe C, Silver H, O'Brien D, eds. *Current Pediatric Diagnosis and Treatment.* 5th ed. Los Altos, CA: Lange; 1978.
11. Silver H, Peterson R, Rumack B. Drug therapy. In: Kempe C, Silver H, O'Brien D, eds. *Current Pediatric Diagnosis and Treatment.* 6th ed. Los Altos, CA: Lange; 1980.
12. Long acting barbiturates. In: Rumack BH, ed. *POISINDEX.* Englewood, CO: Micromedex; 1980.
13. Greenblatt D, Allen M, Noel B. Acute overdosage with benzodiazepine derivatives. *Clin Pharmacol Ther.* 1977;21:497–514.
14. Lansky L. An unusual case of childhood chloral hydrate poisoning. *Am J Dis Child.* 1974;127:275–276.
15. Chazan J, Garella S. Glutethimide intoxication. *Arch Intern Med.* 1971;128:215–219.
16. Adelson L. Fatal intoxication with isopropyl alcohol (rubbing alcohol). *Am J Clin Pathol.* 1962;38:144–151.
17. Westerfield B, Blovin R. Ethchlorvynol intoxication. *South Med J.* 1977;70:1019–1020.
18. Maddock K, Bloomer H. Meprobamate overdosage. *JAMA.* 1967;201:999–1003.
19. Opiates and narcotics. In: Rumack BH, ed. *POISINDEX.* Englewood, CO: Micromedex; 1980.
20. Steiman G, Woerpel R, Sherard E. Treatment of accidental sodium valproate overdose with an opiate antagonist. *Ann Neurol.* 1979;6:274.
21. Browne T. Valproic acid. *N Engl J Med.* 1980;302:661–666.
22. Moore M, Phillipi P. Clonidine overdose. *Lancet.* 1976;2:694.
23. Saperia J. Clonidine overdose. *Br Med J.* 1975;4:580.
24. Biggs J, Spiker D, Petit J. Tricyclic antidepressant overdoses—incidence of symptoms. *JAMA.* 1977;238:135–138.
25. Goldfrank L, Bresnitz E. Phenothiazines. *Hosp Physician.* 1979;15:42–53.
26. Matthew H, Proudfoot A, Brown S. Mandrax poisoning: conservative management of 116 patients. *Br Med J.* 1968;2:101–102.
27. Brown S, Goenechea S. Methaqualone: metabolic, kinetic and clinical pharmacologic observations. *Clin Pharmacol Ther.* 1973;14:314–324.
28. Aronow R, Done A. Phencyclidine overdose: an emerging concept of management. *JACEP.* 1978;7:56–59.
29. Teitelbaum D, Ott J. Acute strychnine intoxication. *Clin Toxicol.* 1970;3:267–273.
30. Gay G, Rappolt R, Inaba D. Cocaine. *Clin Toxicol.* 1975;8:149–178.
31. Haddad L. 1978: cocaine in perspective. *JACEP.* 1979;8:374–376.
32. Reigart J, Brueggeman L, Keil J. Sodium fluoroacetate poisoning. *Am J Dis Child.* 1975;129:1224–1226.
33. Hart J, Wallace J. The adverse effects of amphetamines. *Clin Toxicol.* 1975;8:179–190.
34. Kalant H, Kalant O. Death in amphetamine users: causes and rates. *Can Med Assoc J.* 1975;112:299–304.
35. Tenckhoff H, Sherrard D, Hickman R. Acute diphenylhydantoin intoxication. *Am J Dis Child.* 1968;116:422–425.
36. McLellan D, Swash M. Choreoathetosis and encephalopathy induced by phenytoin. *Br Med J.* 1974;2:204–205.
37. Lovejoy F, Mitchell A, Goldman P. The management of propoxyphene poisoning. *J Pediatr.* 1974;85:98–100.
38. Salzberg M, Gallagher E. Propranolol overdose. *Ann Emerg Med.* 1980;9:26–27.
39. Lagerfelt J, Matell G. Attempted suicide with 5.1 grams of propranolol. *Acta Med Scand.* 1976;199:517–518.
40. Sullivan J, Peterson RG, Rumack BH. Carbamazepine toxicity in acute overdose: serial blood levels and clinical presentations. *Neurology.* 1981;31:621–624.
41. Stewart R. Cyanide poisoning. *Clin Toxicol.* 1974;7:561–564.
42. Mascarenhas B, Geller A, Goodman A. Cyanide poisoning. Medical emergency. *N Y State J Med.* 1969;69:1782–1784.
43. Gordon E. Carbon monoxide encephalopathy. *Br Med J.* 1965;1:12–32.
44. Winter P, Miller J. Carbon monoxide poisoning. *JAMA.* 1976;236:1502–1504.
45. Grossman R, Hamilton R, Morse B. Nontraumatic rhabdomyolysis and acute renal failure. *N Engl J Med.* 1974;291:807–811.
46. Ralph D. Rhabdomyolysis and acute renal failure. *JACEP.* 1978;7:103–106.
47. Myers R, Linberg S, Cowley R. Carbon monoxide poisoning: the injury and its treatment. *JACEP.* 1979;8:479–484.
48. Finley J, VanBeek A, Glover J. Myonecrosis complicating carbon monoxide poisoning. *J Trauma.* 1977;17:536–539.
49. Teehan B, Maher J, Carey J. Acute ethchlorvynol (Placidyl®) intoxication. *Ann Intern Med.* 1970;72:875–882.
50. Burton W, Vender J, Shapiro B. Adult respiratory distress syndrome after Placidyl® abuse. *Crit Care Med.* 1980;8:48–49.
51. Duberstein J, Kaufman D. A clinical study of an epidemic of heroin intoxication and heroin induced pulmonary edema. *Am J Med.* 1971;51:704–714.
52. Katz S, Aberman A, Fraud V. Heroin pulmonary edema: evidence of increased pulmonary capillary permeability. *Am Rev Respir Dis.* 1972;106:472–474.
53. Bogartz L, Miller W. Pulmonary edema associated with propoxyphene intoxication. *JAMA.* 1971;215:259–262.
54. Tweedale M. Salicylate and pulmonary edema. *Ann Intern Med.* 1974;81:710.
55. Bowers RE, Brigham K, Owen P. Salicylate pulmonary edema: the mechanism in sheep and review of the clinical literature. *Am Rev Respir Dis.* 1977;115:261–268.
56. Glauser F, Egan P, Miller J. The effect of salicylate infusion on the alveolar epithelial membrane in the isolated perfused lung. *Crit Care Med.* 1978;6:181–184.
57. Grant M, ed. *Toxicology of the Eye.* 2nd ed. Springfield, IL: Thomas; 1974.
58. Jaffe J. Narcotic analgesics. In: Goodman L, Gilman A, eds. *The Pharmacological Basis of Therapeutics.* 4th ed. New York: Macmillan; 1970.
59. Rumack B, Temple A. Lomotil poisoning. *Pediatrics.* 1974;53:495–500.

60. Vaucher Y, Lightner E, Walson P. Theophylline poisoning. *J Pediatr.* 1977;90:827–830.
61. Zwillich C, Sutton F, Neff T. Theophylline induced seizures in adults—correlation with serum concentrations. *Ann Intern Med.* 1975;82:784–787.
62. Sullivan J. Caffeine poisoning in an infant. *J Pediatr.* 1977;90:1022–1023.
63. Petery J, Rennert O. Arsenic poisoning in childhood. *Clin Toxicol.* 1970;3:519–526.
64. Kline T. Myocardial changes in lead poisoning. *Am J Dis Child.* 1960;99:48–54.
65. Gustafson A, Svensson S, Ugaander L. Cardiac arrhythmias in chloral hydrate poisoning. *Acta Med Scand.* 1977;201:227–230.
66. MacFaul R, Miller G. Clonidine poisoning in children. *Lancet.* 1977;1:1266–1267.
67. Kibler L, Gazes P. Effect of clonidine on atrioventricular conduction. *JAMA.* 1977;238:1930–1932.
68. Harrisson J, Ambrus J, Ambrus C. Acute poisoning with sodium fluoroacetate. *JAMA.* 1952;149:1520–1523.
69. Salzberg M, Gallagher E. Propranolol overdose. *Ann Emerg Med.* 1980;9:26–27.
70. Reuler J. Hypothermia: pathophysiology, clinical setting and management. *Ann Intern Med.* 1978;89:519–527.
71. Stine R. Accidental hypothermia. *Ann Emerg Med.* 1977;6:413–416.
72. Goldfrank L, Kirstein R. Emergency management of hypothermia. *Hosp Physician.* 1979;1:47–52.
73. Noble J, Matthew H. Acute poisoning by tricyclic antidepressants: clinical features and management of 100 patients. *Clin Toxicol.* 1969;2:403–421.
74. Subin H, Weil M. Shock associated with barbiturate intoxication. *JAMA.* 1971;215:263–268.
75. Myers R, Linberg S, Crowley R. Carbon monoxide poisoning—the injury and its treatment. *JACEP.* 1979;8:479–484.
76. Temple A. Pathophysiology of aspirin overdosage toxicity with implications for management. *Pediatrics.* 1978;62(suppl):873–879.
77. Hamilton A, Hardy H. Pesticides. In: *Industrial Toxicology.* 3rd ed. Littleton, MA: Publishing Science Group; 1974.
78. Comroe J. Manifestations of pulmonary disease. In: *Physiology of Respiration.* Chicago: Year Book Medical; 1970.
79. Harris J, Rumack B, Peterson R. Methemoglobinemia resulting from absorption of nitrates. *JAMA.* 1979;242:2869–2871.
80. Hamilton A, Hardy H. Aromatic nitro and amino compounds. In: *Industrial Toxicology.* 3rd ed. Littleton, MA: Publishing Science Group; 1974.
81. Green E, Zimmerman R, Ghurabi W. Phenazopyridine hydrochloride toxicity: a cause of drug-induced methemoglobinemia. *Ann Emerg Med.* 1979;8:426–431.
82. Potter J, Hillman J. Benzocaine-induced methemoglobinemia. *Ann Emerg Med.* 1979;8:26–27.
83. Leavell B, Thorup O. Hemolytic anemia. In: *Fundamentals of Clinical Hematology.* Philadelphia: Saunders; 1971.
84. Cartwright G. Methemoglobinemia and sulfhemoglobinemia. In: *Harrison's Principles of Internal Medicine.* 6th ed. New York: McGraw-Hill; 1970.
85. Clay K, Murphy R. On the metabolic acidosis of ethylene glycol intoxication. *Toxicol Appl Pharmacol.* 1977;39:39–49.
86. Isselbacher K. Metabolic and hepatic effects of alcohol. *N Engl J Med.* 1977;296:612–616.
87. Terman D, Teitelbaum D. Isoniazid self poisoning. *Neurology.* 1970;20:299–303.
88. James J. Acute iron poisoning: assessment of severity and prognosis. *J Pediatr.* 1970;77:117–119.
89. Kittel J. Paraldehyde toxicity. *Hosp Pharm.* 1973;8:263–265.
90. Taher S, Anderson R, McCartney R. Renal tubular acidosis associated with toluene sniffing. *N Engl J Med.* 1974;290:765–768.
91. Fischman C, Oster J. Toxic effects of toluene—a new cause of high anion gap metabolic acidosis. *JAMA.* 1979;241:1713–1715.
92. Rasmussen S, Kirstensen M. Choreoathetosis during phenytoin treatment. *Acta Med Scand.* 1977;201:239–241.
93. Kooiker J, Sumi S. Movement disorder as a manifestation of diphenylhydantoin intoxication. *Neurology.* 1974;24:68–71.
94. Tenckhoff H, Sherrard D, Hickman R. Acute diphenylhydantoin intoxication. *Am J Dis Child.* 1968;116:422–425.
95. Burks J, Walker J, Rumack B. Tricyclic antidepressant poisoning—reversal of coma, choreoathetosis and myoclonus with physostigmine. *JAMA.* 1974;230:1405–1406.
96. Browder A, Joselow M, Louria D. The problem of lead poisoning. *Medicine.* 1973;52:121–139.
97. Gerstner H, Huff J. Selected case histories and epidemiologic examples of human mercury poisoning. *Clin Toxicol.* 1977;11:131–150.
98. Saran B, Gaind R. Lithium. *Clin Toxicol.* 1973;6:257–269.
99. Burns R, Lerner S. Phencyclidine deaths. *JACEP.* 1978;7:135–141.
100. Haddad L. 1978—cocaine in perspective. *JACEP.* 1979;8:374–376.
101. Gay G, Inaba D, Sheppard C. Cocaine—history, epidemiology, human pharmacology, and treatment. *Clin Toxicol.* 1975;8:149–178.
102. Hart J, Wallace J. The adverse effects of amphetamines. *Clin Toxicol.* 1975;8:179–190.
103. Reyes-Jacang A, Wenzl J. Antihistamine toxicity in children. *Clin Pediatr.* 1969;8:297–299.
104. Hooper R, Conner C, Rumack B. Acute poisoning from over-the-counter sleep preparations. *JACEP.* 1979;8:98–100.
105. Binns H, et al. Gasoline contact burns. *JACEP.* 1978;7:404–405.
106. Fredriksson T. Percutaneous absorption of parathian and paraoxon. *Arch Environ Health.* 1961;3:67–70.
107. Hayes W, ed.: *Toxicology of Pesticides.* Baltimore: Williams & Wilkins; 1975.
108. Manno B, Mano J. Toxicology of ipecac—a review. *Clin Toxicol.* 1977;10:221–242.
109. Morgan A, Polak A. The excretion of salicylate in salicylate poisoning. *Clin Sci.* 1971;41:475–484.
110. Bloomer H. A critical evaluation of diuresis in the treatment of barbiturate intoxication. *J Lab Clin Med.* 1966;67:898–905.
111. Innes I, Nickerson M. Sympathomimetic drugs. In: Goodman L, Gilman A, eds. *The Pharmacologic Basis of Therapeutics.* New York: Macmillan; 1975.
112. Gibson T, Nelson H. Drug kinetics and artificial kidneys. *Clin Pharmacokinet.* 1977;2:403–426.
113. Watonabe A. Pharmacokinetic aspects of the dialysis of drugs. *Drug Intell Clin Pharm.* 1977;2:407–417.
114. Pond S, Rosenburg J, Benowitz N. Pharmacokinetics of hemoperfusion for drug overdose. *Clin Pharmacokinet.* 1979;4:329–354.
115. Winchester J, Gelfand M, Knepshield J. Dialysis and hemoperfusion of poisons and drugs. *Trans Am Soc Artif Intern Organs.* 1977;23:762–842.
116. Jaffe L. Carbon monoxide in the environment—sources, characteristics, and fate of atmospheric carbon monoxide. *Ann N Y Acad Sci.* 1970;174:76–88.
117. Ayres S, Giannelli S, Mueller H. Myocardial and systemic responses to carboxyhemoglobin. *Ann N Y Acad Sci.* 1970;175:268–293.
118. Winter P, Miller J. Carbon monoxide poisoning. *JAMA.* 1976;236:1502–1504.

119. Anderson R, Allensworth D, DeGroot W. Myocardial toxicity from carbon monoxide poisoning. *Ann Intern Med.* 1967;67:1172–1182.
120. Garland H, Pearce J. Neurological complications of carbon monoxide poisoning. *Q J Med.* 1967;36:445–455.
121. Ginsberg M, Myers R. Fetal brain injury after maternal carbon monoxide intoxication. *Neurology.* 1976;26:15–23.
122. Ratney R, Wegman D, Elkins H. In vivo conversion of methylene chloride to carbon monoxide. *Arch Environ Health.* 1974; 28:223–226.
123. Way J, Sylvester D, Morgan R. Recent perspectives on the toxicodynamic basis of cyanide antagonism. *Fundam Appl Toxicol.* 1984;4:S231–S239.
124. Cerami A, Allen A, Graziano J. Pharmacology of cyanate—general effects on experimental animals. *J Pharmacol Exp Ther.* 1973; 185:653–666.
125. Evans L. Cobalt compounds as antidotes for hydrocyanic acid. *Br J Pharmacol.* 1964;23:455–475.
126. Milby T. Prevention and management of organophosphate poisoning. *JAMA.* 1971;216:2131–2133.
127. Namba T, Nolte C, Jackrel J. Poisoning due to organophosphate insecticides—acute and chronic manifestations. *Am J Med.* 1971; 50:475–492.
128. Richards A. Malathion poisoning successfully treated with large doses of atropine. *Can Med Assoc J.* 1964;91:82–83.
129. Organophosphates. In: Rumack B, ed. *POISINDEX.* Englewood, CO: Micromedex; 1980.
130. Quinby G. Further therapeutic experience with pralidoximes in organic phosphorus poisoning. *JAMA.* 1964;187:111–118.
131. Berkowitz B. The relationship of pharmacokinetics to pharmacological activity: morphine, methadone, and naloxone. *Clin Pharmacokinet.* 1976;1:219–230.
132. Moore R, Rumack B, Conner C. Naloxone—underdosage after narcotic poisoning. *Am J Dis Child.* 1980;134:156–158.
133. Sesso A, Rodzvilla J. Naloxone therapy in a seven month old with methadone poisoning. *Clin Pediatr.* 1975;14:388–389.
134. Lovejoy F, Mitchell A, Goldman P. The management of propoxyphene poisoning. *J Pediatr.* 1974;85:98–100.
135. Jasinski D, Martin W, Haertzen C. The human pharmacology and abuse potential of N-allylnoroxymorphone (naloxone). *J Pharmacol Exp Ther.* 1967;157:420–426.
136. Rumack B. Anticholinergic poisoning—treatment with physostigmine. *Pediatrics.* 1973;52:449–551.
137. Lee J, Turndoff H, Poppers P. Physostigmine reversal of antihistamine induced excitement and depression. *Anesthesiology.* 1975;43:683–684.
138. Nattel S, Bayne L, Ruedy J. Physostigmine in coma due to drug overdose. *Clin Pharmacol Ther.* 1979;25:96–102.
139. Schanker L. Drug absorption. In: LaDu B, Mandel H, Way E, eds. *Fundamentals of Drug Metabolism and Drug Distribution.* Baltimore: Williams & Wilkins; 1971.
140. Levine R. Factors affecting gastrointestinal absorption of drugs. *Dig Dis.* 1970;15:171–188.
141. Rowland M. Drug administration and regimens. In: Melmon K, Morrelli H, eds. *Clinical Pharmacology—Basic Principles in Therapeutics.* New York: Macmillan; 1972.
142. Nimmo W. Drugs, diseases and altered gastric emptying. *Clin Pharmacokinet.* 1976;1:189–203.
143. Hug C. Pharmacokinetics of drugs administered intravenously. *Anesth Analg.* 1978;57:704–723.
144. Curry S. *Drug Disposition and Pharmacokinetics.* London: Blackwell; 1977.
145. Morselli P. Clinical pharmacokinetics in neonates. *Clin Pharmacokinet.* 1976;1:81–98.
146. Levy G. Clinical pharmacokinetics of aspirin. *Pediatrics.* 1978; 62(suppl):867–871.
147. Rane A. Urinary excretion of diphenylhydantoin metabolites in newborn infants. *J Pediatr.* 1974;85:543–545.
148. Rane A, Garle M, Borga O. Plasma disappearance of transplacentally transferred diphenylhydantoin in the newborn studied by mass fragmentography. *Clin Pharmacol Ther.* 1974;15:39–45.
149. Ehrnebo M, Agurell S, Jalling B. Age differences in drug binding by plasma proteins—studies on human fetuses, neonates, and adults. *Eur J Clin Pharmacol.* 1971;3:189–193.
150. Rane A, Wilson J. Clinical pharmacokinetics in infants and children. *Clin Pharmacokinet.* 1976;1:2–24.
151. Peterson R. Pharmacologic considerations for the newborn and premature. In: Aldrete J, Stanley T, eds. *Trends in Intravenous Anesthesia.* Chicago: Year Book Medical; 1980.
152. Peterson R, Simmons M, Rumack B. Pharmacology of furosemide in the premature newborn infant. *Pediatrics.* 1980;97:139–143.
153. Greenblatt D, Sellers E, Shader R. Drug disposition in old age. *N Engl J Med.* 1982;306:1081–1088.
154. Crooks J, O'Malley K, Stevenson I. Pharmacokinetics in the elderly. *Clin Pharmacokinet.* 1976;1:280–296.
155. Mitenko P, Ogilvie R. Rational intravenous doses of theophylline. *N Engl J Med.* 1973;289:600–603.
156. McDonald J, Turk J, Dietzler D. Theophylline toxicity. *Clin Chem.* 1978;24:1603–1608.
157. Arnman K, Carlstrom S, Thorell J. The effect of norepinephrine and theophylline on blood glucose, plasma free fatty acids, plasma glycerol and plasma insulin in normal subjects. *Acta Med Scand.* 1975;197:271–274.
158. Eldridge F, Salzer J. Effect of respiratory alkalosis on blood lactate and pyruvate in humans. *J Appl Physiol.* 1967;22:461–468.
159. Emmett M, Narrins R. Clinical use of the anion gap. *Medicine.* 1977;56:38–54.
160. Lesko L. Dose dependent elimination kinetics of theophylline. *Clin Pharmacokinet.* 1979;4:449–459.
161. Kadlec G, Jarboe C, Pollard S. Acute theophylline intoxication—biphasic first order elimination kinetics in a child. *Ann Allergy.* 1978;41:337–339.
162. Diafsky K, Sitar D, Rangno R. Theophylline kinetics in acute pulmonary edema. *Clin Pharmacol Ther.* 1978;21:310–316.
163. Snodgrass W, Sawyer D, Conner C. Asymptomatic theophylline overdose. *Drug Intell Clin Pharm.* 1980;14:783.
164. Slaughter R, Green L, Kohli R. Hemodialysis clearance of theophylline. *Ther Drug Monit.* 1982;4:191–193.
165. Russo M. Management of theophylline intoxication with charcoal column hemoperfusion. *N Engl J Med.* 1979;300:24–26.
166. Radomski L, Park G, Goldberg M. Model for theophylline overdose treatment with oral activated charcoal. *Clin Pharmacol Ther.* 1984;35:402–408.
167. Biberstein M, Ziegler M, Ward D. Use of β-blockade and hemoperfusion for acute theophylline poisoning. *West J Med.* 1984; 141:485–490.
168. Hall K, Dobson K, Dalton J. Metabolic abnormalities associated with intentional theophylline overdose. *Ann Intern Med.* 1984; 101:457–462.
169. Vohra J, Burrows G, Hurst D. The effect of toxic and therapeutic doses of tricyclic antidepressant drugs on intracardiac conduction. *Eur J Cardiol.* 1975;3:219–227.
170. Biggs J, Spiker D, Petit J. Tricyclic antidepressant overdose—incidence of symptoms. *JAMA.* 1977;238:135–138.

171. Brown T, Barker G, Dunlop M. The use of sodium bicarbonate in the treatment of tricyclic antidepressant induced arrhythmias. *Anesth Intensive Care.* 1973;1:203–210.
172. Brown T. Tricyclic antidepressant overdosage—experimental studies on the management of circulatory complications. *Clin Toxicol.* 1976;9:255–272.
173. Kingston M. Hyperventilation in tricyclic antidepressant poisoning. *Crit Care Med.* 1979;7:550–551.
174. Hoffman J, McElroy C. Bicarbonate therapy for dysrhythmia and hypotension in tricyclic antidepressant overdose. *West J Med.* 1981;134:60–64.
175. Bessen H, Niemann J, Haskell R. *West J Med.* 1983;139:373–376.
176. Molloy D, Penner S, Rabson J. Use of sodium bicarbonate to treat tricyclic antidepressant-induced arrhythmias in a patient with alkolosis. *Can Med Assoc J.* 1984;130:1457–1459.
177. Levit A, Sullivan J, Owens M. Amitriptyline plasma protein binding: Effects of plasma pH and relevance to clinical overdose. *Am J Emerg Med.* 1986;4:121–125.
178. Denson D, Coyle D, Thompson G. Bupivaccine protein binding in the term parturient—effects of lactic acidosis. *Clin Pharmacol Ther.* 1983;35:702–709.
179. Javaid J, Hendricks K, Davis J. High affinity binding of tricyclic antidepressants to human plasma involves alpha-1 acid glycoproteins. *Pyschol Pharmacol Bull.* 1983;19:655–658.
180. Javaid J, Hendricks K, Davis J. Alpha-1 acid glycoprotein involvement in high affinity binding of tricyclic antidepressants to human plasma. *Biochem Pharmacol.* 1983;32:1149–1153.
181. Borga O, Azarnoff D, Forshell G. Plasma protein binding of tricyclic antidepressants in man. *Biochem Pharmacol.* 1969;18:2135–2143.
182. Frelich D, Girdina E. Imipramine binding to alpha-1 acid glycoprotein in normal subjects and cardiac patients. *Clin Pharmacol Ther.* 1984;35:670–674.
183. Pentel P, Benowitz N. Effects of blood pH on desipramine toxicity in the rat. *Vet Hum Toxicol.* 1982;24(suppl):196.
184. Roberts R, Mueller S, Lauer R. Propranolol in the treatment of cardiac arrhythmias associated with amitriptyline intoxication. *J Pediatr.* 1973;82:65–67.
185. Tobis J, Aronow W. Effect of amitriptyline antidotes on repetitive extrasystole threshold. *Clin Pharmacol Ther.* 1980;27:602–606.
186. Boehnert M, Lovejoy F. The effect of phenytoin on cardiac conduction and ventricular arrhythmias in acute tricyclic antidepressant overdose. *Vet Hum Toxicol.* 1985;28:297. Abstract.
187. Sullivan JB, Fisher JG. Antidepressant poisoning: an increasing problem with ongoing controversies. *Emerg Med Rep.* 1984;5: 197–204.
188. Comstock T, Watson W, Jennison T. Severe amitriptyline intoxication and the use of charcoal hemoperfusion. *Clin Pharm.* 1983;2:85–88.
189. Asbach H, Holz F, Mohring K. Lipid hemodialysis versus charcoal hemoperfusion in imipramine poisoning. *Clin Toxicol.* 1977;11:211–219.
190. Lydiard R, Gelenberg A. Amoxapine—an antidepressant with some neuroleptic properties—a review of its chemistry, animal pharmacology and toxicology, human pharmacology, and clinical efficacy. *Pharmacotherapy.* 1981;1:163–177.
191. Fugate-Hunt A, Zander J, Lesar T. Adverse reactions due to dopamine blockade by amoxapine—a case report and review of the literature. *Pharmacotherapy.* 1984;4:35–39.
192. Kulig K, Runack B, Sullivan J. Amoxapine overdose—coma and seizures without cardiotoxic effects. *JAMA.* 1982;248:1092–1094.
193. Litovitz T, Troutman W. Amoxapine overdose—seizures and fatalities. *JAMA.* 1983;250:1069–1071.
194. Wells B, Gelenberg A. Chemistry, pharmacology, pharmacokinetics, adverse effects, and efficacy of the antidepressant maprotaline hydrochloride pharmacotherapy. *Pharmacotherapy.* 1981;1:121–139.
195. Park J, Proudfoot A. Acute poisoning with maprotaline hydrochloride. *Br Med J.* 1977;1:1573. Letter.
196. Crome P, Newman B. Poisoning with maprotaline and mianserin. *Br Med J.* 1977;2:260. Letter.
197. Jukes A. Maprotaline (ludiomil): side effects and overdosage. *J Int Med Res.* 1975;3(suppl 2):126–131.
198. Goergotas A, Forsell T, Mann J. Trazodone hydrochloride: a wide spectrum antidepressant with a unique pharmacologic profile. *Pharmacotherapy.* 1982;2:255–265.
199. Lesar T, Kingston R, Dahms R. Trazodone overdose. *Ann Emerg Med.* 1983;12:221–223.
200. Henry J, Ali C, Coldwell R. Acute trazadone poisoning—clinical signs and plasma concentrations. *Psychopathology.* 1984;17(suppl 2):77–81.
201. Root I, Ohlson G. Trazodone overdose—report of two cases. *J Anal Toxicol.* 1984;8:91–94.
202. Gabow P, Clay K, Sullivan J. Organic acids in ethylene glycol intoxication. *Ann Intern Med.* 1986;105:16–20.
203. Parry M, Wallach R. Ethylene glycol poisoning. *Am J Med.* 1974;57:143–149.
204. Amat-Martin G, Tphly T, McMartin K. Methyl alcohol poisoning—development of a model for ocular toxicity in methyl alcohol poisoning using the rhesus monkey. *Arch Ophthalmol.* 1977;95:1847–1850.
205. Hayreh M, Hayreh S, Baumbach G. Methyl alcohol poisoning—ocular toxicity. *Arch Ophthalmol.* 1977;95:1851–1858.
206. McLean D, Jacobs H, Mielke B. Methanol poisoning—a clinical and pathological study. *Ann Neurol.* 1979;8:161–167.
207. Aquilonius S, Bergstrom K, Enoksson P. Cerebral computed tomography in methanol intoxication. *J Comput Assist Tomogr.* 1980;4:425–428.
208. Wagner J, Wilkinson P, Sedman A. Elimination of alcohol from human blood. *J Pharm Sci.* 1976;65:152–154.
209. Tobin M, Lianoa E. Hemodialysis for methanol intoxication. *J Dialysis.* 1979;3:97–106.
210. Brem J, Pereli E, Gopalan S. Salicylism, hyperventilation, and the central nervous system. *J Pediatr.* 1973;83:264–266.
211. Hill J. Salicylate intoxication. *N Engl J Med.* 1973;288:1110–1113.
212. Spector R, Lorenzo A. The transport and metabolism of salicylate in the central nervous system—in vivo studies. *J Pharmacol Exp Ther.* 1973;185:276–286.
213. Hill J. Experimental salicylate poisoning—observations on the effects of altering blood pH on tissue and plasma salicylate concentrations. *Pediatrics.* 1971;47:658–665.
214. Levy G. Pharmacokinetics of salicylate elimination in man. *J Pharm Sci.* 1965;54:959–967.
215. Done A. Salicylate intoxication—significance of measurements of salicylate in blood cases of acute ingestion. *Pediatrics.* 1960;26:800–807.
216. Mitchell J, Thorgeirsson S, Potter W. Acetaminophen-induced hepatic injury—protective role of glutathione in man and rationale for therapy. *Clin Pharmacol Ther.* 1974;16:676–684.
217. Rumack B, Peterson R. Acetaminophen overdose—incidence diagnosis and management in 416 patients. *Pediatrics.* 1978;62(suppl):898–903.
218. Rumack B, Matthew H. Acetaminophen poisoning and toxicity. *Pediatrics.* 1975;55:871–876.
219. Neuvonen P. Bioavailability of phenytoin: clinical pharmacokinetic and therapeutic implications. *Clin Pharmacokinet.* 1979;4:91–103.

220. Richens A. Clinical pharmacokinetics of phenytoin. *Clin Pharmacokinet.* 1979;4:153–169.
221. Matthew H, Lawson A. Acute barbiturate poisoning—a review of two years experience. *Q J Med.* 1966;35:539–551.
222. Shubin H, Weil M. Shock associated with barbiturate intoxication. *JAMA.* 1971;215:263–268.
223. Bloomer H. A critical evaluation of diuresis in the treatment of barbiturate intoxication. *J Lab Clin Med.* 1966;67:898–905.
224. Kevey R, Pitlick W, Troupin A. Pharmacokinetics of carbamazepine in normal man. *Clin Pharmacol Ther.* 1975;17:657–668.
225. DeZeeuw R, Westenberg H, VanDerkleijn. An unusual case of carbamazepine poisoning with a near fatal relapse after two days. *Clin Toxicol.* 1979;14:263–269.
226. Rawlins M, Collste P, Bertilsson L. Distribution and elimination kinetics of carbamazepine. *Eur J Clin Pharmacol.* 1975;8:91–96.
227. Gugler Rand von Unruh G. Clinical pharmacokinetics of valproic acid. *Clin Pharmacokinet.* 1980;5:67–83.
228. Browne T. Valproic acid. *N Engl J Med.* 1980;302:661–666.
229. Suchy F, Balistreri W, Buchino J. Acute hepatic failure associated with the use of sodium valproate. *N Engl J Med.* 1979;300:962–966.
230. Weber W, Hein D. Clinical pharmacokinetics of isoniazid. *Clin Pharmacokinet.* 1979;4:401–422.
231. Hyatt H. Acute poisoning from overdose of isoniazid. *Am J Dis Child.* 1961;102:106–110.
232. Thornton W. Sleep aids and sedatives. *JACEP.* 1977;6:408–412.
233. McEwen J. Phenylpropanolamine—associated hypertension after use of "over-the-counter" appetite-suppressant products. *Med J Aust.* 1983;2:71–73.
234. Greenblatt D, Shader R. Pharmacokinetic understanding of antianxiety drug therapy. *South Med J.* 1978;71:2–9.
235. Greenblatt D, Allen M, Noel B. Acute overdosage with benzodiazepine derivatives. *Clin Pharmacol Ther.* 1977;21:497–514.
236. Finkle S, McCloskey KL, Goodman L. Diazepam and drug-associated deaths—a survey in the United States and Canada. *JAMA.* 1979;242:429–434.
237. Busto V, Kaplan H, Sellers E. Benzodiazepine associated emergencies in Toronto. *Am J Psychiatr.* 1980;137:224–227.
238. Sellers EM, Holloway MR. Drug kinetics and alcohol ingestion. *Clin Pharmacokinet.* 1978;3:440–452.
239. Olson K, Yin L, Osterloh J. Coma caused by trivial triazolam overdose. *Am J Emerg Med.*
240. Hofer P, Scollo-Lavizzari G. Benzodiazepine antagonist Ro 15-1788 in self-poisoning—diagnostic and therapeutic use. *Arch Intern Med.* 1985;145:663–664.
241. Lynn R, Honig C, Jatlow P. Resin hemoperfusion for treatment of ethchlorvynol overdose. *Ann Intern Med.* 1979;91:549–553.
242. Benowitz N, Abolin C, Tozer T. Resin hemoperfusion in ethchlorvynol overdose. *Clin Pharmacol Ther.* 1980;27:236–242.
243. Maher J. Determinants of serum half-life of glutethimide in intoxicated patients. *J Pharmacol Exp Ther.* 1970;174:450–455.
244. Wright N, Roscue P. Acute glutethimide poisoning—conservative management of 31 patients. *JAMA.* 1970;214:1704–1706.
245. Stalker N, Gambertoglio A, Fukumitsu C. Acute massive chloral hydrate intoxication treated with hemodialysis—a clinical pharmacokinetic analysis. *J Clin Pharmacol.* 1978;12:136–142.
246. Weissberg M. *Dangerous Secrets—Maladaptive Responses to Stress.* New York: Norton; 1983.
247. Haberman P, Baden M. Alcoholism and violent death. *Q J Stud Alcohol.* 1974;35:221–223.
248. Holinger P. Violent deaths among the young—recent trends in suicide, homicide, and accidents. *Am J Psychiatr.* 1979;136:1144–1147.
249. Cummins L. Hypoglycemia and convulsions in children following alcohol ingestion. *J Pediatr.* 1961;58:23–26.
250. Goldfrank L, Starke C. Metabolic acidosis in the alcoholic. *Hosp Physician.* 1979;4:34–38.
251. Sellers EM, Holloway MR. Drug kinetics and alcohol ingestion. *Clin Pharmacokinet.* 1978;3:440–452.
252. Smith TW, Butler VP, Haber E. Treatment of life-threatening digitalis intoxication with digoxin specific F(ab) antibody fragments. *N Engl J Med.* 1982;307:1357–1362.
253. Smith TW, Haber E, Yeatman L. Reversal of advanced digoxin intoxication with F(ab) fragments of digoxin-specific antibodies. *N Engl J Med.* 1976;294:797–800.
254. Ochs HR, Smith TW. Reversal of advanced digitoxin toxicity and modification of pharmacokinetics by specific antibodies and Fab fragments. *J Clin Invest.* 1977;60:1303–1313.
255. Sullivan JB, Russell FE. Isolation, quantitation, and subclassing of Igb antibody to crotalidae venom by affinity chromatography and protein electrophoresis. *Toxicon.* 1983;3:429–432.
256. Russell FE, Sullivan JB, Egen NB. Preparation of a new antivenin by affinity chromatography. *Am J Trop Med Hyg.* 1985;34:141–150.
257. Landrigan PJ. Occupational and community exposures to toxic metals: lead, cadmium, mercury, and arsenic. *West J Med.* 1982;137:531–539.
258. Kreiss K, Feldman R, Niles C. Neurologic evaluations of a population exposed to arsenic in Alaskan wellwater. *Arch Environ Health.* 1983;38:116–121.
259. Terrill J, Montgomery R, Reinhardt C. Toxic gases from fires. *Science.* 1978;200:1343–1347.
260. Hartzell G, Parkman S, Switzer W. Toxic products from fires. *Am J Indus Hyg.* 1983;44:248–255.

30. Oncology in the Emergency Department

MARC BORENSTEIN, MD, FACEP

Among the many causes of death in the United States, cancer is second only to heart disease. Despite many advances in both its treatment and prevention, cancer remains a feared disease. The anxiety and apprehension that surround cancer are felt not only by patients and their families, but by many health care professionals as well. The social stigma associated with a diagnosis of cancer has lessened, but cancer is still a disease that causes considerable unease.

As a result, health care professionals may hesitate to ask patients about important symptoms, and patients may be afraid or embarrassed to volunteer important information. Many factors can compound this problem in the emergency department: (1) patients usually do not know the emergency department personnel; (2) patients may feel that their problem is less important than that of another patient in the emergency department; (3) time constraints may hinder emergency department evaluations; and (4) the emergency department physical plant may lack sufficient privacy to facilitate discussion.

In addition to the psychosocial factors that inhibit a thorough evaluation of the oncology patient, the database itself is voluminous and frequently changing. There has been a marked increase in the amount and sophistication of the technology used in the diagnosis and treatment of cancer. Today at least 100 medications can be included under the broad category of chemotherapy. Most have the potential to produce serious, possibly life-threatening complications. In addition, a large number of uncommon infections are now seen as complications of both cancer and its treatment. Many organisms that are nonpathogenic in the normal host can rapidly disseminate and be fatal in the cancer patient. In a patient with cancer, it is often difficult to determine whether clinical deterioration is due to the cancer, another process such as infection, or the treatment itself. As a result, diagnostic confirmation with tissue biopsy is often imperative.

Health care professionals sometimes wrongly assume that patients with cancer do not have actual emergencies. It is essential to remember that many patients with cancer have a stable or minimally progressive illness. There may be many months or years of high-quality, productive life ahead. Even if a cancer patient's life expectancy is short, the quality of that time is highly dependent on minimizing preventable complications. In addition, emergency department personnel evaluating cancer patients must remember that other acute processes unrelated to the cancer problem can occur, such as appendicitis or myocardial infarction.

When a decline in the cancer patient's clinical status is due to a reversible process, failure to recognize the early signs and/or symptoms of such a process could result in premature disability or death. For example, it would be tragic if an ambulatory patient with stable breast carcinoma developed paraplegia because the diagnosis of spinal cord compression was not entertained or pursued in its early stages when cord function could still be preserved.

Overall, emergency department personnel are often required to evaluate cancer patients and, as the "front line," make vital interventions in the early stages of an oncologic emergency. Thorough understanding of oncologic emergencies is essential to ensure that emergency department personnel key historical and physical findings will be obtained, that the appropriate diagnostic tests will be performed, that emergency therapy will be initiated, and that consultants will be promptly involved. In the final analysis, discovery comes only to the prepared mind.

NEUROLOGIC EMERGENCIES

Raised Intracranial Pressure

In patients over age 35 to 40, raised intracranial pressure is most often due to metastatic disease involving the brain parenchyma. This may be the result of (1) distant spread from a known primary site actively being treated, and therefore, representing progression of the disease; (2) distant spread from an unknown, symptomatically silent primary site representing the first manifestation of neoplastic disease in the patient; (3) distant spread from a previously treated primary site representing a first recurrence in a patient who had previously appeared clinically free of disease. In patients under age 35, raised intracranial pressure is more commonly due to primary brain tumors.

Despite the many etiologies of raised intracranial pressure, there are general principles of diagnosis and management that can be used effectively by emergency physicians. As in other emergency medical situations, the emergency physician must first respond to the severity of the clinical presentation. Two distinct categories of illness can be defined:

1. The patient has a new symptom or constellation of symptoms referable to the central nervous system, but is in no clinical distress.
2. The patient is acutely ill due to problems such as coma, seizures, and/or major neurologic deficits.

Approach to the Stable, Symptomatic Patient

When evaluating a patient with a known cancer problem that is actively being treated or in remission, it is necessary to have a high index of suspicion. Symptoms can be mild and may be of a few days' duration. Symptoms may appear after a long disease-free interval or following an apparent "cure." Headache, which occurs in 50% of patients, is the most frequent presenting symptom. Even if relieved with aspirin or acetaminophen, this symptom must be regarded as ominous when it is daily, progressive, and/or occurring with a nocturnal or early morning component.

Patients may present with an area of focal weakness (40%) or difficulty with gait (20%). Mental status changes occur in 30% of patients and include lapses in memory, confusion, and changes in behavior.

In the patient without a previous history of cancer, assessing the significance of symptoms can be very difficult. It is important to remember that, most often, the duration of symptoms is longer and the course is more insidious. In patients with headache due to primary brain tumor, careful questioning will usually reveal a progressive symptom pattern occurring over 3 to 6 months.

A careful physical examination is mandatory because subtle neurologic deficits may be found that are not reflected by the patient's symptoms. Changes in the mental status exam are present in 75% to 80% of patients and weakness may be detected in 65% to 75%. Other important findings that occur less frequently include sensory deficits (25%), ataxia (25%), and papilledema (25%).

Standard laboratory tests available to the emergency physician are not generally helpful. Skull radiographs may reveal metastases to the calvarium, demineralization of the sella turcica, or shifts in pineal calcification. In adults, the yield is very low. However, in the child or early teenager, craniopharyngioma is the most common primary brain tumor and its characteristic calcifications in the region of the sella turcica are often seen. Computed tomography (CT) or magnetic resonance imaging (MRI) are the procedures of choice and should be scheduled in consultation with the patient's physician or consulting neurologist, usually on a nonemergency, outpatient basis.

The use of corticosteroids in this setting should not be undertaken by the emergency physician prior to specialty consultation. In some settings, corticosteroids may render small tumors less accessible to CT scanning due to the loss of enhancing edema. When indicated, prednisone, 60 mg/day in two or three divided doses is preferred. Parenteral corticosteroids are not indicated unless there is significant nausea and/or vomiting. Other preparations such as dexamethasone or methylprednisolone have no advantages over prednisone for most patients and are substantially more expensive. In cases where very high doses of corticosteroids are being used, usually due to progression of symptoms on lower doses, dexamethasone is generally preferred because it is impractical to give the equivalent of 100 mg of dexamethasone in the form of another corticosteroid. In the absence of seizures, anticonvulsant therapy as a prophylactic measure is not indicated.

Definitive therapy is usually whole brain radiation. Corticosteroid therapy should precede this by 48 hours to minimize the possibility of secondary cerebral edema. Surgical excision is generally limited to (1) solitary metastatic lesions that present following a long disease-free interval, particularly in radioresistant tumors; (2) primary brain tumors accessible to surgical resection; or (3) cases in which the diagnosis is unclear, particularly when nonneoplastic etiologies are possible.

Approach to the Acutely Ill Patient

In this setting, the patient may be actively seizing, postictal, comatose, or have signs of cerebellar herniation and brainstem compression. The basic principles of resuscitation apply. First establish and secure the airway, assure adequate ventilation, and maintain cardiac function. The patient should be monitored at all times and an intravenous (IV) line of 0.9% saline should be started in a secure location at a kvo rate.

Arterial blood gas samples are needed serially to assess acid-base balance and adequacy of oxygenation. Blood sample analysis should include hemoglobin (Hgb), hematocrit (Hct), white blood cell count (WBC), prothrombin time (PT), partial prothrombin time (PTT), platelets, electrolytes, blood urea nitrogen (BUN), glucose, creatinine, carbon dioxide, calcium, and drug screening.

If altered mental status, coma, and/or seizures are present, the patient should receive standard IV doses of dextrose (25 to 50 g), naloxone (2 mg), and thiamine (100 mg) rapidly. Active seizures may be brought under control acutely with IV diazepam, 0.1 mg/kg, or lorazepam. This may be repeated in 5 to 10 minutes if necessary. Since respiratory arrest can occur suddenly in this setting, experienced personnel and appropriate equipment should be immediately available. Diphenylhydantoin loading to a total dose of 15 to 18 mg/kg is used for further control. An initial bolus of 16 to 20 mg of dexamethasone is given IV. When there are signs of impending herniation, additional measures include intubation with hyperventilation to a Pco_2 of 25 to 30, mannitol, 1 mg/kg IV as a 20% solution, and furosemide, 40 to 80 mg/kg IV. Neurologic consultation and immediate CT scanning are indicated.

Spinal Cord Compression

Over 97% of spinal cord compression secondary to malignant disease is the result of extradural compression by metastatic tumor either involving the vertebral bodies or extending through the intervertebral foramina from retroperitoneal lymph nodes or paravertebral soft-tissue masses. Compression from intramedullary metastases is rare, estimated to occur in 1% to 3% of patients, and is associated with a uniformly poor prognosis, even with therapy. Often, the diagnosis of intramedullary metastases is confirmed only at postmortem examination.

Extradural spinal cord compression is a true oncologic emergency. This is because even subtle neurologic deficits can progress rapidly over hours or a few days to total paraplegia and, unfortunately, once paraplegic, the patient has only a 7% or less chance for regaining ambulation. In addition, the chances for remaining fully ambulatory decrease substantially with any signs of neurologic deficit and less than half of patients with significant weakness or loss of anal sphincter tone retain full ambulation.

Even in patients with a progressive cancer illness, the early detection and successful treatment of spinal cord compression can have an enormous positive impact on the remaining quality of life. This point is re-emphasized because there is a great difference between spending three or four months bedridden and spending that same time fully ambulatory.

The major challenge in the diagnosis of spinal cord compression is that when the condition has the greatest potential for response to therapy, neurologic deficits are absent. Many physicians do not appreciate that this is when the true emergency exists. A normal neurologic exam can impart a false sense of security because, while not outwardly apparent, spinal cord compression is there, nonetheless, like a time-bomb in need of rapid defusing.

Therefore, the time for a sense of urgency and high index of suspicion is in the "calm before the storm." In this regard, the emergency physician can play a leading role in the early detection of spinal cord compression, and a vital part in preserving ambulatory function for the cancer patient.

Pain is present in at least 85% to 90% of patients and in most cases this symptom precedes the findings of clinically apparent myelopathy. Most often the pain is progressive over many weeks to months and remains relatively localized to the region of metastatic involvement. There may be a radicular component with either unilateral or bilateral radiation, the latter being more common with compression of the thoracic spine. Subsequently neurologic symptoms and signs of myelopathy begin. These include numbness, paresthesias, weakness, and bowel and/or bladder dysfunction. Careful physical examination may reveal spinal percussion tenderness, reflex diminution, muscular weakness, or sensory changes.

Although pain may present as a relatively stable symptom over long periods of time, the appearance of neurologic disturbances can herald the beginning of a rapid progression to paralysis over several hours to days. Therefore, diagnostic tests and therapeutic interventions must proceed on an emergency basis when neurologic disturbances are documented.

Plain films of the portion of the spine that is symptomatic should be obtained in the emergency department for all patients with a history of active or previously treated cancer, even if the physical exam is normal. If the radiographs are abnormal, disclosing either lytic or blastic changes, myelography is indicated. This should be arranged in conjunction with the patient's private physician and appropriate consultants in oncology, neurology, neurosurgery, and radiology. Although the specific consultant disciplines involved may vary at different institutions, it is important to emphasize that the management of spinal cord compression requires a team effort. An emergency department protocol that will ensure a smooth and rapid mobilization of these specialized, diverse elements should be established. If the neurologic exam is abnormal, myelography must be performed immediately. If the neurologic exam is normal, it may be scheduled for the next working day. In either case, neurosurgery should be involved early because some patients with complete block have a rapid deterioration after the myelogram and may require emergency surgical decompression.

Observation of the patient without myelography is reasonable only when the neurologic exam and plain films are normal or the neurologic exam is abnormal but limited to the extent of a plexopathy and the films are normal. All patients with findings of radiculopathy or myelopathy should proceed to myelography. In uncertain cases, CT scanning or MRI may identify lesions not visualized on plain films or standard tomography. This is particularly important in cases of paravertebral mass with extension through the intervertebral foramina (eg, lymphoma).

Following diagnosis, treatment with corticosteroids is initiated immediately. Currently, dexamethasone, 100 mg/day in four divided doses, is recommended with rapid tapering over several days. This should be given IV initially followed by oral administration as tapering proceeds.

In the past there has been considerable controversy over the relative merits of radiation therapy alone compared with surgical decompression followed by radiation therapy. In general, radiation therapy alone provides results as good as surgical therapy followed by radiation. Therefore, radiation therapy alone is the preferred approach for treatment of spinal cord compression. Surgical therapy is reserved for the following specific situations:

1. No tissue diagnosis of malignancy has been made previously or the spinal cord compression represents an assumed first recurrence of malignancy and the exact etiology is unknown or uncertain.
2. The tumor type is strongly resistant to radiation therapy.
3. There has been a relapse following previous radiation therapy and no further radiation can be delivered to the tissues.
4. Progression of symptoms occurs over 1 to 3 days despite adequate radiation delivery.

The initial approach in the emergency department must be individualized to the severity of the presenting picture. In patients with mild signs and symptoms, admission to the hospital can be arranged for diagnostic and therapeutic procedures. In this setting, chest radiography, electrocardiography (ECG), arterial blood gases, and complete blood chemistries should be obtained. Soft tissue radiographs of the neck will help define the upper trachea. Definitive therapy depends on the tumor histology and location. Surgical resection, radiation therapy, or bronchoscopic laser therapy are all possible modalities.

In cases of severe respiratory distress, surgical consultation should be obtained immediately to assist in airway management. The presence of obstructing tumor can make airway access extremely difficult regardless of the technique employed. Intubation, cricothyrotomy, and formal tracheostomy can all be hazardous or unsuccessful, even in experienced hands. Fortunately, acute tracheal compression necessitating invasive airway management is a rare event.

Cardiac Tamponade

The approach to acute cardiac tamponade in the oncology patient does not differ from the approach utilized in patients with nononcologic disease. Evaluation and therapy of cardiac tamponade in the emergency department should proceed at a pace consistent with the degree of clinical severity. The signs, symptoms, and laboratory findings in the oncology patient parallel those in the nononcology patient.

Acute pericardiocentesis performed in the emergency department can be life saving in critical situations. It is imperative that the pericardial fluid obtained be sent for cytology and cultures. It must be remembered that tamponading pericardial fluid can be the result of nonmalignant etiologies such as infection or radiation pericarditis.

In less severe cases where nontamponading pericardial fluid is suspected on the basis of history, physical, chest radiography, and ECG findings, oncologic and cardiologic consultation should be obtained for echocardiogram and definitive diagnostic studies in the hospital.

SURGICAL EMERGENCIES

Pathologic Fractures

Metastatic disease to bone can occur in the bone marrow, the bone cortex, or both. The most common cancers to involve bone are lung, breast, prostate, kidney, melanoma, and myeloma. If not recognized early, bone metastases can have an enormous negative impact on the quality of life remaining for a cancer patient.

With a progressive osseous metastatic process, there is loss of bony cortex. Architectural strength is diminished and the patient is at risk for fracture. Often this can occur with minimal or no trauma. This is especially true when weight-bearing bones of the pelvic girdle, spine, and legs are involved. Fractures can result in serious disability and pain. Resultant loss of ambulation can then contribute to further complications such as pulmonary emboli, hypercalcemia, decubitus ulcers, infections, and depression.

The emergency physician can play an important role in the early diagnosis of bony metastatic disease. Patients may present in the emergency department with symptoms that they are describing for the first time to a health professional. It is essential that the emergency physician be aware of those symptoms that may reflect underlying osseous metastases and initiate the appropriate diagnostic studies at the time of the initial emergency visit.

Most often, pain will be the presenting symptom. It will generally be localized to the involved region. There may be a radicular component when spinal vertebral bodies are involved. The pain is progressive, often nocturnal, and occurs at rest. It has usually been present for weeks to months, evolving insidiously. Patients may describe a steady, deep, aching feeling that may improve somewhat with activity. Physical examination may reveal bony percussion tenderness. Pain of this type should never be attributed to simple degenerative joint disease or muscles in any patient with a known history of active or previously treated cancer. Even in patients with no history of oncologic disease, this pattern is worrisome and should not be taken lightly.

Skeletal radiographs of the painful areas should be obtained in the emergency department. Two views at 90° angles from each other are mandatory to ensure optimal visualization. Specialized views may be necessary in complex anatomic regions. Tomograms or coned-down views are valuable techniques that are available on an emergency basis. CT scan will often reveal osseous destruction not readily apparent on plain radiographs. Abnormalities may include lytic, blastic or mixed lesions, loss of vertebral pedicles or spinous processes, and vertebral body collapse.

Further evidence of bone marrow involvement may be reflected by leukoerythroblastic changes on the peripheral smear or an anemia. Hypercalcemia may be present and the serum calcium level should be checked.

When lytic lesions have destroyed greater than 25% of the cortical width of the weight-bearing long bones, orthopedic consultation should be obtained on an emergency basis. These lesions of the femur often require immediate prophylactic surgical stabilization. Destructive metastatic lesions of the cervical spine can be unstable and may require halo casting.

Obstruction

Gastrointestinal Obstructions

Obstructions in the gastrointestinal tract can occur at the level of the esophagus, the gastric outlet, and the small or large bowel. Esophageal lesions progress slowly and rarely present as emergencies. More often there is an insidious history of dysphagia, progressing from liquids to solids, often accompanied by weight loss with a background of heavy alcohol intake and smoking.

Gastric outlet obstruction may be due to benign etiologies such as peptic ulcer disease with scarring and edema or gastric carcinoma. Regardless of etiology, the initial emergency department management is the same. The following basic principles also apply to small or large bowel obstruction.

After history and physical assessment, the emergency physician should obtain a complete blood count with differential, amylase, urinalysis, chemistries, and abdominal obstruction series radiographs (flat, upright, and posteroanterior chest views). The patient should be given nothing by mouth and IV fluids should be started for both replacement and maintenance with correction of any electrolyte imbalances. Nasogastric decompression is initiated and surgical consultation obtained. In most cases, surgical therapy is required for definitive management of malignant obstruction.

Genitourinary Obstructions

Typically, obstruction is the result of extrinsic compression of the ureters by direct extension of pelvic tumor masses. Gynecologic malignancies (cervix and ovary), genitourinary malignancies (testicular with retroperitoneal lymph node invasion, prostate), and colonic malignancies are the types most often involved.

Signs and symptoms may include flank pain, hematuria (gross or microscopic), fever, anorexia, nausea, and associated symptoms of azotemia. A mass may be noted on abdominal, rectal, or pelvic exam. Basic studies obtained in the emergency department include complete blood count, electrolytes, BUN, creatinine, abdominal radiographs, and urinalysis. Consultations should be obtained with urology and oncology.

Specific interventions will depend on the individual clinical setting. Ureteral obstruction as a late complication of advanced, previously treated cervical carcinoma may not warrant further invasive procedures. On the other hand, a patient with ureteral obstruction secondary to a metastatic testicular germ cell tumor involving the retroperitoneal lymph nodes would require surgical placement of ureteral stents and aggressive chemotherapy, possibly including hyperalimentation.

INFECTIOUS EMERGENCIES

Fever and Granulocytopenia

Despite the many advances that have taken place in the diagnosis and treatment of oncologic disease, infection continues to be the most serious complication in cancer patients and is the most common cause of death. Although infection may occur as a terminal event in a patient with widespread metastatic disease, it frequently occurs early in the course of the cancer. Often it is associated with the initial induction phase of treatment. When the underlying malignancy is highly responsive to therapy, prevention or successful treatment of a complicating infection becomes crucial to the patient's survival and chance for complete remission.

It is extremely important that all emergency health care personnel recognize the significance of fever in the cancer patient and act with an appropriate sense of urgency. A thorough diagnostic evaluation must be completed within 2 to 4 hours and immediately followed by antibiotic therapy.

There are many factors that contribute to the cancer patient's propensity toward infection. Radiation therapy, chemotherapy, and the malignant process itself can all cause bone marrow suppression or destruction and subsequent granulocytopenia. In addition, the body's natural barriers are lost, allowing host flora (often hospital-acquired) to penetrate mucous membranes. The patient may be clinically debilitated and nutritionally compromised.

The lack of granulocytes causes a marked decrease in the host inflammatory response. Signs of cellulitis or abscess formation may be subtle or absent. Production of purulent material is decreased. There may be less cough and/or sputum than expected. The fever response is due to the release of endogenous pyrogens from fixed macrophages of the liver, spleen, and lungs and is therefore not generally diminished by neutropenia. Signs of pneumonia may be absent on physical exam and the chest radiograph may not disclose an infiltrate. Urinary tract infections may present as frequency without dysuria. Pyuria may be decreased.

At times, delineating the exact etiology of fever in the oncology patient is difficult because transfusion reactions, chemotherapy reactions, and the underlying malignancy can all cause a febrile host response. However, as the number of granulocytes decreases, the risk of infection increases and becomes especially pronounced at absolute granulocyte counts of 500/mm^3 or less. Fever in this setting, particularly if equal to or greater than 101°F (38.3°C), must be assumed to be secondary to infection.

The emergency physician must obtain a careful history and physical assessment, paying particular attention to areas that might be overlooked in the patient with nonmalignant disease and normal granulocytes. This should include examination of the gingiva, axillae, groin, and rectum. Diagnostic studies must include three sets of blood cultures for aerobic, anaerobic, and fungal organisms, urinalysis and culture, throat culture, chest radiographs, PT, activated PTT (APTT), platelet count, and chemistries. Surveillance cultures of the nose, gingiva, and rectum are recommended more often for febrile patients with hematologic malignancies than for those with solid tumors. In patients with accessible fluid such as ascites or pleural effusions, diagnostic samples should be obtained for Gram stain and culture. When central nervous system changes are present, CT scanning and lumbar puncture are indicated.

A sputum sample, if obtainable, should be sent for Gram's stain and culture even though results are often difficult to interpret due to the frequent absence of granulocytes. Use of transtracheal aspiration for obtaining a reliable sputum sample is controversial and will depend on local experience. It should be emphasized that invasive procedures are often necessary to establish a correct diagnosis in cases with pulmonary infiltrates. This is because the malignancy, its treatment (either with chemotherapy or radiation therapy), or infection can account for the infiltrates. Depending on the individual case, this may be accomplished by transbronchial biopsy, percutaneous thin-needle aspiration, or open-lung biopsy.

Broad-spectrum, bactericidal, antibiotics should be started in high doses. Despite the introduction of many broad-spectrum single agents, general preference is still for the use of two or three synergistic agents. There is no single-best combination, but most regimens include an aminoglycoside and a carboxy or extended-spectrum penicillin. Additional agents may be added for specific situations: cotrimoxazole for *Pneumocystis,* erythromycin for *Legionella,* metronidazole for anaerobes, vancomycin for methicillin-resistant staphylococci, and third-generation cephalosporins (ceftadizime, ceftrizyone) when aminoglycosides are contraindicated or when meningitis is suspected. In some cases, antifungal agents may be appropriate. Oncologic consultation should be obtained before initiation of antibiotic therapy. If a hospital bed for admission is not immediately available, antibiotic therapy should be started in the emergency department.

METABOLIC EMERGENCIES

Hypercalcemia

Hypercalcemia is a problem that is frequently encountered in patients with cancer. Several factors contribute to this:

1. In some patients, paraneoplastic syndromes result in ectopic production of parathyroid hormone–like hormones. This is especially notable in epidermoid (squamous cell) carcinoma of the lung.
2. There is calcium resorption from bone secondary to lytic metastases and osteoclastic factors. This is common in multiple myeloma, lymphoma, breast, and non–small cell lung cancer. In contrast, osteoblastic metastases are rarely associated with hypercalcemia.
3. Tumor release of prostaglandins has been shown to enhance bone resorption experimentally. This may be of limited significance in clinical practice, however.
4. Cancer patients often spend prolonged periods of time in bed due to pain, weakness, and/or disability secondary to the malignant process or its treatment.

In addition, dehydration, an exacerbating factor in hypercalcemia, may be present due to decreased fluid intake, poor nutrition, anorexia, nausea, vomiting, and diarrhea secondary to the malignant process or its treatment.

The severity of the patient's clinical picture will depend primarily on the rate of the rising calcium level. Rapid changes can produce marked symptoms at modest serum calcium elevations (12.0 to 12.5 mg/dL). Slowly progressive, chronic elevations to levels of 15 mg/dL, however, may be tolerated by the patient with relatively mild symptoms. The emergency physician should be thoroughly familiar with the many symptoms that can occur with hypercalcemia: fatigue, weakness, anorexia, nausea, vomiting, constipation, polyuria, polydipsia, lethargy, and confusion. At the extreme, hypercalcemia can produce coma and life-threatening changes in cardiac function.

Emergency Department Management of Severe Hypercalcemia

1. If the patient presents with coma, the basic principles of coma management apply. Airway, breathing, and cardiac function must be assured. Dextrose, naloxone, and thiamine should be given. Cardiac monitoring should be utilized continuously while the patient is in the emergency department.
2. Complete blood count, electrolytes, BUN, glucose, calcium, phosphorus, magnesium, and albumin levels are drawn immediately. PT, APTT, platelet count, and toxicology studies are obtained as clinically indicated.
3. A chest radiograph, ECG, and urinalysis are obtained.
4. Accurate recording of input and output is essential. A Foley catheter will be necessary in obtunded or comatose patients.
5. IV hydration with normal saline is started at 200 to 250 mL/hour (4 to 6 L/day). This corrects dehydration and promotes a saline calciuresis. Furosemide, 1 mg/kg (40 to 80 mg), is given IV push to enhance this process. In older patients, or when there is known underlying cardiovascular illness, central venous pressure or Swan-Ganz pulmonary wedge pressure measurements may be needed. Electrolyte balance must be carefully maintained. Replacement must be guided by serial serum electrolyte determinations.
6. In the alert patient, oral phosphates such as Fleets Phospho-Soda, 5 to 15 mL/day may be given to bind calcium in the gut. Diarrhea is a common side effect, particularly if higher doses are used. Diphenoxylate may be given to control this.

Oncologic consultation should be promptly obtained and the patient admitted to the hospital. Additional measures for hypercalcemia, not generally part of the initial emergency department management include administration of mithramycin and corticosteroids. Mithramycin was initially developed as a chemotherapeutic agent. However, it soon became more useful for its side effect of hypocalcemia. The usual dose is 25 μ/kg IV and it should be reserved for hypercalcemia secondary to malignancy. Significant hypocalcemic effects begin approximately 12 to 48 hours after administration. It may be repeated every 2 to 5 days but the total number of doses is generally limited to less than eight due to myelosuppression, notably thrombocytopenia.

Corticosteroids can be especially helpful in the management of hypercalcemia secondary to breast carcinoma, multiple myeloma, and lymphoma. Onset of action is approximately 24 to 48 hours after administration. Prednisone, 50 to 100 mg/day, is given by mouth in divided doses. IV corticosteroids may be given to those patients unable to tolerate oral medications. In part, the hypocalcemic effect of corticosteroids is due to their antitumor activity in these particular neoplasms, and they may be part of the planned chemotherapeutic regimen. For this reason, the emergency physician should not initiate steroid therapy without oncologic consultation.

Ultimately, the successful treatment of hypercalcemia in malignancy depends on treatment of the underlying neoplasm. When this is possible, major improvements in the patient's quality of life can be expected.

Syndrome of Inappropriate Antidiuretic Hormone (ADH) and Hyponatremia

In patients with cancer, hyponatremia is most often due to the elaboration of ectopic ADH or ADH-like hormones. Less frequently, it is due to brain metastases or secondary to vicristine or cyclophosphamide. This leads to increased water retention, decreased serum osmolality, and dilutional hyponatremia. Most often, this syndrome is seen in association with small cell lung cancer.

With mild to moderate hyponatremia, patients may be asymptomatic or have vague constitutional symptoms such as weakness, malaise, nausea, and/or anorexia. However, with severe hyponatremia (usually less than 120 mEq/L) or a rapid rate of development, patients may develop seizures and mental status changes with confusion, stupor, and coma.

Initial tests obtained in the emergency department include chest radiographs, ECG, electrolytes, glucose, BUN, creatinine, and urinalysis. In addition, determinations of the serum osmolality, urine osmolality, and spot urine sodium concentration are needed.

The diagnosis is confirmed when the urine osmolality is inappropriately high (ie, not maximally dilute at a time when the serum osmolality is low). In addition, the urine spot sodium concentration is inappropriately high at a time when the serum sodium concentration is low. Diuretic therapy can confound the interpretation of these tests, and there should be no evidence of dehydration or edema on physical exam. The patient should have normal renal, adrenal, and thyroid function.

Treatment of the underlying malignancy is necessary to ultimately reverse this condition. In mild to moderate cases, water restriction of 750 to 1000 mL/day may be sufficient until antineoplastic therapy becomes effective. Demeclocycline, 300 mg, taken orally four times per day, has been shown to produce a nephrogenic diabetes insipidus and is, therefore, effective in further controlling the syndrome of inappropriate ADH secretion.

Severe cases represent a true medical emergency. Patients will require continuous cardiac monitoring, arterial blood gases, accurate input and output monitoring, frequent serial electrolyte determinations, and hourly urinometer readings. Furosemide, 1 mg/kg IV push, should be given and IV normal saline initiated at a rate consistent with urinary losses. Electrolyte losses are replaced with KCl. Three percent saline may also be used cautiously in addition to or in place of 0.9% saline, but there is a greater risk of fluid overload. In older patients, or when there is known underlying cardiovascular disease, central venous pressure or Swan-Ganz pulmonary wedge pressure readings should be carefully followed. Seizures, if recurrent, should be treated with IV diphenylhydantoin.

Acute Adrenal Insufficiency (Adrenal Crisis)

Although acute adrenal insufficiency is uncommon, its presence must not be overlooked because it represents a true medical emergency that is life threatening if not treated early. Cancer patients may be predisposed to this complication for several reasons: (1) Metastatic disease may involve the adrenals, eliminating the patient's ability to respond to stress with increased corticosteroid output. Lung cancer, especially the small cell type, breast cancer, and malignant melanoma often metastasize to the adrenals. (2) Many cancer patients have been on long-term corticosteroid therapy and in times of stress their adrenals may be unable to produce adequate corticosteroids. (3) Some patients, particularly those with breast cancer may be taking aminoglutethimide which blocks corticosteroid production in the adrenals, thus creating a "medical adrenalectomy."

The key signs and symptoms include weakness, fever, nausea, vomiting, abdominal pain, hypotension, dehydration, and confusion. In severe cases, frank shock is present. Complete blood count, electrolytes, BUN, and glucose will usually show the following abnormalities: hyperkalemia, hyponatremia, hypoglycemia, and azotemia. Plasma cortisol, chest radiographs, ECG, urinalysis with culture, and blood cultures should be obtained.

Intravenous 5% dextrose in normal saline should be started and 250 mg hydrocortisone sodium succinate given intravenously and immediately, followed by 100 mg IV every 6 hours. Underlying infection must be treated vigorously and careful fluid and electrolyte balance must be maintained.

ACUTE COMPLICATIONS OF TREATMENT

Radiation Therapy

Radiation Pneumonitis

Acute radiation pneumonitis most often occurs 1 to 3 months after completion of radiation therapy. Dyspnea and dyspnea on exertion are common presenting symptoms. Cough is usually nonproductive and the presence of purulent sputum should alert the examiner to the possibility of superimposed infection. The WBC is not generally helpful in the differential diagnosis. Most often, it is moderately elevated.

The most helpful finding in establishing the diagnosis of radiation pneumonitis is the chest radiograph. Infiltrates with sharply defined borders corresponding to the radiation ports are very strong evidence in favor of radiation pneumonitis.

At times, the diagnosis will be unclear. Infiltrates from malignancy, particularly when there is lymphangitic spread, infection, and toxic reactions from chemotherapy can all mimic those of radiation pneumonitis. Sputum Gram stain may help to support the diagnosis of bacterial infection in some cases, but in many situations, tissue biopsy will be required.

In the emergency department, arterial blood gases should be obtained and oxygen administered as needed to correct hypoxemia. Following oncology consultation, patients with severe symptoms should be admitted to the hospital for definitive diagnosis and therapy. In most cases, corticosteroid therapy (prednisone, 40 to 60 mg/day by mouth) is initiated and subsequently tapered after symptomatic improvement.

Radiation Enteritis

The bowel mucosa is very sensitive to the effects of ionizing radiation. Radiation enteritis is characterized by nausea, vomiting, diarrhea, and crampy abdominal pain. In severe cases, gastrointestinal bleeding can occur, but this is unusual. More often the stool is positive for occult blood without gross melena or hematochezia.

Mild cases of radiation enteritis are not likely to be seen in the emergency department, but patients in severe distress will benefit from IV fluids, antiemetics, and antidiarrheal agents. With treatment in the emergency department, many patients will be able to remain outpatients. Those who are debilitated and/or toxic may be admitted to the hospital for prolonged treatment.

Chemotherapy

Pulmonary Toxicity

Many chemotherapy agents can produce toxic pulmonary effects. Bleomycin, methotrexate, procarbazine, mitomycin-C, and nitrosoureas are the most frequent offenders. In general, these reactions are uncommon, but with bleomycin and the nitrosoureas, toxicity is dose related. The pathologic changes of diffuse interstitial pulmonary fibrosis are typical in most cases.

Patients may present with progressive dyspnea (both at rest and on exertion), nonproductive cough, and fatigue. Dry, crackling rales are often heard on physical exam. The varying infiltrates seen on chest films can be compatible with the underlying malignant process or infection. In acutely ill patients biopsy may be necessary to establish the diagnosis. Supportive care should be initiated in the emergency department. Oxygen should be given when arterial blood gases reveal hypoxemia. Corticosteroids are often used, but their efficacy has not been documented. Outcome is variable. In some patients the process abates after cessation of the offending drug, but in other cases progressive pulmonary insufficiency ensues, which may be fatal.

Cardiac Toxicity

The most common antineoplastic drugs to adversely affect the heart are the anthracyclines: doxorubicin (Adriamycin) and daunorubicin. Both drugs can produce a congestive cardiomyopathy that is dose related. In addition, prior mediastinal radiation therapy can potentiate the propensity to develop this complication.

The clinical picture is one of congestive heart failure with dyspnea (both at rest and on exertion), fatigue, orthopnea, nonproductive cough, and swelling of the lower extremities. Physical examination confirms the presence of congestive failure with tachycardia, peripheral edema, pulmonary rales, neck vein distention, S3, and cardiomegaly. In severe cases, acute pulmonary edema may develop. Treatment is with conventional diuretics and cardiac glycosides. The response is variable.

Gastrointestinal Toxicity

Nausea and vomiting are the two side effects of chemotherapy that are almost always feared by the cancer patient. Many antineoplastic agents are associated with this, and in some cases nausea and vomiting can be profound and prolonged. It should be remembered, however, that nausea and vomiting are symptoms and can, at times, be related to the underlying malignant process or nonmalignant abdominal disease such as acute cholecystitis or pancreatitis.

When the emergency physician is confronted with this problem, it is important that careful history and physical assessment and ancillary laboratory studies appropriate to the clinical presentation be performed prior to attributing these symptoms to chemotherapy. IV fluids should be given in severe cases and electrolyte balance maintained. In the acute setting, prochlorperazine (Compazine) may be given parenterally in doses of 5 to 15 mg. Haloperidol (Haldol), 1 to 2 mg intramuscularly, may also be effective.

Patients should be examined carefully for signs of mucositis. This can be very serious, predisposing patients to infection through loss of natural barriers. This is especially dangerous when leukopenia is also present. Diarrhea and/or hematochezia may occur which, in turn, can lead to dehydration, anemia, and electrolyte imbalance. In addition, *Candida*, which often colonizes the gastrointestinal tract of cancer patients, can become an invasive pathogen when mucosal membranes are damaged.

It should be noted that vincristine can cause an autonomic nerve dysfunction leading to abdominal pain and constipation. Oncology consultation should be obtained because some patients can develop a severe ileus that would require hospitalization.

Bone Marrow Toxicity

This topic is mentioned briefly to alert the emergency physician to the times when marrow elements are especially likely to be abnormal. Most antineoplastic agents adversely affect the bone marrow because they kill dividing cells. Following administration of one or several agents, a predictable drop in the WBC and platelet count occurs. The red blood cell count tends to remain stable because the red blood cell half-life is 120 days. The half-life of the platelet, however, is 5 to 7 days, and that of the granulocyte is only 6 hours. As the effects of the chemotherapy wear off, there is a recovery phase in the marrow and a return to normal WBC and platelet count. During this time, the activity of the marrow may "overshoot" the normal values and a leukemoid reaction may be observed.

In most cases, the lowest points in the WBC and platelet count (ie, the nadirs) occur 10 to 14 days after the chemotherapy has been given. When evaluating an oncology patient, it is important that the emergency physician determine the time of the last administration of chemotherapy agents. This will help to clarify if abnormal counts are on the way down or past the time of the nadir and on the way up. Clearly, patients in the former category are at higher risk for further problems.

HEMATOLOGIC EMERGENCIES

Hemorrhage

The cancer patient may present in the emergency department with acute bleeding that is uncontrollable and/or massive. Two factors contribute to this:

1. In some patients with advanced disease that is no longer responsive to antineoplastic therapy, the physician may be unable to stop the bleeding process. Often this is encountered in disseminated intravascular coagulation (DIC) secondary to a malignancy that has progressed despite repeated chemotherapy treatments.
2. In some cases, tumor erosion into a major vessel can produce rapid, exsanguinating hemorrhage. This may be accompanied by massive hemoptysis and/or hematemesis. In patients where no further effective treatments are available, uncontrolled bleeding may be the terminal event.

In these situations, attention must be directed toward patient comfort. It must be recognized that severe or uncontrollable hemorrhage can be frightening for both the patient and physician. If readily available, hospice care personnel should be consulted. Their ability to assist the patient and family in the emergency department can be invaluable.

When confronted with acute hemorrhage in the oncology patient, the emergency physician should determine if the bleeding is due to thrombocytopenia or platelet dysfunction, DIC, or a coagulation defect. Mucosal bleeding is almost always due to a qualitative and/or quantitative platelet defect. Coagulopathies usually result in deep tissue bleeding such as hemarthrosis or retroperitoneal hemorrhage.

Initial laboratory studies should include CBC, type and cross-match, platelet count, bleeding time, PT, APTT, thrombin time, fibrin split products, and examination of the peripheral smear. If bleeding is severe, the blood bank should be notified of the possible need for whole blood, packed cells, fresh frozen plasma, and/or platelets. A careful assessment of all medications (over-the-counter and prescription) and the patient's nutritional status is essential. A thorough evaluation should be carried out to exclude infection, sepsis, or tumor progression.

Decreased platelets may be the result of immune destruction, consumption during DIC, or loss of megakaryocyte production. Decreased production is the most commonly encountered etiology and is usually due to bone marrow replacement by tumor or destruction following chemotherapy and/or radiation therapy. In many cases, a bone marrow examination is necessary to clarify the diagnosis, and even with low platelet counts, this can generally be performed safely.

Serious bleeding secondary to thrombocytopenia is rare when the platelet count is above $25,000/mm^3$, unless there is an associated qualitative defect or coagulopathy. Platelet transfusions may be initiated in cases of severe thrombocytopenia. When thrombocytopenia is due to myelosuppression, platelet transfusions are effective, and are utilized until marrow recovery occurs. One unit generally raises the count by $10,000/mm^3$. Typically 4 to 6 U are given per transfusion. In cases of immune destruction, platelet transfusions are generally not helpful because the donor platelets are destroyed rapidly after entry into the host. For this reason, bone marrow examination and antiplatelet antibodies determinations are essential to the diagnostic work-up of thrombocytopenia not clearly due to the myelosuppressive effects of chemotherapy.

Treatment of DIC is complicated and requires hematologic consultation. The use of heparin is controversial and can result in bleeding episodes. Furthermore, the treatment of DIC may require a consolidated approach utilizing chemotherapy and/or radiation therapy directed at the underlying malignant process. Acid-base disturbances must be corrected and infection treated. Treatment of coagulation disorders depends on the specific deficiencies. In most cases, however, fresh frozen plasma can be utilized when uncontrolled bleeding is present.

Thrombosis

The association of migratory thrombophlebitis and gastrointestinal malignancy (Trousseau's syndrome) has been well documented. While adenocarcinomas of the gastrointestinal tract are most often associated with this phenomenon, it has been described in carcinomas of other organs such as breast and prostate.

The emergency physician should suspect occult carcinoma when evaluating a patient with a history of migratory episodes of thrombophlebitis and/or episodes of thrombophlebitis occurring in unusual locations such as the upper extremities or axillary veins. This is particularly true when the patient has no associated medical conditions that would predispose to thrombophlebitis.

Initial management of thrombophlebitis in the setting of malignancy does not differ from the general management of thrombophlebitis. It should be noted, however, that higher doses of heparin are often required, and exacerbations are common when patients are subsequently placed on coumadin therapy. In addition, it is important to initiate therapy against the underlying malignant process. This may enable the thrombophlebitis to come under control.

CARDIOPULMONARY EMERGENCIES

SVC Obstruction

When venous return from the superior vena cava (SVC) is obstructed, either from extrinsic compression or intrinsic (intraluminal) blockage, a clinical syndrome results that is marked by facial and upper body swelling, edema, and venous distention. Dyspnea and tachypnea are often present with cough, dysphagia, and headache occurring less frequently. Back pain is not typically a symptom of SVC syndrome, and when present should alert the physician to the possibility of concomitant spinal cord compression.

Forty to 50 years ago, most cases of SVC obstruction were due to nonmalignant etiologies. Thoracic aortic aneurysms accounted for one-third of all cases with an additional one-third caused by such problems as infection (particularly tuberculosis), chronic fibrosis or mediastinitis. Since the 1950s, there has been a progressive decrease in benign etiologies to the point that today they account for only 5% to 15% of all cases. During this same time period, there has been a marked increase in malignant etiologies which now account for 85% to 95% of all cases. Primarily, this has been the result of a sharp increase in the incidence of lung cancer which now accounts for 70% to 80% of all cases. Lymphoma (10% to 15%) and metastatic tumors (5% to 10%), notably breast and testicular, comprise the remaining malignant etiologies. Unlike neurologic emergencies which often occur in previously diagnosed patients, the SVC syndrome may be the presenting feature of malignancy.

Historically, it was thought that patients with mental obtundation and marked plethora of the head and neck would rapidly progress to coma, convulsions, and death. This led to the generally held opinion that SVC obstruction represented a severe oncologic emergency necessitating rapid empirical treatment prior to definitive diagnosis.

Several important concepts have changed in the understanding of SVC obstruction and its management. First, it is now appreciated that in the vast majority of cases, SVC obstruction does not represent a life-threatening emergency. Contrary to previous thinking, there is time in all but the severest cases to make an adequate tissue diagnosis. The prognosis in SVC obstruction is a function of the underlying etiology. Patients with a rapidly progressive, treatment-resistant tumor will have a rapidly progressive clinical demise. However, those with a treatable malignancy or benign etiology will have a good long-term outlook. Severe respiratory compromise is unlikely in the absence of acute tracheal compression, and seizures have not been documented to occur in the absence of intracranial metastatic disease.

Second, it has become clear that establishing a diagnosis with tissue biopsy is safer than previously realized. Although increased bleeding secondary to elevated venous pressure is a relative contraindication, invasive procedures have resulted in few complications when performed by experienced operators. In addition, it has become increasingly more important to establish a specific tissue diagnosis because today the most common etiologies of SVC obstruction are highly treatable, with either chemotherapy or radiation therapy or both. Currently, small cell lung carcinoma is the single most common etiology of SVC obstruction (40% of all cases). It is highly responsive to polychemotherapy and most oncologists would prefer chemotherapy to radiation therapy as the initial treatment of SVC obstruction due to small cell lung carcinoma. Clearly, treatment planning in these situations is impossible without adequate definition of the specific malignancy.

Overall, the emergency physician should approach SVC syndrome as a true emergency even when the initial presentation appears subtle. Immediate oncologic consultation is indicated because symptoms may progress rapidly and, in most cases, diagnostic studies must be performed without delay.

Initial Emergency Department Management

In patients suspected of having SVC obstruction the following studies should be obtained: chest radiographs, arterial blood gases, ECG, CBC, coagulation studies, and chemistries. If the patient is in distress, an IV line of 5% dextrose in water at kvo rate and cardiac monitoring should be started. When hypoxemia is documented, appropriate concentrations of oxygen should be initiated. Oncology consultation should be obtained and the patient admitted to the hospital.

Temporizing measures include diuretics (furosemide, 40 to 60 mg IV push) and corticosteroids (dexamethasone, 16 mg/day in four divided doses). These should be initiated after oncologic consultation.

Specific diagnostic tests must be individualized to the patient's clinical presentation. In experienced hands the following procedures have been shown to be safe and valuable in establishing the diagnosis: sputum cytology, pleural fluid cytology, pleural biopsy, bronchoscopy with bronchial washings and biopsy, lymph node biopsy, bone marrow biopsy (bilateral iliac crests), mediastinoscopy with biopsy, and limited thoracotomy (Chamberlain procedure).

Acute Tracheal Obstruction

Obstruction of the trachea can be secondary to extrinsic compression by a tumor mass. Intrinsic luminal narrowing may occur when there is direct tracheal tumor invasion or a primary tracheal tumor, most often of the squamous epithelium.

Regardless of etiology, the presenting picture in the emergency department will be similar. Symptoms include dyspnea, cough, hemoptysis, dysphagia, neck and/or chest pain, and marked apprehension. Hoarseness may be a sign of tumor involvement of the recurrent laryngeal nerve. Physical examination will usually reveal inspiratory stridor, tachypnea, wheezing, and labored breathing. Symptoms and signs of hypoxemia may also be present in severe cases.

SUGGESTED READINGS

Ahmann FR. A reassessment of the clinical importance of the superior vena caval syndrome. *J Clin Oncol.* 1984;2:961–969.

Carter SK, Glatstein E, Livingston RB. *Principles of Cancer Treatment.* New York: McGraw-Hill; 1982.

Casciato DA, Lowitz BB. *Manual of Bedside Oncology.* Boston: Little, Brown; 1983.

DeVita VT, Hellman S, Rosenberg SA. *Cancer, Principles and Practice of Oncology.* 3rd ed. Philadelphia: Lippincott; 1989.

Mousa AR, Schimpff SC, Robson ML. *Comprehensive Textbook of Oncology.* 2nd ed. Baltimore: Williams & Wilkins; 1991.

Parish JM, et al. Etiologic considerations in the superior vena caval syndrome. *Mayo Clin Proc.* 1981;56:407–413.

Perry MC, guest ed. Toxicity of chemotherapy. *Semin Oncol.* 1982;9:1–154.

Portlock CS, Goffinett DR. *Manual of Clinical Problems in Oncology.* Boston: Little, Brown; 1980.

Posner JB. Management of central nervous system metastases. *Semin Oncol.* 1977;4:81–91.

Rodichok LD, et al. Early diagnosis of spinal epidural metastases. *Am J Med*. 1981;70:1181–1187.

Rodriguez M, DiNapoli RP. Spinal cord compression. *Mayo Clin Proc*. 1980;55:442–448.

Seigal LJ, Longo DL. The control of chemotherapy-induced emesis. *Ann Intern Med*. 1981;95:352–359.

Stewart AF. Therapy of malignancy-associated hypercalcemia—1983. *Am J Med*. 1983;74:475–480.

Yarbro JW, ed. Oncologic emergencies. *Semin Oncol*. 1989;16:461–594.

Yarbro JW, Bornstein RS, eds. *Oncologic Emergencies*. New York: Grune & Stratton; 1981.

31. Pediatric Cardiopulmonary Resuscitation

JAMES E. PIEROG, MD, FACEP

Pediatric cardiopulmonary resuscitation (CPR) differs from its adult counterpart in several important aspects that must be appreciated for a successful outcome. Key differences include the following:

- size—heightened technical skills and a wide range of proportionate equipment are required
- anatomic structure—techniques for successful procedures are different
- etiologies—primary cardiac events are rare, and respiratory causes predominate
- lower incidence—fewer opportunities exist for developing competency and skill
- drugs and their dosages—differences in effects, complications, and dilutions must be considered on the basis of weight

One of the cornerstones of care in CPR is the rapid establishment of an adequate airway and effective ventilation. This is particularly important in pediatric CPR because of the prevalence of respiratory disorders as the primary insult (Table 31-1) and the fact that successful resuscitation from respiratory arrest is much more common than resuscitation from cardiac arrest. Unlike adult cardiorespiratory arrests, where cardiac causes predominate and rapid reversal of ventricular tachycardia/ventricular fibrillation (VF) may result in normal neurologic function, children rarely arrest from a primary cardiac event. Childhood arrest is usually secondary to a respiratory event or multisystem organ failure. By the time young, healthy hearts arrest, the hypoxic neurologic insult is so overwhelming that resuscitation is rarely effective.

Gillis et al[1] showed in a review of in-hospital resuscitation reports that survival rates for respiratory and cardiac arrests were 44% and 9%, respectively. Moreover, Friesen et al,[2] in a Canadian study of pediatric CPR, showed a dramatic difference in survival between respiratory and cardiac arrests: 40% and 3%, respectively.

Hypoxia and acidosis generated by respiratory failure (with or without circulatory compromise) lead directly to cardiovascular insufficiency. With the establishment of an adequate airway and ventilation, it is not uncommon for bradycardia and hypotension to improve rapidly and often to be completely reversed. Although respiratory causes predominate, there are diverse causes of pediatric cardiopulmonary collapse (Table 31-1). Regardless of the cause, the final common pathway is usually profound acidosis and hypoxia. For some time, attention has been directed to the predominance of respiratory and circulatory dysfunction as major causes of cardiopulmonary arrest.[3,4] Recently,[5] application of this knowledge has led to emphasis on prearrest assessment with anticipatory intervention and ventilation techniques in hopes of reducing the generally dismal results of pediatric CPR in the full arrest state.

AIRWAY

The pliability of the pediatric trachea (lack of firm cartilaginous rings) can cause airway obstruction with excessive

Table 31-1 Pediatric Cardiac Arrest: Etiologies

Respiratory
    Upper airway obstruction: laryngotracheitis, acute supraglottitis, membranous tracheitis, trauma, foreign body, tongue
    Small airways disease: infection, status asthmaticus, trauma, aspiration, submersion injury, toxic inhalation, pulmonary edema, pneumothorax
Shock
    Hypovolemic, distributive, cardiogenic
Near-miss sudden infant death syndrome
Congenital
    Cardiac, respiratory tract, central nervous system
Poisoning
    Primarily narcotics (including maternal), sedatives-hypnotics, anticholinergics, salicylates
Cardiac
    Myocarditis, dysrhythmias, conduction defects
Central nervous system
    Infections, trauma, neuromuscular disorders

hyperextension maneuvers. The sniffing position (neck slightly flexed on the shoulders with the head slightly extended on the neck) provides the best anatomic alignment for opening the airway. This position is easily achieved by placing a small rolled towel or hand under the child's occiput for elevation. The head tilt and chin lift are effective maneuvers in children and often are all that is necessary adequately to open the airway and stimulate ventilation.

If head or neck injury is present or suspected, proper cervical immobilization is indicated. The jaw thrust maneuver is substituted for the head tilt/chin lift as the procedure of choice for opening the airway. Jaw thrust without head tilt appears to be the safest technique for opening the airway when cervical spine or cord injury is suspected or apparent. Manual in-line cervical traction is recommended by the American Heart Association and the American Academy of Pediatrics in their conjoint *Textbook of Pediatric Advanced Life Support*[5] for patients in whom head or neck injury is suspected. They suggest that "manual in-line cervical traction must be maintained until cervical spine injury is excluded or the neck is properly immobilized."[5(p12)] Furthermore, manual in-line cervical traction is recommended by the American College of Surgeons' Advanced Trauma Life Support course as a safe procedure for orotracheal intubation in patients whose cervical spine status is unknown. Recently, Rosen[6] and others[7,8] have challenged the rationale for such practice. At present, it seems prudent to immobilize the cervical spine in the neutral position without manual in-line cervical traction until further definitive studies are available.

Liquids, particulate matter, and foreign bodies may be removed by suctioning or using Magill forceps under direct laryngoscopic visualization. Blind finger sweeps in the pediatric population are fraught with the danger of potentially pushing a supraglottic foreign body into the glottic opening.

Pooling of liquids (blood, mucus, or secretions) in the posterior oropharynx can be facilitated by placing the child in the head-down (Trendelenburg) position. In this position the secretions can be suctioned gently, thereby avoiding the potential complications of aspiration and airway obstruction. With the newer mechanical gurneys, this position is easily achieved by raising the foot and lowering the head ends, respectively. Excessively aggressive suctioning of the posterior pharynx is condemned, because it may cause bleeding and swelling with airway compromise or may stimulate a vagally mediated bradycardia. Parasympathetic responses can be exaggerated in the pediatric population, and laryngoscopy or suctioning that is well tolerated in adults can lead to vagally induced asystole in children. Constant cardiac monitoring and gentle technique are mainstays in avoiding excessive vagal stimulation.

Three infectious causes need special consideration when one is managing the airway. These are viral laryngotracheitis (croup), bacterial tracheobronchitis (membranous tracheitis), and acute supraglottitis (epiglottitis). All three are capable of producing upper airway obstruction and respiratory arrest leading to cardiovascular collapse. Considerable misunderstanding surrounds the management of these conditions, especially acute supraglottitis. If these conditions are suspected, immediate confirmation is required by direct visualization (oropharyngeal examination, direct laryngoscopy, or fiberoptic nasolaryngoscopy).[9,10] It has been repeatedly stressed in textbooks and review articles that upper airway manipulation can result in irreversible upper airway obstruction. Support for this belief is confined to a few isolated anecdotal case reports. The theory for this belief is that the mobile, inflamed epiglottis is aspirated into the glottic opening, causing an irreversible obstruction. Dunbar[11] has shown with cineradiographic studies, however, that the epiglottis is immobile in all phases of respiration. Furthermore, in cases of respiratory arrest with acute supraglottitis it is well documented that ventilation by bag-valve-mask (BVM) is a successful therapeutic option.[12,13] BVM ventilation should be employed as a temporizing measure in situations of respiratory arrest until an artificial airway (preferably endotracheal intubation) can be established. Two helpful mechanisms to enhance successful BVM support are dismantling the pop-off valve and using two people to perform BVM ventilation.

The mechanism of upper airway obstruction or acute respiratory failure with acute supraglottitis is, more realistically, acute laryngospasm secondary to hypoxia, hypercarbia, or irritation from secretions; exhaustion; or obstruction from secretions or edema.[9]

Direct visualization not only will lead to a rapid, safe, and accurate diagnosis but also will confirm the presence or absence of a supraglottic foreign body. If the diagnosis of acute supraglottitis is made, placement of an artificial airway is mandatory because of the explosive natural history of the disease with progression to complete upper airway obstruction. In skilled hands, endotracheal intubation may be accomplished as soon as the condition is diagnosed. Less-experienced clinicians should, appropriately, summon an airway specialist.

In respiratory or cardiac arrest situations, mouth-to-mouth or BVM ventilation may adequately temporize until an artificial airway is placed. Successful BVM ventilation has been reported in cases of acute supraglottitis in Cincinnati, Ohio and in San Diego, Torrance, and Orange, California.[9,10,12,13] BVM ventilation should be attempted and, if successful, should be continued until an artificial airway is placed.

Emergency surgical techniques should not be resorted to until BVM ventilation and orotracheal intubation have been attempted. The disastrous results of emergency surgical airway procedures in acute supraglottitis are well documented in the literature. An emergency pediatric tracheostomy, even in skilled, experienced hands, is a time-consuming and difficult procedure.

In a literature review of 44 patients with confirmed acute supraglottitis who presented in respiratory or cardiac arrest, 43 were successfully orotracheally intubated.[14-32] It is clear from the literature and personal experience that upper airway obstruction from infectious causes (including acute supraglottitis) with impending respiratory failure should be managed as any other type of respiratory insufficiency; that is, with BVM ventilation and subsequent endotracheal intubation. Only if medical intervention is unsuccessful should surgical techniques be resorted to.

BREATHING

If opening the airway and positioning the patient do not result in adequate ventilation, then two slow breaths (1.0 to 1.5 seconds per breath) should be given with a pause between the breaths so that the rescuer can inhale. The breaths should be given with sufficient volume to expand the patient's chest without distending the stomach. In infants the rescuer's mouth covers the patient's nose and mouth, forming a tight seal. In larger children only the mouth is covered, and the nose is pinched with the thumb and index finger with the hand that is maintaining proper (head tilt) position. If available, one-way pocket masks in appropriate pediatric sizes to form a seal should replace mouth-to-mouth technique. Adequate ventilation must be confirmed by watching the chest wall rise symmetrically.

As soon as availability permits, breathing with a BVM should be instituted. Appropriately sized, clear, washable plastic masks that conform to the face are preferred. The proper size mask will be used to form a tight seal on the face and should be positioned from the nasal bridge, avoiding pressure on the eyes, to the cleft between the lower lip and the chin. A tight fit is mandatory for adequate inspired oxygen concentration (Fio_2) with assisted or controlled ventilation. In infants and toddlers the mask can be effectively applied by the one-handed head tilt/chin lift maneuver if one is careful to avoid compressing the airway with the fingertips. In older children, those who prove difficult to ventilate, or those with anatomic variants, the two-person procedure with one person holding the mask to the face with both hands and the second person ventilating may be necessary to achieve a good seal and proper ventilation.[33]

Concern over excessive artificial airway pressures with resultant barotrauma (pneumothorax, tension pneumothorax, and pneumomediastinum) probably results in significant underventilation in many patients. With smaller children and infants, greater airway pressures may be necessary to overcome the resistance to air flow produced by the smaller airways. A good clinical measure of adequate ventilation is gentle chest expansion. By carefully observing chest wall movement and manually sensing pressure on the self-inflating bag during BVM ventilation, the caregiver should be able to avoid underventilation and overventilation pressures. Improper positioning is a common cause of inadequate ventilation, and position should be checked immediately if any problems arise. If the head tilt/chin lift is adjusted and judged to be adequate, the patient's head may need to be moved gently through a range of extension to find the best position. Hyperextension must be avoided because the pliable trachea may collapse if this extreme position is attained. If rescue breathing does not produce adequate chest expansion despite opening of the airway, positioning, and delivery of appropriate ventilation pressures, measures for correcting foreign body obstruction should be undertaken immediately.

Foreign Bodies

Foreign body aspiration is a common problem in the pediatric age group. The vast majority of deaths (90%) from foreign body aspiration and airway obstruction are in the age group younger than 5 years. Sudden onset of respiratory distress, coughing, gagging, drooling, cyanosis, and respiratory noise should be considered secondary to foreign body until a foreign body is ruled out. Forceful coughing should be encouraged if spontaneous ventilation is effective. If ventilation is ineffective, active airway intervention is immediately required. In-hospital treatment relies on direct laryngoscopy and removal of the offending supraglottic foreign body with Magill forceps.

Complete obstruction with subglottic foreign bodies rapidly causes arrest. Controversial methodology surrounds their removal. The American Heart Association and the American Academy of Pediatrics continue to recommend using a combination of four back blows and four chest thrusts to expel upper airway foreign bodies in infants (younger than 1 year) if the "cough is ineffective and/or there is increased respiratory difficulty accompanied by stridor."[5(p16)] Abdominal thrusts are recommended in the older child but are associated with the potential problem of abdominal organ

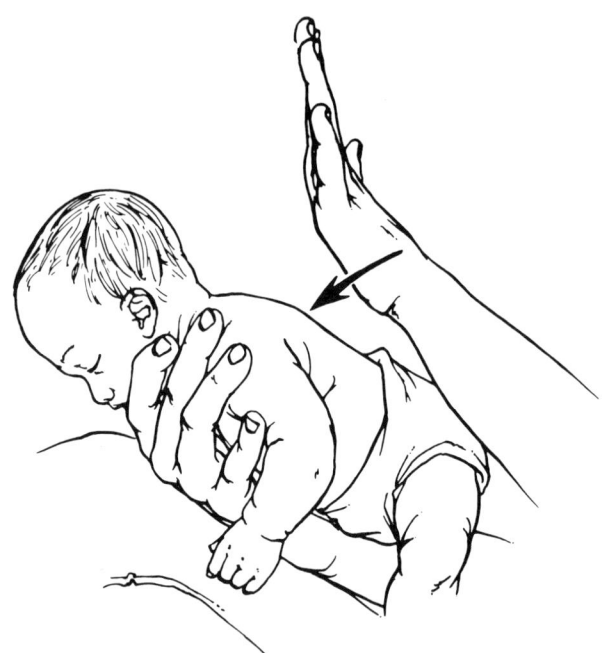

Figure 31-1 Proper positioning for back blows when complete obstruction by a foreign body is suspected in infants.

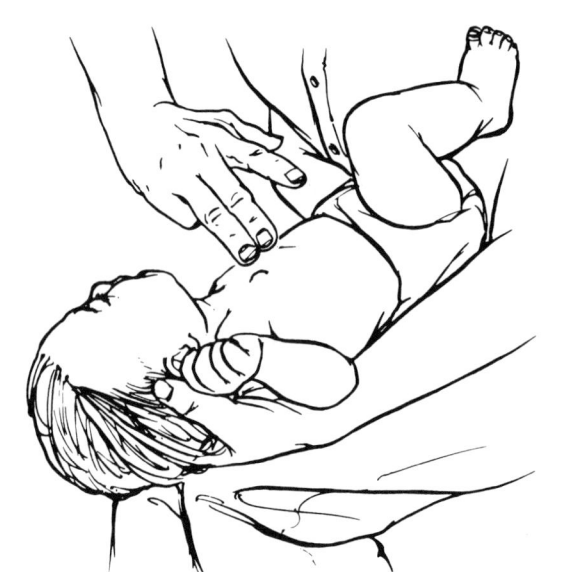

Figure 31-2 Proper positioning for chest thrusts when complete obstruction by a foreign body is suspected in infants.

injury.[34] Many studies, however, have warned of the dangers of back blows in the choking child. In the upright child, back blows may cause displacement of a supraglottic foreign body into the glottic opening. In the child held in the head-down position, a subglottic foreign body may be dislodged against the glottic opening by forceful back blows. In both situations, complete airway obstruction could follow.

Day et al[35] used a model method to compare the forces generated on a supraglottic foreign body by the Heimlich abdominal thrust and back blows. Back blows generated less pressure than the Heimlich maneuver in both young adults and pediatric models in the seated position. Furthermore, back blows straightened the spine and threw the head and neck forward and upward. The resulting mechanics of the back blow could force a supraglottic foreign body farther down the airway if the blow is delivered to a child in the seated or upright position.

The Heimlich technique is a powerful maneuver. Clinical experience and scientific experimentation have shown it to be an effective and relatively safe procedure in life-threatening upper airway obstructions from foreign bodies. Potential injuries to abdominal viscera with the abdominal thrust pale in significance compared to the threat of complete airway obstruction. Reported incidences of actual abdominal injury are quite low (less than 1%). To date the American Heart Association and the American Academy of Pediatrics continue to recommend the use of back blows and chest thrusts in the infant up to 1 year of age (Figs. 31-1 and 31-2) when complete obstruction by a foreign body is suspected.[5]

Oxygen

Providing supplemental oxygen in high concentrations is exceedingly important during resuscitation to help combat hypoxia. Because cardiac output during chest compressions is markedly decreased (to 25% to 30%), oxygen delivery to the tissue beds will be severely reduced. High levels of exogenous oxygen will increase arterial oxygenation and limit tissue hypoxia.

Supplemental oxygen should be supplied to any patient in the arrest situation, in any situation where hypoxemia is suspected, and in situations that may lead to hypoxemia (asthma, infectious upper airway obstruction, foreign body, trauma, or pneumonia). Preoxygenation and postoxygenation with airway suctioning and endotracheal intubation are uniformly mentioned but rarely complied with. Strict adherence results in a wider safety margin and lessens adverse cardiovascular effects.

Oxygen in high concentrations should not be withheld for fear of oxygen toxicity or suppression of the oxygen drive. The Fio_2 can be increased in mouth-to-mouth breathing by placing a nasal cannula with supplemental oxygen on the rescuer or tubing from an oxygen source in the rescuer's mouth. With BVM ventilation, high-flow oxygen (10-15 L/min), and a self-inflating bag with a gas reservoir surrounding the intake valves, oxygen levels of 95% can be delivered.

Airway Adjuncts

The oropharyngeal airway is a commonly used device in adults, but its use in the child is limited to the unconscious patient. Potential problems with its use include stimulation of the gag reflex with vomiting and aspiration, improper placement pushing the tongue posteriorly and causing upper

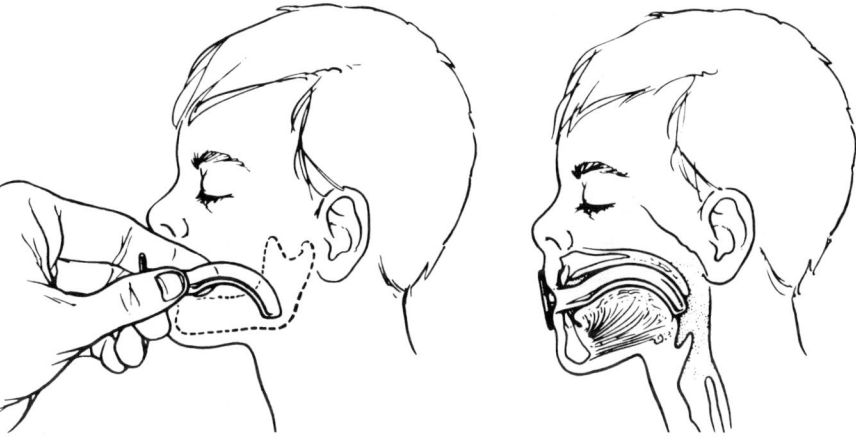

Figure 31-3 Appropriate choice of size and placement of the oropharyngeal airway.

airway obstruction, difficulty in finding the proper size (Fig. 31-3), and trauma to pediatric soft tissues.

A nasopharyngeal airway, when placed after topical application of a vasoconstrictor, anesthetic, and lubricant, is less traumatic and better tolerated in conscious patients. The proper size is determined by the distance from the nasal tip to the tragus of the ear. Bleeding from hypertrophied adenoidal tissue and intraluminal obstruction are problems that can be minimized by gentle technique, avoidance of small tubes, and frequent suctioning.

Ventilation

In unconscious patients who are unable to protect their airway from aspiration and in those with persistent respiratory insufficiency, endotracheal intubation is the airway of choice.

Adequate preparation and delicacy in technique are of prime importance in pediatric intubation. Cardiac monitoring is mandatory for any child. Suction devices, both Yankuer for oropharyngeal tubes and small French catheters for endotracheal tubes, should be available for intubation. Stimulation of vagal reflexes during posterior pharyngeal, laryngeal, or endotracheal suctioning or manipulation may result in marked bradycardia to the point of asystole. An assistant must monitor the heart rate during these procedures and call for immediate cessation of the attempt when the heart rate falls below 80 beat/min. Use of atropine should be considered when the heart rate does not respond to BVM oxygenation. Unless BVM ventilation is impossible, the patient should be preoxygenated with 100% oxygen for 1 to 3 minutes before the intubation attempt.

In children younger than 8 years, straight, uncuffed endotracheal tubes should be used. The taper-shoulder endotracheal tubes (Cole) are contraindicated because they provide only a narrow airway with high resistance that is easily obstructed, have problems holding a curved shape, and have increased contact with and irritation of vocal cords. Because the narrowest airway diameter in young children is at the level of the cricoid cartilage, this anatomically serves as a cuff for children younger than 8 years. Tube size may be determined by the following formula:

$$D = \frac{16 + A}{4}$$

where D is the internal diameter of the tube (in millimeters) and A is the child's age (in years). A clinically useful way of approximating tube size is to select a tube size equal to the width of the patient's little finger or the width of a single external nare. Some individuals prefer to display a size chart near the airway equipment in the resuscitation room (Table 31-2). These methods of choosing tube size serve only as guides. Tubes 0.5 mm larger and 0.5 mm smaller than the size determined should be laid out before the intubation attempt. A flexible yet firm stylet that does not extend beyond the tip of the endotracheal tube is an important adjunct that makes intubation much easier.

Depending on the preference of the intubator, either a straight (Miller) or curved (MacIntosh) laryngoscope blade may be used. In infants and young children the straight blade is probably more effective because of anatomic considerations (small mandible, large tongue, anterior and cephalad position of the epiglottis). Appropriate airway equipment sizes for pediatric patients are noted in Table 31-2. A pencil-handle laryngoscope provides the intubator with a small instrument for the delicate procedure. It can be handled with the thumb and index finger of one hand, thus allowing the long and ring fingers to grip and elevate the chin. The little finger is free to depress the cricoid cartilage. The Sellick maneuver[36,37] is performed by applying digital pressure to the cricoid cartilage, thus moving the cartilaginous ring posteriorly and compressing the esophagus against the cervical spine. Care must be taken not to use excessive force or the trachea may be compressed, obstructing the airway. Advantages of this technique include prevention of gastric regurgitation into the airway; limitation of gastric distension during BVM ventilation; and alignment of the oral, pha-

Table 31-2 Equipment Guidelines According to Age and Weight

Type of Ventilation	Equipment Size					
	Premature (1.0–2.5 kg)	Neonate (2.5–4.0 kg)	6 Months (7.0 kg)	1–2 Years (10–12 kg)	5 Years (16–18 kg)	8–10 Years (24–30 kg)
Airway—oral	Infant (00)	Infant/small (0)	Small (1)	Small (2)	Medium (3)	Medium/large (4/5)
Breathing						
Self-inflating bag	Infant	Infant	Child	Child	Child	Child/adult
Oxygen by ventilation mask	Premature	Neonate	Infant/child	Child	Child	Small adult
Endotracheal tube	2.5–3.0 (uncuffed)	3.0–3.5 (uncuffed)	3.5–4.0 (uncuffed)	4.0–4.5 (uncuffed)	5.0–5.5 (uncuffed)	5.5–6.5 (cuffed)
Laryngoscope blade	0 (straight)	1 (straight)	1 (straight)	1–2 (straight)	2 (straight or curved)	2–3 (straight or curved)
Suction/stylet (F)	6–8/6	8/6	8–10/6	10/6	14/14	14/14

Source: Reprinted with permission from *Textbook of Pediatric Advanced Life Support.* Dallas: American Heart Association, 1988.

ryngeal, and tracheal axes, facilitating tracheal intubation. Pressure is removed once intubation is accomplished.

The small size of the laryngoscope handle and gripping with only two fingers serve as constant reminders of the delicacy of the procedure and the need for good technique to succeed in the intubation. With the patient in the sniffing position without hyperextension (Fig. 31-4), the laryngoscope blade is inserted on the right and moves the tongue to the left. The curved MacIntosh blade is placed in the vallecula, whereas the straight Miller blade is placed under the epiglottis. The laryngoscope is then elevated gently to expose the glottis. Depression of the cricoid cartilage with the operator's little finger or by an assistant helps bring the glottis into view. Gentle lifting of the laryngoscope along the axis of the handle and elevation of the child's head on a small pad may facilitate vision of the glottis. Rotating the laryngoscope in one hand at the wrist uses the lips, teeth, or gums as a fulcrum; this is poor technique and guarantees unnecessary trauma to the patient in the form of bleeding, bruising, lacerations, and fractured teeth.

Additional tricks include advancing the tube from the right corner of the mouth, preserving vision of the glottis as the tube passes through the vocal cords, stopping at the vocal cord marker, and moving the intubator's head away from the patient, thus maintaining stereoscopic vision of oral, pharyngeal, and tracheal axes and greatly enhancing the chances for successful intubation by preserving visibility of the glottis.

Monitoring of cardiac activity, pulse oximetry, and avoidance of excessive head flexion or extension are mandatory during the procedure. Bradycardia, decreasing oxygen saturation, or dysrhythmias during the attempt necessitate immediate cessation and reoxygenation with BVM. The recommended time limit for an intubation attempt is 30 seconds. Unrestrained head movement can result in considerable endotracheal tube movement and should be minimized. Excessive head flexion will displace the tube toward the carina, and extension will tend to move the tube cephalad and cause accidental extubation.

After intubation, correct tube placement must be ensured. Clinically, this can be done by observing for symmetric chest wall elevation with ventilation, auscultating for equal breath sounds in both axillae (not over the anterior chest because transmitted breath sounds from the opposite side or

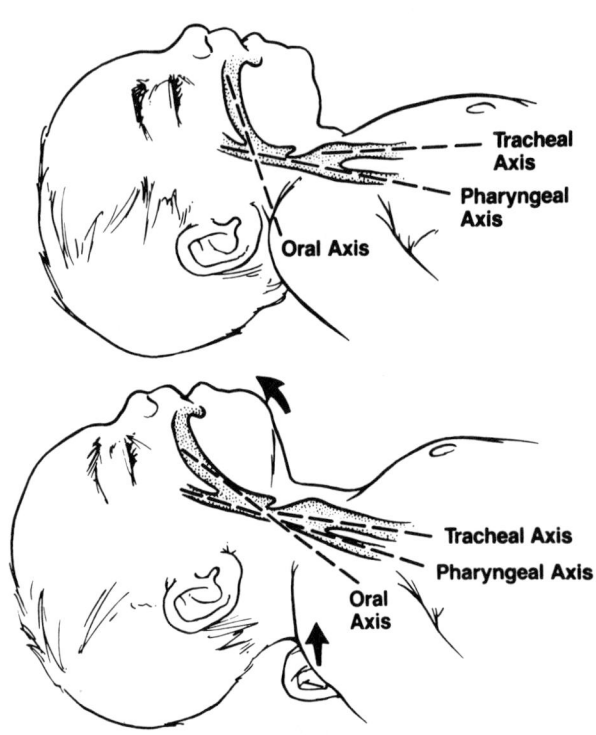

Figure 31-4 Placing the child in the sniffing position to facilitate visualization of the glottis and placement of the endotracheal tube.

esophagus may be misinterpreted), and checking for absence of air noise in the epigastrium. A postintubation, portable anteroposterior chest radiograph is mandatory to assess tube placement as well as thoracic and upper abdominal structures.

Any problems that develop with ventilation after intubation must be corrected rapidly. A systematic approach must be used to check for and eliminate complications:

1. tube—improper position, obstruction, inappropriate size
2. patient—pneumothorax (simple or tension)
3. equipment—mechanical failure with BVM, connections, pop-off valve, oxygen source

Oxygen Powered Mechanical Breathing Devices

Oxygen powered breathing devices (O_2PBDs) are capable of generating excessive airway pressures for pediatric patients. Current technology is incapable of adequately controlling and monitoring pressures that are delivered. Potential complications of barotrauma (pneumothorax) and gastric distension (vomiting and aspiration) contraindicate the use of O_2PBDs in children.[5]

Mechanical Ventilators

During external chest compression, pressure-cycled ventilators function poorly. These devices tend to terminate prematurely the inspiratory cycle when the chest is externally compressed, resulting in inadequate tidal volumes. Additionally, they pose a technical problem of coordinating ventilation with compression. For these reasons, their use during external chest compression is not recommended.[5]

Ventilators are indicated when circulation has been established but ventilation remains inadequate. Initial guidelines for settings are as follows: tidal volume, 10 to 15 mL/kg; Fio_2, 1.00; inspiratory:expiratory ratio, 1:2; respiration rate, 15/min to 30/min; positive end-expiratory pressure, 2 to 5 cmH_2O. Settings must be adjusted according to clinical assessment of breath sounds and chest elevation as well as serial arterial blood gas determinations.

CIRCULATION

Adequacy of circulation is best assessed by palpation of brachial or femoral pulses. Heart rate is a vital sign that is reproducible and serves as an excellent guide to underlying pathology and response to therapy. Tachycardia is a generalized response to multiple factors (fever, fear, pain, hypoxia, hypercarbia, and hypovolemia). Presence of tachycardia requires investigation, especially when one realizes that the neonate and infant rely almost exclusively on increasing heart rate to increase cardiac output. If tachycardia is inadequate to meet tissue demands, then hypoxia and acidosis result. In a critically ill infant or young child, bradycardia is a sign of impending cardiac arrest. Heart rates less than 80 beat/min in the newborn and symptomatic bradycardia in children require immediate chest compression when ventilation is adequate. In situations where the circulatory status is uncertain, it is prudent to initiate chest compression. Compression rates, ventilation rates, and depth and technique of compression all vary with the child's size and age (Table 31-3). Pulse quality and tissue bed perfusion are important clinical determinants of the adequacy of circulation. Differences in the volume of central and peripheral pulses may be an early sign of hypovolemia and diminished cardiac stroke volume. As hypovolemia progresses (increasing shock), the pulse pressure narrows and the pulse volume decreases, giving rise to a weak and thready pulse.

Adequacy of cardiac output and tissue bed perfusion to skin, brain, and kidneys can be evaluated clinically. Slow capillary refill (>2 seconds), cool digits or limbs, and cyanosis indicate failure of peripheral perfusion. Altered mental status (lethargy, agitation, irritability, and confusion)

Table 31-3 Summary of Basic Life Support Maneuvers in Infants and Children

System	Infant	Child
Airway	Head tilt/chin lift, jaw thrust	Head tilt/chin lift, jaw thrust
Breathing		
Initial	Two breaths at 1.0–1.5 sec/breath	Two breaths at 1.0–1.5 sec/breath
Subsequent	20/min	15/min
Circulation		
Pulse check	Brachial/femoral	Carotid
Compression area	Lower third of sternum	Lower third of sternum
Compressed with	2–3 fingers	Heel of one hand
Depth	0.5–1.0 inch (approximate)	1.0–1.5 inch (approximate)
Rate	At least 100 beat/min	80–100 beat/min
Compression: ventilation ratio	5:1 (pause for ventilation)	5:1 (pause for ventilation)

Source: Reprinted with permission from *Textbook of Pediatric Advanced Life Support.* Dallas: American Heart Association, 1988.

will vary with the degree of failure of perfusion and the age of the patient. Unresponsiveness and hypotonia indicate severe and/or prolonged hypoperfusion. Diminished urinary output is a direct reflection of poor kidney perfusion in the absence of intrinsic renal disease. Placement of an indwelling urinary catheter is necessary for measurement of urinary output. Less than 1 mL/kg/hour in a patient with normal renal function is a sign of decreased renal perfusion.

The adequacy of resuscitation chest compression can be assessed accurately by having one member of the team (usually the team leader) continuously palpate the femoral pulse (brachial pulse in infants). By this means, the team leader will have a constant hands-on appreciation of the adequacy and progress of the arrest situation. Beat-by-beat response to various therapeutic modalities and changing cardiorespiratory status can be determined instantaneously.

Vascular Access

Establishment of a reliable intravenous line during a pediatric arrest can be problematic.[38] Delays in securing an access site are common, even in tertiary care settings. There is hardly any clinical situation where the dictum "any port in a storm" is more applicable. Peripheral lines in the upper and lower extremities as well as the scalp have been traditional favorites. Failing these, the external jugular is usually a reliable site. Central access via the internal jugular by means of the high central approach is relatively safe and effective,[39,40] even in the neonate. Femoral vein access has proved to be a popular central approach. Activity at this site does not interfere with compressions and establishment of an airway. If percutaneous access is not gained rapidly, the intraosseous approach should be attempted.[41]

With the need for rapid vascular access for volume resuscitation in shock states and drug therapy in arrest states, clinicians should prioritize the various access sites available to them. Kanter et al[41] have suggested a protocol for timely vascular access that includes the available types of procedures.

Intraosseous Access

Recently,[41-46] the intraosseous route (proximal tibia or distal femur) has undergone a resurgence of interest and use in emergency situations where venous access is not immediately available for volume resuscitation or medication administration. Advantages of the intraosseous route include the following:

- it is an extremely easy technique
- it can be performed rapidly
- all commonly used resuscitative drugs can be given
- large amounts of fluid can be introduced rapidly
- drugs quickly reach the central circulation

- hypertonic drugs (25% to 50% glucose and sodium bicarbonate) can be administered
- sites of access are physically distant from areas of major activity during an arrest
- the technique can be performed in patients up to 6 years of age
- it has a low complication rate

It has been shown that the intraosseous route is established more quickly than peripheral or cutdown venous access, is safer than central venous access in the pediatric patient, and has a much wider range of acceptable drugs than the endotracheal route.

The ease, rapidity, and utility of the intraosseous route may permit its use as first-line access in situations where physicians experienced in pediatric venous access are not immediately available or are delayed. The needle can always be removed if another line is established, and infusion through the line can increase intravascular volume, making venous access easier to obtain.

Drugs and fluids that have been safely administered by the intraosseous route include epinephrine, dopamine, dobutamine, sodium bicarbonate, calcium gluconate, atropine, lidocaine, insulin, digitalis, heparin, dexamethasone, 50% dextrose, blood, diazepam, diazoxide, phenobarbitol, phenytoin, isoproterenol, pancuronium, and colloids.

Major potential complications include infection (cellulitis, osteomyelitis, and abscess formation), bone injury, and growth plate abnormalities. Large clinical studies from the 1940s, however, showed the procedure to be extremely safe and relatively complication free. Heinild et al[47] demonstrated no cases of osteomyelitis in 944 patients where the needle was placed temporarily for bolus infusions of isotonic solutions. Furthermore, they reported only 5 cases of osteomyelitis in 1000 infusions; these were found only in patients who had prolonged placement (days) and/or administration of hypertonic solutions. Short-term fluid and drug administration, which is the modern recommendation, would seem to limit infectious complications to an acceptable level. To date there have been no clinically significant cases reported of fat emboli or bone particles, despite their documented appearance in postmortem lung specimens.[48]

Spivey et al[49] have shown that intraosseous administration of sodium bicarbonate in pigs has no short- or long-term adverse effects on bone. Furthermore, Brickman et al[50] demonstrated that intraosseous administration of saline and bicarbonate into the tibial physeal growth plates of pigs was without adverse effects on tibia or bone growth. These studies are reassuring, and bone or growth plate may not be adversely affected by this technique. LaFleche et al,[51] however, recently reported a case of a 3-month-old patient who sustained bilateral tibial fractures after unsuccessful intraosseous attempts were made in the midshaft of both tibias with 15-gauge Jamshidi needles.

Papper[52] demonstrated more than 45 years ago that drugs and fluids administered by the intraosseous route appear rapidly in the general circulation and that the circulation times are similar to those achieved by the intravenous route. Shoor et al[53] hold that in long bones abundant marrow sinusoids drain into large medullary venous channels, which empty into the systemic venous system by nutrient and emissary veins. The marrow sinusoids provide noncollapsible veins that are easily accessed even when vasculature is shut down. The investigators used 13-gauge needles in bovine tibia (medial malleoli) and were able to produce initial clinical effects of epinephrine within 17 (± 3) seconds and 90% maximal effect within 45 (± 5) seconds of injection. There was no difference in clinical effect of epinephrine when administered by the intraosseous route in either normotensive or hypotensive states. These investigators were also able to achieve infusion rates of 600 mL/hour by gravity (81 cm high) and of nearly 2500 mL/hour at 300 torr.

Morris et al[54] reconfirmed the ability rapidly to infuse large volumes of fluid to resuscitate rabbits from the shock state. This avenue provides an effective route for fluid resuscitation in the hypovolemic state and has been shown to be useful in the prearrest state.

Various needles have been recommended for intraosseous puncture (eg, hollow intravenous needles, bone marrow needles, and spinal needles); most have one technical problem or another (dull point, too long, awkward to use, easily bent, or plugged core). An excellent needle designed specifically for intraosseous use is the Cook needle (A Cook Group Co, PO Box 489, Bloomington, IN 47402). It is short and sharp and has a large, plastic head that makes application of pressure simple, effective, and safe. Currently available sizes are 16 and 18 gauge. For penetration of the proximal tibia, enter the skin 2 to 3 cm below the tibial tuberosity over the flat, medial aspect of the tibia. Advance the needle with steady pressure and a rotary motion. Successful placement is determined by a palpable give as the needle passes through the bony cortex, the ability of the needle to stand alone, aspiration of marrow into a syringe attached to the needle, or free flow of fluid without subcutaneous infiltration. Currently the intraosseous route is not recommended for children older than 6 years.

Umbilical Access

In newborn resuscitation, it should not be forgotten that the umbilical vessels may remain patent up to 2 weeks after birth. The single, large, floppy, thin-walled umbilical vein provides easy access for a saline-filled catheter (3.5-, 5.0-, or 8.0-French feeding tube), which may be advanced until a free flow of blood can be aspirated. Studies[55] have shown that catheter advancement two thirds the distance between the shoulder's acromion process and the umbilicus (6 to 10 cm) usually places the catheter tip in the inferior vena cava. Blood must be aspirated freely to make sure that the tip is not wedged in the hepatic portal system. If blood cannot be aspirated, repositioning is necessary. Radiographic confirmation of catheter location is mandatory.

Antishock Garments

Pediatric antishock garments have been enlisted to promote venous return to the heart, to decrease flow to the abdomen and legs, and to increase cardiac afterload. These physiologic effects may be helpful in distending upper extremity superficial veins, thereby making venous access easier.

FLUID RESUSCITATION

Normal saline and lactated Ringer solution are acceptable intravenous solutions in the arrest state. Especially in children, the relative frequency of hypovolemia secondary to dehydration or blood loss must not be forgotten. Intravenous infusion of 20 mL of an isotonic solution per kilogram body weight is acceptable for a therapeutic trial of volume replacement. This challenge must be repeated until adequate volume has been restored. When known hemorrhagic loss has occurred, replacement with blood products is indicated in shock states unresponsive to crystalloid therapy. Persistent hypotension in the face of apparently adequate fluid resuscitation should direct the clinician to a reevaluation of ventilation, acid-base status, electrolytes (including glucose and hemoglobin), and potential obstructive problems (cardiac tamponade or tension pneumothorax). If hemodynamic instability persists despite addressing the above problems, a vasopressor such as dopamine is indicated (Table 31-4). Placement of a central venous pressure– or pulmonary artery flow–directed catheter will be helpful in patient monitoring at this point.

DRUGS

Drugs are necessary for correcting hypoxia and metabolic acidosis, improving cardiac rate and contractility, and reversing poor cardiac output. Proper dosages of drugs for resuscitation are based on the child's weight (Table 31-5). Often the weight is not known, and exact measurement is not possible during the resuscitation. Investigators[56] have documented the accuracy of the Broselow tape, a pediatric resuscitation aid for drug dosages and equipment sizes. If the child's age is known, an approximate weight can be determined from the 50th percentile of the standard pediatric weight chart. The weight of a child older than 1 year can be estimated by the following formula:

$$W = 2A + 8$$

where W is the child's weight (in kilograms) and A is the age (in years).

Table 31-4 Pediatric Intravenous Infusions

Add	0.6 mg (3 mL)* of isoproterenol 0.6 mg (0.6 mL)* of epinephrine 60.0 mg (1.5 mL)* of dopamine 60.0 mg (2.4 mL)* of dobutamine 120.0 mg (3 mL)* of lidocaine
To	100 mL of diluent
Infuse	at 1 mL/kg/hour or according to guidelines below
To give	0.1 μg/kg/min isoproterenol 0.1 μg/kg/min epinephrine 10 μg/kg/min dopamine 10 μg/kg/min dobutamine 20 μg/kg/min lidocaine

*Based on the following concentrations: isoproterenol, 0.2 mg/mL; epinephrine, 1:1000 (1 mg/mL); dopamine, 40 mg/mL; dobutamine, 25 mg/mL; lidocaine, 40 mg/mL.

Age	50th Percentile Weight (kg)	Infusion Rate (mL/hour)†
Newborn	3.0	3.0
1 Month	4.0	4.0
3 Months	5.5	5.5
6 Months	7.0	7.0
1 Year	10.0	10.0
2 Years	12.0	12.0
3 Years	14.0	14.0
4 Years	16.0	16.0
5 Years	18.0	18.0
6 Years	20.0	20.0
7 Years	22.0	22.0
8 Years	25.0	25.0
9 Years	28.0	28.0
10 Years	34.0	34.0

†These are starting doses. Adjust concentration to dose and fluid tolerance.

Source: Reprinted with permission from *Textbook of Pediatric Advanced Life Support.* Dallas: American Heart Association, 1988.

Oxygen

Because of the overwhelming tendency of clinicians to rush to drug therapy, it must be stressed repeatedly that effective ventilation in children may completely reverse a deteriorating cardiovascular condition. Use of high concentrations of oxygen to correct or reverse hypoxia is a therapeutic mainstay, and oxygen should always be considered a first-line drug in the treatment of cardiopulmonary arrest. Unrealistic fears of oxygen toxicity and suppression of the oxygen drive (pulmonary disease with carbon dioxide retention) must be put to rest in the setting of CPR.

Sodium Bicarbonate

Hypoperfusion states result in production of lactic acid, which causes variable degrees of metabolic acidosis. Sodium bicarbonate administration is critical in attempts to correct metabolic acidosis. Increased ventilation is required to remove the excessive carbon dioxide formed by sodium bicarbonate administration as well as the elevated P_{CO_2} that is the byproduct of decreased respiration (respiratory acidosis), which is usually present in the prearrest state.

Investigators have recently looked closely at the effects of sodium bicarbonate use. After sodium bicarbonate is given intravenously, carbonic acid is formed and rapidly dissociates into carbon dioxide and diffuses across cell membranes into the cells, where it combines with water to reform carbonic acid. The carbonic acid causes an intracellular acidosis before it dissociates into carbon dioxide and water again. The result of extracellular alkalinization, then, is paradoxically to cause a rapid rise in intracellular acidosis. Intracellular acidosis in the myocardium has a profoundly adverse effect on contractile force. Hyperventilation with the resultant lowering of P_{CO_2} causes a respiratory alkalosis. Routine use of hyperventilation in arrest conditions, especially after the administration of bicarbonate, helps diminish the lowering of intracellular pH by removing the carbon dioxide produced by bicarbonate administration and by further lowering P_{CO_2}, which helps compensate for the metabolic acidosis of the arrest.

The above discussion reaffirms the importance of ventilation and the need to focus attention on P_{CO_2} levels. Other potential problems with sodium bicarbonate are summarized in Table 31-6. The potential problems associated with excessive and rapid bicarbonate administration contradict indiscriminate use. Nevertheless, there is clearly a role for its use in the arrest state if it is given in a precise, rationally calculated manner.[57] If the patient's serum bicarbonate level is known, then the base deficit can be calculated according to the following formula:

$$B = (25 - C)(W)(0.3)$$

where B is the required base deficit (in milliequivalents of sodium bicarbonate), C is the actual concentration of bicarbonate, and W is the child's weight (in kilograms). Half the calculated base deficit may be given intravenously at a slow rate. It is essential to follow the acid-base status with repetitive arterial blood gas determinations.

In those cases where the length of the arrest is unknown and/or laboratory data are not easily or rapidly accessible, empiric sodium bicarbonate can be given in the following manner: 1 mEq/kg initially by intravenous bolus, then 0.5 mEq/kg every 10 minutes (or until blood gas determinations become available).

When one is treating newborns and infants, the standard pediatric solution (8.4% sodium bicarbonate = 1 mEq/mL) must be diluted to avoid the potential complication of hyperosmolarity and intracranial hemorrhage. This can be accomplished by mixing the bicarbonate solution with an equal volume of 5% dextrose or sterile water (1:1) and giving it slowly intravenously.

Table 31-5 Drugs for Pediatric Advanced Cardiac Life Support

Drug	Dose	Supplied	Remarks
Sodium bicarbonate	1–2 mEq/kg	8.4% (1 mEq/mL)	Dilute 1:1 with 5% dextrose in water in newborns Flush line after use Hyperventilate after use
Epinephrine	0.1 mL/kg	1:10,000 (0.1 mg/mL)	Give every 5 minutes in arrest states Avoid 1:1,000 solution unless diluted 10:1 with 5% dextrose in water Avoid intracardiac use
Atropine	0.01 mL/kg	0.1 mg/mL	Give minimum of 0.10 mg
Lidocaine	1 mg/kg	10 mg/mL (1%)	
Naloxone	0.01–0.10 mg/kg	0.4 mg/mL	Initially give 0.01 mg/kg and increase dose to 0.1 mg/kg to 2 mg maximum if no response in 2 minutes Short half-life (30 minutes)
Bretylium	5 mg/kg	500 mg/10 mL	Give slowly (5–10 minutes) May increase by 5 mg/kg to maximum of 30 mg/kg
Calcium chloride 10%	0.2 mL/kg	10 mL (100 mg/mL)	Give slowly Do not combine with bicarbonate Use cautiously in digitalized patients
Glucose	0.5 g/kg; 2 mL/kg 25% dextrose in water	50% dextrose in water	Dilute 1:1 with sterile water to make 25% dextrose in water

Atropine

Atropine is a vagolytic drug that decreases vagal tone in the sinoatrial node and the atrioventricular (AV) conduction system. The resulting effects are to increase rates of discharge and to increase pulse rate. Atropine also has a central effect on the medullary vagal nuclei. Paradoxically, if atropine is given at doses less than 0.10 mg, the central effect will predominate, causing an increase in vagal tone and resulting in AV slowing (lower heart rate). Indications for use include cardiac arrest, symptomatic bradycardia (infants with heart rate < 80 beat/min associated with hypotension or ectopy), second- and third-degree heart block, and slow, narrow, complex ventricular rhythms. Most cases of symptomatic bradycardia in children are secondary to hypoxia.

Table 31-6 Potential Problems with Sodium Bicarbonate Use

Metabolic alkalosis
- Shifting of the oxygen dissociation curve to the left causes decreased oxygen release to the tissues
- Hypokalemia

Volume overload
Hypernatremia
Hyperosmolarity
- Leads to intracranial hemorrhage in infants

Paradoxic central nervous system acidosis
- Leads to postarrest cerebral dysfunction

Inactivation of catecholamines
- Must not mix
- Must flush intravenous lines if using these drugs serially

Precipitation of calcium salts
- Must not mix
- Must flush intravenous lines if using these drugs serially

Addressing ventilation and oxygenation becomes a priority over pharmacologic intervention in the pediatric age group.

Intravenous dosage is 0.01 to 0.03 mg/kg with a minimum of 0.10 mg. The dose may be repeated at 5-minute intervals to a maximal, complete vagolytic dose of 2 mg. Atropine may be given down the endotracheal tube and intraosseously. Complications include atrial and ventricular tachydysrhythmias and paradoxic bradycardia. If atropine is to be used to block bradycardia associated with intubation, it must be remembered that hypoxia-induced bradycardia will be masked.

Epinephrine

Epinephrine (Adrenalin) is an endogenous catecholamine with both α- and β-adrenergic effects. Its effects are extremely complex, partly because of its pharmacology, its dose-related effects, and the reflex cardiovascular changes resulting from its use during arrest, which affect subsequent pharmacodynamics (Table 31-7).

Epinephrine use is indicated in all forms of cardiorespiratory arrest, primarily because of its positive effect of pulse pressure elevation. The α-adrenergic effect (vasocon-

Table 31-7 Cardiovascular Effects of Epinephrine

Increases cardiac rate
Increases systemic vascular resistance
Increases mean arterial pressure
Increases myocardial oxygen demand
Improves myocardial contractile strength
Increases incidence of spontaneous myocardial contractions
Improves amplitude of ventricular fibrillation
Increases chances of defibrillation

striction) is the most important in the arrest state, partly because of the large doses used. The vasoconstrictive effect raises blood pressure and increases coronary artery perfusion pressure. Other indications include fine VF (coarsens VF, making it more susceptible to defibrillation), asystole, idioventricular rhythm, and electromechanical dissociation.

The dose is 0.1 mL/kg (0.01 mg/kg) of a 1:10,000 solution given intravenously or intraosseously. The dose is repeated at 5-minute intervals if the arrest state persists because the half-life is short. Recent case reports and animal studies have suggested that higher doses of epinephrine may restore spontaneous circulation more readily than standard dosages.[58-60] High-dose epinephrine concentrations have varied from 2 to 3 times to 20 times the standard dose. The current American Heart Association Pediatric Advanced Life Support guideline for arrest is, if the initial dose is not effective after 5 minutes, to give at least twice the initial dose.[5] Because of the limited amount of experience regarding optimal dosage, timing of dose, complications, and outcome, firm recommendations for use of high-dose epinephrine in pediatric patients are not currently available.

Epinephrine may be given by the endotracheal route if establishment of venous access is delayed. Although the precise endotracheal dose is not known, it seems reasonable to use at least the same dose that is used intravenously (0.1 mL/kg of a 1:10,000 solution with a 0.5-mL minimum). The technique used for endotracheal administration of epinephrine is as follows:

1. The dose of epinephrine is diluted in 5 to 10 mL of normal saline.
2. Chest compressions are stopped.
3. The dilute solution is injected deeply and directly into the endotracheal tube (a 16- or 18-gauge plastic catheter on the syringe assists deep deposition of the drug and avoids the potential trauma of a steel needle).
4. The operator's finger is placed immediately over the tube adaptor to avoid expulsion of the drug by reflex coughing or chest compressions.
5. The BVM is rapidly reattached to the adaptor of the endotracheal tube.
6. Several ventilations are given in rapid succession for drug dispersal in the pulmonary system.

In the recent past a number of reports have expounded the value of this route of administration.[61-64] More recently, however, Chernow[65] and Quinton[66] and their colleagues have questioned the benefit of epinephrine administration by this route in the arrest state. These investigators further call into question the depot effect; that is, epinephrine continues to be absorbed from the lungs for 15 to 20 minutes, which may cause an adverse cardiovascular effect in the resuscitated patient.

Other important considerations with epinephrine use include the following: Do not use the 1:1000 solution unless it has been diluted 1:10 with normal saline. Also, intracardiac use has fallen into disfavor because of the seriousness of potential complications (hemothorax, pneumothorax, intramyocardial injection resulting in intractable ventricular fibrillation, vascular laceration, cardiac tamponade, dysrhythmia, and interruption of cardiac compression).

Glucose

Hypoglycemia in infants is not uncommon and can result in cardiovascular instability clinically indistinguishable from hypoxemia: decreased peripheral perfusion, sweating, hypotension, and tachycardia. Glycogen reserves are limited in infants, and any stress may cause depletion and resultant hypoglycemia. Rapid blood glucose determination with Dextrostix can identify the potentially devastating problem of hypoglycemia. Age and excessive exposure of the product to air can cause the Dextrostix to give a falsely low reading. Tightly resealing the bottle cap and dating the bottle's label can prevent this problem. Abnormal readings from Dextrostix should be confirmed with a simultaneous glucose determination; abnormal readings (<40 mg/100 mL) in clinically suspicious cases should be treated immediately.

Treatment with 25% dextrose in water (0.25 g/mL) given in a 2 mL/kg intravenous bolus will rapidly reverse hypoglycemia. Further hypoglycemia can be avoided by an infusion of 10% dextrose in water at a rate of 4 mL/kg/hour. Repeated use of 25% dextrose may result in intraventricular hemorrhage in the young infant.

Calcium

Calcium ions have long been known to cause an increase in myocardial contractility. This knowledge has mainly been provided from studies during open-heart surgery in adults. Calcium ions may also enhance ventricular excitability and conduction velocities through ventricular muscle. Theoretical indications for the use of calcium ions include electromechanical dissociation and asystole.[67] Retrospective studies,[68-71] however, have found calcium to be ineffective in altering these rhythms and to have uniformly poor outcomes. Katz and Reuter[72] have suggested that calcium entry into the cell cytoplasm is the final pathway of cell death and that calcium administration may add further insult. Furthermore, Clark and associates[73] have demonstrated a beneficial effect of the calcium channel blockers on myocardial preservation in cardiopulmonary bypass. For these reasons calcium treatment for electromechanical dissociation and asystole is no longer recommended by the American Heart Association.[74]

Asystole and electromechanical dissociation represent severe disruption of cardiac function. If their origins are primarily myocardial, successful resuscitation is rare regardless of the therapeutic modality employed. Treatment consists of effective ventilation and drug use (epinephrine, sodium bicarbonate, and atropine). An aggressive search must be carried out for potentially reversible causes (airway obstruction, cardiac tamponade, tension pneumothorax, severe hypovolemia, massive pulmonary embolism, or severe acidosis); if discovered, these must be treated appropriately.

Indications for calcium use are hypocalcemia, hyperkalemia, hypermagnesemia, and calcium channel blocker toxicity/overdose. Calcium chloride is the preferred solution of calcium because of the immediate availability of ionized calcium. The dosage of calcium chloride (10% = 100 mg/mL) is 0.2 mL/kg (20 mg/kg).

Precautions include slow intravenous administration with continuous cardiac monitoring (rapid injection may cause bradycardia), caution with digitalized patients (may cause sinus bradycardia and/or arrest), avoidance of simultaneous use with bicarbonate, and awareness of the potential of severe soft tissue damage with extravasation. The initial dose may be repeated in 10 minutes if indicated, and further doses should be based on measured deficits of calcium, continuing calcium channel blocking agent toxicity, or hyperkalemia/hypermagnesemia.

DEFIBRILLATION

Because of the rarity of ventricular tachydysrhythmias and VF as terminal events in infants and children (6% to 9% of cases),[75,76] blind defibrillation is not indicated in pulseless patients in this group. Rather, strict attention is focused on effective ventilation and oxygenation, external chest compression, and correction of acidosis. If cardiac monitoring reveals VF, defibrillation should be attempted as soon as possible.

Direct current defibrillators, with electrode paddles (4.5 cm in diameter for infants, 8 and 13 cm for older children) placed on gel pads with one paddle to the right of the sternum at the second rib and the other in the left midclavicular line at the xiphoid level, are the currently recommended type of defibrillator, size of paddles, electrode interface, and electrode placement, respectively. Although the ideal paddle size is not known, the largest electrode that allows good chest contact over its entire surface and good separation of the electrodes is preferred.

Recently, Atkins et al[77] found that the use of adult paddles in children older than 1 year (10 kg) minimized the transthoracic impedance compared to pediatric paddles. By decreasing the transthoracic impedance, larger paddles should require less energy for defibrillation and may improve the success rate of defibrillation and/or cardioversion. Clinical application and further study will verify this interesting finding.

The optimal electrical dose that is high enough to defibrillate most infants and children without causing myocardial damage has not been established. Currently available data,[78] however, suggest an initial dose of 2 W·sec/kg. The dose may be doubled to 4 W·sec/kg if the first attempt fails to defibrillate the heart. If the second attempt is unsuccessful, reassessment of ventilation and acid-base status is appropriate.

Children on digitalis preparations in VF should be defibrillated cautiously. Electrical stimulation potentiates the effect of digitalis, and irreversible cardiac arrest may result. The initial electrical dose should be as low as the defibrillator will allow, with slow increases in the dosage if the initial attempts are unsuccessful.

SPECIAL SITUATIONS

Special situations that need to be addressed and reemphasized in the context of pediatric CPR include hypothermia, hypoglycemia, drug overdose, and hypovolemia.

Hypothermia

Hypothermia (≤35°C) and subnormal temperatures due to poor temperature regulation present potential problems in the care of infants. The neonate and young infant can be thought of as poikilotherms, and their temperature will rapidly approximate that of the environment. Anatomic and physiologic bases for poor temperature regulation include a large surface-to-volume ratio, small amount of fatty insulation, lack of shivering ability, decreased energy stores, and lack of ability to defend against heat loss. Complications of hypothermia can be particularly devastating in the arrest situation and may result in increased oxygen consumption, increased acidosis, production of bradycardia or dysrhythmia, and decreased cardiac output or hypotension.

As the infant matures, it develops mechanisms to combat hypothermia, but treatment aimed at prevention is important and should be undertaken to avoid the serious consequences of a lowered core temperature. Rapid drying of fluids in contact with the skin (secretions, blood, emesis, urine, stool, meconium, and water) will decrease the temperature-lowering effect of evaporation. A radiant heat source and/or warming blanket will help raise body temperature and prevent heat loss (radiation) to the typically cool environment of the emergency department. Care must be taken not to overheat or burn the child with external warming devices. Constant use of and reference to an indwelling rectal thermometer, as well as keeping heat sources an appropriate distance from the infant, should obviate these problems.

CPR of hypothermic infants and children should not be discontinued prematurely. There have been case reports[79–82] of severely hypothermic patients successfully resuscitated without neurologic sequelae after prolonged CPR and warming efforts had resulted in nearly normal temperatures.

Table 31-8 Neonatal Resuscitation Equipment for the Emergency Department

Items That Should Be Readily Accessible	Items That Should Be on the Newborn Resuscitation Tray
Radiant warmer	Bulb syringe
Suction with manometer	DeLee suction trap
Resuscitation bag (250–500 mL)	Endotracheal tubes (2.5, 3.0, and 3.5)
Facemasks (newborn and premature size)	Suction catheters (one 5F and two 8F, each taped to the appropriate endotracheal tube)
Laryngoscope	
Laryngoscope blades (straight 0 and 1)	Endotracheal tube stylet
Medications	Umbilical catheter (5F)
Epinephrine, 1:10,000	Syringe (10 and 20 mL)
Sodium bicarbonate, 4.2%*	Three-way stopcock
Volume expander	Feeding tube (5F and 8F)
	Towels
	Obstetric kit/cord-cutting materials

*If the adult 8.4% solution is the only one available, it should be diluted 1:1 with sterile water.

Hypoglycemia

Hypoglycemia should be considered in all infants in arrest states. Myocardial and cerebral dysfunction is a potential complication of hypoglycemia. These complications are not uncommon because of decreased energy stores in the infant. (See earlier section on "glucose" for measuring techniques and dosing therapy.)

Drug Overdose

The possibility of drug overdose secondary to recreational use, accidental ingestion or overdose, child abuse, or maternal addiction/abuse should not be overlooked. Drug screens from blood, urine, and gastric samples are routinely obtained when the possibility of drug overdose is suspected clinically. Use of naloxone (Narcan) should not be delayed pending the results of toxicologic studies or confirmatory historical evidence. The safety and efficacy of large-dose intravenous naloxone in the pediatric setting has been well documented.[83] Current dose recommendations for naloxone are 0.01 mg/kg initially intravenously followed by 0.1 mg/kg to a maximum of 2 mg if there is no clinical improvement within 2 minutes.

Hypovolemia

Hypovolemic states (vomiting, diarrhea, dehydration, and blood loss) are common and must be considered and treated when suspected. Normal saline or lactated Ringer solution (20 mL/kg) as an intravenous push is safe and potentially life saving. This dose may be repeated if hypotension or signs of impaired perfusion persist. An aggressive approach to fluid resuscitation is encouraged. In a recent study of pediatric patients with septic shock, Carcillo et al[84] found that rapid fluid resuscitation in excess of 40 mL/kg in the first hour of emergency department care was associated with improved survival without increased risk of cardiogenic pulmonary edema. Only after adequate intravascular volume has been restored should all intravenous lines incorporate drip chambers to avoid the possibility of runaway intravenous solutions and resultant volume overload.

NEONATAL RESUSCITATION

Optimal outcome of an unexpected delivery in the emergency department requires advance preparation of specialized equipment, including a readily accessible neonatal resuscitation tray (Table 31-8). Little intervention is necessary in the stabilization of most newborns. After delivery, emphasis should be placed on positioning, drying, warming, tactile stimulation, and gentle suctioning while a rapid cardiopulmonary assessment is performed. Subsequent resuscitation depends on this assessment (Fig. 31-5). Indications for positive-pressure ventilation include apnea, heart rate less than 100 beat/min, and persistent cyanosis in spite of high-concentration blow-by oxygen. Chest compressions should be started when the heart rate is less than 60 beat/min before or after airway intervention. When the heart rate remains less than 80 beat/min after airway intervention and chest compressions, intubation and medications are indicated. Special situations requiring deviation from the usual approach to resuscitation include the infant with

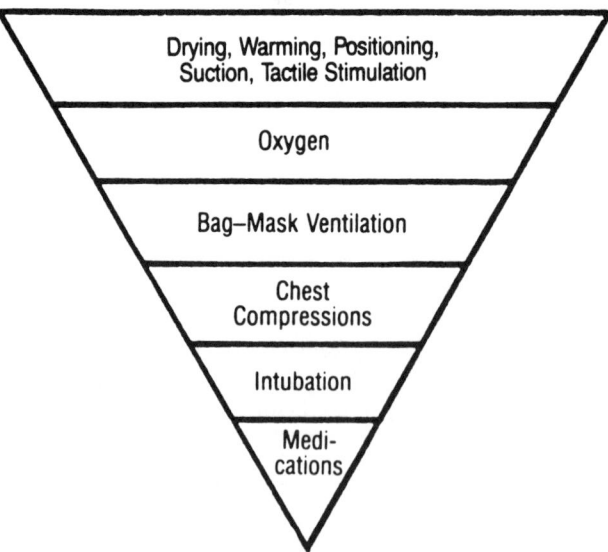

Figure 31-5 Inverted pyramid reflecting relative frequencies of neonatal resuscitation efforts.

meconium-stained fluid and suspected multiple births. If the amniotic fluid is meconium stained, the infant's oropharynx must be suctioned before initiation of spontaneous breathing or positive-pressure ventilation. In addition, in the presence of thick meconium staining, the infant's trachea must be intubated and suctioned immediately upon delivery. These efforts are necessary to avoid the pneumonitis associated with meconium aspiration of the newborn. Multiple equipment set-ups and resuscitation teams should be available for impending multiple births.

CONCLUSION

Pediatric CPR differs from its adult counterpart in several important areas that must be understood to maximize opportunity for success. Persistent arrest situations should be reassessed frequently for underlying causes. Extracardiac causes such as pneumothorax, cardiac tamponade, hypovolemia, hypothermia, hypoglycemia, and overdose need to be evaluated and, if found, treated promptly. Chest and abdominal radiographs aid in assessment of tube position and underlying diagnosis. Initial laboratory evaluation includes baseline blood count, arterial blood gases, electrolytes, and glucose. Drug screening, blood culture, or clotting panel may be helpful in specific cases. The importance of ventilation techniques as well as oxygenation and perfusion status cannot be overemphasized in pediatric cardiac arrest. Careful initial assessment and continuous reassessment are required for optimum outcome.

REFERENCES

1. Gillis J, Dickson D, Reider M, et al. Results of inpatient pediatric resuscitation. *Crit Care Med.* 1986;14:469–471.
2. Friesen RM, Duncan P, Tweed WA, et al. Appraisal pediatric cardiopulmonary resuscitation. *Can Med Assoc J.* 1982;126:1055–1058.
3. Downes JJ, Fulgenicio T, Raphaely RC. Acute respiratory failure in infants and children. *Pediatr Clin North Am.* 1972;19:2:423–445.
4. Crone RK. Acute circulatory failure in children. *Pediatr Clin North Am.* 1980;27:525–538.
5. American Heart Association and American Academy of Pediatrics. *Textbook of Pediatric Advanced Life Support.* Dallas: American Heart Association; 1988.
6. Rosen P. The danger of oral intubation in the unstable cervical spine, a legend in emergency medicine? Presented at the Emergency Medicine Symposium; August 1, 1988; San Diego, CA.
7. Bivins HG, Ford S, Bezmalinovic Z, et al. The effect of axial traction during orotracheal intubation of the trauma victim with an unstable cervical spine. *Ann Emerg Med.* 1988;17:25–29.
8. Majernick TG, Bieniek R, Houston JB, et al. Cervical movement during orotracheal intubation. *Ann Emerg Med.* 1986;15:417–420.
9. Pierog JE. Acute supraglottitis. *Top Emerg Med.* 1981;3:53–66.
10. Diaz JH, Lockhart CH. Early diagnosis and airway management of acute epiglottitis in children. *South Med J.* 1982;75:399–403.
11. Dunbar JS. Epiglottitis and croup. *J Can Assoc Radiol.* 1961;12:86–95.
12. Szold PD, Glicklich M. Children with epiglottitis can be bagged. *Clin Pediatr.* 1976;15:792–793.
13. Glicklich M, Cohen RD, Jona JZ. Steroids and bag and mask ventilation in the treatment of acute epiglottitis. *J Pediatr Surg.* 1979;14:247–251.
14. Adair JC, Ring WH. Management of epiglottitis in children. *Anesth Analg.* 1975;54:622–625.
15. Allen TH, Steven IM. Prolonged nasotracheal intubation in infants and children. *Br J Anaesth.* 1972;44:835–839.
16. Bottenfield GW, Arcinue EL, Sarnaik, et al. Diagnosis and management of acute epiglottitis—report of 90 consecutive cases. *Laryngoscope.* 1980;90:822–825.
17. Breivik H, Klaastad O. Acute epiglottitis in children, review of 27 patients. *Br J Anaesth.* 1978;50:505–509.
18. Davis HW, Gartner JC, Galvis AG, et al. Acute upper airway respiratory obstruction: croup and epiglottitis. *Pediatr Clin North Am.* 1981;28:4:859–880.
19. Eastwood NB. Acute epiglottitis. *Lancet.* 1978;1:205. Letter.
20. Faden HS. Treatment of *Hemophilus influenzae* type B epiglottitis. *Pediatrics.* 1979;63:402–407.
21. Scully RE, Galdabini JJ, McNeely BU. Case records of the Massachusetts General Hospital: case 42-1977. *N Engl J Med.* 1977;297:878–883.
22. Raj PP, Larard DG, Diba YT. Acute epiglottitis in children, a respiratory emergency. *Br J Anaesth.* 1969;41:619–627.
23. Welch DB, Price DG. Acute epiglottitis and severe croup. *Anesthesia.* 1983;38:754–759.
24. Battaglia JD, Lockhart CH. Management of acute epiglottitis by nasotracheal intubation. *Am J Dis Child.* 1975;129:334–336.
25. Balnc VF, Weber ML, Leduc C, et al. Acute epiglottitis in children: management of 27 consecutive cases with nasotracheal intubation with special emphasis on anesthetic considerations. *Can Anaesth Soc J.* 1977;24:1–11.
26. Fearon B, Cinnamond M. Tracheostomy in acute supraglottitis (epiglottitis): the treatment of choice. *Laryngoscope.* 1977;87:879–883.
27. Geraci RP. Acute epiglottitis management with prolonged nasotracheal intubation. *Pediatrics.* 1968;41:143–145.
28. Heldtlander F, Lee F. Treatment of acute epiglottitis in children by long term intubation. *Acta Otolaryngol.* 1973;75:379–381.
29. Schultz RL, Morrison W. Short-term intubation in 200 children with acute epiglottitis. *South Med J.* 1982;75:158–159.
30. Sweeney DE, Allen TH, Steven IM. Acute epiglottitis—management by intubation. *Anaesth Intensive Care.* 1978;1:526–528.
31. Phelan PD, Mullins GC, Laundau LI, et al. The period of nasotracheal intubation in acute epiglottitis. *Anaesth Intensive Care.* 1980;8:402–403.
32. Rapkin RH. Tracheotomy in epiglottitis. *Pediatrics.* 1973;52:428–429.
33. Jesudian MC, Harrison RR, Keenan RL, et al. Bag-valve-mask ventilation: two rescuers are better than one: preliminary report. *Crit Care Med.* 1985;18:122–123.
34. Standards and guidelines for cardiopulmonary resuscitation (CPR) and emergency cardiac care (ECC). *JAMA.* 1980;244:475.
35. Day RL, Crelin ES, Dubois AB. Choking: the Heimlich abdominal thrust vs back blows. An approach to measurement of inertial and aerodynamic forces. *Pediatrics.* 1982;70:113–119.
36. Sellick BA. Cricoid pressure to control regurgitation of stomach contents during induction of anaesthesia. *Lancet.* 1961;2:404–406.
37. Salem MR, Wong AY, Mani M, et al. Efficacy of cricoid pressure in preventing gastric inflation during bag-valve-mask ventilation in pediatric patients. *Anesthesiology.* 1974;40:96–98.

38. Rosetti V, Thompson BM, Aprahamian C, et al. Difficulty and delay in intravascular access in pediatric arrests. *Ann Emerg Med.* 1984;13:406. Abstract.
39. Coté CJ, Jobes DR, Schwartz AJ, et al. Two approaches to cannulation of a child's internal jugular vein. *Anesthesiology.* 1979;50:371–373.
40. Prince SR, Sullivan RL, Hackel A. Percutaneous catheterization of the internal jugular vein in infants and children. *Anesthesiology.* 1976;44:170–174.
41. Kanter RK, Zimmerman JJ, Strauss RH, et al. Pediatric emergency intravenous access: evaluation of a protocol. *Am J Dis Child.* 1986;140:132–134.
42. Spivey WH, Lathers CM, Malone DR, et al. Comparison of intraosseous, central and peripheral routes of sodium bicarbonate administration during CPR in pigs. *Ann Emerg Med.* 1985;14:1135–1140.
43. Rosetti VA, Thompson BM, Miller J, et al. Intraosseous infusion: an alternative route of pediatric intravascular access. *Ann Emerg Med.* 1985;14:885–888.
44. Parrish G, Turkewitz D, Skiendzielewski JJ. Intraosseous infusion in the emergency department. *Am J Emerg Med.* 1986;4:59–63.
45. Berg RA. Emergency infusion of catecholamines into bone marrow. *Am J Dis Child.* 1984;138:810–811.
46. Glaeser PW, Losek JD. Emergency intraosseous infusions in children. *Am J Emerg Med.* 1986;4:34–36.
47. Heinild S, Sondergaard J, Tuvdad F. Bone marrow infusions in childhood: experiences from 1,000 infusions. *J Pediatr.* 1947;30:400–412.
48. Orlowski JP, Julius CJ, Petras RE, et al. The safety of intraosseous infusions: risks of fat and bone marrow emboli to the lungs. *Ann Emerg Med.* 1989;18:1062–1067.
49. Spivey WH, Unger HD, McNamara RM, et al. Effect of intraosseous sodium bicarbonate on bone in swine. *Ann Emerg Med.* 1987;16:773–776.
50. Brickman KR, Rega P, Koltz M, et al. Analysis of growth plate abnormalities following intraosseous infusion through the proximal tibial epiphysis in pigs. *Ann Emerg Med.* 1988;17:121–123.
51. LaFleche FR, Slepin MJ, Vargas J, et al. Iatrogenic bilateral tibial fractures after intraosseous infusion attempts in a 3 month old infant. *Ann Emerg Med.* 1989;18:1099–1101.
52. Papper EM. The bone marrow for injecting fluids and drugs into the general circulation. *Anesthesiology.* 1942;3:307–312.
53. Shoor PM, Berryhill RE, Benumof JL. Intraosseous infusion: pressure-flow relationship and pharmacokinetics. *J Trauma.* 1979;19:772–774.
54. Morris RE, Schonfeld N, Haftel AJ. Treatment of hemorrhagic shock with intraosseous administration of crystalloid fluid in the rabbit model. *Ann Emerg Med.* 1987;16:1321–1324.
55. Amlie R. Care of the newborn in the emergency department. *Top Emerg Med.* 1981;3:7–17.
56. Lubitz DL, Seidel JS, Chameides L, et al. A rapid method for estimating weight and resuscitation drug dosages from length in the pediatric age group. *Ann Emerg Med.* 1988;17:576–581.
57. Gabow P. Sodium bicarbonate. A cure or curse for metabolic acidosis? *J Crit Illness.* 1989;4:18–28.
58. Goetting MG, Paradis NA. High dose epinephrine in refractory pediatric cardiac arrest. *Crit Care Med.* 1989;17:1258–1262.
59. Martin D, Werman HA, Brown CG. Four case studies: high dose epinephrine in cardiac arrest. *Ann Emerg Med.* 1990;19:322–326.
60. Barton C, Callaham M. High dose epinephrine improves the return of spontaneous circulation rates in human victims of cardiac arrest. *Ann Emerg Med.* 1991;20:722–725.
61. Roberts JR, Greenberg MI, Knaub MA, et al. Blood levels following intravenous and endotracheal epinephrine administration. *JACEP.* 1979;8:53–56.
62. Orlowski JP. Pediatric cardiopulmonary resuscitation. *Emerg Med Clin North Am.* 1983;1:1–25.
63. Greenberg MI, Roberts JR, Baskin SI. Use of endotracheally administered epinephrine in a pediatric patient. *Am J Dis Child.* 1981;135:767–768.
64. Lindemann R. Resuscitation of the newborn: endotracheal administration of epinephrine. *Acta Pediatr Scand.* 1984;73:210–212.
65. Chernow B, Holbrook P, D'Angoa DS, et al. Epinephrine absorption after intratracheal administration. *Anesth Analg.* 1984;63:829–832.
66. Quinton DN, O'Byrne G, Aitkenhead AR. Comparison of endotracheal and peripheral intravenous adrenaline in cardiac arrest: is endotracheal route reliable? *Lancet.* 1987;1:828–829.
67. Dembo D. Calcium in advanced life support. *Crit Care Med.* 1981;9:358–359.
68. Steuven HA, Thompson BM, Aprahamian C, et al. Use of calcium in pre-hospital cardiac arrest. *Ann Emerg Med.* 1983;12:136–139.
69. Harrison EE, Amey BD. The use of calcium in cardiac resuscitation. *Am J Emerg Med.* 1983;3:267–273.
70. Iseri LT, Siner EJ, Humphrey SB. Pre-hospital cardiac arrest after arrival of the paramedic unit. *JACEP.* 1977;12:530–535.
71. Steuven HA, Thompson BM, Aprahamian C, et al. Lack of effectiveness of calcium chloride in refractory asystole. *Ann Emerg Med.* 1985;14:630–632.
72. Katz AM, Reuter H. Cellular calcium and cardiac cell death. *Am J Cardiol.* 1979;44:188–190.
73. Clark RE, Christlieb IY, Ferguson TB, et al. The first American trial of nifedipine in cardioplegia. A report of the first 12 month experience. *J Thorac Cardiovasc Surg.* 1981;82:848–859.
74. Standards and guidelines for cardiopulmonary resuscitation (CPR) and emergency cardiac care (ECC). *JAMA.* 1986;255:29–33.
75. Kull Walsh C, Krongrad E. Terminal cardiac electrical activity in pediatric patients. *Am J Cardiol.* 1983;51:557–561.
76. Eisenberg M, Bergner L, Hallstrom A. Epidemiology of cardiac arrest and resuscitation in children. *Ann Emerg Med.* 1983;12:672–674.
77. Atkins DL, Sirna S, Kieso R, et al. Pediatric defibrillation: importance of paddle size in determining transthoracic impedance. *Pediatrics.* 1988;82:914–918.
78. Gutgesell HP, Tacker WA, Geddes LA, et al. Energy dose of ventricular fibrillation of children. *Pediatrics.* 1976;58:898–901.
79. Ferguson J, Epstein F, van de Leuv J. Accidental hypothermia. *Emerg Med Clin North Am.* 1983;1:619–637.
80. Miller JW, Danzl DF, Thomas DM. Urban accidental hypothermia: 135 cases. *Ann Emerg Med.* 1980;9:456–461.
81. Anderson S, Herbring BG, Widman B. Accidental profound hypothermia. *Br J Anaesth.* 1970;42:653–655.
82. Schlissler P, Parker MA, Scott SJ. Profound hypothermia: value of prolonged cardiopulmonary resuscitation. *South Med J.* 1981;74:474–477.
83. Moore RA, Rumak BH, Conner CS, et al. Naloxone-underdosage after narcotic poisoning. *Am J Dis Child.* 1980;134:156–158.
84. Carcillo JA, Davis AL, Zaritsky A. Role of early fluid resuscitation in pediatric septic shock. *JAMA.* 1991;266:1242–1245.

32. Evaluation of Febrile Children Younger Than Two Years of Age

JAMES E. PIEROG, MD, FACEP

Fever in children younger than 2 years of age is a common problem in emergency medicine. As many as 20% to 35% of children presenting to emergency departments have febrile conditions. The majority of febrile illnesses will have a viral etiology, and the diagnosis will usually be apparent on history and physical examination. There are several problems unique to the pediatric population that must be considered, however.

- Some infectious processes may not be accompanied by persistent fever.
- Fever may be caused by noninfectious processes (salicylism, bundling, sickle cell crisis, malignancies, collagen vascular diseases, drug reactions, and central nervous system disorders).
- Hypothermia in infants younger than 3 months (especially younger than 1 month) is associated with a marked increase in the incidence of serious bacterial infections.[1]
- Any temperature elevation greater than 38.5°C in infants younger than 3 months is problematic and may represent a serious bacterial infection despite a benign clinical appearance.[2]
- Children younger than 2 years with fever greater than 38.5°C and no obvious source of infection may have a serious underlying illness (occult bacteremia, meningitis, pyelonephritis, and pneumonia), despite a well appearance.[3–8]

A rapid assessment of all febrile children should begin on their entry to the emergency department. The critically ill child requires immediate intervention and stabilization. The medical history can be obtained as diagnostic and therapeutic procedures are being carried out. A more detailed history and physical examination can be obtained later.

FEVER IN CHILDREN BETWEEN THREE AND TWENTY-FOUR MONTHS OF AGE: THE SPECIAL PROBLEM OF OCCULT BACTEREMIA

Frequency

There have been numerous reports of the problem of unsuspected bacteremia, so-called occult bacteremia (OB), in febrile children younger than 2 years. The frequency of OB in walk-in clinics and pediatric emergency departments is 3% to 7%. Teele et al[4] studied more than 600 consecutive children between 4 weeks and 2 years of age with rectal temperatures greater than 38.3°C and reported a 3.2% incidence of positive blood cultures. McCarthy et al,[8] in a study of 329 patients younger than 2 years with temperatures of 38.3°C or greater found a bacteremic rate of 7.3%. The vast majority of the bacteremic patients (95%) were not suspected on history or physical examination. In another study by McCarthy and associates,[5] when only those children with seemingly minor illnesses (otitis media, upper respiratory tract infection, or fever without apparent source) were reviewed, a 4.7% bacteremic rate was found. Initially it was theorized that these high rates were due to the fact that the studies were gathered from lower socioeconomic groups. The rate of OB in a predominantly middle-class private practice,[9] however, was found to be similar (5.5%) to that in hospital outpatient departments.

Bacteriology

Streptococcus pneumoniae is the most frequent pathogen in OB, occurring in approximately two of three cases. *Hemophilus influenzae* type B is encountered in about 25%, with other pathogens such as *Neisseria meningitidis* and *Salmonella* species accounting for the remainder of cases.

Initial Diagnosis

Upper respiratory tract infections and fever without apparent source are the most common initial diagnoses for patients with OB. Otitis media and pneumonia are also commonly diagnosed. Pharyngitis is an infrequent diagnosis in patients younger than 2 years. An obvious site of infection on initial presentation is found in only 20% of cases with *S pneumoniae* bacteremia,[5] yet more than 90% of culture-proven *H influenzae* cases will have a source of infection that is obvious by examination. As a result of these clinical findings, patients with *H influenzae* bacteremia are much more likely to have antibiotics prescribed when discharged than patients with *S pneumoniae* bacteremia.

Risk Factors

Although no single clinical factor is highly sensitive or specific in identifying those patients with OB, there are some risk factors that should make the clinician acutely aware of the possibility.

Age

Children younger than 24 months clearly have an increased incidence of OB. This fact has been demonstrated repeatedly,[3,4,10,11] with 6- to 18-month-olds being at greatest risk.

Temperature

Despite the fact that there are many studies that correlate increasing temperature with a higher incidence of bacteremia,[3–6,8,12] Surpure[13] was unable to support such a statement in his study of 516 children aged 1 month to 15 years (350 patients younger than 2 years of age) with temperatures greater than 40°C. Unlike McCarthy and Dolan,[12] who found a significant correlation between high fever and bacteremia, Surpure did not demonstrate a relationship between meningitis and fever greater than 41°C. Perhaps Surpure missed cases of OB because in his series blood cultures were drawn in selected situations only, depending on the clinical judgment of the resident physician. The wary clinician should not be concerned over the absolute level of temperature, which may or may not be associated with serious underlying pathology. Rather, he or she should realize that an elevated temperature is a sign of underlying pathology that varies with multiple factors (clothing, ambient temperature, hydration status, antipyretic use, host response, etc) in addition to the disease process itself. A finding of increased temperature, either historically or on review of vital signs, should prompt the clinician to evaluate the patient thoroughly for the possibility of OB or serious underlying bacterial infection. Remember that a parent's or caretaker's subjective or objective report of temperature elevation correlates strongly with a febrile state, regardless of the temperature obtained in the emergency department.

Clinical Judgment

Most clinicians are aware that a febrile infant with a serious illness may not manifest classic physical findings of that illness. Samson[14] demonstrated that 11 of 152 children with bacterial meningitis who were younger than 16 months did not have nuchal rigidity, a bulging fontanelle, altered sensorium, or a positive Brudzinski's sign. Because of the difficulty in eliciting physical findings and the nonspecificity of historical variables, McCarthy et al[15] attempted to identify observational variables on which pediatricians base their instinctive judgment to determine degree of illness in febrile children. Although playfulness was the observational variable with the strongest correlation to illness, the investigators found that attending pediatricians were able to identify only 57% of patients with serious illnesses as moderately or severely ill on assessment. When physical examination was added to the evaluation, 24% of the patients with proven bacterial illness still were not identified. They concluded that instinctive judgment was limited in the accurate assessment of the febrile child. This study is but one of several that address the problem of clinical evaluation of febrile infants. On the one hand, experienced clinicians are adept at accurately assessing sick children[16,17] as well as the vast majority of the well children. Even a thorough predictive model applied by experienced pediatric clinicians,[18] however, that graded observational items (quality of cry, reaction to parent stimulation, mental state variation, color hydration, and response to social overtures) had some limitations. Of the sick children, 92.3% were correctly predicted by the model, and only 2.7% of the patients predicted to be well had serious illness. Although falsely identifying a well patient as sick results in unnecessary diagnostic testing and therapeutic misadventure, not to mention economic burdens, the most distressing problem is missing the sick patient who appears to be well. To date our society and the medical profession will accept excessive false positives in an attempt to identify febrile children with serious illness.

A simple technique called optimal observation is useful in further assessing the febrile child.[19] This technique relies on reported evaluation of the child in a comfortable setting when the child's temperature has been lowered by an antipyretic agent (acetaminophen, 15 mg/kg). The child can be observed serially as the fever abates while he or she is sitting on the caretaker's lap or playing on the gurney. A febrile child who becomes happy, playful, and interactive has a dramatically reduced need for further diagnostic evaluation or treatment, but the child who remains irritable, refuses feeds, and interacts poorly requires further diagnostic and therapeutic intervention.

Despite its limitations, clinical judgment remains the single most important variable in determining which febrile infant has an underlying serious bacterial illness (OB, pneumonia, meningitis, pyelonephritis, septic arthritis, etc).

Laboratory Tests

In an attempt to improve sensitivity in diagnosing OB, many investigators have looked to the laboratory for assistance. The complete blood count (CBC), white blood cell count (WBC), absolute neutrophil count, immature neutrophil count, absolute immature neutrophil count, C-reactive protein (CRP), and erythrocyte sedimentation rate (ESR) have been evaluated in detail.[4,5,8,11] Although bacterial diseases are classically associated with elevated WBC and an increase in both mature and immature neutrophil forms, there are many variables that affect these laboratory tests. Rasmussen and Rasmussen[20] demonstrated conclusively that neither the WBC nor the differential count was predictive of whether an acutely ill child had a bacterial or nonbacterial infection. Factors responsible for altering the classic WBC response to bacteria include bacterial infections that have their own pattern (pertussis, scarlet fever, and *Salmonella* infection), fulminant bacterial infections with leukopenia, medications (corticosteroids and β adrenergics), strenuous exercise, fever, age of the child, duration of infection, endogenous steroid and catecholamine release, and other factors. Morens[21] supported these findings in a review of 328 consecutive children admitted to an infectious disease service. He found that the WBC and differential count could not differentiate between bacterial and nonbacterial disease. Furthermore, of all the abnormal WBC counts and differential counts, only 23% were associated with bacterial disease and 40% with viral disease. Morens recommended caution in interpreting WBC and differential counts and reiterated the multiple factors that affect them. Like Rasmussen and Rasmussen,[20] he suggested other underlying illness in the patient, nature of the infectious agent, and presence of toxin production.

Despite these reports, McGowan[3] and Teele[4] and their colleagues have clearly demonstrated a relationship between increasing WBC ($>10,000/mm^3$) and an increased frequency of OB. McCarthy et al[8] found that a WBC count greater than $15,000/mm^3$ and an ESR greater than 30 mm/hour were the most sensitive laboratory tests in predicting OB. Furthermore, in children younger than 24 months with temperatures greater than 40°C, OB and pneumonia were three times more frequent if the WBC was greater than $15,000/mm^3$ and four times more frequent if the ESR was greater than 30 mm/hour. In an earlier report, however, McCarthy et al[5] found the WBC to be less sensitive in predicting OB because 50% of patients with trivial illnesses and WBCs less than $15,000/mm^3$ had OB.

There is no simple, rapid, accurate test currently available to diagnose OB or underlying bacterial illness. Blood cultures remain the gold standard, but delaying diagnosis for 24 to 28 hours for their result is problematic. The WBC is a simple, readily available, and inexpensive procedure. It is the best test currently available to the clinician. If the clinician realizes its limitations and applies this test appropriately, it may be of utility in assisting with the diagnosis and determining the need for further investigation.

Outcome

Approximately 30% of children with untreated *Streptococcus pneumoniae* bacteremia (diagnosed initially as fever without source, upper respiratory tract infection, or viral syndrome) will become afebrile and asymptomatic within 24 to 48 hours.[7,10] Repeat blood cultures in this group will be sterile. Of these patients, however, 70% to 75% will be unimproved or will have a new focus of infection. Of the unimproved group, 25% to 35% will have persistent bacteremia, and 5% to 10% will develop meningitis. Persistent bacteremia is more common (50% to 76%) with *Hemophilus influenzae* bacteremia,[10,22] as is the development of new foci of infection. Additionally, these patients will have greater rates of meningitis than those with *S pneumoniae* bacteremia.

Presumptive Antibiotics

Presumptive or expectant antibiotics in general, and for those at high risk for OB in particular, have not been enthusiastically embraced by the medical profession. Reasons for this posture include the high incidence of viral infections in this group, fear of producing a partially treated meningitis, and the questionable efficacy of such a practice. Because the outcome of untreated OB can be serious illness, however, it is not to be taken as a trivial condition, even though 25% to 30% of OB cases will resolve spontaneously. Several investigators have looked at the effect of antibiotics in those with risk factors (age, temperature, and WBC or ESR). Bratton et al[7] found an increased chance of clinical improvement in treated compared to untreated patients with OB (80% compared to 30%) as well as a reduction in the incidence of persistent bacteremia from 25% to 4%. Teele et al[10] demonstrated an improved outcome in patients with *S pneumoniae* bacteremia who were initially treated with antibiotics in the form of clinical improvement (80% compared to 31%) and less persistent bacteremia (6% compared to 30%). Improvement was seen in the *H influenzae* group as well. Neither group of investigators demonstrated a decrease in the incidence of meningitis with initial antibiotic treatment.

Jaffe et al[23] described a prospective, randomized, placebo-controlled, double-blind clinical trial of antibiotic administration to treat possible OB in febrile children. The study included 955 children, ages 3 to 36 months, with temperatures greater than 39°C and no focal bacterial infection. The rate of OB was 2.8%, and the incidence of major infectious morbidity was 10.5% in the antibiotic group and 12.5% for the placebo controls. The results of this study led to the conclusion that expectant antibiotics at standard oral doses are not helpful in preventing disease progression in this group. Recently, Baron et al[24] presented a prolonged study with small numbers and a provocative conclusion. The study was a retrospective analysis from a suburban private pediatric practice. The study group included patients, ages 3 to 24 months, with temperatures greater than 39.4°C and non-focal illness. Twenty-three patients with OB (21 with *S pneumoniae* infection) were produced. Of 8 patients (38%) without antibiotics, 3 developed complications (facial cellulitis in 2 and persistent bacteremia in 1). Of 4 patients given standard doses of amoxicillin, 2 also had complications (preseptal cellulitis in 1 and persistent bacteremia in 1). The remaining 11 bacteremic patients were given high-dose amoxicillin (136 to 174 mg/kg/day, mean, 154 mg/kg/day) and, significantly, developed no complications. Although the sample size was small and the results certainly need verification, this study suggests that higher dosages of appropriate antibiotics may be efficacious in the presumptive treatment of OB and may prevent or reduce the rate of complications.

Management

As can be assumed from the preceding discussion, OB in children 3 to 24 months old is surrounded by controversy. Despite refinement, clinical judgment is imperfect. At present there are no specific tests rapidly to detect OB, either clinically or in the laboratory. Controversy surrounds a number of diagnostic and therapeutic options. Clearly, there is no absolutely right management plan for febrile children in this age group, and any number of approaches may be acceptable. The cornerstones of effective care in the uncertain area of OB are caution, re-evaluation, appropriate use of laboratory and consultative support, follow-up in 12 to 24 hours, and immediate return to the emergency department if new findings or deterioration occur.

The following is an acceptable approach:

- If the child has a benign appearance without age or temperature risk factors, routine management is appropriate.
- If the child is between 3 and 24 months of age and has a fever greater than 38.5°C:
  1. perform a complete history and physical examination.
  2. re-examine the child after a period of optimal observation.
  3. if there is a recognizable viral illness, treat accordingly.
  4. if there is a recognizable bacterial infection, treat accordingly. Remember that a focus of infection does not rule out disseminated infection (ie, otitis media). Pre-existing illnesses such as diabetes mellitus, leukemia, lymphoma, sickle cell disease, immunodeficiency, steroid use, or cardiopulmonary disease may require treatment of any fever as sepsis.
  5. if there is an upper respiratory infection, otitis media, pneumonia, or fever with no obvious source, obtain a WBC with or without an ESR. These may be done by fingerstick. If venipuncture is performed, blood cultures may be drawn at the same time and held pending the WBC results.
  6. obtain a urinalysis if there is no source of fever. Collection of the urine specimen is fraught with delay in obtaining the specimen and potential errors of contamination from skin and stool bacteria. If bagged specimens or clinical findings are suggestive of urinary tract infection, then catheterization or suprapubic aspiration is indicated. Nonspecific findings are common in children younger than 2 years with a urinary tract infection and include fever, vomiting, diarrhea, irritability, and poor feeding. Selden et al[25] have demonstrated the high frequency of nonspecific findings with urinary tract infections; in their study 22 of 90 children with urinary tract infections had fever alone as the presenting finding. If pyuria is present, obtain a urine culture and treat accordingly.
  7. obtain a chest radiograph if pneumonia is suspected.
  8. if the WBC is greater than 15,000/mm^3, have a blood culture done.
  9. treat with oral antibiotics if indicated (otitis media, pneumonia, sinusitis, etc). The antibiotic of choice in this situation is usually amoxicillin (40 mg/kg/day in three to four divided doses, possibly 150 mg/kg/day). In areas with high rates of *H influenzae*–ampicillin resistance or penicillin allergy, cefaclor, trimethoprim/sulfamethoxazole, or amoxicillin-clavulanate would be preferable. If

antibiotics are prescribed, initial therapy (usually parenteral) should begin in the emergency department. Manage the child as an outpatient and repeat the physical examination within 6 to 24 hours. It is imperative that the patient's caretakers understand that the child should be returned immediately if his or her condition worsens or new symptoms develop. A definite, scheduled appointment is made to follow and monitor the patient. This may be done with a private physician, a clinic, or the emergency department.

10. if the child appears ill after optimal observation, begin a septic work-up and do a lumbar puncture, especially in children younger than 18 months (neck stiffness and meningismus are unreliable physical findings for meningitis). If the spinal tap is cloudy, begin intravenous antibiotics immediately in the emergency department. If the results of the tap are positive while the patient in is the emergency department, begin intravenous antibiotics before the patient is transported to the ward or intensive care unit. Not to do so subjects the patient to unnecessary delays in treatment,[26] which may increase morbidity and mortality.

Management of Occult Bacteremia

If the cultures are negative, antibiotics may be stopped unless treatment was begun to treat a specific focus or one develops. Follow-up should continue until resolution of the process. If a positive blood culture is identified, management depends on the organism cultured.

If *H influenzae* is cultured, admit, do a complete septic work-up, and begin intravenous antibiotics. If *S pneumoniae* is cultured, re-examine. If the child is afebrile and has a benign appearance, treat with oral antibiotics for 10 days as an outpatient and monitor closely. If the child has evidence of a focal infection and is not toxic, treat in a manner appropriate for the diagnosis. If the child is febrile or symptomatic (even minimally), do a septic work-up, including a repeat blood culture; begin intravenous antibiotics, and admit to an inpatient unit.

EVALUATION OF FEBRILE INFANTS YOUNGER THAN THREE MONTHS

Febrile infants younger than 3 months are at increased risk for serious life-threatening infections. Their immune systems are immature, and they may poorly localize infectious processes, which may lead to disseminated infection. Roberts and Borzy[2] showed a bacteremic rate of nearly 15% in febrile neonates. The infants with bacteremia were indistinguishable from the infants without bacteremia as judged by degree of fever, WBC, differential, or presence of focus of infection. Although clinical judgment was able to detect 8 of 9 bacteremic infants as not well, the investigators believed that missing 1 of 9 bacteremic patients pointed out the limitation of clinical judgment in this age group. Limitation of clinical judgment supported their aggressive approach in performing a complete septic work-up on every febrile infant younger than 3 months, beginning intravenous antibiotics, and hospitalizing every patient until the culture results are known. From these and other findings,[27] it has been the policy of many university and teaching institutions routinely to perform these tasks on every febrile infant. Such dogmatic policy has led to significant overutilization of laboratory and radiologic services as well as unnecessary antibiotic administration and hospitalizations.

Recent reports have demonstrated that serious infections and/or bacteremia occur much less frequently than previously thought. Green et al[28] retrospectively studied 147 infants younger than 2 months with temperatures greater than 37.8°C. In 55 patients who appeared clinically well, all cultures of blood and cerebrospinal fluid (CSF) were negative for pathogens. In another group of 89 patients with a source of fever identified but an uncertain etiologic agent, only 1 patient had a positive blood culture, and there were no positive CSF cultures. Only 3 of 147 patients had obvious bacterial infections on presentation (meningitis, septic arthritis, and pneumonia). An additional 37 patients were studied prospectively. Twenty were safely treated as outpatients without complication, and 17 were admitted to the hospital and either treated with antibiotics or observed. None of the patients appeared ill, and cultures of blood, CSF, or urine obtained from 29 patients were all negative. Despite the low incidence of serious bacterial infections in this study, the management of febrile neonates without routine hospitalization and antibiotics was not simple or uncomplicated. Fully 25% of hospitalized patients with unexplained fever developed a diagnosis within 1 day, and 16% of outpatients evidenced a new diagnosis on follow-up. None of the patients had a delayed diagnosis and treatment, however.

King et al[29] found a 5% incidence of bacteremia or bacterial meningitis in 342 febrile infants younger than 2 months. None of 61 infants in the prospective portion of the study who appeared clinically well developed positive blood or CSF cultures. The investigators found clinical impression to be the most sensitive indicator for absence of serious bacterial infection and considered outpatient management of selected febrile infants appropriate where meticulous clinical evaluation with close follow-up was available.

Dagan et al,[30,31] concerned about iatrogenic complications and severe financial burdens imposed by a universal policy of sepsis work-up and hospitalization, demonstrated an extremely low rate of serious bacterial infections in a low-risk group [absence of deep tissue or skeletal infection or purulent otitis media, normal WBC and differential (5000 to 15,000/mm^3 with < 1,500 band/mm^3), normal urine, and < 25 WBC per high-power field in stool if the patient had diarrhea] who appeared well. In the first study,[30] only 1 of 144 patients in the low-risk group had a bacterial infection (*Salmonella* gastroenteritis); there were no cases of bacteremia or meningitis. In the second study,[31] 148 healthy febrile infants younger than 2 months in the low-risk group were studied. No infants developed a serious bacterial infection. The conclusion of these investigators reiterated that of others: Outpatient management of low-risk febrile infants may be feasible with meticulous and careful, daily follow-up.

From these provocative studies, it is clear that universal admission of febrile neonates may not be the only manner by which to manage this group successfully and that subsets may be better served by a less aggressive, less costly approach. Diagnostic and therapeutic alternatives include use of a sepsis screen,[32] complete septic work-up in the emergency department combined with outpatient management if the evaluation is negative, and limited laboratory work-up in well-appearing neonates with outpatient management and close clinical follow-up.

The clinician should be aware of problems and controversies surrounding the evaluation and treatment of the febrile infant younger than 3 months:

- the actual incidence of serious infection in this age group
- the limitations of clinical evaluation
- the nonspecificity of currently available outpatient laboratory tests (CBC, ESR, CRP)
- the need for a specific, rapid, inexpensive laboratory test accurately to select patients with a serious bacterial infection
- the unnecessary expense and exposure to antibiotics with current policies to hospitalize and empirically treat all patients

Clarification of these problems and a more satisfactory diagnostic and therapeutic approach await further clinical investigation. It appears, however, that the movement for a more rational and practical approach to this controversial problem may be gaining momentum.[33]

Causes of Fever

The most common cause of fever in infants is viral illness acquired from household contacts. Upper respiratory tract infections and acute gastroenteritis are by far the most frequent viral infections. Aseptic (viral) meningitis due to enteroviruses causes fever in infants during summer and fall months. Otitis media, caused mainly by nonencapsulated *H influenzae* and *S pneumoniae*, is frequently found in infants; sepsis and meningitis caused by the same organisms occur much less frequently. Sepsis and meningitis may also be caused by late-onset group B streptococci and *Listeria monocytogenes* acquired during delivery or postnatally. Infants younger than 1 month may contract sepsis from Gram-negative enteric organisms. These enteric pathogens can also cause urinary tract infections, especially in infants with anatomic anomalies of the urinary tract. Skin and soft tissue infections are caused most frequently by *Staphylococcus aureus*. Frequently, the source of fever cannot be determined on initial evaluation, and diagnoses such as probable viral syndrome or rule out sepsis are used.

Clinical Presentation

Signs and symptoms in young, febrile infants are generally nonspecific and include lethargy, irritability, decreased or poor feeding, vomiting, diarrhea, and upper respiratory tract findings. Absence of fever, however, does not eliminate the possibility of a serious infection. Hypothermia (rectal temperature, 34°C or less) has been shown to be common in serious infections. Dagan and Gorodischer[1] demonstrated serious bacterial infection in 27 of 51 (53%) hypothermic infants younger than 3 months. The mortality rate was nearly five times higher in the infected, hypothermic infants. Based on these findings, some clinicians recommend hospitalizing and initiating intravenous antibiotics in all hypothermic infants. A detailed history, including maternal labor and delivery and duration of nursery stay, should be obtained.

Physical examination must include visualization of the tympanic membrane. Cerumen must be removed, so as to see 75% of the tympanic membrane, as its presence does not rule out an underlying otitis media. Schwartz[34] evaluated 279 children with unilateral otitis media and found that nearly 30% required cerumen removal so that the tympanic membrane could be seen and the correct diagnosis made. Neck stiffness is an unreliable physical finding in infants with meningitis, and the younger the child the more unreliable this finding is. Clinical evaluation may be unreliable and has its limitations in identifying all children with underlying serious bacterial infection who appear well. Even so, observational variables such as poor eye contact, decreased playfulness, and limited social smile appear to be the most sensitive indicators of a sick infant.

Laboratory Studies

Compared to the 3- to 24-month age group, in infants a WBC greater than 15,000/mm^3 or an ESR greater than 30 mm/hour are not as useful as predictors of bacteremia or serious illness. A septic work-up, including spinal tap, blood culture, and urine culture, should be done routinely for infants with fever greater than 38.5°C. In the private practice setting, clinicians may decide that a lumbar puncture is not required, especially if the infant appears well and appropriate follow-up is ensured.

A complete septic work-up is recommended if the patient presents to the emergency department. For screening, the bag method for urine collection is adequate, but if sepsis is suspected and antibiotics are to be started then suprapubic aspiration or urethral catheterization is recommended. Even though the yield of positive urinalysis in asymptomatic patients is notoriously low (1.7% in febrile children younger than 5 years), Bauchner et al[35] have shown that 7.4% of febrile children younger than 6 months have bacteriuria. Bacteriuria is rarely found in patients with a non–urinary tract apparent source of infection, and urinalysis and cultures are not recommended in this subset. Work-up of the urinary tract is recommended, however, in those patients diagnosed as having fever without source.

Chest radiographs are routinely ordered on all patients despite the low yield of positive findings. Heulitt et al[36] demonstrated positive chest films in only 5 of 173 febrile neonates without respiratory distress (respiratory rate < 60/min and no cyanosis, chest wall retractions, nasal flaring, rales, grunting, or apnea). All these cases were described as mild, and therapy or duration of hospitalization was not changed. Careful clinical evaluation may eliminate the need for routine chest radiography in febrile neonates who are not in respiratory distress.

Counterimmunoelectrophoresis (CIE) or latex fixation tests may provide rapid identification of specific bacterial antigens (*S pneumoniae, H influenzae*, and group A β-hemolytic streptococci) from urine, serum, or CSF.

Management

A complete septic work-up is in order, including a CBC, ESR, or CRP; routine cultures of urine, blood, and CSF (and stool, nasopharynx, throat, and drainage fluids where applicable); spinal tap; urinalysis; and chest radiograph. Conservative management comprises routine hospitalization and initiation of intravenous antibiotics pending culture results.

As previously discussed, recent reports[28–34] question the necessity to hospitalize all febrile infants. The following criteria may be useful in reaching the decision to treat a febrile infant on an outpatient basis:

- infant older than 1 month
- normal CSF examination and urinalysis with cultures pending
- WBC between 5000/mm³ and 15,000/mm³ with less than 20% immature forms
- a well-appearing infant who is consolable when held or fed and who is responsive to external stimuli
- discussion with a consultant who agrees with the suggested outpatient management
- dependable and scheduled clinical follow-up within 24 hours
- reliable parents or caretakers

When the patient is treated as an outpatient, there should be follow-up within 6 to 24 hours by a clinician. The parents or caretakers must be aware that, if the infant deteriorates or new symptoms and signs develop, they are required to notify the clinician or return for immediate re-evaluation. Infants older than 1 month with otitis media can be managed as outpatients[28] with oral antibiotics as determined by the regional sensitivities of common bacterial pathogens.

Antibiotic Therapy and Observation

Another important decision to make is whether to initiate parenteral antibiotic therapy at the time of hospitalization. Febrile infants may be observed in the hospital without antibiotics if they are well and if frequent examinations by an experienced clinician can be done.

Antibiotic Therapy

The choice of antibiotics is dependent on the age of the infant and the presence or absence of focal infection. Infants with meningitis, documented by lumbar puncture, or a clinical suspicion of sepsis preferably will have antibiotics begun in the emergency department[26] or as soon as possible after cultures have been taken. The currently recommended empiric antibiotics for meningitis and possible sepsis are as follows[37]:

- if age < 1 month: (1) ampicillin, 150 to 200 mg/kg per 24 hours intravenously (every 6 hours), plus gentamicin, 5 mg/kg per 24 hours intravenously (two divided doses every 12 hours) for premature or full-term neonates younger than 1 week and 7.5 mg/kg per 24 hours intravenously (three divided doses every 8 hours) for infants 1 to 4 weeks old or (2) ampicillin (dose as above) plus cefotaxime (Claforan) 50 mg/kg every 8 hours
- if age > 1 month: (1) ampicillin, 200 mg/kg per 24 hours intravenously (four divided doses every 6 hours), plus chloramphenicol 25 mg/kg every 6 hours intravenously or (2) ceftriaxone (Rocephin) 75–100 mg/kg intravenously stat, and 50 mg/kg intravenously every 12 hours or (3) cefotaxime (Claforan) 50 mg intravenously every 8 hours

Cefuroxime is no longer recommended because of occasional treatment failures and relapses.[38] Antibiotics can be discontinued if all cultures are negative at 48 hours.[39]

MENINGITIS

Meningitis, or inflammation of the leptomeningeal covering of the brain, may be a potentially life-threatening infection, as in bacterial meningitis, or it may have an uncomplicated benign course, as in certain viral meningitides. The mortality rate for bacterial meningitis is about 5% to 10%; there is also a high rate of morbidity causing long-term neurologic sequelae. Early diagnosis and immediate institution of therapy are mandatory if morbidity and mortality are to be reduced. The peak incidence of bacterial meningitis is 6 to 12 months of age, with 90% of cases occurring between 1 month and 5 years of age.

Etiology

Purulent or Bacterial Meningitis

The majority of bacterial meningitis cases in children older than 30 days are caused by three pyogenic organisms: *Hemophilus influenzae* type B, *Streptococcus pneumoniae*, and *Neisseria meningitidis*. *Hemophilus influenzae* accounts for more than 60% of bacterial meningitis cases in infants and young children and about 20% of cases in older children. In the neonatal period the predominant organisms responsible for infection include group B streptococci, Gram-negative enteric bacilli, and *Listeria monocytogenes*.

Aseptic Meningitis

Viral meningitis. Coxsackie virus, echoviruses, and mumps viruses are the most frequent causes of viral meningitis. Other viruses less commonly associated are herpes simplex, arbovirus, adenovirus, and lymphocytic choriomeningitis virus.

Granulomatous meningitis. This type of meningitis is caused by *Mycobacterium tuberculosis, Cryptococcus neoformans, Coccidioidomycosis* species, and other fungi.

Less common causes. Less common etiologies include parameningeal infections such as mastoiditis, leptospirosis, lead encephalopathy, and brain abscesses.

Pathogenesis

Hematogenous spread of the organism is by far the most common route of infection. Bacteria spread from the nasopharynx in most cases. Meningitis associated with otitis media generally follows from bacteremia rather than direct extension from the middle ear. Direct extension of bacteria from the parasinuses or mastoids has become a much less frequent cause of meningitis as a result of early, widespread antibiotic use. Skull fracture or a congenital dermal sinus may provide portal of entry for bacteria, especially *S pneumoniae*.

Clinical Manifestations

Clinical findings may be nonspecific, particularly in patients younger than 12 to 18 months, and include fever, vomiting, anorexia, irritability, poor feeding, diarrhea, lethargy, or high-pitched cry. Older children begin to localize the infection and usually complain of headache, photophobia, and neck pain or stiffness. Meningeal signs, including neck pain or stiffness, Brudzinski's sign (knee flexion with rapid neck flexion), and Kernig's sign (pain in the back of the thigh or knee with passive knee extension when the affected hip is flexed to 90°), are usually unreliable findings in children younger than 18 months.[14] Convulsions have been reported in as many as 30% of cases of bacterial meningitis on admission, but often convulsions present in far fewer cases (around 5% to 10%). Fever and seizure, however, may be the only presenting signs in infants with meningitis. Therefore, meningitis must be ruled out by lumbar puncture in most children with a first-time febrile seizure. Interestingly, less than 5% of patients with febrile convulsions will have meningitis as the inciting infection. This percentage is similar to the percentage of patients who have OB associated with febrile convulsions. Chamberlain and Gorman[40] found that 5 of 93 patients (5.4%) with simple febrile consulsions had OB in their series. Pneumococcal bacteremia accounts for nearly 90% of the cases of bacteremia that result in simple febrile convulsions. Belsey[41] noted that 2 of 3 patients with pneumococcal bacteremia presented with simple febrile convulsions; Torphy and Ray[42] reported 5 of 11, Bonadio[43] reported 15 of 17, and Chamberlain and Gorman[44] reported 120 of 133. In the subsets of patients with simple febrile convulsions who are at risk for OB, it seems appropriate to initiate empiric antibiotic therapy that will cover *S pneumoniae*.

Classically a bulging fontanelle is thought to occur with meningitis, but it is a relatively infrequent occurrence. This may be due to earlier recognition of bacterial cases with less resulting effusion and to dehydration secondary to vomiting and decreased fluid intake. Papilledema is a late finding in acute meningitis.

Rashes are not uncommonly associated with a number of etiologic agents in meningitis. Petechiae or purpura may be found with either meningococcal or *H influenzae* type B meningitis. They are most commonly seen on the lower extremities and trunk. The rash may be initially maculopapular. Viral exanthema and enanthema may be seen with enteroviral meningitis.

Diagnosis

Lumbar Puncture

Lumbar puncture is mandatory in establishing the diagnosis of bacterial meningitis. The clinician should not hesitate in performing this relatively simple procedure when confronted with a child in whom the diagnosis of meningitis is considered. A high index of suspicion should always be maintained, and the clinician needs to remember that infections elsewhere in the body do not eliminate the possibility of meningitis.

Increased Intracranial Pressure

In the presence of increased intracranial pressure or papilledema, consultation and/or head computed tomography (CT) should precede the lumbar puncture. If a spinal tap is to be done, a small-bore spinal needle with stylet (21-gauge in children and 23-gauge in infants) should be used, with no more than 2 to 3 mL of spinal fluid being removed for diagnostic studies. In all cases where a strong suspicion of meningitis exists, antibiotics should be administered before CT scanning.

Positioning

One of the keys to a successful and atraumatic tap is adequate positioning and firm restraint by the assistant. Either a sitting or lateral position may be utilized with the following modifications. Weisman et al[45] have shown that the standard lateral knee-chest position in neonates can cause a significant decrease in transcutaneous PaO_2 levels that may persist for as long as 3 minutes after the procedure is completed. The procedure-induced hypoxia was lower if the neonates were placed in the sitting or modified lateral position (on the side with the hips flexed to only 90°). In critically ill neonates, the hypoxic stress induced by a lumbar puncture may be reduced by avoiding the standard curled-like-a-ball position and using either the sitting or the modified lateral position.

Cerebrospinal Fluid Analysis

The basic CSF examination consists of Gram's stain, cultures and sensitivities, CBC and differential, protein and glucose determinations, and, in selected cases, specific rapid bacterial antigen determination techniques. The normal CSF WBC count for neonates and children older than 1 month is up to $22/mm^3$ and $5/mm^3$, respectively.[46] In bacterial meningitis the cell count is usually greater than $1,000/mm^3$ (predominance of polymorphonucleocytes) and may be as high as $60,000/mm^3$. Occasionally, the cell count may be less than $100/mm^3$ if the lumbar puncture is done early in the course of the disease. In viral meningitis, the WBC is $10/mm^3$ to $500/mm^3$, but occasionally (especially with enteroviruses) it may be higher. Mononuclear cells predominate, but early in the course of viral meningitis polymorphonucleocytes are the predominant cells.

Protein is elevated to 100 to 500 mg/dL in bacterial meningitis and is mildly raised to 10 to 50 mg/dL in viral meningitis. CSF glucose is significantly decreased compared to blood glucose in bacterial meningitis. Donald et al[47] studied the relationship between CSF glucose and blood glucose levels in patients with bacterial and aseptic meningitis compared to controls. The ratio of CSF glucose to blood glucose was 0.25, 0.60, and 0.63 for patients with bacterial meningitis, patients with aseptic meningitis, and normal controls, respectively. The suggested lower limits of normal for absolute CSF glucose and the ratio of CSF glucose to blood glucose were 40 mg/dL and 40%, respectively. Traditionally, it has been taught that blood glucose should be measured before lumbar puncture because endogenous epinephrine release from the stress of the lumbar puncture can cause an elevation in blood glucose. Shohat et al[48] demonstrated in a controlled trial that blood glucose levels were not affected by lumbar puncture. The WBC was increased significantly in all patients (from $10,960/mm^3$ to $13,300/mm^3$), however, as a result of the stress of the procedure. It is recommended that blood be drawn before lumbar puncture to avoid the confusing rise in WBC (blood is being drawn anyway, so the glucose might as well be ordered then).

The Gram stain may be helpful in identifying the causative bacteria, but a negative smear occurs in approximately 10% to 15% of culture-proven bacterial meningitis. Rapid antigen detection of *H influenzae*, *S pneumoniae*, *N meningitides*, and group B streptococci may be done by latex agglutination, coagglutination (COA), or CIE tests. A recent multicenter study showed sensitivity and specificity rates of 84% and 100%, respectively, for the Phadebact CSF kit, which utilizes the COA technique, in CSF samples from more than 577 cases of bacterial meningitis in adults and children. Tilton et al[49] have shown that both latex agglutination and COA commercial test kits are more sensitive, overall, than the CIE test (93%, 82%, and 76%, respectively). The use of specially prepared purified antigens and reagents has a profound effect on the reported sensitivity rates in some studies. The rapid antigen detection tests are extremely useful in diagnosing partially treated bacterial meningitis cases where the Gram stains and subsequent cultures may be negative. Negative CSF antigen detection does not rule out bacterial infection, however.

A frequent concern of clinicians is the possibility that previous antibiotic therapy can obscure the diagnosis of meningitis by altering the results of the CSF studies. Blazer et al[50] performed repeat lumbar punctures 44 to 68 hours after intravenous antibiotic therapy was begun on patients with meningitis. Although 97% of the repeat CSF samples were culture negative, 96% had abnormalities of CSF protein, glucose, WBC, and percentage of polymorphonucleocytes in the follow-up sample that were not appreciably different from those in the original sample. This study demonstrates that, if full-dose intravenous antibiotics do not significantly alter CSF parameters, then it is highly unlikely that meningitis partially treated with oral or intramuscular antibiotics will change these parameters and confuse the diagnosis.

Lumbar Puncture in Patients with Bacteremia

The fact that febrile infants with bacteremia who have negative lumbar punctures can later develop meningitis is well known.[11,51] In one study, three patients with normal CSF analyses (negative Gram's stain, culture, and chemistries and less than eight monocytes and one polymorphonucleocyte) and bacteremia returned within 48 hours with meningitis. Teele et al[52] clearly demonstrated the disturbing relationship of performing a lumbar puncture in febrile infants with bacteremia and the subsequent development of meningitis with the same bacterial pathogen found in the blood. Animal studies have shown a much greater incidence of the development of meningitis in bacteremic dogs after penetration of the meninges than in those whose meninges were not manipulated. Reasons proposed for this finding include the following: lumbar puncture as a direct cause; clinical judgment selecting the sicker child in whom meningitis is developing but before the CSF analysis is diagnostic; and advanced bacteremia without meningitis in which the child's ill appearance mandates lumbar puncture.

Despite the implications of these studies, lumbar puncture with CSF analysis is the only method currently available to diagnose meningitis. The seriousness of bacterial meningitis and its high rates of morbidity and mortality demand performance of a spinal tap in any patient in whom the diagnosis is suspected. Teele et al[51] were able to show that patients who were initially treated with empiric antibiotics for possible OB had a much lower rate of subsequent meningitis. Currently, it is a reasonable recommendation empirically to treat febrile infants at risk for OB with appropriate antibiotics in the absence of localized infection.

Other Laboratory Tests

Blood cultures should be obtained routinely. In previously untreated meningitis, positive blood cultures are found in 90%, 80%, and 91% of cases of *H influenzae*, *S pneumoniae*, and *N meningitides* meningitis, respectively. CBC, electrolytes, Gram's stain, and culture of petechial lesions should be requested routinely. Viral isolation and serology as well as CSF, stool, and nasopharyngeal viral studies may be obtained in selected cases.

Management

Antibiotics

Once appropriate cultures and blood have been drawn, an intravenous line should be started. Empiric antibiotic treatment is begun as soon as possible if the diagnosis of bacterial meningitis is entertained; drugs and dosages are the same as for febrile illness (see above). Appropriate antibiotics are chosen later, depending on culture and sensitivities. No antibiotics are necessary if the CSF analysis suggests a viral etiology. If viral meningitis is suspected but there is a polymorphonucleocyte predominance in the CSF, the child may be observed without antibiotics in the hospital. A repeat lumbar puncture may be performed 8 to 12 hours later to clarify the initial diagnostic confusion.

Corticosteroids

Despite the recent use of bactericidal antibiotics, the morbidity and mortality from bacterial meningitis have not improved. The anti-inflammatory effects of corticosteroids and their efficacy in reducing vasogenic brain edema have led investigators to evaluate these drugs as possible adjuncts to antibiotics in patients with bacterial meningitis. A trial of dexamethasone was reported by Lebel et al[52]; dexamethasone (01.5 mg/kg) was given intravenously every 6 hours for 4 days in children with bacterial meningitis. There were significant increases in CSF glucose and decreases in lactate and protein after 24 hours of steroid therapy compared to controls. The steroid-treated patients also became afebrile sooner, and, most important, they were significantly less likely to acquire moderate or severe bilateral sensorineural hearing loss (15.5% compared to 3.3%). These beneficial hearing effects were documented for patients with *H influenzae* meningitis only. On the basis of these findings, and because they held that the advantages far outweigh the disadvantages, the investigators enthusiastically endorsed routine dexamethasone use in infants and children with bacterial meningitis.

In another, more recent study, Lebel et al[53] again addressed the use of dexamethasone. The results were similar to those of the first two trials, with fewer febrile days, improved CSF chemistries, and a lower incidence of unilateral or bilateral moderate or severe hearing impairment in the steroid-treated patients (19% compared to 9%). Magnetic resonance (MR) studies, however, showed no difference between the two groups and did not alter clinical management, and there was no correlation between MR findings and patient outcome. MR imaging was not considered useful in the evaluation of patients with bacterial meningitis.

Most recently, the American Academy of Pediatrics, in the 1991 *Red Book*,[54] has come forth with the following considerations regarding the use of steroids in meningitis:

- Dexamethasone probably reduces the likelihood of deafness after *H influenzae* meningitis.
- The recommended dosage, at present, is 0.6 mg/kg/day in four divided doses given intravenously for the first 4 days of antibiotic treatment.
- If utilized, dexamethasone should be administered at the time of the first dose of antibiotic therapy.
- Dexamethasone therapy should be considered only when the diagnosis of bacterial meningitis has been proven or is strongly suggested on the basis of CSF analysis.
- The utility of dexamethasone in treating pneumococcal or meningococcal meningitis is not yet known.
- Dexamethasone should not be used for suspected or proved aseptic or nonbacterial meningitis.

Supportive Therapy

Vital signs should be monitored. Oral and intravenous fluids should be restricted to two thirds the normal maintenance amount because of the nearly uniform incidence of cerebral edema and syndrome of inappropriate antidiuretic hormone, both of which complicate meningitis. Anticonvulsants, such as phenobarbital (10 to 15 mg/kg) or lorazepam (Ativan) (0.1 mg/kg), may be required to control seizures. With massive cerebral edema and potential brain stem herniation from increased intracranial pressure, intubation with hyperventilation, steroids (dexamethasone, 1 mg/kg initially and 0.25 mg/kg every 6 hours), and mannitol (0.25 g/kg) are indicated.

REFERENCES

1. Dagan R, Gorodischer R. Infections in hypothermic infants younger than 3 months old. *Am J Dis Child*. 1984;138:483–485.
2. Roberts KB, Borzy MS. Fever in the first 8 weeks of life. *Johns Hopkins Med J*. 1977;141:9–13.
3. McGowan JE, Bratton L, Klein JO, et al. Bacteremia in febrile children seen in a "walk-in" pediatric clinic. *N Engl J Med*. 1973;288:1309–1312.
4. Teele D, Pelton S, Grant M, et al. Bacteremia in febrile children under two years of age: results of cultures of blood of 600 consecutive febrile children seen in a walk-in clinic. *J Pediatr*. 1975;87:227–230.
5. McCarthy P, Grundy G, Spiesel S, et al. Bacteremia in children: an outpatient clinical review. *Pediatrics*. 1976;57:861–868.
6. McCarthy P, Dolan T. The serious implication of high fever in infants during their first 3 months. *Clin Pediatr*. 1976;15:794–796.
7. Bratton L, Teele D, Klein JO. Outcome of unsuspected pneumococcemia in children not initially admitted to the hospital. *J Pediatr*. 1977;90:703–706.
8. McCarthy P, Jekel J, Dolan T. Temperature greater than or equal to 40°C in children less than 24 months of age: a prospective study. *Pediatrics*. 1977;59:663–668.
9. Baron M, Fink H. Bacteremia in private pediatric practice. *Pediatrics*. 1980;66:171–175.
10. Teele DW, Marshall R, Klein JO. Unsuspected bacteremia in young children. A common and important problem. *Pediatr Clin North Am*. 1979;26:773–785.
11. Hamrick HJ, Murphy TF. Bacteremia in 28 ambulatory children. Relationship to pneumonitis and meningitis. *Clin Pediatr*. 1978;17:109–112.
12. McCarthy P, Dolan T. Hyperpyrexia in children. *Am J Dis Child*. 1976;130:849–851.
13. Surpure JS. Hyperpyrexia (temperature > 40°C) in children. *JACEP*. 1979;8:130–133.
14. Samson JH. Febrile seizures and purulent meningitis. *JAMA*. 1969;210:1918–1922.
15. McCarthy PL, Jekel JF, Stashwick CA, et al. History and observation variables in assessing febrile children. *Pediatrics*. 1980;65:1090–1095.
16. Waskerlitz S, Berkelhamer J. Outpatient bacteremia: clinical findings in children under two years with initial temperature of 39.5°C or higher. *J Pediatr*. 1981;99:231–233.
17. McCarthy P, Jekel X, Stashwick C. Further definition of history and observational variables in assessing febrile children. *Pediatrics*. 1981;67:687–693.
18. McCarthy PL, Sharpe MR, Spiesel SZ, et al. Observation scales to identify serious illness in febrile children. *Pediatrics*. 1981;67:687–693.
19. McCarthy PL. Controversies in pediatrics: what tests are indicated for the child under 2 with fever. *Pediatr Rev*. 1979;1:51–56.
20. Rasmussen NH, Rasmussen LN. Predictive value of white blood cell count and differential cell count to bacterial infections in children. *Acta Paediatr Scand*. 1982;71:775–778.
21. Morens DM. WBC count and differential. Value in predicting bacterial diseases in children. *Am J Dis Child*. 1979;133:25–27.
22. Marshall R, Teele D, Klein J. Unsuspected bacteremia due to *Hemophilus influenzae*. *J Pediatr*. 1979;95:690–695.
23. Jaffe DM, Tanz RR, Davis AT, et al. Antibiotic administration to treat possible occult bacteremia in febrile children. *N Engl J Med*. 1987;317:1175–1180.
24. Baron MA, Fink HD, Cicchetti DV. Blood cultures in private pediatric practice: an eleven-year experience. *Pediatr Infect Dis J*. 1989;8:2–7.
25. Selden R, Freidman J, Kaplan M. Managing urinary tract infections in children. *Pediatr Annu*. 1981;10:12–24.
26. Talan DA, Guterman JJ, Overturf GD, et al. Analysis of emergency department management of suspected bacterial meningitis. *Ann Emerg Med*. 1989;18:856–862.
27. Berkowitz CD. Fever in infants less than two months of age: spectrum of disease and predictors of outcome. *Pediatr Emerg Care*. 1985;1:128–135.
28. Green JW, Hara C, O'Connor S, et al. Management of febrile outpatient neonates. *Clin Pediatr*. 1981;20:375–380.
29. King JC, Berman ED, Wright PF. Evaluation of fever in infants less than 8 weeks old. *South Med J*. 1987;80:948–952.
30. Dagan R, Powell KR, Hall CB, et al. Identification of infants unlikely to have serious bacterial infection although hospitalized for suspected sepsis. *J Pediatr*. 1985;107:855–860.
31. Dagan R, Sofer S, Phillip M, et al. Ambulatory care of febrile infants younger than 2 months of age classified as being at low risk for having serious bacterial infections. *J Pediatr*. 1988;112:355–360.
32. Philip AG. Decreased use of antibiotics using a neonatal sepsis screening technique. *J Pediatr*. 1981;98:795.
33. Berkowitz CD, Orr DP, Uchiyama N, et al. Variability in the management of the febrile infant under 2 months of age. *J Emerg Med*. 1985;3:345–351.
34. Schwartz RH. Cerumen removal: how necessary is it to diagnose acute otitis media? *Am J Dis Child*. 1985;137:1064.
35. Bauchner H, Phillip B, Dashefsky B, et al. Prevalence of bacteriuria in febrile children. *Pediatr Infect Dis J*. 1987;6:239–242.
36. Heulitt MJ, Ablow RC, Santos CC, et al. Febrile infants less than 3 months old: value of chest radiography. *Radiology*. 1988;167:135–137.
37. Committee on Infectious Disease, American Academy of Pediatrics. Treatment of bacterial meningitis. *Pediatrics*. 1988,81.904–907.
38. McCracken GH, Nelson JD, Kaplan SL, et al. Consensus report: antimicrobial therapy for bacterial meningitis in infants and children. *Pediatr Infect Dis J*. 1987;6:501–505.
39. Pichichero ME, Todd JK. Detection of neonatal bacteremia. *J Pediatr*. 1979;94:958–960.
40. Chamberlain JM, Gorman RL. Occult bacteremia in children with simple febrile seizures. *Am J Dis Child*. 1988;142:1073–1076.

41. Belsey MA. Pneumococcal bacteremia. *Am J Dis Child*. 1967;113: 588–589.
42. Torphy DE, Ray CG. Occult pneumococcal bacteremia. *Am J Dis Child*. 1970;119:336–338.
43. Bonadio WA. Occult bacteremia in children with simple febrile seizures. The pediatric forum. *Am J Dis Child*. 1989;143:273–274.
44. Chamberlain JM, Gorman RL. Occult bacteremia in children with simple febrile convulsion. The pediatric forum. *Am J Dis Child*. 1989;143:274.
45. Weisman LE, Merenstein JB, Steenbarger JR. The effect of lumbar puncture position in sick neonates. *Am J Dis Child*. 1983;137: 1077–1079.
46. Bonadio WA, Bonadio JF. Significance of polymorphonucleocytes in CSF of bacteremic children. *Pediatr Emerg Care*. 1988;4:180–182.
47. Donald DR, Malan C, van der Walt A. Simultaneous determinations of cerebrospinal fluid glucose and blood glucose concentrations in the diagnosis of bacterial meningitis. *J Pediatr*. 1983;103:413–415.
48. Shohat M, Goodman Z, Rogovin H, et al. The effect of lumbar puncture on blood glucose level and leukocyte count in infants. *Clin Pediatr*. 1987;26:477–479.
49. Tilton RC, Dias F, Ryan RW. Comparative evaluation of three commercial products and counterimmunoelectrophoresis for the detection of antigens in cerebrospinal fluid. *J Clin Microbiol*. 1984;20:231–234.
50. Blazer S, Berant M, Alon U. Effect of antibiotic treatment on cerebrospinal fluid. *Am J Clin Pathol*. 1983;80:386–387.
51. Teele DW, Dashefsky B, Rakusan T, et al. Meningitis after lumbar puncture in children with bacteremia. *N Engl J Med*. 1981;305: 1079–1081.
52. Lebel MH, Freij BJ, Syrogiannopoulos GA, et al. Dexamethasone therapy for bacterial meningitis. Results of two double-blind, placebo-controlled trials. *N Engl J Med*. 1988;319:964–972.
53. Lebel MH, Hoyt J, Waagner DC. Magnetic resonance imaging and dexamethasone therapy for bacterial meningitis. *Am J Dis Child*. 1989;143:301–306.
54. Medical Economics Company. *The Red Book*. Oradel, NJ: Medical Economics, 1991.

33. Pediatric Surgical Emergencies

ARTHUR COOPER, MD, FACS, FAAP, FCCM

Physicians entrusted with the care of the acutely ill or injured child must be familiar with a wide variety of infectious, traumatic, congenital, and developmental abnormalities. The principles of management of common medical and surgical emergencies (including resuscitation from respiratory or circulatory failure) are no different in the child than in the adult. What sets the pediatric emergency medical and surgical disciplines apart, therefore, is their recognition and understanding of the unique pathologic conditions that affect the child as well as the numerous anatomic and physiologic differences from the adult patient. It is the aim of this chapter to arm the emergency physician with a practical working knowledge of pediatric surgical emergencies that will facilitate a rational yet common-sense approach to the initial management of the surgically ill or injured child.

MULTIPLE TRAUMA

Trauma is responsible for more deaths among children aged 1 to 14 years (nearly 10,000 annually nationwide) than all other causes combined.[1] The vast majority of these deaths, and approximately 85% of all serious pediatric injuries, are caused by blunt trauma.[2] Motor vehicle and bicycle accidents, which together account for more than one third of these injuries, cause most of the deaths. In contrast, falls, which account for approximately one third of all childhood trauma, are responsible for only a fraction of the deaths. Death from falls occurs most often in urban areas with high-rise dwellings and typically results from falls onto unyielding ground surfaces from unprotected windows five or more stories above street level.[3]

Penetrating trauma, even in children, is due almost exclusively to gunshot and stab wounds.[2] These injuries are still relatively infrequent in the pediatric population even though, as a group, they represent the most lethal of all childhood injuries. Most of these deaths are accidentally inflicted, but the incidence of fatalities is climbing at an alarming rate as more and more of the population have access to firearms. This trend will continue unless the public insists upon gun safety education as a prerequisite to ownership in lieu of some form of gun control. Intentionally inflicted gunshot wounds are also on the increase, whether as the result of assault, as in many of our larger cities,[4] or suicide, which is a growing problem among older children and adolescents.

Mechanisms and Patterns of Injury

The different mechanisms of injury in the child result in specific patterns of injury that also are unique to the pediatric population. Motor vehicle accidents give rise to two distinct syndromes, depending on whether the child is a pedestrian struck by a moving vehicle or an occupant in a moving vehicle that strikes an immovable object. In the former situation, a particular pattern of injuries known as Waddell's triad occurs, which includes fracture of the midshaft of the femur coupled with closed head and torso injuries.[5] In the latter situation, the unrestrained passenger is subject primarily to closed head and cervical spine injuries.[6] For this reason, use of approved child restraint devices is now a legal requirement in most jurisdictions. However, improperly used infant car seats can also result in a deadly constellation of injuries to the upper cervical spine (chiefly odontoid fractures, although hangman fractures, and atlantoaxial and atlantooccipital subluxation, have each been reported).[7,8] Another unique complex of anatomic derangements (truncal ecchymosis, lumbar fractures, perforated or obstructed bowel, and, in rare cases, bursting injuries of the solid viscera of the upper abdomen or traumatic disruption of the diaphragm with subsequent herniation of intestinal contents into the chest) may occur when lap and shoulder belts designed for adults are inappropriately used as restraint devices for children who have outgrown their infant car seats but have not yet reached sufficient size that the lap belt lies comfortably across their anterior superior iliac spines.[9,10] In such children, booster seats should be used together with lap and shoulder belts.

Bicycles, of course, are notoriously associated with serious injury in children. The incidence of severe closed head injury after an unhelmeted fall from a moving bicycle is significant.[11] The design of the handlebar on most children's bicycles is such that the upper abdomen is easily impaled during a fall, often resulting in hematomas and/or lacerations of the spleen or liver or perforations of the gastrointestinal tract.[12] The long distance a child may be thrown when the bicycle and rider are struck by a moving car renders that child particularly vulnerable to severe closed head injury, and because the head usually strikes the ground not straight on but at an angle, cervical spine injuries may occur as well.

The child's endless curiosity and uncanny ability to escape the watchful eye even of the most attentive caretaker are responsible for the much higher incidence of unintentional injuries among children (90% to 95% compared to 65% to 75% in adults).[2] Of the 5% to 10% of childhood injuries that are not the result of exploratory or adventurous behavior, about one third are inflicted by a more mature individual, often an adult.[2] This perpetrator is usually known to the child or the caretaker and perhaps is the caretaker himself or herself. An entire chapter in this section is devoted to the various manifestations of physical child abuse. Several points are emphasized here, however. More than half of all abused children who present with serious injuries are known to the authorities from previous, usually less flagrant, episodes of child abuse and neglect. Delay in seeking appropriate medical attention and physical signs inconsistent with the suggested mechanism of injury are often the only clues to the true etiology of the injuries. Principles of treatment of the injuries themselves are no different than those for other injuries. This is particularly true for severe injuries of the head and abdomen, which constitute the two leading causes of death in both intentional and accidental childhood injuries.[2] Establishing the underlying cause of the injuries is important, but necessary life-sustaining treatment should not be delayed in the interest of facilitating legal intervention.

Serious head trauma and its complications are ultimately responsible for the great majority of the 3% of serious blunt childhood injuries that result in deaths, perhaps as many as 75%.[13] Although late death is clearly related to the severity of the associated brain injury, early death in the head-injured child (ie, death in the field or during transport) is often due to hypoxia associated with the hypopharyngeal soft tissue airway obstruction that may develop when a child loses consciousness. Serious thoracic and abdominal trauma is the second leading cause of pediatric trauma-related mortality, death being due chiefly to irreversible hemorrhagic shock associated with severe laceration(s) of the spleen and liver.[14] Serious thoracic trauma, as an isolated event, is an infrequent cause of death among children. Similarly, serious musculoskeletal trauma virtually never causes death unless it is associated with a severe comminuted pelvic fracture or the rare cervical spine injury, which frequently cannot be detected by X-ray studies.

Anatomic and Physiologic Correlates

Several factors render the child especially vulnerable to serious head injury. The head is proportionately larger than in the adult, ensuring that whenever a child falls from a height or is struck by or thrown from a moving car (the three leading causes of serious childhood injury) the child will land head first. The bones of the head are softer, explaining why the Ping-Pong ball type of depressed skull fracture, which is rarely if ever seen in children of grade school age or older, occurs with some frequency in infants. Further, although it is axiomatic that shock does not coexist with isolated serious closed head trauma, there are two exceptions. One is the case of irreversible brain stem injury, although it is now recognized that many cases previously ascribed to brain stem injury in fact were due to high spinal cord transection.[15] The other occurs in the young infant whose cranial sutures have not yet fused and whose fontanelles remain open. This situation allows potential expansion of the volume of the intracranial vault, which is of limited size in older children and adults, so that intracranial hemorrhage of sufficient magnitude to cause hypotensive shock may, on rare occasions, precede uncal herniation. Finally, because the softer bones of the skull rarely break (allowing forces of impact to be transmitted directly to the intracranial vault), the spectrum of brain injuries observed in the child is quite different from that in the adult. Diffuse injuries, particularly brain swelling due to the arterial vasodilation associated with the loss of cerebral autoregulation,[16] and diffuse axonal shearing, which may be associated with violent acceleration-deceleration injuries, are far more common in childhood than in later years. In contrast to the older child and adult, in young children serious intracranial hemorrhage (eg, subdural and epidural hematomas) is uncommon. If present, these collections sometimes will be of insufficient size to warrant surgical evacuation. It must be noted, however, that bilateral subdural hematomas, particularly as an isolated finding, are suggestive of child abuse. This condition commonly results from tearing of the bridging meningeal veins, which is known to be associated with violent acceleration-deceleration injuries seen in whiplash shaken infant syndrome.

Injuries to the cervical spine are not common in childhood.[17] When such injuries do occur, however, they are far more frequent at levels above those where nerve roots give rise to diaphragmatic innervation (eg, C-1, C-2, and the atlantooccipital junction). This predisposes the child to respiratory arrest as well as paralysis due to anatomic or functional spinal cord transection (partial or complete) when spinal cord trauma occurs. The increased inertial forces associated with rapid head motion and the more horizontal apposition of the cervical vertebrae in childhood appear largely responsible for this somewhat different spectrum of injuries. Locking of the lower cervical vertebrae is extremely rare, whereas subluxation, with or without dislocation, and/or odontoid fractures are more common. Contributing to the increased proportion of high cervical spine fractures in children compared to adults is the relative laxity and elasticity of supporting ligaments. These ligamentous characteristics allow both rotary subluxations of C-2 and the spinal cord injury without radiographic abnormality (SCIWORA) syndrome. SCIWORA is probably caused by marked subluxation and subsequent shearing of the spinal cord without apparent bony injury.[18]

Chest injuries are also uniquely different in childhood. The extreme flexibility of the more cartilaginous ribs that make up the thoracic cage allows enormous forces to be transmitted to the underlying intrathoracic structures. It is not uncommon for a child to sustain severe pulmonary and/or cardiac contusions in the absence of rib fractures or other external signs of trauma such as bruising or petechiae. Although the pediatric patient is somewhat less likely to sustain rib fractures, pneumothorax and/or hemothorax still occur.[14] Moreover, when such injuries are sustained, the exceptional mobility of the mediastinum places the child at greater risk for marked ventilatory and circulatory compromise. Increasing tension impedes both air flow, because of the high intrathoracic pressures, and blood flow, as a result of torsion of the venae cavae at the upper and lower thoracic inlets. It is this vascular obstruction, not hypoxia, that is usually responsible for the sudden circulatory collapse associated with marked tension pneumothorax.

The abdomen of the child is also more vulnerable to injury than that of the adult. Flexible ribs cover less of the abdomen, and thinner layers of muscle and fat provide less protection to the solid viscera of the upper abdomen. In addition, the proportionately larger size of these organs in the child render them particularly vulnerable to injury. The overall small size of the pediatric abdomen predisposes the child to multiple rather than single organ injuries during the dissipation of energy from a blunt force.

Marked gastric dilatation due to air swallowing associated with crying may contribute significantly to ventilatory compromise resulting from limitation of diaphragmatic motion. Other complications include increased risk of aspiration and, in infants and young children, potential circulatory compromise due to vagally mediated dampening of the normal tachycardic response to hypovolemia. Gastric dilatation may also confound the abdominal examination because the associated abdominal tenderness can mimic peritonitis or mask serious intra-abdominal bleeding, which constitute the leading causes of death from abdominal injury.

Children are subject to a unique spectrum of accidental bony injuries. Detailed discussion of the acute management of these, aside from reiterating the need for proper splinting, lies outside the scope of this chapter. Several points require special emphasis, however. The most frequent long bone injuries sustained by the multiply injured pediatric patient are fractures of the femur and tibia.[2] The most common cause of these injuries is the pedestrian–motor vehicle accident, in which the young child briefly escapes the supervision of the caretaker, darts in front of a moving car, and is struck at midthigh level by the bumper and at torso and head level by the hood, resulting in Waddell's triad of injuries. The child is then thrown some 10 to 20 feet by the force of the impact, landing head first. This recognized injury sequence underscores the necessity of carefully evaluating any child who sustains a femur fracture in a pedestrian–motor vehicle accident for head, neck, and torso injuries. Isolated femur fractures are rarely, if ever, associated with significant blood loss in the pediatric age groups. The average drop in hematocrit is only 3%, and the maximum drop usually observed in this type of injury is 6%.[19] Neither drop, in isolation, is sufficient to cause hypotensive or decompensated shock. Thus, if signs of severe shock are observed, a diligent search must be made for another source of bleeding, which usually will be found in the abdomen. Distal metaphyseal and diaphyseal fractures, especially supracondylar fractures, are frequently associated with vascular injuries, particularly intimal disruption. If unrecognized or incorrectly attributed to posttraumatic spasm, these injuries can result in subsequent ischemic complications that may immediately threaten the limb or cause problematic long-term sequelae such as growth retardation of the affected extremity.

The single most important difference between the child and adult trauma patient, however, is the child's unique ability to compensate for the physiologic derangements induced by the traumatic disruption of homeostasis, particularly those related to the circulatory system. The child is capable of mounting an impressive tachycardia to maintain cardiac output. Even more remarkable, however, is the ability of the child to maintain afterload in the hypovolemic state by means of intense peripheral vasoconstriction.[20] This response occurs at the arteriolar level as well as at the arterial level, thus preserving reasonable perfusion of the core organs. This truly extraordinary capacity to preserve vital functions until the last moments of life, however, ultimately proves costly to the organism as a whole. With diversion of blood flow from the less vital peripheral tissues comes anaerobic cellular metabolism and severe lactic acidosis, which markedly increases work of breathing and decreases myocardial contractility, thus limiting the child's ability to sustain a compensatory response for a prolonged period.

It is this fact perhaps more than any other that underscores both the problem and the challenge of caring for the child with serious blunt trauma that is complicated by shock. Maintenance of relatively normal afterload, and hence mean arterial blood pressure (despite significant hypovolemia), leads to what has been called the deceptive presentation of shock in the pediatric age groups. Those unfamiliar with children will tend to underestimate both the degree of blood loss and the severity of the injury in the face of normotensive (compensated) shock. Although the magnitude of the compensatory response in the child is great, however, its duration is short because the overall small size of the blood volume compared to that of the adult provides a smaller margin of safety once shock and acidosis ensue. In this regard, the child may be likened to the sprinter rather than the long distance runner, and it is for this reason that some experts in pediatric trauma call for a "platinum half hour" as the ideal time frame for resuscitation of the pediatric trauma patient as opposed to the "golden hour" that has been advocated for the adult. It is also why the diagnosis and treatment of pediatric shock are based not so much upon abnormalities in the vital signs themselves as on the abnormalities in the physical signs of tissue perfusion. These signs include pale, cool, clammy, or mottled skin; capillary refill time of more than 2 seconds; absent peripheral pulses during simultaneous palpation of the corresponding central pulses; and altered mental status (viz, agitation in early shock and obtundation in late shock). Hypotensive or decompensated shock in the child does not develop until quite late in the downward spiral toward cardiac arrest and implies both that the compensatory mechanisms have already failed and that death of the organism is therefore imminent. Obviously, it is preferable to avoid this situation if at all possible. Doing so requires both that shock be recognized early and that initial treatment be aggressive.

Management Guidelines

The general approach to the pediatric trauma patient is similar to that in the adult. Primary attention is directed to maintenance of airway, breathing, and circulation; treatment of immediately life-threatening chest injuries that may impede successful resuscitation; control of hemorrhage; and treatment of shock. Specific assessment and management should be guided by consensus protocols, such as those contained in the pediatric trauma sections of the American College of Surgeons' *Advanced Trauma Life Support Student Manual*[21] and the American College of Emergency Physicians' and American Academy of Pediatrics' *Advanced Pediatric Life Support Student Manual*.[22] Resuscitation of the child in actual or impending cardiorespiratory arrest should follow the standards set by the American Heart Association and American Academy of Pediatrics, which are outlined in their *Textbook of Pediatric Advanced Life Support*.[23] The first minutes of the trauma response have been accurately depicted as the most important in the seriously injured child's entire hospitalization. It is vitally important, however, that a qualified surgeon experienced in the management of childhood injuries be involved as early as possible in the resuscitation because the major iatrogenic causes of mortality in pediatric trauma are inappropriate resuscitation of head injuries and the failure to recognize and stop internal bleeding in a timely manner.[24,25]

Airway, Breathing, and Cervical Spine

If the child is capable of maintaining his or her own airway, the first step is to supply 100% oxygen via a nonrebreathing mask. If the airway is compromised, it must be opened by means of the modified jaw thrust and a rigid suction device as needed before the child can be given oxygen by mask. If the child is incapable of maintaining spontaneous ventilation, assistance should be provided with 100% oxygen via a properly fitting, clear plastic face mask with a soft or inflatable rim attached to a self-inflating bag-valve device with a reservoir or accumulator. An oropharyngeal airway of appropriate size is added if soft tissue obstruction still impedes adequate gas exchange. The airway must be inserted right-side up to avoid injury to the soft palate.

If this fails to result in effective ventilation as judged by visualization of bilateral chest rise and auscultation of adequate air entry, the child should be intubated immediately. The straight (Miller) laryngoscope blade and an endotracheal tube of the same external diameter as the nares or fifth (little) finger, or selected with the Broselow Resuscitation Tape[26] or the formula $[16 + age (in years)]/4$, are used for this purpose. The child is then hyperventilated with 100% oxygen, again by way of the bag-valve device, as described above. The use of high-pressure oxygen powered breathing devices (demand valve resuscitators) or esophageal obturator airways is contraindicated in children.[27]

The oropharyngeal route is preferred for pediatric intubation. This is so even in the nonapneic but unconscious patient with possible cervical spine trauma because the anterior and cephalad position of the child's larynx makes blind nasotracheal intubation virtually impossible in the emergent setting, not to mention the greater risk of trauma to the large adenoids of the child and subsequent hemorrhage. On occasion, the presence of severe orofacial trauma and/or foreign body obstruction may require direct or fiberoptic laryngoscopy with foreign body removal as necessary and subsequent intubation. Rarely, emergency needle cricothyroidotomy must be performed with a 14- to 16-gauge plastic cannula and a jet insufflator. If the jet system is unavailable, wall oxygen will suffice if the tubing is attached to a Y connector, the open limb of which is intermittently occluded. This procedure should be expediently followed by surgical tracheostomy in the controlled environment of the operating room once the patient has been stabilized.

Regardless of the type of airway used, care must be taken from the first moment of contact with the patient to avoid possible, or further, damage to a potentially injured spinal cord. To this end, cervical spine precautions must be initiated simultaneously with airway control by means of manual in-line spinal stabilization (limitation of cervical motion by means of gentle axial traction).[28] These must be maintained until such time as immobilization is obtained through the application of a semirigid cervical extrication collar of appropriate size is applied. The collar must not be removed until cervical spine films are obtained and interpreted as normal and until the neck has been fully examined for signs of cervical spine fracture or dislocation. At no time does diagnosis of actual or possible cervical spine injury take precedence over establishment and maintenance of a patent airway.

The occasional difficulty encountered in intubating the child while keeping the neck in a neutral position has led some to advocate emergency needle (or surgical) cricothyroidotomy when cervical spine injury is suspected. Few experts in pediatric trauma believe this is necessary except possibly in the case of markedly unstable cervical spine fractures. When a child is placed supine on a completely flat surface, the neck will be slightly flexed because of the prominent occiput.[29] In actual practice, this problem presents little or no difficulty because this slight degree of neck flexion occurs not at the levels at which pediatric cervical spine injury is most likely (ie, C-1 and C-2) but closer to the cervicothoracic junction. Regardless, it is useful to remember this anatomic relationship when difficulty is encountered with orotracheal intubation in the traumatized child: Restoring the child's neck to a truly neutral position by lowering the head of the bed or placing a thin layer of firm padding (eg, folded sheets or blankets) beneath the entire length of the child's body may facilitate intubation without morbidity so long as in-line stabilization is maintained.

Circulation

While ventilation and oxygenation are being established, circulation is addressed. If the patient is in full cardiac arrest, external chest compressions should be begun and intubation performed immediately. Although there are good data to suggest that more effective compressions can be achieved by open chest massage in euvolemic adult patients,[30] the outcome of emergency department thoracotomy in the hypovolemic pediatric blunt trauma patient has been dismal.[31,32] Thus external chest compressions, together with control of external hemorrhage and rapid volume restoration, would seem to be the wiser choice for blunt trauma patients, especially because the cross-clamping of the distal thoracic aorta advocated by some adult trauma surgeons is technically more difficult in the child. Moreover, this technique offers no significant advantage over direct finger compression of the proximal abdominal aorta via laparotomy, which the overwhelming majority of pediatric blunt trauma patients will require if they present in hypotensive or decompensated shock. In contrast, pediatric patients with penetrating chest injuries require immediate thoracotomy if they present in full arrest, as is the case in adults.

Vascular access must be obtained quickly and securely with two large-bore catheters placed at peripheral sites, preferably in the upper extremities (antecubital fossae) given the higher probability of injuries to the abdomen and lower extremities in the child. If such injuries are not suspected, or if venous access cannot be obtained rapidly in the upper extremities, a lower extremity site, particularly the saphenous vein at the ankle, is an acceptable alternative. The intraosseous route, gained with a 15- to 18-gauge Jamshidi bone marrow needle or its equivalent, to obtain access to the venous sinuses of the bone marrow cavity of the proximal tibia may be used as a first step in the child younger than 3 to 6 years if peripheral venous access cannot be established rapidly.[33–35] Failing this, venous access may be obtained via percutaneous cannulation of the femoral vein at the groin or by saphenous vein cutdown at the ankle (if skilled personnel are available), as saphenous vein cutdown at the groin may present an unnecessarily difficult technical challenge in small children, even for those with great experience. Blood samples for type and cross-match are then drawn and sent immediately; blood ordered must be sufficient to allow immediate replacement of half the child's blood volume (0.5 × 80 mL/kg = 40 mL/kg, using the formula 8 + [2 × age in years], or the Broselow Tape[26] to estimate the body weight in kilograms). When perfusion is noted to be compromised, lactated Ringer solution (20 mL/kg) is infused as rapidly as possible once vascular access is obtained.

Primary Survey, Resuscitation, and Monitoring

As airway, breathing, and circulation are being addressed, a rapid primary survey is also performed. This focuses on immediately life-threatening chest injuries, of which tension pneumothorax and massive hemothorax occur most frequently in pediatric multiple trauma patients. Both problems will impede further resuscitative efforts if left untreated, hence require immediate lateral tube thoracostomy without waiting for a confirmatory chest X-ray film; needle decompression (via the second intercostal space on the midclavicular line, just above the third rib) should precede chest tube placement in tension pneumothorax if signs of respiratory distress or shock are present. The child's neurologic status (level of consciousness and pupillary reactions) also should be noted briefly at this time, and neurosurgical consultation obtained as necessary.

Once the primary survey has been completed and immediately life-threatening chest injuries have been treated, a cardiac monitor should be attached to the child and a complete set of vital signs obtained. Knowledge of the normal range of and technique for measuring vital signs in the pediatric age groups is clearly essential for these data to be obtained and interpreted correctly. The lower limit of normal systolic blood pressure in the child is $70 + (2 \times$ age in years) mmHg. The bladder of the cuff used to obtain the measurement must be approximately two thirds as wide as the distance from the axilla to the antecubital fossa for the determination to be accurate. If the child is unconscious (Glasgow Coma Scale ≤ 8) or in respiratory failure and an extended period of hyperventilation is anticipated, an orotracheal airway should be secured at this point, if not already accomplished. Indications for hyperventilation include alveolar hypoventilation, profound metabolic acidemia, and increased intracranial pressure, all of which usually are present in children who are unconscious as a result of severe closed head injury. The presence of profound metabolic acidemia always raises the question of whether treatment with sodium bicarbonate is indicated. In general, it should not be given unless the pH remains below 7.2 despite both aggressive hyperventilation and volume resuscitation because the adverse effect of low pH on myocardial contractility does not reach clinical significance above this level. There are also data to suggest that administration of sodium bicarbonate before adequate ventilation and perfusion have been established may transiently worsen intracellular acidosis.

The need for further volume support is dictated by the child's response to the initial fluid challenge. If vital signs and peripheral perfusion fail to improve as the first crystalloid bolus is given, the line should remain wide open and a second bolus administered immediately. If the child fails to respond after the second bolus, however, or presents in hypotensive (decompensated) shock, it is likely that major (ie, class III or IV) hemorrhage has occurred. In the absence of significant bleeding from an obvious site (eg, open fracture or deep laceration), this degree of hemorrhage can only be due to an unrecognized source in the abdomen or pelvis or, less likely, in the chest. In this situation, blood must be given immediately (type-specific if available or O negative) and the child prepared for the urgent surgical intervention, which almost certainly will be required. To reiterate, the multiply injured child who presents in hypotensive (decompensated) shock, with rare exceptions, will have lost at least 30% to 40% of his or her circulating blood volume and is in mortal danger. This underscores the importance of involving a qualified surgeon experienced in the management of childhood injuries as early as possible during pediatric trauma resuscitation.

By the 3:1 rule, which states that blood is three times more effective than crystalloid as a volume expander, achieving hemodynamic stability after 2×20 mL/kg = 40 mL/kg of lactated Ringer solution has been infused means that less than 25% (about 20 mL/kg) of the circulating blood volume, which normally approaches 80 mL/kg in the small child and infant, has been lost. As stated above, it is within the normal compensatory capacity of most children to tolerate this degree of volume loss.[20] Obviously, every effort should be made to avoid using blood or blood products in such patients because the risk of transmitting the various serum hepatitis and human immunodeficiency viruses, though small, is still real. Once it is recognized that the child will not stabilize unless more than 40 mL/kg of lactated Ringer solution is infused, however, blood must be given immediately. In contrast to the situation with shock from dehydration, volume losses in trauma are usually rapid and ongoing and result not simply in a lack of circulating volume but also in a nearly linear fall in blood oxygen content and carrying capacity as the blood hemoglobin concentration also decreases.

In most instances, the primary survey and resuscitation phases of the trauma response are conducted concurrently. Once the point in the resuscitation phase has been reached when the airway has been secured, a nasogastric tube or orogastric tube, if the former is contraindicated by the presence of severe facial trauma or a cribriform plate fracture, should be inserted to relieve gastric dilatation. A Foley catheter should also be inserted at about this time, particularly if the child has not yet stabilized from the hemodynamic standpoint. Monitoring urine output allows the adequacy of renal, and hence core organ, perfusion in response to therapy to be assessed. Contraindications to Foley catheter placement such as blood at the meatus, discoloration of the scrotum, a high-riding prostate, or obvious fracture of the pubic symphysis mandate that a retrograde urethrogram be obtained as a guide to further management. Ideally, in contrast to adolescents and adults, who must make at least 0.5 mL/kg of urine per hour to be considered nonoliguric, a child must make at least 1.0 mL/kg/hour and an infant at least 1.5 to 2.0 mL/kg/hour. Higher flows will be required in severe crush injuries to prevent deposition of myoglobin in the renal tubules and the subsequent development of acute renal failure.

Adequate circulating blood volume has been achieved when vital signs have normalized (Table 33-1) and signs of inadequate peripheral perfusion are absent. Ideally, the acid-base status, as reflected by determinations of arterial blood gases, serum electrolyte concentrations, and/or plasma lactate levels, should also have corrected by this time. The most reliable early indicator of resuscitation from shock is a normal(izing) mixed venous oxygen saturation. Early insertion

Table 33-1 Reference Values for Normal Vital Signs in Children

Age (years)	Heart Rate (beat/min)	Respiration Rate (breath/min)	Blood Pressure (mmHg)
Birth	110–160	30–60	60–85
0.5	100–140	30–50	70–105
1	100–140	25–35	80–105
2	90–110	20–30	80–105
3	90–110	20–30	80–105
4	80–100	20–30	80–110
5	80–100	20–30	80–110
6	70–100	16–30	80–110
7	70–100	16–30	80–110
8	70–100	16–30	80–110
9–10	70–90	16–20	90–110
11–12	70–90	16–20	90–120
13–15	60–80	16–20	110–135
16–18	60–80	16–20	110–135

of central venous monitoring lines, particularly pulmonary artery catheters, in the emergency department should be avoided, however, because of the difficulty of performing these procedures in small children, the risk of complications, and the fact that the time required to perform these procedures is far better spent attending to more urgent matters. Even so, central venous routes, particularly the femoral vein, must be accessed expediently when attempts at obtaining peripheral venous or intraosseous access have failed. Short, large-bore percutaneous catheters are preferred over long, small-bore catheters for resuscitation purposes. The relatively thin caliber and long length of most such devices significantly increase resistance to flow and make these lines a poor choice for the type of rapid fluid infusion that is usually required to restore circulating volume in hemorrhagic shock. After fluid resuscitation has been accomplished, a short femoral line may be converted to a long central line for monitoring if needed.

If a child fails to improve despite seemingly adequate volume resuscitation, and in the absence of signs to suggest intra-abdominal or pelvic bleeding, other forms of shock (ie, obstructive, cardiogenic, or distributive) must be considered. Has a tension pneumothorax, hemothorax, or cardiac tamponade developed? If so, immediate needle decompression may be required before definitive tube thoracostomy or pericardiotomy and possible cardiorrhaphy. Is there an unrecognized myocardial contusion? Echocardiography and subsequent cardiac enzyme determinations, particularly of the cardiac muscle fraction of creatine phosphokinase, will be required to confirm this diagnosis. Is there a possible spinal cord injury, either spinal shock or frank neurogenic shock due to a partial or complete transection (Brown-Sequard lesion) that initially was missed on physical examination? Such patients commonly will have warm extremities, lower than expected heart rates, and low to normal blood pressures that will not respond to volume resuscitation in the normal fashion, although urinary output is usually preserved.

Such conditions require directed therapy if found. Most children in hypotensive or decompensated shock, however, have unrecognized hemorrhage that can be reversed only if recognized promptly and treated appropriately by means of rapid transfusion and immediate surgical intervention. If surgical intervention is not readily available, use of the pneumatic antishock garment, also known as medical antishock trousers (MAST), may buy time until the surgeon arrives. The device should only be used if it fits, and care must be taken in young children to avoid using the abdominal compartment because this may impede ventilation. Note that, aside from evisceration and impaling objects, the only real contraindication to the use of MAST in profound hypotension is major arterial disruption in the thorax or upper abdomen as a result of deep penetrating or severe blunt injury.[36] Increasing afterload, the mechanism by which MAST appear to work, may seriously accelerate the blood loss in this type of injury, particularly in mild hypotension.[37] MAST are of added benefit in shock resuscitation cases for splinting fractures of the lower extremities and for helping contain the often massive retroperitoneal hemorrhage resulting from the venous oozing that accompanies severe comminuted pelvic fractures.[38] Although the initiation of definitive therapy for hemorrhagic shock occasionally is aided by the device (obtaining venous access in the upper extremities may be facilitated by its use), MAST must never be used in such a way as to delay needed volume resuscitation.[39]

Secondary Survey

As soon as the primary survey has been performed and resuscitation has been initiated, the secondary survey should be undertaken. To be sure that no injuries are missed, this must include both complete exposure of the patient and log-rolling, especially in penetrating trauma. Care must be taken to avoid the subsequent development of hypothermia, however, which worsens acidosis. Blankets, an overbed radiant warmer, and/or intravenous fluids warmed to body temperature can be used to maintain body temperature. A careful head-to-toe examination, as in the adult, is the cornerstone of this phase of the trauma response. The examination addresses all organ systems, including the central and peripheral nervous systems and the musculoskeletal system.

In performing the neurologic examination, particular attention is directed toward careful determination of level of consciousness and Glasgow Coma Scale score, pupillary and corneal reactions, deep tendon reflexes, and rectal sphincter tone. Use of the doll's-eye maneuver to assess the oculocephalic reflex as a test of midbrain function is contraindicated if there is any suspicion of cervical spine trauma (viz, cervical point tenderness, swelling, spasm, torticollis or wry neck; radiographic findings that cannot definitively be called normal; or a mechanism of injury that suggests that cervical spinal cord injury is possible).

It is, of course, also wise to re-evaluate during the secondary survey for signs of immediately or potentially life-threatening chest injuries, which occasionally are subtle and may have been missed during the primary assessment. These include unilaterally decreased breath sounds with hyperresonance (or dullness) to percussion, which suggest pneumothorax (or hemothorax). Both these injuries can be associated with tracheal shift, which is indicative of tension. Muffled heart tones suggest cardiac tamponade. Multiple posterior rib fractures can be associated with flail chest, which is poorly tolerated in children. Potentially penetrating chest wounds suggest the possibility of open pneumothorax.

In the absence of coma the physical examination has long been regarded as a reliable indicator of significant abdominal injury. A distended abdomen in a hemodynamically unstable patient, in the absence of gastric dilatation and significant external hemorrhage, strongly suggests intra-abdominal bleeding. Irritation of the abdominal parietes by chyme, and possibly blood alone, causes marked tenderness and involuntary guarding. Unrelieved gastric distention and fractures of one or more of the lower ribs with concomitant injury to the intercostal nerve may yield similar findings. The absence of bowel sounds may or may not suggest disruption of a hollow viscus, although their presence usually militates against this possibility. Obviously, abdominal wall ecchymosis and/or hematoma may suggest that significant intra-abdominal injury is present as well. The absence of such signs does not guarantee a benign abdomen, however.

Rectal examination, often overlooked in the child trauma patient, may yield valuable information that might otherwise be ignored. The presence of blood, obvious or occult, usually indicates that the rectum or sigmoid colon has been damaged. Bleeding from more proximal sites is unusual, and traumatic hemobilia is a late finding. Anterior rectal tenderness may indicate parietal peritoneal irritation due to intraperitoneal blood or feces. A boggy or high-riding prostate obviously suggests disruption of the urethra and may be the first clue to the diagnosis of pelvic fracture. Loss of sphincter tone suggests the possibility of spinal cord injury or sexual abuse. In the stable patient, proctosigmoidoscopy and/or fluoroscopic studies of the lower gastrointestinal tract with a water-soluble contrast agent may be a useful adjunct if violation of the rectum or sigmoid colon is suspected.

Laboratory and Radiographic Evaluation

Laboratory evaluation is an integral part of the secondary assessment. Serial hematocrits will offer a clue to the extent of blood loss, but the initial value by itself is most often of limited utility. This is because there generally has not been adequate time for equilibration (ie, the shift of fluid from the extracellular space to the vascular compartment that occurs in response to hypovolemia and results in dilutional anemia) to have occurred. If physical and vital signs indicate the presence of shock, however, an initial hematocrit of 30% or less is suggestive of significant hemorrhage and 25% or less of massive hemorrhage.[40]

Elevation in the serum concentration of amylase indicates the presence of injury to the pancreas and possibly the spleen, which is contiguous with the tail of the pancreas. Similarly, elevations of the serum concentrations of the hepatic transaminases suggest injury to the liver.[41,42] Urine that is grossly bloody or is positive for blood by dipstick and/or microscopy (20 or more red blood cells per high power field) suggests renal damage, and indirectly, damage to adjacent organs (there is a high incidence of associated injuries in blunt renal trauma).[43,44] It should be noted that myoglobin, which turns the urine brown, also may yield positive results on dipstick evaluation of the urine. If this should occur, or if significant crush injury is present or suspected, creatine phosphokinase should be measured to determine whether the skeletal muscle fraction is elevated.

A specific trauma series of radiographs, including lateral cervical spine, supine chest, and combined (where possible) supine abdominal and pelvic views, is obtained in the seriously injured child, so long as the patient is improving and obviously will not require immediate transport to the operating room. At no time should radiographic studies take precedence over resuscitation and/or whatever immediate therapy may be required for treatment of life-threatening injuries. Only hemodynamically stable patients should be taken to the radiology department, and then only if the physician accompanies and continuously monitors the child. Arrangements should also be made at this time (ie, before any other films are ordered) to obtain computed tomography (CT) scans of the head, chest, and abdomen as indicated. These must include the administration of dilute meglumine diatrizoate (Hypaque) suspension via the nasogastric tube if the latter study is required[45] (Table 33-2). Once these have been obtained, whatever other films are required may be taken, as indicated by clinical findings (eg, of bruised, tender, swollen, and/or obviously deformed extremities).

Although spectrum of injuries to which the child is subject is somewhat different from that in the adult, the radiographic manifestations of these injuries are similar. Several points

Table 33-2 Doses of Contrast Agents for CT in Children

Intravenous Contrast	Oral Contrast
Meglumine diatrizoate (Hypaque), 60% A small test dose followed by 2 mL/kg intravenous bolus (maximum, 50 mL) and then 50–100 mL by intravenous infusion during scanning	Meglumine diatrizoate (Hypaque), 1.5% Orally or by nasogastric tube 0–2 years, 60 mL 3–5 years, 120 mL 6–9 years, 180 mL >9 years, 300–400 mL

Source: Kane NM, Cronan JJ, Dorfman GS, et al: Pediatric abdominal trauma: evaluation by computed tomography. *Pediatrics* 82: 11–15, 1988.

must be emphasized regarding emergency department interpretation of pediatric plain films, however:

- A normal lateral cervical spine radiograph, which, as in the adult, must show all seven cervical vertebrae plus the top of T-1, does not rule out cervical spine or spinal cord injury. A full cervical spine series consisting, at a minimum, of anteroposterior and odontoid views in addition to the lateral view is required for this purpose; none of these, of course, excludes the possibility of spinal cord injury if the SCIWORA syndrome is present. Individuals responsible for interpreting such films must also be knowledgeable about the radiologic idiosyncrasies of the cervical spine in children (eg, physiologic subluxation, which may be further accentuated if the radiograph is obtained with the cervical extrication collar in place) and the ages at which the various ossification centers and growth plates fully calcify.

- The supine chest film will often show a widened mediastinum suggestive of aortic dissection or tear, both of which are extremely rare in children in contrast to the adult. If the child is hemodynamically stable, if there are no signs of cervical spine injury, and if the lateral cervical spine film is normal, a repeat chest study, preferably a posteroanterior view obtained in a semi-upright or sitting position while the cervical spine is carefully maintained in a neutral position, may obviate the need for aortography if interpreted as normal. CT of the aortic arch, even if obtained immediately after intravenous contrast administration, is rarely definitive enough to be helpful.

- Although the most common radiographic signs of intra-abdominal catastrophe in the child are a ground-glass appearance of the abdominal cavity as a whole, suggesting intra-abdominal bleeding, and medial displacement of the lateral border of the stomach (marked by the nasogastric tube) by the spleen, suggesting splenic laceration and/or hematoma, signs of hollow visceral injuries are much more subtle. Indeed, short of contrast studies, the only clue to duodenal or proximal jejunal hematoma, when a nasogastric tube is in place, may be the relative lack of gas in the proximal small intestine, although this is rarely an early sign. Similarly, disruptions of the duodenum and/or proximal jejunum may be heralded only by tiny retroperitoneal (ie, perirenal) gas shadows on the right side of the abdomen adjacent to and slightly below the liver. Oral contrast studies may or may not demonstrate the injury. Pneumoperitoneum would confirm its presence but is rarely identified on plain films. Detection is sometimes facilitated if air is injected via the nasogastric tube as a radiolucent contrast agent.

The introduction of sophisticated imaging modalities such as nuclear scanning, ultrasonography, and CT to the diagnostic armamentarium has revolutionized the management of pediatric trauma, the definitive treatment of which is frequently nonoperative. This is especially true with respect to lacerations and/or hematomas of, and/or extravasation from, the liver, spleen, and kidneys.[46–48] Despite the extraordinary power of the newer techniques in demonstrating these lesions, as with plain films they have no place in the management of the hemodynamically unstable patient. Further, they are never a substitute for prompt and timely evaluation by a qualified surgeon experienced in the management of pediatric trauma.

CT is best for evaluation of solid visceral injuries, including liver, spleen, and kidneys and, to a lesser extent, the hollow viscera[49]; ultrasonography is best for evaluation of pancreatic injuries and to diagnose the presence of free intraperitoneal blood (especially in the splenic and pelvic fossae).[50] The utility of CT is dependent upon the use of both intravenous and oral contrast agents[45] (Table 33-2). The use of contrast material is contraindicated in patients with histories of anaphylactic reactions to iodinated contrast agents unless they are known to have been successfully pretreated with corticosteroids and/or antihistaminics in preparation for studies requiring their use. The quality of the study also is dependent upon the patient's lying still, which, on occasion, may require the use of neuromuscular blockade (coupled with sedation if the patient is normotensive), provided, of course, that adequate ventilation, oxygenation, and perfusion are continuously maintained, the patient is fully monitored, and personnel capable of managing the airway are in attendance.

CT scans of the head should be obtained for any head injury associated with loss of consciousness and/or fluctuation or decrease in the level of consciousness, a Glasgow Coma Scale score of 14 or less, or signs of increased intracranial pressure (eg, inappropriate slowing of the heart rate or a history of nausea or vomiting). CT scans of the abdomen should be obtained whenever there are signs of internal bleeding (eg, abdominal distention or bruising), shock in the field that responds to volume resuscitation, or a pattern of injuries that suggests that abdominal injury also may have occurred.[51] Note, however, that a patient who remains in shock despite treatment is a candidate for immediate operation, not further study. Ultrasonography is reserved for those cases in which intra-abdominal injury and/or bleeding is suspected and CT scans cannot be obtained because of the lack or failure of equipment or history of allergy to intravenous contrast agents. Nuclear scans, which remain the gold standard for detection of splenic and hepatic injuries,[52] are now reserved for follow-up of solid visceral injuries initially detected by CT.[53] Nuclear scans may also be used for cases in which these injuries are suspected but CT is unavailable and ultrasonography is negative.

The radiographic diagnosis of blunt renal injuries has undergone rapid evolution in recent years. Ultrasonography has become the diagnostic study of choice when information is sought regarding the structural integrity of the kidneys, and nuclear renal perfusion scans have become the first-line test of renal function. Obviously, CT scans of the abdomen, if obtained, will serve to rule in or out major abnormalities and generally will suffice unless minor injuries are suspected that are beyond the resolution of the scanner.[48] Finally, although intravenous urography has been largely supplanted by these newer techniques, it is still used in the situation where isolated blunt renal injury is suspected and there exist neither clinical findings nor a mechanism of injury to suggest that adjacent structures may be damaged. Intravenous urography may also be helpful when urinalysis reveals significant microscopic hematuria (ie, more than 20 or more red blood cells per high power field) and no other reliable test of renal function is immediately available.[41,42] Arteriography is required only for diagnosis of renal pedicle injury in which specific information regarding vascular anatomy is desired in preparation for urgent operation. Such injuries are rare, but a high index of suspicion for this lesion must always be maintained because hematuria, gross or microscopic, is not always present.[54,55]

Acute Management of Injuries

Acute management of the injured child will depend upon the type, extent, and severity of the injuries. In the unstable patient, immediate surgical intervention generally will be required. In the stable patient, definitive therapy will be directed by the appropriate specialists. Regardless, any patient requiring resuscitation (ie, anything more than simple evaluation or wound care) should be admitted to the hospital for observation under the care of a qualified surgeon experienced in the management of childhood injuries. Any such child should be given nothing by mouth in case general anesthesia should be required later. Assuming that both normal hydration at the time of the injury and normalization of both vital signs and perfusion status after resuscitation have been achieved, the child should receive intravenous fluids at the maintenance rate (Table 33-3). An exception is the child with an acute head injury, whose fluids should be administered at two thirds the maintenance rate. Because hypoxia due to inadequate cerebral perfusion is the most common cause of secondary brain injury in all age groups, however, fluid restriction should not be instituted until restoration of a normal circulating blood volume has been ensured.

Acute management of head injuries, so common in the pediatric age groups, deserves special comment. In addition to hyperventilation to a $Paco_2$ of approximately 25 mmHg, which is intended to restore the cerebral blood volume increased by the traumatic loss of cerebral autoregulation to nearly normal levels, and fluid restriction sufficient to achieve a serum osmolality of 310 to 320 mOsm/L, routine treatment consists simply of elevating the head in the midline to approximately 30°. Loop diuretics (furosemide) and osmotic diuretics (mannitol) are rarely required and may be frankly dangerous if given to children who have marginal intravascular volume. For this reason their use should be limited, and they should be given only after a central venous line has been placed for the purpose of pressure monitoring. Mannitol may occasionally be required before central venous pressure monitoring when signs of uncal herniation supervene. The use of high-dose corticosteroids (dexamethasone) is of no proven benefit in children with head injuries, although recent evidence suggests that early administration may be helpful in spinal cord trauma. Barbiturates are frankly contraindicated except as required for the acute management of posttraumatic seizures that do not respond to first-line drugs such as diazepam and/or phenytoin. Placement of an intracranial bolt or catheter for monitoring of intracranial pressure, if desired, is a procedure that should be reserved for the critical care unit rather than the emergency department and, in any event, should be performed only by a qualified neurosurgeon. Likewise, drainage of subdural and epidural hematomas should be accomplished only in the operating room by properly trained and equipped surgical personnel.

Acute management of other injuries in the child is similar to that in the adult except insofar as abdominal injuries are concerned. In particular, treatment of solid visceral injuries in childhood is largely nonoperative although not nonsurgical. This is because a small but significant percentage of children who are managed nonoperatively will eventually require surgery for their liver and/or spleen injuries, especially when the transfusion requirement exceeds half their calculated blood volume (ie, 40 mL/kg). With few exceptions, however, the child who presents in hypotensive or decompensated shock will require immediate surgical intervention, as is also the case in adults.

The majority of children with hepatic and splenic lacerations will go on to heal spontaneously without the need for operation. This renders diagnostic peritoneal lavage unnecessary for most children because the need for operation is based not upon the presence or absence of intraperitoneal blood but upon the ongoing transfusion requirement.[56,57] Lavage is therefore reserved for patients in whom the usual diagnostic modalities of serial physical and laboratory evaluation are unavailable or unreliable. In this category are patients who are unconscious or about to undergo general

Table 33-3 Maintenance Fluid Requirements in Children*

Body Weight (kg)	Daily Fluid Requirement
0–10	100 mL/kg
10–20	1000 mL (first 10 kg) + 50 mL/kg (10–20 kg)
>20	1500 mL (first 20 kg) + 20 mL/kg (>20 kg)

*Holliday-Segar formula.

anesthesia for operative treatment of associated, usually neurosurgical or musculoskeletal, injuries. As in the adult, diagnostic peritoneal lavage has no place in the management of the hemodynamically unstable patient who requires laparotomy for intra-abdominal bleeding because this test will add nothing to what is already known and will serve only to delay definitive surgical therapy.

There may be a role for routine diagnostic peritoneal lavage in children who have sustained injuries, blunt or penetrating, in which the integrity of the bowel possibly has been violated (Table 33-4). Most experts in pediatric trauma, however, hold that frequent serial examination of the child for signs of peritoneal irritation by a qualified surgeon experienced in the management of childhood trauma is probably the more sensitive test.[58] This approach certainly avoids the complications associated with diagnostic peritoneal lavage. It also negates the possibility that later physical or radiographic examinations will be confounded by tenderness resulting from the presence of intraperitoneal blood due to oozing from the puncture site in the abdominal wall or air introduced at the time of the procedure.

Systems Issues

The early care of the injured child is an extraordinarily complex undertaking that requires the active and collegial participation of a large number of prehospital, medical, nursing, and allied health professionals from different disciplines for the outcome to be successful. Although overall direction of the pediatric trauma resuscitation should be the responsibility of the most qualified and experienced individual available (ultimately a trauma surgeon with extensive experience in the management of childhood injuries), the emergency physician will frequently be called upon to lead the resuscitation until this surgeon is present at the bedside. There is clearly no place for turf battles or power struggles when what is at stake is the care, perhaps even the life, of a child. The early care of the injured child is truly a team effort that requires nothing less than the best efforts of all members of that team if the best possible outcome for the child is to be ensured.

The seriously injured child is best cared for in a hospital that has made a strong institutional, financial, and moral commitment to prioritizing the comprehensive care of the injured child, including the abused child.[59] Most full-service general, university, and/or children's hospitals will meet these criteria, and, to the extent possible, seriously injured children should be preferentially transported by properly trained and equipped prehospital personnel to these facilities. These transfers should be in accordance with regional emergency medical services system policies and protocols and formally established trauma center designations and interfacility transfer agreements. Nevertheless, all emergency physicians and departments must have the basic training, skills, personnel, and equipment required at least to stabilize a seriously injured child in preparation for transfer to a definitive care facility. Children should be considered for triage or transfer to a regional trauma center with pediatric expertise if the mechanism of injury suggests that this level of care may be required (Table 33-5) or if the Pediatric Trauma Score,[60] Revised Trauma Score,[61] or Champion Trauma Score[62] suggests that the injuries sustained are of sufficient magnitude to result in serious physiologic derangement (Tables 33-6 and 33-7).

Table 33-4 Criteria for Positive Diagnostic Peritoneal Lavage[58]

Gross blood aspirated
Red blood cells $> 100,000/mm^3$
White blood cells $> 500/mm^3$
Amylase > 175 μg/dL
Food particles present
Microorganisms present
Gram's stain positive
Bile staining positive

Table 33-5 Guidelines for Transfer to a Pediatric Trauma Center[59]

History of injury
  Patient thrown from a moving vehicle
  Falls from $>$ 15 feet
  Extrication time $>$ 20 minutes
  Passenger cabin invaded $>$ 12 inches
  Death of another passenger
  Patient age $<$ 14 years
  Accident in hostile environment (heat, cold water, etc)
Anatomic injuries
  Combined system injury
  Penetrating injury of the groin or neck
  Three or more long bone fractures
  Fractures of the axial skeleton
  Amputation (other than digits)
  Persistent hypotension
  Severe head trauma
  Maxillofacial or upper airway injury
  Central nervous system injury with prolonged loss of
    consciousness, posturing, or paralysis
  Spinal cord injury with neurologic deficit
  Unstable chest injury
  Blunt or penetrating trauma to the chest or abdomen
  Burns (flame or inhalation)
System considerations
  Necessary service or specialist not available
  No beds available
  Need for pediatric intensive care unit
  Multiple casualties
  Family request
  Paramedic judgment
  Severity scores
    Trauma Score 12 or less
    Revised Trauma Score 11 or less
    Pediatric Trauma Score 8 or less

Table 33-6 Pediatric Trauma Score[60]

Patient Characteristics	Pediatric Trauma Score		
	+2	+1	−1
Weight (kg)	>20	10–20	<10
Airway	Normal	Maintained	Unmaintained
Systolic blood pressure (mmHg)	>90	50–90	<50
Central nervous system	Awake	Obtunded	Coma
Open wound	None	Minor	Major
Skeletal trauma	None	Closed	Open, multiple

Table 33-7 Revised Trauma Score[61]

	Revised Trauma Score		
Glasgow Coma Scale Score	Systolic Blood Pressure (mmHg)	Respiratory Rate (breath/min)	Coded Value
13–15	>89	10–29	4
9–12	76–89	>29	3
6–8	50–75	6–9	2
4–5	1–49	1–5	1
3	0	0	0

Medical directors of emergency medical services and systems have special responsibilities to the child trauma patient. First and foremost among these is to ensure safe and rapid transport of the seriously injured child to the appropriate receiving hospital. Although basic life support is the foundation upon which all prehospital trauma care must be based, advanced life support should not be denied the child trauma patient if it is appropriate, if transport time exceeds approximately 20 minutes and will not be prolonged by the provision of advanced life support en route, and if providers are properly trained and equipped to render this level of care to the injured child. Prehospital pediatric trauma care is usually best executed in emergency medical services systems that have specific pediatric involvement and emphasis.

The overall mortality rate for serious pediatric trauma (ie, that requiring treatment in a pediatric trauma center) approaches 2% in the best hands.[2] Although significant improvement in this statistic is unlikely until effective treatments are devised for debilitating central nervous system injury and irreversible hemorrhagic shock, recent research suggests that unnecessary deaths that do occur are usually due not to errors in definitive management but to inadequate or inappropriate resuscitation.[24,25] This emphasizes the need for education and training of emergency personnel in pediatric advanced life support.[23] There is also a growing body of evidence confirming the long-held presumption that children, once seriously injured, do in fact fare better in organized trauma systems in which there is emphasis upon the special needs of children both in the prehospital sector and in the trauma center itself.[63–65] Nevertheless, experts in pediatric injury epidemiology and prevention state that as much as 20% of serious childhood injuries could have been prevented by appropriately targeted public education initiatives.[1] Chief among these are insistence upon use of infant car seats, child booster seats, appropriately worn lap and shoulder belts; bicycle helmets; pedestrian and bicycle and pedestrian safety training; and window-gating in high-rise urban dwellings.

MINOR TRAUMA

Perhaps the most common reason that children present to the emergency department, aside from conditions that traditionally are managed in the pediatrician's office, is minor trauma. Falls account for the vast majority of these injuries. Precise knowledge of the mechanism of the child's injury, coupled with common sense, will help determine which injuries are of a more serious nature and which are less so. Although most such injuries obviously are sustained during the course of play activities, the emergency physician must always be alert to the possibility of child abuse and should keep in mind the fact that bruises in different stages of healing, particularly if they are located on areas of the body that are not commonly injured during play, are highly suggestive of inflicted injury.

Minor head trauma probably is cause for more than its share of anxiety for parent and physician alike. In general, children who sustain blunt trauma to the head sufficient to cause frank loss of consciousness should be admitted for observation, even if the neurologic examination is normal on arrival in the emergency department. Any sign of increased intracranial pressure, including mild drowsiness, nausea, or vomiting, should mandate CT of the head. Skull radiographs are generally of little use in conscious patients and are no longer ordered routinely for medicolegal reasons because it is now recognized that skull fracture is a poor marker of brain injury. Skull radiographs should be obtained, however, as should radiographs of the cervical spine, if either physical examination or the mechanism of injury suggests that bony abnormality is likely.

Soft tissue contusions are treated simply by elevation of the affected part to the extent possible. Ice packs may retard swelling in the immediate postinjury period but may cause hypothermia in small children. Showers, tub baths, warm soaks, or application of a heating pad thereafter several times daily may promote more rapid resorption of blood. Aspirin-containing analgesics should be avoided because they may interfere with platelet function and promote hematoma development.

Closure of lacerations may present special technical problems in children, chiefly because of the inability to restrain a child who is moving or thrashing about. Use of passive restraints such as the Papoose board and involvement of the parent(s) for the psychologic support of the child during suturing may facilitate the performance of these often tedious procedures. The use of topical anesthetic agents such as tetracaine-epinephrine-cocaine or similar cocktails,[66] infiltrative anesthetic agents buffered with sodium bicarbonate to reduce pain,[67] and appropriate sedative agents may also be useful in reducing the anxiety and discomfort traditionally associated with suturing lacerations in children. No special techniques of suturing are required in children that are different from those used in adults, but it is wise to remember the following points:

- The suture material chosen should be strong enough to do the job but of the thinnest diameter and the least reactivity possible in highly visible areas such as the face.
- Sutures should be large enough, placed far apart enough, and tied loosely enough that they are easy to remove and there is not so much tension as to cause "train track" marks.
- Given the uncanny ability of most children to reinjure with great frequency the very areas of their bodies in which their wounds are located, sutures should not be removed from the extremities until it is clear that the wound has healed completely (eg, 2 to 3 weeks).

The use of antibiotics for soft tissue injuries is controversial. Most experts hold that systemic antimicrobial prophylaxis is of little use, and of potential harm, in patients with blunt trauma, even if extensive. Systemic antibiotics are similarly contraindicated in patients with clean incisive wounds and lacerations, particularly of the face and scalp, that are closed promptly (ie, within 4 to 6 hours of injury). Older wounds and/or tetanus-prone wounds probably should be treated with systemic antibiotics as well as aggressive local care, including debridement of devitalized tissue. Obviously tetanus prophylaxis also should be administered if such wounds are present. Tetanus toxoid is appropriate if immunizations are up to date. The addition of tetanus immune globulin is indicated if the immunization series is deficient.

It must be emphasized that the purpose of administering systemic antibiotics is to prevent local infection from becoming systemic, not to treat the primary local infection itself. The importance of appropriate and timely local wound care in preventing local infection cannot be overemphasized. Wounds must be irrigated thoroughly, in the operating room if necessary, with a jet-lavage or pulse-irrigation device and meticulously debrided of foreign matter and devitalized tissue. This approach should be used whether or not primary closure is indicated. All types of penetrating civilian wounds involving the soft tissues but not violating body cavities should be treated in this fashion. Those involving penetration of body cavities or bony injury (ie, open fractures) require the immediate involvement of the appropriate surgical specialist.

BURNS

Conceptually speaking, the early management of severe burns is no different in children than in adults. Several unique pediatric characteristics must be remembered. There is an increased risk of airway obstruction resulting from mucosal swelling in children with inhalation injuries because of the narrower diameter of the airway at all levels. The thinner skin of the child is more easily damaged than that of the adult. The proportionately larger body surface area in the child results in greater evaporative water loss and hence greater cooling. Yet the basic approach to fluid resuscitation is no different inasmuch as the fluid regimen known as the modified Parkland formula is still preferred.

According to this formula, fluid resuscitation in the first 24 hours after a significant burn is with lactated Ringer solution (4 mL/kg per percentage body surface burn per 24 hours). In calculating body surface area, it must be realized that the head is proportionately larger, and the legs proportionately smaller, than in the adult, so that a modified Rule of Nines for infants is used: The head is assumed to account for 18% of total body surface area and the legs for 13.5% each. Between infancy and adulthood body proportions change, and representative burn charts have been developed (Table 33-8). In addition to the burn regimen itself, maintenance fluid containing 5% dextrose must be provided. Fluid intake is titrated according to the status of perfusion and urinary output, which, as in the pediatric trauma patient, must be maintained at a level appropriate for the child's age.

Early management of the burn wounds themselves is similar in children and adults. Debridement of all large bullae, and all small bullae that have broken or are expected to break, with subsequent gentle cleansing with an appropriate agent (eg, chlorhexidine or dilute iodophor) is called for. Dressing with silver sulfadiazine and fine-mesh gauze constitutes fundamental burn wound management. Prophylactic antibiotics are avoided.

As in adults, smaller burns can be managed successfully on an outpatient basis. Criteria for hospital admission and referral to a burn center, however, are somewhat more stringent for children than for adults.[68] Admission is advised for any child with a third-degree burn; a greater than 10% second-degree burn; severe burns of the hand, foot, face, or perineum; or suspicious social factors.

CORROSIVE EXPOSURES

The word *caustic* is often applied to exposure of skin or mucous membranes to a number of noxious chemical compounds, but tissue injury may occur via various mechanisms depending on the nature of the toxic substance. Although the generation of heat often contributes to the injury, corrosive substances generally do not result in classic thermal burns

Table 33-8 Estimation of Body Surface Area Burn by Age[68]

Area	Percentage Body Surface Area					
	Birth to 1 Year	1–4 Years	5–9 Years	10–14 Years	15 Years	Adult
Head	19	17	13	11	9	7
Neck	2	2	2	2	2	2
Anterior trunk	13	13	13	13	13	13
Posterior trunk	13	13	13	13	13	13
Right buttock	2.5	2.5	2.5	2.5	2.5	2.5
Left buttock	2.5	2.5	2.5	2.5	2.5	2.5
Genitalia	1	1	1	1	1	1
Right upper arm	4	4	4	4	4	4
Left upper arm	4	4	4	4	4	4
Right lower arm	3	3	3	3	3	3
Left lower arm	3	3	3	3	3	3
Right hand	2.5	2.5	2.5	2.5	2.5	2.5
Left hand	2.5	2.5	2.5	2.5	2.5	2.5
Right thigh	5.5	6.5	8	8.5	9	9.5
Left thigh	5.5	6.5	8	8.5	9	9.5
Right leg	5	5	5.5	6	6.5	7
Left leg	5	5	5.5	6	6.5	7
Right foot	3.5	3.5	3.5	3.5	3.5	3.5
Left foot	3.5	3.5	3.5	3.5	3.5	3.5

but rather in patterns of tissue injury characteristic of the toxic chemical involved. Management of corrosive injury does not differ appreciably between children and adults. The reader is directed elsewhere in this book for a detailed discussion of these issues. A few comments, however, specifically with regard to corrosive ingestions in children, are in order.

Airway patency must always be the primary concern. This is especially true for children, in whom both the relatively loose application of the tracheal mucosa to the underlying tracheal wall and the narrower diameter of the airway conspire to make airway edema more frequent and potentially more dangerous. The presence of esophageal injury has not been shown to correlate well with the presence or absence of oropharyngeal injury. As many as one third of patients with esophageal injury will not have an associated oropharyngeal injury. Careful analysis, however, has revealed that about half the patients with two or more of the symptoms of drooling, stridor, and vomiting will have significant esophageal injury; those without at least two of these symptoms are unlikely to have sustained such injury.[69] When injury is suspected, esophagoscopy should be performed as soon as practicable (ie, after allowing adequate time for gastric emptying). The purpose of the procedure is to define the extent of the injury and to determine the need for corticosteroid therapy. Esophagoscopy is contraindicated in the presence of severe hypopharyngeal or laryngeal burns or respiratory distress, in which case the patient should first be intubated. In cases of clinically obvious perforation the procedure will not be necessary. If required, esophagoscopy is probably best performed under general anesthesia, particularly if the use of rigid equipment is anticipated.

Initial management of the child with corrosive ingestion is expectant. Obviously, nothing should be given by mouth until such time as a definitive diagnosis can be made and a specific plan of therapy instituted. In the meantime, the child should be supported with appropriate intravenous fluid and electrolytes at about 1.5 times the maintenance rate (requirements will be increased as a result of the inflammation). Blood counts and chemistries should be obtained both as a baseline and in preparation for possible operation. Radiographs of the chest and abdomen should be examined for signs of esophageal and/or gastric perforation. Finally, all forms of gastric decontamination are contraindicated. Induced emesis may reinjure the tissue by secondary exposure to the corrosive agent and/or by mechanical factors. Blind insertion of a lavage tube may perforate a damaged esophageal or gastric wall.

The single exception to this latter rule occurs in the patient who sustains a large-volume, strong acid ingestion and who presents early after ingestion without signs of perforation. In this situation, removal of the acid via a carefully placed nasogastric tube with subsequent instillation of antacids may help avoid the nearly uniformly fatal outcome that has been observed in this setting. The use of an oral sodium bicarbonate solution to neutralize a strong acid ingestion is not recommended because the large volume of carbon dioxide and other gases produced by this and other comparable reactions could easily distend the stomach, leading to gastric perforation, vomiting with secondary esophageal injury, or both. Neutralization, although intellectually appealing, has never been demonstrated to be effective and has been abandoned as a therapy by most toxicologists.

ABDOMINAL PAIN

After trauma, perhaps the most common potential surgical emergency encountered in the child is abdominal pain. Abdominal pain is a common presenting symptom of many childhood illnesses, many of which are extra-abdominal in origin (eg, lower lobe pneumonias). The diagnosis of exclusion for which the pediatric surgeon is most often consulted by the emergency physician, however, is appendicitis. Failure to recognize and promptly treat this disease still results in unnecessary morbidity and mortality, even in this modern age of powerful antibiotics.

Appendicitis

In most cases, the child with appendicitis is of school age or older, although preschoolers and occasionally even infants may be afflicted. As in the adult, the disease typically runs a 36-hour course from onset of symptoms (ie, the last meal taken normally) to perforation. However, the course of the disease may seem shorter in the child than in the adult because the child may not be aware that anything is especially wrong early in the course of the disease or may not be able to express the symptoms sufficiently well to bring them to the consciousness of the caretaker until late in the course of the disease. Indeed, the fact that most children with appendicitis present during the evening hours is hardly surprising when one considers that children are far more comfortable and far better able to express concerns about their bodies to their parents than to school teachers and/or day care givers.

Although most abdominal pain is not caused by appendicitis, evaluation by a surgeon experienced in the management of children is still the most sensitive and specific way to exclude the diagnosis. Abdominal pain that suggests the possibility of appendicitis should therefore be evaluated promptly by such an individual. Early involvement of surgical expertise increases diagnostic accuracy chiefly by providing the opportunity for serial re-examination. It also relieves the emergency physician of the responsibility for establishing the diagnosis, which may be more easily accomplished once the patient is admitted to the hospital.[70]

Anorexia is usually the first symptom to appear and is followed shortly thereafter by periumbilical abdominal pain. Fever begins to develop some 6 to 12 hours later, concurrent with localization of pain to the right lower quadrant. This latter symptom may be difficult to elicit in the younger child, who will tend to localize all pain to the umbilicus. One or more episodes of vomiting, which typically relieve the pain little, if at all, may occur at about this time. The pain then usually increases in intensity until the appendix perforates, when pain may recede somewhat for a few hours before more diffuse abdominal tenderness develops, suggesting regional or generalized peritonitis. Intermittent episodes of diarrhea, more mucousy than watery, may confound the presentation if the inflamed appendix is contiguous with the sigmoid colon.

Few findings will be apparent on physical examination before the pain localizes to the right lower quadrant (ie, the usual anatomic site of the appendix). At that time, significant direct tenderness will be present at McBurney's point, which is located in the right lower quadrant approximately two thirds of the way from the umbilicus to the anterosuperior iliac spine, unless the tip of the appendix is ectopically positioned. Irritation of the abdominal parietes, initially with voluntary guarding and later with involuntary guarding and percussion or rebound tenderness, is pathognomonic of peritonitis. The development of florid generalized peritonitis in the child is heralded not by the boardlike rigidity that is typical of the adult but rather by generalized spasm of the abdominal wall musculature, which occasionally deceives even the experienced examiner. Finally, it should be noted that the peritonitis associated with appendicitis is far more commonly generalized in the child than in the adult. This is primarily because the omentum is not fully developed in early childhood, so that intra-abdominal infections cannot be contained. Indeed, the younger the child, the more common is generalized peritonitis.

Rectal examination is an important part of the evaluation of any patient with suspected appendicitis, child or adult. Unless properly done, however, it may yield little, if any, valuable information. It is usually performed with the child in the dorsolithotomy or lateral knee-chest position and in such a way as to minimize both the discomfort and the sense of violation that so often prevent the examiner from gaining meaningful information. As in the adult, the key points are to determine whether anterior rectal tenderness or a mass is present. It is revealing if tenderness is greater on the right than on the left.

In part because the child generally presents somewhat later in the course of the disease than the adult, and in part because the smaller appendix may develop high intraluminal pressure (and hence transmural gangrene and perforation) more quickly, the incidence of perforated appendicitis is considerably higher in the child than in the adult. The goal of the emergency physician therefore should be to maintain a higher index of suspicion for the disease in the child than in the adult and to have a lower threshold for admission for observation, the purpose of which is to facilitate not just bowel rest but frequent examination.

It is, of course, axiomatic that appendicitis can be present in the child in the absence of fever and leukocytosis. Such instances are rare, however. The physician who concludes on the basis of history and physical examination that the patient probably does not have appendicitis is on reasonably firm ground in excluding this diagnosis if the temperature and white blood cell count are normal. The converse, however, is not true.

Several comments can be made about the use and misuse of laboratory and radiologic evaluation in the diagnosis of appendicitis. First and foremost is that the diagnosis of appendicitis is made, or excluded, chiefly on clinical grounds. Laboratory tests and abdominal radiographs may be helpful in equivocal cases, but they are rarely definitive. Indeed, the greatest virtue of the white blood cell count as a test for appendicitis may be that it gives the surgeon the opportunity for re-examination before committing the patient to early operation or continued observation. Although this statement obviously trivializes the role of the white blood cell count as an adjunctive diagnostic tool, it does make the point that, in the end, it is up to the surgeon to decide, primarily on the basis of experience, whether the child has appendicitis.

Classically the white blood cell count in appendicitis is in the range of 12,000/mm^3 to 16,000/mm^3 with a shift toward less mature neutrophilic forms. However, it is far more useful at the extremes of its range than near the mean. As previously noted, a normal white blood cell count is rare if appendicitis is truly present, particularly if there is a preponderance of lymphocytes, which suggests a viral type of infection. On the other hand, white blood cell counts in excess of 20,000/mm^3, unless there is clinical evidence to suggest perforation with regional or generalized peritonitis, are uncommon in appendicitis and suggest that there may be another cause for the pain (eg, lower lobe pneumonia, urinary tract infection, or even severe gastroenteritis).

So far as radiographic studies are concerned, plain films are seldom needed to establish the diagnosis, even though it is common practice to order such studies as a routine. Thus, they should not be obtained unless the diagnosis cannot be made, or excluded, with reasonable certainty on clinical grounds. This is particularly true in the adolescent girl, on whom a pregnancy test should always be performed before any radiographic study is ordered. The diagnosis of appendicitis is confirmed if a fecolith is present, which is rare. A mass effect in the right lower quadrant and an air-fluid level in the distal small bowel adjacent to the cecum both suggest the diagnosis, but these are not pathognomonic. Finally, contrast studies are never required on an urgent basis and are used primarily to exclude the diagnosis of appendicitis if the child fails either to improve or to deteriorate while under observation in the hospital for 24 to 48 hours.

Other Causes of Right Lower Quadrant Pain

Gastroenteritis, which involves inflammation of the stomach and intestines from any etiology, is the major cause of abdominal pain in childhood. Diarrhea is typically present in cases of gastroenteritis, but this is not always so. Conversely, diarrhea is not usually associated with appendicitis but may form part of the presenting complex of symptoms if the inflamed appendix is juxtaposed to the sigmoid colon. The entity with which acute appendicitis is commonly confused is fecal stasis, which may also cause fever and significant right lower quadrant (ie, cecal) tenderness in the child. The condition of fecal stasis resolves immediately with an enema.

The differential diagnosis of right lower quadrant pain in the school-age child and adolescent also includes a large number of relatively rare conditions that will not be elaborated here. A few conditions must be mentioned, however, because of their proclivity to affect youngsters in greater numbers than adults. These include sickle cell anemia, inflammatory bowel diseases, Meckel's diverticulitis, and torsed ovarian cysts. Increasingly, pelvic inflammatory diseases are being diagnosed in the pediatric population. It is sufficient for the purpose of this chapter simply to call the attention of the reader to these conditions. Further discussion may be found elsewhere in this book and in any of a number of standard pediatric, surgical, and gynecologic texts.

Right Upper Quadrant Pain

Right upper quadrant pain, although rare in childhood, is being seen with greater frequency in adolescence. Peptic ulcer disease is no longer a rarity in this population. The increased frequency of right upper quadrant pain is also due to an apparent increase in symptomatic gallstone disease, which probably is the result of the widespread use of oral contraceptives among teenage girls. The most common cause of right upper quadrant pain in adolescent girls, however, is perihepatitis (ie, Fitz-Hugh–Curtis syndrome), which now is due chiefly to chlamydial, not gonococcal, pelvic inflammatory disease. The emergency physician treating these young women, whose bodies are still developing, must be sensitive to their delicate feelings, the medicolegal idiosyncrasies of the local jurisdiction insofar as confidentiality is concerned; and current medical therapy.

Abdominal Pain in Infancy

Evaluation of abdominal pain in the infant requires both specialized knowledge of and significant experience with the care of children in this age group because of the great variety of illnesses that may present with abdominal pain. Two conditions that are unique to the child are common enough to warrant comment here: infant colic and ileocolic intussusception. The former condition, of course, is benign and limited to the early months of infancy and rarely comes to the attention of either the emergency physician or the surgeon. The latter, with which the former must not be confused, affects infants and children approximately 6 months to 2 years of age and remains a serious cause of unnecessary morbidity and mortality in childhood.

The infant with colic is generally between 6 weeks and 4 to 6 months of age. Classically, the discomfort, which is manifested chiefly by inconsolable crying, is believed to be due to an accumulation of gas in the stomach and intestines. These episodes of intense crying often follow immediately upon feeding, usually of a cow's milk–based formula, and last for 30 to 60 minutes, gradually subsiding as the infant is rocked or burped in the arms of a parent. The automobile ride to the hospital often seems especially therapeutic. The diagnosis of colic is made chiefly by history, although it is clearly a diagnosis of exclusion. The history includes a typical pattern of crying. The remainder of the history and the physical examination, which are best performed after the child is quieted down, must be entirely normal. The diagnosis is supported if switching to a soy-based or partially hydrolyzed cow's milk protein–based formula relieves the problem. In the rare colicky infant who is breast fed, elimination of certain foods such as turnips, lentils, sweet potatoes, or greens from the diet of the lactating mother may be curative.

The child with ileocolic intussusception classically presents with colicky (ie, intermittently crampy) abdominal pain that often is severe enough to cause the infant to draw the knees onto the abdomen during painful episodes. Initially these paroxysms occur some 20 to 30 minutes apart but gradually become more frequent. In between, the child may become progressively more lethargic and often appears pale and/or shocky. As in appendicitis, however, the manifestations of this condition are protean, and a high index of suspicion must be maintained in any infant who presents with abdominal pain or unexplained lethargy.

The classic finding of a currant jelly stool (ie, small amounts of blood mixed with mucus) in the diaper is present probably in no more than half the patients with ileocolic intussusception. The presence of a mass in the right upper quadrant, the right lower quadrant being empty, is perhaps even less common. Fever and abdominal tenderness are not often present, but if they are they suggest the possibility of peritonitis due to transmural infarction. Plain films may or may not suggest the presence of distal small bowel obstruction. If detected, obstruction usually indicates that the condition has been present for some time, particularly if accompanied by bilious vomiting.

The key to the early management of ileocolic intussusception is prompt recognition even of the possibility that this condition may be present. Once it is suspected, a qualified surgeon experienced in the management of children should be consulted immediately. Intravenous access should then be obtained, and the child should be rehydrated, as determined by physical examination, with lactated Ringer solution (20 mL/kg) and then with a solution of 5% dextrose and 0.45% sodium chloride at twice the maintenance rate (Table 33-3). In no case should barium enema be attempted for either diagnosis or treatment by hydrostatic reduction until the surgeon is present at the patient's bedside because of the attendant risk of perforation and the subsequent immediate development of shock due to barium peritonitis. Emergency laparotomy is required following an unsuccessful hydrostatic reduction. After successful hydrostatic reduction, the patient should be admitted for observation.

VOMITING

Most cases of vomiting in infancy and childhood are of the reflux type (ie, due to chalasia of infancy), reflex type (ie, following upon visceral distention), or metabolic type (ie, resulting from derangement of the body's internal milieu). In rare cases, vomiting is due to obstruction. The most common cause of obstructive vomiting in infancy is pyloric stenosis. If the vomiting is bilious, however, more distal obstruction is invariably present. Incarcerated inguinal hernia and malrotation are respectively the most frequent and most dangerous causes of this latter problem.

Pyloric stenosis commonly presents with a progressive history of projectile vomiting after feeding that is never bilious. It typically affects the first-born male child at 4 to 6 weeks of age, although either sex can be affected. The diagnosis is suggested by the history and the existence of hypochloremic metabolic alkalosis with paradoxic aciduria, but is made by palpation of an olive-shaped mass deep in the epigastrium. Considerable experience is generally required to feel this mass, and confirmatory ultrasonography and/or radiographic contrast studies are often required. Surgical treatment is required to repair the lesion. Early treatment consists simply of rehydration, with care being taken to provide adequate amounts of fluid, chloride, and potassium to replace the water and salts lost by repetitive vomiting.

Incarcerated inguinal hernia is the most common cause of intestinal obstruction from the first to the sixth month of life. Although the presence of an irreducible inguinal mass in a colicky infant is the most common presenting sign, bilious vomiting occasionally is present. As in the adult, incarcerated inguinal hernia is a surgical emergency. In contrast to the adult, manual reduction by gentle pressure on the scrotum, directed retrograde through the external inguinal ring, will obviate the need for emergency operation in the great majority of cases. This procedure obviously should be attempted only by a qualified surgeon experienced in the management of children. All such infants are somewhat dehydrated and should receive an intravenous solution of 5% dextrose and 0.45% sodium chloride at twice the maintenance rate in preparation for operative intervention. The key point, however, is to admit all such obstructed infants to the hospital, regardless of whether bedside reduction is successful. This is because a small number of these infants will develop symptoms and signs of intestinal perforation, which, at laparotomy, is always found to be due to ischemic necrosis at the site of the previous incarceration.

A rare but deadly cause of bilious vomiting in all age groups, but especially young infants, is malrotation. Typically, there is a history of poor feeding and intermittent vomiting. Vomiting is usually not projectile in nature, but if malrotation is truly present the vomitus will usually be frankly bile stained. Any history of bilious vomiting should be aggressively worked up with an emergency upper gastrointestinal examination to rule out malrotation unless there is an obvious cause such as incarcerated inguinal hernia. Failure to do so, if midgut volvulus is present, will delay diagnosis and may result in the loss of nearly the entire length of the small bowel, if not death.

DIARRHEA AND CONSTIPATION

Severe diarrhea with dehydration is a common problem in infants, in whom viral infections (most often rotavirus) and bacterial diarrheas (particularly those caused by *Shigella* species) can result in significant water loss. Infectious diarrheas may also affect older children, but *severe* dehydration is an uncommon sequela of these illnesses beyond infancy. Although treatment of milder cases of dehydration can readily be accomplished in most infants with an oral rehydration solution, intravenous rehydration is usually preferred for hospital patients. The immediate problem in most such infants, especially those who present with signs of inadequate peripheral perfusion (hypovolemic shock), is to replace circulating plasma volume.

As with all patients who present in shock, attempts at obtaining venous access in dehydration initially should be made via the peripheral veins. If dehydration is especially severe, it may be necessary to resort to an intraosseous infusion or a percutaneous central venous infusion, usually via a femoral approach. Lactated Ringer solution, given as rapidly as possible in aliquots of 20 mL/kg, is the resuscitation fluid of choice. Generally speaking, if an infant requires more than three such aliquots (60 mL/kg) to restore adequate peripheral perfusion, a central venous line should probably be inserted for pressure monitoring, preferably in the critical care unit, to which the child should be admitted expeditiously. It is important to maintain a high index of suspicion for hypoglycemia in infants with gastroenteritis who have been unable to retain fluid or have been fed solutions deficient in sugar. Hypoglycemia is best treated expectantly by ensuring that the first bolus of crystalloid replacement fluid contains 5% dextrose.

One cause of diarrhea that is often overlooked is the "overflow" diarrhea associated with fecal impaction due to chronic constipation. Such cases typically affect the preschool-age child and are often associated with early and aggressive toilet training. Hospitalization is not infrequently required for manual and chemical disimpaction to break the cycle of abnormal bowel habits that have been acquired at home. This is especially true for the rare patient in whom fecal impaction is complicated by symptoms of partial distal large bowel obstruction.

A number of regimens are available to break the vicious cycle of fecal retention, chronic constipation, and painful defecation that may or may not be followed by overflow diarrhea. All begin with Fleet type enemas (no more than two at least 1 hour apart) and natural laxatives such as prune juice and dietary fiber. Stool softeners and cathartics such as mineral oil usually are not added until later in the course of treatment. All of these patients require careful long-term follow-up by a physician experienced in the management of such problems in children.

The etiology of constipation is functional in the overwhelming majority of cases. However, the diagnosis of Hirschprung's disease, or colonic aganglionosis, should be entertained in any infant presenting with chronic constipation with or without diarrhea, especially if there are signs of sepsis. It should also be considered in any constipated child in whom there has been a history of infrequent stooling from the time of birth. Hirschprung's disease can be fatal if it progresses to enterocolitis, but is virtually excluded by a history of encopresis (soiling, especially at night), which indicates that the internal sphincter is capable of involuntary relaxation.

GASTROINTESTINAL BLEEDING

Severe gastrointestinal bleeding is a rare phenomenon in children. Upper gastrointestinal bleeding is especially rare unless portal hypertension is present. The etiology of portal hypertension in childhood is usually related not to liver disease per se but rather to prehepatic portal venous obstruction. Thus the dismal outcome after massive variceal hemorrhage observed in adults is not characteristic in children. Every effort must therefore be made to resuscitate the child in hemorrhagic shock from variceal hemorrhage as expeditiously as possible.

Massive lower gastrointestinal bleeding in infants and children is also rare. When present, it is most often due to acid-peptic digestion of intestine adjacent to a Meckel diverticulum or intestinal duplication or, even more rarely, to colonic angiodysplasia. Anal fissure is probably the most common cause of rectal bleeding in young infants. Rectal bleeding is most often due to intussusception in older infants and to bacterial enterocolitis in preschool-age children. Inflammatory bowel diseases and juvenile polyps are the common sources of bleeding in school-age children.

Regardless of cause, the basic principles of hemorrhagic shock resuscitation should be followed whenever massive hemorrhage is present, as in the multiple trauma patient. These include rapid establishment of venous access and restoration of circulating blood volume by means of both crystalloid solutions and blood. If bleeding is chronic and/or intermittent, and if signs of inadequate peripheral perfusion are absent, the hematocrit should be measured, and diagnosis and treatment should proceed on either an inpatient or outpatient basis as appropriate. Diagnostic studies such as endoscopy generally should not be attempted in the emergency department but rather after admission. Likewise, studies such as nuclear bleeding scans or Meckel's diverticulum scans should not be performed unless the patient is admitted to the hospital.

FOREIGN BODIES

Most subcutaneous foreign bodies in children can be removed in the emergency department if they can be clearly felt and if the patient is of such an age that infiltrative anesthesia will be tolerated. Foreign bodies in the tracheobronchial tree or gastrointestinal tract are another matter. In the former, bronchoscopy will be required, emergently if there is ventilatory compromise. In the latter, treatment depends upon the type and location of the foreign body.

Generally speaking, foreign bodies of any type that enter the small bowel usually will pass spontaneously and should be allowed to do so. A possible exception is alkaline batteries. Information as to the specific treatment required may be obtained readily from the local poison control center, which maintains up-to-date information about the effects and proper treatment of all types of battery ingestions.

When an occasional foreign body fails to pass the esophagus even after an observation period of 4 to 6 hours or when symptoms of obstruction (ie, drooling, vomiting, or dysphagia) are present, esophagoscopy is usually required. In some centers, in lieu of esophagoscopy, smooth, round objects, such as marbles or coins, are removed under fluoroscopic guidance with a Foley catheter whose balloon has been filled with a radiopaque contrast agent. This procedure should only be attempted, however, if the operator is particularly skilled in this technique and if resuscitation equipment and personnel capable of emergency pediatric airway management are nearby, as there have been anecdotal reports of complete airway obstruction leading to death as a result of wedging of a foreign body below the vocal cords but above the cricoid ring. Sharp foreign bodies, and most batteries, that lie within reach of the flexible upper endoscope (ie, in the esophagus or stomach) should always be removed.

THE ACUTE GROIN AND SCROTUM

Acute conditions of the scrotum and its contents may present with pain, tenderness, swelling, or a mass. They are often confused with conditions arising from the groin proper (ie, hernia and/or hydrocele). The key to distinguishing between these two different but related types of problems is to palpate a normal spermatic cord just below the external inguinal ring (ie, at the level of the pubic tubercle) as the ipsilateral testis is gently pulled toward the contralateral knee. If the cord can be felt with certainty, symptoms and signs can be attributed safely to scrotal pathology. In practice, however, the differential diagnosis can be treacherous and, when in question, should be left to a surgeon with wide experience in the management of such problems in children.

The two main conditions of the groin that may present with an inguinal or inguinoscrotal mass are the inguinal (incomplete) and inguinoscrotal (complete) hernias, and communicating or noncommunicating (physiologic) hydroceles of the tunica vaginalis (testis) or processus vaginalis (spermatic cord). The two types of conditions have a common etiology: persistence of the processus vaginalis, which is a fingerlike projection of the peritoneal membrane that extends through the internal and external inguinal rings adjacent to the spermatic cord as it accompanies the testis to the bottom of the scrotum during the process of descent. The differences between these conditions are related only to the width and length of the processus vaginalis itself.

Narrow-necked processes that admit fluid but not intestine or ovary become hydroceles, and wide-necked processes become hernia sacs when intra-abdominal pressure exceeds the closing pressure of the internal inguinal ring and abdominal viscera extrude. This increase in pressure occurs during crying or a Valsalva maneuver (associated with coughing or stooling), allowing a loop of bowel, most commonly the distal ileum, or, more commonly in a girl, an ovary to enter the hernia sac.

So long as it can be easily and completely reduced by gentle direct finger pressure aimed retrograde through the external inguinal ring, and so long as there are no signs to suggest either incarceration or intestinal obstruction, a scrotal mass almost certainly represents a simple indirect inguinal hernia (direct and femoral hernias are extremely rare in children) that requires no immediate treatment save follow-up with a children's surgeon. Signs of incarceration include erythema, tenderness, and/or true edema of the overlying scrotal or inguinal skin (ie, a *peau d'orange* appearance). Intestinal obstruction should be suspected in the presence of abdominal distention, vomiting (particularly if bilious), and/or constipation. Of course, if the mass cannot be reduced with ease or if any of the signs described above are present, an incarcerated inguinal hernia must be suspected and managed as described above in the section on intestinal obstruction. The only exception to this rule occurs in the infant girl, in whom a freely mobile but irreducible mass with the size and shape of a lima bean is palpated in the groin. In this instance, although the mass is due to an incarcerated inguinal hernia, it is almost certainly an ovary that has become entrapped in the sac of the sliding type of inguinal hernia commonly encountered in infant girls. This condition requires urgent but not emergent repair because the viability of the ovary rarely is threatened.

Hydroceles in infants and children rarely require urgent surgical intervention. Although they are irreducible, they can be fairly reliably, but not conclusively, differentiated from incarcerated inguinal hernias. Hydroceles lack obstructive symptoms and are painless, nontender, and neither erythematous or edematous and can be readily transilluminated. It must be re-emphasized, however, that the key point in differentiating the hydrocele from the incarcerated inguinal hernia, especially if the hydrocele presents acutely or is a hydrocele of the spermatic cord, is palpation of at least a short length of normal spermatic cord between the external inguinal ring and the most cephalad portion of the cystic mass. If this cannot be felt, groin exploration should be performed on an emergent basis by a qualified surgeon experienced in the management of children. The threshold for groin exploration should also be low for hydroceles of the spermatic cord, even when incarcerated inguinal hernia has been ruled out, because these lesions are notorious for producing ischemic necrosis of the testis on rare occasions. Of course, under no circumstances whatever should a cystic inguinal or inguinoscrotal mass be aspirated for diagnosis in the emergency department. Incarcerated hernias occasionally are mistaken for hydroceles and are liable to subsequent perforation at the site of needle puncture, and the needle tract may be seeded in the unlikely event that the fluid that is drained proves to be a malignant effusion.

Most children with hernias and hydroceles will not require immediate surgical consultation. However, all children with testicular pain, tenderness, inflammation, or mass should be evaluated immediately by a properly qualified pediatric, general, or urologic surgeon experienced in the management of the acute scrotum in childhood. The diagnosis that obviously must be excluded is intravaginal testicular torsion (extravaginal torsion is a rare event that virtually never afflicts boys beyond the neonatal period). None of the signs commonly associated with torsion of testicular or epididymal appendages and/or epididymo-orchitis is reliable enough categorically to exclude torsion of the testis proper. Findings consistent with testicular torsion are a high-riding, transversely oriented, tender testis; increased tenderness with elevation of the testis; an absent cremasteric reflex; and absent testicular flow on nuclear scan. A diagnosis of testicular torsion mandates immediate scrotal exploration and bilateral orchidopexy if proven, due to the high incidence of bilaterality associated with anomalies of testicular fixation.

Epididymo-orchitis, which mimicks testicular torsion, is classically associated with a low-riding, vertically oriented, tender testis; decreased pain as the scrotum is elevated, known as Prehn's sign; and normal or increased testicular flow on nuclear scan. Torsion of the testicular and epididymal appendages (ie, the appendices testis and epididymis) can also mimic true testicular torsion as these conditions rarely present with the classic signs of pinpoint tenderness and/or the blue dot sign that is sometimes on transillumination or gross inspection. A good rule of thumb is that, if there is any question of testicular torsion, static and dynamic nuclear scans of the testes should be obtained. If these scans cannot be interpreted conclusively as normal, or if they cannot be obtained immediately (ie, within an hour or so of presentation to the emergency department), scrotal exploration should be performed along with bilateral orchidopexy if testicular torsion is found.

There are numerous other conditions of the inguinoscrotal region that may be confused with the diseases described above. In the groin, these usually will be due to inflammatory conditions such as suppurative or nonsuppurative lymphadenitis, although direct or femoral hernias occasionally will be encountered. In the scrotum, however, traumatic lesions, particularly traumatic hydroceles, and to a lesser extent neoplastic processes are the leading alternative diagnoses. These diagnostic entities are limited nearly exclusively to children of preschool age and older. Traumatic lesions of the scrotum in younger children often indicate child abuse. Neoplastic processes are rare, but any boy who presents with a scrotal mass that cannot be stated definitively to be a congenital or traumatic hydrocele, particularly if he is of preschool age or older, requires urgent sonography of the scrotal sac and immediate referral to a surgeon experienced in the management of diseases of the scrotum and its contents, including testicular and paratesticular tumors, in childhood.

REFERENCES

1. Rice DP, MacKenzie EJ, et al. *Cost of Injury in the United States: A Report to Congress*. San Francisco: Institute for Health and Aging, University of California, and Injury Prevention Center, The Johns Hopkins University, 1989.
2. DiScala C, Gans BM, Barlow B, et al. *National Pediatric Trauma Registry Biannual Report*. Boston: Tufts University Rehabilitation and Childhood Trauma Research and Training Center; 1990.
3. Barlow B, Niemirska M, Gandhi R. Ten years of experience with falls from a height in children. *J Pediatr Surg*. 1983;18:509–511.
4. Barlow B, Niemirska M, Gandhi R. Ten years' experience with pediatric gunshot wounds. *J Pediatr Surg*. 1982;17:927–932.
5. Rang M. *Children's Fractures*. 2nd ed. Philadelphia: Lippincott; 1983.
6. Cristoffel KK, Ranz R. Motor vehicle injury in childhood. *Pediatr Rev*. 1983;4:247–254.
7. Conry BG, Hall CM. Cervical spine fractures and rear car seat restraints. *Arch Dis Child*. 1987;62:1267–1268.
8. Fuchs S, Barthel MJ, Flannery AM, et al. Cervical spine fractures sustained by young children in forward-facing car seats. *Pediatrics*. 1989;84:348–354.
9. Agran PF, Dunkle DE, Winn DG. Injuries to a sample of seat belted children evaluated and treated in a hospital emergency department. *J Trauma*. 1987;27:58–64.
10. Newman KD, Bowman LM, Eichelberger MR. The lap belt complex: intestinal and lumbar spine injury in children. *J Trauma*. 1990;30:1133–1140.
11. Selbst SM, Alexander D, Ruddy R. Bicycle-related injuries. *Am J Dis Child*. 1987;141:140–144.
12. Sparnon AL, Ford WDA. Bicycle handlebar injuries in children. *J Pediatr Surg*. 1986;21:118–119.
13. Tepas JJ, DiScala C, Ramenofsky ML, et al. Mortality and head injury: the pediatric perspective. *J Pediatr Surg*. 1990;25:92–96.
14. Cooper A, Barlow B, DiScala C, et al. Mortality and truncal injury: the pediatric perspective. *J Pediatr Surg*. In press.

15. Bohn D, Armstrong A, Becker L, et al. Cervical spine injuries in children. *J Trauma.* 1990;30:463–469.
16. Bruce DA, Alavi A, Bilaniuk L, et al. Diffuse cerebral swelling following head injury in children: the syndrome of malignant brain edema. *J Neurosurg.* 1981;54:170–178.
17. Kewalramani LS, Kraus JF, Sterling HM. Acute spinal-cord lesions in a pediatric population: epidemiological and clinical features. *Paraplegia.* 1980;18:206–219.
18. Pang D, Pollack IF. Spinal cord injury without radiographic abnormality in children—the SCIWORA syndrome. *J Trauma.* 1989;29: 654–664.
19. Barlow B, Niemirska M, Gandhi R, et al. Response to injury in children with closed femur fractures. *J Trauma.* 1987;27:429–430.
20. Schwaitzberg SD, Bergman KS, Harris BH. A pediatric model of continuous hemorrhage. *J Pediatr Surg.* 1988;23:605–609.
21. American College of Surgeons Committee on Trauma. *Advanced Trauma Life Support Student Manual.* Chicago: American College of Surgeons; 1990.
22. American Academy of Pediatrics and American College of Emergency Physicians Joint Task Force on Advanced Pediatric Life Support. *Advanced Pediatric Life Support.* Dallas: American Academy of Pediatrics and American College of Emergency Physicians; 1989.
23. American Heart Association and American Academy of Pediatrics Working Group on Pediatric Resuscitation: *Textbook of Pediatric Advanced Life Support.* Dallas: American Heart Association; 1988.
24. McKoy C, Bell MJ. Preventable traumatic deaths in children. *J Pediatr Surg.* 1983;18:505–508.
25. Dykes EH, Spence LJ, Young JG, et al. Preventable pediatric trauma deaths in a metropolitan region. *J Pediatr Surg.* 1989;24:107–111.
26. Luten RC, Seidel JS, Lubitz DS, et al. A rapid method for estimating resuscitation drug doses from length in the pediatric age group. *Ann Emerg Med.* 1988;17:576–581.
27. Osborn HH, Kayen D, Horne H, et al. Excess ventilation with oxygen-powered resuscitators. *Am J Emerg Med.* 1984;2:408–413.
28. Cooper A, Foltin G, Tunik M. Airway control in the unconscious child trauma victim: description of a new maneuver. *Pediatr Emerg Care.* In press.
29. Herzenberg JE, Hensinger RN, Dedrick DK, et al. Emergency transport and positioning of young children who have an injury of the cervical spine. *J Bone Joint Surg Am.* 1989;71:15–22.
30. DelGuercio LRM, Feins NR, Cohn JD, et al. Comparison of blood flow during external and internal cardiac massage in man. *Circulation.* 1965;31(suppl 1):171–180.
31. Beaver BL, Colombani PM, Buck JR, et al. Efficacy of emergency room thoracotomy in pediatric trauma. *J Pediatr Surg.* 1987;22: 19–23.
32. Rothenberg SS, Moore EE, Moore FA, et al. Emergency department thoracotomy in children—a critical analysis. *J Trauma.* 1989;29: 1322–1325.
33. Glaeser PW, Losek JD. Emergency intraosseous infusions in children. *Am J Emerg Med.* 1986;4:34–36.
34. Rosetti VA, Thompson BM, Miller J, et al. Intraosseous infusion: an alternative route of pediatric intravascular access. *Ann Emerg Med.* 1985;14:885–888.
35. MacGregor DF, MacNab AJ. Intraosseous fluids in emergencies. *Pediatrics.* 1990;85:386–387.
36. Mattox KL, Bickell W, Pepe PE, et al. Prospective MAST study in 911 patients. *J Trauma.* 1989;29:1104–1112.
37. Cooper A, Barlow B, DiScala C, et al. Efficacy of MAST use in children who present in hypotensive shock. *J Trauma.* In press.
38. Garcia V, Eichelberger M, Ziegler M, et al. Use of military antishock trouser in a child. *J Pediatr Surg.* 1981;16:544–546.
39. Velasco AL, Delgado-Paredes C, Templeton J, et al. Intraosseous infusion of fluids in the initial management of hypovolemic shock in young subjects. *J Pediatr Surg.* 1991;26:4–8.
40. Cooper A, Floyd T, Barlow B, et al. Major blunt abdominal trauma due to child abuse. *J Trauma.* 1988;28:1483–1486.
41. Lieu TA, Fleisher GR, Mahboubi S, et al. Hematuria and clinical findings as indications for intravenous pyelography in pediatric blunt renal trauma. *Pediatrics.* 1988;82:216–222.
42. Fleisher GR. Prospective evaluation of selective criteria for imaging among children with suspected blunt renal trauma. *Pediatr Emerg Care.* 1989;5:8–11.
43. Oldham KT, Guice KS, Kaufman RA, et al. Blunt hepatic injury and elevated hepatic enzymes: a clinical correlation in children. *J Pediatr Surg.* 1984;19:457–461.
44. Hennes HM, Smith DS, Schneider K, et al. Elevated liver transaminase levels in children with blunt abdominal trauma: a predictor of liver injury. *Pediatrics.* 1990;86:87–90.
45. Kane NM, Cronan JJ, Dorfman GS, et al. Pediatric abdominal trauma: evaluation by computed tomography. *Pediatrics.* 1988;82:11–15.
46. Giacomantonio M, Filler RM, Rich RH. Blunt hepatic trauma in children: experience with operative and nonoperative management. *J Pediatr Surg.* 1984;19:519–522.
47. Pearl RH, Wesson DE, Spence LJ, et al. Splenic injury: a 5-year update with improved results and changing criteria for conservative management. *J Pediatr Surg.* 1989;24:121–125.
48. Karp MP, Jewett TC, Kuhn JP, et al. The impact of computed tomography scanning on the child with renal trauma. *J Pediatr Surg.* 1986;21: 617–623.
49. Haftel AJ, Lev R, Mahour GH, et al. Abdominal CT scanning in pediatric blunt trauma. *Ann Emerg Med.* 1988;17:684–689.
50. Gorenstein A, O'Jalpin D, Wesson DE, et al. Blunt injury to the pancreas in children: selective management based on ultrasound. *J Pediatr Surg.* 1987;22:1110–1116.
51. Taylor GA, Eichelberger MR, O'Donnel R, et al. Indications for computed tomography in children with blunt abdominal trauma. *Ann Surg.* 1991;213:212–218.
52. Harris BH, Morse TS, Weidenmier CH, et al. Radioisotope diagnosis of splenic trauma. *J Pediatr Surg.* 1977;12:385–389.
53. Howman-Giles R, Gilday DL, Venugopal S, et al. Splenic trauma—nonoperative management and long-term follow-up by scintiscan. *J Pediatr Surg.* 1978;13:121–128.
54. Kolihova E, Obenbergerova D, Apetaurova B. Total severance of the renal pedicle caused by blunt trauma in children. *Pediatr Radiol.* 1973;1:59–62.
55. Barlow B, Gandhi R. Renal artery thrombosis following blunt trauma. *J Trauma.* 1980;20:614–617.
56. Powell RW, Green JB, Ochsner MG, et al. Peritoneal lavage in pediatric patients sustaining blunt abdominal trauma: a reappraisal. *J Trauma.* 1987;27:6–10.
57. Rothenberg S, Moore EE, Marx JA, et al. Selective management of blunt abdominal trauma in children—the triage role of peritoneal lavage. *J Trauma.* 1987;27:1101–1106.
58. Cobb LM, Vinocur CD, Wagner CW, et al. Intestinal perforation due to blunt trauma in children in an era of increased nonoperative treatment. *J Trauma.* 1986;26:461–463.
59. Harris BH, Barlow BA, Ballantine TV, et al. American Pediatric Surgical Association: principles of pediatric trauma care. *J Pediatr Surg.* 1992;27:423–426.

60. Tepas JJ, Mollitt DL, Talbert JL, et al. The pediatric trauma score as a predictor of injury severity in the injured child. *J Pediatr Surg*. 1987; 22:14–18.
61. Field categorization of trauma patients (field triage). In: American College of Surgeons Committee on Trauma; ed. *Hospital and Prehospital Resources for Optimal Care of the Injured Patient*. Chicago: American College of Surgeons; 1986:15–18.
62. Champion HR, Sacco WJ, Carnazzo AJ, et al. Trauma score. *Crit Care Med*. 1981;9:672–676.
63. Pollack MM, Alexander SR, Clarke N, et al. Improved outcomes from tertiary center pediatric intensive care: a statewide comparison of tertiary and nontertiary facilities. *Crit Care Med*. 1991;19:150–159.
64. Nakayama DK, Copes WS, Sacco W. Differences in trauma care among pediatric and nonpediatric trauma centers. *J Pediatr Surg*. 1992;27:427–431.
65. Cooper A, Barlow B, DiScala C, et al. Efficacy of pediatric trauma care: results of a population-based study. *J Pediatr Surg*. In press.
66. Schaffer DJ. Clinical comparison of TAC anesthesia solutions with and without cocaine. *Ann Emerg Med*. 1985;14:1077–1081.
67. Cristoph RA, Buchanan L, Begalia K, et al. Pain reduction in local anesthetic administration through pH buffering. *Ann Emerg Med*. 1988;17:117–120.
68. Coren CV. Burn injuries in children. *Pediatr Ann*. 1987;16:328–339.
69. Crain EF, Gershel JC, Mezey AP. Caustic ingestions: symptoms as predictors of esophageal injury. *Am J Dis Child*. 1984;138:863–865.
70. Dolgin SE, Beck AR, Tartter PI. The risk of perforation when children with possible appendicitis are observed in the hospital. *Surg Gynecol Obstet*. 1992;175:320–324.

34. Upper Airway Obstruction

MICHAEL G. TUNIK, MD
GEORGE L. FOLTIN, MD

The upper airway in children is vulnerable to occlusion primarily because of its small caliber. To treat children with upper airway obstruction (UAO) in an appropriate and timely manner, the emergency physician requires a knowledge of upper airway anatomy and physiology, an understanding of the causes of UAO and their clinical presentations, as well as an approach to assessment and management.

The upper airway extends from the nasopharynx to the lower mainstem bronchus before its bifurcation. The small caliber of the airway of infants and young children results in greater baseline airway resistance. It is estimated that 1 mm of mucosal swelling of the airway in an infant will result in a 35% decrease in radius.[1] Any condition that causes further narrowing will have two effects. The first is a rise in airway resistance, which results in significantly increased work of breathing. The second effect is that agitation of the child results in turbulence and further increases resistance to the flow of air.[2]

In young infants, who are primarily nasal breathers, the presence of partial obstruction of the nasopharynx from mucosal swelling and secretions secondary to a simple upper respiratory infection may result in a significant increase in the work of breathing and present clinically as retractions. Gentle suctioning of the nasopharynx of these infants often results in a dramatic improvement in their respiratory status.

The tongue of infants and small children occupies a large percentage of the oropharynx. In the pediatric patient with an altered mental status and secondary loss of muscle tone, a high risk of UAO exists when the tongue falls posteriorly, occluding the oropharynx. This problem should guide the initial approach to airway management in the unconscious child. In these children, either the head tilt with chin lift or, when cervical spine injury is suspected, in-line cervical immobilization and a jaw thrust maneuver should be utilized initially to open and maintain the airway.[3]

Preschool-age and young school-age children frequently have enlarged tonsils and adenoids. These structures can be traumatized and may be a source of hemorrhage during procedures such as insertion of an oropharyngeal or nasopharyngeal airway or during intubation. Rarely do the tonsils and adenoids cause acute UAO. When other causes of obstruction of the upper airway in children occur concomitantly, enlarged lymphoid tissue will contribute to the degree of obstruction.

The trachea of young children is an easily distensible membranous tube composed of semiformed cartilaginous rings except for the cricoid ring, which is fully formed from birth and is the narrowest portion of the upper airway. Overextension of the head during airway maneuvers or a foreign body (FB) in the esophagus is sufficient to compress the soft trachea and cause obstruction.[4] FBs located in the airway often lodge at the cricoid ring.

The glottis is cephalad and virtually pharyngeal in location (at the level of the second and third cervical vertebrae). It is possible to view a normal epiglottis when one is examining the oropharynx of a young child. This anatomy results in an acute angle between the base of the tongue and the glottic opening. The pediatric airway is described, therefore, as being more anterior than that of the adult. This results in young children requiring a different head position during delivery of artificial ventilation and during orotracheal intubation.[5]

Table 34-1 Level of Obstruction by Clinical Findings

Level	IS	ES	DR	SD	MV	BC	NV	H	P
Oropharynx	+	−	+−	+	+	−	−	−	−
Nasopharynx	+	−	−	−	−	−	−	−	−
Supraglottic	+	+−	+	+	+	−	+−	+−	+
Glottic	+	+	+−	+−	−	−	+−	+−	−
Subglottic	+	+	−	−	−	+	−	−	−
Esophagus	+	−	+−	+	−	−	−	−	−

Abbreviations: IS, inspiratory stridor; ES, expiratory stridor; DR, drooling; SD, swallowing difficulty; MV, muffled voice; BC, barking cough; NV, no voice; H, hoarseness; P, position preference.

UAO that is chronic and slowly progressive such as that caused by adenoidal hypertrophy may be tolerated until almost total obstruction occurs. Chronic obstructive processes are often discovered when the child's airway is suddenly further occluded by an intercurrent infection.

Acute obstruction of the upper airway in the child is commonly due to FB or infection. Partial obstruction can present with increased work of breathing, usually on inspiration. This can manifest as accessory muscle use, inspiratory stridor, retractions, decreased breath sounds, tachypnea, and tachycardia. More severe obstruction may present with cyanosis, loss of consciousness, absent breath sounds, bradycardia, and eventually agonal breathing and apnea. Certain clinical findings may correlate with the level of the obstruction (Table 34-1).

Stridor or stridulous breathing is a sound made when narrowing of the upper airway from intrinsic or extrinsic causes results in the turbulent flow of air. It may be high or low pitched. When the obstruction is glottic or supraglottic, the stridor is noted primarily on inhalation. When the obstruction is subglottic, the stridor usually occurs during exhalation as well as inhalation. When the portion of the upper airway involved is located in the thorax, then stridor will be produced primarily on exhalation.

Children who present in respiratory distress with obvious inspiratory stridor may be agitated or quiet. In the early stages of airway obstruction the agitation may be due to anxiety over the airway compromise or hypoxia. Hypoxia and subsequent hypercarbia occur as obstruction worsens and are associated with lethargy and loss of consciousness. Critical to the management of these patients is the avoidance of further compromise of their already precarious status until a definitive airway procedure or therapy is provided. All other actions must be weighed against worsening the child's condition through agitation.

GENERAL PRINCIPLES

General principles need to be adhered to in the initial management of the conscious, partially obstructed child. Children who remain conscious and are exchanging air adequately may be kept with the parent, sitting in an upright position, while the parent provides humidified oxygen. It may be helpful to hold the oxygen tubing several inches away from the child's face or to place the end of the tubing through the bottom of a disposable cup and allow the child to "drink from the cup" rather than place a mask directly on the child's face. These maneuvers may help prevent agitation. Other interventions that are often performed automatically on an ill or injured child may be counterproductive in managing partial UAO. These include examining the ears, eyes, or oropharynx; measuring blood pressure; establishing an intravenous (IV) line; obtaining blood gases or other blood tests; and placing the child in a supine position. These procedures may cause agitation and should be avoided.

Children with UAO who have radiographic studies performed or are moved out of the emergency department (ED) (to the operating room or radiology suite) should always have a physician present who is properly equipped and skilled in advanced airway management.

SYMPTOM COMPLEX AND APPROACH TO THERAPY

Children rarely present with complete airway obstruction. When they present with complete UAO or rapidly progress to complete obstruction, optimal intervention requires a preset definitive plan of action, appropriate equipment, and a calm approach. Conscious children who are completely obstructed may present with the following symptoms: They cannot breathe, cough, cry, or speak, and their increased respiratory efforts (severe retractions and accessory muscle use) and agitation are followed quickly by lethargy and loss of consciousness. The clinician should be familiar with current standards for the management of acute airway obstruction in infants and children as contained within Pediatric Advanced Life Support and Advanced Pediatric Life Support curriculum.

SUDDEN UNEXPECTED STRIDOR

Foreign Bodies

FBs are a common cause of sudden UAO, with most of the events occurring in children younger than 5 years. Sixty-five percent of deaths occur in infants younger than 1 year. Common offending agents are foods such as frankfurters, grapes, nuts, and hard candies as well as small objects such as parts from small toys, marbles, coins, and balloons.[6,7] The vast majority of lethal FB aspirations (FBAs) and the nearly lethal events occur out of the reach of trained health professionals. This underscores the importance of prevention and the training of the lay public in strategies to deal with complete airway obstruction from FBs.

In most cases, the child has already expelled the object, or it has moved to a location in the airway that only causes partial obstruction at the time of presentation to an emergency service. A positive history for FBA or a significant history of symptoms associated with aspiration is highly predictive (80% to 95%) of aspiration. A negative history of FBA is poorly predictive and does not exclude the diagnosis.[2,7,8]

Children who present with a positive history of FBA or a history of sudden stridor, choking, coughing, gagging, hoarseness, or drooling should be aggressively evaluated for FBA. Evaluation may include anteroposterior and lateral views of the upper airway extending from the nasopharynx to the carina (include the entire chest and abdomen because FB ingestion/FBA may include multiple FBs). FBs may move and suddenly convert a partial airway obstruction to a complete one. Therefore, radiographs should not delay definitive management and must be performed only in the ED (or other area with appropriate equipment and personnel), where detection and management of worsening obstruction are immediately available. Most FBs are radiolucent, and radiographs may not be sensitive enough to detect all FBs or surrounding soft tissue swelling.[6–8] If an upper airway or esophageal FB is suspected clinically in the absence of or despite negative radiographic studies, then definitive management involves surgical consultation and endoscopic evaluation under general anesthesia.

Children with esophageal FBs may present with symptoms of UAO and swallowing difficulty.[4,8] Evaluation and management should proceed as for suspected laryngotracheal FBs. The usual locations for esophageal FBs are the cricopharyngeal junction, thoracic inlet, aortic arch, and gastroesophageal junction, the last of which is not associated with airway obstruction. In cases of severe obstruction due to an esophageal FB, basic life support airway clearing maneuvers may increase intra-abdominal pressure and move the FB out of the esophagus, relieving the tracheal compression. Endotracheal intubation should be utilized as the definitive procedure to bypass a complete tracheal obstruction due to compression and to obtain an airway. In cases of partial UAO, definitive therapy involves endoscopy and removal under general anesthesia. If airway obstruction is present, Foley balloon catheter removal of esophageal FBs should not be attempted because positioning and sedation may worsen the UAO. General principles of management should apply as the child with FB causing partial airway obstruction is being evaluated.

Spasmodic Croup

Spasmodic croup (SC) is a clinical variant of classic croup that may be associated with upper respiratory infection symptoms; fever is usually absent. The cause is controversial, but a hypersensitivity reaction or viral infection is frequently mentioned. The children are the same age as those with classic croup (3 months to 3 years) and may have a family history of SC. SC usually presents with sudden onset of brassy cough and stridor, predominantly at night.[9] These symptoms usually resolve after several hours without reported morbidity. The younger child who presents to an ED with sudden stridor may initially be evaluated for a potentially serious process (eg, FB) unless the history and response to therapy make this an unlikely diagnosis. Children with SC usually respond to humidification and a quiet environment, but racemic epinephrine (see Croup below) may be utilized if symptoms persist. Children whose symptoms resolve with humidification may be discharged from the ED if parental supervision is deemed adequate.

Anaphylaxis

Any of the structures of the upper airway of the child may swell as a result of acute angioneurotic edema, including the face, tongue, soft palate, and supraglottic structures (epiglottis and aryepiglottic folds); this will result in severe and rapid airway obstruction. Sudden onset, exposure to a sensitizing agent, and the presence of urticaria suggest the diagnosis of anaphylaxis. It is not uncommon for upper and lower airway obstruction to occur simultaneously.

When an allergic etiology for airway compromise is suspected, immediate treatment with epinephrine (1/1,000, 0.01 mg/kg = 0.01 mL/kg subcutaneously, intramuscularly, or intralingually) is indicated.[10] The drug should be given IV slowly as a medicated drip starting at 0.1 µg/kg/min and titrated; this is the optimal route and dosage for concomitant hypotension. Giving the drug at a 1:10,000 dilution (0.1 mL/kg to a maximum of 5 mL) rapidly IV may cause dysrhythmias. Medications including antihistamines (diphenhydramine, 1 to 2 mg/kg IV or intramuscularly) and corticosteroids (hydrocortisone, 4 to 8 mg/kg per dose IV) should be used as adjuncts. H-2 blockers should also be considered for anaphylaxis unresponsive to other measures.[38] In children with a rapid progression of UAO not relieved by epinephrine, preparations for endotracheal intubation should be made. The child should be intubated before complete obstruction of the airway occurs to avoid a situation where an emergent surgical airway may need to be provided. If the progression of the UAO is halted or reversed with epinephrine, patients should be observed in a pediatric intensive care unit (PICU) to detect any subsequent worsening of UAO that may occur.

Dystonic Reactions

Laryngospasm may be a prominent presenting symptom of a dystonic reaction complex that occurs as an extrapyramidal side effect associated with phenothiazine ingestions.[11] A common agent responsible for phenothiazine dystonia is trimethobenzamide (Tigan) rectal suppositories, which are used to control emesis. Children presenting with a history of drug contact and other dystonic signs (torticollis, oculogyric crisis, muscle rigidity, or inability to move an extremity) should be treated with IV diphenhydramine (1 to 2 mg/kg). When laryngospasm causes severe or complete UAO, appropriate airway maneuvers sufficient to obtain a patent airway should be utilized while diphenhydramine is being administered.

Toxic, Caustic, and Thermal Injuries

Inhalation of toxic substances, usually fumes or superheated air from a fire, may cause upper airway swelling and obstruction. The ingestion of caustic substances, such as lye in drain cleaners or crack cocaine,[12] may also cause upper airway damage and obstruction as acute life-threatening complications. Thermal injury from extremely hot liquids (milk heated in a microwave oven) taken through a bottle may also cause a thermal supraglottitis.[13,14] The history will in most cases be useful in determining the cause of the UAO.

Management of these entities depends on the degree of obstruction. With partial obstruction, complete obstruction is possible, and controlled intubation of the trachea may prevent the need for emergent intubation or surgical airway placement. With complete obstruction, therapy should include visualization, bag-valve-mask (BVM) ventilation, or orotracheal intubation, and if these fail a surgical airway should be inserted.

Physical evidence of lye and liquid thermal burns may not be seen in the oropharynx, yet esophageal and supraglottic damage may be present. Esophageal rupture may also occur with caustic ingestions. Although antibiotics and corticosteroids have been advocated, no compelling studies have proven their utility in the early management of thermal, caustic, or toxic upper airway damage.

Neck Trauma

Trauma to the neck is uncommon in young children. UAO may be caused by an expanding hematoma, recurrent laryngeal nerve damage and vocal cord paralysis, and direct injury to the cricoid and tracheal cartilage. A history of trauma and localized pain as well as signs of UAO and dysphonia may be present. Examination of the neck may reveal ecchymosis, swelling, tenderness, subcutaneous air, crepitus, and the absence of the normal contours of the cricoid and thyroid cartilages.[15]

Management of traumatic partial UAO obstruction includes cervical spine immobilization, emergent ENT consultation for flexible laryngoscopy, and determination of the nature and extent of any injuries. Severe or complete UAO should be managed with visualized orotracheal intubation (with in-line cervical immobilization), or if hematoma formation or disruption of the larynx, cricoid, or trachea make intubation impossible then a surgical airway should be obtained.

Hypocalcemic Tetany

Hypocalcemic tetany may be responsible for laryngospasm. Children who are at high risk for hypocalcemia include those with vitamin D deficiency (from inadequate diet, inadequate sun exposure, chronic renal failure, or gastrointestinal malabsorption), hypoproteinemia, acidosis, diuretic abuse, or phosphate loading. They may present with other symptoms or signs including vomiting, irritability, muscle weakness, hyperreflexia, positive Chvostek's and Trousseau's signs, and laboratory evidence of hypocalcemia.

Treatment for symptomatic hypocalcemia and partial UAO should include IV calcium gluconate at 50 to 100 mg/kg (10% calcium gluconate, 0.5 to 1.0 mL/kg) or calcium chloride at 10 to 20 mg/kg (10% calcium chloride, 0.1 to 0.2 mL/kg) over 3 to 5 minutes while the patient is on cardiac monitoring. If during infusion of calcium bradycardia occurs, the infusion rate should be decreased or the drug discontinued. Admission, monitoring, and evaluation for the cause of hypocalcemia are indicated in the PICU setting.

STRIDOR WITH FEVER

The majority of children who present to the ED with stridor do so because of an infectious etiology. Stridor with fever in a child or infant may represent a disease entity that can rapidly lead to complete obstruction of the upper airway. The specific entities that present with stridor and fever are viral laryngotracheitis (croup), supraglottitis, bacterial tracheitis, peritonsillar abscess, retropharyngeal abscess, and diphtheria.

In some cases the differentiation among croup, supraglottitis, and bacterial tracheitis may not be clear on clinical grounds alone.[16] This may occur especially in infants and toddlers. In cases where the child has a temperature greater than 39.4°C, has a toxic appearance, and/or has no brassy, barking cough, it may be prudent to follow the protocol for evaluation of supraglottitis. This means that the child should be accompanied at all times by an individual trained in advanced airway management with equipment for BVM ventilation, intubation, needle cricothyroidotomy, and cricothyroidotomy.

Radiographic studies may differentiate these entities, with the lateral soft tissue view of the neck being the most critical view to obtain. False-positive and false-negative results are possible on the lateral neck view of the epiglottis and aryepiglottic folds.[17] If clinical suspicion of supraglottitis is high, direct visualization is still necessary.

Supraglottitis (Epiglottitis)

Supraglottitis usually presents in older age children, frequently those from 2 to 6 years of age, with the peak age being 4 years. Supraglottitis, however, can occur in infants and adults as well.[18,19] The disease is usually caused by *Hemophilus influenzae* type B, but other pathogens as well as thermal or chemical burns of the glottic region may cause a similar pattern of obstruction. The usual pathology is a cellulitis that involves the epiglottis, aryepiglottic folds, and surrounding tissues. The disease is therefore more aptly named supraglottitis than epiglottitis. The incidence of supraglottitis is decreasing due to the introduction of HIB vaccinations in infants.

Children with supraglottitis classically present less than 12 hours from the onset of symptoms, which include high fever, a muffled (hot potato) voice, pain on swallowing or inability to swallow, inspiratory stridor, a toxic appearance, and occasionally drooling (10% to 20%). If the child is old enough to sit, he or she may be sitting upright in the tripod position (leaning back on the hands with the neck flexed forward, head extended, and mouth open). The child may be quiet and often cooperative and will appear anxious. The disease can present in a more subtle manner with low-grade fever and inspiratory stridor.

Supraglottitis is a true medical emergency because of the high potential for rapid progression to complete airway obstruction. Therefore, every ED should have a protocol (Table 34-2) in place to involve the appropriate ED personnel along with anesthesia and surgical subspecialists in the institution to perform surgical airway procedures in these children.

If supraglottitis is suspected clinically, the diagnosis should be confirmed in the operating room or equivalent area, where a team composed of senior physicians from the ED, anesthesia, and surgical subspecialties can secure the airway under controlled circumstances and make the diagnosis definitively by direct visualization. Conscious children suspected of having supraglottitis should be kept calm. This may be accomplished by having the child sit in a parent's lap. Oxygen may be offered by the parent but should not be forced if the child becomes agitated. Measurement of blood pressure and temperature, examination of the ears, placement of IV lines, blood drawing, and other painful procedures should be delayed until the airway is secured. Simply laying the child down may result in complete airway obstruction.

Experienced physicians may examine a cooperative older child who will voluntarily allow a visual inspection of the oropharynx. A large, swollen epiglottis may be noted at the base of the tongue. Under no circumstances should a tongue blade be inserted, and if the child becomes agitated during any visualization the examination should cease immediately. The inability to visualize the epiglottis in this manner does not rule out the diagnosis.

The emergency physician's primary goal is to trigger the supraglottitis protocol (Table 34-2), mobilize the team, and get the child to the operating room. The child should be accompanied at all times by a physician skilled at high-pressure BVM ventilation, intubation, and needle cri-

Table 34-2 Supraglottitis Treatment Protocol

Avoid agitation and allow the child to maintain a position of comfort (usually sitting in a parent's lap).
Prepare equipment for BVM ventilation, endotracheal intubation, needle cricothyroidotomy, and tracheostomy or cricothyroidotomy.
Call an expert in provision of a surgical airway and a senior anesthesiologist to the ED.
Prepare the operating room.
Accompany the child at all times with equipment and personnel.
If the child experiences sudden airway obstruction, high-pressure BVM is usually effective.
Attempt intubation if BVM fails.
As a last resort, perform needle cricothyroidotomy or other invasive airway procedures.
Take the child to the operating room and confirm the diagnosis visually.
Intubate (nasotracheal preferred) with a small tube to accommodate swelling.
Culture the supraglottic region.
Initiate antibiotic treatment after the airway is secured (ampicillin and chloramphenicol or a third-generation cephalosporin).
Keep the child sedated or paralyzed and consider splinting the arms at the elbows to prevent accidental extubation.
Transfer the child to the PICU.

---

cothyroidotomy who is carrying appropriate equipment. If the child with supraglottitis experiences respiratory arrest, the emergency physician is faced with a challenging airway management situation. These children can be successfully ventilated with a BVM and high pressure.[20,21] It is important to ensure that if the BVM has a pressure release (pop-off valve) it is disabled. Mouth-to-mask ventilation also allows the delivery of high airway pressures. The child's chest may actually have to be compressed to ensure an adequate exhalatory phase once high-pressure ventilations have been initiated.[22]

Intubation should be performed with an endotracheal tube one size smaller than calculated for the child's age or length to accommodate the supraglottic swelling. During intubation, visualization of the glottic opening may be difficult because of the swelling of the supraglottic structures. It may help to compress the chest while looking for air bubbles to reveal the location of the glottic opening.

If intubation attempts fail and high-pressure ventilation is unsuccessful, then a temporizing surgical procedure such as needle cricothyroidotomy may be life saving until a surgical airway (cricothyroidotomy or tracheostomy) can be established.

Croup

Laryngotracheitis (croup) is a respiratory infection that diffusely affects the upper respiratory tract. This entity accounts for 90% of stridor with fever. The subglottic region is most commonly affected, resulting in edematous, inflamed mucosa with a fibrinous exudate. Agents responsi-

Table 34-3 Etiology of Viral Croup

Parainfluenza types 1, 2, 3
Adenovirus
Influenza type B
Respiratory syncytial virus
Mycoplasma pneumoniae
Measles

Table 34-4 Croup Score

Score	0	1	2	3
Stridor	—	When agitated	At rest	Severe
Retraction	None	Mild	Moderate	Severe
Air movement	Normal	Mildly decreased	Moderately decreased	Severely decreased
Color	Normal	Normal	Normal	Cyanotic
Mental state	Normal	Restless when disturbed	Restless at rest	Lethargic

Combined score: ≤5, mild; 6–7, mild to moderate; 8–9, moderate; ≥10, severe. Any category with a score in one category of 3 = severe.

ble for croup are multiple (Table 34-3). The seasonal predominance (winter) is related to the epidemiology of the most common causative agents.[2,23]

Children ages 1 to 3 years are usually affected. They will present after several days of upper respiratory infection symptoms with inspiratory stridor that may only be apparent when the child is agitated or, when UAO is more severe, when the child is at rest. These children will often have a characteristic brassy or barking cough that is almost unique to croup. Low-grade fevers to 38.9°C are common in the course of the disease. Higher temperatures are possible but should stimulate the wary physician to consider carefully other diagnoses. The usual course of the disease is a worsening of symptoms for 3 to 5 days with subsequent resolution, which can take from a few days to several weeks. The vast majority of children tolerate this common disease without significant morbidity, but a small percentage go on to complete UAO.

The more ill a child appears during assessment in the ED, the greater the chance that he or she is at risk for airway obstruction. A number of croup scores have been developed that take into account a constellation of physical findings and allow the clinician to classify the severity of the subglottic obstruction as mild, moderate, or severe (Table 34-4).[24,25]

The most common presentation will be the child with mild croup, who may be treated as an outpatient if he or she is taking oral liquids and is well hydrated and if the physician is comfortable with parent reliability. Cool mist therapy may be suggested. A classic technique is to steam up the bathroom by running a hot shower. The parents can then sit with the child in this home version of a Turkish bath for no more than 5 to 10 minutes at a time. A car ride in the cool night air with the windows slightly open may result in improvement of the child's symptoms. Follow-up within 48 hours should always be arranged if the patient is discharged with instructions to the parents to return if symptoms worsen.

The patient with a mild to moderate croup score can be discharged if he or she improves with cool humidified oxygen therapy, if the parents are reliable, and if the child is older than 6 months. Patients with a moderate croup score (stridor at rest) are treated as inpatients in most institutions. The purpose of admission is to provide pharmacologic therapy and to observe the child who is at risk for progression to airway obstruction. The use of oxygen, cool mist, and racemic epinephrine delivered by nebulizer (Table 34-5) will usually result in symptomatic improvement of the patient for up to 2 hours.[26,27] It is important to remember that a child may experience a return to a pretreatment level of obstruction 1 to 2 hours after therapy. This phenomenon is inaccurately referred to as rebound. It is not the practice in many pediatric centers to discharge a child after treatment with racemic epinephrine. Racemic epinephrine is not believed to shorten the duration of illness. Although the theory is unproved, many believe that a child with severe croup can be successfully carried through the episode with racemic epinephrine therapy as often as every 20 minutes, thus avoiding the need for intubation. L-epinephrine may be substituted for racemic epinephrine (5 mg = 5.0 mL of 1:1000 epinephrine via nebulizer).[26] Corticosteroids in higher doses (Table 34-5) seem to be of benefit in preventing the progression of croup to complete obstruction and may shorten the duration of illness.[27,28] There seem to be no significant complications of use on a short-term basis. If corticosteroids are being considered (usually for the moderately or severely obstructed patient), they should be administered as soon as feasible.

If a child has a severe croup score (10 or higher or a 3 in any single category), it is prudent to admit that child to a PICU setting. Treatment with oxygen, mist, racemic epinephrine, and corticosteroids should be initiated as soon as possible in the ED.

Table 34-5 Drugs for Viral Croup

Drug	Dose	Peak Effect	Duration
Racemic epinephrine	0.5 mL of 2.25% solution in 2.5 mL normal saline	10–30 minutes	2 hours maximum
Dexamethasone	0.6 mg/kg per dose IV or intramuscularly q6 hours × 2		

Children should be intubated electively for respiratory failure (lethargy, inability to maintain respiratory efforts, Po_2 <70 mmHg on 100% oxygen, or Pco_2 >60 mmHg), but this decision is best made in the intensive care setting.[29] Children who develop severe UAO from this disease do not do so suddenly but rather progress gradually over time. If intubation must be performed in the ED, an endotracheal tube 1 mm smaller than that calculated for age or length should be utilized to accommodate the subglottic edema.

Bacterial Tracheitis

Bacterial tracheitis, also referred to as membranous tracheitis, is an infection of the subglottic region. There is controversy over whether this entity exists alone or whether it is a secondary bacterial colonization of a viral laryngotracheobronchitis. This entity occurs in the same age group as croup, but these children usually present with a toxic appearance and high fever. Pus may be produced during spasms of brassy or barking coughing. The stridor may occur during both inspiration and exhalation. These children do not usually splint their airway in a tripod position.[30]

Children with suspected bacterial tracheitis need to be managed as if they had supraglottitis because their airway is at risk for complete obstruction. It is not prudent to attempt to differentiate this entity from supraglottitis before obtaining a definitive airway in the operating room. Upon intubation, a normal epiglottis combined with the presence of pus, inflammation, and in some cases a pseudomembrane in the subglottic region confirms the diagnosis. Cultures most commonly grow *Staphylococcus aureus*, but *Streptococcus* species, *Hemophilus influenzae*, and *Pneumococcus* species are possible. Meticulous endotracheal tube suctioning in a PICU setting will usually maintain artificial airway patency.[30,31]

Retropharyngeal Abscess

Retropharyngeal abscesses are seen predominantly in children younger than 3 years secondary to suppurative cervical lymphadenopathy. Older children may present with this entity after penetrating trauma to the posterior oropharynx. Organisms most commonly implicated are group A β-hemolytic streptococci and *Staphylococcus aureus*. Symptoms include high fever, muffled voice, difficulty in swallowing, drooling, and, less frequently, inspiratory stridor.[32] The difficulty in swallowing and inability to handle secretions, as evidenced by drooling, are more frequent findings than actual upper airway compromise.

Retropharyngeal abscesses can present with meningismus and may be diagnosed initially as possible meningitis. The presentation may also mimic supraglottitis when inspiratory stridor is present. Therefore, it is acceptable to make this diagnosis in the operating room on direct visualization.

Clinically the diagnosis may be made by noting a swelling of the wall of the posterior pharynx. Given the overlap in presentation with supraglottitis, even if the diagnosis is suspected it is prudent first to obtain a lateral neck film that will demonstrate swelling of the prevertebral soft tissue at the level of the pharynx, a normal epiglottis, and normal aryepiglottic folds. Attempts to visualize the oral cavity and posterior pharyngeal wall may be made in an older cooperative child as long as agitation does not ensue.

Definitive therapy involves intraoperative drainage of the abscess after endotracheal intubation has secured the airway. Children with cellulitis but no collection of pus should be treated with antibiotics. Airway management for severe or complete UAO should include endotracheal intubation under direct visualization (to avoid rupture of the abscess). In children with partial airway obstruction who do not demonstrate signs of respiratory failure, meticulous observation with all equipment and personnel on hand to manage severe UAO (a PICU setting) is acceptable.[32,33] Antibiotics should be given for the common organisms (*Staphylococcus aureus*, *Streptococcus* species, and anaerobes).

Peritonsillar Abscess

This entity presents most commonly in adolescents, although it may be seen in children younger than 10 years. It is a severe case of group A β-hemolytic streptococcal tonsillitis resulting in a cellulitis or actual abscess formation in the peritonsillar tissues. Anaerobes and *Staphylococcus aureus* are the usual pathogens.

These young adults usually present with pain on swallowing or the inability to swallow, drooling, a muffled voice, and trismus due to spasm of the pterygoid muscles. Their usual problem is the inability adequately to hydrate themselves. Routine therapy consists of incision and drainage and admission for IV antibiotics.[34] For the rare child with severe airway obstruction, emergent incision and drainage may be performed by the emergency physician with an 18-gauge needle and large-bore suction with the child in the Trendelenburg position to avoid aspiration. Alternatively, severe UAO may be managed by first securing the airway by orotracheal intubation under direct visualization.

Diphtheria

Diphtheria is rarely diagnosed in the United States and Canada as a result of successful immunization programs. Diphtheria is caused by the phage-bearing, exotoxin-producing bacillus *Corynebacterium diphtheriae*; it is a localized inflammatory process with direct invasion and growth of the bacteria resulting in edema and necrosis of the epithelium with formation of a pseudomembrane. Occasionally, inflammation and necrosis of tissue result in dislodgement of the pseudomembrane, resulting in acute UAO.

The early clinical presentation is protean and includes symptoms of malaise, low-grade fever, poor appetite, and sore throat that progresses over several days. Myocarditis as manifested by dysrhythmias and poor contractility and neuritis presenting with paralysis of various cranial and peripheral nerves may also result from the exotoxin. A bull's-neck appearance from swollen anterior cervical lymph nodes may also be apparent. The formation of a pseudomembrane usually starts on the tonsils, palate, or larynx and may spread to other regions. Laryngeal spread is manifested by hoarseness, cough, and other signs that may mimic croup.

The diagnosis should be suspected on clinical grounds (especially with a history of absent immunization), and treatment with antitoxin and antibiotics (penicillin or erythromycin) should be started immediately. Cultures may delay diagnosis up to 24 hours, and Gram's stains are not reliable enough to be definitive.[35]

Severe UAO should be managed with endotracheal intubation; surgical airway procedures should be utilized as a last resort.

THE INFANT WITH STRIDOR

Infants who present to the ED with stridor will frequently have an infectious etiology such as viral croup or, less frequently, supraglottitis as the underlying cause. Occasionally FB may be responsible, and this diagnosis should be considered even in the young infant because older children may offer objects to their younger siblings. Congenital abnormalities of the upper airway (Table 34-6), gastroesophageal reflux, and trauma secondary to intubation[2,36,37] may present after initially being silent when a secondary event, such as a concomitant viral infection, worsens the degree of obstruction with mucosal edema and increased secretions.

Table 34-6 Congenital Causes of Stridor

Nasal
  Choanal atresia
Oral
  Large tongue, small mandible (Pierre Robin syndrome)
Glottic
  Laryngomalacia
  Trauma secondary to intubation
  Vocal cord paralysis
  Recurrent laryngeal nerve damage
  Neck or chest masses
  Brain stem compression
  Arnold-Chiari malformation
  Laryngeal web, cyst, tumor, hemangioma
Trachea
  Subglottic stenosis secondary to intubation
  Hemangioma, papilloma, other tumor
  Aberrant vessels, extrinsic compression
  Tracheomalacia

Table 34-7 Work-Up for the Infant with Stridor

Stabilization of respiratory status and airway
Direct visualization of the glottic opening
Visualization of the subglottis and trachea
Contrast study of the esophagus for external compression
Computed tomography of the chest for aberrant vessels
Angiography to delineate aberrant vessel anatomy
Head computed tomography to evaluate posterior fossa

After initial stabilization, these infants can be evaluated for the underlying cause of UAO if there has been no previous evidence of UAO. The rapidity of the evaluation is dependent on the severity of obstruction. If the infant has a previously diagnosed cause of stridor, attention typically is sought for them when an acute exacerbation of baseline inspiratory stridor occurs.

The most common pre-existing condition causing stridor in infants is laryngomalacia, a congenital pliancy of the laryngeal cartilage that is usually a benign, self-limited entity. The diagnosis may be suspected when stridor is present during crying and resolves when the infant is in the prone position. The child may outgrow this entity in the first 1 to 2 years of life, although tracheostomy may be required for severe cases that involve cyanosis, feeding difficulty, failure to thrive, and aspiration.

The emergency physician is faced with a difficult decision when trying to ascertain whether these infants are significantly compromised compared to baseline and require airway stabilizing maneuvers and/or admission and observation. It is useful to consult the physician who normally cares for these infants. If this consultation is not available, some indications for aggressive airway management include altered mental status, cyanosis or significant desaturation when not agitated (Pao_2 <70 mmHg) on room air, and history of apnea. The saturation determination requires the use of a pulse oximeter because arterial blood gases by their nature result in agitation.

Indications for admission and observation include a parental history of a significant increase in the frequency or severity of inspiratory stridor from baseline as well as associated irritability, difficulty feeding, or difficulty sleeping. The usual approach to the evaluation for the cause of subacute stridor in infants is outlined in Table 34-7.

REFERENCES

1. Holinger PH, Johnston KC. Factors responsible for laryngeal obstruction in infants. *JAMA*. 1950;143:1229–1232.
2. Kulberg A. A clinical approach to upper airway obstruction in infants and children. *Compr Ther*. 1982;8:55–67.
3. Cooper A, Foltin G, Tunik M. Airway control in the unconscious child trauma victim: description of a new maneuver. *Pediatr Emerg Care*. In press.
4. Schunk JE, Corneli H, Bolte R. Pediatric coin ingestions. *Am J Dis Child*. 1989;143:546–548.
5. Chameides L, ed. *Textbook of Pediatric Advanced Life Support*. Dallas: American Heart Association; 1987.

6. Rothman BF, Boekman CR. Foreign bodies in the larynx and tracheobronchial tree in children. A review of 225 cases. *Ann Otol Rhinol Laryngol*. 1980;89:434–436.
7. Kenna MA, Bluestone CD. Foreign bodies in the air and food passages. *Pediatr Rev*. 1988;10:25–30.
8. Losek JD. Diagnostic difficulties of foreign body aspiration in children. *Am J Emerg Med*. 1990;8:348–350.
9. Koren G, Frand M, Barzilay Z, et al. Corticosteroid treatment of laryngotracheitis V spasmodic croup in children. *Am J Dis Child*. 1983;137:941–944.
10. Sheffer AL. Anaphylaxis. *J Allergy Clin Immunol*. 1985;75:227–232.
11. Lee AS. Drug induced dystonic reactions. *JACEP*. 1977;8:367–371.
12. Kharasch S, Vinci R, Reece R. Esophagitis, epiglottitis and cocaine alkaloid ("crack"): "accidental" poisoning or child abuse. *Pediatrics*. 1990;86:117–119.
13. Kulick R, Selbst SM, Baker MD, et al. Thermal epiglottitis after swallowing hot beverages. *Pediatrics*. 1988;81:441–444.
14. Garland JS, Rice TB, Kelly KJ. Airway burns in an infant following aspiration of microwave-heated tea. *Chest*. 1986;90:621–622.
15. Myer CM, Orobello P, Cotton RT, et al. Blunt laryngeal trauma in children. *Laryngoscope*. 1987;97:1043–1048.
16. Mauro RD, Poole SR, Lockhart CH. Differentiation of epiglottitis from laryngotracheitis in the child with stridor. *Am J Dis Child*. 1988;142:679–682.
17. Stankiewicz JA, Bowes AK. Croup and epiglottitis: a radiologic study. *Laryngoscope*. 1985;95:1159–1160.
18. Singer JI, McCabe JB. Epiglottitis at the extremes of age. *Am J Emerg Med*. 1988;6:228–231.
19. Losek JD, Dewitz-Zink B, Melzer-Lange M, et al. Epiglottitis: comparison of signs and symptoms in children less than 2 years old and older. *Ann Emerg Med*. 1990;19:55–58.
20. Szold PD, Glicklich M. Children with epiglottitis can be bagged. *Clin Pediatr*. 1976;15:792–793.
21. Glicklich M, Cohen R, Jona JZ. Steroids and bag and mask ventilation in the treatment of acute epiglottitis. *J Pediatr Surg*. 1979;14:247–251.
22. Eastwood NB. Acute epiglottitis. *Lancet*. 1978;1:205. Letter.
23. Denny FD, Murphy TF, Clyde WA, et al. Croup: an 11 year study in pediatric practice. *Pediatrics*. 1983;71:871–876.
24. Tausig LM, Castro O, Beudray PH, et al. Treatment of laryngotracheobronchitis (croup): use of intermittent positive pressure breathing and racemic epinephrine. *Am J Dis Child*. 1975;129:790–793.
25. Fanconi S, Burger R, Maurer H, et al. Transcutaneous carbon dioxide pressure for monitoring patients with severe croup. *J Pediatr*. 1990;117:701–705.
26. Waisman Y, Klein BL, Boenning DA, et al. Prospective randomized double-blind study comparing L-epinephrine and racemic epinephrine aerosols in the treatment of laryngotracheobronchitis (croup). *Pediatrics*. 1992;89:302–306.
27. Kairys SW, Olmstead EM, O'Connor GT. Steroid treatment of laryngotracheitis: a meta analysis of the evidence from randomized trials. *Pediatrics*. 1989;83:683–693.
28. Super DM, Cartelli NA, Brooks LJ, et al. A prospective randomized double-blind study to evaluate the effect of dexamethasone in acute laryngotracheitis. *J Pediatr*. 1989;115:323–329.
29. McEniery J, Gillis J, Kilham H, et al. Review of intubation in severe laryngotracheobronchitis. *Pediatrics*. 1991;87:847–853.
30. Kasian GF, Bingham WT, Steinberg J, et al. Bacterial tracheitis in children. *Can Med Assoc J*. 1989;140:46–50.
31. Liston LS, Gehrz RC, Leighton G, et al. Bacterial tracheitis. *Am J Dis Child*. 1983;137:764–767.
32. Morrison JE, Pashley NR. Retropharyngeal abscess in children: a ten year review. *Pediatr Emerg Care*. 1988;4:9–11.
33. Thompson JW, Cohen SR, Reddix P. Retropharyngeal abscess in children: a retrospective and historical analysis. *Laryngoscope*. 1988;98:589–592.
34. Dodds B, Maniglia AJ. Peritonsillar and neck abscesses in the pediatric age group. *Laryngoscope*. 1988;98:956–959.
35. Feigin RD, Stechenberg BW. Diphtheria. In: Feigin RD, Cherry JD, eds. *Textbook of Pediatric Infectious Disease*. 3rd ed. Philadelphia: Saunders; 1987:1110–1115.
36. Gonzalez C, Reilly JS, Bluestone CD. Synchronous airway lesions in infancy. *Ann Otol Rhinol Laryngol*. 1987;96:77–80.
37. Nielson DW, Heldt GP, Tooley WH. Stridor and gastroesophageal reflux in infants. *Pediatrics*. 1990;85:1034–1039.
38. Yarbrough JA, Moffitt JE, Brown DA, et al. Cimetidine in the treatment of refractory anaphylaxis. *Ann Allergy*. 1989;63:235–238.

35. Lower Respiratory Tract Disorders in Children

ELISE W. VAN DER JAGT, MD, MPH

Acute respiratory emergencies in the pediatric patient are frightening to the child, the parents, and often to the staff. They are common and may result in significant morbidity and mortality, and they require calm, decisive, and deliberate intervention. Effective management is predicated on familiarity with the unique anatomic and physiologic characteristics of the respiratory tract in the growing infant and child, a knowledge of the most frequent types of airway problems encountered in children, an understanding of the pathophysiology of specific diseases and how they affect the pediatric host, and, most important, the ability accurately to assess the child. Although the differential diagnosis of lower respiratory tract emergencies is lengthy, the purpose of this chapter will be accomplished if the reader gains a clear, logical, and effective approach to the child in acute respiratory distress from lower airway disease or injury.

ANATOMY AND PHYSIOLOGY OF THE LOWER RESPIRATORY TRACT

The lower respiratory tract consists of all structures below the level of the midtrachea: bronchi, bronchioles, and alveoli. In the infant and child these structures are underdeveloped both functionally and anatomically, gradually maturing with growth. This immaturity is reflected in a decreased number of the vital structures necessary for good oxygenation and ventilation. There is less cartilaginous support of major airways, a smaller number of bronchioles and alveoli, a smaller pulmonary vascular bed, and fewer specialized cells required for respiratory function. In addition to this underdeveloped functional state, the small anatomic size of the structures predisposes the infant and child to major difficulty with any kind of illness that makes the airways even smaller. Narrowing of the airway by even a minimal amount increases airway resistance significantly and results in an enormous hindrance to effective oxygenation and ventilation. Besides the differences in the respiratory tract per se, the immature musculoskeletal and central nervous systems alter the effectiveness of the respiratory system. In infants, for example, the diaphragm is the primary muscle of respiration with little contribution from intercostal muscles. Abdominal distention will significantly interfere with diaphragmatic function and, therefore, with ventilation. The muscle fibers in the infantile diaphragm are also more prone to fatigue, resulting in a diminished respiratory reserve when stressed. Optimal air entry may be diminished even further because the compliant infant chest wall prevents adequate chest wall stabilization during inspiration. Finally, the respiratory center has been shown to be less sensitive to hypoxia during the first year of life, thus placing the infant at risk for an inadequate respiratory response. All these factors complicate the way the pediatric patient responds to respiratory illness/injury and must be considered in assessment and management.

PATHOPHYSIOLOGY OF DISEASE

Obstruction of the lower airway anywhere from the bronchi to the alveoli may result in an inability to oxygenate and/or ventilate. Such obstruction may be due to extrinsic compression of part of the airway, such as with a mediastinal mass, or it may result from an intrinsic obstruction, such as occurs with mucus, edema of the mucosa, bronchoconstriction, or excessive fluid in the alveolar spaces. Complete obstruction will result in atelectasis and intrapulmonary shunting. Incomplete obstruction may result in atelectasis and/or air trapping. Intrapulmonary shunting will lead to inadequate oxygen uptake and ultimately tissue hypoxia. Although the older infant and child will respond to hypoxia by increasing respiratory effort (rate and depth) to improve oxygenation, the younger infant may not do so and, in addition, may become bradycardic. The acidosis that results from lack of tissue oxygenation will increase pulmonary vascular resistance, further decreasing the ability to take up oxygen. Although metabolic acidosis will initially stimulate the respiratory center, thereby decreasing Pco_2 and producing a compensatory respiratory alkalosis, fatigue will rapidly intervene with corresponding respiratory depression and hypercarbia. In infants and children such a diminution of ventilation may occur quite abruptly and without warning.

Difficulty in ventilation is usually accompanied by difficulty in oxygenation. One must carefully determine, however, whether the primary problem is inability to oxygenate or inability to ventilate. Usually the young infant or child has an excellent ability to diminish Pco_2 by increasing the rate of breathing. Failure to ventilate adequately, especially in the absence of hypoxia, is due to ventilatory fatigue, respiratory depression, abnormality of the central nervous system (eg, central hypoventilation or metabolic/toxic encephalopathy), or the presence of a neuromuscular disease (eg, Duchenne's muscular dystrophy).

ETIOLOGY

Table 35-1 lists the major etiologies of diseases of the lower respiratory tract. Infections and reactive airway disease are by far the most common problems seen in the emergency department. Injury of the lung from external trauma, aspiration, burns and smoke inhalation, and the hypoxia of near-drowning may have significant mortality and may be complicated by adult respiratory distress syndrome.

There may be times when the primary problem is not underlying lung disease but rather excessive water from other causes. Cardiogenic and neurogenic pulmonary edema are conditions in which the etiology is quite different yet the treatment is somewhat similar [oxygen, decreased fluid intake, application of positive end-expiratory pressure (PEEP), and diuretics].

Of significant importance is the impingement of a mediastinal mass on the major airways. If the major airways (trachea or bronchi) are significantly narrowed, acute radiation therapy and steroids may be required to relieve the obstruction and restore adequate ventilation and oxygen. Intubation, particularly with the use of sedation or muscle relaxation, may actually result in acute airway collapse or obstruction in the effort to secure a safe and effective airway.[1] Extreme caution is to be exercised with these patients.

Table 35-1 Etiology of Lower Airway Emergencies

Infection
  Bronchiolitis
    Respiratory syncytial virus
    Parainfluenza
    Influenza
    Adenovirus
  Viral pneumonia
    Same as for bronchiolitis
  Bacterial pneumonia
    Streptococcus pneumoniae
    Hemophilus influenzae
    Staphylococcus aureus
    Group A streptococci
    Bordetella pertussis
    B parapertussis
    Mycobacterium tuberculosis
  Protozoal pneumonia
    Pneumocystis carinii
Reactive airways disease
  Asthma
  Anaphylaxis
  Bronchopulmonary dysplasia
Injury
  Foreign body/material aspiration
  Near-drowning
  Inhalation injury
  Pulmonary contusion/pneumothorax
  Gastroesophageal reflux
Increased lung water
  Cardiogenic pulmonary edema
  Neurogenic pulmonary edema
  Adult respiratory distress syndrome
Extrapulmonary fluid (pleural effusion)
  Empyema
  Hemothorax
  Chylothorax
  Tumor metastasis
  Nephrotic syndrome
  Inflammatory disease
Neoplastic processes
  Mediastinal mass
  Infiltrative tumor (lymphoma, leukemia)
Congenital/genetic disease
  Cystic fibrosis
  Congenital cysts
  Lung sequestration
Miscellaneous
  Spontaneous pneumothorax

Pleural effusions are usually associated with bacterial pneumonias. Small effusions are unlikely to result in significant respiratory distress, but large pleural effusions, which may be seen with group A streptococcal disease or staphylococcal pneumonia, may impede pulmonary function sufficiently to require rapid removal.

In the congenital/genetic category, cystic fibrosis is the most common, having an incidence of about one case per

2000 population. Exacerbations of the underlying lung disease occur frequently, and children may present with an increased cough, increased sputum, and increased respiratory failure. Complications include atelectasis, hemoptysis, pneumothorax, allergic aspergillosis, and cor pulmonale.

CLINICAL EVALUATION

Abnormalities of respiratory function are reflected by symptoms and signs ranging from subtle changes to obvious severe distress. Meticulous attention to detail during the child's clinical assessment should aid in anticipating any progressive deterioration so that proper therapy may be instituted in a timely fashion.

Respiratory distress occurs when an increased work of breathing is required to maintain the respiratory function necessary to meet the body's requirements. Respiratory failure occurs when respiratory effort cannot maintain adequate respiratory function, either oxygenation or ventilation. It is possible to have respiratory failure without evidence of respiratory distress (eg, neuromuscular disease) or to have respiratory distress without respiratory failure (eg, mild asthma).

1. Signs of increased respiratory effort (Table 35-2)
   - Tachypnea: Normal respiratory rates are shown in Table 35-3. Hypoxia and hypercarbia are sensed by the carotid which sends afferent stimuli to the respiratory center in the medulla. The resulting increase in respiratory rate is designed to restore oxygenation and ventilation to as normal as possible. Although tachypnea is frequently caused by hypoxia and hypercarbia, it may also be secondary to fever, metabolic acidosis, pain, and central nervous system disease.

Table 35-2 Signs of Increased Respiratory Effort

Tachypnea
Tachycardia
Use of accessory muscles
Grunting
Upright position
Anxious facial expression
Open mouth
Diaphoresis
Pulsus paradoxus

Table 35-3 Normal Respiratory Rates

Age Group	Breath/min
Newborn	<60
Infant	<40
Toddler	<30
Child/adolescent	<20

- Tachycardia: Tachycardia may occur for many reasons (fever, pain, heart failure, etc), including a decreased ability to deliver oxygen to the tissues (eg, anemia or hypoxia) or an increased oxygen requirement due to increased work of breathing.

- Use of accessory muscles: Intercostal, subcostal, substernal, suprasternal, and supraclavicular retractions as well as nasal flaring and sternocleidomastoid use all indicate significant distress.

- Grunting: A grunting sound at the end of expiration is commonly seen in infants with respiratory distress. By the infant's closing the glottis during the end of expiration, additional PEEP can be generated to prevent the alveoli from becoming atelectatic. Grunting in the pediatric patient should alert the clinician to the presence of moderate to severe respiratory distress.

- Position of comfort: The more respiratory distress is present, the more likely it is that the child will assume an upright position. This allows for easier expansion of the entire chest, easier depression of the diaphragm, and less impingement of abdominal contents on the thoracic cavity.

- Anxious facial expression: Widened eyes, raised eyebrows, or a furrowed brow suggest anxiety about the adequacy of breathing.

- Open mouth: An open mouth suggests air hunger or inability to breathe through the nose because of nasal obstruction. It also may be associated with an inability to swallow secretions (drooling) for fear of increasing respiratory distress.

- Diaphoresis: This usually indicates severe respiratory distress.

- Pulsus paradoxus: If excessive negative intrathoracic pressure needs to be generated to allow adequate inspiration, venous return increases, right ventricular volume increases, the intraventricular septum deviates to the left and impinges on left ventricular volume, pulmonary venous return to the left atrium decreases, and cardiac output drops. A pulsus paradoxus greater than 20 mmHg (normal, 0 to 10 mmHg) correlates well with severe respiratory distress.[2]

2. Signs of respiratory failure (Table 35-4): It is important that signs of respiratory failure be recognized early even in the absence of respiratory distress.
   - Cyanosis/pallor: Cyanosis occurs when there is an excessive amount of deoxygenated hemoglobin in the tissues. This could occur because of inadequate oxygenation in the lungs or because of inadequate oxygen delivery to the heart. Thus, although cyanosis and pallor can be due to respiratory failure, they may also be due to intracardiac shunting or

Table 35-4 Signs of Respiratory Failure

Cyanosis/pallor
Altered sensorium
Decreased/increased respiratory effort
Head bobbing
Bradycardia/hypotension
Hypercarbia/persistent hypoxia

---

inadequate cardiac output. In the latter case, the cyanosis tends to be peripheral rather than central.
- Altered sensorium: Somnolence may be due to hypercarbia and/or fatigue. In the infant, agitation, irritability, and failure to recognize the parents may be due to hypoxia.
- Decreased respiratory effort: A decrease in air entry, breath sounds, and respiratory rate may indicate significant fatigue and impending failure.
- Head bobbing: An exhausted young child will, during inspiration, flex the neck and let the head fall forward. This is due to contraction of the sternocleidomastoid and scalene musculature without counteractive movement of the posterior cervical chain. This sign is suggestive of imminent complete respiratory failure.
- Bradycardia/hypotension: Bradycardia is an ominous sign that often occurs secondary to hypoxia, particularly in young infants. Although it may also be due to vagal stimulation, hypoxia should be ruled out immediately.
- Abnormal arterial blood gases: An elevated P_{CO_2} and/or a decreasing P_{O_2} suggest failure of ventilation and oxygenation, particularly if abnormalities of respiratory rate are present (tachypnea or bradypnea).

3. Clues to specific etiologies
   - History: In the majority of children, a diagnosis can be made by taking a careful history. Evidence of the following should be sought:
     —Chronic pulmonary disease: asthma, bronchopulmonary dysplasia, cystic fibrosis, chronic aspiration
     —Allergies: may be the cause of bronchospasm
     —Injury: can cause pulmonary contusion/pneumothorax/hemothorax
     —Exposure to infectious diseases
     —Congenital heart disease: may result in pulmonary edema, congestive heart failure, increased risk of morbidity with certain infectious diseases
     —Gastroesophageal reflux: may cause recurrent wheezing from chronic aspiration or an acute sudden, unanticipated massive aspiration[3]
     —Sinusitis or symptoms thereof: may exacerbate wheezing in the asthmatic patient
     —Smoking/drug use: marijuana may cause bronchospasm; narcotic withdrawal may cause pulmonary edema; cocaine inhalation has been associated with pneumothorax/pneumomediastinum
   - Physical examination:
     —Temperature: mild elevations of temperature are common and nonspecific and are frequently secondary to dehydration; elevations to 39°C and higher may indicate infection
     —Rhonchi: indicate secretions in the larger airways
     —Wheezing: most commonly associated with reactive airways disease and bronchopulmonary dysplasia; unilateral wheezing is suggestive of foreign body aspiration or a localized impingement of the bronchus either extrinsically or intrinsically
     —Rales: connote bronchiolar/alveolar disease (pneumonia, bronchiolitis, asthma, pulmonary edema)
     —Asymmetric breath sounds: suggest atelectasis, pneumothorax, effusion
     —Cardiac examination (murmurs, increase in P_2, gallop rhythm): suggest evidence of congenital heart disease or myocarditis with congestive heart failure

LABORATORY EVALUATION

The purpose of laboratory testing is to confirm and refine the diagnosis that has been made after a history has been taken and an examination performed and to aid in determining the priorities of management. Laboratory tests that may prove useful are described below.

Pulse Oximetry

It is most important objectively and accurately to detect hypoxia. The advent of the pulse oximeter has greatly simplified this. A child with an oxygen saturation less than 90% to 92% should receive supplemental oxygen. Young children and infants do best with a flexible sensor, which can be wrapped around a finger or foot. There is an excellent correlation with oxygen saturations measured with a co-oximeter. Poor perfusion, methemoglobinemia, carbon monoxide poisoning, nail polish, and environmental light all interfere with oximetry.

Arterial Blood Gases

Measurement of P_{O_2}, P_{CO_2}, and pH in a sample of arterial blood is the gold standard for the assessment of adequate oxygenation and ventilation. In the infant and child the site most commonly sampled is the radial artery by means of a

23-gauge steel butterfly needle. A Po_2 less than 60 mmHg (oxygen saturation less than 90%) suggests significant hypoxia, and a pH less than 7.30 suggests significant acidosis. Interpretation of the Pco_2 must take into account both the respiratory rate and the underlying disease.

Capillary Blood Gases

In small infants it may be difficult to obtain an arterial blood sample. An arterialized capillary blood gas (CBG) may be used instead, as long as it is obtained in the proper manner. A foot or hand is warmed for 5 minutes with a warm wet compress. Puncture should be made on the medial or lateral distal aspect of the digit because it is here that the digital artery courses. The pH and Pco_2 are fairly reliable and may correlate well with arterial blood gases. A Po_2 less than 60 to 70 mmHg also correlates with arterial Po_2, but below 70 mmHg it cannot be relied on. Recently it has been noted that CBGs do not correlate as well with respiratory status as previously thought. If the CBG shows an excellent pH and Pco_2, it is probably reassuring.

Chest Radiographs

A chest film should be obtained only if one suspects a specific problem: pneumonia, cardiac disease, pneumothorax, lobar atelectasis, pleural effusion, foreign body aspiration (inspiratory and expiratory films), toxic aspiration, near-drowning, or unexplained or severe respiratory distress. It should not be obtained routinely in every asthmatic patient because the yield from this is low.

Complete Blood Count and Differential

A white cell count may be helpful in determining the presence of infection. An elevated white cell count without the presence of a left shift, however, can be seen in response to demargination from elevated circulating catecholamines. The presence of polycythemia may suggest chronic hypoxia. If there is anemia, oxygen carrying capacity will be low, and the child is at higher risk for tissue hypoxia.

Blood Cultures

Blood cultures are indicated when a bacterial process is suspected, even though the yield is low (<20% in bacterial pneumonia).

GENERAL MANAGEMENT

Oxygen

Humidified oxygen should be administered to all children who present with respiratory distress and/or respiratory failure. The application of a pulse oximeter can be a guide in determining the specific Fio_2 that should be given to maintain oxygen saturations of 95% or higher. Optimal methods of oxygen delivery depend on the size and cooperation of the child (Table 35-5). Infants do well with an Oxyhood (only the head should be covered), and an Fio_2 of 90% to 100% can be delivered in this manner. For older children, face masks are often adequate as long as they are tolerated. A plain face mask with a 6-L oxygen flow rate will allow for about 40% to 50% Fio_2. Partial rebreather masks have an attached oxygen reservoir bag out of which the patient inhales oxygen. Up to 70% Fio_2 can be achieved with this. A nonrebreather bag also has an oxygen reservoir bag attached, but no exhaled air enters it (one-way valve), and no air is entrained through the other ports of the mask. In this way 95% to 100% Fio_2 may be administered. If the child becomes anxious from the application of a face mask, the parent should be instructed to hold a hose of 100% humidified oxygen to the child's face. Anxiety may reflect a tenuous state of ventilation or oxygenation, however, and should be taken as a symptom of severe disease.

Table 35-5 Oxygen Administration

Device	Fio_2 (%)
Pediatric nasal prongs (1–4 L/min)	22–50
Pediatric face mask (6–8 L/min)	35–45
Partial rebreather mask/reservoir	35–75
Nonrebreather mask/reservoir	95
Oxyhood (use blender to control percentage)	22–95
Canopy tent	50

On occasion, a child will tolerate only a nasal cannula. These come in pediatric sizes, but the nasal prongs may still be irritating. Trimming the prongs down may improve tolerance. For an infant, flows of 0.5 to 1.0 L may be adequate; for older children, flows of 2 to 6 L should be given. The maximum Fio_2 attained is approximately 40% to 50%.

If the history suggests chronic hypercarbia from chronic pulmonary disease (usually coupled with chronic hypoxemia; eg, cystic fibrosis), it is prudent to keep the Po_2 in the low normal range (60 to 70 mmHg) because excessive oxygen may obliterate the hypoxic respiratory drive. These children depend on a mild degree of hypoxia to stimulate breathing because their carbon dioxide drive is absent.

Position

Most children will, and should be allowed to, position themselves in ways to minimize their work of breathing and maximize their oxygenation/ventilation. Usually this is a sitting position. Infants and children who are developmentally unable to position themselves should be positioned to allow for the least impingement on the thorax. In situations where gastric distention prevents adequate ventilation, the infant may be helped considerably by elevating the chest above the abdomen (30° reverse Trendelenburg).

Temperature

An elevated temperature increases the metabolic rate, increases the production of carbon dioxide, and increases oxygen requirements. It is appropriate to administer acetaminophen (15 mg/kg) for temperatures higher than 38.3°C to reduce the respiratory effort required to keep up with these needs. Defervescence may also allow for a more accurate assessment of respiratory distress without the compounding effect of temperature elevation.

Fluids

Respiratory distress usually results in an increase in insensible water loss (normal pulmonary loss, 10% to 15% of maintenance fluids). In addition, fluid intake is often decreased as the disease progresses. Dehydration may hamper the mobilization of secretions. It is therefore important to assess the state of hydration by evaluating capillary refill, urine output, moistness of mucous membranes, weight (loss), and blood urea nitrogen (elevated). Attempts should be made to give fluids to normalize and maintain the state of hydration but not to overhydrate. Depending on the specific disease process, overhydration may cause pulmonary edema and exacerbate respiratory distress.

Medications

Inhaled Bronchodilators

A trial of inhaled bronchodilator therapy is warranted for any child who exhibits signs of wheezing and/or prolonged expiration. With these drugs, deposition occurs directly in the areas that have disease, so that there are fewer systemic side effects. The majority of bronchodilators are β agonists, which act on the adrenergic system and result in both bronchodilation and pulmonary vasodilation. Depending on the degree of β_2 selectivity, the bronchodilator may also cause β_1 stimulation with concurrent side effects such as tachycardia. As with many adrenergic stimulators, tremors, vomiting, and agitation may occur. A list of the commonly available bronchodilators and their dosages is given in Table 35-6. It is best to choose the most specific and potent bronchodilator available. Albuterol is among the preferred agents because it is the most bronchoselective (β_2 selective) and potent. Although it is long acting, it can be given every 20 minutes without any documented untoward effects. In a child who has significant wheezing and poor air movement, it is safe to give continuous nebulizations of albuterol or terbutaline as long as heart rate is carefully monitored. Serious side effects are unusual, and the drug may obviate the need for intubation. Isoetharine and metaproterenol are bronchoselective and perhaps less potent. It is becoming evident that metered-dose inhaler puffs can be substituted for nebulizer therapy in children capable of coordinating puffs with their breaths or if a spacer is used.

Table 35-6 Bronchodilators*

Drug	Dosage
Albuterol (0.5%)	0.5 mL in 2.5 mL normal saline q20 minutes continuously (may increase to 1 mL)
Terbutaline (1 mg/mL)	0.5 mL in 2.5 mL normal saline q20 minutes continuously (may increase to 1 mL)
Metaproterenol (5%)	0.4 mL in 2.5 mL normal saline q20 minutes
Isoetharine (1%)	0.5 mL in 2.5 mL normal saline q20 minutes

*Arranged from most β_2 selective and potent to least β_2 selective and potent.

Theophylline

Theophylline is a phosphodiesterase inhibitor that has multiple actions. It appears to cause direct bronchodilation, increased diaphragmatic contractility, stimulation of the respiratory center, and mild diuresis. The side effects may be considerable: agitation, tachycardia and dysrhythmia (at blood levels greater than 60 μg/dL), gastrointestinal disturbances, and seizures. Because the therapeutic range lies so close to the toxic range, careful attention must be given to proper dosing. Clearance of the drug is age dependent and is often altered by disease and the presence of other drugs. A loading dose of 5 to 6 mg/kg theophylline (6 to 7 mg/kg of aminophylline) should be given intravenously over 20 minutes and followed immediately by a continuous infusion (Table 35-6). As a rule, for every milligram of theophylline given per kilogram body weight, a rise in the serum level of 2 μg/dL will occur. Because the volume of distribution may vary considerably from child to child, however, a postbolus level should be obtained. If this level is not in the therapeutic range (10 to 20 μg/dL), another bolus should be given on the basis of the known volume of distribution. Additional blood levels should be obtained at steady state (four to five half-lives, about 15 hours) if the child does well or if one suspects theophylline toxicity.

Isoproterenol

Isoproterenol is a potent, pure β agent that has prominent β_1 and β_2 effects, thus resulting in bronchodilation, vasodilation, and an increase in cardiac work (increased chronotropy, inotropy, and dromotropy). It can be used intravenously in those children who would otherwise require intubation and ventilation for severe bronchospasm. Administration of this drug should always be accompanied by the insertion of an arterial line for blood pressure monitoring and by serial cardiac tracings to detect any evidence of ischemia. The starting dosage is 0.05 μg/kg/min and may be increased as long as the heart rate does not exceed 200 beat/min in children and 180 beat/min in adolescents and as long as there is no sign of hypotension or ischemia.

Steroids

Steroids should be considered in reactive airways disease not responding quickly to inhalation treatment. They may also be of some help in adult respiratory distress syndrome. Methylprednisolone at 1 mg/kg intravenously every 6 hours is appropriate, but hydrocortisone as well as dexamethasone have been used.

Diuretics

The use of diuretics should be considered in cardiogenic pulmonary edema, bronchopulmonary dysplasia, adult respiratory distress syndrome, postobstructive pulmonary edema, and neurogenic pulmonary edema. Furosemide is commonly used because it is potent and rapid acting and may have a direct salutary effect on pulmonary tissue. The usual dose is 1 mg/kg intravenously or 2 mg/kg orally.

Antibiotics

Antibiotics should be used when a bacterial infection is strongly suspected. The antibiotics should have as narrow a spectrum as possible so that no resistant organisms develop. Prophylactic antibiotics to prevent pulmonary infection are seldom indicated except in patients with neoplasia, in whom trimethoprim-sulfamethoxazole has been shown to decrease infection with *Pneumocystis carinii*.

Endotracheal Intubation/Mechanical Ventilation

Although the need to intubate and mechanically ventilate a child may not always be clear cut and should be decided on an individual basis, the following should be considered strong indications for this procedure:

- Po_2 <60 mmHg if Fio_2 <60%
- Pco_2 ≥55 mmHg or rising >5 mmHg/hour with pH <7.30
- increasing respiratory distress (and thus increasing chance of fatigue)
- increasing signs of respiratory failure

To avoid hypoxia, aspiration, tissue injury, and psychologic trauma during the intubating procedure, the intubation should be performed by an experienced physician in a controlled fashion with proper sedation, a vagolytic, muscle relaxation, and appropriately sized equipment. A pulse oximeter should be in place and the stomach emptied by nasogastric tube before the procedure begins. Blind nasotracheal intubation is not recommended in the child because good cooperation is required and because the pediatric larynx is more anterior than in the adult larynx.

Once the child is intubated, mechanical ventilation may be initiated as follows:

1. for children weighing 10 kg or less:
   - ventilator: time-cycled, pressure-limited (eg, Sechrist)
   - initial settings:
     peak inspiratory pressure, 25 cmH$_2$O
     PEEP, 3 to 5 cmH$_2$O
     Fio$_2$, 100%
     rate, 20/min to 30/min
     inspiratory time, 0.5 to 0.6 second
   - mode, intermittent mandatory ventilation
2. for children weighing more than 10 kg:
   - ventilator: volume-cycled (eg, Bear Cub, Siemens Servo 900C)
   - initial settings:
     tidal volume, 12 to 15 mL/kg
     PEEP, 3 to 5 cmH$_2$O
     Fio$_2$, 100%
     rate, 20/min
     inspiratory time, 0.6 to 0.75 second
   - mode, synchronized intermittent mandatory ventilation

The child should be observed carefully for adequate or excessive chest rise, good breath sounds peripherally, adequacy of expiratory time (especially if the child has bronchospasm), and good color. The pulse oximeter should be helpful in denoting oxygen saturations less than 95%. An arterial blood gas should be obtained to assess for adequacy of oxygenation and ventilation or the need for hyperventilation to compensate for a metabolic acidosis. If ventilation is inadequate, the rate should be increased unless it becomes obvious that there is an insufficient chest rise (tidal volume); in this case, either the pressure limit on the time-cycled ventilator or the tidal volume on the volume-cycled ventilator should be increased. If oxygenation is inadequate, PEEP should be increased in increments of 2 cmH$_2$O with a reassessment (preferably by arterial blood gas) about 10 to 15 minutes after every change. If oxygenation and ventilation appear to be adequate but the child is agitated, sedation and muscle paralysis may be required to improve the efficiency and safety of ventilation and to decrease the probability of accidental extubation.

ASTHMA

An acute exacerbation of asthma is one of the most common respiratory emergencies seen in pediatrics and may have significant associated morbidity. The disease is characterized by bronchospasm, increased production of bronchial mucus, and increased edema of the airways. It is a chronic disease with acute exacerbations whose etiology is multifactorial, including genetic and environmental contributions. A respiratory tract infection is often the precipitating factor (75% of asthma admissions), but allergies and emotional factors may induce an acute attack as well. Of concern is the fact that the prevalence of asthma has increased over the past two decades (now about 7% of all children), as have hospitalization rates and mortality.[4] Although some of this may be due to a delay in seeking appropriate medical care (secondary to excessive home treatment), many of the factors responsible for this increase are not known.

Pathophysiology

The combination of bronchospasm, excessive mucus production, and edema results in airway obstruction. Airway obstruction leads to variable areas of atelectasis and air trapping because narrowed or occluded airways cause an inability to exhale air fully. Increased effort and anxiety exacerbate the process with more air trapping and hypoxia. Extremely high negative intrathoracic pressures can be generated during inspiration in an effort to open the airways. Increased venous return, pulmonary vascular congestion with pulmonary edema, increased cardiac afterload, and decreased cardiac output result. A prominent pulsus paradoxus is an associated physical finding. Markedly high positive pressures can occur within the airways during exhalation, which in combination with severe air trapping may result in pneumomediastinum or pneumothorax. As the acute episode progresses, hypoxia, metabolic acidosis, and eventual respiratory acidosis occur. Failure to intervene quickly will result in complete decompensation and death.

Clinical Evaluation

History

A brief history should be elicited and should include the number, times, and severity of previous episodes of wheezing (history of intensive care unit admission and intubation). A history of even one episode of respiratory failure places the child in a higher risk group for repeated episodes of respiratory failure.[5] Inquiry should be made as to the presence of underlying pulmonary disease such as bronchopulmonary dysplasia and about all current medications. Particular attention should be paid to the therapies that have been tried at home for this acute episode and to any history of theophylline use (see below).

Physical Examination

Frequent, repeated assessments should be done both to note deterioration and to guide therapy. Characteristically the child is sitting up and in clear respiratory distress, although often verbally minimizing his or her degree of distress. Tachypnea, tachycardia, and increased use of accessory muscles are usually evident. Nasal flaring together with intercostal, subcostal, substernal, and supraclavicular retractions can all be seen in various degrees. Retractions involving the sternocleidomastoid and supraclavicular muscle groups has been correlated with severe distress.[6] The chest is hyperresonant and in the chronic asthmatic child may even be barrel shaped. Careful note should be made of the ability to hear air enter and exit with appropriate expansion of the chest. Failure to hear good air exchange suggests extreme compromise. Somewhat asymmetric breath sounds are not uncommon and probably are due to atelectasis. Striking asymmetry may be suggestive of pneumothorax, however, and should be investigated further. On auscultation, it is well to remember how the severity of disease is reflected in the sounds one hears (Table 35-7).

In the older child, inability to speak in sentences is a helpful measure of severity of illness, as is the inability to cry for the infant. The infant may exhibit grunting at the end of expiration, which is a physiologic attempt to maintain the patency of the airways during expiration. If the child can cooperate, usually by age 6 to 7 years, a peak flow rate should be obtained with a peak flow meter. The effect of emergency department management can then be noted as a change from the measured baseline. If the child has not recovered at least 60% of predicted peak flow after therapy, he or she will probably need to be hospitalized. The absence of cyanosis does not exclude significant hypoxia because cyanosis does not occur until the oxygen saturation is 75% to 80% (Po_2, 40 mmHg) or even lower in the presence of anemia.

The temperature may be mildly elevated (up to 39°C) as a result of dehydration or a concomitant infectious process. Diaphoresis connotes severe respiratory effort rather than fever and portends imminent fulminant respiratory failure. Sensorium changes are common, ranging from anxiety and

Table 35-7 Correlation of Asthma Severity and Auscultation Findings

Severity	Auscultatory Sounds
Minimal	Prolonged expiration with normal air entry
Mild	Prolonged expiration, expiratory wheezing, normal air entry
Moderate	Prolonged expiration, expiratory and inspiratory wheezing, decreased air entry
Severe	Decreased expiratory and inspiratory sounds, minimal to no wheezing, inaudible air entry/exit

agitation (possibly due to hypoxia) to sleepiness (suggestive of hypercarbia).

If the diagnosis of asthma is questionable, physical signs suggestive of allergies can be supportive. Allergies, shiners, chronic clear rhinorrhea, Dennie's lines on the lower eyelid, and eczema may all be suggestive.

Laboratory Evaluation

Pulse oximetry should be applied to all patients to ascertain the degree of initial hypoxia and the adequacy of the oxygen being given. A chest radiograph is not routinely indicated and has not been shown to alter management in the large majority of patients.[7] It should be obtained if one suspects a pneumothorax or significant atelectasis, however, or if there is continued deterioration. Lobar pneumonia is uncommonly seen in status asthmaticus. A cell count and differential need not be done routinely because these rarely give information that will alter management. The white cell count may be elevated because of the demarginating effect of circulating catecholamines. Indications for obtaining a cell count include suspicion of a bacterial infection or the presence of anemia. Eosinophilia may support the diagnosis of asthma. An arterial blood gas should be done on any patient who is ill enough to be admitted or who is not responding to therapy. Ordinarily, the child with mild asthma has a low P_{CO_2} reflecting tachypnea. As less air exchange occurs, the P_{CO_2} will rise first to normal and then to higher than normal values. A normal P_{CO_2} in the face of tachypnea and increased respiratory effort is of major concern and may be evidence of early respiratory failure.

Management

Administer oxygen at a minimum F_{IO_2} of 40% to any child with respiratory distress. Follow the adequacy of oxygenation with a pulse oximeter and/or with blood gas measurements. An inhaled bronchodilator should be given every 15 to 20 minutes, with respiratory reassessment being performed after each to determine patient response. A flow sheet should be kept to monitor blood pressure, heart rate, respiratory rate, degree of retractions, inspiratory and expiratory wheezing, and pulsus paradoxicus. Although albuterol is probably best because of its high β_2 selectivity and high potency, other bronchodilators may be used (see above). Nebulized terbutaline is as effective as albuterol but is more expensive because it is used as an intravenous solution. There is no separate aerosolizable solution of terbutaline available in the United States.

Although subcutaneous epinephrine (1:1000) at 0.01 mL/kg has been the traditional treatment and is still used in many offices that do not have nebulizing capability, aerosolized bronchodilators are currently the treatment of choice. They have been shown to be as effective as epinephrine even in the child with minimal air entry and do not have the systemic side effects associated with epinephrine. In addition, the epinephrine injection is painful, whereas the aerosolized treatment is usually well tolerated.

Table 35-8 Aminophylline Dosage

Age of Patient	Dosage (mg/kg/hour)
<6 months	$\left[\dfrac{0.3 \times \text{age (in weeks)} + 8}{24}\right] \times 1.2$
6 months–9 years	1.1
>9 years	0.9

If there is minimal improvement after two bronchodilator treatments, or if the child is in extremis, an intravenous line should be placed, a theophylline level drawn (if the child has received theophylline previously), and the following given:

- methylprednisolone (Solu-Medrol), 1 mg/kg every 6 hours intravenously (initial dose of 2 mg/kg)
- continuous intravenous aminophylline infusion at the appropriate dosage (Table 35-8)
- aminophylline bolus of 6 mg/kg (theophylline, 5 mg/kg) if no previous theophylline received (if patient has received short-acting theophylline in the previous 6 hours or long-acting theophylline in the previous 12 hours, await level before giving a bolus; if levels are not readily available, give half the loading dose)
- fluids at 1.0 to 1.5 times maintenance to maintain adequate hydration

Many children will respond to two to three inhaled bronchodilator treatments, 2 to 4 hours of aminophylline, and one dose of methylprednisolone. Although these children may be discharged to home, some ongoing therapy should be started because the factors precipitating the acute attack are likely to be present for a number of days, particularly if those factors are infectious or environmental in nature. For children who are on no medications, a long-acting inhaled bronchodilator should be prescribed (albuterol or metaproterenol) for 10 days to 2 weeks. Preferably, the patient should be taught how to use the inhaler in the emergency department. If it is doubtful that the child will be able to cooperate (children younger than 5 years may have difficulty with the motor skills required with an inhaler, although the addition of a spacer may circumvent this problem) or that the parents will comply, an oral preparation of albuterol or metaproterenol should be prescribed. It should be impressed on parents that failure of the child to take the medication may result in another asthma attack. If the child is already on some antiasthmatic therapy, he or she should be given additional medication for 1 to 2 weeks. This may be oral theophylline (16 mg/kg/day for short-acting theophylline) or a short course of steroids. Therapeutic theophylline levels are attained more quickly with short-acting theophylline during the first 24 hours of treatment than with the longer-acting preparation. Prednisone at 2 mg/kg/day up to 60 mg/day divided into two daily doses for 5 to 7 days has been shown to be helpful in preventing a relapse.

If there is no response to these interventions after 2 to 3 hours, the child will need to be admitted for ongoing therapy. If there is continued deterioration in spite of therapy, the child should be aggressively treated with continuously nebulized treatments of albuterol or terbutaline.[8,9] Although some tachycardia may be seen, there are few side effects with this therapy. The same cannot be done with isoetharine or metaproterenol because nausea and vomiting, tremulousness, and tachycardia quickly supervene. Serial arterial blood gases should be obtained and serial pulsus paradoxus measured, and if these show evidence of worsening in spite of therapy the child should be placed on a cardiac monitor and a continuous isoproterenol infusion begun at 0.05 µg/kg/min.[10]

Concomitantly, an arterial line should be placed to monitor blood pressure and to obtain frequent arterial blood gases for evidence of improvement. Isoproterenol may cause hypotension as a result of its potent β effects, particularly if the patient is somewhat dehydrated. Tachycardia is common, and myocardial ischemia (as reflected by ST segment elevation and elevation of myocardial enzymes) may occur; most children will tolerate heart rates up to 200 beat/min (adolescents, up to 180 beat/min) relatively well. A baseline electrocardiogram should be obtained to assess for any evidence of ischemic changes later. The child should be transferred as soon as possible to the pediatric intensive care unit for ongoing monitoring and care. Isoproterenol can be increased by 0.1 µg/kg/min every 15 minutes as necessary until the P_{CO_2} has normalized, provided that maximal heart rates have not been exceeded and that there is no evidence of myocardial ischemia or hypotension.

On occasion, a child may arrive who is in such a serious degree of respiratory failure that intubation and mechanical ventilation should be initiated at once. The intubation should proceed with appropriate sedation and muscle relaxation. A volume ventilator should be used with starting tidal volumes of 12 to 15 mL/kg and relatively low rates to allow for adequate expiratory time. It is prudent to set an upper limit on inspiratory pressure (eg, 50 cmH_2O) to avoid the complications of pneumothorax even though the P_{CO_2} will become somewhat elevated. As long as the child is not hypoxic and pH is greater than 7.30, a slightly elevated P_{CO_2} will be well tolerated.

BRONCHIOLITIS

Bronchiolitis is an infectious inflammatory disease that affects predominantly the lower respiratory tract, including the bronchioles and alveoli. It is most commonly caused by respiratory syncytial virus (RSV) but may be due to parainfluenza virus, influenza virus, adenovirus, and others. Adenovirus has been associated with a severe necrotizing form of bronchiolitis called bronchiolitis obliterans. Bronchiolitis is characteristically seen in children younger than 18 months and occurs most commonly in early winter to midwinter (RSV season). The disease may range from a mild form not unlike the common cold to a severe form resulting in respiratory failure and death. Children with congenital heart disease,[11] bronchopulmonary dysplasia,[12] chronic underlying respiratory disease, and compromised immune function[13] are at highest risk for severe morbidity and mortality.

Pathophysiology

The severe inflammatory response to the infectious agent results in necrosis of the respiratory epithelium, mucosal edema, increased mucus production, and probably some bronchospasm in selected patients. There is resultant plugging, obstruction, and air trapping. Hypoxia and respiratory distress occur secondary to intrapulmonary shunting and difficulty in ventilation. RSV is shed from the respiratory tract, particularly from the conjunctivae and in respiratory secretions. The disease is spread by fomites and, if proper precautions are not taken, can be a major source of nosocomial infections.

Clinical Evaluation

It may be difficult to distinguish bronchiolitis from status asthmaticus. Both may present during the first year of life (20% of asthmatics); both may be associated with low-grade fever, wheeziness, rales, respiratory distress, and hypoxia; and both may have physical signs and symptoms related to the upper respiratory tract. The only information that may be helpful is that history of a previous episode may make reactive airways disease or asthma more likely, as does the occurrence of an episode outside RSV and parainfluenza season. Although in the past bronchiolitis was differentiated from asthma by its failure to respond to bronchodilators, it is now apparent that children with bronchiolitis may also have some degree of bronchospasm that is responsive to bronchodilators.

History

In taking a history, one should ask about the presence of any of the following: congenital heart disease, chronic respiratory disease, recent contact with respiratory illness, history of respiratory distress syndrome and/or prematurity, and previous episode of respiratory distress, asthma, or bronchiolitis.

Symptoms

Bronchiolitis often presents as a minor cold or chest congestion for several days. A clear nasal discharge (rhinorrhea) and low-grade fever are present. A moist or hacking cough is present along with tachypnea or labored breathing. The small infant may have a markedly decreased interest and an unwillingness to drink because of the respiratory distress and coughing spasms. Some infants, however, have few to no respiratory symptoms on presentation but instead present with apnea. This occurs more often in infants younger than 3 months, particularly if they have been born prematurely.

Physical Examination

Most patients will demonstrate pronounced, diffuse rales or wheezing in all lung fields along with prolonged expiration. Other signs of respiratory distress may be present, including severe retractions and use of accessory muscles. Exaggerated periodic breathing may occur, as can apnea, which is a not uncommon presenting symptom of RSV disease even when there is no obvious pulmonary disease. The symptoms can wax and wane, so that the child may look distressed one hour and much improved the next. Hypoxemia commonly occurs and is often associated with a respiratory rate greater than 60/min. One should look for conjunctivitis and concomitant otitis media (RSV has been cultured from the middle ear).

Laboratory Evaluation

An RSV culture of nasal washings or nasopharyngeal swab should be sent, and a rapid fluorescent antibody screen should be done, particularly if it is likely that the child will need to be hospitalized. Finding evidence for RSV will make it easier to cohort patients to prevent nosocomial spread to others and will allow for early treatment with ribavirin. An arterial blood gas, if the child is in moderate distress, will provide objective evidence of difficulties in oxygenation and ventilation. Electrolytes, blood urea nitrogen, and glucose should be measured, and a urinalysis should be performed. An elevated urine specific gravity (>1.025) suggests significant dehydration, which may need correction with intravenous hydration if respiratory distress is great enough to prevent adequate oral intake. Finally, a chest radiograph will indicate the typical pattern of hyperexpansion with diffuse patchy infiltrates most commonly involving the perihilar regions.

Management

Children whose oxygen saturation is greater than 94%, who are in minimal distress, who are able to drink adequately and are well hydrated, and whose parents are reliable may be discharged to home. Good follow-up must be done either by telephone or by a return visit to the primary care physician. Contact between the emergency department physician and the primary care provider is absolutely essential. Children with borderline status either medically or socially should be admitted.

The decision to admit to the hospital is based on the following criteria:

1. hypoxia in room air
2. failure to maintain hydration
3. evidence of respiratory failure, including apnea
4. need for ribavirin in high-risk children
5. unclear or unstable social situation in the presence of a moderately ill child whose condition might become severe enough to warrant admission

In the emergency department, management should be initiated as follows:

1. If by pulse oximetry the oxygen saturation is less than 90%, the child will clearly require supplemental oxygen and hospitalization. Give an Fio_2 to maintain oxygen saturation at greater than 90%. This is usually about 30% Fio_2.
2. Oxygen should be humidified but need not be a mist. In fact, a mist may obscure the patient, making observation more complicated and frightening the child.
3. An arterial blood gas should be obtained for better assessment of ventilation and pH. CBGs may not be accurate.
4. Intravenous fluids are necessary for many children because they are already dehydrated from decreased fluid intake and increased respiratory insensible losses. In patients with marked tachypnea (>60/min to 70/min), attempts at oral intake may be unsuccessful because of excessive work of breathing.

FOREIGN BODY ASPIRATION

Foreign body aspiration should be considered in any child who presents with respiratory distress of either acute or subacute onset. The history may be clear cut, with a witnessed aspiration of a foreign object or substance, or it may be subtle, with the child presenting with a persistent cough, a localized wheeze, or evidence of pneumonia. Most commonly, the child is younger than 2 years and has aspirated one of the following: a peanut, seed (especially watermelon and sunflower), corn, small toy part, candy, balloon, hot dog, grape, or popcorn. Peanuts are especially toxic because of the tremendous inflammatory response that the peanut oil elicits. The foreign body can be aspirated into any part of the airway, with left-sided involvement being more common than right-sided. Right-sided involvement appears to be more common in adults.

In children with marked developmental delay, sudden aspiration of gastric contents from reflux can result in an acute hypoxic episode with chemical pneumonitis. These children may also present with chronic wheezing due to chronic reflux and/or recurrent aspiration of oral secretions.

Clinical Evaluation

Any child suspected of a foreign body aspiration must be managed on the premise that severe airway compromise may occur suddenly. Especially if there is a possibility of a foreign body in the upper airway, the child should not be left alone because unexpected acute airway obstruction may occur. The Heimlich maneuver in children older than 1 year and back blows or chest thrusts in children younger than 1 year may need to be applied urgently.

The majority of patients, if appropriately interviewed, will present with a highly suggestive history. It is most important, therefore, that the clinician maintain a high index of suspicion. In several large series of children with foreign body aspiration, there was a delay in diagnosis in 15% to 18%.[14,15]

History

A positive history can be obtained in more than 90% of children with a foreign body aspiration. Initial symptoms are usually cough, choking, cyanosis, or dyspnea of sudden onset. By the time the child is admitted to the hospital, however, these acute symptoms have lessened, and dyspnea and fever are more common. Hoarseness reliably predicts the presence of the foreign body in the upper airway, as does stridor. Once the object has gone beyond the trachea, however, there may be minimal symptoms, and only the history of an acute event several weeks before presentation may be indicative.

Physical Examination

The physical finding most suggestive of lower airway foreign body aspiration is decreased air entry with subsequent tachypnea, rales, fever, and localized wheezing. Bilaterally decreased breath sounds may suggest a tracheal foreign body.

Laboratory Data

A chest radiograph should be obtained on all patients suspected of having aspirated a foreign body. Although most foreign bodies will not be seen because they are radiolucent (vegetable matter), inspiratory and forced expiratory films may show distal air trapping or a mediastinal shift. If there is a delay in seeking medical attention, atelectasis and/or pulmonary infiltrates are more common. The absence of an abnormal chest film, however, does not rule out a foreign body because in more than a third of children the radiographic findings will be normal,[15] particularly if the child presents soon after an event. Although fluoroscopy is a time-honored diagnostic modality, it is not more sensitive than the chest film. Similarly, some of the newer imaging modalities such as magnetic resonance imaging and computed tomography of the chest add little information.

Management

1. Keep the patient on nothing by mouth.
2. Measure oxygen saturation by pulse oximeter.
3. Use rigid bronchoscopy for removal. If there is marginal historical, physical, or laboratory evidence of a foreign body, flexible bronchoscopy might be done first. It is not possible to remove a foreign body with most flexible bronchoscopes, however, so that another procedure will be needed if a foreign body is found.
4. If the foreign body aspiration has been associated with long-standing symptoms, the use of dexamethasone (0.5 mg/kg every 6 hours) may reduce bronchial swelling. Antibiotics to treat pneumonia and bronchodilators for the 24 hours before bronchoscopy may also facilitate removal.

HYDROCARBON ASPIRATION

Although the preceding discussion refers primarily to solid foreign bodies, a number of children and adolescents present with accidental aspiration of liquids, most importantly gasoline, kerosene, or some other hydrocarbon. The primary toxicity, however, usually relates not to systemic absorption but to a small amount being aspirated into the respiratory tract. Such aspiration leads to a necrotizing chemical pneumonitis for which no treatment is available except supportive care.

If the child becomes symptomatic within 4 to 6 hours of the aspiration, a chest film should be obtained and the child admitted for close observation. Oximetry should be done and supplemental oxygen given as necessary. With significant aspiration, fever is common and does not in itself indicate a bacterial infection. A bacterial superinfection may eventually occur, however, for which antibiotics are indicated (usually clindamycin or penicillin) to cover the common mouth organisms that are likely to have been aspirated along with the hydrocarbon. If the child is asymptomatic on arrival, he or she should be observed for 4 to 6 hours. If no symptoms develop, the child can be discharged home with follow-up by the primary care physician.

PNEUMONIA

Pneumonia is an infection of the pulmonary parenchyma and the alveolar air spaces. Etiologies are multiple and include viruses, bacteria, fungi, rickettsiae, and parasites. Pneumonia in children who do not have underlying chronic disease, who are malnourished, or who have some other deficit in host defense is most often due to a few commonly recognized organisms. These etiologies are primarily related to age and season of the year. Children who are immunocompromised, however, develop pneumonia from organisms that are not common pathogens but rather are opportunistic because of decreased host defenses.

Pneumonia accounts for about 13% of all infectious illnesses and occurs most commonly in the 2- to 4-year age group. Because antibiotics are the cornerstones of treatment of bacterial pneumonia, establishment of the etiology as bacterial or viral is important. Although 50% of children never have a clear etiology established, a number of studies have clarified the major identifiable organisms. During the first week of life, group B streptococcus is a major cause of pneumonia; in the first 3 to 4 months of life, *Chlamydia trachomatis* accounts for 15% to 30% of afebrile pneumonitis cases. Before age 5 years, viruses cause the bulk of the pneumonias. RSV is the chief virus, but parainfluenza virus, influenza virus, rhinovirus, adenovirus, and enterovirus have all been implicated. After age 5 years, *Mycoplasma pneumoniae* is the major pathogen. *Streptococcus pneumoniae* and *Hemophilus influenzae* are the most common bacterial causes beyond early infancy, although the former is much more common than the latter. Although *Staphylococcus aureus* should always be in the differential for bacterial pneumonia, it has become less common in the past 20 years. Complicating the search for etiology is that 25% to 75% of patients may be infected by both a virus and a bacterium.[16]

Clinical Evaluation

History

The key symptoms that should lead one to suspect pneumonia are cough and tachypnea. Fever may be a symptom, but if it is absent, particularly in the first 3 to 6 months of life, the afebrile pneumonitis syndrome, usually caused by *Chlamydia* organisms, should be considered. A description of the cough can be helpful. Spasms of coughing during exhalation are seen with pertussis, parapertussis, adenovirus pneumonia, RSV pneumonia, and even *Chlamydia* infection. The classic inspiratory whoop and cough leading to vomiting is often seen with pertussis but may be absent in infants with the disease. Adequacy of the primary immunization series against pertussis needs to be established. In the older child, a dry hacking cough sometimes leading to vomiting and frequently leading to sleeping problems is characteristic of *M pneumoniae* infection. Fever is not uniformly present.

Inquiry should be made about the presence of respiratory symptoms in anyone who has been in contact with the child. If others are ill with a respiratory illness as well, the child's illness is likely to be viral. Nevertheless, bacterial causes cannot be totally excluded, and even *M pneumoniae* has been known to affect multiple members of the same family. Coughing in other family members, particularly in older adults, should make one consider the possibility of tuberculosis.

Generally, the more acute the onset, the more likely it is that the pneumonia is bacterial. Children who have a low-grade fever (<39°C) for a number of days associated with a dry cough, rhinorrhea, malaise, sore throat, and other non-specific systemic systems usually have a viral pneumonia. Bacterial pneumonias usually present with acute onset (24 to 48 hours) of high fever, toxic appearance, malaise, and tachypnea. These children appear ill, are not playful, and seem tired. There have been a number of studies, however, suggesting that duration of illness before seeking medical attention; fever, nonpulmonary symptoms, and even rales are not consistently reliable in distinguishing bacterial from viral pneumonias. An explanation for this may be concomitant bacterial and viral infections. A key example of this is the influenza epidemic of 1918, in which the majority of deaths were due to superimposed staphylococcal pneumonia.

Because respiratory distress can significantly interfere with oral intake, the child's fluid intake and urine output should be questioned carefully. Failure to maintain oral hydration may provide a clue to the severity of the respiratory distress as well as indicate significant dehydration.

Physical Examination

One should initially observe the child at a distance so as not to frighten him or her and to note evidence of respiratory distress (tachypnea, nasal flaring, retractions, position of comfort, facial expression, and pallor/cyanosis). Tachypnea is probably the most consistent finding with pneumonia. Subsequently, a more detailed examination should be done. Physical findings that increase the probability of pneumonia include fever and the presence on chest examination of localized rales, bronchial breathing, dullness to percussion, and increased vocal fremitus. In young children and infants, rales may not be present. Vocal fremitus can be difficult to elicit but can be assessed during crying in the small child. In spite of all the problems with the physical examination, 80% of the time the diagnosis of pneumonia can be established clinically.

Laboratory Evaluation

The need for chest radiographs is somewhat controversial. It has been reported that if the history, observation, and physical examination are all consistent with pneumonia the findings on chest radiography only alter management in 6% of children. If there are inconsistent findings on history, observation, and physical examination, however, the chest radiographic findings alter therapy in 24% of these children.[17] Certainly, a child who has significant distress, who is suspected of having significant atelectasis or pleural effusion, and in whom it is unclear whether pneumonia exists should have a chest film taken. Bilateral infiltrates usually are associated with viral pneumonias, and lobar pneumonias are characteristically seen with bacterial pneumonia. Bacterial pneumonia can present with bronchopneumonia and interstitial infiltrates, however, and viral pneumonia can present with localized infiltrates or atelectasis (RSV and adenovirus). Pleural effusions are not common in children younger than 2 years and may be seen with *H influenzae* type B (76%),[18] *S aureus*, and pneumococci.[19] Less commonly, large effusions can be seen with *M pneumoniae*, group A streptococci and adenovirus. Pneumatoceles are more common with *S aureus* but can be seen with *H influenzae* or *Streptococcus pneumoniae*.

A white blood cell count may be helpful. If there is a high total count and an absolute band count greater than 2,000, a bacterial etiology is likely. Nevertheless, some viruses, notably adenovirus, may present with a similar picture, and a normal white cell count does not necessarily exclude a bacterial etiology.

If the diagnosis of pneumonia is made and a bacterial etiology seems more likely than a viral one, a blood culture should be drawn. In any case, if antibiotics are prescribed it is prudent to draw a blood culture. Although the positivity rate is low (5% to 20% of bacterial pneumonias), knowledge of the organism can guide therapy, particularly if the child appears to be responding poorly to a specific antibiotic.

Culture of the sputum is notoriously difficult in the young child because sputum is usually swallowed. Nasopharyngeal secretions obtained via a nasal washing or via nasopharyngeal swab, however, may be useful to identify the presence of RSV and *Chlamydia* species by rapid fluorescent antigen test and culture.

Management

Two key questions to be considered in the management of the child with pneumonia are: How should the child be treated, and where should the child be treated (home or the hospital)? Specific treatment categories to be considered are oxygen therapy, antibiotic therapy, and fluid therapy.

The need for oxygen therapy is easily determined with pulse oximetry or an arterial blood gas if there is considerable respiratory effort. The need for fluid therapy can be determined by assessing the state of hydration and capacity for taking fluids orally. The need for antibiotic therapy depends on whether there is strong suspicion of a bacterial pneumonia. Because bacterial pneumonias are treatable and most viral pneumonias are not, it is best to err on the side of treatment. Coverage for pneumococci and *H influenzae* should be done as a minimum for the child younger than 5 years; amoxicillin, ampicillin, or cefaclor is adequate. An initial intramuscular injection of ceftriaxone may be helpful, especially if it is unclear whether the child should be treated in the hospital or at home (see below). Children older than 5 years should also have coverage for *Mycoplasma pneumoniae*. Treatment with erythromycin or erythromycin-sulfamethoxazole (Pediazole) is adequate.

The decision to treat a child in the hospital depends on the degree of illness and whether any of the treatment modalities are available only in the hospital. Major aspects of care that point to hospitalization are the need for oxygen, the likelihood that respiratory distress will significantly and rapidly increase in the next 24 hours, the need for intravenous fluids and/or antibiotics, and the ability of the parents to carry through management at home. The need for oxygen is easily determined (any child whose oxygen saturation is less than 90%). The need for intravenous antibiotics is dependent on the severity of the disease process and, of course, on whether the etiology of the pneumonia is believed to be bacterial or viral. Increasing respiratory distress can usually be followed clinically in the emergency department during several hours of observation, and an arterial blood gas can be obtained if there is doubt (rising Pco_2 is of major concern, especially in the presence of tachypnea). If monitoring by continuous pulse oximetry or an arterial line is deemed necessary, the child should be admitted not only to the hospital but also to an intensive care unit.

If the child is not admitted, contact with the family should be made again in 24 to 48 hours. Most bacterial pneumonias respond to antibiotics within that period of time. If there has been no improvement, the child should be re-evaluated for admission to the hospital and parenteral antibiotics. Antibiotics should generally be continued for 10 days. Although follow-up radiographs have been routine in the past, there is no evidence that if the child becomes asymptomatic without residual problems a chest radiograph is necessary.[20]

MISCELLANEOUS LOWER AIRWAY EMERGENCIES: SPONTANEOUS PNEUMOTHORAX

Sudden pneumothorax should be suspected in any child or adolescent who complains of sudden chest pain and/or shortness of breath. In adults the differential diagnosis includes myocardial infarction and pulmonary embolus, but in children these ordinarily need not be considered. The majority of spontaneous pneumothoraces are idiopathic, but the entity is also known to occur with cystic fibrosis, asthma, tuberculosis, staphylococcal pneumonia, and blunt injury to the chest. In neonates there is a 1% incidence of pneumothorax, presumably as a result of the pressures to which the neonate is exposed during delivery.

Physical signs include tachycardia and tachypnea. Shift of the mediastinum to the opposite side as reflected by tracheal deviation and a decrease in cardiac output (hypotension and poor perfusion) are strongly suggestive of a tension pneumothorax and require immediate evacuation of air by either needle aspiration or a chest tube. High-concentration oxygen should be administered because many of these children will be hypoxic both before and after the pneumothorax. On occasion, evacuation of the pneumothorax with re-expansion of the lung has resulted in unilateral expansion pulmonary edema.

REFERENCES

1. Azizkhan RG, Dudgeon DL, Buck JR, et al. Life-threatening airway obstruction as a complication to the management of mediastinal masses in children. *J Pediatr Surg*. 1985;20:816–822.
2. Galant SP, Groncy CE, Shaw KC. The value of pulsus paradoxus in assessing the child with status asthmaticus. *Pediatrics*. 1978;61:46–51.
3. Orenstein SR, Orenstein DM. Gastroesophageal reflux and respiratory disease in children. *J Pediatr*. 1988;112:847–858.
4. Gergen PJ, Mullally DI, Evans R. National survey of prevalence of asthma among children in the United States, 1976–1980. *Pediatrics*. 1988;81:1–7.
5. Newcomb RW, Akhter J. Respiratory failure from asthma. *Am J Dis Child*. 1988;142:1041–1044.
6. Commey JOO, Levison H. Physical signs in childhood asthma. *Pediatrics*. 1976;58:537–541.
7. Gershel JC, Golman HS, Stein REK, Shelov SP, Ziprkowski M. The usefulness of chest radiographs in first asthma attacks. *N Engl J Med*. 1983;309:336–339.
8. Portnoy J, Aggarwal J. Continuous terbutaline nebulization for the treatment of severe exacerbations of asthma in children. *Ann Allergy*. 1988;60:368–371.
9. Moler FW, Hurwitz ME, Custer JR. Improvement in clinical asthma score and $Paco_2$ in children with severe asthma treated with continuously nebulized terbutaline. *J Allergy Clin Immunol*. 1988;81:1101–1109.
10. Herman JJ, Noah SL, Moody RR. Use of intravenous isoproterenol for status asthmaticus. *Crit Care Med*. 1983;11:716–720.
11. MacDonald NE, Hall CB, Suffin SC, Alexson C, Harris PJ, Manning JA. Respiratory syncytial viral infection in infants with congenital heart disease. *N Engl J Med*. 1982;307:397–400.
12. Groothuis JR, Gutierrez KM, Lauer BA. Respiratory syncytial virus infection in children with bronchopulmonary dysplasia. *Pediatrics*. 1988;82:199–203.
13. Hall CB, Powell KR, MacDonald NF, et al. Respiratory syncytial viral infection in children with compromised immune function. *N Engl J Med*. 1986;315:77–81.
14. Vane DW, Pritchard J, Colville CW, West KW, Eigen H, and Grosfeld JL. Bronchoscopy for aspirated foreign bodies in children. *Arch Surg*. 1988;123:885–888.
15. Laks Y, Barzilay Z. Foreign body aspiration in childhood. *Pediatr Emerg Care*. 1988;4:102–106.
16. Turner RB, Lande AE, Chase P, Hilton N, Weinberg D. Pneumonia in pediatric outpatients: cause and clinical manifestation. *J Pediatr*. 1987;111:194–200.
17. Alario AJ, McCarthy PL, Markowitz R, Kornguth P, Rosenfield N, Leventhal JM. Usefulness of chest radiographs in children with acute lower respiratory tract disease. *J Pediatr*. 1987;111:187–193.
18. Ginsburg CM, Howard JB, Nelson JD. Report of 65 cases of *Haemophilus influenzae* b pneumonia. *Pediatrics*. 1979;64:283–286.
19. Freij BJ, Kusmiesz H, Nelson JD, McCracken GH. Parapneumonic effusions and empyema in hospitalized children: a retrospective review of 227 cases. *Pediatr Infect Dis*. 1984;3:578–591.
20. Grossman LK, Wald ER, Nair P, Papiez J. Roentgenographic follow-up of acute pneumonia in children. *Pediatrics*. 1979;63:300–331.

36. Neurologic Emergencies of Infancy and Childhood

RICHARD M. CANTOR, MD, FAAP, FACEP

THE UNCONSCIOUS CHILD

Altered states of consciousness in infants and children are commonly seen in association with a number of illnesses. Central nervous system (CNS) activity is profoundly dependent on adequate oxygenation and perfusion, components that are often compromised in many disease states. It is evident, therefore, that any aberration in consciousness must be considered of global etiology. Failure to provide adequate emergent care will often result in a worsening of the initial insult and, in some tragic instances, a permanent neurovegetative state.

There are many terms that have been utilized in describing the comatose patient, such as *lethargic, drowsy, stuporous,* and *obtunded.* For the purposes of this chapter, the term *coma* will apply to any decrease in the level of consciousness. A more simple and direct description of level of consciousness is contained within the Glasgow Coma Scale (discussed later). Level of consciousness should be considered an important vital sign in documenting the neurologic status of the unconscious child.

This chapter outlines a rational approach for the evaluation and management of the unconscious pediatric patient. Various etiologies are discussed with emphasis on their relative acuity and probable outcomes. Intervention priorities are reviewed with recommendations for a standardized protocol of management.

Common Etiologies of Unconsciousness

Progressive Intracranial Conditions

Acute epidural hematoma. The accumulation of blood in the epidural space represents a true neurosurgical emergency. The associated head injury is accompanied by radiographic evidence of a skull fracture in up to 75% of cases.[1] In the adult, the classic symptom complex includes a period of unconsciousness that is followed by a lucid interval with subsequent rapid neurologic deterioration as expanding arterial bleeding exerts a mass effect on the brain. This triad is often absent in the child because in many instances the source of bleeding is venous. In the most dramatic presentation, the patient develops signs of central herniation that are often unilateral in deficit.

Subdural hematoma. Usually venous in origin, subdural hematomas occur either acutely or as part of a chronic injury pattern. Infants who are the victims of abuse develop subdural hematomas as part of the shaken baby syndrome, where repeated forceful flexion and extension of the head cause shearing of intracranial bridging veins. Symptom development is subacute and includes irritability, lethargy, poor feeding, and eventual unconsciousness. The presence of a tense fontanelle, papilledema, and in most chronic cases retinal hemorrhages will alert the clinician. Skull fractures are seen in less than 30% of cases. The diagnosis is confirmed by computed tomography (CT).

Generalized cerebral edema. Cerebral edema may occur as a result of any traumatic or anoxic insult to the brain. The neurologic findings are often nonfocal in presentation but, unless monitored carefully, will progressively impair more caudal brain stem/midbrain structures.

Metabolic Emergencies

Hypoglycemia. Glycogen stores in infants and children are often inadequate to meet the metabolic demands incurred in critical illness. Hypoglycemia, if untreated, will further damage viable brain tissue. The rapid correction of this deficiency is therefore of enormous benefit and imparts no great risk to the patient.

Narcotic overdose. Opiate derivatives may be part of an accidental ingestion in the child or a suicide mechanism in the adolescent. The presentation of coma, pinpoint reactive pupils, bradypnea, and bradycardia should alert the clinician. The administration of naloxone is a relatively safe and effective means of treating this overdose.

Meningitis. Cerebrospinal fluid (CSF) infections are most common in children from 3 months to 24 months of age. Causative organisms include *Hemophilus influenzae*, pneumococci, *Neisseria meningitidis*, and group B streptococci. Common symptoms in infancy are hypothermia or hyperthermia, apnea, alterations in consciousness, poor feeding, and paradoxic irritability. The older child presents more classically with fever, nausea and vomiting, neck stiffness, and photophobia. In the context of the comatose patient, if meningitis is suspected it is of paramount importance that antibiotics be administered before a spinal tap is performed; in small infants this procedure may be quite time consuming to complete. It has been shown that CSF results will remain reliable for hours after the administration of antibiotics.

Nonprogressive Metabolic Etiologies

Diabetic ketoacidosis. Approximately 30% of newly diagnosed diabetic children present with diabetic ketoacidosis, and 10% of these children are comatose on presentation. Typical manifestations include polyuria, polydipsia, and weight loss followed by vomiting, dehydration, hyperpnea, and profound lethargy. Diabetic coma has been correlated with the neurologic depression seen in other hyperosmolar states. Reversal of coma is seen after appropriate intensive therapy directed at correction of the fluid deficit, hyperglycemia, and acidosis seen in these patients. An uncommon and often fatal neurologic complication seen during treatment of diabetic ketoacidosis is the development of deepening coma secondary to progressive cerebral edema. A clearcut explanation for this has yet to be provided in the literature.

Hypernatremia. Infants with severe gastroenteritis are subject to profound free water loss as a result of persistent emesis and diarrhea.[2] In addition, insensible losses caused by fever are compounded by the disproportionately large body surface area of infants. Other etiologies include the improper mixing of proprietary formulas and, rarely, diabetes insipidus. Symptoms range from lethargy and irritability to muscle weakness, convulsions, and coma. The mainstay of therapy is gradual intravenous replacement of the deficit with saline solutions to prevent the development of cerebral edema.

Hyponatremia. The overutilization of clear (hypotonic) fluids for oral rehydration in gastroenteritis will lower the serum sodium concentration. A more common cause of hyponatremia is the syndrome of inappropriate antidiuretic hormone secretion (SIADH), a disorder seen in many disease states that often involves the CNS or lung. Symptoms common to all sodium-depleted patients include muscle cramps, lethargy, agitation, decreased reflexes, seizures, and coma. Emergent therapy (if clinically warranted) includes the administration of 3% saline solutions. More commonly, fluid administration is restricted until the primary event is resolved.

Viral encephalitis. Acute viral encephalitis often begins with nonspecific complaints (ie, headache, lethargy, vomiting, and anorexia). A progression to more dramatic neurologic signs, such as confusion, combativeness, hallucinations, coma, and seizures, often occurs. Clinical deterioration may be rapid and focal in some instances. Common organisms include herpes simplex virus, Epstein-Barr virus, togaviruses (arboviruses), measles, rubella, varicella, and mumps virus. CSF results may be normal, so that sophisticated serum and immune testing often is necessary to make the diagnosis. Herpes encephalitis differs in some respects because CT will often demonstrate a temporal lobe anomaly; acyclovir is the drug of choice in herpetic cases.

Reye's syndrome. First described in 1963, Reye's syndrome remains a disorder of unknown etiology. After a prodromal viral illness (usually varicella or influenza), the patient develops pernicious emesis and a spectrum of neurologic insults ranging from lethargy or combativeness to cerebral herniation and death. Patients are usually afebrile and anicteric but have laboratory evidence of hepatic damage manifested by elevated serum glutamic-oxaloacetic and -pyruvic transaminases, prolonged prothrombin time, and, classically, elevated serum ammonia.[3] Hypoglycemia is also a common problem and must be corrected. CSF analysis usually reveals no inflammatory change; elevations in opening pressure confirm the development of cerebral edema. Emergent management of these patients ranges from careful observation and minimal support to invasive neurointensive care with intracranial pressure monitoring.

Postictal states. Many children, after experiencing a convulsion, will remain postictal for up to 30 minutes. After repetitive and severe seizures, however, this neurologic depression may be quite prolonged. This represents a diagnosis of exclusion.

Exogenous poisons. The pediatric population represents more than 60% of the annual reported toxic exposures in the United States. Whether a poisoning is an accidental event in childhood or a part of a suicide attempt in adolescence, the clinician must maintain a high degree of suspicion to make the diagnosis.[4] A list of common toxidromes is provided in Table 36-1.

Emergency Management

The goals of intensive therapy when applied to the comatose child are as follows:

- adherence to basic emergency stabilization (the primary survey)
- emergent neurologic assessment
- recognition and treatment of cerebral herniation
- systematic clinical re-evaluation (the secondary survey)

The Primary Survey

Airway/cervical spine. All comatose patients are at risk for unrecognized cervical trauma. A patent and stable upper airway must be guaranteed while cervical spine precautions are maintained. In this setting, the recommended maneuver for opening the airway is the jaw thrust. Any head extension should be avoided. Clearance of the airway is best provided by the use of a rigid (tonsillar) suction device, even on the smallest of patients.

Breathing. The clinician must not permit any element of hypoxia or hypercapnia to exist in the comatose patient. Any rise in the Pco_2 has been shown to cause an increase in intracranial pressure that will only contribute to the primary CNS insult. A common pitfall in neurointensive stabilization is a delay in intubation of the patient. The placement of an endotracheal tube provides protection from aspiration because many depressed patients have a compromised gag reflex (bulbar injury). In addition, if signs of increased intracranial pressure develop, immediate therapy with hyperventilation is accomplished rapidly. Nasotracheal intubation is advocated by some as the preferred approach in the neck-injured patient. A blind attempt, however, is difficult in the pediatric patient because of the anterior position of the trachea. Nasotracheal intubation is contraindicated in the presence of a basilar skull fracture.

Circulation. Cerebral perfusion is dependent on an adequate mean arterial pressure. In most situations the comatose patient is hemodynamically stable, and in the setting of possible SIADH intravenous fluids are often restricted to prevent subsequent cerebral edema. In the hypotensive comatose patient, however, it is mandatory that fluid administration not be withheld. Fluids of choice should be normotonic (eg, lactated Ringer solution or normal saline with or without dextrose) if clinically indicated.

Table 36-1 Toxidromes

Drug Involved	Findings
Anticholinergics	Agitation; coma; hallucinations; seizures; dilated pupils; warm, dry skin; dry mouth; tachycardia; depressed bowel/urinary function
Opiates	Coma, seizures, pinpoint pupils, tachycardia, bradypnea, hypotension
Cholinergics	Coma, seizures, muscle fasciculations, salivation, lacrimation, urination, defecation, wheezing
Tricyclic antidepressants	Anticholinergic symptoms, coma, dysrhythmias
Sedative-hypnotics	Coma, hypothermia, hypotension
Phenothiazines	Anticholinergic symptoms, hypotension, dystonia, oculogyric crisis, torticollis

Emergent Neurologic Assessment

The primary goal of the neurologic examination is to rule out the presence of impending herniation. In addition, it provides a baseline status against which further examinations may be measured to compare clinical progression. Useful components of this evaluation are listed below.

The Glasgow Coma Scale. As previously mentioned, this is a simple and direct method for identifying patients in need of intensive therapy.[5] A score less than 9 may be indicative of a severe insult; ventilation is often necessary in these patients (Table 36-2).

Motor response. Consciousness requires a functioning reticular activating system (RAS) and both cerebral hemispheres. The response to painful stimuli (sternal rub or subungual pressure) provides an assessment of hemispheric function. Purposeful withdrawal suggests patent cortical function. Hemispheric damage will present with decorticate posturing (arm, wrist, and finger flexion with leg extension). Decerebrate posturing (upper and lower extremity extension) correlates with high pontine and midbrain damage. Brain stem injury renders the patient flaccid with no motor responses.

Cranial nerve testing. Evaluation of cranial nerves III through VIII correlates indirectly with RAS function because both components are located in the pons and midbrain. Pupillary dilation is mediated by sympathetic fibers that travel from the hypothalamus to the cervical cord, terminating in the cervical ganglia. Parasympathetic impulses travel along the third nerve and constrict the pupil. Pinpoint, unreactive pupils (unopposed parasympathetic impulses) are seen

Table 36-2 The Glasgow Coma Scale

Response	Points
Eye opening	
No response	1
Response to pain	2
Response to voice	3
Spontaneously	4
Verbal response	
No response	1
Incomprehensible sounds	2
Inappropriate words	3
Disoriented conversation	4
Oriented and appropriate	5
Motor response	
No response	1
Decerebrate posturing	2
Decorticate posturing	3
Flexion withdrawal	4
Localizes pain	5
Obeys commands	6
Maximum score	15

with pontine lesions. Unreactive midposition pupils indicate disruption of both pathways by a midbrain lesion. A unilateral dilated pupil is one of the hallmarks of uncal herniation, in which the oculomotor nerve is compressed against the posterior cerebral artery by the uncus of the temporal lobe. In general, metabolic coma features reactive pupils, albeit with alteration in size.

The corneal reflex. In the normal patient, corneal stimulation with a cotton swab will cause constriction of the orbicularis oculi and blinking. A consensual response is seen in the unstimulated eye. The pathway consists of afferent (trigeminal nerve) and efferent (facial nerve) components.

Doll-eyes (oculocephalic) reflex/caloric testing. Both reflexes measure cranial nerve VIII (afferent) function, the medial longitudinal fasciculus, and cranial nerve III, IV, and VI pathways (efferent). The doll-eyes maneuver involves turning the patient's head and should never be performed in patients with suspected cervical injury. Caloric testing is safer and provides similar clinical information. Normally, infusion of ice water into the auditory canal induces nystagmus with the slow component toward the cold stimulus and the fast component away from it. Compromise of supratentorial structures abolishes the fast component, which leads to tonic eye deviation toward the cold stimulus. In the case of brain stem damage, the response is absent completely.

Cerebral Herniation

Any increase in intracranial volume can cause displacement of tissue with compression and compromise of function. Herniation, if present, represents a true emergency, and therapy must be immediate. Symptoms of increased intracranial pressure are well documented (Table 36-3). Central herniation symmetrically impairs function in a rostrocaudal manner with eventual brain stem compromise. Uncal herniation often is unilateral and will present with the dramatic development of coma accompanied by a unilaterally dilated unreactive pupil. There are multiple interventions available for the treatment of impending herniation (Table 36-4).[6] Hyperventilation represents a rapid and effective method of lowering intracranial pressure and in many cases will buy time until definitive neurosurgical treatment is begun.

The Secondary Survey

After ruling out reversible emergent conditions, the physician should carefully re-examine the patient in a more comprehensive manner. Paramedics, family members, and old medical records are valuable sources of pertinent historical data. A complete discussion of the physical examination of the comatose patient is provided by Plum and Posner.[7]

Laboratory investigation should include a complete blood count to rule out anemia or infectious diseases. Electrolyte analysis will provide a measure of the anion gap. In addition, a calculation can be made to estimate serum osmolarity, which, when compared with the measured osmolarity, defines the presence of an osmolar gap (seen in poisoning with alcohols). Renal and liver function tests (including serum ammonia) should be obtained. Arterial blood gases are indicated in any critical illness. Serum, urine, and gastric aspirates should be collected and analyzed for the presence of a toxin if clinically warranted. The sequence of radiographic studies (skull and cervical spine films and CT scans) is determined by the progression of symptoms.

STATUS EPILEPTICUS

The child in status epilepticus represents a true medical emergency requiring immediate recognition and institution of vigorous therapeutic modalities. The goal of the emergency physician is the prevention of any mortality and permanent neurologic sequelae.

Definitions

Status epilepticus represents a seizure in its most severe manifestation. It is defined variously in the literature, with one of the more common definitions being a single, generalized convulsion that lasts longer than 30 minutes or recurrent tonic-clonic convulsions occurring so frequently that the patient remains obtunded between seizures. Because there are many divergent opinions regarding a precise definition, it may be assumed that any form of seizure that becomes frequent enough may be considered a form of status epilepticus.

Table 36-3 Common Symptoms and Signs of Elevated Intracranial Pressure

Infants	Children	Infants and Children
Full fontanelle	Headache	Altered states of consciousness
Split sutures	Stiff neck	Persistent emesis
Paradoxic irritability	Photophobia	Cranial nerve involvement (VI and III)
Macrocrania	Papilledema	Setting sun sign
Papilledema		Triad of hypertension, bradycardia, hypoventilation; decorticate or decerebrate posturing

Etiology

The true incidence of pediatric generalized tonic-clonic status epilepticus is unknown. The literature is replete with estimates of its incidence in the adult population (5% to 8%), but pediatric estimates are less precise. In the adult patient, the most common etiology for status epilepticus involves a direct relationship between the precipitation of seizures and changes in ongoing anticonvulsant medication. Other causes in the adult patient include idiopathic causes, the progression of an underlying CNS disease or infection, and the onset of intercurrent illnesses in general.

In one study of 239 epileptic children,[8] nearly half the episodes were idiopathic, and the other half were defined more precisely. Known diagnoses included acute CNS insults (meningitis or encephalitis) and progression of a prior cerebral event (tumor or mass lesion). Within the idiopathic population, there was a clear-cut relationship to the presence of a febrile illness.

Mortality and Morbidity Associated with Status Epilepticus

Current estimates of mortality involved with tonic-clonic seizures range from 3% to 18%. Mortality figures rise dramatically in the pediatric patient if there is the concurrent presence of a cerebral lesion.[8] Without question, however, the most common factor involved in the prevention of morbidity is the provision of constant and sufficient neurointensive care.

Experimental animal models have been used in attempts to describe fully the mechanisms and outcomes involved in the morbidity associated with status epilepticus in children.[9] It has been well demonstrated that selective cell damage occurs in almost all areas of the brain after 60 minutes of seizure activity. What is most disturbing is that, even in the presence of sufficient ventilation and normal acid-base status, these changes are not preventable. These CNS insults are presumably related to the insatiable metabolic demands in effect at the cellular level secondary to the continuous firing of affected neurons. Intracranial oxidants have been demonstrated at the pancellular level.

The clinician is more likely to encounter the late secondary effects of status epilepticus, which include lactic acidosis, elevated intracranial pressure, blood glucose abnormalities, hyperthermia, and dehydration. Pronounced muscular activity places these patients at great risk for the development of myoglobinuria. These complications are summarized in Table 36-5.

Table 36-4 Emergent Management of Increased Intracranial Pressure

Therapy	Dose	Mechanism of Action
Head elevation (30°)		Lowers intracranial venous pressure
Head in midline		Prevents jugular vein compression
Hyperventilation	Reduces Pa_{CO_2} to 20–25 mmHg	Promptly decreases cerebral blood volume and thus intracranial pressure
Mannitol or glycerol	0.5–2.0 g/kg IV	Both agents effect rapid osmotic diuresis
Pentobarbital	1–3 mg/kg (loading dose)	Thought to lower cerebral metabolism; may also have some effect on free radical formation; other barbiturates (phenobarbital) have also been utilized
Dexamethasone	0.2 mg/kg IV	Slow onset of action
Hypothermia (27°–31°C)		Thought to decrease cerebral blood flow and metabolic rate; can cause cardiac dysrhythmias

Table 36-5 Medical Complications of Status Epilepticus

Parameter	Effect	Outcome
Blood pressure	Decrease	Hypotension
P_{O_2}	Decrease	Hypoxia
P_{CO_2}	Increase	Increased intracranial pressure
pH	Decrease	Acidosis
Temperature	Increase	Hyperthermia
Potassium	Increase	Dysrhythmias
Creatine phosphokinase	Increase	Renal failure
Cerebral blood flow	Increase	Cerebral hemorrhage
Cerebral oxygen consumption	Increase	Ischemia

Clinical Intervention in Status Epilepticus

Effective and immediate treatment of the patient with status epilepticus is mandatory to avoid severe brain damage or death. As previously described, there is a direct linear relationship between the temporal aspects of the seizure and the development of secondary ill effects. The emergency department physician must maintain a standardized approach to these patients to remain prepared to care for them. Overall goals include the assurance of adequate cardiorespiratory function, stabilization of metabolic imbalances, and treatment of the underlying cause.

The priorities in the management of a patient with status epilepticus are preservation of the airway, maintenance of ventilation, guarantee of oxygenation, and provision of circulatory support. Most patients with status epilepticus experience hypoxemia and hypercarbia. Strict attention should be paid to the head and neck to prevent aspiration or upper airway obstruction. Ventilation should be guaranteed by the use of a stethoscope rather than by oximetry. The use of an oral airway is recommended. In the presence of poor ventilatory effort, the child must receive mechanical ventilatory assistance in the form of bag-valve-mask ventilation or direct intubation. Some clinicians recommend prophylactic intubation for all patients with status epilepticus to ensure ventilation and to prevent the sequelae of aspiration. The clinician must not underestimate the potential for aspiration in these patients because they are usually in good health before their seizure and in all likelihood have eaten before the seizure. All children should receive 100% oxygen until arterial blood gases can be obtained. Experimental evidence supports this intervention.[10]

After the primary survey, serum should be obtained and tested for levels of anticonvulsants (if indicated), electrolytes, blood urea nitrogen, calcium, and glucose. A complete blood count and differential may be obtained at the same time. Once intravenous access is established, some patients may be candidates for administration of hypertonic glucose solutions. This subset of patients may be identified by Chemstrip analysis or by direct laboratory measurements. In either event, the dose is 2 mL/kg of 25% dextrose in water.

Pharmacologic Interventions

Diazepam

The most commonly utilized anticonvulsant agent in the acute setting is diazepam.[11] Diazepam has a rapid distributive phase (specifically to the CNS) and a relatively low rate of toxicity. The most favorable estimates of control of status epilepticus secondary to diazepam use have been encountered in pediatric patients with seizures of idiopathic ideology (90% success rate). Patients with organic lesions are less responsive to this medication. The major disadvantages of diazepam are its tendency to depress respiration and its short half-life within the CNS. The rapid redistribution of diazepam within the CNS accounts for the frequent recurrence of seizure activity 20 to 30 minutes after the initial injection of the drug.[12] Therefore, control of a convulsive episode after a single dose of diazepam represents only a self-limited period of control. In most patients it will be necessary to follow the initial dose with the institution of therapy with a long-acting anticonvulsant.

The initial recommended dose of diazepam is 0.3 to 0.5 mg/kg administered over a 2-minute period. The dose may be repeated within 5 to 10 minutes if seizure activity persists. Side effects of diazepam include sedation, respiratory suppression and/or arrest, and hypotension. Concomitant use of phenobarbital augments the risk of respiratory depression. The emergency department physician should always remain prepared to provide ventilation for all patients receiving intravenous benzodiazepines. In many patients, respiratory depression will necessitate artificial ventilation until the seizure abates or the patient's own efforts are satisfactory.

Lorazepam

An additional benzodiazepine is available for use in the setting of status epilepticus. Lorazepam has been advocated by some investigators because of its longer duration of action within the CNS.[13] In practice, most investigators have noted the onset of effective seizure control within 2 to 3 minutes. Pharmacologic studies have demonstrated that the peak effect of lorazepam occurs at 45 to 60 minutes and that, compared to diazepam, lorazepam penetrates the blood-brain barrier more slowly. Most investigators recommend the use of lorazepam on the basis of its ability to prevent seizure recurrence for periods ranging from 2 to 72 hours. The drug is administered intravenously over a 2-minute period in doses of 0.05 to 0.25 mg/kg. The most common side effect is drowsiness; respiratory depression is notably absent in most patients.

Phenobarbital

Phenobarbital was once considered the initial agent of choice for the treatment of status epilepticus in children. Advantages of phenobarbital include its long half-life and broad-spectrum effectiveness against many forms of seizure disorder. A major disadvantage is its slow absorption by brain parenchyma, which may delay its anticonvulsant effect for 10 to 20 minutes. The recommended loading dose is 15 to 25 mL/kg, which may be administered intravenously or orally. Intramuscular administration is not recommended. Complications include marked sedation, respiratory depression, hypotension, and shock. The maintenance dose of phenobarbital is 5 mL/kg/day, a regimen that should be instituted 12 to 24 hours after the loading dose is given.

Diphenylhydantoin

Many investigators have recommended the use of phenytoin as the anticonvulsant maintenance medication of choice for the patient in status epilepticus.[14] The major advantage of phenytoin is directly related to its relatively long half-life and the relative lack of CNS depression associated with its use. Phenytoin has an ideal distribution curve; its high lipid solubility promotes rapid and complete absorption within the brain. Pharmacologic investigation has demonstrated an equilibrium between plasma and brain tissue levels within 3 minutes.

Intravenous administration of phenytoin should be limited to a rate less than 50 mL/min. This precaution is necessary because the currently available preparations of phenytoin contain propylene glycol, a known cardiotoxic agent. It is therefore important that heart rate, blood pressure, and the electrocardiogram be monitored during all phenytoin infusions. The initial loading dose is 18 to 25 mg/kg. Subsequent maintenance regimens may be instituted 12 to 24 hours after the initial loading dose.

Summary

Status epilepticus constitutes a true medical emergency in the pediatric patient. A standardized approach to care will greatly diminish the possibility of significant mortality and morbidity associated with this event (Table 36-6). The linear relationship between seizure length and the development of permanent sequelae has been well documented. It is therefore imperative that the emergency physician maintain an aggressive approach to the management of this neurologic emergency.

Table 36-6 Emergency Management of Status Epilepticus

Protect and guarantee the airway.
Support ventilation with bag-valve-mask or endotracheal intubation.
Ensure sufficient perfusion.
Establish intravenous access; obtain serum for glucose (bedside and laboratory measurement), complete blood count, electrolytes, toxicology screen, and anticonvulsant levels (if indicated); calcium, magnesium, and phosphate analysis by clinical indication only.
Administer 2 mL/kg of 25% dextrose in water intravenously.
Administer diazepam, 0.3 mg/kg intravenously over 2 minutes up to 10 mg, or lorazepam, 0.05 mg/kg intravenously over 2 minutes up to 10 mg.
Administer phenytoin, 15 mg/kg intravenously at a rate less than 50 mg/min.
If phenytoin is ineffective, administer phenobarbital, 10 to 15 mg/kg intravenously.
If seizures persist, consider additional phenytoin, paraldehyde, or general anesthesia.

FEBRILE CONVULSIONS

Febrile convulsions represent unique and common forms of seizure disorders encountered in childhood. Three percent to 4% of children experience febrile seizures, and within this group 30% to 40% will have a recurrence at some point. Prospective studies have demonstrated that the likelihood of permanent deleterious educational or behavioral effects is quite low.

Definitions

The National Institutes of Health Consensus Development Conference on Febrile Seizures defined a febrile seizure as an event in infancy or childhood, usually occurring between 3 months and 5 years of age, associated with fever but without evidence of intracranial infection or defined course. Retrospective studies of patients with these paroxysms have assisted clinicians in defining what has come to be known as simple febrile convulsions.[15] A simple febrile convulsion is characterized as a seizure that is generalized and lasts less than 15 minutes.[16] Patients are usually between 6 months and 5 years of age. The patient demonstrates no focal or persistent postictal neurologic deficits. The onset of the seizure usually heralds the onset of the febrile illness within 24 hours. It is important to emphasize that the patients contained within this subset have normal prenatal and neurologic histories. They are therefore characteristically developmentally normal. Intercurrent histories are negative for ingestions or trauma. The family history is often positive for seizures of a similar type, and the electroencephalogram usually does not reveal epileptic activity within this group. The mortality associated with simple febrile seizures is extremely low.

Evaluation

When evaluating the child with a febrile convulsion, it is important that the clinician determine whether other family members have experienced a similar event. Patients are commonly transported by ambulance, and distraught and concerned parents may be the only available historians. The emergency physician is faced with the challenge of obtaining a precise history that accurately defines both the quantity and the quality of the event. It is not uncommon for the parent to overestimate the length of the seizure. Most patients will arrive after the paroxysm has subsided, most often in a variant of a postictal state. In many cases, demonstration of a febrile state in the emergency department will be the first awareness the parents have that their child has an elevated temperature.

Investigators have attempted to determine which of these patients are at risk of having the most serious underlying disorder, that is, a CNS infection. Most agree that these patients are at greater risk for having concurrent intercranial

Table 36-7 Clinical Scenarios Associated with Febrile Convulsions that Favor the Possibility of Serious Illness

Age less than 6 months or more than 5 years
Seizure of undue duration requiring anticonvulsant medications
Focal presentation
Recurrent seizures within the same febrile illness
History of pica and bloody diarrhea
Profoundly ill appearance
Focal deficits on neurologic evaluation

processes compared to the pediatric patient with an afebrile convulsive event.[17] It is therefore recommended that a lumbar puncture be performed on all infants younger than 18 months at the time of their first febrile convulsion.[18]

The clinician is also challenged with precisely defining the cause of the fever in this population. If the physical examination accurately demonstrates the presence of a focal infection (otitis media, cellulitis, or pneumonia), these patients may be classified as having fever with localizing signs. In the clinical setting without seizures, this subset of patients is often treated with appropriate antibiotics and discharged. The febrile convulsive patient without localizing signs should undergo the same standardized approach currently recommended for nonlocalized febrile patients without seizures (ie, blood culture, measurement of peripheral white blood cell count and differential, and, if indicated, urinalysis and culture). Evaluation of serum electrolytes or calcium is often unnecessary except in clinical scenarios that dictate the potential for fluid and electrolyte imbalance. Recommended investigative interventions for patients with complex febrile convulsions are directed toward determining more precisely the underlying intracranial processes[19] (Table 36-7). In the case of young infants or older children with these disorders, CT of the brain is often recommended. This radiographic investigation should be performed with enhancement to aid in identifying either vascular malformations or hyperemic foci. Herpetic encephalitis is often associated with a temporal lobe lesion. Patients with arteriovenous malformations often remain quiescent until the presence of a febrile state converts their static condition into a dynamic one.

Disposition

The main goal of therapy is to treat the cause of the fever. By the time most investigations are completed, most infants and children will have satisfactorily resolved their postictal state and returned to normal levels of consciousness. In cases where the child's mental status is not within acceptable limits after a reasonable period, admission for careful cardiopulmonary and neurologic observation is recommended. Institution of anticonvulsant therapy for the first febrile convulsion is currently not recommended.

REFERENCES

1. Rosman NP, Oppenheimer EY, O'Connor JF. Emergency management of pediatric head injuries. *Emerg Med Clin North Am.* 1983;1:141–152.
2. Finberg L. Treatment of dehydration in infancy. *Pediatr Rev.* 1981; 3:113–116.
3. National Institutes of Health Consensus Conference on Reye's Syndrome. Diagnosis and treatment of Reye's syndrome. *JAMA.* 1981; 139:2441–2448.
4. Mofenson NC, Greensher J. The unknown poison. *Pediatrics.* 1974;54:337–342.
5. Jennett B, Teasdale G. Assessment and outcome after severe brain damage: a practical scale. *Lancet.* 1975;1:480–486.
6. Bruce DA. Management of cerebral edema. *Pediatr Rev.* 1983; 4:217–222.
7. Plum F, Posner JB. *The Diagnosis of Stupor and Coma.* 3rd ed. Philadelphia: Davis; 1982.
8. Aicardi J. Convulsive status epilepticus in infants and children: a study of 239 cases. *Epilepsia.* 1970;11:187–192.
9. Meldrum BS. Physiologic changes during prolonged seizures and epileptic brain damage. *Neuropediatrie.* 1978;9:203–211.
10. Kreisman NR. Cerebral oxygenation during recurrent seizures. *Adv Neurol.* 1983;34:231–235.
11. Delgotta-Esqueta AV. Management of status epilepticus. *N Engl J Med.* 1982;306:1337–1340.
12. Canfield PR. Treatment of status epilepticus in children. *Can Med Assoc J.* 1973;128:671–678.
13. Lacey DJ. Lorazepam for status epilepticus in serial seizures in children: 218 consecutive cases. *Ann Neurol.* 1983;18:412–416.
14. Earnst MP. Complications of intravenous phenytoin for acute treatment of seizures: recommendations for usage. *JAMA.* 1983;249:762–765.
15. Gururaj VJ. Febrile seizures: current concepts. *Clin Pediatr.* 1980; 19:731–738.
16. Bettis DB. Febrile seizures: emergency department diagnosis and treatment. *J Emerg Med.* 1985;2:341–348.
17. Jaffe M. Fever and convulsions: indications for laboratory investigations. *Pediatrics.* 1981;67:729–733.
18. Hirtz DG. Survey on management of febrile seizures. *Am J Dis Child.* 1986;140:909–914.
19. Gerber MA. The child with a "simple" febrile seizure. *Am J Dis Child.* 1981;135:431–435.

37. Child Abuse

CELESTE M. MADDEN, MD, FAAP, FACEP

Historically there has been an evolution in the categorization of child abuse. Early reports in the medical literature described associations of physical and radiologic findings that could not be explained adequately by accidental or medical conditions.[1,2] In spite of intellectual resistance to the horrible possibility, these cases were eventually identified as having been caused by intentional injury and were labeled physical abuse. Since the early reports by Kempe et al[1] and Caffey,[2] the identified types of child abuse have multiplied to include physical abuse of all degrees of severity including homicide, shaken baby syndrome, psychosocial failure to thrive, medical neglect, sexual abuse, emotional deprivation and abuse, intentional poisonings, Munchausen's syndrome by proxy, abandonment, Satanic cult practices, and prenatal substance abuse.

Although child abuse can occur in any socioeconomic, ethnic, or racial group, several high-risk factors have been delineated. Child abuse presents more commonly in situations of family violence, family substance abuse, and poverty with its associated stresses. Children of all ages have been victimized, yet the youngest (infants and toddlers) are most at risk and sustain the most severe injuries. The perpetrator is most likely to be a parent or a parent surrogate in a trusting relationship with the victim.

The scope of the problem is huge. In America available figures indicate that at least 1.0% and 1.5% of children, respectively, are abused and neglected yearly.[3] Annual numbers of reports of suspected abuse or neglect, which are underestimated by virtue of the reporting system, fall somewhere in the range of 2.3 million cases nationwide. National figures of child fatality from abuse or neglect are estimated to be as many as 5,000 deaths per year.[4] The frequency of child abuse cases presenting to emergency departments varies from 1.3% to 10.0%.[5,6] These studies are likely to underestimate the true incidence of cases because reports have been limited to the category of physical abuse and because many cases may never be identified as abuse related.[7]

All states have reporting regulations for health care professionals. Emergency department staff must be aware of these requirements for their own jurisdictions. Failure to report suspected abuse and neglect cases may lead to civil and criminal prosecution of medical staff.[8] Optimal evaluation of child abuse situations includes medical and psychosocial investigations in an emotionally supportive environment. In selected cases, the evaluation is best triaged to another, less chaotic site after the emergency physician has determined that the child is medically and psychologically stable. Under no circumstances should the child be released to an environment that is potentially dangerous.

PHYSICAL ABUSE

In the evaluation of all trauma the physician must make an assessment as to the cause. It is the responsibility of the physician to be aware of the patterns or clinical syndromes of abuse and neglect as well as the typical appearance of accidental injuries of children. This knowledge in combination with the ability to assess a child developmentally will allow the physician to predict the likelihood that a situation is

Table 37-1 Suspicious Historical Indicators

Delay in seeking medical care
Absence of explanation for injury
Contradiction(s) in history of cause
Patient identification of perpetrator
Past history of abuse, neglect, or family violence
History that is inconsistent with the child's developmental age or examination findings
Mechanism of injury that is inconsistent with medical findings

---

abusive or neglectful. Several well-recognized historical red flags of child abuse are presented in Table 37-1. These indicators become more significant in the presence of severe injuries.

The most common manifestation of physical abuse is skin trauma. In a typical series of physically abused children from a children's hospital, bruises were present in 39%, and lacerations, scratches, abrasions, and other skin trauma were found in 41%.[9] Other manifestations seen in the same series were burns (8%), fractures (5%), and head trauma (2%). Some types of child abuse may cause serious injuries yet leave no external markings. These include shaken baby syndrome, poisoning, visceral trauma, and Munchausen's syndrome by proxy.

Bruising

Differentiation of abusive from accidental bruising can be based in large part on the appearance and pattern of markings. Table 37-2 categorizes the usual distribution of bruise site by etiology; no opinion should be based on site alone, however. Bruising or other cutaneous injury to the genitalia is rarely accidental. The color of bruises as representative of the phase of hemoglobin degradation can help in dating the bruise and therefore in checking the reliability of the history. Fresh bruises are red, blue, or purple, and old bruises (6 to 13 days) are green or yellow-brown; it must be remembered that depth of injury and fascial plane involved may alter the classic pattern of bruise resolution.[10]

Skin markings must be analyzed carefully to determine the presence of a pattern such as a bite mark, the outline of a hand or instrument used to inflict the injury (Fig. 37-1), or circumferential markings suggesting tethering injuries. Markings in a repeated or symmetric pattern are unusual in nature and suggest an inflicted etiology. The presence of bruises or lesions in multiple stages of healing, especially when found in areas rarely injured by accidental mechanisms, supports the occurrence of child abuse.

Medical conditions causing bruising or unusual skin markings should be considered during the evaluation. Possible medical diagnoses are mongolian spots; erythema multiforme; Henoch-Schönlein purpura; Ehlers-Danlos syndrome; immune thrombocytopenic purpura; hemophilia; vitamin K deficiency; maculae caeruleae associated with pediculosis; and acquired clotting abnormalities secondary to warfarin or salicylate ingestion, disseminated intravascular coagulation, or oncologic diseases. The diagnosis of these conditions is based on a typical history and laboratory testing in combination with characteristic dermatologic clues associated with the condition.

Occasional mistaken reporting of child abuse has occurred in cases of folk medicine practices among Asians.[11,12] Coining produces symmetric linear petechial lesions when the parent firmly rubs a coin or spoon over the sick child. Moxibustion involves burning tufts of herbs on the skin to draw out illness and produces small scars. In eastern European and Mexican cultures the healing practice of cupping, the placing of a heated cup on the back, may cause circular ecchymoses that have been confused with abuse.[13] Other cases of mistaken reporting have been associated with phytodermatitis secondary to psoralen skin contact.[14] Pigmented skin marks from sun exposure to psoralens in lime, celery, or fig juice innocently placed on the child's skin may mimic inflicted bruises, especially when they appear in the shape of a parent's hand. Once aware of this as a possible etiology, the physician can differentiate these cutaneous lesions from bruises.

Burns

Burns represent the second most common category of injury involving the skin.[15] As in accidental childhood burns, scalding fluids are responsible for the majority of abusive burns. The physician can usually identify an intentional burn from an account of the mechanism of the burn, assessment of the patient's developmental stage, and the distribution of the burn. Some suspicious situations will require a scene investigation, including measurement of the household water temperature. As in bruising, a telltale wound shape may reveal the cause of the burn injury. Immersion or dunking burns, the classic abusive burns, are intentional scald burns that leave a glove and stocking distribution or a water tide mark. A distinct border is created between the burned and the unburned skin as the child is held firmly in the hot liquid. Occasionally a confusing picture can result when the child is held in an unusual position or when the palms,

Table 37-2 Common Locations of Inflicted and Accidental Cutaneous Injuries

Inflicted	Accidental
Upper arms	Shins
Trunk	Iliac crests
Upper legs	Bony prominences of extremities
Sides of face, cheeks	Lower arms
Ears, neck	Prominences of spine
Genitalia	Forehead
Buttocks	Under chin
	Periorbital areas

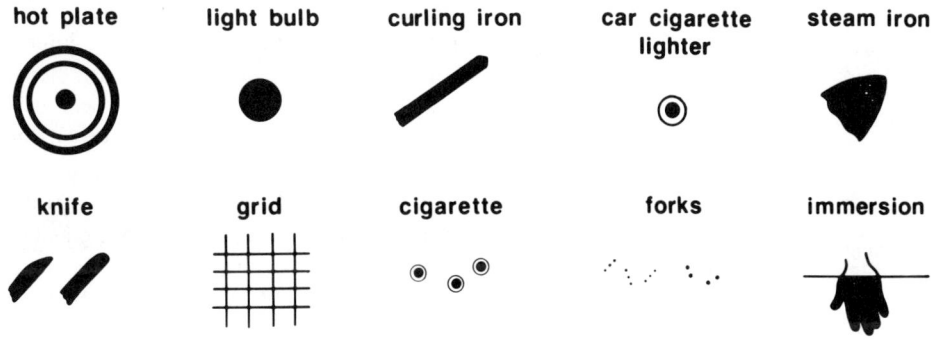

Figure 37-1 Patterns of inflicted injuries.

soles, or parts of the buttock are spared as they are held firmly in contact with the vessel surface and fail to contact the burning liquid long enough to sustain burn injury. Most accidental scald injuries are associated with an asymmetric dribble or splatter burn pattern descending in a waterfall-like distribution from the point of contact.

Particularly suspicious burns are those isolated to the genitalia. It is also unusual for a child accidentally to burn the dorsum of a hand because the palm is the exploring surface.[16] Bilateral hand dorsum burns are highly suspicious as inflicted. Cigarette burns have a characteristic punched-out center with raised borders. This appearance may be altered by superinfection or tangential injury.

A few medical conditions must be distinguished from abusive burns. Bullous impetigo resembles a cigarette burn in its circular configuration, but these lesions are typically not so deep, often appear in clusters of variously sized lesions, and frequently have a delicate collarette of dried skin at their border. Exfoliating dermatologic conditions such as staphylococcal scalded skin syndrome, Stevens-Johnson syndrome, toxic epidermal necrolysis, poststreptococcal peeling, or post–Kawasaki disease peeling can be differentiated by associated historical characteristics or classic patterns of involvement. Psoralen sun hypersensitivity may also mimic skin burns.

Fractures

Documentation of fractures and dislocations in reported cases of abuse ranges from 6% to 55%.[17,18] This broad range may be due to variations in threshold for obtaining radiographic studies, completeness of the study, and sensitivity of technique. The legal impact of identifying fractures in child abuse victims has been recognized. Children with documented fractures are more likely to be removed from the home than victims with negative skeletal evaluations. Kleinman[18] has assigned relative specificities for abuse of children based on location, nature, and chronicity of skeletal injuries (Table 37-3). An important factor in determining the cause of fracture is the consistency of the injury with the purported mechanism as given by the history.

Although shaft fractures are the most common fracture of abuse in all age groups, metaphyseal fractures occur more commonly in infants.[19,20] Metaphyseal fractures are most commonly seen in the distal femur, tibia, and proximal humerus. The mechanism of injury is believed to be axial pulling on the long bone. The fractures were previously referred to as bucket-handle or chip fractures.[21] Metaphyseal fractures frequently occur bilaterally. Kleinman et al[22] recently have elucidated the anatomy and radiologic appearance of these injuries. Histologic examination shows the fracture to consist of a series of microfractures through the bony plane of the metaphyseal primary spongiosa. Radiographic appearance of the fractures may be subtle depending on the X-ray beam angle. In one projection a fracture may appear as a corner chip, whereas in another projection it may be manifested by a transverse fracture across the bone (bucket-handle fracture). The absence of periosteal reaction explains the often subtle appearance and prevents dating of these injuries with a single film. Klein-

Table 37-3 Specificity of Radiologic Findings

High specificity
    Metaphyseal lesions
    Posterior rib fractures
    Scapular fractures
    Spinous process fractures
    Sternal fractures

Moderate specificity*
    Multiple fractures, especially bilateral
    Fractures of different ages
    Epiphyseal separations
    Vertebral body fractures and subluxations
    Digit fractures
    Complex skull fractures

Common but low specificity*
    Clavicular fractures
    Long bone shaft fractures
    Linear skull fractures

*Moderate- and low-specificity lesions become high-specificity lesions when history of trauma is absent or inconsistent with injuries.

Table 37-4 Skeletal Survey in Suspected Infant Abuse

Anteroposterior supine chest (bone technique)
Lateral chest (bone technique in infants)
Anteroposterior humeri
Anteroposterior forearms
Posteroanterior hands
Anteroposterior pelvis
Lateral lumbar spine (in infants)
Anteroposterior femora
Anteroposterior tibiae
Anteroposterior feet
Anteroposterior skull
Lateral skull

Note: All positive sites should be viewed in at least two projections.

man[23] has stated that the likelihood of diagnosis is directly related to the quality of the radiologic studies. He recommends that a careful skeletal survey (Table 37-4) be done with coned views to yield maximum information for diagnosis.

Rib fractures in children are suspicious for abuse. Healthy children with normally mineralized bones rarely fracture their ribs by accidental mechanisms. When they do, the involved forces are great. Rib fractures are similar to metaphyseal fractures in their subtle appearance on plain films. Located most commonly in the costovertebral junction area, acute fractures are masked by the overlying shadows, and even in the healing phase the callus may be overlooked. Bone scan affords a more sensitive test, especially for acute fractures of posterior ribs.[24] This bony injury has been closely associated with the shaken baby syndrome, where multiple fractures (possibly in various stages of healing) and bilateral fractures can be seen. The mechanism is believed to be secondary to compressive force applied to the infant chest, which levers the rib over the transverse process.

Accidental skull fractures in infants falling from short heights such as couches, changing tables, or beds have been characterized as uncomplicated.[25,26] The fractures are simple, linear, nondepressed, and nondiastatic, and the frequency of underlying brain trauma is low. Infants presenting after such an accident generally have no change in their level of consciousness and demonstrate a normal neurologic examination. Unexplained severe head injuries in young children are almost always inflicted.

Spiral fractures of the long bones have been seen in abused children. At one time spiral femoral fractures of childhood were almost always considered abusive in etiology. It was hypothesized that the force required for the injury of such a massive bone could not be mounted by a child alone. More recently it has been determined that weight-bearing children with a rotational injury can accidentally fracture the femur while running or falling.[27] The diagnosis of a spiral femur fracture in a younger (non–weight-bearing) child should continue to prompt a careful developmental history and description of the mechanism of injury. Certain types of humeral fractures may also be suspicious. In a retrospective study of children younger than 3 years, all nonsupracondylar humerus fractures were caused by intentional injury.[27]

Several patterns of injury seem to be strongly associated with child abuse. Fractures involving the sternum, scapulae, or spine have been associated infrequently with accidents in childhood. In the absence of a history of forceful impact, child abuse should be considered. A multiplicity of injuries in various stages of healing and in unusual sites without adequate explanation all add to a high level of concern.

Medical conditions bearing some musculoskeletal similarities to child abuse include osteogenesis imperfecta, Menkes' disease, scurvy, and conditions associated with poor mineralization of bone. Almost all cases of osteogenesis imperfecta can be differentiated by a detailed family history, physical examination, and careful examination of radiographs for characteristic findings. Menkes' disease (copper deficiency) can be diagnosed clinically. An in-depth discussion of the differential diagnosis of skeletal lesions in children has been provided by Brill and Winchester.[28]

Extraskeletal Trauma

Extraskeletal injuries with and without fractures may be seen in child abuse victims. The highest mortality occurs in victims with head injuries. Long-term follow-up of victims has identified a significant associated morbidity of developmental delay and mental retardation.[29,30] The spectrum of injury ranges from hair loss and subcutaneous hematoma to diffuse axonal shearing and intracranial bleeding. Fractures may or may not be present even with the severest of inflicted injuries. As more detail is available through magnetic resonance (MR) imaging, the extent of intracranial lesions is becoming better defined.[23] As group, infants sustain the majority of abusive head injuries and the most severe of these injuries in the spectrum of damage.[31–33]

Shaken baby syndrome is a complex of injuries that frequently includes central nervous system damage, posterior rib and metaphyseal fractures, and retinal hemorrhages.[2,34,35] It occurs in young children, usually younger than 1 year, who have been shaken vigorously and possibly thrown against a surface.[36] The clinical presentation is an infant with apnea, an altered level of consciousness, or seizures that are unexplained. These children may have sustained irreversible brain damage from prolonged periods of anoxia before presenting to the emergency department. Most often physical marks are absent, and the diagnosis is based on the age of the patient, suspicious presentation, and the presence of retinal hemorrhages. Retinal hemorrhages have been reported in 50% to 100% of cases.[35] The diagnosis can be made in their absence. Occasionally other signs of abuse may be found, such as finger and thumb prints left on the victim's chest as it was squeezed. Long bone metaphyseal and rib fractures should be sought carefully by skeletal survey and bone scan. Emergency cranial computed tomography (CT) may reveal various lesions, including subarachnoid hemorrhage, subdural hematoma (classically posterior interhemispheric in location), contusion, and diffuse edema. Spinal cord injury has been recognized in some children with shaken baby syndrome.[37] MR imaging has the ability to define the injuries in more detail than CT, but cost and instability of the patient limit this diagnostic modality during the acute evaluation. Serial CT scans and MR studies have been useful in documenting the timing of injuries as well as in suggesting a significant long-term morbidity in these patients.[38,39]

Intentionally inflicted visceral trauma is predominantly blunt in nature and involves the abdominal structures more frequently than the thoracic organs. Although the associated mortality is high, visceral injuries are an infrequent finding in child abuse cases.[40,41] A pattern of skeletal, visceral, and head injuries is seen predominantly in younger patients as opposed to older patients, in whom visceral injuries are noted more commonly in isolation. The lack of any explanation or an explanation inadequate to account for the degree of force involved is the historical clue to an abusive event.

As in accidental blunt trauma, any organ may be forcefully compressed to the point of rupture. Epigastric trauma occurs most frequently and may involve the pancreas, duodenum, or mesentery. Symptoms of obstruction or pancreatitis may be delayed. Ruptured viscera are uncommon manifestations of accidental childhood mishaps. Not only do perforations occur more commonly among the abused population, but the associated mortality is greater than when the cause is accidental.[42] This increased mortality in the abused population is probably due to the delayed presentation for care until such time as shock from blood loss or peritonitis is irreversible. Ledbetter et al[42] differentiated the abusive situation from the accidental one on the basis of delay in seeking medical care. In that review accidentally injured children were brought to the hospital immediately in 91% of cases, whereas 100% of abused children had a delayed presentation for care. The most commonly damaged solid organ in abuse victims is the liver; this is followed much less commonly by the spleen and kidney. The diagnostic evaluation and management of blunt trauma caused by child abuse does not vary from that for accidental trauma. Kleinman[43] has provided a comprehensive review of the diagnostic imaging of visceral trauma. Surgical management is discussed elsewhere in this section (see Pediatric Surgical Emergencies).

It is important to remember that significant internal damage may have occurred at the hands of the perpetrator in the absence of any cutaneous clues. Discovering the etiology of an injury or confusing symptom complex will certainly be more challenging without a truthful history. The possibility of intentional injury should always be kept in mind, and other telltale signs of abuse should be sought. Experienced emergency physicians are in a unique position to recognize inconsistent mechanisms of injury when examining a seriously injured child.

Unusual Manifestations of Abuse

The emergency physician must be aware of unusual presentations that may represent abusive or neglectful situations. Cases of intentional poisoning and child homicide present to the emergency department. In situations where the developmental skills of the child are inconsistent with the action involved in the poisoning, or when there has been a history of repeated ingestions, the question of intentional poisoning must be raised. Some of the children who come to the emergency department dead on arrival may actually be victims of homicide. A thorough history and physical examination will be necessary to identify these victims. The emergency physician must be aware of the characteristics of shaken baby syndrome and intentional drowning in coming to a final diagnosis.

In a series of child fatalities from a children's hospital emergency department, Showers et al[44] reported that most of the children were younger than 2 years and that 25% had a prior history of abuse or neglect. Head injury was the fatal event in just over half the cases, and blunt abdominal trauma led to death in 12%. Evidence of child abuse on physical examination was lacking in 53% of the cases. From this information, the investigators suggested that the following information be obtained in every series of situation of unexplained pediatric death: a description of the events of the 1 or 2 days preceding the injury or illness; names of all persons living in the home and their relationship to the child; previous injuries, serious illnesses, or deaths among siblings; stresses affecting the family; medical history and development of the child, including behavioral and developmental difficulties; and a thorough psychosocial history of the parent(s). Additionally, all children who die unexpectedly or for unexplained reasons should undergo autopsy. Diagnosis of child homicide will help protect the victim's siblings.

The emergency physician may stumble across a case in which he or she cannot determine a rational medical diagnosis for a child who repeatedly presents to the emergency department with the same symptoms. Meadow[45] described this phenomenon of fabricated or induced illness in children as Munchausen's syndrome by proxy. His cases represent the typical spectrum of medical complaints: apnea, seizures, bleeding, rashes, and fever. Rosenberg[46] described the complex of Munchausen's syndrome of proxy in her review (Table 37-5) and noted that gastrointestinal symptoms were also seen. The overwhelming majority of perpetrators are mothers, with an occasional father, foster mother, or medical caretaker being reported. These mothers are educated and appear remarkably attentive and concerned about their children, but surreptitiously they may be actively bleeding, poisoning, injecting, or suffocating their children. They tend to continue this abuse even in the hospital. More and more

Table 37-5 Munchausen's Syndrome by Proxy

Illness in a child that is simulated or produced by a parent or caretaker
Presentation of the child for medical assessment and care, usually persistently and often resulting in multiple medical procedures
Denial of knowledge by the perpetrator as to the etiology of the child's illness
Acute symptoms and signs that abate when the child is separated from the perpetrator

---

specialists may become involved in the case but fail to arrive at a diagnosis. The diagnosis is usually made when a health care professional familiar with the syndrome becomes aware of the case. Diagnosis from that point involves supervision to catch the perpetrator red handed, directed toxicologic assays for the suspected poison responsible for the victim's symptoms, or documentation of cessation of symptoms with separation from the perpetrator. The perpetrator usually denies the abuse even when the evidence is irrefutable. In situations involving older children, a private interview may not be revealing. At this stage, the child's involvement may be more than passive. The associated mortality approaches 9%. There is significant long-term psychologic morbidity, especially in chronic cases.[46] It is important to discover Munchausen's syndrome by proxy to protect the child from further harm or death. Because the disease may involve more than one child in a family, diagnosis may also prevent future abuse of siblings. Any suspicion on the part of the emergency physician should be communicated to the child's regular physician or the admitting team.

History and Physical Examination in Physical Abuse

As mentioned previously, much of the evidence for child abuse comes from an in-depth history and physical examination. Historical information about an injury must include time of injury, place of injury, mechanism of injury, sequence of events, response to the injury by the caretaker (including explanation for any delay in seeking medical care), persons witnessing the injury, and developmental level of the child. An inappropriate level of parental concern about the child should be objectively noted. The history is best obtained from a witness. In suspicious situations, such as outlined in Table 37-1, it is best to interview each witness and the verbal child separately. If the only witness is absent from the hospital, an effort should be made to interview that person by phone. The history should be taken directly by the physician and recorded carefully. It is helpful for the physician to review the history with the witness so that any inaccuracy can be avoided. Highly suspicious cases may require a scene investigation by child protective services or law enforcement to document the actual physical circumstances surrounding the alleged accident. The physician should be specific about the goals of the scene investigation when discussing the case with law enforcement.

An expanded history including the child's past medical illnesses or surgeries, unusual diet, medications, and family history will be important in differentiating medical causes of bruising and fractures from child abuse. Eliciting a history of previous injuries or poisonings may also be helpful in establishing a pattern consistent with abuse. If during the physical examination suspicious bruises or skin markings are found, a history of their cause and time of occurrence should be noted.

The physical examination should focus on the extent of the injury and an assessment as to whether the injury is consistent with the offered explanation. The location, size, configuration, and color of any bruise (mark) should be noted in the record. Some centers have developed a form that simplifies the process (see Appendix). Characteristic inflicted markings and typical patterns of abusive injuries should be documented. In any situation where a physician is suspicious, a complete physical examination of the child is in order. Growth parameters should be documented, especially if the child appears small for age or undernourished. Careful examination of scalp, ears, retinas, neck folds, genitalia, and hands and feet can yield telltale clues of abusive injuries. Particularly in infants, bones and joints should be palpated for deformity or tenderness. Children presenting with (history of) altered mental status or significant head injury should be assessed quickly for airway, breathing, circulation, and neurologic function. The possibility of concomitant spinal damage should not be overlooked in these patients. In a child with suspected abdominal trauma, serial assessment of vital signs and perfusion status must be performed along with repeated abdominal examinations for peritoneal irritation. When children are critically ill and need rapid intervention for stabilization, it is important to realize the legal need to document the condition of the body upon arrival at the hospital. One of the tasks of the accompanying physician should be to document carefully the extent of injury while the child is being attended to.

Social Intervention and Legal Concerns

At this stage of the visit, most physicians will have made a determination of the likelihood of intentional injury. Although the medical and surgical management of trauma is identical in accidental and abuse cases, the social and legal approach varies. In cases of abuse the social services team of the hospital and the community will need to be activated. Hospital social workers can be helpful in the psychosocial assessment of the family and in informing them of the need to report suspicious injuries to the authorities as required by law.

Physicians must fulfill their legal responsibilities by complying with the reporting procedures of their locality. Child protective services will probably confer with the physician as to the immediate disposition of the child. The disposition will be based on the child's medical condition as well as the estimated risk to the child upon returning home. Before releasing the child from the emergency department, the physician must be convinced that the child will be in a safe environment. If this cannot be guaranteed, the physician has the right to retain the child in protective custody until further investigation of the social situation is completed. Specific guidelines for protective custody vary, so that each physician must be aware of local statutes and hospital policy. Because there exists a risk of concurrent abuse of siblings, it is important for the physician to raise the question of location and safety of the victim's siblings. In cases of suspected child homicide, the physician will want to speak directly with the medical examiner and law enforcement officials as soon as possible. All evidence brought from the scene must be carefully preserved for further investigation. In these circumstances, the child's body should not be handled excessively or washed.

Laboratory Evaluation

The evaluation of an abuse victim is both medically and legally driven. Laboratory testing will be directed toward diagnosing the extent and cause of the trauma. Most patients with cutaneous injury will require a complete blood count and a clotting panel to document normal coagulation. Prothrombin time, partial thromboplastin time, thrombin time, and a platelet count are usually sufficient. Rarely a bleeding time, fibrinogen, and more detailed coagulation testing are indicated. Malnourished patients (failure to thrive) will require a blood count, electrolytes, liver and renal function tests, sedimentation rate, and urine culture as a basic evaluation. Patients with suspected abdominal visceral trauma will require, at a minimum, a screening blood count, amylase, liver function tests, and a urine analysis for gross or occult blood. Further evaluation will depend on these results and the continuing examination of the child. Hennes and associates[47] have reported the correlation of elevated transaminases (aspartateamino transferase >450 IU/L and alanineamino transferase >250 IU/L) with positive liver trauma on CT in blunt trauma. This information is applicable in the suspected abuse victim to rule out significant occult liver injury. Some cases involving possible medical explanations for skin or skeletal manifestations may require specific metabolic analyses to diagnose such diseases as osteogenesis imperfecta, Menkes' syndrome, rickets, scurvy, Ehlers-Danlos syndrome, or others. It is important to remember that medical disease and child abuse may coexist.

Toxicologic assays, serum and urine electrolytes, renal and liver functions, and a coagulation panel may be helpful when poisoning is suspected. The emergency physician will have to select the evaluation in view of the patient's symptom complex. Complicated cases such as Munchausen's syndrome by proxy will require directed use of the toxicology laboratory. In these patients it is best to discuss the suspected poison with the toxicologist or laboratory supervisor to determine the optimal test. Various body fluids, including stomach contents, may reveal the poison. In situations of suspected homicide, it will become important to coordinate laboratory studies with the medical examiner. Some diagnostic tests are more readily available in the university hospital and would be more helpful if performed before postmortem changes occur.

Radiographic Imaging

A number of imaging options are available to emergency physicians in the evaluation of poisoned and traumatized children. Individual tests will be selected according to the same criteria that apply to accidentally injured children. When red flags go up during the assessment of a patient and family, however, the physician may (and should) choose to use imaging studies in a more exploratory manner. For example, the child who presents with a tender distended abdomen without a coherent or consistent history may have abdominal flat plate and upright films taken to document free air. As in the laboratory evaluation, some imaging studies are ordered more for legal documentation of trauma than for actual medical or surgical management. An example is the use of the skeletal survey to document occult skeletal injury.

As numerous imaging techniques have been applied to the evaluations of physically abused children, issues of sensitivity, specificity, availability, interpretability, radiation dose, and cost have been argued. The American Academy of Pediatrics (AAP) Section on Radiology recently released its report on diagnostic imaging guidelines for physicians evaluating child abuse victims.[48] Their recommendations not only address the potential of specific studies in specific clinical situations but include guidelines for technique. The imaging standards suggested must be shared with the radiology services used by emergency physicians to guarantee the highest yield in diagnosis.

It has been recognized by the AAP and others that, although skeletal surveys are infrequently positive, a positive result can be used as irrefutable evidence of child maltreatment. Ellerstein and Norris[49] suggested that the maximal benefit of a skeletal survey in identifying occult trauma is obtained in the nonverbal age group. Certain older children whose ability to communicate is compromised by developmental delay, however, may also benefit from a skeletal survey. These findings are in agreement with the AAP guidelines, which include mandatory screening in suspected abuse of children younger than 2 years and use of clinical judgment in determining the need in older children and in selected cases of neglect and child sexual abuse. The content of the skeletal survey appears in Table 37-4. Each area must be imaged individually with proper technique to detect all fractures, particularly subtle metaphyseal and posterior rib fractures. Skull films should be part of the skeletal survey even when a CT scan or MR study is ordered. Emergency physicians should insist on high-quality films. At all ages, additional films and detail are required for clinically suspicious areas of injury. Surveys are useful in detection of injury as well as in dating the skeletal trauma(s). Repeat surveys or selected views of suspicious areas may be ordered after 1 to 2 weeks to look for callus formation to identify and potentially date fractures. O'Connor and Cohen[50] have provided a comprehensive discussion of the dating of fractures.

The use of bone scintigraphy remains supportive in the diagnosis of occult skeletal trauma. Some injuries, such as rib fractures and early, nondisplaced subtle fractures, are more easily detected by bone scan than plain films. Scan sensitivity is limited in areas of metaphyseal fractures, particularly when these are bilateral, and in spine injuries. Practical matters restricting scan use are availability at all hours, need for vascular access, potential need for sedation, and accuracy in interpretation, particularly in nonpediatric centers. Even when suspicious areas are identified on scan, a plain film will be necessary to delineate further the etiology and to date the finding. Bone scanning therefore remains a powerful but supplemental tool. It is particularly helpful in the case of shaken baby syndrome to identify the entire spectrum of severe skeletal trauma, which might otherwise be missed on plain films.

CT remains the best study in the emergent evaluation of a head injury. Ultrasonography is not sufficiently sensitive to identify all intracranial trauma. Although MR imaging gives greater anatomic detail and is frequently superior in dating injuries, CT will determine the necessity for emergency surgical intervention. At this time, CT has the advantages of accessibility, ease of use with critical patients, ease of interpretation, and lower cost. When MR imaging is used to evaluate head trauma, the physician should be confident that the interpreter is familiar with the norms of the young child's developing brain.

Because of the greater level of detail in MR studies, their use should be advocated in defining as fully as possible the extent of central nervous system damage. It is particularly valuable in suspicious or symptomatic cases when CT reveals little or no pathology. An example is shaken baby syndrome, where MR imaging may delineate bleeding and parenchymal injuries not visualized on CT. Only subarachnoid hemorrhage is equally well defined by CT and MR imaging. Although surgical treatment may be unaffected by additional injuries diagnosed on MR imaging, the legal import of an abnormal MR study may be powerful. It is also in the area of prognosis that MR imaging may have superiority over CT because the extent of chronic residua of inflicted head injuries are more clearly shown by MR studies.[23,48] Both serial CT scans and MR studies can be used to help in dating of injuries. This information will be helpful in cases where ongoing or repeated episodes of abuse are suspected.[38,39] MR imaging may also be applied to the anatomic areas of the orbit and the spine in adding information to CT evaluation of abused children.

The evaluation and management of visceral injuries should follow the usual surgical guidelines as outlined elsewhere in this section (see Pediatric Surgical Emergencies). From a practical standpoint, it may be important for the emergency physician to convey directly to the radiologist the suspicion that the patient has been abused. Once the radiologist is aware, the focus should shift to considering the usual spectrum of inflicted rather than accidental injury. This spectrum includes more intestinal, mesenteric, and pancreatic trauma. The child's serial physical examination, screening laboratory studies, and urinalysis will serve to guide the evaluation further.

Photographic Documentation

Photographic documentation of inflicted trauma is a powerful legal tool. In some jurisdictions photographs must be taken in the evaluation of abused children. The American Medical Association guidelines on evaluation of the child abuse victim include photographic documentation of physical lesions.[51] It is important for the emergency physician to become familiar with local requirements as well as hospital (unit) policy regarding obtaining, developing, identifying, storing, and releasing photographs to the authorities. Obviously, the physician responsible for obtaining the evidence should have a good working knowledge of the equipment available. Ricci[52] provides suggestions for equipment, technique, policy, and identification for physicians (Table 37-6). Because photographs may be destroyed or misplaced, physical evidence must also be noted in the record. Photographs can never substitute for the physician's medical record. Preprinted forms with anatomic diagrams (see Appendix 37-A) may facilitate accurate recording of this information.

Documentation

Because child abuse cases always have the potential for litigation, accurate and complete documentation is neces-

Table 37-6 Suggestions for Photographic Documentation of Child Abuse

Take a photograph with landmarks and one close-up of the lesion alone
Magnify in the original, not in a blow-up
Arrange the subject so that the surface of interest is parallel to the film
Take several shots from different angles and distances
Compose the picture the way you would normally look at the area
Keep the photographer and subject at the same level
Bracket shots if the correct exposure is uncertain
Shoot more slides rather than plan to duplicate
Photograph the patient's face for identification
Take a photograph of the patient's name
Use an uncluttered, neutral-colored background
Shoot only one patient per roll

sary. A detailed medical record serves as a permanent record of the evaluation for any future purpose. The medical report should include the history, physical examination, laboratory and radiology reports, and an assessment and management plan. In critically injured and unstable children, the emergency record may have to be abbreviated. Every attempt should be made by the medical team to complete the history and physical examination while the child is being stabilized. Failing this, the inpatient team should continue the evaluation and documentation process. The medical record of the evaluation should optimally include an assessment of the family by a social work hospital team member. All statements made in any part of the medical record should be objective, truthful, and legible. Any additions or corrections to the record should be dated, timed, and initialed or signed by the individual making the change. Comments made by witnesses and by the victim should be identified and placed in quotations. The record should document the chain of evidence when custody of physical evidence is transferred for legal reasons. This can be done in the nurse's notes or with a specialized form that stays with the medical record. Although the process of documentation is time consuming, a job carefully and completely done will serve both the patient and the physician well in future review of the case.

SEXUAL ABUSE

Sexual abuse has been called the abuse epidemic of the 1980s. Certainly sexual abuse of children occurred before that time, but investigation of the prevalence of the problem in society began to receive attention during the 1980s. Estimates of the magnitude of sexual abuse vary with the methods of study. Commonly accepted figures indicate that approximately one in 10 boys and one in four girls are sexually molested during their childhood. As with physical abuse, disbelief among professionals of the existence of sexual abuse has been a problem. The concept of sexual abuse may strike professionals as even more odious than physical abuse.

Although there exists no unique case model of sexual abuse, it is important for the emergency physician to be aware of the common patterns. Stranger and abduction abuse does happen but accounts for only a small number of incidents. Most sexual abuse of children occurs at the hands of a known teenager or adult. Most cases are considered incestuous in nature. The majority (>85%) of recognized victims are girls. The victim age range extends throughout childhood with peaks in the preverbal and school-age populations. The perpetrator relies on the trusting relationship he or she has with the victim to initiate and continue the abusive relationship. In some cases direct or implied threats are used to maintain the child's secrecy. Many young victims are initially unaware of the abnormality of the relationship because as children they have been conditioned to trust adults and to do what adults tell them to do. Because there are so many pressures on the child not to tell, and because many family members and professionals do not (want to) believe the child, many situations go on for years. The resultant long-term psychologic disturbances have been well documented in the mental health literature.

Unknowing professionals have often expressed doubt. Physicians may be unaware of the dynamics of incestuous abuse. Because most of our knowledge of sexual abuse has been gained in the last 10 years, medical school curricula may be devoid of any training in this area. Physicians are forced to obtain their knowledge from the literature.

Several misconceptions are particularly difficult to overcome. A common one is that perpetrators can be labeled (or protected from labeling) by race, class, profession, or some other social definition. Another is the assumption that when there is no sign of genital trauma abuse did not occur. In fact, experience has repeatedly shown that the examinations in the majority of abused children are normal. Most experts have found less than 25% of examinations of these victims to be abnormal. Even chronically abused children who undergo repetitive penetration can have normal examinations. There are at least two explanations for this situation. Finkel[53] has shown through serial examinations of genital trauma that healing of the genital area is rapid and that scarring is rare. Many times the disclosure and/or the medical examination occurs weeks or months after the last episode of abuse. When fondling, exposure, or orogenital contact represents the predominant abuse, physical findings may persist for less than a few days. From Finkel's work it is clear that damage from even more traumatic forms of assault heals within days to weeks.[53] In short, normal examinations, in isolation, never rule out sexual abuse.

Evaluation

It has been suggested that the emergency department is a suboptimal environment for the evaluation of pediatric sexual abuse. In this population emergent medical and surgical problems are rare. Although physical and sexual trauma can coexist, these circumstances are unlikely in incest, which represents the overwhelming majority of cases. The emphasis in documenting sexual abuse of a child should be placed on a detailed investigative and psychosocial interview and not on the physical examination.[54] Emergency physicians rarely have the training to do this type of interviewing and almost never have the ability to spend the necessary uninterrupted time with the patient in a busy emergency department. Optimal results in interviewing are achieved with a team approach involving specially trained nurses, social workers, and law enforcement officials.[55] In a few hospitals such a team works together with the physician who is involved with the physical examination and collection of evidence. In many situations sexual abuse evaluations can be triaged away from the emergency department to a more appropriate nonacute setting. In this setting it is more likely that the child can be adequately prepared for the examination and that the interview by the specialized team will be productive.

Some sexual abuse cases should be seen immediately, so that evaluation in the emergency department setting is unavoidable. Patients with a history of sexual contact with the perpetrator within the preceding 72 hours should be examined primarily to assess injury and to collect forensic specimens. In postmenarchal victims the indication for pregnancy prevention must also be considered. The cause of active bleeding and severe pain must be assessed expediently. An occasional child will have significant injury requiring surgical attention. A difficult clinical situation is the female victim with active vaginal bleeding. Unless the source of the bleeding can be identified, the child should undergo an examination under anesthesia to achieve sufficient visualization to rule out vaginal hematoma and vaginal tears that could lead to shock from internal blood loss or peritonitis. Psychiatric emergencies include catatonic, suicidal, and homicidal behavior. The emergency department evaluation in these situations is to document the medical stability of the patient and to enlist psychiatric consultation for care. These children will rarely be candidates for full medical and forensic examination until their mental health issues have been addressed. Relative indications for immediate emergency department care include extreme parental anxiety and cases where the safety of the child is in question. Even in these situations, a limited emergency department visit may suffice with triage to the nonacute setting to complete the examination and interview.

History

During the emergency department evaluation of a suspected sexual abuse victim, the physician should conduct a limited investigative interview and a medical history to establish the etiology of the patient's behavioral or physical symptoms. As in physical abuse, several histories may be offered. At a minimum, the (verbal) child and parent(s) can be asked about the reason for the visit. The history from the child may be influenced if a parent is present. A separate interview with the child is best conducted with an understanding demeanor and by encouraging the victim with open-ended questions. Any statements by the child recorded in the medical record in quotations can be considered for legal use. Figure 37-2 includes an example of historical guidelines in evaluating an alleged victim. Although behavioral indicators of child sexual abuse, such as sleep disorders and regressive or aggressive tendencies, have been identified, most of these are nonspecific indicators of stress in childhood. Some behaviors more specific to sexual abuse include inappropriate sexual knowledge or language for age, sexual acts, and excessive masturbation. The physician must be aware of the host of medical problems that, like sexual, may lead to the onset of enuresis, encopresis, genital or rectal bleeding, genital or rectal pain, rashes, or constipation.

Physical Examination

The focus of the physical examination is detecting physical evidence to support a diagnosis of sexual abuse and to distinguish medical conditions that might be mistaken for sexual abuse. Most victims can be guided through a complete physical examination by a supportive physician and assistant. Informing the patient about the examination is helpful in relieving some anxiety. Reassuring the verbal child during the examination that his or her body is not damaged (which is usually true) has been shown to be psychologically beneficial to the patient. No patient should be physically forced or restrained. Sedation may be indicated in some children. The optimal outpatient sedating agent is unknown, but midazolam by various routes has been used to facilitate the examination in traumatized patients. Although the effect of sedation on the examination has not been studied formally, it probably results in relaxation of the circumvaginal and anal muscles. This medication effect must not be misinterpreted as dilation from penetration. Signs of injury anywhere on (or in) the body must be noted. Search the skin for bruises, lacerations, and bite, gag, tether, or other markings. Look for intraoral trauma such as hematoma of the mucous membranes or palatal petechiae.

Examination of the genitalia should document signs of trauma or sexually transmitted diseases. An internal examination in a prepubertal child is almost never necessary. An exception is when there is active vaginal bleeding from an unknown source. A single sensitive internal examination can be done in selected postmenarchal victims. The (prepubertal) genital examination can be performed in the lithotomy (frog leg), lateral decubitus, or knee-chest position or with the child held on the parent's lap. The lithotomy position is the easiest approach and can be used with the technique of labial traction to visualize the hymen and vagina. The knee-chest position is particularly beneficial when one is looking far into the vagina, as for example when a foreign body is suspected. It is important to realize that the examination position and the state of relaxation of the victim will influence the size of the vaginal opening and the appearance of the hymen.[56]

To recognize abnormalities of the genitalia and anus, the physician must be familiar with the normal variants of anatomy. So much attention has been given to the study of the female genitalia in the past 5 years that experts have coined the term *hymenology*. Emergency physicians must take advantage of several excellent publications on the normal and abnormal appearance of the female genitalia.[56-61] The introital diameter or the horizontal diameter of the vaginal opening is associated with sexual abuse of prepubertal girls when it is found to be enlarged for age.[62,63] McCann et al[56] have shown that norms for age will vary with the state of relaxation and position of the patient and with the examination technique. A commentary from Heger and Emans[64] emphasizes the need to avoid basing the entire evaluation of the child on the introital diameter. Over the years of investigation, several hymenal findings have been described that are strongly associated with chronic sexual abuse of girls. These are attenuated or rolled edges, particularly in the posterior hymen; irregular or transected edges; tissue loss; notches between 4 and 8 o'clock in the lithotomy position; and scarring. A few medical conditions (Table 37-7) may be mistaken for sexual abuse.[65] The male victim can also be examined in various positions. In the uncircumcised patient the foreskin must be retracted to examine fully the penis.

External anal examinations for lesions and tone are usually sufficient. When internal trauma, retained foreign body, or extension of condyloma is suspected, a digital rectal examination is indicated. Current studies are in progress to define further the norms with regard to anal tone and spontaneous dilation.

Appendix 37-A contains examples for documenting physical examination findings. The location of genital or anal lesions or trauma is best documented by clock referents. The examination position of the patient must also be noted so that another examiner can relocate the findings.

Forensic Specimens

Sexual molestation of children is almost always a criminal offense. Evidence to prove sexual abuse includes specimens collected to corroborate the victim's or parent's allegations. Some of these specimens are released to law enforcement for analysis, usually in a prepackaged rape kit. If the abuse episode has occurred within 72 hours of the examination, a rape kit should be obtained. Attention has been focused on documentation of foreign materials such as semen, blood, saliva, and hairs; these not only may support the victim's history but also may identify the perpetrator. A Wood's lamp examination is helpful in identifying the presence of seminal fluid on the patient, bed clothes, or clothing. The patient and family should be instructed to bring all clothing or diapers worn at the time of the assault to the hospital to be included in the rape kit. The family should be instructed not to bathe the child before this acute evaluation. Guidelines for legal photography are available.[52] The photographer must be sensitive to the child's emotional state when obtaining these potentially embarrassing photographs. The purpose of the photographs must be explained to children to reassure them that they will not be used for false purposes. DNA testing is a relatively new development in this field, and its applicability is currently limited by cost, accessibility, and legal arguments.[66] Emergency departments should have a standardized rape kit that is acceptable to law enforcement in their jurisdiction. Prepackaging with all the necessary equipment for testing and labeling as well as typed instructions for the completion of the kit are optimal. Collection of specimens for the rape kit can be coordinated with testing for sexually transmitted diseases. As with all legal evidence, a system for chain of evidence must be in effect in the emergency department until law enforcement assumes custody of the specimens.

Table 37-7 Conditions that May Be Confused with Sexual Abuse Trauma

Congenital malformations
Hemangiomas
Urethral prolapse
Straddle injury
Lichen sclerosis
Perianal streptococcal cellulitis

Medical Evaluation

Guidelines for the evaluation of sexually abused children have been published by the AAP Committee on Child Abuse and Neglect.[67] After the history and physical examination, it will be apparent which children will need the services of gynecologists or pediatric surgeons. Few victims will require operative repair. Most of the laboratory testing in child sexual abuse victims is directed toward determining the presence of venereal diseases or other treatable infections and pregnancy. Sexually transmitted diseases are uncommon in pediatric patients, especially when the patients are asymptomatic and a history limited to fondling can be reliably documented. Some sexually transmitted infections can be asymptomatic, however. The AAP Committee on Child Abuse and Neglect recommends that appropriate cultures and serologic tests be obtained when epidemiologically indicated or when the history and/or physical findings suggest the possibility of oral, genital, or rectal contact. When victims are to undergo testing, the usual protocol includes gonorrhea cultures from the throat, genitals, and rectum; chlamydia cultures from the genitals and rectum; and a serologic test for syphilis. The optimal diagnostic technique for chlamydia testing for the child sexual abuse victim is culture, not one of the rapid indirect diagnostic tests. Testing for human immunodeficiency virus, hepatitis B, papillomavirus, herpes, bacterial vaginosis, *Trichomonas* organisms, or other infections is directed by the history of contact, symptoms, and physical findings. The timing of testing must take into account the known incubation periods for specific infections.[68] Additional samples to consider in the care of a victim depend on symptoms and include urine culture, pinworm paddles, and vaginal or anal cultures for bacterial pathogens such as group A streptococci and *Shigella* species.

General guidelines to facilitate the collection of specimens include a coordinated approach with the help of a support person to distract and relax the victim. Collection of vaginal specimens is much less bothersome to the patient if contact with the hymen is avoided as the swab is introduced through the introitus. Microswabs, preferably made of Dacron, should be available for the small victim. Lubrication can be achieved by moistening the swabs with nonbacteriostatic saline, but these swabs should be allowed to air dry before being placed in a rape kit. Venipuncture is best reserved for the end of the evaluation.

Female victims who are imminently pubertal or postpubertal will require pregnancy testing on at least one occasion. Serum samples are preferred. Convalescent syphilis serology may be coordinated with repeat pregnancy testing on a case-by-case basis.

Treatment

Medical treatment of the victim should address repair of injuries, treatment of infection, and consideration of pregnancy prevention. The timing of follow-up appointments will vary from case to case. Unless there is a strong suspicion of a venereal disease at the time of the initial examination, treatment is best delayed until documentation of infection. Recommendations for treatment depend on allergic history, site of infection, and size of the patient.[68] The implications of specific venereal diseases in sexual abuse appear in Table 37-8.[67] In consenting patients who are seen within 72 hours and are determined to be at risk for pregnancy, the oral contraceptive Ovral (2 tablets immediately and 2 tablets in 12 hours) may be prescribed after side effects are discussed. Because this medication is not 100% effective, it will be necessary to arrange for a follow-up pregnancy test. Before the patient is discharged, it is best to review the examination findings, outstanding test results, indications to return to medical care, and follow-up appointments with the family.

Table 37-8 Implications of Commonly Encountered Sexually Transmitted Diseases

Confirmed Infection	Sexual Abuse	Suggested Action
Gonorrhea*	Certain	Report‡
Syphilis*	Certain	Report
Chlamydia*	Probable†	Report
Condyloma acuminatum*	Probable	Report
Trichomonas vaginalis	Probable	Report
Herpes 1 (genital)	Possible	Report§
Herpes 2	Probable	Report
Bacterial vaginosis	Uncertain	Medical follow-up
Candida albicans	Unlikely	Medical follow-up

*If not perinatally acquired.
†Culture is the only reliable diagnostic method.
‡Report to the agency mandated in the community to receive reports of suspected sexual abuse.
§Unless there is a clear history of autoinoculation.

Prepared by the American Academy of Pediatrics Committee on Child Abuse and Neglect (November 1990).

Social management must be coordinated through social services within the hospital and possibly through child protective services. The hospital social worker must assess the family's strengths and ability to protect the victim. Referral of the family to supportive community agencies and available mental health services should be initiated in the emergency department.

The criminal definition of sexual abuse of children will necessitate the early involvement of law enforcement. The emergency department staff must protect the child from multiple, public, and untrained interviews. If possible, an appointment for an investigative interview should be arranged with a special unit trained to work with child victims. Some degree of legal involvement is necessary in attempting to prove the allegation of abuse. The physician can rely on the detailed record of the evaluation for future proceedings. Chadwick[69] has made several recommendations for physicians giving court testimony.

Documentation

Recommendations for documentation in the physical abuse section of this chapter apply to cases of sexual abuse. Any significant historical, physical, or medical findings must be noted. Final assessments of the certainty of abuse are not always possible at the time of patient discharge from the emergency department. Premature judgments on the part of the physician are to be avoided. Under no circumstances should the physician (or court) assume that a normal physical examination proves that a child has not been abused.

CONCLUSION

The evaluations of child abuse are multidimensional and include the need to address medical, social, and legal concerns. These cases are intellectual and emotional challenges to the emergency department staff. It is the responsibility of the physician to recognize the problem, deliver care in a sensitive and supportive environment, and protect the child from further harm.

REFERENCES

1. Kempe CH, Silverman FN, Steele BF, et al. The battered-child syndrome. *JAMA*. 1962;181:17–24.
2. Caffey J. Multiple fractures in long bones of infants suffering from chronic subdural hematoma. *Am J Roentgenol*. 1946;56:163–173.
3. Sedlak AJ. *Study of National Incidence and Prevalence of Child Abuse and Neglect: Final Report*. Washington, DC: ESTAT; 1987.
4. American Humane Association. *Highlights of Official Child Abuse and Neglect Reporting, Annual Report*. Denver: American Humane Association; 1986.
5. Pless IB, Sibald AD, Smith MA, et al. A reappraisal of the frequency of child abuse seen in pediatric emergency rooms. *Child Abuse Neglect*. 1987;11:193–200.

6. Holter JC, Friedman SB. Child abuse: early case findings in the emergency department. *Pediatrics*. 1968;42:128–138.
7. Johnson CF, Apolo J, Joseph JA, et al. Child abuse diagnosis and the emergency department chart. *Pediatr Emerg Care*. 1986;2:6–9.
8. Dobbs D. Legal responsibilities and liabilities when treating child abuse. *Pediatr Emerg Care*. 1986;2:40–44.
9. Johnson CF. Inflicted injury versus accidental injury. *Pediatr Clin North Am*. 1991;37:791–814.
10. Wilson EF. Estimation of the age of cutaneous contusions in child abuse. *Pediatrics*. 1977;60:750–752.
11. Saulsbury FT, Hayden GF. Skin conditions simulating child abuse. *Pediatr Emerg Med*. 1985;1:147–150.
12. Yeatman GW, Shaw C, Barlow MJ, et al. Pseudobattering in Vietnamese children. *Pediatrics*. 1976;58:616–618.
13. Sandler AP, Haynes V. Nonaccidental trauma and medical folk belief: a case of cupping. *Pediatrics*. 1978;61:921–922.
14. Coffman K, Boyce T, Hansen RC. Phytophotodermatitis simulating child abuse. *Am J Dis Child*. 1985;139:239–240.
15. Ellerstein NS. The cutaneous manifestations of child abuse and neglect. *Am J Dis Child*. 1979;133:906–909.
16. Johnson CF, Kaufman KL, Callendar C. The hand as a target organ in child abuse. *Clin Pediatr*. 1990;29:66–72.
17. Johnson CF, Showers J. Injury variables in child abuse. *Child Abuse Neglect*. 1985;9:207–215.
18. Kleinman PK. Skeletal trauma: general considerations. In: Kleinman PK, ed. *Diagnostic Imaging of Child Abuse*. Baltimore: Williams & Wilkins; 1987.
19. Merten DF, Radkowski MA, Leonidas JC. The abused child: a radiologic reappraisal. *Radiology*. 1983;146:377–381.
20. Kleinman PK, Blackbourne BD, Marks SC, et al. Radiologic contributions to the investigation and prosecution of cases of fatal infant abuse. *N Engl J Med*. 1989;320:507–511.
21. Caffey J. Some traumatic lesions in growing bones other than fractures and dislocations: clinical and radiological features. *Br J Radiol*. 1957;30:225–238.
22. Kleinman PK, Marks SC, Blackbourne B. The metaphyseal lesion in abused infants: a radiologic-histopathologic study. *AJR*. 1986;146:895–905.
23. Kleinman PK. Diagnostic imaging in infant abuse. *AJR*. 1990;155:703–712.
24. Smith FW, Gilday DL, Ash JM, et al. Unsuspected costovertebral fractures demonstrated by bone scanning in the child abuse syndrome. *Pediatr Radiol*. 1980;10:103–106.
25. Helfer RE, Slovis TL, Black M. Injuries resulting when small children fall out of bed. *Pediatrics*. 1977;60:533–535.
26. Kravitz H, Driessen G, Gomberg R, et al. Accidental falls from elevated surfaces in infants from birth to one year of age. *Pediatrics*. 1969;44:869–876.
27. Thomas SA, Rosenfield NS, Leventhal JM, et al. Long-bone fractures in young children; distinguishing accidental injuries from child abuse. *Pediatrics*. 1991;88:471–476.
28. Brill PW, Winchester P. Differential diagnosis of child abuse. In: Kleinman PK, ed. *Diagnostic Imaging in Child Abuse*. Baltimore: Williams & Wilkins; 1987:221–241.
29. Elmer E, Gregg GS. Developmental characteristics of abused children. *Pediatrics*. 1967;40:596–602.
30. Martin HP, Beezley P, Conway EF, et al. The development of abused children. Part I. A review of the literature. Part II. Physical, neurological, and intellectual outcome. *Adv Pediatr*. 1974;21:25–73.
31. Billmire ME, Meyers PA. Serious head injury in infants: accidents or abuse? *Pediatrics*. 1985;75:340–342.
32. Sinal S, Ball M. Head trauma due to child abuse: serial computerized tomography in diagnosis and management. *South Med J*. 1987;80:1505–1512.
33. Rivera FP, Kamitsuka MD, Quan L. Injuries to children younger than one year of age. *Pediatrics*. 1988;81:93–97.
34. Ludwig S. Shaken baby syndrome: a review of 20 cases. *Ann Emerg Med*. 1984;13:104–107.
35. Levin A. Ocular manifestations of child abuse. *Ophthalmol Clin North Am*. 1990;3:249–264.
36. Duhaime AC, Gennarelli TA, Thibault LE, et al. The shaken baby syndrome: a clinical, pathological and biomechanical study. *J Neurosurg*. 1987;66:409–415.
37. Hadley MN, Sonntag VK, Rekate HL, et al. The infant whiplash-shake injury syndrome: a clinical and pathological study. *Neurosurgery*. 1989;24:536–540.
38. Zimmerman RA, Bilaniuk LT, Bruce D, et al. Computed tomography of craniocerebral injury in the abused child. *Radiology*. 1979;130:687–690.
39. Alexander RC, Schor DP, Smith WL. Magnetic resonance imaging of intracranial injuries from child abuse. *J Pediatr*. 1986;109:975–979.
40. Merten DF, Osborne RS, Radkowski MA, et al. Craniocerebral trauma in the child abuse syndrome: radiological observations. *Pediatr Radiol*. 1984;14:272–277.
41. Touloukian RJ. Abdominal trauma in childhood. *Surg Gynecol Obstet*. 1968;127:561–568.
42. Ledbetter DJ, Hatch EI, Feldman KW, et al. Diagnostic and surgical implications of child abuse. *Arch Surg*. 1988;123:1101–1105.
43. Kleinman PK. Visceral trauma. In: Kleinman PK, ed. *Diagnostic Imaging of Child Abuse*. Baltimore: Williams & Wilkins; 1987:115–158.
44. Showers J, Apolo J, Thomas J, et al. Fatal child abuse: a two decade review. *Pediatr Emerg Care*. 1985;1:66–70.
45. Meadow R. Munchausen syndrome by proxy. *Arch Dis Child*. 1982;57:92–98.
46. Rosenberg D. Web of deceit: a literature review of Munchausen syndrome by proxy. *Child Abuse Neglect*. 1987;11:547–563.
47. Hennes HM, Smith DS, Schneider K, et al. Elevated liver transaminases in children with blunt abdominal trauma: a predictor of liver injury. *Pediatrics*. 1990;86:87–90.
48. American Academy of Pediatrics Section on Radiology. Diagnostic imaging in child abuse. *Pediatrics*. 1991;87:262–264.
49. Ellerstein NS, Norris KJ. Value of radiologic skeletal survey in assessment of abused children. *Pediatrics*. 1984;74:1075–1078.
50. O'Connor JF, Cohen J. Dating fractures. In: Kleinman PK, ed. *Diagnostic Imaging of Child Abuse*. Baltimore: Williams & Wilkins; 1987:103–114.
51. Council on Scientific Affairs. AMA diagnostic and treatment guidelines concerning child abuse and neglect. *JAMA*. 1985;254:796–800.
52. Ricci L. Photographing the physically abused child—principles and practice. *Am J Dis Child*. 1991;145:275–281.
53. Finkel M. Anogenital trauma in sexually abused children. *Pediatrics*. 1989;84:317–322.
54. Dubowitz H, Black M, Harrington D. The diagnosis of sexual abuse. *Am J Dis Child*. 1992;146:688–693.
55. Jaudes PK, Martone M. Interdisciplinary evaluations of alleged sexual abuse cases. *Pediatrics*. 1992;89:1164–1168.
56. McCann J, Voris J, Simon M, et al. Comparison of genital examination techniques in prepubertal girls. *Pediatrics*. 1990;85:182–187.
57. McCann J, Voris J, Simon M. Genital injuries resulting from sexual abuse: a longitudinal study. *Pediatrics*. 1992;89:307–317.

58. Berenson A, Heger A, Hayes J, et al. Appearance of the hymen in prepubertal girls. *Pediatrics*. 1992;89:387–394.
59. McCann J, Wells R, Simon M, et al. Genital findings in prepubertal girls selected for non abuse: a descriptive study. *Pediatrics*. 1990;86:428–439.
60. Emans SJ. Sexual abuse in girls: what have we learned about genital anatomy? *J Pediatr*. 1992;120:258–260.
61. Chadwick DL, Berkowitz CD, Kerns D, McCann J, Reinhart MA, Strickland S. *Color Atlas of Child Sexual Abuse*. Chicago: Year Book Medical; 1989.
62. Cantwell H. Vaginal inspection as it relates to child sexual abuse in girls under thirteen. *Child Abuse Neglect*. 1983;7:171–176.
63. Cantwell H. Update on vaginal inspection as it relates to child sexual abuse in girls under thirteen. *Child Abuse Neglect*. 1987;11:545–546.
64. Heger A, Emans SJ. Introital diameter as the criterion for sexual abuse. *Pediatrics*. 1990;85:222–223.
65. Bays J, Jenny C. Genital and anal conditions confused with sexual abuse trauma. *Am J Dis Child*. 1990;144:1319–1322.
66. McCabe ER. Applications of DNA fingerprinting in pediatric practice. *J Pediatr*. 1992;120:499–509.
67. American Academy of Pediatrics Committee on Child Abuse and Neglect. Guidelines for the evaluation of sexual abuse of children. *Pediatrics*. 1991;87:254–260.
68. Paradise J. The medical evaluation of the sexually abused child. *Pediatr Clin North Am*. 1990;37:839–862.
69. Chadwick D. Preparation for court testimony in child abuse cases. *Pediatr Clin North Am*. 1990;37:955–970.

APPENDIX 37-A: SUSPECTED ABUSE FORM

Suspected Abuse Form

DATE	PATIENT NAME	HOSPITAL #
AGE	ETHNICITY	Has there been a prior CPS report? ☐ Yes ☐ No

PERSONNEL INVOLVED IN CASE
- Nursing: _____
- Hospital S. W.: _____
- Law Enforcement: _____
- Pediatrics: _____
- Foster care worker: _____
- CPS: _____

NURSES NOTE: TEMP: _____ BP: _____ HR: _____ RR: _____

HT/HT% _____ WT/WT% _____ HC/HC% _____

_____
_____
_____
_____
_____

HISTORY • Delineate if obtained from child, parent, guardian or neighbor - if obtained separately

Chief complaint: _____

Alleged perpetrator:	Perpetrator age:	Relationship to patient:

Site of the incident: ☐ Child's home ☐ Perpetrator's home ☐ Relative/friend's home ☐ Sitter ☐ Public place ☐ Unknown

History of Incident:
(include: interaction with perpetrator, secrecy, circumstances surrounding the disclosure, etc.)

_____
_____
_____
_____
_____

Behavior History:
(include: somatic complaints, increased sex play, masturbation, changes in behavior or sleep, acting out, developmental delay, etc.)

_____
_____
_____
_____
_____

1 of 6

| DATE | PATIENT NAME | HOSPITAL # |

Medical History:
(include: constipation, diarrhea, encopresis, laxative abuse, pruritis, pinworms, straddle injuries, surgeries, vaginal discharge or bleeding, enuresis, dysuria, include an explanation for the injury)

PMH

Medications

Allergies

Family Hx
(number of siblings, ages, relationship of perpetrator)

Social Hx

Patient's MD

SPECIFIC HISTORICAL EVENTS

Relationship of perpetrator:

Number of episodes of abuse: ☐ One ☐ Multiple ☐ Unknown

Date of most recent abuse:

Did the act involve:
☐ Penile-genital contact ☐ Oral-genital contact ☐ Hand-genital contact
☐ Vaginal penetration ☐ Insertion of objects
☐ Penile-anal contact   Did ejaculation occur? ☐ Yes ☐ No
☐ Anal penetration   Was a condom used?   ☐ Yes ☐ No
Body site involved: Date:

Was there loss of consciousness? ☐ Yes ☐ No
For how long?

Are there bruises evident? ☐ Yes ☐ No DESCRIBE ON NEXT PAGE

Since the incident has the patient:
☐ Changed underwear   ☐ Bathed
☐ Eaten/rinsed mouth   ☐ Douched
☐ Urinated/defecated

Is patient menarchal? ☐ ☐ No Onset Age _____

LMP _____   Last intercourse _____
Cycle Length _____   Method of contraception _____

Does patient use contraception? ☐ Yes ☐ No
Method:

DATE	PATIENT NAME	HOSPITAL #

PHYSICAL EXAMINATION

General:
(include: emotional state, condition of body/clothing)

Body Surface and Skin: *give history of etiology on pg 4*
(bruises, lacerations, bite marks, etc.)

Woods lamp exam performed on clothes? ☐ Yes ☐ No   Fluorescence (sperm?) ☐ Yes ☐ No   IF YES, WHICH GARMENT?

on body? ☐ Yes ☐ No   Fluorescence (sperm?) ☐ Yes ☐ No   IF YES, INDICATE WHERE ON DRAWINGS

HEENT oral petechiae, torn frenulum?

CHEST/LUNGS   Breasts:

HEART

ABDOMEN   PULSES

BACK   EXTREMITIES

PERINEUM   *General (friability, ecchymosis, vascularity, discharge, condyloma, vesicles)*

TANNER STAGE:

FEMALES   HYMEN   *annular, crescent, fimbriated, imperforate, microperforations?*

EXAM POSITION ☐ Supine ☐ traction ☐ no traction   ☐ Knee-chest

Are there clefts, notches, bumps, synechiae, assymetry, rounded edges, abrasions, lacerations, adhesions?

Introital diameter: Transverse   mm x Vertical   mm

POSTERIOR FOURCHETTE: *Abrasions, friability, adhesions*

VAGINAL DISCHARGE: *clear, yelllow, green, etc.*

URETHRA   *Discharge, abrasions, etc.*

RECTUM ☐ Supine: ☐ with traction ☐ without traction   ☐ Knee-chest

Anal tone, fissures, discoloration, reflex anal dilatation, size of rectal opening, scars, skin tags, lacerations, funnelling?

DATE	PATIENT NAME	HOSPITAL #	

Describe and number findings such as bruises, lacerations, marks, scars, STD lesions, etc. Include size, shape, color and cause per guardian: **FEMALE:**

NUMBER	DESCRIPTION	CAUSE PER GUARDIAN

MALES   PENIS & SCROTUM *Bruises, etc*

URETHRA   *Discharge, abrasions, etc.*

RECTUM   ☐ Supine: ☐ with traction   ☐ without traction   ☐ Knee-chest
Anal tone, fissures, discoloration, reflex anal dilatation, size of rectal opening, scars, skin tags, lacerations, funnelling?

NUMBER	DESCRIPTION	CAUSE PER GUARDIAN

| DATE | PATIENT NAME | HOSPITAL # |

Describe and number findings such as bruises, lacerations, marks, scars, STD lesions, etc. Include size, shape, color and cause per guardian:

NUMBER	DESCRIPTION	CAUSE PER GUARDIAN

DATE	PATIENT NAME	HOSPITAL #	

Impression: _____

_____

CPS Hotline called? ☐ Yes ☐ No By Whom? _____ Date: _____

Form 2221 filed? ☐ Yes ☐ No By Whom? _____ Date: _____

Patient Discharged to: ☐ Home ☐ Foster Home ☐ Other _____ In Custody of: _____

FOLLOWUP
- C.A.R.E. Clinic appointment card given: Yes ☐ No ☐
- ☐ C.A.R.E. Clinic appointment made for (date) _____
- ☐ E.N.H.A.N.C.E. appointment made for (date) _____
- ☐ Appointment with private M.D. (date) _____

DIAGNOSTIC STUDIES ORDERED

FOR GC:
- ☐ Throat Cx
- ☐ Vaginal/Cervical
- ☐ Urethral Cx
- ☐ Rectal Cx

- ☐ Vaginal KOH prep
- ☐ Vaginal wet prep
- ☐ General vaginal bacterial Cx
- ☐ Vaginal gram stain
- ☐ Clotting functions

FOR CHLAMYDIA:
- ☐ Rectal Cx
- ☐ Vaginal/Cervical Cx
- ☐ Urethral Cx

- ☐ VDRL
- ☐ HIV
- ☐ Pap smear
- ☐ Urine/serum pregnancy test
- ☐ Hep BsAg
- ☐ Urinalysis
- ☐ Urine culture
- ☐ Stool hematest
- ☐ Herpes culture (site: _____)
- ☐ Virapap (HPV)
- ☐ Pin worm prep given to caretaker
- ☐ Sketetal series
- ☐ CT scan
- ☐ Bone scan

☐ Other _____

EVIDENTIARY MATERIAL:
- ☐ Rape Kit: specimens to go to Crime Lab
  Specimens given to _____ Badge # _____ Date/Time _____
- ☐ 35 mm Photos ☐ polaroids ☐ colposcope _____ Date/Time _____

DATE: _____   PHYSICIAN'S SIGNATURE: _____

38. Radiation Emergencies

CHARLES V. POLLACK, JR., MD

Although the lay media and popular cinema may indicate otherwise, the emergency physician's most probable encounter with a radiation injury will not follow a large-scale reactor accident or a thermonuclear explosion. Isolated occupational exposures, often limited to specific parts of the body, are much more characteristic of radiation injuries.

Radiation accidents are indeed rare and complex and too frequently result in patients presenting to a community hospital emergency department that is ill-equipped to handle them. Basic preparation for radiation injuries is not difficult, however, and should be achieved by all hospitals. These patients require prompt evaluation and are rarely of any danger to hospital staff. In addition, facilities located near nuclear power reactors and other large commercial or military sources of radiation should have in place disaster plans specific for large-scale radiation accidents.

PHYSICS AND PATHOPHYSIOLOGY

The term *radiation* encompasses the entire electromagnetic spectrum from ultra–high-frequency γ rays, through visible light, to relatively broad-wavelength microwaves. Nonionizing radiation, including visible light, microwaves, and broadcasting waves for radio, television, and satellite communications, is characterized by low energy. The adverse effects of nonionizing radiation on humans are essentially limited to local heat production and are not discussed further here, but the interested reader is referred to the literature for more information.[1,2]

Ionizing radiation is electromagnetic or particulate in nature and is named for its ability to interact with and form ion pairs in matter. In living tissues, ion formation from water leads to breaks in strands of DNA and RNA and to damaging reactions at the cellular metabolic level. Rapidly dividing cells, such as bone marrow cells and cells lining the gastrointestinal mucosa, are most susceptible to these effects. Types of ionizing radiation include X rays, α and β particles, γ rays, and neutron radiation. There are three important factors that determine the magnitude of an organism's exposure to ionizing radiation: the organism's distance from the source (energy dissipates as the inverse square of the distance), the time spent near the source (to which absorption is directly proportional), and the shielding between the organism and the source of the radiation.

α Particles

α Particles are relatively heavy emissions composed of two protons and two neutrons (identical to the nucleus of a helium atom). Because of their mass and speed, they cannot penetrate the human epidermis. They travel only inches in air from their source. If they are deposited internally, however, the rapid release of energy from α-emitting materials can be quite injurious to cells of the gastrointestinal and pulmonary systems. α Particles are found naturally in rocks and soil. They can be shielded with a piece of paper.

β Particles

β Particles are single electrons. They have relatively low mass and can travel at nearly the speed of light, but they disperse only a few feet in air from their source. β Particles can penetrate tissue more deeply than α particles and primarily cause thermal injuries in both external and internal exposures. They likewise occur naturally in the earth's crust and also are present in the human body from ^{40}K. β Particles can be shielded with a thin sheet of metal.

γ Rays and X Rays

γ Radiation and X rays are not particulate but electromagnetic and massless. They travel in waves at the speed of light. These types of photon radiation are similar; γ rays originate in the atomic nucleus and X rays from the electron cloud. Both can penetrate tissue and deposit energy deeply. Thick layers of concrete or lead are required for shielding. γ Rays frequently accompany the liberation of particulate radiation; β particles are often responsible for the skin damage seen in γ irradiation. Although exposure to X rays generally occurs in the medical or industrial setting, all people are constantly exposed to a low level of γ rays through cosmic radiation.

Neutrons

Exposure to neutron irradiation does not occur naturally but only as a result of nuclear reactions. Neutrons are particulate but carry no electrical charge; they ionize by colliding with atomic nuclei within cells and tissues. Like γ rays, neutrons have strong power to penetrate and are the only type of radiation that can induce radioactivity in sodium, phosphorus, chloride, and other atoms in the body. This radioactivity can be detected in body fluids. Shielding from neutrons requires special concrete, as found in nuclear power plants and munitions factories.

Radiation Dosage

The presence of radiation cannot be sensed by the human body. Special monitors, such as dosimeters and Geiger-Müller tubes, are required to detect, measure, and differentiate between particulate and electromagnetic radiation. The units of measurement of radiation have classically been the rad and the rem. The rad is the unit of absorbed dose of radiant energy that is equal to 100 ergs of energy per gram of absorbing material. The relative biologic effectiveness (RBE) is a measure of the actual biologic damage caused by any particle. The rem is a derived unit equal to the number of rads multiplied by the RBE for the particles of interest. For β particles, X rays, and γ rays, the rad and rem are equivalent.[3] (Most publications now utilize the SI units Gray and Sievert, in which 1 Gy equals 100 rad and 1 Sv equals 100 rem.) For reference, an anteroposterior chest film exposes the patient to 10 mrem (0.0001 Sv or 0.1 mSv); the average annual absorbed background radiation is 75 to 175 mrem; and the 50% lethal dose for whole-body ionizing radiation is 350 to 400 rad (3.5 to 4.0 Gy) if untreated and perhaps 500 to 600 rad (5 to 6 Gy) with intensive support.[4-7] It is estimated that the population in the local area of the Chernobyl nuclear power plant accident received a collective dose of 16,000 Sv.[8]

RADIATION EXPOSURE

Accidental exposure to radiation is rare. Since 1940, approximately 700 patients have been involved in significant radiation accidents, resulting in only 20 reported fatalities worldwide.[9] The criteria for a serious radiation accident are as follows[9]:

- 25 rem (0.25 Sv) or more whole-body irradiation
- 600 rem (6 Sv) or more to the skin
- 75 rem (0.75 Sv) or more to specific organs (eg, the gonads)
- internal contamination of 50% or more of the maximum permissible specific organ burden for each respective radionuclide
- misadministration of radionuclide in a medical environment, provided that any criterion listed above is met

Accidental radiation exposure may be external, either localized or whole body, and may leave external radioactive contamination that must be removed (decontamination). The patient with intact integument is not significantly radioactive and poses minimal, if any, danger to those attending him or her. If a radioactive fragment is embedded in the patient's tissue, however, the fragment could be a source of irradiation to attendants. Exposure may also be internal. The goal of treatment in internal contamination is reduction of the overall body dose (decorporation therapy).

DECONTAMINATION

Most victims of accidental external irradiation will have no significant radionuclide load when seen in the emergency department. At industrial sites where radiation exposure is a potential hazard, decontamination stations and procedures are in place and, unless there is significant associated trauma, are usually implemented before transport to a hospital emergency department. In any event, fear of contamination must never preclude completion of basic stabilization procedures in the acutely injured patient.

On arrival, radiation detecting and monitoring equipment should be immediately employed. Although intact skin does not harbor sufficient radiation to harm attending medical personnel, the patient's clothing should be removed and marked as contaminated. Skin and hair should be thoroughly washed with surgical soap, and radiation detectors should be

Table 38-1 Decontamination Procedures for Victims of Radiation Accidents

General Instructions

- Prepare to receive and treat irradiated patients, gather supplies, establish clean and contaminated treatment areas, review patient treatment protocols.
- Assign staff; preferably a separate staff should be assigned to clean contaminated treatment areas.
- Make sure, before decontamination procedures, that each patient has been medically triaged and deemed stable.
- Collect specimens for radiological survey before and after decontamination, as recommended.
- Monitor patients for radiation contamination before and after decontamination; permanently record the reading levels.
- Transfer decontaminated patients immediately to a clean treatment area to resume medical care.

External Contamination, Whole Body

- Remove all of the patient's clothing and resurvey for radiation. If no radiation is detected, transfer the patient to a clean area and resume medical care. If radiation is detected, proceed with decontamination.
- Decontaminate areas of the body with the highest radiation level. If the body has wounds, seal areas and use separate technique to decontaminate (refer to section dealing with wounds).
- Wash the entire body thoroughly with soap and copious amounts of water; rinse well. Patients who are able to shower should do so. A scrub brush may be used; however, be careful not to abrade the skin.
- Continue procedure until all radiation is removed or until the remaining radiation level is deemed safe.
- Give special attention to hairy body areas and body orifices. Initiate specific procedures if necessary.

External Contamination, Localized

- Cover and protect uncontaminated areas with plastic drapes.
- Cleanse the affected area thoroughly in the same manner as the external contamination, whole-body procedure.
- Continue decontamination until all the radiation is removed or until the remaining radiation level is deemed safe.

External Contamination, Hairy Body Areas

- Cover and protect uncontaminated areas with plastic drapes.
- Do not shave hair; if necessary, it can be cut but abrading the skin must be avoided.
- Continue procedure as for external contamination, localized.

Internal Contamination, Eyes

- Cover and protect uncontaminated areas around the eyes.
- Irrigate eyes thoroughly with water or isotonic saline even though this may induce eye irritation or conjunctivitis.
- Save the irrigant for radiological analysis.

Internal Contamination, Body Orifices

- Determine whether the contamination is in the orifice or on the surrounding area.
- Cover and protect the surrounding areas with plastic drapes.
- Irrigate with copious amounts of water or isotonic solution.
- Use cotton-tipped applicators or sponges to swab the affected areas if contamination persists. Detergent also may be used.
- Continue procedure until all radiation is removed or until the remaining radiation level is deemed safe.

Source: Reprinted from *Radiation and Health: Principles and Practice in Therapy and Disaster Preparedness* (pp 156–158) by AS Bomberger and BA Dannenfelser, Aspen Publishers, Inc., © 1984.

---

used to monitor success. Any dirt or other debris on or around the patient should be regarded as contaminated. Protective clothing and gloves should be worn by attendants and then discarded properly.

All burns and wounds, on the contrary, must be considered contaminated. These must be copiously irrigated, and surgical debridement may be necessary. Retained foreign bodies should be considered a potential hazard to attendants, and there are suggested protocols for their handling.[6,7]

The Joint Commission on Accreditation of Healthcare Organizations requires that all hospitals have procedures for the handling of contaminated patients. These procedures are summarized in Table 38-1. A number of publications are available for reference.[10–14]

LOCALIZED RADIATION INJURY

Localized exposure to ionizing radiation occurs almost exclusively in the occupational setting. These accidents usually involve industrial radiography[15] or accelerator facility accidents[9] and usually affect an upper extremity.[9,15,16] They occur either from direct contact with a source or from exposure to an intense radiation beam. Dosages in these accidents vary widely, but as much as 10,000 rad (100 Gy) has been recorded.[9]

The signs and symptoms of acute radiation syndrome seen in total-body irradiation are conspicuously mild or absent in these cases. The primary effect of localized external irradiation is thermal injury to the skin. The radiation burn develops more slowly than a true thermal burn; early appearances can be deceptive. Ultimate outcome in these injuries is dependent upon the degree of damage to the blood supply of the irradiated area. Burns due to β particles almost always require skin grafting. A useful classification of local radiation injuries is as follows[15]:

- *Type I:* erythema only; equivalent to a first-degree thermal burn. Exposure of the skin to 600 to 1000 rad (6 to

10 Gy) produces erythema and is useful in gauging the dose received and the areas affected. Erythema may not appear until as late as 2 to 3 weeks after exposure. Epilation (loss of hair) occurs at doses as low as 300 rad (3 Gy) but is also delayed. Dry desquamation (scaling) occurs, but medical treatment is not necessary.

- *Type II:* transepidermal injury, or wet desquamation, similar to that seen in a second-degree thermal burn. Erythema develops more quickly than in type I wounds, and blisters appear in 1 to 2 weeks. These injuries result from a brief skin exposure to 1000 to 2000 rad (10 to 20 Gy), and treatment is based on the size, location, and severity of the wound.

- *Type III:* dermal radionecrosis similar to a severe scalding or chemical burn; results from brief exposure to more than 2000 rad (20 Gy) of β particles or γ or X rays. Pain is intense and may be accompanied by tingling paresthesias. Prompt medical attention is required. Gangrene may result from obliteration of vasculature, and skin grafting is usually necessary.

- *Type IV:* chronic radiation dermatitis resulting from frequent exposure of the skin to radiation over many years. This eczemalike condition seldom heals completely, often ulcerates, and is frequently complicated by carcinoma.

Although injury to the extremities is most common, localized radiation injury to other parts of the body (eg, the ocular lens, the thyroid gland, and the gonads) sometimes occurs. Cataract formation, for example, may occur after local irradiation with as little as 200 rad (2 Gy). After a radiation accident, these must be considered and, if indicated, investigated further. Principles of decontamination must be carefully followed for patients exposed to external radiation.

TOTAL-BODY RADIATION INJURY

The critical information needed to treat victims of total-body irradiation is dose: the quantity, quality, and distribution of the radiation exposure.[9] The degree of injury is generally proportional to the dose absorbed. Exposure to less than 100 rad (1 Gy) rarely produces clinical symptoms. Approximately 15% of patients exposed to 100 rad (1 Gy) and almost all patients exposed to 200 rad (2 Gy) will show signs and symptoms of acute radiation syndrome.[17]

Because mechanical dosimetry is not always readily available at the site of radiation injuries, the concept of biologic dosimetry has evolved to enable the examining physician to assess rapidly the approximate magnitude of the irradiation. Indicators of severity (Table 38-2) include the presence of prodromal symptoms, depression of lymphocyte count, and erythema and epilation of the skin.[9] For example, the lymphocyte count at 48 hours after exposure is a good indicator of prognosis. If the lymphocyte count is greater than 1200/mm^3, the prognosis is good; if 300/mm^3 to 1200/mm^3, guarded; if less than 300/mm^3, poor.

Acute radiation syndrome is a progressive series of signs and symptoms that can be divided into four stages: the prodromal stage, the latent stage, the manifest illness stage, and the recovery stage.[17] Prodromal symptoms include nausea and vomiting, anorexia, headache, fatigue, and fever. Onset is usually within 6 hours of exposure and is probably due to acute tissue injury with release of histamine, bradykinins, and other vasoactive substances. More rapid onset of symptoms (within 2 hours) indicates a higher dose, as does persistence of these symptoms for more than 48 hours. Absence of symptoms after 6 hours indicates a probable exposure of 50 rad (0.5 Gy) or less. Skin changes, as described for local injuries, may also be helpful in determination of severity of injury, but again these may be delayed in their appearance even in severe injury.

Table 38-2 Biologic Indicators of Magnitude of Absorbed Dose of Ionizing Radiation

Indicator	Dose	Comment
Nausea and vomiting		
Beginning within 6 hours	>100 rad (1 Gy) total body	
Beginning within 4 hours	>200 rad (2 Gy) total body	
Beginning within 2 hours	>400 rad (4 Gy) total body	
Skin erythema	>1000 rad (10 Gy)	Onset may be delayed
Diarrhea	>400 rad (4 Gy) to abdomen	Occurs at onset of prodrome in severe cases
Ataxia, confusion, coma	>1000 rad (10 Gy)	Must rule out trauma as cause
Lymphocyte count at 48 hours		
>1200/mm^3	100–200 rad (1–2 Gy)	Good prognosis
300/mm^3 to 1200/mm^3	200–400 rad (2–4 Gy)	Fair prognosis
<300/mm^3	>400 rad (4 Gy)	Poor prognosis

Table 38-3 Characteristics of Acute Radiation Syndrome

Total-Body Dose	Prodrome	Latent Stage	Manifest Illness Symptoms	Death Incidence (%)
<200 rad (2 Gy)	Mild, lasting 3–6 hours	>2 weeks	Mild leukopenia, transient sterility in men	None
200–600 rad (2–6 Gy)	Nausea and vomiting within 2–4 hours, lasting <24 hours	1–2 weeks	Hematopoietic: mild to severe leukopenia; requires hospitalization and support; upper dose ranges require bone marrow transplantation	0–75
600–1000 rad (6–10 Gy)	Nausea and vomiting within 1–2 hours, lasting <48 hours	0–7 days	Gastrointestinal: dehydration, early sepsis, hemorrhage	90–100
>1000 rad (10 Gy)	Nausea and vomiting within 1 hour	None	Neurovascular: dehydration, hypotension, disorientation, seizures, coma, erythema, epilation	99–100

The latent stage, in which there is variable resolution of prodromal symptoms, may last for as long as several weeks. The higher the absorbed dose of radiation, the shorter this period and the less complete the relief from symptoms. If the dose was 600 rad (6 Gy) or more, the prodrome may extend into the stage of manifest illness without a discernible latency.

During the stage of manifest illness, symptoms become more specific to the organ systems involved. This specificity is determined by the relative radiosensitivity of the body's tissues and is summarized in Table 38-3. Hematologic changes predominate from doses of 200 to 600 rad (2 to 6 Gy), gastrointestinal illness predominates from 600 to 1000 rad (6 to 10 Gy), and central nervous and cardiovascular system symptoms predominate at doses higher than 1000 rad (10 Gy).

The hematopoietic syndrome is characterized by pancytopenia and is best followed by lymphocyte counts (Fig. 38-1). At this level of exposure, prodromal symptoms usually last 24 hours. Initial leukocyte counts may be elevated as a result of demargination,[5] but the lymphocyte count in the differential will start to decrease. There is usually a latent period of a few days to 3 weeks that is followed by symptoms of pancytopenia such as malaise, dyspnea, opportunistic infection, purpura, and hemorrhage. Patients with bone marrow depression in the absence of gastrointestinal and central nervous system changes may be assumed to have absorbed a sublethal dose, but it must be remembered that patients at the upper end of the hematopoietic syndrome dose range (600 rad) have received an exposure in excess of the human 50% lethal dose and will require intensive support. Bone marrow transplantation within 7 to 10 days of exposure is a possible option for these patients.[18,19]

The gastrointestinal syndrome occurs in patients who have been exposed to 500 to 1000 rad (5 to 10 Gy). The pro-

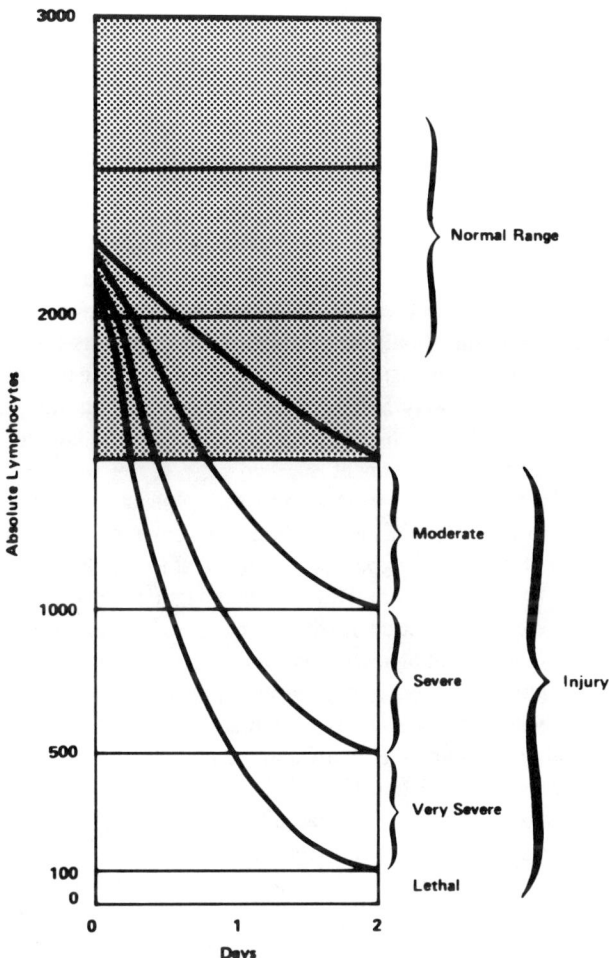

Figure 38-1 Patterns of early lymphocyte count response to total-body irradiation. *Source*: Reprinted from *The Medical Basis for Radiation Accident Preparedness* (p. 299) by KF Hubner and SA Fry with permission of Elsevier Science Publishing Co., © 1980.

dromal phase is abrupt and characterized by diarrhea and vomiting. A short latent period may ensue and is followed by recurrence of symptoms, more severe fluid loss, fever, and prostration. Leukocyte counts rapidly drop to zero. The mucosal cells of the small intestine are as radiosensitive as bone marrow cells and slough precipitously. It is quite unusual for patients to survive this syndrome; death usually results from bloody diarrhea (to which hematopoietic deterioration contributes) and shock within 2 weeks of exposure.

The neurovascular syndrome occurs with total-body irradiation of 1000 to 5000 rad (5 to 10 Gy). At these levels, even the relatively radioresistant neuronal cells are irreparably damaged, and profound hypotension results from direct vascular damage. Death within hours is to be anticipated. Erythema of the skin is generally present, and ataxia and confusion quickly develop. Circulatory collapse, neuromuscular discoordination, and coma ensue before death.

Principles of treatment of radiation accident victims are based on knowledge of these syndromes. Therapy is aimed at support and prevention of complications. Other than decontamination/decorporation, there is no specific treatment for the effects of irradiation. During prodromal and latent periods, rest, hydration, antiemetics, and close hematologic monitoring are indicated. Hospitalization is necessary if the exposure was known to exceed 100 rad (1 Gy), if the lymphocyte count falls below 1200/mm^3, or if intravenous hydration is required. For these patients, prophylactic antimicrobial agents are indicated, but more important is the observance of strict reverse isolation. Complete blood count and differential should be performed every 6 hours for the first 2 days. Transfusions are often necessary. Bone marrow transplantation may be attempted. Treatment with various blocking agents, such as potassium iodide, may be begun in the emergency department.[20–23]

Patients who are triaged into the expectant category require only analgesia and sedation in the emergency department. Patients with exposures estimated at less than 100 rad (1 Gy) generally do not require hospitalization but should be counseled to practice birth control for several months because of potential secondary congenital defects.

Treatment of victims of nuclear explosions is more difficult because of the severity of nonradiation trauma in individual patients and the overwhelming numbers of casualties that must be expected. Only 15% of the energy of a thermonuclear explosion is released as radiation, 5% immediately as γ rays and neutrons and 10% as radioactive fallout.[24] The remainder is dissipated as blast energy (50%) and heat (35%), which result in mechanical and thermal trauma coincident with radiation injury, complicating both initial therapy and ultimate recovery.[6,25]

The true scope of such a disaster is almost unimaginable. Although the care of individual patients with radiation injuries is feasible, large numbers of such patients would quickly outstrip available medical resources. Secondary infection and sepsis would be rampant in patients even at the lower dose range of the hematopoietic syndrome, and patients who might otherwise be salvaged would be lost. In 1983, the American College of Emergency Physicians published a position paper,[26] subsequently the subject of much debate,[27–31] that stated

> attempts to provide for the acute health care needs of the American public following a nuclear war should focus on first aid, sanitation, and essential survival skills. The American College of Emergency Physicians recognizes that no organized medical treatment exists or can currently be developed to meet the public health threat of a thermonuclear war. As with other nontreatable disease threats, prevention is society's only resource.[26(p625)]

The long-term effects of exposure to ionizing radiation, including carcinomas, leukemia, cataracts, and accelerated aging, are not the immediate concern of emergency physicians. A number of studies, however, are available to the interested reader.[32–34]

INTERNAL RADIOACTIVE CONTAMINATION

The emergency physician should treat inhalation, ingestion, skin or wound absorption, or injection of a radioactive substance in much the same way in which any toxic ingestion is treated: by removal, by dilution, and by neutralization.[9] Treatment is particularly critical in internal contamination because the radioactive substance will continue to irradiate tissues until it is physically eliminated or until it naturally decays.

Immediately after internal contamination, there is usually a brief period of time before absorption and cellular uptake of radioactivity. It is during this initial 1 or 2 hours that intervention is crucial. If contamination has occurred by ingestion, gastric emptying, catharsis, or acidification/alkalinization may reduce absorption. Bronchial lavage may remove inhaled particulate matter. All body fluids should be safely retained in clearly labeled containers for subsequent dosimetry and proper disposal.

Regardless of the route of entry, isotope dilution (eg, with potassium iodide) and/or chelation therapy (eg, with zinc or calcium DTPA) are also effective in many radiation poisonings. Reference tables detailing these specific interactions are available[11,20,35] and should be maintained in emergency department files. Nuclear medicine consultation should be expediently sought; assistance is also available by telephone

Table 38-4 Supplies Needed To Prepare the Emergency Department for Victims of Radiation Injuries

I. For Emergency Department Preparation
   A. Rolls of 4-foot-wide plastic sufficient to
      1. Cover floor from ambulance entrance to decontamination room (rolls of paper or sheets can be substituted)
      2. Cover the floor of the decontamination room (rolls of paper or sheets can be substituted)
      3. Prepare several stretchers for contaminated patients
   B. Rolls of 2-inch-wide masking tape to
      1. Secure floor covering
      2. Tape decontamination team's sleeves and cuffs
      3. Cover handles in decontamination room
      4. Make "clean line" at door to decontamination room
   C. Rope to delineate contaminated route from ambulance entrance to decontamination room
   D. "Radioactive" signs to place on rope and on door to decontamination room

II. For Decontamination Room
   A. Decontamination tray, or
   B. Plastic and cotton sheets to make decontamination trough on stretcher
   C. Three 5-gallon containers for wash water
   D. Three large waste containers
   E. Plastic bags to line waste containers
   F. Cotton-tipped applicators
   G. Stoppered glass containers for swabs of contaminated areas
   H. Lead storage containers for stoppered glass containers—obtain from Nuclear Medicine Department
   I. Chart with drawing of patient outline (front and back) for recording of contaminated areas
   J. Clorox®
   K. Lava® soap
   L. Soft scrub brushes
   M. Mixture of ½ Tide®, ½ cornmeal (keep airtight or refrigerate)
   N. 3% hydrogen peroxide

III. For Decontamination Team
   A. Large and extra-large surgical scrub suits
   B. Surgical gowns (waterproof)
   C. Surgical hoods
   D. Surgical masks
   E. Surgical gloves (various sizes)
   F. Waterproof shoe covers
   G. Film badges
   H. Dosimeters

IV. For Radiation Safety Officer
   A. Beta-gamma detector
   B. Alpha detector
   C. Extra batteries for detectors
   D. "Radioactive" tape-labels to mark containers holding contaminated specimens or swabs
   E. "Post-decontamination" tape-labels to mark containers holding relevant swabs

Source: Reprinted with permission from Leonard RB and Ricks RC, Emergency department radiation accident protocol, in *Annals of Emergency Medicine* (1980;9:462–470), copyright © 1980, American College of Emergency Physicians.

(615-481-1000) from the Radiation Emergency Assistance Center and Training Site (REAC/TS) in Oak Ridge, Tennessee.

EMERGENCY DEPARTMENT PREPAREDNESS FOR RADIATION INJURIES

As noted above, all hospitals are required to have plans for receiving and treating victims of radiation injury. Even emergency departments not located in the vicinity of a nuclear power plant or other industry may receive patients from isolated accidents, such as the spillage of radionuclide in a transport vehicle mishap or from within the hospital's own nuclear medicine department.[36] Although such plans must be adapted to individual facilities, the most important aspects are as follows[3,14,37–39]:

- designation of a radiation injury response team of physicians, nurses, and technicians who are knowledgeable in pertinent areas of care; if the hospital is near a nuclear reactor, a radiation physicist from that facility should be included on the response team

- ready availability of supplies needed for receiving and decontaminating irradiated patients (Table 38-4)

- a readily implemented plan for establishing easy patient flow through designated clean and contaminated areas of the department (Fig. 38-2)

- regular drills to check effectiveness of the items above

The National Council on Radiation Protection and Measurements (NCRP) text *Management of Persons Accidentally Contaminated with Radionuclides*[11] should be available to emergency personnel on duty. REAC/TS and other Department of Energy agencies are available for around-the-clock telephone consultation regarding any radiation problem.

For those facilities located near known sources of potential contamination, special consideration must be given to radiation accidents in the formulation of hospital and community disaster and civil defense plans (see Chapter 2, Disaster Management). This may include evacuation plans for the hospital itself.[40–42] It is critical that all emergency personnel be familiar with contingency plans and that these plans be updated regularly.

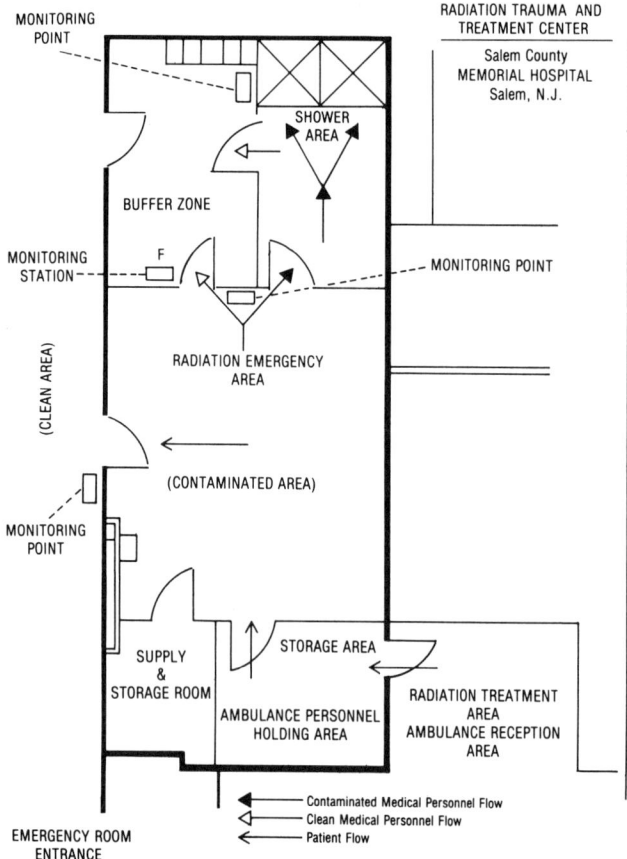

Figure 38-2 Floor plan of emergency area for treatment of radiation injury victims. Reprinted by permission from *HOSPITALS*, vol 53, no 9, May 1, 1979, copyright, 1979, American Hospital Publishing, Inc.

REFERENCES

1. Pollack H. Medical aspects of exposure to radiofrequency radiation including microwaves. *South Med J.* 1983;76:759–765.
2. Tintinalli JE, Krause G, Gursel E. Microwave radiation injury. *Ann Emerg Med.* 1983;12:645–647.
3. Mettler FA, Porter SW. The emergency response to radiation accidents. In: Auerbach PS, Geehr EC, eds. *Management of Wilderness and Environmental Emergencies.* New York: Macmillan; 1983.
4. Cronkite EP. The diagnosis, treatment, and prognosis of human radiation injury from whole-body exposure. *Ann NY Acad Sci.* 1964;114:341–355.
5. Maxfield WS, Hanks GE, Pizzarello DJ, et al. Acute radiation syndrome. In: Dalrymple GV, Gaulden ME, Kollmorgen GM, et al, eds. *Medical Radiation Biology.* Philadelphia: Saunders; 1973.
6. Eiseman B, Bond V. Surgical care of nuclear casualties. *Surg Gynecol Obstet.* 1978;146:877–883.
7. Conklin JJ, Walker RI, Hirsch E. Current concepts in the management of radiation injuries and associated trauma. *Surg Gynecol Obstet.* 1983;156:809–829.
8. Lindell B. Radiation and health. *Bull WHO.* 1987;65:139–148.
9. Mettler FA, Ricks RC. Medical management of radiation accidents. *Contemp Diagn Radiol.* 1982;5:1–6.
10. Mettler FA. Emergency management of radiation accidents. *JACEP.* 1978;7:302–305.
11. National Council on Radiation Protection and Measurements (NCRP). *Management of Persons Accidentally Contaminated with Radionuclides.* Washington, DC: NCRP. NCRP report no 65.
12. Poda GA. Decontamination and decorporation: the clinical experience. In: Hubner KF, Fry SA, eds. *The Medical Basis for Radiation Accident Preparedness.* New York: Elsevier; 1980.
13. Hubner KF. Decontamination procedures and risks to health care personnel. *Bull NY Acad Med.* 1983;59:1119–1128.
14. American Medical Association (AMA). *A Guide to the Hospital Management of Injuries Arising from Exposure to or Involving Ionizing Radiation.* Chicago: AMA; 1984.
15. Saenger EL, Kereiakes JG, Wald N, et al. Clinical course and dosimetry of acute hand injuries to industrial radiographers from multicurie sealed gamma sources. In: Hubner KF, Fry SA, eds. *The Medical Basis for Radiation Accident Preparedness.* New York: Elsevier; 1980.
16. Morse RH. Pain and a radiation accident. *J LA State Med Soc.* 1984;136:16–18.
17. Thoma GE. The diagnosis and management of accidental radiation injury. *J Occup Med.* 1959;1:421–447.
18. Champlin R. Treatment for victims of nuclear accidents: the role of bone marrow transplantation. *Radiat Res.* 1988;113:205–210.
19. Gale RP. The role of bone-marrow transplants after nuclear accidents. *Lancet.* 1988;1:923–926.
20. Lincoln TA. Importance of initial management of persons internally contaminated with radionuclides. *Am Ind Hyg Assoc J.* 1976;37:16–21.
21. Fowinkle EW, Sell SH, Wolle RH. Predistribution of potassium iodide—the Tennessee experience. *Public Health Rep.* 1983;98:123–126.
22. Archer VE. In accidents, give KI promptly. *Health Phys.* 1985;49:1311–1313.
23. Kereiakes JG, Saenger EL, Thomas SR. The reactor accident at Chernobyl: a nuclear medicine practitioner's perspective. *Semin Nucl Med.* 1986;16:224–230.
24. Leaning J, Leaf A. Public health aspects of nuclear war. *Ann Rev Public Health.* 1986;7:411–439.
25. Glasstone S, Dolan PJ. *The Effects of Nuclear Weapons.* Washington, DC: United States Department of Defense and United States Department of Energy; 1977.
26. American College of Emergency Physicians. Nuclear war and emergency health care. *Ann Emerg Med.* 1983;12:635.
27. Maccabee HD, Looney G. On nuclear war and emergency health care. *Ann Emerg Med.* 1984;13:212–213. Letter.
28. Williams SD. On nuclear war and emergency health care. *Ann Emerg Med.* 1984;13:213. Letter.
29. Schwartz AC. On nuclear war and emergency health care. *Ann Emerg Med.* 1984;13:214. Letter.
30. Bock BF. On nuclear war and emergency health care. *Ann Emerg Med.* 1984;13:214. Letter.
31. Magnotto L, Kline JS, Mauer D, et al. On nuclear war and emergency health care. *Ann Emerg Med.* 1984;13:1081–1082. Letter.
32. Upton AC. Radiation carcinogenesis. In: Dalrymple GV, Gaulden ME, Kollmorgen GM, et al, eds. *Medical Radiation Biology.* Philadelphia: Saunders; 1973.
33. Voelz GL, Grier RS, Hempelmann LH. A 37-year medical follow-up of Manhattan Project Pu workers. *Health Phys.* 1985;48:249–259.
34. Dienstbier Z. Long-term effects of nuclear war. *Med War.* 1986;2:251–254.

35. Voelz GL. Current approaches to the management of internally contaminated persons. In: Hubner KF, Fry SA, eds. *The Medical Basis for Radiation Accident Preparedness*. New York: Elsevier; 1980.
36. Leonard RB, Ricks RC. Emergency department radiation accident protocol. *Ann Emerg Med*. 1980;9:462–470.
37. Galvin JM Jr. Hospital makes itself center for treatment of radiation victims. *Hospitals*. 1979;53:37–40.
38. Bomberger AS, Dannenfelser BA. Saint Mary's Hospital radiation accident plan. In: *Radiation and Health: Principles and Practice in Therapy and Disaster Preparedness*. Rockville, MD: Aspen; 1984.
39. Saenger EL. Hospital planning to combat radioactive contamination. *JAMA*. 1963;185:578–581.
40. Bond VP. Medical planning for situations involving large populations. In: Hubner KF, Fry SA, eds. *The Medical Basis for Radiation Accident Preparedness*. New York: Elsevier; 1980.
41. Bomberger AS, Dannenfelser BA. Disaster planning concepts. In: *Radiation and Health: Principles and Practice in Therapy and Disaster Preparedness*. Rockville, MD: Aspen; 1984.
42. Bomberger AS, Dannenfelser BA. Developing radiation disaster plans. In: *Radiation and Health: Principles and Practice in Therapy and Disaster Preparedness*. Rockville, MD: Aspen; 1984.

39. Bites and Stings

ROBERT C. JORDEN, MD, FACEP
CHARLES V. POLLACK, JR., MD

The enormous number of animals and arthropods capable of inflicting injury on humans makes it impossible to cover all types of bites and stings in a single chapter. This discussion is therefore limited to the most common of these injuries, and the reader is referred to a growing literature to pursue more unusual areas of interest.[1-4]

Only injuries caused by animals normally inhabiting the continental United States are included. Injuries from marine animals are covered in Chapter 45, Dangerous Marine Organisms. Those diseases transmitted by the bites and stings of vectors (eg, Lyme disease and malaria) are also addressed in other chapters, with the exception of rabies, which is considered here. The bites of large animals, such as bears, wolves, and cougars, have also been excluded.

DOG BITES

Epidemiology

Numerous studies have indicated that dog bites are becoming truly epidemic in the United States.[5-9,11] The problem is increasingly acute in urban areas, where there are large numbers of unsupervised dogs. Homeless persons living on the streets in American cities are regularly exposed to these animals. The incidence of dog bites in rural areas is also probably much higher than has been reported previously. Additionally, more people are buying and training aggressive dogs for protection of person and property.[12]

The actual magnitude of the dog bite problem in the United States is nonetheless difficult to quantify. The dog population is not known but probably exceeds 50 million and is growing.[12] Dog bites are markedly underreported[9-11,13]; the actual number probably exceeds 1 million per year.[5,12,14] Dog bites represent nearly 90% of all reported animal bites.[10,12,14]

Children are the most frequent victims of dog bites; 40% of victims are between the ages of 5 and 14 years.[7] The reported rate of dog bites in children exceeds the combined rates of all reportable childhood diseases.[13] It has been estimated that nearly 2% of all American children 5 to 9 years of age are bitten annually by dogs.[15] Children are most often the victims of facial bites[6,8,10,14,16-18] because of their size, curiosity, and inexperience with animals. From 1979 through 1988, there were 157 dog bite–related deaths reported in the United States. Seventy percent of these occurred in children younger than 10 years of age.[18]

Overall, most bite wounds occur on the extremities.[6,8,9,10,12,16] Males are bitten by dogs at least twice as often as females.[7,12,19] As many as two fifths of reported dog bites are described by the victim as unprovoked,[16] and the majority are inflicted either by the victim's own dog or by a dog that is well known to the victim.[8,9,11,12,16,20] Larger dogs generally inflict larger wounds and are responsible for most emergency department (ED) visits.[7,8,12,16,17] The annual estimated expense of ED treatment of dog bite wounds exceeds $35 million.[3,6,12] This figure represents only medical expenses; it does not include work losses or damaged clothing and is therefore a conservative estimate.[21]

Nature of Injury

Most dog bites are not serious. Many are only contusions or superficial abrasions. In one series of more than 9000 bites, 6% did not puncture the skin, 55% showed skin punctures only, 32% showed a small skin tear, and only 6% showed a laceration greater than 2.5 cm. Less than 1% of these bites required a plastic surgery consultation.[6]

More severe bites may result in crush injuries, deep puncture wounds and tissue loss, and even death by mauling.[13,22–25] Dogs may bite tissue with a force of 150 to 450 pounds per square inch—easily enough to devitalize tissues and deeply inoculate microorganisms.[9,14]

Two distinct groups of patients seek medical attention for dog and other animal bites. One group presents within 8 to 12 hours of injury because of concern over wound care and rabies or tetanus exposure. The second group presents later with signs and symptoms of infection.[14]

Complications

Infection is by far the most common complication of dog bites. The reported incidence of infection in dog bite wounds has varied widely but is probably 6% to 8%.[7,26–33]

There are two primary risk factors that help predict a higher likelihood of infection in animal bite wounds: the nature of the wound and its location. Puncture wounds exhibit an infection rate double that of lacerations.[9,12,27,33] Likewise, both retrospective and prospective data indicate that hand wounds exhibit the highest rate of infection.

Less significant risk factors include delay in treatment of longer than 12 hours,[12,34] asplenism, diabetes, immune deficiency, use of corticosteroid therapy,[12,33] and patient age less than 2 or more than 50 years.[12,35] Whether or not initial treatment of bites in these patients should be more aggressive from first presentation remains open to debate.[36]

In the majority of cases, the only evidence of dog bite wound infection is a local cellulitis with or without accompanying lymphangitis. In the extremities, however, particularly in the hand and foot, deeper, poorly vascularized tissues in closed spaces, such as tendons, are occasionally infected. Rarely, systemic infection occurs, which can lead to overwhelming sepsis and death. Several case reports of sepsis with *Pasteurella multocida*, DF-2 (a Gram-negative rod), and other organisms attest to the potential for serious morbidity and death.[37–44]

Other forms of infection resulting from dog bites include osteomyelitis,[45,46] tenosynovitis, meningitis,[37] brain abscess,[47] and endocarditis.[48] Although these complications are rare, it is clear that thorough evaluation of dog bites and the judicious use of antibiotics are necessary.

Complications other than infection are uncommon; probably the most significant is disfigurement. Although only 1% of wounds may require care by a plastic surgeon, that number (10,000 or more) is substantial, and many involve facial wounds in which cosmesis, not infection, is the primary treatment consideration.

Psychologic complications of dog bites no doubt occur, but their incidence and seriousness are unknown and debated. Long-lasting personality changes have been documented in small children as a result of severe dog bites.[49] Other investigators have noted few psychologic problems of any significant duration.[11,50]

No data are available to suggest how often tissue loss and subsequent loss of function occur. Dysfunction may also result from infection, particularly in the hand. Fractures of underlying bones rarely occur, although there are several case reports documenting skull fractures as a result of dog bites.[47,51–53]

Treatment

The treatment of dog bite wounds should be individualized to the specific injury and the circumstances of the patient's presentation. Consensus regarding management will probably never be achieved. Nevertheless, treatment guidelines as outlined in Table 39-1 are offered as an approach to dog bites.

Skin Intact

Wounds with intact skin include abrasions and contusions. The protective barrier is violated, but there is no laceration

Table 39-1 Management of Dog Bites

	Cleansing	Irrigation	Debridement	Antibiotics	Suturing	Tetanus and Rabies Precautions
Skin intact	Yes	No	No	No	No	Yes
Facial laceration	Yes	Yes	Yes	Yes	Yes	Yes
Nonfacial laceration	Yes	Yes	Yes	Yes	No	Yes
Puncture	Yes	?	Yes	Yes	No	Yes

per se. These wounds require the least amount of attention. Local care consists of thorough cleansing of the wound with an antiseptic soap. No surgical treatment is indicated, nor are antibiotics. Infection control is limited to tetanus prevention (Table 39-2) and rabies precautions (Table 39-3). All subsequently described wounds also require tetanus prophylaxis and rabies precautions. Analgesia may be necessary, but acetaminophen or ibuprofen is often sufficient. Because local municipal ordinances mandate reporting of dog bite injuries in most states, the proper authorities should be notified.

Lacerations

Cosmetically unimportant wounds are carefully cleansed with an antiseptic solution; high-pressure syringe irrigation is also recommended. Once the wound has been thoroughly cleansed, devitalized tissue should be excised; because dog bite wounds often involve some degree of crush injury and avulsion, debridement is frequently necessary. The emergency physician should perform the minimum trimming and undermining necessary to achieve a good result.[12] The wound is left open and a nonadherent dressing applied.

Table 39-2 Summary Guide to Tetanus Prophylaxis in Routine Wound Management

History of Tetanus Immunization (Doses)	Clean, Minor Wounds		All Other Wounds	
	Td*	TIG†	Td*	TIG†
Uncertain	Yes	No	Yes	Yes
0–1	Yes	No	Yes	Yes
2	Yes	No	Yes	No‡
3 or more	No§	No	No‖	No

*The combined preparations Td, containing both tetanus and diphtheria toxoids, is preferred to tetanus toxoid alone.
†Tetanus immune globulin.
‡Yes, if wound more than 24 hours old.
§Yes, if more than 10 years since last dose.
‖Yes, if more than 5 years since last dose (more frequent boosters are not needed and can accentuate side effects).

Large, gaping wounds may require some modification of this approach. Even in a relatively unimportant cosmetic area, these injuries can be disfiguring. Although there are no data that address this point specifically, a delayed primary closure

Table 39-3 Rabies Precautions and Prophylaxis

The following recommendations are only a guide. In applying them, take into account the animal species involved, the circumstances of the bite or other exposure, the vaccination status of the animal, and presence of rabies in the region. Local or state public health officials should be consulted if questions arise about the need for rabies prophylaxis.			
	Animal species	Condition of animal at time of attack	Treatment of exposed person*
DOMESTIC	Dog and cat	Healthy and available for 10 days of observation	None, unless animal develops rabies†
		Rabid or suspected rabid	RIG‡ and HDCV§
		Unknown (escaped)	Consult public health officials. If treatment is indicated, give RIG‡ and HDCV§
WILD	Skunk, bat, fox, coyote, raccoon, bobcat, and other carnivores	Regard as rabid unless proven negative by laboratory test¶	RIG‡ and HDCV§
OTHER	Livestock, rodents, and lagomorphs (rabbits and hares)	Consider individually. Local and state public health officials should be consulted on questions about the need for rabies prophylaxis. Bites of squirrels, hamsters, guinea pigs, gerbils, chipmunks, rats, mice, other rodents, rabbits, and hares almost never call for antirabies prophylaxis.	

*All bites and wounds should immediately be thoroughly cleansed with soap and water. If antirabies treatment is indicated, both rabies immune globulin (RIG) and human diploid cell rabies vaccine (HDCV) should be given as soon as possible, regardless of the interval from exposure.
†During the usual holding period of 10 days, begin treatment with RIG and vaccine (preferably with HDCV) at first sign of rabies in a dog or cat that has bitten someone. The symptomatic animal should be killed immediately and tested.
‡If RIG is not available, use antirabies serum, equine (ARS). Do not use more than the recommended dosage.
§If HDCV is not available, use duck embryo vaccine (DEV). Local reactions to vaccines are common and do not contraindicate continuing treatment. Discontinue vaccine if fluorescent-antibody (FA) tests of the animal are negative.
¶The animal should be killed and tested as soon as possible. Holding for observation is not recommended.
Source: Reprinted from Rabies Prevention—United States, 1984 *Morbidity Mortality Weekly Rep.* 33:397, 1984.

3 to 5 days after injury may be a reasonable compromise for such a wound.

The use of antibiotics in initial wound management remains debatable. Reference in this regard to antibiotic *prophylaxis* is actually improper; the rationale for giving the treatment is the assumption that the laceration represents a preclinical infection resulting from the combination of traumatized tissue and pathogen inoculation.[12,54] Although a growing prospective literature indicates that empiric antibiotics provide no benefit, all these studies are flawed by an inadequate sample size. They fail to consider wound location as a separate risk factor because the number of wounds in each anatomic location is usually too small to permit conclusive results.

Therefore, based on current data, a recommendation to withhold empiric antibiotics in dog bite lacerations is unwarranted. Specific regimens are listed below. Particularly in more significant wounds, consideration should be given to a parenteral first dose of antibiotics preceding oral therapy to achieve efficacious drug levels in the wound tissue more quickly.[32,33,55] The patient should be instructed to cleanse the wound twice daily with soap and water or peroxide and to return for a wound check in 2 days or sooner if infection develops. Routine culture of a fresh bite wound is not indicated[56–58] but should always be performed if infection is already established (see below).

Table 39-4 Organisms Recovered from Dog Bite Wounds

Actinobacillus species
Bacillus species
Bacteroides species
Blastomyces dermatidis
Brucella canis
CDC alphanumeric group organisms DF-2, M-5, EF-4, IIj, and IIr
Chromobacterium species
Corynebacterium species
Enterobacter cloacae
Eubacterium species
Fusobacterium species
Hemophilus aphrophilus
Leptotrichia bucallis
Micrococcus luteus
Moraxella species
Pasteurella multocida
Peptococcus species
Peptostreptococcus species
Proprionibacterium species
Proteus mirabilis
Pseudomonas fluorescens group
Rabies virus
Staphylococcus aureus
Staphylococcus epidermidis
Streptococcus viridans

Source: Reprinted with permission from Auerbach PS and Morris JA, *Acinetobacter calcoaceticus* infection following a dog bite, in *Journal of Emergency Medical Services* (1987;5:363–366), copyright © 1987, Jems Publishing Co.

Facial wounds are cleansed in the same way, and devitalized tissue is debrided. Wound edges are also excised if necessary. The wound is then closed in a routine fashion, and the patient is started on antibiotics.

The risk of infection after suturing dog bites is not clear. Although some investigators believe that wound closure is a safe practice, others claim that it produces a higher rate of infection. A compromise would allow closure of facial lacerations while leaving all others open. The risk of suturing nonfacial bites is unwarranted because adequate healing can occur by secondary intention. Because unsutured facial lacerations can produce unacceptable scars, however, the risk of suturing these cases seems indicated. Furthermore, the excellent blood supply of the face diminishes the likelihood of infection and provides additional support for closing these wounds.

Puncture Wounds

Puncture wounds are handled uniformly regardless of anatomic location. All wounds are thoroughly cleansed, and any devitalized tissue is excised. The benefit of irrigating puncture wounds is questionable because the egress of fluid is compromised. Deep, forceful irrigation may even be detrimental, allowing for dissemination of bacteria into surrounding tissues. Conversely, irrigation by gravity or superficial jet irrigation can be recommended, although efficacy remains uncertain. All patients are placed on antibiotics and are told to return for a wound check.

Antibiotics

The choice of antibiotics in the management of dog bites is also controversial. Studies of the nasal and oral flora of dogs, compared to organisms cultured from dog bite wounds, have confounded the important issue of which microorganisms are truly pathogenic and which are present only as contaminants. Table 39-4 lists various organisms recovered from dog bite wounds.

In the past, *Pasteurella multocida* has frequently been implicated as the most common cause of dog bite wound infections. Some series have reported a 50% incidence of *P multocida* in infected wounds.[59] Prospective studies, however, have failed to document a preponderance of clinical infections caused by *Pasteurella* species.[14,29,33] Most infections appear to be polymicrobial, and many exhibit complex interactions among microorganisms. In prospective series, no single organism has accounted for more than 15% of infections. *Streptococcus* species, *Staphylococcus aureus*, *Pasteurella* species, and Gram-negative rods named by the Centers for Disease Control alphanumeric grouping (see Table 39-4) are probably the most common etiologic agents in dog bite wound infections,[33] although the distinction between etiology of infection and contamination is difficult to make. The alphanumeric organisms are now commonly reported as the presumed primary pathogens in the most serious dog bite wound infections.[14,33,54,60] Anaerobic bacteria are also often found in these wounds[14,34] but play an undetermined role in pathogenesis.

Such a wide spectrum of microorganisms is difficult to cover adequately with a single agent. Antibiotic selection must be directed at the broadest possible coverage and the best hopes of patient compliance. Most of the commonly cultured pathogens are sensitive to penicillin, the exception being coagulase-positive *Staphylococcus aureus*. Although this species is sensitive to the semisynthetic penicillins such as dicloxacillin, some strains of *P multocida* are not. The latter, however, is sensitive to penicillin, as are the Gram-negative rods (eg, DF-2).

Based on these data, many physicians opt for coverage with both penicillin and dicloxacillin. A first parenteral dose of penicillin, oxacillin, or a cephalosporin such as cefazolin (Ancef) should be considered. Empiric antibiotic treatment of fresh dog bite wounds that are not grossly contaminated should be given for 5 days. Probably the best single-drug coverage for fresh wounds is provided by a cephalosporin such as cephalexin (Keflex, 500 mg every 6 hours). Penicillin-sensitive patients may be given erythromycin. Other investigators have proposed co-trimoxazole,[36] clindamycin,[54] amoxicillin,[61] and tetracycline,[54] but the efficacy of each of these has not been substantiated. The oral quinolone drugs are another potentially useful class of antibiotics.

Although empiric treatment of penetrating dog bites continues to generate controversy, it should be continued until large, well-designed prospective studies can convincingly document a lack of efficacy. The natural rate of infection in dog bites is low, adding to the difficulty of obtaining conclusive data. Meanwhile, because of the ease and relatively low expense of empiric antibiotic coverage, the potentially disabling sequelae of unprevented dog bite infections are unacceptable.

The treatment of established infections of dog bite wounds is less controversial. Infected wounds that have been closed should be opened and irrigated. Initial antibiotic choice, pending culture and sensitivity results, should be based on the Gram stain, with the knowledge that these results are sometimes misleading as a result of mixed flora infection.[56,62] A broad-spectrum antibiotic, such as a cephalosporin, is probably the best choice. Depending on the severity of the infection, the presence of systemic signs, and the location of the wound, the patient may require hospitalization and parenteral antibiotics.

CAT BITES

Epidemiology

Cat bites are much less common than dog bites, accounting for less than 10% of reported animal bites.[12,14,16] Nonetheless, the incidence of cat bites appears to be rising.[14] Women are twice as likely to be bitten by cats as by dogs. The extremities, particularly the hands, are the most common locations of cat bite injuries.[12] Although cat bites have been recognized for many years as a potential source of infection, little attention has been focused on cat bite or scratch injuries.

Nature of Injury

In many ways, cat bites are similar to dog bites. Tissues are disrupted and inoculated with bacteria, and infection is the most common complication of both types of injuries. As in dog bites, various organisms can be cultured from infected cat bites, but the mechanics of cat bites are different from those of dog bites. Cats are smaller animals, do not bite with high pressure, and do not inflict the crush injury that dogs do. Feline teeth are sharper and smaller in diameter and tend to produce deep puncture wounds rather than tearing injuries. The puncture wounds of cat bites, because they are deep, also have a tendency to involve superficial tendons and to penetrate joint spaces.[63,64]

Complications

Infection is much more commonly seen with cat bites than with dog bites. Although cellulitis is most common, more serious infections, including tenosynovitis and osteomyelitis, can occur.[65,66] Retrospective studies have indicated a 20% to 50% infection rate for cat bites.[12,16,26] The pathogenic organisms vary and are often mixed. *Pasteurella multocida* is isolated from cats' oral or nasal mucosa 50% to 80% of the time,[63] but the incidence of *P multocida* in infected cat bites is uncertain. It is known to be a more common cause of infection in cat bites than in dog bites, being found in 80% to 100% of cultured wounds, whether or not they are clinically infected.[16,67] *Pasteurella* species can also cause infections distant from bites, such as septic arthritis,[68] mycotic aneurysm,[69] and overwhelming sepsis.[70] More unusual cat bite wound infectious complications, such as sepsis with the Gram-negative DF-2 bacillus, have also been reported.[71]

Cat scratches have a tendency to become infected even in the absence of bite wounds, which is not true of canine scratch injuries.[72] Cats frequently groom their claws by licking them, and the saliva thus deposited on the claws is assumed to be the source of the infecting bacteria. Again, *P multocida* is a frequent offender; at least one case of fatal *Pasteurella* sepsis has been attributed to a cat scratch.[73] Other diseases, such as cat scratch fever and tularemia, can also be transmitted in this way.[14]

Treatment

The same treatment principles outlined for dog bites apply to cat bites. Wounds should be cleansed, irrigated, and debrided when appropriate. Because cat bites usually consist only of small puncture wounds, little can be done to remove the bacterial inoculum. Empiric antibiotics are recommended for all cat bites that penetrate the skin. Less controversy surrounds this treatment for cat bites than for dog bites because the incidence of infection with the former is significantly higher.

Not all clinicians agree, however, on the choice of antibiotics. Because of the high incidence of *Pasteurella* infection, many recommend penicillin.[12,14,63,72,74] Because *Staphylococcus aureus* and other penicillin-resistant organisms are occasionally found in cat bite wounds, cephalosporins are an alternative first-line drug in cat bite coverage.

For wounds that are grossly infected, Gram stain and cultures should be obtained. Initial treatment should be instituted with a cephalosporin or penicillin, unless the Gram stain is characteristic of a particular organism.

The same precautions and prophylaxis against tetanus and rabies that were recommended for dog bites also apply for cat bites (Tables 39-2 and 39-3). Local municipal ordinances may also mandate reporting of cat bite injuries.

HUMAN BITES

Epidemiology

Human bites occur with a greater frequency than is widely appreciated; the estimated incidence is 10.7 bites per 100,000 population. The incidence in children is higher, but wounds in the pediatric age group tend to be superficial.[75,76] These estimates are certainly low, owing largely to patients' embarrassment regarding human bite injuries.

Overall, the incidence of human bites ranks third behind dog and cat bites compared with bites from other animals.[14,77,78] Bites occur in all anatomic areas with predilection for the upper extremity. Males are most often bitten on the dominant hand[9,14,77,79]; women are frequently bitten on the breast.[9] Children most commonly sustain bite wounds on the face.[75,76] Although accidental bites do occur in adults, in most cases the injury results from an overtly aggressive act.[14]

Nature of Injury

There are two broad categories of human bites: true bites and fight bites. A true bite is an occlusional injury that occurs when tissue is grasped between maxillary and mandibular teeth. Fight bites occur when an assailant strikes another person's mouth, with a laceration resulting from contact with the victim's dentition.

The injury inflicted by an occlusional bite is similar to that of dog bites. Deep puncture wounds are unlikely because humans do not have long fangs, but crush injury, laceration, and tissue loss do occur. Because the majority of bites occur on the hands, there is a significant incidence of traumatic finger tip amputation. Hand bites often violate multiple tissue planes and damage tendons, bones, joint capsules, and articular cartilage.

Fight bites occur by a particular mechanism that is conducive to serious infections. Typically, these lesions are sustained when the striking hand is in a clenched-fist configuration. In this position, the extensor tendon and its underlying bursa are pulled distally over the metacarpophalangeal joint. The result is a deep laceration that can disrupt superficial and deep fasciae, the extensor tendon and its bursa, and the joint capsule. After the injury, the assailant usually extends the fingers, retracting the skin and tendon proximally and sealing the contaminated wound into the deep tissues. If the physician then examines the wound with the patient's fingers extended, the entrance wound into the metacarpophalangeal joint can be missed. This is the most frequently violated joint, followed by the proximal interphalangeal joint.[77,80]

Complications

The most frequent complication of human bites is infection. In fact, many investigators hold that these wounds are more prone to infection than other animal bites. If accurate, this probably reflects the high percentage of hand injuries among human bites rather than greater contamination or a higher virulence of bacteria in the human mouth.[81] Nevertheless, human bites have long been notorious for causing severe infections that lead to functional disability, amputation, sepsis, and even death. These more serious complications have become less frequent with the advent of oral broad-spectrum antibiotics and an increased awareness of the injury.

The infection rate for human bite wounds is not well documented but is probably high, perhaps in excess of 50%.[82] Several factors predispose these injuries to infection; hand anatomy, as discussed, is one factor. Another is delay in seeking treatment.[14,82-88] Victims may not seek help because of embarrassment, the initial innocuous appearance of the wound, or their general socioeconomic status. The problem is compounded when examining physicians do not maintain a high index of suspicion for fight bites, even with a negative stated history. Many studies have documented a poor outcome when human bite injuries are not treated within 12 hours. Conversely, patients seen promptly and treated aggressively rarely develop long-term problems, even in more serious wounds.

The virulence of the infecting bacteria is also a significant factor. As in other animal bites, human bite wound infections are usually mixed, synergistic flora. Streptococci and staphylococci predominate, and *Staphylococcus aureus*, which is usually resistant to penicillin, is a particularly virulent organism in hand infections that may spread rapidly.[89] Similarly, *Eikenella corrodens*, a facultatively anaerobic Gram-negative rod sensitive to penicillin and resistant to diclox-

Table 39-5 Organisms Isolated from Human Bite Wounds

Aerobic	Anaerobic
Streptococcus species	Acidaminococcus species
α-Hemolytic	Actinomyces species
β-Hemolytic	Arachnia propionica
γ-Hemolytic	Bacteroides melaninogenicus
Staphylococcus aureus	Bacteroides intermedius
Staphylococcus epidermidis	Bacteroides ruminicola
Acenitobacter species	Bacteroides oralis
Eikenella corrodens	Bacteroides ureolyticus
Neisseria gonorrhoeae	Other Bacteroides species
Branhamella catarrhalis	Clostridium species
Moraxella species	Eubacterium species
Micrococcus species	Fusobacterium nucleatum
Hemophilus influenzae	Peptostreptococcus anaerobius
Enterobacter cloacae	
Klebsiella pneumoniae	Peptostreptococcus prevotii
Nocardia species	Peptostreptococcus magnus
Corynebacterium species	Other Peptostreptococcus species

Source: Reprinted with permission from Goldstein EJC and Richwald GA, Human and animal bite wounds, in *American Family Physician* (1987;36:101–109), copyright © 1987, American Academy of Family Physicians.

acillin, may produce serious infections in human bites. This organism seems to be particularly associated with infections in intravenous drug abusers.[90–92] Many other organisms have been isolated from human bite wounds (Table 39-5), but, as in animal bites, it is often unclear which organisms grown in culture are actually pathogenic.[9,14,33,67]

The nature of the infections that develop from hand bites, particularly fight bites, has been well established by the work of Kanavel[93] and the study of Mason and Koch.[80] The latter investigators injected barium into and around the metacarpophalangeal joints and documented radiographically how infection is likely to spread. They concluded that several weak points in the joint capsule result in a characteristic spread of infection. Thus the likely sites of infection in hand bites, in decreasing order of frequency, are: the subcutaneous space of the dorsum of the hand, the fascial space of the dorsum of the proximal phalanx, the metacarpophalangeal joint space, the palmar fascial spaces, and the flexor tendon sheaths.

Treatment

Given the potential for serious infection and long-term disability, it is important to recognize the fight bite and to take an aggressive approach in treatment. Any laceration over the metacarpophalangeal joints must be considered a bite wound until proven otherwise. For various reasons, patients may not divulge and may even deliberately conceal the true nature of their injury.

Once an acute injury is identified as a human bite, the next step is to determine whether deep structures have been violated. Thorough cleansing and irrigation with subsequent careful exploration are mandatory. If the bite wound is on the hand, consideration should be given to early consultation with a hand surgeon. Although some surgeons hospitalize and explore all hand wounds,[82,86] others take a more conservative approach.[67,83–85,94] The latter group reserves surgery for grossly infected wounds and for noninfected wounds with foreign body contamination or deep structure damage. It is unanimously agreed that, regardless of a benign appearance, human bites of the hand should never be sutured. Nonsurgical management of the cleansed hand would include empiric antibiotics, elevation, splinting, and careful follow-up.

Human bites that present after the onset of clinical infection are typically inflamed and slightly swollen and may demonstrate a thin, foul-smelling, grayish exudate. In hand wounds, pain on passive range of motion is important to elicit because it may indicate tenosynovitis or joint space infection. Roentgenograms should always be obtained to determine the presence of fractures, retained foreign bodies (especially teeth), air in joints, or periostitis. Infected wounds should undergo Gram stain and culture to help guide therapy, but the initial choice should provide coverage for streptococci and *Staphylococcus aureus*.

A semisynthetic penicillin or a first-generation cephalosporin is a reasonable choice in hand infections but does not provide adequate coverage against *Eikenella corrodens*. A combination of penicillin with one of these antibiotics is probably the best option. Tetracycline or erythromycin should be used in allergic patients, but the former should not be given to children or pregnant women. The first dose of antibiotic should be parenteral to achieve therapeutic levels expeditiously.[33,94]

The management of human bites in other areas of the body is as controversial as dog bite management. Generally, the recommendations for cleansing, irrigation, and debridement in human bites are the same as those for dog bites. Wound closure is recommended only for facial wounds[95]; empiric antibiotics are recommended for all wounds. The antibiotics chosen should be the same as those outlined above for hand bites. Tetanus prophylaxis is recommended, even though tetanus bacteria are rarely found in the human oral flora,[96] because the wound may be contaminated from other sources. Depending on the circumstances surrounding the injury, a social services consultation might be indicated for the patient.

Despite a marked improvement in the outcome of human bite injuries over the years, there is still significant disability associated with some wounds.[84] Hand wounds particularly are associated with long-term sequelae, such as permanently stiff fingers. The importance of early recognition of the nature of the wound, aggressive intervention and early consultation if required, and conscientious follow-up of these patients cannot be overemphasized.

Unusual infections can be transmitted via a human bite. These include syphilis,[97] tuberculosis,[98] actinomycosis,[99] and hepatitis.[100] Transmission of human immunodeficiency virus has been reported but not well substantiated.[101,102] Awareness of these infections is desirable, but routine initial management does not mandate their consideration.

SNAKE BITES

Each year in the United States, 45,000 people sustain snake bite injuries. Of those injuries, only about 8000 are inflicted by poisonous snakes; these result in 15 to 20 deaths.[103,104] Unlike dog, cat, and human bites, in which the primary concern is tissue loss and infection, snake bites are important because of the local and systemic effects of injected venom.

Taxonomy and Physiology

There are 2500 to 3000 species of snakes in the world, 375 of which are venomous. These species are members of five families of poisonous snakes, only two of which are found in the continental United States.

The Crotalidae include the genus *Crotalus* (the rattlesnakes), the genus *Agkistrodon* (cottonmouth and copperhead), and the genus *Sistrurus* (massasauga and pygmy rattlesnake).

The Elapidae include two genera of coral snakes: *Micruroides* (Sonoran) and *Micrurus* (Eastern and Texas).

Each of the 50 states, except Alaska, Hawaii, and Maine, has at least one venomous species.[105] North Carolina has the highest incidence of poisonous snake envenomations in the United States, at a rate of 18 per 100,000 population. Other states with at least 10 envenomations per 100,000 population per year include Arkansas, Florida, Georgia, Louisiana, Mississippi, South Carolina, and Texas.[106,107]

Poisonous snakes deliver their venom by way of fangs. The Crotalidae (pit vipers) have two long, curved, canaliculated, retractable fangs located in the anterior maxilla. In their retracted, resting position, the teeth are tucked up into the mucosa of the upper jaw. In the striking position, the jaws are opened wide and the fangs project forward in a position perpendicular to the maxilla. The snake has control over the movement of the fangs, being able to retract or extend them at will. Each fang is hollow with an anterior opening near its distal tip.

Venom is produced in a modified salivary gland that lies in the soft tissue of the maxilla just below the eye and is delivered to the sheath of each fang by a salivary duct. The sheath forms a pocket around the base of the fang and transmits the venom into the hollow fang. The actual release of venom is controlled by muscles surrounding the venom gland. The innervation of this musculature is separate from that of the biting musculature. Thus the snake has the ability to control the amount of venom injected, independent of the biting process. In addition to the fangs, pit vipers also have two rows of smaller teeth in both the upper and lower jaws. Occasionally, superficial bite wounds caused by these smaller teeth can be seen around the two fang marks. These teeth and the wounds they inflict are of no clinical significance.

The dentition of the coral snakes, the other family of poisonous snakes found in the continental United States, is different from that of the Crotalidae family. The coral snakes also have bilateral maxillary fangs in addition to their smaller dentition, but their fangs are not as long as those of the pit vipers, and they are fixed, not retractable. Their function, however, is the same: the delivery of venom into prey or adversaries.

Epidemiology

Snakes are generally quiet, nonaggressive creatures that rarely seek out adversaries. They bite humans only as a defensive measure. Bites occur most commonly in the snake's natural environment, either when people accidentally stumble into the habitat or when they deliberately disturb a snake. Snakes in captivity, however, are also responsible for a significant number of envenomations. These victims are usually herpetologists, zookeepers, hobbyists, entertainers, or cultists.[103] Snake bites occur five times more commonly in males than in females because of greater occupational and recreational exposure. Half of all snake bites occur in children or young adults, with the highest incidence occurring between the ages of 10 and 19 years. This can probably be attributed to curiosity and naive exploration; an individual's behavior is the major determinant in the possibility of snake bite in an opportune setting.[108] The vast majority of bites (more than 95%) occur on the extremities, with the upper extremities being bitten twice as frequently as the lower extremities.[103]

Snakes are poikilothermic; that is, their body temperature equilibrates with the environment, and they are unable to regulate it. At 8°C (46°F), snakes become motionless, and at 42°C (108°F) they survive for less than 15 minutes. Their optimal temperature range is 27°C to 32°C (81°F to 90°F).[105] Because of these temperature constraints, snakes' activities, and therefore the frequency of snake bites, are subject to seasonal and diurnal temperature variations. The peak season for snake bites is the warmer months, March 15 to October 15; the peak time of day for bites is the evening.[103]

Effects of Venom

As many as 20% of venomous snake bites in the United States show no evidence of envenomation; either no venom is injected with the bite or the venom is sprayed onto the skin before a superficial bite is inflicted.[109] Venoms are complex poisons consisting of some 30 enzymes (mostly hydrolases), peptides, glycoproteins, and other substances.[103,110] Venom serves not only to disable the snake's victim but also to begin digestion.

Knowledge of the pharmacology of venoms and their component parts is far from complete, despite extensive research. In the past, venoms have been labeled and categorized as various toxins (ie, neurotoxins, cardiotoxins, necrotoxins, and hemotoxins). This practice is an oversimplification of the total activity of venoms and may lead to therapeutic errors.[111] Certainly, snake venoms do exhibit these toxic effects, but it is dangerous to assume that a given species has a particular toxic effect to the exclusion of any other.

Persons previously sensitized may have true anaphylactic reactions to snake venoms.[112,113] If the snake fortuitously injects its venom intravenously into the victim, all aspects of venom poisoning may manifest quickly.[114] Otherwise, venom reactions usually follow a progression of local to systemic signs and symptoms, with each step indicating a higher venom load. While recognizing that much overlap of specific toxic effects occurs, it is still convenient to discuss various aspects of venom effects separately.

Local Edema and Necrosis

Soft tissue swelling and local necrosis, a hallmark of pit viper envenomations, are due to a number of venom components. Proteolytic enzymes, trypsinlike hormones that digest tissue protein, have been found in all analyzed crotalid venoms. Venoms with high concentrations of these enzymes cause marked tissue destruction. Pit viper venom also contains a nonproteolytic enzyme that is directly myonecrotic. Collagenase, which digests collagen, and hyaluronidase, which decreases connective tissue viscosity and thus permits further venom penetration, also contribute to tissue necrosis.[111]

Shock

There are several potential causes of shock after pit viper envenomation. Initial hypotension may be attributed to pulmonary and, to a lesser extent, a splanchnic pooling of blood. This pooling is a transient phenomenon that gives way to true hypovolemia and shock secondary to transudation of fluid across endothelium that has been damaged, probably by polypeptides found in the venom. Vasodilation and myocardial depression may also play a role, but the latter is not well established in humans. Renal failure may result from hypotension, although coagulation abnormalities or direct venom toxicity probably also contribute to renal pathology in snake bite victims.[115,116]

Coagulopathy and Hemorrhage

Coagulopathy can result from one of three mechanisms operative in snake venom poisoning: anticoagulation, defibrination, and a procoagulant effect.[103] Venom's procoagulant effect results from stimulation of the clotting cascade at a number of steps. Crotalid venom has been shown to affect factors II, V, IX, and X.[103] In addition, venom contains a thrombinlike enzyme that converts fibrinogen to fibrin. As a result of this enzyme's activity, fibrinogen is consumed, and a secondary fibrinolysis occurs. Fibrin split products are therefore increased. Interestingly, however, platelets are not aggregated, and platelet function remains normal. The net result is a marked hypofibrinogenemia.[103]

Anticoagulant effects of various venoms are also well documented. Venom activity at several sites in the cascade inhibits normal clotting function. The venoms of some *Crotalus* species also have a direct fibrinolytic effect.[103] Hemorrhage secondary to coagulopathy does not generally occur unless there are hemorrhagic factors in the snake's venom, as there are in a number of *Crotalus* species. These factors are nonproteolytic, nonenzymatic proteins that are toxic to the vascular wall. The damage to the endothelial lining leads to bleeding into the vessel wall and surrounding tissues, platelet aggregation, and erythrocyte destruction. The result is significant hemolysis, hemorrhage, and thrombocytopenia.[117,118]

Neurotoxicity

Most *Crotalus* venom is only slightly neurotoxic; the venoms of the coral snakes and the Mojave rattlesnake, however, are severely neurotoxic. The specific component of these venoms that is responsible for the neurotoxicity is not known, although it is thought to be a polypeptide. The mechanism of action is likewise unknown, but it is possibly a nondepolarizing blockade at the neuromuscular junction.[111] The net result is a paralysis that leads to respiratory insufficiency.

Clinical Manifestations of Snake Bites

Snake bites produce various clinical manifestations depending on the species, size, and age of the biting snake; the amount of venom injected; how recently the snake has eaten; the first aid given en route to hospital care; the anatomic location of the bite; and the victim's age and health. The pit vipers account for 98% of all venomous snake bites in the United States, and the signs and symptoms of their bites can be divided into two broad categories: local effects and systemic effects.[103,106,110,117,119–126] As stated earlier, local symptomatology is due to tissue edema and necrosis. The bite wound typically consists of two fang marks that penetrate the surface of the skin. The depth of the wound is variable, but generally the deep fascial layers are not penetrated.

Pain and swelling at the site are almost immediate. The pain caused by the bite itself is probably due to the venom and is not severe. As edema progresses, pain becomes more significant. Swelling usually occurs within 5 minutes, although it may be delayed as long as 15 minutes. If there is no edema present 20 to 30 minutes after the bite, envenomation probably did not occur.[103,120,127] Edema tends to progress rapidly and may continue to spread for as long as 36 hours.

Ecchymosis is common in the area of the bite as well as in contiguous areas.[109,110,127–129] This finding is variable, depending upon the species of the biting snake. Vesicle formation is also related to the snake species. Vesicles appear 8 to 36 hours after envenomation and may be filled with serous fluid or blood.[103,110,129] They rarely appear if antivenin has been administered promptly and in adequate amounts. The administration of adequate antivenin should also prevent the tissue necrosis that, before the advent of antivenin therapy, commonly resulted in tissue destruction.

Systemic symptoms after pit viper bites usually indicate a serious envenomation. Nausea and vomiting are common but may be due, at least in part, to the administration of narcotics. Weakness is a common symptom of severe envenomation,[103,105,110,129] but immediate, transient weakness after snake bite is probably more of an emotional response than a venom reaction.

Numbness and tingling, particularly in the perioral and scalp areas, are frequently seen.[103,105,110] These symptoms may also occur in the fingers and toes or may involve the entire body. They occur early in the course of a bite and indicate significant envenomation.

The presence of a metallic, minty, or rubbery taste in the mouth is a common early symptom of envenomation by several of the crotalid species.[103,110] It also represents significant envenomation. This is a symptom that must be elicited by the examining physician because the patient often does not voice this specific complaint.

Neurologic manifestations of *Crotalus* envenomation may include muscle fasciculations, pinpoint pupils, focal paresis, and, rarely, diffuse paralysis.[110,129] Seizure activity occasionally follows *Crotalus* bites but is probably a result of hypoxia rather than a direct effect of the venom because venom does not cross the blood-brain barrier.[117]

Hemorrhage can be a severe problem in pit viper envenomation.[130] Its presence indicates moderate to severe poisoning, and it may be evident as melena, hematemesis, hemoptysis, hematuria, or epistaxis.[128] Coagulation profiles on these patients are abnormal, and platelet counts may be markedly depressed.[131]

Hypotension, disseminated intravascular coagulation, hemolysis, and rhabdomyolysis may occur in significant pit viper envenomations. Acute renal failure may follow any of these complications.[112,115,116]

The signs and symptoms of Mojave rattlesnake envenomation differ from those of the typical pit viper envenomation. Mojave rattlesnake bites produce little local reaction, even when poisoning is serious. The venom of these snakes contains a potent neurotoxin that can cause paralysis with respiratory arrest.[103,117,120] A possible exception is the bite of the Mojave rattler indigenous to southern Arizona; it produces a predominance of local signs and symptoms rather than neurologic findings.[124] Generally, however, because of the neurotoxic effects of the venom, antivenin administration is recommended for all bites of this species.[103] If early antivenin administration is withheld, close observation is mandatory.

Coral snake poisonings can also be deceptive because local symptoms are lacking and because systemic symptoms may be significantly delayed, even in severe poisonings.[105] Apprehension, giddiness, dyspnea, nausea, salivation, vomiting, and weakness are early symptoms, although they may be delayed for several hours. Bulbar palsy, which is seen in 4 to 7 hours, heralds the onset of a diffuse paralysis that follows in 1 to 2 hours. Once symptoms do occur, progression is rapid.[132,133] An aggressive use of antivenin in coral snake poisoning is therefore recommended.[106,129,134] Coral snake antivenin is effective only in treating the more serious bite of the Eastern coral snake.[134] The venom of the Sonoran coral snake is not neutralized by antivenin, but this snake's envenomations are rarely serious, and treatment is supportive.[134]

Management of Snake Bites

The treatment of snake bite victims occurs in two stages: first aid given at the scene and in transport, and definitive care given after arrival at the hospital. Snake bites are true medical emergencies and merit the same attention as any other life-threatening emergency. The first few hours in the course of envenomation are critical, and delay in treatment can result in serious morbidity and death. The importance of prompt assessment and treatment cannot be overemphasized.

First Aid Management

Recommendations for first aid measures for snake bites vary in the literature. A few simple measures are universally recommended.

Calm the victim. The victim should be removed from the immediate vicinity and instructed to lie down and do as little physical activity as possible because movement may facilitate absorption of venom. The victim should be reassured.

Identify the snake. An effort should be made to identify, as accurately as possible, the offending snake. Although some investigators have recommended killing the snake and bringing it in for identification,[135] this is probably unwise for the inexperienced snake handler. Even dead snakes can bite and envenomate by reflex.[105,120] Instead, the size and certain other identifying characteristics of the snake should be noted (see Appendix 39-A). The snake can usually be found within 20 feet of the site of the incident, even after several hours.[120]

Apply a constricting band. A loosely applied constricting band should be placed above the first joint proximal to the bite or 5 to 10 cm proximal to the wound. Because venom spreads by lymphatic and venous channels,[105,120] the band need not, and should not, occlude arterial flow. The band must be placed within 30 minutes of the bite to be of any value.[106] The wound should be kept in a neutral position, and the band should remain in place until antivenin administration, if necessary, is begun. It should then be removed gradually to prevent liberation of a large bolus of venom. **At no time should a tourniquet be applied**.

Consider incision and suction of the wound. First popularized in the 1920s, incision and suction have been variably recommended and denounced in the literature over the ensuing years.[106] If performed properly within 30 minutes of envenomation, it probably does have therapeutic value. It is not recommended if the victim is less than 1 hour away from definitive care.[129] If incision and suction are deemed appropriate, the two fang marks should be incised in the direction of the strike. The incision should extend only 3 to 6 mm and should penetrate only the skin. Deeper incisions are not necessary and only risk damage to underlying structures.[129] Cruciate incisions or multiple incisions in the area of edema are disfiguring and do not improve the yield of extracted venom. Suction should be applied to the incised area with suction cups supplied in snake bite kits. Oral suction should be used only as a last resort because it contaminates the wound.[129,136]

Immobilize and mark the involved area. The affected body part should be splinted to prevent excessive movement. If edema is noted before arrival at the hospital, the level of swelling should be marked on the skin with a pen along with the time the mark was made. This should be repeated every 15 minutes during transport, thus giving the receiving physician an immediate indication of the degree of envenomation.[137]

Do not apply ice. Cryotherapy is mentioned only to be condemned. Although it was a popular form of therapy in the past, it is now uniformly held to be detrimental. The application of ice enhances tissue ischemia and ultimately causes additional tissue necrosis, possibly resulting in amputation.[129,138]

Evacuate the victim. The final step in the first aid treatment of snake bite, and by far the most important, is evacuation of the victim. First aid is by no means a substitute for definitive medical evaluation and treatment.

Emergency Department Management

The medical management of snake bites is multifaceted, requiring the simultaneous performance of several procedures. The goals of therapy are to prevent further venom absorption, to neutralize what has been absorbed, to prevent and treat complications, and to provide supportive care.

A thorough history. A detailed history regarding the circumstances of the bite must be obtained. Specific details should be sought about the time of injury, the activity of the patient when bitten and after being bitten, the number of bites, and the first aid measures provided. Inquiry about previous bites and allergies, particularly to horse serum, should be made. If the snake was not recovered, the victim must be asked to describe the snake to determine species and size (see Appendix 39-A). A brief review of systems must be performed to determine the presence or absence of any other potentially complicating health problems.

The physician must first allow the patient to relate symptoms and then ask specific questions concerning numbness, tingling, lightheadedness, weakness, nausea, vomiting, and abnormal gustatory sensations. If local swelling is present, it must be determined when it started and how rapidly it has progressed.

Patient examination and laboratory data. Physical examination should emphasize serial vital signs, neurologic function, and the presence and progression of local symptoms. Serial limb measurements can be helpful in monitoring the spread of edema in extremity bites.[123] Careful attention must be paid to distal neurovascular status in affected extremities; detection of pulses may require a Doppler stethoscope. Signs indicative of serious envenomation (above) should be specifically sought.

Blood should be drawn for the following studies: complete blood count including platelet count, electrolytes, blood urea nitrogen and creatinine, and coagulation studies. A urinalysis should be done. Extra blood for future type and cross-match should also be obtained because cross-matching may become difficult as a result of the presence of venom. For more critical patients, arterial blood gases, an electrocardiogram, determination of fibrinogen and fibrin split products levels, and a chest radiograph are indicated. If the history is inadequate, immunologic differentiation of snake species by venom type is possible but not always practical.[139]

Monitoring and supportive measures. The need for supportive measures is based on the vital signs and overall condition of the patient. Stable-appearing patients should be placed in a monitored area and have an intravenous line of lactated Ringer's solution or normal saline started in anticipation of deterioration. More critical patients may require intubation, blood pressure support with fluid and vasopressors, and insertion of central venous or Swan-Ganz catheters. Other general supportive measures include wound cleansing, analgesia, and infection and tetanus prophylaxis. No data exist documenting the need for empiric antibiotic treatment of snake bite victims. Nonetheless, patients with severe local reactions are generally given antibiotics; if so, a broad-spectrum agent such as a cephalosporin should be selected to cover the large variety of aerobic and anaerobic organisms that have been isolated from snake venoms.[103,140,141]

Determination of the need for antivenin. The cornerstone of treatment for snake bites is antivenin. It is effective against

Table 39-6 Classification of Severity of Crotalid Envenomation According to McCollough and Gennaro

Category	Signs
Grade 0	No envenomation
Grade I, minimal	Fang marks, minimal or no local swelling, moderate pain, no systemic signs
Grade II, moderate	More severe and widely distributed edema and pain; possibly local petechiae and ecchymoses; occasionally weakness, nausea and vomiting, and bloody oozing from fang marks
Grade III, severe	Signs of Grades I and II in rapid progression with immediate systemic signs and symptoms
Grade IV, very severe	Sudden pain and rapid swelling that may involve the trunk; ecchymoses and progressive edema; bleb formation; early systemic signs and symptoms; shock, bleeding from body orifices, convulsions, coma, renal failure

Table 39-7 Classification of Severity of Crotalid Envenomation According to Russell

Category	Signs
No envenomation	No local or systemic signs
Minimal	Local swelling, no systemic reactions
Moderate	Swelling progressing beyond the site of the bite and systemic signs and/or laboratory changes, eg, a fall in hematocrit
Severe	Marked local reaction, severe systemic symptoms, and laboratory changes

both the systemic manifestations and the local effects of venom. Antivenin (Crotalidae) Polyvalent, produced by Wyeth Laboratories, is effective against the venom of all North American pit vipers. It is produced from the sera of hyperimmune horses, as is Wyeth antivenin for Eastern coral snake venom.

Antivenin administration is not without risk and should be done only when indicated and only under monitored conditions. The need for antivenin is determined by the severity of the envenomation and the type of snake involved. Although some snake bites always merit antivenin administration (Eastern coral snakes and the Mojave rattlesnake, as mentioned above), with most crotalid species the need for antivenin is determined by the patient's signs and symptoms. Age is also an important determinant, with the very young and the very old being much more sensitive to the effects of venom.[105,128,129] Because venom crosses the placenta, pregnant women are more likely to require antivenin therapy.[142]

Before treatment with antivenin is initiated, it must be determined that the patient was actually envenomated. If the patient has only superficial scratches with no evidence of fang marks, envenomation did not occur. If the patient has fang marks, envenomation may have occurred. The likelihood of envenomation after a bite is species dependent. Cobras, for example, envenomate in only 50% of their bites, whereas rattlesnakes have a 90% envenomation rate.[103] Envenomation, therefore, must be determined by the presence of signs and symptoms other than fang marks.

Two classifications of crotalid envenomations have been developed to determine the severity of the injury and the need for antivenin. The first classification, established by Wood, Hoback, and Green, has subsequently been modified by Parrish as well as by McCollough and Gennaro.[134] There are five categories in this system—0 through IV—corresponding to a nonpenetrating wound through minimal, moderate, severe, and very severe bites. Each category has certain signs and symptoms (Table 39-6). Antivenin is recommended for moderate and severe bites. The second classification is that recommended by Russell[103] and Wingert[143] and uses only four categories: no, minimal, moderate, and severe envenomation (Table 39-7). Antivenin is given for all true envenomations unless the area of swelling is limited to the bite area and there are no systemic symptoms.

It should be noted that, despite general agreement on these principles and classifications, some investigators now recommend using antivenin more sparingly, if at all, because of its significant side effects. They report excellent results even in severe crotalid envenomations treated without neutralization.[144,145] Furthermore, consideration should be given to the types of snakes in a particular geographic region and to the severity of the typical envenomations of these snakes.[145] Although most studies have shown significant efficacy of antivenin in the management of the many manifestations of envenomation,[106,107,110,114,128,131,143,146] it may be wise to withhold it when the anticipated morbidity of envenomation is limited to progressive local swelling.

Antivenin administration. The administration of crotalid antivenin is by the intravenous route only. Intramuscular injections are ineffective; local injections are likewise ineffective and, in the digits, dangerous.[103,120,126,134] Administration should always be preceded by skin testing to determine whether the patient is allergic to horse serum.[126,147] The test is performed by the intradermal injection of 0.02 mL of a 1:10 or 1:100 dilution of the antivenin. If there is no inflammatory reaction or systemic allergic symptoms within 5 to 30 minutes, the test result is negative.[126]

Several important points regarding skin testing should be made. First, skin testing is itself not without risk. Anaphylaxis and death after skin testing have been reported.[148] Second, skin testing may sensitize a patient to horse serum, making future skin testing and antivenin administration dangerous. For this reason, skin testing should be performed only after envenomation has been definitely established and the decision to treat with antivenin has been made.[129,148–151] Third, even a positive skin test does not necessarily preclude antivenin administration in the face of threat to life or limb. In this case, or in the case of a patient who develops allergic symptoms during antivenin therapy even after a negative skin test (10% to 20% in most series[126]), it may be necessary to administer dilute (1:100 or 1:1000) antivenin by slow intravenous infusion with a simultaneous infusion of epinephrine.[103,126,151–154] Less severe reactions may be managed with antihistamines, corticosteroids, and subcutaneous epinephrine[126,155]; some clinicians recommend these latter measures prophylactically.[128,154]

Even under ideal circumstances, antivenin should not be administered in anything but a critical care setting, be it in the ED or the intensive care unit. Although antivenin can be given by intravenous push, most clinicians dilute the desired amount of antivenin 1:4 or 1:10 in normal saline. Infusion should begin slowly to observe for allergic reaction; if no reaction is noted in 15 minutes, the remainder of the solution can be infused over 1 to 2 hours.[137] A second intravenous line should be maintained for fluid resuscitation and the treatment of allergic reactions.

The success of antivenin therapy depends not only on early administration but also on the delivery of an adequate amount. For coral snake poisoning this latter requirement is not difficult to satisfy because 10 vials have been shown to neutralize maximum envenomation completely[126]; 5 vials are recommended for empiric use.[106,129] For crotalids, however, the case is less clear cut. The amount recommended is variable and frequently changes. There is no maximum dose; administration of antivenin must be titrated against clinical indicators such as halting of the progression of swelling or the termination of paresthesias and muscle fasciculations.

Guidelines for antivenin administration, as recommended by Russell,[103] Wingert,[143] and Wingert and Chan[137] are as follows: no envenomation, no antivenin and no skin test; minimal envenomation, 5 vials; moderate envenomation, 10 vials; severe envenomation, 15 vials or more. Children should receive a 50% higher dose. The initial dose can be repeated every 1 to 2 hours as needed.

The optimal time for giving antivenin is within the first 4 hours after the bite. Beyond this time, its efficacy progressively lessens. Venom has been identified in the serum of victims as long as 26 hours after a bite,[103,126] however, which implies that the administration of antivenin even this late may be of benefit.

Other than the immediate complications of anaphylaxis, the major drawback to the administration of antivenin is the subsequent development of serum sickness. This complication is common, with an incidence as high as 75%. It should be anticipated in any patient who is given more than five vials of antivenin.[137,150] Typically, symptoms develop 6 days to 3 weeks after antivenin administration and include malaise, fever, arthralgia, swollen joints, urticaria, lymphadenopathy, and, rarely, peripheral neuritis and meningismus.[120]

Steroid therapy should be initiated at the onset of symptoms and continued until symptoms subside, when the dose should be tapered down and stopped. Severe cases require parenteral medications; outpatient treatment consists of antihistamines plus, if necessary, prednisone (40 to 160 mg/day initially, then tapered; 1 mg/kg/day for children).[121,137]

The use of corticosteroids in the acute management of snake venom poisoning has been advocated in the past.[156,157] Controlled studies in animals, however, have demonstrated no advantage of steroid treatment and in fact suggest a detrimental effect.[158] Based on available data, there is no place for steroids in the management of snake bites. Likewise, low-voltage electric shocks have been recommended for snake bite envenomation.[159,160] This practice has no scientific basis or support and cannot be recommended.[161,162]

Surgical Management

Some experts hold that there is no place at all for surgery in snake bite therapy,[103,107,137] whereas others consider it the mainstay of therapy.[110] Some use surgery as an adjunct to medical management, reserving antivenin as an adjunct only for very serious poisonings.[163] As in most controversial areas of medicine, the correct therapy is not easily identified, probably lies between the two extreme positions, and must be individualized to the patient.

Surgical management includes any or all of the following procedures: incision and suction, excisional therapy with or without extensive debridement, and fasciotomy. Incision and suction are rarely indicated except as a first aid measure immediately after a bite. Excisional therapy is a popular form of treatment that has been practiced for many years. The exact technique of excision varies greatly among clinicians, but most recommend excision of only the skin and any necrotic subcutaneous tissue. The amount of tissue varies from an area 0.5 to 2.5 cm from the fang marks.

Some surgeons take a more aggressive approach.[110,136,164] They advocate making a longitudinal incision into the affected tissue around the bite, excising necrotic tissue, and opening the deep fasciae to inspect the underlying muscle. If necrotic, the muscle is also debrided. The majority of experts, however, are more conservative with fasciotomy and perform it only when vascular compromise is apparent.[125,165,166] Contrary to the claims of some investigators, the development of a compartment syndrome, as determined by pressure measurements, is rare.[107,137,144,146,166] Wholesale application of fasciotomy, especially in a preventive mode, therefore seems unwarranted.

An exception may be made, however, for bites of the fingers. Because of limited space, significant swelling in a digit can result in compromise of distal perfusion and tissue loss. Even when appropriate amounts of antivenin have been given, necrosis may occur. For these finger wounds, some clinicians recommend digital dermotomy.[167] This 5-minute procedure is done in the ED and involves making an incision through the skin from the web space to the level of the middle or distal phalanx. Unlike fasciotomy, this simple procedure does not result in disfigurement and produces a good functional result.

Those opposed to surgical management of snake bites hold that any surgical manipulation is unnecessary if antivenin is properly administered. Those in favor of surgery counter that the hazards of antivenin can be avoided by using excisional therapy and reserving antivenin for only severe envenomations. Both groups argue strongly in support of their position and cite good results from their respective protocols. The controversy may be eased by further research into a more purified antivenin. Gel affinity chromatography methods and development of monoclonal antibodies against venom proteins offer the possibility of a more specific and efficacious antivenin that can be delivered with less foreign, antigenic protein.[168,169] The likelihood of serum sickness and the possibility of anaphylaxis would be reduced, perhaps offering more appeal to those who currently prefer the surgical approach. Although not yet clinically available, this new antivenin is likely to replace the currently used equine serum. Active immunization against snake venom is another potential avenue of research.

ARTHROPOD BITES

Spiders

There are more than 100,000 species of spiders,[170] and all are venomous. Most have short, slender fangs that cannot penetrate human skin.[171] At least 50 species are capable of biting humans, but only a few cause serious problems. Most commonly, a local inflammatory reaction and a minor stinging pain at the time of the bite are the only symptoms, and no specific treatment is required. In the United States, the black widow (*Latrodectus mactans*) and the brown recluse (*Loxosceles reclusa*) are the two species that cause significant morbidity and mortality. In his 10-year survey from 1950 to 1959, Parrish[172] documented 65 deaths in the United States from spider bites. Two of these were attributed to the brown recluse and the remaining 63 to the black widow.

Black Widow

The black widow spider is a small black spider with a characteristic red or yellow hourglass marking on the ventral surface of the abdomen. The body measures roughly 6 mm in diameter, and the maximum leg span is 4 cm.[171] These spiders usually spin their webs in wood piles, under rocks, or in outdoor structures such as garages. Bites in these habitats typically occur on a reaching or prying hand. Occasionally, however, black widows nest in houses; in such cases, victims may sustain bites while in bed or when putting on clothing.[173] Geographically, the black widow is distributed throughout the continental United States but is most common in the southeast and southwest.[171,174] Most bites occur in the late summer and early fall.[175]

Venom. The venom of the black widow spider has not been specifically characterized. It may contain as many as 15 proteins and 5 nonproteins.[173] Only the female can envenomate humans. Like venomous snakes, the black widow can control the release of venom, which is used to paralyze the prey and to begin digestion.

The venom appears to be mainly neurotoxic, with the primary site of action being at the neuromuscular junction. Although studies of the effects of black widow venom on isolated ganglia and neuroeffector junctions have been performed,[176–182] the venom's mechanism of action has not been precisely defined. Nevertheless, black widow venom has been observed to cause an initial massive release of neurotransmitter from the presynaptic membrane, an initial increase in miniature end plate potentials, an inhibition of presynaptic neurotransmitter reuptake, and the inhibition of normal neurotransmission.[171,179–181] On a volume basis, *Latrodectus* venom is a more potent neurotoxin than that of the pit vipers.[175]

Calcium seems to be required for the increased neurotransmitter release.[182,183] Black widow venom has been shown to increase intracellular calcium at the presynaptic nerve terminal, which results in mitochondrial swelling and clumping of neurotransmitter vesicles.[178] The in vivo implications of this are as yet unclear.

Clinical presentation. The clinical course of a person bitten by a black widow spider (the syndrome of latrodectism) is usually benign. At the time of the bite, the patient feels an immediate sharp, stinging pain. This pain frequently causes the patient to kill and retrieve the spider, which aids in the diagnosis. After a few minutes, the pain becomes less severe and more dull in character. Usually, the next and most prominent symptom is muscle cramping. This symptom is delayed in onset, generally by 15 minutes to 2 hours. The cramping can be local initially but usually becomes more generalized with time. If the upper extremity is involved, pleuritic chest pain may be severe, mimicking pulmonary embolism. Bites of the lower extremity tend to produce abdominal wall rigidity and pain, sometimes so severe that it simulates an acute abdomen. Other symptoms frequently elicited from victims of black widow spider bites include nausea, dizziness, headache, anxiety, and weakness.[171,173–175,184] Partial paralysis has been reported.[185]

The signs of latrodectism generally complement the symptoms. Patients appear restless and in pain from their muscle cramps. Muscle spasms and fasciculations generally occur. The bite itself consists of two small punctate wounds surrounded by a small area of inflammation. There is no local necrosis. Other signs that may be seen include ptosis, edema, conjunctivitis, skin rash, pruritis, hypertension, vomiting, and dyspnea.

Victims with serious envenomations become weak, stuporous, and, sometimes, delirious. Seizures can occur, particularly in children. Shock and respiratory depression with their attendant symptomatologies may develop, and death can occur.

Although the duration of symptoms is variable, the intensity of symptoms usually peaks a few hours after the bite and then gradually diminishes. Symptoms usually resolve within 24 hours but may persist for up to 4 days.[172] In some 5% of cases of latrodectism, delayed hypersensitivity reactions occur. Presenting 2 to 3 days postenvenomation, these patients have intense pruritis, with or without ecchymosis, at the site of the bite. There may also be a recurrence of muscle involvement.[106]

The mortality rate in latrodectism is not known. Estimates of 4% to 5% have been reported,[186] but this seems exaggerated if one recalls that only 63 people died in a 10-year period from this spider's bite.[172] Patients generally recover completely from black widow spider bites with no residual sequelae.

Treatment. First aid for a black widow spider bite consists of applying an ice pack to the bitten area. Definitive treatment is primarily symptomatic. The most prominent symptom is muscle cramping, and therapy is aimed at relieving this pain. Intravenous calcium gluconate has been used for this purpose for many years.[173] Although it is not a specific antidote and the physiologic basis for this treatment is unproven, anecdotal literature does support its use.[171,174,175,184,187,188] As noted earlier, black widow venom increases nerve terminal intracellular calcium by allowing extracellular calcium to flow into the cells. Perhaps calcium gluconate replenishes this extracellular calcium, resulting in a cessation of tetanic contractions and fasciculations.

Calcium gluconate (10 mL of a 10% solution) can be given intravenously in 50 to 100 mL of fluid over 10 to 15 minutes. Exact guidelines for administration and dosage have not been established. Hypercalcemia can develop if treatment is overzealous.[189] It is advisable to give no more than two or three ampules in a 2- to 3-hour period and to monitor cardiac function during the infusion. If successful, pain relief is dramatic and usually occurs within minutes after administration.

Muscle relaxants have also been recommended. Methocarbamol [Robaxin, 1 g (10 mL) given intravenously over 5 minutes] may be helpful in relieving symptoms.[107,171,173] The initial bolus can be supplemented with an infusion of 500 to 1000 mg in 250 mL of saline over 1 to 2 hours. If successful, therapy can be continued with oral methocarbamol (500 mg every 6 hours) after the patient has been discharged. Intravenous diazepam (Valium) may be equally effective in doses of 5 to 10 mg every 3 to 4 hours.[107]

Narcotics may be necessary to relieve the painful cramps of latrodectism.[174,188] Meperidine hydrochloride (Demerol) or morphine sulfate may be given. Because the venom itself may cause respiratory depression, however, caution must be exercised in giving narcotics.

Antivenin (Merck, Sharp, and Dohme) is widely available and may be needed to treat or prevent serious complications of latrodectism. Commonly accepted indications for antivenin include the very young and elderly age groups, hypertension or history of hypertension, and acute respiratory distress.[125,173,175,185] Black widow antivenin is a horse serum product and must be administered with the same precautions as those for snake bite antivenin. Skin testing is done before administration, and preparations must be made for the treatment of an allergic or anaphylactic reaction. The dose for adults and children is one vial (2.5 mL of reconstituted antivenin) diluted in 10 to 50 mL of normal saline given intravenously over 15 to 30 minutes.[126,190] Relief of pain is often apparent in minutes, although it may take up to 3 hours. Serum sickness is a possible complication, but it is less likely than in snake bite cases because the amount of spider antivenin given is much smaller.

The optimum treatment for black widow spider bites has not been determined, hence the four treatment alternatives (calcium, muscle relaxants, narcotics, and antivenin) detailed above. Each of these regimens, including antivenin, has a significant failure rate in relieving muscle pain. Even though some investigators claim superiority of one drug over another,[187] it is likely that a combination of the various agents will be necessary to effect relief of symptoms.[174,175]

Admission to the hospital for latrodectism is usually not warranted, except for patients treated with antivenin and those with persistent constitutional symptoms. The elderly and the young should also be observed as inpatients, even if antivenin is not given. The usual patient can be treated successfully by several hours of observation and symptomatic care in the ED with subsequent oral administration of muscle relaxants and/or minor analgesics.

Brown Recluse

The other spider in the United States that can cause significant morbidity and, rarely, mortality is the brown recluse. In reality, there are several *Loxosceles* species in the United States capable of producing necrotic arachnidism, or loxoscelism; the best known and studied of these is the brown recluse, *Loxosceles reclusa*. This spider is light brown in color and has a characteristic dark brown, violin-shaped marking on the dorsum of its thorax, hence the common name brown fiddler or fiddle-back spider. The spider is small, usually 1.0 to 1.5 cm in length and 0.5 to 1.0 cm in width. As the name implies, the spider is not a social animal and tends to remain in dark areas, such as closets and basements.

The recluse spider is generally limited to the southeastern and south central states, although some species of *Loxosceles* have been found in the desert southwest.[191,192] The actual incidence of loxoscelism is unknown, and it is likely that many skin lesions of various etiologies are erroneously attributed to this spider. This tendency toward overdiagnosis has serious medical and legal implications. Consequently, authorities on the subject suggest that a specific diagnosis of recluse spider bite be reserved for those cases in which the biting spider has been recovered and subsequently identified by a qualified expert. Hemagglutinin assays are also available for confirmation.[174] Cases with less compelling evidence should be labeled possible arthropod envenomation.[193,194]

Venom. The most important component of brown recluse venom is an enzyme, sphingomyelinase D. Although not unequivocally proven, this enzyme may be responsible for both the local and systemic effects of the venom.[195–198] Either through direct cytotoxic effects or by mediating an inflammatory reaction through release of intracellular substances, sphingomyelinase D is thought to produce dermonecrosis. Pathologically, this reaction consists of an intense leukocytic infiltration, edema, hemorrhage, and thrombosis.[107,196] Animal models of envenomation utilizing sphingomyelinase D have produced a clinical picture similar to severe loxoscelism including hemolysis, leukocytosis, thrombocytopenia, and complement activation as well as the typical local reaction.

Clinical presentation. The clinical manifestations of the brown recluse bite can be divided into local and systemic effects. The local effects are specifically referred to as necrotic arachnidism. Typically the victim feels no pain, or only a mild stinging sensation, at the time of the bite. Local pain and a blue-gray constrictive halo around the bite are usually the only manifestations in the first several hours.[192,197,199] After 12 to 18 hours a bleb forms, and the ischemic zone spreads. Eventually the center of the zone sinks below the level of the surrounding skin.[197,200] This area progresses to aseptic necrosis, dry gangrene, and eschar formation over the next 5 to 7 days. When the eschar separates, an open ulcer remains.[201] This description is typical of a moderate to severe envenomation; in most cases the bite is trivial, resulting in no tissue loss. At the other end of the spectrum are severe lesions, up to 30 cm or more in diameter, requiring debridement and grafting.[198,202–204] Two characteristics of these bites that help distinguish them from nonnecrotic envenomations are the blue color and the depressed skin level. These findings contrast with the red, raised lesions of more benign bites.[200]

Systemic symptoms of loxoscelism include fever, chills, malaise, nausea, vomiting, and arthralgias. More serious problems, usually seen in children, include disseminated intravascular coagulation, hemolysis, renal failure, and death.[129,192,197,199,205] The reason for the variation in sensitivity to brown recluse bites—from local pain to death—is not known. The serious systemic complications develop only in a minority of cases.

Treatment. No clear approach has emerged as the optimal management for brown recluse bites. No antivenin is available. Because the natural course of these envenomations is so variable, it is difficult to determine whether a given intervention has a true impact on outcome. A number of treatment regimens have been proposed, including drugs (steroids, heparin, and dapsone), early surgical excision, and delayed surgical care. Controversy still exists, but the consensus is against early excision. Poor functional results and animal data showing no clear benefit from early surgery support a more conservative approach.[198,203–207] Animal studies have likewise failed to show any advantage to heparin and steroids in preventing or minimizing local toxicity.[208]

Dapsone has been suggested for necrotic arachnidism because it is effective in other dermatologic disorders characterized by polymorphonuclear leukocyte infiltration. Animal studies have shown an improved outcome with dapsone.[209] Some clinical studies have demonstrated promising results with the use of dapsone both alone and in combination with surgical therapy,[203,204,206] but the data are not yet fully convincing.

First aid for brown recluse bites includes application of ice and thorough cleansing. In the ED, tetanus prophylaxis and a padded splint to prevent further trauma to the bitten area should be provided. Empiric antibiotics are of questionable benefit, although some investigators recommend them.[206] In the absence of any specific, proven treatment, the best approach for local toxicity is a conservative one. If full-thickness skin loss develops, the wound should be debrided and left open for 8 weeks. Subsequent skin grafting may be required.[200,204]

Systemic loxoscelism requires supportive care, including hydration, transfusion, and dialysis in selected cases. Use of steroids is of theoretical value in the early phase of systemic poisoning. Given for no more than 2 days, steroids may help improve a developing coagulopathy.[200,210] No controlled data exist to support this theory.

Scorpions

Scorpionism in the United States is a problem limited to the southwest, particularly to Arizona. Although there are approximately 40 species of scorpions in the United States, only 1—*Centruroides sculpturatus*—possesses a potentially lethal venom. This species is located primarily in Arizona, but it can also be found in some parts of Texas, California, and northern Mexico.[211]

Scorpions are not aggressive creatures and generally sting humans only in self-defense. Scorpion activity varies with temperature and tends to reach a peak in the cool of the evening.[212] It is during this time that most scorpion stings occur. Scorpions do not envenomate by biting, as spiders and snakes do, but by stinging. Venom is produced in a specialized segment of the tail called a telson. A stinger located at the caudal end of the telson delivers the venom into the scorpion's adversary.

Venom

Certain effects of scorpion venoms are species specific and cannot be attributed to all scorpions. The *C sculpturatus* venom is primarily neurotoxic. It contains four neurotoxins[213] that appear to act at neuronal synapses and neuromuscular junctions. Increased sodium permeability of the presynaptic neurons is probably induced, leading to increased acetylcholine release at the neuromuscular junction and causing muscle fasciculations.[214] The clinical significance of these findings is not clear.

Clinical Presentation

The clinical manifestations of scorpionism include a great many symptoms, some of which are helpful diagnostically. Unlike the nonlethal sting of the *Vejovis spinigerus* scorpion, the *C sculpturatus* sting produces no local signs of inflammation and swelling. In fact, the exact site of the sting cannot be determined in most instances, even though one of the most common symptoms is local pain with hyperesthesia.[173,211,215] Another common sign is extreme restlessness and agitation. The agitation is so severe that it may be mistaken for seizure activity.[211] In the series of Rimsza et al,[211] this sign was limited to patients younger than 10 years of age. These investigators also noted roving eye movements, a sign not previously reported, in one third of their patients.[211] Other signs of the *Centruroides* sting, again usually more serious in children than adults, include tachycardia, hypertension, tachypnea, salivation, blurred vision, poor coordination, slurred speech, paresthesias, wheezing, vomiting, stridor, and dysphagia.[129,211] Related scorpion stings can cause direct myocardial toxicity, especially in children, but this has not been demonstrated in *C sculpturatus*.[212,216]

Treatment

The treatment for stings of nonlethal scorpions is symptomatic and nonspecific.[173] The management of *C sculpturatus* stings is also largely symptomatic. In the past, heavy sedation with barbiturates has been recommended to control agitation. This treatment offers no advantage and, in fact, may produce respiratory depression. Measures to support ventilation and blood pressure should be taken as necessary, and analgesia should be provided. Steroids are frequently used for scorpion stings but are of no demonstrable benefit. An as yet unlicensed antivenin has been used in Arizona; its efficacy has not been established.

Mortality from scorpionism is unknown; there have been no reported deaths in the United States since 1968. Stahnke[215] reported that from 1929 to 1948 scorpions were responsible for more deaths in Arizona than any other venomous animal, including rattlesnakes. The improved survival over the past 20 years probably reflects more sophisticated supportive care than a decreased incidence of stings or any change in the nature of the scorpion.[129,211]

The need for tetanus prophylaxis in spider bites and scorpion stings is not clear. Generally, routine tetanus prophylaxis is recommended.

Hymenoptera

The class Hymenoptera contains many stinging and biting insects, but only a few are associated with adverse reactions in humans. These include the honeybee, other bees, the yellowjacket, hornets, wasps, and fire ants.[217,218] Unlike the previously discussed animals that inflict injury by direct trauma, infection, or injection of potent venoms, hymenoptera cause morbidity and mortality by inducing allergic reactions and anaphylaxis. Although these creatures do inject venom into their victims, only in cases of massive numbers of stings does the venom itself produce a serious problem. Rather, the reaction of sensitized patients to the venom is responsible for the deleterious effects of hymenoptera stings.

Epidemiology

It is estimated that approximately 0.4% of the population of the United States is at risk for serious reactions.[219] Most often, sensitive patients give a history of sting reactions that were initially small and progressed to extensive local reactions and, ultimately, to systemic reactions. There are, however, many exceptions to this typical pattern. Some individuals deny any previous stings or report only normal reactions before a serious systemic reaction.[217] Others claim repeated systemic reactions with no evidence of progression or variation. Fifty percent of 2606 sting allergy patients surveyed by the Insect Allergy Committee of the American Academy of Allergy reported no warning of their systemic reactions based on previous stings.[220] This suggests that many people with sting allergy are unprotected simply because they are unaware that they have such an allergy.

Hymenoptera are widely distributed across the United States, although fire ants are mostly limited to the southeast.[221] Stings are likely to occur under various circumstances. People who handle insects, such as beekeepers, are obviously at great risk. Accidental or intentional encroachment on hives or nests also provokes attack and stinging. Walking in meadows or going barefoot in clover patches can result in stings when the insects are disturbed. Other practices that attract hymenoptera and thereby increase the incidence of stinging are wearing brightly colored clothes or sweet-smelling fragrances and eating sweets outdoors.[222]

Venoms

Like other venoms already discussed, hymenoptera venoms are complex poisons. They are delivered by barbs that resemble hypodermic needles. Fire ants can bite as well as sting their victims.[221] Detailed analyses of all hymenoptera venoms are not available, but venoms of the honeybee and wasp are well characterized.[223,224] Biogenic amines (including histamine, dopamine, norepinephrine, and serotonin), proteins, and enzymes (most commonly phospholipase A and hyaluronidase) are all present. Many of these substances are antigenic in humans.[223–228]

Clinical Presentation

The signs and symptoms of hymenoptera stings vary from localized pruritis and erythema to anaphylactic shock and death. The onset of symptoms may be immediate or delayed.

Local reaction. The normal response to a sting is an immediate, sharp, burning pain that is accompanied within a few minutes by edema and pruritis.[217,229] Part of the stinging apparatus may be retained in the victim, particularly if the stinging insect is a honeybee, whose barbed stinger cannot be removed by the bee. The usual local reaction is minimal.

Extensive local reactions may involve an entire extremity. Because the edema is contiguous with the sting site, and because there are no systemic manifestations, these reactions are classed as local; the exception is stings to the tongue or throat, which can quickly cause respiratory distress. It is important to note extensive local reactions because they may indicate increasing sensitivity in the patient and a greater potential risk for systemic reactions with subsequent stings.[220]

Systemic reaction. Systemic allergic reactions vary in severity and symptomatology. Signs and symptoms of mild reactions are histaminergic in nature and include diffuse pruritis, urticarial eruptions, swelling distant from the sting site, and flushing. More severe reactions are manifested by respiratory embarrassment, usually due to either laryngeal edema or severe bronchospasm, and profound hypotension of anaphylaxis resulting in myocardial infarction, brain damage, and renal failure.[217,230,231] Systemic reactions are immediate hypersensitivity reactions mediated by immunoglobulin E (IgE) antibodies.[217]

Delayed reaction. Arbitrarily defined as reactions that begin more than 1 hour after injury, delayed reactions may also be local or systemic. Although most serious anaphylactic reactions occur within the first hour, a significant percentage of serious and fatal reactions are delayed even up to 48 hours. The mechanism for the delay is not well understood, but it may be mediated by basophils through IgE antibodies. It is postulated that the delay is due to the time required for the basophils to migrate to the site of mast cell degranulation (ie, the site where an immediate hypersensitivity reaction has occurred). When IgE-laden basophils do reach that site, they react with residual antigen, causing their own degranulation and the delayed reaction.[232]

Treatment

In the nonsensitive patient, the treatment of hymenoptera stings is nonspecific and symptomatic.[233] In the sting-allergic patient, treatment can be divided into immediate care, prevention of subsequent stings, self-treatment, and hyposensitization.

Immediate treatment varies with the severity of the reaction, but the mainstay of therapy is epinephrine.[234] Other measures indicated in management of anaphylactic shock include airway management and blood pressure support with intravenous fluids and, occasionally, vasopressors (see Chapter 6, Shock). Other specific drugs for counteracting anaphylactic reactions include theophylline, which inhibits the release of vasoactive substances; antihistamines, which counteract the peripheral effects of some of those vasoactive substances; and steroids, whose role is unclear.[234,235] The route of administration and dosages of these agents are determined by the severity of the reaction. It should be emphasized that, although steroids are helpful, they have no immediate beneficial effect. Their action is delayed for several hours, and they must not be given as the sole treatment of anaphylaxis.

Prevention of subsequent stings in sensitized patients is a matter of common sense. Avoiding those activities that are known to increase the risk of being stung is the best recommendation.

Self-treatment for sting-allergic patients involves kits designed for emergency treatment. These kits include a syringe of 1:1000 epinephrine, needles, antihistamine tablets, and a tourniquet. An additional measure is the wearing of a MedicAlert tag. All patients with known sting allergies should be encouraged to wear such tags to ensure prompt consideration of anaphylaxis if they are found unconscious.

Hyposensitization offers the most promising treatment for sting-allergic patients. It is designed to prevent anaphylactic reactions by blocking the interaction of antigen with IgE and the subsequent degranulation of mast cells.[236–239] The procedure is believed to be 95% successful.[237,240] It involves serial intradermal venom injections, which after adequate desensitization must be repeated at monthly intervals. Because hymenoptera stings account for more deaths than any other category of bites and stings discussed in this chapter,[129,218–219,240–242] it is important to have an effective program for the prevention of these anaphylactic reactions.

REFERENCES

1. Callaham ML. Domestic and feral mammalian bites. In: Auerbach PS, Geehr EC, eds. *Management of Wilderness and Environmental Emergencies.* New York: Macmillan; 1983.
2. Klein M. Nondomestic mammalian bites. *Am Fam Physician.* 1985;32:137–141.
3. Paisley JW, Lauer BA. Severe facial injuries to infants due to unprovoked attacks by pet ferrets. *JAMA.* 1988;259;2005–2006.
4. Ordog GJ, Balasubramanium S, Wasserberger J. Rat bites: fifty cases. *Ann Emerg Med.* 1985;144:126–130.
5. Beck AM. The public health implications of urban dogs. *Am J Public Health.* 1975;65:1315–1318.

6. Moore RM, Zehmer RB, Moulthrop JI, et al. Surveillance of animal bite cases in the United States, 1971–1972. *Arch Environ Health.* 1977;32:267–270.
7. Berzon DR, Farber RB, Gordon J, et al. Animal bites in a large city—a report on Baltimore, Maryland. *Am J Public Health.* 1972;62:422–426.
8. Harris D, Imperato PJ, Oken B. Dog bites—an unrecognized epidemic. *Bull NY Acad Med.* 1974;50:981–1000.
9. Goldstein EJC, Richwald GA. Human and animal bite wounds. *Am Fam Physician.* 1987;36:101–109.
10. Daniels TJ. A study of dog bites on the Navajo reservation. *Public Health Rep.* 1986;101:50–59.
11. Beck AM, Jones BA. Unreported dog bites in children. *Public Health Rep.* 1985;100:315–321.
12. Underman AE. Bite wounds inflicted by dogs and cats. *Vet Clin North Am (Small Anim Pract).* 1987;17:195–207.
13. Borchelt PL, Lockwood R, Beck AM, et al. Attacks by packs of dogs involving predation on human beings. *Public Health Rep.* 1983;98:57–66.
14. Rest JG, Goldstein EJC. Management of human and animal bite wounds. *Emerg Clin North Am.* 1985;3:117–126.
15. Beck AM. The epidemiology of animal bite. *Compar Contin Educ Pract Vet.* 1981;3:254–258.
16. Kizer KW. Epidemiologic and clinical aspects of animal bite injuries. *JACEP.* 1979;8:134–141.
17. Thomas PR, Buntine JA. Man's best friend? A review of the Austin Hospital's experience with dog bites. *Med J Aust.* 1987;147:536–540.
18. Sacks JJ, Sattin RW, Bonzo SE. Dog bite–related fatalities from 1979 through 1988. *JAMA.* 1989;262:1489–1492.
19. Jaffe AC. Animal bites. *Pediatr Clin North Am.* 1983;30:405–413.
20. Boenning DA, Fleisher GR, Campos JM. Dog bites in children: epidemiology, microbiology, and penicillin prophylactic therapy. *Am J Emerg Med.* 1983;1:17–21.
21. Berzon DR. Medical costs and other aspects of dog bites in Baltimore. *Public Health Rep.* 1974;89:377–381.
22. Pinckney LE, Kennedy LA. Traumatic deaths from dog attacks in the United States. *Pediatrics.* 1982;69:193–196.
23. Wright JC. Severe attacks by dogs: characteristics of the dogs, the victims, and the attack settings. *Public Health Rep.* 1985;100:55–61.
24. Wiseman NE, Chochinov H, Fraser V. Major dog attack injuries in children. *J Pediatr Surg.* 1983;18:533–536.
25. Baack BR, Kucan JO, Demarest G, et al. Mauling by pit bull terriers: case report. *J Trauma.* 1989;29:517–520.
26. Douglas LG. Bite wounds. *Am Fam Physician.* 1975;11:93–99.
27. Callaham ML. Treatment of common dog bites: infection risk factors. *JACEP.* 1978;7:83–87.
28. Goldstein EJC, Baraff LJ, Meislin H, et al. Animal bites. *JACEP.* 1976;7:417.
29. Callaham M. Prophylactic antibiotics in common dog bite wounds: a controlled study. *Ann Emerg Med.* 1980;9:410–414.
30. Zook AG, Miller M, Van Beek AL, et al. Successful treatment protocol for canine fang injuries. *J Trauma.* 1980;20:243–247.
31. Elenbaas R, McNabney WK, Robinson W, et al. Prophylactic oxacillin in dog-bite wounds. *Ann Emerg Med.* 1982;11:248–251.
32. Rosen RA. The use of antibiotics in the initial management of recent dog-bite wounds. *Am J Emerg Med.* 1985;3:19–23.
33. Callaham M. Controversies in antibiotic choices for bite wounds. *Ann Emerg Med.* 1988;17:1321–1330.
34. Brook I. Microbiology of human and animal bite wounds. *Pediatr Infect Dis J.* 1987;6:29–32.
35. Brown CG, Ashton JJ. Dog bites: the controversy continues. *Am J Emerg Med.* 1985;3:83–84.
36. Jones DA, Stanbridge TN. A clinical trial using co-trimoxazole in an attempt to reduce wound infection rates in dog bite wounds. *Postgrad Med J.* 1985;61:593–594.
37. Bobo RA, Newton EJ. A previously undescribed Gram-negative bacillus causing septicemia and meningitis. *Am J Clin Pathol.* 1976;65:564–569.
38. Butler T, Uyeda CT, Kohler RB, et al. Unidentified Gram-negative rod infection. *Ann Intern Med.* 1977;86:1–5.
39. Findling JW, Pohlmann GP, Rose HD. Fulminant Gram-negative bacillemia (DF-2) following a dog bite in an asplenic woman. *Am J Med.* 1980;68:154–156.
40. Kalb R, Kaplan MH, Tenenbaum MJ. Cutaneous infection of dog bite wounds: association with fulminant DF-2 septicemia. *Am J Med.* 1985;78:687–690.
41. Case 29-1986 of case records of the Massachusetts General Hospital. *N Engl J Med.* 1986;215:241–249.
42. Pers C, Kristiansen JE, Scheibel JH, et al. Fatal septicaemia caused by DF-2 in a previously healthy man. *Scand J Infect Dis.* 1986;18:165–267.
43. Dankner WM, Davis CE, Thompson MA. DF-2 bacteremia following a dog bite in a 4-month-old child. *Pediatr J Infect Dis.* 1987;6:695–696.
44. Job L, Horman JT, Grigor JK, et al. Dysgonic fermenter-2: a clinico-epidemiologic review. *J Emerg Med.* 1989;7:185–192.
45. West M, Gibbs M, Hansman D. *Pasteurella multocida* infection after a dog bite. *Med J Aust.* 1976;1:565–566.
46. Szalay GC, Sommerstein A. Inoculation osteomyelitis secondary to animal bites. *Clin Pediatr.* 1972;11:687–689.
47. Klein DM, Cohen ME. *Pasteurella multocida* brain abscess following perforating cranial dog bite. *J Pediatr.* 1978;92:588–589.
48. Gump DW, Holden RA. Endocarditis caused by a new species of *Pasteurella*. *Ann Intern Med.* 1972;75:275–278.
49. Gislason IL, Call JK. Dog bite in infancy: trauma and personality development. *J Am Acad Child Psychol.* 1982;21:203–207.
50. Voith VL. Prognosis for treatment for aggressive behavior of dogs toward children. *Mod Vet Pract.* 1980;61:939–942.
51. O'Riordan WD, Hubbell DV. Compound depressed skull fracture. *JACEP.* 1976;5:123–124.
52. Wilberger JE, Pang D. Craniocerebral injuries from dog bites. *JAMA.* 1983;249:2685–2688.
53. Kenevan RJ, Rich JD, Gottlieb V, et al. A dog bite injury with involvement of cranial content: case report. *Mil Med.* 1985;150:502–503.
54. Roth RM, Gleckman RA. Human infections derived from dogs. *Postgrad Med.* 1985;77:169–180.
55. Kaluck RS. When best friends bite. *Med J Aust.* 1987;147:527–528.
56. Ordog GJ. The bacteriology of dog bite wounds on initial presentation. *Ann Emerg Med.* 1986;15:1324–1329.
57. Jorden RC. Infection following a dog bite. *J Emerg Med.* 1987;5:431–432.
58. Jones JJ. Routine culture of dog bites. *Ann Emerg Med.* 1987;16:730.
59. Lee MLH, Buhr AJ. Dog-bites and local infection with *Pasteurella septica*. *Br Med J.* 1960;1:169–171.
60. Fumarola D. Increasing evidence for the pathogenic role of DF-2 organisms. *Rev Infect Dis.* 1988;10:668.
61. Goldstein EJC, Reinhardt JF, Marray PM, et al. Outpatient therapy of bite wounds: demographic data, bacteriology, and a prospective, randomized trial of amoxicillin/clavulanic acid versus penicillin ± dicloxacillin. *Int J Dermatol.* 1987;26:123–127.

62. Feder HM, Shanley JD, Barbera JA. Review of 599 patients hospitalized with animal bites. *Pediatr Infect Dis J*. 1987;6:24–28.
63. Veitch JM, Omer GE. Case report: treatment of catbite injuries of the hand. *J Trauma*. 1979;19:201–202.
64. Chapple CR, Fraser AN. *Pasteurella multocida* wound infections: a commonly unrecognized problem in the casualty department. *Injury*. 1986;17:410–411.
65. Pechter EA, Miller TA. Severe osteomyelitis of the wrist following a cat bite. *Hand*. 1983;15:243–245.
66. Bjorkholm B, Eilard T. *Pasteurella multocida* osteomyelitis caused by a cat bite. *J Infect*. 1983;6:175–177.
67. Peeples E, Boswick JA, Scott FA. Wounds of the hand contaminated by human or animal saliva. *J Trauma*. 1980;20:383–389.
68. Orton DW, Fulcher WH. *Pasteurella multocida*: bilateral septic knee joint prostheses from a distant cat bite. *Ann Emerg Med*. 1984;13:1065–1067.
69. Goldstein RW, Goodhart GL, Moore JE. *Pasteurella multocida* infection after cat bite. *N Engl J Med*. 1986;315:460.
70. Jones AGH, Lockton JA. Fatal *Pasteurella multocida* septicaemia following a cat bite in a man without liver disease. *J Infect*. 1987;15:229–235.
71. Carpenter PD, Heppner BT, Gnann JW. DF-2 bacteremia following cat bites: a report of two cases. *Am J Med*. 1987;82:621–623.
72. Tindall JP, Harrison CM. *Pasteurella multocida* infections following animal injuries, especially cat bites. *Arch Dermatol*. 1972;105:412–416.
73. Tessin I, Brorson J-E, Trollfers B. Rapidly fatal *Pasteurella multocida* septicemia in an infant following cat scratch. *Pediatr Infect Dis J*. 1987;6:425–426.
74. Francis DP, Holmes MA, Grandon G. *Pasteurella multocida*. *JAMA*. 1975;233:42–45.
75. Baker MD, Moore SE. Human bites in children: a six-year experience. *Am J Dis Child*. 1987;141:1285–1290.
76. Schweich P, Fleisher G. Human bites in children. *Pediatr Emerg Care*. 1985;1:51–53.
77. Edlich RF, Spengler MD, Rodeheaver GT, et al. Emergency department management of mammalian bites. *Emerg Med Clin North Am*. 1986;4:595–604.
78. Marr JS, Beck AM, Lugo JA. An epidemiologic study of the human bite. *Public Health Rep*. 1979;94:514–521.
79. Lindsey D, Christopher M, Hollenbach J, et al. Natural course of the human bite wound: incidence of infection and complications in 434 bites and 803 lacerations in the same group of patients. *J Trauma*. 1987;27:45–48.
80. Mason M, Koch S. Human bite infections of the hand. *Surg Gynecol Obstet*. 1930;51:591.
81. Boland F. Morsus humanis. *JAMA*. 1941;116:127–131.
82. Mann RJ, et al. Human bites of the hand: twenty years of experience. *J Hand Surg*. 1977;2:97–104.
83. Dreyfuss U, Singer M. Human bites of the hand: a study of one hundred six patients. *J Hand Surg*. 1985;10A:884–889.
84. Chuinard RG, D'Ambrosia RD. Human bite infections of the hand. *J Bone Joint Surg Am*. 1977;59:416–418.
85. McConnell CM, Neale HW. Two-year review of hand infections at a municipal hospital. *Am Surg*. 1979;45:643–646.
86. Malinowski RW, et al. The management of human bite injuries in the hand. *J Trauma*. 1979;19:655–659.
87. Guba AM, Mulliken JB, Hoopes JE. The selection of antibiotics for human bites of the hand. *Plast Reconstr Surg*. 1975;56:538–541.
88. Farmer C, Mann R. Human bite infections of the hand. *South Med J*. 1966;59:515.
89. Karody R, Nash N, Bhasin V. Toxic shock syndrome due to an infected human bite. *Ann Emerg Med*. 1987;17:83–87.
90. Schmidt DR, Heckman JD. *Eikenella corrodens* in human bite infections of the hand. *J Trauma*. 1983;23:478–482.
91. Brooks GF, O'Donoghue M, Rissing JP. *Eikenella corrodens*, a recently recognized pathogen. *Medicine*. 1974;53:325–342.
92. Betos ZJ, Eskestrand TA, Shivaram MS. Deep fasciitis of the biceps region. *J Hand Surg*. 1979;4:378–381.
93. Kanavel AB. *Infections of the Hand*. 6th ed. Philadelphia: Lea & Febiger; 1933.
94. Taylor GA. Management of human bite injuries of the hand. *Can Med Assoc J*. 1985;133:191–192.
95. Earley MJ, Bardsley AF. Human bites: a review. *Br J Plast Surg*. 1984;37:458–462.
96. Robinson IB, Loskin DM. Tetanus of oral origin. *Oral Surg*. 1957;10:831.
97. Owen HR. Chancre complicating laceration of the hand. *Ann Surg*. 1928;8:783.
98. Kankat CT. Direct inoculation of tuberculosis through bite on cheek by tuberculous patient. *Turk Tip Cemiy Meem*. 1946;12:168.
99. Robinson RH. Actinomycosis of the sub-cutaneous tissue of the forearm secondary to a human bite. *JAMA*. 1944;124:1049.
100. MacQuarrie MB, Forghani B, Wolochow DA. Hepatitis B transmitted by a human bite. *JAMA*. 1974;230:723–724.
101. Transmission of HIV by human bite. *Lancet*. 1987;2:522.
102. Shirley LR, Ross SA. Risk of transmission of human immunodeficiency virus by bite of an infected toddler. *J Pediatr*. 1989;114:425–427.
103. Russell FE. *Snake Venom Poisoning*. Philadelphia: Lippincott; 1980.
104. Cone GP. Results of treatment of snakebite in an upstate South Carolina community hospital. *J S C Med Assoc*. 1987;83:587–589.
105. Wingert WA, Wainschel J. Diagnosis and management of envenomation by poisonous snakes. *South Med J*. 1975;68:1015–1026.
106. Winnebarger TR, Allison EJ, Mitchell JM, et al. Snakebite treatment in the 80s. *N C J Med*. 1985;46:572–573.
107. Pennell TC, Babu SS, Meredith JW. The management of snake and spider bites in the southeastern United States. *Am Surg*. 1987;53:198–204.
108. Iserson KV. Incidence of snakebite in wilderness rescue. *JAMA*. 1988;260:1405.
109. Russell FE, et al. Snake venom poisoning in the United States. *JAMA*. 1975;233:341–344.
110. Sprenger TR, Bailey WJ. Snakebite treatment in the United States. *Int J Dermatol*. 1986;25:479–484.
111. Jiminez-Porras JM. Biochemistry of snake venoms. *Clin Toxicol*. 1970;3:389–431.
112. Talpers SS, Bergin JJ. Snakebite: first aid and hospital management. *Kans Med*. 1985;86:155–167.
113. Schmutz J, Stahel E. Anaphylactoid reactions to snakebite. *Lancet*. 1985;2:1306.
114. Davidson TM. Intravenous rattlesnake envenomation. *West J Med*. 1988;148:45–47.
115. George A, Tharakan VT, Solez K. Viper bite poisoning in India: a review with special reference to renal complications. *Renal Failure*. 1987;10:91–99.
116. Mittal BV, Kinare SG, Acharya VN. Renal lesions following viper bites—a study of 14 years. *Ind J Med Res*. 1986;83:642–651.

117. Clement JF, Pietrusko RG. Pit viper snakebite in the United States. *J Fam Pract*. 1978;6:269–279.
118. Hasiba Ute, Rosenbach LM, Rockwell D, et al. DIC-Like syndrome after envenomation by the snake, *Crotalus horridus horridus*. *N Engl J Med*. 1975;292:505–507.
119. Parrish HM, Carr CA. Bites by copperheads (*Agkistrodon contotrix*) in the United States. *JAMA*. 1967;201:107–112.
120. Strickland NE. Snake bites: a review. *J Arkansas Med Soc*. 1976;73:69–77.
121. Wingert WA, Wainschel J. A quick handbook on snake bites. *Med Times*. 1977;105:68–75.
122. Parrish HM, Hayes RH. Hospital management of pit viper venomations. *Clin Toxicol*. 1970;3:501–511.
123. Butner AN. Rattlesnake bites in northern California. *West J Med*. 1983;139:179–183.
124. Hardy DL. Envenomation by the Mojave rattlesnake (*Crotalus scutulatus scutulatus*) in southern Arizona, USA. *Toxicon*. 1983;21:111–118.
125. Kunkel DB. Bites of venomous reptiles. *Emerg Med Clin North Am*. 1984;2:563–577.
126. Otten EJ. Antivenin therapy in the emergency department. *Am J Emerg Med*. 1983;1:83–93.
127. Reid HA, Theakston RDG. The management of snake bite. *Bull WHO*. 1983;61:885–895.
128. Christopher DG, Rodning CB. Crotalidae envenomation. *South Med J*. 1986;79:159–162.
129. Banner W. Bites and stings in the pediatric patient. *Curr Probl Pediatr*. 1988;18:1–69.
130. Saini RK. Haematologic alterations in snake bite poisoning. *Ind J Med Res*. 1985;82:77–82.
131. Riffer E, Curry SC, Gerkin R. Successful treatment with antivenin of marked thrombocytopenia without significant coagulopathy following rattlesnake bite. *Ann Emerg Med*. 1987;16:1297–1299.
132. Parrish HM, Khan MS. Bites by coral snakes: reports of 11 representative cases. *Am J Med Sci*. 1967;77:561–568.
133. Russell FE. First-aid for snake venom poisoning. *Toxicon*. 1976;4:285–289.
134. McCollough NC, Gennaro JF. Treatment of venomous snakebite in the United States. *Clin Toxicol*. 1970;3:483–500.
135. Watt CH. Poisonous snakebite treatment in the United States. *JAMA*. 1978;240:654–656.
136. Glass TG. Early debridement in pit viper bites. *JAMA*. 1976;235:2513–2516.
137. Wingert WA, Chan L. Rattlesnake bites in southern California and rationale for recommended treatment. *West J Med*. 1988;148:37–44.
138. Stewart ME, Greenland S, Hoffman JR, et al. First-aid treatment of poisonous snakebite: are currently recommended practices justified? *Ann Emerg Med*. 1981;10:331–335.
139. Minton SA. Present tests for detection of snake venom: clinical applications. *Ann Emerg Med*. 1987;16:932–937.
140. Goldstein EJD, Citron DM, Gonzalez H, et al. Bacteriology of rattlesnake venom and implications for therapy. *J Infect Dis*. 1979;140:818–821.
141. Russell FE, Ruzic N, Gonzalez H. Effectiveness of Antivenin (Crotalidae) Polyvalent following injection of *Crotalus* venom. *Toxicon*. 1973;71:461–464.
142. James RF. Snake bite in pregnancy. *Lancet*. 1985;2:731.
143. Wingert WA. Rattlesnake bites. *West J Med*. 1984;140:100–101.
144. Ethridge HC. Treatment of poisonous snakebite. *J Miss State Med Assoc*. 1987;28:155–156.
145. Burch JM, Agarwal R, Mattox KL, et al. The treatment of crotalid envenomation without antivenin. *J Trauma*. 1988;28:35–43.
146. Wasserman GS. Wound care of spider and snake envenomations. *Ann Emerg Med*. 1988;17:1331–1335.
147. Wyeth Antivenin (Crotalidae) Polyvalent, package insert. Marietta, PA: Wyeth Laboratories.
148. Spaite D, Dart R, Sullivan JB. Skin testing in cases of possible crotalid envenomation. *Ann Emerg Med*. 1988;17:105–106.
149. White BD, Rodgers GC, Matyunas NJ, et al. Copperhead snakebites reported to the Kentucky regional poison center 1986: epidemiology and treatment suggestions. *J KY Med Assoc*. 1988;86:61–68.
150. Jurkovich GJ, Luterman A, McCullar K, et al. Complications of Crotalidae antivenin therapy. *J Trauma*. 1988;28:1032–1037.
151. Malasit P, Warrell DA, Chanthavanich P, et al. Prediction, prevention, and mechanism of early (anaphylactic) antivenom reactions in victims of snake bites. *Br Med J*. 1986;292:17–20.
152. Buntain WL. Successful venomous snakebite neutralization with massive antivenin infusion in a child. *J Trauma*. 1983;23:1012–1014.
153. Loprinzi CL, Hennessee J, Tamsky L, et al. Snake antivenin administration in a patient allergic to horse serum. *South Med J*. 1983;76:501–502.
154. Otten EJ, McKimm D. Venomous snakebite in a patient allergic to horse serum. *Ann Emerg Med*. 1983;12:624–627.
155. Pollack CV. Rattlesnake bite in a 28-year-old man allergic to antivenin. *Case Stud Emerg Med*. 1989;5:8–11.
156. Cunningham ER, Sabback MS, Smith R, et al. Snakebite: role of corticosteroids as immediate therapy in an animal model. *Am Surg*. 1979;45:757–759.
157. Glass TG. Early debridement in pit viper bite. *Surg Gynecol Obstet*. 1973;136:774–776.
158. Minton SA. Identification of poisonous snakes. *Clin Toxicol*. 1970;3:347–362.
159. Guderian RH, Mackenzie CD, Williams JF. High voltage shock treatment for snake bite. *Lancet*. 1986;2:229.
160. Kroegel C, Buschenfelde K-H. Biological basis for high-voltage shock treatment for snakebite. *Lancet*. 1986;2:1335.
161. Johnson EK, Kardong KV, Mackessy SP. Electric shocks are ineffective in treatment of lethal effects of rattlesnake envenomation in mice. *Toxicon*. 1987;25:1347–1349.
162. Howe NR, Meisenheimer JL. Electric shock does not save snakebitten rats. *Ann Emerg Med*. 1988;17:245–256.
163. Huang TT, Lynch JB, Larson DL, et al. The use of excisional therapy in the management of snakebite. *Ann Surg*. 1974;179:598–607.
164. Henderson BM, Dujon EB. Snake bites in children. *J Pediatr Surg*. 1973;8:729–733.
165. Roberts RS, Csencsitz TA, Heard CW. Upper extremity compartment syndromes following pit viper envenomation. *Clin Orthop*. 1985;193:184–188.
166. Curry SC, Kraner JC, Kunkel DB, et al. Noninvasive vascular studies in management of rattlesnake envenomations to extremities. *Ann Emerg Med*. 1985;14:1081–1084.
167. Watt CH. Treatment of poisonous snakebite with emphasis on digit dermotomy. *South Med J*. 1985;78:694–699.
168. Russell FE, Sullivan JB, Egen NB, et al. Preparation of a new antivenin by affinity chromatography. *Am J Trop Med Hyg*. 1985;34:141–150.
169. Sullivan JB. Past, present, and future immunotherapy of snake venom poisoning. *Ann Emerg Med*. 1987;16:938–944.
170. King LE. Spider bites. *Arch Dermatol*. 1987;123:41–43.
171. Toewe CH. Bug bites and stings. *Am Fam Physician*. 1980;21:90–95.

172. Parrish HM. Analysis of 460 fatalities from venomous animals in the United States. *Am J Med Sci*. 1963;245:129–141.
173. Russell FE. Venomous animal injuries. *Curr Probl Pediatr*. 1973;3:3–47.
174. Timms PK, Gibbons RB. Latrodectism—effects of the black widow spider bite. *West J Med*. 1986;144:315–317.
175. Moss HS, Binder LS. A retrospective review of black widow spider envenomation. *Ann Emerg Med*. 1987;16:188–191.
176. D'Ajello V, Magni F, Bettini S. The effect of the venom of the black widow spider *Latrodectus mactans tredecimguttatus* on the giant neurones of *Periplaneta americana*. *Toxicon*. 1971;9:103–110.
177. Frontali N, Ceccarolli B, Gorio A, et al. Purification of the black widow spider venom of a protein factor causing the depletion of synaptic vesicles at neuromuscular junctions. *J Cell Biol*. 1976;68:462–479.
178. Smith JE, Clark AW, Kuster TA. Suppression by elevated calcium of black widow spider venom activity at frog neuromuscular junctions. *J Neurocytol*. 1977;6:519–539.
179. Rothlin RP, Pardal JF, Pardal MM, et al. Supersensitivity to norepinephrine induced in vitro by crude *Latrodectus mactans* venom in the rabbit ear artery. *Toxicon*. 1977;15:71–74.
180. Pumplin DW, McClure WO. The release of acetylcholine elicited by extracts of black widow spider glands: studies using rat superior cervical ganglia and inhibitors of electrically stimulated release. *J Pharmacol Exp Ther*. 1977;201:312–319.
181. Pinto JE, Rothlin RP, Dagrosa EE, et al. Peripheral adrenergic effect of *Latrodectus mactans* venom. *Toxicon*. 1973;11:395–400.
182. Pardal JF, Granata AR, Barrio A. Influence of calcium on H-noradrenaline release by *Latrodectus antheratus* (black widow spider) venom gland extract in arterial tissues of the rat. *Toxicon*. 1979;17:455–465.
183. Sher E, Gotti C, Pandiella A, et al. Intracellular calcium homeostasis in a human neuroblastoma cell line: modulation by depolarization, cholinergic receptors, and α-latrotoxin. *J Neurochem*. 1988;50:1708–1713.
184. Kobernick M. Black widow spider bite. *Am Fam Physician*. 1984;29:241–245.
185. Sternlicht H, Fosson A. Partial paralysis following a black widow spider bite: case report and review of the literature. *J KY Med Assoc*. 1987;85:531–533.
186. Breland OP. Bionomics and significance of some venomous arthropods. *Cutis*. 1977;19:749–757.
187. Key GF. A comparison of calcium gluconate and methocarbamol (Robaxin) in the treatment of latrodectism (black widow spider envenomation). *Am J Trop Med Hyg*. 1980;30:273–277.
188. Kunkel DB. Arthropod envenomations. *Emerg Med Clin North Am*. 1984;2:579–586.
189. Black widow spider bite. In: Rumack B, ed. *Poisondex*. Englewood, CO: Micromedex; 1981.
190. Antivenin (*Latrodectus mactans*), MSD, package insert. West Point, PA: Merck Sharp & Dohme.
191. Stochosky B. Necrotic arachnidism. *West J Med*. 1979;131:143–148.
192. Hufford DC. The brown recluse spider and necrotic arachnidism: a current review. *J Arkansas Med Soc*. 1977;74:126–129.
193. Russell FE, Gertsch WJ. Letter to the editor. *Toxicon*. 1983;21:337–339.
194. Anderson PC. Letter to the editor. *Toxicon*. 1982;20:533.
195. Rees RS, Nanney LB, Yates RA, et al. Interaction of brown recluse spider venom on cell membranes: the inciting mechanism? *J Invest Dermatol*. 1984;83:270–275.
196. Rees RS, O'Leary JP, King LE. The pathogenesis of systemic loxoscelism following brown recluse spider bites. *J Surg Res*. 1983;35:1–10.
197. Wong RC, Hughes SE, Voorhees JJ. Spider bites. *Arch Dermatol*. 1987;123:98–105.
198. Young VL, Pin P. The brown recluse spider bite. *Ann Plast Surg*. 1988;20:447–452.
199. Madrigal GC, et al. Toxicity from a bite of the brown spider. *Clin Pediatr*. 1972;11:641–644.
200. Anderson PC. Necrotizing spider bites. *Am Fam Physician*. 1982;26:198–203.
201. Burnett JW, Calton GJ, Morgan RJ. Brown recluse spider. *Cutis*. 1985;36:197–198.
202. Foil LD, Norment BR. Review article: envenomation by *Loxosceles reclusa*. *J Med Entomol*. 1979;16:18–25.
203. DeLozier JB, Reaves L, King LE, et al. Brown recluse spider bites of the upper extremity. *South Med J*. 1988;81:181–184.
204. Rees RS, Altenbern DP, Lynch JB, et al. Brown recluse spider bites: a comparison of early surgical excision versus dapsone and delayed surgical excision. *Ann Surg*. 1985;202:659–663.
205. Bernstein B, Ehrlich F. Brown recluse spider bites. *J Emerg Med*. 1986;4:457–462.
206. King LE, Rees RS. Treatment of brown recluse spider bites. *J Am Acad Dermatol*. 1986;14:691–692.
207. Rees R, Campbell D, Rieger E, et al. The diagnosis and treatment of brown recluse spider bites. *Ann Emerg Med*. 1987;16:945–949.
208. Rees R, Shack RB, Withers E, et al. Management of the brown recluse spider bite. *Plast Reconstr Surg*. 1981;68:768–773.
209. King LE Jr, Rees RS. Dapsone treatment of a brown recluse bite. *JAMA*. 1983;250:648.
210. Alario A, Price G, Stahl R, et al. Cutaneous necrosis following a spider bite: a case report and review. *Pediatrics*. 1987;79:618–621.
211. Rimsza ME, Zimmerman DR, Bergeson PS. Scorpion envenomation. *Pediatrics*. 1980;66:298–302.
212. Chaubal CC, Misra NP. Scorpion sting. *Q Med Rev*. 1984;35:1–22.
213. Babin DR, Watt DD, Goos SM, et al. Amino acid sequence of neurotoxin I from *Centruroides sculpturatus* Ewing. *Arch Biochem Biophys*. 1975;166:125–134.
214. Cahalan MD. Modification of sodium channel gating in frog myelinated nerve fibers by *Centruroides sculpturatus* scorpion venom. *J Physiol*. 1975;244:511–534.
215. Stahnke HL. The Arizona scorpion problem. *J Ariz Med Assoc*. 1950;7:23–29.
216. Brand A, Keren A, Kerem E, et al. Myocardial damage after a scorpion sting: long-term echocardiographic follow-up. *Pediatr Cardiol*. 1988;9:59–61.
217. Ewan PW. Allergy to insect stings: a review. *J R Soc Med*. 1985;78:234–239.
218. Barsky HE. Stinging insect allergy. *Postgrad Med*. 1987;82:157–162.
219. Reisman RE. Stinging insect allergy. *J Allergy Immunol*. 1979;64:3–4.
220. Insect Allergy Committee of the American Academy of Allergy: insect sting allergy. *JAMA*. 1965;193:109–114.
221. Stablein JJ, Lockey RF. Adverse reactions to ant stings. *Clin Rev Allergy*. 1987;5:161–175.
222. Frazier CA. The hazards of hymenoptera. *Am Fam Physician*. 1977;15:91–96.

223. Banks BEC, Hanson JM, Sinclair NM. The isolation and identification of noradrenaline and dopamine from the venom of the honeybee, *Apis mellifica*. *Toxicon*. 1976;14:117–125.
224. Habermann E. Bee and wasp venoms. *Science*. 1972;177:314–322.
225. Hoffman DR. Allergens in hymenoptera venom. V. Identification of some of the enzymes and demonstration of multiple allergens in yellow jacket venom. *Ann Allergy*. 1978;40:171-175.
226. Sobotka A, et al. Honeybee venom: phospholipase A as the major allergen. *J Allergy Clin Immunol*. 1974;53:103–104. Abstract.
227. Kemeny DM, Harries MG, Youlten LJF, et al. Antibodies to purified bee venom proteins and peptides. *J Allergy Clin Immunol*. 1983;71:505–514.
228. Engel T, Heinig JH, Weeke ER, et al. Basophil histamine release in insect venom allergy. *Allergy*. 1988;43:132–138.
229. Itkin I. Bee sting. *Am Fam Physician*. 1976;13:124–125.
230. Jones E. Acute myocardial infarction after a wasp sting. *Br Heart J*. 1988;59:506–508.
231. Meszaros I. Transient cerebral ischemic attack caused by hymenoptera stings: the brain as an anaphylactic shock organ. *Eur Neurol*. 1986;25:248–252.
232. Lichtenstein LM, Golden DB. Postscript to bee stings: delayed "serum sickness." *Hosp Pract*. 1983;18:36–46.
233. McLeod LJ, von Witt RJ, Roberts MS. Consequences of wasp stings. *Med J Aust*. 144: 220–221.
234. Barach EM, Nowak RM, Lee TG, et al. Epinephrine for treatment of anaphylactic shock. *JAMA*. 1984;251:2118–2122.
235. Kelly JF, Patterson R. Anaphylaxis. *JAMA*. 1974;227:1431–1436.
236. Lessof MH, Sobotka AK, Lichtenstein LM. Effects of passive antibody in bee venom anaphylaxis. *Johns Hopkins Med J*. 1978;142:1–7.
237. Muller U, Johansson SGO, Streit C. Hymenoptera sting hypersensitivity: IgE, IgG and haemagglutinating antibodies to bee venom constituents in relation to exposure and clinical reaction to bee stings. *Clin Allergy*. 1978;8:267–272.
238. Hoffman DR, Wood CL, Hudson P. Demonstration of IgE and IgG antibodies against venoms in the blood of victims of fatal sting anaphylaxis. *J Allergy Clin Immunol*. 1983;71:193–196.
239. Graft DF. Venom immunotherapy for stinging insect allergy. *Clin Rev Allergy*. 1987;5:149–159.
240. Lichtenstein LM, Valentine MD, Sobotka AK. Insect allergy: the state of the art. *J Allergy Clin Immunol*. 1979;64:5–12.
241. Feingold BF. Allergic reactions to hymenoptera stings. *J Asthma Res*. 1971;9:55–70.
242. Barnard JH. Studies of 400 hymenoptera sting deaths in the United States. *J Allergy Clin Immunol*. 1973;52:259–264.
243. Podgorny G. Snakebite in the United States. *Ann Emerg Med*. 1983;12:651–653.

APPENDIX 39-A: IDENTIFICATION OF SNAKES

In the initial assessment of a snake bite victim, it is important to identify the snake to determine whether it is indeed venomous and, if venomous, the probable severity of envenomation. Some species are more dangerous than others because of their size or the nature of their venom. For example, the eastern diamondback is the largest of the domestic rattlesnakes, and its bite results in some of the most severe envenomations. Patients tend to exaggerate the size of the snakes that bite them; when both fang marks are present, the distance between the marks is an objective indicator of the size of the snake. Up to 8 mm indicates a small snake; 8 to 12 mm, a medium snake; and more than 12 mm, a large snake.[243]

Snake identification can be carried out at two levels. The treating physician can make the distinction between venomous and nonvenomous snakes, and the herpetologist can determine the precise genus and species. The latter should always be sought ultimately, but an expert may not be available for some time; hence the physician's initial decision has greater clinical importance.

Venomous snakes in the United States (pit vipers and coral snakes) can be easily distinguished from nonvenomous snakes by a few simple characteristics. Pit vipers (eg, *Crotalus, Agkistrodon,* and *Sistrurus* species) have the following characteristics:

- the pit, a heat-sensing device that appears as a depression between the eye and nostril
- vertically elliptic pupils
- the rattle (a series of keratin rings not seen in *Agkistrodon* species)
- large anterior retractable maxillary fangs
- a single row of subcaudal plates

The characteristics are contrasted to those of nonvenomous snakes in Fig. 39A-1.

Coral snakes must also be distinguished from nonvenomous snakes that closely resemble them. The key to coral snake identification is knowing the color sequence of

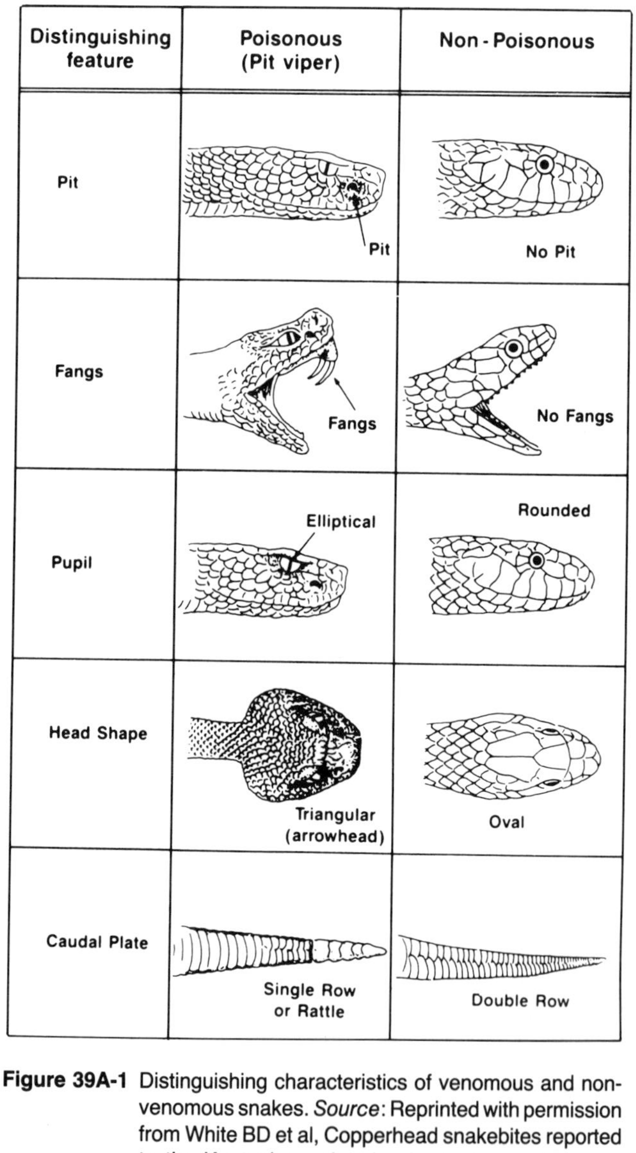

Figure 39A-1 Distinguishing characteristics of venomous and nonvenomous snakes. *Source*: Reprinted with permission from White BD et al, Copperhead snakebites reported to the Kentucky regional poison center 1986: epidemiology and treatment suggestions, in *Journal of the Kentucky Medical Association* (1988;86:65), copyright © 1988, Kentucky Medical Association.

their circumferential bands. The mnemonic "red on yellow, kills a fellow; red on black, venom lack" is useful. That is, if red bands are bordered on either side by yellow bands, the snake is a coral snake; if red is bordered by black, it is a nonvenomous king snake. Coral snakes, in contrast to other venomous snakes, have round pupils and a double row of subcaudal plates.

Nonindigenous snakes are mentioned only as a reminder to obtain a thorough history from the snake bite victim. Snakes normally found only in Africa and Asia are sometimes imported to the United States and kept as exotic pets. Because this is illegal, the patient's history may be deliberately inadequate, and care may be delayed. Furthermore, no specific antivenin for these snakes is readily available. ED personnel should be aware of local resources for herpetologic information (zoos, colleges, poison control centers, etc). In addition, the Arizona Poison and Drug Information Center [in Tucson, (602) 626-6016] keeps an updated log of exotic antivenin stores in zoos and hospitals throughout the country. The generally recommended approach to exotic snake bites is local wound care, supportive care, complete and accurate identification of the snake, and consultation with experts regarding the appropriateness and availability of specific antivenins.[129]

40. Hyperthermia

ERIC A. WEISS, MD

Heat illnesses encompass a spectrum of syndromes ranging from minor reactions such as muscle cramps to heat stroke, a life-threatening emergency. The ramifications of heat illnesses were recorded as long as 2000 years ago, when a Roman army was decimated by heat in 24 BC.[13] In 1743, 11,000 people died during a heat wave in Peking.[1,13] During the 6-day war between Egypt and Israel in 1967, there were more than 20,000 Egyptian casualties from heat stroke. Although heat illness is clearly preventable, thousands of people continue to suffer each year. In the United States more than 4000 people die of heat stroke annually,[2] and it is the second leading cause of death in young athletes.[3] A better understanding of the predisposing factors and mechanisms that produce heat illness, along with the different treatment modalities available, will improve the clinician's recognition and management of this life-threatening environmental emergency.

MECHANISMS FOR ACCUMULATING HEAT

There are both internal and external mechanisms for accumulating heat. Basal metabolic rate that alone can generate a heat load of 65 to 85 kcal/hour.[13] The removal of heat from the body's internal environment is thus obligatory for life. In the absence of heat dissipation, basal metabolism would raise the body temperature by 1.1°C per hour.[1] Moderate work can increase heat production by 500%.[4]

Elevated body temperature imposes its own additional heat load because cellular metabolism increases by 13% for every 1°C rise in body temperature.[29] At 40.5°C, cellular metabolism is 50% above normal.[13] Prolonged exercise can generate more heat than the body can dissipate, resulting in a rise in core temperature. Rectal temperatures of 40° to 42°C have been recorded in trained marathon runners.[5] Status epilepticus or drug overdose (cocaine, metamphetamine) may cause hyperthermia due to sustained or increased muscle activity.

Dehydration plays a significant role in heat illness and may contribute to elevated body temperatures through multiple mechanisms. Dehydration increases the activity of the cellular sodium pump, which accounts for 20% to 45% of the basal metabolic rate.[6] In a study of runners, 5% dehydration was associated with elevated rectal temperatures of 2.5°C compared to controls.[30] Hypovolemia also limits sweating and predisposes to cardiovascular decompensation.

Environmental heat adds to the body's intrinsic heat load and interferes with heat dissipation. When the air temperature is greater than the body temperature, radiant heat gain is possible. An individual standing in the sun may gain 150 kcal/hour.[1]

PREDICTING HEAT STRESS

The best indicator of environmental heat stress is the wet bulb globe temperature (WBGT). The standard dry bulb thermometer temperature by itself is a poor predictor of heat stress because humidity is such an important factor in heat dissipation by sweating. A wet bulb thermometer measures

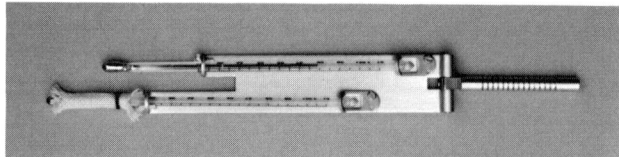

Figure 40-1 Sling psychrometer.

the effect of humidity on temperature. The easiest method of determining the WBGT is with a sling psychrometer (Fig. 40-1). The sling psychrometer has two mercury thermometers attached to an aluminum frame with a hinged handle. The wet bulb thermometer has a wick surrounding the bulb. After the wick is moistened, the psychrometer is slung over the head for approximately 2 minutes. Evaporation occurs in the wick at a rate inversely proportional to the degree of humidity, depressing the wet bulb temperature below that of the dry bulb. This WBGT alone may be used as an indicator of heat stress and as a guide for recommended activity levels (Table 40-1).

The incidence of heat illness increases dramatically when the WBGT approaches 30°C. In a series of 128 gold miners who developed heat stroke, 90% of the cases occurred at WBGTs above 30°C.[12] It is not possible to perform even light work at WBGTs above 32°C, moderately heavy work above 30°C, or strenuous work above 28°C.[12]

MECHANISMS FOR DISSIPATING HEAT

When air temperature is lower than body temperature, radiant heat loss, which is the transferring of heat from the body to a cooler environment, accounts for 65% of cooling.[14] Evaporation, which normally accounts for 30% of cooling, prevails as the only mechanism that the body has to dissipate heat when the ambient temperature exceeds 35°C.[6] When the humidity level exceeds 75%, evaporative heat loss markedly declines. If this condition should occur during a period of high ambient temperature, all mechanisms for heat dissipation are lost, and the potential for heat illness will soar. Sweat that merely drips from the skin and is not evaporated only exacerbates dehydration without providing any cooling benefit. Heat loss through exhaled water vapor, urine, and feces dissipates about 5% of body heat.[13]

PHYSIOLOGIC RESPONSES TO HEAT

In response to heat stress, cutaneous blood vessels dilate to increase the surface cooling area while the splanchnic and renal vascular beds undergo compensatory vasoconstriction.[6] Blood flow increases up to 20-fold as peripheral vascular resistance drops, creating a shunt as high as 4 L/min.[6,7] Thus a tremendous burden is placed on the heart to maintain blood pressure as vascular resistance falls. Cardiac output may quadruple as a result of increases in both stroke volume and heart rate.[27]

Approximately 1 kcal of heat is lost for each 1.7 mL of sweat evaporated.[6] Each liter of completely evaporated sweat cools the body by 580 kcal.[1] Of the two types of sweat glands found in humans, eccrine glands are predominantly responsible for dissipating heat.[7] They exist on all body parts and are most concentrated on the volar surfaces of the hands and feet. Eccrine glands have cholinergic receptors and are blocked by anticholinergic drugs.[7] Sweat volume increases during a heat load and can range from 1 to 2 L/hour to 4 L/hour for short periods in acclimatized individuals.[15]

Physiologic acclimatization to a hot environment is an important adaptive response. It usually requires 8 to 11 days to reach maximum benefit and mandates some amount of daily exercise.[16] Simulating exposure to heat stress by exercising in saunas has been recommended for troops preparing for travel to a hot environment. With acclimatization, sweating is initiated at lower core temperatures, and the sweat rate may more than double. Sodium is conserved in both urine and sweat with concomitant losses of potassium.[17] As acclimatization proceeds, the sodium concentration in sweat decreases from 65 mEq/L to as low as 5 mEq/L.[17] This mechanism, although poorly understood, is thought to be mediated through activation of the renin-angiotensin system with increased production of aldosterone.[9]

Two cardiovascular adaptations that augment delivery of heat from the core to the surface also occur: an increased stroke volume, and a 10% to 25% expansion of plasma volume.[10] An increase in the density of mitochondria per unit muscle, allowing for better oxygen utilization, is a further adaptation.[6]

Table 40-1 Wet-Bulb Globe Temperature (WBGT) and Recommended Activity Levels

WBGT		
°C	°F	Activity
15.6	60	No precautions
19–21	66–70	No precautions provided water, salt and food are easily available
22–24	71–75	Postpone sports practice, avoid hiking
24	76	Lighter practice and work with rest breaks
27	80	No hiking or sports
28	82	Heavy exertion with caution
30	85	Cancel all exertion for unacclimatized persons; avoid sun exposure
31.5	88	Limited brief activity for acclimatized fit personnel only

Source: From Callaham M. *Emergency Management of Heat Ailments.* ACEP-Emergency Physicians Monograph Series, October 1978.

PREDISPOSING FACTORS

The very old and the very young are most likely to suffer heat illness. Because of underlying intrinsic cardiac disease, the elderly are less able to increase and maintain cardiac output in response to a heat load. They also have blunted responses to temperature changes and tend to become dehydrated. Neonates are affected in conditions of excessive heat because they lack thermoregulatory and sweating capabilities. Children produce more metabolic heat per kilogram body weight and sweat proportionately less than adults.[13]

Physical and hormonal problems can increase vulnerability to heat illness. Obese individuals, for example, have more insulation and a smaller ratio of surface area to volume with which to dissipate heat. Hyperthyroidism can markedly increase metabolic rate with a resultant rise in endogenous heat production. Dermatologic disorders, such as cystic fibrosis, scleroderma, and burns affecting large body surface areas, may limit heat dissipation by sweating.

Various medications and drugs of abuse have been implicated in the development of heat illness (Table 40-2). Anticholinergic drugs such as antihistamines, phenothiazines, tricyclic antidepressants, and antispasmodics inhibit sweating and can disrupt normal thermoregulation. β Blockers will inhibit compensatory increases in cardiac output. Amphetamines, PCP, cocaine, and other stimulants can increase muscle activity and produce seizures, resulting in an increased endogenous heat load. Amphetamines and LSD act directly on the hypothalamus to produce elevated temperatures.[50]

The most important predisposing factor to environmental heat illness is dehydration. Therefore, prevention of heat stroke is commensurate with staying well hydrated. Adequate urine output and a "gin clear" color of the urine are gross indicators of adequate hydration.

MINOR HEAT ILLNESS SYNDROMES

Heat Syncope

The diagnosis of heat syncope is made in the context of the appropriate environmental conditions after other causes are ruled out. Heat syncope is a form of postural hypotension resulting from the combined effect of peripheral vasodilation and pooling of blood in the lower extremities as a result of gravity. As in most heat disorders, dehydration is often a contributing factor. Loss of consciousness ensues from inadequate cerebral perfusion. In one study, syncopal episodes occurred in 25% of unacclimatized subjects.[11] These episodes did not appear to be related to thermoregulatory failure because the subjects maintained normal rectal temperatures.

Treatment consists of Trendelenburg positioning, cooling, and fluids when the patient is awake and alert. Hospitalization is usually unnecessary. A careful secondary assessment should be performed after a primary survey to assess for any trauma that may have occurred during the fall.

Table 40-2 Risk Factors Predisposing to Heat Illness

Environment
  High ambient temperature (prevents heat dissipation by radiation)
  High relative humidity (prevents heat dissipation by evaporation)
Age
  Infants (produce more heat and sweat less)
  Elderly (intrinsic heart disease, dehydration, blunted thermoregulation)
Lifestyle
  Military recruits
  Construction and mine workers
  Athletes
Physical factors
  Obesity
  Dehydration
  Lack of sleep
Other illness
  Gastroenteritis (fluid losses)
Drug related
  Anticholinergic effects (atropine, lithium, antihistamines, antispasmodics, tricyclic antidepressants, phenothiazines)
  Inhibited cardiac output (β blockers)
  Disrupted oxidative phosphorylation (salicylates, lithium)
  Disrupted thermoregulation (LSD, phenothiazines)
  Increased muscular activity and seizures (amphetamines, cocaine, PCP)
  Malignant hyperthermia (anesthetic agents, succinylcholine)
  Neuroleptic malignant syndrome (neuroleptics)
  Dehydration (diuretics)

Heat Edema

Peripheral edema is common in unacclimatized travelers during the first few days of exposure to a hot environment. It does not signify an underlying disorder and is self limiting.[13] Diuretics should be avoided because the dehydration that can ensue may predispose the individual to more serious heat illness syndromes.

Prickly Heat

Occasionally an erythematous, papular, pruritic rash will develop on areas of the skin that are kept wet from sweating. This usually occurs in unacclimatized persons and responds to cooling and drying. Antihistamines may help relieve itching.

Heat Cramps

Heat cramps are painful spasmodic muscle cramps that usually occur in heavily exercised muscles. Their onset may occur during exercise or begin after the work has ended.

Although their exact pathogenesis is still debated, a relative deficiency of salt has been postulated.[31] Prevention and treatment consist of replacing both fluids and salt. Mild cases may be treated with oral rehydration solutions that combine 3.5 g of sodium chloride and 1.5 g of potassium chloride in 1 L of drinking water. Severe cases are best managed with intravenous normal saline solutions. Hypertonic saline is not needed. Salt tablets taken by themselves are not recommended; they are gastric irritants and do not treat the hypovolemia that is almost always coexistent.

HEAT EXHAUSTION

Heat exhaustion and heat stroke are often represented as two distinct pathophysiologic entities. This is misleading because with few exceptions they define a continuum of one disease process.[28] A patient with heat exhaustion still maintains the ability to dissipate heat, having not yet decompensated. Such patients are dehydrated and may have elevated temperatures, but in contrast to those with heat stroke central nervous system function is unimpaired.

Common symptoms associated with heat exhaustion are general malaise, headache, nausea, dizziness, loss of appetite, and weakness. Clinical manifestations include vomiting, sinus tachycardia, orthostatic hypotension, diaphoresis, tachypnea, and hyperthermia. Temperature is variable and ranges from normal to 41°C.[34] Because of the nonspecific nature of these symptoms, heat exhaustion remains a diagnosis of exclusion.

Transient renal insufficiency is often characterized by mild elevations of blood urea nitrogen and creatinine with protein and cast formation on urinalysis. This is probably due to decreased renal blood flow, which is common during exercise in the heat.[29] Mild elevations of liver enzymes and creatine phosphokinase often occur.[6]

Treatment is initially aimed at stopping all exertion and moving the patient to a cool, shaded area. Glucose- and salt-containing solutions are administered to reverse dehydration and replace electrolytes. Active cooling techniques similar to those used with heat stroke are recommended for patients with temperatures above 40°C. Generally patients recover rapidly, and hospitalization is not necessary.

HEAT STROKE

Pathophysiology

Environmental heat stroke can be regarded as the end stage of heat exhaustion as compensatory mechanisms for dissipating heat fail. Elucidation of the exact pathophysiology of heat stroke has been limited by the lack of experimental data in humans. The high mortality necessitates immediate cooling and precludes experimental induction of heat stroke in human subjects. Thermoregulatory failure and sweat gland dysfunction were previously thought to be the principal mediating factors. Experimental data in animals and better observations in humans have led to an alternative theory known as the energy depletion model.[28] The proposed model emphasizes overloading of the body's thermoregulatory mechanisms rather than their primary failure. The combination of hypovolemia, hypoglycemia, and increased permeability of the cell membrane to sodium ions resulting in cellular swelling observed in heat stroke supports this theory.[7,28]

Further support for the energy depletion model comes from a recent experiment in rats that were exercised to exhaustion in a hot environment.[18] Initially they were able to maintain normothermia and compensated well. After a prolonged period a drastic peripheral temperature drop occurred that coincided with an explosive rise in core temperature, indicating that compensatory mechanisms had failed and signaling imminent collapse from heat stroke. The preservation of central volume appears to have been a more paramount homeostatic drive overriding heat dissipation effectors, which would have further decreased blood volume.[7,18] This further emphasizes the profound importance of dehydration in the pathogenesis of heat stroke.

Many investigators continue to differentiate two types of heat stroke: classic heat stroke, which develops over a period of days and is seen most commonly in the elderly, and exertional heat stroke, which usually occurs in young exercising individuals over a period of hours. The distinction, however, is more academic than clinically significant, as recognition and treatment remain the same.

Diagnosis

Environmental heat stroke is a diagnosis rendered after excluding other etiologies of hyperthermia. The workup to determine the etiology is begun after cooling is initiated since a delay may result in greater tissue injury (Table 40-3). The diagnosis of heat stroke does not depend on the absence of sweating or hot, dry skin, as is frequently stated. It must be considered in anyone who presents with hyperthermia and an altered mental status or other central nervous system dysfunction regardless of sweating. The cerebellum is highly sensitive to excessive heat, and ataxia is an early finding.[33] Other neurologic signs include irritability, confusion, and disorientation. Later, bizarre behavior and loss of consciousness occur. Generalized seizures, decorticate and decerebrate posturing, and coma will occur if heat stroke is untreated.[42,43]

The presence of sweating does not preclude the diagnosis. In one prospective study, half the patients presenting with full-blown heat stroke were still sweating.[34] Anhydrosis can be a late manifestation due to profound dehydration and necrotic plugging of sweat gland ductules, but its absence

Table 40-3 Differential Diagnosis of Hyperthermia

Meningitis
Encephalitis
Brain abscess
Cerebrovascular accident
Diabetic ketoacidosis
Salicylate toxicity
PCP, cocaine, or amphetamine toxicity
Anticholinergic toxicity
Status epilepticus
Falciparum malaria
Malignant hyperthermia
Neuroleptic malignant syndrome
Thyroid storm
Typhoid fever
Sepsis
Tetanus
Alcohol withdrawal syndrome

should not deter one from diagnosing heat stroke and initiating prompt therapy.

It is not possible to designate arbitrarily a temperature at which heat stroke begins. In one study military recruits were diagnosed with heat exhaustion because they had no central nervous system or other major organ dysfunction despite core temperatures reaching 41.6°C. On the other hand, some recruits with heat stroke who were unconscious and hypotensive had temperatures of 41.0°C.[34]

The exact temperature at which cellular damage begins to occur is still unknown, but clearly cell damage is a function of both the maximum temperature reached and the exposure time at that temperature. Patients with higher temperatures for shorter periods may do better than patients who maintain lower temperatures for longer periods.[22] One case report documented a core temperature of 46.5°C in a patient who made a full neurologic recovery after aggressive cooling.[22]

Cardiovascular manifestations of heat stroke include both hypotension and sinus tachycardia. Tachypnea as a mechanism to dissipate heat and as a result of metabolic acidosis is invariably present early on.[19,27]

Laboratory Findings

Serum glutamic oxaloacetic (SGOT) and glutamic pyruvic transaminases (SGPT) are always elevated in heat stroke. The enzyme levels continue to rise during the subsequent week following heat stroke. SGOT levels in the first 24 hours can be gauged as a prognostic indicator. Less than 1000 IU/L indicates a good prognosis. Values in the high thousands or tens of thousands indicate substantial injury to brain, liver, and kidney and a poorer prognosis.[27]

Electrolyte disorders are usually present but are not diagnostic of heat stroke. Hypokalemia, hyponatremia, hypoglycemia, and hypocalcemia are most common. With rhabdomyolysis, hyperkalemia and CPK elevation occur.

The white blood count is often markedly elevated in heat stroke and does not help to differentiate an infectious etiology.

Coagulation studies including prothrombin time, partial thromboplastin time, platelet count, bleeding time, fibrinogen level, and fibrin split products should be followed closely for the onset of disseminated intravascular coagulation.

Arterial blood gas measurements usually reveal a mixed metabolic acidosis and respiratory alkalosis.[43,49]

Treatment

Prehospital Cooling

The mortality from heat stroke when not promptly and effectively treated approaches 80%.[20] Cooling needs to be initiated in the field and must continue throughout transportation. The faster that cooling is accomplished, the lower is the mortality.[20] Medics should be equipped with thermometers and chemical cold packs. Cold packs placed on the neck, axillae, and groin adjacent to large superficial vessels can produce cooling rates of 0.1°C/min.[21] This technique is almost as effective as submersing the entire body in an ice bath as it is less likely to produce vasoconstriction and shivering, and has the advantage of immediate application in the field.

Evaporative cooling can be initiated by splashing or spraying water over the patient while fanning. If the ambulance is not air conditioned, the windows should be kept open to maximize air flow.

Emergency Department Cooling

In the emergency department, cooling should continue until the core temperature reaches 38.5°C. Various cooling methods and their experimental rates are listed in Table 40-4.

Ice water baths, once the most popular method of cooling, are now rarely used. When evaluated experimentally, immersion in ice water baths resulted in a cooling rate ranging from 0.1°C/min to 0.25°C/min, which is not much better than that achieved with selective cold pack applications.[24,35,36] Vasoconstriction and shivering tend to offset cooling. There are many practical problems with ice water immersion. Few emergency departments have tubs large enough for this purpose. Invasive lines, electrocardiographic monitoring, mechanical ventilation, and complications such as seizures and cardiac dysrhythmias are difficult to manage in a tub. Variations on this method, such as placing sheets presoaked in ice water over patients, have frequently been used with variable success. Reflex vasoconstriction and shivering will slow core cooling with this technique as well. Experiments in dogs suggest that cooling may be just as rapid when patients are immersed in 16°C water as in ice water.[23]

Table 40-4 Experimental Data on Cooling

Method	Cooling Rate (°C/min)	Advantages	Disadvantages
Peritoneal lavage (Dialysate at 6°–10°C)*	0.56	Fast	Time consuming to set up, invasive
Evaporative (15°C water spray, 0.4 M/sec fan, 45°C air)	0.046–0.310	Less shivering, less vasoconstriction, easy to monitor	Requires nonhumid environment
Ice water bath	0.10–0.25	Effective in humid environment	Tub may not be available, difficult management, shivering, vasoconstriction
Iced gastric lavage (iced water at 200 mL/min)*	0.2	Easy and rapid	Aspiration
Ice packs to neck, axillae, groin	0.1	Easy and rapid	
Cold inhaled air by intermittent positive pressure breathing	0.02		

*Animal studies only.

A wide range of cooling rates has been reported with evaporative methods even when identical protocols were used. The most rapid cooling rate achieved in human experimentation was 0.31°C/min, almost three times greater than that achieved with ice baths.[24] The volunteers in this study, however, only had temperatures of 39.5°C before the initiation of cooling. Cooling rates ranging from 0.044 to 0.28°C/min have been reported in other studies of evaporative methods.[24,25,37,38] The degree of vasodilatation and therefore the ability of heat to be transferred to the skin surface, where it can be dissipated by evaporation, may be a significant variable. Wide ranges in cooling times would also be expected to occur because of different thicknesses of subcutaneous fat in patients and different degrees of relative humidity in the treatment environments.

Evaporative cooling works best in a dry, cool environment and depends on an adequate cardiac output to maintain peripheral circulation. When high humidity prevails in the treatment area or when the patient is in profound shock, alternative methods of cooling such as ice-water baths should be used.

Evaporation is further maximized by wetting the skin with warm water instead of cold. This maintains a higher skin-to-air vapor pressure gradient and minimizes vasoconstriction and shivering. Ideally skin temperature should be above 30°C.[24]

Body cooling units have been designed to treat heat stroke patients by evaporative methods. Patients are typically suspended naked on a net over a drainage table while finely atomized water at 15°C is sprayed over the entire body from above and below. Fans are used to circulate air warmed to 45° to 48°C around the body. Air flow is adjusted to maintain a skin temperature of 30°C. With this technique, cooling times of less than 60 minutes can be expected for most heat stroke patients.[24,37] Continuous cardiac monitoring, ventilatory support, and effective management of complications are not impeded by the body cooling unit.

During an annual Mecca pilgrimage, a simplified body cooling unit with a patient trolley and two 35-cm diameter fans was used to treat 25 consecutive heat stroke patients. The mean initial rectal temperature of 42.5°C (range, 40.0° to 43.2°C) was reduced to 39°C in an average time of 40 minutes (range, 20 to 125 minutes), corresponding to an average cooling rate of 0.87°C/min.[37]

More than one modality can be used simultaneously to augment cooling. One group sprayed heat stroke patients with 40°C water from a shower while standing fans were used to circulate air. Ice bags were placed next to the trunk in the axillae and on the chest. This combination lowered temperatures an average of 0.1°C/min in 14 patients, with a maximum rate of 0.15°C/min. The median cooling time for the group was 60 minutes, with a range of 34 to 89 minutes.[38]

Cold water gastric and rectal lavage may be used to augment other cooling modalities but has limited potential as the primary cooling source. In a canine model, iced gastric lavage was found to be half as fast as evaporative cooling.[39] The small surface area for cooling and the relative splanchnic hypoperfusion during heat stroke are the main limiting factors.[26,39]

Although human trials have not been done, in experimental dogs peritoneal lavage has produced the fastest cooling and the greatest survival rates. When a 6°C lavage fluid was used, an average cooling rate of 0.56°C/min was obtained, which was five times faster than the rate with an ice bath.[40] The usefulness of peritoneal lavage is limited by its being both invasive and time consuming to initiate. Its application might be reserved for cases of extreme heat stroke when there is a poor response to noninvasive methods. Lavage has been used successfully in obese individuals, in whom the large amount of subcutaneous fat made surface cooling less effective.

Other Treatment Measures

Concomitant with cooling, the ABCs of resuscitation should be addressed. The airway may need to be protected by endotracheal intubation in obtunded patients, since vomiting and seizures are common. Supplemental oxygen is given since heat stroke produces a hypermetabolic state.

Hypotension in heat stroke victims is common and a consequence of both dehydration and high output failure.[43,45] Fluid deficits range from minimal (1 to 2 L) to severe hydration.[47] Intravenous fluids should be administered as boluses using blood pressure, urine output, and central venous pressure monitoring as a guide. Fluid needs will diminish as cooling proceeds and peripheral vasoconstriction ensues. Overzealous fluid administration combined with heat stroke-induced renal failure can produce acute pulmonary edema.[43]

Normal saline or dextrose (50%) in normal saline is preferred over Ringer's lactate to replace intravascular volume since liver damage may limit lactate metabolism. Pressor agents that produce vasoconstriction will diminish heat loss and should be avoided, if possible, during cooling.[30,43]

Shivering during cooling creates further heat and should be suppressed. Benzodiazepines decrease shivering and help to prevent seizures. Chlorpromazine (25–50 mg IV) will also suppress shivering and has the advantage of decreasing metabolic oxygen consumption and dilating peripheral vessels during cooling.[2]

Although controlled studies are lacking, chlorpromazine has the theoretical disadvantage of lowering the seizure threshold and interfering with thermoregulation.[43,44]

Patients with evidence of rhabdomyolysis (elevated CPK, myoglobinuria) need adequate fluid replacement and urine output (between 50 and 75 cc/hr) to prevent myoglobinuric renal failure.[13] Urinary alkalinization with sodium bicarbonate and administration of intravenous mannitol may help to clear myoglobin and prevent it from precipitating in the renal tubules.[50]

Dantrolene sodium, a skeletal muscle relaxant, effectively treats malignant hyperthermia, which is a familial disorder characterized by muscle rigidity and hyperthermia in response to various anesthetic agents. There is no evidence, however, that dantrolene is beneficial in environmental heat stroke. In a recent canine heat stroke model, dantrolene sodium administration did not alter cooling rates or improve survival when compared with controls.[51]

Antipyretics such as aspirin and acetaminophen are also not beneficial in heat stroke. They lower temperature through the hypothalamic thermoregulatory system, which is elevated by endogenous pyrogens in fever. In heat stroke, cooling mechanisms are overloaded and the hypothalamic set point is unchanged.

Complications of Heat Stroke

Nearly every organ in the body can be damaged by heat stroke. Patients should be admitted to a monitored bed for close observation and treatment.

Central nervous system. Examination of brain tissue after cases of fatal heat stroke has revealed edema, hemorrhages, and neuronal necrosis.[42,44] Seizures occur in almost 50% of heat stroke victims and are best managed with benzodiazepines or barbiturates. Phenytoin is reportedly less effective for heat stroke-related seizures.[13,43]

Liver. Hepatic damage, signaled by elevation of SGOT, SGPT, LDH, and bilirubin, is a hallmark of heat stroke.[19] Enzyme levels may not peak until 2 to 3 days after the heat injury. Later, the patient may develop jaundice and overt hepatic failure.[45]

Kidney. Renal failure occurs in up to 35% of cases and is most likely the combined result of hypoperfusion, direct thermal injury, and myoglobinuria from rhabdomyolysis.[8]

Lung. Noncardiogenic pulmonary edema has been noted in 23% of heat stroke victims during the annual pilgrimages to Mecca[47] and in 58% of autopsy cases of fatal heat stroke.[42] Pulmonary edema may result from thermal injury to the pulmonary vasculature, myocardial dysfunction, or fluid overload, or as a result of disseminated intravascular coagulation.[43]

Coagulopathy. Disseminated intravascular coagulation (DIC) is a common complication of severe heat stroke and portends a poorer prognosis. A number of predisposing factors have been postulated: Thermal inactivation of platelets and clotting factors, heat injury to vascular endothelium producing activation of the clotting cascade, and decrease in clotting factor synthesis due to liver failure.[43,44] Others have postulated that DIC is triggered by activation of heat damaged platelets.[46]

REFERENCES

1. Knochel JP. Environmental heat illness: an eclectic review. *Arch Intern Med*. 1974;137:841.
2. Clowes GHA, O'Donnel TF. Current concepts: heat stroke. *N Engl J Med*. 1974;291(11):564.
3. Knochel JP. Dog days and siriasis. *JAMA*. 1975;233(6):513.
4. Robert Shaw D. Factors in heat stroke. In: Khogali M, Kates JR, eds. *Heat Stroke and Temperature Regulation*. Sydney: Academic Press; 1983.
5. Wyndham CH. Heat stroke and hyperthermia in marathon runners. *Ann NY Acad Sci*. 1977;301:12.
6. Callaham M. Heat illness. In: Rosen P, Baker F, Bakin R, et al. eds. *Emergency Medicine Concepts and Clinical Practice*. St. Louis: CV Mosby; 1988:693–717.
7. Yarbrough BE, Hubbard RW. Heat-related illnesses. In: Auerbach PS, Geehr EC, eds. *Management of Wilderness and Environmental Emergencies*. St. Louis: CV Mosby; 1989:119–143.

8. Tintinnali JE. Heat stroke. *JACEP*. 1976;5:528.
9. Finberg JPM, Berlyne GM. Renin and aldosterone secretion following acute environmental heat exposure. *Isr J Med Sci*. 1976;12(8):844.
10. Appenzelter O. *Physical Training, Heat Acclimatization, and Diet in Heat Stroke*. Sydney: Academic Press; 1983.
11. Lind AR, Leithead CS, McNicol GW. Cardiovascular changes during syncope induced by tilting men in the heat. *J Appl Physiol*. 1968;25:268–276.
12. Kew MC. Temperature regulation in heat stroke in man. *Isr J Med Sci*. 1976;12:759.
13. Stewart CE. Preventing progression of heat injury. *Emerg Med Rep*. 1987;8:16.
14. Eichler A, McFee A, Root H. Heat stroke. *Am J Surg*. 1969;118:855–863.
15. Robinson S. Physiological adjustments to heat. In: Newburgh LH, ed. *Physiology of Heat Regulation and the Science of Clothing*. New York; 1968.
16. William CO, et al. Circulatory and metabolic reactions to work in the heat. *J Appl Physiol*. 1962;17:625.
17. Dill DB, Hall FE, Edwards HT. Changes in composition of sweat during acclimatization to heat. *Am J Physiol*. 1938;123:412.
18. Hubbard RW, Bower WD, Mager M. A study of physiological, pathological and biochemical changes in rats with heat- and/or work-induced disorders. *Isr J Med Sci*. 1976;12(8):884.
19. Shibolet S, Lancaster M, Danon Y. Heat stroke: a review. *Aviat Space Med*. 1976;47:280–301.
20. Bynum GP, et al. Peritoneal lavage cooling in an anesthetized dog heat stroke model. *Aviat Space Environ Med*. 1978;49:799.
21. Hansen PG. Treatment for heat stroke victims. *West J Med*. 1981;134:168.
22. Slovis CM, Anderson GF, Casaloro A. Survival in a heat stroke victim with a core temperature in excess of 46.5C. *Ann Emerg Med*. 1982;11(5):269.
23. Magazanik A, et al. Tap water, an efficient method for cooling heat stroke victims—a model in dogs. *Aviat Space Environ Med*. 1980;5:864.
24. Weiner JS, Khogali M. A physiological body-cooling unit for treatment of heat stroke. *Lancet*. 1980;1:507.
25. Khogali M, Weiner JS. Heat stroke—report on 18 cases. *Lancet*. 1980;1:276.
26. Syveruda S, Barker W, et al. Iced gastric lavage for treatment of heat stroke: efficacy in a canine model. *Ann Emerg Med*. 1984;13(5):35.
27. Schrier RW, Hano J, Keller HI, et al. Renal, metabolic and circulatory responses to heat and exercise: studies in military recruits during summer training. *Ann Intern Med*. 1970;73:213–223.
28. Hubbard RW, et al. Novel approaches to the pathophysiology of heat stroke: the energy depletion model. *Ann Emerg Med*. 1982;16:9,1066–1074.
29. Atkins E. Fever. In: MacBryde C, Blacklaw R, eds. *Signs and symptoms*. New York: JB Lippincott, 1979.
30. Eichler A, McFee A, Root H. Heat stroke. *Am J Surg*. 1965;118:855.
31. Talbot JH, Michelsen J. Heat cramps: a clinical and chemical study. *J Clin Invest*. 1931;12:533.
32. Kew M, Bersohn I, Seftel H, et al. Liver damage in heat stroke. *Am J Med*. 1970;49:192–202.
33. Freeman W, Dumaff S. Cerebellar syndrome following heat stroke. *Arch Neurol Psychiatry*. 1944;51:67–72.
34. Costrini AM, et al. Cardiovascular and metabolic manifestations of heat stroke and severe heat exhaustion. *Am J Med*. 1978;188:463.
35. Ferris EB, et al. Heat stroke: clinical and chemical observations on 44 cases. *J Clin Invest*. 1938;17:249.
36. Saxton CR. Treatment of heat stroke at Parkland Memorial Hospital. *West J Med*. 1980;133:447.
37. Al-Aska, AK, et al. Simplified cooling bed for heat stroke. *Lancet*. 1987;14:381.
38. Graham BS, Lichtenstein MJ, et al. Non-exertional heat stroke: physiologic management and cooling in 14 patients. *Arch Intern Med*. 1986;146:87.
39. White DJ, et al. Evaporation versus iced gastric lavage treatment of heat stroke: comparative efficacy in a canine model. *Crit Care Med*. 1987;15(8):748–750.
40. Bynum GP, et al. Peritoneal lavage cooling in an anesthetized dog heat stroke model. *Aviat Space Environ Med*. 1978;49:799.
41. El-Kassimi FA, Al Mashadani S, Abdullah AK, et al. Adult respiratory distress syndrome and disseminated intravascular coagulation complicating heat stroke. *Chest*. 1986;90(4):571–574.
42. Malamud N, Haymaker W, Custer RP. Heatstroke: a clinicopathologic study of 125 fatal cases. *Milit Med*. 1946;99:397–444.
43. Tek DA, Olshaker JS. Hyperthermia, pulmonary edema and disseminated intravascular coagulation in an 18-year old military recruit. *Ann Emerg Med*. 1990;19:715–722.
44. Shibolet S, Coll R, Gilant T, et al. Heat stroke: its clinical picture and mechanism in 36 cases. *QJ Med*. 1967;36:525–548.
45. Chobanian SJ. Jaundice occurring after resolution of heat stroke. *Ann Emerg Med*. 1983;12(2):102.
46. Mustafa KY, Omer O, Khogali M, et al. Blood coagulation and fibrinolysis in heat stroke. *Br J Hematol*. 1985;61(3):517–23.
47. O'Donnell TF Jr, Clowes GH. The circulatory abnormalities of heat-stroke. *N Engl J Med*. 1972;287:734–737.
48. Stine RJ. Heat illness. *JACEP*. 1979;8:154–160.
49. Geiss P, Marr J. Management of heat injury syndromes. *Symp Crit Care*. 1982;3:1–24.
50. Delaney KA. Heat stroke. *Postgrad Med*. 1992;91(4):379–388.
51. Amsterdam JT, Syverudsa, Barker WJ, et al. Dantrolene sodium for treatment of heat stroke victims: lack of efficacy in a canine model. *Am J Emerg Med*. 1986;4:399–405.

41. Hypothermia

JON W. MILLER., JR., MD, FACEP, FACURP

ACCIDENTAL HYPOTHERMIA

Hypothermia is defined as a decrease from the average 37°C homeothermic core temperature to 35°C or less.[1] Core temperature may be measured in the thoracic aorta, midesophagus, external auditory canal, rectum, or a freshly voided urine specimen,[2–5] in order of descending preference but increasing technical ease. Accidental hypothermia is a subcategory occurring as a spontaneous equilibration toward environmental temperatures resulting from inadequate conservation of heat through insulation or insufficient heat production.[6] Heat is lost through conduction, convection, evaporation, and radiation, in descending rate. The diagnosis of accidental hypothermia specifically excludes iatrogenically induced surgical or therapeutic states.

Accidental hypothermia divides into three subcategories based on rate of heat loss (a function of environmental temperature and physiologic thermoregulatory responses). The three subcategories are as follows:

1. Acute: immersion with heat loss through conduction into a cold (<21°C) fluid in less than 1 hour.
2. Subacute: exposure with heat loss through evaporation, convection, radiation, and decreased thermogenesis occurring over several hours.
3. Gradual: decreased thermogenesis and insulation associated with chronic debilitation occurring over days to weeks, especially in the elderly urban patient.

Note: The section on frostbite was taken from the first edition of this chapter, written by Michael L. Callaham.

Acute Hypothermia

Acute hypothermia is the most publicized and best studied category. It is frequently associated with miraculous recoveries from near-drowning in cold water. Researchers favor it for rapidity of onset. Heat loss is 25 times more rapid in water than in air of the same temperature.[7–9] The information gained from Dachau was obtained in part from cold water immersion.[10] Successive peripheral thermoregulatory defense mechanisms of subcutaneous fat insulation are rapidly overwhelmed. Peripheral vasoconstriction shunts blood to central capacitance vessels. Thermogenesis by shivering is ineffective as skeletal muscles contract. The protective peripheral insulating shell is sacrificed to preserve a central core of vital organs. This process occurs rapidly in children due to their small volume and high surface-to-volume ratio. The child's proportionately larger head increases this rate as 40% of body heat loss occurs above the shoulders.

Metabolism is halted at the cellular level, minimizing depletion of glucose and ATP stores.[11] Decreased cellular respiration minimizes acidosis. The cellular mechanism is preserved intact.

Miraculous resuscitations after 40 minutes of submersion, with good return of neurologic function, are well documented.[12–18]

Neonatal hypothermia deserves special mention. It is probably the least recognized form of acute hypothermia. Noninsulated neonates, still wet from birth, cool quickly by convection, evaporation, and radiation. Heat conduction from core to surface continues relatively unimpeded due to a lack of significant insulation by subcutaneous adipose tissues. Premature or "small for dates" neonates are especially vulnerable. Brain injury, infection, exhaustion, and depressant drugs (phenothiazine, opiates, reserpine) cause further compromise.

Skin sensors rather than hypothalamic temperature sensors initiate norepinephrine-mediated vasoconstriction and nonshivering thermogenesis in brown fat. Physical activity and crying augment heat production.[19]

Absence of crying, anorexia, lethargy, oliguria, abdominal distention, cool skin, edema, peripheral cyanosis, and bradycardia are late and ominous signs of hypothermia. The possibility of sepsis must always be suspected and evaluated.[20,21]

The newborn's zone of thermal neutrality must be maintained to minimize heat loss, dehydration, shock, and even death.[22,23] External warming by radiant lamps and incubators has significantly reduced infant mortality.

Subacute Hypothermia

Subacute hypothermia is commonly associated with exposure and exhaustion in connection with debility, or inadequate insulation from heat loss. This may result from inadequate clothing or loss of insulation due to moisture.[24] Heat is conducted into the clothing and lost through evaporation and convection. Heat may also be conducted into the ground or water.

Thermal challenge is monitored by the hypothalamus. Initial peripheral response to cold is sympathetically induced increase of insulation initiated by cutaneous temperature sensors. Warm blood is shunted away from the surface as peripheral vasoconstriction occurs. Perspiration ceases, decreasing heat lost through evaporation. Piloerection decreases heat lost by convection.[25]

Continued heat loss initiates shivering. Shivering is a nonsynchronous contraction of cutaneous and skeletal muscles. The body metabolism can be raised to a level two to five times normal by this activity.[25,26] The heat generated is not preserved due to loss of insulation and increase of convection following body movement.[25]

Shivering may continue to 26.7°C, depleting the body's ATP and glycogen stores and contributing to dehydration and lactic acidosis.[27] It is replaced by generalized rigidity.

Predisposing factors to subacute hypothermia include physiologic loss of insulation (exfoliative dermatitis, ichthyosis, erythroderma, anorexia nervosa, kwashiorkor, marasmus, and burns), central nervous system compromise due to toxins (opiates, alcohol, barbiturates, phenothiazines, organophosphates, reserpine) or lesions (Parkinsonism, luetic gliosis, stroke, basilar skull fracture, spinal cord lesion above T-1, cerebral neoplasm, agenesis of corpus callosum, Wernicke's encephalopathy, Shapiro's syndrome), endocrine disorders (hypopituitary, hypoadrenal, hypothyroid), metabolic disorders (sepsis, malaria, exhaustion, hypoglycemia, uremia, shock, malnutrition, age), rapid intravenous infusion, and chronic recurrent hypothermia.

Gradual Hypothermia

Gradual hypothermia is also known as urban or domestic hypothermia. It is a disease of debility found in all age groups but especially the extremes of age. Its predilection is toward the elderly poor. Heat loss occurs gradually over weeks to months by evaporation, convection, radiation, decreased heat production due to poor nutrition and inactivity, and loss of insulating subcutaneous adipose tissue. Often the home is cool due to inability to afford fuel. Appreciation of cool environment is lost with increasing age.[28]

Physicians and nursing homes contribute to hypothermia through the administration of behavior-modifying medications of the phenothiazine and barbiturate groups. These medications inhibit hypothalamic thermoregulation and suppress thermogenesis by activity.

Sedentary lifestyle, decreased caloric intake due to diminished appetite, decreased insulation by sweat-permeated light robes, and medication all contribute to hypothermia. Diminished mental acuity may be misdiagnosed as depression, senility, stroke, or medication effect.[29-33]

A unique circumstance not usually seen by physicians is that of salvage or construction divers living in saturation. These people live in chambers under great depths of water for extended periods of time. Decompression difficulties are overcome by replacing the usual 80% nitrogen in the atmosphere with lighter helium. The insulatory properties of nitrogen are sacrificed, and heat is lost at a higher rate through evaporation, respiration, and radiation. The divers are intermittently exposed to cold water outside the living chamber where heat loss occurs through conduction.[34,35]

The commercial diving industry has gone to great lengths to provide heated and insulated diving gear, thermally neutral environment, and high caloric intake to saturation divers.[36]

PHYSIOLOGIC CHANGES ASSOCIATED WITH HYPOTHERMIA

Information on the physiology of cooling is based on extrapolation from nonhuman models, unethical experimentation on starved prisoners of war, military volunteers limited to 35°C as a minimum temperature, or anesthetized surgical patients under total physiologic control. Consistent or frequent changes associated with cooling are presented and discussed by organ system. A synopsis of observations may be reviewed in Table 41-1.

Table 41-1 Symptoms of Hypothermia

°Fahrenheit	°Celsius		°Fahrenheit	°Celsius	
98.6	37	Average body temperature for the adult. Immersion in 5°C fresh water to the neck used to cool subject. Initial gasp of tachypnea, tidal volume, tachycardia transient meiosis—increased blood pressure (140/70–190/103), frequent VPCs but subject not aware of dysrhythmia. Basal metabolism up 500% from normal. After 20 minutes—peripheral vasoconstriction, rapid shallow breathing—core pooling of blood—peripheral numbness well established—pulse variable—blood pressure returning toward control—first signs of rectal temperature drop.	91.8	33.2	Frequent cardiac dysrhythmias, which can go to A-fib. Below this temperature heart resistant to defibrillation.
			87.8	31	Cannot recognize familiar faces. Loss of shivering.
			86	30	Muscle rigidity—entering zone of maximal ventricular irritability—dysarthric speech.
			82.4	28	Pupil dilated—BMR 50% normal.
			80.6	27	Muscle tone lost—flaccid body.
			78.8	26	Definite bradycardia and infrequent shallow respiration. Loss of consciousness.
95	35–35.5	Subject unaware of one third of events around him. Noted loss of tactile sensation—voluntary exposure limits after ten minutes at this temperature—subject frequently does not remember getting out of tub (even under own power). BMR near normal.	77.7	25–24	DTR and vasoconstriction lost (last protective mechanism).
			68	20	No pupillary reflex to light, lowest reading on most thermocouples.
			64.4	18	Flat EEG.
93.2	34	Extreme judgment errors—amnesia to current events (number sequences, time of day after being told)—(may not be present in nonimmersion).	51.9	10.5	Lowest cardiac activity.
			48.2	9	Lowest survival temperature recorded.
			32	0	Water freezes.

Skin

The preceding paragraphs discussed cutaneous vasoconstriction, piloerection, cessation of perspiration, and redistribution of warmed blood to the core capacitance vessels, which allow the formation of an effective insulating shell and warmed heat conserving core.[37–39] Subcutaneous brown adipose tissue of the infant aids in thermogenesis, and white adipose tissue acts as insulation.[19,39,40] Shivering increases heat production up to five times the resting basal metabolic rate in the adult.[25,41,42] Vasoconstriction is lost near 25°C,[43] causing a feeling of warmth. Inappropriate removal of clothing may follow this sensation.[44]

Respiratory System

Respiratory response to induction of hypothermia varies with method of induction. Sudden immersion in cold water elicits an initial involuntary gasp followed by uncontrolled tachypnea. In the submerged victim, drowning, or at least aspiration, is possible. However, if the head remains out of the water, respiratory rate slows with drop of core temperature. Cooling the occipital skull and, thereby, the respiratory center hastens the drop in respiratory rate.[45] These events have not been reported with gradual onset hypothermia. Prolonged or severe hypothermia causes cold bronchorrhea and ciliary immobilization. Bronchodilatation occurs; tidal volume and lung compliance decrease. Pulmonary vascular resistance increases.[46–48]

Carbon dioxide retention, due in part to increased solubility in plasma, is frequently documented.[49,50] Inhibition of oxygen/carbon dioxide diffusion across the alveoli has not been reported. Decreased oxygen secondary to decrease in respiratory rate, tidal volume, and a left shift of the oxyhemoglobin dissociation curve is partially compensated by increased oxygen solubility in plasma.[51] Percentages of oxygen extracted remain unchanged. Reduced metabolic demands may be met by oxygen in solution.

Arterial blood gas machines are calibrated to a 37°C standard. Reported values should be corrected to the temperature of the victim. The formula for correction of pH is $pHt = pH_{38°C} + 0.0147(38 - t)$ where t is the measured temperature. The pH rises 0.0147 for each 1° drop of temperature. The P_{CO_2} drops 4.4% and P_{O_2} 6% per degree.[50,52–54] Precalculated values are shown in Table 41-2.

Acidosis usually corrects spontaneously with rewarming and adequate ventilation.[1,2,51] Correction of metabolic acidosis causes further leftward shift on the oxyhemoglobin dissociation curve. ''Correction'' should be approached with

Table 41-2 Blood Gases in Hypothermia

Temperature		Correction		
(F)	(C)	P_{CO_2}	P_{O_2}	pH
108	42.2	1.25	1.35	.08
106	41.1	1.19	1.26	.06
104	40.0	1.14	1.19	.04
102	38.9	1.08	1.11	.03
98.6	37.0	1.00	1.00	0
95	35.0	.92	.89	+.03
90	32.2	.82	.76	+.07
88	31.1	.78	.72	+.09
86	30.0	.74	.67	+.10
84	28.9	.71	.63	+.12
82	27.8	.68	.59	+.14
80	26.7	.64	.56	+.15
78	25.6	.61	.52	+.17
76	24.4	.59	.49	+.18
74	23.3	.56	.46	+.20
72	22.2	.53	.43	+.22

pH increases 0.008 units per °F fall in temperature.
P_{O_2} decreases 3.3% per °F fall in temperature.
P_{CO_2} decreases 2.4% per °F fall in temperature.

Several excellent reviews on hypothermia have stressed the fact that blood gas results must be corrected for temperature but have failed to provide the correction factors. Based on the work to which these papers refer, the author has calculated the appropriate correction factors and provides them in this table. Note that to obtain corrected P_{O_2} and P_{CO_2}, one multiplies by the appropriate factor, but that for pH, the correction is added.

Source: Reprinted with permission from Wears JL: Blood gases in hypothermia. *JACEP* 8(6):247, 1979.

consideration of altered volumes of distribution. (Rapid changes of pH may induce dysrhythmias.)

Chest roentgenogram should not be affected by hypothermia initially. Pneumonia is a frequently reported postrewarming complication. Most studies now suggest against prophylactic antibiotics although controversy exists.[2,49,51,52–59]

Agonal respiratory efforts may persist after electrocardiographic silence.[10,60]

Cardiac System

Initial circulatory response to rapid immersion is peripheral vasoconstriction, tachycardia (up to 180 beat/min) with frequent premature ventricular contractions (PVC) and elevation of blood pressure. Twenty minutes after immersion, vasoconstriction is well established and blood pressure begins to return toward normal. PVCs become less frequent.[10,45]

The sino-auricular node is most sensitive to hypothermia. Below 32°C atrial flutter and atrial fibrillation can be discerned among shivering artifact. Varying atrioventricular (AV) conduction defects refractory to atropine and vagotomy also begin in this range. Atrial activity has been recorded at 13°C, but usually the AV node or ventricle initiates contractions much sooner due to progressive inactivation of higher pacing centers.[61–69]

Cooling progressively widens the QRS complex (reflecting prolongation of systole) and lengthens the Q-T interval.[61,70–73] T-wave inversion is common. The widely reported junctional point elevation (J-wave) occurring at the end of the QRS complex and beginning of the S-T interval first occurs around 31.5°C (Fig. 41-1).[74–76]

The first reports of its association with hypothermia were made by Tomaszewski (1938) and independently by Osburn (1953).[77–79] Subsequent reports document association with CNS lesions and even as a normal variant.[80] Alterations of ion flux across the cell membrane or, possibly, early repolarization are responsible during hypothermia.[81]

Core temperature below 30°C increases the probability of ventricular fibrillation. Hypoxia, abrupt physical manipulations, sudden postural changes, central line catheter placement, contact with the myocardium, or prolonged attempts at intubation by inept personnel may precipitate ventricular fibrillation.[82–85] Immediate defibrillation with two joules per kilogram should be attempted, despite reports of the heart being "refractory" during hypothermia.

Decreased cardiac output occurs secondary to bradycardia.[86,87] Stroke volume is not affected despite systolic prolongation.[88,89] Peripheral circulation is compromised by loss of volume, through cold diuresis, fluid shifts to the extracellular spaces, increased plasma viscosity, hemoconcentration, and peripheral resistance.[90–93]

Protective peripheral vasoconstriction is lost around 25°C. The lowest documented electrocardiographic activity was recorded at 10.5°C.[65]

Cold-induced cardiac dysrhythmias resolve with rewarming. Attempts to resuscitate hypothermic victims should not be abandoned prior to rewarming to 35°C. "They are not dead until they are warm and dead."

Endocrine System

Endocrine response to cooling is directed by the hypothalamus. Direct sympathetic stimulation of the adrenal medulla initially increases production and release of norepinephrine and epinephrine.[94–97] These catecholamines act in conjunction to increase central production and peripheral conservation of body heat. Production of these catecholamines is transient and drops off sharply.[98]

Acute cold stimulates hypothalamic release of thyrotropin-releasing hormone, which acts at the anterior pituitary causing release of thyroid-stimulating hormone. Thyroid-stimulating hormone stimulates the thyroid to increase production and conversion of tri-iodothyroxine and thyroxine. There is no immediate response to these hormones. Alteration of thermogenesis by thyroid route occurs only in prolonged hypothermia.[1,6,99]

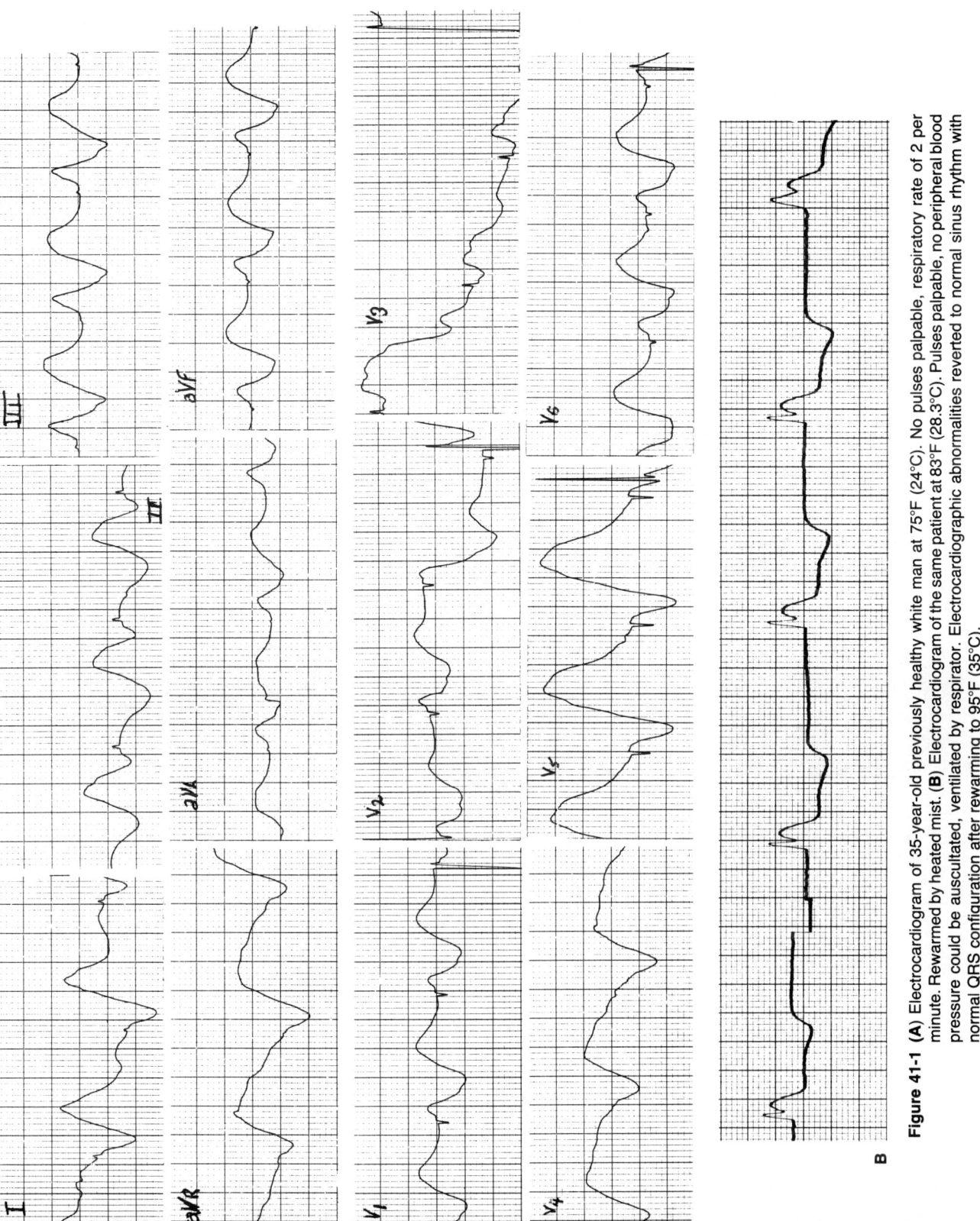

Figure 41-1 (**A**) Electrocardiogram of 35-year-old previously healthy white man at 75°F (24°C). No pulses palpable, respiratory rate of 2 per minute. Rewarmed by heated mist. (**B**) Electrocardiogram of the same patient at 83°F (28.3°C). Pulses palpable, no peripheral blood pressure could be auscultated, ventilated by respirator. Electrocardiographic abnormalities reverted to normal sinus rhythm with normal QRS configuration after rewarming to 95°F (35°C).

Adrenocorticotrophic hormone stimulation of the adrenal center is depressed below 32.2°C.[98] Adrenocortical activity is also directly suppressed by cooling.[100] The decrease of production and release is offset by decreased physiologic demand and hepatic degradation. Cortisol levels are dramatically increased.[101,102]

Insulin production, secretion, and activity are strongly suppressed below 30°C.[103–105] Hypothermic hyperglycemia follows adrenergic gluconeogenesis, decreased transport into the cell, and decreased metabolism.

The posterior pituitary decreases antidiuretic hormone release in response to hypothermia.[106]

Kidneys

Renal response to cold is diuresis. Increased volume in deep capacitance vessels, horizontal position, increased cardiac output, and decreased antidiuretic hormone all contribute to the effect. Decreased glomerular filtration and decreased renal tubular sensitivity to antidiuretic hormone also occur. The net result is excretion of large volumes of urine with low specific gravity (1.002–1.006).[107–109]

Glycosuria is common. Electrolyte disturbances have not been associated with this fluid loss. Myoglobinuria may precipitate acute tubular necrosis as a complication after rewarming. Postrewarming, oliguria, and anuria may require short-term dialysis.[98]

Pancreas

Hyperamylasemia is frequently associated with hypothermia. Pancreatitis is a common sequela of rewarmed victims. Hypothermia may trigger the acute episode of a preexisting chronic condition. The high incidence of alcohol as a precipitating factor to each condition is well documented.[110–114]

Liver

The liver temperature remains 1° to 2°C above rectal temperature. Production and release of glucose and free fatty acids are its initial response to cold. Temperature drop decreases detoxification and conjugation.[115] Liver enzymes may be transiently elevated. Vacuolization and congestion have been reported after severe or prolonged hypothermia.[116]

Central and Peripheral Nervous Systems

Cerebral blood flow decreases 6% to 7% per degree Celsius temperature depression.[117,118] The brain compensates for the decreased flow and relative hypoxia by decreased metabolism and, thereby, reduces oxygen and glucose demands. The decreased metabolism is displayed as a progression of symptoms from dysarthria and amnesia at 34°C to ataxia and stupor near 32°C, and, finally, unconsciousness.[119] Symptoms vary greatly between subjects as heat is lost. The acute hypothermic loses function more rapidly than the gradually cooled victim.

Cooling physically decreases brain and spinal cord volume unless shivering is present, a desirable quality in neurotrauma.[118] Composition of cerebrospinal fluid is unchanged.[120]

Loss of appreciation of sharp and deep pain varies with skin temperature in different methods of cooling.

Deep tendon reflexes are exaggerated down to 32°C due to shivering. Between 32° and 30°C there is a return toward normal with prolongation of both contraction and relaxation phases between 30° and 26°C. The patellar tendon reflex is last to disappear and first to return with rewarming. Babinski's reflex remains downward until 26°C, when it disappears along with gag reflex. Pupillary light response is lost near 20°C. Electroencephalographic activity has not been recorded below 18°C.

Hematologic Response

Hemoconcentration caused by fluid shifts and cold diuresis has already been discussed. Secondary erythrocyte and platelet aggregation in constricted capillary beds with microemboli and microinfarcts is reported.[121]

Hypothermia does not cause hemolysis or drop of hemoglobin or hematocrit. Preexisting predisposing conditions such as gastrointestinal bleed, anemia, and trauma are more likely causes.[122]

The adrenergic stress response to cold causes demargination of leukocytes. Peripheral white blood cell counts of 22,000 µL are common during the initial phases of immersion hypothermia. Leukocytosis of this order would probably be due to trauma or sepsis in gradual or subacute onset hypothermia. Cooling decreases the number of circulating leukocytes by sequestration in core capacitance vessels. The differential of the white blood cell count is not affected by cold.[55]

Platelets are similarly sequestered and possibly inactivated by cold. Disseminated intravascular coagulation is a reported complication of hypothermia.[123,124]

Gastrointestinal System

Decrease in digestive function, including production of gastric fluids and intestinal absorption, occurs with cooling.[55,125] Ileus is a common finding, with constipation the chief complaint. Gastrointestinal hemorrhage and mesenteric necrosis due to microthrombi have also been reported as a postmortem finding.[126–129] Salivation is increased by cooling.[130]

Reproductive System

Research in this area of hypothermia is limited to a single observation of the lowest reported temperature at which a human male has successfully performed intercourse as 30°C.[10] Only one other (quite dissimilar) historic article on this topic is available.[131]

PREHOSPITAL CARE

Hypothermia should be included in the differential diagnosis of all patients with altered sensorium. The index of suspicion should be elevated in all winter- or water-related incidents. Such patients should not be pronounced dead without consideration being given to hypothermia.

Every patient should be considered to have a spinal cord injury. Substitute deep painful stimuli and gentle handling for shake and shout. This can avert further cord injury or precipitation of intractable ventricular fibrillation. A long count may be necessary to detect a shallow pulse or respirations.

Controversy continues regarding initiation of cardiopulmonary resuscitation (CPR) and the rate and depth of compression and ventilation in hypothermia. There is insufficient data available to justify alteration of basic cardiac life support and basic trauma life support protocols.

Severely obtunded patients should be intubated to protect the airway because the gag reflex is suppressed by cold.[1,2,10,51,132–134] Heated, humidified oxygen may then be administered to reverse hypoxia and heat loss. Intubation allows suctioning of cold-induced bronchorrhea. Preoxygenation reduces the risks involved in intubation and suctioning.

Intravenous cannulation and the administration of heated (40°C) nonlactated crystalloid solutions are preferred for volume expansion.[1,46,133] Blood specimens may be obtained simultaneously. Intravenous administration of 5% dextrose in water supplies substrate to reverse hypoglycemia.[134] Oral administration of alcohol or warmed sweet liquids is contraindicated in obtunded patients.[135–141] Naloxone reverses opiate depression.

Wet clothing should be cut from the patient. Insulation can then be applied to prevent additional heat loss. Body-to-body contact or application of a heated plumbed sarong may be employed in the wilderness or during transport to initiate rewarming.[10,142–144] In the prehospital setting insulation and rewarming should continue to the end point of clear mental status, stable vital signs, and sweating.

The urgency of transport should be determined by the patient's underlying or predisposing condition. A bumpy ride may precipitate fatal dysrhythmias in an otherwise stable hypothermic patient.

EMERGENCY DEPARTMENT CARE

Evaluation

Severely hypothermic patients may be stiff and cold but still alive. The severely hypothermic patient's chances of survival correspond with the physician's index of suspicion and experience. Hypothermia often goes undiagnosed in these patients because of the critical nature of other presenting problems. Hypothermia may be the disease or only a symptom of a more complex life-threatening condition. Treat the hypothermia (Table 41-3) but do not assume it to be the only life-threatening condition.

Assessment of vital signs often requires electronic enhancement by Doppler and electrocardiographic monitoring. Most clinical thermometers will not register below 35°C. Obtaining an accurate core temperature requires a low-reading glass laboratory thermometer or thermocouple probe.

Spinal immobilization must be maintained to prevent neurologic injury as well as lethal dysrhythmias. Provide in-line traction while nasotracheally intubating for airway control and suctioning of bronchorrhea. Preoxygenation prevents procedure-induced dysrhythmias.[51,133,134,145–148]

Remaining wet clothing should be carefully cut away to allow physical examination, including neurologic assessment and completion of the Glasgow Coma Scale. Rather

Table 41-3 Hypothermia Protocol

1. Maintain spinal immobilization. Obtain vital signs with Doppler, thermocouple probe, and electronic monitoring if necessary. If viability is in doubt, initiate CPR.
2. Establish and secure patent airway. If patient has rectal temperature less than 32°C and/or is obtunded, preoxygenate and intubate with in-line traction.
3. Carefully cut off wet clothing. Perform physical examination, including neurologic assessment. Place monitor leads. Insulate from further heat loss.
4. Establish intravenous access and obtain samples for complete blood count with platelets and differential, electrolytes, blood urea nitrogen, glucose, amylase, automated chemistry and enzyme profile, prothrombin and partial thromboplastin times, and toxicology screen with emphasis on alcohol, sedatives, and tranquilizers. Test for pregnancy as indicated.
5. Administer intravenous glucose and naloxone if patient is obtunded. Initiate fluid resuscitation.
6. Radiographically assess cervical spine, skull, chest, pelvis, and extremities. Check endotracheal tube and central venous line placement.
7. Perform 12-lead ECG. Preoxygenate and insert nasogastric tube and urinary and arterial catheters. Send arterial blood for analysis.
8. Select and initiate rewarming method.
9. Monitor vital signs, cardiac rhythm, and level of consciousness during rewarming.
10. Cease resuscitation after patient is sweating or if core temperature is 35°C without vital signs.

than being rubbed briskly, the patient should be patted dry. Heated cloth blankets are then applied for head-to-toe insulation. Emphasize insulation of the scalp and neck. Affix electrocardiographic monitor leads, and insert core temperature monitoring probes.

To assist in initiation of intravenous access, peripheral vasoconstriction may be reversed by local application of heat. In moderate and severe cases, large-bore central venous access is generally indicated. This may also be the only source of blood, so collect specimens accordingly. Suggested tests are listed below. Locate the catheter tip in the great vessels outside the heart to prevent ectopic stimulation and fibrillation.[149] As in other shocklike states, only preheated fluids should be infused. Fluids may be heated rapidly in plastic bags or vented plastic bottles through microwave irradiation without contamination.[150]

Crystalloids are generally preferred for volume expansion,[149] although low–molecular weight dextran has been discussed as an alternative.[151–154] Lactated solutions are not advocated because of their poor hepatic metabolism and subsequent promotion of acidosis. Infusion rates are dictated by the patient's vital signs, central venous pressure, neck vein distention, and lung sounds. Volume depletion is generally underestimated. Arterial catheter placement facilitates monitoring of blood pressure and blood gases.

Roentgenographic studies of the cervical spine, skull, chest, pelvis, and extremities should be performed in the emergency department. Placement of the endotracheal tube and central venous catheter tips should be confirmed and documented. Chest studies should be repeated as needed as an adjunct to physical examination.

Evaluation of the standard 12-lead electrocardiogram in severe hypothermia may prove futile (Fig. 41-1). Nonetheless, it should be performed as a baseline study. Document at least four complexes per lead.

After preoxygenation, insert the nasogastric tube into obtunded or severely hypothermic patients to alleviate gastric distention due to ileus. Evaluate the aspirate for blood and toxins, especially alcohol, sedatives, and tranquilizers. Hypothermia delays gastrointestinal motility and absorption, so that even delayed removal enhances resuscitation.[125,155,156]

Urinary bladder catheterization is indicated for initial evaluation of traumatic hematuria and later assessment of perfusion and fluid balance.

Laboratory Studies

Collection and evaluation of samples for the following studies are indicated in assessment of the obtunded or severely hypothermic patient: complete blood count with differential and platelet count; electrolytes; blood urea nitrogen; glucose; prothrombin and partial thromboplastin times; amylase; cardiac enzymes and isoenzymes; toxicology screen of urine, blood, and gastric contents emphasizing alcohol, sedatives, and tranquilizers; and baseline arterial blood gases. Interesting but nonemergent studies include diagnostic thyroid and adrenal functions. Document β–human chorionic gonadotrophin levels in women of childbearing years. You may be treating two patients. Alterations of laboratory values have been discussed.

REWARMING

Overview

Selection of a rewarming method begins with consideration of the optimal rewarming rate and method of attaining that rate with the fewest complications. Optimal methods of rewarming minimize afterdrop and aftershock. Afterdrop is the paradoxic drop in core temperature during rewarming. Peripheral vasoconstriction may be rapidly reversed by some rewarming methods in some individuals. Warmer core blood moves to the peripheral vessels and is cooled. Cooler peripheral blood is returned to the core, where equilibration leads to an apparent drop in temperature. Rapid peripheral vasodilation compounded by inadequate circulatory volume due to cold diuresis and fluid shifts results in further hypotension. Compensatory cardiac response is variable. Heart rate is suppressed by cold, acidosis, and hypoxia as well as prolonged myoneural conduction. Resultant dysrhythmias are more common in moderate than in severe hypothermia.[10] In both cases they are often intractable.

Consider the following variables in selecting a method of rewarming: initial and current vital signs, level of consciousness, predisposing and coexisting conditions, rate and method of cooling, patient's age and physical condition, and the physician's experience with and confidence in the methods available.

Two large comparative studies have been published. Alexander[10] translated the Nazi experiments into English after World War II. His review points out the many internal inconsistencies and contradictions present in that work. Berger[157] reviewed the original documents and confirmed and reiterated many of the discrepancies and inadequacies. Angell[158] addressed the ethics of citing that work. The recent multicenter hypothermia survey reviewed the treatment of 428 cases of accidental hypothermia. Although well conducted and scientifically sound, this survey concluded that treatment must remain individualized.[159]

Sudden vasodilation of peripheral vessels without sufficient circulatory volume due to cold diuresis and fluid shifts causes hypotension. Compensatory increase of cardiac output is compromised by a cold myocardium, which is suddenly deluged by returning cold acidotic blood. In cases of longstanding hypothermia, uncorrected hypoxia, or insufficient substrate ectopy, intractable ventricular fibrillation and death ensue.[10,45] Optimal rates of rewarming minimize this sequence of events.

Slow and Rapid Rewarming

In the chronically debilitated, elderly, or chronically hypothermic patient with normal sensorium, slow rewarming is widely acknowledged to be both safe and effective. This is especially true in the mild to moderate ranges of hypothermia. Steady rise in temperature and improvement in level of consciousness determine the acceptable rate of rewarming. Optimal rates vary from 0.5° to 1°C per hour.[1,6,55,160,161]

Aggressive intervention is demanded by inability spontaneously to raise core temperature, a continued drop in core temperature, deterioration of level of consciousness or vital signs, and onset of ventricular fibrillation. These symptoms indicate exhaustion of substrate or shock from other causes.

The current literature favors rapid rewarming with vigorous volume replacement.[1,32,132,162] Core rewarming methods are gaining in popularity.[29,140,141,143,144,156,163,164]

Rapid rewarming minimizes adenosine triphosphate and glucose depletion by supplying exogenous heat. This reduces anaerobic metabolism and acidosis. Adequate volume resuscitation enhances the body's buffering systems in reversal of acidosis. Decreased acidosis and rapid transition through the range of maximal myocardial irritability reduce the likelihood of ventricular fibrillation. This should theoretically enhance survival.

In early studies the most critical patients were selected for aggressive resuscitation. High mortality rates were common in these cases.[1,114,165] Improved monitoring and rewarming techniques have improved survival by 20% to 100%.[112,132]

Currently Available Methods of Rewarming

The methods of rewarming are shown in Table 41-4 and discussed below.

Passive or Physiologic Rewarming

Passive rewarming is the most widely available and easily practiced form of resuscitation. The patient rewarms through physiologic thermogenesis. Generated heat is conserved through insulation. Blanket changes are held to a minimum to prevent unnecessary heat loss and shivering. The physician supplies intravenous glucose, fluid resuscitation, and monitoring.

Rewarming may occur quickly in a mildly hypothermic, alert, previously healthy patient or not at all in a chronically debilitated individual. An average rise of 0.5°C per hour can be expected with this method.[111] It is generally well tolerated and has no significant side effects. Passive rewarming minimizes afterdrop by gradual reversal of the core shell phenomenon. Survival rates of 55% to 100% have been reported.[132] Failure to rewarm spontaneously or deterioration of the patient's general condition mandates active rewarming.

Table 41-4 Methods of Rewarming

I. Passive Rewarming
Substrates, warm environment, and insulation from further heat loss.

II. Active External Rewarming
Bodily contact, hot water bottles, electric blankets, blankets circulating heated fluids, radiant warmer, "hot rooms," immersion.

III. Active Core Rewarming
Intravenous fluids, gastrointestinal lavage, inhalation of heated humidified oxygen (via mask or intubation), peritoneal lavage, extracorporeal circulation, mediastinal irrigation.

Active External Rewarming

These methods rewarm the patient through radiation or conduction of heat to the skin surface. Rapid fluid shifts are most likely to occur with these methods. Previously healthy young individuals generally tolerate these methods best. Elderly individuals and those with cardiovascular compromise must be stabilized before initiation of external rewarming from moderate or severe hypothermia. Initiate volume replacement and have monitoring and resuscitation equipment, including a defibrillator, available.

In remote rescues the patient is placed between two normothermic volunteers in direct skin-to-skin contact. The group is then insulated, and movement is minimized to prevent heat loss. Sarongs plumbed to circulate heated fluids have been employed for the same purpose.[142]

In the definitive care setting, inguinal and axillary hot water bottles, heated cradles, radiant warmers, electric and plumbed heating blankets, and hot water immersion have been utilized with various degrees of success.[10,114,166-169]

Radiant heaters work well when used to rewarm the neonate. The adult's larger volume-to-surface ratio decreases their effectiveness. Hot water bottles are most effective when applied to large vessels just below the skin surface, as in the axilla, groin, and neck and around the scalp. Local burns have been attributed to direct application of electric blankets or hot packs to the skin.[170,171] Any of these methods may cause premature peripheral vasodilation.

Immersion in 40° to 42.2°C baths can rewarm the patient by up to 7°C per hour. Afterdrop and intractable ventricular fibrillation are classically attributed to immersion rewarming.[10] The physician must also cope with buoyancy, technical difficulty in monitoring, and prevention of aspiration or drowning. Be prepared for rapid extrication before defibrillation.

Survival rates range from 55.4% to 100%.[132] Ideal candidates for active external rewarming are quickly cooled, healthy children and young adults with stable vital signs (Table 41-5). Young and middle-aged patients arriving in ventricular fibrillation or cardiac arrest should be considered candidates for aggressive core rewarming.

Table 41-5 Factors Predictive of Survival in Patients in Full Arrest

Youth
Previously healthy
No acute trauma
Rapid rate of cooling
Cold water (<21°C) immersion of less than 20 minutes

Active Core Rewarming

These methods preferentially supply heat to the organs and great vessels of the thorax and abdomen. Physiologic return of circulation to the extremities rewarms them gradually. The following are methods included in this category: peripheral and central infusion of heated intravenous fluids, nasogastric and colonic irrigation with heated fluids, circulation of heated fluids through a gastric balloon, heated humidified oxygen administered by mask or endotracheal tube, peritoneal lavage with heated dialysates, mediastinal lavage with heated fluids, and extracorporeal circulation. These methods may be used alone or in conjunction with other methods to allow latitude in treatment of complicated cases.

As previously stated, all intravenous fluids should be heated to 40°C before administration. This reduces the body's caloric expenditure to heat the fluid after administration. Fluids administered via peripheral sites cool before reaching the central circulation. Peripheral administration of heated fluids is not an effective method of rewarming.

Central intravenous catheters deliver heated fluids to the core. Catheter placement within the heart may induce transseptal temperature gradients predisposing to ectopy.[172]

Successful rewarming by gastrointestinal lavage with heated fluids has been reported.[173] Adequate data regarding optimal fluid temperature, volume, and recovery of fluids from an atonic gastrointestinal system are not available.

Evaluation of rewarming by inhalation methods is ongoing. Early calculations by Hudson and Robinson[174] predicted an increase of 0.03°C per hour over passive methods with insulation. Later calculations by Meyers et al[175] predicted rates of 0.5°C per hour. Lloyd[176] calculated a total increase of 30% over passive physiologic thermogenesis in a hypothermic patient. Anecdotal case reports document rewarming rates from 0.5°C (equivalent to passive rewarming rates) up to 5.0°C per hour.[51,177]

Prehospital rewarming is possible with portable units that generate heat through the exothermic reaction of soda lime and exhaled carbon dioxide.[128,130] Facial heating by masks reduces shivering. It also increases rewarming of the brain as measured at the tympanic membrane.[137] Rapid rewarming of the medulla increases respiration. The dead space in the semiclosed system recycles carbon dioxide, decreasing to some extent cardiac irritability and respiratory alkalosis. Heat capacitance and conduction of dry air is negligible.

Humidification increases rewarming by water condensation (540 cal/g) and cessation of respiratory heat loss. Condensed water is absorbed through the alveoli into the capillaries without ill effect. It may also be absorbed into the cold-induced bronchorrhea, facilitating its removal.

Nasal or orotracheal intubation facilitates suctioning of secretions. It also facilitates delivery of 40° to 45°C humidified gases to the lower respiratory tract. Rates in one study showed an increase from 0.74° to 1.22°C per hour with intubation.[112]

Generation of 45°C humidified oxygen requires modification of standard equipment to bypass safe upper temperature limits. Frequent calibration, careful monitoring, and proper identification of devices as altered equipment will prevent mishaps. No tracheal burns have been attributed to this technique to date. Survival rates reported for this method range from 73% to 100% when used alone.[132]

Peritoneal lavage is a standard technique for the evaluation of blunt abdominal trauma. It is also used for dialysis in chronic renal failure. With minor modifications in standard technique, it can be used to restore intravascular volume and normal body temperature.[178–183] Standard preparation includes insertion of a nasogastric tube and Foley catheter. A dialysis catheter is placed in one colic gutter, and a second catheter is placed contralaterally. Four to six liters of 40.5° to 42.5°C potassium-free dialysate is then infused and drained through the catheters each hour. It may require 10 to 12 L of dialysate to correct severe hypothermia by this method.

Peritoneal lavage dialyzes aspirin, barbiturates, and glutethimide. Rewarming the liver and kidneys increases toxin metabolism and excretion and normalization of pH.

Contraindications for this procedure include pregnancy, multiple abdominal surgical scars, and obvious abdominal injury requiring surgery. Dialysate should be analyzed for amylase, blood, bile, food, and fecal contamination to rule out blunt trauma.

Bangs and Hamlet[141] report rewarming rates of 8.5°C per hour by this method. Davis and Judfson[185] and Pickering et al[186] report resuscitation from cardiac standstill by peritoneal lavage alone. Survival rate in reported cases ranges from 67% to 100%.[132]

Cardiopulmonary bypass is the definitive resuscitation procedure in hypothermic cardiac arrest. Restoration of oxygenation, circulation, intravascular volume, and acid-base and electrolyte balance can be accomplished while rewarming. If cardiac activity does not return spontaneously, conditions for defibrillation will be optimal.

Cannulization of the iliac vein and femoral artery provides the best emergency access for this procedure. After heparinization, 40° to 42.5°C fluids are circulated at 1 to 3 L/min. Rewarming rates of 10° to 12°C per hour have been reported.[186–188] No data correlating more rapid rates to survival are available.

Machine availability continues to be the restrictive factor for implementation of this procedure. Procedural morbidity includes wound infection, thrombophlebitis, complications of heparinization, hemolysis, and disseminated intravascular coagulation. Associated mortalities are generally attributed to hypothermia and go unreported.

Mediastinal irrigation with heated fluids directly rewarms the heart. This increases conductivity and contractility. In hypothermia this procedure should be reserved for a last ditch effort when the heart remains refractory to less invasive methods of rewarming. If initiated, it should be accompanied by direct cardiac massage. Mortality rates are understandably high considering the indications for the procedure.

Diathermy and gastric balloon methods of rewarming are not widely utilized procedures.

Medications—Generally Approved

1. Oxygen. After securing the airway, high flow administration of humidified oxygen to non-COPD patients is advocated. This increases tissue levels by entering into solution in the plasma bypassing the oxyhemoglobin complex.
2. Intravenous fluids. Crystalloids (5% dextrose in 0.9 normal saline) heated to 40°C should be employed as volume expanders. Blood products can also be warmed to 40°C safely prior to administration. Titrate to blood pressure and central venous pressure readings.
3. Glucose. This can be administered immediately after collection of laboratory samples. Hypoglycemia is a less frequent finding than hyperglycemia. The risk/benefit ratio dictates early administration.
4. Narcan. The reversal of the predisposing cause of ventilatory and CNS depression without reported side effects makes this a well-accepted initial drug.
5. Antidysrhythmics. Most dysrhythmias resolve with rewarming. In the event of ventricular tachycardia or sustained ectopy above 32°C (with adequate oxygenation), the use of lidocaine in doses of 1 mg/kg bolus and a 2:1 drip may be necessary. Caution must be used, as toxicity occurs with decreased metabolism in the liver. Incidental reports of successful chemical defibrillation by bretylium tosylate have come to the author's attention.[189–191] Successful conversion of otherwise refractory ventricular dysrhythmias by intravenous doses of 100 mg/kg have been attributed to magnesium sulfate.[192]
6. Phenothiazines. Administration of intravenous Thorazine in doses of 5 to 10 mg every 30 minutes may be employed to abolish shivering.

Medications—Controversial

1. Corticosteroids. If adrenal insufficiency is suspected, the corticosteroids may be lifesaving. In most cases, blood levels are elevated, so that augmentation is unnecessary.
2. Thyroid replacements. If myxedema is the suspected underlying pathology, or if these are indicated, patient is refractory to rewarming. In the majority of cases, they have no place.
3. Dopamine. Peripheral hypotension may be normal. If a pressor agent is indicated, dopamine is the best candidate due to least cardiac irritability. Early data suggest a central thermoregulatory action.[193,194]
4. Antibiotics. Most authors advocate withholding antibiotics until signs of infection are manifested in the adult. In the neonate and infant, broad-spectrum coverage should be initiated in nonexposure cases due to the high correlation of hypothermia and sepsis.

Contraindicated Until Euthermia

1. Sodium bicarbonate. After correction of arterial blood gases for temperature, most experienced authors propose observation until rewarming to 32° to 35°C prior to administration. In most cases, acidosis resolves with volume and rewarming.
2. Potassium. Supplemental potassium during hypothermia may precipitate dysrhythmias. Most authors wait until 32° to 35°C to avoid complications.
3. Insulin. Insulin is relatively inactivated below 32°C. Early administration subcutaneously may precipitate disastrous hypoglycemia after rewarming. Intravenous administration for normal hypothermic hyperglycemia is not necessary, as reversal occurs with rewarming.
4. Magnesium and calcium. Measured blood levels rise with rewarming. "Prophylactic" administration may result in cardiorespiratory arrest.

Medications—Generally Ineffective or Contraindicated

1. Alcohol. Alcohol is a nonthermogenic anesthetic with the potential for diuresis and hypoglycemia; it may prolong rewarming. The antidysrhythmic properties shown in rat models have not been proven in human subjects to date.[195]
2. Antidysrhythmics. Procainamide precipitates dysrhythmias (ventricular fibrillation). Hydantoins depress conduction and may cause arrest. Quinidine in an acidotic medium may lead to arrest. Digitalis is less effective in hypothermia but may be helpful in mild cases with CHF. Atropine is ineffective against hypothermic bradycardia. Isuprel consistently precipitates fibrillation.
3. Epinephrine. Epinephrine is nonthermogenic in man but useful in arrest situations. Norepinephrine does have some theoretical values worthy of investigation.
4. Amphetamine. This drug has no proven or theoretical application.
5. Vasoconstrictors. These have been shown to have no clear benefit in controlled studies.

6. Vasodilators. These are potentially lethal through precipitation of shock.

CESSATION OF RESUSCITATION

The axiom "They're not dead till they're warm and dead" answers the question of when to cease resuscitation efforts. Young, healthy, rapidly cooled individuals, recovered in a conscious state after brief periods of immersion, and subsequently rapidly transported, should be rewarmed to 35°C and receive all available techniques of advanced life support prior to cessation of efforts. The only definite criterion for death is irreversibility.[196] Electrocardiogram and electroencephalogram are not valid tools for determining death during hypothermia.[197]

PEARLS

1. They are not dead until they are warm (35°C) and dead.
2. Handle gently to avoid dysrhythmia.
3. Clinical thermometers stop at 34°C.
4. Warmed fluids are beneficial in treatment of shock.
5. Preoxygenate prior to procedures.
6. Correct arterial blood gases to temperature.
7. Most dysrhythmias and electrolyte abnormalities will correct by rewarming.
8. Hypothermia goes unrecognized worldwide and year round.
9. Lethargic neonates and burn patients covered with wet sheets and receiving large quantities of fluid need temperature monitoring.
10. Hypothermia is a symptom of potentially lethal pathology. Don't treat the symptom and ignore the disease.

LOCALIZED COLD INJURY*

Chilblains

This entity is commonly seen in climates that are damp and cool for long periods of time. A localized nodule, probably representing a vasculitis, forms on the skin and superficial fatty tissue. These lesions are self-limiting and heal within a few days. Older people with poor circulation may develop ulcerated areas.

Frostnip

This term is given to early and mild frostbite. It is characterized by whitening and pain in the area involved.

---

*Adapted from Callaham ML: Hypothermia, in Kravis TC, Warner CG (eds): *Emergency Medicine,* ed 1. Rockville, MD, Aspen Publishers Inc, 1983, pp 435–436.

Frostbite

Frostbite is the injury and death of localized areas of tissue (most often on the extremities) due to local cold and freezing. Cold conditions cause arteriolar vasoconstriction in the affected part; capillary circulation stops secondary to the increased viscosity and sludging of the blood.[198,199] Eventually the tissues freeze. Ice crystals form within the extracellular space, creating physical damage, hypertonic ECF, and dehydration of cells.[200] Tissue damage is irreversible; pathologic changes include necrosis, with later atrophy, inflammatory changes, and fibroblastic proliferation. The bones may show punched-out lesions near joints.

A number of factors predispose a person to frostbite. Any disorder of the peripheral circulation (such as arteriosclerosis) increases the risk, as does previous frostbite, which seems to permanently damage vasomotor stability. Lack of acclimatization to cold may also be a risk factor, as is race. Blacks suffered a disproportionate share of cold injuries in the Korean War.[6] In addition, type of clothing and activity—particularly wetness and contact with metal, which accelerates heat loss greatly—contribute considerably to the occurrence of frostbite.

The diagnosis of frostbite is relatively simple, although there is as yet no accurate means of determining the true extent of damage on the initial assessment. The first symptoms (which are actually those of frostnip) are a burning pain and whitish discoloration of exposed parts, such as fingers or toes, face, nose, or earlobes. Later a feeling of warmth replaces the pain, and the skin becomes waxy and whitish. As the frostbite becomes deeper the appearance changes little, except that it is firm to the touch and lacks sensation, feeling numb or "heavy." This appearance, combined with a history of cold exposure, makes the diagnosis and excludes other ailments.

The treatment of frostbite in the field, as in the emergency department, is rapid rewarming.[201] In the field this can be accomplished by holding the affected part in the axilla or crotch. Warming in warm water is desirable if the temperature of the bath can be controlled and the resultant pain treated. Great care must be taken to avoid worsening damage by excessive exposure of the numb part to a fire, radiator, or other such heat source.[202] All friction (including the traditional rubbing with snow) must be avoided, as must all weight-bearing. If the leg is thawed or partially thawed, the patient must not walk on it but must be carried; a frostbitten arm must not be used. If this is impossible, it is better to leave it frozen until proper treatment can be assured. Alcohol should be avoided in the field because of its potentiation of hypothermia. Smoking is prohibited due to its deleterious vasoconstrictor effects, which further jeopardize blood supply.

In the emergency department, rewarming is done in a water bath kept at 40° to 42°C. Lower temperature of the bath increases tissue loss; higher may cause thermal burns. Socks or gloves that are frozen on are thawed with the extremity and then carefully removed. The bath is continued until the distal areas of the affected part flush and remain flushed even when removed from the bath. This may take an hour or more. Since it is often very painful, analgesia with morphine or meperidine may be required. Once thawed, the part is protected from any friction or pressure.

Blisters, varying in size, form in minutes to hours; their total absence is a very poor prognostic sign.[203] As in thermal burns, debriding the blisters is controversial, but if punctured they pose an infection risk and should be removed. Systemic hypothermia should be suspected and thoroughly searched for in any victim of frostbite. Transient cyanosis is common in the thawed part, but persistent cyanosis or ischemia despite thawing may indicate a developing compartment syndrome (perhaps due to a fracture, soft tissue sprain, or associated injury). Fasciotomy may be needed if circulation is threatened.

Since depth of injury cannot be initially determined, all but frostnip patients should be hospitalized. Vigorous whirlpool baths in antiseptic solution, with active physical therapy, provide safe debridement and mobilization of joints. Antibiotics should be reserved for actual clinical infection. Tetanus prophylaxis must not be forgotten. The true extent of the damage may not be apparent for weeks, although arterial pulses, Doppler studies, and ^{99m}Tc scans can help demarcate the injury.

As in accidental hypothermia, controversy abounds and few data exist regarding other treatment modalities. Early intra-arterial injection of 0.5 mg of reserpine provides a medical sympathectomy of the affected limb and increases blood flow, thus improving survival of marginal tissue and relieving pain.[204] Phenoxybenzamine, starting at 10 mg/day and increasing to 60 mg/day if needed, does the same thing by the oral route. Heparin has been used with mixed results.[205–208] Early reports using nonsteroidal anti-inflammatory drugs show promising results.[209,210] Fasciotomy may be needed in severe tissue damage if compartment syndromes develop; low–molecular weight dextran is advocated by a few.[211] Surgical sympathectomy also has its advocates, but diathermy and hyperbaric oxygen are not recommended.[212–217] There is little in the way of hard data to support any of these treatments, which appear to be largely a matter of personal experience and preference on the part of their advocates.

REFERENCES

1. Maclean D, Emslie-Smith D. *Accidental Hypothermia*. Philadelphia: Lippincott, 1977.
2. Reuler JB. Hypothermia: pathophysiology clinical settings and management. *Ann Intern Med*. 1978;89:519.
3. Webb GE. Comparison of esophageal and tympanic temperature monitoring during cardiopulmonary bypass. *Anesth Analg*. 1973;52:729.
4. Lilly JK, Boland JP, Zekan S. Urinary bladder temperature monitoring: A new index of core body temperature. *Crit Care Med*. 1980;8:742.
5. Cooper KE, Kenyon JR. A comparison of temperatures measured in the rectum, esophagus and on the surface of the aorta during hypothermia in man. *Br J Surg*. 1957;44:616.
6. Burton A, Edholm O. *Man in Cold Environment*. New York: Hafner; 1969.
7. Beckham EL. Thermal protection during immersion in cold water. *Proc Natl Acad Sci USA*. 1963;1181:247.
8. Beckham EL, Reeves E. Physiological implications as to survival during immersion in water at 75°F. *Aerosp Med*. 1966;37:1136.
9. Golden F. Hypothermia a problem for North Sea industries. *J Soc Occup Med*. 1976;26:85.
10. Alexander L. Treatment of shock from prolonged exposure to cold especially in water. *CIOS*. Item 240, file no 26–37; 1946.
11. Martin DR, et al. Primary cause of unsuccessful liver and heart preservation: cold sensitivity of ATP-ase system. *Am Surg*. 1972;175:111.
12. Betts J. But they wouldn't lie down. *Diver*. 1978;23:478.
13. Hunt PK. Affect and treatment of the "diving reflex." *Can Med Assoc J*. 1974;111:1330.
14. Nemiroff MJ. Resuscitation following cold water near drowning. In: *Proceedings of the 9th International Conference of Underwater Education*, 168. Colton, CA: National Association of Underwater Instructors; 1977.
15. Sekar TS, MacDonnell KF, Namsirikul P, et al. Survival after prolonged submersion in cold water without neurologic sequelae. *Arch Intern Med*. 1980;140:775.
16. Siebke H, Siebke H, Rod T, et al. Survival after 40 minutes submersion without cerebral sequelae. *Lancet*. 1975;1:1275.
17. Theilade D. A danger of fatal misjudgment in hypothermia after immersion. *Anesthesia*. 1977;32:889.
18. Young RSK, Zalneraitis EL, Dooling EC. Neurological outcome in cold water drowning. *JAMA*. 1980;244:1233.
19. Young RSK, Marks KH. Hypothermia and the pediatric patient. In: Pozos RS, Wittmers LE, eds. *The Nature and Treatment of Hypothermia*. Minneapolis: University of Minnesota; 1983.
20. Dagan R, Gorodischer R. Infections in hypothermic infants younger than 3 months old. *Am J Dis Child*. 1984;138:483.
21. El-Radhi AS, et al. Infection in neonatal hypothermia. *Arch Dis Child*. 1983;58:143.
22. Veale WL, Cooper KE, Pittman QJ. Thermoregulation in the newborn. In: Lomax P, Schonbaum E, eds. *Body Temperature*. New York: Dekker; 1979.
23. Prematurity and intrauterine growth retardation. In: Behrman RE, Vaughan VC, eds. *Nelson's Textbook of Pediatrics*. Philadelphia: Saunders; 1983.
24. Siple P. Clothing and climate. In: Newburg RW, ed. *Physiology of Heat Regulation and the Science of Clothing*. New York: Hafner; 1968.
25. Horvath SM, Howell CD. Organ systems in adaptation, the cardiovascular system. In: Dill DB, ed. *Handbook of Physiology*. Washington, DC: American Physiological Society; 1964.
26. Andrews IC, Orkin LR. Environmental cold and man. *Anesthesia*. 1964;25:549.
27. Marcus P. Laboratory comparison of techniques for rewarming hypothermia casualties. *Aviat Space Environ Med*. 1975;46:1236.
28. Collins KJ, et al. Accidental hypothermia and impaired temperature hemostasis in the elderly. *Br Med J*. 1977;2:353.
29. Miller JW, Danzl DF, Thomas DM. Urban hypothermia of the elderly, children, alcoholic and handicapped. Paper presented at the First International Hypothermia Conference; January 23–27, 1980; Kingston, RI.

30. Collins KJ, Exton-Smith AN, Dore C. Urban hypothermia: preferred temperature and thermal perception in old age. *Br Med J*. 1981; 282:175.

31. Cooper KE, Ferguson AV. Thermoregulation and hypothermia in the elderly. In: Pozos RS, Wittmers LE, eds. *The Nature and Treatment of Hypothermia*. Minneapolis: University of Minnesota; 1983.

32. Fox RH, et al. Body temperature in the elderly: a national study of physiological, social and environmental conditions. *Br Med J*. 1973;1:200.

33. Wagner JA, Robinson S, Marino RP. Age and temperature regulation in humans in neutral and cold environments. *J Appl Physiol*. 1974;37:562.

34. Cooper KE. Hypothermia. In: Strauss RH, ed. *Diving Medicine*. New York: Grune & Stratton; 1976.

35. Raymond LW. Temperature regulation in helium-oxygen atmosphere. *Lancet*. 1975;1:807.

36. Webb P. Thermal problems in diving. *The Sixth Undersea Medical Society Workshop*. Bethesda, MD: Undersea Medical Society; 1974.

37. Aschoff J, Wever R. Kern und Schale im Warme Haushalt des Menschen. *Naturwissenschaften*. 1958;20:477.

38. Cooper KE. Regulation of body temperature. *Br J Hosp Med*. 1969;2:1064.

39. Aherne W, Hull D. Brown adipose tissue and heat production in the newborn infant. *J Pathol Bacteriol*. 1966;91:223.

40. Perlstein PH, et al. Adaptation to the cold in the first three days of life. *Pediatrics*. 1974;54:411.

41. Hemingway A. Shivering. *Physiol Rev*. 1963;41:397.

42. Iampietra PF, et al. Heat production from shivering. *J Appl Physiol*. 1960;15:632.

43. O'Hara VS. Hypothermia (a four letter word). Presented at the Sixth International Conference on Underwater Education; October 1974; San Diego, CA.

44. Wedin AB. Cases of parodoxical undressing by people exposed to severe hypothermia. In: Shepard RJ, Itoh S, eds. *Circumpolar Health*. Toronto: Toronto University Press; 1976;61–71.

45. Gagge AP, Herrington LP. Physiological effects of heat and cold. *Annu Rev Physiol*. 1947;9:409.

46. Black PS, Vandevanter S, Cohn LH. Current research review: effects of hypothermia on systemic and organ system metabolism and function. *J Surg Res*. 1976;20:49.

47. Cooper KE, Martin S, Riben P. Respiratory and other responses in subjects immersed in cold water. *J Appl Physiol*. 1976;40:903.

48. Deal CW, Warden JC, Monk I. Effects of hypothermia on lung compliance. *Thorax*. 1970;25:105.

49. Coniam SW. Accidental hypothermia. *Anesthesia*. 1979;34:250.

50. Bradley AF, Stumpfel M, Severinghaus JW. Effects of temperature on pCO_2 and pO_2 of blood in vitro. *J Appl Physiol*. 1956;9:201.

51. Miller JW, Danzl DF, Thomas DM. Urban accidental hypothermia: 135 cases. *Ann Emerg Med*. 1980;9:456.

52. Kelvin GR, Nunn GF. Nomogram for the correction of blood pO_2, pCO_2, pH and base excess for time and temperature. *J Appl Physiol*. 1966;21:1484.

53. Rosenthal TB. Effect of temperature on the pH of blood and plasma in vitro. *J Biol Chem*. 1948;173:25.

54. Severinghaus JW, Stupfel M, Bradley AF. Variations of serum carbonate acid pK^1 with pH and temperature. *J Appl Physiol*. 1956; 9:197.

55. Duguid H, Simpson RG, Stowers JM. Accidental hypothermia. *Lancet*. 1961;2:1213.

56. Irvine RE. Hypothermia. *Mod Geriatr*. 1973;3:464.

57. Maclean D, Morison J, Griffiths PD. Acute pancreatitis and diabetic ketoacidosis in accidental hypothermia and myxodema. *Br Med J*. 1973;4:757.

58. Mills GL. Management of hypothermia in the elderly. Presented at the First World Congress on Intensive Care; June 24–27, 1974; London, England.

59. Petersdorf RG, et al. Study of antibiotic prophylaxis in unconscious patients. *N Engl J Med*. 1957;257:1001.

60. Naizi SA, Lewis FJ. Profound hypothermia in man: report of a case. *Ann Surg*. 1958;147:264.

61. Bigelow WG, Lindsay WK, Greenwood WF. Hypothermia: possible rate in cardiac surgery. *Ann Surg*. 1959;132:948.

62. Fleming PR, Muir FH. Electrocardiographic changes in induced hypothermia in man. *Br Heart J*. 1957;19:59.

63. Gross E, Brockhoff F, Schoedel W. Das Bild der Akuten Unterkuhlung im Tier-Experiment. *Naunyn-Schmiedeberges Arch Exp Pathol Pharmakol*. 1943;201:417.

64. Hicks CE, McCord MC, Blount SG. Electrocardiographic changes associated with hypothermia and circulatory occlusion. *Clin Res Proc*. 1955;3:107.

65. Keatinge WR. *Survival in Cold Water: Physiology and Treatment of Immersion Hypothermia and Drowning*. Philadelphia: Lippincott; 1969.

66. MacLean D, Griffiths PD, Emslie-Smith D. Serum-enzymes in relation to electrocardiographic changes in accidental hypothermia. *Lancet*. 1968;2:1266.

67. Tofler OB. Electrocardiographic changes during profound hypothermia. *Br Heart J*. 1962;24:265.

68. Tysinger DS, Grace JT, Gollan F. Electrocardiogram of dogs surviving 1.5°C. *Am Heart J*. 1955;50:816.

69. Wynne NA, Fuller JA, Szekely P. Electrocardiographic changes in hypothermia. *Br Heart J*. 1960;22:642.

70. Gunton RW, Scott JW, Lougheed WM, et al. Changes in cardiac rhythm and in form of electrocardiogram resulting from induced hypothermia in man. *Am Heart J*. 1956;52:419.

71. Hervey GR. Physiologic changes encountered in hypothermia. *Proc R Soc Med*. 1973;66:1053.

72. Hicks CE, McCord MC, Blount SG. Electrocardiographic changes during hypothermia and circulatory occlusion. *Circulation*. 1956;13:21.

73. Okada M. The cardiac rhythm in accidental hypothermia. *J Electrocardiogr*. 1984;17:123.

74. Okada M, Nishimura F, Yoshino H, et al. The J wave in hypothermia. *J Electrocardiogr*. 1983;16:23.

75. Rothfield EL. Hypothermic hump. *JAMA*. 1970;213:626.

76. Trevino A, Razi B, Beller BM. The characteristic electrocardiogram of accidental hypothermia. *Arch Intern Med*. 1970;127:470.

77. Tomaszewski W. Changements electrocardiographiques observes chez un homme mort de froid. *Arch Mal Coeur Vaisseaux Sang*. 1938;31:525.

78. Osburn JJ. Hypothermia: respiratory and blood pH changes in relation to cardiac function. *Am J Physiol*. 1953;175:389–398.

79. Kennedy WL. Letter to the editor. *Ann Intern Med*. 1980;90:721.

80. Deswit J. Changes simulating hypothermia in the EKG in subarachnoid hemorrhage. *J Electrocardiol*. 1972;5:193.

81. Maclean D, Emslie Smith D. The J-loop of spatial vectorcardiogram in accidental hypothermia in man. *Br Heart J*. 1974;36:621.

82. Covino BG, D'Amato HE. Mechanism of ventricular fibrillation in hypothermia. *Circ Res*. 1962;10:148.

83. Lloyd EL, Mitchell B. Factors affecting the onset of ventricular fibrillation in hypothermia. *J Thorac Cardiovasc Surg*. 1965;49:937.

84. Mouritzen CV, Anderson MN. Mechanism of ventricular fibrillation during hypothermia. *J Thorac Cardiovasc Surg*. 1966;51:585.
85. Swan H, Virtue RW, Blount SG, et al. Hypothermia in surgery. Analysis of 100 clinical cases. *Ann Surg*. 1955;142:382.
86. Rittenhouse EA, Ito DX, Mohri H, et al. Circulatory dynamics during surface induced hypothermia after one hour of cardiac arrest. *J Thorac Cardiovasc Surg*. 1981;61:359.
87. Berne RM. Cardiac dynamics and coronary circulation in hypothermia. *Ann NY Acad Sci*. 1959;80:365.
88. Berne RM. Myocardial function in severe hypothermia. *Circ Res*. 1954;2:90.
89. Kohn LA, Turner JK. Alterations in pulmonary and peripheral vascular resistance in immersion hypothermia. *Circ Res*. 1959;7:366.
90. Eiseman B, Spencer FC. Effects of hypothermia on the flow characteristics of blood. *Surgery*. 1962;52:532.
91. Kanter GS. Hypothermic hemoconcentration. *Am J Physiol*. 1968;214:856.
92. Lofstrom B. Changes in blood volume in induced hypothermia. *Acta Anaesthesiol Scand*. 1957;1:1.
93. Zarins CK, Skinner DB. Circulation in profound hypothermia. *J Surg Res*. 1973;14:97.
94. Felicetta JV, Green WL, Goodner CJ. Decreased adrenal responsiveness in hypothermic patients. *J Clin Endocrinol Metab*. 1980;50:93.
95. Gale CC, Jobin M, Poppe DW, et al. Endocrine thermoregulatory response to isolated hypothalamic cooling in unanesthetized baboons. *Am J Physiol*. 1970;219:193.
96. Hume DM, Egdahl RH. Effect of hypothermia and of cold exposure on adrenal cortical and medullary secretion. *Ann NY Acad Sci*. 1959;80:435.
97. Johnson DG, et al. Plasma norepinephrine responses of man in cold water. *J Appl Physiol*. 1977;43:216.
98. Fruehan AE. Profound hypothermia. *Arch Intern Med*. 1960;106:218.
99. Matthews JA. Thyroid function in accidental hypothermia. *Postgrad Med J*. 1966;42:495.
100. Bernhard WF. The effect of hypothermia on the peripheral serum levels of free 17 hydroxycorticosteroids in the dog and in man. In: Dripps RD, ed. *The Physiology of Induced Hypothermia*. Washington, DC: National Academy of Science; 1956. National Research Council publication 451.
101. Sprunt JG, Maclean D, Browning MCK. Plasma corticosteroid levels in accidental hypothermia. *Lancet*. 1970;1:324.
102. Swan HE, Jenkins D, Helmreich ML. The adrenal cortical response to surgery. III. Changes in plasma and urinary corticosteroid levels during hypothermia in man. *Surgery*. 1957;42:202.
103. Curry DL, Curry KP. Hypothermia and insulin secretion. *Endocrinology*. 1970;87:750.
104. Cooper KE, Ross DN. *Hypothermia in Surgical Practice*. London: Cassell; 1960.
105. Woolf PD, Hollander CS, Mitsuma T, et al. Accidental hypothermia: endocrine function during recovery. *J Clin Endocrin Metab*. 1972;34:460.
106. Wynn V. Some problems of water metabolism following surgery. In: Stoner HB, ed. *Council for International Organizations of Medical Sciences Symposium: The Biological Response to Injury*. Philadelphia: Lippincott; 1960.
107. Morales P, Carbery W, Morello A, et al. Alterations in renal function during hypothermia in man. *Ann Surg*. 1957;145:488.
108. Page L, Kupsinel H, Adams J, et al. Effects of hypothermia on renal function. *Army Med Res Lab Rep*. 1954;152.
109. Segar WE, Riley PA, Barilla TG, et al. Urinary composition during hypothermia. *J Appl Physiol*. 1956;185:528.
110. Fitzgerald FT, Jessop C. Accidental hypothermia: a report of 22 cases and review of the literature. *Adv Intern Med*. 1982;27:127.
111. Laufman H. Profound accidental hypothermia. *JAMA*. 1951;147:1201.
112. Miller JW, Danzl DF. Accidental hypothermia: a survivor of 12 episodes. *J Emerg Med*. 1984;1:407.
113. Symbas PN, Byrd BF, Johnson JS, et al. Influence of hypothermia on pancreatic function. *Ann Surg*. 1961;154:589.
114. Weyman AE, Greenbaum DM, Grace WJ. Accidental hypothermia in an alcoholic population. *Am J Med*. 1974;56:13.
115. Brauer RW, Holloway RJ, Krebs JS, et al. The liver in hypothermia. *Ann NY Acad Sci*. 1959;80:395.
116. Fisher B, Fedor EJ, Lee SH, et al. Some physiological affects of short and long term hypothermia on the liver. *Surgery*. 1956;40:862.
117. Ehrmantraut WR, Tickten HE, Fazekras JF. Cerebral hemodynamics and metabolism in accidental hypothermia. *Arch Intern Med*. 1957;99:57.
118. Rosomoff HL. Pathophysiology of the central nervous system during hypothermia. *Acta Neurochir*. 1964;11(suppl).
119. Fischbeck KH, Simon RP. Neurological manifestations of accidental hypothermia. *Ann Neurol*. 1981;10:384.
120. Dawson H, Spaziani E. Effect of hypothermia on certain aspects of cerebral spinal fluid. *Exp Neurol*. 1962;6:118.
121. Bond TP, Derrick JR, Guess MM. Microcirculation during hypothermia. *Arch Surg*. 1964;89:887.
122. Best R, Syverud S, Nowak RM. Trauma and hypothermia. *Am J Emerg Med*. 1985;3:48.
123. Carden DL, Nowak RM. Disseminated intravascular coagulation in hypothermia. *JAMA*. 1982;247:2099.
124. Mahajan SL, Myers TJ, Baldini MG. Disseminated intravascular coagulation during rewarming following hypothermia. *JAMA*. 1981;245:2517.
125. Salmon PA, Griffen WO, Jensen CB, et al. The effect of hypothermia on intestinal motility. *Surgery*. 1959;46:873.
126. Hirvonin J. Necropsy findings in fatal hypothermia. *Forens Sci*. 1976;8:155.
127. Mant AK. The pathology of hypothermia. In: Simpson K, ed. *Modern Trends in Forensic Medicine*. London: Butterworth; 1967;2.
128. Mant AK. The postmortem diagnosis of hypothermia. *Br J Hosp Med*. 1969;2:1095.
129. Schneider V, Klug E. Tod durch Unterkuhlung. *Z Rechtsmed*. 1980;86:59.
130. Sloan REG, Keatinge WR. Depression of sublingual temperatures by cold saliva. *Br Med J*. 1978;1:718.
131. Of the refrigerant method, in treatment of nymphomania. *US Med Surg J*. 1836;2:323.
132. Danzl DF. Accidental hypothermia. In: Rosen P, ed. *Emergency Medicine, Concepts of Clinical Practice*. St Louis: Mosby; 1983;1.
133. Carden DL. Intubating the hypothermia patient. *Ann Emerg Med*. 1983;12:124.
134. Danzl DF, Thomas DM. Nasotracheal intubation in the emergency department. *Crit Care Med*. 1980;8:677.
135. Southwick FS, Dalglish PH. Recovery after prolonged asystolic cardiac arrest in profound hypothermia. *JAMA*. 1980;243:1250.
136. Guild WJ. Rewarming via the airway (CBRW) of hypothermia in the field? *J R Nav Med Serv*. 1978;64:186.
137. Harnett RM, Obrien EM, Sias FR, et al. Initial treatment of profound accidental hypothermia. *Aviat Space Environ Med*. 1980;51:680.

138. Ledingham IM, Douglas IHS, Routh GS, et al. Central rewarming system for treatment of hypothermia. *Lancet.* 1980;1:1168.
139. Lloyd ELL, Croxten D. Equipment for the provision of airway rewarming and the treatment of accidental hypothermia in patients. *Resuscitation.* 1981;9:61.
140. Lloyd EL, Conliffe NA, Orgel H, et al. Accidental hypothermia: an apparatus for central rewarming as a first aid measure. *Scott Med J.* 1972;17:83.
141. Bangs C, Hamlet M. Out in the cold—management of hypothermia, immersion and frostbite. *Top Emerg Med.* 1980;2:19.
142. Arnold JW, Eichenberger CH. The hydraulic sarong: emergency treatment device for accidental hypothermia. *JACEP.* 1975;4:438.
143. Marcus P. Laboratory comparison and techniques for rewarming hypothermic casualties. *Aviat Space Environ Med.* 1978;49:692.
144. Bangs C, Hamlet MP. Hypothermia and cold injuries. In: Auerbach P, ed. *Management of Wilderness and Environmental Emergencies.* New York: Macmillan; 1983.
145. Ledingham IM, Mone JG. Accidental hypothermia. *Lancet.* 1978;2:391.
146. Pontopidian H, Beecher HK. Progressive loss of protective reflexes in the airway with advances of age. *JAMA.* 1969;174:2209.
147. Tolman KG, Cohen A. Accidental hypothermia. *Can Med Assoc J.* 1970;103:1357.
148. Gillen JP, Vogel MFX, Holterman RK, et al. Ventricular fibrillation during oraltracheal intubation of hypothermic dogs. *Ann Emerg Med.* 1986;15:412.
149. Brantigan CO, Paton BC. Clinical hypothermia; accidental hypothermia and frostbite. In: Goldsmith HS, ed. *Lewis' Practice of Surgery.* New York: Harper & Row; 1978.
150. Gong B. Microwave warming of IV fluids in the management of hypothermia. *Ann Emerg Med.* 1984;13:645.
151. Bolooki H, et al. Comparison of the effect of low molecular weight dextran on blood flow and peripheral resistance during extracorporeal circulation and hypothermia. *J Thorac Cardiovasc Surg.* 1967;54:216.
152. Fukusumi H, Adolph RJ. Effect of dextran exchange upon the immersion hypothermic heart. *J Thorac Cardiovasc Surg.* 1976;59:251.
153. Grossman R, Lewis MJ. The effects of cooling and low molecular weight dextran on blood sludging. *J Surg Res.* 1964;4:360.
154. Long DM, Folkman MJ, McClenathan JE. The use of low molecular weight dextran in extracorporeal circulation: hypothermia and hypercapnia. *J Cardiovasc Surg.* 1963;4:617.
155. Arneil GC, Kerr MM. Severe hypothermia in Glasgow in infants in winter. *Lancet.* 1963;2:756.
156. Davies DM, Millar DM, Miller JA. Accidental hypothermia treated by extracorporeal blood warming. *Lancet.* 1967;1:1036.
157. Berger RL. Nazi science—the Dachau hypothermia experiments. *N Engl J Med.* 1990;322:1435–1440.
158. Angell M. The Nazi hypothermia experiments and unethical research today. *N Engl J Med.* 1990;322:1462–1464.
159. Danzl DF. Multicenter hypothermia survey. *Ann Emerg Med.* 1987;16:1042–1055.
160. Mills WJ. Summary of treatment of the cold injured patient. *Alaska Med.* 1973;15:56.
161. Paulley JW, et al. Old people in the cold. *Br Med J.* 1964;1:425.
162. Fernandez JP, O'Rourke RA, Ewy GA. Rapid external rewarming in accidental hypothermia. *JAMA.* 1970;212:513.
163. Gregory RT, Doolittle WH. Accidental hypothermia. Part II. Clinical implications of experimental studies. *Alaska Med.* 1973;15:48.
164. Zingg W. The management of accidental hypothermia. *Can Med Assoc J.* 1967;96:214.
165. Hudson LD, Conn RD. Accidental hypothermia. Associated diagnoses and prognosis in a common disorder. *JAMA.* 1974;227:37.
166. Frank DH, Robson MC. Accidental hypothermia treated without mortality. *Surg Obstet Gynecol.* 1980;151:379.
167. Freeman J, Pugh L. Hypothermia and mountain accidents. *Int Anesthesiol Clin.* 1969;7:997.
168. Golden FStC. Recognition and treatment of immersion hypothermia. *Proc R Soc Med.* 1973;66:1058.
169. Meriweather WD, Goodman RM. Severe accidental hypothermia with survival after rewarming. *Am J Med.* 1972;53:505.
170. Crino MH, Nagel EL. Thermal burns caused by warming blankets in the operating room. *Anesthesiology.* 1968;29:149.
171. Feldman KW, Morray JP, Schaller RT. Thermal injury caused by hot pack application in hypothermic children. *Am J Emerg Med.* 1985;3:38.
172. Mouritzen CV, Anderson MN. Myocardial temperature gradients and ventricular fibrillation during hypothermia. *J Thorac Cardiovasc Surg.* 1965;49:937.
173. Bristow G, Smith R, Lee J, et al. Resuscitation from cardiopulmonary arrest during accidental hypothermia due to exhaustion and exposure. *Can Med Assoc J.* 1977;117:247.
174. Hudson MC, Robinson GJB. Treatment of accidental hypothermia. *Med J Aust.* 1973;1:410.
175. Meyers RA, Britten JS, Cowley RA. Hypothermia: quantitative aspects of therapy. *JACEP.* 1979;8:523.
176. Lloyd ELL. Accidental hypothermia treated by central rewarming through the airway. *Br J Anaesth.* 1973;45:41.
177. Shields CP, Sixsmith DM. Treatment of moderate to severe hypothermia in the urban setting. *Ann Emerg Med.* 1990;19:1093–1097.
178. Bristow G. Treatment of accidental hypothermia with peritoneal dialysis. *Can Med Assoc J.* 1978;118:768.
179. Desmueles H, Blais C. Accidental hypothermia: treatment of a case using peritoneal irrigation. *Can Anaesth Soc J.* 1979;25:506.
180. Jessen K, Hagelsten JO. Peritoneal dialysis in the treatment of profound accidental hypothermia. *Aviat Space Environ Med.* 1978;49:426.
181. Johnson LA. Accidental hypothermia: peritoneal dialysis. *JACEP.* 1977;6:556.
182. Rueler JB, Parker RA. Peritoneal dialysis in the management of accidental hypothermia. *JAMA.* 1978;21:2289.
183. Soung LS, Swank L, Img TS, et al. Treatment of accidental hypothermia with peritoneal dialysis. *Can Med Assoc J.* 1977;117:1415.
184. Vaamonde CA, Michael UF, Metzger RA, et al. Complications of acute peritoneal dialysis. *J Chron Dis.* 1975;23:637.
185. Davis FM, Judfson JA. Warm peritoneal dialysis in the management of accidental hypothermia: report of five cases. *N Z Med J.* 1981;94:207.
186. Pickering BJ, Bristow GK, Craig DB. Case history 97—core rewarming by peritoneal irrigation in accidental hypothermia with cardiac arrest. *Anesth Analg.* 1977;56:574.
187. Althaus U, Aeberhard P, Schupbach P, et al. Management of profound accidental hypothermia with cardiorespiratory arrest. *Ann Surg.* 1982;195:492.
188. Fell RH, Gunning AJ, Bardhan KD, et al. Severe hypothermia as a result of barbiturate overdose complicated by cardiopulmonary arrest. *Lancet.* 1962;1:392.
189. Wickstrom P, Ruiz E, Lilja GP. Accidental hypothermia. Core rewarming with partial bypass. *Am J Surg.* 1976;131:622.

190. Danzl DF, et al. Chemical ventricular defibrillation in severe accidental hypothermia. *Ann Emerg Med.* 1982;11:698.

191. Dronen S, Nowak RM, Tomlanovich MC. Bretylium tosylate and hypothermic ventricular fibrillation. *Ann Emerg Med.* 1980;9:335.

192. Elenbaas RM, Mattson K, Cole H, et al. Bretylium in hypothermia induced ventricular fibrillation in dogs. *Ann Emerg Med.* 1984;13:994.

193. Buky B. Effect of magnesium on ventricular fibrillation due to hypothermia. *Br J Anaesth.* 1970;42:586.

194. Cox B. Dopamine. In: Lomax P, Schonbaum E, eds. *Body Temperature, Regulation, Drug Effects and Therapeutic Implications.* New York: Dekker; 1979.

195. Nicodemus HF, Chaney RD, Herold R. Hemodynamic effects of inotropes during hypothermia and rapid rewarming. *Crit Care Med.* 1981;9:325.

196. Webb WR, Harrison N, Dodds R, et al. Protective effect of ethyl alcohol in profound hypothermia. *Cryobiology.* 1968;4:290.

197. Gregory RT, Patton JF. Treatment after exposure to cold. *Lancet.* 1972;1:377.

198. Adelstein AM. Certification of hypothermia deaths. *Br Med J.* 1973;851:482.

199. Quintella RF, Krusen H, Essex HE. Studies on frostbite with special reference to treatment and the effect on minute blood vessels. *Am J Physiol.* 1947;149:149.

200. Weatherly-White RCA, Sjostrom B, Paton BC. Experimental studies in cold injury: II. The pathogenesis of frostbite. *J Surg Res.* 1969;4:17.

201. Hanson HE, Goldman RF. Cold injury in man: review of its etiology and discussion of its prediction. *Mil Med.* 1969;134:1307.

202. Bangs CC. Hypothermia and frostbite. *Emerg Clin North Am.* 1984;2:475.

203. Wray RC. Cold injury. In: Zuidema GD, ed. *Management of Trauma.* 3rd ed. Philadelphia: Saunders; 1979.

204. Mills WJ. Summary of treatment of this cold injured patient. Presented at the *Winter Sports Medicine Course;* February 14–21, 1981; Sun Valley, ID.

205. Porter JM. Intra-arterial sympathetic blockade in the treatment of clinical frostbite. *Am J Surg.* 1976;132:625.

206. Lange K, Loewe L. Subcutaneous heparin in the Pitkin menstruum for the treatment of experimental human frostbite. *Surg Obstet Gynecol.* 1946;82:256.

207. Crimson JM. Science in World War II advances. In: *Military Medicine.* Boston: Little, Brown; 1948.

208. Schumacher HB, et al. Studies in experimental frostbite—the effect of heparin in preventing gangrene. *Surgery.* 1947;22:900.

209. Theis FV, O'Connor WR, Wahl FJ. Anticoagulants in acute frostbite. *JAMA.* 1951;146:992.

210. McCauley RH, Hing DN, Robson MC, et al. Frostbite injuries: a rational approach based on the pathophysiology. *J Trauma.* 1983;23:143.

211. Talwar JR, Gulati SM. Nonsteroid anti-inflammatory agents in the management of cold injury. *J Med Res.* 1972;60:1643.

212. Weatherly-White RCA, Paton BC, Sjostrom BL. Experimental studies in cold injury III. Observation on the treatment of frostbite. *Plast Reconstr Surg.* 1965;36:10.

213. Golding MR, Martinez A, deJong P, et al. The role of sympathectomy in frostbite with a review of 68 cases. *Surgery.* 1965;59:774.

214. Mills WJ. Frostbite. A discussion of the problem and a review of an Alaskan experience. *Alaska Med.* 1973;15:27.

215. Mills WJ. Summary of treatment of cold injured patients. *Alaska Med.* 1973;15:56.

216. Schumacker H. Sympathetic interruption in cases of trauma. *Surg Obstet Gynecol.* 1947;84:739.

217. Schumacker HB. Sympathectomy in the treatment of frostbite. *Surg Obstet Gynecol.* 1951;93:727.

42. Altitude-Related Emergencies

MARK A. SELLAND, MD
PETER H. HACKETT, MD

Human residence at high altitude predates the beginning of written history, yet only during the past two centuries has there developed an awareness of the syndromes of maladaptation to high altitude. One of the earliest written descriptions of the effects of high altitude exposure was made in 1590 by a Jesuit priest, Jose de Acosta.[1] While traveling over a 3700-m high pass in Peru, Father de Acosta noted ". . . the element of air is there so subtle and delicate, as it is not proportionable with the breathing of man, which requires a more gross and temperate air. . . ."[1(p14)] Nearly three centuries later, the French physiologist Paul Bert discovered that the administration of oxygen alleviated the symptoms of high altitude sickness. In *La Pression Barometrique*,[2] he described the relationship between hypoxia and decreasing barometric pressure and their role in altitude-related symptoms. These observations were based on his experiments with a decompression chamber to simulate high altitude. In 1913, T.H. Ravenhill[3] published one of the first clinical accounts of mountain sickness, including descriptions of pulmonary and cerebral forms as separate entities, what are now recognized as high altitude pulmonary and cerebral edema.

The medical problems of high altitude have long fascinated respiratory physiologists and are being seen more often by practicing physicians. Caring for the person (usually young and otherwise healthy) with high altitude–related medical problems, which are often rapid in onset and potentially fatal, can be rewarding for the physician who is able to recognize and treat them appropriately.

THE HIGH-ALTITUDE ENVIRONMENT

There is no clear threshold at which altitude illness occurs, but for the purpose of discussing altitude-related illnesses it is relevant to define various altitudes. Colorado and Utah ski resorts, which are located at intermediate altitude (1500 to 3000 m), are popular destinations for low-altitude visitors and have a reported incidence of mountain sickness of 12% to 25%.[4,5] High-altitude regions (3000 to 5500 m) of the world are also accessible to large numbers of people. The Himalayan Kingdom of Nepal issued more than 140,000 trekking permits during a 3-year period from 1984 to 1987; many of these trekkers ventured to altitudes higher than 4000 meters in remote areas far removed from medical care.[6] The summit of Pikes Peak, Colorado (4300 m), which is accessible by automobile, is reached by thousands of visitors each year. At these elevations, oxygen saturation falls below 90%, and the incidence of mountain sickness approaches 50% with overnight exposure. Elevations above 5500 m constitute extreme altitude, which is above the highest level of human inhabitation. At this point, physical deterioration is progressive and exceeds the capacity to acclimatize.[7] Individuals exposed to these altitudes are primarily mountaineers and aviators.

The physiologic stress that occurs at high altitude is due to hypobaric hypoxia. With increasing altitude, oxygen concentration remains constant (21%), but there is a fall in barometric pressure and a resultant decrease in inspired

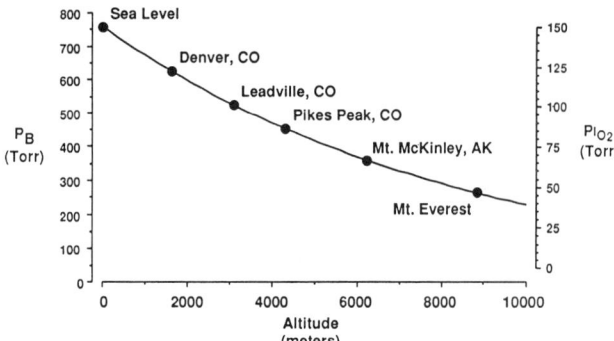

Figure 42-1 Relationship among barometric pressure (P_B), altitude, and inspired oxygen tension (P_{IO_2}).

oxygen tension (Fig. 42-1). In addition to hypoxia, the high-altitude environment places other stresses on the traveler, trekker, skier, and mountaineer. With every 300-m gain in altitude above 3000 m there is a 2°C decrease in temperature. Cold and hypoxia may interact, with hypothermia sometimes being mistaken for acute mountain sickness. Higher insensitive water losses associated with increased ventilation and acclimatization lead to increased water demand and potential dehydration. Through behavioral adaptation, such as the selection of appropriate food, clothing, and shelter, individuals can protect themselves from harsh environments. Adaptation to the diminished oxygen supply at high altitude, however, requires a series of innate physiologic adjustments directed at improving oxygen delivery to the tissues.

ADAPTIVE CHANGES ALONG THE OXYGEN TRANSPORT CHAIN

Effect of High Altitude on Respiration

Within hours of one's arriving at altitude, the process of acclimatization begins.[8] The most important adaptive response is a progressive increase in ventilation over the first few days. This hypoxic ventilatory response is driven by sensitive chemoreceptors located in the carotid body, a highly vascular structure capable of stimulating the central respiratory center in response to changes in arterial oxygenation.[9] This leads to an increase in alveolar oxygen tension and arterial oxygenation at the expense of lowering carbon dioxide, resulting in respiratory alkalosis. The initial increase in ventilation is limited, to some degree, by the respiratory depressant effect of a low arterial carbon dioxide tension (P_{CO_2}).[10] As acclimatization occurs, the renal excretion of bicarbonate increases, partially compensating for the alkalosis and allowing ventilation to increase further.[11]

Generally, persons with a high hypoxic ventilatory response perform better at altitude than those with a blunted response.[12,13] The hyperventilatory response can be extreme, as was demonstrated during the American Medical Research Expedition to Mt Everest in 1981. Measured expired carbon dioxide was approximately 7 torr on the summit (8848 m).[14] Without this degree of hyperventilation, the estimated arterial oxygen tension of 28 torr would have been nearly zero. The ability to increase ventilation is important for the sojourner as well as the elite mountaineer. Individuals who develop acute mountain sickness (AMS) tend to have a smaller hypoxic drive and a lower minute ventilation, higher levels of carbon dioxide, and lower oxygen saturations compared with asymptomatic individuals at the same altitude.[15,16]

Effect of High Altitude on the Pulmonary Circulation and Gas Exchange

The efficient exchange of oxygen and carbon dioxide in the lungs is dependent upon two major components: adequate matching of alveolar ventilation with perfusion (V/Q ratio), and the passive diffusion of gases across the alveolar membrane into the pulmonary capillaries. At rest, V/Q ratio and diffusion capacity are unchanged at altitudes up to 5000 m despite increases in ventilation and higher pulmonary artery pressures, which increase perfusion of the well-ventilated but normally underperfused upper lung zones.[17] When extremes of altitude or heavy exercise are encountered, however, abnormalities of V/Q and diffusion occur, and the alveolar-arterial oxygen gradient widens.[17-19] Impairment of gas exchange under these conditions appears to correlate with the degree of pulmonary hypertension and may be a result of interstitial edema formation; the exact mechanism is unclear, however.[19]

Effect of High Altitude on the Renal System

In response to the respiratory alkalosis, the kidneys increase bicarbonate excretion after 1 to 3 days at approximately 3000 m and with each incremental gain in altitude. The loss of bicarbonate, which is associated with an increase in urine output, permits further reduction in arterial carbon dioxide despite an increased pH. Fluid shifts from the extracellular to the intracellular space and accompanying decreases in plasma volume are associated with an increase in hematocrit, higher serum osmolality, and resetting of the osmoregulatory system, including paradoxic suppression of aldosterone and antidiuretic hormone (ADH) levels.[20,21] Fluid retention and antidiuresis, which occur with impaired acclimatization and AMS, may be related to increases in aldosterone and ADH.[15,22,23]

Hematologic Response to High Altitude

After ascent levels of 2,3-diphosphoglycerate (2,3-DPG) rapidly increase within red cells.[24] This shifts the oxyhemoglobin dissociation curve to the right, favoring the release of oxygen from hemoglobin into the tissues. Within the first few days after ascent, however, an increase in pH secondary to hyperventilation shifts the oxyhemoglobin dissociation curve to the left. This increases the binding affinity of hemoglobin for oxygen, increasing oxygen uptake in the lung. The net result is that 2,3-DPG balances the effects of respiratory alkalosis, so that there is no significant change in the oxyhemoglobin dissociation curve after acclimatization.

Erythropoietin production in the kidney also increases, with peak erythropoietin levels being found in the blood as early as 12 to 48 hours after ascent.[25,26] This results in an increase in hemoglobin production and red cell mass after several days to weeks at altitude. This adaptive response offsets, to some degree, the reduction in arterial saturation by increasing the oxygen-carrying capacity of the blood.

Effect of High Altitude on the Cardiovascular Response

Upon initial ascent, cardiac output increases as a result of an increase in heart rate. Several days later, stroke volume decreases in association with a reduction in plasma volume.[27] Heart rate usually remains elevated at altitude, but it does not compensate completely for the decline in stroke volume, resulting in a decreased cardiac output compared with comparable workloads at low altitude.[28] The heart performs well even at extreme altitude, as was demonstrated during Operation Everest II, a simulated ascent to 8848 m in a hypobaric chamber, which showed no hypoxic depression of myocardial contractility or heart rate during rest and exercise.[29] There is limited information about the effects of hypoxia on systemic blood pressure, but the observed increases are minimal. Dysrhythmias during acute altitude exposure are uncommon.

SYNDROMES OF MALADAPTATION TO HIGH ALTITUDE

Unacclimatized lowlanders who travel above 2500 m are most susceptible to the acute forms of altitude illness. Three major clinical entities exist: AMS, high-altitude pulmonary edema (HAPE), and high-altitude cerebral edema (HACE). These syndromes, often having overlapping features and variable severity, are best considered as a spectrum of disease arising from a common exposure.

AMS

Clinical Presentation

AMS may occur within 4 to 24 hours of ascent to altitude. The clinical presentation includes headache, insomnia, nausea, lassitude, anorexia, dizziness, shortness of breath, and decreased urine output.[22,30–32] Persons with AMS often point to the similarity between their symptoms and those of an alcohol hangover. Dehydration, hypothermia, exhaustion, and carbon monoxide poisoning can cause similar symptoms and should be considered in the differential diagnosis of AMS.

Headache, the most common symptom of mountain sickness, is typically a pounding frontal headache that is usually worse in the morning and with activity. The etiology of altitude headaches may be hypoxia-induced vasodilation of cerebral vessels or increased intracranial pressure, but the mechanism is unclear. Edema of the face and extremities may develop, more often in women, and suggests an inadequate diuresis.[33] The presence of edema without any other symptoms of AMS is considered benign. As acclimatization improves, the edema resolves.

Moderate AMS is characterized by the progression of symptoms, for example a headache unrelieved with nonnarcotic analgesics, nausea with vomiting, and the development of ataxia. Lassitude may impair the performance of routine activities. Exercise intolerance is often out of proportion to that of other members in the group, leading to frequent rests and slow recovery.

The most important risk factors for developing AMS are rate of ascent, altitude gained, and level of acclimatization.[34] Individual acclimatization is variable and cannot be reliably predicted by medical examination or testing before going to altitude. The incidence of AMS does not appear to correlate with age or gender, although children and men may be predisposed to the development of HAPE.[35,36] An individual's level of physical conditioning appears to be unrelated to the ability to acclimatize to high altitude. Well-conditioned athletes often ascend at faster rates than deconditioned individuals, however, which may predispose them to AMS.

As a general guideline, individuals traveling from sea level should spend at least one night at an intermediate altitude before continuing on to higher elevations. Their first day at altitude should be leisurely with minimal exertion. Alcoholic beverages, sleeping aids, and narcotics should be avoided because of the respiratory depression they may cause. A recommended rate of ascent for mountaineers is 300 m/day with a minimum of two nights for every 1000 m above 3000 m.[37] Groups should ascend no faster than the rate at which the slowest member feels well. Individuals with a history of mountain sickness have a tendency for recurrence at a given altitude and should be advised to follow a conservative ascent rate.

Pathophysiology of AMS

AMS is primarily a cerebral syndrome whose features overlap with early or mild forms of HACE, which has led to speculation regarding a common pathophysiologic mechanism. Proposed etiologies for cerebral edema formation include increased cerebral blood flow in response to hypoxic cerebral vasodilatation, which overrides the vasoconstricting effect of a low arterial P_{CO_2}, with overperfusion of capillaries and increased permeability or filtration at the blood-brain barrier.[38] This is often referred to as vasogenic edema. An alternative theory is that hypoxia causes cellular injury, perhaps by damaging the adenosine triphosphate–dependent sodium pump, leading to intracellular (cytotoxic) edema.[39]

Treatment of AMS

The treatment of AMS depends upon the severity of symptoms (Table 42-1). Mild AMS is usually a self-limited illness that improves rapidly with descent. It is not always necessary to descend when symptoms are mild, however; rest and additional acclimatization at the same altitude are often sufficient therapy. The treatment of an altitude headache with nonnarcotic analgesics, such as aspirin or acetaminophen (Tylenol), and rest usually leads to improvement. The empiric use of antiemetics (eg, prochlorperazine or promethazine) may provide symptomatic relief of nausea and allow continued oral hydration. Further ascent should be discontinued until all symptoms of AMS resolve.

The recommended treatment for progressive or moderate AMS is immediate descent.[32,37,40] A descent of as little as 300 to 500 m may result in rapid improvement. Oxygen, if available, is also effective therapy. Low flow rates are usually sufficient to provide symptomatic improvement and will conserve often limited supplies. After recovery at a lower altitude, it is generally safe to ascend again at a rate that allows for adequate acclimatization.

Several pharmacologic agents have been used for the treatment of AMS with variable degrees of success.[41] The corticosteroid dexamethasone (Decadron) has been shown effectively to reduce the symptoms of AMS, although its exact mechanism of action is still unclear.[42,43] It is not recommended for the prophylaxis of AMS because of the unnecessary risk of side effects associated with steroid therapy, but it is effective treatment in emergency situations preceding descent. Treatment with dexamethasone is complicated by the tendency for symptoms to recur after withdrawal of the drug if the patient remains at high altitude.[44]

Acetazolamide (Diamox), a mild diuretic and respiratory stimulant, has been shown to be effective for the prophylaxis of AMS but has not been adequately studied in terms of its efficacy in the treatment of AMS.[45,46] Anecdotal reports, however, suggest that acetazolamide (125 to 250 mg twice a day) reduces the symptoms of mild to moderate AMS. This drug is a carbonic anhydrase inhibitor that decreases the reabsorption of bicarbonate in the kidneys and causes increased bicarbonate excretion and a mild decline in pH, similar to the natural adaptive response in the kidneys. Ventilation increases in response to the lower pH, resulting in improved arterial oxygenation. Acetazolamide also lowers cerebrospinal fluid production and intracranial pressure, which may contribute to its effectiveness in preventing AMS.[47]

Acetazolamide prophylaxis is recommended for individuals making rapid passive ascents above 3000 m (eg, search and rescue personnel flying to high altitude), individuals with a history of recurrent AMS who are planning to travel to altitude, and individuals with periodic breathing during sleep.[41] The recommended dosage is 125 to 250 mg twice a day beginning on the day before ascent and continuing for 2 to 3 days at altitude. Abrupt discontinuation of the drug does not appear to worsen symptoms.[48] Side effects are common, with paresthesias and nausea being most prevalent. Acetazolamide has a sulfa component and is contraindicated in individuals with a history of sulfa sensitivity.

Recently, a portable fabric hyperbaric chamber that is pressurized with a small foot pump has been developed for the treatment of mountain sickness.[49] It can be pressurized up to 110 torr, providing a physiologic descent of approximately 1500 m. Because of its portability, reusability, and effectiveness, this type of chamber has been placed in Hima-

Table 42-1 Treatment of AMS Based on Severity of Illness

Type of Illness	Treatment
Mild AMS	Stop ascent May stay at same altitude as long as symptoms are not progressive Symptomatic treatment with nonnarcotic analgesics and antiemetics Rest and adequate hydration Acetazolamide (125 to 250 mg twice a day) to speed acclimatization
Moderate AMS	Immediate descent for worsening symptoms Low-flow oxygen if available Acetazolamide (250 mg twice a day) or dexamethasone (4 mg every 6 hours) Hyperbaric therapy
HAPE	Immediate descent or evacuation Oxygen Nifedipine (10 mg orally or sublingually every 6 hours) as long as blood pressure remains stable Hyperbaric therapy Continuous positive airway pressure mask Minimal exertion, warmth
HACE	Immediate descent or evacuation Oxygen Dexamethasone (8 mg orally or intravenously, then 4 mg every 6 hours) Hyperbaric therapy
Periodic breathing Periodic breathing during sleep or nocturnal periodic breathing	Acetazolamide (62.5 to 125.0 mg as needed at bedtime)

layan Rescue Association clinics in Nepal and used by high-altitude mountaineering expeditions; there are numerous anecdotal reports of its use in the successful treatment of cases of mountain sickness.[50]

Prevention, through gradual ascent, adequate hydration, and avoidance of respiratory depressants, is still the best form of treatment for mountain sickness. The early recognition of symptoms and appropriate intervention can prevent progression to the life-threatening forms.

HAPE

Clinical Presentation

HAPE is a life-threatening form of noncardiogenic pulmonary edema that may develop in healthy people. The symptoms of HAPE usually occur within 24 to 96 hours of arrival at high altitude. The characteristic presentation includes cough, dyspnea on exertion, and excessive fatigue.[51-53] The physical findings include tachypnea, cyanosis, and rales. In mild HAPE, rales are often inaudible or limited to the right midlung field.

As pulmonary congestion worsens, the individual develops dyspnea at rest, orthopnea, extreme weakness, productive cough, and altered mentation. HAPE may be difficult to differentiate from more common conditions characterized by cough and shortness of breath, such as pulmonary infection, asthma, and congestive heart failure. Neurologic manifestations including headache, vomiting, ataxia, and altered mentation may occur.[52] Untreated, HAPE can progress to florid pulmonary edema with frothy sputum, respiratory failure, and death.

The diagnosis of HAPE is based on the degree of exertional dyspnea, presence of rales, and cyanosis. Chest radiographs, if available, typically show dilatation of the central pulmonary arteries, asymmetric peripheral infiltrates, and a normal cardiac silhouette.[51,54] The electrocardiogram often shows sinus tachycardia and changes consistent with pulmonary hypertension such as right axis deviation, peaked P waves, and a prominent R wave in aVR and V_1.[51,55]

The incidence of HAPE varies from 0.01% to 15% of individuals depending upon rate of ascent, degree of physical activity, and level of acclimatization.[51,56] Observations from Vail, Colorado (2500 m) have shown a higher prevalence among adult male (10 per 100,000) compared to female visitors (0.74 per 100,000).[56] The reason for a higher incidence in men is unclear. Another subset of patients have what is characterized as reentry HAPE.[36] A study done in Leadville, Colorado (3100 m) showed an increased incidence of HAPE among individuals normally residing at high altitude who returned from a brief sojourn to low altitude (less than 2200 m).[35] Their stay at low altitude was as short as 24 hours in some cases. Of the 32 patients studied, 25 were younger than 16 years old, suggesting greater susceptibility to reentry HAPE in children. Finally, individuals with unilateral absence of a pulmonary artery (an uncommon condition) have a strong predisposition for developing HAPE.[57] The presentation of HAPE with unilateral infiltrates on chest radiograph should prompt a diagnostic workup to rule out obstruction or absence of a pulmonary artery.[58]

Pathophysiology of HAPE

HAPE often occurs in fit individuals with no history of cardiac disease. It is a noncardiogenic edema characterized hemodynamically by pulmonary hypertension with normal left ventricular function and normal pulmonary capillary wedge pressures.[59] Proposed mechanisms for the elevated pulmonary artery pressure include hypoxic pulmonary vasoconstriction, excessive circulating catecholamines, and the presence of various vasoactive mediators.[60] In addition to pulmonary hypertension, there is evidence to suggest increased pulmonary capillary permeability. Analysis of bronchoalveolar lavage fluid from individuals with HAPE reveals a large quantity of high–molecular weight proteins, suggesting the presence of a capillary leak.[61] One hypothesis is that uneven hypoxic vasoconstriction of the pulmonary arterioles may lead to overdistension of a portion of the pulmonary capillary bed, impairing endothelial integrity and causing increased permeability.[55,62]

Treatment of HAPE

The treatment of HAPE is directed at improving arterial oxygenation. Any patient with recognizable symptoms of HAPE should descend to a lower altitude. Severe cases with productive cough, marked fatigue, and shortness of breath at rest often require evacuation. Oxygen, if available, should be administered at high flow rates. Oxygen therapy results in improved arterial oxygenation, decreased pulmonary artery pressure, and improved clinical symptoms.[31,53]

A study evaluating 1 to 2 days of bedrest as the only therapy for HAPE in high-altitude residents in Peru showed a significant improvement in symptoms.[63] Both physical exertion and cold exposure heighten the catecholamine response, increasing pulmonary artery pressure and worsening gas exchange.[65] Therefore, bedrest and warmth can be beneficial. Descent and oxygen, in addition to rest and supportive care, are usually sufficient therapy for the majority of patients with HAPE. High-altitude residents with reentry HAPE respond rapidly to oxygen and rest and seldom require descent.[35]

The role of pharmacologic agents in the treatment of HAPE is limited.[53,55] Conventional drugs used to treat cardiogenic pulmonary edema, such as morphine and furosemide (Lasix), are rarely necessary. Indiscriminate diuresis with furosemide may worsen hypovolemia, which is often present in severe HAPE, and may cause hypotension and syncope.[65] Acetazolamide and dexamethasone (Decadron) have not been adequately studied in the treatment of HAPE. Recent studies of nifedipine (Procardia), a calcium-channel antagonist, show improved clinical symptoms, decreased pulmonary hypertension, increased arterial oxygen saturation, and partial resolution of pulmonary infiltrates.[66–68] Until further studies can be performed, the usage of nifedipine should be reserved for extreme emergencies in conjunction with descent.

The use of a continuous positive airway pressure (CPAP) mask as a temporizing measure when descent or oxygen therapy is delayed should be considered.[69] CPAP decreases airway collapse and air trapping, increasing functional residual capacity and improving gas exchange.

Early recognition of the symptoms of HAPE and appropriate therapy will often result in rapid recovery. Fatal cases of HAPE occur when the diagnosis is not made promptly, when descent is delayed, and when oxygen therapy is unavailable. Once an individual has completely recovered, it is often safe to reascend at a rate allowing for adequate acclimatization.

HACE

HACE is an uncommon but extremely severe form of AMS capable of causing coma and death. The clinical presentation includes severe headache, nausea, vomiting, ataxia, and altered levels of consciousness.[39,70,71] Focal neurologic deficits including paresthesias, scotoma, cranial nerve palsies, speech abnormalities, and sensorimotor changes may occur.[71] Ataxia, which is easily tested with the heel-to-toe walk, is present in a high percentage of HACE cases and is a useful indicator of cerebral dysfunction.[71] Reflexes may be hypoactive or hyperactive. Papilledema and retinal hemorrhages may be present upon fundoscopic examination. Mentation may range from irritability to coma.

Several theories regarding the pathogenesis of HACE exist, but the exact mechanism remains unknown. Necropsy results from cases of HACE showed edematous cerebral white matter and widespread hemorrhages.[70] Magnetic resonance imaging scans done recently on two mountain climbers with HACE showed changes consistent with vasogenic edema.[72] Although information is limited, these findings support the concept that hypoxia-induced vasodilatation and increased cerebral blood flow lead to overperfusion and edema formation.

Unrecognized and untreated, HACE may progress to coma and death, sometimes rapidly over a few hours. Initial therapy should be immediate descent to a lower altitude and administration of oxygen at high flow rates. Dexamethasone, an effective agent for the mild cerebral edema of AMS, may also be effective for the treatment of HACE, especially when given early.[7] The initial dose is 8 mg by mouth or injection with 4 mg every 6 hours thereafter until descent or evacuation is completed.

When neurologic disease occurs in healthy individuals at high altitude, it is often in a remote setting, far removed from sophisticated diagnostic equipment. Cerebral edema, the most common cause of severe neurologic symptoms at altitude, is capable of causing diverse and confusing presentations. Strokes, brain tumors, atypical migraine headaches, and Guillain-Barré syndrome have been known to occur or become symptomatic at altitude.[73,74] The differentiation between HACE and primary neurologic disorders may be difficult. Therefore, patients with neurologic symptoms presenting at altitude should undergo a complete neurologic evaluation after descent or evacuation to low altitude.

Other High Altitude–Related Disorders

Periodic Breathing During Sleep

The presence of periodic breathing in sleep, which is characterized by cyclic periods of apnea (Cheyne-Stokes respirations), is common above 4000 m.[75] During sleep at high altitude the respiratory alkalosis that results from increased ventilation inhibits respiratory drive, causing hypoventilation and, in extreme cases, brief periods of apnea. Hyperventilation follows, raising arterial oxygen saturation at the expense of worsening hypocapnea and increasing ventilatory inhibition. This cycle of hyperventilation alternating with hypoventilation or apnea continues throughout the night.

Individuals often complain of frequent waking, a sensation of suffocation, and daytime fatigue. It is not clear what effect periodic breathing has on acclimatization or the development of AMS, but it is generally not considered an indication to descend in the absence of other symptoms of mountain sickness. Interestingly, individuals with a high hypoxic ventilatory response, which is associated with better performance at altitude and a lower incidence of AMS, tend to have a greater incidence of periodic breathing during sleep.

Low doses of acetazolamide (62.5 to 125.0 mg) at bedtime, which stimulates ventilation by increasing bicarbonate excretion and lowering pH, will decrease the frequency of apnea, increase oxygen saturation, and improve the overall quality of sleep.[75–77] There is often great temptation to take sedatives for disturbed sleep. Sedatives, alcohol, and narcotics may further depress ventilation and should be avoided at altitude.

High-Altitude Retinal Hemorrhage

High-altitude retinal hemorrhages are a common occurrence above 4000 m. They may be found throughout the fundus but often spare the macula. Most hemorrhages are asymptomatic, producing no noticeable visual symptoms. Fundoscopic examination reveals tortuous dilated vessels and flame-shaped hemorrhages.[78] The mechanism for hemorrhage formation is unclear, but the pathogenesis may be similar to that of HACE. Hemorrhages involving the macular area with visual deficits are an indication for descent. The hemorrhages usually resolve spontaneously over 1 to 2 weeks, and permanent visual impairment is rare.[79]

Thromboembolic Disease

Cerebral thrombosis, deep vein thrombosis, and pulmonary emboli have all been reported to occur at high altitude. Little is known about their incidence or pathogenesis. Potentiating factors may include dehydration, polycythemia, and hyperviscosity. The treatment for such disorders includes descent and oxygen. After confirmation of the diagnosis, anticoagulation therapy may be initiated.

MEDICAL PROBLEMS AT HIGH ALTITUDE

Modern transportation has made high-altitude environments accessible to a large percentage of the general population. Physicians are often asked for an opinion regarding the safety of altitude exposure in patients with underlying medical conditions.

Persons with impaired gas exchange due to chronic lung disease often experience increased respiratory symptoms as a result of worsening hypoxia with exposure to high altitude. They often have disordered ventilatory drives and abnormal breathing during sleep, which exacerbates hypoxemia. Patients with chronic lung disease may require supplemental oxygen while at altitude. Interestingly, some patients will acually feel better at altitude because of the decreased work of breathing associated with a decrease in air density due to the lower barometric pressure.

Bronchospastic airway disease is often exacerbated by exposure to cold and exertion. Individuals with a history of asthma may develop cough, dyspnea, and wheezing during exercise in the cold, dry air of the mountain environment.[80] The prophylactic use of inhaled bronchodilators before physical activity may prevent wheezing.[81] The use of a face mask to warm inhaled air will decrease the risk of cold-induced bronchospasm.

The risk of a cardiac event in individuals with coronary artery disease who are going to altitude is unknown. Limited studies do not show a greater incidence of cardiac complications at altitude.[82] Initial exposure to high altitude is accompanied by a modest increase in heart rate, blood pressure, and cardiac output as a result of increased activity of the sympathetic nervous system.[83] During this period, exertion should be minimized. As the individual acclimatizes, physical activity may be increased to levels as tolerated. Advice to patients with ischemic heart disease about the risks of high-altitude activities should be based on the stability of their underlying disease.[83,84]

Sickle cell disease occurs in African-Americans who are homozygous for hemoglobin S. Under hypoxic conditions they can develop venoocclusive crises. High-altitude exposure can induce sickling of the red blood cells, resulting in decreased pliability and increased adherence to the endothelium and leading to painful infarcts within the microvasculature of the long bones and splenic, cerebral, pulmonary, and renal vessels.[85] Heterozygotes for hemoglobin S (sickle cell trait) do not usually experience sickle crises unless they have a concomitant hemoglobinopathy, such as hemoglobin SC or hemoglobin S–β-thalassemia. Splenic syndrome, characterized by acute left upper quadrant pain and splenic infarction on exposure to high altitude, may have a higher incidence in whites with sickle trait than in African-Americans.[86] The treatment of sickle cell crisis consists of oxygen and descent, analgesics for pain, and hydration to improve the microcirculation.

Little is known about the effects of acute or brief altitude exposure during pregnancy. There are more extensive data on the effects of continuous altitude exposure on pregnancy in high-altitude residents. Lower infant birth weights, elevated hematocrits, and a higher incidence of neonatal hyperbilirubinemia have been reported.[87] Pregnant women at altitude have a higher incidence of pregnancy-induced hypertension.[87] Until more information is available, pregnant women residing at low altitude should be advised to limit their exposure and to avoid sleeping at altitudes higher than 3000 m.

CHRONIC MOUNTAIN SICKNESS
(Monge's Disease)

Physicians practicing in a high-altitude setting may encounter patients with chronic mountain sickness (CMS). It is a disease of high-altitude dwellers characterized by headache, dyspnea, insomnia, and chronic fatigue.[88] CMS occurs primarily in men and is associated with a blunting of the hypoxic ventilatory response, resulting in chronic hypoxemia and excessive erythropoietin production. Polycythemia is the sine qua non, with hematocrits usually being in excess of 55% and occasionally as high as 80%. The treatment of CMS includes periodic phlebotomy, relocation to a lower altitude, and the use of respiratory stimulants (eg, medroxyprogesterone acetate).[89]

CONCLUSION

The number of people who experience altitude-related illnesses will continue to increase as high mountain regions of the world become increasingly accessible and popular places to live and visit. Physicians are seeing larger numbers of patients with environmental and travel-related medical problems in ambulatory and emergency care settings.

Most altitude illnesses are self-limited, but the severe forms of mountain sickness may present as life-threatening emergencies. In addition to emergency care, the physician may be asked to provide counseling to patients planning a sojourn to altitude. Improved patient knowledge of and ability to recognize the early symptoms of AMS may prevent many of the severe forms from occurring. As our understanding of how altitude affects human physiology expands, new therapies for altitude disorders will develop, and our knowledge of hypoxia-related illnesses in lowlanders will advance.

REFERENCES

1. de Acosta J, West JB, ed, Blount E, Aspley W, trans-eds. *The Naturall and Morall History of the East and West Indies*. Stroudsburg, PA: Hutchinson Ross Publishing; 1981:9–15.
2. Bert P, Hitchcock MA, Hitchcock FA, trans-eds. *La Pression Barometrique*. Columbus, OH: College Book Co; 1943.
3. Ravenhill TH. Some experiences of mountain sickness in the Andes. *J Trop Med Hyg*. 1913;16:313–320.
4. Houston CS. Incidence of acute mountain sickness. *Am Alp J*. 1985;27:162–165.
5. Montgomery AB, Mills J, Luce JM. Incidence of acute mountain sickness at intermediate altitude. *JAMA*. 1989;261:732–734.
6. Shlim DR, Houston R. Helicopter rescues and deaths among trekkers in Nepal. *JAMA*. 1989;261:1017–1019.
7. Hackett PH, Roach RC, Sutton JR. High altitude medicine. In: Auerbach P, Geehr E, eds. *Management of Wilderness and Environmental Emergencies*. St. Louis, MO: Mosby; 1984:1–34.
8. Lenfant C, Sullivan K. Adaptation to high altitude. *N Engl J Med*. 1971;284:1298–1309.
9. Schoene RB. Hypoxic ventilatory response and exercise ventilation at sea level and high altitude. In: West JB, Lahiri S, eds. *High Altitude and Man*. Bethesda, MD: American Physiological Society; 1984:19–30.
10. Huang SY, Alexander JK, Grover RF, et al. Hypocapnia and sustained hypoxia blunt ventilation on arrival at high altitude. *J Appl Physiol*. 1984;56:602–606.
11. Weil JV, Byrne-Quinn E, Sodal IE, et al. Evaluation of hypoxic ventilatory drive—findings at high altitude. *Adv Cardiol*. 1970;5:132–138.
12. Moore LG, Harrison GL, McCullough RE, et al. Low acute hypoxic ventilatory response in acute altitude sickness. *J Appl Physiol*. 1986;60:1407–1412.
13. Schoene RB, Lahiri S, Hackett PH, et al. Relationship of hypoxic ventilatory response to exercise performance on Mount Everest. *J Appl Physiol Respir Environ Exerc Physiol*. 1984;56:1478–1483.
14. West JB. Human physiology at extreme altitudes on Mt Everest. *Science*. 1984;223:784–788.
15. Hackett PH, Rennie D, Hofmeister SE, et al. Fluid retention and relative hypoventilation in acute mountain sickness. *Respiration*. 1982;43:321–329.
16. Matsuzawa Y, Fujimoto K, Kobayashi T, et al. Blunted hypoxic ventilatory drive in subjects susceptible to high-altitude pulmonary edema. *J Appl Physiol*. 1989;66:1152–1157.
17. Gale GE, Torre-Bueno JR, Moon RE, et al. Ventilation-perfusion inequality in normal humans during exercise at sea level and simulated altitude. *J Appl Physiol*. 1985;58:978–988.
18. Torre-Bueno JR, Wagner PD, Saltzman HA, et al. Diffusion limitation in normal humans during exercise at sea level and simulated altitude. *J Appl Physiol*. 1985;58:989–995.
19. Wagner PD, Sutton JR, Reeves JT, et al. Operation Everest II: pulmonary gas exchange during a simulated ascent of Mt Everest. *J Appl Physiol*. 1987;63:2348–2359.
20. Blume FD, Boyer SJ, Braverman LE, et al. Impaired osmoregulation at high altitude. *JAMA*. 1984;252:524–526.
21. Keynes RJ, Smith GW, Slater JDH, et al. Renin and aldosterone at high altitude in man. *J Endocrinol*. 1982;92:131–140.
22. Singh I, Khanna PK, Srivastava MC, et al. Acute mountain sickness. *N Engl J Med*. 1969;280:175–184.
23. Hackett PH, Forsling ML, Milledge J, et al. Release of vasopressin in man at altitude. *Hormones Metab Res*. 1978;10:571.
24. Lenfant C, Torrance JD, Reynafarje C. Shift of the O2-Hb dissociation curve at altitude: mechanism and effect. *J Appl Physiol*. 1971;625–631.
25. Faura J, Ramos J, Reynafarje C, et al. Effect of altitude on erythropoiesis. *Blood*. 1969;33:668–676.
26. Siri BE, Van Dyke DC, Winchell HS, et al. Early erythropoietin, blood, and physiological responses to severe hypoxia in man. *J Appl Physiol*. 1966;21:73–80.
27. Alexander JK, Grover RF. Mechanism of reduced cardiac stroke volume at high altitude. *Clin Cardiol*. 1983;6:301–303.
28. Grover Rf, Weil JV, Reeves JT. Cardiovascular adaptation to exercise at high altitude. *Exerc Sports Sci Rev*. 1986;14:269–302.
29. Reeves JT, Groves BM, Sutton JR, et al. Operation Everest II: preservation of cardiac function at extreme altitude. *J Appl Physiol*. 1987;63:531–539.
30. Hackett PH, Rennie D. Acute mountain sickness. *Semin Respir Med*. 1983;5:132–139.
31. Hultgren HN. High altitude medical problems. *West J Med*. 1979;131:8–23.
32. Johnson TS, Rock PB. Acute mountain sickness. *N Engl J Med*. 1988;319:841–845.
33. Hackett PH, Rennie D. Rales, peripheral edema, retinal hemorrhage and acute mountain sickness. *Am J Med*. 1979;67:214–218.
34. Hackett PH, Rennie D, Levine HD. The incidence, importance, and prophylaxis of acute mountain sickness. *Lancet*. 1976;2:1149–1155.
35. Scoggin CH, Hyers TM, Reeves JT, et al. High-altitude pulmonary edema in the children and young adults of Leadville, Colorado. *N Engl J Med*. 1977;297:1269–1272.
36. Sophocles AM, Bachman J. High-altitude pulmonary edema among visitors to Summit County, Colorado. *J Fam Pract*. 1983;17:1015–1017.
37. Hackett PH. *Mountain Sickness: Prevention, Recognition and Treatment*. New York: American Alpine Club; 1980.
38. Sutton JR, Lassen N. Pathophysiology of acute mountain sickness and high altitude pulmonary oedema: an hypothesis. *Bull Eur Physiopathol Respir*. 1979;15:1045–1052.
39. Houston CS, Dickinson J. Cerebral form of high-altitude illness. *Lancet*. 1975;2:758–761.
40. Shlim DR. Treatment of acute mountain sickness. *N Engl J Med*. 1985;313:891. Letter.
41. Hackett PH, Roach RC. Medical therapy of altitude illness. *Ann Emerg Med*. 1987;16:980–986.
42. Levine BD, Yoshimura K, Kobayashi T, et al. Dexamethasone in the treatment of acute mountain sickness. *N Engl J Med*. 1989;321:1707–1713.
43. Ferrazzini G, Maggiorini M, Kriemler S, et al. Successful treatment of acute mountain sickness with dexamethasone. *Br Med J*. 1987;294:1380–1382.
44. Hackett PH, Roach RC, Wood RA, et al. Dexamethasone for prevention and treatment of acute mountain sickness. *Aviat Space Environ Med*. 1988;59:950–954.
45. Larson EB, Roach RC, Schoene RB, et al. Acute mountain sickness and acetazolamide. *JAMA*. 1982;248:328–332.

46. Greene MK, Kerr AM, McIntosh IB, et al. Acetazolamide in prevention of acute mountain sickness: a double-blind controlled cross-over study. *Br Med J*. 1981;283:811–813.
47. Senay LC, Tolbert DL. Effect of arginine vasopressin, acetazolamide, and angiotensin II on CSF pressure at simulated altitude. *Aviat Space Environ Med*. 1984;55:370–376.
48. Harrison GL, Evans J, Coote J. Discontinuation of acetazolamide after rapid ascent to 4300 meters. In: Sutton JR, Coates G, Remmers JE, eds. *Hypoxia: The Adaptations*. Philadelphia: Decker; 1990:291. Abstract.
49. Gamow RI, Geer GD, Kasic JF, Smith HM. Methods of gas-balance control to be used with a portable hyperbaric chamber in the treatment of high altitude illness. *J Wilderness Med*. 1990;1:165–180.
50. King SJ, Greenlee RR. Successful use of the Gamow Hyperbaric Bag in the treatment of altitude illness on Mount Everest. *J Wilderness Med*. 1990;1:193–202.
51. Singh I, Kapila CC, Khanna PK, et al. High-altitude pulmonary edema. *Lancet*. 1965;1:229–234.
52. Kobayashi T, Koyama S, Kubo K, et al. Clinical features of patients with high-altitude pulmonary edema in Japan. *Chest*. 1987;92:814–821.
53. Hackett PH, Roach RC. High altitude pulmonary edema. *J Wilderness Med*. 1990;1:3–26.
54. Vock P, Fretz C, Franciolli M, et al. High-altitude pulmonary edema: findings at high-altitude chest radiography and physical examination. *Radiology*. 1989;170:661–666.
55. Hultgren HN. High altitude pulmonary edema. In: Staub NC, ed. *Lung Water and Solute Exchange*. New York: Dekker; 1978:437–469.
56. Sophocles AM. High-altitude pulmonary edema in Vail, Colorado, 1975–1982. *West J Med*. 1986;144:569–573.
57. Hackett PH, Creagh CE, Grover RF, et al. High-altitude pulmonary edema in persons without the right pulmonary artery. *N Engl J Med*. 1980;302:1070–1073.
58. Torrington KG. Recurrent high-altitude illness associated with right pulmonary artery occlusion from granulomatous mediastinitis. *Chest*. 1989;96:1422–1423.
59. Kawashima A, Kubo K, Kobayashi T, et al. Hemodynamic responses to acute hypoxia, hypobaria, and exercise in subjects susceptible to high-altitude pulmonary edema. *J Appl Physiol*. 1989;67:1982–1989.
60. Reeves JT, Wagner WW, McMurtry IF, et al. Physiological effects of high altitude on the pulmonary circulation. In: Robertshaw D, ed. *International Review of Physiology: Environmental Physiology III*. Baltimore: University Park Press; 1979;20:289–310.
61. Schoene RB, Hackett PH, Henderson WR, et al. High-altitude pulmonary edema characteristics of lung lavage fluid. *JAMA*. 1986;256:63–69.
62. Schoene RB. High-altitude pulmonary edema: pathophysiology and clinical review. *Ann Emerg Med*. 1987;16:987–992.
63. Marticorena E, Hultgren HN. Evaluation of therapeutic methods in high altitude pulmonary edema. *Am J Cardiol*. 1979;43:307–312.
64. Hasan Nuri MM, Ali Khan MZ, Quraishi MS. High altitude pulmonary oedema—response to exercise and cold on systemic and pulmonary vascular beds. *J Pak Med Assoc*. 1988;38:211–217.
65. Hultgren HN. Furosemide for high altitude pulmonary edema. *JAMA*. 1975;234:589–590. Letter.
66. Oelz O. A case of high-altitude pulmonary edema treated with nifedipine. *JAMA*. 1987;257:780. Letter.
67. Oelz O, Maggiorini M, Ritter M, et al. Nifedipine for high altitude pulmonary oedema. *Lancet*. 1989;2:1241–1244.
68. Hackett PH, Greene ER, Roach RC, et al. Nifedipine for treatment of high altitude pulmonary edema. In: Sutton JR, Coates G, Remmers JE, eds. *Hypoxia: The Adaptations*. Philadelphia: Dekker; 1990:291. Abstract.
69. Schoene RB, Roach RC, Hackett PH, et al. High altitude pulmonary edema and exercise at 4,400 meters on Mount McKinley: effect of expiratory positive airway pressure. *Chest*. 1985;87:330–333.
70. Dickinson JG. High altitude cerebral edema: cerebral acute mountain sickness. *Semin Respir Med*. 1983;5:151–157.
71. Hamilton AJ, Cymerman A, Black PM. High altitude cerebral edema. *Neurosurgery*. 1986;19:841–849.
72. Hackett PH, Yarnell P, Hill RP. MRI in high altitude cerebral edema: evidence for vasogenic edema. In: Sutton JR, Coates G, Remmers JE, eds. *Hypoxia: The Adaptations*. Philadelphia: Decker; 1990:295. Abstract.
73. Shlim DR, Cohen MT. Guillain-Barré syndrome presenting as high-altitude cerebral edema. *N Engl J Med*. 1989;321:545. Letter.
74. Shlim DR, Meijer HJ. Suddenly symptomatic brain tumors at altitude. *Ann Emerg Med*. 1991;20:315–316.
75. Weil JV, Kryger MH, Scoggin CH. Sleep and breathing at high altitude. In: Guilleminault C, ed. *Sleep Apnea Syndromes*. New York: Liss; 1978:119–123.
76. Sutton JR, Houston CS, Mansell AL, et al. Effect of acetazolamide on hypoxemia during sleep at high altitude. *N Engl J Med*. 1979;301:1329–1331.
77. Hackett PH, Roach RC, Harrison GL, et al. Respiratory stimulants and sleep periodic breathing at high altitude. *Am Rev Respir Dis*. 1987;135:896–898.
78. Rennie D, Morrissey J. Retinal changes in himalayan climbers. *Arch Ophthalmol*. 1975;93:395–400.
79. Wiedman M. High altitude retinal hemorrhage. *Arch Ophthalmol*. 1975;93:401–403.
80. McFadden ER, Ingram RH Jr. Exercise-induced asthma: observations on the initiating stimulus. *N Engl J Med*. 1979;301:763–769.
81. Anderson S, Seale JP, Ferris L, et al. An evaluation of pharmacotherapy for exercise-induced asthma. *J Allergy Clin Immunol*. 1975;64:612–624.
82. Grover Rf, Tucker CE, McGroarty SR, et al. The coronary stress of skiing at high altitude. *Arch Intern Med*. 1990;150:1205–1208.
83. Hultgren HN. Coronary heart disease and trekking. *J Wilderness Med*. 1990;1:154–161.
84. Rennie D. Will mountain trekkers have heart attacks? *JAMA*. 1989;261:1045–1046. Editorial.
85. Franklin V. Sickle cell crisis. In: Sutton JR, Jones NL, Houston CS, eds. *Hypoxia: Man at High Altitude*. New York: Thieme Stratton; 1982:177–181.
86. Lane PA, Githens JH. Splenic syndrome at mountain altitudes in sickle cell trait. *JAMA*. 1985;253:2251–2254.
87. Moore LG. Altitude-aggravated illness: examples from pregnancy and prenatal life. *Ann Emerg Med*. 1987;16:965–973.
88. Winslow RM, Monge CC. *Hypoxia, Polycythemia, and Chronic Mountain Sickness*. Baltimore: Johns Hopkins University Press; 1987.
89. Kryger M, McCullough RE, Collins D, et al. Treatment of excessive polycythemia of high altitude with respiratory stimulant drugs. *Am Rev Respir Dis*. 1978;117:455–464.

43. Drowning and Near-Drowning

SHIRLEY A. GRAVES, MD
A. JOSEPH LAYON, MD

No precise statistics exist on the number of persons who nearly drown. Considering, however, that in the 25 years before 1978 patients treated for near-drowning may have numbered more than 1.2 million[1] and that the numbers of people, swimming pools, and boats have steadily increased since 1978, drowning and near-drowning constitute leading causes of morbidity and mortality. More than 7000 deaths result from drowning each year in the United States alone, more than 2000 of these being children.[1a] Indeed, drowning is the third leading cause of death in the United States.[1b] The emergency medical team, however, is concerned with the survivor, the nearly drowned patient.

DEFINITIONS

In 1971, Modell[2,3] defined the terms *drowned* and *near-drowned* and, in 1981, revised these definitions.

To drown, with or without aspiration, is to die while submerged in water. Approximately 10% of drowning victims do not aspirate water but die of respiratory obstruction and asphyxia while submerged.[4] Those who aspirate die from both the asphyxia and the effects of the aspirated water.

To near-drown, with or without aspiration, is to suffocate by submersion in water and to survive, at least temporarily. Approximately 12% of near-drowned persons do not aspirate and suffer only laryngospasm or breath holding, which prevents the aspiration of fluid.[5]

The author thanks Dr. Jerome H. Modell for review of the manuscript and Lynn Dirk for editorial assistance.

Delayed death may occur secondary to near-drowning after an initial, apparently successful resuscitation. Delayed death may be the result of pulmonary injury, infection, or irreversible cerebral injury.

EPIDEMIOLOGY AND ETIOLOGY

Drowning is one of the leading causes of accidental death among young people; the highest incidence occurs during the second decade of life.[6] These victims are generally healthy. Approximately 65% cannot swim. The backyard swimming pool is a particular hazard for the child under 10 years of age.[7] Pearn et al[8] reported an overall annual mortality of 3.1 drownings per 100,000 children in the city and county of Honolulu. The fatality rate in swimming pools, 0.9 per 100,000, is low compared with other studies and may be related to more fencing of pools in Honolulu. The risk of drowning or near-drowning associated with unintended or unsupervised access to an unfenced pool has been estimated at 3.76 times higher than the risk associated with a fenced pool.[8a]

The ability to swim is certainly desirable in the prevention of drowning; however, it is not the only factor. At least 35% of drowned victims can swim,[7] which indicates the importance of other factors, such as regard for safety rules, estimation of one's ability, use of drugs and alcohol during aquatic activities, and physical illnesses (eg, labyrinthitis or pre-existing cardiac disease). Thus, the most important things that could be done to prevent near-drowning are fencing off pools; severely sanctioning intoxicated boaters; and restricting the sale and consumption of alcoholic beverages at pools, beaches, and marinas and around harbors. Perhaps of greatest importance, however, to prevent morbidity and mortality from near-drowning, is instructing the general public in basic cardiac life support.[1a]

Craig[9,10] has documented that hyperventilation before underwater swimming is a dangerous practice. If an individual hyperventilates before underwater swimming, the P_{CO_2} in the blood decreases such that the individual can stay under water longer without feeling the urge to surface and take a breath. Unfortunately, during this time the P_{O_2} also decreases; the individual becomes hypoxemic and unconscious and drowns.

Immersion in cold water causes hypothermia. As body temperature falls, the resultant disorientation and subsequent loss of consciousness can lead to submersion and drowning.[11] If the individual does not drown or near-drown because of the disorientation associated with hypothermia, arrhythmias and even death may occur from the hypothermic effects on the heart. Hypothermia does, of course, decrease oxygen consumption, and cases are reported in the literature of complete recovery after prolonged submersion in cold water.[12] Also, when submerged in cold water, the individual may experience the diving reflex, whereby intense peripheral vasoconstriction occurs, and blood is shunted preferentially to the heart and brain[13] (see Chapter 41, Hypothermia).

Many factors are involved in drowning and near-drowning. Prevention is the most valuable and life-saving measure. For treatment, however, the most important measure is realizing that each near-drowning is a unique event, and, therefore, each case must be evaluated and treated individually.

PATHOLOGY

Autopsies of drowned persons reveal various findings, depending on the amount and type of fluid aspirated, the length of submersion, the degree of hypoxia, the duration of survival, and the effects of therapy. The most extensive changes occur in the lungs and brain.[14]

Gooseflesh, or cutis anserina, and water wrinkling of the palms of the hands and soles of the feet may appear. A pale or plasmalike watery foam, frequently blood-tinged in freshwater victims, may be present in the nose and mouth and may be mixed with mud, debris, or vomitus. This material may also appear in the lower airway.

When the pleura is opened, the lungs frequently appear large, hyperexpanded, and irregularly congested with pink or red mottling. If the patient survives initially but dies later, the lung may show hyaline material in the alveoli, pneumonia, and mechanical injuries such as barotrauma. Microscopic sections of the lung may show alveolar distention, hyaline precipitates, and intra-alveolar hemorrhage (see Chapter 44, Hyperbaric Emergencies).

Changes in the brain vary with the degree and duration of cerebral anoxia. If death occurs within the first few hours or days, brain edema and perivascular hemorrhage may be the only gross changes. With severe anoxia, basal ganglia or midbrain cystic degeneration may appear after a week or two. All of these findings are secondary to anoxia and are not necessarily unique to drowning.

PATHOPHYSIOLOGY

Significant experimental and clinical data obtained since the 1940s have changed our understanding of the pathophysiology of drowning and near-drowning and, thus, have altered the approach to therapy. The evolution of the understanding of the pathophysiology can be divided into three phases: first, serum electrolyte concentrations and blood volume; second, pulmonary and acid-base changes; and third, neurologic damage and brain preservation.

In the 1940s and 1950s, the emphasis in treating the near-drowned patient was on the serum electrolyte concentrations and the blood volume changes that might have occurred.[15,16] However, in the 1960s, Modell and colleagues experimentally and clinically demonstrated that pulmonary insufficiency and acid-base changes were the primary pathophysiology in near-drowned patients.[5,17]

In the late 1970s, concern not only for survival after an anoxic insult but for survival with intact cerebral function led to considerable investigation. Although no controlled studies were done in the area of near-drowning and brain preservation, techniques to preserve the brain were advocated and used by some.[18–20] Subsequently, retrospective review of these therapies and some controlled clinical protocols addressing hypothermia, high-dose barbiturate therapy, and intracranial pressure (ICP) monitoring appeared in the literature.[21–23] Data did not indicate that intact survival rate improved compared with the survival rate of patients treated intensively but without therapy aimed specifically at brain preservation.

Pulmonary, Blood Gas, and Acid-Base Alterations

The most important and immediate consequence of near-drowning is hypoxemia (Fig. 43-1).[5,17,24,25] Hypoxemia may occur whether or not the individual aspirates. As reported by Cot,[4] 10% of drowned humans did not actually aspirate fluid but died secondary to upper airway obstruction. Similarly, 12% of near-drowned victims did not aspirate but suffered hypoxemia from breath holding and laryngospasm.[5] In near-drowning without aspiration, if effective ventilation and circulation can be restored before irreversible cerebral damage occurs, the victim should recover with little or no additional therapy. This situation has been simulated in the laboratory by using dogs anesthetized with barbiturates.[26] When the airway was occluded, the arterial oxygen tension

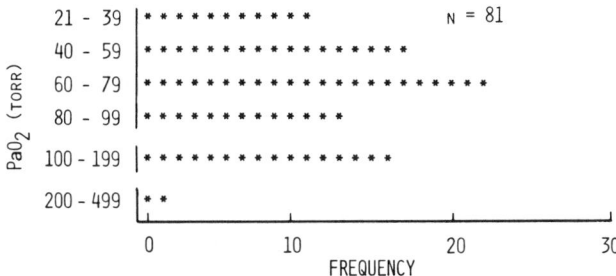

Figure 43-1 Values for Pao₂ on admission to hospital after near-drowning. FIo₂ ranged from 0.2 to 1.0. Each point represents one patient. *Source:* Modell JH, Graves SA, Ketover A: Clinical course of 91 consecutive near-drowning victims. *Chest* 70:232, 1976. Reprinted with permission.

(Pa_{O_2}) decreased from a normal control value of 92 to 40 torr at 1 minute and 4 torr at 5 minutes and the arterial P_{CO_2} increased 3 to 6 torr per minute. Eighty percent of these animals could be successfully resuscitated if they were manually ventilated with room air 5 minutes after tracheal occlusion. Some of the animals required external cardiac massage in addition to the positive pressure ventilation.

If a victim aspirates fluid, then the pulmonary picture is substantially more complicated. Aspiration of even small quantities of water yields significant decreases in Pa_{O_2}.[17,25,27,28] If significant quantities (11 mL/kg) of fresh water or seawater are aspirated, profound hypoxemia occurs within 1 minute and persists for at least 72 hours in surviving animals. This initial hypoxemia is accompanied by hypercarbia and acidosis.[17,25] The hypercarbia is readily reversible once the victim breathes spontaneously or mechanical ventilation is instituted.[5,24] However, the hypoxemia persists and so does the metabolic component of the acidosis.[5,29] Some investigators have been unable to correlate Pa_{O_2} or pH with survival, but these values do indicate the severity of the lesion.[5]

Hypoxia occurs after the aspiration of either fresh water or seawater; however, the physiologic mechanism in each case differs. Seawater is hypertonic (approximately three and one-half times more concentrated than plasma); therefore, fluid is drawn into the alveoli from the circulation in response to this hypertonicity. If 22 mL/kg of seawater is aspirated by dogs, approximately 33 mL/kg can be drained from the lungs by gravity. The result of seawater aspiration is fluid-filled but perfused alveoli.[28,30] Pulmonary surfactant after seawater aspiration has normal surface tension properties. After freshwater aspiration, fluid is absorbed rapidly across the alveolar surface into the circulation and little to no water can be drained from the airway by gravity 3 min later.[27] Fresh water alters surface tension properties of the pulmonary surfactant,[31] which produces unstable alveoli and atelectasis. These poorly ventilated and atelectatic alveoli, in turn, produce ventilation/perfusion mismatching and intrapulmonary shunting (Fig. 43-2).[17] With either freshwater or seawater aspiration, pulmonary compliance decreases, dead space-to-tidal volume ratio and airway resistance increase, and ventilation/perfusion mismatching and intrapulmonary shunting occur.[17,28,32–34] Pulmonary edema occurs secondary to aspiration of either type of water.

It has been demonstrated in the laboratory that the application of positive end-expiratory pressure (PEEP) or continuous positive airway pressure (CPAP) to the airway can significantly improve oxygenation and decrease intrapulmonary shunting after the aspiration of fresh water or seawater. Animals aspirating seawater improved significantly when they breathed spontaneously with CPAP or were mechanically ventilated with PEEP.[30] The animals aspirating fresh water, on the other hand, did not always improve significantly with CPAP alone, but some required positive pressure ventilation also.[35] Both PEEP and CPAP increase functional residual capacity (FRC), improve oxygenation and ventilation/perfusion, and reduce intrapulmonary shunt. Why does the aspiration of fresh water often require positive pressure ventilation in addition to CPAP? One hypothesis is that, because the alteration of surfactant produces unstable alveoli and atelectasis, a high peak inspiratory pressure is necessary to open the alveoli and CPAP is necessary to keep them open.

The near-drowned victim may suffer gastric distention, may vomit, and may aspirate gastric contents, which compounds the pulmonary injury of aspirating water. Gastric distention may also interfere with ventilation (Fig. 43-3). Neurogenic pulmonary edema may also complicate the primary injury.[36]

Although there may be acute and severe pulmonary insufficiency after near-drowning, those who survive the initial

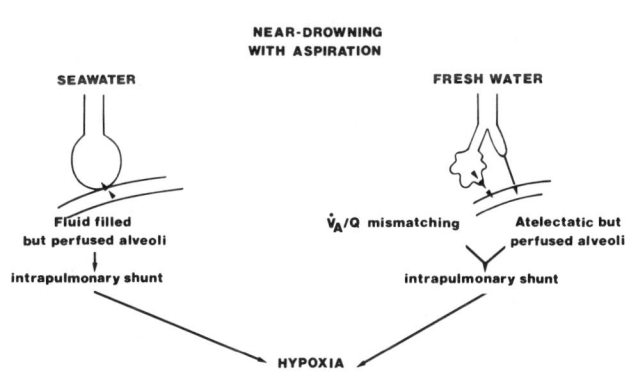

Figure 43-2 Effects of aspiration. After seawater aspiration, fluid fills the alveoli, which produces intrapulmonary shunt. After freshwater aspiration, alteration of surfactant causes partially collapsed and completely atelectatic alveoli, which produces intrapulmonary shunt. Aspiration of either type of water causes hypoxia. $\dot{V}_A/\dot{Q}$, ventilation-to-perfusion ratio.

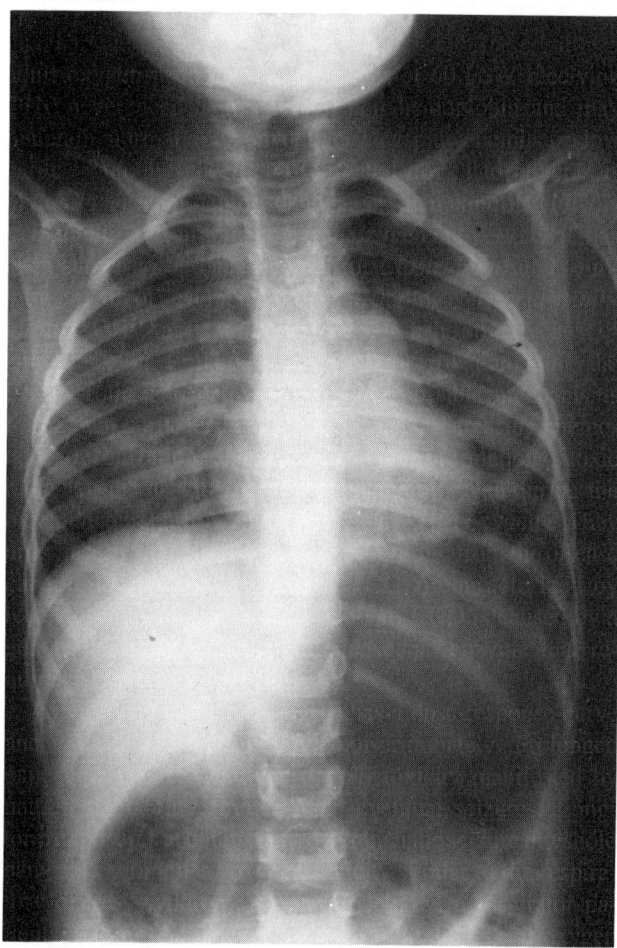

Figure 43-3 Chest roentgenogram of a child postresuscitation. Note the massive gastric distention. This may predispose to vomiting and may also interfere with ventilation.

insult suffer no long-term alteration in pulmonary function as assessed by forced vital capacity in 1 second (FVC_1), functional residual capacity, forced expiratory volume in 1 second (FEV_1), FEV_1/FVC_1, and total lung capacity.[37–38] One study has demonstrated evidence of peripheral airway disease in some near-drowned children.[39]

Serum Electrolyte and Blood Volume Changes

In the 1940s and 1950s, serum electrolyte and blood volume changes were thought to be the primary cause of morbidity and mortality after near-drowning. This phase of understanding the illness and approaching its therapy was based on investigations by Swann and colleagues, who demonstrated significant serum electrolyte and blood volume changes after total immersion of dogs in either seawater or fresh water.[15,16] After total immersion in seawater, animals showed marked increases in serum electrolyte concentrations and in blood density and a decrease in blood volume. If the animals were immersed in fresh water until death, blood density and concentration of extracellular serum electrolyte decreased and blood volume increased. These animals frequently died of ventricular fibrillation in contrast to animals submerged in seawater, none of which suffered ventricular fibrillation.

In the 1960s, Modell and colleagues investigated further the fluid and electrolyte changes after near-drowning and found that these changes, which depend on both the type and the volume of water aspirated, are transient in survivors.[25,27,28] Animals aspirating 22 mL/kg of either fresh or seawater showed no life-threatening changes in serum electrolytes. When 22 mL/kg of fresh water were aspirated, the serum sodium and serum chloride decreased 10 to 20 mEq/L within 3 minutes but returned to normal within 30 minutes. Aspiration of the same quantity of seawater transiently raised these electrolytes 20 to 30 mEq/L. In these animals, potassium concentration rose acutely after the aspiration of either fresh water or seawater. These levels also were not life-threatening and returned to normal within 30 minutes. If 44 mL/kg of fresh water were aspirated, 80% of the animals died of ventricular fibrillation. An analysis of blood from humans drowned in either fresh water or seawater demonstrated similar findings.[40] The 85% who did not have severe changes in serum electrolyte concentrations presumably died of hypoxia and acidosis. On the basis of these data for both drowned and near-drowned animals and humans, survivors probably do not aspirate enough fluid to change electrolytes profoundly but, rather, manifest transient electrolyte changes that revert to normal without specific therapy (Fig. 43-4).[5] The hypotonic fresh water is rapidly absorbed into the circulation after near-drowning[27]; however, in survivors, fluid is rapidly redistributed and hypervolemia is transient. After seawater aspiration, blood volume decreases in proportion to the quantity of fluid aspirated.[28] Drowning

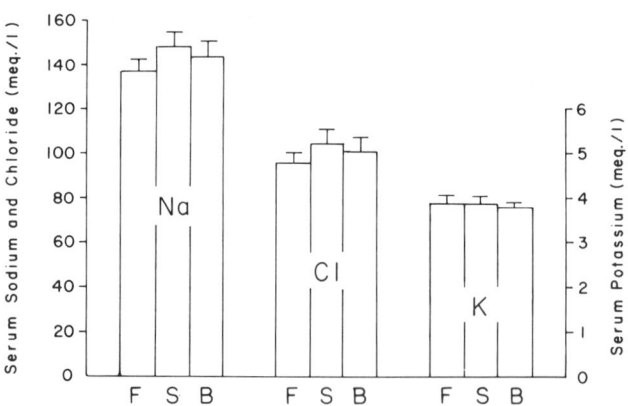

Figure 43-4 Serum concentrations (mean ± SD) of sodium (Na), chloride (Cl), and potassium (K) in patients who suffered near-drowning in fresh (F), sea (S), or brackish (B) water. *Source:* Modell JH, Graves SA, Ketover A: Clinical course of 91 consecutive near-drowning victims. *Chest* 70:234, 1976. Reprinted with permission.

in the Dead Sea, however, can have a more lethal effect on electrolyte concentrations, because swallowing this hypertonic, hypernatremic solution may also result in hypercalcemia and hypermagnesemia with associated cardiac effects documented by electrocardiogram.[40a] Pulmonary edema can occur after freshwater or seawater aspiration and can produce hypovolemia, which may require replacement therapy.

Cardiovascular Changes

Most cardiovascular changes are related to hypoxia and acidosis, which accompany pulmonary insufficiency in the near-drowned victim. The usual situation is cardiovascular stability in the patient without any preexisting cardiovascular compromise. Numerous dysrhythmias have been reported after near-drowning.[7,25,27,28,41–45] Swann and colleagues identified ventricular fibrillation after total immersion in fresh water as a mechanism of death secondary to drowning,[15,16] however, aspiration of this quantity of water by humans is infrequent.[40] Central venous pressure (CVP) increases transiently after the aspiration of either fresh water or seawater[27,28]; if death occurs immediately after the aspiration of large quantities of fresh water, the elevation persists until death.[15,45] Otherwise, the CVP returns to normal after approximately an hour.[25,27] After seawater aspiration, fluid is lost into the lungs and the CVP rapidly decreases and approaches zero.[16]

Cardiac output (CO) transiently falls after the aspiration of fresh water. Controlled mechanical ventilation decreases CO, and this decrease may be accentuated by PEEP.[35] In the dog, if the intravascular volume is augmented with crystalloid, this decrease in CO can be reversed. Contrary to this, inotropic stimulation of the myocardium with dopamine does not restore CO.[46] This lack of effect of dopamine has not been evaluated in near-drowned humans.

Hypothermia may occur secondary to near-drowning and, if the body temperature is below 28°C, dysrhythmias, including ventricular fibrillation, frequently occur[11] (see Chapter 41).

Hematologic Changes

Significant changes in hemoglobin and hematocrit rarely occur in the near-drowned victim.[5] This suggests that near-drowning victims do not aspirate large quantities of fluid. In a retrospective study of 91 consecutive near-drowned patients, hemoglobin (Hb) and hematocrit values were normal, and those of freshwater victims could not be differentiated from those of seawater victims (Fig. 43-5).

When a large volume of fresh water is aspirated and absorbed, hemolysis of red blood cells (RBCs) and hemoglobinemia can occur. Although the hemolysis of RBCs relates to the tonicity of this fluid, the hemolysis increases when combined with hypoxemia. After the IV injection of

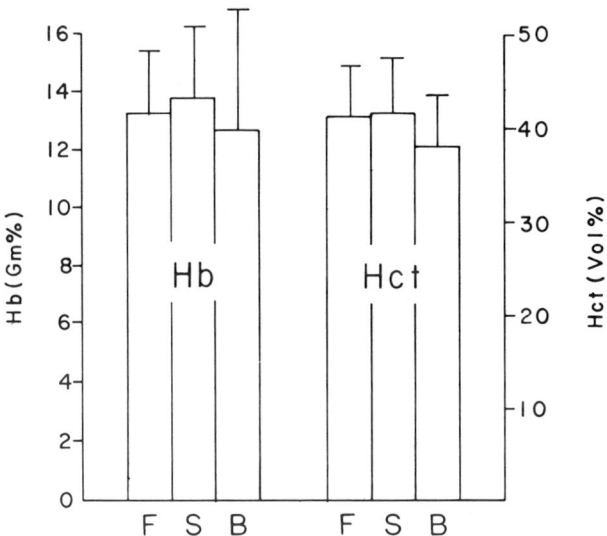

Figure 43-5 Hemoglobin (Hb) levels and hematocrit (Hct) readings (mean ± SD) in patients who suffered near-drowning in fresh (F), sea (S), or brackish (B) water. *Source:* Modell JH, Graves SA, Ketover A: Clinical course of 91 consecutive near-drowning victims. *Chest* 70:234, 1976. Reprinted with permission.

44 mL/kg of fresh water into animals, plasma hemoglobin levels were not significantly elevated as long as the animals were not hypoxemic. When the airway was occluded and the same volume of water infused, plasma Hb concentration exceeded 1000 mg/dL.[26] In near-drowned humans, the plasma Hb level rarely exceed 10 mg/dL; nevertheless, patients with higher levels have reportedly survived without specific therapy for the hemoglobinemia.

Disseminated intravascular coagulation as well as other coagulative disorders in drowned victims have been reported. The etiology of these disorders is unknown but might be related to severe hypoxemia and acidosis, sepsis, shock, or hemolysis of the RBCs with the release of factors that disrupt the coagulative cascade.[47–49] This rarely occurs in a near-drowned patient with no other complications.

Renal Function

When oxygenation and renal perfusion are maintained, renal failure is unusual in the near-drowned patient. This is not to say that such abnormalities cannot occur. There are numerous reports of abnormal findings such as albuminuria, hemoglobinuria, oliguria, anuria, and acute tubular necrosis.[50–54] Any biochemical effects of the absorbed water on the kidney are unknown; however, it seems likely that the abnormalities relate to acidosis, hypoxia, and compromised renal perfusion. Hemoglobinuria is not usually a problem in the near-drowned patient; however, it should be considered a potential problem deserving evaluation.

CNS Changes

Central nervous system compromise may be associated with near-drowning. The underlying cause is likely to be secondary to cerebral hypoxia. The reported incidence of neurologic dysfunction from near-drowning varies considerably, from 0% to 30% of survivors.[5,19,55–57] The high incidence of brain damage reported has led some persons to recommend the consideration of significant neurologic damage before instituting hospital-based intensive care and life support.[56] These same fears led others to pursue aggressive measures for cerebral resuscitation and brain preservation.[18–20]

Pearn and coworkers, attempting to define the best indicator of neurologic outcome, reviewed childhood drownings and near-drownings over a 5-year period.[56] All children who were resuscitated survived without neurologic sequelae; 5 of the 104 children died. Based on these findings, the best indicator of neurologic sequelae was the time elapsed until the first spontaneous gasp during rescue. Most patients who survived made spontaneous respiratory efforts within 2 minutes after removal from the water. The authors concluded that an absence of spontaneous gasps within an hour of rescue indicates that neurologic complications will occur.

Later, to better define the patient at risk of neurologic deficit, two retrospective studies divided the victims of near-drowning into three groups classified according to neurologic status in the emergency department.[20,58] Patients in group 1 arrived at the hospital awake and alert, although they may have suffered cardiopulmonary arrest during the accident and may have required resuscitation at the scene; 100% survived normally.

Group 2 arrived at the hospital with a blunted level of consciousness. These patients were described as lethargic, combative, disoriented, semicomatose, and confused. One hundred percent in one study and 90% in the other survived without neurologic sequelae. Three patients died of pulmonary insufficiency and had no neurologic deficit beforehand. Therapy was directed at pulmonary and cardiac parameters for this group in both studies.

In the third group, comatose patients, one study included adults of whom 73% survived and were normal.[58] In both studies, approximately 44% of children survived with normal function. Patients from one institution received therapy directed primarily at pulmonary and cardiac resuscitation and, in some patients, hyperventilation and steroids.[58] In the other study, therapy was aimed at aggressive cerebral resuscitation including hyperventilation, hyperoxia, fluid restriction and diuresis, hypothermia, muscle paralysis, steroids, and barbiturate coma.[20]

More recent studies[22,23] of near-drowning have failed to show benefit from hypothermia or barbiturate therapy. Additionally, monitoring and control of ICP do not ensure cerebrally intact survival.[21–23] Sustained intracranial hypertension indicates a significant neurologic insult and portends a poor neurologic outcome. The intracranial hypertension appears to result from hypoxia, which may not be accompanied by cerebral ischemia. Not all comatose near-drowned victims with poor outcome have elevated ICP. Recently, a retrospective study looked at prehospital prognostic indicators in pediatric drowning accidents. The best prehospital predictors of death or poor outcome were submersion longer than 10 minutes and resuscitation longer than 25 minutes. Indicators of good outcome were sinus cardiac rhythm, reactive pupils, and responsiveness at the scene.[58a]

It is important that the level of consciousness be documented. The above noted classification of awake, blunted, and comatose is helpful.[20,58] Further classification with the Glasgow Coma Scale, a universally accepted method of scoring brain-injured patients, is recommended. This simplifies assessment of neurologic status and allows comparison of assessment by different examiners on repeat examinations.

DIAGNOSIS AND DIFFERENTIAL DIAGNOSIS

Unlike many medical illnesses, the diagnosis of near-drowning is usually obvious from the history; however, the degree of injury to various organs requires thorough investigation and a complete knowledge of the pathophysiologic changes induced by near-drowning. Also important in assessing the victim is recognizing associated problems.

Although near-drowning may appear to be the only accident, trauma to the head, neck, or other organs may have occurred if the patient fell or was diving into the water. Injuries such as fractures of the neck or back or intracranial hemorrhage must be considered. Whether or not the victim was under the influence of alcohol or drugs at the time of the accident should be ascertained. It is important to know the patient's previous state of health. For example, an older patient may suffer a myocardial infarction while in the water and may aspirate terminally; a diabetic might suffer hypoglycemia, lose consciousness, and near-drown; or the epileptic patient might have a seizure, near-drown, and be postictal or have cerebral depression secondary to cerebral anoxia. As in all serious illnesses, a careful history and a complete physical examination are imperative to determine the extent of the physiologic damage the patient has sustained.

TREATMENT

Prehospital

The outcome of near-drowning depends on the quality of the resuscitation at the scene of the accident. The objective is to maintain oxygenation and acid-base balance. The ABCs of cardiopulmonary resuscitation recommended by the American Heart Association apply to the resuscitation of the near-drowned victim. Safar and coworkers have shown mouth-to-mouth and mouth-to-nose ventilation to be the most effective methods of ventilation in a situation such as near-drowning.[59] If the victim is apneic, hypoxia increases rapidly and the victim may be just a breath away from cardiac arrest. If the rescuer is experienced and a good swimmer, it may be possible to begin mouth-to-mouth ventilation in the water; however, rescuers should not jeopardize themselves or delay resuscitation by attempting a technique in the water that exceeds their abilities.

If the victim remains apneic, mouth-to-mouth ventilation should be replaced with a positive pressure breathing device as soon as available. Hand-operated units are generally preferable to automatic pressure-cycled devices. If pulmonary compliance is decreased, pressure-cycled or pressure-limited devices may fail to deliver an adequate tidal volume. Supplemental oxygen should be supplied as soon as possible.

Heimlich[60] recommended subdiaphragmatic compression to remove aspirated water from the lungs of the near-drowned patient. This author and others[61] do not recommend such a maneuver unless the airway is obstructed by foreign material. This maneuver may even be hazardous if the patient is apneic or has no reflexive airway protection: Swallowed water and gastric contents can be extruded from the stomach and aspirated, which could compound the pulmonary injury. Attempting to remove fresh water from the lungs is futile because it is so rapidly absorbed into the circulation. Seawater is hypertonic, and, in animals resuscitated after the aspiration of large quantities of this type of water, gravitational drainage of the lungs did improve survival.[30] Based on this, if a seawater victim can be resuscitated in a slightly head-down position, some theoretical advantage might be gained; however, it is far more important that rapid and effective artificial ventilation be instituted to restore oxygenation.

If the victim has not aspirated and effective ventilation and oxygenation are restored before permanent circulatory or cerebral hypoxic effects occur, the prognosis for normal recovery is excellent. On the other hand, if water has been aspirated, then pulmonary insufficiency usually ensues and the problem is more complicated. In addition to ventilation, if the patient does not have an effective heartbeat, closed-chest cardiac massage should be instituted immediately.

Many communities have emergency medical personnel who can deliver sophisticated care at the scene. These paramedics and emergency medical technicians can easily replace mouth-to-mouth ventilation with bag-and-mask ventilation or, in some situations, endotracheal intubation. If the rescue personnel are skilled at endotracheal intubation, then the patient who is comatose or apneic or who cannot maintain ventilation should be intubated at the scene. However, it is far better to continue mouth-to-mouth or bag-and-mask positive pressure ventilation when endotracheal intubation proves difficult or impossible or when rescuers are not skilled in performing endotracheal intubation. A rescue team may also be able to establish an intravenous infusion and, if telemetric monitoring and radio contact between the physician and the team are available, additional drugs and therapy may be administered. These advanced life-support procedures should be performed according to established protocol and under the direction of a physician.

If the patient is breathing spontaneously at the time of rescue or begins to breathe after resuscitation, supplemental oxygen should be continued, preferably 100% oxygen through a nonrebreathing mask, and the patient should be transferred to a hospital for further evaluation.

Regardless of how well the patient looks during transport, oxygen should be continued. Respiratory and circulatory assistance should also be continued as dictated by the patient's condition.

If there is a history of diving or trauma or there are physical signs of trauma, cervical spine injury should be suspected and the patient should be treated as though this were the case. These patients should be placed in a cervical collar, and a spine-board should be used for transportation.

Cardiopulmonary and Acid-Base Therapy

The near-drowned patient requires an uninterrupted continuum of care from the time of rescue through the emergency department and to the intensive care unit until vital body functions have stabilized (Fig. 43-6). In the emergency department, immediate assessment of ventilation and circulation is most important. The target organ is the lungs, which makes intensive evaluation for pulmonary insufficiency and its treatment the immediate goal. For other organs to maintain normal function, oxygenation and oxygen delivery must be ensured. The level of ventilatory support required will vary from patient to patient. For example, the spontaneously breathing patient may require only supplemental oxygen, whereas the apneic patient requires immediate endotracheal intubation. One hundred percent oxygen should be continued until arterial blood gas and pH values are determined. The fractional concentration of inspired oxygen (FIO_2), the ventilatory support, and the administration of sodium bicarbonate solution will be dictated by these values as well as by the physical assessment of the patient. Until the results of the arterial blood gas analysis are available, real-time evaluation of oxygenation by pulse oximetry is critically important. If the patient is alert and has a PaO_2 greater than 80 torr while breathing room air, aspiration probably did not occur and observation for 12 to 24 hours is all that is necessary if blood gas values and physical status do not deteriorate.

At the other end of the spectrum, the comatose or apneic patient should be intubated to protect the airway and to provide further ventilatory support. The patient who cannot maintain adequate oxygenation with an FIO_2 of less than 0.4 also requires more aggressive therapy. Application of PEEP or CPAP improves ventilation/perfusion matching and oxygenation.[30,35,62] When the patient is alert and can clear CO_2

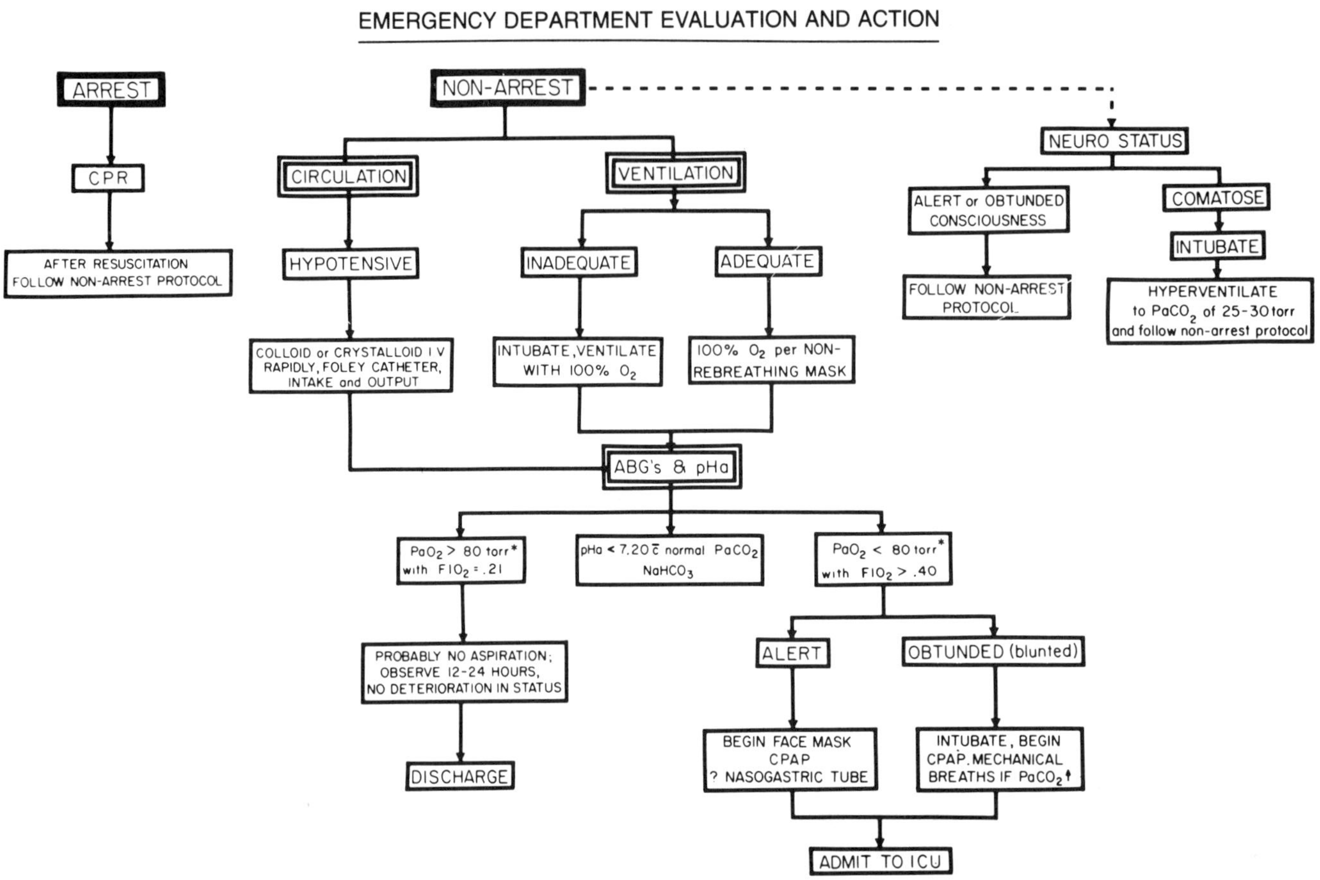

EMERGENCY DEPARTMENT EVALUATION AND ACTION

Figure 43-6 Guidelines for treating the near-drowned patient. See text for details. *Assumes victim had normal arterial blood gas values before near-drowning. CPR, cardiopulmonary resuscitation; ABG's, arterial blood gas values; c̄, with; NaHCO₃, sodium bicarbonate; ICU, intensive care unit.

---

adequately, CPAP may be applied by a special tight-fitting face mask. Most patients easily tolerate 10 to 12 cm H_2O of CPAP applied by this method. We prefer not to administer CPAP by mask at a pressure greater than 10 to 12 cm H_2O, because a higher level risks gastric distention followed by vomiting and pulmonary aspiration of gastric contents. If oxygenation does not improve with this technique, if the patient cannot maintain adequate alveolar ventilation to clear CO_2, if respiration is labored, or if the patient is at high risk of vomiting, the trachea should be intubated. Then CPAP can be increased to improve oxygenation, and mechanical ventilatory breaths can be added.

The degree of venous admixture after near-drowning varies. The exact amount of CPAP each patient will require must be individualized based on therapeutic effect. The optimal level of CPAP is defined by some as the level at which the greatest decrease in intrapulmonary shunting and improvement in ventilation/perfusion ratio are achieved without adversely affecting CO.[63,64] Others simply aim for an acceptable Pao_2 (60 torr or greater with an Fio_2 of 0.40 or less). Our policy is to titrate PEEP/CPAP to the lowest Fio_2 necessary to maintain an acceptable saturation of Hb. Thus, we attempt to keep the Pao_2:Fio_2 ratio ≥300, which is associated with venous admixture <20%, and to keep Fio_2 <0.5, which is nontoxic. Because work of breathing is less with CPAP than PEEP, we recommend CPAP for spontaneously breathing patients. In addition to CPAP, mechanical breaths will occasionally be necessary, not only to maintain $Paco_2$ within a normal range, but also to improve Pao_2, particularly after fresh water aspiration.[35] We prefer that the patient breathe spontaneously if possible because that will enhance venous return and maximize ventilation-to-perfusion matching. When this is only partially possible, intermittent mandatory ventilatory breaths are added; full controlled mechanical ventilation is provided if needed. For the patient who is spontaneously breathing, work imposed by the ventilatory system is minimized by adding pressure support ventilation at approximately 10 cm H_2O.[64a] If controlled ventilation is necessary, CO may be compromised.[35] The addition of PEEP or CPAP at high levels may decrease CO, particularly if hypovolemia is present. Cardiac output may be improved by augmenting intravascular volume with crystalloid, colloid, or, rarely, blood.[46] Spontaneous breaths decrease intrapleural pressure and improve venous return, which helps to maintain CO. Once CPAP has been titrated to optimal oxygenation, interruptions in the expiratory positive airway pressure should be minimized; sudden discontinuation decreases FRC and Pa_{O_2} within seconds. The more severe the pulmonary insufficiency, the more pronounced are these changes and the more difficult it is to restore oxygenation.[65]

Bronchospasm may occur after near-drowning and, if so, should be treated with a bronchodilating agent such as the β-agonist albuterol or the parasympathomimetic glycopyrrolate or both; both may be nebulized. Pulmonary edema may accompany near-drowning with either fresh water or seawater and is best treated with CPAP as just described. Bronchoscopy is not indicated after near-drowning unless solid material has been aspirated.

Steroids should not be used to treat aspiration pneumonitis associated with near-drowning. Animals who have aspirated foodstuff[66] or acid[67-69] or have near-drowned in fresh water[70] show no significant improvement in Pa_{O_2} or in survival with the addition of steroids to therapy. Steroids may actually prevent normal healing after pulmonary injury caused by aspiration of foodstuff.[66] Retrospective analysis of data from near-drowned humans also shows that survival did not improve with steroids.[5]

Prophylactic antibiotics are also not recommended to treat aspiration pneumonitis after near-drowning unless clinical symptoms and cultures indicate an infection. Routine use of antibiotic prophylaxis may actually cause superinfection with resistant organisms. If the patient is intubated, tracheal secretions should be stained and cultured should signs and symptoms of a pulmonary infection occur.

Sodium bicarbonate is indicated to treat persistent metabolic acidosis in a near-drowned patient; we generally do not initiate this therapy unless the arterial pH is <7.2. The dose of bicarbonate to be administered should be based on arterial blood gas values and acid-base balance. The formula for calculating the dose of bicarbonate is

$$\text{sodium bicarbonate (mEq)} = \text{weight (kg)} \times \text{base deficit (mEq/L)} \times 0.20$$

We administer no more than 50% of the calculated dose of bicarbonate at any one time, and we check arterial pH between doses.

Fluid Therapy

Fluid resuscitation is rarely necessary after near-drowning unless pulmonary edema occurs and an excessive loss of fluid results. If hypovolemia does occur, resuscitation with crystalloid, such as lactated Ringer's solution, or colloid is indicated. Ordinarily, only maintenance fluids are required.

If the patient is comatose and has cerebral edema, fluids might actually have to be restricted after the initial resuscitation and evaluation. Data from studies that did not use a near-drowning model may be pertinent, although not directly applicable. Using animal models of hemorrhage without brain injury and of hemodilution to compare the effects on ICP of hypertonic with those of iso/hypotonic resuscitation solutions, one study[70a] did and another did not[70b] report lower ICP with hypertonic solution. One study[70c] in which a focal cryogenic brain injury was induced showed that cerebral blood flow was higher and ICP was lower with hypertonic sodium lactate (500 mOsm/L) than lactated Ringer's solution (270 mOsm/L). The patient's electrolyte changes are usually transient and require no specific therapy; however, persistent imbalances do occur, they should be corrected. Most near-drowned patients do not aspirate enough fluid to cause electrolyte changes that will be evident on arrival at the emergency department.[5] Hyperglycemia should be avoided because it may augment neurologic damage in the brain-injured patient.[70d]

Significant hemolysis of RBCs after near-drowning is extremely rare unless combined with profound hypoxia. If hemoglobinemia and hemoglobinuria occur, consideration should be given to the use of osmotic diuresis to increase urine flow (to ≥1.5 mL/kg per hour) and eliminate plasma Hb. Circulating blood volume must be adequate before the administration of an osmotic diuretic.

CNS Therapy

Although the immediate emphasis of therapy after near-drowning is directed at the lungs and the improvement of oxygenation and oxygen delivery, other organ systems may be affected, particularly if hypoxia has been sustained.[48] The final measure of successful therapy is survival without neurologic deficit. In the emergency department, a careful neurologic examination must be performed. If there is a history of falling or diving, signs of facial trauma, or the patient is comatose, cervical spine injury and intracranial hemorrhage must be ruled out with roentgenography of the cervical spine, CT scan, or, occasionally, arteriography. A cervical collar should be placed on the patient until cervical injury is ruled out. If the patient is alert, then no specific therapy aimed at cerebral salvage is necessary. If the patient has a blunted level of consciousness, therapy aimed at cardiopulmonary resuscitation and improved oxygenation is all that is necessary and should result in survival of 90% to 100% of patients.[20,58]

Treatment of the comatose patient is more complicated. In addition to the guidelines outlined so far, therapy aimed at preserving the brain and decreasing cerebral edema must be considered. Hyperventilation to a Pa_{CO_2} of approximately 25 to 30 torr will reduce cerebral blood flow and cerebral volume and, thereby, will reduce ICP.[71] This is unquestionably indicated if cerebral edema is present and should be started in the emergency department. Other therapy is more controversial. Steroids have been advocated and are used frequently to treat cerebral edema.[72-76] They have not been helpful in treating cerebral edema secondary to global ischemia and hypoxia, however.

At one time, Conn and colleagues[19,20] recommended an aggressive cerebral salvage approach to the comatose, near-drowned patient regardless of the state of ICP. They recommended high-dose barbiturate therapy, induced hypothermia (30°C), muscle paralysis, hyperventilation, diuresis with furosemide, steroids, and a Pao_2 of 150 torr or greater. Later, Conn[77] recommended normothermia or hypothermia (30°C) only when ICP could not be controlled by other means; also, steroids were not used routinely. Bohn et al[22] reviewed retrospectively the effect of hypothermia, barbiturate therapy, and ICP monitoring on outcome of the near-drowned patient. They found no improvement in outcome with hypothermia or barbiturate therapy. Also, there was no clear indication that ICP monitoring affected outcome, and thus they did not recommend ICP monitoring of the near-drowned patient. Nussbaum and Maggi[23] found no improvement in neurologic outcome in flaccid, comatose patients studied prospectively who were treated with or without pentobarbital therapy. Although barbiturates can be useful in reducing ICP, Sarnaik et al[21] found that continuous ICP monitoring, intracranial hypertension prophylaxis, and maintenance of cerebral perfusion pressure at 50 torr did not ensure a favorable outcome in severely comatose children.

In the emergency department, ensuring a patent airway and adequate oxygenation and oxygen delivery constitutes the first line of defense for preserving cerebral integrity. If the patient is comatose, hyperventilation should be started. If seizures occur, they should be treated; phenytoin or other anticonvulsants are appropriate therapy and should be started in the emergency department.

Monitoring

All near-drowned patients must have vital signs (heart rate, blood pressure, respiratory rate, and temperature) monitored. If hypoxemia persists and any type of prolonged support is necessary, ECG and fluid intake and output must also be monitored. Most important is the analysis of arterial blood gases and pH. If multiple determinations are necessary, an arterial catheter facilitates blood sampling.

In addition to arterial blood gases and pH, Hb, Hct, and serum electrolytes should be determined. If the Hct is near normal and the plasma is free of Hb, it is unlikely that the patient has aspirated enough fluid to affect electrolyte concentrations. If hemolysis is present on inspection of the plasma, determination of plasma Hb is indicated. Chest and, if indicated, cervical spine roentgenograms should be obtained. Those patients requiring extensive cardiopulmonary resuscitation should also have baseline coagulation values determined—prothrombin time, partial thromboplastin time, and platelet counts—and a baseline renal metabolic profile performed.

Patients with cardiovascular instability need venous pressure monitoring. Central venous pressure reflects pressure proximal to the right atrium, and monitoring CVP has limited benefit during pulmonary insufficiency and when high levels of expiratory pressure are required. In these situations, a flow-directed, thermistor-tipped pulmonary artery catheter is helpful in assessing pulmonary artery and pulmonary artery occlusion pressures, CO, intrapulmonary shunt, and arteriovenous content difference.[78-80] Multimodality evoked potentials may be helpful after initial resuscitation and stabilization in predicting outcome in comatose children. This is not a test to be used in the emergency department, however.

In summary, therapy must be directed at rapid cardiopulmonary resuscitation as indicated by the victim's condition at the scene of the accident and must be continued uninterrupted until all vital functions are stabilized or death is confirmed. Fear of resuscitating a permanently neurologically damaged patient should not be a consideration as there are reports of intact survival after prolonged submersion and no predictors of outcome that can be used at the time of initial resuscitation are certain. Deciding who should receive subsequent aggressive therapy may be based on combined information such as clinical assessment, coma scale score, and multimodality evoked potentials.[12]

Ambulatory and Follow-Up Care

Patients whose Pao_2 is greater than 80 torr while breathing room air probably did not aspirate. If the patient is alert and, after in-hospital observation for 12 to 24 hours, has no deterioration of physical status or arterial blood gas values, such a patient may be discharged without further follow-up. Always advise the patient to return if any signs of respiratory distress, fever, or other related problems occur within 48 hours of release. If the patient has a normal Pao_2 and a normal chest radiograph and, in addition, is asymptomatic, 6 to 8 hours of observation may be adequate. Each case must be individualized, however, and it is best to err on the side of conservative treatment.

Patients who have minimal alteration of arterial blood gases that rapidly returns to normal during observation or treatment in the intensive care unit should return to a physician familiar with their history after approximately a week, or sooner if problems occur.

Patients who require more prolonged and extensive therapy for respiratory insufficiency, cerebral damage, or damage to other organs require more extensive follow-up, the exact extent of which will depend on the severity of the injury and the residual deficits.

REFERENCES

1. Modell JH. Biology of drowning. *Annu Rev Med.* 1978;29:1–8.
1a. Wintemute GJ. Childhood drowning and near-drowning in the United States. *Am J Dis Child.* 1990;144:663–669.
1b. National Safety Council. *Accident Facts.* Chicago: National Safety Council; 1987.
2. Modell JH, ed. *The Pathophysiology and Treatment of Drowning and Near-Drowning.* Springfield, IL: Thomas; 1971.
3. Modell JH. Drown versus near-drown: a discussion of definitions. *Crit Care Med.* 1981;9:351–352.
4. Cot C. *Les Asphyxies Accidentelles (Submersion, Electrocution, Intoxication Oxycarbonique). Etude Clinique, Therapeutique et Preventive.* Paris: Editions medicales N Maloine; 1931.
5. Modell JH, Graves SA, Ketover A. Clinical course of 91 consecutive near-drowning victims. *Chest.* 1976;70:231–236.
6. Press E, Walker J, Crawford I. An interstate drowning study. *Am J Public Health.* 1968;58:2275–2289.
7. Webster DP. Pool drownings and their prevention. *Public Health Rep.* 1967;82:587–600.
8. Pearn JH, et al. Drowning and near-drowning involving children: a five year total population study from the city and county of Honolulu. *Am J Public Health.* 1979;69:450–454.
8a. Pitt WR, Balanda KP. Childhood drowning and near-drowning in Brisbane: the contribution of domestic pools. *Med J Aust.* 1991;154:661–665.
9. Craig AB Jr. Causes of loss of consciousness during underwater swimming. *J Appl Physiol.* 1961;16:583.
10. Craig AB Jr. Underwater swimming and loss of consciousness. *JAMA.* 1961;176:255–258.
11. Keatinge WR. *Survival in Cold Water: The Physiology and Treatment of Immersion Hypothermia and of Drowning.* Oxford: Blackwell; 1969.
12. Siebke H, Breivek H, Rod T, et al. Survival after 40 minutes' submersion without sequelae. *Lancet.* 1975;1:1275–1277.
13. Gordon BA. Drowning and the diving reflex in man. *Med J Aust.* 1972;2:583–587.
14. Davis JH. Autopsy findings in victims of drowning. In: Modell JH, ed. *The Pathophysiology and Treatment of Drowning and Near-Drowning.* Springfield, IL: Thomas; 1971:74–82.
15. Swann HG, Brucer M. The cardiorespiratory and biochemical events during rapid anoxic death. VI. Fresh water and sea water drowning. *Tex Rep Biol Med.* 1949;7:604–618.
16. Swann HG, Brucer M, Moore C, et al. Fresh water and sea water drowning: a study of the terminal cardiac and biochemical events. *Tex Rep Biol Med.* 1947;5:423–437.
17. Modell JH, Moya F, Williams HD, et al. Changes in blood gases and A-aDO$_2$ during near-drowning. *Anesthesiology.* 1968;29:456–465.
18. Conn AW, Edmonds JF, Barker GA. Near-drowning in cold fresh water: current treatment regimen. *Can Anesth Soc.* 1978;25:259–265.
19. Conn AW, Edmonds JF, Barker GA. Cerebral resuscitation in near-drowning. *Pediatr Clin North Am.* 1979;26:691–701.
20. Conn AW, Montes JE, Barker GA, et al. Cerebral salvage in near-drowning following neurological classification by triage. *Can Anaesth Soc.* 1980;27:201–210.
21. Sarnaik AP, Preston G, Lieh-Lai M, Eisenberry AB. Intracranial pressure and cerebral perfusion pressure in near-drowning. *Crit Care Med.* 1985;13:224–227.
22. Bohn DJ, Biggar WD, Smith CR, Conn AW, Barker GA. Influence of hypothermia, barbiturate therapy, and intracranial pressure monitoring on morbidity and mortality after near-drowning. *Crit Care Med.* 1986;14:529–534.
23. Nussbaum E, Maggi JC. Pentobarbital therapy does not improve neurologic outcome in nearly-drowned, flaccid-comatose children. *Pediatrics.* 1988;81:630–634.
24. Modell JH, et al. Blood gas and electrolyte changes in human near-drowning victims. *JAMA.* 1968;203:337–343.
25. Modell JH, Gaub M, Moya F, et al. Physiologic effects of near-drowning with chlorinated fresh water, distilled water, and isotonic sodium chloride. *Anesthesiology.* 1966;27:33–41.
26. Modell JH, Kuck EJ, Ruiz BC, et al. Effect of intravenous vs aspirated distilled water on serum electrolytes and blood gas tensions. *J Appl Physiol.* 1972;32:579–584.
27. Modell JH, Moya F. Effects of volume of aspirated fluid during chlorinated fresh water drowning. *Anesthesiology.* 1966;27:662.
28. Modell JH, Moya F, Newby EJ, et al. The effects of fluid volume in seawater drowning. *Ann Intern Med.* 1967;67:68–80.
29. Hasan S, Avery WG, Fabian C, et al. Near-drowning in humans. A report of 36 patients. *Chest.* 1971;59:191–197.
30. Modell JH, Calderwood HW, Ruiz BC, et al. Effects of ventilatory patterns on arterial oxygenation after near-drowning in sea water. *Anesthesiology.* 1974;40:376–384.
31. Giammona ST, Modell JH. Drowning by total immersion: effects on pulmonary surfactant of distilled water, isotonic saline and sea water. *Am J Dis Child.* 1967;114:612–616.
32. Colebatch HJH, Halmagyi DFJ. Lung mechanics and resuscitation after fluid aspiration. *J Appl Physiol.* 1961;16:684–696.
33. Colebatch HJH, Halmagyi DFJ. Reflex airway reaction to fluid aspiration. *J Appl Physiol.* 1962;17:787–794.
34. Colebatch HJH, Halmagyi DFJ. Reflex pulmonary hypertension of fresh water aspiration. *J Appl Physiol.* 1963;18:179–185.
35. Bergquist RE, Vogelhut MM, Modell JH, et al. Comparison of ventilatory patterns in the treatment of freshwater near-drowning in dogs. *Anesthesiology.* 1980;52:142–148.
36. Ducker TB, Simmons RL, Anderson RW. Increased intracranial pressure and pulmonary edema. III. The effect of increased intracranial pressure on the cardiovascular hemodynamics of chimpanzees. *J Neurosurg.* 1968;29:475–483.
37. Butt MP, Jalowayski A, Modell JH, et al. Pulmonary function after resuscitation from near-drowning. *Anesthesiology.* 1970;32:275–277.
38. Jenkinson SG, George RB. Serial pulmonary function studies in survivors of near drowning. *Chest.* 1980;77:777–780.
39. Laughlin JJ, Eigen H. Pulmonary function abnormalities in survivors of near drowning. *J Pediatr.* 1982;100:26–30.
40. Modell JH, Davis JH. Electrolyte changes in human drowning victims. *Anesthesiology.* 1969;30:414–420.
40a. Mosseri M, Porath A, Ovsyshcher I, Stone D. Electrocardiographic manifestations of combined hypercalcemia and hypermagnesemia. *J Electrocardiol.* 1990;23:235–241.
41. Fainer DC. Near drowning in sea water and fresh water. *Ann Intern Med.* 1963;59:537–541.
42. Farthmann EH, Davidson AIG. Fresh water drowning at lowered body temperature: an experimental study. *Am J Surg.* 1965;109:410.
43. Lougheed DW, Janes JM, Hall GE. Physiological studies in experimental asphyxia and drowning. *Can Med Assoc.* 1939;40:423–428.
44. Redding JS, Pearson JW. Management of drowning victims. *GP.* 1964;29:100–104.
45. Spitz WU, Blanke RV. Mechanism of death in freshwater drowning. I. An experimental approach to the problem. *Arch Pathol.* 1961;71:661–668.

46. Tabeling BB, Modell JH. Fluid administration increases oxygen delivery during continuous positive pressure ventilation after freshwater near-drowning. *Crit Care Med.* 1983;11:693–696.
47. Culpepper RM. Bleeding diathesis in freshwater drowning. *Ann Intern Med.* 1975;83:675.
48. Hoff BH. Multisystem failure: a review with special reference to drowning. *Crit Care Med.* 1979;7:310–320.
49. Ports RA, Deuel TF. Intravascular coagulation in freshwater submersion: report of 3 cases. *Ann Intern Med.* 1977;87:60–61.
50. Fuller RH. The 1962 Wellcome Prize Essay. Drowning and the post-immersion syndrome. A clinicopathologic study. *Mil Med.* 1963;128:22–36.
51. King RB, Webster IW. A case of recovery from drowning and prolonged anoxia. *Med J Aust.* 1964;1:919–920.
52. Kvittingen TD, Naess A. Recovery from drowning in fresh water. *Br Med J.* 1963;1:1315–1317.
53. Munroe WD. Hemoglobinuria from near-drowning. *J Pediatr.* 1964;64:57–62.
54. Rath CE. Drowning hemoglobinuria. *Blood.* 1953;8:1099–1104.
55. Pearn JH, Bart RD Jr, Yamaoka R. Neurologic sequelae after childhood near-drowning: a total population study from Hawaii. *Pediatrics.* 1979;64:187–191.
56. Pearn JH, Nixon J, Wilkey I. Freshwater drowning and near-drowning accidents involving children: a five-year total population study. *Med J Aust.* 1975;2:942–946.
57. Peterson B. Morbidity of childhood near-drowning. *Pediatrics.* 1962;59:364–370.
58. Modell JH, Graves SA, Kuck EJ. Near-drowning: correlation of level of consciousness and survival. *Can Anaesth Soc J.* 1980;27:211–215.
58a. Quan L, Kinder D. Pediatric submersion; prehospital predictors of outcome. *Pediatrics.* 1992;90:909–913.
59. Safar P, Escarraga LA, Elam JO. A comparison of the mouth-to-mouth and mouth-to-airway methods of artificial respiration with the chest-pressure arm-lift methods. *N Engl J Med.* 1958;258:671–677.
60. Heimlich HJ. The Heimlich maneuver: first treatment for drowning victims. *Emerg Med Serv.* 1981;10:58–61.
61. Ornato JP. The resuscitation of near drowning victims. *JAMA.* 1986;256:875–877.
62. Ruiz BC, Calderwood HW, Modell JH, et al. Effect of ventilatory patterns on arterial oxygenation after near-drowning with fresh water. A comparative study in dogs. *Anesth Analg.* 1973;52:570–576.
63. Downs JB, Klein EF Jr, Modell JH. The effect of incremental PEEP on Pao_2 in patients with respiratory failure. *Anesth Analg.* 1973;52:210–214.
64. Downs JB, Modell JH. Patterns of respiratory support aimed at pathophysiologic conditions. In: Hershey SG, ed. *ASA Refresher Courses in Anesthesiology.* Philadelphia: Lippincott; 1977:5:71–85.
64a. Banner MJ, Kirby RR, Blanch PB. Site of pressure measurement during spontaneous breathing with continuous positive airway pressure—effect on calculating imposed work of breathing. *Crit Care Med.* 1992;20:528–533.
65. Rose DM, Downs JB, Heenan TJ. Temporal responses of functional residual capacity and oxygen tension to changes in positive end-expiratory pressure. *Crit Care Med.* 1981;9:79–82.
66. Wynne JW, Reynolds JC, Hood CL, et al. Steroid therapy for pneumonitis induced in rabbits by aspiration of foodstuff. *Anesthesiology.* 1979;51:11–19.
67. Chapman RL Jr, Downs JB, Modell JH, et al. The ineffectiveness of steroid therapy in treating aspiration of hydrochloric acid. *Arch Surg.* 1974;108:858–861.
68. Chapman RL Jr, Modell JH, Ruiz BC, et al. Effect of continuous positive-pressure ventilation and steroids on aspiration of hydrochloric acid (pH 1.8) in dogs. *Anesth Analg.* 1974;53:556–562.
69. Downs JB, Chapman RL Jr, Modell JH, et al. An evaluation of steroid therapy in aspiration pneumonitis. *Anesthesiology.* 1974;40:129–135.
70. Calderwood HW, Modell JH, Ruiz BC. The ineffectiveness of steroid therapy in treating fresh water near-drowning. *Anesthesiology.* 1975;43:642–650.
70a. Prough DS, Johnson JC, Poole GV Jr, Stullken EH, Johnston WE, Royster R. Effects on intracranial pressure of resuscitation from hemorrhagic shock with hypertonic saline versus lactated Ringer's solution. *Crit Care Med.* 1985;13:407–411.
70b. Ducey JP, Lamiell JM, Gueller GE. Cerebral electrophysiologic effects of resuscitation with hypertonic saline-dextran after hemorrhage. *Crit Care Med.* 1990;18:744–749.
70c. Shackford SR, Zhuang J, Schmoker J. Intravenous fluid tonicity—effect on intracranial pressure, cerebral blood flow and cerebral oxygen delivery in focal brain injury. *J Neurosurg.* 1992;76:91–98.
70d. Lanier WL, Stangland KJ, Scheithauzer BW, Milde JH, Michenfelder JD. The effects of dextrose infusion and head position on neurologic outcome after complete cerebral ischemia in primates—examination of a model. *Anesthesiology.* 1987;66:39–48.
71. Severinghaus JW, Lassen HA. Step hypocapnia to separate arterial from tissue Pco_2 in the regulation of cerebral blood flow. *Circ Res.* 1967;20:272–278.
72. Faupel G, Reulen JH, Müller D, et al. Double-blind study on the effects of steroids on seven closed-head injuries. In: Pappius HM, Feindel W, eds. *Dynamics of Brain Edema.* Berlin: Springer-Verlag; 1976:337–343.
73. Gobiet W, Bock WJ, Liesegang J, et al. Treatment of acute cerebral edema with high dose dexamethasone. In: Beks JW, Bosch DA, Brock M, et al, eds. *Intracranial Pressure III.* Berlin: Springer-Verlag; 1976:231–235.
74. Fishman RA. Brain edema. *N Engl J Med.* 1975;293:706–711.
75. Gudeman SK, Miller JD, Becker DP. Failure of high dose steroid therapy to influence intracranial pressure in patients with severe head injury. *J Neurosurg.* 1979;51:301–306.
76. Dearden NM, Gibson JS, McDowall DG, et al. Effect of high-dose dexamethasone on outcome from severe head injury. *J Neurosurg.* 1986;64:81–88.
77. Conn AW. Fresh water drowning and near-drowning—an update. *Can Anaesth Soc J.* 1984;31:S38–S44.
78. Colgan FJ, Mahoney PD. The effects of major surgery on cardiac output and shunting. *Anesthesiology.* 1969;31:221–231.
79. Gustafson I, Nordstrom L. Central venous Po_2 and open-heart surgery. *Acta Anaesth Scand.* 1970;14(suppl 37):112–113.
80. Swan HJC, et al. Catheterization of the heart in man with use of flow-directed balloon-tipped catheter. *N Engl J Med.* 1970;283:447–451.
80a. Goodwin SR, Freidman WA, Bellefleur M. Is it time to use evoked potentials to predict outcome in comatose children and adults? *Crit Care Med.* 1991;19:518–524.

44. Hyperbaric Emergencies

C. GRESHAM BAYNE, MD

INTRODUCTION

The use of a hyperbaric chamber for medical emergencies has increased dramatically in recent years because of increased availability of facilities and better pathophysiological documentation of the effects of hyperbaric oxygenation (HBO). Prior to 1979, there were fewer than 40 HBO treatment centers in the United States; now there are over 200. These centers are evenly divided between monoplace chambers (Fig. 44-1) and multiplace chambers (Fig. 44-2).

Monoplace Facility

A monoplace chamber provides a convenient and low-cost facility in which a patient is placed recumbent and pressurized with pure oxygen to depths not in excess of 60 feet of sea water (FSW) equivalent. Such chambers can be plugged directly into an existing 50-psi oxygen line, are mobile on wheels, require little maintenance, and are generally well tolerated by patients. Theoretical disadvantages are the flammability hazard of compressed oxygen, which explodes when ignited under 60 FSW pressure; the claustrophobic effect of small spaces; depth limitations; and the inability to access a patient's airway in an emergency.

Multiplace Facility

Multiplace facilities require significantly more capital costs, staffing, and hospital space allocation. Theoretical advantages of multiplace facilities are access directly to patients by inside tenders; reduction in fire hazard, by pressurizing the chamber with air while patients breathe pure oxygen by mask, hood, or endotracheal tube; deeper depth capability; and capability to treat more than one patient at a time. This last characteristic has led to private and Air Force initiatives currently underway to build multimillion dollar chambers capable of pressurizing more than 30 patients on a single dive. By increasing volume, multiplace centers hope to bring costs per dive down to more reasonable levels; current technical fees average over $3.00 per minute in most American chambers.

The controversy over which chamber to install in a given center involves cost, patient selection, and individual preferences. A monoplace chamber can be installed for well under $100,000, whereas a multiplace chamber may cost over $500,000. However, on a per-treatment basis, the ability of a large multiplace chamber to treat 8, 10, or even 30 patients at a time can bring operational costs down below that of monoplace facilities, limited to one treatment at a time. If a facility is designed to treat critical patients and diving accidents, it will be restricted to one patient in the chamber at a time no matter which type is used. Then, the selection is based on the comfort level of the attending clinicians in monitoring such patients remotely. Through-hull penetrators can be used to carry ECG, EEG, and pressure waveform signals to outside monitors. Thus, a patient can be placed in the monoplace chamber with outside monitors equivalent to the intensive care unit.[1] A pressure-cycled ventilator may be placed inside

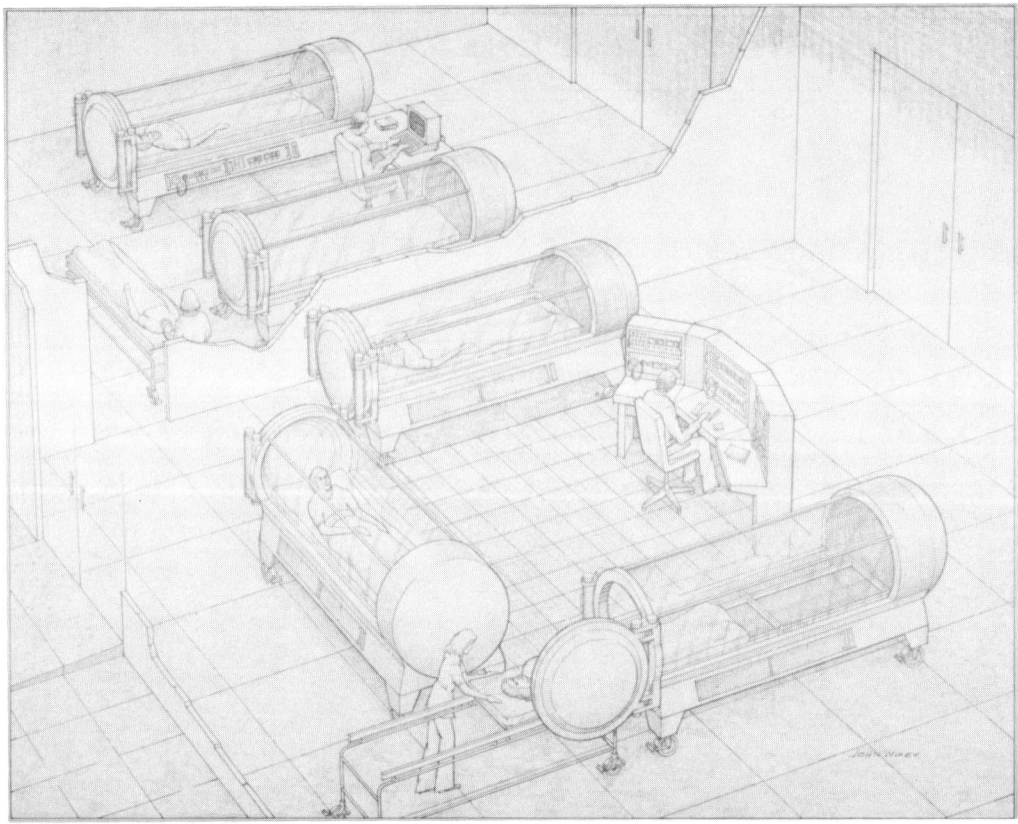

Figure 44-1 Monoplace hyperbaric medical systems with certified single or multiple acrylic pressure chamber console controls. *Source:* Courtesy of Hyperbaric Oxygen Therapy Systems, Inc, San Diego, CA.

the chamber to ventilate the intubated patient. Unlike the multiplace facility, where the attendants are physically beside the patient to avoid problems and correct accidents, monoplace facilities rely on a quick ascent to the surface to retrieve disconnected lines or tubes. The accompanying risk of barotrauma may be moot, since no record exists of a monoplace patient being embolized during a rapid ascent to the surface for such an intervention.

In general, physicians aligned with multiplace facilities tend to endorse them as the best solution to hyperbarics, while those financially restricted in start-up costs tend to espouse the virtues of monoplace facilities. The correct decision is to select the chamber complex fitting a given patient population and financial structure of the hospital. One should be aware that the arguments of attendants at risk in a multiplace chamber, and oxygen toxicity risk being higher in a monoplace chamber, are decidedly inappropriate. The physiology of the treatment is identical except for short air breaks used in the multiplace chambers to reduce oxygen convulsions; however, no increased risk in the small incidence of convulsions has been documented with monoplace chambers. The risks of barotrauma or decompression sickness in multiplace facilities is rendered almost nonexistent by procedures now being used.

PATHOPHYSIOLOGY

The principles involved in HBO therapy are chiefly:

1. Boyle's law compression of gas bubbles
2. increased gaseous resolution of bubbles
3. physiological effects of oxygen under high pressure (OHP)

Boyle's law states simply that at constant temperature the pressure and volume of a gas in an enclosed space are inversely related:

$$P_1V_1 = P_2V_2$$

where P = pressure in atmosphere absolute (ATA) and V = volume in identical units.

As is evident, increasing pressure can decrease volume; however, since it is the intravascular gas that creates most pathology, the radius of a bubble is of more concern. Applying the equation for a sphere ($V = \pi r^2$), it is possible to solve for the radius of a standard one-unit bubble at various treatment depths, as shown in Table 44-1. It is clear that compression deeper than 165 FSW leads to little reduction in

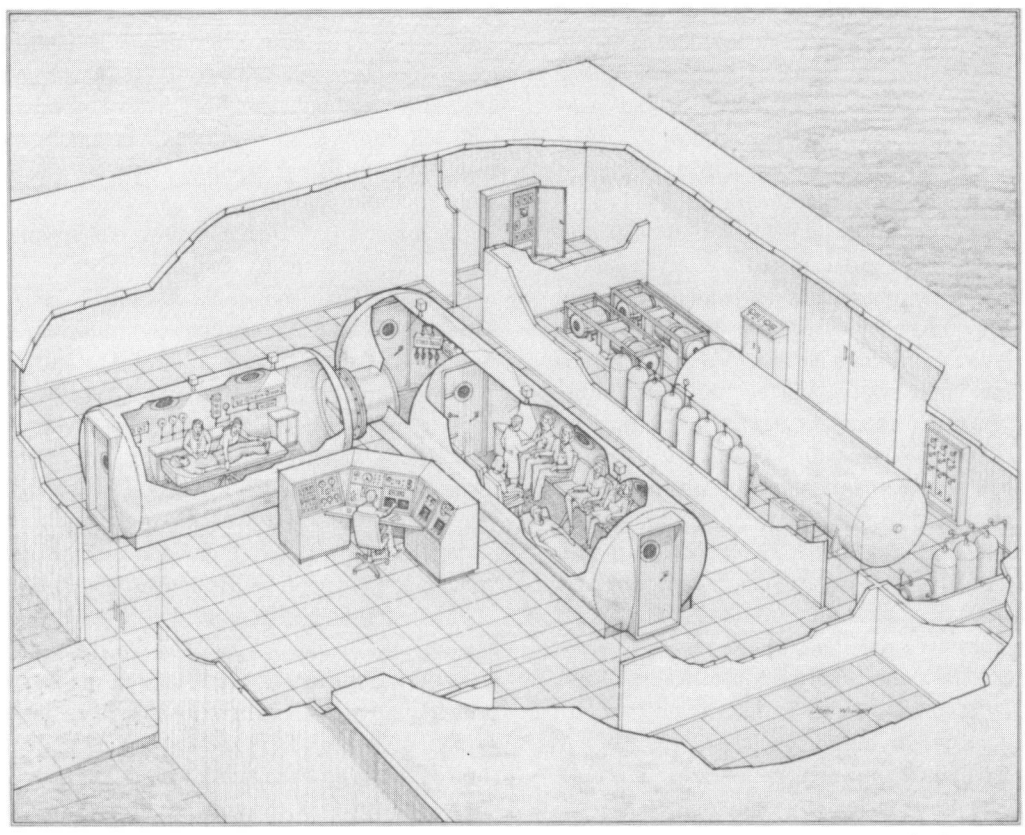

Figure 44-2 Multiplace hyperbaric medical complex including certified clinical treatment and critical care pressure chambers with centralized control. *Source:* Courtesy of Hyperbaric Oxygen Therapy Systems, Inc, San Diego, CA.

bubble diameter. Since these depths are associated with significant decrement in the attendant's performance due to nitrogen narcosis, few HBO centers dive deeper than 165 FSW.

Bubbles introduced into the vascular system by pulmonary barotrauma or iatrogenic misfortune must be resolved by a combination of compression and resolution of the intrabubble gases by diffusion. By placing a patient on pure oxygen, the inert gas partial pressure of the surrounding blood and tissue is reduced by denitrogenation. Concurrently, increased barometric pressure drives the intrabubble inert gas partial pressures up, thereby increasing the diffusion gradient for inert gas from inside to outside the bubble. The net effect is faster resolution of the bubble by diffusion enhancement.

OHP is a potent drug with several important physiological consequences. Increasing the Pa_{O_2} above 2000 mmHg dissolves enough oxygen in human plasma to satisfy the normal

Table 44-1 Relationship of Pressure and Bubble Size

Depth, FSW	Gas Pressure, ATA	Gas Volume, cm³	Bubble Radius, cm	Bubble Diameter, cm	Reduction in Surface Value of Bubble Diameter, %
0	1.00	1.00	0.62	1.24	100.0
33	2.00	0.50	0.49	0.98	79.0
60	2.82	0.35	0.44	0.88	71.0
165	6.00	0.17	0.34	0.68	55.0
198	7.00	0.14	0.32	0.64	52.3

Note that the greatest reductions occur in the initial phases of compression.

adult oxygen needs. Hence, patients at 60 FSW receiving OHP never need to desaturate their hemoglobin and may maintain normal oxygen delivery despite anemia or low cardiac output. Indeed, HBO-treated dogs had better survival (74%) from hemorrhagic shock than controls (17%).[2]

In addition to simple increased oxygen delivery, OHP has been shown to be bacteriocidal for *Clostridium*[3] and to inhibit growth of several anaerobes including *Neisseria meningitidis*.[4] OHP has been shown to increase the effectiveness of antibiotics on certain aerobes possibly by damaging the PABA–folic acid pathway.[5,6] Other possible mechanisms for oxygen's role as an antibiotic include increasing chemotaxis, opsonization, phagocytosis, and the formation of toxic radicals such as superoxides and singlet oxygen during the oxidative burst following phagocytosis. That oxygen is a key drug in combating infections can be inferred from the disease chronic granulomatous disease (CGD) characterized by recurring infections during childhood. CGD is caused by a genetic absence of myeloperoxidase, an enzyme that requires oxygen as a cofactor.

As with any other drug, OHP has a dose-response curve and toxic side effects if used indiscriminately. Prolonged exposures to OHP can cause CNS toxicity manifested by nausea, irritability, tremor, and eventual seizures. Long-term exposures at depths shallower than the seizure threshold can cause pulmonary oxygen toxicity similar to the respiratory distress syndrome of earlier long-term respirator patients. Current experience indicates that the risk of oxygen seizures is about one in 5000 treatments, with pulmonary oxygen toxicity nearly nonexistent on today's tables. Multiplace treatment facilities use air-breathing tenders who become at risk for decompression sickness if their "dives" are not followed and scheduled appropriately. A final complication of therapy is barotrauma or intravenous failure leading to air embolism (to be discussed). This risk is also extraordinarily rare in current HBO centers.

Hyperbaric medicine has advanced dramatically from an earlier checkered history of hucksterism and false claims. Despite the major emphasis on complex, nonhealing wounds providing most centers with their *raison d'être,* several emergency conditions are routinely treated:

1. carbon monoxide poisoning (with neurologic deficit)
2. anaerobic infections
3. decompression sickness
4. air embolism

Carbon Monoxide Poisoning

About half the fatal poisonings that occur each year in the United States are from carbon monoxide.[7] The devastation of this insult is due not so much to the induced anemia (CO binds hemoglobin 200 times more tightly than oxygen), nor to the induced leftward shift of the oxyhemoglobin dissociation curve for unpoisoned hemoglobin, as it is to inhibition of cytochrome a_3 oxidase. This enzyme is required for cellular respiration. In severe CO poisoning, as with cellular anoxia, anaerobic metabolism rapidly creates a base deficit and resultant acidemia. Tissue with high metabolic rates is more susceptible to CO poisoning, hence the presentation with global neurologic deficits.

The importance of understanding the enzymatic inhibition by free CO was demonstrated when experimental dogs transfused with COHb-contaminated blood to a COHb level of 57% to 64% showed no symptoms, whereas controls with similar levels created by inhaling 13% CO died within 1 hour.[8] Since it is the neurological deficit caused by direct cellular toxicity which directs medical care, the serum COHb level by co-oximetry does not necessarily correlate to symptoms. Hence, the COHb level merely documents the presence of poisoning and not the requirement for HBO. Some researchers, however, are recommending HBO for asymptomatic patients with COHb levels over 25%.

The treatment of CO-poisoned patients is often complicated by other emergencies. The patient has often taken an overdose of drugs, has significant ethanolism, or may have been found in a closed, burning space, leading to airways or pulmonary injuries from smoke inhalation. People suffering smoke inhalation from buildings built after about 1955 may have a significant cyanide ingestion from inhaling the byproducts of burning plastic plumbing. Obviously the volume restoration and airways management required by burns takes precedence over HBO management.

When assessing the comatose patient at risk for carbon monoxide intoxication, one should take care to order co-oximetry with the arterial blood gas. A patient with CO poisoning will have a normal Pa_{O_2} unless pulmonary damage has occurred from inhalation of toxins. The %sat oxyhemoglobin level is often calculated from the Dill nomogram and will hence appear normal if not measured directly. Co-oximetry uses a refractometer to measure directly the %sat oxyhemoglobin and carboxyhemoglobin and represents the definitive test. In the absence of co-oximetry, one must be suspicious of the condition of a normotensive patient with a normal Pa_{O_2} and a base deficit in the setting of smoke or exhaust inhalation.

If neurologic symptoms such as confusion, amnesia, ataxia, dysmetria, or lethargy are present in a patient with an elevated COHb level (above 10%), HBO should be instituted. The half-life of CO in humans is approximately 20 minutes using OHP vice 80 minutes with 100% oxygen at atmospheric pressure.[9,10] The clinician must weigh the advantages of the full table against the disadvantage of adding a small but definable dose of pulmonary oxygen toxicity to a patient whose lungs are already injured by smoke and inhalants.

Care must be taken to vent all IVs and fill the endotracheal balloon with saline to avoid barotrauma during the ascent from depth. At the 66 FSW level, the risk of oxygen convulsions is reduced by air-breathing breaks.

In summary, all patients with COHb levels exceeding 10 percent and neurological symptoms beyond the early complaints of nausea and headache should be referred for HBO. Although long-term benefit has not been proven, the rapid resolution of symptoms and removal of CO makes this therapy appropriate if not mandatory. Finally, the failure to use HBO in a patient rendered comatose from CO has been litigated successfully by the patient's relatives.

Anaerobic Infections

Several classifications of life-threatening anaerobic infections exist including necrotizing fasciitis, Meleney's infection, combined synergistic gangrene, and clostridial myonecrosis. When a patient presents with sepsis, hemodynamic instability, and clinical findings suggestive of a synergistic infection involving anaerobes, HBO is indicated as an emergency treatment adjunct. It is important to state that the surgical and infectious disease management of such patients remains primary, with HBO an adjunctive modality added to the regime. One should never expect HBO to change the surgical management of such lesions other than to reduce the amount of tissue to be debrided.

The rationale for anaerobic treatment is supported by HBO augmentation of host defense discussed above, and by direct experiments on clostridial lab models. HBO producing a PO_2 over 250 mmHg stops the alpha-toxin production by *Clostridium perfringens*.[11,12] A PO_2 greater than 1520 mmHg has been shown to kill this organism in culture medium.[3] In an animal model of gas gangrene, the combination of surgery, antibiotics, and HBO gave higher survival than animals treated with any two of the methods listed.[13] In a series of 49 cases of gas gangrene treated with HBO, patients had a survival rate of 73%.[14] This survival rate compares favorably with non-HBO-treated patients with clostridial infections and a survival rate of 55%.[15] In virtually all the clinical reports of clostridial infections, patients presenting in shock or with extensive truncal invasion had a dismal outcome.

The management of patients with anaerobic infections progressing rapidly is tailored for each case. Severely septic patients can be resuscitated in a multiplace chamber while receiving HBO and preparation for the operating room. Antibiotics based on Gram stain and clinical suspicions are started earlier, and radical debridement is the surgical treatment approach. Depending upon the severity of the fasciitis, patients are treated up to three times the first 24 hours, often alternating with operative procedures.

The use of hyperbaric oxygenation in anaerobic infections is not limited to clostridial myonecrosis. Other life-threatening infectious syndromes such as Meleney's ulcer, Fournier's gangrene, and progressive bacterial synergistic gangrene have shown improvement when HBO is added to the clinical treatment involving resuscitation, debridement, and antibiotics. Several possible mechanisms exist to explain the clinical improvement in such aggressive infections. Some 75% of the elderly with necrotizing fasciitis have diabetes; HBO may act by overcoming the ischemic effect of the microangiopathy, promoting neovascularization, reducing interstitial edema, or all three. There may be direct inhibitory or cidal effects of HBO on certain organisms, especially *Bacteroides* species. Reducing interstitial pressure by resorption of tissue gas may allow better blood flow to the infected area. There may be an interruption of the synergism between multiple organisms, especially hemolytic streptococcal species invading a Gram-negative wound.

In complex and rapidly expanding infections producing hypovolemic shock, as evidenced by a metabolic acidosis, HBO consultation by a qualified hyperbarist is indicated. In such cases, HBO will often be of adjunctive value in initial control of the septicemia, control of the fasciitis, demarcation of devitalized tissues, tissue salvage, and ultimate eradication of the infectious organisms. In no case should the use of HBO defer appropriate surgery, antibiotic therapy, or critical care monitoring.[16]

Decompression Sickness

Decompression sickness (DCS) is by nature an extremely hard disease to study. It is uncommon, even in high-density diving areas and, thus, often is initially managed by people ignorant of its potential. It classically presents with vague and nonspecific symptoms frequently suggestive of malingering or minor illness. There are no pathognomonic signs, so the diagnosis may be in question up to the point of recompression.

As with all diseases, diagnosis must await the patient's voluntary solicitation of medical aid, but patients with DCS have traditionally been motivated *not* to seek medical help for many reasons. The US Air Force has a policy of grounding pilots (with loss of flight pay) who experience serious symptoms. Commercial diving supervisors were quick to identify the ''bends prone'' individual and reduce exposures accordingly. Since divers were often paid relative to their depth and bottom time, DCS translated into a loss of income. Perhaps the most common problem is the pervasive philosophy that ''getting bent'' is a sign of weakness. This still-current idea probably goes back to the earlier caisson days, when workers learned to minimize their pain.

Several classifications exist for the subtypes of DCS. For the emergency physician, three presentations are generally seen (colloquial terms are provided in parentheses):

1. limb (bends)
2. cerebral (brain hit)
3. spinal cord (paretic bends)

Table 44-2 Time to Onset of Symptoms in Bounce Divers

Study	% Reporting in 1 hour	% Reporting in 2 hours	% Reporting in 6 hours
Rivera (1964)[18] n = 935	54.7	66.8	86.2
Duffner (1946)[19] n = 113		43.9	71.3
Bayne (1978)[17] n = 50	84.0	92.0	99.0

Limb Bends

Since limb bends by definition has no neurological involvement, pain is the predominant symptom. It has been the author's experience in treating some fifty cases of DCS[17] that the most characteristic finding is an ambiguous or confused history and physical examination. When seen acutely, the limb bends patient has difficulty in localizing or characterizing the pain. When asked to point with one finger, the patient often will use a sweeping motion of the hand, like the patient with abdominal pain secondary to small bowel colic. When asked to describe the pain, the patient is hard pressed to attach a single label such as sharp, dull, or cramplike. Perhaps the only persistent historical factor is that the pain is deepseated. It may be described as piercing or boring, but it is seldom described as superficial.

The vagueness of this history has limited the practitioner's ability to diagnose limb bends throughout the years. The problem of diagnosis is compounded by the lack of physical findings. Seldom is there focal tenderness or pain on specific range of motion. Tricks such as applying a blood pressure cuff or local heat to exacerbate the pain have been used to aid in diagnosis but have no proven rationale. The net result is that a diagnosis of limb bends is subjective. Since no existing data prove that recompression reduces long-term morbidity in limb bends, the true incidence will probably never be known—divers often medicate themselves with aspirin and ethanol until the pain resolves. Furthermore, many limb bends are undoubtedly misdiagnosed as musculoskeletal strains and treated accordingly.

In analyzing US Navy data, it must always be realized that the diagnosis of limb bends *requires* a beneficial response to recompression. Divers with suspected lesions who do not respond to a "trial of pressure" (20 minutes on 100% oxygen at 60 FSW) are sent home with a diagnosis other than DCS. Whether this practice is valid or not is still suspect and certainly affects the reported incidence of limb bends.

Several points should be remembered in the emergency care of divers with pain. First, all that hurts is not simple pain—only bends. Few physicians take the time to test two-point discrimination over the entire body surface area, but those who do are often surprised by the presence of neurological deficits. Second, the disease is known to progress, which means that early treatment of pain-only bends decreases the incidence of serious-symptom disease. Rivera[18] reported 193 cases of muscular weakness with only 8 showing the symptom initially. In addition, he reported 199 cases of numbness or paresthesia with 41 presenting as the initial complaint. Thus, immediate treatment may have prevented these serious symptoms in 343 cases. Finally, it is generally believed that the closer the onset of symptoms is to the end of the dive, the more potential there is for a serious problem to develop. This last statement is difficult to prove, since early treatment prevents progression of the disease and early treatment is more commonly available where deep diving is done. Certainly the time of onset to symptoms is documented in bounce divers with virtually all divers symptomatic within 24 hours postdive (Table 44-2). In an active diving area, one quickly learns to transport and treat aggressively those divers presenting only a few hours after surfacing, and to reserve less urgent philosophies for the pain-only bends presenting 6 to 12 hours postdive.[19]

Cerebral DCS

Involvement of the brain is fortunately rare in divers with decompression sickness. However, when it occurs, it presents with alarming signs such as seizure, blindness, coma, aphasia, apraxia, incoherence, and confusion.

Cerebral DCS is a bizarre disease. Symptoms have been attributed to arterial air embolism via intracardiac shunts, de novo arterial-sided bubbles, cerebral edema, or extravascular bubbles in the brain. It appears to be uncommon in divers, although Fructus[20] reported 23 cases in a series of 67 patients with CNS DCS. The US Air Force emphasizes the relative frequency of cerebral symptoms in altitude DCS, an observation that still remains unexplained. According to US Air Force experience, DCS diving altitude exposures can occur as low as 18,500 feet, but are a significant risk over 25,000 feet.[21] The actual incidence in divers may be far greater than reported, however, because of the difficulty in evaluating vague symptoms such as confusion and fatigue.

Spinal Cord DCS

Spinal cord involvement is generally considered to be the most common serious symptom in divers. As shown in Table 44-3, earlier studies tried to separate the CNS (brain and spinal cord) from the peripheral nervous system (cranial nerves and autonomic nervous system). Following the excellent work of Elliott and Hallenbeck,[22] the pathophysiology of paretic bends appears to be well understood. In their research, the accepted mechanism of retrograde venous thrombosis was shown to cause patchy necrosis of the spinal cord. Their association of spinal cord involvement with pulmonary hypertension (chokes) in the dog model is attractive and fits known anatomical and physiological mechanisms. In the human, however, pulmonary arterial catheterization must be

Table 44-3 Percentage Incidence of Organ System Involved During Illness

	Percent of Divers Affected		
	Rivera[18] (1964)	Behnke[21] (1947)	Duffner[19] (1946)
Bends (localized skeletomuscular pain)	91.8	72.2	85.8
Central nervous system	25.8	10.2	34.4
Peripheral nervous system	21.6		
Skin	14.9	13.6	0.9
Respiratory	2.0	4.0	7.9
Total number of cases	935	159	113

performed before a causal relationship between central venous hypertension and epidural venous thrombosis can be assumed. This relationship is quite important in deciding the fluid management of paretic DCS, as many areas are now indiscriminately hydrating patients with known paretic lesions and provisional cord edema.

Suffice it to say that cord lesions are rare in aviators but account for over half of serious symptoms in divers.[23] These lesions are also associated with pain in 30% of cases.[24] The incidence will obviously depend upon the skill of the investigator and the delay in examination or therapy as pain-only lesions progress.

The predilection for spinal lesions to involve the high lumbar nerve roots was most recently demonstrated among sport divers in whom 62% of all Type II cases involved the lumbar area.[23] The anatomical reason for this grouping may lie in the lack of collateral circulation to the area of the cord supplied by the so-called artery of Adamkiewicz, an end arteriole.

The epidemiology of cord lesions is most important, as it is this group of divers where permanent morbidity becomes most worrisome. At the outset, it must be emphasized that *acute* spinal cord DCS is a different entity from *subacute* cord lesions. An acute lesion, as defined by this author, is one where recompression is provided within 2 hours of symptoms. These cases normally occur in the military, where divers are fit, decompressed according to accepted tables, report their symptoms promptly, and seldom have fixed lesions.[24] It has long been known that delay in recompression reduces the prognosis for complete recovery. In one series of 50 consecutive cases of DCS, 25 of them cord lesions,[17] there were no symptoms or signs after the initial recompression in any of the patients. Since adjunctive therapy was used in only 1 patient and standard US Navy treatment tables applied, the success of this series can be explained by the rapid recompression characteristic of Navy centers.

Acute DCS involving the spinal cord is rare, however, outside the military environment. Most cases have delays in treatment as previously discussed, which create a totally different view of the disease. Although only one civilian death from DCS was reported in 1976, the morbidity of sport diving casualties is widely discussed. Saito[25] reported only four complete cures out of 23 cases of paraplegic DCS following a delay in recompression. Workman[26] reported significant residual disease in 7 of 40 civilian divers treated by the US Navy.

More recently, Kizer[23] reported complete relief in only 58% of 144 diving casualties. His work involving a series of divers treated at the US Navy Underwater Medicine Service at Pearl Harbor from January 1977 to August 1979 is by far the most standardized reference in the literature. Of the total 155 patients studied, 94% were male; 95% were over 20 years of age, with 47% between 20 and 29 years old; 61% had been diving for more than 5 years; 59% had serious (Type II) symptoms; 75% had omitted decompression during their dives; and the average delay between symptom onset increased from 7.4 hours in 1977 to 9.2 hours in 1979. Of interest is the note that only 15% of the patients had had military or commercial dive training.

There emerges the rather bleak picture of the active male diver, poorly trained, presenting hours after his symptoms began, with a significant history of omitted decompression time from his paretic dive(s). The prolonged stasis of blood in his epidural and radicular veins draining a segment of his spinal cord has led to edema and retrograde arterial thrombosis with possible hemorrhagic infarcts of the cord itself. The prognosis for complete recovery is poor. This has been the case with all other therapeutic attempts to reduce morbidity in blunt trauma to the spinal cord when treatment was delayed more than two hours after the accident.

The question is often raised of how long after a lesion occurs should treatment be given. Reports have been made of improvement when recompression was first begun six to eight days postdive. Although such cases are fortunately nonexistent in the US Navy, the author is of the view that treatment should be attempted in virtually all cases arriving at the chamber. Since the therapy, in most hands, has essentially no morbidity, it is hard to justify refusing a trial of pressure.

Treatment of DCS

The treatment of DCS relies upon recognition as the mainstay of therapy. Besides fluid resuscitation of the patient in shock, therapy requires nothing more than application of oxygen (to speed bubble resolution) and transfer of the patient to the nearest multiplace facility. To locate the nearest available chamber and gain access to a hyperbaric physician's advice, two 24-hour phone services are available:

US Air Force (San Antonio, TX)   (512) LEO-FAST
DAN (Divers Alert Network, Durham, NC)   (919) 684-8111

Air Embolism

Most physicians associate intravascular air with divers and cerebral air embolism. However, it is probably more common to see acute cerebral or hemodynamic compromise from therapeutic misadventures or penetrating trauma in major centers. We will discuss this topic based on two separate entities—venous air embolism and systemic (arterial) air embolism.

Venous Air Embolism

Following the discovery of oxygen at the turn of the century, enthusiasm led to intravenous administration of the gas for its therapeutic effects. However, it was soon discovered that infusion rates greater than 20 mL/min led to toxic side effects and the technique was abandoned. These early observations have been expanded to include ingress of gas into the right-side circulation from numerous operations and procedures (see Table 44-4).

Animal studies indicate that both the rate and the amount of gas infused are important in determining the onset of symptoms. Once a critical volume of gas has gained access to the venous circulation, increased pulmonary vascular resistance occurs and right-heart output falls, leading to hypotension and respiratory distress despite clear lung fields.[22] The diagnosis is made based on historical perspective, because the millwheel murmur (Hamman's sign) is frequently absent until dramatic hemodynamic compromise occurs. Other findings such as tachycardia and tachypnea are too nonspecific to alert the clinician to a diagnosis. As venous gas embolism is frequently an intraoperative complication, anesthesiologists have learned to monitor Doppler heart tones and expired CO_2 levels in high-risk patients. The earliest markers of subclinical air embolism are the Doppler phase shift caused by bubbles coursing through the heart and a reduction in end-tidal CO_2 concentration as fresh air in the pulmonary artery is delivered to the lungs. Unfortunately, such monitors are seldom used in the emergency department, where physicians must be suspicious of sudden respiratory distress or hypotension in patients with central line insertion mishaps, penetrating neck and head injuries, or indwelling Hickman catheters.

The treatment of venous gas embolism is as controversial as establishing the diagnosis outside of the emergency department. Certainly, aspiration of air through a central line or pulmonary artery catheter can prove both therapeutic and diagnostic. The recommendation to place patients in the right lateral decubitus (Durant) position is based upon a small dog study in 1942.[27] The theory is that air will gain access more easily to the pulmonary artery by avoiding a right ventricular "vapor lock" in this position. Subsequent studies have shown large variations in the amount of air required to kill a dog in the head-up, head-down, or supine position.[28,29] Failure to remove venous air can lead to activation of various kinins and prostaglandins, then to Hageman factor release and development of either adult respiratory distress syndrome (ARDS) or disseminated intravascular coagulation, or both. I have attended several such patients on the intensive care unit and can attest to the challenge of using high levels of positive end-expiratory pressure (PEEP) to treat ARDS while diffuse permeability defects maintained the patients in hypovolemic shock.

Treatment of gaseous venous embolism remains controversial. The source of air must be managed first by occluding a sucking neck wound with Vaseline gauze or clamping a defective central catheter. When venous gas occurs from an unknown surgical site, anesthesiologists will frequently use 10 cm H_2O end expiratory pressure to raise central venous pressures above ambient. Although little data other than clinical anecdotes exist, one may suppose recompression for acute venous gas embolism will decrease morbidity. By the physiology discussion above, venous bubbles will be resorbed more quickly with immediate reduction in volume gained by initial recompression. Acute emboli are treated initially at 165 FSW by conventional therapy, using air as the medium. Following 30 minutes at depth, the patient is taken to 60 FSW and placed on pure oxygen for final resolution of the bubbles. More advanced hyperbaric centers can now mix gas to provide a 50% oxygen–50% nitrogen mixture to be delivered at a maximum depth of 100 FSW. Such therapy provides a fourfold reduction in bubble volume with an inspired P_{O_2} of over 1500 mmHg to speed bubble resolution by diffusion. As with other conditions, emergency care must continue irrespective of chamber operations.

Arterial Air Embolism

Divers subjected to sudden decompression against a closed glottis (eg, during a panic ascent) are at risk for pulmonary barotrauma. The onset of sudden neurological deficit following *any* decompression event must be considered as arterial air embolism until proven otherwise. Such situations include divers ascending in the water or suddenly surfaced by a passing wave while hanging on an anchor line; pilots explosively decompressed by seal failure at high altitude in a pressurized aircraft; and hyperbaric chamber personnel during ascent, especially if receiving positive-pressure ventilation.

The mechanism of overinflation in divers with subsequent ingress of gas into the pulmonary vein and left heart is not known. Suffice it to say that several factors must be involved:

Table 44-4 Causes of Venous Air Embolism

Craniotomy	Central line placement
Suction curettage	Hyperalimentation
ENT surgery	Penetrating neck injuries
Labor and delivery	Laminectomy
Total hip replacement	Laparoscopy

high peak pressures during inspiration, large lung volumes, and high rate of rise of intrapulmonary pressure. Regional changes in compliance may allow barotrauma during an otherwise normal ascent. Such factors have been implicated in animal studies and clinical observations of divers suffering fatal air embolism after apparently normal ascents.

It is important to recognize the fact that depth or time on the bottom is not important in making a diagnosis of air embolism. A transpulmonic pressure gradient of 90 to 100 mmHg has been shown to rupture the lung in animals and in fresh, unchilled cadavers; this pressure gradient can be exceeded by scuba divers ascending from waist-deep water!

Although the diagnosis is generally apparent by the clinical setting, one should be alert for associated signs and symptoms. Extra-alveolar air may dissect along the pulmonary vessels to the mediastinum, giving rise to inspiratory substernal pressure or chest pain. Further dissection along the pretracheal fascia may lead to subcutaneous crepitus in the supraclavicular fossae or along the lateral chest wall. A pneumothorax may be present, with decreased breath sounds on the affected side. Rare findings include a millwheel crunching heart murmur, tongue geographism from lingual artery embolization, and the presence of intravascular bubbles on fundoscopy. Finally, one should be alert to the possibility of coronary air embolism leading to ischemic heart disease such as arrhythmias or pump failure.

The treatment of arterial air embolism is rather straightforward. To the principles of resuscitation must be added these caveats:

1. Maintain airway pressure as low as possible to prevent further barotrauma and/or embolization.
2. Use the highest oxygen concentration available to speed bubble resolution.
3. Transport in a pressurized aircraft to the nearest recompression facility. Of these rules, the latter is most important, as treatment without recompression has a uniformly dismal outcome.

USE OF HBO IN TRAUMATIC INJURIES

The recent national movement to regionalize trauma patients to a few selected major centers, many of which have hyperbaric centers, has led to a renewed interest in the use of HBO for selected injuries. The ability to supply the normal metabolic needs for oxygen using HBO in the absence of hemoglobin was demonstrated in animals in 1960.[27] Cowley was able to reduce the mortality rate of dogs subjected to hemorrhagic shock from 83% to 26% using oxygen breathed at 3 atmospheres absolute. More recently, Hart has used HBO in the management of severely anemic patients who refused transfusion for religious reasons.[28] With the advent of rapid transport and availability of blood products, such research has found lagging support. As blood becomes more expensive and risks become known from infectious complications with the slow viruses, the use of HBO in conjunction with fluorocarbons may be investigated.

The use of HBO in the treatment of experimental acute cerebral edema and nondisruptive injuries of the spinal cord proved encouraging. Sukoff showed a 50% reduction in intracranial pressure when animals subjected to intracranial balloon inflation were treated with HBO.[29] Numerous small clinical studies have shown equivocal results, however, as early treatment within the first 2 hours appears virtually impossible under current trauma procedural resuscitations. Although cats and dogs subjected to a controlled nondisruptive cord injury showed markedly better return of motor function with HBO,[30,31] clinical trials have also been limited by the delay before initial therapy. At this time, HBO use for traumatic injuries to the central nervous system is not widespread despite its rather excellent pathophysiological rationale.

The use of HBO in extremity injuries is rapidly gaining support. Since HBO stimulates osteogenesis and osteoblastic activity, one might expect the fracture healing time to be reduced. Several animal studies and one uncontrolled human study[32] confirm the observation that HBO can shorten the fracture stabilization time by as much as 30%. The use of HBO in the management of crush injuries and compartment syndromes is becoming widely accepted in the field. The increased tissue oxygenation, reduced compartment pressures, reduced interstitial pressures and bacteriostatic effects are well known and documented.[33]

Once the technical aspects of trauma resuscitation are complete, it is clear that HBO will provide a growing role for adjunctive care in trauma patients. As the number of chambers expands and demands for cost-effective care increase, I am certain that clear-cut protocols for the management of ancillary injuries will emerge.

CONCLUSION

Hyperbaric emergencies constitute an unusual but important group of clinical syndromes wherein prompt recognition in the treatment and transportation of such patients makes a major difference in the outcome. Patients with air embolism, decompression sickness, or carbon monoxide poisoning should be transported with the highest oxygen concentration possible en route to a multiplace chamber. Patients with necrotizing infections should be managed with all appropriate antibiotics, fluids, etc, en route to either a monoplace or multiplace facility.

More than 200 treatment chambers are currently active in the United States. A universal access number available around the clock is located in Durham, North Carolina at the Divers Alert Network (DAN). For up-to-date guidance on transportation, initial management, and referral to a local hyperbaric physician, call DAN at (919) 684-8111.

Although the principles of initial recompression are simple, delivering care in a chamber and using the complex tables requires the expertise of a hyperbaric team to avoid iatrogenic catastrophes. And a final caution: the need for recompression does not obviate the need for good emergency medicine!

REFERENCES

1. Rockswold GL, Ford E, Anderson JR, et al: Patient monitoring in the monoplace hyperbaric chamber. *Hyperbar Oxygen Rev.* 1985; 6:161–168.
2. Cowley RA, Attar S, Esmond W, et al. The utilization of hyperbaric oxygenation in hemorrhagic shock in dogs. In: *Clinical Application of Hyperbaric Oxygen.* New York: Elsevier; 1964:177–181.
3. Kaye D. Effect of hyperbaric oxygenation in clostridia in vitro and in vivo. *Proc Soc Exp Biol Med.* 1967;124:360.
4. Gottlieb SF. Interaction of oxygen, temperature, and drugs on two species of *Neisseria* as concerns the mechanism of oxygen toxicity. In: Water J, Iwa T, eds. *Proceedings of the Fourth International Congress on Hyperbaric Medicine.* Sapporo, Japan: Igaku Shoin; 1970:288–296.
5. Gottlieb SF, Pakman LM. Effect of high oxygen tensions on the growth of selected, aerobic, Gram-negative bacteria. *J Bacteriol.* 1968; 95:1003–1010.
6. Gottlieb SF, Rose NR, Maurizi J, et al. Oxygen inhibition of growth of *Mycobacterium tuberculosis. J Bacteriol.* 1964;87:838–843.
7. McBay AJ. Carbon monoxide poisoning (law-medicine notes). *N Engl J Med.* 1965;272:252.
8. Goldbaum LR, Ramirez RG, Absalom KB. What is the mechanism of carbon monoxide toxicity? *Aviat Space Environ Med.* 1975;46: 1289–1291.
9. Pace N, Stajman E, Walker EL. Acceleration of carbon monoxide elimination in man by high pressure oxygen. *Science.* 1950;111: 652–654.
10. Peterson JE, Stewart RD. Absorption and elimination of carbon monoxide by active young men. *Arch Environ Health.* 1970;21:165–175.
11. Lanphier EH, Brown IW Jr. *Fundamentals of Hyperbaric Medicine.* Washington, DC: National Research Council; 1966.
12. Van Unnik AJM. Inhibition of toxin production in *Clostridium perfringens* in vitro by hyperbaric oxygen. *Antonie Vol Leeuwenhoek.* 1965;31:181.
13. Demello FJ, Haglin JJ, Hitchcock CR. Comparative study of experimental *Clostridium perfringens* infection in dogs treated with antibiotics, surgery, and HBO. *Surgery.* 1973;73:936.
14. Holland JA, Hill GB, Wolfe WG, et al. Experimental and clinical experience with HBO in the treatment of clostridial myonecrosis. *Surgery.* 1975;77:75.
15. Hitchcock CR, Demello FJ, Haglin JJ. Gangrene infection: new approaches to an old disease. *Surg Clin North Am.*1975;55:1403.
16. Bakker DJ. Pure and mixed aerobic and anaerobic soft tissue infections: the classification and role of hyperbaric oxygen in treatment. *Hyperbar Oxygen Rev.* 1985;6:65–96.
17. Bayne CG. Acute decompression sickness: 50 cases. *JACEP.* 1978; 7:351–354.
18. Rivera JC. Decompression sickness among divers: an analysis of 935 cases. *Mil Med.* 1964;129:314–334.
19. Duffner GJ, Van Del Aue OE, Behnke AR. The treatment of decompression sickness: an analysis of 113 cases. *Research Project X-443, Report #3.* Washington, DC: Naval Medical Research Institute; 1946.
20. Fructus X. Treatment of serious decompression sickness. In: *Treatment of Serious Decompression Sickness and Arterial Gas Embolism.* Bethesda, MD: Undersea Medical Society; 1979;37–44. UMS publication 34.
21. Behnke AR. A review of physiologic and clinical data pertaining to decompression sickness. *Research Project X-443, Report #4.* Washington, DC: Naval Medical Research Institute; 1947.
22. Elliott DH, Hallenbeck JM. The pathophysiology of decompression sickness. In: *The Physiology and Medicine of Diving and Compressed Air Work.* London, England: Clowes; 1969:435–455.
23. Kizer WK. Dysbarism in paradise. *Hawaii Med J.* 1980;39:109–116.
24. Slark AG. Treatment of 137 cases of decompression sickness. *Medical Research Council, RN Personnel Research Committee, Report 63/1030.* London; 1962.
25. Saito H. Severe cases of decompression sickness and effects of recompression therapy: a report of 20 years study. In: *Proceedings of the Fourth International Congress on Hyperbaric Medicine.* Baltimore: Williams & Wilkins; 1967:93–99.
26. Workman RD. Treatment of bends with oxygen at high pressure. *Aerosp Med.* 1965;39:1076–1083.
27. Boerema I, et al. Life without blood: a study of the influence of high atmospheric pressure and hypothermia on dilution of blood. *J Cardiovasc Surg.* 1960;1:133.
28. Hart GB. Hyperbaric oxygen in the treatment of acute blood loss anemia. *Hyperbar Oxygen Rev.* 1985;6:189. Abstract.
29. Sukoff MH, Hollin SA, Jacobson JH. The protective effect of hyperbaric oxygenation in experimentally produced cerebral edema and compression. *Surgery.* 1967;62:40–46.
30. Maeda N. Experimental studies on the effect of decompression procedure and hyperbaric oxygenation for the treatment of spinal cord injury. *J Nara Med Assoc.* 1965;16:429–447.
31. Kelly DL, et al. Effects of hyperbaric oxygenation and tissue oxygen studies in experimental paraplegia. *J Neurosurg.* 1972;36:425–429.
32. Wilcox JW, Kolodny SC. Acceleration of healing of maxillary and mandibular osteotomies by use of hyperbaric oxygen. *Oral Surg Oral Med Oral Pathol.* 1976;41:423–429.
33. Strauss MB, Hart GB. Crush injury and the role of hyperbaric oxygen. *Top Emerg Med.* April 1984:9–24.

45. Dangerous Marine Organisms

KENNETH E. SCHULTZ, MD

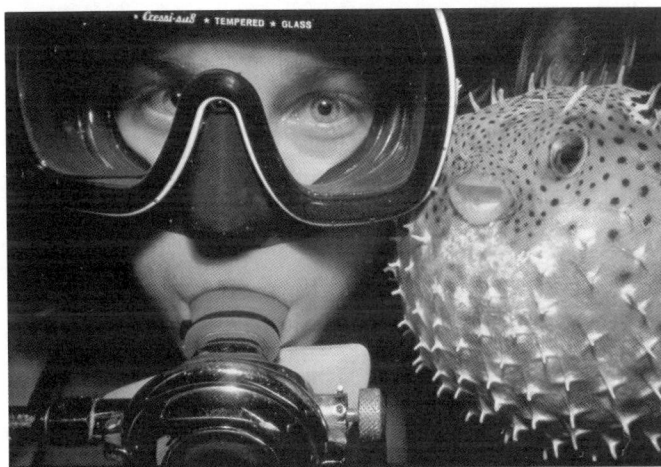

Figure 45-1

The marine environment, in which our earliest ancestors were nurtured, has shaped the evolutionary development of the most beautiful, majestic, and—in many cases—deadly organisms on earth.

When one thinks of dangerous marine life, the usual initial reaction is, "Shark!" However, the majority of illnesses caused by marine life occur through direct contact with or ingestion of a variety of less obviously dangerous organisms. Sims quite accurately describes the broad spectrum of organisms and resultant illnesses.[1]

Dangerous marine life of the oceans ranges in size from minute viruses to large whales, and consists of micro-organisms, plants, and animals. *ANY* marine species which produces human injury or illness may be identified as a dangerous marine organism. Human beings are provided the opportunity to encounter dangerous marine organisms in the native habitat of these organisms while wading (eg, stingray stings), swimming (eg, Portuguese man-of-war stings), snorkeling (eg, coral cuts), scuba diving (eg, moray eel bites), boating (eg, red tide–induced asthma), fishing (eg, fish fin wounds), board surfing (eg, shark bites), body surfing (eg, lyngbya dermatitis), beachcombing (eg, stings from dried-out jellyfish), marine specimen collecting (eg, palythoa intoxication), shellfish harvesting (eg, sea urchin stings), sponge harvesting (eg, sponge poisoning), and shell collecting (eg, sea snake bites). The development of effective technology for maintaining saltwater aquaria has enabled dangerous sea creatures to be brought to public aquaria (where aquarium workers and researchers would be potential victims), private research aquaria (where researchers and aquarium workers would be at risk), and, importantly, home aquaria (where the unwary aquarium enthusiast would be at risk for injury or illness) . . . these aquaria being found scores to thousands of miles *inland* as well as in coastal areas. Home aquariums are sometimes stocked with living venomous "tropical fish" (such as the lionfish *Pterois volitans*), cone shells, sea urchins, moray eels, surgeonfish, and other noxious sea creatures. Aquaria also pose a threat of exotic marine bacterial infections, such as those attributed to *Mycobacterium marinum* and *Pseudomonas cepacia,* for the unprotected person dipping into or changing the aquarium water.

Dangerous marine organisms also affect persons in both coastal and inland areas through the human diet. There are fish and shellfish which, *in the absence of spoilage,* are toxic despite cooking or canning. These ingestion intoxications are endemic in certain areas of the world and include the not so esoteric poisonings such as ciguatera fish poisoning, paralytic shellfish poisoning (PSP), sardine poisoning, pufferfish poisoning, and many others. Travel, scientific research programs, diving expeditions, and war campaigns have brought the unknowing into these endemic areas with resultant fish or shellfish poisoning upon the consumption of toxic species. Inadvertent importation of toxic fish and toxic shellfish has introduced the intoxicating species into the areas well away from the endemic source, although such occurrences are generally uncommon except in a few areas. Inland and coastal scombroid poisoning (by tuna, mahimahi, bonito, sardines, saury, et al), by fresh, frozen, and canned fish and shellfish allergies occur worldwide in many ethnic groups and are presently felt to represent true allergic reactions and not a poisonous ingestion. Bacterial fish and shellfish poisoning will always remain a serious worldwide problem for fresh, frozen, and canned products whenever the prospect of spoilage is not eliminated. The human diet, then, is an example of the opportunity which living and nonliving marine organisms have to produce human illness and injury.

HISTORICAL PERSPECTIVE[2-5]

Historically, poisoning from ingestion of fish has been well recognized, and references to the dangers of eating certain marine organisms, specifically skates and rays, have been found in the writings of early Roman and Greek scholars. The biotoxicological syndrome of ciguatera fish poisoning is described in the *Odyssey* (800 BC). Alexander the Great (356–323 BC), during military campaigns, cautioned his legions to refrain from eating certain species of fish for fear of poisoning. Ch'en T'sang-chi, during the Tang dynasty (618–907 AD), indicated in his writings the danger of eating yellowtail (amberjack), and for centuries yellowtail has been well known to cause human intoxication (ie, ciguatera fish poisoning) after ingestion.

Peter Martyr of Anghera (1457–1526) is credited with the first published reference to ciguatera poisoning in the Americas. One of the earliest reported mass poisonings by ciguatera occurred during the voyage of Pedro Fernandez Quiros in the waters of the southern Pacific off the New Hebrides in 1606. The largest mass outbreak of ciguatera poisoning occurred during the British naval invasion of Mauritius, when the entire fleet of over 1500 men succumbed after eating what appears to have been grouper (*Epinephelus fuscogutatus*).

Sauvages (1758–1790) is credited with the first report of oral intoxication from eating shark (*Squalus catulus*), and on July 23, 1774, one of the most noted outbreaks of ciguatera fish poisoning occurred on Captain James Cook's ship *Resolution*. The crew became ill after ingesting snapper. One of

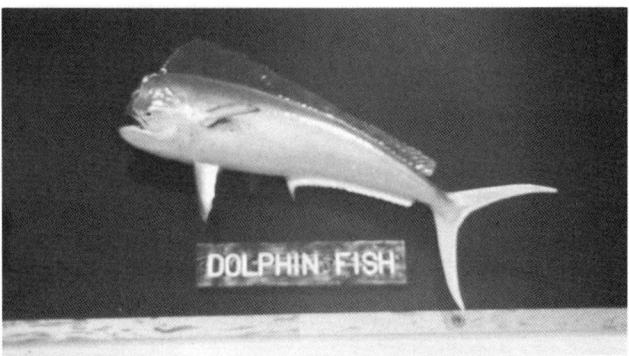

Figure 45-2 Dolphin fish.

the most fascinating accounts of ciguatera fish poisoning occurred on June 8, 1789, after the mutiny on the *Bounty* and the voyage of Captain Bligh. Several of his crew, after being cast adrift in a small lifeboat by the mutineers led by Fletcher Christian, became ill from eating a small dolphin (class Osteichthyes, family Coryphaenidae, genus *Coryphaena*) (Fig. 45-2). This remarkable story is brilliantly outlined by Steinfield and Steinfield.[5]

Buniva in 1803 was the first to comment on the opiatelike effects from a poison found in ratfish (*Chimaeras*), and Chevallier and Duchene (1851) were the first to call attention to cyclostome (hagfishes and lampreys) poisoning. There have been numerous reports of fish poisoning in the 20th century, and from a historical perspective it becomes clear that there have been and will continue to be food-borne diseases caused by the ingestion of poisonous marine organisms.

TRAUMATIC LACERATIONS AND INJURIES

Shark[1,3,4,6-22] (Fig. 45-3)

The frightened cry of "shark" sends chills down the spine of most people, especially those in imminent danger. However, the actual incidence of shark attacks worldwide is less than 100 per year for which the fatality rate is approximately 35%. Of the 250 to 300 species of shark, only 27 species have been definitely implicated in attacks on humans.

Shark attacks seem to be seasonal, occurring with greater frequency in tropical waters where the temperature is above 20°C, and increasing during the late afternoon or evening hours when greater numbers of people are swimming and sharks are more likely to be feeding. Most attacks occur in waist-high water and are generally unprovoked. It is difficult to explain these unprovoked shark attacks, but they may be related to mistaken identity: A shark feeding on a fish may accidentally bite a swimmer's leg. Furthermore, sharks seem to be territorial creatures and may perceive humans as invaders and a threat to their habitats. Unprovoked attacks may be precipitated by blood or commotion in the water, as occurs

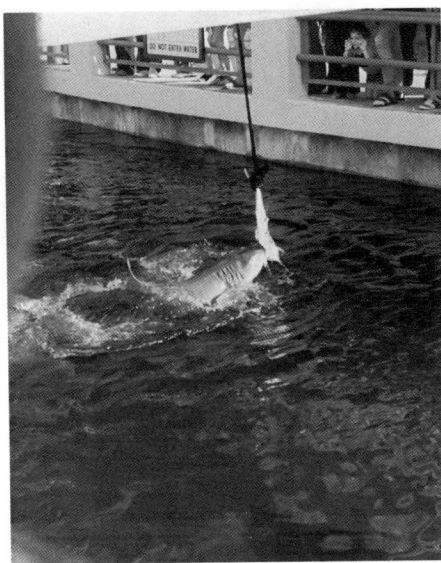

Figure 45-3 A nurse shark feeding at the Miami Seaquarium.

with spear fishing or near-drowning. Drowning victims whose bodies have never been recovered may indeed have been victims of a shark attack.

Provoked attacks certainly occur, usually as a consequence of the provocateur's foolhardiness. The divers who have been attacked have often been teasing, hitting, spearing, riding, and generally annoying the sharks that attack them. Instances of individuals being devoured alive have been documented, but there has been no significant evidence that sharks are true man-eaters that specifically prey on human beings.

The most notorious and frightening instances of shark attacks occurred in sea disasters during World War II. Specifically, on November 28, 1942, in the Indian Ocean south of Africa, the USS *Nova Scotia* was sunk and 1000 men were reported killed by sharks. On July 3, 1945, after the sinking of the USS *Indianapolis*, only 370 men survived out of a crew of 1200; the others died from exposure, drowning, and mass shark attack.

The most dangerous aspect of shark behavior is unpredictability. They may suddenly strike without warning and have been known to attack one individual among a large group of swimmers. Even in the presence of blood and water turbulence, the shark develops "tunnel vision" and becomes oblivious to others splashing about in the bloody water.

Sharks range in size from about 6 inches (*Squaliolus laticautus*) to over 50 feet (the whale shark *Rhinocodan typus*, a plankton eater). The largest of the carnivores is the great white shark *Carcharodon carcharias*, attaining lengths of over 20 feet and weights of over 1000 pounds. There are both freshwater and saltwater sharks, the former being found in freshwater lakes in Nicaragua, Guatemala, and New Guinea.

The chief mechanism of injury inflicted by sharks is their dentition and the powerful force exerted by their jaws. Each jaw has several outer rows of sharp teeth (functional teeth) that are constantly being replaced by the inner rows of teeth (residual teeth). A second system that can inflict injury is their placoid teeth or dermal denticles, which form a sandpaperlike skin known as shagreen. A swimmer or diver brushing against this coarse integumentary layer can sustain severe abrasions or lacerations; this may incite the shark into a full-blown attack because of the victim's agitation and the presence of blood in the water.

Physiologically, sharks have an acute sense of smell, and are able to detect blood measured in parts per billion. Their hearing, combining inner ear labyrinthine structures with pressure-sensing devices along the length of their bodies (lateral lines) and specialized receptors (ampullae of Lorenzini), enables them to detect low-frequency sounds or vibrations miles away.

> When all of the various sensory systems of sharks are taken into consideration, it becomes obvious that the shark is a highly integrated "computerized" sensory marvel possibly without equal either in the aquatic environment or on land.[9]

Of further interest is the fact that neither heart disease nor cancer has ever been detected in sharks. They are cannibalistic, yet repelled by dead sharks, are insensitive to pain, and are extremely difficult to kill.

Killer Whales[1,4,6,9,10] (Fig. 45-4)

The killer whale *Orcinus orca*, one of the largest dolphins, has become very familiar to the public as a result of the motion picture *Orca*, and various marine animal shows. The killer whale has been portrayed as the relentless man-killer and ferocious predator. However, there seems to be no factual justification for the former characterization. Although the killer whale can effectively devour a large sea

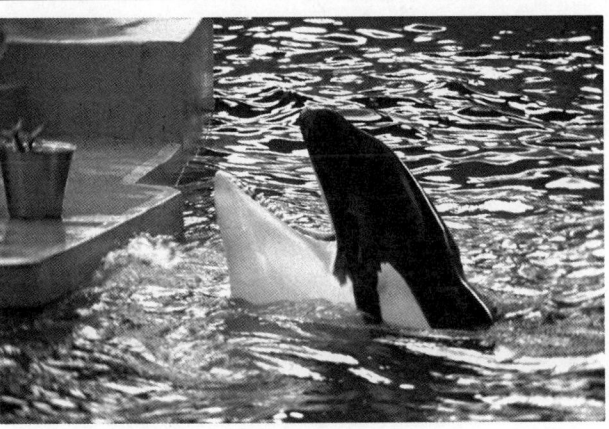

Figure 45-4 Killer whale (*Orcinus orca*).

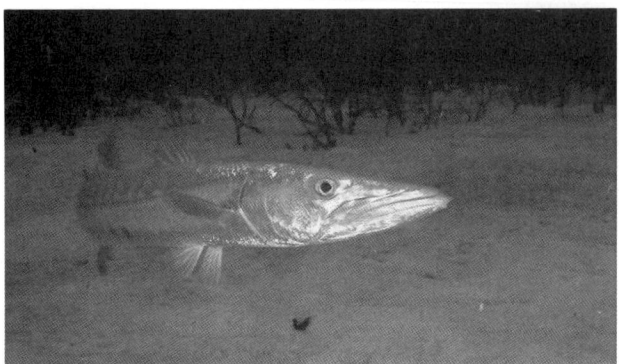

Figure 45-5 *Sphyraena barracuda.* Photo courtesy of Dave Woodward.

lion, it is generally believed to be a case of mistaken identity if a person is attacked. Killer whales are generally found in packs of 40, feeding upon invertebrates as well as sea lions, seals, walrus, birds, and fish. Injuries to human beings can be severe as a consequence of bites or blunt trauma from the animal's use of its body, flippers, or tail.

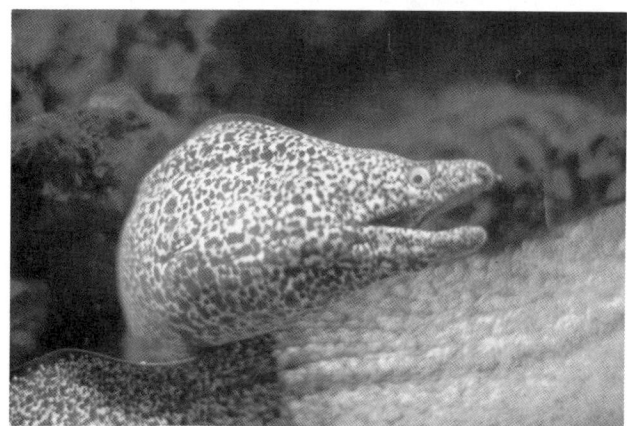

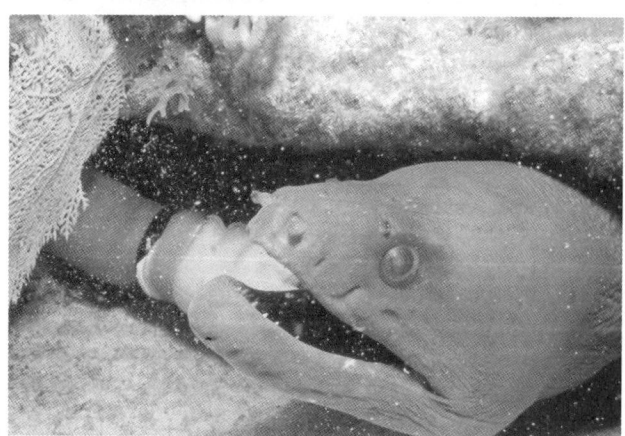

Figure 45-6 (**A**) Spotted moray eel (*Gymnothorax moringa*). (**B**) Green moray eel (*Gymnothorax funibris*).

Barracuda[1,3,4,6,8–13,23] (Fig. 45-5)

Of the approximately 20 species of barracuda, the most dangerous is the great barracuda *Sphyraena barracuda*. They are particularly awesome creatures, having large dangerous canine teeth, and attaining weights of over 100 pounds and lengths of 6 to 8 feet. Barracuda are generally very inquisitive yet seem to be quite timid when approached. Underwater they seem to be constantly observant and wary, and to exhibit an everpresent wolf-like smile. They are attracted to bright, shiny, colorful objects; the metallic reflection from a diver's watch or "sun flash" off a swimmer's bare foot can trigger a lightning-fast attack resulting in a significant laceration, usually consisting of two straight parallel cuts. Luckily, barracuda rarely strike twice.

Moray Eels[1,3,4,6,9,10,24,25] (Fig. 45-6)

Moray eels are similar to barracuda in that they present a very fierce countenance but generally wish to remain unmolested. Moray eels present a double threat to man: the unwary diver may sustain a nasty laceration or fall victim to serious poisoning after ingesting their flesh.

Of the family Muraenidae, approximately 34 species have been described.[24] Moray eels are generally distributed throughout the tropical waters of the world. The most common species in US coastal waters are the green moray *Gymnothorax funibris* (Caribbean Sea south to Brazil), the spotted moray *Gymnothorax moringa* (Gulf of Mexico to Brazil), the *Muraena insularum* (eastern Pacific Ocean), the *Muraena argus* (Gulf of California to Peru), and the *Gymnothorax mordax* (California coast).

Moray eels are rock and reef dwellers, often attaining lengths of 10 feet. Usually they can be seen with their heads protruding from a coral reef, looking extremely forbidding while their jaws open and close rhythmically as water is flushed across their gills. The moray eel has a formidable set of sharp teeth pointing caudad, making it difficult to remove any object unlucky enough to be caught in its viselike grip. In most instances divers are injured when they reach before they look into coral crevices and holes in the reef. Rarely will a moray eel come out of its coral home to attack a diver. If provoked when swimming free, however, the moray can prove to be a very dangerous adversary. Many divers befriend local moray eels and routinely feed them pieces of meat or fish. The novice should refrain from such practices.

Grouper[1,3,4,6,9,10] (Fig. 45-7)

Groupers (family Serranidae) inhabit the tropical waters of the world. Some of the more than 30 species attain lengths of 10 to 12 feet and weights of 300 to 500 pounds. They are very inquisitive, pugnacious creatures, and by their size alone can

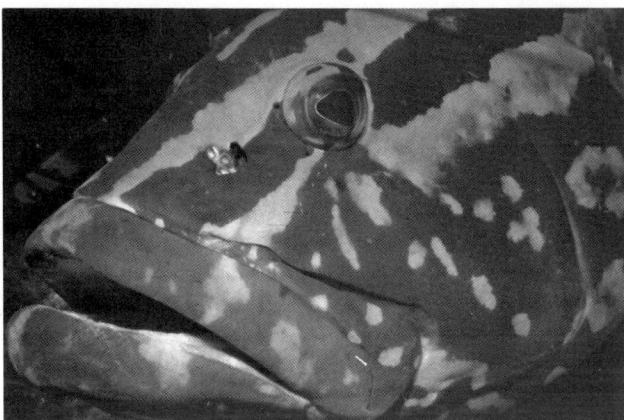

Figure 45-7 Nassau grouper. Generally nonaggressive and playful, especially when being handfed. Larger species can be dangerous because of their size alone. Danger to man can occur as a result of direct trauma or illness from ingestion of their flesh (see ciguatera poisoning).

be menacing. Injuries to humans can be as a consequence of bites from their crushing jaws or damage inflicted by fin contact, such as abrasions, lacerations, and puncture wounds. Most groupers encountered when diving or fishing weigh 2 to 30 pounds. Often after gaining familiarity with friendly divers, the smaller groupers can be petted and fed by hand. Beware, however, because when the food is gone the grouper often goes for ears, fingers, and thighs.

Treatment of Traumatic Lacerations[1,4,7,9–15,19,21,26,27]

The extent of the injury, obviously, depends upon the species of the attacker. Sharks, killer whales, sea lions, seals, and barracudas generally inflict greater damage than moray eels, groupers, crabs, lobsters, and annelid worms (Fig. 45-8). All traumatic wounds are prone to infection. The marine environment (sea water, sea sediment, corals, marine life) contains many microorganisms including a wide variety of bacteria, fungi, parasites, protozoa, and viruses. Thorough wound management with copious irrigation and appropriate debridement is paramount in the successful treatment of minor and extensive injuries. Primary closure of most injuries is desirable but wounds involving deeper structures or displaying contamination with foreign debris may require delayed primary closure or healing by secondary intention and granulation.

Most wounds require local anesthesia or systemic analgesics to permit adequate cleansing and should be treated as follows. All wounds should be thoroughly cleansed before primary closure is effected.

- Provide anesthesia and analgesia as needed.
- Perform aerobic and anaerobic cultures of all wounds.

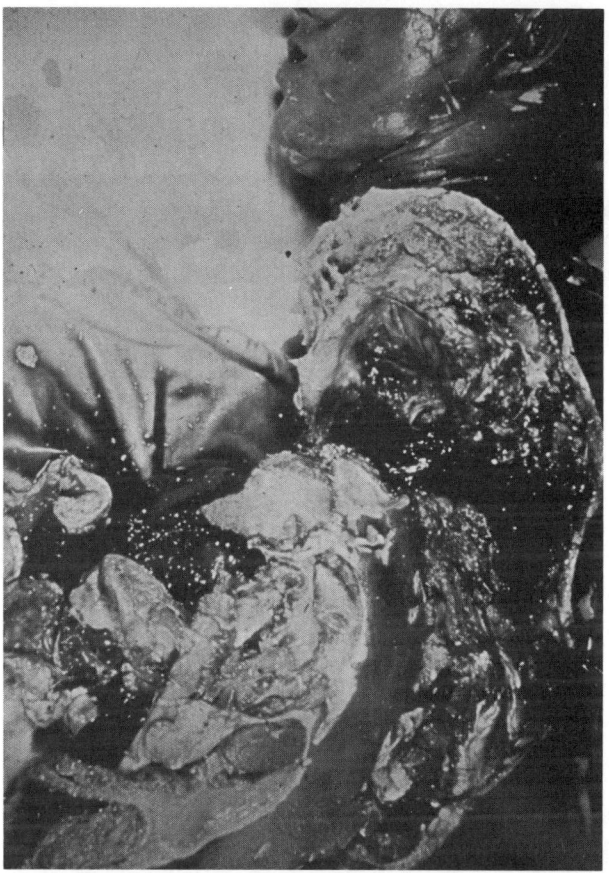

Figure 45-8 This photograph was taken of a diver who was attacked and killed by a shark off the Florida coast. He had been diving alone and in known shark-infested waters. The characteristics of the wounds implicated the attacking species to be that of a hammerhead shark. Photograph courtesy of Dr. Ronald Wright and the Dade County Medical Examiners Office, Miami, Florida.

- Cleanse with 3% hydrogen peroxide (external wounds only). Hydrogen peroxide is excellent for chemical debridement and can be very helpful in removing foreign matter, such as sand or minute pieces of coral, but it kills very few bacteria.
- Irrigate the wound copiously with normal saline.
- Remove all foreign matter, including sand, coral, and (in cases of shark bite) deciduous teeth that may be present in the wound.
- Debride all necrotic tissue.
- Irrigate again with normal saline.
- Take a soft tissue roentgenogram in order to evaluate the effectiveness of decontamination procedures.
- Make every effort to facilitate a primary closure, even if skin grafting is required.

- Provide antitetanus prophylaxis, including tetanus immune globulin.
- Schedule postinjury checkups at 3 and 7 days.

The patient's tetanus immunization status must be ascertained and updated with a booster vaccination if necessary. Passive immunization with tetanus antitoxin must be given to those who have not been fully immunized, or when injuries are extensive or contaminated with significant debris and foreign matter.

Antibiotic ointment such as neosporin or bacitracin can be used although their efficacy is not supported by controlled clinical data. Withholding systemic antibiotics is appropriate in minor lacerations and abrasions, while obtaining initial wound cultures for aerobic and anaerobic organisms may prove helpful if subsequent infection develops. Broad-spectrum antibiotics (which are effective against penicillinase-producing staphylococci and *vibrio* species) should be used for deeper puncture wounds and lacerations or when subcutaneous tissue has been violated or exposed. Examples of useful broad-spectrum antibiotics are penicillins with antistaphylococcal activity as well as second- and third-generation cephalosporins. One also must remember that with marine mammal (eg, seals, sea lions) bites the possibility of rabies infection must be recognized, although the possibility is extremely remote.

Life-threatening wounds are those involving traumatic amputation, significant lacerations involving major vessels, evisceration, and extensive tissue and bone damage. As a consequence, profuse blood loss, hypotension, and shock may ensue. Sterile pressure dressings or clean cloths should be placed over the wounds, and if necessary tourniquets may be used (with appropriate safeguards), or antishock garments. At least two peripheral intravenous (IV) lines, using large-bore intracatheters and infusions of Ringer's lactate or normal saline, should be started. Plasma expanders or blood replacement may be necessary. Wounds of the extremities can be particularly dangerous because of major vessel tears and associated disruption of bone, tendon, and nerve compartments. For proper treatment, most life-threatening wounds require surgical intervention and the talents of several surgical subspecialists.

One must also keep in mind that any person sustaining a significant injury from a bite of a marine organism should also be evaluated for secondary complications of aspiration of sea water, near-drowning, dysbaric accidents, and decompression sickness, as appropriate (see Chapters 43, Drowning and Near-Drowning, and 44, Hyperbaric Emergencies).

Proper initial management of these traumatic injuries may not only save lives but may also decrease the length of hospitalization, prevent recurrent surgical procedures, and lower the incidence of future complications of infection, limitation of motion, and psychological stress.

MARINE ORGANISMS THAT STING

Marine organisms that sting may cause injury with chemical toxins or puncture wounds or both.

Stinging with Spicules

Sponges (Porifera)[1,2,6,9,12,13,28–40]

Of the approximately 4000 known species of sponges only a dozen or so are toxic to humans. The fire sponge, *Tedania ignis,* and *Fibulia nolitangere* inhabit the West Indies. The red moss sponge *Microciona prolifera* is found off the northeast coast of the United States from Cape Cod to South Carolina and causes dermatitis in oyster fishermen and divers. Another interesting dermatitis, known as sponge fishermen's disease, occurs in Mediterranean sponge divers; however, the term is a misnomer. This chemical dermatitis is thought to be caused by a sea anemone *Sagartia rosea,* which adheres to the base of the sponge, and not by a toxin originating in the sponge itself.

Structurally, sponges have minute spicules, composed of silica or calcium carbonate, which bear the chemical toxin. Subcritine, halitoxin (*Haliclonia* spp), and okadaic acid are some of the sponge toxins. When handled, the spicules penetrate the skin, depositing their toxic substances.

Sponge poisoning may present as two distinct clinical syndromes occurring separately or in concert. The first syndrome is a local chemical dermatitis similar to plant-induced contact dermatitis and is characterized by an allergic reaction with a significant pruritic component. Initially, erythema, swelling, a painful stinging sensation (often followed by joint stiffness in the affected extremity), vesicle formation, and skin desquamation occur. This dermatitis often lasts several months. Generalized skin eruptions of erythema multiforme type as well as anaphylactoid reactions can be seen, although they are rare. The second syndrome in sponge contact dermatitis is less inflammatory than the contact allergic dermatitis. The primary clinical symptom is pruritis. This syndrome is thought to be precipitated by the irritating effect of the sponge spicules, which are composed of silica or calcium carbonate.

Treatment consists of removing any remaining spicules with adhesive tape, soaking the affected area with aqueous 5% acetic acid (2 tablespoons of vinegar in a liter of water will suffice) three or four times a day, and using analgesics. Updating tetanus immunization is also necessary. Antibiotics should only be used after definite signs of infection exist and given only after obtaining appropriate specimens or swabs for culture and sensitivity studies. Steroid ointments have not been shown to be effective and indeed may worsen the dermatitis. Intramuscular injection of ACTH has not been dramatically effective. Anaphylactoid reactions and erythema multiforme should be treated in the usual manner according to their severity.

Stinging by Nematocysts[2,6,8–13,31,33,36,38,41–50]

Coelenterates (Coelenterata)[1,2,6,9–13,23,31,33,36,38,41–45,51–63]

Coelenterates are marine organisms comprising three classes: Hydrozoa (hydroids), Scyphozoa (jellyfish), and Anthozoa (sea anemones and sea corals).

Common to all coelenterates is their stinging apparatus or nematocyst (Fig. 45-9). Thousands of nematocysts are found along the tentacles, protuberances, ridges, and oral epidermis of these organisms. The morphologic characteristics of nematocysts have been well documented by Weill.[63] Basically, the nematocyst consists of a pouch-like structure, the cnidoblast, within which rests the venom capsule opening at the operculum. The venom capsule contains a coiled "thread tube" through which the venom is ejected. In some coelenterates, a sensitive receptor, the cnidocil, is located at the tip of the cnidoblast and when touched, signals a sudden opening of the operculum. The coiled thread tube springs forth, inverting the venom sac and injecting toxin into the offending object.

Thus, the unwary prey—whether zooplankton swept by the currents into the waiting embrace of the sea coral (Anthozoa), a small fish darting for safety among the outstretched arms of the sea anemone (Anthozoa), a swimmer's torso embraced by the drifting tentacles of the Portuguese man-of-war (Hydrozoa), or the diver's hand caressed by the deadly, spindly fingers of the sea wasp (Schyphozoa)—becomes the unwitting victim of nature's ever-present intoxication.

The venoms of coelenterates vary in effect from that causing an annoying dermatitis (eg, fire coral *Millipora alcicornis*), to inflicting a sting causing death within minutes (eg, sea wasp *Chironex fleckeri*). In human beings, the variability in degree of toxicity depends upon the coelenterate species involved, its type of nematocyst and potency of its toxin, the dose injected, the extent of tissue exposure, and the victim's sensitivity to the venom.

There is reasonable evidence, additionally, to suggest that allergic reactions play a significant pathophysiologic role in certain types of coelenterate envenomations, particularly those of jellyfish. Case histories in the literature demonstrate that elevated levels of antibodies to specific jellyfish immunoglobulins may persist for several years, that recurrence of clinical cutaneous reactions to jellyfish stings may occur within a few weeks without additional contact with the tentacles, that multiple recurrent eruptions may follow solitary envenomations, that the initial eruption induced by the sting may be delayed by the administration of high doses of systemic corticosteroids, and that immunologic reaction of both B- and T-cell systems can follow jellyfish envenomation. An IgE radioallergosorbent test (RAST) has been developed for coelenterate toxins and shows promise as an accurate indicator of allergic reactions. Much study has been done, and much is currently underway, regarding the chemical nature and structure of coelenterate venom. A detailed discussion of coelenterate toxins and their chemical structure is beyond the scope of this chapter. The reader is advised to review the literature referenced.

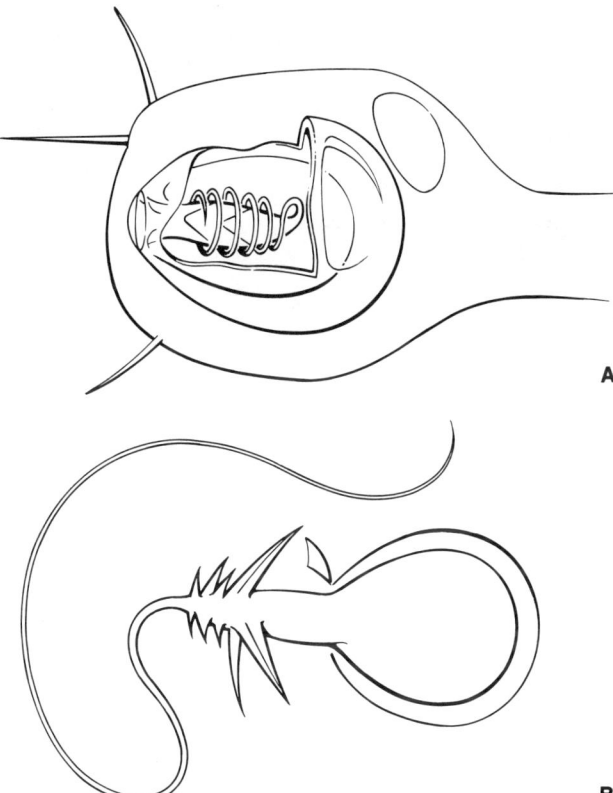

Figure 45-9 Nematocyst or stinging apparatus of coelenterates. **(A)** Undischarged nematocyst. **(B)** Discharged nematocyst. Note the coiled threadlike tube that conveys the venom. Semidiagrammatic. Reprinted with permission from Halstead BW: *Dangerous Marine Animals That Bite, Sting, Shock, Are Nonedible*, ed 2. Centreville, MD, Cornell Maritime Press, Inc, 1980, p 60.

Stinging Hydroids (Hydrozoa)

The class Hydrozoa contains approximately 2700 species, which fall into three basic types.

Stinging Hydroids.[1,2,6,9,10,41] These hydroids grow in plumelike colonies or mosslike colonies (eg, stinging seaweed *Aglaophenia cupresina*) attaching to pilings, rocks, rafts, and shells, and are often mistaken for seaweed.

Hydroid corals (Millepora).[1,2,6,8–10,12,13,31,36,50,64,65] These coral-like organisms live among true corals, having calcareous lime carbonate exoskeletons with thousands of pores within which communicate a network of tiny tentacles containing nematocysts. Colonies may attain beautiful

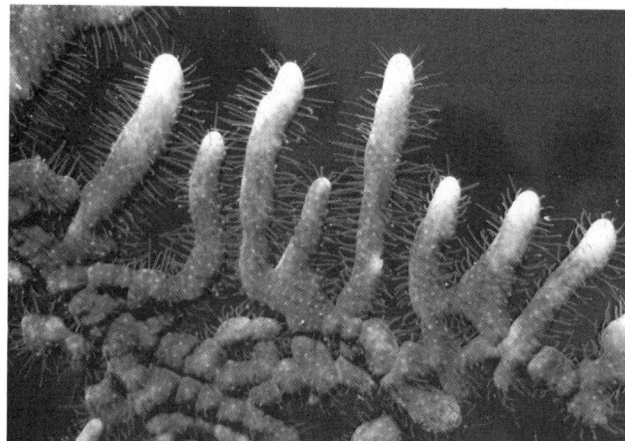

Figure 45-10 Hydroid coral (*Millepora* or fire coral).

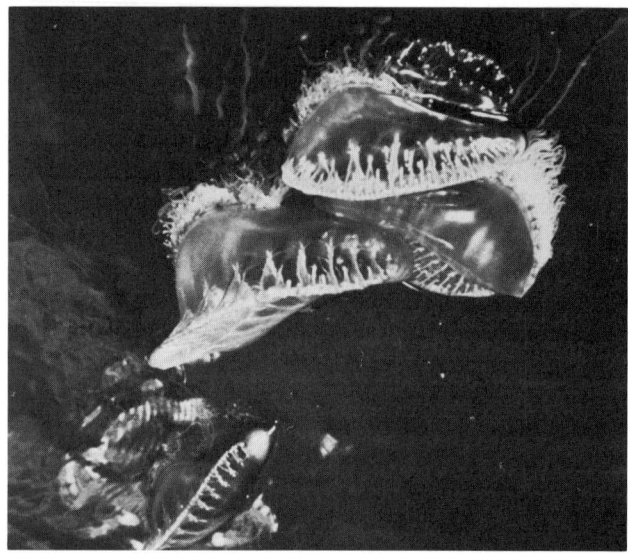

Figure 45-11 Atlantic Portuguese man-of-war (*Physalia physalis*). Courtesy of J.K. Sims, MD.

shapes of varying sizes and are capable of inflicting a fiery sting when touched; thus, the term *stinging fire coral* (Fig. 45-10).

Siphonophores.[1,2,6,8–10,12,13,31,36,38,41,50,66–68] These organisms are free-floating hydroids, such as the well-known Portuguese man-of-war (*Physalia*), having a balloonlike body (pneumatocele) within which are contained several gases: oxygen, nitrogen, carbon monoxide, and carbon dioxide. The pneumatocele, floating on the surface of the water, has numerous tentacles dangling from it that may reach lengths of over 30 feet. These tentacles contain thousands of toxic nematocysts. The Pacific Portuguese man-of-war (*P utriculus*) has a smaller pneumatocele (3 to 5 inches) than the Atlantic Portuguese man-of-war (*P physalis*, Fig. 45-11), whose pneumatocele can attain sizes of 12 to 16 inches.

Symptoms of Hydroid Stings[1,2,6,8–10,12,13,31,33,36,47,50,52,58,66,69,70]

The stinging hydroids and hydroid corals generally are less toxic than the siphonophores (eg, Portuguese man-of-war). Local reactions are common in all hydroid stings but siphonophores can cause significant systemic symptoms with fatal outcomes. Generally speaking, hydroids and hydroid corals produce local reactions, including a stinging, often burning sensation, followed by an urticarial wheal-and-flare reaction, erythema, and edema. These lesions may become hemorrhagic or vesicular, and desquamation of the skin can be severe. Siphonophores produce linear, multilinear, or serpiginous local reactions of edema, erythema, urticarial reactions, petechiae, pruritius, and excruciating pain. Systemic reactions include paresthesias, malaise, headache, abdominal cramps, nausea, vomiting, abdominal rigidity, fever, chills, respiratory distress (including wheezes, stridor, laryngospasm), weakness, pallor, cyanosis, anaphylaxis, cardiovascular collapse, hypotension, shock, and death from cessation of respiratory and cardiac function.

The first human fatality involving envenomation by the Portuguese man-of-war occurred in 1977; a 67-year-old obese woman was swimming in waist-deep water 30 feet off shore at Riviera Beach in an inlet of the Atlantic ocean off Palm Beach, Florida. A detailed description of this case is reported by Stein et al.[71] Of interest, however, is that this patient's serum contained antibodies against jellyfish venom. The studies were performed on serum drawn 5 days after the envenomation. The serum contained high titers of IgG antibody against *Physalia* venom. Low levels of cross-reactive antibody to that against the sea nettle *Chrysaora quinquecirrha* were demonstrated as well.

Jellyfish (Schyphozoa)[1,2,6,8–10,12,13,23,31,33,36,38,41–44,47–49,68,71–81]

Jellyfish are open sea creatures varying in size, shape, and color. They are free-swimming medusae, passively carried about by the currents and winds, but can move vertically by pulsations of their bell-shaped bodies. Approximately 200 species are known to be capable of envenomation by nematocysts. The cubomedusae comprise a group of marine organisms whose venom is among the most lethal in the marine environment. The sea wasp *Chironex fleckeri* or box jelly (*Chiropsalmus quadrigatus, Chirop quadrumanus, Chrysaora quinquecirrha, Carybdea alata, Ca rastoni*) are extremely toxic. *Chir fleckeri* may indeed be the most lethal organism on earth, producing death almost instantaneously. The venom of *Chir fleckeri* is a cardiotoxin, causing cessation of cardiac function. Of further interest is the jellyfish named lion's mane or sea blubber (*Cyanae capillata*), which can attain a diameter several feet across (Fig. 45-12).

Dangerous Marine Organisms 719

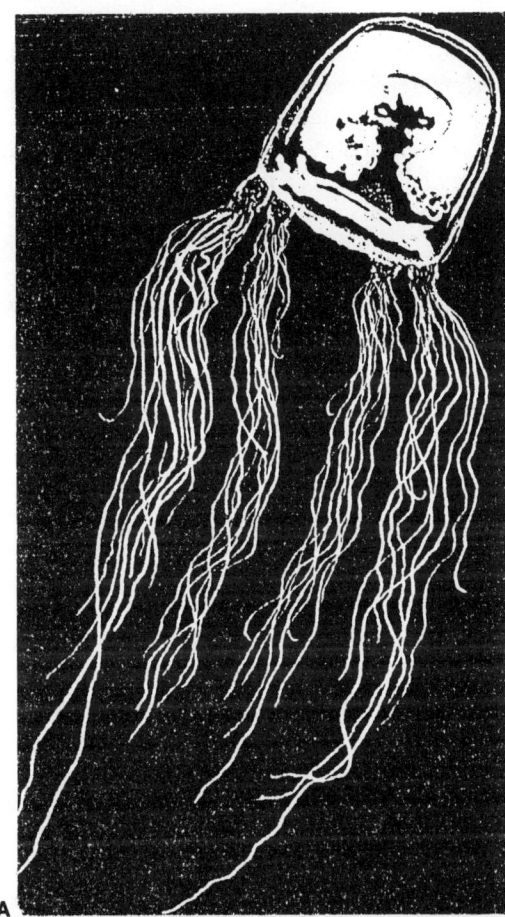

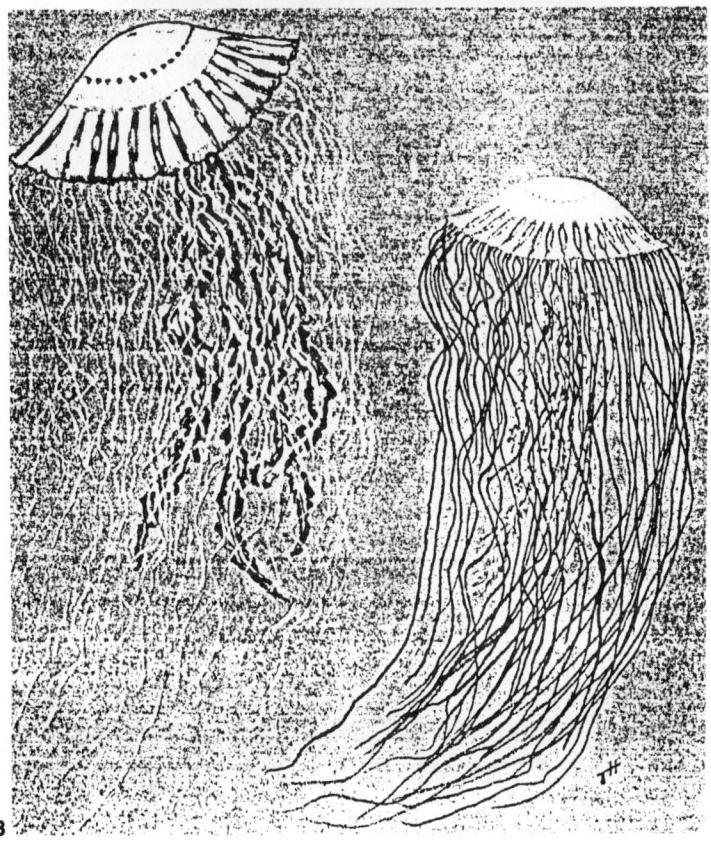

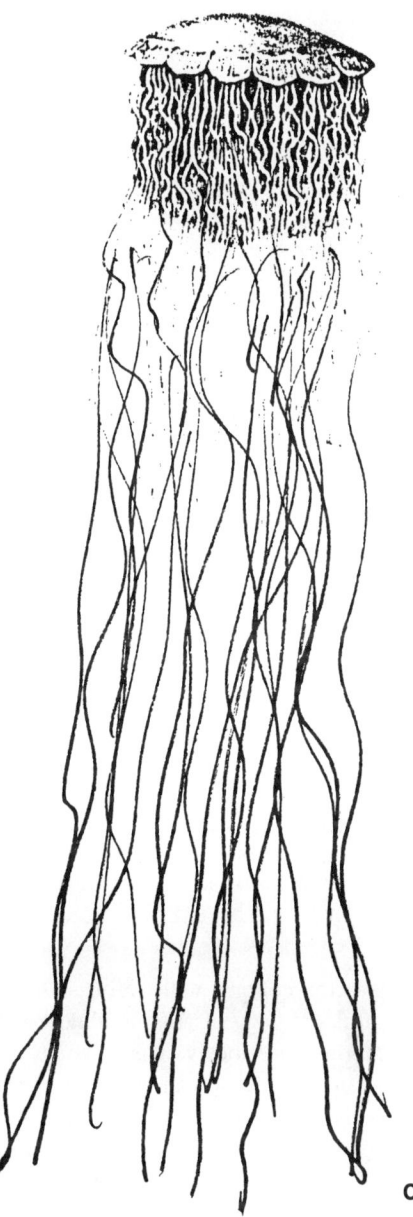

Figure 45-12 (**A**) Sea wasp. *Source:* Reprinted from *Dangerous Sea Creatures: A Complete Guide to Hazardous Marine Life* (p 38) by T Helm with permission of Funk & Wagnalls. (**B**) Atlantic (left) and Pacific sea nettles. *Source:* Reprinted from *Dangerous Sea Creatures: A Complete Guide to Hazardous Marine Life* (p 38) by T Helm with permission of Funk & Wagnalls. (**C**) *Cyanea capillata* (Linnaeus). Diameter of bell, 20 cm. Drawn from a specimen collected in northern California (M. Shirao). *Source:* Reprinted from *Venomous Marine Animals of the World* (p 408) by BW Halstead with permission.

Table 45-1 Local and Systemic Reactions to Jellyfish Stings

Local reactions
  Toxin-induced
    Exaggerated local reaction (angioedema)
    Recurrent reactions
    Delayed persistent reactions (granuloma, indurated nodule)
    Granuloma annulare
    Distant site reactions
    Contact dermatitis
    Papular urticaria
  Long-term reactions
    Keloids
    Pruritic maculopapular scars
    Pigmentation
    Fat atrophy
    Limb necrosis
    Contractions
    Gangrene
Systemic reactions
  Toxin-induced
  Irukandji reaction
Fatal reactions
  Toxin-induced
    Immediate cardiac arrest
    Rapid respiratory arrest
    Delayed renal failure
  Anaphylaxis

Source: Reprinted with permission from Burnett JW et al, Local and systemic reactions from jellyfish stings, in *Clinics in Dermatology* (1987;5[3]:24), Copyright © 1987, JB Lippincott.

Symptoms after contact with jellyfish range from a localized painful stinging sensation to almost instantaneous death, as mentioned previously. The pain may be restricted to the specific area of envenomation or may radiate to other areas of the body, characterized as an excruciating shooting pain and, in cases of the sea wasp, may be so severe as to cause unconsciousness, with subsequent drowning as the cause of death. The local urticarial reaction may progress to vesiculation and necrosis involving the affected area. *Chir fleckeri* produces a specific ladder-type tentacle mark that can be helpful in identifying the sting of this particular jellyfish. Severe systemic reactions consisting of muscle spasms and respiratory distress (from pulmonary edema or pulmonary failure) can be followed by prostration, hypotension, cardiovascular collapse, and death within an average of 15 minutes. Table 45-1 summarizes the local and systemic reactions that may be seen with jellyfish stings. Table 45-2 illustrates clinical characteristics of some coelenterate stings.

Sea Anemones and Sea Corals (Anthozoa)[1,2,6,9,10,12,13,31–33,36,50,82]

The class Anthozoa is subdivided into Alcyonaria (soft corals, sea fans, sea pens, and sea pansies) and Zoantharia (sea anemones and true corals). Sea anemones and true corals belong to the orders Actiniaria and Madreporaria, respectively. The approximately 1000 species of sea anemones generally are sessile carnivores attaching to rocks, coral heads, and crevices of the marine environment. Morphologically, the sea anemone's tentacles are fingerlike projections, having on their surface the majority of the nematocysts. Sea anemones are very beautiful creatures, with their tentacles having variously colored tips (eg, pink, green, and yellow). The toxin injected from nematocysts serves to incapacitate various invertebrates and fish that the creature preys upon. The sea anemone often lives in a symbiotic relationship with the clown fish, which seems to be immune to the sea anemone's venom.

The sea anemone's stings tend to be milder and more localized in their effects than the stings of hydroids and jellyfish. As with stinging hydroids, envenomation causes a painful burning sensation, usually followed by swelling, erythema, and a localized urticarial reaction. Lesions may undergo necrosis and eventually ulcerate, forming multiple abscesses with a purulent discharge. Desquamation of the skin may be severe, and systemic reactions consisting of

Table 45-2 Clinical Characteristics of Some Important Coelenterate Stings[81]

Characteristics of Sting	Physalia	Cubomedusae	Cyanea
Wheal			
Type	Single or replicated line	Multiple lines	Multiple lines
Width	Variable	3 to 7 mm	2 to 3 mm
Pattern	Not regular	Transverse bars	Zig-zag
Duration	1 to 4 hours	2 to 24 hours	0.5 to 1 hour
Pain			
Type	Moderate	Severe	Burning
Duration	0.5 to 2 hours	Many hours	10 to 30 minutes
Necrosis or vesication	Rare	Usual	Rare

Source: Reprinted with permission from Barnes JH, Observations on jellyfish stings in North Queensland, *Med J Aust.* 1960;2:993–999.

nausea, vomiting, abdominal discomfort, general malaise, fever, chills, and prostration may occur.

True corals are one of the primary constituents of the living reef and marine environment. The stony corals with their anemonelike polyps are carnivores that feed basically on zooplankton. Envenomation from corals is usually insignificant. The danger, however, is related to traumatic injury that may become infected if left untreated. Lacerations can ulcerate, resulting in a cellulitis, lymphangitis, and systemic infection. It is well known that coral cuts take a long time to heal. This may be the result of infection by micro-organisms, contamination by coral debris, or envenomation of small amounts of toxin.

Therapy for coral cuts is directed primarily at irrigation and debridement. Coral cuts should initially be scrubbed vigorously with soap and water and then irrigated with a saline solution to remove any foreign material present in the wound. This may prevent secondary infection or the development of a foreign body granuloma. Hydrogen peroxide has also been used in an effort to bubble out coral dust from the wound site. All significant abrasions and wounds should be cultured and then treated with wet to dry dressings of dilute antiseptic agents (povidone-iodine, 1% to 5%). Nontoxic topical antibiotics such as bacitracin are also recommended. Insofar as systemic antibiotic prophylaxis is concerned, current recommendations suggest that patients with normal immune states do not require prophylactic therapy. Compromised hosts should receive a combination of trimethoprim and sulfamethoxazole, ciprofloxacin, or tetracycline to cover marine infections due to such organisms as *Vibrio* or *Alteromonas* species.

Therapy for Nematocyst Stings[1,2,8–13,26,27,31,33,36,41,43,46,47,50,59,60,68,74–76,81,83–89]

Therapy for nematocyst stings consists of pain relief, prevention of envenomation, and treatment of systemic reactions. Morphine sulfate or other opiates may be needed for analgesia. Initial inactivation of nematocysts and prevention of continued discharge has been achieved by utilizing various agents. The literature has few controlled studies and a variety of conflicting results. What is becoming clear, however, is that future therapy for coelenterate envenomation may be species specific. Be that as it may, current guidelines for first aid inactivation of nematocysts and neutralization of toxins suggest immediate rinsing of the wound with sea water. It is important not to use fresh water or to abrade the area by rubbing. Fresh water appears in many cases to stimulate discharge of any nematocysts that have not already fired. Vinegar or acetic acid (3% to 10%) is the agent most highly recommended to inhibit the discharge of nematocysts (particularly *Physalia* and *Chironex* species), reducing pain and resulting in the least skin reaction. A 50% baking soda–saline slurry is suggested as the first line of therapy for Chesapeake Bay sea nettle sting (*Chrysaora quinquecirrha*) and the sea blubber (*Cyanea capillata*). Mentholated spirits (mixed with 90% ethanol and water) and other forms of alcohol, although formerly recommended for first aid measures, have been found to cause massive discharge of nematocysts, increased pain, and severe skin reactions. These substances should be avoided because they may worsen envenomation. Human urine has been found to cause discharge of nematocysts and should not be utilized for first aid measures. Similarly, local heat should not be utilized because it may increase absorption of venom. Ice packs may be used, but when these are applied to the skin avoidance of leakage of fresh water or condensation onto the skin surface is necessary. Other agents utilized and reported to be effective as detoxicants include papain (unseasoned meat tenderizer as a paste), sodium bicarbonate, sugar, olive oil, and dilute ammonium hydroxide. All these agents have variable effectiveness and demonstrate no greater efficacy than vinegar.

Once the wound has been rinsed with salt water and soaked or sprayed with vinegar, the remaining nematocysts must be removed. This may be accomplished by the use of forceps, tweezers, a clamp, pliers, a comb, a stick, or double rubber gloves to prevent envenomation of the rescuer. Any remaining nematocysts may be removed by applying a layer of shaving foam and gently shaving the area. Other substances such as baking soda, diver's talc, or sand and flour mixed with sea water to form a paste can be utilized effectively. After all tentacles have been removed, vinegar should be applied again. Tetanus prophylaxis should be provided as well.

Local therapy using topical and oral steroids and antihistamines has been effective in relieving symptoms and resolving urticarial skin reactions. Epinephrine may be needed for moderate to severe stings as well as anaphylactoid reactions followed by antihistamines such as diphenhydramine in doses of 1 mg/kg intramuscularly or intravenously. Intravenous injections of 5 to 10 mL of a 10% calcium gluconate solution have been effective in relieving muscle spasms. Systemic reactions involving anaphylaxis or neurologic, respiratory, or cardiovascular collapse require appropriate supportive care, including artificial ventilation, use of the MAST suit, IV fluids, epinephrine, high-dose steroids, antihistamines, critical care monitoring, and careful observation.

Antivenom to *Chironex fleckeri* (sea wasp) neutralizes the stings of *Chir fleckeri* and *Chiropsalmus quadrigatus*. This antivenom is available from the Commonwealth Serum Laboratories in Melbourne, Australia. The use of verapamil in patients with hypotension and cardiac dysrhythmia after coelenterate stings may prove efficacious. Effectiveness in humans is unproven, however, and no clinical trials have been performed.

SPINE OR PUNCTURE INJURIES CAUSED BY INVERTEBRATES

Cone Shells[1,2,6,8–10,12,13,27,31,32,36,50,90–93]

Cone shells (phylum Mollusca, class Gastropoda, subclass Prosobranchia, order Archaeogastropoda, suborder Toxoglossa, family Conidae, genus *Conus*) consist of land, fresh water, and marine snails and slugs comprising over 30,000 species. Inhabiting the tropical and subtropical areas of the world, cone shells are univalve mollusks. Cone shells puncture their prey, causing injury by envenomation through a minute harpoonlike tooth. The shells are very colorful and sought by divers, snorkelers, shell collectors, and aquarium enthusiasts, many of whom are unaware of these organisms' lethal natures.

The venom seems to be a multicomponent neurotoxin; its main component is a relatively heat-labile peptide, but quaternary ammonium compounds and amines may be present as well.

Symptoms consist of an initial burning, painful sensation, with local ischemia and cyanosis at the puncture site. However, excruciating pain, pruritus, nausea, and neurologic symptoms of paresthesias, weakness, incoordination, paralysis, dyplopia, dysphagia, dysphonia, aphonia, and coma predominate in the clinical picture. Death is caused by cardiovascular collapse. The sting of *Conus geographus* has been reported to cause death within several hours of envenomation.

Therapy for cone shell envenomation is directed at decreasing pain, preventing local absorption by incision and suction at the puncture site, placing a venoconstrictive tourniquet to limit systemic spread, applying hot water (43° to 46°C) to the affected area to partially inactivate the toxin and to promote bleeding, and supportive care for neurologic and cardiovascular collapse. Respiratory failure (although rare) may occur secondary to muscular paralysis and mechanical ventilatory support may be required. Treatment of shock by the usual methods must be instituted when appropriate. Intravenous 10% calcium gluconate may be helpful in treating pruritus and muscle spasms. Antitetanus prophylaxis and follow-up wound care are also essential for proper management of these injuries.

Sea Urchins[1,2,6,8–10,12,13,26,31,33,36,38,40,50,92,94–98]

Sea urchins are of the phylum Echinodermata. They are free-living nocturnal feeders inhabiting crevices in the coral reef during the day. They can also be found motionless on sandy beaches and ocean bottoms, thereby endangering the unwary wader or swimmer (Fig. 45-13).

Sea urchins have oval, egg-shaped bodies, and their internal organs are encased by a hard shell. Their bodies are covered by several types of venomous and nonvenomous spines that may inflict a painful puncture wound. Sea urchin spines are designated according to size (primary spines are long spindly spines; secondary spines are shorter blunt calcareous spines), and according to location (oral spines are located on the ventral surface, and aboral spines on the dorsal surface). Some species of sea urchins also have tiny venomous pincers called pedicellariae. Venomous sea urchins usually have either spines with venom glands or pedicellariae, but rarely both types of venom apparatus.

Most species of sea urchins have nonvenomous round-tipped spines. However, echinoids of the families Echinothuridae and Diadematidae have long sharp spines that are brittle and very dangerous. The more common sea urchins with toxic spines are the black sea urchin *Diadema antillarum* (West Indies), the white sea urchin *Lythechinus variegatus* (West Indies, North Carolina south to Brazil), and the white sea egg *Tripneustes ventricosus* (West Indies south to Brazil, and the west coast of Africa). Examples of those sea urchins that envenomate through pedicellariae are the sea urchin *Toxopneustes pileolus* (Indo-Pacific and Japan), the sea urchin *T elegans* (Japanese waters), and the sea urchin *Asthenosoma ijimai* (southern Japan to the Moluccan Sea). Contact with sea urchins produces a danger to bathers, swimmers, and divers. Protective gloves, stockings, and flippers may prove inadequate to prevent puncture wounds. Individuals should refrain from handling sea urchins, particularly those with long slender spines and those short-spined urchins with pedicellariae.

Symptoms from sea urchin puncture wounds can be very painful and very difficult to treat. Spines often break off and disintegrate when attempts are made to remove them. Calcareous spines penetrating bone may have to be removed surgically in order to prevent chronic inflammation and infection (Fig. 45-14). Foreign body granuloma may form about sea urchin spines, and pustules with draining sinuses can occur. Spines causing envenomation as well as puncture

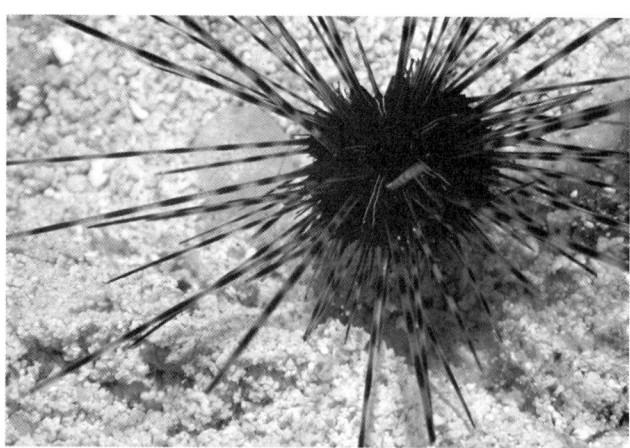

Figure 45-13 Black sea urchin (*Diadema antillarum*).

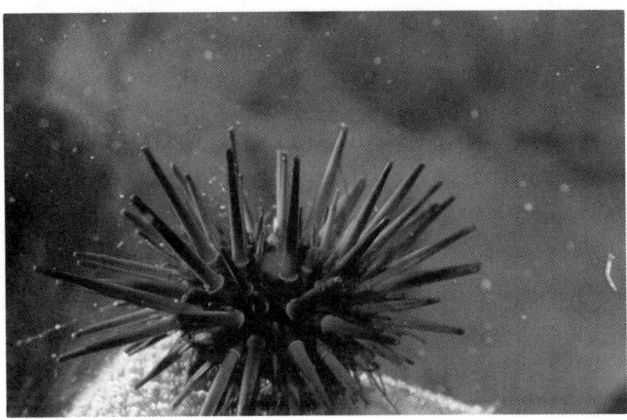

Figure 45-14 Sea urchin demonstrating thick calcareous spines that may puncture bone and require surgical removal.

wounds often produce an aching burrowing type of pain, while pain from envenomation secondary to those urchins with pedicellariae is usually more radiating and severe. Redness, swelling, numbness, paralysis, aphonia, respiratory distress, and anaphylactoid reactions can also occur.

Treatment of sea urchin puncture wounds and envenomation consists of adequate cleansing of the affected area (vinegar soaks may be helpful in dissolving the thin spines, but not the thick calcium carbonate ones) and removal of deeply embedded shorter calcareous spines under local anesthesia. The latter is often necessary to prevent chronic inflammation, draining sinuses, and chronic arthritis. Soaking the affected area in hot water (45° to 50°C) will help to inactivate the heat-labile toxins of venomous urchins, and when necessary the accepted therapy for anaphylactoid symptoms should be instituted. Again, tetanus toxin immunization must be considered, and antibiotic therapy should be withheld until overt signs of infection develop. In addition, specimens should be obtained for proper culture and sensitivity studies.

Starfish, Sea Stars (Asteroidea)[1,2,6,9,10,13,26,31,32,36,38,40,50,92,99]

Starfish are free-living organisms comprising six families (Acanthasteridae, Asteriidae, Asterinidae, Astropectinidae, Echinasteridae, and Solasteridae). The only starfish known to be poisonous, the crown of thorns starfish *Acanthaster planci*, inhabits the Indo-Pacific region from Polynesia to the Red Sea. Starfish in general are star-shaped with a central body and five or more radiating arms. The ventral surface of starfish contains furrows along the arms, from which protrude tubelike structures (tube feet) that enable locomotion, digestion, and sexual function. The dorsal surface contains spines emanating from their hard, calcareous exoskeletons. Starfish have large mouths that can engulf fairly large organisms. *A planci* has played a significant role in the destruction of the coral reefs of the Indo-Pacific. The production of its own venom may be in part the result of ingestion of hydroid coral nematocyst venom.

Wounds inflicted by *A planci* can be very painful, as a result of both traumatic puncture and envenomation injuries. Pain, redness, swelling, nausea, vomiting, and neurologic symptoms of numbness and paralysis are seen. *A planci* thorns contain a red-pink pigment that may stain the tissues, helping to identify injury caused by this venomous organism.

Treatment consists of analgesia, thorough wound cleansing, removal of spines under local anesthesia, immersion of the affected extremity in hot water, 40° to 50°C (to inactivate heat-labile toxins), and careful follow-up in order to detect delayed infections, granuloma formation, cellulitis, lymphangitis, and sepsis.

Bristle Worms (Annelida)[1,2,6,8,9,13,92]

Segmented worms can inflict a lacerating bite with their tough chitinous jaws (eg, the biting reef worm *Eunice aphroditois*). Envenomation, however, may take place through a puncture injury from bristles or setae along the body of the worm, hence the term bristle worm. The setae are paired structures associated with each segment of the worm's body and can inflict a painful sting when touched. The more common bristle worms are the sea mouse *Chloeia viridis*, the fire worm *Eurythöe complanata*, and the bristle worm *Hermodice carunculata* (Fig. 45-15).

Symptoms from contact with bristle worm setae include local pain and minor swelling, and intense itching and numbness that often persist for weeks. Treatment consists of symptomatic relief of pain and immersing the extremity in hot water for 30 minutes, followed by rubbing dilute ammonia or isopropyl alcohol on the wound. After air drying, setae can be removed with adhesive tape. Local anes-

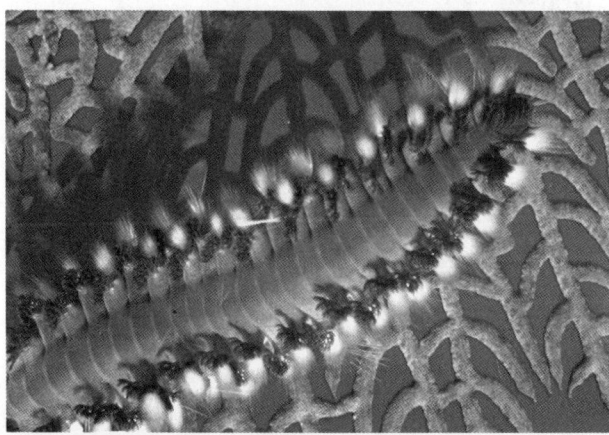

Figure 45-15 Bristle worm (*Eurythöe complanata*).

thetic ointments may be helpful, as well as steroid and antihistamine creams or lotions that may decrease the inflammatory response and intense pruritus. Systemic steroids may be prescribed if inflammation is severe. Prednisone (60 to 80 mg daily) may be employed, and the dosage should be tapered over a 10- to 14-day period. Delayed tissue necrosis and infection must be closely monitored. Antitetanus therapy and careful wound care follow-up should also be provided.

SPINE OR PUNCTURE WOUNDS OF VERTEBRATES

Dogfish Shark[1,4,8,9,26]

Sharks can inflict injury, as previously described, with their sharp teeth and sandpaperlike skin (dermal denticles). In addition, the dogfish shark *Squalus acanthias* and Port Jackson shark can inflict a dangerous spiny puncture wound resulting in a significant laceration as well as a toxic envenomation. The dogfish shark is a slender creature with a pointed snout and high spines anterior to each of its two dorsal fins. Dogfish sharks are relatively small creatures and as adults average 2 to 4 feet in length.

Spine-puncture wounds with envenomation may result in lacerations, hemorrhage, severe radiating pain, erythema, swelling, and serious systemic anaphylactoid reactions in addition to cardiopulmonary and neurologic failure.

Therapy for dogfish shark puncture wounds and envenomation includes general principles of care previously outlined for local wounds, shock, and anaphylactoid reactions. Dogfish shark venom is heat-labile and soaking the affected area in hot water (45° to 50°C) can be very effective in inactivating this toxin. Appropriate use of analgesics is essential and tetanus toxoid immunization should be updated when necessary. Systemic antibiotics having efficacy against penicillinase-producing staphylococcus should probably be used for deep puncture wounds and significant lacerations.

Stingrays[1,4,6,8–13,26,31,33,40,50,92,100–103]

Skates and rays (phylum Chordata, class Chondrichthyes, order Rajiformes) compose the suborder Myliobatoidea and include the families Dasyatidae (stingrays), Potamotrygonidae (river rays), Gymnuridae (butterfly rays), Urolophidae (round stingrays), Myliobatidae (eagle rays), Rhinopteridae (cow-nosed rays), and Mobulidae (devil or manta rays).

Stingrays pose a threat to the bather, swimmer, diver, and fisherman alike (Fig. 45-16). Stingrays vary in size from a few pounds (round stingray *Urolophus halleri*) to over 700 pounds (giant stingray of Australia *Dasyatis brevicaudata*). They inhabit the tropical and subtropical waters of the world, being found usually on sandy bottoms, near shallow reefs, lagoons, river mouths, and inlets. When swimming freely, the stingray generally poses no threat; however, when partially submerged in the sand the stingray is well camouflaged

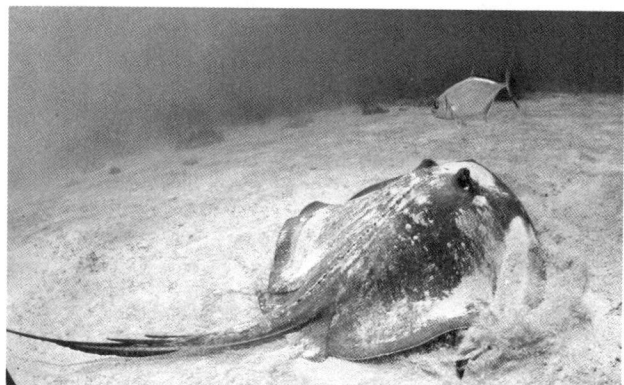

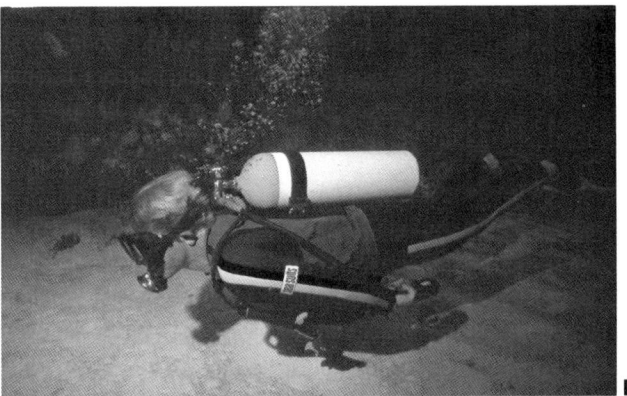

Figure 45-16 (A) Stingray leaving cover of sandy bottom. (B) Diver swimming too close to ocean bottom.

and very difficult to spot (Fig. 45-16A). Only the very observant snorkeler or diver will notice its flat, partially sand-covered body and its vigilant protruding eyes. Divers should refrain from swimming along the ocean bottom (Fig. 45-16B).

The stinging apparatus (caudal appendage) of the stingray consists of a tail from which extends a stinger or spine. There are several types of caudal appendages (gymnurid type, mylibated type, dasyated type, urolophed type) varying according to the development of the spine and its location on the tail.

The gymnurid and mylibated types are poorly developed and usually present limited striking ability. The dasyated and urolophed types are well developed, having muscular tails and caudally placed spines permitting greater whiplike action and striking force.

The stinging spine has sharp recurved teeth along its length, thus forming an organ structurally similar to a fishhook with multiple barbs. The stinging spine is a cartilaginous structure containing grooves along its length harboring the glandular tissue and venom sacs that produce the stingray's toxic venom. The entire spine is covered with an integumentary layer, termed the integumentary sheath.

Injury from stingrays, therefore, consists of a lacerating puncture wound in which pieces of spine, glandular tissue,

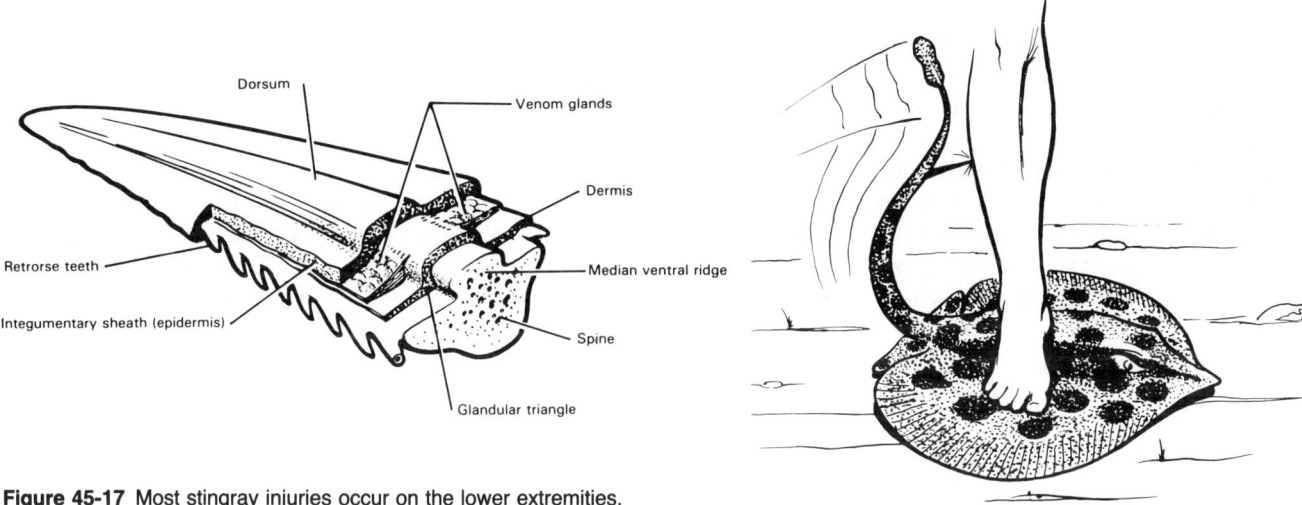

Figure 45-17 Most stingray injuries occur on the lower extremities.

and integumentary sheath may be found. In most instances, wounds occur on the lower extremities when the organism is stepped upon by bathers wading in shallow water (Fig. 45-17). Although rare, deaths have occurred secondary to envenomating abdominal wounds when the victims have fallen off rafts onto a stingray hidden in shallow water along sandy beaches.

Envenomation results from a heat-labile protein toxin. Localized reactions include severe, often excruciating, pain. Numbness may occur, eventually affecting the entire extremity. Systemic reactions include nausea, vomiting, diarrhea, diaphoresis, arrhythmias, cardiovascular collapse, and anaphylactoid reactions.

Pharmacologically, in laboratory animals, the venom seems to have cardiotoxic effects resulting in varying degrees of AV block, ST-T wave changes, cardiac standstill, interventricular conduction defects, ischemia, and premature ventricular contractions (PVCs). Toxicity to the CNS results in depression of medullary respiratory centers, behavioral changes, and convulsive seizures.

Therapy consists of careful wound care. At the scene, the wound should be irrigated with salt water, except in cases of penetrating wounds of the head, chest, or abdomen. Every attempt should be made to remove any remnant of the integumentary sheath in the wound and most importantly, the extremity should be immersed for at least 90 minutes in hot water (45° to 50°C). The hot water inactivates heat-labile toxin, but should not be so hot as to scald the patient. Cryotherapy should never be used.

Emergency department management should include attention to the wound using local infiltration of Xylocaine when necessary. In addition, systemic analgesia is usually required. The spine should be removed at this point. Extensive debridement and copious irrigation removing all foreign matter is often necessary. Drains should be placed prior to closure of extensive lacerations. Simple puncture wounds should not be sutured. In addition to the routine indications for surgery, patients who sustain penetrating abdominal or chest wounds should have exploratory surgery in order to remove intrathoracic or intra-abdominal pieces of integumentary sheath and to permit proper irrigation and debridement of devitalized tissue. Routine management of systemic reactions consisting of hypotension, respiratory depression, and anaphylaxis should be instituted.

All wounds should be cultured for aerobic and anaerobic organisms. In view of empiric evidence that secondary infections are frequent, some investigators suggest the use of prophylactic antibiotics (penicillins combined with a broad-spectrum cephalosporin). Clinical trials studying prophylactic antibiotic therapy do not exist. Tetanus toxoid prophylaxis must be updated when appropriate. Prophylactic use of Benadryl, 50 mg, intramuscularly (IM) in the adult, and methyl prednisolone sodium succinate, 40 mg IM, with oral doses of Benadryl for 24 hours and decreasing oral doses of steroids for 5 days has been recommended for the prevention of anaphylactoid reactions. The most crucial therapeutic aspect in regard to stingray injuries is the inactivation of heat-labile toxin. This in concert with removal of any remaining integumentary sheath and attention to local wound care usually results in uncomplicated wound healing. Those patients not treated as indicated often have problems with subsequent infection, tissue necrosis, and abscess formation, and require extended medical care.

Ratfishes[1,4,6,26]

Ratfishes (class Chondrichthyes, order Chimaerae) are geographically distributed from the north temperate to south temperate zones. They have been found as deep as 1400 fathoms and have been named sea cats. They can inflict a severe bite as well as produce injury and envenomation with their single long tapering dorsal spines. The venom is produced by glandular epithelium located along the spine and covered by an integumentary sheath. Very little is known about the venom of ratfishes.

Medically, symptoms include immediate pain which may lessen over several hours, but continue as a dull ache. Numbness followed by cyanosis and a dark discoloration may develop about the puncture site. Peripherally there is pallor, swelling, arthralgia, and lymphadenopathy. Treatment is similar to that for stingray injuries and the reader is referred to the previous section for details.

Catfishes[1,4,6,8,9,12,13,26,31,33,40,104]

Catfishes (class Osteichthyes, family Siluridae) comprise over 1000 species. Most species vary in size and shape and are found in fresh water while the most venomous, the marine catfish *Plotosus lineatus* is a saltwater inhabitant. Its venom can cause death. The electric catfish *Malapterusus* spp can repel attackers and kill prey by discharging electric currents through the water. The freshwater catfishes of North America include the brownhead *Ictalurus nebulosus,* the Caroline mudtom *Noturus furiosus,* the channel catfish *I punctatus,* the blue catfish *I fucatus,* and the white catfish *I catus*.

The venom glands of catfishes are located along the spines of the dorsal and pectoral fins, which are covered by an integumentary sheath. The stingers are sharp, strong, and easily capable of puncturing skin and muscle (Fig. 45-18). When the integumentary sheath is disrupted venom is released into the wound. The marine catfish's venom appears to have neurotoxic and hemotoxic properties causing muscle spasm, respiratory distress, and death when administered to laboratory animals.

Envenomation in human beings initially involves a severe, throbbing, burning pain which may radiate up the extremity, followed by pallor, swelling, and cyanosis around the puncture site; this is often accompanied by muscle spasms and lymphangitis. Paresthesias at the puncture site may occur and spread to the entire extremity. Systemic symptoms include generalized tremulousness, nausea, vomiting, hypotension, and shock leading to death. In most instances symptoms gradually resolve within a few hours.

Injury most frequently occurs when fishermen are handling catfish caught by rod and reel. Catfish have a very slimy body and are difficult to hold when attempting to remove them from fishhooks. Prevention of injury is critical and is usually possible if these fish are handled with gloves or towels. Fishermen who inadvertently hook a catfish would be advised to simply cut the line.

Initial therapy consists of hot water immersion of the affected extremity (45° to 50°C); care should be taken not to burn the skin. Local wound care and removal of stingers should be done under local anesthesia. Many species of catfish have recurved teeth on their spines which can cause severe lacerations. Proper irrigation and primary wound closure is indicated. If more serious disruption of tissue occurs, drains should be placed prior to wound closure. Systemic analgesia is usually necessary, tetanus toxoid immunization should be updated, and the patient should be placed on broad-spectrum antibiotics having effectiveness against penicillinase-producing staphylococci and *Vibrio* species. Complications of catfish stings include tissue necrosis, gangrene, bacterial infections, foreign body reaction, and peripheral neuropathy.

Weevers[1,4,6,9,12,26,31,40,92,105]

Weevers are small fishes (phylum Chordata, class Osteichthyes, order Perciformes, suborder Percoidei, family Trachinidae), usually not obtaining lengths greater than 18 inches. The species of note are the greater weevers *Trachinus draco* and the lesser weevers *T vipera*. They inhabit inshore waters of the eastern and northern Atlantic Ocean and the Mediterranean and Black seas. They are located in soft, sandy, muddy areas living upon squid, worms, small fish, and crustaceans. Injuries to humans occur while wading or swimming in the areas they inhabit. Weevers are extremely toxic organisms, their venom apparatus being contained in their dorsal and opercular spines. The dorsal spines do not usually number more than seven and contain venom glands covered by an integumentary sheath. Weevers, although sedentary, are easily provoked and can strike very quickly, producing a puncture wound with envenomation.

Envenomation results in immediate local pain of a burning, stabbing, or crushing nature causing the patient to scream in agony, thrash about, and in many cases lose consciousness. The pain may spread to surrounding areas and is often associated with swelling, numbness, edema, and local vesiculation. Systemic symptoms include headache, delirium, nausea, vomiting, dizziness, sweating, cyanosis, arthralgias, lymphadenopathy, cardiac conduction disturbances, seizures, respiratory distress, shock, and death. Sec-

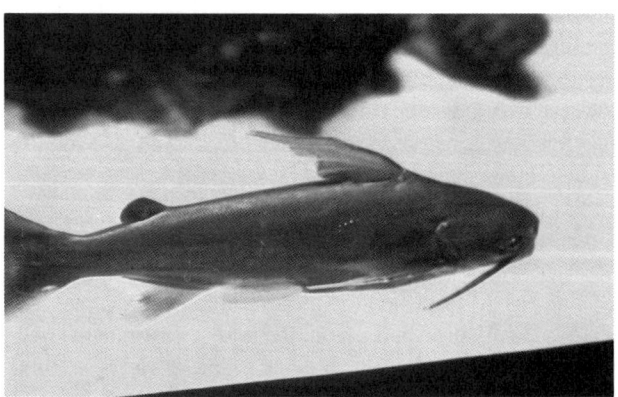

Figure 45-18 Saltwater catfish (*Plotosus lineatus*). Spines contain venom glands covered by an integumentary sheath.

ondary infection and gangrene are not uncommon, and infection has been implicated as the ultimate cause of death in several patients. Full recovery often takes several months.

The venom is thought to contain serotonin as well as epinephrine, norepinephrine, histamine, a cholinesterase, and other proteins.

Since there is no known antidote for the weever's toxins, therapy is directed at symptomatic treatment as outlined for stingray injuries. Analgesia can be a major problem with weever envenomation. Intravenous morphine sulfate has not often been helpful in relieving pain. Intravenous injection of calcium gluconate and Demerol may be helpful as well as local infiltration of Xylocaine or procaine. In addition, in view of the frequent complication of infection, prophylactic antibiotic therapy should be initiated with broad-spectrum antibiotics having efficacy against penicillinase-producing staphylococci and *Vibrio* species.

Scorpionfishes[1,4,6,9,11,12,26,31,32,50,92,106–110]

Scorpionfishes (family Scorpaenidae) comprise several hundred species categorized into three groups according to the anatomy of their venom apparatus: zebrafish type (*Pterois*; Fig. 45-19), scorpionfish type (*Scorpaena*; Fig. 45-20), and stonefish type (*Synanceja*; Fig. 45-21).

Scorpionfishes are generally bottom dwellers inhabiting the rocks and crevices of the ocean floor (hence the term rockfish), but occasionally they can be found buried in the sand (stonefish type) or swimming freely about the coral reef (zebrafish type). They inhabit the temperate and tropical waters of the world, but some species are found in Arctic waters.

Scorpionfishes usually inflict injury during attempts to remove them from fishhooks or nets, after being stepped on by a swimmer's unprotected foot, or while being handled and touched in a home saltwater aquarium. The zebrafish *Pterois volitans* is so beautifully decorated by nature's camouflage that one almost feels compelled to reach out and fondle this venomous creature. *P volitans*, also known as the lionfish, turkeyfish, tigerfish, featherfish, firefish, and scorpionfish, unfortunately, can be found on sale in tropical fish stores throughout the United States. Thousands of these fish are imported from the Philippines each year, ultimately residing in aquaria of tropical fish enthusiasts. Only one case of cardiovascular collapse secondary to *P volitans* envenomation has been documented in the United States to date, and luckily no reported deaths.

The venom apparatus of scorpionfishes is located in dorsal, pectoral, pelvic, and anal fin spines. These spines have extremely sharp points, easily capable of puncturing tissue, glove material, and thin swimfins. Along the spines are venom grooves in which lie venom glands. An integumentary sheath covers the entire glandular and spiny structure. As previously mentioned, the structure of the venom apparatus—that is, fin spines, integumentary sheath, venom

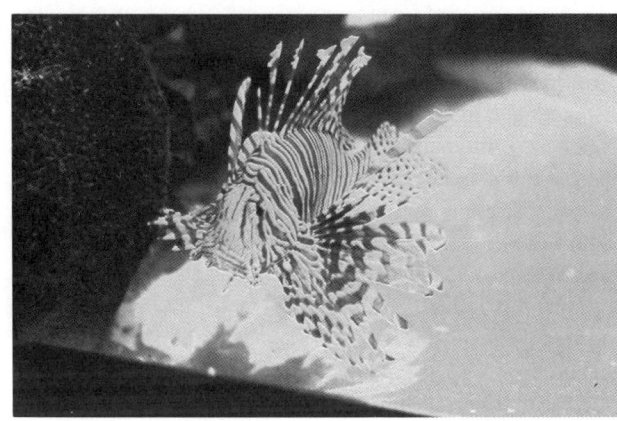

Figure 45-19 Zebrafish.

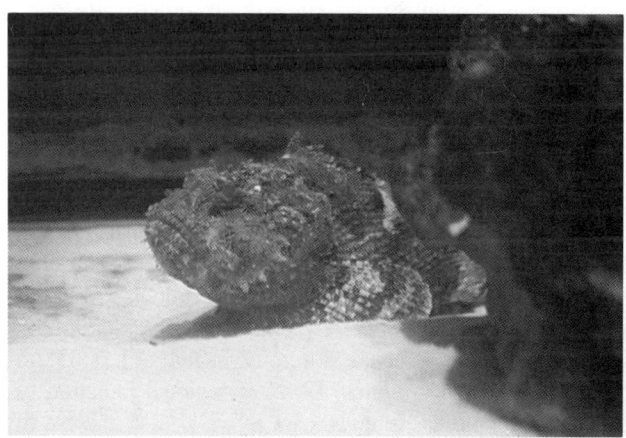

Figure 45-20 Scorpionfish. Scorpionfishes (also called rockfish) are rock dwellers. Venom glands are present in spines that may result in a lethal envenomation.

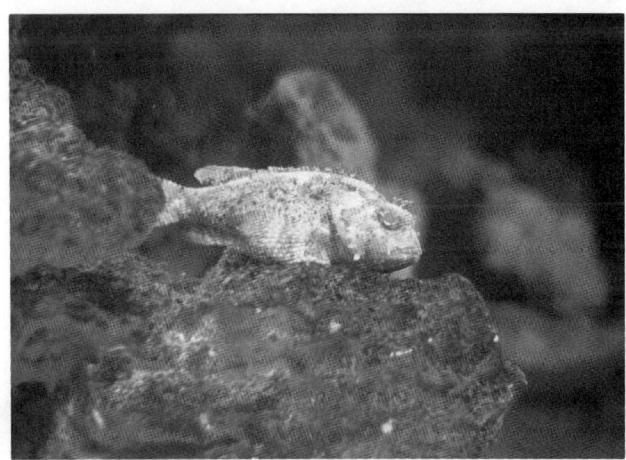

Figure 45-21 Stonefish.

glands, and venom ducts—serves to classify rockfish into three distinct categories.

The venoms of rockfishes contain a variety of proteins and substances that have been defined or characterized. The main component principally responsible for toxic reactions is a nondialyzable heat-stable protein that varies in toxicity according to the species involved. In general, stonefish venom is more potent and more frequently associated with systemic symptoms than scorpionfish or zebrafish venom. However, the lionfish *P volitans* and California scorpionfish *Scorpaena guttata* are capable of producing envenomation comparable to that of stonefish.

Rockfish stings usually cause local reactions of intense pain with radiation followed by swelling, erythema, edema, local cyanosis, and occasionally necrosis and sloughing of the tissues. Life-threatening reactions resulting from systemic absorption of toxin include nausea, vomiting, delirium, lymphangitis, lymphadenopathy, arthralgias, fever, hypotension, cardiovascular collapse, respiratory distress, and death.

Late sequelae of Scorpaenidae envenomation have included neuropathies, infection, skin granulation, and slowly evolving ulceration. A loose proximal constrictive tourniquet may be used in life-threatening envenomation to help prevent further systemic absorption.

Therapy consists of immediate wound irrigation, and encouragement of bleeding from the puncture site in order to remove the toxin and limit systemic absorption. The mainstay of therapy includes inactivation of heat-labile toxin by immersion of the affected extremity in hot water (45° to 50°C) for 30 to 90 minutes. Local or regional injection of anesthetic agents has relieved pain as well. Last, the use of systemic opiates may be required in some patients.

Systemic reactions of hypotension and cardiovascular collapse have been successfully treated with IV fluids and epinephrine. The use of the MAST and adjunctive supportive therapy must be considered in severe reactions. Tetanus toxoid immunization and follow-up wound care may be required. Stonefish Antivenene is very effective in neutralizing all the observable toxic effects of stonefish envenomation. It is available through Commonwealth Laboratories, San Diego's Seaworld, San Francisco's Steinhart Aquarium, and Sea World of Ohio. The initial dose of Stonefish Antivenene is one vial per two stings.

Prevention is the chief consideration in regard to all scorpionfish stings. When diving or snorkeling, one must resist the temptation of reaching into crevices of a coral reef, routinely wear thick gloves while diving, cut fishing lines if scorpionfish are hooked, and refrain from placing hands (even if gloved) in aquaria containing these creatures.

Toadfishes[1,4,8,9,26]

Of the toadfishes (family Batrachoididae) 15 species have been found to be toxic. Toadfishes, ugly and quite repulsive in appearance, inhabit the warm waters of the North American, European, African, southern Australian, and southern South American coastlines. They are also found in the cold waters of the North Sea and off the southern Canadian coast.

Toadfishes are bottom dwellers, preferring turbid water. They are usually found in rock crevices, under debris, hidden by seaweed, or buried in the sand. Their ability to change color gives them superb camouflage, and they are often very difficult to detect. The primary mode of injury is stepping upon these creatures in shallow sandy beach areas.

The highly developed venom apparatus of toadfishes is located on the dorsal and opercular spines. The sting apparatus consists of a hollow spine surrounded by a venom gland and covered almost completely by an integumentary sheath. Very little is known about the toxicology of toadfish venom.

Clinically, the symptoms associated with toadfish stings are stinging, burning, radiating pain accompanied by a typical inflammatory reaction of swelling, redness, and warmth. No known fatalities have been reported from a toadfish sting, and treatment consists of those modalities mentioned in regard to scorpionfish stings. Secondary infection from a toadfish sting may occur and follow-up care should be arranged.

Prevention consists of refraining from wading in sandy beach waters without thick-soled protective foot gear. In addition, a shuffling gait will disturb the sand and often cause a toadfish in the area to move to another location. If caught on hook and line, toadfishes should be released by cutting the line; handling these fishes can prove hazardous.

Surgeonfishes[1,4,6,9,26]

Surgeonfishes (family Ancanthuridae) are so named because of their sharp, lancelike spines located on either side of the tail at the base of the tail fin (Fig. 45-22).

The spine lies within a groove but may extend from the groove pointing cephalad when the fish is disturbed or

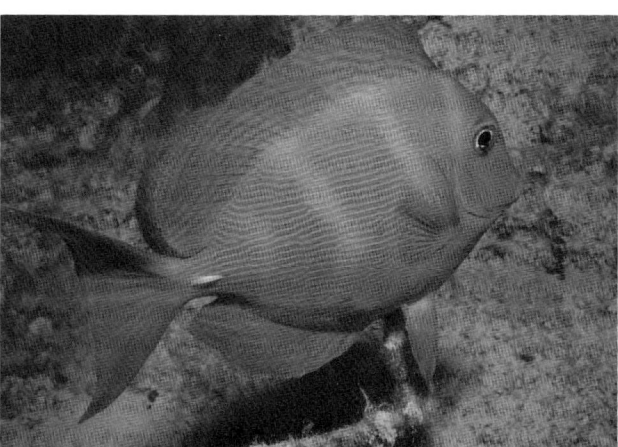

Figure 45-22 Surgeonfish, with lancelike spines, can inflict a nasty laceration.

becomes excited. The spine in relationship to the tail can be likened to a pocket knife when the blade is pulled from the closed position, if one imagines the body of the knife to simulate the tail of the fish, and the attachment of the proximal blade to the knife housing as the caudal part of the tail.

Surgeonfishes are abundant in the coral reefs of tropical waters but rarely pose a threat to swimmers, snorkelers, or divers. Most injuries occur when removing these fish from nets or hooks. In addition, only a few species appear to have venomous spines.

Lacerating, painful wounds can be inflicted by the tail lance. Envenomation may also occur either in association with the tail lance or spines on the caudal peduncle. Symptoms include an intense, radiating pain often lasting for several hours. The pain may continue with varying degrees of severity for up to 1 week. Associated symptoms include local swelling, and occasionally nausea. Treatment is the same as that for stings from scorpionfishes.

Marlin, Sailfish, Swordfish

Game fish can pose a significant danger to fishermen by direct injury or, indirectly, as a result of damage to their boats. Case reports of chest and neck swordfish impalement wounds have been documented. These puncture wounds are not envenomed; however, hemorrhage, tissue injury, and infection pose serious problems. Incidents of huge marlins ramming and puncturing boats below the waterline, although rare, have occurred.

Large game fish must be handled with extreme caution by experienced fishermen using proper equipment. Attempts to handle sworded game fish should only be done after the fish is completely exhausted. Premature boating of these creatures is extremely dangerous and ill-advised.

Miscellaneous Fishes with Venomous Spines[4,6,9,26]

Several other families of fishes have or are reported to have venomous spines, but very little information is available in regard to the toxicological nature of the venom or the anatomy of their venom apparatus. The following is a list of these fishes in phylogenic order:

Common Name	Family Name
Deep sea scaly Dragonfishes	Stomiatidae
Squirrelfishes	Hollocentridae
Leatherbacks (jacks, scard, pompano)	Carangidae
Butterflyfishes	Chaetodontidae
Old wives	Enoplosidae
Majarras	Gerridae
Bugglerfishes	Histiopteridae
Snappers	Lutanidae
Fingerfishes	Monodactylidae
Perches	Percidae
Scats	Scatophagidae
Seabasses	Serranidae
Stargazers	Uranoscopidae
Rabbitfishes	Siganidae
Snake mackerels	Gemphylidae
Sculpins	Cottidae
Searobins	Triglidae
Flying gunardy	Dactylopteridae
Dragonets	Callionymidae
Goosefishes, anglerfishes	Lophiidae

INJURY FROM FANGS

Sea Snakes[1,4,6,8–13,26,31,36,40,92,111–114]

Sea snakes are air-breathing marine reptiles (family Hydrophiodae) comprising about 50 species, 14 of which have been reported to cause human envenomations. Sea snakes inhabit the tropical and subtropical waters of the Indo-Australian seas, and the Indian and Pacific Oceans. There are no sea snakes in North American coastal waters, the Atlantic Ocean, or the Caribbean Sea. The more common dangerous species include[109]:

- Sea snake *Enhydrina schistosa*—Persian Gulf to Cochin China, north coast of Australia.
- Banded sea snake *Hydrophis caerulescens*—Persian Gulf to Japan, Netherlands Indies.
- Hardwick's sea snake *Lapemis hardwicki*—southern Japan to the Merguri Archipelago, northern Australian coast.
- Yellow-bellied sea snake *Pelamis platurus*—eastern Africa, Indo-Australian area, Gulf of Panama.

Sea snakes are extremely venomous creatures capable of inflicting a lethal bite. They pose a significant threat to fishermen and bathers in areas such as Penang, Malaysia, where the incidence is one bite per 270,000 bathing hours. Sea snake bites seem to be more prevalent in turbid water and at river mouths. The incidence may be affected by the time of year and the snake's breeding cycle, during which time they exhibit more aggressive behavior. Bites are most likely to occur when the victim is removing snakes from fishing lines or nets or wading or bathing.

The venom apparatus of sea snakes consists of venom glands, venom ducts, and fangs, the first two being located caudad and ventral to each eye, and the last consisting of one or two pairs located distally in the upper jaw. The venom apparatus of sea snakes is quite primitive in relationship to that of terrestrial snakes. Inflicting a usually painless bite, sea snakes are incapable of dislocating their jaws when striking. Envenomation may be incomplete or may not occur at all. Nevertheless, sea snakes must be considered lethal creatures and appropriate safeguards should be taken when in an aquatic environment inhabited by these serpents.

The venom of sea snakes is considered more toxic than terrestrial snake venom, such as that of rattlesnakes, copperheads, and kraits, but about equal in potency to cobra venom. Toxicologically, one drop of venom is sufficient to kill three adult humans. In animals, sea snake venom causes neurotoxicity acting upon neuromuscular junctions producing paralysis. In human beings, the venom causes myotoxic and hemotoxic effects in addition to neurotoxic symptoms. Sea snake venoms seem to contain a common antigen and, in general, the protein composition is less complex than venoms of other families of snakes. Notably fewer enzymes are contained in sea snake venoms than in venoms of terrestrial snakes.

Pharmacologically, sea snake venoms contain phospholipase $A_2 5'$-nucleotidase, phosphodiesterase, phosphomonoesterase, fibrinogen clotting, hyaluronidase, deoxyribonuclease, acetylcholinesterase, and leucine aminopeptidase, and have thrombinlike activity.

The clinical syndrome of envenomation usually occurs within 30 minutes to 1 hour after the bite. The onset of symptoms can be delayed by 6 to 8 hours, however. Symptoms of envenomation include generalized myalgias, stiffness, euphoria, anxiety, ascending paralysis, flaccidity, ptosis, trismus, dysphagia, nausea, vomiting, dryness of the mouth, thirst, diaphoresis, muscle spasms, fasciculations, cyanosis, mydriasis, hypotension, dysrhythmias, cardiovascular collapse, respiratory arrest, and acute myoglobinuric renal failure. The overall fatality rate is 28%.

Treatment of sea snake bites initially includes proper diagnosis, which is based upon clearly establishing the opportunity for contact with sea snakes, the presence of a painless wound, the presence of fang marks, identification of the snake when possible, and the occurrence of symptoms of envenomation, including early complaints of muscle stiffness, ptosis, paralysis of the legs, and trismus.

Common goals of therapy, as with other types of envenomation injuries, include removal of venom at the site of injury, prevention of absorption of venom, neutralization of toxin, supportive therapy to treat toxic effects, and treatment of secondary complications.

In concert with these therapeutic goals, the recommendations for treatment of sea snake bites with envenomation are:

- Careful consideration of whether a tourniquet should be used. Tourniquets may cause more harm than good. Tourniquets should only be considered if the patient is more than 1 hour from definitive medical care. Local suction is not recommended. Current recommendations are to utilize the pressure-immobilization technique to localize the venom and limit systemic absorption. With a circumferential bandage 15 to 18 cm wide, pressure should be placed over a smaller pad for up to 30 minutes after the bite at a lympathic-venous occlusive pressure of 70 mmHg (without interfering with arterial blood flow).
- Cleansing the wound thoroughly, removing fangs if present.
- Refraining from applying ice to the wound.
- Immobilizing the affected extremity in a dependent position and placing the victim at rest.
- Administering Sea Snake Antivenene (available from the Commonwealth Serum Laboratories, Melbourne, Australia) or any polyvalent snake antivenin containing krait (elapidae) fraction as directed, and only after appropriate skin or conjunctival allergy testing. Antivenin injection continues to be of benefit up to 36 hours after envenomation. Use *Enhydrina schistosa* antivenin first and then *Notechis scutatus* antivenin as a second choice.
- Removing tourniquets upon administration of antivenin.
- Refraining from administering opiates for pain relief; worsening of respiratory status may occur.
- Institution of supportive therapy for hypotension, arrhythmias, respiratory arrest, and renal failure from hemoglobinuria or myoglobinuria.

Two cases of clinically characteristic sea snake envenomation and poisoning (species of sea snake were not identified) in the absence of antivenin were successfully treated with hemodialysis.[114] It is thought that the relatively low molecular weight of sea snake neurotoxins makes them dialyzable, presumably accounting for the effectiveness of hemodialysis.

INJURY FROM BEAKS: OCTOPUSES[1,2,6,8–11,26,31,36,115–122]

Octopuses are strange-looking mollusks of the class Cephalopoda, which includes cuttlefishes and squids. Cephalopods can inflict lacerations, avulsions, or crush injuries by biting and can cause envenomation with their salivary gland toxins, or poisoning, if their flesh is ingested. The following discussion centers upon octopuses but cuttlefishes and squids may produce similar types of injuries, envenomation, and poisoning.

Anatomically, octopuses have a body, within which are situated their eyes and two chitinous jaws that form a sharp beak. The beak is capable of inflicting a serious laceration. Radiating from the body are eight tentacles, having on their ventral surfaces numerous suction cups. The tentacles are used for clinging to and grasping underwater objects and prey. Occasionally, a diver's arm or body may be the object to which the octopus clings, leaving suction marks that are round and erythematous and exhibit petechial hemorrhages.

Octopuses vary in size, the largest reportedly (*Guinness Book of World Records*) weighing 6 to 7 tons and having tentacles reaching lengths of 200 feet. Most venomous octopuses are small, reaching sizes of only 8 to 12 inches.

Usually, octopuses create a minor threat to divers, but the white *Octopus joubini* (Florida) and the blue-ringed octopus *Hapalochlaena maculosus* (Indo-Pacific region) are especially venomous. Three deaths have been reported in Australian waters as a result of bites from *Hapalochlaena* spp. One diver allowed a small octopus of unknown species (*H lunulata?*) to crawl up his arm toward his neck, where he sustained a lethal bite. In spite of artificial ventilation he died within 2 hours of hospitalization.

The venom apparatus of octopuses consists of the anterior and posterior salivary glands, salivary ducts, buccal mass, and two jaws forming a beaklike structure. Envenomation is produced through a laceration caused by the bite. When feeding upon small crabs, however, the octopus apparently releases its toxin near the crab's gill cavity, which results in envenomation in the absence of a bite.

The venom of *H maculosus*, maculotoxin, has been studied and found to be a neurotoxin chemically identical to tetrodotoxin. Maculotoxin selectively blocks nerve action potentials, producing paralysis and causing death from respiratory failure.

Envenomation in humans produces an initial local stinging sensation followed by swelling, redness, warmth, and pruritus at the wound site. Profuse local bleeding may occur and is thought secondary to interference with clotting mechanisms. Systemic reactions include tingling (lips, mouth, and tongue), vomiting, headache, chills, low-grade fever, abdominal pain, anorexia, blurred vision, loss of tactile sensation associated with a floating feeling, seizures, flaccid paralysis, respiratory difficulty, respiratory arrest, and death from respiratory failure.

Therapy of cephalopod bites consists of local suction with a plunger type of device, local irrigation, pressure-immobilization as with sea snake bites, and cone shell envenomation. Heat immersion is not helpful because maculo-toxin is heat stable. There is no antivenin for cephalopod venom. Healing is usually without incident and infection is rare, although delayed cellulitis infrequently occurs. Frequent observation for infection and granuloma formation is warranted and patients should be started on broad-spectrum antibiotics effective against antipenicillinase-producing staphylococci and *Vibrio* species. Tetanus toxoid immunization must be updated as well. Without a known antivenin, respiratory support may play a crucial role in survival after serious envenomation.

Divers should refrain from handling cephalopods so as to prevent injury from bites and envenomation even though the temptation may seem irresistible.

COMMENTS ON ANTIBIOTIC THERAPY[29,40,98,123–140]

The marine environment contains a myriad of pathogenic microorganisms. They tend to be halophilic, heterophilic, motile, and Gram-negative bacilli. Those familiar with injuries involving the marine environment have recognized that these wounds often become infected and are difficult to treat. As mentioned throughout this chapter, wounds occurring in the marine environment often develop into chronic problems, such as granuloma formation, ulceration, and desquamation, that require prolonged treatment. Therapeutic considerations are made more difficult in view of the paucity of clinical information available from scientific study.

In most cases, minor abrasions, lacerations, and puncture wounds do not require prophylactic antibiotic intervention. On the other hand, immunosuppressed patients are at greater risk of infection, especially from *Vibrio* species. The reader is referred to the excellent article by Auerbach et al[140] for a detailed review of the bacteriology of the marine environment.

Current recommendations for antibiotic use in serious wounds and any wound in an immunosuppressed patient (or those with serious liver disease) are oral ciprofloxacin or trimethoprim-sulfamethoxazol. Parenteral antibiotics, if required, initially should include cefoperazone, cefotaxime, ceftazidime, gentamicin, or tobramycin. For fulminant infection, therapy with imipenem and cilastatin should be considered.[40] All wounds, regardless of extent, should be cultured for aerobic and anaerobic microorganisms. Culture media should be supplemented with sodium chloride to permit bacterial growth of marine organisms.[40] Antibiotic therapy as above should be provided pending culture results[40,140] (Table 45-3).

POISONING FROM INGESTING MARINE INVERTEBRATES

Bivalve Mollusks

Bivalve mollusks (clams, oysters, mussels, scallops) are plankton feeders that depend upon extracting food and oxygen from the aquatic environment. These invertebrates siphon and filter large volumes of water; studies of mussels have shown that they can filter up to 20 L of water per day. However, the lack of selectivity in their filtering mechanism unfortunately enables them to concentrate in their visceral organs a significant quantity and wide variety of contaminants pathogenic for humans, including: bacteria, viruses, dinoflagellates, toxic metals, pesticides, hydrocarbons, chemicals, and radioactive material.

Bacteria[1,9,123–144]

Typhoid fever has in the past been linked to the ingestion of raw mollusks, particularly clams and oysters. In 1924 an epidemic of typhoid fever in which approximately 150 died was attributed to the ingestion of contaminated oysters. Contemporary public health surveillance of shellfish harvesting and sanitation programs have essentially eliminated

Table 45-3 Antibiotic Susceptibility of Gram-Negative Marine Bacteria

	Percent of Isolates Susceptible (N = 59)		
	50%	59%–90%	90%
Penicillins			
Ampicillin		X	
Ticarcillin		X	
Azlocillin			X
Mezlocillin			X
Piperacillin			X
Cephalosporins			
First-generation			
Cephalothin	X		
Second-generation			
Cefamandole		X	
Cefoxitin		X	
Third-generation			
Cefoperazone			X
Cefotaxime			X (all)
Ceftazidime			X (all)
Moxalactam			X (all)
Cefsulodin	X		
Aminoglycosides			
Gentamicin		X	
Tobramycin		X	
Amikacin		X	
Aztreonam			X
Chloramphenicol			X (all)
Imipenem			X (all)
Trimeth/Sulfa			X
Trimethoprim		X	
Tetracycline		X	
Fludalanine/Pentizidone		X	

Source: Reprinted with permission from Fisher AA, Water related dermatoses part II: nematocyst dermatitis. *Cutis*. 1980;25:248–249.

Table 45-4 Antibiotics Effective against 90% of Strains of *Vibrio* and *Alteromonas* species

	Vibrio species (35 Isolates)	Alteromonas species (19 Isolates)
Penicillins		
Azlocillin	X	X
Mezlocillin	X	X
Piperacillin	X	X
Ampicillin		X
Ticarcillin		X
Cephalosporins		
Cefotaxime	X	X
Moxalactam	X	X
Cefoperazone	X	X
Ceftazidime	X	X
Cefamandole	X	
Chloramphenicol	X	X
Trimeth/Sulfa	X	X
Aztreonam	X	X
Imipenem	X	X

Pseudomonas species (three isolates) were susceptible to all antibiotics tested.

Deleya species (two isolates) were susceptible to all antibiotics except tetracycline, trimethoprim/sulfamethoxazole.

Source: Reprinted with permission from Auerbach PS, Marine envenomations, *N Engl J Med*. 1991;325:486–493.

the threat of mollusk-borne typhoid fever in the United States.

In spite of current mollusk-associated public health measures, gastroenteritis has continued to plague the world's population, sometimes in epidemic proportions. Gastroenteritis caused by the ingestion of mollusks, fish, and crustaceans (especially shrimp) containing *Vibrio parahemolyticus* produces a clinical syndrome similar to *Salmonella* gastroenteritis. *Vibrio parahemolyticus* is the etiologic agent in the most common type of summer-associated gastroenteritis in Japan; it has been a recognized inhabitant of Japan's coastal waters for some time. *Vibrio parahemolyticus*, and poisoning epidemics as a consequence of its ingestion, have been identified worldwide. These areas include the coastal waters of the United States, the United Kingdom, and Australia and other areas of the Pacific Ocean.

Gastroenteritis produced by *V parahemolyticus* usually follows a 12- to 24-hour incubation period, and clinical symptoms last from 24 to 48 hours, after which time complete resolution is the typical course of events. The symptom complex consists of explosive watery (sometimes bloody) diarrhea, nausea, vomiting, abdominal cramps, fever, headache, prostration, volume depletion, rectosigmoid ulceration, and fecal leukocytosis in severe cases. Although usually a self-limiting process, the disease may cause significant abdominal pain and volume depletion, requiring analgesics and IV administration of fluids and electrolytes. Hospitalization may be required for seriously ill patients. Appropriate stool and blood specimens should be obtained for culture and sensitivity studies prior to the institution of antibiotic therapy. *Vibrio parahemolyticus* is a halophilic (salt-loving) bacterium requiring special bacteriological culture media containing at least 0.5% NaCl, such as TCBS (thiosulfate citrate bile salts sucrose) agar. Table 45-4 gives the in vitro susceptibility of *Vibrio* species to antibiotics.

Vibrio cholera epidemics from ingestion of raw clams and mussels as well as other seafood products has been a problem in some European and Far Eastern countries, particularly Italy and Malaysia. People traveling to countries in which sanitation regulations for shellfish harvesting are ineffective or nonexistent must consider the consequences of eating raw mollusks.

Clostridium botulinum type E has been cultured from coastal waters off the United States and from the eastern oyster but no cases of botulism have been linked to ingestion of fresh mollusks.

Earampamoorthy and Koff[142] rightfully point out that bacterial contamination of mollusks is not limited to those concentrated from the aquatic environment but may also occur during packaging, transportation, storage, repacking, and display of the market product. Improper handling of shellfish may encourage the proliferation of bacteria and the production of toxic products.

Viruses[9,141–154]

Hepatitis is the disease process of major epidemiological importance causally linked to shellfish ingestion. The first recorded outbreak of shellfish-associated hepatitis A infection was reported in Sweden in 1955 in which 600 cases were documented following ingestion of sewage-contaminated oysters. No further cases were reported until 1961 when three major outbreaks of shellfish-associated hepatitis occurred in the United States. Since 1961 sporadic occurrences have been reported in the United States and Germany. Clams are more dangerous than oysters in that they have a greater potential for concentrating hepatitis virus because they are capable of migrating to various aquatic environments, while oysters attach themselves to rocks, permitting more effective surveillance of their environment.

Hepatitis A infection has been associated with steamed clams; studies have shown that the internal temperature at "gaping" is insufficient to kill hepatitis A virus.

Hepatitis B surface antigen (HBsAg) has been isolated from a clam estuary contaminated by the raw sewage of a New England coastal hospital. However, there is no specific data presently to link HBsAg-contaminated shellfish with hepatitis B infection in humans.

A very interesting outbreak of oyster-associated hepatitis B occurred in the spring of 1980 in Baltimore, Maryland, among a 13-member family group who gathered weekly for oyster-eating parties. The oysters were placed in a cooler the nights prior to the parties and were refrigerated overnight until the parties began the following day. The Centers for Disease Control's investigation (reported by Dr Mark Cain April 19, 1982, at the Epidemic-Intelligence Service Conference, Centers for Disease Control, Atlanta, Georgia) revealed that the individual who had cleaned the oysters and placed them in the cooler was a carrier of HBsAg and the index case. It was postulated that traces of his blood (secondary to scrapes and abrasions occurring while cleaning the oysters) had become mixed with the cooler water. Hepatitis B infection occurred in seven individuals and was associated with shucking the oysters that had been placed in the contaminated cooler water. Infection was believed to occur via scrapes and abrasions in the skin of those individuals shucking the oysters, since several family members eating oysters but not shucking did not contract hepatitis B infection. Obviously, this outbreak of hepatitis B was related to circumstances involving oysters but not as a result of oyster-borne infection.

Non-A, non-B hepatitis may also play a role in infections associated with shellfish but information is lacking regarding this possibility.

Those patients who present with symptoms of clinical hepatitis must be questioned as to their history of shellfish ingestion within the 4- to 6-week period preceding the development of symptoms of the disease. The local public health authorities and the Centers for Disease Control (Hepatitis Department, Phoenix, Arizona) should be informed of any patient thought to have shellfish-associated hepatitis.

In addition, patients diagnosed as having shellfish-borne gastroenteritis should receive immune serum globulin (0.6 mg/kg) initially and repeated in 30 days as prophylaxis against hepatitis A. Viral gastroenteritis has been reported as a result of ingestion of contaminated oysters from coastal beds in New South Wales, Australia, and is attributed to infection by the Norwalk virus.

In addition, poliovirus and echovirus have been isolated from shellfish in the Great South Bay, Long Island, New York, although no clinical human infections have been attributed to ingestion of infected mollusks. Other enteric viruses, including enteroviruses, adenoviruses, and reoviruses, are thought to be causally related to shellfish-borne gastroenteritis. Epidemiological data, however, to support this suspicion are lacking. Metcalf[149] points out:

> The virologic dilemma represented involved the formidable technical difficulties encountered in working with those enteric viruses causally associated with shellfish-transmitted enteric disease.... Shellfish virology research needs to take some new directions. A vigorous, imaginative program which places primary emphasis upon these enteric virus pathogens and conditions actually involved in shellfish transmitted disease is needed.... The end result of such a program would be better protection of public health in general, and a possibility that the number of shellfishing waters approved for the taking of shellfish could be increased.

Dinoflagellates[1,2,6,9,50,99,142–144,155–159]

Dinoflagellates (class Mastigophora, order Dinoflagellata) are predominantly free-living, unicellular protozoans forming part of the ocean plankton, synthesizing carbohydrates, proteins, and fats. These one-celled plant-animals when in high concentrations may produce yellow, brown, green, black, blue, red, or milky bioluminescence of the water. The most common color associated with "blooming" of dinoflagellates is red, hence the terms red tide, red current, and red water. The following list indicates the marine dinoflagellates incriminated in human intoxications as a result of shellfish ingestion:

Ptychodiscus brevis (formerly, *Gymnodinium brevis*) (Gulf of Mexico and Florida)

Gymnodinium spp (South Africa)
Gonyaulax actenella (British Columbia)
G catenella (Pacific coast of North America)
G excavata
G grindleyi (Capetown, South Africa)
G tamarensis (eastern coast of North America)
Pyrodinium bahamense (Port Moresby, New Guinea)
P phoneus (Belgium, North Sea)
Exuviaella mariae-lebouriae (Japan, British Columbia, California)

Those dinoflagellates suspected of causing human intoxication are:

Glenodinium foliaceum (Baltic Sea)
Amphidinium spp (warm and cool temperate waters)
Cochlodinium catenatum (California, Japan)
Gymnodinium galatheanum (Walvis Bay, southwest Africa)
Gy mikomoti (Japan)
Gy splendens (Washington, British Columbia)
Gy veneficum (English Channel)
Noctiluca scinitillans (diffuse)
Gonyaulax monilata (Florida)
G polyhedra (southern California, Portugal, Australia)
Heterocapsa triquetra (Baltic Sea)
Peridinium trochoideum (Bay of Guanabara, Rio de Janeiro, Brazil)
Polykrikos schwartzi (Atlantic Ocean, north Baltic and Mediterranean Seas, California coast)
Euviaella baltica (Angola, western Africa)
Prorocentrum micans (California)
Prymnesium parvum (Mediterranean Sea)

Venerupin Shellfish Poisoning[1,2,6,9,62,144]

Venerupin shellfish (order Filibranchia) are found in Japanese, British Columbian, and Californian coastal waters. Venerupin shellfish poisoning has been limited to those mollusks inhabiting and harvested from the brackish waters of certain specific areas of Japan, namely, Lakes Hamana and Kanazawa. The venerupin shellfish producing human intoxication are *Venerupis semidecussata* or *Tapes semidecussata* (Japanese little neck) and *Crassostrea gigas* also known as *Ostrea gigas* (giant Pacific oyster, Japanese oyster). *Dosinia japonica* (Japanese dosinia) has been found to contain venerupin toxin, but no reports of human intoxication from this species of mollusk have been documented.

Venerupin toxin is heat labile and concentrated in the digestive organs and livers of venerupin shellfish. The toxin is believed to be derived from the dinoflagellate *Exuviaella mariae-lobouriae* (previously named *Provocentrum* spp) upon which the shellfish have been feeding.

The syndrome produced by venerupin intoxication usually begins 24 to 48 hours after ingestion of the contaminated mollusks, but the incubation period may extend to one week. It results from a hemorrhagic diathesis combined with liver failure. Initial symptoms include anorexia, abdominal pain, nausea, vomiting, constipation, and headache followed shortly thereafter by bleeding of the gums and nasal passages, petechial hemorrhages, ecchymoses, jaundice, ascites, delirium, coma, and death in 33% of the cases. Laboratory studies reveal anemia, leukocytosis, and abnormalities in blood clotting and liver function tests. Postmortem examinations reveal diffuse liver necrosis with hemorrhage and fatty degeneration as well as congestion and hemorrhage of heart, lung, and gastrointestinal tract.

Therapy consists of activated charcoal combined with purgatives (in a slurry) to prevent absorption and hasten elimination of toxin. Otherwise, supportive care to treat the hemorrhagic diathesis and liver failure is required.

The Japanese government has placed affected areas under quarantine during peak danger periods between January and April in order to prevent outbreaks of venerupin shellfish poisoning.

Paralytic Shellfish Poisoning[1,2,6,8,9,50,51,141–143,158–168]

Paralytic shellfish poisoning (PSP) is produced from ingestion of toxic clams, limpets, and certain shellfish that have been feeding upon toxic dinoflagellates that contain saxitoxin, neosaxitoxin, and/or gonyautoxins, specifically *Gonyaulax* spp (*G acatenella, G catenella, G grindleyi, G tamarensis*), *P bahamense*, and *P phoneus*. Human PSP has a worldwide distribution including North America, Central America, Europe, Africa, Asia, Oceania, and the Pacific Islands.

During warm seasons—encouraged by high light, water temperatures of approximately 10°C, calm seas, water low in nitrogen and phosphorus—these dinoflagellates "bloom," producing bioluminescent tides, commonly called red tides. Dinoflagellate blooms have been associated with large mollusk, fish, and bird kills. At the Merrimack river estuary, Plum Island, off the Massachusetts coast (1972), 95 birds were found dead, and autopsies revealed hemorrhage of their internal organs as well as mollusk shells in their stomachs. The poisoning (initially thought secondary to pesticide spraying of the area) was proved to be from mollusk-borne infestation with the dinoflagellate *G tamarensis*.

The toxin from *G catenella*, saxitoxin, was first isolated from the Alaskan butter clam *Saxidomus giganteus*, from which it received its name. The chemical structure of saxitoxin has been documented as shown in Fig. 45-23. Saxitoxin is similar to a diguanidinium purine resembling guanine. The linear ether moiety causes saxitoxin to resemble some carbamates. The toxic effects of saxitoxin may be related to the fact that guanidiniums may provide firm attachments to cell membranes and cell receptors.

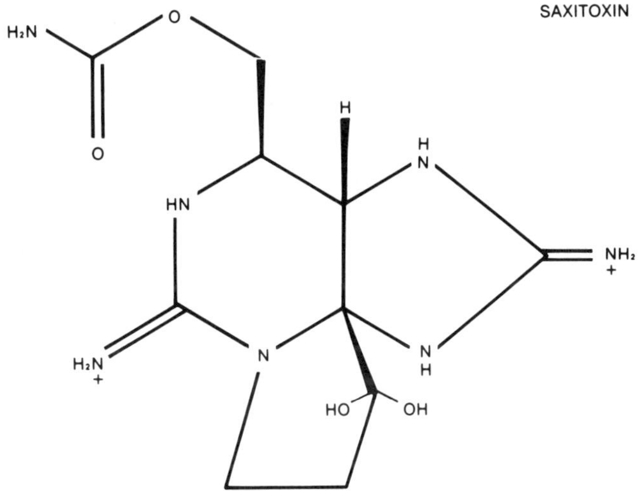

Figure 45-23 Saxitoxin chemical structure.

Saxitoxin is a neurotoxin closely resembling tetrodotoxin but less potent. As Sims[167] points out, saxitoxin behaves as a stimulant for the narcotic receptor (ie, a neuromuscular blocker, catecholamine blocker, ATP blocker, blocker of oxygenation of hemoglobin and the cytochrome system, and urea cycle blocker). Saxitoxin is thought to be 50 times as potent as curare, and an ingestion of as little as 0.5 mg may be lethal. Intraperitoneal injection of bivalve extracts into mice serves as the basis for the bioassay of saxitoxin. A concentration of more than 80 μg per 100 gm of tissue extract is thought dangerous for human consumption. Bioassay for saxitoxin facilitates epidemiological surveillance of shellfish. However, no direct assay is presently available.

The symptoms associated with PSP usually develop within 30 minutes of ingesting the poisonous mollusks. Initially perioral and acral paresthesias, diffuse erythema, nausea, vomiting, diarrhea, and abdominal pain occur, followed by ataxia, muscle weakness, sensations of floating, generalized motor incoordination, dysphonia, dysphagia, vertigo, nystagmus, headache, respiratory distress, and in approximately 8.5% of cases, death from respiratory failure.

Therapy consists initially of purgatives, cathartics (without magnesium, because elevated magnesium levels depress nerve conduction by changing cell membrane potentials, increasing resistance, and therefore, possibly aggravating symptoms of PSP), and saline enemas in order to promote elimination of unabsorbed toxin still present in the GI tract. If vomiting has not occurred, emetics should be administered and gastric lavage should be performed. Administration of IV solutions of normal saline or Ringer's lactate with added electrolytes (as indicated) may be necessary depending upon the patient's vital signs, urine output, and laboratory test results. Observation of the patient's respiratory status is critical.

In the presence of muscle weakness measuring FEV_1 (a portable spirometer can be used) and frequent arterial blood gas analysis to follow $Paco_2$ levels may be extremely helpful in ascertaining when a patient may require mechanical ventilatory assistance. Paresthesias may indicate an alteration in the relationship of ionized and unionized calcium. Since saxitoxin is similar to tetrodotoxin, the latter thought to block sodium channels in nerve membranes, the administration of calcium (as is suggested for neurotoxic shellfish poisoning and ciguatera fish poisoning) may increase the sodium channel blockade, thereby further decreasing neurotransmission of the action potential. Consequently, calcium administration is contraindicated in PSP.

Neurotropic (Neurotoxic) Shellfish Poisoning[1,6,9,99,141,156,159,161,166-169]

Neurotropic shellfish poisoning is caused by the dinoflagellate *Ptychodiscus breve* producing red tides off both the Gulf and Atlantic coasts of Florida. Neurotropic shellfish poisoning is far less severe than paralytic shellfish poisoning and in many ways resembles ciguatera fish poisoning. Symptoms occur within minutes to hours after ingestion of the toxic mollusks and include nausea, vomiting, paresthesias, reversal of hot and cold temperature sensation, diarrhea, ataxia, and rarely, paralysis.

One of the several toxins *P breve* produces has been found to inhibit calcium uptake in endoplasmic reticulum of skeletal muscle. Theoretically this suggests treating severe cases with therapeutic doses of calcium; presently, this hypothesis remains experimental. Another toxin isolated stimulates postganglionic cholinergic nerve fibers and may be responsible for the diarrhea associated with neurotropic shellfish poisoning. Therapy is directed toward eliminating any unabsorbed toxin using those modalities mentioned in reference to paralytic shellfish poisoning.

Ptychodiscus breve is an unarmored dinoflagellate capable of being disrupted in rough surf, thereby becoming aerosolized. This aerosolized mist when breathed by bathers or seashore inhabitants may produce a syndrome comprising copious rhinorrhea, conjunctival irritation, and nonproductive cough. This is usually a transient, rapidly reversible, self-limiting process requiring no therapeutic intervention.

Other Invertebrates[1,2,6,9,62,99,141,144]

Toxic ingestion may be caused by many other invertebrate organisms including univalve mollusks (whelks, ivory shells, turban shells, murex shells, abalone, sea hares), bivalve mollusks (callistin shellfish, Tridacna clam), cephalopods (octopuses, squids, cuttlefishes), and crustaceans (crabs, lobsters, shrimps). A complete description of these poisonings is beyond the scope of this chapter and for further information the reader is directed to the references cited.

POISONING FROM INGESTION OF MARINE VERTEBRATES

Poisonous fishes as defined by Bagnis et al[62] are "... fishes which, when ingested, cause a biotoxication in humans due to a toxic substance present in the fish. Fishes that may become accidentally contaminated by bacterial food pathogens are not included."

Ichthyotoxism is the term used to describe poisoning from ingestion of fish. The major classifications of ichthyotoxism include: ichthyosarcotoxism (poisoning from ingesting a toxin found within the flesh, viscera, or slime), ichthyootoxism (poisoning from ingesting a toxic limited to the gonads), ichthyocrinotoxism (poisoning from ingesting a toxin within or elaborated by glandular structures), and ichthyohematotoxism (poisoning from ingesting a toxin found in the blood).

Ichthyosarcotoxism[3,6,9,62,99,152,170]

Ichthyosarcotoxism is by far the most frequent and dangerous form of ichthyotoxism and poses the greatest public health hazard from ingestion of marine organisms. Halstead[3] classifies ichthyosarcotoxic fish poisoning into: (1) cyclostome poisoning (lampreys, hagfishes), (2) elasmobranch poisoning (sharks, skates, rays), (3) ciguatera poisoning (ciguatoxic fishes), (4) scombroid poisoning (scombroid and non-scombroid fishes), (5) puffer fish poisoning (tetraodontoid fishes), (6) gemphylid poisoning (gemphylidotoxic fishes), and (7) hallucinogenic fish poisoning.

Elasmobranch Poisoning[1,3,6,9,63]

Eating shark flesh has been known to cause a mild gastroenteritis (eg, Greenland shark *Somniosus microcephalus*). Ingestion of shark liver may have lethal consequences, but toxic effects generally produce GI and neurologic symptoms. The composition and nature of the poison is unknown and therapy is purely symptomatic. Abstinence from shark products, unless a particular specimen is definitely known to be nontoxic, is advisable.

Ciguatera Poisoning[1,3,5,6,9,23,50,99,141,143,157,159,161,167,170–203]

The term *ciguatera* was first used by the early Spanish settlers of Cuba. The word is derived from *cigua*, meaning snail, referring to the univalve mollusk *Turbo pica* (class Gastropoda), which is known to produce digestive and nervous disorders when ingested.

Ciguatera poisoning is the most commonly documented and reported poisoning from vertebrate fishes, and in fact is the most common form of food-borne disease related to seafood ingestion in the United States. During the ten-year period 1970 to 1980 the Centers for Disease Control reported 94 outbreaks involving 418 cases of ciguatera poisoning. However, these figures probably do not reflect the true magnitude of the problem. Lawrence and coworkers[184] suggest a ratio of 5 cases per 10,000 population per year as a more accurate estimation of the true incidence of ciguatera poisoning. It is very difficult to obtain data on ciguatera poisoning because minor symptoms may be attributed to a viral gastroenteritis or other enteric food poisoning, physicians and health professionals generally are unfamiliar with the syndrome, and many countries worldwide have no mandatory reporting laws. Furthermore, only over the last few years have papers on ciguatera poisoning been published in the general medical and emergency medical literature to alert physicians to this particular fish-borne illness.

Fishes associated with ciguatera poisoning inhabit the tropical waters of the world extending from 35°N to 34°S latitude. The greatest concentration of ciguatoxic fishes is in the Caribbean and Indo-Pacific. Ciguatoxic fishes are usually reef and bottom dwellers, and those weighing over 10 to 12 pounds are more likely to be toxic. In fact, Hessel and coworkers[192] reported that of the Pacific Ocean red snapper studied, 69% of those weighing over 2.8 kg (6.16 pounds) were found to be toxic, as compared with 18 percent of those under 2.8 kg. Furthermore, there seems to be a higher prevalence of toxicity in those fish whose habitats have been disturbed by natural or man-made destructive forces, such as storms, pier and wharf construction, beach excavations, and dredging.

The following orders of bony fishes (phylum Chordata, class Osteichthyes) have been reported as being ciguatoxic and include some 400 to 500 species[3,9]:

Clupeiformes:	herrings, anchovies
Myctophiformes:	lizardfishes, lanternfishes
Anguilliformes:	true eels, that is, conger eels, moray eels, snake eels
Beloniformes:	needlefishes, halfbeaks
Gasterosteiformes:	trumpetfishes, seahorses
Beryciformes:	squirrelfishes, soldierfishes
Perciformes:	perchlike fishes, that is, surgeonfishes, cardinal fishes, tangs, blennies, jack, pompano, permit, butterflyfishes, bannerfishes, angelfishes, dolphin, silverfishes, gobies, pacific sailfish, sergeant major fishes, grunts, parrotfishes, wahoo, tuna, bonito, king, mackerel, scorpionfishes, grouper, rabbitfishes, barracuda
Bothidae:	flatfishes, for example, flounder
Tetraodontiformes:	filefishes, triggerfishes, cowfishes, puffers, trunkfishes
Batrachoidiformes:	toadfishes
Lophiiformes:	goosefishes, frogfishes

Ciguatera fish poisoning is believed to result from toxins produced from a certain benthic alga dinoflagellate, *Gamberdiscus toxicus,* frequently found on the surface of brown and red seaweed. There is presently confirmed evidence that it produces both ciguatoxin and maitotoxin. The source of ciguatoxin in significant concentration to affect man is a consequence of a multiplicity of environmental factors interwoven with the food chain of marine organisms. Ethnic variations in ciguatera poisoning syndrome seem to be related to dietary intake. Those persons of Chinese or Philippine heritage seem to be more severely affected; those of Hawaiian extraction are least affected.

Present evidence indicates that ciguatoxin is an odorless, colorless, heat-stable, lipid-soluble, acid-stable lipid. Many investigators have tried to elucidate the chemical nature, pharmacokinetics, and properties of toxins associated with ingestion of fish producing the ciguatera syndrome. These toxins include ciguatoxin(s), maitotoxin, lysophosphatidylcholine (maitotoxin-associated hemolysin), scaritoxin(s), and ciguatoxin-associated ATP inhibitor. Additionally, the ciguatera syndrome is not limited to the above named toxins and indeed may be associated with mixed toxin ingestion. Ciguatoxin is unaffected by cooking, freezing, or storage conditions and is not inactivated by gastric juices. These properties, coupled with its tasteless and colorless nature, make prevention of poisoning and detection of ciguatoxic fishes very difficult.

In the effort to detect ciguatoxic fishes, folkloric taboos prohibit eating a lone fish captured from a school, fish products that repel ants or that a pet turtle will not eat, thinly sliced meat not showing a rainbow effect when held up to sunlight, and fish products that tarnish a silver spoon when placed in a cooking pot. Upon close scrutiny, none of these suggestions has proved effective or valid.

Detection of ciguatoxin in tissue of suspected fishes by a radioimmune assay[182] has been possible since 1977. Presently, no methods are available for the detection of ciguatoxin in the blood or secretions of the poisoned victims. Ciguatera poisoning, however, is probably caused by a variety of toxins or other concomitant ichthyosarcotoxic processes, which accounts for the multiplicity of clinical signs, symptoms, and responses to therapy.

The clinical syndrome generally begins within 6 hours after ingestion but can occur as early as 15 minutes or be delayed as much as 30 hours. Approximately 75% of patients have symptoms within the first 12 hours after ingestion of the toxic fish. Initially, acral and perioral tingling, numbness, and prickly and burning sensations occur, followed by headache, vertigo, hypersalivation, metallic taste (rare), nausea, vomiting, watery diarrhea, and abdominal cramps. The GI symptoms may not occur but usually are present and may precede the onset of sensory disturbances.

Neurologic symptoms include the phenomenon of temperature dysesthesias (hot objects feel cold and cold objects feel hot), which usually appears 2 to 5 days after ingestion and is neither pathognomonic nor required for the diagnosis of ciguatera poisoning. However, it is an extremely valuable diagnostic clue. Hyperexcitability manifested as anxiety, nervousness, giddiness, apprehension, restlessness, shouting, hysteria, muscle stiffness or spasms, trismus, fasciculations, hyperreflexia, hallucinations, irrational behavior, generalized seizures, and opisthotonus may give way to fatigue, weakness, ataxia, muscular incoordination, aphonia, hyporeflexia, areflexia, inability to stand, cranial nerve palsies, ptosis, stupor, coma, flaccid paralysis, respiratory muscle paralysis, respiratory failure, and complete adynamism. Cardiovascular symptoms of bradycardia, hypotension, and conduction disturbances with heart block are particularly dangerous and indicative of severe poisoning. Sims points out, "Manifestations of extremely serious ciguatera fish poisoning include the following: severe bradycardia, severe hypotension, convulsions, severe generalized paresthesias, severe hypocalcemia, aphonia, bronchorrhea, unconsciousness, and progressive heart block."[1]

The mortality rate from acute poisoning has been reported from 0% to as high as 80%, depending upon the series of cases reviewed. There have been two deaths in the United States from ciguatera poisoning, both in Hawaii in 1964.[1]

Chronic symptoms of ciguatera poisoning have been well known but generally poorly studied. A wide variety of problems involving cutaneous, GI, neurologic, cardiovascular, genitourinary, and psychic systems can be affected. Chronic symptoms can last for many years and become emotionally and physically debilitating.

Ciguatera poisoning may present as a diffuse multisymptom involvement or as a more limited process with one or more systems predominating. Bagnis in 1968[204] classified ciguatera poisoning according to the predominant symptoms: neurologic symptoms, digestive symptoms, itching, erythema, cardiovascular symptoms, neuromuscular symptoms, and sensory disturbances. This is a useful classification because it may help to predict the course of the patient's illness and degree of aggressiveness required in the therapeutic approach.

Therapy for ciguatera poisoning has included a wide range of modalities, including emetics, gastric lavage, and purgatives for elimination of toxin and prevention of absorption; chlorpromazine as an antiemetic; atropine and 2-PAM for GI, cardiac, and anticholinesterase-like symptoms produced by ciguatoxins; infusions of electrolyte solutions high in calcium, magnesium, potassium, chloride, and bromide, and the administration of EDTA for paresthesias and cardiac and neurologic symptoms; barbiturates, glucocorticoids, and cold showers for itching, paresthesias, and neurologic complaints; magnesium sulfate and sedatives such as phenobarbitol and Valium in order to control insomnia, hyperexcitability, and seizures; and vitamin supplements (particularly B and C complexes) to hasten recovery. All of these regimens have been recommended or condemned for various reasons.

The current therapeutic interventions are based upon the following concepts:

- Ciguatera poisoning is a consequence of multiple toxins and factors.
- Ciguatoxin is not an anticholinesterase.
- Ciguatoxin has been shown to affect sodium membrane permeability and resting membrane potentials by its action as a competitive inhibitor of calcium ions for receptor sites on the nerve membrane.
- The molecular weight of ciguatoxin has been placed at about 1112 ami; proposed molecular formulas fitting this approximate molecular weight are $C_{55-60}H_{75-80}N_{0-3}O_{20-25}$, $C_{53}H_{77}NO_{24}$, and $C_{54}H_{78}O_{24}$. Pharmacologically, the profound shock seen in severe ciguatera poisoning is compatible with maitotoxin hypotensive effects, while ciguatoxin may account for the hypertension effects seen in chronic ciguatera syndrome.
- Polycyclic ethers are apparently responsible for immune sensitization, particularly that related to chronic ciguatera poisoning. Immunologically, T-lymphocyte reaction with polycyclic ethers results in the production of abnormal immunoglobulin E. Theoretically, this prevents mast cell release of serotonin, causing hypotension. This theory is consistent with the hypotensive effects seen in ciguatera syndrome with administration of opiates (ie, morphine is a polycyclic ether). Patients with acute or chronic ciguatera syndrome have demonstrated an intolerance to other substances containing polycyclic ethers such as certain medications and foods. Consideration of these factors plays a significant role in therapeutic interventions in ciguatera poisoning.

In consideration of these factors, the following recommendations are set forth for the treatment of ciguatera poisoning:

- Within 6 to 8 hours after ingestion administer emetics (if vomiting has not occurred) or utilize gastric lavage to promote gastric emptying and elimination of any remaining fish products.
- Administer activated charcoal combined with a non–magnesium-containing cathartic in a slush to promote elimination of toxin.
- Administer atropine, 0.01 to 0.02 mg/kg IV, every 10 minutes if necessary (symptomatic heart rate less than 50 beat/min).
- Administer dopamine infusion, 5 to 20 µg/kg per minute, for severe and prolonged hypotensive episodes or when cardiovascular symptoms predominate. Titrate to systolic blood pressure of 100 to 120 mmHg.
- In patients with significant illness, administer an intravenous infusion of 20% mannitol with a maximum dose of 1 g/kg at 500 mL/hour. Palatox et al[197] studied 24 patients with acute ciguatera poisoning. All were treated with intravenous mannitol and had dramatic clinical improvement. Patients with neurologic symptoms, muscular symptoms, and coma responded dramatically within minutes of infusion. The study was uncontrolled, having been based on empiric observations, and its results must be evaluated with caution. The mechanism of action of mannitol is unclear but may be competitive inhibition of toxin at cell membranes or a direct effect on the toxin, making it inert. Because mannitol is inexpensive and benign, this form of therapy is worth using in patients with significant symptoms. Controlled trials must be performed to explore more adequately what appears to be an important therapeutic modality.
- Administer IV calcium gluconate in doses of 15 mg/kg over 30 minutes, followed by a continuous infusion of 45 to 70 mg/kg of calcium gluconate daily for 5 days or until serum calcium is in mid-normal range. (This is used in severe poisoning to act as a substrate against competitive inhibition of calcium by ciguatoxin.)
- Administer diazepam for hyperexcitability and diazepam and phenytoin for convulsions; do not use barbiturates or paraldehyde.
- Administer IV fluids utilizing normal saline and Ringer's lactate with additional electrolyte solutions, depending upon the patient's vital signs, urine output, amount of vomitus and diarrhea, and the results of laboratory studies.
- Administer large doses of multivitamins and acetaminophen 5 to 10 mg/kg every 6 to 8 hours if necessary for headaches and temperature reversal.
- Administer indomethacin, 25 mg/day or twice a day, for arthralgia or arthritis.
- Provide mechanical ventilatory support and oxygen therapy for respiratory failure.
- Utilize transvenous cardiac pacing in the presence of refractory bradycardia or heart block.
- Provide diet containing no fish, shellfish, alcoholic beverage, or nuts.
- Methdilazine (Tacaryl) 4 mg three or four times a day, has been helpful in controlling the itching associated with chronic symptoms.

While there have been no published studies on utilizing high dose calcium infusions for treatment of ciguatera poisoning, Sims has had encouraging results in several severely poisoned individuals with significant bradycardia, heart block, or hypotension. In life-threatening situations, when all other modalities have been unsuccessful and the patient demonstrates deterioration in spite of routine therapy, high-dose calcium infusions should be considered.

Patients with chronic symptoms should be treated with oral administration of calcium gluconate, multivitamins, and acetaminophen and should refrain from ingesting fish, fish products, shellfish, alcohol, and nuts, all of which have been implicated in producing recurrent episodes of symptoms. Patients also must avoid marijuana, opiates, barbiturates, solvents, herbicides, glues, epoxies, ethers, resins, and cosmetics for at least 6 months and possibly for 12 months. Patients unfortunate enough to sustain a second episode of ciguatera poisoning frequently have more severe symptoms, and it has been postulated that this exaggerated response may be a consequence of immunologic sensitization.

Prevention of illness from ciguatera poisoning involves awareness of the syndrome, refraining from eating fishes in affected areas, ingesting only smaller reef fishes less than 5 pounds, and confirming that the 3 to 5 pound fish fillet, "snapper fingers," or fish sticks, purchased in the market or at a restaurant, are not small fillets or small pieces of a larger fish.

Scombrotoxism[1,3,6,9,62,99,141,143,160,167,205–211]

Scombroid fish poisoning is a consequence of the ingestion of poorly canned, refrigerated, or preserved scombroid fishes (suborder Scombroidei: tuna, albacore, mackerel, kingfish, wahoo, bonito, etc.) or nonscombroid fishes having red skeletal muscle or portions of red skeletal muscle, which have undergone the action of certain bacteria. Recently, mahi-mahi (*Coryphaena hippurus*), a non-scombroid fish, has been implicated in producing scombrotoxism.

This is the only form of ichthyosarcotoxism in which bacteria participate in the poisoning process. The organism usually incriminated in scombroid fish poisoning is *Proteus morgagni*, which is known to contain histadine decarboxylase activity. But *Alcaligenes metalcaligenes*, *Sarcina flara*, *Shigella dysenteriae*, *Clostridium perfringens*, certain *Escherichia coli*, and *Aerobacter aerogenes* have also been found capable of generating histamine. These bacteria, therefore, act upon the histadine in the flesh of the fish, converting it to histamine and a histamine-like substance called saurine, a heat-stable compound which has been found to include histamine dihydrochloride, histamine phosphate, and other substances.

A histamine-like reaction begins within minutes to a few hours after the ingestion of the toxic fish. Interestingly, the ingestion of large doses of histamine in humans does not usually result in poisoning unless the person is taking INH or other GI tract histaminase blockers. Healthy fish usually contain less than 0.1 mg of histamine per 100 g of flesh. Increasing levels of histamine can be measured in fish that are left at room temperature for several hours.

Symptoms of scombroid fish poisoning include a toxic erythema or flushing (particularly involving the face, neck, upper trunk, and conjunctivae) often resembling a sunburn, burning sensation of the mouth and throat, nausea, abdominal cramps, diarrhea, headache, oral blistering, palpitations, dizziness, prostration, chills, thirst, pruritus, blurred vision, urticaria, swelling of the face, increased flatulence, tachycardia, and hyperactive bowel sounds.

The differential diagnosis includes alcohol ingestion associated with chloral hydrate, tyramine, monoamine oxidase inhibitors, Antabuse, and non–alcoholic-related flush syndromes of carcinoid, pheochromocytoma, the Zollinger-Ellison syndrome, and allergy. Other drugs capable of producing flushing are antimuscarinics, histamine releasers (eg, opiates), nicotinic acid, and nitrites, all of which must be considered in the differential diagnosis of flush reactions.

Therapy for scombroid fish poisoning consists of subcutaneous injections of epinephrine, antihistamines IM or IV (diphenhydramine or hydroxyzine) and/or bronchodilators IV if epinephrine and antihistamines are insufficient in relieving bronchospasm. Blakesley[212] reported four patients with scombroid fish poisoning whose symptoms responded within minutes after treatment with an IV infusion of 300 mg of cimetidine given over a 20-minute period. One patient developed a mild hypotensive episode that had coincided with disappearance of his histaminic symptoms. This patient was the only one of the four that had received epinephrine 30 minutes prior to the cimetidine infusion. His hypotension cleared with simple postural maneuvers. The author speculated that blocking histaminic support of blood pressure versus direct effect of cimetidine was the etiologic cause of the hypotension in this patient. All four patients were discharged on a short course of oral cimetidine therapy (eg, 300 mg every 6 hours for 2 days). The author concluded that further study using cimetidine in the treatment of scombroid fish poisoning was warranted. In view of the generally benign nature of short-term cimetidine treatment, it would seem reasonable to use this therapeutic modality if epinephrine and/or antihistamine administration have not been successful in alleviating the patient's symptoms. In order to hasten elimination and prevent absorption of histamine or saurine, emetics and cathartics should be used if vomiting and diarrhea have not occurred spontaneously. Corticosteroids may be required in rare cases.

Scombroid fish poisoning is very difficult to prevent, since surveillance is often lacking, toxins are heat stable, and the fish usually has no abnormal taste. Occasionally, the meat may taste peppery, which should alert the individual to the possibility of spoilage. Fishermen should make every effort to ensure proper refrigeration of their catch, and fish allowed to remain in the sun for more than 2 hours should not be eaten. Furthermore, patients taking certain medications, particularly isoniazid, should refrain from eating scombroid fishes or fish with red skeletal muscle. It has been shown that isoniazid is a potent inhibitor of GI histaminase. Isoniazid in concert with only slightly elevated levels of histamine or saurine in scombroid fishes may have complementary effects, whereas each factor individually may be insufficient to produce poisoning.

Tetrodotoxism[1,3,6,9,62,99,121,141,143, 161–163,167,196,213,214]

Pufferfish poisoning, or tetrodotoxication, is a very rare but serious and often fatal form of ichthyosarcotoxism. Pufferfish poisoning, also known as fugu poisoning, is generally found in the countries surrounding the South Indochina Sea and in Japan. Tetraodontiformes are also found in Californian, African, South American, and Australian waters. Tarichatoxin found in some California newts has been discovered to be identical to tetrodotoxin present in pufferfishes (suborder Gymnodontes). Other terms used to designate tetrodotoxin are: fugu poison, spheroidin, and tetraodontoxin. In Japan, where the fish (Fig. 45-24) is a delicacy, deaths from tetrodotoxism have been reported at 100 per year during the period 1886 to 1958. Public health measures have included the licensing of restaurants and handlers of tetrodon fishes sufficiently knowledgeable to clean and eviscerate the known toxic species without cutting the liver or roe where the toxin is very highly concentrated. In the United States, laws have specifically been established to prevent the sale of tetrodon fishes, markedly reducing the number of poisonings in this country.

Tetrodotoxin acts by reducing membrane permeability to sodium ions by blocking sodium influx and thereby interfering with production of action potentials in certain excitable cells. Other toxins such as saxitoxin may contribute to symptoms.

Pufferfish poisoning produces symptoms within minutes of ingestion, characterized by paresthesias (initially of the mouth, tongue, lips, and face, progressing to involve the extremities and finally producing generalized numbness of the entire body), headache, general malaise, diaphoresis, nausea, vomiting, abdominal pain, dysphagia, and salivation; followed by neurologic symptoms of incoordination, weakness, muscle fasciculations, respiratory paralysis, generalized ascending paralysis, cyanosis, and dermatologic symptoms of blistering and severe scaling of the skin. Hypotension and cardiovascular collapse may occur and the mortality rate may be as high as 60%.

Therapy is directed toward maintaining airway, ventilation, adequate circulatory function, and monitoring and treating dysrhythmias. There is no known antidote for tetrodotoxin and treatment remains symptomatic and empirical.

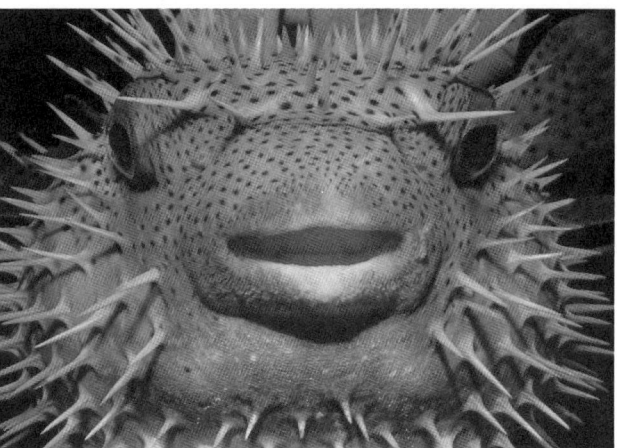

Figure 45-24 Pufferfish.

Sims and Ostman,[215] in their review of emergency diagnosis and management of mild tetrodotoxication, suggest that the narcotic opiate effect of tetrodotoxin might be reversed by the use of naloxone. Additionally, the use of hyperbaric oxygenation might prove valuable because tetrodotoxin appears to react with and bind to cytochrome systems and hemoglobin.

AQUATIC DERMATITIS CAUSED BY MICROORGANISMS[133,216–223]

Dermatologic reactions are common sequelae of contact with dangerous marine life as has been pointed out throughout this chapter. Many topics are beyond the scope of this writing, such as skin disorders from schistosomal organisms, certain annalids (eg, leeches), small crustaceans (eg, sea louse dermatitis), various parasites (eg, cutaneous larva migrans), certain fish (eg, the soap fish *Rypticus saponaceus*).

A few dermatological disorders produced by toxic marine organisms are worthy of further discussion in the ensuing paragraphs.

Toxic Marine Algae[6,133,216–223]

Dermatitis caused by seaweed is classified according to two varieties: the animal plant variety (eg, sea moss) and the marine plant variety (eg, *Microcoleus lyngbyaceus,* formerly *Lyngbya majuscula* Gamont).

Sea moss dermatitis ("Dogger Bank" itch) produces a poison ivy–like eczematous eruption as a result of contact with the seaweed-like animal colony sea-chervil (*Alcyondium hirsutum*). North Sea fishermen are exposed to these organisms as the animals are caught up in fishing nets. Dogger Bank itch typically involves the face and extremities. Initially a transient dermatitis, this eruption becomes progressively more severe with repeated exposure to *A hirsutum*.

Treatment consists of repeated applications of drying agents (eg, dilute solutions of acetic acid), cooling agents (eg, 20% alcohol), and anti-inflammatory agents (eg, potent fluorinated topical corticosteroids). Parenteral steroids (eg, prednisone 20 to 40 mg/day for 2 weeks with decreasing doses) may be necessary in severe reactions.

Stinging seaweed dermatitis is categorized as a marine plant variety dermatitis. Grauer and Arnold[217] (Oahu, Hawaii) in the late 1950s demonstrated that stinging seaweed dermatitis was conclusively shown to be caused by the blue-green algae *Microcoleus lyngbyaceus* (formerly *Lyngbya majuscula* Gamont). *Microcoleus lyngbyaceus* has also been found in Spain, the Bahamas, southeast Florida, and throughout the tropical Pacific and Indian oceans.

Several chemical toxins have been isolated from *M lyngbyaceus*. Two of these toxins have had their chemical structures elucidated. The dermatitis is related to prolonged contact of the seaweed with skin as the seaweed becomes entrapped between the bathing suit and the epidermis. Classically, therefore, stinging seaweed dermatitis is seen in the distribution of the bathing suit. The typical dermatitis occurs a few hours after contact and consists of a burning, itching, stinging sensation. Associated signs include an erythematous, edematous, vesicular eruption often having a scalded appearance which may result in eschar formation. Highly toxic strains may produce inflammatory reactions of the conjunctivae, nasal mucosa, and lips. Generalized edema, pustular folliculitis, and lymphadenopathy may occur as well. Sims et al[218] in 1981 reported the first known case of escharotic stomatitis caused by incomplete ingestion of stinging seaweed (*M lyngbyaceus*). Their patient mistakenly ingested *M lyngbyaceus*, which vaguely resembles edible seaweeds known as "limu." Within seconds of ingestion the patient discarded the seaweed as unpalatable and developed a burning sensation in his mouth. Additional symptoms and signs included an itching, stinging sensation followed by an erythematous, edematous, patchy, scalded appearance of the oral mucosa with hypersalivation. The patient's pain lasted 72 hours and his oral mucosa did not completely heal until 2 weeks after ingestion.

Treatment of stinging seaweed dermatitis consists of active, thorough washing of the affected areas with warm soapy water. Bathing suits should be removed and cleansed as well. Wet compresses utilizing drying agents such as dilute (5%) acetic acid and soothing ointments (eg, vitamins A and D) have proven helpful in some instances. Topical fluorinated corticosteroid preparations as well as parenteral corticosteroids (prednisone 20 to 40 mg/day with decreasing doses over 2 weeks) may be necessary in severe cases.

The patient with escharotic stomatitis reported by Sims et al[218] obtained partial relief by repeated mouth washing with water and sucking on ice cubes. The administration of diphenhydramine, viscous lidocaine, and prednisone were not helpful and proved ineffective in alleviating his symptoms. Sims et al[218] suggest that the mortality and morbidity associated with ingestion of stinging seaweed may be significant in view of the observed mortalities seen in mice force-fed with toxic algae. The authors recommend that complete ingestions producing esophagogastroenteritis should be treated as ingestions of caustic or corrosive materials.

Sea bather's eruption[216] is a self-limiting dermatitis occurring in saltwater bathers and involving covered areas of the body. It has been often confused with cercarial dermatitis (eg, schistosomiasis) but actually it more closely resembles stinging seaweed dermatitis (Table 45-5). The eruption occurs within a few hours after bathing and consists of pruritic, erythematous wheals or papules resembling insect bites. The etiologic agent is unknown.

Treatment consists of soothing creams (eg, calamine lotion) and parenteral antihistamines (eg, diphenhydramine). Corticosteroid therapy is rarely required.

Table 45-5 Dermatological Disorders Produced by Toxic Marine Organisms

Factor	Stinging Seaweed	Swimmer's Itch	Sea Bather's Eruption
Type of water	Salt	Mainly fresh	Salt
Part of body	Covered	Uncovered	Covered
Locale	Hawaii, Spain, Bahamas, Florida, tropical Pacific and Indian oceans	Northern US, Canada (worldwide)	Florida, Cuba, Gulf Coast
Etiology	Blue-green algae (*Microcoleus lyngbyaceus*)	Schistosomes	Unknown
Lesion	Vesicles, papules	Vesicles, papules	Wheal
Treatment	Washing; dilute acetic acid, A&D ointment, topical and parenteral corticosteroids; oral ingestion treat as corrosive	Washing; isopropyl alcohol, calamine lotion, antihistamines, synthetic corticosteroids, topical and systemic antibiotics for secondary infection	Washing; calamine lotion

Source: Blakesley ML: Scombroid poisoning: Prompt resolution of symptoms with cimetidine. *Ann Emerg Med* 12:104–106, 1983.

Dermatitis Caused by Marine Bacteria[134–139,224]:
Mycobacterium marinum

Aronson[224] was the first to isolate *Mycobacterium marinum* as the causative agent producing mycobacterial infections in saltwater fish. Linell and Norden[136] in 1954 identified a new acid-fast bacillus which they named *M balnei*. They published their findings in a monograph entitled "A New Acid-Fast Bacillus Occurring in Swimming Pools and Capable of Producing Skin Lesions in Humans." Later, *M balnei* was found to be identical with *M marinum*.

Mycobacterium marinum is classified as an atypical mycobacterial organism in that (1) it grows rapidly on Löwenstein-Jensen's medium when cultured at 30° to 32°C (in contrast to *M tuberculosis*, which grows optimally at 37°C); (2) it is classified as a photochrome, since its cream-colored colonies turn yellow when exposed to light; (3) it does not produce progressive disease when injected into guinea pigs; and (4) it is resistant to the usual antituberculus drugs such as isonicotinic acid, para-aminosalicylic acid, and streptomycin.

Infections in man occur after exposure in either fresh water or salt water. Sources of infection include swimming pools (hence the term "swimming pool granulomas"), tropical fish tanks, ocean beaches, lakes, and rivers. In addition, Flowers[138] reported a *M marinum* infection as a result of a dolphin bite.

Typically, *M marinum* infections are limited to the cooler acryl skin areas, and bacterial invasion occurs at sites of abraded skin. These organisms can infect deeper structures such as lymphatics and bone. *Mycobacterium marinum* infections have been mistaken for other disease processes such as sporotrichosis, gout, rheumatoid arthritis, and pyogenic infections.

Skin lesions occur within 3 to 4 weeks after exposure. Initially a red papule develops; this eventually increases in size, forming a hard purple nodule commonly 2 cm in diameter. These nodules may ulcerate and become secondarily infected.

Diagnosis is confirmed by culture of a biopsied specimen at 32°C using Löwenstein-Jensen's medium. Drug sensitivities should be performed in order to more clearly define resistant strains.

Mycobacterium marinum infections usually heal spontaneously within 2 to 3 years. Minocycline hydrochloride, ethambutol hydrochloride, rifampin, and cycloserine may be effective in producing symptomatic relief.

OTHER DANGEROUS MARINE ORGANISMS[1–4,6,9,10,24,50,62,99,138,139,141,143]

Many other organisms are dangerous but cannot be described in detail in this chapter. They include poisonous marine turtles; marine mammals such as sea lions, seals, polar bears, and dolphins; marine animals that shock, such as electric rays and eels; parasitic catfish; schistosomal organisms; algae; bacteria; and miscellaneous fishes and reptiles. The reader is referred to the references cited for information regarding these dangerous marine organisms.

REFERENCES

1. Sims JK. *Dangerous Marine Life*. Honolulu: Sims; 1980.
2. Halstead BW. *Poisonous and Venomous Marine Animals: Invertebrates*. Washington, DC: US Government Printing Office; 1965;1.
3. Halstead BW. *Poisonous and Venomous Marine Animals: Vertebrates*. Washington, DC: US Government Printing Office; 1967;2.
4. Halstead BW. *Poisonous and Venomous Marine Animals: Vertebrates*. Washington, DC: US Government Printing Office; 1970;3.
5. Steinfeld AD, Steinfeld HJ. Ciguatera and the voyage of Captain Bligh. *JAMA*. 1974;228:1270–1271.
6. Banner AH. Hazardous marine animals. In: Tedeschi CG, Eckert WG, Tedeschi LG, eds. *Forensic Medicine: A Study in Trauma and Environmental Hazards*. Philadelphia: Saunders; 1977:1378–1429.
7. Davies DH, Campbell GD. The aetiology, clinical pathology and treatment of shark attack. (Based on observations in Natal, South Africa.) *J R Med Serv*. 1962;48:110–136.
8. Ellis MD, ed. *Dangerous Plants, Snakes, Arthropods and Marine Life: Toxicity and Treatment*. Hamilton, IL: Drug Intelligence; 1978.
9. Halstead BW, Courville DA. *Dangerous Marine Animals that Bite, Sting, Shock, Are Nonedible*. 2nd ed. Centreville, MD: Cornell Maritime Press; 1980.
10. Strauss MB, Orris WL. Injuries to divers by marine animals: a simplified approach to recognition and management. *Mil Med*. 1974;139:129–130.
11. Edmonds C. Dangerous marine animals. *Aust Fam Physician*. 1976;5:381–407.
12. Auerbach PS. Hazardous marine animals. *Emerg Med Clin North Am*. 1984;2:531–544.
13. Auerbach PS, Halstead B. Marine hazards: attacks and envenomations. *JEN*. 1982;8:115–122.
14. Charlesworth D. First-aid for shark attack. *SA Nurs J*. 1976;43:24.
15. Burnett JW. Bite wounds. *Cutis*. 1990;45:287.
16. Baldridge HD Jr, Williams J. Shark attack: feeding or fighting? *Mil Med*. 1969;134:130–133.
17. Baldridge HD Jr. Shark repellent: not yet, maybe never. *Mil Med*. 1990;155:358–361.
18. Goodwin NM, White JAM. First aid for shark attack victims. *SA Med J*. 1977;52:981–982.
19. Buck JD, Spotte S, Gadbaw JJ Jr. Bacteriology of the teeth from a great white shark: potential medical implications for shark bite victims. *J Clin Microbiol*. 1984;20:849–851.
20. Welch K, Martini FH. Non-fatal shark attack at Maui. *Hawaii Med J*. 1981;40:95–96.
21. White JAM. Shark attack in Natal. *Injury*. 1975;6:187–194.
22. Pavia AT, Bryan JA, Maher KL, Hester TR, Farmer JJ. *Vibrio carchariae* infection after a shark bite. *Ann Intern Med*. 1989;111:85–86.
23. Morton RA, Burklew MA. Incidence of ciguatera in barracuda from the west coast of Florida. *Toxicon*. 1970;8:317–318.
24. Tinker SW. *Fishes of Hawaii*. Honolulu: Hawaiian Services; 1928.

25. Khlentzos CT. Seventeen cases of poisoning due to ingestion of an eel: *Gymnothorax flavimarginatus*. *Am J Trop Med*. 1950;30:785–793.
26. Sherman RT, Furste W. A guide to prophylaxis against tetanus in wound management. *Am Coll Surg*. 1972.
27. Taylor GD. The otolaryngologic aspects of skin and scuba diving. *Trans Am Laryngol Rhinol Otol Soc*. January 23–24, 1959:409–459.
28. Sims JK, Irei M. Human Hawaiian sponge poisoning. *Hawaii Med J*. 1979;38:263–270.
29. Taylor L. Tetanus from a marine sponge. *J Otolaryngol*. 1958;72:762.
30. Yafee HS. Irritation from red sponge. *N Engl J Med*. 1970;282:51.
31. Kinzer KW. Marine envenomations. *J Toxicol Clin Toxicol*. 1984;21:527–555.
32. Johnston DG, Burger WD. Injury and disease of scuba and skin divers. *Postgrad Med*. 1971;49:134–139.
33. Rosson CL, Tolle SW. Management of marine stings and scrapes. *West J Med*. 1989;150:97–100.
34. Yaffee HS. Regarding poriferal immunology. *Arch Dermatol*. 1972;106:263–264.
35. Southcott RV, Coulter JR. The effects of the southern Australian marine stinging sponges, *Neofibularia mordens* and *Lissodendoryx* sp. *Med J Aust*. 1971;2:895–901.
36. Rosco MD. Cutaneous manifestations of marine animal injuries including diagnosis and treatment. *Cutis*. 1977;19:507–510.
37. Burnett JW, Calton GJ, Morgan RJ. Dermatitis due to stinging sponges. *Cutis*. 1987;39:476.
38. Southcott RV. Human injuries from invertebrate animals in the Australian seas. *Clin Toxicol*. 1970;3:617–636.
39. Russell FE. Sponge injury—traumatic, toxic or allergic? *N Engl J Med*. 1970;282:753–754.
40. Auerbach PS. Marine envenomations. *N Engl J Med*. 1991;325:486–493.
41. Fisher AA. Water related dermatoses part II: nematocyst dermatitis. *Cutis*. 1980;25:248–249.
42. Burnett JW, Calton GJ. Use of IgE antibody determinations in cutaneous coelenterate envenomations. *Cutis*. 1981;27:50–52.
43. Fisher AA. Toxic versus allergic reactions to jellyfish. *Cutis*. 1984;34:450–454.
44. Burnett JW, Hepper KP, Aurelian L. Lymphokine activity in coelenterate envenomation. *Toxicon*. 1986;24:104–107.
45. Burnett JW, Calton GJ. Venomous pelagic coelenterates: chemistry, toxicology, immunology and treatment of their stings. *Toxicon*. 1987;25:581–602.
46. Halstead BW. Coelenterate (cnidarian) stings and wounds. *Clin Dermatol*. 1987;5:8–13.
47. Burnett JW, Calton GJ, Burnett HW, Mandojana RM. Local and systemic reactions from jellyfish stings. *Clin Dermatol*. 1987;5:14–28.
48. Burnett JW. An electron microscopic study of two nematocytes in the tentacle of *Cyanae capillata*. *Chesapeake Sci*. 1971;12:67–71.
49. Burnett JW, Calton CJ. The chemistry and toxicology of some venomous pelagic coelenterates. *Toxicon*. 1977;15:177–196.
50. Manowitz NR, Rosenthal RR. Cutaneous-systemic reactions to toxins and venoms of common marine organisms. *Cutis*. 1979;23:450–454.
51. Burnett JW, Calton GJ. Recurrent eruption following a solitary envenomation by the cnidarian *Stomolophous meleagris*. *Toxicon*. 1985;23:1010–1014.
52. Matusow RJ. Oral inflammatory response to a sting from a Portuguese man-of-war. *JADA*. 1980;100:73–75.
53. Burnett JW, Carrington SC, Kelman SN, Calton GJ. Studies on the serologic response to jellyfish envenomation. *J Am Acad Dermatol*. 1983;9:229–231.
54. Pierard GE, Letot B, Pierard-Franchimont C. Histologic study of delayed reactions to coelenterates. *J Am Acad Dermatol*. 1990;22:599–601.
55. Burnett JW, Hepper KP, Aurelian L, Calton GJ, Gardepe SF. Recurrent eruptions following solitary coelenterate envenomations. *J Am Acad Dermatol*. 1987;17:86–92.
56. Reed KM, Bronstein BR, Baden HP. Delayed and persistent cutaneous reactions to coelenterates. *J Am Acad Dermatol*. 1984;10:462–466.
57. Gaur PK, Calton GJ, Burnett JW. Enzyme-linked immunosorbent assay to detect anti–sea nettle venom antibodies. *Experientia*. 1981;37:1005–1007.
58. Mansson T, Randle HW, Mandojana RM, Calton GJ, Burnett JW. Recurrent cutaneous jellyfish eruptions without envenomation. *Acta Dermatol Venerol (Stockh)*. 1985;65:72–75.
59. Martin JC, Audley I. Cardiac failure following Irukandji envenomation. *Med J Aust*. 1990;153:164–166.
60. Williamson JA, Burnett JW, Fenner PJ, Hach-Wunderle V, Yu Hoe L, Adiga KM. Acute regional vascular insufficiency after jellyfish envenomation. *Med J Aust*. 1988;149:698–701.
61. Fenner PJ, Williamson JA, Burnett JW, et al. The "Irukandji syndrome" and acute pulmonary oedema. *Med J Aust*. 1988;149:150–156.
62. Bagnis R, Berglund F, Elias PS, et al. Problems of toxicants in marine food products (marine biotoxins). *WHO*. 1970;42:69–88.
63. Weill R. Contribution of l'étude des cnidaireset de leurs nematocystes. *Trav Stat Zool Wimbereux*. 1934;10–11.
64. Wittle LW, Middlebrook RE, Lane CE. Isolation and partial purification of a toxin from *Millepora alcicornis*. *Toxicon*. 1971;9:327–331.
65. Wittle LW, Scura ED, Middlebrook RE. Stinging coral (*Millepora tenera*) toxin: a comparison of crude extracts with isolated nematocyst extracts. *Toxicon*. 1974;12:481–486.
66. Speilman FJ, Bowe AB, Watson CB, Klein EF Jr. Acute renal failure as a result of *Physalia physalis* sting. *South Med J*. 1982;75:1425–1426.
67. Arnold HL. Portuguese man-of-war (blue bottle) stings: treatment with papain. *Straub Clin Proc*. 1971;37:30–33.
68. Burnett JW, Calton GJ. Sea nettle and man-of-war venoms: a chemical composition of their venoms and studies on the pathogenesis of the sting. *J Invest Dermatol*. 1974;62:372–377.
69. Weinberg SR. Reactive arthritis following a sting by a Portuguese man-of-war. *J Fl Med Assoc*. 1988;75:280–281.
70. Exton DR. Treatment of *Physalia physalis* envenomation. *Med J Aust*. 1988;149:54.
71. Stein MR, Marraccini JV, Rothchild NE, Burnett JW. Fatal Portuguese man-o-war (*Physalia physalis*) envenomation. *Ann Emerg Med*. 1989;18:212–315.
72. Freeman SE. Actions of *Chironex fleckeri* toxins on cardiac transmembrane potentials. *Toxicon*. 1974;12:395–404.
73. Freeman SE, Turner RJ. Cardiovascular effects of Cnidarian toxins: a comparison of toxins extracted from *Chiropsalmus quadrigatus* and *Chironex fleckeri*. *Toxicon*. 1972;10:31–37.
74. Burnett JW, Calton GJ. Jellyfish envenomation syndromes updated. *Ann Emerg Med*. 1987;16:1000–1005.

75. Williamson JA, Callanan VI. Serious envenomation by the northern Australian box jellyfish (*Chironex fleckeri*). *Med J Aust.* 1980;1:13–15.

76. Burnett JW, Calton GJ. Response of the box jellyfish (*Chironex fleckeri*) cardiotoxin to intravenous administration of verapamil. *Med J Aust.* 1983;2:192–194.

77. Strutton G, Lumley J. Cutaneous light microscopic and ultrastructural changes in a fatal case of jellyfish envenomation. *J Cutan Pathol.* 1988;15:249–255.

78. Drury JK, Noonan JD, Pollock JG, Reid WH. Jellyfish sting with serious hand complications. *Injury.* 1980;12:67–68.

79. Chand RP, Selliah K. Reversible parasympathetic dysautonomia following stinging attributed to the box jellyfish (*Chironex fleckeri*). *Aust NZ J Med.* 1984;14:673–675.

80. Lumley J, Williamson JA, Fenner PJ, Burnett JW, Colquhoun DM. Fatal envenomation by *Chironex fleckeri*, the north Australian box jellyfish: the continuing search for lethal mechanisms. *Med J Aust.* 1988;148:527–534.

81. Barnes JH. Observations on jellyfish stings in north Queensland. *Med J Aust.* 1960;2:993–999.

82. Alsen C, Berress L, Tesseraux I. Toxicities of sea anemone (*Anemonia sulcata*): polypeptides in mammals. *Toxicon.* 1978;16:561–566.

83. Burnett JW, Rubenstein H, Calton GJ. First aid for jellyfish envenomation. *South Med J.* 1983;76:870–872.

84. Fenner PJ, Williamson JA, Blenkin JA. Successful use of *Chironex* antivenom by members of the Queensland Ambulance Transport Brigade. *Med J Aust.* 1989;151:708–710.

85. Burnett JW, Calton GJ. Pharmaceutical effects of various venoms on cutaneous capilary leakage. *Toxicon.* 1986;24:614–617.

86. Exton DR, Fenner PJ, Williamson JA. Cold packs: effective topical analgesia in the treatment of painful stings by *Physalia* and other jellyfish. *Med J Aust.* 1989;151:625–626.

87. Hartwick RJ, Callanan V, Williamson JAH. Disarming the box jellyfish. *Med J Aust.* 1980;1:15–20.

88. Turner B, Sullivan P, Pennefather J. Disarming the bluebottle: treatment of *Physalia* envenomation. *Med J Aust.* 1980;2:394–395.

89. Fenner PJ, Fitzpatrick PF. Experiments with the nematocysts of *Cyanea capillata*. *Med J Aust.* 1986;145:174.

90. Hinegardner RT. The venom apparatus of the cone shell. *Hawaii Med J.* 1958;17:533–556.

91. Kohn AJ. Cone shell stings: recent cases of human injury due to venomous marine snails of the genus *Conus*. *Hawaii Med J.* 1958;17:528–532.

92. Halstead BW. Current status of marine biotoxicology—an overview. *Clin Toxicol.* 1981;18:1–24.

93. Rice RD, Halstead BW. Report of fatal cone shell sting by *Conus geographus* (Linnaeus). *Toxicon.* 1968;5:223–224.

94. Baden HP, Burnett JW. Injuries from sea urchins. *South Med J.* 1977;70:459–460.

95. Cracchiolo A III, Goldberg L. Local and systemic reactions to puncture injuries by the sea urchin spine and the date palm thorn. *Arthritis Rheum.* 1977;20:1206–1212.

96. O'Neal RL, Halstead BW, Howard LD. Injury to human tissues from sea urchin spines. *Calif Med.* 1964;101:199–202.

97. Rocha G, Frago S. Sea urchin granuloma of the skin. *Arch Dermatol.* 1962;85:146–148.

98. Unkles SE. Bacterial flora of the sea urchin *Echinus esulentus*. *Appl Environ Microbiol.* 1977;34:347–359.

99. Goldfrank L, Lewin N, Weisman R. The red snapper. *Hosp Physician.* 1981;17:36–54.

100. Bitseff EL, Garoni WJ, Hardison CD, et al. The management of stingray injuries of the extremities. *South Med J.* April 1970:417–418.

101. Cross TB. A usual stingray injury: the skindiver at risk. *Med J Aust.* 1976;2:947–948.

102. Mullaney PJ. Treatment of stingray wounds. *Clin Toxicol.* 1970;3:613–615.

103. Russell FE, Panos TC, Kang LW, et al. Studies on the mechanism of death from stingray venom: a report of two fatal cases. *Am J Med Sci.* 1958:566–584.

104. Scoggin CH. Catfish stings. *JAMA.* 1975;231:176–177.

105. Russell FE, Emery JA. Venom of the weevers *Trachinus draco* and *Trachinus vipers*. *Ann NY Acad Sci.* 1960;90:805–819.

106. Cameron AM, Endean R. The venom apparatus of the scorpion fish (*Notesthes robusta*). *Toxicon.* 1966;4:111–121.

107. Hunter AE. Lionfish sting—Nevada. *MMWR.* 1979;83–84.

108. Schaffer RC Jr, Carlson RW, Russel FE. Some chemical properties of the venom of the scorpionfish *Scorpaena guttata*. *Toxicon.* 1971;9:69–78.

109. This lion doesn't roar. *JAMA.* 1979;242:17.

110. Weiner S. The production and assay of stonefish antivenene. *Med J Aust.* 1959;15:719.

111. Tu AT. Venoms of hydrophiidae. In: Tu AT, ed. *Venoms, Chemistry and Molecular Biology.* New York: Wiley; 1977:151–177.

112. Tu AT. Biotoxicology of sea snake venoms. *Ann Emerg Med.* 1987;16:1023–1028.

113. Auerbach PS. Clinical therapy of marine envenomation and poisoning. In: Tu AT, ed. *Handbook of Natural Toxins.* New York: Dekker; 1987;3.

114. Sitprija V, Srubbibhadh R, Benjajati C. Haemodialysis in poisoning by sea snake venom. *Br Med J.* 1971;3:218–219.

115. Cage PW, Dulhunty AF. Effects of toxin from the blue ringed octopus (*Hapalochaena maculosa*). In: Martin DF, Padilla GM, eds. *Marine Pharmacognosy.* New York: Academic Press; 1973.

116. Croft JA, Howden MF. Chemistry of maculotoxin: a potent neurotoxin isolated from *Hapalochlaena maculosa*. *Toxicon.* 1972;10:645.

117. Flecker H. Fatal bite from octopus. *Med J Aust.* 1955;2:329–331.

118. Mabbet H. Death of a skindiver. *Aust Skindiv Spearfish Digest.* 1954;13:17.

119. Sheumack DD, Howden MEH, Quinn RJ, et al. Maculotoxin: a neurotoxin from the venom glands of the octopus *Hapalochaena maculosa* identified as tetrodotoxin. *Science.* 1978;199:188–189.

120. Sutherland SK, Brood AJ, Lane WR. Octopus neurotoxins: low molecular weight nonimmunogenic toxins present in the saliva of the blue-ringed octopus. *Toxicon.* 1970;8:249.

121. Sheumack DD, Howden MEH, Spence I, et al. Tetrodotoxin in the blue-ringed octopus. *Med J Aust.* 1978;1:160–161.

122. Trethewie ER. Pharmacological effects of the venom of the common octopus, *Hapalochaena*. *Toxicon.* 1965;3:55.

123. Barlows A, Herman GJ, DeWitt WE. The isolation and identification of *Vibrio cholerae*: a review. *Health Lab Sci.* 1971;8:167–175.

124. Baross J, Liston J. Occurrence of *Vibrio parahemolyticus* and related hemolytic vibrios in marine environment of Washington state. *Appl Microbiol.* 1970;20:179–186.

125. Blake PA, Merson MH, Weaver RE, et al. Disease caused by a marine vibrio: clinical characteristics and epidemiology. *N Engl J Med.* 1979;300:1–5.

126. Bolen JL, Zamiska SA, Greenough WB. Clinical features in enteritis due to *Vibrio parahemolyticus*. *Am J Med.* 1974;57:638–641.

127. Chatterjee BD, Neogy KN, Gorbach SL. Study of *Vibrio parahemolyticus* from cases of diarrhea in Calcutta. *Indian J Med*. 1970;58:234–238.

128. Hollis DG, Weaver RE, Baker CN, et al. Halophilic *Vibrio* species isolated from blood cultures. *J Clin Microbiol*. 1976;3:425–431.

129. Lumsden LL, Hasseltine HE, Leake JP, et al. A typhoid-fever epidemic caused by oyster-borne infection: 1924–1925. *Public Health Rep*. 1925;50 (suppl):1–102.

130. Sakazaki R. Halophilic *Vibrio* infections. In: Riemann H, ed. *Food-Borne Infections and Intoxications*. New York: Academic Press; 1969:115–129.

131. *Vibrio parahemolyticus* gastroenteritis—United States: 1969–1972. *MMWR*. 1973;22:231–232.

132. Kaneko T, Colwell RR. Ecology of *Vibrio parahemolyticus* in Chesapeake Bay. *J Bacteriol*. 1973;113:24–32.

133. Mynderse JS, Moore RE, KashiGrauer FH. Seaweed dermatitis apparently caused by a marine alga-clinical investigative procedure. *Proc Hawaii Acad Sci*. 1959;34:19.

134. Linell, Folke, Norden, et al. Mycobacterium balnei. A new acid-fast bacillus occurring in swimming pools and capable of producing skin lesions in humans. *Acta Tuberc Scand*. 1954;33 (suppl):1–85.

135. Adams RM, Remington JS, Steinberg J, et al. Tropical fish aquariums: a source of *Mycobacterium marinum* infections resembling sporotrichosis. *JAMA*. 1970;211:457–461.

136. Flowers DJ. Human infection due to *Mycobacterium marinum* after a dolphin bite. *J Clin Pathol*. 1970;23:475–477.

137. Williams CS, Riodan DC. *Mycobacterium marinum* (atypical acid fast bacillus) infections of the hand. *J Bone Joint Surg Am*. 1973; 55:1042–1050.

138. Girard SM, Paik YK, Melton RJ, et al. *Clostridium perfringens* cultured from a Hawaiian sardine, *Sardinell marquesensis*. *Hawaii Med J*. 1979;38:317–329.

139. Johnson RM, Katarski ME, Wesirock WP. Correlation of taxonomic criteria for a collection of marine bacteria. *Arch Dermatol*. 1979; 114:1333–1335.

140. Auerbach PS, Vajko DM, Nassos PS, et al. Bacteriology of the marine environment; implications for clinical therapy. *Ann Emerg Med*. 1987;165:643–649.

141. Dembert ML, Strosahl KF, Bumgardner RL. Disease from fish and shellfish ingestion. *Am Fam Physician*. 1981;24:103–108.

142. Earampamoorthy S, Koff RS. Health hazards of bivalve mollusk ingestion. *Ann Intern Med*. 1975;83:107–110.

143. Horwitz MA. Specific diagnosis of food-borne disease. *Gastroenterology*. 1977;73:375–381.

144. McMichael DF. Dangerous marine mollusco. *Bull Postgrad Comm Med Univ Sydney*. 1963: scientific section suppl part III.

145. Follow-up on shellfish-associated hepatitis—southern United States. *MMWR*. 1974;22:388.

146. Koff RS, Sear HS. Internal temperature of steamed clams. *N Engl J Med*. 1967;276:737–739.

147. Mahoney P, Fleischner G, Milliman I, et al. Australian antigen: detection and transmission in shellfish. *Science*. 1974;183:80–81.

148. Mason JO, McClean WR. Infectious hepatitis traced to the consumption of raw oysters: an epidemiologic study. *Am J Hyg*. 1962;73: 90–111.

149. Metcalf TG. Indication of viruses in shellfish growing waters. *Am J Public Health*. 1979;69:1093–1094.

150. Mosley JW, Galabos J. Viral hepatitis. In: Schiff L, ed. *Disease of the Liver*. Philadelphia: Lippincott; 1975:527–528.

151. Murphy AM, Grohmann GS, Christopher PJ, et al. An Australia-wide outbreak of gastroenteritis from oysters caused by Norwalk virus. *Med J Aust*. 1979;329:332.

152. Shellfish-associated hepatitis: Massachusetts. *MMWR*. 1972;21:20.

153. Vaughn JM, Landry EF, Viccale TJ, et al. Survey of human entero virus occurrence in fresh and marine surface waters of Long Island. *Appl Environ Microbiol*. 1979;38:290–296.

154. Collins C. Massachusetts Department of Health: the Red Tide—a public health emergency. *N Engl J Med*. 1973;288:1126–1127.

155. Kim YS, Padilla GM, Martin DF. Effect of *G breve* toxin on calcium uptake and ATPase activity of sarcoplasmic reticulum vesicles. *Toxicon*. 1978;16:495–501.

156. McFarren EF, Tanabe H, Silva FJ, et al. The occurrence of a ciguatera-like poison in oysters, clams and *Gymnodinium breve* cultures. *Toxicon*. 1965;3:111–123.

157. Popkiss ME, Horstman DA, Harpur D. Paralytic shellfish poisoning: a report of 17 cases in Cape Town. *S Afr Med J*. 1979:1017–1023.

158. Akiba. Study of poisoning by *Venerupis semidecussata* and *Ostera gigas* and other poisonous substances (in Japanese, English summary). *Nisshen Igaku*. 1949;36:1–24.

159. Bagden DG. Marine food-borne dinoflagellate toxins. *Int Rev Cytol*. 1983;82:99–150.

160. Hughes JM, Merson MH. Current concepts: fish and shellfish poisoning. *N Engl J Med*. 1976;295:1117–1120.

161. Kao CY. Tetrodotoxin, saxitoxin and their significance in the study of excitation phenomena. *Pharmacol Rev*. 1966;13:997–1049.

162. Narahashi T. Mechanism of action of tetrodotoxin and saxitoxin on excitable membranes. *Fed Proc*. 1972;31:1124–1132.

163. Prakash A, Medcof JC, Tennant AD. *Paralytic Shellfish Poisoning in Eastern Canada*. Ottawa: Fisheries Research Board of Health; 1971.

164. Schantz EJ, Schnoes HK. The structure of saxitoxin. *J Am Chem Soc*. 1975;97:1238–1239.

165. Wong JL, Oesterlin R, Rappoport H. The structure of saxitoxin. *J Am Chem Soc*. 1971;93:7344.

166. Grunfeld Y, Spiegelstein MY. Effects of *Gymnosinium breve* toxin on the smooth muscle of guinea pig ileum. *Br J Pharmacol*. 1974;51: 67–72.

167. Sims JK. A theoretical discourse on the pharmacology of toxic marine ingestions. *Ann Emerg Med*. 1987;16:1006.

168. David SR. Neutralization of saxitoxin by antisaxitoxin in rabbit serum. *Toxicon*. 1985;23:669–675.

169. Trieff NM, Spikes JJ, Ray SM, et al. Isolation and purification of *Gymnodinium breve* toxin. In: de Uries A, Kochva E, eds. *Toxins of Animal and Plant Origin*. New York: Gordon & Breach, 1972: 557–577.

170. Baratta RO, Tanner PA Jr. Ichthyosarcotoxism—ciguatera intoxication. *J Fla Med Assoc*. 1970;57:39–42.

171. Bagnis R, Chanteau S, Chungue E, et al. Origins of ciguatera fish poisoning: a new dinoflagellate *Gambierdiscus toxicus* Adachi and Fukuyo definitively identified as the causal agent. *Toxicon*. 1980; 18:199–208.

172. Adochi R, Fukuyo Y. The tecal structure of a marine toxic dinoflagellate *Gambierdiscus toxicus* gen et sp nov collected in ciguateral endemic areas. *Bull Soc Sci Fish*. 1979;45:67–71.

173. Bagnis R, Kuberslu T, Laugter S. Clinical observations on 3009 cases of ciguatera (fish poisoning) in the South Pacific. *Am J Trop Med Hyg*. 1979;28:1067–1073.

174. Bagnis R. Concerning a fatal case of ciguatera poisoning in the Tuamotu Islands (symposium: marine biotoxicology). *Clin Toxicol*. 1970;3:579–583.

175. Banner AH, Shaw S, Alender C, et al. Fish intoxication: notes on ciguatera—its mode of action and suggested therapy. *South Pac Comm Tech Pap. 141.* 1964.
176. Banner AH. Ciguatera fish poisoning: a symposium—ciguatera in the Pacific. *Hawaii Med J.* 1965;24:353–354.
177. Craig CP. It's always the big ones that get away. *JAMA.* 1980;244:272–273.
178. DeSylva DP, Deichmann WB. Toxins in the food chain. *Dev Toxicol Environ Sci.* 1978;4:433–440.
179. Gelb AM, Mildvan D. Ciguatera fish poisoning, *NY State J Med.* 1979;79:1080–1081.
180. Gudger EW. Poisonous fishes and fish poisonings, with special reference to ciguatera in the West Indies. *Am J Trop Med.* 1930;10:43–45.
181. Heimbecker RO. Ciguatera poisoning: snowbirds beware. *CMA J.* 1979;120:637–638.
182. Hokama Y, Banner AH, Boylan DB. A radioimmunoassay for the detection of ciguatera. *Toxicon.* 1977;15:315–325.
183. Jones HR Jr. Acute ataxia associated with ciguatera-type (grouper) tropical fish poisoning.
184. Lawrence DN, Enriquez MB, Lumish RM, et al. Ciguatera fish poisoning in Miami. *JAMA.* 1980;244:254–258.
185. Li KM. Ciguatera fish poisoning: a cholinesterase inhibitor. *Science.* 1965;147:1580–1581.
186. Okihiro MM, Keenan JP, Ivy AC Jr. Ciguatera fish poisoning with cholinesterase: report of a case. *Hawaii Med J.* 1965;24:354–357.
187. Parc F, Ducousso R, Chanteau S, et al. Problems linked to the ciguatera immunological detection. *Toxicon.* 1979;17 (suppl 1):137.
188. Rayner MD. Mode of action of ciguatera. *Fed Proc.* 1972;31:1139–1145.
189. Russell FE. Short communication: ciguatera poisoning—report of 35 cases. *Toxicon.* 1975;13:383–385.
190. Scheuer PJ, Takahashi W, Tsutsumi, et al. Ciguatera: isolation and chemical nature. *Science.* 1967;155:1267–1268.
191. Teravainen H. Myoneural ultrastructure and cholinesterases after tetrodotoxin treatment. *Acta Physiol Scand.* 1970;79:369–372.
192. Hessel DW, Halstead BW, Peckham NH. Marine biotoxins. I. Ciguatera poison: some biological and chemical aspects. *Ann NY Acad Sci.* 1960;90:788.
193. Ciguatera fish poisoning—Bahamas, Miami. *MMWR.* 1982;31:391–392.
194. Emerson DL, Galbraith RM, McMillan JP, Higerd TB. Preliminary immunologic studies of ciguatera poisoning. *Arch Intern Med.* 1983;143:1931–1933.
195. Anderson BS, Sims JK, Wiebenga NH, Sugi M. The epidemiology of ciguatera fish poisoning in Hawaii, 1975–1981. *Hawaii Med J.* 1983;42:326–334.
196. Bidard JN, Vijverberg HPM, Frelin C, et al. Ciguatoxin is a novel type of Na^+ channel toxin. *J Biol Chem.* 1984;259:8353–8357.
197. Palatox NA, Jain LG, Pinano AZ, Gulick TM, Williams RK, Schatz IJ. Successful treatment of ciguatera fish poisoning with intravenous mannitol. *JAMA.* 1988;259:2740–2742.
198. Tachibana K. *Structural Studies on Marine Toxins.* Honolulu, HI: University of Hawaii; 1980. Thesis.
199. Yasumoto T, Bagins R, Vernoux JP. Toxicity of the surgeonfishes. II. Properties of the principal water-soluble toxin. *Bull Jpn Soc Sci Fish.* 1976;42:359–365.
200. Miyahara JT, Akau CK, Yasumoto T. Effects of ciguatoxin and maitotoxin on the isolated guinea pig atria. *Res Commun Chem Pathol Pharmacol.* 1979;25:177–180.
201. Chungue E, Bagnis R. Isolation of two toxins from a parrotfish, *Scarus gibbus. Toxicon.* 1977;15:89–93.
202. Rayner MD, Szekerczes J. Ciguatoxin: effects on the sodium potassium mediated adenosine triphosphatase of human erythrocyte ghosts. *Toxicol Appl Pharmacol.* 1973;24:489–496.
203. Yosumoto J, Inoue A, Bagnis R, Garcon M. *Bull Jpn Soc Sci Fish.* 1979;45:395–399.
204. Bagnis R. Clinical aspects of ciguatera (fish poisoning) in French Polynesia. *Hawaii Med J.* 1968;28:25–28.
205. Gilbert RJ, Jobbs G, Murray CK, et al. Scombrotoxic fish poisoning: feature of the first 50 incidents to be reported in Britain (1976–1979). *Br Med J.* 1980:71–72.
206. Kim R. Flushing syndrome due to Mahimahi (scombroid fish) poisoning. *Arch Dermatol.* 1979;115:963–965.
207. Merson MH, Beane WB, Gangarosa FJ, et al. Scombroid fish poisoning outbreak traced to commercially canned tuna fish. *JAMA.* 1974;228:1268–1269.
208. Taylor SL, Guthertz LS, Leatherwood M, et al. Histamine production by *Klebsiella pneumoniae* and an incident of scombroid poisoning. *Appl Environ Microbiol.* 1979:274–278.
209. Uragoda CG, Kottagoda SR. Adverse reactions to isoniazid on ingestion of fish with a high histamine content. *Tubercle.* 1977;58:83–89.
210. Uragoda CG. Histamine poisoning in tuberculosis patients on ingestion of tropical fish. *J Trop Med Hyg.* 1978;81:243–245.
211. Zimmer L, Altman R, Thun M, et al. Scombroid poisoning—New Jersey. *MMWR.* 1980;29:106–107.
212. Blakesley ML. Scombroid poisoning: prompt resolution of symptoms with cimetidine. *Ann Emerg Med.* 1983;12:104–106.
213. Burklew MA, Morton RA. The toxicity of Florida gulf puffers, genus *Sphoeroides. Toxicon.* 1971;9:205–210.
214. Torda TA, Sinclair E, Ulyatt DB. Puffer fish (tetrodotoxin) poisoning: clinical record and suggested management. *Med J Aust.* 1973;1:599–602.
215. Sims JK, Ostman DC. Pufferfish poisoning: emergency diagnosis and management of mild human tetrodotoxication. *Ann Emerg Med.* 1986;15:1094–1098.
216. Drayton GE. Aquatic skin disorders. In: Auerbach PS, Geehr EC, eds. *Management of Wilderness and Environmental Emergencies.* New York: Macmillan; 1983:260–269.
217. Arnold HL Jr, Grauer FH, Chu GWTC. Seaweed dermatitis apparently caused by marine alga—clinical observations. *Proc Am Acad Sci.* 1959;34:18–19.
218. Sims JK, Zandee Van Rilland. Escharotic stomatitis caused by the "stinging seaweed." *Hawaii Med J.* 1981;40:243–248.
219. Fogg GE, Stewart WDP, Fay P, et al. *The Blue-Green Algae.* New York: Academic Press; 1973.
220. Habekost RC, Fraser IM, Halstead BW. Toxicology—observations on toxic marine algae. *J Wash Acad Sci.* 1955;45:101–103.
221. Solomon AE, Stroughton RB. Dermatitis from purified sea algae toxin (debromoaplysiatoxin). *Arch Dermatol.* 1979;114:1333–1335.
222. Banner AH. A dermatitis-producing alga in Hawaii: preliminary report. *Hawaii Med J.* 1959;19:33–36.
223. Cardellina JH II, Marner JF, Moore RJ. Seaweed dermatitis: structure of lyngbyatoxin A. *Science.* 1979;204:193–195.
224. Aronson JD. Spontaneous tuberculosis in salt water fish. *J Infect Dis.* 1926;39:315–320.

46. Hazardous Materials

BRENT T. BURTON, MD

In December 1984 the accidental release of more than 25 tons of a toxic gas in Bhopal, India, resulted in the worst chemical disaster in history. This accident caused the deaths of more than 2000 victims and the injury of thousands more. The eventual economic impact from this accident will likely run into hundreds of millions of dollars.[1] The social impact is incalculable. The tragedy of the Bhopal accident profoundly illustrates the potential danger of hazardous substances that are produced, transported, used, and stored near populated areas. Bhopal points out the need to ensure the enforcement of safety standards to prevent such an incident and also to be prepared for the potential mass casualties that may be involved in a large-scale chemical disaster.

There have been ten nuclear accidents in the past quarter century. In April 1986, the worst occurred in a nuclear reactor in Chernobyl, in the Ukraine. Causing untold numbers of deaths and injuries, the meltdown and release of radioactive gases contaminated water and food supplies and sent radioactive clouds into the atmosphere across surrounding continents.

Hazardous materials comprise a vast array of chemicals used in industry for the manufacture of many products. Many chemicals that are utilized in treating diseases, producing energy, or increasing crop yields may have a hazardous potential when improperly used or stored. When they must be transported there is a risk that an accident may result in a spill of toxic substances. There are an average of more than 10,000 hazardous material spills reported to the United States Department of Transportation each year. Highway accidents account for 90% of spills, 8% are on railways, 1% on aircraft, and 1% on waterways. National statistics for industrial spills of hazardous materials are not available, although the total number is probably larger than transportation spills.[2]

Hazardous materials may be defined as substances that are in a quantity and form that may pose an unreasonable risk to health and safety or property when produced, used, stored, or transported for commercial purposes. Military material may also consist of hazardous chemical, radioactive, and biological substances that are produced, transported, and stockpiled for use as weapons. An additional hazard may occur from toxic products of combustion generated from common materials in daily use such as fabrics, plastics, and wood.

There are currently over 60,000 chemical substances in commercial use that are considered potentially hazardous and are regulated by the US Environmental Protection Agency (EPA). Almost 1000 new chemicals are introduced each year of which about 80% do not have adequate toxicity data.[3] Specific toxicity data may not be known concerning some chemicals until they have been used and widely dispersed for decades. An example of this is represented by polychlorinated biphenyls (PCBs), agents that were commonly employed in the production of electrical transformers. These substances were in widespread use for about 30 years until it was learned that they were toxic and were removed from production.

LEGISLATION

The earliest hazardous materials regulations were made by the Association of American Railroads Bureau of Explosives shortly after the Civil War to provide some safety standards for the increasing use of rail transportation of poorly identified and inadequately packaged explosives and ammunition. The federal government began to play a role in producing regulations directed towards protecting human health and safety related to hazardous materials transportation with the development of the Interstate Commerce Commission (ICC) in 1887. In 1908 the ICC was given the responsibility of enforcing the Explosives and Other Dangerous Articles Act. These initial regulations were enacted primarily for rail transport but later evolved to include flammable substances, compressed gases, and other materials transported by rail, highway, water, and air.

The recognition of the possible danger of chemical hazards in our industrialized society resulted in a plethora of legislation in the 1970s aimed at bringing about the formation of several government agencies to control pollution and make the workplace safer. These agencies include the EPA to protect the environment from chemical hazards, the Occupational Safety and Health Administration (OSHA) to set and enforce health and safety standards including safe limits for chemical exposures in the workplace, the National Institute for Occupational Safety and Health (NIOSH) to research information about work-related injuries and illnesses and to recommend standards, and the Consumer Products Safety Commission (CPSC) to protect the health and safety of the general consumer.

Table 46-1 Hazardous Materials Legislation

Legislation	Year
Federal Food, Drug and Cosmetic Act	1938
Federal Insecticide, Fungicide and Rodenticide Act	1947
Atomic Energy Act	1954
Federal Hazardous Substances Act	1960
Coal Mine Health and Safety Act	1969
Hazardous Materials Transportation Control Act	1970
Federal Railroad Safety Act	1970
Poison Prevention Packaging Act	1970
Clear Air Act	1970
Occupational Safety and Health Act	1970
Lead-Based Paint Poisoning Prevention Act	1971
Marine Protection, Research and Sanctuaries Act	1972
Ports and Waterways Safety Act	1972
Federal Water Pollution Control Act	1972
Safe Drinking Water Act	1974
Toxic Substances Control Act	1976
Resources Conservation and Recovery Act	1976
Uranium Mill Tailings Radiation Control Act	1978
Comprehensive Environmental Response, Compensation and Liability Act	1980
Superfund Amendments and Reauthorization Act	1986

Regulation of hazardous material transport was brought under control of the Department of Transportation (DOT) in 1970 by the Hazardous Materials Transportation Control Act, which provides regulation of the quantity and packaging requirements of hazardous materials.

One of the most important pieces of legislation involving regulation of hazardous materials was the Toxic Substances Control Act (TSCA) of 1976. This act gives the EPA the authority to regulate chemicals that present unreasonable risk to health or the environment. Regulatory authority by the EPA includes toxicologic screening of new chemicals before they are introduced into the market and in some cases the power to hold new chemicals off the market if necessary. Implementation of the TSCA by the EPA requires coordination and consistency among government agencies, a need that led to the formation of the Interagency Regulatory Liaison Group providing a link between EPA, OSHA, CPSC, FDA, and the Food Safety and Quality Service.

Federal OSHA Hazard Communication Regulations[4] instituted in November 1985 represent recent legislation regulating hazardous materials. These regulations require chemical manufacturers, employers, importers, and distributors of hazardous materials to provide information to their employees about the hazardous chemicals to which they may be exposed. A hazard communication program consists of information that is available to the employee in the form of labels, material safety data sheets, instruction, and training. This information must provide the employee with the specific names and sources of chemicals, physical and health hazards, safety precautions for handling, route of entry, and emergency first aid.

Substantial new hazardous material emergency planning requirements were introduced upon the passage of Title III of the Superfund Amendments and Reauthorization Act of 1986 (SARA), also known as the Emergency Planning and Community Right-To-Know Act of 1986. The governor of each state must appoint a state emergency response commission with responsibilities for designating emergency planning districts, establishing and supervising local emergency planning committees, reviewing emergency plans, receiving chemical release notifications, and establishing procedures for receiving and processing public requests for information regarding chemical hazards. Title III implementation, as intended, will promote increased preparedness for hazardous material emergencies and will increase public involvement and awareness in the planning process.

Other important legislation relevant to hazardous materials is listed in Table 46-1.

LABELING REQUIREMENTS

The shipper of hazardous materials is responsible for compliance with shipping regulations of the DOT. International shipments must comply with labeling requirements of the importing country and the rules of the International Air Transport Association. The DOT is responsible for regulation of all hazardous material shipments by rail, highway, water, and air according to the Code of Federal Regulations 49,[5] which specifies shipping container requirements and information that must be displayed on a label or placard. Labels are required on all containers of designated hazardous materials that are shipped. They must be in conformance with DOT requirements mandating that specific labels, in the shape of a diamond, be displayed. The diamond-shaped labels and placards are color coded and contain a symbol in the upper corner representing a specific hazard class and a number in the bottom corner representing the UN hazard class (Fig. 46-1). Vehicle placards are similar to labels, but in addition to the information contained in the label, placards

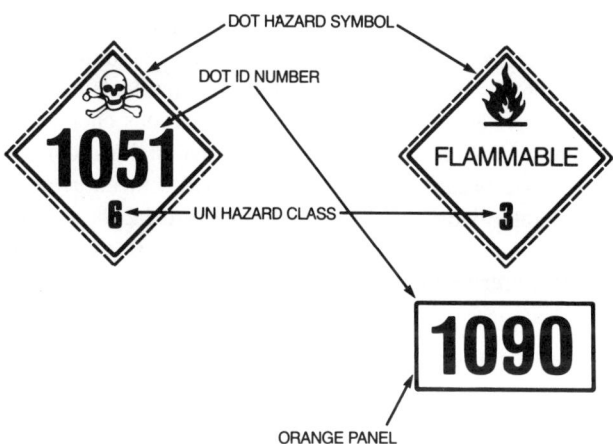

Figure 46-2 Vehicle placards.

contain a four-digit code within the diamond or on an adjacent orange panel (Fig. 46-2) that corresponds to a specific chemical agent referenced in the DOT *Emergency Response Guidebook*.[6] This code system allows for rapid identification of the material in the event of a transportation accident.

A placarding system for buildings that contain hazardous materials has been developed by the National Fire Protection Association (NFPA) for use at facilities where hazardous materials are stored or used. This labeling system utilizes a four-square diamond (Fig. 46-3) that displays numerical codes according to the degree of hazard. A rating scale from 0 (no hazard) to 4 (extremely hazardous) in the categories of health (blue), fire (red), and reactivity (yellow) is displayed in the upper three squares. The lower white square may specify a hazard class or display a "W" to indicate that water extinguishers are incompatible. In the event of a fire or other emergency situation, these placards can be readily seen by firefighters before the building is entered and appropriate protective measures can be instituted.

Some private companies that use or store hazardous materials are incorporating the NFPA symbols and code system into the form of chemical safety data books and hazardous materials safety data sheets that contain emergency information in the event of a hazardous material accident.

Except for DOT regulations on labels and placards for hazardous materials in transit, there is no conformity with

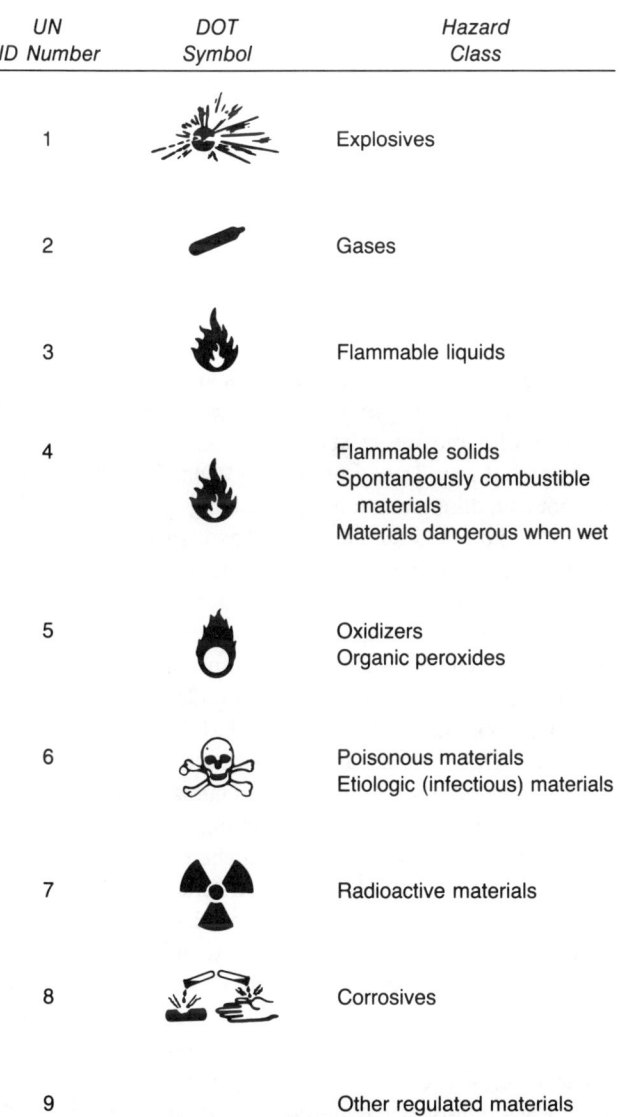

Figure 46-1 Hazard classification system. *Source:* Adapted from *1984 Emergency Response Guidebook*, US Dept of Transportation, publication No P5800.3, 1984.

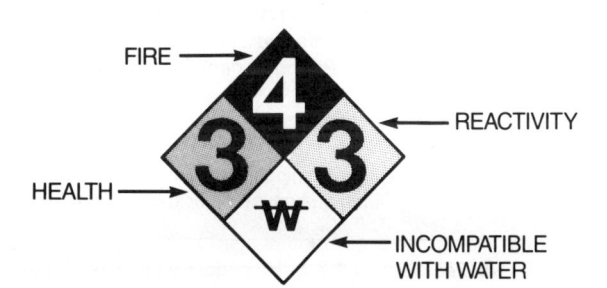

Figure 46-3 NFPA placard.

respect to labels for hazardous materials that are stored or used at the work site. The OSHA Hazard Communication Regulations specify elements that must be implemented in a labeling system for all containers of hazardous chemicals. The label must indicate identity of the material and contain appropriate hazard warnings. This provides manufacturers considerable latitude in formulating hazard labels and the result is a lack of uniformity of labeling practice from one manufacturer to another.

HAZARDOUS MATERIALS RESPONSE SYSTEM

Growing public concern over the escalating number of hazardous materials incidents has led to the development of hazardous materials response (HAZMAT) units consisting of specially trained personnel within fire departments. Hazardous material response specialists, some of whom are trained as paramedics, receive specific training in chemistry, physics, and toxicology in addition to techniques of fire suppression and the use of special equipment applicable to a hazardous material accident.[7]

An effective hazardous materials response unit consists of designated team members assigned specific roles (Table 46-2) and a specially equipped vehicle to respond to a chemical incident. Such a vehicle is equipped with communication equipment including radios to allow communication between team members and the command center at the scene and to provide access to police and fire units. Remote telephone communication at the scene is important for communication with the chemical manufacturer, a poison control center, the Chemical Transportation Emergency Center (CHEMTREC), area hospitals, and other agencies that may require notification or consultation (Table 46-3).

Specialized Equipment

Specialized equipment for detection of toxic substances, personal protection, and material containment and control are needed for a HAZMAT unit. An atmosphere sampling device can be utilized to detect the presence and concentration of up to 62 types of toxic gases in cases of an unknown spill or toxic products of combustion. Special meters are available to assess air-gas mixtures for the potential of explosion. Other specialized equipment includes an infrared detector, smoke bombs to determine wind speed and direction, dye tablets for leak detection, and radiation detection devices. Nonsparking tools are required for entry when the potential of explosion exists.

Control of a spill requires an assortment of plugs, sealing compounds, diking material, neutralizing agents, absorptive agents, and fire retardant foams and extinguishers. For treatment of victims of a hazardous material incident HAZMAT units carry medical equipment necessary for resuscitation, including airway equipment and oxygen, and appropriate antidotes for chemical exposures to specific toxins such as organophosphate insecticides and cyanide.

Full protective clothing is required for HAZMAT responders. This includes appropriate protective gear to prevent inhalation, ingestion, or skin contact with hazardous materials in the form of vapor, liquid, or solid. The usual firefighters' "turnout" clothing will not provide adequate protection against many hazardous materials. Full protective gear when responding to possible toxic hazardous materials incidents includes helmet, gloves, coat, and rubber boots. In some cases an atmosphere-isolating or acid-proof suit may be required for protection. A self-contained breathing apparatus utilizing the nondemand mode should be worn in all instances until it can be determined that the atmosphere is safe. Cartridge-type respirators, gas masks, and demand-type self-contained breathing apparatuses are not safe substitutes and should not be used by HAZMAT responders.[6]

Table 46-2 HAZMAT Team Member Roles

Team leader	Designate team member responsibilities
	Control HAZMAT team at scene
	Act as liaison with fire commander
	Establish entry route
	Determine proper protective gear
Police liaison	Act as liaison with police commander
	Recommend appropriate perimeters
	Perform as member of backup team
	File appropriate reports
Resource Center team member	Notify appropriate officials
	Research hazardous material
	Educate other personnel
	Record all communications
	File appropriate reports
	Monitor and respond to communications
Public information officer	Gather necessary information
	Designate media staging area
	Act as liaison with media
Paramedic	Monitor all team members
	Act as liaison with emergency medical personnel
	Treat victims as necessary
	Recommend decontamination measures
	Notify paramedic physician advisor
	Notify Poison Control Center
Entry team	Contain hazardous material
	Identify materials
	Retrieve shipping papers
	Determine cause of incident

Source: Adapted from Yoder E: Hazardous materials response system. *Top Emerg Med* 7 (1): 1–8, 1985.

Table 46-3 Organizations and Agencies That May Require Notification or Involvement in a Hazardous Material Accident

Local

Police Department
Fire Department
Poison Control Center
Hospital Emergency Departments
Public Utility Commission

State

Police Department (Highway Patrol)
Department of Transportation
Fire Marshal
State OSHA
National Guard
Department of Fish and Wildlife
Department of Energy
Department of Health
Department of Environmental Quality
Office of Emergency Management
Red Cross

Federal

Environmental Protection Agency
National Transportation Safety Board
National Institute of Occupational Safety and Health
Occupational Safety and Health Administration
US Coast Guard
Federal Aviation Agency
US Department of Energy
Federal Emergency Management Agency

Other

CHEMTREC
Chemical Manufacturer and Shipper
Chemical Cleanup Companies

Source: Adapted from Yoder E: Hazardous materials response system. *Top Emerg Med* 7 (1):1–8, 1985.

Prevention

Successful control of hazardous material accidents lies in prevention. A thorough hazard analysis of storage sites, major carriers, and transportation routes during the fire department's yearly fire inspections will identify the amounts and types of materials and compliance with safety and labeling requirements. When this information is incorporated into a computer database, the HAZMAT responder can quickly determine the types of chemicals stored on site in the event of an emergency. Proper placement of NFPA building placards will ensure that in the event of a fire or other incident emergency responders will be able to identify the danger before entering the building. Local transportation routes should be evaluated for accident potential and traffic carrying hazardous materials should be restricted or prohibited from certain dangerous areas such as tunnels. Building diagrams and the location of hazardous materials should be kept on file and contingency plans developed in the event of a fire or hazardous materials incident. Disaster drills that incorporate a hazardous material spill will provide the opportunity to rehearse and critique the community disaster response to such an incident.

Levels of Response

The level of a hazardous material response depends upon the severity of the spill. A level I response occurs when a small amount of a material must be controlled or disposed of and does not present a significant risk. This level of response is also utilized for evaluation of a potentially hazardous situation and is handled by one or two HAZMAT team members. When greater danger exists because of a more toxic substance or larger spill, a level II response occurs. The entire HAZMAT team responds along with local fire and police support. A level II response implies that the materials can be controlled and confined until cleanup occurs. When the materials cannot be contained or the spill presents a significant risk of exposure to toxic substances, a level III response occurs. This results in the commitment of the greatest amount of resources, including the fire department, police, the entire HAZMAT team, and other appropriate personnel.

The highest priority following a hazardous material spill is the protection of human life and safety. The area of the incident should be approached from upwind to protect the responders from exposure to toxic gases. When the first responders arrive at the scene, a dual perimeter is established by securing an inner hot zone surrounded by a decontamination and treatment zone. Only fully protected personnel are allowed inside the inner hot zone. Victims are immediately located outside the danger zone into specific decontamination and treatment areas. Only immediate life-saving treatment is performed within the danger zone (ie, critical airway management). The dimensions of the danger zone will be determined by the properties and toxicity of the substance and also such factors as wind speed and direction and the layout and geography of the scene. Evacuation recommendations, including minimum distances, based on specific substances have been recommended by the DOT. Substances that necessitate immediate evacuation of the surrounding area and corresponding DOT ID Codes are listed in Table 46-4. Evacuation distances of up to 5 miles are recommended depending on the magnitude of the spill and substance. It should not be assumed, however, that if a substance is not listed in this table evacuation is not necessary. Large amounts of less toxic substances may produce an equally large hazard. For example, the toxic gas methyl

Table 46-4 Hazardous Materials Requiring Immediate Evacuation

Substance	DOT ID No	Substance	DOT ID No
Acrolein	1092	Methylamine	1061
Acrylonitrile	1093	Methyl bromide	1062
Ammonia	1005	Methyl chloride	1063
Ammonia solution >44%	2073	Methyl mercaptan	1064
		Methyl sulfate	1595
Boron trifluoride	1008	Nitric acid	2032
Bromine	1744	Nitric oxide	1660
Carbon sulfides	1131	Nitric oxide & nitrogen tetroxide mixture	1975
Chloride of phosphorus	1809		
Chlorine	1017		
Dimethylamine	1032	Nitrogen oxides	1067
Dimethyl sulfate	1595	Perchloromethyl-mercaptan	1670
Epichlorohydrin	2023		
Ethylene imine	1185	Phosgene	1076
Ethylene oxide	1040	Phosphorus trichloride	1809
Fluorine	9192		
Hydrochloric acid	1050	Sulfur dioxide	1079
		Sulfuric acid	1831
Hydrogen chloride	2186	Sulfuric anhydride	1829
Hydrocyanic acid	1051	Sulfur trioxide	1829
		Titanium tetrachloride	1838
Hydrogen sulfide	1053		
Hydrogen fluoride	1052	Trimethylamine	1083

Source: *1984 Emergency Response Guidebook,* US Dept of Transportation, publication No P5800.3, 1983.

isocyanate responsible for the tragedy in Bhopal is not listed in this table.

Judgment regarding the amount of material involved, concentration, physical state, and environmental factors such as terrain and weather conditions should guide decision making with respect to the extent of evacuation. Further technical assistance may be obtained for on-the-scene management from the Chemical Transportation Emergency Center (CHEMTREC; 800-424-9300). Operation of CHEMTREC as an emergency information service is provided as a public service by the Chemical Manufacturers Association. CHEMTREC will provide advice for emergency responders at the scene and will contact the chemical company for further technical advice. The regional Poison Control Center should be contacted by hazardous material responders whenever a significant toxic spill occurs. The Poison Control Center can provide rapid access of toxicological information, including possible acute health effects, decontamination procedures, and treatment recommendations. The Poison Control Center is an excellent resource for notification and coordination of necessary public agencies and hospital emergency departments of incoming patients and potential associated medical problems.[8]

A command post is set up outside the danger zone where representatives of fire, police, and medical personnel coordinate activities under the direction of the incident commander, who is usually the fire chief or senior fire officer.

A specific decontamination zone is designated outside the danger zone where initial medical evaluation and treatment may be performed. Patients should be treated only by adequately protected personnel until the material has been identified and appropriate consultation with a Poison Control Center or other medical authority has been obtained. In the absence of appropriate precautions the health care provider may become contaminated and also require medical care. When multiple victims are involved in a chemical accident it may be necessary to activate the community disaster plan.

As soon as possible the material should be identified by locating the four-digit ID number on the vehicle placard or orange panel that is referenced in the *Emergency Response Guidebook.*[6] Identification should be verified if possible by locating the chemical name on the vehicle's shipping papers. Shipping papers are required on all vehicles transporting hazardous materials, but they may also list other nonhazardous items contained in the shipment. Hazardous materials will be entered on the shipping papers as the first items listed and identified by an "X" in the left column, captioned "HM," or highlighted in a contrasting color. Hazardous material names are followed by a hazard classification (ie, flammable liquid). The letters UN or NA and the DOT four-digit ID code are printed immediately following the chemical name. Shipping papers also include the name, address, and telephone number of the shipper who may be contacted for identification of the material.

In cases of unknown materials or those illegally dumped, a field identification hazardous material protocol (HAZCAT) has been developed for identification based on physical and chemical properties.[9] Until the identity of the material has been determined utilizing testing devices or HAZCAT, the material should be considered dangerous and appropriate safeguards taken.

Transportation regulations do not require vehicle placards for shipments of less than 1000 pounds of many classes of hazardous materials. Therefore, the absence of a vehicle placard does not guarantee that a hazardous material is not present. Also, a vehicle bearing an "EMPTY" placard may still contain dangerous residues of toxic substances and therefore should be approached with caution.

DECONTAMINATION

When indicated, decontamination of victims should occur at the scene in a designated area as soon as possible to reduce exposure to the patient. Substances such as corrosives (acids and alkalis), oxidizers, organophosphates, phenols, halogenated hydrocarbons, organic solvents, and cyanide salts, in addition to other dermally absorbable chemicals, have the highest potential of risk to health care providers if they are not effectively decontaminated. Exposures to toxic gases are unlikely to result in a significant risk of gross contamination. When accomplished at the scene decontamination will confine the area of contamination and greatly reduce the chance of cross-contamination and spread of toxic materials to ambulance personnel, transporting vehicles and equipment, hospital personnel, and treatment rooms. In some cases, health care providers may be severely and permanently injured if proper decontamination has not occurred or proper protective clothing is not utilized.[10] Therefore, the importance of recognizing the need for decontamination and use of proper personal protection must be stressed. Many hospitals are not equipped to perform chemical or radioactive substance decontamination in the emergency department.

The most clearly outlined decontamination procedures have been established for radioactive materials. However, the same principles apply for other nonradioactive hazardous materials. The approach to decontamination should include the following measures:

- Clearly identify the decontamination area. Ideally, it should be separated from the medical treatment area. Only authorized treatment personnel are allowed entry. The number of persons entering the decontamination area should be kept to a minimum.
- Personnel entering the decontamination area are considered contaminated and must leave protective clothing, equipment, etc, in the area before leaving.
- All personnel providing care must wear appropriate protective clothing. A minimum of gown, mask, rubber gloves, and plastic goggles is required. Leather boots and gloves should not be worn for protection because leather absorbs pesticides and other chemicals, and cannot be decontaminated.
- All clothing, shoes, and other items should be removed from the patient, identified, placed in a plastic bag, and should remain in the area until properly discarded or decontaminated. Gowns, towels, and other items used by the patient should also be considered contaminated and not returned for laundering until proven safe to do so.
- Decontamination for some agents such as toxic gases may require simply removing the patient from the source of exposure. Chemicals that are liquid or solid with systemic or dermal toxicity will require aggressive cleansing. Irrigation with plain water will remove 50% to 75% of most contaminants with a single washing.[11] Repeated washings with soap and water will further reduce contamination in some cases to less than 1%.[12] All exposed areas of the patient's body should be washed thoroughly with soap and cool water and rinsed thoroughly. Water temperature may be gradually increased as the washing process continues. Initial use of cool water avoids opening of the skin pores and reduces dermal absorption of the chemical. Waste water used for decontamination should be considered contaminated and should not be discharged into the sewer system without appropriate authorization.
- Wounds should be irrigated copiously with sterile isotonic saline. Some radioactive substances may require irrigation with chelating agents.[13] If radioactive substances are contaminated in a wound the surrounding skin should be covered to prevent spread of radioactivity to other body areas. In some cases surgical debridement may be necessary to remove residual material from the wound.
- Eye exposures should be treated immediately by irrigating the exposed eye with running water for at least 15 minutes.
- Because the effects of a chemical exposure may be delayed, victims should be observed several hours following decontamination for the development of symptoms.

HOSPITAL CARE

Because there are literally thousands of potential chemicals that may be involved in a hazardous material incident it is not possible or reasonable to list each individual chemical and its medical effects and treatment. However, many chemical substances share similar properties and will present with similar medical effects. In all cases, supportive care is the most important aspect of treatment regardless of the specific toxin. Injuries due to hazardous materials will usually occur from exposure to the skin or lungs, resulting in local dermal or pulmonary damage. Absorption from the skin or lungs may result in systemic toxicity involving one or more additional organ systems depending on the type of material (Table 46-5).

Dermal Injury

Liquid and solid materials classified as oxidizers, organic peroxides and corrosives are the most likely to cause dermal and mucosal burns upon direct contact. When ignited, flammable or explosive materials may produce burns in addition to traumatic blast injuries and respiratory injury. Some gases and vapors released in a spill may cause burns to the skin and mucosal surfaces when the concentrations are high. Hydrocarbons may cause skin irritation and occasionally burns because of the defatting nature of the substance. The mechanism that produces a chemical burn is different from that of a thermal burn but the result is similar in character. The most important concern in chemical burn treatment is irrigation of the burn area with copious amounts of water to remove the

Table 46-5 Examples of Common Hazardous Materials Causing Local and/or Systemic Injury

Injury	Material
Local Toxicity	
Dermal/Mucosal	acids
	alkalis
	hydrocarbons
Pulmonary	acid vapors (HCl, HF)
	ammonia
	chloropicrin
	chlorine
	formaldehyde
	hydrocarbons
	nitrogen oxides
	phosgene
	phosphine
	ozone
	sulfur oxides
Systemic Toxicity	
Dermal Absorption	hydrocarbons
	ketones
	organophosphates
	phenols
Pulmonary Absorption	alcohols
	carbon monoxide
	cyanide, acrylonitrile
	hydrogen sulfide
	ketones
	nitrates
	organometallic compounds
	volatile hydrocarbons

Source: Adapted from Wanke LA: Toxic chemical spills. *Top Emerg Med* 7 (5): 15, 1985.

material as soon as possible. Ocular exposures should be treated by irrigating the affected eye for at least 15 minutes with 1 L or more of isotonic saline. Injuries to the eye should be further evaluated with fluorescein and a slit lamp examination and treated with antibiotic ointment and patching when a superficial corneal burn is present. Severe burns require ophthalmologic consultation. Application of acids or bases to a chemical burn in an attempt to neutralize the corrosive substance should not be done, as this practice will increase the exothermic reaction and exacerbate the burn. Following adequate irrigation, chemical burns should receive standard burn therapy, including debridement, antibiotic therapy, sterile dressings, and close follow-up as necessary.

An important exception to standard burn therapy exists for exposures to hydrofluoric acid, a corrosive agent widely used in industry. Exposures to concentrations greater than 50% will cause immediate pain and burning with erythema.[14] Less concentrated solutions may produce delayed symptoms up to 24 hours.[15] Prolonged tissue destruction occurs because the free fluoride ion remains active at the burn site causing continued injury. If the burn area demonstrates evidence of immediate tissue damage or remains painful following irrigation, or if pain develops during the following 24 hours, administration of calcium gluconate is indicated. The burn area should be injected subcutaneously with a 10% calcium gluconate solution using a 30-gauge needle infiltrating 0.5 mL per square centimeter of burn area.[16] For less severe burns a 2.5% calcium gluconate gel may be applied to the burn area instead of subcutaneous infiltration. If the gel is not available it may be prepared by mixing 3.5 g of USP calcium gluconate with 150 g of water-soluble surgical lubricant (eg, K-Y Jelly). After the burn area has been irrigated the gel should be massaged into the wound. The wound may then be covered with a dressing applied to keep the gel in contact with the wound.[17]

Pulmonary Injury

Gases and vapors from liquid materials and aerosolized solid particles may cause pulmonary injury by chemical destruction or irritation of lung tissue. The large surface area of the lungs also provides a route of absorption for chemicals that may have systemic effects (see below). Some gases such as methane, nitrogen, or carbon dioxide do not have irritant properties but may cause asphyxiation when a concentrated exposure results in decreased inspired oxygen tension.

Gases and vapors with primarily irritative effects comprise a diverse group of chemicals that may produce different types of reactions but manifest similar injuries. All respiratory irritants produce inflammation of the mucous membranes and pulmonary tissue. Highly water soluble gases such as chlorine, ammonia, hydrogen chloride, and hydrogen fluoride primarily cause injury of the upper airway. Gases with low water solubility such as phosgene or oxides of nitrogen produce less severe immediate symptoms but may produce a severe, often delayed, pneumonitis because of deeper penetration to the smaller airways and alveoli.

Tear gas agents are pulmonary irritants that are used specifically for their noxious effects in warfare, crowd control, and personal protection. Chloropicrin (CNS) and chloroacetophinone (CN) are the most commonly used agents. The noxious effects of CNS also serve as a method of warning the user when it is added to a toxic, odorless gas such as methyl bromide. The effects of exposure to tear gas agents are usually self-limited but severe exposures may require treatment.

Exposure to respiratory irritants results in symptoms of coughing, choking, burning of the eyes, throat, and lungs, chest pain, headache, nausea, and vomiting. Upper airway obstruction requiring emergency cricothyroidotomy may occur from edema or laryngospasm in the case of severe exposures to water-soluble respiratory irritants. Hemoptysis, bronchospasm, or pulmonary edema may occur from a high dose of an irritant gas.

Physical exam findings include conjunctival inflammation, tearing, and nasal discharge. Respiratory distress and tachypnea, choking, and stridor may indicate impending upper airway obstruction. Breath sounds may be diminished or accompanied by wheezing, rales, or rhonchi. Laboratory data may initially be normal. In symptomatic patients an arterial blood gas, chest roentgenogram, ECG, and spirometry may be helpful as a baseline study and to document pulmonary injury and adequacy of oxygenation. A chest roentgenogram may demonstrate infiltrates or pulmonary edema but may initially be normal. A carboxyhemoglobin level should be obtained in all patients with a history of a significant exposure to methylene chloride or products of combustion.

Treatment for exposure to respiratory irritants is primarily supportive. Symptomatic patients should receive supplemental oxygen pending arterial blood gas results. Respiratory support including endotracheal intubation and artificial ventilation with the use of positive-end expiratory pressure may be required. Patients with evidence of bronchospasm should receive treatment with bronchodilators. Corticosteroids may be administered but are not of proven value under these circumstances.

Systemic Toxins

Chemical substances that are involved in a hazardous material accident or released as a toxic product of combustion may be absorbed through the skin or lungs and produce systemic toxicity. Toxicity may be immediate or delayed with effects upon one or more organ systems. Chemical toxicity from several systemic toxins requires early recognition and specific treatment in addition to the usual supportive measures (see also Chapter 47, Occupational Toxicologic Emergencies).

Cyanide

An extremely toxic substance, cyanide is widely used in industry for many purposes, including extraction of gold from ore, metal plating, fumigants, pesticides, and various chemical processes. Cyanide is released as a toxic product of combustion in half of air samples in fires involving combustion of synthetic materials such as polyurethanes.[18] The related compound acrylonitrile, also used in industry, shares the same toxic properties of cyanide.

Depending on the physical state, cyanide is absorbed by dermal, pulmonary, and oral routes. Early symptoms of exposure may include headache, nausea and vomiting, coughing, giddiness, and dyspnea followed by unconsciousness, convulsions, cardiac arrest, and death.

The diagnosis of cyanide toxicity must be based on historical information and physical and laboratory findings. A history of exposure at the workplace, laboratory, the scene of a fire or a hazardous material accident should suggest the possibility of cyanide toxicity. The classic odor of bitter almonds should not be relied upon since less than half the population is able to detect its presence.[19] There is no specific laboratory test that will provide a rapid and definitive diagnosis. Blood cyanide levels are available in some laboratories but have limited utility for initial treatment decisions because of the prolonged processing time required. Severely intoxicated patients will have a profound metabolic acidosis. Arterial and venous blood gas samples will have similar oxygen content as a result of inhibition of mitochondrial oxidation. Arterial blood gas analysis will demonstrate normal Po_2 and calculated oxygen saturation, but measured oxygen saturation will be reduced as a result of cyanide binding to hemoglobin and displacing oxygen.

Treatment must begin immediately by removing the victim from the source of exposure. In the event of cardiac arrest, cardiopulmonary resuscitation should be performed according to ACLS standards. HAZMAT units should be supplied with cyanide antidote kits (Lilly), which should be administered without delay in cases of known cyanide poisoning. Two ampules of amyl nitrite should be administered every 5 minutes by placing them under a face mask if the patient is spontaneously ventilating or in an ambu bag for positive pressure ventilation. Sodium nitrite and sodium thiosulfate contained in the cyanide kit should then be infused intravenously. Administration of nitrites produces methemoglobin, which competes with cytochrome oxidase for cyanide, allowing restoration of enzyme activity. Sodium thiosulfate converts cyanide to the less toxic sodium thiocyanate.

The cyanide kit should be reserved only for the symptomatic patient and its use should be carefully considered in a case of combined carbon monoxide and cyanide toxicity because induction of methemoglobinemia will further compromise an already diminished oxygen carrying capacity.

Significant toxicity with cyanide will require treatment with intravenous (IV) sodium bicarbonate based on arterial blood gas results. Blood pH monitoring should be done carefully during treatment because of the extreme and often refractory acidosis that occurs with cyanide toxicity.

Treatment with cobalt EDTA and hydroxycobalamin are alternate antidotes for cyanide toxicity but are not currently available in the United States.

Hyperbaric oxygenation has been recommended for use in cyanide poisoning and may be of particular value when carbon monoxide poisoning has occurred concomitantly.[20,21]

Hydrogen Sulfide

Hydrogen sulfide is generated during industrial processing of animal and vegetable matter and in breweries, smelters, sewer sludge, and mining operations. Hydrogen sulfide may also be generated during a fire involving sulfur or sulfur-containing substances. Hydrogen sulfide has a characteristic odor of rotten eggs, but the odor rapidly diminishes with continued exposure as a result of olfactory extinction, a characteristic that may lead the victim, or even the rescuer, to wrongfully believe that the danger no longer exists. The toxicity of hydrogen sulfide is similar to that of cyanide: headache, mucosal irritation, and dyspnea, with progression to cardiac arrest and death. Treatment consists of removing the victim from the source, administration of oxygen, and respiratory support. Administration of amyl nitrite ampules and IV sodium nitrite from the cyanide antidote kit (Lilly) to induce methemoglobinemia will form sulfmethemoglobin, a less toxic substance that can be excreted. Sodium thiosulfate is not given in cases of hydrogen sulfide poisoning.[16]

Carbon Monoxide

Typically, carbon monoxide (CO) poisoning occurs in cases of smoke inhalation. However, poisoning by carbon monoxide may also occur from exposure to methylene chloride, a substance in widespread use as a paint stripper and degreasing agent. Methylene chloride is absorbed by inhalation or dermal exposure and is metabolized to CO.

Early symptoms of carbon monoxide poisoning may include dizziness, headache, dyspnea, cough, chest pain, nausea, and vomiting. At higher levels, confusion, seizures, coma, and cardiac dysrhythmias may occur. Physical examination findings are nonspecific with tachypnea and tachycardia occurring most commonly. The classic "cherry red" skin color is very rare. Retinal hemorrhages may be noted. Neurologic findings usually consist of mental status changes due to brain hypoxia. Arterial blood gas management will often demonstrate a profound metabolic acidosis with a normal Po_2 unless pulmonary oxygen exchange has been damaged as a result of other inhaled toxins. Measured arterial oxygen saturation will be low, although the calculated value will remain normal. A carboxyhemoglobin level should be obtained if any symptoms are present, but frequently this level does not correlate with the severity of the poisoning and should not be used as the sole indicator for therapy decisions.[22]

Treatment for exposure to CO or methylene chloride consists of removal of the victim from the source of exposure, maintenance of the airway, and ventilation with administration of 100% oxygen. The physiologic result of CO poisoning is a functional hypoxemia due to preferential binding of CO to hemoglobin. Administration of 100% oxygen by a nonrebreathing mask will increase oxygen delivery to tissues and reduce the half-life of hemoglobin-bound carbon monoxide from approximately 4 hours to 30 minutes.[23]

If a patient is severely intoxicated with CO and is comatose, has neurological symptoms, myocardial ischemia, or a significant metabolic acidosis, or fails to improve during therapy, hyperbaric oxygen treatment is indicated regardless of the time since exposure[16] (see Chapter 44, Hyperbaric Emergencies).

Halogenated Hydrocarbons and Organic Solvents

Halogenated hydrocarbons and organic solvents are compounds that comprise a large group of substances in common use in industry as cleaning agents, paints, degreasers, and in the production of other compounds (Table 46-6). Hydrocarbons are also the most likely substances to be involved in a transportation accident. Toxicity occurs through inhalation or dermal contact. When these substances are absorbed, acute systemic effects result in primarily CNS and peripheral nervous system toxicity. Depending on the specific toxin, amount, and duration of exposure, acute symptoms may range from fatigue, lethargy and narcosis, headache, numbness, paresthesias, and weakness to unconsciousness and death. Other organ systems affected include the heart, lungs, liver, kidneys, bone marrow, and skin. Acute exposures to these agents should be treated supportively by

Table 46-6 Halogenated Hydrocarbons and Organic Solvents

Aliphatic Hydrocarbons
  butadiene
  cyclohexane
  cyclopropane
  gasoline
  n-hexane
  kerosene
  mineral spirits
  naphtha
  2-nitropropane
  Stoddard's solvent

Aromatic Hydrocarbons
  benzene
  toluene
  xylene
  styrene

Halogenated Hydrocarbons
  carbon tetrachloride
  chlordane
  chloroform
  chlorobromomethane
  ethyl bromide
  ethyl chloride
  heptachlor
  lindane
  methyl bromide
  methyl chloride
  methylene chloride
  dichloroethylene
  trichloroethylene
  tribromoethane
  tetrachloroethylene
  ethylene dichloride
  ethylene dibromide
  chloroprene
  trichloroethane
  tetrachloroethane
  toxaphene

Alcohols
  methyl alcohol
  allyl alcohol
  isopropyl alcohol

Glycols
  methyl cellosolve
  ethylene glycol

Ketones
  acetone
  cyclohexenone
  hexone
  methyl butyl ketone
  methyl ethyl ketone
  methyl (n-amyl) ketone
  5-methyl-3-heptanone

Aldehydes
  formaldehyde
  formic acid
  acrolein

Phenols
  cresol
  phenol
  pentachlorophenol
  2,4-dichlorophenoxy-acetic acid (2,4-D)
  2,4,5-trichlorophenoxy-acetic acid (2,4,5-T)

Other
  boranes
  carbon sulfides
  epichlorohydrin
  N,N-dimethylformamide
  ethylene oxide
  glycidyl ethers
  hydrazines
  mercaptans
  β-propiolactone

decontamination measures and removal from the source of exposure. The airway should be protected and adequate ventilation ensured.

Methyl alcohol and ethylene glycol are examples of organic solvents that require specific treatment in the form of antidotes. Methyl alcohol is a common solvent in a variety of paints, dyes, and stains. Most deaths have occurred by oral ingestion but toxicity may occur by inhalation or dermal absorption.[24] Treatment consists of supportive measures in addition to antidote therapy and hemodialysis. In cases of accidental ingestion, the stomach should be emptied by induction of emesis or gastric lavage. Ethyl alcohol should be administered in sufficient quantity IV or PO to result in a blood ethanol level of 100 mg%. Ethyl alcohol competes for the enzyme alcohol dehydrogenase preventing metabolism of methanol to formic acid and formaldehyde, which are the toxins responsible for metabolic acidosis and visual damage. Hemodialysis is indicated when blood levels of methanol exceed 50 mg% or by the presence of a severe metabolic acidosis.[16]

Ethylene glycol is less of a risk in hazardous materials incidents because it is less volatile and less likely to be absorbed unless vaporized by heating or if it is accidentally or intentionally ingested. The treatment is the same as for methanol.

Organophosphates, Carbamates, and Nerve Gas Agents

Poisoning by such agents as organophosphates, carbamates, and nerve gas results in a cholinergic crisis that is due to excess acetylcholine from blockade of acetyl cholinesterase at the neuromuscular junction. Organophosphates are readily absorbed through the intact skin resulting in signs and symptoms of diaphoresis, hypersecretion, incontinence, nausea and vomiting, dyspnea, and bradycardia. Severe cases of intoxication may result in mental status changes, convulsions, coma, and respiratory arrest.

Treatment consists of establishing an adequate airway and ventilation and providing oxygen. Atropine should be given IV in relatively large doses (2 to 4 mg every 5 minutes) until complete reversal of cholinergic signs results in dry skin and mouth, mydriasis, and tachycardia. Atropine should be repeated as needed for recurrence of cholinergic signs. Pralidoxime (2-PAM) is indicated when organophosphate intoxication is not completely reversed after several doses of atropine. The dosage of 2-PAM is 1.0 g IV in 100 mL of saline over 30 minutes (children, 25 mg/kg).

Nitrates and Related Compounds

Inhalation or dermal absorption of nitrates, nitrites, aniline dyes, nitrobenzene, and dinitrophenol may result in methemoglobinemia. Several drugs are also capable of inducing a methemoglobinemia but are unlikely to be involved in a hazardous material incident. In an instance where firefighters responded to the scene of a fire where isobutyl nitrite was stored, they developed toxic levels of methemoglobin requiring treatment following exposure to the toxic products of combustion.[8]

Symptoms of acute toxicity include a throbbing headache, flushing, dizziness, nausea, and vomiting. Serious toxicity may result in dyspnea, lethargy, and cyanosis. The appearance of an unusual chocolate-brown color of the blood is characteristic of methemoglobinemia.

Treatment consists of administration of 100% oxygen after securing an airway and providing adequate ventilation. Methylene blue is indicated for symptomatic patients or methemoglobin levels greater than 30%. The dose of methylene blue is 1 to 2 mg/kg in a 1% solution over 5 minutes. The dose may be repeated in 1 hour and then every 4 hours as needed.[16]

Organometallic Compounds

Arsine and nickel carbonyl are examples of organometallic compounds that are readily absorbed by the lungs resulting in pulmonary irritation and systemic toxicity.

Arsine exposure results in a severe hemolytic anemia that may be delayed up to 24 hours. Symptoms are nausea, vomiting, dyspnea, headache, and malaise. Jaundice, hematuria, and abdominal pain form the classical triad of presentation for arsine poisoning. Renal failure may occur secondary to hemolysis.[25] Treatment consists of supportive care in addition to alkalinization of the urine, blood transfusion as needed, and monitoring fluid balance. Arsenic chelation is accomplished by administration of dimercaprol initially followed by oral D-penicillamine for five days.[26]

Nickel carbonyl is used in a number of industrial processes and is produced when nickel reacts with carbon monoxide. Symptoms of poisoning are headache, dizziness, weakness, nausea, vomiting, dyspnea, chest pain, chills, and diaphoresis. Symptoms following exposure may be delayed or may progress to respiratory distress as a result of interstitial pneumonitis. The diagnosis of nickel carbonyl toxicity is made by measuring urine or plasma levels of nickel. A urine level greater than 10 μg/dL is an indication for chelation therapy with diethyldithiocarbamate.[27]

Phenols

Pentachlorophenol is an example of a phenol derivative that is widely used as a pesticide and wood preservative. Absorption may occur through dermal and respiratory routes. Dermal exposure has resulted in death.[28] Symptoms of toxicity include irritation of the lungs and mucous membranes, headache, diaphoresis, fever, tachycardia, muscle spasm, abdominal pain, nausea, and vomiting. The mechanism of toxicity occurs from an interaction in oxidative processes resulting in energy release and symptoms of increased metabolic rate.

Laboratory evaluation may demonstrate metabolic acidosis, elevations of alkaline phosphatase, serum creatinine, and BUN (blood urea nitrogen). In severe cases renal failure may occur.

Treatment is primarily supportive. The patient should be removed from the source of exposure and be decontaminated. Supportive measures include maintenance of airway and ventilation and regulation of body temperature. Diuresis may be effective in hastening elimination of PCP in some cases.[29]

RADIOACTIVE MATERIALS

The probability of a serious peacetime nuclear accident is remote. However, wherever radioactive materials are transported or used, the potential for a radiation accident exists. These materials are transported by rail and highway for use in hospitals, nuclear reactors, and weapons for the military. Because of the potential for an accident it is important that prehospital personnel, emergency physicians, and nurses know what to do if such an accident should occur.

The possible types of radiation exposure include particulate radiation in the form of α particles (ionized helium atoms), β particles (electrons), and neutrons. α Particles have little penetrating power and are stopped by paper or skin. β Particles have somewhat more penetrating power and may penetrate subcutaneous tissue. Neutrons have greater energy and require several inches of water to absorb them. When ingested, inhaled, or contaminated in a wound, any of the particulate forms of radiation may become incorporated into body tissue becoming sources of internal radiation.

γ Radiation and X radiation are high-energy forms of nonparticulate radiation that can penetrate deeply, causing damage by ionization of tissue. A victim will not emit radioactivity after removal from the source of gamma radiation.

β and γ radiation are the most widely used radioactive forms and therefore the most likely to be involved in a transportation or industrial accident. It is unlikely in the absence of an explosive accident that radiation will produce immediate symptoms unless the dose received is very high. The time of onset, severity, and type of symptoms correlate with the severity of exposure. Doses of less than 100 rem usually do not cause acute symptoms (the dose of a chest radiograph is approximately 10 millirem). At a dose of 200 rem, nausea and diarrhea may occur at 2 to 4 hours after exposure, but usually symptoms do not persist for more than 2 days. A dose range from 200 to 600 rem will cause gastroenteritis within 2 hours after exposure. At this dose level, the lymphocyte and neutrophil count falls within 24 hours. At exposure levels above 600 rem symptoms occur earlier, are more severe, and longer lasting, with death more probable.[30]

Prehospital management and treatment should follow the same guidelines as with other hazardous material incidents, utilizing proper approach to the area, personal protective equipment, evacuation, and decontamination. All personnel at the scene should wear dosimeters that register an accumulated dose of radioactivity, and the scene should be monitored and surveyed for safe triage and decontamination areas. Even the treatment of severely exposed patients has not resulted in dangerous doses of radiation to health care providers when proper procedures were followed.[31] Safety factors for emergency responders include minimizing time of exposure and maximizing distance from the source. Doubling the distance from the source will reduce exposure fourfold. Use of shielding material, personal protective clothing, and respiratory protection will also reduce exposure risk. The recommended maximum dose during a rescue operation is 100 rem, which may occur not more than once in a rescuer's life.

As with any hazardous material incident, proper decontamination of radioactive materials should be accomplished prior to transport when possible and the patient's condition is stable. Most facilities that handle radioactive materials will have a decontamination and first aid station where the victim will often be able to decontaminate himself or herself when other traumatic injuries are not present. It is most likely that contamination will be limited to a small area of the body, but total body contamination is possible.

Most hospitals do not have specific decontamination facilities, although to conform to guidelines of the Joint Commission on the Accreditation of Healthcare Organizations, a designated area, usually the emergency department, must be available in the event of such an emergency. If decontamination has not been accomplished prior to arrival it must be done at the hospital location. In any event, the patient should be considered contaminated until radioactive monitoring has proven otherwise. Although contamination control should be given a high priority, the patient's medical management should not be compromised to proceed with decontamination. The route from the ambulance to the treatment area should be roped off and labeled and the floors covered with plastic to avoid spread of contamination. The ventilation system in the treatment area should be turned off to avoid airborne contamination of other hospital areas. Upon arrival at the hospital, the patient should be admitted to an isolated area to avoid possible spread of contamination. During decontamination, levels of radioactivity should be measured and further cleansing performed if measurable levels persist.

General guidelines for decontamination are discussed above. Detailed protocols for decontamination of radioactive substances are available.[32] Laboratory tests should include a baseline CBC with differential, platelet count, and coagulation studies. There are likely several governmental and private organizations that will require notification and may be able to supply expert help (see Table 46-3). The Department of Energy maintains a regional office with 24-hour assistance available for help in case of a radiation accident. Also the Radiation Emergency Assistance Center/Training Site

(REAC/TS) provides 24-hour emergency access for consultation in the event of a radiation accident at (615) 576-3131 or (615) 482-2441.

REFERENCES

1. *US News and World Report.* December 17, 1984.
2. Wanke LA. Toxic chemical spills. *Top Emerg Med.* 1985;7:9–19.
3. Emou L. Study confirms paucity of chemical toxicity data. *Chem Eng News.* 1984;62:12.
4. *Federal OSHA Hazard Communication Regulations.* Subpart 1910 of Title 29 CFR 1910.1200. Washington, DC: US Government Printing Office; 1984.
5. *Federal Code of Federal Regulations 49.* Subparts 100 to 177. Washington, DC: US Government Printing Office; 1984.
6. *1984 Emergency Response Guidebook.* Washington, DC: US Dept of Transportation; 1983. DOT publication no P5800.3.
7. Yoder E. Hazardous material response system. *Top Emerg Med.* 1985;7:1–8.
8. Tong TG, Joe G, Morse LH, et al. A poison center experience with environmental emergencies. *Vet Hum Toxicol.* 1983;25(suppl 1):29–33.
9. Turkington RP. *HAZCAT—A Hazardous Materials Identification and Classification Kit for In-Field Use.* San Francisco: CAL/OSHA; 1984.
10. Barr SJ. Chemical warfare agents. *Top Emerg Med.* 1985;7:62–70.
11. Nishiyama H, VanTuinen RJ, Lukes SJ, et al. Survey of ^{99m}Tc contamination of laboratory personnel: hand decontamination. *Radiology.* 1980;137:549–555.
12. Merrick MV, Simpson JD, Liddell S. Skin decontamination—a comparison of four methods. *Br J Radiol.* 1982;55:317–318.
13. Wittlake WA. Radiation exposure. *Top Emerg Med.* 1985;7:53–67.
14. Iverson RE, Lamb DR, Madison MS. Hydrofluoric acid burns. *Plast Reconstruct Surg.* 1971;48:107–112.
15. Dibble DG, Iverson RE, Jones W, et al. HF burns of the hands. *J Bone Joint Surg Am.* 1970;52:931–936.
16. Rumack BH, ed. *POISINDEX.* Englewood, CO: Micromedex; 1985.
17. Brown TD. The treatment of hydrofluoric acid burns. *J Soc Occup Med.* 1974;24:80–89.
18. Gold A, Burgess WA, Clougherty EV. Exposure of firefighters to toxic air contaminants. *Am Ind Hyg Assoc J.* 1978;39:534–539.
19. Bonnichsen R, Maely AC. Poisoning by volatile compounds. *J Forens Sci.* 1966;11:516–527.
20. Trapp W, Lepawsky M. 100% survival in fire—life-threatening acute cyanide poisoning victims treated by a therapeutic spectrum including hyperbaric oxygen. Read before the Eighth Annual Conference in the Clinical Application of Hyperbaric Oxygen; June 8–10, 1983; Long Beach, CA.
21. Litovitz TL, Larkin RF, Myers RAM. Cyanide poisoning treated with hyperbaric oxygen. *Am J Emerg Med.* 1983;1:94–101.
22. Burney RE, Wu S, Nemiroff MJ, et al. Mass carbon monoxide poisoning: clinical effects and results of treatment in 184 victims. *Ann Emerg Med.* 1982;11:394–399.
23. Jackson DL, Menges H. Accidental carbon monoxide poisoning. *JAMA.* 1980;243:772–774.
24. Gimenez ER, Vallejo NE, Roy E, et al. Percutaneous alcohol intoxication. *Clin Toxicol.* 1968;1:39.
25. Fowler BA, Weissberg JB. Arsine poisoning. *N Engl J Med.* 1974;291:1171–1174.
26. Peterson RG, Rumack BH. D-Penicillamine therapy of acute arsenic poisoning. *J Pediatr.* 1977;91:661.
27. Sunderman FW Sr. The treatment of acute nickel carbonyl poisoning with sodium diethyldithiocarbamate. *Ann Clin Res.* 1971;3:182–185.
28. Truhaut R, Vitte G, Boussemart E, et al. Occupational poisoning in the wood industry, observations on two fatal cases. *Arch Mal Prof.* 1952;13:567.
29. Young JF, Haley TJ. A pharmacokinetic study of pentachlorophenol poisoning and the effect of forced diuresis. *Chem Toxicol.* 1978;12:41.
30. Glasstone S. *The Effects of Nuclear Weapons.* Washington, DC: US Government Printing Office; 1962.
31. Hubner KF. Decontamination procedures and risks to health care personnel. *Bull NY Acad Med.* 1983;59:1119–1128.
32. Leonard RB, Ricks RC. Emergency department radiation accident protocol. *Ann Emerg Med.* 1980;9:462–470.

47. Occupational Toxicologic Emergencies

ROBERT HARRISON, MD, MPH

The United States Bureau of Labor Statistics estimates that over 4.8 million work injuries and illnesses severe enough to cause a lost work day occurred in 1982.[1] The National Institute for Occupational Safety and Health (NIOSH) estimates that at least 10 million persons suffer traumatic injuries on the job each year, with at least 3 million severe injuries and at least 10,000 fatalities.[2] Of all lost-time injuries and illnesses, only 2% are considered illnesses. Nevertheless, this accounts for over 100,000 reported cases.

During the first nine months of 1982, of approximately 100 million workers, an estimated 2.4 million patients with occupational injuries were treated in hospital emergency departments in the continental United States.[3] Lacerations, contusions, abrasions, strains, and sprains account for over 65% of reported cases (Table 47-1). Finger injuries account for 749,000, or 25% of all occupational injuries, with an estimated 1.6% resulting in amputation. Health Interview Survey data suggest that about 36% of all job-related injuries are treated in hospital emergency departments, with the remainder seen in physicians' offices, worksite medical facilities, and local industrial medical clinics.[4]

The treatment of occupational injuries does not differ from the treatment of nonoccupational trauma. The frequency of occupational injuries seen in emergency facilities depends on the proximity of high-risk industries, particularly manufacturing. Mining and quarrying, agriculture, and construction consistently have the highest rates of traumatic death; occupations with high injury and illness rates generally involve the use of moving machinery (Table 47-2). Of interest, male workers aged 18 to 19 years appear at highest risk of job-related injury requiring treatment, particularly during the summer months.[3]

No estimate is available for the number of nontraumatic occupational illnesses seen yearly by emergency personnel in hospital emergency departments and clinics. Disorders associated with repetitive trauma (tendinitis, nerve entrapment disorders, bursitis, and back strain) account for the largest percentage of reportable occupational illnesses; skin diseases account for the next largest percentage (Table 47-3). Respiratory conditions due to toxic agents include exposure to gases, vapors, or irritating dusts that may result in lost time. If exposure is brief or low level, no lost time may occur and the incident will go unreported. One study has indicated that less than 5% of all occupational illness is reported.[5]

As the use of chemicals by industry has grown, the treatment of toxic chemical exposures has posed a growing challenge for emergency personnel. Over 70,000 chemicals are in use, with thousands of new ones introduced each year. Although many states now require disclosure of product ingredients, little information is yet available concerning the location and identity of toxic chemicals in the community. Several large-scale disasters involving toxic chemicals have alerted emergency response personnel to the potential hazards to surrounding communities and to the response teams themselves, and "hazardous materials teams" have been formed in many cities and towns.

The increasing use of synthetic materials has resulted in several instances of injury and death due to deadly products of their combustion. Hundreds of toxic chemicals may be

Table 47-1 Leading Causes of Occupational Injury, May 1981–May 1982*

Leading Categories	Number of Cases	Percentage
Laceration	723,800	24.4
Contusions, abrasions	694,300	23.4
Strain, sprain	534,200	18.0
Puncture	179,600	6.0
Fracture	166,100	5.6
All others	674,000	23.0
Total	2,972,000	100.0

*Based on a representative sample of hospital emergency departments.

Source: Adapted with permission from Coleman PJ: Injury surveillance: A review of data sources used by the division of safety research. *Scand J Work Environ Health* 9:130, 1983.

Table 47-2 Injury and Illness Rates: Leading Industries, United States, 1989*

Industry	Rank	Incidence Rate**
Ship building and repairing	1	45.8
Meat packing plants	2	35.1
Structural wood members, nec	3	30.4
Prefabricated wood buildings	4	27.9
Gray and ductile iron foundries	5	27.7
Automotive stampings	6	27.6
Truck trailers	7	27.6
Motor vehicles and car bodies	8	26.6
Canned and cured fish and seafoods	9	25.9
Household cooking equipment	10	25.9

*Injuries and illnesses requiring loss of one day or greater from work.
**Per 100 full-time workers.

Source: Occupational Injuries and Illnesses in the United States by Industry, 1989. US Department of Labor, Bureau of Labor Statistics, 1991.

Table 47-3 Occupational Illness, United States 1989*

Category of Illness	Number (thousands)
Skin diseases	66.7
Dust diseases of the lung	2.4
Respiratory conditions due to toxic agents	22.3
Poisoning	5.2
Disorders due to physical agents	17.4
Disorders associated with repetitive trauma	150.9
All other	32.8
Total	297.7

*Illnesses requiring loss of one day or greater from work.

Source: Occupational Injuries and Illnesses in the United States by Industry, 1989. US Department of Labor, Bureau of Labor Statistics, 1991.

released with the potential to cause respiratory damage and systemic toxicity leading to death. Both industrial workers and firefighters are at risk.

It is impossible for emergency personnel to become familiar with the toxicology of thousands of chemicals. Fortunately, the majority of toxic chemical exposures are to chemicals in common use, and are most likely to cause toxic injury due to gas or vapor inhalation. Several chemicals have systemic effects with which the emergency practitioner must be familiar. Although treatment may range from supportive to the institution of definitive therapy, general principles apply in the management of all toxic chemical exposures. By classifying toxic gases by their properties, the majority of chemical exposures can be readily identified and then effectively managed.

PRINCIPLES OF MANAGEMENT

The evaluation and treatment of all occupational toxicological emergencies involve several basic principles (Table 47-4). For workplace exposures, the key to hazard evaluation is the estimation of dose. Several factors are critical: route of exposure (skin absorption, inhalation, or ingestion), length of exposure, and the physical-chemical properties of the material. The first two factors are ascertained by a brief *occupational history,* the last factor by *identification of the toxic substance.*

A description of the work environment is critical. The treating practitioner must know how long the patient was working prior to the incident and what the work entailed. The circumstances of the incident may not always be known in detail, especially if the victim is acutely ill. If any co-workers were present, they should be questioned. As accidents may result from unusual procedures or unscheduled maintenance, this should be noted. The patient should be questioned as to the use of protective clothing or respiratory equipment. Protective clothing may not be adequate to protect the worker from chemicals such as solvents or polyhalogenated compounds, and significant skin absorption can take place. Respiratory protection may have been insufficient or inappropriate for the material involved. Contaminated clothing or respiratory protection may have been discarded at the workplace prior to arrival in the emergency department; if the exact nature of exposure is unknown, these items should be placed in plastic bags and saved for further analysis.

A brief history must not interfere with the immediate *decontamination* of the patient. If the history reveals direct contact with liquid or gas, or obvious clothing or skin contamination has occurred, then removal of residual chemical

Table 47-4 General Principles of Management of Occupational Emergencies

Brief occupational history
    Work process: source and extent of exposure
    Unusual procedures
    Protective clothing
    Respiratory protection
Decontamination
Identification of toxic substance

must be immediately begun. All contaminated outer clothes and undergarments must be removed, placed in impermeable plastic bags, and sealed to prevent further exposure to both patient and hospital personnel. The patient should then be washed with soap and water to remove any residual skin contamination. Gloves and protective gowns should be worn by hospital personnel to avoid secondary exposure. A recent case of ethylene dibromide exposure has underscored the need to protect hospital personnel when treating the poisoned victim.[6]

The identification of the toxic substance, along with its physical-chemical properties and toxicology, is necessary to estimate potential dose and anticipated effects. This in turn should be used to guide subsequent treatment. If the victim is unable to provide this information, co-workers may be available. Unfortunately, many times the identity of the substance is not known by the victim or co-worker; if the victim is unsure or the exposure is unknown, the emergency practitioner must contact the employee's workplace and speak with the manager, shift supervisor, health and safety officer, or other responsible personnel. In small workplaces where health and safety precautions may not be adequate, or where proprietary products are used, the precise composition of the substance may not be known. If brand name or other identifying information is available, the product manufacturer may have additional information.

Many states now require product information to be made available to employees, their designated representatives, and health care personnel.[7] Material Safety Data Sheets contain information about product composition and physical-chemical properties. Health effects and guidelines for treatment are often outlined. Employers or product manufacturers should be able to verbally supply this information to hospital emergency personnel.

Chemical containers may have labels that list both product constituents and the risk of exposure to eyes, skin, or lungs. Sometimes an emergency telephone number is printed that can be called in the event of an accident.

Toxic exposure may occur to emergency personnel responding to spills or explosions on the highways or from rail accidents. The manifest, or record of cargo, should be used to identify the material. Sometimes the point of destination can be contacted to provide further information about truck or tanker contents.

Inhalation of toxic gas may sometimes be due to complex mixtures of chemicals that result from controlled processes or from unexpected chemical reactions. In some cases, it may be impossible to know with certainty the constituents of a gas from an explosion or chain reaction. Combustion of a chemical may result in more toxic chemicals, such as in the formation of dibenzofurans from polychlorinated biphenyls or hydrogen cyanide from synthetic materials. Chemical engineers or research personnel may be of some help, but there are times when the source of inhalation injury is never identified.

Once the toxic substance has been identified, supportive or specific therapy is guided by the particular acute or delayed effects of the toxin. In addition to the sources of information described above, the local or regional poison control center should be contacted for assistance in management.

The clinician should be aware that other life-threatening conditions may complicate an occupational toxicologic emergency. Concomitant trauma, hyperthermia, and the presence of medical illnesses such as diabetes, alcohol withdrawal, or drug abuse must be considered in the initial management of patients with acute exposures.

TOXIC GAS INHALATION

Injury that is due to toxic gas inhalation represents the major type of occupational toxicologic emergency (see also Chapter 46, Hazardous Materials). Although there are a wide variety of industrial processes and toxic gases employed, noxious gases can be classified by type of insult: physical asphyxiant, chemical asphyxiant, and direct irritant. Because a wide variety of both systemic poisons and pulmonary irritants are formed during the combustion of synthetic materials, the management of toxic smoke inhalation is considered separately.

Physical Asphyxiants

A physical asphyxiant is any gas that produces tissue anoxia by mechanical displacement of oxygen from the environment. Thus symptoms from exposure to physical asphyxiants are likely to occur from high concentrations of toxic gas within an enclosed space. Symptoms of asphyxia are due to decreased oxygen tension in the blood and tissues: headache, hyperventilation, nausea, confusion, loss of consciousness, apnea, and death. At high concentrations of gas, unconsciousness may occur within minutes.

Normally the atmosphere contains 21% by volume of oxygen; at 16.5% to 21% oxygen human beings are asymptomatic. Lower concentration of oxygen in inspired air causes tachypnea, tachycardia, and slight incoordination. At oxygen concentrations of less than 6%, convulsions followed by apnea and cardiac arrest will occur within minutes. If the metabolic demand for oxygen is increased, as in strenuous occupations, symptoms of tissue hypoxia will develop more quickly.

In a 3-year period from 1984 to 1986, almost 9% of 4756 deaths investigated by the Federal Occupational Safety and Health Administration were due to asphyxiation or poisoning.[8] Of these, the most common physical asphyxiants were methane, nitrogen, and carbon dioxide (Table 47-5). Utility workers entering manholes and oil field workers in fracturing tanks appear to have the highest risk of asphyxiation. Many deaths by asphyxiation involve co-workers or other persons attempting to rescue a victim.[9]

Treatment of asphyxia that is due to a simple asphyxiant is straightforward: removal of the individual from the source of exposure and immediate administration of oxygen. If cardiopulmonary collapse has occurred, general life support measures must be instituted. If tissue damage resulting from hypoxia has occurred, careful monitoring is required for late cardiac, hepatic, renal, or central nervous system complications.

Nitrogen

Nitrogen is a clear, colorless gas that is toxic only when it has lowered the relative atmospheric concentration of oxygen or when it is released in the blood as bubbles as in decompression sickness. It is the main component of air, comprising 79% by volume. In hyperbaric environments such as caissons or tunnels, nitrogen can cause a narcotic reaction with decreased ability to work and mood changes. A rapid decrease in pressure may cause nitrogen gas to leave solution and cause circulatory impairment and local tissue damage (the "bends" or "chokes"). Individuals in occupations such as deep-sea commercial diving and caisson and tunnel work may be subject to the complications of hyperbaric environments.

Nitrogen gas is used in many industrial processes, such as in the production of ammonia and other chemicals, and in liquid form as a cooling solution. It is used to displace oxygen or explosive gases from confined spaces. A high concentration of nitrogen gas may be encountered in underground mines; when accompanied by carbon dioxide in coal mines, the combination is known as "black damp."

Carbon Dioxide

Carbon dioxide is a clear, odorless gas that can be used in its gaseous, liquid, or solid form. It is used as a gas in the textile, leather, and chemical industries, in food preservation, in welding, as a fire extinguisher, or as an inert gas to reduce explosive or flammable hazard. It is also encountered in the fermentation of wines and beer and in grain elevators and silos as a result of carbohydrate fermentation. As a liquid, it is used as a fire extinguisher or refrigerant or in the

Table 47-5 Physical Asphyxiants

Nitrogen
Carbon dioxide
Methane (natural gas)
Ethane
Argon, neon, helium

production of dry ice. The solid form of carbon dioxide is dry ice, primarily used as a refrigerant.

Exposure to concentrations of greater than 10% by volume of carbon dioxide can cause unconsciousness and death within minutes. Respiratory rate is increased at concentrations of 2%, and noticeable subjective distress may occur at concentrations of 5%.[10,11] Carbon dioxide is heavier than air and thus will be encountered in the lower reaches of confined spaces.

Reported deaths due to carbon dioxide poisoning have occurred as a result of the fermentation of carbohydrates in brewery vats and grain silos and from the accumulation of gas following mine fires.[12]

Methane and Ethane

Both methane and ethane are low–molecular weight hydrocarbons that are colorless and odorless. Mercaptan is usually added to methane, which imparts a characteristic odor and thus a warning of exposure. Methane is the principal component of natural gas (85%) and is formed from decaying organic matter as from swamps ("marsh gas"). Natural gas is used primarily as a heating fuel and in the manufacture of many chemicals such as hydrocarbon fuels, acetylene, and formaldehyde. Ethane is a small component of natural gas (9%) and is also used as a refrigerant.

Methane is lighter than air and so accumulates in the upper part of a confined space. Explosion may often occur before death by asphyxiation. Deaths by methane poisoning may represent suicides with natural gas, or they may be due to entry into confined spaces such as manure pits.[13] Explosions in underground mines are principally due to the accumulation of methane above the explosive limit.

Chemical Asphyxiants

A chemical asphyxiant is defined as a substance that causes toxicity by producing tissue hypoxia from interference with oxygen delivery or utilization. Carbon monoxide combines with hemoglobin to form carboxyhemoglobin and interferes with oxygen delivery, while both hydrogen cyanide and hydrogen sulfide interfere with the function of oxidative enzymes and impair oxygen utilization.

Carbon Monoxide

Carbon monoxide is a colorless, odorless gas that is produced from incomplete combustion of carbon-containing material. The toxicity and treatment of carbon monoxide poisoning have been reviewed recently.[14–16] Common environmental sources of carbon monoxide are the internal combustion engine and the home heating unit and water heater. The gasoline-powered internal combustion engine is the largest single source of carbon monoxide in the ambient air, with concentrations reaching a maximum during heavy commuting times in early morning and evening.

The increasing use of kerosene space heaters because of rising energy costs in the 1970s led to more reported cases of unsuspected carbon monoxide poisoning.[17,18] Space heaters in campers and recreational vehicles also can be a hazard.

Occupational exposure to carbon monoxide can be encountered in foundries, petroleum refineries, paper mills, steel mills, and in the manufacture of formaldehyde.[19] The use of gasoline-powered forklifts or other machinery, particularly in warehouses or enclosed spaces, is also a source of carbon monoxide. Individuals in occupations at particular risk are firefighters, traffic control workers, and garage attendants.

An estimated 10,000 persons seek medical attention or lose at least 1 day of normal activity each year through carbon monoxide exposure, and at least 1500 individuals a year die of accidental exposure.[20] Carbon monoxide poisoning is the most common cause of poisoning in the United States. Of 11,547 unintentional carbon monoxide deaths over a 10-year period (1979–1988), 57% were caused by motor vehicles, and 10% were due to stoves or fireplaces; 1.6% were due to industrial processes. Rates were highest among African-Americans and the elderly and in high-altitude and cold states. Rates declined steadily over this period, possibly as a result of stricter environmental and regulatory standards.[21] Cases of carbon monoxide poisoning have been reported from the use of gasoline-powered machinery in indoor ice-skating rinks and the operation of heavy equipment in the holds of ships.[22] Carbon monoxide exposure was thought to have contributed to the deaths of two workmen with pre-existing coronary artery disease.[23] Accidental venting of furnace exhaust containing carbon monoxide caused exposure of 184 students and teachers at a public high school.[24] An improperly vented furnace in a newly renovated, well-insulated house caused nighttime carbon monoxide poisoning of a family of six.[25]

The main ingredient in paint remover, methylene dichloride (dichloromethane), is rapidly metabolized in vivo to carbon monoxide. Experimental volunteer exposure to methylene dichloride solvent resulted in significant absorption of solvent, prompt metabolism to carbon monoxide, and elevated carboxyhemoglobin levels for several hours following exposure.[26] Painters, furniture strippers, and degreasers may be exposed to this volatile solvent and are at risk for complications of carbon monoxide toxicity.[27,28]

The toxicity of carbon monoxide is due to the avid affinity of carbon monoxide for hemoglobin, approximately 240 times that of oxygen. By competing with oxygen for binding sites on hemoglobin, the oxyhemoglobin saturation is decreased. In addition to the decrease in the amount of oxygen that can be carried by hemoglobin, the oxyhemoglobin dissociation curve is shifted to the left. This decreases the oxygen tension at which oxygen molecules are dissociated from hemoglobin and therefore decreases the driving pressure for diffusion of oxygen into tissues.

Carbon monoxide has also been demonstrated to bind to myoglobin, possibly contributing to poor cardiac function and ischemia, and may also affect the mitochondrial cytochrome oxidase system, impairing respiration at the cellular level.[29–31]

Normal endogenous production of carbon monoxide results in a carboxyhemoglobin level of approximately 0.7%.[32] Smoke from cigarettes contains 3% to 6% carbon monoxide, or an average exposure of 400 parts per million during inhalation. By comparison, the workplace standard allowed by the Occupational Safety and Health Administration is 50 parts per million, while NIOSH recommends an 8-hour average of 35 parts per million with a ceiling limit of 200 parts per million.[33] A two-pack-per-day cigarette smoker may have carboxyhemoglobin levels of 5% to 7%.[32]

The symptoms of acute carbon monoxide exposure are generally associated with varying levels of carboxyhemoglobin (Table 47-6). Carbon monoxide is eliminated through the lungs with a one-half reduction in carboxyhemoglobin level in approximately 4 hours. If delay occurs in measuring carboxyhemoglobin, or if oxygen has been administered before measurement, the carboxyhemoglobin level may be falsely low. Qualitative tests for carboxyhemoglobin are sensitive only for levels greater than 20% and so may miss low-level exposures with subacute poisoning. Traffic

Table 47-6 Symptomatology Associated with Carbon Monoxide Poisoning

% CO in Atmosphere	% COHb in Blood	Signs and Symptoms
	0–10	None (angina may be noted in patients with CAD)
0.007	10–20	Slight headache, exercise angina, exertional dyspnea
0.012	20–30	Throbbing headache, moderate exercise dyspnea
0.022	30–40	Severe headache, nausea, vomiting, weakness, visual disturbance, impaired judgment
0.035–0.052	40–50	Syncope, tachycardia, tachypnea,
	50–60	coma, convulsions,
0.195	70–80	Death

Source: Goldfrank L, Bresnitz EA, Weisman RS, Lewin NA: The inhaled agents and other disorders of oxygen transport, in Hansen W (ed): *Toxic Emergencies.* New York, Churchill Livingstone Inc, 1984.

policemen or garage workers may suffer acute recurring episodes throughout the day, but may have low or normal carboxyhemoglobin levels if measured after their shifts.[34]

Continuous exposure to 50 parts per million carbon monoxide (0.005%) over an 8-hour period leads to an equilibrium value of 5% carboxyhemoglobin. If physical exercise is performed, the time to equilibrium is shortened. Changes in psychomotor performance can be detected at these levels, and time to onset of angina in patients with pre-existing coronary artery disease is shortened.[32]

When carboxyhemoglobin levels exceed 10%, headache is noted; at 20% to 30% carboxyhemoglobin, nausea, weakness, and dizziness occur. As carboxyhemoglobin levels exceed 30%, visual disturbance and impaired judgment are noted. Above 40%, syncope and collapse are frequent, while convulsions and deaths usually occur at concentrations above 50%.

Heart and brain tissue are the most sensitive to oxygen deprivation, and these organs account for the major toxic manifestations. In addition to curtailing exercise tolerance, carboxyhemoglobin concentrations above 9% can lead to ischemic electrocardiographic changes, dysrhythmias, and myocardial infarction.[32,35] Clinical evidence of myocardial toxicity can occur immediately or can be delayed for several days. Acutely, central nervous system changes due to hypoxia can be nonspecific: headache, vomiting, dizziness, and fatigue. Group exposures can be mistaken for food poisoning.[36] Symptoms of carbon monoxide poisoning have been confused with those of viral syndromes.[37] If severe anoxia has occurred, a variety of residual neurological sequelae may result, including dystonia, ataxia, and disturbances in cognitive function and personality. The basal ganglia appear to be the most severely affected.[38]

Other manifestations of carbon monoxide poisoning include flame-shaped retinal hemorrhage and bullous skin lesions. The cherry-red coloring of skin and mucous membranes is an unreliable sign as it may be absent in subacute or acute poisoning.[39]

The Pa_{O_2} of blood will remain nearly normal in carbon monoxide poisoning, but the O_2 content of blood will fall as oxygen is replaced by carbon monoxide on the hemoglobin molecules. Therefore, determination of Pa_{O_2} is of little diagnostic value in carbon monoxide poisoning.

Diagnosis. The diagnosis of carbon monoxide poisoning is most reliably made by the spectrophotometric measurement of carboxyhemoglobin in the blood or by direct measurement of carboxyhemoglobin saturation with a co-oximeter. Qualitative tests are unreliable and relatively insensitive compared with the spectrophotometric method.[40] Psychometric testing has been used as a sensitive measure of neurologic effects.[41] It must be stressed that a low or normal carboxyhemoglobin level does not rule out toxicity due to carbon monoxide exposure, particularly if there has been a delay in obtaining the carboxyhemoglobin level or if treatment with oxygen has occurred. Routine carboxyhemoglobin or carbon monoxide breath test screening of emergency department admissions is not recommended.[42,43]

Treatment: prehospital. The treatment of choice for carbon monoxide poisoning is the highest possible concentration of oxygen. The half-life of carboxyhemoglobin is reduced to 40 minutes when breathing 100% oxygen. Emergency paramedical personnel should immediately administer 100% oxygen by tight-fitting mask or endotracheal tube, without waiting for carboxyhemoglobin levels. Thereafter, a sample of whole blood should be obtained for later analysis of carboxyhemoglobin.

Treatment: emergency department. The kinetics of carbon monoxide exposure depend on the ventilatory rate, inspired O_2 partial pressure, and pattern and length of carbon monoxide exposure. Therefore, the use of back-extrapolation to determine the maximum carboxyhemoglobin level is not recommended. The morbidity and mortality from carbon monoxide exposure also have not been found to correlate well with carboxyhemoglobin level.[44] Clinical signs and symptoms have been found to correlate with carboxyhemoglobin levels only at low levels of carbon monoxide exposure, and there is no direct correlation between the carboxyhemoglobin level and severity of symptoms.[44,45] If not already obtained, blood should be drawn and sent for carboxyhemoglobin level, complete blood count, BUN, creatinine, cardiac enzymes, and glucose. A β-hCG pregnancy test is recommended for all women of child-bearing age.[46] Arterial blood gases should be drawn to assess acid-base balance. An ECG and chest radiograph should be obtained even in cases of mild carbon monoxide poisoning because myocardial and pulmonary toxicity does not correlate well with carboxyhemoglobin levels. ECG abnormalities include ischemic ST-T wave abnormalities, infarction patterns, dysrhythmias, and conduction system abnormalities. Hospitalization is needed for adults with a carboxyhemoglobin level greater than 25%, children with a carboxyhemoglobin level greater than 15%, adults with a history of heart disease or who are pregnant and have a carboxyhemoglobin level greater than 15%; any symptomatic pregnant woman, patients with a metabolic acidosis or ECG changes, and patients with neuropsychiatric symptoms, abnormal thermoregulation, or a Pa_{O_2} less than 60 mmHg.[46]

Endotracheal intubation should be considered when signs of severe hypoxia are present (loss of consciousness or coma). Repeat carboxyhemoglobin levels must be obtained at periodic intervals. There may be poor correlation between persistence of symptoms and carboxyhemoglobin levels. This may be due to residual anoxic encephalopathy or possibly persistent cellular poisoning by carbon monoxide attached to cytochrome oxidase. For patients with no neurological symptoms, the end point of treatment should be a carboxyhemoglobin level of less than 5%.

Mild metabolic acidemia should not be treated, since acidemia has a beneficial effect on oxygen delivery by shifting the oxyhemoglobin dissociation curve to the right.

Although not conclusively demonstrated, the use of oxygen under hyperbaric conditions is recommended for symptomatic cases of carbon monoxide poisoning[47] or cases with a carboxyhemoglobin level in excess of 25%.[48–51] Oxygen administered at 3 atmospheres will reduce the half-life of carboxyhemoglobin to approximately 23 minutes. If hyperbaric treatment is not available or is delayed, oxygen treatment by mask or endotracheal tube must be instituted immediately. In patients with neurological signs or cardiac complications, oxygen delivery to hypoxic tissues may be improved with hyperbaric oxygen and recovery quickened. One recent large case series suggests that patients with severe myocardial or neurologic symptoms from carbon monoxide poisoning could be managed safely with hyperbaric oxygen treatment. Complications of emesis, agitation, seizures, hypotension, and cardiac dysrhythmia must be carefully managed.[52] Pneumothorax, air embolism, tympanic membrane rupture, and sinus trauma are complications of hyperbaric oxygen therapy.[51,53]

Induced hypothermia, steroids, exchange transfusion, or perfluorocarbon administration are of unproven value.

Delayed symptoms of carbon monoxide poisoning have included a wide variety of neurologic abnormalities including personality changes, learning disabilities, dementia, and organic brain syndromes.

Hydrogen Cyanide

Hydrogen cyanide is a colorless liquid or gas that is in widespread industrial use. The sodium and potassium salts of cyanides are used in metallurgy for the extraction of gold and silver salts from ores and in the electroplating of metals. Hydrogen cyanide is used as a fumigant and in the chemical synthesis of synthetic fibers, plastics, and nitriles. Cyanide gas may be generated in blast furnaces, gas works, and coke ovens.[19] When cyanide salts come into contact with any acid, hydrogen cyanide vapor is released, which is a potential hazard for laboratory workers. Combustion of various plastics such as polyurethanes will liberate hydrogen cyanide upon pyrolysis, a risk to firefighters. Historical reports of poisoning have been recorded in the fumigation of warehouses, buildings, and ships and from contact with cyanide solution.[54]

Acrylonitrile (vinyl cyanide) is used in the manufacture of acrylic fibers, rubbers and plastics, and as a pesticide fumigant. When absorbed through skin contact or inhalation, acrylonitrile is biotransformed in the liver to thiocyanate and cyanide.[55] Acetonitrile (methyl cyanide), used as an extractant for animal and vegetable oils and as a solvent in the pharmaceutical industry, is also metabolized to cyanide.

Nonoccupational sources of cyanide exposure include the ingestion of fruit pits and laetrile, the latter used for alternative cancer therapy. Sodium nitroprusside, used in the management of acute hypertensive emergencies or shock, will liberate cyanide as a metabolic product. Cyanide is also released as a product of tobacco combustion and can be measured in cigarette smoke.

Cyanide is readily absorbed through the skin and mucous membranes and by inhalation. Hydrocyanic acid vapors cause the most rapid onset of toxicity. Alkali salts of cyanide are toxic only when ingested, and effects can be delayed because of gastrointestinal absorption. The toxic effect of cyanide is due to the inhibition of cytochrome oxidase, the terminal oxidase of the mitochondrial respiratory chain. As a result, oxidative metabolism and phosphorylation are compromised and peripheral tissue oxygen tensions rise. The unloading gradient for oxyhemoglobin is decreased, accounting for the clinical observation of high venous oxygen content (the "arterialization" of venous blood). As aerobic metabolism is halted, pyruvate is reduced to lactate and a lactic acidosis ensues.

Cyanide directly stimulates chemoreceptors in the aorta and carotid artery, causing hyperpnea. High doses of cyanide will interfere with brain metabolism and cause respiratory arrest within minutes, even while cardiac activity continues.[56]

The occupational exposure limit to hydrogen cyanide is 10 parts per million as a time-weighted average over an 8-hour day; 130 parts per million can be lethal. Exposure to 300 parts per million hydrogen cyanide over several minutes will be rapidly fatal.[54]

Acutely, cyanide intoxication causes central nervous system effects, with headache, dizziness, weakness, opisthotonos, trismus, confusion, flushing, tachycardia, and tachypnea. Severe anxiety can mimic the early symptoms of cyanide poisoning, presenting a difficult diagnostic challenge.[57] Respiratory symptoms initially include tachypnea and dyspnea progressing to respiratory depression with hypoventilation and apnea. Transient hypertension may be followed by reflex bradycardia and sinus dysrhythmia and tachycardia with hypotension.[58] If large amounts of cyanide have been absorbed, respiratory arrest, convulsions, coma, and death may occur within a few minutes.

Subacute cyanide intoxication after weeks to months of lower-dose exposure may cause symptoms of headache, dizziness, nausea, and vomiting. These symptoms are similar to those with short-term, high-dose exposures and suggest an inhibitory effect on cellular enzyme systems.[59] Contact with cyanide salts may also cause direct respiratory, mucous membrane, and skin irritation, as well as skin burns from the caustic solution.[54]

Diagnosis. The diagnosis of cyanide poisoning relies on a high index of suspicion in the patient with altered mental status and an appropriate history of exposure or ingestion. An odor of bitter almonds is a classic sign, although less than 50% of individuals may be able to smell this.[60] Fundal veins and arteries may appear equally red.

Unfortunately, no test is available for the rapid diagnosis of cyanide intoxication. Lavage or emesis fluid should be saved for qualitative laboratory analysis for cyanide. Unexplained metabolic acidosis and abolition of the arterial-venous oxygen difference are clues to the diagnosis, although they are unreliable. An acyanotic patient with unexplained hypotension, bradycardia, acidosis, and rapid onset of coma may have cyanide poisoning. The whole blood cyanide level is the definitive test of intoxication but is not readily available for emergency department use. A whole blood cyanide level less than 0.2 µg/mL usually does not result in symptoms, although cigarette smokers may be asymptomatic at levels less than 0.4 µg/mL. The median lethal dose is above 2 µg/mL.[61] Plasma thiocyanate levels correlate poorly with cyanide intoxication, and their measurement is not recommended.[58]

Treatment: prehospital. Treatment must be instituted immediately if the diagnosis of cyanide poisoning is suspected (Table 47-7). Initial treatment is supportive and must include airway support, 100% oxygen, cardiac monitoring, intravenous fluids, and sodium bicarbonate if acidosis is present. If ingestion has occurred, gastric lavage should be performed or emesis induced. Activated charcoal in standard doses is recommended for routine use in ingestions.[62]

Specific therapy for cyanide poisoning is initially directed at the production of methemoglobin, which competes with the cytochrome oxidase system for binding of cyanide. Methemoglobin levels of 25% to 30% should be induced. Workplaces with cyanide exposure should have cyanide kits available containing amyl nitrite, and these should be carried by paramedical personnel. The Lilly cyanide kit (no M-76) is approved for use in the United States. Amyl nitrite, available in ampules and in cyanide kits with sodium nitrite and sodium thiosulfate, is administered immediately by inhalation. Amyl nitrite will produce only up to 5% methemoglobin and is not adequate alone. Doses of amyl nitrite sufficient to produce higher levels of methemoglobin will cause excessive hypotension.

Treatment: emergency department. As soon as it is available, administer sodium nitrite, 10 mL of a 3% solution intravenously at 2.5 to 5.0 mL/min over 2 to 3 minutes with a modified dose to children of 0.2 mL/kg. This should produce a methemoglobinemia of about 20%.[63]

Sodium thiosulfate should be administered immediately following sodium nitrite, intravenously as 12.5 mg of a 25% solution over 10 minutes. Thiosulfate serves as a substrate for the enzyme rhodanase, providing sulfur groups to convert cyanide into the less toxic thiocyanate, which can be excreted in the urine.

The use of sodium nitrite is not without risk, as an excess can cause marked methemoglobinemia, hypotension, hypoxia, and vascular collapse.[60] Levels of methemoglobin should be monitored and should not exceed 40%. Patients should be observed for 24 to 48 hours; subsequent doses of sodium nitrite and sodium thiosulfate should be approximately 50% of the initial doses. Inhalation of 100% oxygen may be of value in enhancing tissue oxygen delivery and increasing the conversion of cyanide to thiocyanate by thiosulfate.[34,54]

Other antidotes have been proposed for cyanide poisoning. Hydroxycobalamin (Vitamin B_{12}) is thought to bind to cyanide and form cyanocobalamin, and has been used successfully in Europe. The low toxicity of hydroxycobalamin seems to offer an advantage over sodium nitrite.[60]

Dicobalt EDTA will bind cyanide by chelation and is commercially available in Europe. It may cause hypotension and pruritus and has not been widely used in this country.

Hyperbaric oxygen therapy, if available, has been recommended as an adjunct in the treatment of cyanide poisoning. Its use is supported by case reports and animal data, but it has not been of proven value in humans.[62]

Hydrogen Sulfide

Hydrogen sulfide is a colorless gas with a characteristic rotten-egg odor.[64] It has a very low olfactory threshold at 0.02 part per million, but olfactory fatigue can occur at concentrations of 100 to 150 parts per million, decreasing the warning properties.[65] Hydrogen sulfide is used industrially in the leather industry, in the production of viscose rayon and cellophane, in the Kraft process for making chemical pulp from wood, and in the manufacture of gas or coke from coal. It is present in most volcanic gases and in "sulfur springs."[66] Release of hydrogen sulfide gas may occur from high sulfur crude oil at oil refineries during removal of sulfur compounds. Hydrogen sulfide is produced in the manufacture of carbon disulfide, pesticides, and grease and fatty-acid making processes.[67] Hydrogen sulfide is generated during the decomposition of sulfur-containing organic material and so can be found in gas wells and sewers.[68] It is known as "stink damp" when found in mines extending through sulfurous rock.[69]

Acutely, hydrogen sulfide is a respiratory irritant at low concentrations of up to 100 parts per million, causing conjunctival irritation, lacrimation, rhinitis, and cough.[67] Prolonged exposure to concentrations above 300 parts per million may cause pulmonary edema.

At higher levels, hydrogen sulfide acts as a cellular poison by inhibiting cytochrome oxidase and interfering with oxidative metabolism.[65] Exposure to 300 parts per million for 0.5 to 1 hour can result in dizziness, confusion, and headache, followed by loss of consciousness and respiratory

---

Table 47-7 Management of Cyanide Poisoning

1. Ventilate with 100% oxygen by ambu bag. Perform CPR if necessary.
2. Inhalation of amyl nitrite pearls 15 to 30 seconds every minute.
3. 300 mg or 10 mL 3% sodium nitrite IV at 2.5 to 5 mL/min.
4. 12.5 g or 50 mL 25% sodium thiosulfate IV.

arrest. Levels of 1000 parts per million will cause nearly instant coma and death.[63] Fatalities due to hydrogen sulfide have been reported from entry into an underground manure tank,[69,70] and several cases have been reported from entry into confined spaces containing sewer gas.[65] Hydrogen sulfide gas is heavier than air and so accumulates at the bottom of a confined space.

The diagnosis of hydrogen sulfide poisoning relies on the clinical symptoms and appropriate history. Although not routinely available, blood sulfide levels can be measured.[71,72] The treatment of hydrogen sulfide intoxication proceeds with the same urgency as for hydrogen cyanide, and general supportive measures are similar. Pretreatment with sodium nitrite protects animals from hydrogen sulfide toxicity,[34] and one author has documented success in a human intoxication.[65] The formation of methemoglobin will reverse the effects of hydrogen sulfide poisoning by competitively binding the sulfide anion and forming sulfmethemoglobin, which can be metabolized and excreted. As with cyanide, treatment should be instituted with inhalation of amyl nitrite followed by infusion of 10 mL of a 3% solution of sodium nitrite over 2 to 4 minutes. Although one case has been reported using sodium thiosulfate for the treatment of hydrogen sulfide poisoning,[73] it is not generally recommended.[34]

Although complete recovery is usual after hydrogen sulfide poisoning, permanent neurologic sequelae have been reported.[74]

Irritant Gases

Irritant gases (Table 47-8) cause pulmonary damage by direct injury of the upper and lower respiratory tract.[75,76] The severity of injury depends upon the length of exposure, concentration of the irritant, and physical-chemical properties of the material. More water-soluble irritants, such as ammonia, formaldehyde, and chlorine, cause upper airway injury and burning and watery eyes or cough. These symptoms usually limit exposure and prevent lower respiratory tract damage.

Relatively water-insoluble gases such as phosgene and nitrogen dioxide can cause injury to lower bronchioles and alveoli, leading to sputum production, chest pain, dyspnea, or pulmonary edema. Respiratory failure and death from pulmonary edema may ensue if not promptly treated. Over 2000 deaths occurred in Bhopal, India, as a result of a potent lower respiratory irritant, methyl isocyanate.[77]

The treatment of injury due to irritant gases is supportive. Conjunctival irritation should be treated with copious irrigation with water or saline and the eyes examined with fluorescein for corneal defects. Upper airway swelling and inflammation may necessitate endotracheal intubation or cricothyrotomy if complete obstruction occurs. Oxygen should be delivered by nasal cannula or face mask, or if pulmonary injury leads to severe hypoxemia, by mechanical ventilation.

Table 47-8 Irritant Gases

Chlorine
Phosgene
Ammonia
Nitrogen dioxide
Ozone
Sulfur dioxide
Phosphine
Formaldehyde
Hydrogen chloride

Pulmonary edema may require positive pressure in addition to mechanical ventilation and judicious use of fluids with central pressure monitoring. A chest roentgenogram should be obtained, although pulmonary edema due to less soluble gases may be delayed for several hours. If bronchospasm is present, bronchodilators may be of value. Prophylactic antibiotics should be avoided. Corticosteroids have been employed, but with the possible exception of nitrogen dioxide inhalation, their use is not well established.[78]

Chlorine

Molecular chlorine is a highly reactive gas whose deployment during World War I in 1915 initiated modern chemical warfare. It is greenish-yellow in color and has a pungent odor with a low odor threshold and good warning properties. It is used in the bleaching of paper and wood pulp, in the production of plastics and resins, in textile and household bleaches, in detinning and dezincing iron, and as a disinfecting agent for drinking water and sewage.[19] It is usually transported as a pressurized liquid, although if containers rupture, exposure is to the gaseous form. Exposure after spillage can be prolonged, as chlorine is denser than air and can remain at ground level.

The household mixture of dilute hypochlorite solution with acidic chemicals, as in the combination of bleach with lavatory cleaners, can result in the formation of chlorine gas and subsequent inhalation injury.[79] Industrial accidents have occurred from gas leaks and explosions, while both worker and community exposures have occurred from transportation mishaps.[63,80]

The severity of injury due to chlorine gas is related to the concentration of the gas, the duration of exposure, and the water content of the tissues exposed. Chlorine will react with water to form hypochlorite and hydrochloric acid, which are extremely irritating to respiratory tissues. Exposure to chlorine gas at several parts per million will cause eye and throat irritation within minutes. High-level exposure of several hundred to several thousand parts per million will cause intense burning of the eyes, nose, and throat, followed shortly thereafter by cough, shortness of breath, whitish sputum production, and substernal pain. Severe exposure may result in pulmonary edema, hypoxemia, and respiratory failure.[81]

Individuals with mild exposure without symptoms should be advised to seek medical attention if problems develop over the next 12 to 24 hours. As the toxic effects of chlorine exposure are immediate, this is unlikely to occur. Victims with breathlessness, chest pain, severe cough, and frothy sputum production, or with hypoxemia and/or infiltrates on chest film, should be admitted to the hospital for observation and treatment as outlined above.

Pulmonary function studies may show an obstructive pattern in the few months following hospitalization for pulmonary injury, and subsequent follow-up studies have shown a greater than expected decline in pulmonary function over several years.[75,82–85] Workers with repeated acute chlorine gas exposures have had a greater decline in FEV_1/FVC ratio and a greater prevalence of respiratory symptoms.[86,87]

Phosgene

Phosgene is a colorless gas with a sweet odor similar to musty hay or freshly cut corn. It is estimated to be 10 times as toxic as chlorine gas.[63] As with chlorine, it is heavier than air and accumulates in the lower parts of a confined space or low to the ground. It is estimated that 80% of the deaths due to gas during World War I were due to phosgene. Industrially, it is used in the production of isocyanates and in the manufacture of dyestuffs and pharmaceuticals. The combustion of polyurethane may also produce phosgene, a risk to firefighters. Phosgene results whenever a volatile chlorinated compound comes into contact with a flame or hot metal, and so welders may be exposed when encountering chlorinated solvents with high-temperature arc welding. Degreasers containing chlorinated solvents may liberate phosgene if in contact with a hot metal surface.

Unfortunately, the irritant properties of phosgene are not sufficient to give warning of hazardous concentrations, as the sweet or musty odor is only detectable at 0.5 to 1.0 part per million, well above the recommended threshold limit value of 0.1 part per million.[88] Phosgene is relatively insoluble in water and is thus only a minor upper respiratory irritant. Exposure in animals to as little as 0.2 part per million for 5 days caused delayed onset of pulmonary edema in 41%,[89] while the acute lethal concentration in man has been estimated at 30 parts per million for several minutes.[90] Phosgene reacts with membrane water and is hydrolyzed over several hours to hydrochloric acid and carbon dioxide, which results in increased capillary permeability with release of lipooxygenase products.[91] Several industrial inhalation injuries have been reported.[92–94]

The concentration of gas is often unknown in acute exposures, but burning eyes and cough should occur at 5 to 10 parts per million. Following exposure, a latent period of 30 minutes to several hours typically elapses before the onset of pulmonary edema.[90] Unless a clear history of brief low-dose exposure has occurred, it is prudent to observe patients for at least eight hours following phosgene inhalation and to obtain a chest roentgenogram before discharge. Patients with eye, nose, or pharyngeal irritation, dyspnea, cough, or sputum production should be hospitalized and observed closely for 12 to 24 hours for the development of progressive pulmonary edema.[90]

Ammonia

Ammonia is a colorless gas with a distinctive pungent odor at room temperature and pressure.[95] It is widely used as fertilizer in the form of anhydrous or aqua ammonia or as the source of nitrogen for dry fertilizers. As it has a low boiling point and is easily liquified, it is used in refrigeration systems. Ammonia is also used in the manufacture of nitric acid, synthetic fibers, dyes, and plastics, and in the petroleum refining, chemical, and pharmaceutical industries.[96]

The odor threshold for ammonia is well below the least amount causing mucous membrane irritation. Ammonia exposures below 50 parts per million are unlikely to cause adverse effects.[95] Ammonia gas readily reacts with water to form an alkaline solution that will cause tissue necrosis and burns of skin or mucous membranes. Ammonia thus is primarily an upper respiratory irritant, and with its good warning properties, will provoke the exposed individual to escape quickly from exposure. Mild to moderate exposure to the gas will cause headache, nausea, vomiting, burning of the throat, and substernal pain. If anhydrous ammonia is splashed on the eyes or skin, it can result in severe burns and corneal damage.[19]

Acute industrial poisoning from ammonia usually results from the sudden accidental release of the liquid or gas, often in connection with the installation or repair of refrigeration equipment or in the chemical or fertilizer industries.[97] Several cases of fatal or near-fatal ammonia gas poisoning have been described involving farm ammonia tanks,[98] a railway car derailment,[99] a refrigerant coolant tank,[100] and an ammonia refrigeration plant.[101]

High concentrations of ammonia gas can cause diffuse tracheobronchitis and peripheral airway damage with bronchiolitis and pulmonary edema. Respiratory failure may ensue rapidly over several hours and require mechanical ventilation and positive airway pressure. Most victims of ammonia inhalation recover, but deaths due to respiratory failure have been reported.[102,103] Persistent bronchiectasis and hyperreactive airways have been reported in survivors of toxic ammonia inhalations.[99,100] Extensive cylindrical and saccular bronchiectasis was found on autopsy in a victim of ammonia gas inhalation who died 3 years after exposure.[104]

Nitrogen Dioxide

Nitrogen dioxide is one of the oxides of nitrogen, which include the anesthetic gas nitrous oxide and the colorless gas nitric oxide. Nitric oxide rapidly reacts with atmospheric oxygen to form nitrogen dioxide, a reddish-brown gas with a characteristic odor.[19] Both nitric oxide and nitrogen dioxide are formed when nitric acid reacts with reducing agents as well as by combustion of nitrogen-containing materials. The contact of nitric acid with organic matter produces nitrogen oxides and is an essential part of many industrial processes. Nitric acid is the second most important industrial acid, and nitric acid mist almost always contains nitrogen oxide gases.[12]

The potential for occupational exposure exists during the manufacture of nitric and sulfuric acids, explosives, fertilizers, cellulose compounds, and dyes. Exposure may also occur during metal etching and photoengraving and the cleaning of copper and brass. Nitric oxide is produced in welding arcs and flames and is rapidly oxidized to nitrogen dioxide. Oxides of nitrogen are found in exhaust from gasoline and diesel-powered machinery and may be a risk to coalminers as a result of blasting. Silo gases contain nitrogen dioxide and nitric oxide, in addition to carbon dioxide, and a unique clinical presentation in farmers is known as silo-filler's disease.[105] Firefighters are also at risk for exposure as a result of nitrocellulose combustion.[106]

The odor threshold for nitrogen dioxide is 0.5 part per million, and permissible occupational exposure is set at 5.0 parts per million.[19] Nitrogen dioxide is poorly soluble in water and thus primarily causes lower airway damage. Symptoms of mucous membrane irritation will occur at 15 to 25 parts per million, while acute pulmonary edema may follow exposure at 50 to 100 parts per million.[106] Severe respiratory toxicity due to nitrogen dioxide exposure has been reported from metal plating, detonation of explosives, a chemical plant leak, and silos.[105,107–111]

The mildest form of nitrogen dioxide toxicity results in cough, dyspnea, headache, and nausea, without clinically obvious pulmonary damage or permanent sequelae. At high concentrations of nitrogen dioxide, several clinical responses have been observed. Respiratory failure may occur within hours from laryngospasm or acute pulmonary edema, generally after very heavy exposure from a serious accident. The usual course of overexposure is one of delayed symptoms where respiratory distress develops after a period of several hours. Those surviving the initial effects may recover but after several weeks develop bronchiolitis fibrosa obliterans, a destructive process involving peripheral respiratory bronchioles. Persistent pulmonary function abnormality is uncommon, however.[112]

Methemoglobinemia will result if nitric oxide exposure occurs with nitrogen dioxide. Levels of 2% to 3% have been reported in arc welders and greater than 40% in silo-fillers.[112] Methemoglobin is hemoglobin with iron in the heme moiety oxidized to the ferric (Fe^{3+}) state. Because of this additional positive charge, the molecule is unable to carry oxygen.

Any patient with significant exposure to nitrogen dioxide should be hospitalized and observed for 48 hours for the development of respiratory distress. Although no controlled trials have been performed, high-dose corticosteroids have been reported to be of benefit in reducing the severity and length of respiratory illness due to nitrogen dioxide.[110] Methemoglobin should be measured, and if levels exceed 40% or the patient has a decreased level of consciousness, methylene blue should be administered IV at a dose of 1 to 2 mg/kg body weight (0.1 to 0.2 mL/kg) as a 1% solution over 5 minutes. If cyanosis persists after 1 hour, a repeat dose should be given. Total dose should not exceed 7 mg/kg.[40] As symptoms from bronchiolitis obliterans may occur in several weeks, close follow-up is recommended.

Other Irritant Gases

Ozone is a bluish gas with a characteristic pungent odor that is detectable at less than 0.1 part per million. It is a powerful oxidant that is relatively insoluble in water. Ozone is a major constituent of photochemical smog and is found naturally in the atmosphere as a result of the action of solar radiation and electrical storms.[19] Ozone can often be detected in the cabins of commercial aircraft at levels in excess of the recommended occupational exposure limit of 0.1 part per million.[63] Occupational exposure may occur during electric arc welding shielded by inert gases such as argon and helium; from disinfectants for food in cold storage rooms; in bleaching textiles, waxes, flour, mineral oils, and sugar; and in the rapid drying of varnishes and printing inks.[19]

Prolonged exercise during exposure to ozone at ambient air levels may lead to reversible symptoms of substernal chest discomfort, cough, and shortness of breath associated with a decline in FEV_1.[114,115] Pulmonary edema has been reported in workers exposed to ozone while arc welding.[12]

Sulfur dioxide is a colorless gas with a pungent odor that is widely used in the manufacture of sulfuric acid and sodium sulfite and in many other processes such as bleaching, fumigation, and refrigeration. It is generated as a byproduct of paper manufacturing and petroleum refining, and large quantities are produced in the smelting of sulfide ores of lead, zinc, iron, and copper.[12]

Sulfur dioxide is very soluble in water, forming sulfurous acid on contact with moist membranes.[88] Approximately 90% of inhaled sulfur dioxide is absorbed in the upper respiratory tract, and therefore sulfur dioxide will cause almost immediate coughing with significant exposure. The odor of sulfur dioxide is detectable at 0.3 to 10.0 parts per million. Irritation of the conjunctivae and nasal mucosa occurs between 5 and 10 parts per million, and parenchymal lung damage occurs above 50 parts per million.[76] Increased macrophage activity in bronchoalveolar lavage fluid has been detected with experimental exposures as low as 8 parts per million.[116] Long-term exposure to less than 1.5 parts per million of sulfur dioxide has been associated with increased symptoms of cough, phlegm, wheezing, and exertional dyspnea.[117] If an accident occurs and exposure over the recommended exposure limit of 5 parts per million results, this property of sulfur dioxide should prevent pulmonary injury if escape is possible. Acute high-dose exposures leading to severe injury are unusual, but have been reported from a sulfur fire in a ship hold, among commercial fishermen exposed to sodium bisulfite, and at a paper mill.[12] Upper airway injury predominated in these cases.

Asthmatics and individuals with underlying bronchial hyperreactivity may be more susceptible to low-level exposure to sulfur dioxide. Increases in airway resistance have been shown during exercise in asthmatics exposed to 0.1 part per million of sulfur dioxide.[113] Asthmatic individuals who work in industries with sulfur dioxide exposure may present with work-related exacerbations of asthma due to this effect. Long-term pulmonary sequelae of acute exposures to sulfur dioxide have been reported.[118]

Phosphine is a colorless gas with the odor of decaying fish. Exposure may occur either when acid or water comes into contact with metallic phosphides used in grain fumigation or during the generation of acetylene from impure calcium carbide.[19] Phosphine gas is widely used as a dopant in the manufacture of semiconductor integrated circuits, where the risk of exposure involves accidental release of compressed gas.[119] Lower-dose exposures result in upper respiratory irritation, while pulmonary edema has been noted in scattered case reports.[88]

Toxic Gases from Fires

Pulmonary insufficiency due to smoke inhalation is a major cause of fire-related deaths, accounting for about 80% of the approximately 8000 fatalities per year in the United States.[120] Firefighters are at particular risk as they are routinely exposed to hazardous fire and smoke. Three large hotel fires in 1980 and 1981 drew attention to the role of toxic smoke and hot gases in the death of the victims. Epidemiological evidence has shown that 80% of residential fire victims die from carbon monoxide poisoning or carbon monoxide poisoning plus contributory factors such as heart disease, alcohol, or burns.[121] Cyanide and other gases may contribute significantly to mortality. In addition, analysis of postmortem samples from victims of the MGM Grand Hotel fire in 1980 revealed that two-thirds had carboxyhemoglobin levels of less than 60%, suggesting that other toxic gases contributed to the deaths.[122]

Smoke is a suspension of small particles in hot air and gases. The composition of gases and particulates depends on the combustion materials, temperature, and concentration of oxygen.[121] Smoke at fire scenes can contain from 0.1% to 10% carbon monoxide; a 2-minute exposure during heavy exertion (as in firefighting) to 2% carbon monoxide can result in a lethal carboxyhemoglobin level of 60%.[123]

The thermal decomposition of materials such as polyvinyl chloride, polyurethane, nylon, cotton, and wool result in

Table 47-9 Toxic Products of Combustion

Substance	Toxic Products of Combustion
Wood, cotton, newspaper	Acrolein, acetaldehyde, formaldehyde, acetic acid, formic acid
Polyvinyl chloride	Hydrogen chloride, phosgene, chlorine
Petroleum products	Acrolein, acetic acid, formic acid
Nitrocellulose film	Oxides of nitrogen, acetic acid, formic acid
Polyurethane	Isocyanate, hydrogen cyanide
Polyfluorocarbons (Teflon)	Octafluoroisobutylene
Melamine resins	Ammonia, hydrogen cyanide
Polyester resins	Hydrogen chloride

Source: Adapted with permission from Coleman DL: Smoke inhalation. *West J Med* 135:300–309, 1981.

highly toxic gases that can cause both direct pulmonary injury and chemical asphyxia (Table 47-9). Hydrogen chloride, phosgene, ammonia, and acrolein are irritants that in high doses cause pulmonary edema. Hydrogen chloride is liberated from the combustion of acrylics and polyvinyl chloride, a common electrical wiring insulating material. Firefighters are exposed to smoldering plastics and synthetics from furniture, floor and wall coverings, textiles, and building materials. The "overhaul phase" when firefighters may have removed their self-contained breathing apparatus may be hazardous because of continued emission of toxic smoke and fumes.[124] Persistent respiratory problems among firefighters exposed to polyvinyl chloride has been reported.[125]

Hydrogen cyanide may be liberated from the thermal degradation of polyurethane and polyacrylonitrile. In one study, cyanide levels were higher than normal in 78% of fire deaths in the area of Glasgow, Scotland, and were in the lethal range in 12%.[126] Cyanide is usually detected along with elevated carboxyhemoglobin, and documented cases of fire death due to hydrogen cyanide alone are rare. There may be a synergistic effect of carbon monoxide and hydrogen cyanide in lowering the threshold for ventricular fibrillation.

Management of Smoke Inhalation

The management of smoke inhalation must be directed at the thermal and chemical injury as well as the systemic toxicity from carbon monoxide and cyanide (Table 47-10). The management of smoke inhalation has been the subject of recent reviews.[127–132] Smoke inhalation injury should be suspected in any patient with a history of being burned in a confined space.[130] Carbon monoxide intoxication should always be suspected in the fire victim and 100% oxygen immediately administered. Carboxyhemoglobin should be measured directly in all patients, although it may be normal if

Table 47-10 Management of the Smoke Inhalation Victim

Initial Evaluation

History
  Circumstances of injury?
  What material was burned?
  Steam exposure?
  Prior cardiopulmonary or CNS disease?
  Respiratory, cardiac, or CNS symptoms present?
Physical Examination
  Tachypnea
  Facial, oropharyngeal, nasal hair burns
  Hoarseness, stridor, wheezing, rales, rhonchi
  Abnormal cardiovascular or neurological findings
  Burn extent and other injuries
Laboratory
  Arterial blood gas
  Chest radiography
  Electrocardiogram
  Bedside spirometry
  Sputum for carbonaceous material
  Carboxyhemoglobin
  Cyanide level (if cyanide poisoning suspected)

Treatment

Assessment of airway patency
  Laryngoscopy
  Intubation if indicated
Humidified supplemental oxygen
Bronchodilators for bronchospasm
Replacement of fluid losses
Sputum Gram stain and antibiotics if indicated
Corticosteroids for severe bronchospasm

Source: Adapted with permission from Coleman DL: Smoke inhalation. *West J Med* 135:300–309, 1981.

oxygen therapy has been given prior to arrival in the emergency department.

Thermal injury as a result of temperatures 150°C or higher can result in burns to the face, oropharynx, and nasopharynx. Thermal damage is usually limited to the upper airway because, by the time smoke has reached the trachea, it has cooled and does not result in thermal damage. The likelihood of pulmonary inhalation injury is suggested by the presence of facial burns, singed nasal hairs, hoarseness, cough, dyspnea, and exposure in an enclosed space.[123] Airway or parenchymal injury should be strongly suspected in the presence of cutaneous burns. The presence of wheezing, rales, and carbonaceous sputum is an important sign.[133] The chest radiograph is usually normal in the early phase of inhalation injury, although it should be taken as a baseline. Arterial blood gases should be measured but also may be within normal limits and not predictive of subsequent pulmonary complications. Direct visualization of the larynx, trachea, and bronchus by fiberoptic bronchoscopy or direct laryngoscopy may identify patients with laryngeal edema who require intubation.[134,135]

Radioactive xenon lung scanning with a long washout phase has been used to predict subsequent respiratory complications, although false-positive scans may be found with pre-existing bronchitis, bronchiectasis, asthma, or pneumonia.[136] Fiberoptic bronchoscopy can identify airway inflammation, mucosal necrosis, the presence of soot and charring in the upper airway, and the likelihood of upper airway obstruction due to tracheal edema. Fiberoptic bronchoscopy and radioactive xenon scanning are 93% accurate in diagnosing inhalation injury.[132] Routine use of bronchoscopy or radioactive xenon scanning is not recommended, however.[130,137] Patients with a history of smoke inhalation and hoarseness, stridor, difficulty with phonation, tachypnea, wheezing, or rhonchi should have immediate laryngoscopy or bronchoscopy, and patients with laryngeal edema should be intubated.[123]

Patients with hypoxemia and bronchoconstriction should be treated with supplemental oxygen and bronchodilators. Airflow obstruction should be measured with simple spirometry. Mechanical ventilation may be required for patients with severe pulmonary edema, laryngeal obstruction, or difficulty handling secretions. Positive pressure may be necessary to maintain adequate oxygenation. Measurements of pulmonary capillary wedge pressure should guide fluid management. Corticosteroids should be reserved for use in patients with severe bronchospasm unresponsive to other bronchodilating agents. Because infection is so prevalent in burn patients with lung injury, daily sputum Gram stains should be done and treatment instituted if positive. Prophylactic antibiotics are not recommended.[133]

Cyanide toxicity may be suspected in a fire inhalation victim with unexplained metabolic acidosis and suggestive symptoms. After a blood cyanide level is drawn, treatment should be instituted immediately as described above.

Hospitalization is required in the presence of significant thermal burns or other injuries, physical findings suggestive of pulmonary injury, cardiac or central nervous system symptoms or signs, and abnormal chest radiograph, blood gases, carboxyhemoglobin, or pulmonary function tests.[123] The majority of smoke inhalation victims will manifest pulmonary injury within 12 to 24 hours after exposure, and so a period of observation at least this long is advised.[138] Permanent lung injury, including bronchiectasis and nonspecific airway hyperresponsiveness, has been documented after acute smoke inhalation.[139]

SYSTEMIC TOXINS

Several agents can cause systemic toxicity as a result of pulmonary or skin exposure. Unlike the chemical asphyxiants, clinical symptoms are due to a variety of mechanisms aside from tissue hypoxia.

Volatile Hydrocarbons

The organic solvents encompass a huge number of compounds that are used in practically every industry. The toxicity varies widely depending on physical or chemical properties, degree and duration of exposure, metabolic products, and site of organ damage. The organic solvents can be classified as aliphatic, aromatic, halogenated hydrocarbons, alcohols and glycols, ketones, plastics and epoxies, phenols and cresols. Exposure to all of these occurs primarily through inhalation and skin contact; nonpolar solvents are generally well absorbed through the dermal layer of the skin and significant toxicity can result from this route.

In general, emergencies as a result of hydrocarbon exposure will involve central nervous system depression from the narcotic action of nonpolar compounds. Overexposure to all solvents will acutely result in dizziness, headache, confusion, and drowsiness, followed by lethargy, coma, and respiratory arrest if escape is not immediate. Acute central nervous system symptoms generally resolve within 24 hours, although persistent vestibular and cognitive dysfunction has been reported after acute solvent intoxication.[140] Several solvents may also be associated with other systemic symptoms, which, on presentation to the emergency department, may be of importance to the treating physician.[141]

Among the aliphatic hydrocarbons, compounds containing 5 to 16 carbons are pharmacologically more active and result in narcosis.

Acutely, aromatic hydrocarbons such as *toluene* and *benzene* can cause renal and hepatic damage in large concentrations. Among the halogenated hydrocarbons, *carbon tetrachloride*, *chloroform*, and *2-nitropropane* are acutely hepatotoxic in addition to their anesthetic properties. *Methyl bromide*, a colorless, odorless gas with poor warning properties, is widely used as a fumigant. Acute exposure has resulted in deaths due to pulmonary edema, while chronic exposure may result in neurobehavioral symptoms.[142] *Trichloroethylene* and *tetrachloroethylene* are widely used as degreasing agents and have been implicated in sudden deaths due to ventricular dysrhythmias in workers as well as recreational drug abusers.[143,144] Acute overexposure to *ethylene dibromide*, used in grain fumigation, has caused deaths due to massive tissue necrosis.[6]

Among the alcohols and glycols, *methyl alcohol* (wood alcohol or methanol) is used in the manufacture of formaldehyde and other chemical derivatives and is a component in duplicating fluids, paint removers, stains, and varnishes. Industrial exposure can result in skin and pulmonary absorption with headaches, gait disturbance, weakness, nausea, vomiting, and inebriation. Blurriness and decreased vision with changes in color perception are common symptoms and are thought to result from formate, a metabolic product of methanol. *Methyl cellosolve* and *ethyl cellosolve*, two common glycol ethers, are components of photoresists used in the manufacture of integrated circuits and have been associated with bone marrow depression in addition to central nervous system depression.[145,146]

Formaldehyde, one of the common ketones, is a potent upper respiratory irritant that may aggravate underlying bronchial hyperreactivity.[147] Another ketone, *methyl n-butyl ketone,* has caused peripheral neuropathy in fabric workers and spray painters.[63]

Arsine and Stibine

Arsine is a highly toxic, colorless gas with a mild garlic odor. It is water soluble and readily absorbed through the respiratory tract. Arsine is generated when inorganic arsenic compounds contact sources of nascent hydrogen, as may occur in the chemical, smelting, and refining industry. Exposure to arsine has also been reported from galvanizing, soldering, and lead-plating operations. Arsine may be generated in lead-acid battery manufacture when lead-arsenic alloy comes into contact with acid.[148] Sewage fungi can also generate arsine in the presence of arsenic.[149] Arsine gas is used widely as a dopant in the manufacture of semiconductor chips.

Many cases of arsine poisoning due to accidental generation of the gas have been reported in the literature. Intoxication has been described from spraying water on slag metal, cleaning an industrial drain containing acid, purifying lead alloys, and reclaiming metal from flue dust. Arsine poisoning has occurred from enclosed spaces in the course of cleaning tanks and vats containing arsenic contaminants.[149] Two deaths have recently been reported from arsine gas used in the manufacture of semiconductors.[150,151]

The current standard for occupational exposure to arsine is 0.05 part per million averaged over an 8-hour work day. Exposure to 250 parts per million is instantly lethal, while exposure to 25 to 50 parts per million for 0.5 hour can be fatal.[149] Arsine causes rapid intravascular hemolysis of red blood cells. Arsine binds to hemoglobin with subsequent hemolysis, perhaps because of liberation of intracellular arsenic or binding to essential sulfhydryl groups necessary for cellular respiration.[152] Initial manifestations of arsine poisoning begin 2 to 36 hours after inhalation, with constitutional symptoms of headache, malaise, weakness, dizziness, and dyspnea followed by abdominal pain, nausea, and vomiting. These acute symptoms are followed in 4 to 6 hours by the passage of urine darkened by hemoglobin. Jaundice appears after 24 to 48 hours. The triad of abdominal pain, hematuria, and jaundice is characteristic of arsine poisoning, although all of these signs may not necessarily be present.[152] Acute exposure to high concentrations may also result in pulmonary edema.

Physical examination may reveal a bronze skin color and enlarged liver. Laboratory tests show a picture of hemolytic anemia, elevated plasma hemoglobin, and hemoglobinuria. A history of arsine exposure with a plasma hemoglobin of greater than 1.5% confirms the diagnosis of arsine poisoning. Urinary arsenic levels are not useful in the initial management of acute exposures, although they should be obtained to corroborate the diagnosis. Urinary arsenic levels have been reported as high as 2 mg/L (normal, less than 50 μg/dL).[152]

The treatment of choice for arsine poisoning is exchange transfusion. One author has recommended transfusion if serum hemoglobin is greater than 1.5%.[153] Renal dialysis should be instituted for acute renal failure. Hemolysis may continue for up to 4 days because of nondialyzable arsenic.[152] Death usually results from renal failure. Chelating agents are not recommended.

Stibine is produced accidentally from the generation of nascent hydrogen in the presence of antimony, and exposure can occur in metallurgical, welding, or cutting operations.[19] No recent cases of stibine poisoning have been reported. Like arsine, its toxic effect is due to hemolysis by binding to red blood cells. Treatment of stibine poisoning is similar to that for arsine.

Organophosphate Pesticides

Originally developed for use as a nerve gas during the 1930s, organophosphate pesticides are currently widely used in agriculture because of their insecticidal activity and relatively short environmental half-life. The workforce exposed to organophosphates includes the estimated 2.5 million migrant farm workers, as well as applicators, loaders, flaggers, and ground support crew. Workers in pesticide manufacturing industries are also at risk for exposure, as are pesticide formulating workers and structural pest control applicators.[63]

Organophosphate pesticides are highly lipid soluble and are effectively absorbed by skin, lungs, and gastrointestinal tract. In the occupational setting, dermal exposure is generally more important. The most common incidence of poisoning has been among agricultural workers during or shortly after spraying of crops. Organophosphates act as irreversible inhibitors of the enzyme acetylcholinesterase, resulting in an increase in endogenous acetylcholine at synaptic sites. Acetylcholinesterase is the neurotransmitter at parasympathetic and myoneural junctions and at autonomic ganglia. The clinical presentation of organophosphate poisoning is predictable from the biochemical mechanism of action, with signs and symptoms that mimic the muscarinic, nicotinic, and central nervous system actions of acetylcholine (Table 47-11).

The time interval between exposure and the onset of symptoms varies with the route and degree of exposure, but symptoms generally begin within 12 hours and always within 24 hours.[154] After inhalation of vapors or aerosols, symptoms of eye and respiratory tract irritation occur within minutes. With ingestion, gastric irritation will initially cause nausea and vomiting. With mild poisoning, symptoms

Table 47-11 Signs and Symptoms of Organophosphate Poisoning

Muscarinic Manifestations	
Bronchial tree	Chest tightness, wheezing, dyspnea, bronchial secretions, cough
GI tract	Nausea, vomiting, abdominal cramps, diarrhea, tenesmus, incontinence
Sweat glands	Increased sweating
Salivary glands	Increased salivation
Lacrimal glands	Increased lacrimation
Cardiovascular	Bradycardia, fall in blood pressure
Pupils	Miosis, occasionally unequal
Ciliary body	Blurring of vision
Bladder	Frequency, incontinence
Nicotinic Manifestations	
Striated muscle	Twitching, fasciculation, cramp, weakness, respiratory paralysis
Sympathetic ganglia	Pallor, tachycardia, elevation in blood pressure
Central Nervous System Manifestations	Giddiness, tension, anxiety, restlessness, headache, tremor, drowsiness, difficulty in concentrating, slurred speech, confusion, ataxia, generalized weakness, convulsions, coma, respiratory depression, hypotension

Source: Adapted with permission from Namba T, Nolte CT, Jackrel J, Grob D: Poisoning due to organophosphate insecticides: Acute and chronic manifestations. *Amer J Med* 50:475–492, 1971.

include chest tightness, increased sweating and salivation, nausea, vomiting, diarrhea, and abdominal cramps. With moderate to severe intoxication, coughing, wheezing, increased bronchial secretions, and pupillary constriction occur. Hypotension and involuntary urination and defecation are signs of severe poisoning.

Nicotinic effects result from accumulation of acetylcholine at the endings of motor nerves to smooth muscles and autonomic ganglia. Early signs are weakness and easy fatigue, followed by involuntary twitching, fasciculations, and cramps; and in severe cases, paralysis of respiratory muscles. Central nervous system effects of acetylcholine are responsible for slurred speech, ataxia, depression of respiratory and circulatory centers, convulsions, and central respiratory paralysis. Nicotinic action at autonomic ganglia may in severe intoxication mask the muscarinic action on the heart and result in tachycardia.[34]

Diagnosis

The diagnosis of organophosphate poisoning is made by the appropriate history together with compatible signs and symptoms and the measurement of plasma and/or red blood cell cholinesterase. Red blood cell cholinesterase (true cholinesterase) levels show a wide variation in normal values, and therefore pre-exposure baseline values are critical in the interpretation of single samples. Enzyme depression is usually apparent immediately after, or within 12 to 24 hours of, significant absorption of organophosphate. In acute poisoning, approximately 25% of red blood cell cholinesterase inhibition is evidence that excessive absorption took place.[155] With more chronic exposure, mild symptoms may not correlate with depression of cholinesterase activity, and total inhibition of plasma cholinesterase has been noted in the absence of overt signs of poisoning.[34,156]

About 3% of individuals have a genetically determined low level of plasma cholinesterase. These atypical cholinesterases can be detected in vitro by the inhibitor dibucaine; the degree of inhibition is expressed as the "dibucaine number." These individuals are particularly susceptible to the action of organophosphates. Plasma cholinesterase may also be decreased with advanced liver disease, malnutrition, and chronic alcoholism and may be elevated in the nephrotic syndrome and hyperthyroidism.[155] Red blood cell cholinesterase more closely reflects the degree of inhibition of synaptic cholinesterase and is less likely to be influenced by other factors. Plasma cholinesterase is measured more simply and accurately; given these factors, both red blood cell and plasma cholinesterase should be measured.[157]

Treatment

All patients with suspected or documented organophosphate poisoning should be hospitalized. Treatment of organophosphate poisoning must not be delayed while awaiting laboratory confirmation of decreased cholinesterase. Because of rapid and continuous skin absorption, decontamination of the victim must be done immediately by removal of all clothing and washing the skin with soap and water. Maintenance of a clear airway and adequate oxygenation is critical, as copious secretions, hypoxemia, and skeletal muscle paralysis are the usual causes of death in severe cases. Intubation and mechanical ventilation may be necessary.

Atropine is given as the specific antagonist of the muscarinic effects of excess cholinesterase. It is not adequate for the nicotinic manifestations (muscle weakness, twitching, and respiratory depression), and it does not reverse the binding of organophosphate to acetylcholinesterase. Atropine should be administered intravenously, 2 to 4 mg every 5 to 15 minutes until atropinization is achieved with tachycardia, flushing, dry mouth, and/or dilated pupils. The effects of atropine begin in 1 to 2 minutes and are maximal in 8 minutes. Atropine should be given in repeated doses for 12 hours or longer depending on the severity of the poisoning. As much as several hundred milligrams of atropine may have to be administered over a 24-hour period.

Pralidoxime chloride (Protopam chloride or 2-PAM) should be given in conjunction with atropine, 1 g IV slowly at no more than 0.5 mg/min. 2-PAM promotes the breaking of the bond between acetylcholinesterase and the phosphorus moiety derived from the pesticide. The effectiveness of 2-PAM in reversing cholinesterase inhibition is dependent on its early administration following poisoning, because the "aged" phosphorylated enzyme is resistant to reactivation after 12 to 24 hours. The effects of 2-PAM occur within 10 to 40 minutes with recovery of weakness and decrease in fasciculations and other primary nicotinic symptoms. 2-PAM should be repeated in 1 to 2 hours if needed, then at 10- to 12-hour intervals thereafter. When clinical symptoms recur in patients with severe poisoning, 2-PAM should be infused at a rate of up to 0.5 mg/hour.[154]

Morphine, aminophylline, or theophylline are not recommended, as they have weak anti-acetylcholinesterase activity. Valium, 5 to 10 mg intravenously, may be given for convulsions unresponsive to atropine and 2-PAM.[156]

Red blood cell cholinesterase regenerates at a rate of approximately 1% per day, and plasma cholinesterase at a rate of 25% in 5 to 7 days; therefore acetylcholinesterase levels are not particularly useful clinically in following patients after acute poisoning, as symptomatic recovery occurs while enzyme levels are still decreased. However, individuals should not be allowed to return to work until blood cholinesterase activity has reached the pre-exposure value or, if no baseline cholinesterase is available, the normal range.

REFERENCES

1. United States Bureau of Labor Statistics. *Occupational Injuries and Illnesses in the United States by Industry, 1982*. Washington, DC: US Government Printing Office; 1984.
2. Leading work-related diseases and injuries—United States. *MMWR*. 1984;33:213.
3. Surveillance of occupational injuries treated in hospital emergency rooms—United States. *MMWR*. 1983;32:89.
4. Ries P. Episodes of persons injured: United States, 1975. *Advance Data*. 1978;18:1–12.
5. Discher DP, Kleinman GD, Foster FJ. *Pilot Study for the Development of an Occupational Disease Surveillance Method*. NIOSH Publication no 75–162, 1975.
6. Letz GA, Pond SM, Osterloh JD, et al. Two fatalities after acute occupational exposure to ethylene dibromide. *JAMA*. 1984;252:248–253.
7. Himmelstein JS, Frumkin H. The right to know about toxic exposures: implications for physicians. *N Engl J Med*. 1985;312:687–690.
8. Surada A, Agnew J. Deaths from asphyxiation and poisoning at work in the United States 1984-6. *Br J Ind Med*. 1989;46:541–546.
9. National Institutes for Occupational Safety and Health. *A Guide to Safety in Confined Spaces*. Morgantown, West Virginia. DHHS Publication no 87-113, 1987.
10. National Institute for Occupational Safety and Health. *Occupational Exposure to Carbon Dioxide*. DHEW Publication no 76–194, 1976.
11. Patty FA, ed. *Industrial Hygiene and Toxicology*. 3rd ed. New York: Wiley Interscience; 1978.
12. Hamilton A, Hardy H. *Industrial Toxicology*. Littleton, MA: Wright; 1983.

13. Fatalities attributed to methane asphyxia in manure waste pits—Ohio, Michigan, 1989. *MMWR.* 1989;38:583–586.
14. Ilano AL, Raffin TA. Management of carbon monoxide poisoning. *Chest.* 1990;97:165–169.
15. Thom SR, Keim LW. Carbon monoxide poisoning: a review of epidemiology, pathophysiology, clinical findings, and treatment options including hyperbaric oxygen therapy. *Clin Toxicol.* 1989;27:141–156.
16. Penny DG. Acute carbon monoxide poisoning: animal models: a review. *Toxicology.* 1990;62:123–160.
17. Fisher J, Rubin K. Occult carbon monoxide poisoning. *Arch Intern Med.* 1982;142:1270–1271.
18. Thompson M, Henry JA. Carbon monoxide poisoning: poisons unit experience over five years. *Hum Toxicol.* 1983;2:335–338.
19. Key M, Henschel A, Butler J, et al. *Occupational Diseases: A Guide to Their Recognition.* DHEW Publication no 77–181, 1978.
20. Carbon monoxide intoxication associated with use of a gasoline-powered resurfacing machine at an ice-skating rink—Pennsylvania. *MMWR.* 1984;33:49–51.
21. Cobb N, Etzel RA. Unintentional carbon monoxide–related deaths in the United States, 1979 through 1988. *JAMA.* 1991;266:659–663.
22. Whorton MD. Carbon monoxide intoxication: a review of 14 patients. *JACEP.* 1976;5:505–509.
23. Atkins EH, Baker EL. Exacerbation of coronary artery disease by occupational carbon monoxide exposure: a report of two fatalities and a review of the literature. *Am J Ind Med.* 1985;7:73–79.
24. Burney RE, Wu S, Nemiroff MJ. Mass carbon monoxide poisoning: clinical effects and results of treatment in 184 victims. *Ann Emerg Med.* 1982;11:394–399.
25. Carbon monoxide poisoning—South Dakota. *MMWR.* 1985;34:113–114.
26. Stewart RD, Hake CL. Paint-remover hazard. *JAMA.* 1976;235:398–401.
27. Rioux JP, Myers RA. Methylene chloride poisoning: a paradigmatic review. *J Emerg Med.* 1988;6:227–238.
28. Rudge FW. Treatment of methylene chloride induced carbon monoxide poisoning with hyperbaric oxygenation. *Mil Med.* 1990;155:570–572.
29. Goldbaum LR, Orellano T, Dergal E. Mechanism of the toxic action of carbon monoxide. *Ann Clin Lab Sci.* 1976;6:372–376.
30. Somogyi E, Balogh I, Bubanyi G, et al. New findings concerning the pathogenesis of acute carbon monoxide poisoning. *Am J Forens Med Pathol.* 1981;2:31.
31. Yokoyama K: Effect of perfluoro chemical emulsion in acute carbon monoxide poisoning in rats. *Jpn J Surg.* 1978;4:342–352.
32. Turino G. Effect of carbon monoxide on the cardiorespiratory system. *Circulation.* 1981;63:253A–259A.
33. NIOSH recommendations for occupational standards. *MMWR.* 1984;32 (suppl):1S–22S.
34. Doull J, Klassen CD, Amdur MO. *Casarett and Doull's Toxicology.* New York: Macmillan; 1980.
35. Marius-Nunez AL. Myocardial infarction with normal coronary arteries after acute exposure to carbon monoxide. *Chest.* 1990;97:491–494.
36. Castle SP, Lapham SC, Troutman WG. Carbon monoxide intoxication: diagnostic considerations. *JAMA.* 1984;251:2350.
37. Kirkpatrick JN. Occult carbon monoxide poisoning. *West J Med.* 1987;146:52–56.
38. Smith JS, Brandon S. Morbidity from acute carbon monoxide poisoning at a three year followup. *Br Med J.* 1973;1:319–321.
39. Grace TW, Platt FW. Subacute carbon monoxide poisoning: another great imitator. *JAMA.* 1981;246:1698–1700.
40. Hansen W, ed. *Toxic Emergencies.* New York: Churchill Livingstone; 1984.
41. Myers RA, Britten JS. Are arterial blood gases of value in treatment decisions for carbon monoxide poisoning? *Crit Care Med.* 1989;17:139–142.
42. Heckerling PS, Leikin JB, Maturen A, Terzian CG, Segarra DP. Screening hospital admissions from the emergency department for occult carbon monoxide poisoning. *Am J Emerg Med.* 1990;8:301–304.
43. Turnbull TL, Hart RG, Strange GR, et al. Emergency department screening for unsuspected carbon monoxide exposure. *Ann Emerg Med.* 1988;17:478–483.
44. Thom SR. Smoke inhalation. *Emerg Med Clin North Am.* 1989;7:371–387.
45. Davis SM, Levy RC. High carboxyhemoglobin level without acute or chronic findings. *J Emerg Med.* 1984;1:539–542.
46. Goldfrank LR, Lewin NA, Kirstein RH, Weisman RS, Flomenbaum NE. Carbon monoxide. In: Goldfrank LR, ed. *Goldfrank's Toxicologic Emergencies.* Norwalk, CT: Appleton-Century-Crofts; 1990.
47. Myers RAM, Snyder SK, Linberg S, Cowley RA. Value of hyperbaric oxygen in suspected carbon monoxide poisoning. *JAMA.* 1981;246:2478–2480.
48. Kindwall EP. Carbon monoxide poisoning and cyanide poisoning. *HBO Rev.* 1980;1:115–122.
49. Proudfoot AT. Carbon monoxide poisoning—recent advances. *Acta Clin Belg.* 1990;13:61–68.
50. Risk-benefit analysis in chest medicine: some defenders of hyperbaric medicine. *Chest.* 1988;94:414–416.
51. Grim PS, Gottlieb LJ, Boddle A, Batson E. Hyperbaric oxygen therapy. *JAMA.* 1990;263:2216–2220.
52. Sloan EP, Murphy DG, Hart R, et al. Complications and protocol considerations in carbon monoxide–poisoned patients who require hyperbaric oxygen therapy: report from a ten-year experience. *Ann Emerg Med.* 1989;18:629–634.
53. Murphy DG, Sloan EP, Hart RG, Narasimhan K, Barreca RS. Tension pneumothorax associated with hyperbaric oxygen therapy. *Am J Emerg Med.* 1991;9:176–179.
54. National Institute for Occupational Safety and Health. *Occupational Exposure to Hydrogen Cyanide.* DHEW Publication no 77–108, 1977.
55. Nerlan DE, Benz FW, Babiuk C. Effects of cysteine isomers and derivatives on acute acrylonitrile toxicity. *Drug Metab. Rev.* 1989;20:233–246.
56. Way J. Cyanide intoxication and its mechanism of antagonism. *Annu Rev Pharmacol Toxicol.* 1984;24:451–481.
57. Edwards AC, Thomas ID. Cyanide poisoning. *Lancet.* 1978;1:92.
58. Kulig KW, Ballantyne B. *Cyanide toxicity.* Washington, DC: Agency for Toxic Substances and Disease Research, US Department of Health and Human Services; 1991.
59. Blanc P, Hogan M, Mallin K, et al. Cyanide intoxication among silver-reclaiming workers. *JAMA.* 1985;253:367–371.
60. Graham DL, Laman D, Theodore J, et al. Acute cyanide poisoning complicated by lactic acidosis and pulmonary edema. *Arch Intern Med.* 1977;137:1051–1055.
61. Arena JM. *Poisoning.* 3rd ed. Springfield, IL: Thomas; 1974.
62. Goldfrank LR, Bresnitz EA. Toxic inhalants, including cyanide. In: Goldfrank LR, ed. *Goldfrank's Toxicologic Emergencies.* Norwalk, CT: Appleton-Century-Crofts; 1990.

63. Rom WN. *Environmental and Occupational Medicine*. Boston: Little, Brown; 1983.
64. Glass DC. A review of the health effects of hydrogen sulphide exposure. *Ann Occup Hyg*. 1990;34:323–327.
65. Stine RJ, Slosberg B, Beacham BE. Hydrogen sulfide intoxication: a case report and discussion of treatment. *Ann Intern Med*. 1976;85:756–758.
66. National Institute for Occupational Safety and Health. *Occupational Exposure to Hydrogen Sulfide*. DHEW Publication no 77–158, 1977.
67. Beauchamp RO, Bus JS, Popp JA, et al. A critical review of the literature on hydrogen sulfide toxicity. *CRC Rev Toxicol*. 1984;13:25–97.
68. Smith RP, Gosselin RE. Hydrogen sulfide poisoning. *JOM*. 1979;21:93–97.
69. Osbern LN, Crapo RO. Dung lung: a report of toxic exposure to manure. *Ann Intern Med*. 1981;95:312–314.
70. Parra O, Monso E, Gallego M, Morera J. Inhalation of hydrogen sulphide: a case of subacute manifestations and long term sequelae. *Br J Ind Med*. 1991;48:286–287.
71. McAnnelley BH, Lowry WT, Oliver RD. Determination of inorganic sulfide and cyanide in blood using specific ion electrodes: application to the investigation of hydrogen sulfide and cyanide poisoning. *J Analyt Toxicol*. 1979;3:111.
72. Jappinen P, Tenhunen R. Hydrogen sulphide poisoning: blood sulphide concentration and changes in haem metabolism. *Br J Ind Med*. 1990;47:283–285.
73. Peters JW. Hydrogen sulfide poisoning in a hospital setting. *JAMA*. 1981;246:1588–1589.
74. Tvedt B, Skyberg K, Aaserud O, Hobblesland A, Mathieson T. Brain damage caused by hydrogen sulfide: a followup study of six patients. *Am J Ind Med*. 1991;20:91–101.
75. Wegman DH, Eisen EA. Acute irritants: more than a nuisance. *Chest*. 1990;97:773–775.
76. Schwartz DA. Acute inhalational injury. *Occup Med*. 1987;2:297–319.
77. Gas deaths in India exceed 1000, with thousands hurt. *New York Times*. December 5, 1984.
78. Horvath EP, doPico GA, Barbee RA, et al. Nitrogen dioxide-induced pulmonary disease: five new cases and a review of the literature. *JOM*. 1978;20:103–110.
79. Gapany-Gapanavicius M, Yellin A, Almog S, et al. Pneumomediastinum: a complication of chlorine exposure from mixing household cleaning agents. *JAMA*. 1982;248:349–350.
80. Chlorine poisoning. *Lancet*. 1984;1:321–322. Editorial.
81. Kaufman J, Burkons D. Clinical, roentgenographic, and physiologic effects of acute chlorine exposure. *Arch Environ Health*. 1971;23:29–34.
82. Hasan FM, Hehshan A, Fuleihan F. Resolution of pulmonary dysfunction following acute chlorine exposure. *Arch Environ Health*. 1983;38:76–80.
83. Beach FXM, Jones ES, Scarrow GD. Respiratory effects of chlorine gas. *Br J Ind Med*. 1969;26:231–236.
84. Kowitz TA, Reba RC, Parker RT. Effects of chlorine gas on respiratory function. *Arch Environ Health*. 1967;14:545–558.
85. Schwartz DA, Smith DD, Lakshminarayan S. The pulmonary sequelae associated with accidental inhalation of chlorine gas. *Chest*. 1990;97:820–825.
86. First-aid reports of acute chlorine gassing among pulpmill workers as predictors of lung health consequences. *Am J Ind Med*. 1991;20:71–81.
87. Kennedy SM, Enarson DA, Janssen RG, Chan-Yeung M. Lung health consequences of reported accidental chlorine gas exposures among pulpmill workers. *Am Rev Respir Dis*. 1991;143:74–79.
88. Proctor NH, Hughes JP. *Chemical Hazards of the Workplace*. Philadelphia: Lippincott; 1978.
89. Cucinell SA, Arsenal E. Review of the toxicity of long-term phosgene exposure. *Arch Environ Health*. 1974;28:272–275.
90. Diller WF. Medical phosgene problems and their possible solution. *JOM*. 1978;20:189–193.
91. Guo YL, Kennedy TP, Michael JR, et al. Mechanism of phosgene-induced lung toxicity: role of arachidonate mediators. *J Appl Physiol*. 1990;69:1615–1622.
92. Bradley BL, Unger KM. Phosgene inhalation: a case report. *Tex Med*. 1982;78:51–53.
93. Everett ED, Overholt EL. Phosgene poisoning. *JAMA*. 1969;205:103–105.
94. Fabre M, Boudet F, Boe M, et al. Intoxications par le Phosgene. *Toxicol Eur Res*. 1983;5:185–188.
95. Swontinsky RB, Chase KH. Health effects of exposure to ammonia: scant information. *Am J Ind Med*. 1990;17:515–521.
96. National Institute for Occupational Safety and Health. *Occupational Exposure to Ammonia*. DHEW Publication no 74–136, 1974.
97. Millea TP, Kucan JO, Smoot EC. Anhydrous ammonia injuries. *J Burn Care Rehabil*. 1989;10:448–453.
98. Levy DM, Divertie MB, Litzow TJ, et al. Ammonia burns of the face and respiratory tract. *JAMA*. 1964;190:873–876.
99. Kass I, Zamel N, Dobry CA, et al. Bronchiectasis following ammonia burns of the respiratory tract: a review of two cases. *Chest*. 1972;62:282–285.
100. Flury KE, Dines DE, Rodarte JR, et al. Airway obstruction due to inhalation of ammonia. *Mayo Clin Proc*. 1983;58:389–393.
101. Weiser JR, Mackenroth T. Acute inhalatory mass ammonia intoxication with fatal course. *Exp Pathol*. 1989;37:291–295.
102. Price SK, Hughes JE, Morrison SC, et al. Fatal ammonia inhalation: a case report with autopsy findings. *SA Med J*. 1983;64:952–955.
103. Montague JJ, MacNeil AM. Mass ammonia inhalation. *Chest*. 1980;77:496–498.
104. Hoeffler HB, Schweppe HI, Greenberg SD. Bronchiectasis following pulmonary ammonia burn. *Arch Pathol Lab Med*. 1982;106:686–687.
105. Douglas WW, Hepper NG, Colby TV. *Mayo Clin Proc*. 1989;64:291–304.
106. National Institute for Occupational Safety and Health. *Occupational Exposure to Oxides of Nitrogen*. DHEW Publication no 76–149, 1976.
107. Fleming GM, Chester EH, Montenegro HD. Dysfunction of small airways following pulmonary injury due to nitrogen dioxide. *Chest*. 1979;75:720.
108. Muller B. Nitrogen dioxide intoxication after a mining accident. *Respiration*. 1969;26:249–261.
109. Tse RL, Bockman AA. Nitrogen dioxide toxicity: report of four cases in firemen. *JAMA*. 1970;212:1341–1344.
110. Morrow PE. Toxicological data on NOX: an overview. *Environ Res*. 1984;34:205–227.
111. Ramirez RJ, Dowell AR. Silo-filler's disease: nitrogen dioxide-induced lung injury. *Ann Intern Med*. 1971;74:569–576.
112. Fleetham JA. Methemoglobinemia and the oxides of nitrogen. *N Engl J Med*. 1978;298:1130.

113. Sheppard D, Saisho A, Nadel J. Exercise increases sulfur dioxide-induced bronchoconstriction in asthmatic subjects. *ARRD*. 1981;123:486.
114. Kinney PL, Ware JH, Spengler JD, Dockery DW, Speizer FE, Ferris BG. Short-term pulmonary function change in association with ozone levels. *Am Rev Respir Dis*. 1989;139:56–61.
115. Lippman M. Effects of ozone on respiratory function and structure. *Annu Rev Public Health*. 1989;10:49–67.
116. Sandstrom T, Stjernberg N, Anderson MC, Kolmodin-Hedman B, Lundgren R, Angstrom T. Is the short-term limit value for sulphur dioxide exposure safe? Effects of controlled chamber exposure investigated with bronchoalveolar lavage. *Br J Ind Med*. 1989;46:200–203.
117. Osterman JW, Greaves IA, Smith TJ, Hammond SK, Robins JM, Theriault G. Respiratory symptoms associated with low level sulphur dioxide exposure in silicon carbide production workers. *Br J Ind Med*. 1989;46:629–635.
118. Rabinovitch S, Greyson ND, Weiser W, Hoffstein V. Clinical and laboratory features of acute sulfur dioxide inhalation poisoning: two-year followup. *Am Rev Respir Dis*. 1989;139:556–558.
119. Wade R. *Semiconductor Industry Study, 1981*. California Department of Industrial Relations, Division of Occupational Safety and Health, 1982.
120. Crapo RO. Smoke-inhalation injuries. *JAMA*. 1981;246:1694–1696.
121. Terrill JB, Montgomery RR, Reinhardt CF. Toxic gases from fires. *Science*. 1978;200:1343–1347.
122. Birky M, Malek D, Paabo M. Study of biological samples obtained from victims of MGM Grand Hotel fire. *Anal Toxicol*. 1983;7:265–271.
123. Coleman D. Smoke inhalation. *West J Med*. 1981;135:300–309.
124. Dyer RF, Esch VH. Polyvinyl chloride toxicity in fires: hydrogen chloride toxicity in fire fighters. *JAMA*. 1976;235:393–397.
125. Markowitz JS, Gutterman EM, Schwartz S, Link B, Gorman SM. Acute health effects among firefighters exposed to a polyvinyl chloride (PVC) fire. *Am J Epidemiol*. 1989;129:1023–1031.
126. Anderson RA, Harland WA. Fire deaths in the Glasgow area (III): the role of hydrogen cyanide. *Med Sci Law*. 1982;22:35–40.
127. Haponik EF. Smoke inhalation. *Am Rev Respir Dis*. 1988;138:1060–1063.
128. Kinsella J. Smoke inhalation. *Burns*. 1988;14:269–279.
129. Prien T, Traber DL. Toxic smoke compounds and inhalation injury—a review. *Burns*. 1988;14:451–460.
130. Heimbach DM, Waeckerle JF. Inhalation injuries. *Ann Emerg Med*. 1988;17:1316–1320.
131. Young CJ, Moss J. Smoke inhalation: diagnosis and treatment. *J Clin Anesth*. 1989;1:377–386.
132. Pruitt BA, Cioffi WG, Shimazu T, Ikeuchi H, Mason AD. Evaluation and management of patients with inhalation injury. *J Trauma*. 1990;30:S63–S68.
133. Fein A, Leff A, Hopewell PC. Pathophysiology and management of the complications resulting from fire and the inhaled products of combustion: review of the literature. *Crit Care Med*. 1980;8:94–98.
134. Moylan JA, Chan C. Inhalation injury—an increasing problem. *Ann Surg*. 1978;188:34–37.
135. Wanner A, Cutchavaree A. Early recognition of upper airway obstruction following smoke inhalation. *ARRD*. 1973;108:1421–1422.
136. Agee RN, Long JM, Hunt JL, et al. Use of 133-Xenon in early diagnosis of inhalation injury. *J Trauma*. 1976;16:218–224.
137. Clark WR, Bonaventura M, Myers W. Smoke inhalation and airway management at a regional burn unit: 1974–1983. Part 1: diagnosis and consequences of smoke inhalation. *J Burn Care Rehabil*. 1989;10:52–62.
138. Mellins RB, Park S. Respiratory complications of smoke inhalation in victims of fires. *J Pediatr*. 1975;87:1–7.
139. Moisan TC. Prolonged asthma after smoke inhalation: a report of three cases and a review of previous reports. *J Occup Med*. 1991;33:458–461.
140. Hodgson MJ, Furman J, Ryan C, Durrant J, Kern E. Encephalopathy and vestibulopathy following short-term hydrocarbon exposure. *J Occup Med*. 1989;31:51–54.
141. Flanagan RJ, Ruprah M, Meredith TJ, Ramsey JD. An introduction to the clinical toxicology of volatile substances. *Drug Safety*. 1990;5:359–383.
142. Hine CH. Methyl bromide poisoning: a report of ten cases. *JOM*. 1969;11:1.
143. King GS, Smialek JE, Troutman WG. Sudden death in adolescents resulting from the inhalation of typewriter correction fluid. *JAMA*. 1985;253:1604–1606.
144. Klinefeld M, Tabershaw IR. Trichloroethylene toxicity: a report of five fatal cases. *Arch Ind Hyg*. 1954;10:134.
145. Cohen R. Reversible subacute ethylene glycol monomethyl ether toxicity associated with microfilm production: a case report. *Am J Ind Med*. 1984;6:441–446.
146. Cullen MR, Rado T, Waldron JA, et al. Bone marrow injury in lithographers exposed to glycol ethers. *Arch Environ Health*. 1983;38:347–353.
147. Frigas E, Filley WV, Reed CE. Bronchial challenge with formaldehyde gas: lack of bronchoconstriction in 13 patients suspected of having formaldehyde-induced asthma. *Mayo Clin Proc*. 1984;59:295–298.
148. Landrigan PJ, Costello RJ, Stringer WT. Occupational exposure to arsine: an epidemiological reappraisal of current standards. *Scand J Work Environ Health*. 1982;8:169–177.
149. National Institute for Occupational Safety and Health. *Arsine (Arsenic Hydride) Poisoning in the Workplace*. DHEW Publication no 79–142, 1979.
150. Blake A. MIT technician dies on the job; chemical fumes are suspected. *Boston Globe*. June 16, 1982.
151. Hamilton R. M/A-Com worker dies of poisoning: possible suicide. *Boston Bus J*. July 2–8, 1984.
152. Fowler BA, Weissberg JB. Arsine poisoning. *N Engl J Med*. 1974;291:1171–1174.
153. Pinto SS. Arsine poisoning: Evaluation of the acute phase. *JOM*. 1976;18:633–635.
154. Namba T, Nolte CT, Jackrel J, et al. Poisoning due to organophosphate insecticides: acute and chronic manifestations. *Am J Med*. 1971;50:475–492.
155. Morgan DP. *Recognition and Management of Pesticide Poisonings*. US Environmental Protection Agency no 540/9–80–005, 1982.
156. Hayes W. *Pesticides in Man*. Baltimore: Williams & Wilkins; 1982.
157. Lauwerys R. *Industrial Chemical Exposure: Guidelines for Biological Monitoring*. Davis, CA: Biomedical Publications; 1983.

48. Substance Abuse

CARL KLINGELBERGER, MD
DANIEL SHINE, MD

The chapter begins with an overview of the social and national implications of substance abuse, followed by a discussion of the general topics relevant to these substances. It concludes with a review of each class of drug and the obstetrical and neonatal complications of drug abuse. Although the emergent medical aspects of illicit substance abuse are the primary focus, consideration of its societal impact is of paramount importance. The solution to this national crisis will not be a medical solution, but a combined effort by the major elements of society.

The socioeconomic ramifications of substance abuse are of tremendous national and international importance. The use of illicit drugs adversely affects almost every nation by causing human suffering and personal destruction, draining precious economic resources, and fueling a violent crime epidemic. During the past 20 years, few problems in the United States have risen to such national recognition. No other topic in medicine has been labeled a threat to national security or become a multibillion dollar business for organized crime. In 1980, it was estimated that United States citizens spent $79 billion on the purchase of illicit substances.[1] The trade in and use of illicit substances have been associated with the majority of violent crimes committed and become a new mission for the US military to defend against and the impetus for a number of social programs attempting to combat its societal impact. The export of cocaine is the major industry for organized criminal elements of several South American nations; citizens in regions of the former Soviet Union, facing economic disaster, have turned to the export of opium as a source of revenue.

Millions of families have been affected by illicit substance use. Family members have become drug addicts, casualties of drug-related motor vehicle accidents, or victims of violent crime connected with drug trafficking. It is impossible to assess accurately the true damage that has been wrought by the most recent cocaine epidemic of the 1980s in terms of potential lifetime productivity lost, deterioration of the infrastructure of major segments of society, and the accelerated spread of the acquired immunodeficiency syndrome (AIDS) epidemic. Although statistics from the National Institute of Drug Abuse indicate that we have past the peak of this epidemic, little comfort can be taken in this knowledge as long as millions of Americans are still using cocaine and other illicit substances daily and violent crime continues to plague our cities.

The significant substances of abuse are ethanol, tobacco, and illicit drugs. Alcohol and tobacco will not be dealt with in any detail in this chapter except to demonstrate a comparison of relative usage rates. Table 48-1 represents the population estimates derived from the 1991 National Household Survey on Drug Abuse.[2] This is a voluntary survey of 32,594 individuals representing a total population of 202.9 million people and does not include institutionalized or homeless people, which implies that these estimates are undoubtedly below the actual numbers. The National Household Survey has been conducted for 11 years. It provides information on prevalence, trends, and correlates of drug use. Table 48-2 provides data on the drug usage over the past year and past month for 1991[2] thereby allowing estimates of "regular" users of each illicit substance.

Table 48-1 1991 Household Survey of Substance Usage (millions)†

Drug	Past Year	Past Month
Alcohol	138.2	103.2
Tobacco	74.7	61.7
Illicit drugs*	26.1	12.6

*Illicit drug is defined as marijuana, nonmedical use of psychotherapeutics, inhalants, cocaine, hallucinogens, and heroin.
†Survey was conducted based on sample size of 32,594 for a total population estimate of 202.8 million.

Table 48-2 1991 Household Survey of Substance Usage (millions)†

Drug	Past Year	Past Month
Any illicit drug	26.1	12.6
Marijuana	19.5	9.7
Cocaine (includes crack)	6.4	1.9
Crack	1.0	0.5
Inhalants	2.9	1.2
Hallucinogens (includes PCP and LSD)	2.8	0.7
Psychotherapeutics*	13.3	3.7
Stimulants	2.7	0.7
Sedatives	2.1	0.7
Tranquilizers	3.4	0.9
Analgesics	5.1	1.4
Heroin	0.7	—

*Psychotherapeutics include nonmedical use of sedatives, tranquilizers, stimulants, or analgesics.
†This survey does not account for substance abusers outside of households (ie, institutionalized or homeless). Therefore there is a built-in underestimation of true prevalence.
PCP, phencyclidine; LSD, lysergic acid diethylamide.

Certain general trends have been observed based on this and other studies. The use of illicit drugs, alcohol, and cigarettes peaked during the late 1970s. Marijuana use was highest in the late 1970s, decreased throughout the 1980s, and in 1990 was at a level similar to or lower than the early 1970s. Cocaine use peaked during the period of 1979 to 1985 and has currently diminished. In 1990 the rates of cocaine use were similar to those of the early 1970s. Heroin use in 1990 was found in fewer than 1% of the household population but may be artificially low because of sampling error.

Alcohol and tobacco pose a greater liability to our society than illicit drugs because of their widespread usage. Cigarettes alone account for approximately 430,000 deaths per year in the United States.[3] The portion of the health care dollar that is spent on the medical, surgical, and psychiatric complications of alcohol, tobacco, and illicit substance abuse far exceeds the amount spent on all other medical maladies combined. The key to solving this complex problem lies in being able to prevent addiction to these substances. The focus of this preventive effort must be the youth of the United States.

TERMINOLOGY

The following definitions of terms and criteria for the diagnosis of substance dependence will be useful background information to review before proceeding with the ensuing sections of this chapter.

Drug abuse (substance abuse) are terms used interchangeably and refer to the use, usually by self-administration, of psychoactive drugs in a manner that adversely affects the individual's medical, psychosocial, or economic well-being. Drugs of abuse are commonly categorized as stimulants, opioids, sedatives, psychedelics, inhalants, and alcohol.

Addiction focuses on an established pattern of drug abuse in which the physical aspects of tolerance and abstinence are present.

Tolerance is manifested by a diminished response to a constant dose of a drug, reflecting changes in the pharmacodynamic and cellular mechanisms.

Cross-tolerance is the capacity of a tolerant individual to have a diminished response to a different drug as though prior tolerance had been developed. An example of cross-tolerance is the alcoholic who requires a larger than normal dose of benzodiazepine to achieve the normally expected sedative effects. Cross-tolerance is usually observed between drugs of the same class.

Withdrawal syndrome (abstinence syndrome) is a constellation of symptoms chronologically following the abstinence or decreasing utilization of the drug on which the patient has become dependent.

Illicit drugs are those drugs obtained illegally as well as those substances obtained by prescription but used for unaccepted medical purposes.

Physical dependence is a physiologic state produced by repeated drug use and requiring continued administration of the drug or a predictable group of clinical, biochemical, and toxicologic manifestations will occur.

Psychological dependence is the overwhelming drive to continue taking a drug in the hope of achieving pleasure or avoiding discomfort associated with abstinence.

According to the Diagnostic and Statistical Manual of Mental Disorders (DSM-III), *substance dependence or addiction* is diagnosed when a patient has at least three of the nine characteristic symptoms listed in Table 48-3, and those symptoms have persisted for at least 1 month or have recurred frequently over a prolonged period.[4,5]

Psychoactive *substance abuse* is a term applied in DSM-III to those individuals *not* meeting the criteria in Table 48-3

Table 48-3 Characteristic Symptoms of Substance Dependence[4,5]*

1. Substance often taken in larger amounts or for a longer period than intended.
2. Persistent desire or one or more unsuccessful efforts to reduce or control substance use.
3. Much time spent obtaining the substance, taking it, or recovering from its effects.
4. Recurrent use in physically hazardous situations or frequent intoxication or withdrawal symptoms.
5. Important social, occupational, or recreational activities forsaken or restricted because of substance use.
6. Continued use despite a persistent or recurrent social, psychological, or physical problem that is caused or exacerbated by the substance.
7. Marked tolerance: need for markedly increased amounts of the substance to achieve intoxication or desired effect or markedly diminished effect with continued use of the same amount.
8. Characteristic withdrawal symptoms.
9. Substances often taken to relieve or avoid withdrawal symptoms.

*Source: Taken from Sci Am Med 13:VI, p 1, 1991.

Table 48-4 The Medical, Surgical, and Psychiatric Complications of Drug Abuse[6]

Infectious complications	Endocarditis, hepatitis, cellulitis, cutaneous abscesses, aspiration pneumonia, AIDS, tuberculosis, other sexually transmitted diseases, osteomyelitis, septic arthritis, tetanus, botulism, malaria
Cardiovascular	Pulmonary embolus, thrombophlebitis, cerebrovascular accident, myocardial infarction, dysrhythmia, sudden death, pulmonary edema, cardiomyopathy
Trauma	Violent crime, industrial accidents, motor vehicular accidents
Psychiatric	Drug-induced psychoses, depression, suicidal/homicidal, or withdrawal
Other	Rhabdomyolysis, acute renal failure, disseminated intravascular coagulation

but who have a maladaptive pattern of substance use indicated by the following:

1. continued use despite a persistent or recurrent social, occupational, psychological, or physical problem that is caused or exacerbated by the substance,
2. recurrent use in situations that are physically hazardous, such as driving while intoxicated.[4,5]

THE SUBSTANCE ABUSER

Drug abusers are often difficult patients, medically and personally. The emergency department is frequently their principal source of medical care, and complaints may be acute or chronic. Patients may present with any of the medical, surgical, or psychiatric complications listed in Table 48-4.[6]

The physician evaluating a drug abuser must take into account which drug or drugs were used. Polydrug abuse confounds the difficulties in patient evaluation because of the interactive and often additive effects of multiple drugs. It is conservatively estimated that 2 million Americans are polydrug abusers.[7] The physician must also consider the chronicity of drug abuse; the age of the patient; the route of drug administration; the toxicity of the drug as well as the possible adulterants, substitutes, and diluents; the potential illnesses that may be masked by the abused drug; and the possibility that the patient is feigning illness in an effort to support his/her drug habit.

Substance abusers have a chronic state of ill health secondary to poor nutrition; poor hygiene; high-risk practices of parenteral drug usage; promiscuous sexual practices; and the effects of the drug itself on the cardiovascular, neurologic, and immune system. Violent death, however, has been demonstrated to be the leading cause of death among drug users. A study in New York City noted that 45% of those individuals autopsied and found to be cocaine users died as a result of violent crime.[8]

In approaching diagnostic problems of such diversity and complexity, the physician must seek a good working relationship with the patient. This may be difficult to impossible with the "street-wise" addict who tends to be resentful of authority, have low self-esteem, be deceitful, manipulative, and explosive.

Random violence and violent crime have been demonstrated to have a strong relationship with alcohol, phencyclidine (PCP), amphetamine, and cocaine use.[6] The picture of the multiply tattooed, intoxicated sociopath threatening harm to the entire medical staff of an emergency department is an all too familiar scenario in the inner city. Even without this to contend with, drug use in and of itself connotes serious disruption and maladaption in the life of the patient. Psychiatric referral should be considered for all patients presenting to the emergency department with a complication of illicit drug use.

Physicians are often judgmental about their patients' life styles, annoyed by the chronicity of problems presented for immediate attention, and doubtful about the patients' willingness to comply with whatever treatment may be prescribed or referral arranged. There is no simple or universal solution to each potentiality that may be encountered. The physician must attempt to suppress any personal feelings engendered by the substance-abusing patient, maintain control of the situation by not allowing events to transpire that may be dangerous to the other patients, the medical staff, or the patient under the influence of an illicit substance. This control may be as simple as gentle reassurance or as difficult as using security guards or physical and/or chemical restraints. The approach must be comprehensive in the evaluation of these patients. They often present with altered mental status and every effort must be made to understand the etiology of that alteration.

Despite the problems, care given to drug abusers can be thorough and the system of referral effective. Certainly, drug abuse is a chronic, relapsing condition that is difficult to treat. However, even when definitive cure is not effected by pharmacologic and psychosocial therapy, success is often achieved in stabilization of the patient's drug use, reversal of antisocial behavior, and intervention in potentially life-threatening crises. For these reasons it is essential not only that drug abuse be identified but also that abusers be referred for treatment.

Before discussing the various classes of abused substances and the medical complications associated with each drug, a review of the problems that are common to drug abuse regardless of class of substance is presented. In particular a discussion of the problems associated with the processing and synthesis of illicit substances, the complications of parenteral substance abuse, and the current technology for toxicologic screening.

ADULTERANTS, SUBSTITUTES, AND DILUENTS

The use of illicit substances is comparable to Russian roulette. Not only are the drugs themselves dangerous, they are frequently mixed with multiple other substances that have even greater toxicity. The adage "let the buyer beware" could have been coined for the potential substance abuser.[9] There are no controls governing what substances are sold as heroin, cocaine, methamphetamine, or any of the other illicit substances. The unsuspecting drug user may be exposed to multiple toxins with risk for significant morbidity and mortality. One review of "street-grade" marijuana found samples containing PCP, insect spray, and dried shredded cow manure.[8] Although not necessarily fatal when inhaled, each of these substances has the potential to cause unexpected adverse effects.

Impurities of manufacture refer to new chemicals that arise during the synthesis of a drug in clandestine laboratories.[10] The most recent, very morbid example of this type of impurity is 1-methyl-4-phenyl-1,2,3,6-tetrahydropyridine (MPTP) (discussed in the section on designer drugs), which can produce irreversible neurologic damage.

Adulterants are added in the attempt to simulate a desired effect of the illicit drug. Lidocaine is one of the more common adulterants added to cocaine and heroin samples. Procaine and tetracaine are other local anesthetics that have been used. These drugs in toxic doses can lead to cardiac dysrhythmias, hypotension, and cardiac arrest. Stimulant drugs added to cocaine and amphetamine are caffeine, ephedrine, pseudoephedrine, (PCP), and phenylpropanolamine (PPA). Each of these adulterants can be dangerous in overdose. PPA is an α-adrenergic agonist that can generate a severe hypertensive response. Caffeine can cause abdominal cramps, nausea, vomiting, tonic posturing, coma, seizures, and behavioral disturbances.[9] PCP is the most common pharmacologically active substance found in street drugs and has a long history of causing violent toxic psychoses.[9]

Other toxins added to street drugs are quinine, quinidine, arsenic, and strychnine. Quinine was first used as a heroin adulterant in the early 1940s to combat the malaria epidemic among intravenous drug users in New York City. It remains the adulterant of choice for heroin and cocaine. Quinine poisoning has occurred frequently and has been implicated as a possible cause of a number of heroin- and cocaine-associated deaths. Quinine can lead to visual disturbances, cardiac conduction defects, dysrhythmias, hypotension, and thrombocytopenia. Quinidine has more cardiac toxicity than quinine and is less frequently found in street drugs. Arsenic and strychnine have both been used as cocaine adulterants and have accounted for an unknown number of deaths.

Diluents are substances added to street drugs with the intent to increase the bulk of the substance. Sugars, starches, cellulose, and talc are used. Cellulose and talc are particularly problematic because of the foreign body reactions that occur in the end-organs in which these substances lodge. Pulmonary granulomatosis from talc or cotton particles may cause pulmonary hypertension and cor pulmonale. Acute pulmonary angiitis has been associated with intravenous injection of the cellulose fillers found in oral preparations.

COMPLICATIONS OF INTRAVENOUS SUBSTANCE USE

Parenteral drug users are at risk for a wide range of complications because of exposure to multiple infectious diseases, the locations chosen for injection, and the activity of the illicit substances injected. The infectious disease risk is increased in the chronic substance abuser because of a depressed immune response to potential infection secondary to poor nutritional status and a drug-induced decrease in cell-mediated immunity.[11]

Several practices that chronic substance abusers employ place them at increased risk for infectious disease. The apparatus used to prepare the drug for injection is nonsterile and frequently shared by multiple individuals leading to the spread of communicable diseases. Parenteral injection frequency can be markedly increased in the "binging" cocaine and amphetamine abusers. The frequency of injection, lack of nutritional support, and poor personal hygiene all contribute to an increased incidence of acquiring an infectious disease. The bacterial infections common in intravenous drug users usually result from the skin and oral flora and only rarely from bacterial contamination of the drug. *Staphylococcus aureus* and *Pseudomonas aeruginosa* are the two most common bacterial pathogens in this patient population.

The following are the more common problems precipitated by parenteral drug abuse.

AIDS was first described in five homosexual men in Los Angeles diagnosed with *Pneumocystis pneumonii* pneumonia in 1981.[12] By December 1991, a cumulative total of 206,392 cases of AIDS had been reported to the Centers for Disease Control.[13] Of these cases approximately 27% were intravenous drug users, making this group second only to the homosexual community as the largest group at-risk for AIDS in the United States.[14] It is estimated that there may be an additional 1 to 1.5 million people who are infected with the human immunodeficiency virus type 1 (HIV-1) virus but have not yet manifested signs of the disease. Transmission of the AIDS virus via blood, blood products, vaginal and cervical secretions, semen, placenta, and transplanted organs and tissue has been documented.[15] The increase in AIDS in the intravenous drug using community has led to a significant increase of this disease in both children born to intravenous drug–using women and the sexual partners of HIV-1–infected drug users.

Characteristically drug abusers who have AIDS present with pulmonary, central nervous system (CNS), or disseminated opportunistic infections. The most common infection is *Pneumocystis carinii* pneumonia, characterized by the gradual onset of shortness of breath, fever, cough (often productive), interstitial infiltrates, hypoxemia at rest or after exercise, and pneumothorax. Other common infections are cerebral toxoplasmosis or cryptococcosis and disseminated mycobacterial, cytomegalovirus, fungal, or herpesvirus infections.[16]

Drug abusers who have used parenteral drugs within 5 years and who present to the emergency department with fever, shortness of breath, new onset of seizures, unexplained altered mental status, or severe headache should be suspected of having AIDS, particularly if there is a history of oral thrush, herpes zoster, fatigue, diarrhea, lymphadenopathy or hair loss.[17,18]

Infective endocarditis was previously reported in intravenous heroin abusers but is now more frequent in intravenous cocaine abusers. Although infective endocarditis is most common in chronic drug abusers, it must be strongly considered in any parenteral drug abuser who presents with a fever.[19] The patient frequently develops right-sided disease involving the tricuspid valve, although the pulmonic and mitral valves are also common sites. Chest pain and cough are two prominent presenting symptoms in more than 50% of addicts with infective endocarditis and represent the pulmonary complications common in tricuspid valve involvement.[20] Septic emboli to the brain may result in ischemic infarct or brain abscess. Emboli to the kidneys or liver cause multiple abscesses. Septic pulmonary emboli can lead to pulmonary hypertension, empyema, bronchopleural fistulae, and pneumothorax. Congestive heart failure will develop with significant valvular destruction and may require surgical intervention with valvular replacement to salvage the patient.[19]

In the febrile intravenous drug abuser, a thorough physical evaluation should be performed and evaluation with aerobic and anaerobic bacterial and fungal blood cultures should be obtained. A chest radiograph with multiple pulmonic infiltrates in this setting is highly suggestive of tricuspid or, less frequently, pulmonic valve endocarditis. An echocardiogram may be helpful in diagnosing vegetative valvular lesions. Right-sided infective endocarditis may not present with a murmur on physical examination and may also be difficult to visualize on a echocardiogram. Most authorities recommend empiric antibiotic therapy with nafcillin plus gentamicin if the clinical picture is consistent with infective endocarditis. If the patient is penicillin allergic or there is concern about methicillin-resistant *Staphylococcus aureus*, vancomycin and gentamicin are recommended.[21] Although most of these patients recover from their initial bout of endocarditis, 20 to 40% develop recurrent infective endocarditis due to continued parenteral drug abuse.[19]

Hepatitis B is estimated to have infected more than 80% of intravenous drug abusers.[22] This is a point worth emphasizing to the health care providers who work with these patients and have not been immunized with the hepatitis B vaccine. It is a highly effective vaccine against a disease that still claims the lives of 200 to 300 occupationally exposed health care providers each year.[23]

Osteomyelitis most frequently occurs in the vertebral column and in particular the lumbar spine. *Pseudomonas aeruginosa* is the pathogen in 80% of the cases.[22] Pseudomonas osteomyelitis is, in fact, almost uniquely a disease of drug abusers. The illness may present blandly with localized pain and tenderness in a drug abuser who is apparently simulating pathology to obtain drugs.[24]

Septic arthritis may occur in the pelvic girdle, extremities, and sternoclavicular joints. As many as 88% of the cases are of bacterial etiology, but fungal and mycobacterial infections also are not uncommon.[25] Its location is often related to sites of injection. Involvement of the sternoclavicular joint is considered pathognomonic of intravenous drug abuse.[22]

Other infectious diseases include meningitis, epidural abscess, endophthalmitis, septic thrombophlebitis, skin abscess, cellulitis, necrotizing fasciitis, gas gangrene, tetanus, tuberculosis, aspiration pneumonia, opportunistic infections (cytomegalovirus, toxoplasmosis, cryptococcosis, and atypical mycobacterium), and malaria (rare today).

Noninfectious complications include inadvertent arterial injection with severe vasospasm and thrombosis secondary to the direct activity of the drug to cause vasospasm (cocaine and amphetamine) or the pH of the solution (alkaline pH of barbiturates) resulting in ischemic necrosis in extremities. Pneumothorax has developed from lung puncture attempting to inject internal jugular or subclavian veins.

"Cotton fever" is an acute illness lasting less than 24 hours and manifested by fever, myalgias, and abdominal cramps. It is caused by the intravenous injection of cotton fibers. Cotton fever is especially likely to occur in users who are boiling previously used cotton or cigarette filters to release trapped heroin.[10,26]

TOXICOLOGIC SCREENING IN THE EMERGENCY DEPARTMENT

The evaluation of patients presenting with possible drug intoxication requires the physician to acquire historical data from the patient, friends, and family if available; conduct a thorough physical examination; possess knowledge of the common toxidromes that are associated with various illicit substances; and when necessary obtain toxicologic screening tests to support his suspicions.

If possible, informed voluntary consent must be obtained when performing urine tests on any person over 18 years of age. In true emergencies this can be waived if the patient is comatose, having seizures, exhibiting signs of toxic psychosis, or determined to be otherwise mentally incompetent.[27]

The availability of obtaining "stat" toxicologic screens has increased considerably during the past 10 years. The tests used today are more sensitive and more specific. An understanding of the more commonly available tests may be useful to the emergency physician, in particular, the capabilities and limitations of the laboratory to identify the multiple toxins available. The following are the common technologies available in most hospitals and the utility of these tests.

Chemical spot tests are initial, rapid screening tests for specific drugs. The basis of the tests is a chemical reaction between the illicit drug in a urine specimen and specific reagents. These tests are well suited to the emergency department because of the rapid turnaround time and the simplicity involved in performing them.[28] Tests are available for PCP, methadone, chloral hydrate, ethchlorvynol, tricyclics, salicylates, acetaminophen, and phenothiazines.

Immunoassay tests can provide toxicologic results within 1 to 2 hours and are based on the ability of drug-specific antibody to bind to labeled drug. There are enzyme-linked (EIA) or (EMIT); fluorescent-linked (FPIA); and radio-iodine-linked immunoassays (RIA). The tests are usually performed on urine specimens, but there are manufacturer's modifications to allow testing on serum as well.[28]

Thin-layer chromatography (TLC) requires a pH-dependent extraction, followed by purification and concentration of the drugs in the specimen. This layering out of the various drugs allows identification. It is used in many emergency medical facilities for toxicologic screening. TLC can usually provide results within approximately 3 to 4 hours turnaround time.

The features of specific drugs that determine which tests are both specific and sensitive are as follows.[27]

- *Marijuana.* Intensely lipophilic, can usually be detected in serum for only 1 to 2 hours after use. The urine will remain positive for about 1 to 3 days. Immunoassay test of the urine is sensitive, specific, and rapid for cannabinoids (marijuana).
- *Cocaine.* Metabolites, specifically benzoylecgonine, persist in the urine for approximately 48 hours. Immunoassay test of the urine is sensitive, specific, and rapid for cocaine.
- *PCP.* Excreted in the urine for 2 to 3 days after use. Immunoassay tests are now employed for PCP and can detect urine concentrations of 75 ng/mL or less. There have been false positives reported by the EIA test in patients taking some sympathomimetic cold preparations (ie, Rondec or Dimetapp).
- *Hallucinogenic drugs.* LSD is now detectable by RIA. Mescaline and psilocybin can be detected by TLC.
- *Amphetamines.* Either immunoassay or TLC is used to detect amphetamines. The following common drugs will cause a positive reaction for amphetamine: ephedrine, pseudoephedrine, PPA, theophylline-containing bronchodilators, and phenmetrazine. There are now RIA and FPIA methods that are more specific for amphetamines.
- *Opioids.* Immunoassay tests are most commonly employed to detect opium, morphine, codeine, and other morphine or codeine analogues. Large poppy seeds or dextromethorphan (ie, Robitussin-DM) ingestions can also yield a positive result when screening for opioids. Methadone and the new "designer" fentanyl analogues, however, will not give a positive result on opioid immunoassay test.

The tests described above are screening tests. When indicated, confirmatory tests can be done that are highly specific using gas chromatography-mass spectrometry. This test allows for drug separation by the gas chromatograph and molecular identification by the mass spectrometer. It is considered the gold standard of toxicologic analysis and offers the specificity required for toxicologic confirmation.

SYMPATHOMIMETICS

The 1980s was the decade in which drugs in this class accounted for the major share of the illicit drug market. Cocaine became the predominant substance of abuse in the United States by the mid 1980s. In 1987, crystal meth-

Table 48-5 Sympathomimetics[30,31]

Over-the-counter products
   Phenylpropanolamine (PPA)
   Phenylephrine
   Ephedrine
   Pseudoephedrine
   Caffeine

Hallucinogenic amphetamines
   3,4,5-Trimethoxyamphetamine (TMA)
   Dimethoxyamphetamine (DOM/STP)
   Methylenedioxyamphetamine (MDA)
   Methylenedioxymethamphetamine (MDMA)
   Methylenedioxyethamphetamine (MDEA)

Others
   Cocaine
   Phencyclidine (PCP)
   Nicotine

Plants
   Ma huang (ephedrine)
   Khat
   Cacao (caffeine)
   Cola nuts (caffeine)

Amphetamine and derivatives
   Amphetamine
   Methamphetamine
   Methylphenidate (Ritalin)
   Phenmetrazine (Preludin)
   Benzphetamine
   Mephentermine
   Phenylisopropylamine (Benzedrine)

Table 48-6 Signs and Symptoms/Complications of Sympathomimetic Toxicity[30]

Organ System	Sign/Symptom/Complication
Central nervous system	Agitation, anxiety, delusions, hallucinations, paranoia, seizures headache, transient ischemic attack, cerebrovascular accident, coma, mydriasis, tremor, encephalopathy
Cardiovascular	Hypertension, sinus tachycardia, bradycardia*, atrioventricular block*, chest pain supraventricular tachyarrhythmia, ventricular tachyarrhythmia, myocardial ischemia/infarction, aortic dissection, pneumopericardium, mesenteric ischemia
Other	Hyperthermia, rhabdomyolysis, disseminated intravascular coagulation, acute renal failure, pneumomediastinum, pneumothorax, infectious complications, nasal septal necrosis, hepatotoxicity, traumatic injury, pulmonary edema, pulmonary hypertension, bronchiolitis obliterans, alveolar hemorrhage, pneumonitis, thermal injury to the airway

*Predominantly α-agonist.

amphetamine began to establish a strong foothold in the illicit drug trade on the West Coast.[29] These substances belong to a broad class of drugs that generate responses similar to those induced by catecholamines. They produce cortical arousal and sympathetic stimulation. During the acute response, the user experiences a heightened alertness, euphoria, and enhanced psychomotor activity that is variously described as feelings of omnipotence, excitation, or calm. These agents stimulate α- and β-adrenergic receptors responsible for the increased sympathetic nervous system activity. They also activate dopaminergic and serotonergic receptors that mediate the CNS response in varying degrees. If alpha stimulation is the primary effect of the drug, then hypertension and possibly bradycardia will be the major abnormalities. PPA is an example of a primarily α-agonist stimulant. Table 48-5 is a list of the more common drugs with sympathomimetic characteristics.[30,31]

The signs and symptoms and complications of sympathomimetic toxicity are summarized in Table 48-6. They can be divided into CNS, cardiovascular, and neuromuscular effects. This class of drug is abused for its CNS effects, in particular, the ability to maintain wakefulness and alertness, and experience a euphoric effect.

Cocaine

Cocaine became the third most popular substance of abuse in the 1980s. Alcohol and marijuana were first and second, respectively. In 1986, visits related to cocaine use became the most common of all illicit drug-associated visits to emergency departments. This popularity was due, in large part, to the development and widespread distribution of free-base (crack) cocaine. An estimated 30 to 50 tons of cocaine are brought into the United States each year. Its street value is approximately $50 billion.[32] It is not, however, a new substance of abuse.

Cocaine is a naturally occurring alkaloid obtained from the leaves of two species of the South American coca plant. *Erythroxylon coca* from the highlands of the Andes in Ecuador, Peru, and Bolivia and *Erythroxylon novogranatense* from the mountainous regions of Colombia.[33] The human experience with cocaine dates back at least to 5000 B.C. The Incas used the coca leaf for its ability to increase productivity and performance of their soldiers and workers.[33] In 1857, Albert Niemann, a German chemist at the University of Göttingen, isolated cocaine from the coca leaf and introduced it to the civilized world. In 1863, a new wine advertised as a tonic and restorative appeared in the cafés of Paris. It was called "Vin Mariani" and contained 6 mg of cocaine per ounce. Needless to say, it was an immediate success. Thomas Edison, Robert Louis Stevenson, Jules Verne, and Pope Leo XIII were a few well-known figures at that time who commented on the rejuvenating effects of this wine.[34] Sigmund Freud became interested in cocaine in 1884 and published his work with the drug in *Uber Cocaine*, in which he advocated the drug as a cure for morphine addiction as well as a variety of other problems including dyspepsia, fatigue, hysteria, and headaches.[34] William Stewart Halsted, a noted American surgeon, became the first recorded cocaine-impaired physician, secondary to his self-experimentation with the drug as a local anesthetic agent.[33] Freud, who wrote "a small dose lifted me to the heights in a wonderful fashion," also fell prey to cocaine dependency.[33] The first recorded cocaine-related cardiac arrest was reported in the *British Journal of Medicine* in 1886.[34] Slowly the dangers of cocaine became more well-known, and in 1914, the Harrison Narcotic Act forbade its use in proprietary medicines.[35] In the 1960s and early 1970s interest in all types of illicit substances was rekindled and cocaine abuse began to resurface. In 1973, two US national commissions declared that cocaine caused little dependency, but in the 1980s this opinion was proven to be incorrect.[36] There are an estimated 30 million Americans who have used cocaine. In 1986, cocaine use was the most frequent drug-related cause of emergency department visits. It ranked third after opioids and drugs combined with alcohol as causes of drug-related mortality.[37] Cocaine usage reached its peak in the mid 1980s with the widespread availability of inexpensive crystallized alkaloidal cocaine (crack or free-base). Abuse of cocaine is beginning to taper off but, based on 1991 statistics, is still a significant societal, as well as medical, problem. In 1991, there were 606,000 Americans using cocaine at least once a week, and complications from its use resulted in an estimated 47,000 emergency department visits in the United States that year.[34]

Pharmacology

Cocaine is transported into the United States from South America as a hydrochloride salt. The hydrochloride salt is a 70% to 90%-pure, water-soluble, white, and crystalline powder. It is derived by hydroxylation and benzoylation from the coca leaf. Cocaine is a topical anesthetic and potent CNS stimulant. It prevents the reuptake of norepinephrine and dopamine at the adrenergic nerve terminals as well as potentiates the tyramine-facilitated release of norepinephrine from the adrenergic nerve terminals.[38] The hydrochloride salt may be sniffed or injected intravenously.

Free-base or crack cocaine is a colorless, odorless, crystalline substance prepared by at least two methods. The more complex method is to dissolve the cocaine hydrochloride salt in water and industrial strength alkali. Free cocaine is left in solution to which ether is added. The ether-cocaine supernatant is suctioned off and the ether allowed to evaporate, with free-base cocaine remaining. The second method uses a slightly different technique with cocaine hydrochloride salt, baking soda, and boiling the solution.[7] Crack cocaine is water insoluble and cannot be injected or nasally insufflated (snorted). It can be smoked, however, leading to absorption into the pulmonary circulation and bypassing the liver. The pharmacokinetics for this inhalational route of administration is very similar to intravenous administration. Ingested cocaine hydrochloride is absorbed slowly but to the same extent as if snorted, and absorption is mainly from the duodenum.[39] Massive ingestion by users swallowing bags of cocaine to avoid arrest ("body stuffers") has resulted in deaths.[40] The median lethal dose of cocaine by oral ingestion is 500 mg.

Effects are almost immediate by any route other than oral, and there appears to be concentration in the CNS after intravenous injection. Plasma half-life is approximately 1 hour, and effects usually last 1 or 2 hours when cocaine is sniffed. Cocaine is metabolized by esterases in the blood and liver to several detectable urinary by-products. Benzoylecgonine is the urinary by-product that is the basis for the urinary drug screen for cocaine. Although excretion of unchanged cocaine in the urine is dependent on urine pH, it is not an important phenomenon in detoxification.[41] Tolerance to the effects of cocaine may be considerable and is said to be lost only after a long period.

It is common practice to use cocaine and alcohol together. In the presence of ethanol, cocaine is metabolized by hepatic transformation to cocaethylene. Cocaethylene produces an intense dopaminergic effect that not only increases the euphoria but the toxicity and duration of the symptoms as well. Cocaethylene remains active in the body 7 hours after the last traces of cocaine have disappeared. The risk of sudden death is 25 times greater in persons who abuse both cocaine and alcohol.[42]

The fatal dose of cocaine varies according to the route of administration, the baseline health of the individual, and the adulterants and other toxins the patient is taking. A dose of 1.4 g by insufflation, 700 to 800 mg by intravenous or subcutaneous injection, or inhalation in a 70-kg patient is often fatal.[43]

Cocaine has bona fide clinical application. It is the topical anesthetic of choice for nose, mouth, and throat procedures and is used in the topical TAC (tetracaine, adrenaline, cocaine) anesthetics utilized for laceration repair. Cocaine is also a potent vasoconstrictor and decongestant, making it an ideal drug for treating patients with epistaxis or who require passage of any tubes through the nasal passage.

Clinical Presentation

Prior to 1985, the primary medical complications of cocaine use requiring admission were infectious processes secondary to parenteral abuse. With the development of crack, the complications requiring admission rapidly and dramatically changed. In one study of thoses patients admitted after smoking crack cocaine, 40% had cardiovascular complications, 53% had neurologic complications, and 63% had psychiatric complications.[43] The leading cause of death of cocaine abusers, however, is not a medical complication, but a traumatic complication. A review of 935 patients dying with cocaine in their bodies in Manhattan in 1981 revealed that 53% died because of homicide, suicide, or traumatic accident.[44] Homicide was the cause of death of 38% of the 935 patients.

There are numerous reports of the cardiovascular complications of cocaine. There are now more than 100 reported cases of myocardial infarction associated with cocaine abuse. It has also precipitated sudden cardiac death, hypertensive emergencies, myocardial ischemia, myocarditis, cardiac dysrhythmias, cardiomyopathy, aortic dissection, vasculitis, and superficial thrombophlebitis.[45] Cocaine increases the myocardial oxygen consumption by increasing heart rate and blood pressure. It causes coronary artery vasospasm and increases platelet aggregation leading to greater potential for intracoronary thrombosis. The average age of patients presenting with cocaine-induced myocardial infarction varies between 30 and 36 years. The initial electrocardiogram is the most sensitive indicator of which patient will go on to develop acute myocardial infarction, regardless of how many cases are diagnosed strictly on the basis of cardiac enzymes.[46] The likelihood of developing acute myocardial infarction was independent of the route of administration even though higher blood levels are obtained by intravenous use or smoking crack. This might imply that other mechanisms are significant in the development of coronary thrombosis such as platelet aggregation, coagulation, and injury to vascular endothelium.[46] Myocarditis is usually found in chronic abusers and believed to be secondary to a direct toxic effect of cocaine on the myocardium or a possible hypersensitivity mechanism.[47] Any patient less than 45 years of age presenting to an emergency department with chest pain of a cardiac etiology should be asked about possible cocaine usage as part of the cardiac risk factor history.

Respiratory complications have become more common with the advent of crack cocaine. Diffuse alveolar damage with decreased diffusing capacity, alveolar hemorrhage, pulmonary infiltrates secondary to immune-mediated inflammatory cell infiltration, bronchiolitis obliterans, pneumothorax, pneumomediastinum, pulmonary artery medial hypertrophy, and thermal injury to the airway.[48]

The neurologic complications of cocaine abuse are equally devastating for the generally young population who abuse this drug. Subarachnoid hemorrhage and intracerebral bleeding occur with the sudden onset of severe headache usually minutes after cocaine use. The majority of cases appear to be secondary to rupture of a preexisting arteriovenous malformation or cerebral aneurysm. Ischemic cerebrovascular accidents have occurred either secondary to severe vasospasm or cerebral vasculitis. Transient ischemic attacks also occur, probably secondary to temporary cerebral vasospasm. Cocaine-induced seizures have been recognized for many years. They are commonly generalized tonic-clonic seizures and may be a lethal complication if not rapidly controlled. Cutting agents such as lidocaine, procaine, PCP, amphetamines, and quinidine that have been mixed in with the cocaine all lower the seizure threshold. The high lipid solubility of cocaine leads to a rapid rise in the drug's concentration in the brain and ultimately causes seizure activity.

Cocaine may also trigger migraine headaches because of its sympathomimetic effects.[49]

The psychiatric complications of cocaine abuse vary within an abuser over time. The complications of acute intoxication with high-dose, repetitive usage (binging) are impaired judgment, extreme psychomotor activation, compulsively repeated actions, irritability, severe transient panic, and paranoid psychosis. These complications may lead to accidents, violent crime, or atypical sexual behavior.

The abstinence syndrome is considered to have two primary phases: the crash and the withdrawal. The crash immediately follows the binge. It is most severe in chronic abusers and consists of depression, agitation, anxiety, and stimulant craving, which gives way to sleep craving. Patients will often resort to using alcohol or other sedatives to induce sleep during this phase. Hypersomnolence and hyperphagia during the brief periods of wakefulness follow. Suicidal behavior may occur during this phase. The withdrawal occurs after the crash in chronic abusers. Anergia, anhedonia, and depression are its hallmarks. These symptoms may gradually increase after 12 to 96 hours of abstinence. An intense craving for cocaine recurs to put an end to this dysphoric state. It is postulated that these symptoms are secondary to dopamine and norepinephrine depletion and gradually will subside after 6 to 18 weeks.[50]

Rhabdomyolysis with acute renal failure, severe liver dysfunction, and disseminated intravascular coagulation has been reported in multiple patients with cocaine intoxication.[51-53] The proposed etiologies for rhabdomyolysis are possible muscle injury due to ischemia, hyperthermia, or trauma. Other reported complications of cocaine abuse are a heatstroke-like syndrome, intestinal infarction, and nasoseptal necrosis. Infectious complications of parenteral drug abuse are discussed in an earlier section of this chapter, (complications of intravenous substance use).

Amphetamine

Amphetamine was synthesized in 1887 and methamphetamine in 1914.[9] Amphetamine was introduced in the 1930s as an inhalant (Benzedrine) to counter rhinitis and asthma but quickly became recognized as a euphoriant and anorectic.[54] Amphetamines were found to counter narcolepsy and fatigue, induce anorexia, and promote weight loss. In small doses they are euphorogenic, elevating mood and producing feelings of well-being. These latter effects have led to widespread abuse. During World War II, amphetamines were used to counter fatigue in the military forces of the United States, Japan, and Germany and increase productivity in their civilian work forces. After the war, there was widespread abuse of amphetamines in Japan, necessitating a major law enforcement initiative by the Japanese to control the problem.[55] In the 1950s, despite increasing federal controls, amphetamines were used by students, athletes, shift workers, and truck drivers to maintain wakefulness and increase energy. The other amphetamines (methamphetamine, dextroamphetamine, and amphetamine) were placed on Schedule II (drugs that have medical use, but significant abuse potential). The US Food and Drug Administration (FDA) restricted legal use to hyperkinetic behavior in children, narcolepsy, and short-term appetite suppression.[55]

In the past several years there has been a dramatic increase in amphetamine abuse in the form of crystal methamphetamine ("ice"). Crystal methamphetamine was first synthesized in the Far East and gained wide acceptance by the drug culture in Hawaii.[10] In the late 1980s it became a popular drug of abuse in California and the West Coast. Its popularity stems from the extremely rapid onset of euphoria, comparable to that of crack cocaine, longer duration of action, and an inhalational versus intravenous route of administration.

Pharmacology

Amphetamine (Benzedrine) is actually a single compound called phenylisopropylamine. In common use it refers to a group of compounds that are structurally related including methamphetamine, dextroamphetamine, phentermine, and synthetic amphetamine analogues. Methamphetamine HCl is easily synthesized in crude "kitchen" laboratories. Once this water-soluble compound is produced, it can be boiled in a process similar to that which yields rock candy from sugar, resulting in the formation of crystal methamphetamine, ("ice"), which is volatile and rapidly absorbed into the pulmonary circulation when smoked.[10]

It is believed that amphetamines and their derivatives produce the observed clinical effects by reducing reuptake of dopamine and norepinephrine at the nerve terminals. The hallucinogenic amphetamines are thought to have potent serotonin antagonist properties that account for the hallucinogenic effects.[55] Amphetamines have strong CNS effects with a longer duration of action than cocaine. Chronic use leads to psychological dependence. Physical withdrawal is mild compared with the opioids and sedative-hypnotic abstinence syndromes. Intravenous use was found to produce more intense feelings than oral administration. A "rush," which consists of euphoria, increased alertness, heightened sexual awareness, and a sense of power, is experienced. Tolerance to the central and peripheral effects is considerable, developing rapidly and leading the amphetamine abuser to inject more frequently with increasing doses to achieve the same level of euphoria. Chronic users may require 10 to 20 times the usual starting dose. The abuser gets into a cycle of "speed (methamphetamine) binging" or a "speed run" with repetitive injections lasting several days. The dose may increase to as much as 5 g per day.[55] During this time the individual does not eat, bathe, or sleep. Finally, the patient becomes exhausted or runs out of drug and crashes in a manner similar to the crack cocaine abuser. During the crash, the individual may sleep for 24 to 48 hours, wake up, eat ravenously, and sleep some more. Abstinence occurs within days of withdrawal, and although physical signs are few, there is a predictable period of lethargy, abnormal sleep patterns, and, often, craving for sedatives. During this period, which may persist for several months, patients frequently suffer from a depression that responds in some cases to tricyclic antidepressants, but may be complicated by suicide attempts.

Amphetamine is both metabolized in the liver and excreted unchanged by the kidneys. It is not known whether the metabolites are centrally active; however, formation of a false neurotransmitter may be partly responsible for the marked tolerance that develops to the peripheral adrenergic effects. Plasma half-life varies from 8 to 30 hours, depending on the pH of the urine, and the amphetamine may be found in alkaline urine as long as 1 week following a large dose.[56]

With the advent of crystal methamphetamine, the route of administration has predominantly changed to inhalation of the drug-laden smoke. Although this reduces the complications associated with parenteral drug abuse, there is an increased tendency to use more of the drug via this route, and the risks of overdose and toxicity are increased.

Clinical Presentation

The amphetamine-abusing patient presents in a manner similar to that of the cocaine-abusing patient. There are signs and symptoms of sympathetic overdrive. The mildly intoxicated amphetamine abuser presents with dizziness, headache, restlessness, irritability, and insomnia. With more severe intoxication chest discomfort, nausea, and abdominal pain may occur. Psychiatric symptoms are often prominent, with hallucinations in any sensory modality. Paranoid delusions, a hallmark of chronic stimulant abuse, may be present and tend to last for days, weeks, or even longer than the acute paranoid disorders of cocaine-induced psychosis, which may resolve within hours.[57] Short- and long-term memory are intact, and the response of these patients to the fact that they are experiencing hallucinations is more often one of concern than is the case in schizophrenia. The precipitation of acute paranoid schizophrenia by stimulant abuse is a well-described event and must be differentiated from a toxic, and therefore transient, psychosis.[58]

On examination the intoxicated patient is oriented. Typically there is mydriasis, increased blood pressure and pulse, flushing, tremor, diaphoresis, pallor, dry mouth, and hyperreflexia. Bruxism may be noted.

The severely intoxicated amphetamine abuser may present with delirium, hyperthermia, rhabdomyolysis, seizures, hypertensive emergency, cardiac dysrhythmias, myocardial infarction, coma, and focal neurologic deficits.

In the evaluation of patients suspected of sympathomimetic overdose, the following differential diagnoses should be kept in mind: chronic paranoid states, stimulant-precipitated nontoxic schizophrenia, hyperthyroid crisis, pheochromocytoma, and other drug ingestions (principally hallucinogens). History and urine testing are the best methods of making the diagnosis. Signs of chronic abuse such as needle tracks, extreme weight loss, and stereotypic movements such as picking at the skin may be helpful clues. When the diagnosis of stimulant overdose is made, consideration should be given to the possibility that other substances, especially opiates, may also be present.

The laboratory workup of moderate to severe overdose should include baseline electrolytes, renal and liver function tests, clotting parameters, and urinanalysis for cells, myoglobin (in the presence of high fever), and drugs. The screening laboratory should be notified that amphetamine, benzoylecgonine (cocaine's metabolite), and methylphenidate are specifically being sought. An electrocardiogram and thyroid function tests may also be helpful.

Management of Sympathomimetic Intoxication

There are several potential life-threats that must be evaluated and managed in patients who present with sympathomimetic intoxication. Most patients do not require specific treatment and after a period of observation become asymptomatic. The management is similar regardless of whether the patient is using cocaine or amphetamines. The most common serious life-threats are inadequate airway/ventilation, coma, hypertensive emergencies, cerebrovascular emergencies, cardiac dysrhythmias, myocardial ischemia/infarction, generalized seizures, hyperthermia, rhabdomyolysis, and toxic psychosis. Table 48-7 presents a

Table 48-7 Treatment of Sympathomimetic Toxicity[9,59]

Hypertension	Quiet setting, benzodiazepines (diazepam 0.1–0.2 mg/kg IV or lorazepam 0.1 mg/kg IV to maximum of 4 mg) Phentolamine 0.05–0.1 µg/kg per minute IV or Nitroprusside 0.5–5 µg/kg per minute IV		Lidocaine 1 mg/kg IV bolus, then 2–4 mg per minute IV infusion. If the modalities described above are unsuccessful, lidocaine may be beneficial with the caution that it may induce seizures or increase conduction delay.
Cardiac dysrhythmia			
Supraventricular	Supplemental oxygen, sedation with benzodiazepines Verapamil 0.075–0.15 mg/kg IV bolus or Labetalol 5 mg IV increments or Esmolol 0.5 mg/kg IV bolus over 1 minute, followed by 0.05 mg/kg per minute infusion. If tachycardia persists, rebolus with same dose and increase infusion incrementally to maximum of 0.25 mg/kg per minute (controversial).	Seizures	Diazepam 0.1–0.2 mg/kg IV bolus Lorazepam 0.1 mg/kg IV bolus If benzodiazepines ineffective in terminating seizure: Phenobarbital 15–20 mg/kg IV load over no less than 30 minutes or Phenytoin 15–20 mg/kg IV load over no less than 30 minutes If phenobarbital ineffective in terminating seizures: Rapid sequence induction with sodium thiopental and vecuronium (0.1–0.3 mg/kg) and endotracheal intubation with mechanical ventilation (intensive care unit admission with continuous EEG monitoring will be required)
Ventricular	Supplemental oxygen, sedation with benzodiazepines 1. Unstable: cardiovert 2. Stable Labetalol 5 mg IV increments or Esmolol as described above (controversial) or Sodium bicarbonate 1 mEq/kg IV bolus and consider continuous bicarbonate infusion	Toxic psychosis	Sedatives: benzodiazepines usually effective. Haloperidol 5–10 mg IM/IV may be used but can lower seizure threshold

IV, intravenous; EEG, electroencephalogram; IM, intramuscular.

review of some specific measures recommended in the management of sympathomimetic toxicity.[9,59]

If the patient ingested sympathomimetics by mouth, activated charcoal may be helpful in decreasing the absorption of the drug. "Body packers," professional drug smugglers who swallow dozens of carefully wrapped bags of cocaine, or other substances, to avoid detection, and "body stuffers" who quickly swallows several bags of cocaine or crystal methamphetamine to avoid arrest are at greatest risk for massive overdoses. If these patients are initially asymptomatic, it is reasonable to give them a standard initial dose of activated charcoal (1 g/kg) and repeat one half the dose every 2 hours. Additionally, whole bowel irrigation with GoLYTELY or Colyte at a dose of 1 to 2 L/hour for adults or 500 mL/hour for children by mouth or nasogastric tube may be undertaken to remove the bags of drug from the gut.[60] If the patients are symptomatic suggesting rupture of one or more bags, the patient should be stabilized to control tachycardia, hypertension, seizures, and myocardial ischemia as necessary and activated charcoal should be administered. If the ingested amount is greater than 10 g of cocaine, surgical evaluation for exploratory laparotomy and removal is recommended.[60]

The patient with coma secondary to sympathomimetic intoxication may be unresponsive for multiple reasons. The patient may have had a seizure, a cerebrovascular accident, or a polydrug effect or be in the crash phase of sympathomimetic abuse. Regardless of the etiology of the coma, if the patient fails to respond to the initial coma protocol of glucose, thiamine, and naloxone, endotracheal intubation is indicated to protect the airway.

The patient who presents with hypertension may need only observation if asymptomatic and blood pressure is less than 170/100 mmHg. If the patient is symptomatic or the blood pressure is greater than 170/100 mmHg, it should be controlled. Initially, provide the patient with a reasonably quiet environment and low doses of benzodiazepine. Benzodiazepines blunt sympathetic tone through their γ-aminobutyric acid (GABA) agonist activity.[61] Agents that are nonselective β-adrenergic blockers may produce the deleterious effect of paradoxically increasing the patient's blood pressure by uncovering an unopposed α-adrenergic effect leading to vasoconstriction and exacerbation of coronary artery spasm.[62] The β- and α-adrenergic blocking agent labetalol has been proposed as the ideal drug in the setting of cocaine-induced hypertension or myocardial ischemia. It is recommended in the setting of tachydysrhythmias and myocardial ischemia and infarction. Labetalol must be used with the understanding that it has a 7:1 ratio of β- to α-adrenergic blocking effect.[59] This may lead to the same increase in vasospasm that is of concern with the nonselective β-adrenergic blockers. However, if the patient receives benzodiazepine sedation before labetalol is administered, there is a significant reduction in the unopposed alpha stimulation. An alternative is the α-adrenergic blocker, phentolamine, which has been found to be very effective in reducing blood pressure in titrated doses of 2 to 10 mg intravenously. Nitroprusside is also an effective agent and allows blood pressure control in a titratable fashion.

Cerebrovascular emergencies may require initial protection of the airway and management of hypertension. After these supportive measures have been instituted, a diagnostic evaluation to determine whether the patient has had an ischemic or cerebral hemorrhage insult is necessary. If a hemorrhagic infarct occurred, immediate neurosurgical consultation is recommended to determine whether angiography and/or surgical intervention is advisable. During this evaluation the patient's blood pressure and cardiovascular status should be monitored and preparations made to manage possible seizures.

The best agents to control cardiac dysrhythmias with the least potential morbidity is the subject of some controversy. Supraventricular tachycardias may be successfully approached with supplemental oxygen, benzodiazepine sedation, cooling if febrile, and either a calcium channel blocker, diltiazem or verapamil, or a combined α/β-blocker (labetalol). Esmolol, a short-acting β_1-blocker has been successfully used for supraventricular dysrhythmias with the cautions discussed above for β-blockers in this setting. Ventricular dysrhythmias can also occur. Oxygenation and sedation in the stable patient are useful first steps. Labetalol and calcium channel blockers have been used with success. Lidocaine has to be used with caution because of risk of increasing the seizure threshold and augmenting the stimulant's type I antidysrhythmic properties exacerbating cardiac conduction abnormalities.[59] There has also been a recent report that sodium bicarbonate administration has been effective in reversing wide-complex tachydysrhythmias precipitated by cocaine abuse.[63]

Myocardial ischemia/infarction is managed in the standard manner with oxygen supplementation provided to all patients in this category. Cardiac monitoring and continuous vital-sign monitoring are indicated. Aspirin in a 160 mg dose will help to combat the tendency toward platelet aggregation. Nitrates are effective in relieving cocaine-induced coronary spasm. Calcium channel blockers remain somewhat controversial, but appear to be helpful in combating coronary artery vasospasm. Small doses of intravenous phentolamine (1 to 2 mg) have been used successfully and pharmacologically make sense to relieve the alpha-mediated component of vasospasm.[64] Morphine is useful for pain relief, and benzodiazepines are helpful in alleviating any psychomotor agitation. Haloperidol is contraindicated in this setting because of its adverse effects on dopamine-2 receptors producing increased circulating catecholamines. β-blockers and mixed α/β-blockers are contraindicated because of the potential for unopposed α-adrenergic stimulation. Thrombolysis is also controversial and carries an increased risk in the setting of hypertension for intracranial hemorrhage.

Patients who have uncomplicated, nonfocal, cocaine-related seizures of short duration do not generally require anticonvulsant therapy.[65] When anticonvulsants are required for prolonged seizure activity, the benzodiazepines are the preferred initial choice. Both diazepam and lorazepam have been effective. Occasionally, the benzodiazepines will be ineffective and phenytoin will be required. If the patient continues to have seizures after phenytoin is administered, then general anesthesia is indicated.

Hyperthermia in the setting of sympathomimetic intoxication is usually diagnosed with a core temperature greater than 39°C. Rapid external cooling with exposure, wet towels, and fans blowing across the patient is usually effective. If necessary, internal cooling can be performed with nasogastric lavage, Foley catheter lavage, and cool intravenous fluids.

Acute rhabdomyolysis has been reported in both cocaine and amphetamine intoxication. It occurs in patients with significant sympathomimetic intoxication. History, serum creatinine phosphokinase levels, and a urine screen for myoglobin help to make the diagnosis. Urinary acidification to increase the elimination of amphetamines is contraindicated because it predisposes the patient to develop renal compromise if rhabdomyolysis is present. The treatment of rhabdomyolysis involves alkalinizing the urine and maintaining increased urinary output with fluids and mannitol.

Toxic psychosis is most commonly noted after a single, large dose of cocaine or amphetamine or in the long-term chronic abuser. It closely resembles paranoid schizophrenia and may be mistakenly diagnosed as such. Haloperidol continues to be the drug of choice as long as there is no evidence of myocardial ischemia/infarction.

Most sympathomimetics (except for caffeine) have a very large volume of distribution and are very lipophilic, so that extracorporeal drug removal is ineffective. Patients with hemodynamic compromise or seizures from caffeine overdose should be treated with charcoal hemoperfusion.

Several therapeutic protocols have been designed to assist the chronic cocaine abusers through the abstinence syndrome. The bromocriptine-desipramine protocol was designed to decrease the dysphoria and cocaine craving, which has been believed to be secondary to dopamine-receptor supersensitivity. Bromocriptine and desipramine have both been shown to induce dopamine receptor subsensitivity.[66] Carbamazepine has recently also been used with some success in the treatment of crack cocaine addiction.[67]

Methylphenidate

Methylphenidate (Ritalin) is an amphetamine derivative used in the treatment of pediatric hyperkinesis, narcolepsy, and occasionally depression. Parenteral abuse is most common among intravenous opioid users. Oral abuse has also been reported. Methylphenidate is completely absorbed after ingestion, reaching peak levels in approximately 2 hours. The half-life of the parent compound is only 1 to 2 hours, but metabolites are apparently psychoactive and have half-lives of approximately 7 hours. Subjective effects may last as long as 12 hours. The drug is de-esterified in the liver, and the products are excreted by the kidneys. Methylphenidate is available as 5-, 10-, and 20-mg tablets.[68]

OPIOIDS

Opioids are defined as all drugs, either synthetic or naturally occurring, that have either opium-like or morphine-like pharmacologic activity. Opiate refers only to those drugs derived from the opium poppy *Papaver somniferum*.[69] The opium poppy contains the natural alkaloids morphine and codeine. The semisynthetic opioid drugs derived from morphine are heroin, hydromorphone (Dilaudid), oxymorphone (Numorphan), and oxycodone (in Percodan). The synthetic opioids are meperidine (Demerol), methadone (Dolophine), paregoric, diphenoxylate (in Lomotil), fentanyl (Sublimaze), and propoxyphene (Darvon). Pentazocine (Talwin) is a nonopioid substance that can produce an opioid-like dependence. There are currently approximately 700,000 opioid addicts in the United States.[2] Dependence develops in approximately 50% of the individuals who engage in opioid abuse.[5] The preferred drugs are heroin and methadone, accounting for the bulk of abused drugs in this class.

Opioid pharmacologic activity is similar to that of the endogenous opioid-like substances enkephalins and endorphins, which are produced by the neuronal cells. Both the endogenous substances and opioids act at various receptor sites in the nervous system to produce their pharmacologic effect. The following four receptor sites mediate the analgesic and euphoric effects of this class of drugs[69]:

- μ: considered most important for supraspinal analgesia
  μ_1: supraspinal analgesia
  μ_2: opioid-induced respiratory depression, gastrointestinal tract motility, and cardiovascular effects such as bradycardia and hypotension
- κ: mediates analgesia, important for spinal analgesia
- δ: mediates analgesia, important for spinal analgesia
- σ: mediates dysphoria and psychotomimetic effects

The morphine-like agonist drugs act primarily on the μ and κ receptors to alter pain perception. All of the opioids also have CNS effects that include sedation and mood changes in addition to the analgesic effect. The opioid antagonist naloxone is a competitive inhibitor occupying, but not activating, the receptors.

Opioid abusers are likely to be involved with multiple drugs of abuse, often combining different classes of substances. The combination of heroin and cocaine ("speedball") is an example of the dangerous polypharmacy that has resulted in a number of fatalities. Other popular combinations are opioids plus ethanol and benzodiazepines. Although all opioids produce similar syndromes of intoxication and abstinence, the time courses, routes of administration, and associated complications differ. Knowledge of the different commonly used opioids is therefore of value.

Pharmacology

Heroin

Heroin (diacetylmorphine) as it is purchased on the street varies greatly in purity and in the substances with which it is adulterated. One study found the average concentration of heroin in street samples to be approximately 3%.[70] It is commonly "cut" with quinine, lactose, mannitol, and, occasionally, barbiturates.

Heroin comes from a variety of different locations with a wide range of purity. "Mexican Brown" and Turkish heroin are approximately 15% pure, generally cheaper, and more likely to contain vegetable matter than white heroin from the Far East. "Indian Pink," "Penang Pink," and "China White" are much purer forms of heroin and the user's preferred types.[55] The exact place of origin of a heroin sample can frequently be determined by inspection and chromatographic techniques.[71]

Heroin may be powdered, crystalline, or clumped and is usually sold as fractions of a gram or as dollar amounts (eg, a "quarter" is $25 worth, a "dime" is $10). A heroin abuser with a particularly large habit may use 10 or more quarters a day in five or six injections. A user with a "chippy" (modest habit) may use a dime several times a week. Regular recreational use of heroin by nondependent individuals is also not uncommon.[72]

Before being injected, the heroin is mixed with water of variable purity to which lemon juice is sometimes added to enhance solubility. The mixture is then heated in a spoon or bottle cap ("cooker") over a flame and often strained through cotton or a cigarette filter (which may, at a time of need, be itself heated in water to release trapped heroin). The solution is then injected either intravenously or subcutaneously. Heroin may also be insufflated ("snorted") or liquefied on a hot surface (such as tin foil over a candle) and fumes inhaled ("chasing the dragon"). Heroin is, however, largely inactive when ingested because of the considerable first-pass hepatic metabolism.

Heroin is probably inactive at CNS sites until hydrolyzed to active metabolites by serum esterases (of which a red cell–associated enzyme is the most important).[73,74] Although its half-life in the serum is only between 3 and 20 minutes, heroin is more lipophilic than morphine and may be preferentially concentrated in the CNS, where its active metabolites, 6-monoacetylmorphine (MAM) and morphine, then act.[75,76] Tolerance is developed over time in the habitual user to the extent that the dose required in the habitual user to prevent withdrawal might be lethal in the nontolerant patient. MAM is metabolized in the liver to morphine, which is conjugated with glucuronic acid and excreted in the urine. Neither morphine nor MAM is importantly bound to plasma proteins.

Methadone

Methadone (Dolophine) that is diverted from maintenance and detoxification programs is sold for approximately $1 per milligram on the street. It comes as a 40-mg scored orange diskette ("biscuit") mixed with cellulose to form a sludge in water that is said to discourage parenteral use. The methadone is, however, easily filtered with household apparatus. Methadone also comes as 5- and 10-mg Dolophine tablets ("Dolies" or "Dollies"), as a syrup (10 mg/mL), and as a solution (10 mg/mL).

Unlike most other opiates, methadone is well absorbed from the gastrointestinal tract and undergoes little first-pass metabolism. Parenterally, a single dose of methadone is slightly more potent than morphine on a weight basis, but by the oral route methadone is far more potent than heroin or morphine.[77] Peak levels occur between 2 and 4 hours after ingestion. Methadone is long acting, with a half-life of approximately a day. The drug is highly protein bound and has a large volume of distribution. Methadone is both metabolized in the liver and excreted unchanged in the urine. Plasma levels at steady state vary considerably from patient to patient and from day to day.[78] Acidification of the urine produces a statistically significant, but probably not clinically important, increase in clearance of parent drug.[79] Patients on methadone maintenance programs may be receiving more than 100 mg/day.[80]

Meperidine

Meperidine (Demerol) is not a common street narcotic but is a common substance abused by health care professionals. Its duration of action is 2 to 4 hours compared with morphine's 4- to 5-hour duration of action. Demerol comes as injectable solutions of 2.5, 5.0, 7.5, and 10.0% and as 50- and 100-mg tablets. Meperidine toxicity is characterized by respiratory depression, pupillary dilation, hyperactive reflexes, and convulsions.

Normeperidine is an active metabolite of meperidine. It has greater CNS excitatory potential than meperidine. Accumulated high plasma levels can result in agitation, tremor, myoclonus, and seizures.[69] Normeperidine is eliminated through renal excretion and further metabolization. Factors that allow accumulation are its long half-life (15 to 30 hours), repetitive oral administration, renal compromise, and use of other drugs that increase the N-demethylation of meperidine to normeperidine (phenytoin, phenobarbital, and chlorpromazine). It is not recommended for prolonged analgesia in patients with renal insufficiency, neoplasms, or sickle cell crises. Twitches and tremors occur at lower plasma levels than seizures and myoclonus may be a precursor to seizure activity.[81] Although naloxone reverses all signs of opioid overdose due to meperidine, it does not protect against seizures and cannot be recommended for the treatment of normeperidine-induced seizures.[69]

Propoxyphene

Propoxyphene (Darvon) is a common street drug that is obtainable as the napsylate (Darvon-N) and the more soluble hydrochloride (Darvon). Propoxyphene is a weak opioid related to methadone. It is irritating to the veins and often taken orally by patients on methadone maintenance programs to "boost the methadone dose," an effect for which there is some scientific evidence since propoxyphene may inhibit methadone metabolism.[82] Propoxyphene is metabolized in the liver and has a variable half-life of 3 to 8 hours. In overdose it produces signs of opioid toxicity but may also cause cardiac conduction defects and generalized seizures. The seizures may occur as early as 15 minutes after ingestion and result in status epilepticus.[83] The cardiac conduction defects include transient bundle branch blocks, QRS prolongation, and ST-T wave abnormalities.[69] It does not completely reverse syndromes of abstinence from more potent opioids and itself produces only mild dependence, even after high-dose intravenous use. Large doses of naloxone may be required to reverse the CNS depression caused by propoxyphene.[69] Naloxone will not reverse the cardiotoxic effects of the drug or prevent generalized seizures.

Percodan

Percodan (a combination of oxycodone, aspirin, phenacetin, and caffeine) and Percocet (oxycodone and acetaminophen) are common street narcotics. Although insoluble, Percodan may be crushed, shaken into a suspension, and injected intravenously ("cold shake"). Oxycodone is approximately 50% absorbed from the gastrointestinal tract. Its half-life is approximately 2 hours, and elimination occurs through the liver and kidneys. It is not uncommon for abusers to take 30 or 40 tablets a day and to present with signs of salicylism, acetaminophen-induced hepatic damage, gastrointestinal hemorrhage, and local complications of "cold shaking," such as phlebitis, cellulitis, and skin abscesses.

Pentazocine

Pentazocine (Talwin) has properties of both a narcotic agonist and antagonist. It can produce withdrawal symptoms in persons dependent on more powerful opioids. Pentazocine can cause mild dependence in those who use it regularly.[84] It is a common street drug in the West and Midwest, where oral use together with tripelennamine, an antihistamine ("Ts and blues") occurs.[85] It also has been injected intravenously as an inexpensive substitute for heroin. This intravenous combination produces similar but somewhat milder effects than heroin. There is significant morbidity to the intravenous use of Talwin and tripelennamine because of the microcrystalline cellulose and talc binders used in preparing these medications. Diffuse microemboli resulting in pulmonary morbidity, cerebral infarction, skin necrosis and ulcers, and membranoproliferative glomerulonephritis have been reported.[69] Manufacturers have attempted to discourage intravenous Talwin abuse by mixing naloxone with the Talwin. Because individuals dependent on more powerful opioids may suffer abstinence after taking a partial agonist such as pentazocine, opioid abusers will frequently give a history of allergy to Talwin. This history may be a clue to the diagnosis of opioid abuse, as true allergy is not common.

Lomotil

Lomotil is an antidiarrheal preparation with diphenoxylate and atropine. Although not a common substance of abuse, it has been responsible for a number of accidental overdoses, particularly in young children. It causes an initial anticholinergic syndrome with flushing, tachycardia, hyperthermia, lethargy, hallucinations, urinary retention, and seizures. The atropine also leads to delayed gastrointestinal absorption of the diphenoxylate and subsequently delayed onset of the opioid toxic effects. It is recommended that young children be observed in a monitored setting for 24 hours after the ingestion of Lomotil.[69] Repetitive doses of activated charcoal are also recommended to reduce absorption.

Intoxication and Overdose

Opioid intoxication causes feelings of pleasant drowsiness and contentment. The user may describe a warm sensation in the abdomen and chest. Many chronic users claim that opioids produce in them only remission from abstinence symptoms, but signs of intoxication are often present. For several seconds following intravenous injection, heroin and other powerful opioids produce intense euphoria ("rush" or "flash"), which may be accompanied by nausea and vomiting but is nevertheless pleasurable.[86]

Opioid intoxication is generally recognizable as a triad of respiratory depression, miosis, and CNS depression. Other accompanying physical findings are hypothermia, hypotension, bradycardia, hyporeflexia, and decreased bowel activity. The toxic effects are mediated through stimulation of the μ and κ receptors. The clinical picture is often confused by the pharmacologic activity of adulterants, contaminants, and other drugs intentionally taken with the opioid. Miosis may not always be present in opioid toxicity because of hypoxia, naloxone administration in the field, and congestants that counter the effect of the opioids. Mydriasis or normal pupils can also occur after overdose with meperidine, morphine, propoxyphene, and pentazocine.[69]

Despite reports of an increased prevalence of depression among heroin users, suicide is not particularly common, and overdose is usually accidental, a result of unexpectedly potent heroin or waning tolerance. The use of pharmaceutical grade opioid by heroin users tolerant to poor quality street drugs may produce overdose. Conversely, narcotic overdose is less severe in methadone-treated opioid abusers because of the consistent tolerance that daily methadone confers.

It appears that there are two overdose syndromes. The first results in death within minutes. The mechanism of this is still speculative and may be multifactorial. The various hypotheses range from a hypersensitivity reaction to the effect of adulterants or a synergistic effect of coingesting alcohol or barbiturates. This sudden death syndrome occurs mainly among heroin and ''designer'' opioid users. The patient develops fulminant pulmonary edema, respiratory failure, hypoxia, and ultimately cardiac arrest and death. The etiology of this noncardiogenic pulmonary edema is still unclear. One proposal is that it is secondary to ventilatory compromise resulting in precapillary pulmonary hypertension, increased capillary permeability, and fluid leak.[69]

The second type of overdose syndrome may occur after use of any opioid. Coma develops over minutes after parenteral use and over hours following oral ingestion. There is the classic picture of constricted pupils, shallow and infrequent respiration, hypotension, and occasionally pulmonary edema. Death results from hypoxia.[87]

The diagnosis of opioid overdose should be considered in any patient who is obtunded. Even trauma sufficient to account for unconsciousness may have been associated with opioid overdose. It is still rational to recommend the routine use of naloxone in all patients in whom the cause of coma is in doubt. Naloxone is a pure opioid antagonist that acts by competitive inhibition at the opioid receptor sites. The effect of naloxone on opioid-intoxicated patients is predictable, immediate (peak effect in approximately 5 minutes), and usually striking. Naloxone is therefore both diagnostic and therapeutic.[88]

Before giving naloxone, pupil size, respiratory rate and depth, blood pressure, and pulse should be noted. A 2.0-mg dose of naloxone should be given by rapid intravenous injection in adults or 0.1 mg/kg in infants and children. Patients in whom one of these parameters changes without a change in coma grade should be given an additional 2.0 mg every 3 minutes until a total of 10 mg is administered in the adult patient. In the pediatric patient the amount of repetitive dosing is not firmly established. It is reasonable to repeat the 0.1 mg/kg dose once or twice. Although 2.0 mg will reverse most opioid intoxications, propoxyphene, codeine, diphenoxylate, and pentazocine are examples of opioids that may require more.[69]

Naloxone can be administered intravenously, intralingually, and endotracheally in an emergent situation. Onset of action is approximately 1 to 2 minutes by any of these routes. It is effectively absorbed via the pulmonary vasculature and can be instilled through an endotracheal tube at the same dose as intravenously but in a 5 to 10-mL volume to ensure distribution into the lower airways. It is also effective by the intramuscular route, although peak effect may not occur for 15 to 30 minutes.[89]

Although response to naloxone is the best sign of opioid intoxication, evidence of chronic abuse may point to the diagnosis. Skin findings, sometimes hidden in tattoos, are usually present on parenteral heroin and cocaine users. Parallel punctate scars on either side of the vein (''tram lines'') or a single row following the center of the vein (''tracks'') are characteristic. Palpable sclerotic veins with overlying hyperpigmentation are sometimes found. Dried blood on the skin may indicate recent injection. Opioid-induced histamine release occasionally causes localized urticaria (as well as the risk of laryngeal edema).

The finding of a large number of recent injection marks and/or evidence of severe and widespread phlebitis suggests cocaine rather than heroin abuse. Cocaine has a much shorter duration of action than heroin and is usually taken more frequently.

Signs of chronic venous insufficiency and obliteration of lymph channels are often present (puffy hands or feet), and digital clubbing has recently been described as a common finding of uncertain cause.[90] Healed ulcers and abscesses from subcutaneous administration (''skin popping,'' ''skinning'') or attempted intravenous injections (''misses'') may also be seen. Digital amputations from arterial injections are not rare.

Bronchospasm has been associated with both intravenous and inhaled heroin. Dyspnea and wheezing may occur a few days to months after heroin use and are associated with eosinophils in the sputum. Bronchospasm is believed to be either an allergic reaction to heroin, adulterants, or bronchial hyperactivity to a foreign substance.[91] The spleen is sometimes enlarged and firm in chronic parenteral drug users. This finding, however, should not be dismissed as merely a marker for drug abuse until the possibility of an occult splenic abscess has been considered.[92] Acute rhabdomyolysis with renal failure is occasionally noted in these patients and may be secondary to seizure activity, prolonged immobility, or use of sympathomimetic substances with the opioid.

Other neurologic sequelae of opioid overdose, apart from coma, include vaso-occlusive syndromes of the middle cerebral artery and anterior spinal artery. The patient presents with signs of middle cerebral artery infarction or a spinal cord syndrome. Arteriography reveals unexplained occlusions in these patients.[93,94]

Once considered, the diagnosis of uncomplicated opioid overdose is not difficult to make, and a rapid, complete response to naloxone obviates the need for further investigation. If, however, no response or only a partial response to naloxone occurs, complicating factors, such as mixed overdose, postictal confusion, sepsis, or cerebral anoxia (from hypoventilation, pulmonary edema, dysrhythmia, or shock), become necessary considerations.

Depressed mental status and miosis can be caused by a number of drugs (clonidine, organophosphates, carbamates, phenothiazines, PCP, and sedative-hypnotics). There are usually several other signs and symptoms of each drug that allow for differentiation. Pontine hemorrhage is also a cause of coma and miosis. These patients generally have accompanying neurogenic hyperventilation and significant neurologic deficits.

Mixed overdoses and those complicated by neurologic deficits require further workup with urine screening, electroencephalogram (EEG), and computed tomography (CT).

When signs of chronic heroin use are present in an obtunded patient who responds only partially to naloxone, the following differential diagnoses of drug abuse related coma should be searched for:

- seizure
- tetanus
- sepsis with or without cerebral emboli
- neurologic sequelae of hepatitis
- cerebral angiitis (associated with amphetamine and methylphenidate abuse or as part of the leukocytoclastic angiitis described in opioid abuse)
- uremia from heroin-induced glomerulopathy, secondary amyloidosis, or rhabdomyolysis with acute tubular necrosis
- shock following gastrointestinal hemorrhage from Percodan ingestion, perforation of an abdominal viscus, or pancreatitis, any of which may be masked by opioid analgesia
- internal bleeding from heroin- or quinine-induced thrombocytopenia
- the effects of other drugs, including those with which the heroin may have been cut (see Chapter 57, Coma).

Proper airway management and the use of naloxone are the key therapeutic interventions in the management of opioid overdose. Gastrointestinal decontamination is important in patients who have ingested long-acting opioids such as methadone, MS-Contin, and Lomotil and in "body stuffers" or "body packers" who have large quantities of opioids in their gastrointestinal tract. All patients with oral ingestions, regardless of the opioid, should receive activated charcoal. Dialysis and hemoperfusion are not of benefit.

The patient who arrives in the emergency department with a decreased level of consciousness and hypoventilation can usually safely tolerate assisted ventilations with bag-valve mask until naloxone is administered. If the patient does not respond or no intravenous access can be obtained, it is prudent to endotracheally intubate the patient for airway protection and to allow adequate ventilations. The treatment of opioid-induced noncardiogenic pulmonary edema is adequate oxygenation and ventilation. This often requires endotracheal intubation and positive end-expiratory pressure ventilation until resolution occurs. Infiltrates and blood gases usually improve by the end of 2 days, although pulmonary function tests may be abnormal for weeks.[95] In addition, overdose with propoxyphene or meperidine may require intubation in order to perform lavage if the risk of seizures or dysrhythmia is thought to be significant.

The half-life of naloxone is approximately 45 minutes, and its effects wear off after 60 to 90 minutes. On the other hand, the CNS depressant effects of long-acting opioids may last considerably longer following large ingestions, particularly with overdoses of methadone or sustained-release morphine (MS-Contin). A continuous naloxone infusion may be the best approach in these cases. The hourly infusion rate can be initially approximated by giving two thirds the amount of naloxone it took to reverse respiratory depression.[69] Once it has been shown that naloxone completely reverses coma, it is no longer necessary (and may, from a management standpoint, be undesirable) to keep the patient fully awake while the opioid is metabolized.[88]

The abrupt withdrawal precipitated by naloxone may be accompanied by rage or even psychosis. These reactions usually subside in 20 to 30 minutes as the effect of naloxone decreases. However, the patient should not be allowed to leave the hospital until it is clear that further naloxone is unnecessary. There are case reports of pulmonary edema and hypertensive reactions following abrupt reversal of opioid-induced coma.[96]

Opioid overdoses may result in hypotension, which usually responds to naloxone and intravenous fluids. Urinary retention requiring bladder catheterization and fecal impaction may also occur.

A blood count, clotting studies, measurement of blood gases, liver and renal function tests, an electrocardiogram, a chest roentgenogram, and assessment of electrolytes and blood sugar should be included in the initial assessment of the serious opioid overdose. If Percodan or Percocet ingestion is suspected, early measurement of salicylate and 4-hour (after ingestion) measurement of acetaminophen levels in plasma is important. Plasma opioid levels are not useful in estimating prognosis because tolerance to opioids, not their concentration in the blood, determines the clinical state. Detection of opioids in urine may be helpful in some cases. Since hydrolysis of morphine from its glucuronide conjugate improves sensitivity of testing, the laboratory should be notified when heroin is being sought. Treatment of opioid overdose should not, however, await laboratory confirmation.[97]

Findings that encourage hospitalization of the patient with opioid toxicity include (1) a history of drug screen documenting overdose with a long-acting opioid, (2) a partial response to naloxone, (3) a history or drug screen suggesting multiple drugs, and (4) the presence of serious medical problems related or unrelated to the overdose. It is unlawful to deny admission to a drug addict because of his or her addiction.

Abstinence Syndromes

Daily administration of potent opioids for 2 to 3 weeks can produce tolerance and, upon deprivation, a marked abstinence syndrome.[98] Since its first detailed clinical description 50 years ago, the opioid abstinence syndrome has been well studied.

The withdrawal from opioids begins approximately 8 to 12 hours after the last dose of the drug. It begins with anxiety, drug craving, irritability, insomnia, dilated pupils, rhinorrhea, lacrimation, sweating, and slightly elevated temperature. At approximately 48 to 72 hours of abstinence, nausea, vomiting, diarrhea, abdominal pain, weakness, tachycardia, hypertension, myalgias, muscle spasms, and piloerection (gooseflesh) occur. The withdrawal syndrome gradually resolves over 7 to 14 days.[5] If the individual was addicted to long-acting opioids such as methadone, the withdrawal syndrome will be delayed approximately 24 to 48 hours and usually be somewhat less intense but more prolonged, lasting 2 to 3 weeks.

Opioid abstinence syndromes, although uncomfortable, are almost always benign and self-limited, unlike the sedative-hypnotic drug and ethanol withdrawal syndromes, which may be life-threatening. Seizures, delirium, and high fever should not be attributed to opioid withdrawal if they occur.[99] The patient may have multiple drug addictions and be withdrawing from ethanol or a sedative-hypnotic agent. Sepsis and CNS infection should also be considered in the differential diagnosis and be aggressively evaluated.

When it is difficult but important to differentiate sedative or alcohol from opiate abstinence, a trial dose of a short-acting barbiturate (eg, 200 mg oral pentobarbital, repeated in 2 hours, if necessary) may be helpful. This maneuver will not reverse signs of opioid abstinence, but will markedly improve sedative or alcohol abstinence. Similarly, small doses of a short-acting opiate (eg, 5 to 10 mg morphine subcutaneously) will improve only the signs of opioid abstinence.

Opioid abusers may submit to invasive procedures, even laparotomy, in order to obtain narcotics, so it is important that abstinence be recognized. Other conditions in the differential diagnosis are viral respiratory and gastrointestinal syndromes, tetanus, endocarditis, osteomyelitis, diabetic ketoacidosis, and abdominal conditions of surgical importance. If the opioid-abusing patient presents with a bona fide medical emergency requiring admission or surgery, no attempt at detoxification is recommended acutely. Patients should be placed on maintenance doses of methadone throughout their illness.[36] These patients may require significant doses of other analgesics to control pain; methadone alone will not be effective. Pentazocine, butorphanol, and nalbuphine are contraindicated because their narcotic antagonist effects may precipitate withdrawal.[5]

There are four primary drugs used to treat opioid addiction: methadone, buprenorphine, clonidine, and naltrexone. They are used in maintenance and detoxification programs to transition the addict from parenterally administered agents such as heroin, meperidine, or fentanyl.

Methadone is a pure μ-receptor (morphine-like) agonist, which in sufficient doses acts to reduce craving for opioids and produces cross-tolerance to the effects of other opioids. It has been used for maintenance and detoxification programs since 1965.[100] Methadone can be orally administered, which makes it ideal for outpatient detoxification, and has been credited with decreasing the spread of HIV-1 infection among opioid addicts who have enrolled in the program.

If a patient presents to the emergency department with signs and symptoms of opioid withdrawal, 5 to 10 mg of methadone intramuscularly will be effective in relieving the withdrawal symptoms in the majority of individuals regardless of the amount of heroin or methadone the patient generally takes.[36] In the setting of withdrawal with vomiting and diarrhea, the intramuscular route provides a more reliable level of drug uptake than oral administration. A daily dose of 25 to 60 mg will generally be adequate to blunt the desire for opioids.[101] Once abstinence is under control, a methadone-tapering program has enjoyed some success in helping the opioid addict remain off drugs.

Clonidine is not an opioid but an α_2-adrenergic agonist that acts on the CNS to block adrenergic responses to opioid deprivation and has been successful in suppressing the symptoms of opioid withdrawal. Clonidine has been abused by some patients in conjunction with methadone, diazepam, and alcohol to produce enhanced euphoric effects.[5] When used, clonidine can be titrated to effect by giving 0.1 mg orally every half-hour until the patient feels better, side effects (particularly hypotension) become prohibitive, or six tablets have been given without effect. Clonidine is not equally effective in all patients or for all symptoms and must frequently be given in doses that provoke fatigue, dry mouth, and postural dizziness. Clonidine occasionally causes hallucinations, a finding that may be confusing in a drug abuser.

Naltrexone, approved in 1983, is a relatively long-acting, competitive antagonist at the μ receptor. It has been used to maintain abstinence in detoxified opioid addicts with varying degrees of success.[101] A major side effect of naltrexone is elevation of liver enzymes. Liver enzymes should be monitored in patients receiving naltrexone.[5] A clonidine-naltrexone protocol for acute opioid detoxification has been utilized with some success.

Buprenorphine is a partial μ receptor agonist that produces morphine-like subjective effects and cross-tolerance to other opioids. It may have advantages over methadone in that in increasing doses, there is not a corresponding increase in respiratory depression or sedation. In a recent study, 8 mg/day of buprenorphine was as effective as 60 mg/day of methadone in preventing illicit opioid use among a group of opioid addicts.[101] The most recent recommendation has been a transition heroin and methadone addicts to buprenorphine and then bring them through a short 1- to 3-day naltrexone withdrawal with clonidine to ameliorate the withdrawal symptoms.[102]

Unfortunately, even successful withdrawal of opioids almost never produces a lasting cure. In addition to treatment of abstinence, it is essential that patients receive adequate referral for definitive therapy, whether chemical (methadone, buprenorphine, or naltrexone maintenance) or drug-free (counseling, therapeutic community, day treatment, inpatient rehabilitation). It is illegal for a practitioner or hospital to undertake opioid maintenance therapy of drug dependence on an outpatient basis without prior approval. Even the one-time treatment of abstinence using an opioid should be approached with caution and knowledge of state law. In most states the emergency physician may not prescribe opioids to a known abuser without notifying the health department and may not under any circumstances dispense opioids for longer than 3 consecutive days.

Specialized facilities prepared to treat opioid dependence with drugs and/or psychotherapy offer the best hope of long-term remission. Referral is therefore an important function of emergency treatment of opioid abstinence. Aggressive intervention by social workers, counselors, or nurses skilled in interviewing techniques is more likely to result in adequate follow-up than is referral by the emergency physician. Close cooperation between social service and emergency department staffs is necessary for a successful referral system.

DESIGNER DRUGS

Designer drugs are substances intended for recreational use that are derivatives of approved drugs in an effort to circumvent existing legal restrictions. There are two general classes of designer drugs: the hallucinogenic amphetamines, 3,4-methylenedioxyamphetamine (MDA) and 3,4-methylenedioxymethamphetamine (MDMA), and the synthetic opioid derivatives, which are derivatives of fentanyl or meperidine.

MDMA is not a new drug. It was first synthesized in 1914, and the US Army conducted research involving the hallucinogenic amphetamines during the 1950s.[9,103] No therapeutic utility was found for these drugs and the US FDA subsequently listed them as Schedule I drugs along with heroin and lysergic acid diethylamide (LSD).

They are synthesized by halogenating or substituting one or more methoxy groups on the benzene ring of amphetamine.[55] Disturbing reports from Britain regarding MDMA ("Ecstasy") use in the setting of all-night "rave" dance parties have begun to surface over the past 2 years. The British have reported at least 15 deaths attributable to MDMA. Most commonly the individuals have been consuming alcohol, participating in vigorous dancing for hours in overcrowded night clubs, and taking Ecstasy tablets to produce a hallucinogenic experience.[103] The British "rave" culture has been exported to the United States and has experienced popularity in the areas of Los Angeles and San Francisco in California. MDMA abuse has also been part of the "rave" dances in California.[104] In overdose the difference between other sympathomimetic toxicity and hallucinogenic amphetamine toxicity is small. These patients present with tachycardia, hypertension, hyperthermia, diaphoresis, mydriasis, agitation, muscle rigidity, and hyperreflexia. Death usually results from dysrhythmias,[105,106] intracerebral hemorrhage, or a heatstroke syndrome with acute rhabdomyolysis, renal failure, disseminated intravascular coagulation, and ultimately multisystem organ failure and death.[107] The British have identified seven cases of Ecstasy-induced hepatotoxicity in young people presenting with jaundice and hepatomegaly.[108] It is currently unclear whether this represents an idiosyncratic reaction or a toxic effect from a metabolite of MDMA. MDMA use has also been associated with the development of chronic psychosis.[109-111]

The fentanyl analogues have been the cause of at least 100 fatal overdoses in the past 5 years. "China White" (originally the name of pure heroin from the Far East) is the name given to the new potent analogues of fentanyl that began to appear on the streets in California in 1979.[112] α-Methyl fentanyl was the initial analogue of fentanyl and is credited with causing most of the early deaths prior to 1984. In 1984, 3-methylfentanyl (TMF) was recognized as the cause of most of the deaths between 1984 and 1985 in the western United States.[112] TMF is the most potent of the fentanyl analogues. It is 6000 times more potent than morphine and 1000 to 2000 times more potent than heroin.[113] It produces more analgesia than euphoria, but the euphoria is longer lasting than the sensation produced by heroin, accounting for its popularity.[69] It is very difficult to detect because it is effective in microgram quantities. In 1986–1988, fatalities were noted in Pennsylvania secondary to TMF, indicating the spread of this illicit substance to the East Coast. The cause of death is respiratory depression and the treatment is aggressive airway management and very often large doses of naloxone to maintain effective ventilation.

In 1979, it was recognized that a meperidine analogue called MPTP was responsible for a chemically induced parkinsonism.[114] MPTP is a compound that was accidentally produced in an effort to synthesize 1-methyl-4-phenyl-4-propionoxypiperidine (MPPP), a meperidine analogue sold on the streets for intravenous narcotic abuse. MPTP is metabolized by the monoamine oxidase system in the brain to a toxic metabolite that has been demonstrated to irreversibly destroy the cells in the substantia nigra of the brain producing a rapid and severe parkinsonian syndrome.

The narcotic combination of MPTP-MPPP produces a burning sensation when injected followed by an atypical disorienting and dysphoric "high" quite different from the experience with opioids.[69] In approximately 1 week, the initial symptoms begin to appear. The MPTP syndrome differs from Parkinson's disease in that MPTP selectively destroys only the nigrostriatal dopamine neurons and does not have the diffuse involvement of many other areas of the brain.[115] Patients with the MPTP-induced parkinsonism have a syndrome of hypokinesia, speaking difficulty, cogwheel rigidity, tremor, flexed posture, loss of postural reflexes, and drooling. These patients are sometimes referred to as "frozen" addicts. This syndrome differs from Parkinson's disease in that they do not develop the dementia, cerebellar instability, autonomic impairment, or pyramidal tract deficits. The MPTP parkinsonism syndrome is permanent, but patients are being successfully treated with levodopa and carbidopa to correct the dopamine deficiency present.[115]

SEDATIVE-HYPNOTICS

Sedative-hypnotic drugs, although chemically heterogeneous, produce similar clinical effects, degrees of tolerance, and abstinence syndromes. Most are anticonvulsants and antispasmodics and have similar effects on the EEG. They all produce a degree of relaxation, somnolence, and, in toxic quantities, coma. Moreover, one sedative abolishes the abstinence syndrome caused by withdrawal of others (the phenomenon of cross-tolerance) with the possible exception of the benzodiazepine alprazolam. It appears unique in that other sedative-hypnotics do not block the appearance of an abstinence syndrome when alprazolam is abruptly discontinued.[7] Although sedatives are conveniently discussed as a group, it should be realized that important differences exist among these drugs in their toxic manifestations and liability to abuse.

Table 48-8 lists the more common sedative-hypnotic drugs by class and the relative elimination half-lives of each drug. The data suggest that many of the sedatives remain in the system for days after ingestion. These data are particularly important when viewed with the knowledge that sedative abusers frequently abuse alcohol, compounding the effects of these intermediate- and long-acting drugs.

The earliest sedatives used were the bromides and chloral hydrate introduced in the 1800s. The barbiturates were synthesized in the early 1900s and became the predominant sedative-hypnotic until the 1960s when the benzodiazepines were marketed.[16] Benzodiazepines are now some of the most commonly prescribed drugs in the world and half of all exposures to sedative-hypnotic drugs reported to American poison control centers are drugs from this class.[55]

The sedative abuser is usually introduced to the drug later in life than abusers of other types of substances. Sedatives

Table 48-8 Common Sedative-Hypnotics with Elimination Half-Lives[16,55]

Type	Elimination Half-Life (hours)
Barbiturates	
Short-acting	
Pentobarbital (Nembutal, Pentobarbitone)	20–30
Secobarbital (Seconal, Quinalbarbitone)	22–29
Intermediate-acting	
Amobarbital (Amytal, Amylobarbitone)	15–40
Butabarbital (Butisol)	34–42
Long-acting	
Phenobarbital (Luminal)	48–144
Benzodiazepines	
Ultrashort-acting	
Midazolam (Versed)	2–5
Temazepam (Restoril)	10
Triazolam (Halcion)	1.7–3
Short-acting	
Alprazolam (Xanax)	11–14
Lorazepam (Ativan)	10–20
Oxazepam (Serax)	3–21
Long-acting	
Chlordiazepoxide (Librium)	5–30
Clonazepam (Clonopin)	10–50
Clorazepate (Tranxene)	36–200
Diazepam (Valium)	20–50
Flurazepam (Dalmane)	50–100
Prazepam (Centrax)	26–200
Others	
Chloral hydrate (Noctec)	8–12
Ethchlorvynol (Placidyl)	25
Glutethimide (Doriden)	10–12
Meprobamate (Miltown)	8–12
Methaqualone (Quaalude)	20–50

are more commonly obtained by prescription than from illegal factories and more commonly taken orally than parenterally. They may also be using sedatives to offset abstinence symptoms from other drugs, particularly stimulants. The "disinhibition" euphoria produced by sedatives may be sought by the stimulant addict to counteract a severe underlying depression. Sedative-hypnotic abusers tend to have more vehicular and industrial accidents, remain chronically intoxicated, and have poor personal hygiene and nutritional status and increased incidence of suicide. A small percentage of sedative-hypnotic abusers parenterally inject the drugs and face the same risks discussed earlier in this chapter.

Pharmacology

Barbiturates

Barbiturates are not such common drugs of abuse as they were previously. They have been primarily replaced by the benzodiazepines. Barbiturates may be short-, intermediate-, or long-acting, but abuse is usually limited to intermediate-acting compounds because they produce a greater degree of euphoria than the longer acting barbiturates. The most commonly abused barbiturates are secobarbital (Seconal), pentobarbital (Nembutal), amobarbital (with secobarbital as Tuinal), and butalbital (Fiorinal and others).

These drugs are bitter white powders, soluble in hot water and alcohol, and completely absorbed within 4 hours from the gastrointestinal tract and distributed throughout the body water. Barbiturates of this type are minimally bound to plasma proteins. They are metabolized by the liver to inactive compounds that are excreted in the urine. Excretion is not importantly enhanced by alteration of urine pH, unlike the excretion of phenobarbital, a long-acting barbiturate. The half-lives of intermediate-acting barbiturates are 12 to 24 hours, but duration of effect depends greatly on redistribution within the body. In new users, sleep lasts 6 to 8 hours after usual doses, but an effect on performance of complex tasks may be demonstrated for as long as 24 hours. After 4 to 6 weeks of daily use, usual doses produce little hypnotic effect.[116]

Tolerance develops both acutely and chronically. In acute overdose, patients may emerge from coma at plasma levels of drug that would otherwise render them unconscious. Tolerance to chronic dosing develops over weeks of daily use but is less pronounced than for opioids. The induction of hepatic microsomal enzymes (which may also influence metabolism of many other drugs) is partly responsible for tolerance. Tolerance to the euphoric effect is not accompanied by the same level of tolerance to a lethal dose (ie, there is a reduction in the margin of safety).

Benzodiazepines

Benzodiazepines are an ever-expanding group of antianxiety and hypnotic compounds. Unlike other sedatives, benzodiazepines can produce anxiolysis at concentrations that do not induce lethargy. Also unlike other sedatives, these compounds act on a group of specific receptors in the CNS stimulating the GABA pathways and causing sedation, anxiolysis, and striated muscle relaxation.

Benzodiazepines are very commonly prescribed because they are excellent anxiolytics without the significant risks of cardiorespiratory or CNS depression of the barbiturates. They are relatively safe drugs in overdose because of an apparent rapid adaptation to high blood levels.[55]

Like barbiturates, benzodiazepines may be short-, intermediate-, or long-acting. (Refer to Table 48-8 for the list of benzodiazepines currently available.) All of these compounds, except possibly alprazolam (for which a specific antidepressant role has been suggested), produce similar effects.[117] Abstinence syndromes do occur after prolonged usage and tend to be more severe with the short-acting compounds.[118] Idiosyncratic rage reactions have been reported for most benzodiazepines.

Duration of action depends on speed of redistribution and routes of metabolism. For the most part short- and intermediate-acting benzodiazepines are metabolized to inactive glucuronides that are rapidly excreted in the urine (triazolam and alprazolam are exceptions). They have half-lives of 2 to 20 hours. Long-acting benzodiazepines are oxidized, usually to psychoactive desmethyl compounds. These drugs or their active metabolites have half-lives measured in days that increase linearly with age and are significantly affected by liver disease.[119,120]

Benzodiazepines are completely absorbed, although with variable rapidity, by the oral route. Intramuscular absorption is erratic except for lorazepam. These drugs are almost entirely bound to plasma proteins and do not induce hepatic enzymes.

Methaqualone

Methaqualone (Quaalude, Sopor), introduced as a safe, nonaddicting, barbiturate substitute in 1965, gained popularity because of its reputation for causing intoxication without drowsiness and for acting as an aphrodisiac. It has been withdrawn from the market because of widespread abuse and mortality secondary to severe respiratory depression when combined with ethanol.[7] Like barbiturates, methaqualone is a sedative-hypnotic and anticonvulsant with the ability to reduce inhibitions and sexual performance. It is also an antitussive and may enhance opioid analgesia.

Methaqualone is a lipophilic white powder, soluble in alcohol but not water, that is completely absorbed within 2 hours with a large volume of distribution. There is considerable binding to tissues. The drug is metabolized by microsomal liver enzymes (which it also stimulates) to compounds that are probably inactive and are excreted in urine and bile. Plasma half-life is about 19 hours, but because of redistribution in the body, sleep lasts only 5 to 6 hours after usual doses. Tolerance is moderate.

Glutethimide

Glutethimide (Doriden) was introduced in the United States as a barbiturate substitute in 1965. It is a sedative with some antiemetic properties. In overdose it can produce a prolonged, fluctuating coma with cerebral edema, pulmonary edema, seizures, and apnea.[55] Glutethimide can present with signs of an anticholinergic toxidrome with pupillary dilation, ileus, urinary retention, and warm, dry skin. It is no longer as commonly abused as other sedative-hypnotics. During the 1980s, there were some combinations of codeine and glutethimide, called "packs," "loads," or "sets," sold as oral substitutes for heroin on the East Coast.[121,122]

It is poorly water soluble and absorbed erratically by the oral route. Highly variable peak plasma levels are attained after 1 to 6 hours. Binding to plasma proteins is minimal, and the drug is distributed largely in fat. Metabolism is hepatic with formation of inactive products and a 4-hydroxy metabolite that appears to contribute to the toxicity of glutethimide.[123] Half-life is approximately 12 hours but may be longer in overdose. Redistribution, however, is largely responsible for termination of hypnosis after 4 to 8 hours in new users at usual doses.

Moderate tolerance develops to the effects of glutethimide. Signs of toxicity and abstinence may resemble each other (seizure and tremors), and signs of spontaneous abstinence without a change in drug intake can occur in chronic users. This phenomenon may be due to fluctuating plasma levels associated with erratic absorption or to toxicity of the active metabolite.[124] Glutethimide markedly stimulates hepatic enzymes.

Ethchlorvynol

Ethchlorvynol (Placidyl), introduced in 1955, is an anticonvulsant and sedative-hypnotic that is rapidly absorbed (maximum plasma levels in approximately 1 hour). Clinical effects are brief after usual doses, probably because of rapid redistribution, and its half-life is 5 to 6 hours due to rapid hepatic metabolism. In overdose, coma may be prolonged, with respiratory depression, hypotension, hypothermia, and relative bradycardia.[55] Copious secretions may occur reminiscent of organophosphate poisoning. Hepatic enzyme saturation may prolong half-life to more than 100 hours.[125] Induction of hepatic enzymes does not appear to occur.

The packaging of ethchlorvynol as a liquid-filled gelatin capsule facilitates parenteral use. Intravenous doses of 1.5 g have caused serious poisoning. Moderate tolerance occurs, and prolonged psychosis has been reported after abstinence.

Meprobamate

Meprobamate (Miltown and others), introduced in the 1950s, is no longer a commonly prescribed anxiolytic or sedative. It has been replaced by the benzodiazepines. The drug is well absorbed within 4 hours after usual doses but may form gastric concretions in overdose. Rate of absorption also depends on the formulation.[126] Meprobamate is liver metabolized to inactive products and induces microsomal enzymes; its half-life is approximately 11 hours after usual doses.

Chloral Hydrate

Chloral hydrate (Noctec and others) is often considered a mild soporific, but it can produce marked tolerance and an abstinence syndrome resembling delirium tremens. In overdose, cardiac dysrhythmias, renal failure, jaundice, gastrointestinal bleeding, and respiratory depression occur.[127,128] Chloral hydrate is rapidly absorbed and converted to the active trichloroethanol. This compound is metabolized by the liver with a half-life of approximately 8 hours. Trichloroethanol both stimulates hepatic microsomal enzymes and displaces many drugs from plasma proteins.

Overdose and Intoxication

Sedative intoxication resembles alcohol inebriation and presents as either euphoria or more commonly in the emergency department as respiratory, cardiovascular, and CNS depression. The nonbarbiturate sedatives characteristically cause less respiratory depression and more marked cardiovascular effects than barbiturates. Alcohol intoxication frequently occurs with sedative overdose and synergistically exacerbates the physiologic response to the sedatives. An apparently trivial sedative overdose in the presence of alcohol may result in a severely compromised patient. Although Table 48-9 is provided to point out some of the unique features in the clinical presentation of sedative overdose, the emergency physician's initial approach to the patient will be the same regardless of the agent used.

All comatose patients presenting with a history suggestive of sedative overdose must be approached with an open mind to the possibility of other metabolic or systemic etiologies of coma. The sequence of events to be considered in the resuscitation of each patient is as follows: airway evaluation and control, ventilatory and cardiovascular support, hemodynamic monitoring as necessary, further diagnostic studies to rule out other causes of coma, gut decontamination, forced/alkaline diuresis, and hemodialysis or charcoal hemoperfusion.

Airway Evaluation and Control

If the patient is comatose and unresponsive to painful stimulus, ventilations may be initially supported with 100% oxygen via bag-valve mask while an intravenous line is established, electrocardiographic monitoring is begun, bedside blood glucose is checked, and glucose (as necessary), naloxone, and thiamine are administered. If the history suggests a benzodiazepine overdose, a specific antidote, flumazenil, is now available. It is a selective inhibitor of the central effects of benzodiazepines, specifically CNS and respiratory depression.[129,130] In the setting of isolated benzodiazepine overdose, flumazenil effectively reverses coma within 1 to 2 minutes. In a chronic benzodiazepine user, it may precipitate a withdrawal syndrome. Flumazenil has been associated with at least one death in a patient with both benzodiazepine and tricyclic antidepressant overdose.[131] The patient died from refractory status epilepticus after administration of this benzodiazepine reversal agent. It is recommended to give flumazenil at an initial dose of 0.1 to 0.2 mg intravenously followed by 0.1 mg every minute to a total dose of 2.0 mg.[132] A continuous infusion of 0.1 to 0.2 mg/hour may be indicated in cases where long-acting benzodiazepines have been ingested to prevent lapse back into coma.[133]

Endotracheal intubation is indicated if there is no response to this initial intervention, if the patient is unable to manage his orotracheal secretions or is in acute respiratory/circulatory failure.

Table 48-9 Differential Signs of Sedative-Hypnotic Overdose[55,122]

Sedative-Hypnotic	Clinical Signs
Barbiturates	Respiratory and cardiovascular depression, flaccid muscle tone, vesiculobullous lesions*, hypothermia, noncardiogenic pulmonary edema
Benzodiazepines	Generally milder CNS depression with response to painful stimuli, occasional paradoxical excitatory reaction
Methaqualone	Myoclonus, hyperreflexia, hypertonicity, seizures, prolonged coma, extravasation of blood (purpura, gastrointestinal bleeding, retinal hemorrhage)
Glutethimide	Anticholinergic syndrome (with pupillary dilation), seizures, cyclical prolonged coma, papilledema and cerebral edema, pulmonary complications
Meprobamate	Fluctuating coma, meprobamate bezoar formation, hypotension, pulmonary edema
Ethchlorvynol	Prolonged, deep coma; sweet, aromatic breath odor; respiratory depression; noncardiogenic pulmonary edema; prolonged apnea; bradycardia
Chloral hydrate	CNS, respiratory, and cardiovascular depression; cardiac dysrhythmias; gastritis; urticaria, eczema, purpura, bullae; radiopaque tablets on radiograph; odor of "pears" on breath

*Although dermal bullous lesions are commonly described in barbiturate overdose, they have also been reported in ethchlorvynol, glutethimide, meprobamate, and methaqualone overdose.

Ventilatory Support

If the patient is hypoxemic and/or hypoventilatory, mechanical ventilation with an initial 100% FIO_2 is essential to prevent further compromise and circulatory collapse. The patient may also present in acute pulmonary edema with respiratory failure. Frequently this is a noncardiogenic pulmonary edema that will require mechanical ventilation with positive end-expiratory pressure support.

Cardiovascular Failure

Sedative-hypnotics have several effects leading to decreased cardiac output, hypotension, and cardiac dysrhythmias. These drugs can decrease right ventricular filling and cardiac output as a result of peripheral vasodilation. Cardiac output is also decreased by a direct myocardial depressant effect. Additionally, chloral hydrate overdose sensitizes the myocardium to catecholamines inducing cardiac dysrhythmias.

The initial management of the hypotensive sedative overdose patient is to volume resuscitate the patient with intravenous crystalloid. In the young, otherwise healthy individual 500 mL boluses up to 1 to 2 L total can be given with sequential assessments to monitor response. In the elderly or in patients with known cardiac or renal compromise, a more conservative approach with 200 mL boluses and careful monitoring is indicated. A Foley catheter should be inserted to monitor urine output. If there is no improvement to the initial volume resuscitation, then vasopressors may be started with the goal of raising the systolic blood pressure to 90 to 100 mmHg. Dopamine at an initial dose of 2 to 5 μg/kg per minute or Levophed at 2 to 8 μg/min has each been used with success. Caution must be exercised in the patient with chloral hydrate overdose because of the tendency to develop cardiac dysrhythmias. Lidocaine or phenytoin are usually successful in treating these dysrhythmias.[122]

Hemodynamic Monitoring

Arterial line and central venous pressure monitoring is indicated for those patients requiring mechanical ventilation and vasopressor support. Invasive monitoring is generally instituted in the emergency department when it is unclear what the patient's hemodynamic status is or when it is anticipated that the patient will require monitoring in the emergency department for a prolonged period of time. It is particularly important in the elderly patient or the patient with cardiac or renal compromise antecedent to the overdose. Swan-Ganz catheter placement is preferred to monitor cardiac output and pulmonary capillary wedge pressure but is not commonly available in the emergency department.

Other Diagnostic Studies

The comatose patient should always be approached with a complete differential diagnosis. Sedative-hypnotic ingestion may be only a part of the total picture and not the true life-threat to the patient. A metabolic screen, a search for other toxins, a sepsis workup, and concern about a possible intracranial bleed should be vigorously pursued.

Gut Decontamination

The best technique of gut decontamination is controversial based on the results of recent studies questioning the efficacy of traditional methods. Most of the sedative hypnotics delay gastric emptying, in some cases as long as 12 hours postingestion. Meprobamate has the tendency to form pill concretions or bezoars in the stomach.[55] Gastric emptying is generally indicated in those patients presenting with sedative-hypnotic overdose. Ipecac may be administered to those patients who present within an hour of ingestion and are alert or only minimally sedated at the time of presentation. Gastric lavage with prior endotracheal intubation is preferred in the patient who is comatose or unable to manage secretions. In the patient with a gag reflex who is somewhat responsive and cooperative, gastric lavage may be performed in the head down, left lateral decubitus position with close monitoring of respiratory and mental status and continuous pulse oxymetry. After gut emptying, activated charcoal (1 g/kg) is given to the patient. Pulse charcoal doses (0.5 g/kg every 2 to 4 hours) are indicated in overdose secondary to barbiturates and meprobamate.[122] Its utility in other sedative-hypnotics is unclear at this time.

Forced/Alkaline Diuresis

Diuresis should not be attempted in the hemodynamically unstable patient with hypotension, shock, or pulmonary edema. Alkaline diuresis is effective in overdose with long-acting but not short- or intermediate-acting barbiturates. Forced diuresis with saline and furosemide has been shown to be effective with meprobamate overdose.[55]

Hemodialysis and Charcoal Hemoperfusion

Table 48-10 reviews the indications for hemodialysis and hemoperfusion in sedative hypnotic overdose.[55,122] The vast majority of sedative overdoses recover with supportive therapy and do not require either of these modalities of treatment. Hemodialysis is generally less effective than charcoal hemoperfusion in removing the sedatives.

Abstinence Syndromes

Severe barbiturate abstinence syndromes resemble delirium tremens but occur over a longer period. Abstinence syndromes may occur after abrupt withdrawal of intermediate-acting barbiturates taken in daily doses exceeding 400 to 800 mg. Characteristically, the patient seems to improve for 12 to 16 hours as signs of intoxication resolve. Apprehension and weakness then gradually appear. Insomnia, abdominal pain, nausea, and vomiting occur within 24 hours, and weight loss may ultimately be marked. Tachycardia and hypertension are characteristic. Seizures occur in a large number of barbiturate addicts taking more than 1 g daily. The seizures may be multiple and appear at any time during the first 5 days. Seizures are most common, however, between the first and second days. Clonic and athetoid movements are also seen, and the EEG may be abnormal for 2 weeks.

Onset of delirium usually follows the appearance of seizures, occurring between the third and seventh days. Both auditory and (more commonly) visual hallucinations may be present, and patients usually become disoriented. Psychotic manifestations may abate within 3 to 4 days but may also be prolonged for several weeks.[134]

Abstinence from nonbarbiturate sedatives causes identical signs and symptoms; their time of onset and duration is a function of the duration of action of the drug. Minimal daily drug use sufficient for the development of abstinence syndromes is not clearly established. Meprobamate causes marked abstinence in the majority of patients using 3 to 6 g daily for longer than 6 weeks and in some patients taking 2 to 2.5 g daily for 9 months. Glutethimide can produce abstinence after doses of 2.5 g daily for 3 months. Ethchlorvynol has produced seizures after chronic use of 2 g/day. Lower doses of these drugs produce milder syndromes of abstinence.[135]

Benzodiazepine withdrawal generally occurs with the abrupt cessation of a benzodiazepine that has been taken in high doses for a prolonged period of time. Doses of 100 to 600 mg/day of chlordiazepoxide or 120 mg/day of diazepam for several weeks have resulted in abstinence seizures and psychosis.[136] Signs normally do not occur for several days to 2 weeks after discontinuing the drug. A sudden withdrawal syndrome can be iatrogenically produced by administering flumazenil to a benzodiazepine-dependent patient.

Like delirium tremens sedative abstinence is easier to prevent than to treat. In advanced abstinence, the use of phenothiazines and butyrophenones such as haloperidol can cause impairment of thermoregulation and seizures.[137] Phenytoin may prevent alcohol abstinence seizures but is not effective in the treatment of sedative abstinence seizures.[138]

Table 48-10 Hemodialysis and Charcoal Hemoperfusion in Sedative-Hypnotic Overdose[55,122]

Sedative-Hypnotic	Indications
Barbiturates	Prolonged coma not responding to supportive therapy, multisystem organ failure, or potentially lethal dose: phenobarbital 6–10 g; secobarbital, pentobarbital 2–3 g; amobarbital, butabarbital 2–3 g and blood level >10–15 mg/dL Hemodialysis: long-acting barbiturates Hemoperfusion: short and intermediate acting barbiturates
Methaqualone	Prolonged coma with life-threatening complications, potentially lethal dose: 8–20 g or blood levels >40 μg/mL Hemoperfusion: more effective than hemodialysis
Glutethimide	Prolonged coma with multisystem organ failure, potentially lethal dose: >10 g or blood level >4 mg/dL Hemoperfusion: more effective than hemodialysis
Meprobamate	Prolonged coma with multisystem organ failure, potentially lethal dose: >40 g or blood level >10 mg/dL Hemoperfusion: more effective than hemodialysis
Ethchlorvynol	Supportive measures fail to stabilize the patient, blood levels >150 μg/mL Hemoperfusion: more effective than hemodialysis
Chloral hydrate	Supportive measures fail to stabilize patient, potentially lethal dose: 5–10 g Hemodialysis or hemoperfusion: effectively removes the active metabolite trichloroethanol

There are no data as to its prophylactic effectiveness in humans.

The use of barbiturates is time tested in the prophylaxis and treatment of sedative abstinence. In established abstinence, intermediate-acting barbiturates should be given in small doses (200 mg) but at frequent intervals (every 30 to 60 minutes) until the patient is calm but not oversedated. When oral therapy is impossible, the intramuscular route may be used.[139] After control of symptoms is obtained, the patient may be transferred to long-acting phenobarbital as described below.

The prevention of sedative abstinence syndromes depends on an estimate of the patient's chronic daily drug use. History is often unreliable, and challenge with oral pentobarbital is a safe method of quantitating daily sedative requirements: 200 mg is given orally every 30 to 60 minutes until signs of mild intoxication occur (ataxia, nystagmus, dysarthria, somnolence). The total dose given may then be used as an estimate of the patient's daily barbiturate needs. Detoxification should proceed either by tapering the dose of pentobarbital (given on a thrice daily schedule) or, preferably, by transferring the patient to phenobarbital.[140]

Phenobarbital has a long half-life (48 to 96 hours in the adult) and a wide margin of safety.[141] It has been found to substitute reliably for pentobarbital when 30 mg is given daily for each 100 mg of pentobarbital required during challenge testing. After 3 or 4 days, tapering at a rate of 10% per day can begin.

INHALANTS

Inhalants may be anesthetic agents or organic solvents. The most commonly abused anesthetic agent is nitrous oxide. It is used frequently by medical personnel having access to it. Nitrous oxide is an odorless, colorless gas that produces both euphoria and analgesia. It is rapidly effective and its effect abruptly ceases within three or four tidal volumes of room air. Abusers may inhale deeply from pressurized cylinders and then hold their breath with the potential barotrauma of pneumothorax or pneumomediastinum.[142]

The properties of the most commonly abused inhalants are as follows: (1) contain hydrocarbons, (2) produce a euphoric effect, (3) have minimal or no irritation when inhaled, (4) are gaseous or rapidly evaporate at room temperature, and (5) are highly lipophilic with rapid absorption into the circulation from the lungs and distribution to the brain.

The use of organic solvents as euphoric agents became widespread in the 1960s among lower socioeconomic urban teenagers who were seeking an inexpensive, easily available intoxicant. Common household products such as cleaning fluids, paint thinners, glues, typewriter correction fluid (trichloroethane), toluene, and acetone met the above requirements and became the most commonly abused agents.[142] Gay males and heterosexual teens have used the alkyl nitrites as aphrodisiacs. Industrial workers tend to inhale solvents in the workplace, and American Indians choosing inhalant abuse have historically used gasoline.[142]

Pharmacologic tolerance to these substances usually does not occur. No specific abstinence syndromes apart from craving have been described. Because of their lipid solubility and the route of administration, a small amount of the substance is all that is required to produce an effect in a few seconds. The intoxication produced is similar to sedative-hypnotic or ethanol intoxication. Elimination of these agents occurs through a combination of pulmonary and renal excretion and hepatic metabolism. Some agents have active metabolites that are eliminated only after several days.

Solvents are usually sniffed directly from their containers, from a saturated rag or a plastic or paper bag. Nitrites are available in cotton-wrapped ampules designed to be crushed. The use of heat to raise vapor pressure and large bowls to increase dispersion has been reported. Oral and parenteral use is rare but often rapidly fatal. Most inhaled solvents are mixtures of several substances.

The emergency presentation of inhalant abuse is likely to involve toxic effects related to chronic use or complications of acute intoxication rather than overdose or abstinence. Chronic gasoline sniffing may present with delirium lasting several weeks and accompanied by choreiform movements.[143] Prolonged delirium and congestive cardiomyopathy have both been reported after chronic trichloroethylene exposure.[144,145] Toluene, trichloroethylene, and carbon tetrachloride have been reported to produce hepatitis, pancreatitis, and renal tubular lesions after chronic use. Alcohol use may sensitize the liver to solvent toxicity by facilitating entry to the hepatocyte or competing for metabolic enzymes.[146–149] Aplastic anemia and myeloid metaplasia have occurred after chronic sniffing of hydrocarbons, principally benzene, and the risk may be greater in those with sickle cell disease. Contaminants or additives may also cause complications. Lead toxicity is a recognized consequence of gasoline inhalation.[150] Metal fragments in fluorocarbons have caused pulmonary fibrosis.[151]

Some of the common inhalants are described in more detail below; however, virtually any lipid-soluble substance with a high vapor pressure has psychoactive properties.

Toluene is found in household, plastic, and model cements, lacquer thinner, and gasoline. It is an aromatic hydrocarbon. In chronic high-dose exposures (ie, glue sniffers), it has been associated with sudden death from dysrhythmia and conduction disturbances. Acutely, it produces drowsiness, headache, dizziness, nausea, vomiting, abdominal pain, gastritis, ataxia, and confusion.[142] Chronically, it is associated with permanent cerebellar ataxia, chronic encephalopathy, headaches, and personality changes.[55,152]

Hexane and other *aliphatic hydrocarbons* are present in gasoline, glues, and thinner used in rubber, pharmaceutical, and perfume industries. Intentional abusers may develop a peripheral neuropathy with distal paresthesias and pain, muscular weakness, and fatigue.[153] The CNS effects are headache, nausea, anorexia, confusion, stupor, and coma.[55]

Fluorocarbons, such as carbon tetrachloride, dihydrodifluoromethane, and trichloroflumethane, are constituents of aerosols, refrigerants, and cleaning fluids. Several cases of sudden death have occurred from inhalation abuse of aerosols containing Freon.[55] The exact cause of death is probably secondary to cardiac dysrhythmia.

Acetone is an aliphatic hydrocarbon present in fingernail polish, cements, and paint remover. Acetone has a relatively low toxicity. Heavy exposure causes initial CNS excitement followed by lethargy, stupor, and coma. Patients develop an intoxication similar to ethanol intoxication. Acetone vapor is mildly irritating to mucous membranes. Acetone intoxication can be diagnosed by the classic odor on the breath and ketones in the urine.[55]

Naphtha is found in lighter fluids and cleaning solutions. Intoxication leads to narcosis.[55]

Nitrites are not solvents or psychoactive compounds. Isobutyl, butyl, and amyl nitrites can cause methemoglobinemia, cyanosis, and hypotension.[55] Their central effects depend on their cardiovascular actions. Nitrites, principally amyl and isobutyl nitrite, are often sold in jars under the guise of room deodorants to avoid drug laws.

Overdose and Intoxication

Intoxication with solvents resembles alcohol inebriation. Initially euphoria, dizziness, and auditory or visual hallucinations are typical. The patient may be observed to sneeze or cough, vomit, and avoid bright light. Flushing is common, but pupillary response is inconsistent. In the second stage tinnitus, confusion, diplopia, and blurred vision are prominent. The patient may appear pale and disoriented. In the third stage there is further mental clouding. Nystagmus, ataxia, slurred speech, and diminished reflexes appear. Inhalant intoxication is distinguished from alcohol intoxication by the characteristic odors, the rapidity with which stages evolve, and the presence of hallucinations.[154]

Acute delirium is best treated supportively with fresh air and avoidance of both excessive stimulation and ambiguous stimuli (such as dark rooms or whispering). The patient should not be left alone, but sedatives are rarely needed.

Inhalant intoxication occasionally presents as suffocation or sudden death. Tightly fitting masks or bags may render the patient unconscious with the device still in place. Trichloroethylene and fluorinated refrigerants were the substances most often implicated in more than 100 sudden deaths from inhalant abuse between 1960 and 1970.[155] The association of stress or strenuous activity with sudden death suggests that solvents may sensitize the heart to the dysrhythmogenic actions of catecholamines. Hypotensive episodes should be treated with volume resuscitation and not sympathomimetics if at all possible.

Nitrite intoxication causes vasodilation with a fall in blood pressure and pooling of blood in dependent parts. Intoxication is rapid and brief and consists of light-headedness, an intensification of sounds, and a throbbing headache. Nitrites also have a reputation as aphrodisiacs. Signs include flushing, fainting, and hypotension. Patients with cardiovascular disease that may become decompensated by drastic changes in venous return or systemic blood pressure are at risk from nitrite use.

Nitrites are particularly popular among male homosexuals, possibly because of the drug's action in relaxing the anal sphincter. The known immunosuppressive effect of isobutyl nitrite and the high prevalence of nitrite use among homosexuals who develop AIDS have led to speculation that nitrite use is casually related to AIDS or simply a marker for promiscuity.[156]

A dose-related response to nitrites is the formation of methemoglobin. The mechanism by which a strong reducing agent affects this oxidation is obscure. Methemoglobin levels may reach 20% after recreational inhalation and may be much higher following oral ingestion. Infants and patients with anemia or heart disease are at particular risk for hypoxemia. The occasional patient with hemaglobinopathy or familial deficiency in hemoglobin reductase is also at risk.[157]

Cyanosis unresponsive to oxygen in a patient without pulmonary or cardiac disease suggests methemoglobinemia. Treatment, however, should be reserved for stuporous or comatose patients, because spontaneous reduction of methemoglobin occurs within 1 to 3 days. Methylene blue (1 to 2 mg/kg given intravenously for 5 minutes as a 1% solution) is the treatment of choice. A second dose of 2 mg/kg may be given after an hour if needed, but the total dose should not exceed 7 mg/kg. The aim is to improve tissue oxygenation, not to abolish cyanosis, which may be present at low levels of methemoglobin.[158]

HALLUCINOGENS

Hallucinogens form a chemically heterogeneous group of substances that predictably alter perceptions of surroundings, body image, and time. They produce impaired reality testing; illusions; kaleidoscopic visual, auditory, and tactile hallucinations. They also share with other psychoactive compounds the ability to alter mood, thought, and behavior. Hallucinogens may bring forth feelings of introspection and depersonalization. There is no evidence of a withdrawal syndrome with any of these agents.[7]

These drugs can be grouped into several classes by chemical structure. The indole group contains LSD, psylocibin, morning glory seeds, dimethyltryptamine (DMT), diethyltryptamine (DET), and dipropyltryptamine (DPT). The phenylethylamine group contains peyote, mescaline, dimethoxymethylamphetamine (DOM, STP). Marijuana and PCP, the two hallucinogens of greatest importance in the emergency department, do not fall into either the indole or phenylethylamine group and in fact produce hallucinations only rarely.[159,160]

There has been a steady scientific interest in hallucinogens as models of and treatments for schizophrenia and as agents useful in the study of neurotransmission and hormonal organization in the brain. At the same time, there has been a rapid decline in the recreational popularity of these substances. The two exceptions to the generally waning interest in hallucinogens are PCP and marijuana.

Marijuana appears to have found a permanent place in many segments of American society as a mild euphoriant of recreational use and occasional abuse. In the United States approximately 9.7 million people were estimated to use marijuana at least once a month and approximately 5.3 million people used it once a week during 1991.[2] The ubiquitous presence of PCP in street drugs sold under various, more exotic names seems to be more a result of the drug's potency and ease of manufacture than any real public demand. PCP, marijuana, and, as a representative of other hallucinogens, LSD will be discussed.

PCP

PCP is the principal constituent of many substances sold illegally as LSD, tetrahydrocannabinol (THC), the major active compound in marijuana and hashish, psilocybin, mescaline, peyote, and cocaine. It is also sold as "angel dust," "hog," and multiple other street names. Originally developed as a short-acting dissociative anesthetic in 1957, PCP was dropped because of postanesthetic dysphoric effects that could last for several days. It was subsequently used for a short time as a veterinary anesthetic but was discontinued. Ketamine (Ketalar) is a related dissociative anesthetic that is currently used throughout the United States without the adverse effects of PCP.

In pure form, PCP is a glistening white powder, soluble in water and alcohol. Street samples may be sold as an off-white powder, as tablets of various colors, as a liquid, or sprinkled on "joints" of marijuana or parsley. PCP may be sniffed, ingested, and occasionally injected intravenously; however, smoking is the most common route of administration.

PCP is an analgesic with sympathomimetic, anticholinergic, and CNS stimulant and depressant properties. It is rapidly absorbed by any route and may undergo reexcretion into the stomach and bile. PCP is highly lipid soluble with a volume of distribution of 6.2 L/kg.[161] It accumulates in the adipose tissue of the brain and is primarily metabolized by the liver. Its half-life varies between 7 hours and 3 days.

The major hydroxy metabolite does not appear to be active and is excreted in the urine.[161,162]

Coma after high doses may persist for 12 hours and psychosis for several days.[163] In overdose the presence of a toxic by-product of synthesis may cause bloody diarrhea and vomiting.[164]

Overdose and Intoxication

Patients with PCP intoxication are generally seen in the emergency department because of altered mental status, violent behavior, toxic psychosis, or trauma, often self-inflicted. They are at risk to develop medical complications that include intracranial hemorrhage, seizures, aspiration pneumonia, apnea, cardiac arrest, rhabdomyolysis, acute renal failure, and hyperthermia.[165] Most authors consider doses higher than 10 mg or plasma levels higher than 100 µg/L as likely to produce serious intoxication. The psychiatric and toxic effects tend to be dose and level related. Doses of 100 to 200 mg have caused death.[163] Symptoms of intoxication begin within minutes to several hours after acute dosing, but psychiatric symptoms may have an insidious onset in chronic abuse. Low-dose intoxication produces euphoria, lability of mood, concreteness of thought, confusion, and distortions in body image. True hallucinations are unusual. With increasing dose, marked anxiety, hyperacusis, hostility, depersonalization, and ultimately a cataleptic or stuporous state (often with the eyes open) are seen.[164]

Physical signs are characteristic. Low doses usually produce hypertension and an increase in respiratory rate and depth. At higher doses hypotension may occur, but hyperpnea usually persists until coma is advanced or convulsions supervene. Hyperreflexia and muscular rigidity are common even in coma. Pharyngeal reflexes may be increased, making endotracheal intubation difficult. Corneal reflexes, however, are usually depressed, and ptosis may be seen. Purposeless movements, grimacing and sucking, ataxia, or catatonia may occur. Diminished pain perception is striking. Pupils may be constricted or in midposition, but light reflexes are decreased. Marked horizontal and vertical nystagmus occurs on testing after low doses and in the primary position after higher doses. Hypersalivation and diaphoresis occur occasionally. After serious overdoses, dysrhythmias and shock result in part from the drug's direct myocardial action.

Low-dose manifestations may be distinguished from other hallucinogen intoxications by the absence of hallucinations or dilated pupils and by the presence of ataxia and nystagmus. Moderate overdoses of PCP can be distinguished from sedative poisoning by the presence of hypertension, hyperpyrexia, and hyperpnea. Some nonbarbiturate sedatives may, however, also cause hypertension and fever. High-dose intoxication with PCP may be difficult to distinguish from other causes of coma with convulsions. A history of any hallucinogen use in an agitated or mute patient should suggest PCP intoxication.

Laboratory workup should include urine drug screening and plasma levels if possible. The drug may also be present in high concentration in vomitus or gastric aspirate. The laboratory should be notified that PCP is being sought. In advanced overdose, cardiac monitoring, renal function tests, urinalysis, and close observation of temperature are essential.

Treatment of mild overdose consists of observation in a dimly lit, quiet room. Talking the patient down is probably useless in PCP intoxication. Ear plugs have been used to minimize sensory stimulation in noisy emergency departments. Phenothiazines may produce hypotension, intensify anticholinergic manifestations, and increase the risk of seizures. Benzodiazepines can be used if necessary for mild to moderate agitation. If the patient is severely agitated, restraints with mummification wrappings will reduce the chance of self-inflicted injury, and chemical restraint with haloperidol (5 to 10 mg intramuscularly/intravenously every hour) will generally be effective. The use of haloperidol in this setting has not been associated with any significant complications.

The decision to remove PCP from the gastrointestinal tract depends on balancing the risks of stimulation with the benefit of improved elimination of the drug. PCP undergoes enterohepatic circulation with reexcretion into the gut. Pulse charcoal administration (20 to 50 g every 2 to 4 hours) is indicated to trap as much PCP in the gut as possible. Acidification of the urine is no longer recommended because of the potential exacerbation of myoglobinuric renal failure with urinary acidification.[161] Maintenance of normal urine output is recommended and should be monitored in major intoxications. PCP has a diuretic action at low concentrations but may cause oliguria at higher ones.

Treatment of severe overdose necessitates removal of the drug and may require therapy for seizures, hypertension, hyperpyrexia, dysrhythmia, and rhabdomyolysis. Seizures and opisthotonos should be treated with diazepam or lorazepam. Hypertension appears to be caused by α-adrenergic properties of PCP and may respond best to phentolamine (5.0 mg intravenously). Nitroprusside may also be used. Hyperpyrexia should be vigorously treated with the usual means. Hypotension generally will be responsive to crystalloid boluses. If volume replacement is ineffective, then vasopressors are indicated. Respiratory distress requires intubation, which should be performed by an experienced practitioner prepared to encounter pharyngeal spasm and an increased gag reflex. PCP has been found to inhibit pseudocholinesterase and may prolong the action of succinyl choline given to facilitate intubation.[163] Rhabdomyolysis and myoglobinuria should be looked for with serum creatine phosphokinase determinations and urinanalysis and, if present, treatment with adequate intravenous fluids, mannitol, and bicarbonate is indicated. Hemodialysis and hemoperfusion have not been helpful because of the large volume of distribution of the drug.[161]

Severe psychiatric reactions to PCP may require hospitalization for several days. The insidious development of psychosis that may persist for several weeks is a rare complication of chronic PCP abuse. Few of the chronic abusers who develop psychosis have a history of psychiatric disorders, but poor ego strength and inadequate adjustment to family, work, and school appear to be common. Unlike LSD-precipitated psychosis, the illness is accompanied by neurologic disturbances (chiefly nystagmus), severity is dose related, and resolution follows a predictable course. Phenothiazines and haloperidol appear to be effective.[166]

Marijuana

Marijuana remains the most commonly abused illicit substance in the United States despite the fact that its use has steadily declined since the late 1970s. Cannabis, a term that refers inclusively to both marijuana and hashish, has been used for medicinal and recreational purposes since 2327 B.C. in China's Nung dynasty.[167] Marijuana refers to the dessicated leaves and flowers of the plant *Cannabis sativa*. Hashish is the dried resin made from the flower tops, and hashish oil is a very potent dark extract obtained from the plant. Cannabis has historically been used for medicinal purposes as an antiemetic, appetite stimulant, analgesic, sedative, antidepressant, bronchodilator, and antimigraine agent.[167] Currently cannabis research is directed toward the treatment of glaucoma, seizures, pain, and anxiety.

The principal psychoactive constituent of cannabis is delta-9-THC. Marijuana is approximately 2 to 20% THC, and hashish 15 to 20% THC.[168] THC interacts with noradrenergic, dopaminergic, serotonergic, cholinergic, and GABAergic neurotransmitters.[167] It has both barbiturate and opioid-like effects. THC partially diminishes the opioid withdrawal syndrome and has some cross-tolerance with ethanol. Tolerance develops within a short period of time to both the psychoactive and autonomic effects of THC.[169] Chronic abusers will experience a withdrawal syndrome of irritability, anorexia, tremor, and cholinergic signs.[170]

Cannabis may be smoked in "joints" or ingested. After smoking, effects begin within a few minutes and last for 1 or 2 hours. When ingested, cannabis produces effects within 1 hour that last for 6 hours. Ingested cannabis is absorbed about one third as completely as when smoked, but effects appear to occur at lower plasma concentrations.[171]

Inhaled THC is approximately 10 to 50% absorbed, extensively bound to plasma proteins, partially metabolized by the liver and lung to psychoactive products, and excreted as inactive metabolites in the urine and bile.[172] Ingested THC is only 3 to 6% absorbed.[172] Cessation of the drug's effects is due to redistribution, mainly into fat, and not to metabolism. The half-life of THC is long (18 to 48 hours).

Cannabis has been extensively studied because of the enormous popularity of the drug. Derivatives of THC appear to hold great promise as antiemetics[173] and may have a place in the treatment of glaucoma.[174] Unlike PCP, cannabis produces CNS effects that depend a good deal on the user's expectation and experience. Effects are also much milder and briefer. Overdose is rare despite wide variation in the potency of cannabis preparation and lethal doses are unknown in humans. The emergency physician may encounter acute intoxication as an incidental finding or in the inexperienced user. Medical complications in the chronic user and (rarely) poisoning after parenteral use of cannabis may also present to the emergency department. In patients with cardiovascular disease, intoxication can produce decompensation by inhibiting sympathetic reflexes and raising the concentration of circulating catecholamines.[175]

Government attempts to destroy *Cannabis sativa* plants have included spraying with paraquat and other herbicides. Paraquat is concentrated in the lung, where, in sufficient concentration, it can produce pulmonary fibrosis with severe respiratory insufficiency. Patients in whom paraquat poisoning occurs should be treated promptly and vigorously.[176] Dysphoric reactions to cannabis, however, are unlikely to be due to contamination with herbicide.

Overdose and Intoxication

After one or two "joints" (50 to 1500 mg of marijuana or 5 to 150 mg of THC), cannabis typically produces euphoria, suggestibility, relaxation, appetite stimulation, hilarity, and subtle changes in visual and auditory perceptions. Sedation and dysphoria are alternative reactions in some users. At larger doses, confusion, paranoid ideation, and depersonalization may emerge, particularly in the inexperienced user. Marijuana smoking can exacerbate preexisting schizophrenia and toxic psychosis has been reported.[177]

On examination, the mildly intoxicated patient may be talkative and gregarious or withdrawn and anxious, depending often on the perceived threat of the environment. There are usually slight tachycardia, dry and injected conjunctivae, and, occasionally, a mild tremor. The pupil size is not consistent. With more marked intoxication, postural changes in blood pressure, paranoid behavior, ataxia, confusion, and (rarely) hallucinations may be seen.

Intravenous injection of cannabis represents an exception to the generally benign presentation of intoxication. Onset of symptoms is immediate, with throbbing headache, chills, abdominal pain, vomiting, myalgias, and weakness. These symptoms may persist for several days. On examination tachycardia, extreme hypotension, and fever may be found. Hyporeflexia and muscle weakness are characteristic, but the sensorium is usually clear. Hypoglycemia, thrombocytopenia, cardiac injury, hepatitis, pancreatitis, and transient renal failure may all complicate the course.[178]

Treatment of cannabis toxicity depends on symptoms. The mildly intoxicated, anxious patient needs only friendly, but not condescending, reassurance. Small oral doses of diazepam or a short-acting barbiturate may be used if necessary in the moderately intoxicated patient. Parenteral overdoses are likely to require intensive care. Attention to volume repletion, treatment of cardiac dysrhythmias, maintenance of adequate blood sugar, and attention to renal function, hemostasis, and body temperature form the basis of therapy. The prognosis is good.

LSD

LSD ("acid") is an amine alkaloid with predominantly central effects chemically related to the other lysergic acid derivative ergot. LSD belongs to a group of drugs called psychedelics, which produce perceptual distortions. Other members of this group are mescaline, psilocybin, and the hallucinogenic amphetamines (see section on designer drugs).[179] LSD is believed to produce its effect by inhibition of serotonergic neurons in the brain, which result in stimulation of limbic and visual areas of the forebrain. A second, dopaminergic action of LSD may modulate the intensity of these effects and possibly accounts for the extraordinary potency of the drug. The usual "street dose" is 100 to 250 μg. LSD is well absorbed and reaches peak plasma levels approximately 1 hour after ingestion. It may also be injected parenterally.

Clinical effects are maximal after 2 to 5 hours. The half-life is known to be about 3 hours, but investigations of the products and routes of elimination are conflicting. Clinical effects usually last approximately 12 hours. Street LSD is sold as tablets or capsules, on blotting paper or sugar. It is often diluted with PCP, amphetamine, or strychnine.

Tolerance to the hallucinogenic properties of LSD occurs very rapidly, possibly with the first dose. Patients tolerant to LSD are also tolerant to mescaline and psilocybin. There is no known abstinence syndrome, and tolerance is rapidly lost.[180]

Overdose and Intoxication

LSD produces perceptual, cognitive, affective, and somatic changes in a roughly dose-related fashion. Perceptual changes include intensification of colors and sound, blending of sensory modalities called synesthesia (ie, seeing sounds), visual hallucinations, and disturbances in the appreciation of time. Cognitive effects include depersonalization, suggestibility, and problems with logical thought and reality testing. Affective disturbances consist of marked swings in mood from euphoria to panic. Somatic sensations may include dizziness, weakness, nausea, tremor, and blurred vision.

On examination, the intoxicated patient shows signs of centrally mediated sympathetic activity with 6- to 8-mm pupillary dilation, vasoconstriction, and poverty of expression or loose associations. There may be diffuse muscle weakness and mild hyperthermia. In massive overdoses coma, hypertension, respiratory arrest, tachycardia, hyperthermia, and coagulopathy may occur.[179]

Emergency presentation of LSD abuse is likely to involve dysphoric reactions. Such reactions include "bad trips," LSD-precipitated psychosis, and "flashbacks." Distinguishing among these entities is often impossible on presentation, and the diagnosis is commonly retrospective. A "bad trip" is a panic state occurring during intoxication and characterized by frightening hallucinations, feelings of losing control, fear that the effects are permanent, and loss of insight in the presence of a clear sensorium. Bad trips occur in the novice or the chronic user whose previous experiences may have been pleasant.

Unlike a bad trip, toxic LSD psychosis more typically presents with auditory hallucinations in the absence of panic. These reactions appear to be more common in chronic users, in those with preexisting personality disturbance, and among patients taking LSD in stressful surroundings. Psychotic reactions appear to be more common with LSD than mescaline. The psychosis subsides within 24 hours.[181]

It is unclear whether LSD-precipitated psychosis represents an idiosyncratic reaction or the unmasking of a previously subclinical schizophrenia. These reactions are uncommon but may be prolonged when they occur. They are indistinguishable at the outset from toxic psychosis.

Flashbacks are spontaneous recurrences, usually during times of stress, of previous LSD experiences. They are more commonly dysphoric than pleasurable and may last several hours. Recurrences over several months are not uncommon.

Treatment of bad trips consists of sensory deprivation and reassurance ("talking down") combined with orientation. If necessary, oral doses of diazepam or phenothiazines may be used. Psychotic reactions, both toxic and drug precipitated, respond to phenothiazines. Flashbacks usually do not require treatment apart from reassurance.

THE INNOCENT BYSTANDER: THE NEWBORN

The devastating spread of AIDS to the newborn infants of intravenous drug–abusing mothers has already been discussed. There are, however, other significant neonatal sequelae of maternal drug abuse. The most commonly used drugs during pregnancy are ethanol, tobacco, marijuana, cocaine, heroin, and methadone. Each drug crosses the placenta or has active metabolites that cross the placenta. Often the fetus is exposed to several of these drugs on a regular basis during pregnancy. Each exerts an adverse effect on the developing fetus and newborn infant.

In New York City it is estimated that 3 to 5% of the newborns delivered in municipal hospitals were exposed to heroin or methadone in utero.[182] Opioid-exposed infants are generally small for gestational age with smaller head circumference, delayed developmental milestones, a five- to 10-fold increase in sudden infant death syndrome, and a 21% incidence of strabismus.[183] Sudden maternal withdrawal from opioids in the third trimester of pregnancy can result in fetal hyperactivity, hypoxia, and death.

After birth, the infant of the opioid-addicted mother will require close observation and treatment for neonatal withdrawal. The infant may become irritable, tremulous, and hypertonic; develop repetitive yawning and a high-pitched cry; and demonstrate marked sucking of the hands. In more severe forms of untreated withdrawal, the neonate develops seizures, respiratory distress, apneic episodes, fever, diaphoresis, and sleeplessness. These infants can be treated with supportive care and the opioid paregoric to prevent sudden withdrawal.[183]

The cocaine-abusing mother runs the significant risk of spontaneous abortion, abruptio placenta, premature labor, stillbirth, and precipitous delivery. After birth the neonate will demonstrate a withdrawal syndrome with disturbed sleep/wake cycle, poor feeding, tremulousness, and hyperreflexia. Cocaine intoxication has also precipitated fetal intracranial hemorrhage and neonatal death. The effects of methamphetamine abuse are similar to those of cocaine abuse.

Marijuana appears to be the least toxic of the common drugs of abuse. There have not been associated abnormalities of gestational length, neonatal birth weight, or duration of labor. Exposed neonates have demonstrated tremulousness, increased startle response, and altered visual response.[183]

REFERENCES

1. Williamson RS. International illicit drug traffic: the United States response. *Bull Narc*. 1983;35:33.
2. National Institute on Drug Abuse. *National Household Survey on Drug Abuse-Population Estimates 1991*. Washington, DC: US Department of Health and Human Services; 1991.
3. Centers for Disease Control. Smoking-attributable mortality and years of potential life lost: United States, 1988. *MMWR*. 1991;40:62–71.
4. *Diagnostic and Statistical Manual of Mental Disorders*. Rev 3rd ed. Washington, DC: American Psychiatric Association; 1987.
5. Jenike MA. Drug abuse. *Sci Am Med*. 1991;13:VI.
6. Hoffman RS, Goldfrank LR. The impact of drug abuse and addiction on society. *Emerg Med Clin North Am*. 1990;8:3.
7. Ungar JR, Schwartz GR, Levine DG. Drug and substance abuse emergencies. In: Schwartz GR, ed. *Principles and Practice of Emergency Medicine*. 3rd ed. Malvern, PA: Lea & Febiger; 1992; 3055–3074.
8. Schwartz RH. Marijuana: a crude drug with a spectrum of underappreciated toxicity. *Pediatrics*. 1984;73:455.
9. Schauben JL. Adulterants and substitutes. *Emerg Med Clin North Am*. 1990;8:3.
10. Shesser R, Jotte R, Olshaker J. The contribution of impurities to the acute morbidity of illegal drug use. *Am J Emerg Med*. 1991;9:4.
11. Perez-Castrillon JL, Perez-Arellano JL, Garcia Palomo JD, Jimenez-Lopez A, Decastro S. Opioids depress in vitro human monocyte chemotaxis. *Immunopharmacology*. 1992;23: 57–61.
12. Centers for Disease Control. Pneumocystis pneumonia—Los Angeles. *MMWR*. 1981;30:250–252.

13. Centers for Disease Control. The second 100,000 cases of acquired immunodeficiency syndrome—United States. *MMWR*. 1992;41:28–29.
14. Hahn RA, Onorato IM, Jones TS, Dougherty J. Prevalence of HIV infection among intravenous drug users in the United States. *JAMA*. 1989;261:2677.
15. Kelen GD, Fleetwood D. HIV infection and intravenous drug users. *Emerg Med Clin North Am*. 1990;8:3.
16. Shine D. Clinical presentation of AIDS in drug abusers. *Adv Alcohol Subst Abuse*. 1985–86;5:25.
17. Klein RS, Harris CA, Small CB, et al. Oral candidiasis in high risk patients as the initial manifestation of the acquired immunodeficiency syndrome. *N Engl J Med*. 1984;311:354.
18. Geller SM, Stimmel B. Diagnostic confusion from lymphatic lesions in heroin addicts. *Ann Intern Med*. 1973;78:703.
19. Roberts R, Slovis CM. Endocarditis in intravenous drug abusers. *Emerg Med Clin North Am*. 1990;8:3:665–681.
20. Chambers HF, Korzeniowski OM, Sande MA. *Staphylococcus aureus* endocarditis: clinical manifestations in addicts and nonaddicts. *Medicine*. 1983;62:170–177.
21. Craven DE, Rixinger AL, Goularte TA, et al. Methicillin-resistant *Staphylococcus aureus* bacteremia linked to intravenous drug abusers using a "shooting gallery." *Am J Med*. 1986;80:770–776.
22. Shepherd SM, Druckenbrod GG, Haywood YC. Other infectious complications in intravenous drug users. *Emerg Med Clin North Am*. 1990;8:3:683–692.
23. Centers for Disease Control. Guidelines for prevention of transmission of human immunodeficiency virus and hepatitis B virus to healthcare and public-safety workers. *MMWR*. 1989;38:S6.
24. Holzman R, Bishko F. Osteomyelitis in heroin addicts. *Ann Intern Med*. 1971;75:693.
25. Roca RP, Yoshikawa TT. Primary skeletal infections in heroin users: a clinical characterization, diagnosis, and therapy. *Clin Orthop*. 1979;144:238.
26. Shragg T. "Cotton fever" in narcotic addicts. *J Am Coll Emerg Physicians*. 1978;7:279.
27. Schwartz RH. Urine testing in the detection of drugs of abuse. *Arch Intern Med*. 1988;148:2407–2412.
28. Osterloh JD. Utility and reality of emergency toxicologic testing. *Emerg Med Clin North Am*. 1990;8:3:693–723.
29. Derlet RW, Heischober B. Methamphetamine: stimulant of the 1990's? *West J Med*. 1990;153:625–628.
30. Aaron CK. Sympathomimetics. *Emerg Med Clin North Am*. 1990;8:3:513–526.
31. McMullen MJ. Sympathomimetic toxidrome. In: Rosen P, Barkin RM, eds. *Emergency Medicine Concepts and Clinical Practice*. 3rd ed. St. Louis, MO: Mosby Year Book; 1992;2659–2673.
32. Abelson HI, Miller JD. A decade of trends in cocaine use in the household population. *NIDA Res Monogr*. 1985;61:35–49.
33. Van Dyke C, Byck R. Cocaine. *Sci Am*. 1982;246:128–154.
34. Randall T. Cocaine deaths reported for century or more. *JAMA*. 1992;267:8:1045–1046.
35. Spivey WH, Euerle B. Neurologic complications of cocaine abuse. *Ann Emerg Med*. 1990;19:12:1422–1428.
36. Chiang WK, Goldfrank LR. Substance withdrawal. *Emerg Med Clin North Am*. 1990;8:3:613–631.
37. MacDonald DI. Cocaine leads emergency department drug visits. *JAMA*. 1987;258:2029.
38. Isner JM, Chokshi SK. Cocaine and vasospasm. *N Engl J Med*. 1989;321:1604–1606.
39. Wilkinson P, Van Dyke C, Jatlow P, et al. Intranasal and oral cocaine kinetics. *Clin Pharmacol Ther*. 1980;27:386.
40. Suarez I, Abelardo A, Lester J. Cocaine-condom ingestion. *JAMA*. 1977;238:1218.
41. Javaids J, Fischman M, Schuster C, et al. Cocaine plasma concentration: relation to physiological and subjective effects in humans. *Science*. 1978;202:227.
42. Randall T. Cocaine, alcohol mix in body to form even longer lasting, more lethal drug. *JAMA*. 1992;267:8:1043–1044.
43. Rubin RB. Neugarten J. Medical complications of cocaine: changes in pattern of use and spectrum of complications. *Clin Toxicol*. 1992;30:1–12.
44. Tardiff K, Gross EM, Messner SF. A study of homicides in Manhattan, 1981. *Am J Public Health*. 1986;76:139.
45. Goldfrank LR, Hoffman RS. The cardiovascular effects of cocaine. *Ann Emerg Med*. 1991;20:165–175.
46. Amin M, Gabelman G, Karpel J, Buttrick P. Acute myocardial infarction and chest pain after cocaine use. *Am J Cardiol*. 1990;66:1434–1437.
47. Bunn WH, Giannini AJ. Cardiovascular complications of cocaine abuse. *Am Family Physician*. 1992;46:3:769–773.
48. Forrester J, Steele AW, Waldron JA, et al. Crack lung: an acute pulmonary syndrome with a spectrum of clinical and histopathological findings. *Am Rev Respir Dis*. 1990;142:462–467.
49. Satel SL, Gawin FH. Migrainelike headache and cocaine use. *JAMA*. 1989;261:2995–2996.
50. Gawin FH, Ellinwood EH. Cocaine and other stimulants. *N Engl J Med*. 1988;318:1173–1182.
51. Roth D, Alarcon FJ, Fernandez JA, et al. Acute rhabdomyolysis associated with cocaine intoxication. *N Engl J Med*. 1988;319:673–677.
52. Welch RD, Todd K, Krause GS. Incidence of cocaine-associated rhabdomyolysis. *Ann Emerg Med*. 1991;20:154–157.
53. Singhal PC, et al. Rhabdomyolysis and acute renal failure associated with cocaine abuse. *Clin Toxicol*. 1990;28:321.
54. Snyder SH. *Drugs and the Brain*. New York: Scientific American Books; 1986;130–131.
55. Ellenhorn M, Barceloux D. *Medical Toxicology: Diagnosis and treatment of Human Poisoning*. New York: Elsevier Science; 1988.
56. Davis J, et al. Effects of urinary pH on amphetamine metabolism. *Ann N Y Acad Sci*. 1971;179:493.
57. Jackson JG. Hazards of smokable methamphetamine. *N Engl J Med*. 1989;321:907.
58. Ellinwood E. Amphetamine psychosis. *J Nerv Ment Dis*. 1967;144:273.
59. Goldfrank LR, Hoffman RS. The cardiovascular effects of cocaine. *Ann Emerg Med*. 1991;20:2:165–175.
60. Hoffman R. Drug dealers who swallow the evidence. *Clin Toxicol Update*. 1990;3:2:1.
61. Weiner N. Drugs that inhibit adrenergic nerves and block adrenergic receptors. In: Gilman AG, Goodman LS, eds. *The Pharmacologic Basis of Therapeutics*. 6th ed. New York: Macmillan; 1980:307.
62. Ramoska E, Sacchetti AD. Propranolol-induced hypertension in treatment of cocaine intoxication. *Ann Emerg Med*. 1985;14:1112–1113.
63. Parker RP, Beckman KJ, Bauman JL, et al. Sodium bicarbonate reverses cocaine-induced conduction defects. *Circulation*. 1989;80(suppl II):15.
64. Hollander JE, Carter WA, Hoffman RS. Use of phentolamine for cocaine-induced myocardial ischemia. *N Engl J Med*. 1992;327:5:361.

65. Holland R, Marx J, Earnest MP, Ranniger S. Grand mal seizures temporally related to cocaine use: clinical and diagnostic features. *Ann Emerg Med.* 1992;21:7:772–776.
66. Giannini AJ, Billett W. Bromocriptine-desipramine protocol in treatment of cocaine addiction. *J Clin Pharmacol.* 1987;27:549–554.
67. Halikas JA, Kuhn KL, Crea FS. Treatment of crack cocaine use with carbamazepine. *Am J Drug Alcohol Abuse.* 1992;18:45–56.
68. Bartlett M, Egger H. Disposition and metabolism of methylphenidate in dog and man. *Fed Proc.* 1972;31:537.
69. Ford M, Hoffman RS, Goldfrank LR. Opioids and designer drugs. *Emerg Med Clin North Am.* 1990;8:3:495–511.
70. Brown J, Malone M. Status of drug quality in the street-drug market. *Clin Toxicol.* 1976;9:145.
71. Oneil P, Baker P, Gough T. Illicitly imported heroin products: some physical and chemical features indicative of their origin. *J Forensic Sci.* 1984;29:888.
72. *Nat Inst Drug Abuse Res Monogr* Ser. 1985;35(chap 4):60–62.
73. Inturrisi CE, Schultz M, Shin S, et al. Evidence from opiate binding studies that heroin acts throughout its metabolites. *Life Sci.* 1983;33(suppl 1):773.
74. Owen J, Nakatsu K. Diacetylmorphine (heroin) hydrolases in human blood. *Can J Physiol Pharmacol.* 1983;61:870.
75. Way E, Young J, Kemp J. Metabolism of heroin and its pharmacologic implications. *Bull Narc.* 1965;17:25.
76. Inturrisi CE, Max M, Foley K, et al. The pharmacokinetics of heroin in patients with chronic pain. *N Engl J Med.* 1984;310:1213.
77. Beaver W, Wallenstein S, Houde R, et al. A clinical comparison of the analgesic effects of methadone and morphine administered intramuscularly, and of orally and parenterally administered methadone. *Clin Pharmacol Ther.* 1967;8:415.
78. Verebely K, Volavka J, Mule S, et al. Methadone in man: pharmacokinetic and excretion studies in acute and chronic dosing. *Clin Pharmacol Ther.* 1975;18:180.
79. Bellward G, et al. Methadone maintenance: effect of urinary pH on renal clearance in chronic high and low doses. *Clin Pharmacol Ther.* 1977;22:92.
80. Havassy B, Tschann J. Chronic heroin use during methadone treatment: a test of the efficacy of high maintenance doses. *Addict Behav.* 1984;9:57.
81. Goetting MG, Thirman MJ. Neurotoxicity of meperidine. *Ann Emerg Med.* 1985;14:1007.
82. Kreek MJ, Gutjahr CL, Garfield SW, et al. Drug interactions with methadone. *Ann N Y Acad Sci.* 1976;281:350.
83. Tennant FS. Complications of propoxyphene abuse. *Arch Intern Med.* 1973;132:191.
84. Jasinski D, Martin W, Hoeldtke R. Effects of short- and long-term administration of pentazocine in man. *Clin Pharmacol Ther.* 1970;11:385.
85. Wadley C, Stillie G. Pentazocine (Talwin) and tripelennamine (Pyribenzamine): a new drug abuse combination or just a revival? *Int J Addict.* 1980;15:1285.
86. Burroughs W. *Junky.* New York: Penguin; 1977.
87. Greene M, Luke J, Dupont R. Acute opiate overdose: a preliminary report on mechanism of death. In: *Proceedings of the Fifth National Conference on Methadone Therapy.* New York and Washington, DC, National Association for the Prevention of Addiction to Narcotics, 1973.
88. Jasinski J, Martin W, Haertzen C. The human pharmacology and abuse potential of N-allylnoroxymorphone (naloxone). *J Pharmacol Exp Ther.* 1967;157:420.
89. Berkowitz B. The relationship of pharmacokinetics to pharmacologic activity: morphine, methadone, and naloxone. *Clin Pharmacokinet.* 1976;1:219.
90. Chotkowski LA. Clubbing of the fingers in heroin addicts. *N Engl J Med.* 1984;311:262.
91. Santos-Sastre S del L, Capote-Gil F, Gonzales-Castro A. Airway obstruction and heroin inhalation (letter). *Lancet.* 1986;2:1158.
92. Fry D, Richardson J, Flint L. Occult splenic abscess: an unrecognized complication of heroin abuse. *Surgery.* 1978;84:650.
93. Challenor Y, Brust J, Baden M. Neurological complications of addiction to heroin. *Bull N Y Acad Med.* 1973;49:4.
94. Krause GS. Brown-Séquard syndrome following heroin injection. *Ann Emerg Med.* 1983;12:581.
95. Frand U, Shim C, Williams H. Heroin induced pulmonary edema. *Ann Intern Med.* 1972;77:29.
96. Tanara G. Hypertensive reaction to naloxone. *JAMA.* 1974;288:25.
97. Inglefinger J, Isaacson G, Shine D. Inadequacy of laboratory diagnosis of overdose. *Clin Pharmacol Ther.* 1981;23:456.
98. Fraser H, Isbell H, Van Horn C. Effects of morphine and diaminophenyl thiazole (daptazole). *Anesthesiology.* 1957;18:531.
99. Goldfrank LR, Flomenbaum NE, Lewin NA, et al. Withdrawal. In: Goldfrank LR, ed. *Goldfrank's Toxicology Emergencies.* Norwalk CT: Appleton-Century-Crofts; 1986;494–505.
100. Dole VP, Nyswander M. A medical treatment for diacetylmorphine (heroin) addiction: a clinical trial with methadone hydrochloride. *JAMA.* 1965;193:80–84.
101. Johnson RE, Jaffe JH, Fudala PJ. A controlled trial of buprenorphine treatment for opioid dependence. *JAMA.* 1992;267:20:2750–2759.
102. Stine SM, Kosten TR. Use of drug combinations in treatment of opioid withdrawal. *J Clin Psychopharmacol.* 1992;12:3:203–209.
103. Randall T. Ecstasy-fueled "rave" parties become dances of death for English youths. *JAMA.* 1992;268:12:1505–1506.
104. Randall T. "Rave" scene, Ecstasy use, leap Atlantic. *JAMA.* 1992;268:12:1506.
105. Dowling GP, McDonough ET, Bost RO. "Eve" and "Ecstasy." A report on five deaths associated with the use of MDEA and MDMA. *JAMA.* 1987;257:1615–1617.
106. Suarez RV, Reimersma R. "Ecstasy" and sudden cardiac death. *Am J Forensic Med Pathol.* 1985;9:339–341.
107. Screaton GR, Cairns HS, Sarner M, et al. Hyperpyrexia and rhabdomyolysis after MDMA ("ecstasy") abuse. *Lancet.* 1992;339:677–678.
108. Henry JA, Jeffreys KJ, Dawling S. Toxicity and deaths from 3,4-methylenedioxymethamphetamine ("ecstasy"). *Lancet.* 1992;340:384–387.
109. McGuire P, Fahy T. Chronic paranoid psychosis after misuse of MDMA ("ecstasy"). *BMJ.* 1991;302:697.
110. Schifano F. Chronic atypical psychosis associated with MDMA ("ecstasy") abuse. *Lancet.* 1991;338:1335.
111. Creighton FJ, Black DL, Hyde CE. "Ecstasy" psychosis and flashbacks. *Br J Psychiatry.* 1991;159:713–715.
112. Martin ML, Hecker J, Clark RF, et al. China white in the eastern U.S. emergency department experience. *Ann Emerg Med.* 1989;18:446–447.
113. Hibbs J, Perper J, Winek CL. An outbreak of designer drug-related deaths in Pennsylvania. *JAMA.* 1991;265:1011–1013.
114. Davis GC, Williams AC, Markey SP, et al. Chronic parkinsonism secondary to intravenous injection of meperidine analogues. *Psychiatry Res.* 1979;1:249–254.

115. Burns RS, LeWitt PA, Ebert M, et al. The clinical syndrome of striatal dopamine deficiency. *N Engl J Med.* 1985;312:1418–1421.
116. Goodman L, Gilman A, eds. *The Pharmacologic Basis of Therapeutics.* 5th ed. New York: Macmillan; 1975.
117. Draper R, Daly I. Alprazolam and amitriptyline: a double blind comparison of anxiolytic and antidepressant activity. *Ir Med J.* 1983; 76:453.
118. Tyrer P, Rutherford D, Huggett T. Benzodiazepine withdrawal symptoms and propranolol. *Lancet.* 1981;1:520.
119. Choice of benzodiazepines. *Med Lett Drugs Ther.* 1981;23:41.
120. Klotz U. The effects of age and liver disease on the disposition and elimination of diazepam in adult man. *J Clin Invest.* 1974;55:347.
121. Bender FM, Cooper JV, Dreyfus R. Fatalities associated with an acute overdose of glutethimide (Doriden) and codeine. *Vet Hum Toxicol.* 1988;30:332–333.
122. Baltarowich LL. Sedative-hypnotics. In: Rosen P, Barkin RM, eds. *Emergency Medicine Concepts and Clinical Practice.* 3rd ed. St Louis, MO: Mosby Year Book; 1992.
123. Curry S. Disposition of glutethimide in man. *Clin Pharmacol Ther.* 1971;12:849.
124. Hansen A. Glutethimide poisoning. *N Engl J Med.* 1975;202:250.
125. Teehan B. Acute ethchlorvinol intoxication. *Ann Intern Med.* 1970; 72:875.
126. Heyman J, Krumholtz W, Merlis S. The influence of different pharmaceutical preparations of meprobamate on the rate of absorption in humans. *Curr Ther Res.* 1962;4:416.
127. Gustafson A, Svensson S, Ugander L. Cardiac arrhythmias in chloral hydrate poisoning. *Acta Med Scand.* 1977;201:227.
128. Marshall E, Owens A. Absorption, excretion, and metabolic rate of chloral hydrate and trichloroethanol. *Bull Johns Hopkins Hosp.* 1954; 95:1.
129. Hunkeler W, Mohler H, Pieri L, et al. Selective antagonists of benzodiazepines. *Nature.* 1981;290:514–516.
130. Votey SR, Bosse GM, Bayer MJ, Hoffman JR. Flumazenil: a new benzodiazepine antagonist. *Ann Emerg Med.* 1991;20:2:181–188.
131. Burr W, Sundham P. Death after flumazenil. *BMJ.* 1989;298:1713.
132. Klotz U, Kanto J. Pharmacokinetics and clinical use of flumazenil. *Clin Pharmacokinet.* 1988;14:1.
133. Hofer P, Scollo-Lavizzari G. Benzodiazepine antagonist Ro 15-1788 in self-poisoning: diagnostic and therapeutic use. *Arch Intern Med.* 1985;145:663.
134. Isbell H. Chronic barbiturate intoxication, an experimental study. *Arch Neurol Psychiatry.* 1950;64:1.
135. Essig C. Newer sedative drugs that can cause states of intoxication and dependence of the barbiturate type. *JAMA.* 1966;196:714.
136. Hollister L, Motzenbecker P, Degan R. Withdrawal reactions from chlordiazepoxide. *Psychopharmacologia.* 1961;2:63.
137. Greenblatt D. Fatal hyperthermia following haloperidol therapy of sedative-hypnotic withdrawal. *J Clin Psychiatry.* 1978;39:673.
138. Okamoto M, Rosenberg H, Boisse N. Evaluation of anticonvulsants in barbiturate withdrawal. *J Pharmacol Exp Ther.* 1977;200:479.
139. Wikler A. Diagnosis and treatment of drug dependence of the barbiturate type. *Am J Psychiatry.* 1968;125:758.
140. Smith D, Wesson D. Phenobarbital technique for treatment of barbiturate dependence. *Arch Gen Psychiatry.* 1971;24:56.
141. Waddell W, Butler T. The distribution and excretion of phenobarbital. *J Clin Invest.* 1956;36:1217.
142. Linden C. Volatile substances of abuse. *Emerg Med Clin North Am.* 1990;8:3:559–579.
143. Carrol H, Abel G. Chronic gasoline inhalation. *South Med J.* 1971; 28:203.
144. Ikeda M. Excretion kinetics of urinary metabolites in a patient addicted to trichlorethylene. *Br J Ind Med.* 1971;28:203.
145. Mee A, Wright P. Congestive cardiomyopathy in association with solvent abuse. *J R Soc Med.* 1980;73:671.
146. Cornish H, Adefuin J. Ethanol potentiation of halogenated aliphatic solvent toxicity. *Am Ind Hyg Assoc J.* 1966;27:57.
147. Clearfield H. Hepatorenal toxicity from sniffing spot remover. *Am J Dig Dis.* 1970;15:851.
148. Dorden W, Chipman D. Gasoline sniffing complicated by acute carbon tetrachloride poisoning. *Arch Intern Med.* 1967;119:371.
149. Taher S, Anderson R, McCartney R, et al. Renal tubular acidosis associated with toluene sniffing. *N Engl J Med.* 1974;290:765.
150. Boecks R, Postl B, Coodin F. Gasoline sniffing and tetraethyl lead poisoning in children. *Pediatrics.* 1972;60:140.
151. Smith H. Inhalation of volatile substances. *Pharm Chem Newslett.* 1976;5:1.
152. Brabski D. Toluene sniffing producing cerebellar degeneration. *Am J Psychiatry.* 1961;118:461.
153. Gonzalez E, Downey J. Polyneuropathy in a glue sniffer. *Arch Phys Med Rehabil.* 1972;53:333.
154. Wyse G. Deliberate inhalation of volatile hydrocarbons: a review. *Can Med Assoc J.* 1973;108:71.
155. Bass M. Sudden sniffing death. *JAMA.* 1970;212:2075.
156. Inhalation-induced immunosuppression: sniffing out the volatile nitrite-AIDS connection (Editorial). *Pharmacotherapy.* 1984;4:235.
157. Blush not with nitrates (Editorial). *Ann Intern Med.* 1980;92:700.
158. Smith R, Olson M. Drug induced methemoglobinemia. *Semin Hematol.* 1973;10:253.
159. Davies B, Beech H. The effect of 1-arylcyclohexylamine (Serenyl) on twelve normal volunteers. *J Ment Sci.* 1960;106:912.
160. Ohisson A. Plasma delta-9-tetrahydrocannabinol concentrations and clinical effects after oral and intravenous administration and smoking. *Clin Pharmacol Ther.* 1980;28:409.
161. Baldridge EB, Bessen HA. Phencyclidine. *Emerg Med Clin North Am.* 1990;8:3:541–550.
162. Morgan J, Solomon J. Phencyclidine: clinical pharmacology and toxicity. *N Y State J Med.* 1978;2035.
163. Burns R. Phencyclidine-states of acute intoxication and fatalities. *West J Med.* 1975;123:345.
164. Showalter C, Thornton W. Clinical pharmacology of phencyclidine toxicity. *Am J Psychiatry.* 1977;134:11.
165. Cogen F. Phencyclidine-associated acute rhabdomyolysis. *Ann Intern Med.* 1978;88:210.
166. Fauman B. Psychiatric sequelae of phencyclidine abuse. *Clin Toxicol.* 1976;9:529.
167. Selden BS, Clark RF, Curry SC. Marijuana. *Emerg Med Clin North Am.* 1990;8:3:527–539.
168. Rizlin R, Gupta R, Lundberg G. Delta-9-tetrahydrocannabinol levels in street samples of marijuana and hashish: correlation to user reactions. *Clin Toxicol.* 1979;15:45.
169. Jones RT, Benowitz NL, Herning RI. Clinical relevance of cannabis tolerance and dependence. *J Clin Pharmacol.* 1981;21:143S–152S.
170. Nahas GG. Cannabis: toxicological properties and epidemiological aspects. *Med J Aust.* 1986;145:82–87.
171. Lemberger L. Delta-9-tetrahydrocannabinol: metabolism and disposition in long-term marijuana smokers. *Science.* 1971;173:72.

172. Mason AP, McBay AJ. Cannabis: pharmacology and interpretation of effects. *J Forensic Sci.* 1985;30:615–631.
173. Sallan S, Zinberg N, Frei E. Antiemetic effect of delta-9-THC in patients receiving cancer chemotherapy. *N Engl J Med.* 1975;293:795.
174. Helper R. *The Pharmacology of Marijuana.* March Press; 1976:815.
175. Beaconsfield P, Ginsberg J, Raimsbury R. Marijuana smoking: cardiovascular effects in man and possible mechanisms. *N Engl J Med.* 1972;287:209.
176. In paraquat poisoning—persevere (Editorial). *Emerg Med.* 1976;185.
177. Weil A. Adverse reactions to marijuana-classification and suggested treatment. *N Engl J Med.* 1970;282:997.
178. Mims R, Lee J. Adverse effects of intravenous cannabis tea. *J Natl Med Assoc.* 1977;69:491.
179. Kulig K. LSD. *Emerg Med Clin North Am.* 1990;8:3:551–558.
180. Sullivan A. The fate of LSD in the body: forensic considerations. *J Forensic Sci Soc.* 1978;18:89.
181. Hollister L. *Handbook of Psychopharmacology.* New York: Plenum; 1978:389.
182. Zelson C. Infant of the addicted mother. *N Engl J Med.* 1973;288:1393–1395.
183. Levy M, Koren G. Obstetric and neonatal effects of drugs of abuse. *Emerg Med Clin North Am.* 1990;8:3:633–652.

49. Alcohol Problems

WILLIAM D. CLARK, MD

Mr A is a 38-year-old man who comes to the emergency department for a cough. The examining physician notes the odor of alcohol, a tremor, and a degree of hyperactivity. Mr B, aged 43, comes to the emergency department for an ankle sprain sustained during a fall on the stairs to his cellar. The examining physician orders a blood alcohol level, which is 275 mg/dL. Ms C is a 27-year-old nurse in the respiratory intensive care unit at another hospital, who is brought in for an overdose of diazepam. Questioning reveals that this is a suicide attempt and that she has been confused and depressed over the past several months, regularly drinking heavily. Mr D, a skid row man, visits the emergency department daily for unclear reasons. He is loud, inconsiderate, conniving, scruffy, and generally a nuisance. Professor E presents with a classical perforated peptic ulcer. While he is being prepared for surgery, he confides to the nurse that his wife's drinking has been the center of a family conflict. The couple has been engaged in an escalating cycle of sadomasochistic behavior which is interrupted only by his attacks of abdominal pain. Mr F is 15 years old, very intoxicated, and was slightly injured in an auto driven into a guardrail by an intoxicated friend.

Alcoholism prevalence is high, affecting 5% to 10% of adults, depending on geography and the criteria used for definition of illness.[1] Mortality figures dramatize the human toll: the leading causes of death among 25- to 44-year-old white men are accidents, homicide, suicide, and cirrhosis of the liver (among Black men hypertension is fourth and cirrhosis fifth). Each of these problems has been shown to be directly related to alcoholism. In addition, alcohol-related illnesses account for a large number of visits to all emergency departments,[2,3] and 10% of all deaths in the United States may be related to alcohol.[4]

Specific problems addressed in this chapter include metabolism and effects of alcohol, management of alcohol intoxication and overdose, the withdrawal syndromes, patients who are unexpectedly discovered to need attention for alcoholism, people who come for crisis counseling, and screening medical exams ("clearance").

THE DISEASE CONCEPT

The fundamental lesion in alcoholism is a repetitive but inconsistent and sometimes unpredictable loss of control of drinking that produces symptoms of serious dysfunction or disability, frequently including physical addiction. The afflicted person usually denies the presence of the illness for prolonged periods. Since Jellinek wrote *The Disease Concept of Alcoholism* in 1960,[5] a controversy has raged about the disease idea.[6-11] The conceptualization herein suggests that the physician approach persons with alcoholism as if they had a disease, and use familiar techniques to establish a diagnosis, initiate treatment, and encourage a fruitful physician-patient relationship.

What are the essential elements of this concept, and do they take account of available scientific data on the nature of alcoholism? Does the concept encourage the maintenance and development of human dignity and mutual self-respect between patient and care giver, and does it explain the repetitively self-destructive behaviors? The central idea in this concept is that persons with the alcoholism syndrome are unable to control their intake of alcohol. The lack of control is incomplete, inconsistent, and insidiously deceptive; sometimes the person can abstain and at other times drink in a controlled fashion. However, using a year as a time frame, the person sometimes drinks more than intended, or drinks when he or she had not intended to drink, and suffers as a result. The frequency and amount of uncontrolled drinking determine the severity and spectrum of symptoms. Some manifestations of alcoholism vary in response to socioeconomic factors; thus the lawyer, psychiatrist, active housewife, or retired clerk present distinct complaints. It is not clear whether differential susceptibility or differences in amount of alcohol account for individual variability in medical complaints, such as liver disease, pancreatitis, and delirium tremens.[12]

The essence of the alcoholism syndrome is similar to tobacco dependence, aspirin dependence, compulsive eating, or severe nail-biting. However, the pharmacologic properties of this sedative and addictive drug produce grave consequences as the amount of intake increases. Heavier drinking is higher-risk drinking, although factors other than quantity of intake may be critical for the progression to alcoholism.

The disease concept suggests a discontinuity between alcoholic drinking and healthy drinking. No one sets out to develop alcoholism or to become "hooked" on alcohol (nor does the smoker set out to develop lung cancer). The nascent alcoholic person may begin drinking for the usual reasons. Whatever the factors that promote heavy drinking, as the amount and frequency of intake increases, some people intermittently fail to control their intake. A dependence develops, the person begins to drink for unclear reasons, and is now drinking alcoholically, with serious consequences.[13] The pharmacology of alcohol is one reason for the transition from the person who is controlling his or her drinking to the drinking controlling the person. Other factors are less clearly understood,[14] but the qualitative as well as quantitative difference between alcoholic drinking and healthy drinking is emphasized by the disease concept.

The disease concept serves as a reminder that the disorder has a "life of its own." The syndrome is integrated into the totality of a person's physical, emotional, and social being, while retaining some degree of independence. Diabetes may become visible or worsen during depression or infection, but is not caused by these factors; alcoholism is similarly independent and interdependent. The disease concept reminds care givers that addictive drinking will not disappear without a direct approach any more than diabetes is cured by psychotherapy, better environmental conditions, exercise of will power, or not eating carbohydrates.

Three major hypotheses have been investigated in order to understand the etiology of alcoholism: the sociocultural, the biochemical-genetic, and the psychological. None has been effective at explaining *the* cause of alcoholism. A review summarizes the data as follows:

> No explanation that involves a single class of etiological factors seems adequate to account for what is most likely an "overdetermined" disorder with multiple causes and a complex developmental course.[15]

Like other illnesses such as hypertension, or even infectious diseases such as tuberculosis, a continuum of causal factors is usually present. Another way of stating this is to state two aspects of its unpredictability. First, if conditions are right, any person who drinks alcohol has the potential to move into alcoholic drinking; no regular drinker is invulnerable to this disease. Second, which of 100 drinkers will develop alcoholism cannot specifically be predicted, just as it is impossible to predict which individual smokers will develop cancer. Recent long-term follow-up studies of healthy populations confirm these ideas.[16,17]

Thus, available evidence suggests that the concept of alcoholism as a disease should be accepted. The disease model provides a framework for understanding the destructive dependence exhibited by millions of Americans who seek physical, emotional, and spiritual assistance from physicians. Current data suggest that the fundamental lesion (inconsistent inability to control alcohol intake) is determined or conditioned by an array of etiologic factors that differs from person to person. The disease concept will not be proved or disproved; it is a way of looking at certain facts and ideas that is helpful but not subject to a rational or logical proof per se. Physicians and others who adopt the illness model can condemn bad behaviors while simultaneously addressing the afflicted person with dignity and respect instead of repugnance stemming from a moral model.[11] For patients, accepting responsibility for entering treatment is facilitated when physicians join them in blaming the disease, not the person, for despicable behavior.

ALCOHOL METABOLISM

A background in the physiology and metabolism of alcohol is helpful, and definitions are important in developing a consistent approach. A standard drink is 1½ oz of liquor (about 40% alcohol), 12 oz of beer (about 5%), or 5 oz of table wine (about 12%). Each of these servings contains approximately the same amount of alcohol (1½ × 0.40 = 12 × 0.05 = 5 × 0.12). Patients seldom report drinks in standardized terms; one's "drink" is another's quart of beer or pint of whiskey or double highball with beer chaser, greatly confounding history-taking. Blood alcohol peaks 30 to 40 minutes after a person with an empty stomach takes a drink of alcohol. The height of this peak depends slightly on individual factors, but drinking three to four drinks quickly on an empty stomach typically elevates the standard (70-kg) person's blood alcohol level (BAL) to about 100 mg/dL, legally set as the limit for drunkenness in many states.

Responses to the first drink or two vary, but once a BAL of 100 mg/dL is achieved, individual differences are minimal and the manifestations are solely due to the pharmacologic effect of the drug on the central nervous system (CNS). At this level all persons show some signs of inebriation, namely, slurred speech, uncoordinated gait, poor judgment, and emotional lability. Hepatic alcohol dehydrogenases (ADH) metabolize alcohol, lowering the BAL 15 to 25 mg/dL per hour—a rate not substantially affected by total dose or the starting BAL. Thus, recovery from mild intoxication (100 mg/dL) requires 2 to 3 hours (BAL of 50 mg/dL), and about 5 hours for complete elimination. Metabolic rate differs from person to person and the range of rates in a given group (white men, for example) is much wider than any between group differences (men and women, or Indians and Italians, for example).[18]

Although the oxidizing capacity of ADH does not change with regular exposure to alcohol, the liver's microsomal enzyme oxidizing system (MEOS) does become activated, producing metabolic rates at the high end (25 mg/dL per hour).[19] However, even people with longstanding alcoholism do not exceed this metabolic rate.

ALCOHOL TOLERANCE

The clinical effects of alcohol tolerance are dramatic and striking. Moreover, diagnostic assessment is incomplete if tolerance effects are ignored. The diminished effects of high alcohol levels noted in tolerant persons are produced by nerve tissue adaption. As stated, a BAL of 100 mg/dL produces signs of inebriation in any nontolerant person, whereas the tolerant person may behave in a normal fashion even at very high alcohol levels. For instance, one person who acted soberly and denied drinking had a BAL of 568 mg/dL, a datum which settled the immediate issue (whether the person had been drinking) and also established the diagnosis of alcoholism.

This very dramatic example emphasizes the fact that the person who is tolerant does indeed perform many basic functions well because of the ability of the nervous tissue to adapt to the presence of alcohol. However, judgment, emotional responses, and interpersonal relationships remain impaired, inappropriate, or shallow. The person who has a BAL of over 100 mg/dL but appears sober is tolerant, and usually has alcoholism. This is likely to be the case for Mr B from the introduction. Typically, Mr B and other tolerant patients do not show signs of intoxication at the usual blood levels, but the apparent sobriety in spite of the high BAL may mask a serious cognitive and emotional deficit. The cover-up may be so effective as to mislead experienced physicians[3] if they fail to note the odor of alcohol. The person who says, "Oh, I just had a drink before I came in," is surprisingly often taken at face value, when the "drink" may have been a pint of whiskey or a bottle of sherry!

INTOXICATION AND OVERDOSE

Intoxication and overdose of alcohol is frequently encountered in emergency departments but seldom on other services. All degrees of intoxication may produce serious problems, from coma to disruptive behavior. Moreover, a single patient may frustrate emergency department staff for many hours during expression of the various problems associated with different levels of inebriation. Life support may be necessary, or suturing impossible, or the patient's unruly behavior may disturb staff or patients. Nurse C from the introduction represents a fairly typical situation.

In addition, too often the staff denies that these patients have alcoholism, not recognizing that perhaps 90% of adults who appear drunk in emergency departments do have alcoholism. Although good statistics are not available on this point, it should be apparent that the alcoholic 10% of the population who are frequently drunk (for illustrative purposes assume a conservative average of once a week) should account for more intoxication-related problems than the 60% of the population who are healthy drinkers, infrequently drunk (assume once a year on average). Thus from a hypothetical population of 100, 30 abstainers yield no episodes of drunkenness, 60 healthy drinkers yield 60 episodes, and 10 alcoholics, 520 episodes per year. Additionally the healthy drinkers seldom become as intoxicated and are more often drinking in controlled environments (where someone else can drive, for example). If health care staff understand that healthy drinkers who "have had one too many" only rarely appear in emergency departments, they can more realistically adjust their attitudes, expectations, and treatment approach.

A comatose person with a BAL of 400 mg/dL may require the supports needed with any sedative overdose, including intubation and ventilatory assistance. The patient would likely awaken gradually at a BAL of 200 to 250 mg/dL 6 to 8 hours after the initial measurement. Rapid infusion of intravenous (IV) fructose will increase the degradation rate of ethanol. However, the increase is limited to 20% to 25% (or less if the rate is already maximal because of steady exposure) so that this treatment is not clinically useful.[20] Furthermore, large volumes of fluids must be given, increasing the possibility of fluid or electrolyte disturbances.

Behavior of intoxicated individuals, such as Mr F, shows features well known to emergency department staff. Such people are usually disruptive, often obnoxious, sometimes combative and destructive, and always difficult to control. Often, they are brought to the emergency department against their wishes (by police or friends); or else they may have some specific needs, such as getting off the streets, finding a meal or a warm friendly place; or they may simply be looking for whatever attention is available. What they seek, then, is not what the staff is equipped to deliver, resulting in escalating friction. Furthermore, staff behavior must be adjusted to the reality that negative attention is as valuable to the intoxicated attention-seeker as positive attention.

Staff sometimes believe that patients are totally out of control, but everyone has observed that patients respond very differently to the arrival of a police officer or an attractive nurse. These strikingly different responses clearly demonstrate that staff behavior may have dramatic influences on patients' behavior. Furthermore, patients must be held responsible for their actions even while "out of control." Appropriate limits can be set by knowledgeable staff even though the situation is tense, other matters press for attention, and time is frequently limited. Helpful generalizations concerning appropriate staff behaviors are difficult, but some useful procedures for setting limits can be described.

One typical frustrating situation involves the arrival in the emergency department of a "regular" whose disruptive routines are well known from frequent visits. Careful observation of the objectionable behaviors often discloses ones that are subject to modification through alterations in staff behavior. Physicians and nurses should find protected conference time for considered discussions; only careful planning can result in a coordinated approach and development of a satisfactory management plan. This process of identifying behaviors and developing management plans has been described in a publication from the Addiction Research Foundation.[21]

The violent or agitated patient often responds to skillful "talking down" in a calm environment. However, safety of everyone concerned, including staff, other patients, and the inebriate, must be the primary consideration. Adoption of a nonthreatening posture and attitude allowing the patient to ventilate rather than trying to induce sober or responsible behavior is a helpful start. Offering a cigarette, coffee, or a doughnut sometimes turns wrath and agitation miraculously into tranquility, again demonstrating that emotional lability is a regular feature of drunkenness.

Keeping the patient seated is a helpful strategy and minimizes the potential for violence. However, physical or chemical restraints may be needed to protect personnel or the patient. If physical restraints are used, chemical restraints are usually indicated, except in the case of severe head trauma. Intramuscular (IM) chlorpromazine in doses of 25 to 100 mg will control most situations. It is prudent to start with 25 mg, increasing subsequent doses as necessary. The hypotensive effects of this drug are as dramatic as the sedative effects; thus, patients should be kept supine. Diazepam given in 5-mg IV doses is also effective. Neither drug should be given unless staff are prepared to provide respiratory assistance; this is an unstable situation where good judgment is necessary in weighing the potential dangers of violence against those of additional sedation.

Patients whose lacerations have been sutured or who have no other serious medical problems are often left to sober up in emergency departments. They should always be restrained on stretchers since they may wake up unexpectedly. Caffeine is commonly administered, but may cause a more dangerous situation by producing a slightly more awake inebriate who is as uncoordinated and who has as poor judgment as previously.

After sobering up (if treatment for withdrawal is not indicated), the patient will be discharged from the emergency department. Before dismissal, all patients should have some counseling, with emphasis on a few principles. First, any patient in a blackout state which may persist well into his or her apparent "sobering up" phase will retain little of what is said; therefore any messages must be brief and must be simple. This is true also of the serious cognitive and emotional disarray (short of blackouts) present in many intoxicated people.

Patients who are not regular visitors to emergency departments feel guilty and ashamed of their behavior. Universally such patients are fearful and anxious, and often seriously depressed. Because of these feelings and low self-esteem, they remember the tone of an interview much better than its content. Thus, the discussion must be couched in supportive terms. Frequently, a brief diagnostic interview makes it clear that the patient has alcoholism. The discussion must directly and supportively address this diagnosis, just as would be the case if cancer or diabetes had been discovered. Psychiatric support for Nurse C after her overdose should include these principles. Further guidelines for counseling are included in the section on crisis counseling, below.

Development of working relationships with community alcoholism treatment facilities is useful. Working with "wet drop-in" centers, overnight shelters, and detoxification facilities of various kinds facilitates the effective and appropriate discharge of patients who otherwise might clog the emergency department for many hours, and even then leave with inappropriate treatment plans.

ADDICTION AND WITHDRAWAL

The presence of a withdrawal syndrome associated with daily intake of alcohol defines physical addiction to alcohol. Daily heavy drinking inevitably produces addiction and a subsequent withdrawal syndrome. The pioneering work of Isbell and colleagues demonstrated that this process can occur after a few weeks of steady, heavy drinking in people who had no prior history of alcohol addiction.[22] The clinical manifestations of the withdrawal syndrome suggest that the CNS becomes hyperactive as it recovers from an oversedated state and adjusts to absence of alcohol. Proposed mechanisms for the addiction/withdrawal process have included enzyme induction and receptor proliferation; more recently, membrane alterations; and most recently of all, endorphin stimulation within central nervous tissue.[23,24]

It should be remembered that many alcoholic people who experience great suffering and dysfunction because of episodic drunkenness or erratic abuse patterns never develop the daily drinking pattern that produces addiction. Professor E's wife, whose episodes of intoxication always produce conflict, might be included in this group. A clear example of this situation is the person who drinks only from Friday through Sunday. Although severe adverse consequences (aggressiveness and abuse, or Monday absences) may be apparent, the brain fully recovers from Monday through Thursday and the molecular changes in nervous tissue that produce the withdrawal syndrome will not develop unless the person moves to a pattern of daily drinking. On the other hand, it is true that the physically addicted state is a serious health consequence; therefore, any person who experiences withdrawal symptoms must have alcoholism.

Intoxication and withdrawal appear to be more "shades of gray" than black-or-white, clearly separable states, at least in addicted drinkers. Clinically, unless the alcohol level is rising, the person is in withdrawal. From the viewpoint of the CNS, a falling alcohol level is always interpreted as the "last" drink. The CNS has no way to know whether another dose of alcohol will be taken in an hour, a day, a week, or never. Furthermore, the presence of tolerance means that symptoms and signs of intoxication are unusual. The person must drink very large quantities to become clinically intoxicated. These phenomena have been studied in research units by administering alcohol in a programmed fashion to a person who has been addicted. After a few weeks of sobriety alcohol is given in controlled doses for 16 hours. If alcohol is then withheld withdrawal symptoms can be demonstrated. During the next 24-hour cycle (16 hours drinking and 8 hours off) withdrawal symptoms worsen. By the third cycle, the person has withdrawal symptoms constantly between drinks, worsening steadily as drinking continues.[25] The brain seems to have a "memory circuit" for the addiction syndrome.

Thus, symptoms do not just occur when people cease drinking, but severe symptoms are a regular occurrence during the time that a person is still drinking. At first, heavier drinking may overcome the symptoms, but such factors as gastritis, families, and lack of funds limit the amounts one can drink. Therefore, people actively drinking heavily may arrive in the emergency department with withdrawal symptoms, even severe syndromes. Clinicians must remember that neither recent heavy drinking, nor alcohol on the breath, nor a very elevated BAL rules out delirium tremens.

DIFFERENTIAL DIAGNOSIS OF WITHDRAWAL SYMPTOMS

Occasionally, the differential diagnosis of the withdrawal syndromes is challenging. Paradoxically, intoxication may be difficult to distinguish from withdrawal. As previously discussed, as a drinking episode is lengthened, the time spent not in withdrawal is shortened, and drunkenness may be fleeting. Aggressive and anxious behaviors may be similar during drunkenness or withdrawal. One distinguishing feature is that emotional lability is more dramatic when the individual is inebriated than during withdrawal. A second feature is that the agitation of drunkenness usually worsens with talking, whereas the agitation of withdrawal often responds and improves with "talking down." Finally, if intoxicated people are left alone they may quiet down or go to sleep, whereas people in withdrawal may calm down while alone, but they do not drop off to sleep.

Wernicke-Korsakoff's syndrome may confuse some observers because the "global confusional state" appears similar to the delirium of delirium tremens.[26] Distinguishing features include dramatically less agitation for the degree of confusion during Wernicke's disease and the presence of ocular, cerebellar, and peripheral nerve findings. Patients with hepatic failure who are delirious are usually more somnolent than agitated, and asterixis is present. If spider angiomata, ascites, and jaundice are absent, this diagnosis may be missed.

Acute schizophrenic syndromes typically show fewer autonomic findings and more fixed hallucinations and delusions, but in the individual patient accurate differential diagnosis is sometimes impossible. The history of alcohol intake is essential, but final diagnosis may be delayed seven to ten days while the clinical course is observed.

Subdural hematoma, a frequent concomitant of alcoholism, often shows focal neurologic signs and usually has a more waxing and waning course than does delirium tremens. Because focal signs are not prominent or are overlooked, the subdural is too often missed.[27]

Meningitis, pneumonia, and cerebral vascular accidents can also cause difficulty in diagnosis if atypical syndromes are present, and this demonstrates the need to consider the spectrum of diseases, especially metabolic (uremia, hyponatremia) and toxic (bromides, steroids, amphetamines, psychedelics), that may cause delirium.[27] Withdrawal from other drugs may be concomitant with alcohol withdrawal, but because these patients believe that they require specific appropriate treatment, they often give history correctly, so drug withdrawal is not mistaken for alcohol withdrawal. In people who abuse barbiturates or benzodiazepines with alcohol, the differentiation between withdrawal syndromes may be impossible in the emergency department. Blood levels of barbiturates and a test dose of barbiturate assist in determining appropriate therapy; however, initial treatment of minor tranquilizer withdrawal is not different from alcohol withdrawal treatment (see Chapter 48, Substance Abuse).

WITHDRAWAL SYNDROMES

Mild Withdrawal

The variety of clinical presentations of alcohol withdrawal is well known to most physicians.[23,28] The problems of mild to moderate severity have their onset within minutes to hours after the last drink. Symptoms include tremors, sweating, anxiety, nervousness, agitation, vague fears, stomach upset with nausea and pain, and extreme difficulty sleeping. Hallucinations occur frequently in mild withdrawal. Symptoms peak at 24 hours and then gradually decline over two to four days. Recognition of this syndrome is not difficult in the emergency department if the history of alcohol intake is apparent, as in Mr A from the introduction. Treatment for mild withdrawal is straightforward.

Safe, efficacious pharmacotherapy is available and should be initiated in the emergency department. The pros and cons of many drugs suggested for this purpose are briefly considered.

Alcohol

Alcohol itself has been used by some physicians and, of course, by many patients who attempt self-treatment by "tapering off." Unfortunately, alcohol is a short-acting drug and is hard to control. It is also psychologically difficult for the patient to take or for nurses to administer. Furthermore, physicians rarely prescribe adequate amounts of alcohol, perhaps because of lack of understanding of the data already presented regarding the complex interrelationships among intoxication, addiction, tolerance, and withdrawal symptoms. Finally, continuing damage to the heart, brain, liver, bone marrow, and immune systems is promoted by alcohol. All of these considerations make it inappropriate to prescribe alcohol in any circumstance in the treatment of alcohol withdrawal syndromes. Effective drugs are available that:

1. are longer acting and thus provide smoother symptom relief
2. are cross-tolerant in the CNS itself
3. are not toxic to alcohol-affected organs

Chlordiazepoxide

The prototypical drug used for mild to moderate alcohol withdrawal is chlordiazepoxide.[28] Chlordiazepoxide has an effective half-life of more than 24 hours. Its onset of action is in about 2 hours and peak action does not occur until 6 to 8 hours after a dose. When administered in adequate dosage during the first 24 hours after the onset of withdrawal symptoms and tapered rapidly, its pharmacokinetics are ideal for the treatment of alcohol withdrawal. In the emergency department in otherwise uncomplicated patients the oral administration of 25 to 75 mg is an appropriate starting dose. Follow-up doses of 25 to 100 mg every 4 to 6 hours are given. IM chlordiazepoxide is contraindicated because of unreliable absorption from muscle sites. For average severity 150 to 250 mg in the initial 24 hours is typical, with 75 to 100 mg given in the second 24 hours, and 25 to 50 mg in the third 24 hours. The prolonged excretion results in a gradual decline in blood levels during days 4 to 7 or 8. Protocols in which the entire treatment dose is administered during the first few hours have been tested. Because of the long half-life, subsequent doses are not needed. Chlordiazepoxide is very inexpensive.[29,30]

Phenobarbital

Phenobarbital is an effective drug for patients who are allergic to chlordiazepoxide or if a nasogastric tube or severe GI symptoms prevent the administration of chlordiazepoxide. It should be given in approximately milligram equivalent doses to chlordiazepoxide and can be given intramuscularly.

Oxazepam

Oxazepam has effects similar to chlordiazepoxide but is shorter acting and effectively eliminated in the presence of cirrhosis or acute hepatitis.[31] Thus, it has some theoretical advantages in the setting of known liver disease. Therefore, if a shorter-acting drug is desired in the presence of head trauma or other CNS problems, oxazepam is probably the drug of choice. The starting dose should be 30 to 60 mg, and then 15 to 30 mg every 4 to 6 hours.

Paraldehyde

Paraldehyde was the drug of choice for many years. This drug, although probably the most dramatic and effective in relief of alcohol withdrawal symptoms, should nonetheless not be used. It is dangerous because of acidosis (from outdated lots) and rectal strictures. It is very short-acting and thus produces extreme swings in symptom relief; the short period of action and high potency result in rapid addiction to it. There is disagreement as to whether its odor and taste are objectionable, but it is definitely inconvenient to administer.

Other Drugs and Magnesium

Recent studies show that atenolol and other β-blockers may diminish the doses of benzodiazepines required; however, in consideration of their mechanism of action, β-blockers seem unlikely to replace the benzodiazepines as the treatment of choice for alcohol withdrawal.[28]

A careful study has laid to rest the idea that magnesium treatment, even in patients with very low initial levels, is effective therapy for withdrawal.[32] Other tranquilizers, sedatives, and carbamazepine[33] have been shown to be efficacious, but have little to recommend them in terms of effectiveness, convenience, safety, or cost.

Outpatient Treatment of Mild Alcohol Withdrawal

The initiation of outpatient detoxification regimens in the emergency department may prove helpful and cost effective.[34] Necessary prerequisites for ambulatory management are an environment where a responsible person can be alert for the development of complications (which occur infrequently but may not be recognized by the patient) and the ability to return for followup. If, in addition, circumstances suggest that mild withdrawal is likely, the use of an outpatient detoxification regimen is inexpensive and enlists patients and their family or friends in the early phases of treatment. The patient is given 50 to 100 mg of chlordiazepoxide, and the responsible person is given instructions to give 25 to 50 mg by mouth every 4 to 6 hours depending on the severity of symptoms. Not more than 150 mg should be given to take home. At follow-up the next day, medication can be given for 1 to 2 days and the patient can then enter a longer-term treatment program. If the patient drinks, outpatient treatment has failed, and admission for withdrawal is necessary.

Alcoholic Hallucinosis

So-called alcoholic hallucinosis is a variant mild to moderately severe withdrawal syndrome. The patient typically has very few autonomic signs and may have mild to absent tremor and anxiety but be hallucinating vigorously. Hallucinations begin while drinking or immediately after intake ceases. Hallucinations are frightening, but *not* an indication of severe withdrawal by themselves. This syndrome responds well to the usual drug schedules, and does not need special treatment except for reassurance of patient, family, and friends.

Delirium Tremens

Severe alcohol withdrawal is a complication justifiably feared among patients and physicians. This terrifying disease carries a mortality currently between 5% and 10% in the best circumstances. The onset is classically stated as 72 hours after the last drink of alcohol[35]; however, as previously described, delirium tremens may develop with no apparent change in drinking pattern.[25] Therefore, patients may appear in the emergency department who are drinking heavily and are also in active delirium tremens.

Onset may be abrupt and precipitous, or vague and insidious; the symptoms peak in 1 to 8 hours. Delirium is the hallmark, while other symptoms mimic those listed for mild withdrawal. Hallucinations are usually but not invariably present and autonomic dysfunctions are typically severe, sometimes including hyperventilation (with severe alkalosis), tachycardia, hyperthermia 40.5° to 41°C, and hypertension.

The variability of presentations is confusing to the neophyte; agitation can be minor or extreme, autonomic abnormalities completely absent or dramatic, while derangements of thought content can be minor or as serious as in acute paranoid schizophrenia. The diagnosis is often missed in those patients who have dramatic auditory or visual hallucinations, no autonomic abnormality and little of the violent anxiety and agitation usually associated with delirium tremens. However, the patients with the worst prognosis are those with striking autonomic findings; in particular, hyperventilation and alkalosis are associated with a poor outcome. This may be because of hypersensitivity of the medullary respiratory center to pharmacotherapeutic agents as well as to carbon dioxide.[28]

Severity and duration are difficult to predict. Extremely heavy uninterrupted drinking [for example, 3 quarts (3 L) of whiskey daily for 4 months] and past episodes of delirium correlate with more severe symptoms, but not invariably. "Impending" delirium tremens is a term of little clinical usefulness. If delirium is present, treatment for delirium tremens should be promptly started. If delirium is absent, treatment for mild withdrawal is appropriate. The response over the next 1 to 2 hours will determine subsequent treatment.

Treatment must be initiated promptly in the emergency department. The use of drugs cross-tolerant to alcohol in delirium tremens is not particularly helpful. Apparently a "threshold" is crossed, after which the excitation is no longer specifically relieved by alcohol or cross-tolerant drugs. The ideal drug should possess strong sedative and anti-psychotic properties. The drug whose efficacy has been most convincingly proved by appropriately controlled study is diazepam.[36] Ten milligrams should be administered intravenously over several minutes and then 5 mg given every 5 minutes intravenously until the patient becomes calm. Doses higher than 150 mg may be necessary to induce a calm state. Maintenance doses of 5 mg IV as often as necessary are then given. The point of treatment is to calm patients enough that restraints are not necessary, except to preserve the IV line. Patients should not be comatose, but drowsy and easily aroused. Treatment suppresses symptoms but has never been shown to have an effect on the duration of delirium tremens.

Mild cases of delirium tremens with few autonomic signs and minimum agitation may respond to high doses of oxazepam or haloperidol; however, these should not be used as first-line drugs. These drugs are of low potency for this illness, thus delaying efficacious treatment in some patients.

As previously discussed, alcohol has no role in the treatment of delirium tremens.

Seizures

The patient who presents to the emergency department with alcohol withdrawal seizures raises many issues. The diagnosis of alcohol withdrawal may be unclear if the history is scanty, which is often the case when the patient's cognitive function is compromised during the postictal state. Furthermore, some patients have a seizure as the sole manifestation of withdrawal. In such cases, absence of the typical shakes, sweating, anxiety, and so forth increases the diagnostic difficulty. Alcohol withdrawal seizures are generalized convulsive seizures, typically occurring 24 hours after the last drink. However, early and late seizures (5 to 7 days is common and 14 days possible) do occur.[37,38]

The presence of seizures does not predict severity of other withdrawal symptoms, but in patients who also have delirium tremens, withdrawal seizures precede the onset of delirium tremens. Seizures may be single or multiple, but no controlled data are available regarding efficacy of anticonvulsive treatment after the first seizure. If more than one seizure occurs, the second may follow by as few as one or as many as 8 hours. The data on usefulness of prophylactic treatment against seizures in patients known to be undergoing alcohol withdrawal conflict; thus some physicians use phenytoin if a history of seizures during prior episodes of withdrawal is present, while others do not give medication. Hospital admission is appropriate for patients who have not had prior seizures, so that appropriate diagnostic measures may be undertaken and patients and families counseled in an environment where the patient can be observed. In particular, the diagnosis of alcoholism can be pursued and an appropriate introduction to alcoholism treatment established. Patients should be held under observation for at least eight hours after any withdrawal seizure. Considering the above statements, patients should never be discharged from the emergency department with anticonvulsants, with or without previous withdrawal seizure history.

EMERGENCY DEPARTMENT DIAGNOSIS OF ALCOHOLISM

Many people who do not appear at first glance intoxicated or in withdrawal may have alcoholism. Typical clues for the examiner include the odor of alcohol, the nature of the situation (aggressive behavior, home accident, suicide attempt); or the presence of tremor or anxiety (such as Mr A or B or Ms C). These nonspecific signs should alert staff to consider a possible diagnosis of alcoholism.

The alcoholic patient is likely to be anxious, negative, defensive, and difficult to interview. While attempting to clarify the situation, the interviewer must be sensitive to the patient's concerns, individualize the approach, and remember that the patient is already in pain if alcoholism is present. In the absence of alcoholism, on the other hand, patients will not be offended by a brief and skillful exploration for other symptoms of alcoholism. A simple screening test is available which is adequate for initial interviews. The CAGE (a mnemonic) test is designed to ascertain whether the patient has experienced poor control or adverse consequences of drinking, and what feedback has been received regarding drinking:

CAGE Screening Test for Alcoholism[39]

Have you ever felt the need to	**C**ut down on drinking?
Have you ever felt	**A**nnoyed by criticism of drinking?
Have you ever had	**G**uilty feelings about drinking?
Have you ever taken a morning	**E**ye opener?

Note that the test does not focus on alcohol (as in how much or how often), but on the person and his or her relationship to alcohol. If these problems are present, there is a high probability of alcoholism. Further confirmation can be obtained by using other structured interview devices to explore both the person's preoccupation with drinking (or not drinking) and other associated adverse consequences. Many physicians find mnemonic devices to be useful memory aids; HALT, BUMP, and FATAL DTs make use of this technique (see Appendix 49-A).[40]

Many professionals express skepticism regarding the value of such efforts. However, every interview has therapeutic content, and health care staff generally strive to achieve maximum benefit from their encounters with patients. Consider for a moment the alternatives for interactions with patients in whom some clue to a diagnosis of alcoholism is present.

First, one might do nothing; however, this "conspiracy of silence" is frequently developed to a fine art by the patient's friends and family. Additional silence on the part of physicians and nurses will never be helpful. Waiting for something to happen or for the patient to recognize or acknowledge the problem is courting another accident, pancreatitis, overdose, or violent episode.

A second approach might be to chastise the patient for self-abusive behavior, to criticize the patient for disrupting others' lives, or to issue a reminder that more drinking will "rot out your liver." This approach is perceived as mean and nasty by the patient and amplifies feelings of guilt, shame, and low self-esteem. Patients often strike back with their own hostile, angry criticism, thus generating another futile imbroglio.

A third alternative is to pursue a rational and caring approach in spite of the apparent futility of a desperate and emotionally negative, tense situation. Whether the eventual yield is high or low, the last approach has a chance of being helpful and also has the virtue of feeling good to the provider, who has thus made a positive effort which calls upon our most human and humanitarian inclinations. Moreover, the outlook for these patients is not hopeless,[41] and care givers should not feel helpless about their role. The visit to the emergency department may be only a tiny episode in the patient's life, but may have profound consequences if problems are confronted in a professional manner. Every crack in the wall of denial has the potential to bring it down and begin the recovery process, resulting in the achievement of abstinence from alcohol and the eventual recovery from its destructive effects.

EMERGENCY DEPARTMENT CRISIS COUNSELING

Some patients with alcoholism will be asking for help, either as the "chief complaint" or after a screening interview such as the CAGE test. Since patients may have little idea what alcoholism treatment is, they often ask for *help,* unable to be more specific. The usual options are limited to participating in a withdrawal program, beginning a program of outpatient counseling, or going directly to Alcoholics Anonymous (AA). The skillful staff person will assist the patient in a brief exploration of the appropriateness of these options. Most important is the ability to listen carefully to the patient's thoughts and feelings regarding perception of the illness process, ability to ask for people to help, and commitment to doing something at the present time.[40]

During this process, tone and style are probably more important than logic and rationale. The patient's behavior is more important than what he or she thinks at this stage and the counselor should not surrender to the tendency to present the most logical, rational, and incontrovertible argument possible. The interpretation must be individualized so as to assist the patient to effect positive behaviors after leaving the emergency department. Openness, simplicity, and a forthright acknowledgment of the facts will make it safe for the patient.

Thus, the initiation of treatment is a straightforward empathic discussion of the diagnosis, abstinence, and available avenues for treatment. This process is usually painful to the patient (and often to the care giver) but not harmful. Remembering the distinction between pain and harm will help the care giver maintain courage and empathy while assisting patients to accept the obvious facts and take appropriate action. This kind of confrontation can foster a transition into a more explicitly therapeutic relationship.

Most patients are reluctant to consider entering treatment, and especially to join AA.[42] All patients and most care givers have misconceptions about the nature and operation of AA. It is free, available 24 hours, easy to find, and totally and exclusively committed to facilitating recovery of people with alcoholism. Its use should be encouraged far more frequently than is presently the case, and in spite of the patient's objections. This is where gentle, skillful, supportive counseling can be of most use. Frequently, the patient who finally gets to AA says essentially (as Mr B did during his eventual recovery), "I spent so many years avoiding AA, trying every other avenue, and not willing to face the problem head on. If only my doctor had been more forceful in getting me to start going to AA. . . ."

When patients seem disinclined to discuss the available options, the talk should be kept brief (10 minutes or less). Long discussions about the patient's perceptions of why he or she drinks too much, details regarding difficulties with job, family, and so on represent misguided attempts to be helpful, and produce frustration and anger in the care giver. Even while apparently rational, patients may be in a blackout, and recall little or nothing a few hours later. Thus, a personalized, empathic, and supportive discussion of presently available alternatives will suffice, and keeping several AA principles in mind will help the counselor to be concise and straightforward; namely, "keep it simple," "don't drink today," "easy does it."

For patients whose illness is more advanced or for people who repeatedly come to the emergency department, an even more simplified approach may be necessary. In skid row situations like Mr D's, the focus usually is on finding an appropriate (and swift) placement. Local facilities differ, but patients will usually go to a withdrawal unit or a shelter and sobering-up station.[21] Adjusting expectations to match the reality of the chronicity of the illness can be helpful when care givers must repetitively manage the problems of chronic public inebriates. Acknowledging that a night off the streets or a warm meal with supplemental vitamins in the presence of someone who cares may be the best intervention facilitates making speedy arrangements in a positive frame of mind. Care givers make similar short-term plans for patients with end-stage chronic lung disease or debilitating cancers when there is small likelihood of interrupting the course of the disease. In short, care givers must focus on the similarities to other chronic diseases, and "patch" and bandage in whatever human ways are possible under trying circumstances. An extended discussion of specific treatment principles applicable to office practice is available.[40]

"CLEARING" FOR DETOXIFICATION

Frequently, units that offer lower levels of care than the acute hospital request that emergency personnel "clear" patients for discharge to that facility, often a detoxification unit. Patients who have acknowledged the presence of alcoholism may wish to enter a therapeutic setting where withdrawal can proceed safely in skilled hands, and in a fashion integrated with a comprehensive program for alcoholism treatment. Many detoxification units have minimum medical coverage, and require that patients be declared fit for a stay in such an environment. Emergency physicians should have a definite paradigm in mind to facilitate this examination.

When a patient is intoxicated or agitated, it behooves examiners to be brief and direct without being superficial. In addition to open-ended questions (the "what's the main problem now?" sort), certain specific questions can be used to establish a high probability that the patient does not have serious acute problems and can direct the emphasis of the physical examination. An adequate screening relies heavily on history and vital signs rather than a comprehensive physical examination, and a competent job can be expeditiously done with minimum facilities (see Appendix 49-B). The most serious and prevalent problems to be considered include metabolic disorders, neurologic complications such as Wernicke's syndrome and subdural hematoma, serious bleeding, pneumonia, and decompensated liver disease.

The recent drinking history determines the likelihood of a serious withdrawal syndrome and the likelihood of other medical complications.[22,23,25] At highest risk is the person who has been drinking steadily for months, often previously not known to have alcoholism. The patient's prior experience with delirium tremens and seizures and the use of medications, particularly sedatives or tranquilizers, are relevant to withdrawal risk. Has the patient considered or attempted suicide? Does the patient know of serious liver disease, and has a liver biopsy ever been done? Are abdominal symptoms so severe as to suggest pancreatitis; has the patient recently vomited blood? (See Appendix 49-B.)

Serious GI bleeding is uncommon, and when significant is usually the presenting complaint. For these statistical reasons, the lengthy practice of placing a nasogastric tube and obtaining a hematocrit and stool guaiac for patients who say during a screening history that they have recently vomited blood has been revised. The patient is asked about vomiting and retching since the reported episode of hematemesis. If the response is positive, and the vomitus was free of blood on one or more occasions, the likelihood of serious bleeding is minimal. If the patient has not vomited since the hematemesis, postural vital signs are taken and the abdomen is examined. If the abdominal exam does not show hyperactive bowel sounds, and postural vital signs are normal, no further work-up is done. Positive results call for the usual protocol, including passage of a nasogastric tube, hematocrit, observation for a period of time, and so on. Thus, since most people in alcohol withdrawal whose hematemesis is only apparent after direct questioning do not have serious bleeding, protocols that facilitate treatment while minimizing the time and discomfort should be used (see Chapter 28, Gastrointestinal Emergencies).

The intake of other sedative or intoxicating drugs is problematic. Alcohol withdrawal is more serious than withdrawal from other sedatives and tranquilizers, except for barbiturate addiction. Most patients who abuse other sedatives and tranquilizers can be safely managed in an alcohol "drying-out" facility; moreover, transfer to a hospital can be arranged if the later onset (typically 5 to 10 days) of tranquilizer withdrawal syndromes ensues. Abuse of benzodiazepines has increased, and continues to be a troublesome problem (see Chapter 48, Substance Abuse).

The physical examination should be directed toward ascertaining that the patient is likely to be safe over the next several days. The vital signs should never be neglected. Fever means that the patient must be examined in detail including a white blood cell count, chest roentgenogram, and other diagnostic tests as indicated. Tachycardia and hypertension are common but their presence need only be carefully noted; hypotension requires thorough examination. Examination of the sclerae for icterus and the eyes for nystagmus or paresis is mandatory. All patients should be checked for asterixis ("liver flap"), and gait should be checked for symmetry. Although many patients are staggering and detailed testing is not possible, the presence of a consistently asymmetric gait is a warning that more thorough neurologic examination is necessary. Observation of a symmetric gait and unremarkable neurologic examination suggests that hidden trauma in the trunk and legs is unlikely.

Mental status is of course important, but difficult to describe since the range of behavior during intoxication and withdrawal syndromes is quite wide. The most common mistake is failing to take account of a severely depressed level of consciousness that might indicate hepatic decompensation, overdose, or other metabolic derangement. The observer should be well enough trained to ascertain that the patient's mental status is consistent with drunkenness or withdrawal.

The psychiatric states of schizophrenia and manic depressive illness are too frequently diagnosed. Many observers fail to acknowledge that a diagnosis of psychiatric illness can rarely be made until the acute effects of alcohol intoxication and withdrawal diminish. In patients with bona fide psychiatric decompensation, it may be difficult or impossible to distinguish which problem is producing the presenting symptoms, and the decision to place the patient in a psychiatric, medical, or alcoholism unit must be based on evaluation of the individual case and on local policies concerning these matters.

Two metabolic problems especially relevant to the management of patients with alcoholism are hypoglycemia and acidosis. Alcohol-induced hypoglycemia was described 20 years ago; patients with poor food intake and binge drinking sometimes arrived with profound hypoglycemia. Investigations have shown that the inhibition of hepatic gluconeogenetic pathways by alcohol during glycogen-depleted fasting states is partly responsible for the hypoglycemia.[43] If unrecognized, this serious condition may produce irreversible brain damage. This problem should be considered and treated with 50% glucose IV before definitive laboratory data are available in comatose patients and in patients whose degree of somnolence appears inconsistent with other signs of intoxication. Because acute Wernicke's syndrome may worsen with the administration of 50% glucose (glucose metabolism requires thiamine), thiamine must be given before IV glucose. Although few patients have both Wernicke's and hypoglycemia, thiamine can be life-saving, and is harmless in other conditions.

An equally important problem is the presence of metabolic acidosis. The pathophysiology of this syndrome is not entirely clear, but the clinical picture is one of more or less severe acidosis with variable amounts of ketosis and higher or lower lactate levels.[44] The determination of arterial pH and electrolytes is essential for patients whose clinical condition is severe or where clinical findings are not completely consistent with intoxication or withdrawal. It must be emphasized that clinical indications of acidosis do not always include Kussmaul respirations and hypotension; most cases are discovered because the patient's general condition requires the determination of electrolytes or blood gases (see Chapter 21, Acid-Base Disturbances).

Alcohol affects the metabolism of many drugs.[45] Some are eliminated more rapidly (barbiturates, meprobamate); others show delayed metabolism (warfarin). In other circumstances alcohol interferes with the action of a substance (folic acid), or may potentiate the toxic effects of a drug (acetaminophen). The list is extensive, and the clinician must remember to check this list whenever the clinical situation warrants.

Paraprofessional personnel, nurses, or physicians' assistants can easily perform the screening examination. If the volume of patients with alcohol-related problems is sufficient, it may be cost effective for paraprofessionals to make initial decisions for patients with alcohol-related complaints. Often such personnel become better trained in alcoholism counseling and know community facilities more intimately. They can thus provide more appropriate management than the busy emergency physician.

REFERENCES

1. Kamerow D, Pincus H, MacDonald D. Alcohol abuse, other drug abuse, and mental disorders in medical practice. *JAMA*. 1986;255:2054–2057.
2. Skinner H, Holt S, Schuller R, et al. Identification of alcohol abuse using laboratory tests and a history of trauma. *Ann Intern Med*. 1984;101:847–851.
3. Holts AM, et al. Alcohol and the emergency service patient. *Br Med J*. 1980;281:638–664.
4. *Sixth Report to US Congress on Alcohol and Health*. Washington, DC: US Dept of Health and Human Services; 1987.
5. Jellinek EM. *The Disease Concept of Alcoholism*. New Haven, CT: Hillhouse; 1960.
6. Keller M. The disease concept of alcoholism, revisited. *J Stud Alcohol*. 1976;37:1694–1717.
7. Vaillant G. We should retain the disease concept of alcoholism. *Harv Med Sch Ment Health Lett*. 1990;6:4–6.
8. Ludwig A. *Understanding the Alcoholic's Mind: The Nature of Craving and How To Control It*. New York: Oxford; 1988.
9. Fingarette H. We should reject the disease concept of alcoholism. *Harv Med Sch Mental Health Lett*. 1990;6:4–6.
10. Vaillant G. *Natural History of Alcoholism*. Cambridge, MA: Harvard University Press; 1983.
11. Bean M. Clinical implications of models of recovery from alcoholism. *Adv Alcohol Subst Abuse*. 1983;3:91–104.
12. Schenker S, Speeg K. Risk of alcohol intake in men and women. *N Engl J Med*. 1990;322:127–129.
13. Bacon S. The process of addiction to alcohol. *Q J Stud Alcohol*. 1973;34:1–27.
14. Stabenau J. Additive independent factors that predict risk for alcoholism. *J Stud Alcohol*. 1990;51:164–174.
15. Armor DJ, Polich JM, Stambul HB. *Alcoholism and Treatment*. New York: Wiley; 1978.
16. Vaillant G, Milofsky E. The etiology of alcoholism—a prospective viewpoint. *Am Psychol*. 1982;37:494–503.
17. Vaillant G, Brighton J, McArthur C. Physicians' use of mood altering drugs: a 20-year follow-up report. *N Engl J Med*. 1970;282:365–370.
18. Thacker SB, Veech RL, Vernon A, et al. Genetic and biochemical factors relevant to alcoholism. *Alcohol Clin Exp Res*. 1984;8:375–383.
19. Lieber C. Biochemical and molecular basis of alcohol-induced injury to liver and other tissues. *N Engl J Med*. 1988;319:1639–1650.
20. Woods H, Alberti K. Dangers of intravenous fructose. *Lancet*. 1972;2:1354–1357.
21. Cox A. Management of intoxicated and disruptive patients. In: *Emergency Department Training Manual*. Toronto: Addiction Research Foundation; 1979.
22. Isbell N, Fraser HF, Wikler A, et al. An experimental study of the etiology of "rum fits" and delirium tremens. *Q J Stud Alcohol*. 1955;16:1–33.
23. Sellers E, Kalant H. Alcohol withdrawal and delirium tremens. In: Pattison E, Kaufman E, eds. *Encyclopedic Handbook of Alcoholism*. New York: Gardner; 1982:147–166.
24. Tabakoff B, Hoffman P, Valverius P, et al. Characteristics of receptors and enzymes in brains of human alcoholics. *Alcohol*. 1985;2:419–423.
25. Gross M, Lewis E, Best S, et al. Quantitative changes associated with signs and symptoms of acute alcohol withdrawal: incidence, severity, and circadian effects in experimental studies of alcoholics. In: Gross M, ed. *Alcohol Intoxication and Withdrawal*. New York: Plenum; 1975:615–631.
26. Victor M, Adams R, Collins G. *The Wernicke-Korsakoff Syndrome: A Clinical and Pathological Study of 245 Patients, 82 with Post-Mortem Examinations*, 2nd ed., revised. Philadelphia: Davis; 1989.
27. Plum F, Posner J. *Diagnosis of Stupor and Coma*. 2nd ed. Philadelphia: Davis; 1980.
28. Turner R, Lichstein P, Peden J, et al. Alcohol withdrawal syndromes. A review of pathophysiology, clinical presentation, and treatment. *J Gen Intern Med*. 1989;4:432–444.
29. Sellers E. Alcohol, barbiturate and benzodiazepine withdrawal syndromes: clinical management. *Can Med Assoc J*. 1988;139:113–120.
30. Wilson A, Vulcano B. Double blind trial of alprazolam and chlordiazepoxide in management of acute ethanol withdrawal syndrome. *Alcohol Clin Exp Res*. 1985;9:23–27.
31. Rosenbloom A. Optimizing drug treatment of alcohol withdrawal. *Am J Med*. 1986;81:901–904.
32. Wilson A, Vulcano B. Double-blind placebo-controlled trial of magnesium sulfate in the ethanol withdrawal syndrome. *Alcohol Clin Exp Res*. 1984;8:542–545.

33. Stuppaeck C, Pycha R, Miller C, et al. Carbamazepine versus oxazepam in the treatment of alcohol withdrawal: a double-blind study. *Alcohol Alcoholism*. 1992;27:153–158.

34. Hayashida M, Alterman A, McLellan T, et al. Comparative effectiveness and costs of inpatient and outpatient detoxification of patients with mild-to-moderate alcohol withdrawal syndrome. *N Engl J Med*. 1989; 320:358–365.

35. Victor M, Adams R. The effect of alcohol on the nervous system. *Res Publ Assoc Nerv Ment Dis*. 1953;32:526–673.

36. Thompson W, Johnson A, Maddrey W. Diazepam and paraldehyde for treatment of severe delirium tremens: a controlled trial. *Ann Intern Med*. 1975;82:175–180.

37. Ng S, Hauser W, Brust J, et al. Alcohol consumption and withdrawal in new-onset seizures. *N Engl J Med*. 1988;319:666–673.

38. Alldredge B, Lowenstein D, Simon R. Placebo-controlled trial of intravenous diphenylhydantoin for short-term treatment of alcohol withdrawal seizures. *Am J Med*. 1989;87:645–648.

39. Ewing J, Mayfield D. CAGE. *Am J Psychiatr*. 1974;131:1121–1122.

40. Clark W. The generalist and alcoholism: dilemmas and progress. In: Noble J, ed. *Textbook of General Medicine and Primary Care*. Boston: Little, Brown; 1987.

41. Vaillant G, Clark W, Cyrus C, et al. Prospective study of alcoholism treatment: an eight-year follow-up. *Am J Med*. 1983;75:455–463.

42. Zinberg N, Fraser K. The role of the social setting in the prevention and treatment of alcoholism. In: Mendelson J, Mello N, eds. *Diagnosis and Treatment of Alcoholism*. New York: McGraw-Hill; 1979: 374–382.

43. Wilson N, Brown P, Juul S, et al. Glucose turnover and metabolic and hormonal changes in ethanol induced hypoglycemia. *Br Med J*. 1981; 282:849–853.

44. Wrenn K, Slovis C, Minion G, et al. The syndrome of alcoholic ketoacidosis. *Am J Med*. 1991;91:119–128.

45. Sexias F. Alcohol and its drug interactions. *Ann Intern Med*. 1975;83: 86–92.

APPENDIX 49-A: QUESTIONS TO ASSESS PREOCCUPATION WITH ALCOHOL AND ADVERSE CONSEQUENCES

HALT

Do you usually drink to get **H**igh?
Do you sometimes drink **A**lone?
Have you found yourself **L**ooking forward to drinking?
Have you noticed an increased **T**olerance for alcohol?

BUMP

Do you have **B**lackouts?
Have you found yourself using alcohol in an **U**nplanned way?
Do you drink for **M**edicinal reasons?
Do you work at **P**rotecting your supply of alcohol?

Notes:

High: for example, drinking doubles, rapidly, before the occasion
Looking forward: when your mind should be otherwise occupied
Blackouts (or, have blackouts increased in frequency?): loss of memory for events which occurred while drinking
Unplanned: drink more than intended, or drink when had planned not to
Medicinal: as a panacea for any feeling state; anxious, stressed, depressed, etc.
Protecting: getting alcohol "just in case" company comes, for the weekend, etc., in an obsessional way

FATAL DTs

Family history of alcohol problems
Alcoholics Anonymous **A**ttendance
Thoughts of having alcoholism
Attempts or thoughts of suicide
Legal problems
Depressed, down, or discouraged
Tranquilizer or disulfiram use

APPENDIX 49-B: EMERGENCY DEPARTMENT OR WALK-IN SERVICE SCREENING EXAMINATION

Patient name _____

A. History
  1. Uninterrupted drinking for how long?
  2. Last drink when?
  3. Last time sober (no alcohol) 1 month or more?
  4. Previous detoxifications (yes, no)? Most recently (where, when)?

A. History (continued)   No   Yes*
  DTs in past?
  Fits? seizures?
  Liver trouble?
  Hematemesis today?
  Taking pills/meds?
  Chronic illnesses?
  Other important symptoms/problems?

B. Physical Examination   No   Yes*
  Head trauma?
  Jaundice?
  Pupils not reactive?
  Asterixis?
  Consciousness unusual?†
  Orientation not O.K.?
  Hallucination?
  Agitation severe?
  Gait not symmetric?
  Other important findings?

C. Vital Signs
  Pulse   ‡if > 120
  Respirations   ‡if > 24
  BP   ‡if > 160/110
                   or < 100/70
  Temperature   ‡if > 99.9

D. Laboratory Exam
  1. None done
  2. CBC _____ Chemistry _____‡
     X-ray _____ ECG _____

E. Conclusion/Summary
My screening examination at this time reveals the following:
  _____ 1. Everything consistent with drunkenness/withdrawal in an otherwise healthy individual.
  _____ 2. Evidence of other acute problems manageable at a free-standing unit.
  _____ 3. Evidence of chronic problems which seem stable at this time.*

Date _____ Time _____ Signed _____
                              Checked _____M.D.

*If you check "yes," use the back of this form for documenting details.
†Not consistent with drunkenness/withdrawal.
‡Give details on back of this form.
  Source: The Cambridge and Somerville Program for Alcoholism Rehabilitation, Inc.

50. Depression and Suicidal Feelings and Behaviors

THOMAS F. McGEE, PhD

Depressive feelings are relatively common and are experienced by all segments of the population. Seemingly less common, suicidal feelings are probably far more prevalent than is generally recognized. Both depressive and suicidal feelings can have serious and even tragic consequences if not accurately diagnosed and treated. Moreover, there are no clear-cut patterns to suggest when, how, and where a depressed or suicidal individual or his or her family or friends may seek assistance. As noted by Hankoff et al[1] and Leff-Simon et al,[2] given the emergency department's ready availability, multifaceted treatment characteristics, and hospital relatedness it is likely that an increasing number of individuals experiencing depressive or suicidal feelings, or both, present there for initial treatment. Intervening with such individuals in an emergency department can be challenging, frustrating, and time consuming, and often such patients may stimulate impatience, anger, and hostility in emergency department personnel. Yet there can be little doubt as to the central importance and preventive role an emergency department can play in intervention and treatment of such individuals.

EVALUATION OF DEPRESSION

Depression is a very common affective state, and most people experience at least moderate depressive feelings at some point in their lives. Cancro[3] makes the following observations:

Conservative estimates place the number of people who in any given year experience a depressive episode, which is potentially diagnosable, at between ten and twenty million. In the United States, one in twenty persons is actually diagnosed as having a significant depression at least once in their lifetime.

Depression usually involves a sense of emotional pain and suffering by the patient and his or her family. Depression appears closely related to unexpressed or unresolved anger, and there is probably considerable truth in the observation that depression represents anger turned inward. Depression may become manifest in a variety of ways, and not all individuals are able to directly identify and acknowledge feelings of depression. Feelings of depression may be experienced somatically or in relation to bodily functions. Depressive feelings may also gain primary expression in a variety of indirect ways, such as through family or marital conflicts or excessive alcohol intake.

Depressive feelings or states may range from normal "being down in the dumps" to psychotic levels which are often accompanied by intellectual and emotional retardation and disorganization and delusional thinking. Individuals experiencing normal feelings of depression, which are readily explainable and relatively short in duration, appear in the emergency department infrequently, while individuals experiencing more serious feelings of depression probably appear with greater frequency.

Intervention in the emergency department usually involves a careful assessment of the nature and seriousness of the individual's depression. Treatment alternatives include brief counseling and discharge from the emergency department, a referral for outpatient psychotherapy, the prescription of antidepressant medication coupled with a referral for outpatient psychotherapy, and immediate hospitalization on a psychiatric inpatient service. In the assessment of depression one must evaluate not only the level and intensity of the depressive feelings, but also the individual's potential to cope with these feelings. One must also evaluate the presence and strength of the patient's familial and social network, as these are vital in coping with depression.

Causes of Depressive Phenomena

As suggested above, if depressive phenomena are placed on a continuum, they might range from normal, reasonably resolvable states, such as "being down in the dumps," to psychotic levels of depression, which may involve significant distortion of reality, delusional thinking, and the potential to be life-threatening. Moreover, it is normal to experience feelings of depression in relation to certain events (eg, the death of a loved one, the diagnosis of a serious illness). Causes of depression do not lend themselves to such a clear continuum. It is commonly assumed that both genetic and emotional factors play a role in contributing to depression. From an emotional perspective, it is generally assumed that loss, either real or imagined, and stress, either negative or positive, are implicated in the onset of depression.

To illustrate the range of depressive phenomena, some frequently encountered precipitants of depression are cited: loss of or separation from a loved one, loss of livelihood, financial loss or reversal, work-related demotion or promotion, serious illness or decline in physical status. Another level of precipitants might include postpartum depression, drug- or alcohol-related depression, or illness-induced depression, such as hepatitis.

Levels of Depressive Phenomena

The *Diagnostic and Statistical Manual of Mental Disorders* (DSM III)[4] distinguishes among several levels and types of depressive phenomena. The following portion of this discussion, which is presented in summary form, is drawn primarily from DSM III. In DSM III, a number of levels of depression are subsumed under affective disorders. This category is divided into major affective disorders, other specific affective disorders, and atypical affective disorders.

Major Affective Disorders

Bipolar disorder. Major affective disorders include bipolar disorder and major depression, which are distinguished by whether or not there has ever been a manic episode.

Major depressive episode. The essential feature is either a dysphoric mood, usually depression, or loss of interest or pleasure in all or almost all usual activities and pastimes. This disturbance is prominent, relatively persistent, and associated with other symptoms of the depressive syndrome. These symptoms include appetite disturbance, change in weight, sleep disturbance, psychomotor agitation or retardation, decreased energy, feelings of worthlessness or guilt, difficulty concentrating or thinking, and thoughts of death or suicide or suicidal attempts.

Other Specific Affective Disorders

Cyclothymic disorder. The essential feature is a chronic mood disturbance of at least two years' duration, involving numerous periods of depression and hypomania, but not of sufficient severity and duration to meet the criteria for a major depressive or a manic episode.

Dysthymic disorder (depressive neurosis). The essential feature is a chronic disturbance of mood involving either depressed mood or loss of interest or pleasure in usual activities and pastimes, and associated symptoms, but not of sufficient severity and duration to meet the criteria for a major depressive episode. For adults, 2 years' duration is required; for children and adolescents, 1 year is sufficient.

Atypical Affective Disorders

Atypical bipolar disorder. This is a residual category for individuals with manic features that cannot be classified as bipolar disorder or as cyclothymic disorder. For example, an individual who previously had a major depressive episode and now has an episode of illness with some manic features (hypomanic episode), but not of sufficient severity and duration to meet the criteria for a manic episode. Such cases have been referred to as "bipolar II."

Atypical depression. This is a residual category for individuals with depressive symptoms who cannot be diagnosed as having a major or other specified affective disorder or adjustment disorder. Examples include the following:

- A distinct and sustained episode of the full depressive syndrome in an individual with schizophrenia, residual type, that develops without an activation of the psychotic symptoms.
- A disorder that fulfills the criteria for dysthymic disorder. However, there have been intermittent periods of normal mood lasting more than a few months.
- A brief episode of depression that does not meet the criteria for a major affective disorder and that is apparently not reactive to psychosocial stress, so that it cannot be classified as an adjustment disorder.

In addition to the above subcategories of affective disorders, DSM III describes two additional types of depressive phenomena that may come to the attention of the emergency department. One of these is called adjustment disorder with depressed mood and is subsumed under adjustment disorders; the other is called uncomplicated bereavement.

Adjustment disorder with depressed mood. This category should be used when the predominant manifestation involves such symptoms as depressed mood, tearfulness, and hopelessness. The major differential diagnosis is with major depression and uncomplicated bereavement.

Uncomplicated bereavement. This type of depressive phenomena is subsumed under codes not attributable to a mental disorder that are a focus of attention or treatment. This type of depression is probably encountered on occasion in the emergency department. This category can be used when a focus of attention or treatment is a normal reaction to the death of a loved one (bereavement).

A full depressive syndrome frequently is a normal reaction to such a loss, with feelings of depression and such associated symptoms as poor appetite, weight loss, and insomnia. However, morbid preoccupation with worthlessness, prolonged and marked functional impairment, and marked psychomotor retardation are uncommon and suggest that the bereavement is complicated by the development of a major depression.

In uncomplicated bereavement, guilt, if present, is chiefly about things done or not done at the time of the death by the survivor; thoughts of death are usually limited to the individual's thinking that he or she would be better off dead or that he or she should have died with the person who died. The individual with uncomplicated bereavement generally regards the feeling of depressed mood as "normal," although he or she may seek professional help for relief of such associated symptoms as insomnia or anorexia.

The reaction to the loss may not be immediate, but rarely occurs after the first 2 or 3 months. The duration of "normal" bereavement varies considerably among different subcultural groups.

DIFFERENTIAL DIAGNOSIS OF DEPRESSIVE PHENOMENA

As suggested above, there is considerable overlap among various types and levels of depression. Accordingly, when an individual who is depressed appears in the emergency department, an immediate task of the emergency physician is to accurately diagnose the acuteness, level, and seriousness of the depression. This implies that a tentative diagnosis must be made among the different levels of depression described above. In establishing this diagnosis, the emergency physician should review the nature and extent of the depressive symptoms, particularly the vegetative symptoms, such as recent changes in weight, persistent sleep disturbance, reduced appetite, loss of interest including reduced sexual interest, unexplainable feelings of fatigue, and the extent to which feelings of futility and hopelessness, reduced feelings of self-worth, etc., are present. In addition, the emergency physician should carefully review the presence or absence of previous depressive episodes, the length of time the depressive symptoms have been present, the extent to which these symptoms appear to be disabling to the patient, and the patient's resources to cope with the depressive feelings.

A differential diagnosis among the various levels of depression must also include a careful assessment of the patient's suicidal potential. Georgotas[5] indicates that the suicidal risk for depressed individuals is approximately 30 times greater than that of the general population. Lehman[6] also makes the following observation:

> Suicidal thoughts are present in most, if not all, moderately to severely depressed patients, probably in at least 70 percent of them. The danger of suicide must always be considered to be present in virtually every depressed patient—if not today, then perhaps tomorrow or next week. Suicide risk is greatest among those patients who express more or less complete hopelessness.

If a serious or potentially life-threatening depressive disorder appears to be present, the treatment should be oriented toward immediate psychiatric inpatient care. If the depressive disorder appears less serious, and the patient presents minimal suicidal potential, initial treatment should start in the emergency department. If the second alternative is chosen, strong and active efforts should be made to have the patient engage in outpatient psychotherapy as soon as possible following discharge from the emergency department. A more detailed description of these treatment alternatives follows.

INTERVENTION AND FOLLOW-UP TREATMENT OF DEPRESSIVE PHENOMENA

Following a detailed assessment and differential diagnosis of the patient's level of depression, there are several different types of intervention that can be made in the emergency department. In choosing the type of intervention, it is important that strong efforts be made to link it to follow-up treatment.

Referral for Inpatient Psychiatric Hospitalization

If the patient is viewed as seriously depressed, manifests significant suicidal potential, and appears unable to function adequately within a familial, social, and vocational milieu, psychiatric hospitalization is indicated. This is particularly true if the patient presents a prior history of serious depressive episodes or prior self-destructive attempts. In cases of severe depression, psychiatric hospitalization is legally mandated in many states, particularly if the patient poses a clear and imminent suicidal danger. The following section of this chapter, Evaluation of Suicidal Feelings and Behaviors, examines this issue in greater detail.

Institution of Antidepressant Medication and Referral for Outpatient Psychotherapy

If the patient demonstrates a significant level of depression, but presents minimal suicidal potential, it is often appropriate to prescribe a limited amount of antidepressant medication. When this approach is chosen, it is very important that the amount of medication be limited, and that the patient be referred for outpatient psychotherapy. If antidepressant medication is prescribed by the emergency physician, the amount should be limited not only to exercise appropriate caution against future suicidal attempts, but also to enhance the possibility that the patient will follow through expeditiously with outpatient treatment.

Referral for Outpatient Psychotherapy

If the patient is diagnosed as depressed, but requires neither psychiatric hospitalization nor immediate antidepressant medication, it is very appropriate to make a referral for outpatient psychotherapy. If the patient has experienced sufficient emotional pain in connection with feelings of depression to seek assistance in an emergency department, it is likely that he or she requires some type of immediate, consistent psychotherapeutic intervention, at least on a short-term basis. There is little contention as to the efficacy of antidepressant medication in the treatment of depression; however, depressive feelings or states such as those described above are generally resolved more adequately if outpatient psychotherapy plays a central role in the post–emergency department treatment plan. This viewpoint is stated very clearly by Cancro[3]:

> The unfortunate schism between psychosocial and biological treatments has tended to result in many patients being treated in a less-than-optimal fashion. There is, in fact, no conflict between these approaches. Virtually all affective disordered patients require both psychosocial and somatic intervention. The patient who responds to a tricyclic anti-depressant but does not make appropriate corrections in his or her life-style is at an increased risk for relapse. A strong and supportive social network can have an important prophylactic effect without the dangers of long-term maintenance therapy with an anti-depressant.

When a patient experiencing depression is referred for outpatient psychotherapy, the referral should be made to a facility or to a professional where the patient can be seen as soon as possible. Such effective linkage and rapid follow-up tend to capitalize on the intervention made in the emergency department and often heighten the patient's sense of openness and responsiveness toward psychotherapeutic intervention.

In all three levels of intervention into depressive phenomena in the emergency department described above, the active involvement of family members or other members of the patient's interpersonal support system will often enhance the intervention. Gerson and Bassuk[7] suggest that the availability or lack of such a support system has a most important effect on disposition within the emergency department. There can be little doubt that the presence of such a support system will enhance the patient's follow-through for outpatient psychotherapeutic treatment.

EVALUATION OF SUICIDAL FEELINGS AND BEHAVIORS

Currently, suicide is considered to be among the ten leading causes of death. According to Lehman,[6]

> Approximately 30,000 persons commit suicide every year in the United States alone. It has been estimated that only about five percent of all completed suicides are for rational, nondepressive reasons and that at least 40 to 50 percent of all suicides are committed by patients suffering from major depressions.

This is undoubtedly a conservative figure, as a significant number of suicides are listed as accidents, or are otherwise not reported as suicides. The risk for suicide tends to increase with age, although the suicide rate is growing with particular rapidity in younger persons 15 to 24 years of age. Suicide risk also appears to be correlated with marital status, and individuals who are single, separated, divorced, or widowed represent a somewhat higher suicidal risk than married persons, particularly those who are parents. It is also noteworthy that men appear to commit suicide three times as often as women, although women appear to attempt suicide twice as often as men.

As may be inferred from the above remarks, suicide and suicidal behaviors constitute a serious public health problem. As Farberow and Shneidman[8] observed, suicidal actions constitute a "cry for help" as they often represent a culmination of the suffering and anguish and the pleas for response that are expressed by suicidally prone individuals. The emergency department has become a primary site where individuals who have thus "cried for help" appear for initial intervention. Individuals who have made active suicidal attempts are those who are probably most often thought of in relation to an emergency department. Frequently, such individuals are brought to the emergency department by the police or paramedics; on occasion they may be brought by friends or relatives. However, such individuals are not the only type of suicidal individuals who present in emergency departments. The range of suicidal individuals who present at an emergency department may include the following, among others: individuals who appear seriously depressed and somatically preoccupied, but who deny overt suicidal thoughts or feelings; individuals who are experiencing suicidal feelings which they can acknowledge; individuals who present subsequent to a clear and direct suicidal attempt; and individuals who have made disguised suicidal attempts. All of these types of suicidal individuals must be carefully assessed for continued suicidal potential. Obviously, if the patient has made a suicidal attempt and his or her physical condition merits immediate medical attention, this must take precedence in treatment. *However, no patient in any of the above categories should be discharged from the emergency department or the hospital without careful assessment for continued suicidal potential.* As noted earlier, in many states the emergency physician has a legal obligation to have the suicidal individual placed on a psychiatric inpatient unit if he or she presents a clear, continuing, and imminent suicidal danger.

Suicidal individuals who present at emergency departments may be regarded with special feelings, at least initially. The suicidally prone individual may elicit initial reactions of avoidance, if not anger, on the part of emergency department personnel. With respect to anger, Anderson[9] suggests that emergency department personnel are oriented toward saving lives; they may react adversely when confronted with a patient who has attempted to take, or is thinking of taking, his or her life. With respect to avoidance, we have all experienced feelings of depression, and have probably all experienced some suicidal thoughts. Moreover, we are all subject to having had acquaintances, friends, or family members who have attempted or committed suicide. As a consequence, the suicidal patient may arouse negative feelings or reactions in emergency department personnel. This may result in a tendency to avoid dealing actively and directly with such patients. An associated tendency may be to avoid direct inquiry and immediate assessment with the suicidal patient; yet, this approach is essential in accurately assessing and treating suicidal patients. However, the evaluation of the suicidal patient is rarely easy, given factors such as the nature and the extent of the patient's physical injuries, if any, level of emotional agitation, occasional overt denial of suicidal ideation, and lack of responsiveness or cooperation.

The emergency physician should treat the potentially suicidal patient with great seriousness. In addition to attention, suicidal actions often represent a covert plea for control. Accordingly, if suicidal feelings or actions are not assessed accurately and treated effectively, the individual is quite likely to attempt suicide again, sometimes in the immediate future. Indeed, there have been occasions where individuals have committed suicide immediately following discharge from an emergency department. While previous suicidal attempts are not an absolute predictor of future attempts, a higher percentage of completed suicides occur in individuals who have made previous attempts.[10] These factors underscore the need for the emergency physician to take any indication of suicidal thinking or behavior seriously, and to assess such thinking or behavior carefully. This can be done directly by emergency department personnel, or with psychiatric or psychological consultation, if available in the emergency department. In this effort it is generally wise to err on the side of caution, despite occasional manipulative patients who know how to exploit the medical and legal obligations of the emergency physician with the hope of inappropriately gaining hospital admission or medication.

As suggested in the preceding discussion of depression, some of the primary elements of suicidal evaluation include an assessment of the patient's vegetative signs, the presence of a recent loss or losses, and presence of recent stresses, including perceived medical stresses, previous attempts at suicide, family history with respect to suicide, and the existence of a suicide plan to carry out the suicidal threats. With respect to suicidal evaluation, Georgotas[5] stresses the following clinical features usually associated with increased suicidal risks:

1. personal history of suicidal attempts
2. intense suicidal drive
3. history of acting out as the main expression of anxiety
4. lack of family or social support
5. significant losses
6. hostility
7. intense guilt
8. anhedonia
9. bipolar patients switching rapidly from manic to depressed phase
10. well-established refractoriness to previous treatments

TYPES OF SUICIDAL IDEATION OR BEHAVIOR

The following sections provide a brief discussion of four broad categories of suicidally prone individuals who appear in emergency departments. The first two categories consist of patients who have suicidal feelings and ideation, but who are seeking help in the emergency department prior to making a suicidal attempt. They include patients who present with behavior and symptoms that are not explicitly suicidal, and those who can acknowledge experiencing suicidal feelings. The other two categories consist of patients who present in the emergency department subsequent to a suicidal attempt; they are as follows: patients who present following a clear and direct suicidal attempt, and patients who present having made disguised suicidal attempts.

Patients Whose Behavior and Symptoms Are Not Explicitly Suicidal

As indicated in the discussion of depression, some individuals may present in the emergency department with vegetative signs of depression, but overtly deny suicidal feelings or intent. In part this may relate to efforts to suppress or deny depressive and suicidal feelings. Such patients may reflect vague but persistent somatic complaints accompanied by moderate to strong somatic preoccupations, including possible fears of a fatal illness. Such patients may have a history of recent, recurrent visits to physicians or emergency departments, which they perceive as having been of little help. With these patients it is as though they are communicating suicidal feelings somatically. A careful examination of the patient's emotional status will often reveal the presence of serious feelings of depression. Such an examination also may lead to diagnostically corroborative information such as seriously reduced feelings of self-worth, a pervasive sense of guilt, strong feelings of futility and hopelessness, and an impending sense of doom.

Sometimes referred to as a "smiling depression," the suicidal potential of this type of patient is relatively difficult to assess. As a result of suppression and denial, such a patient may be unable to acknowledge depressive and suicidal feelings to himself or herself, let alone to the emergency physician. Such a patient may be struggling with unconscious or submeditated suicidal feelings which, if undiagnosed and untreated, often result in seemingly impulsive suicidal attempts or "accidents" that are actually suicidal attempts.

When such a patient is encountered in the emergency department, the choice of treatment is usually between immediate psychiatric hospitalization or referral for rapid involvement in outpatient psychotherapy. This choice depends not only on the severity of the suicidal potential, but also the degree to which the individual can begin to more openly acknowledge and discuss depressive and suicidal feelings. If such acknowledgment and increased openness emerge in response to intervention in the emergency department, if the patient is able to provide reasonable assurance that he or she will not attempt suicide imminently, and if the patient has a reasonably good familial or interpersonal support system, and shows good motivation for outpatient psychotherapy, then referral for rapid involvement in outpatient psychotherapy is probably indicated. Conversely, if acknowledgment and increased openness with respect to suicidal feelings do not occur, and if the patient appears to continue to have a significant degree of suicide potential, psychiatric inpatient care is indicated.

Patients Who Are Experiencing Feelings That They Can Acknowledge

Patients who can acknowledge suicidal feelings tend to be more easy to assess than those in the previous category. Although ability to acknowledge and identify suicidal feelings facilitates assessment, it does not necessarily diminish suicidal potential. It is well established that many individuals who talk about suicide attempt suicide. However, due to the patient's ability to acknowledge suicidal feelings and ideation, assessment in the emergency department can often proceed more smoothly and directly. An important aspect of assessment with this type of patient relates to the presence or absence of a suicide plan. As suggested by Hatton and Valente,[11] "This plan can be vague or clear, general or specific, and reflect on a practical level the intensity of the client's distress." If a suicide plan exists, four major elements must be examined in evaluating its seriousness: method, availability, specificity, and lethality.

If the patient's suicidal potential diminishes significantly with intervention in the emergency department, and if he or she has reasonably good familial or interpersonal support, and no suicide plan or a poorly developed one, referral for rapid involvement in outpatient psychotherapy is probably indicated. If such initial resolution does not occur in response to intervention in the emergency department and if a reasonably well developed suicide plan appears present, psychiatric inpatient care is indicated.

Patients Who Present After a Clear and Direct Suicidal Attempt

Patients who have attempted suicide and appear in the emergency department may represent a wide variety of suicidal behaviors (eg, alcohol, drug or poison ingestion or injection, carbon monoxide or gas poisoning, drowning attempts, electrocution attempts, hanging attempts, jumping or falling, slashing, stabbing and cutting, shooting, or vehicular accidents). Such behaviors vary with respect to seriousness and lethality, and when confronted with a patient who has made such an attempt, a primary task of the emergency physician is to make a determination about these factors.

Obviously, intervention in such cases depends on both the medical status and continuing suicidal potential of the patient. By the time some suicidal patients enter the emergency department, their life is seriously threatened, and it is not unusual for patients who have attempted suicide to be pronounced dead on arrival at the emergency department. If the patient's life appears that it can be sustained, transfer to a medical intensive care unit is frequently indicated, following resuscitation in the emergency department. In addition to continued treatment and monitoring of the patient's medical condition, placement in a medical intensive care unit often exercises an important psychological effect on the patient in that it may help him or her comprehend more fully the seriousness of the suicide attempt.

When the patient's condition does not represent a medical emergency (eg, superficial scratches on the wrist or the ingestion of a few aspirin), and if the emergency physician determines that the patient no longer constitutes a clear and imminent suicidal risk, the patient may be discharged from the emergency department. Discharge of such a patient should take place only after careful psychiatric or psychological consultation with respect to continued suicidal potential. In such situations the institution of immediate outpatient psychotherapy may be strongly encouraged as follow-up to emergency treatment as noted in the preceding section.

Disguised Suicidal Attempts

Disguised suicidal attempts are probably far more prevalent than recognized. Such suicidal attempts appear to be closely related to a variety of "accidents." Indeed, if the term "accidental" were to precede most of the methods of suicide mentioned above, one would have a comparatively complete list of actions that may involve disguised suicidal attempts. Disguised suicidal attempts are not always easy to recognize; however, if the emergency physician senses a degree of suspicion or unusualness about an "accident" or its victim(s), further investigation as to the emotional status of the victim(s) and the circumstances of the accident is usually indicated. If the patient's medical condition is stable, and if questions about a possible suicidal attempt are difficult to resolve, immediate consultation with a psychiatrist or psychologist can often assist in this resolution.

Case Presentation

The following case of a disguised suicidal attempt is presented to illustrate some of the complexities associated with the assessment and intervention of suicidal behavior in the emergency department.

> A man in his middle 40s was brought to the emergency department following an automobile accident that involved only his vehicle. He sustained only minor physical injuries, but upon examination, it was observed that his speech was rambling and that he appeared emotionally agitated. On continued assessment, the patient revealed strong feelings of guilt and markedly diminished feelings of self-worth. Eventually, he remarked that he wished he had been killed in the accident, and it became apparent that the patient was seriously suicidal. During consultation with the patient in the emergency department a psychologist was informed that the patient's wife had recently learned that he had been abusing his stepson. After this abuse had been reported to the authorities, the patient had attempted suicide by driving his car off the road. The suicidal attempt appeared to have been impulsive, as the patient had no well-organized suicide plan, had not prepared a suicide note, and had no previous history of suicidal attempts.

Following intervention in the emergency department, the patient was transferred for brief inpatient psychiatric care, and a combination of individual and family psychotherapy was instituted as part of his hospital treatment. Following hospital discharge, the patient and his family continued in this outpatient psychotherapeutic program for a relatively long period of time with generally positive results, and no further child abuse occurred. No further suicidal ideation had been observed and no further suicidal actions had occurred when this patient and his family terminated psychotherapy after approximately 2 years.

CONCLUSION

As suggested in the preceding discussion, it is relatively common for individuals to appear in the emergency department seeking relief from and assistance with a wide range of depressive and suicidal feelings and behaviors. Given that depressive and suicidal feelings often occur or are exacerbated in combination with life crises, and as the emergency department is increasingly regarded as a primary, readily available source of help for individuals undergoing such crises, the following comments seem pertinent.

One of the more significant observations associated with crisis theory suggests that at times of life crisis, many individuals experience a heightened willingness to examine emotional conflicts that relate to the crisis. The emergency department and its personnel, as suggested by Bartolucci and Drayer,[12] along with mental health professionals, will continue to play a most important role in assisting in the resolution of life crises which contribute to or exacerbate depressive and suicidal feelings and behaviors. An interpersonally responsive and psychologically oriented emergency department can and should play a vital role in positively affecting the lives of individuals who seek help as a consequence of depression and suicidal feelings and actions.

REFERENCES

1. Hankoff LD, Mischoff MT, Tomlinson KE, Joyce SA. A program of crisis intervention in the emergency medical setting. *Am J Psychiatr*. 1974;131:47–50.
2. Leff-Simon SI, Slaikeu KA, Hansen K. Crisis intervention in hospital emergency rooms. In: Slaikeu KA, ed. *Crisis Intervention: A Handbook for Practice and Research*. Boston: Allyn & Bacon; 1984:229–239.
3. Cancro R. Overview of affective disorders. In: Kaplan HI, Sadock BJ, eds. *Comprehensive Textbook of Psychiatry*. 4th ed. Baltimore: Williams & Wilkins; 1985:760–764.
4. American Psychiatric Association. *Diagnostic and Statistical Manual of Mental Disorders*. 3rd ed. Washington, DC: American Psychiatric Association; 1980.
5. Georgotas A. Affective disorders: pharmacotherapy. In: Kaplan HI, Sadock BJ, eds. *Comprehensive Textbook of Psychiatry*. 4th ed. Baltimore: Williams & Wilkins; 1985:821–833.

6. Lehman HE. Affective disorders: clinical features. In: Kaplan HI, Sadock BJ, eds. *Comprehensive Textbook of Psychiatry*. 4th ed. Baltimore: Williams & Wilkins; 1985:786–811.
7. Gerson S, Bassuk E. Psychiatric emergencies: an overview. *Am J Psychiatr*. 1980;137:1–12.
8. Farberow NL, Shneidman ES. *The Cry for Help*. New York: McGraw-Hill; 1961.
9. Anderson WH. Psychiatric emergencies. In: Wilkins EW et al, eds. *MGH Textbook of Emergency Medicine*. 2nd ed. Baltimore: Williams & Wilkins; 1983:402–414.
10. Robins E. Psychiatric emergencies. In: Kaplan HI, Sadock BJ, eds. *Comprehensive Textbook of Psychiatry*. 4th ed. Baltimore: Williams & Wilkins; 1985:1311–1316.
11. Hatton CL, Valente SM. Assessment of suicidal risk. In: Hatton CL, Valente SM, eds. *Suicide Assessment and Intervention*. 2nd ed. Norwalk, CT: Appleton-Century-Crofts; 1984:61–83.
12. Bartolucci G, Drayer CS. An overview of crisis intervention in the emergency room of general hospitals. *Am J Psychiatr*. 1973;130:953–960.

51. Domestic Violence

TINA M.H. BLAIR, MD, FACEP
CARMEN GERMAINE WARNER, MSN, RN, FAAN

Until relatively recently, domestic violence (DV) was seen by both the general public and professionals (law enforcement and health care providers) as rare and occurring only among substance abusers, the poor, minority groups, or pathologic relationships. We now know it is the result of the interaction of many cultural, social, and psychologic factors and can happen to anyone.[1]

There are four major subsets of DV, although virtually any combination of these can exist. This chapter deals in depth only with the first three. Spouse abuse is intentional (or assumed to be so) physically, emotionally, or sexually violent or abusive behavior by one partner toward the other half of any intimate relationship [we shall call the male half of any intimate, social relationship the husband (includes spouse, ex-husbands, and past or current boyfriends, fiances, or lovers) and the female half the wife (although legal marriage need not be present)]. The battering syndrome is physical violence against a woman by a social partner. Elder abuse, which need not involve actual violence, is any misuse or maltreatment of a senior citizen. Child abuse is discussed in Chapter 37.

In this chapter we will employ the following definitions, which were compiled from a variety of sources. Verbal abuse results from comments that hurt and interfere with one's ability to deal successfully with others. Minor physical abuse includes pushing, shoving, grabbing, slapping, or throwing objects at another. Severe physical abuse is hitting another with a fist or an object, kicking, biting, tying up, beating, or threatening with or using a gun, knife, or other lethal instrument.

Although opinions differ as to the extent or frequency of mistreatment necessary to define domestic abuse or violence, we shall consider even one episode, regardless of why it is mentioned (ie, chief complaint, incidental finding, or the result of probing), that reaches professional attention (medical practitioner, counselor, social worker, or police) significant and an expression of DV.

Together, these abusive situations create a major health problem of epidemic proportions. Although family members probably have been battering one another as long as there have been families, and child abuse has been a known problem for decades, health practitioners did not recognize violence against a spouse or elder as a health problem until the late 1970s, and society as a whole has yet to come to terms with these situations.

Only in the past 15 years have studies attempted to determine the prevalence of DV, but it has not been easy to do so. Often disguised, ignored, and even accepted as understandable behavior, DV is all the more difficult to quantify and study.[2,3] Professionals also share in misconceptions that violence is rare and confined mainly to the poor, substance abusers, and the insane[4] or to unusually disturbed families in which violence is seen as fulfilling masochistic needs of the wife and necessary for equilibrium.[5]

EXTENT OF THE PROBLEM

Because it is impossible to know the true incidence of DV, the following are estimates from a number of sources and should be considered only guesses. Until every victim tells someone who reports to an agency keeping records, the incidence will continue to be estimated. Different studies that used different definitions and methods and, therefore, yielded variable results account for the broad ranges. It is of note that most of the information comes from records of those already seeking help [ie, crime reports, police files, and emergency department (ED) records]. Because DV is one of the most underreported of all societal or medical entities, however, any extrapolations could be highly erroneous. Although statistical adjustments are made by those who have collected data to attempt to make the numbers generalizable to the population at large, these maneuvers may actually further overestimate or underestimate the incidence.

Factors associated with lethality include the presence of children, prior threats of murder, existence of weapons, threats of retaliation, isolation, pathologic jealousy, use of drugs and/or alcohol, escalation of violence, and failure of support systems.[1]

- One third to two thirds of all families (perhaps more in other social pairings[6]) experience some form of violence.[7]
- A group of 218 men in an alcohol treatment program were asked if they abused a partner. More than a third admitted doing so in the last year, and a fifth reported committing serious assaults. When 33 of their female partners were interviewed, however, they were almost twice as likely to report assault.[8]
- Domestic disputes account for the highest number of police calls.[9]
- A woman is beaten by a male intimate about every 7.4 seconds,[10] and one third have major physical damage,[6] but only 4% present with injuries.[10]
- Of all abused partners, 16% are abused before cohabitation.[11]
- Battering appears to be the most common cause of injury to women, exceeding motor vehicle accidents, rapes, and muggings combined.[2,3]
- One quarter to one third of all American women (perhaps two thirds if separated or divorced) will experience some physical violence, and one sixth to one half will be beaten more than once by a social partner.[7,11–13]
- Of respondents to a 1981 survey of married couples, 26% admitted there had been violence in the prior year, and up to 60% of men or women had experienced it at some time.[2,3]
- Of all women who visit an ED with any complaint, 22% to 35% are there because of abuse (either directly or as a result of stress[2,3]), and 16% to 50% of those with injuries received them from a mate,[14,15] but only 17% of abused women are seen in an emergency department.[14]

Table 51-1 Factors Associated with Lethality of DV[14]

Children in the home
Batterer threatens to kill spouse
Presence of a weapon
Threat of retaliation
Isolation
Pathologic jealousy in spouse
Use of drugs and/or alcohol
Escalation of violence
Failure of multiple support systems

- Of all rapes of women older than 30 years, 50% are part of the battering syndrome.
- Of all murders in the United States, 17% to 50% are committed within the family,[2,3,7,12,14] and 13% (50% of familial murders[14]) are committed by spouses (Table 51-1).
- Of all female homicides, 25% (>4000) in the United States are from battering.[6]
- Of all female victims older than 15 years, 34% to 40% are killed by a mate.[2,3]
- In 1989, 106 Canadian women were killed; 11 were killed in August and September of 1990 in greater Montreal.[15]
- Police may be called five times or more before a homicide actually occurs.[6]
- Of all male homicides, 10% are by wives.[5]
- The number of American women who die from family violence in a 5-year period equals the number of American fatalities in the Viet Nam war.[16]
- Most domestic assaults occur when there has been repeated violence,[2,3] and it continues and worsens far more often than it stops. Rather than being isolated events, beatings tend to recur and escalate.[10] Of these victims, 75% will be abused again.[2,3]
- Of female psychiatric patients, 62% to 67% claim abuse.[15]
- Of all obstetric patients, 37% are abused during pregnancy.[2,3]
- In Canada, for every 10,000 reports of DV, only two men are convicted.[17]
- Of American elderly, 4% are abused or neglected, and there is a 10% increase per year. This is only slightly less often than children, but one third of child abuse cases are reported whereas only one fifth of elder abuse cases are reported.[18]

BARRIERS TO IDENTIFICATION AND TREATMENT

Despite the increased awareness of DV and an expanded understanding of the related dynamics and influencing factors, there still are numerous inhibitors that affect the quality of care provided in the ED and retard and impede intervention. Specific inhibitors that exist between us and these patients are discussed below.[19]

Reasons for Misdiagnosis

Because the ED is always open, it becomes a sanctuary for all sorts of people, including all types of victims. We see the results of DV daily, although much of it is probably unrecognized. Reasons we fail to make a correct diagnosis include the following:

- Our own prejudices and misconceptions blind us.
- The correct origin of the injuries and true reason for the visit are not always known.

  1. Some patients provide an accurate description of the incident, causative factors, and resulting impact; others mask, defend, and deny the reality and implications of the problem.
  2. Many do not report incidents for a variety of reasons, such as fear of reprisal, a belief that nothing can be done, concern that they could not support themselves and their children if their husband were arrested, and frustration and feelings of isolation when help is sought.[2,3,10]

- Emergency personnel often are neither as suspicious nor as astute as they should be.

  1. When the victim does not state exactly what happened, only 5% to 10% of cases are suspected or diagnosed in the ED.[20]
  2. Warshaw[21] in 1987 found 52 patients in 2 weeks who were seriously (85% moderately severe to severe and almost 10% life threatening) and unquestionably injured deliberately. Notes indicated, however, that physicians rarely asked questions showing their awareness of the abuse risk.

- We do not look beyond the obvious injuries (too busy, preoccupied, callous) for the real reasons for the visit; we prefer to treat the physical damage and not address the cause.[2,3]

  1. "I'm not a cop or a social worker. I'm here to treat the body. Their other problems need a psychiatrist."[2,3] This is not the right approach, however, because it adds to feelings that she is responsible and fails to deal with the real issue.[14]
  2. We recognize abuse but do not intervene because we are unsure of what to do or believe our efforts will not help.[14]
  3. We prefer to respond to sequelae (depression, drug abuse, suicide attempts, alcoholism) even when records indicate that problems arose after the battering began.[22]
  4. Physicians almost never ask about violence, and psychiatrists are only interested if it happened in a dream, rarely asking about real-life violence.[2,3]
  5. We prefer to medicate to satisfy medical obligations but do not face the implications of what or why we are medicating. This medical model fosters a detachment that protects physicians from awareness of their own feelings and also those of their patients.[2,3]

- ED limitations prevent complete assessment of patients.

  1. Volume of patients and relative understaffing result in limited time for each patient encounter and, therefore, minimal and problem-oriented history and physical examination.
  2. Past records are often not available, and when they are there is usually no time to read them in depth.
  3. Inadequate staff education and lack of dedicated personnel or resources for victims are further limitations.
  4. Staff are unfamiliar with community resources.
  5. There is a lack of resources during off hours (when most victims come in).
  6. There is no specific protocol. Education of both victims and health care providers can help. A Canadian study showed that the number of identified victims increased by 1500% via education and a staff protocol.[15]

A lack of acknowledgment of abusive experiences can be itself damaging, lead to the development of later psychopathology, increase victim isolation, and discourage victims' efforts to leave an abusive situation.[2,3] Much can be done in terms of identifying the problem and providing acknowledgment that it is a real problem, not something she deserves, and not necessarily something she can change. Acknowledging injuries as abuse without being shocked or judgmental tells the patient it is safe to talk about it. By ignoring abuse, you not only send a message that no help is available but return the victim to a potentially fatal situation. One study[21] showed that the physician failed to determine the woman's relationship to her assailant (75%) and did not obtain a psychosocial history, ask about prior sexual or physical abuse or living arrangements, or address further safety (90%). Most battered women are discharged from the

ED back to the same situation without any arrangements made for protection.[2,3]

Family Sanctity

Historically, the family's right to privacy has been rigorously protected in all spheres, making us reluctant to invade family boundaries. Patients are hesitant to reveal family-centered problems, choosing instead to handle domestic disputes within the home. Consequently, professionals confronted with DV may succumb to the dangerous belief that the sanctity of the family dictates noninvolvement. A better approach is to recognize that the members of a dysfunctional unit may not be able to help themselves without assistance from a skilled outsider.

Historical Precedent

There is a historical precedent for wives being treated as chattel, making them acceptable targets for corporal punishment. Consequently, an abused woman is not viewed as having a problem other than her unwillingness to fulfill the obligation to please the man who owns her. If we excuse violence because the victim asked for it, we unwittingly sabotage treatment. Professionals must help victims distinguish between violent acts (always totally unacceptable) and contributing factors over which they have some control.

Definition of Violence

Those chronically exposed to extreme forms of violence at work or in their personal life may become impervious to less violent acts. A slashed arm is minor compared to a gunshot wound. Likewise, a kick in the abdomen is trivial compared with the slashed arm. Therefore, those who are repeatedly roughly shaken and pinched may not be seen by themselves or others as victims of violence at all. This is detrimental to prevention, early identification, and treatment.

A corollary is the patient's tendency to use nonspecific descriptors and minimizing language to deny the seriousness of the situation. We must be aware of this and anticipate, recognize, interpret, and question further.

A classic example is the woman who reports, "I yelled at my husband, and then we had a fight." After persistent questions requiring her to specify details, it is learned that she yelled obscenities after he chased and threatened to kill her. The fight consisted of his kicking and punching her in the head, chest, and abdomen.

The Patient

Victims of DV often impede helping agencies from mobilizing on their behalf. Along with requests for assistance, they simultaneously exhibit overwhelming dependency, passivity, and even open resistance to change. This can frustrate independent, self-motivated, efficient problem-solving professionals.

The thought of leaving a known but oppressive environment causes a state of ambivalence that may be interpreted as disinterest or laziness rather than an immobilizing psychic conflict. At first, she tries to find ways to decrease the violence while maintaining the relationship. Later she realizes that she cannot do anything about his violence; all she can do is leave. Even this does not ensure that the violence will stop because separation often increases the risk of violent acts.[23]

The female victim fears leaving a relationship for several reasons:

- belief that she is incapable of surviving outside it
- fear of retribution by the assailant
- intolerable thoughts of single parenthood
- fears for her partner's self-destruction if she leaves
- desire to continue the relationship (marriage)
- expectation and hope that the abuser will change if she tries harder
- hope that things will improve[17]
- belief that the situation is not serious

Simultaneously, she fears remaining in the relationship:

- can no longer cope with its chronic, unpredictable stress
- values children's well-being
- dreads continuing a potentially lethal (to self, children, parents, or pets) situation[7]
- would like a better life or more freedom

Element of Blame

Because it is unsettling to believe that events beyond our control can influence us in destructive ways, we deny that the innocent may be victimized and rationalize that they must be blamed for their misfortunes.

We must assist the victim and others to distinguish between blameability and responsibility. The fact that a woman chooses a series of abusive mates is not a cause for blame. Masochistic behavior should not be reinforced by subtly implying that it is her fault for choosing such partners. Rather, we must communicate to these women that they can get help in regaining control over their lives.

Professional Impotence

A lack of education regarding current useful approaches to DV victims, the general underdeveloped state of the art, and a lack of community resources contribute to our feelings of inadequacy.

Thoughts of helplessness may be particularly aroused when we are treating a patient who has been in a violent situation for years and has already made several unsuccessful attempts to get help. Although this type of patient might appear to have a poorer prognosis than one seeking help for the first time, many who eventually do leave are older, have been in the situation longer, and have sought help before.

Common Response

Caring for victims of DV can produce strong responses from well-meaning but naive care givers. Overreaction may frighten them into silence or cause them to defend the assailant. For the victim to recognize, express, and channel anger constructively, it is important to be nonjudgmental.

Although an open discussion is uncomfortable for all, it can actually help the patient. Women who are plagued by the sequelae of DV are relieved to know they have one problem, not two (ie, DV and a serious illness). It is a big relief when physicians confirm their suspicion that it is in fact the violence that is the cause of most of their symptoms.[2,3]

Until a better method is invented, we must be prepared to ask direct questions; if we do not ask the questions, we will never get the answers.

EXCUSING THE ASSAILANT

DV incidents may evoke pity and compassion for assailants. They will almost always be extremely sorry and beg forgiveness. This honeymoon period never lasts.

Observation of their solicitous concern and apologetic behavior toward victims may result in your encouraging the couple to continue the relationship despite evidence of a long history of abuse. Recommending counseling while they continue living together is a risky option at best. Certainly, the assailant requires professional help, but this in no way diminishes the patient's need to be extricated from the abusive situation.

DOMESTIC VIOLENCE IS A HEALTH PROBLEM

Because DV is an ongoing, escalating problem that puts the victim at risk for more injuries[2,3] and can become a terminal illness if not treated appropriately, we must be aware of the subtle signs and symptoms of early stages and provide support, counseling, and shelter. Up to 8 to 12 years may elapse before the extent of the problem is known, and often this is only after a homicide.[6]

DV begets other problems, and for our interventions to be effective we must be aware of these problems.[2,3] Several studies have shown that victims of abuse utilize medical resources (ED physicians and many other providers) for all of the resultant injuries and stress-related disorders far more than their unabused peers.

- Abused women have more gynecologic and chronic pain complaints and presumably utilize more medical services for them.[22,24]
- The following conservative estimates of the cost of DV are given in 1980 dollars and are probably 10 to 40 times understated[2,3,14]:

  1. >$44 million per year (direct medical)
  2. >21,000 hospitalizations (>99,800 days)
  3. >28,700 ED and >39,000 physician visits/year
  4. indirect costs include >175,000 lost work days
  5. inestimable property damage

- Not only are the victim and assailant involved in the problem, but the long-term effects on children witnesses are now beginning to surface.[25-33]
- More than a third of the children of battered women are also abused physically or sexually.[7] Sometimes it is by the same man; sometimes it is by the woman.[30] The etiology of the relationship between spouse and child abuse is not known, but stress is a likely candidate. Whenever there is a lot of stress in a family, all members are at a higher risk of abuse.[7]
- Battering precipitates 25% of suicide attempts by all women and 50% of those by black women.

THE BATTERING SYNDROME

The battering syndrome is a constellation of injuries that are chronologically progressive in severity and are inflicted on a woman by a social partner. It starts with verbal or psychologic abuse and progresses to minor injuries. Later, there is emotional distress, anxiety, depression, substance misuse, suicide attempts, and more significant trauma. At any time victims may attempt to seek help, often unsuccessfully. There are no reliable profiles. The syndrome is seen in all socioeconomic, racial, religious, cultural, and geographic groups. Key components are listed below.[6]

- Psychosomatic complaints (as a means of seeking help) may occur, often with increasing severity and frequency

  1. may result in victims being inappropriately labeled hysterical, ED abusers, or drug seekers[6]
  2. multiple problems or ill-defined symptoms (headache, insomnia, choking sensation, hyperventilation, or chest, back, or pelvic pain)[10]

- Injuries have inadequate or inconsistent explanations[6]

  1. reluctant, vague, or changing[34]
  2. unwilling to give specific, logical details, and explanation may not match or account for the damage[10,35]
  3. may attempt explanation in hesitant, embarrassed, or evasive manner[10]
  4. tries to minimize or deny violence (to psychologically survive the situation)

- A dominating, intimidating, accompanying man may stay close and answer all questions[10]

  1. tells the story or keeps interrupting to get it straight[6]
  2. often very cooperative and wants to give history and answer for the patient[6]
  3. patient does not appear to need to say much because he said it all[6]

- Deterioration eventually occurs[6]

  1. increasing psychiatric symptoms (depression, anxiety, panic attacks, suicide attempts, substance abuse)
  2. spontaneous or self-induced abortions (often multiple)
  3. increasingly severe trauma (at first bruises or a bloody nose, later scars, burns, cuts, fractures, or multiple new and old injuries)[10]
  4. medical record may show a pattern of accidents or notes indicating suspicious injuries[10]

- Agents (alcohol, prescription drugs, street drugs) are often used to escape reality, resulting in suicide attempts, substance misuse, and child abuse[6]

  1. battered women are 16 times more likely to abuse alcohol[2,3,20] and 9 times more likely to abuse drugs[10]; this is usually the result and not the cause of the violence[10]
  2. in a group of 501 women attending a public prenatal clinic, those who admitted to being abused (98) were more likely to be divorced or separated, of greater parity, smokers, drinkers, or admitted users of illicit drugs than those who denied violence[36]
  3. it is estimated that 45% of women in alcohol treatment units started out as battered and turned to alcohol to cope or escape[2,3]
  4. 10% of battered women abuse or overutilize drugs; these are usually the sedatives, hypnotics, or analgesics that are prescribed to alleviate the anxiety and pain of living with violence[2,3]

- Affect may be inappropriate to the injury (ie, hysterical over a bruised arm or extremely calm after being severely beaten)

There are several typical stages[10] consisting of escalation and de-escalation followed by variable periods of calm.

- Escalation phase: increasing tension, verbal disputes, and minor battering.
- Triggering incident: results in violence ranging from a single blow to prolonged physical (beatings, imprisonment), emotional, and sexual abuse.
- Cooling-off (honeymoon) period: abuser often shows remorse or attempts to explain the behavior (alcohol, a bad day at work). Abuser:

  1. promises to change
  2. often apologizes and/or gives gifts
  3. may profess love and beg forgiveness, which rekindles hope in the victim
  4. may accept help; without it, the violent behavior is almost certain to recur
  5. gives way to violence as gifts and apologies are no longer needed to convince the victim to stay

- Entrapment:

  1. victim feels increasingly trapped by fear, intimidation, and lack of options
  2. victim may eventually lose hope, believing there is no way out
  3. depression, substance abuse, and suicide attempts begin to emerge as secondary problems
  4. if victim seeks medical help, she may be stigmatized or even blamed for the abuse and referred for psychiatric evaluation

MISCONCEPTIONS AND REALITIES

For many, the tragedy of DV becomes real only when it touches our own lives. Until then, misconceptions dominate each encounter.

- Female DV is not common. (In >70% of domestic disturbance calls the female is the complainant,[37] and 95% of abused spouses are women.[38])
- Male partners are not beaten by female partners. (The number of husbands battered by wives equals the number of wives abused by husbands.[39])
- DV is a lower-class, minority, unemployed phenomenon. (It occurs in all classes and occupations; in fact, the higher the education level, the greater the acceptance.[37])

- Occasional family disputes result in minor slaps and shakings. (7.0% of wives and 0.6% of husbands sustain serious injuries.[40])
- The victim must have done or said something to precipitate the assault. (77% of women surveyed in one study stated that the assault was not preceded by a verbal confrontation.[37])
- Aggression is inherent in some natures. (Violence and aggression result from conditioning, reinforcement, and learned behavior.[41])
- Victims do not have to remain in bad situations. (Family commitment, financial needs, fear, and loneliness contribute to a need to stay.[37])
- Only women with psychologic problems would stay in an abusive relationship. (Abusers create binds that are difficult to escape despite multiple attempts at extrication.[10])
- Abusers are mentally ill. (There are no supporting data.)
- Battered women are masochists. (Victims do not want to be harmed.[6])
- Alcoholism and other substance abuse on the part of the victim cause the battering. (Problems stem from long-standing abuse, stigmatization, violence escalation, inappropriate referrals, and frustration with legal, health, and social service agencies.[10])
- Victims do not want to talk about problems unless they bring them up; if you ask too many questions, they will become defensive. (Victims, for all sorts of reasons including past bad experiences with nonbelievers, may not be able to bring up the subject but often welcome an opportunity to speak when a care giver asks questions.)

LEGAL IMPLICATIONS

The legal aspects of DV are similar to those of rape, and we need to understand and participate in the legal process. Each state has specific regulations, and you should be familiar with yours. In some states (but not all), battering must be reported even if the victim does not wish to press charges.[6] If this epidemic of violence is to be halted, all care givers need to be well educated as to family violence and be willing and prepared to become involved.[17]

Assault and battery against nonrelatives are crimes, but assault and battery are not always viewed as such when they occur within a family. A stay in jail may be needed to fully convince a perpetrator that what was done is wrong. Police cooperation is variable, however, and you may need to inform the district attorney.

Evidence must be preserved carefully whenever possible (see Chapter 80, Rape and Sexual Assault). Clothing with tears or blood stains should be placed in a sealed, properly labeled and handled paper bag. If there are visible injuries, ask the patient's permission to take photographs, and keep them in a sealed envelope.[10]

The victim may need support and encouragement to press charges. In many states, unless this is done the police will not make an arrest. If the victim is unable to convict a perpetrator for abuse, if she gets a restraining order the abuser can be prosecuted for violation of it. A lack of desire to press charges may really be a protective mechanism, however. No one can ever fully understand the risk the victim faces as well as she does. Sometimes such an order puts her in more danger[10] (Table 51-2).

Table 51-2 Determination of the Need for Legal Information[14]

Has the battered woman ever sought help in order to stop the battering?
Is she familiar with the Protection Against Abuse Act?*
  Has she used it in the past?
  Was it effective in decreasing her contact with the battering spouse?
  If no, were the police called to enforce the court order?
  Did the police provide adequate protection?
Has the battered woman filed a criminal complaint against the batterer?
  Was the case heard?
  If yes, what was the outcome?
  If no, why? Did the battered woman drop charges?
Does the woman want to pursue either the criminal or civil legal procedures at this time? If yes, give her specific written instructions of what needs to be done.
Regardless of her answer to the question above, give her the name and phone number of a contact person for legal help.

*In states that do not have a Protection Against Abuse Act, a criminal complaint can be filed with the district attorney's permission.

THEORIES OF DOMESTIC VIOLENCE

Several theories attempt to explain why DV occurs. In reality, any explosive situation probably results from the interplay of many factors.

Conflict theory states that violence is a means of bringing about change and, thereby, of maintaining the viability of a social unit.[42] Struggles are normal and necessary parts of individual growth and societal development. Because conflict and tension are felt by many to be detrimental to group cohesiveness, this is not a popular view. Rejection of this theory, however, perpetuates the idealized myth of familial love and gentleness that, although useful in preserving the integrity of an important institution, prevents recognition and analysis of the widespread occurrence of DV.[43]

Cultural theory emphasizes approval of violence in a society's value system and the social norms that describe under what circumstances it can be used. Violent outbursts are rationalized on the basis of stereotypes (some societies express themselves physically more often than others) and norms within a particular group. Approval of physical punishment also permits all types of abuse. If we tolerate violence within certain groups, however, we may fail to intervene with those whose need may be the greatest.

Psychopathology theory argues that DV is the result of the psychologic disturbance of one member. Despite the fact that investigators[44-46] have identified a psychopathologic abusive nature, there is strong opposition to this theory[47] because only a small portion of violent people are mentally or organically ill.

General systems theory sees abuse as a systemic product rather than as a result of an individual's pathology. Positive feedback produces an upward spiral of violence, and negative feedback dampens and helps maintain the violence level within tolerable limits. As noted by Straus,[48] violence tends to increase through such processes as:

- labeling persons as violent, thus encouraging them to play out the violent role through the expectations of others
- creating a secondary conflict over the use of violence to settle the original argument
- reinforcing violence if the aggressor achieves desired results
- developing role expectations and self-concepts (ie, being tough)

Any of these circumstances may perpetuate violence, which will then stabilize via dampening processes or escalate until the family is destroyed by divorce, desertion, or murder.[49]

Several studies point out the possibility that interaction contributes to a violent outcome.[50,51] In one, involving communication patterns of a sample of abusive couples, Gage[52] found that both members of the couple regarded themselves as victims responding justifiably to provocation on the part of the other.

Most investigators see the roles as fixed: The man is the perpetrator, and the woman is the victim. This is understandable if the injured party is the only informant. When both are interviewed, a different story may surface. Violence is a continuum. On one end is mutual combat in which both are aggressors. On the other end is an innocent woman victimized by a man. Because the truth is probably somewhere in between, violent couples should be viewed together and methods found to interrupt the cycle.[53] Although abuse is never an excusable form of conflict resolution no matter to whom it is directed, both parties must understand that both share some responsibility. If we intervene sensitively, it is hoped that they can learn better ways of problem solving.[52]

Status inconsistency theory maintains that violence is most common in families in which the classically dominant members fail to possess the superior skills, talents, or resources expected of them.

Resource theory states that violence is a resource that is used to achieve desired ends when others (money, respect, shared goals, or love) are absent or insufficient.[49] Although DV occurs at all income levels, it is felt that there is more aggression in those families that have financial stress.[5] Straus et al[54] showed that families at or below the poverty level had a violence rate 500% greater than rates among the well off. Barnes[55] states that low-income women are conditioned to fight for survival and are more likely to physically fight back. Wives from working-class families appear to have stronger resources, less fear, and more control over their lives than middle-class women.[56]

Income levels are not a good indicator of violent behavior, (ie, it can happen to anyone), although a greater percentage of violence occurs in families having lower-prestige jobs than their neighbors,[47] and some investigators hold that financial stress is a significant factor.[50] Prevalence is equal in the upper and middle classes. Data are more readily available for the poor, however, because the poor utilize public services more frequently.[56] Because they are more countable, it appears as if there is a higher incidence when there is not.

Middle- and upper-class women are concerned about society's reaction and maintain taboos against taking husbands to court, calling the police, or admitting they have been battered. It is impossible to know the exact number of white, middle-class, and upper-class victims because many see private physicians who do not report these cases. This gap in the data perpetuates the misconception that DV happens to the poor or minorities.[2,3]

Economic decline parallels a rise in DV along with a decrease in supportive agencies and services. EDs (open 24 hours and not requiring payment in advance or even at discharge) have been the only outlet for those who otherwise might seek help from public agencies.[1]

Currently the most common belief is that DV is learned and passed from one generation to the next. Most victims either were abused as children or saw violence between their parents.[7] Bergmann[30] suggested that child abuse is associated with spouse abuse when the victim is also the more passive parent, who then retaliates upon the child. Poteat[7] found that women were eight times more likely to abuse children when they were in an abusive relationship.

CHARACTERISTICS AFFECTING ABUSE

ED personnel are responsible for educating all patients about their condition and preventive measures. Victims of DV are no exception. Note the following characteristics in assessing a family unit that may generate violent behavior:

- amount of time spent with each other (time at risk)
- diversification and range of interests and activities: the greater the areas of interaction, the greater the potential for conflict

- activity overlap: can cause potential competition
- intensity level of emotional involvement: activities that are central to family interaction involve more frustration
- presumed right of members to influence others: comments and suggestions are more fully exchanged among family members
- men and women often have different views on the same subject
- family roles are usually assigned on the basis of age and sex rather than ability, opportunity, or interest
- membership choice: involuntary for children and only semivoluntary for spouses; commitment to family is basically strong, and even without legalities it is difficult to end a marriage
- family privacy: insulates the unit from others

Awareness of some of these characteristics should help you understand the existence of family conflict despite displayed evidence of interpersonal support and love. This, together with crisis intervention skills and awareness of community services, is a critical part of the assessment and intervention process.

PROFILE OF AN ABUSED WOMAN

Although portions of this profile are helpful for many patients, each situation should be assessed individually.

- masking of true causes of injuries, or pain without obvious damage[10]
- bilateral or multiple injuries at different sites not logically connected; isolated extremity injuries (unless multiple) that may be inconsistent with the history are not typical[10]
- central location is typical (face, head, chest, breasts, abdomen, genitalia)[10]; accidental trauma more often involves the periphery
- recurrent ED admissions
- recurrent soft tissue injuries
- injuries to specific parts of body (Table 51-3)
- identification as being accident prone, or returns with "I had another fall"[6]
- previously abused physically
- suicide attempts
- prior rape by husband, boyfriend, or unknown assailant; abused women are reported victims of rape by boyfriends and husbands eight times more frequently than nonabused women
- complaints of chronic pain without an apparent organic cause and other problems associated with chronic stress (often mean fear of impending or actual abuse; more common than physical injuries)[10]

Table 51-3 Body Indicators of Trauma

Domestic Violence Trauma	Nondomestic Violence Trauma
Head	Forearm
Face	Wrist
Chest	Hands
Breast	Lower legs
Abdomen	Ankle
Buttocks	Feet
Back	
Bodily injury during pregnancy	

1. trouble with breathing
2. headaches
3. sleep disorders (especially a fear of falling asleep)[6]
4. abdominal, muscle, and joint pain
5. atypical chest pain
6. pelvic pain complaints, vaginal infections, and/or dyspareunia[24]
7. eating problems, anorexia, nausea, vomiting, functional bowel disease
8. depression paranoia, anxiety, panic attacks, hyperventilation[6]

- witnessed abuse of a parent or sexually abused as a child
- misuse of alcohol or drugs by parent or partner
- requests for pain medication or tranquilizers
- unstable marriage
- real or suspected child abuse (where there is a battered woman, there is a 50% chance of child abuse, now or later)[6]
- special notation should be made of any injury during pregnancy because the first abuse episode often occurs then[6,10]

1. pregnancy increases risk by a factor of 3
2. commonest sites: breasts, chest, and abdomen
3. a pending or completed miscarriage frequently occurs in battered women, who have a miscarriage rate of 25% (the rate is 6.6% if not abused)
4. abused women of all socioeconomic backgrounds choose a legal abortion more frequently than non-abused women
5. divorce or separation sought during pregnancy
6. more abuse in less educated women (perhaps better educated women tend to marry men with a better education, coping skills, and self-image[11])

PROFILE OF AN ABUSED MAN

The profile of an abused man is less defined than that of a woman. The actual incidence of male abuse is a complete unknown because men are reluctant reporters. Until men openly seek assistance, it will be impossible to assess the extent of the problem. Use the list below only as a basis for further questioning:

- injuries primarily on legs, back, head, or shoulders
- damage reflects use of a hard or sharp object rather than bruising or beating with fists
- serious injuries requiring immediate attention are possible
- maintains a strong, rigid expectation of each partner's specific role
- body size or shape not relevant to type or degree of trauma
- indicates on questioning that verbal aggression led to physical aggression
- battered men tend to see their relationships more positively and request help less often
- some injuries may actually be inflicted in self-defense by the woman

PROFILE OF AN ABUSER

Because little is known about women who abuse men, the following applies only to men[11]:

- less formal education
- less education than their partner
- poor impulse control (anger, alcohol or chemical abuse)
- stress (usually financial)

PSYCHOLOGIC ASPECTS OF ABUSE

Little is known about the complex psychologic aspects of DV. No one patient will have all these characteristics, but they could be used as indicators of potential abusive problems in both men and women. Victims of long-term violence may still suffer emotional abuse even after the actual battering ceases (eg, he may no longer need to be physical to get her to behave).

The abused have a high risk of mental illness[2,3]; a third are depressed, and suicide attempts are common. Of all female suicide attempters, 26% are battered; most attempts are gestures rather than fatal or nearly successful attempts. In a study of 100 abused women, 71 reported taking antidepressants or tranquilizers, 21 were diagnosed as depressed, and 34 had poisoned themselves. Other factors common to these women were as follows[2,3]:

- all had disastrous marriages
- 58% had not experienced a traditional courtship and engagement
- 85% had had premarital sex without using contraceptives
- 60% were pregnant before marriage
- 25% were abused before marriage

Although these data are from one study, other features that identify the abused include the following:

- low self-esteem
- dependent and fearful of loss of support
- few friends
- terrible sense of insecurity
- afraid to be alone
- passive personality, apparently unable to resist abuse but strong enough usually to prevent being killed
- believes all myths about battered relationships
- strongly believes in family unit
- accepts responsibility for the batterer's actions
- suffers from guilt, yet denies the terror and anger felt
- has severe stress reactions with psychophysical complaints
- uses sex as a way to establish intimacy
- believes that no one will be able to resolve the predicament except herself

Victims are often psychologically and physically debilitated by the time they seek help and thus lack the energy to reflect objectively on their past or to conceive of an improved future. It is only through persistent professional help that they can restore their resources sufficiently to choose healthy alternatives.[21]

Because the problem of DV is often unidentified and without effective intervention, many victims have a history of repeated and frustrated attempts at seeking help. Such well-known patients are often seen skeptically and given analgesics or tranquilizers.[21]

A battered woman's emotional response can be misunderstood if standard psychologic techniques are used without consideration of the normal response to the stress of chronic victimization.[14]

SPECIAL CONSIDERATIONS WITH THE ABUSED ELDER

Elderly abuse is increasing in recognition, identification, and intervention. As the percentage of the aged increases, so will the amount of abuse against them. As with the other forms of abuse, this involves not single attacks but recurring events. There are several forms of abuse that should be identified and reported[18]:

- *physical abuse*: corporal punishment, beatings, sexual assault, and constraint
- *fiduciary abuse/exploitation*: stealing money or property or using an elder's resources for personal gain
- *neglect*: deprivation of food and water; failure to assist in personal hygiene, provide health care, protect from health and safety hazards (ranges from being unable to meet needs to maliciousness)
- *abandonment*: desertion by anyone responsible for care and custody
- *psychologic abuse*: social isolation, derogation, infantilization, verbal threats

Although any elderly person is potentially at risk, there are some common patterns[18] (Table 51-4):

- Men are battered and abused, but women older than 75 years are more often victims.
- Most victims are widowed and socially isolated.
- Most have cognitive and/or physical impairments.
- Victims usually live at home and have needs that exceed family abilities.
- Many are not in the home out of love; their caretakers have other motives:
  1. responsibility
  2. greed (dependent on victim for financial support or housing)
  3. unable to afford an alternative

Abusers have the following characteristics in common:

- They are usually female because most of those providing care, despite the relationship, are younger women.
- As caretakers, children are most likely followed by grandchildren, spouse, siblings, and unrelated caretakers who are:
  1. younger than 50 years
  2. ill prepared or reluctant to provide care
  3. frequently experiencing some form of stress (ie, alcoholism, illness, marital discord, job loss)
  4. involved in a past or current abusive situation

Factors contributing to the vulnerability of older people are that they are:

- less mobile than younger individuals
- dependent on the individual inflicting the abuse
- financially exploited by those caring for them
- being physically beaten as well as mentally abused

Table 51-4 Indicators of Possible Abuse or Neglect[18]

Conflicting or implausible accounts regarding injuries
Patients or caretaker has a history of "doctor shopping"
Prolonged interval between the trauma or illness and presentation for care
Inadequate or unsafe conditions in the home
Brought to the ED by someone other than the primary caretaker
Patient is not given an opportunity to speak or be examined alone
History of similar episodes or other suspicious injuries in the past
Bruises and welts on trunk, arms, or legs (usually in various states of healing) or unusual patterns that might reflect the use of an instrument, human bites, or confinement with ropes or chains
Thermal injuries (hot or cold) with suspicious shapes and locations
Head injuries, lacerations, facial abrasions, and trauma to the eyes
Suspect neglect if the examination shows improper care of medical problems, untreated injuries, poor hygiene, dehydration, or poor nutrition
Psychosocial indicators include extreme withdrawal or agitation, infantile behavior, depression, and expression of ambivalent feelings toward family

- being abused by individuals who themselves have serious problems
- afflicted with age-related diseases that may make their care more difficult
- unable to leave their present living situation
- afraid that they will be sent to a nursing home
- fearful of being left alone
- not suited for presently designed shelters

Findings suspicious for abuse or neglect are listed in Table 51-4. Because an adequate history of abuse is frequently not obtainable from the patient, the most important aspect of diagnosis is understanding the physical signs.[18]

The proper course of action depends on the type of abuse, the severity of injuries, and the caretaker's interest in improving conditions. The first step is to explore the situation to determine whether there are possibilities such as respite care, homemaker services, home nursing, day programs, or accessible transportation. Although the family is often the source of abuse, it is still potentially the most nurturing source of long-term care. Efforts should be directed toward assisting the stressed caregiver to cope with the role and prevent abuse-potentiating situations. Adult abuse reporting is mandatory in all but 9 states. Specifically, 17 states have reporting laws covering abused individuals older than 60 years, and 21 have laws protecting the elderly.

Hospitalization is warranted in high-risk situations. It provides the opportunity to define the actual care needs and to arrange for necessary services, but the victim has the right to refuse admission. On discharge from the ED, follow-up arrangements must be made immediately with guarantee of a home visit by a visiting nurse or social worker.[18]

MANAGEMENT OF VICTIMS OF DOMESTIC VIOLENCE

Abused women seek medical attention more frequently than women who are not abused. Because this patient-physician interaction is often the sole confidential contact possible for them, we must properly assess and manage these patients.[23]

Assessment

Part of a complete evaluation of abused patients is seeking the real reason why they chose to be seen at that time for that problem. Whenever a woman or a child appears in the ED at an odd hour for a simple or nonacute complaint, consider abuse as the etiology and the visit a means of escape. (See Fig. 51-1.)

Despite recognition that the abused are increasingly seeking medical attention, we must remember that not all will openly identify themselves as victims. In fact, it is common for them to disguise apparent trauma and to attribute it to other unrelated incidents, and we must use other assessment techniques and be detectives. To do this well, we must understand the following factors:

- Make sure you get any information that other staff members might have obtained.
  1. The first one who spoke with the victim may have gotten the real or best story. Later, realizing the implications of what she said, the victim may change her story.
  2. The receptionist might have seen the way that the abuser really treated her[6] and how the couple interacted.
- Interview victims alone in a safe, secure, private area so that they can speak frankly.[10]
- Assure them of the confidentiality of any information.[10]
- Old records are important to identify trends.
  1. Look for similar injuries that may reveal a pattern and help you diagnose abuse. Confronting the patient with this may also help overcome defenses.[34]
  2. Ask if the patient has been seen elsewhere, and contact the other facilities.
  3. Look for other odd accidents that are becoming progressively more severe.

Environmental Assessment

Note the following:

- condition on arrival: hesitant or open with personnel and level of comfort displayed by patient toward others
- alone or accompanied by another (who?)
- interaction between patient and accompanying others
- time span between incident and ED admission
- existing lines of communication between patient and mate
- relationship of this incident to existing life stressors
- comparison of this incident with previous abuse visits

Physical Abuse Assessment

The assessment for physical abuse should include a search for:

- repeated abuse on certain body parts (ie, head and face)
- recurrence of injuries and bruises on body parts usually covered by clothing (ie, buttocks, thighs, breasts, chest, abdomen)
- fractures of the nose, ribs, jaw, and arms
- soreness and general body pain from being hurled or shoved

The entire body should be examined.

- Ask the patient to disrobe.
- If, for example, she has a broken arm, she might not mention the multiple bruises on her back, the bite mark on her shoulder, and so forth.
- Note old and new injuries.
- If sexual assault is suspected, a pelvic examination is necessary.

Emotional Assessment

Assess the patient for emotional problems,[55] such as evidence and level of fear, anger, guilt, depression; lack of confidence or self-esteem; shame; or despair. Observe her for a tendency to misdirect her feelings with physical destruction rather than verbalize them.

Specific Questioning Techniques

Those who have an information base about DV victims may be better able to manage not only the patients who openly admit to being abused but also those who mask the truth. Do not be reluctant to inquire directly about the nature of injuries because you assume that the victim does not want a discussion. On the contrary, patients who have been abused are frightened, lonely, overwhelmed, and embarrassed and desperately need to share their dilemma with someone. This is evident even when they deny its reality. Often victims will be relieved that someone asked and will readily provide more information.[10] Ask direct questions in an empathetic, concerned, nonjudgmental, nonthreatening manner, being aware of your voice and body language. One study showed

1. Date of Assault _____ .

2. Statement of Complaint (use patient's own words):

3. Description of Assault (use patient's own words):
   a. Specific detail and chronology of assault:
   b. Pain and symptoms mentioned:

4. Check physical findings:

	Contusions	Abrasions	Lacerations	Bleeding	Fracture	Other (Specify)
Head						
Ears						
Nose						
Cheeks						
Mouth						
Neck						
Shoulders						
Arms						
Hands						
Chest						
Back						
Abdomen						
Genitalia						
Buttocks						
Legs						
Feet						

5. Describe presence of trauma. Indicate location, appearance, and size. Indicate possible source such as teeth, cigarette burns, etc.:

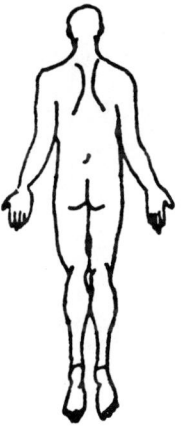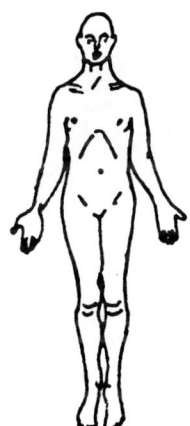

6. Internal injury:

7. Previous assaults (describe injuries and treatment):

8. Additional comments:

9. Assessment:

10. Consultations (service and consultant):

Figure 51-1 Domestic violence victim's assessment and treatment report. *Source:* Goldberg W, Carey A: Domestic violence victims in the emergency setting. *Top Emerg Med* 3:71–73, 1982.

Mental Health Consultant

	Specific Comments

I. *History of Current Abusive Relationship*
  A. Relationship to assailant (circle):
    Married   Friend
    Divorced   Ex-friend
      Separated
  B. Living arrangement (circle):
    Cohabit   Separate
  C. Length of relationship:
  D. Onset of abuse:
  E. Frequency of abuse:
    1) How often:
    2) Abuse pattern is (circle):
      Increasing   Staying the same
        Decreasing
  F. Types of abuse (circle):
    Verbal   Mobility Restriction
    Battering   Phone Restriction
    Sexual   Economic
      Other (specify)
  G. Instruments of abuse (circle):
    Gun   Fire
    Knife   Hot substance
    Blunt object   Cord
      Other (specify)
  H. Descriptive quality of assault (circle):
    Ritualistic   Slow rise in tension
    Impulsive   Other (specify)
  I. Coincidental Factors:	

	Victim	Assailant
Alcohol		
Drugs		
Argument		
Omission		
Commission		
Other (specify)		

  J. Behavior after assault(s) (circle):
    Reconciliation   Terminate relationship
    Leave scene   Contact friend
    Contact relative   Other (specify)
  K. Attempts to leave relationship (describe):
  L. Supportive resources (circle):
    Family   Employer
    Friends   Other (specify)
  M. The overall relationship is changing in the following way (circle):
    Much worse   Better
    Worse   Much better
      Same

II. *Education Level* (circle highest):
1 2 3 4 5 6 7 8 9 10 11 12
GED
Post High School (specify) _____
Graduate Education (specify) _____
Other Education (specify) _____

III. *Employment Summary*
Current: _____
Past: _____

IV. *Children*

Name	Sex	Date of Birth	Place of Residence	Well Being	Comments

Figure 51-1 continued

V. *Summary of Past Abusive Relationships*
   A. Adult: _____
   B. Child: _____

VI. *Mental Status* (circle)
   above average intelligence   average intelligence   below average intelligence   mentally retarded   alert   disoriented
   short-term memory intact   long-term memory intact   depressed   elated   fearful   angry   flat   passive   demanding
   manipulative   labile   apathetic   agitated   bizarre   poverty of ideas   flight of ideas   loose associations   delusional
   paranoid   suicidal   homicidal   drug abuse   alcohol abuse
   Additional comments:

VII. *Alternative Place(s) of Residence*   _____ Yes   _____ No
   Name: Name:
   Address: Address:
   Telephone: Telephone:

VIII. *Contact Person(s)*
   Name: Name:
   Address: Address:
   Telephone: Telephone:
   Relationship: Relationship:

IX. *Victim's Goals*
   A. Short-term:
   B. Long-term:

X. *Assessment*
   A. Present danger: D. Readiness for intervention:
   B. Problem solving ability: E. General impressions:
   C. Needs:

XI. *Recommendations*

XII. *Victim's Plan* (if known)
                                                                    _____
XIII. *Final Disposition*   Signature

Figure 51-1 continued

---

that by ED personnel asking simple, direct, and specific questions, the number of identified DV victims increased from 6% to 30%.[14]

Ideally, we should ask directly about abuse in all patient encounters because DV is ubiquitous.[10] A nonthreatening line of questioning might include the following[10]:

- How much do you smoke?
- How much do you drink?
- How are things at home?
- Are you safe there?
- I'm really worried that you're under a lot of stress. What's going on at home?
- We all have disagreements. When you and your partner argue, have you ever been physically hurt or threatened?

    1. Many tell me they argue with their mates and later state that they have been beaten. Could this be happening to you?
    2. What happens when you have a fight with your partner?
    3. Are you being beaten?
    4. Have you ever been hurt?
    5. Are you frightened?
    6. Do your verbal fights also include physical contact?
    7. Have there been any times during your relationship when you have had physical fights?

- How do you express your feelings with your mate?
- Have you ever been in a relationship in which you have been hit, punched, kicked, or hurt in any way? Are you in such a relationship now?
- How does your mate act when he is drinking? Is he verbally or physically abusive?
- You have mentioned that your mate loses his temper with the children. How are things between the two of you?
- You seem to have some special concern about your mate. Can you tell me more about this? Are you fearful? Has he ever hurt you?
- Sometimes when mates are overprotective and as jealous as you describe, they react strongly and use physical force. Is this happening in your situation?
- I notice you have a number of bruises. Would you tell me how they happened?
- Do you feel that you have to adjust your behavior to avoid conflict with your mate?

Table 51-5 Structured Interview for Use with Battered Women[13]

How were you hurt?
Has this happened before?
When did it first happen?
How badly have you been hurt in the past?
Was a weapon involved? Is there a weapon in the house? What kind?
Who lives in the home?
What are the children's ages?
Are the children in danger?
Hae they been hit or hurt by him?
How badly have they been?
Have you ever told anyone about this before? Is so, who?
What have you done in the past to protect yourself?
What have you done in the past to get help?
Have you ever called the police?
If yes, when, and what did they say/do?
Did you report this incident to the police? If not, why not?
If yes, what precinct?
What did they say?
Have you ever obtained a protective order?
Have you ever tried to press charges this time or before?
Does your boyfriend/husband have a criminal record?
Has he beaten up or hurt other people?
Has he threatened to kill you?
Has he tried to kill you?
What did he do?
Are you afraid to go home?
Where can you go?
Have you ever called Women Against Abuse, Women in Crisis, etc?
If yes, do you have a contact there? Who?

Carefully choose your words.[6] Victims may not feel that they were abused but would perhaps admit to being hit: "I'm concerned about these injuries and wonder if you might have gotten them from someone's hitting you." Tell victims that they are not alone. It is a common, tragic problem, but help is available. Leave your card or a pamphlet and say there are people who could help: "You need not talk now if you do not want to." Once abuse is established, assess the victim's safety by asking about it[2,3] (Table 51-5).

Finally, ask about the following:

- extent of the violence and whether weapons have been involved
- whether the children are threatened, in danger, or abused
- whether there is a safe place to go
- whether they are afraid for their lives
- whether they have considered a plan to kill the abuser

THE INTERVENTION PROCESS

For many victims, arrival at the ED is their first contact with any system. The initial support, understanding, and sensitivity provided by us will greatly influence whether they will obtain and maintain contact with law enforcement, social services, and the health care system. Regardless of the length of the ED visit, it is essential for us to provide materials about referrals and filing a complaint.

There should be one staff member with whom the victim can develop an attachment. The title (nurse, crisis or social worker, volunteer, chaplain, or physician) is not as important as that person's commitment to both the victim and the process. If you involve more than just the physician and nurse, trust is more likely to occur.[34]

The greater our understanding of current problems confronting these patients, the easier it will be to design and implement appropriate management methods. The following guidelines may assist in assessing and designing a referral and evaluation process.

- Obtain pertinent data from the patient, family, friends, law enforcement personnel, community violence advocates, and first responders.
- Identify DV, and name it as a problem. Acknowledge that you have the same concerns that the victim has and that you know this is a serious problem.[2,3]

  1. Simply recognizing the problem and talking helps empower victims to do something further about their situation.
  2. Inform victims that abuse is not their fault.[34]
  3. Remind them that battering rarely happens once and that the risk of worse injury increases with time.[34]

- Do not alienate victims by being judgmental or accusatory; it is important to believe victims.[11]

  1. Comments such as "Why don't you leave?" or "I can't believe he'd do this" lower self-esteem and place blame on the victim. The result may be that she does not come back to you or see anyone else.[11]
  2. Support their decisions about how best to end the violence and deal with the situation.[2,3]

- Provide information about resources, and document this.

ED intervention with DV victims should include identification; details of the abusive history to create a realistic view of the past, present, and future; exploration of treatment options; and documentation of the process to promote continuity of care.[1]

Immediate stabilization of and intervention with these patients are necessary, and the cause of the injuries as well as the cure must be recognized. Special considerations include the following:

- Admit and attend to the patient immediately.
- Maintain total privacy for patient, family, and friends.

- Establish an environment of honesty, support, and trust.
- Stress the importance and worth of self.
- Gather information as privately as possible.
- Perform the proper history and physical examination.
- Recognize the importance and legal requirements of photographs, patient teaching, and consent forms.
- Understand the psychologic state of the victim as different from that of other patients.
- Remain cognizant of nonverbal behavior. If personnel are hostile or biased, replace them with ones who are open and comfortable dealing with these patients. Document verbal and nonverbal interactions along with staff impressions and reactions.
- Provide specific intervention for trauma-related problems.
- Notify appropriate authorities if rape, stabbing, or gunshot wound has occurred.
- Record the patient's emotional state in addition to her physical appearance.

If the patient desires to leave, at least try to design a system of escape from the abuse situation if the need should arise and include the following:

- safety of the home
- alternative place to stay
- getting important documents (ie, marriage license, birth certificates, passports, bank books, credit cards) out of the house
- where she can get help

Abuse will not be cured in one visit; arrange follow-up.[11]

Documentation is important; be thorough and descriptive, and use the patient's own words. List specific injuries in the diagnosis, and include "alleged abuse by _____" when patients state that they have been abused or if denial of abuse continues despite direct questions.

Words Mask Abuse

We often use passive, disembodied phrases that disregard the interaction of the batterer and the victim.[11] In one study, "hit by lead pipe," "blow to head by stick with nail in it," and "hit on left wrist with jackhammer" were given as injury mechanisms without any mention of either who did it or the circumstances of the attack.[11]

Warshaw[21] says that this medical shorthand is an important shaper of how physicians learn to organize their thinking and that it obscures the etiology and meaning of the symptoms. It also sends a message to the victim that the instrument and the injury are all that are important.[11]

The only place where documentation is contraindicated is on any record that the victim would need for personal use (ie, discharge instructions) that could fall into the hands of the abuser.[1]

Design

Designing systems for establishing and coordinating priorities of care and preparing personnel, equipment, and procedures are critical requirements. Steps involved include the following (although few, if any, facilities could do all these, most could do at least some):

- Develop a special DV team to be on call and a network of resources to activate immediately.
- Design and develop a management protocol.
- Conduct staff training and development, incorporating the knowledge and skills contained in the established protocol. Topics to be covered include:
  1. commonalities of social violence and DV
  2. theoretical concept of violent behavior (misconceptions, trends, and current studies)
  3. family systems theory
  4. recommended techniques for assessment and management, communications, interviewing, and networking with law enforcement and justice, legal, and community support systems.
- Require certification of personnel.
- Develop a monitoring system.
- Incorporate an evaluation and feedback component and standards of quality care.

Referral and Networking Procedures

We must assess the need for admission, transfer, or referral. Regardless of the disposition, contact hospital social services to see the patient while she is still in the ED (but do not expect them to come unless it is part of their job description; Table 51-6). Whenever possible, contact referral agencies yourself; if you rely on the victim to do it later, it may not get done.

Table 51-6 Follow-Up Plan for Battered Women[13]

Determine the need for emergency shelter and work with woman in analyzing whether the plan for emergency shelter is adequate.
Develop a concrete plan for mobilizing help when violence erupts at home.
Design long-term planning process with scheduled follow-up visit within the week.
Give woman the name and phone number of a contact person with the local group working with battered women (eg, Women Against Abuse, Women in Crisis, etc).
Give woman the name and phone number of a contact person who can help her navigate through the legal process when necessary.
If children are at risk, involve the Child Neglect/Abuse Team in the institution and file an official report of suspected child abuse.

Consider transfer to a psychiatric or rehabilitation facility or a shelter or community center, and assist the patient in contacting (in private) crisis hotlines and law enforcement. Some or all of the following resources can be mobilized:

- facilities for birth control, abortion, and tubal ligation
- medical and mental health care
- social service agencies for financial aid, child protective services, food stamps, clothing, day care, housing, and emergency shelter
- criminal justice agencies for protection against further violence
- legal aid for assistance with warrants, court procedures, separation, and divorce agreements
- vocational rehabilitation agencies for financial assistance and information about educational pursuits, job training, and employment counseling
- women's or men's groups for information, support, and shelter

In addition, patient and family teaching sessions can be incorporated into follow-up care.

There should be overnight protection so that the victim need not stay in the abusive environment. A stay in the ED or hospitalization may be needed if there are no relatives (victims may be isolated from them) or shelters available. Chronic victims may feel that they are not worthy of help.[34] Remember to ask whether there are children who need protection.

CONCLUSION

ED professionals have witnessed an increase in the number of DV patients and have experienced a consciousness raising that has alerted them not only to the sensitivities of this problem but also to the indicators leading to proper assessment and intervention techniques.

The professional growth occurring during these past years has not been without its barriers and resistance. Those who are experiencing similar personal situations try to avoid caring for these patients because of the inner struggle it presents; others unfamiliar with the reality of this problem find these patients to be time consuming and annoying.

DV is underreported and underrecognized despite immense medical, social, psychologic, and emotional costs. Recognizing victims and direct questioning about the possibility of DV are the first steps in identification and treatment. Be alert to signs of abuse even with patient denial. Treatment of the medical and surgical problems is just the first step. Documentation of injuries serves the victims and future physicians. Reporting to authorities should only be done if it is legally required or if the victim requests.[57]

With the increase in recommended approaches for physical management comes the importance of understanding and implementing psychologic and sociologic considerations. Only through a consistent network of approaches addressing the total patient can there be any opportunity for rectifying the situation and preventing further violent episodes.

REFERENCES

1. Goldberg WG, Tomlanovich MC. Domestic violence victims in the emergency department. *JAMA*. 1984;51:3259–3264.
2. Randall T. Domestic violence begets other problems of which physicians may be aware to be effective [news]. *JAMA*. 1990;264(8):940, 943–944.
3. Randall T. Domestic violence intervention calls for more than treating injuries [news]. *JAMA*. 1990;264(8):939–940.
4. Nichols WC. Understanding family violence: an orientation for family therapists. *Contemp Fam Ther*. 1986;8:188–207.
5. Hilberman E. Overview: the "wife-beater's wife" reconsidered. *Am J Psychiatry*. 1980;137:1336–1347.
6. Borenstein M, Blair T. Domestic violence. In: Blair T, ed. *Introduction to Emergency Medicine* (National Medical Student Series). Malvern, Pa: Harwall, (in press).
7. Poteat GM, Grossnickle WF, Cope JG, Wynne DC. Psychometric properties of the Wife Abuse Inventory. *J Clin Psychol*. 1990; 46(6):828–834.
8. Gondolf EW, Foster RA. Wife assault among VA alcohol rehabilitation patients. *Hosp Commun Psychiatry*. 1991;421(1):74–79.
9. Stephens DW. Domestic assault: the police response. In: Roy M, ed. *Battered Women: A Psychosociological Study of Domestic Violence*. New York: Van Nostrand Reinhold; 1977:18–23.
10. The battered woman: breaking the cycle of abuse. *Emerg Med*. 1989;June 15:104–115.
11. Rath A, Daniel G, et al. Rates of domestic violence against adult women by men partners. *JABFP*. 1989;2(4):227–233.
12. Pagelow MD. *Family Violence*. New York, N.Y.: Praeger; 1984.
13. McLeer S, Anwar R. The role of emergency physician in the prevention of domestic violence. *Ann Emerg Med*. 1987;16:1155–1161.
14. McLeer SV, Anwar R, Herman S, et al. Education is not enough: a systems failure in protecting battered women. *Ann Emerg Med*. 1989;18:651–653.
15. Bain JE. Wife assault: physicians cannot ignore it [editorial]. *Can Med Assoc J*. 1990;144(3):283–284.
16. Domestic violence. *AMA News*. 1991;34(41):.
17. Sullivan P. NB physicians sent hard-hitting discussion paper on wife abuse. *Can Med Assoc J*. 1989;143(3).
18. Jones J, Blair T. Geriatric Abuse. In: Blair T, ed. *Introduction to Emergency Medicine* (National Medical Student Series). Malvern, Pa.: Harwall (in press).
19. Goldberg W, Carey A. Domestic violence victims in the emergency setting. *Topics Emerg Med*. 1982;3:65–76.
20. Goldberg WG, Tomlanovich MC. Domestic violence victims in the emergency department: new findings. *JAMA*. 1984;251(24): 3259–3264.
21. Warshaw C. *Gender and Society*. 1989;3:506–517.
22. Rapkin AJ, Kames LD, Darke LL, Stampler FM, Naliboff BD. History of physical and sexual abuse in women with chronic pelvic pain. *Obstet Gynecol*. 1990;76(1):92–96.

23. Filicraft A. Battered women: an emergency room epidemiology with a description of a clinical syndrome and critique of therapeutics. Testimony before Subcommittee on Domestic and International Scientific Planning, Analyses, and Cooperation. Washington, D.C., February 18, 1978.
24. Schei B. Psychosocial factors in pelvic pain: a controlled study of women living in physically abusive relationships. *Acta Obstet Gynecol Scand*. 1990;69(1):67–71.
25. Cummings JS, Pelligrini DS, Notarius CI, Cummings EM. Children's responses to angry adult behavior as a function of marital distress and history of interparent hostility. *Child Dev*. 1989;60(5):1035–1043.
26. Fantuzzo JW, DePaola LM, Lambert L, Martino T, Anderson G, Sutton S. Effects of interparental violence on the psychological adjustment and competencies of young children. *J Consult Clin Psychol*. 1991;59(2):258–265.
27. Gage RB. Consequences of children's exposure to spouse abuse. *Pediatr Nurs*. 1990;16(3):258–260.
28. Jouriles EN, LeCompte SH. Husbands' aggression toward wives, and mothers' and fathers' aggression toward children: moderating effects of child gender. *J Consult Clin Psychol*. 1991;59(1):190–192.
29. Holden GW, Ritchie KL. Linking extreme marital discord, child rearing, and child behavior problems: evidence from battered women. *Child Dev*. 1991;62(2):311–327.
30. Bergman B, Brisman B. Battered wives—measures by the social and medical services. *Postgrad Med J*. 1990;66(771):28–33.
31. Hershorn M, Rosenbaum A. Children of marital violence: a closer look at the unintended victims. *Am J Orthopsychiatry*. 1985;55:260–266.
32. Jaffe P, Wolfe D, Wilson S, Zak L. Similarities in behavioral and social maladjustment among child victims and witnesses to family violence. *Am J Orthopsychiatry*. 1986;56:142–146.
33. Wolfe D, Jaffe P, Wilson S, Zak L. Children of battered women: the relation of child behavior to family violence and maternal stress. *J Consult Clin Psychol*. 1985;53:657–665.
34. Ludwig S. The abused adult. In: Callahan ML, ed. *Decision Making in Emergency Medicine*. St. Louis: Mosby Year Book; 1992.
35. Brown C, Van Ripen M. The battered woman. *Nursing Grand Rounds* presentation UNMC, 1989.
36. Berenson AB, Stiglich NJ, Wilkinson GS, Anderson GD. Drug abuse and other risk factors for physical abuse in pregnancy among white non-Hispanic, black, and Hispanic women. *Am J Obstet Gynecol*. 1991;164(6, pt. 1):1491–1496; discussion, 1496–1499.
37. Appleton W. The battered woman syndrome. *Ann Emerg Med*. 1990;9:84–91.
38. Bureau of Justice Statistics. *Criminal Victimization in the United States*, 1982 (Publication no. NCJ-92820). Washington, DC: U.S. Dept. of Justice; 1984.
39. Bay Area Hospital Conference on Sexual Assault. *Medical Protocol for Victims of Sexual Assault*. Queen's Bench Foundation; 1976:4.
40. Steinmetz SK. The battered husband syndrome. *Victimology*. 1978;2:499–509.
41. Brazil J. Violence: dynamics of learned behavior. In: Warner CG, ed. *Conflict Intervention in Social and Domestic Violence*. Bowie, Md.: Brady; 1981:19–36.
42. Steinmetz SK, Straus MA, eds. *Violence in the Family*. New York, N.Y.: Dodd, Mead; 1974.
43. Gil DG. Violence against children. *J Marriage Fam*. 1971;33:637–648.
44. Young L. Parents who hate. In: Steinmetz SK, Straus MA, eds. *Violence in the Family*. New York, N.Y.: Dodd, Mead; 1974:187–189.
45. Steele BF, Pallach CB. A psychiatric study of parents who abuse infants and small children. In: Hefler RE, Kempe CH, eds. *The Battered Child*. Chicago: University of Chicago Press; 1968:89–134.
46. Kempe CH, Silverman FN, Steele BF, et al. Battered child syndrome. *JAMA*. 1962;181:17–24.
47. Gelles RJ. Child abuse as psychopathology: a sociological critique and reformulation. *Am J Orthopsychiatry*. 1973;43:611–621.
48. Straus MA. A general systems theory approach to a theory of violence between family members. *Soc Sci Info*. 1973;12:105–123.
49. Goode WJ. Force and violence in the family. *J Marriage Fam*. 1971;33:624–636.
50. Finkelhor D, Gelles R, Hotaling GT, Straus M, eds. *The Dark Side of Families: Current Family Violence Research*. Beverly Hills, Ca.:Sage Publications; 1983.
51. Neidig PH, Freidman DH. *Spouse Abuse: A Treatment Program for Couples*. Champaign, Il.: Research Press; 1984.
52. Gage RB. Letter. *Pediatr Nurs*. 1990;16(6).
53. Gage RB. Examining the dynamics of spouse abuse: an alternative view. *Nurse Pract*. 1991;16(4):11–16.
54. Straus M, Geles R, Steinmetz SK. *Behind Closed Doors: a survey of family violence in America*. New York, N.Y.: Doubleday; 1980.
55. Barnes SL. Psychosocial aspects of wife abuse in the United States. *Emotional First Aid*. 1991;2:29–36.
56. Davidson T. *Conjugal Crime: Understanding and Changing the Wife-Beating Pattern*. New York, N.Y.: Hawthorne Books; 1978.
57. Hult DM. Spouse abuse: care goes beyond the office door. *Postgrad Med J*. 1990;98(2):130–135.

52. Emotional and Spiritual Support

ANN R. SCHREIER, MSN, RN

Emergency care requires the ability to prioritize and make quick decisions. Frequently time pressures, acuity level, constraints of the professional role, and the organization of the unit make it difficult to provide the emotional and spiritual support the client needs. Although emotional and spiritual needs may be present, they are frequently viewed as separate problems of a lower priority. In reality, they are just another dimension of the total patient problem and can function to facilitate or detract from the health care interventions being provided.

Although it may appear easier to delegate the emotional and spiritual care to others or to give it such a low priority that it is never addressed, it is a fact that patients are whole human beings. Even if we fragment their care, they will continue to interact with us and with their environment as whole beings: body, mind, and spirit. Emotional and spiritual support can and should be an integral part of the care available to any patient or family requiring emergency treatment. This is possible only when the focus of the care giver moves from the presenting problem to the patient as a whole.

HOLISTIC MODEL FOR CARE

Modern medicine with its increasingly complex technology and extensive specialization has played a significant role in fragmenting and depersonalizing patients in the process of providing care. A holistic model for health care seeks to return the person to his or her appropriate status as a unified and integrated human being. Viewing the patient as whole and integrated not only is essential to providing total care but honors the complexity of human existence and the understanding that we are more than the sum of our parts.[1]

In the first half of the 20th century, the philosopher Teilhard de Chardin spoke of the "within" of an individual. The "within" can be defined as the interior organizing principle of an organism. It is the principle of unification that makes a thing what it is. It is not precisely a physical energy, but it is what gives energy its pattern. Teilhard stated that modern science by its nature analyzes and breaks things into its parts. The organizing reality or "within" of a thing, however, cannot be ascertained simply by analyzing the parts. Thus science, by its own limitations, misses the whole of a reality.[2]

Griffin[3] believes that the modern world view, under which the natural sciences and modern medicine have flourished, has been heavily influenced by Cartesian dualism, which creates a false separation between mind and matter. This dualism has led to certain understandings about the natural world: that it is mechanistic, materialistic, and nonanimistic; that all experience comes to us through our sense organs and hence is limited to the types of experience that these senses are able to perceive, namely the physical; and that there is no divine presence in the world, which is a natural conclusion from the first two assumptions. These three understandings, or perhaps misunderstandings, largely account for the modern world view's inability to explain the complexities and richness of human experience.

All dimensions of human life—biologic, psychologic, sociologic, and spiritual—are interrelated. Each dimension

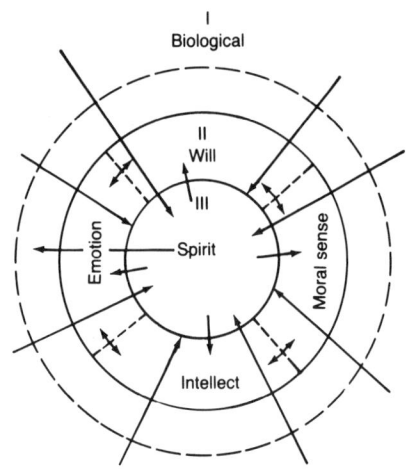

I. Biological: Five senses, world-conscious.
II. Psychosocial: Soul, self-conscious; self-identity.
III. Spirit: God-conscious, relatedness to deity. Incoming arrows are examples of life experiences penetrating the spirit:
  Via intellect: unanswered philosophical and religious questions.
  Via emotion: relationships of love and hate.
  Via will: decisions regarding job, marriage, divorce, births, deaths, deity.
  Via moral sense: support of personal convictions or inability to support personal convictions.
Outgoing arrows are examples of spirit responses:
  Via intellect: statements of affirmation or doubt about God.
  Via emotion: joy, peace, fear, loneliness, anxiety.
  Via will: decisiveness or instability.
  Via moral sense: integrity or guilt.
  Via biological: energetic activity or perhaps illness related to stress (i.e., peptic ulcer, ulcerative colitis, overindulgences in food and drugs).

Figure 52-1 Conceptual model of nature of man. *Source:* Reprinted with permission from Beland IL, Passos J: *Clinical Nursing: Pathophysiological and Psychosocial Approaches*, ed 3. New York, Macmillan, p. 1087, 1975. Copyright © 1975 by Macmillan Publishing Co., Inc.

infiltrates and affects all other dimensions and cannot be adequately dissected out without the loss of its true context. When a person is ill, his or her total being is involved. For the sake of discussion, a three-dimensional model will be used, where human beings can be thought of as consisting of three aspects: spirit, mind, and body (Fig. 52-1).

The innermost human dimension is the spirit which is the guiding force within each individual. The spirit contains the presence of the Absolute Source (God) who constantly and continuously generates life into the entire human being. The spirit contains the basic spiritual principles of love and wisdom from which everything originates and is transmitted to the other human dimensions.

The intermediate human dimension is the mind. This area constitutes the unique mentality or soul of the individual. Human will, reasoning, understanding, intellect, knowledge, intuition, higher feelings, memories, emotions, and moral sense are all part of the mind.

The outermost human dimension is the body. The body contains everything related to bodily functions and to senses, beliefs, attitudes, perceptions, exterior memory, and all physiologic and biological functions.[4]

Holistic care requires an understanding and appreciation for all of the human dimensions and for their interrelatedness. Nothing can happen in one dimension of an individual without it having repercussions in the other dimensions. Change, from within or without, affects this system of interrelatedness, calling for constant modifications in order to maintain equilibrium.

Optimal health can be described as the positive balance of the three dimensions of spirit, mind, and body. When there is an imbalance in one dimension the other two dimensions are affected, and therefore the individual as a whole is placed in disequilibrium. Disequilibrium frequently leads to illness and disease. Emergency care is intimately involved in the restoration of equilibrium. Restoring the physical balance is usually the primary focus of emergency treatment, though it must not be forgotten that the psychosocial and spiritual dimensions may also require intervention.

Holistic care in the emergency setting requires a perception of the elements of the human body, mind, and spirit that enhances the objective scientific approaches of care and addresses the subjective qualitative factors.[1]

EMOTIONAL NEEDS IN CRISIS

For most people, a visit to an emergency department is a stressful event that is frequently associated with crisis and/or loss. Stress is defined as any event that involves the deprivation of some basic psychospiritual or physical need. Stress is a component of every crisis. However, stress in and of itself does not constitute a crisis. To be considered a crisis, the stress must create a state of disequilibrium that the individual cannot correct through his or her usual problem-solving activities or coping skills.[5] When one's familiar coping abilities fail to reestablish equilibrium, the stress of the unmet need rises unchecked. Four characteristic phases in the development of a crisis are[6]:

1. The patient faces a stressful situation and his or her habitual problem-solving responses are mobilized.
2. Efforts to cope with the stress fail and feelings of frustration, anxiety, confusion, anger, and ineffectuality occur. At this stage some degree of disorganization of functioning occurs.
3. Feelings of inner disturbance escalate and help to mobilize additional coping resources. Crisis counseling helps in this stage by supplementing and supporting the indi-

vidual's latent coping skills. Emergency personnel can have tremendous impact at this stage.
4. If unresolved, the stress of the unmet need and the inner disorganization can escalate to a point where a personality break may occur.

The person in crisis needs immediate help aimed at restoring equilibrium. Crisis care involves short-term intervention focused on the immediate problem. It is a "Band-Aid" for the stressful situation and not therapy for deep-seated psychological problems.[5] Referral for long-term therapy may be an appropriate part of crisis counseling.

Dynamics of Crises

Before exploring means of handling people in crisis, it may be useful to have a clear understanding of the scope and dynamics of crises and the relationship between crisis and grief. There are two categories of crises: developmental (or maturational) and accidental (or situational).[5,6]

Developmental crises occur as the natural consequence of going through growth stages. Each growth stage challenges the ego, and builds on the learning acquired in earlier phases. The transitions between stages of growth are periods of heightened anxiety and crisis when the person is pulled forward by maturational forces and backward by security. Developmental crises are a normal and integral part of growth. They include birth, going to school, adolescence, leaving home, entering a vocation, engagement, adjustment to marriage or singlehood, pregnancy, parenthood, middle-age crisis, loss of parents, menopause, retirement, death of one's spouse, death of friends, and one's own impending death.[6] Most individuals are able to successfully handle the pressures of developmental crises through use of familiar coping skills. However, individuals who have developed weak or inadequate coping abilities, and individuals who have experienced multiple developmental crises, or a combination of developmental and accidental crises over a short period of time are likely to present for emergency care.

Accidental crises can occur at any age and at any time, and are precipitated by the unexpected loss of something that is regarded as essential in getting one's needs met. Accidental crises include personal injury and illness, an accident, surgery, mental illness, alcoholism, a physical handicap, an unwanted pregnancy, a divorce, a loss of status and respect, a natural disaster such as a flood or earthquake, or social problems such as economic depression, unemployment, and war.[6]

Any event entailing a loss or requiring a significant change produces an emotionally hazardous situation and can lead to crisis. Furthermore, crises can be triggered by both positive as well as negative occurrences.[6] In people who seek emergency help, there is frequently a series of recent changes or losses. A series of stressful events within a limited time span can have a cumulative effect. It is wise to ask people in crisis what other significant changes, transitions, or losses they have had in recent months, for a series of crises may be taxing their coping skills and intensifying their need for nurturing and support.

Dynamics of Grief

Crisis and grief are closely linked; the core experience in both is loss. A loss or threat of loss is an essential ingredient in both crisis and grief. Traditionally grief reactions are associated with death, although some form of grief reaction follows any significant loss, change, transition, or crisis. Grief reactions imply crisis, but crises do not have to involve grief.

Like the stages in crisis development, the stages of the grieving process involve a set of responses designed to restore personal equilibrium[6]:

1. shock, denial, and disbelief: involves a reluctance to acknowledge the reality of the situation
2. anger, hostility: can also involve rage, resentment, and envy; angry feelings are frequently displaced and/or projected outward
3. guilt feelings
4. anxiety and depression
5. acceptance of the loss: involves the surrendering of emotional ties and readjustment
6. integration: involves giving meaning to and learning from the loss
7. extension: involves reaching out to assist and help others with similar loss.

Due to the nature of emergency care, the later stages of the grief process, namely acceptance, integration, and extension, are not usually seen by the staff. However, the earlier stages, especially shock and denial, anger, and guilt, are frequently seen in the emergency department and may be misinterpreted. The stages of grieving are not rigid categories, and people experiencing grief frequently vacillate between the stages. The behavior of all people experiencing any kind of loss or threat of loss needs to be viewed in terms of the grieving process.

Death or any of the losses precipitated by an emergency department admission (including loss of control, self-esteem, etc) can throw the patient or family into the shock/denial stage of the grieving process. Even patients who have been dealing with a chronic or terminal illness can respond with disbelief when complications arise. Because these people may have had a longer time to adjust to their situation, their coping skills may appear more sophisticated than those of a person experiencing sudden trauma, but it is grief just the same.

The health professional needs to understand that the use of shock or denial is an emotional defense against overwhelming pain. Denial is a normal early response to loss. It should be understood that even though the use of denial may appear to be a suboptimal or unrealistic way of coping, it meets the need of the person using it to buffer the pain.[7]

During the shock/denial stage the patient and/or family will be unable to see the situation clearly. The health professional should expect people utilizing shock and denial to have difficulty in making decisions. At this time they usually depend on other family members or hospital personnel for input and guidance on what to do during the crisis. Reducing problems to their simplest elements and giving the patient or family limited aspects or small portions to work on assists them in relieving feelings of helplessness. Supportive listening and appropriate touch are also helpful in this stage.[7]

The grieving individual or family can exhibit other behaviors associated with the grieving process while in the emergency department. Anger is a normal part of the grief response and surfaces sooner or later. Anger and hostility are usually projected outward onto "expendable" people, which allows for the intense feelings to be expressed without jeopardizing the primary support system.[8] The hospital staff is frequently the target of this displaced anger.

Anger focused inward is frequently heard in statements of guilt or anxiety. "If only . . . ," "Why didn't I . . . ," and "I should have . . ." are statements that convey underlying guilt. Fear, helplessness, frustration, and anxiety can complicate the grief reaction seen in the emergency department. The acute nature of the emergency department allows the staff to see the patient or family only in the crisis-response stages of the grief process, a time at which the patient's behavior can be dramatically altered as he or she attempts to cope.

Grief and Death*

Most cultures throughout the world and throughout history have had some sort of mechanism for coping with the dynamics of death. The United States, however, is in a period of cultural development in which there is no readily identifiable pattern for dealing with death.[8] The manner of dying and grieving has changed radically in recent years due to our highly mobile and technological society. Dying is a significantly different event than it was one or two generations ago. As a result, grievers have to struggle through their grief without benefit of sanctioned behaviors. This has led many to hang on to cultural or religious standards for guidance in matters of disposing of the body and resolving grief.

When a patient dies, the family essentially becomes the patient. After the death, the family needs to perceive support and caring by the staff as the multitude of hospital routines surrounding death and disposal of the body are carried out.[8] Family and friends should be escorted to a private area, preferably near the emergency department. The importance of designating a private room for families in crisis cannot be overemphasized.

If life-saving measures are still in progress, someone should be designated as the liaison between the treatment room and the family. The family should be provided with as many details as possible in an effort to prepare them for what is to come. Following death, grievers seek for and sort out the details of their experience. Conveying information in an honest and caring manner makes this part of the grief work easier.[8]

The physician should make every effort to be present when the family is told of a death.[8] Although it is an unpleasant responsibility, the authority of the physician in matters of life and death lends credibility to the news. In consideration of the family, as well as the staff, the news of death should be relayed to the family as soon as possible.

There is no easy way to tell someone of the death of a loved one. Directness and honesty help. A simple statement such as "I am sorry, your son is dead" conveys the news accurately.[4] The only word for *dead* is *dead*. Words or phrases like expired, deceased, passed away, didn't make it, are substitutes that health care workers use to convey death, but frequently they do not convey the finality that the family needs to hear.[8]

Individual reactions to the news of death, however, can vary widely. All are proper, and none is a measure of the love the individual had for the dead person.[8] Some grievers cry, wail, and throw themselves on the body. Others become anesthetized and act mechanically. Still others engage in constant activity, taking care of the details, comforting others, assuming responsibility, and seeking to keep themselves in control. All of these are normal responses to grief.

Two of the most important things for grief resolution that the health care professional can give are permission and forgiveness.

> Grievers need permission to cry, to be angry, and to talk about the loss. They must learn to forgive the dead person for causing the pain, to forgive family and friends for difficulties arising during the stress, and most of all to forgive themselves for real or imagined guilt concerning their relationship with the deceased.[8]

Some people, particularly children, deal with increments of their grief and only for short periods of time.

> For a short time they will express intense grief and just as quickly they will return to play. Adults show a lack of understanding of child growth and development when they say, "It's so nice to be children; see how quickly they forget." Do not be misled. A child never forgets a primary grief. It is essential that children be involved in all grief processes.[8]

---

*This section is based on Grief and Loss by Clarice Schultz in *Emergency Medicine*, ed 1, 1983.

If adults show confidence that the child has the inner resources to deal with it, the child learns there is nothing wrong with having feelings of great sadness. If children are denied the opportunity to grieve, they will imagine occurrences that are far worse than any reality they might experience.[8]

Viewing of the body by the family is an important aspect of grief work because it results in a perceptual confirmation of the death. Most people who do not view the body at the time of death or in the emergency department are sorry later. Until they see and touch the lifeless body the news is too unbelievable to accept.[8] Seeing the body helps to set the grief work into motion.

Some individuals will state that they are not interested in viewing the body. It is wise to explore this refusal with the person. Many are afraid of what they might see or how the body may look. Some are afraid of confronting themselves with the reality of the death. As one person put it, "I wanted to see him, but I wanted to see him alive not dead." After discussing it and allowing a suitable period of time to elapse, the staff must honor the person's refusal. Realize, however, that one refusal does not speak for the whole family. Other relatives of the deceased may need to spend time with the body. Grief work can be facilitated by one member of the family who has seen the body and can share what they saw and reassure the other grievers.[8]

Though some families choose not to view the body, countless others become angry because they are advised not to see the body due to severe injuries. Later, however, they find that these injuries were actually minor compared to what they had imagined. Advice against viewing the body or misinformation about the extent of the injuries should be avoided, for it denies the family the right to choose the most appropriate means for them to cope.[8]

Seeing the body at peace brings solace to most grievers. Thus, the staff should take care in preparing the body. Immediately after death, the head of the cart or bed should be elevated slightly to prevent pooling of blood in the head and face. Tubes and equipment may be removed but do not need to be put away. The presence of equipment can be comforting, for it signifies that extraordinary efforts were used in an attempt to save the life.[8]

Every effort should be made to have a portion of the body uncovered during the viewing, even in cases of severe injury. For example, if the face has been badly damaged, the hands of a loved one can remain uncovered and will be readily recognizable to the family. Clean bandages should be applied to any mutilated parts of the body. The body should be placed with the least damaged side toward the door. Check that the hands are in a restful position, the head is on the pillow, and the sheets are neatly arranged.[8]

If the hospital has a private viewing room, it should be used. When the family views the body they should be encouraged to touch the body, to talk to the body, and to tell the body how they feel. It should be suggested that they say goodbye to the body before they leave. Many people feel embarrassed to talk to or touch the body and may need prompting or permission from the staff. Role modeling by the staff is an effective way of giving permission. Having a staff member caress the arms, stroke the hair, and initiate conversation with the body allows the family to behave similarly.[8]

Many people wish to have time alone with their loved one. If possible, give the family private time with the body. Tell them where you will be and ask them to notify you when they leave. When the family is ready to leave, again express your concern and sympathy.[8]

If the body has been severely mutilated, the staff may need to spend time with the family identifying possessions. For example, a lock of hair can be given to the family, jewelry can be identified, and roentgenograms can be shown. As much time should be spent with identifying possessions as would have been spent in viewing the body. All information possible should be shared with the family, for this is all that they have.[8]

Some people donate the body to science as a means of escaping the need for dealing with the rituals and routines of disposing of the body. The final disposition frequently brings a sense of completion to the family.[8] When the body is donated this sense of completeness may be missing and this can retard the grief work.

Many families express sorrow that they were not asked to donate organs of their dead loved one. Many people find comfort in knowing that a part of someone they loved is improving the life of another. Often they had discussed the donation of organs with the dead person and had planned to do so, but in the disorientation of the crisis, it was forgotten. If handled sensitively, medical personnel need not be reluctant to approach the family with this type of request.[8]

Grief and the Emergency Department Staff

Experiencing loss and death with patients can be draining and is a source of burnout for staff working in high-risk areas, like the emergency department. On units where large amounts of time and energy are spent on life-saving tasks, death is a sign that those efforts have been futile. To the health care worker, death is usually an unwelcome event that can arouse feelings of helplessness and failure. Death challenges the professional image and values of workers who focus on saving or prolonging life. It robs the health care worker of feelings of usefulness and being in control.

The death of a patient triggers not only a grief response to the loss of that individual, but a grief response for the loss of our aspirations and desires as professionals. It provides a dose of reality. As health care workers, we really do not have control over life and death. We simply provide an environment in which health may be facilitated. We control the environment and not the outcome. Health care workers who believe that they control the outcome may have difficulty in

Table 52-1 Staff Grieving Process

Stage	Behavior
Shock/denial	Overly efficient Preoccupied with job functions Avoidance of family except for routine information
Anger	Criticizing or lashing out at co-workers Anger at family's behavior
Guilt	Blaming self for not responding quickly enough, asking the right questions, dealing with the situation properly, etc. Feeling responsible for the outcome
Anxiety/depression	Preoccupation with replaying the event and finding ways to have altered the outcome Sense of emptiness or disillusionment about the job
Acceptance	Compassion for patient, family, and staff Can discuss death and show feelings of pain and loss appropriately

Source: Patricia S: Supporting survivors of unexpected death. In *Nursing Skillbook Series: Using Crisis Intervention.* Springhouse, PA, Intermed Communications, Inc, 1982.

coping with death. It is an event inconsistent with their belief.

The death of a patient evokes a grief response from the health care workers who have worked most closely with the patient. Table 52-1 illustrates some of the feelings and behaviors that staff members may exhibit as they move through their grief.[7] To deal with dying and death effectively, staff members must confront their own feelings about it. Staff members that have unresolved grief of their own may be particularly disturbed by the death of a patient.

The significance of a supportive staff cannot be overrated on medical units that have a high mortality rate. Sharing feelings with co-workers is one good way of gaining perspective.[7] Covering or providing relief for staff members who are temporarily having difficulty coping is important to the emotional well-being of the entire unit.

SPIRITUAL NEEDS EXPERIENCED IN CRISIS

Many health care workers relegate the patient's spiritual needs to a superficial acquaintance with specific rites, rituals, and beliefs of religion. Though spiritual needs may be associated with religion, spiritual needs are really an expression of more profound and universal concerns experienced by everyone.

Spirituality can be defined as that dimension of a person that is concerned with ultimate ends and values. Spirituality contains religious as well as existential and psychologic aspects. O'Brien[9] defines spirituality "as relating to the nonmaterial forces or elements within man. Spirituality is that which inspires in one the desire to transcend the realm of the material."

The 1971 White House Conference on Aging defined the spiritual dimension as pertaining to "man's inner resources especially his ultimate concerns, the basic value around which all other values are focused, the central philosophy of life, which guides a person's conduct, the supernatural and nonmaterial dimensions of human nature."[10,11]

The term *spirituality* can be assigned many meanings and definitions. In describing the diversity of meanings, Stoll[12] points to a number of ways in which spirituality is understood:

- as the core of one's being and personhood
- as being concerned with the meaning and purpose of one's existence
- as an experience of God as a transcendent and personal being
- as an intangible motivation moving one toward the ultimate values of love, meaning, hope, wisdom, and truth
- as a peak or supreme experience
- as a trust relationship with or in the transcendent that provides meaning to one's life

In attempting to conceptualize spirituality, three categories have emerged: spiritual distress, spiritual needs, and spiritual well-being.[10,12]

Spiritual Distress

Spiritual distress has been defined as "a disruption in the life principle which pervades a person's entire being and which integrates and transcends one's biological nature."[10]

The critical characteristic of spiritual distress as defined by the North American Nursing Diagnosis Association is the patient's expression of concern with the meaning of his or her life/death or belief system. Other characteristics include[12]:

- anger toward God
- questions regarding the meaning of suffering
- verbalization of inner conflict about one's beliefs
- verbalization of concerns with the relationship with one's deity
- questions regarding the meaning of one's own existence
- inability to participate in one's usual religious practices
- seeking out of spiritual assistance
- questions about the moral or ethical implications of one's therapeutic regimen
- gallows humor
- displacement of anger toward religious representatives

- nightmares or sleep disturbance
- alteration of behavior or mood evidenced by anger, crying, withdrawal, preoccupation, anxiety, hostility, or apathy

In keeping with the medical model, the nursing diagnosis of spiritual distress is problem oriented and based on pathology. It presupposes a previous state of spiritual well-being without an adequate understanding of what constitutes spiritual well-being for that particular patient.

Spiritual Needs

Hess and Stoll have defined spiritual needs as factors necessary to establish and maintain a relationship with God, however "God" is defined by the individual. They define five spiritual needs: forgiveness, love, hope, trust, and meaning and purpose in life.

Fish and Shelley[13] identify three spiritual needs: the need for meaning and purpose, the need for love and relatedness, and the need for forgiveness. Clinebell[6] states that human spiritual needs can be viewed as fitting into four general categories:

1. the need for meaning and purpose in life
2. the need to give love
3. the need to receive love
4. the need for hope and creativity

O'Brien[9] defines spiritual needs as "involving any essential variables required for the support and viability of that element which inspires in man the desire to transcend the realm of the material."

Although there is no definitive list of spiritual needs, there are two aspects of these needs that are worthy of discussion: the need for a transcendent relationship with a God figure (as defined by the individual), also known as religiosity; and the need meaningfully to live one's life with oneself and others in keeping with one's relationship to God, also defined as existential concerns.[12]

Spiritual Well-Being

Spiritual well-being has been defined as "the affirmation of life in a relationship with God, self, community, and environment that nurtures and celebrates wholeness."[10–12]

Ellison[11] believes that spiritual well-being involves a religious (religiosity) and a psychosocial (existential) component. The religious component refers to a sense of well-being that one has in relation to God and is described as the vertical dimension, implying a transcendent relationship with God. The psychosocial component refers to a sense of life purpose and life satisfaction with no reference to anything specifically religious. This is known as the horizontal dimension or existential well-being.

Ellison[11] believes that the spiritual dimension synthesizes the total personality and provides a sense of direction and order. It is the integrative force behind the mind and body and thus affects both mental and physical well-being. The question concerning spiritual well-being is not whether it is present but to what degree it is present and how health professionals can enhance the degree of spiritual well-being of a patient.

Religiosity

It is recognized that psychodynamically there are different ways of being religious. The two most popular ways of looking at religiosity have been proposed by Batson and Ventis.[14] Allport[14] distinguishes between extrinsic and intrinsic religion. The extrinsic religious orientation is one in which religion is used to justify self-centered ends in a strictly utilitarian way for one's safety, social standing, and solace and for endorsing one's chosen way of life. By contrast, the intrinsic religious orientation is one in which religious commitments are carefully thought out and taken seriously as a major goal in life. The internal religious orientation regards faith as a supreme value in its own right. "The extrinsically motivated individual uses his religion, whereas the intrinsically motivated lives his."[14]

Spilka[14] offers another way of distinguishing between religious orientations by comparing consensual and committed religion. Committed religion is defined as a discerning, highly differentiated, candid, open, self-critical, abstract, and relational approach to religious questions. Consensual religion is the opposite of this.

The models of Allport and Spilka provide a two-dimensional analysis of the role of religion in the life of a believer. A three-dimensional analysis of religious orientation has been proposed by Clark.[14] To the two previously discussed dimensions, Clark adds a third: religion as a quest. Individuals who approach religion as a quest are involved in an open-ended, critical struggle with existential questions. They attempt honestly to face existential questions in all their complexity while resisting clear-cut pat answers provided by religious dogma. It is probable that the quest orientation is psychologically more adaptive than the other two orientations.

Spiritual Concerns During Crisis

When patients or families talk about their responses to illness, suffering, and crisis, the meaning of their lives, and their "when the chips are down" attitudes, they are asking for help with spiritual questions.[6]

Dealing with such patients is a bilevel process of helping the person cope with the immediate crisis and encouraging him or her to examine the underlying value-related spiritual questions that the current situation has evoked. Helping patients and families face the problems of inadequate meanings and distorted or destructive values and lifestyles begins to address some of the factors that keep patients and families in self-destructive and unhealthy modes of existence.

People in crisis frequently perceive the spiritual issues in their experience. The common questions "Why is this happening?" and "Why now?" speak to spiritual concerns, raising the issues of meaning and purpose.[1] When death is involved, the question of the meaning and purpose of life is crucial to the survivors.

Illness, crisis, and death have no meaning in and of themselves. It is the person experiencing the crisis who gives it meaning.[1] People who have no faith or belief in a god frequently view their experiences and gain their meanings through a psychological perspective. Individuals who have a faith or belief in a god may seek to understand the psychological impact, but will also turn to their relationship with their god to explain and give meaning to what is happening.

People have different personal beliefs and experiences with what they perceive as God. *God* can be defined as whatever the person holds to be the highest or ultimate value in life.[1] In Christian religions the ultimate value is *agape* or unconditional love (love which demands nothing). The life of Jesus Christ exemplifies this spiritual principle. In some of the eastern religions there is no supreme being defined as God. Instead, God is perceived as a state of being and true reality that is not a person.

How God is perceived is not as important as the role that perception plays in the person's life. The person who believes that God is a very real being, involved in human experience, and providing opportunities for growth in even the most devastating situations will experience illness, crisis, and death in a much different way than the person who thinks of God only in an emergency or crisis with the hopes of being saved or spared. For some, God remains a nonentity even in times of crisis.

Emergency situations can be times of real spiritual crisis where persons feel that the significant meanings or values of their lives are being threatened or are lost.[1] They may feel abandoned by their god. Emergencies can also be a time of tremendous spiritual growth and reliance on one's faith for help and support.

Assessment

An assessment of the patient or family's spiritual needs can be divided into four areas of concern: the person's concept of God or deity; the person's source of strength, hope, and meaning; the significance of religious practices and rituals to the person; and the person's perceived relationship between his or her spiritual beliefs and his or her health.[15]

An assessment of the spiritual needs can start with a few very basic questions. A simple question, such as, "Do you have a faith?" opens the door for the patient to begin expressing his or her spiritual needs. This question is benign because it does not imply religion or a specific concept of God. A more direct method would be to ask the patient how important religion or God is to him or her. Other questions that can facilitate the assessment of the patient's spiritual beliefs are[6,15]:

- Does God or a deity function in your personal life? How?
- Does what is happening to you now have any meaning for you in terms of your faith?
- Do you have a philosophy of life that helps you through the hard times?
- When you need help, what comforts and supports you best?
- Do your values and beliefs provide you with the strength to deal with crisis, loss, and death?
- Do your values and beliefs provide you with a sense of hope?
- Are religious practices and rituals important to you? Would you like your pastor or the hospital chaplain called?
- Is prayer, meditation, or reading of sacred books or writings, like the Bible, important to you? Would it help now? Would you like to pray together?
- Do your values and beliefs help or hinder your health, mental and emotional well-being, and relationships to others?

Religious Resources

Religious resources can be tremendously helpful when used appropriately. This is usually seen as, but is not exclusively, the domain of the chaplain. When using religious resources it is wise to consider the following[6]:

1. Use religious resources only after the patient and family's feelings and attitudes about religion are determined. Patients who have no value for prayer or scripture can be easily alienated by a well-intentioned health care worker or chaplain.
2. Ask if spiritual support would be meaningful. This shows respect for the patient's feelings and beliefs. If it is important to the patient it may be appropriate to call a chaplain. Several Bibles or inspirational books kept on the unit can be used with patients and families that wish that type of support.
3. With patients requesting spiritual intervention, allow the patient and family the opportunity to use prayer and religious materials as a means of catharsis. Be willing to allow any thoughts or feelings triggered by religious practices to be expressed.
4. Never feel that religious words or resources need to be used with patients experiencing spiritual needs. God is continually active in all relationships, whether or not formal religious resources are used. Discussing with the patients their concerns about how their beliefs are being affected by the situation may be the most prac-

tical means of handling some patients. Guided imagery, relaxation techniques, and right-brain communication can be excellent substitutes for prayer.

Health care workers should be sensitive to the attitudes and beliefs of various religious groups. Understanding a patient's religious beliefs can dramatically affect how the staff perceives the patient and the type of care appropriate for that patient.

For example, many orthodox and fundamentalist groups believe that illness and disease are a divine punishment or test of faith. The guilt associated with being punished can tremendously affect the patient's response to treatment.[16]

Some religious groups, such as the Christian Scientists, deny the reality of discomfort spiritually, emotionally, and physically. Strict adherents to this faith avoid medical consultation, deny need for treatment, and rely on church practitioners for health concerns. They rarely enter the traditional medical system and may suffer tremendous feelings of personal and spiritual failure if they need to surrender to the medical staff.[16]

Some religious groups support modern medicine but object to specific practices. The Seventh Day Adventist Church urges its members to avoid drugs unless absolutely necessary. Many churches, notably the Roman Catholic Church, Greek Orthodox Church, and Jehovah's Witnesses, oppose abortion, regardless of the medical reason or risk to the mother.[16] Many Hindus consider the loss of a limb as a sign of wrongdoing from a previous life. Orthodox Jews and some Roman Catholics require burial of an amputated limb.[16] Jehovah's Witnesses oppose transfusions and transplants, as well as medications that require blood for their manufacture. They do, however, approve of certain intravenous feedings.

Anointing, laying on of hands, confession, communion, observance of the Sabbath and holy days, and restrictions in diet or physical appearance are issues that vary from religion to religion. The best way of determining the patient's needs on these issues is to ask the patient or family.

BELIEFS AND PRACTICES OF VARIOUS RELIGIOUS GROUPS*

Adventists (Seventh Day Adventist, Advent Christian Church)

Beliefs

The dead are only asleep and will be physically resurrected on Christ's return. Some believe in divine healing and practice anointing with oil and the use of prayer. The Bible is interpreted literally.

---

*Sources: Pumphrey, J: Recognizing your patients' spiritual needs. *Nursing 77*, December 1977; Carson, VB: *Spiritual Dimensions of Nursing Practice*, 1989.

Practices

Baptism by immersion for adults only. Dedication services for children if requested. No alcohol, coffee, tea, tobacco, narcotics, or stimulants. No special practices surrounding death. Many groups prohibit the eating of meat, and most avoid pork. Some oppose the use of hypnosis. Saturday is the Sabbath.

Armenian

Beliefs

No conflict between the Church and medicine.

Practices

Baptism by immersion 8 days after birth, followed by immediate confirmation. Communion performed as last rites. Advocate laying on of hands. Fasting during Lent and 6 hours before communion.

Baha'i

Beliefs

No conflict between the Church and medicine. Spiritual health and physical health are interrelated. Prayer and fasting, if permissible, are essential adjuncts to medical healing.

Practices

No baptism or last rites. Alcohol and drugs permitted only with physician's orders.

Baptist (More than 27 Different Groups in the United States)

Beliefs

The Bible is the supreme authority. Some groups have difficulty with medicine because it accepts the theory of evolution. Most groups believe that God works through the physician.

Practices

Baptism of only believers by immersion. No infant baptism. Abstinence from alcohol, coffee, and tea for many groups. Belief in laying on of hands. Prayer with clergy important to family if death is involved.

Buddhist

Beliefs

No conflict between the Church and medicine. Illness is a trial to aid the development of the soul.

Practices

Some groups discourage use of alcohol, tobacco, and drugs. Last rite chanting is often practiced at the bedside soon after death. The body is cremated. Holy days for some groups: January 1 and 16, February 15, March 21, April 8, May 21, July 15, September 1 and 23, December 8 and 31.

Christian Scientist

Beliefs

Deny the existence of illness. Sickness and sin are the errors of the human mind and can be eliminated by spiritual truth, not by drugs or medicines. Many will refuse all medical treatment.

Practices

Have their own practitioners and nurses who administer support and health care. No infant baptism. No alcohol, coffee, tea, tobacco, or other drugs. No blood transfusions. Vaccines and autopsies only when required by law. No biopsies. Organ donation is unlikely but is considered a personal decision. No last rites. Cremation and burial both acceptable.

Church of Christ

Beliefs

No conflict between the Church and medicine, but a recognition of human limitations of medicine.

Practices

Communion, anointing with oil, and laying on of hands by the minister for healing. No alcohol. No last rites. Baptism by immersion after age eight. No objections to medical treatment on the Sabbath (Sunday).

Church of God

Beliefs

Divine healing is through prayer, though more liberal groups do not prohibit medical therapy at the same time. Speaking in tongues is part of the mystical experience.

Practices

No alcohol or tobacco. No baptism at birth. No last rites. No cremation.

Church of Jesus Christ of Latter-Day Saints (Mormon)

Beliefs

Divine healing through laying on of hands, though medical therapy not prohibited. Strong tradition of revelation through visions.

Practices

Baptism by immersion after age 8. No cremation. Baptism and preaching of the Gospel to the dead. No alcohol, coffee, tea, or tobacco. Sparing use of meats. Special undergarments worn. Sacrament of the Last Supper administered on Sunday.

Disciples of Christ (Christian Church)

Beliefs

No conflict between the Church and medicine.

Practices

No infant baptism, but a dedication service may be requested. Believers baptized by immersion. Communion is central to Sunday worship and may be provided by the pastor in the hospital. No special practices surrounding death. Church elders as well as clergy may provide spiritual support.

Eastern Orthodox

Beliefs

No conflict between the Church and medicine.

Practices

Baptism within 40 days of birth. Baptism is by immersion followed by immediate confirmation. Last rites are obligatory. Cremation is discouraged. Anointing of the sick is a form of healing by prayer. Hospitalized persons are exempt from fasting. Christmas is celebrated on January 7 and the New Year on January 14.

Episcopal (Anglican)

Beliefs

No conflict between the Church and medicine.

Practices

Infant baptism. Baptism is urgent if the newborn is likely to die. Last rites are not mandatory. Some groups believe in spiritual healing. Some abstain from meat on Friday and fast before communion.

Grace Brethren (Church of the Brethren)

Beliefs

No conflict between the Church and medicine.

Practices

No infant baptism, but may have a dedication service for children. Baptism by immersion for only those old enough to profess faith. Anointing of the sick for physical and spiritual healing. No last rites, but clergy to be notified for counsel and prayer at the time of death. Abstinence from alcohol, tobacco, and illicit drugs. Cremation permitted. Stillborn infants are buried.

Greek Orthodox

Beliefs

No conflict between the Church and medicine. Oppose euthanasia; every effort should be made to preserve life until terminated by God.

Practices

Baptism within 40 days of birth is essential. Communion is considered last rites. Autopsies and cremation discouraged. Fasting from meat and some dairy products on Wednesday, Friday, and during Lent. Holy Communion and Holy Unction can be provided by a priest on request.

Hindu

Beliefs

Most groups accept modern medical practices.

Practices

Prescribed rites follow death: priest ties a thread around the neck or wrist signifying a blessing, priest pours water into the mouth of the corpse, family washes the body. Particular about who touches the dead. Bodies are cremated. Some conditions, like loss of limb, represent sins from a previous life. Many dietary restrictions, dependent on the sect.

Jehovah's Witnesses

Beliefs

Oppose "false teachings" of other religions, which often extends to medicine. Attempt to convert others.

Practices

No infant baptism. No last rites. Use of alcohol and tobacco is discouraged. Cremation is acceptable. Autopsy is by personal decision. Opposed to abortion and blood transfusions. Organ transplants are optional, but if performed the organ must be cleaned with a nonblood solution.

Judaism

Beliefs

No conflict between the Church and medicine. Ill persons are required to seek medical assistance. Someone should be with the person when the soul leaves the body, so that family and/or friends should be allowed to stay with critically ill patients.

Practices

Male circumcision on day 8 after birth. Fetus, organs, body parts, and tissues must be buried. Abortion permitted only to save the life of the mother. Kosher dietary laws include no mixing of milk and meat at a meal, no eating of animals not slaughtered in accordance with Jewish law, use of separate cooking utensils for meat and milk products, 24-hour fast during Yom Kippur (although exceptions can be made for medical reasons), no leavened products during Passover. Opposed to euthanasia, autopsy, and cremation. Donation or transplantation requires consultation with rabbi. Sabbath is from sunset Friday to sunset Saturday; medical or surgical procedures should be postponed during this time if possible. In case of impending death, Psalms 23, 103, and 139 may be read. Last words heard should be "Hear O Israel, the Lord is our God, the Lord is One." After death the body should be untouched for 8 to 30 minutes. Preparation of the body after death should be by an Orthodox person or the Jewish Burial Society. Burial within 24 hours. No burial on the Sabbath (Saturday).

Lutheran (10 Different Branches)

Beliefs

No conflict between the Church and medicine.

Practices

Baptism 6 to 8 weeks after birth by immersion or sprinkling with water. Last rites optional. Anointing may be requested.

Mennonite (12 Different Groups)

Beliefs

No conflict between the Church and medicine. Deep concern for self-determination and avoidance of treatments that affect the individual personality or will. A nonsacramental church.

Practices

No infant baptism (baptism in teens). A child may be dedicated at the request of the parents. No last rites, communion, or other sacraments. Abstinence from alcohol. Prayer is highly important in times of crisis. Women may wear head coverings during hospitalization.

Methodist (More than 20 Different Groups)

Beliefs

Divine judgment: The good will be rewarded and the evil punished. Ministers counsel but do not hear confession.

Practices

Baptism for children and adults. Communion may be requested. Scripture reading and prayer are important at the time of death. Donation of organs is encouraged.

Moravian

Beliefs

Disease is not a form of divine punishment, although breaking from God can lead to physical problems.

Practices

Infant baptism. No last rites. Do not believe that life should be extended at all costs, but the patient should be kept comfortable. Communion and laying on of hands may be requested.

Muslim (Moslem, Islam)

Beliefs

Conservative groups can have a fatalistic view that can affect compliance with therapy.

Practices

No baptism. Fetuses aborted after 130 days must be buried according to custom. Abortion forbidden. Women are not allowed to sign consent forms. Patient must confess sins and beg forgiveness before death in the presence of the family. The family washes and prepares the body, then turns it toward Mecca. Only family or friends may prepare the body. Health care workers may be allowed to prepare the body if they wear gloves. No autopsies or removal of body parts unless required by law. Burial as soon as possible after death. No cremation. Donation of organs not allowed. No alcohol or pork products eaten. Daylight fast during Ramadan (ninth month of the Islamic year). The Koran must not be touched by anyone ritually unclean. Nothing may be placed on top of the Koran. Certain items of jewelry, such as bangles, may have religious significance and should not be removed.

Native American

Beliefs

There are approximately 300 different tribal groups each with its own nature-oriented religion. Disease has two principal forms: the presence of a material object in the body and the absence of the soul from the body. Protection against disease occurs through the use of superhuman powers.

Practices

Most native American religions have elements of magic, folklore, disease treatment, and herbal medicine. Medicine men and shamans perform the symbolic rites against disease.

Nazarene

Beliefs

No conflict between the Church and medicine. Believe in divine healing but not exclusive of medical treatment.

Practices

Baptism optional, not considered a saving sacrament. No last rites. Cremation permitted. Stillborns are buried. Communion and laying on of hands by pastor as a means of grace. No alcohol or tobacco.

Pentecostal (Assembly of God, Foursquare Church)

Beliefs

Illness considered an intrusion of Satan. Deliverance from illness is provided in atonement. Pray for divine intervention for self and others when ill.

Practices

Baptism by immersion after age of accountability. No last rites. Divine healing through anointing, prayer, and laying on of hands. No alcohol, tobacco, or illicit drugs. No eating of strangled animals or anything to which blood has been added. May refuse pork products.

Presbyterian (10 Different Groups)

Beliefs

Science to be utilized for relief of suffering and is recognized as a gift from God. Full forgiveness through repentance for any illness connected with a sin.

Practices

Infant baptism. Last rites not a sacrament and involve reading of scripture and prayer. Communion may be requested.

Quaker (Friends)

Beliefs

No creed, so that there is a diversity of personal beliefs. Pacifists. God is in every person and can be approached directly. Emphasis on individual choice and decision making.

Practices

No baptism at birth. No rituals surrounding death. Leave decision making up to the individual. Most Quakers avoid alcohol and drugs.

Roman Catholic

Beliefs

No conflict between the Church and medicine except for the issue of abortion on demand. Donation or transplantation of organs permitted if no harm is done to the donor.

Practices

Infant baptism is mandatory. Emergency baptism for neonates with a poor prognosis, stillborns, and fetuses if not clinically dead (determined by evidence of tissue necrosis). Last rites or anointing of the sick mandatory. Some dioceses require that amputated limbs be buried. Fasting and abstinence from meat on Ash Wednesday and Good Friday (obligatory fasting is excused during hospitalization).

Russian Orthodox

Beliefs

No conflict between the Church and medicine.

Practices

Baptism by priest only. No autopsies, embalming, or cremation. After death, arms are crossed with fingers set in a cross. Clothing of dead must be of natural fiber to decompose faster. Male patients not to be shaved unless absolutely necessary. Cross necklace worn and is important and should be left in place. Abstinence from meat and dairy products on Wednesday and Friday and during Lent.

Salvation Army

Beliefs

No conflict between the Church and medicine except for the issue of abortion on demand. Bible seen as the only rule for one's faith.

Practices

Infant dedication ceremony. No particular baptism, communion, or death practices.

Unitarian (Universalist)

Beliefs

Reason and practicality are most important. Each person has the right to approach values individually. Some may prefer not to have clergy visit if they are assuming responsibility for themselves.

Practices

Baptism by choice and without a trinitarian formula. Dedication of children. No official sacraments. Cremation often preferred to burial. Attitudes toward immortality vary widely. Organ donation advocated.

NONMEDICAL METHODS OF HEALING

The idea of divine healing has long been a part of the Judeo-Christian tradition. In light of the fact that Jewish and Christian traditions are predominant in Western culture, it may be helpful for health professionals to have some understanding of what is meant by the term *divine* or *spiritual healing*.

In a secular society, nontheists usually believe that healing is due to the forces of nature or is the result of human effort (or both). Theists, on the other hand, believe that God is responsible for healing. Theists generally fall into two categories: traditional and postmodern. Traditional theists attribute all healing solely to God. Postmodern theists do not attribute healing solely to God but see it as the conjoined action of God and human effort.[17]

Traditional theism usually espouses the following beliefs regarding divine healing:

- By virtue of God's omnipotence, God is capable of healing any and all human afflictions.
- When healing occurs, it is the result of God's direct intervention, which may include circumventing or overriding preexisting laws of healing.
- It is frequently necessary for individuals to petition God to become a recipient of divine healing.
- Human faith plays a critical role in all forms of divine healing.
- When God's healing does occur, it happens immediately.

In contrast, a postmodern view of divine healing concludes the following[17]:

- Despite God's tremendous power, there are limits to what God can heal unilaterally.
- God does not heal by divine intervention in the sense of using extraordinary means but rather by supporting the natural laws of healing that have already been established by God.
- Petitioning God for healing is rarely required.
- Faith, although critical in some instances, is not an essential ingredient in most forms of divine healing.
- Healing is seldom an immediate event.

Postmodern theists see humans as being in a relationship with and participating with God. As such, the postmodern position sees humans as co-healers with God. This does not imply that God's power and human power are equivalent but rather that God and humanity are in a relationship that requires input from both sides.[17]

In discussing present-day nonmedical methods of healing, Weatherhead[18] states that the art of healing is not the exclusive province of medicine. He avoids use of the term *spiritual* or *divine healing* because it implies a distinction or separation between the various forms of healing. "All healing is of God. No man has ever healed another. All he has done is cooperate with God either on the physical, psychical, or spiritual levels of man's personality."[18]

Weatherhead[18] lists the following as methods of nonmedical healing:

- methods that involve suggestion: hypnosis and autosuggestion
- methods that involve psychic abilities: spiritualism and odic forces
- methods involving the Church: healing missions, laying on of hands, intercession for the sick, confession, and psychotherapeutic conversations

Methods involving suggestion are currently employed by health professionals and are detailed in the next section. Methods of nonmedical healing that involve psychic abilities include various PSI phenomena as studied in the field of parapsychology. One of the most famous cases is that of Oskar Estebany, who claimed the ability to heal by the laying on of hands. He was involved in a set of experiments at McGill University in Montreal, Canada. In the first experiment superficial wounds were made on the backs of mice, some of which were treated by Estebany, who held them in a container for two 15-minute periods daily until the wounds healed. Control mice were placed in similar containers and either were left untreated or were treated in the identical manner as those in the Estebany group except by persons making no claim of having a gift of healing. The results showed that the rate of wound healing was significantly faster in the group treated by Estebany than in the other two groups. A second experiment involved the rate of growth of barley seeds in containers held by Estebany, in containers held by a person claiming no gift of healing, and in containers not held. Again, the containers held by Estebany showed a significant increase in the rate of barley growth compared with the other types of containers.[19]

The methods of nonmedical healing that Weatherhead[18] lists as involving the Church are essentially methods that utilize the power of ritual. Illness is an alienating and fragmenting experience, an experience of liminality. Rituals assist people in a liminal state to reframe and reassemble their lives into new patterns of significance. Rituals allow for the expression of "an immediate human future and at the same time [contain] a pledge of an eschatological future from which all life takes its ultimate meaning."[20] The most common rituals that accompany illness are the laying on of hands and anointing with oil.

On the level of religious experience, laying on of hands is an act of identification, aggregation, and restoration that has a multiplicity of meanings in various religious traditions. In the First Testament it represents the coalescing of two themes: that a person is able to communicate his or her numen (spirit) to another through rituals of bodily touching, and that the person's hand is a symbol of his or her personal power. Thus the laying on of hands symbolizes the transmission of life force or divine force from one person to another. This power-laden gesture is used to represent a divinely enacted blessing, which could include the restoration of health.

The Second Testament cites Jesus as performing healing miracles through the laying on of hands. The laying on of hands in the Second Testament contains the same fundamental concepts as in the First Testament except that the rite is acted out in the name of that Lord and symbolizes the transmission of the power of the Holy Spirit.

The laying on of hands provides to the believer the hope not only of bodily healing but of the healing of the total person who is fractured and alienated and has lost a sense of the future. It does this through the symbolic renewal of the promise of both an individual and an eschatological future, not in denial of one's mortality but in confrontation with it.[19] The laying on of hands is also a gesture of reconciliation; through its implicit statement of the acceptability of the sick person, it may release the patient from any guilt or worthlessness that may have been self-imposed.

Anointing with oil is symbolically similar to the laying on of hands. They both are rituals of touch, have a common history, and are used in the rituals of initiation, ordination, and healing. In both the First and Second Testaments oil was used in religious rites and as a medicinal remedy.

TECHNIQUES FOR PSYCHOSPIRITUAL SUPPORT*

During crisis patients need comfort and support. How this is provided depends entirely on the patient. The patient is responsible for conveying his or her needs to the health care worker, but in crisis many patients are unable to articulate what they need. Thus, the health care worker must have skills designed to help the patients define their needs.

The necessary skills relate to the ability to communicate. Some of these skills involve general principles of communication, like effective listening and joint exploration. Other techniques, such as right-brain techniques, require more

---

*This section was based on Emotional and Spiritual Support by Ruth Stoll in *Emergency Medicine*, ed 1, 1983.

specialized skills for dealing with psychospiritual needs and crisis situations.

Therapeutic Use of Self

Some people are able to provide support more effectively than others. These people tend to be highly intuitive and sensitive individuals who are able to use themselves as instruments of care. Therapeutic use of self requires knowledge of and comfort with one's identity. It requires a profound understanding of the human condition, one's spiritual values, and one's philosophy on life, illness, and suffering, and an ability to help others find meaning in their situation.[1] People who use themselves therapeutically are able to facilitate growth, even in crisis.

The therapeutic use of self implies a self-awareness and sensitivity to one's own behavior and the effect of that behavior on others.[1] This involves an awareness of the possibility of countertransference. Countertransference is the development of particular feelings toward a patient because the patient represents a significant figure from the health care worker's past.[21] Countertransference is an unconscious process. Being aware of one's personal strengths and weaknesses and being alert for development of this phenomenon is essential in therapeutic use of self.

Working out one's unresolved problems in the work setting is an inappropriate use of self and can be detrimental to the patient. Unconscious communication of detachment, defensiveness, or impatience may be ways that the health care worker protects himself or herself against sensory overload and painful involvement with patients. However, these can be interpreted by patients as rejection, which undermines the patient's self-esteem and causes him or her to withdraw.[1] Nonverbal communication, including body language, voice inflections, and choice of certain words, are aspects of care that can be used in either a positive therapeutic fashion or in a negative nontherapeutic way. The use of nonverbal communication is generally left to the discretion of the health care worker and is at the core of therapeutic use of self. Health care workers need to be aware of their own needs and coping behaviors and must be willing to develop alternate coping strategies when their behavior interferes with their ability to help.[1] Recognizing one's unspoken messages to patients and families is a vital part of being supportive.

Health care workers cannot give what they do not possess.[1] Assessing one's personal strengths, limitations, capacities, resources, and susceptibility to pain and crisis and then planning for development of knowledge and skills in areas of deficit is important for growth within one's role. Health care workers, therefore, must be willing to work on themselves for the ultimate benefit of those they aid. For mastering the healing arts, self-exploration and self-confrontation are as important as learning skills and reading the literature.

Communication: Listening and Responding

Patients in crisis are frequently unable to communicate their needs clearly or adequately to hospital personnel. Thus, a major component of providing psychospiritual support is to pay attention to the patients' verbal and nonverbal behavior and help them see, organize, and interpret this information in a more objective manner that allows them to articulate their needs. This requires the attention and concentration of the health care worker on the patient and his or her problems. It requires that the health care worker listen to the patient and reflect what he or she is saying. Sometimes this can be done quickly, other times it requires an investment of time that the staff does not have. When time is not available, the worker should honestly acknowledge this to the patient and state clearly what help is possible. It may be possible to return at a later time or to provide another resource. The staff and the patient should know the boundaries of the help available; this knowledge provides security.[1]

Listening allows the patient to verbalize feelings and reactions, to understand, and to be understood. It is an active process whereby the health care worker tries to see things from the patient's point of view. It requires the use of more than one sense. It means making eye contact, observing body movements, body position, and underlying messages, relevant omissions, and patterns or themes. Touch can be used to "listen" to physiologic reactions, such as trembling, body rigidity, or cold, clammy hands.[1]

In conjunction with listening, the health care worker must respond to the patient. Responses should be tailored to what the health care worker wishes to learn or convey. The basic types of responses include the following[6]:

- *supportive:* to reassure and reduce the patient's anxiety
- *interpretive:* to impart meaning, explain why, or teach
- *probing:* to seek further information or discuss a point further
- *evaluating:* to indicate that a judgment has been or is being made about the patient or his or her condition
- *advising:* to recommend certain actions, approaches, beliefs, or attitudes
- *understanding:* to communicate understanding or seek clarification of what is happening to ensure that the health care worker does understand

Thus, listening includes paraphrasing and clarifying what is said. This does not mean parroting what has been said in a mindless manner but seeking to understand what is meant.[1] It is important for the health care worker to validate what is heard, seen, and felt from the patient to be certain that the interpretation is accurate.

One of the largest barriers to sensitive listening and responding is selective hearing. Selective hearing occurs when the health care worker hears only what he or she wants to hear. This happens frequently when strong emotions, such as anger and despair, or spiritual needs are expressed by the patient.[1]

Effective listening allows the patients to share at whatever level is comfortable for them. The levels at which communication occur are those of facts, opinions, and feelings. The level of feelings is the closest to disclosure of the real person.[1]

Initial remarks, such as "It must really hurt," "You really look concerned; let's talk about it," or "What helps you cope?" facilitate patient exploration. If the patient appears receptive, the health care worker can provide an opportunity to externalize and sort out the feelings and thoughts of the patient. Open-ended questions and reassuring gestures or phrases encourage the patient or family to continue recounting events and perceptions. Through this process, patients begin to recognize their situation. They may be able to shed their denial or acknowledge the pain of their loss. The health care worker can be a sounding board, helping the patient confront reality.[1]

The health care worker is in a key position to encourage hope within the patient. "Hope is the ability to see a way through, to have a sense of confidence that there is an anchor or that there are some alternative options and possibilities."[1] When a patient is in an emergency situation and in crisis, hope may be lost. It is impossible to see beyond the present moment, and that experience may be overwhelming. Depression and despair are likely to occur. Realistic hope is the mobilization of available resources so that action can be taken to reorganize one's life.[1]

Hope is fostered under conditions of mutuality. Patients derive a sense of hope from the health care worker who believes in their abilities and encourages them. Setting short-term achievable goals with patients increases hope:

> This may mean planning the next hour: Who should be called? Were children left alone? What hospital routines and procedures must be done? Allowing patients to participate in the decision-making processes and actions enhances feelings of hope.[1]

Special Communication Techniques

Specialized communication techniques that employ the use of the right side of the brain are powerful treatment modalities. Though use of right-brain communication is in no way new, it has only recently been used in the medical setting. Right-brain treatment techniques are effective clinical tools that require a degree of skill and practice. The techniques must be learned and practiced before they can be effective.

Right-brain communication techniques stem from studies done on the functions of the left and right hemispheres of the brain. The left brain performs rational, analytical functions and the right brain metaphorical, synthesizing, and holistic functions. As a result people communicate through two quite different languages: precise, logical left brain expression and figurative, metaphorical right-brain talk.[22]

An important function of the right brain is to synthesize each person's life experiences into a holistic image unique to that person. The individual then uses that image to interpret and make sense of reality. The person perceives life through that image and responds to the world on the basis of perceptions colored by that image. For a person's responses to change there must be a change in that personal image. Those changes occur through right-brain communication.[22]

As with most clinical intervention, use of the right-brain techniques require that a therapeutic rapport be established with the patient. Thus, skill with the more traditional communication skills and therapeutic use of self is essential.

NEUROLINGUISTIC PROGRAMMING

Neurolinguistic programming (NLP) is a relatively new approach to understanding communication. NLP has as its base the disciplines of linguistics and psychiatry.[23] NLP is concerned with the manner in which individuals take in and make sense of information. Although NLP believes that there are four sensory modes used for accessing and processing information, only three are used for verbal communication. These are: visual, auditory, and kinesthetic. Most people tend to favor one mode, though they will use all three to some extent. Highly effective communicators tend to be proficient in the use of all three modes and can move from one to another with relative ease.[23]

The selection of words that people use when explaining or describing a situation gives a strong clue as to which mode they prefer. People who are highly visual will tend to process information using words such as *see*, *view*, *imagine*, and *look* when they converse. People who are highly auditory will use language such as *hear*, *take in*, *sounds like*, and *listen* in their descriptions. Kinesthetic people use words such as *feel*, *stir*, *sharpen*, and *soften* when they converse.[24] By listening to the patient's choice of words the health care worker can determine the patient's representational system. Then in responding to the patient, he or she can select words that match the patient's representational system. This increases the possibility of establishing rapport with the patient.

The health care worker needs to be aware of his or her own predominant mode of perceiving and processing information, then work at learning how to switch to the other modes so that they may be used when communicating with patients. The mirroring of the words of a patient's representational system is a powerful therapeutic tool. An example of how to communicate in each of the three representational systems using the same thought follows[23]:

1. *Visual:* I can see that you are much better. You look good. Your eyes are clear. Your appearance has certainly changed.
2. *Auditory:* I can hear from the sound of your voice that you are better. Talking with you now is quite different from an hour ago. You really sound good.
3. *Kinesthetic:* You seem to be feeling much better. You're holding your head up. Your grasp is firmer. You have a good hold on things.

NLP is a method for improving and expanding effective communication. Matching your verbal responses to the patient's representational system increases the probability of establishing a therapeutic rapport, helping patients express their needs and assisting them in understanding what is happening. Table 52-2 gives some word choices particular to each of the three sensory modes.

Pacing and Leading

An excellent adjunct to matching the patient's verbal behavior is the matching of nonverbal behavior through techniques such as pacing and leading.[25] Pacing is the attempt to gradually change aspects of patients' behavior by getting them to follow the lead of the health care worker. For example the first attempt would be to subtly match the patient's body position and speech pattern (matching). Then, slowly and smoothly the health care worker begins to change his position and posture and observe if the patient is following (pacing). If not, the health care worker returns to matching and then after a while attempts a different behavior change. If the patient begins to follow the pacing, it is then called leading.

The experience of pain and crisis lends itself nicely to the use of matching, pacing, and leading. For example, if a patient is writhing in pain and screaming, "I hurt! I hurt! Oh God, I hurt!" the health care worker can move in on that patient, touch him or her, and in a loud voice state "You hurt! You hurt! God, you hurt!" (matching). The matching of the patient's words, voice tone, and body position can continue as long as necessary for the patient to realize that the hurt is being communicated. Pacing can then begin. "You wish it would stop hurting. Maybe it won't hurt so much in a minute. Maybe it will stop hurting soon, just lie still." The pacing helps to establish that the patient's desire for the pain to decrease has been communicated. It also expresses protection for the patient (lie still). As the health care worker continues with verbal pacing, the voice should decrease in volume and become softer, and the body position should relax. This constitutes nonverbal pacing.[25]

Watch for feedback from the patient. Is he or she more relaxed, quieter, calmer? Is he or she taking the lead? If not, return to matching.[25] Use a different set of suggestions when pacing is done for the second time. "You wish it would stop hurting. You want some medicine for the pain. Maybe the pain will let up while we wait for the doctor." Pacing is not an exact science and may require several attempts before a suggestion is given to which the patient will respond.

Matching, pacing, and leading are special skills that improve with knowledge and practice. They begin with the experience of the patient, and require the health care worker to give clear, firm, and simply stated assistance. They allow the health care worker to lead the patient to a calmer experience through therapeutic suggestion.

Hypersuggestion and Hypnosis

Pain and crisis lead to a state of hypersuggestibility. Matching, pacing, and leading techniques capitalize on this, but techniques of hypnosis can also make use of the suggestibility brought about by the crisis.

Hypnosis and the legalities surrounding the use of hypnosis still remain controversial in today's society.[26] Caution should be exercised when working with patients who are in a state of hypersuggestibility that no attempt is made to work on the psychodynamics of the patient. In the emergency care setting the only appropriate use of hypnotic techniques is to restore the security and equilibrium of the patient.

There are gray areas in the use and definition of hypnosis. Usually as long as the word *hypnosis* is not used, or traditional induction techniques are not employed, no claim can be made that the patient was hypnotized. Many of the phenomena associated with hypnosis and hypersuggestibility are present during crisis and can be capitalized on for the benefit of the patient. Some of the phenomena that might be seen in the emergency setting are as follows[26]:

Table 52-2 Word Choices in NLP

Visual	Auditory	Kinesthetic
see	listen	feel
observe	hear	turn
view	gripe	thin-skinned
perceive	hassle	tender
discern	attend	stir
sight	give an ear to	excite
discover	get	arouse
notice	eavesdrop	sharpen
distinguish	hang on every word	sore spot
recognize	take in	itch
imagine	overhear	creeps
look	register	sting
catch sight of	reach	tingle
behold	hearsay	shudder

Source: Knowles R: Through neuro-linguistic programming. *Am J Nurs*, July 1983.

- *Figures of authority:* For many people, the presence or the reassuring word or touch of a physician, nurse, priest, or other health care worker who appears to be in authority is all that is required for the patient to accept that everything will be taken care of and that there is hope. Using phrases such as "I've treated similar cases as this with great success," or when accurate, "Everything is going well" or even "Everything is all right" if said sincerely will be readily accepted by patients. Be careful not to say things that are not accurate for they will readily accept them also.

- *Shock:* If the condition is severe enough to create emotional shock, the patient will experience extreme heightened suggestibility. Speaking in a loud, authoritative voice (almost shouting) to a hysterical patient "unless you do as I say you will continue to hurt [lose blood, require restraints, or whatever the situation warrants]" capitalizes on the shock for an instant, which is usually long enough to tell the person to lie flat, breathe deeply, "do as I say and it will hurt less," etc. The suggestion is usually accepted and more merciful techniques can be employed after equilibrium is established.

- *Time distortion:* Time can appear to speed up or slow down depending on the situation. When things are fun, time moves quickly. When people are in crisis they tend to feel every agonizing moment. Being aware of this, the attention of the patient can be diverted to more pleasant things.

    When his or her condition improves, the patient will only intermittently realize that he or she is spending less time in pain. Bring this to the attention of the patient with such phrases as "You must be feeling better. Your pain is not lasting as long nor is it as intense as when we started talking."

- *Disassociation:* The ability to remove oneself from the situation or externalize the pain or suffering is greater with heightened suggestibility. The health care worker can ask the patient to take the pain elsewhere such as by squeezing the hand. Suggesting that "the harder you squeeze my hand the less pain you will feel," or "as your hand squeeze gets weaker and weaker the pain is getting less and less," takes the patient's pain from the affected area, to the hand, and out of the focus of the mind. A subtle suggestion can be planted at that time that if the pain should be too severe a towel roll, pillow, padded siderail, etc, can be squeezed and the pain will minimize.

As with any of the modalities discussed, the health care worker is only as good with the techniques as the amount of time spent studying and practicing them. This is particularly true of suggestion and hypnosis.

Therapeutic Metaphors

The left brain performs rational and analytic functions. The right brain provides the synthesizing, creative, and holistic functions. Metaphors are right-brain ways of talking about an experience. For example, thanks to our right brain we understand that an "underdog" is not a dog hiding under something. We understand that "feeling like a lead weight" is a representation of an experience and not an actuality.[27]

Metaphoric or right-brain communication can be used clinically to give the patient another perceptual avenue for coping with the situation. There are many techniques for metaphoric communication, some of which have been discussed in the preceding sections on hypersuggestibility and NLP. Others that can be practically used in the emergency setting include relating various stories and using guided imagery, visualization, meditation, or prayer.[22]

Anecdotes, Stories, and Parables

The metaphoric mind translates vague, impersonal stories into that which is important for the individual. Health care workers have long used success stories about other patients to motivate without realizing they were using a right-brain phenomenon. Using anecdotes about "other" patients or "other" situations or experiences can serve as a vehicle for helping the patient make sense of his or her experience.[27] For example: "I had a patient in here just a few weeks ago who had a problem similar to yours. . . . It was interesting how he dealt with it. What he did was . . ."

The Bible is a wealth of metaphoric communication in the form of stories, psalms, and parables, which can be read to a patient seeking spiritual support. The sustaining presence of God is communicated, for example, in the familiar words of the nineteenth and twenty-third psalms.[22] The Bible can be used for its therapeutic metaphors to provide strength to people seeking spiritual reassurance.

Guided Imagery, Visualization, Meditation, and Prayer

The mind has the capacity to calm and relax the body, mind, and spirit and thus facilitate the healing process. Techniques for doing this include relaxation techniques, guided imagery, and visualization. Imagery and visualization when used in conjunction with meaningful religious symbols become meditation or prayer.

An illustration of the use of several techniques follows. The relaxation techniques are used as preludes to set the stage for effective use of imagery, meditation, and prayer.

Relaxation.[6] [/ This mark means pause.] Close your eyes and be aware of your breathing./ Slow your breathing./ As you breathe you begin to relax./ Allow any tension to flow out as you exhale./ With each breath your muscles relax more and more./ Any pain or body sensation can be used by your mind to relax more and more,/ deeper and deeper./ Any sounds you hear can be used to relax you more and more./ Any ideas or feelings that come into your mind can relax you more all the time./ As your breath slows, think the word "calm" as you inhale and "peace" as you exhale,/"calm" as you inhale and "peace" as you exhale.

Guided imagery. Imagine yourself on a sunny, warm beach./ Feel the warmth of the sun on your body./ Feel the warm sand between your toes./ Feel the gentle sea breeze in your hair and on your face./ Experience the blue sky and the call of the seagulls./ Lie on the warm sand and allow the sun to engulf you./ Feel the warmth and strength of the sun [drying up the congestion, soothing and taking away the pain, shrinking the swelling or whatever suggestion is appropriate for that particular patient]./ Experience the inner peace of lying in the sun./ You may remain there for as long as you choose even as care is being given to you.

Meditation and prayer.[6] As you relax more and more, the spaces between your breaths will gradually lengthen./ You will feel increasingly quiet and peaceful./ Let yourself experience this inner serenity./ Choose a religious or spiritual symbol that has meaning for you. This may be the dove of peace, the cross, the Star of David, the burning bush, the Good Shepherd, the everlasting arms, a mandala, or whatever you choose./ If you have difficulty selecting a symbol, try concentrating on the brilliant white Light of God./ Form a picture of the symbol in your mind./ Focus your full attention on this symbol./ Allow that picture to flow through your entire being—from the top of your head to the bottom of your feet./ Release all of your problems to the Lord as you allow this picture to move throughout your body. If you choose to pray directly to God you may do so at this time./ You may do this silently or out loud.

If the health care worker wishes to pray with the patient it may also be done at this time. The prayer does not need to be long or involved for those uncomfortable with praying with patients. For example, "We ask you, Lord, to watch over Mary Smith. Give her the strength and aid she needs to handle this problem."

By its very nature emergency care is time limited. Thus, the emotional and spiritual interventions provided in the emergency department need to be viewed as only one segment of an ongoing process toward wholeness for that patient. In assisting our patients in their move toward greater wholeness we need to view our contribution, regardless of how brief, as significant. The simplest of words or actions have the capacity for changing an entire course of events. The intentional use of self is the key to psychospiritual support.

REFERENCES

1. Stoll R. Emotional and spiritual support. In: Kravis T, Warner C, eds. *Emergency Medicine*. Rockville, MD: Aspen; 1983.
2. Heaney J. *The Sacred and the Psychic*. New York: Paulist Press; 1984.
3. Griffin D. Charles Hartshorne's postmodern theology. In: Kane R, Phillips S, eds. *Hartshorne Process Philosophy and Theology*. Albany, NY: SUNY Press; 1989.
4. Francuch P. *Fundamentals of Human Spirituality*. Santa Barbara, CA: Spiritual Advisory Press; 1982.
5. Johnson R. Recognizing people in crisis. In: *Nursing Skillbook Series: Using Crisis Intervention Wisely*. Springhouse, PA: Intermed Communications; 1982.
6. Clinebell H. *Basic Types of Pastoral Care and Counseling*. Nashville: Abingdon; 1984.
7. Sharer P. Supporting behaviors of unexpected death. In: *Nursing Skillbook Series: Using Crisis Intervention Wisely*. Springhouse, PA: Intermed Communications; 1982.
8. Schulz C. Grief and loss. In: Kravis T, Warner C, eds. *Emergency Medicine*. Rockville, MD: Aspen; 1983.
9. O'Brien ME. The need for spiritual integrity. In: Yura H, Walsh MB, eds. *Human Needs and the Nursing Process*. Norwalk, CT: Appleton-Century-Crofts; 1982.
10. Ryan JE. Selecting an instrument to measure spiritual distress. *Oncol Nurs Forum*. 1985;12.
11. Ellison CW. Spiritual well being: conceptualization and measurement. *J Psychol Theol*. 1983;11:341–348.
12. Stoll R. The essence of spirituality. In: Carson VB, ed. *Spiritual Dimensions of Nursing Practice*. Philadelphia, PA: Saunders; 1989.
13. Fish S, Shelley JA. *Spiritual Care: The Nurse's Role*. Downers Grove, IL: InterVarsity; 1983.
14. Batson C, Ventis W. *The Religious Experience: A Social-Psychological Perspective*. New York: Oxford University Press; 1982.
15. Stoll R. Guidelines for spiritual assessment. *Am J Nurs*. 1979.
16. Pumphrey J. Recognizing your patient's spiritual needs. *Nurs 77*. 1977.
17. Ford P. *The Structure and Dynamics of Divine Healing*. Claremont, CA: Center for Process Studies; 1990.
18. Weatherhead L. Present-day non-medical methods of healing. In: Crowlesmith J, ed. *Religion and Medicine*. London: Epworth; 1962.
19. Ebon M. *Handbook of Parapsychology*. New York: Signet; 1978.
20. Glen MJ. Sickness and symbol: the promise of the future. *Worship*. 1980;54.
21. Solomon P, Patch V. *Handbook of Psychiatry*. Los Altos, CA: Lange Medical; 1974.
22. Anderson D. *New Approaches to Family Pastoral Care*. Philadelphia: Fortress; 1980.
23. Brockopp D. What is NLP? *Am J Nurs*. 1983.
24. Knowles R. Through neuro-linguistic programming. *Am J Nurs*. 1983.
25. Cotanch P. *Diversion Therapy*. Durham, NC: Duke University; Thesis.
26. Greene D. Use of hypnosis. Unpublished lecture notes.
27. Gordon D. *Therapeutic Metaphors*. Cupertino, CA: Meta; 1978.

53. Pain Management

*GARY SPARGER, RN, MSN, CEN, MICN
K. SUE HOYT, RN, MSN, CEN
ROLAND HEIDENHOFER, MD, FACEP

DEFINITION OF PAIN

Pain is defined as a feeling of distress caused by stimulation of specialized nerve endings. Most pain is caused by injury or inflammation. Therefore pain has a purpose: it acts as a warning device. Pain is a subjective response in conscious humans, many times manifesting itself with outward symptoms such as facial grimaces or posture changes. The receptors for the stimulus of pain are located in myelinated and unmyelinated nerve fibers abundantly distributed near the surface of the body. Internal organs, such as the lungs and uterus, have few receptors and are relatively insensitive to painful stimuli. The distribution of pain receptors in the mucosa of the intestinal tract is similar to that in the skin, which is very sensitive to painful stimuli. Superficial pain is perceived when the stimulus reaches the cutaneous receptors near the body surface. It is felt as a sudden sharp pain at the site of stimulation. Deep pain arises from stimulation of receptors in such internal structures as muscles and viscera. Pain emanating from these internal structures tends to be of longer duration, duller in sensation, and less localized.

When pain receptors are stimulated, impulses are transmitted along nerve fibers that become the spinal ganglia. The receptors travel upward along nerve fibers to the thalamus. Pain impulses are synthesized, and it is then that the individual becomes aware of the painful stimulus. Impulses are then transmitted to the sensory portion of the cerebral cortex, where the pain is analyzed by the brain. The pain's location and density are determined at that time. Reactions to pain are physical and psychological.

It is important to remember that pain is subjective and that it is what patients tell us they feel. It can be classified in a number of ways. A widely accepted classification is that of acute versus chronic pain.

Acute Pain

Acute pain is defined as an episode of pain lasting from 1 second to less than 6 months. Organic diseases or injury account for acute pain. Acute pain tends to warn of tissue damage or the need for convalescence. Examples of this type of pain would be an individual who is involved in a motor vehicle accident and sustains a traumatic injury to a lower extremity or a patient who comes to the emergency department complaining of abdominal pain from an acute appendicitis. Acute pain frequently results from a sudden onset injury and can range from a small laceration or minor bruise to a major chest injury.

The management of acute pain ranges from no treatment to analgesic medication or other forms of invasive methods, which are discussed in this chapter.

Chronic Pain

Chronic pain is defined as a feeling of distress or uncomfortableness lasting for 6 months or longer. It is classified as limited, intermittent, or persistent pain. Examples of this might include intractable low back pain or pain felt by a cancer patient. The patient with chronic pain often exhibits signs of depression and assumes the role of being sick.

---

*In loving memory, January 9, 1991.

Benign pain patients, hypochondriacs, often experience interpersonal and behavioral conflicts related to the pain complaint. Patients with chronic pain related to an actual disease process seem to complain less and function better despite their pain.

Management of chronic pain is a challenge to health care providers. Noninvasive and invasive methods of pain control are administered in patients with chronic pain and will be discussed later in this chapter.

Limited Pain

Limited pain involves physical pathology. Examples of limited pain include the pain of cancer and slow healing injuries, as in burns or muscular tears.

Intermittent Pain

Intermittent pain implies by definition that the individual experiences pain but also has periods where there is no pain. Physical pathophysiology may exist. Examples of intermittent pain are migraine headaches that occur on an intermittent basis.

Persistent Pain

Persistent pain occurs daily. It is also known as chronic benign pain. The most common example of persistent pain is low back pain.

Prolonged Pain

A pain term that has recently gained popularity in its usage is *prolonged pain*. Prolonged pain is used to refer to a significant duration of pain that does not fit the accepted definitions of acute or chronic pain. It includes pain of varying durations which may be from several weeks to several years.

PAIN THEORIES

Gate Control Theory

The Gate Control Theory was proposed by R. Melzack and P. Wall in the late 1960s.[1] It was the most comprehensive pain relief model and was widely accepted into the early 1970s. It became a way to conceptualize the theoretical basis of pain at that time. The Gate Control Theory stated that the transmission of potentially painful impulses could be modulated by what was known as a "gating" mechanism. The theory postulated that when the gate was open, painful impulses flowed through easily; when the gate was closed, no pain impulses could get through. It also stated that the gate could be partially open with some pain impulses passing through.

The location of the gating mechanism was in the substantia gelatinosa in the dorsal horn of the spinal cord. Activity in the peripheral nervous system and/or central nervous system could potentially alter the opening and closing of the gate.

Nature of the Gate

The transmission of potentially painful impulses to the level of conscious awareness may be affected by this gating mechanism, which may be located in the spinal cord level of the central nervous system. The structures involved include the spinal cord, nerve fibers, brain stem, cerebral cortex, and thalamus. No pain or decreased intensity of pain resulted from (1) closing of the gate by activity of the large diameter nerve fibers which is caused by skin stimulation, (2) inhibitory impulses from the brain stem caused by a sufficient or maximum sensory input arriving through distraction or guided imagery, or (3) inhibitory impulses from the cerebral cortex and thalamus caused by anxiety reduction based on learning when the pain will end and how to relieve it.

Pain results from opening the gate by activity in the small diameter nerve fibers. This opening occurs by tissue damage facilitory impulses from the brain stem caused by input from a monotonous environment, or facilitory impulses from the cerebral cortex and thalamus caused by fear that the intensity of pain will escalate and will be associated with death. This, according to the gate theory, was the nature of the gate, the structures involved, and how it was felt that pain either did or did not occur.

Major Contributions of Theory

An integrated conceptual pain relief model was the major contribution of the Gate Control Theory. It explained individual differences in the pain experience. Additionally it brought about a conceptualization of the categories of activity that formed a theoretical basis for the development of future pain relief models. Although in practice the gate control theory is rarely used, it did have some basis as one of the first pain theories.

Theoretical Limitations

The Gate Control Theory relied heavily on complex neurophysiologic processes, which was its most questionable aspect. In 1976 Wall and Melzack[1] restated much of the information regarding these complex neurophysiologic processes involved in the Gate Control Theory. A portion of the Gate Control Theory that is still used in clinical practice includes the general categories of activity that may contribute to pain relief. This includes such measures as cutaneous stimulation, guided imagery, and basic accurate information about the cause and relief of pain which provides the patient with a sense of control. In any event, the Gate Control Theory provided researchers with some general concepts regarding pain, its definition, how it occurred, and how pain relief occurred.

Endorphins

An additional pain theory that has gained acceptance in the medical community is the endogenous pain control mechanism. Although this theory is not new, much remains unknown about what occurs. It is evident that the reaction to pain and its control within the nervous system can be affected not only by exogenous or outside influence on the nervous system but also through endogenous substances from the nervous system acting on itself. Electrostimulation in several areas of the brain and spinal cord can greatly reduce or almost block pain signals transmitted to the brain.

Endorphins, opiatelike substances that are produced and found in the hypothalamus and the pituitary gland, are thought to activate portions of the brain's analgesic system. They can effect significant decrease in the perception of pain and also provide analgesia. Endorphins may also inhibit brain transmission of pain at other points in the brain pathway, such as at the reticular activating system, the thalamus, and in the gut. Therefore, in times of stress the body produces these endogenous substances in an attempt to nullify the painful stimuli of the stress and allow the body to overcome or tolerate the stress insult to which it is subjected. The discovery of endorphins has not led to the development of new pharmacologic therapies for pain relief, but it has resulted in the use of spinal intrathecal and epidural morphine for pain control.

ASSESSMENT METHODS

History and Physical Exam

As the medical practitioner knows, a good history will elicit 90% of the findings in the physical exam. In the case of pain, this is especially true. The practitioner obviously wants to validate findings in relation to this chief complaint of pain. As the physical exam is undertaken and the history is being pursued, it is important to obtain specific information by asking the patient the following:

1. Where is your pain today? (location)
2. How long have you had this pain? (duration)
3. Describe the pain. (quality)
4. What kinds of things increase your pain? (aggravating factors)
5. What kinds of things take away your pain? (relieving factors)
6. When did this pain first occur? (onset)
7. Can you rate this pain on a scale of 1 to 10? (intensity)
8. How have you dealt with this pain in the past? (history)
9. Are you currently using any methods of pain relief and what are they? (medications, biofeedback, cutaneous stimulation, etc)

Pain Communication

It is important to note that there are cultural differences that also occur in individuals who are complaining of pain. For example, the native American population tends to be very stoic in the complaint of pain. Some people frequently deny pain or painful experiences because they consider this inappropriate behavior. There are also others who exaggerate their pain. The practitioner must remember that the authority for pain lies with the patient. If the patient claims to be in pain, whether it is real or imagined, then he or she is in pain. There are many misconceptions hampering pain assessment and many prejudices regarding a patient's pain. Who really is the authority about pain? If a patient complains of a subjective experience, then the patient should be the authority about the pain experienced. Pain is whatever the experiencing person says it is, existing whenever the patient says it does.[2] The assumption then is that the patient must be believed. Physicians are uneasy about believing patients' statements regarding pain because of the lack of objective evidence. Physicians also deal with many malingerers in the emergency department; hence, a distrust develops between client and physician. Pain is also associated with secondary gain, meaning any practical advantages that result from having the symptom, for example, financial compensation or preferred treatment by significant others.

Regardless of these issues it is important to note the subjective complaint of pain during the physical exam and in the history-taking component of care.

Situational Factors Affecting Pain Perception

There are many factors in the emergency department that affect the patient's pain and the perception of that pain: the type of patient presenting with pain, the practitioner treating that patient for pain, the personnel and/or staff also treating that patient, the surroundings, and environment. The way the patient is initially greeted may have an effect on the patient's pain perception as well. In a busy emergency department, the priorities given to one patient over another may be a situational factor affecting pain perception. It is important to be aware of these factors when determining appropriate treatment of patients for pain.

TREATMENT OF PAIN

The decision to treat pain in the emergency department and the tendency to undertreat patients in pain are common among practitioners. Patients frequently become "regulars" in emergency departments and the tendency is to undertreat these patients, who may actually be in chronic pain. Many times patients with intermittent or persistent pain will currently be on medications, and it is difficult for the physician to decide how much is too much in relation to the ordering of medications. Another patient who is difficult to treat is the cancer patient or the patient in sickle cell crisis who frequently requires administration of large amounts of medication to achieve pain relief. Regardless of what the pain is, it is the responsibility of the practitioner ordering the type of pain relief or suggesting certain pain methods to be aware of these tendencies to undertreat the patient.

PAIN MANAGEMENT

Pharmacology

The relief of pain in the emergency department is a challenge for the practitioner. The pharmacologic approach is often the treatment of choice in the emergency setting and may involve a variety of medications and routes of administration. Analgesics, which relieve pain without producing loss of consciousness and reflex activity, are frequently administered in the emergency department. Analgesics act in several ways: by elevating the pain threshold, by altering the attitude or mood of the patient from one of concern to one of detachment, promoting a sense of well-being or a mild euphoria, and by producing sedative effects.

The search for an ideal analgesic continues, but it is difficult to find one that has all the desired effects. Ideally, the drug should be potent so that it will provide maximum pain relief, not cause dependence, exhibit a minimum of side effects, not cause tolerance to develop, act promptly and over a long period of time with a minimum amount of sedation, and be relatively inexpensive. Examples of analgesics include opium and its derivatives, related synthetic compounds, and the nonnarcotic analgesics.

Nonnarcotic Analgesics

Nonnarcotic analgesic agents act on pain regardless of its origin, are usually safe, and do not lead to tolerance or addiction. Their action may begin within minutes and last for a few hours. The nonnarcotic analgesic is frequently used in the emergency department to treat minor aches and pains such as toothache, musculoskeletal pain, and headache.

Nonnarcotic analgesics are often classified as either simple analgesics or anti-inflammatory drugs. Table 53-1 provides a list of medications commonly used to treat minor pain and inflammation.

Simple analgesics. The simple analgesics provide pain relief only and are commonly used to treat intermittent pain. Administration is most often by the oral route and taken as

Table 53-1 Simple Analgesics and Anti-Inflammatory Drugs Used To Treat Minor to Moderate Pain

Aspirin	Indoprofen
Azapropazone	Mefenamic acid
Diflunisal	Naproxen
Fenbufen	Naproxen sodium
Fenoprofen	Paracetamol
Flurbiprofen	Prioxicam
Ibuprofen	Zomepirac
Indomethacin	

needed by the patient. There is no need to prescribe simple analgesics on a regular basis; they should be taken only as needed.

Effectiveness, tolerance, safety, convenience, and cost should be considered when determining the treatment of choice for a particular individual. Side effects, although often minor, must also be considered when prescribing analgesics. Analgesics are frequently used in attempting suicide and unfortunately are often effective.

Nonsteroidal anti-inflammatory drugs. Nonsteroidal anti-inflammatory drugs are ideal for treating most musculoskeletal pain because of their anti-inflammatory properties. Table 53-2 lists some nonsteroidal anti-inflammatory drugs and appropriate doses. Drugs in this class all relieve pain and stiffness. Relief of symptoms usually occurs within 24 hours of initiation of treatment. These drugs also reduce swelling and warmth for an extended period of time, up to 3 weeks.

Although choice of drug is an important aspect of pain management, there is minimal difference between the most effective and least effective nonsteroidal anti-inflammatory drug. The most commonly associated side effect, often dose related, is gastrointestinal (GI) disturbances and indigestion. A more serious complication—gastric bleeding—may occur with high-dose, long-term therapy with aspirin. Safety first is a good rule to follow when prescribing this class of medication.

Narcotic Analgesics

Narcotic analgesics are used to treat moderate to severe pain, usually on a short-term basis due to the potential for drug dependence. The narcotic agents may be classified as either nonsynthetic or synthetic.

The nonsynthetic narcotic analgesics—opiates—are derived from the hardened dry juice of the unripe seed capsule of the poppy. The active ingredients of opium are alkaloids of which there are some 20 variations. The three opiates most widely used in the practice of medicine are morphine, codeine, and papaverine. Table 53-3 lists some of the selected effects of the opiates and the potency of analgesic action of morphine, codeine, Dilaudid, and papaverine.

The effects of opium result mostly from the morphine it contains. Morphine exhibits a narcotic action which results

Table 53-2 A Selection of Nonsteroidal Anti-Inflammatory Drugs with Appropriate Dosages

Approved Name	Trade Name	Dosage
Aspirin	(Various)	600 to 900 mg qds or 600 mg as required for pain
Azapropazone	Rheumox	600 mg bid
Benorylate	Benoral	10 mL (4 g) bid os suspension or 1.5 g tid using tablets
Choline magnesium trisalicylate	Trilisate	1 g bid for osteoarthritis; 1.5 g bid for rheumatoid arthritis
Diclofenac	Voltaren	50 mg mane 100 mg nocte or 50 mg tid
Dilfunisal	Dolobid	500 mg stat then 250 or 500 mg bid
Fenbufen	Lederfen	300 mg mane 600 mg nocte Night doses only may be enough
Fenclofenac	Flenac	300 mg bid
Fenoprofen	Nalfon	600 mg tid or 300 mg as required for pain
Feprazone	Methrazone	200 mg bid
Flurbiprofen	Ansaid	50 mg mane 100 mg nocte
Flufenamic acid	Meralen	200 mg tid
Ibuprofen	Motrin	400 mg tid or 400 mg as needed for pain
Indomethacin	Indocin	25 mg tid, 75–100 mg at night for night pain/morning stiffness
Indomethacin (slow release)	Indocin SR	75 mg nocte or bid
Indoprofen	Flosint	200 mg tid or 200 mg as needed for pain
Ketoprofen	Orudis	100 mg bid
Meclofenamate sodium	Meclomen	50–100 mg tid or qid
Mefenamic acid	Ponstel	500 mg tid or 500 mg as needed for pain
Naproxen	Naprosyn	500 mg bid
Phenylbutazone	Butazolidin	100 mg tid, not more than 7 days
Piroxicam	Feldene	20 mg od morning or night
Sulindac	Clinoril	200 mg bid
Tolmetin sodium	Tolectin	400 mg tid
Zomepirac	Zomax	100 mg tid or 100 mg as needed for pain

bid = twice a day
mane = in the morning
tid = three times a day
nocte = at night
od = oral dose

Source: Adapted with permission from Wall P, Melzack R: *Textbook of Pain.* New York, Churchill Livingstone, Inc.

in analgesia and sleep. Its dependence liability is explained by its ability to cause a relatively intense euphoria. The exact mode of action is still unknown. Morphine's greatest effect is its relief of pain, and when used in large enough doses it will abolish almost all forms of pain. It continues to be the most valuable analgesic in medicine. In small doses, morphine has little or no effect on the motor areas of the brain. It does, however, have a highly selective action on the respiratory center causing depressed respirations, which is one of its major side effects.

Synthetic narcotic analgesics grew out of the need to provide the ideal analgesic without causing respiratory depression and drug dependence. There are various synthetic narcotic analgesics used for pain relief and these can be found in Table 53-4.

Synthetic narcotic analgesics include the drugs meperidine and methadone. Meperidine is used primarily as a substitute for morphine to produce analgesia. When so used it has the advantage of producing much less sedation. It does not, however, take the place of morphine for the relief of severe pain. It is quick acting and of short duration.

Narcotic Antagonists

The three most common antinarcotic drugs utilized in medicine today are nalorphine, levorphanol tartrate, and the newer, most commonly used drug naloxone (Narcan). Narcan is an important narcotic antagonist that reverses the respiratory depressant action of narcotics such as morphine, meperidine, and methadone. An important feature of the pharmacology of Narcan is its lack of respiratory depressant action and its failure to cause sedation or analgesia. It is a pure narcotic antagonist. Doses range from 0.4 to 4.0 mg in adults and 0.01 to 0.03 mg/kg in children for single intravenous doses repeated as necessary. Continuous infusion of 0.4 to 0.8 mg/hour also may be given.

Placebos

Placebos have been used at times in patients as an effective method of pain reduction. The term *placebo* is derived from a Latin word meaning "I shall please."[3] Recently the placebo has been used as a control in drug research designed to diagnose psychogenic versus somatogenic pain. The effectiveness of a particular medication was evaluated by comparing it with a placebo preparation in double-blind studies. However, a true and positive placebo response cannot be used to diagnose pain as psychogenic rather than somatogenic. A positive placebo response may occur in relation to the treatment of many conditions and symptoms, including that of pain. Placebos have been used to effectively increase appetite, induce sleep, treat bleeding ulcers, increase sexual desire, decrease nausea, relieve allergies, remove skin blemishes, and lower blood pressure. Side effects and toxic reactions do occur in response to placebos ranging from nasal

Table 53-3 Selected Effects of Opiates

	Morphine	Codeine	Dilaudid	Papaverine
Potency of analgesic action	Potent	One sixth to one tenth that of morphine	Ten times more potent than morphine	None
Effects				
Respiration	Markedly depressed Carbon dioxide retention	Depression one fourth that of morphine	Like morphine	None or slight bronchial relaxation
Gastrointestinal	Decreased activity, spasm, and constipation	Like morphine but less prominent	Like morphine but less constipating	Relaxes
Biliary	Increased intrabiliary pressure Possibility of spasm	Less intense spasms than from morphine	Like codeine	Relaxes
Genitourinary				
Ureters	Possibility of spasms Increased tone, decreased motility	Increased tone, decreased motility	Like morphine	Relaxes
Bladder	Increased sphincter tone Retention of urine	Increased tone, decreased motility	Like morphine	Relaxes
Uterus	Tone increased Contractions decreased	Not significant	Like morphine	None
Eyes	Pupil constriction	Less than morphine	Like morphine	None
Cerebral	Stimulation of vomiting center—nausea and vomiting Depressed cough center Cortical sedation Rise in pain threshold Euphoria	Less than morphine Large doses required to produce euphoria	Less than morphine	None

Source: Reprinted with permission from Hahn AB, Barkin RL, Oestreich SJK: *Pharmacology in Nursing*, ed 15. St. Louis, CV Mosby, p 144, 1982.

stuffiness, dizziness, and diarrhea, to more serious addiction and anaphylactoid reaction.

Placebo responses, whether they are intended or the side effects of intended reactions, are not imaginary. They are also not restricted to subjective reports by the individual. Patients can respond to a placebo with objective measurable physiologic changes over which they could have had no direct effect of conscious control because they do not know the placebo medication is being received.

Hypnotics and Sedatives

Hypnotics are drugs that produce sleep, while sedatives relieve anxiety. The only difference between a hypnotic and a sedative action is one of degree. Therefore, the term *hypnotic* or *sedative* is dose dependent.

Barbiturates. The barbiturates were among the first drugs to be synthesized for hypnotic and sedative use. Barbiturates have been shown to depress the neurons and synapses of the ascending reticular formation of the brain stem, and this effect may be responsible for the reduction in electrical activity of the cortex. The ascending reticular formation receives stimuli from all parts of the body and relays impulses to the cortex, thus promoting wakefulness and alertness. Depression of the ascending reticular formation, therefore, decreases cortical stimuli and thus reduces the stimuli for wakefulness and alertness. There is evidence that the barbiturates act at all levels of the central nervous system. All of barbiturates used clinically depress the motor cortex of the brain when administered in large doses. However, drugs such as phenobarbital, mephobarbital, and mepharbital exert a selective action on the motor cortex even in small doses. This explains their anticonvulsant use. See Table 53-5 regarding the dosage administration and length of action of barbiturates.

Phenobarbital is an example of a barbiturate producing hypnotic or sedative effect; secobarbital is a short-acting barbiturate, more active than barbital and given in correspondingly smaller doses. Small doses produce a sedative effect, larger doses produce a hypnotic effect. Pentobarbital is the most widely used of the short-acting barbiturates.

Nonbarbiturate hypnotics and sedatives. Although several nonbarbiturate sedatives and hypnotics are available, it should be emphasized that all are habit forming, may cause physical dependence, and are subject to physical abuse. Examples of the nonbarbiturate group include ethchlorvynol (Placidyl), ethinamate (Valmid), glutethimide (Doriden),

Table 53-4 Selected Effects of Some Synthetic Narcotic Analgesics

	Meperidine (Demerol)	Methadone	Levorphanol (Levo-Dromoran)
Analgesic potency	Between that of codeine (60 mg) and morphine (15 mg)	Like morphine	Four to eight times that of morphine Hypnotic effect similar to morphine
Action			
Onset	10 to 15 minutes	10 to 15 minutes	15 to 45 minutes (intramuscular)
Duration	2 to 4 hours (intramuscular)	4 to 6 hours	2 to 5 hours
Effects			
Respiratory	Mild depression Bronchodilation Sometimes bronchospasm	Depression—similar to morphine Bronchial constriction	Depression—like morphine Apnea caused by overdose
Gastrointestinal	Decreased motility Spasm No constipation effect	Increased tone Decreased motility Spasms—like morphine	Decreased motility Spasms Moderate constipation
Genitourinary			
Ureters	Decreased motility and tone	Spasms—like morphine	
Bladder	Increased tone Retention uncommon		
Kidney	Not significant Some decrease in urinary output	Antidiuretic action Reduced urinary output	Reduced urinary output
Uterus	Decreased tone and contractions	No relief of pain of labor or uterine contractions	Reduced motility
Eyes	No pupil change with therapeutic dose Blurred vision	Miosis with large dose	Miosis
Salivary glands	Moderate decrease in secretions Dryness of mouth	Stimulation Slight increase in secretions	
Cerebral	Euphoria Mild depression Drowsiness Dizziness Giddiness	Not significant with therapeutic dose Cortical depression with large doses	

Source: Reprinted with permission from Hahn AB, Barkin RL, Oestreich SJK: *Pharmacology in Nursing,* ed 15. St Louis, CV Mosby, p 153, 1982.

Table 53-5 Dosage, Administration, and Length of Action of Barbiturates

Preparation	Usual Adult Dose	Usual Method of Administration	Relative Length of Action
*Barbital; barbitone sodium	300 mg (gr 5)	Oral	Long
*Phenobarbital; phenobarbitone	30 to 100 mg (gr ½ to 1½)	Oral	Long
Mephobarbital (Mebaral)	400 to 600 mg (gr 6 to 10)	Oral	Long
Metharbital (Gemonil)	100 mg (gr 1½)	Oral	Long
*Amobarbital (Amytal)	100 mg (gr 1½)	Oral	Intermediate
Aprobarbital (Alurate)	60 to 120 mg (gr 1 to 2)	Oral	Intermediate
Butabarbital sodium (Butisol Sodium)	8 to 60 mg (gr ⅛ to 1)	Oral	Intermediate
Pentobarbital sodium (Nembutal Sodium); pentobarbitone sodium	100 mg (gr 1½)	Oral, rectal	Short
Secobarbital sodium (Seconal); quinalbarbitone sodium	100 to 200 mg (gr 1½ to 3)	Oral, rectal	Short
Sodium hexobarbital	2 to 4 mL 10%	Intravenous	Ultrashort
Thiopental sodium (Pentothal Sodium); thiopentone sodium	2 to 3 mL 2.5% in 10 to 15 seconds; repeated in 30 seconds as required	Intravenous	Ultrashort

*Sodium salts are available.
Source: Reprinted with permission from Hahn AB, Barkin RL, Oestreich SJK: *Pharmacology in Nursing,* ed 15. St Louis, CV Mosby, p 170, 1982.

and flurazepam hydrochloride (Dalmane). These drugs are used at times in conjunction with analgesic medications to enhance or increase the amount of pain relief in the patient.

Other hypnotics. There are a number of hypnotics that were almost abandoned when the barbiturates became popular, but seem to be gradually regaining some of their lost popularity. They include chloral hydrate, chloral betaine, paraldehyde, and the bromide group.

Local Anesthesia and Regional Blocks

Local anesthesia refers to a loss of sensation in a restricted or regional part of the body, primarily by affecting some portion of the peripheral nervous system. Local anesthetics do not alter the state of consciousness.

Local anesthetics applied to body surfaces and injected about nerves are used primarily to prevent pain during a surgical procedure. They are also used in the treatment of pain associated with trauma or disease. Drugs interfere with the initiation and transmission of nerve impulses by mechanisms based on biochemical and physical changes. A good way to explain the action is to relate anesthetic activity to the transmission of the nerve impulse. Local anesthesia has continued to be useful for the following reasons: (1) it is simple to use; (2) the methods are economical; (3) the agent is injectable and nonexplosive; (4) the equipment required is minimal; and (5) some of the undesirable effects of general anesthesia can be avoided and a localized area of the body can be operated on without any loss of consciousness. The methods are ideal for ambulatory patients for brief and superficial operations and in situations in which recently ingested food poses a threat of regurgitation or aspiration. Local anesthetics include topical agents that are used primarily on the surface of a mucous membrane such as the nasal mucosa, urethra, vaginal mucosa, and oral mucosa. In addition, the agent may be applied to superficial wounds to effect local anesthesia. An example would be tetracaine, adrenaline, and cocaine (TAC).

Local infiltration, the most common form of local anesthesia, is the injection of a drug subcutaneously at the surgical area and results in anesthesia of the skin and underlying subcutaneous structures. Indications for use would be superficial and subcutaneous lacerations. Table 53-6 lists the local anesthetic agents more commonly used in the emergency department, their clinical characteristics, and dosage.

The mechanism of action of local anesthetic agents is primarily through a membrane stabilization by blocking the influx of sodium. It also increases the threshold for electrical excitation and decreases the rate of rise of the action potential, therefore decreasing the velocity of the nerve conduction. In addition, extinction of the action potential can occur and thereby cause total nerve conduction block. The susceptibility of nerve fibers to local anesthetics is inversely related to the diameter of the nerve. For instance, the larger the nerve, the harder to block that nerve.

Duration of action of the local anesthetic agents varies. For example, procaine will last approximately 1 hour, lidocaine will last 1.5 hours, tetracaine approximately 3 hours, and mepivacaine and bupivacaine last in excess of 3 hours. Epinephrine can be used to decrease the absorption rate of the local anesthetic from the area in which it is injected by inducing vasoconstriction. Its use should be avoided in areas of potential ischemic injury (eg, in areas of tissue nourished by an end-arteriolar blood supply, such as the pinna, nasal alae, penis, or digits).

The side effects of local anesthetics can include primarily a localized supersensitivity reaction to generalized anaphylactic reaction. In addition, cardiovascular depression with decreased force of ventricular contraction may occur and central nervous system convulsions may result from the use of local anesthetic agents. Treatment for reactions to local anesthetic agents include: (1) discontinuation of the drug; (2) use of epinephrine and/or diphenhydramine (Benadryl) in treating the local and/or systemic reaction; (3) in the event of convulsions or seizures, barbiturates or Valium may be given intravenously to halt the seizure activity; and (4) in the event of cardiovascular depression, supplemental oxygen

Table 53-6 Clinical Characteristics and Dosage of Local Anesthetics

	Procaine (Novocaine)	2-Chloroprocaine (Nesacaine)	Lidocaine (Xylocaine)	Mepivacaine (Carbocaine)	Prilocaine (Citanest)	Tetracaine (Pontocaine)	Bupivacaine (Marcaine)	Etidocaine (Duranest)
Latency (speed of onset)	Moderate	Fast	Fast	Moderate	Moderate	Very slow	Fast	Very fast
Penetrance (diffusibility)	Moderate	Marked	Marked	Moderate	Moderate	Poor	Moderate	Moderate
Duration	Short	Very short	Moderate	Moderate	Moderate	Long	Long	Long
Optimal concentrations (%)								
Infiltration	0.5	0.5	0.25	0.25	0.25	0.05	0.05	0.1
Spinal nerve and plexus block	1.5 to 2	1.0 to 2	0.5 to 1.0	0.5 to 1.0	0.5 to 1.0	0.1 to 0.2	0.25 to 0.5	0.5 to 1.0
Maximum amount (mg/kg)	12	15	6	6	6	2	2	2

Source: Reprinted with permission from Wall P, Melzack R: *Textbook of Pain.* New York, Churchill Livingstone Inc, 1984.

Table 53-7 Classification of Local Anesthetics

Ester Group	Amide Group
Tetracaine (Pontocaine)	Mepivacaine (Carbocaine)
Benoxinate HCl	Lidocaine (Xylocaine)
Cocaine	Bupivacaine (Marcaine)
Ethylaminobenzoate (Benzocaine)	Prilocaine (Citanest)
Procaine (Novocaine)	

and circulatory support should be provided as clinically indicated.

The occurrence of allergies to local anesthetic agents is a not infrequent problem encountered in the emergency department. The intelligent choice of an alternative local anesthetic agent requires an understanding of the pharmacology of the available agents. (Refer to Table 53-7 to see pharmacologic classifications.) If a patient is allergic to an ester he or she may not be allergic to an amide. An appropriate decision can be made based on the above information.

The occurrence of drug allergy to both amide and ester groups, although rare, is nevertheless a possibility. In this case the astute clinician will not be stumped and will still be able to effect adequate local anesthesia through the use of diphenhydramine, which can be locally infiltrated. Apparently the antihistamines have the general structural features necessary for local anesthesia without sharing the specific antigenic determinants of the conventional drugs.

Regional nerve blocks affect conduction block at a peripheral nerve. Indications for use would be the need for anesthesia in an area that would be too large to be accomplished with local infiltration. The method of administration is injection of the medication around a regional nerve root or trunk, thereby providing anesthesia to the areas supplied by that nerve (for instance, block of the brachial plexus).

Intercostal Block

The intercostal nerve block is extremely effective in relieving severe pain associated with rib and sternum fractures, dislocation of the costocondral junction, slipped rib cartilage, contusion chest pain, pleurisy, and acute herpes zoster. It is the most useful procedure for the relief of severe post-traumatic and postinfectious pain in the thoracic or abdominal wall. Intercostal block significantly increases the duration of pain relief over that accomplished with segmental epidural block.

The most important complication of intercostal blocks is the development of pneumothorax. Only the experienced practitioner should attempt an intercostal nerve block.

Epidural Anesthesia

Another example of local anesthesia would be an epidural block, in which the medication is placed in the epidural or peridural space that bathes the nerve sheaths. Epidural local anesthetics have been used for many years, but only recently has epidural narcotic analgesia been attempted. The epidural space, extending from the base of the skull to the sacral hiatus, is a convenient repository for drugs that can block impulses to the cord. The epidural route does not physically breach the meninges; therefore, the risk of meningitis is reduced and the headache from cerebral spinal fluid leakage does not occur. Again, only the experienced practitioner should attempt an epidural block.

Spinal anesthesia, although rarely if ever used in the emergency department, is mentioned only as a matter of completeness. In this case, the drug is administered via the subarachnoid fluid.

Topical Anesthetic Agents for Emergency Department Use

TAC is a liquid topical anesthetic agent containing tetracaine hydrochloride 0.5%, adrenaline 1:2000, and cocaine 11.8% that has been used effectively in the repair of minor skin lacerations. The use of TAC in the emergency department was first reported by Pryor et al.[4] Since that time it has been used extensively in emergency departments throughout the United States. Individual studies by Schaffer,[5] White et al,[6] and Crabbe et al[7] have demonstrated that the anesthetic effectiveness of TAC is superior to that of the individual components used in TAC. The original reason why the specific concentrations (tetracaine hydrochloride 0.5%, adrenaline 1:2000, and cocaine 11.8%) were chosen is unclear and appears arbitrary. Bonadio and Wagner[8] have successfully used half-strength TAC (tetracaine 0.25%, adrenaline 1:4000, and cocaine 5.9%) to demonstrate its therapeutic effectiveness and safety in diminishing the risk of potential systemic toxicity due to the absorption of the component medications of TAC. Also, numerous studies have been performed documenting its successful use,[9,10] especially for lacerations located on the face and head in the pediatric age group.[11]

The advantages of TAC include painless application (appreciated by pediatric patients and their parents), absence of any tissue distortion (enhancing accurate tissue approximation), improved patient cooperation, and ease and effectiveness of application. In general, the dose of TAC has varied from 1 to 3 mL (0.09 mL/kg) to 3 to 5 mL of standard-strength TAC to a maximum of 3 mL of half-strength TAC. Its application to the wound has involved either direct instillation within the inner margins of the wound in a gravity-dependent position or application of a 2 × 2 cm saturated gauze pad for 10 to 20 minutes. A second dose has also been used, but this probably would ensure that most children would be exposed to a cocaine dose higher than that accepted for adults.

Despite reported acclaim for its use, TAC as a local anesthetic is not without complications due to its component drugs, primarily cocaine. Adverse reactions to TAC have been reported, including a fatality in a 7-month-old girl and seizures in four other children (6 months to 6 years in age).[12-15] Review of these cases reveals that TAC was inappropriately used (inadvertently coming in contact with oral mucous membranes). In addition, clumsy application allowed TAC to drip into the nose and to be licked by the child. In one case, a TAC-soaked cotton pledget was sucked by a child into the posterior pharynx. Prescribing inconsistencies and lack of protocols regarding amount of drug, duration of application, and location of use will contribute to future potential complications.[15]

The disadvantages of TAC include individual anesthetic components that are highly potent, rapid systemic absorption with potential for systemic toxicity, use by individuals who may be unfamiliar with its pharmacologic properties, and inconsistent dosage guidelines. Considering the reported cases of toxic reactions associated with the use of TAC, it should not be used for laceration of the pinna, nasal alae, penis, digits, mucosal surfaces, or burned skin. Also, patients with seizure disorder or cardiac dysrhythmia and patients with a likelihood of sniffing or swallowing the solution should be excluded from receiving TAC.

TAC is an effective topical anesthetic for the repair of nonmucosal lacerations of the head and neck that is seemingly well accepted by patients. It has a low incidence of toxic reactions and wound infections.

General Anesthesia

General anesthetics affect pain control through altering the state of consciousness, inducing narcosis, stupor, or loss of consciousness. The general anesthetics in use today can be divided into inhalation and intravenous classifications. The inhalation general anesthetics can be divided into gaseous agents, including nitrous oxide, ethylene, cyclopropane, and volatile agents, which include ether, halothane, methoxyflurane, enflurane, isoflurane, and trichloroethylene. The only inhalation agent currently used in the emergency department is nitrous oxide, which will be discussed in detail because of its applications in this setting.

Nitrous oxide is a fairly potent analgesic with 30% to 50% concentration being comparable with 10 mg of morphine given intramuscularly. Individual responses vary, therefore the ideal concentration of nitrous oxide required to produce analgesia should be determined by titration against response. The effects of nitrous oxide are rapidly reversed through discontinuation and administration of 100% oxygen via mask or nasal cannula.

The administration of 50% nitrous oxide and 50% oxygen is a recommended pain management modality for use in the emergency department and other ambulatory settings. In some parts of the world the 50% mixture is supplied in premixed cylinders as Entonox. A device that conveniently and safely delivers 50% nitrous oxide and 50% oxygen (Nitronox) is available for emergency use. Nitronox is self-administered by the patient through the use of a hand-held mask, enabling the patient to determine the amount of Nitronox administered and prevent possible overdose. As the patient achieves analgesia the hand falls away from the mask, the mask falls from the face, and administration ceases.

The purpose of Nitronox administration is to provide analgesia in patients who present to the emergency department suffering from pain, whose mental status is not deterred, and whose physical condition does not contradict its use. Contraindications to the administration of Nitronox are:

1. altered mental status (eg, head injury, sedation, intoxication)
2. severe maxillofacial injuries
3. pneumothorax, pneumomediastinum, or any other condition where nonphysiologic free air may exist
4. diving injuries
5. chronic obstruction pulmonary disease, carbon dioxide retention states, dyspnea of undetermined origin
6. asthma
7. pregnancy
8. recent cardiovascular accident
9. aplastic anemia
10. recent reconstructive ear surgery
11. under the age of 1 year

Indications for the use of nitrous oxide in the emergency department are extensive and continue to increase as practitioners become aware of the beneficial results, safety, and convenience. Indications may include:

- incision and drainage
- wound cleaning/debridement
- renal calculi
- cardiac pain
- abdominal pain while awaiting consultation
- orthopedic maneuvers
- sickle cell crisis

The most important aspect of nitrous oxide administration in the emergency department is that it is for self-administration only and that it is never administered without the combination of oxygen. The abuse of nitrous oxide by emergency personnel is an issue of concern. Staff education and some mechanism to monitor the use of nitrous oxide is recommended.

The intravenous general anesthetic agents include alterflurbarbiturates which are thiopental sodium (Pentothal), thiamylal (Surital), and methohexital (Brevital). Other agents include Innovar, Droperidol, and ketamine. Note as a matter of curiosity, ketamine produces a dissociative analgesia. It produces sleep, but before this stage is reached, the patient will appear dissociated from his or her environment. It has a profound analgesic effect and produces profound cardiovascular stimulation. It should be used with caution in patients with heart disease, especially coronary artery disease. Postoperatively the patient may have vivid dreams and hallucinations, especially if he or she is in a noisy environment.

ALTERNATIVE PAIN MANAGEMENT MODALITIES

In addition to pharmacologic management of pain, noninvasive techniques are gaining popularity and increased acceptance. Psychological or physical methods may possibly trigger pain modulating systems such as naturally occurring endorphins. Pain alleviation in certain situations may result from acupuncture or transcutaneous electric stimulation. Pain control may also result from forms of suggestion, either hypnosis or placebo therapy. Alternative pain management modalities are considered noninvasive techniques.

The main treatment of acute pain will continue to be traditional methods including narcotic and non-narcotic drugs and anesthetic agents. In selected patient populations noninvasive techniques may provide significant pain relief or augment other treatment modalities. A major key to the success of alternative pain management modalities is patient desire and willingness to cooperate. Several major categories of alternative pain relief modalities will be discussed in this chapter.

Psychotherapy

Distraction

One such noninvasive pain relief method is distraction. Distraction may be appropriately utilized in the emergency department in certain situations and with a specific patient population. Distraction is defined as focusing attention on something other than the pain sensation. This frequently occurs with young children as we give them stuffed animals, toys, and brightly colored pictures on walls. Distraction is reported as a sensory shielding, where one's self is protected from the pain sensation by focusing on sensations unrelated to pain. The successful use of distraction requires finding a stimulus that will distract a particular patient.

Guided Imagery

Guided imagery is useful in pain management to decrease the intensity of pain, to totally eliminate it, or to temporarily anesthetize the painful area. Imagery ideally involves any or all of the senses: vision, hearing, movement, touch, smell, and taste. Guided imagery may be viewed as capturing one's daydreams or using the imagination. It therefore is a purposeful or therapeutic use of images. Many individuals have used guided imagery when in a very hot environment and, in attempting to be less uncomfortable, have imagined white powdery snow on high mountains or jumping into an icy mountain stream.

Hypnosis

Hypnosis has been widely and successfully used in the treatment of acute and chronic pain. Hypnosis is thought to result in distortions of perception, memory, or mood that occurs in relation to appropriate suggestions. Hypnosis may be referred to as an altered state of consciousness, believed-in imaging, role enactment, fantasy absorption, or focused attention.

The use of hypnotic suggestion or hypnosis is not a modality for frequent use in the emergency department. There are patients who have attained the ability of self-hypnosis through previous experience. This ability may prove beneficial to particular patients experiencing pain.

Relaxation Techniques

Relaxation response is a physiologic response resulting from many various techniques. Generally, relaxation is thought of as mental and physical freedom from tension or stress. Relaxation techniques consist of specific procedures to promote a state of freedom from anxiety and skeletal muscle tension. Although many procedures exist, meditation and autogenic training are two that might be most appropriate for use in the emergency department.

Meditation

Meditation involves concentration or focusing attention on a single thought or task. Breathing slowly and totally concentrating on taking deep slow breaths is a form of meditation. Most relaxation techniques include some form of meditation.

Autogenic Training

Voluntary self-regulation or self-generated therapy is accomplished through autogenic training. In this form of relaxation technique, the patient must possess a "let it happen" attitude. Autogenic training consists of a conscious but silent repetition of phrases about the body's physiological state. It might be referred to as a positive attitude about one's physiologic and psychological state of being. An example of a phrase is "every day, in every way, I am getting better and better."

Cutaneous Stimulation

Cutaneous stimulation as a treatment to control pain is a concept that has existed for centuries. Aches and pains have been relieved by simple therapies such as rubbing, massage, scratching, and application of heat and cold. Cutaneous stimulation is defined as stimulating the patient's skin for the purpose of relieving pain. It is well known that one pain can sometimes be relieved by inflicting another, possibly greater, pain. For this discussion only noninjurious cutaneous stimulation methods will be included.

Pressure

The application of pressure is an almost intuitive response to injury and pain. Pressure not only tends to relieve pain but also controls bleeding and may constitute preventive pain relief if it prevents the development of painful swelling. Pressure may be applied in various ways; using the entire hand or the heel of the hand, with both hands to encircle an extremity, or with the ball of the thumb, fingertips, or knuckles.

Acupressure is a form of pressure application for pain relief. This is thought of as acupuncture without the use of needles. It consists of applying pressure and/or massage to the traditional acupuncture points.

Massage

Massage, rubbing a painful body part, is another method of cutaneous stimulation that is used almost instinctively to relieve pain. Massage is felt to result in muscle relaxation and sedation to some extent.

Vibration

Vibration has not been used much to relieve pain except possibly by patients in their homes. It is felt that vibration has implications for successful pain relief. Vibration may be provided through use of inexpensive hand-held electric or battery powered devices. The use of vibration may have great potential for pain alleviation which has not yet been tried.

Heat/Cold Stimulation

Heat and cold applications to produce cutaneous stimulation have been effective in reducing muscle spasms and decreasing pain. Generally, when either heat or cold is applied to the skin, the pain threshold is elevated. Table 53-8 indicates the different effects of heat and cold application. Also, the patient's preference for heat or cold therapy should be considered whenever possible.

Transcutaneous Electrical Nerve Stimulation and Transcutaneous Nerve Stimulation

Peripheral nerve stimulation can be applied either transcutaneously or via implanted electrodes. For use in the emergency department transcutaneous electric nerve stimulation (TENS), also referred to as transcutaneous nerve stimulation, will be discussed. TENS is the procedure of applying controlled, low-voltage electrical impulses to the nervous system by passing an electric current through the skin via electrodes.

Indications for the use of TENS are extensive, and therapeutic success is widely acclaimed. C. Norman Shealy, in Mannheimer's *Clinical Transcutaneous Electrical Nerve Stimulation,* states that

> TENS is completely safe and it can be used universally, subject to instruction and the caution that it not be used in cases of persistent pain without medical advice. Most certainly, it should be standard in every emergency department. My feeling is that it should be used in every single pain state and it should be the very first treatment for acute pain, even before any drugs.[16]

Table 53-8 Effects of Cutaneous Stimulation with Heat and Cold

Response	Heat	Cold
Inflammation	Increased	Decreased
Blood flow	Increased	Decreased
Edema	Increased	Decreased
Hemorrhage	Increased	Decreased
Stiffness in rheumatoid conditions	Decreased	Increased

TENS may be used alone as the sole treatment of pain or in conjunction with other clinical management modalities. The use of TENS in the alleviation of pain in the emergency department holds great promise for success.

ROLE OF THE EMERGENCY PRACTITIONER IN THE TREATMENT OF PAIN

Pain is the primary factor that causes the patient to seek medical attention. Frequently the initial source for medical care occurs in the emergency department. Pain is a subjective complaint, and the patient's statement of pain must be believed. The emergency practitioner should remember that pain is what the patient tells us he or she feels. It often is a warning signal, but it is always subjective, often without evidence of objective data to substantiate the complaint.

Pain, as a subjective complaint, is a symptom that can provide both helpful and misleading information. It is therefore imperative that the emergency patient provide as much information as possible and the emergency practitioner conduct a thorough evaluation to determine the cause or pathology of the pain.

The goal of pain management in the emergency department is to initiate a treatment program designed to correct the pathology, control or alleviate the pain, and prevent its recurrence. This may seem to be an impossible task to be accomplished during a brief visit. The important aspect to remember is the *initiation* of a comprehensive treatment program. The emergency patient complaining of pain, either acute or chronic, depends on the emergency practitioner to know what to do to help and to be willing to help. This help involves not only alleviation of pain at that moment but also the initiation of therapeutic modalities to correct the pathology, control pain, and prevent its recurrence.

The trend in the emergency setting is often to undertreat pain. This is understandable when considering the nature of this practitioner–patient interaction. The interaction is of a short duration and is episodic, frequently a one-time encounter. A rapport of trust is not developed and it is often difficult to believe the stated need for pain relief. While the dangerous overuse of narcotic analgesics does occur in some cases, the overall trend is toward the undertreatment of acute pain and cancer pain. Additional reasons for underuse include:

- lack of knowledge about narcotic analgesic pharmacology
- use of standard rather than individually determined doses
- fear of causing respiratory depression
- fear of causing addiction
- fear of events outside control of emergency practitioner (eg, complication at home)
- other fears about narcotic analgesics
- previous experiences with abusers and addicts

The intent of this chapter is not to suggest that all pain be treated in the emergency department, but to provide awareness of various aspects of pain and its alleviation which will enable the emergency practitioner to respond appropriately to the needs of the patient experiencing pain. It is important to be aware of cultural differences, situational factors, and personal experiences that influence the management of pain.

FUTURE DIRECTIONS

Pain is a subjective feeling of discomfort and distress, which is caused by stimulation of specialized nerve endings. Most pain is associated with injury or inflammation and therefore has a purpose; it acts as a warning device. Pain problems in America support a multibillion-dollar industry annually. More over-the-counter medications are sold for pain relief than for any other reason. Yet there remains uncertainty about how to assess and evaluate pain, determining individual perceptions, and use appropriate treatment modalities for the management of pain.

One direction being taken in the field of pain is the increased interest and desire to fully understand the concept of pain. This includes interest in the ability not only to objectively measure pain but also to successfully relieve pain. Although drugs will continue to be the mainstay in the management of pain, the trend toward adjunctive therapy with alternative methods continues to increase.

Society is beginning to develop and cherish a "take control of oneself" attitude. This pertains to the management of pain as well as other health care issues. Individuals desire an increased, or at least perceived, control over bodily processes and social life. This can be accomplished as one feels more control over perceptions of pain. For these reasons it is thought that the management of pain will involve increasing utilization of alternative methods such as psychotherapy, relaxation techniques, and various forms of cutaneous stimulation.

Another trend in progressive pain management seems to be the use of transcutaneous electric nerve stimulation (TENS). This modality has experienced an extremely notable success rate and is becoming widely accepted as an appropriate management of both chronic and acute pain. Because TENS is a noninvasive and safe method for pain relief, it is ideal for use in the emergency department.

The use of inhalation agents, such as 50% nitrous oxide and 50% oxygen (Nitronox), in the management of pain is gaining acceptance from emergency practitioners and patients alike. Successful results occur in the alleviation of pain associated with particular disease processes and various aspects of wound care. Nitronox is for self-administration only and therefore provides the patient with a perceived sense of control and involvement in the treatment regimen.

There is no one panacea for the relief of pain, and probably there never will be one. What is likely to occur is a better understanding of pain and its underlying cause. Also expected is the concurrent use of commonly accepted treatment modalities in conjunction with newer alternative management modalities.

Management of pain in the emergency department will continue to present a challenge to the emergency physician. With an increased awareness of one's own perceptions about pain and pain relief, one is more likely to initiate appropriate treatment modalities.

REFERENCES

1. Wall P, Melzack R. *Textbook of Pain*. New York: Churchill Livingstone; 1984.
2. Smith G, Covino B. *Acute Pain*. London: Butterworth; 1985.
3. McCaffery M. *Nursing Management of the Patient with Pain*. Philadelphia: Lippincott; 1979.
4. Pryor GJ, Kilpatrick WR, Opp AR. Local anesthesia in minor lacerations: topical TAC versus lidocaine infiltration. *Ann Emerg Med.* 1980;9:568–571.
5. Schaffer DJ. Clinical comparison of TAC anesthetic solutions with and without cocaine. *Ann Emerg Med.* 1985;14:1077–1080.

6. White WB, Iserson KV, Criss E. Topical anesthesia for laceration repair: tetracaine versus TAC (tetracaine, adrenaline, and cocaine). *Am J Emerg Med.* 1986;4:319–322.
7. Crabbe LH, Ernst AA, Winsemius DK, Bragdon R. Comparison of tetracaine, adrenaline, and cocaine with cocaine alone for topical anesthesia. *Ann Emerg Med.* 1990;19:51–54.
8. Bonadio WA, Wagner V. Half-strength TAC topical anesthetic. *Clin Pediatr.* 1988;27:495–498.
9. Hegenbarth MA, Altieri MF, et al. Comparison of topical tetracaine, adrenaline, and cocaine anesthesia with lidocaine infiltration for repair of lacerations in children. *Ann Emerg Med.* 1990;19:63–67.
10. Cannon CR, Chouteau S, Hutchinson K. Topically applied tetracaine, adrenaline, and cocaine in the repair of traumatic wounds of the head and neck. *Otol Head Neck Surg.* 1989;100:1:78–79.
11. Bonadio WA, Wagner V. Efficacy of TAC topical anesthetic for repair of pediatric lacerations. *Am J Dis Child.* 1988;142:203–205.
12. Mofenson HC, Caraccio TR. Tack up a warning on TAC. *Am J Dis Child.* 1989;143:519–520.
13. Dailey RH. Fatality secondary to misuse of TAC solution. *Ann Emerg Med.* 1988;17:159–160.
14. Daya MR, et al. Recurrent seizures following mucosal application of TAC. *Ann Emerg Med.* 1988;17:646–648.
15. Tipton GA, et al. Topical TAC (tetracaine, adrenaline, cocaine) solution for local anesthesia in children. *South Med J.* 1989;82:1344–1346.
16. Kwako J, Shealy C. Psychologic considerations in the management of pain. In: Mannheimer J, Lampe G, eds. *Clinical Transcutaneous Electrical Nerve Stimulation.* Philadelphia, Davis; 1984.

BIBLIOGRAPHY

Barker W, et al. Damage to tissue defenses by a topical anesthetic agent. *Ann Emerg Med.* 1982;11:307–310.

Bergersen B. *Pharmacology in Nursing.* 13th ed. St Louis, MO: Mosby; 1976.

Kerr F. *The Pain Book.* Englewood Cliffs, NJ: Prentice-Hall; 1981.

Stimmel B. *Pain, Analgesia, and Addiction: The Pharmacologic Treatment of Pain.* New York: Raven; 1983.

54. Head Injuries

ANTHONY J. CAPUTY, MD
KOUROSH B. AFSHAR, MD

Head trauma of variable severity constitutes a substantial portion of the admissions to every emergency department. Every 15 seconds someone receives a head injury in the United States. The total number of head injuries is estimated to be 2 million per year. Motor vehicle accidents represent half of all traumatic brain injuries, with the remaining half being accounted for by falls, assaults, industrial accidents, and sport injuries. Traumatic brain injury is the leading cause of death and disability in children and young adults, with child abuse being responsible for the majority of head injuries in infants. Of those patients who survive a head injury, up to 90,000 will be disabled.

Prompt and sophisticated emergency treatment of a head-injured patient is of paramount importance in minimizing further brain injury arising from the secondary effects of hypoxemia or ischemia and thereby in reducing the degree of disability and mortality associated with head injuries.

ACUTE EVALUATION AND RESUSCITATION

On-Site Emergency Medical Services

Rapid and definitive prehospital care is essential. The cascade of injury, hypoxemia, and ischemia, which results in mortality and devastating disability, can be interrupted by prompt, skillful care rendered in the early minutes after a head injury. The brain has a limited reserve capacity and depends on continuous blood flow and oxygenation for its metabolic demands. A direct brain injury may result from the initial trauma, but secondary insults may have an even more profound effect on the patient's neurologic outcome than the initial trauma. The predominant secondary insults are those associated with ischemia or hypoxia.

The immediate on-site goals are the basics of all trauma life support: airway, breathing, and circulation.

- Airway: The airway must be evaluated, any obstruction cleared, and an oropharyngeal or nasopharyngeal airway inserted. Vomiting is common in head-injured patients and may occur at any time without warning. Vomiting is more frequent after drug or alcohol intoxication. Precautions must be taken to prevent aspiration.
- Breathing: Ventilation must be established and maintained. An oxygen mask should be applied with an oxygen flow rate of 10 to 20 L/min.
- Circulation: Circulation must be evaluated and maintained to promote cerebral perfusion. Ischemia from inadequate cerebral perfusion is due to systemic hypotension (systolic blood pressure <90 mmHg) and/or intracranial hypertension. If there is no carotid pulse, then cardiopulmonary resuscitation should be initiated. Venous access should be obtained. If the blood pressure is stable and greater than 100 mmHg in the adult or 70 mmHg in the child, then a "keep open" flow rate of lactated Ringer's solution should be maintained to avoid an exacerbation of cerebral edema. If, however, the blood pressure is unstable and/or there are signs of

excessive blood loss, then a higher rate may be used to prevent circulatory compromise.

A basic physical assessment and stabilization should be undertaken as soon as the airway, ventilation, and circulation parameters have been stabilized. All wounds should be covered with sterile gauze and supported. If a foreign body has penetrated the skull, it should be stabilized in position, and no attempt should be made to remove it. All external bleeding should be controlled. The head and neck should be immobilized in a neutral position to avoid any kinking of the jugular vein. All patients with head injuries are presumed to have sustained a cervical spine injury until proven otherwise. The head should be elevated above the level of the heart by 30°. This is done by supporting the trunk and elevating from the hip, thereby preventing flexion of the cervical or thoracic spine. Head elevation will be precluded if the blood pressure is not stable. Inspect and palpate to define any other areas of injury to the chest, abdomen, or extremities.

A neurologic examination is done concurrently with the assessment of other injuries. The level of consciousness can be quickly evaluated by determining the following: Is the patient alert, oriented, aware of the situation, and able to converse? Can the patient follow simple commands? Can the patient move all the extremities to command or, if not to command, to a painful stimulus? Check the pupil size and reaction to light. Record the initial Glasgow Coma Scale (GSC) value (Table 54-1). The vital signs and the neurologic examination should be repeated every 5 minutes until the patient is stable and ready for transport and thereafter at 10-minute intervals.

The history of the injury and the patient's medical history should be obtained from the patient or from observers at the accident scene. Information about the accident, the mechanism of the injury, and the site events before the arrival of the emergency medical service team should be obtained and documented. The patient's medical history, medication history, and drug allergies should also be documented.

In preparation for transport, serial vital signs and neurologic examinations should be recorded and must be stable. The optimal form of transport is that which takes the least amount of time to transfer a patient to a trauma facility. In some communities helicopters have been shown to be of great benefit. The patient with a severe head injury should be transferred to a level I or II trauma center. If the vital signs or neurologic examination are unstable, however, the patient may be transported to a nontrauma facility. This would be the best course of action for a patient in whom systemic stabilization is of primary importance and the head injury is less preeminent. In patients with progressive neurologic deterioration, however, rapid transport to a trauma center with neurosurgical capabilities would be the most prudent and effective treatment. The intermediate transport of these patients to facilities without a computed tomography (CT) scanner or neurological services should be avoided.

Management in the Emergency Department

Treatment must be initiated immediately after a head injury. Secondary insults from hypoxemia or ischemia must be minimized. Defining surgical lesions rapidly is important and would allow the neurosurgeon to render treatment early in the acute phase, which is critical to the outcome of the head-injured patient. The speed and efficiency of the emergency physician in stabilizing and evaluating the patient and in organizing the treatment plan are of cornerstone importance in reducing the mortality and disability associated with head injuries.

Evaluation and Stabilization

The basics of life support must be reassessed immediately on the patient's admission to the emergency department. The airway, ventilation, and circulation are the prime concerns of the emergency department personnel during the first minutes after admission. Treatment directed at the head injury may not take place until the basic resuscitation is complete and the vital functions have stabilized. As with the on-site resuscitation, all patients with head injuries must be presumed to have a cervical spine injury until proven otherwise, and the stability of the cervical spine should not be compromised.

Airway

Transient respiratory arrest is common after a concussive head injury, and prolonged apnea may be the cause of death at the scene. In the emergency department the upper airway must be inspected and cleared of all foreign bodies and secretions. Vomiting is common after a head injury and more frequent when alcohol has been consumed.

Although an oral airway or oxygen mask can provide some protection of an airway, airway integrity is more consistently guaranteed by the passage of a cuffed endotracheal tube. All patients who are unable to follow commands and who are not verbalizing should be intubated immediately. These patients have a severe brain injury and are often found to have an intracranial mass-producing lesion. In addition to airway protection and the prevention of hypoxemia, it may be necessary to provide hyperventilation to reduce intracranial pressure (ICP). Nasotracheal intubation has often been used to prevent excessive neck manipulation in patients in whom a cervical spine injury has not been ruled out. Nasal intubation is no longer indicated because of the risk of upper airway hemorrhage and/or brain injury or contamination in cases with skull base fractures. Oral intubation can be accomplished without compromising spinal stability, but it is often difficult in the combative patient. Occasionally, a short-acting paralytic agent is used. A prolonged postintubation paralysis precludes ongoing neurologic assessment, however.

If the airway is not obstructed and is anatomically normal and if the patient is hemodynamically stable, then intubation with a rapid sequence technique may be undertaken. For this to be accomplished, two members of the anesthesia team should be present as well as a third physician from the emergency or neurosurgery team to stabilize the neck in axial traction. After preoxygenation for 4 to 5 minutes, lidocaine (1.0 to 1.5 mg/kg) is administered intravenously. Thiopental (3 to 5 mg/kg) and succinylcholine (1.0 to 1.5 mg/kg) are then administered intravenously in rapid sequence, and, with cricoid pressure, the intubation is completed. Equipment for ventilation and suctioning should be present, and instrument sets for an urgent tracheostomy or cricothyroidotomy should be available.

Intubation with rapid sequence induction and the use of succinylcholine is controversial. Nevertheless, this technique may prove to be acceptable when weighed against the effects of prolonged hypoxemia or ischemia. Nondepolarizing agents such as vecuronium (0.15 mg/kg) may also be used. In severely unresponsive patients, pretreatment with lidocaine alone to reduce ICP may be sufficient. In patients with severe maxillofacial disruptions in whom orotracheal or nasotracheal intubation is not possible, a tracheostomy should be performed.

Once intubation has been achieved and the cuff inflated, 100% oxygen should be started until blood gases can be checked and Fio_2 adjustments made. The patient should also be hyperventilated down to a Pco_2 of 25 mmHg to assist in lowering ICP.

The stomach should be emptied with a number 18 French sump tube by insertion via the nasogastric or orogastric route. Care must be taken in the placement of the nasogastric tubes to avoid intracranial passage through open fractures at the skull base.

Respiration

The injured brain requires a high level of oxygen to prevent further damage. Significant hypoxemia can occur without outward physical signs. All patients should have a high flow (10 to 12 L/min) of humidified oxygen. Arterial blood gas measurements should be done quickly, and even mild hypoxemia or hypercapnia should be avoided. Other injuries to the airway, thorax, abdomen, or spine that may restrict respirations should be noted. Aspiration after head injuries is common.

If in a moderately head-injured patient there is a significant amount of respiratory distress (Pco_2 >40 mmHg and Pco_2 <80 mmHg) the patient should be intubated. Pulse oximetry measurements may be useful in the ongoing monitoring of patients to provide early intervention and correction of hypoxia.

Circulation

While the airway is being established and secured, venous access should be obtained. A large-bore venous catheter (16-gauge or larger) or a central venous catheter should be inserted. On occasion a venous cutdown may be necessary. Laboratory tests including complete blood count, prothrombin time/partial thromboplastin time, blood chemistries, toxicology screen, and type and cross should be obtained. Systemic hypotension is virtually never the result of a primary brain injury except in patients who have received massive brain stem injury in whom all homeostatic mechanisms have been lost and who are considered neurologically dead and in infants with open cranial sutures and expansible skulls.

PATHOPHYSIOLOGY (PRIMARY AND SECONDARY INJURIES)

The initial insult will leave the brain susceptible to further injury from secondary sources. The hallmark of intracranial pathology is cerebral edema. Cerebral edema may be the result of cell disruption and a breakdown of the normal homeostatic sodium-potassium pumping mechanisms, a breakdown of the normal blood-brain barrier, or an intracranial mass with resultant elevation of ICP and venous outflow obstruction. The magnitude of the permanent brain injury after head trauma is defined by the extent of the primary injury and the degree of further compromise by secondary insults.

The primary brain injury occurs at the moment when the head is struck by an outside force. This can occur from a motor vehicle accident with an acceleration/deceleration injury, it can be from blunt force after an assault, or it can be from a penetrating projectile injury.

There can be considerable local injury (coup) or remote injury (contracoup) from the movement of the brain inside the calvarium. The primary insult results in cell loss and permanent damage. A zone of dysfunctional cells surrounds the permanently damaged cells. These dysfunctional cells have been injured but are not mechanically disrupted.[1] If the cells' extracellular environment is physiologically optimized, the secondary damage can be minimized, and many of these cells will recover.

A secondary brain injury may occur after the initial injury. It is usually the result of a series of pathophysiologic events that were set into motion by the primary injury. These secondary brain injuries are most often due to hypoxia and ischemia (secondary to systemic hypotension and/or intracranial hypertension). In normal circumstances the brain has an intrinsic ability to regulate its own blood flow and to maintain a constant supply of glucose and oxygen to meet its metabolic demands. Cerebral blood flow is maintained at a constant level throughout the mean arterial blood pressure range of 50 to 180 mmHg. The maintenance of an adequate (70 to 110 mmHg) cerebral perfusion pressure is essential in avoiding ischemia after a brain injury. Cerebral perfusion pressure is defined as mean arterial blood pressure minus ICP. With an injury, however, this autoregulation may be impaired, and cerebral blood flow can respond passively to the systemic blood pressure in the affected regions of the brain. In addition, a disruption of the blood-brain barrier in head-injured patients results in increased capillary permeability. Thus a hydrostatic gradient may develop as a consequence of increased cerebral blood flow (secondary to loss of autoregulation) and a leaky blood-brain barrier, which results in the formation of cerebral edema.

After a brain injury from trauma a cascade of pathologic events is initiated. The initial insult leads to local cerebral vascular dilatation and loss of autoregulation. This in turn causes a passive increase in cerebral blood flow with resulting edema and subsequent expansion of the area of injury. Therapeutic measures to interrupt this cascade and contain the area of damage are the primary concern of the emergency department personnel.

Hypoxemia and cerebral ischemia can be prevented by providing an adequate airway at the scene of the accident by mouth-to-mouth resuscitation, mask ventilation, or endotracheal intubation. Hypotension can be treated by vigorous fluid replacement. Increased ICP can be controlled by hyperventilation, head elevation to 30°, and/or osmotic agents. It is also important that the treatment not be overzealous. For example, fluid overloading may increase cerebral edema and ischemia. Vigorous hyperventilation (P_{CO_2} <25 mmHg) can result in paradoxic vasoconstriction, further aggravating cerebral ischemia. Severe hypertension (systemic blood pressure >180 mmHg) can further compound cerebral edema and possibly exacerbate an underlying intracranial hematoma. Aggressive diuresis with an osmotic agent can result in unwarranted hypotension.

EXAMINATION: NEUROLOGIC

After the patient has been stabilized from a cardiopulmonary standpoint, an initial neurologic assessment should be performed rapidly. It is important to note the various factors in addition to traumatic intracranial injury that can impair consciousness, such as hypoxia, hypotension, toxic and metabolic states, seizures, stroke, tumor, and infection. These factors should be kept in mind along with the many other variables that may be accounting for a patient's state of altered consciousness.

Neurologic injury can produce a diffuse dysfunction that can impair the level of consciousness or produce a focal area of dysfunction, or both. This neurologic examination should include the history of the injury, inspection for external trauma, and evaluation of the level of consciousness and memory. Further evaluation of pupillary responses, eye movement, cranial nerves, and motor activity is used to complete an initial baseline examination; more detailed neurologic testing can be performed as the situation allows.

The most commonly used system to describe a patient's level of consciousness is the GCS (see Table 54-1). This is a relatively simple, reproducible system that all examiners can use to quantify a patient's level of consciousness. This scale assigns a numerical value for eye opening and verbal and motor responses. The score provides a quick assessment of the patient's neurologic status and provides a baseline for following the patient's clinical course.

The best eye opening response reflects the minimum command, sound, or painful stimulus that will cause the patient to open the eye(s). If there is an injury or swelling in the orbital area, the test is not valid.

The best verbal response is based on the patient's level of communication after being maximally aroused. Five points are given if the patient is able to carry on a conversation and is oriented to name, place, date, and the situation; 4 points reflect a confused conversation or disorientation; 3 points are assigned when the patient cannot sustain a conversation and utters intelligible words in a disorganized fashion; 2 points may be given for sounds or moans that are not recognized as words; and 1 point is given for no sound even with a noxious stimuli. If the patient cannot respond because of intubation or aphasia, then the test score is not valid.

The best motor response reflects the highest level of motor activity after the patient is maximally aroused. Six points are given if the patient follows specific motor commands. Additional testing to grade strength may also be done. For the test to be accurate, a spinal cord injury must be excluded, and the stimulus must be sufficiently noxious. Five points reflect the patient's attempt to localize a painful stimulus. Various types of noxious stimuli are applied (ie, sternal rub, deep trapezius pressure, or supraorbital pressure). The patient should attempt to find the noxious stimulus and to ward off or intercept it. The patient may attempt to grasp the examiner's hand and even to reach across the midline of the torso. Four points may be given if the patient withdraws an extremity in response to a noxious stimuli. The patient does not attempt to localize and ward off the stimulus. The response is usually elicited by deep nail bed pressure. All four extremities are examined and

Table 54-1 Glasgow Coma Scale

Eye opening
    4—Spontaneous
    3—To speech and sound
    2—To pain
    1—None
Verbal
    5—Alert, oriented
    4—Confused conversation
    3—Inappropriate words
    2—Incomprehensible sounds
    1—None
Motor
    6—Obeys commands
    5—Localizes pain
    4—Withdraws to pain
    3—Flexor response to pain
    2—Extensor response to pain
    1—None

variations noted. Three points are given for an abnormal flexion response or decorticate posturing, which consists of flexion of the arm, wrist, and fingers with adduction of the shoulders and extension and plantar flexion of the lower extremities.[2] Two points are given for an abnormal extension response posture. The abnormal extension response or decerebrate posture consists of shoulder adduction and internal rotation with the arms stiffly extended and abducted and the legs stiffly extended with the feet plantar flexed. One point is given for no motor response.

It is generally accepted that a decorticate posture indicates a relatively better prognosis than a decerebrate posture in the presence of a mass lesion. Classically, it has been believed that the distinction between decorticate and decerebrate posturing localizes the lesion to the level of the midcollicular region in the midbrain. Lesions rostral to the midbrain result in decorticate posturing, and lesions caudal to the midbrain produce decerebrate posturing. This correlation in structural brain damage does not always exist.[3] Abnormal posturing can result from various causes such as anoxia, hypoglycemia, drug intoxication, and seizures. Therefore, the GCS provides the examiner with a simple construct by which the temporal course of a patient's level of consciousness can be followed reliably.

Focal neurologic signs are as important in the neurologic examination as the level of consciousness. The pupil examination provides a measure of focal changes. One must carefully document the size, shape, symmetry, and response to light of both pupils. An inadequate light source is the most common source of nonreactive pupils. Temporal or uncal lobe herniation can be deduced if there is an enlargement of an ipsilateral pupil that reacts sluggishly. This situation can be a sign of a surgical mass lesion. Metabolic encephalopathies and diencephalic transtentorial herniation can cause bilateral small reactive pupils. Large, fixed, midposition pupils are consistent with midbrain damage or diffuse anoxic damage. Pinpoint pupils are found in patients with pontine damage. It is also important to understand pharmacologic effects on the pupils. Atropine and scopolamine can cause fixed and dilated pupils. Eye drops such as those used in glaucoma patients must be considered in the differential diagnosis of dilated pupils. Opiates can cause pinpoint pupils similar to those in patients with pontine damage. Other pupillary findings in a comatose patient include the following:

- hippus, which is a rhythmic dilation and contraction of the pupil of unknown significance. This phenomenon can also occur in the alert and awake patient.
- afferent pupillary defect (Marcus-Gunn pupil), which can be elicited by the swinging flashlight test. In normal individuals brisk constriction of both pupils can be obtained by rapid alternating stimulation of the pupils. With this defect the affected pupil, once stimulated in this fashion, exhibits a slow constriction that is followed

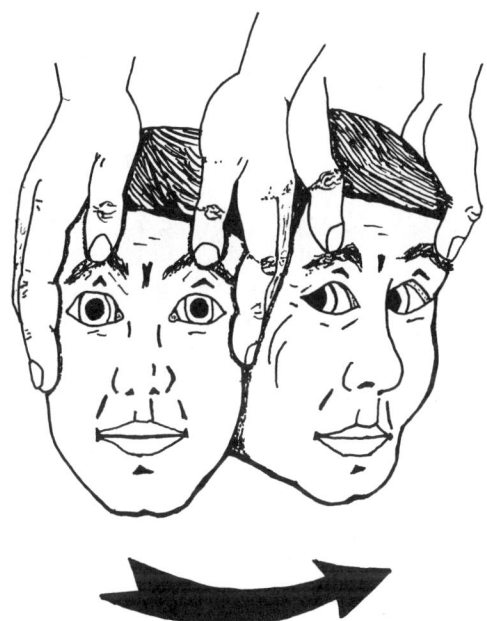

Figure 54-1 Oculocephalic reflex.

by dilation. This pupillary escape phenomenon can occur in lesions or injuries to the retina, optic nerve, or optic chiasm. In the presence of opacification of the ocular media, this test is not reliable.

Eye movements provide information about the functional integrity of the brain stem. It is known that horizontal fast (saccadic) eye movements are controlled in the paramedian pontine reticular formation at the level of the pontomedullary junction. If there is any damage to this region, horizontal eye movements will be impaired. In an unconscious patient horizontal eye movements can be elicited by the oculocephalic or oculovestibular responses. The oculocephalic maneuver (doll's eyes) is performed by raising the patient's head 30° from the supine position and briskly rotating the head in the horizontal plane (Fig. 54-1). In the normal response, both eyes will move conjugately in a direction opposite the direction of the head movement. If there is any brain stem damage, the eyes will move dysconjugately or there will be no movement. In most trauma settings this maneuver is ill advised because the patient can have an occult underlying cervical spine injury. Oculovestibular response or caloric stimulation is accomplished by raising the head 30° and irrigating the external ear canal with 20 to 30 mL of iced saline. The normal response is ipsilateral tonic deviation in an unconscious patient, usually seen within 1 minute (Fig. 54-2). If no response is seen, a larger volume of iced saline (100 mL) should be used. If there is disruption of brain stem integrity, the eyes will move dysconjugately or have no response at all. It is important to examine the ear canals before irrigation. If there is rupture of the tympanic membrane or otorrhea, irrigation is contraindicated. Debris or

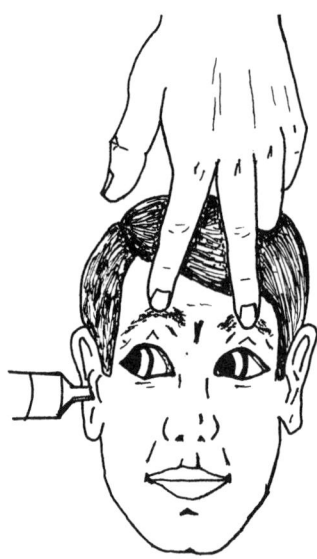

Figure 54-2 Oculovestibular reflex.

cerumen may limit the effectiveness of caloric response and should be cleared before irrigation. The physician should be aware that certain drugs such as barbiturates can impair the oculocephalic or oculovestibular response.

The cranial nerve examination can provide additional information about focal brain stem function in a comatose patient. The corneal reflex checks the integrity of the fifth and seventh cranial nerves both ipsilaterally and contralaterally. This test is performed by applying a wisp of cotton to each cornea and observing the blink response, which should be symmetric. Any asymmetry noted in this response could be indicative of underlying brain stem injury. The remaining cranial nerves should be examined as dictated by the patient's level of consciousness. Testing the lower cranial nerves by the gag reflex could cause vomiting and potential aspiration. External signs of head injury can reveal possible basilar skull fractures such as hemotympanum, ecchymois over the mastoid process (Battle's sign), and periorbital ecchymosis (raccoon eyes). In patients who are intubated, sedated, and paralyzed, the pupillary response is the only clinical parameter that may be followed other than vital signs in regard to central nervous system function.

If the patient is alert and cooperative, a more detailed neurologic examination can be performed. A facial nerve injury can be indicated by widened palpebral fissures or loss of the nasolabial fold. This abnormality may be secondary to a contused or lacerated seventh cranial nerve from a temporal bone fracture.

The motor examination in the awake and alert patient is straightforward, but in the unconscious or uncooperative patient it may be difficult. Evaluation of strength can best be accomplished by observation after application of noxious stimulation. Asymmetry of movement or reflexes is a key indicator that a pathologic lesion may exist.

EXAMINATION: EXTRACRANIAL

Many head-injured patients have sustained significant injuries to the chest, abdomen, spine, or long bones. Often these injuries can be life threatening and command immediate attention.

Respiratory System

Facial or neck injuries can cause areas of swelling that compromise the upper airway. Intubation is often difficult and should be performed in a controlled manner. A tracheostomy may be necessary. A chest injury with a pneumothorax or a spine injury with loss of intercostal muscle support may restrict ventilation. Aspiration is a significant occurrence in patients with a severe head injury. A chest radiograph should be obtained routinely.

Cardiovascular System

Trauma patients are in a hyperdynamic state and often can have fluctuations in blood pressure. Cardiac injuries or injuries to the great vessels in the chest or abdomen may occur. Injury to the carotid artery should be considered in association with a neck injury.

Gastrointestinal-Urinary System

Abdominal tenderness to palpation, guarding, or rigidity should be attributed to abdominal injuries. Virtually all trauma patients have full stomachs and are at risk for vomiting and aspiration. The patient should be assessed for traumatic kidney, bladder, or urethral injuries.

Musculoskeletal System

Long bone and pelvic injuries are common. These injuries should be defined and appropriate stabilizing measures taken. Pain to palpation of the spinous processes of the cervical, thoracic, or lumbar spine may indicate an acute injury. All unresponsive patients should be presumed to have sustained a spine injury, and measures should be taken to support and stabilize the spine.

RADIOLOGIC AND LABORATORY TESTS

Upon arrival of a head-injured patient at the emergency department, the following routine laboratory studies should be obtained immediately during the stabilization phase:

- complete blood cell count
- chemistries, including renal function tests
- glucose level
- serum osmolality

- arterial blood gases (if indicated)
- toxicology screen

The following radiographic studies should be obtained:

- cervical spine (cross-table lateral): These films are to be reviewed by an experienced radiologist and neurosurgeon before a patient's neck is moved. A systematic approach should be used when examining these films, and the following should be looked for:

  1. prevertebral anterior soft tissue swelling (abnormal in adults if greater than 6 mm at the inferior edge of C-2 or if greater than 22 mm at the inferior edge of C-6)
  2. on the lateral view, the predental space (atlas to anterior dens; abnormal if greater than 3 mm)
  3. bony alignment (should be anatomic)
  4. bony fractures or compressions
  5. facet fractures and rotation
  6. C-7 and T-1 (swimmer's view or CT scan if necessary; cervical spine stability is not ensured with a single cross-table lateral view, but if there is no abnormality the patient can be moved for more complete studies)

- chest: This film is important to rule out associated injuries of the chest such as pneumothorax, lung contusion, aortic dissection, thoracic fractures, or malpositions of the endotracheal tube.
- skull: The use of the skull radiograph in head trauma has been supplanted by CT. Nevertheless, the skull film may be useful in the final evaluation of awake, alert patients with mild head injuries. Approximately 3% of these patients have been found to deteriorate in spite of a normal initial neurologic examination. In this group an abnormal skull film has been associated with a high probability that the patient will go on to require a neurosurgical procedure.[4] Although no fracture pattern is pathognomonic of a developing intracranial hematoma, fractures crossing the middle meningeal groove or dural venous sinuses warrant close observation and a head CT scan. Intracranial air or air-fluid levels in the paranasal sinuses could indicate a basal skull fracture.
- other views: Abdominal, pelvic, and extremity films are performed as clinically indicated.

TREATMENT

Positioning

Elevating the head to 30° significantly reduces ICP without compromising cerebral perfusion pressure, cardiac output, or cerebral blood flow.[5] It is also important to keep the neck in straight alignment to prevent kinking of the internal jugular vein. Kinking of the internal jugular vein impedes the venous outflow of the cerebral circulation, resulting in increased ICP.

Hyperventilation

The most effective means to reduce ICP in the acute setting of the head-injured patient is hyperventilation. Hyperventilation reduces the Pco_2 by causing a cerebral arteriolar vasoconstriction. This reduces the total blood volume in the cerebral circulation, thus resulting in a decrease in ICP. Pco_2 should be maintained in the 25- to 30-mmHg range. Overzealous hyperventilation (<25 mmHg) should be avoided as it could result in ischemia.

Dehydration

Mannitol is the most widely accepted agent used to decrease ICP. The mechanism of action has been debated throughout the literature. It is generally thought that mannitol establishes an osmotic gradient between the plasma and the brain, resulting in a shift of water out of the brain and therefore a fall in ICP.[6] Other studies have shown that, in addition to the dehydrating effect, a decrease in blood viscosity after mannitol administration causes a vasoconstriction secondary to improved oxygen transport, thus resulting in a decrease in ICP.[7]

In the trauma setting, if a patient's neurologic status declines or if the patient develops a dilated pupil, mannitol should be given. The current recommended dose is 1.0 to 1.5 g/kg by intravenous bolus. Serum osmolality is usually kept at 290 to 310 mOsm/L depending on ICP.

Some investigators have recommended the use of furosemide in addition to mannitol.[1] A brisker diuresis can be obtained with the two agents used in combination. With this therapy, rapid electrolyte losses and hypotension can occur, and therefore aggressive fluid and electrolyte replacement must be instituted.

Steroids

The efficacy of steroids in head-injured patients has been a controversial issue in the literature. Studies in the late 1970s showed that a high dose of steroids reduced the mortality rate in head-injured patients.[1] When these studies were scrutinized, however, deficiencies in the study designs were found; furthermore, the reduction in mortality was a reflection of an increase in vegetative survivals. Further studies in the early and late 1980s showed that high-dose steroids have no statistically significant effect on morbidity, mortality, or intracranial ICP.[8–10] Thus steroids have no proven role in the management of the head-injured patient.

Barbiturates

Barbiturates have been reported to protect the brain against ischemia and to lower ICP. The pharmacologic and biochemical mechanism responsible for this protection is currently unknown. The clinical use of high-dose barbiturates in the severely head-injured patient has not been shown to be of any benefit.[9,11,12] Barbiturates may benefit a small group of patients (usually young patients) who have failed the traditional forms of therapy (hyperventilation and dehydration). These patients initially present in good neurologic status and then deteriorate secondary to uncontrolled increased ICP. One recommended dose for barbiturate is 5 to 10 mg/kg intravenously and then 1 to 3 mg/kg/hour as a maintenance dosage until a burst-suppression pattern is achieved on electroencephalography.[12]

Anticonvulsants

The use of phenytoin is required in all head-injured patients who are intubated and paralyzed in the emergency department because clinically evident seizure activity could be masked by paralysis. The recommended initial loading dose of 15 mg/kg intravenously is followed by a maintenance dosage of 100 mg intravenously every 8 hours. The effectiveness of anticonvulsants in the awake head-injured patient has been controversial, however, and many controlled studies have shown inconclusive results. A recent randomized double-blind study[13] determined that phenytoin reduces seizures only during the first week after severe head injury.

Intracranial Pressure Monitoring

ICP monitoring should be considered in the acute setting for the patients most at risk for developing increased ICP. The following groups of patients are at the highest risk:

- those with a GCS value of 8 or less
- those with CT findings consistent with increased ICP (diffuse cerebral edema, obliteration of basal cisterns, or midline shift) and who had periods of hypoxia and ischemia
- those whose CT scans appear normal but who remain comatose and are older than 40 years, have pathologic motor posturing, have a systolic blood pressure less than 90 mmHg, or are recovering after cardiopulmonary resuscitation

Various forms of ICP monitoring devices are available. These include ventriculostomy, subarachnoid bolt, and, more recently, fiberoptic systems. The last of these may be used in the subarachnoid space, intraparenchymal tissue, or ventricles.

HEAD INJURY: COMPONENTS

Scalp and Skull Injuries

Scalp lacerations are one of the most common injuries to the head. A thorough examination of the scalp must be performed in all head-injured patients. The hair should be shaved as necessary to visualize areas of suspected injury. After the laceration is localized, digital pressure can be applied for hemostasis, and the hair should be shaved about 2 cm from the margins of the wound. These lacerations should be irrigated vigorously with 1 L of sterile normal saline and then carefully explored and debrided under sterile conditions. During exploration the underlying bone should be assessed for fractures. The physician may then close the wound primarily if no fracture is detected. The galea is first reapproximated with 2-0 Vicryl absorbable structure in a simple inverted fashion, and the skin is approximated with 3-0 nonabsorbable suture (nylon). For cosmesis, areas on the forehead should be sutured with a 5-0 nylon suture. Tetanus prophylaxis is given as clinically indicated.

A fracture may be discovered while one is inspecting a laceration. This is considered an open skull fracture. A depressed skull fracture is diagnosed when a fragment has been depressed by the width of the adjacent skull. Open depressed skull fractures should be treated by operative debridement of the wound, elevation of depressed fragments, and exploration of the dura. Nondepressed open or closed skull fractures need no surgical intervention. The use of antibiotics is recommended for open depressed skull fractures. Nafcillin (2 g intravenously) is given before surgical intervention and is followed by 5 to 7 days of nafcillin (2 g intravenously every 6 hours).

Basilar skull fractures are usually diagnosed indirectly from the clinical examination. Signs of basilar skull fractures include hemotympanum, rhinorrhea, otorrhea, raccoon eyes, and Battle's sign. Raccoon eyes and Battle's sign usually do not appear until 24 hours after the injury and therefore cannot be relied upon in the early stages of the evaluation of head-injured patients. Basilar skull fractures are usually located in the petrous portion of the temporal bone or in the floor of the anterior cranial fossa involving the cribriform plate and/or orbital roof. These fractures can cause cranial nerve deficits. A petrous temporal bone fracture can involve the seventh and eighth cranial nerves. An anterior cranial fossa fracture can result in anosmia. Plain skull films usually have a poor yield in demonstrating basilar skull fractures. CT scan with bone window images can usually detect these fractures, but a normal scan cannot exclude the diagnosis of basilar skull fracture. If a basilar skull fracture is associated with rhinorrhea or otorrhea, prophylactic antibiotics are not recommended. These patients warrant admission. The usual treatment for cerebrospinal fluid leaks is to have the patient elevate the head to 30° and avoid coughing, sneezing, or straining. Most leaks (greater than 90%) will stop spontaneously with conservative treatment. A documented case of meningitis should be treated with appropriate antibiotics as dictated by cerebrospinal fluid cultures.

A subgaleal hematoma is a collection of blood between the galea and pericranium. This is commonly seen in young children. The hematoma can spread across suture lines and appear quite extensive. The hematoma will enlarge as it liquefies. No surgical treatment is necessary, and the mass will disappear in 1 to 3 weeks. These lesions are not usually associated with fractures except in children younger than 1 year. These infants may have a linear nondisplaced skull fracture that requires no treatment. Occasionally the collection may become so large that the infant may become anemic, and hospital admission to monitor serial hematocrit is required.

Penetrating and Projectile Injuries

Penetrating injuries of the head are considered low-velocity injuries and will damage only those structures in the path of the object. Penetrating injuries are often caused by stab wounds from, for example, a knife or an ice pick. If this object remains in a patient's head, it should not be removed in the emergency department. Plain skull films are obtained as well as CT scans of head. A neurosurgeon must be consulted immediately and the operating room prepared. The usual resuscitation protocols also apply in this situation, as in all other head injuries. Prophylactic antibiotics should be instituted immediately (nafcillin, 2 g intravenously every 6 hours or vancomycin, 500 mg intravenously every 6 hours).

Projectile injuries are high-velocity injuries compared to penetrating injuries. They are often caused by gunshot wounds. The projectiles not only directly damage brain tissue in their path but also impart a significant amount of kinetic energy to the surrounding tissue, which can be more destructive over a larger area by creating a shock wave effect. The standard head injury resuscitation applies, including prophylactic antibiotics. On the basis of the outcome of a recent prospective study, all patients with a cranial gunshot wound should initially receive aggressive resuscitation, and a CT scan should be performed when patients are stable.[14] Those patients with GCS values of 5 or less and with no operable hematoma present should not receive any further aggressive therapy. Those patients with a GCS value greater than 5 should undergo aggressive therapy, surgical exploration, and debridement. Poor outcomes have been noted in patients who have GCS values of 5 or less, transventricular injuries, diffuse bihemispheric injuries, or a unilateral dominant hemispheric injury.

Closed Head Injuries

A closed head injury may cause a diffuse disruption of the neural architecture and be manifested as edema, or it may be associated with a variable degree of intracranial hemorrhage. Traumatic intracranial hematomas can be divided into epidural, subdural, intraparenchymal, and subarachnoid types.

Epidural Hematoma

Epidural hematomas usually occur when there is an associated fracture of the cranial vault. The temporal bone is most commonly involved near the middle meningeal vessels. These hematomas result from direct impact injuries. Classically, it was thought that these epidural hematomas resulted from a tear of the middle meningeal artery, but the middle meningeal vein also may frequently be the primary site of the hemorrhage.[1] Other sources of epidural hematoma include the diploic veins, the dural venous sinuses, and venous tributaries. Patients usually present with a history of a loss of consciousness from which they recover uneventfully; this is followed by a lucid interval that deteriorates into a coma. This description is not universal, and various other clinical presentations can be seen depending on the location of the hematoma, its rate of expansion, and the degree of underlying parenchymal damage.

The usual CT scan appearance demonstrates a hyperdense biconvex or lenticular lesion in the epidural space that does not cross suture lines and is associated with a bony fracture. Occasionally, if a CT scan is performed early in the patient's evaluation, an epidural hematoma may not be present. The hematoma may evolve subsequently while the patient is awaiting a further diagnostic work-up. This again emphasizes the need for frequent serial neurologic examinations. Epidural hematomas are usually not associated with underlying parenchymal injury and therefore often have a more favorable prognosis compared to subdural hematomas.

Subdural Hematomas

Subdural hematomas usually result from injury to the cortical bridging vessels on the surface of the brain. These traumatic hematomas tend to occur with acceleration/deceleration injuries with rotation, such as occur in falls. Subdural hematomas are usually associated with an underlying brain injury such as a contusion or laceration. These patients have sustained a significant brain injury, which accounts for their adverse outcome. Mortality rates are in the 60% to 90% range despite major advances in the management of head injury. The following factors significantly affect mortality and functional survival: age, sex, presenting GCS value, hypotension, hypoxia, and timing of operative intervention. The timing of surgery has been a controversial issue. Recently, it has been shown that the timing of interventions does not affect morbidity or mortality.[15] The prevailing philosophy, however, is that the expeditious removal of a subdural hematoma is still warranted to prevent secondary insult from edema.

An acute subdural hematoma usually appears as a hyperdense lesion conforming to the cortical surface, but it can occasionally resemble an epidural hematoma. There is 15% to 20% incidence of bilateral subdural hematomas in head-injured patients. Sometimes isodense hematomas can occur. In these cases a contrast CT scan or magnetic resonance scan may be helpful.

Intraparenchymal Hematomas

These lesions occur secondary to a crush injury (contusion) or laceration of the cortex and white matter. It is generally held that these injuries result from acceleration/deceleration and rotational forces, which cause movement of the brain against the irregular surfaces of the anterior cranial and middle fossae (for example, the cribriform plate or the petrous ridge of the temporal bone). If the brain contusion or hematoma lies directly underneath the point of impact, one refers to this as a coup injury. In contrast, a contracoup injury is in a remote part of the brain, usually opposite the point of impact. The most common sites of injury are the tip and basal surface of the frontal and temporal lobes.

Intraparenchymal hematomas appear as high-density lesions on CT scan, usually in the white matter and occasionally surrounded by a low-density region of edema. Those lesions causing mass effect and increased ICP require immediate aggressive surgical management. Clinical presentation again is determined by location, size, edema, and extent of injury. Delayed posttraumatic hematomas can occur up to 1 week after injury. If there is a change in neurologic status or ICP, a repeat CT scan is warranted. This phenomenon is believed to occur secondary to breakthrough bleeding as a result of a loss of autoregulation and a breakdown of the blood-brain barrier.

Subarachnoid Hemorrhage

This entity is the most common hemorrhagic lesion after head injury. The presence of a small amount of subarachnoid blood has no prognostic significance, but large amounts may exacerbate cerebral vasospasm in the head-injured patient. Subarachnoid hemorrhage may also result in the development of hydrocephalus. The CT scan reveals high-density lesions with blood distributed along cortical sulci, interhemispheric fissures, and basal cisterns.

DISPOSITION

Patients admitted to the emergency department after a head injury have variable severities of injury ranging from a minor head bump to irreversible coma and brain death.

Patients with mild head injury are awake, alert, and conversant on admission to the emergency department. They are oriented and aware of their circumstances. In many instances there may have been a brief loss of consciousness, and they may be amnestic for the events surrounding the accident. They may have complaints of headache, nausea, or vomiting.

Approximately 3% of patients in the mild head injury group (GCS 13 to 15) have been found to deteriorate and require a neurosurgical procedure in spite of a normal initial neurologic examination and alert level of consciousness.[4] An abnormal skull radiograph usually correlates well with an abnormal head CT scan and is associated with a higher probability that the patient will require a neurosurgical procedure. It is unusual for a patient with a GCS value of 15 and a normal skull film or head CT scan to require surgery for intracranial pathology.

A patient with a mild head injury should be observed with serial neurologic examinations. Skull radiographs or a CT scan of the head should be obtained. If the neurologic examination, including memory, is not improving, and/or if there is an abnormality on the head CT scan or skull film, then the neurosurgeon should evaluate the patient, and the patient should be admitted to the hospital for continued observation. Patients who do not meet the admission criteria may be discharged from the emergency department with a reliable adult companion and with specific written instructions and follow-up clinic appointments.

The criteria for admitting a mild head injury patient who is apparently awake, alert, and oriented are as follows:

- progressive deterioration in level of consciousness
- sustained amnesia with the inability to form new memory
- history of a significant loss of consciousness
- severe intractable headache
- skull fracture or abnormal head CT scan
- cerebrospinal fluid leak (rhinorrhea or otorrhea)
- systemic symptoms or injuries that would require a hospital admission
- alcohol or drug intoxication
- children younger than 5 years with paroxysms of agitation or vomiting

Patients with moderate to severe head injury have sustained a significant neurologic injury and will have a GCS value less than 13, or alternatively they may be alert but with a focal neurologic deficit. These patients require hospital admission for continued observation and treatment. Patients who are unable to follow commands should be intubated immediately. A patient with a GCS value less than 8 should have ICP monitoring. Rapid and definitive medical and, if indicated, neurosurgical treatment should be instituted.

OUTCOME

It is difficult to predict a patient's final outcome after a head injury. Clinical data that include age, GCS, pupillary reaction, eye movement, and pathologic motor posturing have often been relied upon. The prompt treatment of a surgical lesion has also been evaluated with respect to outcome. Predictive information has also been proposed from data from CT scans and sensory, auditory, and visual evoked potentials.[16]

The most important factor in improving a patient's outcome is the prevention of secondary brain injury. Hypoxemia and ischemia must be minimized. In a review of a group of head-injured patients who were initially talking after a head injury and who subsequently died, it was concluded that avoidable factors had occurred that contributed to the deaths. These factors included hypoxemia, hypotension, delay in treatment, sepsis, and seizures.[17]

The most significant advance in the management of head injuries has been made in the area of emergency services. The rapid response and scrupulous attention to the details of resuscitation both at the scene and in the emergency department, with immediate correction of hypoxemia or hypotension coupled with rapid surgical intervention to remove a mass lesion and aggressive treatment of elevated ICP, have resulted in an increasing number of head-injured patients with a satisfactory recovery.[18]

Delayed complications may occur after a head injury. Injuries to the cervical spine are common after a head injury, and proper precautions must be taken. Seizures also can occur after any head injury. They are more common after a penetrating injury and are more frequent in patients with a focal motor deficit or mass lesion. Phenytoin is useful in reducing early seizures. The seizure frequency in the first year after the trauma is predictive of the future severity of seizures.[13] Rhinorrhea or otorrhea is common after a basilar skull fracture and occurs in 2% to 3% of head injuries. The majority of cerebrospinal fluid leaks will stop spontaneously within 1 to 2 weeks. It is not recommended that antibiotics be used prophylactically. Surgical procedures to correct persistent leaks can be performed.

REFERENCES

1. Becker DP. Common themes in head injury. In: Becker DP, Gudeman SK, eds. *Textbook of Head Injury*. Philadelphia: Saunders; 1989:1–6.
2. Plum F, Posner JB. *Diagnosis of Stupor and Coma*. Philadelphia: Davis; 1982:65–70.
3. Marshall LF, Marshall SB. Medical management of intracranial pressure. In: Cooper PR, ed. *Head Injury*. Baltimore: Williams & Wilkins; 1987:185–186.
4. Dacey RG, Alvers WM, Rimel RW. Neurosurgical complications after apparently minor head injury. Assessment of risk in a series of 610 patients. *J Neurosurg*. 1986;65:203–210.
5. Feldman Z, Kanter MJ, Robertson CS, et al. Effect of head elevation on intracranial pressure, cerebral perfusion pressure, in head injured patients. *J Neurosurg*. 1992;76:207–211.
6. Narayan RK. Emergency room management of the head-injured patient. In: Becker DP, Gudeman SK, eds. *Textbook of Head Injury*. Philadelphia: Saunders; 1989:50–51.
7. Muizelaar JP, Lutz HA, Becker DP. Effect of mannitol on intracranial pressure, cerebral blood flow, and correlation with pressure autoregulation in head injured patients. *J Neurosurg*. 1984;61:700–706.
8. Braakman R, Shouten HJA, Dishoeck MB, et al. Megadose steroids in severe head injury. Results of a prospective double-blind clinical trial. *J Neurosurg*. 1983;58:326–330.
9. Clifton GL. Controversies in medical management of head injury. *Clin Neurosurg*. 1988;34:587–600.
10. Deardon NM, Gibson JS, McDowall DG, et al. Effect of high-dose dexamethasone on outcome from severe head injury. *J Neurosurg*. 1986;58:326–330.
11. Piat JH, Schiff SJ. High dose barbiturate therapy in neurosurgery and intensive care. *Neurosurgery*. 1984;15:427–444.
12. Ward JD, Becker DP, Miller JP, et al. Failure of prophylactic barbiturate coma in the treatment of severe head injury. *J Neurosurg*. 1985;62:383–388.
13. Tempkin NR, Dikmen SS, Willensky AJ, et al. A randomized, double-blind study of phenytoin for the prevention of post-traumatic seizures. *N Engl J Med*. 1990;323:497–502.
14. Grahm TW, Williams FC, Harrington TH, Spetzler RF. Civilian gunshot wounds to the head: a prospective study. *Neurosurgery*. 1990;27:696–700.
15. Wilbeger JE, Harris M, Diamond DL. Acute subdural hematoma: morbidity and mortality related to timing of operative intervention. *J Trauma*. 1990;30:733–736.
16. Eisenberg HM. Outcome after head injury: general considerations. In: Becker DP, Povleshock JT, eds. *Central Nervous System Status Report*. Bethesda, MD: National Institutes of Health; 1985:271–280.
17. Rose J, Valtoness S, Jennett B. Avoidable factors contributing to death after head injury. *Br Med J*. 1977;2:615–617.
18. Cooper PR. Delayed brain injury: secondary insults. In: Becker DP, Povleshock JT, eds. *Central Nervous System Status Report*. Bethesda, MD: National Institutes of Health; 1985:217–228.

55. Cervical Spine Injuries

DAVID J. DULA, MD, FACEP

Traumatic injuries to the cervical spine must be recognized as soon as possible and managed properly if the catastrophic complications of such injuries are to be avoided. Conservative estimates place the number of serious spinal cord injuries at approximately 5000 per year, with an additional number of spinal injuries that do not involve the cord.[1] Statistics show that less than 50% of the patients with significant injury to the bony cervical spine have injuries to the cord. Of cord injuries, less than 50% are complete injuries (total loss of cord function distal to the lesion); the majority are partial (some remaining cord function distal to the lesion) and these patients have an excellent prognosis for recovery.[2]

It is estimated that up to 10% of patients with an underlying cervical spine injury develop paralysis as the result of unprotected manipulation of the head and neck during their initial medical care.[3] Because of the devastating nature of spinal cord injuries and the prolonged disability that results, it is vital to develop a system of care for such patients that will prevent any additional cord injury and provide the best chance for recovery. To achieve this goal, emergency care personnel must be trained to recognize and treat injuries of the cervical spine. Of special importance is the detection of partial cord injuries, because these injuries are the most difficult to detect and have the greatest potential for recovery. The development and utilization of regional spinal cord centers, along with good prehospital and emergency department care, provide patients with cord injuries optimal care.

ANATOMY

The cervical spine is composed of seven vertebrae; the first, the atlas, articulates with the occipital condyles superiorly and the odontoid process and superior facets of the second vertebra body inferiorly. It is a ringlike structure and is different from the other six cervical vertebrae in that it has no vertebral body. The remaining six cervical vertebrae have a vertebral body, pedicles, laminae, and a spinous process (Fig. 55-1). The second cervical vertebra, the axis, has a bony strut (the odontoid) attached to its vertebral body that permits both stable articulation with the atlas and rotational mobility. The remaining cervical vertebrae articulate with each other by way of the facet joints.

The ligamentous structures of the cervical spine are vitally important to its stability. The major ligaments include the supraspinous ligament and the interspinous ligament, the articular capsule of the facet joints, the ligamentum flavum, the posterior longitudinal ligament, the anterior longitudinal ligament, and the transverse ligament (Fig. 55-2). The anterior longitudinal ligament is a strong, narrow band of dense fibers connected to tissue that is attached to the anterior margins of the vertebral body and the intervertebral disks; it maintains stability when the cervical spine is extended. The posterior longitudinal ligament courses along the posterior aspect of the vertebral bodies and disks and forms the ante-

---

I would like to give special thanks to Donna Rentzel for her help and encouragement in preparing this manuscript and to James Schmidt for his help in providing the illustrations used in this chapter.

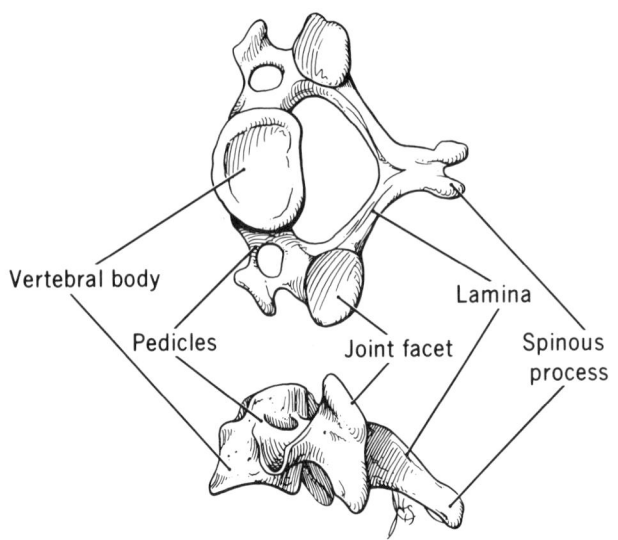

Figure 55-1 Anatomy of the cervical vertebrae.

rior boundary of the spinal canal. The capsular ligament is a thin, loose structure that attaches to the margins of the articular processes of the facet joints. The ligamentum flavum is a thick, dense ligament that connects with the lamina of each vertebral body and forms the posterior ligamentous margin of the spinal canal. The supraspinous ligament and the interspinous ligament connect the spinous processes of the vertebral bodies and impart stability to the cervical spine during flexion maneuvers. The transverse ligament maintains the odontoid in its fixed position within the atlas.

The combination of these vertebrae and ligaments allows the cervical spine to maintain its stability despite its high degree of mobility.

PATHOPHYSIOLOGY

Traumatic injuries to the bony cervical spine and cervical cord are often interrelated (Table 55-1). However, to understand the different injuries that can occur to the cervical spine and cord, it is easier to consider them separate entities.

Cervical Spine Injuries

Trauma to the cervical spine from either direct or inertial forces most commonly results from motor vehicle accidents, but such an injury can also occur in falls, sports, and incidents involving projectiles (Table 55-2). Inertial forces play a prominent role in an automobile accident, for example, when the driver is wearing a shoulder harness and a seatbelt.

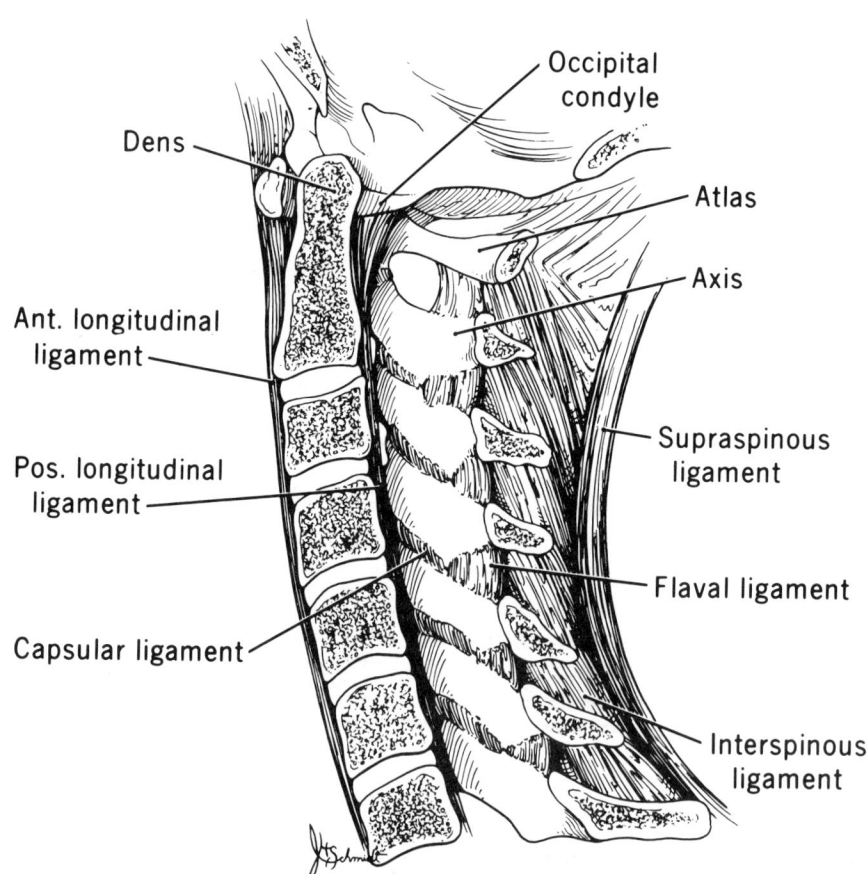

Figure 55-2 Ligamentous anatomy of the cervical spine.

Cervical Spine Injuries   905

Table 55-1 Relation of Cervical Spine Injuries to Cervical Cord Injuries

Type of Spine Injury	Number	(%)	Total Cord	Partial Cord
Stable fracture	20	(22)	9	3
Unstable fracture	63	(69)	19	13
No fracture	8	(9)	0	8
Total	91	(100)	19 (21%)	24 (26%)

Table 55-2 Trauma to Cervical Spine

	Number	Percent
Auto	65	62.5
Falls	24	23.0
Motorcycle	5	4.8
Dive	5	4.8
Sport	2	1.0
Missile	1	1.0
Other	2	1.9

The thorax is secured to the seat of the car, whereas the head and neck remain mobile and are subjected to inertial forces that may result in a flexion or extension injury to the cervical spine.[4] Whether the cervical spine is traumatized from a direct blow or from an inertial event, the injury results from a combination of several forces—flexion, rotation, compression, and extension.

A. Flexion Injuries
   1. Anterior subluxation
   2. Bilateral interfacetal dislocation
   3. Clay shoveler's fracture
   4. Flexion tear-drop fracture
B. Rotation Injuries
   1. Unilateral interfacetal dislocation
C. Vertical Compression Injuries
   1. Bursting fracture
      a. Jefferson fracture of atlas
      b. Burst fracture, lower cervical vertebrae
D. Extension Injuries
   1. Extension tear-drop fracture
   2. Hangman's fracture (deceleration, hyperextension)

These forces may cause injury to either the ligaments or the osseous structures of the cervical spine.

Flexion injuries to the cervical spine may disrupt the posterior longitudinal ligament, resulting in various degrees of anterior subluxation and cervical instability. A severe flexion force may produce additional subluxation and dislocation of the facet joints (Fig. 55-3). When the posterior longitudinal ligament tears, separation or fanning of the spinous processes results, an important finding that can be seen on the lateral cervical spine roentgenogram. A simple wedge fracture or teardrop fracture of the vertebral body results from compressive forces exerted on the anterior portion of the vertebral body during extreme flexion (Fig. 55-4).

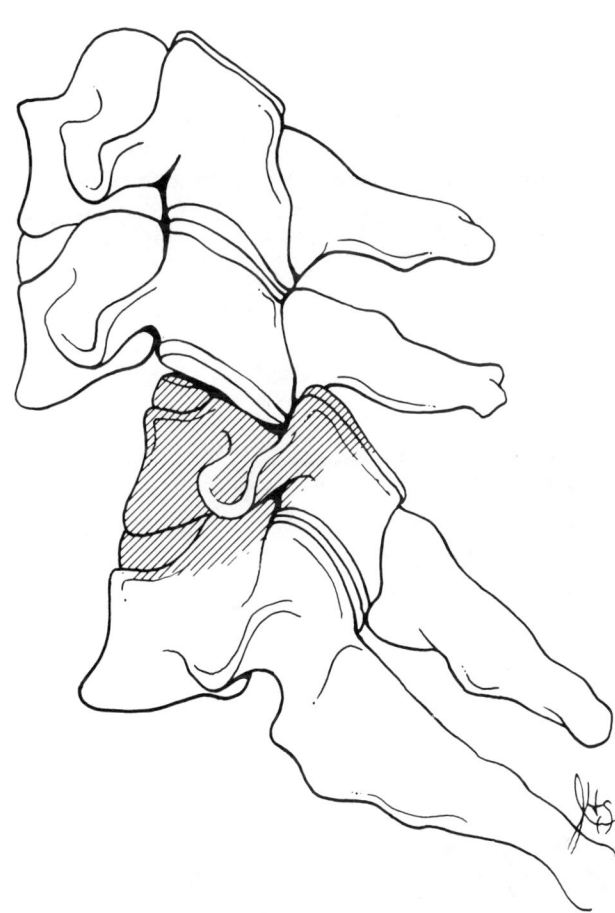

Figure 55-3 Interlocking articular facets.

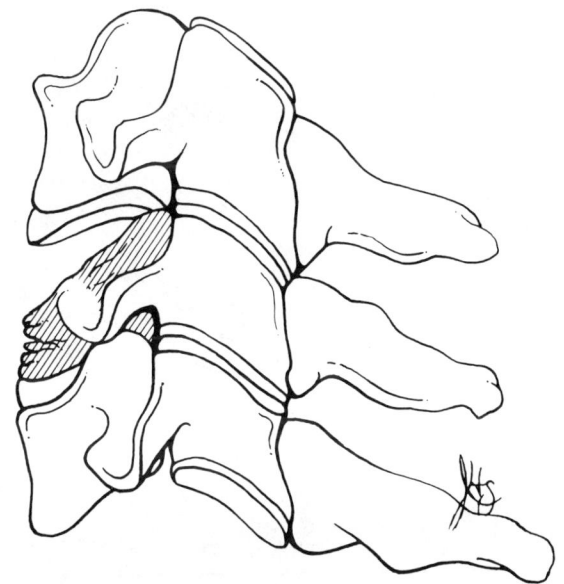

Figure 55-4 Wedge fracture of a cervical vertebra.

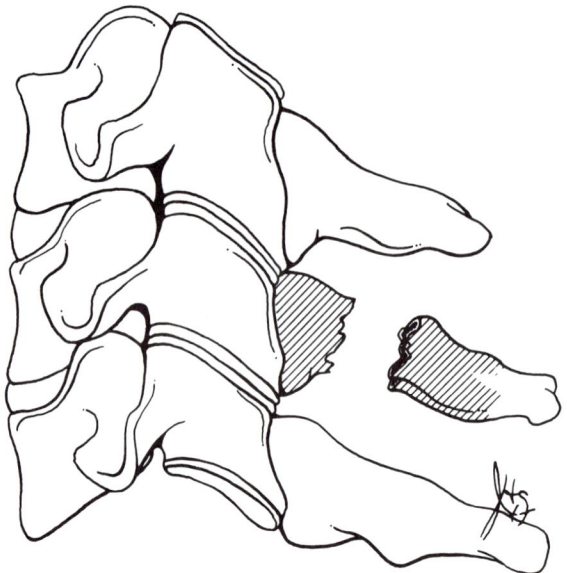

Figure 55-5 Clay shoveler's fracture.

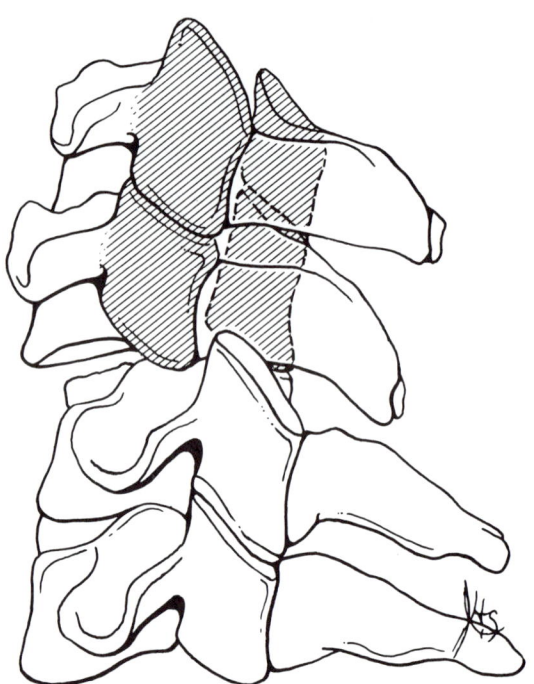

Figure 55-6 Unilateral locked facet.

A clay shoveler's fracture (Fig. 55-5) is defined as an avulsion type of fracture of the proximal portion of the spinous process, usually occurring at C-6, C-7, or T-1 as a result of an abrupt flexion of the head against the tensed posterior ligaments.

A flexion-rotation mechanism of injury may result in a unilateral facet dislocation. This injury occurs when the flexion force is great enough to cause one facet to move across its adjacent inferior facet and come to rest in a dislocated position (Fig. 55-6). The posterior ligament complex and capsule of the involved joint is disrupted, and the posterior longitudinal ligament is partially disrupted. In this position, the vertebral bodies are locked, however, and the fracture is therefore considered to be stable.

A compressive force to the cervical spine results in several classical injuries, such as a Jefferson fracture of the atlas (Fig. 55-7). This injury is the result of a force transmitted

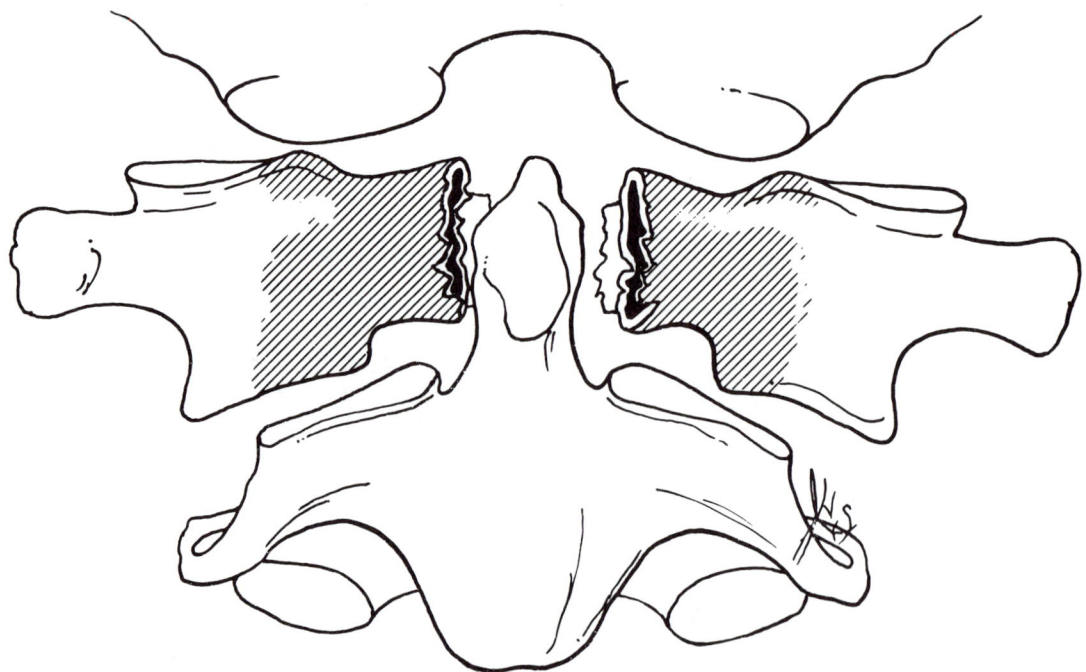

Figure 55-7 Jefferson fracture with bursting of the ringlike structure of the atlas.

through the occiput to the lateral masses of the atlas. The force drives the articular masses laterally, producing bilateral fractures of both the anterior and posterior arches of C-1, and disrupting the transverse atlantal ligament. A bursting fracture of the lower cervical bodies may result from vertical compression forces transmitted to the cervical spine (Fig. 55-8). This is the result of the nucleus pulposus being imploded into the vertebral body, resulting in the characteristic comminuted fracture of the cervical vertebral body. The posterior fragments of the vertebral body are usually displaced posteriorly.

Extension injuries of the cervical spine frequently cause injuries to the cord without evidence of injury to the cervical vertebrae. Buckling of the ligamentum flavum posteriorly and compression of the cord against the spurs of the vertebral body anteriorly cause a temporary compression of the cord (Fig. 55-9). Additionally, hyperextension of the neck can cause fracture dislocations of the cervical spine, posterior atlantal arch fractures, or extension teardrop fractures of the cervical spine. The teardrop deformity results from an avulsion of bone by the stressed anterior longitudinal ligament during extension (Fig. 55-10). Another type of hyperextension injury is the hangman's fracture, which derives its name from the fact that its pathologic skeletal characteristics are similar to those caused by judicial hanging.[5] This fracture is a bilateral fracture of the pedicles of the axis associated with a subluxation of C-2 on C-3 (Fig. 55-11).

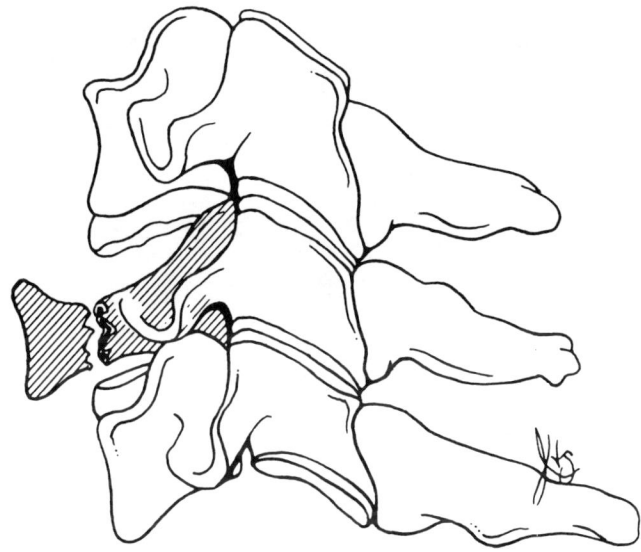

Figure 55-8 Bursting fracture of a cervical vertebra.

Shearing forces acting on the first and second vertebrae may cause fracture of the odontoid and/or disruption of the transverse ligament—the fibrous band that retains the odontoid in its proper anatomical position within the ring of the atlas (Fig. 55-12). These injuries are highly unstable and require immediate care to prevent injury to the cord.

Figure 55-9 Mechanism of cord compression in hyperextension injuries of the cervical spine.

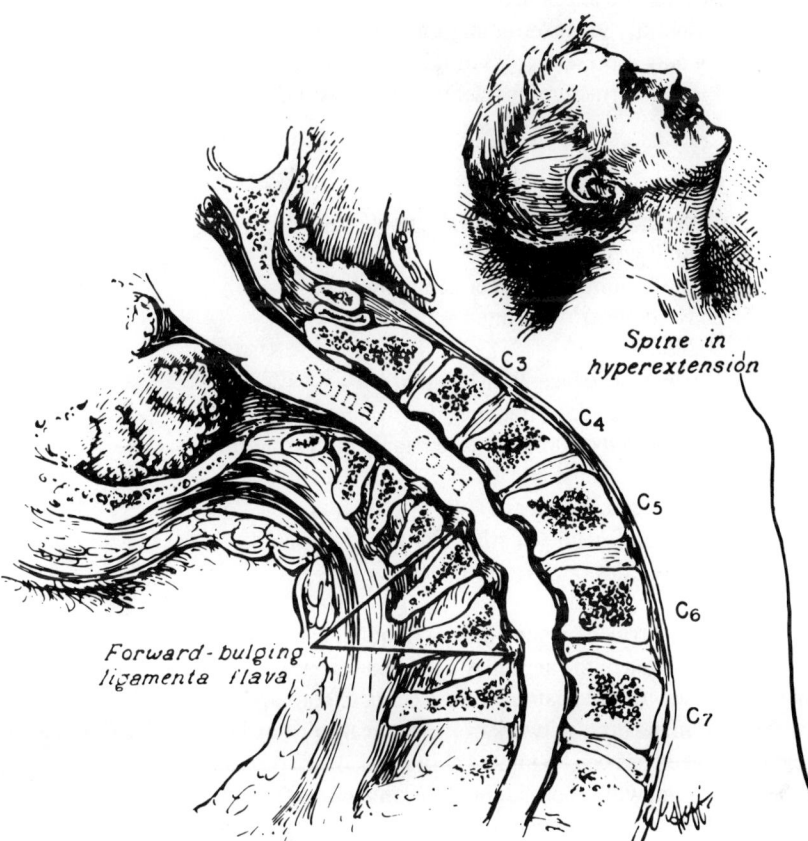

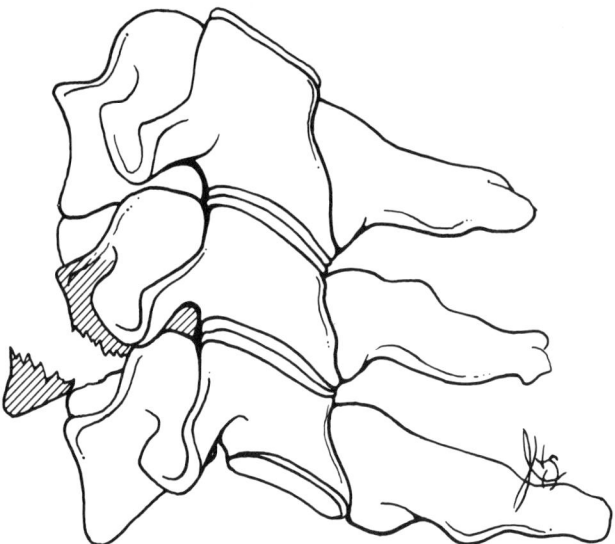

Figure 55-10 Teardrop fracture of the cervical vertebrae.

Other types of fractures, dislocations, and subluxations can best be understood in relation to the anatomical structures involved. It is difficult to determine with certainty whether any cervical fracture is stable or unstable, and a realistic approach may be to divide types of fractures into those that have a high probability of being stable and those that have a high probability of being unstable. Some cervical spine injuries may be unstable only in certain positions, such as flexion instability in posterior longitudinal ligament tears, while others may represent gross instability in any position, such as hangman's fracture or fractures of the odontoid.

A. Stable
1. Anterior subluxation
2. Unilateral interfacetal dislocation
3. Simple wedge fracture
4. Burst fracture, lower cervical vertebrae
5. Clay shoveler's fracture

B. Unstable
1. Bilateral interfacetal dislocation
2. Flexion tear-drop fracture
3. Extension tear-drop fracture (stable in flexion, unstable in extension)
4. Hangman's fracture
5. Jefferson fracture of atlas
6. Hyperextension fracture-dislocation

Even stable cervical spine injuries require care, since exaggerated motion of the neck may exacerbate a partial cord injury. A review of the anatomy of the cervical cord and its position within the bony network of the cervical spine makes it clear how the cord can be injured (Fig. 55-13). Disruption of the bony framework, herniation of disk material, or compromise of the vascular supply to the cord may all result in an insult to the cervical cord. Hyperextension may temporarily compress the cord. Inertial forces acting on the cervical cord may result in areas of contusion to the cord, while a severe injury may result in anatomical transection of the cord.

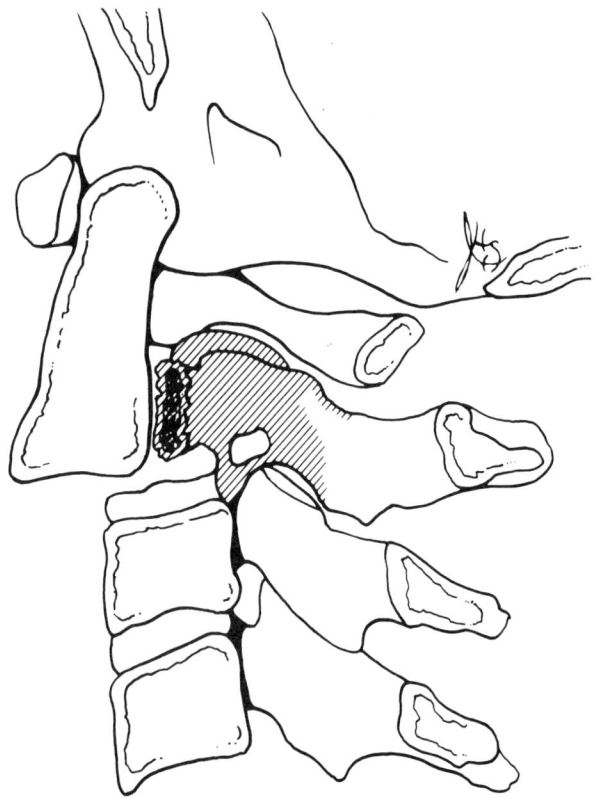

Figure 55-11 Hangman's fracture with anterior subluxation of C-2 on C-3 and bilateral pedicle fractures of C-2.

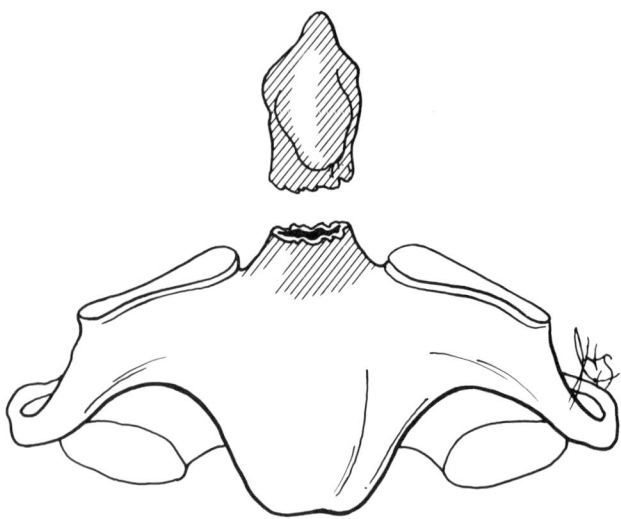

Figure 55-12 Fracture of the odontoid.

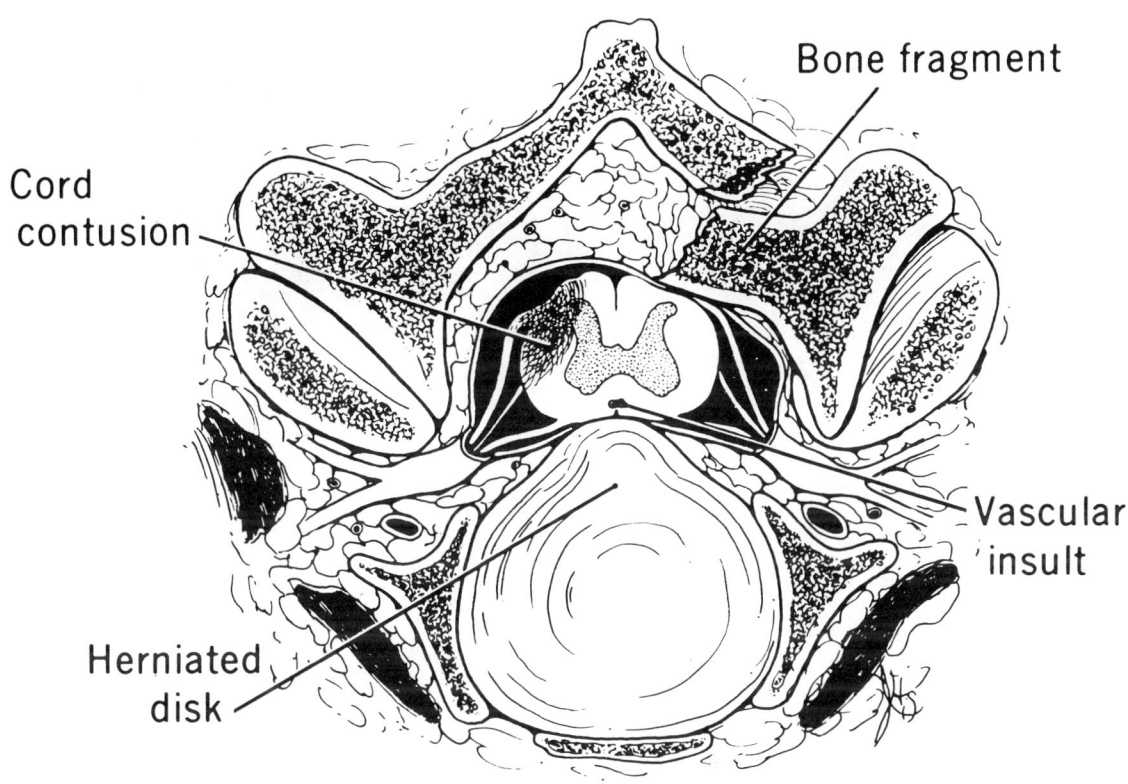

Figure 55-13 Mechanisms of cord injury associated with trauma.

Cervical Cord Injuries

The variety of clinical conditions that result from trauma to the cervical cord can be classified as partial or complete cord injuries, depending on the degree of damage to the cord. A *complete* cord injury is defined as the absence of any sensory, motor, or autonomic neurologic function below the level of the lesion.[6] A *partial* cord injury is defined as a partial loss of cord function below the level of the lesion, ie, some sensory, motor, or autonomic nervous system function remains. In a study of 91 cases of injury to the cervical spine, the cord was injured in 47% of the cases; 21% were complete cord injuries, whereas 26% were partial.[2]

Partial cord injuries can be further subgrouped into three major clinical presentations: (1) central cord injury, (2) anterior cord injury, and (3) the Brown-Séquard syndrome. Central cord injury results in motor weakness of the arms greater than that in the legs, loss of urinary bladder function, and varying degrees of sensory loss secondary to the injury.[7] The anterior cord injury is characterized by an immediate paralysis with hypoesthesia and hypalgesia up to the level of the lesion, although touch, motion, position, and vibratory sensation are spared.[8] The Brown-Séquard syndrome results from a cord injury that impairs motor function on one side of the body and pain and temperature perception on the contralateral side of the body below the level of the lesion.[9] An anatomical analysis of the cervical cord (Fig. 55-14) shows that total disruption or necrosis of the cervical cord and thus of all pathways through the cord results in complete loss of sensation, motor function, and autonomic nervous system function below the level of this lesion. The most evident autonomic effects are the absence of sweating, difficulties with vasomotor control, and priapism.

The acute central cord syndrome is caused most often by hyperextension of the cervical spine; injury to the cord results from posterior compression by bulging of the ligamentum flavum and anterior compression by the vertebral bodies (see Fig. 55-9). The unique pattern of muscle weakness, combined with a history of hyperextension of the cervical spine, should make the emergency physician highly suspicious of this entity. This lesion is associated with varying degrees of edema and/or contusion, hemorrhage, or necrosis of the central portion of the cord. Since fibers in the lateral cortical spinal tract are laminated with the upper extremity fibers, which are located medially, and the lower extremity fibers are located more peripherally, the fibers supplying motor function to the arms are more susceptible to this type of injury (Fig. 55-15). The recovery from this injury usually follows the same laminar pattern in that leg strength is recovered before arm strength; finger and fine hand movements are usually the last to be recovered. Depending on the amount of central cord destruction, the degree of recovery may vary. The neurologic deficit may have occurred at the time of the injury and may have already cleared by the time

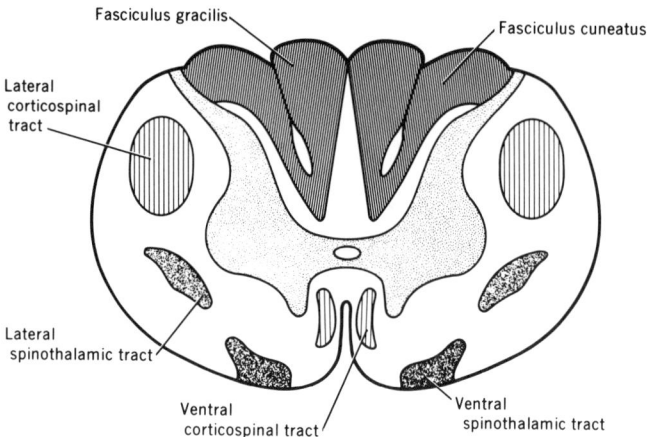

Figure 55-14 Anatomy of the cervical cord.

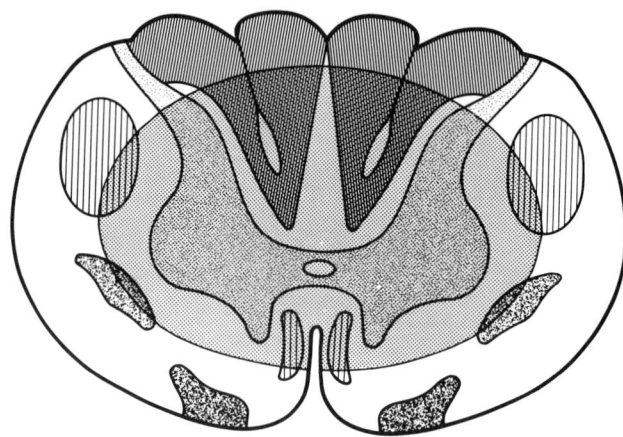

Figure 55-15 Central cord syndrome.

emergency care personnel arrive. This is especially common with football players, who may have only temporary paresthesias or dysesthesias of the hands after suffering an injury to the neck.[10]

The differential diagnosis of the central cord injury should include cruciate paralysis of Bell and a bilateral brachial plexus injury. Cruciate paralysis results from an injury to the atlanto-occipital area with subsequent injury to the cord in the area of the pyramidal decussation.[9] A lesion in this area presents a clinical picture similar to that of the central cord syndrome. For this reason, roentgenograms of the odontoid are important in the evaluation of physical findings consistent with a central cord injury. Bilateral brachial plexus injury may also simulate a central cord injury, although the neurologic deficit in this entity is confined to the nerve roots and is usually associated with absence of deep tendon reflexes.

The syndrome of acute anterior spinal cord injury usually results from compressive forces to the anterior portion of the cord by either a bony fragment or a herniated disk. The clinical findings of this lesion can be explained by noting the area of the cord that is injured (Fig. 55-16). The uninjured area is that of the posterior columns, which are the tracts that convey touch, motion, position, and vibratory sense. This lesion may occur in the absence of any fracture or dislocation; for example, it may be caused by a herniated disk.

The Brown-Séquard syndrome can also be explained by observing the area of cord that is injured and the tracts that have been disrupted (Fig. 55-17). Since sensory tracts cross at the cord level and motor tracts cross at the pyramidal decussation, a lesion of this type results in a loss of sensation and temperature sense on one side of the body (contralateral to the cord lesion) and a resultant weakness on the opposite side of the body (ipsilateral to the lesion).[11] This lesion may result from a lateral compressive force to the cervical cord as a result of disk or bony disruption of the cervical spine.

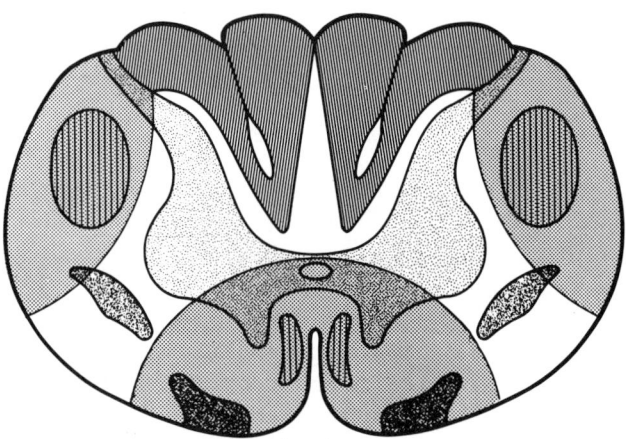

Figure 55-16 Anterior cord syndrome.

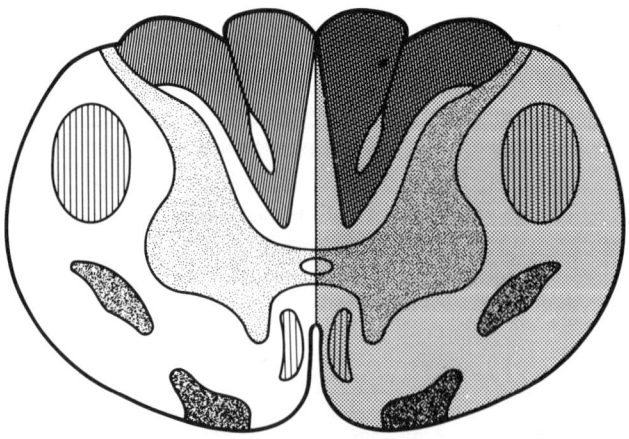

Figure 55-17 Brown-Séquard syndrome.

DIFFERENTIAL DIAGNOSIS

Other entities that may be considered in the differential diagnosis of cervical cord injuries are hysterical paralysis and brachial plexus injuries. Hysterical paralysis may be difficult to distinguish from an acute cervical cord injury, especially when the complex clinical manifestations of the partial cord syndromes are considered. In hysterical paralysis, the motor and sensory deficits usually do not follow any known anatomical patterns, but caution must be used to exclude any possibility of a partial cord syndrome. In true cord injuries, reflexes are usually lost; however, they are retained in hysterical paralysis.[12] If the patient has a weakness of one leg, the Hoover test may be applied; the physician places a hand below each of the patient's heels, and the patient is asked to raise the paralyzed leg. If the nonparalyzed leg is not pushed down against the hand during such an effort, the patient is not trying to lift the so-called paralyzed leg, and the suspicions of hysteria are strengthened.[12]

Traumatic injuries to the brachial plexus may mimic a cord injury. The injury may be partial or complete, and the patient may have a sensory and motor deficit that corresponds to the injured nerve roots. Rarely, bilateral brachial plexus injury may be difficult to distinguish from a central cord injury. With brachial plexus injuries, however, the deficit should be confined to the extremity of the injured brachial plexus, and there should be no true cord deficit demonstrated on neurologic examination.[13,14]

Nontraumatic conditions may also cause spinal cord injury and should be considered in patients with acute spinal cord injuries. For example, ischemia of the spinal cord may occur because atherosclerotic disease, thrombosis, or dissection of the thoracic aorta has occluded the spinal cord circulation.[11] An oncologic emergency may arise when a tumor encroaches on the spinal cord and causes neurologic dysfunction. This condition may manifest itself suddenly, and its consequences may be devastating if it is not diagnosed and treated rapidly.[15] Hematomas may occur around the spinal cord, especially in patients receiving anticoagulants, and cause spinal cord compression.[16] Osteoarthritis and ankylosing spondylitis of the cervical spine may cause bony encroachment on the spinal cord and make it more susceptible to injury, even from trivial trauma.[12,17]

CLINICAL MANIFESTATIONS

The condition of patients with traumatic injuries to the cervical spine should be evaluated by an appropriate history and physical examination. The physician should suspect cervical spine injury in any patient who suffers significant trauma, especially one who has suffered injury to the head or neck or who has lost consciousness. The absence of a head injury does not exclude a cervical spine injury, however; those wearing shoulder harnesses may be protected from injury to the head, although the inertial forces may cause flexion or extension injuries to the cervical spine.[4] Complaints of neck pain, stiffness, paresthesias, or radicular pain of the extremities may indicate cervical spine injury. The ability of patients to walk after their accident does not exclude the possibility of significant cervical spine or cervical cord injury, as 17% of patients with serious injury to the cervical spine have been reported walking at the scene of their accident.[2]

Palpation of the spinous processes of the cervical spine may reveal significant tenderness or deformity that may make the emergency physician suspect cervical spine injury. In addition to examining patients for possible bony injuries to the cervical spine, the clinician must check for any evidence of cord injury. Cursory examinations are to be condemned, as they may reveal only a total cord injury and miss the partial cord injury. Physical examination must include examination of the motor and sensory functions of the cord. Strength of the arms and legs must be assessed and any differences in strength noted. A quick sensory examination can be performed to determine any level of sensory deficit. Once the examination has been completed, the findings should indicate whether there has been any cord injury.

RADIOLOGY

Early roentgenogram evaluation of the cervical spine is an important step in the management of the traumatized patient and should be done in all trauma patients unless they are alert, have no alcohol or drugs to impair their level of consciousness, and have no neck pain or tenderness.[18] It should be done in a way that permits adequate evaluation of all seven cervical vertebrae without adding further insult to a potentially unstable cervical spine. This goal can be met by performing a portable cross table lateral roentgenogram of the cervical spine with downward traction on the patient's arms (Fig. 55-18).[19] A cross table lateral view, anterior-posterior view, and view of the odontoid constitute a minimum roentgenologic evaluation of the cervical spine, as 17% to 25% of injuries to the cervical spine may be missed by limiting studies to the cross table lateral view alone.[20] In patients with a suspected neck injury, a full cervical spine series should be taken—including careful flexion and extension views if the spine is stable—as only with these latter roentgenograms can ligamentous injuries be fully evaluated.[19] Tomography and scan of the cervical spine by computed tomography (CT) are useful adjuncts in the radiologic evaluation of the cervical spine when findings on routine studies are equivocal.

In general, roentgenogram evaluation may underestimate the degree of injury as ligamentous injury may be difficult to detect and cord injury may be present despite a negative

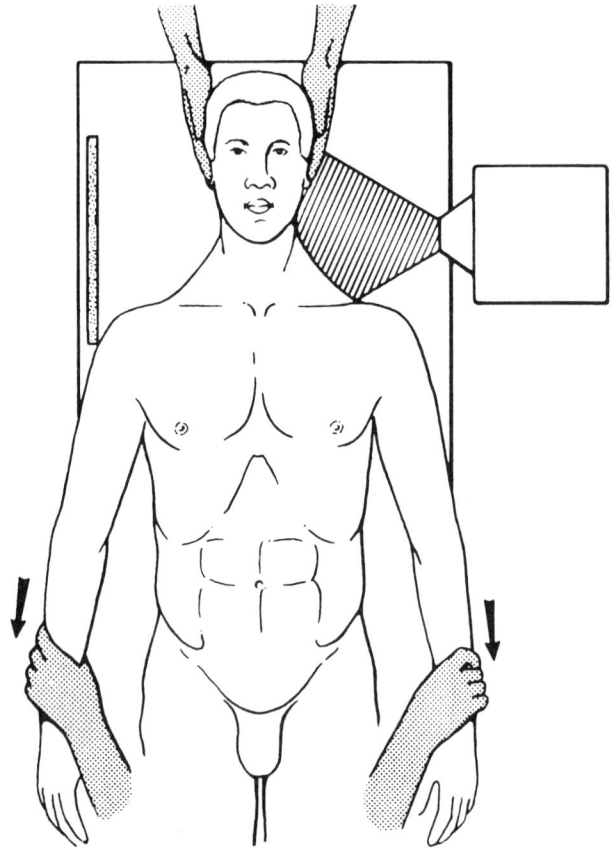

Figure 55-18 Method of obtaining lateral roentgenogram of the cervical spine with downward traction on the patient's arms to expose all seven cervical vertebrae.

roentgenogram (see Table 55-1). In cases of suspected cord injury, magnetic resonance imaging is most effective in demonstrating spinal cord pathology.

SPECIAL PROBLEMS

Immediate problems associated with cervical cord injuries include disorders of temperature regulation and blood pressure control. In the normal, intact nervous system, alterations in body temperature can be corrected by impulses traveling through the autonomic nervous system under the control of the thermal regulatory center in the hypothalamus. These impulses are conducted mainly by the sympathetic nervous system, which is involved in vasomotor control of blood vessels in the skin, muscular shivering, and sweating. Disturbances of thermal regulation seem to be most prominent with lesions at the T-8 level and above. A patient with a nervous system intact to the T-8 level retains sufficient thermal regulatory response to maintain an adequate body temperature, despite fluctuations in the ambient temperature.[21] The disturbances of thermal regulatory mechanisms in patients with spinal cord injuries make them prone to both hypothermia and hyperthermia, but the former is more common. Patients with spinal cord lesions below the cervical level are at much less risk for thermal regulatory disorders not only because they have more active voluntary muscle, but also because they retain some normal sympathetic activity related to sweating and vasomotor control.

Hypothermia is considered a core body temperature at or below 35°C (95°F).[22] Severe hypothermia is particularly likely to occur soon after injury to the spinal cord as a result of the cutaneous vasodilatation and subsequent heat loss that takes place during this stage of the injury (see Chapter 41, Hypothermia).

Hyperthermia may occur after spinal cord transection and is likely to develop in hot climates or in the presence of infection. Hyperthermia occurs because of the body's inability to lose body heat through the vasodilatation and sweating that is normally mediated by the sympathetic nervous system. Although sweating and heat loss may occur in the skin that is still normally innervated, thus allowing some degree of temperature control, this limited degree of thermoregulation may not be sufficient to maintain a normal body temperature[21] (see Chapter 40, Hyperthermia). Clinical management involves recognizing that substantial alterations in body temperature may occur in patients with spinal injuries. A temperature probe that records wide fluctuations in core body temperature is extremely useful.

Hypothermia is best treated by passive rewarming measures when it is mild and the patient is stable; active rewarming measures, such as the use of a heated aerosol oxygen mask, may be needed if the hypothermia is severe, however.[21] Treatment for mild hyperthermia requires keeping the patient in a cool place, while severe cases, those with core body temperatures above 40.5°C (104.9°F), may require immediate treatment similar to that used in managing heat stroke. When the patient's body temperature is stabilized, the patient should be warned that precautions to prevent the recurrence of hypothermia or hyperthermia must be taken.

Cervical cord injuries may also disrupt the normal blood pressure regulation owing to the loss of sympathetic innervation distal to the cord lesion.[23] As a result, severe orthostatic hypotension may occur in ''spinal man'' and result in syncope in the head-up posture. This phenomenon usually diminishes with time as the body adapts to the hypotensive change caused by the head-up position. Any symptomatology or severe orthostatic hypotensive change that occurs can be quickly resolved by putting the patient in the supine position.

Although patients with cervical cord injuries have a lower resting blood pressure, they manifest paroxysmal increases in blood pressure during certain physiologic stimuli, such as defecation, urinary bladder distention, muscle spasms, distention of the rectum, or cutaneous stimuli. This rise in blood pressure, which may be associated with sweating, flushing of the face, and headache, was described as a distinct syndrome by Head and Riddoch in 1917.[16] Known as *autonomic hyperreflexia* or *autonomic dysreflexia*, it appears to be the result of an exaggerated reflex of the sympathetic nervous system in victims of spinal cord injury. Autonomic dysreflexia can have damaging effects on the body and requires urgent treatment. The most important therapeutic measure is to alleviate the precipitating causes. This would entail emptying the urinary bladder correctly, preventing fecal impactions, and treating severe muscle spasms with diazepam (Valium).[22] If the precipitating cause cannot be identified and removed, then the head-up position may be used to help lower the blood pressure. In severe cases, an infusion of selected pharmacologic may be carefully used to control blood pressure (see Chapter 65, Hypertensive Emergencies).

Hypoventilation may result from cervical cord injury because innervation to the intrathoracic and accessory musculature of respiration may be lost. Patients must rely on the diaphragm, which is innervated by the phrenic nerve, as their only muscle of breathing. This results in diaphragmatic breathing, that is, abdominal raising and chest retraction during inspiration and the reverse during expiration.

TREATMENT

It is vital that all emergency care personnel maintain a high index of suspicion regarding cervical spine injuries. Initial management begins in the field, where stabilization of the cervical spine is most important in the prehospital care of these patients. This may be accomplished by use of long or short spine boards, a cervical collar, and/or sandbags. The combination of a rigid plastic collar and short spinal board provides the most practical and effective method to immobilize the cervical spine.[24-26] Patients with injury to the cervical cord may require urgent airway support since they may develop an ileus that will predispose them to vomiting and subsequent aspiration. For these reasons, cervical spine immobilization should be accomplished in a way that permits personnel to deal rapidly with life-threatening problems, such as airway compromise or respiratory failure.

The patient should be kept flat to avoid problems associated with neurogenic shock, which frequently results from the loss of vasomotor control that occurs when a cervical cord injury has disrupted the autonomic nervous system. Such patients are extremely sensitive to change in position and may become hypotensive if placed in a head-up or seated position. In addition, the body temperature should be monitored in order to detect hyperthermia or hypothermia. Care should be taken to avoid having the patient lie on hard objects in order to avoid the development of pressure sores.

When the patient arrives in the emergency department, stabilization of the cervical spine should be continued while care for the airway, respiratory system, and cardiovascular system is provided. A history of any neurologic deficit and any changes during transport should be obtained from the EMS personnel. A physical examination should be done in the emergency department to detect partial cord injury, for this is the most common type of cord injury. Injury to the cervical spine often occurs without neurologic deficit, and stabilization of the cervical spine should be continued even though the patient shows no sign of cervical cord injury. Furthermore, although the cervical spine roentgenograms may be normal, the possibility of cord injury still exists. It has been reported that 10 of 91 patients in a retrospective study had cord injury without any evidence of bony damage to the cervical spine.[2] Unnecessary manipulation of the head and neck should be avoided until the condition of the cord is fully evaluated. Endotracheal intubation if required can be accomplished by either nasotracheal intubation or oral tracheal intubation, using a laryngoscope and manual immobilization of the head to maintain the axis of the cervical spine. If these measures are unsuccessful, a cricothyrotomy or intubation of the trachea over a fiberoptic laryngoscope can be considered.

Once instability of the cervical spine is diagnosed, a more permanent means of stabilization is required. An easy, effective procedure that can be performed in the emergency department is the application of Gardner-Wells tongs with about 10 to 15 pounds of traction.[27,28] Hypotension resulting from neurogenic shock can usually be resolved by putting the patient in a flat or slight degree of Trendelenburg position. Respiratory insufficiency is common and may require timely ventilatory support as dictated by the patient's clinical status, arterial blood gas levels, and spirometry. Gastrointestinal ileus requires the use of a nasogastric tube to empty gastric contents and reduce the risk of aspiration. Urinary retention requires the use of a Foley catheter, and measures should be instituted early to prevent development of decubital ulcers. There is evidence to suggest that steroids are of value in the treatment of spinal cord injury, and their use is advocated.[29] Such therapy should be initiated in the emergency department as a bolus of 30 mg/kg of methylprednisolone followed by an infusion of 5.4 mg/kg for 23 hours.[29] Definitive care of such patients should be provided by neurosurgical and/or orthopedic subspecialties at a trauma center. Referral of such patients to a regional spinal cord center for management of their acute problems and rehabilitation is ideal.

REFERENCES

1. Talbot HS. Spinal cord injury. *Arch Surg*. 1971;102:539–540.
2. Dula DJ. Trauma to the cervical spine. *JACEP*. 1979;8:504–506.
3. Rogers WA. Fractures and dislocations of the cervical spine: an end result study. *J Bone Joint Surg Am*. 1957;39:341.
4. Huelke DF. Cervical fractures and fracture dislocations sustained without head impact. *J Trauma*. 1978;18:533–538.
5. Wood JF. The ideal lesion produced by judicial hanging. *Lancet*. 1913;1:53.
6. Stauffer ES. Diagnosis and prognosis of acute cervical spinal cord injury. *Clin Orthop*. 1975;112:9–15.
7. Schneider RD, Charie G, Pantek H. The syndrome of acute central cervical spinal cord injury. *J Neurosurg*. 1954;11:546–577.

8. Schneider RD. The syndrome of acute anterior spinal cord injury. *J Neurosurg.* 1955;12:95–122.
9. Schneider RD, Crosby EC. Traumatic spinal cord syndromes and their management. *J Clin Neurosurg.* 1972;20:424–492.
10. Maroon JC. Burning hands in football spinal cord injuries. *JAMA.* 1977;238:2049–2051.
11. Vick NA. *Grinker's Neurology.* Springfield, IL: Thomas; 1976.
12. Youmans JR, ed. *Neurological Surgery.* 3rd ed. Philadelphia: Saunders; 1973;1049–1066.
13. Taylor E. Traumatic intradural avulsion of nerve roots of the brachial plexus. *Brain.* 1962;85:579–602.
14. Dula DJ. Traumatic avulsion injury of the brachial plexus. *Ann Emerg Med.* 1981;10:45–48.
15. Nissenblatt MJ. Oncologic emergencies. *Am Fam Physician.* 1979; 20:104–114.
16. Head H, Riddoch G. The autonomic bladder, excessive sweating and some other reflex conditions in gross injuries of the spinal cord. *Brain.* 1917;40:188–263.
17. McCarty DJ. *Arthritis in Allied Conditions.* 9th ed. Philadelphia: Lea & Febiger; 1979.
18. Fischer RP. Cervical radiographic evaluation of alert patients following blunt trauma. *Ann Emerg Med.* 1984;13:905–907.
19. Kimball M, Sachagello CR. Avoiding a pitfall in resuscitation: the painless cervical fracture. *South Med J.* 1977;70:477–478.
20. Shaffer MA, Doris PE. Limitation of the cross table lateral view in detecting cervical spine injuries. *Ann Emerg Med.* 1981;10:508–513.
21. Johnson RH. Temperature regulation and spinal cord injuries. In: Vinken PJ, Bruyn GW, eds. *Handbook of Clinical Neurology.* Amsterdam: North Holland; 1976;26:355–373.
22. Reulen JB. Hypothermia: pathophysiology, clinical setting and management. *Ann Intern Med.* 1978;89:519–527.
23. Frankel H, Mathias C. Cardiovascular systems in tetraplegia and paraplegia. In: Vinken PJ, Bruyn GW, eds. *Handbook of Clinical Neurology.* Amsterdam: North Holland; 1976;26:313–334.
24. Podosky S, Baroff L, Simon R, et al. Efficacy of cervical spine immobilization methods. *J Trauma.* 1983;23:461–464.
25. Graziano AF, et al. A radiographic comparison of prehospital cervical immobilization methods. *Ann Emerg Med.* 1987;16:1127–1131.
26. McCabe JB, Knowland DJ. Comparison of the effectiveness of different cervical spine immobilization collars. *Ann Emerg Med.* 1986; 15:50–53.
27. Schwartz GR. *Principles and Practice of Emergency Medicine.* Philadelphia: Saunders; 1978.
28. Gardner WJ. The principles of spring-loaded points for cervical traction. *J Neurosurg.* 1973;39:543.
29. Bracken MB, et al. A randomized controlled trial of methylprednisone or naloxone in the treatment of acute spinal cord injury. *N Engl J Med.* 1990;322:1405–1411.

SUGGESTED READINGS

Gerlock AJ, Kirchner SG, Heller RM, et al. *Advanced Exercises in Diagnostic Radiology—The Cervical Spine in Trauma.* Philadelphia: Saunders; 1978.

Harris JH Jr. *The Radiology of Acute Cervical Spine Trauma.* Baltimore: Williams & Wilkins; 1978.

Rockwood CA Jr, Green DP. *Fractures.* Philadelphia: Lippincott; 1975;2.

Vinken PJ, Bruyn GW. *Handbook of Clinical Neurology—Injuries of the Spine and Spinal Cord, Part I.* Amsterdam: North Holland; 1976.

Vinken PJ, Bruyn GW. *Handbook of Clinical Neurology—Injuries of the Spine and Spinal Cord, Part II.* Amsterdam: North Holland; 1976.

Youmans JR. *Neurological Surgery.* Philadelphia: Saunders; 1973;2.

56. Headache

JAMES SANTIAGO GRISOLÍA, MD

Head and facial pain are among the most common afflictions of humankind, ranking as the seventh leading complaint among ambulatory care encounters in the United States.[1] Although most headaches result from benign causes, headache may on occasion herald many serious processes. Despite the unlikelihood of serious neurologic sequelae, from the patient's perspective the pain of a severe migraine attack may be devastating and seem to require the most urgent attention. These contradictions set the stage for frequent conflicts between patient and emergency staff, making headache management both commonplace and yet anxiety provoking for the emergency physician.

ETIOLOGY OF PRIMARY HEADACHE DISORDERS

Headaches may be grouped into primary and secondary (or symptomatic) headache disorders. The first group includes so-called vascular and tension headaches (Table 56-1), where organic head pain arises in the absence of any discoverable pathology. The second group includes various cerebral and systemic diseases that may present with headache as a cardinal sign.

In contrast to our detailed empiric knowledge concerning headache, our theoretical understanding lies in total disarray. The classic distinction between vascular headache and muscle tension headache may be preserved to facilitate communication with colleagues, but since the late 1970s growing evidence suggests that the factors underlying vascular headaches are not vascular and that muscle tension headaches produce less muscle tension than migraines.

In the 1930s, Wolff[2] performed experiments in human volunteers that supported a vascular theory for migraine headaches. The concept evolved that the migrainous aura results from vasospasm of intracranial arteries, particularly those in the circle of Willis. This vasospasm then leads to vasodilation of the extracranial arteries of the scalp and/or face, leading to the actual head pain. More recent work, especially by Olsen and colleagues[3] in Europe, demonstrates a significant discordance between cerebral blood flow (as

Table 56-1 Clinical Features of Typical Vascular and Tension Headache

Feature*	Vascular Headache	Tension Headache
Pain onset	Abrupt	Gradual
Pain quality	Throbbing	Pressure
Associated neurologic symptoms	Yes	No
Nausea, autonomic symptoms	Yes	No
Location	Unilateral	Bilateral, bandlike with neck pain
Duration	<24 hours	Days to years

*These features describe prototype headache attacks. Most patients describe mixed vascular and tension features with some variation from one attack to the next.

measured by xenon blood flow studies) and clinical symptoms. Neurologic auras such as visual phenomena, hemiparesis, or dysarthria actually begin before the reduction of blood flow in the appropriate cortical area, and their cessation does not appear to correspond to resolution of blood flow abnormalities. Additionally, no consistent blood flow changes could be demonstrated for common migraine patients. These discrepancies prompted the suggestion that migraine involves a primary neurogenic phenomenon similar to cortical spreading depression of Leao,[3] and subsequent work by other investigators has attempted to correlate dysfunction in brain stem monoamine neurotransmitter systems[4] or trigeminal nerve nuclei[5] with some secondary vascular disturbance. Under this hypothesis the neurogenic process would be the primary disturbance, with the vascular disturbance being a secondary and inconsistent accompanying factor not necessarily required either for pain or for transient neurologic symptoms. Although the work of Oleson and colleagues[3] has been criticized recently,[6] many investigators continue to hold that the vascular hypothesis fails to explain the full range of symptoms and findings in migraine and related headache.

Tension headaches were once believed to result from ischemia or abnormal tension in muscles, and Wolff[2] found some support for this in studies reproducing a tensionlike headache in volunteers receiving injections of hypertonic saline in the neck muscles. Biofeedback studies have consistently found increased electromyographic activity in both migraine and tension headache patients, however, and often the degree of increase is higher in migraine patients.[7] Attempts to show increased depression, anxiety, or other psychogenic features in tension headache patients have failed consistently to distinguish them from vascular headache patients, and recent epidemiologic evidence supports the likelihood that so-called tension and vascular headaches form part of a single spectrum with the possibility of a single underlying mechanism for both types of headache.

Vascular headache may be divided into common migraine, classic migraine, and a number of special syndromes. Despite theoretical confusion, it is worthwhile to retain familiarity with the terms because the clinical entities are clearly delineated in many patients, although they are blurred in others. Classic migraine is a headache that is unilateral, episodic, often throbbing, accompanied by nausea, and preceded by neurologic symptoms (aura). Common migraine denotes a headache that is unilateral, often throbbing, and accompanied by nausea but no aura. In the newest international Headache Classification, the terms ''classic migraine'' and ''common migraine'' are replaced by ''migraine with aura'' and ''migraine without aura,'' respectively. Cluster headache is a persistently unilateral, intense, boring, periorbital pain accompanied by Horner's syndrome that follows a characteristic temporal pattern. Attacks occur in clusters of several weeks' duration, during which the headache occurs once or several times per day until the cluster abates. Typically there is a symptom-free period of several weeks to months before a new cluster begins. Carotidynia refers to a pain of the lower face that is usually nonthrobbing and is accompanied by tenderness of the carotid artery in the neck. Pressure on the artery may intensify pain in the face.

Complicated migraine describes persistence of neurologic symptoms/signs beyond the attack of pain. These neurologic defects may persist for hours, for days, or permanently and may correlate with persistent filling defects on cerebral angiography. Confusional migraine, ophthalmoplegic migraine, and hemiplegic migraine all refer to different neurologic findings that may accompany classic migraine and may or may not persist as complicated migraine. On occasion, abdominal pain, nausea, confusion, or focal neurologic symptoms may occur in the absence of headache yet with the same presumed pathogenesis. These attacks are sometimes referred to as migraine equivalents and remain in the differential diagnosis of stroke, transient ischemic attacks, and partial seizures, especially in younger patients. The absence of a definitive diagnostic test for vascular headache makes the diagnosis of migraine equivalent difficult to confirm, but the occurrence of similar episodes (ie, hemiparesis, dysarthria, and the like) at other times with a typical vascular headache strongly supports the diagnosis. In older patients or in middle-aged patients with significant atherosclerotic risk factors, the diagnosis of migraine equivalent should generally be one of exclusion.

The prototypic tension headache, also called muscle contraction headache, is a nonthrobbing, continuous pain in a band distribution around the head that may persist for days, weeks, or years and is not accompanied by nausea, visual blurring, scintillations, vertigo, or any other neurologic symptoms. Close examination of headache histories will reveal some vascular features (such as throbbing, abrupt onset, nausea, photophobia, and unilaterality of neurologic symptoms) in most patients with so-called tension headaches, lending force to the argument that vascular and tension headaches form a continuous spectrum. Also noteworthy is the coexistence of both vascular and tension headache episodes in the same patients, often with improvement in both headache types on the same medication.

ETIOLOGY OF SECONDARY HEADACHE DISORDERS

In considering secondary causes of headache, our theoretical understanding rests on much firmer ground. Many of the secondary causes of headache can be understood in terms of certain structures in the head and neck that are demonstrably pain sensitive. Pain receptors in the temporomandibular joint (TMJ), dental pulp, mucosal lining of the sinuses, periostea of the cervical vertebrae, and the skull itself are all important in the genesis of pain syndromes. Many intracranial processes cause pain through direct traction or irritation of the pain-sensitive blood vessels and meninges at the base of the brain, although at times a stroke, brain tumor, or other intracranial process appears quite capable of triggering a headache with fairly typical vascular features, presumably by activating the same mechanisms involved in primary headache disorders.

Sinusitis

Sinusitis causes a dull, usually nonthrobbing pain over the forehead or cheeks. In the case of acute sinusitis the maxillae or frontal bones are tender over the involved sinus, and a purulent intranasal discharge is evident to the patient or on nasal examination. Chronic sinusitis presents more subtly and is considerably overused by laypersons and physicians alike as an explanation for primary headache disorder. The diagnosis of sinus headache should be regarded with suspicion until the basis for the original diagnosis is clearly understood. If sinus radiographs are positive for chronic changes ipsilateral to the pain, a course of appropriate antibiotics is not harmful, but a specific attack on a primary headache disorder should not be delayed if obvious vascular features are present.

Temporomandibular Joint Dysfunction

Dental pathology usually is obvious as a cause of facial pain, but in the area of TMJ dysfunction both false-positive and false-negative errors are common. When TMJ dysfunction is contributory, the pain typically extends down to involve the preauricular and mandibular areas. The pain increases with chewing, and nocturnal bruxism, clicking, and locking of the jaw may also occur. Supportive examination findings include limitation in jaw opening (less than three fingerbreadths' excursion), visible serrations on the tongue margins due to pressure against the teeth, and audible jaw clicks that may be auscultated with a stethoscope over the joint.

Cervical Pain

Cervical osteoarthritis and ligamentous spraining injuries most frequently cause pain localized to the neck itself. This pain may provoke secondary tension or vascular headache, usually localized to the posterior head and bilateral or lateralized. Rarely, the head pain may so predominate that the neck complaints are not obvious. Specific inquiry and/or assessment of cervical range of motion may then disclose cervical disease as an important precipitant. Ice, heat, muscle relaxants, physical therapy, or other modalities may then help the head pain as well as the neck pain.

Ophthalmologic Disease

Although minor degrees of eye strain commonly cause minor headache, on rare occasions ophthalmologic complaints may provoke medically significant head or eye pain, often by precipitating attacks of a primary headache disorder. Refraction errors and strabismus most often precipitate headache when a patient is reading or studying, but narrow angle glaucoma may cause orbital pain unrelated to use of the eyes and is associated with decreased visual acuity, conjunctival injection, and corneal edema. An ophthalmologist should be consulted immediately.

Temporal Arteritis

Among systemic illnesses, a few deserve mention as potential causes of head pain. Temporal arteritis is an inflammatory systemic arteritis affecting primarily the branches of the external carotid artery. It may present with lateralized or bilateral temporal pain and pronounced local tenderness over the affected arteries, especially the superficial temporal branch of the external carotid. Because the arteritis may progress to blindness, stroke, or myocardial infarction if untreated, this disorder assumes great importance despite its rarity. For this reason, an erythrocyte sedimentation rate (ESR) should be obtained on all acute headache patients older than 60 years. If positive, a temporal artery biopsy should be performed urgently for diagnosis. In elderly patients with classic examination findings, a biopsy should be performed even in the presence of a normal or minimally elevated ESR because on rare occasions the ESR may be normal in this condition. Presumptive steroid therapy should be initiated while one is awaiting the biopsy results. Steroids may be started up to 24 hours before biopsy without danger of normalizing the pathology.

Systemic Illness

Other systemic illnesses may cause head pain without direct involvement of the nervous system. Fever or systemic infection, including common viral infections, may provoke head pain as a result of nonspecified toxic factors, although direct central nervous system invasion (meningitis or brain abscess) must always be considered in the differential diagnosis. Hypertension does not generally cause headache until diastolic pressure reaches 130 mmHg,[8] generally as a result of an acute crisis such as hypertensive encephalopathy, pheochromocytoma, or toxemia of pregnancy.

Hypercarbia may cause headache in the setting of severe chronic obstructive pulmonary disease, possibly as a result of a vasodilatory effect on cerebral vessels. Sleep apnea may provoke daytime headache, presumably via the same mechanism. Carbon monoxide poisoning gives headache as an early symptom. Headache characterizes altitude sickness. Hypothyroidism may also cause headache.

Medications

A number of medications may cause headache, including oral contraceptives, female hormones, nitrates, hydralazine and other vasodilating compounds, calcium channel blockers, alcohol, antihistamines, decongestants, sympathomimetics, nicotinic acid, histamine, perhexiline, theophylline, terbutaline, bromocryptine, dopamine, nonsteroidal anti-inflammatory drugs, antidepressants, and ranitidine.[9] Monoamine oxidase inhibitors give headache in conjunction with tyramine or other sympathomimetics. Withdrawal of amphetamines, ergotamine, caffeine, β blockers, antidepressants, methysergide, or benzodiazepines may provoke headache.

Cerebral Aneurysm

Among intracranial processes, perhaps the most dreaded cause of headache is cerebral aneurysm. At times the clinical distinction between severe primary headache and mild subarachnoid hemorrhage may prove difficult, and the disastrous yet potentially treatable implications of cerebral aneurysm create considerable anxiety regarding liability issues, much more so than meningitis or brain tumor, for example.

Cerebral aneurysms generally result from congenital weakness in the media and elastica of the cerebral arteries, resulting in a gradual enlargement and outpouching of the arterial wall. These are found most commonly at branch points of the major cerebral arteries (mycotic aneurysms are found more distally in the cerebral arteries and atherosclerotic aneurysms in the basilar artery, but these entities rarely present with subarachnoid hemorrhage in an otherwise healthy subject). Congenital aneurysms most often present with subarachnoid hemorrhage in patients in their late 20s through their 60s or later. As much as 15% of aneurysmal ruptures prove fatal before hospital admission,[10] but the remainder may have effects ranging from devastating to rather subtle. Premonitory headaches occurring before a major rupture can result from miniscule bleeds, although some may well result from abrupt distention of the aneurysmal wall because pain-sensitive nerve endings are documented to innervate the arteries in the circle of Willis. Many of the minor premonitory headaches are mild and nondescript enough that the patient does not seek medical attention, but the presentation of a herald bleed should be assiduously sought among all patients presenting to the emergency department with headache.

Factors that should warn of the possibility of subarachnoid bleed include abrupt apoplectic onset of the headache, which is distinct in quality from any previous headache and is easily the worst headache of the patient's life. Frequently this headache hits so abruptly that the patient falls shaken to the ground, briefly stunned or even unconscious. Ruptured aneurysm patients may present to the emergency department obtunded or comatose; the presence of a mild degree of sleepiness or confusion in a headache patient is perfectly compatible with a severe migraine but also represents the mildest end of the clinical spectrum of subarachnoid bleed. Meningismus as well as the photophobia and nausea more characteristic of migraine may be found on physical examination. Focal neurologic findings are rare because the blood spreads throughout the subarachnoid space, causing diffuse symptoms through irritation of the parenchyma and meninges at the base of the brain. One major exception to the lack of focal findings is a partial third nerve palsy associated with posterior communicating aneurysms, which are so located that they frequently compress the ipsilateral third nerve as it emerges from the brain stem. Isolated pupil dilation is more common than ptosis or diplopia because the pupillary fibers lie on the outside of the nerve and are most vulnerable to compressive lesions. Focal findings may occur several days after a subarachnoid hemorrhage as a result of intense vasospasm in the circle of Willis vessels; stroke will occur in the territory of the affected vessels.

If subarachnoid bleed is considered, then an urgent computed tomography (CT) scan of the head without contrast should be obtained. To date, magnetic resonance (MR) imaging is less sensitive for detecting blood, particularly in the subarachnoid space. If the CT scan is negative but the clinical picture strongly suggests a bleed, then an atraumatic lumbar puncture should be performed. Angiography is generally not performed unless the CT or spinal tap documents blood, although under rare circumstances the clinical suspicion may be high enough to justify it. Subarachnoid blood may also result from trauma, arteriovenous malformation, or metastases, but the history, examination, or CT scan will disclose these possibilities. If doubt remains, a contrast CT scan will define the latter two possibilities in the vast majority of cases.

Chronic Subdural Hematoma

Chronic subdural hematoma may present with a dull, persistent headache and no lateralizing findings as a result of the diffuse spread of blood and fluid in the subdural space; headache and somnolence are caused by diffuse pressure, and hemiparesis appears late in the course. Particularly in elderly patients, the trauma needed to cause a subdural bleed may be so trivial as to be forgotten, and this entity remains in the differential diagnosis of any headache that is gradually progressive over days to months. Among younger patients with prior insults resulting in brain atrophy, subdural bleeds also occur with higher frequency. Atrophic brain regions tend to pull away from the overlying meninges, placing more tension on the veins bridging the subdural space and predisposing to subdural bleed. With late-generation CT or MR imaging, the isodense subdural collection is less easily missed than with earlier CT, but the presence of bilateral isodense subdurals in an elderly patient still may lay a trap for the unwary.

Pseudotumor Cerebri

Pseudotumor cerebri presents with headache and bilateral papilledema resulting from a diffuse brain swelling phenomenon that is poorly understood. CT scan shows slitlike ventricles and establishes the absence of mass lesions or hydrocephalus. Lumbar puncture temporarily relieves the increased intracranial pressure, and medical therapy may include steroids, glycerol, acetazolamide, or other agents. Young obese women demonstrate a predisposition toward this condition, possibly reflecting the importance of hormonal mechanisms in its pathogenesis. Other entities that may provoke pseudotumor include oral contraceptives, tetracycline, nalidixic acid, nitrofurantoin, ketamine, nitrous oxide, hypervitaminosis A, etretinate, danazol, amiodarone, ampicillin, minocycline, thyroxine, steroids, or steroid withdrawal.[9]

Lumbar Puncture Headache

Headache after lumbar puncture may present with mixed vascular and tension features, but prompt relief with lying down is characteristic. Headache complicates as much as 10% to 15% of spinal taps, and most controlled series show no preventive effect from enforced bed rest after the procedure. Pain results from a persistent cerebrospinal fluid leak with resultant traction on the meninges in the upright position. Bed rest after the headache onset does improve the chance of spontaneous resolution, and for refractory cases epidural blood patching offers excellent relief.

Infectious Etiologies

Acute meningitis presents with headache, photophobia, neck stiffness, and fever. Acute bacterial meningitis rarely presents subtly and constitutes a true medical emergency. Lumbar puncture should not be delayed until CT scanning or other special studies are performed, and empiric antibiotics (usually penicillin and cefotaxime or penicillin and chloramphenicol) should be started immediately after the spinal fluid is obtained. Acute viral meningitis may result in a similar picture, although a less intense prostration is more common. If focal findings or minimal neck stiffness are present, especially with risk factors for brain abscess (congenital heart disease, intravenous drug abuse, cavitary lung disease, and severe untreated dental or sinus/otic infection), then a CT scan should be obtained with and without contrast; an ill-advised spinal tap in the presence of an acute brain abscess may result in brain herniation.

A number of infections may produce a chronic meningitis with less intense but progressive headache, confusion, variable fever, meningismus, and peripheral leukocytosis. These include tuberculosis, cysticercosis, cryptococcosis, and coccidioidomycosis, all of which may present in immunocompetent hosts. In a chronic clinical picture, neurologic consultation and inpatient admission will probably be required for complete diagnosis, but a contrast CT or MR scan with a subsequent generous lumbar puncture (assuming that there are no contraindications on CT or MR scan) will be integral to the work-up. Initiation of antibiotic/antiparasitic therapy is rarely urgent.

Immunocompromised hosts, especially patients with acquired immunodeficiency syndrome, are seen in emergency departments with greater frequency. Even acute bacterial meningitis can present with subtle clinical symptoms in these patients, and a high degree of suspicion for infectious or neoplastic complications must be maintained with any complaint of headache, mild confusion, or any symptom referrable to the nervous system. Isolated headache, even a mild headache without other symptoms or neurologic signs, should be investigated by lumbar puncture and contrast CT or MR imaging in the significantly immunocompromised host.

Brain Tumors

Brain tumors, either primary or metastatic, present with headache that is typically insidiously progressive and often worse in the middle of the night, with leaning over, or on Valsalva maneuver, as a result of intracranial pressure dynamics. A completely normal neurologic examination is distinctly unusual, although the abnormalities may be subtle and consist of no more than slight confusion or mental dullness. Contrast CT will pick up all but the most subtle lesions, although MR imaging is more sensitive for small or multiple lesions and for assessing the extent of edema. Dexamethasone may help the meningeal traction component of this headache by reducing edema, but additional prophylactic therapy for vascular headache is sometimes helpful in addition to therapy directed at the tumor itself.

Postconcussion Headache

Posttraumatic or postconcussion headache results commonly from motor vehicle accidents and many other types of head trauma, both major and minor. Although the underlying mechanisms are controversial (and probably multiple), the headaches resulting from minor head trauma are clinically indistinguishable from primary headache disorder, often having mixed vascular and tension features. The head pain may be part of a broader postconcussion syndrome, which may include dizziness, confusion, memory loss, and depression. These headaches are most often unaccompanied by any tangible evidence of abnormality on CT, MR imaging, or other diagnostic imaging studies, although they may coexist with subdural, subarachnoid, or intracerebral hemorrhage or contusion. The diagnostic work-up is directed toward excluding these more serious processes by CT or MR imaging, evaluating for serious concomitant neck pathology with plain cervical spine films, and then initiating therapy as for a primary headache disorder. Most patients with postconcussion headache will improve within days to weeks of the injury, but some will have prolonged or lifelong headaches. Litigation may be a factor in prolonging disability, but most recent studies in this area suggest that the limiting factors are organic rather than psychogenic in most patients.[11]

Stroke

Ischemic stroke is characterized by the abrupt or progressive onset of a focal neurologic deficit and may be accompanied by a major or minor degree of headache in about one third of cases. Although headache may attend conventional strokes as a result of thromboembolic disease, if the head pain is especially prominent an ESR and a noncontrast CT scan should be done to exclude temporal arteritis and intracerebral hemorrhage, respectively.

Prominent neck pain associated with acute stroke is classically associated with carotid dissection, although thrombosis and other local conditions affecting the artery may also cause local pain.

Facial Pain

Facial pain carries a slightly different differential diagnosis than head pain. Primary vascular headache is still prominent, and facial migraine may occur with or without pain elsewhere in the head. Cluster headache and carotidynia both involve facial pain, and less defined vascular headaches occur even more frequently. The term *atypical facial pain* was classically used to signify psychogenic facial pain, and regrettably this term has become confusing because some clinicians now use it to refer to patients with organic facial pain of vascular origin whereas others still reserve the term to identify the ever-shrinking group of patients who truly seem to have psychogenic disturbances. Maxillary sinusitis, dental pain, TMJ dysfunction, and temporal arteritis all remain in the differential diagnosis.

Especially important among causes of facial pain is trigeminal neuralgia or tic douloureux. This pain is clinically distinct from other types of facial pain in that it is brief, sharp, lancinating, and electrical. The pain is confined to one or two subdivisions of the trigeminal cutaneous territory and characteristically is triggered by local stimulation of facial sensory fibers, such as occurs incidentally with talking, eating, shaving, or other activities. This pain usually strikes intensely, so much so that patients spontaneously give up the inciting activity, even eating at times, until their pain is controlled.

The pain of trigeminal neuralgia arises from local damage to the cranial nerve as it leaves the brain stem. If this damage permits lateral conduction between parallel nerve fibers, the conditions are set up for re-entrant electrical discharges, which reverberate within the trigeminal ganglion until an intense burst of pain is felt. This characteristic lancinating pain arises by a similar mechanism in other cranial and peripheral nerves. Glossopharyngeal, nervus intermedius, and occipital neuralgias are felt in the sensory territories of the involved nerves in the throat, ear, and occiput. When a classic lancinating pain is described, carbamazepine, phenytoin, or baclofen most often help. When these medications fail, local injection or surgical decompression of the nerve may be required.

Many vascular or tension pains felt in the occiput are erroneously diagnosed as occipital neuralgia and therefore show little or no change with attempts to block the nerve with local anesthetic or steroid injections. Such injections may be useful in true occipital neuralgia because the greater or lesser occipital branches may easily be irritated where they exit through the cervical fascia.

Psychogenic Headache

Psychogenic headache is included as a category in most headache classifications. To some extent this label is misleading because most organic headache disorders are strongly influenced by emotional factors yet relatively few headaches can be clearly demonstrated to be entirely psychogenic. In the emergency department, the most troubling form of psychogenic headache is the factitious headache used to obtain narcotics. Many legitimate headache patients are falsely accused of narcotic-seeking behavior, and few narcotic abusers are regularly able to obtain narcotics in the absence of pathology, but this is clearly a function of local socioeconomic conditions and vigilance by the emergency staff. The best solution is in all cases to avoid giving narcotics whenever possible, but particularly in questionable cases. Factitious headache may rarely be used for other types of secondary gain, including litigation issues or to manipulate psychodynamic issues within the family or social group. Other types of psychogenic headache include bizarre descriptions of head sensations, which may be seen in psychosis, or the refractory, relentless tension headache seen with depression, which is usually accompanied by multiple somatic complaints. Although these psychogenic factors rarely stand alone, they commonly complicate primary headache disorders.

The approach to the psychogenic headache patient begins with some effort to diagnose the apparent underlying psychiatric condition and the formulation of an appropriate disposition and treatment plan for this aspect. A separate decision should then be made as to whether the head symptoms can be explained entirely as functional or whether a separate organic headache disorder exists. Unless the headache clearly represents neither a primary nor a secondary headache disorder, appropriate work-up and treatment must be arranged. Emphasis should be given to the use of effective, nonnarcotic agents in complex cases with appropriate referral to psychiatric, neurologic, or other specialists as indicated. Coupled with a sympathetic, nonjudgmental, but firm demeanor, this approach will avoid most conflicts with patients and staff.

EVALUATION OF THE ACUTE HEADACHE PATIENT

History and Physical Examination

Correct headache diagnosis must be based on the history because few useful clues typically arise from examination or diagnostic studies. A brief but thorough history of the presenting complaint should include the location, quality, and frequency of the pain; duration of the overall problem (as well as of each individual attack of headache); associated nausea or neurologic symptoms; precipitating and relieving factors; and overall progression or improvement in the condition. Prior head pain that the patient may consider irrelevant must be uncovered. Work-up and prior therapy for the current headaches should be reviewed briefly, as should other medical, traumatic, otorhinolaryngologic, or dental conditions and family history of head pain.

The physical examination should be goal directed. In all patients, include the following items:

- blood pressure and temperature
- mental status, including level of consciousness and orientation (if the patient is inattentive, distractable, or confused, digit span and memory for three objects should be added as well as other mental status examinations as needed)
- trauma, including hematoma/scalp edema, lacerations, raccoon eyes, Battle's sign, hemotympanum, and cervical range of motion
- cranial nerves, including ocular fundus, visual fields by confrontation, pupils, extraocular motions, facial asymmetry, and dysarthria
- muscle strength and coordination by rapid alternating movements
- muscle strength reflexes with careful attention to asymmetry or Babinski's sign
- nuchal rigidity (when this is due to meningeal irritation, neck flexion is significantly more painful than rotation in other directions; Kernig's and Brudzinski's signs are confirmatory)

This basic examination should be supplemented with other studies as indicated, including visual acuity, ocular tonometry, palpation (sinuses, carotids, superficial temporal arteries, cranial and cervical muscles, and so forth), and inspection (nasopharynx, oropharynx, tympanic membranes, otorrhea, rhinorrhea, and TMJ range of motion).

Warning Factors in Headache Evaluation

Warning factors suggesting the possibility of a serious underlying cause of headache include fever, diastolic blood pressure greater than 130 mmHg, a relatively short history of headache, elderly at onset of headache, progressive worsening of headache, persistent pain on one side of the head without any contralateral attacks, abrupt onset of the worst headache of the patient's life, onset with exercise, confusion that is evident to the observer, meningismus, or focal abnormalities on the neurologic or ear, nose, and throat examination. History of immunosuppression also arouses concern. Most of these features may be seen on occasion with primary headache disorders, but they raise the possibility of an underlying problem with secondary headaches. In contrast, headache that recurs over a long duration in a young patient or headache that is nonprogressive, building rather than abrupt in onset, capable of switching from one side of the head to the other, and unaccompanied by any abnormalities of mental status, neurologic examination, or ear, nose, and throat examination is likely to be a benign primary headache disorder.

Laboratory Studies

Diagnostic work-up should include an ESR in any elderly patient. A CT or MR study is appropriate if enough of the warning signs mentioned above are found. Although neurodiagnostic imaging studies are rarely positive in headache patients, this consideration must be balanced against liability concerns and patient reassurance. If a patient has had a previous CT or MR study, no additional studies should be required unless the symptoms or examination findings show major changes from those noted previously (recall that a migraine history does not indemnify the patient against a future ruptured aneurysm). Lumbar puncture should only be considered if the patient is immunocompromised, has a history suggestive of subarachnoid bleed with a negative CT scan, or has findings suggestive of acute or chronic meningitis. Other studies including cervical spine films, sinus films, and angiography are only used when prompted by appropriate historical or examination findings. If a CT scan is ordered, neither sinus films nor skull films should be requested because all pertinent information will be obtained from the head CT, especially when instructions for bone windows are given to the radiology technician.

Table 56-2 Parenteral Abortive Agents for Acute Headache

Medication*	Typical Dose	Remarks
Meperidine	50–100 mg IM	Narcotic agent; sedating
Chlorpromazine	25–50 mg IM	Sedation ± pain relief; dystonia, blood pressure effects possible
Prochlorperazine	5 mg IV	Pain and nausea relief; dystonia possible
Metaclopramide	10 mg IV	Nausea ± pain relief; dystonia possible
Dihydroergotamine	0.5–1.0 mg IV or SQ 0.5–1.5 mg IM	Pain and nausea relief; pregnancy and other contraindications

*These agents are representative of many others that have been used; particularly, most narcotic agents may be used interchangeably in equivalent dosages. Monitoring and other precautions vary, and appropriate drug references should be consulted before unfamiliar agents are used.

Table 56-3 Some Prophylactic Agents for Primary Headache

Agent*	Starting Dosage	Final Dosage	Remarks
Propranolol	40 mg twice a day	240 mg daily	Fatigue
Imipramine	50 mg nightly	200 mg nightly	Sedation
Verapamil	80 mg twice a day	480 mg daily	6-week trial
Cyproheptadine	2 mg three times a day	4 mg three times a day	Sedation
Methysergide	2 mg twice a day	2 mg four times a day	Fibrosis, vasospasm

*These agents are representative of the major classes of prophylactic agents. Other β blockers, calcium channel blockers, and serotonergic antidepressants may be effective as well. All agents should be initiated at the starting doses listed above (lower doses should be used in the elderly and in other sensitive individuals) and gradually increased to attain final doses unless limiting side effects or maximal headache relief occur with a lower dose. The final dose is that sufficient to guarantee an adequate trial and is not the maximum dose permissible. Consult appropriate texts for more information.

THERAPY FOR ACUTE HEADACHE

Acute Abortive Therapy

Acute headache attacks may be treated with abortive or prophylactic therapy. If the acute headache is quite severe, then parenteral abortive agents may be advisable both for their greater biologic activity and to avoid malabsorption due to vomiting and other autonomic dysmotility phenomena resulting from the attack itself (Tables 56-2 and 56-3).

Narcotics are effective for some patients with headache, although many patients find that their particular headache is not helped by this type of pain relief. Often an agent such as meperidine is given along with an antinausea agent such as hydroxyzine or promethazine. The advantages of adequate pain relief, rapid onset, and familiarity of the narcotic to both emergency staff and patient must be weighed against several important disadvantages. In the patient with frequent headaches, narcotic agents have a short half-life with a significant potential for rebound headache (discussed in more detail below). Additional problems of addiction and habituation also exist, although these are unlikely to become serious issues as long as parenteral narcotics are administered sporadically by health care providers only. The rare patient who juggles multiple emergency departments to hide the frequency of his or her visits is more likely to have a rebounding organic headache than a true abuse problem, but such patients must be handled within firm limits and preferably with only nonnarcotic agents.

Among abortive agents, several nonnarcotic agents may be useful even for the severe vascular or tension headache presenting to the emergency department. Dihydroergotamine is a parenterally administered ergot preparation that is generally quite effective in headaches with a clear vascular component; it has much greater efficacy than other ergotamine preparations and has the same (or slightly decreased) side effects of nausea, peripheral vasoconstriction, and so forth. Various protocols exist, but the drug is quite effective when administered intravenously or subcutaneously in doses of 0.5 to 1.0 mg or intramuscularly in doses up to 1.5 to 2.0 mg. Particularly with the intravenous route, pretreatment for nausea is desirable (metaclopramide, 10 mg intravenously is a convenient and effective agent). Because of its vasoconstrictive and other side effects, dihydroergotamine should never be used in pregnancy and only with extreme caution in the presence of hypertension, coronary artery disease, or peripheral atherosclerotic disease.

Other agents may be helpful in selected patients. Metaclopramide itself, in addition to its useful antinausea properties, has an analgesic effect against headache when given by the intravenous route. Most of the antinausea agents have some intrinsic antiheadache effect, and chlorpromazine (25 to 50 mg intramuscularly) may be effective for sedation and to some extent for pain. Orthostasis and other side effects such as dystonic reactions occur rarely. Sedation alone is an adequate goal for many patients with acute primary headache attacks because most headache patients are not over the attack until they have slept it off. The once common practice of using parenteral barbiturates or benzodiazepines for acute headache should be restricted, however, and never should be done on a chronic basis except as below. Oxygen by mask has value in breaking acute cluster headaches and a few other acute vascular headaches. Sublingual or inhaled ergotamine may be useful in selected patients; by these routes the drug enters the bloodstream faster than by the oral route without loss due to emesis. Unlike dihydroergotamine, ergotamine rapidly loses its effectiveness after the acute onset and is more useful when taken at home at the onset of pain or, better yet, during the prodrome. In experienced hands, acupuncture is strikingly effective at aborting acute headache but seems to have no prophylactic value for most patients.

Although not yet commercially available as of this writing, sumatriptan has proved effective against migraine in clinical trials. For example, a multicenter trial found 70% pain relief with 6 mg subcutaneously.[12]

Oral Abortive Agents

For patients with infrequent attacks of pain or for those who are just beginning prophylactic therapy, prescription of an oral agent to abort acute headaches assists immeasurably in improving quality of life. Because of the chronic, recurrent nature of headache, addictive drugs should be avoided except in unusual patients under the continuing care of an outpatient physician. Rather than acetaminophen with codeine, for example, any of the nonsteroidal anti-inflammatory drugs can often be used abortively for minor headaches. Ergotamine can be given sublingually, orally, or via inhaler for acute attacks, with the first route being preferred to speed absorption. This agent must be used at the onset of headache or during the prodrome for maximum benefit, and a maximum dose of 10 to 12 mg/week should only be exceeded under close supervision. Isometheptate (Midrin) is an effective agent that clearly works in both vascular and tension headache and is relatively free of side effects. For many patients this is the agent of choice. Butalbital preparations are helpful for many patients. The low intrinsic addiction potential of this barbiturate is rarely a problem but must be kept in mind.

Prednisone (40 to 60 mg daily) is sometimes used over a course of 3 to 10 days to break an acute series of headaches. The mechanism of action is obscure, but the drug seems to be useful in vascular headaches and some tension headaches as well. This treatment is not useful for infrequent or isolated headache because the medication needs at least 24 to 48 hours to work, but for a new onset of headache (or a recent exacerbation of a chronic disorder) it may be extremely useful. Prednisone is especially useful in cluster headache. As with other suppressive pain therapy, this treatment should not be used unless an adequate diagnosis has been established.

Rebound Headache with Abortive Therapy

A critical issue is the concept of the rebound headache. When headache is frequent or continuous, repeated use of any short-acting compound tends to bring transient relief that is followed by a rebound phenomenon with a worsening of the headache, creating a vicious cycle that considerably complicates management and can render all prophylactic regimens ineffective. Physicians become alarmed when patients use butalbital or narcotics to excess, but from the point of view of controlling the headache any short-acting agents, including aspirin, ergotamine, isometheptate, or caffeine, may prove equally deleterious. Parenteral dihydroergotamine seems to be (at least in most patients) an exception to this rule, and in the hands of experienced clinicians it is sometimes used around the clock on an inpatient or outpatient basis to break the rebound cycle.

Headache and Pregnancy

An exception to the proscription against narcotics occurs in pregnancy. Although many primary headache disorders remit during pregnancy, others worsen for all or part of gestation. Teratogenicity becomes the overriding concern, and codeine or occasionally stronger narcotics are used for the duration of pregnancy. The oxytocic effect of oral ergotamine is controversial (parenteral ergot compounds clearly cause uterine contraction), and some obstetricians use oral ergotamine during pregnancy, but concerns regarding vasospastic effects, nausea, uterine contraction, and possible teratogenicity prevent most clinicians from using this agent. Prophylactic therapy is generally avoided, although β blockers may be used cautiously. Prednisone is not teratogenic and a course of 5–10 days or so may be used to reduce frequent, severe headache.

Prophylactic Therapy

In the emergency department, emphasis is appropriately given to excluding dangerous causes of headache and administering treatment for acute pain. Depending on the physician's interest and local referral arrangements, it may also be desirable to start prophylactic therapy for primary headache disorders. Most preventive therapy for headache requires at least 1 to 2 weeks to become effective (6 weeks for calcium channel blockers) but provides the cornerstone for effective therapy of most recurrent headache. Infrequent headaches do not require preventive therapy (unless fixed neurologic residua result more than once), but the critical frequency for deciding to begin prophylaxis is an individual decision depending on lifestyle, degree of prostration with each headache, patient attitudes toward taking medication, patient compliance, and so forth.

Multiple agents may be effective against headache, and it may not be terribly helpful to differentiate vascular from so-called tension headache in prescribing medication. Agents are selected according to side effects and interaction with other concomitant medications or illness and particularly to avoid repeated trials of an agent that has already been adequately tried. Adequate trial is emphasized because many physicians try medications for too short a time or in inadequate doses to permit an intelligent assessment of efficacy. A good rule of thumb for most medications is a 2- to 3-week trial with at least 2 weeks at maximum dose (or maximum tolerated dose if dose-related side effects limit use); calcium channel blockers require a 6-week trial.

Antidepressant Medications

Antidepressants are extremely effective agents. The antiheadache effect is clearly separable from the antidepressant effect and probably reflects modification of monoamine neurotransmitter traffic at the level of the brain stem, in the arterial wall, or both. Many clinicians hold that these agents not only are valuable for vascular headache but may be the most helpful agents in tension or mixed headache.

In general, the serotonergic agents appear more effective, and within this group side effects then become the decisive factor. Many studies have been done with amitriptyline, but this compound is severely limited by its sedation and anticholinergic side effects. Imipramine is at least as effective for most patients and is much better tolerated, although sedation, insomnia, dry mouth, constipation, palpitations, myoclonus, and nausea still occasionally supervene. This agent should be started at 25 mg nightly in the elderly or 50 mg in younger patients, building every several days as tolerated until the headaches are controlled or until a nightly dose of 200 to 300 mg is attained. Earlier literature suggesting no additional benefit beyond 50 to 75 mg daily was incorrect. Fluoxetine is a novel agent that has a low side effect profile, but it also has the disadvantage of being expensive. Its effect does not appear to overlap entirely with the effects of older antidepressant agents, and ineffectiveness of fluoxetine for a given patient should not exclude a trial of conventional agents, or vice versa. This agent should be started at 20 mg every morning (usually activating rather than sedating) and should build rapidly to a dose of 60 mg in a young person. The elderly may not tolerate higher doses.

β-Blocking Agents

β Blockers are quite effective against primary headaches of all types. Propranolol may be built rapidly to a daily dose of 240 mg; it has the infrequent side effects of exercise intolerance, impotence, and hypotension. If partial benefit is noted at lower doses, this agent may be built to higher daily doses in selected patients. Other agents such as nadolol and atenolol may be worth trying if fatigue or other central effects are limiting because these agents are less lipid soluble and less likely to cross the blood-brain barrier. These agents should be avoided in patients with pronounced focal neurologic deficits because of the theoretical risk of promoting cerebral vasospasm.

Calcium Channel Blockers

Calcium channel blockers recently have gained prominence in managing primary headache disorders. Verapamil has been well studied and is generally well tolerated in young people, with nausea, hypotension, and constipation being infrequent side effects. In patients with intrinsic cardiac disease, exacerbation of conduction defects or congestive heart failure may occur. A maximum dose of 480 mg daily should be reached rather quickly in view of the long trial needed to determine effectiveness. Nifedipine and other agents are also used occasionally with good results. The vasodilating properties of verapamil and nifedipine offer theoretical protection against residual neurologic deficits but also sometimes result in paradoxic increase in head pain, which occurs promptly and obviously on beginning the medications.

Miscellaneous Agents

Cyproheptadine is a useful prophylactic medication that is particularly effective in childhood migraine. The limiting side effect is sedation, but standard doses of 4 mg three times a day may not be required for all patients, especially children. Valproic acid, used as an anticonvulsant, recently has been used successfully in headache prophylaxis. The dose may be rapidly increased to 1500 to 3000 mg daily in divided doses, with nausea, tremor, and weight gain prominent among its side effects. Hepatitis and neutropenia/thrombocytopenia are rare complications. Methysergide is a serotonin-blocking agent that carries great effectiveness against vascular headache, but severe side effects limit its use to experienced clinicians. Vasospastic phenomena, confusional states, and retroperitoneal fibrosis are some of the most important side effects, and the fibrotic changes may provoke emergency presentations with cardiac, pulmonary, or renal complications.

A number of other agents are used prophylactically for primary headache, but most of them are second- or third-line agents at best. Biofeedback training, relaxation therapy, and various nonmedication therapies may be equally useful in either vascular or tension headaches. As noted earlier, acupuncture generally has no prophylactic value against headache.

PATIENT EDUCATION

The effectiveness of headache education in the emergency department is limited by many practical considerations, but several points should be emphasized in the interest of both the emergency staff and the patient. The extent and direction of the discussion will depend on the patient, the physician, the time available, and any confusional state induced by the headache and/or medication. Written handout sheets may be useful to emphasize certain points.

Table 56-4 Some Dietary Precipitants of Headache

Alcohol	Pork
Aged cheese	Canned figs
Pickled herring	Onions
Cured meats	Bananas
Sodium glutamate	Pizza
Skipped meals	Tea, Coffee
Chocolate	Soft drinks
Sour cream	Avocado
Yogurt	Chicken livers
Nuts	Raised bread
Broad bean pods	Seafood

Because many physicians as well as patients overemphasize the concept of tension in tension headache, it relieves the patient's guilt to confirm that a primary headache disorder is an organic condition. Although the headache may be influenced by stress and emotional factors, this is also true of heart attacks, asthma, and peptic ulcer disease. This improves the patient's confidence in medical care, shifting the emphasis away from pointless psychodynamic speculation yet affirming the patient's responsibility to analyze immediate stressors that may affect the headaches.

Other precipitating factors should be searched for by both patient and physician, including the effect of diet, glare, allergy, alcohol, contraceptives, and changes in sleep cycle. Some vascular headache patients thrive on minute details and should not be permitted to invest excessive concern in elucidating precipitating factors, but inquiry for major precipitants is appropriate. Elimination diets should not be undertaken wholesale but only to watch for effects of those items shown in Table 56-4.

To avoid unnecessary emergency department visits, the patient should be told clearly that once dangerous causes of headache have been eliminated the pain is not a sign of damage. Often the pain of vascular headache is so intense and anxiety provoking that it is difficult for patients to understand this unless they are told clearly, often more than once. Many patients, once they understand that nothing will explode or rupture if they have a severe headache, finally grasp why the medical world seems to treat their obviously life-threatening headache with nonchalance and even a little deprecation. This reduces the number of return visits and reduces patient-staff conflicts significantly. Family members may need to be told this as well to avoid manipulation by the patient.

The patient should be told that abortive headache medication should be used as early as possible for infrequent headaches because it usually is easiest to break the acute headache in its early minutes or even during the prodromal stage. For frequent headaches, abortive therapy should still be taken early, but frequent abortive use must be curtailed as quickly as possible to avoid rebound headache and a vicious cycle. The best way of eliminating abortive therapy is to begin effective prophylactic therapy, phasing out abortive therapy as prophylaxis begins to take effect. Depending on the patient, more or less emphasis should be given to the ineffectiveness and dangers of repetitive narcotic use.

REFERENCES

1. Ries PW. *Current Estimates from the National Health Interview Survey, United States 1984*. Washington, DC: Dept of Health and Human Services; 1986. Vital and Health Statistics Series 10, no 156, Dept of Health and Human Services publication (PHS) 86-1584.
2. Wolff HG. *Headache and Other Head Pain*. 2nd ed. New York: Oxford University Press; 1963.
3. Oleson J, Larsen B, Lauritzen M. Focal hyperemia followed by spreading oligemia and impaired activation of rCBF in classic migraine. *Ann Neurol*. 1981;9:344–352.
4. Raskin N, Hosobuchi Y, Lamb S. Headache may arise from perturbation of brain. *Headache*. 1987;27:416–420.
5. Moskowitz MA. The neurobiology of vascular head pain. *Ann Neurol*. 1984;16:157–168.
6. Olsen TS, Friberg L, Lassen NA. Ischemia may be the primary cause of the neurologic deficits in classic migraine. *Arch Neurol*. 1987;44:156–161.
7. Philips C. Tension headache: theoretical problems. *Behav Res Ther*. 1978;16:249–261.
8. Bedran RH, Weir RJ, McGuiness JB. Hypertension and headache. *Scott Med J*. 1970;15:48–51.
9. Mastaglia F. Iatrogenic (drug-induced) disorders of the nervous system. In: Aminoff M, ed. *Neurology and General Medicine*. New York: Churchill Livingstone; 1989:507–527.
10. Ljunggren B, Saveland H, Brandt L, et al. Aneurysmal subarachnoid hemorrhage: total annual outcome in 1.46 million population. *Surg Neurol*. 1984;22:435–438.
11. Rimel RW, Giordani B, Barth JT, et al. Disability caused by minor head injury. *Neurosurgery*. 1981;9:221–228.
12. Cady RK, Wendt JK, Kirchner JR, et al. Treatment of acute migraine with subcutaneous sumatriptan. *JAMA*. 1991;265:2831–2835.

57. Coma

MARK SMITH, MD

Clinicians use a rich and precise vocabulary to describe a patient's physical findings, but they rarely describe the mental landscape with the same vividness and clarity. The categories of "altered mental status" and "altered level of consciousness" are commonly used to describe any of a wide variety of deviations from the lucid and aware state that constitutes normal mentation. Coma is but one of many forms of "altered mental status." Prior to discussing the pathophysiology, assessment, etiology, and management of coma, it is worthwhile embedding the term in this broader context.

Coma is a state of pathologic and nonwillful unresponsiveness in which the patient lies quietly with his or her eyes closed. As a clinical entity, coma lies at one end of the spectrum of the acute confusional state, which is defined as a state in which the patient is unable to think with his or her customary speed and clarity. Confusion thus implies a problem with cognition; confused patients have deficits of orientation, attention, and knowledge.

There are two broad classes of patients who fit into the category of acute confusional state: those falling into the stupor–coma spectrum and those falling into the agitated–delirium spectrum. Confusion is the symptom shared by patients from both groups. The prototypical patient in the stupor–coma category is the patient with a sedative-hypnotic drug overdose. Such patients are characterized by a paucity of psychomotor activity, absence of a vivid mental world of hallucinations, lack of autonomic hyperactivity, and a reduced state of alertness and attentiveness. Such patients pass from inattentiveness through stupor and into coma. The prototypical patient falling in the agitated–delirium category of the acute confusional state is the patient with delirium tremens. These patients show increased psychomotor activity, pronounced tendency to hallucinate, a great degree of autonomic hyperactivity, and an increased level of alertness and attentiveness. In most instances, patients in this category do not progress to coma.

ANATOMY OF CONSCIOUSNESS

Two parts of the central nervous system contribute to the awake and aware state that comprises consciousness: the brain stem and the cerebral cortex. The cerebral cortex is responsible for the content of consciousness; without the cortex there is no meaningful interaction with the environment. The brain stem supplies the nonspecific background arousal state that forms the substrate on which the content of consciousness is built. Its presence is a necessary but not specific condition for consciousness to occur.

A person in the normal nonsleeping state is ordinarily awake and aware. Wakefulness (synonymous with arousal or alertness) is a function of the ascending reticular activating system of the brain stem, a fuzzily demarcated section of periaqueductal gray matter beginning in the pons and extending through the midbrain into the thalamus. An awake patient has his or her eyes open. Awareness, by contrast, implies that the person has meaningful interaction with his or her environment, ie, is able to respond appropriately to stimuli. The anatomic site of awareness is the cerebral cortex. The commonly recorded two-part observation that a patient is "awake and alert" is redundant; these two terms are synonymous. A more correct terminology that reflects the underlying anatomy and is richer in content is that the patient is "awake and aware" or "awake and lucid."

Different neurologic functions reside in different parts of the central nervous system. Eye opening is a brain stem function; speech is a cerebral cortex function. Scales to assess level of consciousness interrogate the different parts of the central nervous system and measure the intactness of those functions that they control.

Without the substrate of a working reticular activating system in the brain stem (i.e., without wakefulness or arousal), there can be no manifest cortical activity (ie, awareness). No person can be aware but not awake. The converse, however, is not true. The persistent vegetative state is a condition of a dead cortex and a living brain stem. These patients are awake but are not aware. They spontaneously open their eyes, move their eyes around, have sleep-wake cycles, but lack any meaningful or purposeful interaction with their environment. They do not respond to verbal commands; they do not speak; they do not respond appropriately to pain. Because of their spontaneous eye opening and eye movements, such patients may appear to be "conscious" to the lay observer. This condition of the persistent vegetative state is usually seen after recovery from a severe head injury or from an anoxic cerebral insult and occurs because the brain stem is more resilient to injury than are the cerebral cortices.

The locked-in syndrome is another state that may be confused with the comatose state. In the locked-in syndrome, there is a functioning cortex but only a partially functioning brain stem. The patient is conscious because both the cerebral cortex and the ascending reticular activating system of the brain stem are intact. However, the brain stem's descending corticospinal and corticobulbar tracts are interrupted; these tracts are necessary for extremity movement and lower cranial nerve function. The patient lies mute, still, quadriplegic, and facially motionless but fully awake and aware. The patient's only means of communicating with the external environment is through vertical eye movements and eyelid blinking.

A patient in coma must either have damage to the ascending reticular activating system of the brain stem or have bilateral cortical dysfunction. Damage to only one of the cerebral hemispheres will not cause coma. The brain stem can be damaged by direct destruction (by trauma, hemorrhage, ischemia), secondary destruction (by pressure or traction from the supratentorial compartment), or diffuse depression (by metabolic problems). Bilateral cerebral cortex dysfunction is caused either by seizure activity or by diffuse metabolic insult, although in the latter case there is probably brain stem dysfunction as well. In cases of diffuse metabolic depression, it is difficult to state with certainty whether the comatose state results from the cerebral cortex insult or from the brain stem insult. Because the patient in coma has his or her eyes closed, and because the brain stem reticular activating system is the anatomic site for eyelid opening, coma may be thought of, at least at first approximation, as a brain stem problem.

SCALES TO ASSESS RESPONSIVENESS

Measurements of Responsiveness

Terms such as "obtundation" and "stupor" mean different things to different clinicians. These terms lack both precision and interobserver reliability. It is preferable to describe a patient's state of consciousness in terms of his or her state of responsiveness, ie, what it is that the patient does in response to a particular stimulus.

The AVPU grid provides the template for all of the scales that measure responsiveness:

A = alert and aware and responding normally
V = responding to verbal stimulation
P = responding to painful or noxious stimulation
U = unresponsive to any stimulation

Reasonable methods of applying a painful or noxious stimulus are nailbed pressure to fingers or toes, supraorbital ridge pressure, trapezius muscle pressure, sternal rub, and nasal or nasopharyngeal tickle. Squeezing the nipples or testicles is not reasonable. Note that insertion of a cotton-tipped applicator or a nasopharyngeal airway into the nose provides a noxious but not painful method of stimulation and is an excellent means of arousing a patient.

The Glasgow Coma Scale represents a refinement of the AVPU grid. Although initially conceived to be used in the assessment of the neurotrauma patient, the Glasgow Coma Scale can be used as a way of grading any patient with an acute confusional state. There are three components to the Glasgow Coma Scale: verbal behavior, eye opening, and motor response. Each component assesses a different aspect of the central nervous system. Best verbal response provides a window into the cerebral cortex; best eye opening response provides a window into the brain stem; and best motor response interrogates both the cerebral cortices and the brain stem, specifically the corticospinal tract.

Glasgow Coma Scale

Best Verbal Response

5 = alert, aware, lucid, oriented, converses normally
4 = confused but talks in sentences
3 = uses words, but no sentences; incoherent
2 = moans and groans; no words
1 = silent

Verbal response is assessed using whatever stimulus is required to produce the response. If the patient talks spontaneously, there is no need to provide either painful or verbal stimulation. Best verbal response is a window into the cerebral cortex.

Eye-Opening Response

4 = opens eyes spontaneously
3 = opens eyes to verbal stimulus
2 = opens eyes to painful or noxious stimulus
1 = does not open eyes

The eye-opening response is a window into the brain stem.

Best Motor Response

6 = moves spontaneously or in response to commands
5 = localizes to noxious stimulus
4 = withdraws to noxious stimulus
3 = abnormal flexor response (decorticate posturing)
2 = abnormal extensor response (decerebrate posturing)
1 = no motor response to noxious stimulus

Best motor response provides a window into both the cerebral cortex and the brain stem. The presence of purposeful movement implies a functioning cortex. The abnormal flexor response (upper extremity flexed, lower extremity extended and internally rotated) implies a functioning brain stem with a lesion around the diencephalon (thalamus). The abnormal extensor response (both upper and lower extremities extended and internally rotated) implies a midbrain or high pontine lesion but a functioning mid and lower brain stem. Absence of any extremity motor response suggests either a damaged lower brain stem or a corticospinal tract injury in the cervical spine.

The scores assessed on each of the three components of the Glasgow Coma Scale are traditionally summed to form a total score (with an awake and lucid patient scoring 15 and a patient who is brain dead scoring 3). It is far more important to record the actual responses in each of the components of the scale than it is to report the number that represents the sum of the three scores. The Glasgow Coma Scale can be assessed in 30 to 45 seconds, has excellent interobserver reliability, and can be used as an index to follow the patient's response to therapy.

CAUSES OF UNRESPONSIVENESS

The primary overriding question that needs to be answered by the emergency physician evaluating an unresponsive patient is whether the cause of the unresponsive state is structural or metabolic. Does the patient need immediate radiologic evaluation of the brain with computerized tomography (CT) to define the precise structural lesion, or does the patient need rapid correction of a significant metabolic perturbation?

Structural Lesions

The brain is divided by the tentorium cerebelli, a double layer of dura, into a supratentorial and a subtentorial compartment. Above the dura sits the diencephalon (thalamus and hypothalamus) and the frontal, parietal, and temporal lobes of the cerebral cortex. Below the tentorium sits the brain stem (midbrain, pons, and medulla) and the cerebellum. An oval opening in the tentorium called the "incisura" or "tentorial notch" permits passage and connection of the brain stem to the diencephalon. The midbrain occupies the anterior portion of the tentorial notch; the superior part of the cerebellum occupies the posterior portion. On the anterior portion of the brain stem sits the basilar artery. On each side of the incisura sits the uncus of the temporal lobe.

Structural lesions cause unresponsiveness by either direct or indirect damage to the reticular activating system of the brain stem and not by direct destruction of cortical material. Therefore, for a supratentorial lesion to cause coma, it must produce compression on the brain stem or on blood vessels supplying the brain stem. It does so by one of two transtentorial herniation syndromes: uncal herniation or central herniation. The cranial cavity can permit only a limited amount of expansion of its contents before displacement of structures occurs. Such expansion may be a result of hemorrhage, either traumatic or nontraumatic, or other space-occupying lesion, located either intracranially or in the subarachnoid, subdural, or epidural spaces.

In the central herniation syndrome, the thalamus and midbrain are pushed caudally through the tentorial notch. In the uncal herniation syndrome, the uncus of the temporal lobe dislocates medially, pushes on the adjacent midbrain that is sitting in the tentorial notch, and compresses it against the contralateral incisural edge. At the same time, the uncus presses on the oculomotor nerve, which is coursing along the surface of the tentorium, causing a sluggishly reactive and dilated pupil. In both transtentorial herniation syndromes, there may be damage to brain stem arteries and veins and compression of the aqueductal system that results in further edema, swelling, intracranial hypertension, brain stem hemorrhage, and consequent central nervous system dysfunction.

The common supratentorial structural lesions that cause coma are intracerebral hemorrhage, subarachnoid hemorrhage, subdural hematoma, cerebral edema, and epidural hematoma. In addition, any lesion causing acute obstructive hydrocephalus can cause unresponsiveness.

Subtentorial lesions cause unresponsiveness by either direct or indirect damage to the reticular activating system. Direct damage usually results from hemorrhage into or ischemia of the midbrain and pontine structures. Subtentorial lesions in the posterior fossa (eg, cerebellar hemorrhage) can injure the brain stem by secondary destruction from compression, caused by direct pressure on the tegmentum of the pons, by upward herniation of the cerebellum through the tentorial notch, or by downward herniation of the cerebellar tonsils through the foramen magnum, which compresses and displaces the medulla. Posterior fossa lesions can also cause an acute obstructive hydrocephalus via pressure on the cerebral aqueduct and fourth ventricle.

Clues to the presence of a structural lesion must be assiduously sought. Although not all structural lesions are traumatic, all traumatic lesions are structural. Therefore, all unresponsive patients must be carefully assessed for signs of trauma. The clues to the presence of a structural lesion are:

1. history of trauma
2. history of previous structural lesion
3. sudden onset of unresponsiveness (a time course that suggests hemorrhage)
4. physical examination evidence of trauma, in particular head trauma:
    a. scalp contusion
    b. retroauricular hematoma (Battle sign)
    c. raccoon eyes
    d. hemotympanum
5. presence of focal or lateralizing neurologic signs:
    a. asymmetrically reactive pupils
    b. asymmetric weakness or flaccidity
    c. asymmetric plantar reflex (least reliable)
6. neuroanatomical consistency, ie, all neurologic signs and symptoms can be explained by a lesion at a single site in the central nervous system
7. evidence of progressive rostro-caudal deterioration over time.

All unresponsive patients in whom a structural lesion is suspected need to have a CT or magnetic resonance (MR) scan of their brain. Most structural lesions are visible on head CT, but some, such as a brain stem infarction or a small subarachnoid hemorrhage, are not. Brain stem infarction is visible on MRI. Patients with structural lesions need to have hypoxemia corrected, need to be evaluated for the possibility of operative intervention, and may need vigorous therapy aimed at reducing elevated intracranial pressure (by hyperventilation to promote cerebral vascular constriction and administration of dehydrating agents such as mannitol). In some structural lesions, the most notable being certain cases of subarachnoid hemorrhage, pathologic cerebral vasoconstriction rather than elevated intracranial pressure may be causing the unresponsive state. In these cases, hyperventilation would not be indicated. If endotracheal intubation of a patient with a structural lesion is performed, it should be done in a controlled manner that minimizes any increases in intracranial pressure, using sedating drugs, lidocaine, and muscle paralyzing agents.

Some structural lesions may cause no localizing signs. In some cases of subarachnoid hemorrhage, there may be only bilateral extensor plantar reflexes or abnormal posturing. Suddenness of onset is the clue. The diagnostic modality of choice for a suspected subarachnoid hemorrhage is the CT scan. Only if the CT scan is negative should a lumbar puncture be performed.

Metabolic Lesions

A host of different metabolic insults can result in unresponsiveness. Whether that unresponsiveness is secondary to diffuse depression of both cerebral cortices or whether it is due to depression of the ascending reticular activating system of the brain stem is not a settled question.

Common and uncommon metabolic causes of unresponsiveness are hypoxemia, hypercarbia, hypoglycemia and hyperglycemia, shock, intoxications and poisonings, infection (sepsis, meningitis, encephalitis), hypothermia and hyperthermia, acidemia or alkalemia, hyponatremia and hypernatremia, hypercalcemia, uremia, hepatic encephalopathy, myxedema, seizures, postictal state, eclampsia, Reye's syndrome, hyperviscosity syndrome, thrombotic thrombocytopenic purpura, and, Wernicke's encephalopathy.

Clues to the presence of a metabolic cause of coma are:

1. absence of evidence for a structural lesion:
    a. no signs of trauma
    b. no lateralizing signs (although certain metabolic diseases such as hypoglycemia and hyperglycemia and hepatic encephalopathy may generate localizing signs)
    c. no neuroanatomic consistency
2. pupillary reactivity preserved (in the absence of drugs that affect pupillary size)
3. presence of asterixis, tremor, or myoclonus.

In some cases, the structural–metabolic distinction may be blurred. A patient's structural lesion may not be sufficient by itself to cause a substantial change in that patient's level of consciousness but may cause a seizure that, along with the subsequent postictal state, becomes the proximate cause of the unresponsiveness.

Psychogenic Unresponsiveness

Some patients may present with unresponsiveness that is neither structural nor metabolic in origin, but rather has a psychiatric or psychogenic basis. There are several clues to the presence of this feigning of unresponsiveness:

1. The eyelids, when pulled open, close actively instead of shutting in the slow, smooth glide of the organically unresponsive patient.

2. The arm, when upraised over the patient's head and then released, may arc gently over the patient's head or fall conveniently to his or her side instead of striking the face. Care must be taken when performing this maneuver because of the potential damage the dropped arm may cause to the nose.
3. The patient may not respond to the usual forms of painful noxious stimulation but may awaken either to an ammonia pearl placed under his or her nose or by gentle nasopharyngeal stimulation with either a cotton swab or a nasopharyngeal airway.

The one stimulus to which a psychogenically unresponsive patient cannot feign a response is caloric stimulation. Doll's eyes may not be present on movement of the head (see next section) but cold caloric stimulation always results in both a fast and slow component of nystagmus, implying both cortical and brain stem activity. No one can willfully resist the cold caloric stimulus. Any truly unresponsive patient will have the fast component of nystagmus absent.

NEUROLOGIC EVALUATION OF THE UNRESPONSIVE PATIENT

There are five neurologic parameters which should be assessed in all unresponsive patients:

1. level of consciousness
2. motor function
3. respiration pattern
4. pupillary size and reactivity
5. extraocular movements

Level of consciousness and motor function are assessed using the Glasgow Coma Scale. The presence of pathologic reflexes (Babinski) should be considered part of the motor examination and may indicate a structural lesion. Pupillary signs and extraocular movements will be discussed at length in the subsequent section.

The pattern of respiration is traditionally considered to be a clue to the location of a structural lesion but in actuality is rarely of substantive diagnostic help. Recognized abnormal patterns of respiration are Cheyne-Stokes, hyperventilation, apneustic, and ataxic. The Cheyne-Stokes pattern occurs in a variety of metabolic conditions (eg, severe congestive heart failure); its presence in a patient with a structural lesion suggests damage to the cerebral hemispheres or diencephalon with an intact brain stem. Hyperventilation patterns of respiration (ie, central neurogenic hyperventilation) had traditionally been thought to represent low midbrain or upper pons damage; current thinking is that the entity of central neurogenic hyperventilation is rare if not nonexistent and that the hyperventilation seen with a structural neurologic lesion occurs because of subclinical neurogenic pulmonary edema. In apneustic breathing there is a pause at the end of inspiration; this pattern suggests mid to low pontine damage with an intact medulla. It is seen more often in pontine hemorrhage than in herniation syndromes. In ataxic breathing there is irregularity of both depth and rate of respiration, which suggests damage to the medulla.

EYE SIGNS IN THE UNRESPONSIVE PATIENT

There are four key observations to be made about the eyes in an unresponsive patient: eyelid opening, fundi, pupillary size and reactivity, and, intactness of extraocular movements.

Eyelid Opening

If the patient opens his or her eyes spontaneously or to stimuli, then the ascending reticular activating system is at least partially working. Eyelid opening is one of the three responses assayed as part of the Glasgow Coma Scale. There is one metabolic abnormality that can affect eyelid position in an unusual manner: severe phencyclidine intoxication can produce a mute patient with a blank stare.

Fundoscopic Examination

Fundoscopic examination may reveal papilledema indicative of intracranial hypertension, retinal hemorrhages indicative of systemic hypertensive encephalopathy, and subhyaloid hemorrhages indicative of a subarachnoid hemorrhage (these appear as a puff of red in the fundus).

Pupillary Size and Reactivity

The assessment of pupillary size and reactivity provides two very important pieces of information. First, pupillary reactivity helps to distinguish metabolic from structural lesions. In general, the pupillary light reflex is preserved in all cases of metabolic coma. Second, asymmetry of pupillary size and/or lack of reactivity is a sensitive indicator of cortical herniation syndromes and of direct brain stem destruction.

The pupillary light reflex has, as its afferent, cranial nerve II, and, as its efferent, cranial nerve III. The resting and reactive tone of the pupil results from the dynamic tension between the parasympathetic pupilloconstrictor muscle and the sympathetic pupillodilator muscle. Pupillodilation is controlled by the sympathetic nervous system. This system has a long intracranial and extracranial journey. It begins in the hypothalamus, courses down the brain stem, synapses at the first three thoracic vertebrae, synapses again at the superior cervical ganglion, travels with the internal carotid artery, and then enters the orbit with the ophthalmic and then nasociliary branch of the trigeminal nerve to reach the pupillodilator muscle.

The parasympathetic control of pupilloconstriction begins in the Edinger-Westphal nucleus located in the midbrain, emerges as cranial nerve III, which courses outside the brain stem between the posterior cerebral and superior cerebellar arteries (where it is vulnerable to compression by a posterior communicating artery aneurysm), spins around the tentorial notch on top of the tentorium cerebelli (where it is susceptible to pressure from a herniating uncus), and then courses through the dura into the cavernous sinus and then into the orbit.

Lesions of cranial nerve III result in dysfunction of pupilloconstriction and therefore produce a dilated, sluggishly reactive, and then fixed pupil. Cranial nerve III controls, in addition, four of the six extraocular muscles as well as the levator palpebrae muscle, which provides eyelid opening. A complete third nerve lesion therefore results in a dilated pupil, a ptotic eyelid, and an abducted and depressed eyelid. The Edinger-Westphal nucleus and the intra-brainstem course of cranial nerve III lie close to the reticular activating system; because of this close proximity, it is unlikely that there will be substantial destruction of the reticular activating system without pupilloconstriction being affected.

Compression of the third cranial nerve outside the brain stem by a herniating uncus or an expanding aneurysm results first in dysfunction of pupilloconstriction prior to dysfunction of extraocular movements or eyelid opening. The pupilloconstrictor fibers in the third nerve are located more peripherally and thus are more susceptible to pressure. Conversely, diabetic third nerve neuropathy affects extraocular movements but generally spares the pupil. Patients who have a dilated pupil secondary to transtentorial herniation usually have an abnormal mental status to go along with their pupillary inequality. A patient who is complaining of a headache and has a dilated and unreactive pupil but is awake and lucid either has an aneurysm of the posterior communicating artery or has local globe pathology such as an acute glaucoma attack.

Damage at different sites in the brain stem results in characteristic pupillary patterns. A lesion in the midbrain destroys both the pupilloconstrictor third nerve pathway and the descending sympathetic fibers. Therefore, midbrain destruction results in midposition pupils that are nonreactive. These are the true pupils of death with neither pupilloconstrictor nor pupillodilator input. A lesion in the pons destroys the descending sympathetic tracts but leaves intact the parasympathetic innervation, which has already exited at the midbrain level. There is thus unopposed pupilloconstriction resulting in the pinpoint pupils of pontine destruction. When a pupil dilates as part of the uncal herniation syndrome, the dilated pupil is almost always on the same side as the herniating uncus, because the mechanism for dilation is compression of cranial nerve III as it courses along the tentorium. Weakness of the contralateral arm and leg may accompany the pupillary sign either because of direct brain stem damage to the descending corticospinal tract or because of damage to the ipsilateral frontal motor strip. Sometimes the patient's weakness appears on the same side as the dilated pupil. This represents a Kernohan's notch syndrome in which the contralateral cerebral peduncle is compressed against the incisural edge of the tentorium.

In a patient with an acute confusional state, unequal pupils that react differentially to light represent evidence of a structural lesion in the brain until proven otherwise. Differential reactivity is the key finding; pupils that are asymmetric in size but briskly reactive usually represent physiologic anisocoria, which is a normal finding in many patients. Patients with metabolically caused coma may have signs suggestive of lower brain stem dysfunction, such as absent respirations or flaccid muscle tone, but their pupillary reactivity is invariably preserved. This "neuroanatomic inconsistency," so called because the motor signs and respirations suggest brain stem damage, whereas the pupillary exam suggests an intact brain stem, is one of the diagnostic clues to a metabolic cause of coma. In a patient who has a unilateral nonreactive pupil, there are several noncentral nervous system causes of a nonresponsive pupil that must be ruled out: local globe trauma, acute glaucoma, iritis, and inadvertent administration of a sympathomimetic during nasotracheal intubation with the drug traveling retrograde from the nose through the nasolacrimal duct.

Certain drugs cause characteristic alterations in pupillary size. The drugs that cause miosis are opiates (with meperidine the least miosis inducing), organophosphate and other anticholinesterase pesticides, pilocarpine and other antiglaucoma eye drops, barbiturates, ethanol, and some phenothiazines. The drugs that cause mydriasis are agents with anticholinergic potency (tricyclic antidepressants, antihistamines, phenothiazines, over-the-counter sleep preparations, and certain plants), sympathomimetics such as amphetamines and cocaine, and glutethimide.

Extraocular Movements

A patient who can conjugately move his or her eyes in a horizontal direction has proved the intactness of cranial nerve III in the midbrain (supplying the medial rectus and adducting the eye) and of cranial nerve VI in the pons (supplying the lateral rectus and abducting the eye), as well as the connections between these two nerves—the medial longitudinal fasciculus. The reason for the great interest and emphasis on eye movement is not the eye movements themselves; people could train themselves to turn their heads instead of moving their eyes. Rather, the eye movement system covers a large amount of territory in the brain stem and is located next to the ascending reticular activating system. Demonstrating the intactness of conjugate gaze gives a clean bill of health to a large territory of central brain stem.

If the patient spontaneously looks to the right and to the left or does so upon command, then these key eye movement pathways are demonstrated to be intact, and no more eye movement testing need be carried out. If, however, the patient is lying with the eyes pointed straight ahead, then maneuvers must be used to elicit either the oculocephalic (doll's eyes) or oculovestibular (caloric stimulation) reflex.

The doll's eyes reflex is elicited by rapidly rotating the head of the patient to the right or to the left and observing the position of the eyes. If the eyes stay fixed with respect to the orbits, ie, move with the head as it is turned, then doll's eyes are said to be absent and the intactness of conjugate gaze has not been demonstrated. If the eyes move with respect to the orbit but stay fixed with respect to the room, then the intactness of the conjugate gaze has been demonstrated and doll's eyes are said to be present. A patient whose brain stem is not functioning will not have doll's eyes. A patient whose cortex is not functioning but whose brain stem is functioning will have doll's eyes. However, the patient who has cortical function (either because the unresponsiveness is psychogenic in origin or because the degree of brain injury is not that great) may be able to effect a cortical override of the doll's eyes reflex. Unless the examiner is astute and follows the oculocephalic maneuver with oculovestibular testing, he or she may be misled into overestimating the degree of unresponsiveness of the patient. Elicitation of the oculocephalic reflex should not be attempted if there is any possibility the patient has a cervical spine injury. Any unresponsive patient whose history is uncertain therefore needs radiographic evaluation of the cervical spine prior to moving the head.

The oculovestibular reflex (caloric stimulation) is more potent than the oculocephalic reflex in eliciting conjugate gaze. This reflex is elicited by injecting ice water into the external ear canal with the purpose of stimulating the semicircular canals. The horizontal semicircular canal is the most lateral of the three canals, and therefore the most easily stimulated. If the patient is placed 30 degrees up from the supine position, the horizontal semicircular canal will be situated vertically and gravity will help reinforce the response. The tympanic membrane should be checked for absence of perforation and the external canal checked for absence of wax. Ten mL of cold water should then be injected into the ear canal with a flexible plastic catheter (the clear plastic connecting tubing from a butterfly needle has the correct size and flexibility).

There are three possible responses to the instillation of this cold water stimulus. A patient who has an intact brain stem and an intact cortex will have nystagmus, with the fast component directed away from the side of the cold water stimulus and the slow component directed toward it. In the patient who has a depressed cortex but a functioning brain stem, only the slow component will be present, and there will be tonic deviation of the eyes toward the side of the cold stimulus. Intactness of conjugate gaze and hence intactness of the brain stem has been demonstrated. If the patient's brain stem pathways are not functioning, then the eyes will remain pointed straight ahead. Successful caloric stimulation depends also, of course, on an intact afferent, which is cranial nerve VIII.

A patient with an isolated nuclear palsy (either cranial nerve III or cranial nerve VI) will have deviation of the eye, either medially or laterally, at rest. A patient with an isolated medial longitudinal fasciculus lesion (as in multiple sclerosis) will have eyes that are pointed straight ahead at rest, but there will be paralysis of adduction (moving medially) of the ipsilateral (to the medial longitudinal fasciculus) eye and nystagmus of the abducting eye on attempts at conjugate lateral gaze. Certain drugs cause nystagmus that may be elicited on attempts at lateral or vertical gaze; the four most important are phenytoin, ethanol, barbiturates, and phencyclidine.

MANAGEMENT OF THE UNRESPONSIVE PATIENT

The standard principles of patient assessment and intervention apply when managing the unresponsive patient:

1. Assess vital signs first. Until proven otherwise, an unresponsive patient is unresponsive because of no ventilation, profound hypotension, or tachy- or brady-dysrhythmia.
2. Protect the neck. All unresponsive patients are presumed to have a traumatic cause of unresponsiveness unless the history clearly contraindicates and so should have the cervical spine secured and a cervical spine roentgenogram ordered.
3. Assess the patient's level of consciousness, using the three components of the Glasgow Coma Scale.

    The assessment and management of the unresponsive patient is one of the classical patient care problems in emergency medicine. Rigorous attention to following the basic steps outlined above will ensure that the proper diagnosis is made and that morbidity and mortality are minimized. More patient care mistakes are made because basic procedures are not followed than because the esoteric diagnosis or intervention is missed.
4. Perform a bedside test of serum glucose or administer 25 g of dextrose IV (50 cc of 50 percent dextrose).
5. Take the temperature. The patient's temperature may provide a clue to one of several causes of unresponsiveness: hypothermia, hyperthermia, infection, myxedema, and certain intoxications. It is frequently the forgotten vital sign.
6. Perform a focused neurologic examination: level of consciousness, pupil size and reactivity, extraocular

movements, motor function and posturing, and respiration pattern.
7. Perform a more detailed physical examination. Look for the clues to a structural lesion that were outlined above, in particular look for signs of trauma. Look for evidence of intravenous drug use. Look for skin lesions that may suggest a metabolic cause of the unresponsive state, such as the petechiae of thrombotic thrombocytopenic purpura or disseminated intravesicular coagulation secondary to sepsis, or the characteristic rash of meningococcemia or pneumococcemia.
8. Consider administration of intravenous naloxone and thiamine. If there is any depression of respiration or presence of small pupils or any possibility of a narcotic overdose, 1.2 to 2.0 mg of naloxone is administered. Certain drugs, such as pentazocine or propoxyphene, may require higher doses of naloxone for antagonism. There is no contraindication to naloxone, and some clinicians administer it to all unresponsive patients. It is both diagnostic and therapeutic. It is not unreasonable to administer thiamine to all unresponsive patients in whom the cause of the unresponsiveness is uncertain. Wernicke's encephalopathy is an extremely rare cause of coma, but is totally reversible if treated with thiamine. Physostigmine, an acetylcholinesterase inhibitor, should not be administered as a diagnostic or therapeutic agent to unresponsive patients because of the potential risk of bradycardia and seizures. This represents a change in standard practice from the late 1970s. Physostigmine is now used only as a second line agent in cases of suspected anticholinergic poisoning; even in those cases the indications for its use are very strict.
9. If a metabolic cause of the unresponsive state is suspected, draw a set of diagnostic tests to identify the cause of metabolic coma. The following tests are appropriate in the initial workup of the patient with unresponsiveness of unknown cause: glucose, electrolytes, calcium, BUN, hemoglobin/hematocrit, white blood count, platelet count, ethanol level, arterial blood gas, and urine analysis. If there is possibility of the relevant clinical entity, additional tests may be ordered: appropriate toxicology assays (urine or blood, depending on the agent suspected), or a test of liver function (coagulation assay or transaminase level).
10. Reassess the patient frequently along the parameters outlined in step 6.
11. Initiate appropriate therapy for a structural lesion if one is suspected. Perform controlled endotracheal intubation and hyperventilate to a pCO_2 of 25 to 30 mm Hg if indicated. Precede the intubation with administration of agents that minimize increases in intracranial pressure.
12. Obtain a CT or MR scan of the brain if there is any suspicion of a structural lesion.

BIBLIOGRAPHY

Adams R, Victor M. *Principles of Neurology,* 4th ed. New York: McGraw-Hill, 1989.

DeMyer W. *Technique of the Neurologic Examination,* 4th ed. New York: McGraw-Hill, 1992.

Plum F, Posner J. *The Diagnosis of Stupor and Coma,* 3rd ed. Philadelphia: FA Davis, 1980.

Wilson JD, Braunwald E, Isselbacher KJ, Petersdorf RG, Martin JB, Fauci AS, Root RK. *Harrison's Principles of Internal Medicine, 12th ed.* New York: McGraw-Hill, 1991.

58. Cerebrovascular Accident

RON M. WALLS, MD, FRCPC

The designation cerebrovascular accident (CVA, stroke) is applied to all pathologic processes involving the blood vessels and circulation that arise in the absence of trauma and that lead to the relatively abrupt onset of an abnormality in the structure or function of the brain. Although the incidence of CVA is decreasing, presumably due to increased awareness of the causative role of hypertension, it remains the third leading cause of morbidity and death in the United States.

CLASSIFICATION

Cerebrovascular accidents fall into two categories: ischemic and hemorrhagic (Table 58-1). Ischemic CVAs are further subdivided by three etiologies: (1) thrombosis, (2) embolism, and (3) low flow state. Whether a CVA is ischemic or hemorrhagic, damage to the brain arises via one or both of the following mechanisms:

1. interruption of adequate blood flow to a particular area of the brain, resulting in ischemic damage
2. insult to the structural integrity of the brain as a result of hemorrhage or edema, leading to compression of tissue with secondary compromise of oxygen delivery

Cerebrovascular disease may involve large vessels, small vessels, or both. Depending on the vessels involved, and the type of injury (ischemic versus hemorrhagic), identifiable patterns of brain injury result. Differentiation between these categories and localization of the area of the brain injury will determine the appropriate diagnostic and therapeutic intervention.

Table 58-1 Classification of CVA

Ischemic	Hemorrhagic
Thrombotic	Subarachnoid hemorrhage
Anterior circulation	Intracerebral hemorrhage
Posterior circulation	Cerebellar hemorrhage
Lacunar	
Embolic	
Anterior circulation	
Posterior circulation	

RISK FACTORS

The two cardinal risk factors for stroke are diabetes mellitus and hypertension (systolic or diastolic). Other factors, including cigarette smoking, hyperlipidemia, vascular disease in another body system (eg, coronary artery disease, claudication), and familial predisposition may also represent increased risks for the development of CVA. Patients with cardiac chamber enlargement, valvular disease, and certain dysrhythmias (especially atrial fibrillation) are at increased risk for embolic stroke regardless of the condition of their cerebral vasculature.

This chapter is reprinted from the second edition of *Emergency Medicine*.

INITIAL EVALUATION

Patients with CVA may present anywhere on a spectrum from mild, subtle neurologic deficits to coma with massive brain injury and impending herniation. The history of the onset and progression of the neurologic deficit must be unambiguously obtained. This may require interviewing family members, attendants, and ambulance personnel in addition to the patient. This is of paramount importance in determining the type of CVA that has occurred. Thrombotic strokes usually present with gradual onset of a variably progressive neurologic deficit, which often waxes and wanes over the first few hours and usually begins at rest or while asleep. Decreased level of consciousness and headache, if present, are usually mild, except in cases of massive stroke, as in total occlusion of the internal carotid artery in patients with poor collateral circulation. Sudden, dramatic neurologic deficits are usually the result of embolism or hemorrhage. These two conditions can be further differentiated by the presence of depressed mental status and headache, which argue strongly in favor of hemorrhage. Risk factors for thrombotic or embolic stroke should be sought. All medications, especially cardiovascular and anticoagulant drugs, should be noted. A general physical examination, including a meticulous cardiovascular assessment, should precede a detailed neurologic evaluation. In severe cases, resuscitation of the patient and treatment of increased intracranial pressure may preempt all but a cursory initial examination. Rapid determination of the blood glucose level (eg, with Dextrostix) and administration of opiate antagonists should be performed early in these cases. Profound alteration of mental status should raise the suspicion of intracranial hemorrhage or of a nonvascular event, since ischemic brain injury is rarely accompanied by markedly depressed consciousness. Following initial physical assessment and stabilization, all patients must undergo a thorough, organized neurologic examination. Further evaluation and treatment will be dictated by these findings.

CEREBROVASCULAR ANATOMY

There are two distinct, yet interconnected, vascular systems supplying the brain. The carotid, or anterior, system is the major supplier of blood to the cerebral hemispheres. The vertebrobasilar, or posterior, system is the major supplier of the brain stem and cerebellum.

Anterior Circulation

The internal carotid artery arises from the common carotid artery at its bifurcation, near the angle of the mandible. It ascends through the base of the skull, gives off the ophthalmic artery, and rises to anastomose with its contralateral fellow via the anterior communicating artery. At this point also, a posterior communicating artery is given off (forming an anastomosis with the ipsilateral posterior cerebral artery of the posterior system), and the major portion of the vessel continues as the middle cerebral artery, supplying the largest portion of the cerebral hemisphere.

Posterior Circulation

The vertebral artery arises from the subclavian artery and ascends via the transverse processes of the cervical vertebrae, through the foramen magnum, supplying the brain stem and cerebellum. At the junction of the medulla and pons, the artery joins its opposite fellow to form the basilar artery. The basilar artery ascends along the brain stem, giving off various branches, and then divides to form the two posterior cerebral vessels, which communicate, via the posterior communicating arteries, with the carotid system. The posterior cerebral vessels continue on to supply the upper brain stem, portions of the temporal lobe, and the median occipital lobe, including the visual cortex.

Collateral Circulation

The caliber and flow characteristics of the communicating arteries, which interconnect the anterior and posterior circulations, have great individual variability. This variability is responsible for the large range of deficits produced by occlusion of any one of the major vessels. Identical levels of obstruction may produce dense hemiplegia in one individual, while leaving another entirely asymptomatic. The degree of recovery from the initial neurologic deficit associated with the CVA is also largely dependent on the function of this collateral system.

PATTERNS OF CVA

Depending on the location of the vascular event and the status of the collateral circulation, certain patterns of neurologic deficit are associated with disruption of the various intracranial vessels. The most important clinical tasks include the following:

1. Determine that a CVA has occurred and whether it is thrombotic, embolic, or hemorrhagic.
2. Determine the vascular system involved (ie, anterior versus posterior circulation).
3. Determine which side the lesion is on.

The answers to these three questions will determine the best approach to the patient. The distinguishing features in the presentation of ischemic versus hemorrhagic and of embolic versus thrombotic stroke have been discussed. Determination of whether the CVA involves the anterior or posterior circulation, and which side the lesion is on, requires a knowl-

Table 58-2 Anterior versus Posterior CVA

Findings Supporting Anterior Lesions	Findings Supporting Posterior Lesions	Not Helpful
Aphasia	Crossed findings (eg, ipsilateral facial deficit with contralateral body deficit)	Hemiparesis alone
Hemiparesis with ipsilateral sensory deficit		Hemiparesis or hemisensory loss with hemianopsia
Hemiparesis with sudden contralateral blindness	Cranial nerve signs	
	Cerebellar signs	
	True central vertigo	
	Hemianopsia alone	
	Dysconjugate gaze or pupillary abnormality	
	Bilateral findings	
	Depressed level of consciousness	

edge of the neurologic functions associated with the various areas of the brain supplied by these vessels.

Features that differentiate between lesions of the anterior circulation and those of the posterior circulation are summarized in Table 58-2. Once the major circulatory system has been identified, it may be possible to identify the specific vessel involved, although this does not necessarily have any impact on the management of the patient.

MAJOR NEUROVASCULAR SYNDROMES

Ischemic CVA

Middle Cerebral Artery Syndrome

Occlusion of the middle cerebral artery without adequate collateral perfusion will result in the following picture:

- contralateral hemiparesis
- contralateral hemisensory loss
- aphasia (if the left, or rarely right, hemisphere is involved)
- homonymous hemianopsia
- anosognosia (if the right, or rarely left, hemisphere is involved)

Internal Carotid Artery Syndrome

Occlusion of the internal carotid artery will generally lead to the following:

- all of the features of the middle cerebral artery syndrome
- sudden loss of vision on the side opposite the hemiparesis (due to occlusion of the ophthalmic artery)
- stupor or coma secondary to the large mass of the involved brain
- symptoms and signs consistent with anterior cerebral artery occlusion, if collateral circulation via the circle of Willis is inadequate

Anterior Cerebral Artery Syndrome

Occlusion of the anterior cerebral artery will generally lead to symptoms and signs only if the occlusion is distal to the anterior communicating artery, since collateral flow is almost invariably adequate. The clinical picture is as follows:

- hemiparesis of the contralateral side, with foot and leg affected most severely and the face usually spared
- hemisensory deficit of the contralateral foot and leg
- contralateral grasp and sucking reflex
- various degrees of "frontal lobe syndrome," with apathy, blunting of personality, and inability to identify objects correctly

Posterior Cerebral Artery Syndrome

Occlusion of the posterior cerebral artery leads to the following:

- homonymous hemianopsia involving the contralateral visual field
- contralateral hemisensory deficit without persistent motor deficit
- short-term memory loss
- amnesic aphasia, especially of colors (inability to name an object, despite being able to describe and use it correctly)
- alexia with or without agraphia
- extrapyramidal movement disorders, such as hemiballismus

Vertebral Artery Syndrome

Occlusion of the vertebral artery results in varying degrees of damage to the medulla oblongata, producing a highly variable clinical syndrome. The lateral medullary syndrome is the most familiar of these, and includes the features listed below:

- pain and temperature sensory deficit of the ipsilateral face and contralateral body
- ipsilateral Horner's syndrome

- deficits of cranial nerves IX and X, resulting in ipsilateral loss of the gag reflex, hoarseness, and dysphagia
- vertigo, nausea, vomiting, nystagmus
- ipsilateral ataxia

Rarely, the medial medullary syndrome is seen, including contralateral hemiparalysis of the body, contralateral loss of position and vibration sense, and ipsilateral paralysis of the tongue.

Basilar Artery Syndrome

The basilar artery gives off branches to the pons, cerebellar peduncles, and cerebellar hemispheres. Complete occlusion of the basilar artery produces quadriplegia, multiple cranial nerve abnormalities, and coma (secondary to involvement of the reticular activating system). More often, the occlusion involves branches of the basilar artery, and the resultant syndrome will depend entirely on which branch is involved. There are a number of commonly recognized basilar branch syndromes:

- If the paramedian arteries, which supply the medial pons, are obstructed, the clinical syndrome is dominated by contralateral hemiplegia and extraocular movement abnormalities (usually internuclear ophthalmoplegia or a conjugate gaze palsy).
- If the short circumferential arteries, which supply the lateral pons, are obstructed, the syndrome consists primarily of contralateral sensory deficits.
- If the long circumferential arteries, which supply the cerebellum, are obstructed, the picture is one of ipsilateral cerebellar dysfunction with or without pontine findings.

Lacunar CVA

When small arteries, which penetrate the brain to supply a discrete area, become obstructed, isolated infarction ensues. Subsequent healing processes result in resorption of the infarcted tissue, leaving a small cavity, or lacuna. Depending on the location of the obstruction, the entire event may be clinically inapparent or may result in dramatic neurologic deficit. Because of the small amount of tissue involved, prognosis for recovery is usually excellent. Although any area of the brain may be affected, certain common syndromes have been identified:

- Internal capsule or pontine occlusion may result in isolated hemiparesis or hemiplegia.
- Thalamic involvement may manifest with a pure, isolated hemisensory deficit.
- Pontine injury may manifest as a dysarthria—clumsy hand syndrome.
- Midbrain lesions may cause hemiparesis with cerebellar ataxia.

Management of Ischemic CVA

Management of the patient with ischemic CVA has three major goals:

1. general evaluation and resuscitation of the patient
2. correction of underlying abnormalities
3. preservation of brain function

CVA patients are often elderly and prone to bone injury. If a fall occurred as a result of the stroke, the patient may have sustained a fractured hip, pelvis, ribs, or spine. If there is any question that trauma to the spine may have occurred, the patient should be appropriately immobilized on a long backboard until radiographic and physical examination exclude this injury. A careful physical examination will generally detect most other injuries, and radiographs should be obtained as needed.

Acute or chronic hypertensive vascular disease may result in pulmonary edema or myocardial ischemia. This should be evaluated by history, physical examination, radiography, and electrocardiography. The patient's volume status should be ascertained and corrected with crystalloid if necessary. Determination of the blood glucose value in all patients should be an early priority. Hypoglycemia should be rapidly corrected. Preservation of brain function is a relatively unexplored area of medicine. A short time after the CVA occurs, a portion of the brain will die and will not be retrievable. However, depending on the state of the collateral circulation, there may be another large area of brain tissue surrounding this that is at jeopardy but potentially salvageable. Emergency management of the stroke patient should be conducted in such a way as to optimize the chances for recovery of this threatened brain tissue. This requires attention to the fundamental requirements of brain cells.

First, perfusion must be optimized. Underperfused brain tissue will be damaged, even if all other factors are ideal. Three factors related to perfusion need to be considered: (1) hypotension, (2) hypertension, and (3) increased intracranial pressure.

If the patient is hypotensive, the cause of the hypotension must be ascertained. Rapid determination of hematocrit may indicate hemorrhage or hemoconcentration. Hypotension secondary to hemorrhage is unusual, and the gastrointestinal tract is the most frequent site of the blood loss. Examination of stool for blood and passage of a nasogastric tube may be indicated. Usually, the hypotension is the result of dehydration and should be corrected with crystalloid. CVA is not a contraindication to the administration of normal saline or lactated Ringer's solution if the blood pressure is low on the basis of dehydration. Cardiogenic shock will usually be apparent on physical examination and mandates the use of pressors rather than volume expanders. Blood products are rarely indicated. Occasionally, the patient's mental status will improve dramatically with restoration of adequate circulating volume.

Management of hypertension is a little more controversial. Many of these patients have chronic hypertension, which is modestly elevated at presentation. It is generally agreed that modest elevations of blood pressure should not be corrected, since overcorrection may result in underperfusion of the ischemic brain tissue. As a rule of thumb, systolic blood pressures up to 200 or 210 mmHg and diastolic pressures of 100 to 120 mmHg should be managed by close observation only. Pressures in this range are unlikely to jeopardize the patient, and normalization over several hours is the rule. If the patient is on chronic antihypertensive medication, however, this therapy should be continued. More severe elevations in blood pressure should prompt treatment, and in the vast majority of circumstances, intravenous nitroprusside infusion is the method of choice. Use of oral, sublingual, intramuscular, transdermal, or intravenous "push" agents may result in precipitous decline of blood pressure, which may be difficult to manage.

Significant increase in intracranial pressure is seen most often in hemorrhagic CVA, and management of this entity is discussed below.

Simultaneous with the management of brain perfusion, adequate supply of glucose and oxygen to the brain must be ensured. If the serum glucose level reads low on a dipstick test, intravenous glucose should be administered at once. The 30- to 60-minute delay engendered by waiting for laboratory confirmation of the hypoglycemia is unacceptable.

All patients, except those with chronic carbon dioxide retention, should receive oxygen by nasal cannula or mask. If arterial blood gases show the Po_2 to be in a normal range (>75 mmHg), administration of additional oxygen is unlikely to benefit the patient, however.

Finally, cardiac rate and rhythm must also be assessed. Tachydysrhythmias or bradydysrhythmias that compromise cardiac output must be treated. Cardiogenic shock may be at the root of the low flow state that led to the CVA, and appropriate monitoring and pressors should be used. Computed tomography (CT) will, for the most part, fail to demonstrate ischemic infarction acutely. The area of injury will become apparent on CT scan a number of days later (Fig. 58-1). Determination of serum electrolytes and a complete blood cell count should be performed in all cases. Coagulation profiles, serum calcium, toxicology screens, and other studies are indicated for many, but not all, patients.

Hemorrhagic CVA

Subarachnoid Hemorrhage

The most common cause of subarachnoid hemorrhage (SAH) is rupture of an aneurysm arising from the circle of Willis. These so-called berry aneurysms are small saccular structures that are most often found at a point of bifurcation of the major cerebral vasculature. It is believed that the aneurysm develops as a result of a congenital defect in the wall of the artery, which over years dilates to a size of 1 to 3 cm. This gradual development accounts for the paucity of aneurysmal ruptures prior to the third or fourth decade of life. Occasionally, the aneurysm will develop in such a location that it presses on adjacent cranial nerves (especially the third to sixth cranial nerves) and presents as an isolated nerve palsy. More often, the presence of the aneurysm becomes apparent only when rupture leads to an intracranial catastrophe.

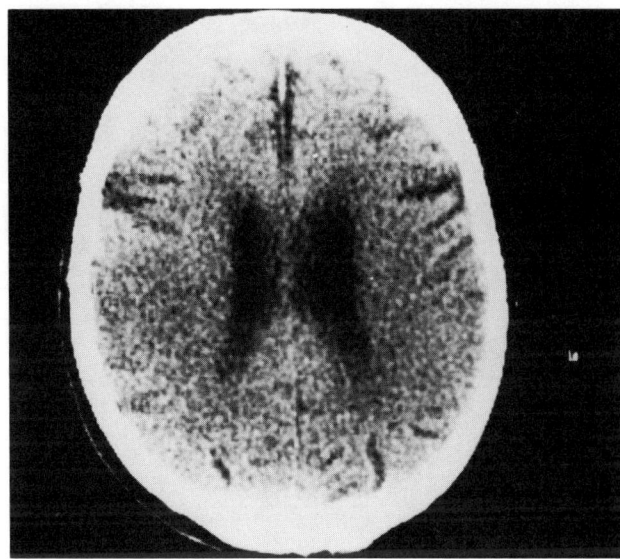
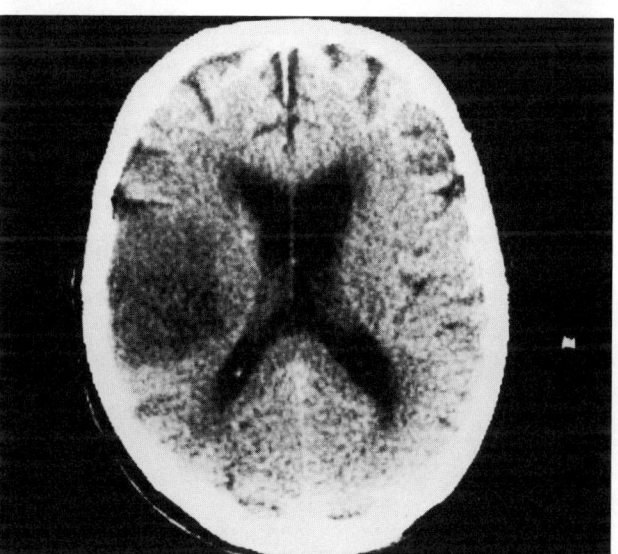

Figure 58-1 (A) Essentially normal noncontrast head CT scan of patient who presented with left-sided neurologic deficit. History was consistent with ischemic CVA. (B) Same patient as in A. This noncontrast scan was obtained 5 days later and shows a large lucency in the right parietal area, consistent with ischemic infarct.

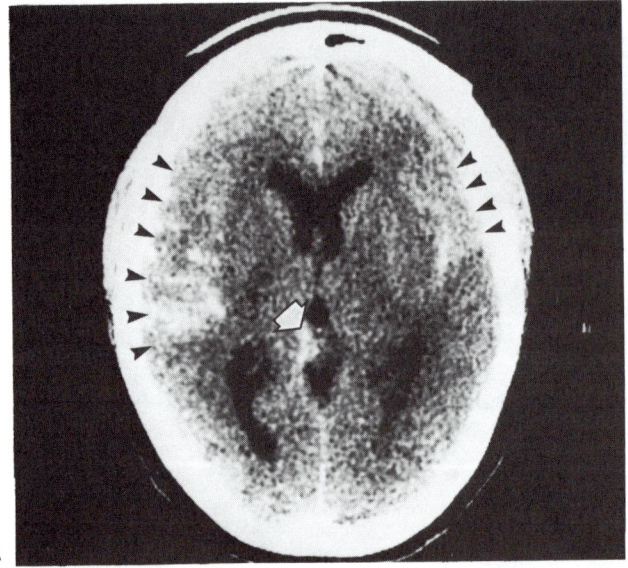

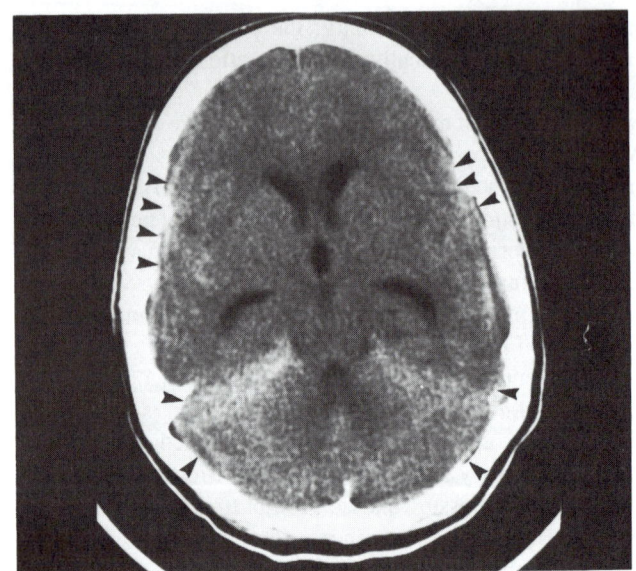

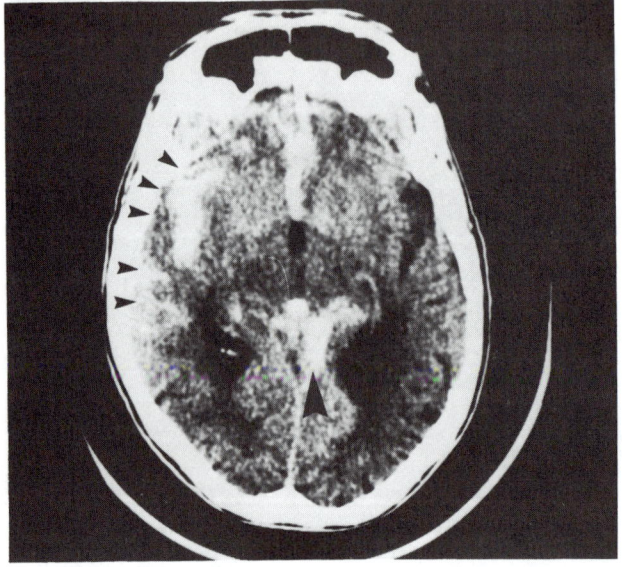

Figure 58-2 (**A**) Noncontrast head CT scan showing increased density in sulci (narrow arrows) and third ventricle (wide arrow) consistent with recent subarachnoid hemorrhage. (**B**) Noncontrast head CT scan showing blood in the sylvian fissures (narrow arrows) and outlining the tentorium (wide arrows). The tentorium is normally not readily visible on a noncontrast scan. (**C**) Noncontrast head CT scan of subarachnoid hemorrhage with blood in the sylvian fissure (narrow arrows) and sulci (wide arrows). Additional intracerebral hemorrhage (solid arrow) is seen posterior to the third ventricle, and ventricular size is increased, consistent with hydrocephalus.

The onset of symptoms following rupture is varied. Relatively sudden onset of severe headache, often with alteration of mental status or frank syncope, is common. The headache usually arises during exertion, such as straining at stool, sexual intercourse, or athletic activity. Some patients will experience unheralded syncope, followed by the gradual evolution of severe headache. Meningismus is frequent but not invariable. Photophobia is common. Rarely will the patient have a completely normal, alert mental status. In severe cases, the hemorrhage may be so massive that the patient becomes rapidly comatose and dies despite appropriate intervention.

On the other hand, some patients will present with a relatively benign appearance and moderate symptomatology and may be misdiagnosed as having migraine or tension headache. A number of patients, if able to provide a history, will describe a headache of lesser severity in the two to three weeks preceding their current presentation. This is believed to represent a "warning bleed," or small, self-limited leaking of blood from the aneurysm.

The vast majority of patients will not have focal neurologic deficits, unless massive hemorrhage with impending herniation has occurred. This distinguishes subarachnoid hemorrhage from intracerebral hemorrhage, the latter most often presenting with headache and focal neurologic findings.

Suspicion of subarachnoid hemorrhage mandates performance of a CT scan of the brain (Fig. 58-2). In the majority of cases, the diagnosis can be secured in this manner. Contrast medium is usually not necessary. A negative CT scan does not exclude SAH, however. If the diagnosis is still in doubt following CT scan, the patient should undergo diagnostic lumbar puncture. The lumbar puncture will generally show a modest elevation in opening pressure, and the cerebrospinal fluid (CSF) will, in most cases, be grossly bloody. Red blood cell counts will range from a few hundred to a million or more cells per cubic millimeter. The ratio of red to white blood cells will generally mirror that of the peripheral blood, although a reactive leukocytosis of the CSF may be seen. Centrifugation of the specimen will usually demonstrate xanthochromia of the supernatant. Xanthochromia develops within about four hours of the introduction of blood into the CSF; therefore, the specimen should be centrifuged and observed immediately to avoid confusion between SAH and a traumatic spinal tap. Xanthochromia may also develop as a result of high concentrations of protein (>150 mg/dL) in the CSF, so protein should be measured to ensure that the observed xanthochromia is indeed due to blood breakdown. Judicious use of sedation and local anesthesia during the lumbar puncture is important. If SAH has occurred, all attempts must be made to keep the patient quiet and comfortable during the procedure, and after.

The role of clinical suspicion in the timely diagnosis of subarachnoid hemorrhage cannot be overstressed. The reduction in morbidity afforded by the early diagnosis and successful treatment of intracranial aneurysm in a single case more than offsets the cost of negative CT scans and lumbar punctures in patients who are ultimately diagnosed with another form of headache.

The primary goal in the management of subarachnoid hemorrhage is prevention of additional bleeding, which is often fatal. Immediate neurosurgical consultation is mandatory. The patient should be kept quiet, preferably in a dimly lit room, and must be observed constantly. The head of the bed should be elevated 20° to 30°. If arterial hypertension is present, it should be lowered to a range similar to that described for ischemic CVA (see above). Sedation and analgesia should be achieved using barbiturates or benzodiazepines and narcotics. If seizures occur, the patient should be loaded with 15 to 17 mg/kg of phenytoin. Further seizure activity may require phenobarbital. The use of aminocaproic acid (Amicar) remains controversial. Advocates believe that lysis of the hemostatic clot is impeded by this agent. In general, such therapy should only be administered in consultation with the neurosurgeon who will be assuming ultimate care of the patient. Most patients will be admitted for a period of stabilization, followed by angiography and surgery 7 to 10 days after presentation.

Intracerebral Hemorrhage

Unlike subarachnoid hemorrhage, in which blood accumulates in the subarachnoid space, intracerebral hemorrhage involves bleeding into the brain parenchyma. This results in a mass effect and fairly prompt development of neurologic deficit. Patients with this condition are generally somewhat younger than those who sustain thrombotic stroke, and pre-

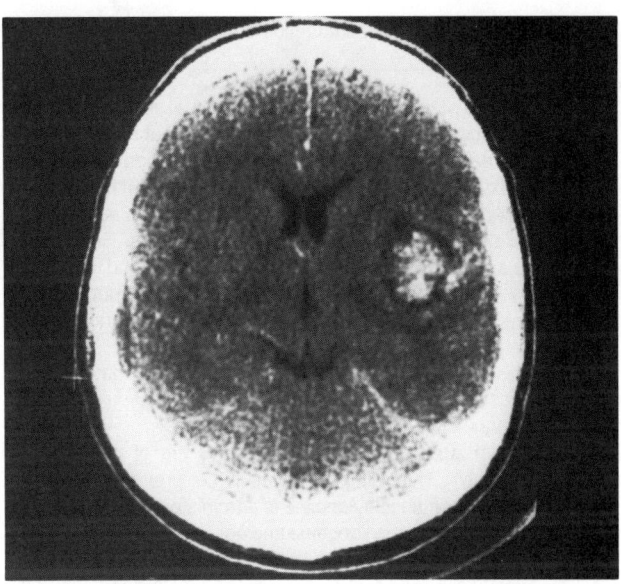

Figure 58-3 Noncontrast head CT scan. Note intracerebral hematoma of left parietal lobe.

existing hypertension (usually essential) is present virtually 100% of the time. The onset and severity of symptoms are variable. Almost all patients will complain of headache or a pressure sensation within the head. This is accompanied, or closely followed, by a progressive neurologic deficit. Depending on the severity and location of the hemorrhage, rapid development of coma, followed by herniation and death, may occur. Unlike subarachnoid hemorrhage, which presents as headache and alteration of mental status, intracerebral hemorrhage is almost invariably associated with focal findings on neurologic examination. These findings will vary from mild hemiparesis to dense hemiplegia with signs of tentorial herniation.

The management of intracerebral hemorrhage, in most cases, must proceed on the basis of a provisional diagnosis. CT scan must be obtained early in the course (Fig. 58-3), but therapy for increased intracranial pressure, control of hypertension, and general resuscitation of the patient should not be delayed for radiographic confirmation of the intracranial catastrophe. Rapid control of blood pressure is essential. Systolic pressures greater than 200 mmHg or diastolic pressures greater than 120 mmHg should be treated. As in thrombotic stroke, the agent of choice is nitroprusside by intravenous infusion. An arterial line is usually required. Care must be taken to avoid excessive lowering of the blood pressure, which might compromise perfusion of the compressed areas of brain adjacent to the mass of the hemorrhage. Blood pressures in the vicinity of 160 mmHg systolic and 100 mmHg diastolic should be targeted. If signs of increased intracranial pressure are present, treatment should be instituted immediately. Elevated intracranial pressure is a relative contraindication to nasotracheal intubation, since

Table 58-3 Rapid Sequence Intubation of Adults

1. Prepare the patient and the area. Ensure that suction apparatus and all equipment are in working order and that back-up equipment is readily available. Preoxygenate the patient by providing 100% oxygen for 5 minutes of normal breathing. If time is of the essence, have the patient breathe 100% oxygen as deeply as possible for a minimum of three to five breaths. Have instruments available for bag ventilation of the patient and for surgical airway maneuvers in the event that intubation is not possible.
2. Ensure that one, or preferably two, reliable intravenous routes are established.
3. Administer 1.0 to 1.5 mg/kg of lidocaine intravenously. This is believed to attenuate the rise in intracranial pressure that may accompany intubation.
4. Administer precurarizing dosage of 1.0 mg of pancuronium intravenously. This will greatly diminish or prevent muscle fasciculation when succinylcholine is administered.
5. Wait 2 minutes for the lidocaine and pancuronium to take effect. The patient should continue preoxygenation.
6. Administer 1.5 mg/kg of succinylcholine by intravenous push, followed by 5 mg/kg of a short-acting barbiturate, such as sodium thiopental. Observe the patient's respirations. As the patient ceases breathing spontaneously, gentle pressure should be applied to the cricoid cartilage by an assistant. This prevents passive regurgitation of gastric contents up the esophagus. Pressure should continue until the endotracheal tube is in position with the cuff inflated. If the patient actively vomits, pressure must be immediately released to prevent esophageal injury.
7. Approximately 45 seconds after the succinylcholine has been administered, check the state of paralysis of the patient's mandible. When relaxation has been achieved, orally intubate the patient, inflate the endotracheal tube cuff, and confirm the tube position by auscultation of both lung fields and the stomach. Once the airway is secured, cricoid pressure may be released.
8. At no time should the patient have ventilations assisted by mask prior to the intubation, since risk of gastric aspiration is greatly increased by this maneuver. If intubation is unsuccessful, however, ventilate the patient by mask for 30 seconds; then repeat the intubation attempt.

sharp rises in the intracranial pressure may result. Consequently, the patient should be orally intubated using a rapid sequence technique. It is recommended that patients with elevated intracranial pressure receive 1 to 1.5 mg/kg of lidocaine intravenously 2 to 3 minutes prior to intubation. The remainder of the technique essentially consists of standard rapid sequence induction of anesthesia, followed by orotracheal intubation. *Thorough familiarity with this technique is the responsibility of all physicians caring for critically ill patients.* A summary of rapid sequence intubation is provided in Table 58-3. Once intubation is achieved, the patient should be hyperventilated to achieve an arterial P_{CO_2} of 25 to 30 mmHg. Mannitol, furosemide (Lasix), and dexamethasone (Decadron) may be administered as desired or indicated. Additional sedation should be given, and the patient should be paralyzed and maintained on a ventilator. Once the patient is stable, a CT scan should be immediately obtained. Extravascular blood will generally be readily visu-

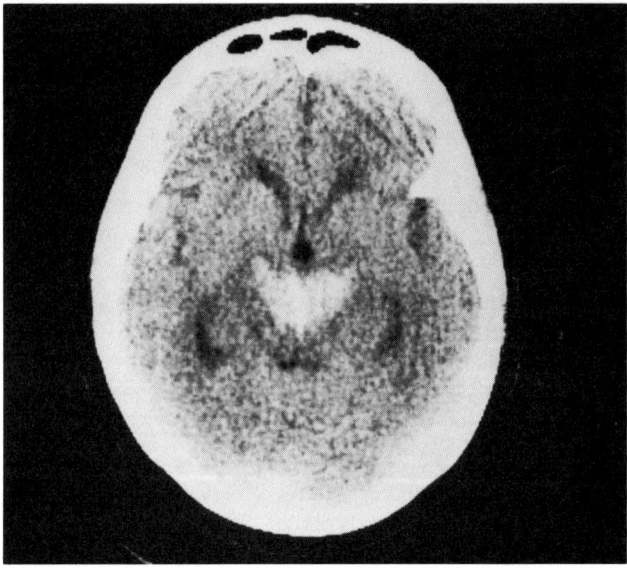

Figure 58-4 Brain stem (midbrain) hematoma.

alized on the unenhanced CT scan (Fig. 58-4), and significant mass effect may also be present. Often, blood will also be visualized within the ventricular system. Lumbar puncture is generally unnecessary in the diagnosis of intracerebral hemorrhage and should be avoided in patients with increased intracranial pressure. If lumbar puncture is performed, however, the opening pressure will be elevated and the fluid will usually be bloody, with the blood having reached the subarachnoid space via the ventricular system. Once the diagnosis of intracerebral hemorrhage has been made, immediate neurosurgical consultation should be obtained.

Cerebellar Hemorrhage

Cerebellar hemorrhage is a true neurosurgical emergency. The location of the hemorrhage adjacent to the brain stem leads to early compromise of respiratory and cardiovascular centers and death. Rapid surgical intervention is critical to the outcome of these patients. Generally, the patients will have hypertension of long standing and will present with severe occipital headache, nausea and vomiting, vertigo, and ataxia. Focal neurologic signs and cranial nerve deficits will usually not be found, although the profound ataxia will often preclude unassisted walking. CT scan must be performed immediately, and appropriate measures must be readied to deal with respiratory or cardiac arrest during the scan. The radiologist should be informed that the purpose of the scan is to evaluate the patient for cerebellar hematoma, since special cuts may be necessary to visualize the area adequately. Once diagnosed, the patient should be taken to surgery to evacuate the hematoma without delay, since deterioration may be sudden and catastrophic. In a small number of cases in which the diagnosis is believed to be clinically certain, or if CT scanning is going to engender an unusually long delay in definitive therapy, the patient should undergo craniotomy without prior radiographic study. These patients are also often profoundly hypertensive, and blood pressure should be managed as outlined for ischemic stroke.

Transient Ischemic Attack (TIA)

Transient ischemic attacks consist of brief, self-limited focal neurologic deficits that are caused by cerebrovascular disease. TIAs may be embolic or thrombotic, and the deficit arises quickly and then resolves over the next 12 to 24 hours, or less. The symptoms may be subtle (transient loss of vision in one eye) or dramatic (hemiparesis) and are almost invariably accompanied by normal mentation. Findings on examination will depend entirely on the area of the brain involved. Often, the patient is already improving or normal prior to medical examination. The use of CT scan in TIA should be limited to those cases in which hemorrhage or a nonvascular CNS event needs to be ruled out. Routine scanning in patients with uncomplicated TIA will generally not contribute to management. Emergency department evaluation should focus on determining whether a TIA has occurred, and which circulation is involved (see Table 58-2). Not all patients with TIA need to be admitted to the hospital, but such decisions must take into account the wishes of the patient's physician, the patient, and the family and the certainty of the diagnosis. Virtually all "first time" TIA patients should be admitted for detailed evaluation. Additionally, patients whose TIAs have changed in frequency or pattern, or whose symptoms are not resolving, should be admitted. Fewer than half of patients presenting with a first TIA will go on to have a CVA over the next several years, but this likelihood is unpredictable in each individual case. Decisions concerning anticoagulation, antiplatelet therapy, or surgery involve life-long consequences for the patient and should not be addressed in the emergency department setting.

THE ROLE OF ANTICOAGULATION

The indications for anticoagulation in the acute management of CVA have sharply diminished over the past decade. In general, anticoagulation therapy is now only considered in a small number of cases for specific indications. It is important to consider this modality in consultation with the neurologist or neurosurgeon who will care for the patient, since opinion is sharply divided on this issue. There are two situations wherein anticoagulation might be of benefit to the patient:

1. *Stroke in evolution*. This situation is represented by the patient who presents with a neurologic deficit that appears to be worsening over a period of observation. If anticoagulation is to be of benefit, it must be begun before the stroke is completed. However, prior to anticoagulation, CT must be performed to ensure that the CVA is not hemorrhagic. Anticoagulation is absolutely contraindicated in the presence of hemorrhagic stroke. Even when the CT scan fails to demonstrate hemorrhage, a risk of promoting or exacerbating hemorrhage remains. This "double-edged sword" aspect of anticoagulation cannot be overstressed. The decision to begin heparin must be highly individualized.
2. *Embolic stroke*. Patients who present with a history and examination consistent with embolic stroke, who have a clear source of emboli (eg, chronic atrial fibrillation), and whose CT scan fails to demonstrate hemorrhage are candidates for anticoagulation. The same caveats as for stroke in evolution apply.

SPECIAL DIAGNOSTIC CONSIDERATIONS

Angiography

The role of angiography in the evaluation of cerebrovascular disease is in a state of evolution. At present, there are few indications for angiography during the emergency department phase of the patient's care. CT scanning, as discussed previously, has largely replaced angiography in the emergency evaluation of CVA. If CT scanning is not available, the decision must be made whether to proceed with angiography or to transfer the patient to a facility where CT is available. These decisions must be individualized and must be made in conjunction with the neurologist or neurosurgeon who will ultimately assume care of the patient.

Magnetic Resonance Imaging

Magnetic resonance imaging (MRI) is the newest technology available for the evaluation of patients with suspected CNS disease. Unlike the CT scan, MRI can detect brain infarction early in the patient's course. Since there is no specific therapy for this condition, however, this capability is of limited merit. MRI is very insensitive for cerebral or subarachnoid hemorrhage during the early phases of evaluation, and thus at the present time, CT scanning remains the method of choice for the evaluation of these conditions. An additional role for MRI, however, is in the acute evaluation of the posterior fossa and brain stem of patients who have a normal CT scan but are suspected of infarcts in these regions.

CONCLUSION

The myriad presentations of CVA make these entities a diagnostic challenge. Knowledge of the anatomy of the cerebral vasculature, patterns of CVA, appropriate interventions, and management of complications is a critical part of the emergency physicians' skill armamentarium. Timely evaluation of these patients and skillful therapeutic management will ensure optimal outcome in the majority of patients.

BIBLIOGRAPHY

Earnest MP. Emergency diagnosis and management of brain infarctions and hemorrhages. In: Earnest MP, ed. *Neurologic Emergencies*. New York: Churchill Livingstone; 1983.

Ferguson GG. Physical factors in the initiation, growth, and rupture of human intracranial saccular aneurysms. *J Neurosurg*. 1972;37:666.

Kinkel WR, Jacobs L. Computerized axial transverse tomography in cerebrovascular disease. *Neurology*. 1976;26:924.

Mutlu N, Berry RG, Alpers BJ. Massive cerebral hemorrhage—clinical and pathological correlations. *Arch Neurol*. 1963;8:74.

Ramirez-Lassipas M. Antifibrinolytic therapy in subarachnoid hemorrhage caused by ruptured intracranial aneurysm. *Neurology*. 1981;31:316.

Toole JF, Yuson CP, Janeway R. Transient ischemic attacks: a study of 225 patients. *Neurology*. 1978;28:746.

VanGijn J, VanDongen KJ. Computerized tomography in subarachnoid hemorrhage: differences between patients with and without an aneurysm on angiography. *Neurology*. 1980;30:538.

59. Seizures

GREGG HUSK, MD

APPROACH TO THE PATIENT WITH SEIZURES

Seizures commonly result in an emergency department visit. Approximately 1 million Americans suffer from epilepsy,[1] and a seizure is the presenting symptom in 2% to 4% of emergency visits. In one patient, a generalized seizure may represent life-threatening trauma; yet in another patient, it may be an isolated fit that briefly interrupts a normal life span. The emergency physician must quickly identify the critically ill patient; attempt to define etiology and reversible precipitants; make therapeutic decisions, often based on little history; and decide on inpatient or outpatient management.

The initial contact with the patient and witnesses offers an important opportunity to obtain a history. What is called a seizure may be a simple faint or syncope from a profound bradycardia. Hence, exactly what is observed is of key importance. Medications (and compliance), past medical history, and trauma, either before or during the seizure, should be elicited. Seizures are dramatic events that have a variety of presentations, each of which requires a particular approach (Table 59-1).

DEFINITIONS

A *seizure* is a temporary alteration in behavior due to abnormal electrical activity in the brain. *Epilepsy* refers to spontaneously recurring seizures. It can be classified as *idiopathic* when no cause is identified or as *symptomatic* when there is a known underlying condition. In adults *generalized tonic-clonic* seizures (grand mal) are most common. In these the patient suddenly loses organized postural tone and becomes unresponsive; there follows a sequence of extensor tone and apnea lasting seconds, followed by bilateral clonic motions lasting a few minutes. This sequence is followed by a period of depressed consciousness with stertorous breathing that resolves over minutes. Repetitive generalized tonic-clonic seizures without interictal recovery of consciousness is termed *convulsive status epilepticus*.

MECHANISMS OF MORBIDITY

Patients with generalized seizures can be injured in a number of ways. The cause of the seizure (eg, an intracerebral hemorrhage) may carry short-term morbidity. The seizure itself, by depriving the patient of normal protective movements, may result in burns, drowning, or a variety of traumatic injuries. Vomiting with aspiration can lead to pneumonia. With frequent seizures, intellectual deterioration can occur. In a study of sudden deaths in patients with epilepsy, 10% of sudden deaths were from defined complications of seizures (head injury, bathtub drowning, and aspiration).[2] The majority of the sudden deaths were in young men with symptomatic epilepsy who had low anticonvulsant levels. Eighty percent of the patients demonstrated pulmonary edema.

With convulsive status, there are additional risks.[3–6] Disorganized neuronal activity with resultant increased cerebral oxygen consumption[7] is coupled with poorly coordinated

Table 59-1 Etiologies of Generalized Convulsive Seizures

Idiopathic generalized convulsive epilepsy is called *primary epilepsy*; epilepsy caused by central nervous system or systemic processes is called *secondary epilepsy*. Central nervous system processes that can lead to epilepsy are

- Birth injuries
- Trauma
- Craniotomy
- Infection (meningitis, encephalitis, tuberculosis)
- Tumor
- Subarachnoid hemorrhage
- Cerebrovascular accident (CVA)

Systemic processes that can cause seizures include

- Medication withdrawal in an epileptic
- Hypoglycemia
- Uremia
- Hyponatremia
- Hypocalcemia
- Hypoxia
- Drug ingestions
- Drug withdrawal
- Malignant hypertension
- Toxemia
- Fever

respiratory motions and upper airway obstruction from secretions or the tongue. Hypoxia may result in brain damage with cerebral edema. Increased motor activity can cause hyperthermia, which can lead to a cascade of complications. Electrolyte disturbances and profound acid-base abnormalities are common. Hypotension and dysrhythmias can be produced by hypoxia, acidosis, and hypovolemia. Pathologists often find evidence of anoxic encephalopathy, in addition to a predisposing structural lesion. Morbidity and mortality have been described within the first 30 minutes of convulsive status, although most patients succumb after many hours of uncontrolled seizures.[3–5]

CONVULSIVE STATUS EPILEPTICUS

Clinicians recognize convulsive status separate and apart from isolated seizures because of the 3% to 15% hospital mortality and the substantial long-term morbidity that these patients sustain.[3–6] Most often, convulsive status is associated with a definable etiology or precipitant. Hence, symptomatic epilepsy is more likely to result in status than is idiopathic epilepsy. In recent years, medication noncompliance[4,6] has been recognized as a common precipitant of status. Because clonic motions depend on the integrity of cortical neurons and subcortical pathways, many patients with large destructive lesions or major metabolic abnormalities may appear to have focal (partial) seizures and coma[6]—the emergency clinician must recognize this as true grand mal status and treat it accordingly.

Diagnostic questions are generally interspersed with therapeutic interventions. At the outset, the primary examiner should dispatch someone to obtain a history from witnesses, relatives, or friends. The patency of the patient's airway should be ensured and the vital signs measured. Oxygen (100%) should be administered by rebreather mask. Ensuring the adequacy of ventilation and oxygenation in these patients cannot be stressed too much—they commonly have a respiratory acidosis and may be hypoxemic. Although the timing of endotracheal intubation is often debated, it becomes more pressing with the passage of time and the administration of drugs that are respiratory depressants. Many clinicians intubate early, the interictal period being used of necessity. An intravenous line is established, and blood is drawn to determine glucose, sodium, urea, anticonvulsant, and calcium levels. Fifty milliliters of a 50% glucose mixture (D_5W) are given intravenously, and 100 mg of thiamine is administered intramuscularly (IM). Arterial blood gases are measured to ensure adequate oxygenation and to assess acid-base status.

The clinician must then shift attention to the control of ongoing seizure activity. The ideal drug controls seizures rapidly, has no sedative properties that cloud the return to a premorbid mental state, and has no major short-term side effects. Most clinicians use diazepam followed by phenytoin. If barbiturate withdrawal is suspected, phenobarbital is a first choice; otherwise, its sedative and respiratory depressant effects have led many clinicians to consider it a second-line drug. Diazepam given at 2.5 mg/min aborts seizures in the majority of patients. It can cause respiratory depression and occasionally hypotension, so the vital signs must be monitored during its administration. Patients who initially respond to diazepam may have a resumption of seizures within 15 to 60 minutes as a result of redistribution of diazepam from brain to other organs. To avoid this phenytoin[8] may be added—a loading dose is given intravenously at 25 to 50 mg/min up to a total dose of 18 mg/kg. Bradycardia, hypotension, and occasionally respiratory depression may complicate[9] the rapid infusion. Electrocardiographic monitoring and frequent checking of the patient's vital signs minimize risks. Phenytoin's solubility in aqueous solutions is marginal, but it may be given dissolved in 500 mL of normal saline. Because of erratic absorption, phenytoin should not be administered intramuscularly. Dosage modifications should be made if the patient is known to be currently taking the drug or if seizures are controlled at a lower total dose. Other clinicians prefer intravenous lorazepam (1 to 4 mg in 2 minutes up to a total dose of 9 mg) because of its

Table 59-2 Intravenous Drugs Useful in Status Epilepticus

Drug	Dosage Adult	Dosage Pediatric	Precautions	Miscellaneous
Phenytoin	50 mg/min up to 1 g	15–20 mg/kg given evenly over 20 minutes	Hypotension; bradycardia; rarely, respiratory depression; need to monitor heart and vital signs	Given IV through rapidly flowing line, with normal saline, avoiding extravasation
Diazepam	5–15 mg at a rate of 2.5 mg/min	0.3 mg/kg at a rate of 0.5–2 mg/min	Respiratory depression; occasional hypotension; need to monitor vital signs	Side effects much more common if phenobarbital is also given
Lorazepam	1–4 mg by slow push q5 minutes up to 9 mg	0.1 mg/kg over 2 minutes	Respiratory depression	
Phenobarbital	100 mg/min up to 20 mg/kg	10–20 mg/kg over 20 minutes	Respiratory depression; hypotension; need to monitor vital signs	Drug of choice if barbiturate withdrawal is suspected
Paraldehyde	1 mL/mg (4% solution)		Occasional hypotension	Can be used only with glass syringes and metal needles
Lidocaine	100 mg IV over 2 minutes		Very rarely causes heart block	

apparently longer duration of action (its side effect profile is similar to that of diazepam).[10] Convulsive status will be controlled in most patients with the diazepam-phenytoin regimen outlined above. In a patient who continues to seize, the trachea should be intubated, and phenobarbital[11,12] may be administered intravenously at a rate of 50 to 100 mg/min until seizures stop or to a total dose of 20 mg/kg. An alternative regimen is to administer diazepam[8] by continuous infusion at a rate of 8 mg/hour. Lidocaine,[13] paraldehyde,[13] and general anesthesia[14] are subsequent therapeutic options (see Table 59-2 for dosage guidelines).

When convulsive status is controlled, etiology can be investigated. The laboratory results may provide a clue, and specific therapy may succeed in an occasional patient when anticonvulsants have failed (eg, in hyponatremia). A general physical examination is performed, with special attention directed to the temperature, blood pressure, possible trauma, evidence of drug abuse, and tumor. A funduscopic examination may show signs of increased intracranial pressure. The neurologic examination may suggest an underlying structural lesion, such as tumor or cardiovascular accident (CVA), or multiple areas of dysfunction, as in drug ingestion or encephalitis. If meningitis is suspected because of fever combined with meningeal signs or a petechial eruption, a lumbar puncture should be performed immediately.

Although a cerebrospinal fluid pleocytosis (often polymorphonuclear) has been described in patients with seizures[15] and convulsive status[6] who have no underlying infectious or inflammatory meningeal process, patients with a pleocytosis (or a positive Gram stain) should be treated for meningitis pending culture results. In some settings the lumbar puncture should be deferred until a computerized tomographic (CT) scan of the head is performed in order to minimize the risk of inducing transtentorial herniation.

The pace of drug administration and work-up must respect the pace of morbid events. As mentioned above, mortality and morbidity are most common in status that continues for hours. This has encouraged some to suggest that phenytoin alone should be the first-line drug, and yet, morbidity and, occasionally, death are seen even when status is successfully aborted within the first hour. In addition, the practical problems of placing and maintaining a stable intravenous catheter at a tightly controlled infusion rate support a role for diazepam. This is particularly true for prehospital therapy, in which a 20-minute loading regimen for phenytoin is particularly undesirable.

There are few distinctions between the prehospital and emergency department priorities in the treatment of convulsive status. The airway management skills of EMT-paramedics are generally excellent, so that potential side effects of field treatment can be effectively managed. The general guidelines listed above are applicable in the field. Certainly, airway management, oxygen administration, assessment of the vital signs, placement of an intravenous line, obtaining blood for glucose determination, and the subsequent administration of D_5W are mandatory. Diazepam should be considered when transport times are long or the status has persisted for one-half hour.

ISOLATED GENERALIZED TONIC-CLONIC SEIZURES

A patient who has had a single generalized tonic-clonic seizure and remains confused or comatose should be assessed for airway patency, vital signs, and D_5W and naloxone should be administered after venous blood has been drawn for glucose determination. In the case of a patient whose level of consciousness returns to normal, both patient and any witnesses should be interviewed in an attempt to identify an aura, a focal motor or sensory convulsive activity, the duration of the convulsion and postictal state, and incontinence. These answers will help to establish whether a seizure did occur and whether a focal onset was noted. Etiologic inquiries should address pre-existent medical conditions, specifically diabetes and renal disease; medication history; barbiturate, alcohol, or other drug ingestions; head trauma; operations; CVA; tumor; and headaches. Cocaine and amphetamine use may produce single grand mal seizures or grand mal status.[16] If the patient is known to have epilepsy, questions on medication compliance and prior evaluation should be included, as well as whether the patient sustained injuries during the seizure.

The patient should be asked about risk factors for acquired immunodeficiency syndrome. A seizure[17] may be the first sign of illness in a patient infected with human immunodeficiency virus (HIV), and such seizures have a broad differential diagnosis (CNS toxoplasmosis; HIV encephalopathy; CNS lymphoma; cryptococcal, tuberculous, or aseptic meningitis). Such patients should be hospitalized for evaluation. Thus, questions should concern etiology, precipitants, and complications.

The physical examination addresses the same areas. Is there evidence of dysfunction that establishes an etiologic diagnosis or the presence of complications? If the patient is known to be epileptic, the examination should include measurement of vital signs; a survey for trauma; an assessment of the patient's level of consciousness, memory, and orientation; and an examination of the cranial nerves. Muscle strength and cerebellar function can be screened by means of an upper extremity drift test, an assessment of tandem gait, finger-to-nose test, and a Romberg maneuver. Discovery of any abnormalities mandates more detailed testing. A patient with a first seizure requires a full neurologic examination. The decision to hospitalize adult patients with a first seizure is based on the observation[18] that 10% of patients who have their first seizure after age 20 have an underlying brain tumor. This remains a possible etiology even with a normal neurologic examination. Studies[19] suggest that a much smaller fraction, perhaps 1% to 2% of patients, have a tumor as the underlying cause of a first seizure in adulthood—if the examination and history are nonfocal. Many experts hospitalize adults with first seizures. This allows for the initiation of drug therapy, as well as the performance of diagnostic studies, such as a CT scan, an electroencephalogram (EEG), and, if no mass lesion is found, a lumbar puncture. A partial seizure mandates an inpatient work-up, because the prevalence of tumor is higher[18] in these patients.

If a patient with known epilepsy is brought to the emergency department for a rare breakthrough seizure, the drug regimen should not be changed. The patient should be carefully questioned about alcohol use. Even a single evening of heavy social drinking[18] may increase the likelihood of a seizure during the withdrawal period. Measuring the levels of anticonvulsants and providing this information to the patient's primary physician is the usual disposition for these patients. Patients with frequent generalized seizures or patients who are noncompliant may require a dosage adjustment; at times a new medication may be necessary. If possible, the change in medication should be made after consultation with the patient's primary physician. Patients with repetitive convulsions (with interictal recovery of consciousness), may benefit from a slow intravenous infusion of phenytoin, or the intramuscular administration of phenobarbital. Parenteral injection may be preferred, as it may take hours[20] for phenobarbital or phenytoin to achieve peak blood levels after oral administration. Table 59-3 describes the most commonly used oral anticonvulsants.

SEIZURES ASSOCIATED WITH DRUG WITHDRAWAL

Although the theory is somewhat controversial,[21] most clinicians hold that generalized tonic-clonic seizures may occur as part of the early alcohol withdrawal syndrome. This usually occurs in patients who have drunk heavily for some weeks. Ninety percent of patients who have seizures due to withdrawal have the seizures from 6 to 48 hours after a decrease in alcohol consumption. Most often, these patients have one to four seizures with interictal recovery of consciousness. Convulsive status epilepticus is uncommon in alcohol withdrawal seizures, but alcohol withdrawal may facilitate the development of status in patients with prior head trauma or cerebrovascular disease or who are intermittently compliant with respect to anticonvulsive medicines. In 84% of patients studied with multiple seizures, the interval between the first and last seizure was less than 6 hours.[22] Many such patients are tremulous and agitated. Some patients who seize will develop delirium tremens, usually after a lucid interval.

How does this information help us to treat the individual patient? The general recommendations for airway management, assessment of vital signs, routine administration of D_5W and thiamine for patients who are seizing or postictal remain valid. Binge drinking places the patient at risk for hypoglycemia as well as withdrawal seizures.

In the history and examination, one should search for alternative etiologies for seizures. A cautious examination,

Table 59-3 Oral Anticonvulsants

Drug	Indication	Daily Dose and Dosing Frequency	Therapeutic Level	Adverse Effects
Phenytoin	GCS,PS	4–8 mg/kg divided in 1–3 doses	10–20 µg/mL	Sedation, ataxia, rash, hepatic dysfunction
Phenobarbital	GCS,PS absence, febrile	1–6 mg/kg divided in 1–2 doses	10–25 µg/mL	Sedation, ataxia, paradoxical hyperactivity in children
Primidone	GCS,PS	5–20 mg/kg divided in 3 or 4 doses	5–10 µg/mL (active metabolites are also present)	Sedation, ataxia, rash
Carbamazepine	GCS,PS	10–20 mg/kg divided in 3 or 4 doses	6–8 µg/mL	Sedation, leukopenia, dizziness, diplopia, hepatic dysfunction
Valproic acid	GCS,PS	15–60 mg/kg in 3 doses	50–100 µg/mL	Nausea, sedation, ataxia, hepatic dysfunction
Ethosuximide	Absence	20–30 mg/kg in 2 doses	40–100 µg/mL	Nausea, sedation, bone marrow depression

GCS = Generalized Convulsive Seizures   PS = Partial Seizures
Source: Goodman AG, Gilman LS, Gilman L: *The Pharmacologic Basis of Therapeutics,* ed 6. New York, Macmillan Publishing Co Inc, 1980.

with attention to focal deficits, is of great value[23] in separating patients with a neurosurgically treatable cause of seizures from those patients with simple withdrawal seizures.

Alcoholic patients with seizures should be hospitalized on an acute medical service if they have fever, evidence of significant head trauma or focal neurological dysfunction, a depressed sensorium, more than four seizures, evidence of severe early alcohol withdrawal, or delirium tremens. Patients who do not meet these criteria should be observed for six hours, the period of greatest risk for further seizures. No anticonvulsants should be given if the seizure is nonfocal. The high frequency of delirium tremens following alcohol withdrawal seizures argues for detoxification and administration of benzodiazepines, since these medications appear to reduce the risk of seizures. Among 2200 patients without prior seizures[24] who underwent inpatient detoxification with benzodiazepines alone, only 4 had seizures. For patients who have sustained generalized seizures, observation and treatment of coexisting early withdrawal with benzodiazepines is recommended. Barbiturate withdrawal results in convulsive status more frequently than does alcohol withdrawal. Patients should be hospitalized on a medical service. A similar syndrome has been described with many other sedative drugs.

ABSENCE SEIZURES

Children between the ages of 4 and 12 may have brief lapses of consciousness without loss of posture. Often there is no motor activity, although some children have eye blinking, lip smacking, or isolated clonic activity. These episodes usually last from 5 to 30 seconds and are followed by an immediate return to normal orientation. However, the seizures may occur so frequently as to interfere with scholastic performance. Most patients have a remission by age 20 if they have not developed generalized tonic-clonic seizures. If this diagnosis is suspected, an EEG may provide confirmation. Valproic acid, ethosuximide, clonazepam, or trimethadione may prove useful in controlling the seizures.

PARTIAL SEIZURES

Some patients have sensory symptoms, focal motor seizures, or a disturbance of consciousness associated with bizarre behavior. The latter, partial complex seizures, are often followed by postictal confusion. These disturbances generally last from seconds to a few minutes. Many of these patients also have generalized convulsive seizures. Even if a partial clonic seizure continues uninterrupted for hours (*epilepsia partialis continua*), the short-term risk is small and the patient may be treated in a leisurely fashion with oral medicines or a slow intravenous infusion.

With a focal seizure, the abnormal activity may remain localized; spread transcortically generating additional symptoms; or spread to diencephalic structures, giving rise to a generalized tonic-clonic seizure with a focal onset. The oral drugs useful in treatment of tonic-clonic seizures are also useful for partial seizures. The work-up for a patient with a new focal seizure is done on an inpatient basis because such seizures strongly suggest focal brain disease.

FEBRILE SEIZURES

Up to 5% of children between the ages of 6 months and 5 years have a seizure associated with a febrile illness. These are typically generalized and brief, and the history and examination usually do not demonstrate neurologic disease. Most commonly the seizure is precipitated by a viral illness or otitis media. In children below 2 years of age, the emergency physician should routinely perform a spinal tap, as meningitis can be difficult to exclude clinically in this age group. Certain factors[25] identifiable at the time of the emergency department visit allow an assessment of the probability of subsequent epilepsy. Children with complicated seizures (repetitive seizures, seizures that last for more than 15 minutes, or partial seizures); a family history of nonfebrile seizures; and a previous neurologic abnormality in the child each increase the chance of subsequent development of epilepsy. Anticonvulsant therapy with phenobarbital is controversial, and the decision regarding its implementation belongs to the patient's primary physician. Emergency department therapy consists of cooling the child with antipyretics and sponging, and ruling out the presence of a bacterial infection.

REFERENCES

1. Epilepsy Foundation of America. *Basic Statistics on the Epilepsies*. Philadelphia: Davis; 1975.
2. Leetsma JE, Walczak T, Hughes JR, et al. A prospective study on sudden unexpected death in epilepsy. *Ann Neurol*. 1989;26:195–203.
3. Oxbury JM, Whitty CW. Causes and consequences of status epilepticus in adults. *Brain*. 1971;94:733–744.
4. Hunter RA. Status epilepticus—history, incidence, problems. *Epilepsia*. 1959;1:162–188.
5. Rowan AJ, Scott DF. Major status epilepticus. *Acta Neurol Scand*. 1970;46:573–584.
6. Aminoff MJ, Simon RP. Status epilepticus—causes, clinical features and consequences in 98 patients. *Am J Med*. 1980;69:657–665.
7. Duffy TE. Cerebral energy metabolism during experimental status epilepticus. *J Neurochem*. 1975;24:925–934.
8. Delgado-Escueta AV, Enrile-Bascal F. Combination therapy for status epilepticus: intravenous diazepam and phenytoin. *Adv Neurol*. 1983;34:477–485.
9. Earnest MP, Marx JA, Drury LR. Complications of IV phenytoin for acute treatment of seizures. *JAMA*. 1983;249:762–765.
10. Levy RJ, Krall RL. Treatment of status epilepticus with lorazepam. *Arch Neurol*. 1984;41:605–611.
11. Goldberg MA, McIntyre HB. Barbiturates in the treatment of status epilepticus. *Adv Neurol*. 1983;34:499–504.
12. Shaner DM, McCurdy SA, Herring MO, et al. Treatment of status epilepticus: a prospective comparison of diazepam and phenytoin versus phenobarbital and optional phenytoin. *Neurology*. 1988;38:202–207.
13. Browne TR. Paraldehyde, chlormethiazole, and lidocaine for treatment of status epilepticus. *Adv Neurol*. 1983;34:509–517.
14. Opitz A, Marshall M, Degen R, Koch D. General anesthesia in patients with epilepsy and status epilepticus. *Adv Neurol*. 1983;34:531–535.
15. Prokesch RC, Rimland D, Petrini JL, et al. CSF pleocytosis after seizures. *South Med J*. 1983;76:322–327.
16. Alldredge BK, Lowenstein DH, Simon RP. Seizures associated with recreational drug abuse. *Neurology*. 1989;39:1037–1039.
17. Holtzman DM, Kaku DA, So YT. New-onset seizures associated with human immunodeficiency virus infection: causation and clinical features in 100 cases. *Am J Med*. 1989;87:173–177.
18. Solomon GE, Kutt H, Plum F. *Clinical Management of Seizures. A Guide for the Physician*. 2nd ed. Philadelphia: Saunders; 1983.
19. Livingston S. Etiologic factors in adult convulsions. *N Engl J Med*. 1956;254:1211–1216.
20. Penry JK, Newmark JE. The use of antiepileptic drugs. *Ann Intern Med*. 1979;90:207–218.
21. Ng SK, Hauser WA, Brust JC, et al. Alcohol consumption and withdrawal in new-onset seizures. *N Engl J Med*. 1988;319:666–672.
22. Victor M. The role of alcohol in the production of seizures. *Mod Probl Pharmacopsychiatr*. 1970;4:185–199.
23. Victor M. A study of epilepsy in the alcoholic patient. In: Locke S, ed. *Modern Neurology*. Boston: Little, Brown; 1969.
24. Feussner JR, Linfors EW, Blessing CL, et al. Computerized tomography brain scanning in alcohol withdrawal seizures. *Ann Intern Med*. 1981;94:519–522.
25. Sampliner R, Iber F. Diphenylhydantoin control of alcohol withdrawal seizures. *JAMA*. 1974;230:1430–1432.
26. Nelson KB, Ellenberg JH. Predictors of epilepsy in children who have experienced febrile convulsions. *N Engl J Med*. 1976;295:1029–1033.

SUGGESTED READING

Delgado-Escueta AV, Wasterlain C, Treiman DM, et al. Management of status epilepticus. *N Engl J Med*. 1982;306:1337–1340.

60. The Confused Patient

GREGG HUSK, MD

Bizarre behavior or confused speech may reflect a wide variety of underlying disturbances, ranging from schizophrenia to acute liver failure. An approach that respects the morbid nature of the possible etiologies is required. The clinician must be able to deal with an incoherent patient presenting with no available history, as well as a patient brought by a relative who can detail past history and chronicle the course of the presenting symptoms. The patient may cooperate for an examination or violently resist all attempts at interactions. Management decisions are often based on the presenting syndrome rather than a specific etiologic diagnosis. Drugs may be given, diagnostic tests may be performed, and a disposition may be made before establishing an etiologic diagnosis.

When dealing with a confused patient in the emergency department, it is critically important to distinguish between patients who are suffering from a *psychiatric* illness (schizophrenia or an affective disorder) and those who are suffering from an *organic* illness (delirium or dementia; Fig. 60-1). Delirium is often difficult to distinguish from schizophrenia or mania, and depression may be confused with dementia. The initial portion of this chapter deals with the acute confusional states with clouding of consciousness, and the latter portion discusses patients presenting with confusion in the presence of a clear sensorium.

ACUTE CONFUSIONAL STATES

The most common serious error made with acute confusional states is to ascribe the patient's condition to a psychiatric state based on limited data, and to transfer the patient to a psychiatric facility. These hospitals often lack medical or neurological consultants. Unless the history and examination speak strongly for a psychiatric diagnosis, initial hospitalization in a medical facility is indicated since significant short-term mortality and morbidity occur with much greater frequency in patients with organic brain disease than in those with psychiatric illness.

The history may help with this distinction. Relatives, police, or ambulance crew might provide needed details. The patient's age at the onset of dysfunction can be a guide. A first schizophrenic break is unusual after the age of 45. Delirium tends to be short lived, generally lasting a few days, whereas the schizophrenic patient may have a history of months to years of delusional thinking. Although an individual episode of mania may last a few days, the patient may have had prior episodes or periods of depression. Eliciting a history of drug, alcohol, or medication use, chronic medical

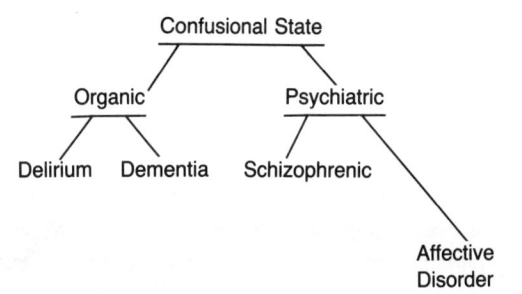

Figure 60-1 Algorithm for approach to the confused patient.

Table 60-1 Mental Status Exam in Acute Confusional States

	Delirium	Schizophrenia	Mania
Level of consciousness	Fluctuating	Normal	Normal
Orientation	Disoriented—time > place > person	Oriented	Oriented
Perceptions	Visual hallucinations	Auditory hallucinations common	Hallucinations uncommon
Thought process and content	Train of thought difficult to follow; thought often dominated by frightening visual hallucinations	Grossly distorted, complicated delusions	Flight of ideas, grandiose
Affect	Labile; fear often predominates	Low-level emotional response, considering patient's expressed plight	Elated, expansive, may be irritable

or psychiatric problems, or hospitalizations helps the examiner to construct a hypothesis of organic or psychiatric disease.

The vital signs are assessed. Any abnormality should raise the suspicion of delirium.

The mental status exam is the cornerstone of the differentiation of psychiatric and organic confusional states. This exam seeks to formally profile a patient's level of cognitive and emotional functioning. Psychiatric disease tends to disrupt particular spheres of function, leaving other areas unscathed. Organic mental syndromes tend to affect mental functions diffusely. Certain disease states (eg, thiamine deficiency leading to amnestic syndrome) produce more selective dysfunction, but the most common diagnostic dilemma arises in a patient who has agitation and profound cognitive impairment.

The examination begins with a description of the patient's level of arousal. Any depression of consciousness will affect performance on other aspects of the exam and strongly suggests organic disease. Orientation to surroundings should be assessed. Most schizophrenic and manic patients retain orientation to time, place, and person. At times pronounced inattention, or a delusional construct may produce errors. With organic diseases disorientation to time is most readily lost, and spatial disorientation is common. Disorientation to person is rare in delirious states.

Attention can be checked by asking the patient to demonstrate a particular sign every time a specific number is spoken by the examiner. Inattention is common in organic and psychiatric confusional states. Its assessment helps the examiner determine the accuracy of subsequent testing.

Memory may be checked by asking the patient about events of public record. The patient should be asked to remember three unrelated words for five minutes. Cortical function can be further checked by arithmetical problems and by copying and producing drawings.

The examiner should evaluate the accuracy of the patient's perceptions. Inquiry into the cause of the patient's frightened appearance may encourage the patient to describe illusions or hallucinations. The examiner should ask the patient about voices speaking to or about him or her. Does the patient experience his or her own thoughts being spoken aloud? Auditory hallucinations are very common in schizophrenia. In delirious patients visual hallucinations are common and patients frequently misidentify visual experience (illusions).

The interviewer should attempt to characterize the patient's thought process and content. Can the examiner follow the patient's train of thought? The schizophrenic commonly presents systematized delusions, reproducible at different phases of the interview. They may be patently absurd. The manic patient may speak quickly, moving from one idea to another with alacrity. The delirious patient may move from one notion to another without understandable transitions, and the content is usually simpler, more based in immediate sensory experience (or hallucination), and often accompanied by the fear one would expect given the patient's experience.

The mental status exam will correctly classify the majority of patients. Other diagnostic possibilities may not be identified by this brief exam (eg, a patient with a fluent aphasia who is frustrated and agitated may appear delirious). Table 60-1 lists the most useful distinctions in mental status testing of the archetypal schizophrenic, manic, and delirious patient.

The remainder of the neurological exam may elicit signs of an organic disease (tremor, asterixis, focal deficits, papilledema). The general examination may suggest a specific area of dysfunction (eg, fever, marked hypertension, stigmata of chronic liver disease, meningismus).

Lab tests are rarely useful in the distinction. EEGs can help to make this initial categorization but is rarely available to emergency departments. Blood tests can help to confirm many metabolic and toxic insults, but they cannot be used to rule out all organic etiologies. The lumbar puncture serves as the initial test if bacterial meningitis is suspected. The CT scan can confirm bleeding, mass lesions, and cerebral atrophy.

The patient with a depressed sensorium may be hypoglycemic, hypoxemic, or hypotensive. After the vital signs are checked, blood should be drawn for glucose, electrolytes, urea, calcium, and D_5W should be administered. An arterial blood gas should be drawn and if hypoxemia is suspected the patient should be placed on supplemental oxygen. These therapies are administered early in the work-up of confused patients, as they are safe, and a delay of minutes in the metabolic support of the brain may result in irreversible damage.

DELIRIUM AND OTHER ACUTE CONFUSIONAL STATES

A patient is said to be delirious if there is evidence of grossly distorted perceptions in the setting of physical, autonomic, and emotional overactivity. The delirious patient seems unable to persistently attend to a given stimulus. Physical overactivity is characteristic, with the patient rarely resting and almost never sleeping. Lability of affect is often striking, with the patient demonstrating elation, terror, grief, all within the span of a few minutes. Tachycardia, orthostatic hypotension, and diaphoresis are common. Often the patient articulates distorted or imagined perceptions (illusions or hallucinations).

Abundant speech, at times engaging the examiner, at times directed at imagined beings, is common. The patient may not cooperate for any verbal interchange, yet minutes later may allow a brief examination. Disorientation to time and place is typical with the patient usually preserving a sense of identity. Attention, memory, numerical calculations, and judgment are all disturbed. The patient may volunteer gross perceptual abnormalities. Visual hallucinations are characteristic.

ETIOLOGIES

For many of the conditions listed below stupor or coma is a more common presentation. The conditions are described here since collectively they are responsible for a large fraction of patients with acute confusional states, and therapy based on a precise etiologic diagnosis may be required.

Infection

Systemic and central nervous system infections can result in confusion. Most often this takes the form of a delirium, although patients may show a depressed sensorium. Bacterial sepsis, meningitis,[1] pneumonia, and viral encephalitis[2,3] are the common causes. The temperature, the general appearance of the patient, and the white blood cell count are the most important clues suggesting this category of diagnosis.

In addition to an altered sensorium, patients with meningitis frequently have a stiff neck, nausea, vomiting, and seizures. A petechial eruption is common in meningococcal meningitis.[1] Patients with bacterial meningitis can present with symptoms evolving over days but some 10% to 20% of patients will present with symptoms evolving over hours interrupting an upper respiratory infection. In patients presenting with rapidly progressive symptoms, therapy should be begun within minutes, as soon as blood and CSF have been obtained for culture. In patients over 6 years old penicillin 50,000 u/kg (up to 2 million units) q4h IV should be begun. In patients 2 months to 6 years, chloramphenicol 25 mg/kg IV q6h and ampicillin 50 mg/kg IV q4h should be started. In neonates, or older patients with high risk for gram-negative and staphylococcus aureus infection (penetrating trauma to CNS or immunosuppression), oxacillin 25 mg/kg IV q6h, chloramphenicol 25 mg/kg IV q6h, gentamicin 1.5 mg/kg IM q8h are initiated. This rush to early therapy is justified in patients presenting acutely by the high risk of death within the first 24 hours. In patients who have a more subacute onset of symptoms, who do not appear critically ill, one can do a more careful physical examination, and the CSF can be examined microscopically and biochemically. The CSF should be spun and the sediment Gram stained even in the absence of WBC count. A CSF WBC >1200 per mm^3 with a poly predominance, a glucose <40 mg% and protein >100 are characteristic of bacterial meningitis, but the CSF findings in bacterial, tuberculous, viral, and partially treated bacterial meningitis overlap with sufficient frequency[4] that it is rarely justified to withhold therapy in a patient solely on the basis of the initial CSF examination.

Metabolic Disturbances

As a rule metabolic disturbances produce confusion, with a depressed sensorium and no lateralizing findings. Hypoxia can at times produce a delirium. Hypoglycemia merits special concern as it is common, and routine therapy of the confused patient with D_5W is safe and effective. Plum and Posner[5] found a number of patients with hypoglycemia who presented with lateralizing neurological findings. Marked hyperglycemia with hyperosmolarity[5] and diabetic ketoacidosis commonly present with confusion.

Acute changes in serum sodium are likely to cause confusion. This usually occurs with substantial abnormalities[5] (sodium less than 128 mEq/L[6,7] or greater than 160 mEq/L). Hypercalcemia can produce polyuria, constipation, dehydration, and a confused state.[5] Renal failure and liver disease often declare themselves by confusion rather than by other presentations. Asterixis can be seen with almost any of the metabolic encephalopathies.

Disorders of Thermoregulation

Profound alterations of body temperature may produce a confusional state. This can be a direct consequence of the body temperature or of the disease process that produced the altered temperature. With hypothermia a depression of consciousness is common with body temperature below 27°C[8] and a confusional state with mild hypothermia should raise the examiner's suspicion of hypoglycemia, hypothyroidism, head trauma complicated by exposure, or drug-induced hypothermia. To allow for recognition of hypothermia the thermometer must be shaken down completely. If the patient does not raise the thermometer's recording, a thermometer with an expanded temperature scale should be used. Therapy entails general metabolic support (D_5W, O_2, monitoring), therapy of coexisting disorders (drug ingestion, trauma), and rewarming. Methods of rewarming are controversial. For severe hypothermia many would choose rewarming with 42° to 43.5°C peritoneal dialysate and warmed inhaled oxygen.[8]

Hyperpyrexia can cause a confusional state, seizures, or coma. Exposure, exertion, and bacterial infection are the most common precipitants. Rapid patient cooling to 38.5°C with the aid of a bathtub or ice and skin massage, monitoring, and a careful search for a bacterial infection are the mainstays of therapy.

Drug Ingestions

Most young patients with an acute confusional state are manifesting a drug effect. The history may be useful, but specific details of the quantity and identity of the ingested drug are in error as often as they are accurate. The physical examination may suggest a specific clinical syndrome. The findings of tachycardia, dry skin, fever, large unreactive pupils, and visual hallucinations strongly suggest a centrally acting anticholineric drug (eg, amitryptyline). Delirium with tachycardia, large reactive pupils, moist skin, and hypertension suggests sympathomimetic ingestion (eg, cocaine). The management of the patient with an acute confusional state who has used cocaine is particularly difficult. These patients may have a broad differential diagnosis,[9,10] including postictal delirium, cocaine psychosis, subarachnoid hemorrhage or intraparenchymal hemorrhage, lethargy secondary to extreme sleep deprivation, or one of the myriad defined complications of acquired immunodeficiency syndrome. These patients should be rapidly sedated with an intravenous benzodiazepine so that these diagnostic issues can be addressed.

Complete reversal of the abnormal sensorium with administration of naloxone suggests an acute intoxication with a narcotic. Partial arousal suggests a mixed ingestion where a narcotic is acutely ingested *or* nonspecific arousal in a patient who is habituated to narcotics, in whom naloxone produced acute painful withdrawal. At times blood or urine tests can help in diagnosis and management of ingestion.

In the elderly, drug intoxication is often accidental and an etiologic diagnosis is often delayed. In one series of 73 patients with salicylism, the diagnosis was delayed in 20.[11] Eight of these patients were admitted with a diagnosis of encephalopathy of unknown origin or alcohol withdrawal. A *complete* medication history is indispensable. Making a diagnosis of a drug ingestion can allow for the institution of general supportive therapy and at times specific measures are indicated.

Drug Withdrawal

In patients with narcotic withdrawal the sensorium is clear. In early alcohol withdrawal the patient is usually coherent. Intermittent visual or auditory hallucinations may interrupt the patient's lucid state. The patient may be tremulus and diaphoretic. This presentation is usually hours to a few days following a decrease in alcohol consumption. Late alcohol withdrawal, or delirium tremens, usually presents three to five days after decreased consumption.[12,13] The patient shows physical, autonomic, and emotional overactivity, is hallucinating, and often verbalizes fearful perceptions. He or she may be febrile. This may be due to physical overactivity but at times the fever provides a clue to an underlying disease process that precipitated the alcohol withdrawal. A traumatic or infectious precipitant should be diligently pursued, for patients presenting with delirium tremens and a serious infection have a particularly high mortality. A benzodiazepine should be administered to produce mild sedation. Barbiturate and other sedative hypnotics can produce a similar withdrawal state.

Trauma

Patients sustaining a concussion can show a delirious behavior while recovering.[5] Patients with extra-axial collections of blood within the subdural or epidural space tend to show changes in level of consciousness out of proportion to focal findings. A confusional state, usually with a depressed sensorium, is common. The pupillary findings and progressive deterioration of arousal indicate the critical state of the patient's health. A CT scan provides diagnostic confirmation and guidance in the planning of neurosurgical therapy. With chronic subdural hematomas, there may be no history of trauma and the findings evolve more insidiously. These patients often have a history of headache and progressive cognitive dysfunction.

Postictal Confusion

Confusional states are common after grand mal or psychomotor seizures. The diagnosis is usually established by history coupled with a rapid return to a normal sensorium. If the sensorium remains disturbed or deteriorates, alternative diagnoses (eg, a head injury or medication intoxication) should be entertained.

Wernicke-Korsakoff Syndrome

Chronic alcoholics and other malnourished patients can demonstrate an acute confusional state due to thiamine deficiency.[13] Extraocular palsies, nystagmus, or truncal or appendicular ataxia are commonly associated. Reversal of the eye findings and acute confusional state reward prompt therapy, whereas death may penalize diagnostic delay. Even with the prompt administration of thiamine (50 mg IM) these patients are often left with residual memory impairments.[14]

Subarachnoid Hemorrhage

Although the abrupt onset of a severe headache is the most important diagnostic clue to a subarachnoid hemorrhage, the diagnosis is frequently missed. In one series[15] of 182 patients, the initial diagnosis was incorrect in 41 patients. Five of these patients demonstrated an acute confusional state. If a subarachnoid hemorrhage is suspected in a comatose patient or a patient with focal neurologic deficits, a CT scan should be the first study.[16] This may well indicate the diagnosis of subarachnoid hemorrhage, and will allow an assessment of the risk of lumbar puncture. If no CT scan is available and the patient has no focal deficits, papilledema, or depressed level of consciousness, a lumbar puncture should be performed, looking for blood and xanthochromia.

Focal Brain Disease

Occasionally, strokes, brain tumors, or brain abscesses can produce apparent confusion. Usually, a detailed examination will demonstrate the focal nature of the process. As mentioned above, this is often secondary to a fluent aphasia.

PATIENT ASSESSMENT

Once the diagnosis of delirium is made, the physician must attend to the general support of the patient, the support of brain metabolism, and the elucidation of an etiologic diagnosis. The vital signs are assessed—any abnormality will color the pace and direction of the evaluation. Attempts should be made to explain all procedures to the patient. The physician should draw blood for glucose, electrolytes, urea, and calcium, and D_5W should be administered. Thiamine should be given if the patient appears malnourished or is a known alcoholic. If hypoxemia is suspected, an arterial blood gas should be drawn and the patient placed on supplemental oxygen.

With the level of evaluation outlined above, the clinician can usually be confident that the patient is manifesting a toxic metabolic encephalopathy or delirium, and often a specific diagnosis can be made. The early diagnosis of an acute confusional state allows for both specific therapy to avoid irreversible brain injury and general supportive therapy to limit complications common to all delirious states (aspiration pneumonia, brachial plexus injuries, electrolyte changes, volume depletion). For severely agitated patients intravenous haloperidol,[17] lorazepam, or diazepam may be used. Intravenous haloperidol has been used in combination with intravenous lorazepam.[18]

If the patient will not cooperate for an evaluation, the physician should consider sedation. If alcohol or sedative-hypnotic withdrawal is suspected as an etiology, diazepam is a reasonable choice—otherwise haloperidol is commonly used (Table 60-2).

The patient whose initial evaluation suggests delirium should have a lumbar puncture. If the examination is focal, a CT scan should be the initial test (see Table 60-2). One can withhold these tests if the history and examination strongly suggest a specific diagnosis and the patient is improving with appropriate therapy. The general management of delirious patients provides for specific therapy, cautious sedation, restraints to prevent the patient from major injury, careful attention to fluid and electrolyte balance, and early diagnosis of complications.

PSYCHIATRIC CONFUSIONAL STATES

The schizophrenic patient may resemble the patient with delirium. Anxiety may generate hyperactivity, tachycardia, sweating. Most often these patients are oriented. Disturbances of orientation are often bizarre, or may be seen in the schizophrenic who is grossly inattentive.

The patient commonly shows a decrease in affective responses. Distressing social circumstances or frightening hallucinations may be reported in an unemotional tone. The examiner may note little emotional resonance as the patient describes his or her plight.

Auditory hallucinations are common. The patient may experience his or her own thoughts spoken aloud or may hear other voices offering commentary on the patient's behavior. At times the voices instruct the patient to perform violent acts towards himself or herself or others. This is a marker for future violent behavior and such patients with command hallucinations should be hospitalized.

Certain types of delusions are commonly seen in schizophrenics. The feeling of being taken over by an outside force, of having thoughts placed in one's mind by others or withdrawn by others, and of believing that others can read one's mind are characteristic. A wide variety of delusions are also seen. Often they are complicated, bizarre, and the patient adheres to the delusion throughout the interview despite evidence to the contrary.

At times patients with mania may present with acute confusional states. These patients most often have an increase in social behavior and may demonstrate elevated, expansive mood. They may also express irritability when the world will not conform to their expectations. The examiner is usually able to follow the patient's train of thought although all too rapid. The break from reality is linked to the patient's grandiose notion of self and persecutory delusions. Hallucinations are less frequent than in schizophrenia but auditory hallucinations may occur. There may be a history of similar episodes often with interspersed episodes of depression.

Table 60-2 Sedation of the Agitated Patient

Drug	Dosage	Side Effects	Miscellaneous
Haloperidol	5 mg oral concentrate or IM q 30 minutes	Hypotension, acute dystonia	Lower dose (1 to 2 mg) in elderly
Chlorpromazine	25 to 50 mg oral concentrate or IM q 30 minutes	Hypotension, acute dystonia, sedation	
Diazepam	5 mg IV q 5 to 10 minutes	Respiratory depression	Useful in alcohol withdrawal
Lorazepam	1 mg slow IV push qs minutes up to 9 mg	Respiratory depression	
Meperidine	50 mg IV q 10 minutes	Respiratory depression, hypotension, vomiting, decreased sensorium	Sedative effects antagonized by Narcan; drug of choice for sedation for CT scan

The initial steps in therapy are similar irrespective of the exact etiologic diagnosis. Verbal reassurance, a quiet environment, and a relaxed interviewer may do much to calm the patient who is grossly disconnected from reality. If agitation persists and the patient cannot be interviewed and examined, tranquilization should be considered. Table 60-2 lists doses of commonly used neuroleptics. Oral concentrate doses or IM doses can be administered. In addition to acute dystonias, hypotension or sedation may occur. The vital signs should be rechecked before each dose. The neuroleptics will not eliminate all of the patient's symptoms, but they may help to reduce the overt anxiety and agitation.

Admission guidelines are difficult to delineate because much depends on the patient's social support system, the availability of outpatient psychiatric facilities, as well as the patient's psychiatric diagnosis and functional status. Certainly, a patient should be hospitalized if he or she is experiencing command hallucinations, having a first episode of psychosis, remains unable to care for self despite tranquilization, is judged to be a threat to self or others, or if there is any question regarding diagnosis.

DEMENTIA AND DEPRESSION

Dementia refers to a loss of cognitive faculties sufficient to impair social or occupational functioning.[19] Most often this is a slowly progressive impairment. A history from the patient is often distorted because of the cognitive impairments and the patient's passion to remain intellectually complete. A history from a second party may be invaluable.

The prevalence of dementia is ill defined. Katzman,[20] using data from European surveys, suggests that 4% of adults above the age of 65 are unable to care for themselves because of dementia, and another 11% have deterioration of function but still perform their activities of daily living. Dementia is less common in younger people, but still represents a significant public health problem.

Dementia is not a diagnosis—rather it is a clinical syndrome. The clinician faces two major tasks when asked to evaluate a patient with progressive intellectual deterioration: (1) Does the patient have a dementia? (2) Can a treatable etiology be discovered?

Is the Patient Demented?

To attempt to establish a diagnosis of dementia in an emergency department setting is most difficult. Many patients are not brought to the hospital because of their cognitive impairments, but rather for another medical problem (which may be a complication of the intellectual dysfunction). The need for a history indicative of dysfunction in the patient's home or job environment is important, as acute medical illness commonly compromises intellectual functioning in elderly patients—a dysfunction which resolves as the illness is treated. Charting the time course of dysfunction is useful as dysfunction that spans years is suggestive of a dementing disease, and the onset of dementia is usually in patients beyond the age of 55 years.

Particularly characteristic is impairment of memory. But the abnormalities tend to be much more general, with impairment of attention, constructional capacity, and judgment being commonplace. Family members may volunteer that the patient's personality has changed. The mental status examination should be carried out formally. Patients with slowly progressive dysfunction can often cover up these defects with social pleasantries and in mild cases the examiner may miss defects that have hampered functioning in demanding social or occupational situations. Testing should proceed in the hierarchical fashion discussed previously. If the history and examination are concordant, a presumed diagnosis is justified and the examiner can initiate a search for a reversible etiology.

Nonetheless, the diagnosis is fraught with hazard. Marsden and Harrison[21] noted that 14% of 106 patients admitted to a hospital for evaluation of dementia had a different discharge diagnosis. These patients had been previously evaluated by a psychiatrist or neurologist. Depression was the most common diagnosis in this group of 15 patients. If one looks at long-term follow-up studies to evaluate the accuracy of the diagnosis, the need for caution is underscored. In a series[22] of 52 patients with hospital discharge diagnosis of presenile dementia, 16 were noted to not merit a diagnosis of dementia at follow-up 5 to 15 years later. Affective illness was present in the majority of these patients. Yet another example[23,24] is that of a 56-year-old woman with many years of depressive illness who was evaluated for a 1-year history of memory impairment. The evaluation was extensive including clinical examination, psychiatric testing, skull radiography, pneumoencephalography, EEG, CSF profile, blood chemistries, iodinated albumin cisternography. She escaped brain biopsy only through the randomization process. Yet at follow-up five years later, she was the caretaker for her invalid husband and functioning independently. With this degree of uncertainty, the emergency clinician must be loath to tattoo the label of irreversible dementia on a patient.

The term pseudodementia has been coined to remind us of the importance of depression masquerading as dementia. Certain features[25] should augment one's suspicion of a depressive etiology. Often these patients have a past history of depression. They may vociferously complain of their memory impairment. The mood disturbance is often prominent prior to the cognitive dysfunction. The mental status exam may show spotty areas of dysfunction with memory most severely affected.

The diagnosis of dementia is perilous. Emergency clinicians should make a presumptive diagnosis if an independent history supports past cognitive dysfunction and the examination shows multiple areas of dysfunction. If the patient is acutely ill, evaluation of cognitive function may mislead the examiner, and an arrangement should be made for the patient to be re-examined at a later date.

If a Presumed Diagnosis of Dementia Is Justified, Can a Reversible Etiology Be Defined?

Most patients with dementia do not have a reversible etiology. Alzheimer's disease, a clinicopathologic entity of unknown etiology, is responsible for dementia in the majority of these patients. Multi-infarct dementia—where treatment of risk factors for stroke may arrest further deterioration—is probably the second most common etiology.

The general history and examination may be useful. Elderly patients may take medications that produce a dementia. A thorough medication history is in order, as salicylates,[11] sedative-hypnotics, antihypertensives,[25] and neuroleptics[26] have been implicated. Diuretics can produce electrolyte disturbances that produce a dementia. Are there coexisting symptoms of hypercalcemia? Does the patient have symptoms of hyperthyroidism or hypothyroidism? Are there symptoms of liver or renal disease? Has the patient had

Table 60-3 Etiologies of Dementia and Laboratory Clues to Reversible Etiologies

*Hypothyroidism	Thyroid function test
*Chronic liver disease	Liver profile
*B_{12} deficiency	Serum B_{12} level
*Syphilis	Blood and CSF VDRL
*Chronic meningitis	CSF cell count, culture, chemical, cytological, and immunological studies
*Chronic subdural hematoma	CT scan
*CNS mass lesion (tumor, abscess)	CT scan
*Hydrocephalus	CT scan
*Uremia	BUN
*Hypoglycemia	Glucose
Alzheimer's disease	
Multi-infarct dementia	

*Potentially reversible etiology

symptoms of central nervous system dysfunction—stroke, weakness, gait abnormality, incontinence, headache? The presence of ataxia of gait, urinary incontinence, and dementia suggests normal pressure hydrocephalus. The general exam may show signs of the reversible etiologies. The neurologic examination may show the residual of multiple cerebral infarcts, papilledema, or asterixis. Frontal release signs are common to many of the dementing diseases.

Despite the plethora of clinical guides, most patients will be without an etiologic diagnosis. Laboratory screening can be justified by the noninvasive nature of these tests and the high cost of missing the diagnosis of reversible etiology. Table 60-3 outlines the reversible etiologies and the laboratory techniques used to make a diagnosis.

The decision to admit patients with presumed dementia stems more from the patient's social support symptoms than the degree of intellectual impairment. If the patient will be brought for follow-up and social supports suggest that the patient will not injure himself or herself at home, then an outpatient work-up is desirable. For patients with nocturnal wandering, gentle sedation with low doses of haloperidol (1 to 2 mg orally) just before sleep may be useful.

REFERENCES

1. Swartz M, Dodge P. Bacterial meningitis, A review of selected aspects. *N Engl J Med*. 1965;272:725–731, 779–787, 842–848, 898–902.
2. Olson L, Buescher E, Artenstein M, Parkman P. Herpes virus infections of the human central nervous system. *N Engl J Med*. 1967;277:1271–1277.
3. Meyer H, Johnson R, Crawford I, et al. Central nervous system syndromes of "viral" etiology. *Am J Med*. 1960;29:334–347.
4. Karandanis D, Shulman J. Recent survey of infectious meningitis in adults: review of laboratory findings in bacterial tuberculosis and aseptic meningitis. *South Med J*. 1976;69:449–457.

5. Plum F, Posner J. *The Diagnosis of Stupor and Coma*. 3rd ed. Philadelphia: Davis; 1980.
6. Arieff A, Llach F, Massry S. Neurological manifestations of hyponatremia: Correlation with brain water and electrolytes. *Medicine*. 1976;55:121–129.
7. Burnell G, Foster T. Psychosis with low sodium syndrome. *Am J Psychiatr*. 1972;128:1313–1314.
8. Reuler J. Hypothermia: pathophysiology, clinical settings, and management. *Ann Intern Med*. 1978;89:519–527.
9. Lowenstein DH, Massa SM, Rowbotham MC. Acute neurologic and psychiatric complications associated with cocaine abuse. *Am J Med*. 1987;83:841–846.
10. Rowbotham MC. Neurologic aspects of cocaine abuse. *West J Med*. 1988;149:442–448.
11. Anderson R, Potts D, Gabow P, et al. Unrecognized adult salicylate intoxication. *Ann Intern Med*. 1976;85:745–748.
12. Victor M. Treatment of alcoholic intoxication and withdrawal syndrome. *Psychosom Med*. 1966;28:636–650.
13. Victor M, Adams R. The effect of alcohol on the nervous system. *Res Publ Assoc Res Nerv Ment Dis*. 1952;32:526–573.
14. Victor M, Adams R. *The Wernicke-Korsakoff Syndrome*. Philadelphia: Davis; 1971.
15. Adams H, Jergenson D, Kassel N, et al. Pitfalls in the recognition of subarachnoid hemorrhage. *JAMA*. 1980;244:794–796.
16. Weisburg L. Computerized tomography in the diagnosis of intracranial disease. *Ann Intern Med*. 1979;91:87–105.
17. Clinton JE, Sterner S, Stelmachers Z, et al. Haloperidol for sedation of disruptive emergency department patients. *Ann Emerg Med*. 1987;16:319–322.
18. Adams F. Emergency intravenous sedation of the delirious, medically ill patient. *J Clin Psychiatr*. 1988;49(suppl):22–27.
19. American Psychiatric Association. *Diagnostic and Statistical Manual of Mental Disorders*. 3rd ed. Washington, DC: American Psychiatric Association; 1980.
20. Katzman R. The prevalence and malignancy of Alzheimer disease. *Arch Neurol*. 1976;33:217–218.
21. Marsden C, Harrison M. Outcome of investigation of patients with presenile dementia. *Br Med J*. 1972;2:249–252.
22. Ron M, Toone B, Garraldo M, Lishman W. Diagnostic accuracy in presenile dementia. *Br J Psychiatr*. 1979;134:161–168.
23. Lijtmaer H, Fuld P, Katzman R. Prevalence and malignancy of Alzheimer disease. *Arch Neurol*. 1976;33:304.
24. Coblentz J, Mattis S, Zingesser L, et al. Presenile dementia. *Arch Neurol*. 1973;29:299–308.
25. Thornton W. Dementia induced by methyldopa with haloperidol. *N Engl J Med*. 1976;244:1222.
26. Wells C. Pseudodementia. *Am J Psychiatr*. 1979;136:895–900.

GENERAL REFERENCE

Strub R, Black F. *The Mental Status Examination in Neurology*. Philadelphia: Davis; 1977.

61. Syncope

GREGG HUSK, MD

Emergency physicians agonize over decisions they make about patients who have fainted. Syncope may be the presenting feature of a life-threatening illness or it may represent an insignificant punctuation mark in the life of a healthy person. Until recently, most authors have stressed the need for making a precise diagnosis in patients who have fainted. Although this is often possible, the cause of syncope may remain obscure in up to 50% of patients,[1-4] even after extensive inpatient evaluation and long-term follow-up. Despite this uncertainty, prognostic information has become available that allows for a more rational approach to treating these difficult patients. The emergency clinician's most pressing task is to identify and hospitalize those patients who have a life-threatening cause for syncope. A careful history, physical, and selected laboratory tests may result in a secure diagnosis in many patients. Many patients may be safely referred for outpatient follow-up—including some in whom the etiology of syncope is uncertain.

Syncope is defined as a transient loss of consciousness accompanied by an inability to maintain postural tone. A significant fraction of young patients report a prior syncopal episode.[5,6] Yet fainting is sufficiently disturbing that it commonly results in an emergency department visit—almost 1% of emergency department visits[3] are precipitated by a syncopal episode. Table 61-1 portrays the causes that should be considered in a diagnostic work-up. A detailed history and examination are the central pillars of the diagnostic approach to these patients.

CARDIOVASCULAR SYNCOPE

A sudden reduction in cerebral blood flow may cause a loss of consciousness. A dysrhythmia or a primary hemodynamic disturbance may culminate in this decrease in cerebral perfusion.

Aortic Outflow Obstruction

Patients with aortic outflow obstruction, from aortic stenosis[7,8] or hypertrophic cardiomyopathy[9,10] may faint. These patients may have dysrhythmias that impair cardiac output. Physical exertion, with its resultant decrease in the vascular resistance of the exercising skeletal muscles, can threaten cerebral blood flow in these patients with a low maximal cardiac output. The history may reveal a prior diagnosis, angina, or exertional dyspnea. The physical examination may reveal diagnostic or suspicious features. Patients with hypertrophic cardiomyopathy may have a bisfiriens pulse, and a harsh systolic murmur heard along the left sternal border or at the apex that increases with standing or a Valsalva maneuver. Some patients also have a murmur of mitral regurgitation. Patients with aortic stenosis often demonstrate a decreased carotid upstroke and a harsh systolic murmur that radiates into the neck. The ECG in both conditions may reveal evidence of left ventricular hypertrophy. In the elderly, the features on physical examination are often not diagnostic. A history of exertional syncope and any

Table 61–1 Causes of Syncope

I. *Cardiovascular*

   Dysrhythmias
      Bradydysrhythmias
      Tachydysrhythmias
   Limitation of cardiac output
      Aortic stenosis, obstructive cardiomyopathy, atrial myxoma, myocardial infarction, pulmonary embolus, aortic dissection, pulmonary hypertension, pulmonary stenosis, tetralogy of Fallot, pericardial tamponade
   Miscellaneous carotid sinus syncope

II. *Noncardiovascular*

   Vasodepressor
   Orthostatic
      Drug induced
      Hypovolemia
      Autonomic dysfunction (diabetes, Shy-Drager syndrome)
   Seizure
   Situational micturition, cough, defecation
   Miscellaneous CNS and cerebrovascular
      Subarachnoid hemorrhage, subclavian steal syndrome, TIA
   Metabolic
      Hypoglycemia, hypoxia, carbon monoxide poisoning

III. *Syncope of Unclear Etiology*

---

systolic murmur in the elderly merits additional diagnostic tests. Patients with pulmonic stenosis, tetralogy of Fallot, and pulmonary hypertension may also experience exertional syncope.

Pulmonary Emboli

Some 13% of patients with pulmonary emboli[11,12] faint at the onset of their symptoms. Most of these patients have risk factors (bedrest, congestive heart failure, lower extremity injury or immobilization, pregnancy or oral contraceptives, cancer, or recent surgery). Pleuritic pain is frequent, and 95% of patients have a respiratory rate of at least 16. Arterial hypoxemia is common, but arterial desaturation is seen in many patients who have only the disease risk factors. A chest roentgenogram may demonstrate a peripheral infiltrate or an effusion. Syncope is most common in those patients with massive pulmonary emboli—hypotension and pronounced hypoxemia are frequent findings. Despite this, failure to diagnose pulmonary emboli has led to emergency department discharge and resultant subsequent death.[3]

Aortic Dissection

Aortic dissection generally causes severe pain,[13] but painless dissection complicated by syncope has been described.[14] Hypertension, pain traveling along the course of the aorta, pulse asymmetries, evidence of tissue ischemia (skin mottling or demarcation, paralysis or anesthesia secondary to spinal cord ischemia, stroke, myocardial infarction, oliguria, or anuria) are all common. The chest roentgenogram is abnormal in the majority of patients,[15] revealing widening of the aortic knob, tracheal deviation to the right, a pleural effusion, or an abnormal aortic contour. Syncope seems most common in patients with proximal dissections, complicated by aortic insufficiency and pericardial tamponade (secondary to blood dissecting into the pericardium from the proximal aorta).

Myocardial Infarction

Myocardial infarction may produce syncope from dysrhythmias or pump failure. Rarely, myocardial infarction may be complicated by septal or free-wall rupture resulting in syncope from pump failure or pericardial tamponade.

Dysrhythmias

Dysrhythmias that compromise cardiac output can cause syncope. Bradydysrhythmias include sinus bradycardia, complete heart block, sinus arrest, or sinoatrial exit block. Mobitz II second-degree heart block, although it usually does not threaten cerebral blood flow, indicates a sufficiently fragile atrioventricular conduction that the patient is likely to have intermittent complete heart block. Tachydysrhythmias that may critically impair cardiac output include supraventricular tachydysrhythmias, ventricular tachycardia, or paroxysmal ventricular fibrillation. The accuracy of the diagnosis of syncope due to dysrhythmias is limited because of the intermittent nature of dysrhythmias as well as the frequent occurrence of asymptomatic dysrhythmias in elderly patients.

Syncope due to dysrhythmias usually presents with a minimal warning period.[2] The patient may have a history of cardiac disease or symptoms that suggest cardiac disease. Monitoring in the emergency department or the routine electrocardiogram frequently assists in establishing a diagnosis—about 75% of patients ultimately judged to have cardiovascular syncope have the diagnosis established by emergency department data.[4] In the remaining patients, the diagnosis is established by ambulatory or intensive care unit monitoring, exercise testing, or invasive electrophysiological studies.

NONCARDIOVASCULAR SYNCOPE

Vasodepressor Syncope

Patients with vasodepressor syncope give a history of a severe psychological or physical stress immediately before the syncope. Venipuncture, severe pain, a frightening experience, or standing in a hot, crowded environment are typical precipitants. The patient has a warning that things are awry—lightheadedness, graying out of the vision, extreme weakness, pallor, mydriasis, sweating, and epigastric distress may be seen. The warning period can last several minutes. Most patients note their symptoms in an upright or sitting position. The loss of consciousness is typically brief, and hypotonic, although brief clonic, or tonic-clonic activity is seen in a significant minority of patients. In contrast with the case of true seizures, the patient recovers consciousness quickly, but may continue to feel weak and remain pale for several minutes—especially upon sitting or standing. During the warning period, these patients manifest a tachycardia, but a bradycardia is regularly observed[16] at the time of syncope. There is a lowered systemic vascular resistance without the expected reflex increase in cardiac output—culminating in a decrease in cerebral perfusion. Atropine can reverse the bradycardia, but many patients remain hypotensive—hence the name *vasodepressor* is preferable to the term *vasovagal*.

Orthostatic Syncope

Orthostatic syncope may be due to hypovolemia, drug effect, or autonomic dysfunction. Bleeding may be evident or occult (gastrointestinal bleeding and intraperitoneal bleeding from a ruptured ectopic pregnancy are the major concerns). Drugs may cause venous pooling (eg, nitrates), vasodilatation (eg, prazosin) or may interfere with postural reflexes (eg, imipramine). Anaphylactic reactions may result in hypotension and syncope. Autonomic dysfunction may be due to a defined disease (eg, diabetes), or it may be idiopathic (eg, Shy-Drager syndrome).

Seizures

Patients with tonic-clonic seizures or focal seizures with secondary generalization may present with syncope. Retrograde amnesia may cloud the memory of the focal onset. Patients with seizures may recall a warning period, the aura, which may be confused with the prodromal phase of vasodepressor syncope. A history from a witness, a postictal state, a focal neurological examination, incontinence, tongue biting, or an anion gap metabolic acidosis may suggest the diagnosis.

Situational Syncope

Syncope while urinating, defecating, or coughing is classified as situational syncope only if there is a history of the activity during or immediately preceding the syncope, *and* no other explanation for syncope is found. Micturition syncope[17] occurs most commonly in men who have ingested alcohol, arise from a recumbent position quickly to void, and faint during or just after urinating. Cough syncope again favors men who drink alcohol. Most have a chronic lung disease, and the syncopal episode occurs after a paroxysm of coughing. Defecation syncope occurs after straining at stool. In a series of syncope due to pulmonary emboli,[12] fully one quarter of the patients described fainting upon defecation—hence the caveat to exclude other causes of syncope.

Miscellaneous CNS and Cerebrovascular Diseases

Subarachnoid hemorrhage may result in syncope. Although the headache usually dominates the clinical picture, diagnostic errors occur.[18] Transient ischemic attacks may threaten the circulation to the ascending reticular activating system and hence cause a loss of consciousness. The vast majority of these patients have additional symptoms[19] (ataxia, diplopia, or dizziness). Most cases of syncope and focal neurological findings are due to seizures.

The subclavian steal syndrome occurs in patients with an occlusion of the subclavian artery proximal to the origin of the vertebral artery. If the patient exercises the arm on the affected side, its vascular resistance falls, and the vertebrobasilar circulation may be threatened by retrograde blood flow through the ipsilateral vertebral artery into the subclavian artery. The diagnosis is suggested by a history of syncope, ataxia, diplopia, or vertigo upon arm exercise.[20] Pulse or blood pressure asymmetries between the arms and an infraclavicular bruit provide strong support. Angiography can confirm the diagnosis.

Metabolic Diseases

Any process that temporarily interferes with the delivery of vital metabolic substrate to the central nervous system can result in syncope. Hypoglycemia, hypoxemia, carbon monoxide poisoning may produce a self-limited syncopal state.

Syncope of Unknown Etiology

In many patients, a cause of syncope cannot be established, even after intensive emergency department, inpatient, and follow-up evaluation. Such patients have a low mortality, and exhaustive testing rarely produces a therapeutic intervention.[21] Unfortunately, cardiovascular syncope, which has a high 1-year mortality, cannot be reliably excluded in an emergency department evaluation. In one study, a cardiovascular cause of syncope was identified at the time of admission in 74% of those patients in whom it was ultimately established.[4] In other studies, however, more than 50% of the patients with cardiovascular syncope were so classified only after prolonged ECG monitoring.[1,22] One should be particularly circumspect in assigning this diagnosis in elderly patients after an emergency department evaluation, given the high likelihood of a cardiovascular cause of syncope.[22]

DIAGNOSTIC EVALUATION

History

A minute-by-minute chronicle of the events spanning the syncopal episode is of key importance in the diagnosis of situational and vasodepressor syncope. Exertional syncope suggests an obstructive lesion limiting cardiac output, and syncope with arm exercise suggests the subclavian steal syndrome. Recreational drugs,[23] prescription, and over-the-counter medications may cause syncope. Anaphylaxis, bradydysrhythmias or tachydysrhythmias, orthostatic hypotension, hypoglycemia, or seizures may be secondary to medications. A complete drug history detailing recent medications and drugs is essential.

Focal neurologic symptoms may lead to the diagnosis of a posterior circulation transient ischemic attack (TIA), or more often a seizure. The neurological findings of most TIAs last less than 15 minutes,[24] and postictal focality is commonly measured in minutes—hence the history may be the only clue to diagnosis.

Physical Examination

The vital signs should be assessed. Febrile illnesses predispose to syncope and treatable disease may be overlooked if the temperature is not measured. The respiratory rate should be counted. Although tachypnea is common in patients who have fainted, persistent tachypnea should raise the possibility of pulmonary embolus. The blood pressure and heart rate should be measured in the supine and upright position. Although precise ranges of normal have not been established for elderly patients (or for patients on various combinations of medications), a decrease in systolic blood pressure of >25 mmHg (or to a level <90 mmHg) or the development of syncope or dizziness identifies an orthostatic condition. In these patients the examination must look further for occult hypovolemia—gastrointestinal bleeding and ectopic pregnancy should be considered.

The carotid pulse should be assessed. The examiner should listen for murmurs, and if a systolic murmur is heard, the examiner should assess the change in the murmur with standing and a Valsalva maneuver. Carotid sinus massage may be safely performed in elderly patients with no manifest cardiovascular or cerebrovascular disease—a period of asystole for >3 seconds or a decrease in blood pressure of >50 mmHg suggests carotid sinus hypersensitivity.[25]

The neurological examination may show postictal confusion or focal neurological dysfunction. Finally, the physician should assess the patient for injuries resulting from the syncopal episode.

Laboratory Assessment

With the exception of the electrocardiogram and ambulatory ECG monitoring, the laboratory has little to offer the average patient with syncope. Careful evaluation of the utility of routine complete blood count, glucose, electrolyte, calcium measurements has indicated that large sums may be expended with little diagnostic benefit.[2,3] Of course, selected tests are essential in patients where clinical suspicion exists, but routine screening should be discouraged. A patient with evident bleeding or orthostatic changes in vital signs would have a hematocrit measured. Syncope in a patient on insulin or oral hypoglycemic agents is an indication for a glucose measurement. Serum sodium and potassium should be checked in a patient on diuretics. At times a decreased bicarbonate has provided a clue that a seizure has occurred, but this finding is not specific for seizures, and this abnormality tends to resolve within an hour.

The initial ECG identifies a cardiovascular cause for syncope in a significant fraction of patients. It may document a dysrhythmia, a myocardial infarction, conduction disturbances, or a prolonged QT interval. In approximately 25% of those patients with cardiovascular syncope, the initial ECG provided strong evidence for the diagnosis.[1,3] The importance of identifying this subgroup of patients suggests that an ECG should be done on all patients when the initial history and physical examination do not establish a noncardiovascular diagnosis.

The selection of ambulatory or intensive care unit monitoring is controversial. Most patients do not have symptoms during the period of monitoring, so the finding of a pristine monitoring report does not exclude dysrhythmias. Asymptomatic dysrhythmias are common during monitoring. In healthy adults between the ages of 60 and 85, 13% have paroxysmal supraventricular tachycardia, and 50% demonstrate complex ventricular dysrhythmias[26] (including 4% with ventricular tachycardia). Despite these limitations, monitoring is the diagnostic modality that most frequently implicates dysrhythmias in patients with cardiovascular syncope. Inpatient or ambulatory monitoring should be considered in patients with an uncertain diagnosis. The duration of monitoring is undefined[27]—although most patients demonstrate their dysrhythmias within 24 hours of monitoring.

Additional studies may lead to cardiovascular diagnoses in selected patients. Exercise testing,[28] while less sensitive than ambulatory monitoring, may demonstrate evidence of ischemia or provoke dysrhythmias. Electrophysiological testing[29] has led to diagnoses and successful therapeutic strategies in certain patients. Consensus regarding its role remains elusive. This technique may fail to identify patients with intermittent high-grade heart block resulting in syncope.[29] Patients with syncope that remains undiagnosed after noninvasive evaluation in the presence of organic heart dis-

Table 61-2 Diagnostic Criteria

Cardiovascular Syncope

Myocardial infarction—typical evolution of ECG and enzymes
Dysrhythmias—Documentation of symptomatic bradydysrhythmias or tachydysrhythmias or asymptomatic V tach, Mobitz II, complete heart block, sinus pause >3 seconds
Obstruction to cardiac output—evidence on catheterization of AS, hypertrophic cardiomyopathy, pulmonary stenosis, atrial myxoma, pulmonary emboli
Carotid sinus syncope—asystole >3 seconds or a drop in systolic BP >50 mmHg with carotid massage

Noncardiovascular Syncope

Vasodepressor syncope—loss of consciousness in the setting of severe pain, a real or perceived threat of injury, or severe emotional distress

Orthostatic syncope—if the systolic blood pressure drops upon standing more than 25 mmHg or to a level <90 mmHg with associated symptoms of dizziness or syncope

Seizure disorder—a witnessed seizure or a postictal state

Situational syncope—syncope during or just after micturition, defecation, or a bout of coughing for which no other explanation is found

---

ease or with frequent syncopal episodes seem to be the best candidates for such testing.

Some patients who do not give a history of a situational precipitant characteristic of vasodepressor syncope have neurally mediated hypotension and bradycardia. Some of these patients may have no initial orthostatic change in their vital signs but will develop hypotension and bradycardia if subjected to a tilt test. This test is not well standardized. The patient is placed on a table that tilts to an 80° angle, and the patient's vital signs, ECG, and sense of well-being are monitored for 10 to 60 minutes. A positive inotropic effect of catecholamines combined with a decreased central blood volume may result in an increased afferent vagal activity from receptors in the ventricle, with resultant bradycardia and hypotension. A modification of the tilt test, adding an isoproterenol infusion, has been shown to produce hypotension, bradycardia, and syncope in a significant fraction of patients with recurrent syncope and no evident cause on conventional and electrophysiologic testing.[30]

Diagnostic criteria have emerged from several research studies[1-4] that show promise in guiding the judgments that emergency clinicians make (Table 61-2). Although the diagnostic standards vary somewhat from study to study, each group has identified a substantial minority of patients that cannot be given a diagnosis. Longitudinal studies reveal that over a 1-year follow-up the cause of syncope remains unknown in most of these patients, and that they have a 6% to 12% 1-year mortality (versus an 18% to 33% mortality in patients with cardiovascular syncope).

Much of this mortality is due to comorbid diseases, and these patients have a lower incidence of sudden death than patients given an assigned noncardiovascular cause of syncope. Hence, if we could confidently assign diagnostic criteria after an emergency department evaluation, we could hospitalize those patients who required interventions.

Unfortunately, patients cannot be reliably placed in the category of syncope of unknown etiology after an emergency department evaluation. Despite this, the low hospital mortality[31] for patients who do not require active interventions in the emergency department and the availability of ambulatory electrocardiographic monitoring argue that an outpatient monitoring is appropriate for many patients. Monitoring in an intensive care unit should be reserved for patients with a defined cardiovascular etiology, those with a suspected acute myocardial infarction, and older patients with a short warning period.

REFERENCES

1. Kapoor WN, Karpf M, Wieand S, et al. A prospective evaluation and follow-up of patients with syncope. *N Engl J Med*. 1983;309:197–204.
2. Martin GJ, Adams SL, Martin HG, et al. Prospective evaluation of syncope. *Ann Emerg Med*. 1984;13:499–504.
3. Day SC, Cook EF, Funkenstein H, et al. Evaluation and outcome of emergency room patients with transient loss of consciousness. *Am J Med*. 1982;73:15–23.
4. Silverstein MD, Singer DE, Mulley AG, et al. Patients with syncope admitted to medical intensive care units. *JAMA*. 1982;248:1185–1189.
5. Williams RL, Allen PD. Loss of consciousness: incidence, causes, and electroencephalographic findings. *Aerosp Med*. 1962;33:545–551.
6. Savage DD, Corwin L, McGee DL, et al. Epidemiologic features of isolated syncope: the Framingham study. *Stroke*. 1985;16:626–629.
7. Ross J, Braunwald E. Aortic stenosis. *Circulation*. 1968;38(suppl 5):61–67.
8. Schwartz LS, Goldfischer J, Sprague GJ, et al. Syncope and sudden death in aortic stenosis. *Am J Cardiol*. 1969;23:647–658.
9. McKenna W, Harris L, Deanfield J. Syncope in hypertrophic cardiomyopathy. *Br Heart J*. 1982;47:177–179.
10. Kowey PR, Eisenberg R, Engel TR. Sustained arrhythmias in obstructive cardiomyopathy. *N Engl J Med*. 1984;310:1566–1569.
11. Bell WR, Simon TL, De Mets DL. The clinical features of massive and submassive pulmonary emboli. *Am J Med*. 1977;62:355–360.
12. Thames MD, Alpert JS, Dalen JE. Syncope in patients with pulmonary embolism. *JAMA*. 1977;238:2509–2511.
13. Slater ES, De Sanctis RW. The clinical recognition of dissecting aortic aneurysm. *Am J Med*. 1976;60:625–633.
14. Kuhlmann TP, Powers RD. Painless aortic dissection: an unusual cause of syncope. *Ann Emerg Med*. 1984;13:549–551.
15. Earnest F, Muhm UR, Sheedy PF. Roentgenographic findings in thoracic aortic dissection. *Mayo Clin Proc*. 1979;54:43–50.
16. Epstein SE, Stampfer M, Beiser GD. Role of the capacitance and resistance vessels in vasovagal syncope. *Circulation*. 1968;37:524–531.
17. Lyle CB, Monroe JT, Flinn DE, et al. Micturition syncope. *N Engl J Med*. 1961;265:982–986.
18. Adams HP, Jergenson DD, Kassell NF, Sahs AL. Pitfalls in the recognition of subarachnoid hemorrhage. *JAMA*. 1980;244:794–796.

19. Futty DE, Conneally M, Dyken ML, et al. Cooperative study of hospital frequency and character of transient ischemic attacks. V. Symptom analysis. *JAMA*. 1977;238:2386–2390.
20. Fields WS, Lemak NA. Joint study of extracranial arterial occlusion. III. Subclavian steal—A review of 168 cases. *JAMA*. 1972;222:1139–1143.
21. Kapoor WN, Karpf M, Maher Y, et al. Syncope of unknown origin. The need for a more cost-effective approach to its diagnostic evaluation. *JAMA*. 1982;247:2687–2691.
22. Kapoor W, Snustad D, Peterson J, et al. Syncope in the elderly. *Am J Med*. 1986;80:419–428.
23. Lowenstein DH, Massa SM, Rowbotham MC, et al. Acute neurologic and psychiatric complications associated with cocaine abuse. *Am J Med*. 1987;83:841–846.
24. Dyken ML, Conneally M, Haerer AF, et al. Cooperative study of hospital frequency and character of transient ischemic attacks. I. Background organization and clinical survey. *JAMA*. 1977;237:882–886.
25. Coplan NL, Schweitzer P. Carotid sinus hypersensitivity. *Am J Med*. 1984;77:561–565.
26. Fleg JL, Kennedy HL. Cardiac arrhythmias in a healthy elderly population. *Chest*. 1982;81:302–307.
27. Kapoor W, Karpf M, Levey G. Issues in evaluating patients with syncope. *Ann Intern Med*. 1984;100:755–757.
28. Boudoulas H, Schaal SF, Lewis RP, Robinson JL. Superiority of 24 hour outpatient monitoring over multi-stage exercise testing for the evaluation of syncope. *J Electrocardiol*. 1979;12:103–108.
29. Fujimura O, Yee R, Klein GH, et al. The diagnostic sensitivity of electrophysiologic testing in patients with syncope caused by transient bradycardia. *N Engl J Med*. 1989;321:1703–1707.
30. Almquist A, Goldenberg IF, Milstein S, et al. Provocation of bradycardia and hypotension by isoproterenol and upright posture in patients with unexplained syncope. *N Engl J Med*. 1989;320:346–351.
31. Thibault GE, Mulley AG, Barnett GO, et al. Medical intensive care: indications, interventions, and outcomes. *N Engl J Med*. 1980;302:938–942.

62. Acute Myocardial Infarction

LESTER B. JACOBSON, MD, FACC, FACP

Coronary artery disease continues to affect a large segment of the American population. Some patients are asymptomatic, but others suffer from angina pectoris, congestive heart failure, and dysrhythmias. Both asymptomatic and symptomatic patients are at risk for acute myocardial infarction and sudden death, events that occur with frightening unpredictability. While the statistical likelihood that patients with coronary artery disease will suffer acute myocardial infarction within a specified time period can be predicted from the responses of their ST segments and blood pressure to treadmill exercise testing, the occurrence and time of occurrence of the event in an *individual* patient cannot be prognosticated.

Acute myocardial infarction is a dramatic event. Neither the clinical course nor the short- and long-term prognoses can be predicted in an individual at the time of its onset. Patients with acute myocardial infarction are generally impressed with their symptoms, and those around the patients are generally impressed by their critically ill appearance. The gravity of the situation is underscored by the seriousness of purpose exhibited by the physician and other health care personnel in attendance. Their attentiveness reflects their appreciation of the fact that patients with acute myocardial infarction can suddenly and unpredictably develop catastrophic, potentially fatal dysrhythmias that require immediate treatment.

PATHOGENESIS OF ACUTE MYOCARDIAL INFARCTION

Myocardial ischemia occurs when the myocardial oxygen demand, the amount of oxygen needed per minute per gram of cardiac tissue to maintain the functional and structural integrity of the heart, exceeds the oxygen supply to the myocardium for a period of time. Myocardial infarction occurs when this demand exceeds supply for so long a time—generally several minutes—that necrosis of cardiac tissue occurs.

Three major determinants account for about 80% of the myocardial oxygen demand: (1) the heart rate, (2) the contractile state of ventricular muscle, and (3) the left ventricular wall tension. Wall tension is directly proportional to the product of the pressure developed within the left ventricular myocardium and the radius of the left ventricle as it generates pressure; it is inversely proportional to the left ventricular wall thickness.

Myocardial oxygen supply also has three major determinants: (1) the coronary blood flow, (2) the oxygen-carrying capacity of the blood, and (3) the shape of the hemoglobin-oxygen dissociation curve. The coronary blood flow depends on the size of the coronary arteries, which may be altered by anatomical stenoses and vasomotor influences; the coronary vascular resistance; and the aortic and left ventricular pressures during diastole. The oxygen-carrying capacity of the

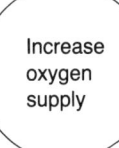

Figure 62-1 Interventions that alter the size of an experimental myocardial infarction.[6]

blood depends predominantly on the hemoglobin concentration. The shape of the hemoglobin-oxygen dissociation curve depends on metabolic factors.

While almost all patients (more than 95%) who suffer an acute myocardial infarction have significant anatomical stenoses in the coronary artery distribution to the infarcted myocardium, a few such patients have normal coronary arteries. In view of this latter finding, it has been suggested that prolonged, severe vasoconstriction of the vessel, thromboembolism, or in situ thrombosis with subsequent lysis of the thrombus is the mechanism of infarction in some individuals. Constriction of a coronary artery to such a degree that little or no blood flows through it, spasm, has been documented to occur in normal as well as in pathologically (atherosclerotically) narrowed vessels.[1,2] Spasm may occur spontaneously, as a result of mechanical stimulation (eg, catheter), or in response to specific pharmacologic agents, of which ergonovine maleate is the most commonly used.

It is difficult to know exactly why acute myocardial infarction occurs when it does in patients with coronary artery disease, for the overwhelming majority of patients have the infarction at times of inactivity, when there is no clear increase in the myocardial oxygen demand. Thus, it has been hypothesized that the event is initiated by a decrease in myocardial oxygen supply, presumably because of a decrease in coronary blood flow. It is not possible in an individual patient to identify the exact event(s) responsible for diminished flow, but the most plausible mechanism is a decrease in the size of the supplying artery lumen because of intraluminal thrombus formation,[3,4] dissection into the base of an atherosclerotic plaque, or an increase in vasomotor tone that causes vasoconstriction.

It has been discovered during the past two decades that myocardial infarction evolves over a period of several hours and that the size of the infarction is not determined at the time of the onset of the event.[5] Rather, extensive laboratory studies in experimental animals have shown that the size of an evolving myocardial infarction may be altered by maneuvers and medications that change the balance between myocardial oxygen demand and supply. Interventions that decrease demand or increase supply lessen the size of an evolving infarct, while those that increase demand or decrease supply increase the size of the necrotic area (Fig. 62-1). Clinical studies aimed at determining the applicability of these principles to acute myocardial infarction in humans have demonstrated that the acute administration of thrombolytic agents, nitroglycerin, aspirin, heparin and beta-blocking drugs, alone or in combination, effects reductions in morbidity and mortality in acute myocardial infarction, but that other interventions do not.[6,7]

CONSEQUENCES OF MYOCARDIAL ISCHEMIA

The metabolic abnormalities that occur with myocardial ischemia result in dramatic alterations in the electrical and mechanical properties of the heart. Changes in conduction velocities and refractory periods of cardiac electrical tissue predispose to the development of ventricular dysrhythmias and may result in intraventricular and atrioventricular (AV) conduction abnormalities. Changes in mechanical properties of the heart, such as an increase in the stiffness of the myocardium in diastole or a tendency for cardiac muscle to expand rather than contract during mechanical systole, contribute to the increase in left ventricular diastolic pressure and the decrease in left ventricular stroke volume that accompany myocardial ischemia.

SYMPTOMS OF ACUTE MYOCARDIAL ISCHEMIA AND INFARCTION

Patients with acute myocardial ischemia and infarction may or may not have symptoms to suggest what is occurring. The classic symptom is a discomfort that, in most patients, is located in the precordial area, but may be located in the epigastrium, the neck, the mandible, the shoulders, the arms, or the back. The discomfort is usually described as a pressure, tightness, or weightlike feeling; however, it may be described as a true pain with an aching or sharp, stabbing quality. Occasional patients complain of gastrointestinal symptoms that they commonly term "indigestion."

Some patients with acute myocardial infarction simply collapse and die suddenly before any symptoms occur. Others complain of a feeling of weakness that may be mild to profound. Lightheadedness, with or without an awareness of cardiac activity, diaphoresis, nausea, vomiting, and a sense of impending doom are also commonly described symptoms. In rare instances, the abrupt onset of congestive heart failure symptoms may be the only manifestation of acute myocardial infarction.

PHYSICAL EXAMINATION FINDINGS

Patients with acute myocardial infarction usually appear seriously ill and uncomfortable. If their cardiac output is low, they may have an ashen, dusky coloration, and their skin may be cool and clammy. These signs, which are attributable to the large amounts of catecholamines secreted in response to the hemodynamic and psychological stresses of the event, may be masked to variable degrees in patients taking adrenergic blocking or depleting medications, such as atenolol, metoprolol, propranolol, and reserpine. Patients with acute myocardial infarction may be tachypneic. If so, they generally breathe small tidal volumes rapidly in response to pulmonary congestion and/or emotional stress.

The pulse may be rapid, normal, or slow, depending on the hemodynamic stress of the event, the responses of the autonomic nervous system, and the ability of the cardiac conduction system to respond to the hemodynamic and metabolic stimuli. The arterial pulses may be bounding, normal, or thready, depending on the stroke volume. The blood pressure (BP) may be high, normal, or low, depending on the cardiac output and the systemic vascular resistance. The jugular venous pressure may be high, normal, or low, depending on the circulating blood volume, the venous tone, and the cardiac performance.

The heart, on palpation, may be normal size or large. Its movement may seem to be normal or abnormal, depending on its condition prior to the acute infarction and on the anatomical and functional magnitude, as well as the location, of the evolving infarction. A fourth heart sound is commonly heard; in the presence of congestive heart failure, a third heart sound may also be audible. When the heart rate is rapid, the third and fourth heart sounds may fuse into a single sound and result in a triple cadence termed a *summation gallop*. Mitral insufficiency, typically across the posterior mitral valve leaflet, may occur as a result of ischemia or infarction that involves, generally, the inferior wall of the left ventricle, but may involve a papillary muscle itself. The resultant murmur may be pansystolic, midsystolic, or late systolic, depending on the systolic timing and the severity of the left ventricular-wall motion abnormality. The mitral insufficiency murmur may be heard best at the base of the heart, at the left lower sternal edge, or at the apex; in contrast, the murmur of rheumatic mitral insufficiency, which is due almost exclusively to regurgitation across the anterior mitral valve leaflet, is almost always heard best at the apex. Ventricular septal rupture, a rare event in the early hours of acute myocardial infarction, may be recognized by a harsh, loud pansystolic murmur that is heard best at the left lower sternal edge and is accompanied by a prominent thrill in the area where the murmur is heard with maximum intensity.

A pericardial rub attributable to acute myocardial infarction only rarely occurs in the first hours of an infarction, although it commonly occurs during the second through fourth days of the event. As rubs are generally heard only in patients whose infarction involves the epicardium, they are most commonly heard in patients whose electrocardiograms (ECGs) suggest transmural myocardial infarction (ie, show pathologic Q waves in addition to abnormalities of the ST segments and T waves). However, pericardial rubs are occasionally heard in patients whose ECGs do not show evidence of transmural myocardial infarction, presumably because transmural and epicardial infarctions are not always accompanied by pathologic Q waves.

ECG Evidence of Acute Myocardial Infarction

Specific ECG findings that suggest the presence of acute myocardial ischemia or infarction include peaked T waves, elevations and depression of the ST segments, pathologic Q waves, T-wave inversions, and atrioventricular and/or intraventricular conduction abnormalities. One of the earliest ECG abnormalities in acute myocardial infarction is a change in the contour and amplitude of the T wave, which may become tall and sharply peaked. This *hyperacute* pattern usually lasts for only a few minutes and is not generally seen because patients rarely have ECGs taken in the early minutes of an acute myocardial infarction (Fig. 62-2). ST segment elevations that are convex upward define the epicardial injury pattern, which is a reliable sign of extensive ischemic myocardial injury (Fig. 62-3). Leads vectorially opposite to those exhibiting ST elevations often show ST

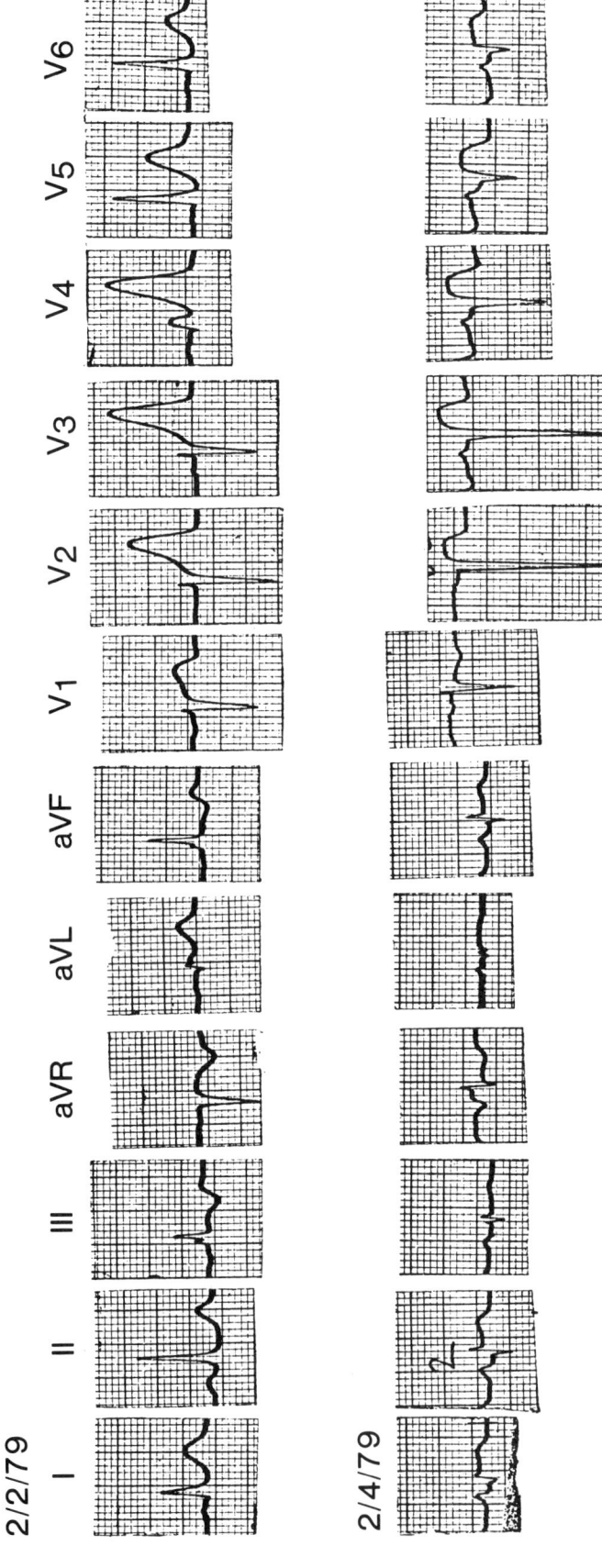

Figure 62-2 ECGs showing evolution of an acute myocardial infarction from the hyperacute T-wave pattern (*top*) to the pathologic Q-wave and ST segment and T-wave abnormality pattern (*bottom*). *Note:* The 12-lead ECG at top was recorded from a patient about 20 minutes after the onset of symptoms suggesting acute myocardial infarction. Leads V_2 through V_5 most clearly display the prominent hyperacute T-wave contours. The T waves in leads I, aVL, and V_6 are also abnormally tall, but less so. The 12-lead ECG (bottom), which was recorded 2 days later in the same patient, shows pathologic Q waves and ST segment and T-wave abnormalities indicating transmural infarction of myocardium seen by the leads in which the hyperacute T-wave abnormalities had been present. (ECG shown at 96% of original.)

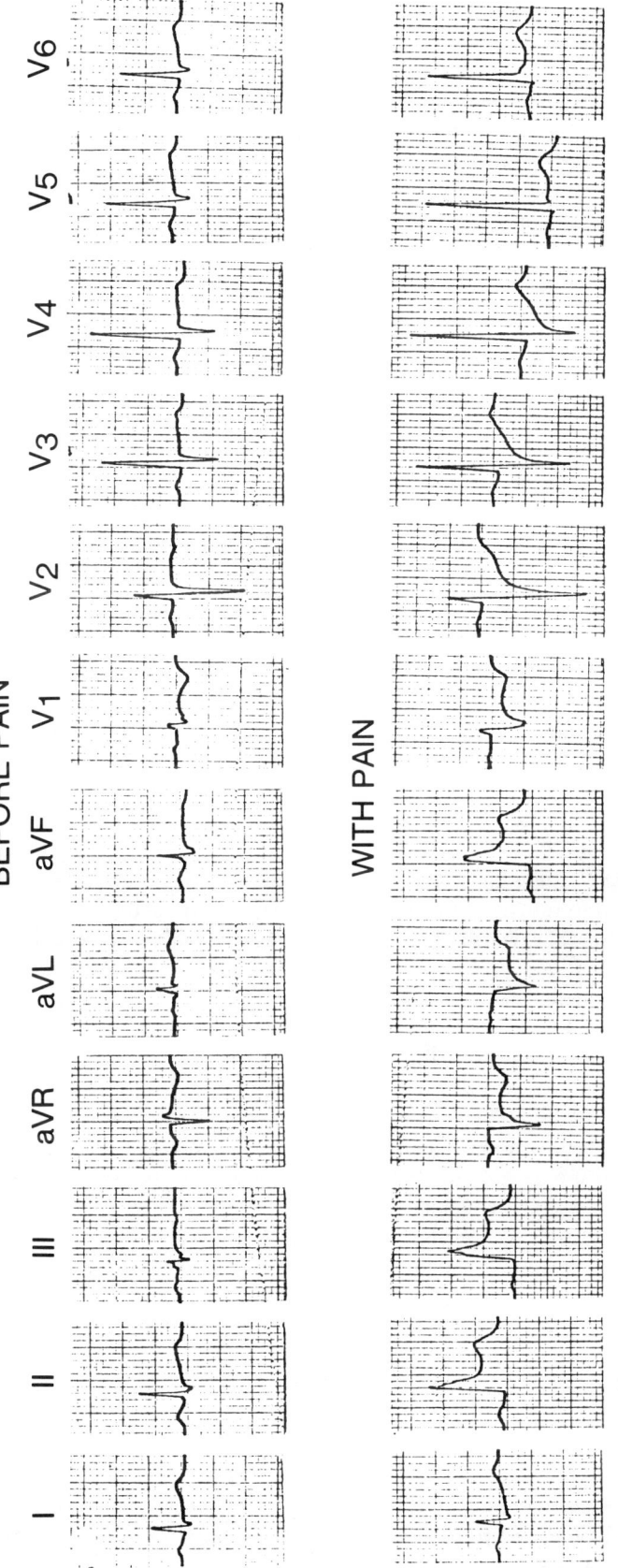

Figure 62-3 ECGs of patient with reversible myocardial ischemia due to coronary artery spasm. *Note:* These 12-lead ECGs were recorded from a 54-year-old man with normal coronary angiogram before and after (*top*) and during (*bottom*) an episode of reversible myocardial ischemia due to coronary artery spasm. During the pain, the ST segments in leads II, III, aVF, and V_6 are markedly elevated, displaying the epicardial injury pattern. Leads I, aVR, aVL, and V_1 through V_4 show reciprocal ST segment depression. Only minor T-wave abnormalities are present in the top tracing. (ECG shown at 93% of original.)

depressions, which are termed reciprocal changes or abnormalities. In some patients, the ST segment depressions are more marked than the ST segment elevations (Fig. 62-4); and changes in the contours of T waves may or may not accompany ST segment changes. In other patients, especially those with previous myocardial infarctions or with left ventricular hypertrophy, changes in previously abnormal ST segments may be the only ECG evidence of acute ischemia or infarction (Fig. 62-5).

In some patients, changes in the direction of T waves may be the only signs of myocardial ischemia and infarction. If the T waves were initially normal, the ECG may show only T-wave inversion; however, if the T waves were initially abnormal, then the ECG may look more "normal" despite the occurrence of a new ischemic event (Fig. 62-6).

Pathologic Q waves, which reflect the absence of cardiac electrical activity from those portions of the heart "seen" by the leads in which they occur, may appear within 8 to 24 hours of the onset of symptoms of acute myocardial infarction (Fig. 62-2, bottom). However, as pathologic Q waves rarely appear earlier than 8 hours after the onset of symptoms, such Q waves in an ECG recorded shortly after the onset of symptoms suggest that a myocardial infarction has occurred earlier, but this does not help assess whether or not a new infarction is occurring. ECGs showing pathologic Q waves are said to indicate transmural infarction, because the presence of Q waves correlates anatomically with infarction that extends from the endocardium through the epicardium (ie, is transmural).

Certain ECG patterns make it difficult, if not impossible, to confirm an acute myocardial infarction electrocardiographically. In patients whose ventricular rhythm is completely paced by an artificial cardiac-pacing system, the QRST complexes may show little, if any, change when infarction occurs. This may also be the case when a myocardial infarction has occurred previously (Fig. 62-5). Difficulty also arises when no previous tracings are available for comparison in a patient with Wolff-Parkinson-White syndrome, in whom atrioventricular conduction occurs exclusively via the accessory atrioventricular conduction pathway, for in such patients the ECG may show dramatic QRST abnormalities even in the absence of an ischemic event (Fig. 62-7). In patients whose ECGs show left bundle branch block prior to the onset of acute myocardial infarction, changes of variable degrees usually occur in the ST segment and T-wave contours during the acute event. However, the ST segments and T waves usually return to their preinfarction contours as the infarction evolves, and new Q waves do not usually appear. Thus, in a patient with left bundle branch block, an ECG taken before an infarction may be identical to one taken after the infarction. In contrast, patterns indicating right bundle branch block or left anterior fascicular block occurring prior to, or developing in the course of, acute myocardial infarction do not interfere with the evolution of the typical ECG abnormalities associated with the event (Fig. 62-8).

Complicating the ECG interpretation of myocardial infarction are the occurrences of ECG patterns that simulate ischemic events although the patients' coronary arteries and myocardium are structurally normal. As mentioned earlier, one such pattern occurs in patients with accessory atrioventricular conduction pathways. When AV conduction occurs via the accessory pathway, a negatively directed delta wave may simulate a pathologic Q wave and prompt the incorrect diagnosis of myocardial infarction (Fig. 62-9). Another complicating pattern is seen in patients with intermittent left bundle branch block; when intraventricular conduction is normal, the T waves in the anterior precordial leads may at times have deeply inverted, symmetrical contours like those seen in anterior wall ischemic events (Fig. 62-10). A third pattern occurs in patients whose ventricles have been paced for periods of hours to years. In such patients, the nonpaced QRS complexes that are stimulated by supraventricular impulses may show ST segment and T-wave contour abnormalities suggesting an ischemic event (Fig. 62-11). The mechanism of the development of such postpacing T-wave changes remains unclear.

In some patients, the development of bundle branch or fascicle blocks, or of first-, second-, or third-degree AV block may be a clue to the occurrence of acute myocardial infarction.

While virtually any dysrhythmia may occur in the presence of acute myocardial infarction, the only dysrhythmia that is essentially diagnostic of this event is the so-called accelerated idioventricular rhythm. (See Chapter 63, Fig. 63-24.)

Serum Enzyme Levels

Determination of the serum levels of enzymes that originate in the myocardium may help establish the presence of recent myocardial necrosis. The enzymes commonly measured are the creatine kinase (CK), and lactic dehydrogenase (LDH). As shown in Fig. 62-12, however, the time courses of the levels of these enzymes is such that all may be within normal limits within the first several hours of acute myocardial infarction. Furthermore, CK also exists in skeletal muscle, brain, and kidney; and LDH, in red blood cells, skeletal muscle, kidney, and liver. Therefore, elevations in the serum levels of one or more of these enzymes may reflect skeletal muscle, cerebral, renal, hepatic, or erythrocyte injury rather than myocardial necrosis. A firm diagnosis of evolving myocardial infarction may require determination of the serum levels of the myocardium-specific isoenzymes (CK-MB and LDH_1), measurements that are more expensive and usually take several hours to perform. For these reasons, the decision

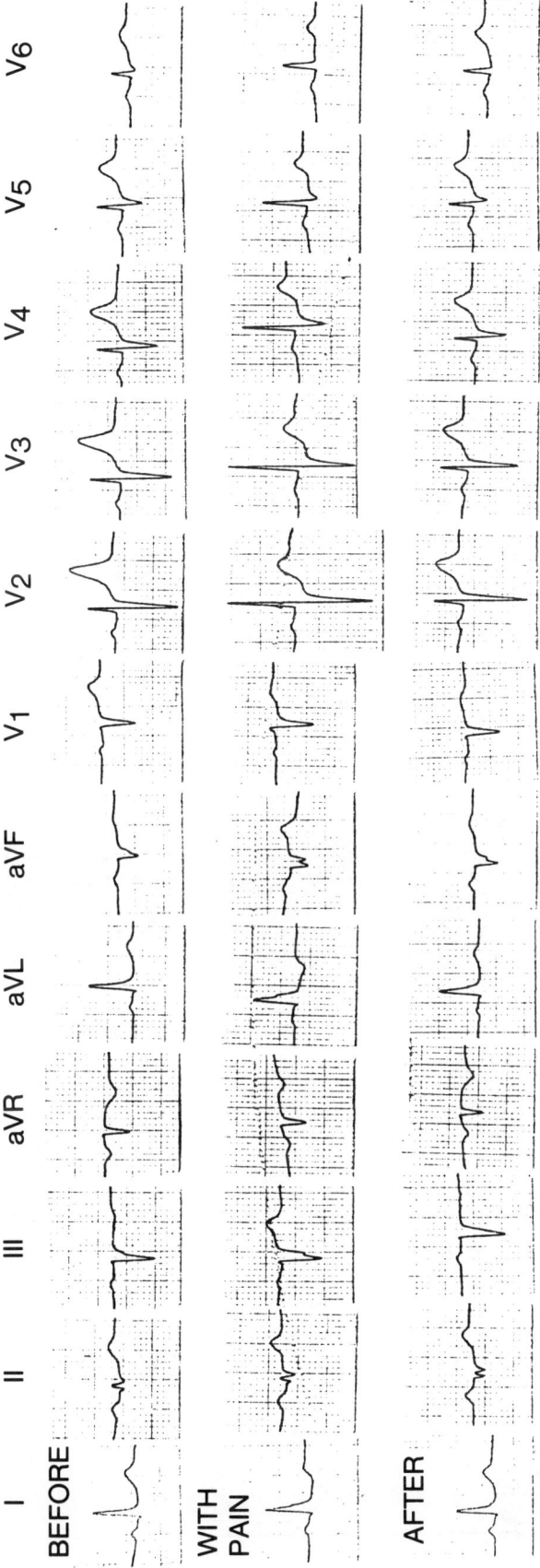

Figure 62-4 ECGs showing transient depressions of ST segments and diminutions in the T-wave amplitudes during myocardial ischemia. *Note:* These 12-lead ECGs were recorded from a 58-year-old man with severe three-vessel coronary artery disease before (*top*), during (*middle*), and after (*bottom*) an episode of nocturnal chest discomfort. During pain, transient depression of the ST segment and diminution in the T-wave amplitude occur in leads I, aVL, and V_2 through V_4. Both ST segment and T-wave contours return to baseline following relief of the chest discomfort. (ECG shown at 84% of original.)

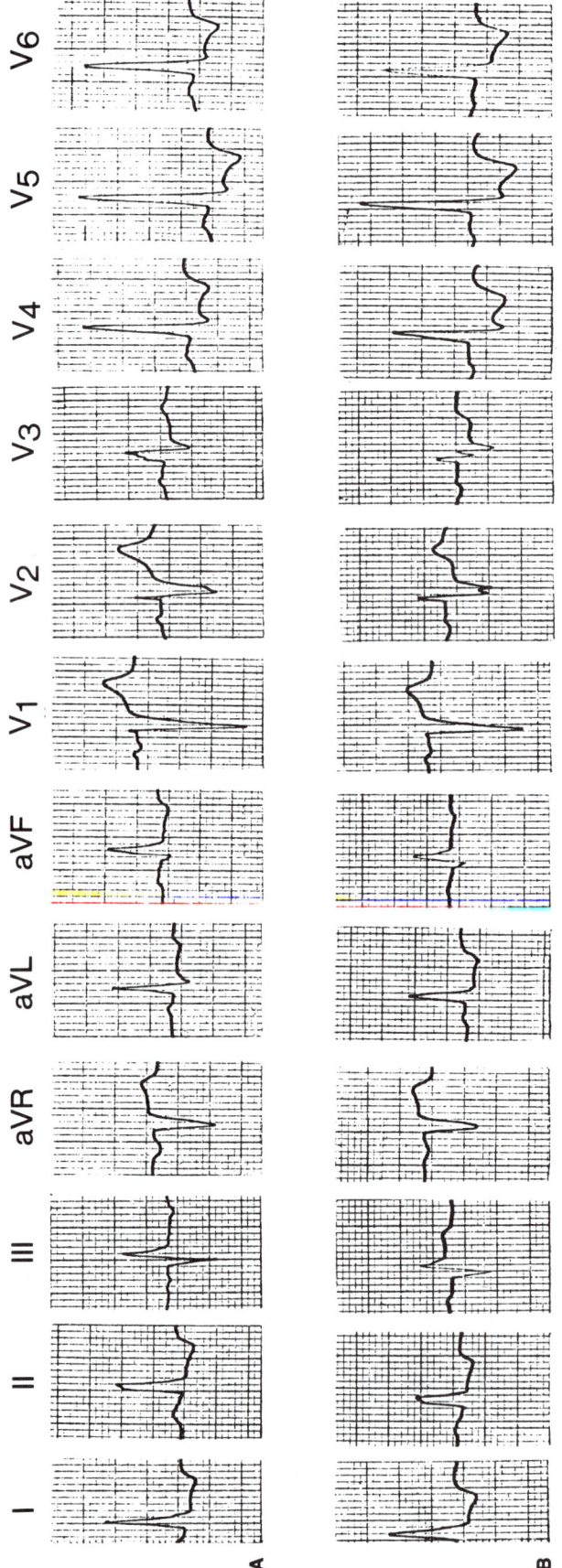

Figure 62-5 ECGs showing changes in ST segment contours as the only manifestations of acute myocardial infarction. *Note:* These 12-lead ECGs were recorded from a man with hypertension and previous myocardial infarctions at a time when he was feeling quite well (*A*) and 2 weeks later, several hours after the onset of symptoms suggesting acute myocardial infarction (*B*). The ST segments in the later ECG are much more depressed in leads I, aVL, and V_2 through V_5. The patient died 2 days later in profound heart failure. At autopsy, extensive evolving myocardial infarction was found. (ECG shown at 95% of original.)

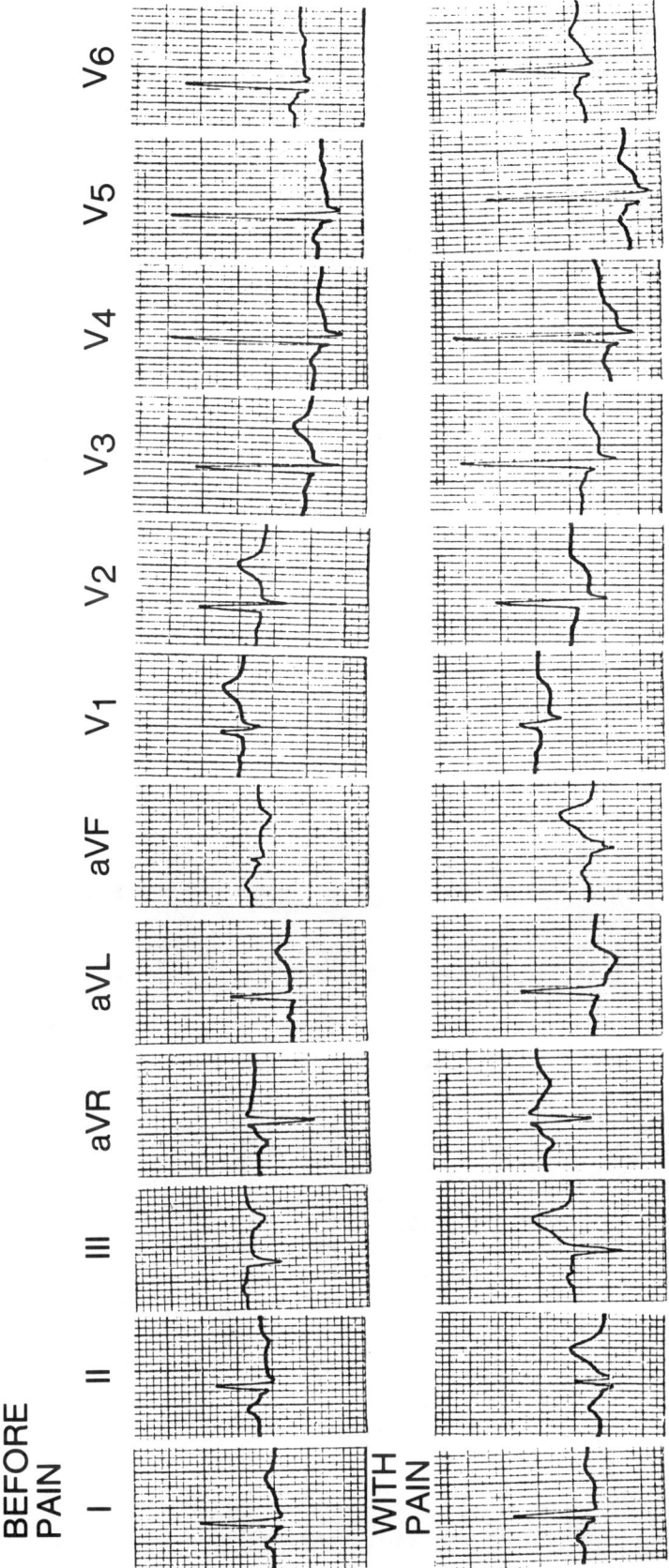

Figure 62-6 ECGs showing changes in Q waves, ST segments, and T waves during pain of myocardial ischemia. *Note:* These 12-lead ECGs were recorded before (*top*) and during (*bottom*) chest discomfort in a 48-year-old man with acute inferior and true posterior wall myocardial infarction 3 days earlier. The top strip, showing Q waves and ST segment and T-wave abnormalities in leads II, III, and aVF, as well as $R > S$ with an upright T-wave in lead V_1, is compatible with inferior wall and true posterior wall myocardial infarctions of uncertain age. During pain of myocardial ischemia, ST segment and T-wave changes occur in all leads, and the T-wave direction becomes "normal" in the inferiorly directed leads and in lead V_1.

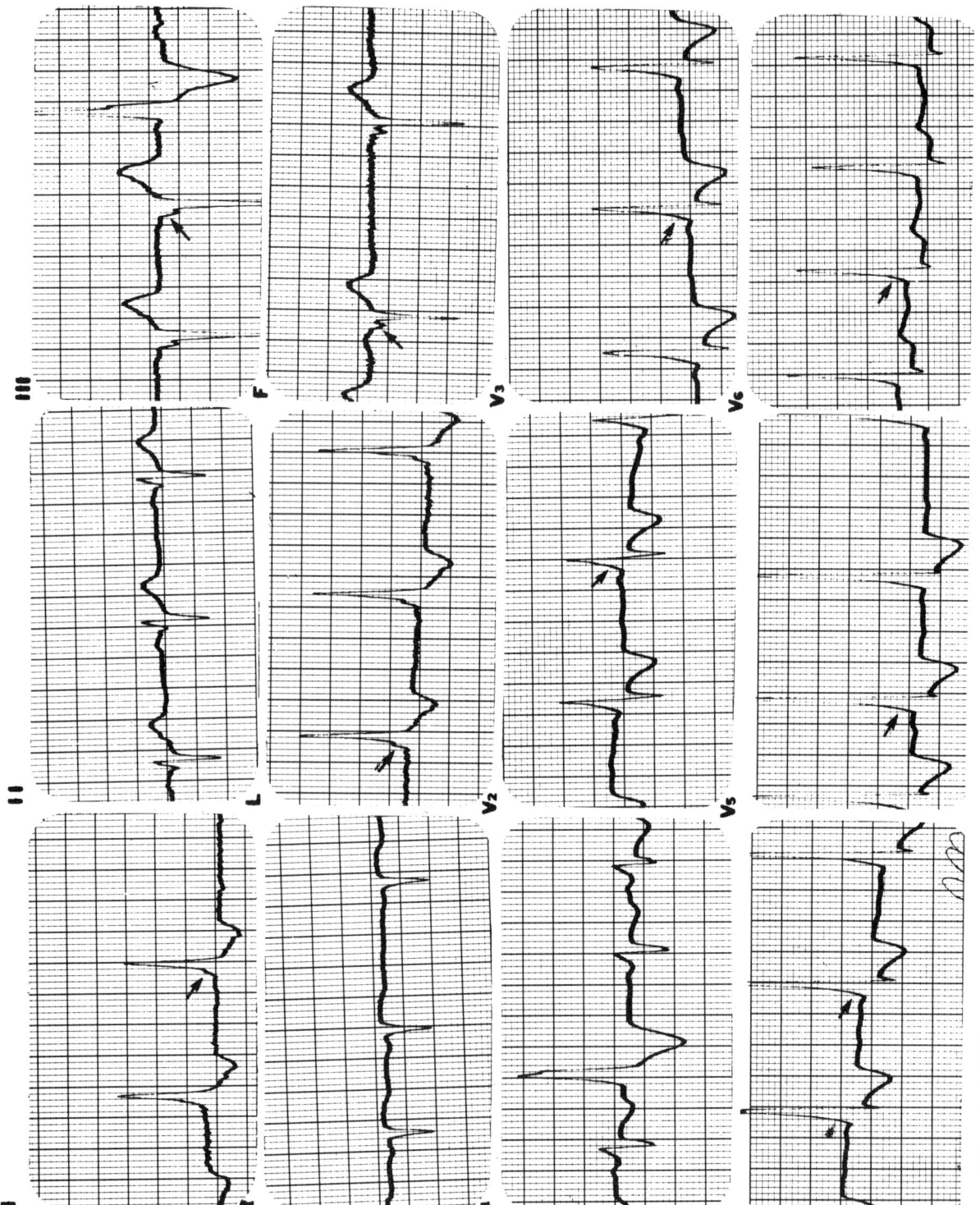

Figure 62-7 ECGs showing QRST abnormalities in a patient with Wolff-Parkinson-White syndrome during accessory pathway conduction. *Note:* This 12-lead ECG was recorded from a 67-year-old woman with angina pectoris and Wolff-Parkinson-White syndrome during accessory pathway conduction. The PR interval is at the lower limit of normal (0.12 second), the QRS duration is abnormally long (0.13 second), and delta waves (*arrows*) are present. The dramatic ST segment and T-wave abnormalities might simply reflect an abnormal sequence of ventricular repolarization resulting from the abnormal sequence of ventricular activation via the accessory pathway, but they could conceivably reflect myocardial ischemia.

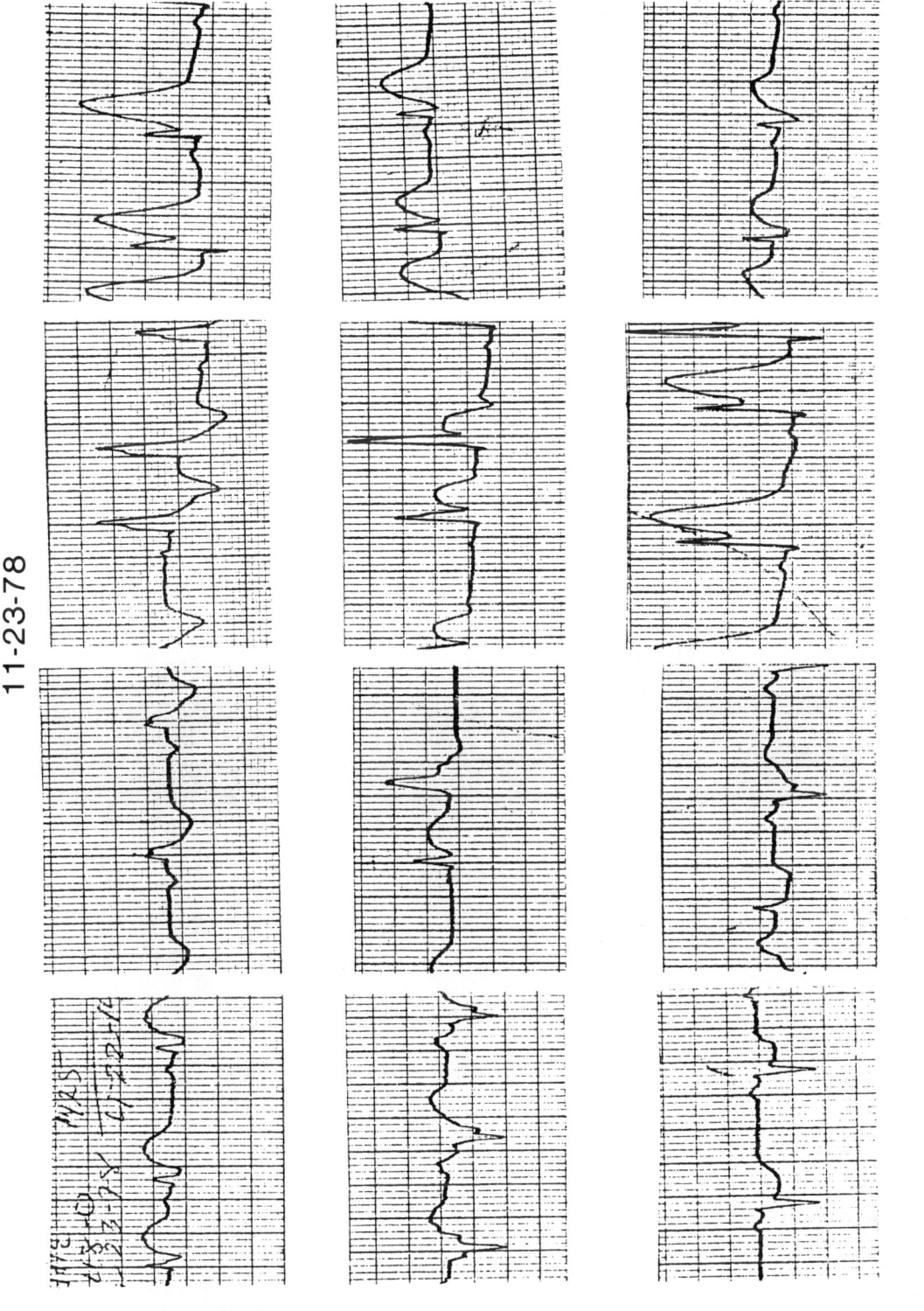

Figure 62-8 ECGs showing evolutionary changes of acute myocardial infarction in patient with pre-existing right bundle branch block and left anterior fascicular block. *Note:* These 12-lead ECGs were recorded from a patient with pre-existing right bundle branch block and left axis deviation attributable to left anterior fascicle block (A) 3 hours after the onset of symptoms suggesting acute myocardial infarction and (B) 15 days later. Despite the intraventricular conduction abnormalities, extensive ST segment elevations reflecting ischemic injury are seen in A, and pathologic Q waves and ST elevations and T-wave inversions indicative of transmural anterior wall myocardial infarction are clearly seen in B.

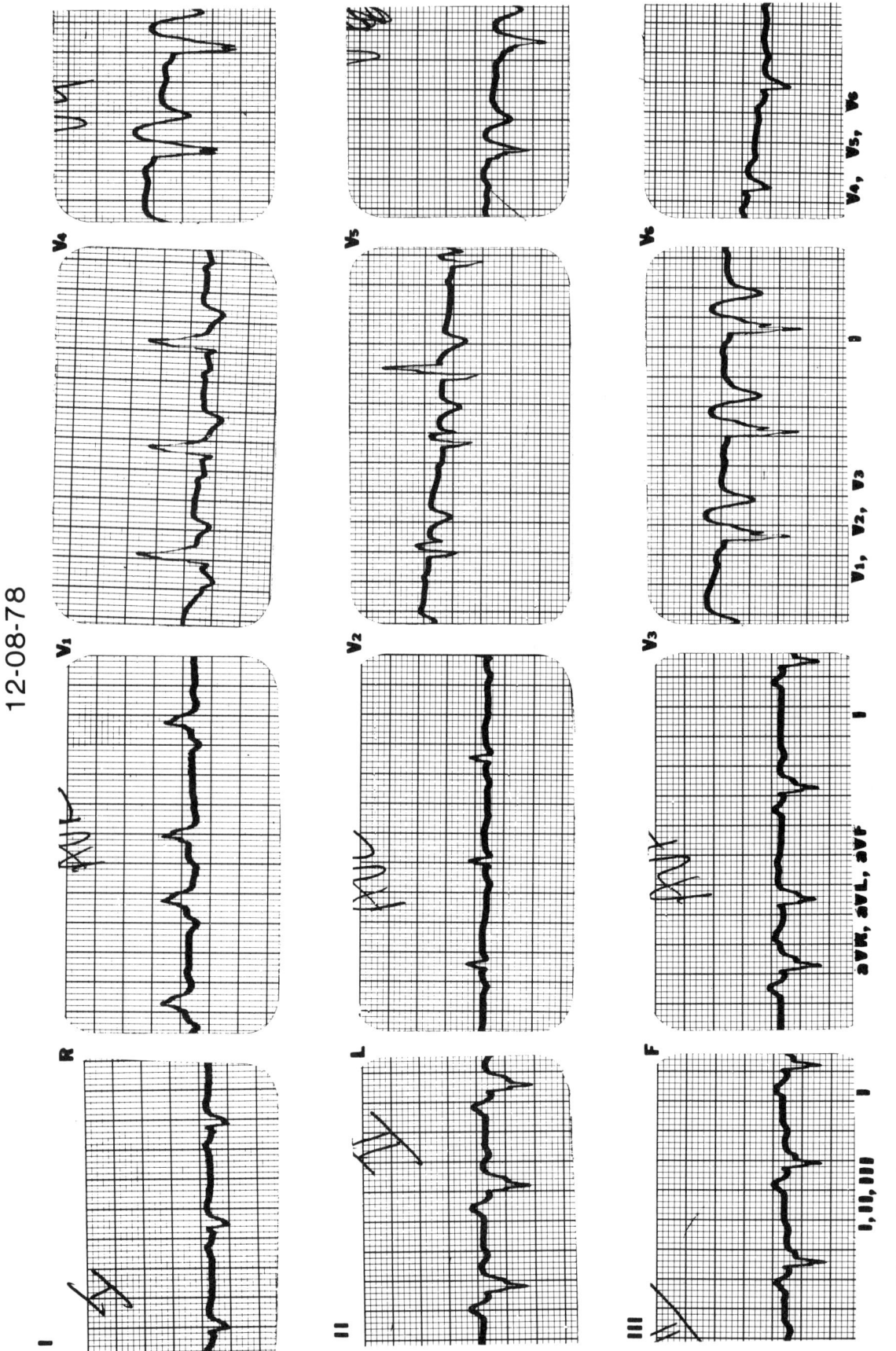

Figure 62-8 continued

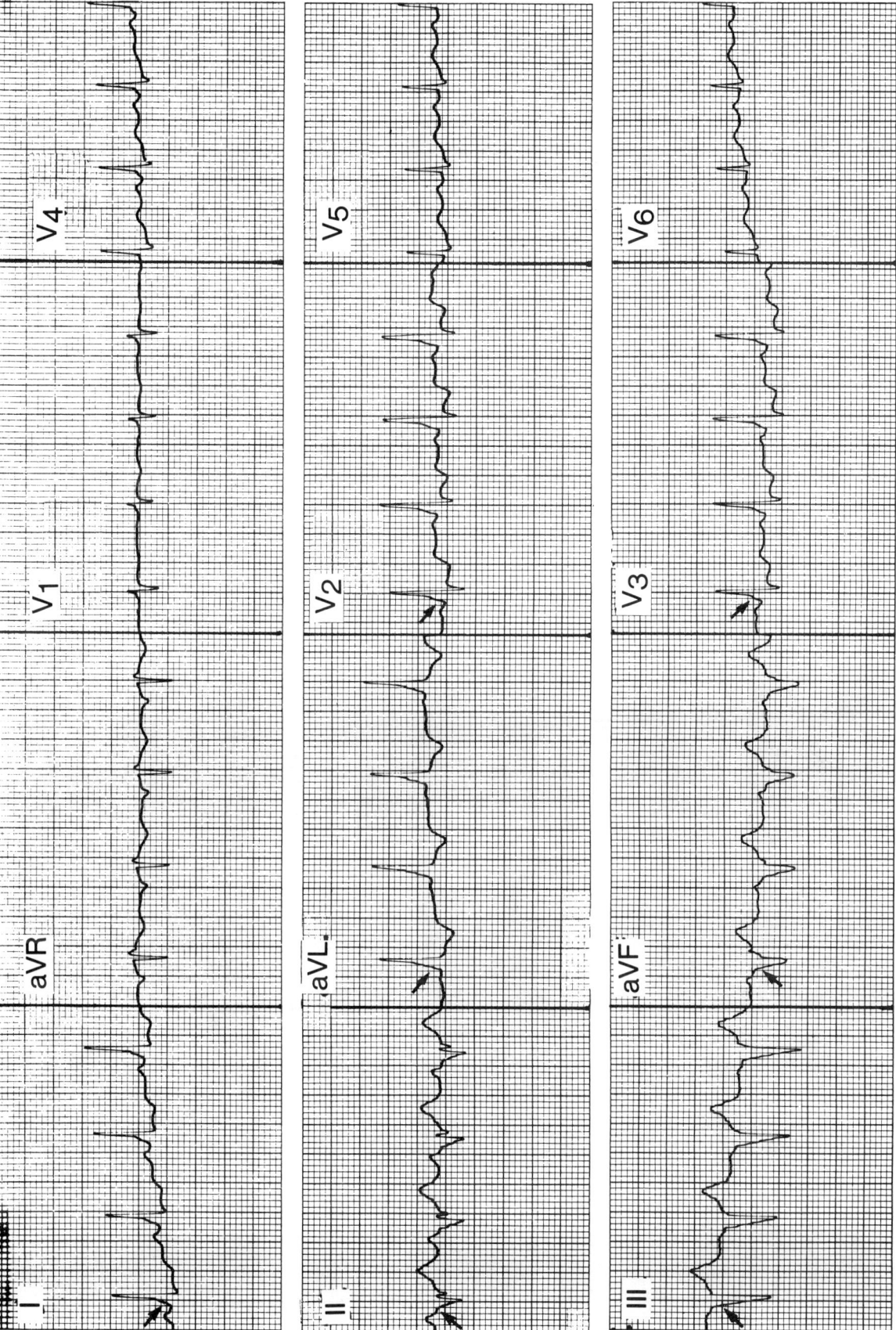

Figure 62-9 ECG showing pseudoinfarction pattern in a patient with Wolff-Parkinson-White syndrome. *Note:* This 12-lead ECG was recorded from an asymptomatic 30-year-old man with an accessory atrioventricular conduction pathway that allows ventricular pre-excitation. The PR interval is abnormally short (0.11 second), the QRS duration is abnormally long (0.12 second), and delta waves (*arrows*) are present. The negatively directed delta waves in leads II, III, and aVF simulate pathologic Q waves and suggest myocardial infarction. As this patient has no evidence of coronary artery disease or myocardial infarction, the pattern is referred to as a pseudoinfarction pattern.

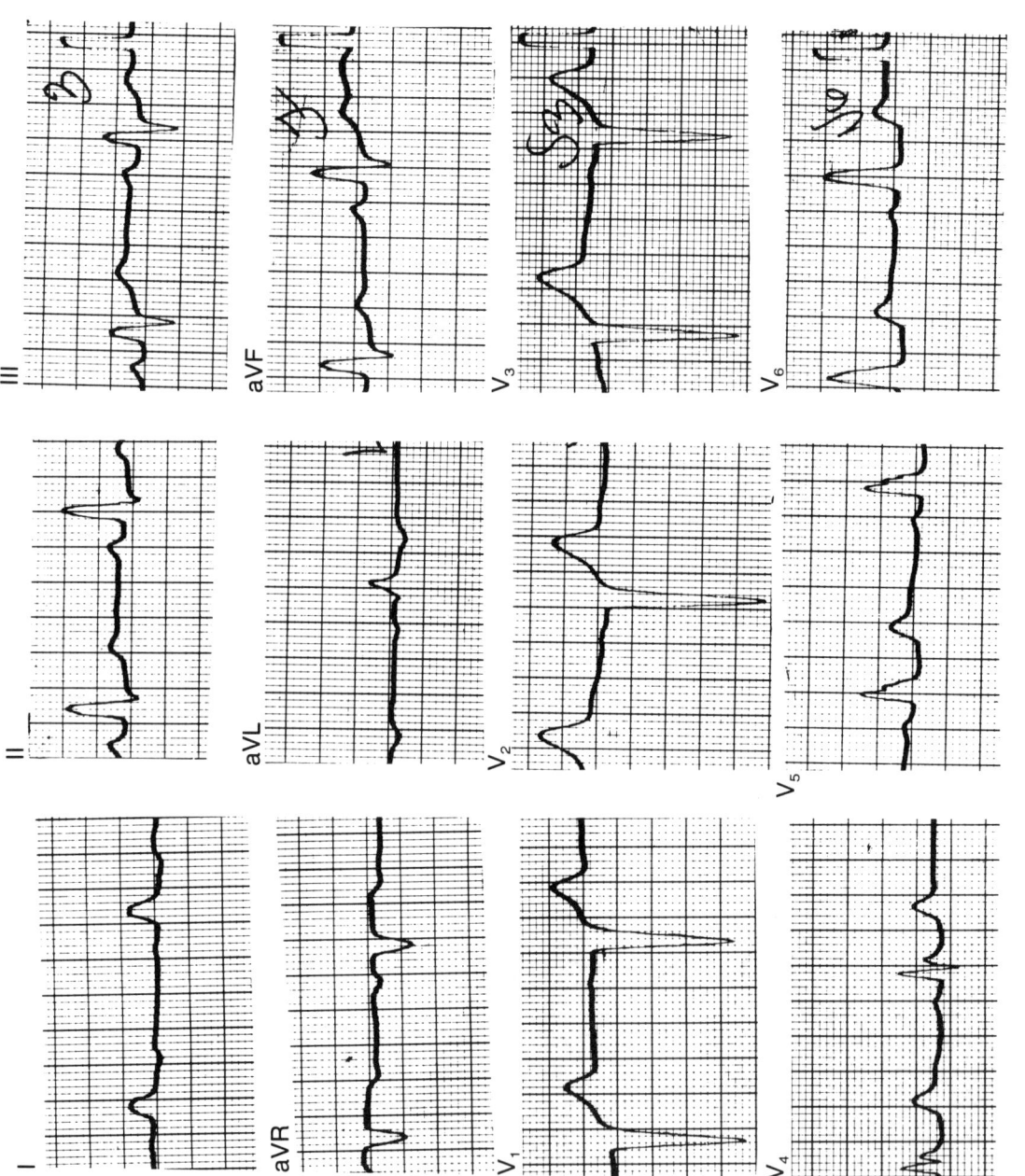

Figure 62-10 ECGs in a patient with intermittent left bundle branch block. *Note:* These ECGs were recorded from a 70-year-old woman with intermittent left bundle branch block and no evidence of coronary artery disease. *A:* This 12-lead ECG was recorded during left bundle branch block. *B:* Twelve-lead ECG during normal intraventricular conduction shows nonspecific T-wave contour abnormalities, most suggesting an ischemic process, in leads V_2 and V_3. *C:* Lead V_2 shows the transition from normal to left bundle branch block type of intraventricular conduction pattern.

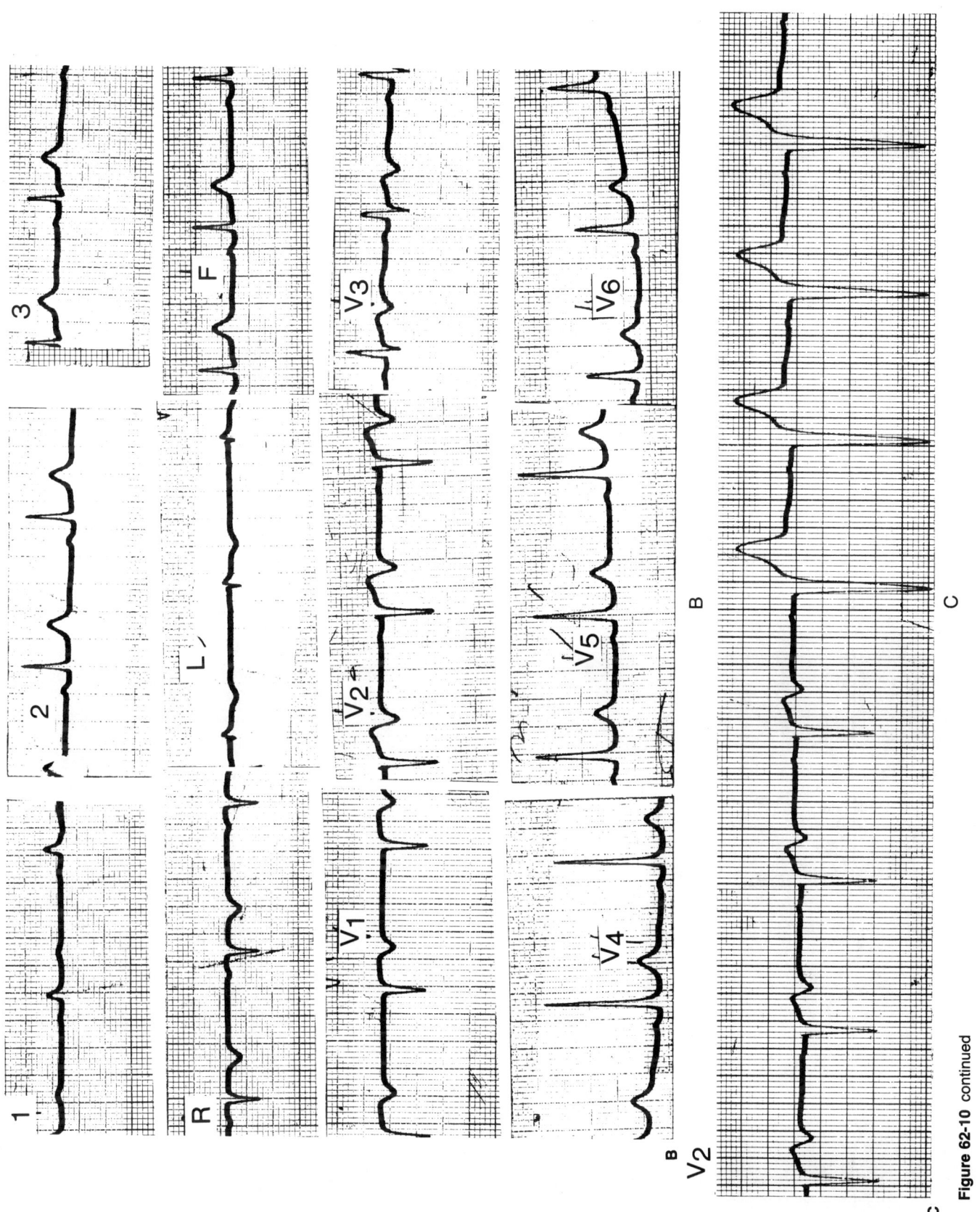

Figure 62-10 continued

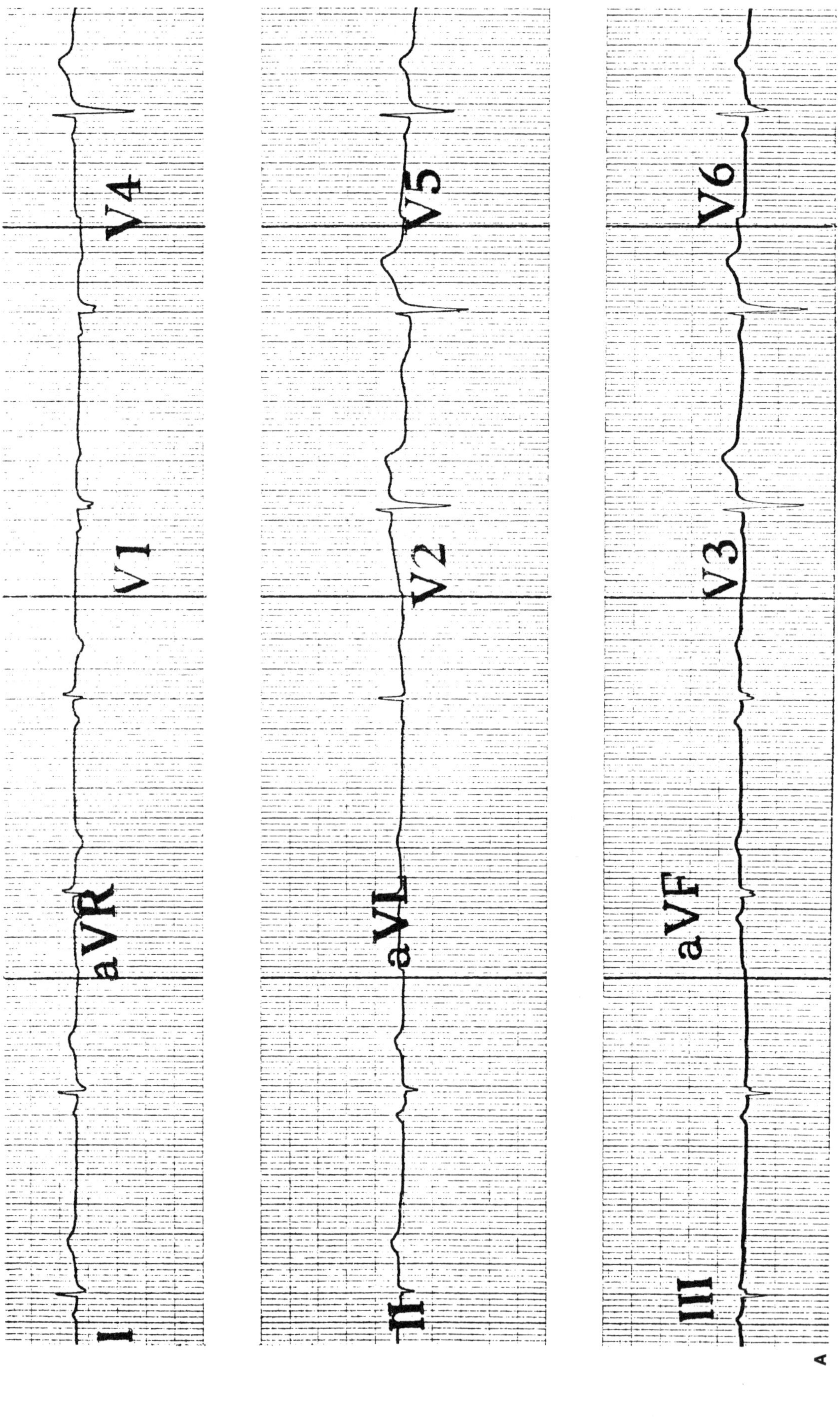

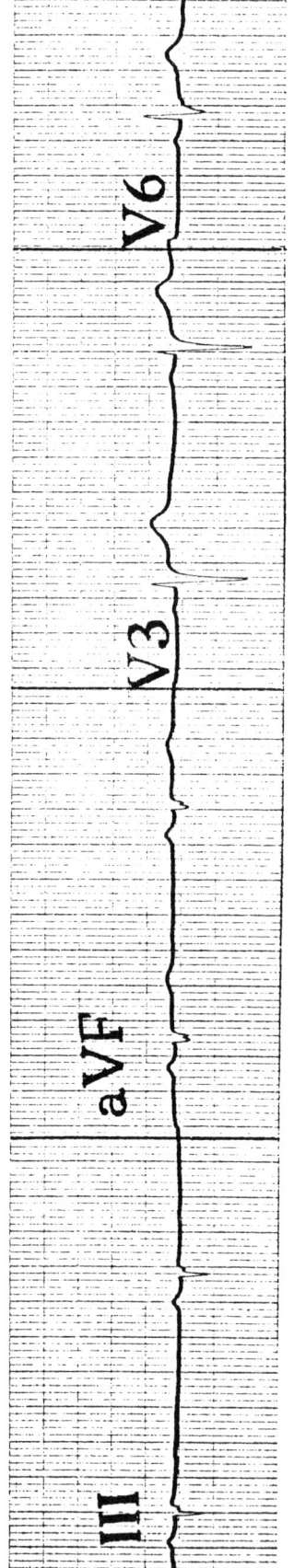

Figure 62-11 ECGs illustrating the phenomenon of postpacing T-wave changes. *Note:* These 12-lead ECGs were recorded from a 72-year-old woman before (*A*) and 1 week after (*B*) implantation of a permanent demand right ventricular endocardial pacing system. The nonspecific inversion of the T waves in leads II, III, aVF, and V_3 through V_6 suggests an interval ischemic process, although none had occurred. Such T-wave abnormalities occurring following a period of ventricular pacing are termed postpacing T-wave changes.

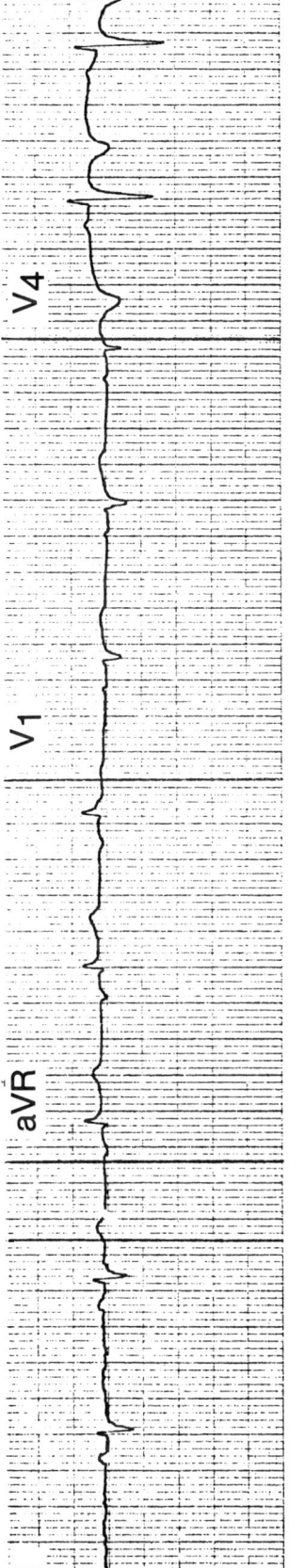
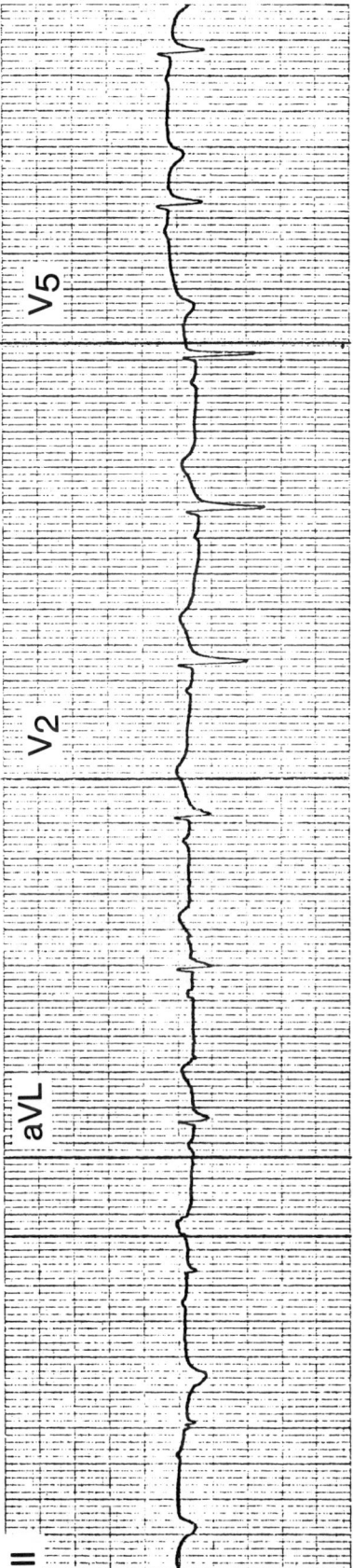
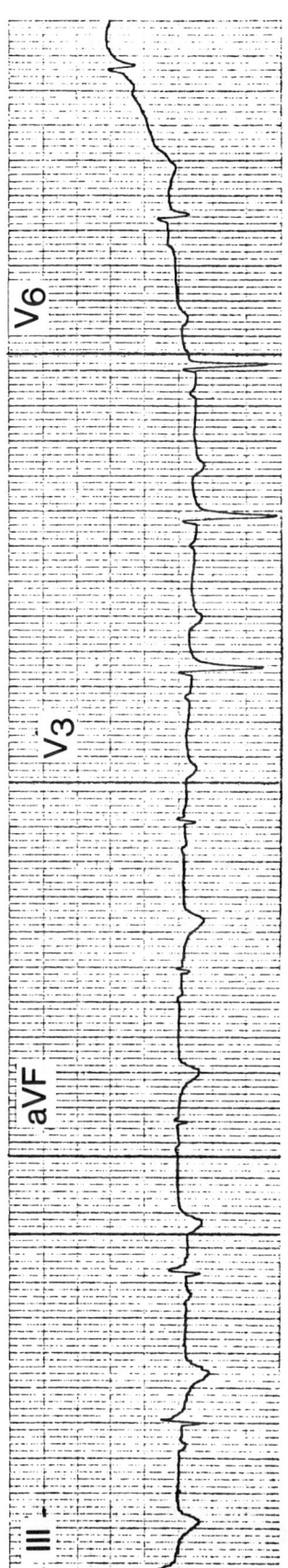

Figure 62-11 continued

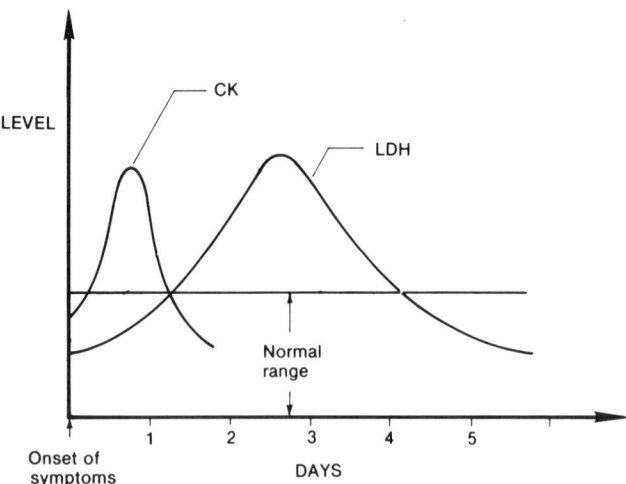

Figure 62-12 Time courses of serum enzyme levels in a patient with acute myocardial infarction.

to admit a patient to the hospital with a suspected acute myocardial infarction should not depend on the results of serum enzyme determinations alone.

EMERGENCY DEPARTMENT MANAGEMENT OF THE PATIENT WITH ACUTE MYOCARDIAL INFARCTION

Cardinal in the management of the patient with acute myocardial infarction is early consideration of the diagnosis, for the overwhelming majority of deaths from infarction occur within the first 3 to 4 hours of the onset of symptoms.

Clearly, a confident and reassuring manner on the part of the physician and other health care personnel who are attending the patient will be of inestimable value in the management of the patient's anxiety and discomfort. The physician should discuss the suspected diagnosis with the patient in simple terms, stating that, since the patient is in the hospital and under close observation, the outlook for survival and meaningful recovery is excellent. It should be explained that medications will be given to relieve the symptoms until they disappear spontaneously within the ensuing 12 to 24 hours and that plans are being made for admission to the coronary care unit as soon as practical. The usual treatments and environment to which the patient will be subjected in the coronary care unit should also be discussed. Once the diagnosis has been established or is considered likely, attention must be directed toward (1) reestablishment of blood flow in the infarct-related artery by the administration of a thrombolytic agent; (2) minimization of infarct size by the administration of nitrates and beta blockers; (3) detection and treatment of dysrhythmias; (4) relief of symptoms; and (5) maintenance of adequate circulation.

REESTABLISHMENT OF BLOOD FLOW IN THE INFARCT-RELATED ARTERY

Coronary angiograms performed in patients in the first few hours of the onset of symptoms of acute myocardial infarction have demonstrated total occlusion of most of the arteries perfusing the infarcting myocardium and subtotal occlusion in most of the remainder. Intracoronary administration of nitroglycerine has effected the opening of only a small minority (less than 5%) of such acutely occluded vessels, suggesting that coronary vasospasm is not a critically important mechanism of the occlusion. However, thrombolytic agents have been demonstrated to effect restoration of blood flow in the majority (about 75%) of totally occluded arteries in this setting, suggesting that thrombosis is the major event precipitating acute myocardial infarction. When administered intravenously, streptokinase, and the two other currently available thrombolytic agents, recombinant tissue type plasminogen activator (r-TPA, Activase®) and APSAC (anistreplase, EMINASE®), will achieve reperfusion of 60% to 80% of infarct-related arteries and will result in reductions in infarct size; incidences of cardiogenic shock, ventricular tachycardia, and ventricular fibrillation; and rates of mortality. The earlier the thrombolytic agent is given, the better the results will be. Thus, thrombolytic therapy has become an essential part of the emergency department management of patients with acute myocardial infarction.

Patients with symptoms of acute myocardial infarction and ECG abnormalities suggesting epicardial injury (Figs. 62-2, 62-3, 62-8, 62-13, and 62-15) may be given sublingual or intravenous nitroglycerine. If symptoms and ECG abnormalities do not resolve within minutes, such patients may be given thrombolytic therapy, so long as they do not have contraindications to the use of such drugs, such as recent intracerebral processes (eg, stroke, tumor, brain surgery), recent operations or trauma of any sort, or bleeding diatheses due to hematologic or other processes (peptic ulcer, hematuria, etc). Streptokinase, the least expensive of these agents, but the one most likely to cause significant hypotension, may be given intravenously in a dose of 750,000 to 1,500,000 units over 30 to 60 minutes, but many cardiologists feel that such patients should be given diphenhydramine (Benadryl®) and a corticosteroid intravenously before the streptokinase is given to minimize the effects of possible allergic reaction. The most expensive, least allergenic, and possibly the most effective of these three agents, r-TPA, may be given intravenously in a 6 to 10 mg "push" dose, followed by 50 to 54 mg over the next 1 hour, and 40 mg over the ensuing 2 hours. Anistreplase, the most recently released of these agents, may be given intravenously over a period of 2 to 5 minutes. Many authorities also recommend having all patients who are to receive thrombolytic therapy chew a 325 mg aspirin tablet as soon as the decision to use thrombolytic therapy is made, since ongoing studies suggest that aspirin minimizes the incidence of coronary artery reocclusion after successful thrombolysis.

If a diagnosis of acute myocardial infarction can be accurately established and patients accurately evaluated in the prehospital phase, thrombolytic therapy will probably become a routine part of the prehospital management of patients with this potentially devastating event.

Patency of acutely totally occluded coronary arteries can also be achieved mechanically in the majority of instances by percutaneous transluminal coronary angioplasty (PTCA). However, studies of immediate PTCA performed in the presence of thrombolytic therapy have demonstrated that patient survival and infarct size are not better than, and may be worse than, when thrombolytic therapy is used alone. Studies comparing the results of PTCA alone with those of thrombolytic therapy alone are now underway.

MINIMIZATION OF INFARCT SIZE

Nitroglycerin

The effects of nitroglycerin in patients with acute myocardial infarction have been clearly defined. When administered sublingually, this medication may act in one or two ways: (1) it may dilate systemic veins, causing venous pooling and decreased venous return to the heart; (2) it may dilate coronary arteries and thereby, perhaps, relieve obstruction in a vessel that has been totally occluded by a functional constriction in an area of severe anatomical stenosis. The systemic venodilating effect tends to decrease myocardial oxygen demand by decreasing preload and wall tension; the coronary arterial dilating effect tends to increase coronary blood flow. Both effects should be beneficial to the patient with acute myocardial infarction. When administered intravenously, nitroglycerin may additionally effect arteriolar dilatation. The potential risks of nitroglycerin administration are hypotension and vasovagal episodes, both of which may unpredictably accompany its use. It is still unclear whether nitroglycerin contributes to relief of chest discomfort associated with acute myocardial infarction, although it does help to relieve chest discomfort due to reversible myocardial ischemia (ie, angina pectoris). Its cautious use in acute myocardial infarction has become routine since its effectiveness in reducing mortality in acute myocardial infarction has been established.[6]

Beta-blocking drugs are competitive inhibitors of catecholamines with $beta_1$ and $beta_2$ properties. Their cardiovascular effects include effecting slower heart rate by depressing sinus node function, depressing AV nodal function, decreasing contractile state, and lowering the blood pressure. Beta-blocking drugs have been demonstrated to decrease the size of an acute myocardial infarction and the incidences of ventricular tachycardia and ventricular fibrillation and to increase the survival of patients with an acute myocardial infarction. These medications are most useful and least risky for acute myocardial infarction patients with hypertension, sinus tachycardia, high cardiac output, and reasonably well-preserved left ventricular function. They are ill-advised in the settings of slow sinus rates, AV nodal conduction disturbances, congestive heart failure, and significantly depressed left ventricular function. They are clearly contraindicated in patients with active bronchospastic lung disease. Lopressor, a $beta_1$ selective blocking agent that is the most commonly used beta blocker in acute myocardial infarction, is generally administered in 5-mg boluses IV 5 minutes apart for a total dose of 15 mg, as long as adverse effects do not occur during its administration. This medication is probably most effective if used as early as possible.

MANAGEMENT OF DYSRHYTHMIAS

Because dysrhythmia is the most common cause of death from acute myocardial infarction, the cardiac rhythm must be continuously monitored. Intravenous access should be achieved immediately in case rapid antiarrhythmic medication administration is subsequently required. An electrical defibrillator should be positioned in close proximity to the patient. (See Chapter 68, Cardiopulmonary Resuscitation.)

Although initial experiences with cardiac rhythm monitoring of patients with acute myocardial infarction suggested that the occurrence of ventricular tachycardia and ventricular fibrillation could be anticipated from the occurrence of premature ventricular complexes, more recent studies suggest that they more commonly occur without any "warning" dysrhythmia. This has prompted the practice of administering prophylactic lidocaine to all patients with documented or strongly suspected acute myocardial infarction. However, since subsequent studies have shown a statistically significant increase in mortality in patients given lidocaine prophylactically, the routine administration of this drug in acute myocardial infarction is thought to be ill-advised.[8] However, if premature ventricular complexes do occur, and especially if they are frequent, or occur in pairs or runs, lidocaine is administered intravenously (IV) in an initial bolus dose of 1 to 1.5 mg/kg over approximately 1 to 3 minutes; then an IV infusion of about 30 µg/kg/minute is started. For the average 70-kg person, this translates into an initial dose of 70 to 100 mg and a continuous infusion of about 2 mg/minute. Lidocaine in these doses may prevent the occurrence of ventricular tachycardia and fibrillation without much risk of serious side effects.

If premature ventricular complexes persist despite these doses of lidocaine, a repeat bolus of 1 to 1.5 mg/kg (70 to 100 mg) over 1 to 3 minutes and an increase in the rate of infusion to about 55 µg/kg/minute (4 mg/minute) is advised. However, these quantities of lidocaine may induce serious side effects, such as tinnitus, acute loss of hearing, diplopia, blurred vision, paresthesias, lightheadedness, disorientation, twitching, convulsions, respiratory depression, and hypotension.

If premature ventricular complexes or brief (ie, several seconds) runs of ventricular tachycardia occur even after the patient has received the above-mentioned doses of lidocaine, then procainamide is administered intravenously in a loading dose of about 5 to 15 mg/kg (350 to 1000 mg for the 70-kg person) at a rate of about 25 to 50 mg/minute. After the loading dose has been given, the procainamide may be administered by continuous IV infusion at a rate of about 30 to 40 µg/kg/minute (2 to 3 mg/minute for the 70-kg person). Usually, the only serious side effect encountered with the IV administration of procainamide is hypotension. As the hypotension is usually due to vasodilatation, it is generally successfully reversed by slowing the rate at which the medication is being given or by stopping it altogether. In rare instances, however, restoration of adequate blood pressure may require the administration of IV fluids or vasoconstrictor-positive inotropic medications, such as dopamine, dobutamine, and norepinephrine.

If ventricular tachycardia occurs prior to the administration of antidysrhythmic medication, the lidocaine or procainamide should be administered in the previously discussed dosages so long as the patient's hemodynamic state is adequate. During this time, a sharp blow may be given to the precordium, for this maneuver occasionally terminates ventricular tachycardia. If ventricular tachycardia persists despite the IV administration of lidocaine and procainamide, and despite the precordial blow, then direct current cardioversion is in order. The patient should be given the minimum amount of IV diazepam (Valium), Midazolam (Versed), or thiopental (Pentothal) needed to achieve amnesia. If the patient is hemodynamically stable, a 10 to 50 watt-second electrical discharge synchronized to the QRS complex may be applied across the chest, as it will usually terminate the ventricular tachycardia and restore sinus rhythm. However, if ventricular tachycardia is causing severe hemodynamic deterioration, a 400 watt-second *nonsynchronized* discharge should be applied across the chest. If this shock precipitates ventricular fibrillation, the ventricular fibrillation can usually be terminated by immediately repeating the 400 watt-second nonsynchronized discharge.

If ventricular fibrillation that occurs spontaneously or in response to an attempted electrical termination of ventricular tachycardia cannot be terminated with repeated 400 watt-second nonsynchronized electrical discharges, then chemical defibrillation may be attempted by giving bretylium tosylate (Bretylol), 5 to 10 mg/kg (about 350 to 700 mg for the 70-kg person), IV as rapidly as possible while the patient is treated for cardiac arrest with closed chest cardiac massage, respiratory support, correction of metabolic abnormalities, and repeated precordial shocks. If ventricular fibrillation still cannot be terminated, or if it recurs after initial termination, another dose of bretylium, 5 mg/kg (about 350 mg), may be given IV as rapidly as possible. Doses of up to 10 mg/kg (about 700 mg) may be given rapidly every 15 to 30 minutes, up to a total dose of 30 mg/kg (about 2100 mg) before the medication is considered ineffective.

Bretylium tosylate may also be useful in preventing and treating premature ventricular contractions (PVCs), and in preventing recurrences of ventricular tachycardia and ventricular fibrillation when lidocaine and procainamide fail to do so. In this situation, it is recommended that a loading dose of 5 to 10 mg/kg (350 to 700 mg) be given IV over a period of more than 8 minutes; the slow rate of administration is aimed at minimizing the nausea and vomiting that may occur with more rapid injection. Maintenance dosage may be given by continuous IV infusion at rates of 1 to 2 mg/minute or by six hourly boluses of 5 to 10 mg/kg (350 to 700 mg) over a period of more than 8 minutes.

Bretylium tosylate administration may initially result in transient increases in blood pressure and ventricular ectopy, usually lasting for periods of several minutes. The drug's most serious undesirable effect is significant hypotension, which may occur with dosages inadequate for suppression of ventricular dysrhythmias; since this effect is due to vasodilatation, it is often exacerbated by the upright position. For these reasons, it seems prudent to restrict use of this medication to the treatment of hospitalized patients, except in the prehospital treatment of intractable and recurrent ventricular fibrillation.

Slowing of the sinus rate often occurs within minutes to hours after the onset of acute myocardial infarction involving, usually, the inferior wall of the heart. The mechanism is presumably enhanced parasympathetic input into the sinus node, for appropriate acceleration of sinus rate usually follows atropine administration. Therefore, if slow sinus rates are contributing to inappropriately low cardiac output or blood pressure, or to the predisposition to ventricular dysrhythmias, atropine may be administered rapidly IV in doses of 0.5 to 2 mg. A few reported instances in which ventricular fibrillation occurred soon after the IV administration of atropine to patients with acute myocardial infarction should not preclude the use of this medication when slow heart rates are responsible for significant problems.[9] If cardiac standstill (an event that carries about an 85% mortality) occurs, the treatment of cardiac arrest should be commenced.

Disadvantageously slow ventricular rates may also occur in the early hours of acute myocardial infarction because of second- and third-degree atrioventricular block. The appearance of second-degree atrioventricular block heralds the onset of complete atrioventricular block, which may occur within minutes to hours. In inferior wall infarction, the site of atrioventricular block is usually the atrioventricular node, and the second-degree atrioventricular block is of the Mobitz Type I (Wenckebach) variety; during complete atrioventricular block, the emerging escape pacemaker usually originates within the atrioventricular junction (His bundle) and has an automatic rate of about 35 to 45 beats/minute (Figs. 62-13 and 62-14). If the ventricular rate occurring during the second- or third-degree AV block in inferior wall myocardial infarction is judged to be inadequately slow, atropine, 0.5 to 2 mg IV "push," or isoproterenol, 0.5 to 4 µg/minute by continuous IV infusion may be administered. Either medication may effect either an improvement in atrioventricular conduction or a mild to modest acceleration of the junctional rhythm. However, serious consideration should be given to establishing temporary demand ventricular pacing, which is the safest and most effective therapeutic modality for ensuring adequate ventricular rates in this setting in which the conduction disturbance is almost always transient and the left ventricular performance is not usually severely depressed.

In anterior wall myocardial infarction, the sites of second- and third-degree atrioventricular block are usually the proximal portions of the bundle branches that lie within the infarcting myocardium. The second-degree atrioventricular block is Mobitz Type II; during complete atrioventricular block, the emerging escape pacemaker originates in the distal portion of a bundle branch or fascicle, or in Purkinje fibers, and usually has a dangerously slow rate of about 20 to 40 beats/minute (Fig. 62-15). While isoproterenol administered in doses of 0.5 to 4 µg/minute by continuous IV infusion may rarely improve atrioventricular conduction or increase the rate of the escape pacemaker to an adequate level, this medication should be used only as a temporizing measure—a temporary ventricular pacing system should be established with dispatch. The majority of patients with anterior wall myocardial infarction complicated by complete atrioventricular block have cardiogenic shock related to extensive myocardial necrosis; thus, the mortality rate in these patients is high even when bradycardia is prevented by pacing.

In complete heart block with depressed left ventricular function in acute inferior or anterior wall myocardial infarction, sychronized atrial and ventricular (ie, dual chamber), pacing may be more hemodynamically advantageous than ventricular pacing alone.

MANAGEMENT OF SYMPTOMS

Most patients with acute myocardial infarction suffer chest discomfort that may be only bothersome, but more commonly is quite severe. Relief of the discomfort and alleviation of the anxiety that usually accompany acute myocardial infarction are important not only for humanitarian reasons, but also for medical reasons. A reduction in pain and anxiety results in a decrease in the secretion of catecholamines, which predispose to dysrhythmias and increase myocardial oxygen demand by increasing heart rate, contractile state, and wall tension (via their peripheral vasoconstrictive effects).

Morphine sulfate continues to be the most widely used analgesic for patients with acute myocardial infarction and is generally administered IV in doses of 2 to 3 mg every 4 to 5 minutes until pain relief is adequate or until blood pressure falls to undesirably low levels. Usually, 8 to 25 mg are required as an effective initial dose. Meperidine hydrochloride (Demerol) is also widely used in this setting and is generally administered IV in doses of 15 to 20 mg every 4 to 5 minutes to the same end points. Both morphine sulfate and Demerol must be used with great caution in patients who have hypotension and/or bradycardia, for these medications may exacerbate the abnormalities. Furthermore, presumably because of their effects on vagal nuclei, both medications may result in bradycardia, hypotension, nausea, and vomiting. These drug-induced problems can generally be reversed within seconds to minutes by the IV administration of atropine in doses of 0.5 to 2 mg. Atropine appears to be more effective than the phenothiazine antiemetic medications in abolishing nausea related to the administration of morphine and Demerol; clinical experience suggests that this medication does not measurably increase the predisposition to ventricular tachycardia and fibrillation.

Diazepam (Valium) may be useful in the management of the patient who manifests an unacceptably high level of anxiety despite adequate relief of chest discomfort. In the acute situation, this medication may be administered IV in doses of 1 to 5 mg at a rate no more than 1 mg every 2 to 3 minutes. More rapid IV administration may result in hypotension, respiratory arrest, obtundation, and undesirably long periods of oversedation. In the less acute situation, Valium may be given orally in doses of 2 to 10 mg, depending on the level of anxiety, the age of the patient, the presence of associated diseases that might alter metabolism of the medication, and the hemodynamic state.

Currently, the sublingual, transcutaneous, and IV administration of nitroglycerin is gaining wider usage in patients with acute myocardial infarction. The theory is that nitroglycerin may favorably alter the balance between myocardial oxygen supply and demand and thereby diminish the area of myocardial ischemia and the chest discomfort related to the ischemia. While the beneficial effect of nitroglycerin in the relief of chest discomfort due to reversible myocardial ischemia is clearly documented, its effectiveness in relieving chest discomfort in patients with acute myocardial infarction is still unclear.

MAINTENANCE OF ADEQUATE CIRCULATION

The prime function of the cardiovascular system is to provide adequate blood flow at appropriate perfusion pressure to the tissues of the body. The cardiac output (ie, the volume of blood ejected into the circulation by the heart in a minute's time) is the product of the stroke volume (ie, the

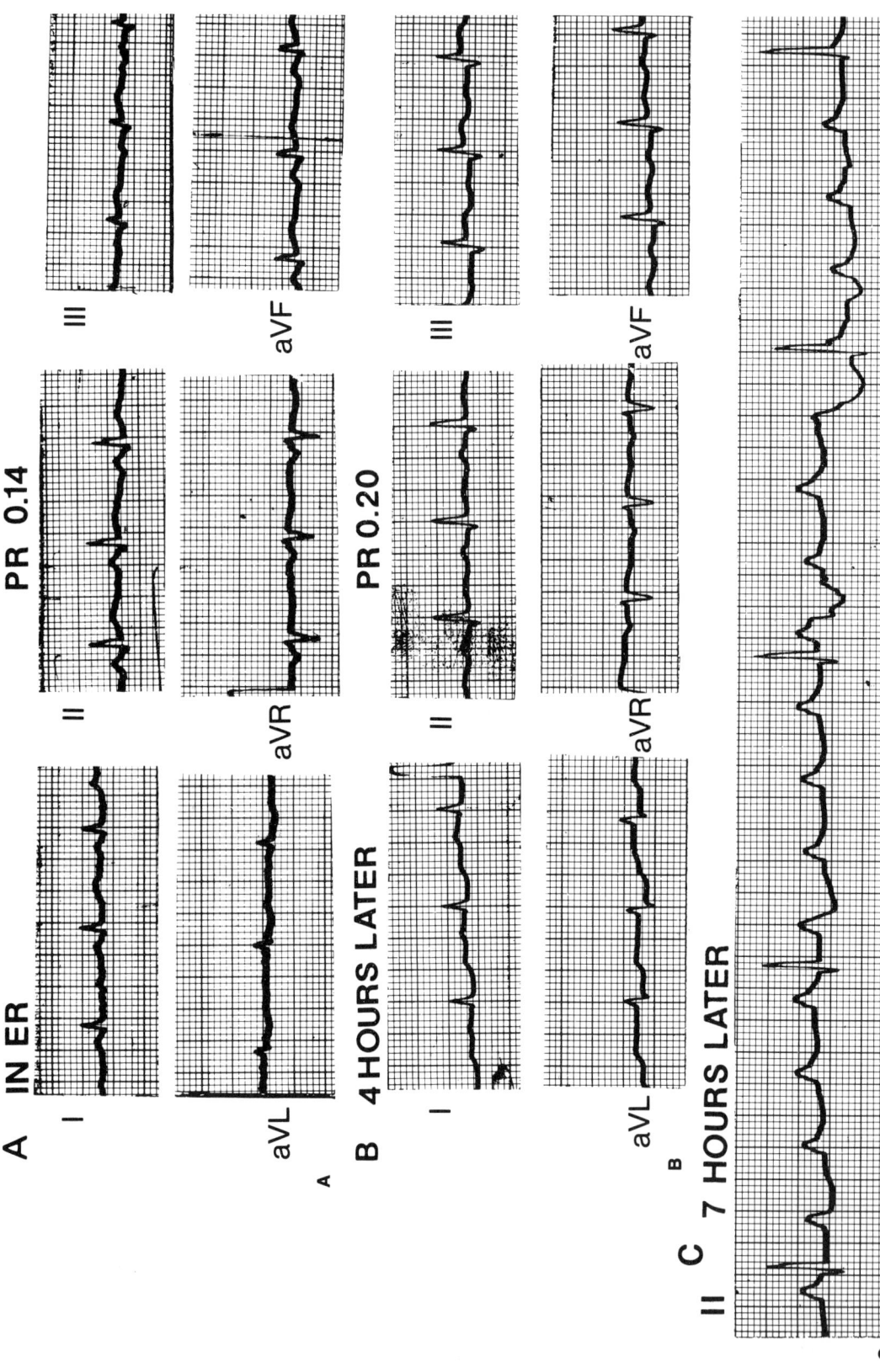

Figure 62-13 ECGs from a patient with acute inferior wall myocardial infarction. *Note:* These ECGs were recorded from a 44-year-old man with an acute inferior wall myocardial infarction. *A:* When the patient was first seen in the emergency department, there were mild ST segment elevations in leads II and III, and mild ST segment depressions in leads V_2 and V_3, compatible with an acute ischemic process. *B:* The same leads, recorded 4 hours later, show more dramatic ST segment abnormalities and document an increase in the PR interval from 0.14 to 0.20 seconds. *C:* Seven hours later, there is complete atrioventricular block with a junctional rhythm occurring at a rate of about 31 beats/minute. The sinus rate is now very rapid, about 130 beats/minute, because atropine and isoproterenol have been administered in an unsuccessful attempt to improve AV conduction and to increase the rate of the junctional rhythm.

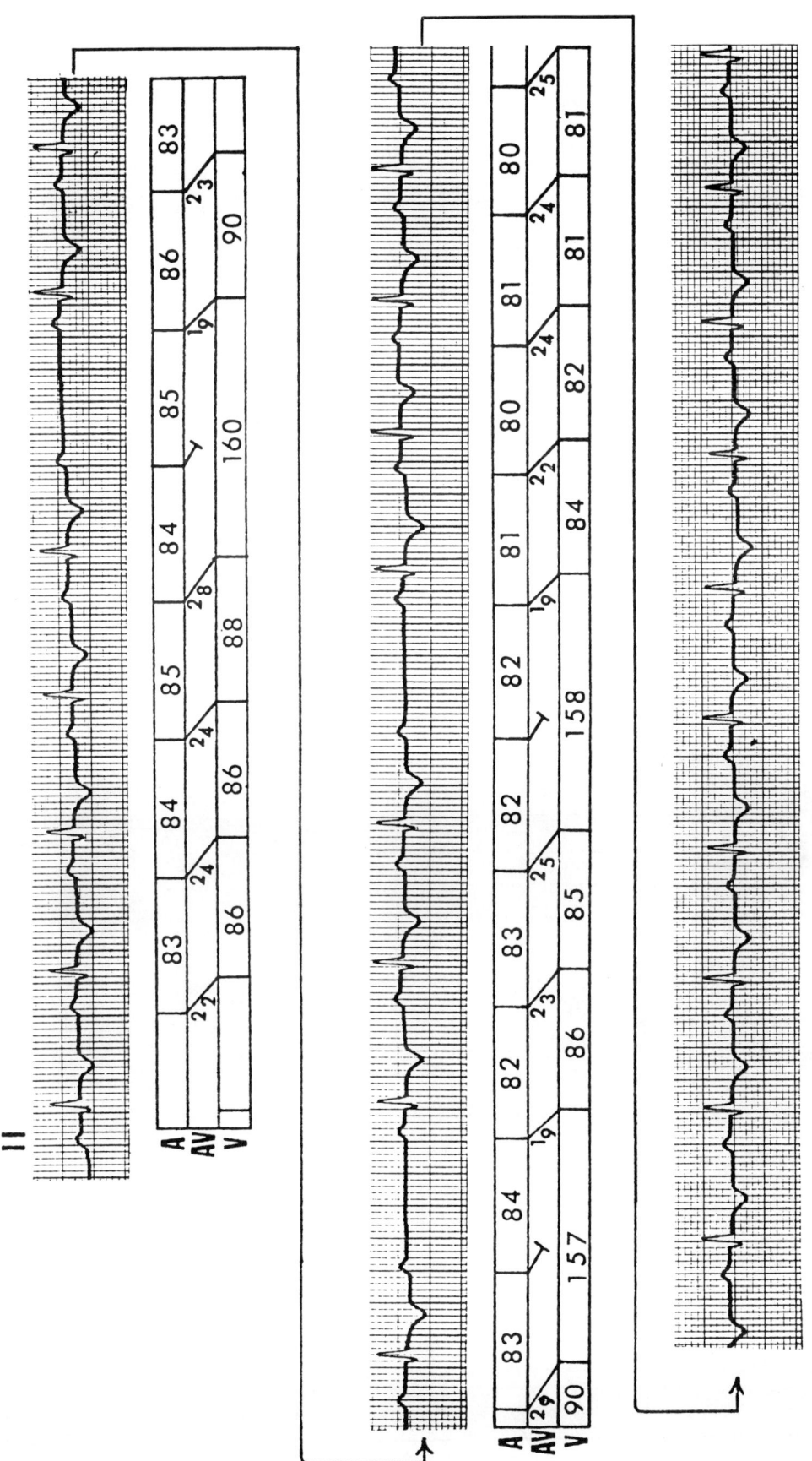

Figure 62-14 AV Wenckebach periods occurring in a man with an inferior wall myocardial infarction. *Note:* These three continuous strips were recorded 9 days later from the same patient whose ECGs are displayed in Figure 62-13. Atrioventricular conduction has returned, but there are periods of Mobitz Type I (Wenckebach) second-degree atrioventricular block. *Source:* Reprinted by permission of Elsevier Science Publishing Co Inc from Jacobson LB, Goldschlager N: *Arrhythmias: Case Studies.* Copyright 1978 by Medical Examination Publishing Co Inc.

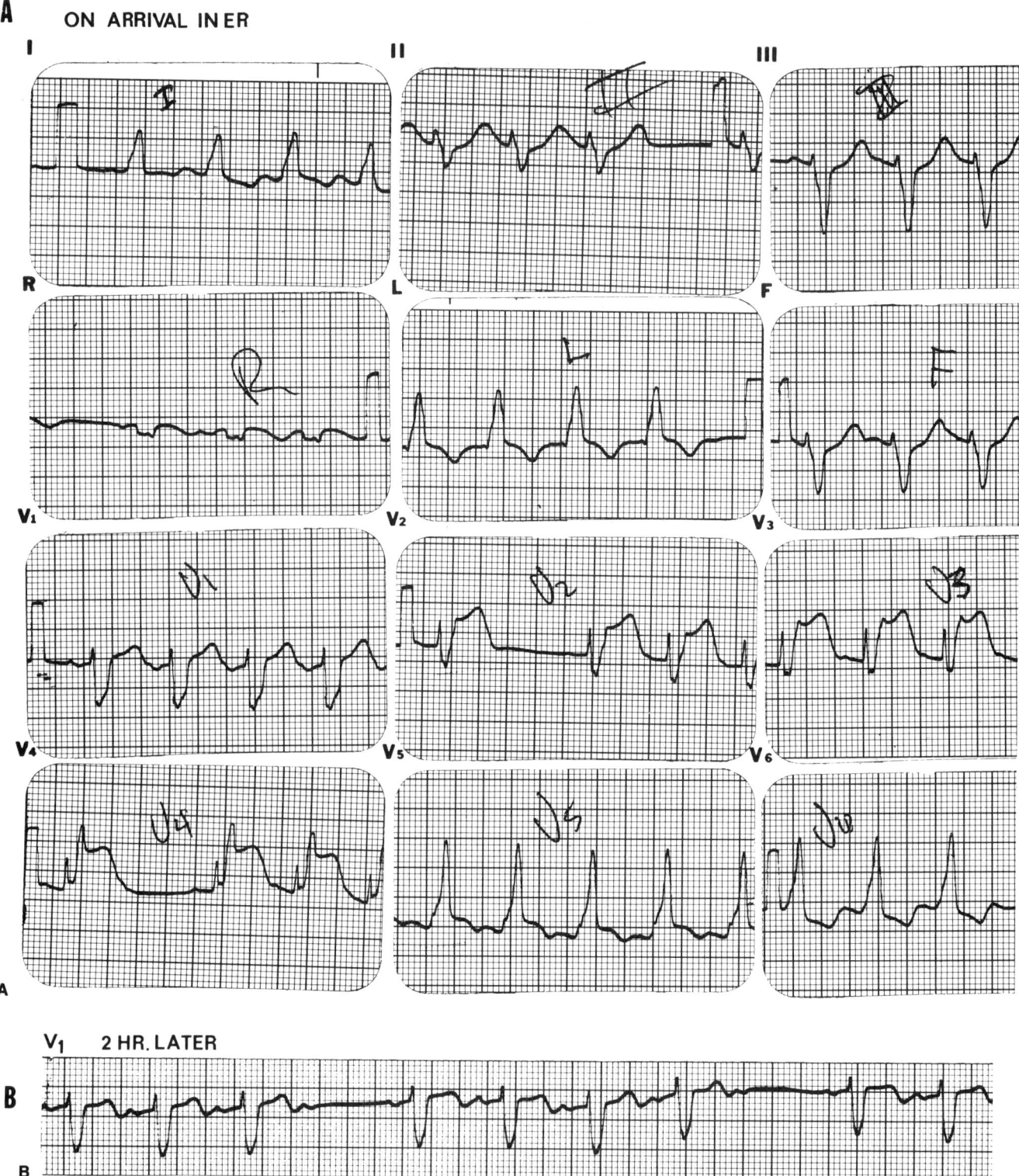

Figure 62-15 ECGs from a patient with acute anterior wall myocardial infarction. *Note:* These ECGs were recorded from a 72-year-old woman with acute anterior wall myocardial infarction. *A:* This 12-lead ECG, which was recorded shortly after the patient's arrival in the emergency department, shows an extensive anterior wall injury pattern, suggesting the acute infarction. In addition, there is left bundle branch block with left axis deviation and pauses in QRS rhythm due to Mobitz Type II second-degree atrioventricular block. *B:* Two hours later, the sinus rate is slightly slower, allowing the Mobitz Type II block to be seen more clearly. *C:* Six hours later, there is complete atrioventricular block with a ventricular escape rhythm occurring at a rate of about 58 beats/minute. The somewhat rapid rate of this escape rhythm (which, showing a right bundle branch block pattern, probably originates near the left bundle branch) is probably contributed to by the high doses of isoproterenol and dopamine that the patient was receiving to support her circulation.

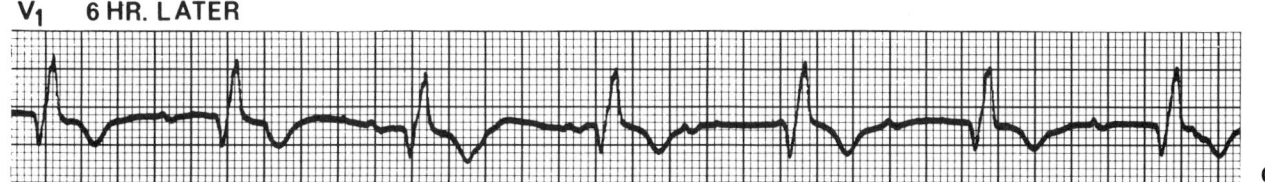

Figure 62-15 continued

volume of blood ejected by the left ventricle with each systole) and the heart rate. The systemic arterial blood pressure is the product of the cardiac output and the total systemic arterial resistance (TSR). The complex mechanisms that regulate heart rate, stroke volume, and TSR may be dramatically altered by endogenous physiologic events such as occur with acute myocardial infarction and by therapeutic interventions.

In sinus rhythm, heart rate depends on the intrinsic function of the sinus node and on the responses of the sinus node to neurohumoral autonomic nervous system traffic. Sympathetic stimuli increase and parasympathetic stimuli decrease the automatic firing rate of the sinus node, while beta-adrenergic blocking agents slow and parasympatholytic agents accelerate it. Thus, heart rate can be altered by modifying the autonomic milieu.

TSR is determined by the sum total of the cross-sectional areas of arterioles perfusing all body tissues. The size of an arteriole perfusing a particular tissue is regulated by the relative influences of vasoconstrictor and vasodilator stimuli acting in response to events that may originate within or distant from the particular tissue. As the stimuli mediating local vascular events may be neurohumoral transmitters (eg, adrenalin, noradrenalin, acetylcholine) released by the autonomic nervous system or vasoactive materials (eg, adenosine, histamine, hydrogen ion, potassium, angiotensin) produced by metabolic events, therapeutic alteration of TSR generally involves the administration of medications that antagonize the effects of endogenous vasoactive materials.

Left ventricular performance has three major determinants: (1) the preload, (2) the contractile state, and (3) the afterload. The preload is the size, or volume, of the left ventricle at end diastole, when the myocardium begins to develop its systolic tension. The end diastolic volume is highly dependent on the circulating blood volume, the systemic venous tone, and the TSR, the diastolic volume being higher when blood volume is elevated and venous tone and TSR are high and lower when blood volume is decreased and venous tone and TSR are low. The contractile state of the left ventricular myocardium will be defined below. The afterload is the tension that the left ventricular myocardium must generate in order to open the aortic valve and eject blood into the aorta. Left ventricular wall tension is inversely proportional to the thickness of the left ventricular myocardium, and it is directly proportional to the product of the pressure generated by the left ventricle and its radius during preejection and ejection periods. Because left ventricular wall tension is related to the size of the left ventricle, it follows that afterload is dependent on preload. Furthermore, as the pressure that the left ventricle must generate is directly related to the diastolic pressure in the aorta at the onset of ejection, it follows that afterload is highly dependent on TSR.

The relationship of stroke volume to preload, contractile state, and afterload is shown in the ventricular function curves of Figs. 62-16 through 62-18. In Fig. 62-16, the contractile state of the left ventricle is defined in terms of stroke volume and end diastolic volume. At any end diastolic volume, the greater the stroke volume, the better the contractile state of the left ventricle. Figure 62-16 also illustrates the Frank-Starling phenomenon, that stroke volume increases with increments in end diastolic volume in both normal and depressed contractile states. However, for a given increment in end diastolic volume, the increment in stroke volume is greater with better contractile function.

Acute myocardial ischemia and infarction, by reducing the amount of functioning left ventricular myocardium, depresses left ventricular performance; the left ventricle then operates on a ventricular function curve that lies below that on which it was operating prior to the ischemic event. The degree of depression of left ventricular performance is generally proportional to the amount of infarcted tissue, although the location of the infarction also appears to be important. Patients with anterior wall infarction appear to have a greater degree of depression of left ventricular performance than patients with inferior wall infarction of comparable magnitude, as estimated by CKMB determinations and by histopathologic and histochemical studies. This difference in degree of depression in left ventricular performance seemingly related to the location of the infarct more likely reflects the fact that in an anterior wall infarction, the process involves almost exclusively left ventricular myocardium, while in inferior wall infarction there is less left ventricular involvement and more right ventricular involvement, the latter rarely of significant magnitude to cause clinically significant right ventricular dysfunction.

The closed circles in the normal and depressed ventricular functional curves of Fig. 62-16 represent the stroke volume and end diastolic volume usually present in the basal resting state of patients with normal and chronically depressed left ventricular contractile function. The left ventricle with

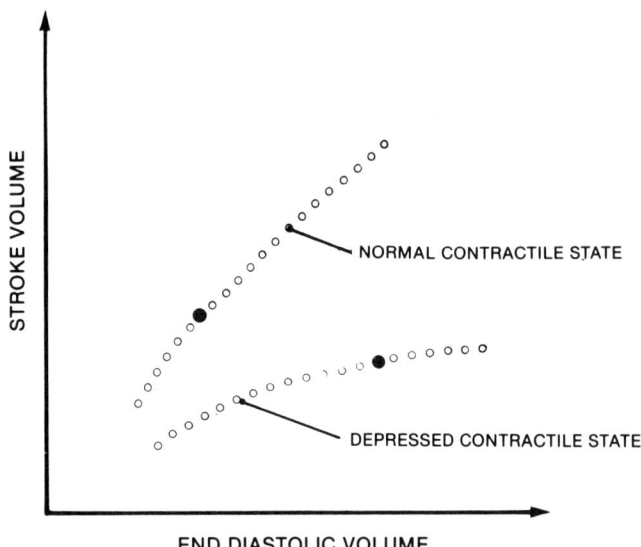

Figure 62-16 Ventricular function curves. *Note:* Ventricular function curves, constructed by plotting left ventricular stroke volume as a function of left ventricular end diastolic volume, illustrate the Frank-Starling mechanism of cardiac performance and define the contractile state of the left ventricle. The function curve of the left ventricle with depressed contractile state is flatter than and lies below that of the left ventricle with normal contractile state. The large, closed circles on each curve represent the stroke volume and end diastolic volume at which left ventricles with normal and depressed contractile states usually function in the basal resting state. The left ventricle with depressed contractile state usually operates at a higher end diastolic volume yet ejects a smaller stroke volume than the left ventricle with normal contractile state.

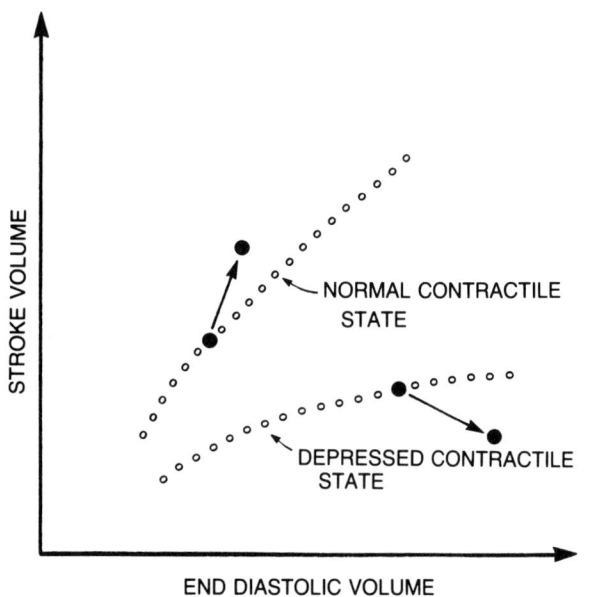

Figure 62-17 Ventricular function curves showing the effects of increasing afterload on the relationship of stroke volume to end diastolic volume. *Note:* Ventricular function curves showing the effects of increasing afterload (by increasing arteriolar resistance) on end diastolic volume (EDV) and stroke volume (SV). Regardless of the contractile state of the left ventricle, increasing the afterload results in a larger end diastolic volume. However, whereas the increment in end diastolic volume effects an increase in stroke volume if the left ventricle has normal contractile function, it effects a decrease in stroke volume if the left ventricle has depressed contractile function.

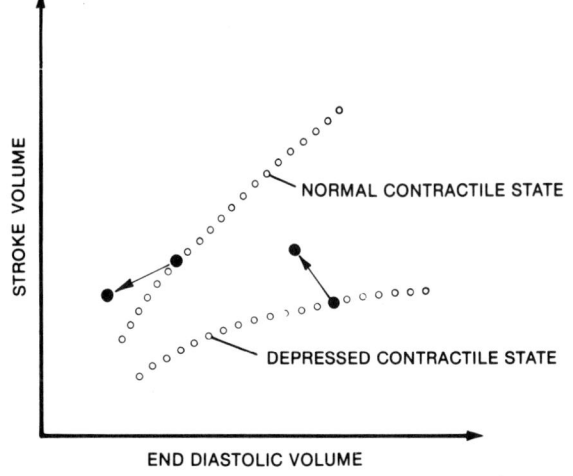

Figure 62-18 Ventricular function curves showing the effects of decreasing afterload on the relationship of stroke volume to end diastolic volume. *Note:* Ventricular function curves showing the effects of decreasing afterload (by decreasing arteriolar resistance) on EDV and SV. Regardless of the contractile state of the left ventricle, decreasing afterload results in a smaller end diastolic volume. However, whereas the decrement in end diastolic volume effects a slight decrease in stroke volume when left ventricular contractile state is normal, it effects an increase in stroke volume when left ventricular contractile state is depressed.

depressed contractile state generally performs at an end diastolic volume that is much larger than normal, yet ejects a stroke volume that is somewhat less than normal. Presumably, the left ventricle operates at the larger end diastolic volume in an attempt to normalize stroke volume. However, functioning at high end diastolic volume has deleterious consequences. Figure 62-19 displays the exponential relationship of diastolic left ventricular pressure to the diastolic volume of the chamber. When the left ventricular diastolic volume is normal, left ventricular diastolic pressure is low. As diastolic volume increases above normal, the diastolic pressure rises; the greater the initial volume, the greater will be the increment in pressure for a given increment in volume. At high diastolic volume, even small increments in volume result in dramatic rises in diastolic pressure to extremely high levels. As pressure in the pulmonary veins must exceed the diastolic left ventricular pressure if blood is to flow in the proper direction, the pulmonary venous pressure may rise to levels at which pulmonary congestion and pulmonary edema occur.

The exponential shape of the diastolic pressure-volume curve has important therapeutic implications, for at very high filling pressures even small decrements in diastolic volume, which may be achieved by venodilatation, diuresis, phlebotomy, or reduction in TSR, dramatically decrease left ventricular diastolic and pulmonary venous pressures. Acute myocardial infarction generally causes a shift of the left ventricular diastolic pressure-volume curve upward and to the left. The magnitude of the displacement is roughly proportional to the magnitude of infarcted tissue. Thus, at any given diastolic volume, diastolic pressure is higher with an ischemic event than it was prior to the event. The larger the infarcted area, the greater the increment in pressure.

The ventricular function curves in Fig. 62-17 display the relationships of stroke volume and end diastolic volume to increases in afterload achieved by raising TSR. Such increases in afterload effect increases in end diastolic volume regardless of the contractile state of the left ventricle. However, the rise in end diastolic volume is accompanied by an increase in stroke volume when contractile state is normal, but by a decrease in stroke volume when contractile state is depressed. Reducing afterload by lowering the TSR has the opposite effects, as shown in Fig. 62-18. While it results in a reduction in end diastolic volume, regardless of the contractile state, the reduction in end diastolic volume is accompanied by a fall in stroke volume when the contractile state is normal, and by a rise in stroke volume when the contractile state is depressed. Reducing TSR is the most effective intervention for lowering the diastolic pressure in and increasing the stroke volume from a left ventricle with depressed contractile state that is operating at high end diastolic volume.

Essential in the management of the patient with acute myocardial infarction is the achievement and maintenance of a hemodynamic state in which tissue perfusion is adequate and pulmonary venous pressure is not unduly elevated. The

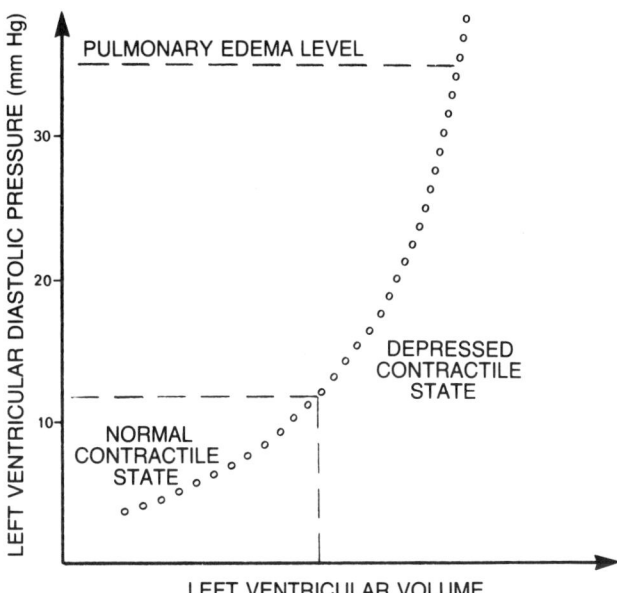

Figure 62-19 Exponential relationship of pressure to volume in the left ventricle during diastole. *Note:* The left ventricle with normal contractile state operates at lower diastolic volume and, therefore, at lower diastolic pressure than does the left ventricle with depressed contractile state. For a given increment in volume, the increment in pressure is greater if the initial volume is higher.

adequacy of tissue perfusion is generally assessed by measurement of the arterial blood pressure, palpation of the central (femoral and carotid) and peripheral (brachial, radial, tibial) pulses to determine their volume and contour, by examination of the skin on the trunk and on the extremities to assess its temperature and to observe its color, by verbal interaction with the patient to evaluate cerebral function (which reflects cerebral blood flow), and by measurement of urine output (which reflects renal perfusion). If the blood pressure is normal; the pulses of normal contour and volume; the skin pink, warm, and dry; the patient responding clearly and making urine, tissue perfusion may be judged to be adequate. On the other hand, if the blood pressure is low; the pulse thready; the skin pale, cool, and moist; the patient lethargic; and the urine output low, tissue perfusion is clearly inadequate.

Clinical assessment of the level of the pulmonary venous pressure is at best crude, as the physician is only able to observe the respiratory pattern and to examine the chest. Generally, if the respiratory pattern and the results of the chest examination are normal, the pulmonary venous pressure is probably not extremely high; if signs and symptoms of pulmonary edema are present, the pulmonary venous pressure is usually extremely elevated (greater than 30 mmHg). However, the respiratory pattern and the results of the chest examination may be normal when the pulmonary venous pressure is significantly elevated (25 to 30 mmHg) or even extremely low (less than 6 mmHg). Also, when cardiac output is very low, and especially if acidemia is present, a patient may be tachypneic and dyspneic even when the pulmonary venous pressure is very low. Furthermore, the chest radiograph is of relatively little value in assessing the pulmonary venous pressure, partly because radiologic abnormalities often do not appear until several hours after a rise in and do not disappear until several days after a fall in the pulmonary venous pressure. For these reasons, and because the pulmonary venous pressure may be dramatically and abruptly altered by spontaneous or therapy-induced changes in left ventricular performance, TSR, venous tone, and circulating blood volume, accurate measurements of pulmonary venous pressure require direct measurement of the pulmonary artery wedge pressure. For this purpose, a balloon-tipped end-hole catheter (eg, the Swan-Ganz catheter) is most commonly used. (See Chapter 86, Atlas of Emergency Procedures.)

Because the changes in hemodynamic state that accompany acute myocardial infarction depend on a multitude of interrelated factors, such as the circulating blood volume, the size of the infarction, the left ventricular performance prior to the event, and the autonomic nervous system responses to the event (ie, in terms of altering heart rate, systemic venous tone, and TSR), frequent thorough re-evaluations of the patient are essential.

MANAGEMENT OF HYPOTENSION AND INADEQUATE CARDIAC OUTPUT

Hypotension often occurs in the early hours of acute myocardial infarction, and its management depends on its mechanism. When hypotension reflects vasodilatation and bradycardia due to inappropriately high parasympathetic nervous system activity, atropine in doses of 1 to 2 mg IV usually resolves the problem. Leg raising and the IV administration of intravascular volume-expanding fluids, such as normal saline, are helpful when vasodilatation and/or volume depletion is the mechanism. When hypotension occurs in the presence of normal heart rate and normal to elevated circulating blood volume and venous tone, the hypotension presumably reflects depressed left ventricular performance. In this case, the cautious administration of dopamine (Intropin), a catecholamine with very strong alpha (ie, peripheral vasoconstricting), very strong beta$_1$ (ie, cardiac stimulating), and moderately strong beta$_2$ (ie, peripheral vasodilating) properties, may be used to raise the arterial blood pressure to an acceptable level. Dopamine is administered by continuous IV infusion, beginning with 2 to 5 μg/kg/minute (150 to 350 μg/minute) and increasing the dose every 1 to 2 minutes until either an acceptable arterial pressure is achieved or a dose of about 50 μg/kg/minute (3500 μg/minute) is reached. Higher doses do not generally improve the hemodynamic state and may predispose the patient to ventricular dysrhythmias. When hypotension persists despite an adequate heart rate, normal to high circulating blood volume, adequate venous tone, and the administration of dopamine, norepinephrine (Levophed) may be given.

Norepinephrine, a catecholamine with very strong alpha and beta$_1$ properties but no beta$_2$ activity, is administered by continuous IV infusion, starting with a dose of 1 to 2 μg/minute. The dose is increased by about 0.5 μg/minute every 3 to 4 minutes until either an adequate arterial blood pressure is achieved or a dose of 10 μg/minute is reached. Doses of norepinephrine in excess of 10 μg/minute are not likely to improve the hemodynamic state and may produce such severe vasoconstriction that the cardiac output falls and perfusion of vital organs is dramatically reduced. As both norepinephrine and dopamine may cause tissue necrosis if they extravasate, these medications are delivered into the central, rather than the peripheral, venous circulation.

Dobutamine (Dobutrex) is a synthetic catecholamine with very weak alpha, very strong beta$_1$, and moderately strong beta$_2$ properties. It has been shown to increase cardiac output and arterial blood pressure significantly when administered to patients who have low cardiac output and high intracardiac filling pressures in the settings of cardiac surgery and chronic left ventricular dysfunction of various etiologies.[10,11] While it has been documented to have similar beneficial effects in patients with acute myocardial infarction who are not hypotensive and whose cardiac outputs are not very low, documentation of its effects in acute myocardial infarction complicated by hypotension and severely depressed cardiac output is presently inadequate.[12] Normovolemic patients who remain hypotensive despite high doses of dopamine, dobutamine, and norepinephrine have a very poor prognosis, because left ventricular performance is usually severely depressed. But mechanical complications such as ventricular septal rupture, cardiac rupture, or acute severe mitral regurgitation may be the major factor responsible for the low blood pressure. These possibilities can usually be rapidly and accurately evaluated with 2-D echocardiography and Doppler studies.

A somewhat unusual case of hypotension and inadequate cardiac output in the presence of high systemic venous pressure is infarction involving predominantly right ventricular myocardium. In this instance, the pulmonary venous pressure may be very low, presumably because the right ventricle cannot adequately eject blood through the pulmonary circulation into the left ventricle. Management involves IV fluid administration in volumes that ensure enough blood is delivered to the left ventricle to increase the left ventricular stroke volume and the IV administration of dobutamine. Although the presence of right ventricular infarction can often be established in the first 10 hours of acute myocardial infarction by the finding of ST elevations of 0.1 mV or greater in the right precordial leads V3R or V4R, the diagnosis of right ventricular infarction as the cause of hypotension can be made *only* by direct measurements of intracardiac filling pressures. Acute right ventricular infarction occurs almost exclusively in patients having an acute *inferior* wall infarction.

MANAGEMENT OF CONGESTIVE HEART FAILURE

Acute myocardial ischemia and infarction may so profoundly depress left ventricular performance that left ventricular end diastolic pressure rises dramatically and results in pulmonary congestion or even pulmonary edema. The severe depression of left ventricular performance may be due to a very large area of ischemia in a previously normal heart or to a small area of ischemia in a heart that previously had been functioning poorly. Patients with severe pulmonary venous hypertension are generally tachypneic and dyspneic because the interstitial and intra-alveolar edema results in abnormal lung compliance. If pulmonary edema is severe, blood gas exchange may be markedly impaired, resulting in severe hypoxemia and even hypercapnia. Patients with congestive heart failure may have high, normal, or low cardiac output, depending on the circulating blood volume, the systemic vascular resistance, and the degree to which left ventricular function is depressed. Those with dramatically low cardiac output and high intracardiac filling pressure qualify as having cardiogenic shock. (See Chapter 64, Congestive Heart Failure.)

Treatment of the patient with pulmonary congestion involves ensuring adequate blood gases by the administration of

1. supplemental inspired oxygen
2. diuretics (such as Lasix, 20- to 80-mg IV push) in order to decrease the circulating blood volume, lower intracardiac filling pressures, and draw the intra-alveolar and pulmonary interstitial fluid back into the circulation
3. venodilators (such as sublingually administered nitroglycerin or isosorbide dinitrate or intravenously administered nitroglycerin or Lasix) in order to diminish venous return to the heart and thereby diminish intracardiac filling pressures
4. arteriolar dilating agents such as sodium nitroprusside or trimethaphan camphorsulfonate (Arfonad) to reduce the impedance to left ventricular ejection, especially in the presence of hypertension or mitral regurgitation

Rotating tourniquets may be applied to the extremities to diminish venous return. The exact medications and maneuvers used should be selected on the basis of the severity of the pulmonary congestion, the degree of depression of cardiac output, and the arterial pressure. In the most ominous situation of extensive pulmonary edema with respiratory depression, assisted or controlled ventilation with endotracheal intubation is appropriate.

Sodium nitroprusside (Nipride) is a fast acting, potent vasodilator that alters both venous and arteriolar tone. Its venodilating effect allows rapid lowering of intracardiac filling pressures; its arteriolar dilating effect rapidly lowers the impedance to left ventricular ejection, making it extremely useful in increasing forward stroke volume and reducing regurgitant volume when there is mitral insufficiency. It is also extremely useful in the treatment of pulmonary edema in the hypertensive patient. This medication is most widely used, however, in the management of acutely ill patients with high intracardiac filling pressures, low cardiac output, and poor left ventricular performance attributable to acute myocardial infarction or to a period of cardiopulmonary bypass during cardiac surgery.

Sodium nitroprusside is administered by continuous IV infusion, starting with a dose of 0.5 µg/kg/minute (35 µg/minute) and increasing the dose by about 0.5 µg/kg/minute every 5 to 10 minutes until the desired hemodynamic state is achieved or until the arterial pressure becomes undesirably low. In order to allow recognition of the achievement of an optimum hemodynamic state, and to avoid reaching an even more deleterious state than that present prior to administering this medication, it is essential to continuously monitor the arterial pressure and the left ventricular filling pressure (ie, mean pulmonary artery wedge or pulmonary artery diastolic pressure). The maximum recommended dose of sodium nitroprusside is 10 µg/kg/minute (700 µg/minute), for doses in excess of this may result in tinnitus, blurred vision, and delirium related to thiocyanate toxicity. Higher doses than this may cause cyanide poisoning.

MANAGEMENT OF HYPERTENSION

A small percentage of patients with acute myocardial infarction have abnormally elevated blood pressure, which predisposes them to cardiac rupture and may increase the size of the evolving infarct by increasing myocardial oxygen demand. In many patients, the hypertension occurs in response to pain and anxiety, and the blood pressure falls to normal levels as analgesic medications relieve the pain and anxiety. When rapid lowering of the blood pressure is felt to be advisable, the cautious IV administration of Nipride or Arfonad may lower blood pressure to a desirable level within minutes. Continuous monitoring of arterial pressure with an intra-arterial catheter is advised when such potent antihypertensive agents are used, although frequent non-invasive measurements of BP using an automated device may suffice in many instances. In general, the hypertension that occurs in acute myocardial infarction lasts for only a few hours; thus, the oral or intramuscular administration of antihypertensive medications is inadvisable. Absorption may make them unavailable when needed, or their effects may become apparent at a time when they are not needed and are even perhaps detrimental.

Beta-blocking drugs may be used to effectively lower blood pressure in hypertensive patients with adequate left ventricular function who do not have pulmonary congestion, slow heart rate, or AV conduction disturbances. Esmolol, a rapidly acting beta blocker, and metoprolol, a medium rapidly acting beta blocker, are selective $beta_1$ blocking drugs commonly used intravenously to acutely lower blood pressure in acute myocardial infarction.

THERAPY OF DEBATABLE VALUE IN ACUTE MYOCARDIAL INFARCTION

Supplemental Inspired Oxygen

The administration of supplemental inspired oxygen to the patient with acute myocardial infarction is a tradition likely to continue, even though its clinical benefit is unproved. However, it appears to be justified by the fact that hypoxemia is common in these patients. The hypoxemia generally reflects ventilation-perfusion ratio abnormalities within the lung. These abnormalities may be the result of (1) pulmonary interstitial and intra-alveolar edema; (2) the rapid, small tidal-volume respiratory pattern that occurs as a response to the discomfort or anxiety of the situation, or to pulmonary congestion or edema; and (3) the low pulmonary blood flow that may occur in the presence of low cardiac output or hypotension.

The aim of supplemental inspired oxygen administration is to ensure "adequate oxygenation," which generally means a systemic arterial oxygen saturation of greater than 95% (pO_2 greater than 70 mmHg). Experimental studies of the effects of arterial oxygen tension on the size of an experimentally induced acute myocardial infarction suggest that the size of the infarct can be diminished when arterial oxygen tension is greater than normal. This beneficial effect has yet to be documented in the clinical setting, however. Of course, the administration of supplemental inspired oxygen to the patient with chronic obstructive pulmonary disease may result in CO_2 narcosis, so its use in such patients with acute myocardial infarction must be closely monitored.

TRANSFER TO THE CORONARY CARE UNIT

Patients with suspected or documented acute myocardial infarction should be transferred to the coronary care unit (CCU) as soon as the CCU staff is prepared to assume responsibility for their care, but only when they are stable enough for the transfer. Patients who are having recurrent ventricular tachycardia or fibrillation that requires repeated electrical conversions should not be transferred, for the CCU offers no advantage over the emergency department in the management of a patient requiring almost continuous resuscitation.

Cardiac arrest occurs all too often in transit from the emergency department to the CCU, and the disadvantages of resuscitating a patient in a hallway or elevator are minimized if a transfer routine has been well rehearsed. Specifically, there must be at least two persons trained in cardiopulmonary resuscitation with the patient. The cardiac rhythm must be clearly displayed on an oscilloscope that is constantly in view of the accompanying personnel. Some monitoring devices generate an audible pulse of sound whenever a QRS complex is sensed, allowing auditory as well as visual monitoring of cardiac rhythm. The patient must be able to exercise reasonable self-control and to cooperate, or else be adequately sedated; the patient must not be thrashing about because of the risk of interfering with the ECG monitoring and with treatment. A portable defibrillator with electrode jelly must be placed on the bed or gurney so that it is immediately accessible if needed. An IV infusion must be functioning, and medications, such as lidocaine, atropine, and sodium bicarbonate must be readily available in clearly marked syringes. A portable oxygen tank, as well as equipment for endotracheal and nasotracheal intubation and for suction, must accompany the patient. The CCU staff should be informed of the time the patient departs from the emergency department in order to make themselves immediately available when the patient arrives.

REFERENCES

1. Maseri A, Severi S, DeNes M, et al. "Variant" angina: one aspect of a continuous spectrum of vasospastic myocardial ischemia. Pathogenetic mechanisms, estimated incidence and clinical and coronary arteriographic findings in 138 patients. *Am J Cardiol*. 1978;42:1019–1035.
2. Gunther S, Muller JE, Mudge GH Jr, et al. Therapy of coronary vasoconstriction in patients with coronary artery disease. *Am J Cardiol*. 1981;47:157–162.
3. Rentrop P, Blanke H, Karsch KR, et al. Selective intracoronary thrombolysis in acute myocardial infarction and unstable angina pectoris. *Circulation*. 1981;63:307–317.
4. Alderman EL, Jutzy KR, Berte LE, et al. Randomized comparison of intravenous versus intracoronary streptokinase for myocardial infarction. *Am J Cardiol*. 1984;54:14–19.
5. Braunwald E, Sobel BE. Coronary blood flow and myocardial ischemia. In: Braunwald E, ed. *Heart Disease*. Philadelphia: WB Saunders Co; 1992:1161–1199.
6. Yusif S, Sleight P, Held P, McMahon S. Routine medical management of acute myocardial infarction. Lessons from overviews of recent randomized controlled trials. *Circulation*. 1990;82(suppl II):117–134.
7. Yusef S, Peto R, Louis J, Colins R, Sleight P. Beta blockade during and after acute myocardial infarction. An overview of the randomized trials. *Prog Cardiovasc Dis*. 1985;17:335–371.
8. Hine LK, Laird N, Hewitt P, Chalmers TC. Meta-analytic evidence against prophylactic use of lidocaine in acute myocardial infarction. *Arch Intern Med*. 1989;149:2694–2698.

9. Massumi RA, Mason DT, Amsterdam EA, et al. Ventricular fibrillation and tachycardia after intravenous atropine for treatment of bradycardia. *N Engl J Med.* 1972;287:336.
10. Leier CV, Webel J, Bush CA. The cardiovascular effects of the continuous infusion of dobutamine in patients with severe cardiac failure. *Circulation.* 1977;56:468–472.
11. Bendersky R, Chatterjee K, Parmley WW, et al. Dobutamine in chronic ischemic heart failure: alterations in left ventricular function and coronary hemodynamics. *Am J Cardiol.* 1981;48:555–558.
12. Gillespie TA, Ambos HD, Sobel BE, et al. Effects of dobutamine in patients with acute myocardial infarction. *Am J Cardiol.* 1977;39:588–594.

63. Disturbances in Cardiac Rhythm

LESTER B. JACOBSON, MD, FACC, FACP

Disturbances in cardiac rhythm are among the most common problems seen by emergency physicians today. Dysrhythmias may occur in infants as well as in the elderly, and in otherwise healthy persons as well as in the chronically or seriously ill. The dysrhythmia may be of no clinical significance, or it may be of catastrophic proportions. Faced with a patient who may be having dysrhythmias, the emergency physician must (1) determine whether the patient has a dysrhythmia at that moment and, if not, assess the likelihood that the patient has had a dysrhythmia in the recent past or is likely to have one in the near future; (2) establish an accurate electrocardiographic diagnosis of the dysrhythmia; (3) predict the clinical course of the dysrhythmia in the individual patient; and (4) plan a course of management based on these considerations and on the patient's clinical condition and underlying cardiovascular status.

SYMPTOMS ATTRIBUTABLE TO DYSRHYTHMIAS

Many symptoms are attributable to dysrhythmias. Some patients simply have an awareness of cardiac action, commonly termed *palpitation*. The sensation may be a single pumping feeling in the chest that is due to premature beating, a fluttering in the chest that reflects premature beats occurring in rapid succession, cardiac irregularity that is due to the irregularity of the underlying rhythm as in atrial fibrillation, or a pounding in the chest that may occur with slow as well as rapid heart rates. It is clear that the regularity or irregularity and the rapidity or slowness of the rhythm, as sensed by the patient, may have little relationship to the exact cardiac cadence that is occurring.

Some patients with dysrhythmias may be totally unaware of cardiac action, but rather complain of transient presyncope (lightheadedness, dimming of vision, nausea, loss of balance) or frank syncope. Others complain of paroxysmal or persistent and progressive shortness of breath, with or without signs and symptoms of obvious congestive heart failure. Still others experience chest discomfort suggesting myocardial ischemia. Some patients with dysrhythmias, be they rapid or slow, paroxysmal or sustained, have no symptoms; rather, their dysrhythmia may have been detected on a routine examination or a routine electrocardiographic tracing.

HEMODYNAMIC CONSEQUENCES OF CARDIAC DYSRHYTHMIAS

While an awareness of cardiac action may be the major reason that a patient with a dysrhythmia seeks medical assistance, it is the hemodynamic consequence of the dysrhythmia that determines the morbidity and mortality associated with it. The prime function of the cardiovascular system is to provide adequate blood flow at appropriate perfusion pressure to the tissues of the body. The cardiac output (ie, the volume of blood ejected into the circulation by the heart in a minute's time) is the product of the volume of blood ejected with each systole [stroke volume (SV)] and the heart rate (HR). Thus, maintenance of adequate cardiac output requires an adequate stroke volume times heart rate product. Arterial blood pressure is the product of the cardiac output and the total systemic resistance (TSR). Thus, maintenance of adequate arterial pressure requires maintenance of an adequate SV × HR × TSR product.

As the ability of the heart to increase stroke volume is limited, a dramatic fall in heart rate (generally from normal to less than 30 to 40 beats/minute) may result in a sudden fall in cardiac output and, therefore, in blood pressure. Also, with the sudden onset of tachycardia (either supraventricular or ventricular) the stroke volume may fall so dramatically that cardiac output and, thus, blood pressure may fall to catastrophically low levels before reflex adjustments in capacitance (venous) and resistance (arteriolar) vessels can be made. The compensatory mechanisms include an increase in venous tone, which will increase intracardiac volume and thus stroke volume, and an increase in arteriolar resistance, which will increase the blood pressure.

In an individual patient, the hemodynamic consequences of and the symptoms related to a cardiac rhythm disturbance depend on many factors. These include the rate of the dysrhythmia, the atrial and ventricular relationships during the dysrhythmia, the functional state of the heart, the presence of coronary artery and cerebral vascular disease, the extracellular fluid volume, the patient's posture and level of consciousness at the time the dysrhythmia occurs, and the ability of the autonomic nervous system to make rapid adjustments to the alteration in cardiac rhythm, a response that may be vitally affected by vasoactive medications, such as vasodilator and antihypertensive agents. Symptoms attributable to the hemodynamic consequences of cardiac dysrhythmias may be separated into three categories: (1) presyncope, syncope, and seizure, which reflect a sudden catastrophic fall in cerebral blood flow; (2) chest discomfort, which reflects myocardial ischemia; (3) dyspnea, which reflects pulmonary congestion due to high pulmonary venous pressure.

THE CARDIAC CONDUCTION SYSTEM

The cardiac conduction system may be viewed as having two portions. The upper, or supraventricular, part consists of the sinus node and the atrioventricular (AV) junction, which is comprised of the AV node and the bundle of His. The lower, or intraventricular, part consists of the bundle branches and their fascicles, which terminate in the Purkinje fibers that activate the ventricular myocardium.

Under normal circumstances, the sinus node, which lies at the junction of the superior vena cava with the right atrium, has the most rapid automatic firing rate of all cardiac electrical tissues. Thus, the cardiac depolarization process is normally initiated by electrical impulses arising in the sinus node. Impulses exiting the sinus node enter the right atrium, where they initiate an orderly sequence of depolarization of both right and left atrial tissue, right atrial activation beginning about 0.01 seconds before left atrial activation. The contour and duration of normal P waves reflect the normal atrial activation sequence. Abnormal anatomical sequences of atrial depolarization may result in P waves with contours and durations that differ from the norm.

Impulses traversing atrial tissue reach and enter the superior portion of the AV node, which lies near the tricuspid valve in the lower portion of the interatrial septum and the upper portion of the interventricular septum. It is still unclear whether atrial impulses travel from the sinus node to the AV node solely in atrial muscle or whether they also travel in specialized conduction pathways termed *internodal tracts*. The impulses travel in orderly fashion from the upper to the lower portion of the AV node. At the inferior portion of the AV node, the impulses enter the bundle of His, through which they travel to enter fibers of the right and left bundle branches. Fibers of the right bundle branch, which functionally consists of one fascicle, terminate in right ventricular myocardium. Fibers of the left bundle branch, which functionally consists of anterior, posterior, and sometimes septal fascicles, terminate in left ventricular and interventricular septal myocardium. Under normal circumstances, ventricular tissue is depolarized by impulses arriving via both right and left bundle branches. Ventricular activation by the left bundle branch fibers begins about 0.03 to 0.04 seconds before that by the right bundle branch fibers.

Ventricular tissue is initially depolarized simultaneously in three distinct areas: (1) the central portion of the left side of the interventricular septum, (2) the paraseptal anterior free left ventricular wall, and (3) the paraseptal posterior left ventricular wall. The depolarization process then spreads to involve the right side of the interventricular septum, the free right ventricular and free left ventricular walls, and finally the high lateral and posterior portions of the left ventricle. The contour and duration of normal QRS complexes reflect the normal anatomical sequence of ventricular activation. Abnormal sequences of ventricular depolarization may produce QRS complexes with contours and durations that differ from the norm.

Some patients have, in addition to the normal AV node-His-Purkinje system, another (accessory) pathway connecting atrial to ventricular tissue. Some accessory AV conduction pathways are capable of transmitting impulses from atrium to ventricle as well as from ventricle to atrium, while others can conduct impulses in only one direction. The tissue that comprises the accessory AV conduction pathways usually has properties similar to those of His-Purkinje system tissue and very different from those of normal AV nodal tissue. Consequently, accessory AV conduction pathways may be able to conduct impulses more rapidly or in more rapid succession than the normal AV conduction system. (For further discussion of accessory AV conduction pathways, see The Wolff-Parkinson-White Syndrome.)

DIAGNOSIS OF THE DYSRHYTHMIA

Accurate diagnosis of a dysrhythmia is facilitated by first defining the ventricular (QRS) rhythm, then defining the atrial rhythm, and, finally, determining the relationships between the ventricular and atrial rhythms. From a practical point of view, it is helpful to determine whether a dysrhythmia consists of ectopic beats, a bradycardia, or a tachycardia; and then whether the dysrhythmia arises in supraventricular (sinus node, atrium, AV node, His bundle) or ventricular (bundle branch, Purkinje fiber) tissue. However, the emergency physician facing a patient who appears to be seriously ill because of a dysrhythmia that is not clearly definable may have to make an educated guess concerning the type of dysrhythmia. In this endeavor, the clinical setting of the patient is of utmost importance, because specific dysrhythmias occur with greater frequency in specific clinical settings. Table 63-1 indicates the dysrhythmias that are more likely or less likely to occur in specific clinical settings.

ECTOPIC BEATS

P waves or QRS complexes that are stimulated by impulses arising outside the sinus node are termed *ectopic* complexes or beats. The contours of P waves or QRS complexes initiated by ectopic impulses generally differ from the norm because the ectopic impulse results in an abnormal anatomical sequence of atrial or ventricular activation. The duration of an ectopic P wave is generally similar to that of a sinus-stimulated P wave, presumably because both sinus impulses and ectopic atrial impulses initially activate one small area from which depolarization must spread throughout atrial tissue. The duration of an ectopic QRS complex, however, is generally longer than normal, because it takes longer for all ventricular tissue to be activated when depolarization is initiated at a single site than it does when several different areas are activated almost simultaneously, as normally occurs with initial ventricular depolarization via the bundle branches.

Atrial (Supraventricular) Premature Complexes or Beats

Ectopic atrial beats may occur one at a time as isolated events, in pairs, or in brief runs. They may initiate supraventricular tachydysrhythmias, or a brief or prolonged period of cardiac standstill. It is crucial to determine whether the ectopic atrial beat is premature indicating abnormal atrial irritability, or whether it occurs after a pause in atrial rhythm and thus reflects an escape mechanism that prevents prolonged pauses in rhythm.

An atrial premature complex (APC) can be recognized in the surface electrocardiogram (ECG) by the appearance of a P wave before the next sinus P wave is expected to occur (Fig. 63-1). While prematurity is quite easy to define when the sinus rhythm is reasonably regular, the presence of dramatic sinus arrhythmia makes the diagnosis of prematurity more difficult. The contours and axes of premature P waves are usually different from those of sinus P waves unless the premature atrial impulse arises in or near the sinus node, in which case it resembles the sinus P wave. The identification of a premature P wave may be difficult if the P wave falls in the ST segment or TU wave of the preceding QRSTU complex and is obscured by it, or if the sequence of atrial depolarization causes the P wave to be diminutive or isoelectric in the surface ECG lead being examined. Thus, it may be necessary to record more than one surface ECG lead in order to see premature P waves accurately (Fig. 63-1).

Table 63-1 Arrhythmias Encountered in Specific Clinical Settings

Clinical Setting	More Likely	Less Likely
Acute myocardial infarction	PVCs, VT, VF, AV block	Atrial FIB, flutter, APCs, PSVT
Sick sinus syndrome	Sinus arrest, pauses, atrial FIB, flutter, APCs, PSVT	PVCs, VT, VF, AV block
Wolff-Parkinson-White syndrome	PSVT, atrial FIB, flutter	VT, VF, AV block

Key: APCs, atrial premature complexes; AV, atrioventricular; FIB, fibrillation; PSVT, paroxysmal supraventricular tachycardia; PVCs, premature ventricular complexes; VF, ventricular fibrillation; VT, ventricular tachycardia.

While isolated APCs may be bothersome to the patient because they cause an unpleasant awareness of cardiac action, they are rarely of great hemodynamic consequence *per se*. Rather, their significance relates to the ability of the APCs to initiate sustained atrial tachydysrhythmias, such as fibrillation (FIB), paroxysmal supraventricular tachycardia (PSVT), and flutter (Fig. 63-2) and to the ability of the patient's cardiovascular system to tolerate the tachydysrhythmias. The emergency physician must (1) assess possible factors predisposing the patient to a supraventricular tachydysrhythmia, (2) determine the underlying cardiovascular status of the patient to help predict whether an atrial tachydysrhythmia will result in significant problems, and (3) then decide what specific management is appropriate for that individual patient.

The physician confronted by the patient with even isolated APCs, however, should attempt to evaluate the factors predisposing to the ectopy. In some patients, the APCs may simply be a reflection of anxiety or emotional stress. In others, they may be a reflection of (1) large left-atrial volume or high left-atrial pressure, as commonly seen in atrial septal defect, left ventricular hypertrophy, mitral stenosis, mitral

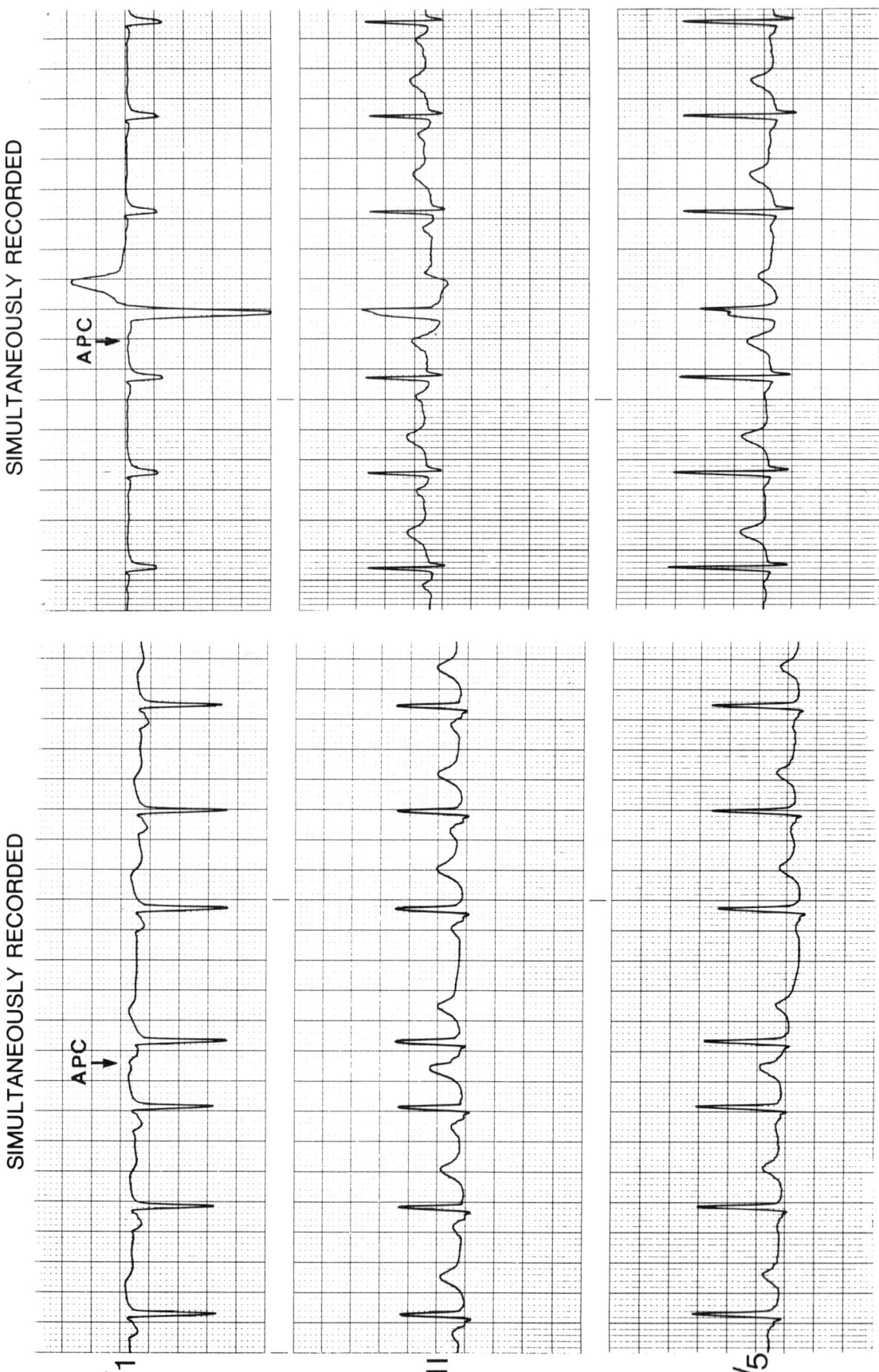

Figure 63-1 ECGs showing atrial premature complexes. *Note:* The ECG in *A* shows an atrial premature complex (APC) stimulating a QRS complex that has a contour essentially identical to that of the sinus-stimulated QRS complexes. In *B*, an APC stimulates a QRS complex with a left bundle branch block pattern, whereas sinus-stimulated QRS complexes have normal contours. In *A*, the APC is clearly seen in leads V_1 and II, but not in lead V_5; in *B*, the APC is clearly seen only in lead V_1.

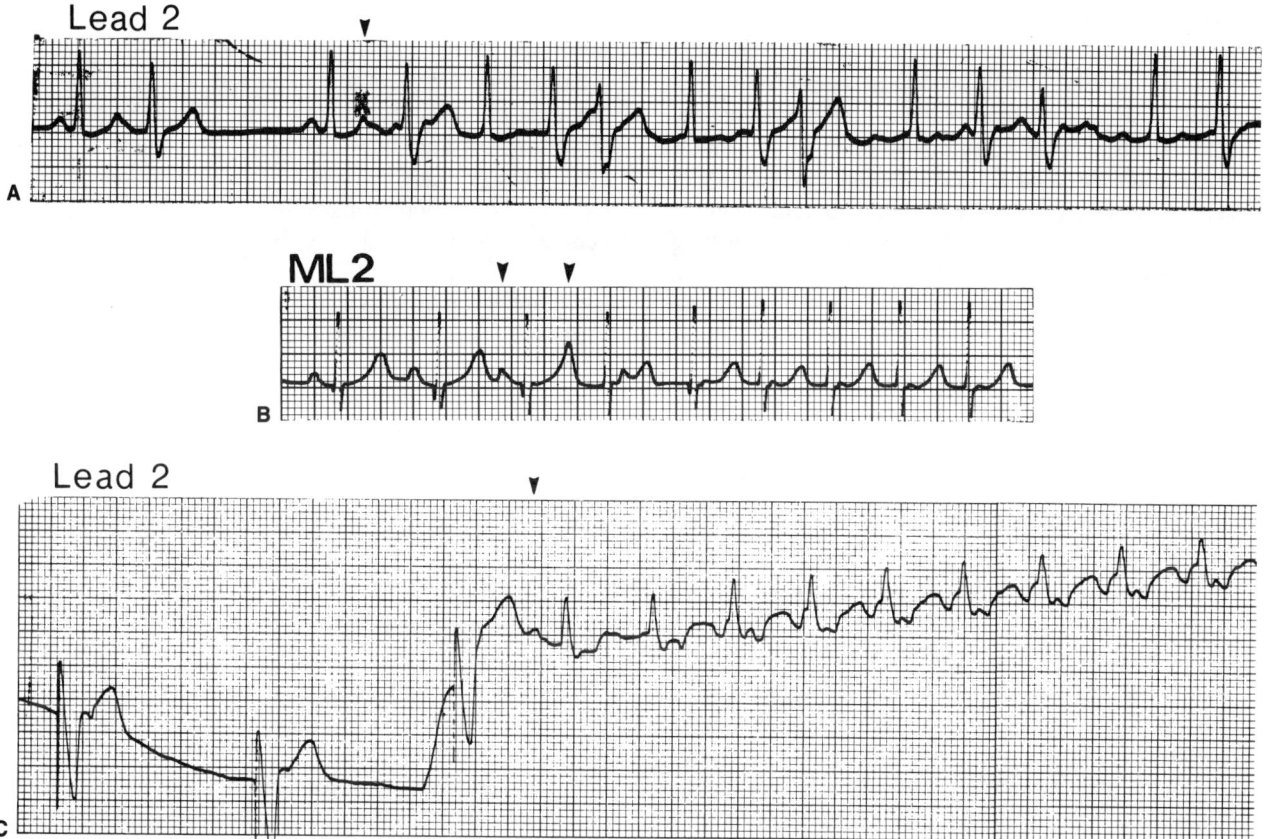

Figure 63-2 ECGs showing the onsets of three atrial tachydysrhythmias. *A:* An atrial premature beat (*arrow*) initiates atrial fibrillation. *B:* Sustained AV nodal reentrant paroxysmal supraventricular tachycardia is established following two atrial premature beats (*arrows*). *C:* An atrial premature complex (*arrow*) initiates atrial flutter, during which there is 2:1 AV conduction. (ECG at 90% of original.)

insufficiency, or congestive heart failure; or (2) large right-atrial volume or high right-atrial pressure, as commonly seen in atrial septal defect, right ventricular hypertrophy, and chronic obstructive pulmonary disease. Furthermore, because of their stimulant effects, alcoholic beverages, caffeine, cigarette smoking, and medications such as thyroid hormone, bronchodilators, and sympathomimetic amines may be contributory factors. Finally, APCs may reflect pericardial irritation or inflammation, as may occur in acute myocardial infarction or renal failure, and primary pericarditis of other various etiologies. Patients who tolerate atrial tachydysrhythmias poorly include

- those with mitral stenosis in whom the rapid ventricular rate may result in dramatic elevation of left atrial pressure and the precipitation of pulmonary edema, and in whom the ineffective atrial mechanical activity may predispose to thromboembolism
- those with severe congestive heart failure or severe left ventricular hypertrophy (such as is seen with valvular aortic stenosis and hypertrophic cardiomyopathy) who need the properly timed atrial contribution to ventricular filling to maintain adequate left ventricular performance
- those with the bradycardia-tachycardia variant of the sick sinus syndrome in whom termination of tachycardia is followed by prolonged cardiac standstill
- those with rapidly conducting accessory AV conduction pathways.

Management of the patient with APCs must be based on the total clinical picture. If anxiety or sleep deprivation is playing a major role in an otherwise healthy patient, a supportive discussion and possibly a minor tranquilizer or soporific medication might be appropriately prescribed. Discontinuation of stimulants should be advised and dosages of potentially inciting medications reduced. Therapeutic maneuvers aimed at controlling congestive heart failure should be optimized. In some patients with mitral stenosis, aortic stenosis, or idiopathic hypertrophic subaortic stenosis, the onset of APCs raises the possibility that the mechanical cardiac lesion is serious enough to warrant consideration of cardiac surgery. Thus, thorough cardiologic evaluation is advisable at this time.

Several antidysrhythmic medications are available for treating the patient with APCs. As the treatment of APCs is rarely an emergency, the oral route of administration is preferred. Quinidine preparations, procainamide (Pronestyl, Procan-SR), propranolol (Inderal), and disopyramide (Norpace) are all reported to be effective in suppressing atrial premature beats. In recent years flecainide (Tambocor) has been approved for effective prevention of PSVT in patients with good left ventricular function and no coronary artery disease. As the relative efficacy of these different agents in suppressing APCs is unclear, selection of a specific drug generally depends on the potential side effects of the drug in an individual patient, the necessary dosage schedule, and the cost. For example, a beta-blocking medication, such as propranolol, would be ill-advised for the patient with bronchospastic lung disease, poor left ventricular function, or insulin-dependent brittle diabetes mellitus; but it is often extremely effective and well tolerated by young, otherwise healthy patients with APCs. Disopyramide, which may have a significant depressant effect on cardiac performance, would be ill-advised for the patient with poor left ventricular function; furthermore, its anticholinergic properties often cause urinary retention in older males and constipation in older patients of both sexes. Quinidine preparations may cause significant diarrhea. Procainamide preparations must be administered at 4- to 6-hour intervals to achieve consistent, effective serum levels. On long-term administration they result in positive antinuclear antibody and lupus erythematosus cell tests in a high percentage of patients, and a bothersome, often prolonged, lupus-like polyarthritis in a few of them.

Flecainide should *not* be used in patients with previous myocardial infarction, for when this medication was administered to patients with recent myocardial infarction and PVCs in the Chronic Arrhythmia Suppression Trial (CAST) study, patients taking this medication and having effective suppression of their PVCs have higher incidences of sudden cardiac death and other coronary events than patients taking placebos.

Supraventricular beats may originate in the AV junction as well as in the atrium. An AV-junctional premature beat (JPC) may be recognized by the premature occurrence of a normal-appearing QRS complex with, quite frequently, an abnormal-appearing P wave either preceding it at an unusually short interval (less than 0.11 seconds) or occurring within it or shortly after it. The abnormal contour and axis of the P wave reflect the abnormal sequence of atrial depolarization that is due to the initiation of atrial activity near the upper portion of the AV node, well away from the sinus node. Junctional premature complexes appear to occur much less frequently than APCs, but their clinical significance and management do not appear to be different from those of APCs.

Ventricular Ectopic Beats

Impulses arising in the bundle branches or in ventricular tissue stimulate QRS complexes that are called ventricular ectopic beats (VEBs). VEBs may be recognized by their abnormal, often bizarre contours and by their prolonged duration (Fig. 63-3). When VEBs follow normal QRS complexes at intervals shorter than expected on the basis of the preceding rhythm, they are called *premature* ventricular complexes or beats (PVCs). When they follow pauses in QRS rhythm of more than about 1.2 seconds, they are called ventricular *escape* complexes or beats.

PVCs may arise in both healthy and diseased hearts. They commonly occur in association with ischemia, hypokalemia, digitalis excess, hypoxemia, congestive heart failure, and during the administration of catecholamines, sympathomimetic amines, phenothiazines, and tricyclic antidepressants. PVCs may occur singly, in pairs, or in brief runs, and they may initiate paroxysmal or sustained ventricular tachycardia or ventricular fibrillation (Figs. 63-3 and 63-4).

While isolated PVCs may cause an unpleasant awareness of cardiac action, they generally do not contribute to hemodynamic deterioration unless they occur very frequently. Such might be the case in a bigeminal rhythm in which a PVC follows each sinus beat at an interval so brief that the PVC is mechanically ineffective (ie, does not produce adequate stroke volume) (Fig. 63-3, D). PVCs generally assume clinical importance when they initiate repetitive ventricular beating, sustained ventricular tachycardia, and ventricular fibrillation, hemodynamically disadvantageous and often disastrous rhythms that occur only rarely in the absence of heart disease—although the heart disease may not be clinically apparent prior to the occurrence of the catastrophic dysrhythmia. So, faced with a patient having PVCs, the emergency physician must attempt to determine whether the patient has cardiac disease. In this pursuit, it is essential to obtain both a detailed medical history and a family history, to perform a thorough physical examination, and to review a 12-lead ECG. In selected patients, a chest radiograph, echocardiogram, ambulatory monitoring, and a treadmill exercise test may be necessary.

Antidysrhythmic medication should not be prescribed for patients with asymptomatic PVCs if there is no evidence of cardiac disease; it may be offered to normal patients with significantly symptomatic PVCs after discussing with them the potential benefits and risks of specific antidysrhythmic medications. Asymptomatic or symptomatic PVCs in a patient with a history or symptoms of coronary artery disease, especially left ventricular aneurysm, should probably be looked upon as a potentially serious problem. However, even in these settings, one cannot strongly recommend treatment with specific antidysrhythmic medication, for it has never been proven that suppression of PVCs with antidysrhythmic medications will prevent sudden death from ventricular tachycardia or ventricular fibrillation. Such medications have been shown to be proarrhythmic, ie, to increase the frequency, duration, rate, and severity of ventricular arrhythmias.[1,2] If hypomagnesemia, hypokalemia, hypox-

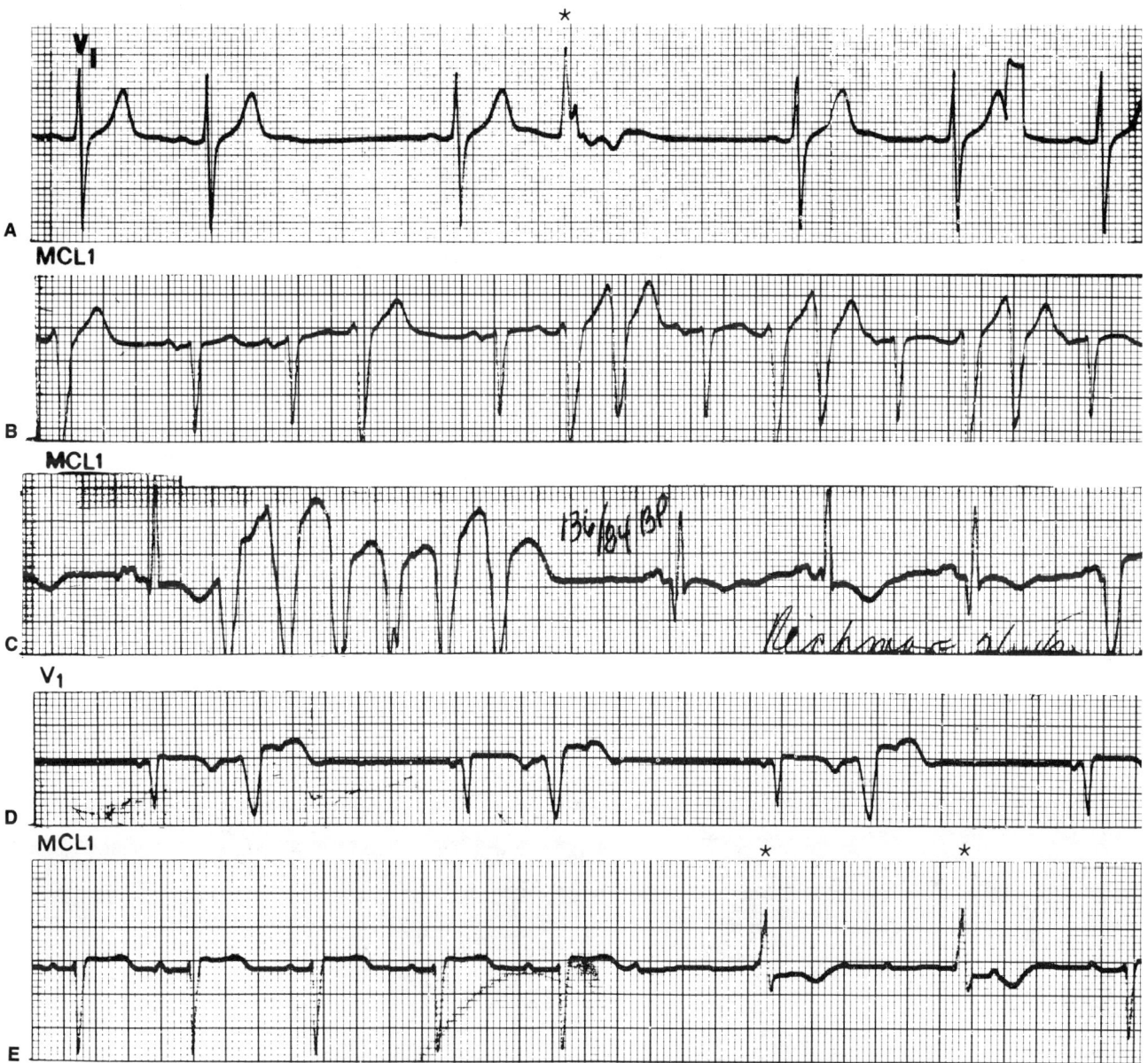

Figure 63-3 ECGs showing ventricular ectopic beats. *A:* The fourth QRS complex (*asterisk*) is a premature ventricular complex (PVC). *B:* PVCs are occurring both singly and in pairs. *C:* A brief (1.8 second) run of ventricular premature beats at a rate of about 170/minute. *D:* Bigeminal rhythm in which a PVC follows each sinus-stimulated (or AV junction-stimulated) QRS complex. *E:* Ventricular escape beats (*asterisks*) terminate pauses in QRS rhythm occasioned by a brief period of AV block.

emia, congestive heart failure, or medications (eg, digitalis, phenothiazines, tricyclic antidepressants) are clearly playing a role, they should be appropriately treated before specific antidysrhythmic medication is administered. Patients with unstable angina pectoris and PVCs should probably be admitted to the hospital for observation of their cardiac rhythm while antimyocardial ischemia management is commenced.

PVCs are very common in patients with the *mitral valve prolapse,* or *click-murmur,* syndrome. In these patients, the mitral valve and/or its supporting structures typically have abnormalities that may be detected clinically by the presence of one or more systolic clicks and a systolic murmur; the click(s) and murmur may vary in intensity and timing with changes in body position, as well as in response to respiration and vasoactive medications, such as amyl nitrite. Sudden death has been reported to occur in a small number of patients with the mitral valve prolapse syndrome, suggesting that a fatal ventricuar dysrhythmia was initiated by the PVCs. However, the reported high frequency with which mitral valve prolapse has been detected echocardiographically and the small number of patients with this syndrome who suffer sudden death make it as yet unclear whether it is advisable to treat asymptomatic (or even symptomatic) isolated PVCs in

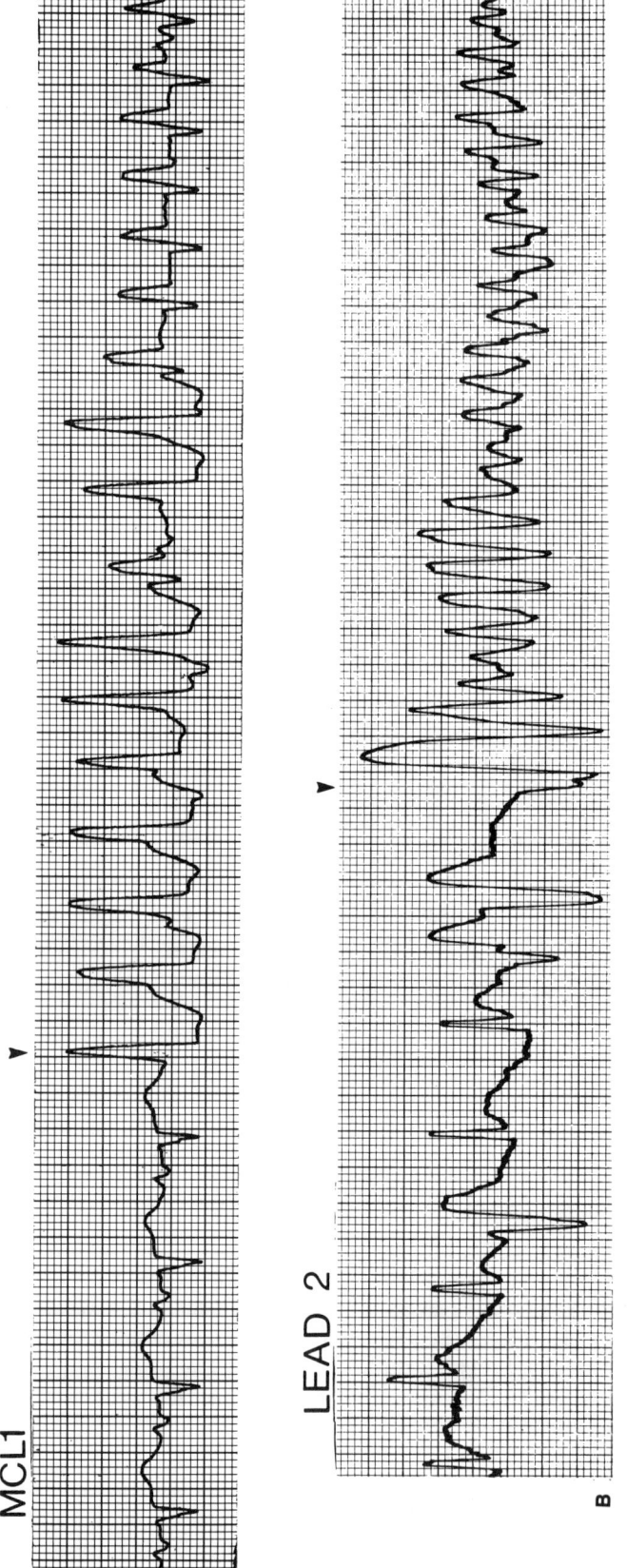

Figure 63-4 ECGs showing the onsets of ventricular tachycardia and ventricular fibrillation. *A*: Premature ventricular complex (*arrow*) initiates sustained ventricular tachycardia during which there is AV dissociation. *B*: premature ventricular complex (*arrow*) initiates ventricular fibrillation.

these patients. As the few patients with mitral valve prolapse reported to have died suddenly had either dramatic anatomical abnormalities of the mitral valve apparatus, long QTU intervals, or nonspecific ST segment and T-wave abnormalities in the inferior and lateral precordial leads of a resting ECG, it would seem reasonable to prescribe specific antidysrhythmic medication to patients with mitral valve prolapse syndrome and isolated PVCs *if* they have physical examination or echocardiographic evidence of dramatic anatomic abnormalities of the mitral apparatus, or these ECG abnormalities.[3]

PVCs may initiate serious ventricular dysrhythmias in patients whose ECGs show long QTU intervals. A few patients with long QTU intervals may have a congenital predisposition to this abnormality, and some of them may have congenital hearing loss, a history of recurrent episodes of presyncope or syncope, and a family history of unheralded sudden death in childhood, young adulthood, or early middle age, usually associated with emotional events. However, the majority of patients with long QTU intervals either have coronary artery disease, hypokalemia, or mitral valve prolapse syndrome; or they are taking phenothiazines, tricyclic antidepressants, quinidine, procainamide, or disopyramide.

As a general principle, treatment of a patient with PVCs is initially directed at correcting metabolic, hemodynamic, and drug-related abnormalities, unless the PVCs are presently initiating hemodynamically deleterious dysrhythmias, in which case specific antidysrhythmic medication might be administered immediately. Antidysrhythmic medications may be administered orally or intravenously, depending on the urgency of the clinical situation and the specific drug selected. The choice of a specific medication depends on the predicted effectiveness and potential side effects of the drug, the route of administration available, the dosage schedule, and the clinical condition of the patient. Beta-blocking medications, such as propranolol, metoprolol* (Lopressor), atenolol* (Tenormon), and nadolol (Corgard), would be ill-advised for the patient with poor left ventricular function, congestive heart failure, sick sinus syndrome, AV-nodal conduction abnormalities, and bronchospastic lung disease; but they might be useful in the otherwise healthy patient, the anxious patient, the thyrotoxic patient or the patient with mitral valve prolapse syndrome. Administration of quinidine and procainamide might be dangerous in the patient with long QTU intervals, for these medications may lengthen the interval even further and thereby worsen ventricular dysrhythmias. Furthermore, because recent studies suggest that the administration of a quinidine preparation to a patient on digoxin may result in a dramatic rise in the serum digoxin level and an increase in ventricular dysrhythmias, particular care must be taken to administer digoxin less frequently and/or in lower dosage than normal to a patient who is to be started on quinidine, and quinidine should not be given to a patient with digitalis-related ventricular dysrhythmias.[4] Disopyramide, also, is best avoided in long QTU syndromes, as it has been reported to lengthen the QTU interval, and to result in more serious ventricular dysrhythmias in this situation. It is also prudent not to use disopyramide in the presence of severe congestive heart failure and poor left ventricular performance, as it has been reported to cause even more profound depression of left ventricular performance in such patients. Lidocaine is generally the drug of choice when rapid suppression of PVCs is in order, as in the patient with acute myocardial infarction (see Chapter 62, Acute Myocardial Infarction); it usually has few side effects if administered in the recommended dosages. PVCs suppressed by lidocaine are likely, at the 90% level of probability, to be suppressed by one or both of the orally effective lidocaine derivatives mexilitine (Mexitil) and tocainamide (Tocainide). Diphenylhydantoin (Dilantin) is reported to be effective in suppressing PVCs in patients with long QTU intervals, and in patients whose PVCs are digitalis-induced or digitalis-related. As mentioned above, flecainide should *not* be used to suppress PVCs in patients with recent myocardial infarction. Its safety in treating patients without coronary artery disease is currently unproven.

PARASYSTOLE

While the occurrence of most premature ectopic beats is somehow dependent on the basic underlying rhythm, the occurrence of some premature beats is totally independent of the basic underlying rhythm. The concurrent occurrence of two independent rhythms within the same part of the heart is termed *parasystole,* and the complexes stimulated by the ectopic impulses comprise the *parasystolic rhythm.* Parasystolic rhythms most commonly originate in ventricular tissue, although they occasionally arise in the atrium or AV junction. A parasystolic focus generates impulses at constant intervals, regardless of the underlying rhythm; whenever an impulse finds surrounding tissue in a nonrefractory state, it initiates depolarization of the tissue. The parasystolic focus cannot be entered or depolarized by impulses arising outside it, a property termed *protection,* which allows the focus to remain independent of the underlying rhythm.

Parasystolic beats may be recognized by their occurrence at regular intervals and by their temporal independence from the underlying rhythm, which results in (1) variable coupling intervals of the parasystolic complexes to the complexes of the underlying rhythm; (2) consecutive parasystolic complexes occurring at intervals that are multiples of a common interval; and (3) the frequent appearance of fusion complexes in which both a parasystolic impulse and an impulse of the underlying rhythm contribute to ventricular activation (Fig. 63-5). Obviously, long rhythm strips are necessary to establish the diagnosis of a parasystolic rhythm. Accurate

---

*Metoprolol and atenolol may be used with caution in patients with bronchospastic lung disease.

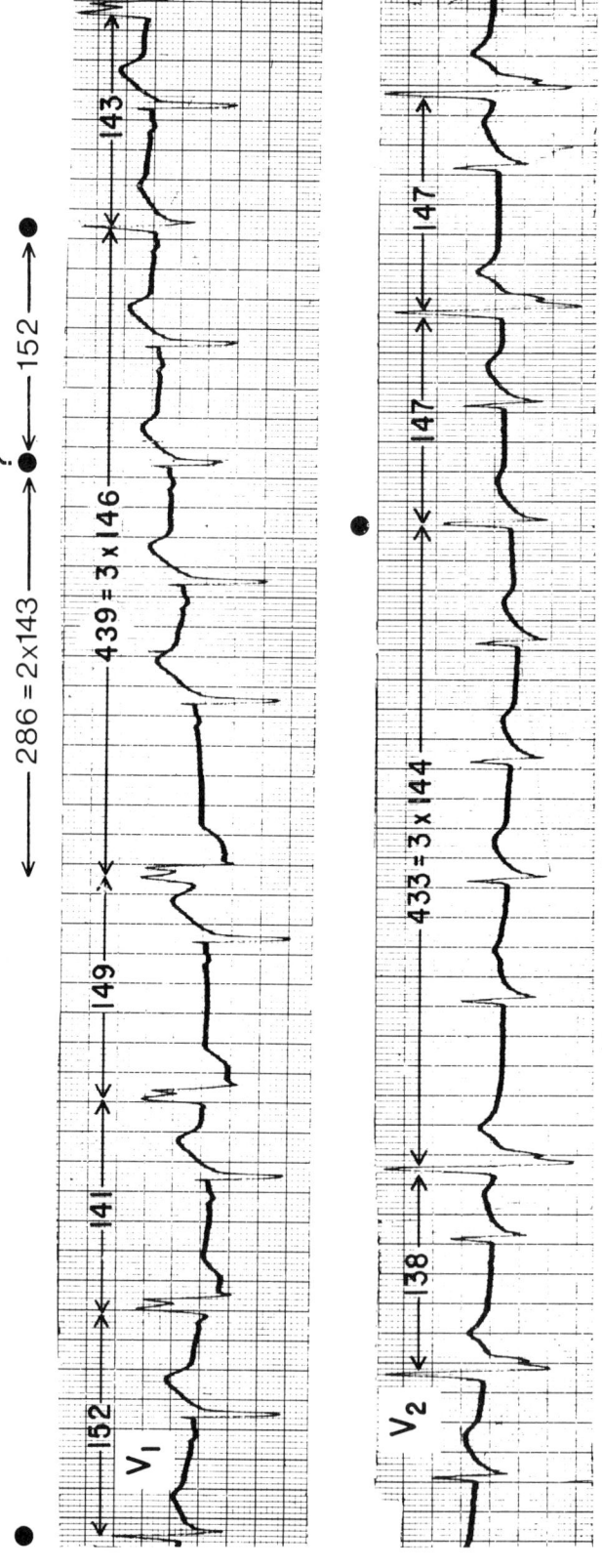

Figure 63-5 ECGs showing ventricular parasystole. *Note:* The wide, bizarre QRS complexes occurring at variable coupling intervals and at intervals that are multiples of a common interval establish the diagnosis of ventricular parasystole. Fusion complexes (●) occur frequently. Times noted are the intervals in hundredths of a second between consecutive parasystolic complexes. (ECG at 81% of original.)

diagnosis of parasystole is important, for ventricular parasystolic beats have *never* been reported to precipitate ventricular fibrillation, and only once have they been reported to initiate ventricular tachycardia.[5] Thus, they are generally of little hemodynamic significance and ought to be treated only if they are causing symptoms. When treatment (ie, suppression) of a parasystolic rhythm is felt to be appropriate, the usual antidysrhythmic medications may be prescribed.

ABERRATION VS. ECTOPY

The typical contour, axis, and duration of QRS complexes reflect the normal anatomical ventricular activation sequence via both left and right bundle branches.ABnormal sequences of ventricular activation may result in QRS complexes that have abnormal contours and durations. The adjective *aberrant* means deviating or straying from normal; in its strictest sense, then, the phrase *aberrant intraventricular conduction* refers to impulses that activate the ventricular myocardium in an abnormal temporal sequence, resulting in an abnormal anatomical sequence of ventricular depolarization. This abnormal course of events may be manifested on surface ECG tracings by the appearance of a QRS complex that differs from normal in contour, duration, or mean frontal plane axis. In this sense, aberrant intraventricular conduction could be initiated by impulses arising in supraventricular *or* in ventricular tissue. In clinical practice, however, the term *aberrant intraventricular conduction* is generally reserved for the phenomenon in which a supraventricular (sinus, atrial, or junctional) impulse activates the ventricles in an abnormal sequence, resulting in a QRS complex with a contour different from those generally stimulated by supraventricular impulses *in that same patient*—regardless of whether or not the patient's usual QRS complexes are of normal or abnormal contour or duration. It is *not* used to describe abnormal QRS complexes that result from ectopic impulse formation within the ventricles themselves, even though such ectopic impulses result in an abnormal sequence of ventricular activation.

Application of the adjective *aberrant* to an unusual appearing QRS complex indicates that the complex is stimulated by an impulse arising in supraventricular rather than ventricular tissue. In fact, the concept of aberrant intraventricular conduction assumes clinical relevance because it is critically important prognostically and therapeutically to know whether an abnormal QRS complex results from aberrant intraventricular conduction of a supraventricular impulse or from ectopic ventricular impulse formation.

Aberrant intraventricular conduction of a supraventricular impulse occurs when a supraventricular impulse reaches the intraventricular conduction system (the bundle branches and their fascicles) at a time when one or more portions of the system cannot conduct the impulse either as rapidly as usual or at all, because it is still refractory (ie, still recovering its excitability from having been recently depolarized). Thus, ventricular activation occurs via those portions of the intraventricular conduction system that are nonrefractory when the supraventricular impulse reaches them. The contours of aberrantly conducted supraventricular impulses generally show rather characteristic right bundle-branch block, left bundle-branch block, or left anterior fascicle-block patterns, probably because the proximal portions of the bundle branches (or fascicles) have the longest refractory periods of the intraventricular conduction-system tissue. In contrast, PVCs generally do *not* have a pure bundle branch block or fascicle block contour, but are more bizarre because ectopic ventricular-impulse formation usually results in an anatomical sequence of ventricular depolarization different from that occurring in bundle branch or fascicle blocks (Fig. 63-6, D and E). Furthermore, PVCs are usually wider than QRS complexes with pure bundle branch or fascicle block patterns, probably because depolarization of the entire mass of ventricular myocardium from one small area of peripheral Purkinje fiber takes more time than does depolarization from a bundle branch or fascicle which depolarizes several areas of ventricular myocardium almost simultaneously. In the unusual event that an ectopic ventricular impulse arises in the proximal portion of a bundle branch or fascicle, the contour of the resultant PVC may have a pure bundle branch or fascicle block pattern (Fig. 63-6, F). In this instance, the contour of the abnormal QRS complex does not accurately reflect the mechanism of its occurrence.

In the presence of sinus rhythm, evaluation of the P wave preceding an abnormal premature QRS complex may be helpful in the differential diagnosis of aberration versus ectopy. When a premature abnormal QRS complex is preceded by a *premature* P wave, the QRS complex is most likely to be supraventricular in origin, either stimulated by the preceding P wave or by an AV junctional impulse that has initiated depolarization of the atrium before the ventricles. It is always possible, of course, to explain a premature P wave preceding a premature abnormal QRS complex as the result of the fortuitous occurrence of sequential atrial and ventricular ectopic impulses, but this seems to occur only very rarely. Impulses arising in the intraventricular conduction system activate ventricular tissue well in advance of atrial tissue, since the atrium can be reached only after the impulse retrogradely traverses the AV node, which conducts impulses much more slowly than does the intraventricular conduction system. Thus, when a PVC causes atrial activation, the resultant P wave generally falls within, or follows, the PVC. Preceding P-wave criteria obviously are useless in the presence of atrial fibrillation in which atrial activity is so rapid and disorganized that the relationships of atrial to ventricular activity cannot be defined.

In the presence of atrial fibrillation, the differential diagnosis of aberration versus ectopy is facilitated by an evaluation of the relationship of the coupling interval of the abnormal QRS complex (ie, the interval between the abnor-

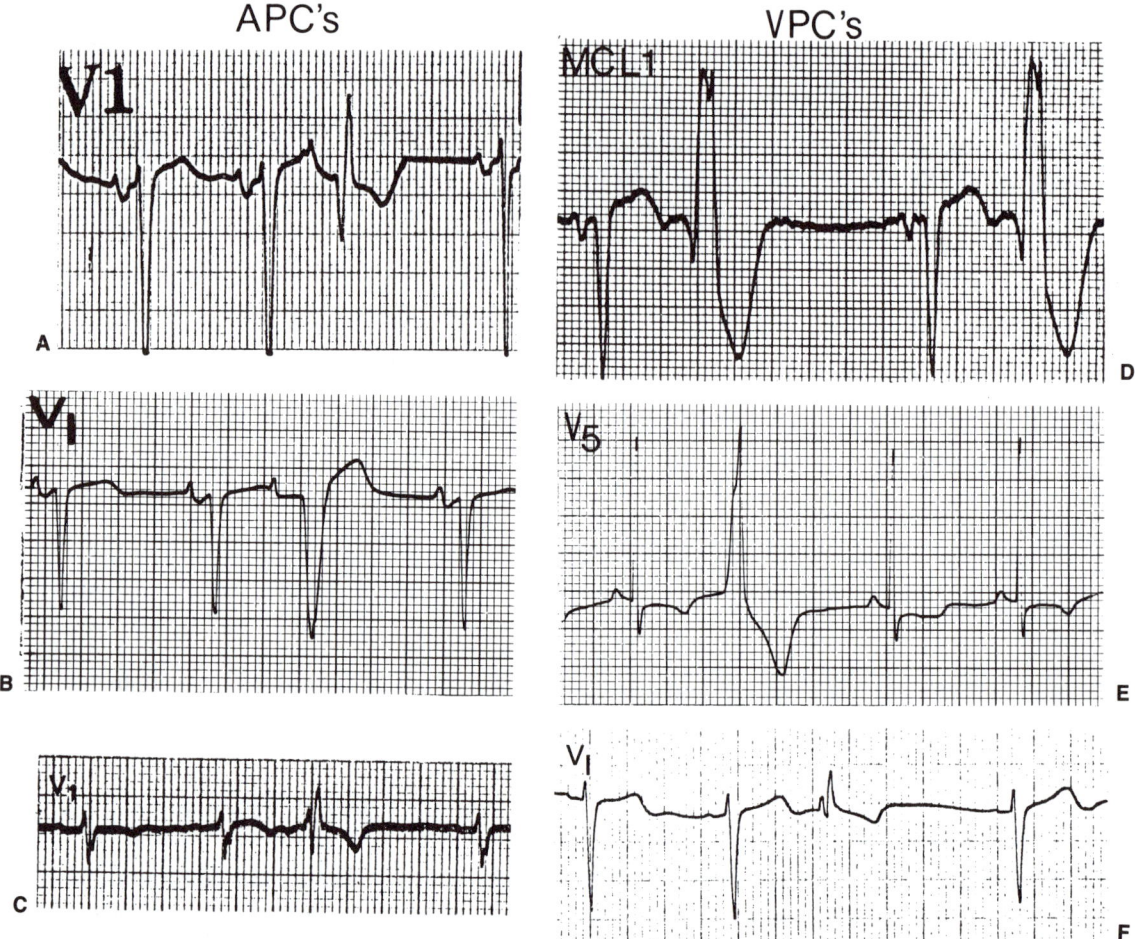

Figure 63-6 ECGs showing atrial and ventricular premature complexes. Tracings show atrial premature complexes (APCs) conducted with right bundle branch block (*A*), left bundle branch block (*B*), and mild right bundle branch conduction delay patterns (*C*). The ventricular premature complexes (VPCs) in (*D* and *E*) probably originated in distal Purkinje fibers. The VPC in *F* probably originated within the left bundle branch, as it has a "pure" right bundle branch conduction delay pattern and is only mildly widened.

mal QRS complex and the immediately preceding typical one) and the preceding cycle length (ie, the interval between the two QRS complexes immediately preceding the abnormal QRS complex in question). As the refractory periods of different portions of the intraventricular conduction system are set on a beat-to-beat basis and shorten with increasing heart rate (ie, following shorter R-R intervals), an abnormal QRS complex occurring at a coupling interval longer than the preceding cycle length is more likely to be due to ectopic ventricular impulse formation than to aberrant intraventricular conduction of an atrial fibrillatory impulse. In contrast, a wide QRS complex occurring at a short coupling interval relative to the preceding cycle length is more likely to be due to aberrant intraventricular conduction. If the preceding cycle length is *very* long, however, the propensity for ventricular ectopy is enhanced, a phenomenon termed the *rule of bigeminy*. Ventricular ectopy is also likely to be the mechanism of essentially identical abnormal QRS complexes occurring at *constant* coupling intervals, despite variable preceding cycle lengths during atrial fibrillation. The term *Ashman phenomenon* refers to a brief run, during rapid atrial rhythms, of aberrantly conducted supraventricular impulses that simulate ventricular tachycardia. The first abnormal QRS complex in such a run usually occurs at a short coupling interval relative to the preceding cycle length. Figure 63-7 displays several rhythm strips that illustrate these points.

BRADYDYSRHYTHMIAS*

While it is well recognized that heart rates in the range of 40 to 50 beats/minute may occur in normal, healthy adults and that heart rates as low as 30 beats/minute may be seen in

---

*Portions of this section have, with permission of the publisher, been modified and reprinted from Jacobson LB, Lester RM, Scheinman MM: Management of acute bundle branch block and bradyarrhythmias. *Med Clin North Am* 63:93, 1979.

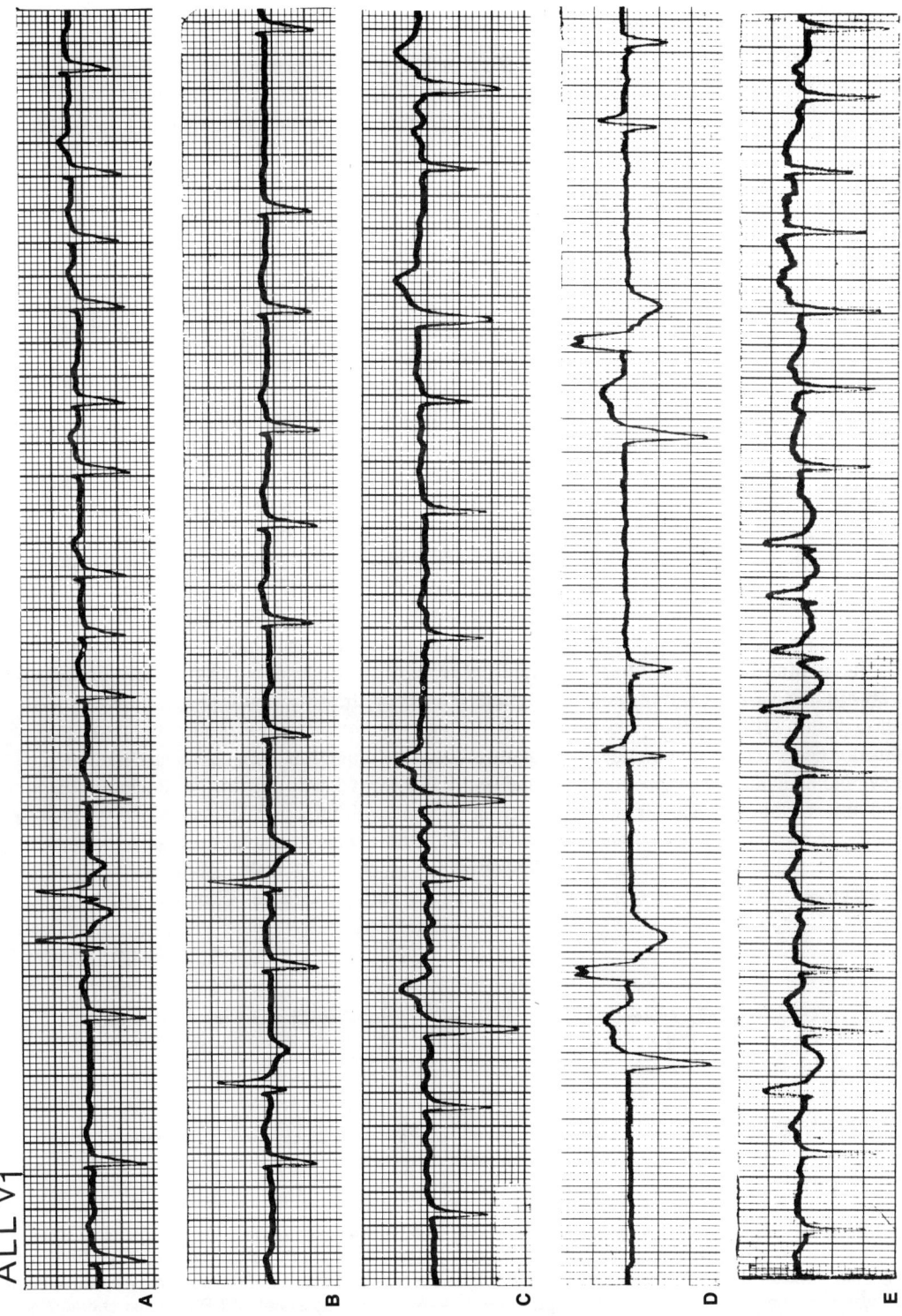

Figure 63-7 *Note:* In all strips, the atrial rhythm is fibrillation. In *A* and *B*, the rsR' complexes occur at short coupling intervals relative to the preceding cycle lengths and have a "pure" right bundle branch block-type pattern, suggesting they reflect aberrantly conducted fibrillatory impulses. In *C*, the wide QRS complexes are most likely ventricular ectopic beats because although they occur at short coupling intervals relative to the preceding cycle lengths, the coupling intervals are identical. In *D*, there is a bigeminal rhythm in which the QRS complexes that terminate very long pauses are followed by different and even more bizarre QRS complexes that occur at short cycle lengths. The QRS complexes occurring at short cycle length are probably ventricular ectopic beats because their contours are very abnormal and because they occur at short coupling intervals after QRS complexes that terminate very long pauses. The events in *D* illustrate the *rule of bigeminy*. In the middle of strip *E*, an abnormal QRS complex occurring at a short coupling interval relative to the preceding cycle length is followed by a run of three similarly abnormal QRS complexes. This brief run of aberrantly conducted supraventricular impulses that simulate ventricular tachycardia illustrates the *Ashman phenomenon*.

very well trained athletes, a sudden fall in heart rate to these levels or pauses in ventricular rhythm lasting more than a few seconds may have serious, even disastrous, clinical consequences. The presyncopal symptoms, syncope, seizure, and sudden death that may occur at times of bradycardia reflect inadequate cerebral perfusion resulting from low cardiac output and low systemic arterial blood pressure.

An acute fall in ventricular rate may occur because of failure of either impulse formation or impulse conduction (Table 63-2). When the sinus node does not activate the atrium, either because the sinus impulse is not generated appropriately (ie, sinus arrest) or because the generated impulse cannot be conducted into the atrium (ie, sinoatrial exit block), subsidiary automatic tissue in the AV junctional area would be expected to terminate the pause within 1 to 2 seconds by generating a stable rhythm that would gradually increase its rate to about 45 to 55 beats/minute. Following resumption of an atrial rhythm whose rate exceeds the junctional rate, the lower AV-junctional pacemaker would be overdriven and would then become dormant. This expected course of events is shown in Fig. 63-8. If, however, the AV-junctional tissue fails to generate an impulse, automatic tissue in the fascicles or Purkinje fibers of the intraventricular conduction system would be expected to begin to initiate ventricular activation within a few seconds and to maintain a stable rhythm at a rate of about 30 to 40 beats/minute. Thus, clinically important bradycardias would not be expected to follow the sudden cessation of sinus or atrial activity, because of the availability of subsidiary pacemakers. This is not always the case, however, and prolonged cardiac standstill may ensue (Fig. 63-9).

Since patients in whom the expected escape rhythm does occur are not likely to be symptomatic and, therefore, not likely to come under clinical observation, it is unclear how often the expected AV-junctional escape mechanism prevents clinically symptomatic bradycardia related to sinus or atrial arrest, or sinoatrial exit block. Prolonged junctional arrest in patients with sinus arrest or sinoatrial exit block may be related to concomitant disease in the approaches to and body of the AV node and His bundle, and/or to increased parasympathetic traffic or decreased sympathetic traffic into this subsidiary automatic tissue.

Table 63-2 Mechanisms of Bradycardias

Abnormal Impulse Formation	Abnormal Impulse Conduction
Sinus arrest	Sinoatrial exit block
Spontaneous	AV nodal block
Following termination of tachycardias	His-Purkinje system block
Artificial cardiac pacemaker malfunction	

Source: Modified and reprinted with permission from Jacobson LB, Lester RM, Scheinman MM: Management of acute bundle branch block and bradyarrhythmias. *Med Clin North Am* 63:93, 1979.

Sudden Sinus or Atrial Standstill

A diagnosis of sinus or atrial standstill is established by the sudden disappearance from the electrocardiogram of atrial activity (ie, P waves, flutter waves, or fibrillatory waves). Sinoatrial exit block should be suspected when the length of a pause in sinus rhythm is a multiple of the spontaneous sinus cycle length at that time (Fig. 63-10). When the pause is not a multiple of the spontaneous sinus-cycle length, the pause is referred to as a sinus pause or, when overly prolonged, a period of sinus or atrial standstill, or arrest (Fig. 63-9).

While these bradydysrhythmias may be associated with acute myocardial infarction or electrical termination of atrial and ventricular tachydysrhythmias, they are most commonly seen in patients with the so-called sick sinus syndrome, in which APCs, atrial tachydysrhythmias, slow sinus rhythm, sinoatrial exit block, and sinus arrest may occur at different times. In many patients with sick sinus syndrome, the occur-

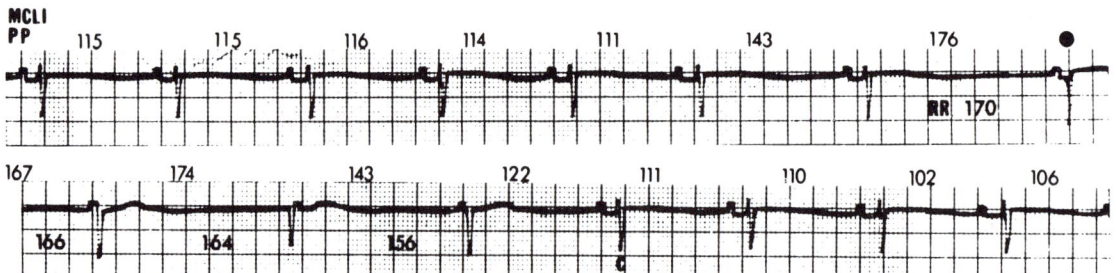

Figure 63-8 Continuous ECG strips showing the expected response to sinus slowing. *Note:* In the top strip, the sinus rate suddenly slows (PP intervals lengthen), and a junctional escape beat (●) terminates the resultant pause. The first three QRS complexes in the bottom strip are dissociated from the P waves and are junctional escape beats. These escape beats occur at progressively shorter intervals, demonstrating the warm-up phenomenon of a subsidiary pacemaker. As sinus rate accelerates (PP intervals shorten), sinus impulses again capture the ventricles. *C* denotes the first capture beat that reintroduces AV association. Numbers denote time in hundredths of a second. (*Source:* Reprinted with permission from Jacobson LB, Lester RM, Scheinman MM: Management of acute bundle branch block and bradyarrhythmias. *Med Clin North Am* 63:93, 1979.)

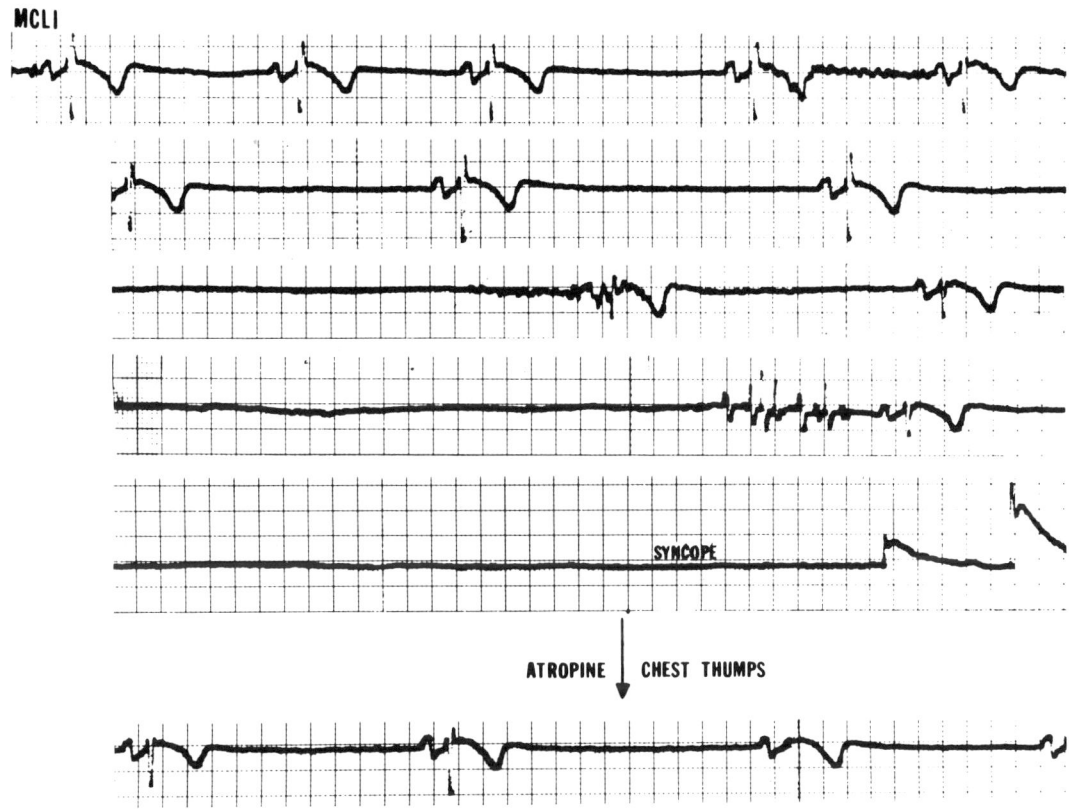

Figure 63-9 ECGs showing sinus slowing followed by cardiac standstill, but no escape rhythm. *Note:* The top five continuous ECG strips show profound sinus slowing and sinus arrest or atrial standstill, followed by complete cardiac standstill. No escape beats appear despite a pause of at least 10 seconds. Following blows to the precordium and the intravenous administration of atropine, very slow sinus rhythm (at a rate of about 20 beats/minute) resumes, as shown in the bottom strip. (*Source:* Reprinted with permission from Jacobson LB, Lester RM, Scheinman MM: Management of acute bundle branch block and bradyarrhythmias. Med Clin North Am 63:93, 1979.)

rence of atrial standstill is totally unpredictable (Fig. 63-9), while in other patients it may predictably follow the spontaneous cessation of an atrial tachydysrhythmia (Fig. 63-11). Regardless of the events preceding atrial standstill in the sick sinus syndrome, the period of asystole rarely lasts more than 5 to 10 seconds and is usually terminated by atrial or junctional complexes. Sudden death is not common in patients with sick sinus syndrome because the bradycardia that occurs is usually neither profound nor persistent.

The management of the patient with transient sinus or atrial standstill involves stimulating the sinus node or AV-junctional automatic tissues so that they will generate impulses. This can usually be achieved with one or more blows to the lower sternal area or by alteration of the autonomic nervous-system traffic into these pacemaker tissues. Parasympathetic stimuli and beta-adrenergic blocking agents slow the automatic rate of the sinus node and decrease the ability of sinus impulses to traverse the sinoatrial junction into atrial tissue; while parasympatholytic agents and beta-adrenergic stimulating agents enhance sinus node automaticity and the ability of a sinus impulse to traverse the sinoatrial junction. Thus, it might be expected that intravenously (IV) administered atropine or isoproterenol would be effective in managing sinus arrest or atrial standstill in patients with recurrent bouts of bradycardia; however, the time required to administer these medications often exceeds the period of cardiac standstill, which is usually terminated by spontaneously occurring supraventricular rhythms, making the use of such medications unsatisfactory in an emergency. Atropine is generally administered in a dose of 1 to 2 mg IV as rapidly as possible, while isoproterenol is administered in a dose of 1 to 3 μg/minute by continuous IV infusion of a solution containing 1 mg isoproterenol in 250 mL of 5 percent dextrose in water. Because some patients with sick sinus syndrome have blunted responses to autonomic interventions, these medications are often ineffective even in clinically significant bradycardias. In such instances, the institution of temporary atrial or ventricular pacing is required immediately to ensure an adequate heart rate. Permanent atrial and/or ventricular pacing is the only reliable and effective treatment for the patient with recurrent clinically significant supraventricular bradydysrhythmias.

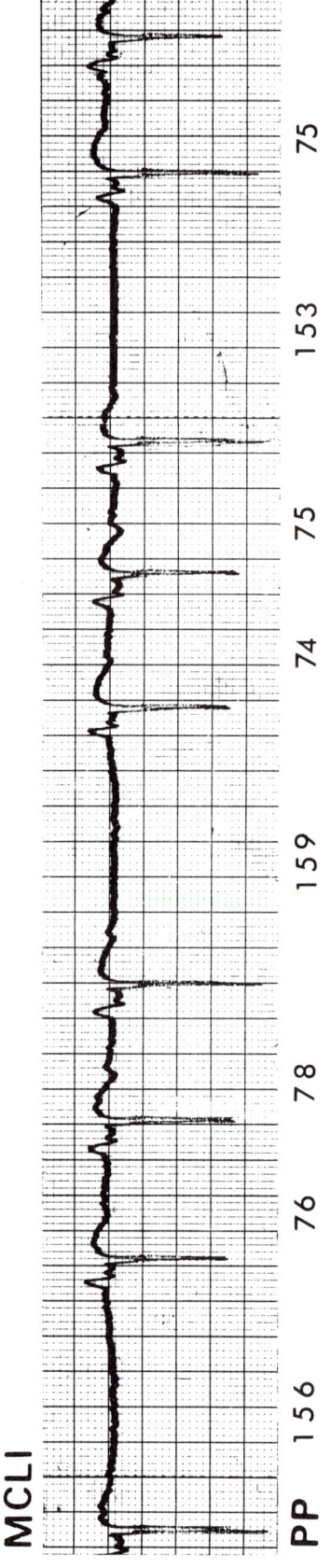

Figure 63-10 ECG showing 4:3 sinoatrial exit block. *Note:* The group beating is attributable to 4:3 sinoatrial exit block, for the PP intervals during the pauses are almost exactly twice the shorter PP intervals. Times are in hundredths of a second. (*Source:* Reprinted by permission of Elsevier Science Publishing Co Inc from Jacobson LB, Goldschlager N: *Arrhythmias: Case Studies.* Copyright 1978 by Medical Examination Publishing Co Inc.)

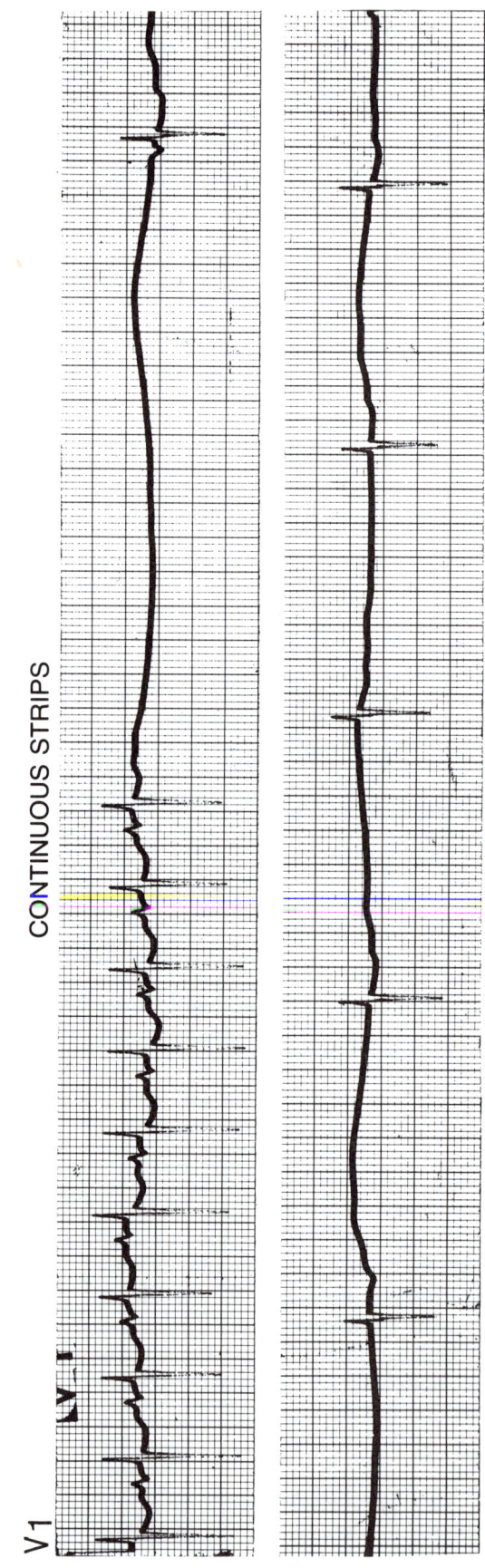

Figure 63-11 ECG showing transient cardiac standstill after termination of a supraventricular tachydysrhythmia. *Note:* Following spontaneous termination of a supraventricular tachydysrhythmia, there is a 3.9-second period of cardiac standstill that is terminated by a junctional or atrial escape beat. About 3.6 seconds later, there emerges a junctional escape rhythm that gradually increases its rate until, in the next to the last beat in the bottom strip, it is suppressed by emergence of a more rapid atrial rhythm. These strips were recorded from a patient with the bradycardia-tachycardia variant of the sick sinus syndrome.

Atrioventricular (AV) Block

Abnormalities in conduction of impulses from atrium to ventricle are termed AV blocks. AV blocks are categorized as first degree (1°), second degree (2°), or third degree (3°); the higher the degree of block, the greater the impairment in AV conduction. First-degree AV block is said to be present when all sinus impulses are conducted to the ventricles, but AV conduction takes longer than normal. Thus, the presence of 1° AV block is recognized when all P waves are followed by QRS complexes that they stimulate, but the PR interval exceeds 0.20 seconds.

In 2° AV block, some, but not all, sinus impulses are conducted into the ventricles. Second-degree AV block is recognized by the intermittent failure of a QRS complex to follow a sinus P wave. Second-degree AV blocks are divided into Mobitz Types I and II. Mobitz Type I 2° AV block, also known as a Wenckebach Type 2° AV block, is characterized by progressive PR-interval prolongation in the conducted beats preceding the sinus P wave that fails to stimulate a QRS complex (Fig. 63-12, A). Mobitz Type II 2° AV block is characterized by constancy of the PR intervals in the beats preceding and following the nonconducted sinus P wave (Fig. 63-12, B). Mobitz Type I block is almost always due to depressed conduction in the AV node, while Mobitz Type II block is almost always due to depressed conduction in the His bundle or in the bundle branches. The term *high-grade 2° AV block* refers to the failure of two or more consecutive sinus P waves to be conducted to the ventricles; this may occur when the block is Mobitz Type I or II. First- and second-degree AV blocks are defined only when the atrial rhythm is sinus.

Third-degree or complete AV block is said to be present when atrial impulses are never able to be conducted to the ventricles. In this event, the ventricular rhythm must be stimulated by impulses arising in automatic tissue below the level of block, which may be in the AV node, the His bundle, or the proximal portions of the bundle branches. Such escape rhythms are usually regular and have rates of 30 to 50 beats/minute. QRS rhythms arising in the AV junction (His bundle) generally have more normal contours and more rapid rates than those arising in the bundle branches or in Purkinje fibers. Third-degree AV block is recognized by the occurrence of a QRS rhythm that is temporally independent of the atrial rhythm, even though atrial impulses occur at times when they would normally be able to traverse the AV conduction system. The total independence of atrial and ventricular rhythms allows the diagnosis of third-degree AV block to be made regardless of whether the atrial rhythm is sinus, fibrillation, flutter, or ectopic tachycardia (Fig. 63-13).

When there is a sudden failure of impulse conduction from atrium to ventricle (ie, when there is AV block) there will be a pause in ventricular rhythm until either AV conduction resumes (Fig. 63-14, A) or an escape rhythm emerges (Fig. 63-14, B). It is at the time of onset of AV block and of cessation of firing of an escape pacemaker that patients with paroxysmal or chronic AV block may experience presyncope, syncope, seizure, or sudden death. The severity of the symptoms is roughly related to the duration of ventricular standstill, the rate and stability of the emerging escape rhythm, the posture and activities of the patient at the time, and the presence of cardiovascular disease.

When AV block occurs within the AV node, the emerging escape pacemaker usually arises in the His bundle. Such junctional pacemakers usually emerge within a few seconds and initiate a stable rhythm at a rate of about 40 to 50 beats/minute. When AV block occurs within or below the His bundle, however, the emerging pacemaker must arise in the fascicles or Purkinje fibers of the intraventricular conduction system. Such *infra-Hisian* pacemakers usually take several seconds to emerge, initiate a rhythm at a rate of about 20 to 40 beats/minute, and may unpredictably cease to fire for many seconds for no apparent reason.

While transvenous ventricular pacing is the safest, most effective, and most reliable therapy for bradycardia related to AV block, attempts to establish temporary pacing in an emergency department that has no fluoroscopy capability is impractical and risky. Thus, the emergency management of the patient with paroxysmal or persistent AV block generally involves attempts to ensure an adequate ventricular rate by administering medications that enhance AV conduction or increase the rate and stability of the escape pacemaker.

When the site of AV block is in the AV node, AV conduction can usually be improved by atropine and isoproterenol; both medications, but especially the latter, may also increase the rate of a junctional pacemaker. Thus, in Wenckebach (Type I) second-degree AV block and complete AV block that occurs in acute inferior-wall myocardial infarction or with digitalis excess, atropine and isoproterenol may result in more rapid ventricular rates (Fig. 63-15, A). When the site of the AV block is within or below the His bundle, as in Mobitz Type II second-degree AV block or complete AV block that occurs in acute anterior-wall myocardial infarction, isoproterenol, but not atropine, might increase the ventricular rate (Fig. 63-15, B).

Although atropine and isoproterenol *may* be useful in increasing ventricular rate in AV block, their administration should be viewed as a temporizing measure to be used while plans are being made for the institution of ventricular pacing. In the most urgent situation of ventricular standstill, "blind" attempts to achieve ventricular pacing may be made with a standard or a balloon-tip "flow-directed" electrode catheter inserted into a vein, or with a wire electrode inserted percutaneously through the chest wall or subxiphoid area into the right or left ventricular chambers.

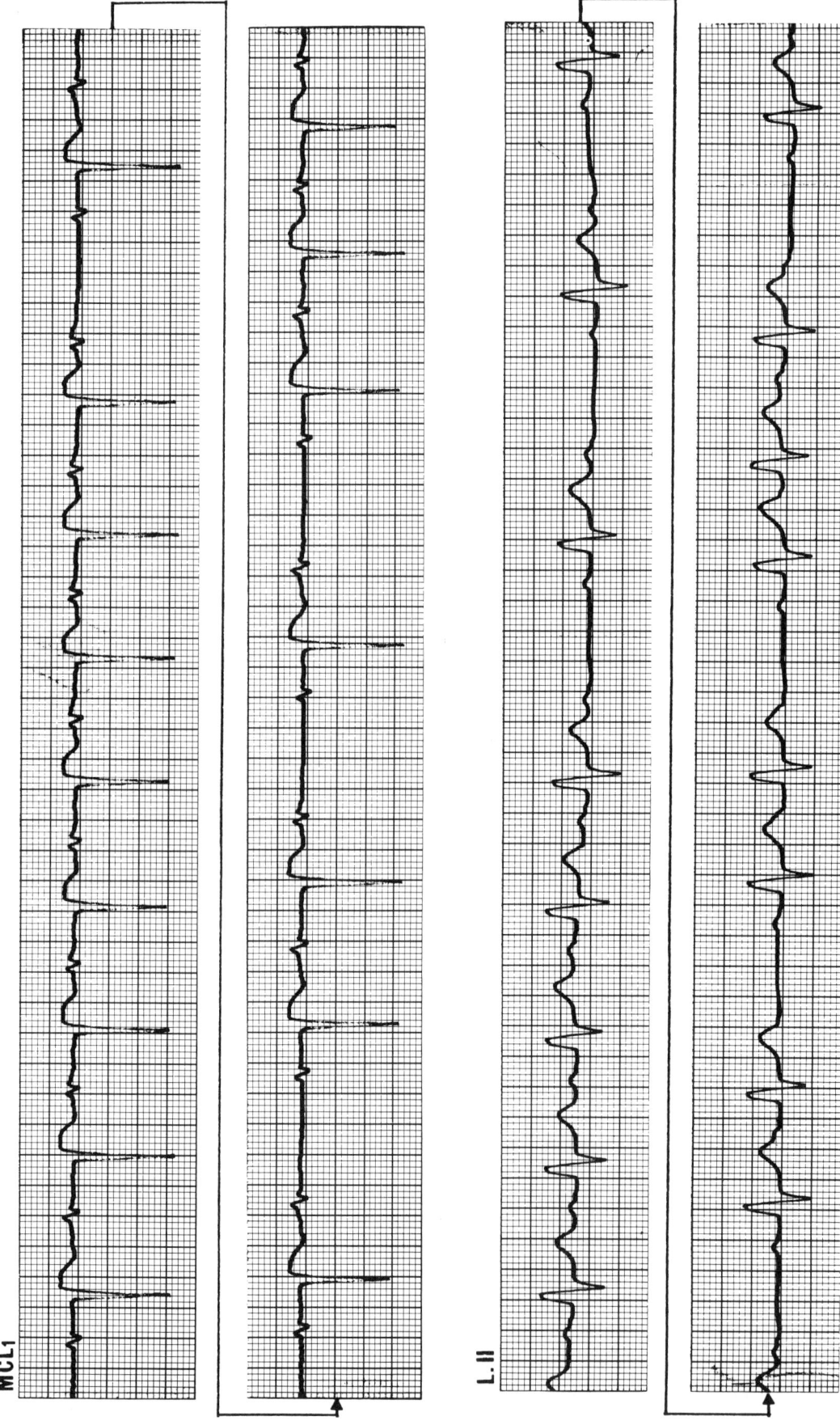

Figure 63-12 ECGs showing Mobitz Types I and II second-degree AV blocks. *A:* These two continuous-lead MCL1 rhythm strips were recorded from a 74-year-old woman with digitalis intoxication. Sinus P waves, which occur with regularity at a rate of about 72 beats/minute, intermittently fail to stimulate QRS complexes. The progressive PR-interval prolongation in the conducted beats that precede the nonconducted P waves establishes the diagnosis of Mobitz Type I or Wenckebach Type second-degree AV block. *B:* These two continuous-lead II rhythm strips were recorded from an 82-year-old woman with paroxysmal presyncopal symptoms and dyspnea. Sinus P waves occur with reasonable regularity, but they intermittently fail to stimulate QRS complexes. The constancy of the PR intervals in the conducted beats that precede and follow the blocked P waves establishes the diagnosis of Mobitz Type II second-degree AV block. During the period of block, there is some mild irregularity in the P-wave rhythm, perhaps owing to autonomic nervous system mediated beat-to-beat changes in sinus rate or to the occurrence of atrial premature complexes.

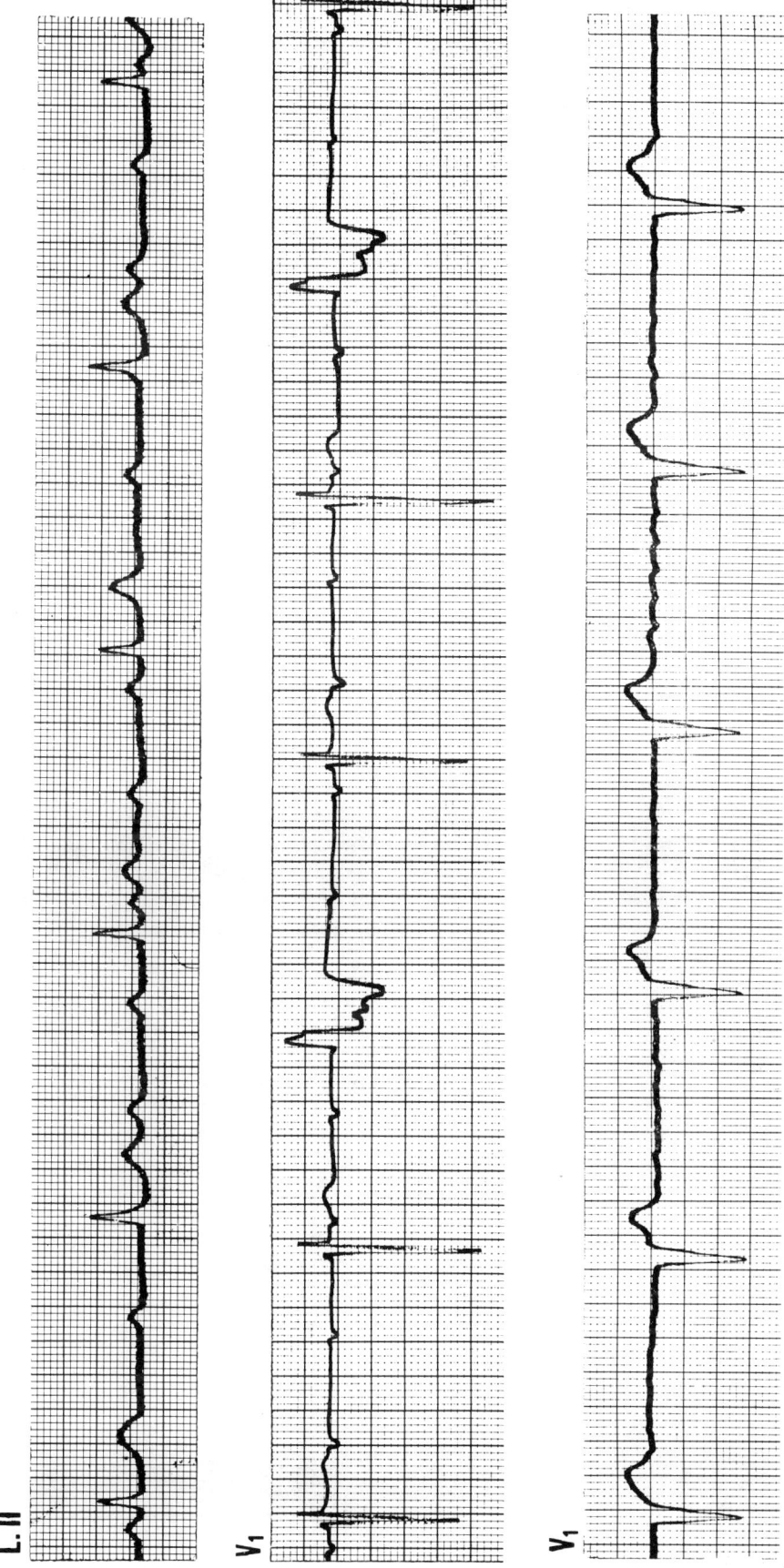

Figure 63-13 ECGs from three patients with complete AV block. *Note:* These three patients have AV dissociation due to complete AV block. *A:* This strip was recorded from a 15-year-old boy with acute rheumatic fever. The atrial rhythm is sinus. The QRS complexes, which occur with regularity at a rate of about 32 beats/minute, have normal contours, except when P waves are superimposed upon them. The normal QRS contours suggest that this escape rhythm arises in the AV junction (His bundle). *B:* This strip was recorded from an 82-year-old woman with recent onset of weakness, fatigue, paroxysmal lightheadedness, and congestive heart failure. The atrial rhythm is sinus. There is group beating of the QRS complexes; two escape complexes which have a right bundle branch block-type contour, indicating that they probably originate near the left bundle branch, are followed by a ventricular ectopic beat. The average ventricular rate is about 40 beats/minute. *C:* This strip was recorded from a 66-year-old man with chronic atrial fibrillation and complete AV block contributed to by digoxin. The QRS complexes, which occur with regularity at a rate of about 39 beats/minute, show a left bundle branch block pattern, suggesting that they originate in or near the right bundle branch.

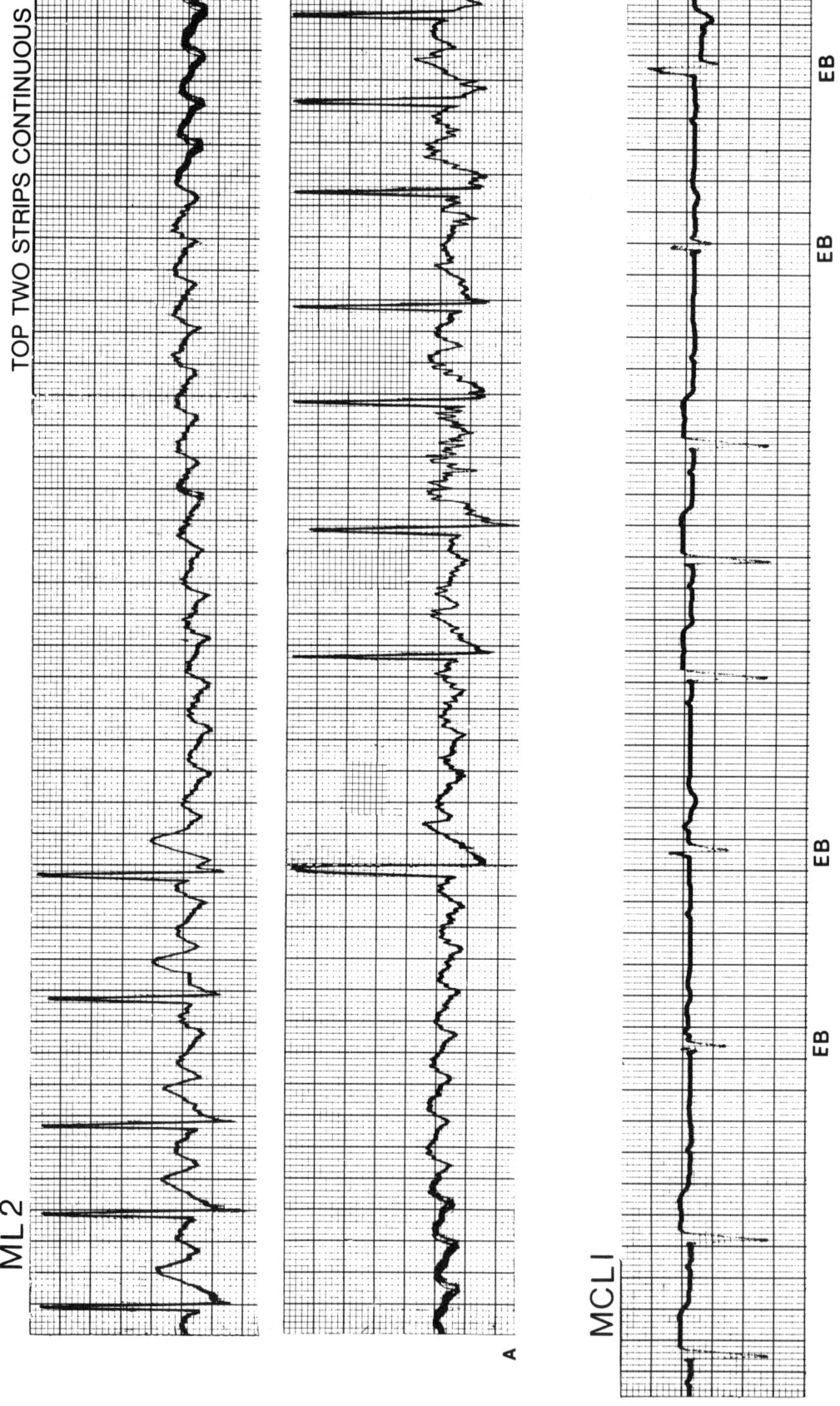

Figure 63-14 ECGs showing transient AV block. *A:* During atrial flutter, a 9-second period of ventricular standstill due to AV block is terminated when AV conduction resumes. *B:* Pauses in QRS rhythm occasioned by periods of Mobitz Type II second-degree AV block are terminated by fascicular or ventricular escape beats (*EB*).

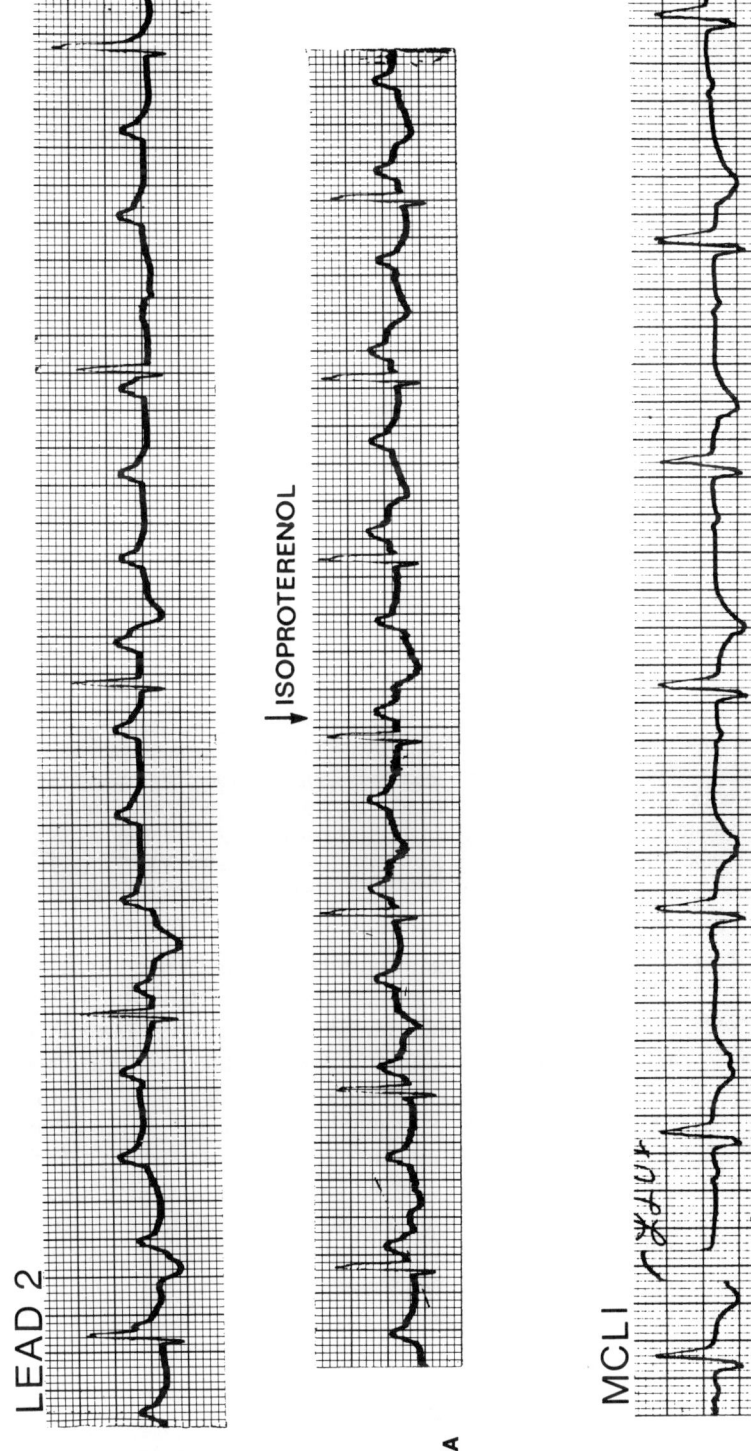
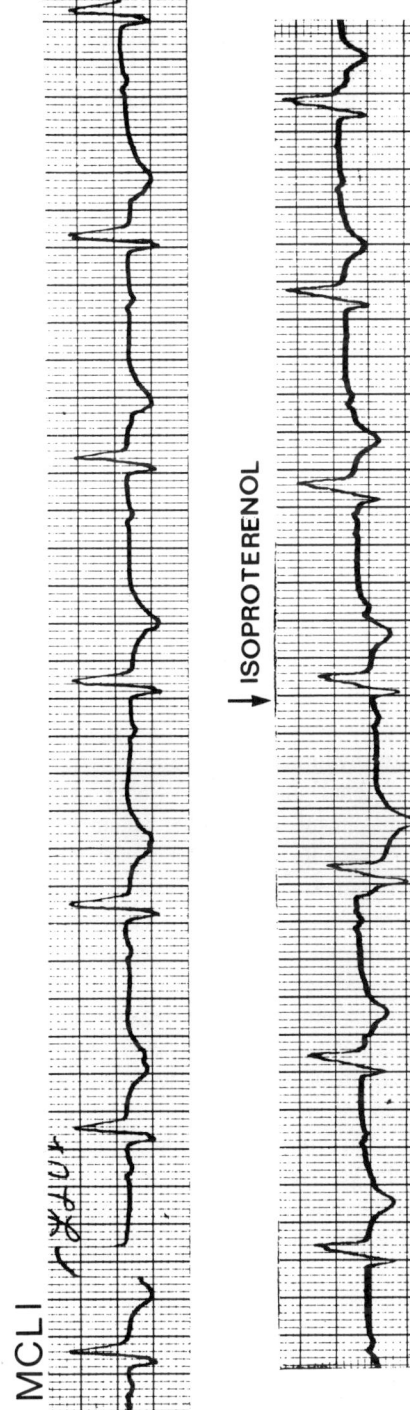

TACHYDYSRHYTHMIAS

Tachycardia is said to be present when the rate of a rhythm exceeds a particular, but arbitrarily chosen, limit. Tachycardias may be clinically significant because of the adverse hemodynamic effects of the rapid heart rate and, often, the accompanying changes in atrial and ventricular contraction sequences; or because of their ability to degenerate into even more rapid and, therefore, more hemodynamically disadvantageous dysrhythmias.

The management of the patient with a tachydysrhythmia depends on the immediate hemodynamic effects of the dysrhythmia, the projected clinical course of the dysrhythmia with and without specific therapeutic interventions, the underlying cardiovascular status of the patient, and the nature of the dysrhythmia itself. It is, therefore, critical in evaluating a patient with a tachydysrhythmia to answer the following questions:

1. Is the tachydysrhythmia causing a serious problem at the moment, or is its continuation likely to do so?
2. What, exactly, is the tachydysrhythmia?
3. What is the patient's underlying cardiovascular status; does the patient have evidence of heart disease?
4. What is the most prudent way to terminate the dysrhythmia or to attenuate its adverse effects?

Supraventricular Tachydysrhythmias

Supraventricular tachydysrhythmias are unusually rapid rhythms that arise in sinus nodal, atrial, or AV-junctional tissue. The dysrhythmia may result from either enhanced automaticity or reentry within supraventricular tissue. In supraventricular tachydysrhythmias, the ventricular rhythm is stimulated by supraventricular impulses. The tachydysrhythmias may have adverse hemodynamic effects because the resultant ventricular rate is quite rapid, because atrial contraction becomes ineffective, and/or because the normal atrial and ventricular contraction sequence has been lost. Essential to the management of patients with supraventricular tachydysrhythmias is an assessment of the relative significance of these factors, for therapeutic maneuvers aimed simply at slowing the ventricular rate may be quite different from those aimed at terminating the tachydysrhythmia in order to restore the normal atrial and ventricular contraction sequence.

The specific supraventricular tachydysrhythmias are

- sinus tachycardia
- ectopic atrial tachycardia (EAT)
- multifocal atrial tachycardia (MAT)
- atrial fibrillation
- atrial flutter
- paroxysmal supraventricular tachycardia (PSVT)
- nonparoxysmal junctional tachycardia (NPJT)

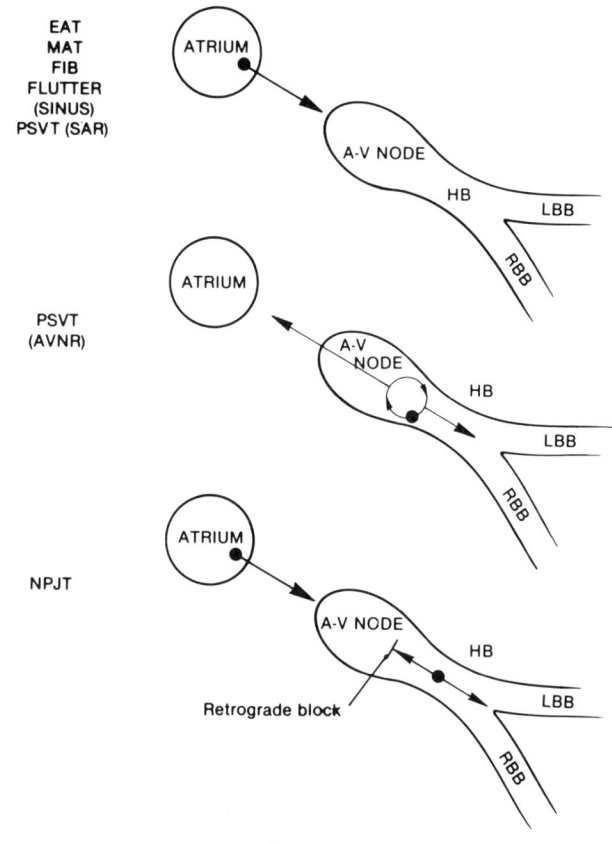

Figure 63-16 Mechanisms of supraventricular tachydysrhythmias. Key: *AVNR*, AV nodal reentry; *EAT*, ectopic atrial tachycardia; *FIB*, fibrillation; *HB*, His bundle; *LBB*, left bundle branch; *MAT*, multifocal atrial tachycardia; *NPJT*, nonparoxysmal junctional tachycardia; *PSVT*, paroxysmal supraventricular tachycardia; *RBB*, right bundle branch; *SAR*, sinoatrial reentry.

The mechanistic similarities and differences of these tachydysrhythmias have important diagnostic and therapeutic implications (Fig. 63-16). For example, in most supraventricular tachydysrhythmias, a rapid independent atrial rhythm stimulates the ventricular rhythm. In paroxysmal supraventricular tachycardia (PSVT) due to the mechanism of AV nodal reentry (AVNR), however, both atrial and ventricular rhythms are dependent on AV nodal reentrant impulses. In nonparoxysmal junctional tachycardia, the atrial rhythm is independent of the more rapid AV junctional pacemaker that stimulates the ventricular rhythm; but, because of retrograde AV-nodal conduction block, the junctional impulse cannot stimulate the atrium.

Sinus Tachycardia

The sinus node is strongly influenced by the autonomic nervous system, circulating catecholamines, the temperature of the circulating blood, and thyroid hormone. The automatic firing rate of the sinus node is increased by stimulation of the sympathetic portion of the autonomic nervous system, as well as by circulating catecholamines, elevation of body temperature, and thyroid hormone. Its automatic firing rate is decreased by stimulation of the parasympathetic nervous system, beta-adrenergic blocking agents, decrement in body temperature, and deficiency of thyroid hormone.

Sinus rhythm at rates in excess of 100 beats/minute in normothermic adults is said to be abnormal; this tachydysrhythmia is termed *sinus tachycardia*. Since the normal sinus mechanism is operating, sinus tachycardia is a dysrhythmia only by virtue of its rate. Thus, sinus tachycardia should not be looked upon as a dysrhythmia *per se*, but rather as a response to certain events. It is the responsibility of the physician to search for the specific event causing the tachycardia.

Sinus tachycardia is commonly seen in patients with infection, heart failure, acute anxiety reactions, asthmatic attacks, and intravascular volume depletion that is, most often, due to hemorrhage or gastrointestinal fluid loss. In some patients, medications such as thyroid hormone, bronchodilators, or vasodilators (eg, hydralazine hydrochloride) contribute to the rapid rate. Rarely, sinus tachycardia at rates as high as about 140 beats/minute may occur chronically for no identifiable reason. Only in the rarest instances, for example, thyrotoxicosis, are specific medications (generally beta-blocking agents) administered in an attempt to slow the heart rate.

Ectopic Atrial Tachycardia

Ectopic atrial tachycardia (EAT) is a rare dysrhythmia in which an ectopic atrial pacemaker discharges at a reasonably constant and rapid rate. While in most clinically encountered ectopic atrial tachycardias, the atrial rate is in the range of 160 to 190 beats/minute, cases have been observed in which the atrial rate is only slightly more than 100 beats/minute, or as rapid as about 240 beats/minute. Most ectopic atrial tachycardias are seen in patients with severe heart disease during a period of profound congestive heart failure; in some patients, it may be a manifestation of digitalis excess.

The ventricular (QRS) rate and rhythm in ectopic atrial tachycardia depend on conduction of the atrial impulses through the AV conduction system, the slowest conducting portion of which is almost always the AV node. At times, there may be consistent 1:1 or 2:1 AV conduction; at other times, AV Wenckebach periods (eg, 3:2, 4:3, 5:4) may occur (Fig. 63-17, A). The AV-conduction ratio generally depends on the atrial rate, conduction being "better" at lower atrial rates, and on the conduction properties of the AV node, which can be altered by medications and by autonomic nervous-system traffic.

The P waves in ectopic atrial tachycardia are generally of abnormal contour and duration, being sharply pointed and narrow (Fig. 63-17, B). When the atrial rate is rapid and 1:1 AV conduction is present, P waves may not be seen easily. However, when AV conduction is less than 1:1, as may occur spontaneously or in response to carotid sinus massage or medication (eg, edrophonium chloride [Tensilon], verapamil, adenosine, or digitalis), P waves may be clearly seen.

The adverse hemodynamic effects of ectopic atrial tachycardia relate predominantly to the rapidity of the ventricular rate, for the *atrial kick* is maintained by the organized atrial rhythm. When AV conduction is 1:1, the patient may be profoundly ill, and treatment aimed at slowing the ventricular rate by slowing AV nodal conduction is in order. If digoxin is *not* the cause of the dysrhythmia, then digoxin may be given, preferably intravenously, in doses of 0.125 to 0.375 mg. Even if the dysrhythmia *is* digoxin-related, more digoxin may be given to slow the ventricular rate when AV conduction is 1:1. However, it should be administered only in very small doses of about 0.0675 to 0.125 mg. It should be used simply to achieve slower ventricular rate while the heart failure, which predisposes to the ectopic atrial tachycardia, is brought under control. Beta-blocking agents, and verapamil or diltiazem, calcium-blocking agents, should rarely, if ever, be used in these patients, as they may worsen the already usually profound heart-failure state.

If AV conduction of the ectopic atrial tachycardia is 2:1, the ventricular rate is usually about 100 beats/minute and the rhythm *per se* is not a problem. Such patients probably should be admitted to the hospital for treatment of heart failure, however, and for monitoring of the cardiac rhythm, especially if digoxin is causing or contributing to the dysrhythmia. Digoxin should *not* be given to patients with ectopic atrial tachycardia when the AV-conduction ratio is 2:1 or greater, for such an intervention may result in higher grades of AV block and in ventricular dysrhythmias that are often fatal.

If due to digoxin excess, ectopic atrial tachycardia may be terminated by the cautious IV or oral administration of potassium chloride (KCl), even if the serum potassium level is normal. KCl usually produces a gradual slowing of the atrial rate by about 10 to 20 beats/minute, an event that has the undesirable effect of increasing the tendency for AV conduction to become 1:1. However, while the resultant increase in ventricular rate may worsen the patient's hemodynamic state, the deterioration is usually transient, for the ectopic atrial tachycardia generally terminates shortly (minutes to an hour or so) after such slowing of the atrial rate. Direct current cardioversion of ectopic atrial tachycardia, especially if digitalis-related, is ill-advised because of the severe, and occasionally disastrous ventricular dysrhythmias that may follow.

Multifocal (Chaotic) Atrial Tachycardia

Multifocal atrial tachycardia is characterized by the occurrence, during sinus rhythm, of APCs of several contours at rapid rates, at variable coupling intervals, and in salvos (Fig. 63-18). The APCs may be conducted normally or aberrantly, or they may be blocked within the AV conduction system.

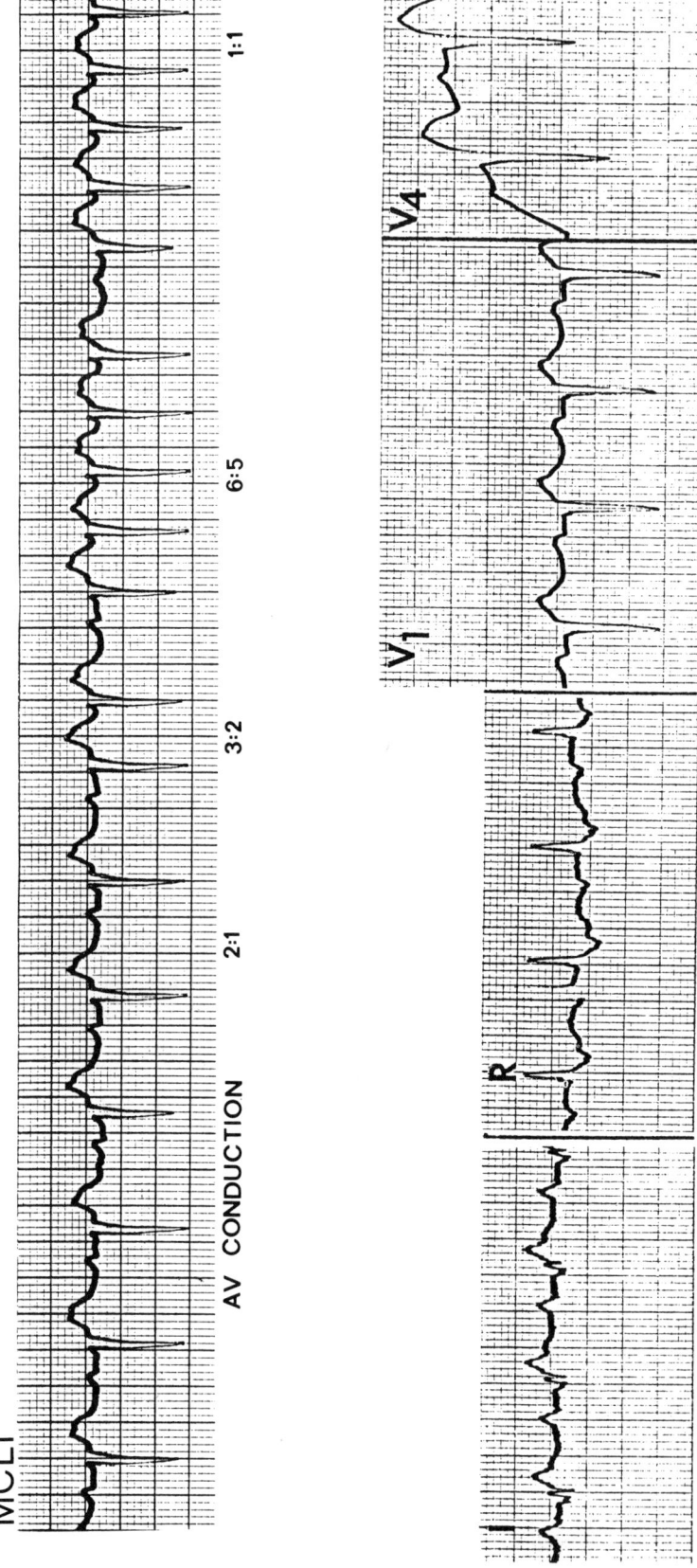

Figure 63-17 ECGs showing ectopic atrial tachycardia. *A*: Rhythm strip recorded during ectopic atrial tachycardia shows the effects of variable AV conduction on the QRS rhythm. *B*: Twelve-lead ECG recorded from the same patient whose rhythm strip is seen in *A* shows consistent 2:1 AV conduction and abnormal P-wave contours. This tracing also shows extensive anterior-wall myocardial infarction and left axis deviation attributable to left-anterior fascicle block.

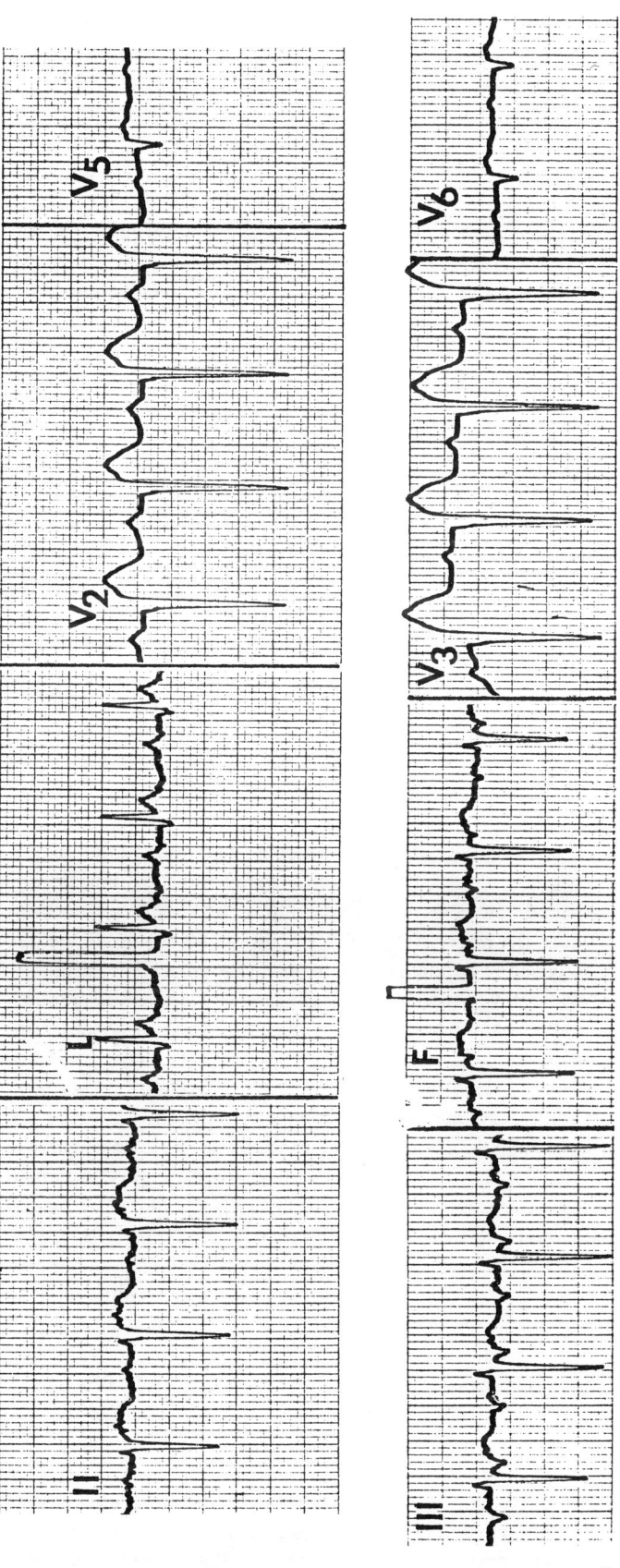

Figure 63-17 continued

Figure 63-18 ECG showing multifocal atrial tachycardia. *Note:* The occurrence of P waves of several different contours at variable and brief intervals establishes the diagnosis of multifocal atrial tachycardia. The variability in the contours of the QRS complexes reflects different degrees of aberrant intraventricular conduction.

Multifocal atrial tachycardia is seen almost exclusively in patients with respiratory failure related to acute and chronic pulmonary disease, although it occasionally occurs in patients with end-stage heart disease. Hypoxemia, acidemia, hypercapnia, and the high state of sympathetic stimulation attributable to abnormal respiratory function are predisposing factors. The rhythm presumably reflects high right-atrial pressures and volumes that occur in those patients with severe right-ventricular hypertension. The rhythm *per se* is rarely, if ever, of hemodynamic consequence. Rather, it is a marker of the precarious respiratory status of the patient, and it mandates immediate attention to the respiratory problem. Therapy is directed at improving the arterial blood-gas levels and correcting metabolic abnormalities, which may require the use of bronchodilators, supplemental inspired oxygen, antibiotics, chest percussion and postural drainage, and even assisted or controlled ventilation with a respirator. As the arterial blood gas and metabolic abnormalities improve, multifocal atrial tachycardia typically abates and disappears, occasionally leaving isolated APCs. Specific antidysrhythmic medications should not be administered to these patients, because their blood gas and metabolic abnormalities predispose them to the toxic effects of these medications, though verapamil may be effective in slowing the ventricular rate in MAT. (See Chapter 72, Obstructive Airway Disease.)

Atrial Fibrillation

Atrial fibrillation is characterized by a fine or coarse irregular baseline, which reflects disorganized atrial activity, and, in the presence of adequate AV conduction, an irregularly irregular ventricular (QRS) rhythm attributable to more or less random temporal conduction of the fibrillatory impulses through the AV conduction system (see Figs. 63-7 and 63-16). The rate of the ventricular rhythm in atrial fibrillation is determined by the conduction properties of the AV node, which may be altered by medications and by changes in autonomic nervous-system traffic. In the presence of normal AV nodal function, the ventricular rate during atrial fibrillation is in the range of 160 to 180 beats/minute; when AV nodal function is depressed, the ventricular rate is slower. In patients with accessory AV-conduction pathways that conduct rapidly and have short refractory periods, the ventricular response during atrial fibrillation may be much faster, occasionally as rapid as 300 beats/minute (see discussion of Wolff-Parkinson-White syndrome).

Although atrial fibrillation may occur episodically in otherwise healthy patients, it is generally seen in patients with structural cardiac disease and/or progressive degenerative disease of the supraventricular portion of the cardiac conduction system. The rapid ventricular rate associated with atrial fibrillation generally results in symptoms and in hemodynamic deterioration, and the loss of the atrial contribution to ventricular filling may dramatically depress ventricular performance in patients with left ventricular hypertrophy or with significant left-ventricular dysfunction. In still other patients, especially those with large left atria, mitral stenosis, idiopathic hypertrophic subaortic stenosis, and congestive heart failure, atrial fibrillation predisposes to the formation of left atrial thrombi and, therefore, to arterial embolism.

Management of the patient with atrial fibrillation begins with an assessment of the relative deleterious effects of the rapid ventricular rate and the loss of atrial contraction on the hemodynamic state, the reversibility of the circumstances that predisposed to or precipitated the onset of the dysrhythmia, and the likelihood that sinus rhythm can be restored and maintained. The aim of treatment is to convert the atrial rhythm to sinus, but if this is not advisable or not likely to be accomplished, to slow the *resting* ventricular rate to about 70 to 80 beats/minute and to prevent excessively rapid ventricular rates from occurring with effort.

If the patient with atrial fibrillation and rapid ventricular rate is critically ill, because of either the rapid rate itself or the loss of atrial contraction, direct-current cardioversion to sinus rhythm may be attempted and can usually be achieved with a 100 to 400 (but occasionally only a 50) watt-second electrical discharge, which should be synchronized to the spontaneous QRS complexes. In the less seriously ill patient, the oral or IV administration of digoxin will generally effect slowing of the ventricular response, but usually requires many hours to do so. The IV administration of beta-blocking drugs such as esmolol, metoprolol, and propranolol, and of calcium-blocking drugs such as verapamil and diltiazem will usually slow the ventricular rate dramatically within minutes. However, beta- and calcium-blocking drugs are ill-advised in hypotensive patients and in patients with significant left ventricular dysfunction and congestive heart failure. However, the heightened sympathetic nervous system stimulation that is often present in patients with congestive heart failure, acute or recent myocardial infarction, pericarditis, pulmonary embolus, or pulmonary parenchymal processes may oppose the rate-slowing effect of these medications. Atrial fibrillation of recent onset may abruptly terminate spontaneously, or as the ventricular response slows in response to medications. If atrial fibrillation persists despite achievement of a reasonably slow ventricular rate, plans should be made to perform direct-current cardioversion. Quinidine or procainamide should be administered in the usual therapeutic doses for 24 to 48 hours prior to the electrical-conversion attempt, for these medications may themselves convert the rhythm to sinus (or to atrial flutter). Furthermore, they seem to aid in maintaining sinus rhythm once it is restored. It is inadvisable to attempt direct-current cardioversion in the presence of electrolyte, metabolic, or blood-gas abnormalities, or digitalis excess, because more serious dysrhythmias may emerge within seconds to minutes after the electrical discharge. It is often difficult to restore and impossible to maintain sinus rhythm if right or left atrial

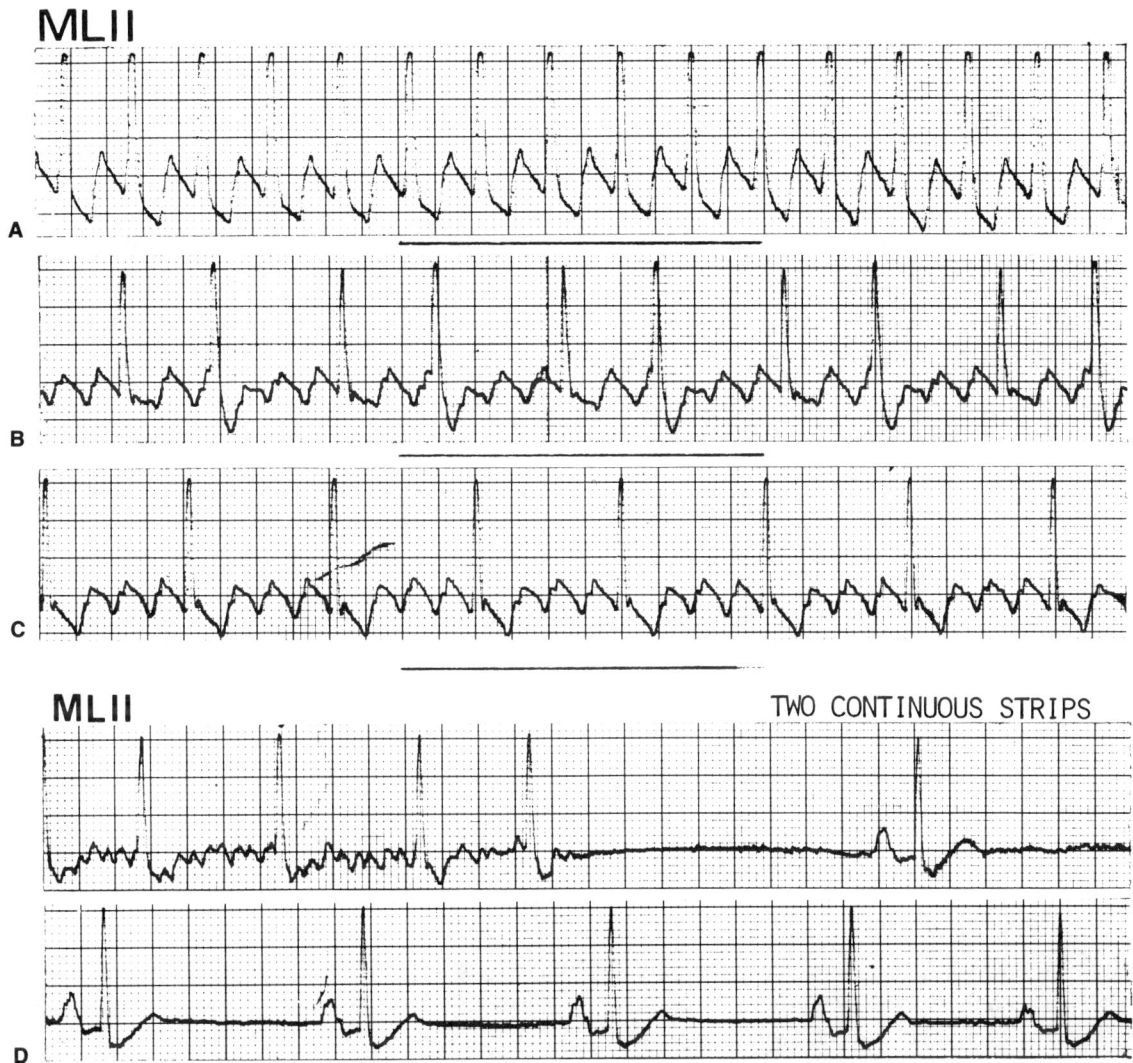

Figure 63-19 ECGs showing effects of digoxin and propranolol in atrial flutter. *Note:* A, B, and C were recorded serially, following the oral administration of digoxin and propranolol to a patient with atrial flutter. These medications effect a change in AV conduction from 2:1 in A to 4:1 in C. About 2 hours after the strip in C was recorded, the strips in D were recorded; they show the spontaneous termination of atrial flutter to cardiac standstill and the resumption of sinus rhythm that gradually increases in rate.

enlargement is extreme, or if the fibrillation has persisted for more than a few months. As conversion to sinus rhythm in patients with severe mitral valve disease, idiopathic hypertrophic subaortic stenosis, and low cardiac output from any cause courts the disaster of systemic embolism from a left atrial thrombus, many cardiologists feel that such patients should be anticoagulated for at least a few weeks prior to any conversion attempt if the atrial fibrillation has been present for more than 48 to 72 hours.

It may be necessary to manage atrial fibrillation differently in patients with accessory AV-conduction pathways, for the accessory pathway is composed of tissue with properties different from those of AV nodal tissue and much more like those of His-Purkinje system tissue. If AV conduction is occurring predominantly by the accessory pathway, digitalis, beta-blocking medications, and verapamil are usually *not* effective in slowing ventricular rate, but procainamide, quinidine, or disopyramide might be. (This topic is discussed in more detail in the section on the Wolff-Parkinson-White syndrome.)

Atrial Flutter

Atrial flutter is recognized by the regular occurrence of saw-tooth contour waves, seen best in leads II, III, and aVF of the surface ECG (Figs. 63-14, A, and 63-19). The usual rate of these flutter waves is about 300/minute, but it may be as slow as 200/minute or as rapid as 340/minute. The ventricular rate and rhythm in atrial flutter depend on conduction of the flutter impulses through the AV node. In most clinical circumstances and at most flutter rates, the normal AV node conducts every other flutter impulse into the ventricles, resulting in the regular appearance of QRS complexes of the usual contour at a rate exactly one-half the flutter rate. Diseased AV nodes conduct the flutter impulses less well, and the resultant ventricular rate is slower. One-to-one AV conduction of flutter impulses may be seen in infants, in patients with accessory AV-conduction pathways that have short refractory periods (see Wolff-Parkinson-White Syndrome), and in patients with relatively slow flutter rates of about 220 to 240 per minute. AV nodal conduction of the flutter impulses may be enhanced by beta-adrenergic stimulating drugs, bronchodilators, and vagolytic medications or maneuvers; it may be depressed by digitalis glycosides, parasympathetic stimulation, vagotonic medications and maneuvers, beta-adrenergic blocking agents, and the calcium-blocking drugs verapamil and diltiazem.

Atrial flutter generally occurs in patients with structural cardiac disease, but it may be the only manifestation of disease of the sinus node and atrial tissues, in which case it would be considered a manifestation of the sick sinus syndrome. Atrial flutter generally causes hemodynamic deterioration by virtue of the rapid ventricular rates that usually accompany it, although loss of the atrial contribution to ventricular filling may contribute to the deterioration in patients with poor left-ventricular function and left ventricular hypertrophy. Management of the patient with atrial flutter is aimed at terminating the dysrhythmia or at slowing the ventricular response by administration of medications that slow AV nodal conduction and by withdrawal of medications that enhance it. The exact management program chosen depends on the hemodynamic state of the patient at the time, the patient's underlying cardiovascular state, and the medication that the patient has taken up to that point. Atrial flutter can generally be terminated by direct-current cardioversion with electrical discharges of 10 to 100 watt-seconds. In the patient with 1:1 AV conduction, the patient who has a rapid ventricular rate and is tolerating it poorly, and the patient who has no other cardiac disease and in whom converting the dysrhythmia in advance of medication administration seems to carry little risk, electrical conversion is advisable as the initial therapeutic intervention.

The ventricular response to atrial flutter, like that to atrial fibrillation, may be slowed with digitalis preparations, beta-blocking agents, diltiazem and verapamil, but the latter three are best avoided in patients with poor left-ventricular function, for they may precipitate or worsen congestive heart failure. These medications and verapamil may be given intravenously or orally; the route of administration is chosen on the basis of the speed with which slowing of the ventricular rate is desired. The dosage of propranolol required to slow the ventricular rate is in the range of 5 to 10 mg orally three times daily, much lower than that needed for treatment of angina pectoris or hypertension. Patients who present with atrial flutter with 2:1 AV conduction but have no problems may be given oral digitalis, beta blockers, or verapamil and sent home from the emergency department to return for follow-up, while sicker patients might best be managed by monitoring their cardiac rhythm in a holding area of the emergency department or in the hospital.

As AV nodal blocking drugs are administered to the patient in atrial flutter, the AV-conduction ratio generally changes from 2:1 to a bigeminal rhythm in which the average AV-conduction ratio is 3:1 (Fig. 63-19). During this bigeminal rhythm, the shorter R-R intervals are slightly longer than the R-R intervals during 2:1 AV conduction, and the longer intervals are slightly shorter than twice the R-R intervals during 2:1 AV conduction. Further administration of these medications results in predominantly 4:1 AV conduction and a perfectly regular ventricular response at a rate of about 70 to 80 beats/minute. When the average AV-conduction ratio is 3:1 or 4:1, quinidine or procainamide may be administered in the usual therapeutic doses for 24 to 48 hours. These medications may convert the atrial flutter to sinus rhythm, and they seem to aid in the maintenance of sinus rhythm once it is achieved. However, both quinidine and procainamide often slow the flutter rate slightly before they convert the rhythm. If they are given to patients whose flutter rates are initially relatively slow (less than about 260/minute), they may slow the atrial rate to a rate at which the AV node can conduct every flutter impulse, resulting in 1:1 AV conduction with a dangerously rapid ventricular rate. Thus, before quinidine or procainamide is administered to patients with relatively slow flutter rates, it is advisable to depress AV nodal conduction, as evidenced by an average AV-conduction ratio of 3:1 or 4:1, with the AV nodal blocking medications. Occasionally, during the administration of digitalis, beta-blocking agents, verapamil, quinidine, or procainamide, or following a low-energy (less than about 75 watt-second) electrical discharge, atrial flutter may convert to atrial fibrillation; in this case, management of that specific dysrhythmia must be undertaken, but often terminates spontaneously within seconds to minutes of its onset.

Paroxysmal Supraventricular Tachycardia

The term *paroxysmal supraventricular tachycardia* (PSVT) refers to a rapid regular rhythm that, in the overwhelming majority of patients, is due to reentry within the AV node. On occasion, however, it may be caused by reentry within the sinus node or atrial tissue. In patients with accessory AV-conduction pathways, the mechanism of PSVT usually involves conduction from atrium to ventricle via one of the two pathways, and from ventricle to atrium via the other pathway.

PSVT is recognized in the surface ECG by the regular occurrence of QRS complexes at rates in the range of 140 to 220/minute, usually between 160 and 170/minute

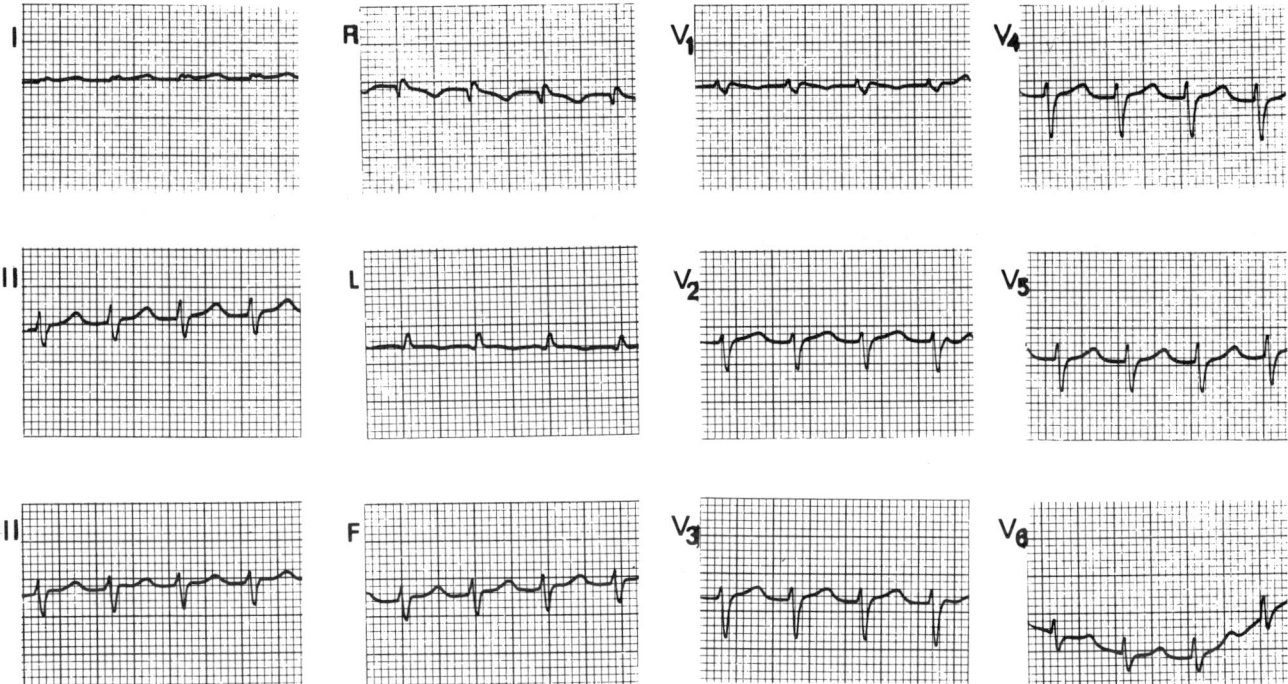

Figure 63-20 ECG showing AV nodal reentrant PSVT. *Note:* This 12-lead ECG was recorded from a patient during an episode of AV nodal reentrant PSVT. P waves are not clearly identifiable, because they fall within the QRS complexes.

(Fig. 63-20). The QRS complexes are usually identical to sinus-stimulated QRS complexes in that same patient, although they may be different on occasion because of aberrant intraventricular conduction of the supraventricular impulses. When PSVT occurs in patients with accessory AV-conduction pathways, the supraventricular impulse usually enters ventricular tissue via the normal AV node-His-Purkinje system pathway and returns to the atrium via the accessory pathway, and then reenters the AV node; thus, the QRS complexes are usually normal. Rarely, the directions of conduction in the two pathways are reversed; in this instance, the QRS complexes may be very wide and bizarre because ventricular activation is initiated via the accessory pathway in an area well away from those areas in which the His-Purkinje system normally initiates ventricular activation. When the rate of PSVT is above 200 beats/minute, it is likely that an accessory pathway is involved in the reentry circuit.

In AV nodal reentrant PSVT, the AV node behaves as if it has two pathways that are isolated from each other in the mid-portion of the node, but are joined together in the upper portion of the node, near the atrium, and in the lower portion of the node, near the His bundle (Fig. 63-21). During PSVT, one AV nodal-conduction pathway transmits impulses from the upper portion of the node to the lower portion of the node; from that point it may enter both the His bundle, from which it can activate the ventricles, and the lower portion of the other AV nodal pathway in which it travels retrogradely to the upper portion of the AV node; at this point it can both enter the atrium to stimulate a P wave and *reenter* the upper portion of the other AV nodal pathway to begin another cycle.

In PSVT due to AV nodal reentry or to accessory pathway reentry, both atrial and ventricular rhythms are dependent on maintenance of the reentry circuit; thus, there is *always* a 1:1 relationship of P waves to QRS complexes. When sinus node or intra-atrial reentry is the mechanism of PSVT, however,

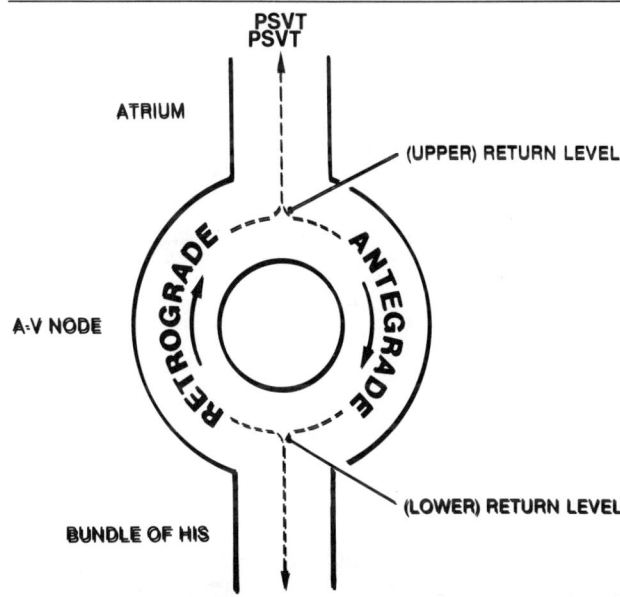

Figure 63-21 Movement of electrical impulses during AV nodal reentrant PSVT.

the ventricular rhythm depends on the atrial rate and on the conduction properties of the AV node. At times of 1:1 AV conduction, there is a 1:1 relationship between P waves and QRS complexes; but at other times, when AV conduction is depressed, the ventricular rate is less than the atrial rate.

In AV nodal reentrant PSVT, the P waves usually fall within or close to the QRS complexes and are obscured by them (Fig. 63-20). In accessory pathway reentry PSVT, the P waves usually occur outside of (later than) the QRS complexes and are thus somewhat easier to identify (Fig. 63-22). In sinus node or intra-atrial reentry PSVT with 1:1 AV conduction, the P waves precede the QRS complexes at intervals that are generally normal to only mildly prolonged.

Patients with PSVT generally complain of rapid heart action. The occurrence of other symptoms depends on the hemodynamic effects of the tachycardia and the underlying cardiovascular status of the patient. In most patients, the deleterious hemodynamic effects result from the rapid heart rate and, in AV nodal reentrant PSVT, also from the loss of the normal atrial and ventricular contraction sequences because of the simultaneous activation of atria and ventricles. It is not unusual at the onset of PSVT for the patient—even a healthy one—to have presyncope or syncope if the rate of the tachycardia is very rapid and the ability of the cardiovascular system to adjust to sudden decreases in stroke volume and blood pressure is depressed.

The rate of AV nodal reentrant and accessory pathway reentrant PSVT is determined by the conduction velocities of the tissues that comprise the reentrant circuit; the dysrhythmia persists only when the impulses travel in the reentrant pathways at specific velocities. Alterations of the conduction velocities and refractory periods of the reentrant pathways may interrupt the circus movement and, thus, terminate PSVT. In fact, PSVT is generally terminated by administering medications or by inducing changes in autonomic nervous-system traffic that alter conduction velocities or refractory periods of the reentrant pathways. The following medications and maneuvers are commonly used in attempts to terminate PSVT:

- Adenocard (adenosine)
- vagal stimulation: carotid sinus massage, Valsalva's maneuver
- parasympathetic stimulating agents: Tensilon
- alpha-adrenergic stimulating agents: Vasoxyl, Aramine, Neo-Synephrine
- calcium-blocking agents: verapamil
- beta-adrenergic blocking agents: Inderal, Lopressor, Brevibloc
- digitalis preparations
- procainamide preparations
- quinidine preparations
- Norpace
- lidocaine
- direct-current cardioversion

Carotid sinus massage, Valsalva's maneuver, and elevation of the blood pressure with sympathomimetic amines such as methoxamine hydrochloride (Vasoxyl), metaraminol (Aramine), or phenylephrine hydrochloride (Neo-Synephrine), result in sympathetic withdrawal from, and the increased parasympathetic traffic into, the AV nodal reentrant pathways; such changes may lengthen the refractory period and/or slow conduction or effect a block of one or both pathways, thus interrupting the circus movement and terminating the dysrhythmia. Tensilon, a rapidly acting but short-lived cholinesterase inhibitor, allows the sudden build up of large quantities of acetylcholine within the AV node, transiently blocking impulse conduction in one or both pathways and terminating the circus movement. Verapamil, a calcium-blocking agent, acts by directly slowing conduction in AV nodal pathways. Adenosine, the newest material used to terminate PSVT, is a naturally occurring nucleoside that slows conduction through and probably lengthens the refractory period of the AV node. Digitalis preparations probably act both by stimulating increased parasympathetic traffic into and by directly depressing conduction through the AV node. Beta-blocking agents, such as propranolol hydrochloride (Inderal), esmolol (Brevibloc), and metoprolol tartrate (Lopressor), act by slowing conduction and lengthening refractory periods in AV nodal pathways by virtue of their ability to block the effects of catecholamines. Quinidine, procainamide, and disopyramide (Norpace) are capable of slowing conduction and lengthening refractory period in retrogradely conducting AV nodal pathways and in antegradely and retrogradely conducting accessory AV-conduction pathways; thus, they may be extremely effective in terminating PSVT that is due either to AV nodal reentry or to accessory pathway reentry. Lidocaine may be effective in terminating PSVT due to accessory pathway reentry, for it is capable of suppressing conduction in some accessory pathways.

The specific treatment selected for an individual depends on the potential effectiveness, the potential risk, and the simplicity of administering the therapy. For example, carotid sinus massage may quickly and effectively terminate PSVT in a young, healthy adult, but it may result in a cerebrovascular accident (CVA) in an older individual with extracranial cerebrovascular disease. Carotid sinus massage, Valsalva's maneuver, and Tensilon may be ineffective when the arterial blood pressure is low (ie, less than 110 mmHg systolic), but each may rapidly terminate PSVT when the blood pressure is normal, or is pharmacologically increased to 140 to 180 mmHg systolic. Such an elevation in blood pressure may be achieved by the administration of sympathomimetic amines, preferably at a slow rate, measuring blood pressure frequently to avoid an excessive elevation,

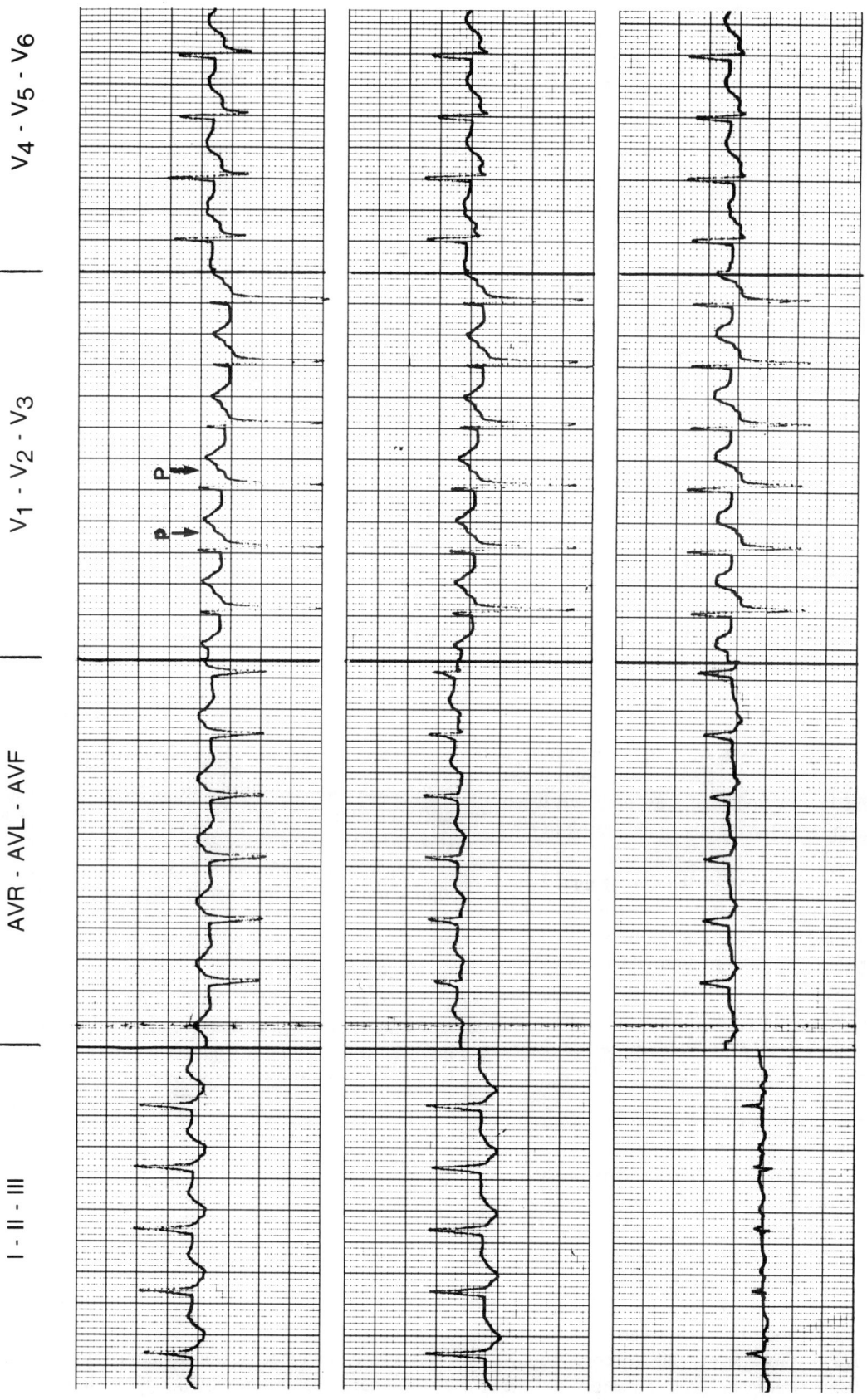

Figure 63-22 ECGs showing PSVT due to accessory pathway reentry. *Note:* This 12-lead ECG was recorded during PSVT in a patient with an accessory AV-conduction pathway and Wolff-Parkinson-White syndrome. The P waves fall well after the QRS complexes, whereas in AV nodal reentrant PSVT (Fig. 63-20) the P waves fall within the QRS complexes. The QRS complexes in this tracing are normal because the ventricles are activated normally via the AV node and His-Purkinje system.

which may have disastrous consequences in patients with coronary artery disease, cerebrovascular disease, or severe left ventricular dysfunction. Occasionally, elevation of the blood pressure itself terminates PSVT, and there is no need for a vagal maneuver. Tensilon is best avoided in the asthmatic, in whom it may initiate bronchospasm, and in the patient with acute or chronic gastrointestinal disease, in whom it may induce nausea, vomiting, abdominal cramping, or evacuation of the bowels. Adenosine, verapamil, and beta-blocking medications are best avoided in patients with sick sinus syndrome in whom it may dramatically prolong the period of standstill that follows termination of PSVT; the latter two are also best avoided in patients with poor ventricular function. Adenosine should also not be used in patients chronically taking disopyramide (Norpace), for this antidysrhythmic medication inhibits the cellular uptake of adenosine and may, therefore, make its effects more prolonged and more profound. Digoxin and verapamil are best avoided in the patient with Wolff-Parkinson-White syndrome *if* the patient has a history of atrial fibrillation and rapid ventricular rates because of rapid accessory-pathway conduction, for these medications may enhance AV conduction if atrial fibrillation occurs. Lidocaine is likely to be effective only when a limb of the reentrant circuit is an accessory pathway, but its IV administration in a dosage of 50 to 150 mg is generally quite safe, so long as the patient does not have an antegradely conducting accessory pathway with fast conduction velocity and short refractory period. Procainamide is extremely effective in terminating PSVT due to AV nodal reentry, as it blocks conduction in the retrogradely conducting AV nodal pathway; however, when administered intravenously too rapidly, it may result in profound hypotension. Direct-current cardioversion can be safely used to terminate PSVT regardless of the underlying mechanism, but it requires some form of anesthesia. Occasionally, attempts at electrical conversion of PSVT result in atrial fibrillation rather than sinus rhythm, in which case the atrial fibrillation must be managed, but often terminates spontaneously within seconds to minutes of its onset.

As PSVT tends to be recurrent and is initiated by APCs and PVCs, it is important to consider prescribing chronic antidysrhythmic therapy for suppression of ectopic beats in patients who have frequent or poorly tolerated episodes of the dysrhythmia. Furthermore, before they are sent home from the emergency department, such patients might be taught how to perform carotid sinus massage, Valsalva's maneuver, and other vagal stimulatory maneuvers. They may also be advised to take specific medications in specific dosage schedules in an attempt to terminate the dysrhythmia shortly after its onset and thus avoid a trip to the hospital. If an accessory AV-conduction pathway is clearly involved in the PSVT, thorough cardiologic evaluation seems appropriate, for catheter ablation techniques can safely and effectively render the accessory pathway permanently nonfunctional.

Nonparoxysmal Junctional Tachycardia

A rarely encountered dysrhythmia, nonparoxysmal junctional tachycardia is due to acceleration of the automatic rate of an AV-junctional pacemaker (Fig. 63-16). In order for this accelerated pacemaker to emerge during sinus rhythm, it must have a more rapid rate of discharge than the sinus node at the time; usually, the junctional rate is just slightly in excess of the sinus rate. In the presence of atrial fibrillation or flutter, or ectopic atrial tachycardia, the junctional rhythm emerges only when there is such high-grade AV block that the interval between consecutive atrial impulses traversing the AV node and reaching the AV-junctional (His bundle) pacemaker exceeds the escape interval of the junctional pacemaker. This dysrhythmia is generally seen only in the presence of digitalis excess and in very ill patients in the early hours after cardiac surgery.

Nonparoxysmal junctional tachycardia can be recognized by the regular occurrence of QRS complexes that are usually normal for the patient (Fig. 63-23). Typically, there is a retrograde conduction block of these junctional impulses, so retrograde atrial activation does not occur (Fig. 63-16). However, antegrade conduction of sinus or atrial impulses through the AV node is usually possible, although it may be depressed. If antegrade AV conduction is normal, atrial impulses reaching the AV-junctional pacemaker before it is set to discharge are conducted through the AV junction and into the ventricles to stimulate a QRS complex that will occur prematurely. The premature QRS complex may have a contour identical to that of the usual QRS complexes if intraventricular conduction of this impulse is normal, but a different contour if intraventricular conduction is aberrant (Fig. 63-23).

Nonparoxysmal junctional tachycardia *per se* causes only mild to moderate hemodynamic deterioration, attributable to the intermittent loss of the atrial contribution to ventricular filling due to the AV dissociation resulting from the junctional automatic rate exceeding the sinus rate. As digitalis excess is the cause of this dysrhythmia in most patients seen in the emergency department, management of the patient involves withdrawing digitalis. Continued digitalis administration to patients with nonparoxysmal junctional tachycardia may result in an increase in the rate of the dysrhythmia and may be followed by ventricular tachycardia and ventricular fibrillation. It may be prudent to hospitalize these patients for cardiac-rhythm monitoring until the dysrhythmia disappears.

Ventricular Tachydysrhythmias

Accelerated Idioventricular Rhythm

Accelerated idioventricular rhythm (AIVR) is recognized by the emergence, during slowing of the sinus rate or during the slow phase of sinus arrhythmia, of wide and abnormal (but generally not very bizarre) QRS complexes that occur

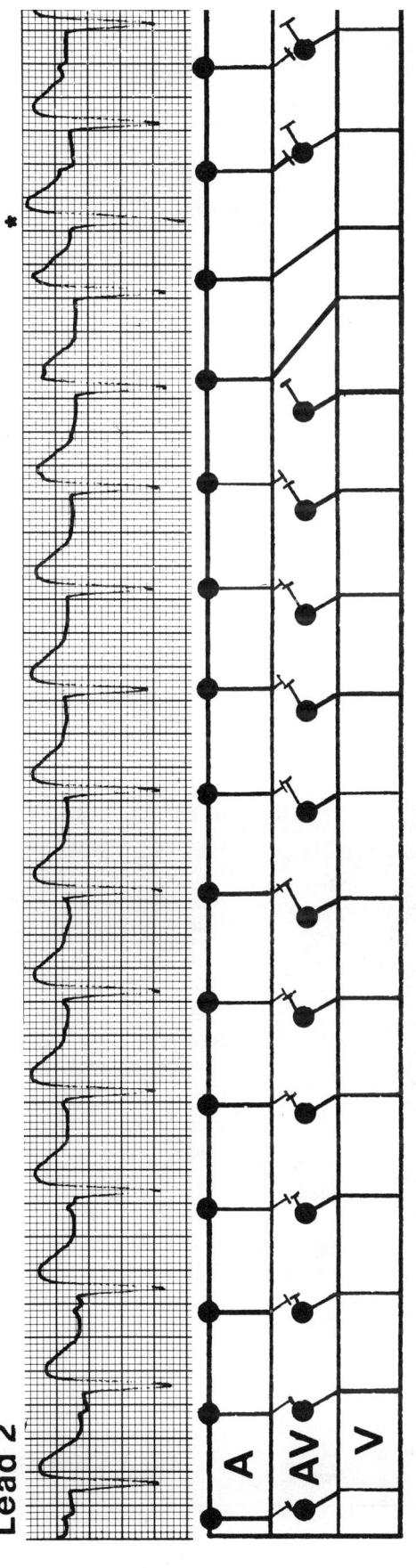

Figure 63-23 ECG showing nonparoxysmal junctional tachycardia in a patient with digoxin excess. *Note:* The independent atrial rhythm is able to capture the ventricles only when the P wave falls shortly after the QRS complex. The wider QRS complex near the end of the strip (*asterisk*) is an aberrantly conducted sinus beat. The closed circles (●) in the ladder diagram represent impulse formation in the sinus node (*top line*) and AV junction (*middle panel*). The vertical lines represent impulse conduction through the atria (A) and ventricles (V), while the slanted lines represent conduction through the AV node and His bundle (AV).

with regularity and are dissociated from the atrial rhythm (P waves) (Fig. 63-24). Fusion QRS complexes, which reflect activation of the ventricles by both the sinus impulse and the ectopic ventricular impulse, typically occur at the times of emergence and disappearance of the abnormally wide QRS complexes. Generally, AIVR will disappear when the sinus rate increases to the point that it consistently exceeds the escape rate of the AIVR.

AIVR occurs almost exclusively in acute myocardial infarction, usually during the initial hours or days of the event. It is felt to reflect enhanced automaticity within the ischemic myocardium that bridges infarcted and normal tissue. AIVR does *not* degenerate into ventricular fibrillation, and does *not* cause hemodynamic deterioration because of its rate, which is very close to the prevailing sinus rate at the time of its appearance. However, in patients with significant left-ventricular dysfunction it may result in a mild to profound fall in blood pressure resulting from the loss of the atrial contribution to ventricular filling that occurs during transient AV dissociation. If the fall in blood pressure is felt to be clinically disadvantageous, the AIVR can generally be suppressed by increasing the sinus rate with intravenously administered atropine (0.5 to 1 mg), a phenomenon termed *overdrive suppression*. Generally, AIVR is most clinically significant because it indicates that acute myocardial necrosis has occurred within hours to days of its appearance.

Ventricular Tachycardia

Ventricular tachycardia (VT) is defined as the occurrence of at least three PVCs in a row at a rate in excess of 100/minute. Ventricular tachycardia is almost uniformly initiated by PVCs; it may be sustained, lasting minutes to days, or nonsustained, lasting several seconds to a minute or so and terminating spontaneously (Figs. 63-4, A, and 63-25). The QRS complexes during ventricular tachycardia may vary in contour from mildly abnormal to very bizarre; the more bizarre complexes usually occur at more rapid rates, in specific clinical settings, and in enlarged hearts. In sustained ventricular tachycardia, the QRS rhythm is generally perfectly regular; in nonsustained ventricular tachycardia, especially if rapid, the QRS complexes usually occur at variable intervals that are often very difficult to accurately measure.

The majority of patients with ventricular tachycardia have an awareness of abnormal cardiac action. Although most patients with ventricular tachycardia are symptomatic, some are totally asymptomatic and the tachycardia is unexpectedly detected on routine physical or electrocardiographic examination. In some, the rapid ventricular rate and the absence of the normal atrial and ventricular contraction sequence may result in such dramatic falls in cardiac output and blood pressure that the patient experiences profound weakness, presyncope, syncope, shortness of breath, and chest discomfort that suggests myocardial infarction. Recognition of ventricular tachycardia is of critical importance because it may degenerate into ventricular fibrillation and thus lead to circulatory arrest.

Ventricular tachycardia occurs most commonly in patients with cardiac disease, particularly coronary artery disease. It may occur in the initial seconds to days following acute myocardial infarction, or weeks to years afterwards as a manifestation of recurrent ischemia or infarction, or ventricular aneurysm. In a patient with coronary artery disease, runs of abnormally wide QRS complexes must be considered ventricular tachycardia until proved otherwise; however, they must be differentiated from AIVR and from supraventricular impulses with aberrant intraventricular conduction. In some patients, ventricular tachycardia may be a manifestation of digitalis excess, hypokalemia, or an idiosyncratic effect of quinidine, other antiarrhythmic drugs, phenothiazines, or tricyclic antidepressants (*infra vide*).

Management of the patient with sustained ventricular tachycardia involves termination of the tachycardia and prevention of its recurrence.* If the patient is on the verge of or has already suffered cardiovascular collapse, direct-current countershock, preferably synchronized to the QRS complex, is the therapy most likely to restore sinus rhythm (Fig. 63-26, A). The energies needed to terminate sustained ventricular tachycardia may be as low as about 10 watt-seconds, although much higher energy levels are sometimes required. For the patient with cardiovascular collapse, an initial high-energy (200 to 400 watt-second) discharge is advisable. Closed-chest cardiac massage may be used to support the circulation until the electrical discharge can be administered. Many patients with hemodynamically significant ventricular tachycardia may be hypoxemic or acidemic, and correction of these abnormalities may improve the chances for successful termination of ventricular tachycardia and prevention of its recurrence.

In the less seriously ill patient with ventricular tachycardia, the IV administration of lidocaine (50 to 150 mg over 30 seconds to 5 minutes), or procainamide (50 mg/minute up to a dose of about 1000 mg) may terminate the dysrhythmia (Fig. 63-26, B). In the patient with recurrent ventricular tachycardia that is neither suppressed nor terminated by lidocaine or procainamide, bretylium tosylate (Bretylol) may be administered (see Chapter 62). Once sinus rhythm has been restored, medication aimed at suppressing PVCs, such as lidocaine, procainamide, quinidine, bretylium, or disopyramide, may be started, the specific medication and route of administration to be based on the patient's clinical condition, the likelihood that ventricular tachycardia will recur, and the hemodynamic effects of the tachycardia in the individual patient.

Paroxysms of self-terminating ventricular tachycardia may occur in patients whose ECGs show long QTU intervals (Fig. 63-27). In some of these patients, the long QTU inter-

---

*For a detailed discussion of the pharmacologic treatment of ventricular dysrhythmias associated with acute myocardial infarction, see Chapter 62, Acute Myocardial Infarction.

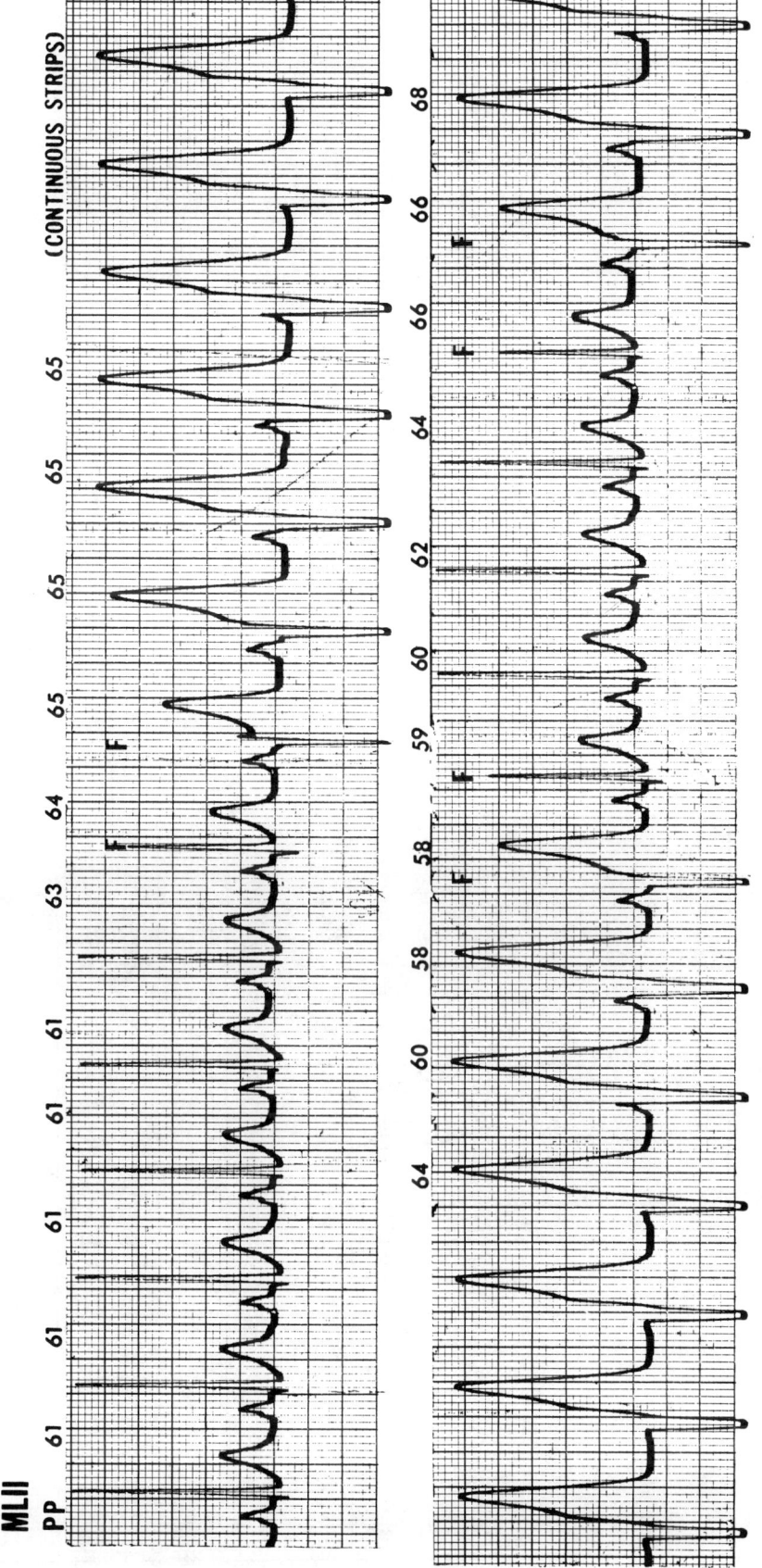

Figure 63-24 ECGs showing AIVR. *Note:* These strips, showing AIVR, were recorded from a patient with acute anterior-wall myocardial infarction. The intervals between sinus P waves (PP) are in hundredths of a second. In the top strip, as the sinus rate slows (ie, PP intervals lengthen) there appears a wide but reasonably organized and regularly occurring ventricular rhythm at a rate close to the sinus rate. Near the end of the top strip, the P waves disappear within the QRS complexes. In the bottom strip, the P waves reappear as the sinus rate accelerates; for a few seconds, they stimulate QRS complexes. When the sinus rate again slows, however, the wide, regular ventricular rhythm reappears. At the time of transition from one rhythm to another, the ventricles are activated by both sinus and ventricular impulses, resulting in fusion beats (F).

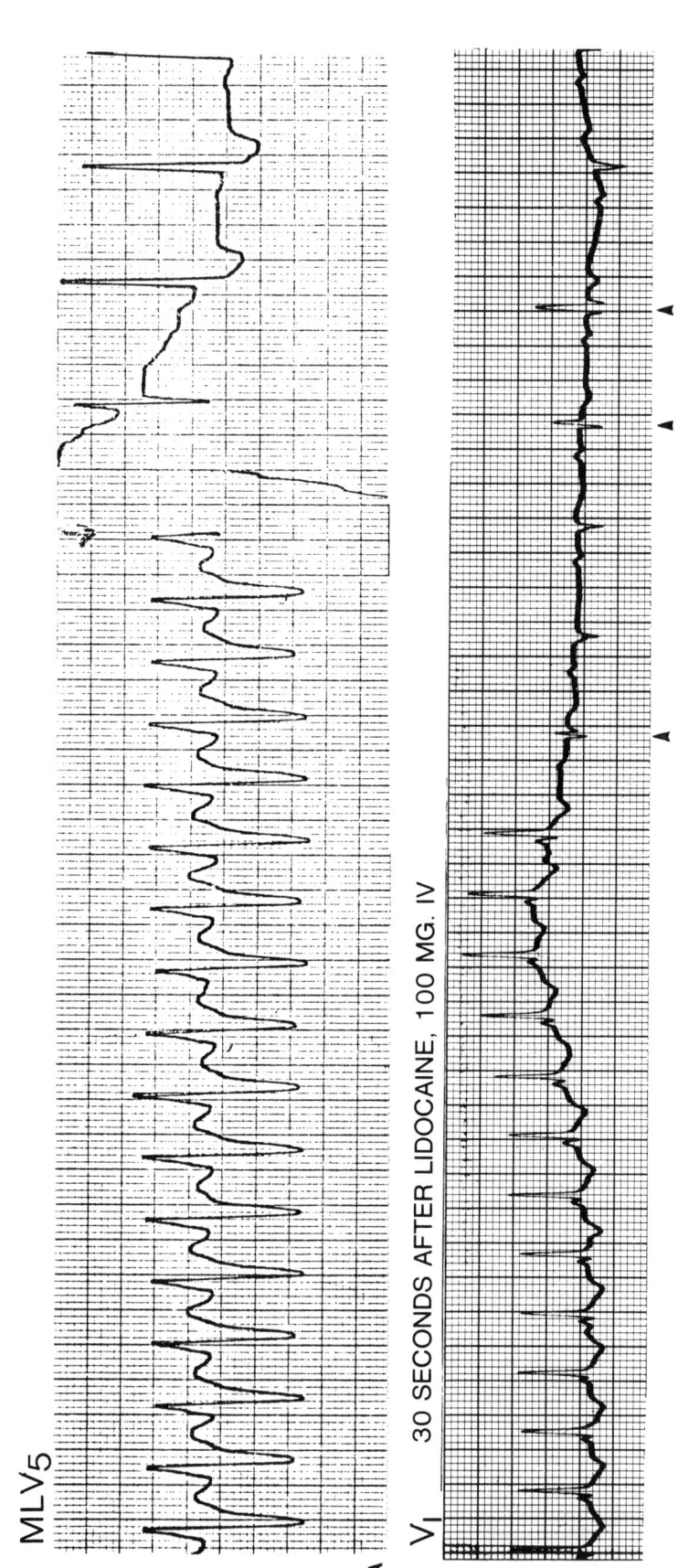

Figure 63-25 ECG showing nonsustained ventricular tachycardia. *Note:* Two brief runs of ventricular tachycardia are each initiated by premature ventricular complexes (*arrows*) that fall in the T waves of sinus-stimulated QRS complexes. *Source:* Reprinted by permission of Elsevier Science Publishing Co Inc from Jacobson LB, Goldschlager N: *Arrhythmias: Case Studies.* Copyright 1978 by Medical Examination Publishing Co Inc.

Figure 63-26 ECGs showing terminations of sustained ventricular tachycardias. *A:* Sustained ventricular tachycardia at a rate of about 167 beats/minute is converted to sinus rhythm at a rate of about 90 beats/minute by a 15 watt-second synchronized direct-current electrical precordial discharge. *B:* Sustained ventricular tachycardia at a rate of about 170 beats/minute is terminated by the IV administration of lidocaine. Following termination of the ventricular tachycardia, the underlying atrial rhythm stimulates the QRS complexes. Some PVCs occur in the first few seconds after termination, and as they fall in late diastole result in fusion complexes (*arrows*).

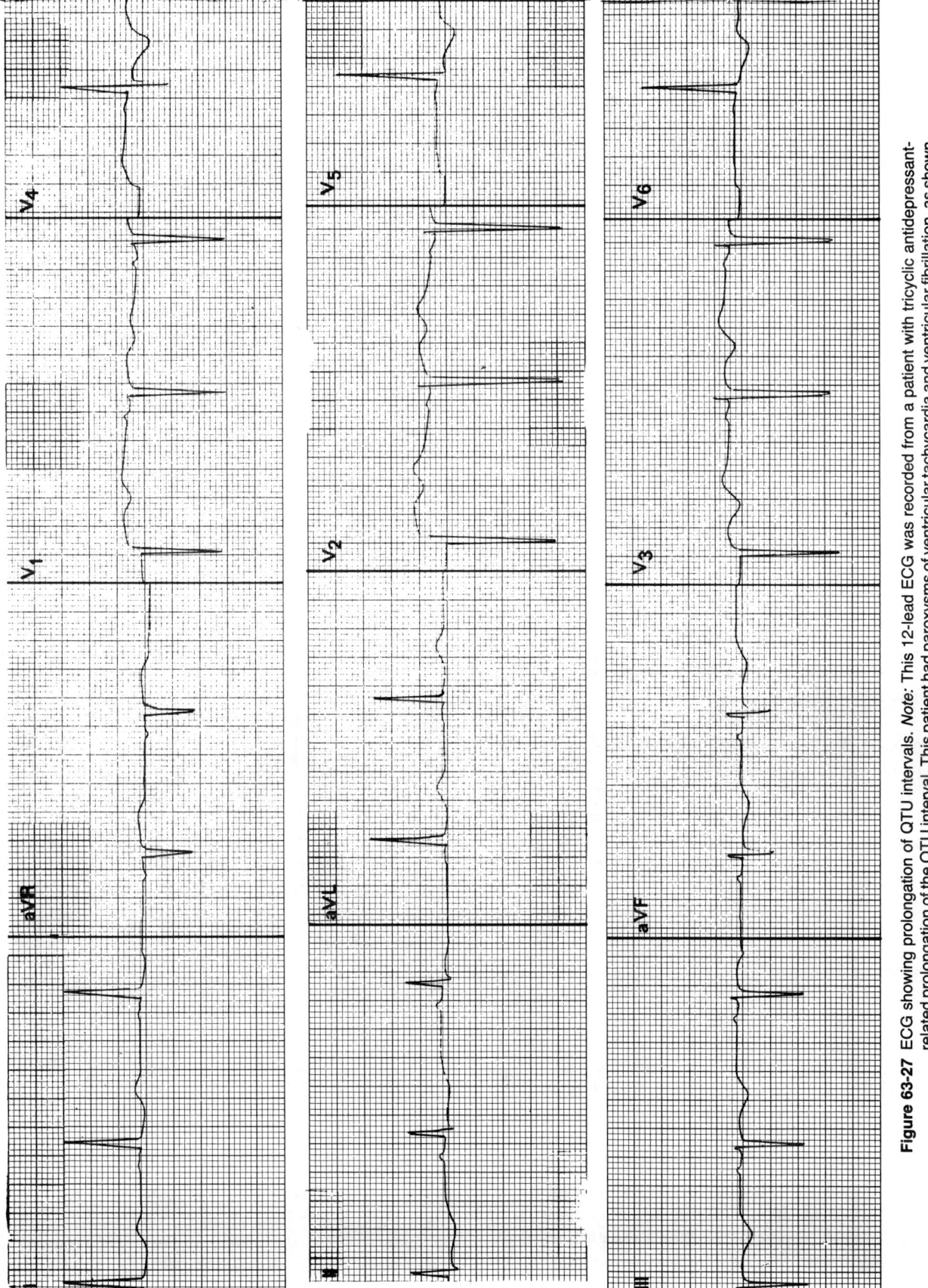

Figure 63-27 ECG showing prolongation of QTU intervals. *Note:* This 12-lead ECG was recorded from a patient with tricyclic antidepressant-related prolongation of the QTU interval. This patient had paroxysms of ventricular tachycardia and ventricular fibrillation, as shown in Fig. 63-28.

val is congenital and familial and may be associated with deafness; in others, it may be acquired, as a result of hypokalemia, coronary artery disease, or the administration of tricyclic antidepressants, phenothiazines, and antidysrhythmic medications (ie, quinidine preparations, procainamide, and disopyramide). The runs of QRS complexes comprising ventricular tachycardia in association with long QTU intervals have a characteristic morphology termed *torsades de pointes*. This term describes the gradual and cyclic transition in the directions of the QRS complexes from upright to biphasic to inverted and vice versa (Fig. 63-28). It is critical to identify *torsades de pointes* and self-terminating paroxysms of ventricular fibrillation related to the long QTU interval, for the administration of quinidine, procainamide, or disopyramide to these patients may prolong the QTU interval even more, facilitating the appearance of ventricular tachycardia and increasing its severity. These patients must be managed by withdrawal of medications that may be contributing to the long QTU interval; by correction of hypokalemia, if present; and by the administration of lidocaine, diphenylhydantoin, or propranolol, in that order of preference. Occasionally, repeated electrical terminations of the dysrhythmia may be required while the reversible abnormalities are being corrected. If the heart rate is very slow, both atrial and ventricular overdrive pacing may decrease the predisposition to the PVCs that initiate *torsades de pointes*. Atrial, but not ventricular, overdrive pacing may be helpful in shortening the QTU interval.

When ventricular tachycardia is due to digitalis excess, termination of the dysrhythmia by direct-current cardioversion is often followed by more serious ventricular dysrhythmias and even ventricular fibrillation. Thus, it is preferable to attempt to terminate ventricular tachycardia with IV lidocaine or procainamide in this setting. Furthermore, as hypokalemia and/or hypomagnesemia is often present in such patients, management might include correction of these abnormalities by the cautious administration of KCl or magnesium sulfate.

Ventricular Fibrillation

Ventricular fibrillation (VF), the most common cause of sudden death from acute myocardial ischemia and infarction, is recognized in the surface ECG by the absence of identifiable QRST complexes and by the presence of irregular oscillating electrical activity that may be fine or coarse (Figs. 63-4, B, and 63-29). Ventricular fibrillation may be induced during electrical conversion of ventricular tachycardia, even when there has been appropriate synchronization of the electrical discharge to the QRS complex; it also may occur in the setting of long QTU intervals. As ventricular fibrillation is a mechanically useless rhythm that results in circulatory arrest, it must be terminated if the patient is to survive. Defibrillation is best achieved using nonsynchronized direct-current precordial countershock at high (approximately 200 to 400 watt-second) energy levels (Fig. 63-29, B). If defibrillation does not occur after two or three maximum energy direct-current discharges, it may reflect the presence of hypoxemia, acidemia, or hyperkalemia, and closed-chest cardiac massage should be performed while attempts are made to correct the abnormalities. Alternatively, bretylium tosylate may be given by rapid IV injection in an attempt to achieve a *chemical defibrillation*. When electrical defibrillation has failed despite correction of metabolic abnormalities, this medication may terminate the ventricular fibrillation and allow restoration of an effective cardiac rhythm. (See Chapter 62.)

Regular, Wide QRS Tachycardias

The regular, rapid occurrence of abnormally wide QRS complexes could reflect PSVT with aberrant intraventricular conduction of supraventricular impulses or sustained ventricular tachycardia. As these cardiac-rhythm disturbances may have dramatically different clinical significance and respond to very different therapies, differential diagnosis is crucial, though often difficult. As shown in Table 63-3, the rate of the QRS complexes during tachycardia is not generally helpful in determining whether the rhythm is supraventricular or ventricular in origin. The wider and more bizarre the QRS complexes, and the more superior and rightward the mean frontal-plane axis of the complexes, the more likely the rhythm is to be ventricular tachycardia. The identification of atrial and ventricular relationships during tachycardia is extremely helpful in the differential diagnosis; although there are 1:1 atrial and ventricular relationships in virtually all episodes of PSVT and in many episodes of ventricular tachycardia, the finding of AV dissociation excludes the diagnosis of PSVT and establishes the diagnosis of ventricular tachycardia. Examination of ECGs taken prior to the tachycardia may assist in differential diagnosis. If the contours of sinus-stimulated QRS complexes are *identical* to the wide, bizarre QRS complexes that occur during tachycardia, the diagnosis of PSVT is almost certain. The clinical history may also be helpful; if a patient with regular tachycardia at a rate of about 160 to 170 beats/minute has had similar episodes over a period of years, the dysrhythmia is almost

Table 63-3 Differential Diagnosis of Regular Wide QRS Tachycardia

	Ventricular Tachycardia	PSVT
Rate	130–180 (100–200)	140–180 (120–220)
QRS contours	Often bizarre	Rarely bizarre
QRS axis	Superior, rightward	Usually normal
P:QRS relationships	1:1, 1:2, dissociated	1:1 almost exclusively

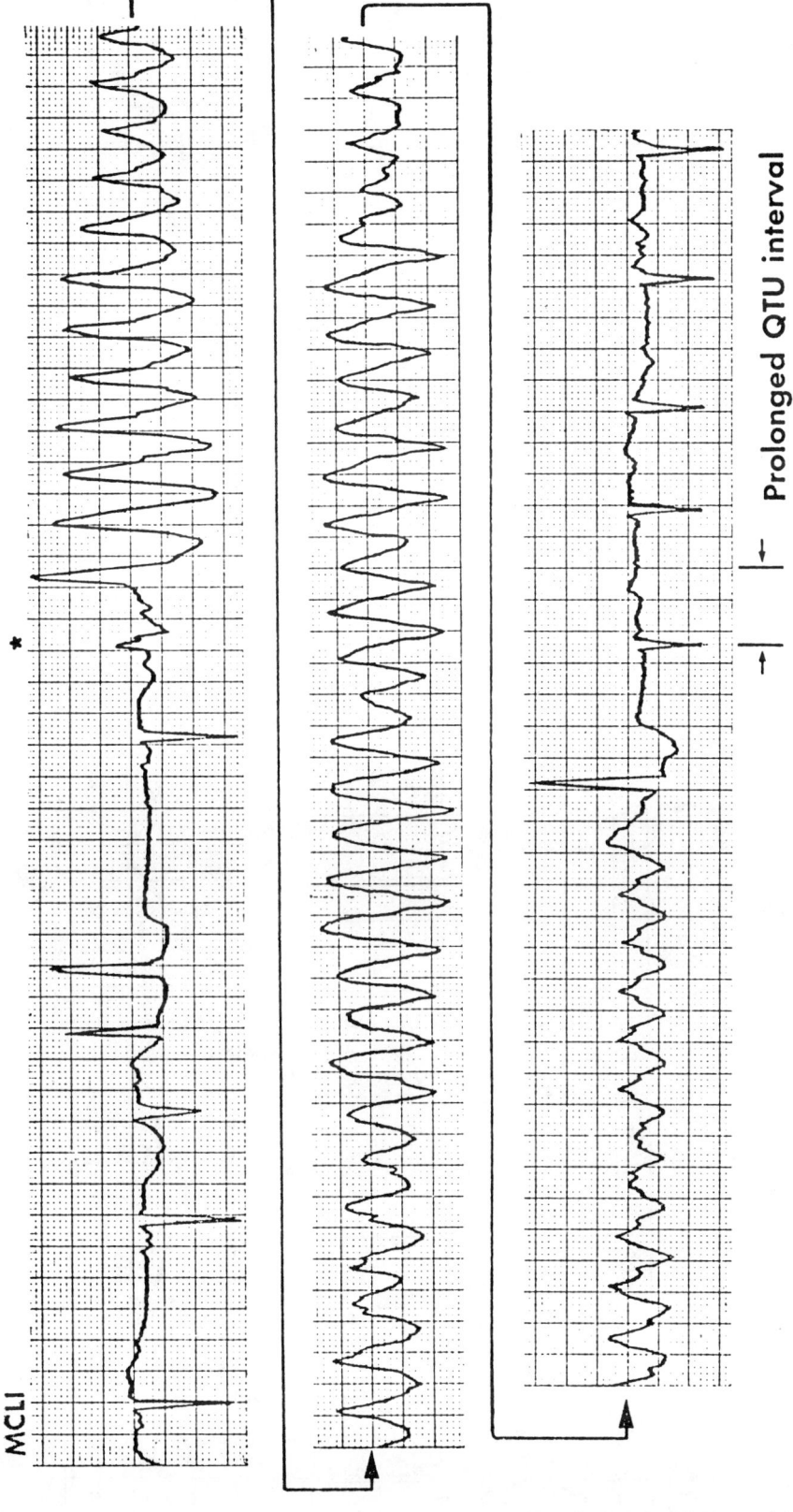

Figure 63-28 ECG showing *torsade de pointes*. *Note:* These strips were recorded from the same patient whose 12-lead ECG appears in Fig. 63-27. Beginning in the top strip, two sinus beats are followed by three PVCs. There then appears a sinus beat, in the U wave of which falls a PVC *(asterisk)*, which initiates a 17-second run of bizarre ventricular tachycardia at a rate of about 200 beats/minute. This tachycardia terminates spontaneously, and sinus rhythm resumes. During tachycardia, the QRS complexes are initially upright, then equiphasic, and then inverted. This alternation in direction then repeats itself.

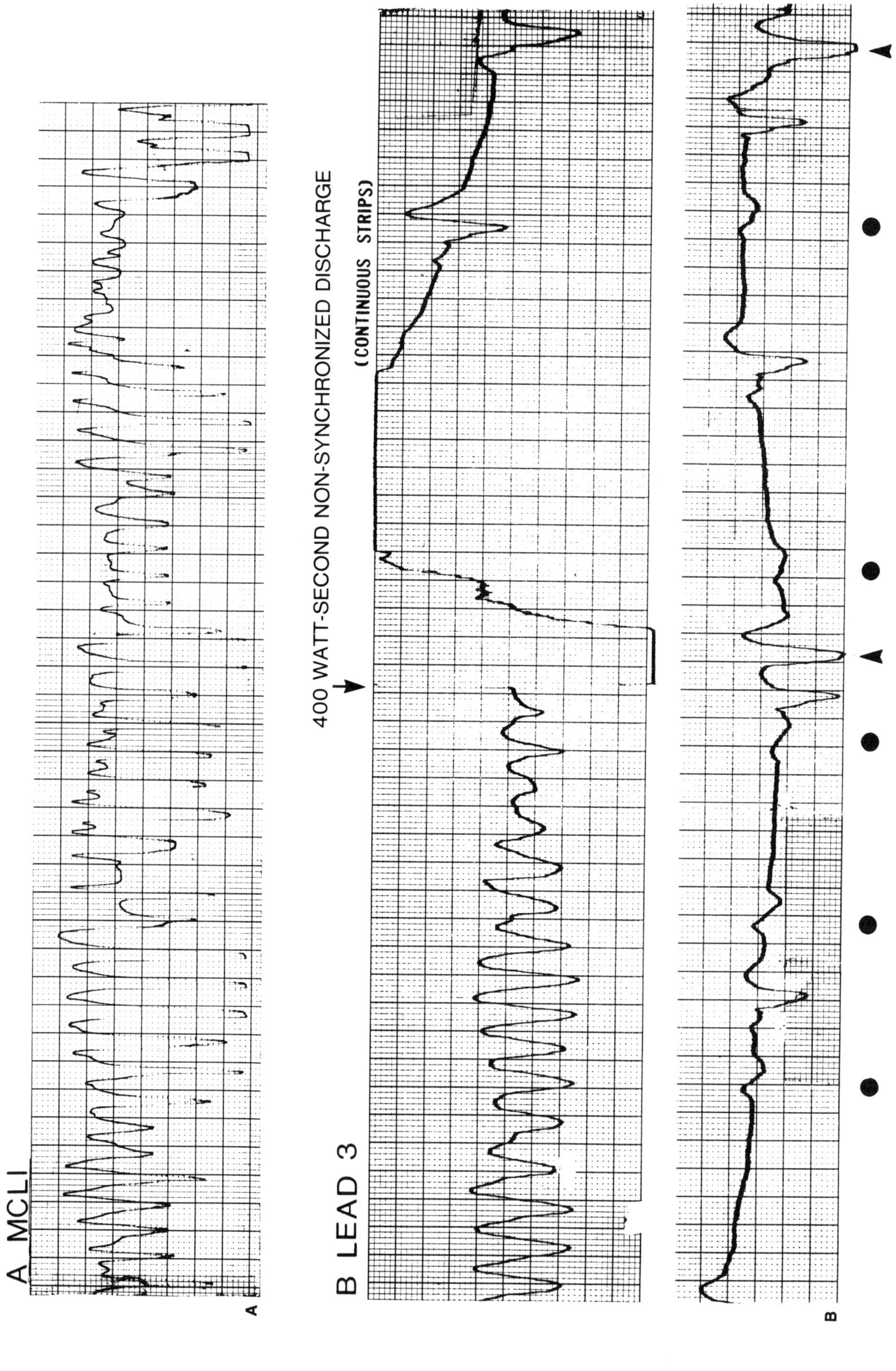

Figure 63-29 ECGs showing ventricular fibrillation. *A*: This ECG shows coarse, rapid, irregular electrical activity representing ventricular fibrillation in a patient with acute inferior-wall myocardial infarction. *B*: These two continuous strips show the termination of ventricular fibrillation by a 400 watt-second nonsynchronized electrical discharge. Following termination of ventricular fibrillation, slow sinus rhythm with premature ventricular beats (*arrows*) appears. The unusual deflections identified by the closed circles (●) are attributable to the manual closed-chest cardiac compression that is being performed at the time.

certainly PSVT. Figures 63-30 and 63-31 display 12-lead ECGs during PSVT with aberrant intraventricular conduction and during ventricular tachycardia, respectively.

Faced with a patient who has a rapid, regular, wide QRS tachycardia with 1:1 atrial and ventricular relationships, the emergency physician may perform a number of maneuvers that might have both diagnostic and therapeutic effects. Carotid sinus massage and the IV administration of Tensilon, adenosine, or verapamil may terminate PSVT but would not be likely to terminate ventricular tachycardia. Lidocaine may terminate ventricular tachycardia and, occasionally, PSVT when one of the reentry pathways is an accessory pathway that has properties like those of bundle branch and Purkinje fibers. Elevation of the blood pressure with sympathomimetic amines may terminate both PSVT and ventricular tachycardia and is therefore of little diagnostic help, but it would be useful if it terminated the dysrhythmia. So, the emergency physician faced with a patient whose wide QRS tachycardia could be either supraventricular or ventricular in origin may find it valuable to apply carotid sinus massage or to inject Tensilon, adenosine, or lidocaine intravenously to see the effect on the rhythm. Verapamil should not be administered if the patient clearly has heart disease and the rhythm is likely to be ventricular tachycardia, for its vasodilator and myocardial depressant effects may exacerbate hypotension and congestive heart failure and may precipitate cardiogenic shock and circulatory arrest.

THE WOLFF-PARKINSON-WHITE SYNDROME

Some patients have, in addition to the normal AV node-His-Purkinje system pathway connecting atria to ventricles, another AV-conduction pathway. Such accessory AV-conduction pathways usually enter ventricular tissue well away from the areas in which ventricular activation is normally initiated, and are capable of conducting impulses more rapidly than is the AV node. Thus, QRS complexes stimulated by supraventricular impulses entering the ventricles via an accessory AV-conduction pathway are grossly abnormal, typically showing a slow initial deflection (the delta wave) and an abnormally long duration, typically greater than 0.12 seconds. The PR interval in these patients is often shorter than normal and typically less than 0.12 seconds, presumably because the impulse can travel from atrium to ventricle more rapidly via the accessory pathway than via the AV node-His-Purkinje system. Figure 63-32 shows a 12-lead ECG recorded from a patient with an accessory AV-conduction pathway during sinus rhythm with accessory pathway conduction. Patients with accessory AV-conduction pathways and supraventricular tachydysrhythmias are said to have the Wolff-Parkinson-White syndrome. In addition to PSVT, these patients may experience atrial flutter and fibrillation.

As accessory AV-conduction pathways exhibit electrophysiologic properties like those of bundle branches and Purkinje fibers, they have conduction velocities, refractory periods, and responses to antidysrhythmic medications that usually differ dramatically from those of the normal AV conduction system, which contains the relatively slowly conducting AV node. Specifically, accessory pathways may have such rapid conduction velocities and such short refractory periods that they are capable of conducting impulses from atrium to ventricle at rates in excess of 300/minute. While quinidine, procainamide, and disopyramide generally lengthen refractory periods of, and slow conduction velocities in accessory pathways, beta-blocking agents, digoxin, and verapamil generally do not. In fact, digoxin and verapamil commonly effect a slight shortening of the refractory period of an accessory pathway which has a very brief refractory period to begin with. When atrial fibrillation and flutter occur with accessory pathway conduction that results in ventricular rates above 240 beats/minute, digoxin, verapamil, and beta-blocking drugs usually do not slow the ventricular rate; on occasion, digoxin and verapamil may even increase the already dangerously rapid rate. Quinidine, procainamide, and disopyramide, however, generally do slow the ventricular rate. Thus, in the presence of atrial flutter and fibrillation with rapid ventricular rates attributable to accessory pathway conduction, the IV administration of procainamide may help to slow the ventricular rate. However, if the patient is experiencing or is on the verge of experiencing cardiovascular collapse, direct-current cardioversion at the energy levels usually used for atrial flutter and fibrillation is a more appropriate therapy; it is probably less risky than the IV administration of quinidine, procainamide, or disopyramide to such critically ill patients. Such patients should have a thorough cardiologic evaluation because catheter ablation techniques can safely and effectively render the accessory pathway permanently nonfunctional.

Accessory pathway conduction during atrial fibrillation is recognized by the occurrence of wide, very bizarre QRS complexes at irregularly irregular intervals (Fig. 63-33). Accessory pathway conduction in atrial flutter with 1:1 AV conduction can be recognized by the regular occurrence of wide and very bizarre but essentially identical QRS complexes at rates of about 300/minute, well in excess of the rates of most sustained ventricular tachycardias. Atrial flutter with 1:1 AV conduction via an accessory pathway is more likely than ventricular tachycardia if the patient is a young adult, has no other symptoms of heart disease, and has a history of recurrent episodes of tachycardia, such as PSVT.

In most patients with Wolff-Parkinson-White syndrome, the mechanism of PSVT usually, but not always, involves a reentrant impulse traveling from atrium to ventricle via the normal AV node-His-Purkinje system pathway and from ventricle to atrium via the accessory pathway. Thus, during

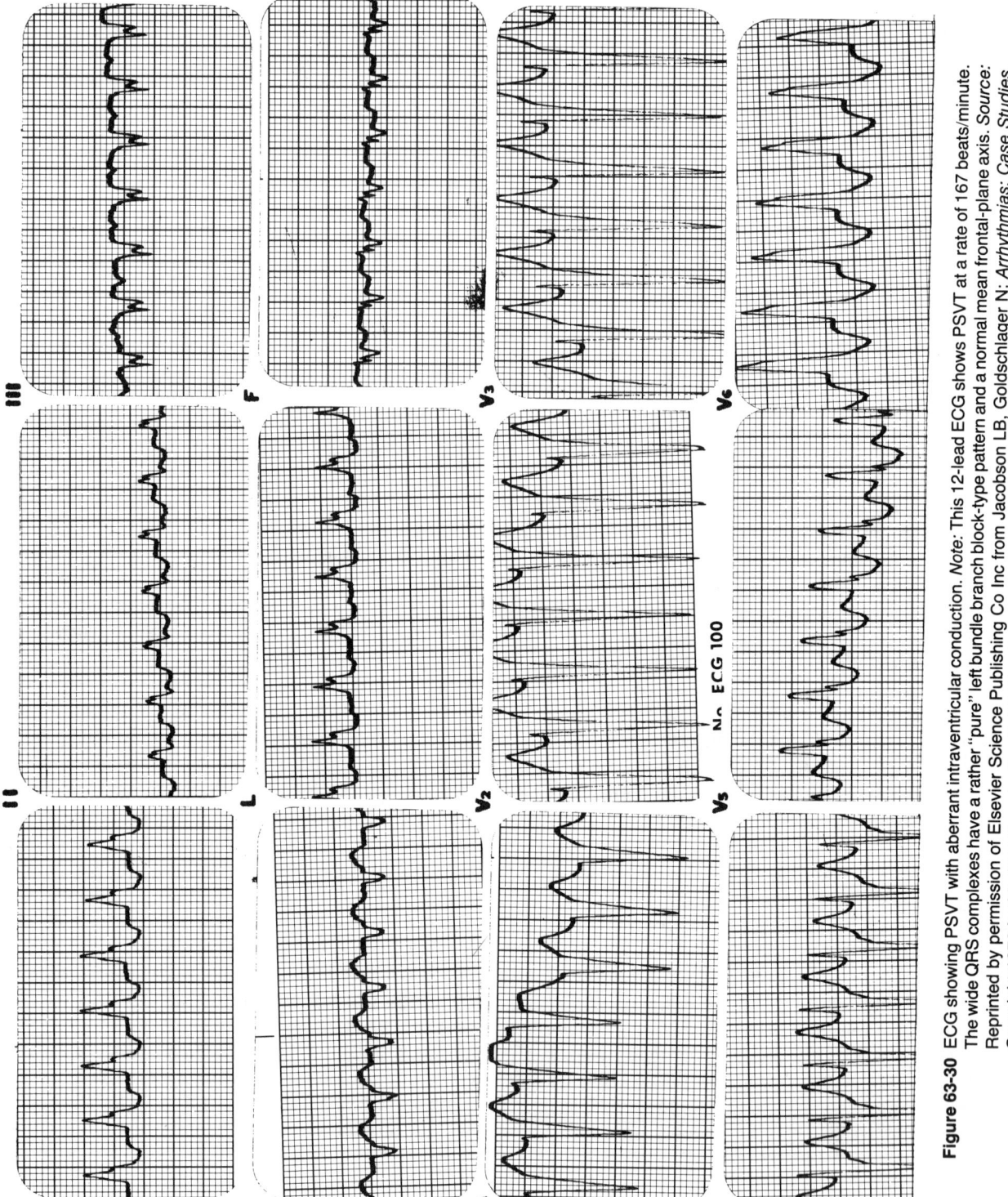

Figure 63-30 ECG showing PSVT with aberrant intraventricular conduction. *Note:* This 12-lead ECG shows PSVT at a rate of 167 beats/minute. The wide QRS complexes have a rather "pure" left bundle branch block-type pattern and a normal mean frontal-plane axis. *Source:* Reprinted by permission of Elsevier Science Publishing Co Inc from Jacobson LB, Goldschlager N: *Arrhythmias: Case Studies.* Copyright 1978 by Medical Examination Publishing Co Inc.

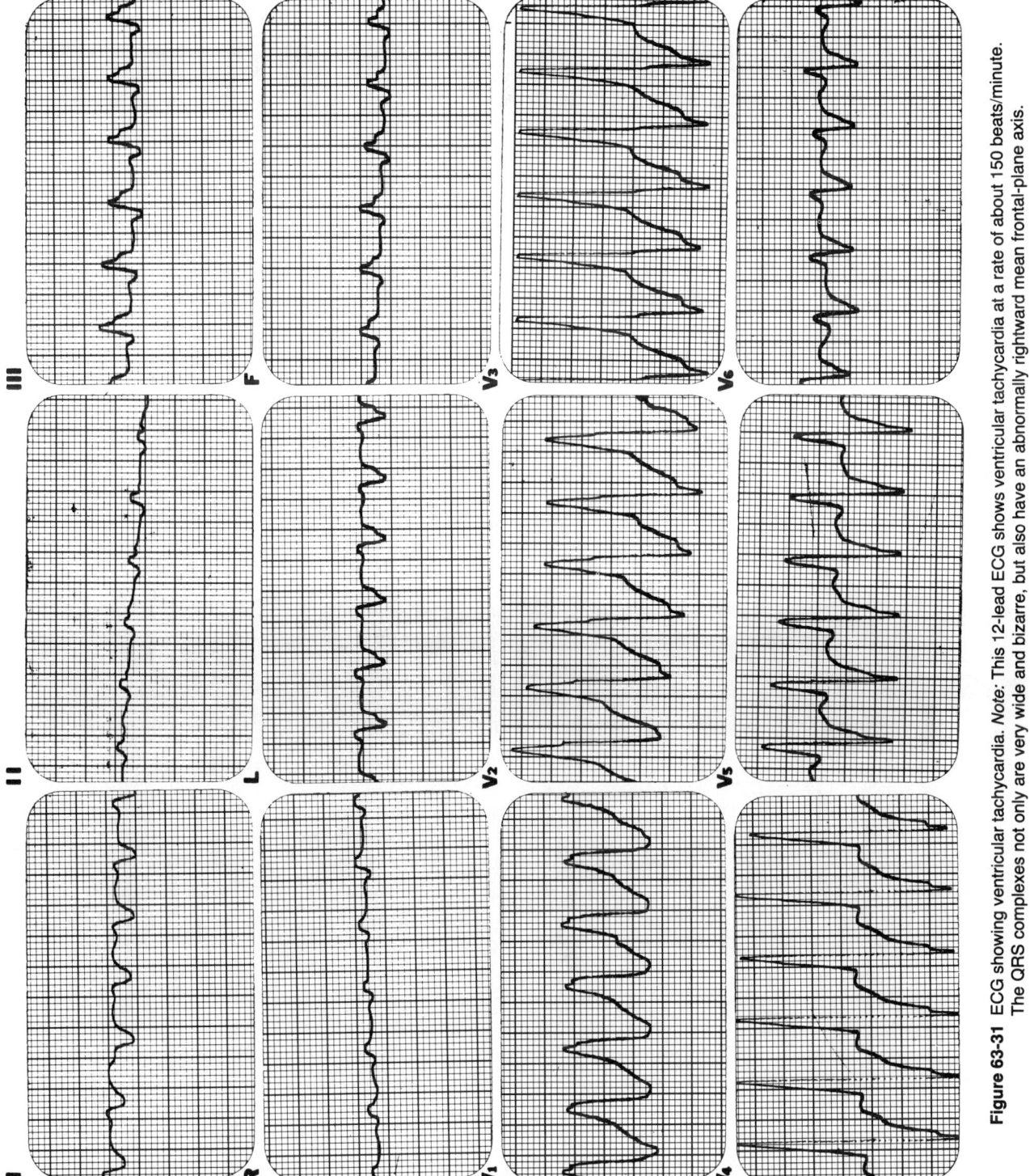

Figure 63-31 ECG showing ventricular tachycardia. *Note:* This 12-lead ECG shows ventricular tachycardia at a rate of about 150 beats/minute. The QRS complexes not only are very wide and bizarre, but also have an abnormally rightward mean frontal-plane axis.

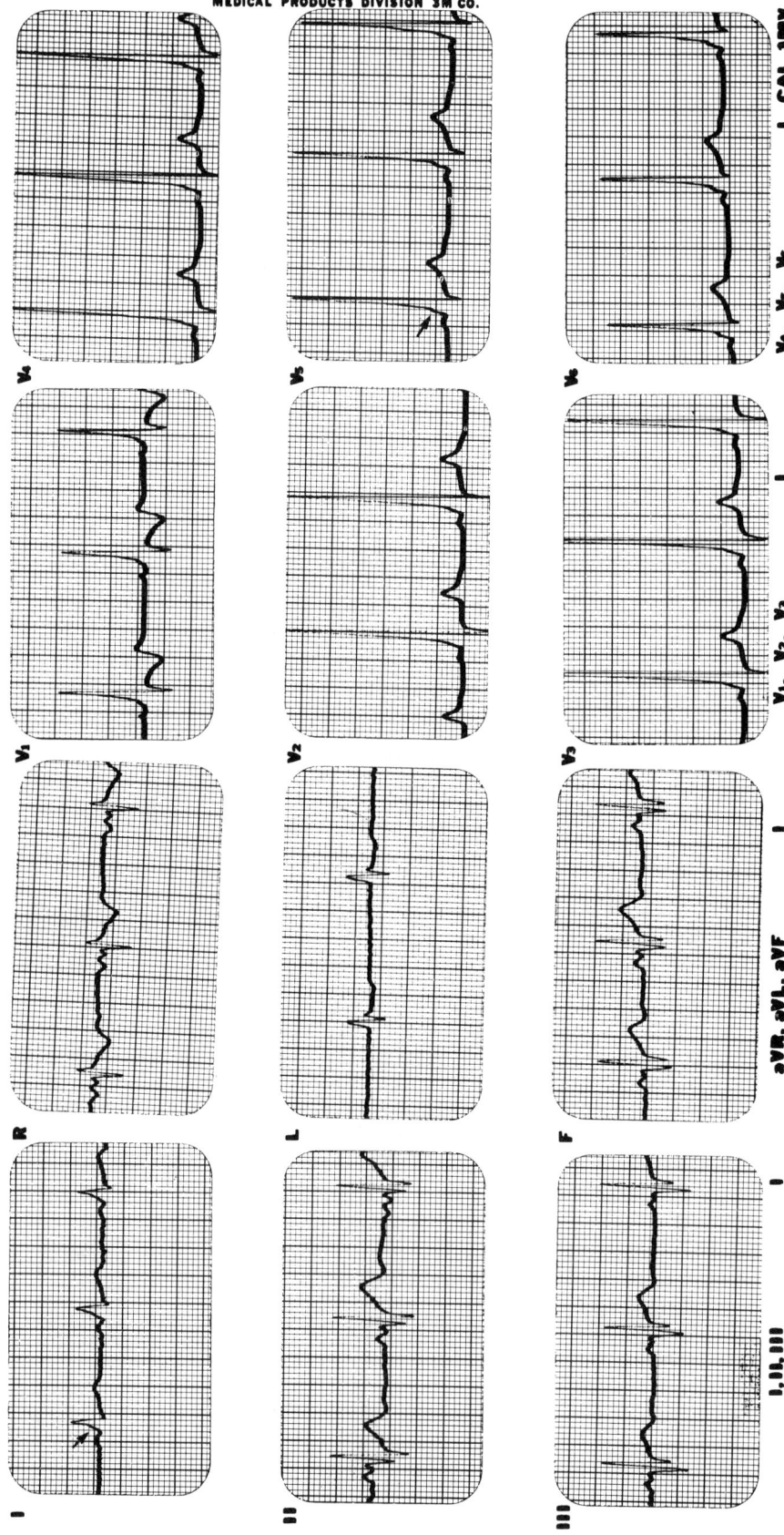

Figure 63-32 ECG from a patient with Wolff-Parkinson-White syndrome. *Note:* This 12-lead ECG recorded from a patient with Wolff-Parkinson-White syndrome shows the short PR interval, the wide QRS complexes, and the delta waves, two of which are indicated by the arrows (leads I and V₅). (ECG is at 81% of original.)

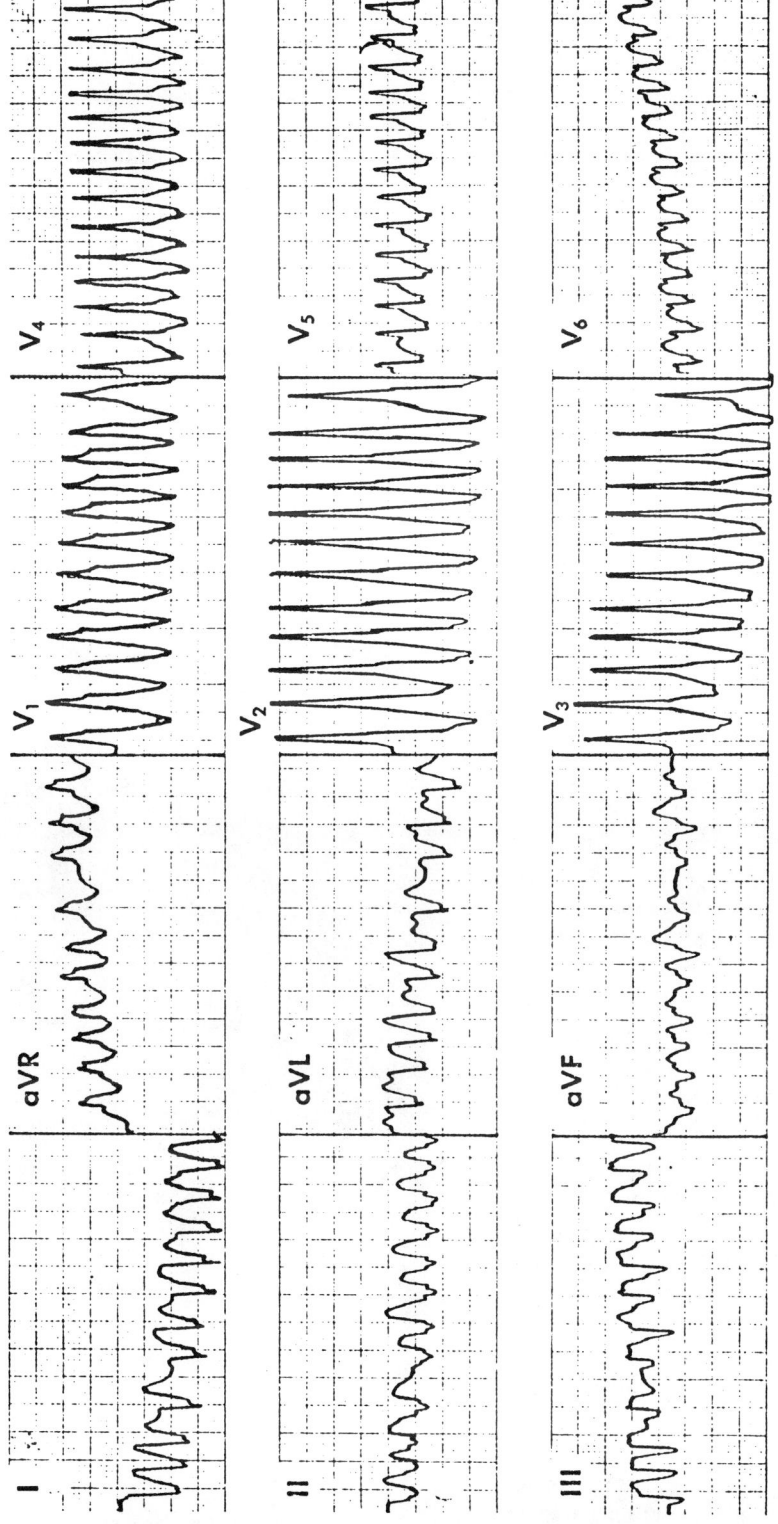

Figure 63-33 ECG showing atrial fibrillation in a patient with Wolff-Parkinson-White syndrome. *Note:* This 12-lead ECG was recorded from a patient with Wolff-Parkinson-White syndrome during atrial fibrillation. The very wide bizarre QRS complexes that occur at irregular intervals at an average rate of about 280/minute reflect ventricular activation via the accessory AV-conduction pathway, which obviously has a very short refractory period.

PSVT, the QRS complexes usually have normal contours (Fig. 63-22). PSVT may be terminated by maneuvers or medications that slow conduction through or lengthen refractory periods of the normal and/or the accessory AV conduction pathways. Carotid sinus massage, Tensilon, verapamil, adenosine, Valsalva's maneuver, beta-adrenergic blocking agents, and sympathomimetic amines that increase arterial blood pressure may terminate PSVT by slowing conduction through or lengthening refractory period of the AV node and may be used in doses similar to those used in PSVT in patients without accessory pathways. Lidocaine, procainamide, quinidine, and disopyramide may terminate PSVT by slowing conduction in the accessory pathway. As lidocaine is the safest, most rapidly acting, and simplest to administer, a 50- to 125-mg bolus of this medication might be the first therapeutic maneuver. While digoxin may terminate PSVT by slowing conduction in the AV node, some authorities feel it should not be used in the presence of antegradely conducting accessory pathways because it may enhance accessory pathway conduction and thus increase the ventricular rate if the rhythm changes from PSVT to atrial fibrillation or flutter, which not uncommonly occurs. Recent reports suggest that such undesirable events may also follow the administration of lidocaine and verapamil in this setting.

PERMANENT CARDIAC-PACING SYSTEMS

Most patients with permanent artificial cardiac-pacing systems have had the system implanted for prevention or treatment of bradycardias. Because bradycardias are the functional manifestations of disease processes that are usually progressive, the abnormality in cardiac rhythm present after months to years of pacing may be more profound than that present before pacing was instituted. Thus, failure of a permanent cardiac-pacing system may result in profound bradycardia with catastrophic consequences. The appearance or recurrence of symptoms suggesting bradycardia in a patient with a permanent cardiac-pacing system raises the strong possibility that the pacing system has malfunctioned or failed.

Cardiac-pacing systems consist of two parts, a pacemaker generator and a lead system (Fig. 63-34). The pacemaker generator contains the energy source of the system and the electronic components necessary to generate the electrical impulses (pacing stimuli) that depolarize the heart and to sense spontaneous cardiac electrical activity. The lead system, which carries electrical impulses from the pacemaker generator to the heart and spontaneous cardiac electrical activity from the heart to the sensing circuit within the pacemaker generator, consists of an insulated wire. At one end of this wire is a metallic pin that inserts into the pacemaker generator; at the other end is a bare metallic surface (the electrode) that makes contact with cardiac muscle.

The emission of a pacing stimulus into body tissues is recorded on the surface ECG as a sharp deflection of very brief duration, termed a *pacing artifact* (Fig. 63-35). When pacing artifacts initiate ventricular activation, they are seen at the onset of the QRS complex. The interval at which pacing stimuli are emitted from a pacemaker generator is termed the *pacing,* or *automatic, interval* of the device; the corresponding rate is termed the *pacing,* or *automatic, rate* (Fig. 63-35). The rate of many pacemaker generators may be changed noninvasively by application of a small "programmer" onto the skin overlying the generator. Most pacemaker generators implanted since 1988 are said to be "rate responsive," for they alter their pacing rates in response to changing body needs for cardiac output. These changing needs are "perceived" by detection of skeletal muscle activity, changes in thoracic impedance, or changes in the temperature of blood returning to the right atrium or right ventricle that occur when patients perform activities that increase oxygen consumption.

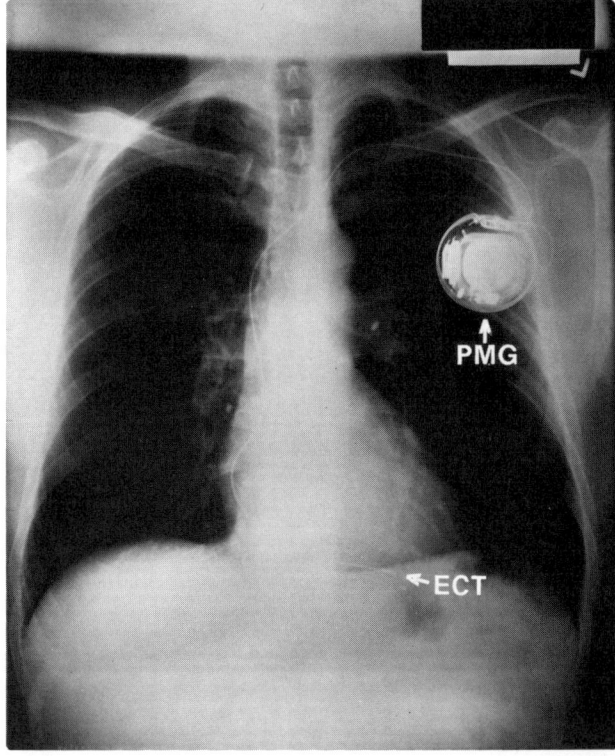

Figure 63-34 Radiograph showing permanent transvenous-ventricular pacing system. *Note:* This posteroanterior chest radiograph of a patient with a permanent transvenous-ventricular pacing system shows that the lead, an electrode catheter, has been introduced into the left cephalic vein. The electrode catheter tip (*ECT*) lies in the apex of the right ventricle, and the pacemaker generator (*PMG*) lies in the left infraclavicular area.

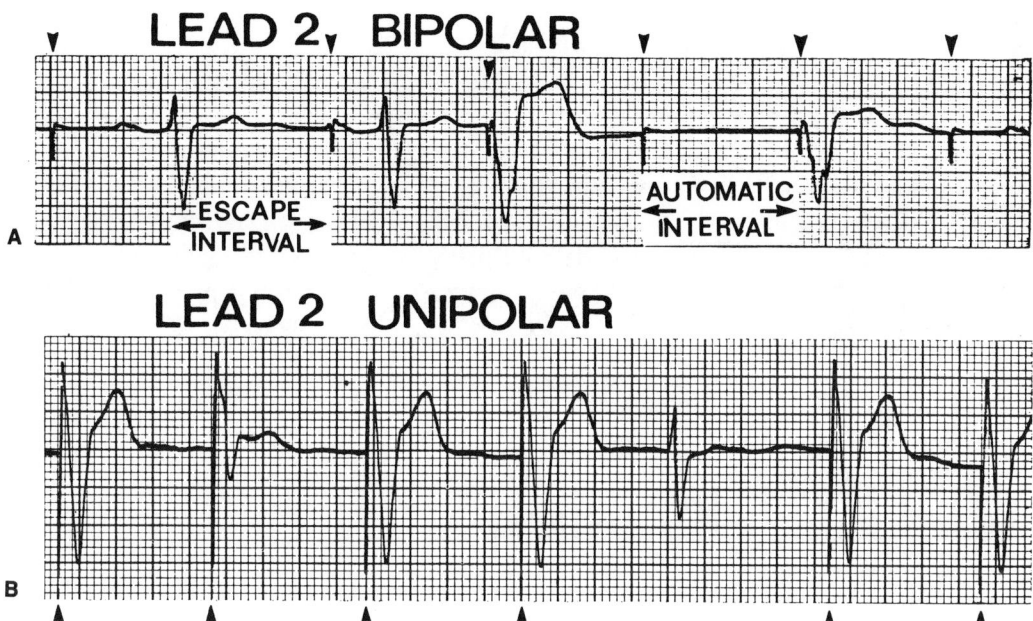

Figure 63-35 ECGs showing pacing artifacts. *Note:* These lead 2 rhythm strips from two different patients display pacing artifacts (*arrows*). The bipolar pacing artifacts *(A)* are small relative to the QRS complexes that they stimulate, while the unipolar pacing artifacts *(B)* are larger and distort the onsets of the QRS complexes that they stimulate. In *A*, the first, second, fourth, and sixth pacing artifacts do not stimulate QRS complexes because the energy output of the pacing system in this patient was intermittently too low to activate the ventricles. The second QRS complex is not sensed, but does not reflect "faulty sensing," for this complex falls within the sensing refractory period of this pacemaker generator.

Pacing systems may fail to function properly because of energy-source depletion, electronic-component failure, fracture or insulation break within the lead system, a change in the interface between the electrode portion of the lead system and the myocardium with which it makes contact, and interaction between the pacing system and high-energy radiation fields. As a discussion of all types of permanent cardiac-pacing systems is beyond the scope of this chapter, a detailed evaluation of only permanent-demand ventricular pacing systems—those most widely implanted—is presented. A brief discussion of dual-chamber pacing is presented at the end of this chapter. A technique for the insertion of a pacemaker is reviewed in Chapter 86, Atlas of Emergency Procedures.

Permanent-Demand Ventricular Pacing Systems

Permanent-demand ventricular pacing systems are designed to emit pacing stimuli only when spontaneous cardiac electrical activity is not sensed within a specific time interval, termed the *escape interval* (Figs. 63-35 and 63-36). Pacing stimuli are not emitted if spontaneous QRS complexes are sensed at intervals shorter than the escape interval. However, in order to keep the pacemaker generator from sensing a portion of a paced QRST complex or the later portion of a spontaneous QRST complex, the initial portion of which has already been sensed, the sensing circuit of a demand pacemaker generator is designed not to process incoming signals for a specific time interval after the emission of a pacing stimulus or after the sensing of spontaneous cardiac electrical activity. The duration of this *sensing refractory period* is generally in the range of 300 ± 75 milliseconds, but it varies among pacemaker generators.

Figure 63-35, *A* illustrates the sensing refractory period. In this strip, the first two QRS complexes are stimulated by the P waves that precede them; the last two QRS complexes are paced. The first QRS complex must have been sensed, for a pacing artifact follows its onset at an interval of about 0.88 seconds, slightly longer than the pacemaker generator escape interval of about 0.84 seconds. However, the second QRS complex must *not* have been sensed, for a pacing artifact follows its onset at an interval much shorter than the escape interval (0.58 seconds versus 0.84 seconds). This second QRS complex was not sensed because it fell about 0.26 seconds after emission of the second pacing stimulus, within the 0.32 ± 0.05 second sensing refractory period of this pacemaker generator. The first QRS complex was sensed because it has its onset about 0.64 seconds after the first pacing artifact, well after the sensing refractory period of 0.32 ± 0.05 seconds had elapsed.

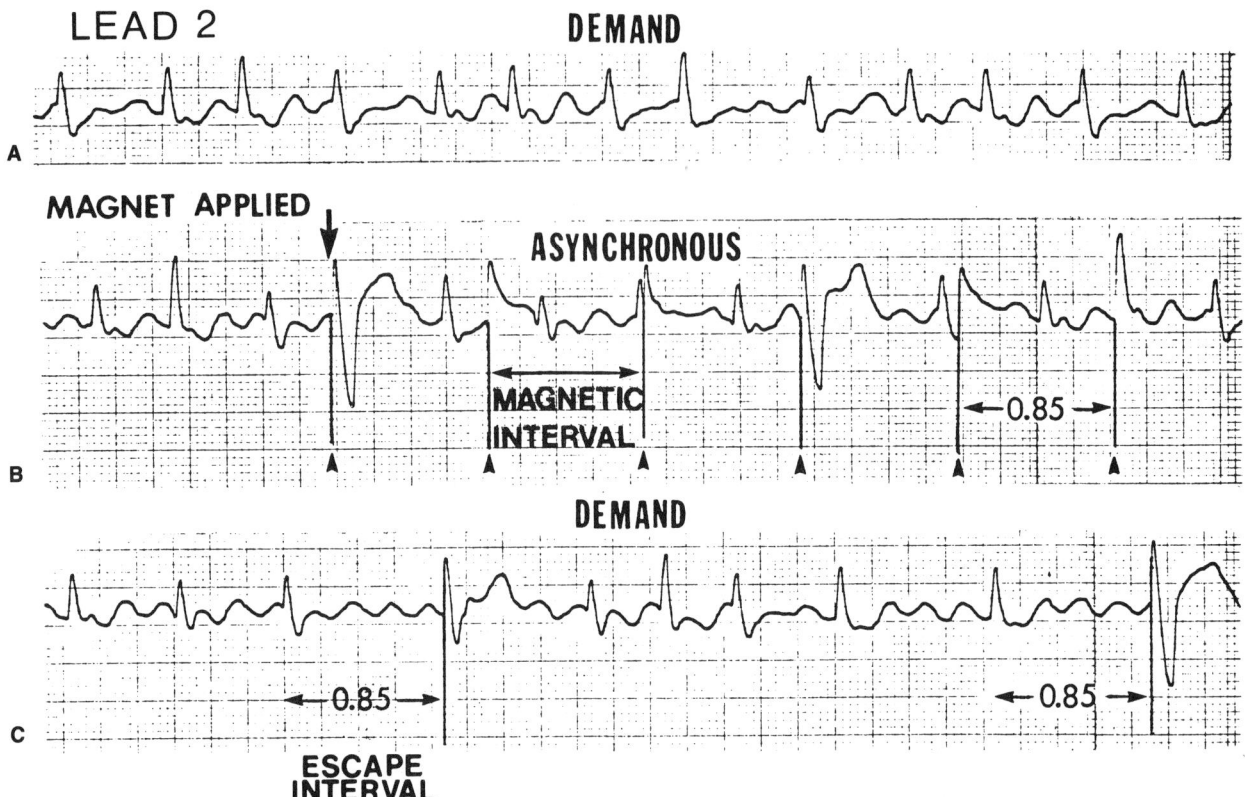

Figure 63-36 ECGs showing normal function of a permanent-demand ventricular pacing system. *Note:* These three lead 2 rhythm strips were recorded from a patient with a permanent-demand ventricular pacing system. The atrial rhythm is fibrillation in all three strips. *A:* Pacing artifacts are not seen, as the intervals between spontaneous QRS complexes never exceed the escape interval (0.85 seconds) of the pacemaker generator. *B:* Application of the magnet onto the skin overlying the pacemaker generator results in the emission of pacing stimuli at regular intervals of 0.85 seconds. The first, fourth, and sixth pacing artifacts initiate or contribute to ventricular activation, but the others do not because they fall within the refractory period of ventricular tissue. *C:* Recorded at a later time, pacing artifacts appear when the intervals between spontaneously occurring QRS complexes exceed the pacemaker-generator escape interval.

In order to permit an evaluation of pacing function when the rate of the spontaneous QRS rhythm exceeds the demand pacing rate of the pacemaker generator, all demand ventricular-pacemaker generators are designed to emit pacing stimuli at regular intervals without regard for the underlying rhythm (ie, to function in an *asynchronous* or *fixed rate* mode) when a specifically designed magnet is placed on the skin overlying the pacemaker generator (Fig. 63-36). The rate at which pacing stimuli are emitted when a magnet overlies the pacemaker generator is called the magnetic rate. The magnetic rate may be similar to, identical to, or faster than the pacing (automatic) rate during demand function, depending on the design specifications of the pacemaker generator. The pacemaker generator is usually designed such that the magnetic rate either decreases linearly with energy source depletion or shows a quantum decrement when energy source depletion is extreme. Thus, accurate assessment of pacing-system function requires a thorough knowledge of the design specifications of the particular pacemaker generator being evaluated.

In the evaluation of pacing-system function, the occurrence of specific ECG phenomena generally allows an accurate diagnosis of the mechanism of the abnormality. For example, the failure of pacing artifacts to be recorded in the ECG at a time when the spontaneous ventricular rate is lower than the expected demand pacing rate indicates abnormal pacing-system function (Fig. 63-37, A). There may be no pacing artifacts because (a) the pacemaker-generator energy source is depleted to the point where the demand pacing rate has fallen below the spontaneous ventricular rate at that time; (b) the energy source is depleted to the point where not enough is left to emit a pacing stimulus; (c) electronic circuitry malfunction is prohibiting the generation or emission of stimuli from the pacemaker generator; (d) complete fracture of the lead system is preventing the emitted stimuli from reaching body fluids, which they must do if pacing artifacts are to be detected in the surface ECG; (e) the pacemaker generator is sensing, and being recycled by, signals other than spontaneous QRS complexes, so-called spurious signals. Application of the magnet over the pacemaker gener-

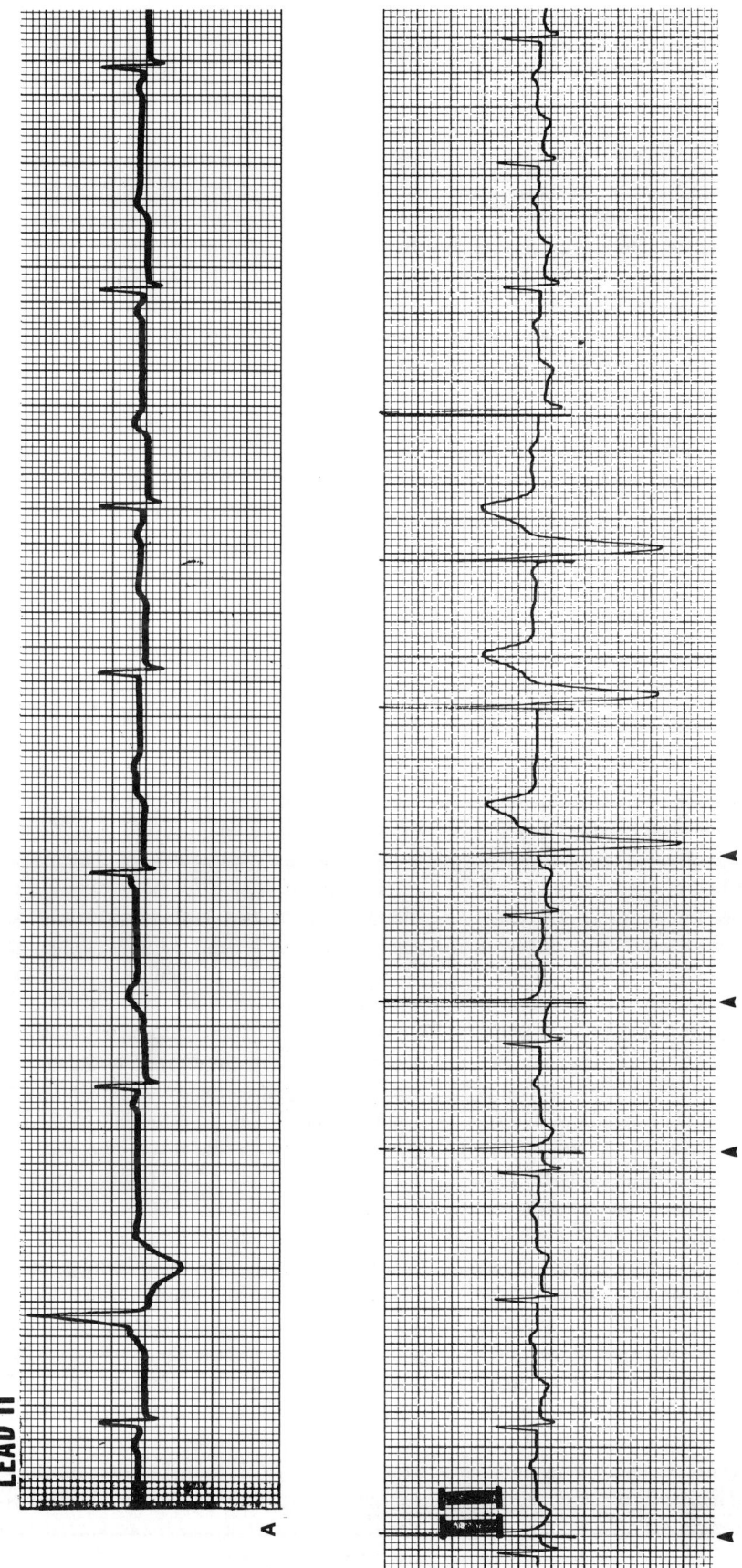

Figure 63-37 ECGs showing malfunction of demand ventricular pacing systems. *A:* This ECG was recorded from a patient with a demand ventricular pacing system that has an escape interval of 0.82 seconds. The failure of pacing artifacts to appear in this strip, in which almost all RR intervals exceed 0.82 seconds, indicates that pacing stimuli are not reaching body fluids. In this patient, there was a fracture in the lead close to the pacemaker generator. *B:* This ECG was recorded from a patient with a demand ventricular pacing system that has an escape interval of about 0.88 seconds. The appearance of some pacing artifacts *(arrows)* at intervals less than 0.88 seconds following spontaneous QRS complexes indicates intermittent failure to sense spontaneous QRS complexes. In this patient, the malfunction was related to suboptimal position of the electrode catheter tip within the right ventricle.

ator would result in the appearance of pacing artifacts only if explanations (a) and (e) were correct. If (a) were correct, the pacing artifacts would appear at a rate slower than the usual magnetic rate of the pacemaker generator; if (e) were correct, the pacing artifacts would occur at the expected magnetic rate. Explanation (d) may be evaluated by the technique of radioauscultation, which involves placing the antenna of a portable FM radio over the pacemaker generator, tuning the dial between stations, and placing the amplitude at maximum level. Because a pacing stimulus that originates within the pacemaker generator emits radio frequency signals even if the pacing stimulus does not exit from the pacemaker generator or the lead system, a "click" can be heard on the radio speaker every time a pacing stimulus is generated. Thus, when a pacemaker generator is emitting impulses appropriately but pacing artifacts are not seen on the surface ECG, radioauscultation may allow the diagnosis of lead fracture to be established.

If pacing artifacts are being emitted at a rate faster than that expected on the basis of the pacemaker-generator design specifications and programmed parameters, a phenomenon termed *runaway,* electronic component or circuitry failure is the mechanism of the abnormal function.

If pacing artifacts follow spontaneous QRS complexes at intervals shorter than the escape interval of the pacing system, the QRS complexes in question are not being sensed appropriately (Fig. 63-37, B). Such a failure is usually due to suboptimal location of the electrodes within the heart; the amplitude of spontaneous ventricular electrical activity (ie, the QRS complexes) that is reaching the pacemaker-generator sensing circuit is too small to be detected by it. This problem usually occurs because the tip of an electrode catheter changes position within the heart. Rarely, it occurs as a transient phenomenon in patients with acute myocardial infarction, presumably because the infarction temporarily alters spontaneous ventricular activity so that it no longer has the amplitude and frequency required for sensing.

If pacing artifacts occur at the expected escape interval or at the expected magnetic rate following application of a magnet over the pacemaker generator, but do not consistently stimulate QRS complexes despite falling outside of the expected refractory period of ventricular tissue, the energy of the stimulus may be said to be too low to activate ventricular tissue (Fig. 63-35, A). Pacing stimuli may fail to initiate ventricular activation because the energy output of the pacemaker generator is extremely low, because the myocardium surrounding the pacing electrode has an extremely high threshold for stimulation, or because there is an inappropriately large distance between the electrode and the myocardium, perhaps because the electrode has moved from its original position. Such *threshold problems* can generally be accurately evaluated and effectively resolved noninvasively if the pacemaker generator's energy output is programmable, as most devices have been for the past several years.

Management of Patients with Malfunction of a Permanent-Demand Ventricular Pacing System

When no pacing stimuli appear despite a slow spontaneous ventricular rhythm, a magnet should be placed over the pacemaker generator to see if it is sensing spurious signals. If it is, the pacing system will function in an asynchronous or fixed-rate mode, emitting pacing stimuli at regular intervals. If the emitted stimuli capture the ventricles, an adequate ventricular rate will be ensured. If this maneuver does not result in the appearance of pacing artifacts, attempts may be made to increase the generally slow spontaneous ventricular rhythm by cautious IV administration of isoproterenol in the case of second- and third-degree AV block, and by IV administration of atropine in the case of slow sinus rhythms with or without Mobitz Type I (Wenckebach) second-degree AV block. Establishing a temporary ventricular pacing system would, of course, ensure adequate ventricular rates.

When the pacing system is a runaway and the resultant ventricular rate is dangerously rapid, it *may* be possible to noninvasively reprogram the pacemaker-generator energy output to a level below stimulation threshold, but if this cannot be achieved, then surgical interruption of the pacing system by opening the pacemaker pocket *under sterile conditions* and detaching the lead from the pacemaker generator is required to terminate the rapid rhythm. However, plans must be made to ensure an adequate ventricular rate following interruption of the runaway pacing system, for profound cardiac standstill may ensue. An adequate rate may be achieved most expeditiously by immediately connecting the implanted lead to an external (temporary) pacemaker generator. The connection should be sterile so that the implanted lead system can be utilized with the new pacemaker generator that will be implanted to reestablish permanent ventricular pacing.

When failure to sense is occurring, the possibility exists that a pacing stimulus emitted in the vulnerable period of a spontaneous QRS complex will initiate repetitive ventricular beating, ventricular tachycardia, or ventricular fibrillation. In the absence of acute myocardial ischemia or infarction, however, the chance of this is quite small. Furthermore, it is possible that lidocaine or procainamide may increase the threshold for repetitive beating in this situation. If pacing stimuli are causing repetitive beating the generator may be reprogrammed to a higher sensitivity. If sensing is still inadequate and the patient has a reliable underlying spontaneous QRS rhythm, the energy output can be reprogrammed to a value so low (ie, subthreshold) that ventricular capture will not occur. However, if the spontaneous QRS rhythm is not adequate to allow pacing to be terminated, then reprogramming the pacing rate to a higher level may "overdrive suppress" the spontaneous QRS rhythm that has not been appropriately sensed. However, surgical revision of the pacing system may be necessary to achieve reliable pacing-system function.

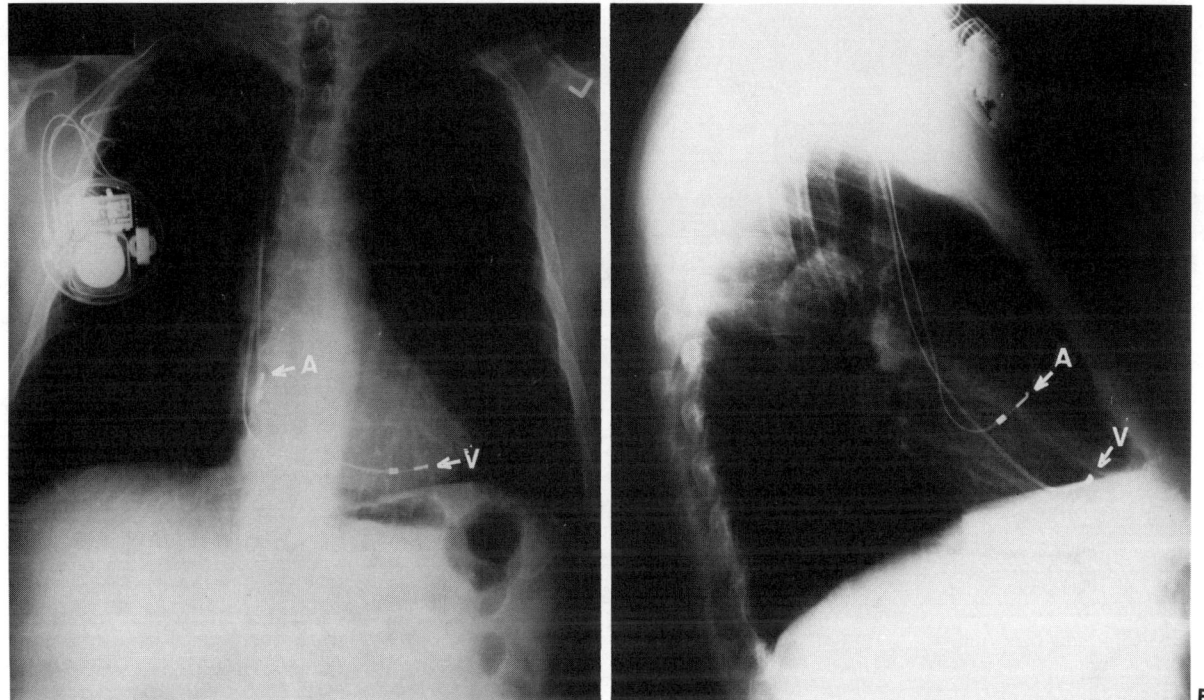

Figure 63-38 Posterior-anterior and lateral chest radiographs of a patient with a transvenous bipolar dual-chamber pacing system. The atrial electrode catheter tip, designated by the letter "A," is located in the right atrial appendage. The tip of the ventricular electrode catheter, designated by the letter "V," is located in the right ventricular apex. The pacemaker generator is located in the right infraclavicular fossa.

For threshold problems that cannot be adequately managed by reprogramming the pacemaker-generator energy output to its maximum, the cautious IV administration of isoproterenol may lower the threshold and allow an otherwise subthreshold pacing stimulus to activate the ventricles. Of course, insertion of a temporary transvenous ventricular pacing system would ensure an adequate ventricular rate.

The exact emergency management of the patient with pacing-system malfunction depends on the specific pacing-system problem, the resultant cardiac rhythm, and the patient's hemodynamic state at that time. In general, therapy involves watchful waiting if the underlying rhythm is stable and adequate, immediate interruption of the pacing system if there is a runaway phenomenon, the IV administration of isoproterenol or the insertion of a temporary transvenous pacing system if profound bradycardia is present, the IV administration of isoproterenol if Mobitz Type II second-degree AV block is present, and the IV administration of atropine if slow sinus rhythm with or without Mobitz Type I (Wenckebach) second-degree AV block is present.

Over the past several years, as the hemodynamic importance of maintaining the normal atrial and ventricular contraction sequence has become more clearly appreciated, and as technical advances have effected improvements in the reliability and ease of implantation of atrial electrode catheters, pacemakers that function in atrium as well as in ventricle are becoming more widely used. Such *dual-chamber* pacemakers are usually set to function in the *dual demand,* or *DDD* mode, in which both atrium and ventricle may be sensed and paced. Such pacing systems ensure a minimum atrial-pacing rate, ensure synchronization of the QRS complex to paced and spontaneous P waves, and allow the ventricular rate to increase directly with the atrial rate. Most recently manufactured pacemaker generators are also "rate responsive," allowing increments in the paced atrial and ventricular rates to occur during physical activities. Figure 63-38 displays PA and lateral chest radiographs of a patient with a dual-chamber pacing system in which bipolar electrode catheters are located with their tips in the right atrial appendage, and in the right ventricular apex.

Figure 63-39 displays four rhythm strips from patients with dual-chamber pacing systems functioning in the DDD mode. In strip A, in which the spontaneous sinus rate is about 75/minute, all P waves are spontaneous, but all QRS complexes, which are synchronized to the preceding P waves at PR intervals of about 0.20 seconds, are paced, because the spontaneous PR interval is longer than the pacemaker AV interval. In strip B, all P waves are paced at the atrial demand rate of about 75/minute, because the patient's spontaneous sinus rate is less than this. All of the QRS complexes, which follow the atrial pacing artifacts by about 0.20 seconds, are stimulated by the paced P waves, because at this time the

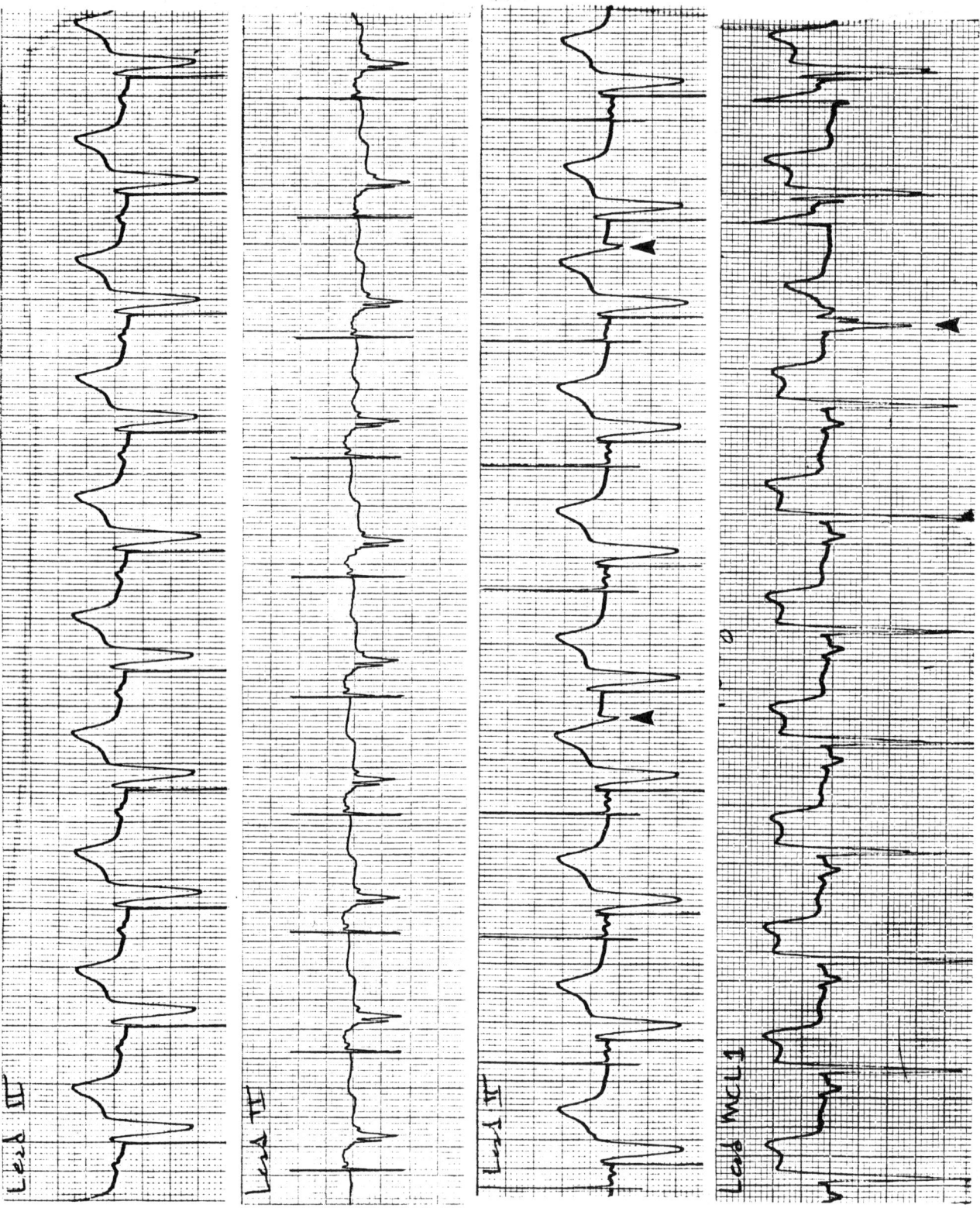

Figure 63-39 Four rhythm strips recorded from patients with dual-chamber pacing systems operating in the dual-demand mode.

spontaneous PR interval is shorter than the pacemaker AV interval.

In strip C, all QRS complexes are paced, and are synchronized to the P waves that precede them, indicating that the spontaneous AV-conduction time exceeds the pacemaker AV interval. The first four P waves are paced, because the spontaneous intersinus interval at this time is longer than the interval corresponding to the pacemaker-demand atrial rate. The fifth P wave, designated by the first arrowhead, is an atrial premature complex that must have been sensed, for it is followed at the pacemaker AV interval by a paced QRS complex. The pause in atrial rhythm following the APC is terminated by a paced P wave, because the sinus node escape interval at this time is longer than the pacemaker escape interval. The following two P waves are also paced, but then another APC, shown at the second arrowhead, occurs and again triggers a paced QRS complex at the pacemaker AV interval. The pause following this APC is, as shown earlier in this strip, terminated by a paced atrial complex.

In strip D, eight spontaneous PQRST complexes are followed by a premature ventricular complex, designated by the arrowhead. An on-time sinus P wave falls at the very end of the premature QRS complex and runs into the beginning of the ST segment. This P wave is obviously not sensed, for if it had been sensed a ventricular pacing artifact would have followed it at the pacemaker AV interval. Rather, the pause occasioned by the PVC is terminated by an atrial pacing artifact that stimulates a difficult to observe P wave, following which a ventricular pacing stimulus is emitted to stimulate a QRS complex. The fact that the QRS complex looks very similar to the spontaneous QRS complexes preceding the PVC indicates that these complexes are probably not pure paced QRS complexes, but rather are fusion complexes in which ventricular activation is contributed to by both the ventricular pacing stimulus and by the paced P wave. An identically paced PQRST complex ends the strip.

REFERENCES

1. Zipes DP. Proarrhythmic effects of antiarrhythmic drugs. *Am J Cardiol*. 1987;59:26E–31E.
2. Podrid PJ, Lampert S, Graboys TB, Blatt CM, Lown B. Aggravation of arrhythmia by antiarrhythmic drugs—incidence and predictors. *Am J Cardiol*. 1987;59:38E–44E.
3. Devereux RB, Perloff JK, Reichek N, et al. Mitral valve prolapse. *Circulation*. 1976;54:3–14.
4. Leahey EB Jr, Bigger JT Jr, Butler VP Jr, et al. Quinidine-digoxin interaction: time course and pharmacokinetics. *Am J Cardiol*. 1981;48:1141–1146.
5. Jacobson LB. Spontaneous ventricular parasystole initiating ventricular tachycardia. *J Electrocardiol*. 1973;6:63–70.

64. Congestive Heart Failure

RICHARD G. FRIEDMAN, MD, FACC

The dyspneic patient presents a diagnostic and therapeutic challenge to the emergency physician. The correct diagnosis and therapy can rapidly change an anxious, frightened, critically ill patient into a calm, asymptomatic one. Incorrect or inadequate therapy can just as easily make the patient profoundly worse. Since congestive heart failure (CHF) is the most common etiology of dyspnea in emergency department patients with infiltrates on their chest roentgenograms,[1] it is important for the physician to be thoroughly familiar with its diagnosis and management. A physician must quickly decide the most pressing problems and determine whether the patient is safe or in immediate danger. This approach is similar for any medical emergency. While examining the patient and obtaining a history and laboratory data base, the physician or paramedic in the field should already be deciding the most likely etiology of the dyspnea. Is it cardiac, pulmonary, psychogenic, or caused by a less commonly diagnosed disorder? Conservative therapy should be initiated as soon as possible, and definitive therapy should be started once the diagnosis is established. An approach to the diagnosis and management of the patient with CHF will be presented here, along with a brief review of the pathophysiology that leads to the common signs and symptoms of CHF.

DEFINITION

Heart failure refers to any condition in which an alteration in myocardial function results in the heart's inability to circulate enough oxygenated blood to meet the body's metabolic needs during rest or exercise.[2,3] Congestion is found in the organs that are in the anatomic circuit located behind the failing ventricle. In right-sided CHF, the liver is engorged with fluid; while in predominant left-sided CHF, the lungs may be engorged.

CHF may be an acute or chronic condition. Either form involves some element of elevated ventricular filling pressures, but the rate of rise and the ability for compensatory mechanisms to increase cardiac output will determine the level of symptoms that the patient will experience. Compensatory mechanisms involved in regulating cardiac output are outlined below[3,4]:

I. Cardiac
   A. Ventricular hypertrophy
   B. Ventricular dilatation (Frank-Starling mechanism)
   C. Sympathetic nervous system
      1. Heart rate
      2. Contractility (inotropic state of the heart)
II. Peripheral circulation
   A. Venous constriction
   B. Arteriolar constriction
III. Renal
   A. Increased sodium retention (increases preload)
   B. Inappropriate secretion of antidiuretic hormone

The functional class of the patient with CHF is based on the relationship of symptoms of CHF to the activity level of the individual. According to the New York Heart Association classification the functional classes of CHF include[4]:

- *Class I:* normal basal output in the absence of circulatory congestion. Lesser degrees of myocardial dysfunction such as hypertrophy without failure may be seen. No symptoms are noted at rest or with activity.
- *Class II:* moderate elevations of systemic and pulmonary venous pressures. Symptoms may occur with greater than normal activity.
- *Class III:* compensated CHF. The resting cardiac output is normal with excessive elevation of pulmonary venous pressure. Symptoms may occur with normal levels of activity.
- *Class IV:* decompensated CHF. Inability of the heart to maintain basal cardiac output. Symptoms occur at rest.

In chronic compensated CHF, the left ventricular end-diastolic pressure (LVEDP) and end-diastolic volume may be elevated, which causes the heart to operate at a different point on the Frank-Starling curve.[5] The increased diastolic myocardial stretch developed as a result of the increased LVEDP causes an increase in forward stroke volume as the diastolic reserve is tapped, but this is at the expense of increased filling pressures, which may result in symptoms of dyspnea and congestion with any increased demands.[5] Similarly, flow to the central nervous system and heart may be maintained through sympathetic nervous system mediated arteriolar and venous vasoconstriction and tachycardia at the expense of decreased peripheral blood flow to the skin, splanchnic, and renal beds.[4,5] All the compensatory mechanisms listed previously can lead to the classic symptoms of CHF, which include dyspnea, tachycardia, diaphoresis, paroxysmal nocturnal dyspnea, orthopnea, vasoconstriction, and edema if increased metabolic demands are made on the compensated ventricle.[6] In acute CHF, either the insult occurs so rapidly that the compensatory mechanisms cannot handle the situation or the mechanisms were already being utilized chronically and no reserve capacity remained. Patients seeking aid in the emergency department will usually have some element of decompensated CHF. Patients with class I or II CHF will most often be asymptomatic and are managed as outpatients without emergency care. If, however, there is increased metabolic demand, CHF can decompensate and symptoms are apparent. In decompensated left-sided CHF, forward flow can no longer be maintained adequately even at rest, and any increased demand on the circulatory system may cause fluid to move from the edematous pulmonary interstitium and into the alveolar sacs, resulting in pulmonary edema.[7] In the most severe form of heart failure, cardiogenic shock, the heart fails to perfuse the tissues, and all compensatory mechanisms are inadequate or have failed.

This chapter will focus on those forms of heart failure that result from a defect in the myocardium and will not deal at length with CHF caused by acute volume overload, high output failure that results from increased peripheral demands, or diastolic dysfunction in which the ventricles fail to receive blood under low pressures.[21]

PATHOPHYSIOLOGY

Cardiac function is predominantly determined by the following interrelated parameters[6,8,9]:

- afterload, defined as the resistance to forward flow from the ventricle or the intraventricular systolic tension developed during ejection
- preload, the Frank-Starling mechanism or the diastolic stretch of myocardial fibers
- heart rate
- contractility, defined as the inotropic state of the heart
- normal temporal sequence of segmental contraction of the ventricle
- lusitrophy, improved diastolic function through increased rate of ventricular relaxation.

Any condition that significantly alters any of these parameters or their interrelationship may result in decreased forward blood flow consistent with CHF. Various pathologic mechanisms that can give rise to CHF and conditions that are associated with them are listed in Table 64-1.

Ideally, the therapy for CHF is linked to its etiology. If the problem is increased afterload from systemic hypertension, then afterload reducing agents would be a logical measure. If increased preload is present, then diuresis or peripheral venous pooling would be helpful. If the CHF is caused by decreased contractility, then inotropic agents are useful. However, if the problem is cardiac tamponade or hypovolemia, the use of diuretics would be potentially harmful. In a patient with a high-output heart failure with a diminished afterload, further afterload reduction might be injurious.

Availability of the flow-directed pulmonary artery catheter allows the clinician to determine the precise pathophysiology at the patient's bedside. Since treatment varies with the etiology of the CHF, it is often useful to pass a Swan-Ganz catheter. Direct pressure measurements can be made in the right atrium, right ventricle, and pulmonary artery. The pulmonary-artery wedge pressure approximates the left atrial pressure, which approximates the LVEDP, which represents preload. Clinical conditions causing CHF that have typical findings with a Swan-Ganz catheter are listed in Table 64-2. In general, interstitial edema is present in the lungs with a pulmonary-artery wedge pressure of 13 to 20 mmHg, symptoms of CHF develop at a pressure of 20 to 24 mmHg, and pulmonary edema occurs with a pressure greater than 25 mmHg.[7] In chronic situations, higher levels of the pulmonary-artery wedge pressure may be compensatory and may not be associated with symptoms at rest.

Table 64-1 Pathophysiologic Mechanisms Causing CHF

Mechanism	Associated Conditions
Global decrease in contractility	Cardiomyopathy Hypothermia Infiltrative disorders Ischemia Metabolic disorders Myocarditis Toxins
Regional decrease in contractility	Ischemia Trauma
Decreased quantity of myocardium	Infarction
Increased afterload	Aortic stenosis Coarctation of the aorta Hypertension Idiopathic hypertrophic subvalvular aortic stenosis Pulmonary stenosis Tricuspid stenosis
Increased forward flow with volume overload	Aortic regurgitation Mitral regurgitation Tricuspid regurgitation Ventricular septal defect
Dyssynergy of contraction	Aneurysm Atrioventricular dissociation
Inadequate heart rate	Disorders of rhythm and conduction
Decreased return of blood to heart	Cardiac rupture Constriction Hypovolemia Restriction Tamponade Vena cava obstruction
High output failure with increased peripheral demand	Anemia Arteriovenous communication Beri-beri Hyperthermia Hyperthyroidism Paget's disease Sepsis
Abnormal anatomy	Congenital heart disease
Inability to handle volume	Iatrogenic volume overload
Obstruction to atrial emptying	Cor triatriatum Left or right atrial myxoma Left or right atrial thrombus Mitral stenosis
Diastolic dysfunction	Constrictive pericarditis Restrictive cardiomyopathy Tricuspid or mitral stenosis Acute volume overload Dilated cardiomyopathy Advanced hypertrophy Flash pulmonary edema, secondary to myocardial ischemia[21,22]

Table 64-2 Pulmonary Artery Flow–Directed Catheter Findings in Conditions Causing CHF

Condition	Finding
Constriction or restriction	Equalization within 5 mmHg of the diastolic right and left ventricle pressures with RA mean and PAW
Right ventricular infarction	↑ RA, ↑ RV, normal or ↓ PAW, normal or ↓ PA
Pulmonary hypertension	↑ PA, normal PAW
Left ventricular infarction	↑ PAW, ↑ RA
Hypovolemia	↓ RA, ↓ PAW
Mitral regurgitation	V wave in PAW tracing
Tricuspid regurgitation	↑ V wave in RA tracing
Noncardiac pulmonary edema	All pressures normal or decreased

Note: ↑, increased; ↓, decreased; PA, pulmonary artery pressure; PAW, pulmonary artery wedge pressure; RA, right atrial pressure.

The Swan-Ganz catheter can also be used to measure cardiac output by thermal dilution, and the cardiac index can be calculated. Serial saturation samples can be obtained to determine whether an intracardiac shunt may be present. Simultaneous pulmonary artery and arterial saturation samples and a hemoglobin value may be used to determine the arteriovenous oxygen (AVO_2) difference. The AVO_2 difference is the amount of oxygen extracted from the blood as it passes through the tissues and is important in validating the cardiac output measurements. Tissue perfusion will not correlate with cardiac output in all cases. If cardiac output is normal or elevated but the red blood cells hold onto oxygen more avidly than usual, the AVO_2 difference would be narrow, reflecting a lack of perfusion independent of the cardiac output. Conditions that may cause increased avidity for oxygen by the red blood cell include hypophosphatemia, hypothermia, alkalosis, carbon monoxide poisoning, methemoglobinemia, sepsis, and some hemoglobinopathies.

Other valuable measurements that may be calculated with the use of a Swan-Ganz catheter and an arterial line include the systemic vascular resistance, which reflects afterload, and pulmonary vascular resistance. Swan-Ganz fiberoptic catheters provide continuous determination of oxygen saturation and allow cardiac output determination by green dye as well as by thermal dilution. (See Chapter 72, Obstructive Airway Disease for a technique used in inserting the Swan-Ganz catheter.)

DIAGNOSIS

Accurate and rapid diagnosis is crucial to ensure the comfort and safety of the dyspneic patient. As the patient is evaluated, any prehospital treatment that may alter the physical findings must be considered.[10] When first entering the patient's room, one should watch the patient carefully and make the following observations:

- Is the patient sitting or lying? If lying, is the patient either less dyspneic or so hypoxic that he or she may be semistuporous and unable to sit up?
- What does the cardiac monitor show?
- What is the respiratory rate, and are the accessory muscles of respiration being used?
- Is the patient cyanotic?
- Is there evidence of diaphoresis or peripheral edema?
- When questioned, is the patient gasping for breath or able to speak freely?

If the history is inadequate, the physician should consult friends, relatives, the old hospital chart, and the private physician as soon as possible.

While examining the patient, emergency care personnel must look for findings that may suggest an etiology for the patient's dyspnea:

- What are the vital signs?
- Is there evidence of a paradoxical pulse that may suggest chronic obstructive pulmonary disease (COPD), tamponade, pericardial effusion, constriction, or restriction?
- Is there a mechanical alternating pulse suggestive of tamponade?
- Are there postural blood-pressure changes suggestive of hypovolemia?
- On auscultatory examination, is there an S_3 gallop rhythm? If so, is it right- or left-sided in origin?
- Are there murmurs, suggestive of aortic stenosis, idiopathic hypertrophic subvalvular aortic stenosis, pulmonic stenosis, tricuspid stenosis, or mitral stenosis, or of regurgitation with increased volume overload such as mitral, tricuspid, aortic, or pulmonary regurgitation?
- Is there any evidence of congenital heart disease or a murmur suggestive of a ventricular septal defect or other intracardiac shunt?
- Are there any unusual findings such as a pericardial knock suggestive of constrictive disease?
- Are the heart sounds faint, suggestive of pericardial effusion, or do the peripheral pulses decrease with inspiration when inspecting the neck?
- Is there jugular venous distention or a positive hepatojugular reflux?
- Is there a large V wave or cannon wave suggestive of tricuspid regurgitation or atrioventricular dissociation?
- Is Kussmaul's sign, found in COPD, cor pulmonale, right ventricular infarction, or constriction, present?
- On ausculation of the lungs, are there rales or wheezes?
- Is there evidence of pleural effusion?
- Is there any suggestion of a pneumothorax or of foreign body aspirations that might cause dyspnea?
- Are there physical findings of hyperthyroidism, arteriovenous fistulas, dialysis shunts, sepsis, or any other systemic disorders that can lead to CHF?

Observation of the patient and completion of the examination outlined above should take only a few moments, and the examiner should quickly be able to determine whether a primary cardiac problem is involved or whether the CHF is secondary to a problem in another oxygen system. While the patient is being examined, routine measures should be performed simultaneously if not already done en route to the hospital. These include establishing an intravenous line and an airway, administering supplemental low flow oxygen (see Chapter 72), starting cardiac monitoring, and administering diuretics, morphine sulfate, and lidocaine, if indicated. An ECG, chest radiograph, arterial blood-gas values, and baseline laboratory data (including sodium, potassium, carbon dioxide, chloride, creatinine, creatine phosphokinase, lactic dehydrogenase, magnesium, phosphorus, and a urinalysis) should be obtained as soon as possible. An emergent two-dimensional color flow Doppler echocardiogram can assess systolic and diastolic function, valvular heart disease, intracardiac shunts, constrictive pericarditis, pulmonary hypertension, pericardial effusions, and right ventricular function.[23,24] Conservative therapy should be started immediately and should be directed by new data as available.

TREATMENT

Treatment of CHF can be divided into five phases: (1) conservative measures to ensure oxygenation and make the patient comfortable; (2) elimination of the underlying etiology; (3) classic therapy including digitalis and diuretics; (4) optimizing preload, afterload, and inotropic states (Table 64-3),[6,11–20] and (5) unusual techniques, including intraaortic balloon pumping, phlebotomy, and artificial pacing.

When confronted with a dyspneic patient, it is important to eliminate any reversible causes of CHF or dyspnea. A careful, rapid physical examination may reveal any evidence of tamponade or cardiac dysrhythmias or may point to noncardiac causes of dyspnea, including pneumothorax or airway obstruction. (See Section XI, Alterations of Respiratory System Functions.) The laboratory data may show electrolyte abnormalities that may depress myocardial function. Arterial blood-gas values may suggest a pulmonary embolus, and the radiograph may reveal pulmonary infarction. An attempt should be made to reverse any underlying cause of CHF or conditions that mimic it while temporary therapy is continued.

Table 64-3 Drugs Used in Congestive Heart Failure

Drug	Route	Dose	Effects
Aminophylline	IV	2.75 mg/kg IV	Decreased bronchospasm Mild inotropic effect
Amrinone	IV	0.75 mg/kg loading dose	Improved diastolic function Positive inotropic effect
Bumetanide	IV Oral	0.25–2 mg 0.5–2 mg	Diuresis
Captopril	Oral	25- to 150-mg initial dose	Arterial and venous dilatation
Chlorthiazide	IV Oral	500 mg 500–1000 mg	Potentiates effects of loop diuretics
Digoxin	IV or oral	0.5-mg loading dose	Increased contractility Increased cardiac output Reflex decrease in peripheral vasoconstriction
Dobutamine	IV	2.5–15 μg/kg/min	Increased contractility Increased cardiac output
Dopamine	IV	2–5 μg/kg/min; up to 30 mg/kg/min	Increased contractility Increased cardiac output Vasodilatation of renal vascular bed
Enalapril	IV Oral	0.625–1.25 mg 2.5–5 mg	Arterial and venous dilatation
Ethacrynic acid	IV or oral	50 mg	Diuresis
Furosemide	IV or oral	10–100 mg	Diuresis Increased peripheral venous capacitance
Hydralazine	IV Oral	20–50 mg 25–200 mg	Arterial dilatation Reflex tachycardia not found when treating CHF
Isoproterenol	IV	Starting at 1–3 μg/min	Increased contractility Increased heart rate β-mediated vasodilatation
Isosorbide dinitrate	Sublingual Oral	5–20 mg 10–60 mg	Venodilatation Slight arterial dilatation
Lisinopril	Oral	5–10 mg	Arterial and venous dilatation
Metolazone	Oral	2.5–10 mg/day	Potentiates effect of loop diuretics
Minoxidil	Oral	10–40 mg/day	Arterial dilatation
Morphine	IV	2- to 3-mg increments	Decreased anxiety Decreased preload
Nifedipine	Oral	10–40 mg	Mild arterial and venous dilatation
Nitroglycerin	IV Sublingual Topical Oral	5–100 μg/min and titrate to effect 1/150 grain 1/2–1 inch or 5-mg patch 10–40 mg	Venodilatation Slight arterial dilatation
Nitroprusside	IV	20–300 μg/min	Arterial and venous dilatation
Prazosin	Oral	1–10 mg	Arterial and venous dilatation

Conservative initial measures that may be started in the field include establishment of an airway and administration of supplemental oxygen. If there is any history or suspicion of chronic lung disease, then low-flow oxygen at 1 to 2 L/minute should be used until the patient is in a fully monitored setting where endotracheal intubation equipment is available. An intravenous line should be established and maintained at a keep-open rate. All medications should be given intravenously if possible. Intramuscular injections may cause an elevation in creatine phosphokinase, which may confuse the early diagnosis of a myocardial infarction. Vasoconstriction to the skin may decrease absorption of intramuscular injections. Oral medications may be erratically absorbed secondary to bowel edema or decreased splanchnic blood flow. Morphine sulfate may be given intravenously in doses of 2 to 3 mg to decrease anxiety and reduce preload. An initial intravenous dose of a diuretic such as furosemide, 20 to 40 mg, may be given. Furosemide increases venous capacitance peripherally and reduces preload even before diuresis begins. If there does not appear to be an acute myocardial infarction and the patient is not already on digitalis, then digoxin, 0.5 mg, may be given intravenously. If wheezing is present, aminophylline may be given intravenously with a loading dose of 2.75 mg/kg over 20 to 30 minutes, but watch for inappropriate tachycardia. Lidocaine may be given as a 75- to 100-mg intravenous bolus for ventricular ectopy and may be repeated if necessary. (See Chapter 62, Acute Myocardial Infarction.) If available, rotating tourniquets may be used to reduce preload. While therapy is continuing, the patient should be in a comfortable position (usually sitting up) and all laboratory specimens should be obtained, the rest of the history should be taken, and the physical examination should be completed. If there is an inadequate response to the loop diuretic, the dose may be repeated or increased, or 250 to 500 mg of chlorthiazide may be given IV to potentiate diuresis.

While the patient is being evaluated and conservative measures are in progress, an effort should be directed at reversing any obvious underlying condition. If severe bradycardia is present, consider insertion of a temporary transvenous pacemaker or the use of an external temporary pacemaker. An AV-sequential pacemaker is preferable, since it preserves AV synchrony. If rapid atrial fibrillation or supraventricular tachycardia are present, and refractory to medications, consider synchronized electrical cardioversion.

In recent years, treatment of CHF has been expanded to include manipulation of contractility, preload, and afterload. If forward flow is restricted by increased afterload, arteriolar vasodilators including nitroprusside, hydralazine, prazosin, and captopril may be useful. While hydralazine is a pure arteriolar vasodilator, nitroprusside and prazosin predominantly dilate the arterial bed but also dilate the venous beds. Nitroglycerin and isosorbide dinitrate predominantly dilate the venous beds and decrease preload. The inotropic agents, dopamine and dobutamine, may decrease preload and afterload indirectly by increasing cardiac output and decreasing reflex vasoconstriction and directly by β-mediated vasodilatation.[12] Amrinone may improve diastolic dysfunction and provide a positive inotropic effect.[25,26] If hypovolemia is clinically suspected, a volume challenge of 250 mL of normal saline given intravenously over 20 to 30 minutes may be used, while urine output, blood pressure, and central venous pressure are monitored.

The rational use of potent vasodilators or inotropic agents and volume administration is best managed by hemodynamic measurements obtained by pulmonary artery catheter and an arterial line. A simple central venous-pressure line may give erroneous information regarding filling pressures. The doses of the most commonly used agents in congestive heart failure that are currently available are listed in Table 64-3.

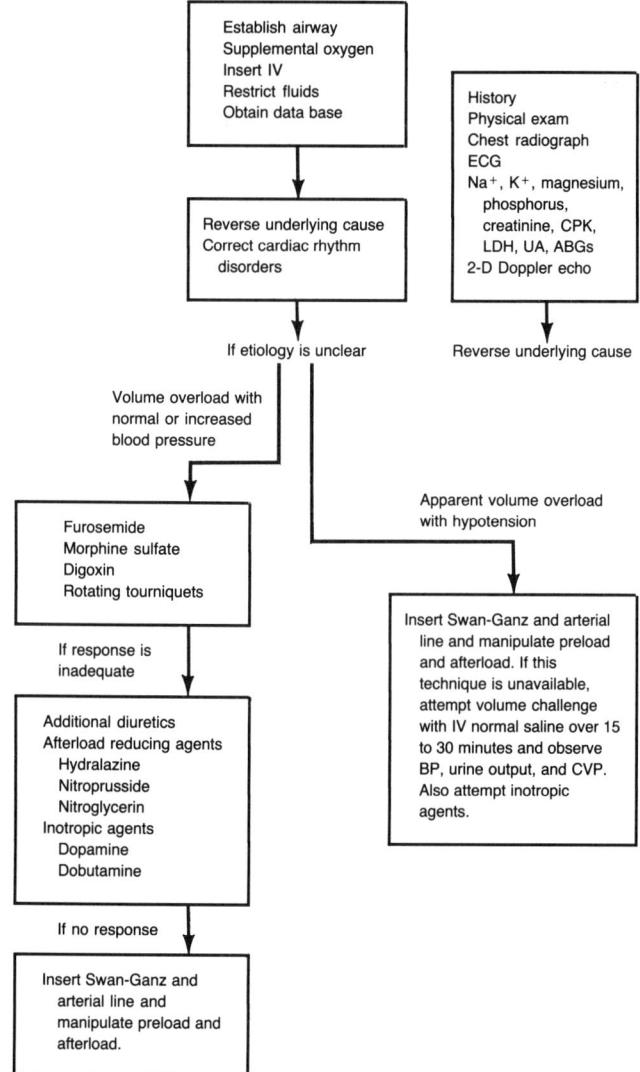

Figure 64-1 Emergency treatment of congestive heart failure.

SUMMARY

CHF refers to any condition that results in failure of the myocardium to pump enough oxygenated blood to maintain tissue perfusion. The body has several mechanisms that are invoked to maintain cardiac output, and the signs and symptoms of CHF may be a part of these reflex mechanisms. The patient who presents in the emergency department with congestive heart failure should have a careful history and physical examination, and an adequate data base should be obtained while conservative therapy is being administered. Definitive therapy is based on the underlying etiology. Current therapy of CHF based on decreased contractility consists of fluid and salt restriction, oxygen, diuretics, and digitalis. Vasodilators, inotropic agents, and mechanical support may be useful in certain situations. Early use of a Swan-Ganz catheter may help in the differential diagnosis and may direct therapy so that the CHF may be treated effectively with minimal risk to the patient. A decision algorithm for guidance in the treatment of congestive heart failure is found in Figure 64-1.

REFERENCES

1. Gerard S. Shortness of breath in emergency room patients. *Radiol Clin North Am*. 1978;16:113–121.
2. Mantle J, et al. Advances in the treatment of heart failure. *Cardiovasc Clin*. 1981;2:49–64.
3. Mason DT. The failing heart. *DM*. January 1977.
4. Mason DT, et al. Alternations of hemodynamics and myocardial mechanics in patients with congestive heart failure: pathophysiologic mechanisms and assessment of cardiac function and ventricular contractility. *Prog Cardiovasc Dis*. 1970;12:507–557.
5. Weber KT, Janick JS. The heart as a muscle-pump system and the concept of heart failure. *Am Heart J*. 1979;98:371–384.
6. Zelis R, et al. Circulatory dynamics in the normal and failing heart. *Ann Rev Physiol*. 1981;43:455–476.
7. Smulyan H, et al. Pulmonary effects of heart failure. *Surg Clin North Am*. 1974;54:1077–1087.
8. Kaplan S. New aspects of management of congestive heart failure. *Cardiovasc Clin*. 1981;22:293–299.
9. Cohn JN. Vasodilator therapy of congestive heart failure. *Adv Intern Med*. 1980;26:293–315.
10. McManus WF, et al. Prehospital advanced emergency care: a potential pitfall. *J Trauma*. 1978;18:305-307.
11. Atkinson AB. Captopril in the treatment of clinical hypertension and cardiac failure. *Lancet*. 1979;2:836–839.
12. Goldberg L, et al. Newer catecholamines for treatment of heart failure and shock: an update on dopamine and a first look at dobutamine. *Prog Cardiovasc Dis*. 1977;14:327–340.
13. Chatterjee K, Parmley W. The role of vasodilation therapy on heart failure. *Prog Cardiovasc Dis*. 1977;14:301–325.
14. Mason DT. Afterload reduction and cardiac performance. *Am J Med*. 1978;65:106–125.
15. Watanabe AM. Recent advances in knowledge about beta adrenergic receptors: application to clinical cardiology. *J Am Coll Cardiol*. 1983;1:82.
16. Krikler D, Rowland E. Clinical value of calcium antagonists in treatment of cardiovascular disorders. *J Am Coll Cardiol*. 1983;1:355–364.
17. Romankiewicz JA, et al. Captopril: an update review of its pharmacological properties and therapeutic efficacy in congestive heart failure. *Drugs*. 1983;25:6–40.
18. Massie B. Myocardial hypertrophy and cardiac failure: a complex interrelationship. *Am J Med*. 1983;75(3A):67–74.
19. Zsoter T. Vasodilators. *Can Med Assoc J*. 1983;129:424–432.
20. Braunwald E, Colluci WS. Vasodilator therapy of heart failure. Has the promissory note been paid? *N Engl J Med*. 1984;310:459–461.
21. Grossman W. Diastolic dysfunction and congestive heart failure. *Circulation*. 1990;81(suppl III):III.1–III.7.
22. Dougherty AH, Naccarelli GV, Gray EL, et al. Congestive heart failure with normal systolic function. *Am J Cardiol*. 1984;54:778–782.
23. DeMaria AN, Bommer W, Lee G, et al. Value and limitations of two dimensional echocardiography in assessment of cardiomyopathy. *Am J Cardiol*. 1980;46:1224–1231.
24. Soufer R, Wohlgelernter D, Vita N, et al. Intact systolic left ventricular function in clinical congestive heart failure. *Am J Cardiol*. 1985;55:1032–1036.
25. Silver PJ. Biochemical aspects of inhibition of cardiovascular low (K_m) cyclic adenosine monophosphate phosphodiesterase. *Am J Cardiol*. 1989;63(suppl):2A–8A.
26. Hood WB Jr. Controlled and uncontrolled studies of phosphodiesterase III inhibitors in contemporary cardiovascular medicine. *Am J Cardiol*. 1989;63(suppl):46A–53A.

65. Hypertensive Emergencies

HOWARD A. BESSEN, MD, FACEP

The emergency physician is frequently called upon to evaluate and manage patients with hypertension. Prompt and aggressive therapy may be indicated, but overtreatment may lead to significant morbidity. Although nitroprusside remains the drug of choice for most hypertensive emergencies, a number of recently described treatment modalities and newly available antihypertensive agents can now be used in the emergency department.

DEFINITIONS

The term *hypertensive emergency* implies the presence of acute central nervous system, cardiopulmonary, or renal dysfunction; the conditions likely to be seen in the emergency department are listed in Table 65-1. With any of these conditions, the patient is at risk for irreversible end-organ damage within minutes to hours if the blood pressure (BP) is not reduced, and immediate therapy with rapid-acting agents is indicated. Several authors have used the term *hypertensive urgency* to describe situations with significant elevation of the BP but without acute end-organ damage. It is unclear that this situation is truly urgent, and the need to acutely lower the BP in this setting has not been demonstrated.

The terms *accelerated* and *malignant hypertension* are sometimes used to describe hypertensive emergencies. However, more proper use of these terms denotes a clinical syndrome with a variable rate of progression, in which immediate blood pressure reduction may not be indicated (see below).

It should be emphasized that it is the presence or absence of acute target organ dysfunction that determines the need for rapid lowering of the BP. Marked elevation of BP alone does not constitute a hypertensive emergency, and chronic end-organ damage generally does not require acute reduction of BP.

Table 65-1 Hypertensive Emergencies

Accelerated and malignant hypertension (some cases)
Hypertensive encephalopathy
Intracranial hemorrhage
Thromboembolic stroke with severe hypertension
Acute left ventricular failure
Acute cardiac ischemia
Acute aortic dissection
Eclampsia
Catecholamine-induced hypertension*

*Sympathomimetic drug overdose, pheochromocytoma crisis, tyramine or sympathomimetic amine ingestion in patient taking monoamine oxidase inhibitors, clonidine withdrawal syndrome.

ETIOLOGY

Prompt therapy of hypertensive emergencies is necessary for a favorable outcome; identification of precipitating factors may be helpful but is of secondary importance.

Most hypertensive emergencies arise in patients with untreated or poorly controlled essential hypertension. Hypertension and its sequelae may also occur as a result of renal vascular disease or intrinsic renal disease (glomerulonephritis, interstitial nephritis), or as a complication of pregnancy or the use of oral contraceptives. Catecholamine-excess states, such as pheochromocytoma crisis and ingestion of tyramine or sympathomimetic amines in a patient taking monoamine oxidase inhibitors, present an uncommon but dramatic clinical picture; a similar presentation may be seen in patients who take overdoses of sympathomimetic drugs, or during withdrawal from clonidine. Other relatively uncommon conditions underlying hypertensive emergencies include collagen vascular diseases (polyarteritis nodosa, scleroderma), thyroid storm, primary hyperaldosteronism, and Cushing's disease. Finally, an elevation of systemic BP may occur as a reflex response to intracranial hypertension of any cause.

PATHOLOGY, PATHOGENESIS, AND PATHOPHYSIOLOGY

Pathologically, severe hypertension with end-organ damage is characterized by fibrinoid necrosis of arteriolar walls. The exact mechanisms responsible for the development of the vascular lesions remain unclear, but the end result is damage to the brain, cardiovascular system, and kidneys.

In patients with chronic hypertension, certain adaptive mechanisms may serve to prevent damage to the brain and other organs. Normally, cerebral blood flow is maintained within a narrow range by the process of autoregulation. This takes place through cerebral arteriolar constriction when BP rises and arteriolar dilation when BP falls. In normotensive individuals, autoregulation maintains a constant cerebral blood flow when mean arterial pressures range from 60 to 160 mmHg. In chronic hypertensives, the autoregulatory curve is shifted to the right (Fig. 65-1). While this may protect the brain against the effects of chronic hypertension, it also predisposes the patient to developing cerebral hypoperfusion at pressures that would be tolerated by normal individuals. Overaggressive therapy of hypertension may thus lead to cerebral ischemia and infarction, even at relatively "normal" BP.

On the other hand, patients with a rapid onset of hypertension, such as those with acute glomerulonephritis, preeclampsia or eclampsia, or catecholamine-excess states, may develop end-organ dysfunction with relatively moderate BP elevations. These patients may safely have their BP lowered into the normal range. Thus, both the absolute magnitude of the arterial pressure and the rate of development of hypertension influence the severity of the clinical situation and the potential complications of therapy.

DIAGNOSIS

The diagnosis of hypertensive emergencies is largely clinical, supplemented by radiologic and laboratory data. While the definitive diagnosis of certain hypertensive

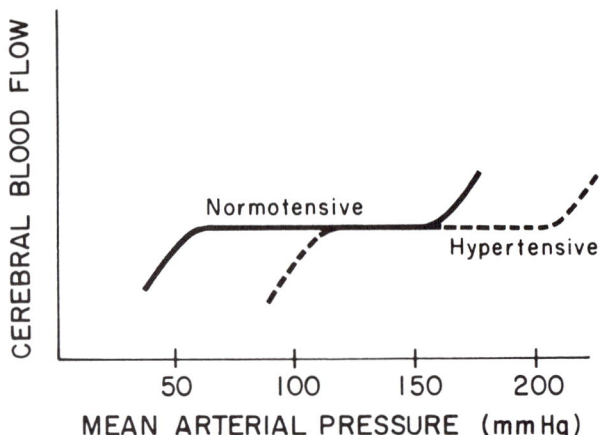

Figure 65-1 Autoregulation of cerebral blood flow in normotensive and chronic hypertensive individuals. *Source:* Adapted with permission from Strandgaard S et al: Autoregulation of brain circulation in severe arterial hypertension. *Br Med J* 1: 507–510, 1973.

emergencies (for example, intracranial hemorrhage and aortic dissection) usually requires radiologic confirmation, a presumptive diagnosis may be made and therapy may be initiated in the emergency department. Again, the key to assessing the hypertensive patient is a careful clinical evaluation for target organ dysfunction.

History and physical examination should be directed toward identifying or excluding those entities listed in Table 65-1. History from the patient or relatives may reveal chest pain, shortness of breath, or a change in mental status. Physical examination should include a search for retinopathy, signs of congestive heart failure, and neurologic abnormalities. Laboratory studies may show anemia (secondary to microangiopathic hemolysis or chronic renal disease), azotemia, proteinuria and/or hematuria, radiographic evidence of congestive heart failure, and ECG evidence of left ventricular hypertrophy (LVH). It should be remembered, however, that some of these abnormalities (retinopathy, anemia, renal dysfunction, LVH) may represent chronic changes that are not indications for acute BP reduction.

ANTIHYPERTENSIVE MEDICATIONS

Nitroprusside

For several years, sodium nitroprusside has been considered the antihypertensive agent of choice for most hypertensive emergencies. Nitroprusside is a potent arteriolar and venous dilator and is effective in virtually all patients with acute hypertension. It has a rapid (within seconds) onset of action and is easily titratable to the desired BP. Nitroprusside is administered by constant intravenous (IV) infusion at a dose (for adults) of 30 to 500 μg/min. Practically, this may be achieved by mixing 50 mg of the drug in 250 mL D_5W and beginning the infusion at 10 microdrops per minute (10 mL/hour). The infusion rate is then increased every few minutes until the desired end point is achieved.

The main adverse effect of nitroprusside relates to its powerful antihypertensive action: if not carefully monitored, patients may develop hypotension and impaired organ perfusion. This potential complication may occur more often in the emergency department than in a more controlled setting such as the ICU. The patient's BP and clinical status must be closely monitored, and the inability to frequently assess the patient is a contraindication to the use of nitroprusside. BP monitoring is optimally achieved with an intra-arterial catheter, but patients may be effectively managed in the emergency department with frequent auscultation of the BP or with automated BP measuring devices. Because nitroprusside has a very short duration of action, hypotension will usually resolve promptly when the infusion is slowed or discontinued. As compared with diazoxide and hydralazine, reflex cardiac stimulation accompanying the use of nitroprusside is usually not marked; it is, however, an important consideration in patients with aortic dissection (see below).

Nitroglycerin

Like nitroprusside, IV nitroglycerin is rapid, short-lived, and titratable. It is a more potent venous than arteriolar dilator, but nitroglycerin does cause significant arteriolar dilation, especially at higher doses. It is administered by constant IV infusion beginning at a dose of 10 µg/min; as with nitroprusside, the infusion rate is gradually increased until the desired effect is achieved. Doses greater than 250 to 300 µg/min are rarely necessary. As with nitroprusside, patients receiving IV nitroglycerin must be closely and carefully monitored.

Although nitroprusside is a more potent antihypertensive, nitroglycerin may dilate coronary collateral vessels and improve perfusion to ischemic myocardium to a greater degree than nitroprusside (the data on the subject are not conclusive). Nitroglycerin is also effective in the management of congestive heart failure. Thus the primary role of IV nitroglycerin in hypertensive emergencies is in the treatment of cardiovascular complications such as angina, myocardial infarction, and congestive heart failure.

Nifedipine

The calcium-channel blocking agents cause relaxation of vascular smooth muscle, vasodilation, and consequent reduction of BP. Although all the calcium-channel blockers have been used in the treatment of acute hypertension, nifedipine has the greatest effect on systemic vascular resistance and the least depressant effect on cardiac conduction and contractility. Hence nifedipine is usually chosen over the other calcium-channel blockers in the emergent treatment of hypertension.

Nifedipine may be given orally or sublingually. With sublingual administration absorption of the drug is fairly poor, so that the oral route is generally preferable. If a very rapid effect is desired, "bite-and-swallow" administration may be employed: The patient bites into the capsule to break it and then swallows the capsule and its contents. This method obviates a potential delay in effect associated with the time for dissolution of the capsule in the stomach. The initial dose is 10 mg, which may be repeated in 1 hour, if necessary; maximal BP reduction is achieved within 30 to 60 minutes. The drug's hypotensive effect lasts 3 to 5 hours. The effect on heart rate is variable; some patients develop significant reflex tachycardia after receiving nifedipine, while others have little or no increase in cardiac rate.

Clinical experience with nifedipine has shown that it is usually effective in the treatment of hypertensive emergencies, and few significant side effects have been reported. Several features make it an attractive agent for the treatment of hypertensive emergencies. Its effect is rapid, and the magnitude of the BP drop is proportional to the pretreatment BP; marked hypotension is rarely seen. Patients do not require constant BP monitoring, as is necessary with nitroprusside. It is an effective agent for long-term BP control; for this purpose, a sustained-release preparation allows once-a-day dosing.

Nifedipine is convenient to use and generally efficacious. It should be remembered, however, that the drug's effects cannot be controlled as closely as those of IV agents and that nifedipine has the potential to cause hypotension, possibly resulting in complications such as stroke or myocardial infarction. Its exact place in the management of acute hypertension and hypertensive emergencies remains uncertain. The future availability of newer, IV calcium-channel blockers may allow titrated BP lowering in a more controlled fashion.

Labetalol

Labetalol is a combined α- and β-adrenergic blocking agent; the β blockade is noncardioselective and more potent than the α blockade. It is available in both oral and parenteral forms for the treatment of hypertension. The maximal BP lowering effect is seen 1 to 3 hours after oral administration of the drug and within 5 to 10 minutes after intravenous injection; IV therapy is thus required for rapid BP lowering in hypertensive emergencies.

The combination of α- and β-adrenergic blockade offers certain advantages over pure β blockers or vasodilators. Systemic vascular resistance and arterial pressure are reduced, but reflex tachycardia does not occur; a slight (but not marked) decrease in heart rate is commonly seen. Cardiac output is usually well maintained.

In hypertensive emergencies, labetalol may be administered in multiple bolus injections or as a constant intravenous infusion. The former method is somewhat more suitable to the emergency department. Twenty milligrams are given IV over 2 minutes, followed by 40 to 80 mg every 10 to 15 minutes until reaching the desired blood pressure. Alternatively, a constant infusion beginning at a rate of 2 mg/min may be given, with the infusion being stopped as soon as a satisfactory BP response has occurred; this may take from 15 minutes to 2 hours. The maximal total dose by either method is 300 mg.

Duration of response is highly variable. BP generally begins to rise within 2 to 6 hours after completion of parenteral therapy, although individual patients may be controlled for as long as 24 hours. The availability of oral labetalol facilitates a smooth transition to long-term therapy after acute BP control with the intravenous preparation.

Treatment with intravenous labetalol is successful in the majority of patients. A response rate between 80% and 90% can be expected, although some clinical trials have shown less success in patients previously treated with β blockers. The drug should not be used in patients with conditions contraindicating β blockade, namely bronchospastic pulmonary disease, congestive heart failure or cardiogenic shock, and significant bradycardia or heart block.

Diazoxide

Diazoxide, an arteriolar dilator with little (if any) effect on veins, was formerly considered a first-line drug in the treatment of hypertensive emergencies. Although it is usually effective, diazoxide's potential complications are significant and frequently preclude its use.

The traditional dose of diazoxide was 300 mg given by rapid IV bolus injection to achieve a high serum concentration and to overcome the drug's avid protein binding. When administered in this way, diazoxide rapidly lowers the BP, with the maximal hypotensive effect being reached within 5 minutes. After this, the BP gradually returns to baseline over the next 3 to 15 hours, allowing the initiation of therapy with oral agents after the initial BP reduction.

Bolus doses of 300 mg cause sudden falls in BP that may not be tolerated by chronically hypertensive patients. Also, the magnitude of the BP drop is somewhat unpredictable; significant hypotension may result. The hypotension may be long lasting and may lead to irreversible morbidity from cerebral or myocardial ischemia.

Because of the potential problems with "standard-dose" diazoxide therapy, other methods of administration have been evaluated and have generally been successful. Bolus injections of smaller doses (50 to 150 mg at a time) allow some degree of individual dose titration. The dose may be repeated every 5 to 15 minutes until the desired BP is achieved. Alternatively, diazoxide may be given by constant IV effusion. A larger dose may be required (probably because of increased protein binding), but the resultant fall in BP is more smooth and gradual than that seen with bolus injections. The drug is given undiluted or mixed with a small amount of IV fluid at a rate of 15 to 30 mg/min until the goal BP is reached; the infusion is then discontinued. Adequate BP reduction generally takes from 20 to 40 minutes by this method.

Diazoxide given by any method may cause a significant reflex increase in heart rate and cardiac output; the resultant increase in myocardial oxygen demand may be deleterious to patients with coronary artery disease. It is also potentially dangerous in patients with cerebrovascular disease, and the drug should not be used in patients with aortic dissection.

Because of its potential complications, diazoxide should rarely be a first-line agent in the emergency department. A possible exception is for the treatment of hypertensive emergencies in children, in whom the drug is fairly safe and unlikely to cause complications such as cardiac ischemia. In this setting, bolus injections of 1 to 3 mg/kg given every 5 to 15 minutes until adequate BP reduction has been achieved are generally safe and effective.

Trimethaphan

Trimethaphan is a ganglionic blocking agent that produces both arteriolar and venous dilation. It has a very rapid onset and offset of action (Table 65-2) and must be given by constant IV infusion. Like nitroprusside, it requires continuous patient monitoring.

The side effects of trimethaphan may be significant. Small increases in infusion rate may cause marked falls in blood pressure, emphasizing the need for constant patient supervision. Parasympatholytic effects may cause ileus, urinary retention, and visual impairment, although these effects are unusual with short-term administration of the drug. At high doses, respiratory depression or arrest may occur.

Because of its drawbacks and the availability of more convenient drugs, trimethaphan is rarely used except in patients with acute aortic dissection. Trimethaphan's hypotensive effect is accompanied by a decrease in the force and velocity of left ventricular ejection, and reflex tachycardia does not occur. These properties are desirable when trying to reduce the forces that propagate dissection of the aorta. Even in this setting, trimethaphan should be considered a second-line agent (see below).

A trimethaphan infusion can be administered by mixing 500 mg of the drug in 500 mL of IV fluid, beginning the infusion at 30 microdrops per minute (30 mL/hour or 0.5 mg/min). As with nitroprusside, the infusion rate is gradually increased until reaching the desired BP. The effect of trimethaphan is much greater in the upright position; high doses may be required in the supine patient.

Hydralazine

Parenteral hydralazine has been used in the treatment of hypertensive emergencies but has largely been replaced by other drugs. Its main disadvantage is a variable and unpre-

Table 65-2 Drug Therapy of Hypertensive Emergencies

Drug	Dosage and Administration*	Onset	Peak (Time Course)	Duration
Nitroprusside	30–500 mcg/min Mix 50 mg/250 mL D_5W; begin infusion at 10 microdrops/min (10 mL/hr) and titrate to desired BP	<1 min	1–2 min	<5 min after infusion discontinued
Nitroglycerin	10–250 mcg/min Mix 50 mg/250 mL D_5W; begin infusion at 3 microdrops/min (3 mL/hr) and titrate to desired effect	<1 min	2–5 min	<5 min after infusion discontinued
Nifedipine	10 mg orally, sublingually, or "bite-and-swallow" (see text). Repeat dose in 60 min if necessary	5–20 min	30–60 min	3–5 hr
Labetalol	20 mg IV, then 40–80 mg every 10–15 min until BP controlled; up to total dose of 300 mg	<5 min	5–10 min	2–6 hr (highly variable)
	Constant infusion, beginning at 2 mg/min and gradually increased, until BP controlled; up to total dose of 300 mg		See text	
Diazoxide	50–150 mg rapid IV bolus every 5–15 min until BP controlled	1–2 min	2–5 min	3–15 hr
	Constant infusion at 15–30 mg/min until BP controlled		See text	
Trimethaphan	0.5–6 mg/min. Mix 500 mg/500 mL D_5W; begin infusion at 30 microdrops/min (30 mL/hr) and titrate to desired BP	1–2 min	2–5 min	5–10 min after infusion discontinued
Hydralazine	5–25 mg IV	10–30 min	20–40 min	3–8 hr
Clonidine	0.1–0.2 mg orally, then 0.1 mg every hr to desired BP; up to total dose of 0.8 mg (see text)	30–60 min	2–4 hr	6–12 hr

*Dosages listed are for adult patients of average body weight.

dictable degree of hypotensive effect. Some patients show very little response to hydralazine, while in others an exaggerated BP drop is seen. As with diazoxide, marked reflex cardiac stimulation can occur. In addition, hydralazine's onset of action is somewhat delayed (10 to 30 minutes) compared to the onset of other IV agents used for acute BP reduction.

At present, the main indication for the use of hydralazine is severe pre-eclampsia or eclampsia, in which there is considerable experience with the use of this drug. The required dosage is highly variable. In the pregnant woman, an initial dose of 5 mg IV may be followed by 5 to 25 mg every 20 to 30 minutes until a satisfactory BP response has occurred. If bothersome tachycardia or palpitations develop, the addition of a β-adrenergic blocker may be helpful.

Clonidine

Clonidine is the only oral agent aside from nifedipine that has been evaluated for acute BP reduction in large numbers of patients. Its central α-agonist effect decreases sympathetic tone to the heart and peripheral vessels, thus lowering the BP.

Clonidine begins to lower the BP within 30 to 60 minutes, with a peak effect in 2 to 4 hours and a duration of 6 to 12 hours. It has generally been given in a regimen using 0.1 to 0.2 mg initially followed by 0.1 mg every hour until the target BP is reached. This regimen is successful in most patients, and the decline in BP is usually smooth and gradual. Long-term therapy can then be instituted.

Several disadvantages of oral clonidine should be noted. The relatively slow BP control with this drug makes it inappropriate for most hypertensive emergencies. Sedation is a frequent complication of clonidine loading (30% to 60% of patients); this could potentially interfere with the neurologic assessment of the patient. Clonidine is effective for long-term BP control, but severe hypertension may occur if the drug is abruptly discontinued. Also, with the commonly used hourly clonidine regimen, additional drug is given before the peak effect of the previous dose is achieved; cumulative drug effect may then cause hypotension.

Administration of clonidine is appropriate for patients who will receive long-term therapy with this drug, although the need for acute loading is uncertain. It is also effective in patients with rebound hypertension after clonidine withdrawal. For other patients, alternative agents should be given.

ADJUNCTIVE AGENTS

β Blockers

While β blockers are effective agents in the long-term management of chronic hypertension, they have relatively little acute effect on BP. Their primary indication in the treatment of hypertensive emergencies is to prevent or abolish the reflex cardiac stimulation that can occur with the use of other drugs. This may be important in patients with coronary artery disease, who may not tolerate the increase in myocardial oxygen demand accompanying treatment with potent vasodilators. In patients with acute aortic dissection, myocardial contractility must be reduced (see below), and propranolol or other β blockers are convenient and effective for this purpose. Contraindications to β blockade have been discussed (see section on labetalol).

Furosemide

Controversy exists regarding the use of potent diuretics in the acute treatment of hypertension. There is evidence that many patients presenting with hypertensive emergencies are sodium and volume depleted, and may actually be harmed by treatment with diuretics. On the other hand, many of the agents used to rapidly reduce BP cause salt and water retention, which can be prevented or treated with furosemide. The efficacy of antihypertensive agents may be enhanced with the concomitant administration of a diuretic.

Diuretics will often be necessary to maintain BP control, but they are rarely needed in the emergency department to achieve initial reduction of BP. They are clearly indicated in the treatment of edematous states; otherwise, their use in the emergency department should be cautious and based on a clinical exam that excludes hypovolemia.

Furosemide is quite ineffective as a single-agent therapy for acute hypertension, and its use in this fashion is to be discouraged. BP is reliably diminished only with large (greater than 120 mg) doses of the drug, and even then the onset of the hypotensive effect is delayed for 30 to 45 minutes.

TREATMENT

General Considerations

The emergency department management of hypertension requires careful consideration of the patient's clinical status. In true hypertensive emergencies (Table 65-1), prompt therapy is necessary to prevent irreversible organ damage. On the other hand, the potential hazards of using potent antihypertensive medications have been increasingly recognized, and the dangers of the hypertensive state must be weighed against the risks of therapy. Cerebral or myocardial ischemia may be precipitated if the BP is reduced rapidly or excessively.

In general, only acute end-organ damage mandates acute reduction of BP, and less aggressive therapy is indicated in patients without such effects. Each patient's response to therapy must be carefully followed, as there is much variation in the magnitude of BP elevation required to produce symptoms and in the amount of BP reduction tolerated without complications. As explained above, chronically hypertensive patients may tolerate excessive lowering of the BP quite poorly.

Prehospital Care

Hypertensive emergencies lend themselves poorly to prehospital therapy; intervention should generally await the patient's arrival at the hospital. Some of the potent antihypertensive agents necessary to manage hypertensive emergencies are difficult to administer in a prehospital setting, and all require closer patient monitoring than may be feasible for prehospital personnel.

Medications used for prehospital care vary from system to system, but specific antihypertensive agents are often not available. Nifedipine is perhaps the most reasonable choice for prehospital therapy, but its efficacy and safety in this setting have not been evaluated in large numbers of patients. Sublingual nitroglycerin is an effective therapy for angina and congestive heart failure; when these are associated with hypertension, nitroglycerin is a logical therapeutic choice. Because of its predominantly preload-reducing properties, sublingual nitroglycerin cannot be expected to be effective for other hypertensive emergencies, although its use for hypertension in the prehospital setting has not been studied. As previously discussed, furosemide is a poor choice for the acute treatment of hypertension except in patients with volume overload (eg, congestive heart failure).

In general, it is safer to wait until the patient arrives in the emergency department to begin treatment. Clinical evaluation will determine whether or not the patient requires acute therapy for hypertension. If such therapy is required, careful minute-to-minute monitoring will be necessary; this can rarely be accomplished in the field.

SPECIFIC HYPERTENSIVE EMERGENCIES

Accelerated and Malignant Hypertension

The terms *accelerated* and *malignant hypertension* describe a clinical syndrome characterized by severe BP elevation and progressive target organ damage. These terms are often used interchangeably, although some authors require the presence of papilledema for the diagnosis of malignant hypertension.

Presenting complaints are fairly nonspecific, consisting of headache, nausea, malaise, and sometimes visual changes. The diastolic BP is usually at least 130 mmHg, unless the development of hypertension has been particularly rapid. Grade III (hemorrhages and exudates) or grade IV (papilledema) retinopathy is almost always seen. Anemia and evidence of renal dysfunction may be present. If untreated, accelerated and malignant hypertension have an extremely poor prognosis, with progressive end-organ damage, renal failure, and death occurring within months.

Malignant hypertension may be complicated by any of the other conditions listed in Table 65-1. When this is the case, rapid lowering of the BP is necessary. Rapid control is also indicated when retinal lesions cause acute visual loss or when there is evidence of rapidly deteriorating renal function.

However, not all cases of accelerated and malignant hypertension need to be treated as hypertensive emergencies, and therapy must be individualized. Although most patients should be admitted to the hospital for observation of their response to therapy, many patients with "uncomplicated" malignant hypertension can be treated with oral agents. This is a condition that produces morbidity over days to weeks or months, and it may not be necessary or desirable to achieve rapid BP control. Intensive oral therapy with BP reduction over a period of several days is usually appropriate for patients without complications dictating immediate BP control.

Hypertensive Encephalopathy

Hypertensive encephalopathy is a syndrome of diffuse cerebral dysfunction whose pathogenesis is still poorly understood. Clinically, it is characterized by a variable combination of headache, nausea and vomiting, retinopathy, and neurologic abnormalities including confusion, alterations in consciousness, sensory and motor deficits, visual impairment, and sometimes seizures. A severe headache is often the initial symptom; this is followed in hours to days by other features of the syndrome. Neurologic deficits are sometimes focal and are often transient; seizures may be focal or generalized. If untreated, the disease progresses to coma and irreversible brain damage or death.

It is important to note that the patient with hypertension and neurologic findings may also have a cerebral infarction or embolus, intracranial (intracerebral or subarachnoid) hemorrhage, an intracranial mass lesion, or encephalopathy due to a CNS infection, drug ingestion, or uremia (Table 65-3).

Certain clinical features may help to establish or exclude the diagnosis of hypertensive encephalopathy. Symptoms of this disorder usually develop gradually and progressively over a period of hours to days; a rapid onset of neurologic impairment is more consistent with a cerebral infarction or embolus, or intracranial hemorrhage. Severe headache is a characteristic feature of hypertensive encephalopathy and some other conditions listed in Table 65-3, but it is not common in patients with thrombotic or embolic strokes. Focal neurologic findings may be due to hypertensive encephalopathy but are more suggestive of focal lesions (infarction, embolus, hemorrhage, or mass). A careful

Table 65-3 Differential Diagnosis of Hypertensive Encephalopathy

Stroke
Intracranial hemorrhage
Intracranial mass
CNS infection
Toxic encephalopathy
Uremic encephalopathy

clinical and laboratory evaluation should help to exclude other entities in the differential diagnosis.

The diagnosis of hypertensive encephalopathy should be considered tentative until other potential etiologies of the symptom complex have been excluded. Clinically, this may present a difficult problem for the emergency physician; a complete diagnostic work-up can be time consuming, and prompt therapy is necessary to halt the progression of hypertension encephalopathy. The most expeditious way to confirm the diagnosis is to demonstrate a response to antihypertensive therapy. If hypertensive encephalopathy cannot be ruled out in the emergency department, the patient's BP should be lowered, taking care not to induce hypotension and its resultant cerebral ischemia. The diagnosis of hypertensive encephalopathy should be questioned if the patient's signs and symptoms fail to respond to the reduction of BP. Neurologic abnormalities may resolve within an hour, although recovery may be slower in patients in whom treatment has been delayed many hours after the onset of symptoms.

A dramatic response to antihypertensive therapy virtually establishes the diagnosis of hypertensive encephalopathy. Patients with the other conditions listed in Table 65-3 will fail to improve when the BP is lowered.

Intracranial Hemorrhage

While it is clear that hypertension is a major risk factor for the development of strokes, the optimal management of hypertension in the patient who has sustained an acute intracranial hemorrhage (or an acute thrombotic or embolic stroke) is much less clear. An improved outcome with antihypertensive therapy has not been conclusively demonstrated in any study. Moreover, some degree of hypertension may actually be protective to the brain. A high systemic BP may be needed to ensure cerebral perfusion in the patient with elevated intracranial pressure or cerebral vasospasm, both of which may occur after intracranial hemorrhage. Nonetheless, most authorities feel that extremely high BP may lead to further clinical deterioration and they recommend lowering the BP while scrupulously avoiding hypotension.

A reasonable end point is a diastolic BP of approximately 100 to 110 mmHg, although some recommend more vigorous BP reduction in patients with acute bleeding. Short-acting, easily titratable agents (usually nitroprusside) should be used in these patients, and the clinical response to therapy should be carefully followed. If neurologic deterioration occurs when the BP is lowered, the dose of nitroprusside must be decreased and the BP allowed to rise to a level that restores the previous degree of cerebral function.

Acute Left Ventricular Failure or Acute Cardiac Ischemia

Hypertension raises the workload of the myocardium and may precipitate or contribute to left ventricular failure or myocardial ischemia. Alternatively, patients with acute respiratory distress or angina often have high levels of circulating catecholamines with resultant hypertension. It is often difficult to determine whether hypertension is the primary problem or a reflection of the patient's distress. Practically, if these patients remain hypertensive after receiving conventional therapy (see Chapters 62, Acute Myocardial Infarction, and 64, Congestive Heart Failure), specific antihypertensive therapy should be initiated.

Acute Aortic Dissection

Dissection of the aorta is a rapidly lethal condition, with half of the patients dying within 48 hours of symptom onset if not properly treated. The main complications (and causes of death) are rupture of the aorta (usually into the pericardium or pleural space), occlusion of aortic branch arteries, and aortic valve insufficiency.

Severe chest pain of acute onset is the usual presenting symptom; other presentations include neurologic abnormalities, congestive heart failure, syncope, and pulse loss with ischemia in the distribution of the involved artery. Typical findings include various combinations of hypertension, pulse deficits, an aortic insufficiency murmur, and neurologic deficits. It should be noted, however, that while aortic dissection is classically considered a hypertensive emergency, many patients with acute dissection are not hypertensive at the time of presentation, and that patients with cardiac tamponade, aortic rupture with hypovolemia, or massive aortic insufficiency may present with hypotension. Presumptive diagnosis is made clinically, based on history, physical examination, and chest radiographic abnormalities. A detailed discussion of aortic dissection may be found in Chapter 67, Heart and Great Vessel Emergencies.

Definitive diagnosis is made by aortography, computed tomography (CT) scanning of the thoracic aorta, or echocardiography, but emergent treatment must begin as soon as the diagnosis is suspected. Even a short delay in initiating therapy may cause further damage to the aorta. Dissections are propagated not only by hypertension but by the force of the left ventricular impulse; therapy must be directed at reducing both the BP and cardiac contractility. This can be accomplished with either a combination of a β blocker and nitroprusside or with trimethaphan alone. The reflex cardiac stimulation accompanying treatment with nitroprusside alone may actually worsen the dissection, and concomitant β blockade is mandatory.

The β blocker–nitroprusside regimen is preferable in patients without contraindications to β blockade. The β blocker is given in incremental intravenous doses until clinical β blockade is achieved (usually this means a heart rate less than 60 beat/min). A nitroprusside infusion is titrated to decrease the systolic BP to approximately 90 to 120 mmHg. This BP is only a guideline, however; adequate vital organ perfusion must be maintained. Evidence of impaired cerebral, cardiac, or renal perfusion may indicate that the BP has been lowered too far (although these complications may be caused by the dissection itself). Labetalol will also lower both BP and contractility and would appear to be a sound therapeutic choice, although there is very little clinical experience with labetalol in patients with aortic dissection. An infusion of trimethaphan alone can be used in patients who will not tolerate β blockade; the blood pressure is titrated down as with nitroprusside.

Definitive diagnosis is sought only after control of blood pressure, contractility, and pain. Further medical or surgical management depends on a number of factors, including the specific type of dissection, and is discussed in Chapter 67.

Eclampsia

A pregnant woman with hypertension, edema, proteinuria, and seizures or other neurologic abnormalities is at risk for maternal as well as fetal morbidity and mortality. Traditional antihypertensive therapy has been with parenteral hydralazine, which is usually effective. Other drugs, such as labetalol, nifedipine, and diazoxide, have also been used with good results. Care must be taken with the use of diazoxide, as patients with pregnancy-induced hypertension may be very sensitive to small doses of this drug. Nitroprusside is usually avoided because of fear of fetal cyanide or thiocyanate toxicity. This concern may be unfounded and should not preclude the use of nitroprusside if the mother is critically ill. All patients should also receive parenteral magnesium sulfate. Hypertension in pregnancy is discussed in detail in Chapter 79, Obstetric and Gynecologic Emergencies.

Catecholamine-Induced Hypertension

Markedly elevated catecholamine activity can cause a dramatic clinical syndrome with severe hypertension, tachycardia, and diaphoresis. The patient may be agitated and complain of severe headache and palpitations. This syndrome may occur in sympathomimetic drug overdose, in pheochromocytoma crisis, in patients taking monoamine oxidase inhibitors who ingest tyramine or sympathomimetic amines, and sometimes during withdrawal from clonidine. Hypertension in this setting is caused by peripheral vasoconstriction mediated by α-adrenergic stimulation as well as by tachycardia and incompletely understood central mechanisms.

In patients with hypertension caused by stimulant drugs such as cocaine, sedation may be all that is needed to lower the BP. If the BP remains elevated after adequate sedation, specific antihypertensive agents can be administered. It should be noted that most patients with stimulant drug toxicity are not chronically hypertensive, and their BP can be safely lowered into the normal range.

Catecholamine crises can be treated with either the α-blocking agent phentolamine, with vasodilating drugs such as nitroprusside or nifedipine, or possibly with labetalol. If phentolamine is used, an IV test dose of 0.5 to 1.0 mg should be given to assure that hypotension does not occur. If this is tolerated, 5 mg can be given every 5 minutes until the BP is controlled, and repeated as necessary to maintain control. Some physicians prefer nitroprusside for continuous, precise BP control. Tachycardia or cardiac dysrhythmias can be treated with β-blocking agents, but only after treatment with phentolamine or vasodilators (to avoid unopposed α-mediated vasoconstriction). Because of its α-blocking properties, labetalol is probably safer than pure β blockers in this regard. Even labetalol could theoretically worsen hypertension because it is a more potent β than α blocker. In clinical practice, however, this has not been a common problem, and some investigators advocate the use of labetalol as single-agent therapy to treat both hypertension and tachycardia. If clonidine rebound is suspected, reinstitution of clonidine therapy may be effective, but more rapid BP control can be achieved with phentolamine or nitroprusside.

BIBLIOGRAPHY

1988 Joint National Committee. The 1988 report of the Joint National Committee on detection, evaluation, and treatment of high blood pressure. *Arch Intern Med.* 1988;148:1023–1038.

Atkin SH, Jaker MA, Beaty P, et al. Oral labetalol versus oral clonidine in the emergency treatment of severe hypertension. *Am J Med Sci.* 1992;303:9–15.

Anderson RJ, Hart GR, Crumpler CP, et al. Oral clonidine loading in hypertensive urgencies. *JAMA.* 1981;246:848–850.

Calhoun DA, Oparil S. Treatment of hypertensive crisis. *N Engl J Med.* 1990;323:1177–1183.

Chung M, Reitberg DP, Gaffney M, et al. Clinical pharmacokinetics of nifedipine gastrointestinal therapeutic system: a controlled-release formulation of nifedipine. *Am J Med.* 1987;83(suppl 6B):10–14.

Cohn JN, Burke LP. Nitroprusside. *Ann Intern Med.* 1979;91:752–757.

Cressman MD, Gifford RW. Hypertension and stroke. *J Am Coll Cardiol.* 1983;1:521–527.

Cressman MD, Vidt DG, Gifford RW, et al. Intravenous labetalol in the management of severe hypertension and hypertensive emergencies. *Am Heart J.* 1984;107:980–985.

Dilmen U, Caglar K, Senses A, et al. Nifedipine in hypertensive emergencies of children. *Am J Dis Child.* 1983;137:1162–1165.

Doroghazi RM, Slater EE. *Aortic Dissection.* New York, NY: McGraw-Hill Book Co; 1983.

Dunn FG. Hypertension and myocardial infarction. *J Am Coll Cardiol.* 1983;1:528–532.

Ellrodt AG, Ault MJ, Riedinger MS, et al. Efficacy and safety of sublingual nifedipine in hypertensive emergencies. *Am J Med.* 1985;79(suppl 4A):19–25.

Fenakel K, Fenakel G, Appelman Z, et al. Nifedipine in the treatment of severe preeclampsia. *Obstet Gynecol.* 1991;77:331–337.

Ferguson RK, Vlasses PH. Hypertensive emergencies and urgencies. *JAMA.* 1986;255:1607–1613.

Frishman WH, Weinberg P, Peled HB, et al. Calcium entry blockers for the treatment of severe hypertension and hypertensive crisis. *Am J Med.* 1984;77(suppl 2B):35–45.

Garrett BN, Kaplan NM: Efficacy of slow infusion of diazoxide in the treatment of severe hypertension without organ hypoperfusion. *Am Heart J.* 1982;103:390–394.

Gifford RW, Westbrook E. Hypertensive encephalopathy: mechanisms, clinical features, and treatment. *Prog Cardiovasc Dis.* 1974;17:115–124.

Gifford RW. Effect of reducing elevated blood pressure on cerebral circulation. *Hypertension.* 1983;5(suppl III):17–20.

Gonzalez ER, Peterson MA, Racht EM, et al. Dose-response evaluation of oral labetalol in patients presenting to the emergency department with accelerated hypertension. *Ann Emerg Med.* 1991;20:333–338.

Haft JI, Litterer WE. Chewing nifedipine to rapidly treat hypertension. *Arch Intern Med.* 1984;144:2357–2359.

Healton EB, Brust JC, Feinfeld DA, Thomson GE. Hypertensive encephalopathy and the neurologic manifestations of malignant hypertension. *Neurology.* 1982;32:127–132.

Hill NS, Antman EM, Green LH, et al. Intravenous nitroglycerin: a review of pharmacology, indications, therapeutic effects and complications. *Chest.* 1981;79:69–76.

Houston MC. Treatment of severe hypertension and hypertensive crises with nifedipine. *West J Med.* 1987;146:701–704.

Houston MC. Treatment of hypertensive emergencies and urgencies with oral clonidine loading and titration: a review. *Arch Intern Med.* 1986;146:586–589.

Houston MC. The comparative effects of clonidine hydrochloride and nifedipine in the treatment of hypertensive crises. *Am Heart J.* 1988;115:152–159.

Houston M. Hypertensive emergencies and urgencies: pathophysiology and clinical aspects. *Am Heart J.* 1986;111:205–210.

Jaker M, Atkin S, Soto M, et al. Oral nifedipine vs. oral clonidine in the treatment of urgent hypertension. *Arch Intern Med.* 1989;149:260–265.

Koch-Weser J. Diazoxide. *N Engl J Med.* 1976;294:1271–1273.

Lavin P. Management of hypertension in patients with acute stroke. *Arch Intern Med.* 1986;146:66–68.

Lebel M, Langlois S, Belleau LJ, et al. Labetalol infusion in hypertensive emergencies. *Clin Pharmacol Ther.* 1985;37:615–618.

Lindheimer MD, Katz AI. Hypertension in pregnancy. *N Engl J Med.* 1985;313:675–680.

Lowenstein J. Clonidine. *Ann Intern Med.* 1980;92:74–77.

McAllister RG. Kinetics and dynamics of nifedipine after oral and sublingual doses. *Am J Med.* 1986;81(suppl 6A):2–5.

McRae RP, Liebson PR. Hypertensive crisis. *Med Clin North Am.* 1986;70:749–767.

O'Mailia JJ, Sander GE, Giles TD. Nifedipine-associated myocardial ischemia or infarction in the treatment of hypertensive urgencies. *Ann Intern Med.* 1987;107:185–186.

Ram CVS, Kaplan NM. Individual titration of diazoxide dosage in the treatment of severe hypertension. *Am J Cardiol*. 1979;43:627–630.

Spitalewitz S, Porush JG, Oguagha C. Use of oral clonidine for rapid titration of blood pressure in severe hypertension. *Chest*. 1983;83 (suppl):404–407.

Strandgaard S, Olesen J, Skinhoj E, et al. Autoregulation of brain circulation in severe arterial hypertension. *Br Med J*. 1973;1:507–510.

Walters BNJ, Redman CWG. Treatment of severe pregnancy-associated hypertension with the calcium antagonist nifedipine. *Br J Obstet Gynecol*. 1984;91:330–336.

Wilson DJ, Wallin JD, Vlachakis ND, et al. Intravenous labetalol in the treatment of severe hypertension and hypertensive emergencies. *Am J Med*. 1983;75(4A):95–102.

Zeller KR, Kuhnert LV, Matthews C. Rapid reduction of severe asymptomatic hypertension: a prospective, controlled trial. *Arch Intern Med*. 1989;149:2186–2189.

66. Vascular Emergencies

JAMES B. ALEXANDER, MD
ANTHONY J. DELROSSI, MD
JONATHAN H. CILLEY, JR., MD

Trauma is the leading killer of adults under the age of 65. Death in the first hours following injury is frequently the direct result of bleeding or inadequate ventilatory support. In patients experiencing life-threatening hemorrhage, disruption of a major blood vessel must be suspected, and management should proceed accordingly.

The initial steps in the evaluation and management of any injured patient are identical. Adequate ventilation must be maintained, exsanguinating hemorrhage controlled, and circulation restored. Vascular injury may thwart even these fundamentals. There may be brisk bleeding from laceration of a peripheral vessel or shock secondary to massive hemorrhage from disruption of a vessel into a body cavity. Visible bleeding is best controlled by direct pressure. In extraordinary circumstances, the application of a tourniquet may be required to provide adequate control on the way to the operating room. Blind clamping of the bleeding wound is to be avoided at all times.

Shock unresponsive to massive fluid administration is an indication for immediate surgical intervention. This is best carried out in the operating room with either emergent laparotomy or thoracotomy, depending on the clinical situation. On occasion, regardless of the likely site of injury, left anterolateral thoracotomy and cross-clamping of the descending thoracic aorta may be a life-saving initial step in resuscitation.[1] In the patient in extremis, it may even be necessary to perform a resuscitative thoracotomy in the emergency department in order to maintain vital signs until the patient can be transported to the operating room. However, this is a "last ditch" maneuver, and over three-fourths of the patients will die despite its application.[2-4]

Military antishock trousers (MAST) have been advocated to both tamponade hemorrhage and restore intravascular volume. Because of their theoretical attractiveness and ease of application, they have achieved widespread acceptance. Nonetheless, they are not a substitute for direct pressure on a lacerated vessel. They may be relatively contraindicated in a patient with an arterial injury because the rapid restoration of central vascular volume may actually produce hypertension. Additionally, the application of the MAST garment is associated with an increase in afterload. Both of these consequences of MAST application may destabilize the clot from a transiently contained arterial disruption and produce a precipitous deterioration in a previously compensated patient.[5]

In the discussion that follows, we will focus on arterial injuries. Concomitant venous injuries are also important, and these will be mentioned in association with the adjacent artery where appropriate. With a few notable exceptions (eg, the vena cava and the portal vein), most isolated venous injuries either do not bleed much or are readily controlled with simple pressure. No doubt many isolated venous injuries go unrecognized. Most diagnosed venous injuries are found during exploration for a simultaneous arterial injury.

PATHOPHYSIOLOGY

An artery consists of three concentric layers. The innermost layer, the intima, is the most fragile. The intima is composed of endothelial cells that line the lumen of the artery and the underlying basement membrane. The endothelial cells are in constant contact with the flowing stream of blood and exert a variety of influences to maintain blood in its liquid form and prevent clotting. Loss of this fragile inner layer exposes the underlying deeper layers, which lack the anticoagulant properties of the endothelial cells, thereby promoting thrombus formation. In addition, endothelial cells release a factor (known simply as endothelial cell-derived relaxing factor) that keeps the surrounding muscular layer relaxed so that the arteries remain well dilated.[6] Damage to the endothelial cells inhibits the release of this factor, with resulting tightening of the muscular layer and vasoconstriction. Thus, when an artery is injured the thrombogenic surface and vasoconstriction are important homeostatic mechanisms that promote sealing of the severed artery and prevent exsanguination.

The middle arterial layer is the media. This consists of a concentric arrangement of smooth muscle cells. The smooth muscle cells relax and contract and thereby regulate the luminal diameter of the artery. This function is, in turn, integral to the regulation of the velocity and volume of blood flow, as well as to the maintenance of the blood pressure.

As previously mentioned, concentric contraction of the media results in vasoconstriction, which will, in turn, promote hemostasis. On the other hand, a longitudinal laceration of a vessel will be pulled open by the contraction of the media on either side of the laceration, thereby making hemostasis more difficult.

The outermost layer of the arterial wall, the adventitia, is the strongest. It can contain the arterial pressure, at least for a while, even if the two inner layers have been disrupted. It consists of fibrous collagen and provides a tough outer sheath for the arterial tube. In patients sustaining blunt injury with disruption of the more delicate inner layers, an intact adventitia may be lifesaving.

Blood vessels may sustain either penetrating or blunt injury. In penetrating trauma, a missile first encounters the adventitia and then may penetrate a variable distance into the media or intima. If sufficient force is present to reach the artery and penetrate the adventitia, the less resilient media and intima usually yield as well. This produces a full-thickness injury with the escape of blood outside the vessel. Bleeding, hematoma, pseudoaneurysm, or arteriovenous fistula is the result.

When subjected to the shear stresses of a blunt injury, an artery tears from the inside. The intima tears first as it is the most fragile. Depending on the magnitude of the shear stresses placed upon the vessel, the tear may extend for a variable depth into the arterial wall through the media and even through the adventitia. This tear may or may not be circumferential. Because of the exposure of the thrombogenic subintimal tissues, clot often fills in the luminal rent. This may produce a filling defect within the lumen of the vessel but provides little strength to reinforce the weakened segment.

Regardless of the mechanism of injury, the sine qua non of vascular injury is a luminal defect. A hematoma in the wall of

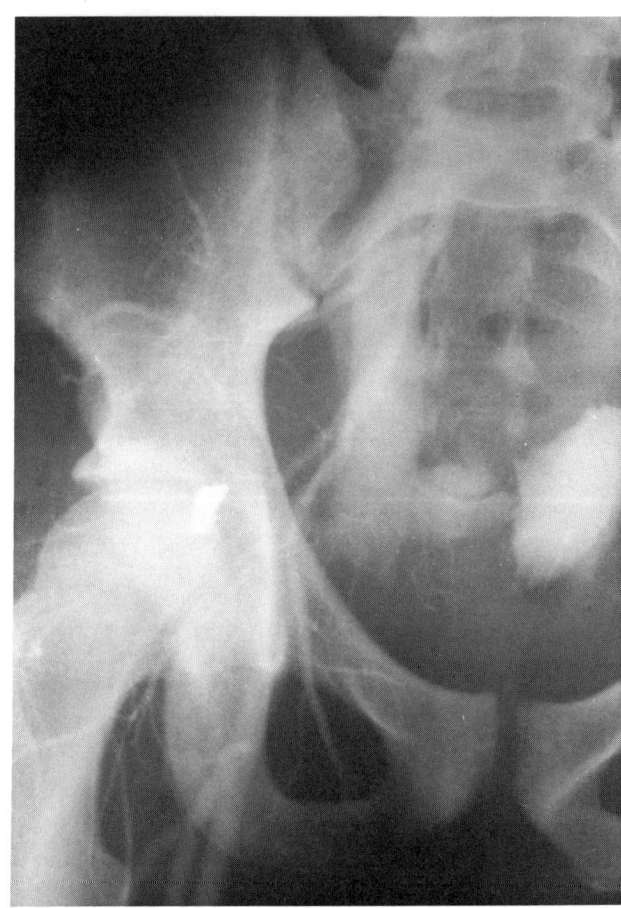

Figure 66-1 Arteriogram of a gunshot wound to the right groin with formation of an acute arteriovenous fistula between the common femoral artery and vein. Note early opacification with dye of the right external iliac vein.

a vessel is usually seen at surgical exploration in association with a clinically significant vascular injury, but this is not an essential finding. It follows that vascular injury is most reliably diagnosed by methods that are sensitive to defects in the luminal surface. Arteriography is the "gold standard" in this regard. Other diagnostic tools such as computed tomography (CT) and magnetic resonance imaging have yet to find a place in the diagnosis of vascular trauma.

Similarly, methods that rely on hemodynamic effects, such as the palpation of pulses, auscultation of bruits or Doppler signals, determination of systolic occlusion pressures and indices, or plethysmographic techniques, are not nearly as sensitive or specific. The absence of pulses, the presence of bruits, and such should be looked for, and these signs should heighten the suspicion of an arterial injury; however, their absence does not rule out a significant injury. When vascular trauma is suspected, it is mandatory that the injury be excluded or confirmed by arteriography.

Acute arteriovenous fistula is the consequence of a penetrating injury that involves both an artery and the adjacent vein (Fig. 66-1). Massive bleeding is rarely a problem because the artery "bleeds" into the low-pressure, low-resistance venous circuit. Distal pulses may be normal, or they may be weak or absent. Venous engorgement, especially distal to the site of injury, may be noted. A bruit and sometimes a thrill may be appreciated over the site of injury. With a very large caliber, high-flow arteriovenous fistula, acute congestive heart failure can be precipitated by right ventricular overload.[7] If the penetrating object is a bullet, it may embolize from its venous entry site to the lungs.[8]

Recent reports have suggested that not all documented arterial injuries require intervention.[9,10] However, traumatic arteriovenous fistulas and pseudoaneurysms do not generally resolve without operative correction. Limited intimal defects in major arteries that are not associated with hemodynamic compromise have remained stable or even healed with time. At the moment, sufficient numbers of patients with adequate long-term follow-up are not available to recommend this as standard practice. Clearly, the decision not to repair an injured, major artery presupposes a reliable patient and close long-term follow-up. This may be difficult to assure in the traumatically injured population. At this time, the recommendation must remain that any recognized major arterial injury should be promptly repaired. The decision to follow an asymptomatic arterial defect should be limited to well-organized, prospective study protocols at specialized centers.

THORAX

Penetrating Thoracic Injuries

Although generally well protected within the rib cage, the aorta and great vessels are vulnerable to exsanguinating injury from penetrating chest wounds. Exposed on either side by the pleural cavities, there is little opportunity for tamponade once a mediastinal vessel has been lacerated. Therefore, all but the smallest penetrating wounds involving a major thoracic vessel may result in fatal hemorrhage in the field.

The patient with a penetrating chest wound should have an ipsilateral tube thoracostomy. The initial evacuation of large quantities of blood may increase the suspicion of a significant vascular injury but is not pathognomonic. Hemodynamically stable patients should be observed for further bleeding. If blood pressure cannot be maintained above 90 mmHg, the patient should go directly to the operating room for thoracotomy. The threshold for surgical intervention for continued bleeding after the placement of a thoracostomy tube varies with the clinical setting and index of suspicion. Bleeding of more than 250 mL/h is excessive, and the patient should be taken to the operating room expeditiously. On the other hand, bleeding of less than 150 mL/h can generally be watched with the expectation that the bleeding will diminish over the next 6 to 12 hours. In the stable patient with intermediate levels of bleeding from the chest, it is usually reasonable to watch for the first 3 to 4 hours to determine whether the bleeding will persist or diminish following re-expansion of the lung.

In a patient with persistent bleeding after tube thoracostomy, thoracotomy should be performed. This procedure usually reveals hemorrhage from the chest wall or lung parenchyma. Bleeding intercostal vessels are simply oversewn. Injured lung parenchyma is debrided or excised to achieve hemostasis. Wedge resection is usually sufficient, although occasionally a formal anatomic excision may be warranted. If injury to a major artery or vein is discovered, it should be repaired. In penetrating thoracic injuries, this will most likely be a relatively small laceration and will usually be amenable to direct suture repair.

Blunt Thoracic Injuries

Patients with blunt chest injury frequently present difficult management problems because they may have sustained significant injuries to multiple organ systems. The vascular injury resulting from blunt trauma may be less obvious and, therefore, requires a higher index of suspicion. The most frequent mechanism of injury is acute deceleration in association with a motor vehicle accident. This results from a vehicle's forward motion being abruptly halted by encountering an oncoming vehicle or a stationary object. The thoracic cage comes to a sudden stop while the thoracic aorta continues forward within it. The aortic arch is tethered to the bony thorax by the great vessels and ligamentum arteriosum. The descending thoracic aorta is relatively less fixed than the arch. Therefore, the aortic isthmus becomes a focus of significant sheer stress and is the most frequent site of aortic disruption in blunt chest injury (Fig. 66-2).[11]

A patient sustaining blunt thoracic trauma may present with a hemothorax, seen as a pleural effusion on admission chest x-ray film. As in the patient who has suffered a penetrating injury, tube thoracostomy is appropriate as an initial procedure, and subsequent indications for thoracotomy for bleeding are similar. On the other hand, arterial disruption may occur, with the blood contained by the outer layer of adventitia. In this case, there may be little or no initial bleeding. Nonetheless, significant risk of delayed hemorrhage or thrombosis is present. The diagnosis may be suggested by diminished or absent pulses, a bruit, or a tense supraclavicular hematoma. However, physical examination does not delineate the injury. There are several findings on upright anteroposterior chest x-ray film that may suggest the diagnosis (Table 66-1).[12] Their presence should serve as an indication for arteriography to confirm or exclude a thoracic vascular lesion (Fig. 66-3).

An exsanguinating abdominal injury such as a shattered spleen may require attention prior to repair of a contained arterial injury in the chest. Nonetheless, if the diagnosis is

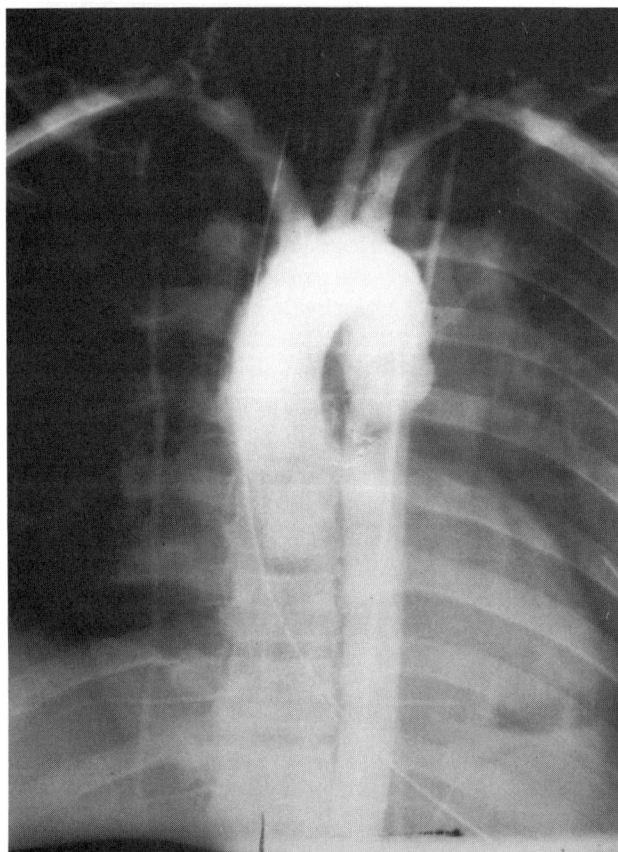

Figure 66-2 Aortogram of a patient sustaining a blunt chest injury demonstrating aortic disruption at the level of the isthmus.

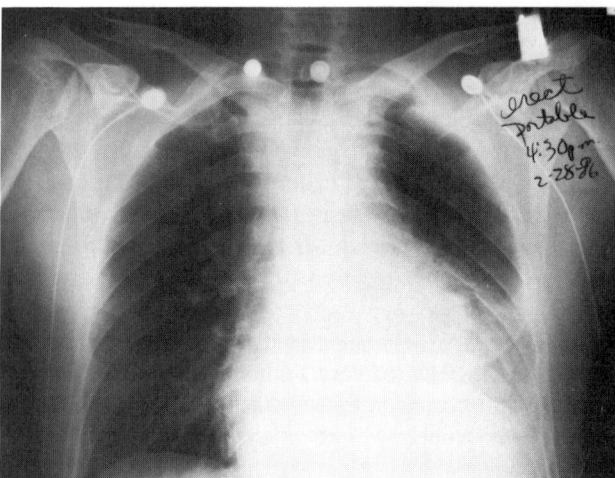

Figure 66-3 Erect admission chest x-ray film of the same patient as in Fig. 66-2.

suspected, it is prudent to prepare the operative field so that access to the chest is available should the patient become hypotensive after abdominal bleeding has been controlled.

Several different incisions may be selected, depending on the exact site of injury. Median sternotomy with a variety of extensions is an excellent approach for the ascending aorta, proximal aortic arch, and great vessels. However, the distal arch and descending aorta, including the origin of the left subclavian artery, are best approached through a left thoracotomy. Preoperative arteriography is invaluable in defining the exact anatomy of the injury so that a correct incision may be selected.

ABDOMEN

Penetrating Abdominal Injuries

Penetrating abdominal injuries mandate surgical exploration. Local exploration of the wound may be needed to ascertain penetration of the fascia, but once fascial penetration has been determined surgical exploration is warranted. No further work-up of the abdomen is indicated. There is no need for peritoneal lavage, CT scan of the abdomen, or arteriography of the abdominal vessels. At laparotomy, injury to the aorta, vena cava, or mesenteric or visceral vessels may be discovered. Repair is tailored to the nature of the injury and must take account of any associated damage to intra-abdominal organs. The details of specific repairs are beyond the scope of this chapter.

Blunt Abdominal Injuries

Essentially the same principles apply to abdominal vascular trauma secondary to blunt or penetrating injury. Intra-abdominal bleeding will necessitate laparotomy. If the source is a major vessel, this will need to be dealt with appropriately. On the other hand, exploration may reveal a retroperitoneal hematoma. All retroperitoneal hematomas above the pelvic brim found at laparotomy should be explored to exclude a significant vascular injury.

The important exception to the exploration of retroperitoneal hematomas is a pelvic hematoma in a patient with a pelvic fracture. Pelvic fractures can result in massive hemorrhage from presacral veins and cancellous bone. Once begun, the bleeding can prove to be unstoppable. Bleeding

Table 66-1 Radiographic Signs of Aortic Injury

1. Mediastinal width > 8 cm
2. Mediastinum to chest ratio > 1:4
3. Aortic contour abnormality
4. Aortopulmonary window opacification
5. Left main stem of bronchus depression (>140°)
6. Tracheal deviation
7. Nasogastric tube deviation
8. Apical cap
9. Paraspinal line widening
10. Right paratracheal stripe > 0.5 cm
11. Left hemothorax

from a pelvic fracture is best controlled by pelvic fixation. If a femoral pulse is absent, arteriography prior to the exploration is the safest course. Occasionally, extravasation of contrast material can be demonstrated from a branch of the hypogastric artery. This can be embolized by the transcatheter technique at the time of arteriography.

The other indication of an intra-abdominal vascular injury is failure of visualization of one or both kidneys on contrast urography. This may be noted on an intravenous pyelogram for hematuria, as part of computed tomography of the abdomen with intravenous contrast agent, or at the end of an arteriographic study being performed for other reasons. Regardless, the next diagnostic study should be arteriography of the abdominal aorta and renal arteries bilaterally. If a renal artery injury is confirmed with loss of renal perfusion, prompt repair should be undertaken. If primary repair cannot be accomplished, saphenous vein interposition grafting or even renal autotransplantation may be required. However, if there is arterial injury without apparent hemodynamic compromise, expectant management is preferable.[13] If exploration is undertaken, the prospect for renal salvage following renal artery injury is poor. Especially if there is concomitant renal parenchymal injury, there is a high likelihood of nephrectomy being required at operation.

EXTREMITIES

Penetrating Extremity Injuries

Significant arterial injury may be suspected following a penetrating extremity wound as a consequence of brisk arterial bleeding from the wound; a tense, expanding, or pulsatile hematoma; diminished or absent distal pulses; or a bruit over the injury. Any penetrating wound in close proximity to a major artery should be suspect, even in the absence of specific signs or symptoms. It is preferable to diagnose arterial injury prior to thrombosis and the loss of distal pulses since it is easier to repair. Diagnosis is confirmed by arteriography. This may simply be a one-shot arteriogram in the emergency department or operating room without the need for formal arteriography.[14]

The greatest determinant of long-term salvage and function of the extremity is usually not repair of the vascular injury. In most cases, the vessels can be adequately repaired. However, massive soft tissue injury and especially major nerve damage may result in a useless extremity with little or no rehabilitation potential.[15] Therefore, although meticulous vascular repair is essential to the salvage of a useful extremity, it is only the first step and is by no means sufficient in itself.

Blunt Extremity Injuries

Vascular injury resulting from blunt trauma to the extremities is most commonly associated with fracture of the adjacent bones. There may be coolness of the extremity distally, with diminished or absent pulses. Frequently, pulses and perfusion can be restored by stabilizing the extremity in proper osseous alignment. The return of pulses does not exclude an underlying arterial injury but does ensure that there is adequate perfusion while further diagnostic studies and therapeutic interventions are undertaken. If there is a markedly displaced fracture in a region where a major artery travels in close proximity, it is prudent to obtain an arteriogram to exclude an intimal flap even if pulses are normal.

The classic example occurs in posterior dislocations of the knee. Approximately 10% of patients sustaining this injury may have concomitant injury to the popliteal artery.[16] Therefore, any patient having a posterior dislocation of the knee or a similar adjacent injury such as a tibial plateau fracture or distal femur fracture should be considered for arteriography even if pulses are present. If pulses are diminished or absent, arteriography is mandatory (Fig. 66-4).

The principles of treatment of blunt extremity injuries are similar to those of penetrating injuries. Because of the nature of a blunt injury, it is more likely that a long segment of

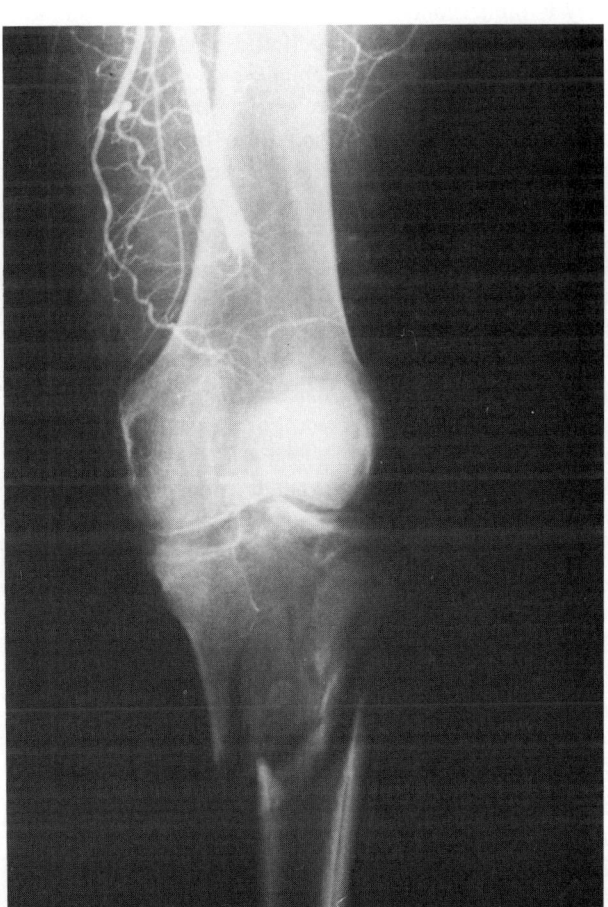

Figure 66-4 Arteriogram of a patient sustaining a tibial plateau fracture as a consequence of an automobile bumper injury. Note complete occlusion of the popliteal artery.

the artery will be contused, requiring graft replacement. Saphenous vein is the graft of choice. There is a high incidence of compartment syndrome following revascularization, no doubt because of the cumulative effects of the crushing soft tissue injury of the blunt trauma followed by the ischemia and reperfusion as a consequence of the vascular injury. Accordingly, there should be a low threshold for performing fasciotomy of all muscular compartments. Even if this necessitates turning a closed fracture into an open one, it is preferable to the permanent loss of neuromuscular function as a consequence of inadequate treatment of a compartment syndrome.

NECK

Penetrating Neck Injuries

There is some controversy regarding whether patients with penetrating wounds in the neck should be subjected to a battery of diagnostic studies or routinely taken to the operating room for immediate exploration.[17–19] However, as regards potential vascular injuries in the neck, this controversy is limited only to a very select group of penetrating wounds, those limited to zone II. The neck may be divided into three vertical regions referred to as zones I to III.[20] Zone I, the base of the neck, extends from the top of the clavicle up a distance of 2 in. Zone III extends from the angle of the mandible up. Zone II is the region between the other two areas.

Depending on the philosophy of the surgeon and the clinical presentation, patients with zone II injuries may be taken to the operating room for exploration or may undergo arteriography first (Fig. 66-5). With zone I penetrating injuries, arteriography must be performed prior to surgery unless the patient is too unstable because the injury may involve the great vessels and require control at the level of the aortic arch. Matters are further complicated by the fact that control of the origin of the innominate or left carotid artery is readily obtained through a median sternotomy, but control of the left subclavian artery is difficult. If the arteriogram shows that control of the left subclavian near its origin is required, left thoracotomy may be an optimal approach, but this precludes exposure to the proximal arch. At times, a median sternotomy incision with a perpendicular left third interspace incision may be required.

Similarly, because distal control may be difficult or impossible to obtain, injuries in zone III mandate arteriography prior to exploration.[21] An injury of the distal internal carotid artery may require special maneuvers such as anterior subluxation of the mandible to achieve adequate exposure. If the vertebral artery is injured near the base of the skull, it may be preferable to manage this nonoperatively or even to choose transcatheter embolization rather than surgical exploration. A reckless approach to injury of these vessels can result in surgical disaster.

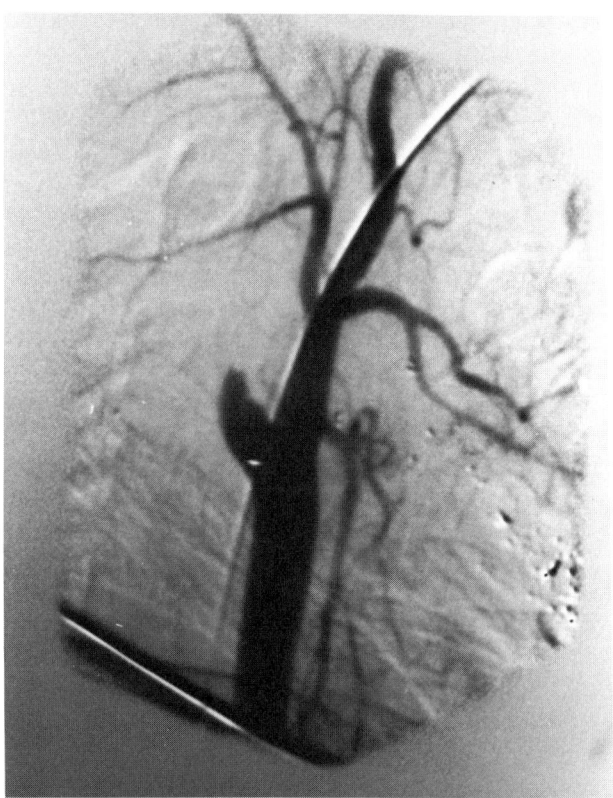

Figure 66-5 Arteriogram of the right carotid artery in a patient sustaining a shotgun wound to the neck. Note complete occlusion of the proximal internal carotid artery. This was repaired by primary end-to-end reanastomosis.

Blunt Neck Injuries

Bleeding is generally not as great a problem with blunt as with penetrating injuries to the neck. However, intimal disruption with hemodynamically significant intimal flaps and complete vessel occlusion secondary to thrombosis may produce a reduction of blood flow to the brain, with resulting neurologic deficit. The clinical picture is clouded by the fact that significant blunt trauma to the neck is frequently accompanied by significant trauma to the head, with the possibility of brain injury.

An absent carotid pulse is a clear-cut indication for four-vessel cerebral arteriography. On the other hand, if there is no pulse deficit, a patient presenting with blunt injury to the head and neck associated with a neurologic deficit would ordinarily be taken first to CT for intracranial evaluation. If findings on the CT scan do not adequately account for the neurologic deficit, consideration must be given to the possibility of a vascular injury. Specifically, if the patient appears alert and responsive but with a focal, unilateral neurologic deficit not adequately accounted for by intracranial pathologic findings on CT scan, arteriography should be performed.

There is some controversy surrounding the repair of the extracranial vessels supplying the brain.[22,23] The concern is that re-establishment of normal arterial pressure to an area of brain that has sustained a recent infarct may result in increased edema of the injured tissue or even frank bleeding into the area of infarction. In general, if the patient has sustained a massive infarction with a markedly reduced mental status or coma, operative intervention should be deferred. On the other hand, the asymptomatic patient or one with circumscribed, focal neurologic findings should be promptly explored if an arterial injury is documented.

INTRA-ARTERIAL INJECTION OF FOREIGN SUBSTANCES

The rising use of illicit drugs, especially by parenteral routes, has resulted in an increased frequency of intra-arterial injection of foreign substances. The drugs themselves may be highly irritating to the endothelium. This is further compounded by the fact that most available illicit drugs are mixed with a variety of "inert" compounds such as cornstarch or talc and are not generally prepared in a sterile fashion, being at times mixed with tap water or even saliva.

Distal embolization with occlusion of small end arteries may result. In addition, severe vasospasm is commonly noted. Arteriography is indicated to exclude a correctable lesion such as an intimal flap at the site of injection or a large occluding embolus or thrombus amenable to surgical removal. Unfortunately, correctable lesions are rarely found. If the typical picture of pruned distal vessels and intense vasospasm is seen at arteriography, the physician should be prepared to commence the intra-arterial administration of vasodilating drugs such as papaverine. In addition, the sublingual administration of 10 mg of nifedepine may be a useful adjunct.

These patients are best treated with supportive therapy, including maintaining the limb in a neutral position and avoiding all further trauma. Avoiding β-blockers, caffeine, and nicotine is prudent. The patient must not smoke. There is no proven benefit of sympathectomy. However, if the leg is the site of injection, the placement of an epidural catheter will provide both a convenient form of pain control in the acute phase and maximal available dilatation resulting from temporary autonomic denervation. The development of a compartment syndrome is possible, and early fasciotomy should be performed if this complication develops.[24]

Revascularization is usually not possible. Amputation is best deferred until the acute phase is past and the level of demarcation is well defined. Debridement and amputation of clearly infarcted tissue is then warranted, although it may be equally acceptable to permit autoamputation of the ends of digits or soft tissue eschars.

SEQUELAE OF VASCULAR INJURY

The specific complications of vascular trauma are a consequence of acute ischemia and reperfusion of the organs and tissues supplied by the vessel injured. Therefore, depending on the site of injury, these include stroke, ischemic hepatitis, hemorrhagic gastritis, acalculous cholecystitis, ischemic pancreatitis, intestinal ischemia, acute renal failure secondary to acute tubular necrosis from renal ischemia or myoglobinuria from infarcted muscle, paraparesis or paraplegia from spinal cord ischemia, and compartment syndrome. The best way to manage these complications is to avoid them by limiting the period of ischemia as much as possible.

SUMMARY

Patients sustaining major injuries in any anatomic region are at risk for significant vascular trauma. The vascular injury is not always immediately apparent and, therefore, a high index of suspicion must be maintained. The complications of a normal arteriogram are trivial compared to those of the missed arterial injury.

Once the vascular lesion has been documented, expeditious surgical intervention is warranted. If there is no active bleeding, other, more urgent lesions may be attended to first. Nonetheless, unnecessary delay should be avoided.

Injury to major blood vessels can result in crippling morbidity and even mortality if not expertly treated during the first few hours after the injury. However, for the most part these injuries are imminently manageable with the expectation that normal perfusion can be restored. The diagnosis and management of vascular trauma is challenging but extremely rewarding. The successful management of the patient with a vascular injury is the measure of an expert emergency medical team.

REFERENCES

1. Jones TK, Barnhart GR, Greenfield LJ. Cardiopulmonary arrest following penetrating trauma: guidelines for emergency hospital management of presumed exsanguination. *J Trauma*. 1987;27:24.
2. Baker CC, Thomas AN, Trunkey DD. The role of emergency room thoracotomy in trauma. *J Trauma*. 1980;20:848.
3. Cogbill TH, Moore EE, Millikan JS, Cleveland HC. Rationale for selective application of emergency department thoracotomy in trauma. *J Trauma*. 1983;23:453.
4. Washington B, Wilson RF, Sterger Z, Bassett JS. Emergency thoracotomy: a four-year review. *Ann Thorac Surg*. 1985;40:188.
5. Mattox KL. Thoracic vascular trauma. *J Vasc Surg*. 1988;7:725.
6. Vanhoutte PM, Rubany GM, Miller VM, Houston DS. Modulation of vascular smooth muscle contraction by the endothelium. *Annu Rev Physiol*. 1986;48:307.
7. Frykberg ER, Vines FS, Alexander RH: The natural history of clinically occult arterial injuries: a prospective evaluation. *J Trauma*. 1989; 29:577.
8. Michelassi F, Pietrabissa A, Ferrari M, et al. Bullet emboli to the systemic and venous circulation. *Surgery*. 1990;107:239–245.
9. Dennis JW, Frykberg ER, Crump JM, et al. New perspectives on the management of penetrating proximity extremity trauma. *Proc ISCVS*. 1989;39:40.
10. Cammack V, Rapport RL, Paul RJ, et al. Deceleration injuries of the thoracic aorta. *Arch Surg*. 1959;79:244.

11. Woodring JH, Loh FK, Kryscio RJ. Mediastinal hemorrhage: an evaluation of radiologic manifestations. *Radiology*. 1984;151:15.
12. Mattox KL, Holzman M, Pickard LR, et al. Clamp/repair: a safe technique for treatment of blunt injury to the descending thoracic aorta. *Ann Thorac Surg*. 1985;40:456.
13. Kaufman JL, Dinerstein CR, Shah DM, Leather RP. Renal artery intimal flaps after blunt trauma: indications for nonoperative therapy. *J Vasc Surg*. 1988;8:33.
14. O'Gorman RB, Feliciano DV. Arteriography performed in the emergency center. *Am J Surg*. 1986;152:323.
15. Menzoian JD, Doyle JE, Cantelmo NL, et al. A comprehensive approach to extremity vascular trauma. *Arch Surg*. 1985;120:801.
16. Lefrac EA. Knee dislocation. *Arch Surg*. 1976;111:1021.
17. Obeid FN, Haddad GS, Horst HM, Biuns BA. A critical reappraisal of a mandatory exploration policy for penetrating wounds of the neck. *Surg Gynecol Obstet*. 1985;160:517.
18. Ayuyao AM, Kaledz YL, Parsa MH, Freeman HP. Penetrating neck wounds. *Ann Surg*. 1985;202:563.
19. Bishova RA, Pasch AR, Douglas DD, et al. The necessity of mandatory exploration of penetrating zone II neck injuries. *Surgery*. 1986;100:655.
20. McSwain NE. Penetrating neck wounds: major advances in the 1980's. In: Maull KI, Cleveland HC, Strauch GO, et al, eds. *Advances in Trauma*. Chicago, Ill: Year Book Medical Publishers; 1986;1:135.
21. Sclafani SJA, Panetta T, Goldstein AS, et al. The management of arterial injuries caused by penetration of zone III of the neck. *J Trauma*. 1985;25:871.
22. Richardson JD, Simpson C, Miller FB. Management of carotid artery trauma. *Surgery*. 1988;104:673.
23. Demetriades D, Skalkides J, Sofianos C, et al. Carotid artery injuries: experience with 124 cases. *J Trauma*. 1989;29:91.
24. Cohen SM. Accidental intra-arterial injection of drugs. *Lancet*. 1948;2:361.

67. Heart and Great Vessel Emergencies

ANTHONY J. DELROSSI, MD
JONATHAN H. CILLEY, JR., MD
JAMES B. ALEXANDER, MD

GENERAL PRINCIPLES

Heart and great vessel injuries are usually catastrophic and require immediate attention. Traumatic injuries such as penetrating wounds to the heart are readily apparent, and their magnitude is usually appreciated. However, cardiac tamponade can be a difficult diagnosis to make, especially when not associated with chest trauma. Therefore, a careful initial assessment of the patient is essential. In traumatic cases, single versus multiple organ involvement must be established early, and the mechanism of injury noted. If the patient is involved in a motor vehicle accident, it is important to determine if the patient was restrained. Deceleration injuries are far more common than initially thought, and many seriously injured patients arrive in the emergency department alive because of rapid evacuation from the crash site.

Emergencies involving the heart and great vessels exclusive of myocardial infarction are usually secondary to trauma. A rapid, thorough physical examination is essential, with note taken of any obvious penetrating injuries, bruises, or crepitant areas over the chest wall. Particular attention must be paid to neck vein distention since this is especially important in cardiac tamponade. All pulses must be felt and recorded because avulsions or occlusions of the great vessels can alter the circulation in one or more extremities. Obviously, assessment of the hemodynamic status takes precedence. Vital signs are recorded and mental status is noted.

Hypotension and/or hypoxia can cause agitation and confusion and must be distinguished from associated head trauma.

Regardless of whether the injury to the heart is penetrating or blunt, the consequences will be hemorrhage, cardiac tamponade, or myocardial infarction, the latter secondary to myocardial contusions and/or coronary artery injuries with secondary infarction. Injuries to the aorta are usually secondary to deceleration, with resultant tearing of the aorta at the isthmus just distal to the left subclavian artery. The second most common site of injury is just above the coronary ostia. Dissection of the aorta is the most frequent nontraumatic emergency and usually begins just above the coronary ostia and progresses to the iliac bifurcation. However, a second type of dissection may involve the aorta just distal to the left subclavian artery, where the dissecting hematoma begins and progresses distally.

Resuscitation is begun immediately, even before the nature of the injury has been completely assessed. Access to the venous circulation must be accomplished promptly either by peripheral IV, a central venous catheter, or venous cutdown. The saphenous vein at the ankle can be a useful site in the acute setting. Arterial access via a femoral or radial artery catheter is established for continuous blood pressure monitoring and analysis of blood gases. Blood for type and crossmatching and for standard laboratory determinations (ie, hematocrit, hemoglobin, electrolytes, and BUN), is drawn and sent.

CARDIAC EMERGENCIES

Ascertaining the precise area of the heart injured is very important. Although the heart is centrally located immediately beneath the sternum, injuries can occur from wounds that enter from below the costal cartilages or posteriorly in the vertebral area.

The right atrium and ventricle lie to the right of the sternum and are anterior, whereas the left atrium and ventricle are located posteriorly. The apex of the left ventricle is behind the fifth interspace and extends to the midclavicular line. Penetrating injuries to the heart can be made by low-velocity instruments such as knives, screwdrivers, or ice picks. Gunshot or shotgun blasts are classified as high-velocity injuries and usually cause more extensive tissue damage. As expected, because of its anterior location, the right ventricle is more frequently injured than the left ventricle. In approximately 50% of cases, the right ventricle is the site of injury, whereas the left ventricle is injured in approximately 25%.[1] The right and left atrium follow, respectively, in the incidence of injuries. In approximately one-third of traumatic injuries, more than one chamber is involved. Fortunately, injuries to the coronary arteries occur in only 5% of patients, with the left anterior descending artery the most frequently damaged. This artery follows a course just immediately beneath the sternum and slightly to its left.[2] Isolated valvular and septal injuries occur, but their frequency is low.

Hemorrhage from the traumatized myocardium may be confined to the rigid pericardial sac. If the mechanism of injury is severe, however, blood may drain into the mediastinum or pleural spaces. The emergency physician must recognize the signs of hypovolemic shock. Initially, patients present with only a rapid pulse, slight changes in mental status, pallor, and normal blood pressure. Gradually, hypotension ensues, the extremities become cool, and respirations become shallow and rapid. Immediate volume resuscitation is critical if these patients are to survive.

Emergency Department Thoracotomy

Patients often arrive in the emergency department in a "lifeless" condition. Examination may reveal a penetrating wound with no discernible vital signs except electrical activity on the electrocardiogram. These patients are often immediately intubated and placed on ventilatory support. Again, rapid assessment as to the nature of the injury must be made. Entrance and exit wounds in these paients are observed, and those that are within the boundaries of the cardiac silhouette should be considered for emergency department thoracotomy.[3-5] The type of incision is related to the location of the entrance wound and the specific offending agent. Stab wounds on the left side of the chest usually require a left thoracotomy. However, a gunshot wound on the left side may exit in the right hemithorax, and a midline incision may be necessary to expose all chambers of the heart. Alternately, an incision starting in the left fifth intercostal space and carried across the sternum into the right chest and its corresponding intercostal space will provide access to the entire heart, including the vena cava (Fig. 67-1). The latter incision is favored by many trauma surgeons since a bilateral thoracotomy incision across the midline affords exposure to the heart as well as the hila of both lungs.[6,7] Both pleural spaces can be evacuated, and injuries to the hila or lung tissue controlled.

Few instruments are needed to expose the heart, especially if a left thoracotomy incision is made. However, a midline incision through the sternum usually requires a sternal saw or a lebsche knife, either of which should be immediately available in any emergency department that expects to see this kind of trauma.

Once visualized, the pericardium can be incised, with complete relief of tamponade. Once the pericardium is opened, hemorrhage can be controlled, and the heart can be manually compressed if pulseless. Electrocountershock can be used to convert ventricular dysrhythmias or ventricular fibrillation to a sinus mechanism. Finally, epinephrine can be given directly into the aortic root if necessary.

Care should be used to avoid injury to the friable right ventricle during manual cardiac resuscitation. Injury to the phrenic nerve must be avoided since it courses on the lateral aspect of the pericardium.

Once the pericardium is opened, volume can be administered directly into the heart; depending on the exposure, either the right atrium or the right ventricle may be used. Rapid assessment of the injury must be made, and the bleeding controlled with digital compression (Fig. 67-2). Finger control of ventricular bleeding is all that is usually necessary. However, an alternate strategy is to place a Foley cathe-

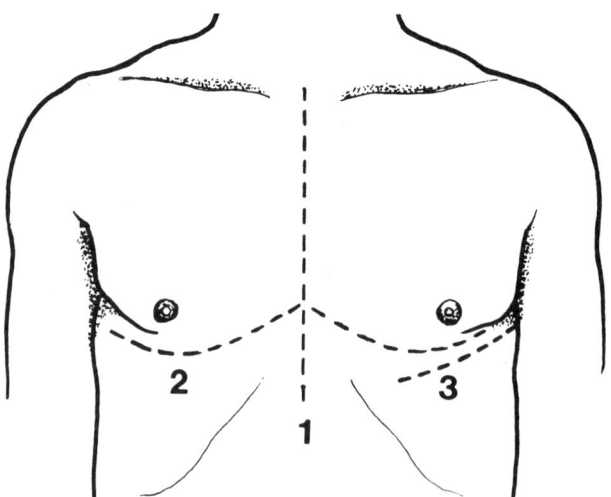

Figure 67-1 Incision 1 is a median sternotomy providing access to the entire heart. Incision 2 is a right-sided thoracotomy. Incision 3 is a standard left-sided thoracotomy, which can be extended across the midline to expose both pleural spaces.

Sometimes, temporary occlusion of the descending thoracic aorta will provide more efficient circulation to the heart and brain in patients who are severely hypovolemic. The descending thoracic aorta is usually visualized in its anterior location to the vertebral bodies, especially when a left thoracotomy incision has been made. The aorta is mobilized and then occluded with a nontraumatic vascular clamp at the level of the diaphragm. This allows increased blood flow to the coronary and cerebral circulation until more effective circulation can be established. Care must be used when placing the aorta cross-clamp at this level. The esophagus is adjacent to the aorta and may be included in the clamp, causing a laceration.

Some authors have reported good survival rates with successfully repaired cardiac wounds. In the more stable patients (ie, those who are alert prior to surgery), the survival rate for penetrating injuries to the heart is approximately 70% to 80%.[2,6] The best results are obtained in those with simple stab wounds. Those with high-velocity injuries such as gunshot wounds sustain a 70% mortality. Nevertheless, patients who undergo emergency room thoracotomy because of a "lifeless" state but are not in ventricular fibrillation have a 20% survival rate.[10]

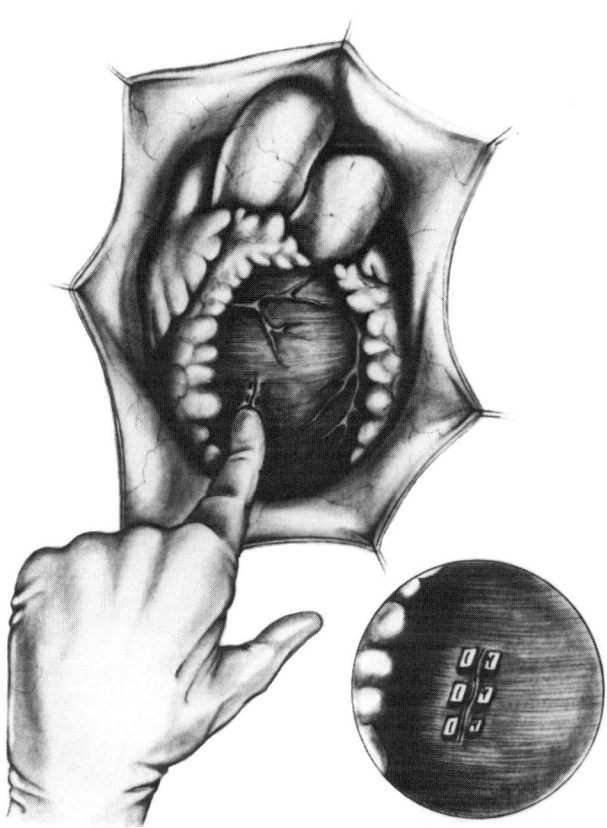

Figure 67-2 Digital compression of a myocardial laceration with suture closure.

ter through the cardiac wound and inflate the balloon (Fig. 67-3). This often serves as an occlusive device for hemorrhage control. In right-sided injuries, it also serves as a site for rapid fluid infusion.[8] Most injuries to the ventricular chambers can be managed successfully by simple suture repair using a nonabsorbable suture over Teflon pledgets. These pledgets are used to buttress friable muscle. Atrial injuries are best managed by using a nontraumatic vascular clamp to occlude the tear, which can then be closed with nonabsorbable suture. Tears of the venae cavae are usually quite extensive and require complicated surgical techniques.[9] Unfortunately, mobilization of the heart will kink the venae cavae and impede venous return. Therefore, these patients must be transported to the operating room as rapidly as possible. Once there, it may be necessary to use cardiopulmonary bypass for complex lesions, especially if the injury is located on the posterior aspect of the heart or the vena cava. However, cardiopulmonary bypass is contraindicated in multiply injured patients because total body heparinization is required. In this setting, when the heart is beating and the patient is exsanguinating rapidly, temporary occlusion of both venae cavae for 2 to 3 minutes can be performed by the physician. By limiting inflow to the heart, the physician gains the time to place a suture accurately and obtain better control of the hemorrhage.

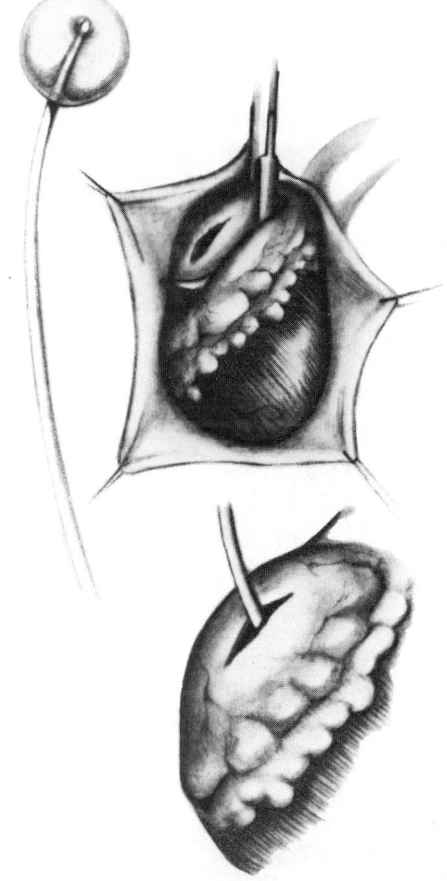

Figure 67-3 A torn right atrium and the insertion of a Foley catheter for control of hemorrhage.

Pericardial Tamponade

The pericardial sac is composed of fibrous tissue and is relatively nondistensible. The sac itself contains approximately 50 mL of serous fluid. In traumatic injuries to the heart, the blood may be contained in the rigid pericardial space with clot preventing its exit through the slit in the pericardium, and tamponade will ensue. If the normal volume of pericardial fluid is rapidly expanded to approximately 150 to 200 mL, diastolic filling is impaired and systolic blood pressure and cardiac output will decrease (Fig. 67-4). Subsequently, organ perfusion fails and death becomes imminent.

Classically, pericardial tamponade consists of a triad of hypotension, distant heart sounds, and venous hypertension. However, this is present in only 60% of patients presenting with penetrating injuries.[11] The remaining cases are associated with hypotension and decreased venous pressure due to associated profound bleeding, usually into the pleural cavities. A paradoxical pulse with a decrease in systolic pressure of greater than 20 mmHg is often helpful in determining the presence of tamponade. However, this is absent in many cases and is generally unreliable in the acute setting. A more reliable parameter is a narrow pulse pressure with a normal diastolic pressure and a low systolic pressure.[11]

Patients with suspected pericardial tamponade should be treated with immediate resuscitative procedures. Central venous pressure monitoring should be obtained, and a Foley catheter inserted for measurement of urinary output. Accurate measurements of the central venous pressure (CVP) are very helpful, and a pressure of greater than 15 cmH$_2$O is often diagnostic. However, a low CVP does not rule out cardiac tamponade.

Other diagnostic studies are often unreliable and time consuming. Chest radiographs, especially a supine film, will show only a wide cardiac silhouette. However, such a film is useful in determining the location of the central venous pressure catheter, the tip of the endotracheal tube, and also the presence or absence of a hemothorax or pneumothorax. Fluoroscopy and electrocardiography are of little value in the acute setting. Echocardiography in hemodynamically stable patients is very helpful and may aid in the diagnosis of tamponade.

Emergency pericardiocentesis is recommended by some in the acute setting.[12] The withdrawal of only a few milliliters of nonclotting blood from the pericardial cavity may be lifesaving. However, a negative pericardiocentesis does not rule out the diagnosis of tamponade.

The technique is simple and requires only a few minutes. A large-bore needle (gauge, 14 to 16) attached to a syringe is positioned at an angle of 45° from the chest wall with the tip directed toward the left shoulder (Fig. 67-5). The xiphoid is noted, and the needle is advanced under the costal cartilage at this level.[13]

Determination of the location of the pericardial space can be aided by the attachment of an indifferent electrode to the hub of the needle and observation of changes in the electrocardiographic complexes when the myocardium is encountered. Aspiration of nonclotting blood is diagnostic, but if rapid bleeding occurs this may not be a reliable finding. If one is confident that the pericardial cavity has been reached, a small plastic tube may be inserted over a guidewire and left in position to drain residual blood until a more definitive evacuation can be accomplished.

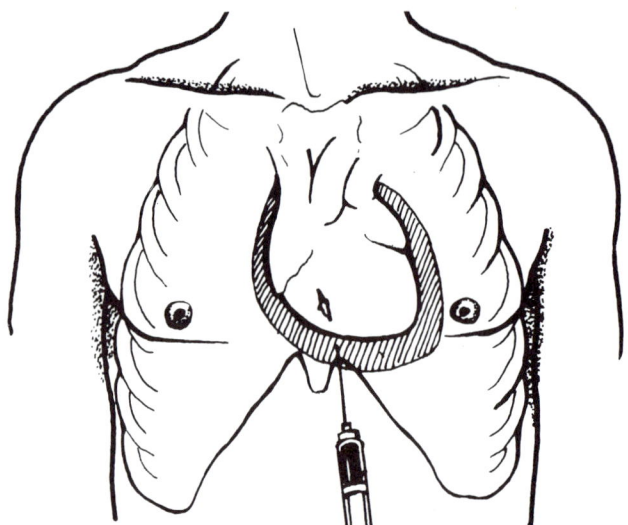

Figure 67-5 Pericardiocentesis with removal of nonclotting blood from around the heart.

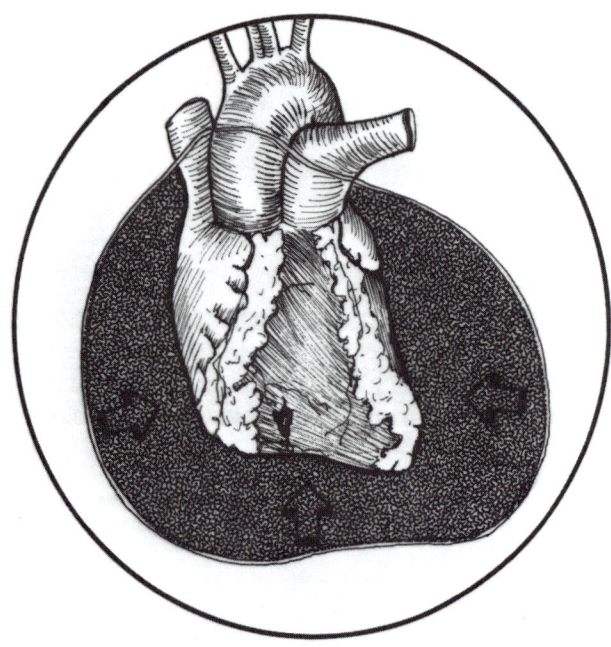

Figure 67-4 Diastolic compression of the ventricles in cardiac tamponade.

An alternate approach would be to make an incision over the xiphoid process and open the space just above the diaphragm. The pericardial sac will be visible and can be opened quickly with the relief of tamponade. A chest tube can then be positioned to drain any residual accumulation. Unfortunately, once the pericardium is opened, massive hemorrhage may ensue; because of the limited exposure, it may be difficult to control the myocardial laceration. In this setting, an emergency thoracotomy is indicated or, whenever possible, subxiphoid exploration should be done in the operating room with a thoracic surgeon present.

Blunt Injuries to the Heart

Surprisingly, the most common cause of death in motor vehicle accidents is blunt injury to the heart, which is often unsuspected. The exact incidence of myocardial injury may vary from 15% to 75% of accident victims.[14] Myocardial contusion is a common finding, and severe injuries to other organs often mask the myocardial damage. This frequently occurs in steering wheel injuries, but the heart may also be injured by rapid rises in intra-abdominal and intrathoracic pressures, as seen in falls from great heights.

Myocardial contusion is the most common injury to the traumatized heart, and its diagnosis is often difficult because the signs are variable. Approximately 25% of patients sustaining chest injury will have myocardial contusion as diagnosed by serial electrocardiogram.[15] The injury itself can vary from epicardial bruising to transmural myocardial infarction. In fact, differentiation from acute myocardial infarction is impossible since the histologic picture is the same. Of course, many patients with myocardial contusion have normally patent coronary arteries.

On presentation to the emergency department, most patients with myocardial contusion complain of chest pain. These patients often give a history of rapid deceleration with the chest coming in contact with the relatively fixed steering wheel, or they have been thrown from the vehicle completely, hitting other stationary objects. The pain that they feel is therefore similar to anginal pain in both its location and its intensity. However, this pain is not relieved by nitroglycerin or other nitrates. Other nonspecific symptoms are nausea, vomiting, and palpitations. Tachycardia is frequently observed but can also be associated with other injuries. However, tachycardia in a patient with no significant injuries is suggestive of myocardial contusion. Bruises over the anterior chest wall and especially fractures of the sternum are additionally suggestive.

The management of patients with a suspected myocardial contusion is aimed at control of hypotension by appropriate volume replacement and correction of hypoxia by intubation if necessary. A central venous pressure catheter and a Swan-Ganz catheter should be inserted, and serial electrocardiograms and CK-MB isoenzyme determinations for myocardial injury should be obtained.[15] These can be done at the time of initial blood sampling. Radionuclide imaging has been advocated by some to demonstrate the area of myocardial contusion. Unfortunately, it is diagnostic only for full-thickness injuries; in mildly contused areas, it is nonspecific. A multiple gaited acquisition (MUGA) scan is also not specific enough to diagnose myocardial contusion.

Ventricular dysrhythmias should be treated immediately with lidocaine as a bolus and then as an infusion. As in most traumatic injuries, anticoagulation must be avoided since hemorrhage may ensue elsewhere. All patients with myocardial contusion as a suspected diagnosis should be admitted and followed closely because of complications such as fatal dysrhythmias and congestive heart failure. The overall prognosis for the majority of patients with myocardial contusion is good.

Besides contusion, frank myocardial rupture can occur, and it is usually associated with compressive injuries. The site of rupture may be the free wall, the ventricular septum, or the valve components themselves. Rupture in the free wall can be contained by the pericardial cavity should the sac be intact; however, the sac may also rupture, leading to bleeding into the mediastinum or pleural spaces. Patients presenting with pericardial tamponade should be treated with needle aspiration and then an immediate thoracotomy. Repair can be accomplished in selected cases by simple suture. However, when large areas of the myocardium are injured, survival is unusual.

AORTIC INJURIES

Aortic emergencies are either traumatic, with resultant aortic disruption, or acute aortic dissection. Acute aortic dissections are one of the most common aneurysms of the aorta. The lesion has been estimated to have an incidence of 10 to 20 cases per million population per year in the United States. Dissections are really advancing hematomas that begin with an initial intimal tear and then propagate along the length of the aorta in varying degrees.

The pathophysiology of nontraumatic aortic dissection includes medial degeneration, as in cystic medial necrosis, which is seen in approximately 20% of cases. The disease entity is also associated with Marfan's syndrome, bicuspid aortic valves, aortic coarctation, pregnancy, Turner's syndrome, and occasionally with open heart surgery at the site of aortic cannulation. Classification of these injuries is based on the location of the intimal tear. DeBakey classified these lesions as types I, II, and III. The current terminology includes type A, which represents a combination of types I and II and is associated with tears that have their origin in the ascending aorta. This is present in 65% of cases. Type B comprises the rest and is associated with tears that begin at the level of the left subclavian artery and progress distally. The advancing hematoma starts as an intimal tear and shears the media into two layers with a false channel that progresses and can either rupture freely into the pleural space or cause pericardial tamponade. If the hematoma compresses the coronary arteries, myocardial ischemia occurs. The progressive hematoma can disrupt the aortic valve, and severe aortic insufficiency may develop. Finally, when the dissection is propagated in the distal aorta, the mesenteric vessels may be part of the false lumen, reducing the blood supply. This sets up small bowel infarction as well as renal insufficiency.

The diagnosis of acute aortic dissection may be difficult to make. The symptoms vary, but most commonly the acute onset of excruciating pain is associated with the initial tear. If the dissection begins in the ascending aorta, pain tends to radiate to the anterior chest wall. As the hematoma advances, the pain will shift to the midback. Differential diagnosis is often myocardial infarction versus pulmonary embolus. As the hematoma advances, various organs may be involved and the picture of an acute abdomen may be a prevalent sign. Many patients are hypertensive, especially if the dissection begins at the level of the left subclavian artery. Forty percent of patients have aortic insufficiency and, additionally, 25% have pericardial tamponade with a shocklike picture.[16] Approximately 10% suffer a completed stroke secondary to the shearing off of the cerebral circulation. Patients who present with the characteristic onset of severe chest and back pain associated with differential pulses and hypertension should be considered to have an aortic dissection.

An initial electrocardiogram in the emergency department may help rule out the diagnosis of myocardial infarction. A chest radiograph will often show a widened mediastinum; however, this is not specific. A computed tomographic study is useful, and echocardiography may reveal an intimal flap and entry point. The definitive diagnosis is made by arteriography with demonstration of the two lumens and the intimal tear.

Initial treatment includes the institution of an IV, insertion of a Foley catheter, and measurement of central venous pressure and arterial pressure. Patients who are hypertensive should be treated initially with a combination of nitroprusside and propranolol. The latter is used to decrease the stroke work of the left ventricle and limit the advancement of the hematoma. The blood pressure should be maintained at approximately 100 mmHg systolic or just enough to allow a urinary output of 0.5 mL/kg/h. Arterial pressure must be monitored continuously when sodium nitroprusside is administered to prevent severe hypotension.

The overall prognosis for untreated aortic dissections is grim. Approximately 60% of patients with type A dissection will die within the first 24 hours, and 90% will be dead within 3 months. Type B has a more favorable prognosis, and a 25% mortality will be noted. Treatment is left in the hands of a cardiothoracic surgeon, and virtually all type A dissections should be considered surgical emergencies unless there are severe disturbances of the central nervous system. Type B dissections can be treated medically or surgically, depending upon the presence or absence of symptoms. Control of hypertension, alleviation of pain, and preservation of adequate urinary output in patients with no other organ involvement preclude surgical intervention. These patients may be treated medically with a satisfactory outcome.

REFERENCES

1. Robbs J, Baker L. Cardiovascular trauma. *Curr Probl Surg*. 1984;21:4.
2. Harley E, Mayfield W. Cardiac injuries. In: Blaisdell, Trunkey DD, eds. *Trauma Management*, III: *Cervicothoracic Trauma*. New York, NY: Thieme Inc; 1986.
3. Ivatury RR, Nallathambi MN, Rohman M, Stahl WM. Penetrating cardiac trauma: quantifying the severity of anatomic and physiologic injury. *Ann Surg*. 1987;205:61–66.
4. Evans J, Gray LA Jr, Rayner A, et al. Principles for the management of penetrating cardiac wounds. *Ann Surg*. 1979;189:777.
5. Tavares S, Hankins JR, Moulton AL, et al. Management of penetrating cardiac injuries: the role of emergency room thoracotomy. *Ann Thorac Surg*. 1984;38:183–187.
6. Baker CC, Thomas AN, Trunkey DD. The role of emergency room thoracotomy in trauma. *J Trauma*. 1980;20:848.
7. Symbas PN, Harlaftis N, Waldo WG. Penetrating cardiac wounds: a comparison of different therapeutic methods. *Ann Surg*. 1976;83:377.
8. Wilson SM, Au FC. In extremis use of a Foley catheter in a cardiac stab wound. *J Trauma*. 1986;26:400–402.
9. Richardson DJ, Flint LM, Snow NJ, et al. Management of transmediastinal gunshot wounds. *Surgery*. 1981;90:671–676.
10. Mattox KL, Koch LV, Beall AC, DeBakey ME. Logistics and technical consideration in the treatment of the wounded heart. *Circulation*. 1975;51:1212.
11. Moreno C, Moore EE, Majure JA, Hopeman AR. Pericardial tamponade: a critical determinant for survival following penetrating cardiac wounds. *J Trauma*. 1986;26:9.
12. Evans J, Gray LA, Rayner A, Fulton RL. Principles for management of penetrating cardiac wounds. *Ann Surg*. 1979;189:777–784.
13. Breaux EP, DuPont JB, Albert HM, et al. Cardiac tamponade following penetrating mediastinal injuries: improved survival with early pericardiocentesis. *J Trauma*. 1979;19:461.
14. Symbas PN. Major injuries: heart injuries from blunt trauma. In: Grillo, Eschapasse, eds. *International Trends in General Thoracic Surgery*. Philadelphia, Pa.: WB Saunders Co; 1987; 2.
15. Tenzer ML. The spectrum of myocardial contusion: a review. *J Trauma*. 1985;25:620–627.
16. Kirklin JW, Barratt-Boyes BG. Acute aortic dissection. In: *Cardiac Surgery*. New York, NY: John Wiley & Sons Inc; 1986.

68. Cardiopulmonary Resuscitation

ALAN D. GUERCI, MD

Cardiopulmonary resuscitation (CPR) encompasses a series of efforts aimed at the delivery of adequate amounts of oxygenated blood to the brain and heart until effective, spontaneous circulation can be restored. It is the cornerstone of a strategy that includes defibrillation and drug therapy and that has been proven effective both in and out of hospitals. This chapter will focus on the basic mechanics of CPR and a series of related issues: the characteristics of patients who experience cardiac arrest, the physiology of external chest compression, defibrillation and drug therapy, and the outcome of resuscitative efforts.

SUDDEN CARDIAC DEATH: THE MAGNITUDE OF THE PROBLEM

More than 250,000 Americans will die suddenly this year. Although there is some disagreement over the best definition of sudden death, one fact is established beyond doubt: the shorter the interval between the onset of symptoms and death, the higher the likelihood of heart disease. In Kuller's landmark study, among patients who died within 24 hours of the onset of symptoms, approximately 60% of deaths were attributed to heart disease.[1] In another study, 91% of deaths within 1 hour of the onset of symptoms were due to heart disease.[2]

The overwhelming majority of sudden deaths are the result of acute and chronic coronary artery disease. More than half the deaths due to acute myocardial infarction occur before presentation to a hospital. An even larger number of sudden deaths are the result of advanced multivessel disease without evidence of acute infarction. Some of these patients have acute ischemia without necrosis; others have old infarcts and re-entrant ventricular tachyarrhythmias without acute ischemia.[3-5] Valvular heart disease, primary myocardial disease, and noncardiac disease, such as massive pulmonary embolism or intracranial hemorrhage, account for a relatively small number of sudden deaths.

The majority of cardiac arrest victims can be characterized with regard to one additional feature. The first recorded rhythm is most commonly a ventricular tachyarrhythmia, particularly ventricular fibrillation.[4-6] As will be discussed later, this observation supports the policy of blind defibrillation in cases in which an electrocardiograph is not immediately available.

BASIC LIFE SUPPORT

In its most basic form, CPR consists of the establishment of unresponsiveness and the ABCs of airway, breathing, and chest compression.

Unresponsiveness

Not all unresponsiveness is due to cardiac arrest. In fact, as every wary clinician knows, not all apparent unresponsiveness is even true unresponsiveness. The discomfort and potential risk of performing CPR on the nonarrested patient necessitate establishing unresponsiveness as the first step in any resuscitative effort. This can usually be ascertained by firmly shaking and shouting at the patient. If the patient does not respond, the rescuer is strongly advised to call for help or to instruct bystanders to activate the nearest available emergency medical system. Even under the best of circumstances, CPR is rarely a definitive form of therapy, and the prompt recruitment of trained and equipped personnel is critical to a successful outcome.

Airway Function

The sequence of airway, breathing, and chest compression is based on the assumption that prolonged circulation of unoxygenated blood is of no value to arrest victims. Judging from the outcome of cases of unrecognized esophageal intubation, from which death or survival with severe brain damage almost invariably ensues, this assumption seems valid. However, neither the maximal permissible delay in ventilation nor the minimal ventilatory requirements have been established for CPR. Moreover, chest compression is easily taught and remembered, whereas airway management is difficult to learn and remember, and mouth-to-mouth ventilation is specifically regarded by lay persons as a means of transmission of disease. Thus, although American Heart Association recommendations call for the establishment of ventilation prior to chest compression in single-rescuer CPR, chest compression without ventilation may be beneficial in situations in which the arrival of persons skilled in airway management is expected in 2 or 3 minutes.[7] In addition, airway obstruction should not delay chest compression when two rescuers are present.

Following confirmation of unresponsiveness, the rescuer must determine whether the patient is breathing. The rescuer can accomplish this by placing his or her ear and cheek next to the victim's mouth and nostrils. At the same time that the rescuer is listening and feeling for breathing, the rescuer can observe the victim's neck and chest wall. Movement of the diaphragm or retraction of intercostal spaces or suprasternal soft tissue without air moving through the nose or mouth suggests airway obstruction.

Because the tongue often falls back into the oropharynx in supine arrest victims, creating upper airway obstruction, it is generally advisable to position the airway at the same time that one looks, listens, and feels for breathing. The only exception to this rule is with trauma victims in whom head and facial injuries or other circumstances suggest the possibility of cervical spine fracture. In cases of suspected cervical spine injury, the jaw thrust should be used without extending the neck (see below).

Several maneuvers can be used to position the airway properly. The first and simplest of these is the head tilt (Fig. 68-1). One hand is placed under the victim's neck; the other is placed on the victim's forehead. The neck is then lifted gently while the head is tilted back. If this does not restore spontaneous breathing, the rescuer should provide mouth-to-mouth breathing or some other form of positive-pressure ventilation. High resistance to ventilation or failure of the chest wall to rise during ventilation provides presumptive evidence of airway obstruction. Obstruction of the oropharynx by the tongue is still the most likely problem, and efforts should be made to reposition the airway. If repetition of the head tilt is unsuccessful, the head tilt-chin lift may be employed. While the forehead is pressed back with one hand (as in the head tilt), the chin or lower jaw is lifted forward (Fig. 68-2). This brings the lower jaw into rough apposition with the upper jaw (without closing the mouth) and should pull the base of the tongue out of the upper airway. If the head tilt-chin lift maneuver fails to open the airway, the jaw thrust, with or without head tilt, may be used. Using both hands, the rescuer places his or her thumbs on either side of the forehead and the remaining fingers of each hand under the angles of each side of the jaw. The mandible is then displaced forward while tilting the head back or, in the case of suspected neck injury, while supporting and stabilizing the head.

Airway Obstruction

If, after all efforts to position the head and upper airway properly, ventilation is still met by high resistance and the absence of chest expansion, the rescuer must initiate another series of steps to relieve airway obstruction. The American Heart Association has issued a statement on airway obstruc-

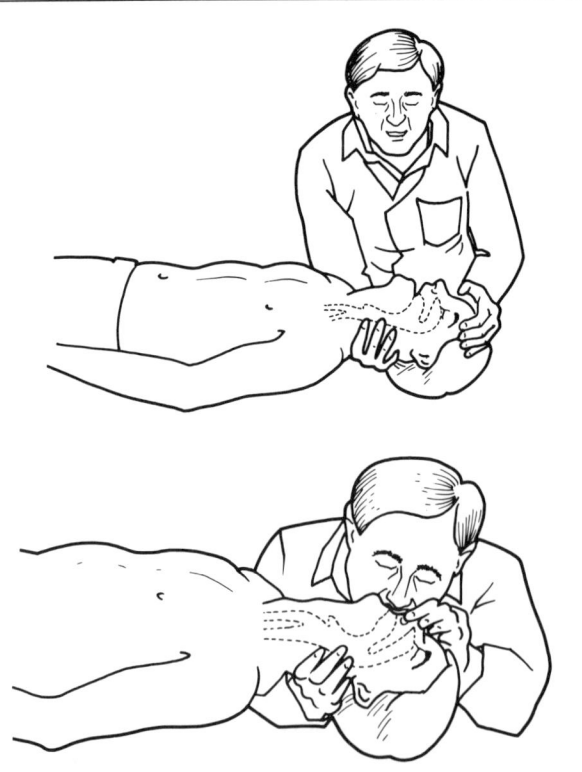

Figure 68-1 Cardiopulmonary resuscitation method 1, head tilt-neck lift.

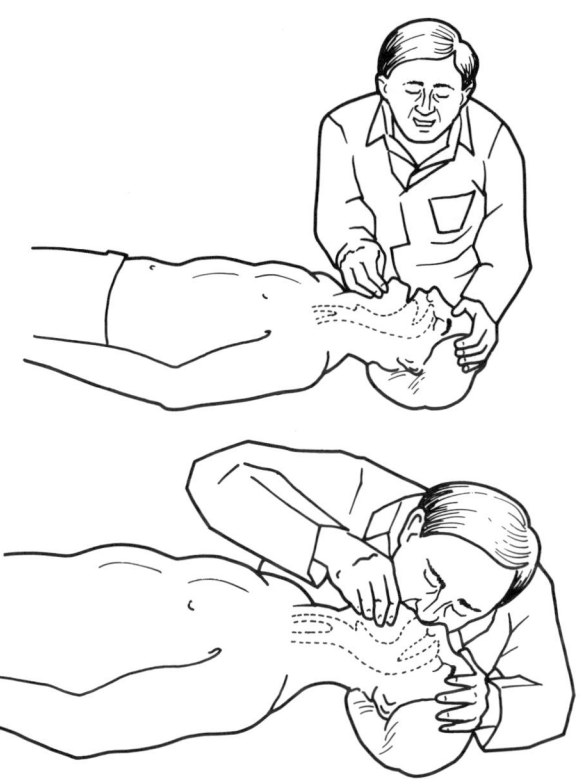

Figure 68-2 Cardiopulmonary resuscitation method 2, head tilt-chin lift.

tion that embodies several important principles but that also seems in several instances to be intended primarily for use by lay persons in an out-of-hospital setting.[8] For example, potential rescuers are advised never to place their fingers in the mouths of conscious victims of upper airway obstruction. Foreign body obstruction at the level of the oropharynx can be made worse by an unskilled hand, and the jaw muscles of an adult, capable of generating several hundred pounds of force, can inflict severe injury. While this rule is worthy of observation by lay people, it is perhaps best regarded as a general guideline by medical personnel. Intervention by persons skilled in the use of a laryngoscope, blunt forceps, and suction apparatus prior to loss of consciousness (and the profound hypoxia and respiratory acidosis it represents) would seem to be in the victim's interest. Likewise, the American Heart Association recommends that potential rescuers not interfere with efforts made by a conscious patient with an upper airway obstruction if the victim can still speak or cough forcefully. If the patient cannot speak or emits only feeble crowing sounds, the following sequence of efforts, designed to dislodge the object, raise intrathoracic pressure, and expel the foreign body, is recommended. First, using the palm of one hand, the rescuer applies four sharp blows to the back between the scapulae. These should be forceful enough to necessitate supporting the victim's chest with the other hand. If the four back blows fail, the Heimlich maneuver should be performed. Approaching the victim from behind, the rescuer places both arms around the victim's body. A fist is made with one hand, with the thumb pressed against the upper abdomen, just below the xiphoid process. The other hand grasps the first, and the rescuer abruptly and forcefully pulls both hands into the upper abdominal wall. If necessary, the Heimlich maneuver is repeated three more times. The sequence of four vigorous back blows and four Heimlich maneuvers is to be repeated until the obstruction is relieved or the patient loses consciousness. Again, these are sensible rules for nonmedical personnel but probably should not be construed as completely restricting the activity of persons trained in airway management.

The Heimlich maneuver is not used in unconscious patients with airway obstruction. Instead, the rescuer kneels beside the victim and rolls the victim on his or her side, facing the rescuer. While supporting the victim against his or her knee, the rescuer applies four back blows. Next, the victim is placed in the supine position, and the rescuer quickly delivers four abdominal thrusts. These are performed by kneeling beside the victim, putting the heel of one hand against the upper abdominal wall (just below the xiphoid process), placing the second hand on top of the first, and driving both hands under the xiphoid (ie, in a cephalad and posterior direction). Alternatively, the rescuer may deliver four chest thrusts. These are identical to the chest compressions used in cardiopulmonary resuscitation (see below) and are particularly recommended for pregnant women and the massively obese. Only after completing four back blows and four abdominal or chest thrusts in the unconscious victim is the rescuer advised to place his or her hands in the victim's mouth. The head is turned to the side, and the rescuer sweeps across the posterior oropharynx with several fingers. At this point the rescuer should reposition the airway and attempt to ventilate the victim. If the lungs are successfully aerated, the rescuer proceeds with ventilation and chest compression. If ventilation is still met with resistance, the rescuer should return to the cycle of four back blows, four abdominal or chest thrusts, and a finger sweep, followed by yet another attempt at ventilation.

Breathing

Once airway patency is established, the rescuer should take a deep breath, pinch the victim's nostrils, form a tight mouth-to-mouth seal, and forcibly exhale. This should be repeated for a total of two deep ventilations. In cases of facial trauma, it may be advisable to position the airway, close the mouth, and ventilate the victim with mouth-to-nose breathing. Although the pattern of subsequent ventilations varies according to the number of rescuers, the mechanics of ventilation remain the same. In one-rescuer CPR, two ventilations are provided after every 15 chest compressions. In two-rescuer CPR, a single ventilation is interposed between the fifth and first chest compressions of each five-beat cycle.

Chest Compression

Hemodynamics of External Compression

Kouwenhoven, Jude, and Knickerbocker, the developers of external chest compression, assumed but never actually proved that blood flows during CPR because of direct compression of the heart between the sternum and the vertebral column.[9] Despite a few early objections,[10,11] the direct cardiac compression mechanism was soon accepted and went unchallenged for more than a decade. Subsequent findings have cast doubt on the hypothesis of direct cardiac compression. First, Criley and his associates demonstrated that consciousness could be maintained for up to 40 seconds during ventricular fibrillation by rapid and vigorous coughing.[12] Second, chest compression in large animals produces increases in pressure of similar magnitude in a variety of sites throughout the thorax: right atrium, pulmonary artery, left ventricle, aorta, esophagus, and lateral pleural space.[13–16] Intrathoracic pressure is efficiently transmitted to the carotid artery, but reflux of blood (and pressure) up the jugular vein is prevented by venous valves at the thoracic inlet.[15–17] As a result, an extrathoracic arteriovenous pressure gradient is established during chest compression, and blood flows in proportion to this pressure gradient. Together, these data indicate that (1) chest compression produces a generalized elevation of intrathoracic pressure, (2) blood flows during chest compression because of the creation of extrathoracic arteriovenous pressure gradients, and (3) because there is no pressure gradient across the heart during chest compression, the heart is a conduit, not a pump, during CPR.

Despite the abundance of data demonstrating that increased intrathoracic pressure provides the motive force for blood flow during CPR in a variety of animal species, the hemodynamics of external chest compression are less well characterized in humans (Fig. 68-3). Several lines of evidence indicate that the intrathoracic pressure mechanism is operative and possibly dominant in humans as well. First, Criley's observations on cough clearly show that intrathoracic pressure fluctuations can move substantial amounts of blood. Second, the studies of Werner and his associates, who performed two-dimensional echocardiography during CPR in humans, showed that the mitral valve is open during chest compression.[18] This result is incompatible with selective compression of the left ventricle. At the same time, this is the expected result if the intrathoracic pressure mechanism is operative, because a column of blood extending from pulmonary veins to the aorta is propelled into the periphery during chest compression and the mitral valve remains open.[15] Third, several characteristics of blood pressure and flow during CPR also suggest that the intrathoracic pressure mechanism accounts for blood flow in humans.

Understanding these features of the circulation requires some theoretical considerations. First, assume that chest compression always produces cardiac compression. We will then idealize cardiac compression as a volume pump; that is, if the force of chest compression is constant, then the amount of cardiac compression and stroke volume will be constant. The behavior of such a system is analogous to the beating heart. Assuming (as seems to be the case) that preload and afterload remain constant, increased chest compression force, like increased contractility, will increase stroke volume, arterial flow, and pressure. Decreased compression force will be associated with a reduction in stroke volume, blood flow, and blood pressure. Increasing compression rate while keeping compression force constant will also raise arterial flow and pressure because a constant stroke volume will be pumped into the arterial tree at an increased frequency. Finally, arterial pressure in the volume pump system will be insensitive to the duration of chest compression because the heart will be evacuated of blood as soon as the

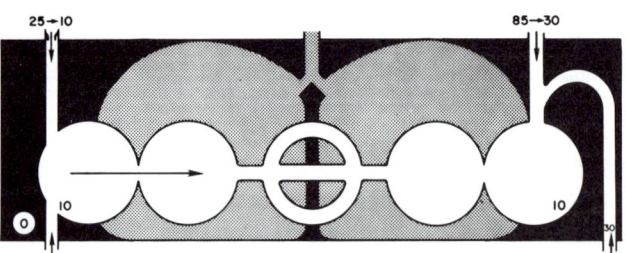
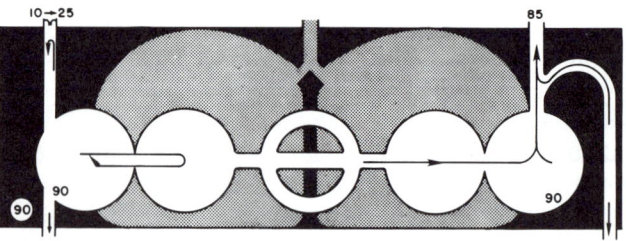

Figure 68-3 Diagrammatic representation of the hemodynamics of CPR. **A**: During chest compression, pressure in the pleural space and right and left heart rise by similar amounts. Ninety mmHg is a representative figure. Intrathoracic pressure is efficiently transmitted to the carotid artery (85 mmHg), but venous valves prevent retrograde blood flow up the jugular (10 to 25 mmHg). In response to the extrathoracic arteriovenous pressure gradient, a column of blood extending from pulmonary veins to the aorta (heavy arrow) moves toward the head. Because there are no venous valves in the inferior vena cava, substantial arteriovenous pressure gradients are not established in the abdomen, and lesser amounts of blood move down the descending aorta. Although some blood moves down the inferior vena cava, stasis predominates in the right heart and great veins. Extrathoracic jugular pressure actually increases because of antegrade flow across capillary beds while the valve remains closed. **B**: During the release phase all intrathoracic pressures fall toward zero. A large amount of blood enters the chest via the superior vena cava, and blood in the right heart moves across the lungs. Substantial amounts of blood return to the thoracic aorta from extrathoracic large arteries. This retrograde flow, together with aortic capacitance, determines aortic "diastolic" pressure.

sternum is fully depressed. Prolongation of sternal compression beyond the time necessary to achieve maximal sternal displacement will not increase blood flow.

On the other hand, if blood circulates during CPR as a result of fluctuations in intrathoracic pressure, the effects of varying compression rate and duration would be the opposite of those observed in the volume pump system. Blood flow due to increased intrathoracic pressure will be referred to as a pressure pump, and its behavior will be analyzed with respect to compression force, rate, and duration. Compression force is a major independent variable in the pressure pump system, just as in the volume pump system. However, instead of producing a predictable stroke volume, the force applied to the chest will simply pressurize the thorax. Stroke volume is a secondary phenomenon, dependent on compression force (peak pressure), duration of force (time during which blood can move in accordance with pressure gradients), peripheral resistance, and the availability of transferable blood that can be moved from the thorax into the periphery during each chest compression. A pressure pump is therefore dependent on duty cycle (the duration of compression expressed as a percentage of each compression-release cycle), that is, the amount of time during which pressurized intrathoracic blood can move into the periphery rather than the rate. Thus, both the volume pump and the pressure pump are dependent on the force of compression, but the behavior of each system varies markedly in relation to compression rate and duration.

Blood pressure and flow have been studied as a function of variable compression rates and duration in both animals and humans, and the data strongly support the intrathoracic pressure (pressure pump) hypothesis. In animal studies, blood pressure and flow are insensitive to changes in rate from a range of 40 to 150 if the duty cycle is held constant. On the other hand, blood pressure and flow are highly dependent on duty cycle. Cerebral and myocardial perfusion are maximized at duty cycles of 40% to 50%.[19] In humans, over a range of rates from 40 to 80 compressions per minute, arterial flow increased substantially as duty cycle was increased from a range of 30% to 40% up to 50% to 60%.[20] At the same time, when duty cycle was held constant, arterial pressure was unchanged when rate was increased from 60 to 150 compressions per minute.[21] These results are consistent with predictions based on the pressure pump model and incompatible with the volume pump (direct cardiac compression).

In contrast to these data, recent transesophageal echocardiographic observations indicate that direct cardiac compression occurs in at least some humans undergoing sternal compression.[21a] In view of the apparent lack of rate dependence of arterial pressure, the clinical implications of these observations are uncertain.

The renewal of interest in the physiology of blood flow during chest compression has led to a number of modifications of conventional resuscitative techniques in recent years. These include simultaneous compression-ventilation CPR,[22] vest CPR,[16,23] rapid impulse CPR,[24] the use of abdominal binding and military antishock trousers,[25,26] and abdominal counterpulsation[27] and active compression-decompression CPR.[27a] In general, these interventions attempt to increase intrathoracic pressure or manipulate arterial capacitance and resistance in an effort to improve vital organ perfusion. What is their role in resuscitation? To answer this question, two considerations must be kept in mind. First, none of these techniques has been proven superior to conventional CPR in an adequately controlled, randomized, prospective trial. Second, the intrathoracic pressure and direct cardiac compression hypotheses are not mutually exclusive. Both depend above all on vigorous chest compression. The current recommendation for rate, 80 to 100 per minute, was chosen because there is a natural tendency to compress the chest for 300 to 350 milliseconds at this rate (duty cycle 50%). This seems to provide maximal or near maximal cerebral and coronary perfusion. Departures from conventional techniques should be regarded as experimental and should not routinely be applied except where on-line measurement of central venous and arterial pressures permit immediate detection of benefit or detriment to perfusion pressure gradients and gas exchange. Because aortic and right atrial pressures increase by similar amounts during chest compression, coronary perfusion pressure gradients (mean aortic pressure less mean right atrial pressure) are small and myocardial blood flow is near zero.[13,28,29] Even under the best circumstances, when vigorous chest compression and the administration of vasoconstrictors succeed in establishing substantial aortic-right atrial "diastolic" gradients, coronary perfusion probably never exceeds ischemic thresholds.[22] As a result, most (if not all) CPR is accompanied by progressive myocardial metabolic deterioration.

Practical Aspects

Once the victim of cardiac arrest has been ventilated, the rescuer must determine whether the heart is beating effectively. The fingertips of one hand should be positioned into the groove between the cricoid cartilage (Adam's apple) and the sternomastoid muscle, and the rescuer should attempt to feel the carotid pulse. If no pulse is detected in 5 to 10 seconds, chest compression should be initiated immediately. The heel of one hand is placed over the lower half of the sternum, the second hand is placed on the first, and the chest is compressed by 1.5 to 2 in. Fifteen compressions should be delivered over the next 10 seconds, followed by two rapid ventilations, and the cycle of 15 compressions and two ventilations should be repeated.

After 1 minute of CPR and at approximately 5-minute intervals thereafter, rescuers should pause briefly and attempt to determine whether spontaneous breathing or an effective heart beat has been restored. Where doubt exists as to the effectiveness of the victim's own cardiorespiratory efforts, ventilation, external chest compression, or both should be resumed. In addition, interruptions of CPR for re-evaluation or transportation of the victim should, for obvious reasons, be kept as brief as possible. Finally, in view of the hemodynamic considerations discussed above, every effort should be made to ensure the proper depth and duration of chest compression. Except where arterial pressure increases as a function of compression rate (a result that would indicate direct cardiac compression), minor deviations from recommended compression rates do not seem to be critical and should not draw attention away from other more important mechanical and therapeutic aspects of resuscitation.

Resuscitation of Infants

In general, the approach to airway obstruction and the ABCs of CPR in infants closely resembles the resuscitation of adults. Maneuvers to relieve airway obstruction in the conscious victim should be initiated only in the presence of persistent incomplete or complete airway obstruction. Back blows remain the initial step and are delivered while supporting the head in the hand and straddling the infant over the rescuer's forearm. The head should be pointed down and four back blows applied rapidly and forcefully between the shoulder blades. If these are unsuccessful in relieving the obstruction, the infant should be rolled over so that its back is on the forearm. The head remains below the thorax, supported by the rescuer's hand. Four chest thrusts are delivered to the midsternum in the same manner as in external chest compression. The four back blows and four chest thrusts should be repeated until the obstruction is relieved or the infant loses consciousness. If the infant does lose consciousness, a finger sweep is performed at the end of each series of back blows and chest thrusts. In addition, care must be taken not to hyperextend the neck of the infant while positioning the head for positive-pressure ventilation, since hyperextension may close the airway.

As in the case of an adult, the procedure for resuscitation of an infant in cardiac arrest consists of the determination of unconsciousness and the ABCs of airway, breathing, and chest compression. Positive-pressure ventilation is best accomplished by forming a seal around the infant's mouth and nose. Two breaths are then delivered in rapid succession. The tidal volume should be sufficient to produce unequivocal expansion of the chest. For the next step, determination of pulselessness, the rescuer is advised to palpate the brachial artery, since its pulsations are generally more prominent than those of the carotid artery of infants. Chest compression is performed with two fingers depressing the midsternum by 0.5 to 1 inches while supporting the infant with the other hand and forearm. The rate of chest compression is at least 100 per minute, and one ventilation is supplied for every fifth chest compression without slowing the cadence. As in the case of cardiac arrest in adults, it is advisable to re-evaluate the victim at the end of the first minute of CPR and periodically thereafter.

ADVANCED CARDIAC LIFE SUPPORT

Detailed discussion of advanced cardiac life support (ACLS) is beyond the scope of this chapter, and the interested reader is referred to the American Heart Association's *Textbook of Advanced Cardiac Life Support*.[30,31] This section will therefore focus on several aspects of defibrillation and drug therapy and on the approach to several common dysrhythmias.

Defibrillation

Ventricular tachyarrhythmias, particularly ventricular fibrillation, account for most inpatient and outpatient cardiac arrests.[32] Defibrillation has been shown repeatedly to be the single most effective treatment in the entire armamentarium of ACLS.[7,33] Since even the most vigorous CPR is accompanied by progressive myocardial ischemia and since two or three defibrillatory discharges are not known to be harmful to arrested patients with bradyarrhythmias, defibrillation should be performed without delay in cases of cardiac arrest in which an electrocardiograph is not immediately available.[34]

The purpose of electrical countershock in any tachyarrhythmia is to depolarize the heart synchronously. In this way the tachycardia is interrupted and an opportunity is created for uniform repolarization of the heart and subsequent re-emergence of normal pacemaker activity. In practice, the amount of energy required to accomplish this depends on the actual rhythm, the size of the patient, the size of the heart, the metabolic status of the myocardium, and the ionic and pharmacologic milieu that surround the heart.

Several points must be observed if countershock is to be safe and successful. First, paddles should be placed on the chest in such a way as to maximize current flow through the heart. The usual approach is to place one paddle at the right upper sternal border and the other slightly inferolateral to the cardiac apex. An acceptable alternative is anterior-posterior paddle placement. The anterior paddle is placed over the left precordium, and the posterior paddle is positioned along the inferomedial portion of either scapula. In this way current moves directly through the heart in its route from the charged to the ground paddle. Firm pressure (approximately 5 kg) and sufficient electrolyte gel should be applied to each paddle to minimize the electrical resistance of the skin. Saline-soaked pads have a higher resistance but are still an effective alternative to electrolyte gel. Isopropyl alcohol, frequently (and inappropriately) used to establish contact between leads and skin for electrocardiographic recordings, should never be used as a conductive medium for countershock.

Resistance through alcohol is high, and the heat generated by the electrical discharge may cause fire or an explosion.

Several other rules govern the use of a defibrillator. First, synchronization of electrical discharge to R waves is vital to the safe termination of supraventricular tachyarrhythmias and is recommended for the termination of ventricular tachycardia. The advantage of synchronization is that it avoids electrical discharge on the T wave, when dispersion of refractoriness could allow re-entry at the ventricular level and consequent worsening of the arrhythmia to ventricular tachycardia or ventricular fibrillation. At the same time, it must be remembered that a defibrillator set in the synchronization mode will not discharge during ventricular fibrillation, for there are no R waves for the device to sense, a prerequisite to discharge. This also means that a charged defibrillator set in the asynchronous mode can be discharged immediately, whereas a fully charged defibrillator in the synchronous mode requires one or two R-R intervals to identify R waves.

Drug Therapy

The successful management of most cardiac arrests requires consideration of the deranged circulatory physiology during CPR and of the specific properties of the drugs that are used. Delivery of drugs from peripheral or central intravenous access sites to the heart and systemic arteries requires 1 to 2 minutes, a time frame that must be kept in mind when assessing drug effects or initiating therapies dependent on drug effect. In addition, several drugs, particularly epinephrine and lidocaine, can be administered through an endotracheal tube if intravenous access has not been secured. The recommended dose for endotracheal administration of drugs is 2 to 2.5 times the intravenous dose diluted in 10 mL of distilled water or normal saline.

Catecholamines

Catecholamines are used during cardiac arrest for their positive chronotropic, positive dromotropic, and positive inotropic effects. The use of drugs with potent β-adrenergic effects, such as epinephrine, in patients with severe bradyarrhythmias or electromechanical dissociation thus speaks for itself. Less obvious but more important are the peripheral vasoconstrictive effects of epinephrine in cardiac arrest. In high doses, epinephrine reduces blood flow to nonessential vascular beds, raises aortic and carotid pressure, increases myocardial and cerebral perfusion, and increases survival from experimental cardiac arrest.[22,35–37] β-Adrenergic blockade has no influence on the salutary effects of epinephrine, whereas α-adrenergic blockade abolishes the benefit of epinephrine.[38]

These observations raise important questions about the optimal dose of epinephrine or alternative sympathomimetics in cardiac arrest. The current American Heart Association guidelines call for the use of 1.0 mg of epinephrine at 3- to 5-minute intervals in patients requiring CPR to support their circulation. In two randomized clinical trials, higher doses of epinephrine did not improve either survival or neurologic status in adult victims of cardiac arrest.[39,40] Nevertheless, higher doses of epinephrine (0.1 mg/kg) are permitted later in arrest, on the grounds that if 1 mg of epinephrine fails to promote resuscitation early in arrest, it is even less likely to promote resuscitation later in the arrest, when acidosis and ischemia are more severe.

Recognition of the role of intense α-adrenergic stimulation in the generation of coronary and cerebral perfusion pressure had led to interest in the use of pure or predominant α-agonists such as phenylephrine or methoxamine as a substitute for epinephrine, particularly in fibrillatory arrest, in which the β effects of epinephrine are known to increase myocardial oxygen demand.[41] These studies have not demonstrated the superiority of phenylephrine over epinephrine, however, and there is some suggestion that methoxamine may be less effective than epinephrine.[42,43] Therefore, epinephrine remains the pressor of choice during cardiac arrest.

Antiarrhythmics

Four drugs (lidocaine, bretylium, procainamide, and atropine) occupy a central position in the pharmacologic approach to resuscitation. Lidocaine offers the dual advantages of efficacy in the treatment of ventricular tachyarrhythmias and ease of administration. It should be given as an initial bolus of 1 mg/kg, followed by 0.5 mg/kg at 8-minute intervals up to a total dose of 3 mg/kg. Like the loading regimen for conscious patients (1 mg/kg at 8-minute intervals up to a total of 3 mg/kg), the loading regimen for lidocaine provides therapeutic serum levels as soon as the first dose is administered. However, it differs from the regimen for conscious patients in two important ways. The regimen is slower because the distributive phase of lidocaine is prolonged during cardiac arrest.[44] In addition, since hepatic blood flow is negligible during CPR,[22] lidocaine metabolism may be ignored. Once a patient is fully loaded with lidocaine, the patient will remain fully loaded as long as cardiac arrest persists. A lidocaine infusion is therefore unnecessary during cardiac arrest but should be started if lidocaine promotes resuscitation.

Bretylium tosylate first promotes and then blocks norepinephrine release from postganglionic neurons. The net effect is a reduction of the dispersion of refractoriness of cardiac tissue.[45] For patients in cardiac arrest, bretylium can be administered as a 500-mg or a 7-mg/kg bolus, followed by 1 g every 10 minutes up to a total of 2.5 g. It should be given slowly to conscious patients, such as those with nonhypotensive ventricular tachycardia, because bolus administration may cause nausea and vomiting.

Bretylium appears to be as effective as lidocaine in cardiac arrest,[46,47] but is considered a second-line drug because it reduces blood pressure, complicating postarrest care. If bretylium is to be given in cardiac arrest, it should probably be given early, for it has a slow onset of action.

Procainamide, which slows conduction velocity and prolongs refractoriness, is also effective in the treatment of ventricular tachycardia and ventricular fibrillation. Doses of 100 mg can be administered over 2 to 3 minutes every 5 minutes up to a total of 1 g. Hypotension and prolongation of QRS duration by 50% constitute alternative end points. Procainamide can also be administered by continuous intravenous infusion; 2 to 4 mg/min is the usual dose range.

The vagolytic effects of atropine make it useful in severe supraventricular bradyarrhythmias and atrioventricular block due to conduction block in the AV node. Atropine may also be helpful in asystole. Two milligrams is a complete parasympatholytic dose. In full arrest situations, it is recommended that atropine be given in 1-mg boluses at 5-minute intervals. In conscious patients with heart block, smaller doses are preferred. As many as four 0.5-mg doses, spaced at 5-minute intervals, may be given.

Magnesium sulfate (2 g IV) may reduce mortality in acute myocardial infarction and is effective in undulating ventricular tachycardia (torsades de pointes) with prolonged QT interval. It is not effective in torsades de pointes without prolongation of the QT interval.[31]

Propranolol, not frequently called for in cardiac arrest, should be considered in one special situation. When acute myocardial ischemia is complicated by recurrent ventricular fibrillation or tachycardia refractory to conventional antiarrhythmics, intravenous propranolol may be effective. Increments of 1 mg may be given intravenously every 1 to 2 minutes up to a total of 0.1 mg/kg (or 10 mg). Severe left ventricular failure between episodes of fibrillation constitutes a contraindication to this approach.

Sodium Bicarbonate

Although metabolic acidosis, which invariably accompanies prolonged cardiac arrest, depresses contractile performance and reduces the ventricular fibrillation threshold,[48,49] sodium bicarbonate has had no effect on outcome from resuscitation in studies in which coronary perfusion pressure has been controlled.[50–52] This failure is due to the inability of the small amounts of bicarbonate that can be delivered to the heart to reverse the intense intracellular acidosis.[52a,52b,53]

Moderate hyperventilation is the preferred treatment for mild to moderate metabolic acidosis accompanying cardiac arrest. Use of sodium bicarbonate is permitted, but its use should be guided by arterial blood gas determinations whenever possible. The total dosage probably should not exceed 2 mEq/kg.[54,55]

Arrhythmias

Ventricular Fibrillation

In cases of monitored ventricular fibrillation, a precordial blow should be delivered immediately. If the blow fails to defibrillate the patient or if the arrest is unmonitored, help should be summoned and CPR should be performed only long enough to obtain a defibrillator. The patient should be given nonsynchronized precordial countershock starting at 200 J. If this fails to restore an adequate rhythm or if no monitoring is available and the patient remains pulseless and unresponsive, a 300-J shock should be delivered immediately. If the second shock fails, a 400-J shock should be administered. If this fails, CPR should be reinstituted and intravenous access obtained. Epinephrine should be given as soon as possible. One to 3 minutes later defibrillation should be attempted again with 400 J. If this fails, the patient should receive a loading dose of lidocaine and/or bretylium. Epinephrine and bicarbonate should be given according to the recommendations outlined in the previous section. Defibrillation with 400 J should be repeated after each pharmacologic intervention.

Ventricular Tachycardia

The approach to ventricular tachycardia is similar to that for ventricular fibrillation, with the exceptions that conscious patients should be sedated prior to cardioversion, lower energy levels often suffice, and antiarrhythmic therapy sometimes precedes cardioversion. As in ventricular fibrillation, a precordial thump is recommended as the initial step for all patients, conscious or unconscious. The thump often converts ventricular tachycardia to sinus rhythm but may also induce ventricular fibrillation. Thus, if the patient is conscious and tolerating the rhythm, it is probably best to defer the chest thump until a defibrillator is available. For conscious patients, lidocaine is generally preferred because the first dose (1 mg/kg) can be delivered over 30 to 60 seconds and because most patients can receive a loading dose within 10 minutes. Providing a conscious patient with a starting dose of bretylium takes 8 to 10 minutes, whereas providing a loading dose of procainamide to a patient may take more than 30 minutes; consequently, bretylium and procainamide are considered second-line agents by most authorities. Time should be taken to sedate patients who remain conscious but who do not tolerate the tachycardia (eg, the development of pulmonary edema) prior to cardioversion.

As in the case of ventricular fibrillation, immediate precordial countershock with 200 J is recommended for unconscious patients in ventricular tachycardia. If the patient has a pulse and if blood pressure is higher than that which can ordinarily be obtained with CPR, the therapeutic strategy consists of rapid loading with antiarrhythmic medications and repeated countershocks. If the patient is pulseless or profoundly hypotensive, the approach is exactly the same as that for ventricular fibrillation: CPR, epinephrine, antiarrhythmics, and repeated attempts at electrical cardioversion.

Asystole

As a rule, asystole is a manifestation of the most extreme forms of acute and chronic heart disease and, with the exception of asphyxial arrests, mortality approaches 100%. The therapeutic approach consists of direct chronotropic stimulation with catecholamines, vagolytic medication (atropine), and, if appropriate, transvenous or transthoracic pacing. The goal of these interventions is the stimulation of electrical activity accompanied by effective mechanical activity. Epinephrine, 1 mg or more every 5 minutes, is the preferred drug because it is a potent vasoconstrictor as well as a potent chronotrope. As such, it will maximize coronary perfusion during CPR while stimulating cardiac pacemaking tissues. Because excess vagal tone rarely causes prolonged suppression of cardiac pacemaker tissues, atropine is not the mainstay of therapy. Nevertheless, it may be helpful and should be given in a fully vagolytic dose (ie, 2 mg over 5 to 10 minutes). Sodium bicarbonate may be given according to the guidelines discussed under "Drug Therapy." As in the case of ventricular tachyarrhythmias, CPR is not ordinarily a definitive therapy for asystole. Although vigorous chest compression and effective ventilation are essential to a successful outcome, their role is to support the circulation while drug therapy or pacing is instituted. When asystole is due to complete heart block, the ventricles may contract in response to chest thumps. "Thump pacing" may be effective until temporary pacing can be established. Also, fine ventricular fibrillation can masquerade as asystole. Thus, when asystole does not respond to the usual measures, at least one attempt at defibrillation should be considered.

Electromechanical Dissociation

Electromechanical dissociation is a condition in which cardiac electrical activity is present but effective mechanical activity is totally or virtually absent. Ventricular rates are often low, but, by definition, the hypotension is out of proportion to the heart rate. When electromechanical dissociation is myocardial in origin, successful resuscitation is unusual. Consequently, the diagnosis of electromechanical dissociation should prompt a search for more treatable, extramyocardial causes. These include airway obstruction, cardiac tamponade, tension pneumothorax, severe hypovolemia (almost always due to hemorrhage), massive pulmonary embolism, and possibly severe acidosis. Treatment therefore consists of CPR plus the following: (1) careful evaluation of ventilation and oxygenation, (2) administration of epinephrine and perhaps sodium bicarbonate and calcium chloride, (3) consideration of volume infusion, and (4) consideration of pericardiocentesis. Although tension pneumothorax requires a chest tube, the lung can usually be temporarily decompressed by inserting a small needle (eg, 20 or 22 gauge) into the pleural space. Epinephrine is used for its positive inotropic and vasoconstrictive effects. Any use of bicarbonate should be accompanied by aggressive ventilation to prevent further depression of contractility by the carbon dioxide that is generated. Calcium chloride (10%), another positive inotrope, can be given in a dose of 5 to 10 mL every 5 minutes but has never been shown to affect the long-term outcome from routine arrest situations. It may be of value in patients with suspected overdose of calcium channel blockers, hyperkalemia, or recent massive blood transfusion. In the latter case, the citrate anticoagulant in transfused blood binds calcium-depressing ventricular function. In cases in which a patient's intravascular volume status is unknown, it is probably well to give at least 500 to 1000 mL of normal saline during resuscitative efforts. Finally, pericardiocentesis can be accomplished by inserting a long needle into the subxiphoid area and directing it toward the left shoulder at a 30° to 45° angle to the skin. The needle should be advanced under suction until fluid (blood or effusion) is withdrawn. At least 40 mL should be removed and the patient reassessed. In view of the high mortality rate in electromechanical dissociation, clinicians should never hesitate to attempt early pericardiocentesis when tamponade is a reasonable diagnostic possibility.

MISCELLANEOUS CONSIDERATIONS

Postresuscitation Dysrhythmias

Virtually any rhythm may follow resuscitation. Of these, sinus tachycardia is perhaps the most common and is usually an appropriate physiologic response to the acidosis, catecholamine excess, and depressed cardiac performance of the arrest. It usually resolves after a short time and is usually best left alone. The approach to sinus tachycardia illustrates a key point in the treatment of postresuscitation arrhythmias: effective management requires consideration of the underlying cause and clinical significance of the specific rhythm disturbance.

When patients are resuscitated from ventricular tachyarrhythmias, one or more antiarrhythmics should be given until the inciting event has resolved or the patient's condition has stabilized.

Open Chest Massage

Open chest massage is a more effective means of circulating blood than is external chest compression,[56,57] but this superiority must be weighed against the morbidity of emergency thoracotomy under incompletely sterile conditions. Open chest massage should be considered in young, witnessed arrest victims who have not responded to brief periods of basic and advanced life support—that is, patients likely to be in good overall health who have not sustained irreversible brain damage.

Is Resuscitation Worthwhile?

The widespread application of resuscitative techniques has led to public concern over the possibility of meaningless prolongation of the lives of large numbers of cardiac arrest victims. In fact, the record of resuscitation is a remarkable success story, and the number of patients who linger on in vegetative states is quite small. In a comparison of outcomes among areas with different levels of out-of-hospital support, only 6% of patients attended to by emergency medical technicians (who performed only CPR) were discharged alive. By contrast, the discharge rate was 22% among arrest victims cared for by paramedics authorized to defibrillate, intubate, and administer drugs. Response times were similar for both groups. In a follow-up study, conversion of rescue services from emergency medical technician to paramedic level reduced time from collapse to delivery of definitive therapy from an average of 27.5 to 7.7 minutes. Short-term survival (ie, hospital admission) increased from 19% to 34%, and long-term survival (ie, hospital discharge) increased from 7% to 17% ($P < .01$ for both). For ventricular fibrillation, discharge rates rose from 15% to 28% ($P < .05$).[58] Thus, on-the-scene delivery of definitive care has been shown to be of vital importance. At the same time, the provision of basic life support by lay persons also can improve survival. In Ohio, when CPR was initiated by bystanders, hospital discharge rates increased from 8% to 36%. In Seattle, bystander initiation of CPR raised long-term survival rates from 21% to 43%.[59] Whereas 21 of 38 patients who survived cardiac arrest without bystander CPR had obvious neurologic deficits, only 1 of 27 survivors of bystander-initiated CPR had gross deficits. Indeed, in Seattle, if an arrest was witnessed, if CPR was initiated by a bystander, if paramedics arrived within 4 minutes of collapse, and if the initial rhythm was ventricular fibrillation, approximately 70% of victims were long-term survivors.[60]

Among hospitalized patients, where survival correlates with severity of illness and with probability of long-term survival independent of the index arrest, resuscitation rates are somewhat lower. Nevertheless, short-term survival rates in excess of 40% are commonly reported, and hospital discharge rates may exceed 10%. The median survival time for those who were short-term survivors was only 6 days in one study (ie, patients destined to die did not languish in intensive care units or chronic care facilities for excessive periods), whereas approximately 80% of long-term survivors were alive 6 months later.[32] In three quarters of these patients, memory was intact. In a review of the Seattle experience, 81% of long-term survivors were reported as alive at 6 months and 49% at 4 years. This latter figure compares with 4-year survival rates of 80% for age-adjusted controls and 66% for age-adjusted infarct survivors. Ninety percent of long-term survivors were able to return home, and nearly three quarters of those working prior to arrest were able to return to work.[60] Thus, CPR and allied measures, if promptly and properly applied, have saved and should continue to save the lives of thousands of people annually without burdening society with a massive load of agonizing and costly disability.

REFERENCES

1. Kuller L. Sudden and unexpected non-traumatic deaths in adults: a review of epidemiological and clinical studies. *J Chronic Dis.* 1966; 18:1165–1192.
2. Spain DM, Bradess VA, Mohr C. Coronary atherosclerosis as a cause of unexpected and unexplained death. *JAMA.* 1960;174:384–388.
3. Perper JA, Kuller LH, Cooper M. Arteriosclerosis of coronary arteries in sudden, unexpected death. *Circulation.* 1975;52(suppl 3):27–33.
4. Liberthson RR, Nagel EL, Hirschman JC, et al. Pathophysiologic observations in prehospital ventricular fibrillation and sudden cardiac death. *Circulation.* 1974;49:790–797.
5. Reichenbach D, Moss N, Meyer E. Pathology of the heart in sudden cardiac death. *Am J Cardiol.* 1977;39:865–872.
6. Bigger JT, Dresdale RJ, Heissenbuttel RH, et al. Ventricular arrhythmias in ischemic heart disease: mechanism, prevalence, significance, and management. *Prog Cardiovasc Dis.* 1977;19:255–300.
7. Cobb LA, Hallstrom AP. Community based cardiopulmonary resuscitation. *Ann NY Acad Sci.* 1982;382:330–341.
8. *First Aid for Foreign Body Obstruction of the Airway.* Dallas, Tex: American Heart Association; 1976.
9. Kouwenhoven WB, Jude JR, Knickerbocker GG. Closed-chest cardiac massage. *JAMA.* 1960;73:1064–1067.
10. Weale FE, Rothwell-Jackson RL. The efficiency of cardiac massage. *Lancet.* 1962;1:990–992.
11. MacKenzie GJ, Taylor SH, McDonald AH, et al. Hemodynamic effects of external cardiac compression. *Lancet.* 1964;1:1342–1345.
12. Criley JM, Blaufuss AH, Kissel GL. Cough-induced cardiac compression. *JAMA.* 1976;236:1246–1250.
13. Rudikoff MT, Maughan WL, Effron M, et al. Mechanisms of blood flow during cardiopulmonary resuscitation. *Circulation.* 1980; 61:258–265.
14. Chandra N, Guerci A, Weisfeldt ML, et al. Contrasts between intrathoracic pressures during external chest compression and cardiac massage. *Crit Care Med.* 1981;9:789–792.
15. Niemann JT, Roseborough JR, Hausknecht M, et al. Pressure synchronized cineangiography during experimental cardiopulmonary resuscitation. *Circulation.* 1981;64:985–991.
16. D'Agostini E. Mechanics of the pleural space. *Physiol Rev.* 1972; 52:57–128.
17. Yin FCP, Cohen JM, Tsitlik J, et al. Role of carotid artery resistance to collapse during high intrathoracic pressure CPR. *Am J Physiol.* 1982; 243:H285–H287.
18. Werner JA, Greene HL, Janko CL, et al. Visualization of cardiac valve motion during external chest compression using two-dimensional echocardiography. *Circulation.* 1981;63:1417–1423.
19. Halperin HR, Tsitlik JE, Guerci A, et al. Optimization of myocardial and cerebral flow during cardiopulmonary resuscitation. *J Am Coll Cardiol.* 1984;3:595. Abstract.

20. Taylor GJ, Tucker WM, Greene HL, et al. Importance of prolonged compression during cardiopulmonary resuscitation. *N Engl J Med.* 1977;296:1515–1517.
21. Halperin HR, Tsitlik JE, Guerci AD, et al. Determinants of blood flow to vital organs during cardiopulmonary resuscitation in dogs. *Circulation.* 1986;73:539–550.
21a. Tucker KJ, Cohen TJ, Redberg RF, Schiller NB, Callaham ML. Active compression-decompression resuscitation: effect on left ventricular volume and transmitral flow (abstract). *Circulation.* 1992;86:I234.
22. Michael JR, Guerci AD, Koehler RC, et al. Mechanisms by which epinephrine augments cerebral and myocardial perfusion during cardiopulmonary resuscitation in dogs. *Circulation.* 1984;69:822–835.
23. Halperin H, Guerci A, Chandra N. Vest inflation without simultaneous ventilation during cardiac arrest in dogs: improved survival from prolonged cardiopulmonary resuscitation. *Circulation.* 1986;74:1407–1415.
24. Maier GW, Tyson GS, Olsen CO, et al. The physiology of external cardiac massage: high impulse cardiopulmonary resuscitation. *Circulation.* 1984;70:86–101.
25. Koehler RC, Chandra N, Guerci AD, et al. Augmentation of cerebral perfusion by simultaneous chest compression and lung inflation with abdominal binding after cardiac arrest in dogs. *Circulation.* 1983;67:266–275.
26. Mahoney BD, Mirick MJ. Efficacy of pneumatic trousers in refractory prehospital cardiopulmonary arrest. *Ann Emerg Med.* 1983;12:8–12.
27. Sack JB, Kesselbrenner MB, Bregman D. Survival from in-hospital cardiac arrest with interposed adbominal counterpulsation during cardiopulmonary resuscitation. *JAMA.* 1992;267:379–385.
27a. Cohen TJ, Tucker KJ, Lurie KG, et al. Active compression-decompression: a new method of cardiopulmonary resuscitation. *JAMA.* 1992;267:2916–2923.
28. Ditchey RV, Winkler JV, Rhodes CA. Relative lack of coronary blood flow during closed chest resuscitation in dogs. *Circulation.* 1982;66:297–302.
29. Chandra N, Weisfeldt ML, Tsitlik J, et al. Augmentation of carotid flow during cardiopulmonary resuscitation by ventilation at high airway pressure simultaneously with chest compression. *Am J Cardiol.* 1981;48:1053–1063.
29a. Paradis HA, Martin GB, Rivers EP, et al. Coronary perfusion pressure and the return of spontaneous circulation in human cardiopulmonary resuscitation. *JAMA.* 1990;263:1106–1113.
30. *Textbook of Advanced Cardiac Life Support.* 2nd ed. Dallas, Tex: American Heart Association; 1987.
31. Guidelines for cardiopulmonary resuscitation and emergency cardiac care. *JAMA.* 1992;268:2171–2299.
32. Bedell SE, Delbanes TL, Cook EF, et al. Survival after cardiopulmonary resuscitation. *N Engl J Med.* 1983;309:569–576.
33. Eisenberg M, Bergner L, Hallstram A. Paramedic programs and out-of-hospital cardiac arrest: factors associated with successful resuscitation. *Am J Public Health.* 1979;69:30–38.
34. Grace WJ, Nolte CJ. Blind defibrillation. In: *Proceedings of the National Conference on Standards for CPR and Emergency Cardiac Care.* May 1973:67–68.
35. Pearson JW, Redding JS. Influence of peripheral vascular tone on cardiac resuscitation. *Anesth Analg.* 1965;44:746–750.
36. Redding JS, Pearson JW. Evaluation of drugs for cardiac resuscitation. *Anesthesiology.* 1963;24:203–207.
37. Pearson JW, Redding JS. The role of epinephrine in cardiac resuscitation. *Anesth Analg.* 1963;42:599–606.
38. Yakaitis RW, Oho CW, Blitt CD. Relative importance of alpha and beta adrenergic receptors during resuscitation. *Crit Care Med.* 1979;7:293–296.
39. Stiell IG, Hebert PC, Weitzman BN, et al. High dose epinephrine in cardiac arrest. *N Engl J Med.* 1992;327:1045–1050.
40. Brown CG, Martin DR, Pepe PE, et al. A comparison of standard-dose and high-dose epinephrine in cardiac arrest outside the hospital. *N Engl J Med.* 1992;327:1051–1055.
41. Ditchey RV, Lindenfeld J. Failure of epinephrine to improve the balance between myocardial oxygen supply and demand during closed chest resuscitation in dogs. *Circulation.* 1988;78:382–389.
42. Kronenberg MW, McCain RW, Boncek RJ, et al. Effects of methoxamine and phenylephrine on left ventricular contractility in rabbits. *J Am Coll Cardiol.* 1989;14:1350–1358.
43. Brown CG, Taylor RB, Werman HA, et al. Myocardial oxygen delivery/consumption during cardiopulmonary resuscitation: a comparison of epinephrine and phenylephrine. *Ann Emerg Med.* 1988;17:302–308.
44. Chow MSS, Ronfeld RA, Ruffett D, et al. Lidocaine pharmacokinetics during cardiac arrest and external cardiopulmonary resuscitation. *Am Heart J.* 1981;102:799–802.
45. Koch-Weser J. Drug therapy: bretylium. *N Engl J Med.* 1979;300:473–477.
46. Haynes RE, Chinn TL, Copass MK, et al. Comparison of bretylium tosylate and lidocaine in the management of out of hospital ventricular fibrillation: a randomized clinical trial. *Am J Cardiol.* 1981;48:353–356.
47. Olson DW, Thompson BM, Darin JC, et al. A randomized comparison study of bretylium tosylate and lidocaine in resuscitation of patients from out-of-hospital ventricular fibrillation in a paramedic system. *Ann Emerg Med.* 1984;13:807–810.
48. Gerst PH, Fleming WH, Maln JR. Increased susceptibility of the heart to ventricular fibrillation during metabolic acidosis. *Circ Res.* 1966;19:63–70.
49. Cingolani HE, Faulkner SL, Mattiazzi AR, et al. Depression of human myocardial contractility with "respiratory" and "metabolic" acidosis. *Surgery.* 1975;77:427–432.
50. Guerci AD, Chandra N, Johnson E, et al. Failure of sodium bicarbonate to improve resuscitation from ventricular fibrillation in dogs. *Circulation.* 1986;74(4):75–79.
51. von Planta M, Gudipati C, Weil MH, Kraus LJ, Rackow EC. Effects of trometamine and sodium bicarbonate buffers during cardiac resuscitation. *J Clin Pharmacol.* 1988;28:594–599.
52. Gazmuri RJ, von Planta M, Weil MH, Rackow EC. Cardiac effects of carbon dioxide-consuming and carbon dioxide-generating buffers during cardiopulmonary resuscitation. *J Am Coll Cardiol.* 1990;15:482–490.
52a. von Planta M, Weil MH, Gazmuri RJ, Bisera J, Rackow EC. Myocardial acidosis associated with CO_2 production during cardiac arrest and resuscitation. *Circulation.* 1989;80:684–692.
52b. Kette F, Weil MH, von Planta M, Gazmuri RJ, Rackow EC. Buffer agents do not reverse intramyocardial acidosis during cardiac resuscitation. *Circulation.* 1990;81:1660–1666.
53. Weisfeldt ML, Bishop RL, Greene HL. Effects of pH and pCO_2 on performance of ischemic myocardium. In: Roy PE, Rona G, eds. *Recent Advances in Studies on Cardiac Structure and Metabolism.* Baltimore, Md: University Park Press; 1975:10.
54. Bishop RL, Weisfeldt ML. Sodium bicarbonate administration during cardiac arrest: effect on arterial pH, PCO_2, and osmolality. *JAMA.* 1976;235:506–509.
55. Mattar JA, Weil MH, Shubin H, et al. Cardiac arrest in the critically ill, II: hyperosmolal states following cardiac arrest. *Am J Med.* 1974;56:162–168.
56. Weiser FM, Adler LN, Kuhn LA. Hemodynamic effects of closed and open chest cardiac resuscitation in normal dogs and those with acute myocardial infarction. *Am J Cardiol.* 1962;10:555–561.

57. Del Guercio LR, Feins NR, Cohn JD, et al. Comparison of blood flow during external and internal cardiac massage in man. *Circulation*. 1965;31(suppl 1):171–180.
58. Thompson RG, Hallstram AP, Cobb LA. Bystander initiated cardiopulmonary resuscitation in the management of ventricular fibrillation. *Ann Intern Med*.1979;90:737–740.
59. Eisenberg M, Hallstrom A, Bergner L. The ACLS score: predicting survival from out-of-hospital cardiac arrest. *JAMA*. 1981;246:50–52.
60. Cobb LS, Baum RS, Alvarez H. Resuscitation from out-of-hospital ventricular fibrillation: four year follow-up. *Circulation*. 1975;52 (suppl 3):223–228.

69. Dyspnea and Pulmonary Edema

GEORGE L. STERNBACH, MD, FACEP

DYSPNEA

Shortness of breath or difficulty in breathing is a symptom of a variety of illnesses and conditions. The cause of dyspnea may be primarily respiratory, cardiac, neuromuscular, metabolic (eg, acidosis), hematologic (anemia), or psychogenic (primary hyperventilation) (see Table 69-1). The stage at which dyspnea is experienced varies from individual to individual. In a person with normal breathing capacity, a large increase in ventilation may be required to produce dyspnea. On the other hand, a relatively small ventilatory increase from the normal state may induce shortness of breath in an individual with a low breathing capacity.

Patients can experience dyspnea even when 70% of their maximum breathing capacity is not in use.[1] Dyspnea results from increased respiratory work and respiratory muscle dysfunction. The elastic resistance of the lung to stretch, airway resistance to gas flow, and tissue friction must be overcome in the work of breathing. At normal respiratory rates, elastic resistance is the most significant of these factors; at rates higher than 15 breaths per minute, however, resistance to flow in the airways assumes greater importance.

When muscular work is increased, the amount of oxygen required is increased. The oxygen costs of breathing itself increase disproportionately with increased ventilation. The resting state oxygen requirement may be trebled in patients who are tachypneic as a result of pulmonary vascular congestion.

Of the systemic stimuli to the respirator control center, the most profound is arterial CO_2 tension. An increase in P_{CO_2} of 1.5 mmHg from the normal level of 40 may cause a doubling of ventilation. Other factors that significantly influence ventilation are pH and arterial oxygen tension. Dyspnea in patients with chronic respiratory disease is well correlated with breathing reserve, which is the amount of ventilatory capacity available in excess of actual ventilation. The patient with pulmonary edema experiences dyspnea for a variety of reasons, even when breathing reserve is well maintained.

Assessment of the patient with respiratory distress is frequently a challenging process, and a certain degree of flexibility is required. The approach to the dyspneic patient involves a systematic assessment. Assurance of a patent airway, assistance of ventilation, and application of oxygen are initial priorities. Such interventions always take precedence over diagnostic assessment and need to be instituted before detailed evaluation is undertaken.

Rapid history taking and directed physical examination are the starting points for establishing the diagnosis. The history should include details of the rapidity of onset and the duration of dyspnea, the inciting events (such as inhalation of toxic substances), and prior respiratory illness. The presence of associated symptoms such as fever, cough, and sputum production should be determined.

The application of a transcutaneous oximeter is useful to provide continuous monitoring of the patient with respiratory difficulty, this being a noninvasive method of assessing hemoglobin saturation. The determinations of hemoglobin saturation obtained by transcutaneous oximetry compare closely to arterial saturation. Levels of 91% correspond roughly to a Pa_{O_2} of 60 mmHg. Saturation levels of 85% and below reflect severe hypoxemia.[2]

Table 69-1 Causes of Dyspnea

Airway Obstruction
  angioedema
  croup
  epiglottitis
  bacterial tracheitis
  tumor
  foreign body
Respiratory Cause
  aspiration
  asthma
  COPD exacerbation
  thoracic trauma
  pneumonia
  pneumothorax
  pleural effusion
  adult respiratory distress syndrome
  malignancy
  toxic inhalation
Cardiovascular Cause
  congestive heart failure
  cardiac tamponade
  coronary ischemia
  cardiac dysrhythmia
  pulmonary embolism
Neuromuscular Cause
  amyotrophic lateral sclerosis
  Guillain-Barré syndrome
  myasthenia gravis
Metabolic Cause
  metabolic acidosis
  anaphylaxis
  hyperthyroidism
  sepsis
  shock
  salicylate intoxication
Hematologic Cause
  anemia
Psychogenic Cause
  primary hyperventilation syndrome

Measurement of arterial blood gases is frequently necessary in the evaluation of patients presenting to the emergency department with dyspnea. For those with severe respiratory distress or dyspnea of uncertain origin, blood gases should be performed. Patients with antecedent cardiac or respiratory disease presenting with dyspnea should also have blood gas analysis.

The alveolar-arterial (A-a) oxygen gradient may be calculated from the blood gas results. The formula for A-a gradient is:

$$\text{A-a gradient} = [150 - (1.2 \times P_{CO_2})] - \text{arterial } P_{O_2}$$

This is accurate at sea level, where the alveolar partial pressure of oxygen is 150 mmHg. There is normally a gradient of 5 to 20 mmHg on the basis of physiologic shunting. Patients in whom hypoxemia is caused by alveolar hypoventilation (such as occurs with drug overdose or neuromuscular disease) have a normal A-a gradient. When hypoxemia is produced by ventilation-perfusion mismatch, right-to-left shunting, and diffusion barrier (as typically occur in chronic obstructive pulmonary disease [COPD], parenchymal lung disease, and pulmonary embolism), the A-a gradient is increased.

The chest radiograph is often of great value in elucidating the cause of dyspnea. It should be obtained in most cases. Diagnostic radiographic findings can be expected in certain conditions (eg, pneumonia, pulmonary edema, pneumothorax), but the chest radiograph may be entirely normal even when significant illness is present. The case of pulmonary embolism is a notable example.

The mere presence of radiographic abnormalities does not necessarily assure that a given illness is producing an episode of dyspnea. For example, the radiograph of the patient with COPD will manifest various abnormalities. However, a particular episode of dyspnea may be unrelated to that chronic illness. Furthermore, the presence of chronic radiographic changes in such instances may render less apparent a superimposed acute process. Chest radiographic findings may also evolve over time and be absent at the time of initial emergency department presentation (as in aspiration or toxic inhalation, for example).

Additional diagnostic evaluation may be necessary to determine the cause of dyspnea in selected cases. An electrocardiogram, spirometry measurements, a ventilation-perfusion lung scan, or a pulmonary arteriogram may be required, as dictated by the clinical findings and presentation.

CARDIOGENIC PULMONARY EDEMA

Failure of the left ventricle to eject a normal amount of blood, which causes fluid to accumulate in the pulmonary interstitium, alveoli, bronchioles, and bronchi, may produce cardiogenic pulmonary edema. In 1819, Laennec defined pulmonary edema as "an infiltration of serum into the pulmonary tissue, carried to a degree such that it significantly diminishes permeability to air."[3] Paroxysmal nocturnal dyspnea is probably a milder, self-limited form of pulmonary edema. When bronchospasm is a prominent component, an episode may be referred to as "cardiac asthma," but this condition is not a distinct entity on the basis of its pathophysiology or etiology. (See Chapter 64, Congestive Heart Failure.)

Etiology

Acute pulmonary edema may be precipitated by a number of factors, including the following:

- acute myocardial infarction
- pulmonary embolism
- cardiac dysrhythmias

- myocarditis
- overhydration
- uncontrolled hypertension
- thyrotoxicosis

The most common cause of acute pulmonary edema is coronary artery disease.[4] Acute myocardial infarction frequently causes pulmonary edema, especially if myocardial damage is extensive. Pulmonary edema may be an early or late complication of myocardial infarction and is often the presenting form, particularly among elderly patients. It is also a frequent presenting form of acute myocardial infarction in hypertensive patients, even though uncontrolled hypertension is not now as common a cause of acute pulmonary edema as it was in the past. (See Chapter 62, Acute Myocardial Infarction.)

Pulmonary edema accompanies the terminal stages of chronic renal failure. It occurs in patients on hemodialysis, even those whose disease is relatively stable. (See Chapter 78, Renal Failure.)

Stenosis of either the mitral or aortic valves may cause pulmonary edema, but mitral or aortic insufficiency is a more common cause. Acute severe aortic insufficiency is most often the result of bacterial endocarditis, dissecting aortic aneurysm, spontaneous rupture of an abnormal aortic leaflet, or blunt chest trauma. Of these, bacterial endocarditis is by far the most frequent cause.[5] Acute mitral insufficiency is usually the consequence of rupture of the chordae tendineae or papillary muscles. Chordae tendineae rupture may be due to rheumatic valvular disease, bacterial endocarditis, or blunt thoracic trauma. Rupture of a papillary muscle is most frequently a complication of acute myocardial infarction.[5]

Pathology

At autopsy, the lungs are noted to be heavy and pale or hemorrhagic. The normal tissue elasticity is lacking, and the lungs pit when pressure is applied. Frothy fluid emanates from the cut edges of the lungs, as well as from the bronchi.

Pathophysiology

An increase in hydrostatic pressure, caused by left ventricular failure or fluid overload, is the first step in the pathogenesis of pulmonary edema. Fluid begins to leave the vascular space when the capillary hydrostatic pressure exceeds the colloid osmotic pressure. Initially, the fluid collects in the perivascular interstitial connective tissue. Edema becomes significant when the rate of transudation exceeds the ability of the pulmonary lymphatics to remove fluid from the lung. As fluid continues to accumulate, it fills the alveolar spaces; it becomes more difficult to inflate the lungs, owing to diminished lung volume and reduced elasticity. Because of the nonuniform distribution of edema within the lungs, areas that are poorly ventilated are perfused, resulting in arteriovenous shunting. Peribronchial and bronchiolar edema results in narrowing and eventual collapse of small airways. This leads to increased resistance to air flow in both inspiration and expiration.

Systemic arterial pressure is usually elevated. Cardiac output may be normal, decreased, or increased. Left ventricular end-diastolic pressure is markedly increased, resulting in an elevated pulmonary capillary wedge pressure that changes pulmonary regional blood flow. The apical portions of the lung, normally underperfused, receive more than their normal flow of blood.

Arterial CO_2 tension depends on the balance between alveolar ventilation in the affected and unaffected regions of the lungs. In many patients, the P_{CO_2} is normal or low, reflecting increased total ventilation.[6] With extensive pulmonary edema or significant underlying pulmonary disease, alveolar hypoventilation occurs, resulting in CO_2 retention. Hypoxemia of a moderate or severe degree is almost invariably present.

Narrowing, obstruction, or closure of small airways results from increased interstitial pressure. Edema of the bronchial mucosa and reflex bronchospasm add to changes in air flow dynamics. In severe pulmonary edema, fluid-filled conducting airways also reduce air flow.

Diagnosis

Patients are usually anxious or restless during the early phase of pulmonary edema. They may be struck by a profound sensation of suffocation, which forces them to sit upright in order to breathe. In a severe attack, patients may be drowsy, uncooperative, or stuporous. The skin is cool and clammy, and cyanosis may be evident. The blood pressure is characteristically slightly elevated; the pulse, rapid and thready. The presence of hypotension in the face of pulmonary edema—systolic blood pressure of less than 150 mmHg—may be an ominous sign and correlates poorly with survival.[7] Pulsus alternans may be present. The respiration rate is 30 to 40 breaths per minute. A Cheyne-Stokes respiratory pattern is occasionally evident.

The jugular veins are distended, and hepatojugular reflux is usually present. The chest examination may reveal only a few crepitations during the early phase of the illness. Typically, however, bubbling rales and wheezes are heard diffusely over the lung fields. Cardiac auscultation is difficult because of the volume of the respiratory sounds. A third heart sound may be audible.

In pulmonary edema caused by acute aortic insufficiency, the classic peripheral signs of chronic aortic insufficiency—such as Corrigan's pulse—are absent. This is because the signs of chronic insufficiency are the result of wide pulse pressure, which is not present in the acute condition. The aortic insufficiency murmur is short, typically ending in mid-diastole. A soft systolic aortic flow murmur may be heard.

The patient is acutely, severely ill, and tachycardia is a consistent finding.

The patient with acute mitral insufficiency secondary to ruptured chordae tendineae displays the characteristic murmur of mitral insufficiency. It is commonly crescendo-decrescendo, however, rather than holosystolic. The murmur is heard at the apex and radiates to the left axilla or posterior left hemithorax. The precordium is hyperdynamic. A third heart sound is invariably present.[8] Echocardiography may be a useful diagnostic procedure.

Rupture of a papillary muscle may produce a similar clinical picture, although the murmur may be soft or even absent. The diagnosis is suggested by the abrupt appearance of heart failure in a patient during the first week following acute myocardial infarction.

The chest roentgenogram is a valuable tool in the diagnosis of pulmonary edema. The earliest radiographic change is dilatation of the upper lobe vessels.[9] This is a reliable finding on an upright roentgenogram only, however, as redistribution of blood to the upper lobe vessels is seen on the supine chest roentgenogram of the well patient.[10] The next most important early finding is an increase in interstitial markings. Kerley A and B lines represent interlobular septa distended with edema fluid.[10] Kerley B lines are 1 to 2 cm long and appear perpendicular to the costal, diaphragmatic, or mediastinal pleura; Kerley A lines are longer and more centrally located.

Edema of the connective tissue surrounding the bronchi and blood vessels causes blurring of normally sharp vascular margins and later peribronchial and perivascular cuffing. As edema progresses to alveolar flooding, the roentgenogram shows dense opacification of the central portions of the lung fields with symmetric infiltrates that spare the periphery. Patchy, asymmetric, or unilateral patterns are commonly seen. Cardiomegaly is frequently present.

Radiographic changes have been found to be closely correlated to pulmonary capillary wedge pressure in many cases of acute pulmonary edema. At a pressure of less than 12 mmHg, the roentgenogram is normal; when the pressure reaches 12 to 18 mmHg, upper lobe vascular redistribution occurs; at 18 to 22 mmHg, evidence of interstitial edema appears; and at pressures greater than 25 to 30 mmHg, the full radiographic pattern of pulmonary edema is manifest.[11]

Differential Diagnosis

Entities that should be considered in the differential diagnosis include acute respiratory failure due to chronic obstructive pulmonary disease; acute infectious, toxic, or aspiration pneumonitis; pulmonary embolus; and pneumothorax. History, physical examination, and chest roentgenogram generally provide sufficient information for the physician to make distinctions. The most difficult differentiation is that between pulmonary edema and acute respiratory failure in a patient with chronic obstructive airway disease; not only may physical findings be similar (eg, dyspnea, tachycardia, cyanosis, rales, and wheezes) but the presence of pre-existing disease may so alter pulmonary architecture that the radiographic appearance of pulmonary edema is atypical. Areas of lung that have lost their vascularity, for example, do not display the classic radiographic findings of pulmonary edema.

Noncardiogenic pulmonary edema and the adult respiratory distress syndrome should also be considered in the differential diagnosis. Although these entities do not produce cardiomegaly or the typical radiographic findings of cardiogenic pulmonary edema, differentiation may be difficult on clinical grounds.

Treatment

Prehospital treatment of cardiogenic pulmonary edema has as its therapeutic goals the improvement of oxygenation and the reduction of cardiac work load. To these ends, it involves the proper positioning of the patient, cardiac monitoring, the administration of oxygen, the application of rotating tourniquets, and the use of diuretics and morphine. The patient should be placed in a sitting position with the legs dependent because this position increases lung volume and vital capacity, decreases venous return to the heart, and diminishes the work of respiration. In fact, patients themselves will assume this position, if they are able to do so.

The patient should be monitored for the appearance of cardiac dysrhythmias. Oxygen should be administered by nasal cannula or mask at a rate of 4 to 6 L/min to augment oxygen delivery to ischemic tissues. (A lower flow rate should be considered in the patient with concomitant or suspected chronic obstructive pulmonary disease.) Because a large portion of hypoxemia in pulmonary edema is due to arteriovenous shunting, however, hypoxemia will not be corrected by the inhalation of supplemental oxygen alone.

Rotating tourniquets may be applied to the extremities in an effort to reduce venous return and thereby diminish central blood volume. The tourniquets are to be applied at greater than venous but less than arterial pressure. The tourniquet on one extremity should be released every 20 minutes. The application of tourniquets may be detrimental to the hypotensive patient, however. Although rotating tourniquets have traditionally been used in the therapy of acute pulmonary edema, their value has been increasingly questioned. The application of rotating tourniquets to patients with pulmonary edema has failed to demonstrate significant reduction in pulmonary artery and pulmonary capillary pressures.[12]

The beneficial effects of morphine in pulmonary edema are incompletely understood. It is known that, by dilating the capacitance vessels of the peripheral venous bed, morphine reduces venous return to the central circulation. This diminishes the preload—ventricular diastolic filling pressure—of the heart. In addition, morphine has a sedative effect, decreases musculoskeletal and respiratory activity, and has mild arterial vasodilating effects. Five to 10 mg should be administered intravenously and the subsequent dosage adjusted as needed. Consequent hypotension or respiratory depression may be reversed by the administration of naloxone hydrochloride.

Diuretic agents reduce the fluid volume of the body by renal excretion. Furosemide (Lasix), the agent of choice, effects a diuresis that begins about 20 minutes after intravenous administration. A more immediate effect of this drug is a reduction of pulmonary arterial and capillary wedge pressures, probably as a result of systemic venous dilatation.[13] Thus, furosemide may be used even in patients with chronic renal failure, in whom a profound diuresis is not expected. The usual initial dose is 20 to 40 mg intravenously, although a higher initial dose (80 to 100 mg) may be given to patients with renal insufficiency. If no diuretic effect is noted within 20 minutes of administration, the dose should be doubled. Alternatively, bumetanide (Bumex), 2 mg intravenously, may be given. The pharmacologic effects of this diuretic resemble those of furosemide.[14]

Emergency department treatment should continue as described to improve oxygenation and reduce cardiac work load. If bronchospasm is a prominent feature, aminophylline may be administered. An intravenous loading dose of 5.6 mg/kg should be given, followed by an infusion of 0.35 mg/kg/h. Care must be taken in monitoring the patient to whom maintenance aminophylline is administered. Toxic levels may be attained because of poor metabolism of the drug in heart failure, the consequence of poor hepatic function. (A further discussion of this drug is found in Chapter 72, Obstructive Airway Disease.)

Oxygen should be administered, and this may be passed through 50% ethyl alcohol if substantial frothy sputum is present. The alcohol vapor has an antifoaming action that may improve gas exchange through the airways. In some cases, suction may be an equally efficient method of sputum elimination.

Intermittent positive-pressure breathing (IPPB) is effective in the treatment of pulmonary edema, probably because it impedes venous return to the heart by increasing intrathoracic pressure. In addition, IPPB may help to regulate respirations, provide more uniform ventilation, and decrease arteriovenous shunting. The presence of severe respiratory acidosis is an indication for IPPB or continuous positive-pressure breathing.[6] Endotracheal intubation should be considered if the Po_2 cannot be maintained about 50 mmHg with the methods that have been mentioned or if there is persistent severe CO_2 retention. (See Chapter 74, Respiratory Failure.)

Nitroglycerin may be used for both its peripheral venous and arterial dilating actions. Although it is primarily a venodilator, its modest arterial dilating effect may substantially improve cardiac output in the presence of severe heart failure.[15] The dosage is 0.3 to 0.6 mg sublingually or 1 to 4 in of ointment applied topically. Nitroglycerin may be detrimental to patients with hypotension because it can reduce coronary perfusion pressure, potentially enhancing myocardial ischemia.[16]

Potent vasodilators may be used to reduce resistance to ventricular ejection—afterload—in instances of intractable pulmonary edema. This results in an increased ejection fraction and improved cardiac output. The drug of choice is sodium nitroprusside, a short-acting drug that dilates both arterial and venous vessels. The required dosage varies, but intravenous infusion should be begun at 20 μg/min and adjusted as needed.[17] Profound hypotension is the result of overmedication. Therefore, blood pressure should be monitored closely, preferably by means of an indwelling arterial catheter.

The administration of nifedipine, 10 mg sublingually, in pulmonary edema results in lowering of systolic and diastolic blood pressure, reduction of peripheral vascular resistance, and increase in cardiac output.[18] Effects on blood pressure begin to appear approximately 20 minutes after sublingual administration.

Phlebotomy may be a useful treatment for difficult cases, especially in patients with chronic renal failure. Preferably via a blood bank phlebotomy apparatus, 300 to 500 mL of blood should be removed rapidly. If the patient is anemic, the cellular components may be banked and reinfused at a later time. Care must be taken, as phlebotomy may produce hypotension.

Once the primary goals of therapy have been achieved, efforts should be continued to improve cardiac contractility, to monitor and maintain the stability of the patient's condition, and to ascertain an etiology for the episode of acute heart failure. Digoxin has long been considered the drug of choice for increasing cardiac contractility. However, it does not raise cardiac output rapidly enough to be of use as a primary drug in pulmonary edema. Even the benefit of adding digitalis to a diuretic regimen in the patient with chronic congestive heart failure has been questioned.[19] Digoxin seems to be most useful in patients with pulmonary edema due to severe mitral stenosis in whom atrial fibrillation and a rapid ventricular rate are present. The benefit in the patient in sinus rhythm is less clear.

The use of digitalis in the immediate postmyocardial infarction period is controversial. Digitalis may decrease myocardial oxygen requirements and improve subendocardial oxygen delivery by reducing left ventricular filling pressure. On the other hand, the drug increases myocardial oxygen demands by virtue of its inotropic action and may produce direct coronary vasoconstriction. The administration of cardiac glycosides should probably be delayed in the patient with acute myocardial infarction. However, it has been demonstrated that digitalis can be administered safely in such patients without demonstrably increasing myocardial infarction size.[20]

The patient should be admitted to a coronary or intensive care unit for monitoring and further treatment. Certain patients benefit from early surgery. The patient with aortic insufficiency and intractable heart failure requires early valve replacement, even if infection is present.[21] In acute mitral insufficiency, surgery is often not urgent, and the patient's heart failure may be treated by conventional means and afterload reduction. Antibiotics should be instituted in endocarditis. Cardiac catheterization may indicate whether surgical intervention is needed.[5]

NONCARDIOGENIC PULMONARY EDEMA

Noncardiogenic pulmonary edema is characterized by increased pulmonary alveolar and interstitial fluid accumulation without left ventricular failure. This entity is addressed only briefly here, being discussed more completely in Chapter 74.

Etiology

Noncardiogenic pulmonary edema can result from a wide variety of systemic and pulmonary insults.

- airway obstruction
- central nervous system lesions
- diabetic ketoacidosis
- drugs
- fat embolus
- gastric content aspiration
- high altitude
- hypoglycemia
- infection/sepsis
- near-drowning
- organophosphate insecticides
- pancreatitis
- paraquat ingestion
- lung re-expansion
- trauma
- pulmonary embolus
- smoke inhalation
- transfusion reaction
- toxic inhalation
- uremia

Numerous medications cause pulmonary edema in either overdose or therapeutic use.[22-29]

- barbiturates
- chlordiazepoxide hydrochloride (Librium)
- ethchlorvynol (Placidyl)
- methaqualone-diphenhydramine (Mandrax)
- opiate analgesics
- pentazocine (Talwin)
- propoxyphene hydrochloride (Darvon)
- salicylates
- thiazide diuretics

Pathology

The major pathologic finding in noncardiogenic pulmonary edema is excess fluid in the alveolar and interstitial spaces. The common feature of noncardiogenic pulmonary edema is damage to the alveolar-capillary membrane. This results in increased permeability and exudation of fluid into the interstitial and alveolar spaces. The earliest pathologic findings in animal models is sequestration of leukocytes within the pulmonary microvasculature.[30] The leukocytes, having caused focal endothelial damage, subsequently migrate into the interstitium. In the initial phase of the syndrome, there are areas of petechial hemorrhage, edema, and lobar consolidation. Later in the course, hyaline membranes, marked capillary congestion, and gross pulmonary edema are seen. If the patient survives, edema and hyaline membranes decrease, and interstitial fibrosis ultimately ensues. In some patients a portion of the fibrosis resolves over time.

Pathophysiology

Noncardiogenic pulmonary edema follows injury to either the alveolar epithelium or the vascular endothelium. The sequence of injury production is complex. In some instances the inciting injury is the result of direct pulmonary tissue damage (as is caused by gastric content aspiration or toxic inhalation). In other cases the initiating insult is more indirect. Such indirect damage induces the activation of either the coagulation or complement cascade, which in turn leads to the chemoattraction of neutrophils into the lungs.[31]

The role of neutrophils in the pathogenesis of noncardiogenic pulmonary edema has been viewed as focal. Increased numbers of neutrophils have been found in the lungs,[32] and activated neutrophils are also present in the blood.[33] Activated neutrophils are thought to constitute a major factor in pathogenesis, displaying increased chemotactic activity and the ability to generate toxic oxygen-derived free radicals.[34,35]

Many factors have been implicated as causing pulmonary endothelial injury. These include arachidonic acid metabolites, fibrin and fibrin degradation products, complement, histamine, serotonin, and bradykinin. Release of these substances may involve neutrophils, pulmonary endothelium, platelets, and macrophages. Once a destructive sequence is initiated in noncardiogenic pulmonary edema, it is likely to be self-perpetuating, with capillary endothelial and epithelial damage producing the release of additional toxic substances.

Diagnosis

The clinical picture is one of respiratory distress with a variety of other findings. Cardiomegaly and jugular venous distention are not present as a rule. The patient may experience inspiratory chest pain or substernal discomfort, tachypnea, and a dry or productive cough. Cyanosis, tachycardia, hyperpnea, and hypotension may be present. Wheezing, rhonchi, or crepitant rales may be audible diffusely over both lungs, or such findings may be localized to portions of the thorax. Determination of arterial blood gas levels usually reveals hypoxemia and respiratory alkalosis.

The chest roentgenogram of a patient with noncardiogenic pulmonary edema typically shows bilateral pulmonary vascular congestion and infiltrates, along with a cardiac silhouette of normal size. Many variants may be seen, however, including asymmetric and unilateral patterns. Although a normal cardiac silhouette is characteristic, the picture may be confused by pre-existing cardiomegaly.

The severity of pulmonary edema seen on the chest roentgenogram roughly parallels the clinical severity of the condition. Patchy, irregular, unilateral or bilateral infiltrates are seen in mild cases, most prominently in the midlung areas. In more severe cases, the infiltrates may entirely fill both lung fields.

Differential Diagnosis

With noncardiogenic pulmonary edema, the differential diagnosis is that of any patient in acute respiratory distress. It includes those entities listed in the differential diagnosis of cardiogenic pulmonary edema.

Treatment

Given the variety of conditions that cause noncardiogenic pulmonary edema, individualization of therapy is essential. When there is a clearly defined underlying condition, primary attention must be directed toward treatment of that condition. For example, airway obstruction should be overcome, intracranial lesions evacuated, sepsis treated, narcotic antagonists administered, or metabolic abnormalities corrected, as indicated. In the face of hypovolemia, resuscitation with crystalloid solutions is probably preferable to the use of colloids, as colloid infusion may increase the water content of the lung.

Traditional therapeutic modalities useful in cardiogenic pulmonary edema—diuretics, morphine, and rotating tourniquets—have no place in the treatment of noncardiogenic pulmonary edema. Diuretics particularly may exacerbate the course of this condition, causing hypovolemia and hypotension.[36]

The mainstays of treatment for noncardiogenic pulmonary edema are oxygen administration and—when necessary—mechanical ventilation. Oxygen reduces pulmonary artery pressure, a prime factor in increased pulmonary vascular permeability. Mechanical ventilation enhances oxygenation and reduces atelectasis. A volume-cycled respirator is preferred. A large tidal volume (12 to 15 mL/kg) should be used to reduce the likelihood of atelectasis. Reduction of tidal volume is advisable if the peak inspiratory pressure exceeds 50 cmH_2O.[37] Assisted mechanical ventilation or intermittent mandatory ventilation is recommended as the primary ventilatory mode over controlled mechanical ventilation, in which no spontaneous patient respiration is allowed.[36,38] Positive end-expiratory pressure (PEEP) may be used to increase functional residual capacity, increase pulmonary compliance, and reduce pulmonary arteriovenous shunting. This therapeutic modality should be added to mechanical ventilation specifically to achieve these goals, rather than to reduce pulmonary edema directly, because it effects no primary reduction in pulmonary water content even when it significantly improves pulmonary function. Although PEEP is extensively utilized, issues have been raised regarding its influence on outcome.[39,40]

The prognosis for the patient with noncardiogenic pulmonary edema varies greatly, depending on the underlying cause. In some instances, the course is predictably benign; in others, fatalities are common. Mild forms of high-altitude pulmonary edema, for example, have been successfully treated with bed rest alone.[41] With appropriate management, patients with noncardiogenic pulmonary edema may eventually recover normal pulmonary function, even after an episode of severe respiratory impairment.

REFERENCES

1. Baldwin ED, Cournand A, Richards DW Jr. Pulmonary insufficiency. *Medicine Baltimore*. 1948;27:243–278.
2. Jones J, Heiselman D, Cannon L, et al. Continuous emergency department monitoring of arterial saturation in adult patients with respiratory distress. *Ann Emerg Med*. 1988;17:463–466.
3. Nowakowski JF. Acute alveolar edema. *Emerg Med Clin North Am*. 1983;1:313–343.
4. Jackson F. Pulmonary oedema. *Practitioner*. 1977;219:656–663.
5. Simpson PC Jr, Bristow JD. Recognition and management of emergencies in valvular heart disease. *Med Clin North Am*. 1979;63:155–172.
6. Robin ED, Cross CE, Zelis R. Pulmonary edema. *N Engl J Med*. 1973;288:292–304.
7. Plotnick GD, Kelemen MH, Garrett RB, et al. Acute cardiogenic pulmonary edema in the elderly: factors predicting in-hospital and one-year mortality. *South Med J*. 1982;75:565–569.
8. Luther RR, Meyers SN. Acute mitral insufficiency secondary to ruptured chordae tendineae. *Arch Intern Med*. 1974;134:568–578.
9. Cunningham JH, Richardson RH, Smith JD. Interstitial pulmonary edema. *Heart Lung*. 1977;6:617–623.
10. Grainger RG. The radiological diagnosis of interstitial pulmonary oedema. *Br J Radiol*. 1977;50:161–163.
11. McHugh TJ, Forrester JS, Adler L, et al. Pulmonary vascular congestion in acute myocardial infarction: a hemodynamic and radiologic correlation. *Ann Intern Med*. 1972;76:29–33.
12. Bertel O, Steiner A. Rotating tourniquets do not work in acute congestive heart failure and pulmonary oedema. *Lancet*. 1980;2:762.

13. Biddle TL, Yu PN. Effect of furosemide on hemodynamics and lung water in acute pulmonary edema secondary to myocardial infarction. *Am J Cardiol*. 1979;43:86–90.
14. Brater DC, Chennavasin P, Day B, et al. Bumetanide and furosemide. *Clin Pharmacol Ther*. 1983;34:207–213.
15. Cohn JN, Franciosa JA. Vasodilator therapy of cardiac failure, I. *N Engl J Med*. 1977;297:27–31.
16. Bussmann WD, Schupp D. Effect of sublingual nitroglycerin in emergency treatment of severe pulmonary edema. *Am J Cardiol*. 1978;41:931–936.
17. Cohn JN, Franciosa JA. Vasodilator therapy of cardiac failure, II. *N Engl J Med*. 1977;297:254–258.
18. Polese A, Fiorentini C, Gauzzi MD. Clinical use of a calcium antagonist (nifedipine) in acute pulmonary edema. *Am J Med*. 1979;66:825–830.
19. Poole-Wilson PA. Digitalis: dead or alive? *Cardiology*. 1988;75(suppl 1):103–109.
20. Morrison J, Coromilas J, Robbins M, et al. Digitalis and myocardial infarction in man. *Circulation*. 1980;62:8–16.
21. Morganroth J, Perloff JK, Zelois SM, et al. Acute severe aortic regurgitation. *Ann Intern Med*. 1977;87:223–232.
22. Schoenfeld MR. Acute pulmonary edema caused by barbiturate poisoning. *Angiology*. 1964;15:445–453.
23. Bogartz LJ, Miller WC. Pulmonary edema associated with propoxyphene intoxication. *JAMA*. 1971;215:259–262.
24. Glauser FL, Smith WR, Caldwell A, et al. Ethchlorvynol (Placidyl)-induced pulmonary edema. *Ann Intern Med*. 1976;84:46–48.
25. Oh TE, Gordon TP, Burden PW. Unilateral pulmonary oedema and 'Mandrax' poisoning. *Anaesthesia*. 1978;33:719–721.
26. Richman S, Harris RD. Acute pulmonary edema associated with Librium abuse. *Radiology*. 1972;103:57–58.
27. Davis PR, Burch RE. Pulmonary edema and salicylate intoxication. *Ann Intern Med*. 1974;80:553–554.
28. Bowers RE, Brigham KL, Owen PJ. Salicylate pulmonary edema: the mechanism in sheep and review of the clinical literature. *Am Rev Respir Dis*. 1977;115:261–268.
29. Halpern M, Rho YM. Deaths from narcotism in New York City. *NY State J Med*. 1966;63:2391–2408.
30. Yeston NS, Niehoff JM. Trauma and pulmonary insufficiency: mediators and modulators of adult respiratory distress syndrome. *Int Anesthesiol Clin*. 1987;25:91–116.
31. Hammerschmidt DE, Weaver LJ, Hudson LD, et al. Association of complement activation and elevated plasma-C5a with adult respiratory distress syndrome. *Lancet*. 1980;1:947–949.
32. Bachofen M, Weibel ER. Structural alterations of lung parenchyma in the adult respiratory distress syndrome. *Clin Chest Med*. 1982;3:35–56.
33. Zimmerman GA, Renzetti AD, Hill HR. Functional and metabolic activity of granulocytes from patients with adult respiratory distress syndrome. *Am Rev Respir Dis*. 1983;127:290–300.
34. Ward PA, Johnson KL, Til GO. Current concepts regarding adult respiratory distress syndrome. *Ann Emerg Med*. 1984;14:724–728.
35. Rinaldo JE. Mediation of ARDS by leukocytes: clinical evidence and implications for therapy. *Chest*. 1986;89:590–593.
36. Hultgren HN. Furosemide for high altitude pulmonary edema. *JAMA*. 1975;234:589–590.
37. Stevens JH, Raffin TA. Adult respiratory distress syndrome, II: management. *Postgrad Med J*. 1984;60:573–576.
38. Hudson LD. Ventilatory management of patients with adult respiratory distress syndrome. *Semin Respir Med*. 1981;2:128–139.
39. Pepe PE, Hudson LD, Carrico CJ. Early application of positive end-expiratory pressure in patients at risk for the adult respiratory-distress syndrome. *N Engl J Med*. 1984;311:281–286.
40. Springer RR, Stevens PM. The influence of PEEP on survival of patients in respiratory failure. *Am J Med*. 1979;66:196–200.
41. Marticorena E, Hultgren HN. Evaluation of therapeutic methods in high altitude pulmonary edema. *Am J Cardiol*. 1979;43:307–312.

70. Airway Management

LINDA NORDEMAN, MD
EMILY J. LUCID, MD, FACEP

Airway management is the first consideration in the evaluation and treatment of every seriously ill patient. After only 5 minutes of anoxia the central nervous system undergoes irreversible injury. Therefore, rapid and effective airway management is of prime importance to all emergency physicians. Advances in technology and the training of emergency personnel have led to more effective and efficient patient management.

ASSESSMENT

Airway management begins with airway assessment. It may take only seconds to obtain the information needed to make appropriate interventions. Vital information regarding airway patency and level of consciousness can be gained from the patient's ability to respond verbally. If time permits, a thorough history including onset and duration of symptoms, medications, and previous history of airway disease and its severity should be obtained. Observation and auscultation reveal respiratory rate, pattern, sounds, and effort. Assessment is an ongoing process, and intervention is based on the patient's current respiratory status.

BASIC AIRWAY MANAGEMENT

Supplemental Oxygen

Any disease process resulting in hypoxia or exacerbated by hypoxia should be treated with supplemental oxygen. Patients who have spontaneous respirations and intact protective airway reflexes and those not requiring ventilatory support may receive supplemental oxygen via a nasal canula or by one of a variety of oxygen masks. The goal of therapy is to maintain an oxygen saturation of greater than or equal to 90% and a Pao_2 of greater than or equal to 60 mmHg. Multiple oxygen delivery devices have various oxygen delivery capabilities (Table 70–1).

During the administration of supplemental oxygen to patients with chronic obstructive pulmonary disease, care must be taken to avoid depression of the respiratory drive. However, oxygen should never be completely withheld from these patients. In patients with severe hypoxia or in need of ventilatory assistance, any desired oxygen concentration can be delivered through an endotracheal tube.

Partial Airways

As a patient's level of consciousness declines, the airway can become occluded by the tongue if it falls posteriorly against the pharyngeal wall. This obstruction can be relieved by the chin lift or jaw thrust maneuver. A partial artificial airway, such as the nasopharyngeal or oropharyngeal airway, can also be used to relieve the obstruction.

The nasopharyngeal airway, or nasal trumpet, is a flexible rubber tube that is inserted through the nose and extends into the hypopharynx. The distal aspect elevates the tongue from the posterior pharyngeal wall. An anesthetic lubricant should be applied to the airway prior to insertion. The tip is beveled and, during insertion, the bevel should be directed toward the

Table 70-1 Oxygen Delivery Devices and Their Capabilities

Device	Flow Rate, L/min	F_IO_2, O_2%
Nasal canula*	1–4	24–33
Simple mask	6–12	35–50
Partial rebreather	6–12	60–90
Nonrebreather†	6–8	up to 100
with reservoir bag	10–16	
Venturi‡		24, 28, 31
		35, 40, 50

*Each liter per minute provides an additional 2% to 3% F_IO_2
†For use in patients at risk for CO_2 retention
‡Can deliver precise O_2 concentrations

septum to avoid injury to the turbinates. The nasal airway is well tolerated by alert patients and can be used as an adjunct to suctioning and in preparation of the nares for nasal intubation.

The oropharyngeal airway can be used only in patients without protective airway reflexes. These patients require endotracheal intubation, and use of the oral airway should be very limited. The oropharyngeal airway elevates the tongue and prevents it from resting against the palate. It can also be used to prevent clenching of the teeth against an orally placed endotracheal tube and to facilitate oropharyngeal suctioning.

Bag-Valve-Mask

Effective oxygenation and ventilation can be achieved by use of the bag-valve-mask (B-V-M) device. This device consists of a self-inflating bag that can be connected to an oxygen source, a valve that allows air flow during manual, positive-pressure ventilation as well as during spontaneous respiration, and a mask that provides an airway seal. Proper use of the B-V-M requires a patent airway and a tight mask fit. The total volume of the bag is 1.5 to 2 L. This volume should not be emptied into the airway rapidly as this can result in excessive airway pressure and pneumothorax. The tidal volume should approximate 10 to 15 mL/kg. Prior to endotracheal intubation, the airway should be opened and cleared, and oxygenation should be provided. In patients with depressed respirations, oxygenation is achieved by manual ventilation using a B-V-M device.

Esophageal Airways

The esophageal obturator airway (EOA) is a tube used for intubation of the esophagus. It is constructed with perforations at the level of the hypopharynx to provide ventilation of the lungs. The tube is closed and cuffed at the distal (esophageal) end to prevent gastric distention and aspiration. A mask is connected to the proximal end and provides an airway seal. It may be possible to achieve effective tidal volumes and adequate PaO_2 with proper use of the EOA.

However, use of the EOA is controversial.[1,2] It has lost much of its initial popularity and is currently used infrequently. Endotracheal intubation provides definitive airway control, and use of the EOA should be confined to the prehospital setting in situations in which endotracheal intubation is not available.

Removal of the EOA induces vomiting. Therefore, endotracheal intubation should be accomplished before EOA removal. Complications encountered with use of this device include complete airway obstruction with inadvertent tracheal intubation, esophageal rupture, and aspiration upon removal. To achieve an adequate airway seal, one must flex the neck. For this reason, the EOA is contraindicated in trauma patients.

The esophageal tracheal combitube (ETC) is a new airway designed with two lumens to allow ventilation whether the device is placed in the esophagus or the trachea. It is a combination EOA and endotracheal (ET) tube.[3] The mask of the EOA is replaced by a pharyngeal balloon that provides an airway seal. It is inserted blindly and the balloon is inflated. Because the esophagus is more likely to be intubated with blind insertion, the bag is attached to the EOA connector. Auscultation of breath sounds near the axilla and observation of chest movement with ventilation confirm esophageal placement of the ETC. If these signs are absent and air exchange is heard over the epigastrium, the bag is attached to the endotracheal connector. Placement is confirmed by auscultation and observation with manual ventilations. The ETC is not a substitute for the endotracheal tube; however, in situations in which direct endotracheal intubation is not available, this may serve as an effective alternative to the bag-valve-mask device or the EOA.

ADVANCED AIRWAY MANAGEMENT— ENDOTRACHEAL INTUBATION

Indications

Endotracheal intubation provides a secure, patent airway through which oxygenation and ventilation can be achieved. It is often lifesaving and is a skill that all emergency physicians should be comfortable performing. The point at which endotracheal intubation should be undertaken, however, is not always clear. Several established indications for endotracheal intubation will be discussed.

1. Ventilatory support
   (a) Positive-pressure ventilation
   (b) Administration of high concentrations of oxygen
2. Maintenance of a patent airway
3. Protection of the airway from aspiration
4. Tracheobronchial suctioning
5. Facilitation of emergency investigations
6. Administration of medications

Ventilatory Support

Ventilatory support is required by patients with respiratory failure. These are patients with severe hypoxia refractory to supplemental oxygen or with severe hypercapnia associated with progressive respiratory acidosis and physical exhaustion. Blood gas determination may aid in the decision to intubate (Table 70-2). However, clinical evidence of hypoxia (anxiety, cyanosis), hypercapnia (somnolence), or exhaustion is an indication to intubate prior to blood gas evaluation.

The ET tube provides a conduit through which ventilatory support and end-expiratory manipulations can be provided. Adult endotracheal tubes are cuffed, providing an airway seal so that positive-pressure ventilation can be administered. In addition, end-expiratory maneuvers (ie, PEEP) can be provided to increase oxygenation.

Maintenance of a Patent Airway

Patients at risk for upper airway obstruction require endotracheal intubation to preserve airway patency. This situation is frequently encountered as part of a larger emergency, and it must be remembered that airway management is the first priority. Loss of airway patency may result from relaxation of the pharyngeal muscles or obstruction by the tongue in patients with an altered level of consciousness from any cause. Airway patency may be jeopardized by swelling of intrinsic airway structures or by those adjacent to the airway. For example, infectious processes such as epiglottitis or abscess formation, swelling secondary to anaphylaxis, inhalational burns, tumors, direct laryngeal trauma, or bleeding with hematoma formation can result in encroachment on the airway.

Initial treatment is directed at clearing any potential obstruction. Suctioning, removal of foreign bodies, and manual opening of the airway (chin lift, jaw thrust) may relieve an airway obstruction. A partial airway may maintain patency temporarily so that oxygenation and ventilation can be achieved. If airway obstruction has not been relieved or if the patient is at risk for recurrent obstruction, endotracheal intubation should be performed. In cases of severe upper airway trauma or edema or if intubation cannot be achieved, an emergency surgical airway should be performed.

Protection of the Airway

Patients with loss of the protective airway reflexes (cough and gag) are at risk of aspiration. Those at particular risk are patients with an altered level of consciousness. As the level of consciousness decreases, the protective airway reflexes are lost in a descending order. Initially the gag and swallowing reflexes mediated by cranial nerve IX, the glossopharyngeal nerve, are attenuated and lost. As the process advances, the laryngeal reflex and more distally the cough reflex, both mediated by cranial nerve X, the vagus nerve, are lost. As this occurs the patient's risk of aspiration increases. Also at risk is the patient with an ingestion in whom a large orogastric tube has been placed for gastric lavage. The large tubes mechanically interfere with the protective airway reflexes, thereby increasing the risk of aspiration. Intubation with a cuffed endotracheal tube provides a sealed airway and prevents aspiration.

Table 70-2 Indications for Intubation

Clinical Setting	RR	O_2Sat*	Pa_{O_2}*	Pa_{CO_2}	pH
Acute respiratory failure	>30–40	<90	<50	>50	<7.3
Acute exacerbation of chronic respiratory failure	>30–40		<35–40		<7.2

*On supplemental O_2

Suction

In patients who are unable to clear their lower airway, the placement of an endotracheal tube provides a conduit through which aggressive suctioning can be performed. This alone is seldom sufficient cause for intubation on an emergent basis. This group of patients, however, frequently requires ventilatory support or airway protection as well as aggressive pulmonary toilet and may require intubation for multiple reasons.

Facilitation of Emergency Evaluation

Uncooperative patients may require aggressive evaluation that may be impossible to perform without sedation and/or paralysis. Endotracheal intubation secures a patent airway and allows ventilation so that sedation can be undertaken safely.

Administration of Medications

The tracheobronchial tree provides a large and effective absorptive surface. In emergent situations in which an airway is needed and in which IV access may be difficult to obtain, several medications may be administered endotracheally. These medications include epinephrine, lidocaine, naloxone, diazepam, atropine, and steroids.[4]

Preparation of the Patient for Intubation

The patient should be well oxygenated before intubation as cardiac arrest may result from intubation attempts in a hypoxic patient. Oxygen may be supplied by a high-flow mask in patients who have spontaneous respirations or manually by a B-V-M device in apneic patients. Suction equipment should be available and functioning, and the airway should be cleared of all secretions, emesis, and blood.

Table 70-3 Time Line in Rapid Sequence Induction

Medication	± Nondepolarizing muscle relaxer* ± Lidocaine, 1.0 mg/kg ± Atropine, 0.01 mg/kg	Succinylcholine, 1–1.5 mg/kg ± Thiopental, 3–5 mg/kg or ± Midazolam, 0.3 mg/kg				Long action muscle relaxer† Sedative‡
Time	−3 min	0	45 s	60 s	3 min	6 min
Procedure	Premedication	Induction	Sellick maneuver	Intubation	Bag or surgical airway if unsuccessful intubation	

*d-Tubocurarine, 3 mg; or vecuronium, 1 mg; or pancuronium, 1 mg
†Vecuronium, 0.1 mg/kg (duration of action, 25–40 min), or pancuronium, 0.1 mg/kg (duration of action, 80 min)
‡Valium

Intubation results in transient tachycardia, hypertension, and increased intracranial pressure. This may be detrimental to patients with severe hypertension, coronary artery disease, head trauma, or an intracranial space-occupying lesion. Lidocaine (1 mg/kg), administered intravenously or laryngotracheally just before intubation, may blunt the cardiovascular response and the rise in intracranial pressure.[5,6]

Topical Anesthetic

Topical anesthesia particularly for nasotracheal intubation will make this procedure easier to perform and better tolerated by the patient. Prior to nasal intubation the mucous membrane of the nose and posterior pharynx should be anesthetized. In addition, the nasal mucosa should be treated with a vasoconstrictor. Topical cocaine or topical lidocaine (4% or 10%) plus a vasoconstricting medication should be applied. This can be achieved via nasal pledgets or over a nasal airway. In addition, anesthetic spray can be applied to the supraglottic structures through a nasal trumpet.

Although rarely indicated, anesthesia of the subglottic structures and upper trachea can be achieved with a transtracheal injection. With the patient supine, a 22 or 23 gauge needle is advanced through the cricothyroid membrane. When air is aspirated 2 to 4 mL of 2% to 4% topical lidocaine is injected.[7] This may cause uncontrollable coughing until the tissues are anesthetized, and it should not be used in patients with cervical spine or head injuries.

Sedation

IV sedation for intubation may be useful in select patients. Extreme care must be used as sedation decreases respiratory drive and increases the risk of aspiration. Benzodiazepines with or without narcotics are generally used. This combination is synergistic, and careful monitoring must be performed at all times. Adequate sedation is generally thought to be achieved when the patient is sleepy but responds to verbal commands. Diazepam (Valium) in 2.5-mg increments or midazolam (Versed) in 0.5-mg increments is administered intravenously. Morphine sulfate (1- to 3-mg increments) or fentanyl (25- to 50-μg increments) can be added. Intractable hypotension refractory to vasopressor and fluid administration may occur in response to large doses of benzodiazepine. Therefore, they should be used judiciously in this setting.

Rapid Sequence Intubation

The technique of rapid sequence intubation (Table 70-3) utilizes muscle relaxation (succinylcholine) and sedation (sodium thiopental or midazolam) to facilitate orotracheal intubation.[8–10] This technique is particularly useful in combative patients with severe head injuries. If orotracheal intubation is unsuccessful, however, a surgical airway may become necessary.

The patient is preoxygenated with 100% oxygen. Manual ventilation should be avoided as it results in gastric distention and increased risk of vomiting and aspiration. If time allows, a nondepolarizing muscle relaxer (d-tubocurarine, 3 mg; vecuronium, 1 mg; or pancuronium, 1 mg) can be administered intravenously 2 to 3 minutes before induction to reduce the fasciculations associated with succinylcholine. Children younger than 8 years develop significant bradycardia with the administration of succinylcholine. Therefore, young children should be premedicated with atropine, 0.01 mg/kg IV. In addition, atropine should be readily available for use in adults if needed. Lidocaine, 1 mg/kg, may be administered 2 to 3 minutes before intubation in head-injured patients in an attempt to blunt the rise in intracranial pressure.

Sedation is achieved using thiopental, 3 to 5 mg/kg, or midazolam, 0.3 mg/kg, intravenously. Sodium thiopental blunts the rise in intracranial pressure associated with intubation and is the agent of choice in patients with head injuries. The depolarizing agent, succinylcholine (1.0 to 1.5 mg/kg),

Table 70-4 Neuromuscular Blocking Agents

Agent	Intubating Dose, mg/kg	Onset of Action*	Duration of Action, min	Pretreatment Dose, mg/kg	Comments
Depolarizing					
Succinylcholine	1.0 adult 2.0 children	30–60 s	3–10		May cause bradycardia (particularly in children); therefore, pretreat with atropine, 0.01 mg/kg in children and as needed in adults. Causes fasciculations; therefore, pretreat with nondepolarizing agent† if time allows. Induces transient K^+ efflux from cells, with an exaggerated response in patients with severe burns, massive muscle trauma, or recent motor neuropathies. May trigger malignant hyperthermia. Increases intraocular pressure.
Nondepolarizing†					
Curare	0.5	1–5 min	40–60	0.05	May cause dose-related hypotension.
Pancuronium	0.05–0.2	1–3 min	60–90	0.02	May cause tachycardia and hypertension.
Vecuronium	0.05–0.2	1–2 min	40–120	0.02	
Atacurium	0.4	2–3 min	45–60		Has fewest cardiovascular effects.

*Marked variability exists.
†Subparalyzing dose is given 3 minutes before induction with succinylcholine to prevent fasciculations. Pretreatment is unnecessary in children less than 5 years of age.

is administered intravenously to achieve muscle relaxation. Allow 45 seconds after the administration of succinylcholine before attempting intubation. The Sellick maneuver is performed when the patient becomes unresponsive. Pressure is applied to the cricoid cartilage, occluding the esophagus and preventing passive regurgitation. Cricoid pressure is released only after intubation is achieved and the endotracheal cuff is inflated. If the patient develops active vomiting, this maneuver is interrupted, cricoid pressure is released, and the patient is aggressively suctioned.

If intubation is unsuccessful after 3 minutes, the patient should be manually ventilated with a B-V-M device. Adequate preoxygenation before induction allows 4 minutes to elapse before hypoxia ensues. In addition, the partial pressure of CO_2 increases at a rate of 3 to 4 mmHg/minute after an initial rise of 6 mmHg during the first minute. This results in a rise of only 12 mmHg after 3 minutes of apnea. The effects of succinylcholine last for approximately 6 minutes, after which spontaneous respirations will return. Therefore, if intubation is unsuccessful and adequate oxygenation can be achieved by manual ventilation, the need for a surgical airway may be avoided. However, if adequate mask ventilation is not achieved, a surgical cricothyroidotomy becomes necessary.

The longer-acting muscle relaxers can be used for induction in cases in which succinylcholine is contraindicated (massive muscle trauma, burns, penetrating ocular injuries, or hyperkalemia). Because their duration of action is prolonged (Table 70-4), a surgical airway will be necessary if intubation cannot be achieved. If succinylcholine is used for induction and prolonged paralysis is then desired, an additional muscle relaxer will be required because the effect of succinylcholine begins to diminish in 6 minutes.

Equipment

Equipment should be accessible and always in operating condition. Prior to use, all equipment should rapidly be checked. Suction equipment should be connected and functioning. Both a tonsil tip and a flexible catheter should be available. The laryngoscope consists of a handle and a blade. The handle can be fitted with a variety of blade types and sizes. The two most commonly used blades are the curved MacIntosh, which is inserted into the vallecula, and the straight Miller, which is inserted beneath the laryngeal surface of the epiglottis. Elevation of the laryngoscope in an upward, forward, lifting motion exposes the vocal cords.

The endotracheal tube itself is a conduit for oxygenation, ventilation, and suctioning, and it provides a patent airway. It does, however, increase dead space and may increase resistance to air flow. The smaller the diameter of the tube, the greater the resistance it produces. The tubes are made of a nontoxic material and the size is based on the internal diameter. Generally a size 7 to 7.5 is appropriate for a woman and a size 8 to 8.5 is appropriate for a man. The tubes for adults have high-volume, low-pressure cuffs at the distal ends. This provides an airway seal without producing mucosal ischemia. Pediatric tubes, for use in patients younger than 8 years, are not cuffed. In children the cricoid cartilage is the narrowest part of the airway and provides an adequate seal if the proper size tube is used. The appropriate pediatric tube size can be calculated by use of the formula $4 + age/4$.

In addition to the standard tubes, there are several specialized tubes. The Endotrol tube has a stylet-type system built into the tube itself. Proximally, there is a trigger that, when pulled, changes the curvature of the tube. This tube is particularly helpful in blind nasal intubations but can be used for difficult oral intubations as well. Anode tubes have a wire reinforcement in the tube wall. This tube resists bending and collapse.

Stylets are malleable metal stents that can change the curvature of the endotracheal tube when inserted through the tube. Care must be taken to keep the distal end of the stylet within the tube to prevent mucosal injury.

Magill forceps are used during nasal intubation to guide the tube through the cords. The endotracheal tube is passed through the nares and advanced into the oropharynx. Direct laryngoscopy is then performed. The tube is gripped with the forceps just proximal to the cuff. An assistant advances the tube at the nose as the intubator directs it, by use of the forceps, through the cords.

The lighted stylet is a battery-operated device with a light bulb at the distal end. It is used as a guide in blind intubations. The light transilluminates the neck when it passes through the glottis. An endotracheal tube is then passed over the stylet, and the stylet is removed.

The fiberoptic bronchoscope can also be used as a stent over which an endotracheal tube can be placed. It allows visualization of the airway without use of the laryngoscope. It is very useful in cases of difficult intubation; however, its use requires considerable skill. A size 4.5 or larger endotracheal tube is required to fit over the bronchoscope.

Technique

The actual technique of intubation is discussed in detail in the subsequent atlas of emergency procedures. A brief overview is presented here. Intubation should always be preceded by oxygenation, and all necessary equipment should be available and functioning.

Intubation can be achieved by the oral or nasal route (Table 70-5). Oral intubation can be accomplished in a more rapid manner, with a slightly larger tube, and in an apneic patient. Therefore, in a resuscitation, the oral route is the only option. In less emergent situations, blind nasal intubation may be preferred. This is better tolerated by the patient, and the tube is more easily stabilized in this location. Contraindications to nasal intubation include bleeding diathesis and basilar skull fracture with a nasal cerebrospinal fluid (CSF) leak.

Table 70-5 Recommendations for Orotracheal versus Nasotracheal Intubation

Condition	Orotracheal	Nasotracheal
Rapid intubation	X	
Larger diameter tube	X	
Apneic patient	X	
Bleeding diathesis	X	
Basilar skull fracture	X	
Better stabilization		X
Better tolerated (awake patient)		X
Mandibular-cervical problems		X

Oral Intubation

If the cervical spine is clear, the patient is placed in the sniffing position so that the mouth, pharynx, and larynx are aligned. The neck is flexed, and the head is extended at the atlanto-occipital joint. The mouth is opened with the right hand using the scissors maneuver. The laryngoscope is held in the left hand, and the blade is inserted into the mouth, displacing the soft tissues to the left. The blade tip (MacIntosh) is advanced into the vallecula, the epiglottis is elevated, and the cords are exposed by lifting the handle in an upward, forward direction with the wrist held straight. The laryngoscope should not be used as a lever. With the right hand, the endotracheal tube can be guided through the cords. After the cuff passes the cords, the tube is advanced an additional 3 cm. The cuff is inflated using 5 to 8 mL of air. The cuffs are designed as high-volume, low-pressure devices to avoid tissue ischemia. Cuff pressure should be less than 25 mmHg. Using the Miller blade, the same procedure is followed, with the exception of blade placement. The Miller blade tip is inserted beneath the epiglottis, elevating it against the posterior aspect of the tongue, thus exposing the cords.

This procedure should be completed in 20 seconds. Once the tube is in place, inflate the balloon, confirm proper placement, and secure the tube. If difficulty is encountered, oxygenate and ventilate the patient before a second attempt is made. Intubation is not considered complete until correct placement of the endotracheal tube is confirmed. There are several confirmatory techniques. None is 100% reliable and a question regarding any of these should prompt further evaluation. Auscultation of the chest bilaterally and of the epigastrium is the most practical method of confirmation. Breath sound should be audible laterally near the axilla and nearly absent over the epigastrium. The chest wall should be observed to move symmetrically with ventilations, and compliance to ventilation should be consistent with the clinical condition. In patients without severe bronchospasm, adult respiratory distress syndrome (ARDS), or other severe restrictive diseases, compliance to ventilation should be low.

Immediately after intubation, if a clear endotracheal tube is used, condensation will be seen with expiratory flow. In an awake patient, vocal silence and a harsh cough usually follow endotracheal intubation. The most reliable technique is use of an end-tidal CO_2 monitor (capnometer). A rise in the carbon dioxide concentration from inspired to expired air from 0.04% to 5–6% as measured by a capnometer is confirmation of proper placement. Two types of capnometers are available. The standard capnometer commonly used during anesthesia requires several minutes to warm up before it can be used. It will display the actual carbon dioxide concentration or a wave pattern representing the change in CO_2 concentration with inspiration and expiration. Although it is very accurate, the warm-up time required may make it impractical when confirmation of endotracheal tube placement is emergent. An alternative is the colorimetric capnometer. It is a disposable piece of equipment that changes color as the concentration of carbon dioxide rises during expiration. No warm-up time is required with this colorimetric capnometer.

If properly positioned, the tube measurement at the incisors should be 22 to 24 cm in men and 20 to 22 cm in women. A chest x-ray film (CXR) should follow all emergency intubations. The tip of the tube should be between the clavicle and the carina. The patient's clinical status should be monitored. Signs of hypoxia or hemodynamic instability should prompt re-evaluation of the airway. If a question remains as to proper tube placement, direct visualization with a laryngoscope or bronchoscope should be employed.

Failed oral intubation. Unsuccessful intubation in patients with normal anatomy is due to faulty technique. Some of the errors encountered with oral intubation are listed.

- Improper positioning of the patient's head, with improper alignment of the mouth, pharynx, and larynx
- Inadequate oral access
- Inadequate displacement of the soft tissues
- Levering of the laryngoscope
- Overzealousness and rushing
- Overly cautious technique

Common errors include the improper positioning of the patient, inadequate oral access, and improper use of the laryngoscope. Operator anxiety resulting in overcautiousness or, conversely, overzealousness can result in failed intubation.

Complications. During laryngoscopy, the laryngoscope can cause traumatic injury to the lips, the mucous membranes of the oropharynx, and/or the teeth.[12] Care should be taken to watch for entrapment of the soft tissues and to avoid levering of the laryngoscope against the maxilla.

Hypoxemia resulting from improper preoxygenation, aspiration, the inability to rapidly intubate, or intubation of the right main bronchus or esophagus can result in devastating consequences. The patient should be adequately oxygenated and suction equipment should be available and functioning before any intubation attempt. After intubation, proper tube placement should always be confirmed.

Laryngoscopy and intubation produce transient tachycardia, hypertension, and an increase in intracranial pressure. In normal patients, these transient changes rarely have detrimental effects; however, in patients with severe coronary artery disease or intracranial disease these effects may be more significant. Attempts to blunt these responses, as previously described, may be helpful.

Difficult Intubation

There are many processes that can lead to a difficult intubation.[13–14a]

- Short, thick neck
- Protruding incisors
- Maxillary overgrowth
- High arched palate
- Macrognathia
- Poor mobility at the temporomandibular joint
- Decreased ability to extend the neck
  1. Rheumatoid arthritis
  2. Ankylosing spondylitis
  3. Suspected cervical spine injury
- Submental or submandibular swelling
- Goiter
- Neck carcinoma

Even in the most skilled hands, approximately 1% to 3% of attempted intubations are impossible using traditional techniques. If endotracheal intubation cannot be achieved by conventional measures, several options remain.[15]

A lighted stylet (light wand)[16–18] can be used for blind oral intubations in awake patients. The light transilluminates the neck when it enters the trachea. The endotracheal tube is then advanced over the stylet. Because a laryngoscope is not used, this technique is useful when access to the oropharynx is limited or visualization of the cords is difficult.

Fiberoptic laryngoscopy,[19] bronchoscopy, and intubation are now used frequently if intubation is anticipated to be difficult. Fiberoptic technique can be used for either nasal or oral intubation. It is very effective; to become proficient with this technique, however, significant training and practice are required.

To perform fiberoptic-assisted intubation, the flexible end of the bronchoscope is placed through the endotracheal tube and is advanced into the oropharynx. As the scope is advanced, the operator watches through the handle piece for the epiglottis and cords to come into view. The tip is advanced through the cords, the endotracheal tube is passed over the scope, and the scope is removed.

Unresponsive patients may be successfully intubated using a digital approach.[20] This procedure should be performed only if direct laryngoscopy has failed. The intubator places his or her index and middle fingers in the patient's mouth over the posterior aspect of the tongue until the posterior aspect of the epiglottis is palpable. The tube is then passed between the fingers into the trachea.

Nasal Intubation

Direct laryngoscopy is poorly tolerated by awake patients. The blind nasal approach is an alternative method of endotracheal intubation.[21,22] The procedure should be explained to the patient. The patient's nostril should be anesthetized and lubricated with a topical anesthetic and vasoconstrictor. The tube size is 0.5 to 1 mm smaller than that used for oral intubation. The endotracheal tube is introduced into the nostril with the bevel toward the septum, guided posteriorly, and advanced into the oropharynx. With the intubator's ear placed adjacent to the open end of the tube, the tube is advanced while the operator listens and feels for breath sounds. When the tube enters the trachea (during inspiration), the patient coughs and is unable to phonate. When properly positioned, the tube measurement at the nostril will be 25 to 27 cm, approximately 3 cm further than an orally placed tube. Placement confirmation as previously described is performed and the tube is secured. This method is more difficult and time consuming than oral intubation; however, it may be better tolerated by the awake patient.

SURGICAL AIRWAYS

The need to establish an emergent surgical airway is uncommon and associated with significant morbidity and mortality. It is most commonly required when less invasive methods of airway management are contraindicated or have failed. The situations in which an emergent surgical airway may be required are listed.

- Trauma
  1. Direct airway trauma
     (a) Severe airway burns
     (b) Penetrating injury to the upper airway or larynx
     (c) Crush injury to the larynx
  2. Indirect trauma
     (a) Severe maxillary-mandibular disruption
     (b) Large hematomas of the head or neck
- Infection
  1. Abscess of the head or neck
  2. Epiglottitis
- Upper airway foreign body
- Anatomic abnormalities

The emergency physician, although infrequently faced with this situation, must be familiar with the techniques of surgical airway management. In emergent situations, the cricothyroidotomy is the procedure of choice.

Needle Cricothyroidotomy

Although the needle cricothyroidotomy is rarely indicated, it is the procedure of choice in children requiring a surgical airway. The patient is preoxygenated with 100% oxygen. If no cervical injury is suspected, the neck is extended and the cricothyroid membrane is palpated between the thyroid and the cricoid cartilages. If the patient is awake and time permits, the skin is anesthetized in the midline over the cricothyroid membrane. A 14 gauge catheter over needle is inserted through the cricothyroid membrane in the midline at a slight caudad angle. The physician aspirates as inserting until air return is noted. The catheter is advanced and the needle is removed.

Oxygenation may now be achieved by one of two methods. A high-pressure jet ventilator can be used to administer intermittent "breaths."[23] The jet ventilator is connected to the catheter by high-pressure tubing. The chest is observed for excursion with each "breath." A stopcock, release valve, or Y-connector should be inserted into the system to allow intermittent passive exhalation. A second alternative is to oxygenate the patient using a B-V-M device. The B-V-M is connected to the catheter by a 3-mL syringe and a 15-mm adapter from a size 7.5 endotracheal tube.

The needle cricothyroidotomy provides only a very temporary airway and cannot be used for longer than 20 to 30 minutes. Exhalation is incomplete, dependent on a partially patent upper airway and results in significant hypercapnia after this amount of time. Complications of this procedure include the production of a pneumothorax or pneumomediastinum, perforation of the esophagus, hypoventilation, air embolism, and infection.

Surgical Cricothyroidotomy

A surgical cricothyroidotomy will provide an adequate airway until a formal tracheostomy can be performed. It is the procedure of choice when an emergent surgical airway is necessary.[24,25] A vertical midline incision is made through the skin and subcutaneous tissue overlying the cricothyroid membrane. A transverse incision is then made through the membrane. Tracheostomy hooks are used to pull the cartilaginous rings anteriorly, and a Trousseau dilator is inserted through the membrane into the trachea. A tracheostomy (Shiley size 4 to 6) or endotracheal (size 7) tube is then guided into the trachea, and the hooks and Trousseau dilator are removed. Tube placement is confirmed and the tube is secured. In children younger than 6 to 8 years, the cricothyroid space is too small to accommodate an adequate airway; therefore, this procedure is contraindicated in young children.

Retrograde Intubation

In cases in which the upper airway is patent but attempted intubation has failed, an endotracheal tube may be inserted using a retrograde catheter.[26,27] The cricothyroid membrane is percutaneously punctured. A guidewire is introduced through the needle into the trachea, and the needle is removed. The guidewire or a long, flexible catheter over the guidewire is advanced in a cephalad direction until it is visible in the oropharynx. Using a Magills forceps, the distal end of the wire (or catheter) is pulled out of the mouth. An endotracheal tube is advanced over the wire and the wire is removed. Tube placement is confirmed and the patient is ventilated. This procedure should be used only when conventional intubation techniques have failed and fiberoptic intubation is not available.

Tracheostomy

An emergent tracheostomy is rarely indicated. Only in situations involving direct laryngeal trauma or severe subglottic stenosis will a surgical cricothyroidotomy be ineffective. To perform an emergency tracheostomy, a deep vertical incision is made from the cricoid cartilage to the sternal notch. Several tracheal rings are cut, and an endotracheal or tracheostomy tube is inserted and secured. The extensive bleeding that results from this procedure is addressed only after the airway is secured and the patient is being ventilated.

REFERENCES

1. Don Michael TA. The role of the esophageal obturator airway in cardiopulmonary resuscitation. *Circulation*. 1986;74(suppl IV):IV-134–IV-137.
2. Goldenberg IF, Campion BC, Seibold CM, et al. Morbidity and mortality in patients receiving the esophageal obturator airway and endotracheal tube in prehospital cardiopulmonary arrest. *Minn Med*. 1986;69:707–713.
3. Frass M, Frenzer R, Rauscha F, et al. Evaluation of the esophageal tracheal combitube in cardiopulmonary resuscitation. *Crit Care Med*. 1986;15:609–611.
4. Greenberg MI. Endotracheal drugs: state of the art. *Ann Emerg Med*. 1984;13:789.
5. Derbyshire DR, Smith G, Achola KJ. Effect of topical lignocaine on the sympatho adrenal responses to tracheal intubation. *Br J Anaesth*. 1987;58:300.
6. Hartigain ML, Cleary JL, Schaffer DW. A comparison of pretreatment regimens for minimizing the hemodynamic response to blind nasotracheal intubation. *Can Anesth Soc J*. 1984;31:497.
7. Curran J, Hamilton C, Taylor T. Topical analgesia before tracheal intubation. *Anaesthesia*. 1975;30:765.
8. Batlan DE, Zaid GJ, Johnston WC. Neuromuscular blockade in the emergency department. *J Emerg Med*. 1987;5:225–232.
9. Morris IR. Pharmacologic aids to intubation and the rapid sequence induction. *Emerg Med Clin North Am*. 1988;6:753–768.
10. Talucci RC, Shaikh KA, Schwab CW. Rapid sequence induction with oral endotracheal intubation in the multiply injured patient. *Am Surg*. 1988;54:185–187.
11. Thompson JD, Fish S, Ruiz E. Succinylcholine for endotracheal intubation. *Ann Emerg Med*. 1982;11:526.
12. Blanc VF, Tremblay NAG. Complications of tracheal intubation: classification with a review of the literature. *Anesth Analg*. 1974;53:202–213.
13. McIntyre JWR. The difficult tracheal intubation. *Can J Anaesth*. 1987;34:204–213.
13a. Ament R. A systematic approach to the difficult intubation. *Anesth Rev*. 1989;5:12.
14. Bennett JR. Difficulties in emergency airway management. *Mo Med*. 1988;85:591–595.
14a. Samsoon GLT, Young JRB. Difficult tracheal intubation: a retrospective study. *Anaesthesia*. 1987;42:487–490.
15. Iserson KV, Sanders AB, Kabach K. Difficult intubations: aids and alternatives. *Am Fam Physician*. 1985;31(3):99.
16. Ducrow M. Throwing light on blind intubation. *Anaesthesia*. 1978;33:827–829.
17. Stewart RD, LaRosee A, Stoy WA, et al. Use of a lighted stylet to confirm correct endotracheal tube placement. *Chest*. 1987;92:900–903.
18. Ellis DG, Steward RD, Kaplan RM, et al. Success rates of blind orotracheal intubation using a transillumination technique with a light stylet. *Ann Emerg Med*. 1986;15:138–142.
19. Delaney KA, Hessler R. Emergency flexible fiberoptic nasotracheal intubation: a report of 60 cases. *Ann Emerg Med*. 1988;17:919–926.
20. Hardwick WC, Bluhm D. Digital intubation. *J Emerg Med*. 1984;1:317–320.
21. Baraka A. Blind nasotracheal intubation: the lost art. *MEJ Anaesth*. 1978;5(1):3–6.
22. Danzl DF, Thomas DM. Nasotracheal intubations in the emergency department. *Crit Care Med*. 1980;8:677–682.
23. Attia RR, Battit GE, Murphy JD. Transtracheal ventilation. *JAMA*. 1975;234:1152–1153.
24. Kress TD, Balasubramaniam S. Cricothyroidotomy. *Ann Emerg Med*. 1982;11:197–201.
25. McGill J, Clinton JE, Ruiz E. Cricothyroidotomy in the emergency department. *Ann Emerg Med*. 1982;11:361–364.
26. Bourke D, Levesque PR. Modification of retrograde guide for endotracheal intubation. *Anesth Analg*. 1974;53:1013–1014.
27. McNamara R. Retrograde intubation of the trachea. *Ann Emerg Med*. 1987;16:680–682.

BIBLIOGRAPHY

Dorsch JA, Dorsch SE. *Understanding Anesthesia Equipment*. 2nd ed. Baltimore, Md: Williams & Wilkins Co.; 1984.

Finucane BT, Santora AH. *Principles of Airway Management*. Philadelphia, Pa: FA Davis Co; 1988.

Hochbaum SR. Emergency airway management. *Emerg Med Clin North Am*. 1986;4:411–425.

Roberts JT. Fundamentals of tracheal intubation. New York, NY: Grune & Stratton; 1983.

Safar P, Bircher N. *Cardiopulmonary Cerebral Resuscitation*. 3rd ed. Philadelphia, Pa: WB Saunders Co; 1988.

71. Croup and Epiglottitis

RONALD N. ROTHENBERG, MD, FACEP

One of the most frightening situations in emergency medicine is the presentation of a child with upper airway compromise. Although the cause may be relatively benign, as in spasmodic croup or mild laryngotracheitis, patients with epiglottitis may develop sudden respiratory arrest. This chapter encompasses croup, epiglottitis, and bacterial tracheitis in children and epiglottitis in adults.

There are many controversies in the diagnosis and management of croup and epiglottitis. In the past, direct visualization of the epiglottis was strongly discouraged. However, many authors currently recommend direct visualization to diagnose croup accurately and rule out acute epiglottitis. Other points of controversy include the role of racemic epinephrine in croup, the timing of intubation in epiglottitis, and differences in the management of childhood versus adult epiglottitis. The following discussion covers the recognition and treatment of these disorders.

CROUP

Croup syndrome is defined as the triad of inspiratory stridor, cough, and hoarseness. There are three patterns.

1. *Laryngotracheitis*. This viral illness has an upper respiratory infection (URI) prodrome, low-grade fever, barking cough, and inspiratory stridor.
2. *Spasmodic croup*. This possibly allergic or possibly viral illness manifests with a sudden attack of inspiratory stridor, usually at night. Usually where there is no URI prodrome or fever, the course is self-limited, and repeat episodes are common.
3. *Bacterial tracheitis or membranous croup*. This bacterial infection of the subglottic region has symptoms similar to those of laryngotracheitis but with high fever, toxicity, and the potential for severe airway obstruction.

Laryngotracheitis

Laryngotracheitis (LT) is an acute inflammation of the subglottic airway, which can include the larynx, the trachea, and occasionally the bronchi. LT is the most common cause of upper airway obstruction in children.

Etiology

Parainfluenza viruses are the most frequent causes of LT. Influenza A virus, respiratory syncytial virus, adenovirus, paramyxovirus, and other viruses have been reported.[1,1a]

Pathology

There is subglottic swelling and a sticky exudate in the narrowest point of the airway. The larynx, trachea, and mainstem bronchi may be involved, but the supraglottic region is not. The airway obstruction that can be seen in LT is produced by the increase in resistance to airflow caused by

Table 71-1 Croup versus Epiglottitis

	Croup	Epiglottitis
Etiology	Parainfluenza	H. influenzae
Age	½ to 3 y	3 to 7 y
Onset	24 to 72 h	6 to 24 h
Toxicity	Mild to moderate	Marked
Drooling	Unusual	Frequent
Cough	Frequent	Rare
Hoarseness	Frequent	Rare

the decreased diameter of the airway; 1 mm of circumferential swelling produces a 75% reduction in a corresponding cross-sectional area of a neonate's larynx.[2] The larger airway of the adult still has room for airflow after 1 to 2 mm of circumferential swelling. The tenacious exudate further compromises the narrowed airway.

Clinical Observations[1,3]

The classic age group is 6 months to 3 years, but cases have been reported from 2 months to adult. The age range could be helpful in differentiating LT from acute epiglottitis (AE), since the classic age range for AE is 3 to 6 years (Table 71-1). With both illnesses, however, there is considerable overlap in age groups of patients. LT is seen in males about twice as often as females. Increased incidence is seen during winter months and during epidemics.[1a]

The typical picture includes a preceding URI and a gradual onset over 24 hours. A croupy cough resembling a seal bark is usually present. The patient's voice may be hoarse. Inspiratory and expiratory stridor is caused by the turbulent airflow. Low-grade fever is present. The epiglottis is normal in size, shape, and color. Respiratory distress can range from minimal to severe to respiratory arrest from complete obstruction. Retractions indicate respiratory distress, and they can become progressively worse as the illness progresses. Once fatigue overcomes the child, decreasing retractions may give the false impression that the patient is improving. Tachycardia may be a sign of hypoxemia.

Laboratory Findings

Laboratory studies are not necessary for the diagnosis of LT. In questionable cases, they may be helpful. The white blood cell (WBC) count and differential are usually normal or slightly elevated.[1a] Arterial blood gases may be normal or indicate hypoxemia. Hypercarbia and acidosis are signs of severe airway compromise and are seen only with severe cases. Pulse oximetry is a useful addition to clinical evaluation of a child with croup, especially if the O_2 saturation is consistently high or low. However, a correlation between outcome and O_2 saturation has not been demonstrated. Oxygen saturation may be inaccurate due to movement artifacts

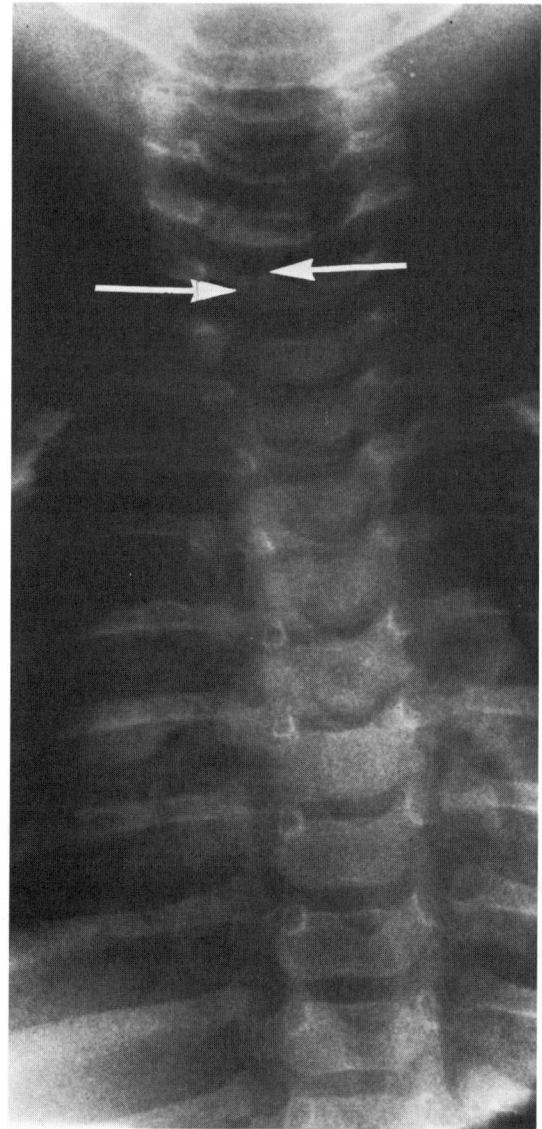

Figure 71-1 AP roentgenogram of the neck showing subglottic edema in a patient with croup, the "steeple sign." *Source:* Reprinted from Kravis TC. Obstructive lung diseases. In Kravis TC, Warner CG, eds. *Emergency Medicine: A Comprehensive Review.* 1st ed. 1983; 833.

in a restless child.[4a,4b] Although radiographs are not necessary to make the diagnosis of LT, certain characteristic x-ray signs may be helpful in atypical or confusing cases. On a normal anteriorposterior radiograph of the neck, the tracheal air column will appear to have shoulders or be in the shape of a Gothic arch. With LT, the air column will be narrowed and pointed as in a Byzantine arch, the steeple sign (Fig. 71-1). On a lateral neck radiograph, the subglottic region will be blurred or narrowed; the epiglottis will be normal; and, if there is significant obstruction, the hypopharynx will be ballooned.[4]

Diagnosis

The clinical picture of LT including history and physical exam (normal epiglottis) should suggest the diagnosis. As mentioned above, laboratory studies might be useful in atypical cases but are not routinely required. Acute epiglottitis, bacterial tracheitis, and other causes of upper airway obstruction listed in the differential diagnosis section should be considered in the differential diagnosis. The only completely reliable way to rule out acute epiglottitis is to visualize the epiglottis (somewhat controversial). Diagnosis made by age group, history, physical, and lab only without visualizing the epiglottis will occasionally miss acute epiglottitis. (See section on AE for suggested plan for visualization of epiglottis.) Posteroanterior and lateral neck radiographs will at times be inconclusive and subject to varying interpretations.[5] If a patient does not respond to the usual treatment (see below), suspect another diagnosis.

Treatment

Any patient with upper airway compromise should be closely observed because his or her condition can change rapidly.

Prehospital. Although there have never been any controlled studies documenting its efficacy, the use of mist is a traditional treatment for laryngotracheitis.[6] Since moist air may decrease the subglottic swelling, it is sometimes recommended that the child's parents can turn on the hot water in the bathroom and sit with the child there. Time should not be wasted if the child has any respiratory distress, stridor, or retractions since definitive therapy will be delayed. During transport by emergency medical technicians, the child with respiratory distress or retractions should receive humidified O_2, if this can be administered without agitating the child.

Emergency department. In the emergency department, cool mist can be administered and the child observed. A croup tent can make the child difficult to observe and should not be used in the emergency department. If the patient improves and there are no signs of respiratory distress while at rest (stridor, retractions, tachycardia), he or she can be sent home after about an hour of observation, provided that the family is reliable and relatively rapid return to the emergency department is possible in cases of deteriorating condition (Table 71-2). Many patients with LT will be in the mild category described above.

Racemic epinephrine. If there is moderate to severe respiratory distress initially or no improvement with mist, the patient should be given humidified O_2 at 40% FiO_2 via mask and treated with racemic epinephrine via nebulizer. The dose is 0.5 mL of 2.25% racemic epinephrine in 3.5 mL saline. The mechanism of action is theorized to be via the α-adrenergic effect, which may shrink the edematous subglottic mucosa, and possibly the β-adrenergic effect, which may reduce laryngospasm or tracheal muscle constriction. There have been many controversies surrounding the use of racemic epinephrine. Racemic epinephrine does not alter the course of LT but provides temporary relief of the upper airway compromise. Since the disease is usually self-limited, this will get the child through the more serious phase. Westley and Brooks[7] compared racemic epinephrine to saline and found significant improvement at 10 to 30 minutes with racemic epinephrine. The overall duration of the illness was not changed, and at 120 minutes after treatment the control group and treated group had similar clinical findings.

In the past, the usual recommendation was to admit all children who had received racemic epinephrine since the overall duration of the illness was not changed and there was concern over a possible "rebound" phenomenon of the child becoming worse after the racemic epinephrine had worn off. Despite this previous recommendation, it is safe to discharge children who have received racemic epinephrine if the following precautions are followed. They are observed for 2 hours following the treatment with racemic epinephrine and

Table 71-2 Croup Score

	0	1	2	3
Stridor	None	Only with agitation	Mild at rest	Severe at rest
Retraction	None	Mild	Moderate	Severe
Air entry	Normal	Mild decrease	Moderate decrease	Marked decrease
Color	Normal	Not applicable	Not applicable	Cyanotic
Level of consciousness	Normal	Restless when disturbed	Restless when undisturbed	Lethargic

Management by Score

	Score $\leq$ 6	Outpatient	
	Score $\geq$ 7	Admit	
	Any one category with score of 3	Admit	

Modified from Taussig et al. Treatment of laryngotracheitis (croup): use of intermittent positive pressure breathing and racemic epinephrine. *Am J Dis Child.* 1975;129:790.

are free of stridor and retractions; they are being discharged with reliable parents and have a reliable means for returning to the emergency department. Although racemic epinephrine does not appear to change the duration of LT, corticosteroids do decrease duration and severity (see next section below) and should be used in children who require racemic epinephrine. Kelley and Simon report a study of 50 children with croup (LT) who were treated with racemic epinephrine and discharged after 2 hours without complication. Most of these children received corticosteroids. If there are stridor or retractions or other signs of dyspnea after 2 hours, repeat treatment with racemic epinephrine is indicated, and the child should be admitted.[4a,7a,7b,12]

If there is no improvement with racemic epinephrine, another diagnosis should be considered, especially acute epiglottitis or bacterial tracheitis. Racemic epinephrine is an equal mixture of *l* and *d* isomers where *l*-epinephrine is the active component. A dose of 5.0 mL of *l*-epinephrine 1:1000 (regular epinephrine) is equivalent to 0.5 mL of racemic epinephrine (2.2%) and has been shown to be equally effective and safe.[8,8a] Subcutaneous epinephrine is not effective for treatment of laryngotracheitis. Racemic epinephrine is not effective for treatment of acute epiglottitis.

Corticosteroids. The use of corticosteroids in LT has been controversial in the past.[9–13] There is excellent evidence from controlled double-blind studies that a single dose of dexamethasone, 0.6 mg/kg intramuscularly (IM), leads to faster recovery, shorter hospital stay, and less need for airway intervention.[13] All children who require racemic epinephrine should be treated with dexamethasone 0.6 mg/kg IM or IV or an equivalent dose of corticosteroid. In children intubated for LT, prednisolone, 1 mg/kg twice daily, has been shown to decrease the duration of intubation and the need for reintubation.[13a]

Antibiotics. Since LT is a viral disease, antibiotics are not effective. There is evidence, however, that bacterial tracheitis may be a complication of viral LT. Because of this, there may be a role for antistaphylococcal antibiotics when bacterial tracheitis is considered (higher fever, toxicity, WBC) or when the diagnosis is in doubt. This point needs further clarification.[14,15]

Intubation. Intubation is rarely required for treatment of LT (3% of admitted patients), but it is lifesaving if the patient's respiratory distress is not improving. If respiratory distress is becoming worse despite the use of racemic epinephrine, the diagnosis of LT may be incorrect; the patient may in fact have acute epiglottitis or bacterial tracheitis and require intubation.

Other indications for endotracheal intubation include increasing lethargy or exhaustion, obtundation, cyanosis with FiO_2 40%, increasing PCO_2, and possibly requiring racemic epinephrine treatment more than once per hour.[2] Recent increases in the need for intubation in LT may have arisen because these patients actually have bacterial tracheitis.[16]

Spasmodic Croup

Spasmodic croup (SC) should be considered when there is no fever and no URI prodrome and there is a history of repeat episodes. The terminology is confusing, since some physicians use the term SC as a synonym for acute laryngotracheitis. Attacks usually occur at night. There is no fine dividing line between the presentations of SC and LT. The pathogenesis is unclear; allergic and viral roles as well as mucosal drying and swelling have been implicated. SC may not have a different etiology, however, and may only represent the mild end of the clinical spectrum of acute laryngotracheitis.[17] Most patients do well with just cool mist, and the stridor and retractions clear. If racemic epinephrine is required, the patient should be treated as having LT.

Bacterial Tracheitis[11,12,18,19,19a]

Bacterial tracheitis (BT) or membranous laryngotracheobronchitis is a bacterial infection of the subglottic trachea presenting as a severe toxic form of LT.

Etiology

Coagulase-positive *Staphylococcus aureus* is the most frequent organism cultured from the subglottic trachea. Group A streptococcus, *Haemophilus influenzae* type B, β-hemolytic streptococcus, *Moraxella (Branhamella) catarrhalis*, and *Streptococcus pneumoniae* have also been reported.[20,21] BT had been described in the 1940s but was reintroduced to medicine in reports by Jones et al[18] and Han et al[24] in 1979.

Pathology

There is mucosal swelling and airway narrowing at the level of the cricoid accompanied by thick purulent secretions causing airway compromise. Since most BT cases are seen during increases in the frequency of LT episodes and parainfluenza viruses are frequently cultured from the subglottic trachea in these patients, it appears that BT may be caused by a bacterial invasion of the subglottic mucosa after it has been damaged by LT. Toxic shock syndrome has been reported secondary to BT caused by *staphylococcus aureus*.[21a]

Clinical Observations

The picture of BT is similar to LT but more severe, and it may resemble acute epiglottitis. There is usually a URI followed by a croupy cough. The patient appears sicker than the LT patient and may have high fever and toxicity. The usual age group is 6 months to 10 years. Case reports of BT in adults have been published.[22,23] Inspiratory stridor is present and may be severe. There is usually leukocytosis and left shift. Radiograph shows a normal epiglottis and a narrowed subglottic region, as with LT. A membrane may be seen on lateral neck radiograph in the subglottic region.[24,24a]

Treatment

Prehospital. As with LT, the patient should be given humidified oxygen via mask, along with calm reassurance.

Emergency department. Endotracheal intubation is necessary for suctioning purulent tracheal secretions. The phenomenon of pus shooting out of the end of the endotracheal tube (ET) has been reported.[14] Racemic epinephrine may possibly be effective if administered after intubation and suctioning. Gram stains and cultures should be obtained, and the patient should be treated with antibiotics appropriate to cover *Staphylococcus aureus* and *Haemophilus influenzae*. Once the airway is assured with endotracheal intubation, some authors have a preference for maintaining the airway with tracheostomy. The thick secretions may be better suctioned, and improved survival and fewer complications can result.[11] If an emergency airway is required in the emergency department, endotracheal intubation is the airway of choice. The airway can be converted to a tracheostomy in the controlled setting of the operating room afterward. There is significant risk for upper airway obstruction with BT, and this illness must be considered as being as life-threatening as AE.[19a]

ACUTE EPIGLOTTITIS

AE is an acute inflammatory swelling of the supraglottic structures of the larynx, which can produce upper airway compromise. The vocal cords and subglottic region are not involved. Supraglottitis is a more accurate term and is preferred by some authors. The epiglottis, aryepiglottic folds, ventricular bands, pharynx, and arytenoid cartilages can be involved. Thick secretions can add to the upper airway compromise. Toxicity and bacteremia are present, and blood cultures are positive in over 80% of pediatric patients. The incidence of AE is rare compared to croup (1:400).[25]

Etiology

In children the causative agent is almost exclusively *Haemophilus influenzae* type B although (rarely) other bacteria have been cultured.[17] Children with epiglottitis and positive epiglottis cultures for group A streptococci have also been reported.[25a] Caustics, gasoline, or thermal injury to the epiglottis can produce a similar clinical picture of upper airway compromise.[26]

Pathology

There is an acute inflammatory swelling of the supraglottic cartilages of the larynx. Rarely, the epiglottis may be normal. The infection of the supraglottic structures probably arises from direct invasion of *Haemophilus influenzae* type B with bacteremia following. The inflammation spreads through the supraglottic structures, which have a loosely attached mucous membrane, but stops at the vocal cords, owing to the tightly adherent mucosa. Hence, supraglottic and subglottic inflammation does not spread below or above the cords.[17] AE was not recognized as a distinct illness until the 1930s and 1940s; it was included in the broad category of "croup." The detailed description of George Washington's final illness and demise provides strong evidence that the first president of the United States died from AE.[27]

Clinical Observations

The classical age group of children with AE is 3 to 7 years, but in the past decade there has been an increasing awareness of the significant percentage of infants less than 2 years old (25% of children in one study)[28] and adults. The time course of epiglottitis is dreadfully rapid, and complete obstruction and respiratory arrest can occur at any minute. The duration of the illness prior to presenting in the emergency department is almost always less than 24 hours and often less than 6 hours.[29] It is the most frightening illness in pediatrics, for the child, the parents, and the physician. Mortality was close to 100% in the era prior to antibiotics and artificial airways.[30]

The child appears toxic and has an ashen grey color. Respiratory distress is the most frequent symptom. There is high fever. Children with AE can present with cyanosis and shock as well as stridor.[31] There will usually be inspiratory stridor and retractions. The child, if old enough, may complain of a sore throat. Drooling may indicate that there is too much pain to permit swallowing. The voice may be clear or it may be muffled. Vomiting is sometimes a prominent symptom; the enlarged epiglottis presumably stimulates the gag reflex. Classically, the child will sit upright with chin thrust forward, the tripod position (Figs. 71-2 and 71-3). This posture apparently maximizes the compromised airway. When the mouth is open, a fiery red epiglottis may be prominent (see Fig. 71-4).

Although diagnosis of a patient with the classic signs and symptoms of AE is not difficult, occasional patients are seen in the emergency department with minimal initial signs and symptoms, if the patient is seen very early in the time course. As mentioned in the section above on LT, there is a grey zone of signs and symptoms and infrequently a child with the clinical picture of AE will actually have LT. Rarely, symptoms that are associated with LT such as hoarseness or croupy cough are reported with AE.[32]

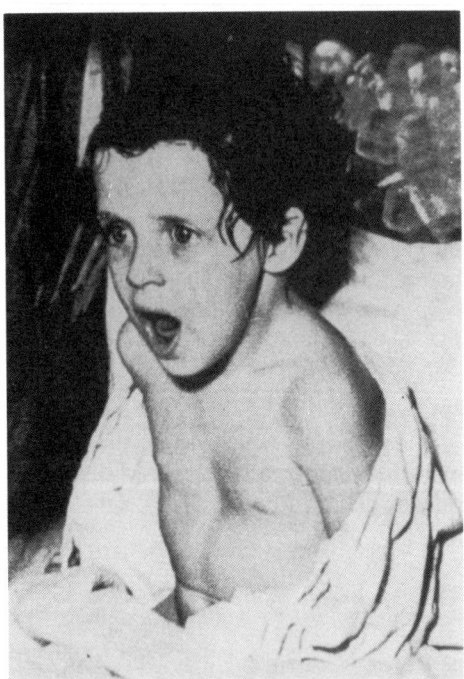

Figure 71-2 Typical appearance of a child with AE. Note child sitting up, mouth open, anxious look. *Source:* Reproduced with Permission from Fearon B. Acute laryngotracheobronchitis in infancy and childhood. *Pediatr Clin North Am.* 1962;9(4):1095.

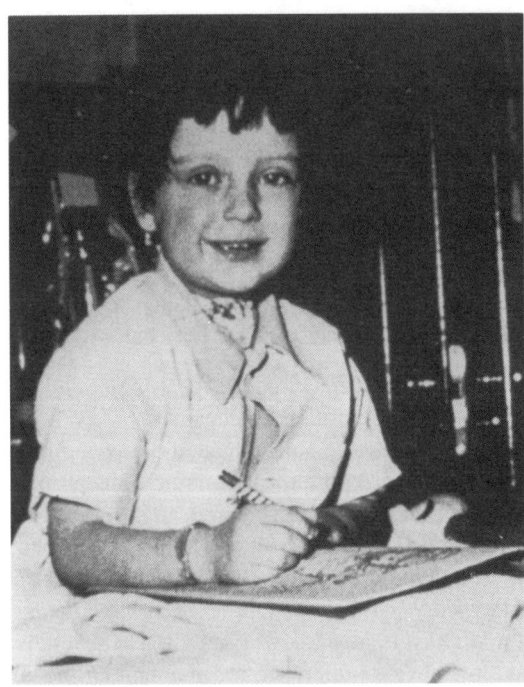

Figure 71-3 The same child in the preceding figure, 48 hours later, with artificial airway (tracheostomy). *Source:* Reproduced with Permission from Fearon B. Acute laryngotracheobronchitis in infancy and childhood. *Pediatr Clin North Am.* 1962;9(4):1095.

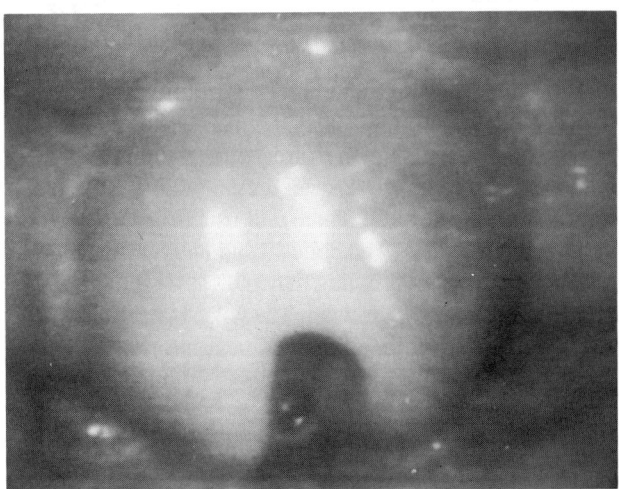

Figure 71-4 Massive swelling of epiglottis and copious secretions. *Source:* Courtesy of University of California at San Diego School of Medicine.

Children with AE less than 2 years of age may occasionally present with atypical signs and symptoms such as croupy cough, URI history, absent or low-grade fever, or a prolonged prodrome. In children less than 6 months of age there is a possible association with parainfluenza virus.[33–36] Since there is less awareness of AE in the younger age group, diagnoses and lifesaving airway intervention may be delayed.

A syndrome of pulmonary edema[37–39] has been reported in AE. After intubation (and in one report before intubation) there is increasing dyspnea and cyanosis. Arterial blood gases show hypoxemia, and chest radiograph shows a pulmonary edema pattern with a normal heart size. Without the full syndrome of pulmonary edema, there is evidence of lower respiratory tract involvement in AE reflected by a decrease in arterial/alveolar oxygen ratio even after intubation.[40] An abnormal chest radiograph is found in 25% of patients. The mechanism for this noncardiac pulmonary edema is believed to be that inspiratory indrawing effort leads to increasing negative pleural pressure, which creates increased pulmonary interstitial fluid volume. Injury to capillary walls due to hypoxia may also be a factor. Hypoxemia can be present even after the upper airway obstruction is relieved with an airway. This syndrome can also be seen with other causes of upper airway obstruction such as LT, severe tonsillitis, or aspirated foreign body.[41]

Associated Infections

Haemophilus influenzae is such an invasive organism that associated infections are not uncommon. Molteni[42] reported that pneumonia, cervical adenitis, and otitis media are often seen and, rarely, meningitis and that septic arthritis is associated with AE; therefore, thorough evaluation of the patient is necessary, keeping in mind extraepiglottic infections.

Treatment

Respiratory Arrest

Before discussing diagnosis and prehospital and emergency department treatment of AE, the initial treatment of respiratory arrest must be stressed. A patient with respiratory arrest from AE can be ventilated with bag-valve-mask technique.[43–45] To overcome the increased resistance to airflow, the pop-off valve on the bag may have to be held down, or an adult bag may be required. Even though this is usually "contraindicated," whatever is necessary to ventilate the child can be lifesaving.

Formerly it was thought that a child with respiratory arrest or "complete obstruction" could not be ventilated by mask because the epiglottis completely filled the airway. Since many were afraid to attempt intubation, last ditch tracheostomies were performed. This technique resulted in many deaths and children with anoxic brain damage. Ventilation by positive pressure, mask, and even mouth to mouth can result in successful resuscitation without neurologic sequelae. The extreme example of this principle was illustrated in a study where children with AE were not intubated but supported with mask and positive-pressure ventilation with 100% survival. In light of the overwhelming evidence that obstruction can occur at any moment, endotracheal intubation still remains the safest method of managing an airway in these patients. If a physician, nurse, or paramedic who is untrained in intubation or one who does not have the necessary equipment must treat a child who appears to be obstructed from AE, the patient can be ventilated until a more definitive airway can be established.

Prehospital

If AE is suspected, the child should be transported to the emergency department quickly but calmly. If the patient is being referred from a physician's office, the physician should accompany the patient along with the paramedics with equipment necessary for airway support.[18] Care should be taken not to agitate the child because agitation, fighting, and struggling can lead to sudden "complete obstruction" and respiratory arrest. The child should be given humidified O_2 via mask as tolerated. Establishment of an IV line can distress the child and waste valuable time and should not be done in the field. A child who is in a sitting position should not be forced to lie down, since respiratory arrest can be precipitated. As discussed previously, bag-mask ventilation can be lifesaving in cases of respiratory arrest and can buy time until an airway is established. If bag-mask ventilation is not effective and intubation is not available or successful, cricothyrotomy or percutaneous transtracheal ventilation can be lifesaving.

Emergency Department

One of the most controversial topics in emergency medicine and pediatrics is the approach to the diagnosis and treatment of acute epiglottitis in the emergency department. There is agreement that acute epiglottitis is a life-threatening emergency and that the conservative lifesaving treatment is the establishment of an artificial airway by endotracheal intubation. Also, there is agreement that needless procedures and airway manipulation must be avoided. Before the patient can be treated appropriately the diagnosis must be considered and other illnesses ruled out. The clinical picture can suggest AE, but to establish the diagnosis many authors recommend that the epiglottis should be visualized. The physician needs a plan to evaluate the epiglottis safely and deal with complications and provide an airway when necessary. The plan described below has been useful for the author. Care should be taken not to agitate the child unnecessarily, and distressing procedures such as arterial blood gases and venipuncture should be withheld until the airway is secured.

An algorithm (Fig. 71-5) for evaluation and treatment of AE in the emergency department is explained below.

1. If respiratory arrest or upper airway obstruction has occurred, ventilate with bag and mask with 100% O_2 and intubate endotracheally.

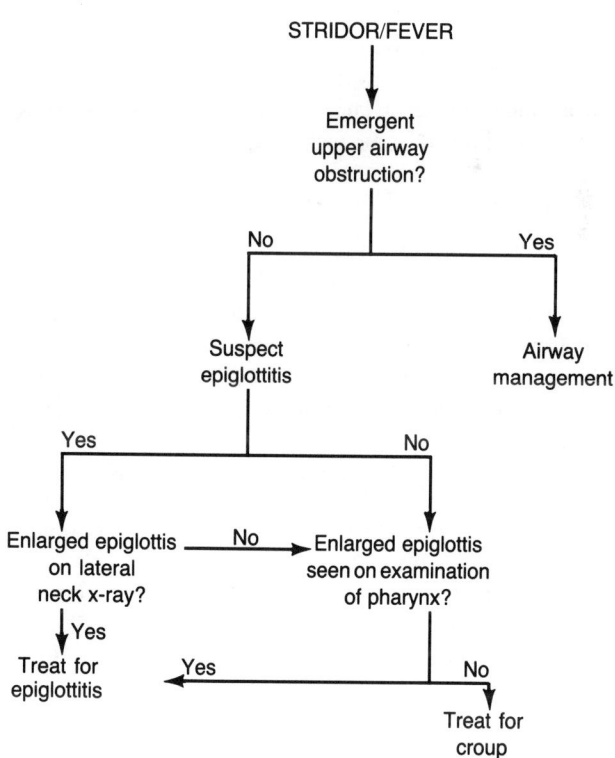

Figure 71-5 Approach to the Child with Stridor and Fever. *Source:* Reprinted with Permission from Fleisher G. Infectious disease emergencies. In: Fleisher G, Ludwig S, eds. *Textbook of Pediatric Emergency Medicine.* 2nd ed. Baltimore, Md: Williams & Wilkins Co; 1988:438.

2. When airway obstruction is imminent, suggested by cyanosis, exhaustion, lethargy, and increased respiratory distress, ventilate with bag and mask with 100% O_2, sedate, paralyze, and intubate endotracheally. There is controversy over sedation. Sedation can cause the exhausted patient to have a respiratory arrest, but that can be treated by proceeding with the intubation. Attempts at intubating a struggling, thrashing patient can be difficult or impossible; therefore an IV line should be established to administer sedation. With the patient paralyzed or adequately sedated, the intubation can proceed in a calm and controlled manner. Options include titrating morphine diazepam or midazolam until the child is sufficiently sedated to intubate. If necessary, the morphine can be reversed with naloxone. Another approach is rapid sequence intubation (see Chapter 70, Airway Management) with succinylcholine (1.5 to 2 mg/kg IV) or vecuronium (0.1 to 0.3 mg/kg IV). If the patient cannot be successfully intubated or manually ventilated, a surgical airway becomes necessary. In weighing the advantages and disadvantages, the awake patient should be sedated or paralyzed. The child should not be forced to lie down during the initial evaluation. However, when the physician is ready and able to intubate, it is necessary to have the child in the supine position. In the operating room, inhalational anesthetics can be administered—with the patient in a sitting position if necessary.

3. If the diagnosis of epiglottitis is only suspected and no signs of significant airway obstruction are present, then two possible approaches are available: (1) direct pharyngoscopy with a tongue blade or laryngoscope and (2) lateral neck radiograph with soft-tissue technique.

Sequential Method

Mauro et al. described a sequential method for visualizing the epiglottis and differentiating AE from LT in the child with stridor.[46] In this study, the diagnosis assigned prior to inspection of the epiglottis was incorrect in 2 of 6 patients with AE and 3 of 149 children with LT. Of the 6 patients with AE, there were no complications resulting from the direct pharyngoscopy. The sequence includes progressively more aggressive techniques for visualizing the epiglottis.

1. Examine the pharynx with light alone by asking the child to open his or her mouth.
2. Use a light and a wooden tongue depressor with the child sitting.
3. Use a laryngoscope (curved blade) with the child sitting.
4. Use a laryngoscope with the child supine.

Additional studies concur with the safety of direct pharyngoscopy.[47,48] Flexible fiber optic endoscopy is another technique that can be used safely to visualize the epiglottis.[48a]

There are anecdotal reports of upper airway obstruction after sticking a tongue depressor in the mouth of a child with suspected AE. Since upper airway obstruction is part of the natural course of this illness, it is possible that obstruction may not be related to the tongue blade. The inflamed epiglottis has been shown to be rigid, and it does not "flop down" into the glottis. Theories presented to explain this phenomenon of obstruction after pharyngeal manipulation include aspiration of secretions, laryngospasm, exhaustion, increased swelling of supraglottic structures, and vagal reflexes.

If AE is strongly suspected, the physician must remain with the child constantly. All resuscitation equipment must be ready: laryngoscope, endotracheal tubes (ETs) of the estimated size and smaller sizes, and cricothyrotomy equipment. The child should be preoxygenated with 100% O_2 for 5 minutes via mask. A curved laryngoscope blade (MacIntosh no. 2) can be used; the tongue should be depressed gently until the epiglottis can be seen. Care should be taken not to touch the epiglottis.

If epiglottitis is present (a swollen, bright red epiglottis with surrounding edema and erythema), the child can be intubated under the most controlled conditions. If the epiglottis is normal, another diagnosis must be considered. It is rarely possible to have supraglottitis without epiglottitis, and a normal epiglottis does not completely rule out a life-threatening upper airway obstruction and the potential need for endotracheal intubation.

Lateral Neck Radiograph[49]

The danger of the lateral neck radiograph lies in (1) abandoning the child to the radiology department and (2) wasting time while obtaining the radiograph for a child who needs to be intubated. There is less danger if the physician is with the child constantly and all airway resuscitation equipment is with the physician and patient so that there is no delay in providing an airway for a child on the verge of obstruction. The radiograph can be obtained by portable technique, allowing the child to remain sitting in the emergency department.[50]

The radiograph should be performed with soft-tissue technique, and the patient's chin should be in the extended position. A normal epiglottis has the shape of a little finger, and a swollen epiglottis in acute epiglottitis has the shape of a rounded thumb[51] (Figs. 71-6 through 71-12). Also, with AE the aryepiglottic folds are thickened and the vallecula and pyriform sinus are obliterated. At times the radiographs are difficult to interpret conclusively. Other potential causes of upper airway compromise may be identified on the lateral neck radiograph, such as radiopaque foreign bodies, retropharyngeal abscess, the subglottic narrowing seen with LT or BT, or the membrane sometimes seen with BT. If the lateral neck radiograph appears normal, the physician can proceed with direct pharyngoscopy for confirmation that the epiglottis and other supraglottic structures are normal. If AE is diagnosed, the physician can prepare for intubation.

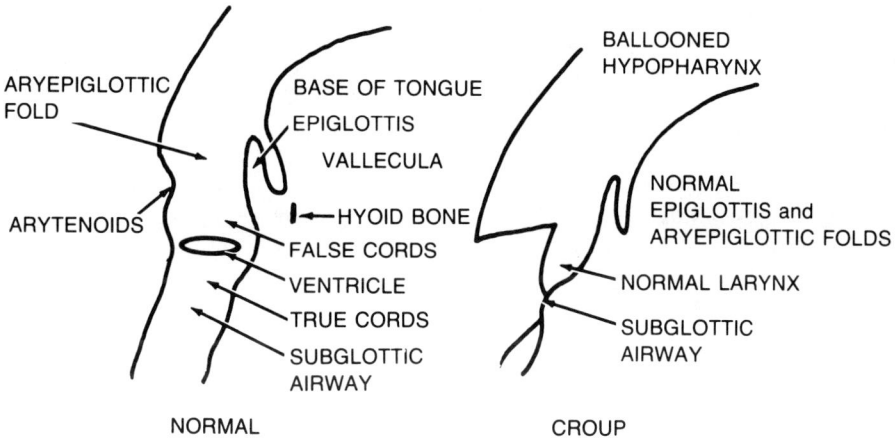

Figure 71-6 Diagram of upper airway: normal versus croup.

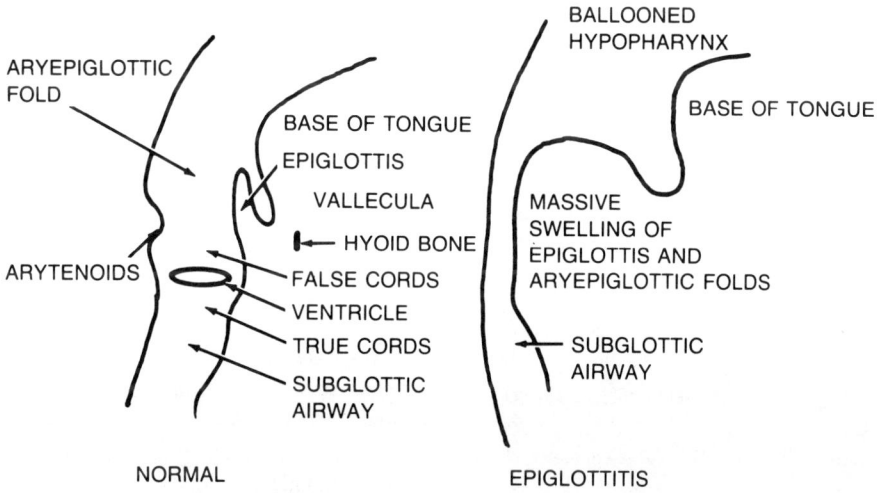

Figure 71-7 Diagram of upper airway: normal anatomy versus acute epiglottitis.

Intubation

The most experienced physician should intubate the child with AE under the most controlled circumstances. In a large medical center/teaching hospital, this may be a pediatric anesthesiologist intubating the child in the operating room. However, in a community hospital the child may have to be intubated by the emergency physician. Consultants should be called when the child arrives in the emergency department if AE is suspected, but time should not be wasted by failing to establish the diagnosis and intubate a child who requires an airway. Children with AE can be intubated successfully by physicians with experience in intubation—although intubation may be more difficult than usual because of the supraglottic swelling. Some suggestions for intubating the child with AE include the following: Preoxygenate the patient with 100% oxygen with a bag-mask if necessary. Choose an ET 1 to 2 mm smaller than the usual tube size for the patient. If the epiglottis cannot be lifted out of the way by the laryngoscope, try pushing it to the side. If ready and able to intubate the child, you may sedate with IV morphine or diazepam or proceed with rapid sequence induction with a sedative and a neuromuscular blocking agent. If the glottis is not well seen, try looking for air bubbles.

If unable to intubate the child successfully, ventilate with bag-mask with 100% oxygen and consider needle cricothyrotomy. Percutaneous transtracheal ventilation with a #14 or greater plastic catheter and high-flow oxygen given intermittently or ventilation with a plastic catheter hooked up to a 3.5-mm ET adapter with rapid bag ventilation may be lifesaving and buy time. To ventilate an adult via percutaneous transtracheal ventilation with a plastic catheter, "wall" oxygen at 50 psi is necessary.[52] Cricothyrotomy with incision and insertion of an endotracheal or tracheotomy tube is difficult to accomplish in children younger than 8 years. Ideally, no child who has arrived alive in the emer-

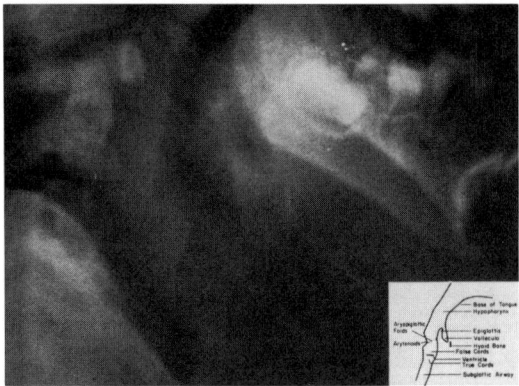

Figure 71-8 Lateral inspiratory airway film demonstrating normal supraglottic, glottic, and subglottic structures clearly outlined in contrast by the air column. The ventricle and true and false cords, though not clearly shown in this reproduction, are often visible on the roentgenogram. *Source:* Reproduced with Permission from Poole CA, Altman DH. Acute epiglottitis in children. *Radiology.* 1963;80(5):798.

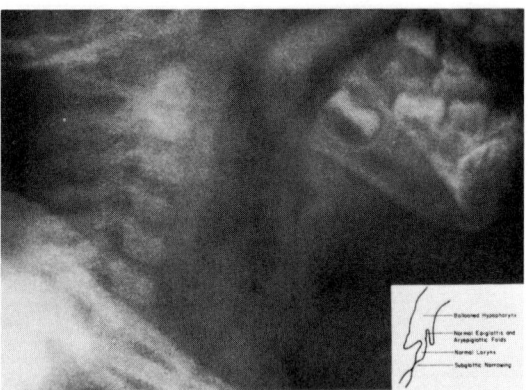

Figure 71-9 Changes seen in "croup" or laryngotracheobronchitis. The supraglottic and glottic structures are normal. There is marked subglottic edema with slight ballooning of the hypopharynx, indicating inspiratory obstruction. *Source:* Reproduced with Permission from Poole CA, Altman DH. Acute epiglottitis in children. *Radiology.* 1963;80(5):798.

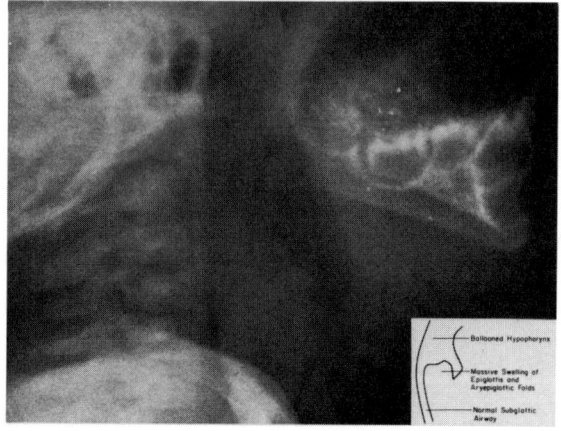

Figure 71-10 Characteristic changes of acute epiglottitis, with massive swelling of the epiglottis and aryepiglottic folds. The swelling stops abruptly at the glottis, which is normal. The hypopharynx is ballooned above the area of obstruction, and the subglottic region is normal. *Source:* Reproduced with Permission from Poole CA, Altman DH. Acute epiglottitis in children. *Radiology.* 1963;80(5):798.

gency department should die from upper airway obstruction, since needle cricothyroidotomy and transtracheal ventilation should always be possible.

Nasotracheal intubation. A nasotracheal tube (NT) is better tolerated than an ET, but in an emergency an ET should be inserted to provide an airway. The ET can be exchanged for an NT under controlled conditions (eg, the operating room).

Intubation versus tracheostomy. Tracheostomy[26,32,53–55] had been the main method of providing an airway in AE prior to the mid-1970s. Slash tracheostomies done in emergency fashion to children with AE resulted in many children with anoxic brain damage. For a tracheostomy to be done safely, an ET should be in place first.

Since the child can be extubated in 24 to 72 hours, why do a tracheostomy with its associated morbidity and even mortality? Most children are treated with intubation instead of tracheostomy today. Possible advantages of a tracheostomy over intubation include easier nursing care (suctioning, etc), less chance of accidental extubation, and easier reinsertion if the tube is dislodged.

Treatment of Pulmonary Edema[23,24]

Because of the potential for hypoxemia even after the airway obstruction is relieved, patients should be treated with 30% humidified oxygen after intubation. If there is evidence of pulmonary edema, the patient may be treated with mechanical ventilation, increased FiO_2, and positive end-expiratory pressure (PEEP).

Laboratory Findings

The WBC count will be increased with a shift to the left. A chest radiograph should be obtained to rule out infiltrates, pulmonary edema, or pneumothorax and to assess ET position. Blood cultures should be obtained—there is a high incidence (80%) of positive cultures, and it is essential to know the sensitivities of the *Haemophilus influenzae* type B (HIB).

After the airway is assured, arterial blood gases should be obtained to assess ventilation and oxygenation. Procedures

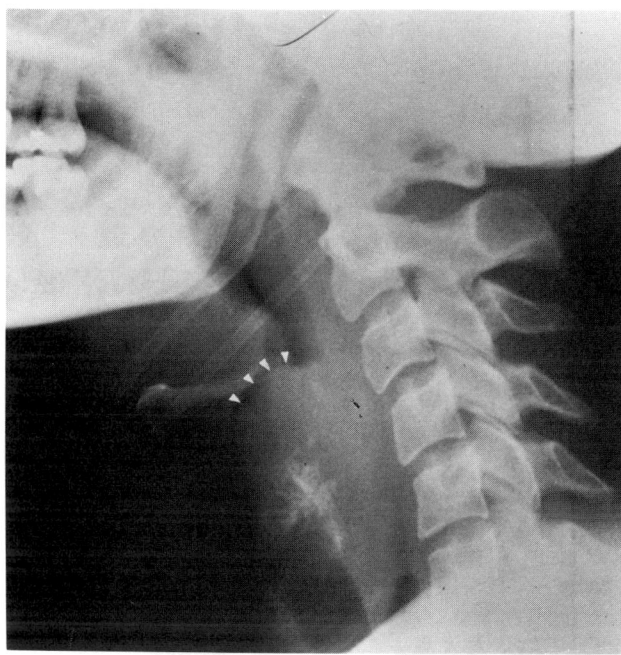

Figure 71-11 Lateral roentgenogram of the structures in the neck demonstrating enlargement of the epiglottis and arytenoids. *Source:* Reprinted from Kravis TC. Obstructive lung diseases. In: Kravis TC, Warner CG, eds. *Emergency Medicine: A Comprehensive Review*, 1st ed. 1983;833.

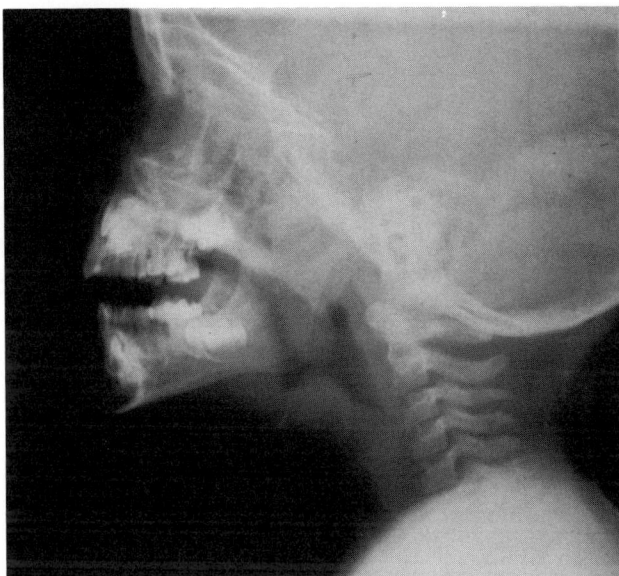

Figure 71-12 Xerogram of 22-year-old man with complaint: I need pain medicine for my throat. No respiratory symptoms or stridor. HIB on blood culture. Note enlarged thumb-shaped epiglottis but no ballooning or hypopharynx (not enough swelling to cause compromised airway . . . yet).

that can agitate the child should be avoided until an airway is provided. Pulse oximetry decreases the need for repeated blood gases and allows the treating physician to make rapid adjustments in oxygen delivery.

Drugs

Antibiotics. Antibiotics must effectively cover HIB. Ceftriaxone, 100 mg/kg/day, or cefotaxime, 100 mg/kg/day, are considered drugs of choice. Up-to-date knowledge of HIB sensitivities is required for the physician to make the most appropriate choice of initial antibiotics.

Corticosteroids. Although there are no controlled studies demonstrating the effectiveness of corticosteroids in AE, they are used by many clinicians who claim that the epiglottis inflammation decreases more rapidly when corticosteroids are used.[28] Dexamethasone, 0.6 mg/kg IV, can be used as an initial dose.

Continued Care

The patient is observed in the intensive care unit. Antibiotics are continued for 7 to 10 days. The epiglottis should be inspected daily, and the patient can be extubated when the epiglottis is no longer swollen or as long as there is a physician standing by with airway resuscitation equipment to reintubate the patient if necessary. The child can usually be extubated in 24 to 72 hours.

EPIGLOTTITIS IN ADULTS[56]

Etiology

HIB is the organism most frequently cultured from the blood in adult epiglottitis, but there is a much lower incidence of positive blood cultures (10% to 20%) compared with children (70% to 90%). As stressed by Fontanarosa et al.,[57] adult epiglottitis does not appear to be a uniform disease but presents in two clinical patterns. The more severe course, which has a rapid onset and frequent upper airway compromise, is associated with positive cultures and hence appears to be due to HIB infection. The milder course has a slower onset, a lower incidence of upper airway obstruction, and no identifiable pathogen; it may be viral in origin.[40,58] Shapiro et al. pointed out that only the more severe cases of adult epiglottitis are reported and that many of the milder cases may go completely unnoticed since laryngoscopy is not generally performed on all cases of pharyngitis. This would bias the reporting toward a more severe description of the illness.[57,59]

Other bacteria that have been isolated include *Streptococcus* group A, *Streptococcus pneumoniae*, *Staphylococcus pyogenes*, and *Haemophilus parainfluenzae*. Interestingly, a report by Glode et al.[38] presented five adults with HIB AE,

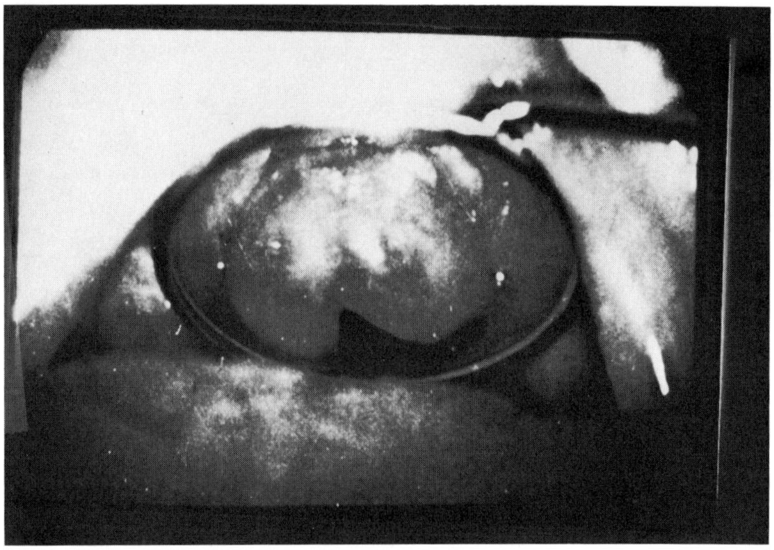

Figure 71-13 AE as seen on indirect laryngoscopy. *Source:* Courtesy of James E. Pierog, MD.

all of whom cared for children colonized with HIB; two of the children had HIB meningitis.[60,61]

There is an acute inflammatory swelling of the epiglottis and the supraglottic structures of the larynx. As with children the term supraglottitis is more accurate due to the involvement of the supraglottic structures and the fact that the epiglottis itself may not be inflamed.[59]

Clinical Observations[62]

AE was considered an extremely rare illness in adults prior to the mid-1970s. Over the past 20 years there has been a dramatic increase in reported cases, which may reflect an actual increase in the incidence of the disease or increased awareness of physicians, especially of the milder cases. An estimate of the incidence of the disease has been 9.7 cases per million adults per year.[63] Despite the increasing incidence and reporting, AE occurs in adults more often than most physicians realize. Since the introduction of HIB vaccines, AE is becoming increasingly rare in children, and if a physician practices in an area where most children are immunized, he or she is more likely to see AE in adults than children. The typical patient may be sent home with a penicillin prescription for presumed β-hemolytic streptococcus type A pharyngitis—only to return with respiratory distress (or DOA).[64]

The time course in adults is usually slower than in children. The typical patient presents after 1 to 2 days of progressively worsening symptoms, although presentation may be delayed up to 1 week. There may be a correlation with a shorter prodrome and more severe symptoms and airway compromise.[59,65] The patient complains of a painful sore throat (see Fig. 71-12) and dysphagia. Pain is usually out of proportion to the physical findings, and only mild erythema is seen in the pharynx. There may be inability to swallow the saliva due to the pain on swallowing, resulting in drooling. The voice may be muffled but is not hoarse. Gentle movement of the larynx may be very painful. There is usually fever. There may or may not be respiratory distress. Of the patients without respiratory distress, some will proceed to airway compromise as the illness progresses.

Diagnosis

A high index of suspicion must be maintained to diagnose AE in adults. All adults who complain of painful sore throat and who do not have adequate physical findings to explain the symptoms (eg, enlarged tonsils with exudate, peritonsillar abscess) should have the epiglottis visualized. Indirect laryngoscopy and flexible nasoendoscopy[59,66] are safe procedures with cooperative adults (Fig. 71-13). Lateral neck radiograph can be useful if the epiglottis cannot be visualized by indirect laryngoscopy. The same precautions mentioned in the section on AE in children must be kept in mind.

Treatment

Less than 50% of adults will require an artificial airway. As with children, exhaustion, cyanosis, and increasing respiratory distress should alert the physician to the need for prompt intubation. Although almost all children with AE require intubation, adults who present without any signs of respiratory difficulty can be treated with antibiotics effective for HIB in an intensive care setting where intubation can be performed if necessary.

Blood cultures should be obtained prior to antibiotic administration. All adults with AE should be admitted to the hospital because even minimal cases can progress rapidly. The need for intubation may vary in urgency. Respiratory arrest requires immediate ventilation and intubation, and severe symptoms require sedation or paralysis and intubation. Patients with milder symptoms can be observed. The patient should be endotracheally intubated in the emergency situation, and the ET can be converted to an NT under controlled conditions. If time permits, the patient can be nasotracheally intubated in the operating room.[67] If an airway cannot be established by endotracheal intubation, cricothyrotomy can be lifesaving.

Initial antibiotic treatment should provide coverage for HIB. Ceftriaxone or cefotaxime can be used. As with children there are no double-blind studies documenting the efficacy of corticosteroid use, but many clinicians feel that there is more rapid resolution of the supraglottic swelling with a large dose of corticosteroids given upon presentation. The recommended corticosteroid dose is dexamethasone, 12 mg IV.

Epiglottitis in AIDS Patients[68]

A series of cases of adult epiglottitis in patients with acquired immunodeficiency has been reported. These patients had a history of malaise, dysphagia, and odynophagia leading to rapidly progressive airway obstruction. All patients required intubation. On flexible fiberoptic laryngoscopy the epiglottis was noted to be pale and floppy with associated supraglottic edema. Organisms cultured from the epiglottis included *S. aureus, S. pneumoniae, S. viridans,* and *Streptococcus epidemicus.*

Differential Diagnosis

Other conditions can cause upper airway compromise or obstruction and can produce a clinical picture similar to that of croup and epiglottitis.

Tonsillar swelling from acute tonsillitis, acute mononucleosis, or peritonsillar abscess can produce stridor and a compromised airway.

Uvulitis[69] secondary to angioedema[70] or infection can produce a compromised upper airway. Acute epiglottitis has been reported to coexist with acute uvulitis.[71]

Foreign body[72] aspiration may produce an episode of coughing and gagging, but this may go unnoticed if the child is not observed during the incident. The child may present acutely or several days later with stridor, cough, or wheezing. Esophageal foreign bodies can compress the upper airway and produce stridor.[73]

Angioneurotic edema of the larynx may cause the patient to present with stridor. There is usually a sudden onset and there may be other signs of angioedema such as urticaria and periorbital edema. The patient is afebrile and may have a hoarse voice. There may be dyspnea and dysphagia. The epiglottis appears pale and swollen on laryngoscopy. Lateral neck radiography may show enlargement of the retropharyngeal space as well as the epiglottis. Treatment includes maintaining the airway with intubation if needed as well as epinephrine (subcutaneous or intravenous), nebulized racemic epinephrine, antihistamines, and corticosteroids IV.

Retropharyngeal abscess is usually seen in children 6 months to 4 years old. There is usually a URI prodrome. The child may present with fever, torticollis, or a stiff neck. There may be respiratory distress, stridor, or dysphagia. Lateral neck radiography will show an increase in the width of the prevertebral space. An air/fluid level can be seen with perforation of the hypopharynx or esophagus and communication into the retropharyngeal space. Treatment consists of airway maintenance, surgical drainage, and antibiotic coverage.[24a,74,75]

Laryngeal diphtheria may present a picture similar to that of croup or epiglottitis. Many patients seen in emergency departments are unimmunized. In laryngeal diphtheria, the onset of the obstructive phase is relatively slow and there may be progressive hoarseness over 2 to 3 days. If the membrane is only on the cords, there is usually not much systemic absorption of toxin and systemic involvement because of the small surface area involved. If there is a diphtheritic membrane in the pharynx as well, there may be greater systemic toxicity.

Ingestion of caustics such as lye or of gasoline[76] can cause inflammation of the epiglottis and upper airway obstruction. Thermal injuries from hot beverages, superheated steam, or smoking crack cocaine can produce the same clinical picture. Tumors such as subglottic hemangiomas can present with attacks similar to laryngotracheitis. Laryngeal papillomas can produce hoarseness and stridor.

Congenital conditions such as laryngeal and pharyngeal cysts usually present in the first few months of life and can present with stridor.

REFERENCES

1. Goldhagen JL. Croup: pathogenesis and management. *J Emerg Med*. 1983;1:3–11.
1a. Sendi K, et al. Tracheitis: outcome of 1,700 cases presenting to the emergency department during two years. *J Otolaryngol*. 1992; 21(1):20–24.
2. Clark WD, et al. Epiglottitis and laryngotracheobronchitis. *Am Fam Physician*. 1983;28:139.
3. Denny FW, et al. Croup: an 11-year study in a pediatric practice. *Pediatrics*. 1983;71:871.
4. Mills JL, et al. The usefulness of lateral neck roentgenograms in laryngotracheobronchitis. *Am J Dis Child*. 1979;133:1140–1142.
4a. Quan L. Diagnosis and treatment of croup. *Am Fam Physician*. 1992;46(3):747–755.
4b. Stoney PJ, Chakrabarti MK. Experience of pulse oximetry in children with croup. *J Laryngol Otol*. 1991;105(4):295–298.
5. Mellis CM. Lateral neck x-rays: useful or dangerous in acute infective upper airways obstruction. *Aust Fam Physician*. 1987;16:1490–1491.
6. Couriel JM. Management of croup. *Arch Dis Child*. 1988;1305–1308.
7. Westley CR. Brooks: Nebulized racemic epinephrine by IPPB for the treatment of croup. *Am J Dis Child*. 1978;132.
7a. Kelley PB, Simon JR. Racemic epinephrine in croup and disposition. *Am J Emerg Med*. 1992;10:181–183.

7b. Corneli HM, Bolte RG. Outpatient use of racemic epinephrine in croup. *Am Fam Physician*. 1992;46(3):683–684.

8. Remington S, Meakin G. Nebulised adrenaline 1:1000 in the treatment of croup. *Anesthesia*. 1986;41:923–926.

8a. Waisman Y, Klein BL, Boenning DA, Young GM, Chamberlain JM, O'Donnell R, Ochsenschlager DW. Prospective randomized double-blind study comparing L-epinephrine and racemic epinephrine aerosols in the treatment of laryngotracheitis (croup). *Pediatrics*. 1992;89(2):302–306.

9. Tunnessen W, Feinstein A. The steroid-croup controversy: an analytic review of methodologic problems. *Pediatr Pharmacol Ther*. 1980;96:751–755.

10. Leipzig B, et al. A prospective randomized study to determine the efficacy of steroids in treatment of croup. *J Pediatr*. 1979;94:194–196.

11. Koren G. Corticosteroid treatment of laryngotracheitis V spasmodic croup in children. *Am J Dis Child*. 1983;137:941.

12. Kuusela A, Vesikari T. A randomized double-blind, placebo-controlled trial of dexamethasone and racemic epinephrine in the treatment of croup. *Acta Paediatr Scand*. 1988;77:99.

13. Super DM, et al. A prospective randomized double-blind study to evaluate the effect of dexamethasone in acute laryngotracheitis. *J Pediatr*. 1989;115:323–329.

13a. Tibballs J, Shann FA, Landau LI. Placebo-controlled trial of prednisolone in children intubated for croup. *Lancet*. 1992;340(8822):745–748.

14. Liston S, et al. Bacterial tracheitis. *Am J Dis Child*. 1983;137:764–767.

15. Edwards K, et al. Bacterial tracheitis as a complication of viral croup. *Pediatr Infect Dis*. 1983;2:390–391.

16. Sofer S, Chernick V. Increased need for tracheal intubation for croup in relation to bacterial tracheitis. *Can Med Assoc J*. 1983;128:160–161.

17. Slonick NS. Treatment of croup: a critical review. *Am J Dis Child*. 1989;143:1045–1049.

18. Jones R, et al. Bacterial tracheitis. *JAMA*. 1979;242:721–726.

19. Liston S, et al. Bacterial tracheitis. *Arch Otolaryngol*. 1981;107:561–564.

19a. Gallagher PG, Myer CM. An approach to the diagnosis and treatment of membranous laryngotracheobronchitis in infants and children. *Pediatr Emerg Care*. 1991;7(6):337–342.

20. Ernst TN, Philp M. Bacterial tracheitis caused by *Branhamella catarrhalis*. *Pediatr Infect Dis J*. 1987;6:574.

21. Bass JL, et al. Bacterial tracheitis caused by *Branhamella catarrhalis*. *Pediatr Infect Dis J*. 1990;5:171–172.

21a. Surh L, et al. Staphylococcal tracheitis and toxic shock syndrome in a young child. *J Pediatr*. 1984;105:585–587.

22. Johnson JT, Liston SL. Bacterial tracheitis in adults. *Arch Otolaryngol Head Neck Surg*. 1987;113:204–205.

23. Ruddy J. Bacterial tracheitis in a young adult. *J Laryngol Otol*. 1988;102:656–657.

24. Han B, et al. Membranous laryngotracheobronchitis (membranous croup). *Am J Roentgenol*. 1978;133:53–57.

24a. Lichenstein R. Retropharyngeal cellulitis: an unusual cause of respiratory distress in infancy. *Pediatr Emerg Care*. 1990;6(2):138–139.

25. Selbst S. Epiglottitis. *Am J Emerg Med*. 1983;3:342–350.

25a. Novotny W, Faden H, Mosovich L. Emergence of invasive group A streptococcal disease among young children. *Clin Pediatr*. 1992;31(10):596–601.

26. Kulick RM, et al. Thermal epiglottitis after swallowing hot beverages. *Pediatrics*. 1988;81:441–444.

27. Scheidemandel HHE. Did George Washington die of quinsy? *Arch Otolaryngol Head Neck Surg*. 1976;102:519–521.

28. Losek JD, et al. Epiglottitis: comparison of signs and symptoms in children less than 2 years old and older. *Ann Emerg Med*. 1990;19:55–58.

29. Willis RJ, Rowland TW. The early management of acute epiglottitis: a survey of current practice. *J Emerg Med*. 1984;2:13–16.

30. Grodin M. Epiglottitis. *J Emerg Med*. 1983;1:13–19.

31. Daum RS, et al. Epiglottitis (supraglottitis). In: *Textbook of Pediatric Infectious Disease*. 1981:138–146.

32. Bass JW, et al. Acute epiglottitis, a surgical emergency. *JAMA*. 1974;229:671–675.

33. Singer JI, McCabe JB. Epiglottitis at extremes of age. *Am J Emerg Med*. 1988;6:228–231.

34. Brilli RJ, et al. Epiglottitis in infants less than two years of age. *Pediatr Emerg Care*. 1989;5:16–21.

35. Goldhagen JL. Supraglottitis in three young infants. *Pediatr Emerg Care*. 1989;5:175–177.

36. Goldhagen JL. Supraglottitis in three young infants. *Pediatr Infect Dis J*. 1990;5:175–177.

37. Soliman MG, et al. Epiglottitis and pulmonary oedema in children. *Can Anaesth Soc J*. 1978;25.

38. Lee SC, et al. Epiglottitis presenting as acute pulmonary edema. *Ann Emerg Med*. 1984;14:60–62.

39. Sofer S, et al. Pulmonary edema following relief of upper airway obstruction. *Chest*. 1984;86:401.

40. Costigan DC, Newth CJ. Respiratory status of children with and without an artificial airway. *Am J Dis Child*. 1983;137:139–141.

41. Izsak E. Pulmonary edema due to acute upper airway obstruction from aspirated foreign body. *Pediatr Emerg Care*. 1987;2:235–236.

42. Molteni RA. Epiglottitis: incidence of extraepiglotic infection: report of 72 cases and review of the literature. *Pediatrics*. 1976;58.

43. Blanc VF, et al. Acute epiglottitis in children: management of 27 consecutive cases with nasotracheal intubation. *Can Anaesth Soc J*. 1977.

44. Szold P, Glicklich M. Children with epiglottitis can be bagged. *Clin Pediatr (Phila)*. 1976;792–793.

45. Glicklich M, et al. Steroids and bag and mask ventilation in the treatment of acute epiglottitis. *J Pediatr Surg*. 1979;14:247–250.

46. Mauro RD, et al. Differentiation of epiglottitis from laryngotracheitis in the child with stridor. *Am J Dis Child*. 1988;142:679.

47. Diaz J, Lockhart C. Early diagnosis and airway management of acute epiglottitis in children. *South Med J*. 1982;75:399–401.

48. Diaz J. Controversies in the diagnosis and management of common upper airway infections. *ER Rep*. 1983;4:25.

48a. Cunningham M. The old and new of acute laryngotracheal infections. *Clin Pediatr*. 1992;(Jan):56–64.

49. Rapkin RH. The diagnosis of epiglottitis: simplicity and reliability of radiographs of the neck in the differential diagnosis of the croup syndrome. *J Pediatr*. 1972;80:96–98.

50. Milko DA, et al. Nasotracheal intubation in the treatment of acute epiglottitis. *Pediatrics*. 1974;53:674–677.

51. Podgore JR. The "thumb sign" and "little finger sign" in acute epiglottitis. *J Pediatr*. 1976;88:154–155.

52. Stewart RD. Manual translaryngeal jet ventilation. *Emerg Med Clin North Am*. 1989;7:1.

53. Oh TH, et al. Comparison of nasotracheal intubation and tracheostomy in management of acute epiglottitis. *Anesthesiology*. 1977;46:214–216.
54. Gross CW. Medical management, nasotracheal intubation, and tracheotomy in the treatment of upper airway obstruction in children. *Symp Pediatr Otorhinolaryngol*. 1977;10.
55. Kenny JF, et al. Meningitis due to *Haemophilus influenzae* type b resistant to both ampicillin and chloramphenicol. *Pediatrics*. 1980;66:14–16.
55a. Knight GJ, Harris MA, Parbari M, O'Callaghan MJ, Masters IB. Single daily dose ceftriaxone therapy in epiglottitis. *J Paediatr Child Health*. 1992;28(3):220–222.
56. Hawkings DB, et al. Acute epiglottitis in adults. *Laryngoscope*. 1973;83:1211–1220.
57. Fontanarosa PB, et al. Adult epiglottitis. *J Emerg Med*. 1989;7:223–231.
58. Grattan-Smith T, et al. Viral supraglottitis. *J Pediatr*. 1987;110(3).
59. Shapiro J, et al. Adult supraglottitis, a prospective analysis. *JAMA*. 1988;259:563–567.
60. Cohen EL. Epiglottitis in the adult. *Postgrad Med*. 1984;75:309–311.
61. Mustoe T, Strome M. Adult epiglottitis. *Am J Otolaryngol*. 1983;4:393–399.
62. Andreassen B, et al. Acute epiglottitis in adults: a management protocol based on a 17-year material. *Acta Anaesth Scand*. 1984;28:155–157.
63. Mayo Smith MF, et al. Acute epiglottitis in adults. *N Engl J Med*. 1986;314:1133–1186.
64. Scully RE, ed. Case records of the Massachusetts General Hospital. *N Engl J Med*. 1977;297:878–882.
65. Deeb ZE, et al. Acute epiglottitis in the adult. *Laryngoscope*. 1985;95:289–291.
66. Cox GJ, et al. The use of flexible nasoendoscopy in adults with acute epiglottitis. *Ann R Coll Surg Engl*. 1988;70:361–362.
67. Wurtele P. Nasotracheal intubation—a modality in the management of acute epiglottitis in adults. *J Otolaryngol*. 1984;13:118–121.
68. Rothstein SG, et al. Epiglottitis in AIDS patients. *Laryngoscope*. 1989;99:389–392.
69. Kotloff KL, Wald ER. Uvulitis in children. *Pediatr Infect Dis*. 1983;2:393–399.
70. Evans TC, Roberge RJ. Quincke's disease of the uvula. *Am J Emerg Med*. 1987;5:211–216.
71. Rapkin RH. Simultaneous uvulitis and epiglottitis. *JAMA*. 1980;243:1843.
72. Blazer S, et al. Foreign body in the airway. *Am J Dis Child*. 1980;134:68–69.
73. Esclamado RM, Richardson MA. Laryngotracheal foreign bodies in children. *Am J Dis Child*. 1987;141.
74. Brook I. Microbiology of retropharyngeal abscesses in children. *Am J Dis Child*. 1987;141:202–294.
75. Morrison JE, et al. Retropharyngeal abscesses in children: a 10 year review. *Pediatr Emerg Care*. 1988;4(1).
76. Grufferman S, Walker FW. Supraglottitis following gasoline ingestion. *Ann Emerg Med*. 1982;11:368–370.

72. Obstructive Airway Disease

MICHAEL R. SAYRE, MD, FACEP
BRIAN CARLIN, MD, FCCP

The emergency physician is frequently faced with the problem of a patient who has a chief complaint of "shortness of breath." Often the physical examination reveals the presence of wheezing. In these cases the differential diagnosis includes many diseases, but among the most common are the obstructive airway diseases.

Generally the obstructive airway diseases are divided into asthma and chronic obstructive pulmonary disease (COPD). In reality, however, these are different disorders, although they share many of the same treatment modalities. COPD in particular is a continuum of disease from emphysema to chronic bronchitis.

Defining these diseases has proven to be problematic. The American Thoracic Society wrote definitions in 1962.[1] However, these definitions have been modified by new knowledge. Asthma may be defined as a clinical disorder in which there are wide variation in and reversible resistance to bronchial airflow. This definition fails to account for the inflammatory component of the disease, while it does account for the physiologic changes in the bronchial smooth muscle. Chronic bronchitis is also defined as a clinical disorder in which the patient has a chronic cough with mucous production that is not responsive to treatment. The 1962 American Thoracic Society definition of emphysema as an anatomic disorder with destruction of the alveolar walls is still a workable explanation.[1]

While these definitions have stood the test of time and are used as the basis for defining these disorders in most research endeavors, other definitions are possible and may better reflect prognosis. It is important that research trials make an effort to clearly define patient characteristics.[2]

Obstructive airway diseases are common among adults. The prevalence of asthma is approximately 2.6% of the general population and the incidence is approximately 2.1/1000 per year.[3] In rural Sweden the lifetime prevalence of asthma among children was 5.1%,[4] and the overall Swedish prevalence was 4%.[5] There is evidence, however, that the incidence of asthma may be increasing. In 1980, 2% of Michigan Medicaid patients had asthma; in 1986, this percentage had increased to 2.8%.[6] In this population the prevalence of asthma decreased during late adolescence and early adulthood but increased thereafter (Fig. 72-1).[6]

Asthma can cause significant morbidity and mortality. While in some areas this morbidity is low (eg, in Sweden), there were not a significant number of school days lost by asthmatics (only 13% lost more than 5 days in 6 months);[7] in other areas the morbidity is higher. Recently there has been an increase in the number of admissions to the hospital for children with asthma without much increase in mortality.[8,9] However, there is some evidence that the overall death rate for asthma, although low, has been increasing in recent years, especially in blacks. In the United States the age-adjusted death rate from asthma for whites increased from 0.8/100,000 in 1979 to 1.0 in 1984. In blacks the rate increased from 1.9 in 1979 to 2.6 in 1984.[10] Worldwide there is a large variation among death rates by country (Fig. 72-2). There has been an overall small increase in mortality, but this increase may be due to changes in diagnosis.[11] It is currently thought that most deaths from asthma are due to inadequate assessment and treatment of the disease as opposed to overaggressive treatment.[12] In addition, there is a seasonal variation in asthma severity, with approx-

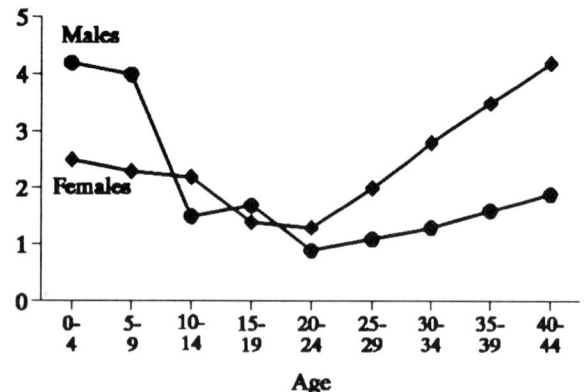

Figure 72-1 Average annual prevalence of asthma in the Michigan Medicaid population for 1980–1986. *Source:* Gerstmann BB, et al. Prevalence and treatment of asthma in the Michigan Medicaid population younger than 45 years, 1980–1986. *J Allergy Clin Immunol.* 1989;83:1032–1039, with permission.

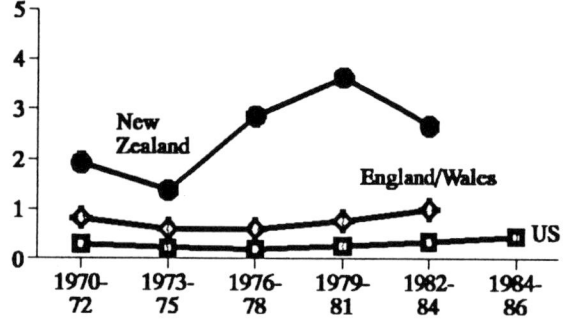

Figure 72-2 Asthma mortality by 3-year periods. *Source:* Adapted from Jackson R, et al. International trends in asthma mortality: 1970–1985. *Chest.* 1988;94:914–918, with permission.

imately 50% more hospitalizations in December than in July.[13]

The chief risk factor for adult asthma is low income, which explains the racial prevalence differences; age and cigarette smoking are not related to the development of asthma, nor is there a significantly increased risk of death.[3] Another study confirmed that smoking was not a strong predictor of asthma in adults.[14] However, an important epidemiologic influence for the development of asthma in children may be passive smoking. Several studies demonstrated an increased risk associated with maternal smoking.[15,16] A history of episodes of bronchiolitis was somewhat predictive of wheezing at age 8 but no longer at age 13.[15] While the meaning of the finding is not entirely clear, respiratory therapists were found to have about a four-time higher incidence of developing asthma after entering their profession when compared to other health-care technicians.[17]

COPD is a disease confined mainly to older adults. In 1986, approximately 15 million Americans suffered from COPD and 71,099 died (Fig. 72-3).[18] Overall mortality rates of adults with COPD depend on whether the patient's disease is due to asthma in the absence of smoking (10-year survival, 85%) or due to nonatopic COPD with a history of smoking (10-year survival, 40%).[2] Shorter term survival is most closely related to the level of arterial O_2 and CO_2.[19]

PATHOGENESIS

Asthma

The pathogenesis of these diseases is complex. In asthma, extrinsic and intrinsic sources or in many instances a combination of both are often involved. These extrinsic sources (eg, dust mite, western red cedar) and other "indoor pollutants" may play a role in the development of some cases of asthma.[20,21] As many as 11% of Olympic athletes have exercise-induced bronchospasm, which is another cause of asthma.[22] Occupational exposure can also be important.[23] Research findings suggest a strong allergic factor in asthma in younger but not older adults.[24] In addition, there is a group of adult patients with severe asthma, aspirin sensitivity, nasal polyposis, and sinusitis.

COPD

The main cause of emphysema and chronic bronchitis is cigarette smoking, and at least 82% of COPD deaths are attributable to smoking.[18,25] There are many factors that may influence the development of COPD, including arc welding[26] and air pollution.[27] Deficiency of α_1 antitrypsin, a protease inhibitor, is responsible for the development of emphysema in some people.

EMERGENCY DEPARTMENT DIAGNOSIS

History

As is usually the case, the most important part of the evaluation of a patient with obstructive airway disease is the history. The physician should direct questions to the duration and onset of symptoms, time of year, concomitant illnesses, work/exposure history, exercise, and sputum production. The new onset of airway obstruction suggested by respiratory distress has a long differential diagnosis (Table 72-1). In addition, the history should include an inquiry about previous hospital and intensive care stays and previous endotracheal intubations.[28]

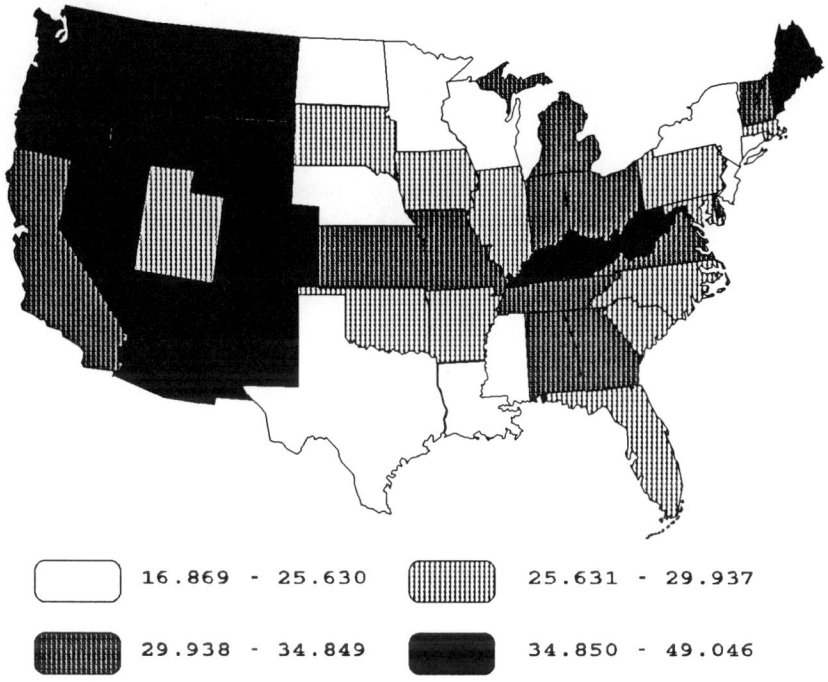

Figure 72-3 Age-adjusted COPD mortality rates per 100,000 population—United States, 1986. *Source: MMWR.* 1989;38:549.

16.869 - 25.630   25.631 - 29.937
29.938 - 34.849   34.850 - 49.046

A medications history is also critical. It is especially important to note whether the medicines are taken chronically or have just been taken during this exacerbation of the condition, as well as the timing of the last dose. The response, or lack thereof, to the usual medication regimen is very important to help determine the severity of the exacerbation. The use of oxygen and steroids also should be specifically addressed. The examiner should assess how well the patient can use an aerosol inhaler, as many patients will not be able to use metered-dose inhalers (MDI) properly.[29]

Table 72-1 Differential Diagnosis of Respiratory Distress

1. Exacerbation of obstructive airway disease
2. Central airway obstruction (foreign body, endobronchial lesion, laryngeal edema)
3. Cardiac failure
4. Pulmonary embolism
5. Vasculitis syndromes
6. Acute inhalational bronchitis (silo filler's lung, etc)
7. Acute tracheal compression (mediastinal mass)
8. Hysteria
9. Carcinoid syndrome
10. Cholinergic poisoning
11. Pneumonitis
12. Spontaneous pneumothorax
13. Acute drug reaction
14. Aspiration

Source: Ramsdell JW, Drucker RD. Obstructive airways disease, in: Kravis TC, Warner CG, eds. *Emergency Medicine*, 2nd ed.

Physical Exam

A patient with bronchospasm typically presents with symptoms of dyspnea and wheezing. In mild exacerbations there is a prolongation of forced expiratory time and wheezing on expiration. As the airway obstruction worsens, there is a further prolongation of forced expiratory time and wheezing on both expiration and inspiration. Severe bronchospasm will allow little air movement and thus less wheezing. Thus, it is important to assess overall air movement in the patient who has little or no wheezing. Tachycardia (rate >120/minute) and the presence of a pulsus paradoxus (a drop in systolic blood pressure of more than 12 mmHg with inspiration) are marks of a severe exacerbation.[30,31] Finally, as the degree of airway obstruction worsens, respiratory muscle fatigue manifested by an increase in respiratory rate, accessory muscle (eg, sternomastoid) use, respiratory alterans (alternating abdominal and thoracic breathing), and paradoxic movements of the chest and abdominal musculature will occur.[31]

Diagnostic Tests

In situations in which there is any question regarding the patient's gas exchange and/or response to treatment, chest radiographs, pulmonary function tests, and serial arterial blood gas (ABG) measurements are helpful. In patients with underlying baseline gas exchange abnormalities, comparison of current with previous ABGs is also helpful in the patient assessment.

Chest Roentgenography

The chest radiograph in the patient with obstructive lung disease may detect pneumonia, atelectasis, mass lesion, or spontaneous pneumothorax. The development of a pneumothorax is associated with significant mortality.[32] Clearly, the known asthmatic patient who is having a typical exacerbation does not require a chest radiograph unless there is failure to respond to treatment. Nearly all patients with a new onset of wheezing or with an exacerbation of COPD should have a chest radiograph.

Pulmonary Function Tests

During an episode of bronchospasm there is a reduction in the forced vital capacity (FVC), the forced expiratory volume in 1 second (FEV_1), and the FEV_1/FVC ratio. Although there are standards for assessment of underlying airway dysfunction, obtaining these measurements is often not feasible in the emergency department setting because of the inaccessibility of equipment necessary to perform the testing.

There will also be a reduction in peak expiratory rate (PEFR). The measurement of PEFR can be easily made with a small hand-held device. The measurement of PEFR upon arrival to the emergency department and after therapy is important in the assessment and in many instances can assist in the decision as to whether hospitalization is necessary. Asthmatic patients with a pretreatment PEFR <100 L/minute and post-treatment PEFR <300 L/minute or those that have a <60-L/minute increase in PEFR after therapy often will require hospitalization.[33]

Arterial Blood Gases and Cutaneous Oximetry

The degree of ventilatory insufficiency and hypoxemia associated with exacerbations of airway disease can be only assessed by measurement of ABGs. Initially, the patient with mild airway obstruction will have hypocarbia, a respiratory alkalosis, and a preserved PaO_2 with an elevated alveolar-arterial (A-a) gradient. As the obstruction worsens, hypoxemia worsens and the A-a gradient widens. As ventilatory insufficiency ensues, CO_2 retention and a respiratory acidosis will occur. Several studies have shown a good predictive value for normal ABGs in those COPD patients who have a PEFR >25% of the predicted value[34] or a PEFR >200 L/minute associated with an O_2 saturation (measured by oximetry) greater than 90%.[35]

THERAPY

Emergency physicians tend to think of asthma and emphysema/bronchitis as a single disease entity because the treatments are very similar. We will consider the therapeutic agents available for the treatment of these disorders and then describe how one might apply the treatments to each.

Although many treatments have been used in the past, ranging from various herbal remedies to acupuncture,[36] the inhaled route of drug administration is preferred whenever possible.[29] In children with an acute asthma attack enrolled in a double-blind trial, either inhaled albuterol or terbutaline was just as effective as subcutaneous epinephrine in improving vital signs and pulmonary function, with an increase in side effects in patients given epinephrine (eg, vomiting, tremor, palpitations).[37,38] In fact, whereas administration of medication by nebulizer has been the mainstay of treatment, administration by MDI can provide just as effective relief if given frequently enough and administered correctly. In a well-controlled study of emergency department patients with severe airflow obstruction, there was no difference in efficacy between 15 mg of nebulized metaproterenol and 1.95 mg (three puffs) of metaproterenol delivered by an MDI with a spacer device.[39] Since many patients do not use MDIs properly, the use of a spacer device may aid the patient with coordination of the actuation of the MDI with a properly timed inspiratory effort.[40] A suggested protocol is inhalation of four puffs over 2 minutes, using a spacer device, followed by one puff every minute until dyspnea is relieved or until unpleasant tremor occurs. Powder inhaler systems are now available and may replace the MDIs because they do not require the same degree of coordination[41]; however, their use in the emergency department has yet to be studied.

Oxygen

Oxygen therapy is of vital importance in the treatment of hypoxemia associated with asthma and COPD. In an asthmatic exacerbation, the hypoxemia is rarely life threatening and is easily corrected with the administration of supplemental oxygen. Bronchodilator therapy may cause a transient widening of the A-a gradient for oxygen,[42] and it is thus reasonable to administer low-flow oxygen to all asthmatics during acute management.[43]

In a COPD exacerbation, hypoxemia is the most lethal complication because of the resultant effects of hypoxemia on the cardiovascular system. Administration of supplemental oxygen with monitoring of either arterial oxygen tension or arterial oxygen saturation is important.

Oxygen can be administered by one of several means. Nasal prongs are probably the most comfortable means to administer low-flow oxygen. However, the magnitude of the subsequent increase in FiO_2 is unknown, being determined primarily by the patient's ventilatory pattern. Administration by a Venturi mask may affect the delivery of a known concentration of oxygen, whereas administration by a face mask with a reservoir device (nonrebreather or partial rebreather masks) may afford the delivery of higher concentrations of oxygen. Unfortunately, mask therapy does not allow the patient to eat without removing the mask and may be uncomfortable due to excessive warmth. Should adequate oxygenation not be possible by any of the above means, then intubation and mechanical ventilation are indicated.

Sympathomimetics

Sympathomimetics are agents that stimulate the α- and β-adrenergic receptors, and their effects depend on which receptors are stimulated. Stimulation of the β_2-receptor produces bronchodilation by relaxation of the bronchial smooth muscle, and drugs that specifically stimulate this receptor are particularly useful in the treatment of obstructive airway disease. Various forms of sympathomimetics are currently being used in the treatment of acute exacerbations of airway obstruction.

Epinephrine

Epinephrine stimulates all α- and β-receptors, thus leading not only to bronchodilation but also to tachycardia, restlessness, and hypertension. Despite the lack of receptor selectivity, the mean heart rate in a group of young asthmatic patients (18- to 45-year-olds) with acute attacks treated with epinephrine was not significantly different from pretreatment values.[44] Interestingly, in one study of subcutaneous epinephrine in older asthmatics without active cardiovascular disease, there was no difference in adverse reactions to epinephrine administration between those asthmatics over age 40 compared to those under age 40.[45] The authors then went on to advocate subcutaneous epinephrine over the use of aerosolized β-agonist therapy on the basis of reduced cost with the subcutaneous epinephrine, although they did not compare the relative safety of these two treatments in their own trial. They also failed to consider the cost advantage of the use of an MDI system with a spacer instead of hand-held nebulizer treatment.[45] In summary, the literature supports the safety of subcutaneous epinephrine for asthma in children or younger adults without concomitant illness.

One specific situation in which subcutaneous epinephrine is often administered is when the bronchospasm is a result of anaphylaxis. In this instance the α-adrenergic properties of the drug are useful to reverse the associated systemic symptoms, particularly hypotension. A dose of 0.3 mL (1:1000 solution) administered subcutaneously (adults) and repeated at 20-minute intervals up to three doses or 0.01 mL/kg (1:1000 solution) up to 0.3 mL (children) is effective in producing bronchodilation.[46] However, the optimal dosing schedule beyond the first hour is unknown.

In patients with acute exacerbations of COPD, the use of epinephrine should be avoided altogether because of the increased incidence of side effects, as it offers little advantage to inhaled β-adrenergic agonist therapy.[47] Taking all evidence together, we believe that aerosolized β-agonist therapy is preferable to subcutaneous epinephrine or terbutaline in the treatment of acute exacerbations of obstructive airway disease.

Isoproterenol/Isoetharine

These drugs are sympathomimetic and possess greater β than α activity compared to epinephrine, thus sharing the β_1 toxicity of epinephrine. Isoetharine possesses less β_1 activity than does isoproterenol. Either may be administered in nebulized (0.5 mL of 0.5% isoproterenol solutions or 0.5 mL of 1% isoetharine solution in 2 mL of saline) or MDI form. Administration of these drugs should be accompanied by cardiac monitoring in those patients at risk for cardiac side effects.

Terbutaline

Terbutaline is a β_2-agonist that may be administered subcutaneously, via aerosol, or orally. Subcutaneous administration (0.25 mg) has been shown to produce twice the bronchodilator effect, with a longer duration of action, than the same dose of epinephrine, in a pediatric population.[48] In the inhaled form (1 to 4 mg in 2 to 3 mL of saline), it is less potent than albuterol but has a longer duration of action.[49] The parenteral form may be useful when inhalation of medication is not feasible and is preferred over epinephrine. The tablet form is not particularly useful in the acute setting.

Other β_2-Selective Agonists

Various other β_2-selective agonists are currently available (metaproterenol, albuterol, fenoterol, bitolterol) and differ minimally according to their onset and duration of action. Many are available in tablet, syrup, MDI, and solution form. Inhalation therapy provides the most effective mode of administration in patients with acute exacerbations of obstructive airway disease and can be given by either an MDI with a spacer or a nebulizer. For those patients who cannot tolerate this route of administration, either syrup or tablet forms may be used, but their usefulness in the acute setting is limited.

Table 72-2 demonstrates that there is little difference between the commonly used agents (metaproterenol and albuterol). Recent experience indicates that a β-agonist can be given every 20 to 30 minutes by inhalation up to the development of undesirable effects (tremor, palpitations) or a total of three to four treatments.

Table 72-2 Pharmacokinetics of Inhaled β-Agonist Drugs

Agent	Onset of Action	Time to Peak Effect	Duration of Action	Usual Inhaled Dose
Albuterol	5 min	60 min	3–4 h	0.5 mL of 0.5% solution*
Isoetharine		5–15 min	1–4 h	0.5 mL of 1% solution†
Isoproterenol		5–15 min	1–2 h	0.5 mL of 0.5% solution*
Metaproterenol	5 min	60 min	2–6 h	0.3 mL of 5% solution†
Terbutaline	5 min	1–2 h	4 h	2 puffs MDI*

*Physician's Desk Reference.
†American Society of Hospital Pharmacists. AHFS Drug Information 1992, Bethesda, MD.

Methylxanthines

Theophylline and aminophylline are methylxanthines that closely resemble caffeine in chemical structure and pharmacologic activity. Although initially believed to act via phosphodiesterase inhibition, their mechanism of action is unknown.[50] Aminophylline was previously considered the standard of care in the treatment of patients with exacerbations of asthma or COPD, but there is little evidence of its efficacy in these situations. Several recent studies have shown no increase in benefit (either in bronchodilation or symptoms) derived from the addition of theophylline to treatment with inhaled metaproterenol (in asthmatic patients) or to treatment with inhaled metaproterenol, intravenous methylprednisolone, antibiotic, and oxygen (in patients with COPD).[51,52]

The addition of aminophylline to a β-agonist does produce an increase in gastrointestinal (nausea, vomiting) side effects,[52] and cardiac dysrhythmias (sinus and supraventricular tachycardia).[53] Therefore, there seems to be little reason to use aminophylline in the acute setting.

When used, a loading dose of 6 mg/kg over 30 minutes followed by a continuous drip of 1 mg/kg/hour can be administered. With the variability in the drug's metabolism, a dosage increase must be made in patients who are smokers and a dosage decrease in patients who are elderly or have congestive heart failure. In addition, a dosage decrease may be in order for patients who are taking erythromycin, ciprofloxacin, oral contraceptives, or cimetidine as these drugs decrease theophylline clearance; a dosage increase is often needed for those who are taking phenytoin, phenobarbital, or carbamazepine. With the ease of measurement of serum theophylline levels, the doses can be adjusted on a frequent, as-needed basis.

Anticholinergic Agents

Anticholinergic agents (atropine sulfate, ipratropium bromide) produce bronchodilation by blocking cholinergic receptors. Atropine is of limited value due to its short half-life and frequent side effects, whereas ipratropium, a quaternary salt derivative of atropine, is of value due to its longer half-life and fewer side effects. In a randomized, double-blind study of asthmatics, the combination of nebulized ipratropium and an inhaled β-agonist (fenoterol) was more effective in producing an improvement in FEV_1 and clinical symptoms than either agent given alone (Figs. 72-4 and 72-5).[54] Whether the addition of ipratropium confers more benefit than would be afforded by simply increasing the dose of the β-agonist is unknown.[55] Ipratropium is currently available in the United States in an MDI, but not in a solution form. Ipratropium is approved by the FDA for maintenance treatment in COPD patients. The usual dose is two puffs (36 μg) four times daily.

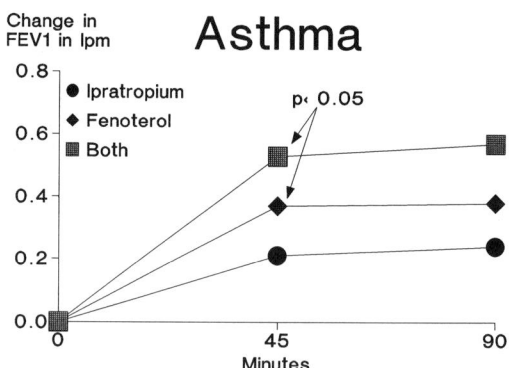

Figure 72-4 Mean increase in FEV_1 above baseline (N=148). *Source:* Rebuck AS, et al. Nebulized anticholinergic and sympathomimetic treatment of asthma and chronic obstructive airways disease in the emergency room. *Am J Med.* 1987;82:59–64, with permission.

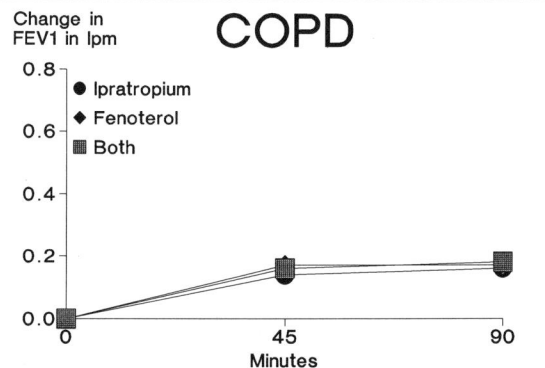

Figure 72-5 Mean increase in FEV_1 above baseline (N=51). *Source:* Rebuck AS, et al. Nebulized anticholinergic and sympathomimetic treatment of asthma and chronic obstructive airways disease in the emergency room. *Am J Med.* 1987;82:59–64, with permission.

Mechanical Ventilation

Some patients in status asthmaticus will not respond to vigorous treatment with medications and will require mechanical ventilation. Asphyxia is the primary cause of death in severe asthma, and most deaths from asthma occur within 8 hours of the onset of the attack.[12] Therefore, the emergency physician must be prepared to intubate and manage the severe asthmatic aggressively. Despite needing mechanical assistance to breathe, the prognosis is still fairly good.[56] Children admitted to a pediatric intensive care unit with asthma required mechanical ventilation approximately 33% of the time; of those children who needed mechanical ventilation, however, 7.5% die.[57]

External chest compression of patients with severe asthma has been described as a treatment for assisting ventilation in emergency situations.[58] This technique may be lifesaving for the patient with severe asthma who cannot expire normally or who has a respiratory arrest. Two rescuers are needed. The first artificially ventilates the patient. The second gives a sustained firm squeeze to the lower chest wall at the end of inflation.[58]

Although patients with COPD are successfully weaned from the ventilator in the majority (75%) of cases, many (62%) die within 1 year.[59] Unfortunately, at the time of intubation, there seem to be few, if any, reliable clinical predictors of those likely to survive.[60]

Indications for the initiation of mechanical ventilation include frank respiratory arrest; impending respiratory muscle failure as suggested by diaphragmatic fatigue, with paradoxic motion of the chest and abdominal walls; sustained or progressive rise in arterial carbon dioxide tension; obtundation; or prolonged severe airway obstruction. Initial ventilator settings should be a tidal volume of 10 to 15 mL/kg, an FiO_2 of 70% to 100%, and a back-up rate (assist control) of 8 to 10. Frequent adjustments may be necessary in the first several hours and should be based on patient comfort and ABG measurements. Attention to peak airway pressure is required to reduce potential barotrauma (pneumothorax, pneumomediastinum). In some instances, sedation and/or anesthesia may be necessary.

Antibiotics

Respiratory infections are frequent triggers of exacerbations of asthma and COPD.[61] Viruses are the major triggers, but bacterial pathogens may play a role.[62] Antibiotic therapy in patients with exacerbations of asthma should be reserved for those patients with a documented bacterial pulmonary infection or purulent sinusitis. Therapy with amoxicillin, trimethoprim-sulfamethoxazole, or erythromycin can be initiated in the emergency setting after appropriate cultures have been obtained.

For the patient with an acute COPD exacerbation, a recent study compared 2-week courses of antibiotics with placebo and found a higher success rate in the patients treated with antibiotics in terms of resolution of infection, rapid recovery of peak flow, and lower rate of clinical deterioration.[63] Common bacterial pathogens colonizing the sputum of a patient with COPD are *Haemophilus influenzae* (37% to 65%), *Streptococcus pneumoniae* (17% to 27%), and *Moraxella (Branhamella)* (5% to 26%).[61] Antibiotic therapy with amoxicillin, tetracycline, trimethoprim-sulfamethoxazole, a second-generation cephalosporin, or erythromycin (if an atypical infection such as *Legionella pneumophilia* is suspected) should be instituted after appropriate cultures (cultures less useful for bronchitis than pneumonia) have been obtained.

Magnesium

The use of magnesium in the treatment of patients with asthma has recently come to the attention of many clinicians. Actually this is not a new idea, as Mg^{2+} was used more than 50 years ago for treatment of asthma.[64,65] Unfortunately, the serum Mg^{2+} level is an imperfect guide to the patient's actual total body Mg^{2+} content since only 1% of Mg^{2+} is found in the serum. If the serum Mg^{2+} level is low, then the patient has Mg^{2+} deficiency; if the level is normal, however, the patient may still be symptomatic secondary to intracellular Mg^{2+} deficiency.[66]

In a double-blind, placebo-controlled trial of acute asthmatics with a poor response to nebulized β-agonists, 1.2 g of Mg^{2+} administered intravenously was shown to increase PEFR (225 to 297 L/minute) more than placebo (208 to 216 L/minute).[67] Another study, although not blinded, also demonstrated rapid bronchodilation in both mild and severe asthmatics following intravenous Mg^{2+} infusion.[68] However, the exact mechanism of the effect of Mg^{2+} in reactive airway disease remains unclear.

Magnesium may be administered as an intravenous infusion of 2 g in 100 mL of normal saline solution over about 20 minutes. In patients with normal renal function, this dose is relatively free of adverse reactions. High doses have been associated with respiratory depression and even death. If too much Mg^{2+} is inadvertently administered, its effects can be tempered by the intravenous administration of calcium salts.

Steroids

Steroids have long been used in the emergency treatment of exacerbations of asthma and COPD. While the exact mechanism of action is unknown, the important effects are to suppress inflammation,[69] to prevent and reverse the late-phase allergic reaction and the subsequent development of increased airway hyperreactivity, and to reduce mucus secretion.[70] By whatever mechanism, corticosteroids reduce the mucosal edema and excessive bronchial secretions, thereby reducing airway obstruction.[71]

Several studies, using various formulations and doses of drugs, have demonstrated that a short course of corticosteroids shortens the duration and severity of severe asthmatic exacerbations and that very early use prevents hospitalizations.[72–74] A recent study failed to show any decrease in admission rate or overall duration of treatment for acute asthma exacerbations following intravenous steroid administration.[75] One should be careful not to conclude that the steroids offered no benefit, but merely that the benefit may be delayed longer than other studies have demonstrated.[76] Although 125 mg of intravenous methylprednisolone (Solu-Medrol) has been used, there is evidence that oral methylprednisolone is as effective as the intravenous form in patients with moderate exacerbations of airway obstruction.[77] Methylprednisolone (0.5 mg/kg) improved airflow more than placebo when added to standard therapy in patients with COPD and acute respiratory insufficiency.[78]

Benefits have also been shown in the initiation of corticosteroids upon discharge home from the emergency department. Reduction in the rate of "relapses" from recur-

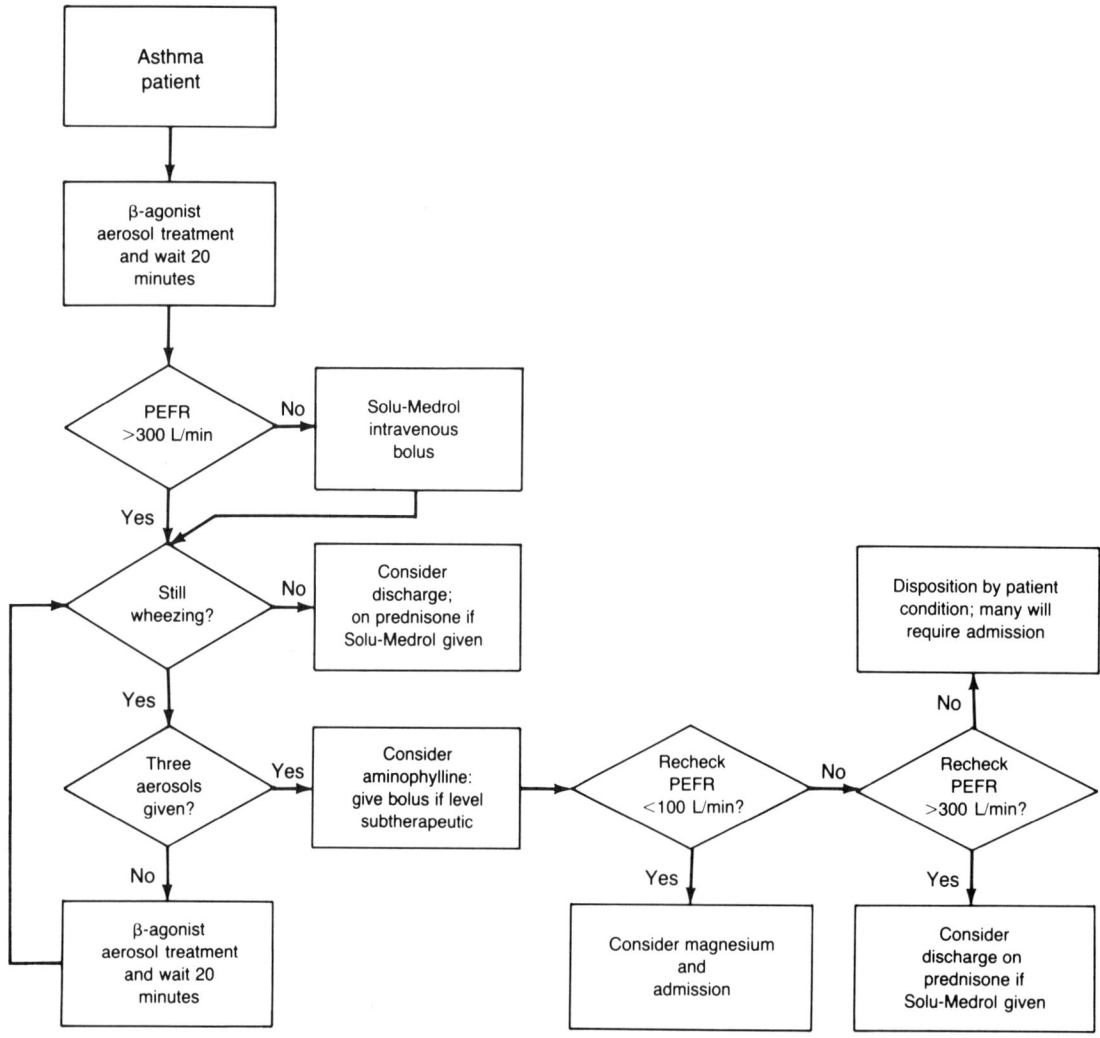

Figure 72-6 Management algorithm for acute asthma attacks.

rent asthma was shown in a controlled trial in which patients received an 8-day tapering course of methylprednisolone.[79] Although there has been little research on the optimal dose and duration of outpatient corticosteroid therapy, several strategies have been proposed: (1) initial administration of 80 mg of prednisone daily with a taper over 3 to 7 days, (2) 0.75 to 1.0 mg/kg/day for 1 to 2 weeks followed by a tapering dose for another 1 to 2 weeks, or (3) 80 mg of repository methylprednisolone (Depo-Medrol) administered intramuscularly.[80–82] Although used in chronic treatment, the utility of inhaled corticosteroids in acute exacerbations of asthma or COPD has not been reported.

Potential Therapies

Calcium channel blockers have also been investigated as possible smooth muscle relaxants for the treatment of bronchospasm. In one small study, nifedipine was compared with albuterol and placebo (all administered orally) in patients with chronic stable asthma. There was a slight but statistically significant improvement in FEV_1 in the nifedipine group compared with the placebo group. However, albuterol was about twice as effective as nifedipine in improving the FEV_1.[83] Although currently not approved for the treatment of bronchospasm, these drugs may be useful in those patients who have concurrent cardiac disease or hypertension.

DISPOSITION

Often one of the most difficult decisions in the care of an acute exacerbation of asthma or COPD is the decision to admit the patient to the hospital or to discharge to home. Using a patient's symptoms alone as a guide to therapy can result in undertreatment or relapse. In general, hospitalization should be strongly considered in those patients who fail to improve promptly after therapy or those who repeatedly require emergency department therapy. Management algorithms are helpful (Figs. 72-6 and 72-7).

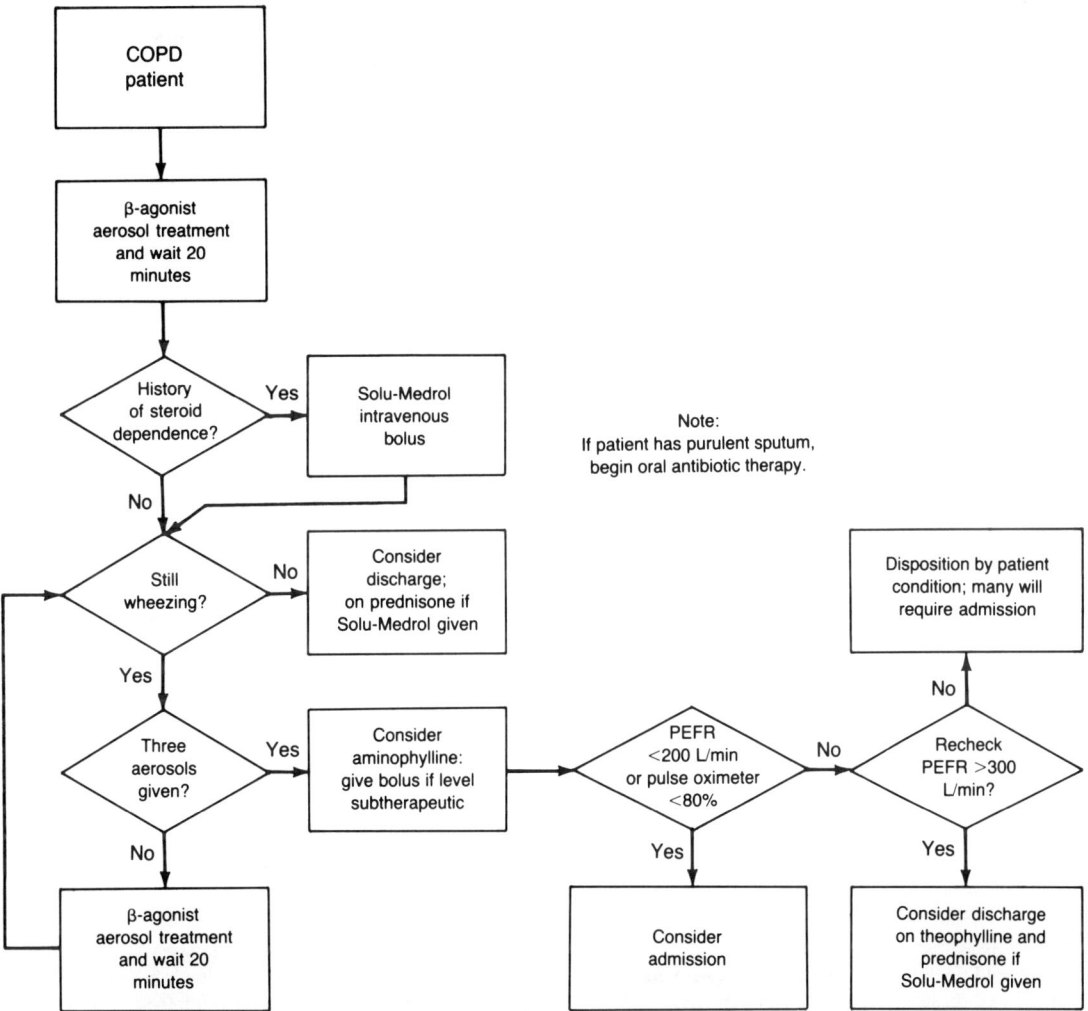

Figure 72-7 Management algorithm for acute COPD exacerbations.

An accurate history, a careful physical examination, and the use of various tests, including chest roentgenography, ABG measurements, and spirometry, will assist in this decision. The longer the patient has been symptomatic, the more likely it is that outpatient management will be unsuccessful. If the patient has required frequent past hospitalizations, has required mechanical ventilation during a previous exacerbation, or has been taking more than the usual amount of medication with poor results, then hospitalization is needed.

The physical examination may be difficult to interpret as the signs may not accurately reflect the severity of the airway obstruction.[84] The presence of wheezing, central cyanosis, confusion, pulsus paradoxus, tachycardia, and/or tachypnea may be indicative of more severe disease and consideration for hospitalization should be made.[85]

Laboratory data will provide further assistance in the determination of need for hospitalization of the asthmatic. The chest radiograph in most asthmatic attacks will be normal or show hyperinflation, but other underlying problems may be revealed, including pneumonia, pneumothorax, or pneumomediastinum, and in these instances hospitalization should be undertaken. If ABG measurements show severe hypoxemia or an arterial carbon dioxide tension above 40 mmHg, further observation is warranted. Spirometry will add additional information. Specific values have been used to determine admission (eg, a post-treatment PEFR <300 L/minute or a FEV_1 <2.1 L),[86] but the patient's failure to improve significantly after therapy is more worrisome than an absolute value of either PEFR or FEV_1.

In those patients who are not hospitalized, adequate follow-up is extremely important. A specific follow-up plan, changes in the maintenance medication regimen, the use of the inhaled β_2-adrenergic agonist on a regular basis, and the use of oral corticosteroids are all very important parts of the outpatient treatment plan.

The above considerations for the determination of admission have been studied in patients with acute exacerbations of asthma, and similar considerations apply to the patient with an exacerbation of COPD. The patient's prior history along with the severity of the underlying illness and comparison of current and previous ABG measurements are helpful, whereas the use of a PEFR or FEV_1 measurement is not as helpful.

A useful rule of thumb is that the patient with obstructive lung disease should leave the emergency department using at least one more drug than when the patient arrived. Using these guidelines, emergency physicians can improve quality of care received by a patient with obstructive lung disease in a given community.

REFERENCES

1. American Thoracic Society. Chronic bronchitis, asthma and pulmonary emphysema: a statement by the committee on diagnostic standards for nontuberculous respiratory disease. *Am Rev Respir Dis.* 1962; 85:762–768.
2. Burrows B, Bloom JW, Traver GA, Cline MG. The course and prognosis of different forms of chronic airway obstruction in a sample from the general population. *N Engl J Med.* 1987;317:1309–1314.
3. McWhorter WP, Polis MA, Kaslow RA. Occurrence, predictors, and consequences of adult asthma in NHANESI and follow-up survey. *Am Rev Respir Dis.* 1989;139:721–724.
4. Holmgren D, Aberg N, Lindberg U, Engstrom I. Childhood asthma in a rural county. *Allergy.* 1989;44:256–259.
5. Braback L, Kalvesten L, Sundstrom G. Prevalence of bronchial asthma among schoolchildren in a Swedish district. *Acta Paediatr Scand.* 1988;77:821–825.
6. Gerstman BB, Bosco LA, Tomita DK, Gross TP, Shaw MM. Prevalence and treatment of asthma in the Michigan Medicaid patient population younger than 45 years, 1980–1986. *J Allergy Clin Immunol.* 1989; 83:1032–1039.
7. Braback L, Kalvesten L. Asthma in schoolchildren: factors influencing morbidity in a Swedish survey. *Acta Paediatr Scand.* 1988;77: 826–830.
8. Richards W. Hospitalization of children with status asthmaticus: a review. *Pediatrics.* 1989;84:111–118.
9. Friday GA, Fireman P. Morbidity and mortality of asthma. *Pediatr Clin North Am.* 1988;35:1149–1162.
10. Sly RM. Mortality from asthma, 1979–1984. *J Allergy Clin Immunol.* 1988;82:705–717.
11. Jackson R, Sears MR, Beaglehole R, Rea HH. International trends in asthma mortality: 1970 to 1985. *Chest.* 1988;94:914–918.
12. Benatar SR. Fatal asthma. *N Engl J Med.* 1986;314:423–429.
13. Weiss KB. Seasonal trends in US asthma hospitalizations and mortality. *JAMA.* 1990;263:2323–2328.
14. Vesterinen E, Kaprio J, Koskenvuo M. Prospective study of asthma in relation to smoking habits among 14,729 adults. *Thorax.* 1988;43: 534–539.
15. McConnochie KM, Roghmann KJ. Wheezing at 8 and 13 years: changing importance of bronchiolitis and passive smoking. *Pediatr Pulmonol.* 1989;6:138–146.
16. Murray AB, Morrison BJ. Passive smoking and the seasonal difference of severity of asthma in children. *Chest.* 1988;94:701–708.
17. Kern DG, Frumkin H. Asthma in respiratory therapists. *Ann Intern Med.* 1989;110:767–773.
18. Centers for Disease Control. Chronic disease reports: chronic obstructive pulmonary disease mortality—United States, 1986. *MMWR.* 1989; 38:549–552.
19. France AJ, Prescott RJ, Biernacki W, Muir AL, MacNee W. Does right ventricular function predict survival in patients with chronic obstructive lung disease? *Thorax.* 1988;43:621–626.
20. Turner KJ, Stewart GA, Woolcock AJ, Green W, Alpers MP. Relationship between mite densities and the prevalence of asthma: comparative studies in two populations in the Eastern Highlands of Papua New Guinea. *Clin Allergy.* 1988;18:331–340.
21. Chapman MD, Pollart SM, Luczynska CM, Platts Mills TA. Hidden allergic factors in the etiology of asthma. *Chest.* 1988;94:185-190.
22. Pierson WE, Voy RO. Exercise-induced bronchospasm in the XXIII summer Olympic games. *N Engl Reg Allergy Proc.* 1988;9:209–213.
23. Chan-Young M, Lam S. Occupational asthma. *Am Rev Respir Dis.* 1986;133:686–703.
24. Pollart SM, Chapman MD, Fiocco GP, Rose G, Platts Mills TA. Epidemiology of acute asthma: IgE antibodies to common inhalant allergens as a risk factor for emergency room visits. *J Allergy Clin Immunol.* 1989;83:875–882.
25. Vial WC. Cigarette smoking and lung disease. *Am J Med Sci.* 1986; 291:130–142.
26. Kilburn KH, Warshaw RH. Pulmonary functional impairment from years of arc welding. *Am J Med.* 1989;87:62–69.
27. Kamat SR, Doshi VB. Sequential health effect study in relation to air pollution in Bombay, India. *Eur J Epidemiol.* 1987;3:265–277.
28. Newcomb RW, Akhter J. Respiratory failure from asthma: a marker for children with high morbidity and mortality. *Am J Dis Child.* 1988; 142:1041–1044.
29. Hill LS. The inhaled route of drug administration in the therapy of asthma. *Br J Clin Prac.* 1988;42:313–315.
30. Rebuck AS, Pengally LD. Development of pulsus paradoxus in the presence of airway obstruction. *N Engl J Med.* 1973;288:66–69.
31. Franklin PK. Review of acute severe asthma. *West J Med.* 1989; 150:552–556.
32. Videm V, Pillgram Larsen, Ellingsen O, Andersen G, Ovrum E. Spontaneous pneumothorax in chronic obstructive pulmonary disease: complications, treatment and recurrences. *Eur J Respir Dis.* 1987; 71:365–371.
33. Nowak RM, Pensler MI, Sarker DD, et al. Comparison of peak expiratory flow and FEV_1 admission criteria for acute bronchial asthma. *Ann Emerg Med.* 1982;11:64–69.
34. Martin TG, Elenbaas RM, Pingleton SH. Use of peak expiratory flow rates to eliminate unnecessary arterial blood gases in acute asthma. *Ann Emerg Med.* 1982;11:70–73.
35. Young GP. Ability of spirometry and oximetry to guide use of arterial blood gases in acute exacerbations of chronic obstructive pulmonary disease. *Ann Emerg Med.* 1990;19:481. Abstract.
36. Tandon MK, Soh PF. Comparison of real and placebo acupuncture in histamine-induced asthma: a double-blind crossover study. *Chest.* 1989;96:102–105.
37. Becker AB, Nelson NA, Simons FER. Inhaled salbutamol (albuterol) vs injected epinephrine in the treatment of acute asthma in children. *Pediatrics.* 1983;102:465–469.
38. Uden DI, Goetz DR, Kohen DP, Fifield GC. Comparison of nebulized terbutaline and subcutaneous epinephrine in the treatment of acute asthma. *Ann Emerg Med.* 1985;14:229–232.
39. Salzman GA, Steele M, Elenbaas R. A comparison of two delivery methods for aerosolized metaproterenol in the treatment of asthmatics in the emergency room. *Chest.* 1987;92(suppl):123S.
40. Benton G, Thomas RC, Nickerson BG, McQuitty JC, Okikawa J. Experience with a metered-dose inhaler with a spacer in the pediatric emergency department. *Am J Dis Child.* 1989;143:678–681.

41. Osterman K, Norborg AM, Stahl E. A multiple dose powder inhaler (Turbuhaler) compared with a conventional aerosol: an acceptance study in asthmatics. *Allergy.* 1989;44:294–297.
42. Ingram RH Jr, Krumpe PE, Duffell GM, Maniscalco B. Ventilation-perfusion changes after aerosolized isoproterenol in asthma. *Am Rev Respir Dis.* 1970;101:364–370.
43. Ballester E, Roca J, Ramis L, Wagner PO, Rodriguez-Roisin R. Pulmonary gas exchange in severe chronic asthma: response to 100% oxygen and salbutamol. *Am Rev Respir Dis.* 1990;141:558–562.
44. Rossing TH, Fanta CH, Goldstein DH, Snapper JR, McFadden ER Jr. Emergency therapy of asthma: comparison of the acute effects of parenteral and inhaled sympathomimetics and infused aminophylline. *Am Rev Respir Dis.* 1980;122:365–371.
45. Cydulka R, Davison R, Grammer L, Parker M, Matthews J IV. The use of epinephrine in the treatment of older asthmatics. *Ann Emerg Med.* 1988;17:322–326.
46. Karetsky MS. Acute asthma: the use of subcutaneous epinephrine in therapy. *Ann Allergy.* 1980;44:12–14.
47. Pancorbo S, Fifield G, Davies S, et al. Subcutaneous epinephrine versus nebulized terbutaline in the emergency treatment of asthma. *Clin Pharm.* 1983;2:45–48.
48. Sly RM, Badiei B, Faciane J. Comparison of subcutaneous terbutaline with epinephrine in the treatment of asthma in children. *J Allergy Clin Immunol.* 1977;59:128–135.
49. Harris JB, Ahrens RC, Annis L, et al. Relative potencies and rates of decline in effect of inhaled albuterol and terbutaline. *J Allergy Clin Immunol.* 1986;77:147.
50. Bergstrand H. Phosphodiesterase inhibitions and theophylline. *Eur J Respir Dis.* 1980;61(suppl 109):37–44.
51. Siegel D, Sheppard D, Gelb A, et al. Aminophylline increases the toxicity but not the efficacy of an inhaled beta-adrenergic agonist in the treatment of acute exacerbations of asthma. *Am Rev Respir Dis.* 1985;132:283–286.
52. Rice KL, Leatherman JW, Duane PG, et al. Aminophylline for acute exacerbations of chronic obstructive pulmonary disease: a controlled trial. *Ann Intern Med.* 1987;107:305–309.
53. Josephson GW, Kennedy HL, MacKensie EJ, et al. Cardiac dysrhythmia during the treatment of acute asthma: a comparison of two treatment regimens by a double-blind protocol. *Chest.* 1980;78:429–435.
54. Rebuck AS, Chapman KR, Abboud R, et al. Nebulized anticholinergic and sympathomimetic treatment of asthma and chronic obstructive airway disease in the emergency room. *Am J Med.* 1987;82:59–64.
55. Easton PA, Jadue C, Dhingru S, et al. A comparison of the bronchodilating effects of a beta-2-adrenergic agent (albuterol) and an anticholinergic agent (iprotropium bromide) given by aerosol alone or in sequence. *N Engl J Med.* 1986;315:735–739.
56. Franklin PK. Review of acute severe asthma. *West J Med.* 1989;150:552–556.
57. Stein R, Canny GJ, Bohn DJ, Reisman JJ, Levison H. Severe acute asthma in a pediatric intensive care unit: six years' experience. *Pediatrics.* 1989;83:1023–1028.
58. Fisher MM, Bowey CJ, Ladd Hudson K. External chest compression in acute asthma: a preliminary study. *Crit Care Med.* 1989;17:686–687.
59. Menzies R, Gibbons W, Goldberg P. Determinants of weaning and survival among patients with COPD who require mechanical ventilation for acute respiratory failure. *Chest.* 1989;95:398–405.
60. Kaelin RM, Assimacopoulos A, Chevrolet JC. Failure to predict six-month survival of patients with COPD requiring mechanical ventilation by analysis of simple indices: a prospective study. *Chest.* 1987;92:971–978.
61. Davies BI, Maesen FP. The epidemiology of respiratory tract pathogens in southern Netherlands. *Eur Respir J.* 1988;1:415–420.
62. Busse WW. The precipitation of asthma by upper respiratory infections. *Chest.* 1985;87(suppl):44S–48S.
63. Anthonisen NR, Manfreda J, Warren CPW, et al. Antibiotic therapy in exacerbations of chronic obstructive pulmonary disease. *Ann Intern Med.* 1987;106:196–204.
64. Rosella JC, Plá JC. Magnesium sulfate in crisis of asthma. *Prena Med Argent.* 1936;23:1677.
65. Haury VG. Blood serum magnesium in bronchial asthma and its treatment by the administration of magnesium sulfate. *J Lab Clin Med.* 1940;25:340–344.
66. Reinhart RA. Magnesium metabolism: a review with special reference to the relationship between intracellular content and serum levels. *Arch Intern Med.* 1988;148:2415–2420.
67. Skobeloff EM, Spivey WH, McNamara RM, Greenspon L. Intravenous magnesium sulfate for the treatment of acute asthma in the emergency department. *JAMA.* 1989;262:1210–1213.
68. Okayama H, Aikawa T, Okayama M, Sasaki H, Mue S, Takishima T. Bronchodilating effect of intravenous magnesium sulfate in bronchial asthma. *JAMA.* 1987;257:1076–1078.
69. Haynes RD Jr, Murad F. Adrenocorticotropic hormone: adrenocortical steroids and their synthetic analogs. In: Goodman A, Goodman L, Gilman A, eds. *The Pharmacologic Basis of Therapeutics.* 6th ed. New York: Macmillan, 1980:1466–1496.
70. Kaliner M. Mechanisms of glucocorticosteroid action in bronchial asthma. *J Allergy Clin Immunol.* 1985;76:845–851.
71. Morris HG. Mechanisms of action and therapeutic use of corticosteroids in asthma. *J Allergy Clin Immunol.* 1985;75:1–13.
72. Fanta CH, Rossing TH, McFadden ER. Glucocorticoids in acute asthma. *Am J Med.* 1983;74:845–851.
73. Fiel SB, Swartz MA, Glanz K, et al. Efficacy of short-term corticosteroid therapy in outpatient treatment of acute bronchial asthma. *Am J Med.* 1983;75:259–262.
74. Littenberg B, Gluck EH. A controlled trial of methylprednisolone in the emergency treatment of acute asthma. *N Engl J Med.* 1986;314:150–152.
75. Stein LM, Cole RP. Early administration of corticosteroids in emergency room treatment of acute asthma. *Ann Intern Med.* 1990;112:822–827.
76. Reed CE, Hunt LW. The emergency visit and management of asthma. *Ann Intern Med.* 1990;112:801–802. Editorial.
77. Ratto D, Alfaro C, Sipsey J, Glovsky MM, Sharma OP. Are intravenous corticosteroids required in status asthmaticus? *JAMA.* 1988;260:527–529.
78. Albert RK, Martin TR, Lewis SW. Controlled clinical trial of methylprednisolone in patients with chronic bronchitis and acute respiratory insufficiency. *Ann Intern Med.* 1980;92:753–758.
79. Fiel SB, Swartz MA, Glanz K, Francis ME. Efficacy of short-term corticosteroid therapy in outpatient treatment of acute bronchial asthma. *Am J Med.* 1983;75:259–262.
80. Bone RC. Step care for asthma. *JAMA.* 1988;260:543.
81. Barker AG. Strategies in managing asthma. *West J Med.* 1989;150:303–308.
82. Hoffman IB, Fiel SB. Oral vs. repository corticosteroid therapy in acute asthma. *Chest.* 1988;93:11–13.
83. Schwartzstein RS, Fanta CH. Orally administered nifedipine in chronic stable asthma. *Am Rev Respir Dis.* 1986;134:262–265.
84. Carden DL, Nowak RM, Sarkar D, Tomlanovich MC. Vital signs including pulsus paradoxus in the assessment of acute bronchial asthma. *Ann Emerg Med.* 1983;12:29–32.

85. Fischl MA, Pitchenik A, Gardner LB. An index predicting relapse and need for hospitalization in patients with acute bronchial asthma. *N Engl J Med*. 1981;305:783–789.

86. Nowak RM, Tomlanovich MC, Sarkar DD, et al. Arterial blood gas and pulmonary function testing in acute bronchial asthma: predicting patient outcomes. *JAMA*. 1983;149:2043.

73. Pulmonary Embolism

CHARLES M. SHUFFLEBARGER, MD
D. KIM ZAISER, MD, FACEP

Acute pulmonary thromboembolism is among the most difficult conditions to evaluate in emergency medicine. Although the true incidence of pulmonary embolism (PE) is uncertain, it is accepted as the primary or contributing cause in hundreds of thousands of deaths annually. The symptoms of PE are variable and are dependent on factors including size of embolism, prior cardiopulmonary disease, and the patient's general condition. The signs and symptoms are also nonspecific and may be attributed to a variety of common conditions such as pneumonia, myocardial infarction, or exacerbation of obstructive lung disease. The commonly available ancillary diagnostic aids such as arterial blood gases, electrocardiography, and chest radiography offer little predictive value. More definitive tests are hampered by controversy in utility with high rates of inconclusive findings, low positive predictive value, and high cost. The definitive test, pulmonary angiography, is invasive, is associated with a low but finite morbidity and mortality, and requires technical facilities and expertise not widely available on an emergency basis.

Thus, the practitioner is faced, on a daily basis, with patients who may suffer from acute pulmonary embolism but has limited diagnostic options available to arrive at a definitive diagnosis.

HISTORY

Although Virchow[1] is generally considered the first to describe pulmonary thromboembolism, pathologists preceding him had long described the presence of pulmonary artery clot in postmortem examinations.[2] These early necropists considered the thrombus to have arisen in situ (primary pulmonary thrombosis). In the mid 1800s, Virchow[1] first described the basic tenets of the pathology of pulmonary embolism, which are still accepted today. Specifically, he described thrombosis arising from the large caudal veins and propagating proximally, eventually dislodging and embolizing, causing occlusion of pulmonary vessels.

Despite recognition of the high frequency of occurrence of pulmonary thromboembolism, little progress in the premortem diagnosis of this ailment was made during the next 75 years. In 1908, Trendelenburg first reported attempted surgical pulmonary embolectomy in three patients with acute massive pulmonary thromboembolism, all of whom died.[3] Kirschner performed the first successful embolectomy using this technique in 1924.[4] Heparin as a systemic anticoagulant for the prevention of venous thrombosis was introduced in 1916 by MacLean[5] and was demonstrated to be efficacious in the treatment of pulmonary thromboembolism by Bauer in 1959.[6]

Since then, important strides in the administration and monitoring of systemic anticoagulation have been made and thrombolytic therapy has been developed. Finally, surgical ligation of the inferior vena cava (IVC) for control of refractory deep venous thrombosis (DVT) with embolization has been largely supplemented by less invasive IVC filter devices.[7,8]

During the past 30 years, significant advancement in the diagnosis of pulmonary thromboembolism has been made.

Wagner introduced radioactive pulmonary perfusion scanning in 1964[9] and reported a complementary role for xenon inhalation scans (ventilatory scanning) in 1968.[10] More recently, the diagnosis of lower extremity and iliofemoral DVT has been revolutionized by the addition of nuclear scans, duplex ultrasound venography, radioactive labeled fibrinogen uptake studies, and impedance plethysmography to the cumbersome standard contrast venogram. Thus, most cases of DVT may now be diagnosed relatively noninvasively.

EPIDEMIOLOGY

Despite recognition of pulmonary thromboembolism as a major cause of morbidity or mortality, its true incidence is unknown. In a well-controlled study of the incidence and natural history of pulmonary thromboembolism in 1975, Dalen and Alpert estimated that 630,000 victims suffered pulmonary thromboembolism annually.[11] One autopsy study employing exhaustive criteria for defining the presence of a pulmonary thromboembolism that had occurred at any time during one's life placed the incidence at 64%.[12] Yet some feel that pulmonary embolism is overdiagnosed and overtreated, citing the frequency of significant complications of therapy of presumed pulmonary thromboembolism.[13] Although postmortem series may indeed overestimate the incidence of pulmonary thromboembolism, aggressive search for the ailment is still mandatory. It is estimated that one-third of deaths from PE occur within 1 hour of embolization and, of the remaining deaths, 90% occur before the diagnosis is established.[13] Anticoagulation can decrease the overall mortality from about 30%[11] to 8%.[14] Because greater than 90% of pulmonary emboli occur in patients with a risk factor (Table 73-1) for DVT, aggressive evaluation for PE is especially mandatory in this group so that early treatment is initiated and mortality reduced.

PATHOPHYSIOLOGY

Pulmonary embolism results from detachment and migration of a deep vein thrombus in the vast majority of cases. Therefore, the pathophysiology of acute pulmonary embolism is primarily the process of thrombogenesis. This includes stasis, activation of clotting factors, and, to a lesser degree, vessel wall damage. Once embolization has occurred, processes including fibrinolysis, vascular and hemodynamic reflexes, and alterations of pulmonary mechanics act to produce the clinical manifestations of acute PE.

Stasis and the activation of clotting factors are the necessary components of thrombus formation. Prolonged sitting, bed rest, immobilization, and elevated right ventricular filling pressures are factors that may contribute to stasis, particularly in the lower extremities. Intimal damage to vessels

Table 73-1 Major Risk Factors for Pulmonary Embolism

Deep venous thrombosis
Advanced age
Congestive heart failure
Chronic obstructive pulmonary disease
Malignancy
Immobilization
   Prolonged bed rest
   Prolonged travel
   Orthopedic immobilization
Recent surgery, especially pelvic and lower extremity orthopedic procedures
Trauma, especially involving the pelvis or lower extremities
Peripartum state
Hypercoaguable states
Obesity
Oral contraceptive use

was thought to play a crucial role in thrombogenesis until recently when several experiments have shown that even major vessel injury does not routinely result in thrombus formation, even if accompanied by stasis.[15,16]

The most important direct cause of thrombus generation is the presence of activated clotting factors. This is the common denominator for the majority of risk factors for DVT. Stasis decreases the clearance of activated clotting factors, thereby elevating their concentration in the affected vessel. Likewise, minor trauma to the lower extremities transiently increases the activity of the coagulation cascade.

The role of the fibrinolytic system has yet to be completely elucidated, although several interesting findings have been reported. The fibrinolytic activity of the blood after venous stasis is lower in patients with thrombosis than in controls.[17] This is most likely secondary to elevated levels of a tissue plasminogen activator inhibitor.[18] The walls of the veins of the upper extremities have higher fibrinolytic activity than those of the lower extremities. This may explain why thrombi are less commonly found in the vessels draining into the superior vena cava. Trauma and surgery both result in a period of decreased fibrinolytic activity which may contribute to the formation of venous thrombi.[19]

It is probably a combination of factors such as stasis, increased thrombin formation by activated clotting factors, and decreased fibrinolysis which result in thrombus formation. Therefore, efforts to prevent venous thrombi and pulmonary embolism are aimed at minimizing stasis, reducing thrombin formation (eg, by heparin), and increasing fibrinolytic activity (eg, by streptokinase, urokinase, or tissue plasminogen activator).

Pulmonary emboli arise from DVT in the lower extremities in 80% to 90% of cases. Thrombus formation usually begins in the deep veins of the calf and propagates proximally. Less commonly, procedures such as hip replacement or pelvic surgery may cause thrombi to originate in the femoral or pelvic veins. Although deep venous thrombosis of the upper extremities is rare, up to 35% may embolize.[20] The remainder of PEs originate from the right cardiac chambers.

Regardless of the site of origin, when the thrombus detaches it migrates rapidly through the venous system to the lungs. The right lower lobe is the most frequently involved site. When the embolus lodges in the pulmonary arterial tree, it partially or completely obstructs blood flow distally with resultant vascular, hemodynamic, pulmonary parenchymal, and airway effects.

Vascular and hemodynamic consequences must be considered together. When a portion of the blood flow to the lungs is obstructed by an embolus, there is an effective decrease in the cross-sectional area of the pulmonary arterial bed. This results in an increase in pulmonary vascular resistance. Approximately 30% to 50% of the vascular bed must be occluded before pulmonary hypertension occurs. To compensate for the increased resistance, pulmonary arterial pressure must rise to maintain adequate blood flow, thus increasing right ventricular work. If the embolus is massive, occluding greater than 50% of pulmonary arterial flow, or if the patient has pre-existing heart or lung disease, the rapid onset of pulmonary hypertension and increased demand on the right heart may result in right ventricular failure and reduction in left ventricular output.

The release of vasoactive amines such as serotonin from the platelets in a fresh pulmonary embolus may add to the hemodynamic effects caused by embolic mechanical obstruction by inducing additional pulmonary arterial vasoconstriction, further increasing right ventricular work. The vasoconstriction shunts blood away from the embolized lung segment. Other areas of the lung become relatively overperfused and underventilated, resulting in an increased alveolar-arterial oxygen gradient.

Pulmonary infarction is not a common hemodynamic consequence of pulmonary embolism, occurring in less than 10% of embolic events. The reasons for this are twofold. First, it is unusual for an embolus to occlude a vessel totally. Incomplete occlusion permits adequate flow to perfuse the distal lung parenchyma. Second, the pulmonary parenchyma receives oxygen from the alveoli and the bronchial arteries in addition to the pulmonary arteries. It is rare that compromise of the pulmonary arterial flow is sufficient to cause infarction in patients with a normal ventilatory status and normal bronchial arterial flow.

Pulmonary embolism results in alterations of lung mechanics, ventilation, and gas exchange. There is an immediate increase in the amount of alveolar dead space; that is, alveoli are ventilated but not perfused, resulting in an abnormally high arterial-alveolar carbon dioxide gradient. Diminished alveolar P_{CO_2} in the ventilated but unperfused area, regional hypoxia, and release of humoral agents from the embolus itself all contribute to effecting a compensatory local pneumoconstriction involving the bronchioles and alveolar ducts. This decreases the functional size of the alveolar dead space.

Pulmonary occlusion results in changes within the lung parenchyma. Hypoxia-induced loss of surfactant causes local alveolar collapse within approximately 24 hours. Surfactant loss and the release of humoral agents that increase vascular permeability lead to the development of an area of hemorrhagic congestion distal to the site of the embolus.

The clinical consequences of the vascular, hemodynamic, airway, and pulmonary parenchymal changes of PE will be determined by the presence of pre-existing heart or lung disease. Underlying cardiopulmonary disease may reduce the size of the pulmonary vascular bed, diminish the work capacity of the right ventricle, or adversely affect gas exchange at the alveolar level. Arterial hypoxemia is common but not universal in PE, depending on the degree of arterial obstruction and the ability of the patient adequately to ventilate the remainder of the normally perfused parenchyma. Approximately 12% of patients with PE will have a Pa_{O_2} of >80 mmHg,[21,22] and 6% will have a Pa_{O_2} of >90 mmHg.

The resolution of a pulmonary embolus occurs by fibrinolysis or organization. A young thrombus can be dissolved within hours by fibrinolysis initiated by fibrinolytic activator in the pulmonary arterial wall. Older thrombi or those organized prior to embolization resolve by organization. This process is much slower, taking several weeks to occur, and results in at least some residual arterial obstruction. Perfusion data reflect this variability in rate of resolution. Perfusion studies normalize within 12 to 24 hours in many patients, but in others defects may persist for weeks.[23]

CLINICAL MANIFESTATIONS

Most data regarding the sensitivity of clinical signs and symptoms of pulmonary embolism have been derived from studies of symptomatic patients. Since the incidence of asymptomatic pulmonary embolism may be relatively high (83% of patients with angiographically documented pulmonary embolism after hip replacement were asymptomatic),[24] the sensitivity of the following findings may be greatly overestimated.

Dyspnea secondary to pneumoconstriction and the increase in alveolar dead space is the most frequent symptom reported, occuring in over 80% of patients with pulmonary embolism. In many patients, it is the only symptom. Pleuritic chest pain is the second most common symptom, occurring in approximately 60% to 70% of cases. The pain is usually located laterally and is not necessarily associated with pulmonary infarction. The etiology is unclear, but pulmonary vascular congestion and irritation of the parietal pleura have been postulated as causes. Although pleuritic pain is considered classic, the pain is frequently dull and substernal, making it difficult to differentiate from angina or myocardial infarction based upon the character of the pain.

Apprehension is the third most common symptom but is nonspecific, especially in the emergency department setting

Table 73-2 Symptoms of Acute Pulmonary Embolism

Symptom	Wolfe[50] (N = 1000)	Bell[51] (N = 327)	UPET[21] (N = 160)	Henry Ford Hospital[22] (N = 112)
Dyspnea	77%	84%	81%	87%
Chest pain	63	88	72	59
Apprehension		59		
Cough		53	54	27
Hemoptysis	26	30	34	22
Sweats		27		
Syncope		13		13
Altered mental status	23			
Calf pain				14
Palpitations				8

Table 73-3 Signs of Acute Pulmonary Embolism

	Wolfe[50] (N = 1000)	Bell[51] (N = 327)	UPET[21] (N = 160)	Henry Ford Hospital[22] (N = 112)
Pulse > 100	59%	44%	43%	67%
Respiratory rate > 16	38	92	88	81
Rales	42	58	54	46
Accentuated P_2 sound	11	53	54	16
Temperature > 37.8°C	43	43	42	14
Phlebitis	23	32	34	
S_4 gallop		34*		11
S_3 gallop				8
Diaphoresis		36		
Edema		24		
Murmur		23		
Cyanosis	9	19		
Elevated central venous pressure	18			12
Shock	11			13
Pleural friction rub				4

*This study did not differentiate between S_3 and S_4 gallops.

where most patients have at least some degree of anxiety. Cough, hemoptysis, syncope, and nonpleuritic chest pain are recorded less frequently (Table 73-2). Hemoptysis occurs due to congestive atelectasis or pulmonary infarction. Syncope, caused by marked reduction of cardiac output or hypoxia, suggests massive pulmonary embolism.

Tachypnea is the most frequent physical sign (Table 73-3) associated with a PE and results from the pathophysiologic changes (increased alveolar dead space and pneumoconstriction) discussed previously. Tachycardia is another common but nonspecific sign. Both tachypnea and tachycardia may be transient and may not be present by the time the patient arrives in the emergency department. Rales, secondary to local atelectasis, are found in approximately half of patients with PE. Wheezing is uncommon but may be found as a result of localized pneumoconstriction.

Occasionally, signs generated by the hemodynamic effects of the embolus on the pulmonary circulation may be appreciated. These include an increase in the loudness of S_2P, a right ventricular S_3, and jugular venous distention. These are more likely to be found in patients with massive pulmonary emboli or in those with pre-existing cardiac disease. Rarely, a massive embolism that produces partial obstruction of a large pulmonary artery may result in a new systolic or diastolic murmur over the second left intercostal space or an intrascapular bruit.

Low-grade fever occurs frequently as a result of acute PE; however, fever may be as high as 40°C and may persist for several days.[25] The fever is caused by infarction, local tissue necrosis, hemorrhage, or inflammatory changes. Pleural rubs are most frequently heard over the lower lobes where emboli are most common. Clinical evidence of DVT is present in only one third to one half of patients with pulmonary embolism, so that absence of such evidence is not helpful in excluding PE.

The clinical history and physical findings in PE are usually nonspecific. However, when such signs and symptoms are found in a patient who is at risk for PE, further evaluation is mandatory.

DIAGNOSTIC STUDIES

Chest Radiography

The chest x-ray film is abnormal in the majority of patients with PE.[26] Unfortunately, the radiographic manifestations are nonspecific. The most commonly seen abnormalities are volume loss, diaphragmatic elevation, atelectasis, and a small unilateral pleural effusion.[26] Signs more specific for PE, such as pulmonic arterial dilatation, regional oligemia with a distinct "cut-off" of the pulmonary vasculature (Westermark's sign), and a pleura-based rounded density convex to the hilum (Hampton's hump) occur much less frequently. The greatest value of chest radiography in the evaluation of possible PE is to exclude those other diagnoses that have more specific radiographic findings.

Electrocardiography

The electrocardiogram (ECG) is usually nondiagnostic in acute pulmonary thromboembolism.[27] Sinus tachycardia is the most common ECG finding. Other changes more specific for pulmonary thromboembolism including the $S_1 Q_3 T_3$ pattern (exaggerated S wave in lead I with a Q wave and T wave inversion in lead III), right ventricular strain pattern, T-wave inversions in the right precordial leads, and new right bundle branch block occur less frequently. These changes usually occur in cases in which right heart pressures are more markedly elevated.[27] The principal utility of the ECG in patients with suspected pulmonary thromboembolism lies in its ability to exclude other diagnoses, such as acute myocardial ischemia and pericarditis.

Arterial Blood Gases

Arterial blood gases are frequently employed to screen for the possibility of acute PE. Shunting and reflex changes may result in arterial hypoxemia and hypocarbia. Thus, the arterial-alveolar gradient is nearly always increased above normal. A retrospective analysis of 78 patients with angiographically documented pulmonary thromboembolism found hypocapnea in 93% and increased arterial-alveolar gradient in 95%. Only one patient had neither.[28]

Of course, similar changes in arterial blood gas partial pressures may be found in a variety of common cardiopulmonary disorders and, although normal arterial blood gases values do not entirely exclude the diagnosis of acute PE, in most scenarios normal results should lead toward other diagnoses.

Serum LDH, SGOT, and Bilirubin

In the past, the triad of elevated lactate dehydrogenase (LDH), serum glutamic oxaloacetate transaminase (SGOT), and bilirubin was felt to be specific for PE. Critical review has shown these findings to be both insensitive and nonspecific for the diagnosis. They offer little diagnostic utility when evaluating for pulmonary thromboembolism.

Radioactive Lung Scans

When introduced in 1964 by Wagner,[9,10] radioactive lung scanning seemed to offer a noninvasive method for diagnosing PE. Greater scrutiny has demonstrated a high proportion of inconclusive (low, intermediate, or indeterminate probability) results. In these cases further testing is usually necessary. Still, these scans are a mainstay in the evaluation of possible PE.

A pulmonary perfusion scan is performed by intravenously injecting isotope-labeled albumin and then obtaining multiple-plane scans. The isotope aggregates in the pulmonary microvasculature, so that the scan image is directly determined by the regional pulmonary blood flow. Because embolism interrupts normal flow, patients with PE will have abnormal perfusion scans. A normal perfusion scan rules out PE[29,30] (Figs. 73-1 and 73-2).

Pulmonary blood flow is affected by a variety of cardiopulmonary disorders in addition to PE. Most importantly, chronic obstructive pulmonary disease and left ventricular

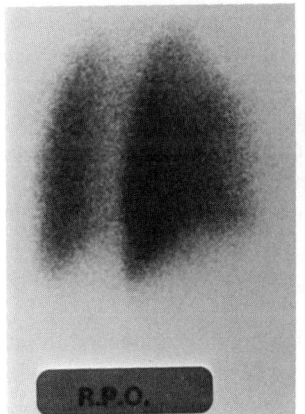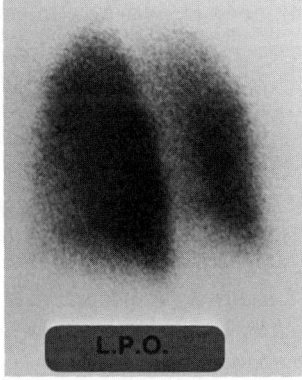

Figure 73-1 Normal pulmonary perfusion scan. **Left:** 47.7 seconds, 430 K. **Right:** 47.7 seconds, 521 K. Emission is homogeneous throughout both lungs. *Source*: Courtesy of Dr. Mustafa Adatepe, Division of Nuclear Medicine, Allegheny General Hospital.

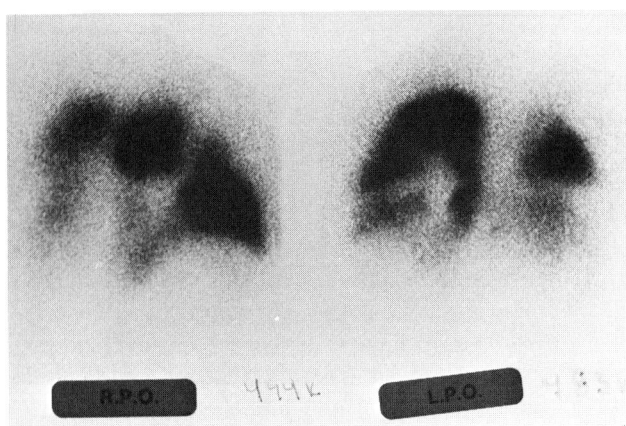

Figure 73-2 Perfusion scan in a patient with PE. Multiple segmental defects are seen. *Source*: Courtesy of Dr. Mustafa Adatepe, Division of Nuclear Medicine, Allegheny General Hospital.

Table 73-4 Scheme for Interpretation of Ventilation-Perfusion Lung Scan

Interpretation	Pattern	Frequency of Pulmonary Embolism, %
Normal Probability of PE	Normal perfusion	0
Low	Small V-Q mismatches	0
	Focal V-Q matches with no corresponding radiographic abnormalities	4.8
	Perfusion defects substantially smaller than radiographic abnormalities	7.7
Intermediate	Diffuse, severe airway obstruction	20
	Matched perfusion defects and radiographic abnormalities	27
	Single moderate V-Q mismatch without corresponding radiographic abnormality	33
High	Perfusion defects substantially larger than radiographic abnormalities	87
	1 or more large or 2 or more moderate-sized V-Q mismatches with no corresponding radiographic abnormalities	92

Source: Biello D et al. Ventilation-perfusion studies in suspected pulmonary embolism. *AJR Am J Roentgenol.* 1979;133:1033. © 1979.

myocardial dysfunction commonly result in abnormal lung perfusion scans and complicate the interpretation of the test.

The specificity of pulmonary perfusion scans is improved when correlated with chest radiography and xenon-133 ventilation scan results.[26,31] Because acute embolism does not substantially affect regional ventilation, a pattern of abnormal flow with normal ventilation within a region is more suggestive of PE than of other diagnoses. Anderson demonstrated that the addition of ventilation scans significantly improves both the sensitivity and specificity of scan interpretation, especially in patients with underlying obstructive disease. A scheme for interpretation of ventilation-perfusion lung scans suggested by Biello is given in Table 73-4.

The greatest utility of the radioactive lung scan is to rule out PE, since a normal perfusion scan is associated with a 0% incidence of PE.[30,31] Furthermore, it is important to realize that the probability of PE is dependent not only on the scan results but also on the degree to which embolus is suggested by clinical evidence. The patient in whom there is relatively little clinical suspicion for PE may require more support for the diagnosis than a "high" probability scan result before subjection to the risks of systemic anticoagulation. Similarly, the patient with classic risk factors, signs, and symptoms of PE may have a high probability of the diagnosis even if scan results are of "low" or "intermediate" probabilities. Thus, nuclear medicine scans should augment rather than replace clinical judgment.

Along with nonspecificity, the greatest drawback to the use of ventilation-perfusion scans is the large proportion of equivocal results. Becker et al. found that 59% of scans in their series were of low, intermediate, or indeterminate probability.[32] Because such findings are insufficient to exclude or diagnose PE reliably, further study is required in most such patients. Even high-probability scans carry a 10% false-positive rate, causing some to argue that even these patients require angiographic confirmation to prevent unnecessary exposure to the hazards of anticoagulation.[33] Under such philosophy, the utility of the perfusion scan would be limited to guiding the angiographic evaluation.

Pulmonary Angiography

Pulmonary angiography is the accepted reference method for diagnosing PE. Direct radiographic demonstration of pulmonary arterial filling defects is considered definitive. Angiographic sensitivity is improved by performing selective or subselective cannulations and injections and by "coning down" views. Emboli as small as 0.5 mm may be detected by this technique. Smaller emboli are clinically inconsequential (Figs. 73-3 and 73-4).

The disadvantages of pulmonary angiography lie with its invasive nature and its requirement for advanced equipment and technical expertise. The overall complication rate is about 4%, with cardiac perforation, dysrhythmia, and

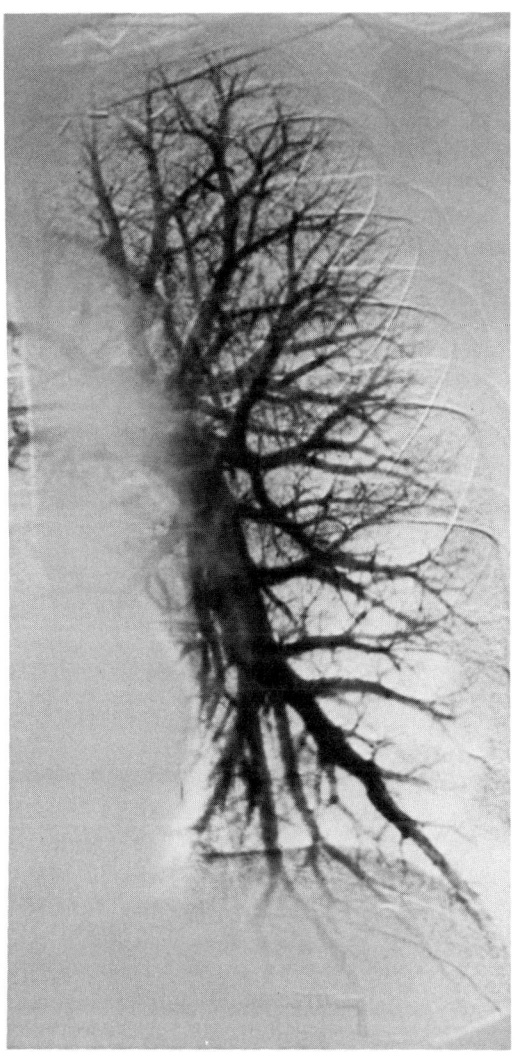

Figure 73-3 Normal pulmonary angiogram. *Source*: Courtesy of Dr. F. Contractor, Department of Radiology, Allegheny General Hospital.

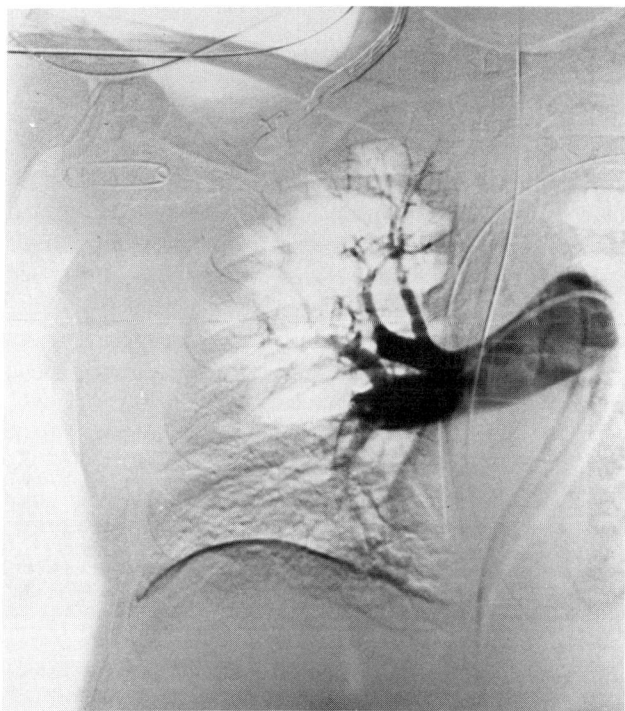

Figure 73-4 Pulmonary angiogram in patient with PE. Defects are noted in the lower lobe artery, and peripheral vessels are nonvisualized. *Source*: Courtesy of Dr. F. Contractor, Department of Radiology, Allegheny General Hospital.

allergic reaction to contrast as the most common problems encountered.[34] The mortality is approximately 0.2%, with most deaths occurring in patients with underlying obstructive pulmonary disease and resultant elevation of right ventricular pressures.[35] Unfortunately, it is in this group that nuclear medicine scans are most commonly nondiagnostic.

Diagnosis of Venous Thrombosis

An alternative approach to diagnosing pulmonary embolism is to search for the venous thrombosis that is the embolic source. The rationale for this approach is that discovery of thrombosis usually warrants full anticoagulation. Therefore, even though the diagnosis of PE may remain only presumptive, the treatment remains the same. The availability of newer, less invasive modalities for the diagnosis of lower-extremity DVT has intensified interest in this approach.

Currently available noninvasive tests for caudal DVT include ^{125}I-labeled fibrinogen scan, Doppler ultrasonography, B-mode ultrasonography, and impedance plethysmography. In the emergency setting, fibrinogen uptake scanning is of limited value because of excessive time requirements.[35] Doppler studies are hampered by a lack of sufficient sensitivity and a lack of objective end points.[36,37]

Real-time B-mode ultrasonography is a sensitive means for the detection of DVT in the femoral and popliteal systems. In comparison with contrast venography, femoral and popliteal thrombosis may be identified with a sensitivity of 95% to 100% and a specificity of 97% to 100%, using a lack of compressibility as the sole criterion for diagnosis.[38] For calf vein thrombosis the sensitivity is much lower but, when evaluating for PE, DVT isolated to these veins appears to be inconsequential.[39] B-mode sonography is also less sensitive for the diagnosis of iliac vein thrombosis.[38]

Impedance plethysmography (IPG) is another accurate method for diagnosing proximal vein thrombosis of the lower extremity. IPG relies on identification of vein distensibility to identify a lack of thrombus. When clot is present, IPG detects a lack of the normally demonstrable increase in blood volume in the extremity when blood pressure cuffs are inflated and released by showing a blunted response in electrical impedance. Like B-mode sonography, IPG is a sensitive means of identifying proximal vein clot while calf vein thrombosis frequently escapes detection.[40,41] Serial IPG tests that remain normal are reported to rule out "clinically significant" DVT even if calf vein thrombosis is present.[41] IPG requires less technical expertise and the equipment is less expensive than B-mode ultrasound.

Contrast venography is the standard reference method for diagnosing DVT. This technique is invasive, painful, and subject to interpretive error. Most importantly, it is in itself phlebitic. Its use should be reserved for cases in which noninvasive studies are not available or are nondiagnostic.

Failure to detect lower-extremity DVT does not rule out PE. DVT in the legs might escape detection by the above modes. A large single thrombus might embolize in toto, leaving no residual vein thrombus. As previously mentioned, other sources such as the heart, the renal veins, the IVC, and the upper extremities are the source of a finite percentage of emboli. Therefore, when evaluating for possible PE, the search for DVT is meaningful only when thrombosis is discovered.

MEDICAL THERAPY

Systemic Anticoagulation

The initial treatment of most patients with acute PE is systemic anticoagulation with heparin. Heparin acts by inhibiting the coagulation cascade and preventing the formation or propagation of thrombus. Because there is no effect on formed clot, heparin inhibits recurrent embolization but does not treat clot that has previously embolized.

The goal of heparin therapy is to maintain the activated partial thromboplastin time at 1.5 to 2.5 times the control. An initial dose of 5,000 to 10,000 U followed by continuous infusion at 1000 to 1500 U (25 U/kg) per hour is employed, frequently monitoring the partial thromboplastin time to allow dosage adjustment. Heparin is administered for 7 to 10 days with initiation of oral anticoagulation with coumadin several days prior to the discontinuation of heparin.

Heparin is contraindicated in patients with an allergy to the drug or with a history of recent or active bleeding, a bleeding disorder, thrombocytopenia, severe hypertension, peptic ulcer disease, recent stroke, or recent major surgery. The most common and severe complication, a major bleeding episode, occurs in less than 2% of patients. Heparin causes mild thrombocytopenia in 25% of those treated, though clinically significant thrombocytopenia is much more rare.[42]

Fibrinolytic Therapy

The role of fibrinolytic therapy in acute PE remains incompletely defined. When the National Heart and Lung Institute first designed a trial to evaluate the thrombolytic efficacy of urokinase, PE was chosen as the study model.[21] The resultant Urokinase in Pulmonary Embolism Trial demonstrated that urokinase results in a more rapid normalization of clinical and hemodynamic variables compared to heparin therapy alone, especially in cases of large emboli, but the 2-week mortality was not improved and there was a significantly higher rate of bleeding complications in the urokinase-treated group. Still, descriptive reports of dramatic improvement after fibrinolytic therapy[43–45] have fostered continued interest in the use of these drugs in certain patients. A recent study comparing urokinase therapy with tissue plasminogen activator showed that tissue plasminogen activator had greater efficacy and fewer complications than urokinase in patients with PE.[46] Although this research may suggest an expanded role for thrombolytic therapy of PE, this treatment is currently proven only to improve initial perfusion and hemodynamics more effectively than heparin alone. At this time the use of fibrinolytic drugs should be considered primarily for patients with severe hemodynamic derangement.

SURGICAL TREATMENT

Surgical intervention is not usually necessary in the treatment of PE. However, there are instances when emergency embolectomy or vena caval disruption may be indicated.

Pulmonary embolectomy may be performed in patients with shock secondary to massive PE. Documentation of the embolus by lung scan or angiography is required since a myocardial infarction may be difficult to distinguish from a PE by clinical signs and symptoms alone. Surgical embolectomy carries a high mortality rate (up to 11% in patients who did not have a cardiac arrest prior to surgery and over 64% in those who did[47]) and, therefore, should be used selectively. Although no clear guidelines exist, it is reasonable to initiate thrombolytic therapy in those patients who present with symptoms indicating a massive PE and consider embolectomy in those few who continue to demonstrate hemodynamic deterioration.

Approximately 5% of patients with a pulmonary embolus have recurrent emboli while adequately anticoagulated, have a significant bleeding episode while anticoagulated, or have specific contraindications to anticoagulation. In these cases, femoral vein ligation or interruption of the IVC may be necessary to prevent recurrent embolization. The Greenfield filter is the intraluminal device most frequently utilized to prevent proximal migration of thrombi. Placement requires a minor operative procedure during which a catheter containing the filter is directed from the internal jugular or femoral vein into the IVC. The filter is then opened, like an umbrella. Tiny points on the ends of the "spokes" of the filter catch on the vein walls to prevent proximal migration of the filter. Unfortunately, the incidence of caval thrombosis is 5% and that of recurrent symptomatic pulmonary embolus is 2%.[48]

A bird's nest filter, recently developed, can be placed percutaneously using local anesthesia and fluoroscopy.

Caval thrombosis has occurred in 2.9% of the patients and recurrent thromboembolism in 2.7%.[49]

Additional complications of IVC intraluminal devices include stasis changes, improper placement of the device (eg, in the renal vein), vessel perforation, and breakage or proximal migration of the device. Since emboli can originate in the heart, hepatic veins, or upper extremities, it is important to document a thrombus in the lower extremities or IVC before the patient is subjected to this procedure.

Finally, the direct surgical approaches to IVC disruption are ligation (total occlusion) or plication (partial occlusion). Each procedure carries a mortality of approximately 10%, a 4% risk of recurrent emboli, and a 20% incidence of stasis sequelae.[47]

In summary, it is rare that surgical intervention is necessary in the treatment of PE. These procedures have significant morbidity and should be used only when deemed absolutely necessary. Although the emergency physician may not be involved in the decision-making process, it is important to know what options are available in the long-term management of the patient with PE.

SUMMARY

PE occurs commonly but is often difficult to diagnose. The key to successfully identifying the patient with acute PE lies in obtaining an accurate history—elucidating any risk factors for PE and eliciting symptoms that are consistent with the diagnosis. Physical exam and routine emergency lab tests such as chest radiography, electrocardiography, and arterial blood gases may support the clinical impression but are rarely definitive. In most cases, a more specific procedure such as a ventilation-perfusion scan or pulmonary angiography is necessary to confirm the diagnosis. Presumptive treatment should be avoided since the complications of systemic anticoagulation are common and potentially fatal. Thrombolytic therapy improves the early hemodynamic parameters in patients with large emboli but has not been shown to improve survival. When medical therapy is contraindicated or fails to prevent recurrent embolization, surgical intervention is necessary.

REFERENCES

1. Virchow R. *Die Cellularpathologie in ihrer Begrudung auf physiologische und pathologische Gewebelehre.* Berlin: A Hirschwald; 1958.
2. Cruveilhier J. *Anatomie Pathologique de Corps Humain.* Paris: JB Bailliere; 1829–1842.
3. Trendelenburg F. Ueber die operative Behandlung der Embolie der Lungenarterie. *Arch Klin Chir.* 1908;86:686.
4. Kirschner M. Ein durch die Trendelenburgsche Operation geheilter Fall von Embolie der Arterien pulmonalis. *Arch Klin Chir.* 1924;133:312.
5. MacLean J. The thromboplastin action of cephalin. *Am J Physiol.* 1916;41:250.
6. Bauer G. The introduction of heparin therapy in cases of early thrombosis. *Circulation.* 1959;19:108.
7. Eicholter P, Schenk WG. Prophylaxis of pulmonary embolism: a new experimental approach with initial results. *Arch Surg.* 1968;97:348.
8. Greenfield LJ, McCurdy JR, Brown PP, et al. A new intracaval filter permitting continued flow and resolution of emboli. *Surgery.* 1973;73:599.
9. Wagner HN, Sabiston DC, Ilio M, et al. Regional pulmonary blood flow in man by radioisotope scanning. *JAMA.* 1964;187:601.
10. Wagner HN, Strauss HW. Radioactive xenon in the differential diagnosis of pulmonary embolism. *Radiology.* 1968;91:1168.
11. Dalen JE, Alpert JS. Natural history of pulmonary embolism. *Prog Cardiovasc Dis.* 1975;17:259.
12. Freidman D, Suyemoto J, Wessler S. Frequency of thromboembolism in man. *N Engl J Med.* 1965;272:1278.
13. Robin E. Overdiagnosis of pulmonary embolism: the emperor may have no clothes. *Ann Intern Med.* 1977;87:775.
14. Alpert JS, Smith R, Carlson J, et al. Mortality in patients treated for pulmonary embolism. *JAMA.* 1976;236:1477.
15. Aaronson DL, Thomas DP. Experimental studies on venous thrombosis: effect of anticoagulants, procoagulants, and vessel contusion. *Thromb Haemost.* 1985;54:866.
16. Thomas DP, Merton RE, Wood RD, et al. The relationship between vessel wall injury and venous thrombosis: an experimental study. *Br J Haematol.* 1985;59:449.
17. Pandolfi M, Isacson S, Nilsson IM. Low fibrinolytic activity in the walls of veins in patients with thrombosis. *Acta Med Scand.* 1969;186:1.
18. Bergsdorf N, Nilsson T, Wallen P. An enzyme-linked immunosorbent assay for determination of tissue plasminogen activator applied to patients with thromboembolic disease. *Thromb Haemost.* 1983;50:740.
19. Bloom AL, Thomas DP. *Hemostasis and Thrombosis.* New York, NY: Churchill Livingstone; 1987:767–777.
20. Horattas MC, Wright DJ, Fenton AH, et al. Changing concepts of deep venous thrombosis of the upper extremity: report of a series and review of the literature. *Surgery.* 1988;104:567.
21. Urokinase Pulmonary Embolism Trial Group. A national cooperative study. *JAMA.* 1970;214:2163.
22. Leeper KV, Popovich J, Adams D, et al. Clinical manifestations of acute pulmonary embolism: Henry Ford Hospital experience, a five year review. *Henry Ford Hosp Med J.* 1988;36:29.
23. Dalen JE, Banas JS, Brooks HL, et al. Resolution rate of acute pulmonary embolism in man. *N Engl J Med.* 1969;280:1194.
24. Hams WH, McKusiek K, Athanasoulis CS, et al. Detection of pulmonary emboli after total hip replacement using serial $C^{15}O_2$ pulmonary scans. *J Bone Joint Surg [Am].* 1984;66A:1388.
25. Murray HW, Ellis EC, Blumenthal DS, et al. Fever and pulmonary embolism. *Am J Med.* 1979;67:232.
26. Moses DC, Silver TM, Bookstein JJ. The complementary roles of chest radiography, lung scanning, and selective pulmonary angiography in the diagnosis of pulmonary embolism. *Circulation.* 1974;49:179.
27. Stein PD. The electrocardiogram in acute pulmonary embolism. *Prog Cardiovasc Dis.* 1975;17:247.
28. Cvitanic O, Marino PL. Improved use of arterial blood gas analysis in suspected pulmonary embolism. *Chest.* 1989;95:48.
29. Biello DR, Mattar AG, McKnight RC, et al. Ventilation-perfusion studies in suspected pulmonary embolism. *AJR Am J Roentgenol.* 1979;133:1033.

30. Kipper MS, Moser KM, Kortman KE, et al: Longterm follow-up of patients with suspected pulmonary embolism and a normal lung scan. *Chest*. 1982;82:411.
31. Alderson PO, Rujanavech N, Secker-Walker RH, et al. The role of ^{133}Xe ventilation studies in the scintigraphic detection of pulmonary embolism. *Radiology*. 1976;120:633.
32. Becker DM, O'Connell MT, Gelbard MA, et al. Diagnostic variability in suspected pulmonary embolism. *South J Med*. 1988;81:998.
33. Menzoian JO, Williams LF. Is pulmonary angiography essential for the diagnosis of acute pulmonary embolism? *Am J Surg*. 1979;137:543.
34. Mills S, Jackson D, Older R, et al. The incidence, etiologies, and avoidance of complications of pulmonary angiography in a large series. *Radiology*. 1980;136:295.
35. Harris WH, Salzman EW, Anthanasoulis CA, et al. Comparison of ^{125}I-fibrinogen count scanning with phlebography for detection of venous thrombi after elective hip surgery. *N Engl J Med*. 1975;292:665–667.
36. Vogel P, Laing FC, Jeffrey RB, et al. Deep venous thrombosis of the lower extremity: US evaluation. *Radiology*. 1987;163:747–751.
37. Appelman PT, DeJong TE, Lampmann LE. Deep venous thrombosis of the legs: US findings. *Radiology*. 1987;163:743–746.
38. Lensing AWA, Pradoni P, Brandjes D, et al. Detection of deep-vein thrombosis by real-time B-mode ultrasonography. *N Engl J Med*. 1989;320:342.
39. Moser KM, LeMoine JR. Is embolic risk conditioned by location of deep venous thrombosis? *Ann Intern Med*. 1981;94:439.
40. Hull RD, Hirsch J, Carter CJ. Diagnostic efficacy of impedance plethysmography for clinically suspected deep-vein thrombosis. *Ann Intern Med*. 1985;102:21.
41. Huisman MV, Buller HR, Ten Cate JW, et al. Serial impedance plethysmography for suspected deep venous thrombosis in outpatients. *N Engl J Med*. 1986;314:823.
42. O'Reilly RA. Anticoagulant, antithrombotic, and thrombolytic drugs. In: Gilman AG, Goodman LS, Rall TW, Murad F, eds. *The Pharmacological Basis of Therapeutics*. New York, NY: Macmillan Publishing Co; 1985:1338.
43. Petitprez P, Simmoneau G, Cerrina J, et al. Effects of a single bolus of urokinase in patients with life-threatening pulmonary emboli: a descriptive trial. *Circulation*. 1974;70:861.
44. Goldhaber SZ, Markis JE, Meyerovitz MF. Acute pulmonary embolism treated with tissue plasminogen activator. *Lancet*. 1986;2:886.
45. Proano M, Frye RL, Johnson CM, et al. Successful treatment of pulmonary embolism and associated mobile right atrial thrombus with use of a central thrombolytic agent. *Mayo Clin Proc*. 1988;63:1185.
46. Goldhaber SZ, Heit J, Sharma GVRK, et al. Randomized controlled trial of recombinant tissue plasminogen activator versus urokinase in the treatment of acute pulmonary embolism. *Lancet*. 1988;2:293.
47. Gray HH, Morgan JM, Paneth M, et al. Pulmonary embolectomy for acute pulmonary embolism: an analysis of 71 cases. *Br Heart J*. 1988;60:196.
48. Mansour M, Chang AE, Sindelar WF. Interruption of the inferior vena cava for the prevention of recurrent pulmonary embolism. *Am J Surg*. 1985;51:375.
49. Roehm J, Johnsrude I, Barth M, et al. The bird's nest inferior vena cava filter: progress report. *Radiology*. 1988;168:745–749.
50. Wolfe WG, Sabiston DC. *Pulmonary Embolism*. Philadelphia, Pa: WB Saunders Co; 1980.
51. Bell WR, Simon TL, DeMets DL. The clinical features of submassive and massive pulmonary emboli. *Am J Med*. 1977;62:355.

74. Respiratory Failure

REBECCA SEIP, MD
MARCUS L. MARTIN, MD

Acute respiratory failure may be considered one of the true life-threatening conditions presenting to the emergency department. The emergency physician must make quick decisions regarding treatment and airway management and have an understanding of basic pulmonary physiology and mechanics. Knowledge of the different types of respiratory failure, the underlying disease processes, and the precipitating events is also essential.

Respiratory failure may be generally classified as hypoxic or hypercapnic, and the relative severity of each parameter depends on the magnitude of the precipitating event and the degree of underlying lung disease. The etiology of hypoxia or hypercapnia is primarily related to ventilation-perfusion abnormalities or hypoventilation. A general knowledge of pulmonary physiology is thus helpful in understanding the different types of respiratory failure.

The basic lung volumes are illustrated in Figure 74-1. Measurements of the volumes and flow rates are important in determining the type of underlying respiratory disease. In obstructive disease, characterized by increased pulmonary resistance, there is reduction in both the FEV_1 (forced expiratory volume in 1 second), FVC (forced vital capacity), and the FEV_1/FVC ratio. Vital capacity during forced expiration is less than during slow expiration due to premature airway closure. Functional residual capacity (FRC) and residual volume (RV) are usually increased secondary to air trapping. Patients with restrictive disease have reduced lung volumes due to limited lung expansion, and the FVC is decreased. Since airway resistance is normal, the FEV_1 is usually not decreased to the same degree; thus, the FEV_1/FVC ratio is normal or elevated. The FRC and RV are usually reduced.[1] A graph of these volumes and flow rates obtained by pulmonary spirometry illustrates the patterns of ventilation in normal individuals and in obstructive and restrictive diseases (Fig. 74-2).

VENTILATION

Ventilation is the movement of air into the alveoli where gas exchange takes place. A portion of the inspired air is not involved in gas exchange. It consists of the air in the conducting airways (anatomic dead space), which is equal to approximately one third of the total ventilation at rest.[2] There is approximately 150 mL of anatomic dead space per 500 mL of tidal volume,[3] which remains unchanged in lung disease. Alveolar dead space ventilation does vary in disease states. This occurs in two clinical situations: (1) The alveolus is not perfused and therefore inspired air cannot participate in gas exchange. (2) The alveolus has excess ventilation in relation to its perfusion.

DISTRIBUTION OF VENTILATION

There is a vertical gradient of intrapleural pressure that is most negative at the lung apex. Thus, at the beginning of inspiration (from residual volume) the transpleural pressure is the greatest at the apex. An increase in inspiratory force

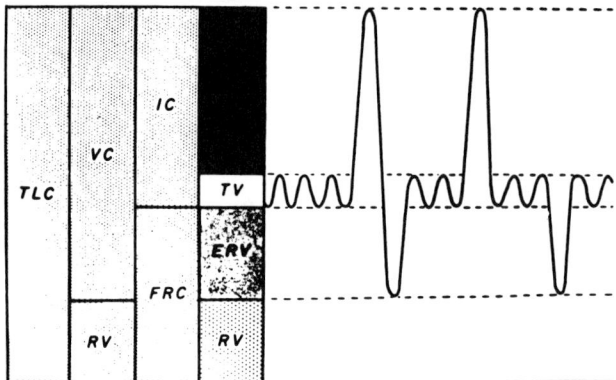

Figure 74-1 Illustration of Lung Volumes. TLC, total lung capacity; VC, vital capacity; RV, residual volume; IC, inspiratory capacity; FRC, functional residual capacity; IRV, inspiratory reserve volume; TV, tidal volume; ERV, expiratory reserve volume. *Source:* Reprinted with permission from Comroe JH et al. *The Lung: Clinical Physiology and Pulmonary Function Tests.* 2nd ed. Chicago, Ill: Mosby-YearBook; 1962.

generates higher transpleural pressure, and before a normal resting volume is reached (FRC), the lower lung zones become better ventilated.[1] Initially, the upper alveoli are more distended and have less capacity to expand while the lower lung alveoli have smaller volumes and are more distensible and compliant. Thus, a greater volume of ventilation is distributed to the lower lung fields. The volume at which the lower alveoli are closed or unventilated is normally less than the FRC. In the aging process and in chronic obstructive pulmonary disease (COPD) the closing volume increases, and closure may occur during normal tidal breathing.[1]

In addition to the vertical gradient of intrapleural pressure, there are other reasons why ventilation is not distributed evenly to all alveoli. The magnitude of the variation depends on the presence and severity of lung disease. Alveolar ventilation is determined by the interaction of resistance and compliance, either of which may vary between alveoli. If alveolar resistance is increased, the time required for the air to flow past the obstruction and completely ventilate the alveolus will increase. So, depending on the inspiratory time, some alveoli may be less well ventilated than others with normal resistance. The inequalities of ventilation are magnified in diseases that increase airway resistance, such as asthma and COPD.[3]

Compliance refers to the distensibility of the alveolus. Alveoli that are easily distensible are more compliant and ventilate more easily than those that are stiff. Compliance is decreased in left ventricular failure, diffuse pulmonary fibrosis, and atelectasis. Compliance is increased in emphysema and old age.[1] In diseases such as emphysema in which the terminal airways are dilated, alveolar dead space increases and effective ventilation decreases.[3]

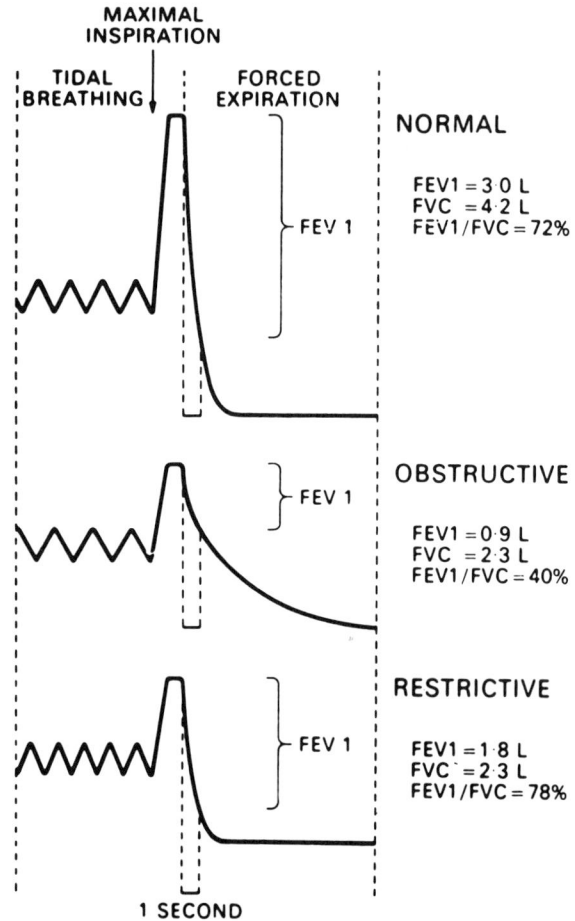

Figure 74-2 Pulmonary function patterns in normal lungs, obstructive disease, and restrictive disease. *Source:* Reprinted with permission from Cole RB. *Essentials of Respiratory Disease.* 2nd ed. Philadelphia, Pa: JB Lippincott Co; 1975.

GAS EXCHANGE

The basic gas exchange unit is the alveolus. The alveoli are lined with a lipoprotein called surfactant that decreases the surface tension, preventing alveolar collapse. Diffusion across the alveolar cell, basement membrane, and endothelial capillary cell usually readily occurs during gas exchange. The gas in the blood entering the alveolar capillaries at rest will equilibrate with the alveolar gas in approximately one third of the time available for exchange. The movement of O_2 across the gradient of high alveolar pressure to low capillary pressure is enhanced by the shape of the oxygen-hemoglobin dissociation curve (Fig. 74-3), ensuring diffusion of most of the O_2 out of the alveoli before the pressures equilibrate. Clinically, limitations of oxygen diffusion may be seen at high altitudes. The lower alveolar oxygen pressure results in a decreased driving pressure between the alveoli and the blood, and the advantage of the shape of the oxygen-hemoglobin dissociation curve is lost. Strenuous

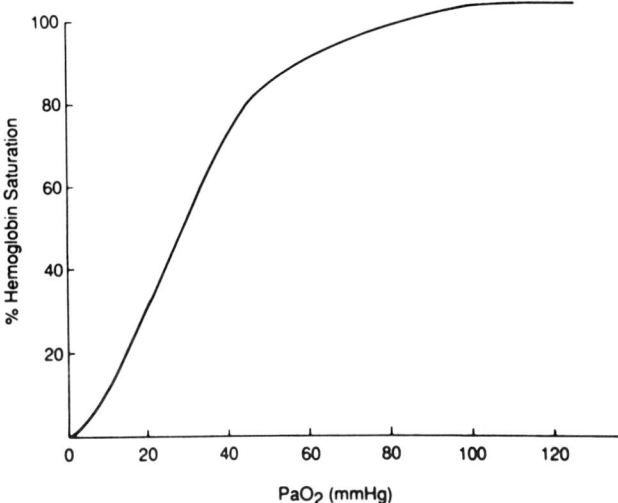

Figure 74-3 Oxygen-hemoglobin dissociation curve.

exercise can exacerbate arterial hypoxemia because of the reduced time the red blood cells spend in the capillary, thus decreasing the time available for diffusion. In diseases in which the alveolar-capillary membrane is thickened (ie, interstitial lung disease), hypoxia at rest is probably not a result of impaired diffusion but is due to co-existing ventilation perfusion abnormalities.[3] However, impaired diffusion across the alveolar capillary membrane may contribute to hypoxemia with exercise.

The rate of diffusion of a gas across a barrier is proportional to the solubility of the gas and inversely proportional to the square root of the molecular weight. Carbon dioxide (CO_2) has a much higher solubility with approximately equivalent molecular weight to O_2; as a result CO_2 diffuses 20 times more rapidly (higher diffusion constant) through tissues than O_2.[4] Despite a significantly smaller diffusion gradient for CO_2 relative to O_2 (5 mm versus 60 mm, respectively), it is generally felt that a clinically significant impairment of CO_2 diffusion is rarely found because of the higher diffusion constant for CO_2.

PERFUSION

The distribution of blood flow in the lung is primarily dependent on hydrostatic pressure variations from top to bottom and the relationship between the pressures of the pulmonary alveoli, arteries, and veins. In general, blood flow increases from the apex to the base.

In the upright position, at the apex of the lung there is no blood flow because the alveolar pressure is greater than the pulmonary artery and venous pressures. In the midlung zones the alveolar pressure is less than the pulmonary arterial pressure but greater than the venous pressure; thus, flow is dependent on the pressure difference between the alveolus and the artery. In the lower lung zones the alveolar pressure is less than both the arterial and the venous pressures, and blood flow is dependent on the arteriovenous pressure difference.

Normal pulmonary arteries are very thin walled with a pulmonary vascular resistance of only one tenth the systemic circulation. Local vascular resistance in the pulmonary bed is in large part a function of surrounding lung volumes. When the lung expands, pulmonary vessels are pulled open, decreasing their vascular resistance.[4]

Pulmonary perfusion may be altered by primary vascular disease or by diseases altering lung parenchymal structure. Blood flow may also be influenced by hypoxia, which causes local vasoconstriction resulting in a diversion of blood to other areas of the lung. A shunt occurs when blood flow effectively bypasses the lung. Normally this occurs with approximately 1% to 2% of the cardiac output.[3] Small amounts of coronary venous blood drain into the left ventricle through the thesbian veins, and some bronchial venous drainage is collected by the pulmonary veins. Abnormally large shunts may occur secondary to congenital right-to-left heart defects, pulmonary arteriovenous anastomoses, or perfusion of unventilated alveoli.

VENTILATION/PERFUSION RATIO

In the normal lung, there are variations in ventilation between individual alveoli and between areas of the lung and similar variations in perfusion. Efficiency of gas exchange depends on the interaction of these two variables known as the ventilation/perfusion (V/Q) ratio. The ratio varies normally between individual alveoli and different areas of the lung due to the previously described variations of its components. The overall V/Q ratio is approximately 1 when the total pulmonary blood flow is 5 L/min and the total alveolar minute ventilation is 5 L. Individual variations have a theoretical range from zero, which indicates perfused, unventilated alveoli, to infinity, which indicates unperfused, ventilated alveoli. In the normal lung most of the ratios vary from 0.6 to 3.0, with an average of approximately 0.85.[3] The V/Q ratios range from a high at the apex toward a lower value at the lung base, where blood flow increases to a greater degree than ventilation.

V/Q mismatch is the most common cause of hypoxia in lung disease.[2] In disease states the normal variations may be magnified, and V/Q inequalities may become very severe. Alveoli with a low V/Q ratio will result in a low blood P_{O_2} concentration and O_2 content. The normal alveoli with a high V/Q ratio, or excess ventilation in relation to perfusion, cannot compensate for alveoli with lower V/Q ratios, due to the shape of the oxyhemoglobin dissociation curve. The hemoglobin molecule is almost fully saturated at a normal P_{O_2}.

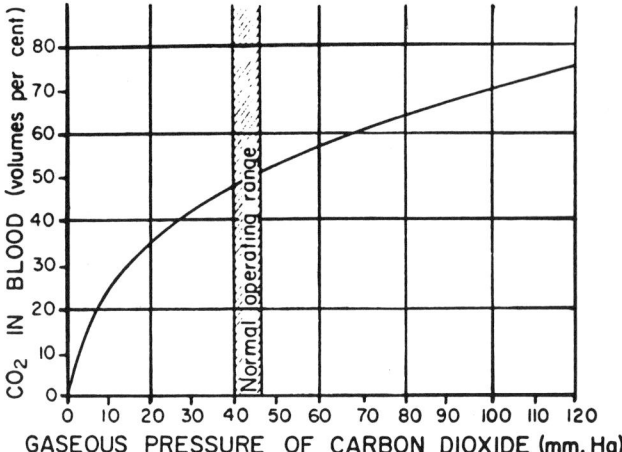

Figure 74-4 Carbon dioxide dissociation curve. *Source:* Reprinted with permission from Guyton AC. *Textbook of Medical Physiology.* 6th ed. Philadelphia, Pa: WB Saunders Co; 1986.

Alveoli with a low V/Q ratio can increase blood P_{CO_2}. However, alveoli with a high V/Q ratio can eliminate excess CO_2 due to the more linear shape of the CO_2 dissociation curve (Fig. 74-4). If the required level of ventilation exceeds the ventilatory reserves of the patient, CO_2 retention may occur.

The alveolar-arterial (A-a) O_2 difference provides an estimate of the V/Q inequality present. An increased A-a gradient ($PA_{O_2} - Pa_{O_2}$) may be the result of either a high or low V/Q ratio. Pure hypoventilation without a V/Q mismatch will have a normal A-a gradient (normal values: age 20, ≤15 mmHg; age 60, 17 ± 11 mmHg). Both V/Q mismatch and a shunt will cause the A-a gradient to increase. PA_{O_2} (alveolar oxygen tension) may be calculated using the following equation.[5,6]

$$PA_{O_2} = PI_{O_2} - \frac{Pa_{CO_2}}{RQ}$$
$$PI_{O_2} = FI_{O_2}(P_B - P_{H_2O})$$
$$= 150 \text{ at sea level on } 21\% \text{ } O_2$$

RQ (respiratory quotient) = 0.8
P_B = barometric pressure (760 mmHg at sea level)
P_{H_2O} = partial pressure of water vapor (47 mmHg)
PI_{O_2} = inspired oxygen tension

V/Q Mismatch

With age there is an increase in ventilation-perfusion mismatching. In diseases such as asthma, COPD, or interstitial fibrosis, low V/Q ratios may result from structural changes of the airways, obstruction, or bronchospasm. A pulmonary embolism causes V/Q mismatching by underperfusion of involved alveoli (high V/Q ratio) and overperfusion of normal areas of the lung (low V/Q ratio).[6]

Shunt

A shunt may reflect an extreme end of the V/Q ratio scale in which the value is zero, meaning ventilation is absent but perfusion is present. In other less extreme cases of low V/Q mismatch, some ventilation is still present. Abnormal shunts in the lung may occur in pulmonary edema, pneumonia, or atelectasis when the alveoli are collapsed or filled with fluid or exudate. Hypoxia may be present and is poorly responsive to oxygen therapy. Supplemental O_2 reaching the normally ventilated portions of the lung cannot compensate for the hypoxia. In contrast, O_2 therapy will usually improve the P_{O_2} to a much greater degree in the presence of V/Q mismatch than in the presence of a shunt. Hypercapnia is rare and may be found only in very large shunts (greater than 50%). However, even in this situation, hypoxia will stimulate hyperventilation, usually keeping the blood P_{CO_2} low.[6]

CONTROL OF VENTILATION

Ventilation is controlled by several chemoreceptors. The peripheral chemoreceptors include the carotid and aortic bodies. The carotid bodies account for most of the ventilatory response to hypoxia and for approximately 30% of the response to hypercapnia. The central chemoreceptors account for most of the response to hypercapnia.[2]

Feedback about the state of the respiratory system is obtained from the intercostals, abdominal musculature, and the diaphragm. Within the lung are various types of receptors that also provide feedback. The stretch receptor is located within the smooth muscle of the proximal and distal airways. Those in the distal airways help regulate the length of inspiration and expiration. Rapidly adapting or irritant receptors are located largely in the proximal airways. They mainly respond during inflation and to the rate of airflow. A decrease in compliance causes an increased response. Bronchial chemoreceptors located in the bronchi respond to substances released during asthma or inflammation and to inhaled irritants resulting in tachypnea, increased secretions, and bronchoconstriction. The J-receptors or juxtacapillary receptors located in the pulmonary interstitium respond to pulmonary congestion. They may produce the pulmonary chemoreflex of apnea, bradycardia, and hypotension.[2]

The overall ventilatory response is controlled by central neural mechanisms in the brain. Central control can be modified by input from the peripheral chemoreceptors, the musculature, and the pulmonary receptors. Central nervous system lesions, trauma, and many drugs can alter central control of respiration. Depression of respiration secondary to severe hypercapnia may occur. In hypercapnic COPD patients, caution must be used with O_2 therapy since the hypoxic drive can be eliminated. However, more recent evidence indicates that the hyperoxia-induced hypercapnia may not be solely due to a depression of the hypoxic drive but may be related to an increased impairment of gas exchange.[7-9]

MUSCULATURE

During inspiration the muscles of the upper airway contract, thus dilating the upper airways. The posterior cricoarytenoid muscle dilates the laryngeal aperture. Other upper airway passages are dilated with stimulation of the alae nasi (nasal dilator), the genioglossus (protrussor muscle of the tongue), and muscles inserting on the hyoid.[2]

During normal breathing the diaphragm is the muscle accounting for the majority of air movement during inspiration. As ventilation rises the intercostal muscles are increasingly activated, and subsequently muscles such as the scalenes and the sternocleidomastoids are recruited. With hyperinflation of the lungs the diaphragm becomes less effective because its fibers are shorter, thus developing less force during contraction, and the advantageous mechanical interactions between the costal and crural parts of the diaphragm are lost.

Expiration occurs mainly due to the elastic recoil of the lungs and the chest wall. During high ventilatory activity or with airway obstruction, the abdominal muscles are utilized, including the internal and external obliques and the transverse and rectus abdominus.

During normal breathing in the supine position, abdominal displacement is more prominent than rib displacement. If the opposite occurs, this could indicate diaphragmatic fatigue or paralysis or increased work of breathing. Respiratory alternans, an alternating pattern of abdominal and rib cage breathing, also indicates inspiratory muscle fatigue. Muscle fatigue with resulting hypercapnia may develop when the work of breathing is increased, as seen with an increased minute ventilation, increased airway resistance, or decreased compliance. Another predisposing factor is a decreased energy supply, which may occur with hypoxia or low cardiac output. Hyperinflation also leads to decreased respiratory efficiency.

Electrolyte imbalances such as hypokalemia or hypophosphatemia can affect muscle function.[2] Neuromuscular disorders or collagen vascular diseases may cause muscle weakness. In patients with chronic disease, a precipitating event such as pneumonia or an increase in airway obstruction may cause an increased work load, with resulting muscle fatigue and hypercapnia.

RESPIRATORY FAILURE

Criteria for Failure

Acute respiratory failure is defined by several parameters. It must develop over a short period (minutes to several days) and is characterized by an inability to adequately oxygenate the blood or remove CO_2. Thus, respiratory failure may be divided into two general groups—hypoxic and hypercapnic.

Arterial blood gases may be used to establish criteria for failure, but the patient's prior blood gas values and the degree of actual change must be taken into account. Hypoxic failure is generally considered to be present when the P_{O_2} is less than 50 mmHg. Below this value hemoglobin oxygen saturation can decrease sharply due to the shape of the oxyhemoglobin dissociation curve. Hypercapnic failure is generally considered to be present when the P_{CO_2} is greater than 50 mmHg.[5] Accompanying this may be a significant respiratory acidosis.

In addition to blood gas evaluation, the diagnosis of acute failure is based on the patient's history and clinical exam. The precipitating events as well as the history of underlying medical illnesses must be elicited. Clinical signs and symptoms are attributable to the acute event (fever and abnormal sputum in a COPD patient with pneumonia or cholinergic signs in a patient with organophosphate poisoning), the chronic underlying disease, and the resulting hypoxia, hypercapnia, or acidosis.

Hypoxia can be clinically manifested in various ways. Cyanosis may be present, although its recognition depends on skin pigmentation, lighting, and hemoglobin levels. Since the degree of cyanosis depends on the amount of reduced hemoglobin, its detection may be difficult in anemic patients. Central nervous system (CNS) symptoms may include restlessness, agitation, confusion, stupor, seizures, and coma. Circulatory effects include initial tachycardia with later arrhythmias and hypotension.

Hypercapnia may cause headache and progressive CNS depression. Cerebral vasodilation and increased intracranial pressure may be present, resulting in cerebral edema and papilledema. A fine tremor of the hands and face or asterixis may occur.[10]

Pulse oximetry and capnography are valuable methods that may be utilized to monitor a patient. However, tissue hypoperfusion may affect the accuracy of pulse oximetry, and, due to the shape of the oxyhemoglobin dissociation curve, large changes in P_{O_2} may occur before being reflected in the saturation values. Capnography measures the carbon dioxide concentration of expired air. This may be used to confirm endotracheal tube placement or to evaluate the arterial P_{CO_2}. The CO_2 value obtained by capnography does not accurately reflect the Pa_{CO_2} when decreased pulmonary (alveolar) perfusion is present.[11]

Etiology of Failure

Hypoxic Failure

Hypoxia is caused primarily by V/Q abnormalities and shunts but also by hypoventilation. Etiologies of hypoxic failure include adult respiratory distress syndrome, pulmonary edema, pulmonary infection, or pulmonary embolus. In addition, tissue hypoxia can occur despite a normal Pao_2. This may be secondary to decreased oxygen carrying capacity (ie, carbon monoxide poisoning or anemia), shock, or interference with oxygen utilization at the tissue level (ie, cyanide poisoning).

Collapsed or fluid-filled airways cause hypoxia via a shunt mechanism. There is no ventilation but blood flow continues, and the A-a gradient increases. In larger shunts there is minimal or only modest response to oxygen therapy even with high concentrations of inspired O_2.[2] Increasing ventilation to the normal lung cannot compensate for the low Po_2 caused by the injured lung due to the shape of the oxyhemoglobin dissociation curve. As a result of the relatively linear shape of the CO_2 elimination curve, increased ventilation to the normal lung can compensate for increases in CO_2, and hypercapnia is not usually a problem. However, if the work of breathing to eliminate CO_2 becomes too high, hypercapnic failure may supervene. In the fluid-filled lung, compliance decreases and the FRC is reduced.[5] Positive end-expiratory pressure helps to increase FRC and may open closed airways.[10]

Hypercapnic Failure

Hypercapnia is caused primarily by hypoventilation and is seen in cases of V/Q mismatch when the work of breathing is increased, resulting in increased energy demands, CO_2 production, and muscle fatigue. Hypercapnic failure may occur in two clinical categories. The first category is patients with no underlying lung disease. Ventilatory abnormalities are primarily due to alveolar hypoventilation. CO_2 retention occurs, as does corresponding hypoxia.[12] The alveolar Po_2 and subsequently the arterial Po_2 decrease, but the A-a gradient is normal. This group includes patients with CNS depression due to trauma or intracerebral disease (ie, tumors, strokes). Many drugs will also cause respiratory depression. More common among these are the anesthetics, opiates, and barbiturates. Toxins such as botulism or the organophosphates may also cause respiratory failure by affecting the respiratory muscles. Status epilepticus and tetanus cause prolonged muscle spasms, which interfere with ventilation. Various neuromuscular disorders that may also affect the respiratory musculature include spinal cord lesions, poliomyelitis, Guillain-Barré syndrome, amyotrophic lateral sclerosis, myasthenia gravis, and the muscular dystrophies. Other etiologies include chest trauma, obesity, and chest wall deformities.

Kyphoscoliosis usually does not cause respiratory compromise until the degree is very severe. The scoliotic component is the more significant determinant. A decrease in lung and primarily chest wall compliance is seen with an increase in the work of breathing. Total lung capacity (TLC) and FRC are decreased. To compensate, a rapid, shallow breathing pattern develops with increased dead space ventilation and alveolar hypoventilation. In ankylosing spondylitis compliance of the chest wall is decreased but respiratory failure is rare. In obesity the chest wall compliance is decreased and the work of breathing is increased. The vital capacity (VC), TLC, FRC, expiratory reserve volume (ERV), and tidal volume are reduced.[2]

Neuromuscular disorders causing respiratory failure affect both the inspiratory and expiratory muscles. Inspiratory capacity, TLC, VC, and ERV are all decreased. Without expiratory muscle function the effectiveness of a cough is limited. The loss of the sigh mechanism and inadequate cough may predispose to atelectasis and further V/Q mismatch.[2]

The second category in which hypercapnic failure occurs is in patients with underlying lung disease. The degree of hypoxia is greater due to V/Q abnormalities. This category includes asthma and COPD.[12] Acute exacerbations may be precipitated by multiple events. The most common of these is infection with bronchitis or pneumonia. The etiologic agent may be viral or bacterial (commonly *Streptococcus pneumonia* or *haemophilus* influenza). Analgesics, sedatives, anesthesia, or abdominal surgery can precipitate acute failure. Other inciting factors include pneumothoraxes or pulmonary emboli.

In this category the hypoxic component of failure is prominent, with varying degrees of hypercapnia. In asthma, hypercapnia is not usually present until late in the course of an exacerbation, while in COPD a chronic hypercapnia may be present with a tendency toward elevations of CO_2 earlier in the course of an exacerbation. The occurrence of bronchial smooth muscle constriction, mucosal edema, and hypersecretion in the asthmatic results in increased airway obstruction and resistance, reduced expiratory flow rates, and hyperinflation. The A-a O_2 gradient may be widened but, in contrast to a pure shunt, relatively small increases in FiO_2 will improve patient oxygenation. With increased work of breathing and subsequent muscle fatigue, hypercapnic failure may intervene. As this is generally a late occurrence in asthma, mechanical ventilation should be considered at this point.

In an acute exacerbation of COPD there is an increase in the V/Q mismatching. The breathing pattern changes, becoming more shallow and rapid. The inspiratory time is shorter with reduced tidal volumes. The respiratory frequency increases, keeping the minute ventilation stable, but there is an increased component of dead space ventilation that results in a decrease in alveolar ventilation.[12] Forceful expiration may cause airway collapse.[1] Chronic hypoxia and hypercapnia are worsened. Hyperinflation and increased airway resistance leading to an increased work load and muscle fatigue may precipitate further CO_2 retention. The A-a O_2 gradient may be widened here also but again responds to small increases in FiO_2.

Management

When a patient presents in acute respiratory failure, the precipitating event must be elicited and specific treatment begun. This might include bronchodilators for asthma or diuretics for pulmonary edema. Clinical assessment of the patient's respiratory status must be initiated immediately. A decision must be made whether to intubate the patient or whether treatment specific for the disease process may be instituted first.

The first goal of treatment is to secure an adequate airway. If the patient is severely hypoventilating or apneic, then tracheal intubation should be performed. However, in a narcotics overdose patient, prompt administration of naloxone may eliminate that need. If the patient has no immediate airway problem, then attention may be directed toward the underlying disease process.

Correction of arterial hypoxia is of primary importance. Assuming that hemoglobin levels and cardiac output are adequate, tissue oxygenation should be improved with the correction of arterial hypoxia. Treatment of the underlying disease process should be initiated. If there is no clinical improvement or if clinical deterioration occurs, then tracheal intubation and mechanical ventilation should be considered. Aside from the obvious situation in which the patient has a severely compromised airway, the exact point at which to initiate mechanical ventilation may not be clear. The patient's clinical appearance may dictate early tracheal intubation (ie, mental status changes, inability to cooperate with the treatment, exhaustion requiring use of accessory muscles, or paradoxic breathing). If the hypoxia, hypercapnia, or respiratory acidosis is extremely severe and cannot be improved or deteriorates with initial treatments, then mechanical ventilation is indicated. In general, the arterial Po_2 should be above 60 to keep the O_2 saturation greater than 90%[2] and the arterial pH should be greater than 7.20. Additional parameters for initiating tracheal intubation may include a respiratory rate > 35/min, VC < 15 mL/kg, FEV_1 < 10 mL/kg, and an inspiratory force of < 25 cmH$_2$O.[13]

CONCLUSION

The emergency physician plays an important role in the diagnosis and treatment of acute respiratory failure. An understanding of pulmonary physiology and the basic categories of respiratory failure is important to deliver appropriate care. Prompt treatment should be initiated based on the identified precipitating events and the underlying disorder. Frequent clinical assessments and pulmonary monitoring (ie, arterial blood gases, pulse oximetry, capnography) must be performed. The emergency physician should then determine whether the patient is responding to treatment or whether tracheal intubation and mechanical ventilation are necessary.

REFERENCES

1. Braunwald E, Isselbacher KJ, Petersdorf RG, Wilson JD, Martin JB, Fanui AS, eds. *Harrison's Principles of Internal Medicine*. 11th ed. New York, NY: McGraw-Hill Book Co; 1987.
2. Fishman AP, ed. *Pulmonary Diseases and Disorders*. 2nd ed. New York, NY: McGraw-Hill Book Co; 1988.
3. Cole RB. *Essentials of Respiratory Disease*. 2nd ed. Philadelphia, Pa: JB Lippincott Co; 1975.
4. West JB. *Respiratory Physiology—the Essentials*. 3rd ed. Baltimore, Md: Williams & Wilkins Co; 1985.
5. Bordow RA, Stool EW, Moser KM, eds. *Manual of Clinical Problems in Pulmonary Medicine with Annotated Key References*. Boston, Mass: Little, Brown & Co; 1980.
6. Danzaker DR, ed. *Cardiopulmonary Critical Care*. Orlando, Fla: Grune & Stratton; 1986.
7. Aubier M, Murciano D, Fournier M, Milic-Emili J, Pariente R, Derenne JP. Central respiratory drive in acute respiratory failure of patients with chronic obstructive pulmonary disease. *Am Rev Respir Dis*. 1980;122:191–199.
8. Aubier M, Murciano D, Fournier M, Milic-Emili J, Pariente R, Derenne JP. Effects of administration of O_2 on ventilation and blood gases in patients with chronic obstructive pulmonary disease during acute respiratory failure. *Am Rev Respir Dis*. 1980;122:747–754.
9. Sassoon CS, Hassell KT, Mahutte CK. Hyperoxic-induced hypercapnia in stable chronic obstructive pulmonary disease. *Am Rev Respir Dis*. 1987;135:907–911.
10. Sykes MC, McNicol MW, Campbell EJM. *Respiratory Failure*. 2nd ed. Oxford, England: Blackwell Scientific Publications; 1976.
11. Timerding BL. Cardiopulmonary monitoring and sudden death. *Topics in Emergency Medicine*. 1989;11(2):14–15.
12. Guenter CA, Welch MH, eds. *Pulmonary Medicine*. 2nd ed. Philadelphia, Pa: JB Lippincott Co; 1982.
13. Pontoppidan H, Geffin B, Lowenstein E. Acute respiratory failure in the adult. *N Engl J Med*. 1972;278:743–752.

75. Miscellaneous Respiratory Emergencies

FRED HARCHELROAD, MD, FACEP, ABMT
DIETRICH JEHLE, MD, FACEP

The majority of respiratory emergencies confronted in the emergency department have been reviewed in the preceding chapters. This chapter will focus on some of the less frequent but nevertheless intriguing respiratory diseases that confront the emergency physician. Despite the low occurrence of these entities, their rapid diagnosis and treatment are as essentially life giving as that of the more common respiratory emergencies.

INHALATION EXPOSURES

Inhalation of pollutants, whether they be gases, liquid droplets, or solid particles, is inescapable as our respirable air is replete with these by-products of our culture.[1,2] Varying parts of the respiratory tract may be directly affected by the size of the inhaled particles, or the entire body may react to the inhaled pollutants if they are not filtered by the respiratory system. Though the final deposition of particles within the respiratory tract depends on size, shape, surface area, hygroscopicity, electrical change, and density,[3] the easiest categorization is by size. The upper airway will filter particles larger than 2 μm; particles between 0.05 μm and 1 μm will be retained by the alveoli; gases will be absorbed through the pulmonary parenchyma (unless they react during transport through the parenchyma), while particles less than 0.05 μm will likely be exhaled. The movement of a gas from air into tissue involves several processes: ventilation, diffusion, and solubility. As ventilation brings the gas inside the respiratory tract, those gases that are very soluble in water will be absorbed in the wet oropharynx and trachea. Gases that are not trapped in this manner will be drawn deeper into the alveoli, where they may diffuse across the alveoli along their concentration gradients.[4]

Inhalation exposures may be divided into three main categories: primary pollutants, secondary pollutants, and hazardous pollutants.[5] Primary pollutants such as carbon monoxide, sulfur oxides, or nitrogen oxides are biologically active compounds whose effects are unchanged by interaction in the air. Secondary pollutants, such as ozone or formaldehyde, require conversion to their active form by elements in the air. Hazardous pollutants, such as asbestos, mercury, or vinyl chloride, are seriously toxic pollutants for which the U.S. government considers no safe threshold to exist.[5] A basic understanding of the chemical properties of these inhalation exposures helps guide the knowledge of the pathophysiology in the subsequent treatment of them.

Carbon Monoxide

Carbon monoxide (CO) is a colorless, odorless, tasteless, nonirritating gas that binds sufficiently well to the heme proteins such as hemoglobin, myoglobin, reduced cytochrome oxidase, reduced cytochromes of the P_{450} type, and tryptophan dioxygenase to inhibit their function.[6] The relative contribution of each of these inhibitions to the clinical scenario of CO inhalation is uncertain. Indeed, it has been proposed that CO could exert some of its toxic effects by adsorbing onto solid surfaces[7] or by causing lipid peroxidation.[8,9]

The mechanism of carbon monoxide binding to hemoglobin was first elucidated by Claude Bernard in 1857[10] and subsequently formalized by the Haldanes in 1895.[11] The Haldane equation

$$\frac{[COHb]}{[HbO_2]} = M \frac{[P_{CO}]}{[P_{O_2}]}$$

formalized by Douglas and the Haldanes in 1912,[12] quantitatively defines the competition between oxygen and carbon monoxide for the same ferrous heme-binding sites on hemoglobin. The affinity constant, M, has the value of 245 at a pH of 7.4. Therefore, if the $P_{CO} = 1/245$ (P_{O_2}), then the blood at equilibrium will be half-saturated with oxygen and half-saturated with carbon monoxide. The affinity constant of carbon monoxide for myoglobin is only 40. As can be seen from Table 75-1, exposure to very low concentrations of CO may lead to high levels of carboxyhemoglobin (COHb), as well as significant clinical signs and symptoms. It should be remembered that these signs and symptoms are very variable, depending on the baseline condition of the person exposed.

Though only 33 deaths secondary to carbon monoxide exposure were reported to the American Association of Poison Control Centers in 1991,[13] an estimated 4,000 deaths per year are caused by carbon monoxide inhalation[14] and 10,000 people per year seek medical attention for this exposure.

Sources of carbon monoxide include the endogenous production from metabolism of the α-methane carbon atom in the protoporphyrin ring during hemoglobin catabolism (which accounts for a blood carboxyhemoglobin level of 0.4% to 0.7%[15]); hemolytic anemias may raise the COHb level to 4% to 8%. Carbon monoxide is produced in vivo during the metabolism of methylene chloride (CH_2Cl_2), a constituent of paint and varnish removers and some degreasing agents. Levels of carboxyhemoglobin following exposure to methylene chloride have been reported as high as 50%.[16]

Though tobacco smokers have chronically elevated COHb levels (up to 9% COHb),[17] even passive inhalation of carbon monoxide occurs when nonsmokers are in the presence of smokers.[18,19] Any source of incomplete combustion will produce carbon monoxide (Table 75-2).

Though carbon monoxide normally appears in the atmosphere at a concentration of less than 0.001% (10 ppm), the threshold limit value is currently set at 35 ppm for an 8-hour work day.[5] Just as the lungs rapidly absorb carbon monoxide, so it is that it is eliminated exclusively through the lungs. The half-life of carboxyhemoglobin is 3 to 4 hours if breathing room air.[20] This is decreased to approximately 40 minutes if ventilation occurs with 100% oxygen and to about 20 minutes with hyperbaric oxygen (100% O_2 at 2.5 atmosphere pressure).

CO toxicity results from tissue hypoxia. This hypoxia occurs not only because CO replaces O_2 in the hemoglobin molecule, but also because it impairs the release of O_2 from Hb to the tissues (shift of oxyhemoglobin dissociation curve to the left). Binding of CO to myocardial myoglobin results in myocardial depression and further tissue ischemia. In vitro, CO binds to cytochrome oxidase, possibly further contributing to tissue hypoxia.[21,22] Pathophysiologically, carbon monoxide affects those organ systems most prone to hypoxia: the cardiovascular and central nervous systems. Within the central nervous system (CNS) one may see edema, perivascular infarct, petechia, and focal necrosis. Bilateral necrosis of the globus pallidus is considered a characteristic CNS lesion following severe CO intoxication. The most severely affected areas are those with the greatest sensitivity to hypoxia: hippocampus, cerebral cortex, substantia nigra, and cerebellum.[23,24] Because of its high oxygen requirements the heart is extremely vulnerable to CO poisoning. Ischemia and patchy myocardial necrosis are commonly seen in patients with pre-existing coronary artery disease and exposure to CO.

The degree of symptoms and tissue hypoxia depends not only on the length and concentration of exposure, but also on

Table 75-1 Symptoms Associated with Varying Levels of Carbon Monoxide Poisoning*

CO in Atmosphere, %	COHb in Blood	Physiological and Subjective Symptoms
0.007	10	No appreciable effect, except shortness of breath on vigorous exertion; possible tightness across the forehead; dilation of cutaneous blood vessels
0.012	20	Shortness of breath on moderate exertion; occasional headache with throbbing in temples
0.022	30	Headache; irritable; easily fatigued; judgment disturbed; possible dizziness; dimness of vision
0.035–0.052	40–50	Headache, confusion; collapse; fainting on exertion
0.080–0.122	60–70	Unconsciousness; intermittent convulsions; respiratory failure, death if exposure is long continued
0.195	80	Rapidly fatal

*Signs and symptoms vary with length of exposure and underlying medical conditions.

Source: Adapted from Winter PM, Miller JN. Carbon monoxide poisoning. *JAMA*. 1976;236:1503. With permission.

Table 75-2 Exogenous Sources of Carbon Monoxide

Automobile exhaust	Charcoal grills
Cigarette smoke	Hibachis
Kerosene, gas, coal heaters	Fire
	Methylene chloride

the metabolic activity during this exposure and the premorbid physical condition of the patient being exposed. For these reasons it is difficult to standardize any correlation between carboxyhemoglobin levels and signs/symptoms. Furthermore, the neuropsychiatric effects are subtle and may not be elicited during a cursory physical exam performed in a busy emergency department.[25,26] The diagnosis of carbon monoxide intoxication is not difficult to make in the comatose person pulled from a garage with the car turned on but no gas in the tank and an arterial blood gas showing a Po_2 of 300 mmHg on 100% O_2 but an O_2 saturation of only 55%. The difficulties arise in the more subtle cases. The effects of carbon monoxide intoxication often mimic other diseases,[27,28] especially in patients presenting with flu-like symptoms (headache, nausea, general malaise) or in children with gastroenteritis.[29] The acute effects on the CNS may present as headache, lethargy, dizziness, agitation, confusion, seizures, or coma. The chronic and delayed effects of CO exposures in the CNS may include apraxia, memory loss, concentration deficits, personality changes, mutism, or parkinsonism.[25,26,30-32] A latent period up to 2 weeks may occur between apparent recovery and the onset of these delayed effects. The acute effects of CO on the cardiovascular system depend on the existence of prior cardiovascular disease. Increased angina may occur with COHb levels as low as 5% to 10%.[33] Hypotension as a result of direct myocardial depression will occur even in healthy subjects. Furthermore, chronic low-level exposure may accelerate atherosclerosis.[5,34]

Carboxyhemoglobin levels (arterial or venous) are used to document exposure and estimate severity. It is imperative to remember that clinical features correlate only roughly with COHb levels. Arterial blood gases will measure a normal Po_2; however a measured percent oxygen saturation will be decreased from that expected (ie, calculated for a given Po_2). Sulfhemoglobinemia and methemoglobinemia also will produce a low measured percent oxygen saturation for a given Po_2. Though hydrogen sulfide may interfere with measurement of COHb, methemoglobinemia will not cause interference. Metabolic acidosis reflects the ischemia and hypoxia of CO poisoning.

Treatment of patients exposed to carbon monoxide consists of supplemental oxygen and evaluation of end-organ damage (ie, heart and CNS). As noted earlier, hyperbaric oxygen (HBO) may decrease the half-life of COHb by a factor of 10 or more. However, the exact role of HBO in the treatment of carbon monoxide intoxication remains controversial.[7,23,26,35-37] Immediate removal from the contaminated environment, control of airway, support of breathing with ventilation, 100% O_2, and the institution of intravenous lines and cardiac monitoring are the initial priorities.[5] The decision to use HBO must be made with regard to the patient's clinical presentation, COHb level, and knowledge of the potential benefits and complications of HBO therapy. The Diving Accident Network at Duke University Medical Center provides a 24-hour hotline (919-684-8111) for the location of hyperbaric oxygen chambers in the United States. HBO therapy should be considered for patients with evidence of severe carbon monoxide poisoning.

1. Any patient with a history of unconsciousness secondary to CO exposure
2. Any symptomatic patient with a COHb level over 25%
3. Any patient with detectable neurologic impairment following CO exposure
4. Any pregnant patient when the COHb level is greater than 15% or if fetal monitoring demonstrates evidence of distress

Other Inhalational Agents

Though carbon monoxide is perhaps the most frequently encountered toxic inhalation exposure, numerous other inhalational agents elicit symptoms for which people present to the emergency department.

Hydrogen sulfide is a heavier-than-air gas with a pungent "rotten eggs" odor detectable at only 0.2 to 0.3 ppm. Mainly found from the decay of organic sulfur-containing products (fish, sewage, manure), it is present occupationally in viscous rayon, silk, and paper mills and in rubber vulcanizing.[38] Hydrogen sulfide, similar to cyanide, inhibits the cytochrome oxidase system.[39] Though respiratory tract and eye irritation are common at levels of 150 to 300 ppm, olfactory paralysis develops at these same levels, and patients may succumb from the resultant anaerobic metabolism without noting any further odor. Acutely, prolonged exposure to high doses affects the CNS: coma, dizziness, nausea, headache, weakness, and seizures.[40] Cardiac signs/symptoms are those expected for any hypoxic insult: arrhythmias and myocardial depression. Treatment includes elimination from further exposure, adequate oxygenation, intravenous sodium nitrite (adult dosage, 300 mg) to produce sulfmethemoglobin, and observation for the development of pulmonary edema.

Metal fume fever (Monday morning fever, zinc shakes, Brazier's disease) is a self-limiting, flu-like illness (chills, high fever, headache, cough, retrosternal chest pain, dyspnea, weakness, and leukocytosis) often preceded by thirst and metallic gustatory sensations that occur 4 to 8 hours after inhalation exposure to metal oxides.[41] Oxides of aluminum, antimony, arsenic, cadmium, cobalt, copper, iron, lead, magnesium, manganese, mercury, nickel, selenium, silver, tin, and zinc have all been reported to produce these symptoms.[42] The exact pathophysiology remains unclear, but both an immunologic mechanism and direct release of endogenous pyrogens have been hypothesized.[42,43] Though initial pulmonary function tests may indicate reduced lung volumes, small airway obstruction, and lowered carbon monoxide diffusing capacity, these abnormalities return to normal within several months.[44] Exposure to the pyrolysis

Table 75-3 Occupational Alveolar and Airway Disease

Source	Workers Affected	Source	Workers Affected
Microbes		**Animals**	
Bacteria		*Ascaris lumbricoides*	Zoologists
Aerobactor cloaceae	Air conditioner, humidifier	Ascidiacea	Oyster culture
Phialophora sp.		Dander	Farmers, fur workers, grooms
Escherichia coli endotoxin	Mill fever—textile workers	Feathers	Turkey and chicken farmers
Pseudomonas sp.	Sewer workers	Insect chitin	
Fungi	Farmer's lung group	*Sitophilus granarius*	Flour
Aspergillus sp.,		Mayfly	Outdoorsmen
Micropolyspora faeni	Farmers	Screwfly	Screw-worm controllers
Aspergillus clavatus	Malt workers	Pancreatic enzymes	Preparation workers
Cladosporium sp.	Combine operators	Rat serum-urine	Laboratory workers
Verticillium sp.		**Chemicals**	
Alternaria sp.		Inorganic	
Micropolyspora faeni		Calcium hydroxide/	Cement workers
Penicillium casei		tricalcium silicate	
Penicillium frequentans		Chromium	Casters
Thermoactinomyces		Vanadium pentoxide	Refinery workers
(*vulgaris*) *sacchari*		Nickel sulfate	Platers
Amoeba		Platinum chloroplatinate	Photographers
Acathamoeba castellani	Air conditioning and humidifier	Tungsten carbide (cobalt)	Hard metal workers
Acathamoeba polyphaga		hard metal	
Naegleria gruberi		Zinc, copper, magnesium fumes	Welders, bronze (metal fume fever)
Plants		Copper sulfate and lime	Vineyard sprayers
Castor bean—ricin	Oil mill	Organic	
Coffee bean	Roasters	Aminoethyl ethanolamine	Solderers
Cotton, hemp, flax, jute, kapok	Textile workers	Chlorinated biphenyls	Transformer manufacturers
Flour dust	Millers	Colophony (pine resin)	Solderers
Grain dust	Farmers	Diisocyanates-toluene, diphenylmethane	Production workers
Gum arabic, gum	Printers	Formalin	Permapress, urethane foam
Papain	Preparation workers	Paraquat	Sprayers
Proteolytic enzymes, *Bacillus subtilus* (subtilus alcalase)	Detergent workers	Penicillin, ampicillin	Production workers, nurses
		Parathion	Sprayers
Tamarind seed powder	Weavers	*p*-Phenylenediame	Solderers
Wood dust—Canadian red cedar, South African boxwood, rosewood (*Dalbergia* sp.)		Piperazine	Chemists
		Polymer fumes (polytetrafluoroethylene)	Teflon manufacture, use
		Synthetic fibers—nylon, polyesters, dacron	Textile workers
		Vinyl chloride (phosgene) (hydrogen chloride)	Meat wrappers (asthma) Firefighters Polymerization plant

Source: Adapted from Last JM. *Maxcy-Roseman: Public Health and Preventive Medicine*. 11th ed. New York, NY: Appleton-Century-Crofts; 1980:620–621.

products of fluorocarbon polymer (Teflon) and fluorinated polyethylene propylene has resulted in the same symptom complex, termed polymer fume fever. Treatment includes recognition of the etiology, assuring adequate oxygenation (supplemental oxygen, sympathomimetic bronchodilators), and observation for the development of hemorrhagic tracheobronchitis or pulmonary edema. Most patients do not require admission to the hospital. As some metals are directly toxic to the lung parenchyma, differentiation between the self-limiting metal fume fever and the initial presentation of a chronic heavy metal pneumonitis may be difficult.

Numerous substances may be inhaled as a consequence of occupational exposure[45,46] (Appendix 75-A). The pulmonary response to these agents may be that of occupational asthma,[47,48] extrinsic allergic alveolitis[49] (Table 75-3), bronchitis[50] (Table 75-4), pneumoconiosis[51] (Table 75-5), or neoplastic disease.[3,52–54] The acute presentation may be that of pleuritic chest pain, dyspnea, noncardiogenic pulmonary edema, hemoptysis, or wheezing. Initial treatment

Table 75-4 Agents That Cause Chronic Bronchitis

Gases	Particles
Aldehydes (acrolein, formaldehyde)	Cement dust
Ammonia	Chromium
Chlorine	Coal mine dust (bronchitis, emphysema)
Chloromethyl methyl ether	Coke oven
Osmium tetroxide	Cotton dust
Phosgene	Diesel exhaust
Toluene diisocyanate	Endotoxin
Vinyl chloride monomer (probable)	Grain dust (wheat, barley)
Oxides of nitrogen (probable)	Pottery dust
	Sodium hydroxide
	Brick dust (probable)
	Cadmium (probable)
	Cobalt (probable)
	Paraquat
	Polychlorinated biphenyls (probable)
	Tungsten carbide (probable)
	Vanadium (probable)
	Western red cedar
	Wood dust

Source: Adapted from Last JM, ed. *Maxcy-Roseman: Public Health and Preventive Medicine*. 11th ed. New York, NY: Appleton-Century-Crofts; 1980:631. With permission.

includes preventing further exposure, maintaining the airway, and assuring adequate oxygenation. Most often, these patients present with an acute exacerbation of a chronic pulmonary disorder. In either case, obtaining a good history is essential, as is assuring timely and appropriate follow-up care.

Smoke

The incomplete combustion of any material may lead to the formation of a large variety of inorganic and organic gases, liquids, and solids. As a suspension of solid or liquid particles in a gas medium (ie, an aerosol), smoke has many different components that can injure the respiratory tract at different places and by different mechanisms. The most common form of smoke inhalation injury is a chemical tracheobronchitis caused by the numerous chemical irritants in smoke.[55] The exact type and severity of injuries are determined by the chemical composition of the smoke, the extent of exposure, and the premorbid condition of the patient. The composition of smoke depends on the type of combustible fuel, the oxygen that is available, and the temperature of the fire.[56] A patient with smoke inhalation may be poisoned with numerous substances that vary with local fire conditions. From a practical point of view, the emergency physician is often confronted with a victim of smoke inhalation with no precise knowledge of the inhaled substance.[57]

Pulmonary injury may be secondary to chemical or thermal injury. Heated, dry air may damage the upper airway; however, because it has a low heat capacity it rarely affects the pulmonary parenchyma. Alternatively, inhaled steam may damage the entire respiratory system.[58] Chemical products may be divided into local irritants or systemic poisons (Table 75-6).

Although soot particles are essentially nontoxic, they produce effects in several ways: (1) They decrease phagocytic action of pulmonary macrophages and overwhelm the mucociliary clearing mechanism, and (2) irritant chemicals may adsorb to the particles. Thus, the particles serve as a carrier to deliver the more noxious agents. The final result is a tracheobronchitis and pulmonary edema.[62] This leads to two types of problems: local pulmonary compromise or systemic hypoxemia.

When inhalation injury and cutaneous burn occur concomitantly, patient mortality is substantial, ranging from 33.7% to 56%.[60,63] However, isolated injury from smoke inhalation, in the majority of cases, results in a self-limited process with less, though still significant, mortality.[64,65]

In actual practice it is impossible to predict which poisons a patient may have inhaled. Any exposure in an enclosed space requires a high index of suspicion for occult pulmonary injury. Loss of consciousness indicates a greater risk of morbidity and mortality from CO and CN poisoning and thus a need for aggressive treatment. There are no uniform criteria for making the diagnosis of smoke inhalation. Any alteration in sensorium is suggestive of hypoxemia that may be secondary to direct asphyxiation or CO poisoning.[57] Facial burns, singed nasal hair, or carbonaceous deposits in the nares or oropharynx suggest underlying pulmonary injury, although their presence or absence cannot be considered a reliable indicator. Stridor, hoarseness, or difficulty with phonation suggests upper airway injury/edema and a need for careful, direct visualization with flexible fiberoptic laryngoscopy.[66-68] Cough, dyspnea, cyanosis, and, on chest auscultation, the presence of rales, wheezes, or rhonchi within 4 to 6 hours following exposure are indicators of poor prognosis.[65,69] The presence of carbonaceous sputum may not be seen for 12 to 24 hours after exposure and may be present in only 40% of those patients with significant pulmonary exposures.[69] Furthermore, its presence does not always indicate clinically significant injury.[66]

Emergency physicians must realize the limitation of the laboratory evaluation of the smoke inhalation victim. Chest radiography is often unremarkable early in the course of smoke injury, yet marked changes (patchy atelectasis and pulmonary edema) will be noticeable 24 hours later. Arterial blood gases (with a carboxyhemoglobin level) may demonstrate hypoxemia associated with respiratory alkalosis.

Table 75-5 Pneumoconiosis: Pathologic and Physiologic Changes

Agent	Type of Pathology	Type of Respiratory Impairment
Silica		
Simple	Nodular fibrosis	Restrictive, diffusion
Complicated	Conglomerate nodular fibrosis	Restrictive, obstructive, diffusion
Hematite	Nodular fibrosis	Restrictive, diffusion
Mixed dusts, iron and silica	Nodular fibrosis (rarely, conglomerate nodular fibrosis)	Restrictive, diffusion
Silicates	Nodular fibrosis (rarely, conglomerate nodular fibrosis)	Restrictive, obstructive
Talc		
Kaolin		
Bentonite		
Diatomite		
Tripoli		
Fuller's earth		
Mica		
Sillimanite		
Cement	Nonspecific bronchitis	Obstructive
Coal		
Simple	Peribronchiolar macules, focal emphysema	Obstructive (small airways)
Complicated	Conglomerate nodular fibrosis	Obstructive, restrictive, diffusion
Graphite	Peribronchiolar macules, focal emphysema	Obstructive (small airways)
Aluminum	Interstitial fibrosis	Restrictive, diffusion
Asbestos	Interstitial fibrosis	Restrictive, diffusion
Beryllium	Interstitial fibrosis (granulomata)	Restrictive, diffusion
Tungsten carbide	Interstitial fibrosis	Restrictive, diffusion
Barium	Simple dust accumulation	None known
Cerium	Simple dust accumulation	None known
Iron	Simple dust accumulation	None known
Tin	Simple dust accumulation	None known
Titanium	Simple dust accumulation	None known

Source: Adapted from Key MM, Henschel AF, Butler J, et al, eds. Occupational Diseases: A Guide to Their Recognition. Washington, DC: US Department of Health, Education and Welfare, US Government Printing Office; 1977:119.

Indeed, hypoxemia and a widened alveolar-arterial (A-a) gradient may be the most reliable indicators of pulmonary injury.[70] Bronchoscopy, although limited by its physical size in assessing distal parenchymal injury, has been used.[67] While xenon scanning[67,71] plus bronchoscopy have increased sensitivity for documenting pulmonary abnormalities, they are not specific for predicting pulmonary dysfunction (25% to 50% of patients with abnormal findings will not develop significant respiratory complications)[57,71] and are not readily available in all emergency departments. Though spirometry may be helpful in the diagnostic work-up

Table 75-6 Common Chemical Products in Smoke

Systemic Poisons	Primary Local Irritants	
CO[59]	Acrolein, aldehydes[60,61]	Hydrochloric acid[59]
CN	Phosgene, isocyanates	Ammonia, nitrogen oxides
HS	Aromatic hydrocarbons	Sulfur oxide

and in assessing therapy for bronchospasm, its usefulness is limited by the need for patient cooperation.[72]

Acute management of smoke inhalation is largely supportive. Airway control during the early postexposure period is focused on the potential of thermal injury.[57] Laryngeal edema develops within the first 2 to 8 hours postexposure,[73] whereas alveolar injuries manifest themselves after 12 to 92 hours.[71] Some evidence suggests that more than the local thermal and chemical irritation from smoke inhalation is responsible for the pathophysiologic changes noted. The white blood cell modulation and degranulation that occur in this injury give rise to phagocyte-generated toxic species that secondarily cause endothelial damage.[60,74] Secondary damage may be exacerbated if the patient is hypovolemic.[75] Supplemental oxygen is the rule in any suspected inhalation injury and must be monitored to maintain adequate arterial oxygenation. Bronchodilator therapy is used as needed for the management of bronchospasm secondary to the acute injury. The use of glucocorticosteroids or prophylactic antibiotics is not recommended at present.[56,76] Any evidence of

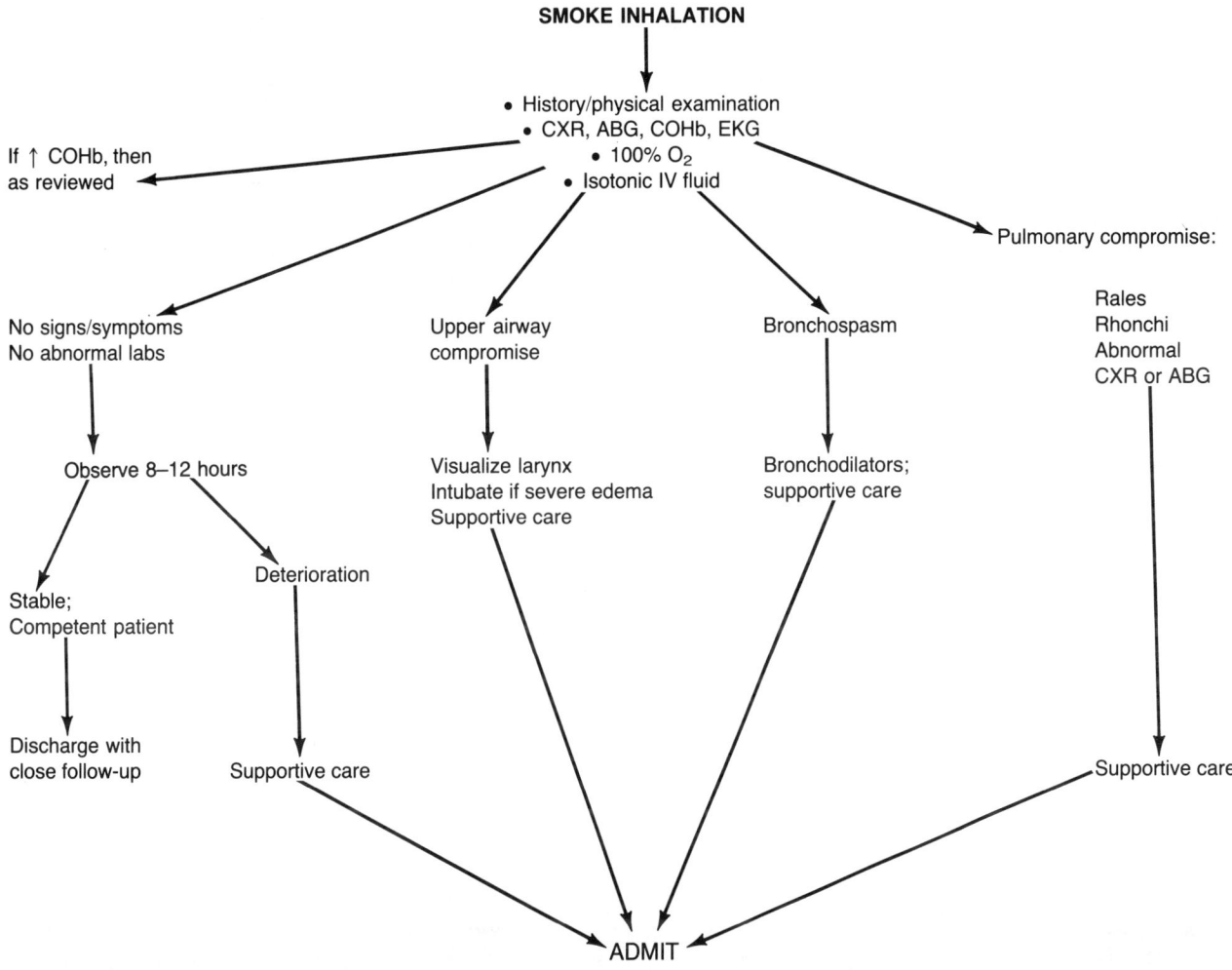

Figure 75-1 Treatment Algorithm for Smoke Inhalation

carbon monoxide intoxication should be treated as previously discussed.

No widely accepted guidelines for admission are known, although conservative management is the best course to follow (Fig. 75-1). Realization that symptoms may not develop for 12 hours implies prolonged observation in the emergency department or explicit and well-understood follow-up instructions for the competent patient to return at the first sign of symptoms.

Aspiration

Aspiration is defined as the presence of any nongaseous material in the tracheobronchial tree. As such it is an inhalational injury and is a common problem for the emergency physician. The pathologic sequelae of pulmonary aspiration are multifactorial and depend on the pH and viscosity of the aspirate, the volume and particulate nature of the material, the bacterial content of the aspirate, and the length of time the aspirate remains in contact with the lung parenchyma.[77-81]

The clinical consequences of pulmonary aspiration of gastric contents were first described in 1946 by Mendelson.[77] Mendelson's syndrome, or toxic aspiration pneumonitis, is synonymous with aspiration of stomach contents with a pH of less than 2.5. However, many of the pathologic sequelae of aspiration are nonspecific and occur regardless of the pH. Significant ventilation-perfusion mismatch and hypoxia occur within seconds as alveoli collapse, airways reflexively close, and interstitial edema develops. Shunting may be extensive and pulmonary compliance will also decrease. The alveolocapillary bed may leak enough fluid to require volume depletion. True bacterial infection is apparent in 3 to 4 days. Whereas hospitalized patients who aspirate most frequently develop infections with gram-negative aerobes (*Pseudomonas, Proteus,* and *E. coli*), community-acquired aspiration pneumonia commonly is secondary to anaerobic bacteria.[80,82]

Multiple factors predispose patients to aspirate (Table 75-7). The most common situations in the emergency department are those in which there is an altered level of

Table 75-7 Common Predisposing Factors in Aspiration-induced Lung Diseases

Altered level of consciousness	Childhood
Drugs	Overfeeding
Metabolic/infectious coma	Ambulating with material in mouth
General anesthesia	
Cerebral vascular accident/tumor	
Trauma	
Seizures	
Gastrointestinal diseases	**Structural**
Gastroesophageal reflux	Tracheostomy
Incompetent swallowing mechanism	Esophageal cancer/stricture
Esophageal cancer	Gastric/small bowel obstruction
Esophageal dysmotility	Bronchogenic carcinoma
Diverticular disease of hypopharynx/esophagus	
Meconium-stained amniotic fluid	
Factors that increase anaerobic mouth flora	**Neurologic/neuromuscular disease**
Gingivitis	Guillain-Barré syndrome
	Multiple sclerosis
	Botulism
	Myasthenia gravis
	Polymyositis
Iatrogenic	
Esophageal obturator airway	
Gastric lavage	
Feeding tubes	
Small volume-high pressure endotracheal tubes	
Forced supine immobilization	

consciousness, whether it is secondary to trauma, drug ingestion, or cerebral vascular accident. The immediate danger of aspiration is complete mechanical obstruction of the tracheobronchial tree, and the emergency physician must be prepared to clear and secure the airway (removal of foreign debris and tracheal intubation) if this occurs. However, prevention of aspiration is the standard to be achieved. Aspiration of bacteria-contaminated fluid may occur in healthy persons during sleep, and a high index of suspicion must be maintained to diagnose this problem.

Dyspnea, tachypnea, tachycardia, cyanosis (evidence of hypoxemia), bronchospasm, frothy sputum, or hypotension may accompany aspiration. Physical examination of the chest may reveal rales, rhonchi, or wheezes. Although the clinical picture may be that of pulmonary edema, left ventricular function is normal and hemodynamic monitoring often demonstrates normal or low right-sided pressures and a high cardiac index. Arterial blood gases will show marked hypoxia with a respiratory alkalosis unless the patient has developed respiratory failure, in which case a combined respiratory and metabolic acidosis will be noted. Radiograph of the chest may show either a diffuse alveolar or interstitial infiltrate or a segmental or lobar infiltrate. Either of these patterns may progress to a widespread pattern of adult respiratory distress syndrome (ARDS). The lower lobe of the right lung is most frequently involved, unless the patient was in the Trendelenburg position when the aspiration occurred. In this instance, infiltrates most likely occur in the axillary segment of the right upper lobe or the apical segment of the right lower lobe.

In the patient at high risk of aspiration, any modality should be used to prevent this occurrence, ranging from placing the patient in a head-down, left lateral decubitus position to tracheal intubation. In the patient who has already aspirated, priorities are to secure the airway and provide adequate oxygenation. This includes positive end-expiratory pressure (PEEP) when oxygenation cannot otherwise be maintained. Massive amounts of particulate matter should be removed by bronchoscopy. Any remaining stomach contents should then be removed by nasogastric tube. Bronchospasm may be treated with sympathomimetic, atropine-like, or corticosteriod aerosols and aminophylline. In severe cases (ie, those requiring tracheal intubation), fluid requirements are best managed by Swan-Ganz catheter measurements. Neither intravenous steroids nor antibiotics are recommended initially.[78,83-85] Bacterial pleuropulmonary infection may develop in 26% to 50% of patients following aspiration of gastric contents.[85] Useful clues indicating the subsequent development of such infection requiring antimicrobial treatment include increasing temperature; new or enlarging pulmonary infiltrates 36 to 48 hours after aspiration; increasing leukocytosis; purulent sputum; and appropriately collected positive cultures and gram-stained material indicating infection.[84,85]

The mortality in patients who aspirate gastric contents has been reported to be as high as 30% to 60%;[78,85,86] however, this is due to the combination of the underlying disease that caused the aspiration with the aspiration itself. More recent studies have shown that the death rate directly attributable to aspiration is close to 10%.[87] Mortality from aspiration is directly related to the extent of pulmonary infiltrate on radiographic exam,[78] the subsequent development of bacterial pleuropulmonary infection,[78,86] and the degree of oxygen transfer dysfunction as measured by the A-a oxygen gradient.[78,87,88] The prevention of aspiration pneumonitis is the most important consideration in the management of patients at risk.

Proper management of any vaginal delivery, but especially the emergent delivery, is to make all attempts to prevent meconium aspiration. A severe chemical pneumonitis may result from meconium aspiration, and this is a significant threat to 20% of the infants born through meconium-stained amniotic fluid. Management includes clearing the nose and pharynx with a bulb syringe after delivery of the head but prior to delivery of the shoulders. If the amniotic fluid is meconium-stained, then the trachea must be suctioned until clear, with an endotracheal tube. Ideally, this should be performed prior to any inspiratory effort, as well as before positive-pressure ventilation is utilized.[89-91]

HEMOPTYSIS

Hemoptysis is a symptom and sign of numerous pathologic processes.[92,93] Such a wide range of diseases necessitates a focused approach on the few likely causes in each clinical setting. Massive hemoptysis requires immediate attention to protect the airway, while nonmassive hemoptysis offers a broad differential diagnosis and time for further evaluation and treatment. We shall deal only with the nontraumatic causes of hemoptysis in this short review.

Massive hemoptysis most commonly refers to expectoration of at least 600 mL of blood in 24 hours;[94,95] however, this accounts for fewer than 5% of the cases referred to chest specialists.[96] The major immediate morbidity from massive hemoptysis is airway obstruction and asphyxiation, though exsanguination has been reported.[97] Most cases of massive hemoptysis are caused by tuberculosis, bronchiectasis, lung abscess (especially aspergillomas[98]), or bronchogenic carcinoma.

Nonmassive hemoptysis may be caused by the same disease processes that cause massive hemoptysis, as well as a whole host of others. Differentiation of the etiology of hemoptysis based on the quantity or quality of blood is neither sensitive nor specific. Also, it is difficult for patients to estimate volumes of blood produced. Table 75-8 lists some of the more common etiologies. Infection is the most common cause of hemoptysis worldwide,[94,99] while bronchitis (viral or bacterial) is the most common infectious cause of nonmassive hemoptysis.[100] The most common organisms that cause hemoptysis include *Staphylococcus*, *Klebsiella*, *Pseudomonas*, and *Aspergillus*.[101] Cancer is considered to be the second most common cause of hemoptysis in all patients, with bronchogenic carcinoma the most common diagnosis. Bronchogenic carcinoma is considered the most common cause of hemoptysis in patients over the age of 40 years.[96]

The first consideration when evaluating a patient who presents with hemoptysis is to determine that the blood is not originating from the nasopharynx or the gastrointestinal tract. Blood from the airway is usually bright red mixed with frothy alkaline sputum, but gastrointestinal blood is usually dark red or black and mixed with food particles and acidic gastric juices. Concomitant emesis while coughing may confuse this standard scenario. Patients who are asymptomatic upon their arrival in the emergency department are more difficult to assess; however, studies to exclude hematemesis (ie, gastric lavage, stool guaiac) are often definitive.

Historic information should be directed toward diseases causing hemoptysis. A smoker over the age of 40 years with a greater than 1-week history of hemoptysis is a likely candidate for carcinoma,[93] while a previously healthy, nonsmoking 20-year-old with acute onset, fever, malaise, and blood-tinged purulent sputum is more likely to be suffering from pneumonia. Pain and dyspnea are common complaints in patients with pulmonary embolism or pneumonia. Concomitant hematuria may suggest Goodpasture's syndrome, *Legionella* pneumonia, or a coagulopathy.[96] Though nasal and sinus pain or bleeding may occur in Wegener's granulomatosis, it is far more common for this to be secondary to upper respiratory tract infection. Parasitic disease as a cause of hemoptysis is extremely rare in the United States; however, this etiology should be considered in those traveling to Third World countries. A pleural lesion (pulmonary infarct, lung abscess, or vasculitis) should be suspected in a patient with pleuritic chest pain, pleural friction rub, and hemoptysis.[93]

Assessment of airway, breathing, and circulation is the most useful function of the physical examination in patients with hemoptysis. Wheezing localized over one lung segment suggests focal obstruction (foreign body, tumor, abscess). Crackles localized to one or both apices are considered pathognomonic of pulmonary tuberculosis.[96] The remainder of the physical examination may provide clues to other less common causes. Oral candidiasis and diffuse lymphadenopathy may suggest infection with the human immunodeficiency virus, while localized adenopathy to the supraclavicular region may suggest cancer. Clubbing of the digits is associated with both chronic lung disease and cancer. Diffuse petechia or ecchymoses give clues that an underlying coagulopathy may be contributing to the hemoptysis.

Laboratory evaluation of all patients with hemoptysis should include chest radiograph and sputum Gram's and acid-fast stain. Other laboratory tests should be guided by the

Table 75-8 Partial Differential Diagnosis of Nontraumatic Hemoptysis

Inflammatory	Neoplastic
Tuberculosis	Bronchogenic carcinoma
Bronchiectasis	Bronchial adenoma
Abscess	
Pneumonia (esp. *Klebsiella*)	
Bronchitis	
Toxic inhalation	

Vascular	Hemorrhagic
Mitral stenosis	Anticoagulant therapy
Left ventricular failure	Hemorrhagic diathesis
Pulmonary thromboembolism	
Pulmonary hypertension	
Arteriovenous malformation	
Pulmonary vasculitis	**Other**
Amyloidosis	Cystic fibrosis
Idiopathic pulmonary hemosiderosis	Foreign body
Eisenmenger's syndrome	Misdiagnosis (ie, nasopharyngeal or gastrointestinal bleeding)

clinical presentation and the findings on chest radiography and sputum examination. Complete blood and platelet count, prothrombin time, and partial thromboplastin time are widely recommended; however, unsuspected coagulopathies are exceedingly rare and these studies may be superfluous for most patients.[96,102] Continuous oximetric measurement of hemoglobin-oxygen saturation is helpful in those patients with massive bleeding, respiratory insufficiency, or the need for surgical intervention to control the bleeding.

Fiberoptic bronchoscopy is a safe and accurate aid to the diagnosis of hemoptysis.[103,104] The timing of bronchoscopy is controversial. Urgent bronchoscopy is more likely to visualize the active bleeding site; however, the diagnostic yield and outcome in patients with nonmassive hemoptysis are not worsened by a delayed (within 24 hours of presentation) procedure.[105] Early bronchoscopy is recommended for those with massive bleeding, respiratory distress, or intracavitary aspergillomas.[95]

Radioisotopic ventilation-perfusion scanning is useful as a diagnostic aid when the clinical presentation suggests a pulmonary embolism. Pulmonary arteriography is the definitive follow-up study.

As with all acutely ill patients the initial approach must be prioritized by the severity of the patient's condition. Patients with massive hemoptysis need emergent radiologic and hematologic evaluation, volume resuscitation, sedation, and both bronchoscopic and surgical evaluation after control of airway and breathing[95,96] (Fig. 75-2). Both rigid and fiberoptic bronchoscopes have utility. The rigid bronchoscope has greater suctioning capability and maintenance of airway control; unfortunately, visualization of the upper lobes is impossible, overall visual range is reduced, and general anesthesia is needed for the rigid bronchoscope. Both types of bronchoscopes allow the passage of Fogarty catheters to tamponade the bleeding segments.[95] The double-lumen Carlen-type endotracheal tube is best placed after the bleeding lung has been identified; however, its use is controversial, especially as the experience with fiberoptic bronchoscopes improves.[95] After the bleeding site is identified, the patient should be placed with the bleeding lung in the dependent position. This decreases the risk of aspiration into the uninvolved lung.

The surgical mortality in patients with massive hemoptysis ranges from 0% to 33%, whereas mortality in the absence of resection ranges from 18% to 85%.[95–97,106] Pre-

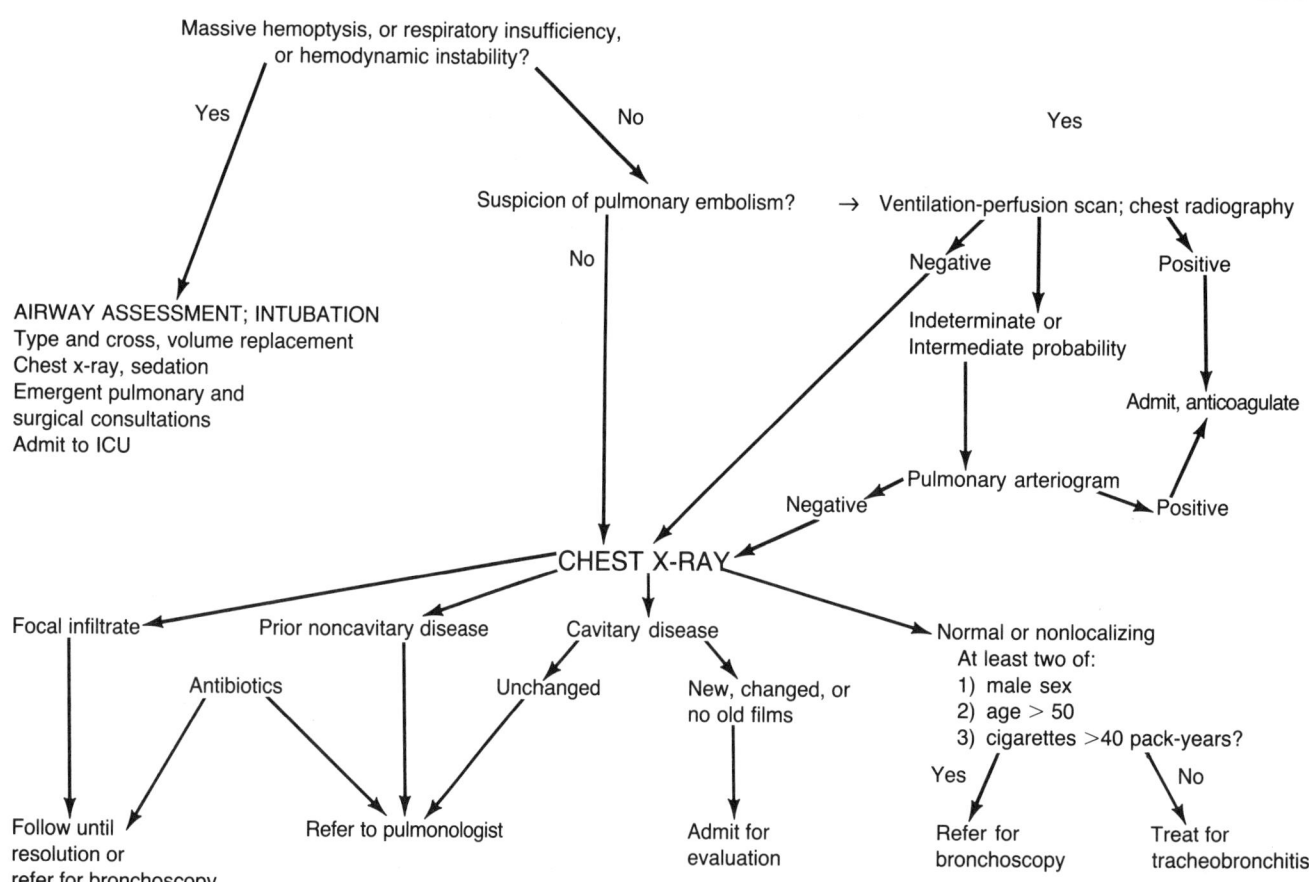

Figure 75-2 Summary Algorithm for Hemoptysis. *Source*: Adapted from Goldman JM. Hemoptysis: emergency assessment and management. *Emerg Med Clin North Am*. 1989;7:336. With permission.

dictors of those patients who will survive massive hemoptysis without surgical intervention are unknown. More recently, experience with embolotherapy suggests that bronchial artery and pulmonary artery embolization and topical thrombin via fiberoptic bronchoscopy may provide adjuncts to surgical resection and its concomitant mortality.[95,107,108]

PLEURAL EFFUSION

The abnormal accumulation of fluid in the pleural space is termed pleural effusion. Under normal conditions there are 5 to 10 mL of clear, alkaline (pH 7.6) fluid in the space between the parietal and visceral pleura. This fluid, which is an ultrafiltrate of plasma, moves from the higher-pressure systemic vessels of the parietal pleura to the lower-pressure visceral circulation, where it is absorbed. There is a net pressure of approximately 10 cmH$_2$O between the parietal and visceral pleural circulations.

Numerous disorders may cause pleural effusions (Table 75-9). These effusions classically are divided into two groups: transudates and exudates. Transudates result from either an increase in hydrostatic pressure or a decrease in plasma colloid osmotic pressure. They are filtrates of plasma containing very little protein. Exudates occur when inflammation or other changes of the pleural surface cause increased capillary permeability or lymphatic obstruction. As such, they contain high amounts of protein. On analysis, any of the three following criteria define an exudative pleural effusion: (1) ratio of pleural fluid lactate dehydrogenase (LDH) to serum LDH greater than 0.6; (2) ratio of pleural fluid protein to serum protein greater than 0.5; and (3) pleural fluid LDH greater than 200 IU/mL.[109,110]

Patients with pleural effusion typically are symptomatic. If the disease process remains localized to the lungs, symptoms often consist of cough, dyspnea, or chest pain.[111] These symptoms will develop as the volume of the effusion reaches 500 mL.[112] However, as many pathologic entities that cause pleural effusions are not localized to the lungs, presenting signs and symptoms are often related to the underlying disease.[113] Asymptomatic pleural effusions do occur, and indeed the spectrum of causes for these is similar to that for symptomatic patients.[114] Pleural effusions secondary to congestive heart failure are seen more commonly in the right hemithorax than in the left.

Physical examination findings are variable but often include decreased breath sounds on the affected side; dullness to percussion and decreased tactile fremitus over the fluid collection; egophany at the superior edge of the effusion; and a pleural rub auscultated throughout respiration but greatest at end inspiration.

A chest radiograph should confirm the clinical suspicion of a pleural effusion. Blunting of the costophrenic angle on an upright posteroanterior (PA) view is observable after 250 mL of fluid collect.[115] A lateral decubitus radiograph with the affected side down helps to confirm the diagnosis and exclude the possibility of a loculated effusion. These views may also be helpful to confirm the presence of small subpulmonic effusions, where the only radiographic findings on a PA chest film may be elevation of the hemidiaphragm or an increase in water density between the apparent lung margin and the gastric air bubble.

A thoracentesis is indicated for all new effusions of uncertain etiology, effusions causing respiratory compromise, and malignant effusions requiring sclerotherapy or antineoplastic treatment. A clinically significant bleeding diathesis is the one contraindication to immediate thoracentesis. For routine thoracentesis performed via the posterior approach, the needle should be inserted immediately superior to the rib margin. This helps prevent damage to the neurovascular bundle. Other complications associated with thoracentesis are perforation of the lung with resultant pneumothorax, re-expansion pulmonary edema resulting in severe hypoxemia, and hepatic or splenic puncture.

If the etiology of the pleural effusion is in question, then the fluid must be sent for laboratory analysis. Analysis should include blood cell count with differential, total protein, glucose, LDH, pH, amylase, cytology, Gram's and acid-fast stain, and cultures for aerobic, anaerobic, and fungal organisms.[109,110,115–118] A red cell count greater than 100,000 cells/mL is seen with malignancy, trauma, or pulmonary embolus. The ratio of pleural fluid glucose to serum glucose normally exceeds 0.5. Lower levels are seen in tuberculosis, empyema, malignancy, and rheumatoid dis-

Table 75-9 Common Causes of Pleural Effusions

Transudates

Congestive heart failure	Cirrhosis with ascites
Nephrotic syndrome	Hypoproteinemia
Acute glomerulonephritis	Myxedema
Acute atelectasis	Peritoneal dialysis
Meigs' syndrome	Superior vena caval obstruction
Sarcoidosis	

Exudates

Tuberculosis	Systemic lupus erythematosus
Lung abscess	Rheumatoid pleuritis
Fungal illness	Sarcoidosis
Parasitic infections	Lymphatic diseases
Bacterial pneumonia	Postradiation
Viral illness	Dressler's syndrome
Rickettsia	Pulmonary infarction
Meigs' syndrome	Chronic atelectasis
Pancreatitis	Uremia
Subphrenic and hepatic abscess	Chylothorax
Whipple's disease	
Esophageal rupture	
Diaphragmatic hernia	
Drug reaction (nitrofurantoin, methysergide, practolol)	

eases. Pleural fluid amylase exceeding 160 somogyi units/dL is associated with pancreatitis, pancreatic pseudocyst, and esophageal rupture. Any purulent effusion (empyema) with a pH less than 7.0 should be treated with chest tube drainage.[118]

Most patients with pleural effusions do not need admission to the hospital for the effusion, but for treatment of their underlying disease. Those with recurrent dyspnea despite thoracentesis, massive effusions, or rapid reaccumulation of fluid may require hospitalization.[115]

EMBOLIC PHENOMENA

Air Embolism

Both venous and arterial air emboli may result in significant morbidity or sudden death. Air entering a central or systemic vein may occur in numerous circumstances: venous cannulation undertaken to supply therapeutic drugs,[119] trauma to any large venous structure[120] (but especially the thorax, neck, or groin), air insufflation to the female genital tract,[121] or surgical procedures, especially in the cranium.[122] It has been suggested that PEEP may decrease the likelihood of venous air emboli occurring during surgical procedures.[123] The morbidity or mortality from venous air emboli results as air bubbles travel from the systemic veins to the right atrium, to the right ventricle, and into the pulmonary arteries. As pulmonary blood flow decreases, pulmonary arterial pressure rises and systemic arterial pressure falls. Adult patients who receive large volumes of air into their venous circulation (greater than 300 mL)[124,125] likely present in severe shock or cardiorespiratory arrest. Those who receive small volumes of air into the venous circulation may present with chest pain, cough, cyanosis, or the "millwheel murmur" (blood flow against air bubbles in the right ventricular outflow tract).[125]

Significant morbidity from arterial air emboli may occur from only 1 mL of air entering the pulmonary veins. Possible scenarios for this include thoracic trauma, surgery, pneumothorax, laser bronchoscopy, positive-pressure ventilation in a neonate, thoracentesis, or dysbaric air embolism from a diving accident.[126–130] As air is ejected from the left ventricle it may pass to the coronary arteries, resulting in cardiac ischemia; to the cerebral arteries, causing a neurologic deficit; or to any systemic arterial bed, with resultant tissue damage. Both immediate and delayed symptoms may occur in these patients and will depend on the vascular bed affected. Dysbaric air embolism (DAE) results from gas bubbles entering the systemic circulation through ruptured pulmonary veins.[131] DAE usually presents immediately after the diver reaches the surface. The brain is by far the most commonly affected organ. The neurologic manifestations are those of any acute stroke syndrome, with asymmetric multiplegias being the most common presentation.

Shock unresponsive to resuscitation, sudden loss of consciousness, seizures, or confusion in a clinical setting conducive to an air/open artery interface are common manifestations of arterial air emboli. These signs may worsen when positive-pressure ventilation is instituted. Other uncommon clinical findings may include air bubbles in the retinal arteries, sharply circumscribed glossal pallor (Liebermeister's sign), or marbling of the skin due to embolization of cutaneous vessels.[126]

The overall mortality may be 50%;[132] however, this will vary with the etiology of air emboli. Recognition of this rare entity is of major importance. Immediate management includes the usual resuscitative measures for shock, as well as placing the patient in the head-down, left lateral decubitus position (Durant's maneuver).[125] This gives the greatest chance for the venous air emboli to float into the right ventricle and away from the right ventricular outflow tract. This allows either gradual dispersal of the large air collection into smaller bubbles, which may be better tolerated by the pulmonary vasculature and parenchyma, or aspiration of the air via a central venous catheter.[122] The pulmonary consequences of venous air embolism occurring during surgery have been reported to be resolved with papaverine.[133] Surgical control of the source may be needed.

If an arterial air embolism is suspected, then the patient should be placed in the Trendelenburg position to allow the emboli to move away from the cerebral and coronary circulation. After the source of the embolic phenomena is controlled, hyperbaric oxygen treatment for recompression may be beneficial, especially for dysbaric injuries,[128,134,135] though it also has been reported beneficial for iatrogenic air embolism.[136] Also, heparin anticoagulation has been advocated for both venous and arterial air embolism to reduce the coincident thromboembolic phenomena, at least when it is not contraindicated by severe trauma.

Fat Embolism

The most common clinical setting in which fat embolism is encountered is that of trauma, with fractures of the long bones, ribs, or pelvis.[137] It also has been described in patients with dysbaric illness, diabetes mellitus, sickle cell disease, chronic alcoholism, and hemorrhagic pancreatitis,[138] as well as in a patient receiving intravenous cyclosporin (believed to be secondary to the drug's excipient).[139] The clinical syndrome of fat emboli occurs whenever fat droplets large enough to occlude capillaries appear in the circulation. The incidence of clinical fat embolism has been reported as 22%[140] in multiple trauma patients; however, autopsy studies have revealed pathologic evidence of fat embolism in 95% of multiple trauma patients.

The clinical findings include hyperthermia, respiratory distress, petechia, retinal fat emboli, and mental status changes. As fat emboli are trapped in the lungs, right atrial and pulmonary artery pressures increase, resulting in signs and symptoms of acute cor pulmonale and ARDS. Thrombocytopenia is a frequent sequela, as the fat droplets stimulate platelet aggregation. Release of vasoactive amines from the platelets and decreased surfactant production from the damaged pneumocytes result in further bronchospasm and hypoxia. Pulmonary embarrassment may be the only evidence of fat emboli in up to 75% of patients who have fat emboli.

Laboratory studies that may help confirm the clinical diagnosis include chest radiograph (patchy infiltrates or diffuse capillary leak), electrocardiogram (right heart strain), elevated serum lipase, decreased platelet count, increased pulmonary artery pressure and pulmonary vascular resistance,[141] and decreased Po_2 on arterial blood gas determination. Alterations in end-tidal CO_2 have not been noted to occur in the presence of fat and marrow emboli.

Prevention and treatment of fat embolism include rapid fixation of fractures[137] and support of hypoxic respiratory insult. Signs and symptoms may occur at any time after the trauma; however, the clinical syndrome associated with fat emboli usually occurs within the first 48 hours after injury.

Cholesterol Embolism

Cholesterol embolization is a rare syndrome that typically presents with skin changes of livedo reticularis and digital necrosis, but which may progress to renal failure, intestinal infarction, and death.[142] Physical disruption of atheromatous plaque (with direct exposure of free cholesterol to the arterial circulation) during invasive vascular procedures is known to trigger the syndrome;[143] however, cholesterol embolization may occur when no obvious physical disruption of the arterial circulation has occurred.[144] It has been reported after the use of thrombolytic agents (ie, streptokinase)[144,145] and is hypothesized to be secondary to disruption of the surface fibrin and thrombus, leading to direct exposure of free cholesterol. Definitive diagnosis requires biopsy evidence of cholesterol clefts in the small arteries of the affected tissue.[142,145] Unfortunately, no therapy exists once the syndrome is initiated other than terminating the precipitating event.

Amniotic Fluid Embolism

Initially described in 1926,[146] amniotic fluid embolism (AFE) is a rare event (1 per 30,000 deliveries) with a high mortality rate.[147] AFE presents as the nonspecific clinical picture of respiratory distress in the peripartum period. Though most cases occur during labor or within several minutes after delivery,[148] reports have extended the time frame to 30 hours postpartum.[147] Cesarean section is a risk factor predisposing to amniotic fluid emboli.

The signs and symptoms of respiratory failure may be the only clinical manifestations, or hypertension and cerebral dysfunction may be more apparent. Rarely, the patient may report unpleasant gustatory sensations as a prodromal manifestation.[148] Confirmation of this diagnosis is made by demonstrating fetal squamous cells in the blood (by May-Grunwald-Giemsa stain) or in the sputum (by Papanicolaou stain).[149,150]

REFERENCES

1. Samet JM, Marbury MC, Spengler JD. Health effects and sources of indoor air pollution, I. *Ann Rev Respir Dis*. 1987;136:1486–1508.
2. Samet JM, Marbury MC, Spengler JD. Health effects and sources of indoor air pollution, II. *Ann Rev Respir Dis*. 1988;137:221–242.
3. Phalen RF. *Inhalation Studies: Foundations and Techniques*. Boca Raton, Fla: CRC Press; 1984:1–31.
4. Morgan MS, Frank R. Uptake of pollutant gases by the respiratory system. In: Brain JD, Proctor DF, Reid LM, eds. *Respiratory Defense Mechanisms*. New York, NY: Marcel Dekker; 1977:chap 6.
5. Ellenhorn MS, Barceloux DG. *Medical Toxicology: Diagnosis and Treatment of Human Poisoning*. New York, NY: Elsevier; 1988.
6. Piantadosi CA. Carbon monoxide, oxygen transport, and oxygen metabolism. *Hyperbaric Med*. 1987;2(1):27–44.
7. Gorman DF. Problems and pitfalls in the use of hyperbaric oxygen for the treatment of poisoned patients. *Med Toxicol Adverse Drug Exp*. 1989;4:393–399.
8. Thom SR. A delayed carbon monoxide induced change in rat brain and its antagonism by hyperbaric oxygen. *Undersea Biomed Res*. 1987;14(suppl 2):40.
9. Thom SR. Antagonism of lipid peroxidation by elevated partial pressures of oxygen. *Undersea Biomed Res*. 1988;15(suppl 1):22.
10. Winter PM, Miller JN. Carbon monoxide poisoning. *JAMA*. 1976;236:1502–1504.
11. Haldane J. The relation of the action of carbonic oxide to oxygen tension. *J Physiol (Lond)*. 1895;18:201–217.
12. Douglas CG, Haldane JS, Haldane JBS. The laws of combination of haemoglobin with carbon monoxide and oxygen. *J Physiol (Lond)*. 1912;44:275–304.
13. Litovitz TL, Schmitz BF, Holm KC. 1991 Annual Report of the American Association of Poison Control Centers National Data Collection System. *Am J Emerg Med*. 1992;10:452–505.
14. Centers for Disease Control. Carbon monoxide intoxication—a preventable environmental health hazard. *MMWR*. 1982;31:529–531.
15. Stewart RD. The effect of carbon monoxide on humans. *Ann Rev Pharmacol*. 1975;15:409–422.
16. Fagin J, Bradley J, Williams D. Carbon monoxide poisoning after accidentally inhaling paint remover. *Br Med J*. 1980;281:1461.
17. Wald N, Idle M, Smith PG, et al. Carboxyhemoglobin levels in smokers of filter and plain cigarettes. *Lancet*. 1977;1:110–112.
18. Seppanen A. Smoking in closed space and its effect on carboxyhemoglobin saturation of smoking and non-smoking subjects. *Ann Clin Res*. 1977;9:281–283.
19. Lam TH. Passive smoking in perspective. *Med Toxicol Adverse Drug Exp*. 1989;4:153–162.
20. Peterson JE, Steward RD. Absorption and elimination of carbon monoxide by inactive young men. *Arch Environ Health*. 1970;21:165–171.

21. Coburn RF. Mechanisms of carbon monoxide toxicity. *Prev Med.* 1979;8:310–322.
22. Meyers RAM, Lindberg SE, Crowley RA, et al. Carbon monoxide poisoning: the injury and its treatment. *JACEP.* 1979;8:479–484.
23. Olson KR. Carbon monoxide poisoning: mechanism, presentation and controversies in management. *J Emerg Med.* 1984;1:233–243.
24. Ginsberg MD. Carbon monoxide intoxication: clinical features, neuropathology, and mechanisms of injury. *Clin Toxicol.* 1985;23:281–288.
25. Klawans HD, Stein RW, Tanner CM, et al. A pure parkinsonism syndrome following acute carbon monoxide intoxication. *Arch Neurol.* 1982;39:302–304.
26. Myers RAM, Snyder SK, Emhoff TA. Subacute sequelae of carbon monoxide poisoning. *Ann Emerg Med.* 1985;14:1163–1167.
27. Grace TW, Platt FW. Subacute carbon monoxide poisoning: another great imitator. *JAMA.* 1981;246:1698–1700.
28. Kirkpatrick JN. Occult carbon monoxide poisoning. *West J Med.* 1987;146:52–56.
29. Gemelli F, Cattani R. Carbon monoxide poisoning in childhood. *Br Med J.* 1985;291:1197.
30. Mofenson HC, Caraccio TR, Brody GM. Carbon monoxide poisoning. *Am J Emerg Med.* 1984;2:254–261.
31. Min SK. A brain syndrome associated with delayed neuropsychiatric sequelae following acute carbon monoxide intoxication. *Acta Psychiatr Scand.* 1986;73:80–86.
32. Smith JS, Brandon S. Morbidity from acute carbon monoxide poisoning at three year follow-up. *Br Med J.* 1973;1:318–321.
33. Rylander R, Vesterlund J. Carbon monoxide criteria. *Scand J Work Environ Health.* 1981;7(suppl 1):17.
34. Atkins EH, Baker EL. Exacerbation of coronary artery disease by occupational carbon monoxide exposure: a report of two fatalities and a review of the literature. *Am J Ind Med.* 1985;7:73–79.
35. Myers RAM, Snyder SK, Linberg S, et al. Value of hyperbaric oxygen in suspected carbon monoxide poisoning. *JAMA.* 1981;246:2478–2480.
36. Matthieu D, Wolf M, Durocher A, et al. Acute carbon monoxide poisoning: risk of late sequelae and treatment by hyperbaric oxygen. *Clin Toxicol.* 1985;23:315–324.
37. Raphael J-C, Elkharrat D, Jars-Guincestre M-C, et al. Trials of normobaric and hyperbaric oxygen for acute carbon monoxide intoxication. *Lancet.* 1989;2:414–418.
38. Milby TH: Hydrogen sulfide intoxication. *J Occup Med.* 1962;4: 431.
39. Nicholls P. The effect of sulphide on cytochrome a_3, isosteric and allosteric shifts of the reduced alpha peak. *Biochim Biophys Acta.* 1975;396:24–35.
40. Burnett WW, King EG, Grace M, et al. Hydrogen sulfide poisoning: review of 5 years experience. *Can Med Assoc J.* 1977;117:1277–1280.
41. Dal A. Metal fume fever. *JACEP.* 1978;7:448–450.
42. Mueller EJ, Seger DC. Metal fume fever: a review. *J Emerg Med.* 1985;2:271–274.
43. McCord CP. Metal fume fever as an immunological disease. *Ind Med Surg.* 1960;29:101–107.
44. Anthony JS, Zamel N, Aberman A. Abnormalities in pulmonary function after brief exposure to toxic metal fumes. *Can Med Assoc J.* 1978;119:586–588.
45. Amdur MO, Doull J, Klaassen CD, eds. *Casarett and Doull's Toxicology: Basic Science of Poisons.* 4th ed. New York, NY: Pergamon; 1991.
46. Done AK. The toxic emergency. *Emerg Med.* 1986;14:196–213.
47. Newman Taylor AJ. Occupational asthma. *Thorax.* 1980;35:241–245.
48. Chen-Yeung M, Lam S. Occupational asthma. *Am Rev Respir Dis.* 1986;133:686–703.
49. Levy MB, Fink JN. Hypersensitivity pneumonitis. *Ann Allergy.* 1985;54:167–171.
50. Last JM, ed. *Maxey—Roseman: Public Health and Preventive Medicine.* 11th ed. New York, NY: Appleton-Century-Crofts; 1980:630–632.
51. Key MM, Henschel AF, Butler J, et al. *Occupational Diseases: A Guide to Their Recognition.* Washington, DC: US Department of Health, Education & Welfare, US Government Printing Office; 1977:116–125.
52. Walker AM, Laughlin JE, Friedlander ER, et al. Projections of asbestos related diseases 1980–2009. *J Occup Med.* 1983;25:409–425.
53. Council on Scientific Affairs. A physician's guide to asbestos-related diseases. *JAMA.* 1984;252:2593–2597.
54. Mossman BT, Bignon J, Conn M, Seaton A, Gee JBL. Asbestos: scientific developments and implications for public policy. *Science.* 1990;247:294–301.
55. Wrobelewski DA, Bower GC. The significance of facial burns in acute smoke inhalation. *Crit Care Med.* 1979;7:335–338.
56. Cornish H, Hahn K, Barth M. Experimental toxicology of pyrolysis and combustion hazards. *Environ Health Perspect.* 1975;11:191–196.
57. Thom SR. Smoke inhalation. *Emerg Med Clin North Am.* 1989;7:371–387.
58. Chu CS. New concepts of pulmonary burn injury. *J Trauma.* 1981;21:958–961.
59. Dyer RF, Esch VH. Polyvinyl chloride toxicity in fires. *JAMA.* 1976;235:393–397.
60. Sharan SR, Heimbach DM, Howard M, Hildebrandt J, Winn RK. Cardiopulmonary responses after spontaneous inhalation of Douglas fire smoke in goats. *J Trauma.* 1988;28:164–170.
61. Terrill JB, Montgomery RR, Reinhardt CF. Toxic gases from fires. *Science.* 1978;200:1343–1347.
62. Stephenson SF, Esrig BC, Polk HC, et al. The pathophysiology of smoke inhalation injury. *Ann Surg.* 1975;182:652–660.
63. Moylan JA. Inhalation injury: a primary determinant of survival following major burns. *J Burn Care Rehabil.* 1981;2:78–84.
64. Robinson NB, Hundson LD, Riem M, et al. Steroid therapy following isolated smoke inhalation injury. *J Trauma.* 1982;22:876–879.
65. Thompson PB, Herndon DN, Traber DL, Abston S. Effect on mortality of inhalation injury. *J Trauma.* 1986;26:163–165.
66. Moylan JA. Inhalation injury. *J Trauma.* 1981;21(suppl):720–721.
67. Horovitz JA. Diagnostic tools for use in smoke inhalation. *J Trauma.* 1981;21(suppl):717–719.
68. Warner A, Cutchavaree A. Early recognition of upper airway obstruction following smoke inhalation. *Am Rev Respir Dis.* 1973;108:1421–1423.
69. DiVincenti FC, Pruitt BA, Reckler JM. Inhalation injuries. *J Trauma.* 1971;11:109–116.
70. Luce EA, Su CT, Hoopes JE. Alveolar-arterial oxygen gradient in the burn patient. *J Trauma.* 1976;16:212–217.
71. Moylan JA, Chan CK. Inhalation injury—an increasing problem. *Ann Surg.* 1978;133:34–37.
72. Whitener DR, Whitener LM, Robertson KJ, et al. Pulmonary function measurements in patients with thermal injury and smoke inhalation. *Am Rev Respir Dis.* 1980;122:731–738.

73. Zikria BA, Sturner WQ, Astarjian NK, et al. Respiratory tract damage in burns: pathophysiology and therapy. *Ann NY Acad Sci.* 1968;150:618–626.
74. Herndon DN, Traber DL, Nichaus GD, et al. The pathophysiology of smoke inhalation injury in the sheep model. *J Trauma.* 1984;24:1044–1051.
75. Herndon DN, Traber DL, Traber LD. The effect of resuscitation on inhalation injury. *Surgery.* 1986;100:248–250.
76. Beeley JM, Crow JC, Jones JG, et al. Mortality and lung histopathology after inhalation lung injury. *Am Rev Respir Dis.* 1988;133:191–196.
77. Mendelson CL. The aspiration of stomach contents into the lungs during obstetric anesthesia. *Am J Obstet Gynecol.* 1946;52:191–205.
78. Cameron JL, Mitchell WH, Zuidema GD. Aspiration pneumonia: clinical outcome following documented aspiration. *Arch Surg.* 1973;106:49–52.
79. Bartlett JG, Gorbach SL, Finegold SM. The bacteriology of aspiration pneumonia. *Am J Med.* 1974;56:202–207.
80. Lorber B, Swenson RM. Bacteriology of aspiration pneumonia. *Ann Intern Med.* 1974;81:329–331.
81. Russin SJ. Pulmonary aspiration: the three syndromes. *Postgrad Med.* 1989;85:155–156, 159–161.
82. Brook I, Finegold SM. Bacteriology of aspiration pneumonia in children. *Pediatrics.* 1980;65:1115–1119.
83. Robertson C. A review of the use of corticosteroids in the management of pulmonary injuries and insults. *Arch Emerg Med.* 1985;2:59.
84. Murray HW. Antimicrobial therapy in pulmonary aspiration. *Am J Med.* 1979;66:188–190.
85. Kirsch CM, Sanders A. Aspiration pneumonia: medical management. *Otolaryngol Clin North Am.* 1988;21:677–689.
86. Lewis RT, Burgess JH, Hampson LG. Cardiorespiratory studies in critical illness: changes in aspiration pneumonitis. *Arch Surg.* 1971;103:335–340.
87. Hickling KG, Howard R. A retrospective survey of treatment and mortality in aspiration pneumonia. *Intensive Care Med.* 1988;14:617–622.
88. Bynum LJ, Pierce AK. Pulmonary aspiration of gastric contents. *Am Rev Respir Dis.* 1976;114:1129–1136.
89. Gregory GA, Gooding CA, Phis RH, Tooley WH. Meconium aspiration in infants: a prospective study. *J Pediatr.* 1974;85:848–852.
90. Linden N, Aranda JV, Tsur M, et al. Need for endotracheal intubation and suction in meconium-stained neonates. *J Pediatr.* 1988;112:613–615.
91. Hageman JR, et al. Delivery room management of meconium staining of the amniotic fluid and the development of meconium aspiration syndrome. *J Perinatol.* 1988;8(2):127–131.
92. American Thoracic Society. The management of hemoptysis. *Am Rev Respir Dis.* 1966;93:471–474.
93. Tisi GM, Braunwald E. Cough and hemoptysis. In: Braunwald E, et al, eds. *Harrison's Principles of Internal Medicine.* New York, NY: McGraw-Hill Book Co; 1987:138–141.
94. Conlan AA, Harwitz SS, Krige L, et al. Massive hemoptysis: review of 123 cases. *J Thorac Cardiovasc Surg.* 1983;85:120–124.
95. Winter SM, Ingbar DH. Massive hemoptysis: pathogenesis and management. *J Intensive Care Med.* 1988;3:171–188.
96. Goldman JM. Hemoptysis: emergency assessment and management. *Emerg Med Clin North Am.* 1989;7:325–338.
97. Garzon AA, Ceviti MM, Golding ME. Exsanguinating hemoptysis. *J Thorac Cardiovasc Surg.* 1982;84:829–933.
98. Jewkes J, Kay PH, Paneth M, et al. Pulmonary aspergilloma: analysis of prognosis in relation to hemoptysis and survey of treatment. *Thorax.* 1983;38:572–578.
99. Israel RH, Poe RH. Hemoptysis. *Clin Chest Med.* 1987;8:197–205.
100. Johnston RN, Lockhart W, Ritchie RT, et al. Hemoptysis. *Br Med J.* 1960;1:592–594.
101. Fisheman AP. Manifestations of respiratory disorders. In: Fishman AP, ed. *Pulmonary Diseases and Disorders.* New York, NY: McGraw-Hill Book Co; 1980:44–83.
102. Suchman AL, Griner PF. Diagnostic uses of the activated partial thromboplastin time and prothrombin time. *Ann Intern Med.* 1986;104:810–816.
103. Poe RH, Israel RH, Marin MG, et al. Utility of fiberoptic bronchoscopy in patients with hemoptysis and a nonlocalizing chest roentgenogram. *Chest.* 1988;92:70–75.
104. Haponik EF, Chin R. Hemoptysis: clinicians' perspectives. *Chest.* 1990;97:469–475.
105. Gong H, Salviatierra C. Clinical efficacy of early and delayed fiberoptic bronchoscopy in patients with hemoptysis. *Am Rev Respir Dis.* 1981;124:221–225.
106. Gourin A, Garzon AA. Operative treatment of massive hemoptysis. *Ann Thorac Surg.* 1974;18:52–60.
107. White RI. Embolotherapy in vascular disease. *Am J Radiol.* 1984;142:27–30.
108. Tsukamoto T, Sasaki H, Nakamura H. Treatment of hemoptysis patients by thrombin and fibrinogen-thrombin infusion therapy using a fiberoptic bronchoscope. *Chest.* 1989;96:473–476.
109. Light RW, Erozan YS, Ball WC, et al. Cells in pleural fluid: their value in differential diagnosis. *Arch Intern Med.* 1973;132:854.
110. Ingram RH Jr. Disease of the pleura, mediastinum, and diaphragm. In: Braunwald E, ed. *Harrison's Principles of Internal Medicine.* 11th ed. New York, NY: McGraw-Hill Book Co; 1987:1123–1125.
111. Light RW. *Pleural Diseases.* Philadelphia, Pa: Lea & Febiger; 1983.
112. Altschule MD. Some neglected aspects of respiratory function in pleural effusions. *Chest.* 1986;89:602.
113. Sahn SA. The pleura. *Am Rev Respir Dis.* 1988;138:184–234.
114. Smyrnios NA, Jederlinic PJ, Irwin RS. Pleural effusion in an asymptomatic patient. *Chest.* 1990;97:192–196.
115. Vukich DJ. Diseases of the pleural space. *Emerg Med Clin North Am.* 1989;7:309–324.
116. Houston MC. Pleural fluid pH: diagnostic, therapeutic and prognostic value. *Am J Surg.* 1987;154:333–337.
117. Jarvi OH, Kunnas RJ, Laito MT, et al. The accuracy and significance of cytologic cancer diagnosis of pleural effusion: a follow-up study of 338 patients. *Acta Cytol.* 1972;16:152.
118. Light RW. Parapneumonic effusions and empyema. *Clin Chest Med.* 1985;6:55–62.
119. Flanagan JP, Gradisar IA, Gross RJ. Air embolus: a lethal complication of subclavian venipuncture. *N Engl J Med.* 1969;281:488–489.
120. Brunicardi FC, Scalea TM, Bernstein MO, Sclafani SSJ, Phillips TF. Air embolism during pulsed saline irrigation of an open pelvic fracture: case report. *J Trauma.* 1989;29:700–701.
121. Gottlieb JD, Ericsson JA, Sweet RB. Venous air embolism: a review. *Anesth Analg.* 1965;44:773–779.
122. Noel TA II. Air embolism removal from both pulmonary artery and right atrium during sitting craniotomy using a new catheter: report of a case. *Anesthesiology.* 1989;70:709–710.
123. Black S, Cucchiara RF, Nishimura RA, Michenfelder JD. Parameters affecting occurrence of paradoxical air embolism. *Anesthesiology.* 1989;71:235–241.

124. Durant TM, Long J, Oppenheime MJ. Pulmonary (venous) air embolism. *Am Heart J*. 1947;33:269–281.

125. Tucker WS Jr. Signs and symptoms of syndromes associated with mill wheel murmurs. *NC Med J*. 1988;49:569–572.

126. Durant TM, Oppenheime MJ, Webster MR. Arterial air embolism. *Am Heart J*. 1949;38:489–500.

127. Kizer KW. Dysbaric cerebral air embolism in Hawaii. *Ann Emerg Med*. 1987;16:535.

128. Bond GF. Arterial gas embolism. In: Davis JC, Hunt TK, eds. *Hyperbaric Oxygen Therapy*. Bethesda, Md: Undersea Medical Society; 1977:141–152.

129. Peachey T, Eason J, Moxham J, Jarvis D, Driver M. Systemic air embolism during laser bronchoscopy. *Anesthesia*. 1988;43:872–875.

130. Lee SK, Transwell AK. Pulmonary vascular air embolism in the newborn. *Arch Dis Child*. 1989;64:507–510.

131. Kizer KW. Dysbarism. In: Tintinalli JE, Krome RC, Ruiz E, eds. *Emergency Medicine: A Comprehensive Study Guide*. New York, NY: McGraw-Hill Book Co; 1992:678–687.

132. Yee ES, Verrien ED, Thomas AN. Management of air embolism in blunt and penetrating thoracic trauma. *J Thorac Cardiovasc Surg*. 1983;85:661–668.

133. Delange JJ, Booij LHDJ, Smelt WLH. Treatment of venous air embolism with papaverine. *Acta Anaesthesiol Scand*. 1989;33:257–259.

134. Kizer KW. Delayed treatment of dysbarism: a retrospective review of 50 cases. *JAMA*. 1982;247:2555.

135. Hart GB. Treatment of decompression illness and air embolism with hyperbaric oxygen. *Aerospace Med*. 1974;45:1190–1193.

136. Massey EW, Moon RE, Shelton D, Camporesi EM. Hyberbaric oxygen therapy of iatrogenic air embolism. *J Hyperbaric Med*. 1990;5:15–21.

137. Riska EB, Myllynen P. Fat embolism in patients with multiple injuries. *J Trauma*. 1982;22:891–894.

138. Oh WH, Mital MA. Fat embolism: current concepts of pathogenesis, diagnosis and treatment. *Orthop Clin North Am*. 1978;9:769–779.

139. Hoefnagels WAJ, Gerritsen EJA, Brouwer OF, Souverijn JHM. Cyclosporin encephalopathy associated with fat embolism induced by the drug's solvent. *Lancet*. 1988;2:901.

140. Sevitt S. The significance and pathology of fat embolism. *Ann Clin Res*. 1977;9:173–180.

141. Byrick RJ, Kay JC, Mullen JB. Capnography is not as sensitive as pulmonary artery pressure monitoring in detecting marrow microembolism. *Anesth Analg*. 1989;68:94–100.

142. Moldveen-Geronimus M, Merriam JC. Cholesterol embolization: from pathologic curiosity to clinical entity. *Circulation*. 1967;35:946–953.

143. Drost H, Bais B, Haan D, Hillers JA. Cholesterol embolization as a complication of left heart catheterization: report of seven cases. *Br Heart J*. 1984;52:339–342.

144. Fine MJ, Kapoor W, Falanga V. Cholesterol embolization syndrome: a review of 221 cases in the English literature. *Angiology*. 1987;38:769–784.

145. Ridker PM, Michel TM. Streptokinase therapy and cholesterol embolization. *Am J Med*. 1989;87:357–358.

146. Meyer JR. Embolia pulmonar amnio-caseosa. *Brasil Med*. 1926;2:301.

147. Anderson DG. Amniotic fluid embolism: a re-evaluation. *Am J Obstet Gynecol*. 1967;98:336.

148. Ricou B, Reper P, Suten PM. Rapid diagnosis of amniotic fluid embolism causing severe pulmonary failure. *Intensive Care Med*. 1989;15:129–131.

149. Masson RG, Ruggieri J, Siddiqui MM. Amniotic fluid embolism: definitive diagnosis in a survivor. *Am Rev Respir Dis*. 1979;120:187.

150. Masson RG, Ruggieri J. Pulmonary microvascular cytology: a new diagnostic application of the pulmonary artery catheter. *Chest*. 1985;88:908.

APPENDIX 75-A: OCCUPATIONAL EXPOSURES

Occupation/Avocation	Toxins
Acid dipper	Arsine, cyanogens, hydrochloric, nitric and sulfuric acid fumes
Acid finishing worker (glass)	*Hydrochloric* acid, sulfuric acid, lead
Agricultural worker	See Farmer
Aircraft mechanic	Alcohols, *chlorinated and other solvents*, gasoline and other fuels, zinc chromate
Aircraft pilot	See Aircraft mechanic
Crop duster	Pesticides and their solvents
Aircraft worker	Cyanides, chromates, fiber glass and resin plastics, *solvents* (especially chlorinated), hydrofluoric acid
Airplane hangar employee	As in other aircraft fields, *carbon monoxide*
Alcohol distiller	Alcohols (including methanol), *amyl* acetate, benzene, mercury, toluene, xylene
Aluminum extraction worker	Aluminum, *hydrofluoric acid*, manganese
Amber worker	*Formaldehyde* (artificial amber), lead
Art-glass worker	Amyl acetate, copper, *hydrofluoric acid, lead* methanol, volatile hydrocarbons (including benzine)
Asbestos products worker	Asbestos, benzene, formaldehyde, toluene, xylene
Automobile worker	Asbestos, chromates, *fiberglass and resin plastics*, gasoline, lead solvents
Radiator cleaner	Borate, isopropanol, *oxalate*, sulfamic acid
Painter	Benzene, lead, *methanol*, zinc
Balloon operator	Arsine, *carbon monoxide*
Barber/beautician	Aliphatic solvents, alkyl sodium sulfates, borates, cadmium, cobalt, copper, detergents, *dyes*, essential oils, lead oxalate (freckle remover), pyrogallol, resorcinol, salicylate, silver, *thioglycolate*
Barometer maker	Mercury
Battery worker	Acids, benzene, mercury, zinc
Blacksmith	*Carbon monoxide* and dioxide, cyanogens, lead

Note: The most important toxins, because of either severity or frequency of toxic effects, are in italics.
Source: Adapted from Done AK. The toxic emergency. *Emerg Med.* 1986;14:196, 201, 205, 209, 213. With permission.

Occupation/Avocation	Toxins
Blast furnace worker	*Carbon dioxide* and monoxide, cyanogens, hydrogen sulfide, phosphine, sulfur dioxide
Bleacher	Caustic alkali, *chlorine*, chromium, *hydrochloric acid*, hydrofluoric acid, *peroxides*, nitric acid, oxalic acid, phosgene, sulfur oxides
Bookbinder	Acetate, arsenic, *formalin*, lead, methanol, oxalate, polyvinyl, solvents
Brass worker (founder)	*Antimony, arsenic*, carbon dioxide and monoxide, copper, lead, phosphorus, sulfur oxides
Brazer	Lead, zinc
Brewer	*Amyl alcohol, carbon dioxide* or monoxide, cobalt formaldehyde, hydrofluoric acid, phenol, sulfuric acid
Brick worker	Carbon monoxide and dioxide, epoxy resins, *hydrofluoric acid, lead, lime*, magnesium, manganese, *silica*, sulfur oxides
Bronzer	Acetone, ammonia amyl acetate, antimony, arsenic, benzene, benzine, cyanides, hydrochloric acid, hydrogen sulfide, lead, manganese, mercury, methanol, sulfur oxides, zinc
Bullet reloader	See Cartridge maker
Burnisher	*Antimony, benzine*, carbon tetrachloride, sulfuric acid, trichlorethylene
Cabinetmaker (see also Painter)	Acetone, *benzine*, bleaches, *methanol, methylene chloride*, resins, solvents, turpentine
Ironwood	*Arsenic*
Candle maker	*Aniline*, borates, chromates, potassium nitrate, sodium hydroxide
Carpenter	See Cabinetmaker
Cartridge maker	Lead, mercury, nitrites
Case hardener	Cyanogens, sodium dichromate or nitrite
Caster	See specific occupation
Cementer (rubber, plastic, etc)	Benzene, benzine, butyl alcohol, carbon disulfide, carbon tetrachloride, methanol, naphtha, tetrachlorethane, trichloroethylene
Cement (Portland) worker	Arsenic, chromates, cobalt, lime, pitch, *silica*
Ceramist	Arsenic, *barium*, carbon monoxide, *chromium*, cobalt, *feldspars*, hydrochloric or hydrofluoric acid, *lead*, manganese, mercury, selenium, *silica*, sulfur oxides, tellurium
Charcoal cook	Carbon *monoxide* or dioxide
Chrome plater (see also Electroplater)	*Chromium*, solvents, sulfuric acid
Coal miner	See Miner
Coal tar worker	*Aniline, creosote, cresol*, cyanogens, naphtha, phenol, pitch
Cobbler	Amyl acetate, aniline, *benzene and related solvents*, benzine, carbon tetrachloride, methanol, plastics
Coke oven worker (see also Coal tar worker)	*Ammonia, benzene, carbon monoxide*, hydrogen sulfide, sulfur oxides
Compositor	*Alkalis, aniline*, antimony, benzine, lead, *solvents*

Occupation/Avocation	Toxins
Construction worker (see also Brick worker, Cabinetmaker, Cement worker, Ceramist, Painter)	*Arsenic, creosote*, gasoline, glass fibers, paint products, *pitch, silica*, solvent
Cosmetic worker	Aniline, *arsenic, mercury*, nitrobenzene, solvents
Dentist	Anesthetics, clove oil, disinfectants, *mercury*
Dockworker	See Longshoreman
Dry cleaner	*Amyl acetate, benzine*, carbon tetrachloride, dichloroethylene, methanol, *naphtha*, oxalate, tetrachloroethane, tetrachlorethylene, *trichloroethylene*, turpentine, waterproofing compounds
Dye maker	*Aniline*, antimony, arsenic, benzine, chlorates, chromates, coal tar products, cresol, *dimethyl sulfate*, ferrocyanides, formaldehyde, lead, manganese, mercury, methanol, nitrobenzene, phenol, titanium, *organotins*
Dyer	Acetone, *aniline,* other *aminobenzene derivatives*, bleaches, mercury, solvents, titanium, zinc
Electric apparatus maker	Asbestos, *epoxy* and *phenolic resins*, solvents
Electroplater	*Antimony, arsenic*, benzine, cadmium, *chromium*, copper, *cyanide*, gold, lead, lime, mercury, nickel, nitrous fumes, potassium hydroxide, silver, sulfuric acid, zinc
Enameler	*Amyl* acetate, antimony, arsenic, chromium, cobalt, lead, nickel, *silica*
Engraver	Acids, alkalis, benzene, copper, cyanide, solvents
Etcher	Acids, alkalis, arsine, *hydrofluoric acid*, nitrous fumes, picric acid
Explosives maker	Acetone, ammonia amyl acetate, mercury, nitrites, *nitroglycerin*, picric acid, TNT
Farmer	Carbon monoxide, *farmer's lung*, fertilizers, pesticides, plants with contact toxicity (poison ivy, sumac, oak, etc), *silo filler's* disease, solvents
Felt hat worker	*Carbon monoxide*, hydrogen peroxide, hydrogen sulfide, *mercury*, methanol, nitrous fumes, *oxalic acid*, sulfuric acid
Fertilizer producer/user	*Ammonia*, arsenic, *calcium cyanamide*, carbon dioxide, castor bean pomace, cyanogens, fluoride, hydrogen sulfide, lime, magnesium, manganese, nitrates, nitric acid, phosphates, sulfur oxides, sulfuric acid
Fire extinguisher maker	Carbon dioxide, chlorobromomethane, *ethyl bromide, ethyl chloride*, ethylene dibromide, methyl bromide, sodium dichromate
Firearms maker	See Explosives maker, Gunsmith
Fireworks maker (see also Explosives maker)	*Antimony, arsenic*, barium, bismuth, mercury, phosphorus, picric acid, thallium
Fish-meal processor	Hydrogen sulfide, *triethylamine*
Foundry worker (see also particular occupation)	Acids, *carbon dioxide* and *monoxide*, lime, resins, *silica*
Furniture polisher	*Amyl* acetate, benzine, chromium, methanol, naphtha, petroleum hydrocarbons, pyridine, rosin, turpentine
Fur processor	*Alum, bleaches*, chromate, dyes formaldehyde, hydrogen sulfide, lime, mercury, nitrous fumes

Occupation/Avocation	Toxins
Galvanizer	Acids, *ammonia*, arsenic, *arsine*, benzine, nitrous fumes, sulfur oxides, trichloroethylene, *zinc*
Garage worker	Benzine, carbon monoxide, detergents, *epoxy resins*, gasoline, glass fibers, lead, paints, solvents
Gardener	Arsenic calcium cyanamide, *fertilizers, fungicides, herbicides, insecticides*, lead, *pesticides*, poisonous plants, venomous insects
Gem/lapidary/jewelry worker	*Arsenic*, asbestos, benzene, bisulfate, borates, cadmium, cyanide, epoxy resins, hydrochloric acid, *hydrofluoric acid*, lead, *mercury* (gold extraction), methanol, methyl salicylate, nitric acid, selenium, silica, sulfur oxides, sulfuric acid, trisodium phosphate, zinc
Glass worker (see also Art-glass worker)	Acids, *arsenic, borates*, carbon monoxide, chlorine, *glass fibers*, hydrofluoric acid, lead, nitrogen oxides, sulfur
Glazer (pottery)	See Ceramist
Gold and silver extractor	*Arsenic, arsine*, bromides, *cyanide*, formaldehyde, hydrofluoric acid, lead, *mercury*
Gunsmith/hunter/marksman (see also Explosives maker)	Cyanide, *kerosene, lead*, magnesium, mercury, nickel, *nitrites, nitrobenzene*, solvents
Bluing	*Chlorate, mercury*, methanol, nitrite, selenium
Browning	Benzine, *cyanide, lead*, petroleum hydrocarbons
Hair dresser	See Barber/beautician
Hunter	See Gunsmith
Ice cream maker	*Ammonia*, carbon dioxide
Ink maker	*Ammonia*, arsenic, benzene, benzine, *chromates, cobalt*, formaldehyde, lead, mercury, *nitrites*, other solvents, silver
Insecticide maker/applier	Solvents as well as specific insecticides
Insulation maker/applier	*Asbestos*, formaldehyde, glass fibers, *silica*
Iron/steel worker	*Arsenic*, cadmium, *carbon monoxide*, hydrofluoric acid, nitrogen oxides, sulfur oxides, *titanium*
Jeweler (see also Gem worker)	Acids, *amyl acetate*, chromates, *cyanide*, mercury, nickel, nitric acid, nitrous fumes, solder fluxes
Lacquer maker/applier	Acetaldehyde, *acetone*, alcohols, *amyl acetate*, benzine, butanone, cresyl phosphate, methylene chloride, solvents
Laundry worker	*Alkaline caustics, bleaches*, chloride, chlorine, detergents, formaldehyde, lime, ozone
Lead smelter	Antimony, *arsenic*, cadmium, carbon monoxide, *lead*, selenium, sulfur oxides, tellurium
Leather worker	Acids, *amyl acetate, barium*, carbon tetrachloride, methanol, trichlorethylene
Tanner	Acetates, acids, *aniline*, arsenic, benzene, carbon dioxide, chromates, cyanide, diethylamine, dyes, formaldehyde, hydrogen sulfide, mercury, *nitrites*, oxalate, picric acid, sodium sulfide, tannin

Occupation/Avocation	Toxins
Linoleum worker	*Amyl acetate, asphalt*, benzene, benzine, carbon tetrachloride, chromates, *dyes*, methanol, resin, solvents
Linotyper	*Antimony*, carbon monoxide, lead
Lithographer	Acids, *aniline*, arsenic, benzene, benzine, chromates, lead, mercury, methanol, nitric acid, *nitrites*, oxalate, tetrachloroethane, turpentine
Longshoreman	Manganese, *various chemicals and fumigants* (depending on cargo), venomous insects and snakes
Match worker	Alkalis, antimony, carbon disulfide, *chlorates, chromates,* hydrogen sulfide, manganese, *phosphorus*
Metal polisher	Acids, *ammonia, benzine, cyanide*, methanol, *naphtha*, oxalates, solvents, trichloroethylene, triethanolamine
Miner (varies with type)	*Asbestos*, carbon dioxide and monoxide, hydrogen sulfide, manganese, nitrogen oxides, *silica, talc*
Mirror maker	Acetaldehyde, *ammonia*, benzene, cyanide, lead, mercury, silver, solvents
Painter	*Acetone, acids*, alkalis, aniline, arsenic, barium, *benzine*, carbon disulfide, carbon tetrachloride, chromates, *lead*, manganese, mercury, methanol, methylene chloride, nitrogen oxides, *solvents*, trichloroethylene, turpentine
Paint maker	Cadmium, *chlorinated diphenyls*, petroleum distillates, titanium, zinc
Paper maker	Acids, acrylamide, *alkalis*, ammonia, amyl acetate, bisulfide, calcium chloride, chromates, DMSO, formaldehyde, hydrofluoric acid, hydrogen sulfide, lead, resins, sulfur oxides, titanium
Petroleum refiner	Acetone, ammonia, arsenic, *benzene, benzine*, gasoline and other petroleum distillates, hydrofluoric acid, *hydrogen sulfide*, nitrites, solvents, sulfur oxides
Photoengraver	Acids, alkalis, *ammonia*, ammonium bichromate, *amyl acetate, benzene*, borates, bromides, chromates, cyanide, ethylene glycol, formaldehyde, hydroquinone, iodine, lead, mercury, methanol, oxalate, pyrogallic acid, silver, *sodium bisulfite*, sodium hypochlorite, sodium sulfite, sodium thiosulfate, tellurium, trichlorethylene, uranium, vanadium
Plastics and resin maker/user	None with finished plastics but unreacted resins are toxic
Plumber	Acids, alkalis, *arsine, carbon monoxide, lead*, solvents, zinc
Pottery worker	See Ceramist
Printer	*Alkalis, aniline, benzine*, carbon tetrachloride, chromates, cyanide, lead, mercury, methanol, tetrachloroethylene, other solvents
Railroad shop/track worker	*Chromates*, contact plant poisons (poison ivy, etc), *creosote*, detergents, dichlorobenzenes, diesel fuel oil, fungicides, herbicides, insecticides, paint, paint strippers, solvents
Rayon worker	*Acetic anhydride*, acids, ammonia, benzine, bleaches, butyl alcohol, *calcium bisulfite*, carbon disulfide, chlorinated diphenyls, cyanogens, *dioxane*, formaldehyde, hydrogen sulfide, methanol, nitrous fumes, solvents, sulfide, sodium sulfite, tetrachlorethane

Occupation/Avocation	Toxins
Refrigeration worker	*Acrolein, ammonia,* carbon dioxide, carbon monoxide, *ethylbromide, ethyl chloride,* glass fiber, *methyl bromide, methyl chloride,* methyl formate, ozone, sulfur oxides
Rubber worker	*Acetaldehyde, acetone,* amyl alcohol, aniline, antimony, arsenic, barium, benzene, benzine, carbon disulfide, carbon tetrachloride, *chloroprene,* chromates, cresol, ethylene dichloride, formaldehyde, lead, magnesium, methanol, nitrogen oxides, *plasticizers, pyridine, silica* solvents, tellurium, zinc
Sewage worker	*Ammonia,* carbon dioxide, chlorine, *hydrogen sulfide,* methane
Shoemaker (see also Leather worker)	*Acetone, adhesives,* ammonia, amyl acetate, amyl alcohol, *aniline and dyes,* benzene, benzine, carbon tetrachloride, methanol, naphtha, plastics, tetrachloroethane, trichloroethylene, waxes
Solderer	*Acids,* antimony, arsenic, *arsine,* borates, cadmium, cyanide, *hydrazine salts, lead,* potassium bifluoride, rosin, zinc
Stone worker	*Lime, silica*
Sugar refiner	Acids, *ammonia, bagasse,* barium, burlap, carbon dioxide, hydrogen sulfide, sulfur oxides
Tannery worker	Acetic acid, acids, alum, ammonia, *amyl acetate, aniline and dyes,* arsenic, benzine, calcium hydrosulfide, chromates, cyanide, dimethylamine, dyes, formaldehyde, hydrogen sulfide, lead, lime, mercury, oxalate, sodium sulfide, solvents, sulfur oxides, tannin
Tar worker	*Arsenic, cresols,* pitch, tar
Taxidermist	*Arsenic,* calcined alum, *mercury,* solvents, tannin, zinc
Upholsterer (see also Lacquer maker)	*Glues, lacquer,* lacquer solvents, methanol
Waterproofer	*Alum,* benzene, *benzine,* carbon tetrachloride, chromates, formaldehyde, melamine, pitch, resins, solvents, tar
Welder	*Arsenic,* benzene, cadmium, chromates, fluoride, lead, manganese, mercury, nitrous fumes, ozone, phosphorus, selenium, *zinc*
Wood preserver	*Arsenic chlorophenols,* chromates, copper compounds, creosote, cresols, dinitrophenols, mercury, pitch, resins, tar, zinc
Woodworker	See Cabinetmaker

76. Chest Trauma

ALAN H. BRADER, MD

Improved prehospital care and rapid transport have presented emergency departments with more severely injured but potentially salvageable patients. With the use of well-planned and practiced resuscitation protocols, it is now possible to save patients with previously lethal thoracic injuries.[1] The recognition and proper management of chest trauma in a critically injured patient are particularly important and can be lifesaving.

A sound working knowledge of potential chest injuries is necessary for the emergency physician to become skilled and comfortable in managing any trauma victim. By following the ABCs of resuscitation, severe cardiorespiratory compromise can be promptly recognized and properly treated.[2] Knowledge and awareness can also reduce the possibility of missing other less urgent thoracic injuries.[3]

EPIDEMIOLOGY OF THORACIC TRAUMA

Thoracic injury is responsible for 25% of deaths from trauma and is a contributing factor for an additional 25% of accident-related deaths.[4] The Major Trauma Outcome Study reported that nearly 31% of all accident patients had chest injuries.[5] Chest trauma is often divided into two categories based on the mechanism of injury—penetrating and nonpenetrating (blunt).

Blunt or nonpenetrating trauma is responsible for the majority of thoracic injuries, with motor vehicle-related accidents being the most common cause.[5] The mortality associated with blunt chest trauma is often related to the number and types of associated injuries. A death rate of 4% to 12% is associated with isolated chest injury, but it increases to 30% to 35% when two or more other body systems are involved.[6] Chest injuries due to blunt trauma are generally not isolated injuries. In one series of 675 hospitalized trauma patients, blunt chest injury was associated with craniocerebral injury (55%), extremity fractures (38%), and abdominal injuries (20%).[3]

Penetrating thoracic trauma is usually caused by knives and low-velocity weapons in civilian practice. Shotgun and impalement injuries are occasionally seen (Fig. 76-1). An important determinant of mortality from penetrating chest trauma is the presence or absence of shock on admission. Approximately 10% of patients with penetrating chest trauma in shock die, while only 1% of penetrating chest trauma patients who are not in shock die.

The location of all entrance and exit wounds is important in determining which intrathoracic structures may be injured. Lateral thoracic wounds in patients who are hemodynamically stable with an initial thoracic blood loss of less than 500 mL from a chest tube usually require no further thoracic intervention.[7] If the penetrating injury is located in the anterior mediastinal or peristernal area, surgical intervention should be considered. Signs of cardiac tamponade, persistent hypotension, or continuing thoracostomy tube blood loss greater than 200 mL/h for more than 4 hours should mandate urgent thoracotomy or sternotomy by a trained surgeon.

Associated intra-abdominal injuries must be considered, especially with missile projectiles or wounds below the nip-

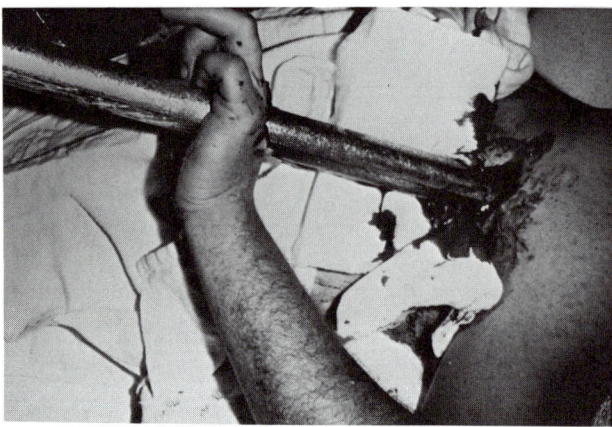

Figure 76-1 Patient impaled with a metal fence pole.

ple line anteriorly and the scapula tip posteriorly. Intra-abdominal injuries occur in 15% of patients with stab wounds and 46% of patients with gunshot wounds to the lower chest.[8]

INITIAL THORACIC TRAUMA ASSESSMENT

The first priorities in any trauma resuscitation are the adequacy of the airway and whether the patient is breathing. One must check the patency of the patient's upper airway and watch the chest wall movement. Simultaneously, an examiner must note the patient's respiratory rate and effort. This is followed by heart and breath sound auscultation over the anterior chest. Rapid palpation of the thoracic wall will determine its integrity and will detect the presence of subcutaneous emphysema. The initial assessment of an injured patient can be accomplished within 30 seconds.[2]

Evaluating a trauma patient for thoracic injuries is only one portion of the total assessment of a multiply injured patient. Fortunately, only a few chest injuries are immediately life-threatening (Table 76-1). All of these conditions can be initially stabilized by an emergency physician.

Other less emergent thoracic injuries that are serious and potentially fatal are listed in Table 76-2. Operative intervention is necessary in only 8% to 15% of cases of blunt thoracic trauma.[2,3] Most thoracic injuries can be treated nonoperatively with thoracostomy tube drainage, volume resuscitation, and proper monitoring.

CHEST WALL TRAUMA

Chest wall injuries can range from relatively simple rib fractures to extensive open chest wounds. Any trauma to the chest wall can impair normal ventilation. The loss of structural integrity or the presence of pain may restrict a patient's ability to breathe.

Table 76-1 Immediate Life-threatening Thoracic Emergencies

Airway obstruction
Tension pneumothorax
Cardiac tamponade
Massive hemorrhage (pleural or mediastinal)
Flail chest
Open pneumothorax

Table 76-2 Serious Thoracic Injuries

Pneumothorax
Tracheobronchial injury
Hemothorax
Esophageal injury
Aortic transection
Myocardial contusion
Diaphragmatic rupture
Pulmonary contusion

Rib Fracture

The most common chest injuries are rib fractures.[9] Physical exam will reveal which rib(s) are injured. Chest radiography may or may not verify a clinician's findings. Since therapy is directed toward the patient's symptoms and not the radiographic imaging of a fracture, rib films are unnecessary. Relief of pain is the goal for treating rib fractures.[10] For minor rib fracture pain, an oral narcotic agent plus a nonsteroidal anti-inflammatory agent is effective. Intercostal nerve blocks or epidural anesthesia is used to control severe pain associated with multiple rib fractures. An elderly patient or a patient with chronic pulmonary disease with one or two rib fractures requires aggressive therapy. By controlling pain effectively, respiratory complications may be prevented.

At one time, first rib fractures were considered hallmarks of significant underlying trauma.[11] Many trauma centers followed a policy of routine aortic arch angiography for patients with first rib fractures, but there is now little evidence to support this practice.[12] Angiography is necessary only for selected patients with a severely displaced first rib fracture, an absent upper extremity pulse, or a brachial plexus injury.[13]

Flail Chest

Flail chest refers to an unstable chest wall segment that is not in continuity with the bony thoracic cage (Fig. 76-2). This means that a rib must be fractured in two locations. Paradoxic motion of the chest wall is observed with spontaneous breathing. During inspiration, the flail rib segment retracts and inhibits normal pleural cavity expansion. Despite the paradoxic flail segment motion and instability, respiratory gas exchange is primarily compromised by the underlying pulmonary contusion. The routine use of endotracheal intubation and ventilatory support for flail chest injuries is not necessary. Artificial ventilation should be based on clinical parameters.[14-16] Therapy should be directed at pulmonary toilet and pain relief. The relatively high morbidity and mortality (12% to 50%) associated with flail chest injuries are often due to the underlying pulmonary contusion, atelectasis, pre-existing pulmonary condition, and concomitant extrathoracic injuries.[17] In addition, objectively measured long-term disability is seen in over 50% of flail chest injury survivors.[18]

Sternal Fracture

Sternal fracture is another common chest wall injury that may result from either a direct or an indirect mechanism. Most sternal fractures occur by direct impact to the anterior chest. Myocardial contusion is also associated with direct sternal injury. However, indirect sternal fractures occur by a flexion-compression mechanism in which the ribs play a role in transmitting the forces from spine to sternum.[19] Because of this mechanism, an association between indirect sternal fractures and spinal injuries has been observed. Careful evaluation for associated spine injuries in patients with sternal fractures is necessary, and vice versa.[20]

Any patient sustaining chest trauma resulting in a sternal fracture, scapular fracture, pulmonary contusion, flail chest, or impaired respiratory effort requires hospitalization. In addition, patients with comorbid diseases and seemingly minor chest wall injuries require admission for treatment and observation. These include elderly individuals with one or more rib fractures, patients with underlying chronic cardiopulmonary disease, and morbidly obese patients.

PULMONARY TRAUMA

The thorax is divided into right and left pleural spaces, separated by the mediastinum. Normally, the lung occupies the pleural space so completely that only a potential space exists. However, in pathologic conditions secondary to trauma, the pleural space can be occupied by air, blood, chyle, or visceral organs. Respiratory and cardiovascular compromise can occur from expansion of the pleural space.

Pneumothorax

A simple pneumothorax is the accumulation of air in the pleural space, which is not under pressure. Blunt or penetrating trauma can cause a pneumothorax. Ninety percent of all pneumothoraces due to blunt chest trauma in adults have associated rib fractures.[21] Hyper-resonance and decreased breath sounds are the most common clinical findings. Occasionally, subcutaneous emphysema is present. The standard

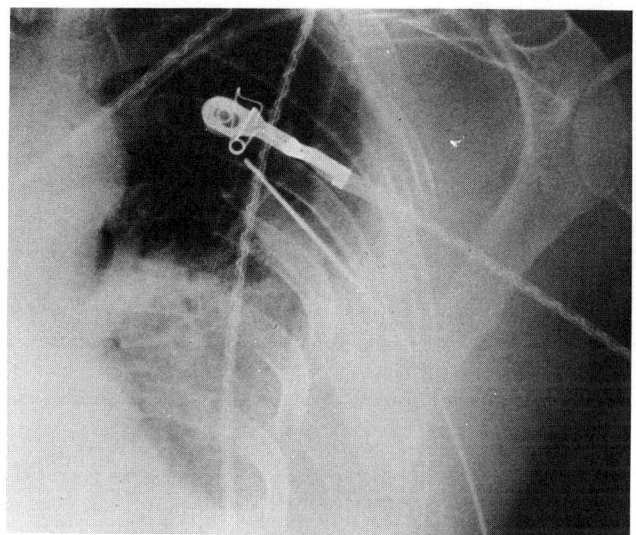
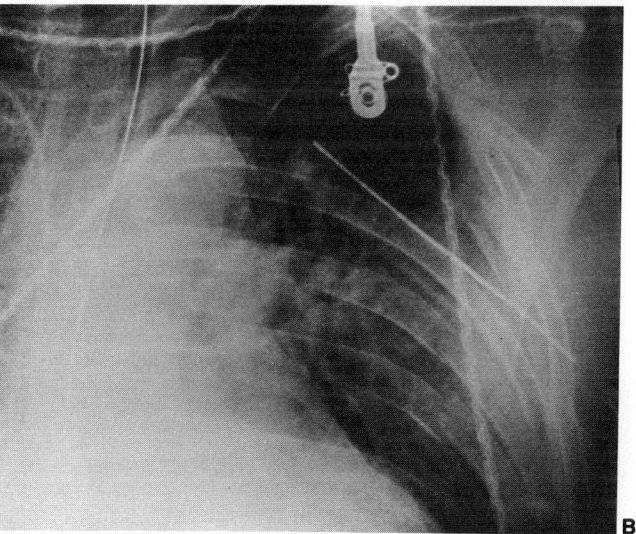

Figure 76-2 Chest radiograph of flail chest segment. **A**, inspiration; **B**, expiration.

treatment of a traumatic pneumothorax is tube thoracostomy. Needle aspiration or clinical observation should be reserved for patients with an isolated minor (<10%) pneumothorax.

Tension Pneumothorax

The accumulation of air under pressure within a pleural space is called a tension pneumothorax. As a result, the lung within the involved hemithorax collapses, and the mediastinum is pushed to the opposite side, with compression of the lung on that side. Both ventilatory exchange and cardiac venous return are impaired.

Progressive deterioration of a patient will occur if the clinical signs of a tension pneumothorax are left unrecognized. Hyper-resonance and decreased breath sounds in the involved hemithorax, hypotension, distended neck veins, and tracheal deviation are all findings associated with a tension pneumothorax. When a tension pneumothorax is suspected on clinical grounds, prompt decompression of the pleural space is necessary to prevent further hypoxic embarrassment and cardiovascular compromise. Percutaneous puncture with a 14 gauge angiocath over the involved hemithorax above the second rib at the midclavicular line will convert a life-threatening tension pneumothorax into a simple pneumothorax. Tube thoracostomy is done following needle decompression to expand the lung fully.

Open Pneumothorax

An open pneumothorax presents as a pneumothorax with a large chest wall defect or as a smaller, open "sucking" chest wound. Because the chest wall continuity is disrupted, intrapleural and atmospheric pressure are at equilibrium. Serious ventilatory embarrassment will occur, since a pressure gradient can no longer be established to promote gas exchange. With a smaller open sucking chest wound, a "one-way flap valve mechanism" will cause a tension pneumothorax.

Management of an open pneumothorax is directed toward restoring chest wall integrity and decompressing the pleural space. In the emergency department, an occlusive dressing should be placed over the defect and a chest tube inserted in the involved pleural space. In the field, a three-corner semiocclusive dressing is placed over the wound, creating a "flutter-valve" system. This stabilizes the patient until a hospital is reached.

Hemothorax

A hemothorax is one of the more common conditions seen with blunt and penetrating thoracic trauma. Causes of a hemothorax include injuries to the lung, intercostal or internal mammary artery, aorta or other great vessels, heart, or diaphragm. Breath sounds are diminished and dullness to percussion is present over the involved hemithorax. A chest radiograph will confirm the presence of a significant hemothorax. The initial treatment of any clinically detectable hemothorax is tube thoracostomy.

The most common cause of a hemothorax is an injury to the lung. The pulmonary vasculature is a low-pressure system; thus, most pulmonary bleeding stops spontaneously and requires only tube thoracostomy drainage. However, injury to any of the major vessels or intercostal or internal mammary arteries usually requires more than simple tube thoracostomy. After the insertion of a chest tube for hemothorax, both the initial amount of blood and subsequent hourly evacuated volumes should be recorded. When the initial amount of blood drained is 1000 to 1500 mL or continues at a rate of 200 mL/h for more than 4 hours, a thoracotomy is indicated.[2,4,21] If a patient is clinically unstable with signs of intrathoracic bleeding, thoracotomy is indicated.

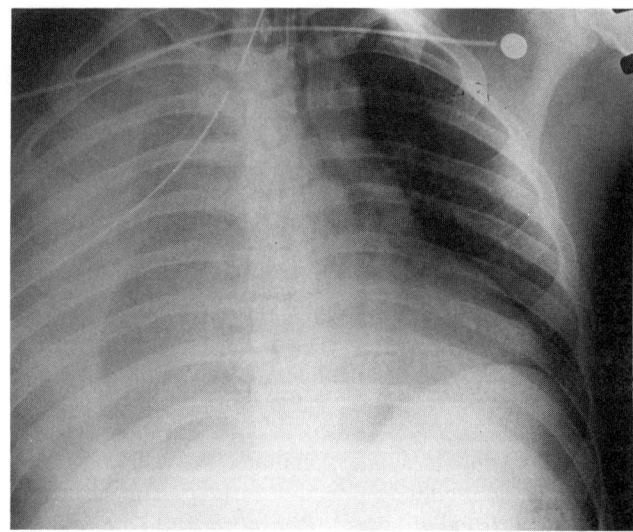

Figure 76-3 Massive right hemothorax in a stab victim with a lacerated right internal mammary artery.

A massive hemothorax (>1500 mL) can represent a life-threatening condition (Fig. 76-3). The physical findings will be similar to a simple hemothorax. Occasionally, a massive hemothorax can mimic a cardiac tamponade or tension pneumothorax. These patients will be hypotensive and have distended neck veins secondary to mediastinal compression. As fluid resuscitation begins, tube thoracostomy should be done to decompress the pleural space of blood and restore effective oxygenation. Emergency thoracotomy is usually necessary to control persistent intrathoracic hemorrhage.

Pulmonary Contusion

A pulmonary contusion is usually caused by high-speed deceleration with direct trauma to the chest wall or a high-velocity gunshot wound to the chest wall or lung. In the past, a pulmonary contusion was defined as an injury to the lung with interstitial and alveolar damage with no significant laceration. However, computed tomography (CT) has shown that the basic component of a pulmonary contusion is a pulmonary laceration surrounded by intra-alveolar hemorrhage without significant interstitial injury.[22,23] Lung lacerations causing pulmonary contusions have been divided into four types based on CT scan appearance: type 1, compression rupture with linear tear; type 2, compression shear; type 3, rib penetration; and type 4, adhesion tears.

Chest radiography is the study of choice to diagnose a pulmonary contusion (Fig. 76-4). Classically, a pulmonary contusion appears within several hours after injury as an infiltrate that does not follow the confines of an anatomic lung segment. The infiltrate may appear (1) irregular with coarse nodular densities, (2) homogeneous, or (3) diffuse and patchy.[24] These radiolucent areas usually disappear within several days. With an isolated pulmonary contusion,

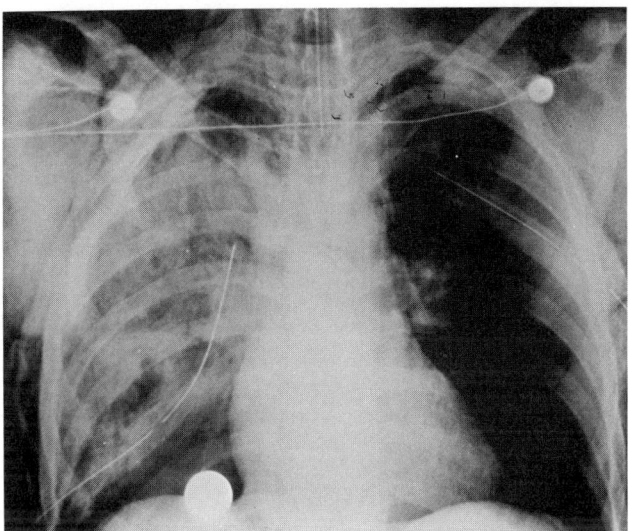

Figure 76-4 Pulmonary contusion of the right lung.

clinical pulmonary findings can often be absent, with minimal effects on lung function.[25] Pulmonary contusions are often difficult to distinguish from gastric aspiration using chest radiographs alone. The prehospital history will help differentiate gastric aspiration from a contusion.

The treatment of minor to moderate pulmonary contusions should be conservative, consisting of supplemental oxygen, chest physiotherapy, and judicious fluid and analgesic administration.[26] Ventilatory support should be reserved for those patients with severe pulmonary contusions based on clinical parameters, not radiographic findings.

MEDIASTINAL TRAUMA

The mediastinum extends from the root of the neck to the diaphragm. It is bounded on either side by the right and left pleural spaces and is centrally located in the thorax. The heart, great vessels, trachea, and esophagus are located in the mediastinum. Injuries to these mediastinal structures may occur by either penetrating or blunt mechanisms. Recognizing the clinical signs of mediastinal injury is important for the prompt, definitive treatment of these injuries.

Cardiac Tamponade

Cardiac tamponade is a life-threatening injury occurring most commonly as a result of penetrating cardiac trauma.[27] Injuries to the great vessels or blunt cardiac trauma may also cause acute cardiac tamponade.

The pericardial sac surrounds the heart and the roots of the great vessels. It lies within the middle mediastinum. Normally, this cavity contains only a small amount of fluid, which acts as a lubricant for heart motion. When injury to the heart occurs, blood can accumulate within this space. This abnormal collection of blood can cause external compression (tamponade) of all heart chambers. Venous return, diastolic chamber filling, and cardiac output are impeded.

Cardiac tamponade is most commonly observed in patients with knife wounds to the heart. Right ventricle injuries are the most common injuries leading to cardiac tamponade. The clinical signs of cardiac tamponade include distant, muffled heart sounds, hypotension, and distended neck veins. These findings constitute Beck's triad. Pulsus paradoxus is also sometimes observed. Unfortunately, these clinical findings are observed in less than 40% of the cases of traumatic cardiac tamponade.[28] In addition the chest radiograph is not a reliable test to diagnose cardiac tamponade.

Surgery should not be delayed for further diagnostic testing in an unstable patient with physical findings suggestive of a cardiac tamponade. In a stable patient, echocardiography, if immediately available, can be used to detect pericardial blood. Pericardiocentesis has a role in attempted stabilization of a patient but not in definitive treatment of cardiac tamponade. False-negative results, up to 23%, have been reported with pericardiocentesis.[29] It has clearly been shown that relying on aspirated unclotted blood to detect a cardiac tamponade is unreliable in an acute setting. A subxiphoid pericardial window may be done prior to thoracotomy to confirm the diagnosis of cardiac tamponade or to decompress the tamponade.[30,31] Other authors argue that a potential cardiac tamponade should not be decompressed by this method unless a thoracotomy or sternotomy can be performed immediately.[28]

The presence of cardiac tamponade appears to have a favorable influence on survival in penetrating cardiac trauma.[32] Survival was 73% with tamponade and only 11% without tamponade. Even though a cardiac tamponade has detrimental cardiovascular effects, it may benefit a patient by temporarily preventing free hemorrhage.

Penetrating Cardiac Injury

The successful management of a penetrating cardiac injury tests the efficiency of a trauma system to its fullest. Despite rapid prehospital transport and immediate definitive care, most studies have a prehospital mortality rate ranging from 50% to 85% for these injuries.[33,34] An anterior precordial wound and hypotension or clinical signs of cardiac tamponade are almost diagnostic of a penetrating cardiac injury. Sixty-five percent of patients who have an upper mediastinal injury require an operation.[35]

Gunshot wounds are the most common form of penetrating cardiac trauma in an urban environment. The frequency of heart chamber injury in cases of penetrating cardiac trauma is: right ventricle, 42.5%; left ventricle, 33%; right atrium, 15.4%; and left atrium, 5.4%. Great vessel injury occurs 5% of the time.[27] The mortality rates for gunshot and knife wounds of the chest range from 14% to 37% and from

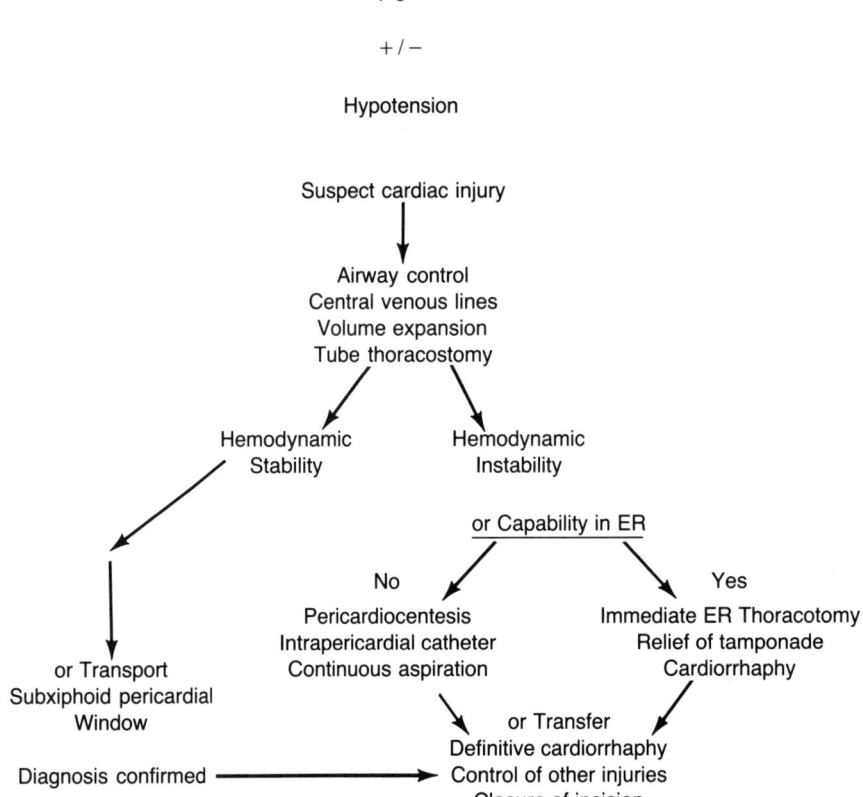

Figure 76-5 Algorithm for the diagnosis and management of penetrating cardiac injuries.

10% to 15%, respectively.[36–38] Multiple cardiac chamber injuries carry a very poor prognosis. An algorithm for the diagnosis and management of penetrating cardiac wounds by Ivatury and Rohman is outlined in Fig. 76-5.

Myocardial Contusion

Myocardial contusion following blunt chest trauma is now more frequently recognized. Evidence of myocardial contusion has been reported in 9% to 76% of patients sustaining major thoracic trauma and in approximately 15% of auto accident victims at autopsy.[39,40] Unfortunately, a good clinical definition that correlates with a histologically contused heart is not available at present.

Making the diagnosis of myocardial contusion is sometimes a difficult diagnostic challenge for the clinician. There is no single test or study that will detect blunt cardiac trauma. The diagnosis is generally based on a constellation of symptoms, clinical signs, and diagnostic studies.[41,42] A rational and detailed approach to the diagnosis and treatment of myocardial contusion is provided in collective review by Tenzer. Currently, electrocardiography (ECG), cardiac isoenzymes, echocardiography, and radioisotope scanning are the only clinical studies available to make this diagnosis. At our institution, the mechanism of injury, ECG, and cardiac isoenzymes are used to triage those individuals with suspected myocardial contusion. Echocardiography is used in patients with CPK-MB values greater than 5% within the first 24 hours of admission. Using echocardiography, a pericardial effusion or acute wall motion abnormalities are taken as evidence for myocardial contusion; these patients undergo intensive care unit monitoring for 48 to 72 hours.[43,44] However, the optimal approach for diagnosing a myocardial contusion is still controversial.[45]

The right ventricle is the most frequently contused heart chamber, and sinus tachycardia is the most common arrhythmia noted.[42,44] Acute complications of myocardial contusion include atrial and ventricular arrhythmias, conduction defects, thromboembolism, pump dysfunction, cardiac chamber rupture, and death.[42,46–50] Several late complications may occur as a result of a myocardial contusion, including ventricular aneurysms, coronary occlusions, thromboembolism, or sinus of Valsalva-right atrial fistula.

Cardiac and hemodynamic monitoring is necessary for a patient with a clinically suspected myocardial contusion. Occasionally, inotropic support is needed for hemodynamic compromise or a pacemaker is necessary for conduction instability. There are several reports of patients temporarily requiring intra-aortic balloon counterpulsation to maintain adequate cardiac output.[51,52] Unlike patients with recent myocardial infarctions, patients with myocardial contusion can safely undergo emergency surgery for associated injuries.[43,53,54]

Great Vessel Injury

Sudden horizontal or vertical deceleration after a motor vehicle accident or a fall from a great height can cause a traumatic aortic rupture or innominate artery avulsion. Seventy percent of patients with traumatic aortic ruptures were ejected from the vehicle, and 45% of aortic injuries were due to a lateral collision at an intersection.[10] Sixteen percent to 36% of the patients who die in automobile accidents at the scene or in transport die from aortic injury.[21,55] An aortic tear from blunt thoracic trauma is fatal at the scene 90% of the time.[2] If untreated, hospitalized patients with a traumatic aortic tear have a 40% to 50% mortality from rupture within the first 24 hours.[56,57]

In horizontal deceleration accidents, the location of an aortic tear in 70% to 95% of patients is just distal to the left subclavian artery at the ligamentum arteriosum. Five percent to 30% of patients rupture in the ascending aorta just above the aortic valve. Rupture of the descending aorta at the level of the diaphragm is rare but does occur.[58–60] In one series, multiple aortic tears were reported in 20% of the patients.[61]

The clinical signs of a transected thoracic aorta include retrosternal or interscapular chest pain, upper extremity hypertension, or a palpable pulse deficit in the lower or upper extremities. It is important to recognize that clinical findings are present in less than one half of patients and up to one third have no evidence of external trauma.[62–64] The initial chest radiograph may display several important clues to the diagnosis of an aortic injury (Table 76-3).[65] A widened mediastinum is the most common radiologic sign associated with thoracic aortic injury (Fig. 76-6). Under age 65, mediastinal widening is the most reliable indicator of traumatic aortic rupture.[66] However, aortic rupture is the cause of mediastinal widening in only 12.5% of patients.[67]

Thoracic aortography remains the gold standard for diagnosis of a thoracic aorta or great vessel injury (Fig. 76-7). The clinical accuracy of chest CT scanning to detect a transected thoracic aorta or great vessel injury is not well established. Currently, there is no large clinical study to support

Table 76-3 Radiologic Signs of a Transected Thoracic Aorta

Widening of the mediastinum
Aortic knob irregularity
Depression of the left mainstem bronchus
Opacification of the aortopulmonary window
Widening of the right paratracheal strip
Deviation of the nasogastric tube to the right
Apical capping
Left hemothorax
Deviation of the trachea to the right

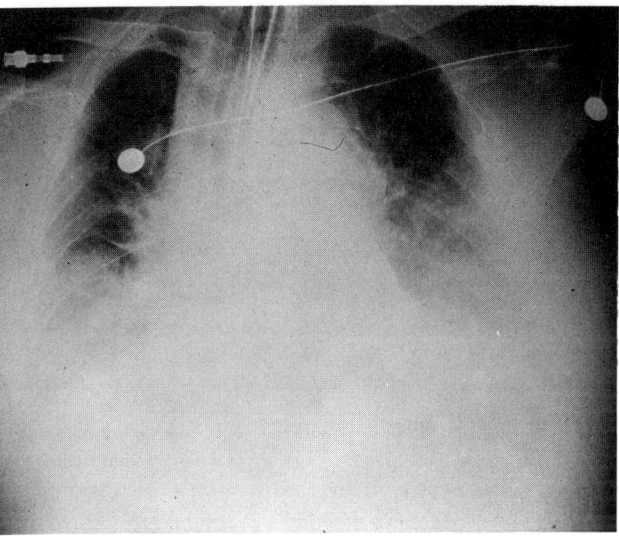

Figure 76-6 Widened mediastinum of a patient with a transected thoracic aorta.

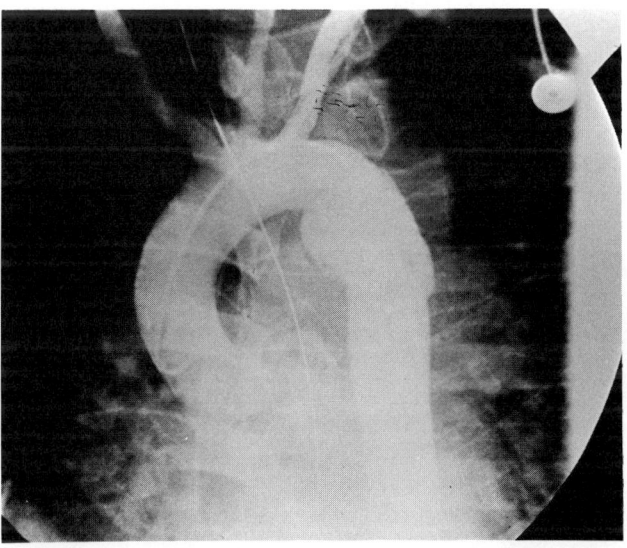

Figure 76-7 Aortogram of a patient with a transected thoracic aorta distal to the left subclavian artery.

CT scanning of the thoracic aorta in trauma. The use of intraarterial digital subtraction angiography to detect great vessel injury is a promising alternative to conventional aortography but requires further clinical testing.[68]

Transesophageal echocardiography (TEE) is another new, exciting modality for the rapid diagnosis of a transected thoracic aorta in a multiple trauma patient. In one study of nontraumatic dissections, TEE correctly identified 93% of cases of thoracic aortic dissection compared with CT scan (54%) and angiography (75%).[69] However, controlled clinical studies will be needed to determine its efficacy in the trauma setting.

Intrathoracic Esophageal Injury

Injuries to the esophagus from external trauma are rare. Penetrating trauma accounts for the majority of external esophageal injuries. Traumatic damage has now superseded iatrogenic perforation as the most common cause of esophageal injury, secondary to the increased number of civilian gunshot injuries.[10] Esophageal injuries are often seen in association with tracheobronchial or great vessel injuries, due to the close proximity of these structures. Cervical esophageal injuries occur more frequently than intrathoracic esophageal injuries.[70] The overall mortality rate in esophageal trauma patients is 20% to 25% and is largely determined by associated injuries.[71]

The diagnosis of esophageal injury can be difficult to make, since other injuries sometimes obscure the clinical findings. Subtle signs such as a small pleural effusion, mediastinal air, or unexplained fever may alert one to the possibility of a thoracic esophageal injury. Any penetrating trauma in the vicinity of the esophagus requires careful evaluation to rule out a potentially devastating injury.

A high index of suspicion is necessary for detecting intrathoracic esophageal injuries. Controversy exists whether barium esophagogram, Gastrografin esophagogram, or esophagoscopy should be the "gold standard" to diagnose esophageal injury.[70–72] Each study has its own advocate, but most authors agree that the combination of esophagogram and esophagoscopy yields the highest sensitivity for nonoperative determination of esophageal injury. Surgical management is necessary once an esophageal injury is recognized, to prevent the sequelae of mediastinitis.

Tracheobronchial Injury

Although tracheobronchial trauma is considered rare, these injuries are being recognized more frequently because of improved prehospital care. Early airway control and rapid transport are crucial for the survival of patients with major airway injuries.

The cervical trachea is much more commonly injured than the intrathoracic trachea. Intrathoracic tracheal injuries usually result from penetrating trauma and often have associated injuries. Complete tracheal separation from blunt trauma results in an almost uniformly fatal outcome. Most of these patients die at the scene of the accident.

The physical and x-ray findings of both tracheal and bronchial injuries include cough, stridor, hemoptysis, dyspnea, mediastinal and cervical subcutaneous emphysema, and pneumothorax. Tension pneumothorax may also result from a tracheobronchial rupture.[73] A persistent high-volume air leak after tube thoracostomy suggests a tracheobronchial injury. Diagnosis of either injury is established by rigid or flexible bronchoscopy. Most bronchial injuries occur within 2 cm of the carina. Nonoperative treatment of distal bronchial tears is usually successful, but surgical intervention is required for all other tracheobronchial injuries.

OTHER THORACIC INJURIES

Diaphragmatic Injuries

Diaphragm injuries can be caused by blunt or penetrating forces. Penetrating wounds below the level of the nipples or scapular tips should alert the clinician to the possibility of a diaphragmatic injury with or without coexistent intraabdominal injuries. Diaphragm injuries from penetrating trauma occur equally between the right and left diaphragm.

Less than 5% of blunt multiple trauma victims have diaphragmatic injuries.[74,75] With blunt abdominal trauma, a sudden rise in the intra-abdominal pressure from external compression ruptures the diaphragm. The point of rupture is usually the left diaphragm (85%). The liver offers some protective effect to the right diaphragm. Diaphragmatic disruption can result in acute respiratory compromise from lung compression.

The diagnosis of an isolated diaphragm injury can be extremely difficult to make. There are no consistent physical findings that are pathognomonic for this injury. Decreased breath sounds on the involved side or the presence of bowel sounds within the chest may be noted. The initial chest x-ray may provide the first clue to a diaphragm injury (Fig. 76-8). A hazy diaphragm contour, abnormal diaphragmatic elevation, coiling of the nasogastric tube behind the cardiac shadow, or bowel gas patterns within the lung fields are seen preoperatively in only 62% of these patients.[76] In another study, 50% of diaphragm injuries were first diagnosed at thoracotomy or laparotomy.[77] CT scan has not proven useful for identification of diaphragm injuries. Occasionally, gastrointestinal contrast studies are employed to outline abnormal bowel patterns within the chest. Feliciano et al. recommended that, whenever a chest tube is inserted in the trauma patient, the diaphragm should be examined for injuries with the operator's index finger.[78]

Delayed diagnosis of a diaphragm injury is not uncommon.[78,79] Serial chest radiographs occasionally reveal a missed diaphragm injury. Once a diaphragm injury is suspected, operative intervention is necessary to prevent pulmonary compromise or bowel strangulation.

Traumatic Asphyxia

Traumatic asphyxia results from severe blunt compressive forces exerted on the chest. The exact etiology of traumatic asphyxia remains unclear, but it is thought to occur from the sudden expulsion of blood from the right ventricle.[80,81] In addition, a closed glottis at the time of impact appears to be an important factor in this condition. This sends blood

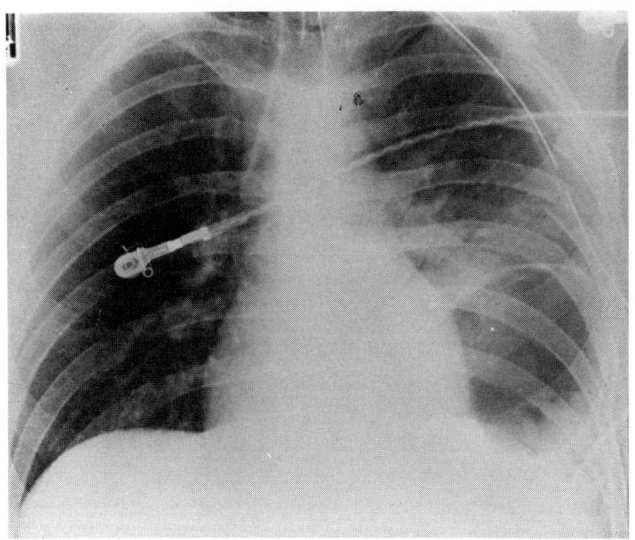

Figure 76-8 Left diaphragm rupture with stomach and spleen found in left pleural space at laparotomy.

rapidly into the valveless great veins of the head and face via the superior vena cava at very high pressures. Interestingly, there is only a slight increase in the inferior vena cava pressure. It is hypothesized that the inferior vena cava is compressed during a Valsalva maneuver, protecting the lower torso from elevated venous pressures and the complications of traumatic asphyxia.[82]

Capillary engorgement with bluish skin discoloration or compressive cyanosis is observed. Ecchymotic petechiae or punctate hemorrhages are seen in the conjunctivae and the mucous membranes of the mouth and throat. Pulmonary parenchymal injury can also be severe. Histologically, a massive pulmonary microembolism syndrome occurs, consisting of fat and bone-marrow embolism.[83] Hematuria, esophageal bleeding, brachial plexus, and spinal cord injury are associated sequelae. About 30% of patients with traumatic asphyxia suffer loss of consciousness, which usually resolves spontaneously within 48 hours.[84]

Despite the severity of the injury mechanism, patients who survive display no long-term disability.[85] Cyanosis, petechiae, swelling, and neurologic impairment are generally not permanent. Survival is usually associated with the severity of other associated injuries. Traumatic asphyxia is rarely an isolated injury.

TREATMENT INTERVENTIONS IN THORACIC TRAUMA

In the management of chest injuries, several procedures may be done in the emergency department setting. Every emergency physician who cares for trauma patients should be adept at these procedures.

Intubation

A selective approach for intubation should be applied for all trauma patients. Supplemental oxygen should be applied to any patient suffering from blunt or penetrating chest trauma, but endotracheal intubation should be done based on the patient's clinical status. At one time, it was felt that all patients suffering from multiple bilateral rib fractures, flail chest, or pulmonary contusion required endotracheal intubation and mechanical ventilation. It has been shown that the severity of the pulmonary injury, number of rib fractures, or age of the patient does not correlate with the need for intubation.[86]

Clinical evidence of respiratory failure, altered mental status, severe maxillofacial or cranial trauma, and obvious surgical intervention are all valid reasons for intubation and mechanical ventilation. Often, an intoxicated or combative patient requires intubation to continue expedient resuscitative efforts. If at all possible, nasal or "fully awake" intubations are to be avoided during a resuscitation. Controlled "rapid-sequence" oral intubation is currently the preferred method for intubation of the trauma patient.

Needle Thoracostomy

Immediate pleural space decompression is necessary for a suspected tension pneumothorax. This can be accomplished rapidly using a 14 gauge intravenous catheter. The catheter is inserted in the second intercostal space in the midclavicular line just superior to the rib. The catheter should remain in place, converting a tension pneumothorax into a simple pneumothorax, until formal tube thoracostomy is done. There is a 10% to 20% chance of causing a pneumothorax with needle thoracostomy in a patient who did not have a pneumothorax.[2]

Thoracostomy Tube Insertion

Thoracostomy tube insertion is done to decompress or drain the pleural space so lung re-expansion and improved ventilation can occur. If the clinical situation permits, tube thoracostomy insertion should be done in a sterile fashion. The site of tube insertion in trauma patients should be the fifth intercostal space along the midaxillary line. A local anesthetic agent is generously infiltrated to create a field block at the site of tube insertion. A 2 to 3 cm incision is made, which is large enough to insert an index finger. No soft tissue dissection is necessary; rather, a controlled puncture of the parietal pleura using a blunt Kelly clamp is done. Once the clamp has penetrated into the pleural space, the clamp is opened widely. Before the thoracostomy tube is inserted, a gloved index finger should be inserted to verify entrance into the pleural space. Any local adhesions can be detected, thereby preventing an inadvertent lung laceration secondary to tube placement. The integrity of the ipsilateral diaphragm may be examined with an index finger.[78] A 32 or 36 French thoracostomy tube should be used for adolescent or adult trauma victims. A larger tube permits rapid pleural space decompression and minimizes the chance of tube blockage. The thoracostomy tube can be guided through the soft-tissue track using a Kelly clamp placed on the tip of the tube. Once the last hole of the tube is within the pleural space, the tube is secured to the skin with 2-0 silk suture.

Complications of Tube Thoracostomy

If a careful method of thoracostomy tube insertion is followed, complications from tube insertion will be minimal. A trocar should never be used to insert a thoracostomy tube. Lung lacerations, cardiac impalement, and pulmonary vessel injuries have been reported with trocar thoracostomy tube insertion.

Two percent to 25% of patients who have an emergency tube thoracostomy develop some form of pulmonary infection.[87] Lack of strict sterile technique, long-term pleural intubation, and incomplete evacuation of hemothoraces will increase the rate of lung-related infections. Routine removal of all emergency thoracostomy tubes and replacement under strict sterile conditions are recommended following the initial resuscitation. The role of prophylactic antibiotics for thoracostomy tubes in blunt and penetrating thoracic trauma is still being debated.[88,89]

Pericardiocentesis/Subxiphoid Pericardial Window

Pericardiocentesis and subxiphoid pericardial window are performed to diagnose and decompress cardiac tamponade. These procedures do not definitively treat this condition. Thoracotomy or median sternotomy should be done promptly by a surgeon if cardiac tamponade is strongly suspected.

While some authors do not believe a role exists for pericardiocentesis in trauma care, the technique will be described in detail for academic purposes. To perform a pericardiocentesis, the xiphoid and subxiphoid area should be prepared in sterile fashion. ECG monitoring is required. A 35-mL syringe and a three-way stopcock are attached to an 18 gauge spinal needle or a 6-in over-the-needle catheter. An alligator clamp is fastened to the hub of the needle and is attached to an ECG chest lead. The skin is punctured with the needle and advanced at a 45° angle to the chest. The needle is directed slowly toward the tip of the left scapula. Any ECG changes during the procedure indicate that the epicardium has been in contact with the needle. When the pericardial sac is entered, blood or serous fluid will be aspirated with the syringe. At the completion of the aspiration, the three-way stopcock is turned off to the patient. The catheter may be left in place and secured to the chest wall for transport to the operating room.

By leaving a catheter in place, continued or repeated pericardial decompression can be performed.

A subxiphoid pericardial window can be performed under local anesthesia much like an open diagnostic peritoneal lavage. A vertical incision is made over the upper epigastrium and xiphoid. The pericardiophrenic membrane is found directly underneath the xiphoid. Two stay sutures are placed in this membrane. The membrane is carefully incised between the stay sutures. This allows direct visualization of the pericardial space. If blood or clot is found, a formal thoracotomy is done immediately.

Emergency Thoracotomy

Emergency thoracotomy is required in special circumstances during the initial assessment and resuscitation of a trauma patient. Four conditions may necessitate immediate thoracotomy[10,90,91]:

1. relief of cardiac tamponade
2. control of hemorrhage
3. control of air embolism
4. shock not responding to aggressive resuscitation

Immediate thoracotomy should be performed only by someone capable of dealing with any injury that could be found once the chest is opened.

A patient may arrive in the emergency department "in extremis" or in cardiac arrest secondary to penetrating or blunt trauma. Emergency thoracotomy has significantly higher successful outcomes for victims of penetrating thoracic trauma than for those of blunt truncal trauma.[92–97] Trauma patients who undergo more than 5 minutes of cardiopulmonary resuscitation prior to arrival at an emergency department do not survive, despite immediate resuscitative thoracotomy.

Emergency thoracotomy is done via a standard left anterolateral incision in the fifth intercostal space. The lung is retracted and the pericardium is opened vertically, anterior to the phrenic nerve. From this approach, tamponade decompression or open cardiac massage can be accomplished. Depending on the clinical situation, the descending aorta may be cross-clamped above the hiatus to improve cerebral perfusion and coronary artery filling. If air embolism is suspected, the ventricles and coronary arteries are aspirated. A left anterolateral incision can be extended across the midline or vertically up the midsternum to control intrathoracic bleeding.

CONCLUSION

Thoracic trauma is a common problem seen by all emergency care providers. As a result of improved prehospital care systems and air ambulances, more patients with life-threatening thoracic injuries are reaching hospital emergency departments alive. The majority of thoracic injuries can be treated nonoperatively, since urgent thoracotomy is required in less than 15% of thoracic injuries. By following a systematic approach for each trauma patient, the physician will recognize potentially lethal thoracic injuries early, will treat them promptly, and will not miss other less serious thoracic injuries.

REFERENCES

1. Shoemaker WC, Corley RD, Liu M, et al. Development and testing of a decision tree for blunt trauma. *Crit Care Med.* 1988;16:1199–1208.
2. Committee on Trauma, American College of Surgeons, Advanced Trauma Life Support Course. *Thoracic Trauma.* Chicago, Ill: American College of Surgeons; 1989:91–104.
3. Glinz W. Priorities in diagnosis and treatment of blunt chest injuries. *Injury.* 1986;17:318–321.
4. Pickard LP, Mattox KL. Thoracic trauma and indications for thoracotomy. In: Mattox KL, Moore EE, Feliciano DV, eds. *Trauma.* East Norwalk, Conn: Appleton & Lange; 1988: chap 22.
5. LoCicero J III, Mattox KL. Epidemiology of chest trauma. *Surg Clin North Am.* 1989;69:15–19.
6. Blair A. Major blunt chest trauma. *Curr Prob Surg.* May 1969;2–64.
7. Siemens R, Polk HC Jr, Gray LA Jr, Fulton RL. Indications for thoracotomy following penetrating thoracic injury. *J Trauma.* 1977;17:493–500.
8. Moore JB, Moore EE, Thompson JS. Abdominal injuries associated with penetrating trauma in the lower chest. *Am J Surg.* 1980;140:724–730.
9. Newman RJ, Jones IS. A prospective study of 413 consecutive car occupants with chest injuries. *J Trauma.* 1984;24:129–135.
10. Mulder DS, Shennib H, Angood P. Thoracic injuries. In: Maull KI, Cleveland HC, Strauch GO, Wolferth CC, eds. *Advances in Trauma.* 1986;1:193–216.
11. Richardson JD, McElvein RB, Trinkle JK. First rib fracture: a hallmark of severe trauma. *Ann Surg.* 1975;181:251–254.
12. Lazrove S, Harley DP, et al. Should all patients with first rib fracture undergo arteriography? *J Thorac Cardiovasc Surg.* 1982;83:532–537.
13. Phillips EH, Rogers WF, Gaspar MR. First rib fracture: incidence of vascular injury and indications for angiography. *Surgery.* 1981;89:42–47.
14. Shackford SR, Smith DE, Zarins CK, Rice CL, Virgilio RW. The management of flail chest: a comparison of ventilatory and nonventilatory treatment. *Am J Surg.* 1976;132:759–769.
15. Trinkle JK, Richardson JD, Franz JL, Grover FL, Arom KV, Holmstrom FM. Management of flail chest without mechanical ventilation. *Ann Thorac Surg.* 1975;19:355–363.
16. Miller HA, Taylor GA, Harrison AW, et al. Management of flail chest. *J Can Med Assoc.* 1983;129:1104–1107.
17. Schaal MA, Fischer RP, Perry JF Jr. The unchanged mortality of flail chest injuries. *J Trauma.* 1979;19:492–496.
18. Landercasper J, Cogbill TH, Lindesmith LA. Long-term disability after flail chest injury. *J Trauma.* 1984;24:410–414.
19. Fowler AW. Flexion-compression injury of the sternum. *J Bone Joint Surg [Br].* 1957;39B:487–497.
20. Jones HK, McBride GG, Mumby RC. Sternal fractures associated with spinal injury. *J Trauma.* 1989;29:360–364.
21. Rutherford RB, Campbell DN. Thoracic injuries. In: Zuidema GD, Rutherford RB, Ballinger WF, eds. *The Management of Trauma.* 4th ed. Philadelphia, Pa: WB Saunders Co; 1985: chap 13.
22. Wagner WB, Crawford WO Jr, Schimpf PP. Classification of parenchymal injuries of the lung. *Am J Roentgenol.* 1988;167:77–82.
23. Wagner RB, Jamieson PM. Pulmonary contusion: evaluation and classification by computed tomography. *Surg Clin North Am.* 1989;69:31–40.
24. Crawford WO Jr. Pulmonary injury in thoracic and nonthoracic trauma. *Radiol Clin North Am.* 1973;11:527.
25. Stevens E, Templeton AW. Traumatic nonpenetrating lung contusion. *Radiology.* 1965;85:247–252.
26. Hallgren RA. Management of patients with lung contusion. *Can J Surg.* 1978;21:523.
27. Karrel R, Shaffer MA, Franaszek JB. Emergency diagnosis, resuscitation, and treatment of acute penetrating cardiac trauma. *Ann Emerg Med.* 1982;11:504–517.
28. Ivatury RR, Rohman M. The injured heart, thoracic trauma. *Surg Clin North Am.* 1989;69:93–110.
29. Sugg WL, Rea WJ, Ecker RR, et al. Penetrating wounds of the heart: an analysis of 459 cases. *J Thorac Cardiovasc Surg.* 1968;56:531–543.
30. Garrison RN, Richardson JD, Fry D. Diagnostic transdiaphragmatic pericardiotomy in thoraco-abdominal trauma. *J Trauma.* 1982;22:147–149.
31. Arom KV, Richardson JD, Webb G, et al. Subxiphoid pericardial window in patients with suspected traumatic pericardial tamponade. *Ann Thorac Surg.* 1977;23:545.
32. Moreno C, Moore EE, Majure JA, Hopeman AR. Pericardial tamponade: a critical determinant for survival following penetrating cardiac wounds. *J Trauma.* 1986;26:821–825.
33. Baker CC, Thomas AN, Trunkey DD. The role of emergency thoracotomy in trauma. *J Trauma.* 1980;20:848–854.
34. Demetriades D, VanderVeen PW. Penetrating injuries of the heart: experience over two years in South America. *J Trauma.* 1983;23:1034–1041.
35. Siemens R, Polk HC Jr, Gray LA Jr, Fulton RL. Indications for thoracotomy following penetrating thoracic injury. *J Trauma.* 1977;17:493–500.
36. Mandal AK, Oparah SS. Unusually low mortality of penetrating wounds of the chest—twelve years experience. *J Thorac Cardiovasc Surg.* 1989;97:119–125.
37. Kish G, Kozloff L, Joseph WL, Adkins PC. Indications for early thoracotomy in the management of chest trauma. *Ann Thorac Surg.* 1976;22:23–28.
38. Beall AC, Crosthwalt RW, Crawford ES, DeBakey ME. Gunshot wounds of the chest: a plea for individualization. *J Trauma.* 1964;4:382–388.
39. Lasky II, Nahum AM, Siegel AW. Cardiac injuries incurred by drivers in automobile accidents. *J Forensic Sci.* 1969;14:13–33.
40. Sigler LH. Traumatic injury to the heart—incidence of its occurrence in forty-two cases of severe accidental bodily injury. *Am Heart J.* 1945;30:459–478.
41. Beggs CW, Helling TS, Evans LL, Hays LV, Kennedy FR, Crouse LJ. Early evaluation of cardiac injury by two-dimensional echocardiography in patients suffering blunt chest trauma. *Ann Emerg Med.* 1987;16:542–545.
42. Tenzer ML. The spectrum of myocardial contusion: a review. *J Trauma.* 1985;25:620–627.

43. Hiatt JR, Yeatman LA Jr, Child JS. The value of echocardiography in blunt chest trauma. *J Trauma.* 1988;28:914–922.
44. Frazee RC, Mucha P Jr, Farnell MB, Miller FA Jr. Objective evaluation of blunt cardiac trauma. *J Trauma.* 1986;26:510–520.
45. Rothstein RJ. Myocardial contusion. *JAMA.* 1983;250:2189–2191.
46. Timberlake GA, McSwain NE Jr. Thromboembolism as a complication of myocardial contusion: a new capricious syndrome. *J Trauma.* 1988; 28:535–540.
47. Ferre GA, Stewart WD. Cardiac contusion. *Clin Orthop.* 1967;53: 123–130.
48. Jackson DH, Murphy GW. Nonpenetrating cardiac trauma. *Mod Concepts Cardiovasc Dis.* 1976;55:123–128.
49. Pomerantz M, Delgado F, Eiseman B. Unsuspected depressed cardiac output following blunt thoracic or abdominal trauma. *Surgery.* 1971;7: 865–871.
50. Calhoon JH, Hoffmann TH, Trinkle JK, Harman PK, Grover FL. Management of blunt rupture of the heart. *J Trauma.* 1986;26: 495–502.
51. Gewertz B, O'Brien C, Kirsh MM. Use of the intraaortic balloon support for refractory low cardiac output in myocardial contusion. *J Trauma.* 1977;17:325–327.
52. Orlando R, Drezner AD. Intra-aortic balloon counterpulsation in blunt cardiac injury. *J Trauma.* 1983;23:424–427.
53. Flancbaum L, Wright J, Siegel JH. Emergency surgery in patients with post-traumatic myocardial contusion. *J Trauma.* 1986;26:795–803.
54. Fabian TC, Mangiante EC, Patterson CR, Payne LW, Issacson ML. Myocardial contusion in blunt trauma: clinical characteristics, means of diagnosis, and implications for patient management. *J Trauma.* 1988; 28:50–57.
55. Greendyke RM. Traumatic rupture of the aorta—special reference to automobile accidents. *JAMA.* 1966;195:527–530.
56. Parmley LF, Mattingly TW, Manion WC, Jahnke EJ Jr. Nonpenetrating traumatic injury of the aorta. *Circulation.* 1958;17:1086–1101.
57. Mattox KL, O'Gorman RB. Injury to the thoracic great vessels, In: Mattox KL, Moore EE, Feliciano DV, eds. *Trauma.* East Norwalk, Conn: Appleton & Lange; 1988:chap 27.
58. Griffith GL, Mattingly WT Jr, Todd EP. Current diagnosis and management of blunt thoracic aortic trauma. *J Ky Med Assoc.* 1981;79: 588.
59. Clarke CP, Brandt PW, Cole DS, Barrett-Boyes BG. Traumatic rupture of the thoracic aorta: diagnosis and treatment. *Br J Surg.* 1967;54: 353.
60. Sevitt S. The mechanisms of traumatic rupture of the thoracic aorta. *Br J Surg.* 1977;64:166–173.
61. Chimoshowski GE, et al. Complete transection of the thoracic aorta secondary to blunt trauma. *Ann Thorac Surg.* 1973;15:536.
62. Mirvis SE, Bidwell JK, Buddemeyer EU, Diaconis JN, Pais SO, Whitley JE. Imaging diagnosis of traumatic aortic rupture: a review and experience at a major trauma center. *Invest Radiol.* 1987;22: 187–196.
63. Kirsh MM, Behrendt DM, Orringer MB, et al. The treatment of acute traumatic rupture of the aorta: a ten-year experience. *Ann Surg.* 1976; 184:308–316.
64. Fox S, Pierce WS, Waldhausen JA. Acute hypertension: its significance in traumatic aortic rupture. *J Thorac Cardiovasc Surg.* 1979;77: 622–625.
65. Woodring JH, Dillon ML. Radiographic manifestations of mediastinal hemorrhage from blunt chest trauma. *Ann Thorac Surg.* 1984;37: 171–178.
66. Gundry SR, Williams S, Burney RE, Cho KJ, MacKenzie JR. Indications for aortography in blunt thoracic trauma: a reassessment. *J Trauma.* 1982;22:664–671.
67. Sandor F. Incidence and significance of traumatic mediastinal haematoma. *Thorax.* 1967;22:43–62.
68. Mirvis SE, Pais SO, Gens DR. Thoracic aortic rupture: advantages of intraarterial digital subtraction angiography. *AJR Am J Roentgenol.* 1986;146:987–991.
69. Gussenhoven EJ, Taams MA, de Jong N, Bos E, Sutherland GR, Roelandt J. Transesophageal echo in the diagnosis of thoracic aortic pathology. *Circulation.* 1988;78(suppl 2):298. Abstract.
70. Glatterer MS Jr, Toon RS, Ellestad C, et al. Management of blunt and penetrating external esophageal trauma. *J Trauma.* 1985;25(8): 784–792.
71. Pate JW. Tracheobronchial and esophageal injuries, thoracic trauma. *Surg Clin North Am.* 1989;69:111–123.
72. DeFore WW Jr, Mattox KL, Hansen HA, Garcia-Rinaldi R, Beall AC Jr, DeBakey ME. Surgical management of penetrating injuries of the esophagus. *Am J Surg.* 1977;134:734–738.
73. Ramzy AI, Rodriguez A. Management of major tracheobronchial ruptures in patients with multiple system trauma. *J Trauma.* 1986;26: 682. Abstract.
74. Cox EF. Blunt abdominal trauma: a five year analysis of 870 patients requiring celiotomy. *Ann Surg.* 1984;199:467–475.
75. Rodriguez-Morales G, Rodriguez A, Shatney CH. Acute rupture of the diaphragm in blunt trauma: analysis of 60 patients. *J Trauma.* 1986; 26:438–444.
76. Christophi C. Diagnosis of traumatic diaphragmatic hernia: analysis of 63 cases. *World J Surg.* 1983;7:277–280.
77. Morgan AS, Flancbaum L, Esposito T, Cox EF. Blunt injury to the diaphragm: an analysis of 44 patients. *J Trauma.* 1986;26:565–568.
78. Feliciano DV, Cruse PA, Mattox KL, et al. Delayed diagnosis of injuries to the diaphragm after penetrating wounds. *J Trauma.* 1988; 28:1135–1144.
79. Hegarty MM, Bryer JV, Angorn IB, et al. Delayed presentation of traumatic diaphragmatic hernia. *Ann Surg.* 1978;188:229–233.
80. Jones MJ, James EC. The management of traumatic asphyxia: case report and literature review. *J Trauma.* 1976;16:235–238.
81. Haller AJ Jr, Donahoo JS. Traumatic asphyxia in children: pathophysiology and management. *J Trauma.* 1971;11:453–457.
82. Thompson AT Jr, Illescas FF, Chiu RC. Why is the lower torso protected in traumatic asphyxia? A new hypothesis. *Ann Thorac Surg.* 1989;47:247–249.
83. Hambeck W, Pueschel K. Death by railway accident: incidence of traumatic asphyxia. *J Trauma.* 1981;21:28–31.
84. Ectors P, Bosschaert T, Vincent G, Franken L. Traumatic asphyxia: an unusual case of traumatic coma and paraplegia—case report. *J Neurosurg.* 1979;51:375–378.
85. Landercasper J, Cogbill TH. Long-term follow-up after traumatic asphyxia. *J Trauma.* 1985;25:838–841.
86. Barone JE, Pizzi WF, Nealon TF, Richman H. Indications for intubation for blunt chest trauma. *J Trauma.* 1986;26:334–338.
87. Eddy AC, Luna GK, Copass M. Empyema thoracis in patients undergoing emergent closed tube thoracostomy for thoracic trauma. *Am J Surg.* 1989;157:494–497.
88. Lo Curto JJ Jr, Tischler CD, Swan KG, et al. Tube thoracostomy and trauma—antibiotics or not? *J Trauma.* 1986;26:1067–1072.
89. Stone HH, Symbas PN, Hooper CA. Cefamandole for prophylaxis against infection in closed tube thoracostomy. *J Trauma.* 1981;21: 975–977.

90. Mattox KL. Indications for thoracotomy: deciding to operate, thoracic trauma. *Surg Clin North Am*. 1989;69:47–58.
91. Demetriades D, Rabinowitz B, Markides M. Indications for thoracotomy in stab injuries of the chest: a prospective study of 543 patients. *Br J Surg*. 1986;73:888–890.
92. Schwab CW, Adcock OT, Max MH. Emergency department thoracotomy (EDT): a 26-month experience using an agonal protocol. *Am Surg*. 1986;52:20–29.
93. Bodai BI, Smith JP, Blaisdell FW. The role of emergency thoracotomy in blunt trauma. *J Trauma*. 1982;22:487–490.
94. Baker CC, Thomas AN, Trunkey DD. The role of emergency room thoracotomy in trauma. *J Trauma*. 1980;20:848–855.
95. Deepak V, Simoni E, Tomlanovich M, et al. Resuscitative thoracotomy for trauma. *Crit Care Med*. 1983;11:226. Abstract.
96. Harnar TJ, Oreskovich MR, Copass MK, et al. Role of emergency thoracotomy in the resuscitation of moribund trauma victims: 100 consecutive cases. *Am J Surg*. 1981;142:96–99.
97. Moore EE, Moore JB, Galloway AC, et al. Post injury thoracotomy in the emergency department: a critical evaluation. *Surgery*. 1979;86:590–598.

77. Common Genitourinary Emergencies

ALEXANDER D. VARGAS, MD, FACS, FRCPC

INJURIES TO THE KIDNEY

Although the kidneys are well protected in the retroperitoneum by the lower ribs, lumbar muscles, and the spine, traumatic injuries are seen frequently in an emergency environment. The etiology and the pathologic classification according to the extent of renal damage are important factors in determining the modality of treatment.

According to the etiology, renal injuries are classified into blunt and penetrating injuries. Blunt injuries most commonly are associated with sudden deceleration of the body. This mechanism usually occurs as a result of an automobile accident or a fall from a height. Direct blows to the abdomen or back may also involve the kidney directly. Penetrating injuries are seen as a result of external violence and usually are caused by gunshot wounds or stab wounds with the point of entrance through the abdomen, flank, or back.

According to the extent of damage, renal injuries may be classified pathologically as follows (Fig. 77-1). In contusions the renal capsule remains intact and the kidney shows ecchymosis and bruising. Occasionally, a subcapsular hematoma develops. Lacerations occur when the renal capsule is torn. The parenchymal defect may be superficial or, on occasion, deep and may involve the calyceal system, resulting in urinary extravasation. Lacerations may be multiple and severe with involvement of the entire kidney. In these cases, the pathologic event is called a shattered kidney. In pedicle injuries the renal artery or vein could be involved as a result of direct injury or, as happens in blunt renal injuries, in the form of an arterial intimal tear, with subsequent formation of a thrombus. Intimal tears occur as a result of sudden deceleration and stretching of the renal artery.

Following a renal injury, varying degrees of intrarenal or extrarenal bleeding may occur. Intrarenal bleeding presents as a subcapsular hematoma or as hematuria. Extrarenal bleeding results in a perirenal hematoma that usually is limited by Gerota's fascia. If the calyceal system is involved, extravasation of urine occurs, resulting in the formation of a urinoma. On rare occasions, a penetrating injury may present as a urinary cutaneous fistula.

Blunt Renal Injuries

Blunt renal injuries are most often sustained in automobile accidents, followed by falls, fighting, football, and crushing and swinging accidents.[1] A review of 252 cases of blunt renal injuries at the Los Angeles County–USC Medical Center revealed that associated injuries were found in 44% of the patients. The viscera most commonly injured were the spleen, liver, and lung.

Clinical Manifestations

Hematuria usually alerts the physician to suspect a renal injury. This sign is found in more than 95% of patients.[1,2] At the Los Angeles County–USC Medical Center, 67% of

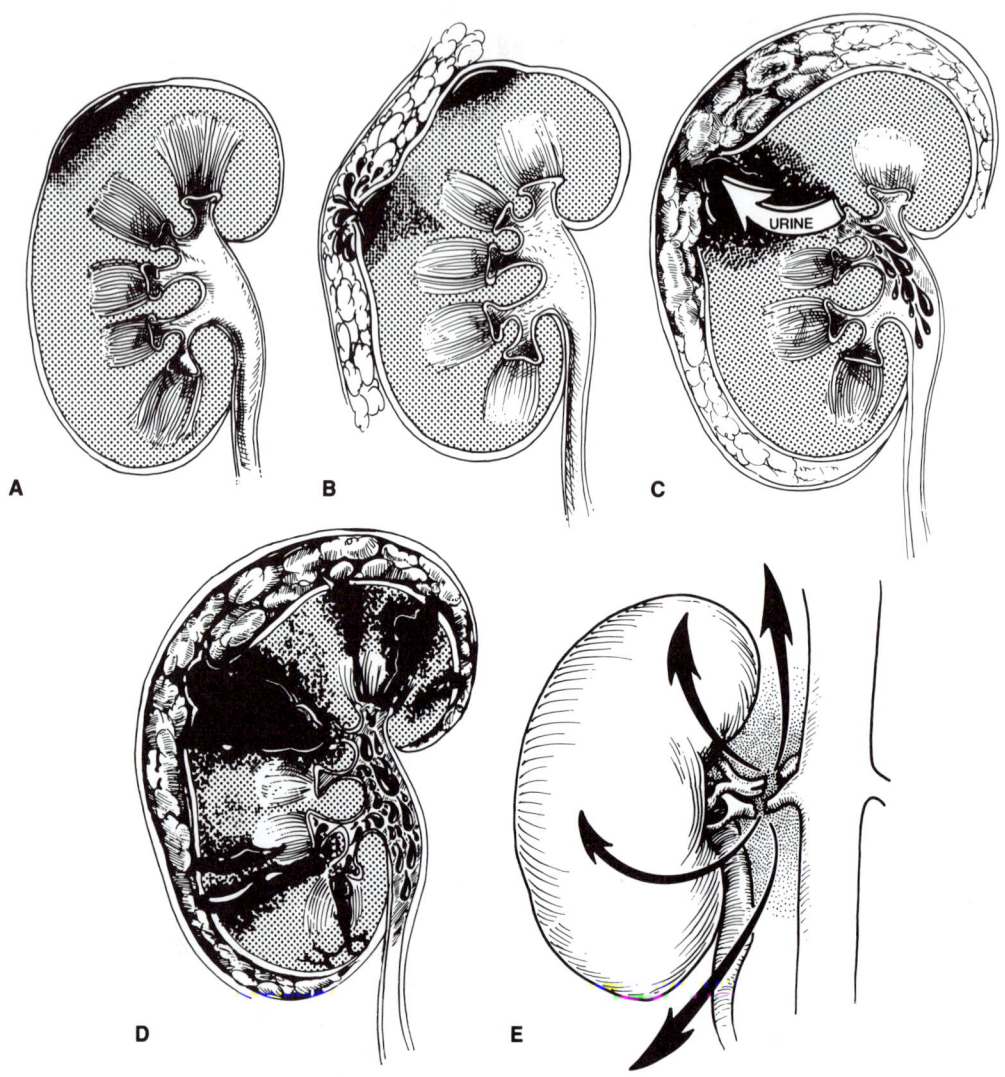

Figure 77-1 Classification of renal injuries. *Note:* **A**, contusion; **B**, superficial laceration; **C**, deep laceration; **D**, shattered kidney; **E**, pedicle injury.

patients presented with gross hematuria and 32% with a microscopic hematuria.

The history surrounding the circumstances of the accident should be thoroughly assessed, taking into consideration the magnitude and characteristics of the accident. The vast majority of patients present with symptoms of flank pain, abdominal pain, or a palpable mass (Table 77-1).

The physical examination most commonly reveals flank or costovertebral pain. Ecchymosis of the flank area or the clinical evidence of a rib fracture may be found. Since abnormal kidneys are more susceptible to renal injuries, assessment of pre-existing renal lesions is important, particularly in the presence of minor trauma with disproportionate renal symptoms. The Los Angeles County–USC Medical Center series indicates an incidence of pre-existing lesions in 3% of the patients.

Radiographic Studies

After clinical stabilization, appropriate radiographic examinations are indicated in the search for associated injuries, particularly of the skull, chest, spine, ribs, and pelvis. If a renal injury is suspected, an excretory urogram should be performed.

Excretory Urography. The excretory urography should be performed by infusion technique or double-dose injection of contrast media. The urogram is abnormal in over 40% of the patients (Fig. 77-2). The most common findings are delayed visualization, extravasation of dye, and renal nonfunction (Table 77-2).

Renal Scan. A renal scan complements the excretory urogram and provides information about renal flow, renal

Table 77-1 Clinical Manifestations in 252 Patients with Blunt Renal Injuries

Symptom	No. Patients	Percent
Flank pain	160	63
Abdominal pain	88	35
Palpable mass	7	3
Gross hematuria	168	67
Microhematuria	80	32
Asymptomatic	4	2

Table 77-2 Results of Excretory Urography in 235 Patients with Blunt Renal Injuries

Result	No. Patients	Percent
Normal	125	53
Delayed excretion	35	15
Extravasation	27	11
Major	9	
Minor	18	
Nonvisualization	10	4
Pre-existing abnormal	8	3
Equivocal	30	13

function, and the existence of parenchymal defects. It is a noninvasive test that unfortunately lacks the detail obtained with renal angiography. It is the test of choice when the excretory urogram is normal or equivocal.

Aortography and Renal Angiography. Aortography and renal angiography without doubt constitute the most accurate test to disclose renal architecture (Fig. 77-3).[3] Since this method is relatively invasive, it is best indicated when the excretory urogram reveals a nonvisualizing kidney, extravasation, or delayed excretion or when there is severe bleeding.

Ultrasonography. Ultrasonography is simple, noninvasive, and of value when the urogram shows a nonvisualizing kidney to assess the presence of a kidney. It may also be extremely helpful to evaluate the extent and course of a retroperitoneal collection.

Retrograde Urography. Retrograde urography is seldom indicated unless a ureteral injury is strongly suspected.

Computed Tomography. Utilizing high-resolution techniques, computed tomography (CT) may reveal lesions not identified by the previously discussed diagnostic tests.

Management

Based on the clinical and radiographic findings, blunt renal injuries may present as a contusion, laceration, shattered kidney, or pedicle injury (Table 77-3). The accurate anatomic definition of the injury dictates the most appropriate treatment.

The vast majority of blunt renal injuries are amenable to conservative treatment. In fact, 88% of the 252 blunt renal injuries reviewed at the Los Angeles County–USC Medical

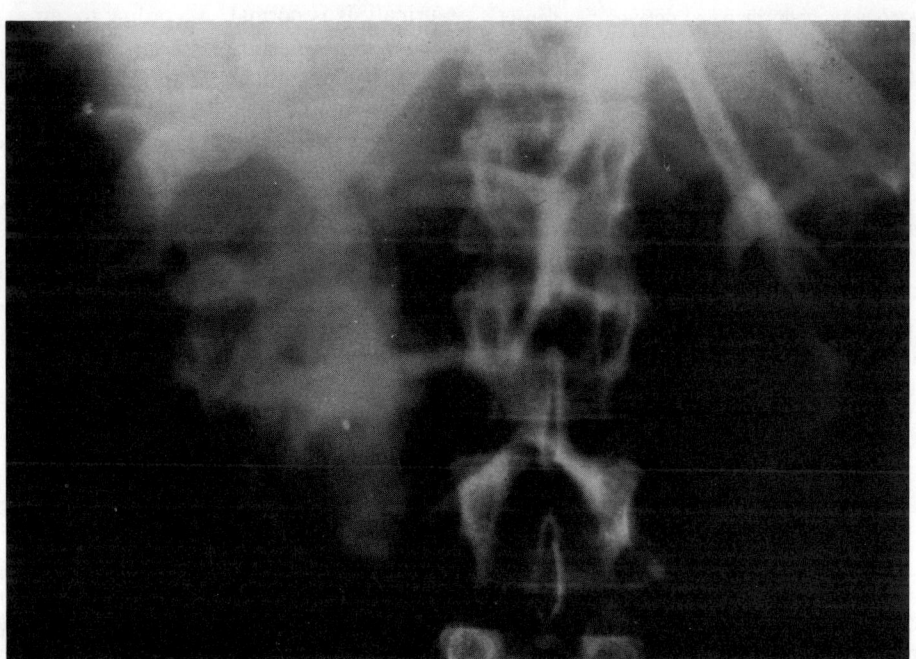

Figure 77-2 Intravenous urogram. *Note:* Extravasation of urine is present on right kidney following blunt trauma.

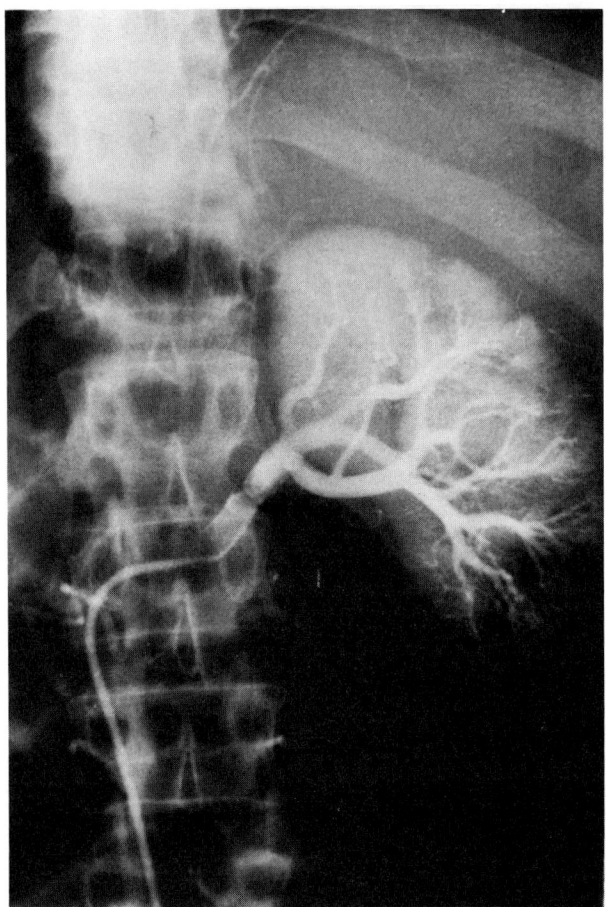

Figure 77-3 Selective angiogram of kidney. *Note:* Arterial injury in the form of an intimal tear of the main renal artery is evident. An intravenous urogram revealed delayed function of the kidney.

Center were treated conservatively. The management will depend on the radiographic evaluation and the clinical condition of the patient.

Medical treatment is based on observation, bed rest until gross hematuria has resolved, and analgesia. Renal exploration is indicated in the following situations: pedicle injuries, extensive parenchymal damage (shattered kidneys), severe recurrent hematuria and/or progressive perirenal hemorrhage, severe urinary extravasation, and expanding hematoma found at the time of laparotomy for associated visceral injuries. If surgical exploration is indicated, mobilization of the kidney should be performed only after the renal pedicle is secured with vascular clamps to prevent renal bleeding that could lead to an unnecessary nephrectomy.[4] After discharge, periodic follow-up is necessary for several months.

Penetrating Renal Injuries

Penetrating renal injuries are usually caused by gunshot or stab wounds. Injuries to the kidney are found in 8% of patients with gunshot wounds and in 6% of patients with stab wounds to the abdomen in large series.[5]

Associated injuries are seen with higher incidence as compared with blunt renal injuries. At the Los Angeles County–USC Medical Center, 94% of 148 patients with penetrating renal injuries had an associated visceral injury.

The injuries caused by gunshot wounds are in direct proportion to the velocity of the missile and also are related to the position and distance of the assailant.[6] On occasion, the bullet is deflected after hitting a bony structure.

Clinical Manifestations

In penetrating renal injuries, the symptoms are usually related to associated intra-abdominal injuries. In the vast majority of patients, there is abdominal or flank pain. It is important to assess the characteristics surrounding the trauma, the relative position of the assailant, and the type of weapon used.

Hematuria may be present and is suggestive of renal or ureteral injury. However, in a significant number of cases urinalysis is normal. According to our experience with 148 cases of penetrating renal injuries, hematuria was absent in 14% of the patients. Other investigators have encountered even a higher incidence of false-negative results of urinalysis.[4] The physician should keep a high index of suspicion when a patient has a penetrating abdominal injury and, if clinically advisable, an excretory urogram should be obtained in all cases of suggested renal injuries.

Initial physical examination will reveal a small entrance wound (and sometimes, a larger exit wound). Generalized abdominal tenderness with or without peritoneal signs is usually present.

Radiographic Studies

After a thorough general evaluation of the patient and after stabilizing the clinical conditions, pertinent radiographic studies are needed.

Excretory Urography. Excretory urography in penetrating renal injuries has a limited accuracy. At the Los Angeles County–USC Medical Center, a false-negative excretory urogram occurs in 40% of patients. Therefore, a normal urogram occasionally may give a false sense of security to

Table 77-3 Types of Renal Injury in 252 Patients with Blunt Trauma

Injury	No. Patients	Percent
Contusions	197	78
Major lacerations	23	9
Minor lacerations	13	5
Shattered kidneys	10	4
Pedicle injuries	9	3

Table 77-4 Results of Excretory Urography in 101 Patients with Penetrating Renal Injuries

Result	No. Patients	Percent
Normal	29	29
Delayed excretion	9	9
Extravasation	14	14
Nonvisualization	6	6
Equivocal	43	42

the surgeon. The excretory urogram findings in this study are seen in Table 77-4. As in cases with blunt renal injuries, an infusion technique or a double-dose injection of contrast medium should be utilized.

Aortography and Renal Angiography. In these cases, as in blunt renal injuries, aortography and renal angiography will demonstrate the renal anatomy with accuracy. In fact, this is the best diagnostic tool available for a thorough assessment in penetrating renal injuries. Unfortunately, since the procedure is relatively invasive and many of these patients are in critical condition, often a surgical exploration to control serious bleeding cannot be delayed and time is not available to perform angiography (Fig. 77-4).

Renal Scan. Renal scanning is noninvasive and may be useful in cases when the excretory urogram is normal or equivocal.

Retrograde Urography. Retrograde urography is indicated only when a ureteral injury is suspected.

Computed Tomography. CT scanning may identify small lesions.

Management

The management of penetrating renal injuries remains controversial. Some investigators advocate surgical exploration in all cases,[4] and others claim that conservatism may lead to the same or even better long-term results.[7,8]

Unquestionably, renal exploration is indicated in serious lacerations, shattered kidneys, or pedicle involvement in an attempt to prevent immediate complications and to preserve renal parenchyma. An important consideration in the planning of management of penetrating renal injuries is the accurate definition of the extent and nature of the renal injury, which can be obtained by renal angiography. In general, stab wounds are more suitable for thorough radiographic evaluation and, in studies at the Los Angeles County–USC Medical Center, 59% of the angiograms were performed in these cases. The pathoanatomic findings in 148 cases treated at the Los Angeles County–USC Medical Center are shown in Table 77-5.

Superficial and moderately deep renal lacerations are successfully treated by conservative measures, provided that the

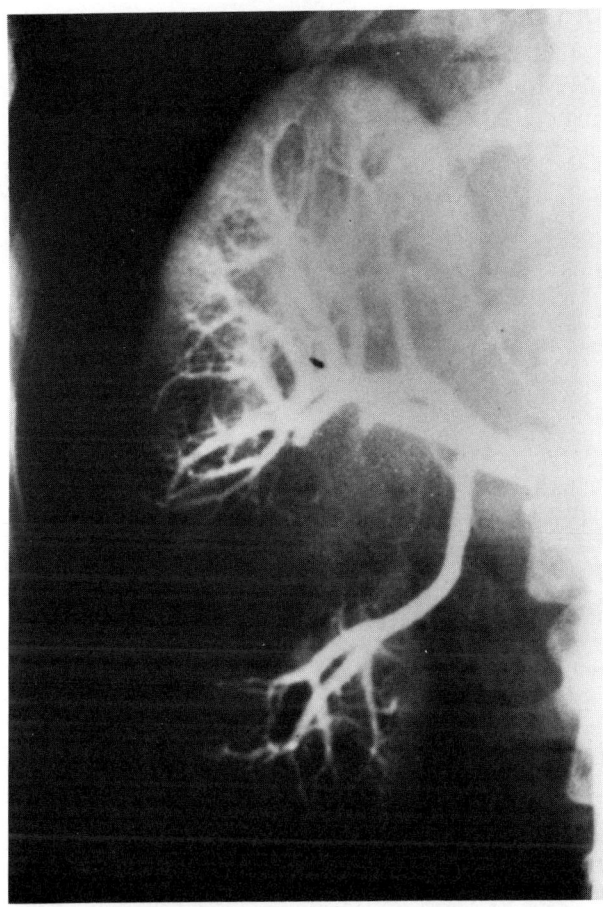

Figure 77-4 Selective angiogram of kidney. *Note:* Deep laceration of the kidney was caused by a gunshot wound.

clinical condition of the patient is stable, angiography indicates no serious vascular derangement, significant urinary extravasation is absent, and on surgical exploration (in a search for unrelated intra-abdominal lesions) the perinephric hematoma is not expanding.

As in blunt renal injuries, renal exploration should be performed after complete control of the renal pedicle to avoid unnecessary bleeding. Periodic follow-up is needed for several months.

Table 77-5 Types of Renal Injury According to Etiology in 148 Patients with Penetrating Trauma

Type of Injury	Gunshot Wound		Stab Wound	
	No. Patients	Percent	No. Patients	Percent
Contusions	4	5		
Lacerations	45	52	60	97
Shattered kidneys	21	24		
Pedicle injuries	16	19	2	3

INJURIES TO THE URETER

By virtue of its size, anatomic position, and relative mobility, the ureter is rarely damaged. When injuries do occur they may be classified as either traumatic or iatrogenic. Early diagnosis is the single most important parameter affecting the success of repair.

Traumatic Ureteral Injuries

The vast majority of traumatic ureteral injuries result from penetrating wounds to the abdomen or the flank. As seen in Table 77-6, results of a study at the Los Angeles County–USC Medical Center indicate that gunshot wounds are responsible for 90% of the cases; stab wounds, 7%; and blunt trauma, 3%. Published figures indicate that 3% to 17% of penetrating abdominal wounds result in ureteral injuries.[9] These injuries predominate in males and are frequently seen in young, active individuals. The proximal or midureter is involved more often in penetrating injuries. However, the distal ureter may be involved in lower abdominal gunshot wounds. Ureteral injuries that result from blunt trauma (fall from heights) occur at the ureteropelvic junction and are usually seen in children. In gunshot wounds the ureteral damage is in direct proportion to the velocity of the missile (blast effect).[6] According to this study, in gunshot wounds, associated visceral intra-abdominal injuries are found in over 90% of the patients. The organs usually involved are the large or small intestine, followed by the liver, large vessels, and pancreas. Stab wounds have a lower incidence of associated injuries, particularly if the entrance is through the flank (50%).

Iatrogenic Ureteral Injuries

The ureter may be injured during an abdominal or a retroperitoneal surgical procedure. However, the majority of injuries occur during pelvic procedures. Occasionally, the injury may be sustained during an endoscopic procedure (eg, catheterization, stone manipulation) (Table 77-6).

The incidence of ureteral injuries in benign gynecologic operations has been reported to be between 0.4% and 2.5%;[10,11] however, for radical pelvic operation it has been described with an incidence as high as 30%.[12] The lower third of the ureter is by far the most predominant portion involved in pelvic operations.

Diagnosis

According to the time at which the ureteral injury is recognized, the diagnosis may be described as occurring during an immediate or delayed period. It is of utmost importance to recognize a ureteral injury at the time of

Table 77-6 Etiology of 111 Ureteral Injuries

Etiology	No. Patients	Percent
Traumatic		
Gunshot wounds	53	90
Stab wounds	4	7
Blunt trauma	2	3
Total	59	100
Iatrogenic		
Ob-gyn procedures	35	67
Urologic procedures	12	23
Endoscopic	5	10
Open	7	13
General surgical procedures	5	10
Total	52	100

Table 77-7 Hematuria in 48 Immediately Recognized Penetrating Ureteral Injuries

Type	No. Patients	Percent
Gross hematuria	11	23
Microhematuria	15	31
None	22	46

presentation in cases of trauma or at the time of the surgical accident in iatrogenic injuries.

The physician should maintain a high level of suspicion in the presence of a gunshot wound or a stab wound to the abdomen or the back. In these cases, specific clinical manifestations are usually not identified in the immediate post-traumatic period, since they are often obscured by the signs and symptoms of other associated visceral injuries. Hematuria may be present and is helpful in making the diagnosis. However, in the author's experience hematuria was absent in 46% of the patients; therefore, a normal urinalysis may be misleading (Table 77-7).

A high-dose excretory urogram is the single most valuable diagnostic study, with an accuracy as high as 90%.[5] Unfortunately, a significant number of these cases remain undiagnosed, since an excretory urogram is not obtained before laparotomy (indicated for associated injuries). The surgeon should then make certain that a ureteral injury has not been sustained by directly visualizing the ureters at the operative field (Fig. 77-5). On occasion, a urine collection may be encountered, suggesting a ureteral compromise. If doubt exists, the intravenous injection of indigo carmine dye is a helpful maneuver to define urinary extravasation.

During a surgical procedure close to the retroperitoneum the ureter may be totally or partially transected, crushed, devascularized, or ligated. Since the ureter is mobile, small, and usually adherent to the posterior peritoneum, the surgeon must always keep a high index of suspicion, particularly when performing a difficult pelvic or abdominal operation.

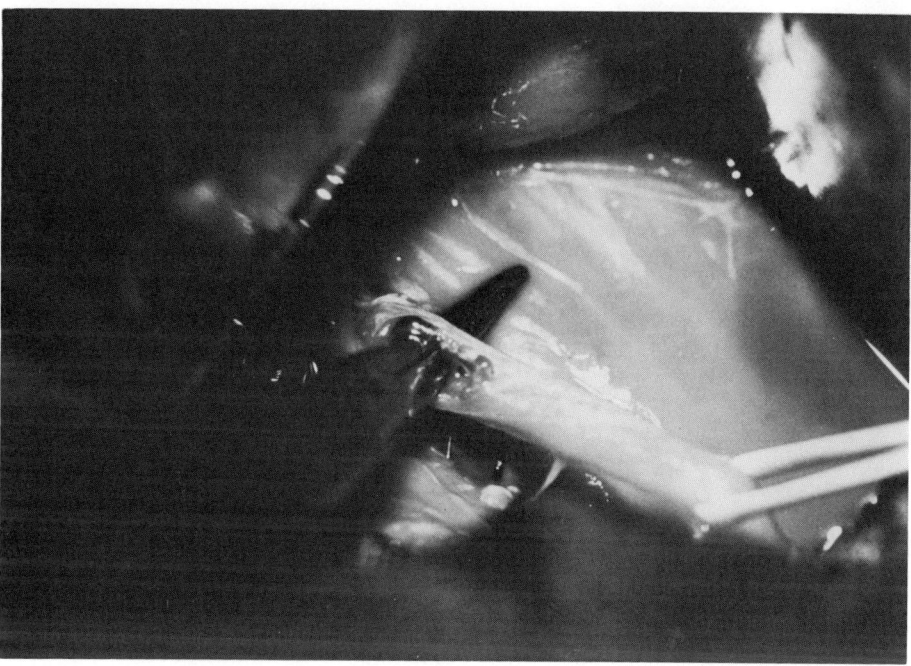

Figure 77-5 Ureteral injury due to gunshot wound.

Preventive measures should be taken if a difficult surgical procedure is anticipated. The placement of ureteral catheters preoperatively may help to prevent a ureteral injury. Undoubtedly, the identification of the ureter as it crosses the operative field is the most optimal preventive surgical maneuver.

The recognition of a significant number of ureteral injuries is delayed. For example, at the Los Angeles County–USC Medical Center the recognition of 19% of the traumatic injuries and 63% of the iatrogenic injuries is delayed (Table 77-8).

As opposed to immediately recognized injuries, the clinical manifestations are more specific in this group of patients, owing to hydronephrosis, tissue inflammation, infection, urinary extravasation, or fistula formation. The most prominent clinical manifestations are pain, fever, hematuria, and/or a palpable mass. A ureterocutaneous or ureterovaginal fistula occurs in a significant number of cases, the majority resulting from iatrogenic injuries (Table 77-9). The excretory urogram followed by a retrograde urogram usually confirms the diagnosis of ureteral injury in these cases.

Management

Once the ureteral injury is recognized, the surgical treatment depends on the location, extent, and type of injury. A meticulous surgical technique must be followed, with adequate debridement of damaged tissue and care to preserve the ureteral vascular supply. Simple maneuvers such as deliga-

Table 77-8 Immediate and Delayed Recognition of 111 Ureteral Injuries

Diagnosis	Traumatic		Iatrogenic	
	No. Patients	Percent	No. Patients	Percent
Immediate	48	81	19	37
Delayed	11	19	33	63

Table 77-9 Delayed Recognition of 44 Ureteral Injuries

Clinical Finding	No. Patients	Percent
Pain and fever	23	52
Ureterocutaneous fistula	8	18
Ureterovaginal fistula	7	16
Palpable mass	2	4.5
Hematuria	2	4.5
Hypertension	1	2
Asymptomatic	5	11

tion or catheter placement may be adequate in certain cases. However, a careful assessment of vascular ureteral supply should be made.

The preferred method of repair of lower third ureteral injuries is ureteroneocystostomy (Fig. 77-6). After adequate mobilization of the proximal ureter to gain sufficient ureteral length, an antireflux subcutaneous tunnel should be

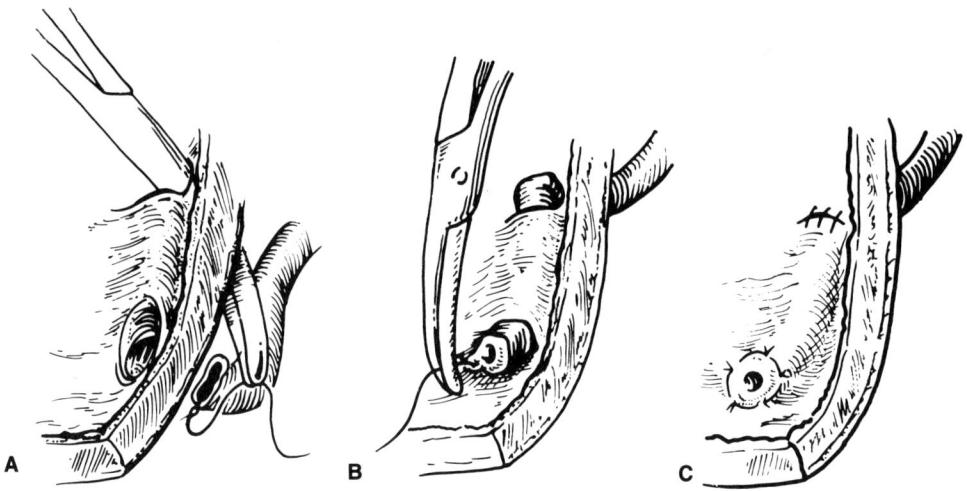

Figure 77-6 Ureteroneocystostomy.

obtained. If an adequate length cannot be obtained, a psoas hitch may be performed.[13] On occasion, a simple end-to-side anastomosis can be safely performed. A Boari flap is an alternative that may successfully bridge a long lower ureteral defect (Fig. 77-7).[14]

An end-to-end ureteral anastomosis is the preferred method to treat injuries to the upper or middle third of the ureter. Adequate debridement, tension-free water-tight anastomosis, and adequate drainage of surrounding tissues are basic principles to be followed. A generous spatulation of the ureteral ends should be performed, and a stent is left indwelling for alignment and drainage (Fig. 77-8).

If a long segment of ureter is resected and an end-to-end anastomosis is not feasible, a transureteroureteral anastomosis, autotransplantation, a posterior vesicle flap, or an ileal ureter may be utilized.[13,15] Occasionally, a nephrectomy is the best alternative, particularly if the patient's clinical condition is less than optimal.

Excellent results are obtained after immediate repair of traumatic or iatrogenic injuries. In injuries in which recognition is delayed, the incidence of failure may be high after repair. At the Los Angeles County–USC Medical Center a failure rate of 20% in this group of patients (9 of 44 cases) has been noted.

INJURIES TO THE BLADDER

Injuries to the bladder are relatively infrequent, since the organ is well protected in the pelvic area. The diagnosis of bladder injury is easily made by radiographic methods; however, a high index of suspicion should be maintained by the physician who initially evaluates the patient. The bladder may be injured during a surgical procedure or by external trauma.

Iatrogenic Injuries

The bladder may be injured during pelvic surgery or urinary instrumentation. Surgical injuries occur more frequently during a difficult operation, particularly when the anatomy is distorted as a result of an inflammatory process, neoplasms, or previous surgery.

Traumatic Injuries

According to the extent of damage, these injuries may be classified into contusions, extraperitoneal rupture, or intraperitoneal rupture. Extraperitoneal rupture usually results from bony fragments penetrating into the vesical wall. Most commonly, this occurs as a result of a pelvic fracture (Fig. 77-9A). Intraperitoneal rupture is seen in patients sustaining a lower abdominal trauma while the bladder is distended with urine. Usually, the rupture occurs at the dome of the bladder and the urine flows freely into the abdominal cavity (Fig. 77-9B).

The most common causes of penetrating injuries to the bladder are gunshot wounds and stab wounds to the lower abdomen. The vast majority of these patients will present with associated intra-abdominal injuries. Small intestinal, rectal, or pelvic vascular structures are most often involved.

Clinical Manifestations

A history of a lower abdominal injury followed by lower abdominal pain and hematuria is usually suggestive of a urinary bladder injury. Hematuria is seen in the vast majority of patients, with an incidence as high as 94%.[16] A fractured pelvis is commonly associated with a bladder injury. If there has been a delay in diagnosis, peritoneal signs may be present.

Common Genitourinary Emergencies 1203

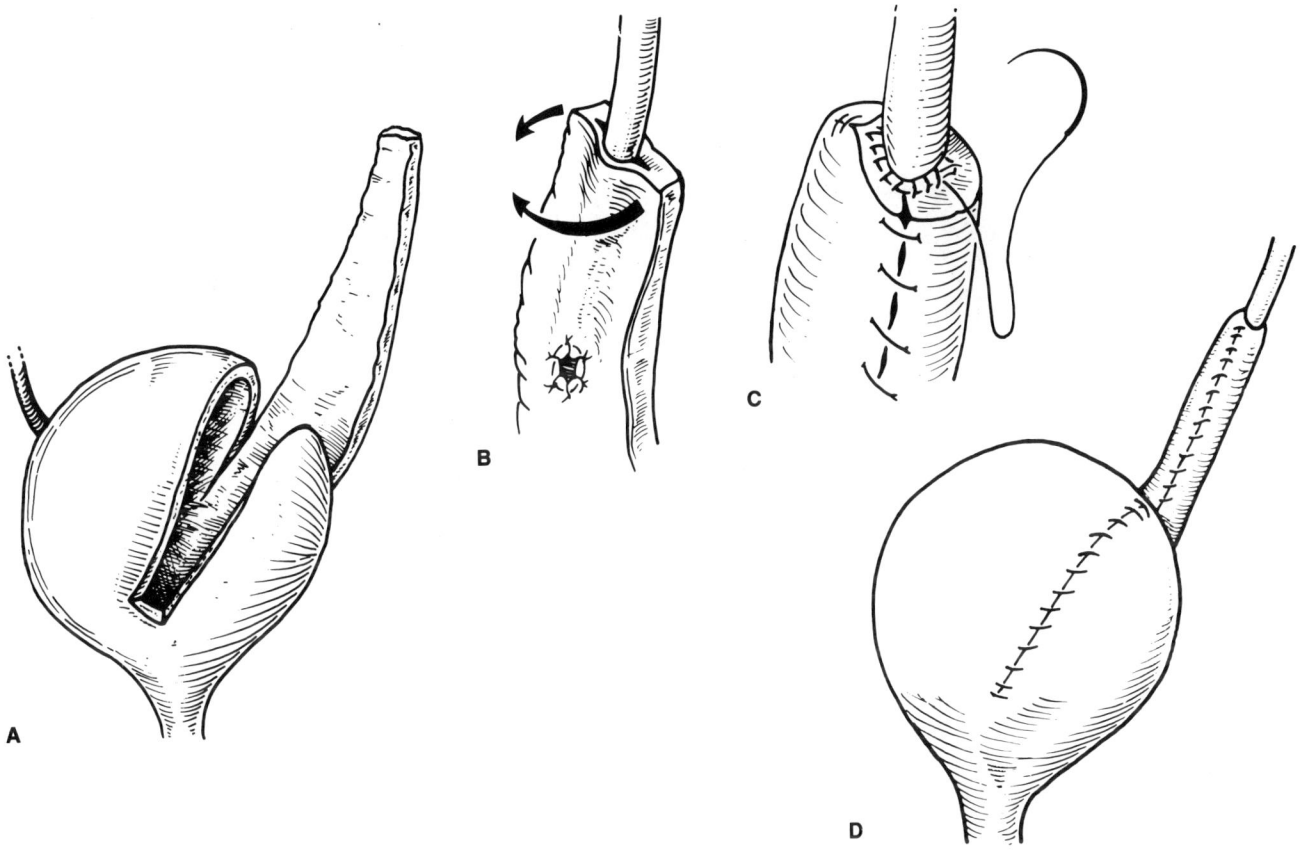

Figure 77-7 Use of Boari flap to repair ureteral injuries.

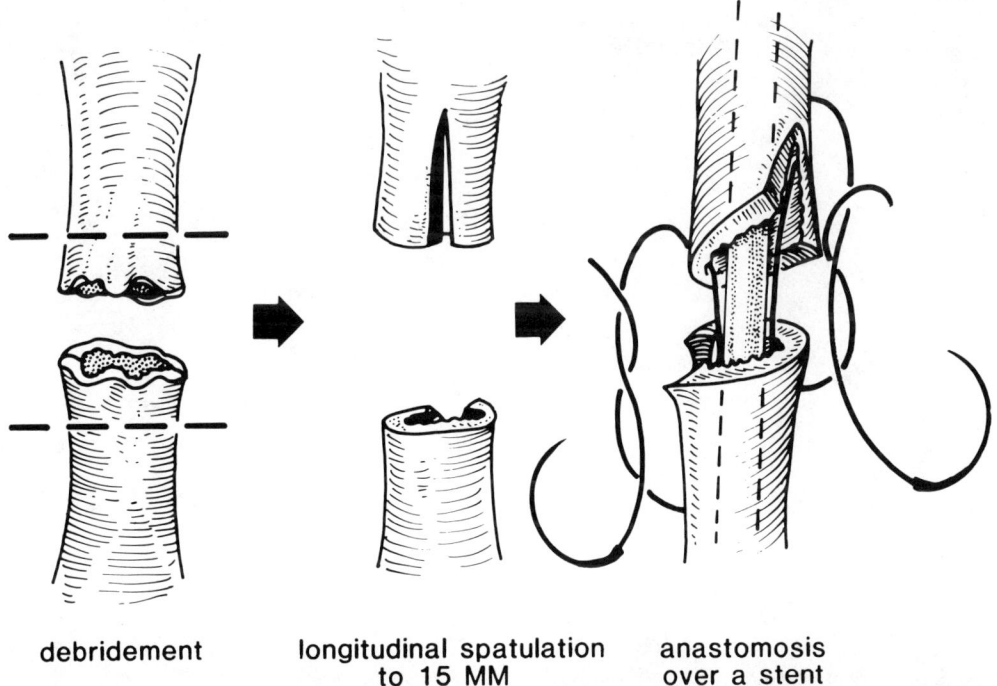

debridement → longitudinal spatulation to 15 MM → anastomosis over a stent

Figure 77-8 End-to-end ureteral anastomosis.

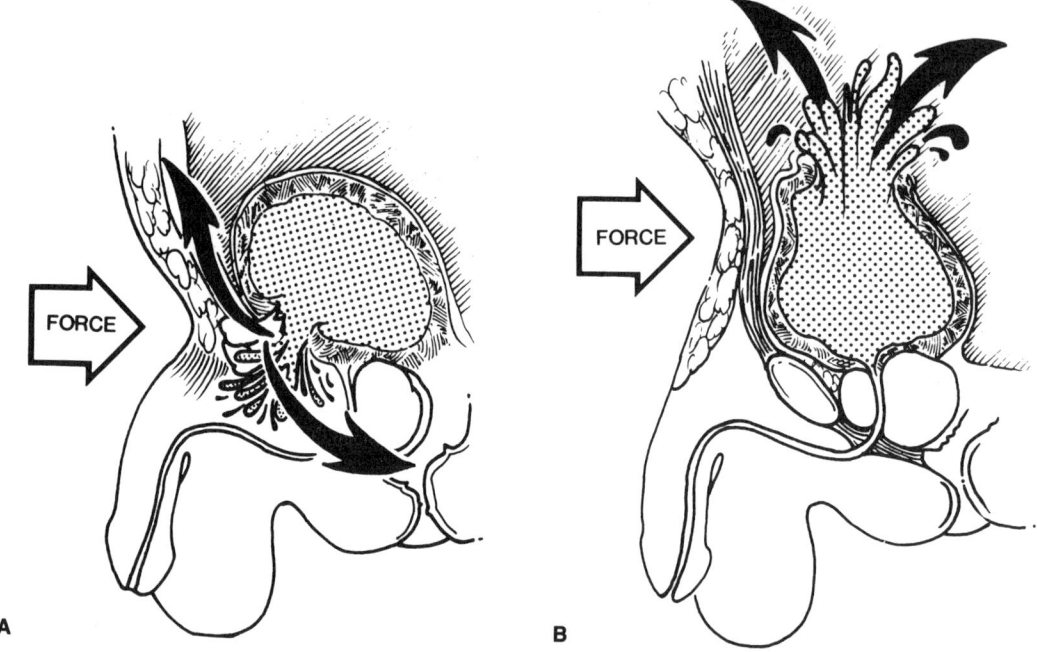

Figure 77-9 Rupture of the bladder. *Note:* **A**, extraperitoneal rupture; **B**, intraperitoneal rupture.

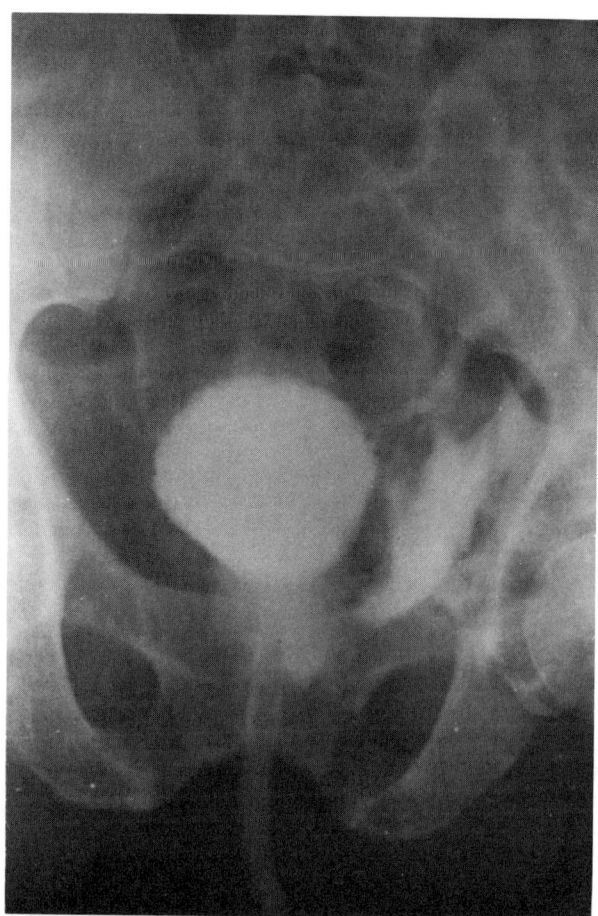

Figure 77-10 Cystogram showing extraperitoneal bladder rupture.

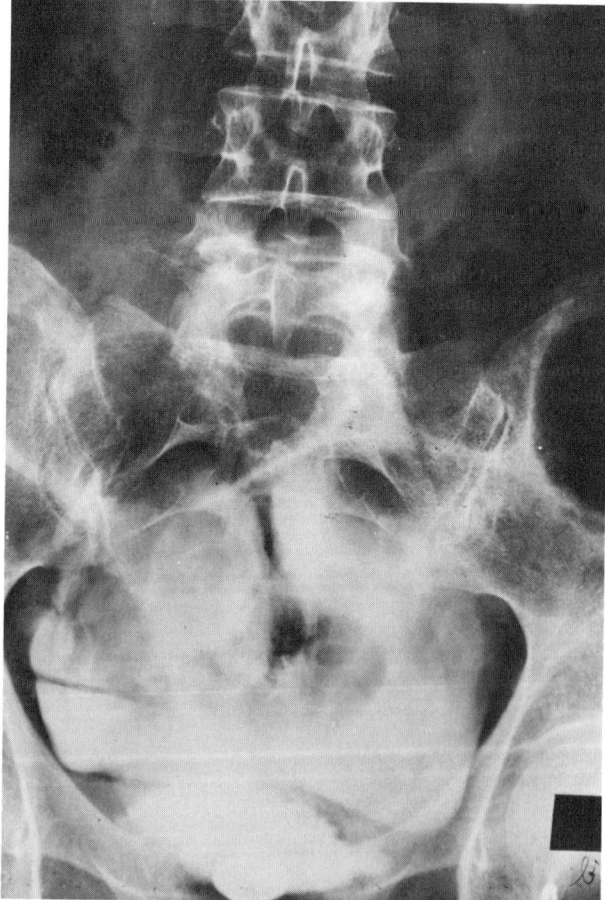

Figure 77-11 Cystogram showing intraperitoneal bladder rupture.

The majority of patients will not be able to urinate because of pain, neurologic disorders, or urinary extravasation. Physical examination may reveal tenderness in the suprapubic area. Ecchymosis of the adjacent skin may be found, and, on occasion, a suprapubic mass develops as a result of extravasation and bleeding.

Diagnosis

A plain roentgenogram may reveal fractures of the pelvic bones. Five percent to 10% of patients with a pelvic fracture will present with a ruptured bladder.[16,17]

A cystogram is the most reliable test to diagnose a bladder rupture. Anteroposterior and oblique views should be performed followed by a drainage film (Figs. 77-10 and 77-11).

When the pelvis is fractured, it is important to obtain a retrograde urethrogram before attempting urethral catheterization to rule out a urethral injury. In these cases, the passage of a catheter may convert a partial urethral laceration into a complete laceration.

Management

After adequate debridement of damaged tissue, immediate repair by anatomic layers with the use of absorbable sutures is the most widely accepted repair in bladder injuries. Bladder rest for 7 to 14 days is preferred by most surgeons, together with appropriate drainage of the perivesical space.

If associated injuries are suspected, it is advisable to explore the abdominal cavity throughout. A suprapubic cystostomy or a urethral catheter is used for vesical drainage. The former is best indicated in the presence of large lacerations and in male patients.

In selected cases, particularly in the presence of an extraperitoneal bladder rupture, the simple placement of a urethral catheter, without surgical exploration, may be utilized with good results.[18,19] At the Los Angeles County–USC Medical Center this approach is used only in small extraperitoneal tears with appropriate antibiotic coverage and judicious observation.

With prompt diagnosis and treatment the prognosis of these injuries is excellent, with minimal morbidity and mortality. However, if the treatment is delayed, a significant incidence of complication and mortality is expected.

INJURIES TO THE URETHRA

Injuries to the urethra are relatively rare. Prompt diagnosis and adequate initial treatment are essential to prevent severe sequelae. In a male patient the clinical implications and management vary with the site of the injury. For this purpose, a separate description of injuries occurring at the membranous urethra, bulbous urethra, and pendulous urethra will follow.

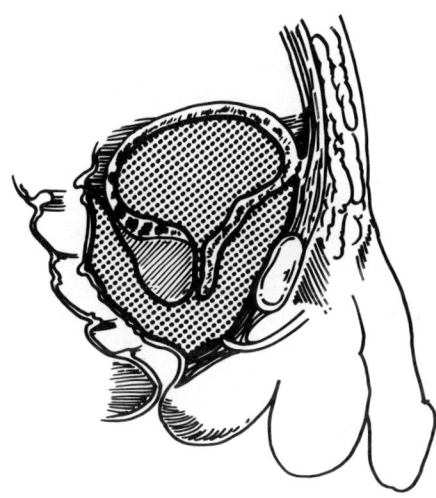

Figure 77-12 Membranous urethral disruption. *Note:* Hemorrhage is confined to the pelvis, above the genitourinary diaphragm.

Injuries to the Membranous Urethra

This type of injury usually presents in the form of a prostatomembranous disruption that is commonly associated with a pelvic fracture. The prostate is separated from its attachments to the genitourinary diaphragm. The laceration may be complete or incomplete. When a complete disruption occurs, the bladder and prostate are displaced upward and the defect is filled with blood clots and urine. Bony fragments may penetrate into the posterior urethra or bladder (Fig. 77-12). Injuries to the posterior urethra also may result from instrumentation, penetrating injuries (gunshot wounds or stab wounds), or iatrogenically during the course of an abdominoperineal rectal resection.

Clinical Manifestations

A history of a severe injury, usually the result of an automobile accident, is always obtained. There may be pain in the lower abdomen and in the perineum. Associated injuries are usually present, and the amount of hemorrhage at the level of the pelvis may be considerable. Urethral bleeding may be present and should alert the physician to the possibility of a urethral injury. The patient commonly is unable to urinate.

The physical examination usually reveals signs of urethral bleeding. There may be tenderness and/or a mass palpable in the suprapubic area due to extravasation, hematoma, or urinary retention. Rectal examination may reveal that the prostate is displaced upward, suggesting a complete prostatomembranous disruption.

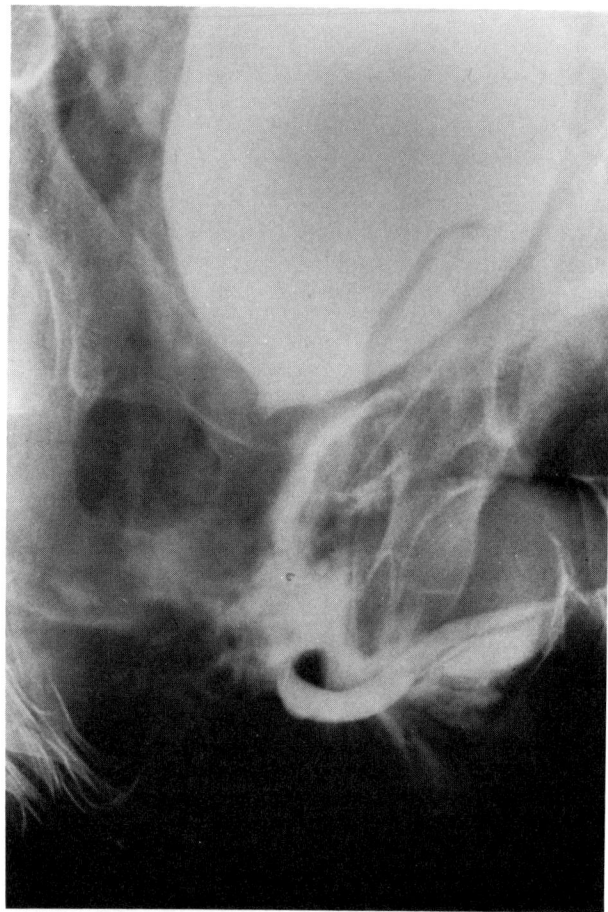

Figure 77-13 Retrograde urethrogram of membranous urethral injury. *Note:* Extensive extravasation of dye at the membranous urethra is shown in a patient with complete urethral disruption secondary to a pelvic procedure.

Management

If a urethral catheter of adequate size can be passed to the bladder, it usually indicates a minor partial laceration and should be left indwelling for 10 to 14 days. Frequently, a more serious laceration occurs and surgical intervention is necessary. Some investigators advocate suprapubic cystostomy for urinary diversion initially, with urethral reconstruction, if needed, performed at a later date.[20] Others advocate early urethral realignment with a perineal traction of the prostate.[21]

At the Los Angeles County–USC Medical Center, these injuries have been managed by the initial placement of a suprapubic cystostomy without attempting to enter the pelvic area. Only in the presence of minimal pelvic hematuria has urethral realignment been attempted 7 days after the injury. The most significant complication is urethral stricture, which may require periodic dilations or surgical correction.

Injuries to the Bulbous Urethra

Most commonly, bulbous urethral injuries result from perineal contusion by falling astride an object. The urethral laceration may be incomplete or complete, with the formation of a perineal hematoma and urinary extravasation. If Buck's fascia is disrupted, the extravasation will be limited only by Colles' fascia with spread to penis, scrotum, and abdominal wall (Fig. 77-14). Injuries to the bulbous urethra may also be caused by instrumentation or penetrating injuries and usually consist of partial tears.

Clinical Manifestations

The history of perineal trauma or instrumentation is usually present. Local pain and urethral bleeding are seen in the

Diagnosis

A pelvic fracture may be evident on a plain roentgenogram. If a urethral disruption is suspected, a retrograde urethrogram should be performed to confirm such diagnosis. Ten to 15 mL of diluted contrast medium is injected per urethra and usually shows extravasation (Fig. 77-13). The excretory urogram may show a tear-drop vesical deformity with upward displacement of the bladder in patients with complete disruption.

A note of caution is in order regarding urethral catheterization. A forceful catheter insertion may convert a partially lacerated urethra into a completely lacerated one. In these cases, if catheterization is advisable, it should be performed by a urologic surgeon under strict sterile conditions. If a catheter is passed to the bladder, it should be left indwelling and its position confirmed radiographically.

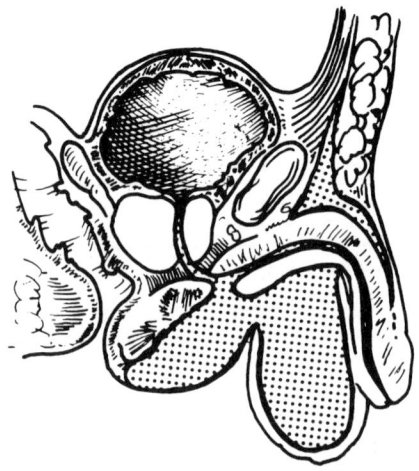

Figure 77-14 Bulbous urethral injury. *Note:* Hemorrhage is below the genitourinary diaphragm and limited by Colles' fascia.

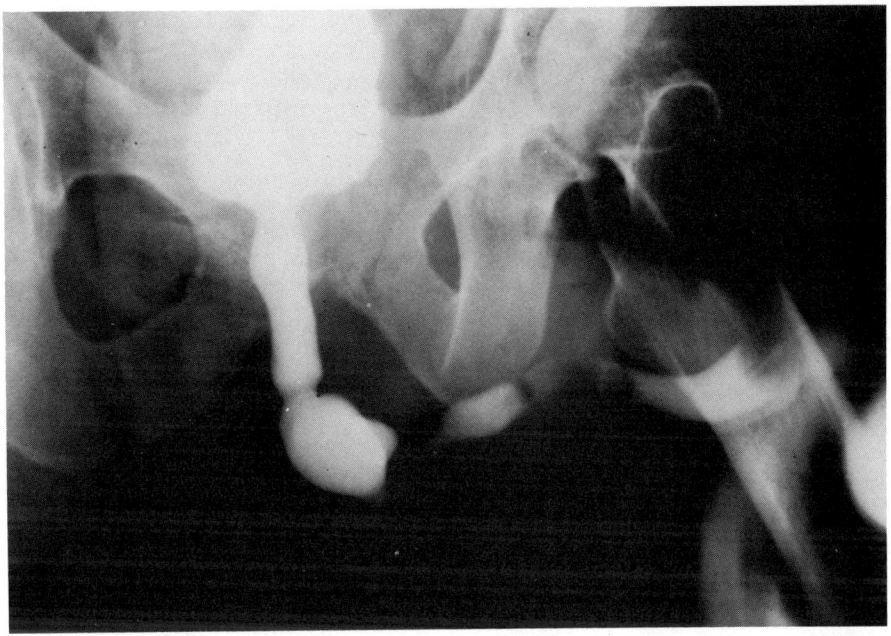

Figure 77-15 Retrograde urethrogram of bulbous urethral injury. *Note:* Bulbous urethra is completely blocked secondary to a straddle injury.

majority of patients. Most commonly, the patient is unable to urinate.

Physical examination reveals tenderness in the perineal region. Edema and extravasation may be palpable in the perineal, penile, or scrotal area or even in the lower abdominal wall. If seen late, signs of inflammation or infection may appear.

Diagnosis

As opposed to membranous urethral injuries, in bulbous urethral lacerations the hemorrhage and urinary extravasation are below the genitourinary diaphragm. The retrograde urethrogram will ascertain the diagnosis with accuracy, showing extravasation at the site of injury (Fig. 77-15).

Management

The initial management of bulbous urethral laceration depends on the extent of the injury. Caution should be used in the passage of a urethral catheter, since a partial injury may be converted into a complete tear. If a catheter is passed, this is left indwelling for 10 to 14 days to allow healing of the laceration. In cases of complete laceration, an end-to-end reanastomosis can be performed; however, the placement of a suprapubic cystostomy has been advocated by the majority of clinical investigators with successful results.[16,22] Subsequently, if a stricture develops, urethral reconstruction is planned several months later. If extensive extravasation is present, drainage of the periurethral area is indicated. This latter approach with the initial placement of a suprapubic cystostomy and urethral reconstruction at a later date if a stricture develops is favored.

Urethral stricture is the most serious complication. Antibiotic coverage may prevent a periurethral infection.

Injuries to the Pendulous Urethra

Most commonly, the pendulous urethra is injured by forceful traumatic instrumentation. Usually, this type of injury is sustained while passing a catheter or a sound in the presence of a stricture.

Penetrating wounds to the penile urethra are rare owing to the extreme mobility of the penis. On occasion, foreign bodies inserted into the urethra, usually for the purpose of masturbation, may injure the penile urethra. As a result, periurethral bleeding and urinary extravasation may occur.

Clinical Manifestations

Urethral bleeding is present in the majority of patients. Varying degrees of penile or scrotal swelling may be seen as a result of extravasation, and the patient may present with urinary retention.

Diagnosis

The diagnosis of an injury to the pendulous urethra is confirmed by a retrograde urethrogram.

Management

Minor mucosal lacerations may be managed conservatively without the passage of a urethral catheter if voiding is normal. A partial laceration may be treated with the passage of a urethral catheter. If significant extravasation occurs, it is advisable to drain the periurethral area. In the presence of a complete urethral rupture, immediate surgical repair with end-to-end anastomosis should be attempted. However, if the clinical conditions are critical, a suprapubic cystostomy should be placed, followed by a urethral reconstruction at a later date.

INJURIES TO THE EXTERNAL GENITALIA

Penile Injuries

Penile injuries are unusual due to the anatomic position and mobility of the penis. The skin, the urethra, or the erectile bodies may be injured.

The penis may be injured by blunt trauma, penetrating trauma, or strangulation. Blunt trauma may be sustained when the penis is flaccid and results in varying degrees of contusion. The most significant blunt injury occurs when the penis is erect and rupture of the corpora cavernosum or the urethra occurs.

Penetrating injuries to the penis may be superficial, with involvement of the skin and subcutaneous tissue, or deep, resulting in a laceration of the corpora cavernosum and/or the urethra. Extensive damage may occur when the genitalia are caught by large industrial machines.

Strangulation occurs as a result of ischemia caused by condoms, catheters, strings, or metal bands around the penis.

Clinical Manifestations

When the corpora cavernosum is fractured, a significant hematoma with associated local deformity is usually present. Occasionally, the urethra is lacerated, resulting in urinary extravasation. The skin commonly shows ecchymosis. On rare occasions, priapism may develop as a result of external trauma.

The extent of laceration will depend on the type of injury and the weapon involved. The urethra, corpora, and skin may be compromised. On rare occasions, the penis may be totally amputated, an event that is usually self-inflicted by mentally ill patients (Figs. 77-16 and 77-17).

Ischemia and necrosis are the complications that result from strangulation of the penis. A metal ring or a string, if found, should be removed immediately.

Management

Simple contusions are successfully treated by conservative measures. Rupture of the corpora cavernosum should be surgically repaired to prevent damage of the erectile function or a penile deformity.

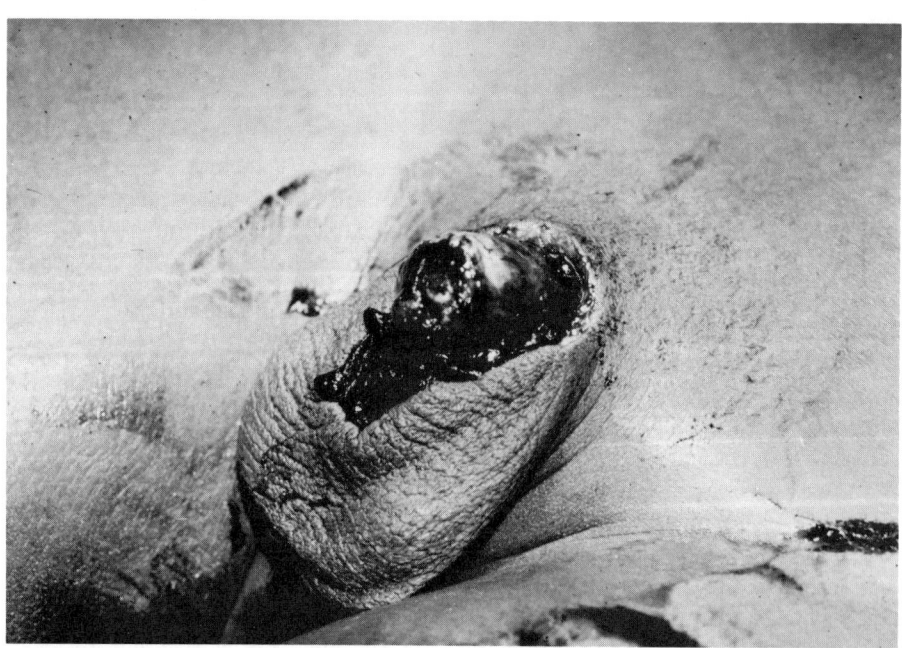

Figure 77-16 Traumatic amputation of the penis in a child.

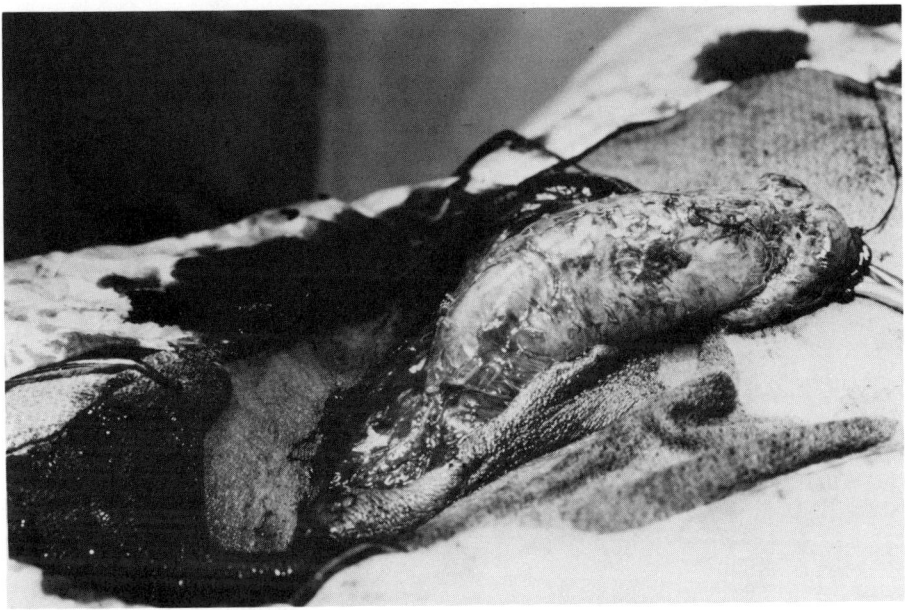

Figure 77-17 Self-inflicted lacerations of penile skin by a mentally ill patient.

In penetrating injuries, it is important to assess fully the extent of the injury. Each structure should be repaired individually, achieving complete hemostasis.

Avulsion of the penile skin may be treated with a split-thickness skin graft when the lesion is extensive. Small lacerations are simply closed with absorbable suture material. If the urethra is compromised, repair should be attempted immediately and a catheter left indwelling for 7 to 10 days.[23]

Complete amputation of the penis should be repaired by reanastomosis with the aid of microsurgical techniques. Successful reanastomosis has been achieved even after several hours of penile amputation.

In patients presenting with penile strangulation, the foreign body around the penis should be removed immediately. A metal band is best removed in the operating room with the patient under anesthesia.

Injuries to the Scrotum and Testicle

Injuries to the scrotum or testicle may be caused by penetrating injuries or blunt trauma. These injuries are uncommon, owing to the mobility and the anatomic position of the scrotum.

Clinical Manifestations

In penetrating injuries it is essential to determine the extent and deepness of the scrotal laceration. A scrotal hematoma is usually present, and if the tunica vaginalis is compromised a hematocele is formed. If the tunica albuginea of the testicle is compromised, seminiferous tubules may be seen extruding from the wound. Local pain associated with nausea and vomiting is common.

In blunt injuries severe pain associated with nausea and vomiting is usually present. The physical examination usually reveals swelling, localized pain, and a scrotal hematoma. The local inflammation and the hematoma formation usually depend on the severity of the injury. If the testicle is ruptured, a hematocele occurs (Fig. 77-18). If the clinical manifestations are disproportionate to the severity of the trauma, the physician should keep in mind the differential diagnosis of epididymitis or testicular torsion.

Management

In penetrating injuries, superficial lacerations are treated by simple skin closure. However, if the laceration is deep, with compromise of the dartos fascia and/or the tunica vaginalis, a thorough debridement, repair, and layered closure are necessary. If the testicle is ruptured, after thorough debridement, it should be repaired by closing the tunica albuginea.

In blunt injuries, prompt surgical exploration is necessary in most cases except if only minimal swelling and tenderness are present. Conservative treatment is based on scrotal elevation, ice packs, and rest for a few days. Scrotal exploration, however, prevents the chance of testicular loss and decreases the mobility to the patient. Extensive avulsions of the scrotal skin should be treated by transposition of the testis into a subcutaneous pouch in the thigh.[24]

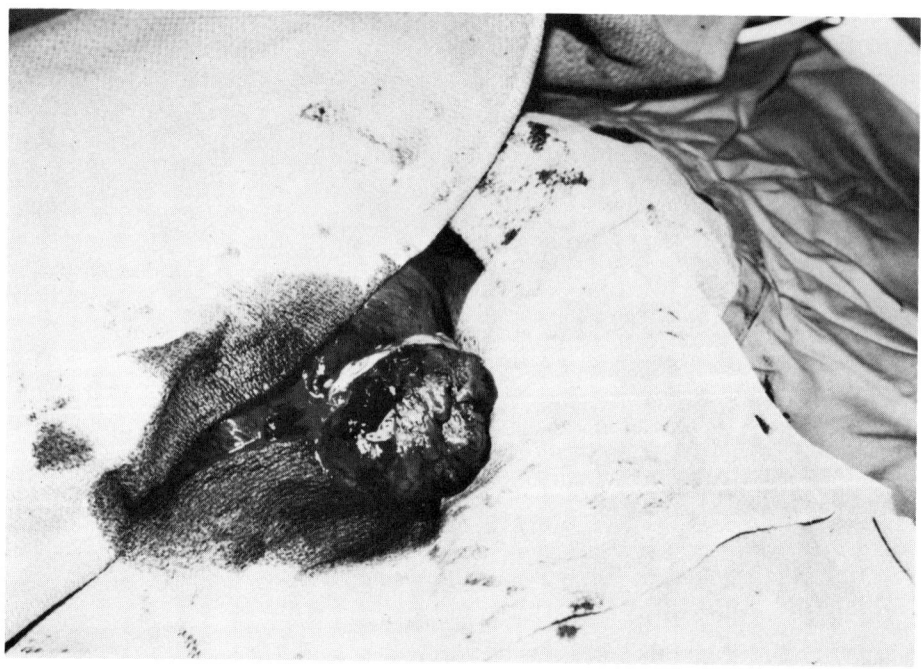

Figure 77-18 Testicular rupture secondary to blunt trauma. *Note:* Seminiferous tubules are seen protruding through the tunica albuginea of the testicle.

ACUTE FLANK PAIN

The emergency physician often sees patients with acute flank pain. In the majority of cases, flank pain is caused by a urinary problem. The pain is usually caused by renal disease or a ureteral obstruction. Renal pain is caused by sudden distention of the capsule that results from hydronephrosis, inflammation, or edema. Ureteral pain occurs as a result of capsular distention combined with periodic smooth muscle spasms.

Ureteral colic is the most common form of flank pain and results from a sudden ureteral obstruction with subsequent hyperperistalsis and smooth muscle spasms.[25] This form of colic is usually due to obstruction caused by a calculus. Ureteral colic may also be caused by hematuria with clots or papillary necrosis. Acute renal pain is caused by acute pyelonephritis, renal rupture, acute hydronephrosis, or an acute vascular disorder.

Clinical Manifestations and Differential Diagnosis

In ureteral colic the pain is usually severe and starts in the flank area, radiating to the lower abdominal quadrant following the course of the ureter. The pain is colicky with periods of relief. Nausea and vomiting may be present. On occasion, the physician may be able to ascertain the location of the obstruction by the characteristics of the pain. If the obstruction occurs in the upper ureter, the pain may radiate to the testicle in men or labia in women since the sensory nerve supply of the upper ureter follows a similar pathway (T11–12). If a stone is close to the bladder, vesical irritability may occur as a result of inflammation at the ureteral orifice.

Physical examination usually reveals pain localized to the costovertebral angle of the side involved. When calculi are present, the urinalysis may show microscopic hematuria and/or crystalluria. When infection occurs, pyuria is usually present. Gross hematuria is present when the etiology is the passage of clots. A flank mass may be palpable in patients with hydronephrosis or tumors. Papillary necrosis is caused by ischemic necrosis of the renal papilla. This disease may be caused by prolonged ingestion of analgesics, diabetes, sickle cell trait, or severe infections.

Patients with acute renal pain usually have constant and less sharp pain than the patient with typical ureteral colic. This pain often radiates along the subcostal area toward the umbilicus and occasionally to the lower abdomen. Sometimes it resembles ureteral colic, making the clinical diagnosis difficult.

Acute pyelonephritis is characterized by sudden flank pain associated with chills and fever. A history of urinary tract infection or ureterovesical reflux may be present. Infundibular obstruction may mimic ureteral colic inasmuch as a similar mechanism occurs with hyperperistalsis and muscle spasms. Intermittent hydronephrosis is usually the result of a congenital malformation causing obstruction at the level of the ureteral pelvic junction; it is usually caused by rapid diuresis. A perinephric abscess frequently originates from a pre-existing renal infection; the history of calculi or obstruction is usually present. On rare occasions a perinephric abscess occurs as a result of hematogenous spread. Spontaneous renal rupture occurs in the presence of pre-existing renal disease and usually is noted in association with hydronephrosis or renal cysts; a history of minor trauma is obtained frequently. Acute renal artery occlusion occurs usually in patients with a history of rheumatic heart disease, arterial fibrillation, or myocardial infarction or after cardiac catheterization. It results from embolic occlusion of the main artery or its branches. Acute renal vein thrombosis is a rare clinical entity that is seen in infants or adults. The most important causes are amyloidosis, perirenal disease, thrombophlebitis, and trauma.

Diagnosis

In the presence of obstruction an excretory urogram will show delayed excretion with a prominent nephrogram effect. A calcified calculus may be seen along the ureteral area; however, when the calculus is radiolucent, the diagnosis will mainly depend on the excretory or retrograde urogram (Fig. 77-19). If the kidney is nonfunctioning, a vascular lesion should be suspected; in these cases a retrograde urogram will show normal upper tracts. A vascular lesion can be confirmed by angiography or venography.

Retrograde urethrography is useful to define the renal architecture, particularly when the excretory urogram is nondiagnostic.

Management

Potent analgesics are usually needed to treat ureteral colic. Because of the magnitude of pain, meperidine (Demerol) or morphine sulfate are the preferred drugs. Proper hydration is important, particularly in patients with calculous disease.

Specific measures depend on the cause of the acute flank pain. A superimposed infection in the presence of obstruction is a particularly alarming situation that necessitates prompt treatment with broad-spectrum antibiotics and urinary drainage.

ACUTE INTRASCROTAL PAIN

Pain within the scrotum is seen frequently in medical practice. Inasmuch as a correct diagnosis will determine the best treatment to follow, the different causes for scrotal pain should be in the mind of the physician who initially evaluates the patient. The most common causes for scrotal pain include acute epididymitis, testicular torsion, acute orchitis, trauma, incarcerated hernia, and torsion of testicular appendages.

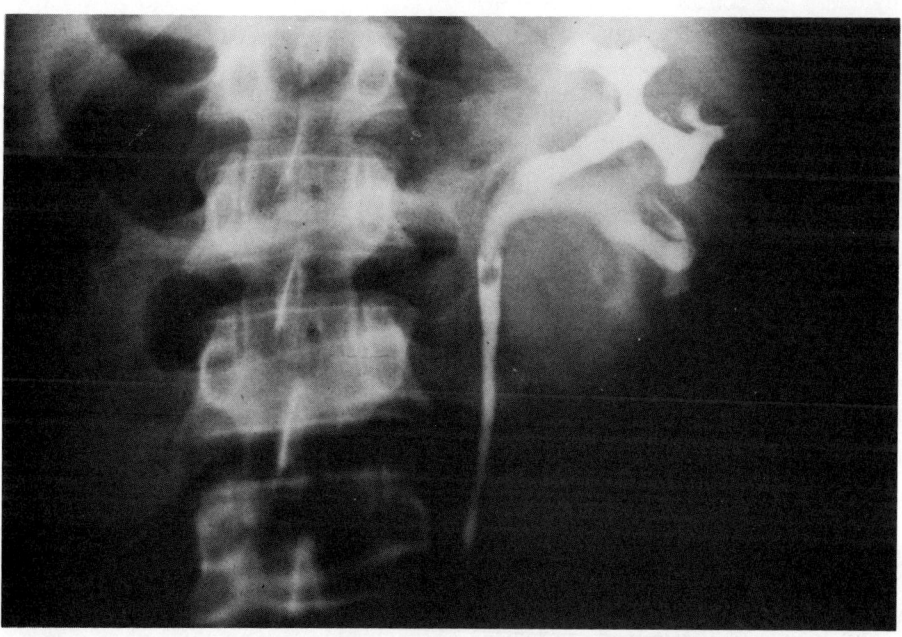

Figure 77-19 Retrograde urogram shows radiolucent calculus in proximal ureter.

Acute Epididymitis

Acute epididymitis implies an acute inflammatory process located within the epididymis. It is rarely seen in childhood and the majority of cases occur in the young adult. Organisms invade the epididymis mainly through the vas deferens and only rarely through a hematogenous or lymphatic route.[26]

Clinical Manifestations

The history of severe physical strain or urethral manipulation may be obtained. Pain is usually severe and develops rapidly. Fever is usually present. On physical examination the scrotum is enlarged and the skin is hyperemic. The epididymis is very tender and indurated. The epididymal induration may be localized in the tail, or it may involve the epididymis or even the testicle (orchioepididymitis). The urine may be infected or there may be evidence of urethral discharge.

Specific Epididymitis. Although several types of specific bacteria and fungus may invade the epididymis and cause various diseases (meningococcosis, blastomycosis, brucellosis, syphilis), two disorders deserve special comment: tuberculosis and gonorrhea.

Tuberculous epididymitis usually follows a prostatic or seminovesicle lesion. The epididymis may contain multiple nodules and "cold abscesses." The vas deferens may appear indurated and beaded. Usually, tuberculous epididymitis follows a subacute or chronic course and an epididymocutaneous fistula may occur.

Gonorrheal epididymitis was a common complication of gonococcal urethritis in the past. It is rarely seen now because of the availability of antibiotics. The epididymis usually appears extremely tender and inflamed. Chills and fever as well as prostration may be present. Symptoms of acute urethritis are usually noted, and there may be a history of urethral discharge.

Nonspecific Epididymitis. Nonspecific epididymitis is usually a purulent type of inflammation caused by common pyogenic bacteria. It often is associated with urinary tract infection, but occasionally the route of contamination is hematogenous. These infections are more apt to suppurate and an abscess may form. A history of trauma may be obtained; however, it is not clear whether this event precipitates epididymal infection.

Differential Diagnosis

On occasion there may be difficulties in differentiating acute epididymitis from torsion of the testicle, testicular tumors, torsion of the testicular appendages, trauma, and mumps orchitis.

Management

Important local measures that provide comfort to the patient include elevation of the scrotum, bed rest, ice packs, analgesics, and anti-inflammatory agents. The antibiotic of choice will depend on the etiology. The bacteria may be isolated by culturing the urine or urethral secretions when present. In nonspecific epididymitis a broad-spectrum antibiotic is recommended for 10 days.

Excellent prognosis is expected after appropriate therapy. Occasionally, an epididymal blockage develops, a situation that may lead to infertility when there is bilateral involvement.

Acute Orchitis

Many infectious diseases may involve the testicle through a hematogenous route. The most common form of orchitis is caused by mumps and occurs only after puberty. It usually involves one testicle, but bilateral involvement can be seen.

Clinical Manifestations

Usually, there is a sudden onset of pain and swelling of the testis. The scrotum becomes edematous and hyperemic. Associated fever is seen in most patients and prostration is marked. Usually, there is clinical evidence of an infectious disease. The testis is usually enlarged and severely tender. The epididymis in most cases cannot be separated from the testis itself, and an acute hydrocele may develop.

Differential Diagnosis

On occasion, it is difficult to differentiate this clinical entity from acute epididymitis or even testicular torsion. The findings of leukocytosis, normal urinalysis, and the clinical evidence of an infectious disease may help in defining the diagnosis.

Management

Bed rest is necessary. The use of scrotal elevation is helpful to relieve the edema and pain. Antibiotics are only indicated when the etiologic agent is a bacterium. Atrophic changes occur in one third to one fourth of the patients and may jeopardize fertility when there is bilateral involvement.[27]

Testicular Torsion

Testicular torsion is a condition in which the testicular circulation is compromised as a result of twisting of the

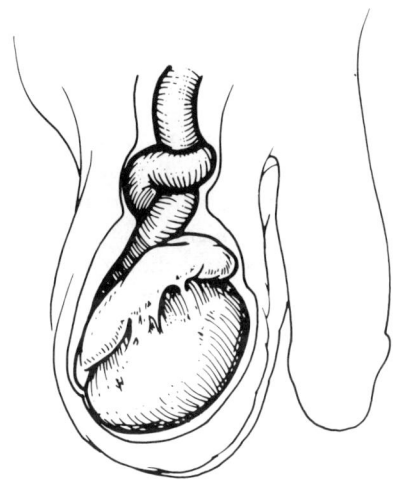

Figure 77-20 Intravaginal form of testicular torsion.

spermatic cord. Two forms may be defined: intravaginal torsion and extravaginal torsion.

Intravaginal Torsion

Intravaginal torsion is the most common intrascrotal disorder in children[28] and results as a consequence of an anomalous suspension of the testicle caused by an overdevelopment of the tunica vaginalis. This type of torsion may occur at any age but is found more often around puberty (Fig. 77-20).

Intrascrotal pain usually is the initial presenting complaint. The pain may develop suddenly; however, on occasion it may be insidious. It may occur during activity or develop during sleep. Testicular torsion may resolve spontaneously and recur later. A past history of a similar episode may be obtained in a significant number of cases.

Physical examination reveals shortening of the spermatic cord, and the testicle often lies higher in the scrotum. The epididymis may be located anteriorly with normal characteristics. Later, both testes and epididymis become involved. The presence of nausea and vomiting together with radiation of the pain into the lower abdomen may be noted.

Testicular torsion may mimic acute epididymitis, torsion of testicular appendages, acute orchitis, incarcerated hernia, or acute hydrocele. Epididymitis occurs in an older age group and is usually accompanied by fever. There may be a history of urinary tract infection. Torsion of the appendix testicle may be impossible to differentiate from testicular torsion. However, occasionally, a tender nodule may be felt at the upper pole of the testicle. Mumps orchitis is usually associated with parotitis. In patients with incarcerated hernia the cord appears thickened and a wide inguinal ring may be felt.

Although occasionally a testicle could be saved after ischemia for as long as 18 hours,[29] most of the surviving testicles had been operated on within 7 hours. The testicle is approached through the scrotum and is untwisted. Warm saline is useful to restore circulation. If the testicle remains ischemic after a period of observation, an orchiectomy should be performed. In all cases an orchiopexy of the contralateral testicle should be performed.

Extravaginal Torsion

Extravaginal torsion is a rare condition that accounts for less than 6% of all testicular torsions.[30] It is seen usually in newborns and, in most instances, the event occurs in utero.

This form of torsion presents as a smooth, firm painless mass that produces thickness and discoloration of the scrotal wall. Usually, diagnosis is simple since testicular tumors are virtually nonexistent in the neonatal period. In most instances at operation the testicle is found to be necrotic, with the torsion at the level of the external inguinal ring. Infarction of the testicle is the rule.

Scrotal exploration with the aim of removing the infarcted testicle is indicated in most cases. Exploration of the opposite side does not appear to be necessary.

ACUTE URINARY RETENTION

Acute urinary retention is the sudden inability to urinate. Except in some cases of neurogenic bladder, it is usually associated with severe lower abdominal discomfort and urgency. This clinical entity is seen frequently in an emergency department environment.

The cause that precipitates urinary retention may be at the level of the urethra or the bladder itself. It may be of acquired or congenital nature. Urethral causes include prostatic obstruction, stricture, urethral valves, trauma, foreign bodies, and extraurethral obstruction. Bladder causes include calculi, tumors, neurogenic dysfunction, ureteroceles, blood clots, and bladder neck contraction.

Pathogenesis

The vast majority of cases presenting as acute urinary retention are due to obstruction at the level of the bladder outlet or the urethra. At times, however, urinary retention is the result of a neurogenic impairment or detrusor imbalance.

In the presence of obstruction, the vesical musculature hypertrophies to overcome the urethral resistance. Soon the bladder will appear grossly trabeculated and the mucosa protrudes through the muscular bundles, forming diverticuli. During this event, two stages may be clearly identified:

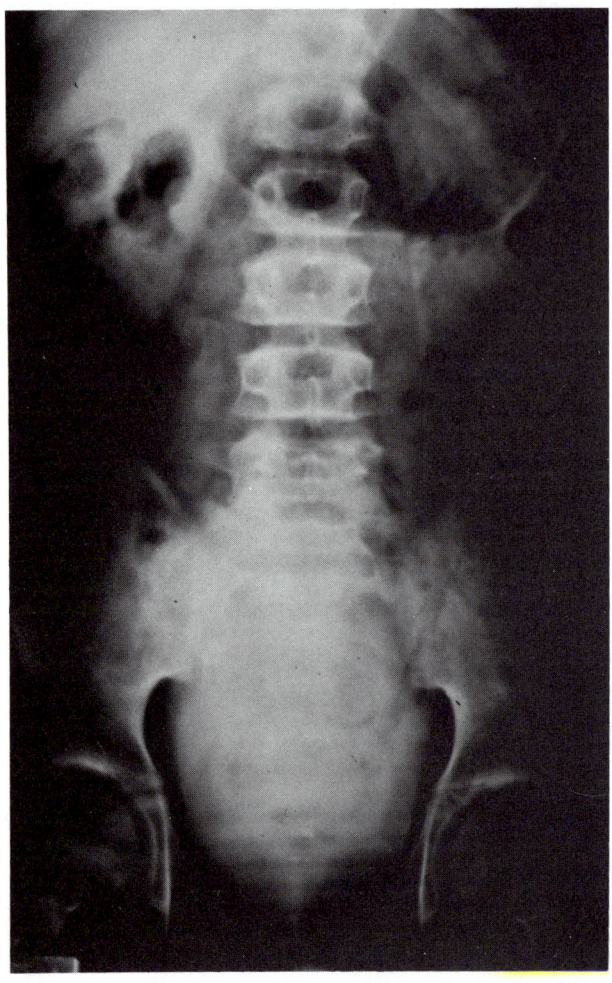

Figure 77-21 Intravenous urogram of child with neurogenic bladder. *Note:* The upper urinary tracts reveal mild ureterectasis and caliectasis.

(1) the stage of compensation, when the bladder is able to empty, and (2) the stage of decompensation that results in increasing amounts of residual urine culminating in urinary retention.[31]

Clinical Manifestations

A thorough clinical history should be obtained in an effort to identify the underlying etiology. In patients with prostatic enlargement, a history of urethritis suggests a possible urethral stricture. A neurologic disorder may be present in a patient with a neurogenic bladder.

The patient is usually in acute distress, except in some cases of neurogenic bladder with sensorial impairment. The pain is located in the lower abdomen and often is associated with severe urgency.

On physical examination the bladder is palpated and percussed above the pubis and close to the umbilical line. Palpation of the urethra may reveal an induration suggestive of a stricture or a calculus. A careful neurologic examination should be performed to rule out a neurogenic component. Rectal examination may reveal an abnormal anal sphincter tonus suggestive of a neurogenic etiology. At the same time, rectal examination may reveal the presence of a pelvic mass or prostatic enlargement.

Laboratory Findings

Gross hematuria with formation of clots may result in urinary retention. The bleeding may occur at a renal, vesical, or prostatic level. A plain abdominal roentgenogram will reveal an enlarged bladder, and spinal deformities (spina bifida) are strongly suggestive of a neurogenic component.

The intravenous urogram is usually diagnostic, revealing a distended bladder and the anatomic conditions of the upper tracts (Fig. 77-21). A retrograde urethrogram is useful when a urethral obstruction is suspected. Finally, instrumental examination with the passage of a catheter is in most cases diagnostic. Cystourethroscopy will accurately assess the anatomy of the lower urinary tract.

Management

The establishment of bladder drainage is the immediate goal. The insertion of a catheter under sterile conditions is usually diagnostic and therapeutic. A small 16F catheter is usually of adequate size except in cases due to clot retention in which a large caliber catheter is preferred with the purpose of thoroughly irrigating the bladder. Catheterization is more difficult to perform in male patients owing to anatomic factors. In the presence of a urethral stricture, care should be taken not to injure the urethral mucosa or cause a false passage that may make further attempts to pass a catheter impossible. An adequate diagnosis is necessary, and in the presence of a urethral stricture, the passage of filliforms and followers is a relatively simple measure that will adequately establish bladder drainage (Fig. 77-22). If drainage cannot be obtained through urethral catheterization, a cystostomy tube (trocar) should be inserted under local anesthesia (Fig. 77-23).[32]

If left untreated, urinary retention will lead to urinary tract infection that may spread throughout the entire urinary system. Bilateral hydronephrosis occurs as a consequence of chronic urinary retention and may result in renal insufficiency.

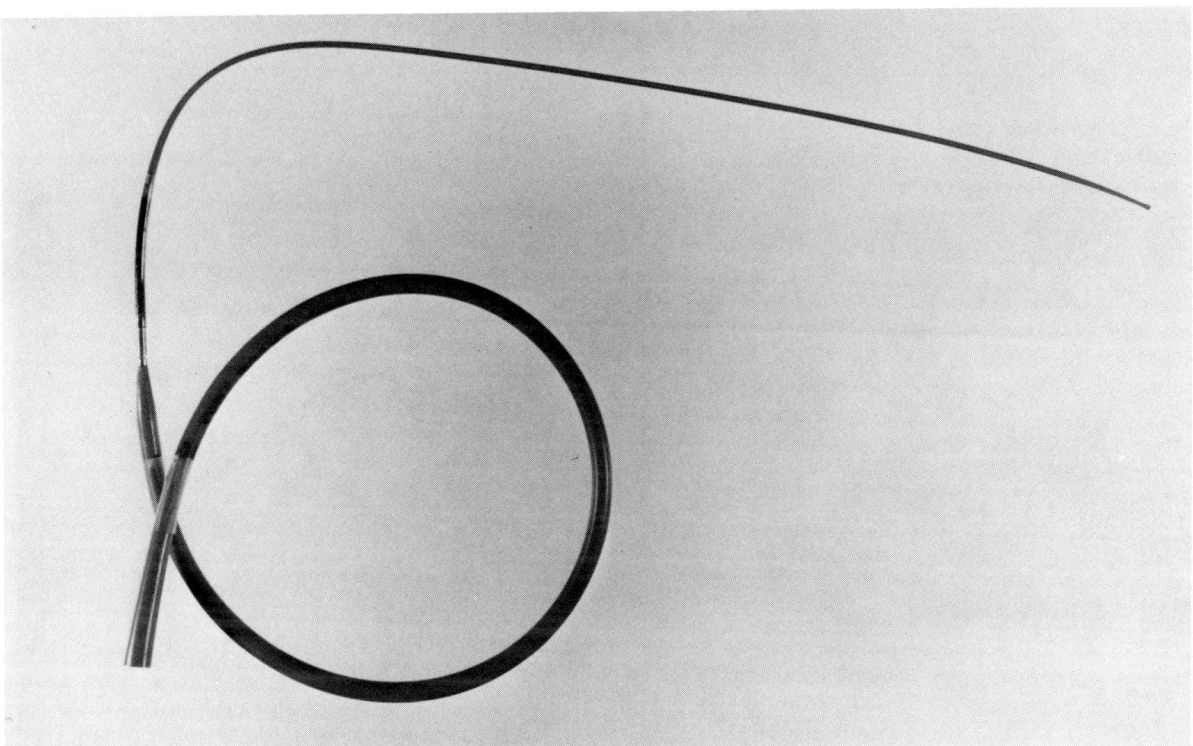

Figure 77-22 Filliform and follower.

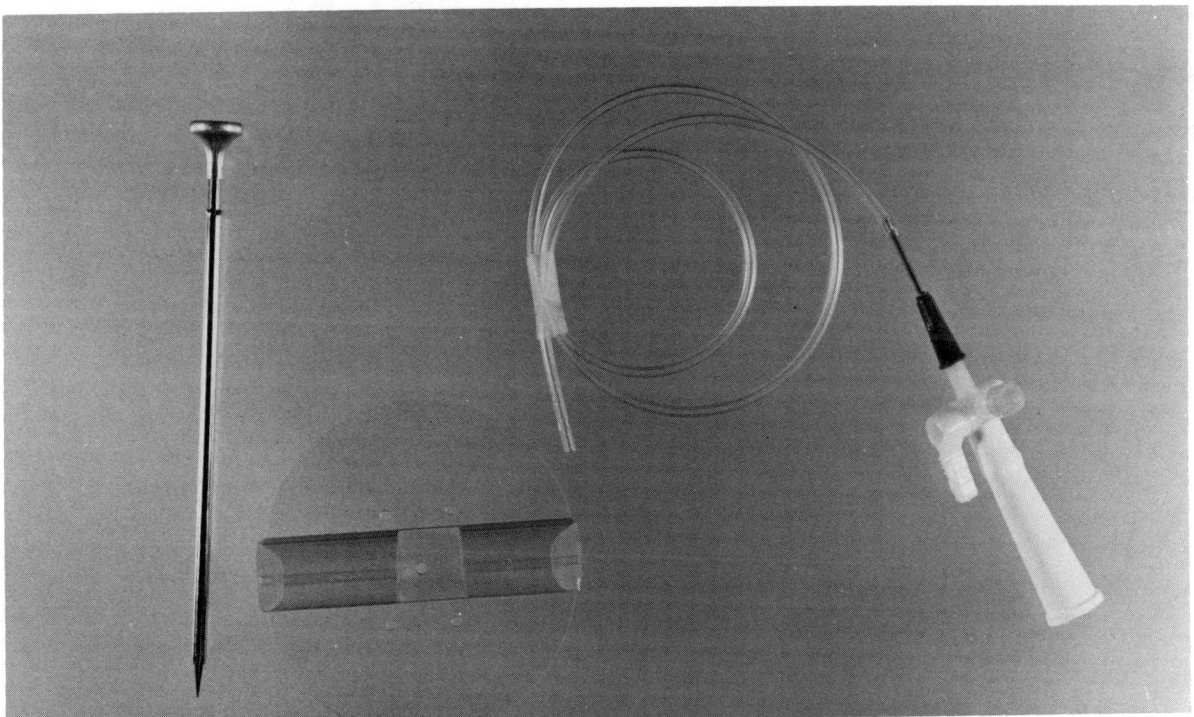

Figure 77-23 Suprapubic cystostomy tube.

REFERENCES

1. Peters PC, Bright TC. Blunt renal injuries. *Urol Clin North Am.* 1977;4:17.
2. Glenn JF, Harvard BM. The injured kidney. *JAMA.* 1960;173:93.
3. Elkin M, Chien-Hsing M, de Paredes RG. Roentgenologic evaluation of renal trauma with emphasis on renal angiography. *AJR Am J Roentgenol.* 1966;98:1.
4. Carlton CE, Scott R, Goldman M. The management of penetrating injuries of the kidney. *J Trauma.* 1968;8:1071.
5. Carlton CE. Injuries of the kidney and ureter. In: Campbell MF, Harrison JH, eds. *Urology.* 4th ed. Philadelphia, Pa: WB Saunders Co; 1978:881.
6. Stutzman RE. Ballistics and the management of ureteral injuries from high velocity missile. *J Urol.* 1977;118:947.
7. Tynberg PLH, Koch WH, Persky LP, Zellinger RH. The management of renal injuries coincident with penetrating wounds of the abdomen. *J Trauma.* 1973;13:502.
8. Peterson WE, Kirakole LU. Renal trauma: when to operate. *Urology.* 1974;3:537.
9. Holden S, Hicks CC, O'Brien DP, Harlan HS, Walker JA, Walton KN. Gunshot wounds of the ureter: a 15-year review of 63 consecutive cases. *J Urol.* 1976;116:562.
10. Newel QU. Injuries to the ureters during pelvic operations. *Ann Surg.* 1939;109:981.
11. Bright TC III, Peters PC. Ureteral injuries secondary to operative procedure: report of 24 cases. *Urology.* 1977;9:22.
12. St. Martin EC. Ureteral injury in gynecologic surgery. *J Urol.* 1953;70:51.
13. Persky LH, Koch WH, Kursch ED. Surgical management of the ureter. In: Campbell MF, Harrison JH, eds. *Urology.* 4th ed. Philadelphia, Pa: WB Saunders Co; 1978:188.
14. Thompson IM. Bladder flap repair of ureteral injuries. *Urol Clin North Am.* 1977;4:51.
15. Vargas AD, Silva E. Mobilization of the ureter by a posterior vesical flap in dogs: preliminary report of a new technique. *Urology.* 1972;107:742.
16. Bright TC III, Peters PC. Injuries to the bladder and urethra. In: Campbell MF, Harrison JH, eds. *Urology.* 4th ed. Philadelphia, Pa: WB Saunders Co; 1978:906.
17. Montie J. Bladder injuries. *Urol Clin North Am.* 1977;4:59.
18. Richardson JR Jr, Leadbetter GS Jr. Nonoperative treatment of ruptured bladder. *J Urol.* 1975;114:213.
19. Mulkey AP, Witherington R. Conservative management of vesical rupture. *Urology.* 1974;4:426.
20. Morehouse DD, McKinnon JK. Posterior urethral injury: etiology, diagnosis, initial management. *Urol Clin North Am.* 1977;4:69.
21. Turner-Warwick R. A personal view of the immediate management of pelvic fracture urethral injuries. *Urol Clin North Am.* 1977;4:81.
22. Roberts M. Injuries to the lower urinary tract. In: Blandy J, ed. *Urology.* London, England: Blackwell Scientific; 1976:954.
23. Culp DA. Genital injuries: etiology and initial management. *Urol Clin North Am.* 1977;4:143.
24. Bright TC, Peters PC. Injuries of the external genitalia. In: Campbell MF, Harrison JH, eds. *Urology.* 4th ed. Philadelphia, Pa: WB Saunders Co; 1978:931.
25. Smith DR. Symptoms of disorder of the genitourinary tract. In: Smith DR, ed. *General Urology.* 9th ed. Los Altos, Calif: Lange Medical Publications; 1975:25.
26. Nickel WR. Other infections and inflammations of the external genitalia. In: Campbell MF, Harrison JH, eds. *Urology.* 4th ed. Philadelphia, Pa: WB Saunders Co; 1978:640.
27. Whitaker RH. Benign disorders of the testicle. In: Blandy J, ed. *Urology.* London, England: Blackwell Scientific; 1976:1182.
28. Allen TD. Disorders of the male external genitalia. In: Kelalis PP, King LR, eds. *Clinical Pediatric Urology.* Philadelphia, Pa: WB Saunders Co; 1976:636.
29. Parker RM, Robison JR. Anatomy and diagnosis of torsion of the testicle. *J Urol.* 1971;106:243.
30. James T. Torsion of the spermatic cord in the first year of life. *Br J Urol.* 1953;25:56.
31. Smith DR. Urinary obstruction and stasis. In: Smith DR, ed. *General Urology.* 8th ed. Los Altos, Calif: Lange Medical Publications; 1975:112.
32. Leadbetter GW. Diagnostic urologic instrumentation. In: Campbell MF, Harrison JH, eds. *Urology.* 4th ed. Philadelphia, Pa: WB Saunders Co; 1978:358.

78. Renal Failure

JONATHAN L. WHITE, MD
JOHN A. MITAS II, MD, FACP
LEONARD G. GOMELLA, MD

The presentation of renal failure may be as varied as the patients who enter the emergency department or who seek care for a seemingly unrelated symptom. For example, renal failure may be diagnosed in the 58-year-old diabetic who recently underwent a diagnostic radiographic procedure; the young expectant mother who arrives with altered mentation, edema, and hypertension; the child with a recent onset of dark urine; the victim of a hit-and-run driver; or the 75th person presenting with weakness after severe vomiting during a viral epidemic or during the hottest week on record. Because of the multiple functions of the kidney (Table 78-1), renal dysfunction must be considered in each of these patients because of different signs or symptoms. Renal failure no longer equates with oliguria[1] but must now be defined as a decrease in renal function, specifically glomerular filtration rate (GFR), with or without oliguria. Current series report that 30% to 60% of patients are nonoliguric.[2] The hallmarks of renal failure are azotemia and the biochemical consequences of decreased GFR, which may include abnormal volume regulation; hyperkalemia, hyperphosphatemia, and hypocalcemia; occasional hyponatremia; metabolic acidosis when the GFR is below 15 mL/minute; and abnormal handling of drugs and metabolites (physiologic and pharmacologic). Although renal failure is not always a true emergency when discovered, it does demand urgent evaluation because it is potentially reversible, many etiologies *are* treatable, and it is associated with a high mortality. Physicians in the emergency department are in a unique position to provide immediate care to victims of severe, traumatic rhabdomyolysis and *prevent* acute renal failure, which previously was virtually a universal sequela of this type of injury.[3]

This chapter presents a workable approach to renal failure, its identification, etiology, and management. Management of the functional abnormalities is considered individually. Although treatment of hyperkalemia and acidemia will not be completed in the emergency department, the recognition of these abnormalities and initiation of therapy may be lifesaving for a patient with renal failure.

ETIOLOGY

Although the recognized causes of renal failure are numerous,[2] they may conveniently be consolidated in the time-honored classification of prerenal, parenchymal, and postrenal causes. Such a classification underscores the concept that many causes are potentially reversible and many are treatable.

The suspicion of renal failure is confirmed by the findings of elevated blood urea nitrogen (BUN) and serum creatinine. The normal values for BUN are 10 to 20 mg/dL and for creatinine up to 1.5 mg/dL (depending on the individual's size and muscle mass). Because a number of factors may influence the concentration of BUN (eg, diet, medications, gastrointestinal hemorrhage, hydration), it is best to consider the creatinine value. Values of 1.6 to 3 or 3.5 mg/dL may be considered representative of "renal insufficiency" (unless

Table 78-1 Functions of the Kidney

Systems Regulated	Examples
Volume regulation	Diuresis or antidiuresis
Acid-base control	H^+ excretion, HCO_3^- reclamation and regeneration
Electrolyte conservation or excretion	Na^+, K^+, Cl^-, Ca^{++}, Mg^{++}, PO_4
Blood pressure regulation	Na^+, volume control; renin-angiotensin-aldosterone; vasodilator systems (prostaglandins, kallikrein-bradykinin)
Excretion of metabolites and waste products	Physiologic and pharmacologic substances
Maintenance of hematocrit	Erythropoietin production or formation
Metabolic	Insulin metabolism, amino acid conservation

there is continued elevation), while values exceeding 3 to 3.5 mg/dL indicate "renal failure." Any of the three classes may cause a markedly elevated serum creatinine, although values of greater than 6 mg/dL are less commonly found in prerenal states and should lead to the consideration of other causes.

Prerenal causes have the common feature of decreased effective arterial volume and decreased renal blood flow, whether true or merely perceived. Although there has been a report of "nonoliguric prerenal failure,"[4] the majority of these patients will manifest oliguria because of an intact renal concentrating mechanism. Oliguria is defined by most nephrologists as a volume insufficient to excrete a maximally concentrated urine (of approximately 1200 mOsm), which contains the waste products, obligate electrolytes, and osmoles that must be excreted daily. Such a volume would be at least 400 mL/day. The entities are multiple but may be roughly divided into cardiovascular, vascular, and hypovolemic states. The former include myocardial infarction, congestive heart failure, and dysrhythmias—all of which lower the cardiac output (or cardiac index)—and mechanical factors such as cardiac tamponade, which reduces filling and cardiac output. Vascular factors such as arterial or venous obstruction may be perceived as low-volume states, as may vascular pooling, which is associated with decreased vascular resistance in states of sepsis or the extreme of acidosis. True hypovolemic causes may be due to renal losses, extrarenal losses, or sequestration. Renal-mediated volume losses may be the result of prior diuretic use or excess, osmotic diuresis associated with uncontrolled diabetes mellitus, or diabetes insipidus. Extrarenal volume losses may occur via the skin (eg, burns or excessive sweating), gastrointestinal tract (eg, nausea, vomiting, diarrhea, hemorrhage), or hemorrhage. Sequestration without true loss occurs in burns, ascites, peritonitis, and occasionally with marked peripheral edema. The importance of these situations is that many are treatable and *if* successfully treated may prevent ischemic renal parenchymal damage from occurring. The major problem in identifying these prerenal states from established parenchymal damage will be discussed in a later section.

The parenchymal causes of renal failure may be subdivided according to the sites of involvement. These sites are vascular, glomerular, and tubular or tubulointerstitial. Only the last of these represents true acute tubular necrosis (ATN), although the term is frequently used (inappropriately) for all forms of parenchymal renal failure. Vasculitis encompasses disorders such as systemic lupus erythematosus, Henoch-Schönlein purpura, large vessel polyarteritis, and small vessel polyarteritis (hypersensitivity angiitis). Scleroderma, Wegener's granulomatosis, and malignant hypertension may present as renal failure owing to their vascular involvement. The glomerulonephritides may be immunologically mediated in bacterial endocarditis,[5] gram-negative abscess,[6] occasional poststreptococcal glomerulonephritis, or rapidly progressive glomerulonephritis (RPGN). RPGN is a clinical syndrome of rapidly decreasing renal function with or without significant proteinuria but accompanied by hematuria and hypertension. Patients with idiopathic RPGN are usually normotensive. Occasionally this is representative of Goodpasture's syndrome, in association with antiglomerular basement membrane antibodies in the serum. The tubular disorders occur as a result of hypercalcemia; hyperuricemia; tubular precipitation of myeloma protein (light chains), uric acid, and sulfonamides; oxalate nephropathy (ethylene glycol ingestion, methoxyflurane, Crohn's disease); and ATN due to ischemia or toxins such as drugs and diagnostic agents. Pregnancy-related renal failure may occur in toxemia or the postpartum state after a normal pregnancy.[7,8] The pathogenesis of pregnancy-related renal failure seems to be a combination of vascular, coagulation, and possible toxin-induced changes to tubules that do not fit neatly into a single category. The hepatorenal syndrome does not fit into any of these categories but consists of a functional derangement characterized by intense renal vasoconstriction but without histologic changes.[9,10] (These kidneys could be transplanted and function normally.)

True ATN includes the ischemic damage resulting from untreated or inappropriately treated prerenal states and direct nephrotoxic damage. Ischemic injury is still the most common etiology of renal failure (and ATN) in adults.[1,2] In contrast, the pediatric patient is much more likely to have glomerulonephritis or the hemolytic-uremic syndrome.[2]

Nephrotoxins are classically considered to be the aminoglycosides, but numerous antibiotics have been recognized to cause ATN, including sulfonamides, cephaloridine, colistin, polymyxin, neomycin, vancomycin, and amphotericin B.[11] These agents do not require prior sensitization, and injury is not strictly dose dependent.[12] In some instances immunologic mechanisms are involved with the use of drugs. The best-delineated association has been methicillin, where there is evidence of antibodies directed against dimethoxypenicilloyl moiety, but other penicillin derivatives have been implicated.[13] Many diagnostic and therapeutic agents other than antibiotics have been identified[14-16] but are too numerous to list. Many environmental agents are capable of causing acute renal failure (ARF), including glycerol compounds, insecticides, many organic solvents, and numerous heavy metals.

Endogenous nephrotoxins may be found in compounds such as myoglobin and hemoglobin, but the "precipitation" of this disorder is not solely nephrotoxic because some other factors such as volume depletion and acidosis may be necessary along with tubular obstruction and tubular cell anoxia.[17,18] Mismatched blood, transfusion reactions, and hemolysis from other causes should be considered. Myoglobinuria commonly follows trauma but perhaps is even more frequent following severe exercise (such as in joggers or unconditioned individuals), heat stroke, prolonged seizures, prolonged coma, and viral myositis.[17,19] The last of these should be considered in older individuals especially.[20,21] Patients with Legionnaire's disease and acute renal failure are being recognized more frequently. Azotemia should be suspected in patients with pneumonia and mental confusion and allegedly is a consequence of rhabdomyolysis or interstitial nephritis.[22,23]

Rhabdomyolysis with myoglobinuria should also be considered in patients with drug abuse—especially those using amphetamines, PCP (phencyclidine), heroin, and strychnine.[24-26] One report even indicates that total parenteral nutrition leading to hypokalemia can induce rhabdomyolysis and severe renal failure.[27]

Contrast materials for radiographic studies deserve special mention. These iodinated agents are commonly in use for a variety of procedures. The agents most frequently involved in nephrotoxicity are employed for excretory urography and angiography, intravenous cholangiography, oral cholecystography, and computed tomography with contrast.[28,29] The agents implicated are sodium diatrizoate, meglumine diatrizoate, meglumine iodipamide, iopanoic acid, and sodium ipodate. Contrast-induced renal failure accounts for approximately 10% of all cases of ARF. Special risk factors for developing dye-induced ATN include increased age, underlying renal disease, insulin-dependent diabetes (especially with onset before age 30 and/or creatinine exceeding 2 mg/dL), dehydration, proteinuria, liver disease, hyperuricemia, and radiographic study with contrast in the preceding 3 days. It is not definitely preventable by drip infusion techniques or by prior rehydration.[30]

Obstructive phenomena occur as a result of intrinsic or extrinsic obstruction. To cause azotemia the obstruction need not be complete but must be at the bladder outlet or bilateral to involve both ureters. If both ureters or collecting systems are not involved, the unobstructed kidney is capable of compensating for the unilateral loss of function. This is an important fact to remember when the diagnostic evaluation is undertaken.

PATHOLOGY

The pathologic features of renal failure vary according to the etiology. In prerenal conditions the renal blood vessels, glomeruli, and tubules are normal. Also, in occasional instances of well-defined clinical ATN, the histology may be totally normal. This emphasizes the point that in ATN there is poor correlation between histologic findings and functional impairment.[31] Focal and minimal tubular damage may be present in patients with severe functional changes. (Conversely, patients without renal failure may have autopsy findings similar to those in patients with ATN.)

The most common histologic findings in ATN depend on whether the damage is ischemic or toxin induced. In the former, tubular necrosis is patchy, with only short segments being affected. The pars recta of the proximal tubule seems to be most vulnerable; however, the proximal convoluted tubule is also commonly involved. The basement membrane may be disrupted at sites of necrosis, and cell rupture may be present. In toxic damage, confluent areas of necrosis are noted in the convoluted and straight portions of the proximal tubule. However, the basement membranes remain intact. Necrotic lesions occur in all nephrons after toxic insult, whereas ischemic injury is patchy. Tubular casts are present in either type and form in the distal tubule. Casts consist of Tamm-Horsfall protein secreted by the thick portion of the ascending limb of the loop of Henle. In this matrix, cellular debris is deposited, forming the characteristic pigmented casts that are finely or coarsely granular and that must be distinguished from red blood cell casts. This can be done by focusing up and down through the cast while viewing through the high-power objective. Granular casts will appear as such, while red blood cell casts are identifiable by the presence of red blood cells at all depths of the matrix, distinguishing them from casts with red blood cells adherent to the exterior. For the histology associated with the various forms of glomerulonephritis or vasculitis, the interested reader is referred elsewhere to more detailed texts.

In obstructive disorders, hydroureter and hydronephrosis ensue. Depending on the duration and completeness, the dilation of the ureter and renal pelvis may be mild to severe. Because glomerular filtration and urine production continue, the dilation is progressive unless a restrictive process prevents dilatation.[32] Patients with the more severe cases may develop dilated collecting ducts, collecting tubules, and even Bowman's spaces with glomerular compression. When the disorder is prolonged, there may be significant loss of renal parenchyma.

PATHOGENESIS AND CLINICAL FEATURES

The prerenal states will result in reduced renal perfusion. This may be due to either real or perceived reductions in circulating volume. As renal blood flow (RBF) and renal plasma flow (RPF) decrease, the GFR falls from a normal of 180 L/day to much lower levels. The duration as well as degree of reduced perfusion may vary considerably between patients without parenchymal damage. During this reduced perfusion the BUN and creatinine concentrations rise. In conditions with diminished total body water, part of this rise is due to hemoconcentration (and can be substantiated by a rise in hematocrit, total protein, and albumen concentrations). Accompanying decreased effective arterial volume there may be reduced clearance to urea, creatinine, and metabolic wastes, leading to retention. As mentioned earlier, the rise in serum creatinine is to values of 6 mg/dL or less in most instances, although there are individual case reports of values of 9 to 10 mg/dL. In states in which the blood pressure is reduced, several factors may play a role, including decreased RPF, reduced perfusion pressure, and reduced filtration. Renal mechanisms to conserve sodium are activated, resulting in marked decreases in urinary sodium excretion. If appropriately treated with volume expansion, increased cardiac filling pressure, or relief of mechanical factors, the BUN and creatinine will return to normal or baseline values.

In glomerulonephritis or vasculitis, inflammation of the capillaries and/or preglomerular vessels alter the hemodynamics, as well as potentially alter the glomerular surface area and filtration.[33]

In one review of the literature of acute renal failure, the results of eight large series (2500 cases) were compiled. Of these cases, 43% were related to surgery and 9% to trauma; 26% occurred in a medical setting, and 13% were pregnancy related.[31] Only 9% were caused by nephrotoxins. A recent prospective evaluation of 2216 patients at risk found an incidence of renal insufficiency of 4.9%, with iatrogenic factors accounting for 55% of all episodes.[34] Of all cases of renal failure, ATN may be the underlying disorder in approximately three fourths. The ischemic causes are those associated with untreated or inadequately treated prerenal disorders with resultant tubular damage. Occasionally, ischemic damage results from very brief periods of hypoperfusion, such as during operative procedures. Decreased perfusion pressure is normally accompanied by autoregulatory changes within the kidney (ie, decreased afferent arteriolar resistance as the mean arteriolar pressure [MAP, diastolic + one-third pulse pressure] falls to 80 mmHg). Total RBF may remain the same but with redistribution to the juxtamedullary cortex, as demonstrated by studies using inert gas washout and microsphere methods. In other studies, RBF may be decreased with a uniform distribution in the cortex, using the same microsphere technique. As the MAP falls still lower (50 to 70 mmHg) the RBF, GFR, and single nephron GFR fall to one half to two thirds of control values and alter the Starling forces. Below 40 to 45 mmHg MAP, single-nephron GFR stops completely in the superficial and deep nephrons.

Significant renal ischemia may occur in the absence of recognized hypotension and with only a modest decrease in cardiac output. This has been demonstrated by experiments using tilt tables or leg tourniquets to decrease the effective blood volume.[31] Although blood pressure may not change, the RPF may fall by more than one third and be accompanied by a fall in GFR and urine flow.

ATN resulting from toxin exposure may occur from any of a number of agents identified.[11,12,14–16,35] However, the factors that establish and maintain renal failure in one patient but not another after similar exposure are multiple and varied. Several experimental models have been devised in an attempt to identify the predominant factor responsible for a decreased GFR. The results vary between agents and among species. It is sufficient to say that vascular and tubular effects are interrelated and play roles of varying importance in each patient. The mechanisms leading to a reduced GFR include diminished RPF, altered glomerular capillary ultrafiltration coefficient (implying altered permeability and/or effective filtering surface area), tubular obstruction, and back-leak.[31,36] The no-reflow phenomenon (ie, cellular swelling preventing normal blood flow) does not appear to have experimental support. In established ATN, iodinated contrast material often yields a dense immediate nephrogram. This material is excreted by glomerular filtration, not by tubular secretion; thus, glomerular filtration continues, although at a lower level. The exact role of the renin-angiotensin system remains unclear. No protection has been noted in attempts to immunize with renin or to utilize angiotensin II blockade or vasodilators. Owing to the proximity of the renin-containing macula densa to the glomerulus, a local role for this system in ischemic and toxin-induced ATN cannot be excluded. Angiotensin II-mediated vasoconstriction may have an important role in the pathogenesis of ARF.

Obstructive uropathy results when intrarenal or extrarenal obstruction alters the normal fall in pressure from kidney to bladder. Common etiologies in men are prostatic hypertrophy or carcinoma, calculi, and urethral strictures. In women, pregnancy, calculi, or malignancy are the most common etiologies. Ureteral strictures as a consequence of radiation therapy or following endoscopic manipulation may also cause obstruction. In children, congenital anomalies should be considered. Continued GFR and urine production lead to increased volume and pressure proximal to the obstruction, whether it is mechanical or functional. RBF and GFR are eventually diminished, owing to increased tubular pressure opposing filtration. Additionally, blood flow is redistributed to the inner cortex while flow to the outer cortex and the inner medulla is reduced.[37]

Intrinsic obstruction should be considered in patients with a history of hematology-oncology disorders. In multiple myeloma, Bence Jones proteinuria seems to be the major determinant of renal failure when associated with infection, hypercalcemia, or dehydration.[38] Patients with leukemia or lymphoma undergoing chemotherapy or irradiation may develop hyperuricemic nephropathy with obstruction when serum uric acid exceeds 20 to 21 mg/dL, urinary uric acid/creatinine exceeds 1.0, and tubular precipitation occurs.[39,40] Obstruction resulting from precipitation of uric acid in the ureters as well as in the tubules is now less common.[40]

DIAGNOSIS

A diagnosis of renal failure must be considered in the appropriate setting if it is to be made. Patients will not readily recognize that they have renal failure and may complain only of pain or generalized malaise. A fairly common presentation is the older adult who simply feels more fatigued or who has unexplained weakness or the younger patient who notes decreased exercise tolerance (with a creatinine of 10 mg/dL). Thus, the symptoms may not point immediately to the kidneys. In the trauma victim, dehydrated patient, or postoperative patient, renal failure comes to mind more readily. Symptoms that should raise the possibility of renal disease include edema of recent onset, scant or dark urine, or the new onset of hypertension. Altered mental status of short duration—confusion, somnolence, sleep disorders, short attention span—should prompt an investigation of renal function. The tests to request initially include BUN and serum creatinine, as well as serum electrolytes (Na^+, K^+, Cl^-, HCO_3^-). Urinalysis should be performed and the urinary sediment examined. If the BUN and creatinine are elevated, the differential considerations must be entertained. The volume status and urine production must be discerned.

How high a BUN or creatinine should be accepted as normal? The BUN value should not exceed 20 mg/dL and the creatinine value should be less than 1.5 mg/dL. Women and men with small frames have somewhat lower values. In pregnancy, values that otherwise would be considered within the normal range are elevated if the BUN value exceeds 13 mg/dL and the creatinine value is greater than 0.8 mg/dL.[41] This is due to the normally increased RBF and GFR that accompany the gravid state. In renal failure, the BUN value rises by 10 to 20 mg/dL each day as the creatinine value increases daily by 0.5 to 1.5 mg/dL. In trauma or severe rhabdomyolysis, these values may increase at a more rapid rate (doubled), with the creatinine value elevated out of proportion to that of the BUN.

Hyperkalemia becomes a risk factor when the GFR is less than 10 mL/min. A rise of 0.5 mEq/L/day or less is expected, but a rise of 1 to 2 mEq/L in a matter of hours is possible in trauma patients.

Acidosis generally occurs as a result of the inability to excrete the acid load of 50 to 100 mEq generated per day. As the GFR falls and tubular function declines, the body is incapable of reclaiming HCO_3^- in the proximal tubule or of regenerating HCO_3^- at the distal tubule. Thus, the serum HCO_3^- concentration falls by 1 to 2 mEq/L each day in patients with uncomplicated conditions and by a more rapid rate if the patient is hypercatabolic. To compensate for the reduced HCO_3^- concentration, CO_2 must be exhaled. However, unmeasured anions begin to accumulate.

A number of secondary problems that ensue are considered individually in the treatment section. Renal failure may involve other organ systems with resultant cardiac arrhythmias, heart failure, or pericarditis; altered mental status, electrocephalographic changes, and asterixis; nausea and vomiting, increased incidence of ulcers, and hemorrhage; respiratory problems related to volume excess; anemia, white blood cell dysfunction, and altered hemostasis; and altered thermoregulation and endocrine function.

Mortality remains high after the onset of renal failure despite the use of hemodialysis, owing to the severity of the underlying illness and current spectrum of disease.[2,42] The major determinants of mortality are infection and the primary illness that precipitated the disorder. It should be remembered that infection is the leading cause of death in ARF. Patients who are at increased risk include older patients, burn victims, those with a large number of complications, and possibly patients with a second episode of ATN.[2,31,42,43] Nonoliguric ATN is not a benign disorder, as claimed in some studies, but does have a mortality of 21% to 26%. Even the recovery or diuretic phase of oliguric ATN is the setting for approximately one fourth of the deaths.

DIFFERENTIAL DIAGNOSIS

Because of the possibility of reversible conditions, it is important to establish as early as possible the category of renal failure in a given patient. Thus, a quick assessment of hydration (effective and total volume status), including cardiac function, and search for an obstructive component must be performed. Historic features such as flank pain or variable urine production suggest obstruction. Has there been a history of nausea and vomiting, diarrhea, limited access to fluids, orthostatic symptoms, dyspnea, angina, orthopnea, arrhythmias, hemorrhage, or documented hypotension during surgery?

A diagnosis of prerenal azotemia is supported by findings of dry skin, dry mucous membranes, low extracellular fluid (ECF) volume, and oliguria. Skin over the forehead or sternum is less susceptible to changes associated with aging and may be used to assess skin turgor. If dependent edema is noted in the legs or presacral area, the patient is not volume deficient. Additionally, "sheet lines" may be assessed over the back—if imprints are made in the skin of a supine patient, it is unusual for total body water to be significantly reduced. For patients in the cardiac care unit, intensive care unit, or trauma unit, the pulmonary capillary wedge (PCW) pressure, cardiac output, and cardiac index can indicate cardiac performance and adequacy of filling pressure. When a more rapid assessment is needed (and realizing that the central venous pressure [CVP] does not perfectly correlate with pulmonary artery diastolic or PCW pressures) the CVP can be used to assess the volume status. If there is *any* consideration of using furosemide or mannitol, it must *first* be established that a patient has an adequate circulating volume. When the CVP is low, a volume challenge should be administered with normal saline, 500 to 1000 mL over 15 to 20 minutes, with a recheck of the CVP at the completion of the infusion and 15 minutes later. Since the intravascular volume is normally one fourth of the ECF and thus one twelfth of the total body water,[44] a solution must be chosen that will not rapidly diffuse throughout the body space, as 5% dextrose and water (D_5W) or hypotonic solutions may. Establishing that the hemodynamic parameters are normal should suggest other etiologies. However, it is not always possible to easily distinguish prerenal causes from parenchymal damage, so a variety of indexes and ratios have been devised that may identify the correct diagnosis.[45,46] These indexes are of greatest use in an oliguric patient who does not have underlying renal insufficiency. It is preferable to assess these indexes without the prior use of diuretics or other agents if possible. The application of these tests will be discussed after the assessment of renal obstruction has been discussed.

This order is appropriate in the usual diagnostic scheme because obstructive uropathy may be the most commonly overlooked diagnosis. Ten percent of cases of ARF may be due to bladder outlet obstruction. Patients with a history of renal calculi, hematuria, diabetes (with or without neurogenic bladder), lymphoma, or malignancy should be considered, but the potential causes are too numerous to list.[37] Precipitation of substances in the ureters such as uric acid should be considered in patients with leukemia or lymphoma who have recently been treated with chemotherapy or radiation. A plain radiograph of the abdomen may provide important diagnostic clues. Renal size may be evaluated and calcifications in the course of the ureters may be seen. Osteoblastic bony lesions, especially in the axial skeleton, may point to the diagnosis of prostate carcinoma and possible ureteric obstruction.

Evaluation for obstruction may be quickly carried out. Percussion and palpation for bladder enlargement and prostatic examination are simple measures. The bladder should be catheterized to rule out lower urinary tract obstruction. This will also allow sterile drainage and sequential accurate determination of urine volume. A urine sample should be used to evaluate electrolytes, uric acid, and urinary creatinine as well as the sediment for crystals (uric acid, sulfa, oxalate) and blood. If there is very little urine in the bladder, the upper tracts must be assessed. Ultrasound can accurately determine renal size and degree of dilation of the ureters and renal pelvis.[47] This procedure has a sensitivity of 98% when used as a screening test. In equivocal cases it may yield a false-positive result, but it will not identify the rare patient with nondilated obstructive uropathy.[32,47] In rare instances, obstructive uropathy may be present without significant hydronephrosis. If clinical suspicion is high, obstruction should be ruled out by other measures such as antegrade or retrograde pyelography or nuclear scan.

If ultrasound is not available, it may be necessary to catheterize one ureter. One ureter is sufficient because a single patent orifice and ureter rules out obstruction as an etiology (since one functioning kidney would be capable of compensating for obstruction of the contralateral side). This approach also avoids the risk of bilateral orifice edema. If an obstruction is found, a catheter can be placed to relieve the obstruction. Percutaneous nephrostomy is a reasonable alternative to alleviate the obstruction while other therapy is rendered. A catheter or nephrostomy may be temporary if hemodialysis can relieve uric acid or myeloma protein precipitation.[40,48]

As parenchymal causes, glomerulonephritis and vasculitis should be suspected when hematuria (especially with red blood cell casts) is present and associated with proteinuria. Although these casts occasionally may be seen in patients with acute interstitial nephritis and rarely with ATN, significant proteinuria (nephrotic range) is most common with glomerulonephritis. Oliguria and hypertension are additional important clues to glomerulonephritis. Acute interstitial nephritis should be considered if there is a history of recent medication use, rash, fever, peripheral eosinophilia, or eosinophils noted in the urine along with hematuria.[49] The kidneys may appear large on ultrasound or an abdominal roentgenogram. For further information the reader should refer to a major nephrology text.

On occasion it is not possible to distinguish which patient has prerenal azotemia or ATN. In this situation, urinary indexes become quite important.[45,46] ATN requires support of the numerous functional deficiencies while the tubules repair themselves (usually over 5 to 10 days), while prerenal causes are potentially reversible. The various ratios and parameters are listed in Table 78-2. Because there is so much overlap using urinary osmolality, ratio of urine to plasma osmolality, and ratio of urine to plasma urea, these indexes are not particularly helpful. Osmolality of the urine depends to a large extent on urea handling, but urea is affected by states of hydration, medications (corticosteroids are catabolic; tetracyclines are antianabolic), gastrointestinal hemorrhage, hepatic function, and diet. Urinary sodium (U_{Na+}) is usually less than 10 mEq/L in prerenal states and greater than 25 mEq/L in 81% of oliguric ATN patients (and 32% of nonoliguric ATN patients). This also is an imperfect test because values of 10 to 25 mEq/L and less than 10 mEq/L were reported in 13% and 6% of one series of oliguric patients, respectively.[31] Using urinary to plasma creatinine ratios, values of greater than or equal to 40:1 are seen in prerenal conditions and less than 10:1 in ATN. This leaves a large potential gray zone, which can be resolved by using a "break point" of 20:1, with the realization that this is usually correct but not always accurate. Improved diagnostic accuracy comes from use of the renal failure index RFI = $(U_{Na+})/(U_{Creat}/P_{Creat})$, which yields values less than 1.0 for

Table 78-2 Useful Urinary and Plasma Parameters in Renal Failure

Test	Prerenal	ATN	Comments
Microscopic evaluation of urine	Normal; occasional hyaline or granular casts	Pigmented casts; epithelial cells	Red blood cell casts suggest glomerulonephritis or acute interstitial nephritis
Concentrating ability			
Specific gravity	>1.015	1.010–1.025	Indistinguishable
Urinary osmolality (mOsm/L)	>500	<350	Considerable overlap
$\frac{\text{Urine osmolality}}{\text{Plasma osmolality}}$	$\frac{2-3}{1}$	<1.1 in oliguric patients <1.2 in nonoliguric patients	Not always reliable
$\frac{\text{Urinary creatinine}}{\text{Plasma creatinine}}$	>40:1	<10:1	Because of large gray zone 20:1 may be more practical division
Urinary sodium (mEq/L)	<10	>25 10–25 <10	In 81% oliguric; 32% nonoliguric In 13% oliguric; 56% nonoliguric In 6% oliguric; 12% nonoliguric
Renal failure index $\frac{(U_{Na+})}{(U_{Creat}/P_{Creat})}$	<1.0	>1.0	Specific volume not needed Most useful in oliguric patients
Fractional excretion of sodium $\frac{(U_{Na+}/P_{Na+})}{(U_{Creat}/P_{Creat})} \times 100$	<1%	>1%	Specific volume not needed Most useful in oliguric patients

prerenal states and greater than 1.0 for ATN. Further refinement considers plasma sodium to determine the fractional excretion of sodium, $FE_{Na} = 100 \; (U_{Na+}/P_{Na+})/(U_{Creat}/P_{Creat})$. Values less than 1% indicate avid sodium reabsorption consistent with prerenal azotemia, while values greater than 1% indicate abnormal tubular handling of sodium seen in acute renal failure. These indexes are useful in mixed disorders in which prerenal causes have been corrected or in which obstruction has been alleviated and yet the clinical state does not improve. In a recent prospective study of 87 patients, 86 were correctly characterized using the FE_{Na}, including those with nonoliguric ATN.[50]

TREATMENT

The treatment of obstruction is the relief of that obstruction via catheter, suprapubic catheter, or percutaneous nephrostomy. After complete or bilateral obstruction is relieved, a marked fluid diuresis may occur. In most cases this diuresis is physiologic and represents the renal response to excrete retained urea, salt, and water. It will be necessary to monitor intake and output closely so that dehydration or vascular collapse does not follow. Special attention should be paid to repletion of K^+, HCO_3^-, and Mg^{++} losses, which may occur with a brisk diuresis. This replacement should prevent severe weakness from hypokalemia, acidosis from HCO_3^- loss, or tetany or cardiac problems secondary to a low Mg^{++} causing hypocalcemia.

"Prerenal" patients should have their volume status normalized if it is truly depleted and optimized if due to cardiac dysfunction. This may involve treatment of dysrhythmias with appropriate medications, use of cardiac pacemakers, digitalization (with levels closely followed due to impaired renal excretion), and hemodynamic monitoring.

Patients with extensive crush injuries appear to benefit from the induction of alkaline solute diuresis immediately upon extrication.[3] This may be accomplished with infusion of lactated Ringer's solution or half-normal saline in D_5W to achieve a urinary pH exceeding 6.5 and a diuresis of 300 mL/hour. Sodium bicarbonate may be added to the infusion to alkalinize the urine, and acetazolamide (Diamox) may be used to keep the arterial pH from exceeding 7.45. Mannitol assists in maintaining the brisk diuresis in some patients when used at a dose of 1 g/kg body mass.

Glomerulonephritis may require corticosteroids, immunosuppressive agents, and even plasmapheresis if it is progressive and unrelenting.[51]

Acute interstitial nephritis accompanied by rash, fever, eosinophilia, or eosinophils in the urine may respond to high-dose corticosteroids (1 to 1.5 mg/kg/day prednisone). Occasionally these patients will require hemodialysis support.

The following recommendations for treatment apply predominantly to the renal parenchymal diseases.

Volume Regulation

Once adequate volume is assured but renal failure persists, it is important not to overload the patient. Furosemide or mannitol occasionally improves the volume of urine production but does not improve the quality of the urine or attendant functions. There is the risk of causing ototoxicity from increasing doses of furosemide as well as hyperosmolality if the mannitol is not excreted. Mannitol is contraindicated when anuria, pulmonary congestion, marked dehydration, or heart failure exists. Either agent may prevent ATN if given prophylactically, especially if given within the first 24 hours after the onset of oliguria, but neither will reverse established ATN.[52] Dopamine in low doses (1 to 3 μg/kg/min) may also be beneficial.

The importance of volume regulation is that too much volume is as bad as too little. Each individual generates 400 mL water daily from endogenous catabolism of proteins and lipids. The administration of 300 to 500 mL more than daily output (plus an additional 100 mL/day for each degree of fever) prevents volume excess. Ideally, the patient should lose 0.5 kg/day. Patients with renal failure may replace body mass (muscle and adipose tissue) with water weight, and this can be significant over long periods. Excessive fluid administration may cause pulmonary edema and difficulty in weaning patients from the ventilator owing to requirements for increased constant positive airway pressure to permit better oxygenation. Data from studies of military personnel in Southeast Asia indicate that pulmonary edema frequently may develop even in patients who have nonoliguric ATN (9 of 14 cases).[53] Patients in precarious hemodynamic status can develop congestive heart failure and will then require medications or dialysis to correct the iatrogenic problem. In other individuals, excess volume may induce hypertension. Ascites may develop and cause wound dehiscence following abdominal surgery. Theoretically, marked peripheral edema could cause an increased fluid phase, slowing mass transfer into and out of cells. Thus, relative restriction of volume can reduce many iatrogenic complications. When possible, fluids should be administered orally for patient comfort and to remove a potential source of infection. Foley catheters should not be used if a patient can void spontaneously or if there is negligible urine output. Despite the best efforts at good catheter care, catheters invite possible infection that may result in death. When the patient enters the polyuric phase, the volume administered should be increased, but one should be cautious not to "chase one's tail." If the volume administered exceeds 2 to 3 L, it is possible that sufficient function has been recovered and the physician is now "driving" the polyuria by the volumes administered. Therefore, after a few days of polyuria, begin decreasing the volume given to 500 mL less than the output.

Acid-Base Disorders

Renal failure is a well-recognized cause of metabolic acidosis. This occurs as a result of the inability of the patient to excrete the daily generated acid load as well as the inability to regenerate HCO_3. Normal adults generate hydrogen ions equal to about 1 mEq/kg/day. In ARF serum bicarbonate can fall from 2 to 15 mEq/day, depending on the degree of catabolism (much higher with trauma or sepsis). The accumulation of sulfate, phosphate, and other organic anions leads to an increased anion gap (normal, 12 ± 2 mEq/L), usually exceeding 15 mEq/L.[54] When the HCO_3 falls, some of the decrement is replaced by chloride. However, when HCO_3 is less than 16 mEq/L, it is advisable to treat the patient with HCO_3 or bicarbonate equivalent. Arterial pH should be measured when the serum bicarbonate falls below 16. Generally, a pH of less than 7.20 should be treated. In extremes of acidosis, the liver and other organs have an intracellular acidosis with impaired conversion of these anions to bicarbonate. In such patients, the optimal replacement is with $NaHCO_3$, either orally or intravenously, to maintain HCO_3 concentration above 18 mEq/L and the arterial pH above 7.20. $NaHCO_3$ must be used cautiously in patients with precarious volume status because of the large sodium load. The rationale of this therapy is to benefit enzyme systems, improve bone metabolism, and aid white blood cell function. An important consideration is that there should be a compensatory respiratory alkalosis. Because compensatory acid-base adjustments never overcorrect, an alkalosis out of proportion to that expected should be considered an early clue to infection or sepsis and should initiate blood cultures and possible antibiotic coverage. Guidelines to follow in assessing mixed acid-base disorders and correction may be found elsewhere. (See Chapter 21, Acid-Base Disturbances.)

Electrolyte Imbalance

Hyperphosphatemia usually develops soon after the onset of ARF. Phosphate retention will cause a corresponding decrease in calcium. This fall in calcium induces the release of parathyroid hormone. It is rare that the hypocalcemia is clinically significant as the ionized calcium is usually normal. However, when the calcium-phosphate product exceeds 70, metastatic calcification may occur in blood vessels, skin, lung, heart, and other sites. When hypocalcemia occurs in states of severe rhabdomyolysis, a rebound *hypercalcemia* should be expected as these deposits mobilize in the recovery phase.[55] Hyperphosphatemia may be controlled by dietary restriction, or phosphate-binding antacids if the patient has an oral intake. (If parenteral alimentation is used, these methods will not be successful.) Since phosphate and potassium accompany each gram of protein at approximately 1 mg and 1 mEq, respectively, the diet may be limited to 40 to 60 g protein to control urea production, hyperphosphatemia, and hyperkalemia. Aluminum hydroxide phosphate binders may be given at the end of each meal to lessen absorption of phosphate from the gastrointestinal tract. The initial doses are Amphojel or Basaljel, 30 mL orally with each meal, or ALternaGEL, 15 mL orally with each meal. The dose may be raised if needed or lessened if the patient becomes hypophosphatemic (less than 2.5 to 3.0 mg/dL) to lessen the risk of severe hypophosphatemia (less than 1.0 mg/dL) and the complications of pulmonary, cardiac, or neurologic dysfunction.[56] Magnesium-containing antacids are contraindicated as phosphate-binding agents, because of the risks of hypermagnesemia, which include death.

Sodium should not be given to excess. One gram of sodium equals 43 mEq, and a 4-g Na$^+$ diet is equivalent to a 10-g salt diet. Less than this quantity is usually required on a daily basis and will avoid increased thirst and volume overload. The dietary needs can be assessed by determining the total urinary losses and the intravenous saline administered and following serum sodium concentrations for the development of hyponatremia or hypernatremia. Hyponatremia is more common, occurring partly as a consequence of obligate urinary sodium loss but more frequently from excessive volume administration.

Serum potassium elevations occur mainly from dietary intake as well as medication, the transfusion of old blood, hematoma resorption, release from injured tissue, and acidosis. Potassium administration should be avoided during the oliguric phase or corrected cautiously if large extrarenal losses are evident. (During periods of polyuria, a marked kaliuresis may occur requiring supplementation.) When hyperkalemia greater than 6.0 mEq/L occurs and electrocardiographic changes are evident, the first treatment should be intravenous 10% calcium gluconate (up to three ampules at a rate of 3 to 5 minutes to administer each with constant electrocardiographic monitoring) to counteract the cardiac effects. (See Chapter 17, Electrolyte Abnormalities.) This may then be followed by two or three ampules of $NaHCO_3$ (50 mEq each), which induces the cellular uptake of potassium within minutes and may last for hours. This treatment may be followed by regular insulin, 1 U/10 kg body weight by intravenous push, followed by a continuous insulin infusion. To prevent hypoglycemia, 2 to 3 g glucose should be given per unit of insulin infused. These measures only temporize and shift potassium to an intracellular location. Therefore, they must be continued until potassium can be removed from the body. This may be accomplished by the use of sodium polystyrene sulfonate (Kayexalate), 15 to 20 g three or four times a day in 20 mL of 70% sorbitol for oral use or 50 g in 50 mL of 70% sorbitol plus 100 mL tap water as a retention enema. The obvious risk of this therapy is significant sodium loading. The ultimate means of potassium removal is via hemodialysis with a potassium-free dialysate. In some trauma cases, dialysis may be required twice daily in addition to other measures to control hyperkalemia.

Hypertension

Hypertension in renal failure is often related to hypervolemia. However, it also may be mediated by a variety of factors, including increased cardiac output, increased activity of the renin-angiotensin system, increased peripheral vascular resistance, autonomic nervous system dysfunction, or a vasodilator deficiency.[57] Control of volume should obviate the need for medications to lower the blood pressure or improve cardiac performance. However, if hypertension is a problem in a previously normotensive individual or if there is a significant risk for a stroke or myocardial infarction, it is imperative to lower the blood pressure. Medications that are used should be titrated to the blood pressure and not to the level of renal function.[57] In renal failure, diuretics usually are not effective; therefore, other agents must be employed such as methyldopa, clonidine, propranolol, hydralazine, prazosin, and terazosin. With either intravenous or oral methyldopa the maximal effect is evident at 4 to 6 hours. Hydralazine may be given intravenously or intramuscularly (at 15 to 25 mg) for rapid effect. Clonidine has the advantages of prompt onset, early maximal effect, and usefulness in moderate and severe hypertension. Because its half-life is prolonged in renal failure, clonidine should be given in the minimal effective dose. Minoxidil and nitroprusside can be used in malignant hypertension even when hemodialysis is necessary to support the patient. If the hypertension is clearly volume mediated, this may be an indication for early hemodialysis. (See Chapter 65, Hypertensive Emergencies.)

Metabolic Disorders

Diet is important in renal failure because patients are frequently catabolic but unable to excrete the metabolic wastes. If the patient can eat, a diet of 20 to 40 g/day of high biologic-value protein may be given. This may be liberalized to 60 g/day as renal function improves or dialysis is initiated. This diet will not give excessive potassium or phosphate as noted earlier. If the patient is unable to eat, 100 g glucose should be given daily to slow protein catabolism. Essential amino acid replacement has been shown to be of benefit in treating renal failure by lowering of the BUN through utilization of urea and possibly enhancing recovery.[58] These amino acids may be given intravenously as Nephramine or orally as Amin-Aid. The daily dose should be gradually increased while glucose, osmolality, and electrolytes are monitored on a daily basis.

Medications may require adjustment of dosage in renal failure as a result of an impaired excretory capacity. Most notably, digitalis compounds and antibiotics should be considered for alteration based on the half-life and route of excretion. Drugs such as gentamicin and carbenicillin (or ticarcillin) used for serious infections may inactivate each other if administered (temporally) closely together.[59] An extremely valuable reference is the updated dosing guidelines for adults with renal failure by Bennett and co-workers.[60] Certain medications should be avoided if possible until resolution has occurred, namely K^+ and Mg^{++} containing drugs, salicylates, and anticoagulants, because of the increased incidence of gastrointestinal hemorrhage in uremia, sulfonamides, and nitrofurantoin. The nonsteroidal anti-inflammatory agents should be avoided until renal function has improved, because there are numerous potential problems in patients with underlying renal disease.[61] Sedatives and hypnotics should be used with extra caution because of prolonged half-lives, altered protein-binding, and volumes of distribution in uremia. Drugs that may be needed include oral phosphate binders, water-soluble vitamins, and folic acid, 1 mg/day, if hemodialysis is employed.

Hematologic Disorders

Anemia is to be expected in patients with renal failure because of decreased erythropoiesis and shortened red blood cell survival. The hematocrit stabilizes at 20% to 25% and rises slowly after recovery. There is usually no need to routinely transfuse these patients. Notable exceptions occur if there is active hemorrhaging or if angina is precipitated. If angina develops, particularly in an older patient, it may be necessary to maintain a hematocrit of 30%. If pulmonary edema or volume overload is present, it may be advantageous to give packed red blood cells during hemodialysis.

Recombinant human erythropoietin is now commonly given to anemic patients on chronic hemodialysis. On maintenance doses a stable hematocrit between 33% and 38% can usually be achieved, eliminating the need for red blood cell transfusion.

White blood cell function is impaired as azotemia worsens; thus, attempts should be made to minimize sources of infection, such as unneeded intravenous lines and urinary catheters. It is best to *expect* infection (especially in the surgical, obstetric, or trauma patient) and be aggressive in treatment as sepsis is the most common cause of death. Hyperosmolality also impairs white blood cell function, and this should be considered when amino acid solutions are employed. Dialysis to improve the uremia and hyperosmolality may be crucial to recovery.

Platelet function and hemostasis become progressively impaired as uremia deepens. Platelets are decreased in number through reduced production as well as utilization; qualitative defects in platelet aggregation and adherence appear as the BUN and creatinine near 100 mg/dL and 10 mg/dL, respectively; coagulation factors may decline, and the bleeding time increases. As the risk of hemorrhage increases, dialysis is often initiated. If possible, medications that inhibit platelet aggregation should be avoided.

Endocrine Disorders

The values for hormone levels frequently appear abnormal in the uremic state owing to altered production, altered metabolism, abnormal protein binding, and alterations in the individual hormonal axis.[62] Thus, an assessment of endocrine function may be misleading unless these factors are taken into account. It is beyond the scope of this discussion to attempt to identify those changes—with one exception: insulin with a molecular weight of 6000 is normally freely filtered at the glomerulus and taken up by the proximal convoluted tubule for catabolism. In uremia, despite what appears to be peripheral resistance to insulin and elevated lipids, insulin catabolism is decreased. Therefore, exogenous insulin may have more of an effect, and attention should be given to decreasing the dose, if necessary, to prevent hypoglycemia.

Indications for Dialysis

Dialytic intervention is indicated in the patient with renal failure when any of the following are noted:

- central nervous system alterations such as altered mentation
- neurologic deficits with a sensory or motor neuropathy
- pericarditis
- hyperkalemia, especially if accompanied by electrocardiographic changes
- BUN value greater than or equal to 100 mg/dL or creatinine value greater than or equal to 10 mg/dL
- massive volume excess
- severe acid-base disorders
- drug overdose

Factors that favor earlier initiation of dialysis include sepsis (with increased catabolism and the need for normal white blood cell function); trauma; diabetes, because of the associated risks; and the need for, or recent completion of, surgery to enhance wound healing, to prevent coagulopathies and hemorrhage, and to minimize the problems of infection and extracellular volume control.

Patients presenting with acute renal failure should be hospitalized until renal function has been recovered, a protracted recovery is evident, or the patients are considered to be chronic hemodialysis or peritoneal dialysis patients. Since some of these patients may require hemodialysis, it is beneficial to the patient to have one arm spared from phlebotomies and intravenous infusions. This will facilitate surgery for an arteriovenous fistula or polytetrafluoroethylene (PTFE) graft. Vessel damage, thrombosis, and phlebitis will also be minimized. Because the number of potential vascular access sites is strictly limited, blood pressures should not be determined in the extremity in which one of these types of access has been placed, owing to the additional risk of stasis leading to thrombosis and loss of the access. The viability of an access can be confirmed by a palpable thrill and audible bruit in the case of arteriovenous fistulas and PTFE grafts. For shunts, an uninterrupted column of blood is visible in all portions of the tubing. (The high flow through these devices may give a high venous return and transmit a bruit to the thorax, simulating a new murmur.) A thrombosed access requires prompt attention from a vascular surgeon.

Hemodialysis offers advantages over peritoneal dialysis; rapid access via femoral catheters, subclavian dialysis catheters, or extremity access as noted above; more rapid clearance of potassium and metabolic wastes; avoidance of respiratory depression and potential volume overload resulting from fluid in the peritoneum; and rapid correction of acid-base disorders. Peritoneal dialysis is preferred in patients in whom hemodynamic instability or hypotension (unsupportable with pressor agents) will not permit safe hemodialysis, in those with severe thrombocytopenia, in patients with a recent myocardial infarction, and in small children.

The morbidity and mortality remain high in renal failure owing to infection and underlying disorders,[2,31,42] but close attention to detail and anticipation of problems with volume overload, infection, and bleeding will improve the chance of survival. Patients with prolonged renal failure (ie, greater than 4 to 6 weeks) have diminished chances of recovery but can be managed by chronic hemodialysis, peritoneal dialysis, or later renal transplantation.

REFERENCES

1. Anderson RJ, Linas SL, Berns AS, et al. Nonoliguric acute renal failure. *N Engl J Med.* 1977;296:1134–1138.
2. Anderson RJ, Schrier RW. Clinical spectrum of oliguric and nonoliguric acute renal failure. In: Brenner BM, Stein JH, eds. *Acute Renal Failure.* New York, NY: Churchill Livingstone; 1980:1–16.
3. Ron D, Taitelman U, Michaelson M, et al. Prevention of acute renal failure in traumatic rhabdomyolysis. *Arch Intern Med.* 1984;144:277–280.
4. Miller PD, Krebs RA, Neal BJ, McIntyre DO. Polyuric prerenal failure. *Arch Intern Med.* 1980;140:907–909.
5. Gutman RA, Striker GF, Gilliland BC, Cutler RE. The immune complex glomerulonephritis of bacterial endocarditis. *Medicine (Baltimore).* 1972;51:1–25.
6. Beaufils M, Morel-Maroger L, Sraer J, Kanfer A, Kourilsky O, Richet G. Acute renal failure of glomerular origin during visceral abscesses. *N Engl J Med.* 1976;295:185–189.
7. Kelleher SP, Berl T. Acute renal failure in pregnancy. *Semin Nephrol.* 1981;1:61–68.
8. Grunfeld JP, Ganeval D, Bournerias F. Acute renal failure in pregnancy. *Kidney Int.* 1980;18:179–191.
9. Conn HO. A rational approach to the hepatorenal syndrome. *Gastroenterology.* 1973;65:321–340.
10. Gordon JA, Anderson RJ. Hepatorenal syndrome. *Semin Nephrol.* 1981;1:37–42.
11. Appel GB, Neu HC. The nephrotoxicity of antimicrobial agents. *N Engl J Med.* 1977;206:663–670, 722–728, 784–787.
12. Moore RD, Smith CR, Lipsky JJ, et al. Risk factors for nephrotoxicity in patients treated with aminoglycosides. *Ann Intern Med.* 1984;100:352–357.
13. Ditlove J, Weidmann P, Bernstein M, et al. Methicillin nephritis. *Medicine (Baltimore).* 1977;56:483–491.
14. Cogan MG. Tubulo-interstitial nephropathies: a pathophysiologic approach. *West J Med.* 1980;132:134–140.
15. Porter GA, Bennett WM. Nephrotoxin-induced acute renal failure. In: Brenner BM, Stein JH, eds. *Acute Renal Failure.* New York, NY: Churchill Livingstone; 1980:123–162.
16. Roxe DM. Toxic nephropathy from diagnostic and therapeutic agents: review and commentary. *Am J Med.* 1980;69:759–766.
17. Knochel JP. Rhabdomyolysis and myoglobinuria. *Semin Nephrol.* 1981;1:75–86.
18. Honda N. Acute renal failure and rhabdomyolysis. *Kidney Int.* 1983;23:888–898.
19. Koffler A, Friedler RM, Massry SG. Acute renal failure due to nontraumatic rhabdomyolysis. *Ann Intern Med.* 1976;85:23–28.
20. Grossman RA, Hamilton RW, Morse BM, Penn AS, Goldberg M. Nontraumatic rhabdomyolysis and acute renal failure. *N Engl J Med.* 1974;291:807–811.
21. Cunningham E, Kohli R, Venuto RC. Influenza-associated myoglobinuric renal failure. *JAMA.* 1979;242:2428–2429.
22. Gartenberg G, Weinstein MP, Fernando NK, et al. Rhabdomyolysis with acute renal failure in legionnaire's disease. *J Med Soc NJ.* 1981;78:119–120.
23. Poulter N, Garbiel R, Porter KA, et al. Acute interstitial nephritis complicating legionnaire's disease. *Clin Nephrol.* 1981;15:216–220.
24. Kendrick WC, Hull AR, Knochel JP. Rhabdomyolysis and shock after intravenous amphetamine administration. *Ann Intern Med.* 1977;86:381–387.
25. Cogen FC, Rigg G, Simmons JL, et al. Phencyclidine-associated acute rhabdomyolysis. *Ann Intern Med.* 1978;88:210–212.
26. Boyd RE, Brennan PT, Deng J-F, et al. Strychnine poisoning: recovery from profound lactic acidosis, hyperthermia, and rhabdomyolysis. *Am J Med.* 1983;74:507–512.
27. Nadel SM, Jackson JW, Ploth DW. Hypokalemic rhabdomyolysis and acute renal failure: occurrence following total parenteral nutrition. *JAMA.* 1979;241:2294–2296.
28. Byrd L, Sherman RL. Radiocontrast-induced acute renal failure: a clinical and pathophysiologic review. *Medicine (Baltimore).* 1979;58:270–279.
29. Harkonen S, Kjellstrand C. Contrast nephropathy. *Am J Nephrol.* 1981;1:69–77.
30. Carvallo A, Rakowski TA, Argy WP, et al. Acute renal failure following drip infusion pyelography. *Am J Med.* 1978;65:38–45.
31. Levinsky NG, Alexander EA, Venkatichalam MA. Acute renal failure. In: Brenner BM, Rector FC, eds. *The Kidney.* 2nd ed. Philadelphia, Pa: WB Saunders Co; 1981;1:1181–1236.
32. Rascoff JH, Golden RA, Spinowitz BS, et al. Nondilated obstructive nephropathy. *Arch Intern Med.* 1983;143:696–698.
33. Blantz RC, Hostetter TH, Brenner BM. Functional adaptations of the kidney to immunological injury. In: Wilson CB, Brenner BM, Stein JH, eds. *Immunologic Mechanisms of Renal Disease.* New York, NY: Churchill Livingstone; 1979:122–143.
34. Hou SH, Bushinsky DA, Wish JB, et al: Hospital-acquired renal insufficiency: a prospective study. *Am J Med.* 1983;74:243–248.
35. Steinman TI, Silva P. Acute renal failure, skin rash, and eosinophilia associated with captopril therapy. *Am J Med.* 1983;75:154–156.
36. Patak RV, Lifschitz MD, Stein JH. Acute renal failure: clinical aspects and pathophysiology. *Cardiovasc Med.* 1979;4:19–38.
37. Wright FS, Howard SS. Obstructive injury. In: Brenner BM, Rector FC, eds. *The Kidney.* 2nd ed. Philadelphia, Pa: WB Saunders Co; 1981;2:2008–2044.
38. Cohen DJ, Sherman WH, Osserman EF, et al. Acute renal failure in patients with multiple myeloma. *Am J Med.* 1984;76:247–256.
39. Kelton J, Kelley WN, Holmes EW. A rapid method for the diagnosis of acute uric acid nephropathy. *Arch Intern Med.* 1978;138:612–615.
40. Kjellstrand CM, Campbell DC, von Hartitzsch B, et al. Hyperuricemic acute renal failure. *Arch Intern Med.* 1974;133:349–359.

41. Lindheimer MD, Katz AI. Renal disease and pregnancy. In: Suki WN, Eknoyan G, eds. *The Kidney in Systemic Disease*, New York, NY: Wiley & Sons; 1976:237–254.

42. Butkus DE. Persistent high mortality in acute renal failure: are we asking the right questions? *Arch Intern Med*. 1983;143:209–211.

43. Planas M, Wachtel T, Frank H, et al. Characterization of acute renal failure in the burned patient. *Arch Intern Med*. 1982;142:2087–2091.

44. Feig PU, McCurdy DK. The hypertonic state. *N Engl J Med*. 1977;297:1444–1454.

45. Espinel CH. The FE_{Na} test: use in the differential diagnosis of acute renal failure. *JAMA*. 1976;236:579–581.

46. Miller TR, Anderson RJ, Linas SL, et al. Urinary diagnostic indices in acute renal failure: a prospective study. *Ann Intern Med*. 1978;89:47–50.

47. Ellenbogen PH, Scheible FW, Talner LB, et al. Sensitivity of gray scale ultrasound in detecting urinary tract obstruction. *AJR Am J Roentgenol*. 1978;130:731–733.

48. Brown WW, Hebert LA, Piering WF, et al. Reversal of chronic end stage renal failure due to myeloma kidney. *Ann Intern Med*. 1979;90:793–794.

49. Linton AL, Clark WF, Driedger AA, et al. Acute interstitial nephritis due to drugs: review of the literature with a report of nine cases. *Ann Intern Med*. 1980;93:735–741.

50. Espinel CH, Gregory AW. Differential diagnosis of acute renal failure. *Clin Nephrol*. 1980;13:73–77.

51. Warren SE, Mitas JA, Golbus SM, et al. Recovery from rapidly progressive glomerulonephritis: improvement after plasmaphresis and immunosuppression. *Arch Intern Med*. 1981;141:175–180.

52. Warren SE, Blantz RC. Mannitol. *Arch Intern Med*. 1981;141:493–497.

53. Lordon RE, Burton JR. Post-traumatic renal failure in military personnel in Southeast Asia: experience at Clark USAF Hospital, Republic of the Philippines. *Am J Med*. 1972;53:137–147.

54. Narins RG, Emmett M. Simple and mixed acid-base disorders: a practical approach. *Medicine (Baltimore)*. 1980;59:161–187.

55. Liu ET, Bristow MR, Stone MJ, et al. Serum myoglobin, ionized calcium, and parathyroid function during rhabdomyolysis. *Arch Intern Med*. 1983;143:154–157.

56. Knochel JP. The pathophysiology and clinical characteristics of severe hypophosphatemia. *Arch Intern Med*. 1977;137:203–220.

57. Mitas JA, O'Connor DT, Stone RA. Hypertension in renal insufficiency: a major therapeutic problem. *Postgrad Med*. 1978;64:113–118.

58. Abel RM, Beck CH, Abbott WM, et al. Improved survival from acute renal failure after treatment with intravenous essential I-amino acids and glucose: results of a prospective double-blind study. *N Engl J Med*. 1973;288:695–699.

59. Weibert R, Keane W, Shapiro F. Carbenicillin inactivation of aminoglycosides in patients with severe renal failure. *Trans Am Soc Artif Int Organs*. 1976;22:439–443.

60. Bennett WM, Aronoff GR, Morrison G, et al. Drug prescribing in renal failure: dosing guidelines for adults. *Am J Kidney Dis*. 1983;3:155–193.

61. Clive DM, Stoff JS. Renal syndromes associated with nonsteroidal antiinflammatory drugs. *N Engl J Med*. 1984;310:563–572.

62. Emmanouel DS, Lindheimer MD, Katz AI. Endocrine abnormalities in chronic renal failure: pathogenetic principles and clinical implications. *Semin Nephrol*. 1981;1:151–175.

79. Obstetric and Gynecologic Emergencies

JOHN J. WILLEMS, MD, FRCS, FACOG
DENNIS E. SANDLER, MD, FACOG

Women bring to the emergency department setting their unique reproductive potential as well as a unique set of reproductive system malfunctions. These singular malfunctions can sometimes be daunting to even the most competent emergency physician. Specialists in obstetrics and gynecology have noted, on occasion, a degree of decompensation in an emergency department suddenly faced with a premature delivery or substantial vaginal bleeding even when that same emergency department can handle a catastrophic myocardial infarction, gunshot wound, third degree burn, or motor vehicle trauma as part of daily routine.

This chapter will discuss symptom-oriented practical guidelines in obstetrics and gynecology that the practicing emergency physician can use to dispel the reproductive mystique of the female patient and put that patient on the same footing for triage and management as any other emergency department (ED) visit. This chapter will not attempt to cover all possible obstetric/gynecologic (OB/GYN) diagnoses. There are many standard specialty texts which perform that function admirably and are readily available for reference. Instead, we will focus on the major presenting symptoms seen most commonly in the emergency department and the algorithms leading to the most important differential diagnoses, together with suggested diagnostic tests and management options. Lastly, the algorithms we recommend are not the only acceptable options but are those that have evolved and worked successfully for us at Scripps Clinic & Research Foundation over the last 10 years.

Before discussing the symptom presentation of specific OB/GYN diagnoses, it is vital to stress the importance of two data points which should be noted on the ED record of every female patient. The first is date of last menstrual period (LMP) and the second is pregnancy test status. The pragmatic emergency physician should have a good answer to the question, "Why am I not ordering a pregnancy test on this patient?" For example, pregnancy after tubal ligation is not unknown and is most frequently ectopic when it occurs. A past history of tubal ligation is, therefore, not an adequate answer particularly if there are any pelvic symptoms such as pain or vaginal bleeding. Second, pregnancy status should be known prior to any radiologic or interventional diagnostic procedure if the stability of the patient's condition permits.

GYNECOLOGIC EMERGENCIES

Pelvic Pain

The most common symptom in female ED patients leading to a gynecologic consultation in our institution is pelvic pain. The process may be acute (6 to 12 hours since onset) or of a more chronic nature with a recent intensification. Initial assessment for triage should include a directed historic review, vital signs, and physical findings that would dictate early surgical intervention. Gynecologic causes of acute pelvic pain include both ectopic pregnancy and pelvic inflammatory disease, which will be discussed separately, as well as ovarian torsion and ovarian cyst rupture. In the case of ovarian torsion, a markedly tender adnexal region with a negative pregnancy test, stable vital signs, and minimally elevated white count point toward torsion. The pain is sudden in onset and constant in nature with some exacerbations noted when the patient moves. Sonography will show a nonspecific adnexal enlargement on the affected side in conjunction with a negligible amount of free intraperitoneal fluid. Ovarian cyst rupture is often seen in the setting of coital trauma and a history of pain onset after an otherwise uneventful coitus is helpful. Clinical presentation can mimic ectopic pregnancy or pelvic inflammatory disease in that the patient can have peritoneal signs including rebound tenderness and a very tender pelvic exam without evidence of a definite mass. The patient will be afebrile, however, and have a negative pregnancy test. Sonography may or may not show an adnexal mass but will show fluid in the pelvis. While most ruptured ovarian cysts will stop bleeding without intervention, if the patient has orthostatic changes in her blood pressure, unstable vital signs, a falling hematocrit, or is anticoagulated, laparoscopy is recommended to evaluate the problem and cauterize the bleeding site as needed. In equivocal cases, overnight hospitalization may be necessary for continued monitoring until a decision regarding surgery can be reached.

Chronic pelvic pain can include cyclic recurrent pain such as mittelschmerz, endometriosis, or adenomyosis. Timing of the onset of pain in relation to the menstrual cycle is a useful point to ascertain. Midcycle pain is usually ovulatory and points toward mittelschmerz. Pain just prior to menses with some relief at onset of menses points towards endometriosis while severe dysmenorrhea is more commonly related to adenomyosis although endometriosis remains a possibility. Physical examination is not specific and laparoscopy is often needed to confirm the diagnosis of endometriosis as well as assess other possible causes of chronic pelvic pain such as chronic pelvic inflammatory disease and pelvic adhesions.

Full evaluation of pelvic pain must also include the nongynecologic causes which every emergency physician is familiar with, including but not limited to appendicitis, diverticulitis, colitis, pancreatitis, cholecystitis, and nephrolithiasis.

Abnormal Vaginal Bleeding

The second most common reason for gynecologic consultation from our emergency department is abnormal vaginal bleeding. Vaginal bleeding can be abnormal based on quantity or timing. Timing can be divided into individual menstrual cycles or stages in a patient's reproductive life. As an example, vaginal bleeding in an 8-year-old is abnormal as is postcoital bleeding, bleeding during pregnancy, or midcycle bleeding. Any bleeding that is excessive in duration, frequency, or amount *for a particular patient* should be considered abnormal and investigated. Bleeding causing hemodynamic instability is always abnormal as is most bleeding leading to anemia.

Initial assessment of the patient with vaginal bleeding includes a rapid check of the patient's vital signs including any postural changes in pulse or blood pressure. Orthostatic decompensation in an otherwise stable patient can lead one to suspect a greater than observed external loss or intra-abdominal hemorrhage from an ectopic pregnancy or a ruptured ovarian cyst. Following the initial physical assessment, historic features regarding timing and quantity of bleeding are discussed. Is this postmenopausal bleeding? Any relationship to coitus? Hormones used? Pain? Knowledge of LMP, history of unprotected intercourse, and pregnancy status are critical at this juncture. If the rapid, sensitive urine pregnancy test is positive, the LMP should indicate the approximate week of gestation. Bleeding in the second and third trimester of pregnancy as disclosed by LMP and abdominal palpation does not require a pregnancy test.

Vaginal bleeding in early pregnancy should lead to the consideration of spontaneous abortion, septic abortion, molar pregnancy, or ectopic pregnancy. Septic abortion must be considered if there is any suspicion that the pregnancy has been tampered with or the uterus instrumented (ie, any mechanical or chemical contamination of the uterine contents). Postabortal endometritis is common and, when associated with retained products of conception, requires surgical intervention. Uterine cramping with a spontaneous abortion can be severe and mimic the abdominal findings of a leaking ectopic pregnancy, whereas the abdominal findings in an unruptured ectopic pregnancy can be entirely benign. Vaginal examination can help with several distinctions. First, it can be ascertained that the blood is coming from the cervical os and not from unsuspected vaginal trauma. Second, if products of conception are seen at the cervical os then the abortion is incomplete and the uterine cavity needs to be emptied. If no products of conception are seen, then the abortion may be threatened, complete, or an ectopic may be present. Palpation of an adnexal mass is not a reliable indicator of ectopic pregnancy because some ovarian enlargement will be present secondary to the corpus luteum. A septic abortion may produce uterine and cervical motion tenderness similar to that found in ectopic pregnancies or pelvic inflammatory disease (PID). At this juncture, ultrasound evaluation is invaluable. In recent years, ultrasound and especially vaginal probe studies have become a critical diagnostic adjunct. Vaginal sonography can demonstrate a viable intrauterine pregnancy at 5 to 6 weeks after the last menstrual period, thereby suggesting threatened as opposed to incomplete abortion. It can also show retained products of conception necessitating a curettage, or it can show the characteristic pattern of a molar pregnancy. If the uterine cavity is empty and there is no adnexal mass either visualized or palpable, then a complete spontaneous abortion is most likely and outpatient follow-up to monitor declining β-human chorionic gonadotropin (BHCG) levels is appropriate. If there is sonographic evidence of fluid in the pelvis or if the sonography is unavailable, serious consideration should be given to culdocentesis.

There has been continuing interest in culdocentesis because of its simplicity and relative accuracy. If a positive pregnancy test is present together with more than 5 mL of nonclotting blood from the cul-de-sac, an ectopic will be found in greater than 90% of cases. Culdocentesis will be positive in about 80% of ectopic pregnancy cases. Of positive studies 62% will be associated with unruptured ectopics and 45% of patients demonstrating positive results will have minimal peritoneal signs at the time of initial evaluation. Culdocentesis can therefore indicate a high probability of ectopic pregnancy even when other physical findings are misleading.[1–3]

Culdocentesis is performed by inserting an 18 gauge spinal needle attached to a glass syringe between the uterosacral ligaments into the cul-de-sac (Fig. 79-1; see also Chapter 86, Atlas of Emergency Procedures). If a plastic syringe is used, any blood obtained should be quickly transferred to a glass tube. The test is positive if >5 mL of nonclotted blood or no fluid at all is obtained. Analysis of several large series of culdocenteses indicates that the procedure rarely leads to complications and is readily learned. However, culdocentesis is contraindicated if there is a fixed mass in the cul-de-sac. While a positive culdocentesis may expedite surgical evaluation, a negative test should not cause delay if other findings are suspicious. Diagnostic laparoscopy can settle a diagnostic dilemma expeditiously. Often the combination of a ruptured corpus luteum can occur with a complete or incomplete spontaneous abortion or an early intra-uterine pregnancy. Laparoscopy is ideal in resolving this issue. Since most ectopics can currently be handled through the laparoscope, even a frankly positive culdocentesis should have laparoscopy as initial operative management as long as the patient is hemodynamically stable.[2,4]

In addition to acute vaginal bleeding, there are the causes of chronic abnormal vaginal bleeding over the course of weeks or months such as uterine leiomyomata (fibroids), adenomyosis, or dysfunctional uterine bleeding related to hormonal dysfunction. With adequate history, the chronic nature should become obvious. However, there may be a superimposed acute aspect in the form of active hemorrhage sufficient to produce hypotension, tachycardia, and anemia. Most chronic bleeding problems can be dealt with as a gynecologic care. This may include intravenous hormone therapy or emergency hysterectomy. Screening laboratory work for chronic vaginal bleeding should always include coagulation studies to exclude possible coagulation disorders such as von Willebrand's disease.

Ectopic Pregnancy

Throughout the gynecologic portion of this chapter, ectopic pregnancy has been emphasized repeatedly. With ectopic

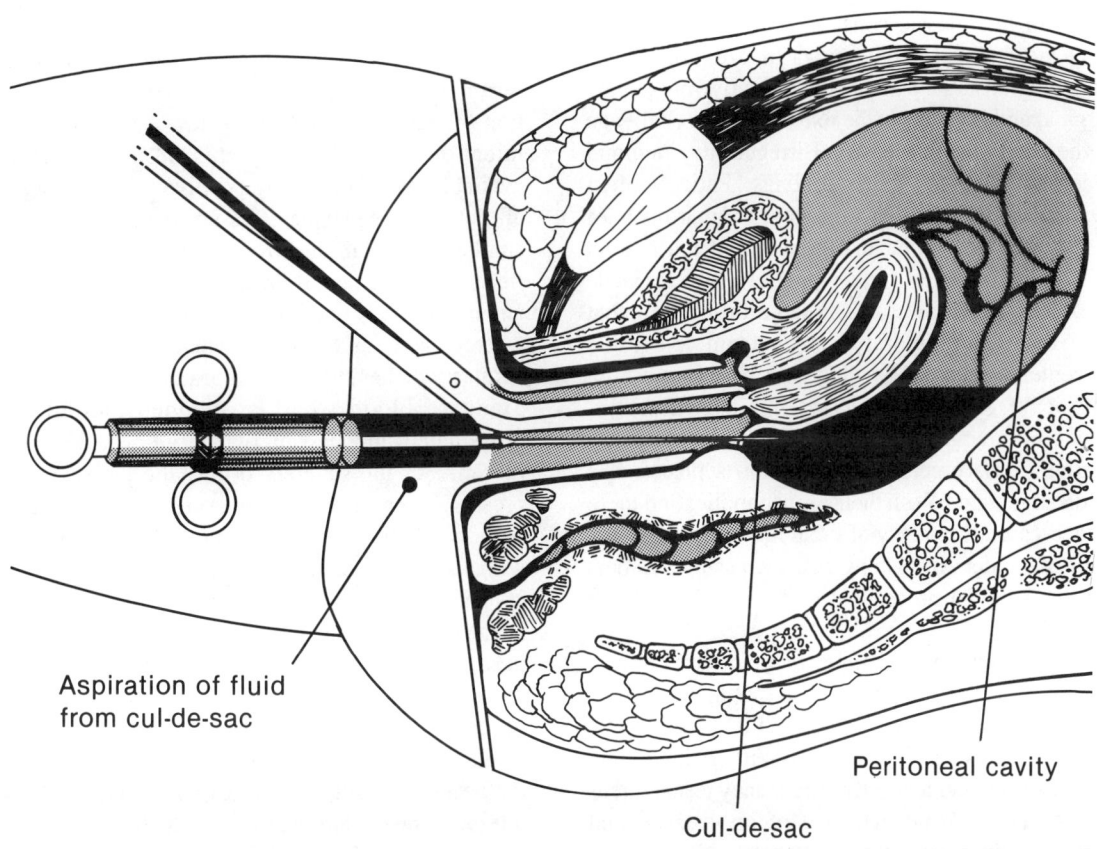

Figure 79-1 Culdocentesis: sagittal, showing aspiration.

pregnancy, one is dealing with a condition whose numbers, as reported to the Centers for Disease Control, have quadrupled between 1970 and 1985. This amounts to more than 78,000 ectopic pregnancies per year in the United States. In the late 1960s ectopic pregnancy accounted for 1 in 200 pregnancies, and it now accounts for almost 2% of all pregnancies, with at least 40 deaths per year reported in the United States.[5]

Reasons for this increased incidence include increased prevalence of sexually transmitted disease, increased numbers of patients with surgery to the fallopian tubes (ie, tubal reanastomosis, tubal ligation, tuboplasty), postabortal pelvic infection, and increased incidence of prior ectopic pregnancy (10% to 20%). Patients with any of these historic markers such as PID need particularly close evaluation. Because of these facts, a high index of suspicion has never been more important or had more clinical utility. Because of these factors, early diagnosis prior to tubal rupture and massive intraperitoneal hemorrhage is critical in the preservation of fertility, and failure to diagnose an ectopic pregnancy can be catastrophic in terms of patient outcome as well as malpractice liability.

When a patient presents with a positive pregnancy test, pelvic or abdominal pain, vaginal bleeding, and an adnexal mass palpable clinically or visualized via sonography, ectopic pregnancy is the diagnosis to confirm or deny. Unfortunately, the patient with an ectopic pregnancy frequently does not present with this classic constellation of findings and there will be no pathognomonic signs or symptoms. The hemodynamically unstable patient with a positive pregnancy test and surgical abdomen is not the real diagnostic challenge but rather the patient with menstrual irregularity, minimal pelvic tenderness, and few other findings. Patients often report one or two visits to an emergency department or physician's office prior to tubal rupture when the correct diagnosis is finally made. If further progress is to be made with the problem of ectopics, this is the time window that must be utilized. Contemporary management of ectopic pregnancy centers around early diagnosis based on a high index of suspicion, sensitive urine or serum BHCG assays, and advances in sonography. Without these tools being rapidly available, the emergency physician is placed at a significant disadvantage. With their proper application there has been a decreased frequency of tubal rupture, with many centers reporting under 20%, along with increasing numbers of conservative surgical procedures performed through the laparoscope.[2,3,6]

The differential diagnosis includes ovarian cyst rupture, ovarian torsion, threatened or incomplete spontaneous abortion, septic abortion, or pelvic infection/PID, and appendicitis should always be considered. With PID, fever, marked leukocytosis, and a negative pregnancy test are generally present. There is no evidence of orthostasis, and uterine size is within normal limits. Appendicitis typically begins with periumbilical pain, more numerous gastrointestinal complaints, more substantial leukocytosis, and fever. It is rarely associated with cervical motion tenderness to the degree seen with ectopic pregnancy or PID, and menstrual abnormality is uncommon, but nonspecific right adnexal tenderness may be present. Adnexal torsion presents with sudden excruciating unilateral lower abdominal pain, with radiation to the anterior and medial thigh. The patient is in marked distress with stable vital signs, a very tender adnexa on pelvic exam, and an adnexal mass clearly seen on sonogram.

As noted, with ectopic pregnancy the clinical presentation can be inconsistent. The patient usually reports a variable period of amenorrhea followed by some pelvic or abdominal pain and irregular bleeding. The patient may or may not "feel pregnant." Tubal rupture is heralded by a marked increase in abdominal or pelvic pain, dizziness, fainting, and pain radiating to the shoulder from intraperitoneal hemorrhage. These symptoms may be precipitated by exertion, coitus, or straining at stool. The clinical picture is one of a pale, distressed woman with cold, clammy skin, a thready pulse, a narrowed pulse pressure, and orthostatic changes in blood pressure. If traumatic hemorrhage can be ruled out, ectopic pregnancy becomes highly likely. Since otherwise healthy young women can tolerate substantial blood loss before a major shift in vital signs, orthostatic blood pressure and pulse changes are a critical point to check since they can alert you to a patient who may rapidly become unstable.

Laboratory evaluation is straightforward. A stat complete blood count (CBC) with sedimentation rate and sensitive serum or urine pregnancy test are ordered. The new generation of sensitive urine pregnancy tests permits rapid determination of pregnancy status in contrast to previously available tests which were positive only in about one half of all ectopic pregnancies. As noted previously, sonography can be invaluable in differentiating early pregnancy events (ie, a threatened abortion with corpus luteum as opposed to an empty uterus with an associated adnexal mass).

Treatment for the hemodynamically unstable patient is similar whether the cause is trauma or ectopic pregnancy. Standard blood work is obtained including type and crossmatch and one or two large-bore IV catheters are placed. For the severely orthostatic patient or if shock is present, a central venous pressure line is also secured. Correction of intravascular volume must be prompt, beginning with Ringer's lactate solution and using a combination of crystalloid and colloid solutions as necessary to maintain adequate perfusion. The patient is placed in Trendelenburg's position and oxygen by mask is begun. Urgent surgical consultation and notification of the operating room are needed so that a surgical suite can be made immediately available with an appropriate operating team together with the necessary equipment to capture, filter, and reinfuse the intraperitoneal blood loss. An elective surgery procedure will need to be deferred until this emergency situation is dealt with. Treatment for the hemodynamically stable ectopic patient begins with diagnostic suspicion and is confirmed with a combination of diagnostic and operative laparoscopy. Linear salpingotomy or partial salpingectomy is the treatment of choice and can be accomplished with laparoscopic techniques on most occasions. Several centers are currently reporting on the use of methotrexate as either primary therapy for ectopic pregnancy or as a second line treatment should there be any residual trophoblastic tissue present after laparoscopic management.[6] This type of treatment requires a motivated and reliable patient. Methotrexate is an evolving therapy at present but since laparoscopy is both diagnostic and curative, we will continue to use it primarily for the near future.

Pelvic Inflammatory Disease

PID is a major health problem in the United States, with 250,000 hospitalized cases in 1985 and at least two million physician office visits that same year diagnosed as acute PID. Subclinical, untreated, undertreated, or asymptomatic pelvic infection is felt to be a major factor not only in the rising tide of venereal disease but also in tubal factor infertility and ectopic pregnancy, both of which have increased dramatically over the last 20 years.[5,7,8] PID is made up of a spectrum of upper genital tract inflammatory disorders including pelvic peritonitis, tubo-ovarian abscess, salpingitis, and endometritis. Antimicrobial regimens for PID are designed to provide empirical, broad-spectrum coverage of the likely etiologic pathogens, including *Neisseria gonorrhoeae*, *Chlamydia trachomatis*, gram-negative bacilli, anaerobes, aerobic streptococci, and *Mycoplasma hominis*. The sexual partners of women with PID should also be treated.

The organism most commonly associated with acute PID is *Neisseria gonorrhoeae*. Up to 85% of women and 15% of men are asymptomatic when infected with gonorrhea. If left untreated, approximately 20% will progress to PID. A symptomatic infected woman may complain of dysuria, frequency, a purulent vaginal discharge, and vulvar pruritus, but most pre-PID patients will have few complaints and will be picked up only if a culture is performed. The cervix, urethra, and anus should be cultured on Thayer Martin or Transgros media. Because of antibiotic-resistant *N. gonorrhoeae*, including penicillinase-producing *N. gonorrhoeae*, tetracycline-resistant *N. gonorrhoeae*, and strains with chromosomally mediated resistance to multiple antibiotics together with the high frequency of chlamydial infections in persons with gonorrhea and the absence of a fast, inexpensive, and highly accurate test for chlamydial infection, the Centers for Disease Control have recommended a regimen for uncomplicated gonorrhea designed to cover chlamydia simultaneously. Ceftriaxone, 250 mg IM once, combined with doxycycline, 100 mg orally two times a day for 7 days, is the current management of choice.

Patients with PID present with lower abdominal pain and fever. Most often the pain begins as a suprapubic dull ache and frequently occurs around the time of menses when pathogenic organisms are more likely to gain access to the upper reproductive tract. With spreading peritonitis, the pain becomes generalized and exacerbated by movement. Patients with chronic PID complain of low back pain and lower abdominal pain which, for reasons noted above, can worsen around menses. Dyspareunia, typically during deep penetration, is common, as is tenesmus and rectal pain during defecation. It is essential to remember that any patient with known or suspected PID may have an ectopic pregnancy and, in fact, history of PID is a known risk factor for ectopic pregnancy. Also, it may be necessary to have a laparoscope and/or sonographic evaluation of the pelvis to rule out appendicitis when the pelvic symptoms are predominantly right-sided. The fact that patients with chronic PID frequently have dysfunctional uterine bleeding secondary to ovarian damage compounds the difficulty in making the correct diagnosis. Fever and chills associated with PID may be slight or marked, depending on the severity of the disease. Tachycardia, dehydration, and leukocytosis with a shift to the left are common. Anorexia, nausea, and vomiting may also play a role in the dehydration. Frequently, an associated anemia of chronic illness is discovered.

Physical examination reveals a febrile, toxic patient in acute distress. She is typically lying on her side in the "fetal position," clutching her lower abdomen. There is abdominal distention with decreased or absent bowel sounds. Suprapubic and bilateral lower quadrant tenderness to palpation is a hallmark of PID. Classic signs of peritoneal irritation (ie, rebound, referred pain, and involuntary muscle guarding) are apparent, especially in the lower quadrants. Upper abdominal signs suggest disseminated intraperitoneal infection. In more severe cases purulent exudate may reach the liver surface via the right paracolic gutter, inciting a perihepatitis with adhesion formation between the capsule of the liver and undersurface of the diaphragm known as the Fitz-Hugh-Curtis syndrome. On pelvic examination, a purulent discharge may be seen coming from the cervical os. The cervix is exquisitely tender to motion, with pain referred bilaterally to the lower abdomen. It is commonly impossible to evaluate the uterus and adnexa secondary to severe pain and guarding, but when examination is possible, the uterus is found to be small and firm. A pelvic sonogram may be needed to assess the presence or absence of a tubo-ovarian abscess. Chronic infection with scarring and adhesion formation produces a fundus that is immobile, commonly retroverted, and slightly tender. A cystic sausage-shaped adnexal mass is a hydrosalpinx, or tubo-ovarian abscess. Fluctuant bulging of the cul-de-sac also heralds the presence of a pelvic abscess. If there is any indication of abscess rupture or septic shock intervening, surgical management will be needed immediately and should be organized while the patient is being rapidly stabilized. A ruptured tubo-ovarian abscess is a true surgical emergency, which formerly carried a mortality rate of 80% to 90%. With appropriate surgical and antibiotic management, mortality is markedly reduced. After a thorough history and physical examination have been completed, intravenous lines are established and correction of hypovolemia and acidosis is begun. Cultures are carefully taken from the cervix for gonorrhea and chlamydia. Urethral and anal cultures should also be sent. Blood is obtained for a CBC, differential, electrolytes, blood culture, and erythrocyte sedimentation rate. Urine specimens are obtained for urinalysis and a rapid, sensitive urine pregnancy test. If the latter is positive, a rethinking of the diagnosis of PID is mandatory; salpingitis is rarely seen concomitant with an intact intrauterine pregnancy, since some protection of the upper genital tract is afforded by the thick cervical mucous plug. Once again, ectopic pregnancy must *always* be ruled out in any patient having lower abdominal pain and a positive pregnancy test.

If an intrauterine device is present, it is removed as soon as adequate serum antibiotic levels are achieved in an attempt to prevent significant bacteremia. If pelvic examination rules out an abscess, it is suggested that a gram stain and culture may be obtained via culdocentesis. With broad-spectrum antibiotic coverage available, this step is not critical. If an abscess is present, culture and placement of drain transvaginally may be achieved by the gynecology or interventional radiology services. Finally, a nasogastric tube is placed when an adynamic ileus results in severe abdominal distention and nausea.

Criteria for hospitalization include a white blood cell count equal to or greater than 16,000, high fever, severe anorexia, nausea, vomiting, dehydration, metabolic derangement, generalized peritonitis, and pelvic abscess. When hospitalization is deemed necessary, the patient is given nothing by mouth and placed on bed rest in semi-Fowler's position so that the infected pelvis remains the most dependent area. Rehydration is continued with restoration of electrolyte balance; analgesics and antipyretics are used as indicated. Both the initial acute attack of PID and acute exacerbations or chronic PID require broad-spectrum coverage of gram-negative and gram-positive aerobic organisms as well as anaerobes. A typical regimen would consist of cefoxitin, 2.0 g IV every 6 hours, with doxycycline, 100 mg every 12 hours orally or IV until afebrile for 48 hours, followed by 2 weeks of outpatient doxycycline therapy. Alternatively, ampicillin, 2.0 g IV every 6 hours, with gentamycin, 2.0 mg/kg stat and 1.5 mg/kg IV every 8 hours, together with clindamycin, 900 mg IV every 8 hours, or metronidazole, 500 mg IV every 6 hours, may be used. Other antibiotics with similar coverage spectra may be substituted as clinically indicated (ie, patient allergies). Response to treatment should be seen within 24 hours. If not, or if the patient's condition deteriorates, thorough reevaluation is indicated and an intraperitoneal abscess ruled out.

With resolution of both fever and peritoneal signs, the pelvic examination is repeated. Patient cooperation will be improved so that a hydrosalpinx or chronic tubo-ovarian abscess missed at the time of initial examination may be palpated. Removal of the pelvic organs is sometimes necessary to control recurrences of chronic PID and its attendant manifestations.

Summary

The emergency physician is faced with several basic decision points when evaluating the female patient. If he or she decides that the problem is most likely gynecologic, then two lists of major differential diagnoses present themselves based on pregnancy status. Ascertaining the LMP, sexual history, and contraceptive usage is helpful together with a sensitive pregnancy test and sonography when indicated. If the patient is pregnant, ectopic gestation must be ruled out and incomplete or threatened abortion considered. If the patient is not pregnant, PID should be ruled out and ovarian cyst rupture or torsion considered. Bleeding in the nonpregnant patient may be dysfunctional or postmenopausal, neoplastic, or related to pelvic/uterine infection. Because of the marked symptom overlap in these conditions, sonography again has an important role to play, as does the liberal use of consultation. With appropriate teamwork between surgeons, both general and gynecologic, and the emergency department, patients with ectopic pregnancies, PID, and appendicitis will receive prompt, accurate triage and care. By evaluating gynecologic problems with a systematic approach, the emergency physician will avoid the majority of diagnostic errors and greatly expedite care of the patient.

OBSTETRIC EMERGENCIES

The previous pages have dealt with what are probably the most perplexing diagnostic dilemmas facing physicians dealing with female patients in the ED setting. It is always challenging to determine whether a certain symptom complex is due to an obstetric or a nonobstetric condition. If pregnant—is the pregnancy viable or nonviable? Intrauterine or extrauterine?

But once the patient has passed the first trimester of gestation, it becomes a simple process to confirm the existence of a viable intrauterine pregnancy. This may be done by the use of a Doppler stethoscope (to auscultate fetal heart tones) or ultrasound. Once confirmed, an intrauterine gestation eliminates a number of diagnostic possibilities associated with the nonpregnant woman. Although this should be quite reassuring to the emergency physician attempting to narrow down the possible differential diagnosis, the ailing obstetric patient is usually met with a great deal of fear and trepidation. Even when physicians become comfortable with the range of diagnoses unique to the obstetric patient, uncertainty arises over the safety of various diagnostic and therapeutic techniques available for use in modern medicine. It will therefore be the goal of the following sections to present a practical, symptom-oriented method for the diagnosis and treatment of the obstetric patient.

Abdominal Pain in Pregnancy

One of the most common and frustrating complaints confronting the emergency physician is the pregnant woman with abdominal pain. The most important consideration should be differentiating pain associated with relatively benign conditions (such as that arising from stretching of the uterine ligaments—the so-called "round ligament pain syndrome") from pain arising from an acute surgical condition (such as appendicitis). Serious fetal and maternal morbidity may arise from a delay in diagnosis and treatment, which may be due to a reluctance to perform radiography or other diagnostic tests. Also, various anatomic and physiologic changes of pregnancy can obscure symptoms and alter test results, thereby making diagnosis difficult. There is always a natural reluctance to subject the pregnant woman to anesthesia or abdominal surgery.

When considering whether or not to perform diagnostic radiography for the evaluation of abdominal pain, common sense dictates that such procedures be kept to a minimum during pregnancy. If, on the other hand, they are deemed necessary to make the proper diagnosis, it is generally felt that the risk of any abnormality arising from radiation is negligible at exposures of 5 rads or less.

There are various physiologic changes that should be kept in mind when interpreting laboratory studies ordered on the pregnant woman. Beginning early in pregnancy, cardiac output increases significantly to maximum levels at around 20 to 24 weeks. Large expansion of the intravascular volume, particularly plasma volume, is one of the hallmarks of normal pregnancy. This increase may be as much as 45% to 55%, with an increase in red cell mass of 20% to 30%. This is manifested by an apparent drop in the hemoglobin concentration and hematocrit. Cardiac output and heart rate are increased. Normal pregnancy is characterized by leukocytosis, due mostly to increased polymorphonuclear leukocytes. It is not uncommon for the leukocyte count to be above 14,000 in late pregnancy. White blood cells and glucose are found in the urine in increased amounts. There may be some increase in alkaline phosphatase and amylase levels and a decrease in blood urea nitrogen and serum creatinine during pregnancy due to an increased glomerular filtration rate.

Anatomic changes during pregnancy to be kept in mind are the enlarging uterus (which may cause displacement of physical findings from their usual location) and marked hydronephrosis (thought to be due to either the effects of progesterone on the smooth musculature or mechanical obstruction). Among the other profound changes that occur in the course of normal gestation are alteration in the physiology of the gastrointestinal system. The global effects of progesterone on the smooth muscle produce depression of tone and action, explaining the increased incidence of regurgitation, delay in stomach and gallbladder emptying, and constipation.

It cannot be emphasized strongly enough that the history, physical examination, and laboratory evaluation of the pregnant patient with abdominal pain must be interpreted in light of the anatomic and physiologic changes of pregnancy and that the presence of the fetus should not deter the physician from the necessary diagnostic and therapeutic interventions. The differential diagnosis should include acute appendicitis, gallbladder disease, pancreatitis, adnexal accidents, intestinal obstruction, pyelonephritis, nephrolithiasis, silent abruption (with no evidence of vaginal bleeding), and labor.

Appendicitis is the most common nonobstetrical complication of pregnancy requiring laparotomy, occurring in 0.07% to 0.18% of all pregnancies. Appendicitis carries a higher risk of perforation in the pregnant state than in the nonpregnant state due to delays in diagnosis and surgery. Common symptoms and signs such as nausea and vomiting are also common symptoms and signs of a normal pregnancy. As pregnancy advances, the appendix is displaced upward and may confound the typical physical findings seen in the nonpregnant patient. On physical examination, the temperature and pulse may be normal in the early stages of the disease and rise only as the condition progresses. The white blood cell count may be normal or slightly elevated. If the diagnosis is suspected, immediate surgical consultation should be obtained. Due to secondary irritation of the uterus, premature labor is a common consequence of appendicitis and should be watched for closely, with liberal use of tocolytic agents. With the use of modern techniques of fetal monitoring, tocolytics, and early diagnosis, the incidence of fetal and maternal morbidity associated with appendicitis has become quite low.[9]

Due to the frequency of cholecystitis and cholelithiasis in reproductive age women, this diagnosis should always be entertained when evaluating the pregnant patient with abdominal pain. Acute cholecystitis complicates approximately 0.08% of pregnancies, with the incidence of cholecystectomy being much less. The gallbladder is relatively hypotonic during pregnancy. There is good evidence to indicate that pregnancy predisposes to the development of cholelithiasis.

Once again, it must be pointed out that many of the symptoms of gallbladder disease mimic the normal symptoms of pregnancy. Acute cholecystitis exhibits itself with pain in the epigastrium and right upper quadrant with upward radiation, nausea and vomiting, and tenderness to palpation. Pain may be of abrupt or gradual onset and is often colicky. A history of fatty food intolerance is helpful when exhibited. Occasionally jaundice occurs. Sonography is often useful as a diagnostic tool in this condition. It is highly accurate and of aid in the diagnosis but should be avoided if at all possible to avoid fetal radiation exposure. An upper gastrointestinal series may also be considered. As a rule, surgery can be avoided in acute cholecystitis although, with more severe disease, surgery is indicated, especially in the face of increasing jaundice.

Intestinal obstruction occurs in approximately 1 in 25,000 pregnancies and once again its diagnosis may be impeded by confusion with typical pregnancy symptoms. History is extremely important in the diagnosis of obstruction, with the most common etiology being previous abdominal surgery and adhesion formation. Volvulus may account for up to 25% of all obstruction cases. Cramping abdominal pain is characteristic of intestinal obstruction, and the rhythmic nature may easily be confused with labor pains. Differential diagnosis is accomplished with the placement of an external uterine tocodynameter, which will reveal no uterine contractions. Auscultation of the abdomen may reveal high-pitched, hyperactive bowel sounds. An abdominal radiograph will indicate obstruction with dilated loops of bowel and air-fluid levels. Advanced cases will show signs of peritonitis on physical examination.

The management of obstruction is the same as in the nonpregnant patient: immediate hospital admission, intravenous fluid and electrolyte replacement, and tube decompression of the intestinal tract. If there is evidence of strangulation or perforation, immediate surgery is required.

Ovarian masses will be seen in approximately 1 in 1000 pregnancies. Most are asymptomatic unless torsion or rupture occurs. With the development of ultrasound, there has been a major increase in the number of pelvic masses detected concurrently with pregnancy. There has also been an increase in the number of masses followed without surgery during pregnancy. It is not uncommon to see benign appearing masses of up to 8 cm in diameter being followed by obstetricians with conservative management. These patients are routinely counseled as to the signs and symptoms of torsion and rupture and told to report immediately to the emergency department should symptoms occur. Patients will typically complain of acute onset of extreme pain on the affected side. With torsion, the pain may be crampy and intermittent with radiation to the flank or thigh. The pain of rupture tends to be more sudden in onset and constant in nature. Examination reveals a tender mass, often with peritoneal signs. The hemoglobin and white blood cell count should be checked and an ultrasound ordered to confirm the diagnosis. Although torsion is a surgical emergency, rupture may be managed expectantly if the patient is hemodynamically stable.

Urinary tract disorders, including acute pyelonephritis and nephrolithiasis, should always be considered in the differential diagnosis of abdominal pain in pregnancy. The physiologic changes of pregnancy cause dilation of the ureters and stasis of urine and therefore predispose the pregnant woman to urinary tract infections and pyelonephritis. Therefore, a urinalysis is probably the most effective test that must always be ordered on the pregnant female with abdominal pain. With pyelonephritis the patient generally complains of chills, fever, flank pain, and frequency or dysuria. Nausea and vomiting are common. The patient often appears acutely ill. Immediate hospitalization is essential due to the frequency of premature labor in inadequately treated patients.

Urolithiasis occurs in 0.4% of pregnancies and patients often present with excruciating pain which may be flank but may also be abdominal in location. Urinalysis will generally show hematuria. Ultrasound and KUB may be helpful, but intravenous pyelograms (IVPs) are generally not required. Surgery is rarely indicated unless urinary tract obstruction or refractory infection is present. In general, treatment consists of intravenous hydration with analgesics and antibiotics if infection is present. Premature labor should always be looked for, with prompt use of tocolytics if necessary.

Placental abruption must also be considered in the differential diagnosis of abdominal pain in pregnancy. Although a great majority of these cases exhibit vaginal bleeding (and therefore will be dealt with later in this chapter), up to 20% will have the hemorrhage concealed—the so-called silent abruption. Because of the lack of bleeding, diagnosis is often delayed. The entire placenta can separate, the fetus die, and the uterus fill with blood in the absence of revealed blood in a very short time. The patient will present with acute onset of abdominal pain, often persisting between contractions, becoming more severe and associated with restlessness and agitation. The fundus is often quite tender to the touch and if there is a considerable amount of concealed bleeding the uterus becomes irritable—often with frequent contractions. A small abruption in the second trimester often times is self-limiting and may be confirmed on ultrasound. After assessing that the patient is hemodynamically stable, with no evidence of coagulopathy, treatment consists of bed rest with serial follow-up evaluations. Treatment of the third trimester abruption is dealt with later in this chapter.

Finally, a discussion of abdominal pain in pregnancy would not be complete without considering what would seem to be the most obvious cause—labor. Although most women approaching their due date are well versed in recognizing the onset of labor, it may surprise the emergency physician to discover that the symptoms of premature labor (defined as labor occurring prior to the completion of 36 weeks of gestation) may be both quite subtle and confusing. Although preterm deliveries represent only 8% to 10% of all births in this country, they are responsible for over 60% of the perinatal morbidity and mortality. Therefore, it is imperative that the emergency physician always rule out premature labor when evaluating the pregnant patient with abdominal pain. The definition of labor is frequent uterine contractions that cause progressive effacement and dilation of the cervix. The simplest way to diagnose premature labor is by assessing the dilation and effacement of the cervix on admission to the emergency department and again after 2 hours of observation. The preterm patient should never receive a digital examination prior to ruling out rupture of membranes. This may be done quickly by performing a sterile speculum examination and checking any fluid coming from the cervical os in two ways. First, a sample of fluid is collected on a sterile Q-tip and placed on nitrazine paper. Since amniotic fluid is alkaline, it will turn the nitrazine paper dark blue. Since blood and other secretions may falsely turn this test positive, it is essential to confirm the diagnosis by examining an air-dried glass slide of a sample of fluid for the typical "ferning" pattern of amniotic fluid. If rupture of membranes is ruled out, digital examination may be performed. If premature labor is suspected or preterm rupture of membranes diagnosed, immediate obstetric consultation should be obtained, with quick transfer to a labor and delivery unit. If transfer is not imminent, the patient should be given the tocolytic terbutaline, 0.25 mg subcutaneously, while awaiting transport.

In review, the evaluation of abdominal pain in the pregnant woman should begin with a detailed history and physical examination. If ultrasound is available it is often immensely helpful in confirming both the viability of the fetus and also the gestational age. Routine laboratory studies should include a CBC, liver function tests, platelet count, and urinalysis. Pelvic examination should be performed initially with a completely sterile speculum examination and then, only after ruling out ruptured membranes, serial cervical checks to rule out premature labor. Most importantly, when deemed necessary for proper evaluation, diagnostic radiography may be judiciously utilized. Finally, if warranted, prompt obstetric or surgical consultation should be obtained to avoid the morbidity associated with delays in diagnosis and treatment.

Vaginal Bleeding in Late Pregnancy

Approximately 3% of pregnancies are complicated by bleeding after the first trimester. The two main causes are abruptio placentae and placenta previa. Other causes that should be ruled out are bloody show, cervicitis/vaginitis, vaginal trauma, cervical carcinoma, or cervical polyps. Regardless of the etiology, all patients should undergo the same evaluation. Vital signs should be taken and, if severe blood loss is suspected, appropriate blood products should be ordered immediately. A history should be taken, including an estimation of the amount of blood loss, the association with any recent activity or trauma, and the accompaniment with any abdominal pain or contractions. The emergency physician's best estimate of gestational age should be determined by taking a menstrual history and noting any previous ultrasound determinations of fetal age. The abdomen should be examined for fundal height, uterine tenderness or contractions, and the presence of fetal heart tones by stethoscope or doptone. Vaginal examination should be delayed until the etiology of the bleeding is clear. If the vaginal bleeding is felt to be minimal or stabilized, then investigation of the cause of bleeding may begin. If the patient is unstable hemodynamically or exhibits profuse bleeding, stabilization should proceed, with placement of at least one large-bore intravenous line, infusion of Ringer's lactate, type and crossmatch for at least 4 U of packed red blood cells, and blood work to include CBC, platelets, and partial thromboplastin time. If coagulopathy is evident, the appropriate blood products should be obtained.

Placenta previa is implantation of the placenta in the lower uterine segment with various degrees of encroachment on the internal cervical os. A central previa is where the internal os is completely covered. A marginal previa is where the placental edge reaches but does not encroach upon the margin of the internal os. Placenta previa occurs in 0.1% to 1% of pregnancies with predisposing factors including advanced maternal age, multiparity, previous uterine incisions, and multiple gestation.

The hallmark of placenta previa is painless vaginal bleeding after 10 weeks gestation. In the gravida patient with this complaint, after the initial assessment as described above, it is essential to locate the placenta with immediate ultrasound evaluation prior to vaginal examination. If a previa exists, even the most gentle cervical examination can cause devastating hemorrhage. If ultrasonography confirms the existence of placenta previa, immediate obstetric consultation should be obtained. When contacting the obstetrician it is essential that the emergency physician provide the patient's gestational age, vital signs, hematocrit, coagulation profile, and the best estimate of the amount of vaginal bleeding. It is generally agreed that the patient with a known previa and vaginal bleeding be observed on an obstetrical unit for at least 24 hours to assure hemodynamic stability and also to rule out the existence of premature labor. If transport to another hospital is necessary, it should be by ambulance or helicopter with appropriate staff attending and also with a large-bore intravenous line infusing Ringer's lactate and appropriate blood products available.

Abruptio placentae is some degree of separation of a normally implanted placenta after 20 weeks gestation. Its incidence varies from 0.2% to 2.4% of all pregnancies. Fifty percent of abruptions occur prior to 36 weeks gestation. There is a risk of recurrence in approximately 11% of patients with a history of previous abruption, and there is a distinct correlation between hypertension in pregnancy and abruption.

The patient with an abruption typically presents with vaginal bleeding preceded by the onset of abdominal pain (although, as noted previously, vaginal bleeding does not always occur). Abdominal examination reveals a uterus that is characteristically tender and irritable, with increased uterine tone between contractions. Immediate evaluation is exactly the same as that for placenta previa, including the placement of a large-bore intravenous line and infusion with Ringer's lactate. Immediate assessment of maternal vital signs should help determine the extent of abruption. Baseline laboratory tests include hematocrit, prothrombin time, partial thromboplastin time, fibrinogen, and fibrin degradation products. Significant coagulopathy accompanies approximately 10% of abruptions because of thromboplastin released from the site of placental injury and secondary activation of the fibrinolytic system. Attention should be given to fundal height and any rapid increase indicating accumulation of blood. Fetal heart tones should be auscultated and ultrasound evaluation performed to rule out the existence of placenta previa. Once ruled out, cervical examination should be performed to assess cervical dilatation and effacement. If the patient is preterm, she should be transported to an appropriate high-risk obstetric center capable of taking care of a preterm infant. Many times, mild abruption is self-limited and can be managed conservatively after maternal/fetal stability is ascertained. Observation for at least 24 hours is necessary, with serial laboratory testing and fetal monitoring. Amniocentesis for lung profile may be considered when the patient is nearing term, with subsequent delivery if mature. If a severe abruption is detected or there is evidence of maternal or fetal instability, delivery becomes necessary, even in the preterm gestation.

In communities where there is a high number of patients who receive no prenatal care, the emergency physician may be called upon to manage patients who deliver outside the hospital. It is, therefore, imperative to be familiar with the management of postpartum hemorrhage. This is defined as a blood loss in excess of 500 mL. The three main causes of uterine hemorrhage are uterine atony, retained placental products, or genital tract lacerations. Rapid assessment is essential since blood loss may be rapid and profuse and transport to an obstetric unit may be impossible. Immediate evaluation of the perineum, vagina, and cervix will reveal any major lacerations, which should be rapidly repaired with dissolvable sutures. Bimanual examination is necessary to detect uterine atony with the finding of a soft, boggy uterus often with blood clots filling the uterine cavity and lower uterine segment. These can be removed manually through the dilated cervix and immediate fundal massage instituted to promote contraction of the uterine musculature. Pitocin infusion should be started with 20 to 40 U in 1000 mL. Ringer's lactate should be run in rapidly. At the time of intravenous placement, blood for hematocrit, platelet count, and coagulation profile should be sent off and appropriate blood products ordered. Should the atony not respond to these initial maneuvers, in the nonhypertensive patient ergotrate or methergine, 0.2 mg IM, should be given. If still unsuccessful, control of postpartum hemorrhage secondary to atony may respond to analogues of prostaglandin $F2^\alpha$ (1 mL administered IM or through the abdominal wall into the myometrium). If still unsuccessful, emergent obstetric consultation is necessary to rule out retained placental products or uterine inversion, necessitating general anesthesia for uterine curettage or repositioning of the uterine fundus.

Trauma in Pregnancy

Accidental injury is estimated to occur in 6% to 7% of all pregnancies and is the leading nonobstetric cause of maternal morbidity. Minor trauma is seldom associated with a poor pregnancy outcome. Severe trauma, on the other hand, requires the knowledge and skills of a combined team including emergency physician, trauma surgeon, obstetrician, and pediatrician. The over-riding principle in the management of the pregnant trauma patient is that "maternal well-being is paramount." Because the most common cause of fetal death is maternal death, initial evaluation and resuscitative efforts should be directed toward the mother.

Initial management priorities are the same as in the nonpregnant patient, that is, ensuring adequate airway and maintaining adequate blood pressure and perfusion. The physiologic changes of pregnancy discussed previously in this chapter must be kept in mind when evaluating physical findings and laboratory results.

Fetal survival should be ascertained promptly in the emergency department. With modern tools such as Doppler and real-time ultrasonography, this question can be resolved quickly. The gravid human uterus is very vulnerable to irritation by physical stimuli. Therefore, abdominal injury may initiate labor. It is important periodically to evaluate the uterus for contractions so that the diagnosis of premature labor may occur promptly, with subsequent treatment. Ultrasonography may be used as a tool not only to ascertain fetal well-being, but also to evaluate placental status. Severe abdominal trauma may cause placental abruption, so it is imperative to look for the presence of hematomas and retroplacental clots. Obstetric consultation should occur as soon as possible to aid in the management of the pregnant trauma patient.

Hypertension in Pregnancy

Hypertensive problems during pregnancy are usually asymptomatic and therefore rarely present themselves in an ED setting. When pregnancy-induced hypertension reaches severe proportions, it is usually accompanied by a symptom complex that should be familiar to any emergency physician. Pre-eclampsia is the development of hypertension with proteinuria and/or edema induced by pregnancy after the 20th week of gestation. Pre-eclampsia is considered severe if one or more of the following signs or symptoms are present: (1) blood pressure readings of at least 160 mmHg systolic or 110 mmHg diastolic pressure on two occasions at least 6 hours apart; (2) proteinuria levels of greater than 5 g in 24 hours or 3+ to 4+ on semiquantitative assay; (3) oliguria of less than 400 mL/24 h; (4) cerebral or visual disturbances such as altered consciousness, headache, scotomata, or blurred vision; (5) pulmonary edema; (6) epigastric or right upper quadrant pain that is persistent; (7) impaired liver function; (8) thrombocytopenia.

Because severe pregnancy-induced hypertension can lead to severe maternal and fetal morbidity and mortality, attention should be paid to any pregnant woman presenting to the ED complaining of persistent dull headache, visual changes such as blurry vision or dark spots in front of eyes, increased swelling (specifically of the hands and face), epigastric or right upper quadrant pain, or any change in mental status.

Immediate evaluation should consist of serial blood pressure measurements with the patient in the left lateral decubitus position, urine dipstick for protein, and laboratory studies including CBC, platelets, and liver and renal function studies. If ultrasound is available, a study of fetal growth is useful as intrauterine growth retardation is also considered to be a sign of severe pre-eclampsia.

If any criteria for severe toxemia are found, immediate obstetric consultation should be obtained and the patient transferred to an obstetric high-risk unit. To prevent the development of eclampsia or seizures, the patient should be started on intravenous magnesium sulfate. Generally a 4- to 6-g bolus over 20 minutes is given, followed by a continuous drip of 2 to 3 g/h. This is administered solely for the prevention of seizures, not blood pressure control. If the patient is found to be hypertensive without criteria indicating severe pre-eclampsia, she should be evaluated by her obstetrician soon because the disease may progress rapidly, hence, the name eclampsia, which is Latin for lightning. Therefore, it becomes imperative to differentiate the diagnosis of pregnancy-induced hypertension from chronic hypertension, since the treatment will vary depending upon the diagnosis.

Medical Conditions in Pregnancy

Since practically any medical condition may exhibit itself during pregnancy, the following is only a partial overview of those conditions most likely to present themselves in an ED setting.

Although genital herpes simplex infections are rarely an obstetric emergency unless present at the time of labor, they are the object of a great deal of maternal anxiety and therefore may present themselves to the ED at any time during pregnancy. The current American College of Obstetricians and Gynecologists guidelines regarding genital herpes infections allow vaginal delivery if there are no visible herpes lesions at the onset of labor.[10] The previous practice of weekly cervical cultures near term has not been proven to be effective in altering the incidence of neonatal herpes infection. Since it is imperative to know which women will be at risk for herpes infection at term, it is important to diagnose those women with perineal lesions during the course of their pregnancy. Although herpes may be present as the typical ulcerated vesicles, it may also take on other forms. Therefore, any suspect perineal lesion seen in the ED should be cultured for the herpes virus to aid in the future obstetric management of that patient. Treatment is symptomatic, since no cure for herpes genitalis exists. Hot sitz baths and compresses are soothing. Topical anesthetics also provide short-term relief. Acyclovir is currently being used to shorten the course of herpes attacks and prophylactically at lower doses but is currently not recommended for use in pregnancy since no adequate controlled studies have been performed. Thus, the safety of this drug during pregnancy is not known, and it should be reserved for life-threatening infections.

Asthma is the most common medical disease coexisting with pregnancy that is seen by emergency physicians. It occurs in 0.4% to 1.3% of pregnancies, with severe asthma requiring hospitalization complicating approximately 0.15% of pregnancies. Status asthmaticus requires immediate attention in the ED. The goal is to ensure adequate oxygenation to the mother and fetus and to break the asthmatic attack. Clinical assessment is no different than that of the nonpregnant patient and includes heart rate, respiratory rate, lung field auscultation, measurement of forced expiratory volume, and chest radiograph (with abdominal shield). Laboratory studies include arterial blood gases, sputum examination, and white blood cell count with differential. The $Paco_2$ is generally decreased due to hyperventilation, and therefore a normal or increased value may imply impending respiratory failure.

The treatment of acute asthma begins with the administration of humidified oxygen by mask and immediate intravenous hydration with 5% dextrose in saline at 200 mL/h. Subcutaneous adrenergic agents remain the first line of drug therapy, with terbutaline (0.25 mg subcutaneously every 20 minutes for three doses) preferred over epinephrine because of its greater β-adrenergic selectivity. This minimizes uterine vessel constriction and provides better uteroplacental blood flow. If the patient does not improve rapidly after the administration of terbutaline or epinephrine, intravenous theophylline should be begun. In a patient who has not been regularly taking aminophylline or theophylline, a loading dose of 5 to 6 mg/kg should be administered over 20 to 30 minutes, followed by a maintenance dose of 0.5 to 0.7 mg/kg/h. Due to the increase in liver enzyme activity during pregnancy, there is more rapid clearance of aminophylline. It is therefore important to determine frequent blood levels during the course of intravenous therapy. As an adjunct to therapy, nebulized bronchoselective non-catecholamine inhalants, such as albuterol, may be given every 4 to 6 hours. Frequent assessment of the arterial blood gases should be used to assess the patient's response during bouts of acute asthma. If no improvement is seen in spite of combined theophylline/β-adrenergic therapy, glucocorticoids should be administered intravenously, with an initial daily dose equivalent to prednisone, 40 to 60 mg/day. Beclomethasone, a corticosteroid, is administered by inhalation with the advantage of relatively little systemic absorption. Although it may be given to allow tapering of systemic steroids, it may also be used in suboptimally controlled patients who have not been receiving prolonged maintenance with oral steroids. If the patient shows evidence of infection on the chest radiograph or sputum smear, antibiotic therapy should be instituted without delay. Most oral antibiotics with the exception of tetracycline derivatives are safe during pregnancy. Sulfa drugs should not be used in the third trimester as they displace bilirubin from binding sites and predispose the newborn to kernicterus. Lastly, in patients unresponsive to the above treatments, a pulmonary specialist should be consulted to assist in management.

When treating medical conditions during pregnancy, the most common question rasied by the emergency physician is Which drugs are safe? Every drug given to the pregnant woman will potentially exert its effect on both the mother and the fetus. Whether or not a drug should be used depends on its possible risk to the fetus and its value or necessity for treatment of the mother. A valuable resource that should be readily available in EDs is *Drugs in Pregnancy and Lactation* by Briggs, Freeman, and Yaffe (Williams & Wilkins Company, Baltimore, 1990). The use of this text combined with judicious obstetric consultation will greatly simplify the job of safely prescribing medications for the emergency physician.

CONCLUSION

In summary, what we have attempted to provide is a guide for the initial evaluation and treatment of gynecologic and obstetric patients seen by the emergency physician. This is a commonsense and systematic approach to the diagnosis and initial treatment of those female patients so often encountered in the ED. By using these principles we hope to alleviate much of the confusion and trepidation that has evolved over the years in dealing with these situations. The physician should have all of the tools necessary for a confident evaluation of the female ED patient so that proper management may ensue and appropriate consultation may be obtained.

REFERENCES

1. Romero R, Copel J, Kadar N, et al. Value of culdocentesis in the diagnosis of ectopic pregnancy. *Obstet Gynecol*. 1985;65:519.
2. Leach R, Ory S. Modern management of ectopic pregnancy. *J Reprod Med*. 1989;34:324.
3. Ectopic pregnancy. *ACOG Tech Bull*. March 1989;126.
4. Vermesh M, Graczykowski J, Sauer M. Re-evaluation of the role of culdocentesis in the management of ectopic pregnancy. *Am J Obstet Gynecol*. 1990;162:411.
5. Centers for Disease Control. Ectopic pregnancy—United States. *MMWR*. 1986;35(17).
6. Ectopic pregnancy. *ACOG Tech Bull*. December 1990;150.
7. Centers for Disease Control. 1989 sexually transmitted disease treatment guidelines. *MMWR*. 1989;38(8).
8. Antimicrobial therapy for gynecologic infections. *ACOG Tech Bull*. March 1991;153.
9. Benrubi G. *Obstetric Emergencies*. New York, NY: Churchill Livingstone; 1990:1–4, 25–44.
10. Perinatal herpes simplex virus infections. *ACOG Tech Bull*. July 1989;122.

80. Rape and Sexual Assault

TINA M. H. BLAIR, MD, FACEP
CARMEN GERMAINE WARNER, MSN, RN, FAAN

Despite achievements in medical science and emergency care, victims of sexual assault often struggle alone. The intimacy and sensitivity of the rape situation, laced with considerable fear, anger, and hostility, produce a very emotional, potentially volatile environment. Victims seek help immediately or at a later time, alone or with police, friends, or family. Physical or emotional damage may be obvious or not manifest for quite some time. The need for an empathetic, thorough, gentle assessment is a challenge unlike that posed by any other patient.

"[Rape victims are] doubly victimized . . . first by the attacker and again by the attitudes of society."[1] This is true for all stages of postrape intervention, but nowhere is the potential invasion of self and dignity more immediate than in the emergency department (ED). It is here that victims reiterate the events, face the fact that the story may be doubted, feel subject to public scrutiny, wait for hours (frequently uninformed and alone), and submit to an embarrassing and potentially traumatizing examination.

Adult men and women* who have suffered the indignity of rape represent very special and unique emergency patients for several reasons.

First, physical injuries require a careful and detailed assessment. Because of the probability of internal trauma, which may be unknown to patients, it is imperative to be thorough. They may not recall being injured and may even be unaware of pain.

Second, there is intense emotional damage that is both complex and real. Apparently inappropriate responses are common and must be understood (see below). This is also a sensitive and frequently difficult situation as a result of a third factor, the personal feelings and reactions of the emergency staff.

The last reason is the fact that rape is a crime. The forensic (legal) aspects require the collection of evidence and the documentation of information. This all must be done correctly if it is to be of use to law enforcement. We must also be aware of the potential need to appear in court. In most states only physical findings are admissible as evidence, but some may allow professional testimony to provide further details. All records must be complete and accurate. Because the required specimens may vary by state, making it impossible for us to list them here, you must be well-versed in your local regulations.

In order to properly care for a rape victim, we must be facile in all aspects of evaluation and treatment, and there must be a cooperative, multidisciplinary approach that includes hospital, police, and counseling personnel.[2] We must first deal with any physical injuries while handling psychologic damage sympathetically. Then we must properly collect and document forensic information and treat and prevent disease or pregnancy. Normal, consensual sexual communication constitutes an expression of giving and sharing, not

---

*Unless we speak of something limited to only one sex, all statements apply to *all* victims.

hostility, aggression, or violence. The pain, fear, humiliation, terror, and degradation of rape are feelings resulting from *violence* and *violation*. Staff must provide sensitivity, gentleness, and support in a manner that will restore the patient's emotional well-being.

MAGNITUDE OF THE PROBLEM

Although the rate of rape appears to be rising faster than any other violent crime, the true incidence is unknown as statistical data reflect only those women who reported it.[3] Surveys indicate a much higher incidence, but their validity could be questioned.

- More than 92,000 rapes were reported in 1988. This is a 1.5% increase over 1987,[4] but these figures are probably only 10% to 25% of the actual incidence.[4-7]
- It is estimated, however, that sexual violation through force, fraud, threat, or intimidation occurs more than 500,000 to 800,000 times per year, and most will know the assailant.
- The risk that a woman may be raped in her lifetime is as high as 1/3 to 1/6.[7]
- Approximately 80% of women are single, divorced, or separated.[9]
- Reported victims range from a few months to more than 90 years old. Most are in their mid-teens to mid-twenties. Significant underreporting occurs in children, estimated at 60% to 90% in one study.[2]
- Drug or alcohol use is frequently involved, and 25% to 30% are mentally deficient or have a history of mental illness.[2]
- Twenty percent to 25% of victims report a prior rape. Those most likely to do so are over 40, black, assaulted by an acquaintance, or have a history of mental illness.[3]
- Complaints of physical trauma vary widely from none to severe injuries, although only about 1% to 2% need hospitalization.[7] Most studies estimate damage at 30% to 50%.[2] A recent international meeting indicated that there is also wide national variation in these numbers, apparently reflecting the overall level of violence in the society.
- Multiple assailants are involved in 20% to 40%.[2]
- Homicide is always a possibility. It appears to be, but cannot be proven, that those who attempt resistance are at increased risk. Original violent or homicidal intent is always a possibility. The following profile is from a series of 41 fatalities.[2]

  - The yearly incidence was 0.14/100,000 population.
  - Death resulted from mechanical asphyxiation by instruments readily available at the scene.
  - Younger women (mean 31 years) were found in isolated areas outdoors and older women (mean 51 years) were found in their homes.
  - Victims weighed less than average females.
  - Binding with ligatures and acute alcoholic intoxication were common.

DEFINITIONS OF RAPE

Rape is not a medical diagnosis but rather a legal term. Specific definitions vary by state and represent the profile of lawmakers and the influence of patient advocates. It is an extremely sensitive issue, and we must be familiar with local interpretations.

In the past, rape was defined (and convictions obtained) emphasizing three integral elements: (1) carnal knowledge of or sexual contact with a woman, (2) lack of consent, and (3) use of force to accomplish the act.[7] These factors were interpreted quite narrowly, with carnal knowledge being vaginal penetration by the penis, lack of consent as forcible resistance, and use of force considered to be violence or the use of a weapon.[9] Because this excluded many types of sexual assault, definitions were broadened or changed to reflect modern reality (see Table 80-1, Definitions).

Professionals may encounter situations that are difficult to explain (ie, involving a social relationship). Completely refraining from interpretation or judgment, we must simply address the presenting physical and emotional trauma. Only the patient and the perpetrator have that right because they were the only ones present. Victims should be assessed with the same attitude as patients with chest pain, who are not questioned whether they really wanted the pain or if they put themselves in the situation deliberately.

Rape includes a large spectrum of criminal sexual acts. It is, therefore, important to ensure proper punishment to design a mechanism by which the reality of the act is accurately reflected. To this end, many states have identified several degrees of rape and created laws allowing juries the flexibility to make appropriate decisions. Changes also reflect the recognition of circumstances that may be extremely dangerous and make it a crime exclusive of the victim's state of mind. These include[21] those items in Table 80-2.[10]

Concomitant with the restructuring of degrees of rape is the need to examine penalties. If a law mandates one that is too harsh, juries may return fewer convictions (ie, an argument *against* mandatory life sentences).

THE REALITY OF RAPE

The ugliness and devastating effects of rape can only be a reality to the victim and those who are close to the victim. Unless we have had the horror invade our lives, it is only

Table 80-1 Definitions

Carnal knowledge: Act of a man having intercourse with a woman. It is not necessary that the vagina be entered or the hymen ruptured. The penis's touching the vulva or labia is sufficient.
Rape: In criminal law, it is unlawful carnal knowledge, forcibly and against another's will.
Simple assault: An attempt to cause bodily harm to another.
Aggravated assault: A perpetrator (who recognizes the seriousness of the act) causes or attempts to cause physical and/or emotional injury.
Sexual assault: Any type of sexual act when committed without the permission of both parties.
Unlawful sexual intercourse (statutory rape): Having sexual intercourse with a female under the age of consent.
Attempted rape: Actions taken by a perpetrator toward completion of an act of rape. He must have been exposed and attempted to subdue and penetrate the victim but was unable to complete the act.
Indecent assault: Touching the private parts of another's body while recognizing that this may cause alarm. It includes contact with the genital area, breasts, or buttocks.
Involuntary sexual intercourse: Forcible vaginal, oral, or anal intercourse without consent, using threat of force, or when the individual is unconscious, mentally deranged, or under the age of 14.
Genital contact: Previously noted as the only type of contact constituting rape. Now contact between the genitals and mouth and anus are included.
Penetration: Now includes fingers, tongue, and foreign objects.
Ejaculation: Has almost disappeared from definitions.
Consent: Definitions are controversial, since it is not only difficult to assess and interpret one's state of mind, but also because there can be little distinction between resistance necessary to negate consent and actions that might cause violence.[20] Consent can only be given by one who is legally competent, awake, not drugged, or intoxicated.
Force: Any sort of intimidation (fraud, fear, authority) is possible, and a weapon need not be involved.
Sexual abuse: Sexual intercourse, molestation, incest, or assault on one unable to provide consent.
Sexual molestation: An act performed by one person on another amounting to noncoital sexual contact without legal consent and with lewd intent. May involve rape or forcible oral and anal sex acts but is most commonly applied to the fondling of a child's genitals.

Table 80-2 Violence Indicators[10]

1. Use of a dangerous weapon
2. Serious injury
3. Attempting the act during the commission of a felony (ie, kidnapping, robbery)
4. Involuntary administration of drugs or alcohol resulting in incapacity
5. Reliance on victim vulnerability (ie, youth, special relationship, intoxication)
6. Use of threats of serious injury or death to the victim or another

Table 80-3 Myths

Rapists are sick and perverted or sexually unfulfilled and carried away suddenly by an uncontrollable urge.
A woman cannot be raped by her husband (yes, she can, but not all places see it as a crime).
Rapists are usually strangers to the victim. (Fifty percent to 75% [especially children] are attacked by someone they know.)
Rapes are interracial. (Races involved reflect the population at large.) Most victims and perpetrators are of the same race. Only 4% involve white men and black women and 3% black men and white women.
Women report rape that is unfounded in order to get attention.
Every woman has rape fantasies.
Rape victims are at fault and probably provoked the attack.
Rape occurs primarily in large cities, dark alleys, warm weather, the evening, and hitchhiking situations; if you stay at home you will be safe.
Rape is a minor crime only affecting a few. (More than 140,000 households were affected by reported cases in 1988, a 21.6% increase over 1987.[3])
It is easy to prosecute rapists. (Rape overall has a four times lower conviction rate.)

"something that happens to another." Although there are numerous factors that help to dispel misconceptions, myths continue to exist in the minds and practice of many (see Table 80-3, Myths). Myths such as only people in lower socioeconomic classes or the young, beautiful, or promiscuous get raped abound. In reality, all societal, income, and occupational levels are involved. Every man, woman, and child is a potential candidate for rape. Recognizing this, there is no way to create categories of "types of victims" more narrowly than "simply being human."

The media have made great commitments to investigation and presentation of factual data, and many organizations have designed educational programs concerning the realities of rape and the appropriate assessment and intervention. Upgraded reporting and management protocols, along with sensitive personnel, encourage more victims (including men, married women, and the elderly) to report the crime.

MEDICAL-LEGAL INTERACTION

It is essential that we coordinate with the criminal justice system to encourage patients, through gentle, supportive management, to continue their efforts throughout the follow-up and prosecutory process and ensure the proper handling of evidence.

Evidence collected following a rape is frequently crucial in the successful identification and prosecution of the perpetrator. This examination (often the initial contact patients have with the system) has a profound effect on their later behavior and healing.

Collection of evidence is the responsibility of law enforcement, even if it is obtained by the medical staff. Despite the value of evidence, it is invalid unless handled properly (ie, via an unbroken custody chain). Procedures for maintaining the integrity of the "chain of evidence" must be followed.

Table 80-4 Evidence Collection Kit and Related Materials[a]

Test	Equipment
Record history and examination	Appropriate forms; paper bags (2): outer garments, underwear; butcher paper to stand on to catch any debris; gloves for handler if not patient; 2 labels
Collection of clothing (look for foreign matter, semen, blood, or secretions)	
Foreign materials on body or hair	Scissors; swabs; containers; labels
Urinalysis	2 containers: pregnancy, if not doing blood, and possible drug screen; 2 labels
Nail scrapings (fingers and toes, if applicable); although not mandatory and may not be useful, tissues or other identifiable materials may be found	Nail file; 2 envelopes; 2 labels
Saliva sample for blood group antigens	Disk or swabs; envelope; label
Oral swab for sperm if applicable	Must be done early if to be valuable; swabs of upper and lower teeth along gumline most useful; 2 swabs; container; label
Miscellaneous droppings	Chux pads to lie on; paper bag; label
Photography (optional and may need specific permission)	Camera (Polaroid is best); film; flash; label
Blood samples	Non alcohol-containing sampling equipment; proper tubes (? HCG [pregnancy], ABO typing, alcohol, ? drugs, VDRL, ?HIV, ?HBV); 7 labels
Pelvic examination	Gloves and other usual equipment; speculum with warm water as lubricant
Pubic hair (should be done by victim)	Combings (looking for those of perpetrator): comb; envelope; label
	Plucked (those confirmed to be from victim) (cutting will not be sufficient in most states number needed varies with protocol); tweezers; envelope; label
Fixed specimens from cervix for sperm morphology	Ayre stick; 2 slides; fixative; slide holder; label; slide marker
Vaginal swabs	Acid phosphatase; ABO antigens; 8 swabs (2 for each test from vaginal orifice and pool); 4 containers or red-topped tubes; normal saline per protocol; 4 labels
Sperm motility from cervix, orifice and pool	3 slides and coverslips; 3 swabs; normal saline **without preservative** and dropper; microscope
Vaginal aspirant from deepest possible source	Angiocath; syringe; label
Vaginal washings if fluid minimal or required by protocol	10 mL normal saline with preservative; aspiration pipette or syringe and angiocath; red-topped tube; label
Anal specimens if indicated	Required supplies will be in kit (time is of the essence): labels; anoscope; materials for washings and/or microscopic evaluation of motile and nonmotile sperm
Cultures of cervix	Gonorrhea; chlamydia
Vaginal or cervical injuries	Toluene blue; ? colposcope
External secretions (foreign material, blood, lubricant, semen)	Wood's lamp (best to use separate set-ups for each location): swabs; normal saline with preservative; red-topped tubes; labels
Suspect	
Blood	ABO; HIV; HBV; VDRL
Urethra	Gonorrhea; Chlamydia; Gram stain
Penile shaft	Vaginal epithelium; fecal stains

[a]Different kits vary as to contents, and different states may have unique requirements.

Everyone handling specimens must not tamper with them. All those involved with the kit or evidence should document their actions in writing (including signatures). It must be locked securely when not in your presence or given to the police.[2] Under normal circumstances, it is given immediately to the police. If police are not present, it should be properly preserved until they arrive. However, this safekeeping should be no longer than 6 hours. (A locked box supplied by the police for this purpose might be useful.)

Evidence is best collected with the help of a prepared kit. Those produced by the Denver, Chicago, and Houston police departments and by crime laboratories are excellent prototypes.[2] Although the contents may vary slightly, they should contain the minimal essentials (see Table 80-4).

Recognizing the environment of a busy ED, the volume of cases, the rotation of personnel, and the sensitive issue of rape itself, it is imperative that a standardized rape protocol listing everything that must be done and allowing space to indicate required data/information and their acquisition be developed. The goal should be that even an inexperienced nurse and physician could do a satisfactory (medical and legal) evaluation by using it.

PREHOSPITAL CARE

First responders establish the foundation for the continued ease of intervention. If there is support, comfort, and a willingness to listen, victims will more easily develop trust and cooperate better with other medical and law enforcement personnel.

Key points for first responders are listed in Table 80-5.

Table 80-5 Duties of First Responders and Prehospital Personnel

Attempt to comfort the victim.
Obtain the needed facts concerning the incident to enable appropriate support.
Relate the importance of reporting the incident to the police if not already contacted.
Make every effort to preserve evidence. Make sure that the victim does not change clothes, eat, drink, take any medication, brush teeth, gargle, urinate, defecate, douche, shower, or delay in going to the ED. (If she/he is informed of the importance of these requests, but still insists on cleaning, respect these wishes.)
Assess injuries and perform essential intervention.
Assist in contacting anyone that victim feels is needed.
Initiate first-stage crisis intervention.
Contact the nearest ED or other appropriate facility.
Accompany the patient.
Establish rapport with the responsible ED staff.
Staying with the victim for a short time is recommended as a means of facilitating a positive and comfortable transition, relating appropriate information, and ensuring constant company.

EMERGENCY DEPARTMENT RESPONSIBILITIES

Rape is a serious crime of assault on the body but even more so on the psyche.[11] Even though the attack was not physically life-threatening, the psychological harm may be devastating to emotional stability. The initial interaction in the ED is equally important as that with the first responder. Here, issues of injury, sexually transmitted diseases (STD), pregnancy, and psychological trauma are first confronted.

Victims may refuse an examination for fear of pain or recollection of the event or may agree only to attend to or evaluate injuries. If this occurs, point out the value and purpose of evidence collection. If adamant opposition continues, thoroughly explain problems regarding eventual legal outcomes and health. Should there be insistence against a procedure, rights must be respected. *Never use force or instill guilt.*

The ED visit, although potentially difficult for all involved, is made easier if protocol guidelines are followed and procedures are explained first in detail. However, because needs and fears of individuals vary, specifics of any protocol are to be seen only as guidelines.

ED rape protocols vary depending on the unique aspects of each facility and local legal requirements. The ultimate privacy, safety, and support of each patient must be foremost. When all personnel share responsibilities, the best possible care is provided. A cooperative effort by staff aids themselves, patients, and families. Despite the fact that care should be administered by one nurse, physician, and counselor, it is important for all to consider the following as opportunities arise:

- Prepare a proper response (following the guidelines below) for all (a limited group is suggested) who might take a phone call from a victim.
- Ensure *immediate attention* to all rape victims, guiding them to a private room with a support person. (A support person is anyone with special training and interest in dealing with rape victims and in coordinating their care. They may be a nurse, special volunteer, social or rape crisis worker, chaplain, or psychiatric staff and should remain with the victim during their entire ED stay.)[2]
- Notify physician and triage nurse of the victim's arrival.
- Assign them priority over all others except life-threatening conditions.
- Even with other emergencies in the ED, someone should ensure that the patient is comfortable and relate reasons for any possible delays.
- Maintain the presence of a nurse (and, if possible, a counselor) throughout the assessment and intervention process.
- Identify patients by proper name or a preassigned code to protect them from further humiliation.
- Inquire if there is pain or bleeding that may need immediate attention. While trying to not damage evidence, assess the presence and severity of any external wounds or internal injuries and the extent, degree, and location of pain.[7]
- If the patient desires the presence of another, make arrangements for aid in the selection. (One who is visibly disturbed may be more upsetting than helpful.)
- Provide maximum emotional support and reduce any potentially traumatizing actions or statements.
- Obtain informed consent for all that is to follow.
- Explain the entire assessment and intervention process, allowing ample time for questions and answers. Inquire about familiarity with pelvic and/or rectal examinations.
- Assess the patient's ability to tolerate the examination (both physically and psychologically).
- Identify each phase of all procedures prior to initiation and explain each step of the process as it is being done.
- Have patient remain dressed in *their* clothes until the examination begins. The police may want photographs of how they appeared initially.
- Arrange for someone to bring in clean clothes.
- Inquire if there are children and who is watching them. If they need attention, obtain assistance from social service, police, or family.
- Explain the possibility of STD and the importance of cultures and treatment.
- Outline the value of pregnancy testing when applicable and explain the patient's options.
- Identify acute anxiety reactions.
- Advise the patient that a rape crisis advocate is available, if desired.

- Recognize the chart as legal evidence and record accurately all statements, procedures, and actions.
- Obtain evidence collection kit and examination set, placing them in the room, out of view, until examination begins. Time is saved and fewer things forgotten if all items (except those needing refrigeration) are assembled in advance (ie, a "super" rape kit).
- Observe, properly collect, and preserve the patient's clothing in a paper bag[12] after having the patient undress while standing on a sheet to collect falling debris. Have only the victim handle items to minimize contamination by sweat or other substances from the staff.[3,7]
- Assist with any photographs as needed.
- Record each step of the evidence collection process.
- Maintain continuity of evidence transmission, ensuring that the proper samples are delivered and received.
- Label each piece of evidence with patient's name; hospital number; day, date, and time of collection; specific material obtained and from where; the collector's name; your name and role in the process; and to whom it was delivered and when.
- Recognize that some tests (ie, pregnancy, cultures) are medical procedures and must be processed in the hospital, while all others are transferred to the police.[13] Note that some may be duplicates if the physician and the police both want the tests.
- Be familiar with crime laboratory proceedings and their requirements in your area.
- After the examination, collect a urine specimen for pregnancy and drugs as indicated. A serum alcohol level might also be useful.
- Supply informational material concerning follow-up instructions, a list of community resources, and a voluntary evaluation form. The patient is not expected to read this now but encouraged to do so later.
- Assess if sedation or counseling is appropriate for the patient or any accompanying persons.
- Follow-up phone call later.

HISTORY AND EXAMINATION

The physician is responsible for (1) *documenting historical details*; (2) *performing a careful examination for injuries*; (3) *assessing and treating injuries promptly and correctly*; (4) *providing emotional support*; (5) *properly collecting evidence*; (6) *maintaining the chain of custody*; (7) *preventing and/or treating STD*; (8) *providing information about possible pregnancy and offering postcoital implantation prevention*; and (9) *arranging for psychological counseling, if desired*.[3] However, many of these tasks could be delegated to a nurse or other staff member. Unfortunately the proper treatment of injuries may delay, disturb, or prevent adequate evidence collection. Having one member of the staff assigned to do this while the rest are involved in the resuscitation might help.

Obtaining an accurate history of the event is essential, not only for a legal case but also for the patient's well-being and integrity. Unfortunately, recollection is similar to reliving, and the patient may be reluctant or have difficulty talking about details that are usually considered intimate. Discussion, however, helps to put it all into perspective. Explain that guilt feelings are normal[14] and that the events were not their fault. If there is a need to ask for embarrassing or upsetting details, specificity and directness on your part will make the questions easier to deal with and answer. Because rape is a crime and not a diagnosis, determining whether it has occurred is done by the courts,[3] not by us. Victims need sympathy and understanding, not moralizing or prejudgment.

Several concepts assist in this process. First, the rationale and value of the history should be slowly and clearly outlined; often a gentle hand and a supportive nature will gain cooperation.

Second, the examination and collection of evidence may be conducted by the physician, with the history recorded when the patient is more stable or, instead of reciting it several times, given once and disseminated appropriately. The needed historical data are outlined in Table 80-6.

Some feel a female physician is preferable to a male for female victims. However, the sex of the examiner is irrelevant; it is the personal attentiveness and interaction that are critical. In fact, it is valuable for females to interact with a supportive, understanding man. This greatly aids in diminishing the "fear of men" that may develop.

Initial reactions vary greatly: both total hysteria (emotional decompensation) and complete tranquility (apparently care-free) are possible. However, most are usually not hysterical, but rather calm and inquisitive. All will need to know details of the examination in order to separate it from the rape. Recording reactions to questions could be helpful later in court action or to evaluate emotional needs. *Do the entire exam with special attention to avoiding pain, trauma, and further humiliation.* Perform a gentle examination, noting all unusual findings (ie, disheveled appearance, torn clothing).[14]

Evidence is used to help to corroborate sexual contact, lack of consent, and identify the assailant and possibly the scene and time of the attack.[15] Although some may be unwilling to prosecute and do not want specimens collected, they should be encouraged to consent now because valid data are impossible after 48 to 72 hours.[3]

The examination is done to treat injuries, prevent disease or pregnancy, and collect forensic evidence. A careful, complete, compulsive examination for documentation and evidence collection and samples is necessary and becomes

Table 80-6 Rape and General History

Health history	Female personal history	General personal history	Rape history	Postrape history
Immunizations: HBV, tetanus	Reactions to estrogens	STD: past, present	Date; time; location	Gargling; brushing teeth; vomiting; douching; urinating; defecating; taking an enema; bathing; showering; sponge bath; changing clothes; tampon use or change; shampoo; drinking; eating; medications
Recent (1 month) illness, injury or trauma: surface, internal	Current birth control	Rectal bleeding or discharge: past, present	Physical surroundings (ie, sand, carpet, grass, leaves, dirt)	
	Sterilization: prior, current		Force used and how: physical violence, weapons, threats, verbal violence, restraints, blindfolds	
	Pregnancy: possibility, early signs	Rectal intercourse in past		
Prescription drugs	Most recent consensual sexual activity: what, when	Prior assaults		
OTC drugs		Oral lacerations or sores: past, present	Number of perpetrators	
Alcohol use	Past pregnancies: dates, outcomes		Alcohol and/or drugs: use, forced use	
Illicit drugs			Loss of consciousness	
Allergies: drugs, topicals, food	Recent gynecologic injury or surgery		Fondling	
	Last normal menstrual period		Use of a foreign body, condom, lubricant	
	Thoughts regarding pregnancy prophylaxis or abortion		Vaginal entry or approach	
			Oral entry or approach	
	Vaginal discharge or infection: present, recent		Anal entry or approach	
			Forced to perform lewd acts	
			Ejaculation, urination, or defecation on the body or in an orifice	
			Did perpetrator claim to be sterile?	

Table 80-7 Physical Examination

General[a]	Female Genitalia	Male Genitalia	Rectal
General demeanor and emotional state	Perineum and thighs (use Wood's light for semen)	Penis: trauma, foreign material, infection	Trauma signs
Vital signs	Vulva carefully for trauma,[b] foreign matter, semen, dirt, blood, pus, grass	Scrotum: trauma, foreign material	Look for presence of lubricant, blood, semen, pus, foreign matter
Physical appearance			
Search skin for possible foreign material	Gently examine the for signs of trauma: introitus, hymen		Anoscopy: trauma; foreign objects, foreign matter; internal: lacerations, bleeding
Collect and label seminal stains, botanicals, glass, plastic, paper, hairs, fibers, dirt, sand, blood	Very carefully assess vaginal area for trauma, signs of foreign objects; internal: lacerations, bleeding		
Upper trunk: breast trauma, sexual maturity	Gently inspect cervix for parity, pregnancy signs, menses, trauma,[c] infection		
Extremities: bruises, fractures, sprains, abrasions, scratches, lacerations, contusions	Collect specimens		
	Gentle bimanual		
Head and neck for trauma	No rectal until after specimen collection if possibility of rectal penetration		

[a]Most physical signs of violence will be found on the face, head, neck, and extremities.
[b]Vaginal or perineal injury will usually be absent.
[c]The culposcope is ideal but not always available; see text.

critical if the case goes to court.[16] This is helped by an understanding of existing statutes and the use of a detailed form.

Each phase of the exam (see Table 80-7) should begin with a step-by-step explanation. Do not undress or put the patient into stirrups until necessary. Put all clothing and hospital sheets and gowns into a *paper* bag (plastic encourages growth of bacteria and mold) and treat like all other evidence.

All vital signs may be elevated because of emotion, injury, anxiety, pain, or hypovolemia, and abnormalities must be pursued as for other patients.

If applicable, aspirate or use a dry cotton swab in the mouth looking for ABO secretor status, and sperm and acid phosphatase. Do this as soon as possible since these substances deteriorate rapidly in the oral environment.

Eight percent to 45% will have some external damage.[13] Abrasions (most often on neck and extremities), contusions (neck, breasts, extremities), ecchymoses, rope burns, human bites (tooth imprints may help identify the assailant[17]), lacerations, and "hickeys" (breasts and neck) are common and must be documented (label with patient's and photographer's names and date and time) (ideally Polaroid photographs or marked on predrawn diagrams [Figs. 80-1 and 80-2]). Look for, document, and take samples of foreign material (leaves, grass, gravel, glass).

Finding semen on skin or clothing can be difficult. Look for lightly crusted spots or fluorescence under a Woods' lamp. Also use the lamp to inspect *all* skin areas (especially perineum, pubic area, and upper thighs). Obtain samples of all fluorescent material (with a saline-moistened cotton swab) but do not attempt to remove from clothes. False positives can occur with nasal drainage, fungi, pus, and soap.[2]

Damage to the head, face, and neck is most common (found in 40% of victims with injuries), with extremity damage next (25%).[18] Choking is a commonly used force, and if hoarseness, crepitus, or laryngeal tenderness are found, evaluate further for laryngeal injury.[2] Take radiographs for bone fractures as indicated.

Abdominal pain means either direct injury or foreign body damage until proven otherwise and evaluate as indicated.

Clip any hairs that appear to have semen. Obtain potential "perpetrator" hairs by combing the pubic area and placing loose ones in a labeled envelope. Hairs can only be identified as to a specific source by viewing growth sheaths or roots and therefore *must* be plucked, despite the apparent barbarity of this act in the immediate postrape phase. (If there is a great deal of difficulty or resistance from the patient [ie, cruel and unusual punishment], this could be delayed. Consult first with the police to ensure that this would later be acceptable as evidence.) Inform the patient of this need. Ask victims if they wish to do this themselves. Grasping close to the skin is less painful. Obtain 12 to 15 (or per your protocol) and place in a separate envelope.[16] Collect fingernail scrapings and place in their container.

Examine the vulva closely for injuries. Remove potential labial semen with a moistened cotton swab and place in its container. Examine and record the condition of the hymen.

Because vaginal or labial mucosal tears may occur, check carefully. In one series, vaginal pain and/or bleeding accompanied every case of vaginal trauma, but in another, these injuries were present in only 20% of injured victims, and 80% of these were mild,[18] whereas a third study found only 16% (most not severe) with damage.[19] However, nearly 50% of elderly victims in another study had genital injuries.[20]

Labial mucosal tears (possibly extending to the rectum if severe) are frequently present in the posterior commissure, particularly in children, virgins, or the elderly.[2] Toluidine

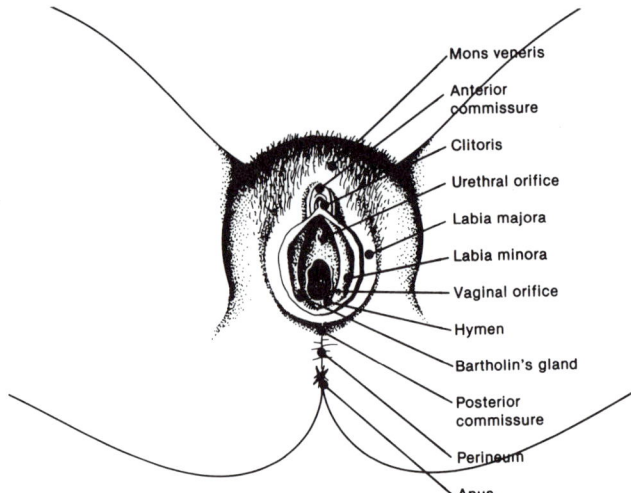

Figure 80-1 Female external anatomy. *Source:* Warner CG, Koerper MJ, Spaulding D, et al: San Diego County Protocol for the Treatment of Rape and Sexual Assault Victims. City of San Diego, Calif, Fall 1978, p 28.

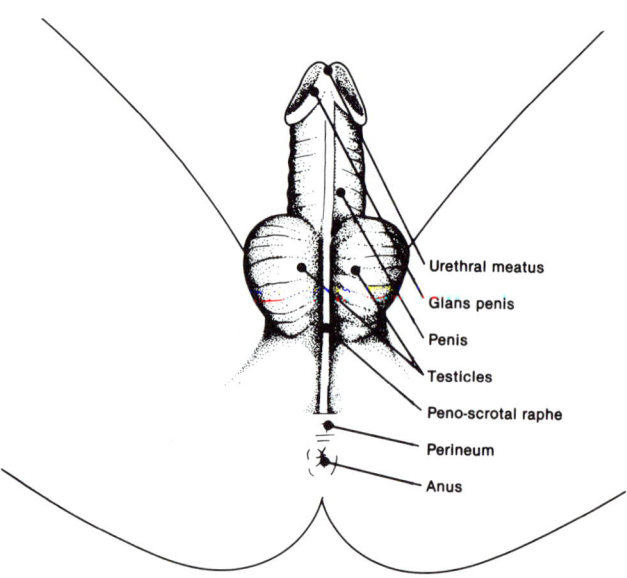

Figure 80-2 Male external anatomy. *Source:* Warner CG, Koerper MJ, Spaulding D, et al: San Diego County Protocol for the Treatment of Rape and Sexual Assault Victims. City of San Diego, Calif, Fall 1978, p 50.

blue applied to the perineum and vagina can greatly increase the detection of small tears. (Apply externally and gently internally and remove excess by gently wiping before inserting speculum because its insertion can itself cause small tears.) Although there can be damage with consensual sex or tampons, rape victims are more likely to stain positive than controls.[7]

Remove all foreign bodies and treat as evidence. Suspect intra-abdominal, vaginal, cervical, and/or uterine damage if any are found.[2]

Perform a speculum examination (using only warm water for lubrication—anything else could destroy potential evidence) to visualize damage and discharge and obtain specimens.

Aspirate or swab secretions that have pooled in the posterior fornix behind the cervix (samples only from the cervical canal may be falsely negative) for sperm and acid phosphatase. Then swab the cervical canal for gonococcal and chlamydial trachomatous cultures.

Some laboratories prefer collection after a 2 to 10 mL of normal saline irrigation of the posterior fornix (place in red top tube). This is also best if there are no apparent secretions. Others prefer a dry swab (placed in a red top tube with 2 mL of normal saline).[2] Distilled water is preferable for ABO and prostatic secretions.[21]

Place some of the material obtained on a glass slide with a drop of warm (body temperature) normal saline (sperm last longer if without preservative) and cover with a coverslip. Examine immediately for motility, trichomonads, and clue cells. Add 10% potassium hydroxide to look for yeast. A positive "whiff" test (fishy odor released when vaginal secretions are mixed with 10% potassium hydroxide) also may indicate bacterial vaginosis. A Pap smear may be done and could be better for finding sperm than other methods.

Collect semen samples for sperm and acid phosphatase. Sperm remain motile in the vagina for 3 to 6 hours and lose motility 2 to 5 minutes after removal. Vaginal nonmotile sperm can be found 7 to 72 hours postejaculation. Sperm are not recovered after 6 hours from the mouth or rectum (and never postdefecation), but are frequently recovered from underwear after anal intercourse.[2]

To the naked eye, the cervix and uterus usually do not appear damaged unless a foreign body was used. However, a study using the colposcope showed that all damage (look for erythema and petechiae as you would in an ordinary examination) may not be apparent.[2] Because colposcopes are expensive and not available in most EDs, their future utility has yet to be determined.

A bimanual examination completes the genital evaluation. Bilateral adnexal tenderness is common, especially if there were multiple attackers or episodes. Document all findings. Consult a gynecologist if there is a great deal of pain or an adnexal mass, which could be the result of a uterine ligament hematoma.[2]

A rectal examination is routine for *all* rape victims. Perform the examination without anesthesia only so far as it is tolerable to the patient. Inspect the anus externally for trauma (abrasions, lacerations, fissures) and check tone (the more lax it is the less likely there will be damage). Injuries result from friction or disproportion between the diameter of the anus and the erect penis or foreign body. If no injuries are seen, either there was no penetration or the victim is homosexual. Other signs of chronic sodomy include decreased sphincter tone, hemorrhoids, and chronic fissures. Using a water-lubricated anoscope (anesthesia may be needed), obtain cultures and look for lacerations, blood, hematomas, semen, ecchymoses, and lubricant. Swab for sperm and acid phosphatase and make air-dried slides. Sources of bleeding should be located, documented, and repaired.

Then inject 10 mL of normal saline into the rectum, allow it to equilibrate for 5 minutes and then aspirate. (Note that if the anus is swollen and tender, this may be all that is possible without sedation/anesthesia and, if at all possible, should not be delayed because of rapid degradation.) The fluid is then examined for sperm and acid phosphatase, although the latter may not be reliable. If a foreign body was used, there is evidence of damage, or your examination is inconclusive, sigmoidoscopy may be needed.[2]

Remember tetanus prophylaxis if indicated (any break in skin or mucosal integrity).

Specific studies needed are listed in Table 80-8 and are discussed in greater detail in the text, as are specific specimens to be collected in Table 80-4.

Table 80-8 Tests

1. **Assessment of injuries** (implies lack of consent)
   Complete blood count and other labs as indicated
   Radiographs as needed
   Photographs
2. **Evaluation of complications or preexisting conditions**
   Culture all involved orifices
      Gonorrhea
      Chlamydia trachomatous
   VDRL
   As indicated
      Pregnancy
      HIV
      ETOH
      Drug screen
3. **Determination of intercourse** (sexual contact)
   Evidence of semen or sperm
   Acid phosphatase
   Vaginal wet mount
   Pap smear
   Any external substances
   Antigen p30
4. **Identify perpetrator**
   ABO antigen typing
      Saliva
      Rectum
      Vaginal fluid
   Hair
   Fingernail scrapings
   DNA typing
   Peptidase-A activity
5. **Follow-up studies**
   VDRL
   Gonorrhea
   Chlamydia
   Pregnancy
   Injuries
   HIV, hepatitis B virus
6. **Photographs**

RISK OF SEXUALLY TRANSMITTED DISEASES

Any STD may be transmitted during an assault. Exact risks are unknown (with individual risk based on known community prevalence) but estimated to be 5% to 10%.[3] The risk of gonorrhea and/or chlamydia appears highest, although hepatitis B virus is most often spread sexually in the United States.[3] It is estimated that the risk is 1/30 for gonorrhea and 1/1000 for syphilis.[22,23] *The patient must be fully informed about the possibility of having contracted an STD and the available modes of treatment*. Include the following: culture for gonorrhea and chlamydia from any sites of real or attempted penetration; draw blood for Venereal Disease Research Laboratory test (VDRL) and possibly human immunodeficiency virus (HIV) (see below) and hepatitis testing.

Evidence of any STD within 24 hours of an assault may represent prior infection.[3] The baseline rate of asymptomatic gonorrhea in females is 5% but varies with different populations.[24] *In children, the presence of any STD should be considered evidence of sexual abuse until proven otherwise*.[24] When a sexually transmitted agent is identified, the positive laboratory report may be required in pending legal action.

Isolation of gonorrhea and chlamydia by culture with confirmation by recognized techniques is the standard. Direct specimen antigen-detection techniques or DNA probes are not recommended unless culture is not available. Because the potential for an inaccurate result is greatest in children, all presumptive isolates from them should be confirmed by at least two tests that involve different principles (ie, biochemical, serologic, enzyme substrate), and nonculture tests are not recommended. Store isolates at $-70°C$ for possible future studies.[24]

Although 90% of women infected with gonorrhea from a rape can be diagnosed with one visit if cultures are obtained from the cervix, urethra, anus, and pharynx, schedule a follow-up in 2 to 3 weeks to repeat gonorrhea and chlamydia tests for cure. There should be a third visit in 3 months for repeat of serologies (VDRL, HIV, and hepatitis B virus)[24] (note that most will not return at all and only a minuscule number will do so twice).

Reassure the patient with information regarding treatment and agencies available for follow-up care. Sexual relations are not safe until it has been determined whether an STD was contracted or prescribed treatment has been successful.

Because follow-up cannot be assured, offer treatment to all victims. Other reasons to treat include victim request, assailant known to be symptomatic or infected, multiple assailants, inability or low likelihood of follow-up, and high community prevalence.[2] The regimen in Table 80-9 is the current (1989) Centers for Disease Control recommendation. Some think, however, that an immediate Betadine or strong vinegar douche will suffice, but most currently believe in standard antibiotic therapy. (Gonorrhea is more difficult to detect in females regardless of the method used, resulting in unrecognized and untreated cases. It is, therefore, strongly recommended that therapy be given and that it includes early lues and chlamydia. Hepatitis prophylaxis is controversial and HIV is discussed in a separate section.) Assailants should be evaluated for STD as far as the law allows.

Antibiotic therapy may disrupt the normal vaginal bacterial balance. A yeast infection may develop but is readily treatable by prescription or with over-the-counter medication. In addition, the assault itself may also have an irritating effect on genital tissues. Female patients must also be informed that a urinary tract infection can result from irritation or injury and that subsequent coitus may be painful. If she experiences an unusual or heavy discharge, sores, dysuria, vaginal pruritus, or prolonged dyspareunia, she should seek prompt medical attention.

HIV TESTING

We should be prepared to discuss the potential danger of acquired immunodeficiency syndrome (AIDS), but what we

Table 80-9 CDC Treatment Guidelines for Gonococcal Infections

Adults and children weighing >100 lb (45 kg)
    Ceftriaxone 250 mg IM
      or
    Amoxicillin 3.0 g PO
      or
    Ampicillin 3.5 g PO
      or
    Procaine penicillin G 4.8 million U IM
      (Each of these regimens except ceftriaxone is accompanied by probenecid 1.0 g PO)
Followed by
    Tetracycline 500 mg PO qid for 7 days
      or
    Doxycycline 100 mg PO bid for 7 days
    Penicillin allergy
      Spectinomycin 2 g IM
        plus
      Erythromycin stearate 500 mg PO qid for 7 days;
      or
      Ciprofloxacin 500 mg PO once
Children weighing <100 lb (45 kg)
    Ceftriaxone 125 mg IM
      or
    Amoxicillin 50 mg/kg (accompanied by probenecid 25 mg/kg PO);
      or
    Procaine penicillin G 100,000 units/kg IM
      plus
    Probenecid 25 mg/kg PO
    Penicillin allergy
      Spectinomycin 40 mg/kg IM
      or
      Tetracycline 40 mg/kg PO qid for 5 days (for children >8 years old)

Source: 1989 STD Treatment. *MMWR* 38 (number 5-8) Sept. 1, 1989.

should do about it is still highly controversial. Although some victims may be very concerned, try to avoid causing unwarranted worry (ie, ask matter-of-fact questions to ascertain perpetrator risk and do not needlessly dwell on the subject). Do not bring it up if you are not prepared to offer *something*, eg, testing, counseling, referral, treatment.

HIV testing in the ED is complicated and controversial because of a lack of proper follow-up. It should be done *only* with a fully informed patient and a specific means of obtaining results and counseling. Some think it should not be done here at all.

Testing is indicated, however, when a victim has signs or symptoms of previously undiagnosed AIDS, the assailant is known or suspected to have AIDS or be HIV positive or engage in high-risk behavior (intravenous drug abuse, homosexual, bought or sold sex, or sex partner of any of these), or the victim requests testing.

Because months elapse before seroconversion (some data indicate that antibodies will develop within 6 months of an exposure in 95% of those who eventually do become infected), it should be repeated in 3 to 6 months.

The exact risk is unknown, but transmission by a single rape has been confirmed.[25,26] Risk is increased with recurrent exposure (ie, child sexual abuse). There are some recent but tentative data indicating the use of postexposure zivodine,[27] but this treatment is unproven, lengthy, and expensive. Immediate douching with strong vinegar has been advocated by some. Because waiting for evidence collection first is too long to wait for this to be effective, a choice of one needs to be made.

SPECIFIC FORENSIC STUDIES

The following studies are used to indicate ejaculation and identify the assailant. Some are used ubiquitously and others are somewhat experimental. You should be aware of which are employed in your area.

Sperm was once the gold standard for determining intercourse, even though the recovery rate was only 20% to 75%. Fifty percent of controls will lose motility in 2 to 3 hours, although most rape examinations will not occur in this time. Whereas nonmotile sperm persist in all at 18 hours and 50% at 72 hours, the normal range of intrafemale sperm decay is 14 hours to 9 days, depending on the study, and probably correlated with the method used. There is little known about anal/rectal sperm survival. One study[7] found dead sperm after 24 hours, but it was rare to find tails after 6 hours.

Because of these variables and many other factors causing false negatives (long delay in seeking care, condom use, azoospermia, vasectomy), new tests have been devised as sensitive indicators of recent intercourse.[7] Determine which are used in your area.

Acid phosphatase is present in high levels in semen (even postvasectomy). Courts now accept its presence as evidence of penetration of the penis, although it is also found in the vagina (normal vaginal is only 1/10 to 1/20 of prostate and laboratories can screen it out), RBC, WBC, platelets, and bone, but a seminal source can be distinguished.[2]

The time period for its detection in the vagina has been reported as 2 to 24 hours with an average of 14 hours.[2,7] Although it decreases more rapidly than sperm, it may correlate better with the time since intercourse than sperm.[7] In one study, 50% of volunteers had significant levels after 9 hours, but by 36 hours none had any.[7] It is of no use in anal or oral intercourse.

A level greater than 20 to 25 King-Armstrong units/mL (or >50 [esp >138] sigma units/mL) usually indicates recent (within 24 hours) coitus.[7] Levels greater than 20 but less than 50 sigma units correlate with intercourse in the past 48 hours.[2] Note different units and be aware of what your facility uses.

Prostatic antigen p30 is a male-specific prostatic glycoprotein that is secreted by seminal epithelial cells. It is an ideal marker because it (1) is highly concentrated in semen, (2) is male-specific, (3) follows a regular pattern of postcoital decline, (4) is reliably detected by an enzyme-linked immunosorbent assay (ELISA), (5) is more sensitive and specific for recent coitus than acid phosphatase, (6) can indicate sexual activity up to 48 hours, (7) can indicate semen with a negative acid phosphatase, (8) is found postvasectomy, and (9) as little as 3 ng/mL of fluid can be detected. It usually lasts 13 to 47 hours (mean 27) as compared to 14 hours for acid phosphatase.[2,7]

MHS-5 (mouse antihuman sperm 5) is a unique monoclonal sperm-coating antigen from seminal vesicles that is present in normal and vasectomized semen and absent in all other tissues or fluids and has no cross-reactivity. There is an ELISA sufficiently sensitive to detect it in 0.75 to 1 ng of seminal protein. Vaginal fluids do not appear to have any effect on it.

There are also four genetic typing markers found in semen: ABO, erythrocyte peptidase A (Pep-A), phosphoglucomutase (PGM), and DNA.

Eighty percent of the population secretes ABO antigens into other body fluids (saliva, tears, sweat, vaginal fluid, semen). If the victim is a secretor, it will match their blood type. If different antigens are found, they may be from the assailant. Obtain specimens from saliva and the posterior fornix. It cannot be used to precisely identify an individual.[2]

Pep-A is common only in black populations. Present in sperm and semen, it follows the same phenotype pattern as blood but is not affected by secretor status. It can be typed (for up to 6 weeks) from a dry semen stain (± sperm) that is free of other body fluids. Activity is absent from vaginal fluid unless there is blood. It cannot be detected on a vaginal swab beyond 3.5 hours postcoitus.[2]

PGM has three subtypes. Activity rapidly decreases and is rarely seen beyond 6 hours. Only DNA typing can positively identify perpetrators (the chance of two nonrelatives having the same DNA pattern is one in a quadrillion). It can be isolated from hair roots, blood, and semen. Sperm DNA has been isolated from a vaginal swab taken 6.5 hours postcoitus.[28] It can also be found in dry semen for at least 1 month, but there must be sperm.[29]

SPECIAL CONSIDERATIONS OF MALE PATIENTS

Rape incidents involving men are extremely traumatic, and it is of the utmost importance that we interact in a sensitive and supportive manner. Males experience many of the same physical and emotional injuries as females, and it is essential that they not be viewed any differently. In fact, the commonalities of all rape patients should be stressed rather than the differences. However, male victims are more stigmatized and may experience greater subsequent guilt and anger.[30]

Because the willingness of men to report rape is at the stage that women were at decades ago, it is essential for all law enforcement and medical personnel to encourage them to report the crime. Use support, sensitivity, and understanding. A few other facts to be noted concerning male rape victims include:

- It is a myth that rapes occur only to male prisoners or that most perpetrators are homosexuals. The overwhelming majority of male rapes are committed by heterosexual men (unknown to the victim) against homosexual men or boys.[31]
- Ten percent of all rape victims are male and comprise approximately 14% of rape victims under 18 years. Girls less than 18 years are one-third of all female victims, but boys less than 18 years are 93.5% of all male victims.[2]
- Male rapes are usually forceful and quite violent, but boys are less apt to be harmed because fear and intimidation by "authority figures" compels passivity.
- The history, examination, and treatment should be the same as for females, with special attention placed on rectal and penile trauma; bleeding or discharge; soreness, infection, or trauma to the mouth or pharynx; internal injuries; and soreness or pain throughout the body.

History-taking is similar to that for women. Tailor the examination to the particulars of the assault. Since the anus is often penetrated with the victim lying prone, search for abrasions on the thorax, abdomen, or knees. Because victims may be subdued by blows to the jaw, face, or abdomen, look for injuries there. Also, if indicated, take swabs (including gonorrhea and chlamydia cultures) of buccal, gingival, and pharyngeal areas even if the patient cleaned his mouth or teeth or ate.

PREGNANCY

Although the chance of pregnancy resulting from a rape is very low (<1% to 5% of those at risk),[13] the possibility of pregnancy must be discussed and "prophylaxis" offered (a 1989 California court ruling stated that this must be *offered* to all even if it is against the philosophy of the physician or hospital[32]) to all with childbearing potential. Alternatives must be presented for the patient to make a fully informed choice. If any option is against the physician's or facility's beliefs, timely referral to another for discussion is acceptable.

First, establish the possibility of pregnancy:

- Is she sterile (tubal ligation or hysterectomy)?
- Has she reached menarche or completed menopause?

If pregnancy is possible, determine:

- What is the length and on what day of her cycle did the rape occur? (Days 10 to 16 are greatest risk for those with a 28-day cycle.)
- What is the current method of birth control, if any?
- Could she already be pregnant? Because 2% to 3% of women who are raped are already pregnant, this must be ruled out. Current urine or serum B human chorionic gonadatropin (hCG) tests are almost equally sensitive (7 or 5 days postimplantation, respectively).

Two general alternatives are available to avoid pregnancy: pharmacologic postcoital implantation prevention and elective abortion. These influence what is done (see Table 80-10).

Table 80-10 Pregnancy Prophylaxis

Do nothing and wait for next period. This will limit further options should a pregnancy result: carry to term or elective abortion.
Repeat hCG in 7 days. If it is negative, the chance of a pregnancy is extremely low; if positive, see above.
Morning-after pill. Rate of failure overall is 1%. All cause nausea and vomiting to some degree. None is effective after 72 hours and all must be begun within that time. Estrogens are contraindicated with a history of pulmonary embolism, deep venous thrombosis, some tumors, etc, although the consequences of such short-term use are unknown.
   Ethinyl estradiol/norgestrel (Ovral): Current drug of choice.
      Dose: two orally immediately, then two in 12 hours.
      Lowest (less than 1%) failure rate.
      Good compliance because of only two doses and minimal side effects.
   Ethinyl estradiol (Estinyl, Femione): 2.5 mg orally immediately, then 2.5 mg bid or 5 mg qd for 5 days.
   Conjugated estrogens (Premarin)
      10 mg orally bid or 30 mg qd for 5 days or 50 mg intravenous qd for 2 days.
      Potentially poor compliance.
Diethylstilbestrol. No longer recommended.

CHILD SEXUAL ABUSE

For in-depth discussion, see Chapter 37. *Sexual misuse* is a better term than *sexual abuse* in reference to children because physical harm is not an integral part of the diagnosis. It refers to "any situation where a child is exposed to sexual stimulation inappropriate for [his/her] age or psychosocial development," with emphasis on the broad range of sexual experiences that may occur, often repeatedly.[7] It includes rape, molestation, and incest. Most victims are premenarchal.

The reported incidence has dramatically increased over the past 5 years, although it is still thought to be greatly underreported. This increase is due in part to greater public awareness, and, unfortunately, also from false accusations. It is estimated that 1% to 3% of all US children are actually victimized.

Children who are molested or raped usually know the assailant. In one study, only 18% were assaulted by strangers, the rest by relatives.[2] Most of the assailants are adult male (93%)[2] neighbors, friends, or "shirt-tail relatives." When the alleged abuser is a relative (see below), fathers, stepfathers, or uncles are most likely.[2] Therefore, most situations are nonviolent and repetitive.

Incest involves a related victim and assailant (usually parent or guardian) who could not legally marry. Father-daughter is the most common, whereas mother-son is the most pathological. Its long-term impact can be poor. Many victims show regressive or antisocial behavior when first seen, and even with therapy, adjustment is not easy.[7]

Because a child's story may not be completely reliable, collect cultures for gonorrhea and chlamydia from the pharynx and rectum as well as the vagina and penis. Prevalence of STD appears relatively low, with chlamydia trachomatous the most frequently found.

Sexual misuse is best handled by an experienced team knowledgeable in dealing with the needs of children, although the emergency physician may be called on to provide a preliminary evaluation. Objectivity must be maintained, and these cases should be handled in the same way as you would any case of alleged child abuse (see Chapter 37).

In virginal victims, pelvic examinations are not done unless an injury or foreign body is suspected. Anesthesia is recommended.

Victim treatment may await results of alleged offender (if available) testing. Remember, however, that this does not preclude perpetrator treatment between the episode(s) and now.

In children, presence of any STD beyond the neonatal period is considered highly suspicious of sexual abuse until proven otherwise. However, there are exceptions: (1) rectal and genital infection with chlamydia trachomatous in young children (up to 3 years) may be due to persistent perinatally acquired infection; (2) bacterial vaginosis can be found in both abused and nonabused children; (3) genital warts, although suggestive, are nonspecific without other evidence of sexual abuse. Therefore, carefully recheck results when the only evidence is an organism or antibodies.[2]

SPECIAL CONSIDERATIONS FOR GERIATRIC PATIENTS

Because of the vulnerability of senior citizens, attacks on them are even more appalling. Factors contributing to vulnerability are included in Table 80-11.

Valid statistics are unavailable because of a lack of reporting. This is due primarily to embarrassment, fear of reprisal, doubt about whether their complaint will be believed, senility, and feeling overwhelmed by the system.

One analysis of rape victims over 50 years of age who did file reports affords a profile of these sexual assaults (Table 80-12). Older victims suffer more severe injuries, especially to genital areas. Aggression, not sexuality, causes the greatest difficulties later, resulting in feelings of isolation, loss of control, and fear.[7]

Psychological Reactions

It is vital that all assisting or questioning of a victim immediately after a sexual assault recognize that there are

---

Table 80-11 Elder Vulnerability

Age and disability
Diminished sensory capacities
Bone and muscle changes
Impaired ability for mobility and self-control
Increased sensitivity of genitourinary organs
Living alone or in an institution
Established daily routines, obvious to the observer
Lack of transportation

Table 80-12 Profile of 78 Raped Patients Over Age 50

Criteria	Percent
Victim lived alone	97
Physical force was used	97
Victim raped in the home	73
Victim raped by a total stranger	68
Rape was associated with theft	65
Victim was actually beaten	50
Victim allowed perpetrator into the home as a repairman, official, or acquaintance	43
Perpetrator gained entrance through window or unlocked door	36
Perpetrator used forcible entry	21

Source: Adapted from information in Davis LJ. Rape and Older Women. In: Warner CG, ed. *Rape and Sexual Assault: Management and Intervention*. Rockville, MD: Aspen, 1980:93–119.

legitimate psychological reactions. The specific characteristics may differ, but psychological trauma is almost always present and must be treated along with medical and evidentiary examinations. Some of the emotional "baggage" that may result include disbelief; both fear of and concern for the rapist; feeling guilt, anger, stupidity, embarrassment, or shame; vulnerability and a sense of loss of control over one's life.[3]

Rape creates an immediate and unanticipated crisis. Mental disorganization, manifested by inconsistencies in the story, incoherence in speech, confusion of numbers, and loss of a sense of time, occurs because it helps victims to psychologically survive the ordeal. It is important to keep these reactions in mind. We may think that those who are disorganized or have controlled reactions or nervous laughter as not telling the truth.

Approaching victims in a caring manner; providing a safe, supportive environment; and legitimizing their experience facilitate the process that follows and aids in restoring mental health. All must be able to recognize shock reactions as normal. Those whom the victim sees first play an important role in eventual psychological resolution. A negative interchange may delay healing, whereas a positive, supportive reaction facilitates not only the process now (ie, examination and investigation), but also the ability to deal with the disaster in the future. Encourage victims to confront the issues and express their feelings.[14]

All too often, when faced with a difficult emotional situation, personnel respond with one of the following common avoidance reactions:

- *Appearing extremely busy*: running in and out of the room without communicating verbally.
- *Leaving the patient completely alone*: finding it easier to deal with rape by avoiding it.
- *Relating to the patient on a very unemotional level*: avoiding any possibility of touching, holding, or caring.

Refraining from the use of dysfunctional modes of communication will prove valuable, save time, and prevent misunderstandings. A few common communication barriers are given in Table 80-13.

It is important to establish good communication and let the patient know that all are caring and supportive. The following are some suggestions to keep in mind during the initial contact.

- *Help patients get in touch with their feelings.* They may be angry, depressed, guilty, dazed, or numb. All are legitimate reactions.
- *Help patients accept their feelings.* Expression of feelings at this time is a healthy way to deal with rape.
- *Be sensitive to nonverbal signals* (eg, posture, fidgeting, shakiness, incoherence in speech).

Table 80-13 Barriers to Communication

Making premature comments and evaluations
Making statements that are too general
Interrupting the patient or family
Talking instead of actively listening
Talking down to patient and family
Asking loaded questions
Placing the blame
Arguing
Displaying irritating listening habits
Repeatedly telling the patient and family what to do

- *Be a receiver*. Listen to patients without judging.
- *Hear the story and take it seriously*. Help legitimize the experience. (Our society often blames victims.)
- *Communicate your stability* by remaining calm and empathic.
- *Establish a common language* and "tune in" to the patient's terminology.

Those who are anxious and fearful naturally react in a way that may seem uncooperative, hostile, or emotional. This may be due to any one or a combination of the following factors: the nature of the assault and its meaning to the victim; their ability to cope; attitudes and responses from significant others and personnel; and the physical setting of the examination. To intervene appropriately and reduce anxiety you must:

- Know and understand the nature of rape/sexual assault.
- Assess how the patient perceives the assault.
- Identify and reinforce the patient's coping abilities.
- Assist "significant others."
- Coordinate care, be an interpreter, advocate if the victim needs assistance, and mobilize community resources.

Another important method of reducing the patient's anxiety is to explain procedures in advance. This includes why it is being done, the specific steps to be followed, how the patient's cooperation will aid in prosecuting the criminal and in his or her own recovery, and what may be done to assist in the procedure. Providing patients with information and eliciting cooperation will also restore their ability to control their own lives and to make decisions after having been rendered helpless and out-of-control by the unanticipated assault.

RAPE TRAUMA SYNDROME[33,34]

Shock and disbelief (rape trauma syndrome [RTS]) is similar to that suffered by victims of any disaster (post-traumatic stress disorder). Characteristic symptoms develop

Table 80-14 Rape Trauma Syndrome[2]

Recurrent, painful recollections or dreams of the event or suddenly acting or feeling as if it were recurring.
Because of anxiety at exposure to situations that symbolize or resemble part of the event, and, therefore, avoidance of thoughts or feelings associated with or that provoke memories, there may be an inability to remember parts of the event.
Decreased interest in important activities and lack of a "future."
Limited range of affect and feeling detached from others.
Sleep disorders and trouble concentrating.
Hypervigilance, irritability, or angry outbursts.

Table 80-15 Social Service

See the victim as quickly as possible.
Communicate with friends, family, or law enforcement to determine the nature of the assault and the victim's condition.
Orient the victim to anticipated proceedings if ED staff have not already done so.
Assist in contacting others, if desired.
Explain the consent forms, their purpose and value.
Encourage patients to relate feelings, discuss the attack, and vent any anger, fear, guilt, or hostility.
Listen.
If a history of the attack obtained, provide this information to the ED staff to minimize repeated questioning.
Explain follow-up care and provide reading material and written instructions.
Assist in arranging follow-up appointments.
Arrange for someone to accompany the patient home or to another place of comfort.
Place a follow-up telephone call in a few days to assess the condition. Maintain contact for at least a year, especially throughout the legal proceedings. The trial may be a greater burden than the assault, causing significant symptoms.[174]

following a psychologically distressing event that is outside the range of usual human experience and usually lasts at least a month.[2] The symptoms are more severe and last longer when the event is caused in some way by a human rather than an uncontrollable act of nature. It consists of acute and long-term phases.

The *acute stage* (disorganization) lasts from a few days to months. There is usually one of two reaction styles, equally distributed.[2]

- *Expressed*: There is demonstrated fear, anger, or anxiety. Specific behaviors may include crying, restlessness, or tenseness.
- *Controlled*: Feelings are masked by a seemingly calm, composed, or subdued affect. Questions are answered in a matter-of-fact manner and there may be inappropriate smiles or laughter.

The *long-term* phase (disorganization-reorganization) begins in about 2 to 3 weeks and may last forever. It is how victims develop coping mechanisms and is characterized by changes in lifestyle, ie, change of residence or telephone number or trips home to parents. Nightmares, phobias (especially of being alone), sexual anxieties, or the end of a relationship are common. In a study of long-term effects of rape, victims were found to be significantly more depressed, anxious, and fearful than controls.[2] Other components are included in Table 80-14.

SOCIAL SERVICE INTERVENTION

The role of a social or rape-crisis worker is most valuable because it affords continuity of and establishes the necessary linkages between initial medical management and follow-up psychological and medical care. It is imperative that they be notified immediately on arrival of a rape victim so that if the emergency staff is busy with life-threatening cases, the patient need not wait unattended.

The assistance of one who is trained to deal with rape victims helps with all stages of the process, including recovery. Counseling and support should be offered as part of the initial evaluation. Special considerations to be followed as part of the social service intervention are noted in Table 80-15.

FOLLOW-UP CARE

Patients without significant physical damage can be discharged to follow-up for injuries, STD, and counseling. There must be a specific follow-up plan and assurance that help is always available. However, most will not return. Patients will recall very little of what is presented to them while in the ED, but an informational brochure, an appointment card, and written instructions placed in a pocket, purse, or wallet can be read later.

Injuries may require home care and/or follow-up. Inform the patient as to how these are to be done and when and where to obtain further care.

In most crisis situations, people can become upset and may be faced with unexpected changes in their lives. Since sexual assault may present a serious threat to patients' safety and well-being, it is understandable that they may experience mental or emotional stress as an after-effect. Also, family and friends may be affected.

The patient needs to be around those who can be supportive and sympathetic. Some women's antirape groups offer woman-to-woman support throughout the procedures. The patient may also wish to seek short- or long-term counseling. Members of the patient's immediate family may also benefit. Sexual problems, nightmares, and phobias can be alleviated with proper care and support from friends, family members, and/or counselors.

Table 80-16 Evaluation Form for Hospital Examination, Laboratory Testing, and Counseling

---

Our concern is that the best possible care be provided to you and other patients of sexual assault. In order to evaluate and improve this program, your suggestions are needed. Please take a few moments to answer these questions and return the form at your convenience. Thank you for your cooperation.

1. Which hospital were you taken to?
   (List available hospitals)

2. Date of hospital exam _____
   Time of hospital exam _____
   Date this application was filled out
   _____

3. Were you left alone at the hospital? _____ If so, for how long? _____
   Did this bother you? _____ Was an explanation provided? _____

4. Please check any of the following areas that were explained to you prior to the procedure.

	Yes	No		Yes	No
• Reason for physical exam	___	___	• Reasons for asking personal questions	___	___
• Collection of evidence process	___	___	• Reasons for lab test(s)	___	___
• Steps in physical exam	___	___	• Possible treatment for venereal disease/pregnancy	___	___
• Other: _____	___	___			

5. Were the following counseling services satisfactory?

	Yes	No	Not given
• Advice on birth control measures	___	___	___
• Advice on the prevention of venereal disease	___	___	___
• Counseling on pregnancy prevention measures	___	___	___
• Other: _____	___	___	___

6. What type of social service counseling did you receive?
   _____ Were you counseled by the hospital social worker?
   _____ Were you referred to outside community resources?
   _____ Were family and friends involved in the counseling?
   Was the counseling satisfactory? Yes _____ No _____

COMMENTS

7. What type of follow-up recommendations were made?
   _____ Medical follow-up care was recommended
   _____ Signs and symptoms to watch for in case of complications were described
   _____ Psychological follow-up care was recommended

8. Did you receive a follow-up call from the hospital? _____ If yes, what did they recommend? _____
   _____

9. Were you pleased with your care and treatment? _____ If not, what did you dislike? _____
   _____

10. What improvements would you suggest for the care of future patients of sexual assault? _____
    _____

11. How did you feel about your interview with the police officer? _____
    _____

    The plain clothes officer? _____
    _____

12. Other comments: _____
    _____

If you feel comfortable signing your name, it would be most helpful, but please recognize that this is not required.

_____

EVALUATION OF RAPE INTERVENTION

The assessment, planning, design, development, and implementation of a rape management program are incomplete without an evaluation. Professionals may have designed a program thought to be ideal, but, in reality, it may not meet the needs of victims. Consequently, each facility should develop and integrate an evaluation and feedback network used to strengthen and reinforce the original goals and objectives of the program.

In addition to personnel assessment, elicit feedback from those receiving care. This type of evaluation should *not* be pursued prior to a 6-week follow-up visit. If social service personnel maintain contact with these patients, the evaluation process would be easily implemented with their assistance. An example of a patient evaluation form is noted in Table 80-16.

REFERENCES

1. Caplan GM. *Rape and Its Victims: A Report for Citizens, Health Facilities and Criminal Justice Agencies*. U.S. Department of Justice, Law Enforcement Assistance Administration, 1975.
2. Drury L, Barkin R. Sexual assault. In: *Emergindex*, 3/90.
3. Beebe DK. Emergency management of the adult female rape victim. *Am Fam Physician*. 1991;43(6):2041–2046.
4. Bureau of Justice Statistics Data Report, 1988. Washington, D.C.: Department of Justice, Bureau of Justice Statistics, 1989.
5. U.S. Department of Justice. *Uniform Crime Reports for the United States*. Washington, D.C.: U.S. Government Printing Office, 1989.
6. Geist RF. Sexually-related trauma. *Emerg Med Clin North Am*. 1988;6:439–466.
7. Hoelzer M. Rape and sexual assault. In: Tintinally JE, ed. *Emergency Medicine, A Comprehensive Study Guide*, 3rd ed. New York, N.Y.: McGraw-Hill; 1987.
8. Hicks J. Sexual assault. In: Michols DH, Eviad JR, eds. *Obstetrics and Gynecology*. Philadelphia, Pa: Harper & Row; 1985:473.
9. Carrow DM. *Rape: Guidelines for a Community Response*. U.S. Department of Justice, Law Enforcement Assistance Administration, National Institute of Law Enforcement and Criminal Justice. January 1980: pp. 130, 170, 253–255.
10. *Forcible Rape: An Analysis of Legal Issues*. U.S. Department of Justice, Law Enforcement Assistance Administration, National Institute of Law Enforcement and Criminal Justice, 1978: pp. 8, 16, 17, 20.
11. Report of the task force to study treatment of the victims of sexual assault. Prince Georges County, Maryland, March 1973.
12. Warner CG, Koerper MJ, Spaulding D, et al., eds. *San Diego County Protocol for the Treatment of Rape and Sexual Assault Victims*. City of San Diego, Fall 1978: pp. 14, 19, 20.
13. Braen GR. Physical assessment and emergency medical management for adult victims of sexual assault. In: Warner CG, ed. *Rape and Sexual Assault: Management and Intervention*. Rockville, Md.: Aspen Publishers; 1980: 57, 60, 69.
14. Patterson DC, Chapin DS. Sexual Assault. In: Wilkins EW Jr, ed. *Emergency Medicine*, 3rd ed. Baltimore, Md.: Williams & Wilkins; 1990:657.
15. Hochbaum SR. The evaluation and treatment of the sexually assaulted patient. *Emerg Med Clin North Am*. 1987;5:601–22 (quoted in Beebe).
16. Hicks DJ, Weissberg MP. Sensitive emergency management of rape victims. *Emerg Med Rep*. 1988;9:113–120.
17. Everett RB, Jimerson GE. The rape victim: a review of 17 consecutive cases. *Obstet Gynecol*. 1977;50:88–90 (cited in *Emergindex*).
18. Tintinally JE, Hoelzer M. Clinical findings and legal resolution in sexual assault. *Ann Emerg Med*. 1985;14:447–453.
19. Cartwright PS. Sexual assault study group. Factors that correlate with injury sustained by survivors of sexual assault. *Obstet Gynecol*. 1987;70:44–46.
20. Cartwright PS, Moore RA. The elderly victim of rape. *South Med J*. 1989;82:988–989.
21. Dunn S. Lavage fluid in sexual-assault examinations (letter). *Can Med Assoc J*. 1988;138:400.
22. Cate W, Blackmore CA. Sexual assault and sexually transmitted diseases. In: Holmes KL, Marsh PA, Sparling PF, Wilsner PJ, eds. *Sexually Transmitted Diseases*. New York, NY.: McGraw-Hill; 1984:119.
23. Forster GE, Pritchard J, Munday PE, et al. Incidence of sexually transmitted diseases in rape victims during 1984. *Genitourin Med*. 1986;62:266–269.
24. Sexually transmitted diseases treatment guidelines. *MMWR*. 1989;38 (suppl 8):1–43.
25. Murphy S, Kitchen V, Harris JRW, et al. Rape and subsequent seroconversion to HIV. *BMJ*. 1989;299:718.
26. Murphy S, Munday PE, Jeffries DJ. Anti-HIV substances for rape victims (letter). *JAMA*. 1989;252:2090–2091.
27. CDC: Public Health Service statement on management of occupational exposure to human immunodeficiency virus regarding zidovudine postexposure use. *MMWR*. 1990;39: no. RR-1.
28. Gill P, Jeffreys AJ, Werrett DJ. Forensic application of DNA 'fingerprints' (letter). *Nature*. 1985;318:577–579.
29. Giusti A, Baird W, Pasquale S, et al. Application of deoxyribonucleic acid (DNA) polymorphisms to the analysis of DNA recovered from sperm. *J Forensic Sci*. 1986;31:409–417.
30. Mezey C, King M. Male victims of sexual assault. *Med Sci Law*. 1987;27:122–124.
31. Groth AN, Burgess AW. Male rape: offenders and victims. *Am J Psychiatry*. 1980;137:806–810.
32. Brushwood DB. Must a Catholic hospital inform a rape victim of the availability of the "morning-after" pill. *Am J Hosp Pharm*. 1990; 47:395–396.
33. Rosenberg MS. Rape crisis syndrome. *Med Aspects Hum Sex*. 1986;20(3):65–71 (cited in Beebe).
34. Burgess AW, Holmstrom LL. Rape trauma syndromes. *Am J Psychiatry*. 1974;131:981–986.

81. Ocular Emergencies

JAMES CABRAL, MD

Within the general medical community, the emergency physician should be considered second only to the ophthalmologist in the ability to manage ocular problems. People living in isolated communities remote from major medical centers may actually look to the emergency physician as the person most competent to manage ocular emergencies. Consequently, the emergency physician must have a thorough understanding of the following factors:

- the eye's gross anatomy as well as the anterior and posterior anatomy as viewed with both a direct ophthalmoscope and a biomicroscope (the slit lamp),[1,2] including the eye muscles and related structures. (See Fig. 81-1.) (See Appendix 81-A for four comprehensive illustrations of the eye and all of its components.)
- the range of ocular tissue response to exogenous infection, to chemical and physical trauma, and to endogenous agents[2-4]
- the types of ocular manifestations and responses to systemic disease[2,5,6]
- the mechanisms and routes of invasion of the ocular tissue by infectious agents[2,5,7,8]
- the bony anatomy of the skull and facial bones examined radiographically and accurately by palpation[1,2]
- the pharmacology and clinical applications of a limited number of ocular drugs[2,5,9]

Certain skills also are essential, including the ability to

- recognize, and to a reasonable extent appraise, ocular inflammatory response in the different regions of the eye and adnexa[5-7]
- obtain an exceptionally well-documented history of ocular trauma, including the circumstances and mechanisms of trauma, as well as the sequence of ocular symptoms that develop during ocular medical disorders[2-5]
- perform a relatively thorough and accurate ocular examination[2,5,6]
- detemine a patient's approximate visual status that may have existed prior to ocular trauma or disease and measure in a reproducible manner visual acuity and at least gross visual fields in the emergency department prior to both instilling ocular medications and manipulating the eye[2]
- communicate ocular history and clinical findings in the jargon of the ophthalmologist (Appendix 81-B)[5,10]
- obtain useful and reliable bacterial specimens for culture and ensure timely and proper inoculation in correct media[8,11-14]
- use commonly available emergency department instruments for both the examination and the treatment of the eye
- gain confidence and skill in a limited number of emergency ocular surgical procedures[3,4]
- prepare an ocular trauma patient for safe transport to another facility[3,4]

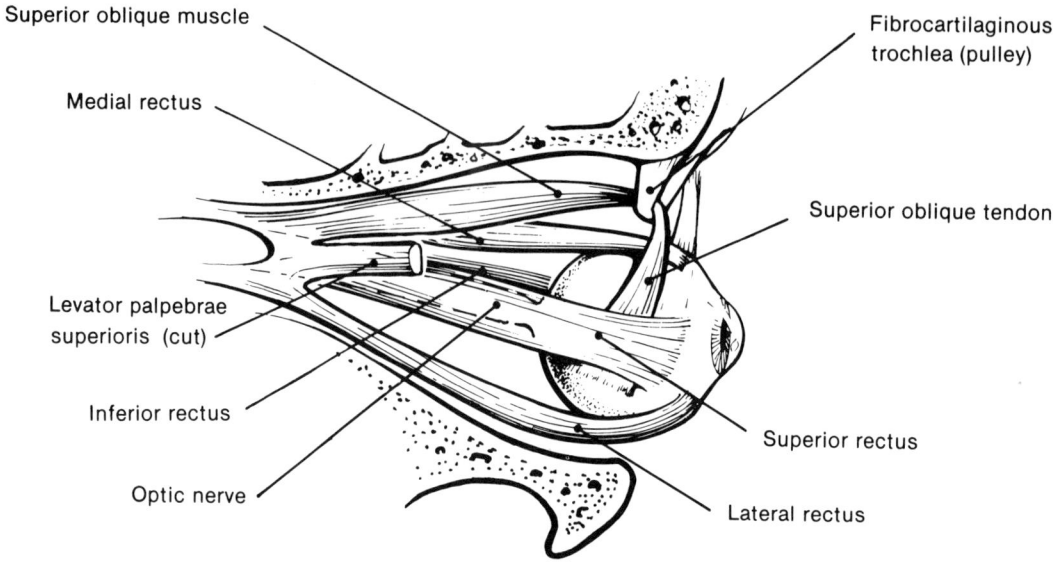

Superior view

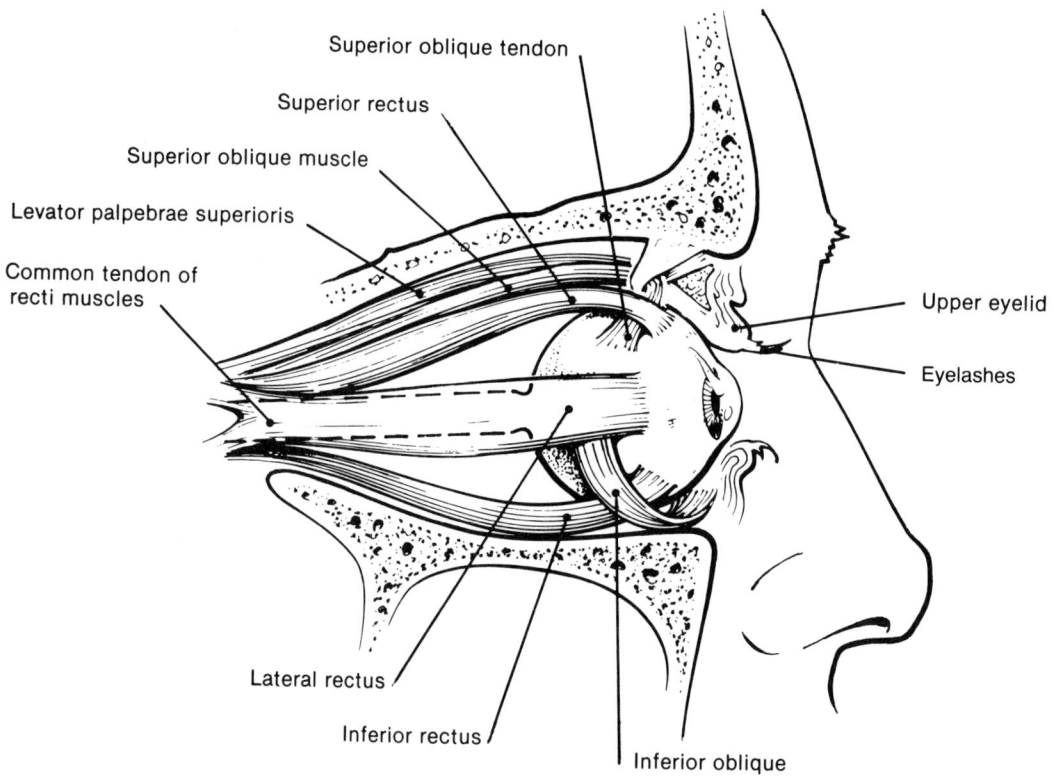

Lateral view

Figure 81-1 Superior and lateral views of right eye showing muscles and related structures.

- develop a high index of suspicion, a fair degree of confidence, and a reasonable degree of caution

THE OCULAR HISTORY

Since no two ocular problems are identical, and since many minor ocular problems are potentially devastating, prehospital care personnel and the emergency physician should approach the ocular emergency with the same open-mindedness and concern with which fever of unknown etiology, chest pain, or acute abdomen is evaluated. Ocular symptoms are frequently precipitated by a systemic disease or by a disorder remote from the eye. Prior to conducting the ocular examination, it is safer, and ultimately more efficient, to approach the patient with the objective of first obtaining, in an orderly manner, a classic history, which should include the following:

- chief complaint
- present illness
- past history of ocular disorders:
  - previous eye diseases
  - surgery, intraocular lens implant
  - infections and inflammations
  - trauma
  - previous use of eyeglasses and approximate age of current eyeglass prescription
  - status of previous visual acuity, noting particularly any history of visual deficit or asymmetry
- list of drug allergies and sensitivities
- list of currently employed drugs, vitamins, and mood-altering substances
- habits of smoking and drinking
- review of systems
- occupation and hazardous exposures, including sports, industry, and hobbies
- time of last oral intake, including nature of food and fluids ingested
- past medical history
- family history of ocular disorders, including specific questions in reference to cataracts, glaucoma, severe refractive errors, retinal detachment, diabetic retinopathy, eye tumors, and severe visual loss

A careful review of Freeman's trauma-history checklist (Table 81-1) will give the emergency physician insight to the extent to which the ophthalmologist may pursue the history of ocular trauma in order to understand the mechanisms of injury, to conduct examinations and special studies, to plan

Table 81-1 Trauma History Checklist

I. Details of Accident
   A. Date
   B. Time
   C. Location
   D. Accidental?
   E. Intentional?
   F. Self-inflicted?
   G. While at work?
   H. Goggles worn?
   I. Glasses worn?
   J. Damage to glasses or goggles or frames?
   K. Names and addresses of witnesses

II. Object Producing Injury
   A. Blunt injury
      1. Description of object
      2. Distance traveled to eye
      3. Direction traveled to eye
   B. Foreign body cases
      1. Suspected composition of foreign body
      2. Single or multiple
      3. Possible contamination
      4. Pathway of foreign body to eye
         a. Distance traveled
         b. Direction traveled
         c. Position of patient's head at impact
         d. Direction of gaze at impact
      5. Tool or machinery involved in producing foreign body
         a. Description of tool or machinery
         b. Composition of tool or machinery
         c. Composition of grinding surface
         d. Possible contamination of surface

III. Events Before Examination
   A. Name and address of other professional personnel examining patient
   B. Previous treatment?
      1. Ocular
      2. Systemic
      3. Antitetanus
   C. Transported
      1. Lying
      2. Sitting
   D. Change in vision
      1. Sudden
      2. Gradual
   E. Time fluid or food last taken by mouth

IV. Visual Status Before Accident
   A. Injured eye
   B. Uninjured eye
   C. Preexisting ocular disease or amblyopia?
   D. Previous ocular surgery?
   E. Family history of ocular disease?

V. Animal Bites
   A. Animal provoked?
   B. Probable location of animal for follow-up

Source: Freeman HM, McDonald PR, Scheie HG: Evaluation and examination of the traumatized eye. In Freeman HM (ed): *Ocular Trauma.* New York, Appleton-Century-Crofts, 1979.

treatment and aftercare, and, if necessary, to prepare for the medical-legal consequences of trauma.[3]

After cardiopulmonary resuscitation and the control of shock, the immediate care of chemical burns of the eye by freshwater irrigation takes priority over all other emergency department procedures and protocols.[15] It is important to remember, however, that preoccupation with an ocular disaster must not cause the physician to overlook a less apparent life-threatening injury or disorder. Treat first the patient, then the eye.

VISUAL ACUITY TESTING

Because in ocular trauma, claims of loss of vision may be associated with future compensation, it is crucial to establish a probable visual status of both of the patient's eyes prior to an accident. The most reliable information is probably obtainable when the patient is distracted during the initial examination in the emergency department rather than later when compensatory reimbursement may influence the patient's recall.

Visual acuity ideally should be measured prior to both the instillation of eye drops and any manipulation of the eyes. Severe ocular discomfort and secondary blepharospasm may necessitate the use of topical anesthetic drops prior to acquiring a reliable visual acuity, which should be obtained in both eyes and preferably with and without eyeglasses. If the patient's eyeglasses are not available, the pinhole visual acuity may also be recorded. If treatment is initiated prior to testing vision, visual loss may be attributed to the therapy itself.

The examining physician must exercise extreme caution in guaranteeing that while testing the vision of one eye, the fellow eye is well covered. Not uncommonly, a patient will innocently perform visual acuity tests while viewing with the "covered" eye and inadvertently deceive the unwary examiner. Reliability of vision testing is further enhanced by testing first the eye with the least visual acuity, thus denying the patient the opportunity to memorize a visual acuity chart or to identify test objects inadvertently.

The successive levels of decreasing distance visual acuity are identified by the terms expressed in Table 81-2. If visual acuity is less than 20/400, the patient should be moved toward the distant visual acuity chart or vice versa until the 20/400 figure is identified. Visual acuity is then recorded as a fraction, the numerator of which is the distance in feet from the chart and the denominator is 400. Thus, if the 20/400 letter is first seen at 10 feet, acuity is recorded as 10/400.

If the patient is confined to a stretcher, it may prove convenient simply to hand-carry the distance visual acuity chart to a point 20 feet distant from the patient, who may turn his or her head to the side to view the chart, which is then rotated 90° in order that the figures may be viewed in a normal manner relative to the patient's immediate posture.

Table 81-2 Distance Visual Acuity

Feet	Metric	Decimal
20/15	6/4.5	1.33
20/20	6/6	1.0
20/25	6/7.5	0.8
20/30	6/9	0.66
20/40	6/12	0.5
20/50	6/15	0.4
20/60	6/18	0.33
20/70	6/21	0.3
20/80	6/24	0.25
20/100	6/30	0.2
20/200	6/60	0.1
20/300	6/90	0.07
20/400	6/120	0.05

C.F. = Counting fingers at _____ feet/meters
H.M. = Hand motion at _____ feet/meters
L.P. & P. = Light perception and projection (identifies direction of light source)
L.P. = Light perception without projection
N.L.P. = No light perception

For this type of patient, every emergency department must be equipped simply to test near visual acuity with a standard type near visual acuity card as illustrated in Fig. 81-2. If standard test charts are not available, one must improvise with a test that is reproducible, such as various sizes of newsprint, telephone directory print, or commonly known small objects held at recorded distances. Confrontation visual fields may be obtained even while the patient remains in either the prone or supine posture and may provide the first indication of an intracranial injury or a retinal detachment.

The uncooperative child or adult who is suspected of having a severe ocular injury may require ocular examination under anesthesia. Common sense may dictate that the examiner not persist in any attempts to perform the classic ocular examination but should pass this responsibility on to the ophthalmologist as soon as possible and record reasons for failing to acquire the visual acuity during the initial phases of management.

EXAMINATION OF THE GLOBE AND CONJUNCTIVAL FORNIX

Exposure of the Globe

Displacing the eyelids to permit direct examination of the globe can be accomplished by lid retraction, eversion, and double eversion. If the examiner suspects a perforated or lacerated globe, pressure on the globe must be avoided at all costs. Prior to manipulation of the injured globe, the globe of the uninjured eye should be gently ballotted through the

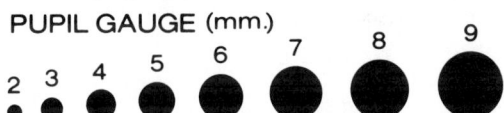

Figure 81-2 Standard type near vision acuity card. *Source:* J.G. Rosenbaum. Reproduced with permission.

uninjured lid to acquire a feel for the normal tension of the globe and the normal resilience of the orbit. If necessary, the same trial examination could be performed on a cooperative emergency assistant. If very gentle ballottement of the injured eye with a delicate finger suggests the presence of hypotony, the examiner must assume the presence of a perforated or ruptured globe and proceed to examine the eye with greater caution.

Retraction of the Upper and Lower Lids

Simultaneous retraction of both the upper and lower lids is accomplished by applying the thumbs to the patient's brow just above the superior orbital rim and to the malar eminence just below the inferior orbital rim, respectively, and *gently* applying pressure away from the globe. Even in a very healthy patient, these bony prominences can be tender. The maneuver can be accomplished, however, very successfully with a minimum amount of pressure.

Eversion of the Upper Lid

Since eversion of the upper lid is usually performed for purposes of removing a superficial foreign body, the physician should be prepared to remove the foreign body immediately on everting the lid. Thus, the patient probably should have received a topical anesthetic. A good source of oblique illumination should be available, preferably held by an assistant. The physician should be wearing a loupe or have an alternate source of magnification available, such as a simple magnifying glass. Immediately at hand should be an instrument such as a moistened cotton-tipped applicator or a jeweler's forceps for removing extremely fine foreign bodies such as tiny splinters of glass or the delicate spines of a cactus. The patient should be comfortably seated at a slit lamp or placed in the supine position and be sufficiently informed to be both confident and helpful to the physician.

Eversion of the upper lid is initiated with the patient gazing downward. The lid is grasped by the central eyelashes and pulled downward with one hand while the physician's second hand applies a cotton-tipped applicator centrally to the upper margin of the tarsus and then gently flips the upper lid to eversion over the applicator tip, which is removed from behind the everted lid and reapplied to stabilize the upper lid margin. The key to success at this point is the patient's cooperation in avoiding blepharospasm and in maintaining a steady downward gaze. Return of the lid to normal position is accomplished by gently pulling the lid outward as the patient assumes an upward gaze.

Double Eversion of the Upper Lid

Double eversion of the upper lid becomes essential in exploring the upper fornix of the conjunctival sac in a search for multiple foreign bodies and the elusive single foreign body. This is accomplished by first simply everting the upper lid and then inserting the blade of a Desmarres retractor behind the already everted lid and then elevating the lid gently away from the globe with rotation of the retractor arm away from the globe and toward the forehead in order to open up the upper fornix. The hand grasping the retractor handle should be resting on the patient's forehead in order to maintain a sustained and gentle traction. The patient must maintain a steady downward gaze. The examiner's second hand can then apply the tip of a moistened cotton-tipped applicator to the upper fornix and very gently retract inferiorly the folds of conjunctiva, thus opening the crevices to expose any small residual foreign bodies and wounds. A readily available

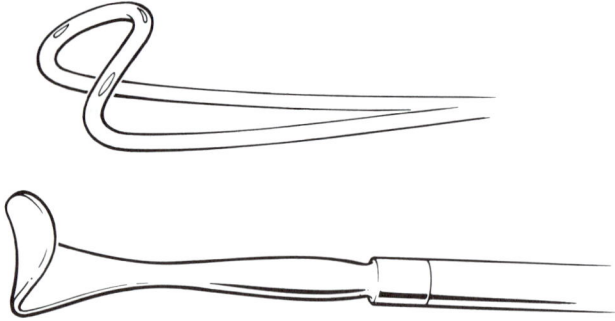

Figure 81-3 Desmarres retractor fashioned from a medium-sized paper clip.

substitute for the Desmarres retractor can be fashioned from a medium-sized or large paper clip (Fig. 81-3).

HERPETIC OCULAR DISEASE

Herpetic ocular disease may present solely in one of the following acute clinical forms:

- "itchy eye"
- "corneal abrasion"
- "corneal foreign body"
- "pink eye"
- primary keratoconjunctivitis (usually in children)
- vesicular ulcerative blepharitis
- blepharoconjunctivitis
- acute follicular conjunctivitis
- coarse epithelial keratitis
- dendritic keratitis
- geographic keratitis
- acute or recurrent iridocyclitis
- panuveitis
- nodular episcleritis
- interstitial keratitis

Although acute ocular herpes usually presents as a combination of these clinical forms, this list serves to emphasize the danger of using topical corticosteroids to treat what may appear to be a less dangerous problem. These clinical forms may present before the appearance of keratitis, or keratitis may never actually appear. It is advisable to examine carefully with magnification any lesions of the lid, lid margins, and conjunctiva in order to detect small or sparse herpetic vesicles.

The signs and symptoms of dendritic keratitis include the following:

- gradual onset of symptoms
- watery ocular discharge
- ocular discomfort varying from a very mild itching sensation to an intense foreign body sensation or irritation
- photophobia of varying degrees
- conspicuous absence of a sudden onset of symptoms from an accurately detailed history in considering a diagnosis of corneal abrasion or a corneal foreign body
- single or clustered, large or small vesicles appearing on the skin, lid margin, or conjunctiva
- punctate keratitis developing into dendritic keratitis within one week
- ciliary and/or conjunctival injection
- conjunctival smears demonstrating lymphocytes, mononuclear cells, and a few polymorphonuclear leukocytes
- markedly reduced corneal sensitivity to light touch when tested with a wisp of cotton (a valuable diagnostic sign that may persist long after the initial dendritic lesion has healed)

The unfavorable manner in which corticosteroids influence herpetic ocular disease is best considered at this point. Topical and systemic corticosteroids do not increase the recurrence of ocular herpes but do increase the severity of spontaneously recurring herpetic infections by enhancing viral replication, enhancing viral penetration of deep corneal tissues by increasing the permeability of stromal ground substance, and inhibiting lymphoid immune response.[14,16] Corticosteroids are therefore contraindicated in the treatment of simple dendritic keratitis and are inadvisable in treating the acute phase of most forms of acute follicular conjunctivitis. Caution should be exercised in applying corticosteroids to eyes that possess corneal scars suggestive of a previous herpetic keratitis.

Prophylactic Therapy

If acute herpetic dermatitis is in close proximity to an otherwise unaffected eye, the patient should instill antiviral ointment or eye drops into the conjunctival sac six times per day until the rash begins to resolve and then twice daily until the skin rash has completely healed. Acceptable antiviral medications might include: trifluorothymidine, also known as trifluridine (Viroptic Ophthalmic Solution); vidarabine (Vira-A Ophthalmic Ointment); and idoxuridine (Stoxil Ophthalmic Solution and Ointment).

If the patient is being treated with systemic corticosteroids concurrent with herpetic keratitis in one eye, it is prudent to administer antiviral drops prophylactically to the uninvolved eye.

When the physician is uncertain but suspects an acute or chronic herpetic process, it is probably safest to document clinical observations carefully, initiate antiviral therapy, and refer the patient to an ophthalmologist as soon as possible.

Treatment of Active Herpetic Keratitis

Since the first physician treating this vision-threatening disorder has the best chance of effecting a permanent cure, the emergency physician should be relatively aggressive and precise in selecting the initial therapeutic regimen and in arranging adequate follow-up care.[12,16] The complications of herpetic ocular disease can be very difficult to manage. The unfavorable effects on vision tend to be cumulative. The therapeutic objectives include the following:

- to eliminate the virus from the epithelium quickly
- to reduce the risk of corneal stromal keratitis and scarring
- to avoid uveitis and glaucoma
- to avoid side effects of treatment

Removal of virus-replicating epithelium is probably safely accomplished only by the physician who is skilled at performing procedures on the cornea with the use of slit-lamp magnification. A topical anesthetic solution is applied to the cornea. It may be advantageous to instill a few drops of an antiviral ophthalmic solution just prior to and just after debridement. It must be emphasized that the objective is to gently debride the infected corneal epithelium, the dendrite, without spreading the infection to adjacent healthy epithelium, and more importantly without damaging the underlying Bowman's membrane. This deeper damage could lead to viral invasion of the stroma and eventually to increased corneal scarring.

Although it is frequently recommended, it may be safer to avoid both wiping the dendrite with a cotton-tipped applicator and scraping with a sharp instrument. A safer instrument might be a semi-sharp, chisel-ended wooden stick, the tip of which has been moistened with a 10% phenol solution.[16]

With the aid of slit-lamp magnification, the physician may identify the infected epithelium by means of fluorescein staining. The involved area may then be gently outlined by scoring the epithelium with the semi-sharp tip of the wooden stick, which is then used to elevate the involved epithelium away from the underlying Bowman's membrane.

The major contraindication to debridement and patching is the coexistence of a nearby herpesvirus reservoir (eg, the vesicles of herpes blepharoconjunctivitis) that can reinfect open corneal wounds.

Until the corneal lesion has healed, antiviral eye drops should be instilled hourly during the day. Antiviral ointments may be employed every 2 hours at night and may be applied to involved areas of the conjunctiva, eyelid, and skin immediately adjacent to the eye. When the corneal lesions have healed, the regimen may be progressively decreased over a 2- to 3-week period.

In general, the eye should not be patched unless debridement has been performed, there is an irregular and uncomfortable corneal wound, and the area to be patched is free of any virus reservoir. Topical antibiotics should be administered in the presence of corneal ulceration, particularly after debridement. The routine prophylactic use of topical antibiotics in the presence of only a dendritic keratitis and in the absence of concurrent corticosteroid therapy should be discouraged. Antibiotic therapy should be specific and when possible based on sensitivity testing.

Cycloplegia for the relief of photophobia, ciliary spasm, and uveitis may be accomplished with one of the following ophthalmic solutions: cyclopentolate hydrochloride 2%, one drop four times daily; scopolamine hydrobromide 0.25%, one drop twice daily; or homatropine 5%, one drop four times daily. Secondary glaucoma may best be controlled with acetazolamide (Diamox), 125 mg to 250 mg, orally four times a day, and with one drop timolol maleate (Timoptic) 0.5% twice daily. Very high initial intraocular pressures may require the use of systemic osmotic agents such as 75 to 100 mL citrus-flavored 50% glycerin served over cracked ice and sipped via a straw or mannitol, 12 to 25 g, administered as a 20% intravenous solution over a 30-minute period.

The use of corticosteroids in the treatment of ocular herpes is generally dangerous and contraindicated in the clinical setting of the emergency department unless the patient is already on a regimen of topical or systemic corticosteroids. In general, the physician should attempt to attain an acute reduction in the dose schedule of corticosteroid therapy, while avoiding the complications associated with a sudden total cessation of corticosteroid therapy. Corticosteroid therapy for the complications of ocular herpes requires considerable judgment and can be safely and effectively administered only under close observation in reliable patients and at times only during hospitalization. This therapy must be conducted by an ophthalmologist.

Oral analgesics, including codeine-containing compounds or synthetic narcotics, may be required for ocular discomfort. Young children may require hand restraint and the application of a shield to both protect the eye and avoid further contamination and spread of infection. Sunglasses and a large-brimmed hat may help to reduce photophobia due to iritis.

The principles of hygiene must be emphasized. The patient should avoid spreading the infection to any personal contacts and should particularly avoid patients who may be immunosuppressed. The physician should be cautious to avoid self-inoculation or inoculation of other patients through contamination of digits or ophthalmic instruments.

The emergency physician should try to ensure follow-up care for the patient, by an ophthalmologist, within 72 hours. This need should be reinforced by instructing the patient on both the complications of the immediate disease and the possibility of developing recurrences within the same eye if proper follow-up care is not sought.

CORNEAL ABRASIONS AND FOREIGN BODIES

Corneal epithelial defects due to corneal abrasions and foreign bodies frequently extend into Bowman's membrane and occasionally into the corneal stroma. Both foreign bodies driven with force and high-speed projectiles may penetrate to the deepest corneal layers and occasionally penetrate to attain the deepest spaces of the globe and orbit.[3,4] This possibility must be suspected when there is a history of high speed, violent force, or explosion and when only one corneal foreign body is identified in the presence of multiple corneal defects. On these occasions, the patient's pupils must be dilated and the eyes examined with indirect ophthalmoscopy and gonioscopy. The emergency physician should obtain radiologic studies when the possibility of an intraocular foreign body exists and should consult a radiologist and ophthalmologist immediately. Moderate to deep corneal wounds are usually associated with some degree of iritis or iridocyclitis. When there is a delay of at least 24 hours between injury and presentation at the emergency department, the wound may have progressed to a bacterial corneal ulcer, if the offending agent was contaminated or if the patient had a concurrent infection.

Because the patient usually experiences a sudden intense sharp pain and foreign body sensation, the exact time of injury can usually be identified. When the patient is vague and uncertain of the exact time of injury, a differential diagnosis should be developed to include viral keratitis, especially herpes simplex keratitis; ultraviolet radiation keratitis; and infections or disorders involving the lid margins. The foreign-body sensation is typically experienced with any corneal epithelial defect and does not require the presence of a true foreign body. The burden of proof remains with the physician who may have to doubly evert the upper lid and carefully examine the upper fornix to rule out a foreign body that may be hidden in the upper folds of the conjunctival sac. Very uncomfortable photophobia and blepharospasm may be induced by a corneal wound, a foreign body, or an iritis.

Although a corneal epithelial defect or foreign body may be grossly visible, the full extent of injury, inflammation, and complications can only be appreciated by examination with magnification and fluorescein stain and topical anesthesia. The emergency physician must be careful not to become distracted by the first readily visible corneal foreign body but to develop the habit of everting both the upper and lower eyelids and examining the fornices to rule out the possibility of a second foreign body that may become masked by topical anesthetic.

The irrigation method of removing superficial particulate or plaquelike foreign bodies requires the use of a syringe or intravenous-type tubing to direct a steady stream of normal saline or balanced salt solution against the edge of the foreign body in order to float the object away from the cornea. This method may be particularly useful when the cornea and conjuctiva are covered by numerous small particulate foreign bodies that are not imbedded. Subsequent examination of the eye may then reveal the presence of a few residual imbedded foreign bodies that must be removed by a different method.

The moistened cotton-tipped applicator is useful for removing individual, very superficial, or only slightly imbedded foreign bodies. The vigorous use of a cotton-tipped applicator may prove more destructive to normal corneal epithelium than the gentle use of a sharper instrument when trying to remove a foreign body that is firmly adherent and more deeply imbedded. In this circumstance, it is less traumatic to directly manipulate the foreign body with a sterile spud or with a modified 21- or 25-gauge hypodermic needle mounted either on a cotton-tipped applicator or on a hypodermic syringe (Fig. 81-4). The tip of the disposable hypodermic needle is modified by forcefully dragging the tip of the needle against the inner sterile surface of the plastic cylinder in which the needle itself is delivered. Under magnification one can bend the scalpel-like tip of the needle 45° to 90° in order to effect the desirable microscopic instrument, which more efficiently permits surgical dissection immediately around the edge of the foreign body and also provides a

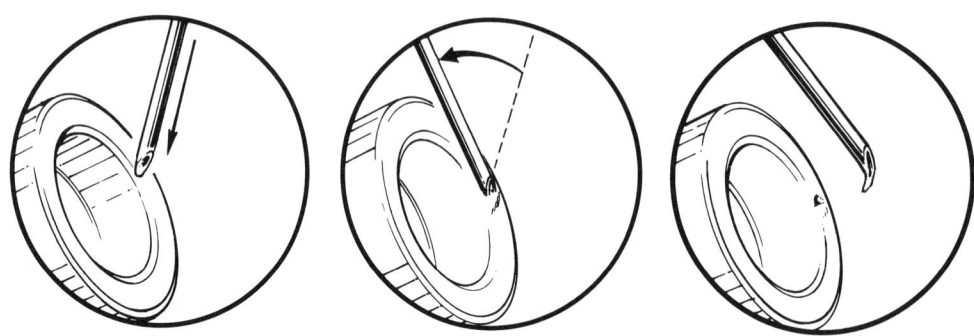

Figure 81-4 Modification of a 21- or 25-gauge needle used to manipulate a foreign body.

surgical blade for excising necrotic tissue and rust. The physician's hand holding such an instrument should be resting on the patient's brow or cheek, while the patient is stabilized against the examining chair or slit lamp. The instrument itself is advanced tangentially to the anterior surface of the cornea in order that the cornea not be perforated in the event that the patient lunges forward during manipulation.

All reasonable attempts should be made to remove a rust ring by sharp and precise dissection during the initial therapy. The ophthalmologist should be consulted immediately, if after a reasonable and cautious effort the foreign body or rust cannot be satisfactorily removed from the visual axis in the center of the cornea. If, however, the rust is distant from the visual axis, the foreign material may be removed more easily within 24 hours, as it is sloughed toward the surface by the inflammatory reaction and by softening of the adjacent corneal tissue. In general, there will be a greater deal of corneal scarring at the site of such a wound.

Because of the frequency with which the emegency physician is called on to treat corneal abrasions and foreign bodies, and because of the possibility of very serious complications that may arise even from an apparently simple corneal abrasion, the physician must strive to be consistently successful and efficient in managing this problem. If the physician's management is cavalier or incomplete, the patient may leave the emergency department feeling briefly relieved and comfortable but may soon experience considerable inconvenience and suffering. The management of corneal abrasions and foreign bodies must span the following objectives:

- relief of acute pain, including foreign-body sensation, photophobia, blepharospasm, and ciliary spasm
- acquisition of a sufficiently accurate history and examination to rule out small occult wounds and intraocular foreign bodies
- detection and safe, efficient removal of anterior segment foreign bodies
- restoration of corneal epithelial integrity
- prevention of infection due to the primary offending agent or that which may arise at the levels of primary care and aftercare
- reduction of ocular inflammatory responses including conjunctivitis, keratitis, and iritis
- reduction of corneal surface abrasion by limiting ocular and lid motility and by reducing friction and adhesion between the lids and globe
- assurance of rapid corneal healing and reduction in ocular inflammation through effective relief of ocular discomfort by local eye care and proper selection of oral medications and effective patient instruction regarding the proper use of medications and the necessity of sound rest and sleep to the healing process

- prevention of severe complication by ensuring timely and appropriate aftercare
- return of the patient to full normal activity as soon as possible

The steps in management of corneal abrasions and foreign bodies are listed below:

1. Obtain a careful ocular history as described earlier.
2. Check and record the visual acuity.
3. Relieve ocular pain and blepharospasm with topical anesthesia.
4. Reevaluate the visual acuity after the patient is comfortable, if the loss of visual acuity seems out of proportion to the apparent injury.
5. Complete the gross, microscopic, and direct fundus examination of both eyes. Be certain to examine the discs and maculas for signs of other ocular disease. *Always examine carefully both fundi of all diabetic patients:* the physician may be the first physician to diagnose diabetic retinopathy and save the patient from total blindness by timely referral to an ophthalmologist.
6. Initiate bacteriologic studies of the corneal wound and foreign bodies if indicated by history and examination.
7. Initiate cycloplegia and mydriasis if history and physical examination suggest the possibility of an intraocular foreign body or other intraocular disorders.
8. Remove foreign bodies of the cornea and conjunctiva by the least traumatic method under the given circumstances.
9. Instill broad-spectrum antibiotic eye drops (Tables 81-3 and 81-4).
10. Perform the dilated eye examination of the fundus by direct and/or indirect ophthalmoscopy as indicated.
11. Instill antibiotic eye drops and apply a light gauze dressing prior to transferring the patient for radiographic studies to rule out foreign bodies and/or bony injury.
12. Review radiographs, preferably with the radiologist, and determine the need for ophthalmologic consultation and/or specialized radiographic studies such as computed tomography (CT).
13. If there is no need for further consultation or special studies, prior to discharge the patient should receive the following local eye care:
    a. Repeat the instillation of topical anesthetic eye drops, such as proparacaine 0.5%.
    b. If homatropine 5% eye drops are used to rest the eye and relieve spasms, advise the patient to anticipate blurred vision for the first 24 to 48 hours after instillation.

Table 81-3 Preparation of Fortified Antibiotic Eye Drops

Antibiotic	Preparation
Penicillin G	1. Remove 5 mL "tears" from a 15-mL tear-substitute squeeze bottle. 2. Add 5 mL "tears" to 1 vial penicillin G (5 million U). 3. Replace 5 mL reconstituted penicillin into tear squeeze bottle (10 mL + 5 mL = 15 mL). 4. Final concentration of penicillin = 333,000 U/mL.
Oxacillin	1. Remove 7 mL "tears" from a 15-mL tear-substitute squeeze bottle. 2. Add 7 mL "tears" to 1 ampul oxacillin (1 g). 3. Replace 7.2 mL reconstituted oxacillin into tear squeeze bottle (8 mL + 7.2 mL = 15.2 mL). 4. Final concentration of oxacillin = 66 mg/mL.
Carbenicillin	1. Reconstitute 1 vial carbenicillin (1 g) with 9.5 mL sterile water. 2. Add 1.0 mL reconstituted carbenicillin into 15-mL tear-substitute squeeze bottle (15 mL + 1 mL = 16 mL). 3. Final concentration of carbenicillin = 6.2 mg/mL.
Ticarcillin	1. Reconstitute 1 vial ticarcillin (1 g) with 10 mL sterile water. 2. Add 1.0 mL reconstituted ticarcillin into 15-mL tear-substitute squeeze bottle. 3. Final concentration of ticarcillin = 6.3 mg/mL.
Cephaloridine	1. Remove 2 mL "tears" from a 15-mL tear-substitute squeeze bottle and discard. 2. Add 2 mL sterile saline to 1 ampul cephaloridine (500 mg). 3. Replace 2.4 mL reconstituted cephaloridine into tear squeeze bottle (13 mL + 2.4 mL = 15.4 mL). 4. Final concentration of cephaloridine = 32 mg/mL.
Cefazolin	1. Remove 2 mL "tears" from a 15-mL tear-substitute squeeze bottle and discard. 2. Add 2 mL sterile saline to 1 ampul cefazolin (500 mg). 3. Replace 2.2 mL reconstituted cefazolin into tear squeeze bottle (13 mL + 2.2 mL = 15.2 mL). 4. Final concentration of cefazolin = 33 mg/mL.
Vancomycin	1. Remove 9 mL "tears" from a 15-mL tear-substitute squeeze bottle and discard. 2. Add 10 mL sterile water to 1 vial vancomycin (500 mg). 3. Replace 10.2 mL of reconstituted vancomycin into tear-substitute squeeze bottle. 4. Final concentration of vancomycin = 31 mg/mL.
Gentamicin	1. Add 2 mL parenteral gentamicin to the 5-mL dropper bottle of commercial ophthalmic gentamicin. 2. Final concentration of gentamicin = 14 mg/mL.
Tobramycin	1. Remove 2 mL "tears" from a 15-mL tear-substitute squeeze bottle and discard. 2. Add 2 mL parenteral tobramycin (80 mg) to tear-substitute squeeze bottle (13 mL + 2 mL = 15 mL). 3. Final concentration of tobramycin = 5 mg/mL.
Amikacin	1. Remove 2 mL "tears" from a 15 mL tear-substitute squeeze bottle and discard. 2. Add 2 mL parenteral amikacin (100 mg) to tear-substitute squeeze bottle (13 mL + 2 mL = 15 mL). 3. Final concentration of amikacin = 6.7 mg/mL.
Bacitracin	1. Remove 9 mL "tears" from a 15-mL tear-substitute squeeze bottle. 2. Add 3 mL "tears" to each of three commercial vials of bacitracin (50,000 U each). 3. Replace 9.6 mL reconstituted bacitracin into tear squeeze bottle (9.6 mL + 6 mL = 15.6 mL). 4. Final concentration of bacitracin = 9,600 U/mL.
Neomycin	1. Remove 2 mL "tears" from a 15-mL tear-substitute squeeze bottle. 2. Add 2 mL "tears" to 1 vial neomycin (500 mg). 3. Replace 2 mL reconstituted neomycin into tear squeeze bottle (13 mL + 2 mL = 15 mL). 4. Final concentration of neomycin = 33 mg/mL.

Source: Baum JL: Antibiotic use in ophthalmology, in Duane TD (ed): *Clinical Ophthalmology.* Hagerstown, Md, Harper & Row, vol 4, chap 26, 1980.

---

c. Use a broad-spectrum antibiotic eye drop such as gentamicin, chloramphenicol, or a combination such as Neosporin.

d. Instill into the conjunctival sac a broad-spectrum antibiotic ointment to lubricate opposing surfaces (Table 81-5).

e. Ask the patient to close the eyelids until completion of the dressing and to avoid attempts to open the eyelids beneath the dressing in order to avoid inverting the eyelids and causing further abrasion by the eyelashes.

f. Apply two gauze dressings to the injured eye. The patient may assist by gently holding the dressings in place.

g. The skin area to which the adhesive tape shall be applied may be cleansed with either acetone or alcohol sponges. If necessary, apply tincture of benzoin to ensure a secure dressing.

Table 81-4 Commercially Available Antibiotic Eye Drops

Antibiotic	Trade Name	Concentration	Preservative
Tetracycline	Achromycin	1%	
Gentamicin	Garamycin	3 mg/mL	Benzalkonium chloride, 1:10,000
Colistin	Coly-Mycin S ophthalmic	1.2 mg/mL	Thimerosal, 0.002%
Sulfacetamide	Belph 10	10%	Thimerosal, 0.005%
	Belph 30	30%	Thimerosal, 0.005%
	Sodium Sulamyd 10%	10%	Methylparaben, 0.5 mg/mL
	Sodium Sulamyd 30%	30%	Propylparaben, 0.1 mg/mL
	Sodium sulfacetamide 10%	10%	Disodium edetate, 0.1%
	Sodium sulfacetamide 30%	30%	Benzalkonium chloride, 0.005%
	Sulfacef-15	15%	Methylparaben, 0.05% Propylparaben, 0.01%
Sulfisoxazole	Gantrisin	4%	Phenylmercuric nitrate, 1:100,000
Chloramphenicol	Chloroptic	0.5%	Chlorobutanol, 0.5%
	Antibiopto	0.5%	
	Ophthochlor	0.5%	
	Econochlor	0.5%	Thimerosal, 0.01%
Polymyxin B-neomycin-gramicidin	Neosporin	Polymyxin B, 5000 U/mL; neomycin sulfate, 2.5 mg/mL; gramicidin, 0.025 mg/mL	Thimerosal, 0.001%
Polymyxin B-neomycin	Polyspectrin	Polymyxin B, 5000 U/mL; neomycin sulfate, 5 mg/mL	Thimerosal, 1:100,000
Polymyxin B-neomycin	Statrol	Polymyxin B, 16,250 U/mL; neomycin sulfate, 3.5 mg/mL	Benzalkonium chloride, 0.004%

Source: Baum JL: Antibiotic use in ophthalmology, in Duane TD (ed): *Clinical Ophthalmology.* Hagerstown, Md, Harper & Row, vol 4, chap 26, 1980.

Table 81-5 Commercially Available Antibiotic Ointments

Antibiotic	Trade Name	Concentration	Preservative
Tetracycline	Achromycin	1%	
Chlortetracycline	Aureomycin	1%	
Gentamicin	Garamycin	3 mg/g	Methylparaben, 0.5 mg/g Propylparaben, 0.1 mg/g
Sulfacetamide	Cetamide	10%	Methylparaben, 0.05% Propylparaben, 0.01%
	Sodium Sulamyd	10%	Methylparaben, 0.5 mg/g Propylparaben, 0.1 mg/g Benzalkonium chloride, 0.25 mg/g
Sulfisoxazole	Gantrisin	4%	Phenylmercuric nitrate, 1:50,000
Chloramphenicol	Chloroptic S.O.P.	1%	Chlorobutanol, 0.5%
	Antibiopto	1%	
	Chloromycetin	1%	
	Econochlor	1%	
Polymyxin B-bacitracin-neomycin	Neosporin	Polymyxin B, 5000 U/g; zinc bacitracin, 400 U/g; neomycin sulfate, 5 mg/g	
Polymyxin B-bacitracin	Polysporin	Polymyxin B sulfate, 10,000 U/g; zinc bacitracin, 500 U/g	
Polymyxin B-bacitracin-neomycin	Polyspectrin S.O.P.	Polymyxin B sulfate, 5000 U/g; zinc bacitracin, 400 U/g; neomycin sulfate, 5 mg/g	Chlorobutanol, 0.5%
Polymyxin B-neomycin	Statrol	Polymyxin B sulfate, 6000 U/g; neomycin sulfate, 3.5 mg/g	Methylparaben, 0.05% Propylparaben, 0.01%

Source: Baum JL: Antibiotic use in ophthalmology, in Duane TD (ed): *Clinical Ophthalmology.* Hagerstown, Md, Harper & Row, vol 4, chap 26, 1980.

h. Prepare three strips of 1-inch paper tape, long enough to extend from the center of the forehead diagonally across the eye to just below the malar bone. Apply the first strip of tape by anchoring it to the forehead. Extend the tape diagonally downward across the eyepatch. With the second hand, draw the skin of the cheek up toward the eye and simultaneously secure the free end of the tape to the cheek. Apply the second and third strips above and below and parallel to the first strip. Tell the patient that the dressing is deliberately applied with tension in order to provide a firm splint to the eye. *Advise the patient that the dressing is to be removed within 24 hours, preferably by an ophthalmologist but definitely by the patient if no physician is seen.*

14. Prescribe oral analgesics equivalent to the efficacy of 5 grains aspirin combined with 30 mg codeine to be administered every 4 to 6 hours for the first 24 hours only.
15. *Under no circumstances should the physician prescribe any form of topical anesthetic.* The sustained use of a topical anesthetic is damaging to the cornea, may mask a corneal ulceration, and may of itself result in corneal opacification, degeneration, and ulceration.
16. Instruct the patient what to do if symptoms develop in the first 18 to 24 hours after discharge from the emergency department.
17. Insist that the patient restrict activities, rest, and preferably obtain as much sleep as possible in the ensuing 24 to 48 hours to facilitate reepithelialization of the cornea and relief of the iritis. To ensure the quality of rest and comfort, the patient should be encouraged to use the analgesics as prescribed.
18. Strongly urge the patient to have follow-up care within 24 hours.
19. Prescribe an antimicrobial eye solution such as sulfacetamide 10% eye drops, gentamicin, or chloramphenicol (Tables 81-3 and 81-4).
20. Instruct the patient of the need for caution since the patient is leaving the emergency department as a one-eyed person and will experience unexpected hazards in driving and using machinery.

LABORATORY AIDS IN THE DIAGNOSIS OF OCULAR INFECTIONS

In the majority of ocular infections, simple culture of the proper specimen and cytologic examination of tissue scrapings or aspirates together with clinical findings are sufficient to obtain a specific or presumptive diagnosis.[8,11] Although laboratory studies are not routinely indicated in obvious situations, laboratory studies should be performed when the diagnosis is in question and are mandatory in the following clinical situations:

- neonatal conjunctivitis (ophthalmia neonatorum)[17]
- corneal ulcers (non-herpetic)[12-14]
- membranous conjunctivitis[2,8]
- hyperacute (very severe) conjunctivitis[2,8]
- post-traumatic/postoperative infection[2]
- unresponsive ocular inflammation or infection
- preseptal and orbital cellulitis[7]
- dacryocystitis[18]
- infections in immunosuppressed patients
- ocular wounds associated with either highly contaminated foreign objects or with concurrent infections[3]
- endophthalmitis[18]

The emergency physician must have a reasonable facility in selecting proper solid and liquid bacteria culture media as well as the most useful stains for cytologic examination of corneal ulcers and conjunctival scrapings.[8,11] Without becoming a bacteriologist, the physician must develop and maintain skills in obtaining reliable specimens for culture, smear, and stain.

The solid culture media are relatively inexpensive and convenient (Table 81-6). The bacterial specimen is easily streaked on a medium's surface with the inoculating swab or spatula (Figs. 81-5 and 81-6). Bacterial growth within the streak is considered positive while growth off the streak is assumed to be a contaminant. Simultaneous cultures from the uninvolved eye permit the physician to roughly quantitate isolated bacteria by comparing the numbers of colony-forming units (cfu) and the confluency of growth between the cfu from different regions of the same eye and by comparing cfu growth with that of the uninvolved eye.[11]

Although blood agar is readily available and inexpensive, chocolate agar is enriched to support the growth of more fastidious pathogens such as *Hemophilus, Gonococcus,* and *Meningococcus.* All bacteria that can be cultured on blood agar may also be cultured on chocolate agar but not vice versa—a culture difference that could be very significant in dealing with acute ocular infections in children. Thayer-Martin medium is an enriched chocolate agar containing antibiotics and antifungals that eliminate contaminants that may inhibit the growth of *Gonococcus,* which is an important advantage in the diagnosis of neonatal and adult conjunctivitis and corneal ulceration.

Lowenstein-Jensen medium is used to isolate mycobacteria, especially *M. tuberculosis,* as well as *Nocardia* organisms. Prior to obtaining the bacterial specimens, at least two tubes of Lowenstein-Jensen media should be prewarmed to room temperature. Immediately after obtaining the bacterial specimen, the culture media must be quickly inoculated and tightly sealed.

Table 81-6 Culture Media in Ocular Microbiology

Suspected Infection	Blood Agar	Chocolate Agar	Thayer-Martin Medium	Lowenstein-Jensen Medium	Cystine-Glucose-Blood Agar	Sabouraud's Agar	Fluid Thioglycolate Medium
Acute bacterial conjunctivitis	+	+ (southern US)					
Blepharitis	+	+				+	
Chronic conjunctivitis	+	+				+	
Hyperacute conjunctivitis (purulent)		+					
Neonatal conjunctivitis		+	+				
Oculoglandular conjunctivitis		+		+	+	+	+
Canaliculitis	+	+				+	+
Dacryocystitis	+	+				+	+
Corneal ulcer	+	+		+*		+	+
Endophthalmitis	+	+		+*		+	+
Orbital cellulitis	+	+		+*		+	+

*If cytology suggests a mycobacterium infection.

Source: Wilson LA, Sexton RR: Laboratory aids in diagnosis, in Duane TD (ed): *Clinical Ophthalmology.* Hagerstown, Md, Harper & Row, vol 4, chap 1, 1980.

Fluid thioglycolate medium is suitable for cultivating strictly anaerobic, microaerophilic, and aerobic organisms that may be obtained from wounds and infections of the conjunctiva, corneal ulcers, lacrimal drainage system, aqueous, and vitreous. If an anaerobic organism is suspected, the specimen must be inoculated as quickly as possible after collection.

Cystine-glucose-blood agar selectively favors the growth of *Pasteurella tularensis*.

Most mycotic corneal ulcers are due to saprophytic fungi, which are inhibited by cycloheximide, a frequent component of fungal media. Cycloheximide must be avoided by selecting a fungal culture media such as Sabouraud's agar that has been fortified, preferably with a yeast extract to provide B-complex vitamins, essential for most fungi, and with antibiotics such as chloramphenicol to suppress bacterial contamination.

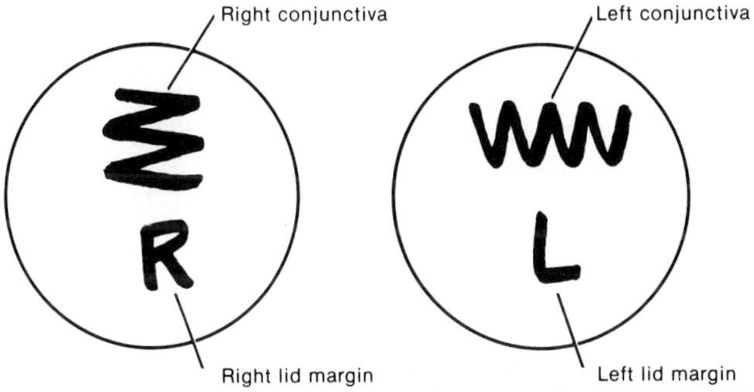

A glucose-peptone-yeast extract broth inoculated with fungal specimen and incubated at 27°C on a gyrotary shaker may demonstrate fungal growth as early as 36 hours after inoculation. Once fungal growth is observed, the fungus should be subcultured promptly to induce sporulation for further identification.

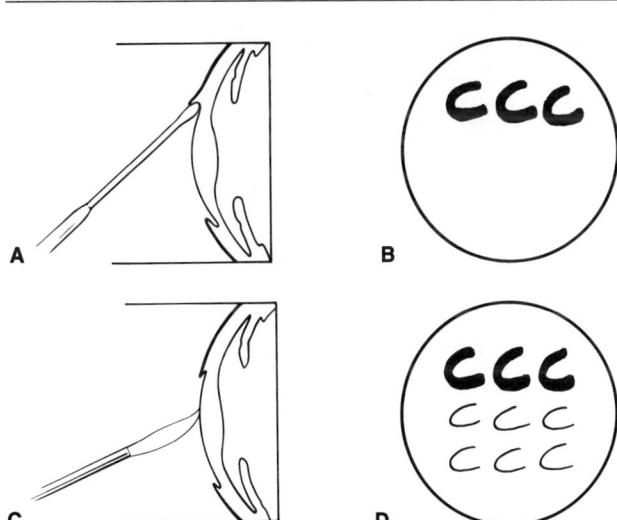

Figure 81-6 Method of sampling of corneal ulcer and inoculation of media. *Note:* (**A**) Initial sampling of a corneal ulcer with a sterile applicator stick. (**B**) Inoculating first row of C streaks with applicator on solid media. (**C**) The corneal ulcer is scraped centrally and at its advancing edges with a sterile, platinum spatula. (**D**) The second and third rows of parallel C streaks are inoculated onto the same solid media as in **B**. *Source:* Wilson LA, Sexton RR: Laboratory aids in diagnosis, in Duane TD (ed): *Clinical Ophthalmology.* Hagerstown, Md, Harper & Row, vol 4, chap 1, 1980.

Figure 81-5 Pattern of inoculating streaks on solid media for routine culture of the right and left eyes. *Source:* Wilson LA, Sexton RR: Laboratory aids in diagnosis, in Duane TD (ed): *Clinical Ophthalmology.* Hagerstown, Md, Harper & Row, vol 4, chap 1, 1980.

Swabs and scrapings for viral culture should be placed in a transport solution such as an antibiotic-treated Hanks' or Earle's balanced salt solution available through a viral laboratory and chilled in ice if it can be inoculated within 6 hours. If culture is to be delayed more than 6 hours, the specimen in the transport solution should be quick-frozen to $-20°C$ and kept frozen during transport to an appropriate laboratory facility.

Tissue scrapings and smears from any infection threatening the eye permit the physician to select the most useful staining techniques for cytologic study in order to determine the nature of the inflammatory response, the morphology of the offending organisms, or morphologic changes in the involved tissues such as the presence of inclusion bodies, multinucleation, and keratinization.

The Giemsa stain (Table 81-7) is the most useful in identifying the type of inflammatory cell response, the status of epithelial cells, the presence or absence of cytoplasmic inclusions, and the identification of hyphal fungal fragments and may therefore be more useful in determining whether a conjunctivitis is bacterial, viral, allergic, or fungal. Gram stain (Table 81-8) is useful to identify the morphologic features of bacteria and fungal hyphal fragments and as such to help determine the cause of conjunctivitis, but it is absolutely indispensable in determining the etiology of corneal ulcers.

Ideally, cytologic study should include both the Giemsa and Gram-stain techniques. When the site of infection is too small to yield a sufficient specimen for multiple cultures and slides, the Gram and Giemsa stains are most likely to yield useful information regarding bacterial, viral, allergic, and fungal etiologies. When only one slide is prepared, however, the emergency physician must exercise caution in selecting the single stain that will be most helpful in the given situation. In dealing with corneal ulcers, priority is always given to the Gram-stained slide.

Typical and atypical mycobacteria are selectively stained by both the older Ziehl-Neelsen acid-fast stain or by high-speed fluorochrome technique combined with fluorescent microscopy.

If sufficient infectious material is available, the physician may seek to identify fungal hyphal fragments by first placing a single drop of 10% or 20% potassium hydroxide on each of two precleaned glass slides. The infected material, obtained with a platinum spatula, is immediately smeared and mixed with the potassium hydroxide on the glass slide and confined to a 1-cm surface area. A coverslip is immediately placed over this mixture, and the borders are sealed with petroleum

Table 81-7 Giemsa Cytology of Conjunctival Scrapings in Acute and Chronic Conjunctivitis

Cytology	Possible Diagnosis
Predominantly polymorphonuclear leukocyte (PMN) response	Fungal and bacterial conjunctivitis Canaliculitis, lacrimal conjunctivitis Neonatal inclusion conjunctivitis Any severe conjunctivitis with inflammatory membrane formation Erythema multiforme Reiter's syndrome Drugs (zinc sulfate, cocaine, silver nitrate) Early benign mucous membrane pemphigoid
Equal number of PMNs and lymphocytes	Presumed *Chlamydia* infection
Equal number of PMNs and lymphocytes plus fewer plasma cells, Leber cells, multinucleated cells with four or fewer nuclei	Trachoma, adult inclusion conjunctivitis
Predominantly mononuclear response (lymphocytes)	Epithelial keratoconjunctivitis Pharyngoconjunctival fever Herpes simplex conjunctivitis Newcastle disease conjunctivitis Toxic conjunctivitis (molluscum contagiosum, idoxuridine, miotics) Acute hemorrhagic conjunctivitis
Eosinophils and eosinophilic granules	Atopic keratoconjunctivitis Vernal conjunctivitis Hay fever conjunctivitis (ocular atopy) Erythema multiforme Benign mucous membrane pemphigoid

Epithelial cell changes
  Cytoplasmic inclusion
  Keratinization
  Increased goblet cells
	
	Definite *Chlamydia* infection
	Xerophthalmia, epithelial plaques, keratoconjunctivitis sicca (severe)
	Keratoconjunctivitis sicca, chronic conjunctivitis

Source: Wilson LA, Sexton RR: Laboratory aids in diagnosis, in Duane TD (ed): *Clinical Ophthalmology.* Hagerstown, Md, Harper & Row, vol 4, chap 1, 1980.

Table 81-8 Gram-Stain Cytology in Conjunctivitis and Corneal Ulcer

Staining Characteristics and Morphology	Most Probable Causative Organism	
	Conjunctivitis	Corneal Ulcer
Gram-positive		
Cocci; singly, in pairs, or in clusters	*Staphylococcus* sp.	*Staphylococcus* sp.
Cocci in chains	*Streptococcus* sp.	*Streptococcus* sp.
Lancet-shaped diplococci	*Pneumococcus*	*Pneumococcus*
Rods	Diphtheroids	*Bacillus* sp., atypical mycobacteria
Filaments	*Actinomyces* sp., fungus	Fungus
Gram-negative		
Diplococci	*Neisseria gonorrhoeae*	*N. gonorrhoeae*
	N. meningitidis	*N. meningitidis*
	N. catarrhalis	
Diplobacilli	*Moraxella* sp.	*Moraxella* sp.
Rods	*Hemophilus* sp.	*Pseudomonas aeruginosa* (until culture proves otherwise)
Filaments	Fungus	Fungus

Source: Wilson LA, Sexton RR: Laboratory aids in diagnosis, in Duane TD (ed): *Clinical Ophthalmology.* Hagerstown, Md, Harper & Row, vol 4, chap 1, 1980.

jelly (Vaseline) to prevent evaporation. The slide should be read immediately. If sufficient biologic material is available, two extra slides may be prepared, with the assistance of the bacteriology technician, and held in reserve for special fungal staining, including the use of Schiff periodic acid and Gormori methenamine-silver stains.

The ideal technique for obtaining culture specimens from the conjunctiva and lid margins employs sterile swabs, moistened with sterile saline or with bacteriologic broth prior to everting the eyelid and wiping the swab along the conjunctival fornix or cul-de-sac.[12] The upper and lower lid margins should be similarly swabbed. All swabs from a single eye are streaked on the same solid-media culture plate in the manner described by Wilson and Sexton (Fig. 81-6) to avoid confusion and to facilitate identifying the origins of the respective cultures.[11] Because the preservatives of topical anesthetic solutions markedly suppress bacterial growth, topical anesthetics should not be employed while obtaining these particular cultures.

Scraping epithelial surfaces for cytologic study requires both the instillation of a topical anesthetic into the conjunctival sac prior to everting the lids and the gentle scraping of the epithelial surface with a platinum spatula that has been flame sterilized and allowed to cool to room temperature.

Scrapings are obtained from the sites of maximum infection and inflammatory response. Gentle scraping is mandatory to avoid conjunctival bleeding. The lid and conjunctival specimens from one eye may each be spread in a thin layer but on different identifiable sections of a single precleaned glass slide, and each should be confined to a 1-cm surface area to facilitate location and identification of organisms. The slide is then air dried for at least 5 minutes prior to immersion in a fixative of 95% methanol for 5 to 10 minutes and then air dried a second time. Final staining may then be performed at the convenience of the physician or laboratory technician.

BACTERIAL CORNEAL ULCERS (BACTERIAL KERATITIS)

The bacterial corneal ulcer (bacterial keratitis) is an active invasion of the cornea by bacteria leading to stromal abscess formation associated with inflammatory findings of variable intensity. Since the cornea's resistance to bacterial invasion is attributable to the integrity of the outer epithelial layer, the cleansing mechanism and barrier protection of the normal eyelid, and the separate functions of the three layers of the precorneal tear film, defects in any one of these three defense mechanisms, whether from a slight injury or from a chronic debilitating disease, will dispose to bacterial corneal ulcers.

The clinical features of bacterial corneal ulcers may include the following[8,12,13]:

- preexisting infection such as a localized anterior-segment ocular infection, an upper respiratory-tract infection, a tracheostomy frequently in a comatose patient, contaminated surgical wounds, and contaminated eye medications and cosmetics
- predisposing disorders debilitating to the cornea specifically or to the patient in general
- epithelial injury and defect
- ulceration occurring within 72 hours of the initial inoculation
- sudden deterioration in visual acuity and in the clinical appearance of the cornea
- intense panconjunctival injection
- severe ocular pain usually, although the discomfort may be minimal or absent in the presence of a preexisting corneal anesthesia
- necrotic grayish stromal infiltrate at the base of an epithelial defect
- surrounding halo of white or gray epithelial and stromal edema
- radiating folds in the posterior cornea and Descemet's membrane
- abundant mucopurulent discharge clinging tenaciously to the ulcer

- central, paracentral, or peripheral localization on the corneal surface; centrally directed advancing ulcer border, undermined by replicating bacteria and overhung by a lip of necrotic stroma; and numerous microabscesses in the anterior corneal stroma
- anterior chamber reaction ranging from a mild flare and cell to an extensive sterile hypopyon and fibrin clot filling the entire anterior chamber and obscuring all iris detail and the fixation of a dense fibrin plaque to the endothelial surface behind the ulcer
- corneal melting (colliquative necrosis of the corneal stroma)
- extensive posterior synechia
- secondary cataract
- herniation of Descemet's membrane through an eroded corneal stromal defect manifest as a shiny black descemetocele
- corneal perforation within 3 to 7 days of injury or inoculation

Because the clinical features of bacterial corneal ulcers are too variable and preclude etiologic diagnosis and a rationale for antimicrobial therapy, a laboratory work-up for corneal ulcers is mandatory and must be approached methodically with considerable clinical discipline.[11–13]

The initial emergency and continued care of corneal ulcers is entirely the province of the ophthalmologist. Most patients with significant ulcers will be hospitalized because of the complex work-up, the intensity of nursing care required, the close monitoring of the clinical course, and the frequency of slit-lamp examinations.

The realities of emergency medicine are such, however, that the emergency physician, particularly in a remote community or military outpost, may not have access to an ophthalmologist and adequate hospital facilities during the first 24 to 72 hours of this crisis. Because of the potential of the bacterial ulcer to involve the entire cornea, to impair vision severely, to perforate the cornea rapidly, and to lead eventually to loss of the globe, it is imperative that the physician be prepared to initiate swift and proper management. Subsequently, complete clinical and laboratory data must accompany the patient when the patient is transferred to the care of the ophthalmologist.

The one procedure most likely to renew and refresh the emergency physician's bacteriologic skills and train him to deal with a wide range of infectious problems is the work-up of a central corneal ulcer, the successful treatment of which is entirely dependent on the meticulous technique and careful preparation in identifying the infecting organism and in initiating specific antimicrobial therapy.[8,11–13,18]

The therapeutic goals include the following:

- identifying the organism
- eliminating the organism
- minimizing the destructive effects of inflammation
- promoting rapid reepithelialization of the cornea

To meet this challenge the physician's knowledge must span the following:

- the bacteria commonly known to cause corneal ulcers
- the Gram-staining characteristics of these bacteria[8]
- the clinical signs suggestive of bacterial corneal ulcer
- a reliable technique for obtaining ulcer material for Gram-stain cytology and culture[8,11,13,18]
- the antimicrobials used topically and subconjunctivally against organisms known commonly to cause bacterial corneal ulcers[13,18]

Recognition of the corneal ulcer as bacterial is based on the Gram-stain cytology of the smeared ulcer scraping. Probable specific etiology and selection of immediate antibiotic therapy are based on the physician's awareness of the common pathogens, the Gram-stain characteristics and morphology, as well as their general antimicrobial sensitivity (Table 81-9). The physician should be quick to employ the services of a bacteriologist or bacteriology laboratory technician and prepare a checklist of desired smears, cultures, equipment, labels and charge slips, and instructions regarding early sensitivity testing.

The most common cause of corneal ulcers in the United States include the following[11]:

- *Pseudomonas aeruginosa:* gram-negative bacillus
- *Staphylococcus aureus:* gram-positive cocci
- *Streptococcus pneumoniae:* gram-negative diplococci
- *Moraxella lacunata:* gram-negative diplobacilli

Less common causes of corneal ulcers include:

- *Staphylococcus epidermidis:* gram-positive cocci
- *Streptococcus viridans:* gram-positive cocci
- *Streptococcus pyogenes:* gram-positive cocci
- Enterobacteriaceae *Escherichia coli, Proteus, Klebsiella pneumoniae, Serratia marcescens):* gram-negative bacilli
- *Neisseria gonorrhoeae:* gram-negative diplococci

Rare causes of corneal ulcers are:

- anaerobic micrococci
- gram-positive bacilli
- nonhemolytic enterococcus *(Streptococcus faecalis)*

Smears and cultures should first be obtained from the conjunctiva, lid margins, and nasolacrimal sac reflux in the involved eye (Fig. 81-6). The cornea is then anesthetized with 0.5% proparacaine hydrochloride, which has less anti-

Table 81-9 Antibiotics of Choice

Organism	First Choice	Alternatives
Gram-positive cocci		
Staphylococcus aureus		
Non-penicillinase producing	Pencillin G	A cephalosporin, clindamycin, vancomycin
Penicillinase producing	Oxacillin, methicillin, nafcillin	A cephalosporin, clindamycin, vancomycin
Streptococcus pyogenes	Penicillin G	Erythromycin
Streptococcus, anaerobic	Penicillin G	Clindamycin, a tetracycline, erythromycin
Streptococcus pneumoniae	Penicillin G	A cephalosporin, erythromycin
Gram-negative cocci		
Neisseria gonorrhoeae	Penicillin G	Spectinomycin, tetracycline
Gram-positive bacilli		
Bacillus anthracis	Penicillin G	Erythromycin, a tetracycline
Clostridium perfringens (welchii)	Penicillin G	Erythromycin, a tetracycline
Corynebacterium diphtheriae	Erythromycin	Penicillin G
Listeria monocytogenes	Ampicillin with or without streptomycin	A tetracycline, erythromycin
Enteric Gram-negative bacilli		
Bacteroides		
Oropharyngeal strains	Penicillin G	Clindamycin, chloramphenicol, ampicillin, a tetracycline
Gastrointestinal strains	Clindamycin	Chloramphenicol, ampicillin, a tetracycline
Enterobacter	Gentamicin	Tobramycin, chloramphenicol, a tetracycline, carbenicillin
Escherichia coli		
Community acquired	Ampicillin	Gentamicin, a tetracycline, a cephalosporin
Hospital acquired	Gentamicin	Ampicillin, carbenicillin, a cephalosporin, tobramycin
Klebsiella pneumoniae	Gentamicin with or without cephalosporin	Tobramycin, a tetracycline, chloramphenicol
Proteus mirabilis	Ampicillin	Amoxicillin, a cephalosporin, gentamicin, tobramycin
Other *Proteus* species	Gentamicin	Tobramycin, carbenicillin, a tetracycline
Serratia	Gentamicin	Kanamycin, chloramphenicol, carbenicillin
Other Gram-negative bacilli		
Acinetobacter (Mima-Herellea)	Gentamicin	Tobramycin, chloramphenicol
Hemophilus influenzae	Chloramphenicol	Ampicillin
Pasteurella multocida	Penicillin G	A tetracycline
Pseudomonas aeruginosa	Carbenicillin or ticarcillin with tobramycin or gentamicin	
Actinomycetes		
Actinomyces israelii (actinomycosis)	Penicillin G	A tetracycline
Nocardia	A sulfonamide	Trimethoprim-sulfamethoxazole

Source: Baum JL: Antibiotic use in ophthalmology, in Duane TD (ed): *Clinical Ophthalmology.* Hagerstown, Md, Harper & Row, vol 4, chap 26, 1980, and modified from *The Medical Letter on Drugs and Therapeutics,* revised edition, 1976.

septic than either cocaine or tetracaine. A sterile, dry Dacron or calcium alginate applicator is touched to the center of the corneal ulcer and is streaked first on bacterial and then on fungal culture plates, effecting an upper row of five C streaks in the manner described by Jones.[12] The applicator tip must not touch the lid margins or conjunctiva. Next, the magnification of the slit lamp or loupes is employed to obtain deeper ulcer scrapings with the platinum spatula applied first to the center of the corneal ulcer and then to advancing edges (Fig. 81-6), yielding material that is then spread on a series of precleaned glass slides for Gram and Giemsa stains and lastly for special stains. In dealing with corneal ulcers priority is always given to the Gram-stained slide.

In a similar manner, the corneal ulcer is scraped again deeper centrally and along the advancing ulcer edge. This material is used to inoculate the solid media, effecting the second and third parallel rows of five C inoculation streaks each. Attempts should be made to obtain scrapings from different depths and different regions of the corneal ulcer. The practice of effecting five C-streaked inoculations for each specimen tends to ensure effective inoculation and results in the highest success rate for culture (Fig. 81-7).[12]

Scrapings should be inoculated on a Lowenstein-Jensen slant to culture mycobacteria, which if cultured on blood agar could be misinterpreted as diphtheroids. Lastly, scrapings obtained for a suspected viral corneal ulceration are

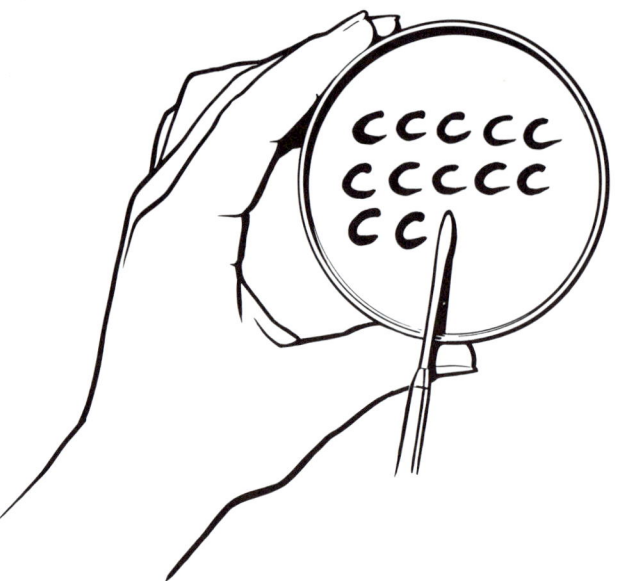

Figure 81-7 Direct inoculation of an agar plate with platinum spatula. *Note:* Each row of C streaks represents a separate corneal scraping. *Source:* Jones DB: Early diagnosis and therapy of bacterial corneal ulcers. *Int Ophthalmol Clin* 1981;13(4):1.

placed in the transport media and prepared as described previously.

Gram-stained cytology of the corneal ulcer is the starting point in both diagnosis and treatment. The presence of organisms confers the infectious etiology. The staining characteristics and morphology permit classification of the organism. Based on this incomplete information on the infecting organism, initial therapy is selected according to the general effectiveness of the specific antibiotic agent against the group of bacteria in general. It must be assumed that the organisms identified by Gram-stained cytology represent the most virulent and resistant within the group.[13] As subsequent laboratory data identify the specific organisms and the antimicrobial sensitivities, drug therapy may be altered to improve clinical response if indicated.[12,13,18]

An alternate regimen for the initial therapy of bacterial corneal ulcers is to employ multiple antibiotics known to be effective against the most virulent bacteria of both the gram-positive and gram-negative groups as outlined by Baum (Tables 81-10 and 81-11).

Within 18 to 24 hours, the preliminary identification of the isolated organisms may be possible by inspection of the culture plates, at which time antimicrobial sensitivity must be initiated even prior to final identification of the organism. The extent of visual impairment is ultimately determined by the severity of the inflammatory response elicited by the invading organism, the degree of pathogenicity of the organism, and the speed with which the organism is eliminated from the cornea. The 1- or 2-day advantage gained by determining the antimicrobial sensitivity early may be the deciding factor in determining the preservation of vision or indeed in preserving the eye.

UVEITIS

Although it is generally sufficient for the emergency physician to diagnose an ocular inflammatory process accurately as a form of uveitis (ie, iritis, cyclitis, iridocyclitis, anterior uveitis, posterior uveitis, panuveitis), it is absolutely mandatory that all patients with any form of uveitis be referred to an ophthalmologist for definitive diagnosis, regardless of whether the uveitis was spontaneous in onset or secondary to an apparent traumatic event. For the welfare of the patient, it is safest for the physician to regard all forms of uveitis as symptomatic of a more serious latent underlying process.

The specific etiologic diagnosis of uveitis requires considerable diagnostic clinical acumen and the use of special diagnostic procedures, such as indirect ophthalmoscopy with scleral depression and contact lens biomicroscopy as well as the selection of laboratory tests.[6] Although many forms of acute uveitis respond without sequelae to a classic regimen, the physician should not accept the responsibility for diagnosing what is apparently an innocent and transient process. This applies particularly to the care of all children and to adults who experience the spontaneous onset of an iritis without apparent cause. Flare and cells, the hallmark of uveitis, may actually be related to any one of the following entities:

- necrotic malignant intraocular tumor
- metastatic tumor
- leukemic infiltration
- transudation and cellular proliferation associated with a primary degenerative process or intraocular infection
- degenerative diseases involving the posterior eye
- retinal tear and retinal detachment
- retinal dystrophies

The emergency physicians who accurately diagnose uveitis, initiate treatment, and make a reasonable effort to ensure proper aftercare have done their duty well. However, the physicians who are able to distinguish accurately between granulomatous and nongranulomatous uveitis in the different regions of the eye have greatly expanded their ophthalmologic skills, thus providing an increased level of competence in the general evaluation of all ocular disorders.

Signs and symptoms of uveitis include the following[6,19]:

- dull ipsilateral aching pain referred to any branch of the trigeminal nerve, but most commonly to the brow and the periorbital region

Table 81-10 Treatment of Bacterial Corneal Ulcers

Initial therapy for all suspected bacterial corneal ulcers
1. Cefazolin, 100 mg (0.75 mL), and gentamicin, 40 mg (1.0 mL), subconjunctivally daily for 4 to 5 days or until culture report and clinical condition suggest change
2. Concentrated drops of cefazolin and gentamicin: 2 drops every 15 to 30 minutes around the clock for 48 hours or until culture report and clinical condition suggest change
3. Cycloplegia
4. Anticollagenase, especially if *Pseudomonas* suspected
   Acetylcysteine (Mucomyst) 20%, 2 drops every 1 to 2 hours
5. Concentrated drops of cefazolin and gentamicin

Subsequent antibiotic therapy for specifically diagnosed bacterial corneal ulcers*
   Staphylococcus (penicillin-sensitive)
     Subconjunctival
       Penicillin G, 0.5–1.0 million U
       If patient is allergic to penicillin, gentamicin, 40 mg (1st choice), *or* cefazolin, 100 mg (if penicillin hypersensitivity unrelated to anaphylaxis or giant urticaria)
     Topical
       Bacitracin, 10,000 U/mL
   Staphylococcus (penicillin-resistant)
     Subconjunctival
       Cefazolin, 100 mg (1st choice), *or* oxacillin, 100 mg, *or* vancomycin, 25 mg
     Topical
       Bacitracin, 10,000 U/mL (1st choice), *or* vancomycin, 33 mg/mL
   Streptococcus (*S. pyogenes, S. viridans,* or *S. pneumoniae*)
     Subconjunctival
       Penicillin G, 0.5–1.0 million U
     Topical
       Bacitracin, 10,000 U/mL
   Enterococcus (*S. faecalis*)
     Subconjunctival
       Penicillin G, 0.5–1.0 million U plus gentamicin or tobramycin, 40 mg (1.0 mL)
     Topical
       Vancomycin, 33 mg/mL
   Pseudomonas
     Subconjunctival
       Tobramycin, 40 mg (1.0 mL) *and* ticarcillin, 100 mg
     Topical
       Tobramycin, 15 mg/mL (1.5%)
       Ticarcillin, 6 mg/mL
   Proteus
     Subconjunctival
       Gentamicin, 40 mg (1st choice), *or* neomycin, 500 mg
     Topical
       Gentamicin, 14 mg/mL, *or* neomycin, 33 mg/mL
   Enterobacter, Escherichia coli, Klebsiella, Acinetobacter (Mima-Herellea)
     Subconjunctival
       Tobramycin, 40 mg (1.0 mL), *or* gentamicin, 40 mg (1.0 mL)
     Topical
       Gentamicin, 14 mg/mL

*Provided the organism is resistant to initial antibiotics, the ulcer continues to worsen, and the pathogen is sensitive to the suggested antibiotics.

Source: Baum JL: Antibiotic use in ophthalmology, in Duane TD (ed): *Clinical Ophthalmology.* Hagerstown, Md, Harper & Row, vol 4, chap 26, 1980.

Table 81-11 Parenteral and Subconjunctival/Retrobulbar Antibiotic Therapy in the Treatment of Bacterial Corneal Ulcers of Endophthalmitis

Generic	Trade Name	Subconjunctival or Retrobulbar	Parenteral
Penicillin G	Multiple	500,000–1 million U, 300–600 mg	2–6 million U every 3–4 hr*
Ampicillin	Multiple	100 mg	2.0 g every 3–4 hr IV*
Methicillin	Staphcillin	75–100 mg	1.5 g every 4 hr*
Oxacillin	Prostaphlin	75–100 mg	2.0–2.5 g every 4 hr*
Nafcillin	Nafcil-Unipen	†	1.5–2.0 g every 4 hr IV*
Carbenicillin	Geopen	100 mg	2.0–4.0 g every 3–4 hr IV*
Ticarcillin	Ticar	100–150 mg	3 g every 4 hr IV*
Cephalothin	Keflin	‡	1.0–2.0 g every 3–4 hr IV
Cephaloridine	Loridine	100 mg	1.0 g every 3–4 hr IM§
Cefazolin	Kefzol, Ancef	100 mg	1.0 g every 4 hr IV*
Cefamandole	Mandol	†	1.5–2.0 g every 4 hr IV*
Cefoxitin	Mefoxin	†	1.5–2.0 g every 4 hr IV*
Bacitracin	Bacitracin	10,000 U	Do not use, too toxic
Clindamycin	Cleocin	150 mg	0.5–1.0 g every 8 hr IV
Gentamicin	Garamycin	20–40 mg	4 mg/kg every 24 hr
Tobramycin	Nebcin	20–40 mg	4 mg/kg every 24 hr
Amikacin	Amikin	†	5 mg/kg every 8 hr IM or IV
Neomycin	Mycifradin	250–500 mg	Do not use, too toxic
Vancomycin	Vancocin	25 mg	Do not use (nephrotoxic and ototoxic)
Chloramphenicol	Chloromycetin	50–100 mg	1 g every 6 hr IV
Tetracycline	Multiple	2.5–5.0 g	—
Doxycycline	Vibramycin	†	50–100 mg every 12 hr IV
Colistin	Coly-Mycin M	25 mg	5 mg/kg every 24 hr IM in 2–4 doses

*Use probenecid, 0.5 g, orally four times a day.
†Undetermined.
‡Very irritating, use cefazolin.
§Maximum of 4 g every 24 hours—nephrotoxic.
Source: Baum JL: Antibiotic use in ophthalmology, in Duane TD (ed): Clinical Ophthalmology. Hagerstown, Md, Harper & Row, vol 4, chap 26, 1980.

- spasmodic sharp pain associated with the pupillary light reflex and due to stimulation of trigeminal nerve pain fibers in the cornea, iris, or ciliary body
- epiphora—excessive tearing from trigeminal irritation
- blurred vision due to cloudiness of the media because of the inflammatory reaction in the aqueous and/or vitreous
- ciliary injection—a violaceous episcleral hyperemia involving the deep ciliary vessels radiating around the limbus and distinguished from conjunctival hyperemia by remaining fixed and not moving when the conjunctiva is manipulated with a cotton-tipped applicator
- altered iris color when compared with the iris color of the uninvolved eye
- smaller pupillary size when compared with the pupil diameter in the uninvolved eye
- flare—a milky homogeneous relucency in the aqueous humor visible across the anterior chamber only when viewed with a narrowed beam of intense light against a dark background free of reflections and examined prior to any attempts at pupil dilation and applanation tonometry (Table 81-12). A flare is due to a transudate of protein across the inflamed uveal tissue and may be graded. "Plasmoid aqueous" signifies a low concentration of fibrin in the anterior chamber. "Plastic aqueous" designates such a high concentration of fibrin as to form a readily visible fibrin clot in the anterior chamber.

Table 81-12 Grading of Flare and Cells in the Anterior Chamber*

Grade	Flare	Cells
½	Not visible	Rare cell
Normal	Normal	Normal
1	Very slight	Occasional cell
1½	Mild	2–7
2	Mild to moderate	8–15
2½		16–30
3	Moderate	Too many to count
3½		Too many to count
4	Severe	Largest number ever seen

*Beam is 15 units wide, using the Haag-Streit 900 slit lamp; length is set at 2 units and is varied to optimum conditions.
Source: Schlaegel TF Jr: Symptoms and signs of uveitis, in Duane TD (ed): Clinical Ophthalmology, Hagerstown, Md, Harper & Row, vol 4, chap 32, 1980.

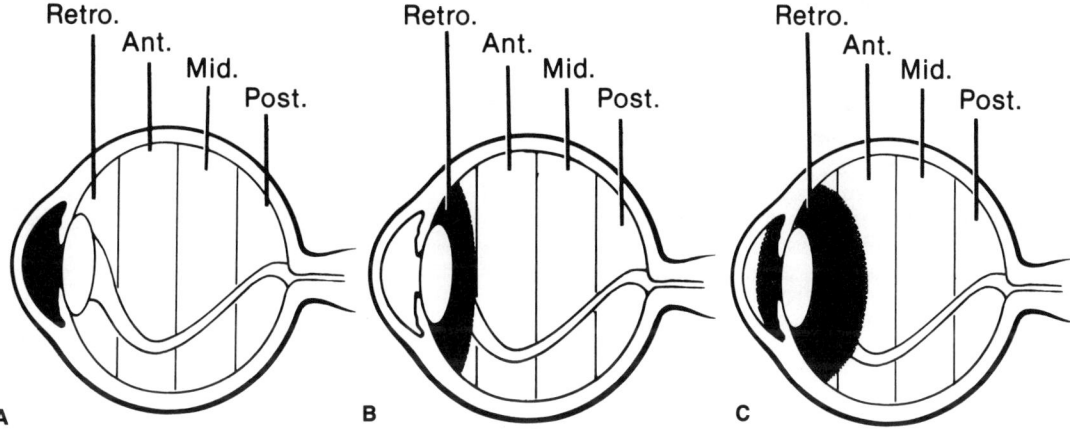

Figure 81-8 Location of inflammatory cells in the diagnosis of uveitis. *Note:* (**A**) Iritis is diagnosed when all or almost all of the cells are found in front of the lens. (**B**) Cyclitis is diagnosed when all or almost all of the cells are found behind the lens in the retrolental or anterior vitreous spaces. (**C**) The most common diagnosis of anterior uveitis is that of iridocyclitis when a roughly equal number of cells is found in front of and behind the lens. *Source:* Schlaegel TF Jr: Symptoms and signs of uveitis, in Duane TD (ed): *Clinical Ophthalmology.* Hagerstown, Md, Harper & Row, vol 4, chap 32, 1980.

- inflammatory cells in the aqueous humor and the retrolental and vitreous spaces (Fig. 81-8). The grading of cell concentration and media haziness in the separate regions of the eye (Tables 81-12 through 81-14) serves to indicate the major location in the inflammatory process and its severity. It should be emphasized that the evaluation of flare, cells, and media haziness is best determined in a darkened examining room by a dark-adapted examiner with intense illumination and both a narrowed and shortened slit beam of the slit lamp. The examiner must make a conscious effort to focus on the finest conceivable detail in the adjacent anatomy in order to focus the individual's eyes properly for the small detail within the media.
- keratic precipitates (KPs)—punctate aggregates of inflammatory cells deposited on the corneal endothelial surface at or below the central cornea. KPs may be graded according to their distribution and composition and are described as being fibrinous, fine, medium, large, giant, hyalinized, "greasy" or "mutton-fat," discrete, coalescent, shrunken, pigmented, and shadow or ghost.
- nodules and precipitates—punctate cellular aggregates of the granulomatous "greasy or mutton-fat" variety detected on the iris surface, pupillary border, the trabecular meshwork, the anterior and posterior hyaloid (vitreous) faces, the anterior vitreous base, or the surface of the retina

Table 81-13 Grading of Inflammation Behind the Lens*

	Grade by Number of Cells	
Grade	Retrolental Space	Anterior or Middle Vitreous
Mild		
½	Questionable	Questionable
1	1–7 cells	1–11 cells
Moderate		
1½	8–13 cells	12–19 cells
2	14–19 cells	20–34 cells
2½	20–25 cells	35–60 cells
Severe		
3	26–60 cells	61–120 cells
3½	Too many to count	
4	Too many to count	

*Long beam, 10 units wide, using the Haag-Streit 900 slit lamp.
Source: Schlaegel TF Jr: Symptoms and signs of uveitis, in Duane TD (ed): *Clinical Ophthalmology.* Hagerstown, Md, Harper & Row, vol 4, chap 32, 1980.

Table 81-14 Vitreous Haze

Grade	Criteria
0	Crystal clear
1	Faint—must focus with direct ophthalmoscope
2	Mild haze
3	Moderate haze
4	Unable to see fundus with direct ophthalmoscope

Source: Kimura SJ, Thygeson P, Hogan MJ: Signs and symptoms of uveitis: II. Classification of the posterior manifestations of uveitis. Published with permission from The American Journal of Ophthalmology 47:171–176. Copyright by The Ophthalmic Publishing Company, 1959.

Table 81-15 Differentiation of Granulomatous and Nongranulomatous Uveitis

Portion of Eye	Granulomatous	Nongranulomatous
Anterior segment	Insidious and mild; eye relatively white	Acute onset of severe inflammation (red eye)
	Nodules are superficial or deep in the iris	No nodules in the iris
	Floccules on the iris (evanescent)	No floccules on the iris
	Greasy exudates on the lens	May be heavy fibrinous exudate on lens
	Medium and large and often mutton-fat (greasy) keratic precipitates if patient is not on cortisone drops, which reduce the size of the keratic precipitate	Small, nongreasy keratic precipitates
Posterior segment	Common in choroid or retina	Rare in choroid or retina
	Heavy vitreous exudate or veils common	No or only fine punctate opacities in the vitreous
	Definite nodular lesion(s)	Diffuse—flat involvement characterized by edema and pigment changes

Source: Schlaegel TF Jr: Symptoms and signs of uveitis, in Duane TD (ed): *Clinical Ophthalmology.* Hagerstown, Md, Harper & Row, vol 4, chap 32, 1980.

- small pupillary size associated with a sluggish pupillary light response due to inflammation and edema of the uveal tissue
- intraocular pressure that tends to be normal or decreased depending on the extent to which the ciliary body is malfunctioning due to the inflammatory cyclitis. The physician must be constantly alert for the possibility of a secondary glaucoma due to obstruction of the trabecular meshwork in an eye that may have been already predisposed to glaucoma.

The prime reason for the physician's attempt to classify uveitis as granulomatous, nongranulomatous, or transitional (ie, possessing features of the previous two forms of uveitis) (Table 81-15) is that the exercise trains the physician to observe, record, and report observations in an accurate, disciplined manner. The secondary gains for the physician include greatly increased ophthalmologic skills and the opportunity to increase diagnostic acumen.

Since it is generally not the role of the emergency physician to pursue the specific etiologic agents that may cause uveitis,[6,20] efforts should be directed at the nonspecific treatment of uveitis with the object of rapidly decreasing the inflammatory process in order to minimize or repair ocular damage and thereby minimize visual loss. Topical corticosteroid therapy remains the most effective method of eliminating the inflammatory process in the most frequent forms of uveitis. This route is more effective and is associated with fewer complications than systemic therapy. Once the physician is committed to the diagnosis of uveitis, topical corticosteroid therapy must be initiated without fear of inducing cataracts or glaucoma in the treated eye. These are problems that are consequent to long-term treatment and are the responsibility of the ophthalmologist attending to the patient's follow-up care. Once the physician is committed to using topical corticosteroids, the physician must be aggressive in prescribing a dose schedule that is sufficient to obtain the desired clinical response (Table 81-16). By being too cautious and employing weaker corticosteroid solutions or a less aggressive dose schedule, the physician could do the patient a disservice. As topical corticosteroids eliminate the inflammatory process, the eye becomes more responsive to other medications and the late complications of uveitis are less likely to ensue.

Mydriatics and cycloplegics (Table 81-17) should be sufficient to provide patient comfort and yet be short acting enough to permit pupil mobility periodically through each

Table 81-16 Principles of Corticosteroid Therapy of the Eye

- Use enough, soon enough, often enough, and long enough to secure the desired results.
- Suppress inflammation until the pathogenic mechanism burns out. Determine the minimum necessary maintenance dose by a process of trial and error. Constantly attempt to decrease the dose by steplike decrements. Continue to reduce it if no relapse occurs. Increase the dose immediately if symptoms of inflammation reappear.
- In therapy that lasts longer than 2 weeks, never stop abruptly at a high dosage. If therapy must be discontinued, attempt to control the decrease with injections while tapering the systemic medication.
- Recognize that the contraindications to systemic corticosteroids apply less to the use of topical or periocular routes, although systemic absorption occurs.
- Realize that the reaction of a specific ocular entity may vary, depending on the route of administration.
- Never start with the assumption that a case is hopeless.
- Do not regard corticosteroids as 12th-hour therapy, but institute them immediately on indication.
- Start with high doses and decrease as the disease responds rather than starting with low doses and working up to the required amount.
- Do not decrease the dosage by some predetermined plan but according to the response of the patient.

Source: Gordon DM: Diseases of the uveal tract. In Gordon DM (ed): *Medical Management of Ocular Disease.* New York, Harper & Row, 1964.

Table 81-17 Mydriatics and Cycloplegics

Parasympatholytic Drugs*	Sympathomimetic Drugs†

Atropine (0.5% to 2.0%): The most powerful cycloplegic available, producing mydriasis and cycloplegia lasting up to 2 weeks. It can be temporarily reversed by 1:100 intracameral acetylcholine.
Indication: Treatment of severe anterior uveitis
Oxyphenonium (Antrenyl) (1% and 5%): Produces a powerful mydriasis lasting up to 4 days and cycloplegia lasting up to 12 days.
Indication: Useful substitute for atropine in sensitive patients.
Hyoscine (Scopolamine) (0.25% and 0.5%): Produces a powerful mydriasis and cycloplegia lasting up to 5 days.
Indication: Treatment of severe anterior uveitis in atropine-sensitive patients
Homatropine (1% to 5%): Mydriasis lasts up to 2 days. It does not cause complete cycloplegia in children. It is augmented by cocaine and reversed by eserine.
Indication: Mild to moderate uveitis
Eucatropine (Euphthalmine) (5% and 10%): Effective mydriatic lasting only 4 hours, producing little cycloplegia.
Indication: Mild anterior uveitis
Cyclopentolate (Mydrilate, Cyclogyl) (0.5% to 2.0%): Short-acting cycloplegic.
Indications: Refraction, maximum cycloplegia occurs within 45 minutes; mild or moderate anterior uveitis. Particularly valuable in patients with heavily pigmented irides.
Tropicamide (Mydriacyl) (1% and 2%): Rapid-acting mydriatic and cycloplegic reaching its maximal activity in 20 minutes and lasting 6 hours. Good for bedtime use in patients with minimal flare and cells.
Indication: Mild anterior uveitis
Ocular side effects:
  There may be blurring of vision and inability to accommodate due to cycloplegia; precipitation of closed-angle glaucoma in patients with narrow angles may occur.
  Contact dermatitis of eyelids occurs in 5% of patients using atropine; it is less common in those using hyoscine.
Systemic side effects:
  Atropine, hyoscine, and (rarely) homatropine may cause dryness and flushing of the skin, thirst, and tachycardia, especially in infants. Delirium and confusion may also occur, particularly in the elderly. These effects are due to systemic absorption and can be prevented by pressing over the lacrimal sac or by tipping the head.
	Phenylephrine (Neo-Synephrine) (10%): Produces mydriasis without cycloplegia within 20 minutes and lasts 3 hours. It is particularly effective when combined with a parasympatholytic mydriatic.
	Indication: Breaking posterior synechias
	Ephedrine (5%): Produces mydriasis within 30 minutes, lasting 3 hours.
	Indication: Ophthalmoscopy
	Hydroxyamphetamine (Paredrine) (1%): Produces mydriasis within 40 minutes.
	Indication: Ophthalmoscopy
	Epinephrine: Poor mydriatic when instilled into the normal eye, but a 1:1000 solution dilates the pupil of a patient with Horner's syndrome.
	Cocaine (2% to 4%): Produces mydriasis within 20 minutes which lasts 2 hours, together with a partial cycloplegia. It augments the action of homatropine and potentiates the action of Neo-Synephrine.
	Indications: Breaking posterior synechias and as a local anesthetic
	Ocular side effects:
	  Precipitation of closed-angle glaucoma in patients with narrow angles; possible occurrence of transient corneal edema with phenylephrine; melanin deposits in the conjunctiva and cornea with epinephrine; macular edema with epinephrine (uncommon); ocular pain and stinging; desiccation of the corneal epithelium with cocaine; and shaking loose pigment floaters into the anterior chambers and the vitreous with phenylephrine have been noted.
	Systemic side effects:
	  The adrenergic drugs may produce tachycardia and palpitations; they should be used with caution in patients with hypertensive cardiovascular disease.
	  Cocaine may produce hyperreflexia, restlessness, delirium, tachycardia, irregular respiration, and chills and fever, all of which result from central nervous system stimulation, which may terminate in convulsions. These side effects may be counteracted by a short-acting barbiturate.

*Parasympatholytics cause pupillary dilatation and paralysis of accommodation by rendering the sphincter pupillae and ciliary muscles insensitive to acetylcholine.
†Sympathomimetics imitate or potentiate the action of epinephrine and produce pupillary dilatation but no cycloplegia.
Note: These drugs potentiate the action of parasympatholytic drugs. Most mydriatics reach their maximum effect by 30 to 60 minutes, although in people with deeply pigmented irides this may take longer.
Source: Kanski JJ: Ophthalmologic synopses: Mydriatics. *Br J Ophthalmol* 1969;53:428.

day's cycle in order to avoid the complications of posterior synechia and a fixed immobile iris. The decision to employ such a long-acting mydriatic as atropine should be the responsibility of the ophthalmologist. The most useful mydriatic is homatropine 5% ophthalmic solution. The most useful topical corticosteroid is prednisolone 1% ophthalmic solution.

Oral analgesics containing a combination of ingredients such as aspirin and codeine might greatly relieve the periorbital pain. The prescription should be limited to cover a 36-hour period, however, to avoid masking a poor clinical response to the primary medications. The salicylate itself is a potent anti-inflammatory agent and will contribute to inhibiting prostaglandin synthetase within the eye.

Although uveitis is typically associated with a normal or decreased intraocular pressure, the emergency physician may unexpectedly be confronted with a secondary glaucoma combined with uveitis. The physician should calmly evaluate the two entities separately. If the patient was known to have glaucoma prior to the onset of an apparent iritis, the inflammation is very likely due to uncontrolled glaucoma per se. Therapy should first be directed at controlling the glaucoma,[21] and the regimen for controlling the glaucoma may indeed include topical corticosteroids, which may enhance the eye's response to the antiglaucoma medications. If the patient has no antecedent history of glaucoma, if the fellow eye gives no suggestion of glaucoma, and if the affected eye does not show signs of an angle-closure glaucoma,[22] it is probably safe to initiate the regimen for uveitis after first initiating control of the glaucoma with oral and/or intravenous hyperosmotic agents, topical timolol 0.5% eye drops, and oral or intravenous carbonic anhydrase inhibitors. When confronted with such a dilemma, the physician should seek the assistance of an ophthalmologist.

Topical antibiotic and antiviral (antiherpetic) eye drops should not be added to the regimen of topical medications, unless there is reasonable suspicion of infection of the external eye or if there is a remote concurrent infection that could inoculate the eye made vulnerable by corticosteroid therapy. Antiviral eye drops should be added to the regimen if the cornea of the affected eye shows the stigmata of old herpes keratitis or if the patient currently has any type of active herpetic infection.

Every reasonable effort should be made to improve the patient's sense of well-being by improving the patient's general health and by a genuine effort at obtaining both mental and physical rest. Through mechanisms yet to be defined, the patient's mental and physical health, apart from any immediate ocular problems, does seem to influence the clinical course of uveitis. Efforts should be made to control and eradicate concurrent infections or inflammatory disorders. Sunglasses and a large-brimmed hat (like a sombrero) may increase the patient's comfort by decreasing the spasmodic pain associated with the pupillary light reflex.

The patient must be advised of the urgency for follow-up care by an ophthalmologist in order to obtain the special diagnostic procedures essential to rule out a more serious underlying ocular disorder that may manifest itself as uveitis. The therapeutic regimen usually requires modification throughout 2 to 4 weeks of treatment during the acute phase. The clinical course of uveitis is unpredictable. Complications of uveitis can devastate the eye and lead to total blindness. The etiologic diagnostic work-up requires the skills and training of an ophthalmologist.

A summary of the nonspecific treatment of uveitis is presented in the following guidelines:

- prednisolone 1% ophthalmic solution, 1 drop every 1 to 2 hours during the waking hours and every 2 to 4 hours at night. To ensure that the patient receives the prescribed dose, the patient must vigorously shake the bottle of corticosteroid ophthalmic solution. To guarantee penetration of the eye by the medication after instilling the eye drops, the lids should be gently closed without squeezing and without blinking for at least 3 minutes. There should be a 3- to 5-minute interval between the instillation of separate eye medications. Ophthalmic solutions should be administered prior to the instillation of any ophthalmic ointments.

- homatropine 5% ophthalmic solution, 1 drop at bedtime only to as frequently as 1 drop every 4 hours according to the severity of the uveitis

- control of glaucoma, particularly pressures in excess of 30 mmHg, with topical drugs specific for either angle-closure or open-angle glaucoma. When the clinical picture is confused by the presence of uveitis, the physician should consider the use of timolol 0.5% twice daily; intravenous acetazolamide, 500 mg (diluted in 5 mL sterile water), followed by 500-mg acetazolamide sequels (1 tablet orally every 12 hours); and hyperosmotic agents including oral glycerol and intravenous mannitol or intravenous urea.

- wearing of sunglasses and a broad-brimmed hat to relieve ocular pain due to the pupillary light reflex

- recommendation of complete and effective mental and physical rest

- use of appropriate topical antibiotic eye drops only in the presence of a concurrent infection of the external eye or one that may be transferred to the eye

- instillation of antiviral (antiherpetic) eye drops if the infected eye shows stigmata of old herpes keratitis or if the patient is currently exposed to any type of active herpetic infection

- appropriate patient referral for control and eradication of any other concurrent infection and inflammatory disorder

- mandatory referral to an ophthalmologist for completion of special diagnostic examinations and aftercare

HYPHEMA

Hyphema, the presence of blood in the anterior chamber, is almost always the consequence of trauma. The rare occurrence of spontaneous hyphema should raise suspicions of physical abuse or of clinically significant preexisting intraocular lesions such as a tumor or vascular anomaly, inflammation, or blood dyscrasias. Even the smallest hyphema should command considerable respect, since there is frequently a more serious latent injury involving other ocular tissues and periocular structures. All hyphemas are particularly challenging because of the lack of an ideal therapeutic regimen and the threats of secondary hemorrhage and of uncontrollable glaucoma, which may suddenly lead to blindness in an eye that initially presented with good vision and an innocent-appearing small hyphema.

The most common site of bleeding in traumatic hyphema is in the anterior chamber angle at the anterior aspect of the ciliary body (70 to 90%) or at the iris root where the iris is in continuity with the ciliary body. Hyphemas usually clear within 5 to 6 days by egress of blood cells and inflammatory debris via the trabecular meshwork and Schlemm's canal. One third of all hyphemas are associated with elevation of intraocular pressure to about 24 mmHg within 24 hours of injury due to the combined effect of direct injury to the filtering trabecular meshwork and to its obstruction by plugs of red cells, platelets, and fibrin. Typically, a period of ocular hypotension ensues between the second and seventh day after injury and is attributed to reduced aqueous production consequent to ciliary body injury. The hypotension is coincident with and may dispose to secondary hemorrhage, which occurs most often between the third and fifth day after trauma.

As ciliary body functions recover, aqueous is again produced, and there is a second rise in intraocular pressure that gradually subsides between the sixth and eighth day as the trabecula filtering apparatus recovers.

Associated with total hyphema, however, there is usually an immediate and simultaneous elevation of intraocular pressure well in excess of 24 mmHg, persisting for an extended period until there is a final delayed resolution of the blood clot. Unfortunately, however, an intractable glaucoma frequently accompanies a total hyphema as a consequence of both extensive damage to the anterior chamber angle and organization by extensive peripheral anterior synechias.

A vitreous hemorrhage may occur simultaneously with a hyphema and be associated with a delayed onset of glaucoma, presenting 1 to 3 months after the initial injury and after apparent resolution of the anterior chamber injury. The delay is attributed to the slow migration of depigmented red blood cells ("ghost cells") passing forward from the vitreous and progressively obstructing the trabecular meshwork.

True secondary hemorrhage in the anterior chamber is indicated by an obvious increase in the amount of bright red blood as distinct from the thin border of brightness appearing at the edge of an old dark blood clot where the clot begins to dissolve between the fourth and sixth days after initial clotting. Secondary bleeding is attributed to the combined effects of ocular hypotension and to the lysis and retraction of the blood clot and fibrin in the originally ruptured blood vessel between the second and seventh days after trauma. The clinical prognosis is generally thought to be worse with secondary bleeding, which occurs at a decreasing incidence with an increase in patient age. The overall incidence of secondary hemorrhage is 25% but increases to 33% in children under the age of 6.[23] Read and Crouch have provided us with a useful grading system for traumatic hyphemas. (See Table 81-18.) Grade III and grade IV hyphemas are associated with a greater incidence of secondary bleeding than are grades I and II. This may well be associated with a greater degree of trauma. The incidence of secondary glaucoma following secondary bleeding is in excess of 50%.

The initial evaluation of traumatic hyphema should be thorough. The mechanism of injury should be carefully documented. The sequence of signs and symptoms that evolved prior to the patient's arrival at the emergency department should be accurately recorded. Antecedent ocular disorders and the prior use of any medications, particularly aspirin, should be carefully documented. Topical anesthesia may be required to allow a patient to open the eyelids and to cooperate with testing. System analgesics should be carefully selected to minimize the chance of inducing nausea and vomiting and should interfere as little as possible with normal coagulation mechanisms. Aspirin compounds are generally contraindicated.

Table 81-18 A Grading System for Traumatic Hyphema

Grade	Fraction of Anterior Chamber Filled by Layered Blood	Clinical Presentation of All Hyphemas	Prognosis for Good Visual Acuity: 20/40 (6/12) or Better
1	Less than one third	58%	80%
2	One third to one half	20%	70%
3	One half to less than total	14%	60%
4	Total "eight ball"	8%	35%

- 75% of all hyphemas result in an acuity of 20/40 or better.
- 25% of all hyphemas result in an acuity of 20/50 or worse:
  - 10% are directly related to the hyphema.
  - 15% are related to associated injury.
  - 60% of hyphema patients below age 6 obtain good vision.
  - The percentage of good visual results increases with patient age.

Source: Read JE, Crouch ER Jr: Trauma: Ruptures and bleeding, in Duane TD (ed): *Clinical Ophthalmology*. Philadelphia, Harper & Row, vol 4, chap 61, 1984.

Visual acuity should be measured with a standard chart or at least by hand motion or finger counting at specific distances. If this is not obtainable, establish the acuity in terms of light projection, color perception, and consensual pupil reaction in the uninjured eye. Abnormal consensual pupil reaction in the uninjured eye in response to light stimulation of the injured eye suggests the possibility of optic nerve and/or retinal damage.

The physician must be accurate and proficient in preparing anterior-segment eye drawings, which include details of the lids, the cornea, iris, pupil, and lens, as well as leakage and levels and character of blood in the anterior chamber. Drawings should accurately reflect the pupil size and shape, iris dialysis, and any other grossly apparent anterior-segment injuries. The intraocular pressure should be gently obtained by applanation or by Schiotz tonometry. Do not attempt to dilate the pupil of the injured eye even when treating a small hyphema unless instructed to do so by an ophthalmologist. Dilation of the pupil may suddenly lead to the development of a total hyphema with tragic consequences. Make every attempt, however, to obtain a direct ocular fundus examination of both eyes through the pupils at their presenting sizes. Special diagnostic technique for evaluation of the fundus should be performed only by the ophthalmologist, who must accept responsibility for manipulating the eye and for dilating the pupils.

Attention should next be directed to periocular and periorbital structures. Determine the presence of any extraordinary conjunctival edema, bleeding, unusual softness of the globe, proptosis, enophthalmos, disturbances in ocular motility, and bony defects of the cranium and facial bones with particular attention to the orbital rim and floor.

Since ocular injuries frequently precipitate drowsiness by unknown mechanisms, it may be essential to rule out intracranial injury and neurologic deficits. The presence of neurologic symptoms and/or a ruptured globe will require radiographic studies to rule out cerebral injury and the presence of intraocular foreign bodies, respectively.

Laboratory studies should include complete blood-cell count, platelet count, prothrombin time, partial thromboplastin time, bleeding time, and sickle cell prep (black patients). If the sickle cell prep is positive, a hemoglobin electrophoresis may be ordered. If there is a possibility that the patient ingested aspirin prior to presentation at the emergency department, the determination of serum salicylate levels may have important clinical as well as medical-legal significance.

Management

The management of hyphema is directed toward preventing and treating the complications of hyphema and toward performing the earliest fundus evaluation that can be safely obtained:

- Minimize recurrent bleeding.
- Minimize secondary glaucoma and its optic atrophy.
- Minimize nonglaucomatous optic atrophy due to associated systemic disease such as sickle cell disease.
- Avoid or minimize blood staining of the cornea.
- Minimize the development of both posterior and peripheral anterior synechias.

Although the ideal treatment of hyphema remains controversial and is the subject of ongoing study at major ophthalmologic institutes, it is fortunate that most hyphemas can be managed successfully by means that are accepted by most ophthalmologists:

1. Restrict patient's activities either by hospitalization or at home. Realistically, this decision must be guided by consideration of economics, patient reliability, and suitability of the home environment. Activity may be as restricted as bedrest with bathroom privileges or be as liberal as modified activities with ambulation.
2. Promote sound rest of the whole patient and of the injured eye. Sedation, if employed, must be judicious and appropriate for the patient's age, size, and personality. It is very likely that excellent primary care, relief of pain, rest, patient education, and justified confidence will provide sufficient sedation. Eye patching may be either single or bilateral but must include the injured eye. Close viewing such as reading and the performance of games must be prohibited during the acute phase of the illness if cycloplegics are not applied to the injured eye. Viewing of remote targets such as television and scenery will relax accommodative effort. The patient may be distracted by appropriate music and television. If bilateral patching is employed, a single patch in the normal eye may be removed at various times during the day for grooming, meals, and for brief entertainment. Analgesia may be obtained initially by topical anesthetics followed by systemic analgesics such as acetaminophen (Tylenol) alone or in combination with codeine or other synthetic narcotics. Every effort must be made to exclude all systemic medications that interfere with platelet aggregation and other coagulation mechanisms. One must particularly avoid aspirin.
3. Protect the injured eye 24 hours per day from further mechanical trauma initially by the application of a metal Fox shield over a single eye patch and subsequently by employing spectacles or sunglasses. Small children may actually require the judicious application of restraints essential to prevent the child from rubbing the injured eye but ideally allowing sufficient freedom to minimize struggling and anxiety. Local treatment must be administered to other simultaneous

ocular complications, particularly to corneal wounds, while avoiding the use of mydriatics and cycloplegics if possible.
4. Avoiding or minimizing rebleeding is first accomplished by the steps noted previously. Attempts to minimize the patient's work effort must also eliminate emotional stress, physical strain, coughing, nausea, vomiting, and constipation as these problems arise. Elevation of the head of the bed by 30° to 45° or the use of multiple pillows will decrease the vascular hydraulic pressure in the globe while simultaneously promoting settling of the blood clot away from the pupil and away from the macula if a vitreous hemorrhage is also present. During the acute phases of the clinical course, a physician must limit or avoid manipulating the globe and iris by the use of cycloplegics, mydriatics, or special diagnostic procedures unless these are strongly indicated by suspicions of ruptured globe, retinal detachment, or intraocular foreign body. Such manipulation and examination should be accomplished only by an ophthalmologist who is prepared to deal with secondary complications such as rebleeding and a total hyphema that might be induced by such manipulation. The incidence of secondary hemorrhage in hyphema has been significantly reduced by preventing normal blood-clot lysis in the traumatized vessels through the systemic administration of aminocaproic acid. It is recommended that aminocaproic acid be employed for hyphemas that occupy 75% or less of the anterior chamber, since the clot may persist, and its retention would be disadvantageous in hyphemas of larger volume.[23] The drug is contraindicated in early pregnancy. The recommended dose is 100 mg/kg every 4 hours (a maximum of 30 g/day) orally for 5 days.
5. Obtain ophthalmologic consultation as soon as practical or possible.
6. Never predict a favorable visual outcome or an uncomplicated clinical course. Trauma that is sufficient to cause a small hyphema is sufficient to be associated with other serious intraocular problems and to lead ultimately to a secondary total hyphema and to intractable glaucoma or to retinal tears and detachment.
7. Document accurately the clinical course, signs, symptoms, and treatment that existed prior to the patient's presentation. Establish an excellent documentation of the initial clinical findings in the emergency department. Thereafter, the physician must thoroughly examine the patient's eye and record observations of the clinical course at least every 12 to 24 hours. Ideally, these observations should include the following:

- intraocular pressure, gently performed by Schiotz or applanation tonometry
- blood staining of the innermost layers of the cornea
- the hyphema in amount, character, and location
- vision as determined by visual acuity testing with a standard chart or if necessary by light perception and projection or by consensual pupillary light reflex if necessary
- the progress of specific symptoms, especially of pain
- the response to medication and the patient's cooperation

Slit-lamp (biomicroscope) evidence for corneal blood stain includes the following:

- The earliest sign of corneal blood staining is the presence of fine, yellow granules in the deepest most posterior layers of the corneal stroma.
- A blurred appearance may be seen in the ordinarily distinct and well-defined fibrillar structure in the posterior layers of the corneal stroma.
- Yellow reflections originating in the fibrinous coagulum in the anterior chamber may be deceptive.

These subtle warnings may precede gross corneal stainings by only 24 to 36 hours and should signal immediate consideration of surgical intervention to avoid gross corneal staining, which alone may impair vision for 6 months to several years. Although corneal staining tends to be proportional to the elevation of intraocular pressure and to the severity of the hyphema, staining may occur rapidly in the presence of lower levels of intraocular pressure and hyphema in the presence of preexisting or newly acquired corneal endothelial damage.

8. Baseline laboratory studies must include complete blood-cell count, platelet count, prothrombin time, partial thromboplastin time, and, particularly, an accurately performed bleeding time. A sickle cell prep must be performed on all blacks. If the prep is positive, a hemoglobin electrophoresis should be ordered. If there is a possibility that the patient ingested aspirin prior to presentation, the determination of a serum salicylate level may have important clinical as well as medical-legal significance.
9. Intraocular pressure elevation must be controlled:
- Pressure elevations between 22 and 35 mmHg are best treated with systemic medications such as acetazolamide (Diamox). The dose schedule for infants is 5 to 10 mg/kg and for children under age 8 is 20 mg/kg/day in four divided doses. For adults, the dosage is 30 mg/kg/day in four divided doses except in those patients with sickle cell trait, sickle

thalassemia, or sickle cell disease, since acetazolamide may promote sickling of erythrocytes by increasing the acidity of aqueous in the anterior chamber. In this group of patients, methazolamide (Neptazane) is preferred.[24]

- For intraocular pressures exceeding 35 mmHg, osmotic agents, particularly mannitol, should be added to the above regimen. Mannitol should be administered intravenously every 12 hours or every 8 hours in patients with extremely high intraocular pressure at a dose of 1.5 mg/kg as a 20% solution administered over a 45-minute period. With these patients, it is mandatory to monitor renal output, blood urea nitrogen, and serum electrolytes. Generally, mannitol is avoided in children because of problems with dehydration. If, however, it is used for children, pediatric consultation should be obtained early, and the child's weight should be monitored several times daily to avoid dangerous dehydration. If orally administered glycerol is employed as an osmotic agent, it should probably be preceded by medications intended to control nausea and vomiting. It should, however, only be considered as a secondary choice in comparison with mannitol.

- Betaxolol HCl 0.5% (Betoptic), levobunolol HCl (Betagan), or timolol maleate (Timoptic) 0.5% when applied topically every 12 hours may sustain a lowering of intraocular pressure. Topical miotics such as pilocarpine should be reserved for continued lowering of the pressures after resolution of the acute phase of hyphema and after the resolution of the traumatic iridocyclitis.

10. Early definition of both therapeutic goals and of the clinical guidelines for timely surgical intervention is essential to the sound management of hyphema, particularly in remote communities where the correct application of these guidelines will dictate the evacuation of the patient to a major medical center sufficiently early in the clinical course to obtain a more favorable visual prognosis through surgery. Fortunately, most hyphemas may be treated medically for the first 3 to 4 days. This would normally allow for telephone communication between the local physician and the ophthalmologist. The following are suggested indications for surgical intervention in the management of hyphema:

- in patients with sickle cell trait or sickle cell disease: intraocular pressure above 35 mmHg for 2 days or more and hyphema of 50% or greater associated with any secondary glaucoma (to prevent optic atrophy, anterior segment ischemia, and central vessel occlusion)

- pressures above 45 mmHg unresponsive to acetazolamide and mannitol and present for at least 48 hours
- microscopic corneal blood staining at any time
- total hyphema of 5 days' duration with the pressures of 25 mmHg or higher (to prevent corneal staining)
- total hyphema with pressures of 35 mmHg or more for 4 days (to prevent optic atrophy)
- hyphemas of more than 50% for more than 8 days (to prevent peripheral anterior synechias and uncontrolled glaucoma)

These guidelines are intended to assist the primary care physician and are conservative modifications of guidelines originally suggested by Read and Crouch [23] for the ophthalmologist.

In considering these guidelines during the early stages of medical management, the local physician managing the hyphema must anticipate time required for patient transportation and the delays associated with hospitalizing a patient at a distant hospital.

GLAUCOMA

Glaucoma is an ocular disorder in which the intraocular pressure, measured by Schiotz or applanation tonometry, is relatively high for the health of the ocular tissues, causing injury, particularly to the nerve fiber layer and ganglion cell layer of the retina and to the nerve fibers and glial cells in the optic disc, resulting in visual field defects and abnormally wide and deep optic disc cupping (glaucomatous optic neuropathy), respectively. In the spectrum of glaucoma patients, different etiologic mechanisms seem to be operating while numerous clinical features are shared. As a consequence, there is controversy regarding the terminology for mechanisms of glaucoma. Incomplete glaucoma syndromes are far more commonly encountered by the emergency physician.

Ocular hypertension is the presence of high intraocular pressure associated with normal optic discs and visual fields. Low tension glaucoma is the presence of normal intraocular pressure associated with a glaucomatous type of optic disc cupping and visual field changes. The emergency physician must regard both categories of patients as glaucoma suspects and refer them in consultation to the ophthalmologist.

The pathogenesis of glaucoma seems to require that across the lamina cribrosa of the optic nerve head there be a pressure gradient sufficient to impede capillary blood flow and axoplasmic intracellular flow within the nerve fiber layer of the retina and optic nerve head. In the hypertensive type of glaucoma, the drainage of aqueous outflow at the trabecular meshwork is impaired and causes an elevation of intraocular pressure. In normotensive glaucoma patients, the posterior choroidal ciliary arteries and arterioles are sufficiently diseased as to provide a low perfusion pressure across the optic nerve head. As a consequence, even normal intraocular pressures are sufficient to cause ischemia of the nervous tissue. In both categories, however, there is damage to the nerve fibers and ganglion cells associated with the optic nerve and retina and this is manifest clinically as glaucomatous cupping and visual field loss.

The following classification of glaucomas[25] is intended to provide emergency physicians with a perspective of the patients and the clinical presentation of glaucomatous eyes and is not intended to require that they become experts in the field of glaucoma. Primary glaucomas result from developmental or degenerative abnormalities affecting the channels of aqueous outflow and are frequently hereditary. Secondary glaucomas arise from injuries and disorders that primarily damage other ocular tissues and only secondarily affect the aqueous outflow channels.

I. Childhood Glaucomas*

These may be present at birth (congenital glaucoma), appear during the first year of life (infantile glaucoma), or arise later during the first two decades of life (juvenile-onset glaucoma). The cause, in most varieties, is a malformation of the trabecular meshwork (developmental glaucoma).

A. Primary congenital or infantile glaucoma
B. Secondary glaucomas in children
   1. Secondary to or associated with other ocular abnormalities
      a. Axenfeld's anomaly
      b. Rieger's syndrome
      c. Peters' anomaly
      d. Sclerocornea
      e. Megalocornea
      f. Aniridia
      g. Angle-closure glaucoma secondary to posterior segment lesions
         (1) Retinoblastoma
         (2) Retrolental fibroplasia
         (3) Persistent hyperplastic primary vitreous
      h. Trauma
      i. Corticosteroid-induced glaucoma
      j. Iritis
      k. Following surgery for congenital cataracts
         (1) Early onset angle-closure glaucoma due to pupillary block from swollen lens remnants
         (2) Late developing open-angle glaucoma

   2. Secondary to systemic diseases
      a. Sturge-Weber syndrome
      b. Neurofibromatosis
      c. Marfan's syndrome
      d. Homocystinuria
      e. Weill-Marchesani syndrome
      f. Lowe's syndrome
      g. Maternal rubella syndrome
      h. Chromosomal disorders
      i. Other rare syndromes and associations

II. Adult Glaucomas
A. Primary open-angle glaucoma
   1. Ocular hypertension
   2. Low tension glaucoma
B. Primary closed-angle glaucoma
   1. Relative pupillary block
   2. Plateau iris
   3. Malignant glaucoma
C. Secondary glaucomas
   1. Exfoliative glaucoma
   2. Pigmentary glaucoma
   3. Corticosteroid-induced glaucoma
   4. Glaucoma associated with iritis
      a. Angle-closure glaucoma
         (1) Posterior synechiae causing pupillary block
         (2) Peripheral anterior synechiae from organization of inflammatory exudate in the chamber angle
      b. Hypertensive uveitis
      c. Glaucomatocyclitic crisis
      d. Fuchs' heterochromic cyclitis
      e. Interstitial keratitis
   5. Glaucoma after trauma
      a. Closed-angle glaucoma from the formation of posterior and anterior synechiae after a penetrating injury
      b. Early onset open-angle glaucoma after a contusion
      c. Glaucoma associated with hyphema
      d. Late onset angle-recession glaucoma
   6. Lens-induced glaucoma
      a. Phacomorphic glaucoma
      b. Phacolytic glaucoma
      c. Microspherophakia
      d. Ectopia lentis
   7. In aphakia
      a. Transient postcataract extraction pressure elevation
         (1) Secondary to the surgery
         (2) Secondary to α-chymotrypsin
         (3) Secondary to corticosteroids
      b. Aphakic pupillary block glaucoma

---

*Source: Phelps CD: Glaucoma general concepts. In Duane TD (ed): Clinical Ophthalmology: Philadelphia, Harper & Row, vol 3, chap 42, 1984.

c. Synechial closed-angle glaucoma, the late result of a postoperative flat anterior chamber
d. Epithelial ingrowth
8. Secondary to high episcleral venous pressure
   a. Carotid-cavernous fistula
   b. Superior vena caval syndrome
   c. Sturge-Weber syndrome
9. Associated with intraocular tumor
10. Neovascular glaucoma
11. Ghost cell glaucoma
12. Iridocorneal endothelial syndrome
    a. Essential iris atrophy
    b. Chandler's syndrome
    c. Cogan-Reese syndrome
13. Posterior polymorphous corneal dystrophy
14. Angle closure secondary to ciliary swelling
    a. After scleral buckling operation
    b. After panretinal photocoagulation with scleritis

The terms *open-* and *closed-angled glaucomas* refer to the anatomical configuration of the anterior chamber angle. In open-angle glaucoma the anterior chamber angle has a normal configuration allowing the aqueous humor direct access to the filtering trabecular meshwork, which unfortunately is less porous or less patent than normal. In closed-angle glaucoma, the iris root is applied to the surface of the filtering trabecular meshwork and denies aqueous normal access to this outflow channel. Angle closure may be partial or complete, intermittent or constant, reversible or permanent.

Fortunately, emergency physicians need not preoccupy themselves with the subtle distinctions in the various types of glaucoma. They must simply be able to identify an acute glaucoma with intraocular hypertension and must declare an ocular emergency and obtain, if possible, immediate ophthalmologic consultation. Primary care physicians must initiate definitive therapy in order to prevent blindness.

The differential diagnosis of an acute glaucoma includes primarily iridocyclitis and acute conjunctivitis. (See Table 81-19.) The patient may be from any age group. Most commonly the patient is an adult presenting with all the classic signs and symptoms of acute angle-closure glaucoma. The pain varies from mild discomfort and fullness to the most intense degree of aching pain referred to the trigeminal nerve distribution. Vision is blurred due to steaminess of the corneal edema, which causes the patient to perceive individual lights as possessing a colored halo. The autonomic nervous stimulation, precipitated by an acute rise in intraocular pressure, may be sufficient to induce severe nausea and vomiting. The secondary abdominal discomfort may be so severe as to overshadow ocular symptoms and cause the patient to present with an acute abdomen. The vagal oculocardiac reflex may produce marked bradycardia and profuse sweating.

Ocular examination reveals a red eye due to conjunctival injection and ciliary flush. The cornea is usually involved with some degree of edema, which can be momentarily cleared by the application of 3 drops of topical glycerin, thereby allowing the examiner a brief time during which he may examine the anterior chamber by oblique illumination to

Table 81-19 Red-Pink Eye: Signs and Symptoms in the Differential Diagnosis*

	Refer (R) to Ophthalmologist	Acute Glaucoma	Acute Iridocyclitis	Keratitis	Bacterial Conjunctivitis	Viral Conjunctivitis	Allergic Conjunctivitis
Ciliary flush	R	1–2	2–3	3	0	0	0
Conjunctival injection		2	2	2	2–3	2–3	1
Corneal haze	R	3	0	1–3	0	0–1	0
Pupil	R	Mid-dilated nonreactive	Small ± irregular	Normal or small	Normal	Normal	Normal
Anterior chamber depth	R	Shallow	Normal	Normal	Normal	Normal	Normal
Intraocular pressure	R	High	Usually low	Normal	Normal	Normal	Normal
Discharge		0	0	0–3	2–3	0–2	0–1
Preauricular node		0	0	0	0	0–1	0
Blurred vision	R	3	1–2	1–3	0	0	0
Pain	R	2–3	2	2	0	0	0
Photophobia	R	1	3	3	0	0	0
Halo	R	2–3	0	0	0	0	0
Itching		0	0	0–1	0	0–1	2–3
Head cold, fever, viral syndrome		0	0	0	0	0–2	0

*Scale of intensity of sign or symptoms = 0 to 3.

determine if the anterior chamber angle is narrow or deep or involved with an apparent pathosis such as rubeosis iridis. In this brief moment, the examiner should quickly examine the eye for other intraocular pathology after attempting a direct examination of the optic disc and macula. The pupil size should be noted. Typically, when the pressure is in excess of 50 mmHg, the pupillary sphincter is paralyzed, and the pupil is mid-dilated and nonreactive to light. Unfortunately, protein leakage may create an aqueous flare, and pigment cells may be seen floating in the anterior chamber. Passive congestion and/or rubeosis may actually cause bleeding in the anterior chamber. These findings do not assist in the differential diagnosis but should not deter the physician. The optic disc may be grossly normal, or it may have become hyperemic and edematous. Significant optic disc cupping is seldom seen except in cases of chronic glaucoma. Unless there is a co-existing conjunctivitis or a viral syndrome, it is unlikely that one would encounter an ocular discharge of lymphadenopathy. Itching is not a typical symptom. Photophobia is not usually significant. Digital palpation will reveal a relatively firm globe by comparison with the fellow eye. Schiotz or applanation tonometry will generally reveal elevated intraocular pressures ranging from 40 to 50 mmHg to pressures exceeding the levels of the instrument.

Primary care physicians must anticipate that they will occasionally encounter a patient with a gradually developing angle-closure glaucoma. A relatively comfortable patient will present with a white eye, clear vision, and intraocular pressures ranging from 40 to 65 mmHg. This is attributable to a gradually increasing but incomplete angle occlusion, which, because of its chronicity, may have resulted in glaucomatous optic disc cupping.

The infant with congenital glaucoma will present with epiphora, photophobia, and blepharospasm.[26] There may be various levels of corneal haziness in proportion to the degree of corneal edema. As the pressure increases and the cornea enlarges, the child may develop, in Descemet's membrane, tears visible as long sweeping gray zones, extending across a great diameter of the cornea in its deepest layer. There may be no evidence of tear duct occlusion. The anterior chamber is typically very deep and a wide optic cup may be present. The eye may be huge. Since most infant corneas measure less than 10.5 mm in horizontal diameter, a corneal diameter in excess of 12 mm is usually diagnostic of congenital glaucoma especially when associated with finding of tears in Descemet's membrane.

The treatment of congenital glaucoma is almost always surgical. A medical regimen may be initiated until an ophthalmologist assumes responsibility for the patient. Treatment should begin as soon as the primary physician diagnoses acute glaucoma:

1. Relief of pain, nausea, and vomiting should begin immediately with the physician's preference for parenteral narcotics and antiemetics.

2. An intravenous route is established for the administration of a carbonic anhydrase inhibitor, acetazolamide (Diamox), 500 mg, over 25 minutes.

3. Infants tolerate acetazolamide in dosages of 5 to 10 mg/kg every 4 to 6 hours.[26] A decrease in intraocular pressure begins within 15 to 30 minutes of administering intravenous acetazolamide, which thereafter may have to be administered in lesser doses at 6-hour intervals. Patients allergic to acetazolamide may tolerate dichlorphenamide (Daranide, Oratrol) available only orally in adult dosages of 50 to 200 mg every 6 to 8 hours. Another alternate oral medication substituting for acetazolamide is methazolamide (Neptazane), administered in adult dosages of 50 to 100 mg every 8 hours.

4. Intravenous hyperosmotic agents should be administered immediately. The intravenous agent of choice is mannitol 20% at 1 to 1.5 g/kg body weight administered over 30 to 45 minutes. Most adults will tolerate very readily an injection of 12.5 g commonly available as a 20% solution in a glass ampule. A clinical response is apparent within 10 to 20 minutes. An alternate intravenous agent is urea, administered as a 20% solution in a dosage of 2 to 7 mL/kg.

5. An oral hyperosmotic agent, glycerol, may be preferable to urea administered intravenously. Glycerol's major disadvantage is its induction of nausea and vomiting. Therefore, the patient should be premedicated with an antiemetic, and ideally the oral solution is administered as a 50% fruit-flavored drink or mixed with a cola drink. The dosage of glycerol is 1 to 1.5 g/kg.

6. Topical glaucoma medications should be initiated immediately. Betagan, Betoptic, timolol 0.5% (Timoptic), or dipivefrin (Propine) should be applied immediately in a dose of 2 drops. Care should be taken that the patient gently close the eye for 10 minutes to facilitate absorption. The patient should be discouraged from blepharospasm or frequent blinking since this may cause loss of the medication and decrease contact time between the cornea and the medication.

7. A miotic, 2% pilocarpine, in a dosage of two drops every 15 minutes for three or four applications, may be started in the first hour. Its effect may not be observed, however, until the intraocular pressure is below 50 mmHg, at which level the paralytic mydriasis is relieved and the pupil sphincter may respond to pilocarpine.

8. Every effort should be made to evacuate the patient to facilities capable of ocular surgery by an ophthalmologist since the continued care of the patient may be very difficult and may require glaucoma surgery. If evacuation is not immediately possible, steps should be taken at least to establish communication with an ophthalmologist.

REFERENCES

1. Wolff E. *Anatomy of the Eye and Orbit*. London, England: HK Lewis & Co; 1968.
2. Duane TD, ed. *Clinical Ophthalmology*. Hagerstown, Md: Harper & Row; 1980:1–13.
3. Freeman HM, McDonald PR, Scheie HG. Evaluation and examination of the traumatized eye. In: Freeman HM, ed. *Ocular Trauma*. Norwalk, Conn: Appleton-Century-Crofts; 1979:1–13.
4. Paton D, Goldberg MF. *Management of Ocular Injuries*. Philadelphia, Pa: WB Saunders Co; 1976.
5. Newell FW, Ernest JT. *Ophthalmology: Principles and Concepts*. St Louis, Mo: CV Mosby Co; 1974.
6. Schlaegel TF Jr. *Essentials of Uveitis*. Boston, Mass: Little, Brown & Co; 1969.
7. Jones DB. Microbial preseptal and orbital cellulitis. In: Duane TD, ed. *Clinical Ophthalmology*. Hagerstown, Md: Harper & Row; 1980;4:chap 25.
8. Fedukowics HB. *External Infections of the Eye*. 2nd ed. Norwalk, Conn: Appleton-Century-Crofts; 1977.
9. Havener WH. *Ocular Pharmacology*. St Louis, Mo: CV Mosby, Co; 1974.
10. Vaughan D, Asbury T. *General Ophthalmology*. Los Altos, Calif: Lange Medical Publications; 1974.
11. Wilson LA, Sexton RR. Laboratory aids in diagnosis. In: Duane TD, ed. *Clinical Ophthalmology*. Hagerstown, Md: Harper & Row; 1980;4:chap 1.
12. Jones DB. Early diagnosis and therapy of bacterial corneal ulcers. *Int Ophthalmol Clin*. 1981;13(4):1.
13. Wilson LA. Bacterial corneal ulcers. In: Duane TD, ed. *Clinical Ophthalmology*. Hagerstown, Md: Harper & Row; 1980;4:chap 18.
14. Pavan-Langston D. *Ocular Viral Disease*. Boston, Mass: Little, Brown & Co; 1975:19–35.
15. Ralph RA. Chemical burns of the eye. In: Duane TD, ed. *Clinical Ophthalmology*. Hagerstown, Md: Harper & Row; 1980;4:chap 28.
16. O'Day DM, Jones BR. Herpes simplex keratitis. In: Duane TD, ed. *Clinical Ophthalmology*. Hagerstown, Md: Harper & Row; 1980;4:chap 19.
17. Chandler JW, Rotkis WM. Ophthalmia neonatorum. In: Duane TD, ed. *Clinical Ophthalmology*. Hagerstown, Md: Harper & Row; 1980;4:chap 6.
18. Baum JL. Antibiotic use in ophthalmology. In: Duane TD, ed. *Clinical Ophthalmology*. Hagerstown, Md: Harper & Row; 1980;4:chap 26.
19. Schlaegel TF Jr. Symptoms and signs of uveitis. In: Duane TD, ed. *Clinical Ophthalmology*. Hagerstown, Md: Harper & Row; 1980;4:chap 32.
20. Schlaegel TF Jr. Nonspecific treatment of uveitis. In: Duane TD, ed. *Clinical Ophthalmology*. Hagerstown, Md: Harper & Row; 1980;4:chap 23.
21. Kolker AE, Hetherington J Jr. *Becker-Shaffer's Diagnosis and Therapy of the Glaucomas*. St Louis, Mo: CV Mosby; 1976.
22. Moses RA, ed. *Adler's Physiology of the Eye: Clinical Application*. St Louis, Mo: CV Mosby; 1981.
23. Read JE, Crouch ER Jr. Trauma: ruptures and bleeding. In: Duane TD, ed. *Clinical Ophthalmology*. Philadelphia, Pa: Harper & Row; 1984:chap 61.
24. Goldberg MF. Sickle erythrocytes, hyphema and secondary glaucoma, I: diagnosis and treatment of sickled erythrocytes in human hyphemas. *Trans Am Ophthalmol Soc*. 1978;76:481.
25. Phelps CD. Glaucoma: general concepts. In: Duane TD, ed. *Clinical Ophthalmology*. Philadelphia, Pa: Harper & Row; 1984;3:chap 42.
26. Kolker A, Hetherington J. *Diagnosis and Therapy of Glaucoma*. St Louis, Mo: CV Mosby; 1976:267–321.

APPENDIX 81-A: ANATOMY OF THE HUMAN EYE

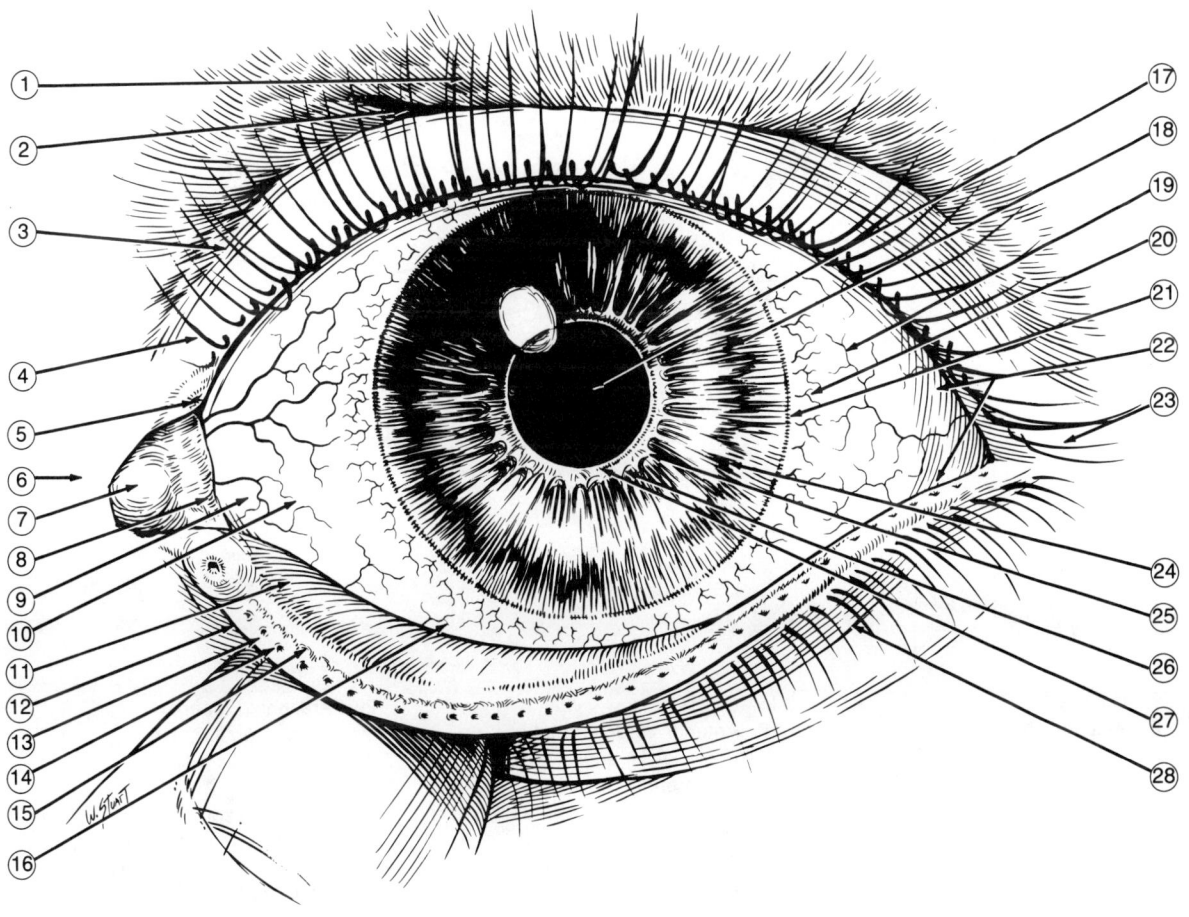

1. Preseptal lid
2. Superior lid crease
3. Pretarsal lid
4. Cilia
5. Superior lacrimal punctum in the lacrimal papilla
6. Medial canthus
7. Caruncle
8. Plica semilunaris
9. Lacrimal lake
10. Bulbar conjunctiva & sclera
11. Palpebral conjunctiva
12. Anterior lid margin
13. Grey line
14. Meibomian gland (oil) openings (tarsal glands)
15. Posterior lid margin
16. Inferior fornix (conjunctival fold)
17. Central (optical) cornea & pupil of iris
18. Paralimbal cornea
19. Conjunctival vessels
20. Ciliary Vessels
21. Limbus
22. Interpalpebral fissure (lid aperture)
23. Lateral canthus
24. Iris (ciliary portion)
25. Iris collarette
26. Iris (pupillary portion)
27. Pupil margin
28. Inferior lid crease

Figure 81A-1 Frontal surface anatomy.

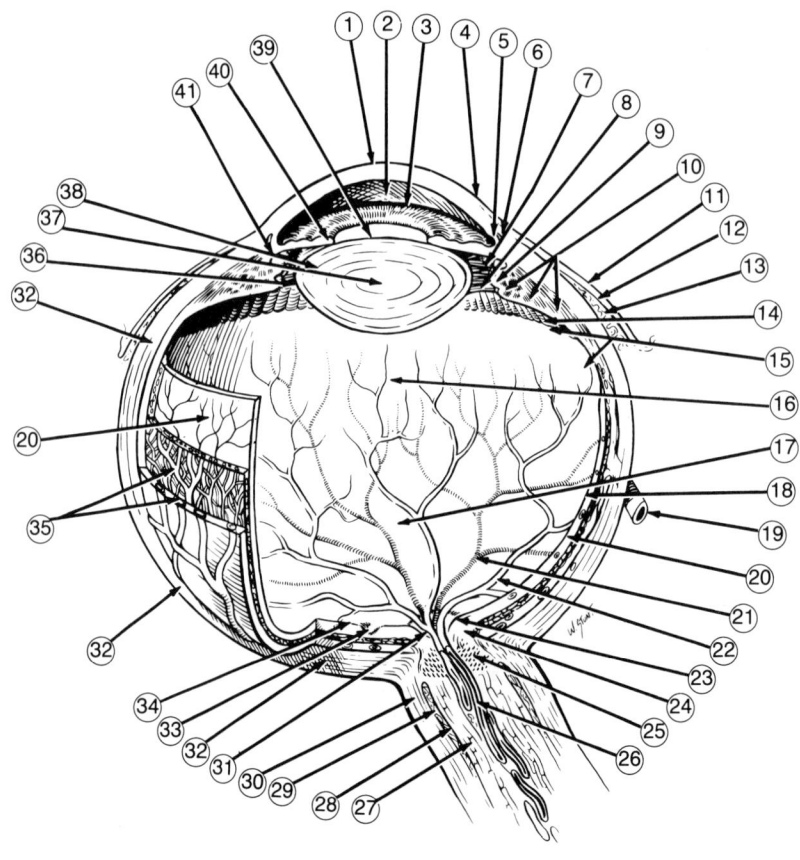

1. Cornea
2. Anterior chamber & aqueous
3. Anterior chamber angle
4. Limbus
5. Schwalbe's line
6. Schlemm's canal
7. Posterior chamber & aqueous
8. Zonules
9. Ciliary processes
10. Ciliary body
11. Bulbar conjunctiva
12. Tenon's fascia
13. Episclera fascia & vessels
14. Pars plana of ciliary body
15. Ora serrata
16. Anterior vitreous (body)
17. Posterior vitreous
18. Vitreoretinal interface
19. A vortex vein
20. Retina
21. Retinal arteries (arterioles)
22. Retinal veins
23. Optic disc rim (margin)
24. Nerve fiber layer
25. Lamina cribrosa (scleral fibers)
26. Central retinal artery & vein
27. Medullated fibers (optic nerve)
28. Pia of optic nerve
29. Arachnoid (space)
30. Dura of optic nerve
31. Cup of optic disc
32. Sclera
33. Fovea, foveola, & umbo (retina)
34. Macula & macula lutea (retina)
35. Choroid & suprachoroid
36. Posterior lens capsule
37. Lens nucleus
38. Lens cortex
39. Anterior lens capsule
40. Pupil margin of iris
41. Iris root
42. Visual axis (line thru #33 & #39)

Figure 81A-2 Internal structures of the human eye and optic nerve.

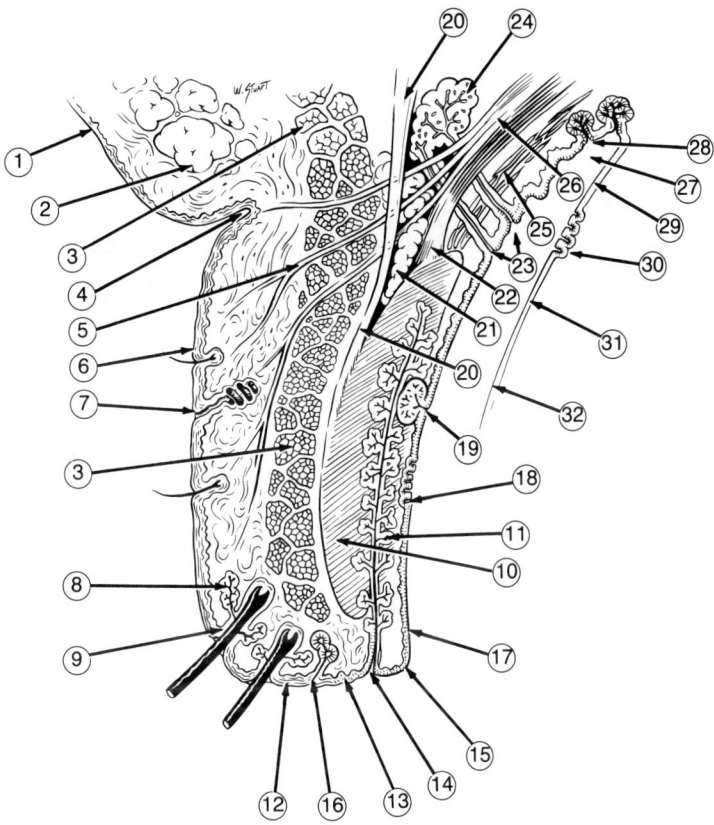

1. Preseptal (orbital) lid
2. Subcutaneous fat & fascia
3. Orbicularis muscle
4. Superior lid crease (furrow)
5. Insertions of aponeurosis of levator palpebrae M. (C.N. III)
6. Pretarsal lid skin
7. Sweat glands of skin
8. Glands of Zeis (sebaceous oil)
9. Hair follicle & cilia
10. Tarsus (tarsal plate)
11. Tarsal (Meibomian) glands (sebaceous oil)
12. Anterior lid margin
13. Grey line (intermarginal sulcus)
14. Duct of tarsal gland
15. Posterior lid margin
16. Glands of Moll (ciliary sweat gland)
17. Tarsal conjunctiva
18. Crypts of Henle (mucin)
19. Glands of Wolfring (accessory Lacrimal)
20. Orbital septum (fascia)
21. Pre-aponeurotic fat (orbital)
22. Tarsal insertion aponeurosis of levator palpebrae superosis M.
23. Secretory ducts of main lacrimal gland
24. Main (orbital portion) lacrimal gland
25. Muller's muscle fibers (sympathetic)
26. Muscular portion levator palpebrae superioris M. (CN III)
27. Upper fornix of conjunctival sac
28. Glands of Krause (access, lacrimal)
29. Bulbar conjunctiva
30. Glands of Manz (mucin)
31. Limbus
32. Corneal epithelium

Figure 81A-3 Sagittal section of upper eyelid and fornix showing mucinous, sebaceous, and lacrimal glands.

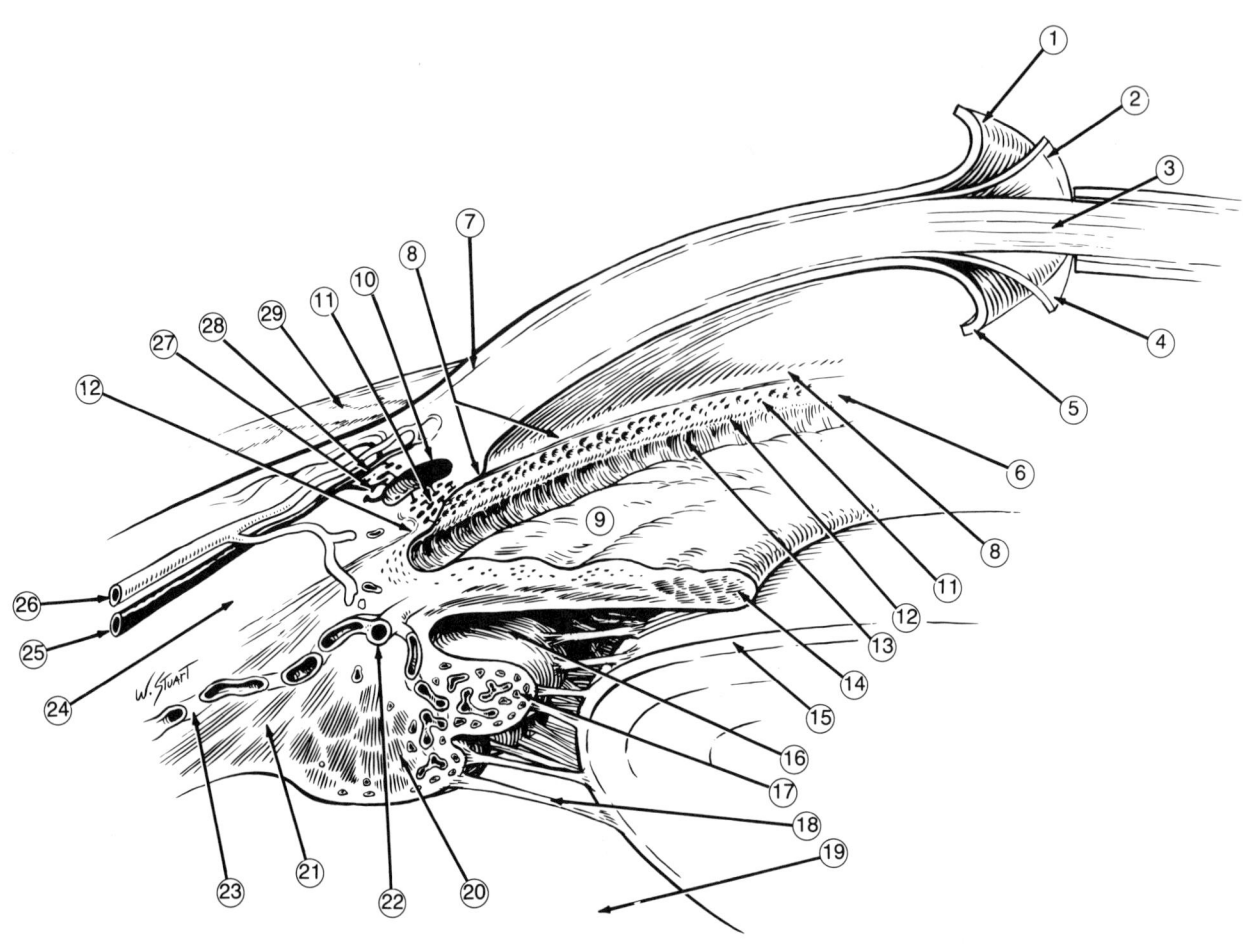

Figure 81A-4 Anterior segment of eye and gonioscopic view of iris, corneal angle.
Anterior Segment of Eye and Gonioscopic View—Iris–Corneal Angle

1. Corneal epithelium
2. Bowman's membrane
3. Corneal stroma
4. Descemet's membrane
5. Corneal endothelium
6. Anterior chamber angle
7. Limbus
8. Schwalbe's line
9. Inlet to anterior chamber angle (iris–corneal angle)
10. Canal of Schlemm
11. Filtering trabecular meshwork
12. Scleral spur
13. Iris processes
14. Pupil margin of iris
15. Lens (anterior capsule)
16. Posterior chamber
17. Ciliary process
18. Zonules
19. Vitreous
20. Circular muscle (ciliary body)
21. Longitudinal muscle (ciliary body)
22. Major arterial circle (ciliary body)
23. Long posterior ciliary artery
24. Sclera
25. Anterior ciliary artery
26. Episcleral venous plexus
27. Collector (aqueous) channels
28. Aqueous veins
29. Bulbar conjunctiva & conjunctival vessels

APPENDIX 81-B: THE TERMINOLOGY OF OCULAR DISORDERS

The list of ocular terms presented below is not very scientific and is not intended to suggest specific etiologies, but these terms are included in the jargon of the ophthalmologist, are very useful, and in a given clinical situation may permit the development of a differential diagnosis and a plan for management. This jargon accurately identifies and immediately communicates to the ophthalmologist the problem confronting the emergency physician, who should strive to employ the terms accurately in order to maintain credibility as a clinician and to establish a strong rapport with ophthalmologic consultants.

All the disturbances of visual acuity listed below must at some time be evaluated with indirect ophthalmoscopy by an ophthalmologist. This particularly applies to such visual disturbances as visual field defects, photopsia or flashes of light, black spots or floaters, amaurosis fugax, sudden blurring of vision, morphopsia, and halos. The list of ocular signs and symptoms includes much of the phraseology employed by emergency patients. The circumstances of emergency medical practice are such that the physician may become insensitive to vague, ill-defined, and apparently nonspecific symptoms. Most ocular symptoms are genuine and have as their basis real ophthalmologic disorders. Malingering and visual hysteria are relatively rare in the general ophthalmologic population, including that of the emergency department practice. Even our most intelligent and reliable patients with as devastating a disorder as retinal detachment or an intraocular tumor may only be able to describe their visual disturbances as a vague, ill-defined monocular or binocular visual disturbance. Because these visual signs and symptoms may reflect a medical disorder remote from the visual system itself, may be induced by medications, or may be related to a serious process within the brain or within the extracortical anatomy of the head, these signs and symptoms can be evaluated and treated appropriately only by an ophthalmologist.

amaurosis fugax—transient, brief, usually recurrent loss of vision in one or both eyes and described by the patient as a graying or darkening of visual images. The cause is usually vascular.
amblyopia—a lazy or weak eye
aniscoria—asymmetry of pupil size associated with either miosis or mydriasis that is congenital or acquired, permanent or transient
asthenopia—eye strain, visual discomfort

black eye
blepharoptosis—drooping upper eyelid
blepharospasm—persistent forcible eyelid closure
blindness (total)—no light perception
blurred vision
burning and itching
color blindness (partial or total)
dimness of vision
diplopia (monocular or binocular)
discharge from eye (serous, mucoid, purulent, fibrinous, bloody)
dry eyes
ectropion—outturning of lid margin
enophthalmos—sunken eye
entropion—inturning of lid margin
epiphora—excessive tearing
exophthalmos—bulging eyes
eyelid flutter (involuntary)—myokymia
floaters—black dots, threads, webs, smoke, crescents, and other silhouetted shapes observed as fixed or drifting across the visual field of one or both eyes periodically or constantly
foreign-body sensation
hallucination (visual)—formed or ill-defined figures
hemorrhage or blood clot—ecchymosis of the lid, subconjunctival hematoma, hyphema
hyperopia—farsightedness
hysteria (visual)
iridescent vision (halos)
lack of depth perception
lagophthalmos—eyelids do not cover the eyeball
leukocoria—a constant or transient appearance of a white image in the pupil of the eye (must be seen by an ophthalmologist)
loss of vision (gradual or sudden, isolated or recurrent, transient or sustained, partial or total)
morphopsia (micropsia, macropsia, or metamorphopsia)
myopia—nearsightedness
nyctalopia—night blindness
nystagmus—an involuntary repetitive movement or rotation of the eye
obscured vision (haziness or cloudiness of vision)
pain (palpebral, bulbar, retrobulbar, orbital or localized to specific regions of the face or head)
photophobia—abnormal or increased sensitivity to light
photopsia—a perception of illumination such as flashes of light, streaks, swirls, or bursts of light

presbyopia—holding newspapers and books at a progressively increasing distance for reading, occurring at the ages of 40 to 55 and associated with a decreased amplitude of accommodation

red or pink eye

strabismus (frequently manifest as "cross-eyed" or "wall-eyed")

swelling

trichiasis—eyelashes directed inward and scratching the globe

vertigo (objective or subjective)

visual field defect (total or partial, unilateral or bilateral, transient, recurrent, constant, positive or negative)

Table 81B-1 Distinguishing Features of Bacterial Preseptal Cellulitis, Orbital Cellulitis Secondary to Sinusitis, and Cavernous Sinus Thrombosis

Finding	Bacterial Preseptal Cellulitis	Orbital Cellulitis Secondary to Sinusitis	Cavernous Sinus Thrombosis
Lid edema	Moderate to marked	Marked	Marked
Color of lids	Red	Red	Blue-purple
Increased warmth of lids	Present	Present	Absent
Proptosis	Absent or slight	Marked	Marked
Chemosis	Moderate	Marked	Moderate
Sensation			
V-1	Normal	May be reduced	Reduced
V-2	Normal	Normal	Reduced
Vision	Normal	May be reduced	Generally reduced
Pupil	Normal	Normal	Dilated, sluggish reaction to light (III paresis)
Motility	Normal	Restricted in proportion to orbital edema	III, IV, VI paresis
Pain on motion	Absent	Present	Absent
Intraocular pressure	Normal	May be elevated	May be elevated
Ophthalmoscopy	Normal	May be normal	Venous congestion Disc edema
Temperature	Normal or slightly elevated	Elevated (102–104°F)	Elevated (102–104°F [38.9–40°C] or above)
White blood cell count	10,000–12,000/cu mm	15,000–20,000/cu mm	Above 15,000/cu mm
Other features	Evidence or trauma Purulent drainage	Radiographic changes of sinusitis Unilateral	Bilateral involvement Progressive loss of consciousness Intracranial complications

Source: Jones DB: Microbial preseptal and orbital cellulitis. In Duane TD (ed): *Clinical Ophthalmology.* Hagerstown, Md, Harper & Row, 1980, vol 4, chap 25.

Table 81B-2 Routes of Infection in Orbital Cellulitis

Exogenous (direct inoculation)
  Post-traumatic
    Puncture wounds
    Retained foreign body
  Postsurgical
    Exploration for tumor
    Retinal reattachment procedure
    Strabismus surgery
Extension from adjacent structures
  Face and lids
    Post-traumatic cellulitis and abscess
    Erysipelas
Paranasal sinuses
  Direct extension through the orbital wall
  Intravascular extension by venous communication
Dental
  Anterior surface of the maxilla
  Maxillary sinus empyema
  Venous connection to the pterygoid plexus
Intracranial
  Extradural abscess through the orbital roof
  Septic cavernous sinus thrombosis
Intraorbital
  Suppurative dacryoadenitis
  Panophthalmitis
Endogenous (metastatic)

Source: Jones DB: Microbial preseptal and orbital cellulitis. In Duane TD (ed): *Clinical Ophthalmology.* Hagerstown, Md, Harper & Row, 1980, vol 4, chap 25.

Table 81B-3 Standard Therapeutic Regimen for the Initial Treatment of Bacterial Endophthalmitis

Organisms in Gram Stain	Intravenous Antibiotics
Gram-positive cocci	Methicillin and penicillin G
Gram-positive rods	Penicillin G
Gram-negative rods	Gentamicin and penicillin G
None	Methicillin, penicillin G, and gentamicin

Source: Jones DB: Microbial preseptal and orbital cellulitis. In Duane TD (ed): *Clinical Ophthalmology.* Hagerstown, Md, Harper & Row, 1980, vol 4, chap 25.

Table 81B-4 Selection of Initial Antibiotics in Post-Traumatic Preseptal Cellulitis

Immediately following diagnosis of bacterial endophthalmitis and anterior chamber and vitreous aspiration for diagnostic purposes, commence therapy as follows:
Intravitreal injection
  Gentamicin, 0.1 mg (100 μg), in 0.1 to 0.2 mL. Following aspiration of fluid from the vitreous for diagnostic purposes, a 22-gauge needle remains in mid vitreous while a new tuberculin syringe containing antibiotic is exchanged and the material slowly injected into mid vitreous. In phakic eyes, both the diagnostic and therapeutic vitreal aspiration and injections are performed behind the lens through a tract made in the sclera 5.5 mm behind the corneal limbus.
Periocular injection
  Gentamicin, 40 mg (1 mL)
  Cefazolin, 100 mg (0.75 mL)
  Injections are made with a disposable tuberculin syringe, 25-gauge, ⅝-inch needle
Systemic
  Gentamicin, 4 mg/kg, IM daily in three divided doses
  Cefazolin, 1.0 g, every 4 to 6 hr, IV
  Probenecid, 0.5 g, orally, four times a day
Twelve hours after the above therapy, repeat the periocular injections of gentamicin and cefazolin and give:
Periocular injection
  Dexamethasone phosphate, 4 mg (1 mL), *or* prednisolone succinate, 25 mg (1 mL)
  Prednisone, 60 mg, orally
The periocular injections are then given daily for 4 to 7 days, each drug in a separate syringe. Systemic antibiotic and corticosteroid therapy is continued for 10 to 14 days. Modify antibiotic therapy if necessary based on clinical condition and results of culture and sensitivity report of anterior chamber and vitreous tap.

Source: Baum JL: Antibiotic use in ophthalmology. In Duane TD (ed): *Clinical Ophthalmology.* Hagerstown, Md, Harper & Row, 1980, vol 4, chap 26.

Table 81B-5 Intraocular Pressures in Millimeters of Mercury for the Four Weights Supplied with Sklar-Schiotz Tonometer

Scale Reading	Plunger Load (In grams)			
	5.5	7.5	10.0	15.0
0	41	59	82	127
.5	38	54	75	118
1.0	35	50	70	109
1.5	32	46	64	101
2.0	29	42	59	94
2.5	27	39	55	88
3.0	24	36	51	82
3.5	22	33	47	76
4.0	21	30	43	71
4.5	19	28	40	66
5.0	17	26	37	62
5.5	16	24	34	58
6.0	15	22	32	54
6.5	13	20	29	50
7.0	12	19	27	46
7.5	11	17	25	43
8.0	10	16	23	40
8.5	9	14	21	38
9.0	9	13	20	35
9.5	8	12	18	32
10.0	7	11	16	30
10.5	6	10	15	27
11.0	6	9	14	25
11.5	5	8	13	23
12.0		8	11	21
12.5		7	10	20
13.0		6	10	18
13.5		6	9	17
14.0		5	8	15
14.5			7	14
15.0			6	13
15.5			6	11
16.0			5	10
16.5				9
17.0				8
17.5				8
18.0				7

Note: This calibration scale includes the latest revisions of the scale adopted January 1955 by the Committee on Standardization of Tonometers of the American Academy of Ophthalmology and Otolaryngology.

82. Ear, Nose, and Throat Emergencies

JANICE BIRNEY, MD
KENNETH KULIG, MD
GORDON GENTA, MD

A significant number of patients presenting to the emergency department have complaints referable to the ears, nose, or throat; yet most emergency physicians have had no formal, in-depth training in otolaryngology. This chapter is presented as an overview of some of the more common otolaryngologic problems seen in the emergency department.

ACUTE SINUSITIS

"Sinus problems" as understood by the lay public are responsible for myriad complaints, including nasal obstruction, headache, fatigue, nasal drainage, halitosis, and many others. True sinusitis refers to infection within one or more of the sinus cavities, usually bacterial, but not infrequently viral or fungal in origin. In general, acute sinusitis is a condition that has caused symptoms for hours to weeks and can usually be managed medically. Symptoms caused by chronic sinusitis have usually been present continually or intermittently for weeks to years. They are often refractory to medical treatment, and patients may require a surgical procedure to establish adequate sinus drainage.

Anatomy and Development

The sinuses are irregular air cavities that lie within bones whose names they carry (Fig. 82-1). Although generally grouped into four pairs (frontal, ethmoidal, maxillary, and sphenoidal), there are about 12 sinuses on each side of the skull. The number is variable and frequently not the same on both sides.[1] Once the sinuses are fully developed (usually by adolescence), over half the circumference of the orbit is surrounded by sinus cavities and separated from them by only a thin plate of bone.[1,2]

The frontal sinus forms a portion of the roof of the orbit and extends posteriorly under the cranial cavity. The ethmoidal sinuses lie roughly between the orbits and the nasal cavities. The extremely thin bone separating the ethmoidal sinus from the orbit is appropriately termed the *lamina papyracea*.[3]

The maxillary sinus underlies the floor of the orbit, is the largest of the sinuses, and is the most frequently involved by an infectious process. The thickness of bone covering the apices of the teeth inferiorly is variable and occasionally absent. Odontogenic infection may be responsible for subsequent maxillary sinusitis in up to 10% of cases.

The sphenoidal sinus occupies the sphenoid bone and may extend into the wings of the sphenoid and even into the clinoid processes. The sphenoidal sinus is only very rarely infected.

The ethmoidal and maxillary sinuses are present at birth, although they are usually filled with amniotic fluid until the newborn is several weeks of age. The frontal sinuses may be detected radiographically after 5 or 6 years of age but are usually clinically significant only after 10 years of age.[4] Up to 20% of normal adults have absent frontal sinuses radiographically. The sphenoidal sinuses are the last to develop, reaching adult size in adolescence.

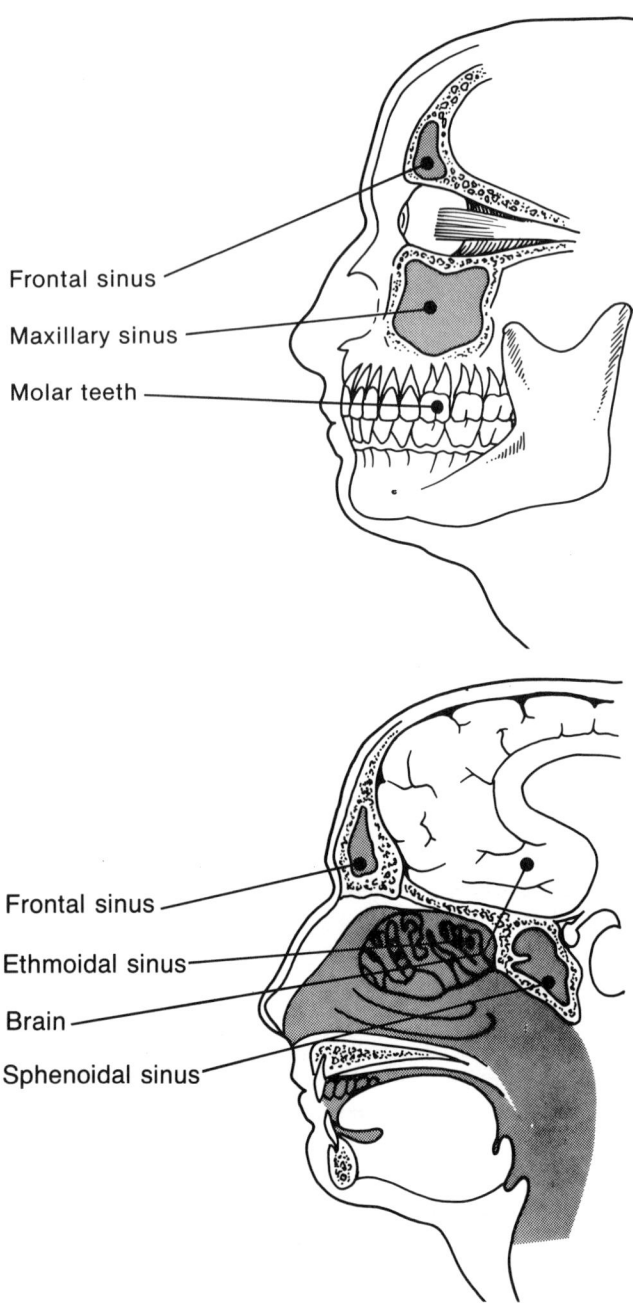

Figure 82-1 The paranasal sinuses.

Of great importance is the venous drainage of the sinuses, from which infection may spread via valveless anastomosing veins to the orbit and also intracranially.[3] This will be further discussed in the section on complications.

The anterior sinuses (frontal, maxillary, and anterior ethmoidal) drain into the middle meatus beneath the middle turbinate. The posterior sinuses (sphenoidal and posterior ethmoidal) drain into the superior meatus and sphenoethmoidal recess. The close proximity of the ostia increases the likelihood of multiple sinus involvement.

Pathophysiology

The vast majority of cases of sinusitis are initiated by an obstruction of some type of the ostium draining that sinus (Table 82-1).[1,5] This most commonly occurs in the maxillary sinus, followed by the ethmoidal, frontal, and sphenoidal sinuses.[5,6] Because of the reasons cited previously, it is more common to have sinusitis involving multiple cavities than an isolated process in one sinus.

The nature of the obstruction, in the vast majority of cases, is related to upper respiratory tract infections and/or allergies, with resultant hyperemic and swollen mucosa surrounding the ostia. Subsequent interference with ciliary action along with mucus accumulation and inflammatory response provide the conditions for bacterial growth. Neoplasms, foreign bodies, and anomalies are other rare causes of obstruction.

Trauma may precipitate sinusitis by similarly interfering with normal mucus clearing and by introducing foreign material into the sinus cavity. Even relatively minor trauma may nevertheless cause a contusion of the sinus mucosa with similar results.[1]

Less common causes of acute sinusitis are also listed in Table 82-1. In many cases no etiology can ever be elucidated. The development of subacute or chronic sinusitis, however, should prompt a vigorous search for rare causes that may radically alter the therapy.

Clinical Manifestations

The most common symptoms seen in acute sinusitis are malaise (which may be pronounced), headache, and occasionally fever.[2] Fever is usually present in one half of patients.[7] It is usually low grade unless a major complication of sinusitis has occurred. There may be a feeling of fullness and/or a dull throbbing pain over the involved area. Sudden movements frequently aggravate the pain, which may be referred to the teeth in the case of maxillary sinusitis.[6] The patient may complain of mucopurulent secretions coming from the nose, usually unilaterally. If the ethmoidal sinuses are involved, loss of vocal resonance may occur. The sense of smell may be lost, or there may be a persistent putrid odor.

Frontal sinusitis may cause the classic symptoms of pain above the eyebrow, which is excruciating in the morning and lessens as the day progresses.[2,5] The patient is reluctant to allow anyone to touch the forehead over the involved area.

Ethmoidal sinusitis, particularly in children, frequently presents as orbital features ranging from mild lid edema to orbital cellulitis or abscess.[3] It is prudent to evaluate every patient with nontraumatic periorbital swelling for sinusitis.

Physical signs found in cases of sinusitis are frequently nondiagnostic but may be pronounced when present. An accurate temperature should always be recorded. Tapping with the finger over the involved sinus may elicit excruciating pain in some individuals, but this sign is frequently

Table 82-1 Etiology of Acute Sinusitis

Obstruction
  Allergic (especially if polyps present)
  Infectious (viral upper respiratory tract infections most common)
  Anatomic (ie, cleft palate, turbinate anomalies)
  Tumors (rare)
  Nasal foreign bodies
  Nasal packing for epistaxis control
  Adenoid hypertrophy

Trauma
  Fracture (ie, orbital blowout)
  Penetrating wounds
  Contusion
  Barotrauma

Dental Infection
  Periodontitis
  Periapical abscess
  Sinus perforation (ie, during tooth extraction)

Altered Immunity
  Hypogammaglobulinemia
  Chemotherapy-induced bone marrow depression
  Other immune deficiencies

Other
  Influenza
  Measles
  Cystic fibrosis
  Sepsis
  Pneumonia (particularly pneumococcal)
  Other pulmonary disease

absent. It is more likely to be found in cases of frontal sinusitis.

Ethmoiditis, as mentioned, often presents with orbital involvement. If this is absent, tenderness between the medial canthus and the bridge of the nose may be found. The ethmoidal sinuses, as is the case with the other sinuses, will rarely be involved by themselves, so that "pinpoint" tenderness is usually absent.

Unless the sinus ostia are completely obstructed, there will often be a mucopurulent discharge from the nose on the involved side, since purulent material under pressure is expelled from the sinus.[6] The absence of discharge, however, is often associated with more severe symptomatology.

Transillumination is often used but is generally not helpful in making the diagnosis.[1,2] Also, chronic mucosal thickening of the sinuses makes transillumination difficult to interpret and thus not very accurate.[1] Congenital absence of one or both frontal sinuses is common, and only the frontal and maxillary sinuses can be successfully transilluminated. With the advent of high-resolution sinus radiography, which is far more accurate diagnostically, transillumination has been employed less frequently. Plain radiographs provide some information about the maxillary and frontal sinuses. The best radiographic evaluation is a limited coronal CT scan, which shows all of the paranasal sinuses and whether the natural ostia are patent.

Laboratory and Radiologic Studies

Since virtually all patients with sinusitis will eventually be placed on antibiotics, it is useful to obtain cultures beforehand if suitable material is available. The most valuable culture material is obtained from the sinus itself, but this necessitates a surgical procedure for retrieval.[8] If frank pus under the turbinates or in the posterior pharynx is present, this may be a good second choice as a site for obtaining cultures, but it is still likely to grow mixed flora.[1,2] It is important to use the smallest swab available to avoid contamination. Obtaining cultures of the anterior nasal secretions is useless and never recommended. The bacteriology of acute sinusitis is further discussed in the section on treatment and in Chapter 25, Infectious Disease Emergencies.

In the case of a febrile toxic-appearing patient, a complete blood-cell count and blood cultures should be obtained. In children with orbital involvement, a lumbar puncture is often recommended even in the absence of meningeal signs, particularly if the frontal sinus is involved, which is more likely to be associated with intracranial extension.[3,5] Whether to do a lumbar puncture is a difficult question with few guidelines available in the literature, and the decision should always be made in conjunction with the consulting services.

Radiographs are always necessary to make the diagnosis of acute sinusitis except in small children in whom they are extremely difficult to interpret. Even in adults the findings are frequently ambiguous and subject to a large degree of interpretation. Paranasal sinusitis is characterized radiographically by a decrease in the air content of the sinuses and by changes in the definition of the bony margins.[4] Initially, the air space is reduced peripherally by edema and inflammation of the mucosal lining. The radiologic findings during this stage of sinusitis are indistinguishable from those of chronic sinusitis or uncomplicated allergy.[1,4]

As the sinus fills with purulent material it becomes more opaque and the radiologic diagnosis becomes more certain. It is essential to remember that differences in depth of the paired sinuses may give a cloudy appearance to the shallower air space even in the absence of disease and that overlying soft tissue swelling (ie, cellulitis) may also cause the appearance of haziness of the sinus. Oblique radiographic projections in this setting may be helpful.[4]

Radiographs in infants and children are particularly difficult to interpret because the small, underdeveloped sinuses may be filled with normal redundant mucosa, leading to a "physiologic cloudiness."[4]

Air-fluid levels are the most valuable radiologic finding when present. These are most common in the large maxillary and frontal sinuses; supine horizontal radiographs may help define an air-fluid level in the sphenoidal and posterior ethmoidal sinuses.[1,6]

Rare radiologic findings secondary to complications of sinusitis include bony involvement characterized by local sclerosis of bony walls of the sinus, as seen in regional chronic osteitis, and bony destruction, as seen in osteomyelitis. The latter is more commonly seen in maxillary sinusitis in children.[3,5] Mucous cysts appear as peripheral thickening of the mucosa surrounding a well-rounded air space. Neoplasms in the paranasal sinuses cause opacity of the air space; secondary sinusitis is common. The use of computed tomography (CT), radiopaque dyes, and other special techniques is occasionally helpful in diagnosing neoplasms, cysts, or bony destruction.

Differential Diagnosis

Although there are many conditions that may mimic acute sinusitis in regard to pain, the diagnosis is generally not difficult to make based on a thorough history and physical examination, along with high-quality radiography. In the differential diagnosis the most common cause of confusion is pain of dental origin.[1] Dental caries, particularly when associated with infection and abscess, not only frequently mimics maxillary sinusitis but also frequently gives rise to it. (See Chapter 85, Dental Emergencies.) The lining of the sinuses may appear thickened on the radiograph even in the absence of sinus infection per se. In difficult cases antral puncture may be required to rule out maxillary sinusitis.

Migraine headaches may mimic frontal sinusitis, but the character and onset of the headache are dissimilar from that seen in sinus headaches.

Trigeminal neuralgia is characterized by severe paroxysms of pain, commonly commencing after a "trigger" stimulus, that follow the distribution of the fifth cranial nerve.

Insect bites may produce local redness and swelling, and if the patient is unaware that such a bite occurred, there may be an initial confusion with sinusitis.

Neoplasms of the sinus usually present as facial pain and are commonly associated with acute sinusitis. Recurrent attacks or nonresolution of sinusitis, along with persistent radiographic abnormalities, suggest the diagnosis. Also, the oral cavity should be carefully examined since dental disease may be an initiating factor in some cases of sinus disease.

Foreign bodies in the nose may cause a persistent nasal discharge, and if any of the ostia are obstructed, may also result in sinusitis. A high index of suspicion and a thorough nasal examination will usually lead to the true diagnosis.

Complications

The incidence of complications of sinusitis has decreased greatly since the advent of the antibiotic era, but complications are still seen and are likely to be seen initially in the emergency department. The fact that the most serious complications are seen in otherwise healthy young people should prompt an aggressive approach.[3] The complications of sinusitis, in descending order of incidence, can be classified as orbital, intracranial, chronic sinusitis and mucocele formation, and osteomyelitis.[1,5]

Ethmoiditis is primarily responsible for the orbital complications seen in acute sinusitis, and this most frequently occurs in children. The degree of orbital involvement comprises a spectrum, beginning with eyelid edema and progressing to frank orbital cellulitis, that may be severe enough to result in limitation of gaze, proptosis, and interference with vision.[1,3,9,10] Sinusitis must always be considered when orbital cellulitis is present, regardless of the history given. Orbital abscess and cavernous sinus thrombosis are the endpoints of this process, the latter associated with an 80% mortality.

Intracranial extension of infection may result in epidural or subdural abscesses, intracranial thrombosis, or frank meningitis. The findings may initially be subtle and secondary to increased intracranial pressure. The presence of sinusitis should be considered in patients with meningitis caused by unusual organisms. (See Chapter 25.)

Chronic sinusitis results from chronic obstruction of the ostia and/or inadequate treatment of acute sinusitis. Once well established, chronic sinusitis usually necessitates a surgical drainage procedure for resolution.[2,6] Mucoceles may result from chronic sinusitis and also may need to be drained. They are generally innocuous but may enlarge and erode surrounding structures.

Osteomyelitis resulting from sinusitis is rare, although before the advent of antibiotics it was relatively common, particularly in children with maxillary sinusitis. Radiography may demonstrate bone erosion and loss of the intrasinus septa. Subperiosteal abscess may result in pain and marked swelling over the involved area (ie, Pott's puffy tumor).

Treatment

Uncomplicated acute sinusitis can be treated on an outpatient basis if careful follow-up is available. Treatment consists of antibiotics, decongestants, and local heat.

An understanding of the bacteriology of sinusitis is essential in choosing antibiotic therapy; unfortunately the literature varies greatly as to the bacteria most commonly responsible for acute sinusitis. Although the percentages vary significantly, organisms most frequently recognized are pneumococcus, *Hemophilus influenzae, Streptococcus, Staphylococcus,* anaerobes, and *Klebsiella*.[1,6,8,11] Although rare, fungal infections are most commonly caused by *Mucor, Candida,* and *Aspergillus. Streptococcus pneumoniae* and *Hemophilus influenzae* account for more than one half of the cases. *Staphylococcus aureus, Streptococcus pyogenes, Branhamella catarrhalis,* and α-hemolytic streptococci account for a smaller portion of cases.[12] *Hemophilus influenzae* and *pneumococcus* combined are probably responsible for the majority of cases of acute sinusitis seen in otherwise healthy adults.[6,8] *Hemophilus* infections are more commonly seen in children. Nosocomial infections associated with tubes in the nasal cavity are most often due to gram-negative *Pseudomonas aeruginosa, Klebsiella pneumoniae,* and *Enterobacter* species.[13] The significance of *Staphylococcus aureus* sinusitis is yet to be ascertained, but its existence is without question. For this reason, dicloxacillin or a cephalosporin is recommended for adults without complications.[1,6] A cephalosporin may be preferable to ensure gram-negative coverage in addition to *Staphylococcus*. Erythromycin may be substituted when the patient is penicillin and cephalosporin sensitive.

Because of the increased likelihood of *Hemophilus influenzae* in children, ampicillin is the drug of choice. The question of sinusitis caused by ampicillin-resistant *Hemophilus influenzae* and other bacteria that are beta-lactamase positive should be treated with appropriate antibiotics (eg, cephalosporin, amoxicillin-clavulanic acid).

In both adults and children with significant complications, therapy with intravenous oxacillin or nafcillin together with ampicillin is indicated.

Oral antibiotics in uncomplicated cases should be continued for 4 to 6 weeks. Referral to an otolaryngologist should be obtained immediately for complicated sinusitis, antibiotic unresponsiveness, or unusual organisms (ie, fungi) on culture when identified.

Topical decongestants promote drainage by shrinking the nasal mucosa surrounding the ostia. Oxymetazoline is probably the most effective, with the least amount of rebound effect. Topical steroid sprays are often helpful if there is an underlying allergic rhinitis. They also decrease the inflammation of the nasal mucosa to help promote drainage.

Local heat seems to be comforting to the patient and may promote sinus drainage. The patient should be advised to avoid swimming, smoking, flying, and physical exertion until the sinusitis has cleared. The possible complications of sinusitis should be explained to the patient so that a return visit can be scheduled should they occur.

The majority of cases of acute sinusitis will respond to the above measures. More difficult cases or those with complications should prompt referral to a specialist.

PERITONSILLAR ABSCESS (QUINSY)

Infection in the tonsil may occasionally extend through the capsule and form an abscess in the potential space between the capsule and the tonsil bed. The resulting "quinsy" is usually unilateral and located anterior and superior to the tonsil so that it is just behind the anterior tonsillar pillar.[14,15] For reasons not well understood, it is rare in children under 12 years of age. It may appear early or late in the course of tonsillitis.

Clinical Manifestations

The classic history is one of gradually increasing severe throat pain, resulting in dysphagia, drooling, and trismus. The pain is usually referred to the ear on the affected side. The patient is febrile, feels miserable, and appears "toxic"; the cervical lymph nodes are enlarged and tender.

Examination is difficult because of the patient's unwillingness to open the mouth. Examining the pharynx, however, confirms the diagnosis. The bright red peritonsillar swelling displaces the uvula to the opposite side, and the soft palate and uvula are edematous. The drooling and toxic appearance may simulate epiglottitis, but quinsy rarely causes stridor. (See Chapter 72, Obstructive Airway Disease.)

Bacteriology

In many instances the patient is already taking antibiotics so that cultures of the abscess contents are frequently negative. In one study of 68 patients, β-hemolytic *Streptococcus* was cultured from 16, α-hemolytic *Streptococcus* from 11, and *Staphylococcus aureus* and *Hemophilus influenzae* from 1 each; thirty-nine cultures were negative. Anaerobes, although known to cause abscesses of the head and neck, were not cultured in this study.[16]

Complications

Although not common, peritonsillar abscess may result in airway compromise secondary to edema around the piriform sinus.[14,15] It also may lead to extension of infection to retropharyngeal or lateral pharyngeal deep-neck infections. Rupture of the abscess may cause complete airway obstruction or pulmonary abscesses and may lead to aspiration of pus. Mediastinitis may occur via extension from the retropharyngeal space or carotid sheath.[16] Extension into the parapharyngeal space may erode the carotid artery or result in thrombophlebitis of the internal jugular vein with intracranial extension.[15] Rheumatic fever or glomerulonephritis may occur.

Treatment

Incision and drainage is always the treatment of choice, and referral to an otolaryngologist is mandatory. The procedure is done using local anesthesia, and the pus is allowed to drain freely out of the mouth. Classically, the tonsils are then removed 4 to 6 weeks later. However, many specialists are now advocating immediate tonsillectomy as a safe procedure that guarantees removal of the entire abscess, thus avoiding a second hospitalization.[16,17]

Once the problem is recognized in the emergency department, appropriate steps should be taken to admit the patient to the hospital with an otolaryngologic referral. Active airway management is seldom necessary; however, if rupture should occur the patient should be sitting upright with the head down, and suction should be employed to remove the pus. (See Chapter 70, Airway Management.)

An intravenous loading dose of aqueous penicillin should be administered, even if the patient is already taking oral antibiotics. An adequate dose for the average adolescent or adult is 600,000 units.

EPISTAXIS

Epistaxis is an extremely common disorder affecting all age-groups. The peak incidence occurs in children/adolescents and the elderly and is much more common during the winter.

Anatomy

The blood supply of the superior septum and superolateral walls is derived from the internal carotid artery via the ethmoidal arteries, while the blood supply of the inferior portion of the septum and turbinates is derived from the external carotid artery via the palatine and sphenopalatine arteries (Figs. 82-2 and 82-3).[18] Kiesselbach's area, the anteroinferior portion of the septum, receives an abundant blood supply from all arteries supplying the nose and is the most common site of epistaxis.[19] The three horizontally placed turbinates are located on the lateral walls of the nose and shield the sinus ostia. Most posterior epistaxis originates in branches of the sphenopalatine artery located posterior to the turbinates.

Pathophysiology

Most cases of epistaxis are anterior in location, so that the source can be either identified and cauterized or controlled by an anterior pack. The causes of anterior epistaxis are quite different from the causes of posterior epistaxis.

The mucosa in the anterior portion of the nose is extremely susceptible to drying, and particularly during the winter months when upper respiratory tract infections are epidemic, the atmospheric humidity is low, and nose-picking is common, the extremely well-vascularized nasal mucosa is apt to break down and bleed. Allergies, environmental irritation, overuse of local decongestants, and habitual use of cocaine all result in a swollen, hyperemic mucosa, which, especially when combined with the previously mentioned factors, is likely to cause epistaxis.

Nasal trauma and fracture frequently result in anterior epistaxis, probably from mucosal tears. The bleeding seen with trauma is often alarmingly profuse initially but self-limited and short in duration.[20]

A rare cause of anterior epistaxis is Rendu-Osler-Weber disease (hereditary hemorrhagic telangiectasia), in which cutaneous and mucosal telangiectasia appear in family members via an autosomal dominant transmission. Recurrent anterior epistaxis with a strong family history of the same is often the first clue to the diagnosis. Replacement of sections of nasal mucosa by skin grafting is sometimes necessary to prevent recurrence.[21,22]

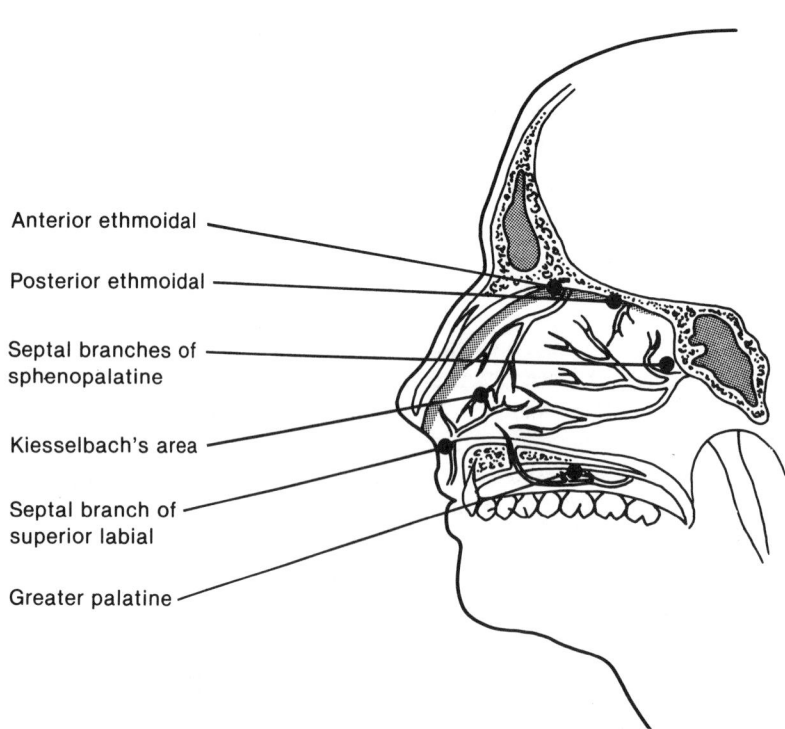

Figure 82-2 Blood supply to the nasal septum.

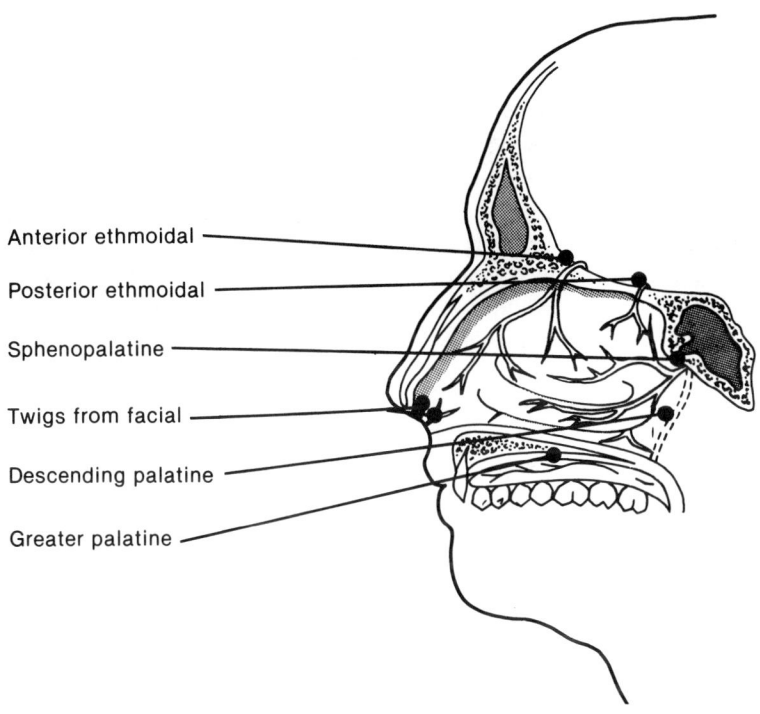

Figure 82-3 Blood supply to the turbinates.

Posterior epistaxis is usually seen in the elderly patient with a history of hypertension and/or atherosclerotic vascular disease.[18,23,24] The nasal arterioles are subject to the same changes seen in the retina,[25] with loss of the tunica media with age and narrowing with circumferential plaques. These vessels in the nose are susceptible to spontaneous rupture and because of loss of their ability to contract continue bleeding.

Coagulopathies only rarely cause epistaxis without evidence of bleeding elsewhere. Epistaxis secondary to a bleeding disorder is usually posterior and often resistant to tamponading attempts.[18,23] Fresh frozen plasma may be required before hemostasis can be achieved.

Other rare causes of posterior epistaxis include pharyngeal and sinus neoplasms and rupture of internal carotid artery aneurysm. The history obtained in these disorders usually suggests the diagnosis.

History and Physical Examination

A brief history can usually be obtained while the equipment needed for a physical examination is being prepared. The most important questions to ask each patient are listed below:

- What is the duration of bleeding and its frequency and amount?
- With the head held horizontally, does blood run down the throat (posterior epistaxis) or out the front of the nose (anterior epistaxis)?
- Is there a past history of hypertension and treatment?
- What is the drug history: anticoagulants, aspirin, anti-inflammatory medications, cocaine?
- Are there any upper respiratory tract infections or allergies, or is there a history of nose-picking?
- Is there a foreign body? Has there been previous surgery or nasal packing that may have resulted in retained material in the nose?
- Is there a family history of epistaxis or bleeding diathesis?
- Is there a history of liver disease or alcoholism?
- Has there been recent nasal trauma?
- In the general medical history, is there anemia or cardiac or pulmonary disease?
- Is there a history of renal disease or leukemia?

These questions are directed at finding an underlying condition responsible for the epistaxis. In most cases no such conditions are found. However, the history will often determine which laboratory studies may need to be ordered and even whether or not admission should be contemplated.

On physical examination, a comment on the overall condition of the patient should be made. Orthostatic vital signs should be obtained, and correction of volume loss begun if the pulse rate increases by more than 15 mmHg or the systolic blood pressure decreases by more than 20 mmHg on standing. In a young male, examination of the nasopharynx should be done to rule out angiofibroma.

The patient with epistaxis is frequently agitated, and sedation with meperidine (Demerol) or diazepam (Valium) often will facilitate the examination. The patient should be seated in front of the examiner with the head and neck in the classic "sniffing position." A bright head lamp or mirror with light source, point suction, bayonet forceps, nasal speculum, gauze sponges, silver nitrate sticks, cotton with anesthetic/vasoconstrictor, and petrolatum gauze should be readily at hand. A quick look into the nose with adequate suctioning may instantly reveal the bleeding site; frequently, however, it is just necessary to anesthetize and vasoconstrict the nasal mucosa with 2% cocaine or a combination of epinephrine or 3% ephedrine and 1% tetracaine (Pontocaine) or 4% lidocaine (Xylocaine). Cotton can be shaped into the proper form by winding it around the bayonet forceps and, when soaked in the solution, inserting it into both sides of the nose. The patient is instructed to pinch the nose, or two tongue blades taped together on one end can be used in a pinching fashion.

Treatment

After a period of 15 minutes the cotton is removed and a thorough examination is conducted. Kiesselbach's area must always be thoroughly searched, since this is the site of the majority of epistaxis. Bleeding vessels here are usually easily cauterized using silver nitrate sticks, which should be gently touched to the septum for only several seconds at a time. Usually more than one stick is required, and all suspicious areas on the septum should be cauterized, because the vasoconstrictor may have temporarily stopped the bleeding from several sources or the actual bleeding source may now be masked.

If the epistaxis is not controlled by the above method, anterior nasal packing is now placed on the bleeding side if the epistaxis is unilateral. Petrolatum gauze saturated with antibiotic ointment inserted in a stairstep fashion with bayonet forceps should result in a nasal pack that will tamponade anterior bleeders. A broad-spectrum antibiotic such as ampicillin or a cephalosporin, and a decongestant, should be given to prevent bacterial sinusitis resulting from a now obstructed sinus ostia. The pack should remain in place for at least 48 hours.

If bleeding into the back of the throat continues, despite placement of what is believed to be an adequate anterior pack, posterior epistaxis can be assumed. Once this diagnosis is made, one must plan on hospital admission for the patient, otolaryngologic referral, an intravenous line, and oxygen. Posterior nasal packing is an invasive procedure that should subsequently be managed only in a hospital setting.[18,19,23]

There are many methods used in placing a posterior pack, but probably the easiest and perhaps the safest is the one that employs the Foley catheter. A #14 French Foley is inserted into the bleeding side until its tip can be seen behind the uvula. The balloon is inflated with 10 mL water, and gentle traction is applied as both nostrils are packed with petrolatum gauze as described for anterior packing. It is imperative that the catheter not touch the skin of the nares as it emerges from the nose, since deforming pressure necrosis of the nose may result. The catheter should be securely taped to the skin of the face to ensure against slippage posteriorly. Antibiotics and a decongestant are indicated to prevent sinusitis. The patient is given supplemental oxygen with a mist mask with 40% O_2 being preferred. The nasopulmonary reflex leading to hypoxia is a common event associated with nasal and nasopharyngeal packs. Thus, arterial blood-gas analysis should be done if there is any evidence of hypoxia.

Laboratory and Radiographic Studies

All patients who have had a history of prolonged epistaxis should at least have their hematocrit determined. This also applies to patients who demonstrate orthostatic changes in their blood pressure or to patients with a serious medical illness. Generally, all elderly patients with epistaxis should have a hematocrit, blood clotting studies, and a platelet count. Information gained from the initial history will usually be the basis on which these studies are obtained. All patients who are admitted with a posterior pack in place should have blood clotting studies determined in addition to their routine-admission laboratory tests and serial hematocrits.

Radiographs of the sinuses are indicated for recurrent epistaxis or for suspected sinusitis by history, particularly if recent nasal packing has been done.

Complications

The majority of the complications of epistaxis are iatrogenic and are not rare. The septum may be perforated during the course of cauterization and subsequently require surgical repair. Nasal packing may force blood into the eustachian tube, the sinus ostia, or the nasolacrimal duct, with resultant pain and possibly infection. Patients with a posterior pack may have a febrile episode secondary to otitis or sinusitis. They may also become hypoxemic even with a patent airway.[26] This is believed to be due to the nasopulmonary reflex.[27]

The most disastrous complication can occur if the packing material slips posteriorly, resulting in complete airway obstruction. Hypovolemic shock is only rarely seen with epistaxis, and if it is present a related event such as rupture of an aortic aneurysm should be sought. Anemia is more common and may be dangerous if it occurs in the presence of concurrent medical illness.

TYMPANIC MEMBRANE PERFORATIONS

Traumatic tympanic membrane perforation is frequently seen in the emergency department setting. Head and neck trauma or ear pain bring the patient to the physician, and routine examination may disclose a perforation. The cause is likely due to compression trauma seen in blows to the ear, overzealous use of cotton swabs and other foreign bodies, water skiing accidents, and instrumentation by a physician. Spontaneous rupture of the eardrum owing to acute or chronic infection generally presents as ear pain and drainage.

Evaluation

Initial evaluation includes pertinent history of the type of trauma and any associated symptoms, such as bloody or clear drainage, vertigo, abnormal taste, tinnitus, hearing loss, and prior ear diseases. Examination begins with careful inspection for other otolaryngologic or head and neck trauma, such as scalp lacerations, Battle's sign, maxillofacial fractures, facial nerve dysfunction, dental malocclusion, and any other obvious injury, including airway and vision (eg, nystagmus). The examination is completed with careful otoscopic visualization of the tympanic membranes, ear canals, and auricles.

The hearing level must be documented prior to any treatment. If formal audiometrics are unavailable, a reasonable screening examination can be done by asking the patient to identify whispered words repeated at 2 to 3 feet from the ear or to distinguish a wristwatch held near the ear as a ticking or humming type. Standard Weber and Rinne tuning fork tests are also excellent screening tests. For medical-legal reasons the results of the audiologic tests should be documented on the patient's chart prior to treatment.

Management

Management begins with a careful cleaning of the ear. This is most easily done with direct vision and suction. Local anesthesia may be required for adequate cleaning. If there is no middle ear damage, observation and good aural hygiene constitute conservative management. Water should be kept out of the ear by using ear plugs or cotton plugs covered with petrolatum. An antibiotic (balanced pH suspension) ear drop is used because of probable contamination of the middle ear. Oral antibiotics and decongestants are used only if there is a concurrent acute infection.

Immediate consultation by the otolaryngologist is necessary if there is severe vertigo, middle ear ossicular disruption, clear fluid drainage (perilymph or cerebrospinal fluid), facial nerve dysfunction, or more than scant bleeding. Eighty percent to 90% of traumatic perforations heal spontaneously with good auditory function. Surgical correction is indicated if the perforation has not healed within 3 to 4 months.[28–32]

FOREIGN BODIES

Foreign bodies of the ear, nose, and throat region are a common emergency department presentation. Problems range from the mild irritation from a foreign body in the ear to a life-threatening situation of respiratory distress caused by airway compromise following aspiration.

Ear

The ear can collect various objects such as beads, cotton tips, insects, beans, welding sparks, and any other conceivable small object. Clinical features include hearing loss, pain, tinnitus, and purulent drainage.

Evaluation begins with an assessment of hearing prior to manipulation. If audiometrics are unavailable, gross screening tests of whisper, watch tick, and tuning forks are recommended. Radiographs are rarely indicated.

Many patients with foreign bodies in their ear may have tried to remove them, and the ear canal may be swollen and tender on presentation. An anxious child who will not cooperate makes extraction of the object difficult. In these cases, sedation or restraint may be necessary. Extraction is best accomplished under the operating microscope or the operating head of a hand-held otoscope. Simple irrigation and suction may accomplish removal, with care being taken not to use extremely hot or cold water. This may elicit the caloric vestibular response, causing the patient to become vertiginous and nauseated. Instruments that are useful are the cerumen curette, a blunt right-angle ear hook, Hartman forceps, and Blake forceps. If the object cannot be grasped directly, the hook is introduced past the foreign body, rotated 90°, then withdrawn pulling the foreign body out (Fig. 82-4).

Certain organic foreign bodies (eg, seeds, beans) may expand and require local anesthesia (four-quadrant block with lidocaine) (Fig. 82-5) for removal. After successful removal of the foreign body, the ear canal and tympanic membrane should be examined for injury. If there is a perforation, follow the guidelines described in the section on tympanic membrane perforation. Ear drops with antibiotics and corticosteroids should be used for several days if there is any bleeding, swelling, or signs of infection. If an insect is trapped in the ear, 70% alcohol or mineral oil is placed in the ear and then the insect is removed.

The otolaryngologist should be consulted if there is a perforation, moderate bleeding, or inexperience in removing foreign bodies from the ear.[33,34]

Nose

Foreign bodies in the nasal passages are more frequently seen in the pediatric age-group, usually children under 6 years of age. The classic presentation of a nasal foreign body is unilateral foul-smelling purulent discharge, unless the child is observed placing the foreign body in the nose. Nasal obstruction secondary to a foreign body may also present as general body odor. Paper, cloth, small toys, jewelry, and sponge remnants are common offenders.

Examination is facilitated by anesthetizing and shrinking the nasal mucosa with 10% cocaine or 2% lidocaine/phenylephrine mixture allowed to cover the nasal mucosa for sev-

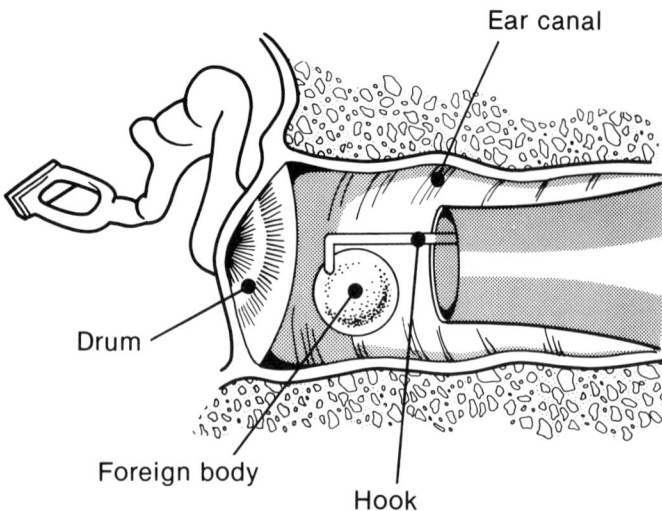

Figure 82-4 Foreign body removal using ear hook.

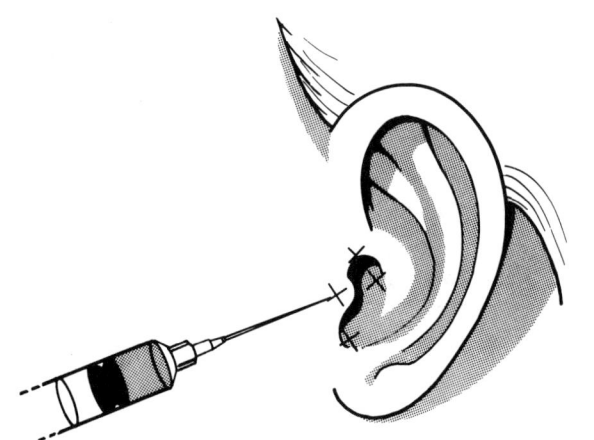

Figure 82-5 Four-quadrant block of ear canal.

eral minutes. A good light source such as a head mirror is helpful for removal. Suction, right-angle hooks, or bayonet forceps are used to deliver the foreign body, being careful not to injure the nasal mucosa. The nasal fiberoptic instruments can also be quite helpful in locating the foreign body in the nasal cavity or nasopharynx. Antibiotics and oral decongestants are useful for 5 to 6 days following removal to clear any obstructive sinusitis.[35,36] Examination of the septum should be done to observe any septal hematomas.

Airway

A foreign body in the throat can be fatal and requires prompt diagnosis and management. Although treatment is usually directed by the otolaryngologist with assistance from the anesthesiologist and pediatrician, the diagnosis and initial care begin in the emergency department. Foreign bodies may lodge in the tracheobronchial tree or the esophagus. Rapid diagnosis is important because both may present with signs of airway distress.

Foreign bodies in the airway are commonly seen in children, in edentulous patients (denture aspiration), and following motor vehicle accidents. Dentures, coins, peanuts, or a large bolus of meat can be aspirated and lodged into any part of the tracheobronchial tree. The Heimlich maneuver has successfully saved many lives from sudden laryngeal obstruction. Immediate tracheostomy is occasionally necessary but is fraught with hazards even in the controlled setting. Several authors prefer emergency cricothyrotomy as an immediate airway-opening measure, which can be converted to a more conventional tracheostomy in the operating room.

In less emergent situations of airway aspiration, the patient may present with a history of coughing, stridor, or wheezing or with a choking sensation after contact with small objects or following an automobile accident. Individuals at high risk include those with seizures, stroke patients, children running with food or other objects in their mouths, or someone who has recently eaten. Tracheobronchial foreign bodies may also present less acutely as a mild upper respiratory tract infection or more chronically as the signs and symptoms of pneumonia. Some studies have indicated that bronchial foreign bodies are more likely to be found in the right mainstem bronchus, owing to its more acute angle with the tracheal axis. Pulmonary foreign bodies may change position and cause a variety of clinical presentations.

Physical examination begins with observation of the patient in the emergency department. Coughing, stridor, cyanosis, a rapid ventilatory rate, wheezing, and asymmetric chest movement with retractions of intercostal spaces may be observed separately or in combination.

When possible, the safest approach is to take anteroposterior and lateral soft tissue radiographs of the neck and chest. Then careful mirror examination of the larynx should be attempted. Many foreign bodies are not radiopaque and the radiograph may be normal. However, films may show obvious foreign bodies, atelectasis, localized hyperinflation, or mediastinal shift.

The degree and location of the obstruction determine the urgency of treatment. As discussed previously, sudden laryngeal obstruction requires removal of the foreign body using the Heimlich maneuver or establishing an artificial airway. Other tracheobronchial foreign bodies require rigid or flexible bronchoscopy as soon as available. More conservative therapy of distal foreign bodies includes chest percussion, dependent drainage, oxygen, and bronchodilator therapy. However, there is the risk of the foreign body dislodging into a more dangerous position in the trachea. As soon as available, there is no substitution for prompt endoscopic evaluation and removal of the foreign body.

Esophagus

Esophageal foreign bodies are frequently less emergent than airway obstructions but can develop into critical conditions if the esophagus is perforated. Small objects such as keys, coins, toys, fish or chicken bones, partial dentures, and a bolus of food make up the majority of esophageal foreign bodies.

History may reveal a motor vehicle accident, a child who suddenly "loses" a coin, or the patient who presents with "something stuck in my throat" after eating. Often there is gagging, choking, excessive salivation and drooling, odynophagia, and dysphagia. There also may be the airway symptoms of dyspnea, wheezing, and cough if the esophageal foreign body pushes anteriorly against the trachea.

Diagnosis should include complete examination of the oral cavity, hypopharynx, and piriform fossae and a general neck examination. With any esophageal foreign body, there is a possibility of an esophageal perforation that can lead to severe mediastinitis and neck abscess. Symptoms include subcutaneous emphysema in the neck, fever, elevated white blood-cell count, decreased mobility of the thyroid cartilage on manipulation, and nuchal rigidity.

Radiographs are the mainstay of diagnosis with anteroposterior and lateral neck and chest views. A radiopaque contrast medium (nonprecipitated) swallowed or a string pledget soaked in the medium can give additional radiographic confirmation. Barium should not be used because it may obscure the object at endoscopy.

Conservative management, with consideration of the object, is to let the foreign body traverse the alimentary canal naturally. Liquids will usually not cause harm, but giving solid food to "push" the object into the stomach is contraindicated.

Endoscopic removal under direct vison is the safest and most reliable method of treatment. A newer method of removal for certain nonjagged esophageal obstructions in children is fluoroscopic removal by passing a Foley catheter beyond the object, inflating the catheter, and then pulling the foreign body out. This method is not entirely without hazard and requires a team experienced in the procedure. Complications include a sudden airway obstruction as the foreign body is flipped into the larynx. In esophageal foreign bodies as in airway foreign bodies, there is no substitution for removal of the object by an experienced endoscopist.[37-42]

ACUTE OTITIS MEDIA

Acute otitis media is one of the more common infectious diseases seen in the ambulatory patient. The highest incidence of infection occurs during the first three years of life.[43]

Clinical Manifestations

The individual with acute otitis often has a preceding upper respiratory tract infection. This is followed by earache, fever, malaise, loss of hearing, and otorrhea. Children may pull at the affected ear and may develop diarrhea and eat poorly. The objective signs of acute otitis include erythema, bulging of any portion of the tympanic membrane, loss of visualization of the bony landmarks, bullae formation, decreased mobility of the membrane on insufflation, and perforation with purulent drainage.

Etiology

The bacterial pathogens of acute otitis have been found to be *Streptococcus pneumoniae* and *Hemophilus influenzae* in 70% of cases cultured, with the latter predominating in children under 5 years of age. *Streptococcus pyogenes, Staphylococcus aureus,* and *Neisseria catarrhalis* are also found. Less often, gram-negative bacteria, anaerobes, and *Mycoplasma* are associated with acute otitis. Although viral upper respiratory tract infections often precede acute ear infections, viral agents are rarely cultured from acute otitic infections.[44,45] The incidence of allergy in acute ear disease is unclear. Tympanocentesis has been the mainstay of diagnosis in the past but can be difficult, time consuming, and potentially dangerous, leading to damage of middle ear structures. Recent studies have shown a high correlation between middle ear and nasopharyngeal cultures.[46,47]

Treatment

The mainstay of therapy for acute otitis media is antibiotics. The choice of drug should include an antibiotic or combination that will eradicate the three primary pathogens. Ampicillin or amoxicillin is effective against pneumococci, most *Hemophilus influenzae*, and group A streptococci. The appropriate dose is administered orally with respect to the weight and age of the patient. The major side effects are allergic reactions and diarrhea. (See Chapter 87, Emergency Drug Index.) Culturing of a purulent discharge obtained after the eardrum bursts or after the nasopharyngeal culture can be used to guide therapy.

In the older patient (over 6 years of age), penicillin is the treatment of choice. The penicillin-allergic patient can be managed with erythromycin or sulfisoxazole.[48] Adjunctive measures in treatment, including nose drops and decongestants, have not consistently been shown to affect treatment or incidence of recurrences. These modalities may be of benefit in the relief of symptoms of the upper respiratory component of the illness. When evaluating otitis media, a middle ear effusion can be quite prolonged after treatment is initiated. After a patient's first episode of otitis media, 70% of children will have a middle ear effusion at 2 weeks, 40% at 1 month, and 20% with fluid at 2 months.[49]

Persistent and recurrent episodes of acute otitis media can be treated with a change from the original antibiotic to a combination drug such as trimethoprimsulfamethoxazole. Once the infection has cleared, a regimen of chemoprophylaxis can be instituted. Studies have shown that chemoprophylaxis reduces the number of episodes of infection.[50]

Unresolved and breakthrough episodes should be referred to the otolaryngologist for audiologic evaluation and possible surgical intervention. Published data now reveal a reduction in the number of infectious episodes when tympanostomy tubes are placed in the ear.[51] Otitis media with tympanostomy tubes in place is treated with medical regimens and antibiotic otic drops.

The major sequelae of acute otitis media are persistent serous otitis media (nonpurulent middle ear fluid with hearing loss) and chronic otitis media (perforation with or without cholesteatoma). These patients should be referred to the otolaryngologist for evaluation.

OTITIS EXTERNA

Anatomy

The external auditory canal in the adult is approximately 24 mm long and ends blindly at the tympanic membrane. The outer third of the canal is supported by cartilage that is continuous with the cartilage of the auricle. The skin lining the cartilaginous canal is thick and contains fine hairs, sebaceous glands, and glands that produce cerumen.[36] The auditory canal is oriented in an oblique direction inferiorly, medially, and anteriorly and also curves slightly superiorly, necessitating upward traction on the auricle for adequate visualization of the tympanic membrane.

The inner bony canal is lined with thin epithelium attached directly to bone. Directly anterior to the ear canal is the temporomandibular joint. Disease or dysfunction of this joint is often perceived as ear pain.

Pathophysiology

Infectious external otitis can be found in all age-groups, in all seasons, and in all climates. However, the incidence increases dramatically during the summer when the disorder can be found frequently among swimmers. *Swimmer's ear* is the popular term for infectious external otitis. (See Chapter 25.)

Predisposing factors include anatomic considerations: narrow ear canal, excessive cerumen, mechanical blockage; traumatic origin: from placing foreign bodies in the canal; and environmental factors: heat, humidity, and conditions brought about by swimming.[52] Skin disease, particularly eczema, likewise predisposes to development of otitis externa.[53] Folliculitis and furuncles, which can develop in the thick skin of the cartilaginous canal, frequently set the stage for bacterial invasion.[54]

The normal ear canal may harbor *Staphylococcus albus* and diphtheroids but no pathogenic organisms.[55] The pathogenesis of infectious external otitis seems most likely to be the introduction of pathogenic organisms into a mechanically traumatized ear canal, which will then allow the growth of these organisms.

The bacteria most commonly cultured from patients with otitis externa are *Pseudomonas aeruginosa, Staphylococcus aureus, Proteus vulgaris,* and non-group-A *Streptococcus*.[52-56] *Aspergillus niger*, which produces a black growth, and *Candida* are infrequent causes of ear canal infection except in tropical climates. The true incidence of viral otitis externa is unknown but is probably very low. There has been at least one case of documented gonococcal otitis externa,[57] a diagnosis suggested by the sexual history obtained and the presence of a urethral discharge.

Malignant otitis externa (also referred to as necrotizing otitis externa) is a particularly severe variant of the disease and is responsible for a high incidence of neurologic sequelae and a high mortality.[58-60] It most frequently occurs in diabetic, elderly adults and is usually caused by *Pseudomonas aeruginosa*. Several case reports describing this entity in children with systemic disease testify to its invasive nature, with a very high incidence of neurologic sequelae, particularly peripheral facial nerve palsy.[61]

Clinical Manifestations

In early or mild acute otitis externa, the patient will most commonly complain of ear pain that is aggravated by opening the mouth widely or by movement of the auricle. There is usually a yellow discharge from the ear, and low-grade fever may be present. Hearing loss or the feeling of a "blocked ear" may be present if the canal is obstructed.

In severe otitis externa, the ear pain will be intense, frequently involving the entire side of the face. Any manipulation of the ear will be excruciating to the patient. High fever may be present, and the purulent discharge may be profuse.

Lymphadenopathy is common in otitis externa, usually involving the preauricular and postauricular, posterior cervical, or occipital nodes. The nodes may be slightly tender.

The epithelium of the ear canal may be so edematous that the tympanic membrane cannot be visualized. A thick discharge, which is often foul smelling, should be obvious. If the tympanic membrane can be visualized, it may be inflamed like the ear canal,[52] but it is usually normal in appearance and mobility. The ear canal will usually appear pale and "soggy" and may be occluded by cerumen and desquamated epithelium. Irrigation of the ear will probably not allow better visualization and may be poorly tolerated by the patient because of the discomfort this procedure may induce.

Otitis externa is for all practical purposes a skin infection and may involve the skin of the auricle, which can become swollen and tender. Pustules and crusting may be present.

In chronic otitis externa, the ear canal is usually excoriated, and itching rather than pain is the most common presenting symptom.⁵² Patients will often attempt to relieve the itching by using a foreign body such as a pencil, often aggravating the condition by further damaging the epithelium.

Malignant external otitis will produce similar local symptoms but may also present as high fever, prostration, cranial nerve palsies, and osteomyelitis, progressing to seizures, coma, and death. The disease must be suspected early in patients with diabetes or other systemic disease and treated aggressively if significant sequelae are to be avoided.

Laboratory Findings

In all cases of otitis externa, cultures of the exudate should be obtained. Routine cultures should be adequate if the offending organism is *Pseudomonas, Staphylococcus, Streptococcus,* or *Proteus.* Fungal cultures may be useful if a candidal rash is present, if the growth on the canal is black (suggesting *Aspergillus niger*), or in cases not responding to antibacterial therapy.

If the local infection is particularly severe and a spread outside the confines of the ear canal is suggested, radiographs of sinuses and mastoids are indicated. A complete blood-cell count and blood cultures should be obtained if the patient appears to be septic, particularly if malignant external otitis is suggested.

Differential Diagnosis

Pain referred to the ear is common in the presence of dental infections, temporomandibular joint problems, and tumors or infections of the pharynx.⁵⁶ Otalgia without an evident cause mandates a thorough otolaryngologic examination, particularly in the elderly, in whom a nasopharyngeal carcinoma may not be readily apparent.

Perhaps the most common confusion arises when otitis media is present with perforation of the tympanic membrane, in which purulent material fills the ear canal. A history of ear trauma, swimming, or prior episodes of otitis externa suggests infection limited to the ear canal. Hearing may be decreased in either otitis media or externa, but tragal palpation should elicit pain only if the ear canal is involved.⁵⁴,⁵⁶ Fever, rhinitis, and sore throat suggest otitis media, while the presence of inflamed lymph nodes is more commonly found in association with otitis externa.

If the tympanic membrane can be visualized, otitis media should not be difficult to diagnose. Likewise, if enough debris can be removed to see the epithelial lining of the ear canal, a normal appearance should be maintained in the presence of otitis media, even with perforation.

The results of bacterial cultures should likewise help make the correct diagnosis. Pneumococcus and *Hemophilus influenzae* are still the most common organisms causing otitis media and are not the cause of typical otitis externa. Confusion may result if *Staphylococcus aureus* is isolated, but the clinical examination is paramount.

Treatment

Treatment of all but the most severe forms of otitis externa consists of heat, analgesia, topical antibiotics (usually with cortisone), and use of an ear wick if the ear canal is swollen and occluded.

Heat seems to provide a good deal of comfort and may be provided by a heat lamp, hot wet compresses, or a heating pad.⁵⁵ Care should be taken not to accidentally burn the auricle. Analgesics should be prescribed according to the degree of pain present. Narcotics may be required in severe cases.

Most otolaryngologists have their own preference for the topical antibiotic of choice. Cortisporin otic solution or suspension, containing polymyxin B, neomycin, and hydrocortisone, is widely used. The use of topical corticosteroids is recommended for their anti-inflammatory effect; the danger of worsening a fungal infection is remote except in tropical climates where fungal otitis externa is common.

The removal of significant amounts of debris from the ear canal employing a point suction is recommended if the ear canal is significantly occluded. The use of a microscope may be required for the procedure to be adequately performed. Irrigation is not generally recommended and is usually very painful for the patient.

Ear wicks consisting of cotton or gauze are useful when the ear canal is occluded; otherwise topical antibiotics cannot reach all of the involved area. The wick may be easily inserted using bayonet forceps and should be kept moistened with the antibiotic at all times. As swelling subsides, the wick will usually fall out of the ear canal spontaneously. If it does not, it should be replaced in 2 to 3 days.

In severe cases of otitis externa, particularly in diabetic patients or in those with severe chronic disease, hospital admission and otolaryngologic referral is recommended.

REFERENCES

1. Ballantyne J, Groves J, eds. *Scott-Brown's Diseases of the Ear, Nose, and Throat.* London, England: JB Lippincott Co; 1971;3:183–213.
2. Adams GL, Boies LR, Paparella MM, eds. *Boies's Fundamentals of Otolaryngology.* 5th ed. Philadelphia, Pa: WB Saunders; 1978.
3. Hawkins DB, Clark RW. Orbital involvement in acute sinusitis. *Clin Pediatr (Phila).* 1977;16:464–471.
4. Caffey J. *Pediatric X-Ray Diagnosis.* Chicago, Ill: Year Book Medical Publishers; 1973;1:104–111.
5. Sheffield RW, Cassisi NJ, Karlan MS. Complications of sinusitis. *Postgrad Med.* 1978;63:93–101.
6. Chapnik JS, Bach MC. Bacterial and fungal infections of the maxillary sinus. *Otolaryngol Clin North Am.* 1976;9:43–54.
7. Gwaltney J. Acute sinusitis in adults. *Am J Otolaryngol.* 1983; 4:422–423.

8. Kinnman J, et al. Bacterial flora in chronic, purulent, maxillary sinusitis. *Acta Otolaryngol (Stockh)*. 1967;64:37–44.
9. Chandler JR, Langenbrunner DJ, Stevens ER. The pathogenesis of orbital complications in acute sinusitis. *Laryngoscope*. 1970;80:1414–1428.
10. Healy GB, Strong MS. Acute periorbital swelling. *Laryngoscope*. 1972;82:1491–1498.
11. Frederick J, Braude A. Anaerobic infection of the paranasal sinuses. *N Engl J Med*. 1974;290:135.
12. Bjorkwall T. Bacteriological examination of maxillary sinusitis: bacterial flora or maxillary antrum. *Acta Otolaryngol (Stockh)*. 1950;83(suppl):33–38.
13. Caplan ES, Hoyt NJ. Nosocomial sinusitis. *JAMA*. 1982;247:639–641.
14. Ballantyne J, Groves J, eds. *Scott-Brown's Diseases of the Ear, Nose, and Throat*. London, England: JB Lippincott Co; 1971;4:113–118.
15. Levit GW. Cervical fascia and deep neck infections. *Laryngoscope*. 1970;80:409–435.
16. McCurdy JA. Peritonsillar abscess: a comparison of treatment by immediate tonsillectomy and internal tonsillectomy. *Arch Otolaryngol (Stockh)*. 1977;103:414–415.
17. Cantrell RW. Quinsy tonsillectomy. *Laryngoscope*. 1976;86:1714–1717.
18. Lingeman RE. Epistaxis. *Am Fam Physician*. 1976;14:79–83.
19. DeWeese DD, et al. Epistaxis: from A to Z in nosebleed control. *Patient Care*. April 30, 1978:66–83.
20. Moran WB. Nasal trauma in children. *Otolaryngol Clin North Am*. 1977;10:95–101.
21. Flessa HC, Glueck HI. Hereditary hemorrhagic telangiectasia (Osler-Weber-Rendu disease). *Arch Otolaryngol (Stockh)*. 1977;103:148–151.
22. McCaffrey TV, et al. Management of epistaxis in hereditary hemorrhagic telangiectasia: a review of 80 cases. *Arch Otolaryngol (Stockh)*. 1977;103:627–630.
23. Jaffe BF. Diseases and surgery of the nose. *Clin Symp*. 1974;26:2–32.
24. Charles R, Corrigan E. Epistaxis and hypertension. *Postgrad Med*. 1977;53:260–261.
25. Ibrashi F, et al. Effect of atherosclerosis and hypertension on arterial epistaxis. *J Laryngol Otol*. 1978;92:877–881.
26. Lin YT, Orkin LR. Arterial hypoxemia in patients with anterior and posterior nasal packings. *Laryngoscope*. 1979;89:140–144.
27. Jacobs JR, Levine LA, Davis H, et al. Posterior packs and nasopulmonary reflex. *Laryngoscope*. 1981;91:279–284.
28. Armstrong BW. Traumatic perforations of the tympanic membrane: observe or repair. *Laryngoscope*. 1972;82:1822–1830.
29. Lee KG. *Essential Otolaryngology*. Garden City, NY: Examination Publishing Co; 1977.
30. Griffin WL. A retrospective study of traumatic tympanic membrane perforations in a clinic practice. *Laryngoscope*. 1979;89:261–283.
31. Juers AL. Traumatic tympanic perforations. *Trans Am Acad Otolaryngol*. 1974;78:261–283.
32. Pulec JL, Kinney SE. Diseases of the tympanic membrane. In: Paparella MM, Shumrick DA, eds. *Otolaryngology*. Philadelphia, Pa: WB Saunders Co; 1979:2.
33. Wood RP. *Handbook of Emergency ENT Care*. Denver, Colo: University of Colorado Medical Center Press; August 1973.
34. English GM. Trauma to the pinna and external auditory canal. In: English GM, ed. *Otolaryngology: A Textbook*. Hagerstown, Md: Harper & Row; 1976.
35. Katz HP, et al. Unusual presentation of nasal foreign body in children. *JAMA*. 1979;241:1496.
36. Deweese DD, Saunders WH. *Textbook of Otolaryngology*. 5th ed. St Louis, Mo: CV Mosby Co; 1977:234.
37. Heimlich HJ. Pop goes the cafe coronary. *Emergency Med*. 1974;6:154–155.
38. Law U, Kosloske AM. Management of tracheobronchial foreign bodies in children: a re-evaluation of postural drainage and bronchoscopy. *Pediatrics*. 1976;58:362–367.
39. Cantrell RW, et al. Foreign body and caustic ingestion: management 1979. *Ann Otol Rhinol Laryngol*. 1979;88:872–879.
40. Ballentyne JJ. *Diseases of the Nose, Throat, and Ear*. 12th ed. Philadelphia, Pa: Lea & Febiger; 1977:chap 60.
41. Jackson C. Foreign bodies in the air and food passages. In: English GM, ed. *Otolaryngology*. Hagerstown, Md: Harper & Row; 1979.
42. Wood RP, Northern JL. *Manual of Otolaryngology, A Symptom-oriented Text*. Baltimore, Md: Williams & Wilkins Co; 1979.
43. Howard JE, et al. Otitis media of infancy and early childhood. *Am J Dis Child*. 1976;130:965–970.
44. Brooke I. Otitis media in children: a prospective study of aerobic and anaerobic bacteriology. *Laryngoscope*. 1979;89:992–997.
45. Fairbanks DNF. Microbiology of ear, nose and throat infections. *Ear Nose Throat J*. 1981;60:6–16.
46. Schwartz R, et al. The nasopharyngeal culture in acute otitis media: a reappraisal of its usefulness. *JAMA*. 1979;241:2170–2173.
47. Proctor B. Etiology of otitis media. In: Wiet RJ, Coulthard SW, eds. *Otitis Media: Proceedings of the Second National Conference on Otitis Media*. Columbus, Ohio: Ross Laboratories; 1979:21–25.
48. Paradise JL. Medical treatment of acute otitis media: a critical essay. In: Wiet RJ, Coulthard SW, eds. *Otitis Media: Proceedings of the Second National Conference on Otitis Media*. Columbus, Ohio: Ross Laboratories; 1979:79–84.
49. Shurin PA. Prevention of otitis media with antimicrobial drugs. In: Wiet RJ, Coulthard SW, eds. *Otitis Media: Proceedings of the Second National Conference on Otitis Media*. Columbus, Ohio: Ross Laboratories; 1979:67–69.
50. Gebhart DE. Tympanostomy tubes in the otitis media prone child. *Laryngoscope*. 1981;91:849–966.
51. Peterkin GA. Otitis externa. *J Laryngol Otol*. 1974;88:15.
52. Mawson SR. *Diseases of the Ear*. Baltimore, Md: Williams & Wilkins Co; 1974:233–241.
53. Farmer HS. A guide for the treatment of external otitis. *Am Fam Physician*. 1980;21:96.
54. DeWeese DD, Saunders WH. *Textbook of Otolaryngology*. St Louis, Mo: CV Mosby Co; 1978:332–339.
55. Walike JW. Management of acute ear infections. *Otol Clin North Am*. 1979;12:439.
56. Pareek SS. Gonococcal otitis externa. *N Engl J Med*. 1979;300:1490.
57. Chandler JR. Malignant external otitis. *Laryngoscope*. 1968;78:1257.
58. Chandler JR. Pathogenesis and treatment of facial paralysis due to malignant external otitis. *Ann Otolaryngol*. 1972;81:648.
59. Schwarz G, Blumenkrantz M, Sundmaker W. Neurologic complications of malignant external otitis. *Neurology*. 1971;21:1077.
60. Sherman P, Black S, Grossman M. Malignant external otitis due to *Pseudomonas aeruginosa* in childhood. *Pediatrics*. 1980;66:782.

83. Laryngeal Emergencies

JANICE BIRNEY, MD
KENNETH KULIG, MD

Trauma to the larynx may be blunt or penetrating, iatrogenic (secondary to endoscopy or intubation) or autogenous (voice abuse), or result from thermal, chemical, or radiation burns (secondary to radiation therapy). In this chapter, emphasis will be placed on blunt laryngeal trauma and its diagnosis and management in the emergency department.

ETIOLOGY

Blunt trauma to the larynx is rare and is most frequently seen as a result of motor vehicle accidents in which severe multisystemic trauma is sustained. (See Chapter 7, Management of the Multisystem-Injured Patient.) The mandible usually protects the larynx, with the head, neck, and face absorbing the major impact force.[1] However, in head-on automobile collisions the craniofacial complex is thrown forward and may strike the windshield, dashboard, or steering wheel. This movement extends the neck and exposes the larynx, which may strike the dashboard or steering wheel and be compressed against the cervical spine.[2] The most susceptible individual is the front seat passenger, followed by the driver.[3] The use of the lap belt without shoulder harness increases the risk of cervical and upper airway injury, since it causes the passenger to flex at the hips and thus extend the neck and chin.[4] One reason for the rarity of treated laryngeal fractures is that the patients often die of complete airway obstruction or related injuries before resuscitation can be instituted.[5]

Other causes of blunt laryngeal trauma include strangulation, fist blows, projectile rocks, and blows received during athletic events. Trailbike, snowmobile, and minibike riders encountering unexpected rope or cable barriers are presenting in increasing numbers with laryngeal trauma.[6]

Penetrating neck trauma has a low incidence of resulting laryngotracheal damage. In three separate series, the incidence of laryngeal or tracheal trauma associated with penetrating cervical wounds was 2%,[7] 9%,[8] and 8%.[9] In the majority of these cases, the wounds are clean, do not involve major destruction of cartilaginous tissue, and are easily repaired at surgery.[7,8]

ANATOMY

The larynx consists of a cartilaginous framework interconnected by ligaments and membranes (Fig. 83-1). The three unpaired cartilages, the cricoid, thyroid, and epiglottis, are the largest and form the foundation of the larynx. The three paired cartilages, the arytenoid, cuneiform, and corniculate, are important in phonation.

The true vocal cords are mucous membranes that cover the vocal ligaments and extend from the arytenoids to the interior midportion of the thyroid cartilage. The fissure between the true cords is frequently termed the *glottis* (rima glottidis).

Easily palpable of the laryngeal structures are the thyroid cartilage (laryngeal prominence, or "Adam's apple"), the cricoid cartilage, and the first two tracheal rings. The hyoid bone, also easily palpable, is not considered a formal part of

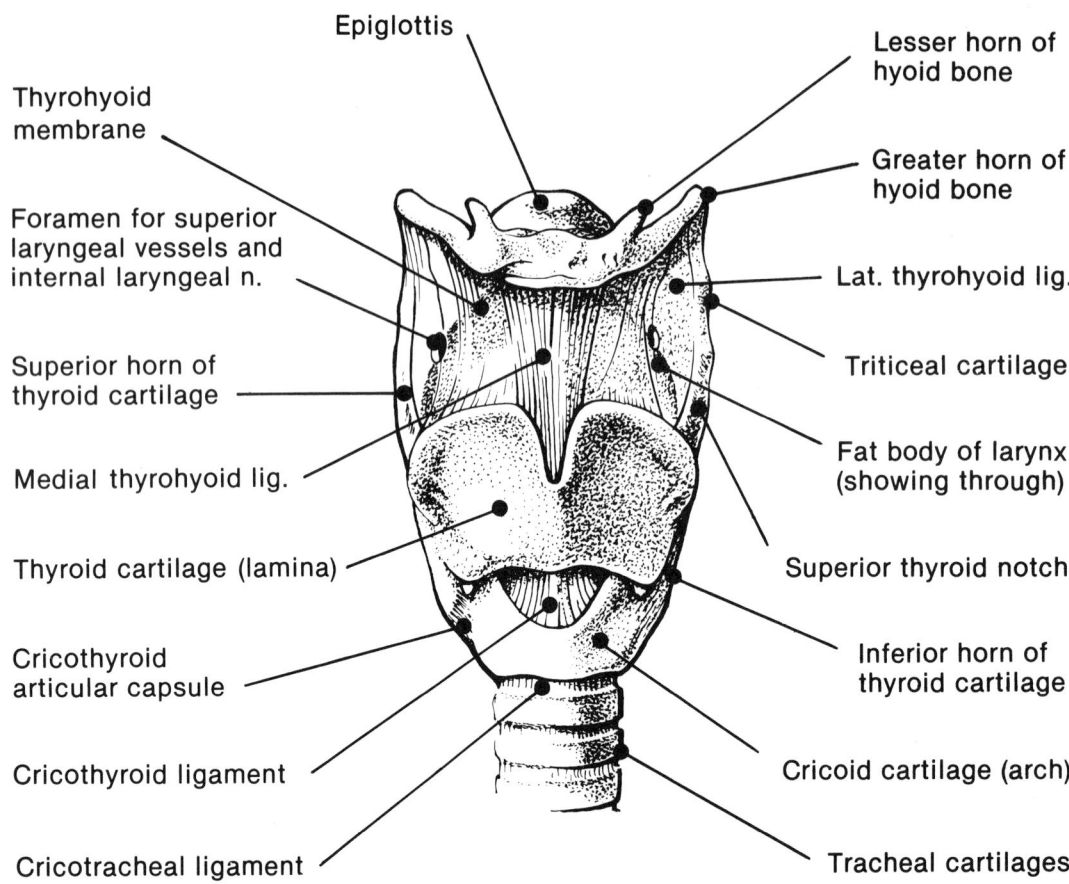

Figure 83-1 The cartilaginous framework of the larynx interconnected by ligaments and membranes.

the laryngeal complex. The cricothyroid ligament, an important access to the lower airway, is felt between the cricoid and thyroid cartilages.

Anatomically, laryngeal trauma may be limited to soft tissue edema and ecchymosis or may extend to mucosal laceration, vocal cord avulsion, linear fracture of the thyroid or cricoid cartilage, arytenoid joint subluxation, recurrent laryngeal nerve contusion or laceration, comminuted fracture of the cartilaginous structures, or complete laryngotracheal disruption.[10] Edema and small hematoma formation in the loose supraglottic tissues is common to almost all laryngeal injuries and will resolve spontaneously and completely in the absence of any other injury.[11] It must be remembered, however, that hematomas can slowly increase in size. Hematomas must be carefully evaluated as they can expand and risk obstruction of the airway.[12]

The most common laryngeal fracture is the vertical midline fracture of the thyroid cartilage (Fig. 83-2).[4,13] The fracture often extends from the thyroid notch to the cricothyroid membrane, and the anterior vocal cord attachments may be avulsed.

Supraglottic injuries include avulsion of the attachments of the epiglottis from the thyroid cartilage or fracture of the epiglottis itself and fractures of the hyoid, which are painful but not dangerous. Infraglottic injuries involve fractures of the cricoid cartilage and possible separation from the upper tracheal rings, which may retract into the upper mediastinum. Associated thyroid cartilage fracture and recurrent laryngeal nerve damage are common.

ASSOCIATED INJURIES

The patient with laryngeal trauma usually also has severe multisystem trauma, including that to the extremities. However, once trauma to the larynx is suspected, several common associated injuries should be vigorously investigated.

Forces great enough to damage the flexible cartilaginous structures in the neck are great enough to damage any cervical structure, including the vertebrae. Fracture-dislocations of C2, C3, and C4 are the most common associated cervical spine injuries.[4] In one series 50% of patients with tracheal transection had associated cervical fractures.[14] The importance of the initial cross-table cervical spine radiograph cannot be over-emphasized in the patient with multiple trauma. (See Chapter 7, Management of the Multisystem-Injured Patient, and Chapter 11, Emergencies of the Vertebral Column.)

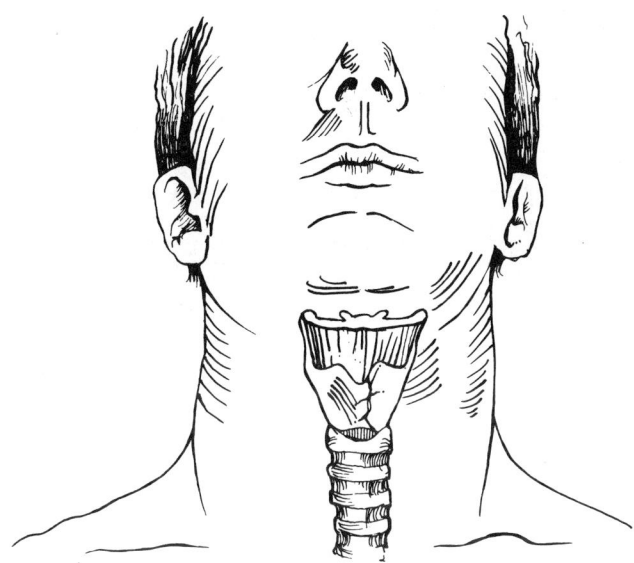

Figure 83-2 Vertical midline fracture of the thyroid cartilage.

Aside from cervical spine fractures, the most common injuries associated with laryngeal trauma are chest trauma, pharyngeal or esophageal laceration, closed head injury, facial fractures, and recurrent laryngeal nerve injury.[3] Associated chest trauma (see Chapter 76, Chest Trauma) is common enough that, especially when it is obvious on physical examination, it is often mistakenly assumed to be the source of the subcutaneous emphysema actually caused by laryngeal disruption.[5,10,14]

Esophageal disruption from blunt cervical trauma has been reported and also should be considered when subcutaneous air is present.[15]

Vascular injuries secondary to blunt cervical trauma are rare and may present later as an aneurysm of an arteriovenous fistula.[14] If vascular injuries are suspected, arteriography should be considered.

In general, blunt trauma to the larynx, esophagus, cervical vertebrae, and chest tends to occur concurrently and may be clinically subtle. For this reason, injuries to each structure must be diligently searched for in the presence of trauma to one of them. Associated head and facial trauma tends to be more obvious at the time of presentation to the emergency department.

CLINICAL MANIFESTATIONS

The presenting symptoms of the patient with laryngeal trauma are often minimal and may be attributed to some other cause.[4,5] When a good history is obtainable and not overshadowed by other major trauma, major complaints will be concerning problems with voice, swallowing, neck pain, and respiratory difficulties.

Dysphonia (change in the quality of voice, almost invariably hoarseness) or aphonia (total loss of voice) may be present in nearly one half of patients. It is usually due to recurrent laryngeal nerve injury, thyroid cartilage fracture, anterior subluxation of the arytenoids, or hematoma in the area of the vocal cords.[4]

Dysphagia (difficulty in swallowing) and odynophagia (pain with swallowing) are both common in laryngeal fractures and can be attributed to distraction of fractured cartilage and/or disrupted tissue during the second stage of swallowing.[4,5] Either symptom can occur without esophageal injury.

The pain caused by neck motion, coughing, or speaking is common and due to distraction of fractured cartilage or damaged tissue. Examination of the cranial nerve should also be done since glossopharyngeal, vagus, and hypoglossal nerve injuries may be associated.

Hemoptysis after laryngeal trauma is very common[3] but also very nonspecific in the patient with facial and cervical trauma who may swallow and/or aspirate blood from the upper airway. True hemoptysis (coughing up blood originating in the lower airway) secondary to trauma is rare.[16,17]

The most threatening symptoms of laryngotracheal damage are those of airway obstruction. (See Chapter 72, Obstructive Airway Disease.) The submucosal tissues of the supraglottic larynx permit rapid accumulation of fluid, and the resulting edema or hematoma formation may obstruct the airway and prevent intubation.[4] For this reason, any subjective feelings of dyspnea or stridor on the part of the patient must be taken seriously and the patient monitored continuously. Not uncommonly, patients develop airway obstruction in the radiology department after their initial evaluation in the emergency department.

The physical findings of laryngeal trauma vary with the extent of injury and with injury to related structures. The most common findings are subcutaneous emphysema, changes in voice, loss of palpable landmarks, and airway obstruction (stridor or dyspnea as manifested by increased respiratory rate, use of accessory muscles, and agitation).[3,4]

Subcutaneous emphysema is almost universally present[14] but may vary from subtle to massive. There appears to be no direct correlation between the amount of subcutaneous emphysema and the size of the mucosal break.[18] It is often mistakenly attributed to a lower airway injury, and the larynx is overlooked.[5] Free air as seen on a soft tissue lateral radiograph of the neck may be the only sign of disruption of the upper airway.[4] The dissection of air from the larynx may spread into the mediastinum and pericardium without air leak elsewhere[10,13] and suggests contamination of deep cervical and thoracic structures by respiratory secretions and saliva.

Over 50% of patients will have some degree of airway obstruction, and although this may be minimal initially, complete obstruction may occur several hours after the injury.[3,4]

The loss of cartilaginous landmarks is common in laryngotracheal injury: the anterior neck may be flattened, and the usual thyroid prominence may not be palpable.[11,13] Vigorous manipulation of the larynx during physical examination, however, is to be avoided, since this may aggravate existing injuries.[14]

The presence of a sucking wound in the neck, particularly after penetrating trauma, is almost always associated with upper airway perforation.[3]

Other less-specific signs include cervical swelling (which may represent large vessel injury), bony crepitus, and anterior neck tenderness. Changes in voice quality have already been mentioned.

It is important to realize that the external appearance of the neck may be quite misleading as far as the degree of laryngotracheal injury is concerned, since dangerous conditions may exist beneath nearly normal-appearing soft tissue.[14,19] A high index of suspicion, a meticulous physical examination, and continued observation are often necessary in assessing the true extent of injury. Indirect (mirror) laryngoscopy or fiberoptic examination of the larynx is often difficult because of pooling of secretions or bleeding.

It has long been recognized that delayed diagnosis and repair of laryngeal fractures dramatically alters the reconstructive potential. Thus, a brief endoscopic examination should be done in most cases of significant blunt trauma.[5] Since the patients often require other surgery, endoscopy can be rapidly accomplished at the beginning of the case.

RADIOGRAPHIC STUDIES

All patients who have sustained injuries to the neck serious enough to suggest a laryngeal injury should have a chest radiograph, cross-table lateral view of the cervical spine, and soft tissue lateral view of the neck.[4,13,19] All three radiographs can be obtained as portables, keeping the unstable patient in the emergency department for observation. As an initial procedure in most patients, particularly if any degree of airway difficulty is present, a soft tissue lateral view of the neck with the cassette placed posteriorly to include the cervical spine should be done. This should demonstrate any subcutaneous emphysema if present (frequently this is unsuspected or obscured by a large hematoma), give a clear view of the laryngeal air column, and demonstrate any instability of the cervical spine that would contraindicate endotracheal intubation.[13,19] The information gained from this one portable radiograph is invaluable should it be necessary to support the patient's airway. At a later time, a complete cervical-spine series should be done in all patients with laryngeal trauma.

The chest radiograph is essential to rule out mediastinal emphysema and any associated injury such as hemothorax or pulmonary contusion. Mediastinal extension of cervical air implies contamination, and the patient should be started on antibiotics and taken to surgery.[13]

The cartilaginous structures in the neck are seen on routine radiographs as indistinct shadows, and the diagnosis of a fracture of the larynx will require special studies, including endoscopy, to confirm the clinical impression. Clues to airway disruption observed on the soft tissue films include emphysema, hyoid bone fracture, supraglottic or subglottic narrowing of the laryngeal air column, prevertebral soft tissue swelling, and flattening of the normal prominence of the thyroid notch.[19,20]

Further radiologic studies of the larynx may include xeroradiography, tomography, fluoroscopy, barium swallow, contrast laryngotracheography, and computed tomographic scanning.[20] Each study offers a different perspective and depends on the skill of the radiologist for performance and interpretation.

MANAGEMENT IN THE EMERGENCY DEPARTMENT

Once laryngotracheal trauma has been recognized, the major decisions faced by emergency personnel are when should active airway support be initiated and should an attempt at endotracheal intubation be made or should tracheostomy be performed? Unfortunately, the literature provides few guidelines for these very difficult questions. In most cases, the true extent of injury is unknown, making any decision for intervention primarily one of clinical judgment and past experience. Attempts at laryngoscopy in the emergency department are controversial; in addition to usually being of questionable benefit, the manipulation required may totally obstruct the patient's airway.[4,5,13]

Several authors have used initial endotracheal intubation with success in laryngeal-trauma patients with respiratory distress.[3,8,21] In one series of 23 patients with trauma to the larynx or trachea, 17 patients were successfully intubated; among these were 3 patients with complete laryngotracheal disruption.[3] The advantages of endotracheal intubation compared with tracheostomy are that it is faster, provides direct visualization of the area of damage, and allows immediate suctioning of the airway. Strong disadvantages include the necessity of neck manipulation when the status of the cervical spine may not be known, the possibility of dislodging the distal end of a complete laryngotracheal disruption, and the hazards of placing a tube through the area of trauma. Endotracheal intubation in these cases is always temporary. Tracheostomy in the operating room under more optimum conditions is performed as soon as possible. With a laryngeal fracture tracheotomy is preferable to endotracheal intubation since a tracheotomy avoids further laryngeal trauma, possible disruption of a precarious airway, and creation of a false lumen or passage.[22]

The disadvantages of immediate tracheostomy in the emergency department are primarily those of technical difficulties in carrying out the procedure, particularly on a patient who may be awake and combative from hypoxemia or other reasons. However, some authors still recommend it as the initial procedure of choice.[4,5,10,13] The procedure has the obvious advantage of requiring minimal cervical manipulation and bypassing the area of trauma (usually).

Nasotracheal intubation in laryngeal trauma is to be condemned as too hazardous, as is cricothyroidotomy.

Perhaps the problem that presents the biggest management dilemma is the awake patient with known laryngeal trauma but with only mild (or even absent) respiratory distress. In closed injuries, it has been the experience of some authors that neither intubation nor tracheostomy were required in this type of case.[14,23] In one series of 22 closed injuries, 13 patients were managed in the hospital without tracheostomy or intubation and all recovered. The majority of these patients were symptomatic, with dysphonia, dysphagia, and emphysema. The management of the traumatized patient in this manner requires that an "attendant" be available constantly at the patient's bedside with an available tracheostomy set. Such practices are probably too risky to be considered adequate treatment for today's trauma patients.

REFERENCES

1. Nahum AM, Siegel AN. Biodynamics of injury to the larynx in automobile collisions. *Ann Otolaryngol*. 1967;76:781–790.
2. Butler RM, Moser FH. The padded dash syndrome: blunt trauma to the larynx and trachea. *Laryngoscope*. 1968;78:1172–1176.
3. Lambert GE, McMurray GT. Laryngotracheal trauma: recognition and management. *J Am Coll Emergency Physicians*. 1976;5:883–887.
4. Zuidema GD, Rutherford RB, Ballinger WF, eds. *The Management of Trauma*. 3rd ed. Philadelphia, Pa: WB Saunders Co; 1979:347–352.
5. Whited RE. Laryngeal fracture in the multiple trauma patient. *Am J Surg*. 1978;136:354–355.
6. Alonso WA, Caruso VG, Roncace EA. Minibikes: a new factor in laryngotracheal trauma. *Ann Otol Rhinol Laryngol*. 1973;82:800–804.
7. Blass DC, James EC, Reed RJ, et al. Penetrating wounds of the neck and upper thorax. *J Trauma*. 1978;18:2–7.
8. Knightly JJ, Swaminathan AP, Rush BF. Management of penetrating wounds of the neck. *Am J Surg*. 1973;126:574–579.
9. Penn I. Penetrating injuries of the neck. *Surg Clin North Am*. 1973;53:6, 1469–1478.
10. Larson DC, Cohn AM. Management of acute laryngeal injury: a critical review. *J Trauma*. 1976;16:858–862.
11. Ballenger JJ. *Diseases of the Nose, Throat, and Ear*. 11th ed. Philadelphia, Pa: Lea & Febiger; 1969:318–335.
12. Boster SR, Martinez SA. Acute airway obstruction in the adult. *Postgrad Med*. 1982;72:61–67.
13. Paparella MM, Shumrich DA, eds. *Otolaryngology*. Philadelphia, Pa: WB Saunders Co; 1973;3:609–615.
14. Fitz-Hugh GS, Wallenborn WM, McGovern F. Injuries of the larynx and cervical trauma. *Ann Otol Rhinol Laryngol*. 1971;80:419–442.
15. Spenler CW, Benfield JR. Esophageal disruption from blunt and penetrating external trauma. *Arch Surg*. 1976;111:663–667.
16. Lyons HA. Differential diagnosis of hemoptysis and its treatment. In: Pierce AK, ed. *Basics of Respiratory Disease*. New York, NY: American Lung Association; 1976;5:2.
17. Wolfe JD, Simmons DH. Hemoptysis: diagnosis and management. *West J Med*. 1977;127:383–390.
18. LeMay SR Jr. Penetrating wounds of the larynx and cervical trachea. *Arch Otolaryngol*. 1971;94:558–565.
19. Greene R, Stark P. Trauma of the larynx and trachea. *Radiol Clin North Am*. 1978;15:309–320.
20. Momose KJ, Macmillan AS. Roentgenologic investigations of the larynx and trachea. *Radiol Clin North Am*. 1978;16:321–341.
21. Sheely CH, Mattox KL, Beall AC. Management of acute cervical tracheal trauma. *Am J Surg*. 1974;128:805–808.
22. Schaeffer SD. Laryngeal fracture. In: Hott G, Mattox D, Gates G, eds. *Decision Making in Otolaryngology*. Philadelphia, Pa: BC Decker; 1984.
23. Chadwick DC. Closed injuries of the larynx and pharynx. *J Laryngol Otol*. 1960;74:306–311.

84. Maxillofacial Injuries

STEPHEN V. CANTRILL, MD, FACEP

Maxillofacial injuries are commonly encountered in the practice of emergency medicine and may run the gamut from a small lip laceration to a facial "crunch" associated with major trauma. The goal of this chapter is to provide guidance for the evaluation and treatment of this wide range of disorders.

There are many possible etiologies for maxillofacial injuries, including motor vehicle accidents, assaults, athletic injuries, home accidents, work-related injuries, animal and human bites, and nonaccidental childhood trauma (child abuse). More than 50% of these injuries, however, are sustained in motor vehicle accidents, and many of these (60% in some series) are associated with additional major trauma.

Maxillofacial injuries mandate special attention because of the importance of the face. The face contains the many important organs needed for seeing, hearing, smelling, breathing, eating, and talking, and the appearance of the structure has a major impact on daily life. Much of an individual's personality is embodied in the face, and any defect detracts from this quality. In working with facial injuries, care is required to avoid leaving any more of a defect than is absolutely necessary.

PATHOPHYSIOLOGY AND CLINICAL CORRELATES

Maxillofacial injuries may be inflicted by sharp or blunt instruments or both. Trauma from a sharp object is more likely to produce only a laceration, while blunt trauma may produce a contusion, avulsion, and/or bony disruption. Maxillofacial injuries resulting from vehicular trauma are usually deceleration injuries that might have been avoided if the patient had used the passenger restraint system available in the automobile. The kinetic energy present in a moving body is a function of the mass of the body times the square of its velocity; it is the dispersion of this energy during deceleration that produces the force that causes the injury. Thus, it is easy to see why the magnitude of the injury can be greatly increased by only a moderate increase in speed.

Patients with major facial trauma, hemorrhage, and airway obstruction may also present with severe, life-threatening injuries to other organ systems. These patients should have their maxillofacial trauma dealt with only to the degree of ensuring a patent airway and controlling the hemorrhage; their other injuries must be evaluated and treated before attention is again given to the facial area. Facial injuries may appear grotesque, but except for airway and bleeding control they rarely present a true emergency. A further complicating factor is that vehicular accident patients are often under the influence of ethanol, thus making accurate evaluation of the patient more difficult. It should be remembered that shock is almost never due to maxillofacial trauma alone; an additional major cause must be sought elsewhere in the body. It should also be noted that any alteration in the level of consciousness in a patient sustaining maxillofacial trauma mandates a thorough evaluation to determine the cause of this finding.

DIAGNOSIS AND TREATMENT

Prehospital Care

The most important component of prehospital care in patients with maxillofacial trauma is the maintenance of a patent airway. The patient's airway can be compromised by bony or cartilaginous disruption or by obstruction of the airway by soft tissue, blood, or a foreign body. After the oropharynx is initially cleared of blood and debris, the method of airway management is a function of the patient's mentation and other suspected injuries. If a cervical spine injury is suspected, as it often is in vehicular trauma, the cervical spine must be immobilized, usually with the patient in a supine position. If the victim is obtunded but not bleeding into the airway, an oropharyngeal or nasopharyngeal airway may be adequate for maintenance of a patent airway. If the patient is comatose or bleeding into the oral cavity, nasotracheal intubation should be considered as long as there is no evidence of mid-face bony disruption, which is a contraindication for this procedure. It should be kept in mind that many paramedic programs do not permit endotracheal intubation or nasotracheal intubation in their accepted list of functions. In the case of respiratory arrest, orotracheal intubation may be necessary. In the rare case in which the patient has also sustained severe laryngeal trauma, a cricothyrotomy may be the only way of establishing an airway. If cervical spine injury is not suspected, the patient may be transported sitting, prone, or in a lateral decubitus position to avoid aspiration. Patients with isolated traumatic eye injuries should be transported in a sitting position.

Control of hemorrhage is second in importance, after ensuring an airway, in patients with maxillofacial trauma. Direct pressure, either by hand or pressure dressings, is almost always adequate in the field. (See Figs. 84-1 and 84-2 for location of blood vessels.) Care must be taken not to further compromise the airway in applying the dressings to the head and face.

Impaled foreign bodies in the face and eye should be stabilized with gauze bandages prior to transport. Those involving *only* the cheek may be safely removed in the field, with finger pressure used to control hemorrhage. All other foreign bodies should be left in place until the patient is in the operating room.

Soft tissue injuries of the facial area should also be given prehospital attention. Large avulsion flaps should have any gross contamination removed by irrigation and then be replaced in their tissue bed. Completely avulsed tissues, especially ears, the nose, or teeth should be retrieved if possible, wrapped in gauze soaked in normal saline, and transported with the patient.

In cases in which the eyes have been in contact with acid or alkali solutions, the eyes should be copiously irrigated on the scene. Any source of running water is adequate for this irrigation.

Emergency care personnel at the scene should also note the mechanism of injury and the position in which the patient was found. This information should be conveyed to those caring for the patient in the emergency department since it is frequently helpful in assessing the patient for other injuries. The patient's mental status both at the time of initial evaluation and during transport should be noted, because closed head trauma frequently accompanies maxillofacial injuries. Any change in mental status without evidence of shock should be assumed to be evidence of closed head trauma until proved otherwise. (See Chapter 7, Management of the Multisystem-Injured Patient.)

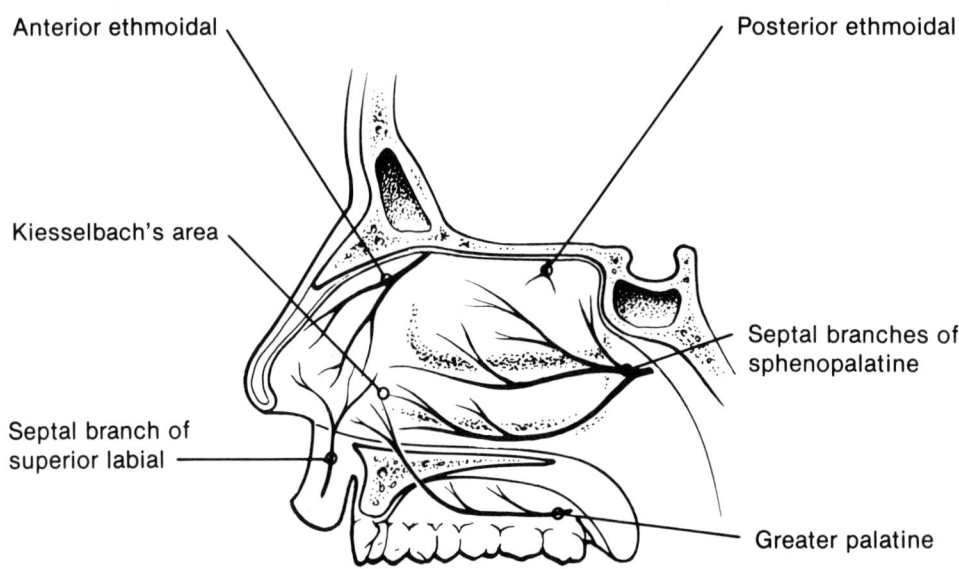

Figure 84-1 Blood supply to the nasal septum.

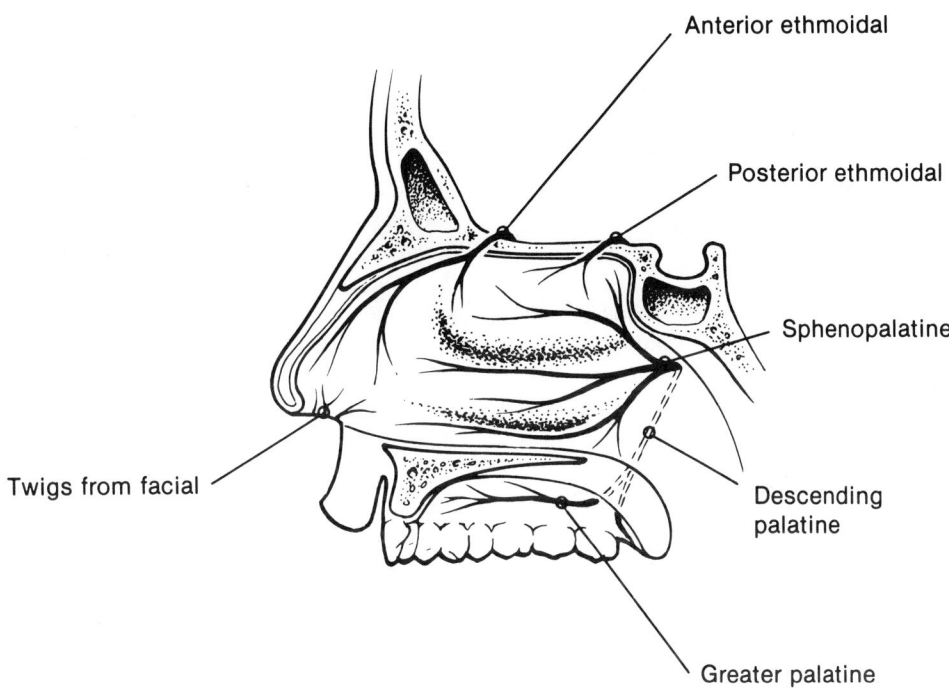

Figure 84-2 Blood supply to the turbinates.

Emergency Department Care

Initial Stabilization and Evaluation

On arrival in the emergency department, the patient may have been stabilized to varying degrees, based on the sophistication of the prehospital care system that was used. The initial care of the patient follows the same protocol as outlined previously. A patent airway must be ensured, with intubation if necessary. A nasotracheal route is preferred if the patient is relatively stable or if there is concern about a possible cervical spine injury. This route, however, is contraindicated if there is any bony disruption of the mid-face. In cases of massive facial and/or laryngeal trauma, a cricothyrotomy may be necessary as a life-saving measure. A true tracheostomy has no place in the emergency department in a "crash" situation, since it is often a very difficult and time-consuming procedure, even under the best of controlled circumstances.

If shock is present, it must be aggressively treated with fluid resuscitation and bleeding control. As noted previously, the presence of shock almost always indicates major trauma to areas other than the face. Head, chest, and abdominal etiologies for the hypotension must be ruled out. The presence of cervical spine trauma must be assumed until disproved in any person with altered mental status due to the trauma or other agents (eg, ethanol). Any alert patient complaining of neck pain or paresthesia should also have the cervical spine immobilized until any injury can be discounted radiographically.

The patient should be completely evaluated for serious life-threatening injury, such as head trauma, before the maxillofacial trauma is evaluated. As noted, most facial hemorrhage can be controlled through direct pressure. Rarely, hemostats may be required to control an isolated bleeder. This should be done only under direct vision to avoid iatrogenic injury to important structures, such as the facial nerve or the parotid duct (Fig. 84-3). After evaluation, most

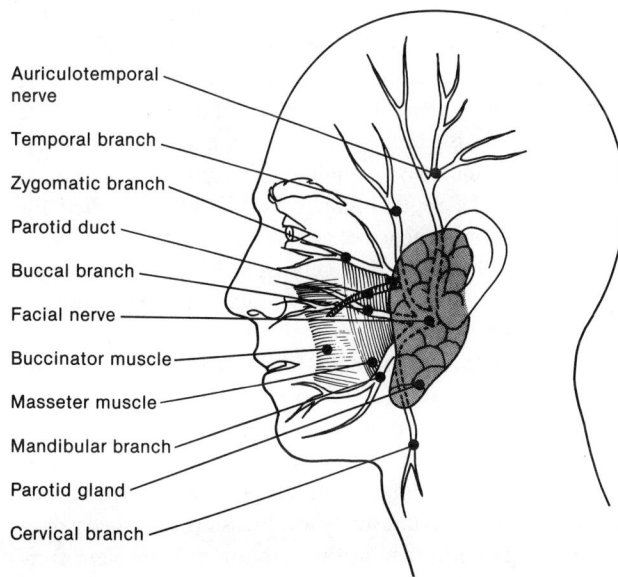

Figure 84-3 Muscles, nerves, and glands of the head.

clean facial lacerations may wait up to 24 hours for definitive care. If this is to be the case, the wound should be irrigated and the tissues placed in rough approximation. Grossly contaminated wounds, animal bites, human bites, and wounds with foreign-body tattooing should be addressed as soon as possible to provide maximum opportunity for a good result.

Evaluation of Maxillofacial Injuries

Much of facial trauma is obvious, but a surprising amount may elude the examining physician unless a thorough, systematic approach to evaluation is made. Since many maxillofacial injuries will be treated by a specialist, the main function of the emergency physician may only be to discover the injury. This is a crucial role. In many cases, if the injury is missed (eg, a tripod fracture of the zygoma), the patient may end up with a healed injury that results in compromised function (eg, diplopia) that may be extremely difficult to correct at a later date.

The evaluation of facial injuries begins with a history. This important source of data is often given short shrift, with unfortunate repercussions. It is important to understand the mechanism of injury to construct a differential diagnosis of what types of injury may have occurred and therefore must be ruled out. If alert, the patient can answer questions about sources of pain, but this may be unreliable since a greater pain (eg, a femur fracture) may override the pain of other injuries. If mandibular trauma is a possibility, the patient should be asked if the dental occlusion feels normal. If it does not, the patient is assumed to have a mandibular fracture until proved otherwise.

Inspection of the facial area is performed, with deformity or asymmetry being sought as indicators of possible bony disruption. Enophthalmos (the sinking of the eye globe posteriorly in the orbit) and loss of consensual gaze should both be checked as indicators of possible disruption of the orbits. The bite should be inspected for malocclusion and the dentition should be inspected for evidence of a step deformity, both implying a mandibular fracture. The area beneath the tongue should also be inspected, since a sublingual hematoma may also indicate a mandibular fracture. If nasal trauma is suspected, the septum should be visually inspected for integrity and for existence of a septal hematoma. Excessive, watery rhinorrhea may be cerebrospinal fluid, indicating a fracture of the cribriform plate. (Glucose determination of the rhinorrhea is not a valid method to differentiate cerebrospinal fluid from other fluids.) All soft tissue injuries must be thoroughly and carefully inspected. Often foreign material may be found deep in the wound, or a fracture may be directly visualized that is not seen on the radiograph. The integrity of the eye globes should be ensured by inspection. By demonstrating an unusually low pressure, tonometry may help in diagnosing penetrating violation. Complete fundoscopic examination, including careful examination of the iris and the anterior chamber, is indicated in all cases of trauma involving the eye. Fluorescein staining should be performed if nonpenetrating corneal injury is a possibility.

Documentation of clinical observations is probably more important regarding the face than elsewhere in the body. In one series, it was noted that 24% of facial injuries resulted in personal litigation. Possible legal questions obviously require the treating physician to be able to reconstruct carefully the nature of the initial injury. Photographs are the best available answer. A camera with instantly developing film provides an easy mechanism for this, with the resultant picture stapled to the patient's record. Careful drawings with measurements should be supplied if photographs are unavailable.

The next step is evaluation of neuromuscular function. Motor function of the facial nerves may be easily evaluated by observing the face in repose and then by asking the patient to bare the teeth, smile, wrinkle the forehead, and close the eyes tightly. Sensory innervation of the three branches (supraorbital, infraorbital, and mental) of the trigeminal nerve should be tested bilaterally. A fracture near the foramina of exit of any of these nerves will frequently present as anesthesia/hypoesthesia in the distribution of that nerve (Fig. 84-4). Extraocular movements should be completely tested as indicators of a possible orbital floor fracture. The patient should be asked about diplopia in each of the directions of movement. Visual acuity should be tested with a Snellen or similar chart if trauma to the eye is suspected. Palpation of the bony structure of the face, the next step, should be done in a systematic fashion (Fig. 84-5). Tenderness, step defects, crepitus, and false motion should all be investigated. Each is an indicator of potential facial fracture. The infraorbital area, the supraorbital ridge, the zygoma, the nasal bones, the lower maxilla, and the mandible should be carefully palpated. Stability of the teeth and the alveolar ridge should be tested by grasping the upper and lower incisors and attempting to move them.

Following the clinical evaluation and if the patient's condition allows, the physician should obtain radiographs, based on clinical suspicion as a result of the mechanism of injury and findings on physical examination. A multitude of radiographic views are possible. The workhorse of facial-bone evaluation is the Waters' projection (Fig. 84-6), which allows evaluation of the maxilla, maxillary sinuses, orbital floors, orbital inferior rims, and zygomas. This view is usually accompanied by posteroanterior and lateral facial-bone views for routine screening. Other specific radiographs that may be indicated include those of the nasal bones, zygomatic arches, and lateral orbits. Mandible views may be ordered also, although Panorex views, if available, will show mandibular fractures more clearly. Fractures, fluid-filled sinuses, herniation of soft tissue into the sinuses, and subcutaneous air should all be investigated. All of these findings indicate probable skeletal disruption.

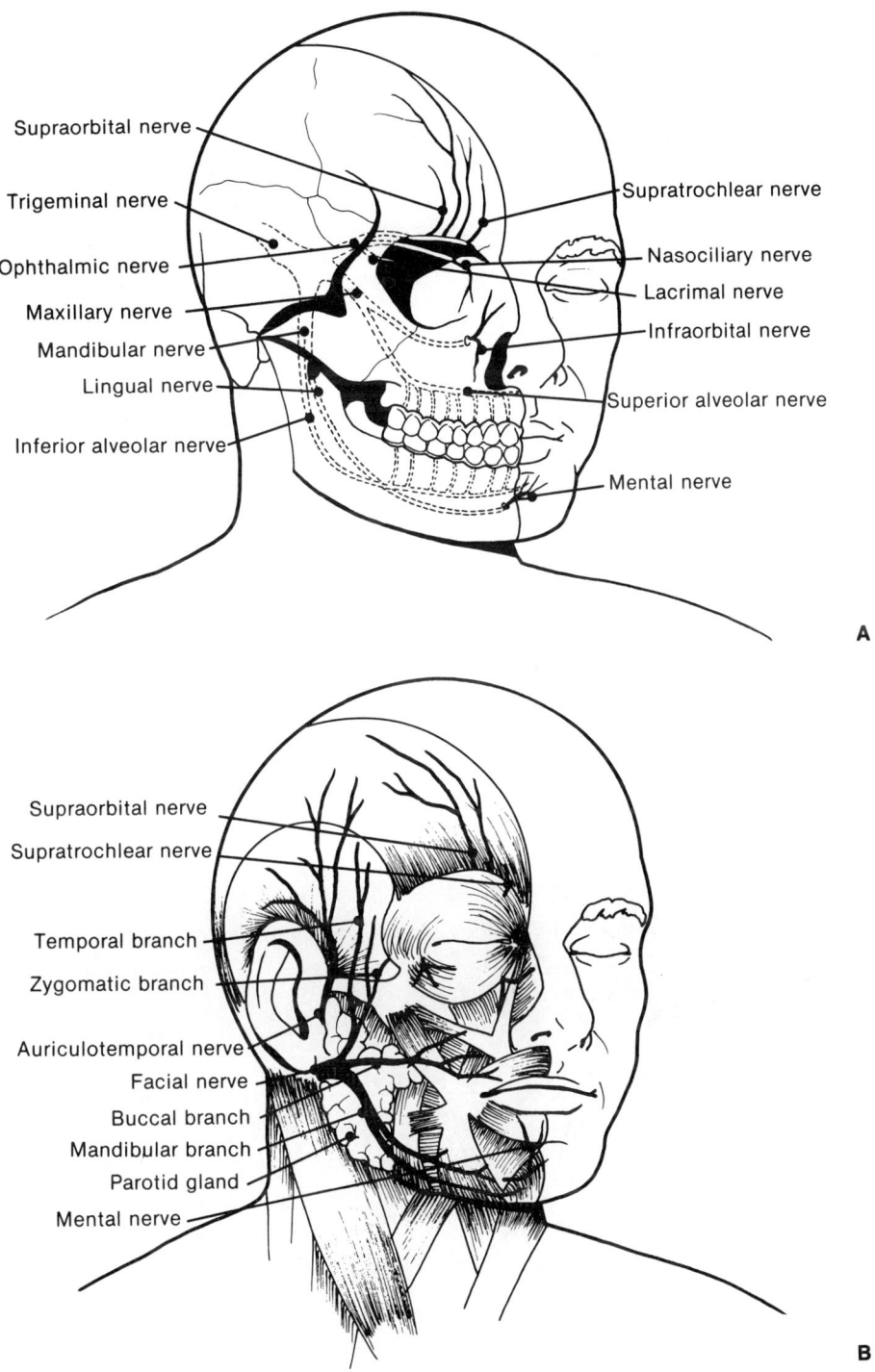

Figure 84-4 A: Trigeminal nerve. B: Facial nerves.

Abnormalities discovered on plain radiographs may be further elucidated by the use of computed tomography (CT) of the facial bones in question. These studies are probably best ordered after consultation with a radiologist, since the usefulness of these modalities is a function of the equipment and experience available in each radiology department.

Use of Consultants

Decisions regarding consultants in maxillofacial trauma are sometimes difficult because of overlapping areas of clinical expertise. Different facial injuries may require consultation with plastic surgeons, otolaryngologists,

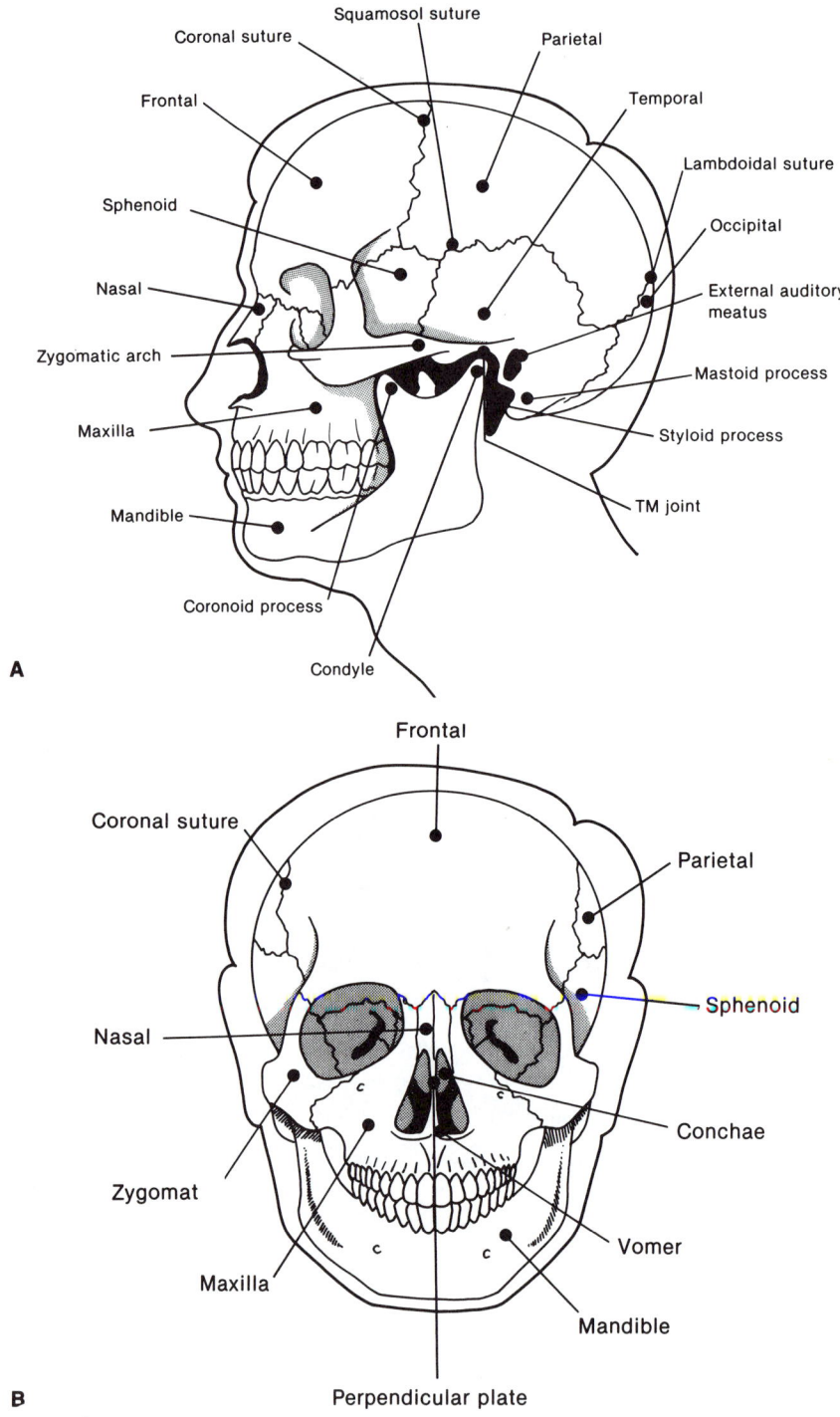

Figure 84-5 Normal skull and facial bones. *Note:* **A**: Sagittal view. **B**: Coronal view.

ophthalmologists, and/or oral surgeons. Some specific recommendations are made in the sections that follow, but it is best for the emergency physician to provide referral based on the interests and capabilities of the specialists immediately available. The decision for referral may at times be difficult, encompassing such factors as the emergency physician's expertise in handling different injuries, the patient load in the emergency department at that time, and the complexity of the injury. Indicators for referral include the necessity of general anesthesia for repair (such as in an uncooperative child), the possibility of nerve transection, the necessity of a delayed primary closure, the requirement that the patient be admitted

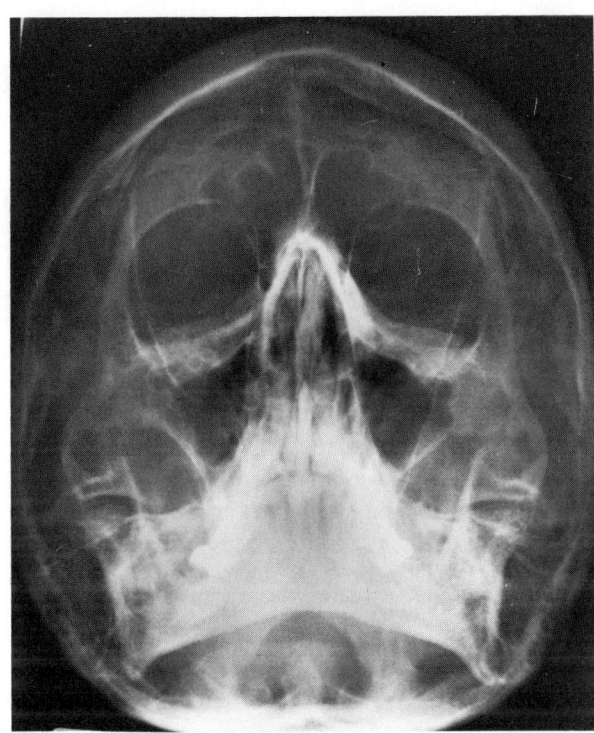

Figure 84-6 View of facial bones. *Note:* Head tilted back (Waters' projection).

due to severe injuries, the necessity of elaborate follow-up, the likelihood for successful repair being low, or the patient asking for a consultation or acting in a litigious manner.

Management of Soft Tissue Injuries

All soft tissue injuries regardless of location require consideration of tetanus prophylaxis. Patients with no history of prior tetanus immunization need treatment with tetanus hyperimmune globulin (Hypertet) as well as initiation of their tetanus immunization series. Patients with up-to-date immunization (within 5 years) but with grossly contaminated wounds probably should also have Hypertet. Normal wounds require only that the patient's last immunization be within the previous 5 to 10 years, with many institutions favoring the 5-year figure. Comatose patients with soft tissue injuries should receive a tetanus immunization.

The decision may be made not to close the soft tissue wound in the emergency department. This is indicated if the patient is unstable from other injuries. In this case, hemostasis should be achieved, the tissues of the wound loosely approximated, the wound covered with saline-soaked gauze, an occlusive dressing applied, and the patient started on antibiotics. Wound age may also be a consideration. Most wounds on the face can be closed up to 24 hours post injury. Older injuries should be referred for delayed primary closure. If the wound contains a foreign body or contamination that cannot be removed, it should not be closed. Severely contaminated wounds (eg, bites, pavement injuries) should be closed only if they are less than 6 hours old. Any wound covering a fracture that will require later reduction should not be closed but rather dressed as noted previously. All injuries that are not closed primarily should be carefully irrigated and dressed, and the patient should be given antibiotics.

Wound anesthesia is usually straightforward in maxillofacial injuries. Local infiltration of 1% lidocaine with 1:100,000 epinephrine will suffice in most cases, although epinephrine should not be used around the ear or the tarsal plate of the eye owing to the relative avascular nature of these structures. Plain lidocaine may also be preferable around large flaps that have tenuous circulation and about the nose. Up to 30 mL of 1% lidocaine and up to 60 mL of 0.5% lidocaine may be used. Infiltration is done with the smallest needle possible through the wound margins. Topical anesthesia with a tetracaine-adrenaline-cocaine mixture (TAC) is advocated by some, but it must be used with care and must not be used near mucous membranes.

Additional anesthesia may be achieved, if necessary, through a regional block. Sensory innervation of the face is illustrated in Figure 84-4. One or 2 mL of 1% lidocaine instilled at the exit foramen of any of the major branches of the trigeminal nerve will produce anesthesia in the distribution of that branch. If both local and regional anesthesia are to be used, the regional block should be done first, with local augmentation supplied where necessary.

Children may require systemic analgesia to facilitate a facial repair. Meperidine (1 mg/kg), a meperidine-promethazine-chlorpromazine combination, or ketamine may be administered intramuscularly. The disadvantages of this approach include the additional time required for the medication to take effect and the necessity of close monitoring of the patient's respiratory status, both during and after the repair. Fentanyl may also be used intravenously to establish sedation in children. Its use also requires careful respiratory monitoring of the patient. A "papoose board" is also advisable for restraint of small children. Care must be used to not overaggressively restrain young children, since this has resulted in respiratory arrest.

Wounds should be cleansed vigorously. Irrigation with a jet stream of normal saline (500 mL nominally) is preferred. Topical anesthesia of wounds requiring scrubbing (eg, those with imbedded material) may be achieved through application of 4% lidocaine solution. To avoid a traumatic tattoo (which requires extensive treatment later for correction), all imbedded material should be removed. Any material not removed by scrubbing should be carefully picked out with a No. 11 scalpel blade or 16-gauge needle.

Following cleansing, the wound should be thoroughly explored for any retained material, fractures of the bony skeleton, or injury to any specialized structures (eg, lacrimal apparatus of the eye). Any devitalized tissue is then debrided, but conservatively so, limited if possible to 1 to 2 mm at the wound edge. Any excision of irreplaceable structures, such as the philtrum (Cupid's bow) of the lip, should be avoided. Clinical judgment is sometimes required to decide if closing a large defect might produce more scarring and deformity than allowing the wound to granulate in, with subsequent plastic revision if necessary. Any beveled wound edges should be revised so the edges of the wound are perpendicular to the surface, resulting in a smaller, smoother scar.

In all but the most superficial of wounds, a layered closure should be performed. The deep layers should be approximated with 4-0 or 5-0 absorbable sutures. The absorbable synthetics are probably superior because they last longer and cause less tissue reaction than chromic sutures. The skin layer is then closed with 5-0 or 6-0 monofilament synthetic nonabsorbable sutures. Landmarks, such as wrinkles, eyebrows, and the vermilion border of the lips should be approximated first to ensure continuity of these highly visible structures. The remainder of the wound may then be closed with interrupted simple or running sutures.

Dressings are usually not required over facial lacerations unless the patient is a child or a large forehead laceration has been repaired. A circumferential head pressure dressing is advisable in the latter case to minimize hematoma formation. Adhesive bandages may be used in an attempt to avoid having a child pick at a wound. In all other cases, a thin layer of water-soluble antibiotic ointment is adequate.

Ongoing wound care consists of two basic principles: (1) keep the wound clean, removing any dried blood or serum with water or saline as needed, and (2) keep the wound soft and pliable, which is done by applying water-soluble antibiotic ointment several times per day. The patient should be informed of signs and symptoms of wound infection. Follow-up arrangements should be made for suture removal (normally in 4 to 6 days). Antibiotic usage during healing is probably only required in heavily contaminated wounds, such as animal or human bites.

Lip Injuries

The most important aspect of repair of lip injuries is the meticulous approximation of the vermilion border. Because infiltration of anesthetic may obliterate this border, the physician may wish to mark this structure on opposite sides of the wound with a small needle scratch prior to infiltration. A layered closure should be employed here if the injury violates the subcutaneous tissue. Violation of the muscular layer (the orbicularis oris) mandates that this tissue be approximated with suture to avoid a defect that will be noticed with lip movement. When placing the skin sutures, the first stitch should approximate the vermilion borders. The skin external to the lip may then be closed with synthetic nonabsorbable sutures. The vermilion section is then closed using fine silk for comfort with lip movement.

Mouth and Tongue Injuries

All but the most insignificant intraoral lacerations should be sutured. To not do so runs the risk of increased scar formation and subsequent functional impairment or a permanent soft tissue defect that may impair oral hygiene. Treatment of tongue lacerations follows the standard of a deep layer of absorbable suture if necessary, followed by a mucosal layer of silk or synthetic absorbable sutures. This exterior layer should have many knots placed to avoid having the tongue untie the suture material. Mucosal lacerations of the mouth are handled in a similar manner. Through-and-through lacerations (eg, through the cheek into the oral cavity) require a three-layered closure. After irrigation, a watertight closure is made of the mucosal surface, using silk or synthetic absorbable sutures. The competency of this layer is tested by irrigating the wound from outside the mouth and checking for solution leaking into the mouth. The subcutaneous tissue and skin are then closed from outside in the standard manner. Patients with through-and-through lacerations and those with significant oral lacerations should have a course of antibiotics: 5 to 7 days of oral penicillin is probably adequate. Oral wound care consists of rinsing the mouth with a mild antiseptic three or four times per day.

The physician should be suspicious of all oral lacerations in the area of the parotid ducts or submandibular ducts. Patency of these structures should be demonstrated by milking the associated salivary gland and watching for flow of saliva from the duct. If there is a question of violation of these structures, the patient should be referred for careful exploration of the area.

Ear Injuries

The major principle in treating ear injuries is the preservation of as much of the cartilaginous structure as possible. Small lacerations may be anesthetized by direct infiltration with lidocaine without epinephrine (due to the relative avascularity). Large defects are best anesthetized by raising a wheal around the base of the entire ear on the scalp. This will anesthetize all but the external canal and the concha, which may be directly infiltrated if necessary.

Injuries involving the cartilage require careful irrigation and closure of the perichondrium with fine absorbable sutures, followed by skin closure. If skin tissue loss does not allow the cartilage to be covered adequately, a consultant should be called in, since the cartilage may be saved in a subcutaneous pocket for later reconstruction. After repair, the ear should be splinted with wet cotton balls molded about the ear and held in place by a circumferential head bandage. Antibiotics are indicated if the perichondrium has been violated owing to the risk of a low-grade chondritis.

Injuries to the ear not violating the skin but causing swelling also require careful attention. The swelling is often a subperichondrial hematoma, which, if not treated, will calcify, forming a "cauliflower ear." This injury is treated by aseptically aspirating the blood and applying a compression dressing, as noted above, for 5 to 7 days.

Eye Injuries

Probably the most common eye injury is the corneal abrasion, an injury to the corneal epithelium due to direct trauma. These lesions are clearly seen with fluorescein stain under a Wood's light. Treatment is straightforward. The eye is anesthetized with topical ophthalmic solution, antibiotic ointment is placed in the eye, and the eye is patched. The patient is discharged with a prescription for oral pain medication and is told to consult an ophthalmologist in 24 hours for reevaluation. The patient should not drive with an eye patched because of the acute loss of binocular vision.

A related corneal injury is superficial keratitis or "flash burn" caused by ultraviolet radiation exposure. This uncomfortable entity is diagnosed by history and fluorescein stain. Treatment is identical for a corneal abrasion with the addition of instillation of a mydriatic (eg, homatropine) before patching to help decrease the patient's discomfort.

Foreign bodies on the surface of the eye require careful inspection after application of topical anesthetic. This evaluation is best done with a slit lamp, although magnifying glasses may be adequate. Careful attention is paid to the entire globe as well as to the conjunctival surfaces of the lids. The upper lid should be everted to allow careful inspection. Most foreign bodies may be removed by a moist cotton-tipped applicator, but some corneal foreign bodies may require sharp removal with an eye spud or a needle. After removal of the object, antibiotic ointment is instilled as above. The eye should be patched with ophthalmologic follow-up in 24 hours.

Chemical burns to the eye represent a true ocular emergency since the action taken immediately following the injury is of extreme importance. The patient's eye should be copiously irrigated immediately after the accident. Specific neutralizing agents should not be used since the heat produced by the chemical reaction could further damage the eye. Immediately after arrival in the emergency department, the patient should have the affected eye locally anesthetized and gently irrigated with normal saline. If the chemical in question is alkali, the irrigation should continue until the pH of the eye returns to 7.0 (as tested by pH paper) since alkali is not inactivated by the tissues (as acid is) and therefore can continue to cause tissue destruction until physically removed. After irrigation, the injured eye should have a mydriatic and antibiotic ointment instilled and a patch applied. All ocular burns require ophthalmologic follow-up. The treatment of severe chemical burns, especially those caused by alkali, should be discussed with an ophthalmologist.

Corneal and scleral lacerations require immediate attention by an ophthalmologist. Nothing should be placed in the eye. It should be covered by a metal protective patch that gently covers the globe. The patient should be admitted to the hospital and kept fasting in the event that surgery is required.

Hyphemas, or gross blood in the anterior chamber due to direct blunt trauma, are not uncommonly seen in the emergency department. Patients with hyphemas should be admitted to the hospital and kept in a 30° head-elevated position to allow the blood to layer out and clot. Bilateral eye patches may help to decrease eye motion.

Intraocular foreign bodies represent a true ocular emergency that may not be appreciated even by the careful examiner. Any patient with ocular trauma from flying material must be assumed to have an intraocular injury until proved otherwise. Intraocular foreign bodies may be difficult to demonstrate if they are not radiodense. Posteroanterior and lateral orbital radiographs will help locate metallic foreign bodies. The localization of nonmetallic foreign bodies may require the assistance of an ophthalmologist. These patients should be admitted to the hospital.

Lacerations of the eyelids are not uncommon. Simple lacerations not involving the lid margin may be closed in the standard layered technique using 6-0 suture material, and the eye is patched. Lacerations involving the lid margin require meticulous technique and are best left for a plastic surgeon or ophthalmologist to repair. If necessary, artificial tears should be used to keep the cornea moist until the lid is repaired. Any laceration near the medial canthus requires that the integrity of the lacrimal apparatus be demonstrated by probing with a nylon or polypropylene suture and making sure it does not appear in the wound. Any violation of this structure requires repair by an ophthalmologist. (See Chapter 81, Ocular Emergencies.)

Eyebrow Injuries

The repair of soft tissue injuries of the eyebrow is straightforward. Debridement should be kept to a minimum. The eyebrow should not be shaved because it is a vital landmark in the repair. Any revision of the wound should be done parallel to the hair follicle roots (as opposed to perpendicular to the skin as is usually the case) to minimize any bald area in the resultant scar. The first sutures should be placed to align the borders of the eyebrow to avoid any step defect.

Nasal Injuries

Nasal injuries include bony and soft tissue injuries. Nasal fractures may result in either lateral or posterior displacement of the bony fragments. Edema, epistaxis, tenderness, deformity, crepitus, and/or hypermobility are part of the clinical presentation. Radiographs are of limited usefulness except for documentation purposes. Gross lateral deformity can sometimes be corrected in the emergency department by lateral pressure. In all cases of documented or suspected fracture, follow-up 5 to 7 days post injury is necessary to evaluate the nose after the swelling subsides. A high index of suspicion should be maintained for nasal fractures in children because the growth potential of the nose may be disrupted by an unrecognized fracture. In children, tenderness, swelling, and post-traumatic epistaxis are sufficient grounds to arrange for follow-up in 3 to 5 days.

In all cases of nasal trauma, the physician must be careful to check for a nasal septum hematoma. This presents as a big, bulging, purple grapelike structure on the septum. If such a lesion is missed, septal necrosis may ensue. Treatment involves a small vertical incision over the hematoma to drain it, an anterior nasal pack to guard against reaccumulation, oral antibiotics, and follow-up by an otolaryngologist or plastic surgeon.

Soft tissue injuries to the nose are best repaired with a combination of regional and local anesthesia. An infraorbital and supratrochlear block may be used. (The supratrochlear nerve is located 1.5 cm medial to the supraorbital foramen.) A layered closure should be used, with careful attention to covering any exposed cartilage and with diligent irrigation after each layer. The nasal skin may be closed with a running subcuticular stitch of absorbable suture material to avoid the common problem of stitch abscesses in this area.

Abrasion/Avulsion Injuries

Facial abrasion/avulsion injuries are commonly seen when the patient's face impacts and skids along a roughened surface, such as highway pavement or a fractured windshield. The result is an area of abrasion with numerous small avulsions, some of which may contain foreign material (eg, gravel, glass). These wounds require vigorous cleansing to avoid traumatic tattooing of the skin. All avulsion wounds require careful inspection and probing to ensure maximum removal of foreign material. In such injuries, it is not uncommon to find shards of glass deeply imbedded in the subcutaneous tissues.

All full-thickness wound areas should be closed with nonabsorbable synthetic suture. Antibiotic gauze should then be applied to the entire area to help in the reepithelization of the wound. Suture removal may be delayed to the seventh day to allow for adequate healing and for the gauze to loosen. The patient should be informed that the resultant healed wound may be uneven and "pebbly." This may be treated at a later date through dermabrasion.

Management of Fractures and Dislocations

Mandibular Fractures

Mandibular fractures are the third most common facial fracture, following nasal and zygomatic fractures. The cardinal sign of a mandibular fracture is dental malocclusion that is either observed or noted when the patient relates that his or her teeth do not "fit right." These patients also have mandibular pain and tenderness. A step in dentition or an ecchymosis in the floor of the mouth are also indicators of fracture of the mandible. Any patient with these signs or symptoms following trauma must have a mandibular fracture ruled out. This is most elegantly done by a Panorex radiograph of the mandible. Failing that, standard anteroposterior and lateral views are obtained.

Because the mandible is a ring-type structure, the traumatic impact may be transmitted about the ring, causing a fracture remote from the site of impact. This also explains the high (50%) incidence of multiple fractures of the mandible.

Most patients with mandibular fractures require admission to the hospital for occlusal fixation. If bony fragments are seen in the mouth or if periodontal bleeding is present near the site of the fracture, the fracture is considered an open fracture. These patients should be started on antibiotic therapy.

Temporomandibular Joint Dislocation

Dislocation of the temporomandibular joint (TMJ) may be seen following trauma or after opening the mouth excessively wide (eg, with a yawn). Unilateral or bilateral dislocations may be present. In either case, the patient is unable to close the mouth and will have moderate TMJ discomfort, which will worsen with the passage of time owing to increased spasm of the muscles of mastication. If the dislocation is secondary to trauma, mandibular radiographs should be obtained prior to reduction to rule out a possible condylar fracture; TMJ dislocation occurs anteriorly and superiorly and is usually easily reduced by reversing this movement. This is accomplished by the physician placing gauze-wrapped thumbs (to avoid injury) on the patient's lower third molars with the fingers curled under the symphysis of the mandible. The mandibular condyles are then levered down with downward pressure on the molars and upward pressure on the symphysis of the mandible. The mandible is then slipped posteriorly for the completed reduction. If difficulty is encountered, diazepam or midazolam may be administered intravenously to help overcome the muscle spasm. Postreduction radiographs are indicated if this is an initial TMJ dislocation for the patient. After reduction, if pain free, the patient may be discharged on a soft diet with instructions to avoid opening the mouth wide. However, if significant spasm or tenderness is present, admission for fixation of the mandible should be considered.

Maxillary Fractures

Maxillary fractures are usually seen as the result of massive facial trauma, frequently coexisting with other life-threatening injuries. These patients present with facial swelling, mid-face mobility to palpation, malocclusion, and/or cerebrospinal-fluid rhinorrhea. Radiographic diagnosis is made by the Waters' and lateral facial-bone views. These fractures were classified, based on location, by Le Fort as Le

Fort I, II, or III fractures (Fig. 84-7). All combinations of these fractures may be seen (eg, a Le Fort I on one side, with a Le Fort II on the other).

Patients with maxillary fractures all require admission to the hospital. Emergency care consists of airway maintenance and ruling out other concomitant injuries. To protect the airway, intubation or, in severe cases, cricothyrotomy may be required. If cerebrospinal-fluid rhinorrhea is present, the patient should be kept in a head-elevated position and started on antibiotic therapy.

Zygomatic Fractures

Zygomatic fractures are often caused by deceleration injuries. A common zygomatic fracture is the tripod fracture with fracture lines at the zygomaticotemporal suture, the zygomaticofrontal suture, and through the infraorbital foramen. These patients may present with a bony step defect, infraorbital hypoesthesia, flatness of the malar eminence, diplopia, or change in consensual gaze. An isolated fracture of the zygomatic arch is often due to a roundhouse punch. These patients have tenderness over the arch and may have painful or limited mandibular movement due to encroachment by the arch on the mandible. Radiographs required to evaluate the zygoma include the Waters' view and the submentovertex view.

All patients with zygomatic fractures require referral for possible elevation and fixation. If mandibular motion is not compromised and in the absence of other injuries, these patients may be followed as outpatients.

Orbital Floor Fractures

Fractures of the orbital floor are commonly seen following application of substantial force to the globe of the eye. This force is transmitted hydraulically to the interior orbit, fracturing the weakest portion, the inframedial area. Because of the architecture of the external orbit, the eye is well protected except from those objects less than 5 cm in radius (eg, a knuckle or handball). As a result of the fracture, the inferior extraocular muscles may become entrapped or the fatty tissue surrounding the globe may herniate into the maxillary sinus. Muscle entrapment gives rise to diplopia and loss of full extraocular movements, especially upward gaze. Herniation of orbital contents may produce enophthalmos or the "hanging drop" sign on the radiograph. The patient may also present with infraorbital hypoesthesia. However, the patient may have none of these findings and still a fracture may be seen on the radiograph. It should be stressed that clouding of a maxillary sinus or an air-fluid level in a maxillary sinus without other explanation must be taken as indirect evidence of an orbital fracture until proved otherwise (Fig. 84-8). These patients all require careful follow-up since operative intervention may be required to ensure proper binocular vision. Immediate admission is usually not indicated.

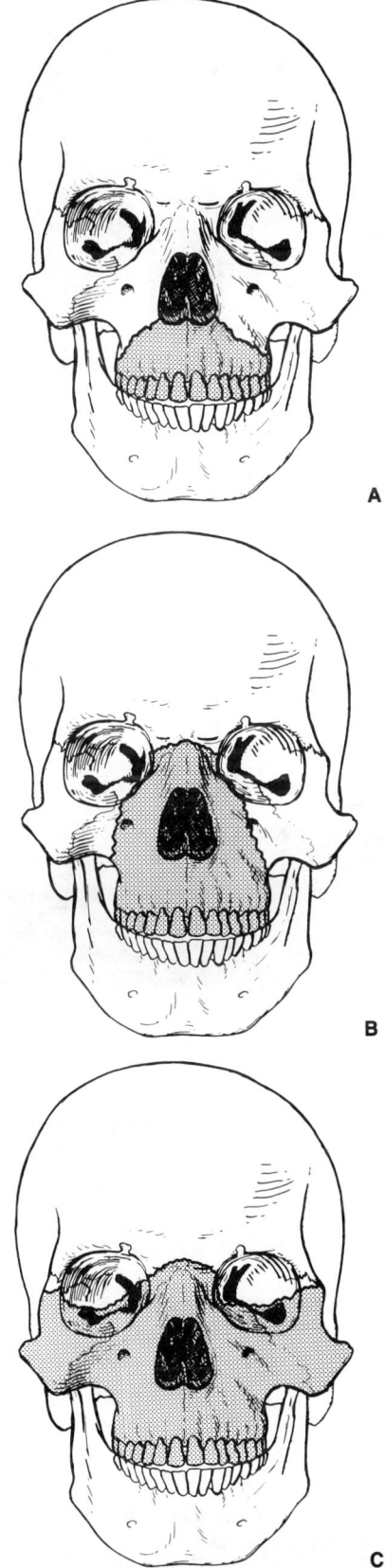

Figure 84-7 Classification of mid-face fractures by Le Fort: **A**: Le Fort I, **B**: II, and **C**: III.

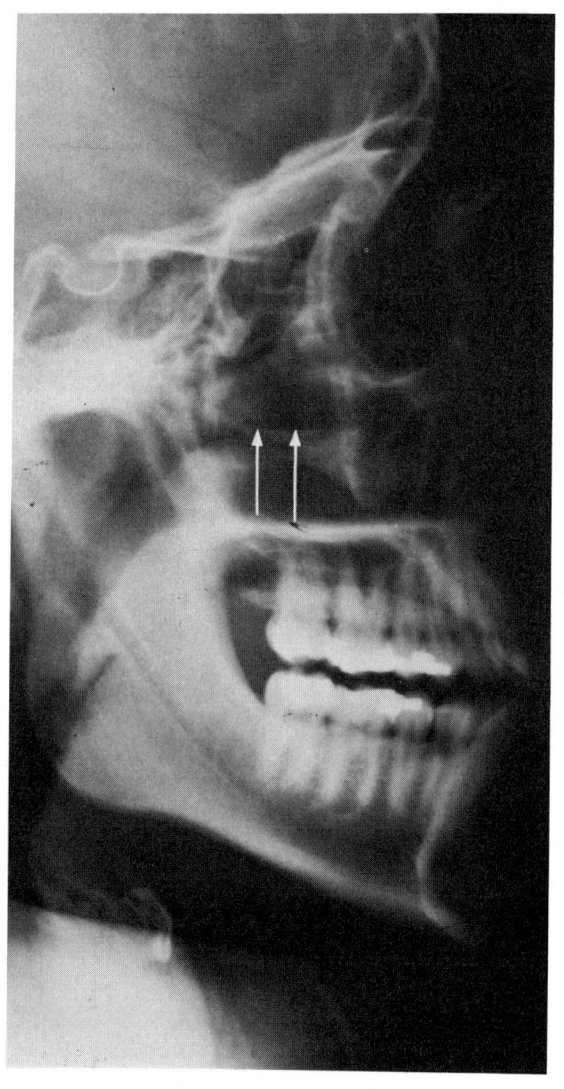
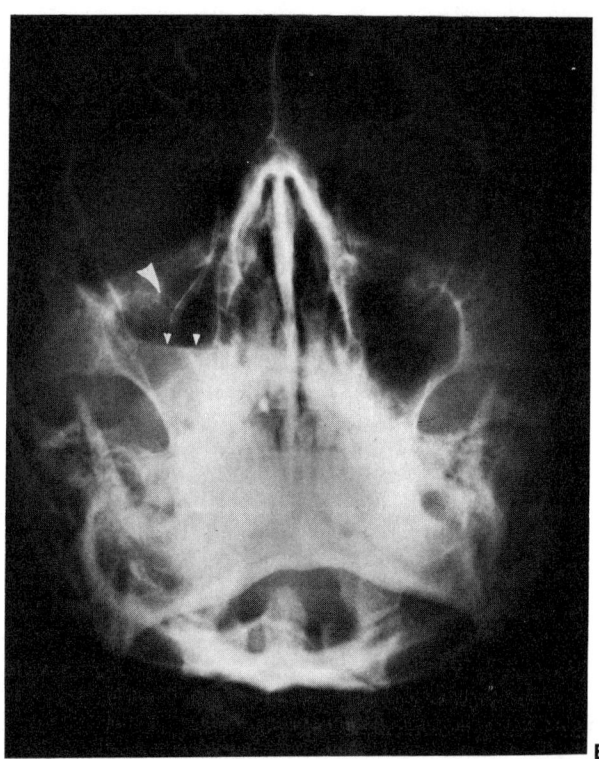

Figure 84-8 A: Upright lateral roentgenogram of the face demonstrating an air-fluid level in the maxillary sinus. **B:** Upright Waters' view roentgenogram of the face. *Note:* The small arrows demonstrate the air-fluid level in the right maxillary sinus shown in *A*. The large arrow points to the herniated orbital contents. The findings suggest a "blowout" fracture of the right orbit.

BIBLIOGRAPHY

Baker SP, Schultz RC. Recurrent problems in emergency room management of maxillofacial injuries. *Clin Plast Surg.* 1975;2:65–71.

Carroll MJ, Hill CM, Mason DA. Facial fractures in children. *Br Dent J.* 1987;163:23–26.

Converse JM, et al. *Reconstructive Plastic Surgery.* Philadelphia, Pa: WB Saunders Co; 1977:2.

Curtis JW. Basic plastic surgical techniques in repair of facial lacerations. *Surg Clin North Am.* 1973;53:33–46.

Dingman RO, Natvig P. *Surgery of Facial Fractures.* Philadelphia, Pa: WB Saunders Co; 1969.

Dolan K, Jacoby C, Smoker W. The radiology of facial fractures. *Radiographics.* 1984;4:4.

Dushoff IM. About face. *Emerg Med.* 1979;11:59–111.

Gentry LR, Smoker WRK. Computed tomography of facial trauma. *Semin Ultrasound CT MR.* 1985;6:129.

Hegenbarth MA, et al. Comparison of topical tetracaine, adrenaline and cocaine anesthesia with lidocaine infiltration for repair of lacerations in children. *Ann Emerg Med.* 1990;19:63–67.

Luce EA, Tubb TD, Moore AM. Review of 1000 major facial fractures and associated injuries. *Plast Reconstruct Surg.* 1979;63:26–30.

Paletta FX. Soft tissue injuries of face and scalp. *Clin Plast Surg.* 1977;4:479–490.

Schultz RC. *Facial Injuries.* 2nd ed. Chicago, Ill: Year Book Medical Publishers; 1977.

Schultz RC, Oldham RJ. An overview of facial injuries. *Surg Clin North Am.* 1977;57:987–1010.

Shepherd SM, Lippe MS. Maxillofacial trauma: evaluation and management by the emergency physician. *Emerg Med Clin North Am.* 1987;5:371–392.

Sinclair D, et al. A retrospective review of the relationship between facial fractures, head injuries, and cervical spine injuries. *J Emerg Med.* 1988;6:109.

Steele MT, et al. Prophylactic penicillin for intraoral wounds. *Ann Emerg Med.* 1989;18:847–852.

Tsai FY, Teal JS, Hieshima GB. *Neuroradiology of Head Trauma.* Baltimore, Md: University Park Press; 1984.

Winspur I. Facial fractures and the ED physician. *Emerg Med Serv.* May/June 1979:31–36.

Zook EG, ed. *The Primary Care of Facial Injuries.* Littleton, Mass: PSG Publishing Co; 1980.

85. Dental Emergencies

JOHN P. KELLY, DMD, MD

Personnel in primary contact with patients seeking emergency care will frequently encounter complaints related to the oropharynx. The widespread prevalence of dental decay and the high incidence of pathology in and about the oral cavity will often result in acute symptoms for which the patient will seek emergency care. The nature of the patient's symptoms or the timing of their onset commonly brings the patient to the nondental practitioner for whom the diseases of the oral cavity are unfamiliar.

With this review of the emergency conditions arising in the teeth, jaws, and oral soft tissues, the emergency care personnel with first contact with the patient will be more confident and capable of appropriate triage, emergency treatment, and definitive referral for continued care. Provision of adequate analgesia and initiation of antibiotic therapy where appropriate are the most critical components of initial emergency care.

ODONTOGENIC INFECTION

Pathology and Pathophysiology

Dental caries is the most prevalent disease in the United States. The action of oral microbes on the teeth in the presence of dietary carbohydrates and in the absence of adequate oral hygiene produces decalcification of enamel and subsequent decay of the underlying dentin. As decay progresses, recognizable patterns of pain will be described by the patient. The sensory receptors of the tooth are solely pain receptors; hence thermal or pressure stimuli are perceived only as painful stimuli by the dental pulp.

Incipient dental decay is only mildly symptomatic, producing mild pain when hot or cold liquids or sweet substances are ingested. The pain may be difficult to localize to an individual tooth, but the minimal and transient nature of the pain rarely brings such a patient to an emergency care facility.

As decay progresses deeper into the dentin and approaches the pulp chamber, the pulp becomes inflamed. The pain becomes considerably more debilitating; it may be stimulated by extremes of temperature, but it may also appear spontaneously and be unremitting, relieved only by therapeutic doses of narcotic analgesics. The same syndrome of pain can be experienced following restorative dental procedures when a filling is placed close to the pulp of the tooth. A fractured tooth can produce the same symptoms. In children, the pulpitis may be reversible; but in adults, the pulp usually becomes necrotic as a result of the inflammatory process.

When the necrotic pulp is infected, pain returns as the first evidence of a developing abscess. The pain in this instance is usually incited or aggravated by hot liquids and relieved by cold. Most often, the patient can localize the pain to a particular tooth with referral of pain from a mandibular tooth to the ear and from a maxillary tooth to the periorbital area. However, paradoxical referral of pain may make it difficult for the patient to determine whether the offending tooth is in the upper or lower jaw. Fever, swelling, and leukocytosis are not seen when the pain arises from a necrotic pulp.

Spread of infection from the necrotic pulp to the alveolar bone surrounding the root of the tooth gives a significant additional finding. The involved tooth is tender to the pressure of biting force; tenderness can be elicited by percussion of the tooth, and the tooth may be mobile. Palpation of the soft tissues overlying the root may reveal fullness, frank swelling, or fluctuance as the abscess proceeds from the alveolus to the surrounding periosteum and adjacent soft tissue planes. The accompanying swelling usually spreads to the submandibular area from an infected mandibular tooth; abscessed maxillary teeth characteristically produce a cellulitis involving the cheek and periorbital tissues. The patient may present with malaise, fever, and leukocytosis.

An untreated alveolar abscess may progress to life-threatening infection if the process reaches the fascial spaces of the floor of the mouth (Ludwig's angina) or the vascular drainage system of the maxilla (cavernous sinus thrombosis). (See Fig. 85-1.)

Painful infection associated with the soft tissues around partially erupted wisdom teeth is a frequently seen condition in the young adult population. In its mildest form, pericoronitis produces symptoms described as "teething." The more severe infections are accompanied by constant, throbbing pain, worsened by attempting to close the teeth together; the patient may be unable to open the mouth, the trismus resulting from spasm of the masticatory muscles adjacent to the mandibular third molars.

Diagnosis

A thorough history is required for evaluation of odontogenic pain and swelling. The various stages of dental infection have such individual historical characteristics that the diagnosis can often be made by addressing the specific questions of the pain's nature, onset, severity, duration, location, radiation, and aggravating and ameliorating factors (Table 85-1).

Initial examination requires comfortable positioning of the patient and a suitable lighting fixture for illuminating the mouth while leaving the examiner's hands free. Inspection of the mouth for fractured, decayed, or extensively restored teeth and inflammation or swelling of the soft tissues is easily accomplished. Palpation of the oral structures and percussion of the teeth with the handle of a dental mirror will aid in localization of the offending tooth; mobility and painful response to percussion are significant findings, as are the nature and location of any swelling.

Unless dental radiography equipment is available in the emergency care location, radiographic studies are best deferred.

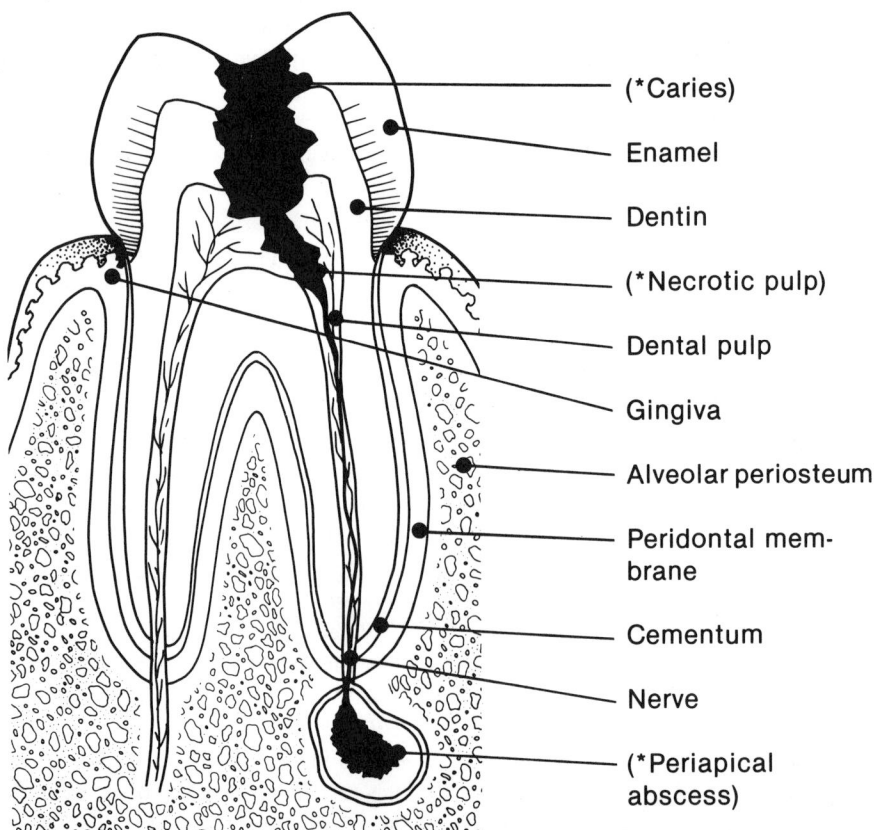

Figure 85-1 Abscessed tooth and gum. *Note:* * denotes abnormal conditions.

Table 85-1 Differential Diagnosis of Dental Pain

Disorder	Pain	Swelling	Emergency Treatment	Definitive Treatment
Decay	Dull; response to heat, cold, sweets	None	Analgesics	Dental restoration
Pulpitis	Sharp; response to heat, cold; may be spontaneous	None	Analgesics	Endodontic treatment or extraction
Pulpal necrosis	Throbbing; response to heat; relieved by cold	None	Analgesics	Endodontic treatment or extraction
Periapical abscess	Throbbing; tender to percussion or chewing	Usually none	Analgesics, antibiotics	Endodontic or surgical treatment
Alveolar abscess	Aching; tender to palpation	Present	Antibiotics, drainage	Surgical treatment

Source: Adapted from Kelly JP: Evaluation of facial pain and swelling, in Goroll AH, May LA, Mullae AG (eds): *Primary Care Medicine.* Philadelphia, JB Lippincott, 1981.

Laboratory studies are not indicated unless the odontogenic infection has produced systemic symptoms. In the latter case, white blood-cell count and differential, blood sugar, and blood cultures may aid in subsequent management.

Differential Diagnosis

Differential diagnosis of odontogenic pain must include the various neuralgias (eg, trigeminal, glossopharyngeal), maxillary sinusitis, salivary gland infection, masticatory muscle spasm, or temporomandibular joint afflictions. The nondental sources of pain often are more chronic; acute exacerbation may lead the patient to seek emergency care, but definitive diagnosis and treatment are better deferred to the neurologist, oral and maxillofacial surgeon, or otorhinolaryngologist.

Treatment

Dental pain from caries, pulpitis, or pulpal necrosis requires referral to a dentist for definitive care; emergency treatment is confined to analgesic prescription. Codeine, oxycodone, or another of the synthetic narcotics in combination with aspirin or acetaminophen will usually be required. There is no evidence to suggest the use of antibiotics for these conditions. Emergency care by the dentist or endodontist may be appropriate.

When dental pain is accompanied by swelling or by the earlier signs of tooth mobility and sensitivity to percussion, initiation of antibiotic treatment is mandatory. The drug of choice is penicillin V, the usual dosage being 250 mg orally every 4 to 6 hours for 10 days. The alternative drug for patients allergic to penicillin is erythromycin in the same dosage. Tetracyclines, ampicillin, the cephalosporins, and other antibiotics have no place in the initial management of odontogenic infection, because the offending organisms are sensitive to penicillin in nearly all cases. A change in antibiotic is only mandated by subsequent sensitivity testing of cultured pathogens.

Treatment of acute pericoronitis associated with the erupting wisdom tooth is initiated with penicillin or erythromycin in the same dosage described above. Frequent mouth rinses with dilute hydrogen peroxide and the extraoral application of warm compresses will help to provide symptomatic relief.

Evaluation by an oral and maxillofacial surgeon is critical for the patient with facial cellulitis to determine the need for incision and drainage, tooth extraction, or other early management. Patients with toxic systemic symptoms or with massive swelling involving the airway may require hospital admission for parenteral antibiotic therapy and definitive care.

DENTOALVEOLAR TRAUMA

Fractured and Avulsed Teeth

The etiology of fractured teeth is similar to the causes of jaw fractures. (See Chapter 84, Maxillofacial Injuries.) They include injuries sustained in motor vehicle accidents, contact sports, and altercations. These minor injuries frequently may be accompanied by more severe problems, but, commonly, they are seen as isolated injuries or as trauma concomitant with such minor wounds as lip and chin lacerations. Hence, triage personnel must be familiar with the appropriate diagnosis and early management of such dental injuries.

Pathophysiology

The anterior teeth are most often those that are fractured or avulsed. The anatomic form of these teeth is a significant factor in their susceptibility, although their exposed location is obviously most important.

Whenever trauma to the anterior mouth is recognized, careful examination of the patient to rule out fractures of the mandibular condyles must be carried out. The condyles are most often fractured by a blow to the chin. Consequently, an innocent-appearing chin laceration or anterior chipped tooth may signify a more serious injury, one that can become much more difficult to manage and treat successfully if it is not recognized at the earliest opportunity.

Diagnosis

Management of chipped teeth will depend on the amount of tooth structure that has been lost (Fig. 85-2). The simple enamel fracture is uncomfortable only to the extent that it presents a sharp or rough surface to the tongue and lip. Loss of enamel and dentin produces mild sensitivity to cold air and liquids. Exposure of the pulp of the tooth is exquisitely painful when the pulp is contacted by cold air or by the tongue or lip.

Teeth that have been loosened by trauma must be evaluated by dental radiographs to determine whether or not the mobility of the teeth is due to fractured roots or to partial avulsion of the tooth from the alveolar bone. Apparent mobility of the teeth is observed when an alveolar segment (teeth and their surrounding bone) is fractured. Complete avulsion of anterior teeth is also common; the preexisting status of the surrounding soft tissues and alveolar bone must be assessed in order to determine the feasibility of replanting the tooth.

Treatment

Minor fractures of enamel or dentin require no emergency treatment; routine dental restorative measures can be carried out to return the teeth to a comfortable and aesthetic condition.

A tooth fractured to the level of the pulp demands immediate attention in order to relieve patient discomfort. If the fracture is above the level of the alveolar bone, then immediate extirpation of the pulp and subsequent endodontic treatment can be carried out. However, if the fracture line extends below the level of the alveolar bone, extraction of the tooth and its root is usually necessary.

Partially avulsed teeth may be repositioned with light finger pressure; local anesthesia may be necessary. Splinting of the teeth to adjacent teeth with wires, arch bars, or other suitable appliances should be carried out by the oral surgeon or dentist as an emergency procedure.

Replantation of completely avulsed teeth should always be attempted unless the condition of the surrounding bone and soft tissues or the patient's general condition makes such a procedure impossible. Prior to replantation, the tooth should be kept clean and moist. The best method of transport for the tooth is in the socket itself, if the patient can be instructed to do so prior to arrival in the emergency department. If the patient is unable to reposition the tooth, the tooth should be carried in the floor of the mouth. When the patient is uncoop-

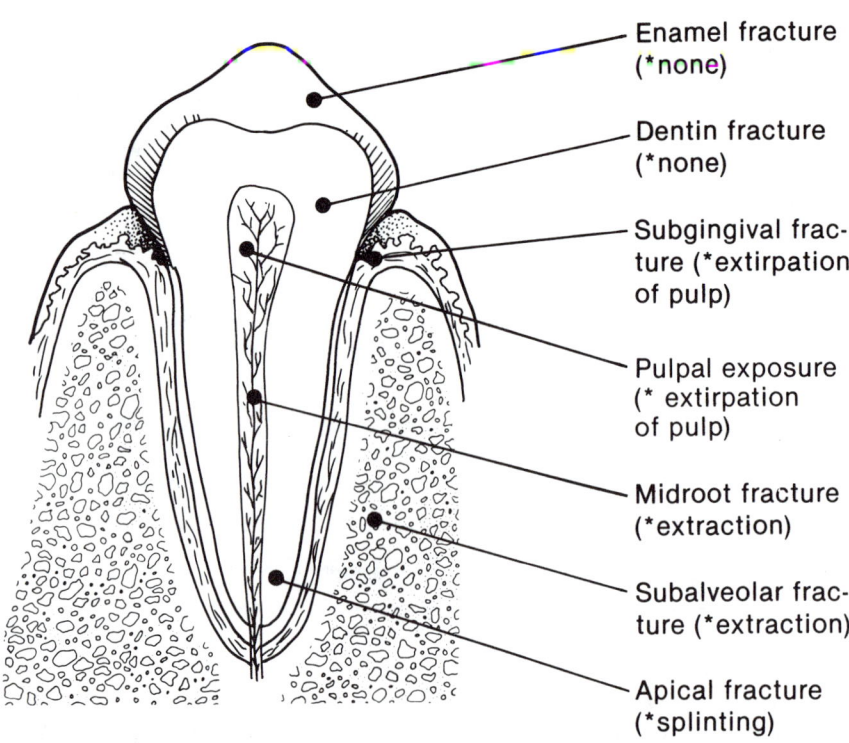

Figure 85-2 Tooth and gum anatomy. *Note:* * denotes recommended emergency treatment.

erative or otherwise unable to transport the tooth in this fashion, the tooth should be wrapped in clean, moistened gauze—it should neither be immersed nor allowed to dry. The oral surgeon should be consulted for definitive replanting and splinting of the tooth.

Fractured primary teeth can be treated in the same fashion described above for permanent teeth. Avulsed deciduous teeth are never replanted; when they are partially avulsed, they will usually require extraction.

Alveolar segment fractures are managed by wiring the teeth in the fractured segment to adjacent stable teeth.

TEMPOROMANDIBULAR JOINT DISLOCATION

Acute emergency conditions relating to the temporomandibular joint are confined to fractures, post-traumatic joint effusion, and dislocations. Fractures of the mandibular condyle have been previously discussed. Joint effusions in the absence of fracture are easily managed with warm compresses and analgesic and anti-inflammatory agents.

Pathophysiology of Dislocation

Dislocation of one or both temporomandibular joints is the result of displacement of the condylar process of the mandible anterior to the articular eminence of the temporal bone. The usual inciting event is a blow received while the mouth is open. Secondary muscle spasm prevents the mandible from returning to its normal position with the condyle in the glenoid fossa posterior to the articular eminence.

Diagnosis

The patient with a dislocated mandible presents with an open mouth that cannot be closed voluntarily; if the dislocation is unilateral, the jaw will be deviated to the opposite side. Because of the inability to close the mouth, the patient may be unable to swallow and, consequently, the common presentation will include drooling of saliva. Pain is a variable symptom with dislocation; in the presence of muscle spasm, pain and tenderness in the masseter muscle will be significant. The dislocated condyle can be palpated as a lateral prominence 1 or 2 cm anterior to the tragus of the ear.

Differential Diagnosis

Extrapyramidal reaction to a wide variety of drugs can produce symptoms similar to those of jaw dislocation. Phenothiazine tranquilizing agents, antihistamines, and antiemetic medications have all been implicated. The clinical signs of dislocation are absent in this instance. An intravenous dose of 50 mg diphenhydramine (Benadryl) produces dramatic resolution of the symptoms.

Acute episodes of the so-called temporomandibular joint disorder are distinguished from dislocation by the inability of the patient to open the mouth in the former condition. Reassurance, analgesics, and referral to an oral surgeon are the only acute measures appropriate for the emergency management of this disorder.

Treatment

Manual reduction of the dislocated mandible is most easily accomplished if it is attempted as soon as possible after the injury.

Relaxation of the patient is essential. In the presence of severe pain from muscle spasm, intramuscular administration of a narcotic, eg, meperidine 50 mg (Demerol), or diazepam 10 mg (Valium), may be necessary to diminish the spasm and allow repositioning of the mandible. A good alternative to parenteral medication is the spraying of ethyl chloride on the skin over the masseter muscle; if the dislocation is not longstanding, this simple measure will often suffice.

The patient should be seated in a simple straight-backed chair placed against a wall so that the patient may brace the back of the head against the wall and so that the person doing the procedure can be directly in front of the patient. Reduction is accomplished by placing an index finger in the buccal sulcus just lateral to the posterior teeth on each side; the fingers should never be placed over the teeth themselves. At the same time, the thumbs are placed extraorally beneath the chin. With the patient applying countertraction against the wall, steady, firm pressure in a downward and forward direction is applied with the thumbs and index fingers. Once sufficient pressure has been exerted to bring the condyle free of the articular eminence, muscular forces will provide the posterior motion necessary to return the condyle to the glenoid fossa. The patient must then be instructed to keep the teeth together while the muscular spasm subsides.

In instances of prolonged dislocation, attempts at simple reduction can only be accomplished with the use of general anesthesia and muscle relaxants.

Following reduction of the dislocation, the patient must limit jaw activity for several days; wide mouth opening and heavy chewing must be avoided. Aspirin or ibuprofen, 300 to 600 mg orally every 4 hours, is recommended for analgesic and anti-inflammatory effects. Patients with chronic or habitual jaw dislocations should be referred to an oral and maxillofacial surgeon for further evaluation.

POSTEXTRACTION BLEEDING

Bleeding following the extraction of teeth is usually effectively managed by applying firm pressure onto gauze sponges placed over the socket. However, rebleeding several hours after the procedure may bring the patient to the emergency department.

Pathophysiology

Postextraction bleeding may result either from local surgical factors or from systemic coagulopathies. Following the removal of a tooth, the socket fills with blood and forms a clot by the familiar mechanisms; the adjacent soft tissues are compressed tightly against the alveolar bone and bleeding stops. Inadequacy of the clot or poor adaptation of the gingival tissues results in prolonged bleeding.

Diagnosis

A succinct history of prior bleeding episodes, concomitant medical problems or symptoms, current or recent drug usage, and familial bleeding problems should be obtained at the outset to determine the possibility of a nonsurgical cause of the bleeding. Hemorrhage occurring several days after extraction is more suggestive of a circulating-factor deficiency than is bleeding several hours after the procedure.

Examination of the patient's mouth requires adequate lighting and suction apparatus. Excess clot must be rubbed or suctioned away so that the socket area can be visualized; in fact, exuberant clot may itself be the cause of prolonged, minor bleeding. A search should be made for any laceration or unsutured incision in the soft tissue adjacent to the socket since these are the most common causes of delayed bleeding; the effects of the vasoconstrictor used with the local anesthetic at the time of extraction may mask the potential for bleeding from minor mucosal interruptions until several hours later.

Treatment

When a systemic cause of bleeding is suspected, appropriate blood studies should be ordered to determine the number and function of platelets and the integrity of the coagulation cascade.

Removal of excessive coagulum and the application of firm pressure over the site of bleeding are the initial therapeutic steps to be taken. When mucosal apposition to the bone is inadequate, or when lacerations can be identified, the placement of sutures (3-0 catgut or silk) will be necessary. The placement of gelatin sponge (Gelfoam) into the socket is occasionally useful in conjunction with suturing; topical thrombin powder, silver nitrate sticks, and other topical hemostatic agents are rarely of any value.

If medical causes of bleeding are diagnosed, subsequent care as an inpatient or on an ambulatory basis can be determined. When the bleeding has been controlled, patients should be instructed to bite firmly on gauze for 20 to 30 minutes, after which the socket is best left untouched. Any food or drink may be taken, but care should be exercised in order to protect the newly formed clot. For the same reason, mouth rinsing and gargling should be avoided for the following 24 hours. Analgesics containing aspirin should not be prescribed if there is any suggestion of a systemic etiology of the bleeding. Sutures are usually removed after 7 days.

MUCOSAL ULCERATIONS

Single or multiple erosive lesions of the oral mucosa are often painful enough for the patient to seek emergency assistance. The more common acute ulcerative conditions of the mouth include aphthous ulcers, herpetic ulcers, Vincent's infection ("trench mouth"), and traumatic ulcerations beneath dental prostheses. Less commonly, erosive lesions of pemphigus, pemphigoid, lupus erythematosus, or lichen planus may be seen. The ulcers associated with oral syphilis or carcinoma are not usually painful; as a result, these diagnoses are rarely made in the emergency department.

Pathophysiology

Aphthous ulcers, which are acutely painful, shallow, well-demarcated lesions of the mucosa of the lip, cheek, or floor of the mouth, have no specifically proved cause. It is currently thought that the lesion results from an autoimmune phenomenon. The condition frequently is associated with periods of emotional stress; young adults are most often afflicted.

Primary herpetic infection, common in the pediatric age-group, produces large clusters of ulcers throughout the mouth, in contrast to the solitary aphthous ulcers. Herpes zoster of the oral cavity results in ulcers along a sharply demarcated area that follows a division of the trigeminal nerve, just as the same infection in other parts of the body follows a dermatome distribution.

Vincent's infection is of bacterial origin and affects the gingival tissues. The gingival papillae between teeth are blunted and ulcerated, and the adjacent gingiva is friable with a gray membranous coating; a foul smell accompanies the condition. Young adults are the usual victims.

Denture sores or traumatic ulcers associated with sharp or broken teeth can usually be identified by direct examination. Carcinoma must be included in the differential diagnosis of the apparently traumatic ulcer.

Treatment

No specific therapy can be offered for aphthous or herpetic ulcerations. Topical anesthetics in liquid or gel form can be used in order to allow the patient to have adequate nutrition. A preparation such as Benzocaine in Orabase offers longer-lasting relief because the vehicle for the topical anesthetic has mucosal-adhering properties and can be recommended for symptomatic relief. Creams and ointments containing corticosteroids offer few advantages and are contraindicated if herpetic infection is suspected.

Penicillin, 250 mg orally every 6 hours for 10 days, is the treatment of choice in patients with systemic signs or symptoms of acute Vincent's infection. Mouth rinses with dilute hydrogen peroxide often improve symptoms and are most effective in eliminating the accumulated gingival debris.

Removal of an irritating dental prosthesis is the only emergency treatment for the painful traumatic ulcer. Referral to a dentist or oral surgeon is required for correction of the inciting cause or for biopsy of the ulcer.

BIBLIOGRAPHY

Chow AW, Roser SM, Brady FA. Orofacial odontogenic infections. *Ann Intern Med*. 1978;88:392.

Guralnick WC, Donoff RB. Oral surgical disorders. In: Wilkins EW, ed. *MGH Textbook of Emergency Medicine*. 2nd ed. Baltimore, Md: Williams & Wilkins Co; 1983:659–667.

Kelly JP. Evaluation of facial pain and swelling. In: Goroll AH, May LA, Mullae AG, eds. *Primary Care Medicine*. Philadelphia, Pa: JB Lippincott Co; 1981:758–762.

86. Atlas of Emergency Procedures

THOMAS CLARKE KRAVIS, MD

1. SUBCLAVIAN VEIN CANNULATION

Indications

A. Determine and monitor central venous pressure.
B. Establish a route for intravenous therapeutic agents, cardiac pacemaker, or Swan-Ganz catheter.
C. Determine the presence of pericardial tamponade, left ventricular heart failure, and shock.

Procedure

Fig. 1-1. Place the patient in a supine, head-down 15° Trendelenburg position. Turn the head 90° to the opposite side of the procedure. Support the shoulders. Prepare and drape in usual sterile manner.

Note: In patients with penetrating wounds of the chest, the side of the injury should be used for the insertion of a central venous line.

Identify the anatomical landmarks: the subclavian vein is anterior to the scalene muscle and courses over the first rib, anterior and inferior to the subclavian artery; it joins the internal jugular vein to form the innominate vein.

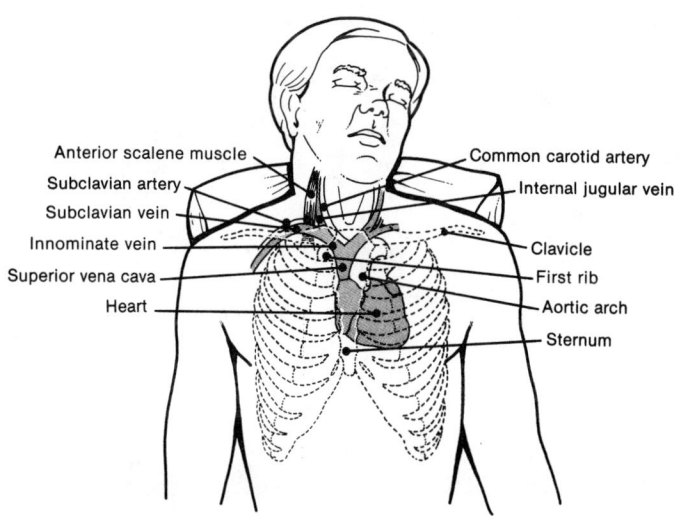

Figure 1-1 Anatomy.

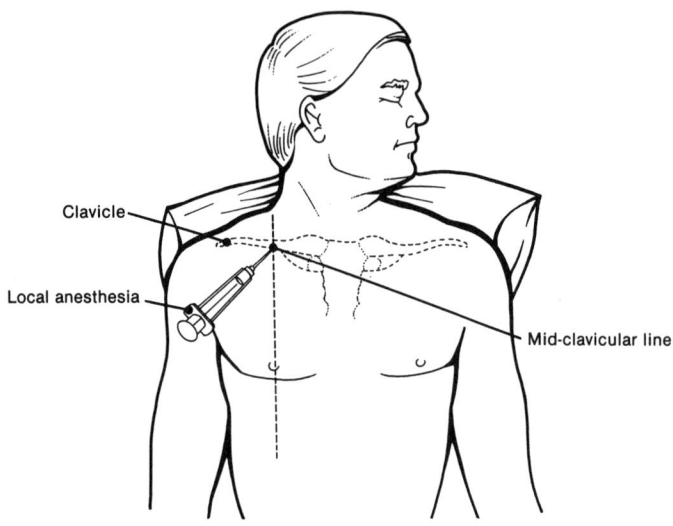

Figure 1-2 Local anesthesia.

Fig. 1-2. Infiltrate 0.5% to 1% lidocaine (Xylocaine) anesthetic one fingerbreadth (2 to 3 cm) below the inferior border of the midpoint of the clavicle. Allow the needle to pass underneath the clavicle.

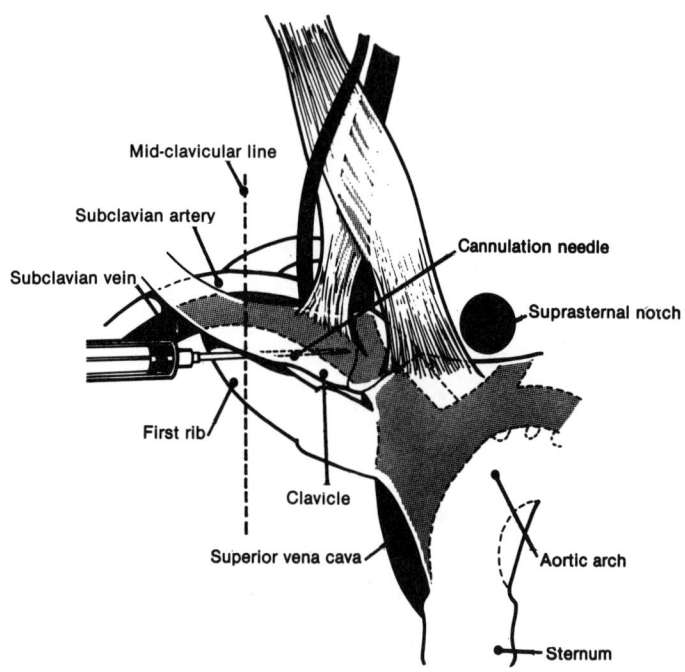

Figure 1-3 Cannulation needle entering subclavian vein.

Fig. 1-3. Attach a sterile 5- to 10-mL syringe filled with sterile saline to the angiocath or cannulation needle being introduced. Insert the needle into the anesthetized puncture site with the bevel of the needle upward; advance the needle toward the suprasternal notch parallel to the line of the lateral one half of the clavicle, maintaining gentle negative pressure on the syringe. After the needle passes the first rib, gently aspirate.

Fig. 1-4. After venous blood can be aspirated freely through the needle, rotate the bevel of the needle clockwise 90° and caudad; remove the syringe and slide the catheter through the needle into the subclavian vein. (If a plastic angiocath is being utilized, remove the needle, keeping the tip of the plastic catheter in the subclavian vein, introduce a flexible straight or J-tipped guide wire through the needle, and gently manipulate the guide wire into the subclavian vein. Advance the plastic catheter over the guide wire; remove the guide wire; reaspirate to confirm presence of free venous blood.)

Note: When the syringe is removed from the needle, instruct the patient to take and hold a deep breath; at the same time, cover the opening of the needle with a sterile-gloved finger to decrease the likelihood of air embolism. If the patient is on a mechanical ventilator, remove the syringe during inspiration. Raise the needle bevel in the anterior caudal position during cannulation. Rotate the patient's head to the ipsilateral side during cannulation, and rotate the needle 360°.

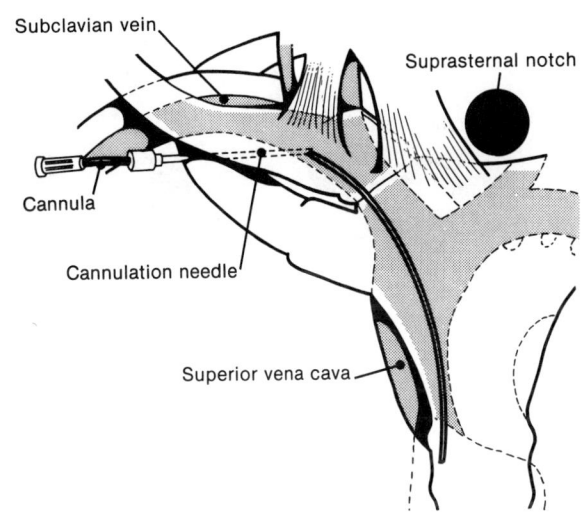

Figure 1-4 Cannula entering cannulation needle into subclavian vein.

Fig. 1-5. Aspirate free venous blood and flush the cannula with normal saline; attach the cannula to the intravenous line.

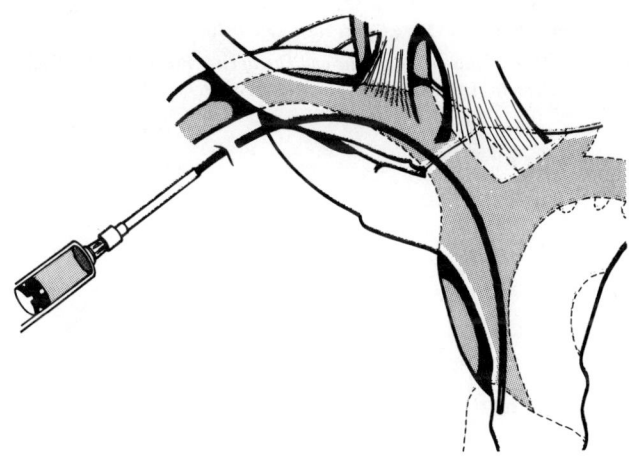

Figure 1-5 Flushing of cannula with saline.

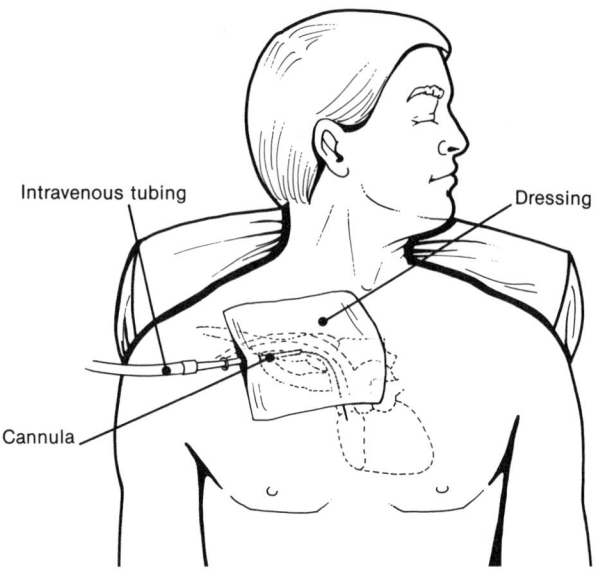

Figure 1-6 Dressing applied.

Fig. 1-6. Secure the needle and tubing to the skin with a single suture—without compressing the catheter lumen—and apply a sterile dressing over the site, using povidone-iodine ointment at the puncture site. Tape the sterile dressing securely to the skin. Return the patient to a supine or head-up position, and obtain a chest radiograph to confirm that the tip of the cannula is located in the lower end of the superior vena cava, outside the right atrium, and at the level of the interspace between the seventh and eighth thoracic vertebrae (ie, 5 cm below the manubrial-sternal junction). Observe for the presence of complications of the procedure (eg, hemothorax, pneumothorax, hematoma, hydrothorax, hydromediastinum, air embolism, subclavian vein thrombosis, catheter embolism, myocardial puncture, or cardiac tamponade).

BIBLIOGRAPHY

Borja AR. Current status of infraclavicular subclavian vein catheterization. *Ann Thorac Surg*. 1972;13:615.

Borja AR, Hinshaw JR. A safe way to perform infraclavicular subclavian vein catheterization. *Surg Gynecol Obstet*. 1970;130:673.

Cosgriff JH. *An Atlas of Diagnostic and Therapeutic Procedures for Emergency Personnel*. Philadelphia, Pa: JB Lippincott Co; 1978.

Keeri-Szanto M. The subclavian vein, a constant and convenient intravenous injection site. *Arch Surg*. 1956;72:179.

McIntyre KM, Lewis AJ, eds. *Textbook of Advanced Cardiac Life Support*. Chicago, Ill: American Heart Association; 1981.

Vander Salm TJ, Cutler BS, Wheeler HB. *Atlas of Bedside Procedures*. Boston, Mass: Little, Brown & Co; 1979.

Wilson JN, Grow JB, DeMong CV, et al. Central venous pressure in optimal blood volume to maintenance. *Arch Surg*. 1962;85:563.

2. INTERNAL JUGULAR VEIN CANNULATION

Indications

A. Determine and monitor central venous pressure.
B. Establish a route for intravenous therapeutic agents, cardiac pacemaker, or Swan-Ganz catheter.
C. Determine the presence of pericardial tamponade, left ventricular heart failure, and shock.

Note: Cannulation of the internal jugular vein may be the method of choice to measure the central venous pressure because of the lower incidence of complications. If hematomas form, they are visible in the neck and compressible, and the procedure provides a direct route to the right atrium when a balloon-tipped flow-directed pulmonary catheter is inserted. The right internal jugular vein is usually chosen, since the right lung is lower than the left and this route does not endanger the thoracic duct. In penetrating wounds of the chest, the central venous catheter should be introduced on the same side as the penetrating injury. An alternative site may be indicated in suspected cervical spine injury.

Procedure

Fig. 2-1. Place the patient in a supine, head-down 15° Trendelenburg position. Turn the head 45° to the opposite side of the procedure.

Prepare and drape the patient in the usual sterile manner. Identify the anatomical landmarks: the internal jugular vein lies lateral to the carotid artery; the sternocleidomastoid muscle overlies the internal jugular vein in the lower half of the neck.

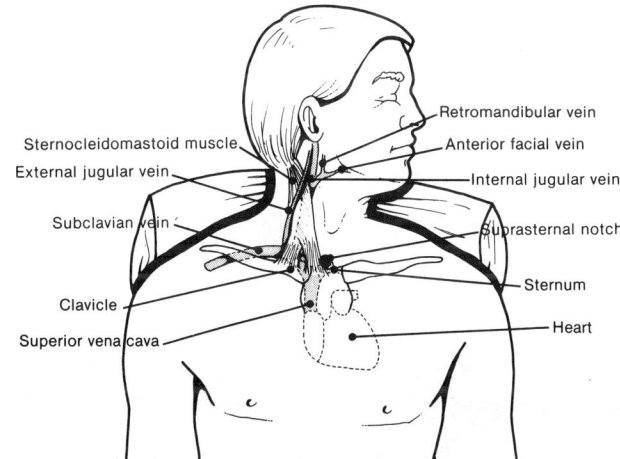

Figure 2-1 Anatomy.

Fig. 2-2. Introduce 0.5% to 1% lidocaine (Xylocaine) at a site under the posterior border of the sternocleidomastoid muscle 4 cm above the clavicle (ie, two to three fingerbreadths), or just above the point at which the external jugular vein crosses the sternocleidomastoid muscle. Attach a 5- to 10-mL syringe filled with sterile saline to the angiocath or cannulation needle being introduced.

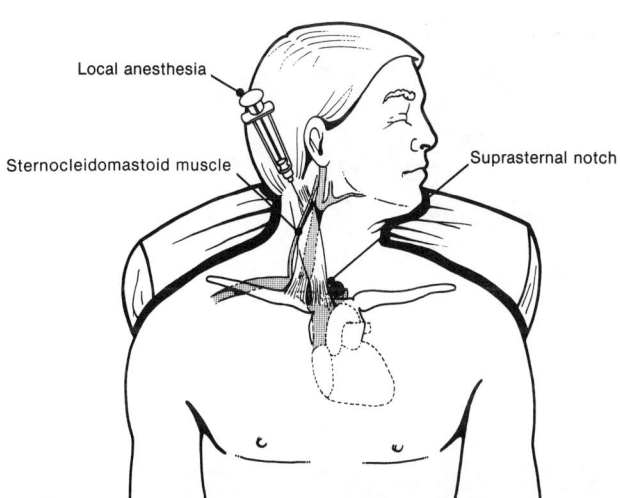

Figure 2-2 Local anesthesia.

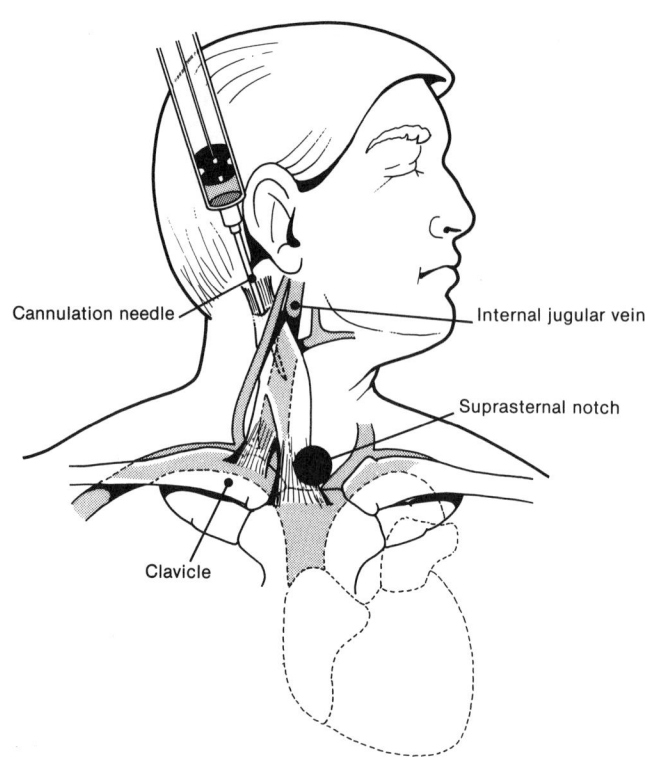

Figure 2-3 Cannulation needle entering internal jugular vein.

Fig. 2-3. Aim the needle caudally and ventrally toward the suprasternal notch underneath the sternocleidomastoid muscle at an angle that is 45° to the sagittal and horizontal planes and 15° forward in the frontal plane; advance and aspirate gently until there is free return of venous blood. Remove the syringe carefully. Have the patient take and hold a deep breath, and, at the same time, cover the top of the needle with a gloved finger.

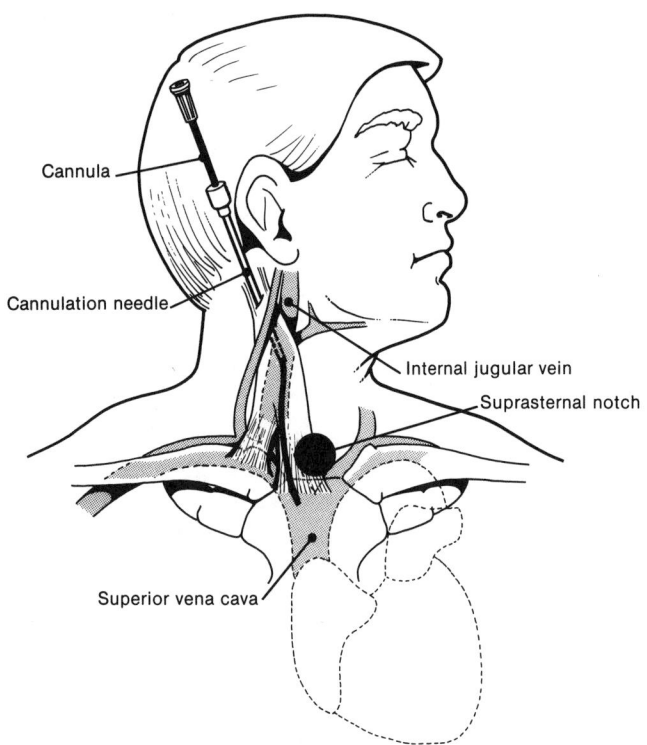

Figure 2-4 Cannula entering cannulation needle into internal jugular vein.

Fig. 2-4. Then introduce the cannula into the needle. Insert the cannula through the needle into the internal jugular vein.

Fig. 2-5. If a plastic angiocath is used, keep the tip of the catheter in the internal jugular vein and withdraw the needle.

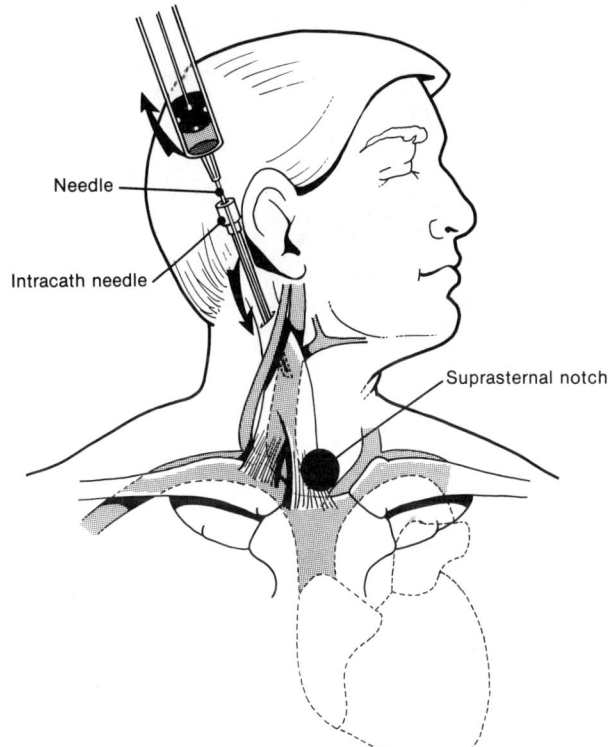

Figure 2-5 Alternate method.

Fig. 2-6. Withdraw needle, aspirate to confirm flow of blood, and flush with saline; attach to intravenous line.

Suture, apply sterile dressing with povidone-iodine ointment, and secure with tape. Obtain chest radiograph to rule out complications and to establish position of the catheter in the superior vena cava (at the level of the seventh and eighth thoracic vertebrae).

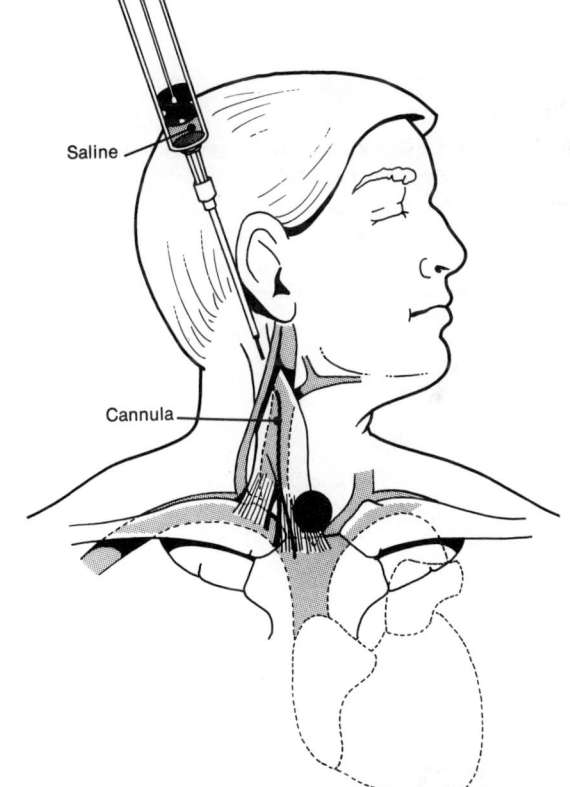

Figure 2-6 Flushing of cannula with saline.

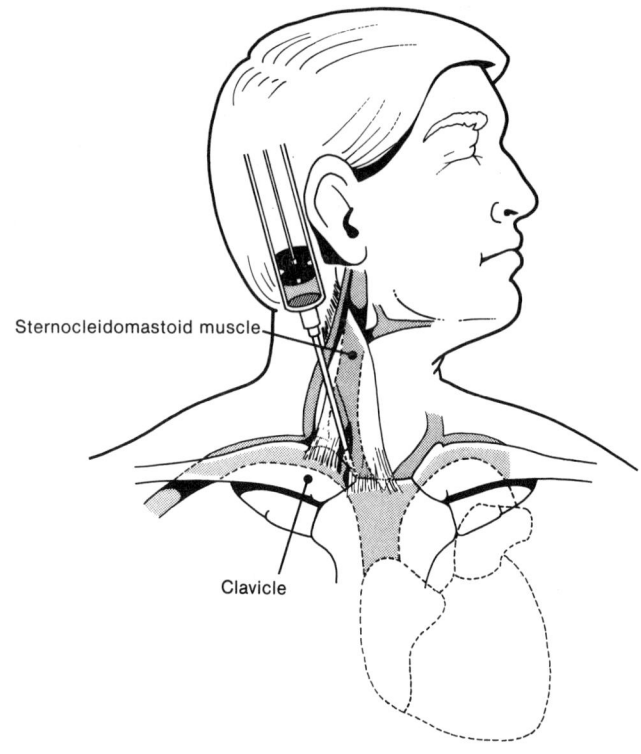

Fig. 2-7. *Note: In the supraclavicular or central technique of internal jugular vein cannulation, the needle is inserted in the apex of the triangle formed by the clavicle and the clavicular and sternal heads of the sternocleidomastoid muscle. The needle is advanced in a sagittal plane 30° posterior and caudad toward the ipsilateral nipple at a 50° angle with the frontal plane. Aspiration is performed until there is free return of venous blood.*

Figure 2-7 Supraclavicular technique.

BIBLIOGRAPHY

Civetta JM, Gabel JC, Gemer M. Internal jugular vein puncture with a margin of safety. *Anesthesiology.* 1972;36:622.

Cosgriff JH. *An Atlas of Diagnostic and Therapeutic Procedures for Emergency Personnel.* Philadelphia, Pa: JB Lippincott Co; 1978.

Daily PO, Griepp RB, Shumway NE. Percutaneous internal jugular vein cannulation. *Arch Surg.* 1970;101:534.

Jernigan WR, et al. Use of the internal jugular vein for placement of central venous catheter. *Surg Gynecol Obstet.* 1970;130:520.

McIntyre KM, Lewis AJ, eds. *Textbook of Advanced Cardiac Life Support.* Chicago, Ill: American Heart Association; 1981.

Vander Salm TJ, Cutler BS, Wheeler HG. *Atlas of Bedside Procedures.* Boston, Mass: Little, Brown & Co; 1979.

3. PULMONARY ARTERY (SWAN-GANZ) CATHETERIZATION

Indications

A. Assess right and left ventricular function (hypovolemic, cardiogenic, and neurogenic shock; pericardial tamponade; pulmonary edema; and pulmonary embolism).

B. Measure pulmonary artery, pulmonary capillary wedge, and right and left atrial pressures.
C. Measure cardiac output.
D. Sample right atrial and pulmonary arterial blood.

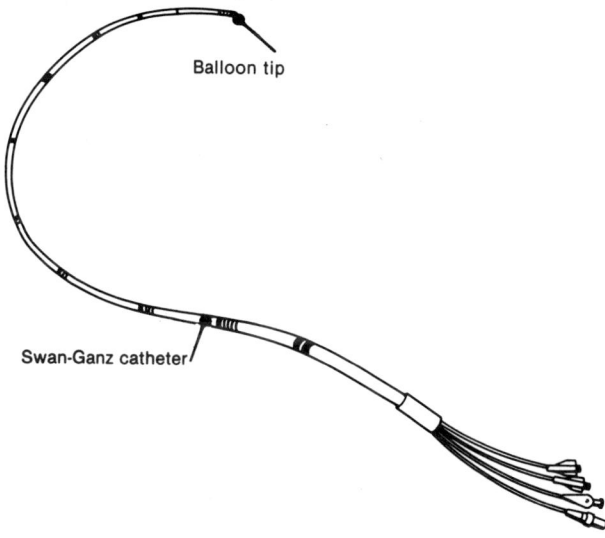

Figure 3-1 Swan-Ganz catheter.

Procedure

Fig. 3-1. Use a Swan-Ganz catheter with flotation balloon; a thermistor hub for measuring cardiac output; a proximal lumen hub to measure right atrial central-venous pressure; a distal lumen hub to measure pulmonary-artery wedge pressure; and rings indicating 10-cm intervals.

Place the patient in the supine 10° to 20° Trendelenburg position. Insert the catheter into the internal jugular vein, using a #16 angiocath (see 2. Internal Jugular Vein Cannulation), or the subclavian, femoral, or medial basilic vein.

Fig. 3-2. Introduce a guide wire into the angiocath.

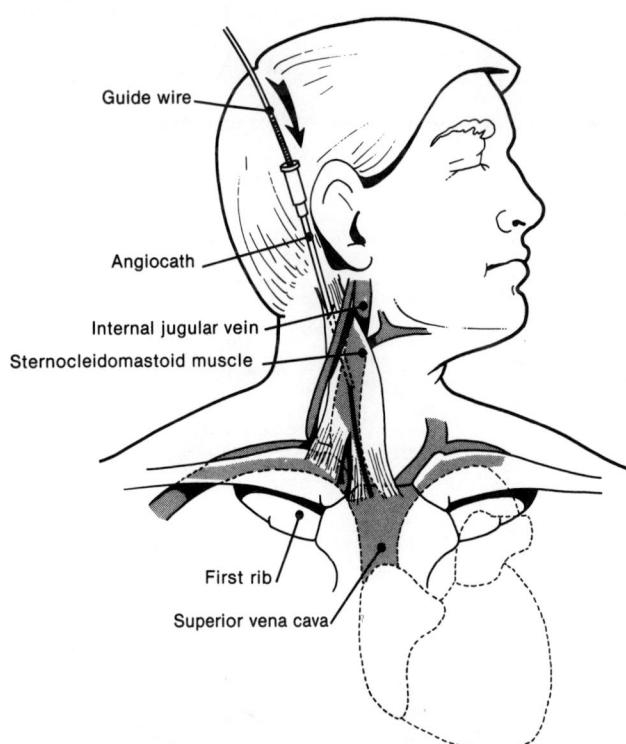

Figure 3-2 Guide wire slides through angiocath.

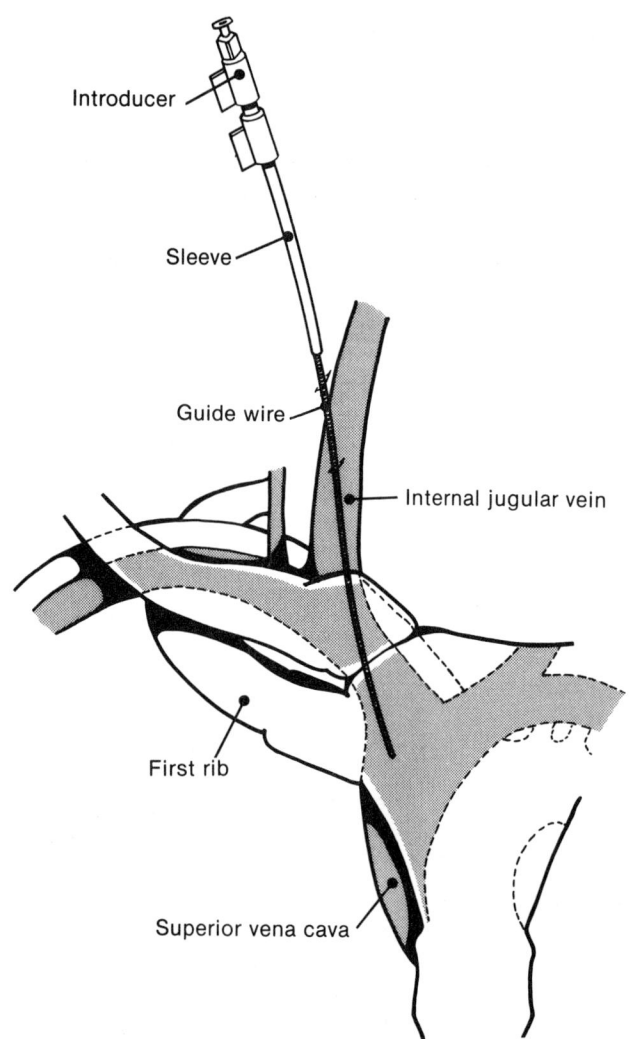

Figure 3-3 Introducer and sleeve replace angiocath.

Figs. 3-3 and 3-4. Remove the angiocath and replace with an introducer and sleeve. Remove the guide wire. Remove the introducer and leave the sleeve in place. A sterile-gloved thumb is placed over the end of the catheter to prevent air embolism and bleeding.

Slide the pulmonary artery catheter through the introducer sleeve.

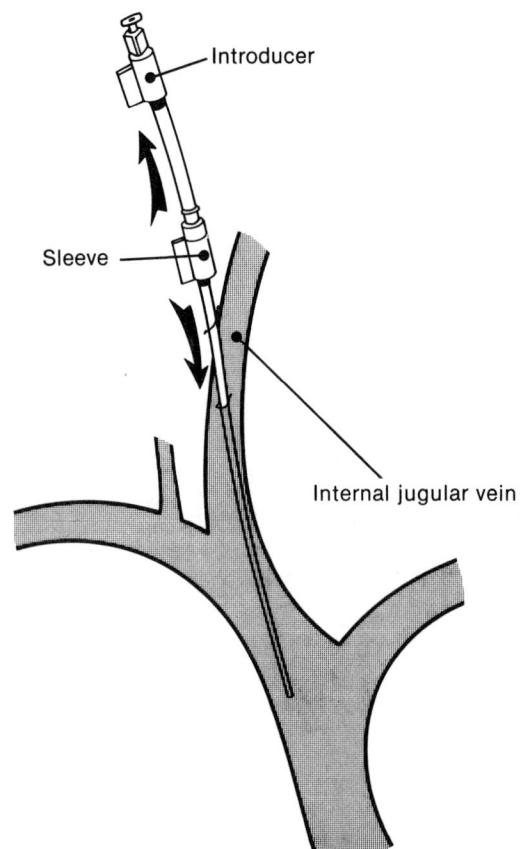

Figure 3-4 Introducer removed.

Fig. 3-5. Advance the catheter centrally 10 to 15 cm into the right atrium. Advance the catheter into the right ventricle.

Attach a three-way stopcock to the tube and flush it with heparinized saline. Note fluctuations on the monitor with the changes in respiration, which indicate the intrathoracic location of the catheter.

Inflate balloon to its full volume (1.25 to 1.50 mL). Observe the characteristic pressure changes. Advance the balloon into the pulmonary artery until the artery is occluded.

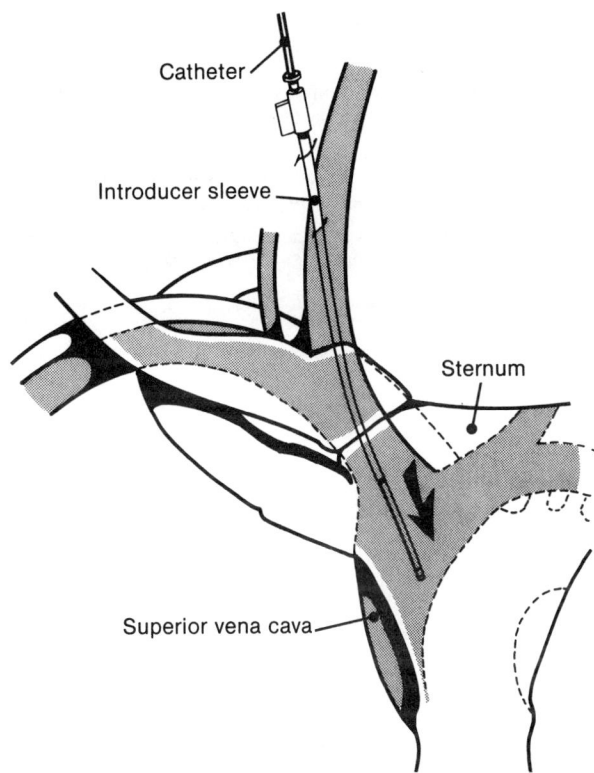

Figure 3-5 Pulmonary artery catheter slides through introducer sleeve.

Fig. 3-6. Confirm that the tip of the catheter is in the pulmonary artery by the characteristic pressure wave on tracing and a chest radiograph. Secure catheter with suture. Commence heparin-saline flush. Apply dressing. Watch for complications of the procedure, such as pneumothorax, thrombosis of veins, pulmonary hemorrhage, cardiac dysrhythmias, endocarditis, fracture of the catheter, and balloon rupture.

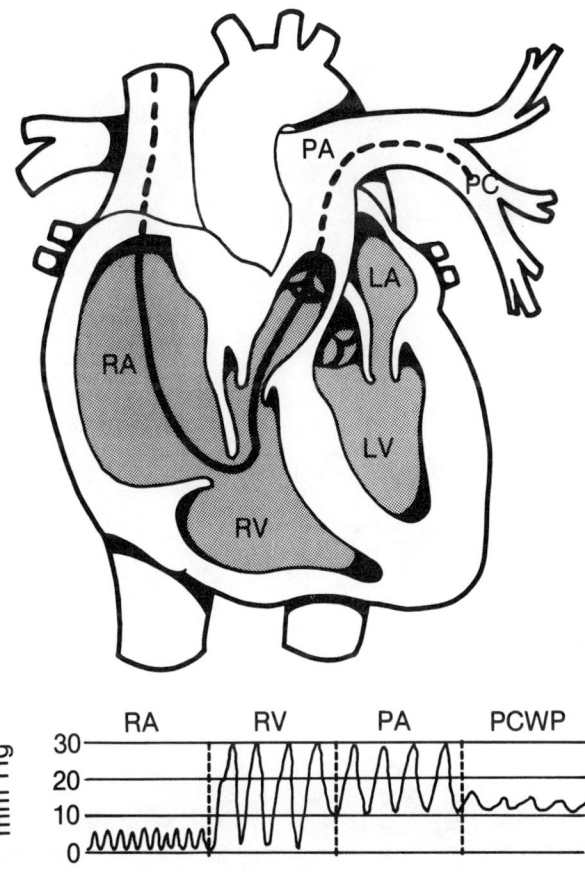

Figure 3-6 Catheter advanced to heart/sequential pressure tracings.

BIBLIOGRAPHY

Anderson WP, Dunegan JF, Knight DC, et al. Rapid estimation of pulmonary extravascular water with an instream catheter. *J Appl Physiol.* 1975;39:843.

Fitzpatrick GF, Hampson LG, Burgess JH. Bedside determination of left atrial pressure. *Can Med Assoc J.* 1972;106:1293.

Foote GA, Schabel SI, Hodges M. Pulmonary complications of the flow-directed balloon-tipped catheter. *N Engl J Med.* 1974;290:927.

McIntyre KM, Lewis AJ, eds. *Textbook of Advanced Life Support.* Chicago, Ill: American Heart Association; 1981.

Swan HJC, Ganz W. Use of balloon flotation catheters in critically ill patients. *Surg Clin North Am.* 1975;55:501.

Swan HJC, Ganz W, Forrester J, et al. Catheterization of the heart in man with use of a flow-directed balloon-tipped catheter. *N Engl J Med.* 1970;283:447.

Vander Salm TJ, Cutler BS, Wheeler HB. *Atlas of Bedside Procedures.* Boston, Mass: Little, Brown & Co; 1979.

4. TEMPORARY TRANSVENOUS PACEMAKER PLACEMENT

Indications

A. Identify hemodynamically compromising dysrhythmias without adequate escape mechanism.
 1. Sinus node dysfunction
 2. Supraventricular bradycardia
 3. Disturbance of atrioventricular conduction
B. Prevent dysrhythmias in association with acute myocardial infarction.
 1. Symptomatic bradycardia, sinoatrial block, and sick sinus syndrome.
 2. Drug-resistant tachydysrhythmias
 3. Right bundle branch block with either left anterior fascicular block or left posterior fascicular block.
 4. Acute onset of Mobitz II second-degree arterioventricular block with anterior myocardial infarction.
 5. Alternating bundle branch block
C. Treat ventricular asystole.
D. Correct malfunction of implanted pacemaker.

Procedure

Fluoroscopic Control of Insertion

Fig. 4-1. Use bipolar semifloating pacing catheter.

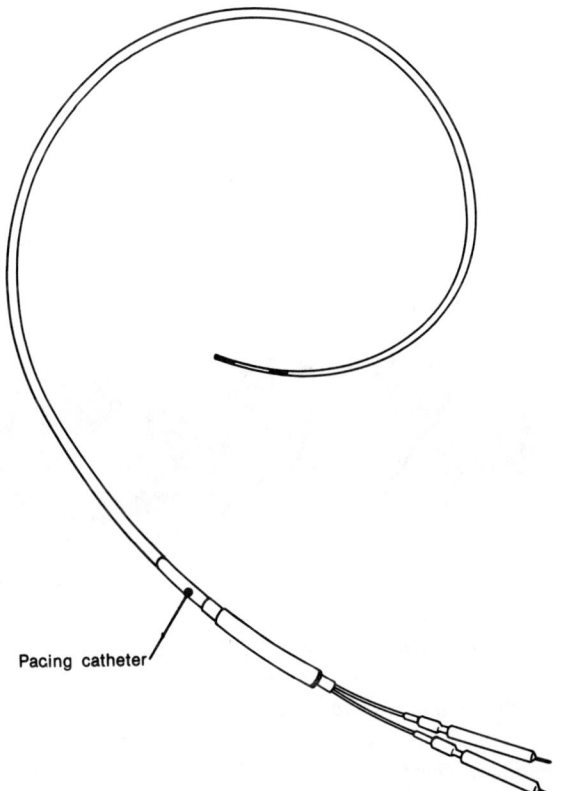

Figure 4-1 Pacing catheter.

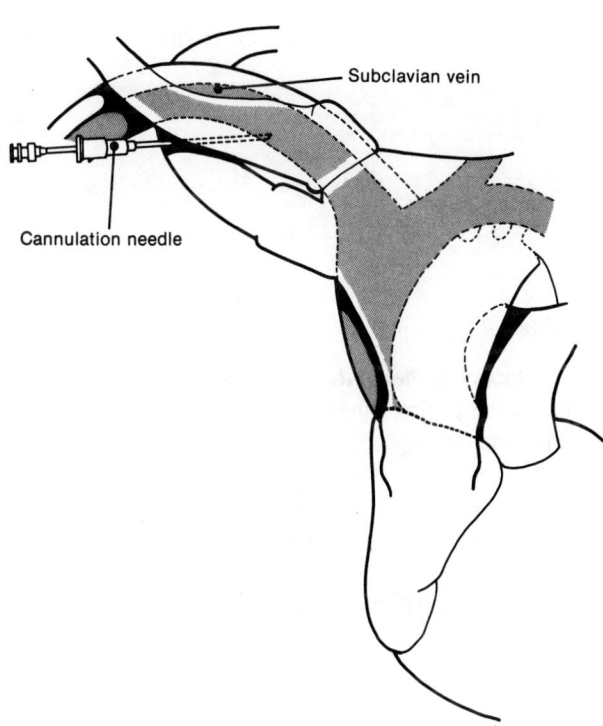

Figure 4-2 Cannulate superior vena cava.

Fig. 4-2. Place the patient in the position for subclavian or internal jugular vein cannulation, and cannulate as previously described. Monitor electrocardiogram (ECG).

Fig. 4-3. Insert the catheter under fluoroscopic control. Introduce the catheter through the superior vena cava into the right atrium with the catheter tip against the lateral wall (Fig. 4-3A). Advance the catheter across the tricuspid valve (Fig. 4-3B). Float the catheter into the pulmonary artery and withdraw to confirm its position in the right ventricle. Advance the catheter tip into the trabeculae of the right ventricle and confirm by fluoroscopy (Fig. 4-3C).

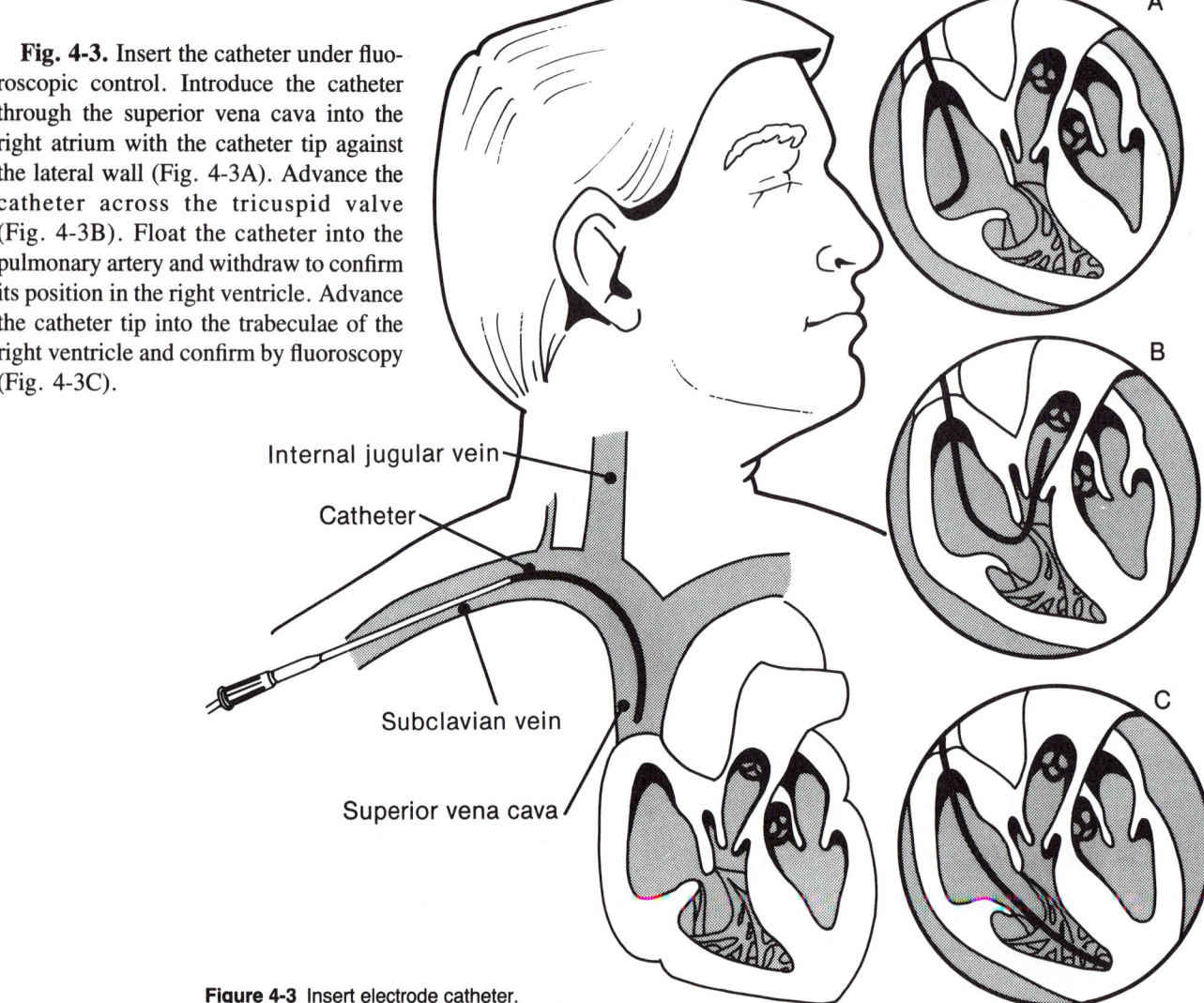

Figure 4-3 Insert electrode catheter.

ECG Control of Insertion

If the electrocatheter is to be introduced under ECG control, attach the pacing catheter to the V lead of a grounded ECG machine, and observe the P wave and QRS configuration during catheter introduction: when the catheter enters the right atrium, two large complexes are observed; as the catheter is advanced across the tricuspid valve into the right ventricle, the amplitude of the P wave decreases, and a large amplitude QRS complex appears.

Blind Insertion

When fluoroscopic or ECG control is not possible, introduce a temporary transvenous pacemaker by the "blind" approach. Introduce the electrocatheter into the superior vena cava, attach it to the external pacemaker generator, and adjust it to a pacing rate of 70 beats/minute at the highest output. Advance the catheter until ventricular pacing is observed.

Note: The electrical thresholds for pacing and sensing are determined immediately after the pacing catheter is positioned. For optimal temporary pacing, the threshold should be below 1 mA; for continuous maintenance pacing, the output should be 5 mA. Alternatively, the generator output can be increased until a pacing spike is immediately followed by a widened QRS complex. A 12-lead ECG with an operative pacemaker will display an ECG pattern suggestive of a left bundle branch-block pattern.

Combined Pulmonary Artery Pressure Monitoring and Temporary Pacing

It is possible to combine pulmonary artery pressure monitoring and temporary pacing with a special Swan-Ganz catheter. After floating the catheter into the wedge position with the electrodes in the atrium and ventricle, choose the best threshold available. This technique allows atrioventricular sequential pacing.

BIBLIOGRAPHY

Atkins JM, Leshin SJ, Blomqvist G, et al. Ventricular conduction blocks and sudden death in acute myocardial infarction: potential indications for pacing. *N Engl J Med.* 1973;288:281.

Castellanos A Jr, Zuckerman W, Berkovits BV. Cardiac pacemakers. In: Harken DE, ed. *Cardiac Surgery.* 2nd ed. Philadelphia, Pa: FA Davis Co; 1971.

Charduck WM. Cardiac pacemakers and heart block. In: Sabiston DE et al, eds. *Gibbon's Surgery of the Chest.* 3rd ed. Philadelphia, Pa: WB Saunders Co, 1976.

Cosgriff JH. *An Atlas of Diagnostic and Therapeutic Procedures for Emergency Personnel.* Philadelphia, Pa: JB Lippincott Co; 1978.

DeSantis RW. Short-term use of intravenous electrode in heart block. *JAMA.* 1963;184:544.

Furman S. Fundamentals of cardiac pacing. *Am Heart J.* 1967;73:261.

Furman S, Escher DJW. *Principles and Techniques of Cardiac Pacing.* New York, NY: Harper & Row; 1970.

Furman S, Schwedel JB, Robinson G, et al. Use of an intracardiac pacemaker in the control of heart block. *Surgery.* 1961;49:98.

Lown B, Kosowsky BD. Artificial cardiac pacemakers I, II, III. *N Engl J Med.* 1970;283:907, 971, 1023.

McIntyre KM, Lewis AJ, eds. *Textbook of Advanced Cardiac Life Support.* Chicago, Ill: American Heart Association; 1981.

Parsonnet V, Zucker R, Gilbert L, et al. An intracardiac bipolar electrode for interim treatment of complete heart block. *Am J Cardiol.* 1962;10:261.

Rubin I, Arbeit SR, Gross H. The electrocardiographic recognition of pacemaker function and failure. *Ann Intern Med.* 1969;71:603.

Schnedel JB, Escher DJW. Transvenous electrical stimulation of the heart. *Ann NY Acad Sci.* 1964;111:972.

Solomon N, Escher DJW. A rapid method for insertion of the pacemaker catheter electrode. *Am Heart J.* 1963;66:717.

Vander Salm TJ, Cutler BS, Wheeler HB. *Atlas of Bedside Procedures.* Boston, Mass: Little, Brown & Co; 1979.

Weale FE. Cardiac resuscitation via jugular vein. *Lancet.* 1959;2:73.

5. CULDOCENTESIS

Indication

Determine the presence of blood or inflammatory fluids in the cul-de-sac.

Procedure

Place the patient in the lithotomy position. Perform pelvic and rectovaginal examinations; insert the speculum; prepare the posterior vagina with povidone-iodine.

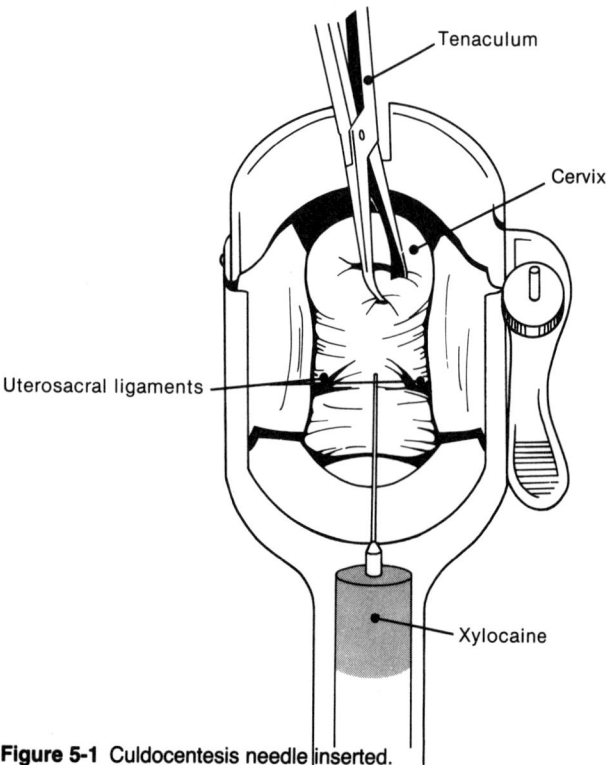

Figure 5-1 Culdocentesis needle inserted.

Fig. 5-1. Gently grasp the posterior lip of the cervix with a tenaculum. Infiltrate 0.5% to 1% lidocaine (Xylocaine) into the cervix in the midline posterior to the vaginal reflection.

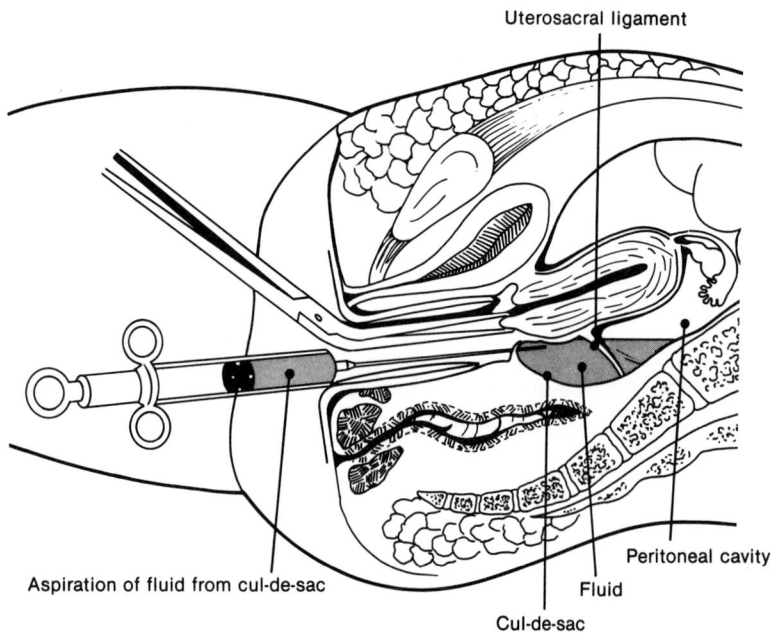

Figure 5-2 Aspirate cul-de-sac.

Fig. 5-2. Insert an 18-gauge spinal needle attached to a glass syringe midline between the uterosacral ligaments and into the apex of the cul-de-sac. Keep the axis of the needle parallel to that of the uterus. Aspirate and place the contents into a glass tube. Examine the fluid: if nonclotting blood is obtained, the test is described as positive; if straw-colored peritoneal fluid is obtained, the test is described as negative. (If no fluid is obtained, the procedure may be repeated.)

BIBLIOGRAPHY

Beacham DW, Beacham WD. Culdocentesis. *New Orleans Med Surg J.* 1951;103:283.

Cosgriff JH. *An Atlas of Diagnostic and Therapeutic Procedures for Emergency Personnel.* Philadelphia, Pa: JB Lippincott Co; 1978.

Decker A. *Culdoscopy.* Philadelphia, Pa: FA Davis Co; 1967.

Halpin TF. Ectopic pregnancy. *Am J Obstet Gynecol.* 1970;106:227.

McGown L, Stein DB, Miller W. Cul-de-sac aspiration for diagnostic cytologic study. *Am J Obstet Gynecol.* 1966;96:413.

Vander Salm TJ, Cutler BS, Wheeler HB. *Atlas of Bedside Procedures.* Boston, Mass: Little, Brown & Co; 1979.

6. PERITONEAL LAVAGE

Indication

Determine the presence of intraperitoneal bleeding or rupture of hollow viscus.

Procedure

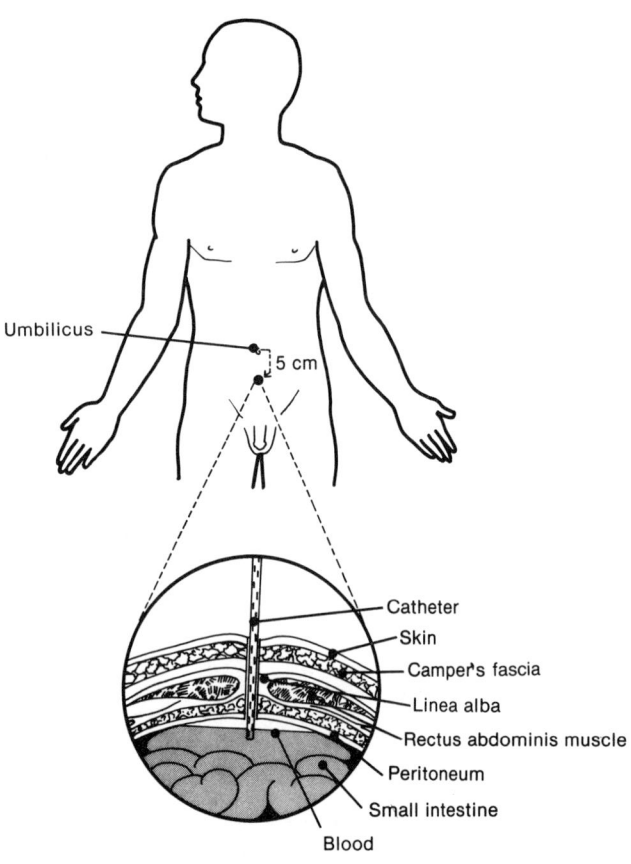

Figure 6-1 Insert catheter into peritoneal cavity.

Fig. 6-1. After the patient has emptied the bladder, place the patient in the supine position. Prepare and drape the patient in the usual sterile manner. Infiltrate 0.5% to 1% lidocaine (Xylocaine) with epinephrine 1:100,000 5 cm below the umbilicus in the midline from the skin to the peritoneum. Do not infiltrate into the peritoneum. Make a horizontal, 5-mm incision in the anesthetized area.

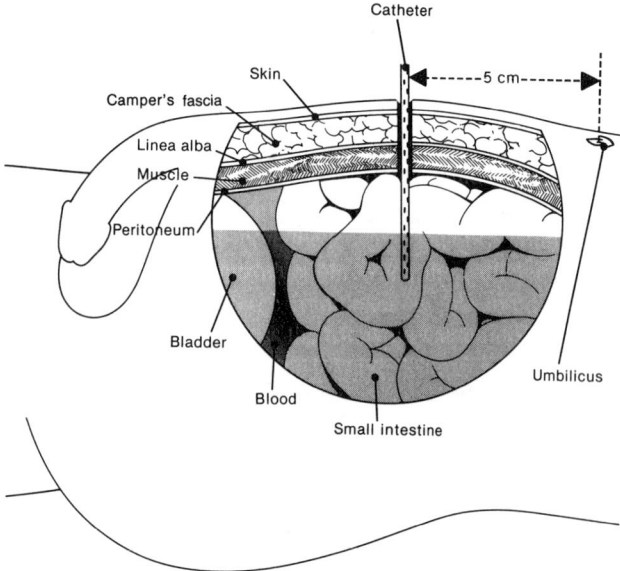

Figure 6-2 Advance catheter.

Fig. 6-2. Insert a trocar-type peritoneal dialysis catheter, with the stylet protruding ⅛ inch (3 mm) through the incision site with the catheter in the midline, perpendicular to the abdominal wall. Have the patient lift the head to tense the abdominal wall. Advance the catheter with one hand while controlling excessive penetration with the other hand. Insert the catheter through the rectus muscle, and penetrate the linea alba through the peritoneum.

Gently advance the catheter retroperitoneally to the suspected site of injury. Remove stylet and immobilize the catheter with a clamp to the abdominal wall.

Aspirate with a syringe. If gross blood or bowel contents are aspirated, the test is definitive. Remove the catheter and apply a sterile dressing. In the absence of these findings, attach the peritoneal catheter to an intravenous line and infuse 10 mL/kg (up to 1 liter) of Ringer's lactate into the peritoneal cavity. If possible, gently roll the patient in order to disperse the fluid.

Fig. 6-3. After five to ten minutes, reattach the intravenous tubing to the vent hole of the intravenous bottle and place the bottle below the level of the patient. Allow gravity to siphon the lavage fluid.

Interpret findings: if the intravenous tubing containing the lavage fluid is held over newspaper print, one of the following statements can be made:

1. No printing can be seen, indicating significant injury.
2. Printing can be seen, but not read, indicating a strong possibility of injury.
3. Fluid is bloody, but printing can be read, an equivocal test result.
4. Fluid is clear, a negative test result.

Alternatively, the test result may be positive if the hematocrit of the fluid obtained is greater than 2%; if the red blood-cell count is greater than $100,000/mm^3$; or the white blood-cell count is greater than $500/mm^3$ (in unspun samples).

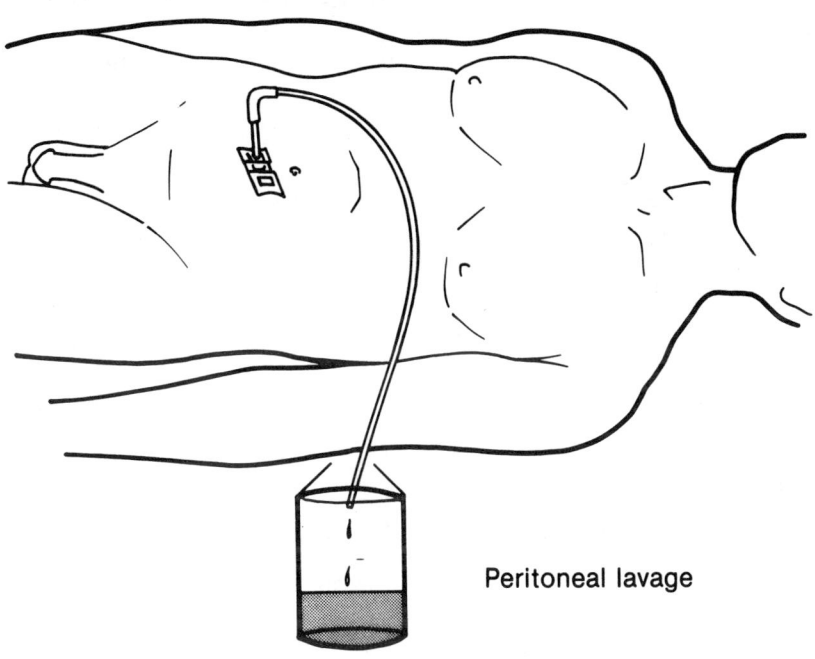

Figure 6-3 Peritoneal lavage.

BIBLIOGRAPHY

Bivins BA, Jona JZ, Belin RP. Diagnostic peritoneal lavage in pediatric trauma. *J Trauma*. 1976;16:739.

Cosgriff JH. *An Atlas of Diagnostic and Therapeutic Procedures for Emergency Personnel*. Philadelphia, Pa: JB Lippincott Co; 1978.

Engrav LH, Benjamin CI, Strate RG, et al. Diagnostic peritoneal lavage in blunt abdominal trauma. *J Trauma*. 1975;15:854.

Jergens ME. Peritoneal lavage. *Am J Surg*. 1977;133:365.

Kazarian KK, Devanesan JD, Mersheimer WL. Diagnostic peritoneal lavage. *NY State J Med*. 1975;75:2145.

Olsen WR, Redman HC, Hildreth DH. Quantitative peritoneal lavage in blunt abdominal trauma. *Arch Surg*. 1972;104:53.

Parvin TS, Smith DE, Asher WM, et al. Effectiveness of peritoneal lavage in blunt abdominal trauma. *Ann Surg*. 1975;181:255.

Perry JF Jr, DeMueles JE, Root HD. Diagnostic peritoneal lavage in blunt abdominal trauma. *Surg Gynecol Obstet*. 1970;131:742.

Root HD, Hauser CW, McKin CR, et al. Diagnostic peritoneal lavage. *Surgery*. 1965;57:633.

Root HD, Keizer PJ, Perry JF Jr. The clinical and experimental aspects of peritoneal response to injury. *Arch Surg*. 1967;95:531.

Sachatello CR, Bivins B. Technic for peritoneal dialysis and diagnostic peritoneal lavage. *Am J Surg*. 1976;131:637.

Vander Salm TJ, Cutler BS, Wheeler HB. *Atlas of Bedside Procedures*. Boston, Mass: Little, Brown & Co; 1979.

7. PERICARDIOCENTESIS (INDIRECT METHOD)

Indication

Identify acute pericardial effusion and tamponade.

Procedure

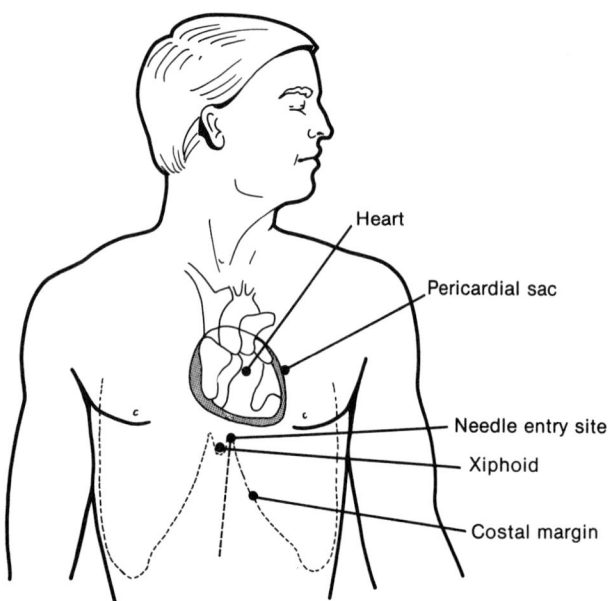

Figure 7-1 Anatomical location.

Fig. 7-1. Position the patient at 60° elevation from the horizontal. Attach ECG leads to the patient. Prepare and drape the patient in the usual sterile manner. Identify the anatomical landmarks: the cardiac apex is 1 cm inside the left cardiac border (the angle between the left costal margin and the xiphoid). Infiltrate 0.5% to 1% lidocaine (Xylocaine) just to the left of the xiphocostal angle, and infiltrate deeply to the costal arch.

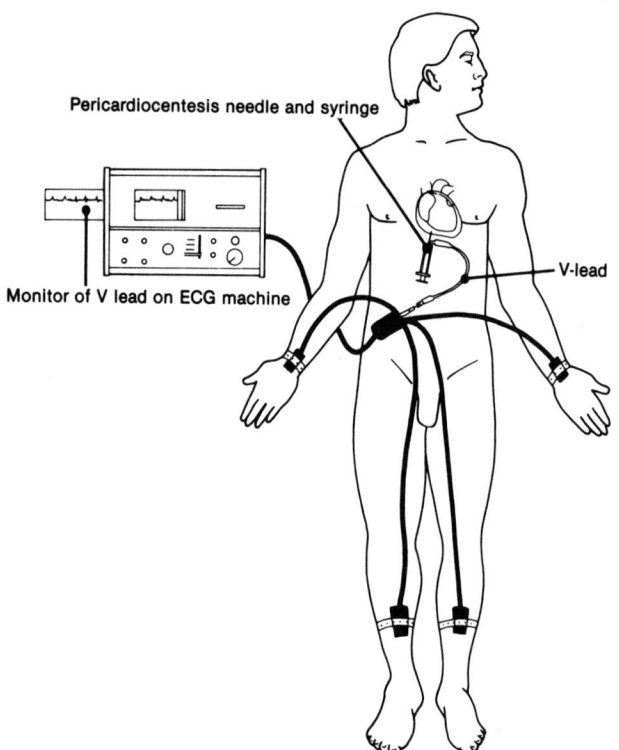

Figure 7-2 Monitor of V lead on ECG machine.

Fig. 7-2. Connect the V lead to a sterile alligator clip, and place the sterile needle on a 10-mL syringe. Insert the needle into the anesthetized tract.

Fig. 7-3. Advance the needle in the direction of the left shoulder while applying slight negative pressure to the attached syringe and continually monitoring the ECG. Advance the needle until the needle suddenly seems to "give," a sensation that signals pericardial penetration. If the ECG develops an "injury current" (ST-segment elevation), which indicates contact with the epicardium, withdraw the needle slightly from the epicardium, simultaneously withdrawing pericardial fluid, if present. Examine the fluid: failure of the blood to clot in a glass tube establishes that the bloody fluid was not obtained from a cardiac chamber. Withdraw fluid until the patient's unstable hemodynamic state has been reversed or until fluid can no longer be aspirated.

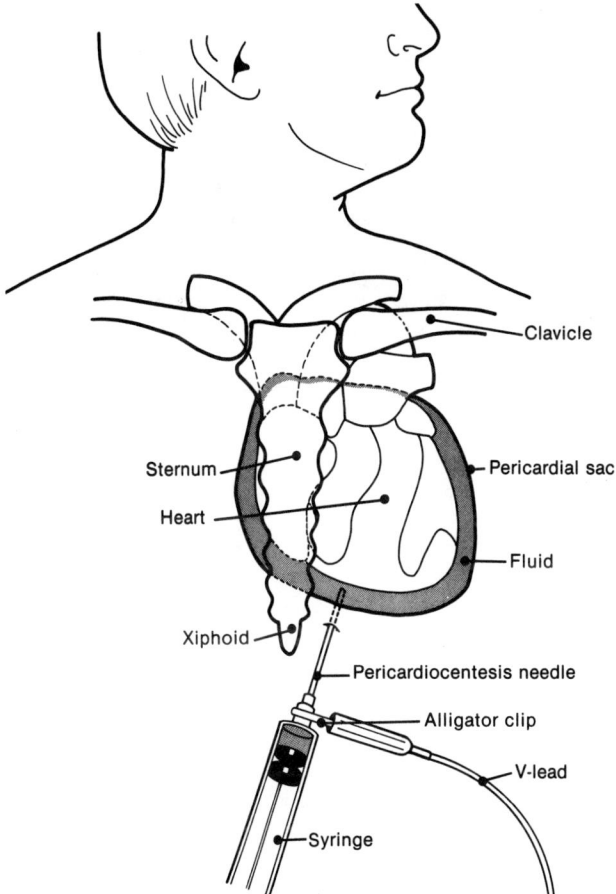

Figure 7-3 Insertion of pericardiocentesis needle.

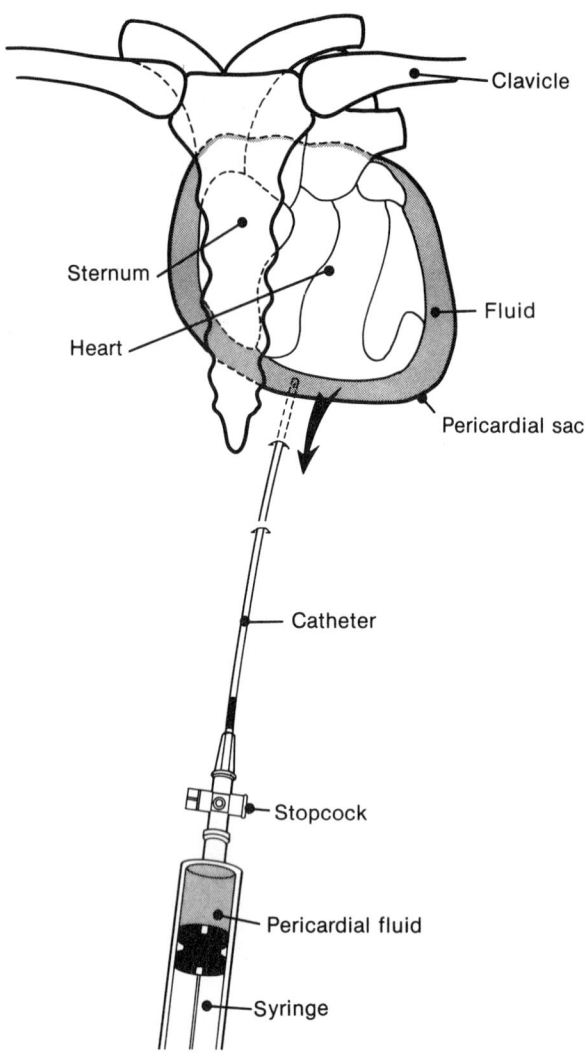

Fig. 7-4. Remove the syringe from the needle, and slide a plastic catheter through the needle into the pericardial space. Utilizing a three-way stopcock, withdraw fluid from the pericardium. Leave the catheter in the pericardial sac for continued drainage if indicated. Alternatively, remove and apply sterile dressing and tape.

Figure 7-4 Catheter insertion.

BIBLIOGRAPHY

Bains MS, Beattie EJ Jr. Cardiac tamponade. *Hosp Med.* 1976;12:47.

Bishop LH Jr, Estes EH Jr, McIntosh HDJ. The electrocardiogram as a safeguard in pericardiocentesis. *JAMA.* 1956;162:264.

Cosgriff JH. *An Atlas of Diagnostic and Therapeutic Procedures for Emergency Personnel.* Philadelphia, Pa: JB Lippincott Co; 1978.

Fredricksen RT, Cohen LS, Mullins CB. Pericardial windows or pericardiocentesis for pericardial effusions. *Am Heart J.* 1971;82:158.

Kilpatrick ZM, Chapman CB. On pericardiocentesis. *Am J Cardiol.* 1965;16:722.

McIntyre KM, Lewis AJ, eds. *Textbook of Advanced Cardiac Life Support.* Chicago, Ill: American Heart Association; 1981.

Neill JR, Hurst JW, Penfold ELJ. A pericardiocentesis electrode. *N Engl J Med.* 1961;264:711.

Schaffer AI. Pericardiocentesis with the aid of a plastic catheter and ECG monitor. *Am J Cardiol.* 1959;4:83.

Simpson JS. *Thoracic Injuries in Care of the Injured Child.* Baltimore, Md: Williams & Wilkins Co; 1975:139.

Spodick DH. Acute cardiac tamponade: pathologic physiology, diagnosis, and management. *Prog Cardiovasc Dis.* 1967;10:64.

Vander Salm TJ, Cutler BS, Wheeler HB. *Atlas of Bedside Procedures.* Boston, Mass: Little, Brown & Co; 1979.

8. DEFIBRILLATION AND ELECTRICAL CARDIOVERSION

Indication

Determine the presence of life-threatening ventricular or atrial dysrhythmias causing hemodynamic compromise.

Procedure

Secure the direct current cardioversion apparatus, and select the appropriate mode and electrical charge required.

Fig. 8-1. Use electrode paste or saline pads to lower electrical impedance. Apply one paddle over the second right intercostal space, just below the right clavicle, and the second paddle over the fifth intercostal space (ie, on the left midaxillary line just lateral to the left nipple). If the patient is conscious and time permits, give diazepam (Valium), 5 to 10 mg, intravenously for sedation, and hyperventilate the patient with supplemental oxygen. Then apply the electrical shock.

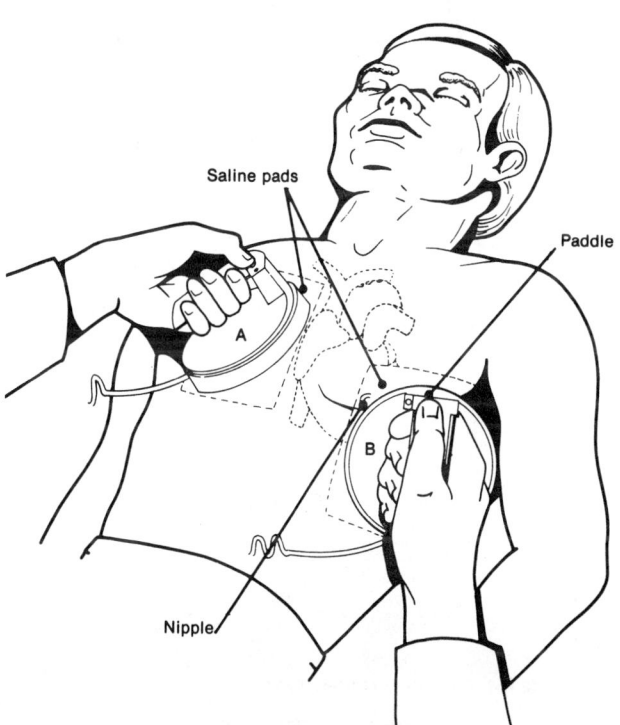

Figure 8-1 Apply paddles.

BIBLIOGRAPHY

Dorney ER. The use of cardioversion and pacemakers in the management of arrhythmias. In: Hurst JW, et al, eds. *The Heart*. 3rd ed. New York, NY: McGraw-Hill Book Co; 1974:558–562.

Lown B, Neuman J, Amarasingham R, et al. Comparison of alternating current with direct current electroshock across the closed chest. *Am J Cardiol*. 1962;10:223.

McIntyre KM, Lewis AJ, eds. *Textbook of Advanced Cardiac Life Support*. Chicago, Ill: American Heart Association; 1981.

Parker MR, ed. Defibrillation and synchronized cardioversion. In: *Advanced Cardiac Life Support*. Chicago, Ill: American Heart Association; 1975.

Resnekov L. Theory and practice of electroversion of cardiac dysrhythmias. *Med Clin North Am*. 1976;60:325.

Vander Salm TJ, Cutler BS, Wheeler HB. *Atlas of Bedside Procedures*. Boston, Mass: Little, Brown & Co; 1979.

9. NASOTRACHEAL SUCTIONING

Indication

Remove secretions or blood from the tracheobronchial tree.

Procedure

Position the patient in the sitting, semisitting, or supine position. Hyperventilate the patient with supplemental oxygen if the patient is in respiratory distress.

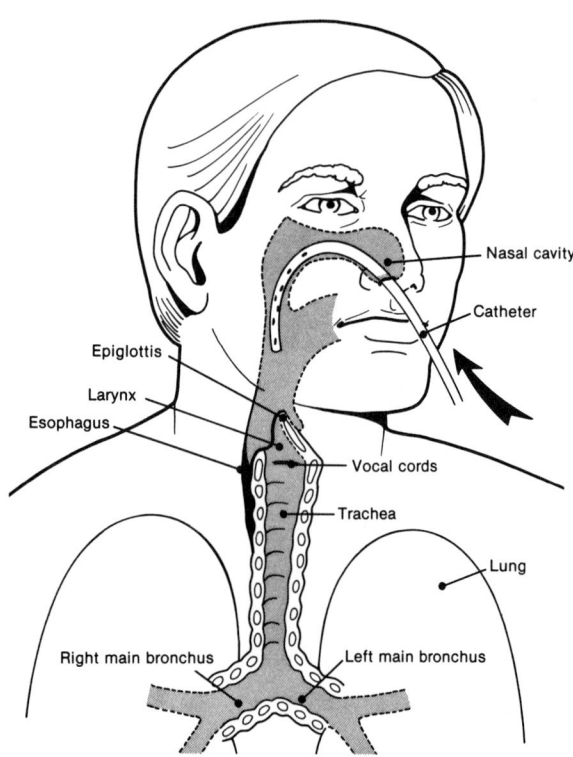

Figure 9-1 Catheter inserted into nose.

Fig. 9-1. Select a sterile, clear, plastic, low-friction, coefficient #14 French suction catheter with adequate side holes. Lubricate the end of the catheter, and introduce it into the patient's nostril. Advance the catheter along the floor of the nose into the hypopharynx. Advance the catheter during inspiration.

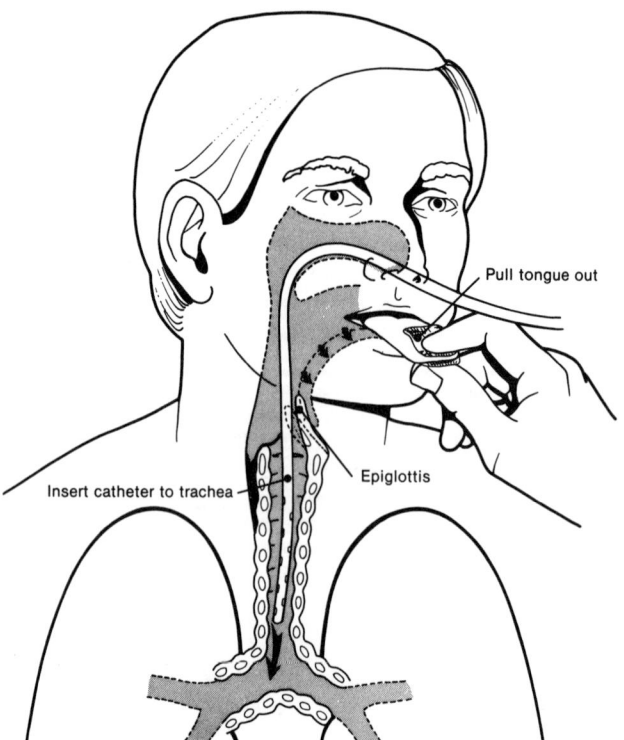

Figure 9-2 Advance catheter into trachea.

Fig. 9-2. Alternatively, gently place light traction with a sterile-gloved hand and gauze on the tongue, pull it forward, and advance the catheter.

Fig. 9-3. Watch for patient coughing or changes in phonation, which suggest that the catheter tip has advanced into the trachea below the vocal cords. Apply suction via the vacuum tube for five to ten seconds at −60 to −80 mmHg. Collect mucus in trap if indicated. Remove catheter.

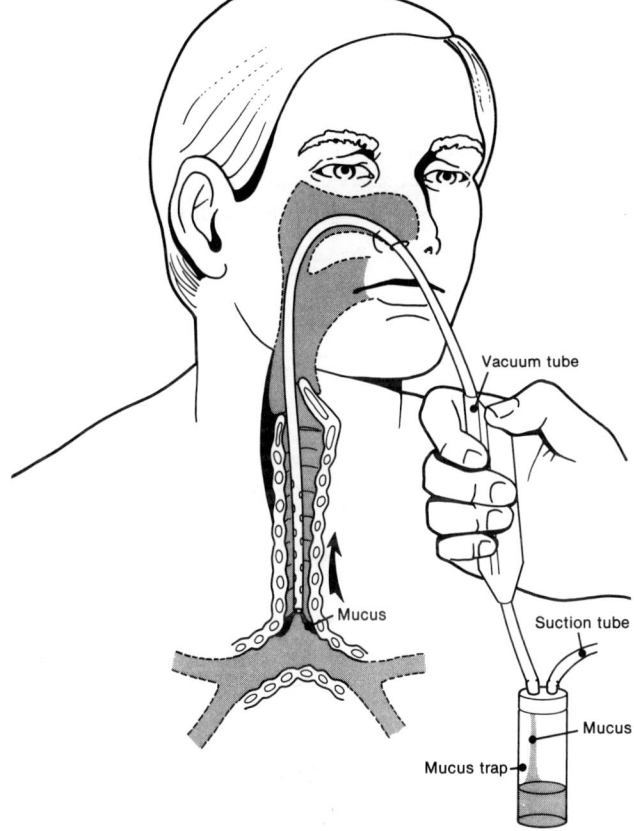

Figure 9-3 Apply suction vacuum.

BIBLIOGRAPHY

Haight C. Intratracheal suction in the management of postoperative pulmonary complications. *Ann Surg*. 1938;107:218.

Shim C, Fine N, Fernandez R, et al. Cardiac arrhythmias resulting from tracheal suctioning. *Ann Intern Med*. 1969;71:1149.

Vander Salm TJ, Cutler BS, Wheeler HB. *Atlas of Bedside Procedures*. Boston, Mass: Little, Brown & Co; 1979.

10. NEEDLE CRICOTHYROID PUNCTURE

Indications

A. Provide an emergency airway when endotracheal intubation is not possible or indicated.
B. Provide an emergency airway when the upper airway is obstructed secondary to trauma or foreign body.

Procedure

Place the patient in the supine position with support under the shoulders.

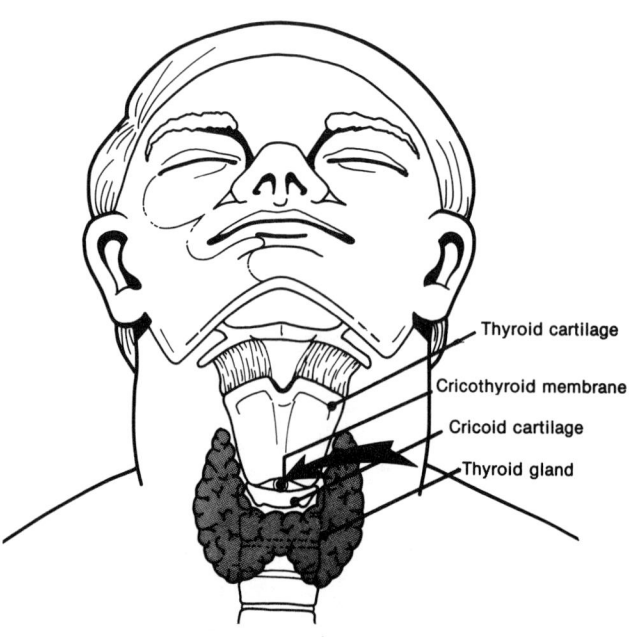

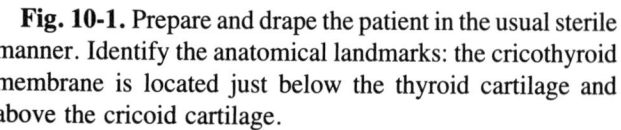

Fig. 10-1. Prepare and drape the patient in the usual sterile manner. Identify the anatomical landmarks: the cricothyroid membrane is located just below the thyroid cartilage and above the cricoid cartilage.

Figure 10-1 Anatomy.

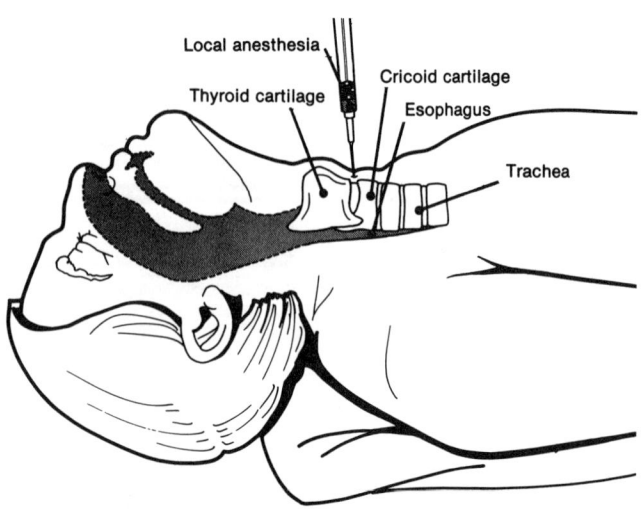

Fig. 10-2. Introduce 0.5% to 1% lidocaine (Xylocaine) in the midline over the cricothyroid membrane.

Figure 10-2 Local anesthesia.

Fig. 10-3. Penetrate the cricothyroid membrane with a 14-gauge intracath needle on the end of an air-filled syringe. Keep the bevel of the needle up, and direct the point of the needle at an angle of 45° to the neck. Aspirate until the presence of air confirms the position of the needle in the trachea. Remove the syringe.

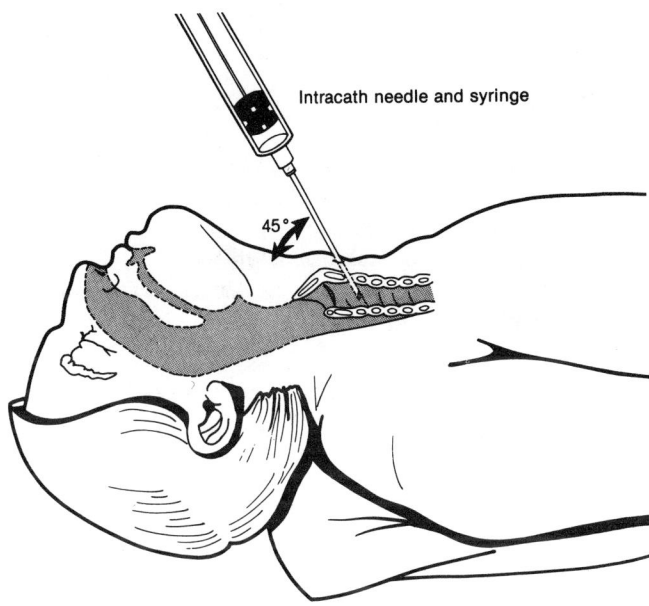

Figure 10-3 Intracath needle punctures cricothyroid membrane.

Fig. 10-4. Thread the catheter through the needle into the trachea. Attach the catheter hub to a 3.0-mm pediatric endotracheal tube adapter.

Apply supplemental oxygen apparatus, via a "Y"-connector at a high flow rate, to the opening of the catheter if the patient is ventilating. Attach to a mechanical ventilatory apparatus if the patient requires ventilatory assistance. A second catheter with a stopcock can be inserted adjacent to the first: with the stopcock closed during inspiration and opened during exhalation, CO_2 can be eliminated. Apply povidone-iodine to wound site and a sterile dressing. Visualize lung inflations and auscultate the chest for adequate ventilations.

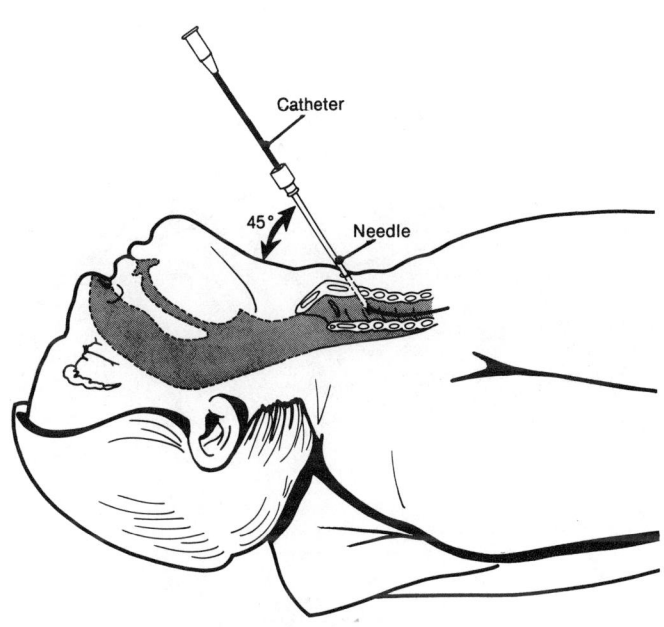

Figure 10-4 Catheter inserted into intracath needle.

BIBLIOGRAPHY

Bartlett JG, Rosenblatt JE, Feingold SM. Percutaneous transtracheal aspiration in the diagnosis of anaerobic pulmonary infection. *Ann Intern Med.* 1973;79:535.

Cosgriff JH. *An Atlas of Diagnostic and Therapeutic Procedures for Emergency Personnel.* Philadelphia, Pa: JB Lippincott Co; 1978.

Craig DB. Transtracheal ventilation. *JAMA.* 1976;235:2082.

Jacobs HB. Emergency percutaneous transtracheal catheter and ventilator. *J Trauma.* 1972;12:50–55.

Jacoby JJ, Hamelburg W, Ziegler CH, et al. Transtracheal resuscitation. *JAMA.* 1956;162:625–628.

Kalinske RW, Parker RH, Brandt D, et al. Diagnostic usefulness and safety of transtracheal aspiration. *N Engl J Med.* 1967;276:604.

Pecora DV. A method of securing uncontaminated tracheal secretions for bacterial examination. *J Thorac Cardiovasc Surg.* 1959;37:653.

Spencer CD, Beaty HN. Complications of transtracheal aspiration. *N Engl J Med.* 1972;286:304.

Vander Salm TJ, Cutler BS, Wheeler HB. *Atlas of Bedside Procedures.* Boston, Mass: Little, Brown & Co; 1979.

11. ENDOTRACHEAL INTUBATION

Indications

A. Maintain an airway in a patient with respiratory or cardiac arrest.
B. Protect against aspiration.
C. Suction the tracheobronchial tree.
D. Provide positive pressure mechanical ventilation.
E. Administer high levels of oxygen.

Caution: Nasotracheal approach is indicated in suspected cervical spine injuries.

Procedure

Test the laryngoscope light and the balloon on the endotracheal tube. Provide supplemental oxygen and/or hyperventilate the patient with oxygen briefly before initiating the procedure.

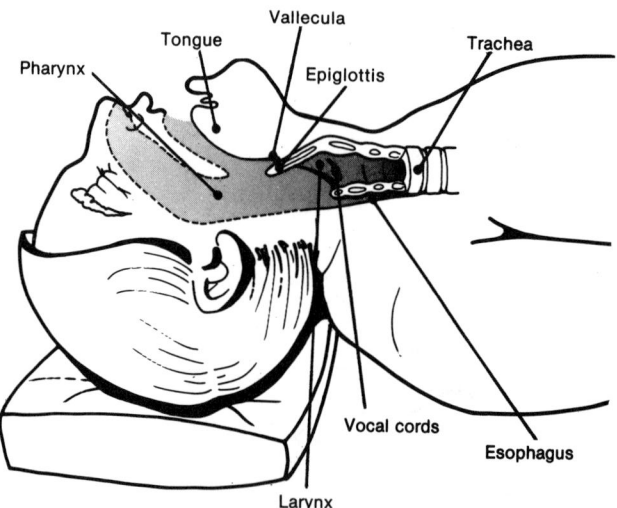

Fig. 11-1. Position the patient in the sniffing position (the neck flexed forward and the head extended backward). If necessary, place a support under the occiput to elevate the head a few centimeters above the horizontal.

Lubricate the tube and stylet, and introduce the metal stylet into the endotracheal tube with the desired tube configuration.

Figure 11-1 Anatomy.

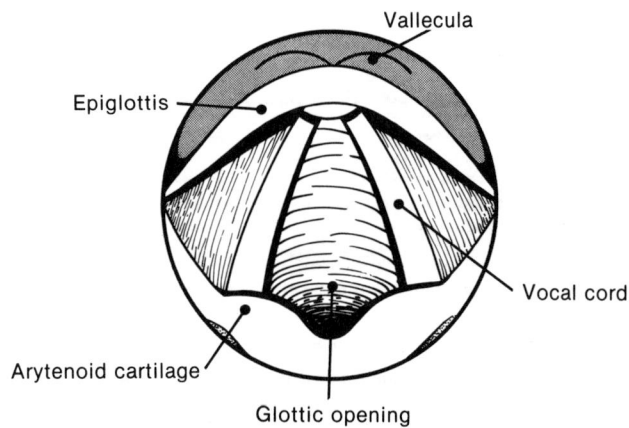

Straight Blade Technique

Fig. 11-2. Insert the laryngoscope blade between the patient's teeth and open the patient's mouth with the right hand. Advance the blade to the right side of the mouth, displacing the tongue to the left, but observe the cords before advancing the tube. Utilizing the laryngoscope, visualize the glottic opening.

Figure 11-2 View through laryngoscope.

Fig. 11-3. Advance the blade to just beyond the tip of the epiglottis. Aim it below the epiglottis.

Exert upward traction on the handle of the laryngoscope, displacing the base of the tongue and the epiglottis anteriorly to expose the glottic opening.

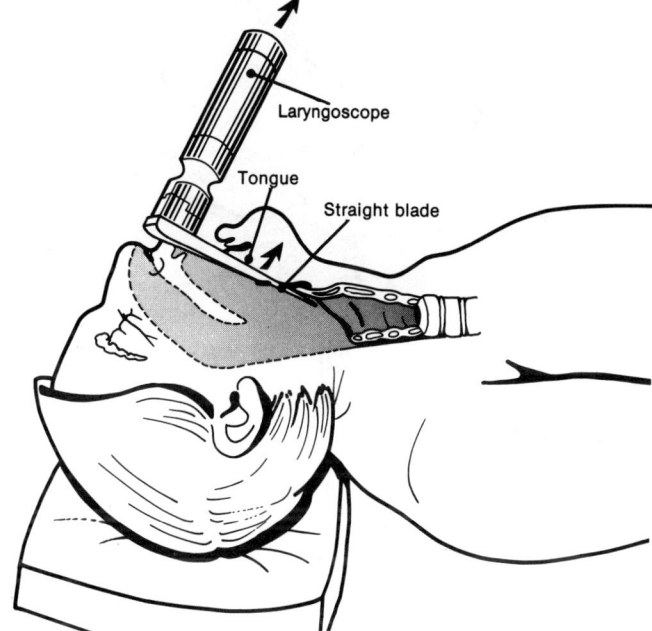

Figure 11-3 Straight blade technique.

Curved Blade Technique

Fig. 11-4. Insert the tip of the blade into the vallecula. Displace the epiglottis anteriorly by upward traction with the tip of the blade. Gently lift the laryngoscope upward and forward at the base of the tongue and epiglottis.

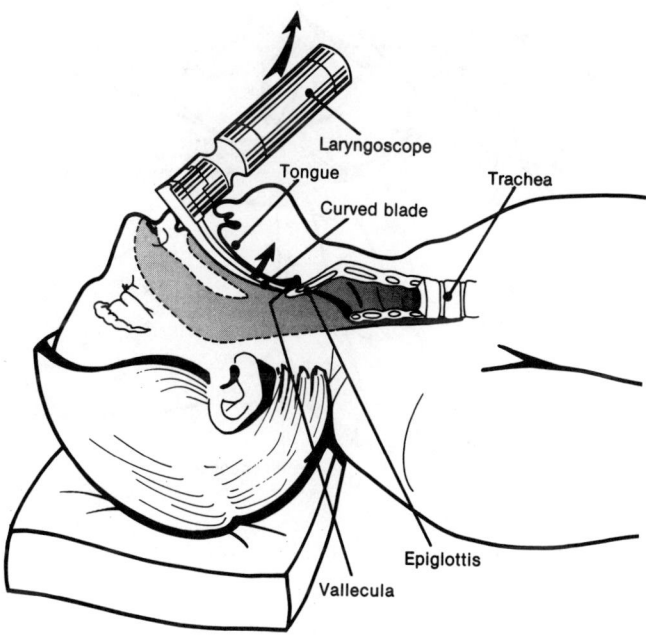

Figure 11-4 Curved blade technique.

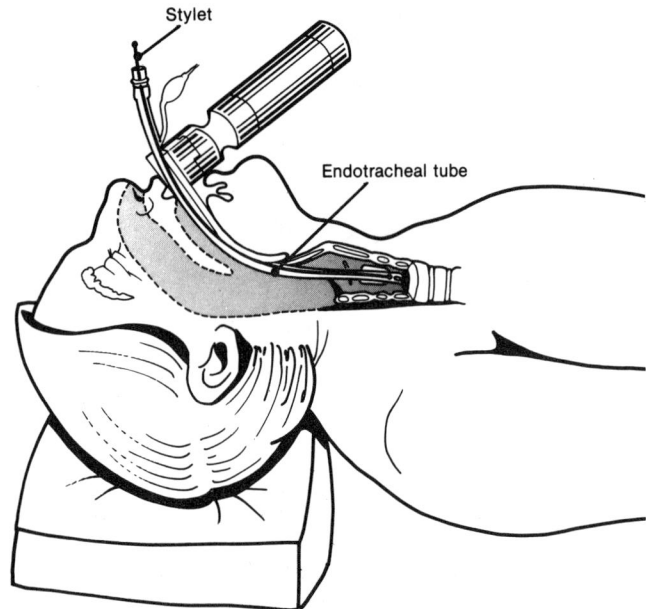

Figure 11-5 Endotracheal tube in place.

Fig. 11-5. As in the straight blade technique, observe the cords before advancing the tube. Advance the endotracheal tube between the vocal cords so that the balloon is just below the cords.

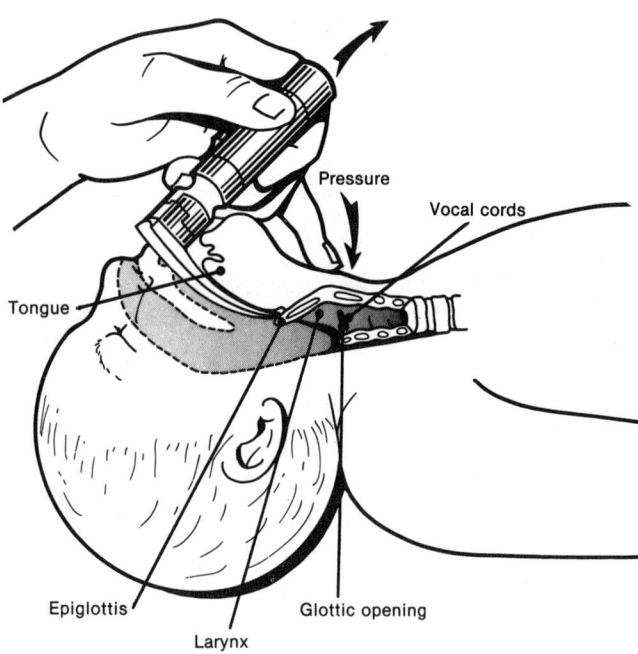

Figure 11-6 Intubation of infant.

Fig. 11-6. In a child or infant, utilizing the curved blade technique and applying pressure over the cricoid cartilage will occlude the upper end of the esophagus (Sellick maneuver) and may facilitate glottic visualization.

Fig. 11-7. Remove the stylet.

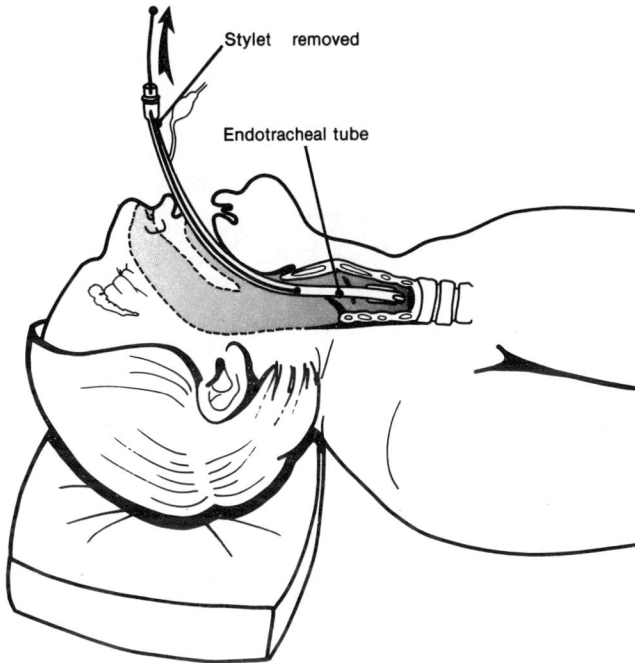

Figure 11-7 Stylet being removed.

Fig. 11-8. Inflate the balloon. Confirm that no air is escaping around the tube by listening at the patient's mouth. Establish that both the right and left lungs are ventilated by auscultating the chest. Attach the tube to a bag valve device or mechanical respirator.

Tape the tube securely. Provide supplemental oxygen or mechanical ventilation as indicated. Obtain a chest radiograph to confirm the position of the endotracheal tube.

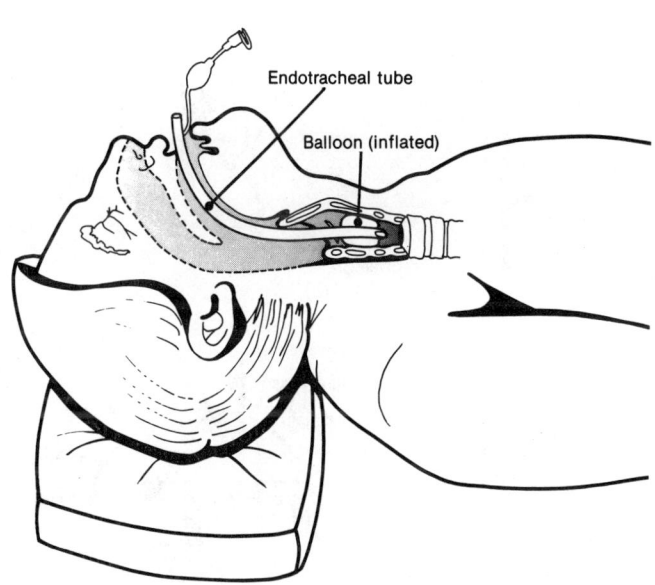

Figure 11-8 Inflate cuff.

BIBLIOGRAPHY

Collins VJ. *Principles of Anesthesiology*. 2nd ed. Philadelphia, Pa: Lea & Febiger; 1976:379.

Dripps R, et al. Intubation of the trachea. In: *Introduction to Anesthesia*. 4th ed. Philadelphia, Pa: WB Saunders Co; 1972:186–199.

Magill IV. Endotracheal anesthesia. *Am J Surg*. 1936;34:450.

McIntyre KM, Lewis AJ, eds. *Textbook of Advanced Cardiac Life Support*. Chicago, Ill: American Heart Association; 1981.

Vander Salm TJ, Cutler BS, Wheeler HB. *Atlas of Bedside Procedures*. Boston, Mass: Little, Brown & Co; 1979.

Waters RM, Rovenstine EA, Guedel AE. Endotracheal anesthesia and its historical developments. *Anesth Analg*. 1933;12:196.

12. CLOSED THORACOSTOMY

Indication

Remove fluid or air from the pleural space.

Procedure

For removal of air by the anterior apical approach, position the patient in the supine position, elevated 30°. Place the patient in the lateral decubitus position if the basilar or lateral apical-tube approach is to be used. Prepare and drape the patient in the usual sterile manner.

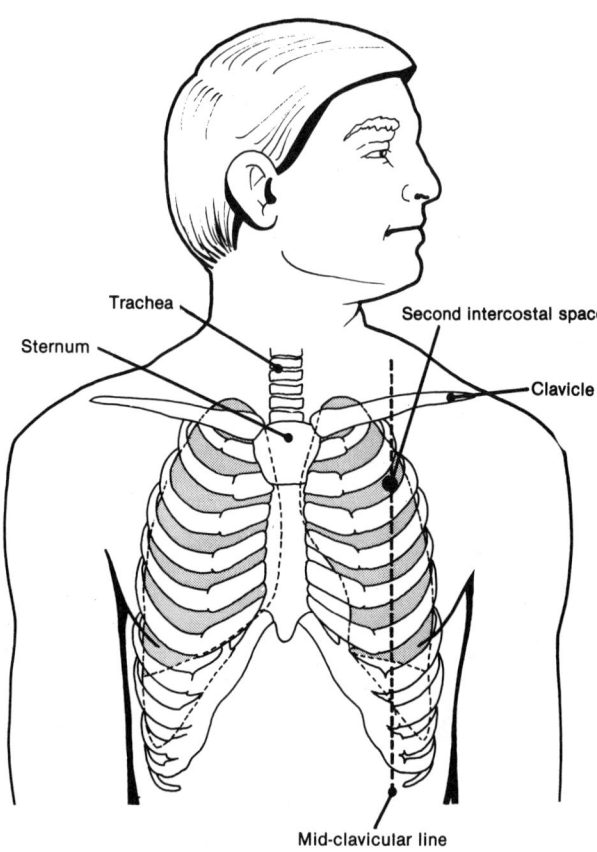

Figure 12-1 Anatomical position.

Fig. 12-1. Identify the anatomical landmarks: the second intercostal space on the midclavicular line or, alternatively, the midaxillary line at the caudal edge of the axillary line.

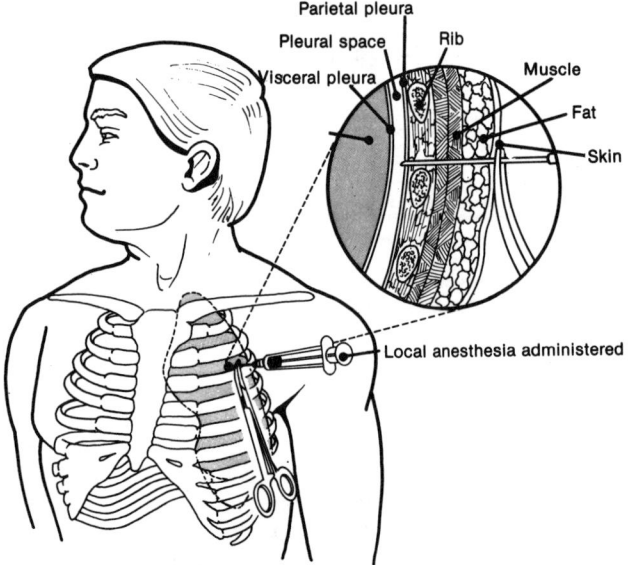

Figure 12-2 Local anesthesia.

Fig. 12-2. Introduce 0.5% to 1% lidocaine (Xylocaine) into the skin muscle and fat to the parietal pleura above the superior border of the rib. Also infiltrate the skin over the next caudal interspace. Aspirate from the pleural space to confirm the presence of fluid or air.

Fig. 12-3. With a #10 scalpel blade, make an incision in the area of the skin previously anesthetized. The space should be large enough to admit the small finger. Introduce a curved clamp into the incision site, and spread the fascia over the superior edge of the rib.

Perforate the pleura and enter the pleural space.

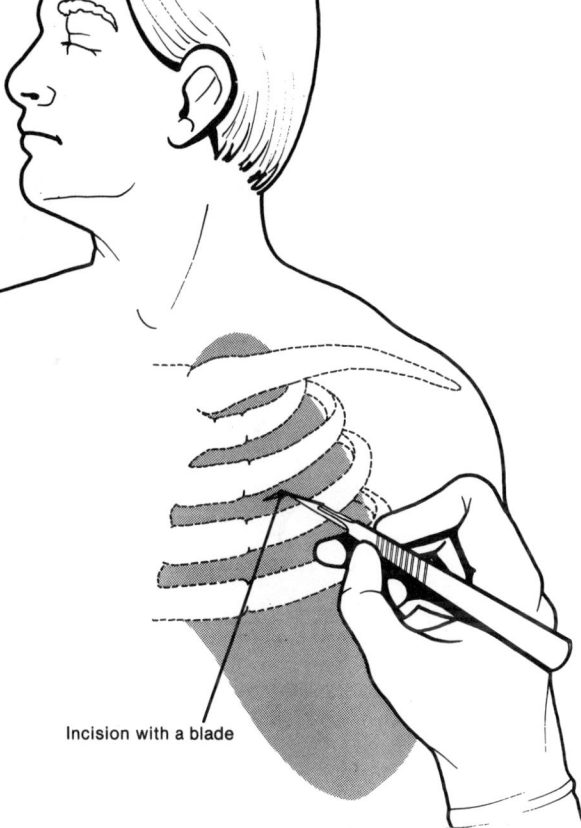

Figure 12-3 Incision of skin.

Fig. 12-4. Introduce the fifth (small) finger into the pleural space to confirm the space and exclude the possibility that lung tissue is against the incision site.

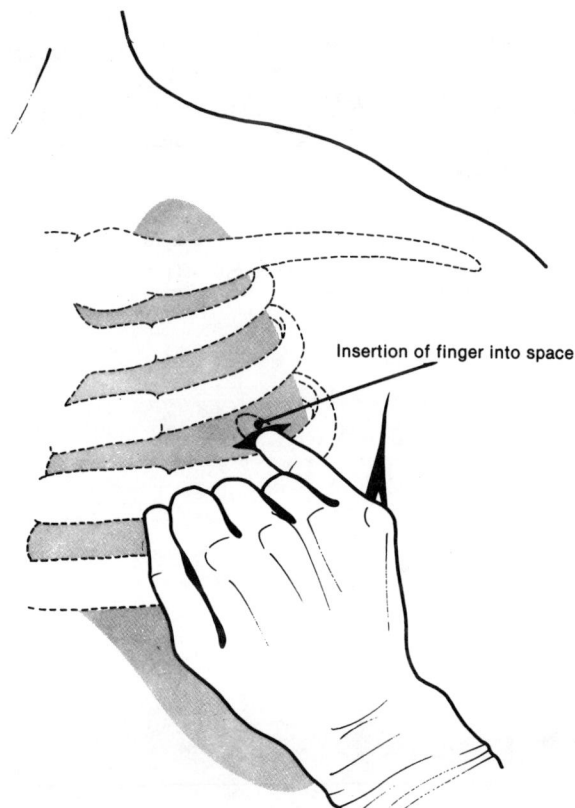

Figure 12-4 Finger in pleural space.

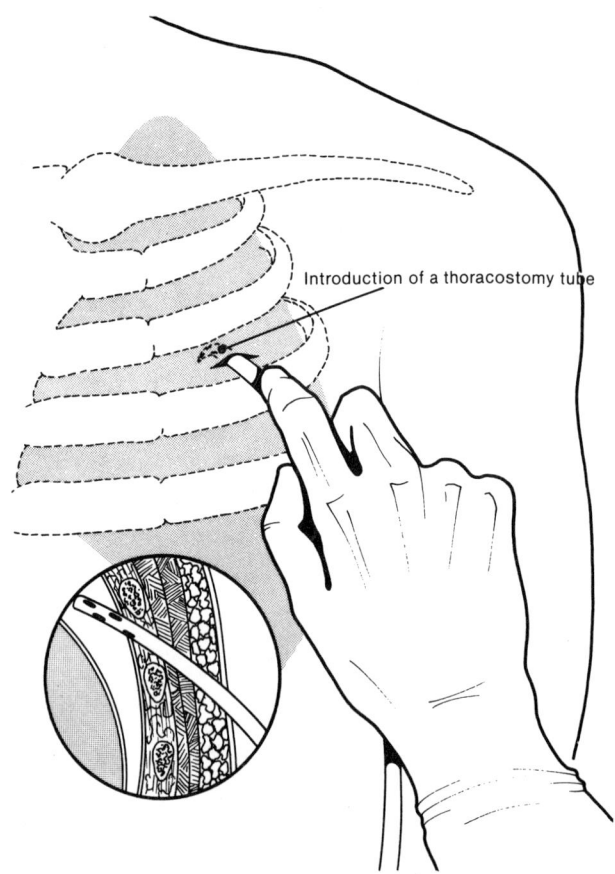

Figure 12-5 Insertion of tube.

Fig. 12-5. Insert the chest tube into the pleural space, advancing the tube toward the lung apex. Attach the chest tube to a water-sealed suction bottle apparatus. Suture the chest tube to the skin of the chest wall. Tape the tube to the chest wall and apply a sterile dressing. Obtain a chest radiograph to confirm the location of the chest tube and the success of therapy.

For treatment of hemothorax, use the sixth or seventh intercostal space on the midaxillary line. After the tube is advanced, position it posteriorly and basally.

BIBLIOGRAPHY

Cosgriff JH. *An Atlas of Diagnostic and Therapeutic Procedures for Emergency Personnel*. Philadelphia, Pa: JB Lippincott Co; 1978.

Gott PH. A simplified method for thoracentesis and pleural fluid drainage. *Am Rev Respir Dis*. 1965;92:295.

Hoffmann L. A modified thoracentesis technique. *Am Rev Respir Dis*. 1964;89:106.

Neptune WB. Thoracentesis. In: Nora PF, ed. *Operative Surgery*. Philadelphia, Pa: Lea & Febiger; 1972:217–218.

Vander Salm TJ, Cutler BS, Wheeler HB. *Atlas of Bedside Procedures*. Boston, Mass: Little, Brown & Co; 1979.

13. ASPIRATION AND INJECTION OF JOINTS, BURSAE, AND TENDONS

Indications

A. Determine the presence of joint effusion.
B. Evacuate hemarthrosis or other effusion.
C. Instill therapeutic agents.

Procedure

Knee Joint

Fig. 13-1A. For the anterior approach, flex the knee to 90°. Insert the needle through the middle of the patellar tendon, directly to the intercondylar notch.

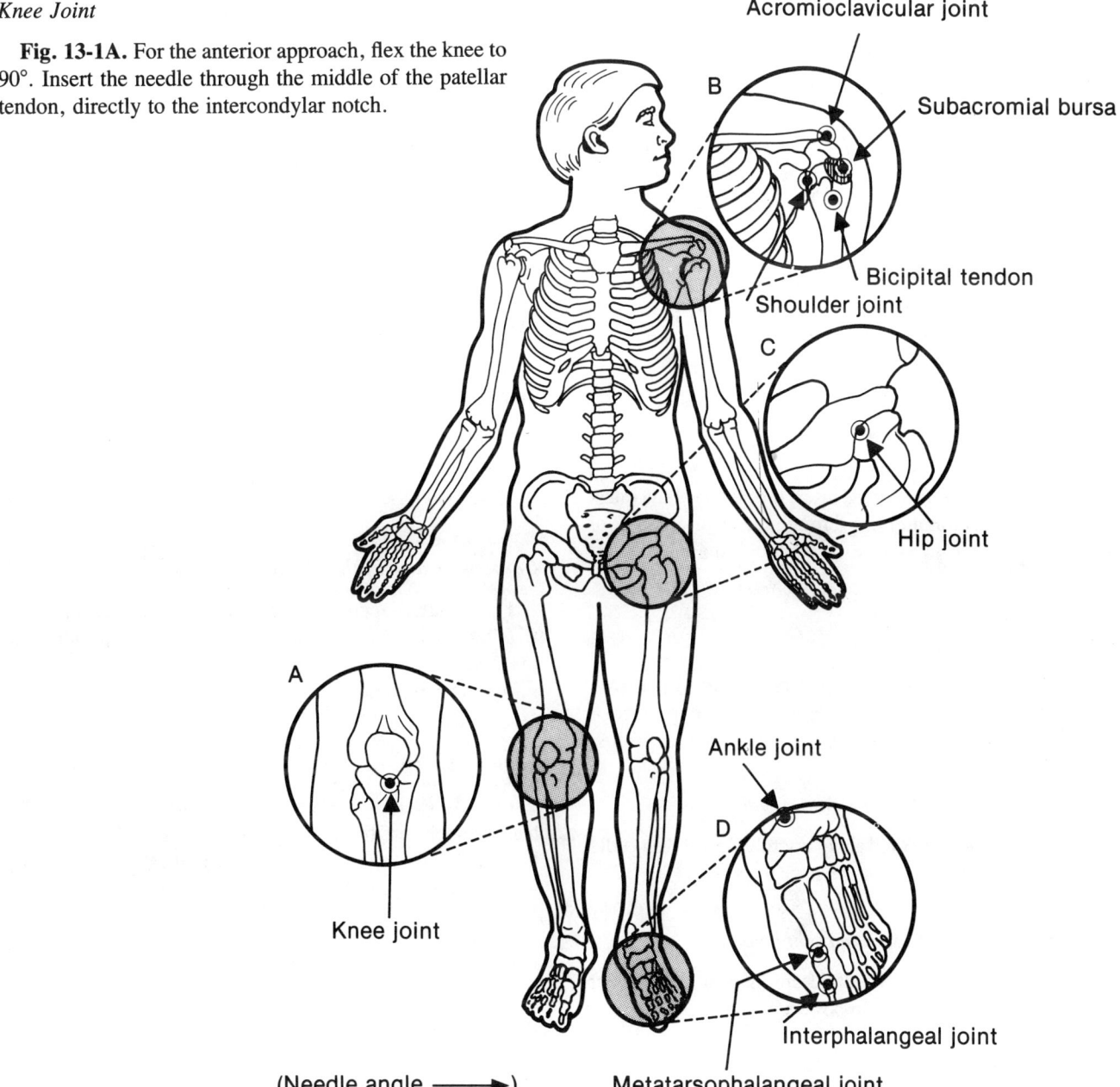

Figure 13-1 Anterior view.

Glenohumeral (Shoulder) Joint

Fig. 13-1B. Place the patient in a sitting position with the arm at the side and the hand across the abdomen. In the anterior technique, insert the needle lateral and inferior to the coracoid; direct it to the anterior rim of the glenoid.

Acromioclavicular Joint

Place the patient in same position as for the glenohumeral joint, and palpate the joint. Insert the needle superiorly; direct it to the lateral end of the clavicle.

Subacromial Bursa

Place the patient in the same position, applying downward traction to the flexed elbow, and insert the needle laterally 1 cm below the tip of the acromion; direct it medially to the bursa.

Bicipital Tendon

With the patient in the same position, insert the needle anteriorly at the point of maximum tenderness; direct the needle to the bicipital groove.

Hip Joint: Anterior Approach

Fig. 13-1C. Place the patient in the supine position, hip straight and in neutral rotation. Insert the needle at the intersection of the parasagittal line through the anterior-superior iliac spine and the transverse line through the pubic symphysis.

Tibiotalar (Ankle) Joint

Fig. 13-1D. Place the foot in the plantarflexed position. Insert the needle medial to the anterior tibial tendon; direct it to the hollow at the anterior margin of the medial malleolus.

Metatarsophalangeal and Interphalangeal Joints

Flex toes to 15° to 20° and apply traction. Insert the needle dorsally, medial or lateral to extensor tendon.

Glenohumeral Joint: Posterior Technique

Fig. 13-2A. Insert the needle 2 cm inferior to posterior angle of acromion; direct it to posterior rim of glenoid.

Radiohumeral (Elbow) Joint

Fig 13-2B. Place the patient in a sitting position, flexing the elbow 90°; pronate the forearm (palm down), and insert the needle between the lateral epicondyle and radial head; direct it medially.

Lateral Epicondyle

Place the patient in a sitting position with the elbow flexed 90°, pronate the forearm, and insert the needle at and directly to the point of maximum tenderness.

Olecranon Bursa

Flex the elbow to 90° and insert the needle at the posterior tip of the olecranon; direct it along the shaft of the ulna.

Hip Joint: Lateral Approach

Fig. 13-2C. Place the patient in the supine position with the hip straight and internally rotated. Insert the needle anterior to the greater trochanter, directly beneath the midportion of Poupart's ligament.

Greater Trochanteric Bursa

Place patient in the same position as for a lateral approach to a hip joint, and insert the needle directly to the point of maximum tenderness.

Metacarpophalangeal and Interphalangeal Joints

Fig. 13-2D. Flex fingers to 15° to 20°, apply traction to finger, and insert the needle dorsally, medial or lateral to extensor tendon.

Carpometacarpal (Thumb) Joint

Fig. 13-2E. Oppose the thumb to little finger, applying traction to the thumb, and insert the needle proximal to prominence of base metacarpal on the palmar side of abductor pollicus tendon.

Radiocarpal (Wrist) Joint

Fig 13-2F. Flex the wrist to 30°, apply traction to the hand, and insert the needle dorsally, distal to the dorsal tubercle, medial to extensor pollicus longus tendon, directly volar to joint.

Knee Joint: Anteromedial Approach

Fig. 13-2G. Place the patient in a supine position with the knee extended. Insert the needle 1 cm medial to patella directly to intercondylar notch.

Anserine Bursa

Extend the knee, and insert the needle directly to the point of maximum tenderness.

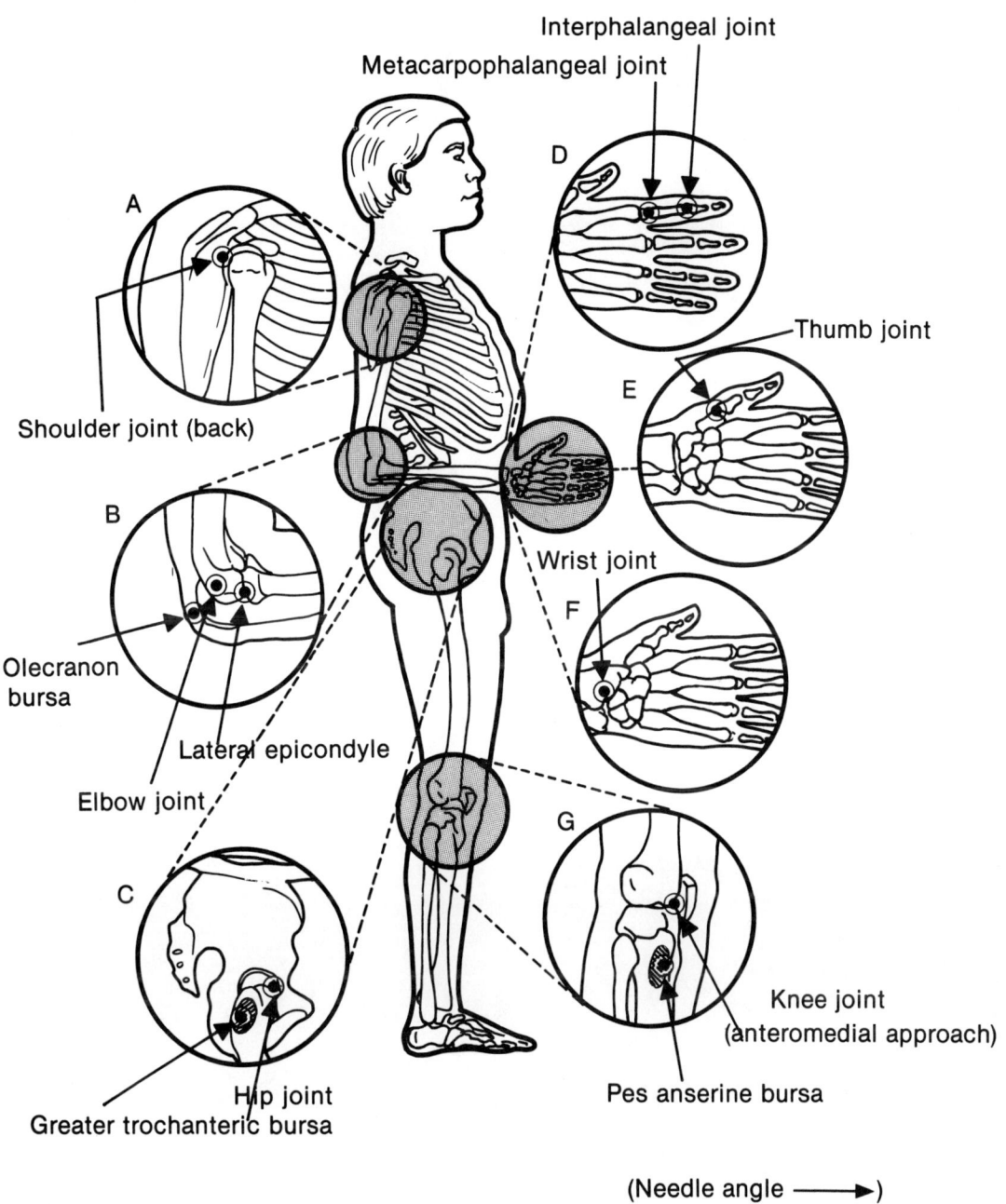

Figure 13-2 Lateral view.

BIBLIOGRAPHY

Calabro JJ. Rheumatoid arthritis. *Ciba Found Symp.* 1971;23:1.

Cosgriff JH. *An Atlas of Diagnostic and Therapeutic Procedures for Emergency Personnel*. Philadelphia, Pa: JB Lippincott Co; 1978.

Hollander JL. *Arthritis and Allied Conditions*. Philadelphia, Pa: Lea & Febiger; 1972:517.

Miller JA. Joint paracentesis from an anatomic point of view, I: shoulder, elbow, wrist and hand. *Surgery.* 1956;40:993.

Miller JA. Joint paracentesis from an anatomic point of view, II: hip, ankle, and foot. *Surgery.* 1957;41:999.

Pruce AM, Miller JA, Berger IR. Anatomic landmarks in joint paracentesis. *Ciba Found Symp.* 1964;16:19.

Steinbrocker OT, Neustadt DH. *Aspiration and Infection Therapy in Arthritis and Musculoskeletal Disorders*. Hagerstown, Md: Harper & Row; 1972.

Sweetnam R. Corticosteroid arthropathy and tendon rupture. *J Bone Joint Surg [Br].* 1969;51:397.

Vander Salm TJ, Cutler BS, Wheeler HB. *Atlas of Bedside Procedures*. Boston, Mass: Little, Brown & Co; 1979.

87. Emergency Drug Index

JOSEPH A. GRILLO, BS Pharm
EDGAR R. GONZALEZ, PharmD

CONTENTS

ANTIARRHYTHMICS, VASOPRESSORS, CARDIAC ARREST MEDICATIONS
- Adenosine 1381
- Amiodarone 1381
- Amrinone Lactate 1382
- Atropine 1382
- Bretylium Tosylate 1382
- Calcium Chloride 1382
- Calcium Gluconate 1383
- Digoxin 1383
- Diltiazem (IV) 1383
- Disopyramide 1384
- Dobutamine 1384
- Dopamine 1384
- Edrophonium 1385
- Epinephrine 1385
- Esmolol 1385
- Isoproterenol 1386
- Lidocaine 1386
- Methoxamine 1387
- Moricizine 1387
- Norepinephrine (Levarterenol) 1387
- Phenytoin (IV) 1388
- Potassium Chloride 1388
- Procainamide 1388
  - Parenteral 1388
  - Oral 1388
  - Sustained Release 1389
- Propafenone 1389
- Propranolol 1389
- Quinidine Gluconate 1390
- Quinidine Sulfate 1390
- Sodium Bicarbonate 1390
- Tromethamine 1391
- Verapamil 1391

ANTIHYPERTENSIVES, ANTIANGINAL AGENTS
- Atenolol 1391
- Captopril 1391
- Clonidine 1392
- Diazoxide 1392
- Diltiazem 1392
- Enalapril 1392
- Enalaprilat 1392
- Guanabenz 1392
- Guanethidine 1393
- Hydralazine 1393
- Isosorbide Dinitrate 1393
- Labetalol (Parenteral) 1393
- Labetalol (Oral) 1394
- α-Methyldopa 1394
- Metoprolol 1394
- Minoxidil 1394
- Nadolol 1395
- Nifedipine 1395
- Nifedipine Extended Release 1395
- Nimodipine 1395
- Nitroglycerin 1395
  - IV 1396
- Papaverine 1396

Prazosin 1396
Reserpine 1396
Sodium Nitroprusside 1397
Timolol 1397
Trimethaphan Camphor Sulfonate 1397
Verapamil (Oral) 1397

ANTICONVULSANTS
Diazepam 1398
Magnesium Sulfate 1398
Paraldehyde 1398
Phenobarbital Sodium 1399
Phenytoin 1399

ANTICOAGULANTS, ANTIFIBRINOLYTICS
Alteplase Recombinant (r-tPA) 1400
ε-Aminocaproic Acid 1400
Anistreplase (APSAC) 1400
Heparin Sodium 1401
Phytonadione 1401
Streptokinase 1402
Ticlopidine 1402
Warfarin Sodium 1403

ANTI-INFLAMMATORY/ANTIGOUT AGENTS
Allopurinol 1403
Colchicine 1403
Diflunisal 1404
Ibuprofen 1404
Indomethacin 1404
Naproxen 1404
Oxyphenbutazone 1405
Phenylbutazone 1405
Probenecid 1405
Sulfinpyrazone 1405

ANTIDEPRESSANTS, ANTIEMETICS, TRANQUILIZERS
Amitriptyline 1406
Buspirone 1406
Chlordiazepoxide 1406
Chlorpromazine 1406
Haloperidol 1407
Ondansetron 1407
Prochlorperazine 1407
Promethazine 1408
Trimethobenzamide 1408

ANTIHISTAMINES/ANTIPRURITICS
Cyproheptadine 1408
Diphenhydramine 1408
Hydroxyzine 1409

AMINOGLYCOSIDE ANTIBIOTICS
Amikacin 1409
Gentamicin 1409
Kanamycin 1410
Neomycin 1410
Netilmicin 1410

Streptomycin 1411
Tobramycin 1411

CEPHALOSPORIN ANTIBIOTICS
Parenterally Administered Cephalosporins
Cefamandole 1412
Cefazolin 1412
Cefonicid 1412
Cefoperazone 1412
Cefotaxime 1412
Cefoxitin 1412
Ceftazidime 1412
Ceftizoxime 1412
Ceftriaxone 1412
Cefuroxime 1412
Cephalothin 1412
Cephapirin 1413
Cephradine 1413
Moxalactam 1413

Orally Administered Cephalosporins
Cefaclor 1413
Cefadroxil 1413
Cefixime 1413
Cefuroxime Axetil 1413
Cephalexin 1413
Cephradine 1413

PENICILLIN AND PENICILLIN DERIVATIVE ANTIBIOTICS
Amoxicillin 1413
Amoxicillin/Clavulanic Acid 1413
Ampicillin 1414
Carbenicillin 1414
Cloxacillin 1414
Dicloxacillin 1415
Methicillin 1415
Mezlocillin Sodium 1415
Nafcillin 1415
Oxacillin 1415
Penicillin G 1416
Penicillin V 1416
Piperacillin 1416
Ticarcillin 1416

SULFONAMIDES
Sulfamethoxazole/Trimethoprim 1417
Sulfisoxazole 1417

TETRACYCLINES
Doxycycline 1417
Tetracycline 1418

MISCELLANEOUS ANTI-INFECTIVES
Acyclovir 1418
Amphotericin B 1418

Chloramphenicol 1419
Ciprofloxacin 1419
Clindamycin 1420
Erythromycin 1420
Fluconazole 1420
Imipenem-Cilastatin 1421
Ketoconazole 1421
Mebendazole 1421
Methenamine Mandelate 1422
Metronidazole 1422
    IV 1422
    Oral 1422
Nitrofurantoin 1422
Norfloxacin 1422
Nystatin 1423
Phenazopyridine 1423
Pyrimethamine 1423
Quinacrine 1423
Rifampin 1423
Spectinomycin 1423
Vancomycin 1424
Zidovudine (AZT) 1424

BRONCHODILATORS, ANTIASTHMATIC AGENTS
Acetylcysteine 1424
Albuterol (Salbutamol) 1425
Aminophylline 1425
    Oral 1425
    Parenteral 1425
Beclomethasone 1426
Ipratropium Bromide 1426
Isoetharine 1426
Isoproterenol 1426
Metaproterenol 1427
Oxtriphylline 1427
Terbutaline 1427
Theophylline 1427
    Sustained Release 1427
    Immediate Action 1427

CORTICOSTEROIDS
Dexamethasone 1428
Fludrocortisone 1429
Hydrocortisone 1429
Methylprednisolone 1429
Prednisone 1429

DIURETICS
Acetazolamide 1429
Amiloride 1430
Bumetanide 1430
Ethacrynic Acid 1430
Furosemide 1430
Glycerol (Glycerin) 1430
Hydrochlorothiazide 1431
Mannitol 1431
Metolazone 1431
Spironolactone 1431
Triamterene 1431

HYPOGLYCEMICS/ANTIHYPOGLYCEMICS
Dextrose (50%) 1432
Glucagon 1432
Insulin 1432

GASTRIC ACID INHIBITORS
Cimetidine 1433
Famotidine 1433
Misoprostol 1433
Omeprazole 1434
Ranitidine 1434
Sucralfate 1434

NARCOTIC AND NON-NARCOTIC ANALGESICS
Acetaminophen 1435
Aspirin 1435
Butorphanol 1435
Codeine 1436
Fentanyl 1436
    Transdermal 1436
Ketorolac Tromethamine 1436
Meperidine HCl 1437
Morphine Sulfate 1437
Pentazocine 1437
Propoxyphene 1437

SEDATIVE-HYPNOTICS
Barbiturates
Amobarbital 1438
Chloral Hydrate 1438
Ethchlorvynol 1439
Flurazepam 1439
Glutethimide 1439
Midazolam 1439
Pentobarbital 1440
Phenobarbital 1440
Secobarbital 1440
Temazepam 1440
Thiopental IV 1440
Triazolam 1440

SKELETAL MUSCLE RELAXANTS
Atracurium 1441
Carisoprodol 1441
Cyclobenzaprine 1441
Dantrolene 1442
Diazepam 1442
Methocarbamol 1443
Pancuronium 1443
Vecuronium 1443

PLASMA VOLUME EXPANDERS
Albumin 1444
Dextran 40, 70, 75 1444
Hetastarch 1444
Plasma Protein Fraction 1445

THYROID/ANTITHYROID AGENTS
Levothyroxine 1445
Propylthiouracil 1445

ERGOT ALKALOIDS, OXYTOCICS, ESTROGENS
Conjugated Estrogens 1445
Ergotamine Tartrate 1446
Methylergonovine Maleate 1446
Methylsergide Maleate 1446
Oxytocin 1446

HEMATINICS
Ferrous Sulfate 1447
Iron Dextran 1447

MISCELLANEOUS AGENTS FOR OVERDOSE TREATMENT
Acetylcysteine 1447
Activated Charcoal 1448
Amyl Nitrite 1448
Deferoxamine 1448
Flumazenil 1448
Ipecac Syrup 1449
Lactulose 1449
Methylene Blue Injection 1449
Naloxone HCl 1449
Physostigmine 1449
Sodium Nitrite 1450
Sodium Polystyrene Sulfonate 1450
Sodium Thiosulfate 1450

Bibliography 1450

Appendix 87-A List of Pharmacologic/Therapeutic Drugs and Agents for Emergency Facilities 1452

ANTIARRHYTHMICS, VASOPRESSORS, CARDIAC ARREST MEDICATIONS

Generic Name: ADENOSINE
Trade Name: Adenocard
Dosage Form: Injection, 6 mg/2 mL
Uses: Adenosine is an endogenous nucleoside with antiarrhythmic properties that result from its ability to slow conduction time through the AV node and interrupt re-entry pathways. It is currently indicated for the treatment of paroxysmal supraventricular tachycardia (PSVT), including Wolff-Parkinson-White syndrome.
Adult Dosage (Parenteral): Rapid IV bolus either directly into a vein or, if given into an IV line, administered as proximal as possible and followed by a rapid saline flush. Initial dosage, 6 mg (over 1–2 seconds). If first dose does not result in elimination of PSVT within 1–2 minutes, then an additional 12-mg rapid IV bolus should be administered. The 12-mg dosage may be repeated a second time if necessary.
Pediatric Dosage (Parenteral): Safety and efficacy not established in children.
Contraindications: Second- or third-degree AV block or sick sinus syndrome (except in patients with an artificial pacemaker); atrial fibrillation; atrial flutter; ventricular tachycardia; hypersensitivity to the drug product.
Precautions: Since adenosine has the potential to cause bronchospasm (rarely) it should be used with caution in patients with a history of asthma.
Adverse Reactions: Most adverse reactions are self-limiting because of adenosine's short half-life (<10 seconds). GI—nausea and metallic taste; CNS—headache, lightheadedness, tingling, numbness, blurred vision; CV—AV block, bradycardia, facial flushing, palpitations, chest pain, hypotension (rare); RESP—bronchospasm (rare), dyspnea, and hyperventilation; other—neck/back pain and throat tightness.
Drug Interactions: With methylxanthines (eg, theophylline, caffeine), may antagonize the effects of adenosine. With carbamazepine, may precipitate higher degrees of AV block when used concomitantly with adenosine. With dipyridamole, potentiates the effects of adenosine.

Generic Name: AMIODARONE
Trade Name: Cordarone
Dosage Form: Tablets, 200 mg
Uses: Class III antiarrhythmic indicated for the treatment of life-threatening recurrent ventricular fibrillation or hemodynamically unstable ventricular tachycardia that does not respond to other antiarrhythmics or when alternative agents are not tolerated. The antiarrhythmic effect is thought to be a result of (1) a prolongation of the action potential duration and refractory period or (2) a noncompetitive α- and β-adrenergic inhibition.
Adult Dosage (Oral): An initial loading regimen of 800–1600 mg/day is administered for 1–3 weeks until a therapeutic response occurs. If the total daily dose is ≥ 1000 mg or if GI intolerance occurs, the daily dose should be divided and administered with meals. When desired arrhythmia control has been attained or if side effects become intolerable, the total daily dose should be reduced to 600–800 mg/day and maintained for 1 month. The dose should then be further reduced to a daily maintenance dose, which can be 200–600 mg/day.
Pediatric Dosage (Oral): Safety and efficacy not established.
Contraindications: Severe sinus node dysfunction, causing marked sinus bradycardia; second- and third-degree AV block; and episodes of bradycardia causing syncope (except when used in conjunction with a pacemaker).
Precautions: Has been shown to decrease the defibrillation threshold acutely and increase the defibrillation threshold after chronic use. Corneal microdeposits (discernible only by slit lamp examination) appear in the majority of adults treated, resulting in visual disturbances (halos and blurred vision) in as many as 10% of the patients treated. Corneal microdeposits are usually reversed upon reduction of the dose or discontinuation of drug therapy. Since amiodarone peripherally inhibits the conversion of thyroxin (T_4) to tri-iodothyronine (T_3) and is itself a source of organic iodine, the potential for hypothyroidism and hyperthyroidism exists. Therefore, thyroid function tests should be measured at baseline and periodically throughout therapy. Amiodarone has also been associated with photosensitization in about 10% of patients treated (may be afforded with sun barrier cream and protective clothing) and a blue-gray skin discoloration after prolonged therapy (slowly reversible upon discontinuation of drug therapy).
Adverse Reactions: Most commonly occur at dosages ≥ 400 mg/day for ≥ 6 months. GI—nausea, vomiting, constipation, anorexia, and abdominal pain; CNS—malaise, fatigue, tremor/abnormal involuntary movements, ataxia, sleep disturbances, headache, peripheral neuropathy, dizziness, and decreased libido; DERM—photosensitization and blue-gray skin discoloration; CV—proarrhythmia, CHF, bradycardia (may respond to dosage reduction), hypotension, and SA node dysfunction; other—abnormal liver function tests, hepatitis and cirrhosis (rare), pulmonary infiltrates and fibrosis, hypothyroidism, hyperthyroidism. *Pulmonary toxicity, CHF, and elevation of liver enzymes require discontinuation of drug therapy.*
Drug Interactions: With oral anticoagulants, an increase in prothrombin time usually requires a reduction in the anticoagulant dose by ½ to ⅓, with careful monitoring of PT. With digoxin, increased digoxin serum levels by as much as 70% can occur, requiring a reduction in the digoxin dose by ½. With quinidine, increased serum levels by 30–50% can occur requiring a reduction in dose by ⅓ to ½ or discontinuance of therapy. With procainamide, increase in both procainamide and NAPA serum levels requires a reduction in dose by ⅓ to ½ or discontinuance of

---

NOTE: Although the authors have been careful to provide general drug administration guidelines that are in agreement with current literature, we suggest that the reader refer to the text itself for specific indications and dosages. We also suggest that appropriate information sources be consulted when dealing with new and unfamiliar drugs. It remains the responsibility of every practitioner to evaluate the appropriateness of a particular opinion in the context of the actual clinical situation and with due consideration to any new developments in the field. A review of pharmacokinetics and drug overdose is found in Chapter 29.

Joseph A. Grillo, BS Pharm
Edgar R. Gonzalez, PharmD

therapy. With phenytoin, serum levels increased by 200–300% require a phenytoin dosage adjustment. With β-blockers and calcium channel antagonists, there is a potential for bradycardia, AV block, and sinus arrest.

Generic Name: AMRINONE LACTATE
Trade Name: Inocor
Dosage Form: Injection (IV), 100 mg/20 mL ampule (5 mg/mL)
Uses: Cardiac inotropic agent and vasodilator given for short-term management of congestive heart failure. At normal dosage ranges, it increases cardiac output, decreases both pulmonary capillary wedge pressure and systemic vascular resistance without significant changes in heart rate or myocardial oxygen consumption.
Adult Dosage (Parenteral): 0.75 mg/kg slow IV bolus over 15–30 min followed by IV infusion of 5–10 μg/kg/min (up to 13 μg/kg/min).
Contraindications: Hypersensitivity to amrinone.
Precautions: Ampules are light-sensitive; do not use solution if particulate matter or marked discoloration is observed. Dilute ampules in NS or non-dextrose–containing IV solutions to a concentration of 1 to 3 mg/mL. Monitor patient's response using cardiac output; blood, central venous, and pulmonary capillary wedge pressures; fluid and electrolyte balances; urine output; and degree of dyspnea or fatigue. Slow or stop infusion if excessive decreases in blood pressure occur. Perform blood platelet counts before and periodically during therapy. Vigorous diuretic therapy may cause insufficient cardiac filling and consequently inadequate responses to amrinone therapy. Use cautiously in patients with hypertrophic subaortic stenosis as it may aggravate outflow tract obstruction. Not recommended for use during acute phase of postmyocardial infarction.
Adverse Reactions: Thrombocytopenia (with platelet count reductions below 100,000/mm^3) has occurred and appears to be related to dosage and duration of therapy. Other reactions include gastric upset, nausea, vomiting, anorexia, abdominal pain, arrhythmias (supraventricular and ventricular), hypotension, chest pain, fever, hypersensitivity reactions, and burning at the site of injection. Some hepatic toxicity with necrosis and enzyme elevations has also been reported (rare).
Drug Interactions: Precipitate forms when furosemide is injected into IV line or amrinone infusion. Do not mix amrinone directly with dextrose solutions.

Generic Name: ATROPINE (Parenteral)
Trade Name: Atropine
Dosage Form: Injection (IV), 1 mg/10 mL preloaded syringe and 0.3–2.0 mg/mL vials
Uses: Anticholinergic, used for treatment of sinus bradycardia (pulse under 60 beats/min) and improvement of atrioventricular conduction.
Adult Dosage (Parenteral): 0.5–1 mg IV push or via endotracheal tube (range: minimum dose, 0.5 mg; maximum dose, 0.04 mg/kg). Doses may be repeated q. 5 min until pulse is over 60 beats/min or 0.04 mg/kg have been given. For improvement of atrioventricular conduction, give 0.8–1.2 mg IV or subcutaneously q. 4h, prn (maximum dosage of 4 mg/day). Endotracheally administered doses should be 2 to 2.5 times the IV dose.
Pediatric Dosage (Parenteral): 0.01–0.03 mg/kg IV or via endotracheal tube; can repeat dose in 5 min (minimum dose, 0.1 mg; maximum dose, 1 mg).
Precautions: Glaucoma, coronary artery disease (1-mg doses may produce ventricular arrhythmias).
Adverse Reactions: Dose-related. Keep IV rate at 1 mg/min or less. Adverse reactions that may occur include the following:
- at 1 mg: tachycardia, dry mouth, pupil dilation
- at 2 mg: increase of symptoms that develop at 1 mg; blurred vision
- at 5 mg: aggravation of symptoms mentioned; speech disturbances; hot, dry skin
- at 10 mg: increased severity of all symptoms; atropine ''flush''; excitement; hallucinations; coma; arrest. (Antidote: physostigmine IV.)

Drug Interactions: Incompatible with sodium bicarbonate.

Generic Name: BRETYLIUM TOSYLATE
Trade Name: Bretylol
Dosage Form: Injection (IV/IM), 500 mg/10 mL ampule (50 mg/mL)
Uses: Adrenergic blocking and antiarrhythmic agent for treatment of life-threatening ventricular arrhythmias, particularly tachycardia and fibrillation refractory to lidocaine. Onset is rapid (within minutes), and duration of action is 6–9 hours.
Adult Dosage (Parenteral): For emergency treatment, 5–10 mg/kg IV push. May repeat with 2 doses of 10 mg/kg up to 15 to 30 min apart (maximum total dosage of 30–35 mg/kg). For prophylaxis, 5–10 mg/kg IV over 8 min, then either repeat bolus dose q. 6h or continuous IV infusion of 1–2 mg/min.
Pediatric Dosage (Parenteral): 5–10 mg/kg/dose, slow IV push; can repeat in 15 to 30 min (maximum cumulative dose, 30 mg/kg).
Precautions: For short-term use only. Follow bolus dose with electrical defibrillation attempt. For conscious patients, give bolus doses slowly (over 8 min). Patient should be weaned from drug over 3 to 5 days. Initial release of norepinephrine caused by bretylium may worsen digitalis-induced arrhythmias. No more than 5 mL should be given in any one IM injection site; avoid repeated IM doses.
Adverse Reactions: Nausea, vomiting, and hypotension after too rapid IV administration. Hypotension (incidence 50%–75%), to which tolerance usually develops, may be treated with dopamine or norepinephrine if supine diastolic blood pressure is less than 75 mmHg. Bradycardia, substernal pressure, and angina have been reported.
Drug Interactions: Should not be mixed with any other medications. Additive hypotension with other ventricular antiarrhythmic medications (eg, lidocaine, procainamide).

Generic Name: CALCIUM CHLORIDE (IV, 10%)
Trade Name: Calcium Chloride
Dosage Form: Injection (IV/intracardiac), 10 mL (10% solution) preloaded syringe (13.6 mEq Ca^{2+})
Uses: Stimulation of myocardial contractility, particularly in states of low cardiac output; treatment of severe hypocalcemia and tetany. (Normal serum calcium level, 4.5–5.5 mEq/L or 9–11 mg/dL).
Adult Dosage (Parenteral): For CPR, 5–10 mL 10% solution slow IV or intracardiac injection.

Pediatric Dosage (Parenteral): 0.2–0.5 mL/kg slow IV push; can repeat dose in 10–20 min as needed.

Contraindications: Relative contraindication in digitalized patients.

Precautions: Should not be given IM or subcutaneously because of risk of tissue necrosis. Rate of calcium ion infusion should not exceed 0.7–1.5 mEq/min (less than 3 mL/min). Caution must be used in digitalized patients. Chloride salt is acidifying; can cause acidosis in newborns and infants.

Adverse Reactions: Most result from too rapid IV administration (toxic serum level of calcium, 15 mg/dL [7.5 mEq/L] or more). Symptoms include tingling sensations, calcium taste, sense of heat waves, vasodilation, bradycardia, arrhythmias, shortened QT intervals, and ventricular fibrillation. Treatment of hypercalcemia includes hydration, IV furosemide, mithramycin, sodium sulfate solutions, or IV phosphates.

Drug Interactions: Physically incompatible with sodium bicarbonate, phosphates, and cephalothin; may precipitate serious arrhythmias in patients receiving digitalis glycosides.

Generic Name: CALCIUM GLUCONATE (IV 10%)
Trade Name: Calcium Gluconate
Dosage Form: Injection (IV/intracardiac), 10 mL 10% solution (4.7 mEq Ca^{2+})
Uses: See calcium chloride. Preferred for pediatric use.
Adult Dosage (Parenteral): For CPR, 10 mL of 10% solution IV or intracardiac. Dosage may be repeated q. 5–10 min prn. For tetany, 10–20 mL 10% solution slow IV over 5–10 min, then IV infusion of 15 mEq Ca^{2+} in D_5W 1000 mL over 4–12 hours.
Pediatric Dosage (Parenteral): 1–2 mL/kg slow IV push (up to 5 mL total dose in premature infants and 10 mL in full-term infants).
Contraindications: See calcium chloride.
Precautions: See calcium chloride.
Adverse Reactions: See calcium chloride.
Drug Interactions: See calcium chloride.

Generic Name: DIGOXIN
Trade Name: Lanoxin
Dosage Forms: Injection (IV/IM), 0.1 mg/mL (pediatric), 0.25 mg/mL (adult); tablets, 0.125 mg, 0.25 mg, 0.5 mg; capsules, 0.05 mg, 0.1 mg, 0.2 mg; oral elixir, 0.05 mg/mL
Uses: Digitalis glycoside for treatment of congestive heart failure, pulmonary edema, and atrial and re-entrant supraventricular arrhythmias.
Digoxin Dosage Parameters:
- therapeutic blood level: 0.8–2 ng/mL
- toxic blood level: 2–3 ng/mL
- half-life: approximately 36 hours (1.5–2.0 days)
- IV doses: 100% absorption (onset, 5–10 min)
- oral doses: 80% absorption (onset, 1–2 hours)
- IM doses: approximately equal to oral doses but painful; no advantage unless other routes are contraindicated.

Adult Dosage (Oral): If patient has been on digitalis for past 2 weeks, one-half digitalizing dose. For digitalization, 0.5–0.75 mg by mouth initially, then 0.25–0.5 mg q. 6–8h until total loading dose is given (usually 1–1.5 mg/d). For maintenance, 0.125–0.5 mg/d.

Adult Dosage (Parenteral): For digitalization, 0.25–0.5 mg IV to start, then 0.25 mg q. 4–6h to full digitalizing dose (0.5–1 mg/d). For maintenance, 0.125–0.5 mg/d IV.

Pediatric Dosage (Oral): (*Note:* All daily maintenance doses are 25%–35% of the digitalizing dose.) The following are digitalizing doses to be divided q. 6h: For a child over 10 years, 10–15 μg/kg; 5 to 10 years, 20–35 μg/kg; 2 to 5 years, 30–40 μg/kg; 1 to 24 months, 35–60 μg/kg; full-term infant, 25–35 μg/kg; premature infant, 20–30 μg/kg.

Pediatric Dosage (Parenteral): (*Note:* All daily maintenance doses are 25%–35% of the digitalizing dose.) The following are digitalizing doses to be given slowly IV, divided q. 6h: For a child over 10 years, 8–12 μg/kg; 5 to 10 years, 15–30 μg/kg; 2 to 5 years, 25–35 μg/kg; 1 to 24 months, 30–50 μg/kg; full-term infant, 20–30 μg/kg; premature infant, 15–25 μg/kg.

Contraindications: Ventricular fibrillation, hypersensitivity to cardiac glycosides (rare).

Precautions: Hypokalemia, hypomagnesemia, and hypercalcemia may predispose or enhance toxicity. "Sick sinus" syndrome, incomplete atrioventricular block, or outflow obstruction in idiopathic hypertrophic subaortic stenosis may worsen. Atrial arrhythmias associated with hypermetabolic and febrile states are particularly resistant. Caution is needed in the presence of renal impairment, premature infants, and patients with severe types of cardiac and pulmonary disease. Digoxin toxicity may mimic many of the arrhythmias it is being used to treat.

Adverse Reactions: Gastric upset with anorexia, nausea, vomiting, diarrhea; visual disturbances such as blurred or yellow vision, diplopia, halos, difficulty in red-green color perception, photophobia; headache, weakness; drowsiness; paresthesias. Various cardiac arrhythmias include paroxysmal atrial tachycardia with or without block, nodal arrhythmias, premature ventricular contractions, bigeminy, and other ventricular arrhythmias.

Drug Interactions: With antacids, decrease in oral absorption of digitalis. With potassium-depleting diuretics and calcium salts, increase in digitalis toxicity. With sympathomimetics, may precipitate/exacerbate digitalis-induced arrhythmias. With β-blockers, may worsen atrioventricular block. With quinidine, may increase digoxin serum levels. With amiodarone, may increase digoxin serum levels.

Generic Name: DILTIAZEM (IV)
Trade Name: Cardizem IV
Dosage Form: Injection, 5 mg/mL in 5 mL (25 mg) and 10 mL (50 mg) vials
Uses: Indicated for the temporary control of rapid ventricular rate in atrial fibrillation or flutter; atrial fibrillation or flutter not associated with an accessory pathway (eg, WPW); and the conversion of paroxysmal supraventricular tachycardia to sinus rhythm.
Adult Dosage (Parenteral): Direct IV bolus—initial dose is 0.25 mg/kg as a bolus administered over 2 min (20 mg, average patient); if response inadequate after 15 min a second bolus may be administered at 0.35 mg/kg over 2 min (25 mg, average patient). Continuous IV infusion—may be instituted immediately following bolus administration; recommended initial infusion rate is 5 to 10 mg/h and may be increased by 5 mg/h increments up to 15 mg/h as needed; dilute 250 mg diltiazem in 250 mL 5% dextrose injection or other suitable diluent and run at

12 mL/h (10 mg/h) to 18 mL/h (15 mg/h); infusions may be maintained up to 24 hours.

Pediatric Dosage: Safety and efficacy not established.

Contraindications: See diltiazem (oral) in the antihypertensives section.

Precautions: See diltiazem (oral). Infusion rates >15 mg/h and duration >24 hours are not recommended. Hypotension can usually be managed by the administration of 0.9% sodium chloride infusion or by placing the patient in the Trendelenburg position.

Adverse Reactions: See diltiazem (oral).

Drug Interactions: See diltiazem (oral).

Generic Name: DISOPYRAMIDE
Trade Name: Norpace
Dosage Form: Capsules, 100 mg and 150 mg
Uses: Antiarrhythmic, similar to quinidine and procainamide used for treatment of ventricular arrhythmias, particularly premature ventricular tachycardia and contractions.

Adult Dosage (Oral): 100–150 mg q. 6h. If loading dose is required, 200–300 mg (usual dosage range, 400–800 mg/d). Therapeutic serum level is 2–4 μg/mL (up to 7 μg/mL). For severe refractory ventricular tachycardia, up to 300–400 mg q. 6h with constant cardiac monitoring.

Pediatric Dosage (Oral): The following are total daily doses to be divided q. 6h: For a child 12 to 18 years, 6–15 mg/kg/d; 4 to 12 years, 10–15 mg/kg/d; 1 to 4 years, 10–20 mg/kg/d; under 1 year, 10–30 mg/kg/d.

Contraindications: Cardiogenic shock, pre-existing second- or third-degree atrioventricular block (if no pacemaker present), torsade de pointes, hypersensitivity to disopyramide.

Precautions: Renal or hepatic insufficiency, pregnancy, lactation, diabetes. Effects are unpredictable in Wolff-Parkinson-White and ''sick sinus'' syndromes. Drug has negative inotropic effect; caution must be used in congestive heart failure and cardiomyopathies. Anticholinergic activity may be prominent and may exacerbate myasthenia gravis, urinary retention, or other conditions aggravated by anticholinergic activity.

Adverse Reactions: Toxic serum levels generally 9 μg/mL or more. Anticholinergic side effects include dry mouth, blurred vision, urinary retention, and gastric upset. Drug may precipitate or worsen congestive heart failure and pre-existing atrioventricular block. Hypoglycemia, generalized malaise, hypotension, CNS derangements, hypersensitivity reactions, and hepatic enzyme changes may occur.

Drug Interactions: With quinidine, procainamide, or propranolol, serious negative inotropic effects and slowed conduction; with oral anticoagulants, possible potentiation of hypoprothrombinemic effects. Disopyramide may potentiate with activity of other anticholinergic agents.

Generic Name: DOBUTAMINE
Trade Name: Dobutrex
Dosage Form: Injection (IV), 250 mg
Uses: Sympathomimetic vasopressor for short-term inotropic support in cardiogenic shock, hemodynamically significant hypotension, and refractory congestive heart failure. It directly stimulates β-adrenergic receptors without causing release of endogenous norepinephrine. Moderate doses decrease preload and have minimal chronotropic and blood pressure effects; high doses can cause tachycardia and decreased peripheral vascular resistance.

Adult Dosage (Parenteral): Administer with controlled infusion device. IV infusion of 2.5 to 10 μg/kg/min (up to 40 μg/kg/min). Suggested dilution is 250 mg/500 mL normal saline or D_5W for a concentration of 500 μg/mL.

Pediatric Dosage: Not established, but IV infusions of 2.5–10 μg/kg/min (up to 40 μg/kg/min) have been used.

Contraindications: Idiopathic hypertrophic subaortic stenosis.

Precautions: Maintain or replace blood volume as necessary. Adjust infusion rates according to heart rate, blood pressure, pulmonary artery wedge pressure, and urine flow. Drug may precipitate or exacerbate ventricular ectopic activity by increasing atrioventricular conduction (digitalize patient if necessary). Pre-existing hypertension may cause exaggerated pressor response. Dobutamine may intensify or extend myocardial ischemia associated with acute myocardial infarction. It may be ineffective in patients who have recently received β-blocking agents.

Adverse Reactions: Dose-related effects seen with doses over 20 μg/kg/min. Ventricular ectopic beats, premature ventricular contractions, chest pain, palpitations, increased heart rate (5–15 beats/min), and increased blood pressure (10–20 mmHg) occur. Atrioventricular conduction is increased.

Drug Interactions: Incompatible with sodium bicarbonate and alkaline solutions, such as aminophylline and phenytoin. Dobutamine and nitroprusside together may result in higher cardiac output and lower pulmonary arterial wedge pressures than when either is used alone. β-Blocking agents may inhibit dobutamine's effects.

Generic Name: DOPAMINE
Trade Name: Intropin
Dosage Forms: Injection (IV), 200-mg ampule, 400-mg vial, premixed solution of 400 mg/250 mL D_5W (1600 μg/mL)
Uses: Sympathomimetic for increasing cardiac output, blood pressure, and urine flow via direct, β_1-receptor stimulation.

Adult Dosage (Parenteral): Suggested IV dilution is 400 mg/250 mL D_5W or 1600 μg/mL. Administer with controlled infusion device. IV infusion at 2–5 μg/kg/min to start; may be increased by 5–10 μg/kg/min up to 50 μg/kg/min. Most patients require 20 μg/kg/min or less, but rates of 50–100 μg/kg/min have been used.

Pediatric Dosage (Parenteral): Safety and efficacy not established but IV infusion range of 2 to 30 μg/kg/min titrated to desired effect has been used.

Contraindications: Pheochromocytoma, uncorrected tachyarrhythmias, or ventricular fibrillation.

Precautions: Hypovolemia should be corrected first or simultaneously. Hypoxia, hypercapnia, and acidosis all reduce dopamine effectiveness. Discolored solutions should not be used. Avoid extravasation of solution. Monitor urine output especially when high doses are used. Use cautiously in the elderly and those patients with cardiovascular disease, hypertension, angina, and hyperthyroidism.

Adverse Reactions: Dose-related. High doses cause renal arterial vasoconstriction with resulting decrease in renal output; also tachycardia and ventricular arrhythmias. Low doses cause vasodilation and hypotension. Occasionally, nausea, vomiting, and angina can occur. Extravasation causes tissue necrosis, ischemia, and gangrene.

Drug Interactions: Incompatible with sodium bicarbonate and other alkaline solutions. Cyclopropane/halogenated hydrocarbon anesthetics sensitize myocardium to arrhythmias; fatal ventricular arrhythmias have occurred. With MAO inhibitors, dopamine should be reduced to one tenth of the usual dose. Phenytoin produces additive bradycardia and hypotension.

Generic Name: EDROPHONIUM
Trade Name: Tensilon
Dosage Form: Injection (IM/IV), 10 mg/mL
Uses: Cholinesterase inhibitor with rapid onset (30–60 s) and brief duration (5–10 min). Used primarily as diagnostic agent for myasthenia gravis and differential diagnosis of cholinergic and myasthenic crisis. Also given postoperatively to reverse effects of nondepolarizing neuromuscular blocking agents. Investigationally, used to terminate paroxysmal supraventricular tachycardias not controlled by vagal maneuvers.
Adult Dosage (Parenteral): For termination of paroxysmal supraventricular tachycardias, 10 mg slow IV bolus or titrate by 2-mg increments (decrease to 5–7 mg for geriatric and digitalized patients). To reverse effects of nondepolarizing neuromuscular blocking agents, 10 mg slow IV over 30–45 s; can repeat q. 5–10 min (up to 40 mg); precede doses with IV atropine.
Contraindications: Asthma.
Precautions: IV atropine and equipment for assisted respiration should be readily available. Reduce dosage in geriatric and digitalized patients. Digitalis may sensitize myocardium to edrophonium. May induce uterine contractions in pregnant women.
Adverse Reactions: "Cholinergic crisis," with nausea, vomiting, diarrhea, blurred vision, increased salivations, bronchospasm, muscle cramps and fasciculations, paralysis, hypotension, bradycardia, cardiac arrest. (Antidote: atropine IV.)

Generic Name: EPINEPHRINE (Injection)
Trade Names: Epinephrine, Adrenalin, Sus-Phrine
Dosage Forms: Injection (subcutaneous), 5 mg/mL (1:200); (IM/subcutaneous/IV), 1 mg/mL (1:1000) ampules; (IV/intracardiac), 1 mg/10 mL (1:10,000) preloaded syringe
Uses: Sympathomimetic used in CPR to coarsen fine ventricular fibrillation before electrical defibrillation. Produces bronchodilation in anaphylactic shock and other hypersensitivity reactions.
Adult Dosage: For CPR, 0.5–1 mg (5–10 mL 1:10,000 solution) IV via endotracheal tube/intracardiac; may be repeated q. 5–10 min prn. For bronchodilation, 0.2–0.5 mL 1:1000 solution subcutaneously. Dose may be repeated in 20 min and again q. 2h, prn; 0.1–0.3 mL of 1:200 suspension (Sus-Phrine) may be given subcutaneously and repeated in 4 hours if needed.
Pediatric Dosage: For CPR, based on available clinical data, the 1 mg (10 mL of a 1:10,000 solution) IV dose of epinephrine should be considered the dose of first choice in cardiac arrest victims. A higher dose of epinephrine (5 mg or approximately 0.1 mg/kg) is considered a class IIb recommendation for use during resuscitation. Therefore, the use of higher doses of epinephrine can neither be recommended nor discouraged. Regardless of which dose of epinephrine is chosen during resuscitation, it is imperative that epinephrine be administered at intervals that do not exceed 3–5 min. If the dose is given by peripheral injection, it should be followed by a 20-mL flush of IV fluid to ensure delivery of drug into the central compartment.

Epinephrine has good bioavailability following endotracheal delivery, if administered properly. Although the optimal dose of epinephrine for endotracheal delivery is unknown, a dose that is at least 2 to 2.5 times the peripheral IV dose may be needed. Intracardiac administration should be used only during open cardiac massage or when other routes of administration are unavailable. Intracardiac injections increase the risk of coronary artery laceration, cardiac tamponade, and pneumothorax and cause interruption of external chest compression and ventilation.

During cardiac arrest epinephrine may also be administered by continuous infusion. The dose should be comparable to the standard IV dose of epinephrine (1 mg q. 3–5 min). This is accomplished by adding 30 mg of epinephrine hydrochloride (30 mL of a 1:1000 solution) to 250 mL of normal saline or D5W to run at 100 mL/hr and titrating to desired hemodynamic end point. Continuous infusions of epinephrine should be administered by central venous access to reduce the risk of extravasation and to ensure good bioavailability.

Epinephrine can also be used as a vasopressor agent for patients who are not in cardiac arrest (eg, symptomatic bradycardia), although it is not a first-line agent. Epinephrine hydrochloride, 1 mg (1 mL of a 1:1000 solution), is added to 500 mL of normal saline or D5W and administered by continuous infusion. The initial dose for adults is 1 µg/min titrated to desired hemodynamic response (2–10 µg/min).

For bronchodilation, 0.01 mL/kg of 1:1000 solution subcutaneously; can repeat dose q. 15–20 min for 2 doses, then q. 4 h as needed; when using Sus-Phrine (1:200), 0.004–0.005 mL/kg subcutaneously as a single dose.
Contraindications: (Excluding CPR use.) Narrow angle (congestive) glaucoma, organic brain damage, shock other than anaphylaxis, coronary insufficiency, labor, hypersensitivity to sympathomimetics.
Precautions: Do not use discolored solutions. Aqueous suspensions and those in oil should never be given IV. Do not give isoproterenol simultaneously or within 1 hour of injection of aqueous epinephrine or within 4 hours of Sus-Phrine. Epinephrine "resistance" or tachyphylaxis can occur. Use cautiously in elderly patients and those with hypertension, cardiovascular disease, hyperthyroidism, angina, diabetes, or chronic emphysema with degenerative heart disease.
Adverse Reactions: Arrhythmias, palpitations, anginal pain, cerebral hemorrhage, pulmonary edema secondary to peripheral vasoconstriction, anxiety, tremor, local tissue necrosis at injection site.
Drug Interactions: Incompatible with calcium salts, sodium bicarbonate, aminophylline, and phenytoin. Simultaneous administration with isoproterenol may induce serious arrhythmias. Halogenated anesthetics/cyclopropane may sensitize myocardium to epinephrine-induced arrhythmias. Cardiac stimulant effect is antagonized by β-blockers.

Generic Name: ESMOLOL
Trade Name: Brevibloc
Dosage Forms: Injection, 2.5 g/10 mL (vial), 100 mg/10 mL (ampule)

Uses: β-selective adrenergic receptor blockade with a rapid onset and short duration of action. Primarily indicated for the control of ventricular response found in the setting of atrial fibrillation or atrial flutter. Other possible indications include conversion of recent-onset atrial fibrillation to normal sinus rhythm, postoperative hypertension, reinstitution of β-blockers postoperatively.

Adult Dosage (Parenteral): Bolus, 0.5–1 mg/kg followed by an infusion of 50 μg/kg/min. If inadequate response within 5 min, repeat bolus and increase maintenance dose to 100 μg/kg/min. Can repeat procedure up to 200–300 μg/kg/min.

Pediatric Dosage: Safety and efficacy not established in children.

Contraindications: Severe bradycardia, greater than first-degree heart block, cardiogenic shock, overt CHF, hypersensitivity to the drug.

Precautions: 2.5 g/10 mL strength is not intended for direct IV administration and should be diluted prior to infusion. Venous irritation and thrombophlebitis are more often associated with infusions containing concentrations greater than 10 mg/mL. Esmolol is not compatible with 5% bicarbonate injection. Caution should be used when abruptly withdrawing this drug and in patients with inadequate cardiac function or a history of asthma.

Adverse Reactions: GI—nausea, vomiting, abdominal pain, and constipation; CNS—dizziness, somnolence, headache, and confusion; CV—hypotension (20–50% of patients, with greatest risk being within the first 30 min of the infusion), bradycardia, chest pain, and heart failure; RESP—bronchospasm and dyspnea; DERM—inflammation and induration at injection site.

Drug Interactions: With verapamil, may result in AV block. With digoxin, increase in digoxin serum levels by 10–20%. With morphine, esmolol serum levels may increase by up to 50%. With metocurine and pancuronium, may prolong neuromuscular blockade.

Generic Name: ISOPROTERENOL (Parenteral)
Trade Name: Isuprel
Dosage Forms: Injection (IM/IV/subcutaneous/intracardiac), 1:5000 ampules, or 1 mg/5 mL; 1:50,000 ampules, or 0.2 mg/10 mL

Uses: Sympathomimetic for treatment of Stokes-Adams syndrome, cardiac arrest, heart block with ventricular arrhythmias. Primarily used to maintain heart rate in third-degree block.

Adult Dosage (Parenteral): As an IV infusion, 2–20 μg/min titrated according to heart rate and rhythm response (up to 40 μg/min). Suggested IV dilution is 1 mg/250 mL D_5W (4 μg/mL).

Pediatric Dosage (Parenteral): As IV bolus injection 0.01–0.03 mg/dose. As an IV infusion, 0.01 μg/kg/min (or 1–3 μg/min) initially, then titrate to response (range, 0.01–1.0 μg/kg/min).

Contraindications: Tachycardia due to digitalis toxicity.

Precautions: May worsen shock by systemic vasodilation. Volume deficits must be corrected first. It increases myocardial oxygen demand. Caution must be used in patients with coronary insufficiency, acute myocardial infarction, diabetes, hyperthyroidism, sensitivity to sympathomimetics. Infusion must be decreased or temporarily discontinued if heart rate rises above 110 beats/min. Light sensitive; discolored solutions should not be used.

Adverse Reactions: Doses sufficient to increase heart rate to more than 130 beats/min may induce ventricular arrhythmias. Other reactions include facial flushing, headache, nausea, vomiting, sweating, nervousness, mild tremor, anginal pain, tachycardia, and palpitations.

Drug Interactions: Incompatible with sodium bicarbonate, aminophylline, phenytoin, other alkaline solutions, and lidocaine. Simultaneous administration with epinephrine may induce serious arrhythmias (see Epinephrine, Precautions). Antagonized by β-blocking agents.

Generic Name: LIDOCAINE (Parenteral)
Trade Name: Xylocaine
Dosage Forms: Injection (IM/IV), 100 mg/5 mL preloaded syringe; 1 g or 2 g for IV infusions; premixed solution of 2 g/500 mL D_5W (4 mg/mL)

Uses: Antiarrhythmic for treatment of ventricular arrhythmias, especially premature extrasystoles and tachycardia.

Adult Dosage (Parenteral): There is extensive literature on the proper way to load and maintain blood levels of lidocaine in an effective suppressive range of 1.5–6.0 μg/mL. For refractory ventricular fibrillation and pulseless ventricular tachycardia, an initial dose of 1.5 mg/kg is suggested for all patients. Cardiac arrest victims may require only a single bolus dose of lidocaine. Plasma lidocaine concentrations should persist within the therapeutic range for a protracted period because of reduced drug clearance from poor blood flow during CPR. Experimental animal models show an alteration in the pharmacokinetics of lidocaine because of reduced liver blood flow during cardiac arrest. Studies during CPR in humans show that lidocaine may produce a therapeutic effect at doses that are considered suboptimal in animal models.

Because of poor blood flow and prolonged circulatory times observed during CPR, only bolus administration of lidocaine should be used in treating patients in cardiac arrest. After restoration of spontaneous circulation, lidocaine should be administered by continuous IV infusion at a rate of 30–50 μg/kg/min (2–4 mg/min). The need for additional bolus doses of lidocaine should be guided by clinical response and by plasma lidocaine concentrations.

In noncardiac arrest situations, an initial bolus of 1.0–1.5 mg/kg followed by a maintenance infusion at a rate of 30–50 μg/kg/min (2–4 mg/min) is required to rapidly achieve therapeutic lidocaine levels. To prevent subtherapeutic plasma lidocaine levels after the initial bolus, a second bolus of 0.5 mg/kg is recommended after 10 min. Additional bolus injections of 0.5–0.75 mg/kg can be given every 5–10 min, if ventricular ectopy persists, to a total dose of 3 mg/kg. The maintenance infusion should be titrated according to clinical needs and plasma lidocaine concentrations.

Lidocaine undergoes blood-flow–dependent hepatic metabolism. Although the loading dose of lidocaine does not need to be reduced, the maintenance dose of lidocaine should be decreased by 50% in the presence of impaired hepatic blood flow (acute myocardial infarction, congestive heart failure, or circulatory shock) because total body clearance of lidocaine is reduced. Elderly patients (ie, >70 years) have a reduced volume of distribution; in such patients the maintenance dose should also be reduced by 50%. Because the half-life of lidocaine is increased after 24–48 hours of continuous infusion therapy, the maintenance dose should be decreased by 50% after 24 hours and the blood level of lidocaine should be monitored closely. In patients with renal failure, there is no need to adjust the dose of lidocaine because its clearance and volume of distribution are unchanged. However, renal failure leads to the accumulation of MEGX and

GX, lidocaine's metabolites, which have little pharmacologic activity but can produce significant neurotoxicity.

Pediatric Dosage (Parenteral): Initial bolus of 1 mg/kg, IV or via endotracheal tube; can be repeated in 5–10 min if necessary (maximum of 5 mg/kg/dose or 100 mg/h). Follow bolus with IV infusion of 10–50 μg/kg/min.

Contraindications: Known hypersensitivity to local anesthetics of amide type. Stokes-Adams syndrome, severe degrees of sinoatrial, atrioventricular, or intraventricular heart block.

Precautions: Caution must be used in atrial flutter/fibrillation with pre-existing rapid ventricular rate. Dosage reductions of 50% may be necessary in cirrhosis, liver failure, cardiogenic shock, advanced heart failure.

Adverse Reactions: Appear to correlate with plasma levels of 5–9 μg/mL (or IV rates of 5 mg/min or repeated IV boluses). CNS symptoms include drowsiness, dizziness, excitement, diplopia, tinnitus, muscle twitching, respiratory depression, and convulsions. Cardiovascular side effects include hypotension, bradycardia, and prolongation of QRS and PR intervals. Hypersensitivity reactions of urticaria, rash, or edema may occur.

Generic Name: METHOXAMINE
Trade Name: Vasoxyl
Dosage Form: Injection (IM/IV), 10 mg/mL and 20 mg/mL
Uses: Vasopressor (α-adrenergic vasoconstriction) that is also used to terminate paroxysmal supraventricular tachycardia.
Dosage (Parenteral): IM, 10–15 mg; IV, 3–5 mg over 5 min, then 10–15 mg IM if indicated. For termination of PSVT, 5–15 mg IV slowly or 10–20 mg IM (rarely used).
Contraindications: Shock due to myocardial infarction or peripheral mesenteric thrombosis.
Precautions: May exacerbate congestive heart failure or myocardial infarction. Caution is required with hyperthyroidism, hypertension, and elderly patients. Volume deficits must be replaced.
Adverse Reactions: Excessive hypertension with severe reflex bradycardia, severe headache, precordial pain, nervousness, dizziness, vomiting, pilomotor response, and severe peripheral and visceral vasoconstriction.
Drug Interactions: β-Blocking agents may increase vasoconstriction. Phenothiazines decrease pressor effect; anticholinergics increase pressor effect.

Generic Name: MORICIZINE
Trade Name: Ethmozine
Dosage Form: Tablets, 200, 250, 300 mg
Uses: Class I antiarrhythmic agent. Electrophysiologically, moricizine both has lidocaine-like class IB properties and also prolongs the PR and QRS times, while leaving the QT interval unchanged. Therefore, moricizine may portray a mixed class IB/IC agent. Indicated for the treatment of documented ventricular arrhythmias such as sustained ventricular tachycardia that, in the judgment of the physician, are life threatening. Because of the proarrhythmic effects of moricizine, its use should be reserved for patients in whom, in the opinion of the physician, the benefits of treatment outweigh the risks.
Adult Dosage (Oral): The dosage of moricizine must be individualized on the basis of antiarrhythmic response and tolerance. Usual adult dosage is between 600 and 900 mg/d, given every 8 hours in three equally divided doses. Within this range the dose can be adjusted as tolerated, in increments of 150 mg/d at 3-day intervals, until desired effect is obtained. Hepatic/renal impairment—Start at ≤600 mg/d and monitor closely, including the measurement of EKG intervals, before dosage adjustment. When transferring from another antiarrhythmic, the previous antiarrhythmics should be withdrawn for 1–2 half-lives before starting moricizine.
Pediatric Dosage (Oral): Not established in children <18 years old.
Contraindications: Patients with pre-existing second- or third-degree AV block and patients with right bundle branch block when associated with left hemiblock unless a pacemaker is present; presence of cardiogenic shock; known hypersensitivity to the drug product.
Precautions: Has not been proven to improve survival in patients with ventricular arrhythmias. When considering therapy, the known proarrhythmic effects of moricizine must be weighed against its possible benefit (proarrhythmic effects can range from an increase in frequency of PVCs to development of a new, more severe ventricular tachycardia). Electrolyte imbalances (hypokalemia, hyperkalemia, or hypomagnesemia) should be corrected prior to initiation of therapy. Use with extreme caution in patients with sick sinus syndrome (eg, sinus bradycardia, sinus pause, or sinus arrest may occur) and pre-existing heart failure. Pacing parameters of artificial pacemakers should be monitored since moricizine's effect on the sensing and pacing thresholds of artificial pacemakers has not been adequately studied.
Adverse Reactions: Most commonly include fatigue, dizziness, paresthesias, headache, and nausea. Other possibly more serious adverse effects include proarrhythmia (both ventricular and supraventricular), conduction defects (AV block, sinus pause, junctional rhythm), cardiac arrest, hypotension, syncope, bradycardia, chest pain, pulmonary embolism, vasodilation, CHF, AMI, cerebrovascular events, dyspnea, drug fever, and blurred vision.
Drug Interactions: With cimetidine, results in a 1.4-fold increase in moricizine serum levels. With digoxin and propranolol, results in a possible additive prolongation of PR interval. With theophylline, results in reduced theophylline clearance by 44–66%.

Generic Name: NOREPINEPHRINE (LEVARTERENOL)
Trade Name: Levophed
Dosage Forms: Injection (IV/intracardiac), 4 mg norepinephrine BASE/4 mL ampule (1 mg/mL)
Uses: Sympathomimetic vasopressor (predominantly direct α-stimulation) for restoration of blood pressure in cardiogenic shock.
Adult Dosage (Parenteral): Average initial infusion rate, 8–12 μg BASE/min, which is then adjusted to maintain systolic blood pressure 80–100 mmHg with an average maintenance infusion of 2–4 μg BASE/min. Dosage range up to 40–50 μg BASE/min has been used. (*Note:* 4–8 mg BASE [1–2 ampules] should be diluted in 500 mL D_5W to a final concentration of 8–16 μg/mL.)
Pediatric Dosage (Parenteral): Initially, 0.05–0.10 μg/kg/min, then titrate to desired effect (usual IV rate, 2 μg/min). Suggested dilution, 0.5–1 mg BASE/500 mL D_5W for a final concentration of 1–2 μg/mL.
Contraindications: Hypotension secondary to uncorrected blood volume deficits, mesenteric or peripheral vascular thrombosis, pregnancy (causes fetal anoxia).
Precautions: Administer infusions with controlled infusion device. Do not mix drug in normal saline alone; do not use brownish-

colored solutions of the drug. Metabolic acidosis must be corrected first because it inhibits cardiovascular response to levarterenol. Tissue necrosis may be caused by vasoconstriction or extravasation; treat with phentolamine infiltration of IV site or by IV infusion. Abrupt stopping of infusion may cause hypotensive relapse, so taper rate gradually.

Adverse Reactions: Headache (first sign of overdose), severe hypertension, reflex bradycardia, decreased cardiac output, weakness, tremor, pallor, anxiety, insomnia.

Drug Interactions: Incompatible with phenytoin, sodium bicarbonate, aminophylline, metaraminol, and ampicillin. Normal saline promotes oxidation of drug. With MAO inhibitors and tricyclic antidepressants it causes severe hypertension. With some anesthetics (eg, cyclopropane and halothane) may sensitize myocardium to arrhythmias.

Generic Name: PHENYTOIN (IV)
Trade Name: Dilantin
Dosage Form: Injection, 50 mg/mL (IV use only recommended)
Uses: Antiarrhythmic agent for suppression of both digitalis-induced tachyarrhythmias (with or without AV block) and ventricular arrhythmias. Also used as anticonvulsant.
Adult Dosage (Parenteral): 100–250 mg q. 5–15 min slow IV up to toxicity or 750–1000 mg. (IV rate not to exceed 50 mg/min.)
Pediatric Dosage (Parenteral): 1–5 mg/kg slow IV (rate not to exceed 25 mg/min); can repeat dose q. 10 to 15 min up to cumulative dose of 1000 mg.
Contraindications: Sinus bradycardia, sinoatrial block, second- and third-degree block, Stokes-Adams syndrome.
Precautions: Should be diluted in normal saline or lactated Ringer's solution only. Mix just prior to use. IV line should be flushed with normal saline after direct IV push to minimize venous irritation.
Adverse Reactions: Rapid IV injection may cause tremors, nystagmus, CNS depression, and cardiovascular collapse. IM administration can cause tissue necrosis, and absorption is erratic.
Drug Interactions: Should not be mixed with any other medications since phenytoin is extremely alkaline (pH 11.5).

Generic Name: POTASSIUM CHLORIDE
Trade Names: KCL, Klorvess, K-Lor, Slow-K, Klotrix
Dosage Forms: Tablets, 8 mEq slow release, 10 mEq slow release; capsules, 8 mEq, 10 mEq; injection, 2 mEq/mL (IV only); oral elixirs/solutions, 10% (20 mEq/15 mL) and 20% (40 mEq/15 mL)
Uses: Potassium and chloride replacement for correction of hypokalemia; used as an adjunct in the management of digitalis toxicity.
Adult Dosage (Oral): 40–60 mEq/d in divided doses (adjust to patient's needs) up to 100–200 mEq/d.
Adult Dosage (Parenteral): Slow IV infusion up to 10 mEq/h if serum potassium less than 2.5 mEq/L. Up to 40 mEq/h if serum potassium less than 2 mEq/L (maximum recommended dose, 400 mEq/d). Constant cardiac monitoring is required with use of high concentrations. For treatment of digitalis toxicity, 10–15 mEq/h for 2–4 hours with constant cardiac monitoring.
Pediatric Dosage (Oral): As needed. Average requirement is 1–3 mEq/kg/d.
Pediatric Dosage (Parenteral): For severe hypokalemia or digitalis toxicity, 0.3 mEq/kg/dose slowly IV over at least 1 hour; monitor with ECG.
Contraindications: Hyperkalemia, impaired renal function with oliguria or azotemia, Addison's disease.
Precautions: Concomitant use of potassium-sparing diuretics. With digitalis, it may induce atrioventricular conduction defects. It is extremely irritating to vein. *Never given IM.*
Adverse Reactions: With oral use, gastric upset, abdominal discomfort, bad taste. With parenteral use, local tissue necrosis. Hyperkalemia must be treated immediately if serum potassium greater than 6.5 mEq/L:

- at 6–8 mEq/L: weakness, fatigue, atrioventricular or intraventricular block, widened QRS complexes
- at 8–9 mEq/L: atrial arrest, neuromuscular paralysis
- over 9 mEq/L: idioventricular rhythms, ventricular tachycardia, fibrillation, asystole

For treatment of hyperkalemia, discontinue all potassium chloride and obtain serum potassium level immediately. IV calcium (unless patient is on digitalis), glucose and insulin infusions, Kayexalate enemas, and dialysis may be given.

Generic Name: PROCAINAMIDE (Parenteral)
Trade Name: Pronestyl
Dosage Forms: Injection (IM/IV), 100 mg/mL; IV only, 500 mg/mL (dilute before use)
Uses: Treatment of ventricular tachycardia, especially that not controlled by lidocaine, or ventricular arrhythmias associated with digitalis toxicity.
Adult Dosage (Parenteral): 100–200 mg IV bolus (at 25–50 mg/min), followed by 100 mg q. 5 min prn (up to 1-g loading dose). If control achieved, initiate IV drip at 1–5 mg/min (2 mg/kg/h). Administer with controlled infusion device.
Pediatric Dosage (Parenteral): 1.5–2.0 mg/kg, slow IV bolus (25 mg/min); can be repeated q. 10–15 min until arrhythmia controlled or 1000 mg has been given. Initial bolus dose can be followed by maintenance IV infusion of 20–80 μg/kg/min.
Contraindications: See procainamide (oral).
Precautions: Do not use amber or darkly discolored solutions. Risk of toxicity increases with IV bolus rates of over 50 mg/min or maintenance IV infusion rates of over 6 mg/min. Stop infusion if QRS complex widens 25% to 50% or systolic blood pressure falls more than 15 mmHg. Use cautiously in those with shock. Reduce dosage (up to 50%) in renal or hepatic impairment, congestive heart failure, or low output cardiac failure. Hypokalemia reduces procainamide's effectiveness. See also procainamide (oral).
Adverse Reactions: See procainamide (oral).
Drug Interactions: See procainamide (oral).

Generic Name: PROCAINAMIDE (Oral)
Trade Names: Pronestyl and Procan
Dosage Forms: Capsules, 250 mg, 375 mg, 500 mg
Uses: Antiarrhythmic agent similar in activity to lidocaine and quinidine for treatment of atrial and ventricular arrhythmias.
Adult Dosage (Oral): Initial therapy with regular, not sustained release, procainamide. For atrial fibrillation, 1–1.25 g to start. Dose may be repeated in 1 hour with 750 mg, then 500 mg–1 g q. 2h until arrhythmia stopped (maximum 4 g/d); for maintenance, 500 mg–1g q. 4–6h. For ventricular tachycardia and premature ventricular contractions, 1 g to start, then 250–500 mg q. 3h.

Pediatric Dosage (Oral): 40–60 mg/kg/d, divided q. 4–6h (up to 1 g/d).

Contraindications: Complete atrioventricular heart block, second- or third-degree atrioventricular block (unless pacemaker present), hypersensitivity to procainamide.

Precautions: Possesses high degree of anticholinergic activity; therefore, caution is needed in myasthenia gravis, glaucoma, and other conditions aggravated by anticholinergic activity. "Vagolytic" effect can increase atrioventricular conduction. It may be necessary to digitalize patient to control ventricular rate during conversion of atrial flutter. Hepatic or renal disease, congestive heart failure, and low output cardiac failure may require 50% dosage reduction. Effectiveness is reduced in hypokalemia.

Adverse Reactions: Symptoms of toxicity occur at plasma levels of 8–16 µg/mL. Cardiac effects include hypotension, widened QRS complexes, PR interval prolongation, heart block, ventricular tachycardia and fibrillation, and asystole. Gastric upset, lupus-like syndrome (positive lupus erythematosus and antinuclear antibody test results, incidence about 50%) with or without symptoms, blood dyscrasias; CNS derangements, including mental depression, weakness, confusion, hallucinations.

Drug Interactions: See disopyramide. Neuromuscular blocking agents and aminoglycosides may be potentiated by procainamide.

Generic Name: PROCAINAMIDE (Sustained Release)
Trade Name: Procan SR
Dosage Forms: Tablets, 250 mg, 500 mg, 750 mg
Uses: See procainamide. Sustained release tablets should be used for preventative maintenance only.
Adult Dosage (Oral): For a person who weighs 50 kg or less, 500 mg q. 6h; for 50–90 kg, 750 mg q. 6h; for over 90 kg, 1 g q. 6h.

Generic Name: PROPAFENONE
Trade Name: Rythmol
Dosage Form: Tablets, 150, 300 mg
Uses: Class IC antiarrhythmic with β-sympatholytic activity about 1/50 the potency of propranolol. Indicated for the treatment of documented life-threatening ventricular arrhythmias such as sustained ventricular tachycardia. Because of the proarrhythmic effects of propafenone, its use should be reserved for patients in whom, in the opinion of the physician, the benefits of treatment outweigh the risks.
Adult Dosage (Oral): Should be individually titrated on the basis of response and tolerance. Usually, treatment is initiated with 150 mg every 8 hours. Dosage may be increased at a minimum of 3- to 4-day intervals to 225 mg every 8 hours and, if necessary, 300 mg every 8 hours. Safety and efficacy have not been fully studied at dosages exceeding 900 mg/d.
Pediatric Dose (Oral): Safety and efficacy have not been established.
Contraindications: Uncontrolled CHF; cardiogenic shock; sinoatrial, AV, and intraventricular disorders of impulse generation or conduction (eg, sick sinus syndrome) in the absence of an artificial pacemaker; bradycardia; marked hypotension; bronchospastic disorders; manifest electrolyte imbalance; hypersensitivity to drug product.
Precautions: When considering therapy, the known proarrhythmic effects of propafenone must be weighed against its possible benefit (proarrhythmic effects can range from an increase in frequency of PVCs to development of a new, more severe ventricular tachycardia). Electrolyte imbalances (hypokalemia, hyperkalemia, or hypomagnesemia) should be corrected prior to initiation of therapy. Use with extreme caution in patients with sick sinus syndrome (eg, sinus bradycardia, sinus pause, or sinus arrest may occur) and pre-existing heart failure. Pacing parameters of artificial pacemakers should be monitored since propafenone's effect on the sensing and pacing thresholds of artificial pacemakers has not been adequately studied. Administer cautiously in patients with hepatic and/or renal impairment. Positive ANA titers have occurred in some patients under treatment. It has been shown to be reversible upon cessation of treatment.

Adverse Reactions: Most common adverse reactions (usually dose related) include dizziness, unusual taste, nausea, vomiting, abdominal discomfort, constipation, blurred vision, weakness, CNS derangements, proarrhythmia (usually manifesting as incessant wide complex ventricular tachycardia), PR and QRS prolongation and conduction block, as well as sinus node dysfunction. CHF may be precipitated. Rare reactions include hepatitis and a positive ANA.

Drug Interactions: With β-blockers, results in an increased β-blocker plasma level due to inhibition of metabolic pathways. With cimetidine, results in an increased propafenone level (up to 20%). With digoxin, results in a dose-related increase in serum digoxin levels from 35–85%. With quinidine, results in an increase in propafenone levels. With warfarin, may result in an increased PT of approximately 25%.

Generic Name: PROPRANOLOL
Trade Name: Inderal
Dosage Forms: Tablets, 10 mg, 20 mg, 40 mg, 80 mg; injection (IV), 1 mg/mL ampule
Uses: β-Adrenergic blocker (both $β_1$ and $β_2$ receptors) for treatment of various atrial and ventricular arrhythmias, particularly those induced by digitalis, sympathomimetics, or excess catecholamine stimulation. Also used for management of angina and hypertension, for prophylaxis of migraine headache, and for reduction of mortality following acute myocardial infarction.
Adult Dosage (Oral): Dosage must be titrated to response. For arrhythmias, 10–40 mg tid or qid. For angina, 10 mg tid initially; maintenance, 160–240 mg/d. For hypertension, 20–40 mg tid (up to 480 mg/d). For migraine prophylaxis, initially 80 mg/d in divided doses; increase in gradual increments until optimal response achieved (usual range, 160–240 mg/d). For prophylaxis of myocardial infarction, 40 mg tid initially, then 60–80 mg tid after 1 month; alternatively, 40 mg qid 1 week after infarct and continue for 1 year.
Adult Dosage (Parenteral): 0.5–3 mg slow IV (1 mg/min or less). Dose may be repeated in 2–5 min, but additional doses should be delayed at least 4 hours. Maximum dose is 10 mg in resistant ventricular fibrillation. Administration rates of more than 1 mg/min may cause severe hypotension and asystole.
Pediatric Dosage (Oral): 0.2–4.0 mg/kg/d in 3 or 4 divided doses.
Pediatric Dosage (Parenteral): 0.05–0.15 mg/kg slowly IV as a single dose (diluted and given over 10 min); can be repeated once in 10 min, then q. 8h, prn.

Contraindications: Congestive heart failure, right ventricular failure due to pulmonary hypertension, cardiogenic shock, sinus bradycardia, bronchial asthma, bronchospasm, heart block greater than first degree, concurrent use of psychotropic agents such as MAO inhibitors, Raynaud's syndrome.

Precautions: Rapid infusion rates may cause asystole; use isoproterenol or atropine to reverse propranolol-induced bradycardia. May precipitate congestive heart failure, severe bradycardia in Wolff-Parkinson-White syndrome, bronchospasm. May mask symptoms of thyrotoxicosis or hypoglycemia. Use cautiously in those with renal or hepatic impairment or acute myocardial infarction.

Adverse Reactions: Bronchospasm, decreased respiratory function, hypotension, bradycardia, atrioventricular block. May precipitate or aggravate congestive heart failure. Hypoglycemia, fatigue, lethargy, vertigo, light-headedness, ataxia, mental derangements, paresthesias, gastric upset, ischemic colitis, mesenteric arterial thrombosis, and hypersensitivity reactions may occur.

Drug Interactions: Potentiates insulin and oral hypoglycemic agents. Antagonizes bronchodilation of theophylline and other bronchodilators. Worsens digitalis- or phenytoin-induced bradycardia. Additive hypotension with barbiturates, narcotics, and phenothiazines.

Generic Name: QUINIDINE GLUCONATE
Trade Name: Quinaglute
Dosage Forms: Tablets, 324 mg; injection (quinidine gluconate) (IM/IV), 80 mg/mL (50 mg BASE/mL)
Uses: Antiarrhythmic agent for atrial arrhythmias and premature ventricular contractions. Parenteral use for treatment of ventricular tachycardia. Long-acting oral forms used for preventive maintenance therapy.
Adult Dosage (Oral): 1–2 tablets (324–648 mg) q. 8–12h.
Adult Dosage (Parenteral): For ventricular tachycardia or premature ventricular contractions, 400–600 mg IM q. 2h as needed; IV, 16 mg/min by infusion (800 mg quinidine gluconate diluted in 50 mL D_5W and administered at 1 mL/min). Infusion should be stopped immediately if tachycardia is controlled, toxicity appears, or significant hypotension and QRS prolongation (over 25%) occur. (Caution: IV use is hazardous.)
Pediatric Dosage (Parenteral): 2–4 mg/kg IM q. 2–4h for 4 or 5 doses. IV use not recommended.
Contraindications: Digitalis toxicity (with atrioventricular conduction disturbances); hypersensitivity or idiosyncratic reaction to quinidine or quinine; heart block (second- or third-degree, complete); ectopic impulses and rhythms resulting from escape mechanisms.
Precautions: Use parenteral doses cautiously. Discontinue drug if prolongation of PR interval, QRS widening over 25%, absence of P waves, or significant hypotension occurs. See also quinidine sulfate.
Adverse Reactions: Toxic serum levels, 8–15 μg/mL. Gastric upset with diarrhea is common. Cinchonism, which includes nausea, vomiting, diarrhea, tinnitus, visual disturbances, and dizziness. Cardiotoxicity, including bradycardia, hypotension, complete heart block with asystole, and idioventricular rhythms. CNS effects of syncope, vertigo, confusion, and delirium. Hypersensitivity reactions, hemolytic anemia, thrombocytopenic purpura, and anaphylaxis.

Drug Interactions: May potentiate action of neuromuscular blocking agents and aminoglycosides. Can increase serum levels of concomitantly administered digoxin. May potentiate hypoprothrombinemia of oral anticoagulants. Phenytoin and phenobarbital may accelerate quinidine's metabolism. Additive anticholinergic effects with atropine and other anticholinergic agents.

Generic Name: QUINIDINE SULFATE (Oral)
Trade Names: Quinidine and others
Dosage Forms: Tablets, 100 mg, 200 mg, 300 mg (sustained release, 300 mg); capsules, 200 mg, 300 mg
Uses: Antiarrhythmic agent for atrial arrhythmias (eg, atrial premature contractions and paroxysmal tachycardia, atrial flutter and fibrillation, paroxysmal supraventricular tachycardia), and premature ventricular contractions.
Adult Dosage (Oral): Therapeutic blood levels, 2–8 μg/mL. For maintenance, 200–300 mg tid or qid. For premature atrial or ventricular contractions, 200–300 mg qid up to 200–400 mg q. 4–6h (maximum 3–4 g/d). For PSVT, 400–600 mg q. 2–3h until paroxysm is terminated (maximum, 3–4 g/d). For conversion of atrial fibrillation, 200 mg q. 2–3h for 5 to 8 doses, then daily doses up to 3–4 g/d until rhythm restored or toxicity seen.
Pediatric Dosage (Oral): 10–30 mg/kg/d in 4 or 5 divided doses.
Contraindications: See quinidine gluconate.
Precautions: Test dose of 200 mg orally or IM recommended before treatment. Renal or hepatic disease may require dosage adjustments. Hypokalemia or hypoxia may cause refractoriness or predispose to quinidine-induced arrhythmias. Caution in myasthenia gravis, bronchial asthma, hyperthyroidism, congestive heart failure, glucose 6-phosphate dehydrogenase (G6PD) deficiency.
Adverse Reactions: See quinidine gluconate.
Drug Interactions: See quinidine gluconate.

Generic Name: SODIUM BICARBONATE (IV)
Trade Name: Sodium Bicarbonate
Dosage Forms: Injection (IV), 50 mEq/50 mL preloaded syringe (8.4%), 10 mEq/10 mL preloaded syringe (pediatric)
Uses: Treatment of metabolic acidosis hyperkalemia, tricyclic antidepressant overdose.
Adult Dosage (Parenteral): 1 mEq/kg IV initially (approximately 1–1.5 ampules), then 0.5 mEq/kg IV q. 10–15 min prn. Repeat doses should be governed by arterial blood gas and pH values. (Note: 3 ampules (150 mL) will raise serum pH approximately 0.05–0.1 unit.)
Pediatric Dosage (Parenteral): 1–2 mEq/kg (at rate less than 10 mL/min); alternatively, 0.3 × kg weight × base deficit (in mEq/L). For newborns and infants, dilute dose 1:1 with water.
Contraindications: (Excluding CPR use.) Respiratory or metabolic alkalosis, edema.
Precautions: Maintain effective alveolar ventilation. Adjust dose on basis of pH, $Paco_2$, and base deficit values. Use cautiously in those with hypertension, congestive heart failure, severe cardiomyopathy, renal impairment. In children under 2 years old, rapid injection rates (over 10 mL/min) can cause hypernatremia, increased CSF pressure, intracranial hemorrhage.
Adverse Reactions: Metabolic alkalosis with consequent impaired oxygen release to tissues, hypokalemia, hypocalcemia, and tetany. Also hypernatremia, edema, circulatory overload, hyper-

osmolality, CSF acidosis, intracranial hemorrhage, and vein irritation.

Drug Interactions: Direct IV admixture incompatible with calcium salts, sympathomimetics, dopamine, hydrocortisone, atropine, and lidocaine.

Generic Name: TROMETHAMINE
Trade Names: THAM, Tris Buffer
Dosage Forms: Injection (IV), 0.3M isotonic solution, 250 mL (when reconstituted)
Uses: Organic buffer used to counteract metabolic acidosis especially when accompanied by respiratory acidosis. Particularly useful for infants and children because it alkalinizes without adding carbon dioxide or excess sodium as does sodium bicarbonate injection.
Adult Dosage (Parenteral): Depends on severity and progression of acidosis. Calculate dose (in mL) according to following formula:

$$\text{mL of } 0.3M \text{ THAM needed} = (\text{wt in kg}) \times \text{base deficit (in mEq/L)}$$

One fourth of calculated dose can be given IV over 5–10 min; the remainder over 4–6 hours (maximum dose should not exceed 40 mL/kg/d).
Pediatric Dosage (Parenteral): Same as adult dosage.
Contraindications: Anuria or uremia, chronic respiratory acidosis, status asthmaticus, pregnancy.
Precautions: Check arterial blood gases and serum pH after about one half of calculated dose is given; avoid raising pH higher than 7.25 to 7.30 as a too rapid rise in pH can cause respiratory depression or arrest by inhibiting the respiratory drive of an acidotic patient. Solutions are highly alkaline (pH, 10.6); administer through a large-bore needle or indwelling venous catheter. Elevate limb receiving the infusion and discontinue infusion if extravasation occurs. Use cautiously in renal impairment (possible hyperkalemia). To minimize hypoglycemia, THAM can be reconstituted with D_5W.
Adverse Reactions: Local reactions include tissue inflammation, necrosis, sloughing, thrombophlebitis, and venospasm. Large doses and/or rapid infusion rates can cause serum hyperosmolality, hypoglycemia, and respiratory depression. Hyperkalemia occurs in renal impairment.
Drug Interactions: Additive respiratory depression with other CNS depressants.

Generic Name: VERAPAMIL (IV)
Trade Names: Calan, Isoptin
Dosage Forms: Injection (IV), 2.5 mg/mL (2-mL ampules)
Uses: Calcium slow-channel blocker used primarily for treatment of supraventricular tachyarrhythmias and control of ventricular rate in atrial flutter/fibrillation.
Adult Dosage (Parenteral): Initial dose of 5 to 10 mg (0.075 to 0.150 mg/kg) slow IV bolus; can repeat with 10 mg in 30 min if necessary. Investigationally, a constant IV infusion of 0.005 mg/kg/min following a loading dose has been given.
Pediatric Dosage: In patients 1–15 years old, 0.1–0.3 mg/kg single IV dose, which may be repeated in 30 min. In patients under 1 year old, 0.1–0.2 mg/kg single IV dose, which may be repeated in 30 min.
Contraindications: As for oral verapamil (see the antihypertensives section). Concurrent administration of IV β-blocking agents.
Precautions: Give IV doses slowly over at least 2 or 3 min. Use cautiously in those with atrioventricular block, congestive heart failure, decompensated cardiac failure, and significant renal or hepatic impairment. May accelerate ventricular rate in atrial fibrillation or flutter.
Adverse Reactions: Hypotension, bradycardia, occasional increase in pulmonary artery wedge pressure, premature ventricular contractions, tachycardia, dizziness, headache, CNS depression. (See also oral verapamil.)
Drug Interactions: See oral verapamil.

ANTIHYPERTENSIVES, ANTIANGINAL AGENTS

Generic Name: ATENOLOL
Trade Name: Tenormin
Dosage Forms: Tablets, 50 mg and 100 mg
Uses: Antihypertensive agent (cardioselective β_1-blocker in low doses). Also used for treatment of chronic stable angina pectoris.
Adult Dosage (Oral): For hypertension, 50 mg daily to start (alone or with a diuretic); can increase in 1 to 2 weeks to 100 mg/d if necessary. Withdraw doses slowly over 1 to 2 weeks if discontinuation is necessary. For chronic stable angina, up to 100 mg/d to maintain resting heart rate at 55–60 beats/min.
Contraindications: See metoprolol.
Precautions: See metoprolol. Renal impairment requires dosage adjustments.
Adverse Reactions: See metoprolol.
Drug Interactions: See metoprolol.

Generic Name: CAPTOPRIL
Trade Name: Capoten
Dosage Forms: Tablets, 12.5 mg, 25 mg, 50 mg, and 100 mg
Uses: Antihypertensive (inhibits angiotensin I-converting enzyme) for treatment of essential, renovascular, and severe refractory hypertension. Also used as adjunct to digitalis and diuretics for management of refractory congestive heart failure.
Adult Dosage (Oral): Initially, 12.5–25 mg tid. Can be increased at 1- to 2-week intervals to maximum of 450 mg/d.
Contraindications: None known.
Precautions: Should be taken on an empty stomach since food reduces drug's gastric absorption by 30 to 40%. Renal impairment (dosage adjustments necessary). Caution in patients with serious autoimmune disease or on therapy with immunosuppressive agents; blood cell counts recommended every 2 weeks for first 3 months, then periodically thereafter. Monitor serum levels of potassium. Use cautiously in patients on vigorous diuretic therapy since salt and volume depletion worsen hypotension (reduce captopril dosage).
Adverse Reactions: Commonly, urticarial rash, fever, loss of taste, and anorexia. Also, tachycardia, chest pain, angioedema, leukopenia, agranulocytosis, neutropenia, pancytopenia, pro-

teinuria, nephrotic syndrome, membranous glomerulopathy, and renal failure. Rarely, serum-sickness type reactions, mouth and peptic ulcers, jaundice, and hepatocellular injury.

Drug Interactions: Additive hypotension with diuretics, nitrates, and other antihypertensives. Hyperkalemia noted with potassium-sparing diuretics.

Generic Name: CLONIDINE
Trade Names: Catapres, Combi-pres (in combination with chlorthalidone)
Dosage Forms: Tablets, 0.1 mg, 0.2 mg
Uses: Antihypertensive agent (acts centrally to decrease sympathetic outflow).
Adult Dosage (Oral): Initially, 0.1 mg bid; increased at weekly intervals by 0.1–0.2 mg to desired response. Maximum dose, 2.4 mg/d.
Precautions: Abrupt withdrawal may cause hypertensive crisis due to sudden catecholamine release; doses should be tapered slowly over 3–7 days. Concomitant administration of tricyclic antidepressants can cause hypertension. Caution required in congestive heart failure, myocardial insufficiency, chronic renal failure, recent myocardial infarction.
Adverse Reactions: Dry mouth, sedation, and drowsiness occur most frequently. Constipation, dizziness, orthostatic hypotension, impotence, and allergic manifestations occur occasionally. Edema, CNS depression and excitement, and increased alcohol sensitivity have been reported.
Drug Interactions: With tricyclic antidepressants, hypertension may result.

Generic Name: DIAZOXIDE (IV)
Trade Name: Hyperstat
Dosage Forms: Injection (IV), 300 mg/20 mL ampules
Uses: Antihypertensive agent for emergency reduction of blood pressure in malignant hypertension.
Adult Dosage (Parenteral): Bolus of 150–300 mg (or 5 mg/kg) rapidly IV (10–30 s), which may be repeated in 30 min; then at 4- to 24-hour intervals prn.
Pediatric Dosage (Parenteral): 5 mg/kg rapidly IV push; can repeat dose in 30 min and at 4- to 24-hour intervals prn. Alternatively, 1–3 mg/kg rapidly IV q. 5–15 min up to maximum of 150 mg (minibolus technique).
Contraindications: Hypersensitivity to thiazides. Treatment of compensatory hypertension associated with aortic coarctation or arteriovenous shunt.
Precautions: Fall in blood pressure cannot be titrated. Tolerance may develop if edema is not prevented by diuretic. Caution is required in diabetes, concomitant use of other vasodilator therapy, and impaired cardiac or cerebral circulation.
Adverse Reactions: Hyperglycemia, salt and water retention, edema, gastric distress, hyperuricemia, hypertrichosis, hypotension, pain at injection site, angina, vertigo, and flushing. (Minibolus technique may provide a more gradual reduction in blood pressure, thus causing fewer circulatory and neurologic risks associated with acute hypotension.)

Generic Name: DILTIAZEM
Trade Name: Cardizem
Dosage Forms: Tablets, 30 mg, 60 mg, and 90 mg
Uses: Calcium-entry blocking agent for treatment of angina pectoris due to coronary artery spasm (variant angina) and for chronic stable angina refractory to nitrates and β-blocking agents.
Adult Dosage (Oral): 30 mg qid to start; can increase at 1- or 2-day intervals, up to 240 mg/d in divided doses.
Contraindications: Sick sinus syndrome (unless functioning pacemaker is present), hypotension (systolic pressure under 90 mmHg), and second- or third-degree atrioventricular block.
Precautions: Potentially serious atrioventricular conduction disturbances and sinus bradycardia in those on concurrent β-blocker therapy. Caution in renal or hepatic impairment. See also nifedipine.
Adverse Reactions: Gastric upset, drowsiness, dizziness, headache, hypotension, syncope, flushing, bradycardia, heart block, palpitations, congestive heart failure, pedal edema, mental confusion, weakness, pruritus, urticaria, and photosensitivity reaction.
Drug Interactions: With β-blockers, atrioventricular conduction disturbances, bradycardia.

Generic Name: ENALAPRIL
Trade Name: Vasotec
Dosage Forms: Tablets, 5 mg, 10 mg, 20 mg
Uses: Angiotensin-converting enzyme inhibitor, similar to captopril, used for treatment of hypertension.
Adult Dosage (Oral): Initially, 5 mg/d (decrease to 2.5 mg/d if diuretics concurrently given). May increase to 10–40 mg/d in single or divided doses bid.
Contraindications: Hypersensitivity to enalapril.
Precautions: See captopril. Also, patients with severe congestive heart failure or renal insufficiency should be followed closely for first 2 weeks whenever a dose of enalapril and/or a diuretic is increased. Discontinue drug if laryngeal stridor or angioedema of face, tongue, or glottis occurs. Gastric absorption of the drug does not appear to be influenced by food.
Adverse Reactions: See captopril.
Drug Interactions: See captopril.

Generic Name: ENALAPRILAT
Trade Name: Vasotec IV
Dosage Form: Injection, 1.25 mg/mL in 1- and 2-mL vials
Adult Dosage (Parenteral): Hypertension—1.25 mg every 6 hours IV over 5 min; may be increased to 5 mg every 6 hours (conversion to oral—start at 5 mg daily, then adjust as needed). Those with renal insufficiency (creatinine clearance < 30 mL/min/1.73 m^2), on dialysis, or on concomitant diuretic therapy may be started at 0.625 mg every 6 hours; if no response seen in 1 hour then may repeat 0.625-mg dose followed by additional doses of 1.25 mg every 6 hours (conversion to oral—start at 2.5 mg daily, then adjust as needed).
Pediatric Dosage (Parenteral): Safety and efficacy not established.

Generic Name: GUANABENZ
Trade Name: Wytensin
Dosage Forms: Tablets, 4 mg and 8 mg
Uses: Antihypertensive (centrally acting, α$_2$-adrenergic agonist) used for treatment of mild to moderate hypertension.

Adult Dosage (Oral): Initially, 4 mg bid. Can be increased by 4- to 8-mg increments at 1- to 2-week intervals to a maximum of 32 mg/d (with or without a diuretic).
Contraindications: Hypersensitivity to guanabenz.
Precautions: Abrupt withdrawal may cause rebound hypertension. Drug-induced drowsiness may impair ability to perform hazardous tasks. Use cautiously in those with severe renal, hepatic, or vascular insufficiency.
Adverse Reactions: Commonly, drowsiness, sedation, dizziness, dry mouth. Also gastric upset, headache, dyspnea, chest pain, palpitations, edema, anxiety, sleep disturbances, nasal congestion, blurred vision, urinary frequency, sexual dysfunction, gynecomastia, muscle aches, and rashes.
Drug Interactions: Concomitant use with CNS depressants causes increased sedation.

Generic Name: GUANETHIDINE
Trade Name: Ismelin
Dosage Forms: Tablets, 10 mg, 25 mg
Uses: Antihypertensive agent for treatment of moderate to severe essential hypertension (depletes catecholamines).
Adult Dosage (Oral): 10 mg initially, increased by 10- to 25-mg increments at 5- to 7-day intervals, depending on response. Usual maintenance dose is 25–50 mg/d.
Pediatric Dosage (Oral): 0.2 mg/kg/d as a single dose; increase at weekly intervals to desired effect and patient tolerance.
Contraindications: Hypersensitivity to guanethidine, use of MAO inhibitors, pheochromocytoma, frank congestive heart failure not due to hypertension.
Precautions: May significantly compromise renal blood flow, causing fluid retention. Caution in renal impairment, congestive heart failure, bronchial asthma, peptic ulcer, coronary insufficiency, cerebral vascular disease.
Adverse Reactions: Frequent dizziness, weakness, diarrhea, bradycardia, syncope, and severe orthostatic hypotension. Occasional inhibition of ejaculation, sodium and fluid retention, and blurred vision.
Drug Interactions: Decreased antihypertensive effect with concomitant use of tricyclic antidepressants, CNS stimulants, and phenothiazines. With MAO inhibitors, hypertensive crisis. With vasopressors, hypertension, risk of cardiac arrhythmias. With reserpine, excessive hypotension and mental depression.

Generic Name: HYDRALAZINE
Trade Name: Apresoline
Dosage Forms: Tablets, 10 mg, 25 mg, 50 mg, 100 mg; injection (IM/IV), 20 mg/mL ampules
Uses: Antihypertensive for treatment of essential hypertension (direct arteriolar vasodilation).
Adult Dosage (Oral): 10 mg qid for first 2–4 days, increased slowly to 25–50 mg qid if necessary (maximum of 200–300 mg/d).
Adult Dosage (Parenteral): 20–40 mg IM or slow IV, repeated q. 4–6h as needed.
Pediatric Dosage (Oral): 0.7–1.0 mg/kg/d in divided doses q. 6–8h; can increase dose every 3 or 4 days to desired effect (maximum dose, 200 mg/d).
Pediatric Dosage (Parenteral): 0.15 mg/kg q. 6h IV or IM; can increase by 0.1 mg/kg q. 6h to desired effect (range, 1–4 mg/kg/d).

Contraindications: Hypersensitivity to hydralazine. Coronary artery disease (may exacerbate angina). Rheumatic mitral valve disease (may precipitate congestive heart failure).
Precautions: Slow acetylators should not receive more than 200 mg/d. β-Blockers may be used to prevent tachycardia. Use cautiously in presence of cerebral vascular accident, severe congestive heart failure, or significant renal impairment.
Adverse Reactions: Primarily dose and duration dependent. Frequently: headache, tachycardia, palpitations, flushing, anorexia, nausea, and dizziness. Occasionally: sweating, nasal congestion, dyspnea, drug fever, rash, blood dyscrasias, and "antipyridoxine" effect of peripheral neuritis (treatable with pyridoxine). Systemic lupus erythematosus may develop, especially with daily doses of 400 mg or more.
Drug Interactions: Additive hypotension with diuretics or other antihypertensive medications.

Generic Name: ISOSORBIDE DINITRATE
Trade Names: Isordil, Sorbitrate
Dosage Forms: Tablets (oral), 5 mg, 10 mg, 20 mg, 30 mg, 40 mg (sustained release); capsules, 40 mg (sustained release); sublingual tablets, 2.5 mg, 5 mg, 10 mg
Uses: Antianginal vasodilator (primarily venodilation) used sublingually for treatment of acute angina pectoris and orally for prophylaxis and long-term management.
Adult Dosage (Oral): 5–30 mg qid (regular tablets); 40 mg (sustained release) q. 6–12h; sublingual, 2.5–10 mg q. 2–3h prn.
Contraindications: Severe postural hypotension. Severe anemia. Hypersensitivity to organic nitrates.
Precautions: See nitroglycerin.
Adverse Reactions: See nitroglycerin.
Drug Interactions: See nitroglycerin.

Generic Name: LABETALOL (Parenteral)
Trade Names: Normodyne, Trandate
Dosage Form: Injection (IV), 100 mg/20 mL ampule (5 mg/mL)
Uses: Antihypertensive agent with combined nonselective β-adrenergic and selective α_1-adrenergic blocking effects, given IV to control blood pressure in severe hypertension and hypertensive emergencies. It produces prompt, but gradual, dose-related decreases in systemic arterial blood pressure and systemic vascular resistance without substantially reducing cardiac output or resting heart rate. In hypertension associated with acute myocardial infarction, however, labetalol decreases cardiac index, pulmonary artery wedge pressure, and heart rate. It does not appear to reduce glomerular filtration rate or renal plasma flow.
Adult Dosage (Parenteral): Repeated injection method: 20 mg (or 0.25 mg/kg) slow IV bolus over 2 min. Can repeat doses of 40–80 mg at 10-min intervals as necessary (up to total dose of 300 mg). Monitor blood pressure immediately before and 5 and 10 min after injection. Continuous infusion method: Dilute to 1 mg/mL concentration in D_5W or NS; infuse solution at 2 mg/min, adjusting according to pressor response.
Contraindications: Overt cardiac failure, cardiogenic shock, greater than first-degree heart block, severe bradycardia, bronchial asthma.
Precautions: Keep patient in supine position during and immediately following (for up to 3 hours) injection. Monitor blood

pressure, ECG, and heart rate during and after completion of infusion or IV injection. Use cautiously in patients with inadequate cardiac function; may precipitate or exacerbate congestive heart failure. In cases of severe hypertension, control infusion rate to avoid decreasing blood pressure too rapidly. Impaired hepatic function may decrease metabolism of labetalol; discontinue drug if jaundice or evidence of hepatic injury occurs. Use cautiously in patients with bronchitis or emphysema.

Adverse Reactions: Frequently, symptomatic postural hypotension, especially if patient is allowed to assume upright position within 3 hours of receiving dose. Also, pain at injection site, dizziness, drowsiness, paresthesias, numbness, tingling of scalp/skin, gastric upset, dyspnea, wheezing, bronchospasm, rashes, pruritis, cholestasis with or without jaundice, elevations in blood urea nitrogen, positive antinuclear antibody titers, and systemic lupuslike syndrome.

Drug Interactions: Antagonizes bronchodilator effects of β-agonist medications. Potentiates hypotensive effect of halothane anesthetic. Physically incompatible with sodium bicarbonate.

Generic Name: LABETALOL (Oral)
Trade Names: Normodyne, Trandate
Dosage Form: Tablets, 100 mg, 200 mg, 300 mg
Uses: See labetalol (Parenteral). Oral doses used for management of hypertension, either alone or with other antihypertensives, especially diuretics.
Adult Dosage (Oral): Initially, 100 mg bid. Can be titrated in increments of 100 mg bid every 2 or 3 days (up to 2400 mg/d). Usual maintenance dose, 400–800 mg/d.
Contraindications: See labetalol (Parenteral).
Precautions: See labetalol (Parenteral) and metoprolol. Although it may be less likely than other β-adrenergic blockers to produce adverse cardiovascular withdrawal reactions (eg, angina, rebound hypertension) following abrupt discontinuance, dosage should be tapered gradually over 1–2 weeks in patients with angina or ischemic heart disease.
Adverse Reactions: See labetalol (Parenteral) and metoprolol.
Drug Interactions: See metoprolol. Also, cimetidine may increase bioavailability of labetalol.

Generic Name: α-METHYLDOPA
Trade Name: Aldomet
Dosage Forms: Tablets, 125 mg, 250 mg, 500 mg; injection (IV only) 250 mg/5 mL
Uses: Antihypertensive agent (acts centrally and also depletes catecholamines by acting as "false" neurotransmitter).
Adult Dosage (Oral): 250 mg bid or tid (up to 3 g/d in two to four divided doses).
Adult Dosage (Parenteral): 250–500 mg (diluted in 100 mL D_5W) given slowly IV over 30–60 min, repeated q. 6h prn (maximum, 4 g/d).
Pediatric Dosage (Oral): Initially, 10 mg/kg/d, divided q. 6h (up to 50 mg/kg/d or 3 g/d).
Pediatric Dosage (Parenteral): Initially, 10 mg/kg/d slowly IV, divided q. 6h (up to 50 mg/kg/d or 3 g/d).
Contraindications: Hypersensitivity to methyldopa. Active hepatic disease, hepatitis, cirrhosis, or liver disorders associated with prior methyldopa therapy.

Precautions: Do not give IM. Administer IV doses slowly to avoid paradoxic hypertension and excessive sedation. Onset of action (3 to 5 hours) too slow for hypertensive crisis management. Oral doses should be slowly increased at weekly intervals. Dosage adjustments are necessary in renal impairment. Use with extreme caution in hepatic impairment.
Adverse Reactions: Transient sedation and drowsiness often occur initially. Occasional vertigo, lactation, dry mouth, nasal stuffiness, gastric upset, postural hypotension, edema, positive Coombs' test, liver damage, drug fever, depression, and impotence may occur. Rarely, hemolytic anemia, thrombocytopenia, and systemic lupus erythematosus.

Generic Name: METOPROLOL
Trade Name: Lopressor
Dosage Forms: Tablets, 50 mg, 100 mg; injection (IV), 5 mg/mL ampules
Uses: $β_1$-Receptor blocking agent used orally for treatment of hypertension and for reduction of cardiovascular mortality after myocardial infarction; given parenterally to reduce cardiovascular mortality in hemodynamically stable patients in the early phase of definite or suspected myocardial infarction.
Adult Dosage (Oral): 50–100 mg bid or tid with meals (range, 100–450 mg/d). If discontinuation is necessary, withdraw doses slowly over 1 or 2 weeks. For reduction of cardiovascular mortality after myocardial infarction, 25–50 mg q. 6h for 48 hours (started 15 min after last IV dose or if parenteral doses not tolerated); thereafter, 100 mg bid for up to 3 months.
Adult Dosage (Parenteral): 5 mg as IV bolus given q. 2–5 min for 3 doses during early phase of definite or suspected myocardial infarction as soon as clinical condition allows.
Contraindications: Sinus bradycardia, heart block greater than first degree, cardiogenic shock, overt congestive heart failure, and right ventricular failure secondary to pulmonary hypertension.
Precautions: During IV administration, monitor heart rate, blood pressure, and ECG carefully. Solutions are light sensitive. Avoid abrupt withdrawal of oral doses; taper gradually. Use cautiously in those with bronchial asthma, congestive heart failure, atrioventricular conduction defects, cardiomegaly, and Raynaud's syndrome. May mask symptoms of hyperthyroidism and labile diabetes. Renal or hepatic impairment requires lengthened dosage intervals.
Adverse Reactions: Fatigue, drowsiness, dizziness, headaches, depression, bronchospasm, shortness of breath, diarrhea, gastric upset, cold extremities, mental disturbances, bradycardia, dry eyes and mucous membranes, rash, pruritus, reversible alopecia, and decreased libido. Abrupt withdrawal may exacerbate angina or lead to myocardial infarction in ischemic heart disease.
Drug Interactions: With digitalis, additive bradycardia and decreased atrioventricular conduction. With sympathomimetics, antagonistic effects. With catecholamine-depleting agents (eg, reserpine), additive effects.

Generic Name: MINOXIDIL
Trade Name: Loniten
Dosage Forms: Tablets, 2.5 mg, 10 mg

Uses: Antihypertensive. Nonadrenergic vasodilator for treatment of severe hypertension not manageable with maximal diuretic doses and other antihypertensive agents.
Adult Dosage (Oral): 5 mg/d to start, increased to 10, 20, then 40 mg/d in single or divided doses (up to 100 mg/d). Usual maintenance dose, 10–40 mg/d.
Pediatric Dosage (Oral): For a child under 12 years old, 0.2 mg/kg/d to start (up to 50 mg/d). Usual maintenance dose, 0.25–1 mg/kg/d. (*Note:* A diuretic [eg, furosemide] should always be prescribed with minoxidil.)
Contraindications: Pheochromocytoma.
Precautions: Congestive heart failure, angina, recent myocardial infarction, renal impairment, patients on dialysis. Too rapid blood pressure control may precipitate cerebrovascular accident or myocardial infarction.
Adverse Reactions: Hypertrichosis (80% incidence), tachycardia, angina (pretreatment with β-blockers or methyldopa required), edema, salt and water retention, rash, pericardial effusion and tamponade.
Drug Interactions: With CNS depressants, sedative-hypnotics, alcohol, and other antihypertensive agents, additive hypotension.

Generic Name: NADOLOL
Trade Name: Corgard
Dosage Forms: Tablets, 40 mg, 80 mg, 120 mg
Uses: Nonselective β-blocker for treatment of angina pectoris and mild to severe hypertension.
Adult Dosage (Oral): 40 mg/d initially, increased prn every 3–7 days. Angina dosage range, 80–240 mg/d; hypertension dosage range, 80–320 mg/d. If discontinuation is necessary, withdraw slowly over 1 to 2 weeks.
Contraindications: See metoprolol.
Precautions: See metoprolol.
Adverse Reactions: See metoprolol.
Drug Interactions: See metoprolol.

Generic Name: NIFEDIPINE
Trade Name: Procardia
Dosage Form: Capsules, 10 mg
Uses: Calcium channel blocker used primarily for treatment of chronic angina and vasospastic (variant) angina.
Adult Dosage (Oral): 10 mg tid to start. (Increase dosage gradually at weekly intervals.) Usual dose, 10–20 mg tid. Coronary artery spasms may require 20–30 mg qid. Maximum recommended daily dose, 120–180 mg.
Contraindications: Known hypersensitivity to nifedipine. Use in pregnancy not established.
Precautions: Single doses of more than 30 mg are not recommended. Frequent clinical assessment is necessary if dosage is to be increased sooner than weekly intervals. May precipitate angina in patients abruptly withdrawn from β-blocking agents. Drug-induced decrease in coronary perfusion associated with lowered diastolic pressure and increased heart rate may worsen angina.
Adverse Reactions: (These are primarily a result of vasodilating effects and are dose-related.) Hypotension, dizziness, lightheadedness, headache, flushing, weakness, peripheral edema. Also gastric upset, nasal and chest congestion with dyspnea, joint stiffness, muscle cramps, nervousness, blurred vision, dermatitis, fever, chills, sexual difficulties, and increased angina.
Drug Interactions: With β-blocking agents, excessive hypotension, congestive heart failure symptoms, and exacerbation of angina.

Generic Name: NIFEDIPINE EXTENDED RELEASE
Trade Name: Procardia XL
Dosage Forms: Extended release tablet (GITS), 30, 60, 90 mg
Uses: See nifedipine (oral); hypertension
Adult Dosage (Oral): 30 to 60 mg once daily initially, then titrate over 7- to 14-day period. Dosages $\geq$ 120 mg/d are not recommended. Angina patients maintained on nifedipine capsules may be switched to the sustained release product at the nearest equivalent total daily dosage.
Pediatric Dosage (Oral): Safety and efficacy not established.
Precautions: See oral; do not chew or divide tablet.

Generic Name: NIMODIPINE
Trade Name: NIMOTOP
Dosage Form: Liquid-filled capsules, 30 mg
Uses: Dihydropyridine calcium channel blocker that causes relaxation in arteriolar and coronary vessels. Nimodipine appears to be more selective for cerebral arterioles. Primarily indicated for the improvement of neurologic deficits due to spasm following subarachnoid hemorrhage from ruptured congenital intracranial aneurysm in patients who are in good neurologic condition postictus.
Adult Dosage (Oral): Therapy should be initiated within 96 hours of subarachnoid hemorrhage at 60 mg every 4 hours for 21 consecutive days. If the capsule cannot be swallowed, the contents may be extracted into a syringe and then administered via nasogastric tube followed by a 30-mL saline flush.
Pediatric Dosage: Safety and efficacy not established.
Contraindications: Hypotension or hypersensitivity to the drug product.
Precautions: Dose should be reduced by ½ in patients with hepatic disease.
Adverse Reactions: GI—dry mouth, dyspepsia, and nausea; CNS—dizziness, headache, somnolence, and paresthesia; CV—flushing, chest pain, palpitations, pedal edema, tachycardia, and rebound vasospasm; other—rash, pedal edema, and myalgias.
Drug Interactions: With antihypertensive agents, can potentiate the vasodilatory and hypotensive response to nimodopine.

Generic Name: NITROGLYCERIN
Trade Names: Nitrostat, Nitrol, Nitro-Bid, Transderm-Nitro, Nitro-Dur
Dosage Forms: Tablets (sublingual), 0.15 mg, 0.3 mg, 0.4 mg, 0.6 mg; ointment, 2%; transdermal disks, 2.5 mg, 5 mg, 10 mg, 15 mg (released over 24 hours); capsules (sustained release), 2.5 mg, 6.5 mg
Uses: Venodilation and coronary artery vasodilation. Used intermittently to prevent or relieve acute attacks of angina pectoris. Sustained release forms available for prophylaxis.

Adult Dosage (Sublingual): 0.15–0.4 mg initially, which may be repeated at 5-min intervals three times. Doses must be individualized; some patients require up to 0.6 mg.

Adult Dosage (Ointment): 0.5–2 in applied q. 3–4h, prn (up to 4–5 in per application).

Adult Dosage (Transdermal Disk): One disk applied to chest q. 24h.

Adult Dosage (Sustained Release): 2.5–6.5 mg PO q. 8–12h.

Contraindications: Hypersensitivity to nitroglycerin, increased intraocular pressure, severe anemia, increased intracranial pressure.

Precautions: Glaucoma, head trauma, cerebral hemorrhage. Concurrent use of drugs and/or conditions that may reduce myocardial oxygen supply or increase oxygen demand. Tablets should be kept in their original container and protected from heat to avoid loss of potency.

Adverse Reactions: Headache, blurred vision, dry mouth, vertigo, weakness, postural hypotension, palpitations, syncope, rash, methemoglobinemia, iatrogenic organic nitrate dependence, and tolerance may develop.

Generic Name: NITROGLYCERIN (IV)
Trade Names: Tridil, Nitroglycerin
Dosage Forms: Injection (IV only), 5 mg/mL in 5-mL and 10-mL vials (must be diluted before use)
Uses: Venodilation to reduce cardiovascular preload and arteriolar dilation to reduce afterload. Used for blood pressure control in perioperative hypertension and during surgical procedures, treatment of congestive heart failure associated with acute myocardial infarction, and treatment of angina pectoris not responding to recommended doses of β-blockers and organic nitrates.
Adult Dosage: (Must be titrated to desired response.) Initially, 5 μg/min. Titrate with increments of 5 μg/min q. 3–5 min until response is seen. If no response at 20 μg/min, titrate with increments of 10–20 μg/min (suggested dilution of 50 mg/250 mL NS or D_5W, for a concentration of 200 μg/mL). Concentrations greater than 400 μg/mL should be avoided because propylene glycol in diluent may precipitate. (*Note:* Drug must be mixed in *glass* IV bottles only and administered through special non-PVC nitroglycerin infusion tubing; 40%–80% of dose may be absorbed by standard PVC IV tubing.)
Contraindications: Hypersensitivity to organic nitrates, uncorrected hypovolemia, increased intracranial pressure, constrictive pericarditis, and pericardial tamponade.
Precautions: Administer with controlled infusion device. Renal and/or hepatic disease. Excessive hypotension may compromise effective coronary perfusion. Attendant risk of ischemia and thrombosis. Paradoxic bradycardia and increased angina pectoris may accompany nitroglycerin-induced hypotension.
Adverse Reactions: Primarily headache, then tachycardia, hypotension, nausea, vomiting, restlessness, apprehension, muscle twitching, retrosternal discomfort, palpitations, vertigo, and abdominal pain.
Drug Interactions: Do not admix with any other medications.

Generic Name: PAPAVERINE
Trade Names: Pavabid, Papaverine
Dosage Forms: Tablets, 30 mg, 60 mg, 100 mg, 200 mg, 500 mg; capsules (sustained release), 150 mg; injection (IV), 30 mg/mL
Uses: Spasmolytic and vasodilating agent for treatment of various obstructive and vasospastic diseases and cerebral vascular insufficiency. Questionable use in treatment of angina.
Adult Dosage (Oral): 150 mg q. 8–12h (sustained release form), up to 300 mg q. 12h.
Adult Dosage (Parenteral): 30–120 mg slow IV, which may be repeated q. 3h, prn (with extreme caution to avoid arrhythmias).
Contraindications: Complete atrioventricular block.
Precautions: Glaucoma. Too rapid IV administration may produce arrhythmias, apnea.
Adverse Reactions: Nausea, gastric upset, abdominal discomfort, drowsiness, headache, flushing of face, hyperhidrosis, tachycardia, tachypnea, hepatic hypersensitivity reactions.

Generic Name: PRAZOSIN
Trade Name: Minipress
Dosage Forms: Capsules, 1 mg, 2 mg, 5 mg
Uses: Antihypertensive agent. Produces direct arteriolar vasodilation and sympatholytic effect that blocks reflex tachycardia.
Adult Dosage (Oral): 1 mg bid or tid (up to 20 mg/d). Usual maintenance dose, 6–15 mg/d, divided q. 8–12h.
Pediatric Dosage (Oral): For a child over 12 years, 1 mg tid (maximum, 20 mg/d).
Precautions: When another antihypertensive agent is added, prazosin dose must be reduced to 1–2 mg tid and retitrated. Initial dose should be limited to 1 mg and increased slowly. Syncope, dizziness, light-headedness, and loss of consciousness may occur within 30–90 min of initial dose or with rapid dosage increases. Severe tachycardia (eg, heart rate greater than 120–160 beats/min) may precede syncopal episode.
Adverse Reactions: See precautions. Also drowsiness, fatigue, gastric upset and disturbances, dry mouth, blurred vision, diaphoresis, tinnitus, nasal congestion, urinary frequency, or incontinence.
Drug Interactions: With CNS depressants, sedative-hypnotics, alcohol, other antihypertensive agents, additive hypotension.

Generic Name: RESERPINE
Trade Name: Serpasil
Dosage Forms: Tablets, 0.1 mg, 0.25 mg, 1 mg; injection (IM), 2.5 mg/mL
Uses: Antihypertensive agent for treatment of mild essential hypertension and hypertension emergencies.
Adult Dosage (Oral): 0.5 mg/d for 1–2 weeks, then 0.1–0.25 mg/d.
Adult Dosage (Parenteral): For hypertensive emergency, 0.5–1 mg IM stat, then 2–4 mg q. 3h prn.
Pediatric Dosage (Oral): 0.02 mg/kg/d, up to a maximum of 2 mg/d.
Pediatric Dosage (Parenteral): For hypertensive crisis, 0.07 mg/kg IM; can be repeated q. 4–6h, prn.
Contraindications: Hypersensitivity to *Rauwolfia* alkaloids. Mental and suicidal depression, electroshock therapy. Peptic ulcer, ulcerative colitis.
Precautions: Parenteral onset slow (1–3 hours). Can cause withdrawal symptoms of depression after high doses. Severe hypotension with IM doses over 0.5 mg. Nasal stuffiness is common, so avoid use in newborns who are obligate nose breathers.

Adverse Reactions: Gastric upset, gastric acid hypersecretion, abdominal pain, diarrhea, anorexia, dry mouth, nasal stuffiness, edema, hypotension, and bradycardia are common. Frequent CNS disturbances include drowsiness, weakness, lethargy, headache, vertigo, depression, and nightmares. Incidence of drug-induced depression seems to be dose related. Large doses can cause parkinsonian syndrome, extrapyramidal reactions, and convulsions.

Drug Interactions: With MAO inhibitors, hypertension may result. With digitalis or quinidinelike drugs, arrhythmias, bradycardia, and angina may occur.

Generic Name: SODIUM NITROPRUSSIDE
Trade Name: Nipride
Dosage Forms: Injection (IV), 50 mg
Uses: Antihypertensive vasodilator (lowers both arterial and venous pressures). Used for treatment of hypertensive crisis. Can be given in combination with vasopressors for management of cardiogenic shock and for preload and afterload reduction. Onset is immediate; duration of action is brief (1 to 10 min).
Adult Dosage (Parenteral): IV infusion at 1–3 μg/kg/min to start (range, 0.5–10 μg/kg/min). Rate should not exceed 10 μg/kg/min or 800 μg/min. Suggested dilution of 50 mg in 250 mL D_5W produces a 200-μg/mL concentration.
Pediatric Dosage (Parenteral): Same as adult dosage.
Contraindications: Arteriovenous shunt, coarctation of aorta.
Precautions: Should be diluted in preservative-free D_5W only; resulting solution must be protected from light. Do not use highly discolored solutions. Solutions must be used fresh and discarded after 24 hours. Administer with controlled infusion device. Monitor blood pressure continuously until stable, then frequently throughout crisis therapy. Metabolized to cyanide and thiocyanate in tissues and liver. Use cautiously in renal and hepatic impairment, vitamin B_{12} deficiency, and hypothyroidism (thiocyanate inhibits iodine uptake).
Adverse Reactions: Thiocyanate toxicity with thiocyanate levels of 50–100 μg/mL. Tinnitus, blurred vision, fatigue, delirium, anorexia, rash, dyspnea, dilated pupils, pink skin color, coma. Also symptoms of rapid reduction in blood pressure (eg, nausea, sweating, headache, palpitations, substernal distress).
Drug Interactions: With dopamine, higher cardiac output, lower pulmonary vascular resistance (synergistic). Should not be mixed with any other medications.

Generic Name: TIMOLOL
Trade Name: Blocadren
Dosage Forms: Tablets, 10 mg and 20 mg
Uses: Antihypertensive (nonselective β-blocker) for treatment of hypertension. Also for prophylactic use to decrease mortality after myocardial infarction.
Adult Dosage (Oral): For hypertension, 10 mg bid (alone or with diuretic) to start; can increase at weekly intervals to 60 mg/d. For infarction prophylaxis, 10 mg bid beginning 1 to 4 weeks after infarction.
Contraindications: See propranolol in the antiarrhythmics section.
Precautions: See propranolol.
Adverse Reactions: See propranolol.
Drug Interactions: See propranolol.

Generic Name: TRIMETHAPHAN CAMPHOR SULFONATE
Trade Name: Arfonad
Dosage Forms: Injection (IV), 500 mg/10 mL (50 mg/mL)
Uses: Antihypertensive. Produces cholinergic and adrenergic blockade.
Adult Dosage (Parenteral): Slow IV infusion (1 g/500 mL D_5W). Initially, 0.5–1 mg/min (0.25–0.5 mL/min); rate adjusted to response. In hypertensive emergency, may increase to 1–15 mg/min.
Contraindications: Hypovolemia, shock, uncorrected anemia, asphyxia, uncorrected respiratory insufficiency.
Precautions: Use cautiously in children; pregnant women; elderly, debilitated patients; patients with hepatic, cardiac, or renal disease, diabetes, degenerate CNS disease, or allergic individuals (drug releases histamine).
Adverse Reactions: All side effects of ganglionic blockade: orthostatic hypotension, tachycardia, urinary retention, constipation, parolytic ileus, angina, dry mouth, gastric upset, cycloplegia, mydriasis, weakness, xerostomia, urticaria, and pruritus.
Drug Interactions: Incompatible with alkaline solutions.

Generic Name: VERAPAMIL (Oral)
Trade Names: Calan, Isoptin
Dosage Forms: Tablets, 80 mg, 120 mg; sustained release, 120 mg, 240 mg
Uses: Calcium slow channel blocker for treatment of angina pectoris, including vasospastic (Prinzmetal's variant), unstable (crescendo), and chronic stable angina.
Adult Dosage (Oral): 80 mg tid to qid to start. Increased at daily or weekly intervals until desired response obtained (24–48 hours recommended between dosage increments). Dosage range, 240–480 mg/d. Once dose stabilized, may switch to daily sustained-release product.
Contraindications: Severe left ventricular dysfunction or congestive heart failure, hypotension (systolic blood pressure under 90 mmHg), cardiogenic shock, "sick sinus" syndrome (except with functioning pacemaker), second- or third-degree atrioventricular block. Concomitant use of β-blockers (relative contraindication).
Precautions: Use cautiously in those with atrioventricular block, congestive heart failure, severe cardiomyopathy, significant renal or hepatic impairment, and concurrent use with β-blockers, which may accelerate ventricular rate in atrial flutter or fibrillation.
Adverse Reactions: Hypotension, pulmonary/peripheral edema, bradycardia, congestive heart failure, atrioventricular block (third-degree), dizziness, headache, fatigue, gastric upset, constipation, elevated liver enzymes. Occasional CNS symptoms include blurred vision, paresthesias, equilibrium disorders, muscle cramps, and syncope.
Drug Interactions: With β-blockers, additive negative inotropic/chronotropic effects, which may be therapeutically useful, however. With digitalis, increases in serum digoxin levels of 50%–75%; possible digitalis toxicity. With antihypertensive agents and quinidine, additive hypotensive effects.

ANTICONVULSANTS

Generic Name: DIAZEPAM (Parenteral)
Trade Name: Valium
Dosage Forms: Injection (IM/IV), 5 mg/mL
Uses: Benzodiazepine derivative given parenterally for control of status epilepticus and other convulsive episodes. Also used to manage anxiety and convulsions associated with acute alcohol withdrawal syndrome. Not recommended for seizure prophylaxis since duration of action is brief.
Adult Dosage (Parenteral): (IV bolus rate should not exceed 5 mg/min). For status epilepticus, 5–10 mg slowly IV; can be repeated q. 10–20 min up to 100 mg/d. For acute alcohol withdrawal, 10 mg slowly IV or IM initially, then 5–10 mg slowly IV or IM q. 20–30 min until patient is calm but not comatose (usually intervals of q. 3–4h are satisfactory). Maximum dosage is 100 mg/d.
Pediatric Dosage (Parenteral): (IV doses should be given slowly over at least 3 min). For acute seizures in a child (1 month to 5 years), 0.2–0.5 mg/kg slowly IV, repeated q. 2–5 min as needed, up to a cumulative maximum dose of 5 mg; for seizures in a child over 5 years, 1–2 mg slowly IV, repeated q. 2–5 min as needed, up to a cumulative maximum dose of 10 mg. Doses can be repeated in 2 to 4 hours (up to 40 mg/d) but longer-acting anticonvulsants should be given after initial control of acute seizures. For febrile seizures, 0.3 mg/kg slowly IV. (*Note:* Doses may be instilled rectally via a rectal tube.)
Contraindications: Hypersensitivity to benzodiazepines. Newborns up to 1 month old, shock, coma, psychosis, and acute alcohol withdrawal seizures if vital signs are depressed. Relative contraindication for prolonged use: acute narrow angle and open angle glaucoma.
Precautions: IV doses should be given slowly undiluted and into the injection port closest to the infusion site; flush IV line after administration of dose. Avoid extravasation or intra-arterial administration. Monitor blood pressure and respiration closely as cumulative dose increases. IV administration can cause severe hypotension. IM doses are slowly and erratically absorbed so they are not recommended for acute seizure control. Use with caution in depressed or suicidal patients. Reduce doses and give cautiously to elderly or debilitated patients, those with hepatic impairment, and infants and children. Higher doses may be required in excessive smokers. May be habit forming and cause barbiturate-like withdrawal symptoms.
Adverse Reactions: From oral use: drowsiness, ataxia, fatigue, vertigo, dizziness, paradoxic hyperexcitation, hallucinations, nightmares (especially in elderly), rash, hepatic abnormalities, jaundice. From parenteral use: tissue necrosis, thrombophlebitis, hypotension, respiratory depression, premature ventricular contractions, laryngospasm, cardiovascular collapse.
Drug Interactions: Do not mix injection with any other medications or aqueous solutions. Additive CNS depression with other CNS depressants. Cimetidine may impair hepatic metabolism of diazepam so excessive sedation may occur.

Generic Name: MAGNESIUM SULFATE (Parenteral)
Trade Name: Magnesium Sulfate
Dosage Forms: Injection (IM/IV), 1 g/2 mL ampule (50%), 5 g/10 mL ampule (50%) (4.06 mEq Mg^{2+}/mL)
Uses: Anticonvulsant for treatment of seizures caused by eclampsia or severe hypomagnesemia; for control of hypertension and convulsions associated with acute nephritis. Also given as electrolyte replacement in magnesium deficiency.
Adult Dosage (Parenteral): For eclampsia or seizures, 4 g IV (diluted in 250 mL D_5W and given over 3 hours); additionally, 4 to 5 g IM into each buttock, followed by 4 to 5 g IM into alternate buttocks q. 4h as needed according to response and absence of magnesium toxicity. Alternatively, 4 g IV (diluted in 250 mL D_5W, given slowly) followed by 1–2 g/h by constant IV infusion. For severe hypomagnesemia, 2 g IM q. 2h for 3 doses, then 1 g IM for 4 doses on first day; on second day, 1 g IM q. 4h for 6 doses; on days 3 to 5, 1 g IM q. 6h. Alternatively for severe hypomagnesemia, 6 g IV (diluted in 1000 mL and given over 3 hours) followed by 10 g/2000 mL of IV solution infused over rest of the day; on days 2 through 5, 6 g/d distributed equally in desired IV fluids via constant infusion.
Pediatric Dosage (Parenteral): For seizures, 100 mg/kg (0.2 mL of 50% solution/kg) IM q. 4–6h as needed. Dose can also be given as a 1% solution slowly IV, half over 20 min, the remainder over 1 hour. For hypomagnesemia, 0.1 to 0.2 mL/kg of a 50% solution IM or slowly IV q. 12h. (Dose can also be added to daily IV solution for infusion.)
Contraindications: Heart block, myocardial damage.
Precautions: Reduce dosages in renal impairment. Maintain adequate hydration and urine output of at least 25 mL/h. IV use is hazardous; infusion rate should not exceed 150 mg/min (1.5 mL/min of a 10% solution). Monitor vital signs and serum magnesium levels closely.
Adverse Reactions: Disappearance of patellar reflex is useful sign of clinical toxicity. Normal serum level, 1.5–2.5 mEq/L. Toxicities correlate well with serum levels:

- at over 4 mEq/L, deep tendon reflexes decrease, hypotension, nausea
- at over 7 mEq/L, CNS depression, muscular weakness, flushing, sweating
- at over 10 mEq/L, loss of deep tendon reflexes, heart block, respiratory paralysis
- at over 12 mEq/L, possibly fatal

Rapid IV administration may produce symptoms of flushing and intense heat in throat and radiating down body. (Antidote: 10–20 mL 10% calcium gluconate over 5–10 min IV.)
Drug Interactions: Incompatible with calcium salts and sodium bicarbonate. Additive CNS depression with other CNS depressants. Diuretics increase excretion of magnesium.

Generic Name: PARALDEHYDE
Trade Name: Paraldehyde
Dosage Forms: Injection (IM/IV), 2 mL, 5 mL, 10 mL ampules; oral solution, 15 mL, 30 mL
Uses: Sedative-hypnotic for management of acute agitation caused by alcohol withdrawal and for control of seizures refractory to other anticonvulsants.
Adult Dosage (Oral): For alcohol withdrawal, 5–10 mL q. 4–6h for 24 hours, then q. 6h. Can be given through nasogastric tube.
Adult Dosage (Rectal): Same as oral dosage but diluted in equal parts of mineral or vegetable oil. For seizures, 0.2 mL/kg as oil retention enema.

Adult Dosage (Parenteral): For seizures, 5–10 mL IM or 0.2–0.4 mL/kg IV (well diluted in 100–250 mL NS).

Pediatric Dosage (Oral/Rectal): 0.15–0.30 mL/kg via nasogastric tube or in equal parts oil given as retention enema; can repeat dose in 1 hour if needed.

Pediatric Dosage (Parenteral): Not recommended. However, 0.15–0.30 mL/kg, well diluted in 100 mL NS and given slowly IV has been used.

Contraindications: (Relative) Bronchopulmonary disease, hepatic insufficiency, gastroenteritis/ulceration.

Precautions: IM use causes sterile abscesses. Use *glass* syringes only. Solution oxidizes rapidly; discard opened bottles after 24 hours. Patients in pain may become severely agitated.

Adverse Reactions: Gastric or rectal mucosal irritation with oral or rectal use. IM doses cause sterile abscesses or sciatic nerve injury. IV use can cause pulmonary hemorrhage or edema, respiratory distress, hypotension, circulatory collapse. Rashes, metabolic acidosis, and liver damage can also occur.

Generic Name: PHENOBARBITAL SODIUM (Parenteral)
Trade Names: Luminal, Phenobarbital Sodium
Dosage Forms: Injection (IV/IM), 65 mg/mL and 130 mg/mL ampules, syringes; 65 to 325 mg/mL vials
Uses: Sedative-hypnotic (barbiturate derivative) given parenterally for control of acute seizure episodes including febrile seizures and status epilepticus. Its long duration of action is useful for preventing the recurrence of convulsions.
Adult Dosage (Parenteral): For status epilepticus, 8–20 mg/kg (up to 1 g) slowly IV, divided into 2 to 4 doses and given at 3- to 60-min intervals. Usual initial dose, 200–600 mg slowly IV, then 120–240 mg IV q. 30–60 min prn.
Pediatric Dosage (Parenteral): For status epilepticus or acute seizures, loading dose of 10–20 mg/kg slowly IV (25–50 mg/min); can repeat q. 30 min with 4–6 mg/kg slowly IV as needed. (*Note:* Repeat doses may not be necessary since loading dose usually achieves therapeutic serum levels quickly.) Maximum cumulative dose, 40 mg/kg/d. For maintenance therapy in seizure prophylaxis, 3–8 mg/kg/d IM or IV, divided q. 12h (dependent on loading dose; measure serum phenobarbital levels). For acute febrile seizures, 2–3 mg/kg IM initially (usually 120 mg); can repeat dose in 20 minutes if needed. For prevention of febrile seizures, 3–5 mg/kg/d in divided doses.
Contraindications: Hypersensitivity to barbiturates, porphyria, and respiratory disease when dyspnea or obstruction is present.
Precautions: Because the onset of action is slow, allow at least 20 min between repeat doses. Administer IV doses slowly (60 mg/min or less). Monitor vital signs frequently during parenteral use. Additive CNS, cardiovascular, and respiratory depressant effects can occur if diazepam was also recently given. Use cautiously and adjust doses in elderly or debilitated patients; those with asthma, severe allergies, severe cardiac disease, and renal or hepatic impairment (causes drug accumulation); and those who are pregnant. Barbiturates may induce paradoxic and excessive hyperexcitability in infants and young children.
Adverse Reactions: IV administration can cause thrombophlebitis, severe respiratory depression, apnea, hypotension, coughing, hiccoughing, laryngospasm, bronchospasm, hypothermia, nausea, and vomiting. Paradoxic excitement and hyperkinetic activity in infants and young children, drowsiness, dizziness, ataxia, CNS depression, hypersensitivity reactions, and skin eruptions can occur. Drug can cause postpartum and neonatal hemorrhage, precipitate acute attacks of porphyria, and worsen hepatic coma (elevates blood ammonia levels). Drug dependence and withdrawal symptoms can occur.
Drug Interactions: Additive CNS depression with other CNS depressants. See also barbiturates in sedative-hypnotic section.

Generic Name: PHENYTOIN
Trade Name: Dilantin
Dosage Forms: Tablets, 50 mg (chewable); capsules, 30 mg, 100 mg; injection, 50 mg/mL (IV use only recommended); oral suspension, 30 mg/5 mL, 125 mg/5 mL
Uses: Anticonvulsant for various types of seizures including grand mal, focal, and psychomotor seizures; antiarrhythmic (see phenytoin IV in section on antiarrhythmics).
Adult Dosage (Oral): Loading dose of 1 g in divided doses over 4 hours, then 300–400 mg/d. This usually achieves therapeutic levels in 8–12 hours.
Adult Dosage (Parenteral): Loading dose of 750–1000 mg slow IV (no faster than 50 mg/min). IM route not recommended because of slow, erratic absorption.
Pediatric Dosage (Oral): Usual maintenance, 5–7 mg/kg/d divided q. 12–24h (up to 300 mg/d). Loading dose method: 500–600 mg divided doses to start, then usual maintenance dose qd. (*Note:* Without a loading dose, steady-state plasma levels are not achieved for 5–15 days. Therapeutic serum levels, 10–20 µg/mL.)
Pediatric Dosage (Parenteral): For status epilepticus, 5–10 mg/kg (slowly IV not to exceed 25 mg/min); repeat doses of 1.5 mg/kg can be given q. 30 min as needed (up to 20 mg/kg/d).
Contraindications: Hypersensitivity to hydantoins.
Precautions: Dilute doses in NS or Ringer's lactate only and mix just prior to use; flush IV line with NS after administration of dose. Give IV doses slowly to avoid cardiovascular collapse. Measure phenytoin serum levels 6 to 12 hours after loading doses. Use cautiously in pregnancy, hepatic impairment, uremia (displacement of phenytoin from protein binding sites), and elderly or severely ill patients. Abrupt withdrawal of doses during maintenance therapy may precipitate seizures.
Adverse Reactions: Frequently dose related. (Toxic serum level, over 20 µg/mL):
- 20–30 µg/mL, nystagmus
- 30–40 µg/mL, ataxia, slurred speech
- over 40 µg/mL, mental confusion, somnolence, lethargy
- over 50 µg/mL, coma, cardiovascular collapse

Also, gastric upset, gum hyperplasia, megaloblastic anemia, reversible lymph node hyperplasia ("pseudolymphoma"), rashes, blood dyscrasias, liver damage, toxic hepatitis, hirsutism, peripheral neuropathy, lupus syndrome, depressed serum folic acid, and vitamin K concentrations with bleeding.
Drug Interactions: Barbiturates may increase phenytoin metabolism, but effect varies and is unpredictable. Oral anticoagulants, disulfiram, and phenylbutazone increase phenytoin toxicity. With chronic alcohol ingestion, anticonvulsant effect is decreased. High doses of tricyclic antidepressants and antipsychotics may increase seizure risk.

ANTICOAGULANTS, ANTIFIBRINOLYTICS

Generic Name: ALTEPLASE RECOMBINANT (r-tPA)
Trade Name: Activase
Dosage Form: Injection, 20 mg and 50 mg vials
Uses: Serene protease that produces a fibrin-enhanced conversion of plasminogen to plasmin primarily at the site of a fibrin clot, resulting in a local fibrinolysis with a relatively limited systemic fibrinogenolysis. Primarily indicated for the management of acute transmural myocardial infarction in adults for the lysis of thrombi-obstructed coronary arteries and in acute massive pulmonary embolism in adults.
Adult Dosage (Parenteral):
- Should be reconstituted with sterile water for injection, without preservatives, to a final concentration of 1 mg/mL (slight foaming is to be expected) and administered within 8 hours. Avoid excessive agitation during dilution (mix by gentle swirling or slow inversion). May be administered as 1 mg/mL or the reconstituted solution may be diluted with an equal volume of 0.9% sodium chloride injection or 5% dextrose injection to yield a concentration of 0.5 mg/mL.
- AMI (standard method)—100 mg total given over 3 hours as 10-mg bolus followed by 50 mg to be infused over the first hour, then the remaining 40 mg infused at a rate of 20 mg/h over the second and third hours. For smaller patients (<65 kg) a dose of 1.25 mg/kg given over 3 hours (in the manner described above) should be substituted.
- AMI (front loading)—100 mg total over 90 minutes as a 15-mg bolus followed by 50 mg over 30 minutes, then the remaining 35 mg over 1 hour (may lead to an even better patency rate).
- Pulmonary embolism—IV infusion of 50 mg over 2 hours followed by an additional 40 mg over the next 4 hours.

Pediatric Dosage: Safety and efficacy not established in children.
Contraindications: Absolute—active ongoing bleeding, stroke or intracranial/intraspinal surgery within 2 months, intracranial neoplasm. Relative—major surgery/biopsy within 10 days, GI bleeding/biopsy within 10 days, recent trauma/prolonged CPR, pregnancy/postpartum state, diabetic retinopathy, uncontrolled arterial hypertension, severe hepatic/renal disease, and active malignancy.
Precautions: Since r-tPA present in blood samples is still pharmacologically active, coagulation tests or measures of fibrinolytic activity performed during therapy may be unreliable unless specific precautions are taken to prevent in vitro artifacts (addition of aprotinin). Half-life may be prolonged in severe hepatic dysfunction. A dosage of 150 mg or greater should not be used as it has been associated with an unacceptable increase in intracranial bleeding with little added benefit to standard dosages. Patient should be monitored for signs of bleeding, especially at the sites of arterial puncture, and for arrhythmias associated with reperfusion (sinus bradycardia, accelerated idioventricular rhythm, PVCs, AV block, and ventricular tachycardia). Serious bleeding requires immediate discontinuance of therapy and application of direct pressure if possible. Fresh-frozen plasma or cryoprecipitate may be used to restore circulating fibrinogen levels. In extreme circumstances, ε-aminocaproic acid (AMICAR) may be considered, although no proven protocols exist for such administration.
Adverse Reactions: Bleeding is the most common complication associated with therapy and may be internal (eg, GI tract, GU tract, or intracranial sites) or superficial (eg, sites of venous cutdowns, arterial puncture, or recent surgery). Others include mild rash, hypotension, reperfusion arrhythmias, and chest pain.
Drug Interactions: While the benefit of heparin and antiplatelet drugs (eg, aspirin) in the setting of AMI has been well established, the increased risk of severe bleeding with concomitant administration of heparin, warfarin, and antiplatelet drugs must be considered. The fibrinolytic activity of r-tPA may be inhibited by AMICAR.

Generic Name: ε-AMINOCAPROIC ACID
Trade Name: Amicar
Dosage Forms: Tablets, 500 mg; injection (IV), 250 mg/mL (5 g/20 mL vial)
Uses: Antifibrinolytic agent for treatment of excessive bleeding resulting from systemic hyperfibrinolysis and urinary fibrinolysis. Used as adjunct to antihemophilic factors VIII and IX to control excessive bleeding in hemophiliacs from the nose and oral cavity. Has been used investigationally to prevent clot lysis and further bleeding in subarachnoid hemorrhage secondary to ruptured aneurysm.
Adult Dosage (Oral): Same as IV dosage.
Adult Dosage (Parenteral): IV infusion (diluted in NS or D_5W) of 4–5 g for first hour, followed by 1 g/h for approximately 8 hours. More than 30 g/d is not recommended.
Pediatric Dosage (Oral): Same as IV dosage.
Pediatric Dosage (Parenteral): Initially, 100 mg/kg/dose slowly IV, then 30 mg/kg/h by continuous IV infusion until bleeding controlled. Maximum dose is 600 mg/kg/d.
Contraindications: Pregnancy (teratogenicity in animals). Evidence of active intravascular clotting process.
Precautions: Rapid IV administration should be avoided. Drug should not be administered without definite diagnosis and/or laboratory findings indicative of hyperfibrinolysis (hyperplasminemia). Do not use in disseminated intravascular coagulation (DIC) without also administering heparin. Use cautiously in cardiac, hepatic, or renal disease.
Adverse Reactions: Rapid IV administration causes hypotension, bradycardia, arrhythmias. Thrombophlebitis with IV administration. Occasional nausea, cramps, diarrhea, hypotension, tinnitus, malaise, nasal and conjunctival congestion, rash, headache, and muscle weakness. Also, intrarenal obstruction and renal impairment from fibrin deposition and glomerular capillary thrombosis may occur.

Generic Name: ANISTREPLASE (APSAC)
Trade Name: Eminase
Dosage Form: Injection, 30 U/vial (refrigerate)
Uses: Plasminogen activator complex that mediates the conversion of plasminogen to plasmin, resulting in the degradation of fibrin clots as well as circulating fibrinogen. APSAC is indicated for the management of acute transmural myocardial infarction in adults for the lysis of thrombi-obstructed coronary arteries.
Adult Dosage (Parenteral): The contents of one vial (30 U) should be reconstituted by slowly adding 5 mL sterile water for injection

and gently rolling the vial to mix the dry powder and fluid (do not shake). The entire contents (30 U) should then be withdrawn from the vial and administered via IV line or vein over 2–5 minutes. If not administered within 30 minutes of reconstitution, discard.

Pediatric Dosage (Parenteral): Safety and efficacy not established in children.

Contraindications: Absolute—active ongoing bleeding, stroke or intracranial/intraspinal surgery within 2 months, intracranial neoplasm. Relative—major surgery/biopsy within 10 days, GI bleeding/biopsy within 10 days, recent trauma/prolonged CPR, pregnancy/postpartum state, diabetic retinopathy, uncontrolled arterial hypertension, severe hepatic/renal disease, active malignancy, hypersensitivity to either APSAC or streptokinase, previous APSAC or streptokinase therapy within 6 months, streptococcal infection within 6 months.

Precautions: Plasma fibrinogen levels are decreased for 24–36 hours. Thrombin time may be prolonged for up to 24 hours. Since APSAC present in blood samples is still pharmacologically active, coagulation tests or measures of fibrinolytic activity performed during therapy may be unreliable unless specific precautions are taken to prevent in vitro artifacts (addition of aprotinin). Since APSAC is a bacteriologic product, anaphylactoid reaction is possible (rare), requiring that supportive therapy such as epinephrine be available when using this agent. Readministration of APSAC should not be performed more than 3 days after initial therapy because antistreptokinase antibodies will have increased to a level sufficient to blunt the thrombolytic effect of the drug. Half-life may be prolonged in severe hepatic dysfunction. Patient should be monitored for signs of bleeding, especially at the sites of arterial puncture, and for arrhythmias associated with reperfusion (sinus bradycardia, accelerated idioventricular rhythm, PVCs, AV block, and ventricular tachycardia). Serious bleeding requires immediate discontinuance of therapy and application of direct pressure if possible. Fresh-frozen plasma or cryoprecipitate may be used to restore circulating fibrinogen levels. In extreme circumstances, ε-aminocaproic acid (AMICAR) may be considered, although no proven protocols exist for such administration.

Adverse Reactions: Bleeding is the most common complication associated with therapy and may be internal (eg, GI tract, GU tract, or intracranial sites) or superficial (eg, sites of venous cutdowns, arterial puncture, or recent surgery). Others include urticaria, itching, flushing, rash, fever, anaphylactic reactions, hypotension, reperfusion arrhythmias, and chest pain.

Drug Interactions: While the benefit of heparin and antiplatelet drugs (eg, aspirin) in the setting of AMI has been well established, the increased risk of severe bleeding with concomitant administration of heparin, warfarin, and antiplatelet drugs must be considered. The fibrinolytic activity of APSAC may be inhibited by AMICAR.

Generic Name: HEPARIN SODIUM
Trade Name: Heparin
Dosage Forms: Injection (IV/subcutaneous), 1000, 5000, 7500, 10,000, 20,000, 40,000 U/mL
Uses: Anticoagulant (see warfarin).
Adult Dosage (Parenteral): Must be titrated to coagulation test responses. Therapeutic effect is 1.5–2.5 times control value using APTT or ACT. Half-life increases with increasing doses.
Adult Dosage (Intermittent IV): 100 U/kg IV q. 4h.
Adult Dosage (Continuous IV infusion): IV bolus of 35–50 U/kg followed by continuous infusion of 900–1200 U/h *or* 5000 U IV bolus, followed by 1000 U/h IV infusion.
Adult Dosage (Subcutaneous): For prophylaxis, 5000 U q. 8–12h.
Pediatric Dosage (Parenteral): As for adult, to yield clotting times of 20–30 min or 2 to 3 times the control value.
Contraindications: Hypersensitivity to heparin, unavailability of suitable blood coagulation tests required for monitoring therapy, conditions predisposing to hemorrhage and bleeding (see warfarin).
Precautions: Avoid IM injections since they can cause hematomas. Subcutaneous injections should be deep; do not massage injection site. Administer continuous IV infusions using a controlled infusion device. Regulate dosage by frequent coagulation tests; for continuous IV therapy, perform APTT immediately before, every 4 hours during early stages of therapy, and daily thereafter; for intermittent IV or subcutaneous therapy, perform APTT before treatment, prior to each dose during early stages of therapy, and daily thereafter. Periodic platelet counts are recommended if therapy is longer than 5 days. Special risk patients include those with hepatic or renal disease, hypertension, and indwelling catheters; women over 60 years old; pregnant patients; and those with conditions that may predispose to bleeding (see warfarin precautions).
Adverse Reactions: Hemorrhage, immune thrombocytopenia (reversible), hypersensitivity reactions (chills, fever, urticaria, anaphylaxis), histamine-like reactions at injection site, delayed transient alopecia, osteoporosis (with long-term use). An acute vasospastic reaction can develop 6–10 days after initiating therapy and can cause pain, ischemia, cyanosis in affected limb, feeling of oppression, tachypnea, chest pain, cyanosis, arthralgia, hypertension, itching or burning of soles of feet, and headache. (This reaction is unresponsive to protamine.) For treatment of heparin overdose, give 1–1.5 mg of 1% protamine sulfate solution, slowly IV, for every 100 U of heparin to be neutralized; if given 30 minutes or more after last heparin dose, about 0.5 mg of protamine per 100 U of heparin is usually sufficient (maximum, 50 mg in any 10-minute period).
Drug Interactions: Antiplatelet drugs that may increase risk of bleeding or hemorrhage include aspirin, dextran, dipyridamole, ibuprofen, indomethacin, oxyphenbutazone, phenylbutazone, and glyceryl guaiacolate. Also coumarin anticoagulants, streptokinase, and urokinase potentiate heparin.

Generic Name: PHYTONADIONE
Trade Names: AquaMephyton, Mephyton, Vitamin K_1
Dosage Forms: Injection (IM/IV/subcutaneous), 1 mg/0.5 mL (neonatal) and 10 mg/mL (AquaMephyton); tablets, 5 mg (Mephyton)
Uses: For treatment of hypoprothrombinemia induced by oral anticoagulants, salicylates and other drugs, broad-spectrum antibiotic therapy, vitamin K deficiency, and severe hepatic disease; also used for prophylaxis and treatment of hemorrhagic disease of the newborn.
Adult Dosage (Oral): For anticoagulant-induced hypoprothrombinemia, 2.5–10 mg as a single dose; can repeat in 12 to 48 hours (larger doses have been used in rare instances). For hypoprothrombinemia from other causes, 2–25 mg initially, then repeated if necessary (up to 50 mg/dose).

Adult Dosage (Parenteral): For anticoagulant-induced hypoprothrombinemia, 2.5–10 mg IM or subcutaneously; can repeat in 6 to 8 hours. When bleeding present or imminent, 10–50 mg slowly IV q. 4h if needed.

Pediatric Dosage (Oral): For prothrombin deficiencies in an older infant or child, 5–10 mg; in a newborn under 1 year, 2 mg.

Pediatric Dosage (Parenteral): For prophylaxis of hemorrhagic disease in newborn, 0.5–1.0 mg IM or subcutaneous as a single dose; for treatment, 1–2 mg IM, subcutaneous, or slow IV. For prothrombin deficiency in an older infant or child, 5–10 mg IM, subcutaneous, or slow IV. For treatment of poisoning with oral anticoagulants, 2–5 mg/kg IM or slowly IV.

Contraindications: Hypersensitivity to phytonadione, bleeding disorders that are not vitamin K dependent, severe hepatic impairment (when repeat doses give unsatisfactory response).

Precautions: Use IV route only when other routes of administration are not feasible. Give IV doses slowly (not to exceed 1 mg/min). Doses may be diluted in D_5W or normal saline only; protect solutions from light. Subcutaneous or IM injections given for hypoprothrombinemia may cause hemorrhage or hematomas at injection site. Since phytonadione may require 3 or more hours to stop bleeding, administration of whole blood or plasma may be indicated if bleeding is severe. High doses may re-expose patient to hazard of intravascular clotting; use lowest effective dose that will not decrease prothrombin time to below the effective anticoagulant level. Use cautiously in premature newborns and jaundiced infants.

Adverse Reactions: With IV use, flushing, dizziness, sweating, muscle cramps, tightness in chest, cyanosis, dyspnea, bronchospasm, rapid and weak pulse, hypotension, shock, cardiac or respiratory arrest, hypersensitivity reactions, and anaphylaxis. With IM or subcutaneous injections, pain, swelling, redness, hematomas. High doses in newborns can cause hyperbilirubinemia, hemolytic anemia, and hemoglobinuria.

Drug Interactions: Antagonizes hypoprothrombinemic effect of oral anticoagulants.

Generic Name: STREPTOKINASE
Trade Name: Kabikinase, Streptase
Dosage Forms: Injection, 250,000; 600,000; 750,000; 1,500,000 IU vials
Uses: Combines with plasminogen to produce an activator complex that mediates the conversion of plasminogen to plasmin, which results in the degradation of fibrin clots as well as circulating fibrinogen. Primarily indicated for the management of acute transmural myocardial infarction in adults for the lysis of thrombi-obstructed coronary arteries, in acute massive pulmonary embolism, deep venous thrombosis, peripheral artery thrombosis, and clearance of occluded AV catheters in adults.

Adult Dosage (Parenteral):
- Reconstitute with 5 mL 0.9% sodium chloride injection or 5% dextrose injection. Avoid shaking, which may cause foaming and flocculation. For use in AV catheter clearance the contents of a 250,000-IU vial should be reconstituted with 2 mL of appropriate diluent.
- AMI (intracoronary)—bolus, 20,000 IU followed by a maintenance infusion of 2000 IU/min for 60 minutes (250,000-IU vial diluted to a total volume of 125 mL).
- AMI (IV)—750,000 to 1.5 million IU administered over 30–60 min (diluted to a total volume of 45 mL) or 750,000 IU given as a 10-min load and the remainder of the 1.5 million units infused over 60 minutes.
- DVT/PE/peripheral artery thrombosis—load with 250,000 IU (IV) over 30 minutes followed by a maintenance infusion of 100,000 IU/h for up to 24–72 hours as dictated by clinical response (the contents of 1.5-million IU vial diluted to a total volume of 90 mL to be run at 6 mL/h).
- AV catheter occlusion—250,000 IU in 2-mL solution; fill catheter for 2 hours, remove, flush with saline solution.

Pediatric Dosage (Parenteral): Safety and efficacy not established in children.

Contraindications: Absolute—active ongoing bleeding, stroke or intracranial/intraspinal surgery within 2 months, intracranial neoplasm. Relative—major surgery/biopsy within 10 days, GI bleeding/biopsy within 10 days, recent trauma/prolonged CPR, pregnancy/postpartum state, diabetic retinopathy, uncontrolled arterial hypertension, severe hepatic/renal disease, active malignancy, hypersensitivity to either APSAC or streptokinase, previous APSAC or streptokinase therapy within 6 months, streptococcal infection within 6 months.

Precautions: Intracoronary infusions offer little benefit over IV therapy in the setting of an AMI. Plasma fibrinogen levels are decreased for 24–36 hours. Thrombin time may be prolonged for up to 24 hours. Since streptokinase activator complex present in blood samples is still pharmacologically active, coagulation tests or measures of fibrinolytic activity performed during therapy may be unreliable unless specific precautions are taken to prevent in vitro artifacts (addition of aprotinin). Since streptokinase is a bacteriologic product, anaphylactoid reaction is possible (rare), requiring that supportive therapy such as epinephrine be available when using this agent. Readministration of streptokinase should not be performed more than 3 days after initial therapy because antistreptokinase antibodies will have increased to a level sufficient to blunt the thrombolytic effect of the drug. Half-life may be prolonged in severe hepatic dysfunction. Patient should be monitored for signs of bleeding, especially at the sites of arterial puncture and for arrhythmias associated with reperfusion (sinus bradycardia, accelerated idioventricular rhythm, PVCs, AV block, and ventricular tachycardia). Serious bleeding requires immediate discontinuance of therapy and application of direct pressure if possible. Fresh-frozen plasma or cryoprecipitate may be used to restore circulating fibrinogen levels. In extreme circumstances, ε-aminocaproic acid (AMICAR) may be considered, although no proven protocols exist for such administration.

Adverse Reactions: Bleeding is the most common complication associated with therapy and may be internal (eg, GI tract, GU tract, or intracranial sites) or superficial (eg, sites of venous cutdowns, arterial puncture, or recent surgery). Others include urticaria, itching, flushing, rash, fever, anaphylactic reactions, hypotension, reperfusion arrhythmias, and chest pain.

Drug Interactions: While the benefit of heparin and antiplatelet drugs (eg, aspirin) in the setting of AMI has been well established, the increased risk of severe bleeding with concomitant administration of heparin, warfarin, and antiplatelet drugs must be considered. The fibrinolytic activity of streptokinase may be inhibited by AMICAR.

Generic Name: TICLOPIDINE
Trade Name: Ticlid
Dosage Form: Tablets, 250 mg

Uses: Platelet aggregation inhibitor. When taken orally, causes a time- and dose-dependent inhibition of both platelet aggregation and release of platelet granule constituents. Indicated to reduce the risk of thrombotic stroke in patients who have experienced stroke and in patients who have had a complete thrombotic stroke in whom aspirin therapy is not possible.

Adult Dosage (Oral): 250 mg taken twice daily with food.

Pediatric Dosage (Oral): Safety and efficacy not established.

Contraindications: Hypersensitivity to drug, presence of hematopoietic disorders such as neutropenia and thrombocytopenia; presence of a hemostatic disorder or active pathologic bleeding; patients with severe liver impairment.

Precautions: Therapy has been associated with severe neutropenia (usually occurring 3 weeks to 3 months after initiation of treatment) and thrombocytopenia requiring the performance of CBCs, white cell differential, and platelet count (for all patients) every 2 weeks for the first 3 months of therapy and then as needed unless absolute neutrophil count had been declining consistently over the first 3 months (then more frequent labs are required). Use with caution in patients with increased risk of bleeding from trauma, surgery, or pathologic conditions. Drug should be discontinued 10–14 days prior to elective surgery. Prolonged bleeding time may be normalized within 2 hours after administration of 20 mg methylprednisolone IV or via platelet transfusion.

Adverse Reactions: Most common adverse reactions include diarrhea, nausea, dyspepsia, rash, GI pain, neutropenia, thrombocytopenia, purpura, vomiting, flatulence, pruritus, dizziness, anorexia, abnormal liver function tests, ecchymosis, epistaxis, hematuria, conjunctival hemorrhage, GI bleeding, and perioperative bleeding.

Drug Interactions: With antacids, results in an 18% decrease in plasma levels of ticlopidine. With cimetidine, results in a decrease in the clearance of ticlopidine. With theophylline, results in an increased theophylline elimination. With phenytoin, not fully studied but administer with caution (possible effect on protein binding—follow phenytoin levels).

Generic Name: WARFARIN SODIUM
Trade Name: Coumadin
Dosage Forms: Tablets, 2 mg, 2.5 mg, 5 mg, 7.5 mg, 10 mg, 25 mg; injection (IM/IV), 50 mg
Uses: Anticoagulant for prophylaxis therapy of venous thrombosis and pulmonary embolism, treatment of atrial fibrillation with embolization, and adjunctive therapy of coronary occlusion and cerebral transient ischemic attacks.

Adult Dosage (Oral): 10–15 mg/d for 2–3 days until desired prothrombin time is reached. Maintenance dosage range, 2–10 mg/d (based on prothrombin time determinations).

Adult Dosage (Parenteral): IM/IV as for oral dosage regimen.

Contraindications: Active bleeding or hemorrhagic tendencies, vitamin K deficiency. Pregnancy, severe hypertension, renal or hepatic disease, acute adrenal hemorrhage or insufficiency, open wounds, visceral carcinoma, gastrointestinal or genitourinary lesions, subacute bacterial endocarditis, recent eye, brain, or spinal cord surgery, retinopathy.

Precautions: Prothrombin time should be determined daily; stools and urine should be examined daily for blood. Altered anticoagulant activity may occur in congestive heart failure, vitamin C and vitamin K deficiencies, alcoholism, fever, diarrhea, severe diabetes and allergic disorders, hyperlipemia, hypothyroidism, edema, hereditary warfarin resistance, and polycythemia vera.

Adverse Reactions: Bleeding, hemorrhage, "purple toes" syndrome, gastric upset, diarrhea, fever, dermatitis, alopecia, hemorrhagic infarction and skin necrosis, priapism, uterine bleeding, ovarian hemorrhage upon ovulation, hematuria. (Treat overdose with vitamin K [phytonadione].)

Drug Interactions: Drugs that may potentiate response include anabolic steroids, chloral hydrate, chloramphenicol, clofibrate, cimetidine, dipyridamole, disulfiram, oxyphenbutazone, phenylbutazone, other nonsteroidal anti-inflammatory agents, thyroid drugs, tricyclic antidepressants, quinine, quinidine, salicylates, streptokinase, urokinase. Drugs that may decrease response include alcohol (chronic ingestion), barbiturates, corticosteroids, glutethimide, meprobamate, estrogens, vitamin K, vitamin C, griseofulvin, and antacids.

ANTI-INFLAMMATORY/ANTIGOUT AGENTS

Generic Name: ALLOPURINOL
Trade Name: Zyloprim
Dosage Forms: Tablets, 100 mg, 300 mg
Uses: Treatment of chronic gout, both primary and secondary, and treatment of primary or secondary uric acid nephropathy.

Adult Dosage (Oral): 100 mg daily to start, followed by weekly increases of 100 mg/d until serum uric acid falls to 6 mg/dL or less or until a maximum of 800 mg/d is reached. Average dose for mild gout is 200–300 mg/d; for moderately severe tophaceous gout, 400–600 mg/d. Doses over 300 mg should be divided.

Pediatric Dosage (Oral): For a child under 6 years, 150 mg/d, adjusted after 48 hours. For a child 6–10 years, 300 mg/d, adjusted after 48 hours.

Contraindications: Children (except for hyperuricemia secondary to malignancy) and location.

Precautions: Prophylactic doses of colchicine should be given with allopurinol for several months, owing to an initial increased risk of gouty attacks. Do not initiate during acute gouty episode. Fluid intake must be sufficient to keep urine output at least 2 L/d. Renal impairment mandates reduced dosage. Caution in hepatic impairment. May be used with salicylates and uricosurics.

Adverse Reactions: Frequently, maculopapular rash occurs, but exfoliative, urticarial, purpuric, and erythema multiforme lesions have also been reported. Severe hypersensitivity reactions include vasculitis and epidermal necrolysis. Gastric upset, drowsiness, and reversible hepatotoxicity are reported. Rarely, alopecia, cataract formation, and bone marrow depression occur.

Drug Interactions: With iron salts, increased hepatic iron concentration and toxicity. With ampicillin, increased incidence of rashes. With dicumerol (but not warfarin), potentiation of anticoagulant effect and bleeding.

Generic Name: COLCHICINE
Trade Name: Colchicine

Dosage Forms: Tablets, 0.5 mg, 0.6 mg; injection (IV), 0.5 mg/mL (2 mL ampule)

Uses: Treatment of acute gouty attack and prophylaxis of chronic gout.

Adult Dosage (Oral): 0.6–1.2 mg initially, then 0.5–0.6 mg q. 1–3h until pain relieved or until gastrointestinal toxicity (up to maximum of 7–8 mg). A 3- to 4-day delay is required before repeating. Maintenance dose, 0.6–1.2 mg orally qd or qod.

Adult Dosage (Parenteral): Initially, 1–3 mg slowly IV (diluted), then 0.5 mg q. 6h (up to 4 mg/d); allow 3–4 days between repeat IV courses.

Contraindications: Hypersensitivity to colchicine; pregnancy; serious gastrointestinal, cardiac, or renal disease.

Precautions: Dilute doses in normal saline only; administer slowly IV over 2–5 min. Do not give IM or subcutaneously. Nausea, vomiting, and diarrhea indicate full therapeutic dose has been attained. Use cautiously in debilitated patients, the elderly, or those with renal, gastric, or cardiac disease.

Adverse Reactions: Primarily nausea, vomiting, and diarrhea. Also hemorrhagic gastroenteritis, alopecia, vascular damage, thrombophlebitis, nephrotoxicity, peripheral neuritis, and paralysis. Prolonged use may cause bone marrow depression with agranulocytosis and aplastic anemia.

Generic Name: DIFLUNISAL
Trade Name: Dolobid
Dosage Forms: Tablets, 250 mg, 500 mg

Uses: Nonsteroidal anti-inflammatory analgesic (long-acting salicylate derivative) for treatment of mild to moderate pain, osteoarthritis, and rheumatoid arthritis.

Adult Dosage (Oral): For mild to moderate pain relief, 500–1000 mg initially, then 250–500 mg q. 8–12h, prn. For arthritis, 250–500 mg bid (maximum, 1500 mg/d).

Contraindications: Hypersensitivity to diflunisal, demonstrated hypersensitivity to aspirin or other nonsteroidal anti-inflammatory agents.

Precautions: Do not crush or chew tablets. Use cautiously in conditions predisposing to fluid retention, renal impairment (adjust dosage), asthma, or upper gastrointestinal tract bleeding or ulcer disease. Inhibits platelet function.

Adverse Reactions: Gastric upset, diarrhea, gastrointestinal bleeding, peptic ulceration, dizziness, drowsiness, nervousness, edema, and tinnitus. Hypersensitivity reactions include rashes, urticaria, rhinitis, dyspnea, and bronchospasm. Also reported are Stevens-Johnson syndrome, acute interstitial nephritis, cholestatic jaundice, visual disturbances, muscle cramps, and paresthesias.

Drug Interactions: With coumarin anticoagulants, increased prothrombin time. With thiazide and loop diuretics, decreased hyperuricemic effect. Antacids and aspirin decrease serum levels of diflunisal. Increases serum levels of acetaminophen and indomethacin.

Generic Name: IBUPROFEN
Trade Name: Motrin
Dosage Forms: Tablets, 200 mg, 300 mg, 400 mg, 600 mg, 800 mg

Uses: Nonsteroidal anti-inflammatory agent for treatment of rheumatoid arthritis and osteoarthritis. Also used as analgesic for mild to moderate pain and primary dysmenorrhea.

Adult Dosage (Oral): For analgesia, 400 mg q. 4–6h with food (up to 2400 mg/d); for arthritis, 300–600 mg tid to qid with food (up to 2400 mg/d).

Contraindications: See indomethacin.
Precautions: See indomethacin.
Adverse Reactions: See indomethacin.
Drug Interactions: See indomethacin.

Generic Name: INDOMETHACIN
Trade Name: Indocin
Dosage Forms: Capsules, 25 mg, 50 mg

Uses: Nonsteroidal anti-inflammatory agent for treatment of many forms of arthritis, including acute gouty arthritis.

Adult Dosage (Oral): 25 mg bid or tid with meals to start, increased by 25 mg at weekly intervals prn (maximum recommended dose, 150–200 mg/d). For acute gouty arthritis, 50 mg tid (maximum dose, 200 mg/d).

Contraindications: Children under 14 years. Pregnancy, lactation, history of gastrointestinal lesions (latent or active). Allergy to aspirin, indomethacin, and other nonsteroidal anti-inflammatory agents if manifested by bronchospastic reactions.

Precautions: See naproxen. Use cautiously in the elderly because of increased risk of ocular and CNS toxicities. May exacerbate epilepsy, psychiatric disorders, or parkinsonism. Inhibits platelet aggregation.

Adverse Reactions: Frequent headache, dizziness, sedation, syncope, tinnitus, severe gastric upset, and mental confusion. Hypersensitivity reactions include mild to severe rash, urticaria, exacerbation of asthma, acute respiratory distress, angioedema, and anaphylaxis. Also psychiatric disturbances, peripheral neuropathy, paresthesias, aggravation of epilepsy or parkinsonism, coma, convulsions, peptic ulceration with perforation and bleeding, gastrointestinal inflammation, edema, hypertension, tachyarrhythmias, nephrotoxicity, jaundice, abnormal results of liver function tests, hepatotoxicity, hyperglycemia, hyperkalemia, and various hearing and ocular disturbances (ocular-corneal deposits). Blood dyscrasias such as agranulocytosis, leukopenia, and bone marrow depression can occur.

Drug Interactions: Probenecid and diflunisal increase indomethacin serum levels. Aspirin exacerbates gastrointestinal upset/bleeding. With oral anticoagulants, possible potentiation of hypoprothrombinemia with increased risk of gastrointestinal bleeding. With diuretics, decreased natriuretic and antihypertensive effects. With β-blockers, decreased antihypertensive effects.

Generic Name: NAPROXEN
Trade Name: Naprosyn
Dosage Forms: Tablets, 250 mg, 375 mg, 500 mg

Uses: Nonsteroidal anti-inflammatory agent for treatment of rheumatoid arthritis, osteoarthritis, and acute gout. Also used as an analgesic for relief of mild to moderate pain, primary dysmenorrhea, and acute tendinitis or bursitis.

Adult Dosage (Oral): For inflammation, 250–375 mg bid with meals. For analgesia or dysmenorrhea, 500 mg initially, then 250 mg q. 6–8h, prn (maximum, 1250 mg/d). For acute gout, 750 mg initially, then 250 mg q. 8h until attack subsides.

Pediatric Dosage (Oral): For juvenile rheumatoid arthritis, 10 mg/kg/d in divided doses, q. 12h.

Contraindications: Hypersensitivity to naproxen, aspirin, or other nonsteroidal anti-inflammatory agents when manifested by asthma, urticaria, bronchospasm.

Precautions: To minimize gastric irritation, give doses with food, milk, or antacids. Inhibits platelet aggregation so use cautiously in those with bleeding disorders or patients on anticoagulant therapy. Use cautiously in renal or hepatic impairment, congestive heart failure, hypertension, lupus erythematosus, mental disorders, gastric or peptic ulcer disease, or the elderly. May cause bronchospasm and respiratory failure in patients sensitive to aspirin. May mask signs of infection or inflammation. Periodic ophthalmic examinations are recommended during prolonged therapy. Drug-induced sedation may impair mental alertness. Do not use aspirin concurrently with naproxen.

Adverse Reactions: Headache, CNS sedation, gastric upset, and depression are frequent but may be less severe than with indomethacin. Other side effects similar to indomethacin may occur.

Drug Interactions: Naproxen metabolite may cause false elevation in assay for urinary 17-ketogenic steroids. With oral anticoagulants, possible increased hypoprothrombinemic effect and gastrointestinal bleeding. (See also indomethacin.) Naproxen can displace albumin-bound drugs from their binding sites thus increasing their serum levels (eg, phenytoin, sulfonylureas, sulfonamides). Aspirin increases excretion of naproxen.

Generic Name: OXYPHENBUTAZONE
Trade Name: Tandearil
Dosage Form: Tablets, 100 mg
Uses: See phenylbutazone.
Adult Dosage (Oral): See phenylbutazone.
Contraindications: See phenylbutazone.
Precautions: See phenylbutazone.
Adverse Reactions: See phenylbutazone.
Drug Interactions: See phenylbutazone.

Generic Name: PHENYLBUTAZONE
Trade Name: Butazolidin
Dosage Form: Tablets, 100 mg
Uses: Anti-inflammatory agent beneficial in treatment of acute attacks of gouty arthritis.
Adult Dosage (Oral): 400 mg initially, then 100 mg q. 4h for 1 week. Maintenance therapy for other anti-inflammatory indications, up to 400 mg/d.
Contraindications: Children under 12 years, senile patients. Phenylbutazone or oxyphenbutazone allergy. Severe renal, hepatic, or cardiac disease, peptic ulcer/gastrointestinal inflammatory disease, thyroid disease, hypertension. Concomitant use of oral anticoagulants. Parotitis, stomatitis, polymyalgia rheumatica, temporal arteritis, blood dyscrasias, systemic edema.
Precautions: To minimize gastric irritation, administer doses with food, milk, or antacids. Use cautiously during first trimester of pregnancy. Therapy in the elderly should be restricted to 1 week since toxicity risk is greater over 40 years of age. Serious blood dyscrasias may occur many weeks after the drug has been withdrawn; therefore, blood cell counts every 2 weeks are recommended. Asthma, peptic ulcer disease, lupus, and bleeding disorders may be aggravated. Visual disturbances such as blurred vision can indicate toxicity. Drug should be discontinued if leukopenia or granulocytopenia is significant.

Adverse Reactions: See naproxen. Serious blood dyscrasias such as agranulocytosis, purpuras, aplastic anemia, and bone marrow depression can occur. Severe hypersensitivity reactions including exfoliative dermatitis, angiitis, and Stevens-Johnson syndrome may also occur.

Drug Interactions: Displaces many protein-bound drugs. With insulin/oral hypoglycemics, potentiation of hypoglycemic effects. Increases serum levels of phenytoin and sulfonamides. With coumarin anticoagulants and heparin, potentiation of anticoagulant effects.

Generic Name: PROBENECID
Trade Name: Benemid
Dosage Forms: Tablets, 500 mg; also in combination with colchicine as ColBENEMID
Uses: Uricosuric agent for treatment of chronic gout and adjuvant to penicillin therapy.
Adult Dosage (Oral): 250 mg bid for 1 week, then 0.5 g bid. As an adjuvant to penicillin therapy, 2 g/day in divided doses. For uncomplicated gonorrhea, single dose of 1 g prior to penicillin dose.
Pediatric Dosage (Oral): As an adjuvant to penicillin therapy in a child under 50 kg, 25 mg/kg/d to start, then 40 mg/kg/d in four divided doses. In a child over 50 kg, same as adult dosage.
Contraindications: Hypersensitivity to probenecid; uric acid kidney stones or blood dyscrasias, acute gouty attacks, salicylate therapy. Do not use in children under 2 years of age.
Precautions: If gout is exacerbated, colchicine should be added. Liberal fluid intake and urine alkalinization recommended. Renal impairment (probably ineffective if glomerular filtration rate is under 30 mL/min). Caution in peptic ulcer disease or G6PD deficiency. Hypersensitivity reactions necessitate discontinuance of drug.
Adverse Reactions: Gastric upset, sore gums, flushing; hypersensitivity reactions (mild to severe) including rash, pruritus, fever; blood dyscrasias (hemolytic anemia, aplastic anemia [rare]). Genitourinary effects, including renal colic, hematuria, uric acid stones, and urinary frequency.
Drug Interactions: Increases plasma concentrations of penicillins, cephalothin, methotrexate, p-aminosalicylic acid, rifampin, indomethacin, sulfonamides, sulfinpyrazone, and sulfonylureas. Salicylates inhibit uricosuric action of probenecid.

Generic Name: SULFINPYRAZONE
Trade Name: Anturane
Dosage Forms: Tablets, 100 mg; capsules, 200 mg
Uses: Uricosuric agent for treatment of chronic or intermittent gouty arthritis.
Adult Dosage (Oral): 100–200 mg bid with meals. Increase over 1 week to 200 mg bid as necessary.
Contraindications: Hypersensitivity to sulfinpyrazone or phenylbutazone (and derivatives). Active peptic ulcer/gastrointestinal ulceration and inflammation. Blood dyscrasias (past or present).
Precautions: See probenecid. Sulfinpyrazone also inhibits platelet aggregation and may increase prothrombin time in patients on oral anticoagulants.
Adverse Reactions: See probenecid, although incidence of rashes may be lower.
Drug Interactions: See probenecid. With anticoagulants, additive hypoprothrombinemia.

ANTIDEPRESSANTS, ANTIEMETICS, TRANQUILIZERS

Generic Name: AMITRIPTYLINE
Trade Names: Elavil, Endep
Dosage Forms: Tablets, 10 mg, 25 mg, 50 mg, 75 mg, 100 mg, 150 mg; injection (IM), 10 mg/mL
Uses: Tricyclic antidepressant.
Adult Dosage (Oral): 75 mg/d, divided doses or single dose at bedtime to start. Dosage may be increased by 25- to 50-mg increments at bedtime to 150 mg/d.
Adult Dosage (Parenteral): 20–30 mg IM qid initially, replaced with oral therapy as soon as possible. (*Note:* Hospitalized patients may require 100 mg/d to start, followed by gradual increases up to 200–300 mg/d.)
Contraindications: Hypersensitivity to amitriptyline. Concomitant MAO inhibitor therapy. Myocardial infarction during acute recovery phase.
Precautions: Has anticholinergic activity, so use with caution in glaucoma (narrow angle), myocardial infarction, urinary retention, cardiovascular disease, and hyperthyroidism. Psychotic, manic-depressive, or suicidal patients may worsen. Hepatic impairment may cause drug accumulation.
Adverse Reactions: Dry mouth, blurred vision, increased intraocular pressure (may precipitate acute attack in narrow angle glaucoma), hypotension, hypertension, tachycardia, palpitations, myocardial infarction, arrhythmias, and heart block. Possible CNS disturbances include excitement, hallucinations, delusions, fatigue, sedation, peripheral neuropathy, ataxia, numbness, and extrapyramidal symptoms. Gastric upset, black tongue, abnormal liver function tests, hepatitis, and allergic reactions (including rash and photosensitivity) may occur.
Drug Interactions: With MAO inhibitors, hyperpyrexia, convulsions, coma, death. With anticholinergics, increased anticholinergic effects. With sympathomimetics, severe hypertension, hyperpyrexia. With alcohol and other CNS depressants, additive CNS depression.

Generic Name: BUSPIRONE
Trade Name: Buspar
Dosage Form: Tablets, 5, 10 mg
Uses: Indicated for the management of anxiety disorders or short-term relief of symptoms of anxiety.
Adult Dosage (Oral): Initially, 15 mg daily (5 mg three times a day), then gradually increase the dose by 5 mg/d every 2–3 days as needed. Do not exceed 60 mg/d.
Pediatric Dosage (Oral): Safety and efficacy not established in children < 18 years of age.
Contraindications: Hypersensitivity to buspirone.
Precautions: Has no established antipsychotic activity. Has shown no potential for abuse. Use with extreme caution in patients with hepatic or renal impairment. Patients should be cautioned as to possible sedative effects. Will not block withdrawal symptoms associated with the discontinuance of benzodiazepine therapy where dependence has occurred. Usually 3–4 weeks are required to see therapeutic response.
Adverse Reactions: Most common include dizziness, headache, nervousness, lightheadedness, excitement, nonspecific chest pain.
Drug Interactions: With haloperidol, may increase haloperidol concentrations. With monoamine oxidase inhibitors, may result in an increased blood pressure. With trazadone, possibly increased hepatic transaminases.

Generic Name: CHLORDIAZEPOXIDE
Trade Name: Librium
Dosage Forms: Capsules, 5 mg, 10 mg, 25 mg; injection (IM/IV), 100 mg
Uses: Benzodiazepine derivative for treatment of moderate to severe anxiety, tension, and alcoholic withdrawal symptoms.
Adult Dosage (Oral): For anxiety, 5–10 mg tid or qid (up to 200 mg/d). For alcohol withdrawal, 50–100 mg repeated prn (up to 300 mg/d).
Adult Dosage (Parenteral): For anxiety, 50–100 mg IM initially, then 25–50 mg tid or qid prn. For alcohol withdrawal, 50–100 mg IM q. 2–4h, prn (up to 300 mg/d).
Contraindications: Hypersensitivity to chlordiazepoxide, shock, comatose states.
Precautions: IM injections are slowly and erratically absorbed; diluting doses with normal saline may improve absorption. For IV injections, normal saline should be used as diluent; infusion should be slow, over 1 minute; observe for hypotension and respiratory depression after IV administration. Maximum parenteral dose recommended is 300 mg in any 6- to 24-hour period. Elderly or debilitated patients should be given one-half doses. Use cautiously in hepatic or renal impairment or in those receiving concomitant psychotherapy. Drug may be habit-forming; barbiturate-like withdrawal symptoms may occur.
Adverse Reactions: Drowsiness, vertigo, ataxia and oversedation (especially in elderly), gastric upset. Hostility reactions, paradoxical excitement, stimulation, acute rage (especially in psychiatric patients); allergic reactions with rash and drug fever, cholestatic jaundice. Parenteral use can cause syncope, hypotension, tachycardia, extrapyramidal symptoms, blurred vision, and respiratory depression.
Drug Interactions: Additive CNS depression with alcohol, tricyclic antidepressants, sedative-hypnotics, MAO inhibitors, and other CNS depressants.

Generic Name: CHLORPROMAZINE
Trade Name: Thorazine
Dosage Forms: Tablets, 10 mg, 25 mg, 50 mg, 100 mg, 200 mg; capsules (sustained release), 30–300 mg; injection (IM/IV), 25 mg/mL; suppositories, 25 mg, 100 mg; syrup, 10 mg/5 mL; oral concentrate, 30 mg/mL, 100 mg/mL
Uses: Phenothiazine antipsychotic tranquilizer. Also used to control nausea and vomiting (except that caused by motion sickness), for treatment of intractable hiccups, and as adjunct in management of tetanus. Small doses can be given to prevent shivering and central pooling when hypothermia must be induced during therapy of intracranial hypertension.
Adult Dosage (Oral): As an antiemetic, 10–25 mg q. 4–6h, prn. For intractable hiccups, 25–50 mg q. 6–8h; switch to IM if symptoms persist for 2 or 3 days. As an antipsychotic, 200–800 mg/d in divided doses.
Adult Dosage (Parenteral): As an antiemetic, 25 mg IM initially; if no hypotension, 25–50 mg IM q. 3–4h, prn. For acute agitation, 25 mg IM stat; can repeat in 1 hour with 25–50 mg. For intractable hiccups, 25–50 mg IM; can follow with 25–50 mg

slow IV if necessary. As adjunct to tetanus therapy, 25–50 mg slowly IV (1 mg/min) or IM q. 6–8h. For control of shivering during induced hypothermia, 0.1–0.2 mg/kg/dose IM or slowly IV.

Pediatric Dosage (Oral): For antiemesis or sedation in a child or infant over 6 months old, 2 mg/kg/d, divided q. 4–6h (up to 0.55 mg/kg/dose).

Pediatric Dosage (Parenteral): As an antiemetic, 0.55 mg/kg/dose deep IM, q. 6–8h. For control of shivering during induced hypothermia, 0.1–0.2 mg/kg/dose IM or IV.

Contraindications: Hypersensitivity to phenothiazines. Circulatory collapse, severe hypotension, CNS depression, comatose states, presence of large amounts of CNS depressants. Bone marrow depression (prolonged therapy).

Precautions: IV injection can cause severe hypotension; administer only to supine patients. Dilute doses at least 1 mg/mL; give slowly, no faster than 1 mg/min. Solution is light sensitive; do not use if extremely yellow. Use cautiously in children because it may cause extrapyramidal symptoms; avoid use in infants under 6 months old and in those patients with Reye's syndrome or other CNS encephalopathies (drug may mask symptoms of these diseases). Reduce doses of narcotics and other CNS depressants by 50%–75% if given concomitantly. Use cautiously in seizure disorders, chronic respiratory disease, asthma, hyperthermia, hepatic or cardiac impairment, myasthenia gravis, and other conditions aggravated by anticholinergic activity. Can suppress cough reflex so patient could aspirate.

Adverse Reactions: CNS sedation and depression, thermoregulatory impairment (hyperpyrexia), lowered convulsive threshold with seizures, cerebral edema, extrapyramidal effects (moderate for chlorpromazine), and tardive dyskinesia. Anticholinergic effects of tachycardia, dry mouth, blurred vision, urinary difficulty, and constipation. Also, orthostatic hypotension (due to α-adrenergic blockade), "quinidine-like" effect on heart, shock-like syndrome, heart block; allergic reactions including cholestatic jaundice, urticaria, rashes, contact dermatitis, and photosensitivity; blood dyscrasias, skin pigmentation, pigmentary retinopathy, gynecomastia, amenorrhea, lupus syndrome, and carbohydrate intolerance.

Drug Interactions: Additive CNS depression with narcotics, sedative-hypnotics, alcohol, other tranquilizers. With alcohol, epinephrine, and antihypertensives, excessive hypotension. With anticonvulsants, lowered convulsive threshold with seizures. Additive anticholinergic effects with other anticholinergic medications.

Generic Name: HALOPERIDOL
Trade Name: Haldol
Dosage Forms: Tablets, 0.5 mg, 1 mg, 2 mg, 5 mg; injection (IM), 5 mg/mL; oral solution, 2 mg/mL
Uses: Antipsychotic tranquilizer (butyrophenone derivative) given parenterally to control acute, severe agitation; used orally for symptomatic management of psychotic disorders, Tourette's disorder, agitation; hyperkinetic activity in children.
Adult Dosage (Oral): 0.5–2 mg bid or tid (up to 3–5 mg tid or more).
Adult Dosage (Parenteral): 2–5 mg IM q. 1–8h, prn.
Pediatric Dosage (Oral): 0.05–0.15 mg/kg/d (maximum 6 mg/d).
Contraindications: Hypersensitivity. Severe toxic CNS depression or comatose states, Parkinson's disease.

Precautions: Reduce dosage in elderly or debilitated patients. Use cautiously in those with severe cardiac disease, thyrotoxicosis, bronchopneumonia, convulsive disorders, or those receiving antiparkinson medications. May cause rapid mood swings to depression in manic-depressive patients. Avoid skin contact when using solutions (contact dermatitis).

Adverse Reactions: High incidence of extrapyramidal symptoms. Other side effects similar to those of phenothiazines. Also causes severe neurotoxicity in patients with thyrotoxicosis; gastric upset, laryngospasm, bronchospasm, dyspnea, anginal pain.

Drug Interactions: With lithium, encephalopathic syndrome characterized by weakness, lethargy, fever, tremulousness, confusion, extrapyramidal symptoms, blood dyscrasias, elevated serum enzymes, and irreversible brain damage. See also chlorpromazine.

Generic Name: ONDANSETRON
Trade Name: Zofran
Dosage Form: Injection, 2 mg/mL in 20 mL multidose vials
Uses: Selective 5-HT$_3$ receptor antagonist used for the prevention of nausea and vomiting associated with cancer chemotherapy.
Adult Dosage (Parenteral): Three 0.15 mg/kg dosages. The first infused over 15 minutes beginning 30 minutes prior to the start of chemotherapy. Subsequent doses are administered at 4 and 8 hours after the first dose. Ondansetron should be diluted in 50 mL of 5% dextrose injection or 0.9% sodium chloride injection prior to administration.
Pediatric Dosage (Parenteral): 4–18 years, treat as adult.
Contraindications: Hypersensitivity to the drug product.
Precautions: No adequate and well-controlled studies in pregnant or lactating women. Therefore, use only if potential benefit justifies the possible risk to the infant or fetus.
Adverse Reactions: Common complaints include diarrhea, headache, akathesia, and acute dystonic reactions (primarily in patients receiving concomitant metoclopramide), transient increase in AST/ALT, constipation, and rash.
Drug Interactions: No clinically significant interactions reported.

Generic Name: PROCHLORPERAZINE
Trade Name: Compazine
Dosage Forms: Tablets, 5 mg, 10 mg; capsules (sustained release), 10 mg, 15 mg, 30 mg, 75 mg; injection (IM/IV), 5 mg/mL; suppositories, 2.5 mg, 5 mg, 25 mg (adult); oral syrup, 5 mg/5 mL; oral concentrate, 10 mg/mL
Uses: Phenothiazine antiemetic for severe nausea and vomiting (except that caused by motion sickness).
Adult Dosage (Oral): 5–10 mg tid or qid (tablets); 10 mg q. 12h (spansules).
Adult Dosage (Rectal): 25 mg bid.
Adult Dosage (Parenteral): 5–10 mg IM or slow IV q. 3–4h, prn (maximum, 40 mg/d).
Pediatric Dosage (Oral/Rectal): For a child over 2 years and over 10 kg, 0.4 mg/kg/d, divided q. 8–12h; usual dose, 2.5 to 5 mg q. 8–12h.
Pediatric Dosage (Parenteral): 0.13 mg/kg/dose IM as a single dose.
Contraindications: Children under 2 years and less than 10 kg; pediatric surgery. See also chlorpromazine.
Precautions: Do not give subcutaneously. IM injections should be made deeply into upper outer quadrant of buttock. IV doses

should be well diluted and administered slowly (rate not to exceed 5 mg/mL/min). Higher incidence of extrapyramidal reactions than with chlorpromazine; especially severe reactions in children so avoid its use in all infants and children if possible. Fever, dehydration, CNS disease, and viral illness can predispose patients to extrapyramidal reactions. See also chlorpromazine.

Adverse Reactions: See chlorpromazine.
Drug Interactions: See chlorpromazine.

Generic Name: PROMETHAZINE
Trade Name: Phenergan
Dosage Forms: Injection (IM/IV), 25 mg/mL, 50 mg/mL; tablets, 12.5 mg, 25 mg, 50 mg; oral syrup, 6.25 mg/mL; rectal suppositories, 25 mg, 50 mg
Uses: Phenothiazine derivative with antihistaminic properties used as an antiemetic (including motion sickness), sedative, antihistamine for various allergic reactions, and as an adjunct to narcotic analgesia.
Adult Dosage (Oral or Rectal): As antiemetic, 25 mg initially, then 12.5–25 mg q. 4–6h as needed; for motion sickness, 25 mg given 30–60 min before departure and repeated q. 8–12h later; for sedation or allergic rhinitis, 25–50 mg at bedtime.
Adult Dosage (Parenteral): As antiemetic, same as oral dosage; as adjunct to opiate analgesics, 25–50 mg IM or IV with reduced dose of narcotic; for sedation, 25–50 mg IM or IV; as antihistamine, 25 mg IM or IV, repeated in 2 hours if needed.
Pediatric Dosage (Oral or Rectal): As antiemetic, 0.25–0.50 mg/kg q. 4–6h as needed; as antihistamine, 0.5 mg/kg at bedtime or divided tid; as preoperative sedative, 0.5–1.0 mg/kg/dose.
Pediatric Dosage (Parenteral): Same as oral or rectal doses, given by deep IM injection.
Contraindications: Hypersensitivity to promethazine, subcutaneous use. See also chlorpromazine.
Precautions: See also chlorpromazine. Give IM injections deeply. Dilute IV doses well and give slowly at rate not to exceed 25 mg/mL/min. Avoid extravasation. Do not give subcutaneously (severe tissue necrosis and irritation). Reduce concomitant doses of barbiturates and narcotics to 50%. Use cautiously in the elderly and in children or infants because of possible extrapyramidal effects. Avoid use in acutely ill or dehydrated children; those with Reye's syndrome; CNS, viral, or hepatic disease; and newborns and young infants. Use cautiously in acute or chronic respiratory impairment (suppresses cough reflex), bronchial asthma, and cardiac or hepatic impairment. Drug-induced drowsiness may impair performance of potentially hazardous activities. Paradoxic hyperexcitability and restlessness may occur when given together with narcotic analgesics to patients in pain.
Adverse Reactions: Drowsiness, dizziness, anticholinergic effects (eg, blurred vision, dry mouth) are common. Extrapyramidal reactions occur less frequently than with chlorpromazine. See also chlorpromazine.
Drug Interactions: See chlorpromazine.

Generic Name: TRIMETHOBENZAMIDE
Trade Name: Tigan
Dosage Forms: Injection (IM), 100 mg/mL; capsules, 100 mg, 250 mg; suppositories, 100 mg (pediatric), 200 mg
Uses: Antiemetic (ethanolamine antihistamine derivative).
Adult Dosage (Oral): 250 mg q. 6–8h, prn.
Adult Dosage (Rectal): 200 mg q. 6–8h, prn.
Adult Dosage (Parenteral): 200 mg IM q. 6–8h, prn.
Pediatric Dosage (Oral): For a child 13–40 kg, 100–200 mg q. 6–8h, prn (or 20 mg/kg/d in divided doses).
Pediatric Dosage (Rectal): For a child 13–40 kg, 100–200 mg q. 6–8h, prn; for a child under 13 kg, 100 mg q. 6–8h, prn (or 15 mg/kg/d in divided doses).
Contraindications: Hypersensitivity to trimethobenzamide; use in premature infants and newborns; use of injection in infants or children; use of suppositories in those allergic to benzocaine or similar local anesthetics.
Precautions: See chlorpromazine.
Adverse Reactions: Pain, burning, redness, itching at IM injection site. Occasional parkinsonian (extrapyramidal) symptoms, hypersensitivity reactions, drowsiness, hypotension. See also chlorpromazine.
Drug Interactions: See chlorpromazine.

ANTIHISTAMINES/ANTIPRURITICS

Generic Name: CYPROHEPTADINE
Trade Name: Periactin
Dosage Forms: Tablets, 4 mg; oral syrup, 2 mg/5 mL
Uses: Antihistamine, antipruritic agent.
Adult Dosage: 4 mg tid or qid (maximum, 0.5 mg/kg/d).
Pediatric Dosage: 0.25 mg/kg/d in 3 or 4 divided doses.
Contraindications: Hypersensitivity to drug, patients on MAO inhibitor therapy, elderly and debilitated patients, newborn and premature infants, conditions aggravated by anticholinergic action (eg, glaucoma, stenosing peptic ulcer).
Precautions: See diphenhydramine. Also may cause increased appetite and weight gain in children. Antiserotonin activity may inhibit adrenocorticotropic hormone release in Cushing's disease. Caution patients about drug-induced drowsiness since it may impair performance of hazardous tasks.
Adverse Reactions: Frequent sedation (less than diphenhydramine), dizziness, disturbed coordination, dry mouth and mucous membranes, thickening of bronchial secretions, epigastric distress. Also hypotension, headache, palpitations, tachycardia, CNS stimulation and depression, rashes, urticaria, blurred vision, urinary retention and frequency, photosensitivity.
Drug Interactions: With alcohol, other CNS depressants, additive CNS depression. With MAO inhibitors, increased anticholinergic side effects.

Generic Name: DIPHENHYDRAMINE
Trade Name: Benadryl
Dosage Forms: Capsules, 25 mg, 50 mg; injection (IM/IV), 10 mg/mL, 50 mg/mL; elixir, 12.5 mg/5 mL
Uses: Antihistamine for treatment of allergic rhinitis, hypersensitivity reactions, drug-induced extrapyramidal reactions, parkinsonism, motion sickness, and emesis. Also used as antitussive and nighttime sleep aid.

Adult Dosage (Oral): 25–50 mg tid or qid. For hypnotic dose, 50–100 mg at bedtime.
Adult Dosage (Parenteral): 10–50 mg IM or IV q. 4–6h (up to 400 mg/d).
Pediatric Dosage (Oral): (Based on 5 mg/kg/d). For a child over 9 kg, 12.5–25 mg q. 6–8h; under 9 kg, 6.25–12.5 mg q. 6–8h.
Pediatric Dosage (Parenteral): 5 mg/kg/d IM (deep) or IV, divided q. 6h (up to 300 mg/d). For extrapyramidal reactions, 1.5 mg/kg slowly IV as a single dose.
Contraindications: Hypersensitivity to diphenhydramine or related compounds (dimenhydrinate). Newborn and premature infants, lactation, patients on MAO inhibitor therapy, conditions aggravated by anticholinergic action (eg, glaucoma).
Precautions: Use cautiously in infants under 2 years old and the elderly over 60 years, patients with bronchial asthma, glaucoma, hyperthyroidism, hypertension, cardiovascular disease, stenosing peptic ulcer, prostatic hypertrophy, and other conditions aggravated by anticholinergic effects. Drug-induced drowsiness can impair performance of hazardous tasks. Paradoxical CNS stimulation can occur in children. May mask signs of drug-induced vestibular toxicity.
Adverse Reactions: See cyproheptadine. Sedation more prominent.
Drug Interactions: See cyproheptadine.

Generic Name: HYDROXYZINE
Trade Names: Vistaril, Atarax
Dosage Forms: Tablets (HCl), 10 mg, 25 mg, 50 mg, 100 mg; capsules (pamoate), 25 mg, 50 mg, 100 mg; injection (IM only), 25 mg, 50 mg, 100 mg; oral suspension, 25 mg/5 mL; oral solution, 10 mg/5 mL
Uses: Antihistamine derivative for symptomatic treatment of anxiety, tension, acute alcohol withdrawal, allergic pruritis, emesis, and motion sickness. Also given with narcotics to reduce opiate analgesic dosage and for preoperative sedation. Effective and safe sedative and antiemetic for children.
Adult Dosage (Oral): For anxiety, 50–100 mg qid. For pruritus, 25–50 mg tid to qid. For preoperative sedation, 50–100 mg.
Adult Dosage (Parenteral): 25–100 mg IM q. 4–6h, prn.
Pediatric Dosage (Oral): 2 mg/kg/d, divided qid (maximum daily dose for a child under 6 years, 50 mg; over 6 years, 100 mg).
Pediatric Dosage (Parenteral): As antiemetic or preoperative sedative, 1.1 mg/kg as single IM dose.
Contraindications: Hypersensitivity to hydroxyzine, early pregnancy.
Precautions: Should not be given IV or subcutaneously. Use Z-track technique for IM injections. Reduce dosage by up to 50% if other CNS depressants are given concomitantly. Drug-induced drowsiness may impair performance of potentially hazardous activities.
Adverse Reactions: Transient drowsiness and dry mouth are common. Involuntary motor activity, tremor, convulsions, urticaria, and rashes occur rarely. Inadvertent subcutaneous, IV, or intra-arterial injection can cause severe gangrene or thrombosis.
Drug Interactions: Alcohol, tricyclic antidepressants, narcotic analgesics, sedative-hypnotics, and other CNS depressants cause increased CNS depression.

AMINOGLYCOSIDE ANTIBIOTICS

Generic Name: AMIKACIN
Trade Name: Amikin
Dosage Forms: Injection (IM/IV), 100 mg, 500 mg, 1 g
Uses: Aminoglycoside antibiotic useful in gentamicin- and kanamycin-resistant infections with gram-negative organisms. Other indications as for gentamicin.
Adult Dosage (Parenteral): For uncomplicated infections, 250 mg IM bid. For moderate to severe infections, 7.5 mg/kg q. 12h or 5 mg/kg q. 8h IM or slow IV. Desirable peak and trough concentrations range from 15–30 µg/mL and <5 µg/mL, respectively.
Pediatric Dosage (Parenteral): In the child and infant, same as adult. For sepsis in the newborn, 10 mg/kg IM or IV to start, then 7.5 mg/kg q. 12h.
Contraindications: Hypersensitivity to amikacin or other aminoglycosides.
Precautions: See gentamicin. If no definite clinical response in 3–5 days, recheck culture and sensitivity. Patient must be adequately hydrated to minimize renal irritation.
Adverse Reactions: See gentamicin.
Drug Interactions: See gentamicin.

Generic Name: GENTAMICIN
Trade Name: Garamycin
Dosage Forms: Topical preparations; injection (IM/IV), 20 mg, 60 mg, 80 mg; intrathecal, 2 mg/mL (2 mL)
Uses: Aminoglycoside antibiotic for serious infections caused by a variety of gram-negative organisms, notably *Pseudomonas*, *Klebsiella-Enterobacter*, and *Serratia*; limited activity against gram-positive organisms but can be used for penicillin-resistant staphylococci. Ineffective against anaerobes; synergistic with penicillin against enterococci (*S. faecalis*).
Adult Dosage (Parenteral): Therapeutic levels, 4–10 µg/mL. Toxic levels, peak concentrations greater than 10–12 µg/mL, and trough concentrations greater than 2 µg/mL. Dose varies with type and severity of infection. Usual dose, 3–5 mg/kg/d IM or IV in divided doses q. 8h (up to 6–8 mg/kg/d). Intrathecal dose, up to 5 mg q. 18–24h, in combination with systemic administration.
Pediatric Dosage (Parenteral): In a child, 2–2.5 mg/kg IM or IV q. 8h; in an infant, 2.5 mg/kg IM or IV q. 8h; in a newborn, 2.5 mg/kg IM or IV q. 12h. Intrathecal dose, 1–2 mg/d with or without systemic administration.
Contraindications: Hypersensitivity to gentamicin (absolute); hypersensitivity to other aminoglycosides (relative).
Precautions: Dilute IV doses to 1 mg/mL or less; administer slowly over 30–60 min. Keep patient well hydrated and maintain adequate urine output during therapy. Monitor renal function and perform urinalysis periodically especially if treatment is over 10 days' duration. Renal impairment requires dosage adjustments. Monitor auditory function periodically during prolonged therapy, use of high doses, or use in elderly or high-risk patients. Use cautiously in those with neuromuscular disorders or those receiv-

ing neuromuscular blocking agents. Culture and sensitivity tests are recommended to ensure bacterial susceptibility to this aminoglycoside; possible cross-allergenicity with other aminoglycosides.

Adverse Reactions: Nephrotoxicity (mild to acute) and ototoxicity (tinnitus, roaring in ears, high-tone auditory impairment, vestibular damage). CNS and neurotoxic effects include lethargy, dizziness, hypotension, visual disturbances, numbness, tingling, muscle twitching, pseudotumor cerebri, convulsions, and neuromuscular blockade with apnea. Also gastrointestinal upset, hypersensitivity reactions, blood dyscrasias, and superinfections.

Drug Interactions: Increased nephrotoxicity with cephalosporins, other aminoglycosides, vancomycin, polymyxin, and potent diuretics. Increased ototoxicity with potent diuretics and other aminoglycosides. Additive neuromuscular blockade with other aminoglycosides, anesthetics, and curariform drugs. Synergistic with carbenicillin, ticarcillin, piperacillin, and mezlocillin against *Pseudomonas* (but avoid direct admixture in same container).

Generic Name: KANAMYCIN
Trade Name: Kantrex
Dosage Forms: Capsules, 500 mg; injection (IM/IV), 75 mg (pediatric), 500 mg, 1 g
Uses: Aminoglycoside antibiotic given orally for preoperative bowel sterilization, adjunctive therapy of hepatic encephalopathy, and treatment of diarrhea caused by enteropathic *Escherichia coli*. Used parenterally for infections caused by staphylococci and susceptible coliform bacteria. *Pseudomonas* and anaerobes are resistant.
Adult Dosage (Oral): For hepatic encephalopathy, 6–12 g orally or rectally as enema daily in divided doses. For bowel sterilization, 1 g every hour for four doses, then 1 g q. 4h for 24 hours.
Adult Dosage (Parenteral): 7.5 mg/kg q. 12h or up to 15 mg/kg/d IM or slow IV infusion in divided doses q. 8–12h (not to exceed 1.5 g/d). Intraperitoneal irrigation should not exceed IM or IV dosage. (Therapeutic blood levels usually 15–25 μg/mL.)
Pediatric Dosage (Oral): For suppression of intestinal bacteria, 50 mg/kg/d in divided doses, q. 4–6h for 5 to 7 days.
Pediatric Dosage (Parenteral): For a child or infant over 1 week old, 15–20 mg/kg/d IM or IV, divided q. 8–12h. For a newborn under 1 week old under 2 kg, 15 mg/kg/d IM or IV, divided q. 12h; if over 2 kg, 20 mg/kg/d IM or IV, divided q. 12h.
Contraindications: See gentamicin.
Precautions: IV use should be avoided (unless IM use not feasible). Administer IV doses slowly over 30–60 min. Prolonged oral use may lead to malabsorption syndrome. Systemic absorption from oral, rectal, or irrigation use may occur in presence of renal impairment or denuded/ulcerated mucosa. For other precautions, see gentamicin. Complete cross-resistance with neomycin.
Adverse Reactions: Primarily ototoxicity with cochlear, vestibular damage, especially with serum levels over 35 μg/mL or with prolonged therapy at lower doses. For other adverse reactions, see gentamicin.
Drug Interactions: See gentamicin. Oral kanamycin may impair gastrointestinal absorption of vitamin K and digitalis.

Generic Name: NEOMYCIN
Trade Names: Mycifradin, Neomycin
Dosage Forms: Tablets, 500 mg; oral solution, 125 mg/5 mL; various topical preparations
Uses: See kanamycin. Also used topically for a variety of skin and eye infections.
Adult Dosage (Oral): For hepatic encephalopathy, 6–8 g (or rectally as enema) in 4 to 6 divided doses for 1–2 days, then decreased to 2–4 g/d in divided doses. For bowel sterilization, 1 g every hour for four doses, then 1 g q. 4h for 24 hours.
Pediatric Dosage (Oral): For diarrhea due to *Escherichia coli*, 100 mg/kg/d, divided q. 6h.
Contraindications: Hypersensitivity to neomycin (absolute); hypersensitivity to other aminoglycosides (relative).
Precautions: See kanamycin.
Adverse Reactions: See kanamycin.
Drug Interactions: See kanamycin.

Generic Name: NETILMICIN
Trade Name: Netromycin
Dosage Forms: Injection (IV/IM), 100 mg/mL in 1.5 mL vials (adult); 25 mg/mL in 2 mL vials (pediatric); 10 mg/mL in 2 mL ampules (neonate)
Uses: Aminoglycoside antibiotic which irreversibly binds to the 30S subunit of bacterial ribosomes, resulting in inhibition of protein synthesis and eventually cell death. Indicated for the treatment of complicated urinary tract infections and serious or life-threatening systemic gram-negative infections. Most notably *Escherichia coli*, *Klebsiella* species, *Proteus* species, and *Pseudomonas aeruginosa*. May be effective in the treatment of serious infections caused by organisms resistant to other aminoglycosides.
Adult Dosage (Parenteral):
- Complicated UTI (normal renal function)—1.5–2 mg/kg (based on lean body weight) IV/IM every 12 hours.
- Serious systemic infections (normal renal function)—1.3–2.2 mg/kg IV/IM every 8 hours or 2–3.25 mg/kg every 12 hours (based on lean body weight).
- Desirable peak and trough concentrations range from 6–10 μg/mL and 0.5–2 μg/mL, respectively.
- In the setting of renal impairment, dosage adjustments based on level of impairment (creatinine clearance) and serum drug concentration should be made. In the absence of serum levels the manufacturer recommends that a loading dose of 1.3–3.25 mg/kg be administered and then subsequent doses be calculated multiplying the appropriate daily dose for normal patients by the fraction obtained when the creatinine clearance of the patient with impaired renal function is divided by the normal creatinine clearance. The adjusted daily dose may be given at 24-hour intervals or divided at 8- or 12-hour intervals, but each dose should not exceed 3.25 mg/kg.
- In patients undergoing hemodialysis, a dose of 2 mg/kg should be administered at the end of each dialysis period until the results of tests measuring serum levels become available, at which time dosage adjustments should be made based on these tests.

Pediatric Dosage (Parenteral): Newborns ($\leq$ 7 days)—2.5 mg/kg/dose load 1 followed by 2 mg/kg/dose every 12 hours. Infants and children—2.5 mg/kg/dose every 8 hours.
Contraindications: Hypersensitivity to netilmicin (absolute) or other aminoglycosides (relative).

Precautions: Because of the neuromuscular blocking effect of aminoglycosides, caution should be used in patients being weaned from mechanical ventilators, with myasthenia gravis, parkinsonism, and botulism. Serum concentrations should be closely monitored in elderly patients, premature infants, and neonates as a state of reduced renal function may exist. Because of reported synergism, many clinicians recommend concomitant use of an extended-spectrum penicillin with antipseudomonal activity (eg, ticarcillin) and an aminoglycoside such as netilmicin for the treatment of serious pseudomonal infections.
Adverse Reactions: See gentamicin.
Drug Interactions: See gentamicin.

Generic Name: STREPTOMYCIN
Dosage Forms: Injection (IM only), 500 mg, 1 g, 5 g
Uses: Aminoglycoside antibiotic for treatment of tuberculosis, bacterial endocarditis (adjunct), tularemia.
Adult Dosage (Parenteral): For tuberculosis, 1 g/d IM to start, then 2 to 3 doses weekly up to 1 year (given with other antituberculars). Usual dose for other infections, 1–2 g IM daily divided q. 12h (maximum, 4 g/d). For bacterial endocarditis, 1 g IM bid for 1 week, then 0.5 g bid IM for 1 week (with penicillin).
Pediatric Dosage (Parenteral): For a child, 20–40 mg/kg/d IM divided q. 6–12h (along with other anti-infectives). Not recommended for infants or newborns.
Contraindications: Hypersensitivity to streptomycin (absolute); hypersensitivity to other aminoglycosides (relative).
Precautions: Not for IV use. Caution in pregnancy, the elderly, renal and auditory impairment, as well as in use with other ototoxic drugs. Therapeutic levels, 25–50 µg/mL. Toxic serum levels, greater than 50 µg/mL.
Adverse Reactions: Vestibular ototoxicity (frequent, sometimes irreversible). Nephrotoxicity, paresthesias, rash, fever, neuromuscular blockade, hepatic necrosis. See also gentamicin.
Drug Interactions: See gentamicin.

Generic Name: TOBRAMYCIN
Trade Name: Nebcin
Dosage Forms: Injection (IM/IV), 20 mg (pediatric), 60 mg, 80 mg
Uses: As for gentamicin, except active against gentamicin-resistant strains of *Pseudomonas*.
Adult Dosage (Parenteral): 3–5 mg/kg/d IM or IV divided q. 8h, depending on severity of infection; should be decreased to 3 mg/kg/d as soon as possible. Desirable peak and trough concentrations range from 3–8 µg/mL and 1–2 µg/mL, respectively.
Pediatric Dosage (Parenteral): For a child, 6.0–7.5 mg/kg/d IM or IV, divided q. 6–8h (up to 10 mg/kg/d); for a premature or full-term newborn, 4 mg/kg/d IM or IV, divided q. 12h.
Contraindications: Hypersensitivity to tobramycin and/or other aminoglycosides.
Precautions: See gentamicin. Higher milligram per kilogram doses and dosage intervals for 4–6 hours may be necessary in children 2 to 18 years old because of the more rapid renal clearance and larger volume of distribution of drug in this age-group.
Adverse Reactions: See gentamicin.
Drug Interactions: See gentamicin.

CEPHALOSPORIN ANTIBIOTICS

Uses: Broad-spectrum class of antibiotics divided into three "generations," based on their activity against gram-negative organisms:
- First-generation cephalosporins: cephalothin (Keflin), cefazolin (Ancef, Kefzol), cephapirin (Cefadyl), cephradine (Anspor, Velosef), cephalexin (Keflex), and cefadroxil (Duricef, Ultracef). Active against most gram-positive cocci, including penicillinase-producing staphylococci (but *not* enterococci or methicillin-resistant *Staphylococcus aureus*). Gram-negative spectrum includes *Escherichia coli*, *Haemophilus influenzae*, *Proteus mirabilis*, and *Klebsiella* species. Useful for treatment of urinary tract, respiratory tract, skin and soft tissue, and bone and joint infections and septicemias caused by susceptible organisms.
- Second-generation cephalosporins: cefamandole (Mandol), cefonicid (Monocid), ceforanide (Precef), cefoxitin (Mefoxin), cefaclor (Ceclor), cefuroxime axetil (Ceftin), and cefuroxime (Zinacef). Gram-positive spectrum similar to first-generation agents; increased activity against gram-negative bacilli. Cefamandole, cefaclor, and cefuroxime are more active against *H. influenzae*; cefoxitin and cefuroxime have improved activity against *Neisseria gonorrhoeae*. Cefoxitin is very effective for infections caused by *Bacteroides fragilis* and other anaerobes. Useful for treatment of intra-abdominal, gynecologic, and serious *H. influenzae* infections and for penicillin-resistant gonorrhea. Cefonicid, having the longest half-life of these, is approved for once-daily dosing.
- Third-generation cephalosporins: cefotaxime (Claforan), ceftizoxime (Cefizox), cefoperazone (Cefobid), cefixime (Suprax), and moxalactam (Moxam). Less active than other cephalosporins against gram-positive cocci but more effective against gram-negative bacilli. Cefoperazone is more active than the others against *Pseudomonas*; all are highly effective against *H. influenzae* and gonococcal infections (including those resistant to penicillin). All third-generation agents appear to penetrate the CSF well. Used for treatment of gram-negative meningitis and intra-abdominal, gynecologic, penicillin-resistant gonococcal, and "mixed" aerobic-anaerobic infections. The long half-life of ceftriaxone permits once-daily dosing for mild to some serious infections.

Contraindications: Hypersensitivity to any cephalosporin.
Precautions: Possible cross-allergenicity with penicillins (7%–10% incidence). Except for cefoperazone, which is metabolized by the liver, all cephalosporins require some dosage adjustments in renal impairment (when creatinine clearance is 50 mL/min or less).
Adverse Reactions: Gastric upset, diarrhea, hypersensitivity reactions, serum sickness (especially with prolonged parenteral use), thrombophlebitis with IV use, eosinophilia and other transient blood dyscrasias, some renal impairment (including increased blood urea nitrogen and serum creatinine levels). Transient rises in liver enzymes may occur, as well as a positive direct Coombs' test, especially in azotemic patients. Superinfections with enterococci and yeasts may occur. (*Note:* Pseudomembranous colitis

and a vitamin K–responsive hypoprothrombinemia with bleeding have been reported particularly with the second- and third-generation cephalosporins. A disulfiram-like reaction may occur when alcohol is ingested after administration of cefamandole, moxalactam, or cefoperazone.)

Drug Interactions: Probenecid increases serum levels of cephalosporins. Aminoglycosides, potent loop diuretics, increase nephrotoxicity.

PARENTERALLY ADMINISTERED CEPHALOSPORINS

Generic Name: CEFAMANDOLE
Trade Name: Mandol
Dosage Forms: Injection (IM/IV), 500 mg, 1 g, 2 g vials
Adult Dosage: 500 mg–1 g IV q. 4–8h (up to 12 g/d); 500 mg–1 g IM q. 8h for uncomplicated urinary tract infections.
Pediatric Dosage: In a child or infant 1 month or older, 50–100 mg/kg/d IM/IV, divided q. 4–8h (maximum of 150 mg/kg/d for severe infections).

Generic Name: CEFAZOLIN
Trade Names: Ancef, Kefzol
Dosage Forms: Injection (IM/IV), 250 mg, 500 mg, 1 g vials
Adult Dosage: 250–500 mg IM q. 8h for mild infections; 500 mg–1 g IV q. 6–8h (up to 12 g/d) for severe infections.
Pediatric Dosage: For a child or infant, 40–80 mg/kg/d IV or IM, divided q. 6–8h; for a newborn under 1 week old, 30–40 mg/kg/d IV or IM, divided q. 12h. (*Note:* Significant biliary levels achieved with cefazolin.)

Generic Name: CEFONICID
Trade Name: Monocid
Dosage Form: Injection (IM/IV)
Adult Dosage (Parenteral): 1–2 g IM or IV q. 24h. For uncomplicated gonorrhea, single 1-g IM dose with or without oral probenecid.

Generic Name: CEFOPERAZONE
Trade Name: Cefobid
Dosage Forms: Injection (IM/IV), 1 g, 2 g vials
Adult Dosage: 2–4 g/d IM or IV, divided q. 12h (up to 12 g/d, divided q. 6–8h). Dosage adjustments required in hepatic but not in renal impairment.
Pediatric Dosage: Not established.

Generic Name: CEFOTAXIME
Trade Name: Claforan
Dosage Forms: Injection (IM/IV), 1 g, 2 g vials
Adult Dosage: 1 g IM or IV q. 12h for uncomplicated urinary tract infection or pneumonia; 1–2 g IV or IM q. 6–8h for moderate to severe infections; 2 g IV q. 4h for life-threatening infections (maximum, 12 g/d).
Pediatric Dosage: For a child over 50 kg, use adult dosages; for a child 1 month to 12 years under 50 kg, 50–200 mg/kg/d IM or IV, divided q. 4–6h. For a newborn (1 to 4 weeks), 25–50 mg/kg IM or IV q. 8h; for a premature or full-term newborn (up to 1 week), 25–50 mg/kg IM or IV q. 12h.

Generic Name: CEFOXITIN
Trade Name: Mefoxin
Dosage Forms: Injection (IM/IV), 1 g, 2 g vials
Adult Dosage: 1 g IM or IV q. 6–8h for uncomplicated infections; 1–2 g IV q. 4–6h for moderate to severe infections (up to 12 g/d).
Pediatric Dosage: For a child or infant over 3 months, 80–160 mg/kg/d IV or IM, divided q. 4–6h (up to 12 g/d); for a newborn, 40 mg/kg/d IV, divided q. 12h.

Generic Name: CEFTAZIDIME
Trade Names: Fortaz, Tazidime
Dosage Forms: Injection (IM/IV), 500 mg, 1 g, 2 g vials
Adult Dosge (Parenteral): 1–2 g IV or IM q. 8h; for more serious infections, 2 g IV q. 8h. For urinary tract infections, 250–500 mg IM or IV q. 8–12h. (*Note:* Less in vitro activity against *Bacteroides* than other third-generation cephalosporins.)
Pediatric Dosage (Parenteral): For a newborn, 30 mg/kg IV q. 12h; for an infant over 1 month and a child up to 12 years, 30–50 mg/kg IV q. 8h (up to 6 g/d); for a child over 12 years, same as adult dosage.

Generic Name: CEFTIZOXIME
Trade Name: Cefizox
Dosage Forms: Injection (IM/IV), 1 g, 2 g vials
Adult Dosage: For urinary tract or moderate infections, 1–3 g/d IM or IV, divided q. 8–12h; for severe infections, 3–6 g/d IM or IV, divided q. 8–12h; for life-threatening infections, 9–12 g/d IV, divided q. 8h.
Pediatric Dosage: Not established.

Generic Name: CEFTRIAXONE
Trade Name: Rocephin
Dosage Forms: Injection (IM/IV), 250 mg, 500 mg, 1 g, 2 g vials
Adult Dosage (Parenteral): 1–2 g q. 24h IM or IV. For more serious infections including CNS infections, 2 g q. 24h IV. For uncomplicated gonorrhea, single 250-mg IM dose; for disseminated gonococcal infection, 1 g IV daily for 7 days.
Pediatric Dosage (Parenteral): For a child over 12 years, same as adult dosage. For a newborn or a child under 12 years (excluding CNS infections), 50–70 mg/kg/d IM or IV, divided q. 12h (maximum, 2 g/d). For CNS infections, 100 mg/kg/d IV, divided q. 12h.

Generic Name: CEFUROXIME
Trade Name: Zinacef
Dosage Forms: Injection (IM/IV), 750 mg, 1.5 g vials
Adult Dosage: For moderate infections, 750 mg IM or IV q. 8h; for serious infections, 1.5 g IV q. 6–8h (up to 9 g/d for meningitis); for gonorrhea, 1.5 g IM with 1 g oral probenecid.
Pediatric Dosage: For a child or infant over 3 months, 50–100 mg/kg/d IM or IV, divided q. 6–8h; for bacterial meningitis, 200–240 mg/kg/d IV, divided q. 6–8h.

Generic Name: CEPHALOTHIN
Trade Name: Keflin
Dosage Forms: Injection (IM/IV), 1 g, 2 g, 4 g vials
Adult Dosage: 500 mg–1 g IV q. 4–6h (up to 12 g/d).
Pediatric Dosage: For a child or infant over 1 month, 80–160 mg/kg/d IV, divided q. 8–12 h. For a newborn up to 1 week old, 40 mg/kg/d IV, divided q. 12h; 1 to 4 weeks old, 60 mg/kg/d IV, divided q. 8h. Avoid IM injections since they are extremely painful.

Generic Name: CEPHAPIRIN
Trade Name: Cefadyl
Dosage Forms: Injection (IM/IV), 500 mg, 1 g, 2 g vials
Adult Dosage: 500 mg–1 g IV q. 4–6h (up to 12 g/d).
Pediatric Dosage: For a child or infant 3 months or older, 40–80 mg/kg/d IV, divided q. 6h.

Generic Name: CEPHRADINE
Trade Name: Velosef
Dosage Forms: Injection (IM/IV), 250 mg, 500 mg, 1 g, 2 g, 4 g
Adult Dosage: 1–2 g IM or IV q. 6h (up to 8 g/d).
Pediatric Dosage: In a child or infant over 1 month, 50–100 mg/kg/d IM or IV, divided q. 6h.

Generic Name: MOXALACTAM
Trade Name: Moxam
Dosage Forms: Injection (IM/IV), 1 g, 2 g vials (Oxa-beta lactam derivative)
Adult Dosage: 500 mg–2 g IM or IV q. 8h for mild to moderate infections; 3–4 g IV q. 8h for severe infections (maximum dose, 12 g/d).
Pediatric Dosage: For a child or infant over 1 month, 50 mg/kg IM or IV q. 6–8h (up to 200 mg/kg/dose for serious infections); for a newborn 1 to 4 weeks, 50 mg/kg IM or IV q. 8h; under 1 week, 50 mg/kg IV q. 12h. (*Note:* for meningitis, loading doses of 100 mg/kg should be given.)

ORALLY ADMINISTERED CEPHALOSPORINS

Generic Name: CEFACLOR
Trade Name: Ceclor
Dosage Forms: Capsules, 250 mg, 500 mg; oral suspension, 125 mg/5 mL, 250 mg/5 mL
Adult Dosage: 250 mg–500 mg PO q. 8h (up to 4 g/d).
Pediatric Dosage: 20 mg/kg/d, divided q. 8h (up to 40 mg/kg/d or 1 g/d for severe infections). Claimed especially useful for ampicillin-resistant *Haemophilus influenzae* in treatment of otitis media.

Generic Name: CEFADROXIL
Trade Names: Duricef, Ultracef
Dosage Form: Capsules, 500 mg
Adult Dosage: 1 g PO qd to bid, depending on severity of urinary tract infection; 1 g/d single dose or divided bid for skin and soft tissue infections.
Pediatric Dosage: For a child or infant over 5 kg, 30 mg/kg/d, divided q. 12–24h.

Generic Name: CEFIXIME
Trade Name: Suprax
Dosage Forms: Tablets, 200 mg, 400 mg; oral suspension, 100 mg/5 mL
Adult Dosage (Oral): 400 mg/d as a single 400-mg tablet or as 200 mg every 12 hours. Has much greater gram-negative activity than second-generation but less than traditional third-generation cephalosporins.
Pediatric Dosage (Oral): 8 mg/kg/d as suspension in a single daily dose or as 4 mg/kg every 12 hours. Children >50 kg or >12 years should be treated as adults.

Generic Name: CEFUROXIME AXETIL
Trade Name: Ceftin
Dosage Form: Tablets, 125 mg, 250 mg, 500 mg
Adult Dosage (Oral): 250–500 mg twice daily (125–250 mg twice daily for uncomplicated UTI).
Pediatric Dosage (Oral): <12 years—125 mg twice daily. Otitis media—<2 years, 125 mg twice daily; ≥2 years, 250 mg twice daily.

Generic Name: CEPHALEXIN
Trade Name: Keflex
Dosage Forms: Capsules, 250 mg, 500 mg; oral suspension, 125 mg/5 mL, 250 mg/5 mL
Adult Dosage: 250–500 mg q. 6h (up to 4 g/d).
Pediatric Dosage: For a child or infant over 1 month, 25–50 mg/kg/d, divided q. 6h (up to 100 mg/kg/d for severe otitis media).

Generic Name: CEPHRADINE
Trade Names: Anspor, Velosef
Dosage Forms: Capsules, 250 mg, 500 mg; oral suspension, 125 mg/5 mL, 250 mg/5 mL
Adult Dosage: 250 mg q. 6h or 500 mg q. 12h PO (up to 4 g/d).
Pediatric Dosage: For a child over 9 months, 25–50 mg/kg/d, divided q. 6–12h (up to 100 mg/kg/d or 4 g/d for severe otitis media infections).

PENICILLIN AND PENICILLIN DERIVATIVE ANTIBIOTICS

Generic Name: AMOXICILLIN
Trade Names: Amoxil, Larotid, Polymox
Dosage Forms: Capsules, 250 mg, 500 mg; oral suspension, 125 mg/5 mL, 250 mg/5 mL; pediatric drops, 50 mg/mL
Uses: See ampicillin. Higher blood levels than ampicillin, owing to better oral absorption.
Adult Dosage (Oral): 250–500 mg q. 8h. For gonorrheal urethritis, 3 g with 1 g probenecid as a single dose.
Pediatric Dosage (Oral): Dependent on severity of infection. For a child weighing 20 kg or more, same as adult; for an infant weighing less than 20 kg, 20–40 mg/kg/d divided q. 8h. For an infant 6–8 kg, 50–100 mg q. 8h; for an infant less than 6 kg, 25–50 mg q. 8h.
Contraindications: Penicillin hypersensitivity.
Precautions: See ampicillin.
Adverse Reactions: See ampicillin, but may produce less diarrhea in children.
Drug Interactions: See ampicillin.

Generic Name: AMOXICILLIN with CLAVULANIC ACID
Trade Name: Augmentin '125', '250', and '500'
Dosage Forms: Tablets, 250 mg, 500 mg (amoxicillin) each with 125 mg clavulanic acid; tablets (chewable), 125 mg, 250 mg (amoxicillin) with 31.25 mg and 62.5 mg clavulanic acid, respectively; oral suspension, 125 mg, 250 mg (amoxicillin) per 5 mL with 31.25 mg and 62.5 mg clavulanic acid per 5 mL, respectively.

Uses: For treatment of lower respiratory, urinary tract, and skin infections; otitis media, and sinusitis caused by susceptible organisms. Particularly useful for infections caused by *Branhamella catarrhalis* (formerly *N. catarrhalis*), *H. influenzae*, *E. coli*, *Klebsiella*, and *Staphylococcus aureus* (including some penicillinase-producers). The synergistic bactericidal effect of clavulanic acid, a β-lactamase enzyme inhibitor, enhances amoxicillin's activity against many strains of β-lactamase-producing bacteria that are resistant to amoxicillin alone.

Adult Dosage (Oral): (based on amoxicillin) 250–500 mg q. 8h.

Pediatric Dosage (Oral): (based on amoxicillin) For a child weighing over 40 kg, same as adult dosage; for a child less than 40 kg, 20–40 mg/kg/d, divided q. 8h (depending on severity of infection).

Contraindications: Hypersensitivity to penicillin, ampicillin, or amoxicillin.

Precautions: See ampicillin. Although active in vitro against many penicillinase-producing staphylococci, it is recommended that those strains resistant to the penicillinase-resistant penicillins should also be considered resistant to amoxicillin with clavulanic acid.

Adverse Reactions: See ampicillin. Also, there seems to be a higher incidence of gastric upset, nausea, vomiting, and diarrhea than with amoxicillin alone (presumably due to the clavulanic acid content).

Drug Interactions: See ampicillin. Although the rationale is unclear, the FDA has stated that disulfiram should not be used concurrently with amoxicillin/clavulanic acid.

Generic Name: AMPICILLIN
Trade Names: Polycillin, Amcill
Dosage Forms: Capsules, 250 mg, 500 mg; injection (IM/IV), 125 mg, 250 mg, 500 mg, 1 g, 2 g; oral suspension, 125 mg/5 mL, 250 mg/5 mL

Uses: Broad-spectrum penicillin-derivative for various infections due to penicillin G-sensitive gram-positive and gram-negative cocci, *Haemophilus influenzae*, *Salmonella*, *Shigella*, *Escherichia coli*, and *Proteus* species (penicillinase-producing staphylococci are resistant). Particularly effective for otitis media and meningitis caused by susceptible *H. influenzae* and for chloramphenicol-resistant typhoid fever.

Adult Dosage (Oral): For mild to moderate infections, 250–500 mg q. 6h. For gonococcal urethritis, 3.5 g with 1 g probenecid as a single dose.

Adult Dosage (Parenteral): For mild to moderate infections, 250–500 mg IM or IV q. 6h; for severe infections, 1–2 g IV q. 4–6h (up to 14 g/d in six to eight divided doses).

Pediatric Dosage (Oral): For a child weighing 20 kg or more, same as adult dosage; for a child weighing less than 20 kg, 50–100 mg/kg/d divided q. 6–8h.

Pediatric Dosage (Parenteral): For a child over 20 kg, same as adult dosage; under 20 kg, 50–100 mg/kg/d IM or IV, divided q. 6h; for severe infections or meningitis, 150–400 mg/kg/d IV, divided q. 3–4h. For a newborn 1 to 4 weeks old, 100 mg/kg/d IM or IV, divided q. 8h; under 1 week old, 100 mg/kg/d IM or IV, divided q. 12h; for meningitis, 200 mg/kg/d IV in divided doses.

Contraindications: Penicillin hypersensitivity.

Precautions: Possible cross-allergenicity with cephalosporins (7%–10% incidence). β-hemolytic *Streptococcus* infections should be treated for at least 10 days. Not active against penicillinase-producing staphylococci. High incidence of rashes when used in patients with infectious mononucleosis or other viral infections.

Adverse Reactions: Gastric upset with oral use, diarrhea, pseudomembranous colitis, black hairy tongue. Hypersensitivity reactions, including "ampicillin rash" (erythematous, maculopapular); superinfections, blood dyscrasias. Neurotoxicity and convulsions with high doses, especially in presence of renal impairment.

Drug Interactions: Probenecid increases ampicillin serum levels. With allopurinol, increased incidence of rashes.

Generic Name: CARBENICILLIN
Trade Names: Geopen, Geocillin, Pyopen
Dosage Forms: Tablets (Geocillin), 382 mg carbenicillin base; injection (IM/IV), 1 g, 2 g, 5 g, 10 g

Uses: Broad-spectrum semisynthetic penicillin active against many gram-positive and gram-negative cocci and gram-negative enteric bacteria, including anaerobes and *Pseudomonas*. (*Klebsiella* and penicillinase-producing staphylococci are resistant.)

Adult Dosage (Oral): For urinary tract infection, 1–2 tablets qid.

Adult Dosage (Parenteral): 1–2 g q. 6h IM for mild to moderate infections; for severe infections, 300–500 mg/kg/d IV in divided doses or continuous infusion (up to 30–40 mg/d).

Pediatric Dosage (Oral): For a child, 50–60 mg/kg/d, divided q. 6h (oral use not recommended, however).

Pediatric Dosage (Parenteral): For mild to moderate infection in a child, 50–200 mg/kg/d IM or IV divided q. 4–6h; for severe infections, 300–500 mg/kg/d IM or IV divided q. 4–6h. For neonatal sepsis, 100 mg/kg IM or IV q. 12h during first week of life; thereafter, 100 mg/kg q. 8h for infants 2 kg or less and q. 6h for infants over 2 kg.

Contraindications: Penicillin hypersensitivity.

Precautions: High sodium content (4.7 mEq Na^+/g). Dosage adjustments necessary for renal or hepatic impairment. Must be well diluted for IV use to reduce incidence of thrombophlebitis. Do not crush tablets (bitter and unpalatable). Gram-negative resistance may develop; culture and sensitivity must be checked frequently.

Adverse Reactions: See penicillin G. Coagulation abnormalities, platelet dysfunction, and bleeding have occurred, especially in the presence of renal impairment. Hypokalemic metabolic alkalosis, fluid overload, anicteric hepatitis, and superinfections with *Klebsiella* or *Serratia* may occur.

Drug Interactions: Synergism with gentamicin or tobramycin may permit a decrease in the dose of carbenicillin. (They cannot be mixed together in same IV, however.) Probenecid increases serum levels of carbenicillin.

Generic Name: CLOXACILLIN
Trade Name: Tegopen
Dosage Forms: Capsules, 250 mg, 500 mg

Uses: Antistaphylococcal (penicillinase-resistant) penicillin derivative.

Adult Dosage (Oral): 250–500 mg q. 6h, before meals; may be doubled in severe infection.

Pediatric Dosage (Oral): For a child weighing 20 kg or more, same as adult dosage. For a child weighing less than 20 kg, 50–100 mg/

kg/d divided q. 6h (higher in severe infections). Not recommended for newborns.
Contraindications: Penicillin hypersensitivity.
Precautions: See methicillin. Methicillin-resistant staphylococci should be considered resistant to cloxacillin.
Adverse Reactions: See oxacillin.
Drug Interactions: See penicillin G.

Generic Name: DICLOXACILLIN
Trade Name: Dynapen, Veracillin
Dosage Forms: Capsules, 125 mg, 250 mg, 500 mg; oral suspension, 62.5 mg/5 mL
Uses: Antistaphylococcal (penicillinase-resistant) penicillin with exceptionally good oral absorption.
Adult Dosage (Oral): 250–500 mg q. 6h, before meals; may be doubled in severe infections.
Pediatric Dosage (Oral): For a child weighing 40 kg or more, same as adult dosage; for a child weighing less than 40 kg, 25–50 mg/kg/d divided q. 6h; may be doubled in severe infections. Not recommended for newborns.
Contraindications: Penicillin hypersensitivity.
Precautions: Methicillin-resistant staphylococci should be considered resistant to dicloxacillin as well. (See also oxacillin.)
Adverse Reactions: See oxacillin and penicillin G.
Drug Interactions: See oxacillin and penicillin G.

Generic Name: METHICILLIN
Trade Name: Staphcillin
Dosage Forms: Injection (IM/IV), 1 g, 4 g, 6 g
Uses: Semisynthetic penicillin for infections due to penicillinase-producing staphylococci.
Adult Dosage (Parenteral): For mild to moderate infections, 1 g q. 4–6h IM/IV. For severe infections, 2 g q. 4–6h IV.
Pediatric Dosage (Parenteral): For a child, 100–300 mg/kg/d IM or IV, divided q. 4–6h. For a newborn over 1 week old, 100–150 mg/kg/d IM or IV, divided q. 6–8h; less than 1 week old, 50–100 mg/kg/d IM or IV, divided q. 12h (up to 400 mg/kg/d for severe infections).
Contraindications: Penicillin hypersensitivity.
Precautions: See penicillin G. Methicillin is a potent inducer of penicillinase so resistance may develop among staphylococci; perform culture and sensitivity tests to ensure susceptibility. Severe renal impairment requires some dosage adjustments; also newborns have slower renal clearance of antistaphylococcal penicillins.
Adverse Reactions: See penicillin G. Also, kidney damage, interstitial nephritis, and reversible bone marrow depression with resulting blood dyscrasias may occur. IV administration can cause thrombophlebitis; IM use causes pain at injection site.
Drug Interactions: See penicillin G.

Generic Name: MEZLOCILLIN SODIUM
Trade Name: Mezlin
Dosage Forms: Injection (IM/IV), 1 g, 2 g, 3 g, 4 g
Uses: Broad-spectrum penicillin active in vitro against a variety of gram-negative and gram-positive cocci (except penicillinase-producing strains) and gram-negative bacteria, including *Klebsiella, Enterobacter, Haemophilus, Escherichia, Serratia, Proteus, Bacteroides* and other anaerobes, and *Pseudomonas*. High activity against enterococci.
Adult Dosage (Parenteral): For uncomplicated infection, 1.5–2 g IM or IV q. 6h. For severe infection, 3 g IV q. 4–6h or 4 g IV q. 6h. (Maximum recommended dosage is 350 mg/kg/d or 24 g/d.)
Pediatric Dosage (Parenteral): For a child over 1 month and under 12 years, 50 mg/kg IV q. 4h. For a newborn less than 2 kg, 75 mg/kg q. 12h for the first week of life, then q. 8h thereafter; over 2 kg, 75 mg/kg q. 12h for the first week of life, then q. 6h thereafter.
Contraindications: Hypersensitivity to penicillin.
Precautions: See penicillin G and carbenicillin. Sodium content, 1.85 mEq/g. *Pseudomonas* can develop resistance rapidly. Culture and sensitivity tests are required for serious infections.
Adverse Reactions: Hypersensitivity reactions, including rashes, urticaria, drug fever, anaphylaxis. Gastric upset with nausea, vomiting, diarrhea reported. Hypokalemia, abnormalities in renal and liver function tests, blood dyscrasias, and abnormal platelet aggregation with bleeding can occur. High doses can cause neuromuscular irritability and seizures. IV use can cause thrombophlebitis; IM injections cause pain.
Drug Interactions: See carbenicillin.

Generic Name: NAFCILLIN
Trade Names: Unipen, Nafcil
Dosage Forms: Tablets, 500 mg; capsules, 250 mg; injection (IM/IV), 500 mg, 1 g, 2 g, 4 g; oral solution, 250 mg/5 mL
Uses: Antistaphylococcal (penicillinase-resistant) penicillin. (Significant biliary concentrations achieved.)
Adult Dosage (Oral): 250 mg–1 g q. 4–6h, on an empty stomach.
Adult Dosage (Parenteral): For mild infections, 500 mg IM q. 4–6h; for moderate to severe infections, 500 mg–2 g IV q. 4–6h.
Pediatric Dosage (Oral): Take on an empty stomach. For a child or older infant, 50–100 mg/kg/d, divided q. 6h; for a newborn, 30–40 mg/kg/d, divided q. 6–8h.
Pediatric Dosage (Parenteral): For a child or older infant, 50–100 mg/kg/d IM or IV, divided q. 4–6h (up to 300 mg/kg/d for severe infections); for a newborn, 40–60 mg/kg/d IM or IV, divided q. 8–12h.
Contraindications: Penicillin hypersensitivity.
Precautions: See methicillin. Methicillin-resistant staphylococci should be considered also resistant to nafcillin. Dosage adjustments are minimal in renal impairment. Avoid extravasation of IV doses (causes severe thrombophlebitis and tissue necrosis).
Adverse Reactions: See oxacillin.
Drug Interactions: See penicillin G.

Generic Name: OXACILLIN
Trade Name: Prostaphlin
Dosage Forms: Capsules, 250 mg, 500 mg; injection IM/IV, 250 mg, 500 mg, 1 g, 2 g, 4 g; oral solution, 250 mg/5 mL
Uses: Antistaphylococcal (penicillinase-resistant) penicillin.
Adult Dosage (Oral): 500 mg to 1 g q. 4–6h, taken on an empty stomach.
Adult Dosage (Parenteral): 250–500 mg IM or IV q. 4–6h for mild to moderate infection; 1–2 g IV q. 4–6h for severe infection.
Pediatric Dosage (Oral): Take on an empty stomach. For a child 40 kg or more, 500 mg q. 4–6 h; less than 40 kg, 50 mg/kg/d, divided q. 4–6h.
Pediatric Dosage (Parenteral): For a child 40 kg or more, 250 mg to 1 g IM or IV, divided q. 4–6h (up to 8 g/d); for a child under 40 kg, 50–100 mg/kg/d IM or IV, divided q. 4–6h (up to 200 mg/

kg/d for severe infections); for a newborn, 25–100 mg/kg/d IV or IM, divided q. 12h for the first week of life, then 100–150 mg/kg/d IV or IM, divided q. 6–8h thereafter.

Contraindications: Penicillin hypersensitivity.

Precautions: See methicillin and penicillin G. Methicillin-resistant strains of staphylococci should be considered resistant to oxacillin. Possible nephrotoxicity in newborns on high doses (over 150 mg/kg/d).

Adverse Reactions: See methicillin and penicillin G. Also hepatic hypersensitivity reactions (cholestatic jaundice, elevated liver enzymes, hepatic dysfunction) may occur.

Drug Interactions: See penicillin G.

Generic Name: PENICILLIN G
Trade Names: Pentids, Penicillin G
Dosage Forms: Tablets, 125 mg (200,000 U), 250 mg (400,000 U), 500 mg (800,000 U); oral suspension, 125 mg/5 mL, 250 mg/5 mL; injection (IM/IV), 1, 5, 20 million U (potassium and sodium salts available); long-acting IM procaine PCN-G, 300,000 U/mL, 600,000 U/mL; benzathine PCN-G, 300,000 U/mL, 600,000 U/mL

Uses: Bactericidal antibiotic for penicillin G-sensitive cocci, syphilis, *Neisseria gonorrhoeae*, *Clostridium*. (Penicillinase-producing staphylococci are resistant.)

Adult Dosage (Oral): 250–500 mg q. 6h, before meals.

Adult Dosage (Parenteral): Depends on type and severity of the infection. For most coccal infections, 1 to 5 million U IV q. 4–6h; for meningitis or endocarditis, up to 30 million U/d IV in divided doses. Usual dosage of procaine PCN-G, 0.6 to 1.2 million U IM q. 12–24h; for benzathine PCN-G, 1.2 to 2.4 million U IM as a single dose.

Pediatric Dosage (Oral): For a child 12 years and older, same as adult dosage; for a child under 12 years, 25,000–100,000 U/kg/d (15–60 mg/kg/d) in 3 to 6 divided doses.

Pediatric Dosage (Parenteral): Depends on type and severity of the infection. In a child or infant, 25,000–250,000 U/kg/d IV, divided q. 4–6h (up to 400,000 U/kg/d for meningitis); in a newborn or premature infant, 50,000 to 100,000 U/kg/d IM or IV, divided q. 12h (if less than 1 week old) and q. 6–8h if over 1 week old. For group B streptococcal infection, use 100,000 to 200,000 U/kg/d; for meningitis, use at least 150,000 to 250,000 U/kg/d. For gonococcal urethritis in a child, procaine PCN-G 100,000 U/kg IM once with 25 mg/kg probenecid PO.

Contraindications: Hypersensitivity to any penicillin.

Precautions: Possible cross-allergenicity with cephalosporins (incidence, 7% to 10%). Inactivated by penicillinase; do culture and sensitivity tests for suspected staphylococcal infections. Treat β-hemolytic streptococcal infections for at least 10 days. Potassium content of potassium salt form, 1.7 mEq/million U; sodium content of sodium salt form, 1.7 mEq/million U. Avoid use of potassium salt form in newborns, premature infants, and renal impairment. High doses of both salts should be used cautiously in the elderly and those with renal or cardiac impairment. Give large IV doses of potassium salt slowly with regard for potassium content.

Adverse Reactions: Oral doses cause occasional gastric upset, diarrhea, and black tongue. IV use can cause thrombophlebitis; sterile abscesses can occur at IM injection sites. Hypersensitivity reactions include various rashes, serum sickness, anaphylaxis, and blood dyscrasias. With high IV doses of potassium salt, hyperkalemia, cardiac arrhythmias, hyperreflexia; with high IV doses of sodium salt, fluid overload, worsening of congestive heart failure. Large IV doses of penicillin, especially in renal impairment, can cause CNS toxicity with seizures. Pseudoanaphylactic reactions and cardiac arrest reported after inadvertent IV administration of procaine PCN-G. Jarisch-Herxheimer reaction can occur during syphilis therapy.

Drug Interactions: Probenecid increases serum levels of penicillins. Synergistic activity with aminoglycosides against enterococci.

Generic Name: PENICILLIN V
Trade Names: V-Cillin K, Pen-Vee K
Dosage Forms: Tablets, 125 mg, 250 mg, 500 mg; oral suspension, 125 mg/5 mL, 250 mg/5 mL
Uses: See penicillin G. Better oral absorption than penicillin G.
Adult Dosage (Oral): See penicillin G.
Pediatric Dosage (Oral): See penicillin G.
Contraindications: See penicillin G.
Precautions: See penicillin G.
Adverse Reactions: See penicillin G.

Generic Name: PIPERACILLIN
Trade Name: Pipracil
Dosage Forms: Injection (IM/IV), 2 g, 3 g, 4 g vials
Uses: Broad-spectrum semisynthetic penicillin with antimicrobial activity similar to mezlocillin.

Adult Dosage (Parenteral): For mild to moderate infections, 6–8 g/d IM or IV, divided q. 6–12h; for severe infections and serious pneumonias, 12–24 mg/d IV, divided q. 4–6h; for uncomplicated gonococcal urethritis, 2 g IM as a single dose, given 30 min after 1 g of oral probenecid.

Pediatric Dosage (Parenteral): Dosages for infants and children under 12 years old are not established. For mild to moderate infections in a child over 12 years, 6 to 8 g/d IM or IV, divided q. 6–12h; for severe infections and serious pneumonias, 12 to 24 g/d IV, divided q. 4–6h.

Contraindications: Hypersensitivity to any penicillin.
Precautions: See mezlocillin.
Adverse Reactions: See mezlocillin.
Drug Interactions: See carbenicillin.

Generic Name: TICARCILLIN
Trade Name: Ticar
Dosage Forms: Injection (IM/IV), 1 g, 3 g, 6 g
Uses: See carbenicillin.

Adult Dosage (Parenteral): For mild to moderate infections, 1 g IM q. 6h or 150 to 200 mg/kg/d IV, divided q. 4–6h; for severe infections, 200 to 300 mg/kg/d IV, divided q. 3–6h (up to 30 g/d).

Pediatric Dosage (Parenteral): In a child weighing less than 40 kg, 50 to 200 mg/kg/d IV, divided q. 4–8 hours, depending on severity of the infection; in a child weighing 40 kg or more, use adult dosage. For sepsis in a newborn under 2 kg, 100 mg/kg IV initially, then 75 mg/kg IV q. 8h for first week of life, then 100 mg/kg IV q. 4h thereafter; if over 2 kg, 100 mg/kg IV initially, then 75–100 mg/kg IV q. 4–6h thereafter.

Contraindications: Penicillin hypersensitivity.
Precautions: See carbenicillin. Sodium content, 5.2–6.5 mEq/g.
Adverse Reactions: See carbenicillin.
Drug Interactions: See carbenicillin.

SULFONAMIDES

Generic Name: SULFAMETHOXAZOLE/TRIMETHOPRIM (SMZ/TMP)

Trade Names: Bactrim, Septra

Dosage Forms: Tablets, 400 mg SMZ/80 mg TMP (single strength), 800 mg SMZ/160 mg TMP (double strength); injection (IV), 400 mg SMZ/80 mg TMP per 5-mL ampules; oral suspension, 200 mg SMZ/40 mg TMP per 5 mL

Uses: Treatment of acute and chronic urinary tract infection, shigellosis, *Pneumocystis carinii* pneumonia, and diarrhea caused by enteropathogenic *Escherichia coli*.

Adult Dosage (Oral): For urinary tract infections, 1 double strength tablet q. 12h for 10–14 days. For shigellosis, same for 5 days; for *P. carinii* pneumonia, 15–20 mg/kg/d (TMP concentration) in divided doses q. 6h for 14 days.

Adult Dosage (Parenteral): Doses are based on TMP concentration. For urinary tract infection, 8–10 mg/kg/d IV divided q. 6h for 10–14 days; for shigellosis, same for 5 days; for *P. carinii* pneumonia, same as oral dosage but given slowly IV over 60–90 min. (Each 5-mL ampule should be diluted in at least 125 mL D_5W.)

Pediatric Dosage (Oral): For above indications in a child or infant over 2 months old, use adult dosages.

Pediatric Dosage (Parenteral): For above indications in a child or infant over 2 months old, use adult dosages.

Contraindications: See sulfisoxazole.

Precautions: See sulfisoxazole.

Adverse Reactions: See sulfisoxazole.

Drug Interactions: See sulfisoxazole.

Generic Name: SULFISOXAZOLE

Trade Name: Gantrisin

Dosage Forms: Tablets, 500 mg; injection (IV), 400 mg/5 mL ampule; oral suspension, 500 mg/5 mL; topical preparations

Uses: Bacteriostatic antibiotic used primarily for acute and chronic urinary tract infections due to susceptible gram-negative urinary pathogens; also used for acute otitis media caused by susceptible strains of *Haemophilus influenzae* and *Streptococcus pneumoniae*. Occasionally given for meningitis caused by susceptible strains of *H. influenzae* or meningococci.

Adult Dosage (Oral): 2–4 g initially, then 4–8 g/d in divided doses q. 4–6h.

Adult Dosage (Parenteral): For meningitis, 50 mg/kg IV initially, then 100 mg/kg/d in divided doses q. 6h in a well-diluted slow IV infusion over 60–90 min.

Pediatric Dosage (Oral): For a child over 2 months, 75 mg/kg initially, then 150 mg/kg/d divided q. 6h (maximum, 6 g/d). Not recommended for newborns.

Pediatric Dosage (Parenteral): For a child over 2 months, same as adult IV dosage.

Contraindications: Hypersensitivity to sulfonamides, pregnancy/lactation, severe renal or hepatic impairment, infants under 2 months old.

Precautions: Maintain adequate fluid intake and urine output; alkalinize urine if it is highly acidic or output is low. Dilute IV doses well; administer slowly and avoid extravasation. Dosage adjustments necessary in significant renal impairment. Give folic acid supplements if megaloblastic anemia develops. Use cautiously in patients with severe allergies or bronchial asthma because of higher sensitivity risk. Use cautiously in renal or hepatic impairment, urinary tract obstruction, glucose-6-phosphate dehydrogenase deficiency, or porphyria. Topical preparations can be sensitizing. Do not use sulfonamides for β-hemolytic streptococcal infections. Possible cross-allergenicity with thiazide diuretics, furosemide, and sulfonylureas.

Adverse Reactions: Gastrointestinal disturbances, stomatitis, folic acid depletion, renal or hepatic damage, hepatitis, kernicterus in newborns, and blood dyscrasias. Can precipitate hemolytic anemia in G6PD-deficient patients and exacerbate porphyria. Hypersensitivity reactions include rashes, photosensitivity, drug fever, lupus-like syndrome, and Stevens-Johnson syndrome. CNS toxicity includes lethargy, headache, peripheral neuropathy, and mental derangements.

Drug Interactions: Can displace many drugs, such as oral anticoagulants, sulfonylureas, and phenytoin from their protein-binding sites to potentiate their activity.

TETRACYCLINES

Generic Name: DOXYCYCLINE

Trade Names: Vibramycin, Vibratabs

Dosage Forms: Tablets, 100 mg; capsules, 100 mg; injection (IV only), 100 mg, 200 mg; oral suspension, 25 mg/5 mL

Uses: See tetracycline. Also used for prevention of traveler's diarrhea caused by enterotoxigenic *Escherichia coli*; effectiveness against anaerobes makes it useful for pelvic inflammatory disease and chlamydial infections.

Adult Dosage (Oral): 100 mg q. 12h for 24 hours, then 100 mg/d (up to 100 mg q. 12h for severe infections); for syphilis, 300 mg/d for 10 days; for gonorrhea, 300 mg stat, then 100 mg bid for 3 days. For prevention of traveler's diarrhea, 200 mg on first day of travel, followed by 100 mg/d for 3 weeks.

Adult Dosage (Parenteral): 200 mg IV initially, then 100–200 mg/d divided q. 12–24h. IV doses should be well diluted in at least 100 mL diluent.

Pediatric Dosage (Oral): For a child over 8 years, 4.4 mg/kg in two divided doses to start, then 2.2 mg/kg/d in single or divided doses; may be increased to 4.4 mg/kg in severe infections.

Pediatric Dosage (Parenteral): In a child over 8 years, 4.4 mg/kg IV in one or two divided doses to start, then 2.2–4.4 mg/kg/d in one or two divided infusions, depending on severity of infection.

Contraindications: Severe hepatic impairment, hypersensitivity to tetracycline, children under 8 years old.

Precautions: For patients with slower renal clearance, give dose q. 24h only. Drug should not be given IM since it causes severe tissue necrosis. See also tetracycline.

Adverse Reactions: See tetracycline. However, not significantly antianabolic as is tetracycline and may not further increase azotemia in renal failure.

Drug Interactions: See tetracycline. Phenytoin can increase doxycycline metabolism.

Generic Name: TETRACYCLINE
Trade Names: Achromycin, Sumycin
Dosage Forms: Capsules, 250 mg, 500 mg; injection (IM), 100 mg, 250 mg (contains 2% procaine); injection (IV), 250 mg, 500 mg; oral syrup, 125 mg/5 mL; topical preparations
Uses: Broad-spectrum antibiotic; useful in penicillin-sensitive patients for infection due to susceptible gram-positive and gram-negative cocci and bacilli, *Rickettsia, Chlamydia*; syphilis, intestinal amebiasis, gonorrhea. Frequently given for treatment and prophylaxis of acne and for acute or chronic bronchitis caused by sensitive *Haemophilus influenzae, Streptococcus pneumoniae,* or *Klebsiella.*
Adult Dosage (Oral): 250–500 mg q. 6–12h on an empty stomach.
Adult Dosage (Parenteral): 250 mg/d IM single or divided doses; 250–500 mg IV q. 6–12h, depending on infection severity (IV solutions for infusion should be well diluted in at least 100 mL of diluent).
Pediatric Dosage (Oral): For a child over 8 years, 25–50 mg/kg/d divided q. 6–12h.
Pediatric Dosage (Parenteral): For a child over 8 years, 10–20 mg/kg/d IV divided q. 6–12h; IM administration not recommended.
Contraindications: Hypersensitivity to any tetracycline, pregnancy, lactation, children under 8 years old.
Precautions: IM injections contain 2% procaine. Use cautiously in renal or hepatic impairment (dosage adjustments necessary). Avoid use during period of bone and tooth development (eg, from birth to 8 years). Do not use outdated tetracyclines (can cause Fanconi's syndrome). Caution patients to avoid prolonged exposure to sunlight when taking tetracyclines. "Antianabolic" effect can cause azotemia, acidosis, and negative nitrogen balance.
Adverse Reactions: Gastric upset, glossitis, black tongue, blood dyscrasias, hyperpigmentation, enterocolitis, photosensitivity, hypersensitivity reactions, candidal superinfections, increased intracranial pressure, pseudotumor cerebri, bulging fontanelles, mottling and discoloration of fetal and children's teeth. Renal impairment may lead to azotemia, nephrotoxicity, hepatotoxicity. Large IV doses can cause fatty infiltration of liver, pancreatic damage, and nephrotoxicity. IV administration causes pain and thrombophlebitis; rapid IV rates can produce nausea, vomiting, fever, chills, and hypotension.
Drug Interactions: Multivalent cations (Fe^{3+}, Mg^{2+}, Ca^{2+}) in food and antacids decrease oral absorption of tetracyclines.

MISCELLANEOUS ANTI-INFECTIVES

Generic Name: ACYCLOVIR
Trade Name: Zovirax
Dosage Forms: Injection (IV), 500 mg; ointment, 5%
Uses: Antiviral agent used topically for initial episodes of genital herpes and mild mucocutaneous herpes simplex infections; given parenterally for initial and recurrent herpes simplex infections in immunocompromised patients and for severe, initial genital herpes infections in nonimmunocompromised patients. Has also been effective in the treatment of disseminated herpes simplex (HSV-1, HSV-2) and herpes zoster (varicella-zoster virus [VZV]) infections.
Adult Dosage (Parenteral): For mucocutaneous herpes simplex infections, 5 mg/kg IV q. 8h for 7 days; for herpes genitalis, same dosage for 5 days. Investigationally, for disseminated VZV infections, 5–15 mg/kg IV q. 8h for 5 to 10 days.
Adult Dosage (Topical): Apply ointment to lesions q. 3h six times a day for 7 days. Use finger cot or rubber glove for application.
Pediatric Dosage (Parenteral): Same as adult dosage.
Pediatric Dosage (Topical): Same as adult dosage.
Contraindications: Hypersensitivity to acyclovir.
Precautions: To minimize thrombophlebitis and vein irritation, dilute IV doses well (concentration should be less than 10 mg/mL); infuse doses slowly over at least 1 hour. Do not refrigerate mixed solutions since they may precipitate. Keep patient well hydrated and maintain a good urine output. Monitor renal function during therapy. Renal impairment requires dosage adjustments. For best clinical results, initiate therapy with acyclovir as soon as possible. Use cautiously in those with diminished renal function, dehydration, or underlying neurologic disease. Widespread repeated use of the ointment has produced viral resistance to acyclovir.
Adverse Reactions: Rapid IV infusion rates (less than 10 min) can cause crystalluria, rises in blood urea nitrogen and serum creatinine, renal tubular damage, and acute renal failure. With IV use, thrombophlebitis and inflammation of injection site, nausea, sweating, headache, hypotension, hematuria, tremors, mental derangements, seizures, coma. With topical use, pruritus, rash, burning and stinging at site of application.
Drug Interactions: Probenecid can decrease renal excretion of acyclovir.

Generic Name: AMPHOTERICIN B
Trade Name: Fungizone
Dosage Forms: Injection, 50 mg (IV); topical preparations
Uses: Antifungal agent for IV or intrathecal use for various disseminated fungal infections, including candidiasis and coccidioidomycosis.
Adult Dosage (Parenteral): 250 µg/kg/d initially as a single dose, slow IV infusion. May be increased by increments of 250 µg/kg/d up to total dose of 1.0 mg/kg/d (usual dose, 50 mg/d). For bladder irrigation, 15–50 mg/d (using up to 5 mg/10 mL concentration in sterile water). For intrathecal use, 300 µg/d or 500 µg two or three times weekly.
Pediatric Dosage (Parenteral): Same adult dosage in milligrams per kilogram.
Contraindications: Hypersensitivity to amphotericin B (unless infection is life threatening).
Precautions: Impaired renal function, pregnancy (safe use not established). Should be diluted in D_5W only, not NS or electrolyte solutions. Recommended IV concentration, no more than 1 mg/10 mL. Solutions are light sensitive; cover container with foil. Dose should be infused over 2–6 hours. Use cautiously in hepatic impairment.
Adverse Reactions: Fever, chills, nausea, headache, vomiting, malaise, injection site pain, and thrombophlebitis are very common during infusing period. Cardiovascular collapse and arrhythmias are possible with rapid IV infusion. Renal tubular acidosis with hypokalemia and hypomagnesemia may occur in

renal impairment (usually reversible). Intrathecal administration may cause peripheral neuritis, convulsions, and chemical meningitis. Blood dyscrasias, muscle or joint pain, peripheral neuropathy, CNS toxicity, and hypersensitivity reactions may also occur.

Drug Interactions: Additive renal toxicity with other nephrotoxic antibiotics; additive hypokalemia with corticosteroids and diuretics.

Generic Name: CHLORAMPHENICOL
Trade Name: Chloromycetin
Dosage Forms: Capsules, 250 mg; injection (IV), 1 g; oral suspension, 150 mg/5 mL
Uses: Broad-spectrum, bacteriostatic antibiotic active against many gram-positive and gram-negative cocci and bacilli, *Chlamydia*, *Rickettsia*, and *Mycoplasma*. Particularly effective for acute typhoid fever, serious *Salmonella* and *Bacteroides* infections, and meningitis caused by *Haemophilus influenzae* (including ampicillin-resistant strains) or *Neisseria meningitidis*. Useful topically for ocular infections.
Adult Dosage (Oral): 50–100 mg/kg/d divided q. 6h to start, decreased to 50 mg/kg/d divided q. 6h as soon as possible.
Adult Dosage (Parenteral): 50 mg/kg/d IV divided q. 6h (average dose, 1 g IV q. 6h).
Pediatric Dosage (Oral): For a child, use adult dosage; for an infant over 2 weeks of age, 25–50 mg/kg/d, divided q. 6–12h; for a newborn less than 2 weeks of age, 25 mg/kg once daily.
Pediatric Dosage (Parenteral): For a child, same as adult dosage (up to 100 mg/kg/d for meningitis); for an infant over 2 weeks of age, 25–50 mg/kg/d IV divided q. 6–12h; for a newborn less than 2 weeks of age, 25 mg/kg IM once daily.
Contraindications: Hypersensitivity to chloramphenicol. Should not be used prophylactically.
Precautions: Should not be given IM because absorption is erratic. Avoid its use during pregnancy and lactation. Hepatic impairment requires dosage adjustments. Use cautiously in premature and newborn infants and in those patients with renal or hepatic impairment. Avoid concurrent therapy with other drugs that can depress bone marrow. Blood studies are recommended initially and every 2 to 3 weeks during therapy. Monitor and maintain serum levels at 10–20 µg/mL.
Adverse Reactions: Blood dyscrasias, bone marrow depression (reversible and irreversible), aplastic anemia (rare), hemolytic anemia in glucose-6-phosphate dehydrogenase deficiency, hypersensitivity, and febrile reactions. Also gastric upset, diarrhea, enterocolitis, stomatitis, and fungal superinfections. CNS neurotoxicity includes headache, delirium, optic neuritis, and peripheral neuropathy. Can cause "gray baby" syndrome (cardiovascular collapse) in newborn and premature infants.
Drug Interactions: With alcohol, disulfiram-like reaction. Increased anticoagulant effect with warfarin and dicumarol. Increased hypoglycemia with sulfonylureas. Chloramphenicol increases toxicity of phenytoin.

Generic Name: CIPROFLOXACIN
Trade Name: Cipro
Dosage Forms: Tablets, 250 mg, 500 mg, 750 mg; injection, 200 mg, 400 mg vials
Uses: Fluroquinolone antibiotic that acts by inhibiting DNA gyrase, which is needed for the synthesis of DNA. Spectrum of activity includes staphylococci (plus MRSA) and most gram-negative aerobes (*Pseudomonas aeruginosa* but not other *Pseudomonas* species); moderate activity against streptococci; inactive against anaerobes. Has been proven effective in the management of complicated urinary tract infections (active against most uropathogens); gastrointestinal infections (*E. coli*, *Salmonella*, *Shigella*, *Yersinia*, *Vibrios*, *Campylobacter* but not *Clostridium difficile*); osteomyelitis (staphylococcal and gram-negative organisms); skin and soft-tissue infections, as well as medical prophylaxis.
Adult Dosage (Oral): UTI—250 to 500 mg every 12 hours; respiratory tract/bone and joint/skin and soft tissue—500 to 750 mg every 12 hours; infectious diarrhea—500 mg every 12 hours. Although duration of therapy depends on the severity of the infection, the usual duration of therapy is 7–14 days; however, bone and joint infection may require therapy for up to 6 weeks or longer. Renal impairment—creatinine clearance (Clcr) >50 mL/min/1.73 m^2, no change; Clcr 30–50 mL/min/1.73 m^2, 250–500 mg every 12 hours; Clcr 5–29 mL/min/1.73 m^2, 250–500 mg every 18 hours; hemodialysis or peritoneal dialysis, 250–500 mg every 24 hours after dialysis.
Adult Dosage (Parenteral): Must be diluted with a suitable IV solution (0.9% sodium chloride or 5% dextrose injection) to a concentration of 1 to 2 mg/mL. Should be administered slowly (over 60 minutes) to minimize venous irritation. UTI—200 to 400 mg IV every 12 hours; respiratory tract/bone and joint/skin and soft tissue—400 mg IV every 12 hours. Renal impairment—Clcr $\geq$30 mL/min/1.73 m^2, usual dose; Clcr 5–29 mL/min/1.73 m^2, 200–400 mg every 18–24 hours; hemodialysis or peritoneal dialysis, 200–400 mg every 24 hours (after dialysis).
Pediatric Dosage (Oral): Not recommended for use in this population.
Contraindications: History of hypersensitivity to ciprofloxacin or the quinolone group of antibiotic agents.
Precautions: Should not be used in children <18 years of age since ciprofloxacin has been shown to cause arthropathy and osteochondrosis in immature animal models. Pregnancy category C—should not be used in pregnant or lactating women. Use with caution in patients with known or suspected CNS disorders (eg, epilepsy). Since rare cases of crystalluria have been reported, patients should be well hydrated whenever possible, urinary alkalinity avoided, and recommended daily dose not exceeded.
Adverse Reactions: Generally well tolerated. Most common adverse effects include GI—nausea, vomiting, abdominal pain, diarrhea; CNS—headache, dizziness, restlessness; and DERM—rash. Other more serious adverse effects (reported in less than 1% of the population studied) include seizures, elevated liver function tests, psychotic reactions, severe hypersensitivity reactions, palpitations, syncope, angina, ventricular ectopy, Stevens-Johnson syndrome, interstitial nephritis, crystalluria, renal failure, pulmonary embolism, agranulocytosis, and cholestatic jaundice.
Drug Interactions: With probenecid, results in a 50% reduction in the renal clearance of ciprofloxacin. With aluminum/magnesium-containing antacids, iron salts, sucralfate, results in decreased bioavailability of ciprofloxacin if administered concurrently. With theophylline, results in an increase in serum theophylline levels and possibly increased seizures.

Generic Name: CLINDAMYCIN
Trade Name: Cleocin
Dosage Forms: Capsules, 75 mg, 150 mg (HCl salt); injection (IM/IV), 300 mg, 600 mg; oral suspension, 75 mg/5 mL
Uses: Alternate antibiotic for penicillin-allergic patients for treatment of staphylococcal infections. Also used for anaerobic infections (outside CNS), particularly those due to *Bacteroides*.
Adult Dosage (Oral): 150–450 mg q. 6h.
Adult Dosage (Parenteral): 600–2700 mg/d IM or IV divided q. 6, 8, or 12h (usual dose, 300–600 mg IV q. 6h). Maximum dose, 4800 mg/d (IV infusion rate not to exceed 30 mg/min).
Pediatric Dosage (Oral): (Based on HCl salt.) For a child or infant over 1 month, 10–25 mg/kg/d, divided q. 6–8h. (Minimum dose is 37.5 mg q. 8h regardless of body weight.)
Pediatric Dosage (Parenteral): For moderately severe infection in a child or infant over 1 month, 10–25 mg/kg/d IM or IV, divided q. 6–8h; for severe infections, 25–40 mg/kg/d IV, divided q. 6h (not less than 300 mg q. 6h).
Contraindications: Hypersensitivity to lincomycin and clindamycin, meningitis (no cerebrospinal fluid diffusion).
Precautions: Avoid use in newborns under 1 month of age. Give oral doses with full glasses of water. Administer IV slowly (30 mg/min or less). Discontinue if significant or persistent diarrhea develops; do differential diagnosis for pseudomembranous colitis. Use cautiously in bronchial asthma (capsules), elderly patients, those with gastrointestinal disease (particularly colitis), severe renal or hepatic impairment, pregnancy, or lactation. Possible cross-resistance with lincomycin and erythromycin.
Adverse Reactions: Gastric upset and esophageal irritation after oral administration, including nausea, vomiting, cramps, diarrhea, severe pseudomembranous colitis (rare with parenteral use and usually reversible on oral drug discontinuation). Also candidal superinfections, hypersensitivity reactions, rashes, jaundice, and blood dyscrasias. Rapid IV administration can cause syncope, hypotension, apnea, thrombophlebitis, pain, and redness at injection site; IM doses can cause sterile abscesses.
Drug Interactions: General anesthetics, neuromuscular blocking agents may cause neuromuscular blockade and respiratory depression. Chloramphenicol and erythromycin antagonize antibacterial effect.

Generic Name: ERYTHROMYCIN
Trade Names: E.E.S., Ilosone, E-Mycin
Dosage Forms: Tablets, 125 mg, 200 mg, 250 mg, 400 mg, 500 mg; capsules, 125 mg, 200 mg, 250 mg, 400 mg, 500 mg; injection (IV only), 500 mg, 1 g; topical preparations; oral suspension, 125 mg/5 mL, 200 mg/5 mL, 250 mg/5 mL, 400 mg/5 mL
Uses: Alternative antibiotic for gram-positive coccal infections in patients allergic to penicillin; effective against penicillin-resistant staphylococci, *Haemophilus influenzae*, *Bordetella pertussis*, *Mycoplasma*, and *Legionella pneumophila*. Also for prophylaxis of rheumatic fever.
Adult Dosage (Oral): 250–500 mg q. 6h before meals (up to 4 g/d).
Adult Dosage (Parenteral): 15–50 mg/kg/d IV divided (usual dose, 500 mg q. 6–8h). Maximum dosage, 4 g/d.
Pediatric Dosage (Oral): For a child or infant over 1 month, 30–50 mg/kg/d divided q. 6h; may be doubled in severe infection.
Pediatric Dosage (Parenteral): For a child or infant over 1 month, same as adult dosage in milligrams per kilogram and dosage interval.
Contraindications: Hypersensitivity to erythromycin; hepatic impairment (estolate form only).
Precautions: IV doses should be well diluted to at least 10 mg/mL; administer slowly over 30–60 min. Use cautiously during pregnancy. Hepatic impairment requires dosage adjustments. Do not give IM.
Adverse Reactions: Gastric upset, cramping, hypersensitivity reactions with rash and urticaria, cholestatic jaundice (estolate form). Thrombophlebitis and pain frequent with IV use. Rare ototoxicity with IV doses greater than 4 g/d.
Drug Interactions: Erythromycin can cause elevated theophylline serum levels and toxicity. With terfenadine, may result in life-threatening arrhythmias.

Generic Name: FLUCONAZOLE
Trade Name: DiFlucan
Dosage Forms: Injection, 200 mg/100 mL, 400 mg/100 mL; tablet, 50 mg, 100 mg, 200 mg
Uses: Synthetic broad-spectrum bis-triazole antifungal agent that selectively inhibits fungal cytochrome P_{450} and sterol C_{14} α-demethylation. Indicated for the treatment of oropharyngeal candidiasis, esophageal candidiasis, and cryptococcal meningitis.
Adult Dosage (Oral): Oropharyngeal candidiasis—200 mg on the first day, followed by 100 mg once daily for at least 2 weeks. Esophageal candidiasis—200 mg on the first day, followed by 100–400 mg daily (based on response) for a minimum of 3 weeks and at least 2 weeks following resolution of symptoms. Systemic candidiasis—400 mg on the first day, followed by 200 mg daily for a minimum of 4 weeks and at least 2 weeks following resolution of symptoms. Cryptococcal meningitis—400 mg on the first day, followed by 200–400 mg daily (based on response) for at least 10–12 weeks after CSF becomes culture negative. The dosage for suppression of relapse of cryptococcal meningitis in patients with AIDS is 200 mg daily. Renal impairment—give initial load (50–400 mg) and then base daily maintenance dose on creatinine clearance (Clcr): Clcr >50 mL/min/1.73 m^2, give 100% of normal dose; Clcr 21–50 mL/min/1.73 m^2, give 50% of normal dose; Clcr 11–20 mL/min/1.73 m^2, give 25% of normal dose; dialysis, give 100% of normal dose after each dialysis period.
Adult Dosage (Parenteral): Since oral absorption of fluconazole is rapid and complete, the daily dose of fluconazole is identical for oral and IV administration.
Pediatric Dosage (Oral and Parenteral): Efficacy has not been established; however, a small number of children (age 3–13 years) have been treated safely with fluconazole using doses of 3–6 mg/kg daily.
Contraindications: Hypersensitivity to fluconazole.
Precautions: Fluconazole should be used with caution in patients hypersensitive to other azole antifungal agents. Since serious hepatic reactions have been reported following the use of fluconazole, liver function tests should be monitored throughout therapy. Dosage adjustment should be made in renal impairment (see adult dosage).
Adverse Reactions: GI—nausea, headache, vomiting, abdominal pain, diarrhea; other—skin rash, hepatic necrosis (rare), and Stevens-Johnson syndrome (rare).

Drug Interactions: With cyclosporin, results in an increase in cyclosporin AUC. With rifampin, results in a decrease in fluconazole half-life and AUC. With warfarin, theophylline, sulfonylureas, and phenytoin, results in increased serum levels of these agents. The inhibitory effects of ciprofloxacin on cytochrome P_{450} are additive to those produced by cimetidine.

Generic Name: IMIPENEM-CILASTATIN
Trade Name: Primaxin
Dosage Forms: Injection, 250, 500 mg vials (IV); 500, 750 mg vials (IM)
Uses: Combination of a thienamycin antibiotic (which inhibits cell wall synthesis) and cilastatin, which inhibits renal dipeptidase (dehydropeptidase-1), thereby preventing the metabolism and decreasing possible renal toxicity of imipenem. Very broad spectrum of activity including most gram-positive and gram-negative aerobes and anaerobes. Usually reserved for serious infections caused by resistant pathogens or mixed aerobic/anaerobic organisms that are susceptible to the drug, including *Staphylococcus* (no MRSA), *Streptococcus*, *E. coli*, *Klebsiella*, *Proteus*, *Enterobacter*, *P. aeruginosa*, and *Bacteroides*.
Adult Dosage (Parenteral): IV—mild infection (fully susceptible), 250 mg q. 6h, (moderately susceptible) 500 mg q. 6h; moderate infection (fully susceptible), 500 mg q. 8h to q. 6h, (moderately susceptible) 500 mg q. 6h to 1 g q. 8h; severe life-threatening infection (fully susceptible), 500 mg q. 6h, (moderately susceptible) 1 g q. 8h to 1 g q. 6h; uncomplicated UTI (fully susceptible), 250 mg q. 6h (moderately susceptible) 250 mg q. 6h; complicated UTI (fully/moderately susceptible), 500 mg q. 6h. Each 250- or 500-mg dose should be infused over 20 to 30 minutes (dosages > 4 g/d are not recommended). IM—lower respiratory/skin and skin structures/gynecologic infections of mild to moderate severity, 500 to 750 mg q. 12h depending on severity; intra-abdominal infection of mild to moderate severity, 750 mg q. 12h (total dosages >1500 mg not recommended). Renal impairment—creatinine clearance (Clcr) > 70 mL/min/1.73 m², no adjustment; 31–70 mL/min/1.73 m² (fully susceptible) 500 mg q. 8h, (moderately susceptible) 500 mg q. 6h; 21–30 mL/min/1.73 m² (fully susceptible) 500 mg q. 12h, (moderately susceptible) 500 mg q. 8h; 6–20 mL/min/1.73 m² (fully susceptible) 250 mg q. 12h, (moderately susceptible) 500 mg q. 12h; 0–5 mL/min/1.73 m² with dialysis (fully susceptible) 250 mg q. 12h, (moderately susceptible) 500 mg q. 12h (dosages should be given after hemodialysis and at 12-hour intervals timed from the end of the dialysis session—do not exceed 2 g/d).
Pediatric Dosage (Parenteral): Neonates—not established. <3 years—100 mg of imipenem per kg per 24 hours divided every 6 hours. >3 years—60 mg of imipenem per kg per 24 hours divided every 6 hours.
Contraindications: Hypersensitivity to any component; IM—hypersensitivity to local anesthetics of the amide type and in patients with severe shock or heart block due to the use of lidocaine HCl as a diluent.
Precautions: Severe CNS adverse experiences (eg, myoclonic activity, confused states, seizures) have been seen primarily in patients with certain risk factors including a history of seizure disorder, renal insufficiency, advanced age, and dosages exceeding recommended daily dosages. Renal function should be monitored throughout therapy. Increased hyperventilation, shakiness, nausea, and vomiting are associated with a rapid infusion.
Adverse Reactions: Similar to other β-lactams (see mezlocillin in the penicillin section); common complaints include nausea, vomiting, thrombophlebitis, rash, and hypotension. Seizures possible, especially in patients with renal dysfunction.
Drug Interactions: With ganciclovir, results in increased generalized seizures.

Generic Name: KETOCONAZOLE
Trade Name: Nizoral
Dosage Form: Tablets, 200 mg
Uses: Broad-spectrum antifungal agent for treatment of mucocutaneous candidiasis, coccidioidomycosis, histoplasmosis, and a variety of resistant dermatophytes. Duration of therapy varies; up to 12 months required for severe infections. (Cannot be used for fungal meningitis because penetration into CSF is poor.)
Adult Dosage (Oral): 200 mg as a single daily dose, initially. Dose may be increased to 400 mg once daily for more severe infections.
Pediatric Dosage (Oral): For a child over 2 years weighing 20 kg or less, 50 mg once daily; for a child 20 to 40 kg, 100 mg once daily; for a child weighing over 40 kg, 200 mg once daily.
Contraindications: Hypersensitivity to ketoconazole.
Precautions: Use should be avoided in nursing mothers. Use cautiously in hepatic impairment. Teratogenic in rodents. Patients with achlorhydria should take tablets with meals or dissolve them in 4 mL 0.1–0.2N HCl and take through a straw to protect tooth enamel.
Adverse Reactions: Most frequently, nausea, vomiting, abdominal pain, and pruritus. Also reported are headache, dizziness, somnolence, fever, chills, photophobia, diarrhea, transient increases in liver enzymes, and idiosyncratic hepatotoxicity.
Drug Interactions: Concomitant administration of antacids, anticholinergics, and H_2-blockers reduce absorption of ketoconazole. (These medications may be given at least 2 hours after ketoconazole.) With terfenadine, may result in life-threatening arrhythmias.

Generic Name: MEBENDAZOLE
Trade Name: Vermox
Dosage Form: Tablets, 100 mg (chewable)
Uses: Anthelminthic for treatment of enterobiasis (pinworm infection), ascariasis (round worm infection), trichuriasis (whipworm infection), and hookworm infections caused by *Necator americanus* and *Ancylostoma duodenale*.
Adult Dosage (Oral): For pinworms, single 100 mg dose that can be repeated in 3 weeks if necessary; for other helminthic infections, 100 mg bid for 3 days; can repeat course in 3 weeks if necessary. Tablets can be swallowed whole, chewed, or crushed and mixed with food.
Pediatric Dosage (Oral): For a child over 2 years old, same as adult dosage.
Contraindications: Hypersensitivity to mebendazole; pregnancy.
Precautions: Cure rates may be lower in patients with massive infections or increased gastrointestinal motility. Stress hygienic precautions to aid in preventing reinfection.
Adverse Reactions: Virtually nontoxic because of poor systemic absorption. Occasional transient diarrhea or abdominal pain in cases of massive infections and expulsion of worms.

Generic Name: METHENAMINE MANDELATE
Trade Name: Mandelamine
Dosage Forms: Tablets, 250 mg, 500 mg, 1 g; granules, 500 mg, 1 g packets; oral suspension, 250 mg/5 mL and 500 mg/mL (Forte)
Uses: For urinary tract infections caused by a variety of gram-positive and gram-negative urinary pathogens.
Adult Dosage (Oral): 1 g q. 6h.
Pediatric Dosage (Oral): Initially, 100 mg/kg/d divided q. 6–8h, then 50 mg/kg/d divided q. 6–8h (maximum, 3 g/d).
Contraindications: Renal insufficiency, conditions in which urine acidification is contraindicated or unattainable.
Precautions: Urinary pH should be maintained at 5.5 or less for maximum antibacterial effect. Do not give concurrently with sulfonamides since sulfa drugs can precipitate in renal tubules in the presence of an acidic urine.
Adverse Reactions: Dysuria with bladder irritation and painful urination caused by methenamine's byproduct, formaldehyde. Also gastric upset, abdominal cramps, occasional rashes, albuminuria, and hematuria.
Drug Interactions: Urinary alkalinizing agents, antacids, carbonic anhydrase inhibitors (eg, acetazolamide), and thiazide diuretics can all alkalinize the urine and decrease methenamine's antibacterial effect.

Generic Name: METRONIDAZOLE (IV)
Trade Name: Flagyl IV RTU
Dosage Form: Injection (IV only), 500 mg/100 mL
Uses: Parenterally for serious infections caused by susceptible anaerobic bacteria, including *Bacteroides* and *Clostridia* species. All aerobic organisms should be considered resistant.
Adult Dosage (Parenteral): Initially, 15 mg/kg over 1 hour by IV infusion, then 7.5 mg/kg q. 6h over 1 hour IV (maximum, 4 g/d). May be changed to oral therapy when conditions warrant (ie, 7.5 mg/kg PO q. 6h).
Pediatric Dosage (Parenteral): Not recommended.
Contraindications: Hypersensitivity to metronidazole or other nitroimidazole derivatives. Should be avoided in pregnancy, especially in the first trimester.
Precautions: Use cautiously in hepatic disease (drug accumulation), pregnancy, lactation, patients with active CNS disease or those prone to blood dyscrasias. Carcinogenic in rodents. Avoid ingestion of alcohol during therapy.
Adverse Reactions: Gastric upset, unpleasant metallic taste, *Candida* superinfections, hypersensitivity reactions, darkened urine, cystitis, leukopenia, thrombophlebitis (IV use only). CNS toxicity includes peripheral neuropathy, seizures, ataxia, vertigo, and syncope.
Drug Interactions: Potentiates warfarin. Alcohol causes disulfiram-like reaction.

Generic Name: METRONIDAZOLE (Oral)
Trade Name: Flagyl
Dosage Form: Tablets, 250 mg
Uses: Trichomonacide also used in treatment of enteritis due to *Giardia lamblia* or intestinal amebiasis.
Adult Dosage (Oral): For trichomoniasis, 2 g single dose, or 250 mg tid for 7 days. For *Giardia lamblia* enteritis, 250 mg tid for 10 days. For intestinal amebiasis, 750 mg tid for 5–10 days.
Pediatric Dosage (Oral): For *Giardia lamblia* enteritis in a child, 15 mg/kg/d divided tid for 10 days. For intestinal amebiasis, 30–50 mg/kg/d divided tid for 10 days.
Contraindications: See metronidazole (IV).
Precautions: See metronidazole (IV).
Adverse Reactions: See metronidazole (IV).
Drug Interactions: Potentiates warfarin. Alcohol causes disulfiram-like reaction.

Generic Name: NITROFURANTOIN
Trade Name: Macrodantin
Dosage Forms: Capsules, 25 mg, 50 mg, 100 mg; oral suspension, 25 mg/5 mL
Uses: Urinary tract infections except those caused by *Pseudomonas* or *Proteus* species.
Adult Dosage (Oral): 50–100 mg qid with food or milk.
Pediatric Dosage (Oral): For a child or infant over 1 month, 5–7 mg/kg/d divided qid with food or milk.
Contraindications: Significant renal impairment, pregnancy at term, infants under 1 month, hypersensitivity to nitrofurantoins.
Precautions: Avoid prolonged therapy (over 14 days). With long-term therapy, possible pulmonary fibrosis or interstitial pneumonitis. Hemolytic anemia in G6PD deficiency. Severe or irreversible peripheral neuropathy in high-risk patients (eg, those with renal impairment, diabetes, debilitation). Maintain adequate hydration and urine output.
Adverse Reactions: Frequent gastric upset, brownish urine, hypersensitivity reactions, blood dyscrasias, severe peripheral neuropathy, diffuse interstitial pneumonitis, pulmonary fibrosis, cholestatic jaundice, hepatitis, transient alopecia.
Drug Interactions: Probenecid and sulfinpyrazone increase serum level of nitrofurantoin. May potentiate action of oral anticoagulants.

Generic Name: NORFLOXACIN
Trade Name: Noroxin
Dosage Form: Tablets, 400 mg
Uses: Fluroquinolone antibiotic that acts by inhibiting DNA gyrase, which is needed for the synthesis of DNA. Indicated for the treatment of adults with complicated and uncomplicated UTI caused by susceptible strains of the following microorganisms: *E. coli*; *K. pneumoniae*; *E. cloacae*; *P. mirabilis*; indole-positive *Proteus* species; *P. aeruginosa*; *C. freundii*; *S aureus*; *S epidermidis*; group D streptococci.
Adult Dosage (Oral): Uncomplicated UTI—400 mg twice daily for 7–10 days; complicated UTI—400 mg twice daily for 10–21 days; renal impairment—patients with Clcr $\leq$ 30 mL/min/1.73 m^2, administer 400 mg once daily for the duration stated above. Doses should be taken 1 hour before or 2 hours after meals.
Pediatric Dosage (Oral): Not recommended for use in this population.
Contraindications: History of hypersensitivity to norfloxacin or the quinolone group of antibiotic agents.
Precautions: See ciprofloxacin.
Adverse Reactions: Generally well tolerated. Most common adverse effects include GI—nausea, vomiting, abdominal pain, diarrhea; CNS—headache, dizziness, somnolence, insomnia; DERM—rash, erythremia; HEME—eosinophilia, leukopenia, neutropenia; and elevated liver function tests. Other more serious

adverse effects (reported rarely) include seizures, arthralgia, hepatitis, crystalluria.

Drug Interactions: With probenecid, results in a 50% reduction in the renal clearance of norfloxacin. With aluminum/magnesium-containing antacids, iron salts, sucralfate, results in decreased bioavailability of norfloxacin if administered concurrently. Norfloxacin may reduce the clearance of theophylline, warfarin, and phenytoin.

Generic Name: NYSTATIN
Trade Names: Mycostatin, Nilstat
Dosage Forms: Tablets, 500,000 U; oral suspension, 100,000 U/mL; topical and vaginal preparations
Uses: Treatment of oral, intestinal, and cutaneous candidiasis.
Adult Dosage (Oral): For oral candidiasis, 4–6 mL oral suspension qid; should be continued at least 48 hours after oral symptoms have cleared. For gastrointestinal candidiasis, 500,000–1 million U tid (tablets). For vaginal candidiasis, one vaginal tablet inserted bid for 2 weeks.
Pediatric Dosage (Oral): For a child or infant, 250,000 U qid; for a newborn, 100,000 U qid.
Contraindications: Not for systemic use. Hypersensitivity to nystatin.
Precautions: Suspension should be retained in mouth as long as possible when treating oral candidiasis. Plaques should be wiped off with gauze prior to drug application. Vaginal tablet should be retained in vagina as long as possible when treating vaginal candidiasis.
Adverse Reactions: Virtually nontoxic. Large doses may cause gastric upset.

Generic Name: PHENAZOPYRIDINE
Trade Name: Pyridium
Dosage Forms: Tablets, 100 mg, 200 mg
Uses: Urinary antiseptic and analgesic.
Adult Dosage (Oral): 100–200 mg tid after meals.
Contraindications: Renal insufficiency or hepatitis.
Precautions: May discolor feces and turn urine reddish orange. Hemolysis in glucose-6-phosphate dehydrogenase deficiency. Yellow skin or sclera if drug accumulates (eg, renal impairment).
Adverse Reactions: Gastric upset, methemoglobinemia, hemolytic anemia (especially with G6PD deficiency), hepatic hypersensitivity reactions.

Generic Name: PYRIMETHAMINE
Trade Name: Daraprim
Dosage Form: Tablets, 25 mg
Uses: Antimalarial agent also used for treatment of toxoplasmosis.
Adult Dosage (Oral): For toxoplasmosis, 50–75 mg/d with 1–4 g of a sulfonamide for 1–3 weeks. Dosage of each drug then reduced by one-half and continued for 4–5 weeks more.
Pediatric Dosage (Oral): For a child, 1 mg/kg/d divided bid with pediatric dose of sulfonamide. After 2–4 days, dose reduced to one-half and continued for 1 month.
Contraindications: Large doses in first trimester of pregnancy.
Precautions: Blood cell counts should be done twice a week while patient is on initial high-dose therapy, every week when dose is reduced. (Pyrimethamine is a folic acid antagonist.)
Adverse Reactions: Gastric upset, anorexia, vomiting, megaloblastic anemia, bone marrow depression with leukopenia and thrombocytopenia. Blood dyscrasias may be treated with 3–9 mg folinic acid IM until blood cell count returns to normal.

Generic Name: QUINACRINE
Trade Name: Atabrine
Dosage Form: Tablets, 100 mg
Uses: Anthelminthic, antimalarial, antiparasitic agent.
Adult Dosage (Oral): 100 mg tid for 5–7 days for *Giardia lamblia* enteritis.
Pediatric Dosage (Oral): For a child, 6–7 mg/kg/d divided tid for 5 days (maximum, 300 mg/d).
Precautions: Patients over 60 years old or those with history of psychosis; pregnancy.
Adverse Reactions: Gastric upset, vomiting, dizziness, headache, toxic psychosis, hypersensitivity reactions, urticaria, blood dyscrasias, ocular disturbances, yellow staining of skin, blue and black nail pigmentation, acute hepatic necrosis.
Drug Interactions: Disulfiram-like effect with alcohol. Primaquin has increased toxicity if given with quinacrine.

Generic Name: RIFAMPIN
Trade Names: Rifadin, Rimactane
Dosage Form: Capsules, 300 mg
Uses: For treatment of tuberculosis, prophylaxis against meningitis caused by sulfonamide-resistant meningococci and *Haemophilus influenzae*. Also used for treatment of *Legionella* pneumonia and carriers of diphtheria or *H. influenzae*. Combined with parenteral vancomycin, it is effective for severe methicillin-resistant staphylococcal infections.
Adult Dosage (Oral): For tuberculosis, 600 mg/d in combination with at least one other antitubercular drug. For meningococcal meningitis prophylaxis, 600 mg bid for 2 days.
Pediatric Dosage (Oral): For tuberculosis in a child or infant over 1 week old, 10–20 mg/kg/d as a single dose (up to 600 mg/d), given in combination with at least one other antitubercular drug; for a newborn (under 1 week), 10 mg/kg/d as a single dose. For meningococcal meningitis prophylaxis in a child (1 to 12 years), 20 mg/kg/d, divided q. 12h for 2 days; in an infant (3 months to 1 year), 10 mg/kg/d, divided q. 12h for 2 days. Using these dosages, treat diphtheria carriers for 7 days, *H. influenzae* carriers for 4 days, and *Legionella* pneumonia for 14 days.
Contraindications: Previous rifampin-associated hepatitis, hypersensitivity to rifampin.
Precautions: May impart a brick-red color to body fluids. Avoid use during lactation and pregnancy, especially first trimester. Use cautiously in hepatic impairment.
Adverse Reactions: More frequent and severe with intermittent high-dose therapy. Gastric disturbances, allergic reactions, subclinical hepatitis, jaundice, and brick-red discoloration of body fluids are frequent. Clinical hepatitis may occur, especially with pre-existing liver disease. Also reported are ''flu-like'' syndrome, visual defects, mental disturbances, blood dyscrasias, hematuria, hemoptysis, decreased hemoglobin levels, superinfections, and nephritis.
Drug Interactions: May decrease effect of oral anticoagulants and oral contraceptives.

Generic Name: SPECTINOMYCIN
Trade Name: Trobicin
Dosage Forms: Injection (IM), 2 g, 4 g

Uses: Treatment of uncomplicated gonorrhea in penicillin-allergic patients; effective against penicillin-resistant *Neisseria gonorrhoeae* and for those infections not responding to other antibiotics. Not effective for syphilis or pharyngeal gonorrhea.

Adult Dosage (Parenteral): 2 g IM as single dose (4 g if resistance is prevalent).

Pediatric Dosage (Parenteral): For a child under 8 years, 40 mg/kg as a single IM dose.

Contraindications: Hypersensitivity to spectinomycin.

Precautions: Give IM injections deeply into upper outer quadrant of gluteal muscle. Avoid use in infants and newborns. May mask or delay symptoms of incubating syphilis; serologic syphilis tests should be done.

Adverse Reactions: Pain at injection site, transient dizziness, nausea, rash, urticaria, chills, fever.

Generic Name: VANCOMYCIN
Trade Name: Vancocin
Dosage Forms: Injection (IV), 500 mg; oral solution 500 mg/6 mL (may use injection preparation orally)

Uses: Bactericidal antibiotic for serious infections caused by gram-positive cocci resistant to less toxic antibiotics. Given parenterally for systemic infections due to enterococci and methicillin-resistant staphylococci; orally, for staphylococcal enterocolitis and antibiotic-induced colitis caused by *Clostridium difficile*.

Adult Dosage (Oral): 500 mg–1 g q. 6h.

Adult Dosage (Parenteral): 2 g/d IV divided q. 6–12h.

Pediatric Dosage (Oral): For enterocolitis in children and newborns, 40–50 mg/kg/d, divided q. 6–12h.

Pediatric Dosage (Parenteral): For a child, 40 mg/kg/d IV, divided q. 6–12h; for an infant or newborn, 10 mg/kg/d IV, divided q. 6–12h.

Contraindications: Renal/auditory impairment, hypersensitivity to vancomycin.

Precautions: Should not be given IM. Dosage adjustments necessary in renal impairment. Dilute IV doses in 100–200 mL of diluent; administer slowly over 30–60 min. To minimize thrombophlebitis, alternate injection sites. Use cautiously in the elderly, in renal impairment, and with concurrent use of other ototoxic or nephrotoxic medications.

Adverse Reactions: Thrombophlebitis, ototoxicity, nephrotoxicity, hypersensitivity reactions, peripheral neuropathy, and leukopenia. Commonly seen is a histamine-like reaction ("red neck" syndrome) with fever, chills, and erythema of upper back and neck. Rapid IV rates can cause shock, cardiovascular collapse, and anaphylaxis.

Drug Interactions: See gentamicin in the aminoglycoside section.

Generic Name: ZIDOVUDINE (AZT)
Trade Name: Retrovir
Dosage Forms: Capsules, 100 mg; syrup, 50 mg/5 mL; injection, 10 mg/mL in 20 mL vial

Uses: Antiretroviral agent that interferes with retroviral RNA-dependent DNA polymerase (reverse transcriptase). Indicated for oral use in adults for the management of HIV infection with evidence of impaired immunity (CD_4 cell count $\leq$ 500/mm^3) and in children > 3 months of age who have HIV-related symptoms or who are asymptomatic with abnormal CD_4 cell counts indicating significant HIV-related immunosuppression. For IV use in adult patients with symptomatic HIV who have a history of cytologically confirmed *Pneumocystis carinii* pneumonia or an absolute CD_4 count of < 200 mm^3 before therapy is begun.

Adult Dosage (Oral): Symptomatic HIV—200 mg every 4 hours around the clock initially and then at 1 month the dose may be reduced to 100 mg every 4 hours. Asymptomatic HIV—100 mg every 4 hours while awake.

Adult Dosage (Parenteral): 1 to 2 mg/kg infused over 1 hour every 4 hours around the clock.

Pediatric Dosage (Oral): 3 months to 12 years—180 mg/m^2 every 6 hours (do not exceed 200 mg every 6 hours).

Contraindications: Life-threatening allergic reactions to the drug product.

Precautions: Dose reduction or interruption may be warranted with significant anemia (hemoglobin < 7.5 g% or reduction of > 25% of baseline) and/or significant granulocytopenia (< 750/mm^3 or a reduction of > 50% from baseline). Avoid rapid infusion or bolus dosing.

Adverse Reactions: Most common include anemia/granulocytopenia (related to CD_4 cell count at onset, dose, and duration of therapy), severe headache, dizziness, malaise, nausea, anorexia, myalgia, insomnia.

Drug Interactions: With acetaminophen, results in an increased granulocytopenia. With drugs that interfere with the number and function of RBC/WBC (eg, dapsone, pentamidine, amphotericin B, flucytosine, pyrimethamine, vincristine, vinblastine, adriamycin, interferon), may result in increased myelosuppression. With probenecid, results in an increase in AZT serum levels.

BRONCHODILATORS, ANTIASTHMATIC AGENTS

Generic Name: ACETYLCYSTEINE
Trade Name: Mucomyst
Dosage Forms: Solution for nebulization, 10%, 20%

Uses: Adjuvant therapy for patients with abnormal viscid or inspissated mucous secretions. Also used for treatment of acetaminophen overdose.

Adult Dosage: For nebulization, 6–10 mL 10% (or 3–5 mL 20%) tid or qid into facemask, mouthpiece, or tracheostomy; for direct instillation, 1–2 mL 10% or 20% every hour prn. For treatment of acetaminophen overdose, 140 mg/kg 20% solution PO or via nasogastric tube to start. Then 70 mg/kg q. 4h for 16 doses (should be given within 12 hours after overdose).

Pediatric Dosage: For nebulization, 1 to 3 mL of 10% solution q. 4–6h, depending on patient tolerance.

Contraindications: Hypersensitivity to acetylcysteine.

Precautions: Refrigerate opened vials or bottles; use within 96 hours after opening. Solutions may discolor slightly (light purple) without loss of potency. Frequent suctioning may be necessary for increased bronchial secretions. Bronchospasm may occur especially in asthmatics and pediatric patients (may be relieved by concurrent administration of inhaled bronchodilator).

Adverse Reactions: Stomatitis, nausea, hemoptysis, rhinorrhea, reversible bronchospasm.

Generic Name: ALBUTEROL (SALBUTAMOL)
Trade Name: Proventil, Ventolin
Dosage Forms: Tablets, 2 mg, 4 mg; metered inhaler, 90 μg/dose
Uses: Bronchodilator (primarily β_2-receptor agonist) similar to metaproterenol.
Adult Dosage (Oral): 2–4 mg tid or qid (up to 32 mg/kg/d).
Adult Dosage (Inhalation): 1–2 inhalations 1 or 2 minutes apart, q. 4–6h, prn.
Pediatric Dosage (Oral): For a child over 12 years, same as adult dosage.
Contraindications: Hypersensitivity to albuterol or to any component of the inhaler.
Precautions: See metaproterenol.
Adverse Reactions: See metaproterenol.
Drug Interactions: See metaproterenol.

Generic Name: AMINOPHYLLINE (Oral)
Trade Names: Aminophyllin, various generics available (dihydrate and anhydrous forms)
Dosage Forms: Tablets, 100 mg, 200 mg; suppositories, 250 mg, 500 mg; oral solution, 105 mg/5 mL; rectal solution, 100 mg/mL
Uses: Bronchodilator (xanthine derivative) for symptomatic treatment of bronchial asthma and reversible bronchospasm.
Adult Dosage: See theophylline (immediate action). Follow dosage guidelines for each condition. To convert to equivalent doses of aminophylline dihydrate, divide recommended theophylline dosage by 0.80; for aminophylline anhydrous, divide by 0.86.
Pediatric Dosage: See theophylline (immediate action). Follow dosage guidelines for each condition. To convert to equivalent doses of aminophylline dihydrate, divide recommended theophylline dosage by 0.80; for aminophylline anhydrous, divide by 0.86.
Contraindications: Hypersensitivity to aminophylline, theophylline, or other xanthine derivatives; active peptic ulcer disease.
Precautions: Give oral doses with meals to minimize gastric irritation. Absorption of rectal suppositories is slow, erratic, and unpredictable. Draw serum samples for peak theophylline level 1 to 2 hours after last dose; if patient experiences toxicity, postpone further doses for at least 6 hours and re-evaluate therapy. Infants and children are especially sensitive to theophylline toxicity (particularly the CNS effects), so use cautiously in newborns, infants, and children. Use cautiously in those with acute myocardial injury or cardiac disease, renal or hepatic impairment, peptic ulcer disease, diabetes mellitus, hyperthyroidism, hypertension, age over 55 years, and concurrent therapy with narcotics. Infants, children, and smokers usually require higher milligram per kilogram dosages. Theophylline has a low therapeutic index; monitor vital signs, response, tolerance, pulmonary function, and theophylline serum levels. Do not attempt to maintain any dose that is not tolerated.
Adverse Reactions: Common are gastric upset, nausea, vomiting, dyspepsia, diarrhea, bitter aftertaste, headache, insomnia, restlessness, and irritability. Also reported are hypersensitivity reactions, hematemesis, and exacerbation of peptic ulcers. Other CNS effects (severe in children) include nervousness, dizziness, vertigo, tinnitus, hyperactive reflexes, muscle twitching, and convulsions. Palpitations, tachycardia, arrhythmias, flushing, sweating, fever, dehydration, thirst, diuresis, hypotension, hyperglycemia, and circulatory failure may occur.
Drug Interactions: Ephedrine, other sympathomimetics, and other xanthine derivatives can cause increased cardiac and CNS toxicity. With β-blockers, decreased bronchodilator effect or antagonism of β-blocking effects. With lithium, increased renal excretion of lithium. Cimetidine, clindamycin, erythromycin, lincomycin, and troleandomycin can reduce theophylline clearance, increase theophylline serum levels and toxicity.

Generic Name: AMINOPHYLLINE (Parenteral)
Trade Name: Aminophyllin
Dosage Form: Injection (IV), 25 mg/mL
Uses: Bronchodilator (xanthine derivative) for relief of acute bronchospasm, pulmonary edema, status asthmaticus; also given for neonatal apnea to stimulate respiration and myocardial contractility; for bronchospasm associated with cystic fibrosis and acute descending respiratory infections.
Dosage (Parenteral): The following doses are for theophylline base; to convert to equivalent amount of aminophylline (theophylline ethylenediamine), divide by 0.8. For patients who have *not* received theophylline in the previous 12 to 24 hours, give a loading dose of 5 mg/kg slowly IV over 30 min. (Obtain serum level 30 min after completion of infusion to determine if additional loading dose is required.) Follow with constant IV infusion according to table:

Initial Maintenance Dosage of Theophylline*

Patient Type	Age	Infusion Rate (mg/kg/h)
Newborn	Up to 24 days	1 mg/kg q. 12h†
	Over 24 days	1.5 mg/kg q. 12h†
Infant	6 to 52 weeks	mg/kg/h = (0.008) × (age in weeks) + 0.21
Child	1 to 9 years	0.8‡
	9 to 12 years	0.7‡
Adolescent		
Smoker	12 to 16 years	0.7‡
Nonsmoker	12 to 16 years	0.5‡
Adult smoker (otherwise healthy)	16 to 50 years	0.5‡
Adult nonsmoker (otherwise healthy)	16 years to elderly	0.4‡§
Cardiac decompensation, cor pulmonale, liver dysfunction (or combination of these)	Over 16 years	0.2‡ǁ

*To achieve target serum concentration of 10 μg/mL. Aminophylline dose = theophylline dose/0.8. Measure serum levels at 4–6 hours, 12 hours, and 24 hours after start of infusion.
†To achieve target serum concentration of 7.5 μg/mL for neonatal apnea.
‡Further dosage reductions may be necessary if patients are also receiving drugs that can decrease theophylline clearance (see drug interactions).
§Not to exceed 900 mg/d unless serum levels indicate need for larger dose.
ǁNot to exceed 400 mg/d unless serum levels indicate need for larger dose.

For patients who *have* received theophylline in the previous 12 to 24 hours, obtain stat serum theophylline measurement; for each desired 1 μg/mL increase in serum level, give 0.5 mg/kg slowly

IV over 30 min; recheck serum level 30 min later for further dosage adjustments. If stat serum theophylline level cannot be obtained, a 2.5 mg/kg dose can be administered with relative safety as long as patient exhibits no signs of theophylline toxicity.

Contraindications: Hypersensitivity to theophylline, aminophylline, or xanthine derivatives.

Precautions: IV doses must be given slowly (20–25 mg/min) to avoid profound hypotension, arrhythmias, and convulsions. Use controlled infusion device for continuous infusions. Do not give doses IM because they are painful and absorption is incomplete. For dosage adjustments when using intermittent IV infusions, draw serum sample for peak theophylline level immediately after completing the infusion; when using a continuous infusion, draw sample at any time during administration. Therapeutic serum levels, 10–20 μg/mL; for neonatal apnea, at least 7.5 μg/mL.

Adverse Reactions: (See also aminophylline, oral). Most are related to plasma levels over 20 μg/mL:
- over 20 μg/mL: nervousness, irritability, headache
- over 40 μg/mL: atrial tachycardia, ventricular arrhythmias
- over 60 μg/mL: seizures, vasomotor collapse.

Too rapid IV administration can cause flushing, headache, dizziness, palpitations, precordial pain, premature ventricular contractions, hypotension, ventricular fibrillation, bradycardia, and cardiac arrest.

Drug Interactions: Unstable at pH below 8. Incompatible with acidic drugs and pressor amines (eg, dopamine, isoproterenol, epinephrine, levarterenol). See also aminophylline, oral.

Generic Name: BECLOMETHASONE
Trade Names: Vanceril, Beclovent
Dosage Form: Metered dose inhaler (42 μg/inhalation)
Uses: Adjunctive treatment of bronchial asthma requiring chronic corticosteroid therapy.
Adult Dosage: Two inhalations tid or qid, or up to 20 inhalations/24 hours, if needed.
Pediatric Dosage: For a child 6–12 years old, one or two inhalations tid or qid, or up to 10 inhalations/24 hours, if needed.
Contraindications: Hypersensitivity to beclomethasone or other components of inhaler. Primary treatment of status asthmaticus or acute asthmatic episodes requiring intensive measures.
Precautions: Fungal infections of mouth common (*Candida, Aspergillus*). Steroid withdrawal symptoms may occur during transfer from systemic steroids to inhaler.
Adverse Reactions: Pulmonary infiltrates with eosinophilia, bronchospasm (rare), hoarseness, dry mouth, suppression of hypothalamic-pituitary-adrenal function.

Generic Name: IPRATROPIUM BROMIDE
Trade Name: Atrovent
Dosage Forms: Metered dose inhaler (18 μg/spray)
Uses: Synthetic quaternary ammonium compound chemically related to atropine. Not readily absorbed systemically following inhalation. Indicated as a bronchodilator for maintenance treatment of bronchospasm associated with chronic bronchitis and emphysema.
Adult Dosage (Inhalation): 2 inhalations (36 μg) four times a day. Patients may take additional inhalations as required; however, do not exceed 12 inhalations in 24 hours.
Pediatric Dosage (Inhalation): Safety and efficacy not established.

Contraindications: Hypersensitivity to atropine or its derivatives.
Precautions: Not indicated for the initial treatment of acute episodes of bronchospasm where rapid response is required. Onset of action slow; maximum effect may not be noted for 45–60 minutes. Use with caution in patients with narrow angle glaucoma, prostatic hypertrophy, or bladder neck obstruction.
Adverse Reactions: Most common adverse reactions include cough, nervousness, nausea, headache, GI distress, dry mouth, blurred vision, irritation from aerosol, exacerbation of symptoms, palpitations, and rash.
Drug Interactions: Ipratropium bromide has been used concomitantly with other drugs, including sympathomimetic bronchodilators, methylxanthines, steroids, and cromolyn sodium, commonly used in the treatment of chronic obstructive pulmonary disease without adverse reactions.

Generic Name: ISOETHARINE
Trade Name: Bronkosol, Bronkometer
Dosage Forms: Metered inhaler, 340 μg/dose; solution for inhalation, 0.25%, 0.5%, 1.0%
Uses: Bronchodilator (β-receptor agonist) similar to isoproterenol and metaproterenol.
Adult Dosage: For administration via intermittent positive-pressure breathing (IPPB) or oxygen aerosolization, 0.5–1.0 mL of a 0.5% solution, diluted in 2.0–2.5 mL of water or saline, given q. 4h; administer each dose over 15–20 min. For metered inhaler, 1 or 2 inhalations, 1 to 2 minutes apart, q. 4h, prn.
Pediatric Dosage: For administration via IPPB or oxygen aerosolization, 0.25–0.5 mL of 0.5% solution, diluted in 2.0–2.5 mL of water or saline, given q. 4h, depending on patient tolerance.
Contraindications: Hypersensitivity to isoetharine or to any component of the inhaler.
Precautions: See isoproterenol (for inhalation). To avoid possibility of cardiac toxicity, do not give isoetharine within 1 hour of aqueous epinephrine injections or within 4 hours of subcutaneous injections of epinephrine suspension.
Adverse Reactions: See isoproterenol (for inhalation).
Drug Interactions: See isoproterenol (for inhalation).

Generic Name: ISOPROTERENOL (For Inhalation)
Trade Names: Isuprel Mistometer, Norisodrine, Aerolone
Dosage Forms: Metered inhaler, 0.25% w/w; solution for nebulization, 0.25% (1:400), 0.50% (1:200), 1.0% (1:100)
Uses: Bronchodilator (nonselective β-agonist) given by inhalation for symptomatic treatment of bronchial asthma and reversible bronchospasm.
Adult Dosage: For metered inhaler, 1 or 2 inhalations taken 1 to 5 minutes apart, q. 3–4h, prn (maximum, 6 inhalations in any hour during a 24-hour period). For solution via hand-bulb nebulizer, 5 to 15 deep inhalations (1:200 solution) or 3 to 7 deep inhalations (1:100 solution), repeated once in 5–10 min if necessary; treatment can be repeated up to five times per day. For administration via intermittent positive pressure breathing (IPPB) apparatus, 0.5 mL (of 1:200 solution), diluted to 2.0–2.5 mL with water or saline and delivered over 15–20 min; can repeat treatment up to five times per day.
Pediatric Dosage: For administration via IPPB apparatus, 0.25 mL (of 1:200 solution) diluted to 2.0–2.5 mL with water or saline and delivered over 10–15 min; can repeat treatment up to five times per day.

Contraindications: Hypersensitivity to isoproterenol, patients with tachyarrhythmias, tachycardia caused by digitalis intoxication.
Precautions: See also parenteral isoproterenol in the antiarrhythmics section. Excessive use can lead to refractoriness or severe paradoxical airway resistance ("lung lock"). May be less effective in patients with severe disturbances in ventilation distribution, status asthmaticus, or abnormal blood gas tensions. Use cautiously in elderly patients, diabetics, those with renal or cardiovascular disease, hypertension, or hyperthyroidism. Discontinue drug if angina, precordial distress, or ventricular arrhythmias occur.
Adverse Reactions: See parenteral isoproterenol.
Drug Interactions: See parenteral isoproterenol.

Generic Name: METAPROTERENOL
Trade Names: Metaprel, Alupent
Dosage Forms: Tablets, 10 mg, 20 mg; solution for nebulization, 5%; oral syrup, 10 mg/5 mL; metered dose inhaler, 0.65 mg/inhalation
Uses: Bronchodilator (primarily β_2-receptor agonist).
Adult Dosage (Oral): 20 mg or 10 mL tid. For metered inhaler, 2 to 3 inhalations q. 3–4h (up to 12 inhalations/day). For nebulization via intermittent positive-pressure breathing (IPPB) apparatus, 0.1 to 0.3 mL of 5% solution, diluted with 2–3 mL saline and administered q. 4–8h (depending on patient tolerance).
Pediatric Dosage (Oral): For a child 6 to 9 years old (less than 27 kg), 10 mg or 5 mL tid or qid. For metered inhaler in a child over 12 years, same as adult dosage. For nebulization via IPPB apparatus, 0.1–0.3 mL of 5% solution, diluted with 2–3 mL saline and administered q. 4–8h (depending on patient tolerance; monitor pulse rate and blood pressure).
Contraindications: Cardiac arrhythmias associated with tachycardia; hypersensitivity to metaproterenol or to any components of inhaler.
Precautions: Use cautiously in the elderly or those patients with hypertension, congestive heart failure, coronary artery disease, hyperthyroidism, diabetes, and sensitivity to sympathomimetics. Monitor heart rate and blood pressure especially in infants and children. To avoid possibility of cardiac toxicity, do not give metaproterenol within 1 hour of aqueous epinephrine or within 4 hours of an injection of epinephrine suspension.
Adverse Reactions: Tachycardia, hypertension, palpitations, nervousness, tremor, gastric upset, bad taste.
Drug Interactions: With sympathomimetic bronchodilators, additive adrenergic effects. Nonselective β-blockers antagonize bronchodilator effect.

Generic Name: OXTRIPHYLLINE
Trade Names: Choledyl, Choledyl SA
Dosage Forms: Tablets, 100 mg, 200 mg; tablets (sustained release), 400 mg, 600 mg; elixir, 100 mg/5 mL; pediatric syrup, 50 mg/5 mL (32 mg anhydrous theophylline/5 mL). Oxtriphylline contains 64% theophylline as choline salt.
Uses: Bronchodilator.
Adult Dosage (Oral): For chronic asthma, usual dose is 200 mg q. 6h (up to 1400 mg/d); using sustained-release tablets, divide daily dosage q. 12h.
Pediatric Dosage (Oral): For chronic asthma in a child 6 months to 9 years, 6.2 to 9.4 mg/kg q. 6h; in a child 9 to 12 years, 6.2–7.8 mg/kg q. 6h; in a child 12 to 16 years, 6.2–7.0 mg/kg q. 6h. Using sustained-release tablets, divide daily dosage every 12 hours.
Contraindications: Pediatric syrup is a theophylline and is contraindicated in theophylline hypersensitivity.
Precautions: See aminophylline.
Adverse Reactions: See aminophylline.
Drug Interactions: See aminophylline.

Generic Name: TERBUTALINE
Trade Names: Bricanyl, Brethine
Dosage Forms: Tablets, 2.5 mg, 5 mg; injection (subcutaneous), 1 mg/mL ampules
Uses: Bronchodilator (β_2-receptor agonist) with a longer duration of activity than metaproterenol.
Adult Dosage (Oral): 2.5–5.0 mg tid (at 6-hour intervals). Recommended maximum dose, 15 mg/d.
Adult Dosage (Parenteral): 0.25 mg subcutaneously in a single dose; may repeat in 15–30 min. (maximum 0.5 mg/4-hour period).
Pediatric Dosage (Oral): For a child over 12 years old, 2.5 mg tid (up to 7.5 mg/d).
Pediatric Dosage (Parenteral): For a child over 12 years, single dose of 3.5–5 µg/kg subcutaneously, but safety not established.
Contraindications: Hypersensitivity to sympathomimetics.
Precautions: Diabetes mellitus, hypertension, hyperthyroidism, cardiac disease, pregnancy, labor.
Adverse Reactions: (Dose-related, usually transient.) Increased heart rate, palpitations, headache, dizziness, nervousness, tremor, nausea, gastric upset, sweating, tinnitus.
Drug Interactions: Propranolol and β-blockers antagonize bronchodilator effects of terbutaline. With other sympathomimetics, additive cardiovascular effects.

Generic Name: THEOPHYLLINE (Sustained Release)
Trade Names: Theo-Dur, Quibron-T, Theo-Dur Sprinkle
Dosage Forms: Tablets, 100 mg, 200 mg, 300 mg; capsules (Sprinkle), 50 mg, 75 mg, 125 mg, 200 mg
Uses: Bronchodilator (see aminophylline, oral)
Adult Dosage (Oral): Initially, 200 mg q. 12h; after 3 days, can be increased as tolerated to 300–400 mg q. 12h.
Pediatric Dosage (Oral): For children 6 years and older. The following doses are to be divided q. 12h: 15 to 20 kg, 200–250 mg/d initially, then 300–400 mg/d; 20 to 30 kg, 300 mg/d initially, then 400–500 mg/d; 30 to 35 kg, 350–400 mg/d initially, then 500–600 mg/d; over 35 kg, 400 mg/d initially, then 600–800 mg/d.
Contraindications: See aminophylline, oral.
Precautions: See aminophylline, oral. Do not chew or crush tablets or capsules; capsules may be swallowed or sprinkled on food immediately before ingestion. The total daily dose may be given q. 8h instead of q. 12h. Check serum theophylline concentrations between 3 and 8 hours after last dose when no doses have been added or missed for at least 3 days.
Adverse Reactions: See aminophylline, oral.
Drug Interactions: See aminophylline, oral.

Generic Name: THEOPHYLLINE (Immediate Action)
Trade Names: Slo-Phyllin, Theolair, Theophylline (Anhydrous)
Dosage Forms: Tablets, 100 mg, 200 mg (Slo-Phyllin); 125 mg, 250 mg (Theolair); elixir, 80 mg/15 mL

Uses: Bronchodilator (see aminophylline, oral).
Dosage (Oral): For acute asthma symptoms in patients *not* currently receiving theophylline products, give loading dose of 6 mg/kg; follow with maintenance doses according to table:

	Maintenance Dose	
	Next 12 hours (mg/kg)	Beyond 12 hours (mg/kg)
Adults		
Young smoker	3.0 q. 4h	3.0 q. 6h
Healthy nonsmoker	3.0 q. 6h	3.0 q. 8h
Older patient; cor pulmonale	2.0 q. 6h	2.0 q. 8h
Patient with congestive heart failure or liver failure	2.0 q. 8h	1.0–2.0 q. 12h
Children		
6 months to 9 years	4.0 q. 4h	4.0 q. 6h
9 to 16 years	3.0 q. 4h	3.0 q. 6h

For acute asthma symptoms in patients currently receiving theophylline products within the past 48 hours: Defer the loading dose if a serum theophylline level can be rapidly obtained; if not, a loading dose of 0.5 mg/kg (for each desired 1 µg/mL increase in serum concentration) may be given provided patient exhibits no symptoms of theophylline toxicity.

For chronic asthma, initially 16 mg/kg/d (maximum, 400 mg/d), divided q. 6–8h; if no patient intolerance, can increase dose by 25% increments at 2- or 3-day intervals to the following maximum amounts: for a child under 9 years, 24 mg/kg/d; child 9 to 12 years, 20 mg/kg/d; child 12 to 16 years, 18 mg/kg/d; child over 16 years and adult, 13 mg/kg/d (maximum, 900 mg/d).

Contraindications: See aminophylline, oral.
Precautions: See aminophylline, oral.
Adverse Reactions: See aminophylline, oral.
Drug Interactions: See aminophylline, oral.

CORTICOSTEROIDS

Uses: Corticosteroids are anti-inflammatory agents for palliative therapy of a variety of disorders, including endocrine, rheumatic, collagen, neoplastic, and respiratory diseases; dermatologic, allergic, and hematologic disorders; renal, gastrointestinal inflammatory disease, and certain inflammatory ocular disorders. Parenterally, corticosteroids are primarily used as adjunctive treatment of shock (including septic), anaphylaxis, status asthmaticus, cerebral edema, and increased intracranial pressure.
Dosage Forms: Topical, parenteral, oral preparations.
Contraindications: Systemic fungal infections, hypersensitivity to individual agents.
Precautions: Short-term high-dose therapy: If possible, limit duration of therapy to 72 hours or less. Prophylactic antacids (q. 2h) may be indicated to prevent formation of peptic or stress ulcers. Prolonged oral or parenteral therapy: Use smallest dosage, for the shortest period of time, that will control symptoms. Administer oral doses with food, milk, or antacids to minimize gastric irritation. Corticosteroids may mask symptoms of and increase severity of bacterial, fungal, or viral infections. Do not give immunizations or vaccines during therapy with large doses as antibody response may be suppressed. Abrupt discontinuance of doses can cause acute adrenal insufficiency; taper dosage gradually over 7 to 10 days. Avoid use during lactation. Emotional instability or psychotic tendencies may be precipitated or aggravated. Increased dosages may be necessary during periods of stress, trauma, and surgery. Use cautiously during pregnancy, peptic ulceration, gastrointestinal perforation, diabetes mellitus, osteoporosis, tuberculosis, chronic or active infections, ocular viral infections, hypertension, congestive heart failure or other cardiovascular disease, convulsive disorders, and psychological disorders. Cirrhosis may enhance corticosteroid effects.
Adverse Reactions: Short-term high-dose therapy: Incidence of side-effects is low. Parenteral doses can cause burning, tingling, pain, or sterile abscesses at injection sites. Prolonged therapy: Peptic ulceration, gastrointestinal hemorrhage, acute pancreatitis, impaired glucose tolerance, hyperglycemia, superinfections, psychosis, increased intracranial pressure with papilledema, convulsions, allergic reactions, cushingoid syndrome, adrenal-pituitary suppression, growth suppression, fluid and electrolyte imbalances (hypokalemia, sodium retention, edema, congestive heart failure), osteoporosis, easy bruising, poor wound healing, petechiae, striae, muscle weakness and wasting, acne, hirsutism, facial erythema, subcapsular cataracts, increased intraocular pressure, menstrual irregularities. Abrupt discontinuance of doses can precipitate acute adrenal insufficiency and steroid withdrawal syndrome (nausea, vomiting, lethargy, headache, myalgia, fever, joint pain, hypotension).
Drug Interactions: With potassium-depleting diuretics, increased risk of hypokalemia; with oral hypoglycemics/insulin, hypoglycemic action antagonized.

Generic Name: DEXAMETHASONE
Trade Name: Decadron
Dosage Forms: Tablets, 0.25 mg, 0.5 mg, 0.75 mg, 1.5 mg, 4 mg; injection (IM/IV), 4 mg/mL, 10 mg/mL; long-acting suspension for IM use, 8 mg/mL (Decadron-LA)
Uses: For oral use, see corticosteroids. Given parenterally for treatment of cerebral edema, shock, status asthmaticus.
Adult Dosage (Oral): 0.75–9 mg/d to start, then titrate dose to lowest clinically effective level.
Adult Dosage (Parenteral): For shock, 1–6 mg/kg as a single IV bolus or up to 40 mg IV q. 4–6h for 24 to 48 hours. For cerebral edema, 10–20 mg IV bolus initially, then 4–6 mg IM or IV q. 6h.
Pediatric Dosage (Oral): For inflammation or allergy, 24–340 µg/kg/d, depending on severity of symptoms; taper doses gradually.
Pediatric Dosage (Parenteral): For cerebral edema, 4 mg IV push initially, then: for infants and children under 5 years, 0.5–1.0 mg IM or IV q. 6h; for children 5 to 10 years, 1.5 mg IM or IV q. 6h; for children over 10 years, 2–4 mg IM or IV q. 6h.
Precautions: High-dose therapy should be continued only until patient's condition stabilizes and usually should not be continued past 48 to 72 hours. Prophylactic antacid therapy may be indicated to prevent peptic or stress ulceration during high-dose therapy. Since corticosteroid peak effects may not become evi-

dent for 12 to 24 hours and maximum neurologic benefits may require 3 or 4 days, it is advisable to include osmotic diuretics (eg, mannitol) in the acute therapy of cerebral edema.

Adverse Reactions: Short-term parenteral administration unlikely to produce harmful effects. Peptic ulcer, burning or tingling in perineal area, paresthesias, ataxia, convulsions, anaphylaxis have occurred. See also corticosteroids.

Generic Name: FLUDROCORTISONE
Trade Name: Florinef
Dosage Form: Tablets, 0.1 mg
Uses: Mineralocorticoid with moderate glucocorticoid effects; for replacement therapy in chronic adrenocortical insufficiency (Addison's disease) and salt-losing forms of congenital adrenogenital syndromes.
Adult Dosage (Oral): 0.05–0.2 mg/d.
Adverse Reactions: Primarily fluid and electrolyte imbalances (eg, edema, hypokalemia, sodium retention, hypertension, cardiac hypertrophy).

Generic Name: HYDROCORTISONE (Sodium Succinate)
Trade Name: Solu-Cortef
Dosage Forms: Injection (IM/IV), 100 mg, 250 mg, 500 mg, 1000 mg
Uses: Corticosteroid with both glucocorticoid and prominent mineralocorticoid effects. Used for replacement therapy in adrenocortical insufficiency; also adjunctive therapy of status asthmaticus, acute hypersensitivity reactions. Massive doses given for life-threatening shock.
Adult Dosage (Parenteral): For shock, 50–150 mg/kg as single IV bolus over several minutes or 30–50 mg/kg IV q. 4–6h. For status asthmaticus or severe hypersensitivity reactions, 100 mg to 1 g IV q. 4–6h, depending on severity of the condition.
Pediatric Dosage (Parenteral): For shock, 25 mg/kg slowly IV, then 12 mg/kg/d IV in divided doses, q. 6–12h. For status asthmaticus/severe allergic reactions, 5–10 mg/kg slowly IV initially, then q. 4–6h as indicated.
Precautions: Give large IV bolus doses over 1 to 10 minutes. See also dexamethasone.
Adverse Reactions: Causes more sodium retention than either methylprednisolone or dexamethasone. See also dexamethasone.

Generic Name: METHYLPREDNISOLONE (Sodium Succinate)
Trade Name: Solu-Medrol
Dosage Forms: Injection (IM/IV), 40 mg, 125 mg, 1000 mg
Uses: Anti-inflammatory corticosteroid lacking significant mineralocorticoid properties. Used for immunosuppression; adjunctive therapy of shock, status asthmaticus, severe allergic reactions.
Adult Dosage (Parenteral): For shock, 30 mg/kg slowly IV over several minutes; can repeat q. 4–6h if indicated. For status asthmaticus/severe allergic reactions, 10–250 mg IV q. 4–6h as needed.
Pediatric Dosage (Parenteral): Based on severity of condition. For shock, 25 mg/kg slowly IV initially, then 12 mg/kg/d IV, divided q. 6–12h (not less than 0.5 mg/kg/d). For other inflammatory conditions, 0.04–0.2 mg/kg/d IV or IM, divided q. 6–12h.
Precautions: Dilute large doses in D_5W or NS for slow IV infusion. See also dexamethasone.
Adverse Reactions: Cardiac arrhythmias and circulatory collapse have been reported, primarily in renal transplant patients, with doses greater than 500 mg IV. Anaphylaxis and allergic reactions have been reported following parenteral corticosteroid therapy.

Generic Name: PREDNISONE
Trade Name: Deltasone
Dosage Forms: Tablets, 1 mg, 2.5 mg, 5 mg, 10 mg, 20 mg, 50 mg
Uses: See corticosteroids.
Adult Dosage (Oral): Total daily dose is variable and depends on the clinical disorder. Oral range is 5–60 mg/d, followed by gradual reduction in dose to lowest level possible to maintain adequate clinical response. Every other day dosage regimen may be used for minimum pituitary-adrenal suppression. For acute asthma, allergy, bronchospasm, 30–60 mg/d (divided doses) tapered over 3–5 days.
Pediatric Dosage (Oral): Pharmacologic replacement dose, 0.5–2.0 mg/kg/d, taken with meals. For asthma, 20–40 mg/d initially, tapering by 5 mg/d until lowest effective dose achieved.
Contraindications: See corticosteroids.
Precautions: See corticosteroids.
Adverse Reactions: See corticosteroids.
Drug Interactions: See corticosteroids.

DIURETICS

Generic Name: ACETAZOLAMIDE
Trade Name: Diamox
Dosage Forms: Tablets, 125 mg, 250 mg; capsules (sustained release), 500 mg; injection (IM/IV), 500 mg
Uses: Carbonic anhydrase inhibitor with weak diuretic action. Used primarily to reduce intraocular pressure for management of primary open angle and other chronic glaucomas. Also used for seizure therapy and for maintenance of an alkaline urine for prophylaxis of uric acid nephropathy.
Adult Dosage (Oral): 250 mg q. 4–6h or 500 mg sustained release capsule q. 12h. For maintenance of alkaline urine, 0.5–1.0 g/d.
Adult Dosage (Parenteral): 500 mg IV or IM initially; may be repeated in 2–4 hours.
Pediatric Dosage (Oral): 10–15 mg/kg/d in divided doses. For chronic anticonvulsant therapy, 5–25 mg/kg/d in divided doses.
Pediatric Dosage (Parenteral): 5–10 mg/kg IV q. 6–8h.
Contraindications: Renal impairment, gout or chronic obstructive pulmonary disease, hypersensitivity to acetazolamide, long-term treatment of chronic noncongestive angle closure glaucoma.
Precautions: Should be avoided during pregnancy (teratogenic in rodents). Possible cross-allergenicity with sulfonamides.
Adverse Reactions: Frequent anorexia, gastric disturbances, malaise, lethargy, and depression. Also paresthesias, headache, dizziness, transient myopia, renal calculus formation and colic, sulfonamide-like nephropathy, hyperuricemia, blood dyscrasias, and hypersensitivity reactions.

Generic Name: AMILORIDE
Trade Name: Midamor
Dosage Form: Tablets, 5 mg
Uses: Potassium-sparing diuretic used as adjunctive treatment with thiazide in congestive heart failure and hypertension.
Adult Dosage (Oral): 5 mg/d with meals (up to 10–20 mg/d). Usually given with other kaliuretic diuretics or antihypertensive agents.
Contraindications: See spironolactone.
Precautions: See spironolactone.
Adverse Reactions: See spironolactone.
Drug Interactions: Decreases lithium excretion so may predispose to lithium toxicity. With potassium salts or spironolactone, hyperkalemia.

Generic Name: BUMETANIDE
Trade Name: Bumex
Dosage Forms: Injection (IM/IV), 0.25 mg/mL; tablets, 0.5 mg and 1.0 mg
Uses: Loop diuretic, similar to furosemide, used for treatment of edema caused by congestive heart failure and hepatic or renal disease. Better absorption of oral doses than with furosemide; no cross-allergenicity with furosemide.
Adult Dosage (Parenteral): 0.5–1.0 mg IM or slowly IV (over 1 to 2 minutes); can repeat q. 2–3h, prn (up to 10 mg/d).
Adult Dosage (Oral): 0.5–2.0 mg/d. Can give additional doses q. 4–5h, up to 10 mg/d (can use alternate-day or intermittent therapy).
Contraindications: See furosemide. (May be used in patients allergic to furosemide.)
Precautions: See furosemide.
Adverse Reactions: See furosemide.
Drug Interactions: See furosemide.

Generic Name: ETHACRYNIC ACID
Trade Name: Edecrin
Dosage Forms: Tablets, 25 mg, 50 mg; injection (IV), 50 mg
Uses: Potent loop diuretic with activity and indications similar to those of furosemide.
Adult Dosage (Oral): 50–100 mg/d (titrated in 25- to 50-mg increments to desired response, up to 200 mg/d).
Adult Dosage (Parenteral): 50 mg or 0.5–1 mg/kg slow IV (over 2–3 min); may be repeated once (maximum dose, 100 mg).
Pediatric Dosage (Oral): For a child, 1–3 mg/kg/d; titrate by 25-mg increments to desired response. Use in infants is not recommended.
Pediatric Dosage (Parenteral): For a child, 0.5–1.0 mg/kg slow IV. Use in infants is not recommended.
Contraindications: Hypersensitivity to ethacrynic acid; anuria; hepatic coma; increasing oliguria, azotemia, electrolyte imbalances; pregnancy; lactation.
Precautions: Give oral doses with meals to minimize gastric irritation. Administer IV doses slowly over several minutes. Do not give IM or subcutaneously. Other precautions as for furosemide. Use in severe renal disease should be discontinued if oliguria, azotemia, or electrolyte imbalances worsen or if ototoxicity develops.
Adverse Reactions: See furosemide and hydrochlorothiazide. However, hearing loss is *more frequent* and often permanent, especially in oliguric patients and those with preexisting auditory impairment. Oral tablets can cause gastric upset and bleeding. IV use frequently causes thrombophlebitis.
Drug Interactions: See hydrochlorothiazide and furosemide.

Generic Name: FUROSEMIDE
Trade Name: Lasix
Dosage Forms: Tablets, 20 mg, 40 mg, 80 mg; injection (IM/IV), 10 mg/mL (20 mg, 40 mg, 100 mg ampules); oral solution, 10 mg/mL
Uses: Potent loop diuretic for treatment of moderate to severe edema, acute pulmonary edema, and hypertension. Also adjunctive treatment of hypercalcemia.
Adult Dosage (Oral): 20–80 mg in morning (usual dose). If no response, may be increased by 20- to 40-mg increments q. 6–8h, prn (up to 600 mg/d has been used).
Adult Dosage (Parenteral): 20–40 mg IM or IV push (over 1–2 min) initially. May be increased by 20-mg increments q. 2h until desired response obtained. Doses up to 4–6 g/d have been used in acute and chronic renal failure. (*Note:* IV administration rate should not exceed 4 mg/min in elderly and renally impaired patients and 15 mg/min in general.)
Pediatric Dosage (Oral): 2 mg/kg to start. May be increased by 1–2 mg/kg q. 6–8h, up to 6 mg/kg/d maximum.
Pediatric Dosage (Parenteral): 1–2 mg/kg IM or slow IV; can be increased by 1 mg/kg/dose q. 2h until desired response (maximum, 6 mg/kg/dose).
Contraindications: Hypersensitivity to furosemide. See also ethacrynic acid.
Precautions: Possible cross-allergenicity with sulfonamides. Caution in severe or progressive renal disease, liver disease or cirrhosis (may precipitate hepatic encephalopathy), newborns and infants, diabetes, gout, patients on digitalis glycosides, or those with severe electrolyte imbalances.
Adverse Reactions: See hydrochlorothiazide. Also tinnitus and reversible or permanent hearing damage has occurred after rapid or large IV doses (generally occurs within 10–20 min after administration).
Drug Interactions: See hydrochlorothiazide. Renal excretion of lithium and salicylates is decreased so possible toxicity from resulting increased serum levels. With aminoglycosides, additive ototoxicity.

Generic Name: GLYCEROL (GLYCERIN)
Trade Names: Glyrol, Osmoglyn
Dosage Forms: Oral solution, 50% v/v, 75% v/v, and 96% v/v
Uses: Osmotic diuretic for lowering intracranial pressure (ICP) during cerebral edema; it is used as an adjunct to mannitol IV for production of chronic diuresis for ICP reduction. Also used to lower intraocular pressure.
Adult Dosage (Oral): 1.0–1.5 g/kg orally or via nasogastric tube q. 6h.
Pediatric Dosage (Oral): 0.5–1.0 g/kg orally or via nasogastric tube q. 6h.
Contraindications: Severe dehydration, intracranial hemorrhage.
Precautions: Nausea and vomiting may be minimized by administering the less concentrated solutions (50% or 75%). Use cautiously in cardiac disease, congestive heart failure, pulmonary

edema, and pre-existing dehydration. May cause a slight hyperglycemia in diabetics.
Adverse Reactions: Commonly, nausea, vomiting, diarrhea, mild headache, dizziness, and thirst. Also dehydration, hyperglycemia, pulmonary edema can occur.
Drug Interactions: May increase insulin requirements in diabetics.

Generic Name: HYDROCHLOROTHIAZIDE (Representative thiazide-type diuretic)
Trade Name: HydroDIURIL
Dosage Forms: Tablets, 25 mg, 50 mg, 100 mg
Uses: Thiazide diuretic for treatment of mild to moderate hypertension and edema.
Adult Dosage (Oral): 50–100 mg/d or bid depending on response (up to 200 mg/d).
Pediatric Dosage (Oral): 2–5 mg/kg/d in two divided doses.
Contraindications: Anuria, mild edema of pregnancy, hypersensitivity to hydrochlorothiazide. Hypersensitivity to other sulfonamides (relative contraindication).
Precautions: Use cautiously in renal or hepatic impairment, gout, diabetes mellitus, asthma, systemic lupus erythematosus. Avoid use in newborns and jaundiced infants. Possible cross-allergenicity with sulfonamides.
Adverse Reactions: Fluid and electrolyte imbalances resulting in dehydration, volume depletion, orthostatic hypotension, hyponatremia, hypokalemia, hypochloremic alkalosis; hyperuricemia, decreased glucose tolerance with hyperglycemia. Also paresthesias, weakness, vertigo, muscle spasm, cramps, gastric upset, azotemia, exacerbation of systemic lupus erythematosus, hyperbilirubinemia, cholestatic jaundice, precipitation of hepatic coma, and blood dyscrasias (rare). Hypersensitivity reactions can include rashes, urticaria, and photosensitivity.
Drug Interactions: With antihypertensive agents, additive effects. With oral hypoglycemics/insulin, hypoglycemic effects antagonized. With steroids, increased risk of hypokalemia. With alcohol and CNS depressants, additive orthostatic hypotension. Thiazides decrease lithium excretion and predispose to lithium toxicity.

Generic Name: MANNITOL
Trade Names: Mannitol, Osmitrol
Dosage Forms: Injection (IV), 5%, 10%, 20% (500 mL bottles), 25% (12.5 g/50 mL vial, ampule)
Uses: Osmotic diuretic for treatment of acute cerebral or ocular edema and promotion of renal excretion of toxins.
Adult Dosage (Parenteral): For cerebral or ocular edema, 1–2 g/kg slow IV over 30–60 min (through in-line filter); for diuresis in toxin excretion, continuous IV infusion of 5%–20% solution to maintain urine output of approximately 100 mL/h. (Maximum dose, 200 g.)
Pediatric Dosage (Parenteral): For cerebral edema, 0.25–0.5 g/kg IV over 30–60 min (15%–20% solution); for diuresis in toxin excretion, 0.25–0.5 g/kg IV (using 5%–10% solution) at a rate to maintain a high urine output.
Contraindications: Anuria or impaired renal function not responding to test dose of 200 mg/kg IV push. Severe pulmonary congestion or edema, congestive heart failure, dehydration; active intracranial bleeding, edema associated with abnormal capillary fragility or membrane permeability.

Precautions: Do not mix with infusing blood. Solutions more concentrated than 15% often crystallize so administer through an in-line filter; use only clear, crystal-free solutions. Monitor urine output, central venous pressure, and serum electrolytes. Use cautiously during pregnancy; use lower dosages in children and infants to avoid rebound cerebral edema. Avoid extravasation.
Adverse Reactions: Headache, nausea, vomiting, chills, dizziness, lethargy, confusion, chest pain, allergic reactions, and convulsions secondary to hyponatremia. Fluid and electrolyte imbalances resulting in fluid overload with pulmonary edema, water intoxication, hypertension, congestive heart failure, rebound cerebral edema, and intraocular hemorrhage. Too rapid diuresis can lead to dehydration and hypovolemia. Tissue necrosis and thrombophlebitis may occur if solution extravasates.

Generic Name: METOLAZONE
Trade Name: Zaroxolyn
Dosage Forms: Tablets, 2.5 mg, 5 mg, 10 mg
Uses: Diuretic agent similar in activity to thiazides potentiates the effect of loop diuretics. Often given with furosemide for treatment of refractory edema.
Adult Dosage (Oral): For edema, 5–10 mg/d. For hypertension, 2.5–5 mg/d. (Maximum daily dose, 20 mg.)
Contraindications: Anuria, hepatic coma or precoma, hypersensitivity to metolazone.
Precautions: See hydrochlorothiazide.
Adverse Reactions: See hydrochlorothiazide.
Drug Interactions: See hydrochlorothiazide.

Generic Name: SPIRONOLACTONE
Trade Name: Aldactone
Dosage Forms: Tablets, 25 mg, 100 mg (also available with hydrochlorothiazide as Aldactazide)
Uses: Potassium-sparing diuretic for treatment of edema associated with congestive heart failure, cirrhosis, and nephrotic syndrome; also given as adjunctive treatment of essential hypertension and primary aldosteronism. Since it causes no hyperuricemia or glucose intolerance, it is useful in patients with gout or diabetes.
Adult Dosage (Oral): For edema or hypertension, 50–100 mg/d in single or divided doses, titrated as necessary. For primary aldosteronism, 100–400 mg/d in divided doses.
Pediatric Dosage (Oral): 1.0–3.3 mg/kg/d in divided doses bid. Adjust after 4–5 days according to response.
Contraindications: Significant renal impairment, anuria, acute renal insufficiency, hyperkalemia.
Precautions: Excessive amounts of high potassium foods or salt substitutes should be avoided, as should prolonged use of aspirin or salicylates.
Adverse Reactions: Hyperkalemia, hyponatremia, other electrolyte disturbances, dehydration, drowsiness, lethargy, headache, mental confusion, gastric upset, diarrhea, rashes, hirsutism, gynecomastia, menstrual irregularities, mild acidosis, elevated blood urea nitrogen.
Drug Interactions: Salicylates antagonize spironolactone activity. With potassium salts or other potassium-sparing diuretics, possible hyperkalemia.

Generic Name: TRIAMTERENE
Trade Name: Dyrenium

Dosage Forms: Capsules, 50 mg, 100 mg (available with hydrochlorothiazide as Dyazide)
Uses: Potassium-sparing diuretic similar to spironolactone.
Adult Dosage (Oral): 100 mg bid after meals (up to 300 mg/d).
Pediatric Dosage (Oral): For a child, 2–4 mg/kg/d initially. May be increased to 6 mg/kg/d in divided doses.

Contraindications: See spironolactone.
Precautions: See spironolactone.
Adverse Reactions: Similar to those with spironolactone, except hyperuricemia is possible. Diabetics are particularly prone to hyperkalemia. Gastric upset is frequent.
Drug Interactions: See amiloride.

HYPOGLYCEMICS/ANTIHYPOGLYCEMICS

Generic Name: DEXTROSE (50%)
Trade Name: 50% Dextrose
Dosage Forms: Injection (IV), 25 g/50 mL (50%) preloaded syringe. Caloric content, 3.4 cal/g.
Uses: Osmotic diuretic; treatment of hypoglycemia.
Adult Dosage (Parenteral): 25–50 mL (12.5–25 g) slow IV push.
Pediatric Dosage (Parenteral): Initially, 1–2 mL/kg (0.5–1.0 g/kg) slow IV bolus over 1 to 2 minutes; can follow with IV infusion of $D_{10}W$ at 4–8 mg/kg/min.
Contraindications: Diabetic coma; intracranial or intraspinal hemorrhage.
Precautions: Extremely hypertonic (2,526 mOsm/L); do not give IM or subcutaneously. IV bolus doses should be given slowly over 1 or 2 minutes (maximum infusion rate without causing glycosuria, 0.5 g/kg/h). Before administration to infants and children, dilute doses 1:1 with water to make $D_{25}W$.
Adverse Reactions: Phlebitis, sclerosis of veins, thrombosis, hyperglycemia, osmotic diuresis.

Generic Name: GLUCAGON
Trade Name: Glucagon
Dosage Forms: Injection (IM/IV/subcutaneous), 1 mg, 10 mg
Uses: Pancreatic hormone used for treatment of severe hypoglycemic reactions and insulin overdose.
Adult Dosage (Parenteral): For hypoglycemia, 1–2 mg IM or subcutaneously; may be repeated once in 15 min. Maximum effects usually occur in 10–15 min.
Pediatric Dosage (Parenteral): 0.03 mg/kg IM or IV; can be repeated in 6–12 hours. For an infant of a diabetic mother, 0.3 mg/kg (300 µg/kg) IM or IV.
Contraindications: Hyperinsulinism
Precautions: Hyperglycemic effect is brief; as soon as patient responds, give supplemental carbohydrates orally or IV. Hyperglycemic response may be reduced in juvenile diabetics, emaciated or malnourished patients, or those with uremia or liver disease. Use cautiously in those with insulin-secreting tumors (rebound hypoglycemia) or pheochromocytoma (hypertension).
Adverse Reactions: Mild hyperglycemia (with rebound hypoglycemia after glucagon stopped), hypokalemia, nausea, vomiting, hypocalcemia. Hypersensitivity reactions are possible since glucagon is a protein of animal origin.

Generic Name: INSULIN
Trade Names: Iletin, Insulin
Dosage Forms: Concentrations of 40, 80, 100 U/mL (pure beef, pure pork, beef-pork mixtures, and semisynthetic human insulins available).

Insulin Type	Onset (hours)	Peak (hours)	Duration (hours)	Route
Rapid				
Regular (CZI)	0.5–1	2–4	5–8	IV/subcutaneous/IM
Semilente	1–3	2–8	12–16	IM/subcutaneous
Intermediate				
Globin Zinc	1–2+	6–10	12–18	IM/subcutaneous
Isophane (NPH)	1–3	6–15	22–24+	IM/subcutaneous
Lente	1–3	6–14	18–24+	IM/subcutaneous
Prolonged				
Protamine Zinc (PZI)	4–6	14–24	36+	IM/subcutaneous
Ultralente	4–6	18–30	36+	IM/subcutaneous

Uses: Regular insulin used for rapid reversal of hyperglycemia in diabetic ketoacidosis (DKA) and hyperglycemia nonketotic coma; also given with glucose infusions for management of hyperkalemia. Intermediate and long-acting insulins used for chronic management of diabetes mellitus.
Adult Dosage (Parenteral): For diabetic maintenance therapy, doses must be titrated to clinical response (usual range, 0.6–1.0 U/kg/d). For diabetic ketoacidosis, using regular insulin: (1) "high-dose" method: 0.5–1.0 U/kg (half by IV push, half by subcutaneous injection), then 0.25–0.5 U/kg subcutaneously q. 2–4h until blood sugar less than 300 mg/dL and plasma ketones negative; (2) "low-dose" method, 0.1–0.5 U/kg IV push, then 0.1 U/kg by continuous IV infusion via controlled infusion device; discontinue infusion and give doses subcutaneously when acidosis improves and blood sugar falls to 300 mg/dL or less; (3) "low-dose" IM method: 0.1–0.5 U/kg IV push, then 0.1 U/kg IM every hour until DKA controlled. Once DKA is under control, give regular insulin subcutaneously (sliding scale) or a longer-acting insulin administered subcutaneously.
Pediatric Dosage (Parenteral): Same as adult dosage for all methods.
Contraindications: Insulin allergy (rare, although desensitization procedures may be warranted in some patients); hypersensitivity to beef or pork (can switch to insulin derived from the opposite source or use the semisynthetic human insulin preparations).
Precautions: Only *regular* insulin can be given IV; use only clear solutions. Insulin adsorbs to surfaces of IV infusion bottles and tubing (albumin, 25% solution, can be added to infusion container to minimize adsorption). Administer IV infusions with controlled infusion device; adjust rates according to hourly blood/urine levels of glucose and acetone. Onset of action of doses given IM or subcutaneously may be delayed in markedly dehydrated or poorly perfused patients. Hyperinsulinism with rebound hypoglycemia may occur in brittle diabetics, use of high doses, or use of IV fluids containing no glucose if given during the later phases of DKA therapy. Patients with renal impairment

or uremia may be more sensitive to insulin's hypoglycemic effect. To minimize lipodystrophy, rotate injection sites, use insulin warmed to room temperature, or switch to highly purified pork or human insulins. Insulin requirements may increase with fever; infection; trauma; surgery; weight gain; reduction in physical activity; hyperthyroidism; and thyroid, estrogen, or corticosteroid medications.

Adverse Reactions: Hypoglycemia (symptoms include bradycardia with hypotension, diaphoresis, nausea, vomiting, hunger, diarrhea, lethargy, hypertension, tachycardia, convulsions, coma). Rebound hyperglycemia, caused by glycogen, catecholamine, and adrenal steroid release, can develop. Local reactions include urticaria, itching, swelling, stinging, insulin allergy (rare), and lipodystrophy. Insulin insensitivity and resistance are sometimes treated with steroids or a switch to another animal or human source insulin.

Drug Interactions: Hypoglycemic effect potentiated by alcohol, MAO inhibitors, salicylates, guanethidine, disopyramide; antagonized by thiazide diuretics, loop diuretics, estrogens, corticosteroids, thyroid hormone, catecholamines. With β-blockers, symptoms of hypoglycemia are masked and carbohydrate intolerance occurs.

GASTRIC ACID INHIBITORS

Generic Name: CIMETIDINE
Trade Name: Tagamet
Dosage Forms: Tablets, 200 mg, 300 mg, 400 mg; oral solution, 300 mg/5 mL; injection (IM/IV), 300 mg/2 mL
Uses: Histamine H_2-receptor antagonist that inhibits gastric acid secretion. For prevention and treatment of active and recurrent duodenal ulcers. Also used in the treatment of pathologic hypersecretory conditions.
Adult Dosage (Oral): For active duodenal ulcer, 300 mg qid with meals and at bedtime, continued for 6–8 weeks (unless healing demonstrated endoscopically); for prevention; 400 mg at bedtime. For hypersecretory condition, 300 mg qid, with meals and at bedtime as long as clinically indicated (up to 2400 mg/d).
Adult Dosage (Parenteral): 300 mg IV (or IM) q. 6h. May be given slow IV push over 1–2 min, but IV piggyback is preferred.
Pediatric Dosage (Oral): For a child over 12 years old, 300 mg q. 6h; under 12 years old, 20–40 mg/kg/d, divided q. 6h.
Pediatric Dosage (Parenteral): For a child over 12 years old, 300 mg IV q. 6h; under 12 years old, 20–40 mg/kg/d IV, divided q. 6h.
Precautions: With severe renal impairment, dosage interval should be adjusted to 12 hours. Elderly and/or severely ill patients may experience increased mental confusion, which is reversible within 48 hours of discontinuing drug.
Adverse Reactions: Dizziness, muscular pain, mild and transient diarrhea, neutropenia, and rash more frequent. Also mental confusion, dizziness, headache, blood dyscrasias, mild gynecomastia, hepatitis, pancreatitis, and interstitial nephritis have been reported. Rapid IV injection may cause cardiac arrhythmias and hypotension.
Drug Interactions: May potentiate hypoprothrombinemic effect of oral anticoagulants. Through hepatic microsomal enzyme suppression, cimetidine can inhibit metabolism and thus potentiate theophylline, phenytoin, diazepam, and propranolol.

Generic Name: FAMOTIDINE
Trade Name: Pepcid
Dosage Forms: Tablet, 20 mg, 40 mg; powder for oral suspension, 40 mg/5 mL; injection, 10 mg/mL, 2 mL single dose, and 4 mL multidose vials
Uses: H_2 receptor antagonist similar to ranitidine. Indicated for the short-term treatment of active duodenal ulcer, benign gastric ulcer, and gastric hypersecretory condition. May be effective in patients unresponsive to or intolerant of cimetidine.
Adult Dosage (Oral): For duodenal or benign gastric ulcer, 20 mg twice daily or 40 mg once daily at bedtime until the ulcer heals or for 4 to 8 weeks. After healing, 20 mg once daily at bedtime as prophylaxis. For other pathologic hypersecretory conditions, 80–160 mg every 6 hours have been used.
Adult Dosage (Parenteral): Dilute 20 mg (2 mL) famotidine with 0.9% sodium chloride injection or other compatible IV solution to a total volume of 5–10 mL and inject IV over not less than 2 minutes every 12 hours. Infusion, 20 mg diluted with 100 mL 5% dextrose injection or other compatible solution and infuse over 15–30 min every 12 hours.
Pediatric Dosage (Oral and Parenteral): Safety and efficacy not established in children.
Contraindications: Hypersensitivity to famotidine or other H_2 antagonists.
Precautions: With severe renal impairment (creatinine clearance < 10 mL/min/1.73 m^2), dosage interval should be adjusted to every 36–48 hours as indicated or a total daily dose reduced to 20 mg at bedtime. Liver function tests should be monitored periodically.
Adverse Reactions: See ranitidine.
Drug Interactions: See ranitidine.

Generic Name: MISOPROSTOL
Trade Name: Cytotec
Dosage Forms: Tablets, 100 μg, 200 μg
Uses: Synthetic prostaglandin E_1 analog with both antisecretory and mucosal protective properties. Indicated for the prevention of NSAID (including aspirin)-induced gastric ulcer in high-risk patients (eg, history of ulcer disease). May be useful in the treatment of duodenal ulcers unresponsive to H_2 antagonists.
Adult Dosage (Oral): 200 μg four times daily with food. If this dosage cannot be tolerated, then 100 μg four times daily may be used. Therapy should last for the duration of NSAID treatment.
Pediatric Dosage (Oral): Safety and efficacy not established.
Contraindications: History of allergy to prostaglandins; pregnancy.
Precautions: Pregnancy category X—misoprostol may cause incomplete miscarriage, uterine contractions, uterine bleeding, and expulsion of products of conception. Does not prevent duodenal ulcers in patients on NSAIDs. Dose-related diarrhea usually develops early in the course of therapy but is for the most part self-limiting. Diarrhea incidence may be minimized by administering the drug after meals and at bedtime and avoiding magnesium-containing antacids.

Adverse Reactions: GI—diarrhea (13–40%), abdominal pain, nausea, flatulence, dyspepsia, vomiting, constipation; OB/GYN—spotting, cramps, hypermenorrhea, dysmenorrhea; other—headache.

Drug Interactions: None of clinical importance reported.

Generic Name: OMEPRAZOLE
Trade Name: Prilosec
Dosage Forms: Capsules, 20 mg
Uses: Suppresses gastric acid secretion by specific inhibition of the H^+/K^+ ATPase (proton pump) enzyme system at the secretory surface of the gastric parietal cell. Indicated for the short-term treatment of active duodenal ulcer, severe erosive esophagitis, poorly responsive symptomatic gastroesophageal reflux disease (GERD), pathologic hypersecretory conditions.
Adult Dosage (Oral): Active duodenal ulcer and GERD—20 mg daily for 4–8 weeks. Pathologic hypersecretory conditions—60 mg once daily initially, then dosage should be individualized to patient need (dosages > 80 mg should be divided). Dosages up to 120 mg three times a day have been used.
Contraindications: None known.
Precautions: Long-term studies in animal models have shown a dose-related increase in gastric carcinoid tumors over time. Pregnancy category C—use only if potential benefit justifies potential risk to the fetus. Bioavailability may be increased in the elderly. Long-term safety awaits further study.
Adverse Reactions: Generally well tolerated. Most common complaints include headache, diarrhea, abdominal pain, nausea, vomiting, dizziness, rash, constipation, cough, flatulence.
Drug Interactions: May potentiate hypoprothrombinemic effect of oral anticoagulants. Through hepatic microsomal enzyme suppression, omeprazole can inhibit metabolism and thus potentiate the effects of diazepam and phenytoin. May interfere with the absorption of drugs where gastric pH is a determinant of bioavailability (eg, ketoconazole).

Generic Name: RANITIDINE
Trade Name: Zantac
Dosage Forms: Tablets, 150 mg, 300 mg; injection (IM/IV), 25 mg/mL; syrup, 15 mg/mL; premixed infusion, 0.5 mg/mL in 100 mL single use plastic container
Uses: Histamine H_2-receptor antagonist similar to cimetidine; used for short-term treatment of active duodenal ulcers and gastric hypersecretory conditions. May be effective in patients unresponsive to and intolerant of cimetidine.
Adult Dosage (Oral): For duodenal or gastric ulcers or gastroesophageal reflux disease (GERD), 150 mg bid or 300 mg once daily at bedtime until ulcer heals or for 4 to 8 weeks; after healing, 150 mg at bedtime as prophylaxis. For other pathologic hypersecretory conditions, 600–900 mg/d in divided doses.
Adult Dosage (Parenteral): 50 mg IM or IV q. 6–8h (maximum, 400 mg/d). Intermittent IV infusion—dilute 50 mg (2 mL) in 100 mL of 5% dextrose injection (or other suitable diluent) and infuse over 15–20 minutes every 6–8 hours. Continuous IV infusion—150 mg (6 mL) ranitidine in 250 mL 5% dextrose (or other suitable diluent) to be delivered at a rate of 10.7 mL/h. Continuous IV infusion for Zollenger-Ellison patients—ranitidine injection in compatible IV solution diluted to a concentration not greater than 2.5 mg/mL; start infusion at 1 mg/kg/h; if after 4 hours either a measured gastric acid output is >10 mEq/h or the patient becomes symptomatic, adjust dose upward in 0.5-mg/kg/h increments and measure acid output; dosages up to 2.5 mg/kg/h have been used.
Pediatric Dosage (Oral): 2–18 years, 37.5 mg/dose or 1.25–2 mg/kg/dose every 12 hours.
Pediatric Dosage (Parenteral): 0.1–0.8 mg/kg/dose every 6–8 hours.
Contraindications: None known.
Precautions: Dosage should be adjusted in renal impairment (give 150 mg/d orally or 50 mg parenterally every 18–24 hours if creatinine clearance is less than 50 mL/min). Use cautiously in hepatic impairment (monitor SGPT enzyme levels).
Adverse Reactions: Headache, dizziness, malaise, constipation, nausea, abdominal pain, rash, transient increases in liver enzymes. Less antiandrogenic than cimetidine so lower incidence of gynecomastia or impotence. Less drug-related mental confusion than with cimetidine.
Drug Interactions: Concomitant administration of oral H_2 antagonists and antacids will decrease the H_2 antagonist absorption; therefore administration should be separated by two hours if possible. Absorption of ketoconazole may be reduced.

Generic Name: SUCRALFATE
Trade Name: Carafate
Dosage Form: Tablets, 1 g
Uses: In the acidic medium of gastric secretions, sucralfate forms an ulcer-adherent complex with proteinaceous exudate forming a protective barrier to hydrogen ion diffusion. Sucralfate promotes prostaglandin synthesis and mucus and bicarbonate secretion in the gut. Sucralfate also binds to bile acids and pepsin. Indicated for the short-term and prophylactic management of duodenal ulcer. Other potential uses include long-term treatment of gastric ulcers, GERD, NSAID and aspirin-induced GI symptoms and mucosal damage, prevention of stress ulcers and GI bleeding in critically ill patients, and oral mucositis. Sucralfate may be used as a phosphate-binding agent.
Adult Dosage (Oral): One gram four times a day on an empty stomach (1 hour before meals and at bedtime) until ulcer heals or for 4 to 8 weeks. After healing, 1 g twice daily as prophylaxis. For treatment of oral mucositis, dissolve 1 tablet in 10–30 mL water and swish and swallow four times daily.
Pediatric Dosage (Oral): Safety and efficacy not established.
Contraindications: None known.
Precautions: Do not use antacids 30 minutes before or after sucralfate. During administration, small amounts of aluminum are absorbed from the GI tract; concomitant use with other aluminum-containing products (eg, antacids) may lead to aluminum accumulation and toxicity in patients with chronic renal failure or receiving dialysis; therefore, use with caution in these patients.
Adverse Reactions: Generally well tolerated; most frequent complaints include constipation, diarrhea, nausea, vomiting, bloating, flatulence, dry mouth, rash, headache, and dizziness.
Drug Interactions: To avoid possible binding of sucralfate to other concomitant drug therapy, other agents should be administered at least 2 hours prior to sucralfate dose (most notably tetracycline, digoxin, phenytoin). Quinolone antibiotics must be administered no less than 2 hours prior to the administration of sucralfate. If this cannot be accomplished, then concurrent administration should be avoided.

NARCOTIC AND NON-NARCOTIC ANALGESICS

Generic Name: ACETAMINOPHEN
Trade Names: Tylenol, Datril, Panadol
Dosage Forms: Tablets, 325 mg, 500 mg; tablets (chewable), 80 mg, 120 mg; capsules, 325 mg, 500 mg; oral elixir, 120 mg/5 mL, 160 mg/5 mL; oral solution, 120 mg/5 mL, 165 mg/5 mL; oral drops, 48 mg/mL, 100 mg/mL; rectal suppositories, 120 mg, 125 mg, 325 mg, 600 mg
Uses: Analgesic and antipyretic agent.
Adult Dosage (Oral or Rectal): 650 mg–1 g q. 4–6h, prn (up to 4 g/d).
Pediatric Dosage (Oral or Rectal): The following are single doses to be given four to five times daily, divided q. 4–6h; children over 11 years old, use adult dosage; 11 years, 480 mg; 9 to 10 years, 400 mg; 6 to 8 years, 320 mg; 4 to 5 years, 240 mg; 2 to 3 years, 160 mg; 1 to 2 years, 120 mg; infants 4 to 11 months, 80 mg; up to 3 months, 40 mg.
Contraindications: None known.
Precautions: For prolonged therapy, use cautiously in those with anemia or cardiac, pulmonary, renal, or hepatic disease.
Adverse Reactions: Nontoxic in normal doses. Can cause blood dyscrasias or hypersensitivity reactions (rashes, urticaria, drug fever, mucosal lesions, laryngeal edema), but incidence is rare. Toxic overdoses exhibit symptoms of nausea, vomiting, malaise, diaphoresis, hepatotoxicity, hepatic necrosis, nephrotoxicity, delirium, thirst, hypoglycemia, methemoglobinemia, CNS depression, vascular collapse, coma, and convulsions. (Overdose treatment, acetylcysteine 20% given orally.)
Drug Interactions: Large doses can cause slightly increased hypothrombinemic effect with oral anticoagulants. With phenothiazines, possible profound hypothermia.

Generic Name: ASPIRIN
Trade Names: Various generics available
Dosage Forms: Tablets, 325 mg, 400 mg, 650 mg (with or without caffeine or antacids); tablets (enteric-coated), 325 mg, 650 mg, 975 mg; timed-release preparations, 486 mg, 650 mg; rectal suppositories, 65–650 mg; chewable tablets, 81 mg (1¼ gr)
Uses: Analgesic, antipyretic, anti-inflammatory agent. Also used as antiplatelet therapy.
Adult Dosage (Oral): For analgesia or antipyresis, 325–650 mg q. 4–6h, prn (up to 4 g/d). Timed-release preparations are given q. 8h; for antiplatelet or antithrombosis therapy, 325–650 mg/d or bid (up to 1300 g/d); for anti-inflammatory effect, 3.6–5.4 g/d, in divided doses.
Adult Dosage (Rectal): For analgesia or antipyresis, 325–650 mg q. 4h, prn (up to 4 g/d).
Pediatric Dosage (Oral): For analgesia or antipyresis in a child 2 to 11 years old, usual dose is 65 mg/kg/d (1.5 g/M²/d), divided q. 4h (up to 5 doses/d and 100 mg/kg/d); for a child over 11 years, same as adult dosage. Alternatively, the following single doses are given q. 4h, up to five times daily: for a child 11 years, 480 mg; 9 to 10 years, 400 mg; 6 to 8 years, 325 mg; 4 to 5 years, 240 mg; 2 to 3 years, 160 mg. For juvenile arthritis in a child weighing 25 kg or less, 60–90 mg/kg/d; in a child over 25 kg, 80–130 mg/kg/d in divided doses.
Pediatric Dosage (Rectal): For analgesia or antipyresis, same as oral dosage.
Contraindications: Hypersensitivity to salicylates, hemophilia, hemorrhagic states, active gastric or peptic ulcer disease, asthma, premature and full-term newborns.
Precautions: Children and infants, particularly if dehydrated or hyperthermic, are especially sensitive to aspirin toxicity; maintain adequate hydration and monitor respirations. Minimize gastric distress by giving doses with food, milk, or full glasses of water. Absorption of rectal suppositories may be slow and incomplete. Use cautiously in peptic ulcer disease, gastritis, coagulation abnormalities, vitamin K deficiencies, renal impairment, and concurrent anticoagulant therapy. Asthma, hay fever, nasal polyps, or multiple allergies may predispose patient to salicylate toxicity. (*Note:* **Use of salicylates in infants and children with varicella infections or influenza-like illness has been associated with increased risk of developing Reye's syndrome.** Until the nature of this association has been clarified, it is strongly recommended that aspirin and other salicylates not be used in infants, children, and teenagers with such infections unless directed by a physician.)
Adverse Reactions: Gastric upset and occult blood loss. "Salicylism," ie, dose-related tinnitus at plasma level of 200–400 μg/mL. Severe or fatal toxicity at over 400 μg/mL or ingestion of 150 mg/kg or more. Symptoms include hearing impairment, tinnitus, visual disturbances, nausea, vomiting, hyperventilation, diaphoresis, vertigo, mental confusion, tachycardia, fever, hemorrhage, oliguria, convulsions, vasomotor depressions, coma, respiratory failure and alkalosis, motor depressions, followed by metabolic and respiratory acidosis (especially in children), and circulatory collapse.
Drug Interactions: With oral anticoagulants, potentiation of bleeding. With alcohol, corticosteroids, nonsteroidal anti-inflammatory agents, increased risk of gastrointestinal ulceration. With probenecid and sufinpyrazone, decreased uricosuria. With phenothiazines, profound hypothermia.

Generic Name: BUTORPHANOL
Trade Name: Stadol
Dosage Forms: Injection (IM/IV) 1 mg/mL, 2 mg/mL
Uses: Non-narcotic analgesic for moderate to severe pain. A 2-mg dose is approximately equal in potency to 10 mg morphine sulfate. Duration of analgesia is 3–4 hours. It also has narcotic-antagonist activity equivalent to ¹⁄₄₀ that of naloxone and 30 times that of pentazocine.
Adult Dosage (Parenteral): 2 mg IM q. 3–4h, prn (range, 1–4 mg q. 3–4h); 1 mg IV q. 3–4h, prn (range, 0.5–2 mg q. 3–4h).
Contraindications: Hypersensitivity to butorphanol. Not recommended for children under 18 years.
Precautions: Caution in respiratory decompensation, renal or hepatic impairment (severe), pregnancy, lactation, head injury and increased intracranial pressure, acute myocardial infarction, ventricular dysfunction, or coronary insufficiency. Possible addiction liability in emotionally unstable individuals or those with history of drug abuse. Because of its narcotic antagonist properties, butorphanol is not recommended for patients physically dependent on narcotics, and it may reduce the effectiveness of previously administered narcotics. Dosage of butorphanol should be reduced when administered concomitantly with phenothiazines and other tranquilizers.

Adverse Reactions: Most frequent include sedation, nausea, clamminess, sweating, headache, vertigo, dizziness, lethargy, and "floating" feeling. Also CNS excitation, including nervousness, unusual dreams, and hallucinations may occur, as well as palpitations, blood pressure changes, elevated cerebral spinal fluid pressure, flushing, cold intolerance, dry mouth, respiratory depression, rashes, hives, diplopia, or blurred vision. (Treatment of overdose: naloxone.)

Drug Interactions: Narcotic withdrawal symptoms with methadone and other narcotics. Increased CNS depression with alcohol, tranquilizers, hypnotics, and other CNS depressants. With pancuronium, conjunctival changes may occur.

Generic Name: CODEINE
Trade Names: Various
Dosage Forms: Tablets, 15 mg, 30 mg, 60 mg; injection (IM/subcutaneous); in combination with other analgesics and antitussives (usually 10 mg codeine per 5 mL)
Uses: Narcotic analgesic for mild to moderate pain. Also given as an antitussive. It has about 1/12 to 1/16 the analgesic potency of morphine sulfate; oral doses are 2/3 as effective as parenteral doses. Onset of action, 15–30 min; duration of analgesia, 4–6 hours.
Adult Dosage (Oral): For analgesia, 15–60 mg q. 4h, prn; for antitussive effect, 5–15 mg q. 4h, prn.
Adult Dosage (Parenteral): 15–60 mg IM or subcutaneous q. 4h, prn.
Pediatric Dosage (Oral): For analgesia, 3 mg/kg/d, divided q. 4h; for antitussive effect, 1–1.5 mg/kg/d in divided doses.
Pediatric Dosage (Parenteral): For analgesia, same as oral dosage.
Contraindications: Hypersensitivity to codeine.
Precautions: See morphine. May have lower addiction potential and lesser toxicity than other narcotics. Avoid IV administration.
Adverse Reactions: Light-headedness, dizziness, sedation, gastric upset, constipation, respiratory depression, pruritus. IV administration has caused anaphylaxis.
Drug Interactions: See morphine.

Generic Name: FENTANYL
Trade Name: Sublimaze
Dosage Forms: Injection, 0.05 mg/mL in 2, 5, 10, and 20 mL ampules
Uses: Narcotic analgesic similar to morphine but 75–125 times more potent. Indicated as an adjunct to local, regional, or inhalational anesthesia; for pain management in potentially hemodynamically unstable patients; as a primary component in nitrous oxide-narcotic-relaxant anesthesia; as the predominant anesthetic in high-dose techniques (eg, cardiac anesthesia); and epidurally for postoperative pain management. Fentanyl has a rapid onset and a brief duration of action.
Adult Dosage (Parenteral): Preoperative sedation/analgesia—1 µg/kg IV/IM. General anesthesia—10 to 30 µg/kg IV. Cardiac surgery—75 to 100 µg/kg IV. Epidural analgesia—bolus, 50 to 100 µg/kg followed by infusion of 1–2 µg/kg/h.
Pediatric Dosage (Parenteral): Anesthesia—50 to 100 µg/kg/dose. Sedation for minor procedures (1 to 3 years old)—2 to 3 µg/kg/dose, may repeat after 30 to 60 minutes as required; (3 to 12 years old)—1 to 2 µg/kg/dose.

Contraindications: Hypersensitivity to narcotics; acute bronchial asthma; upper airway obstruction. Epidural—presence of infection at injection site; bleeding diathesis; parenterally administered corticosteroids within a 2-week period; or other medical conditions that would contraindicate the epidural technique.
Precautions: See morphine. Use with caution in patients with known bradyarrhythmias as fentanyl may produce bradycardia (treatable with atropine). Hemodynamic compromise seldom a problem except occasionally when large doses are used and in the setting of hypotension and/or shock. Respiratory rate, heart rate, blood pressure, and mental status should be monitored. Skeletal muscle rigidity occasionally occurs, resulting in difficulty in ventilation and chest wall compliance (concomitant administration of skeletal muscle relaxants can diminish this reaction). No significant histamine release (even at relatively large doses).
Adverse Reactions: See morphine.
Drug Interactions: See morphine. With benzodiazepines, may result in cardiovascular depression (especially with high-dose fentanyl). With droperidol, may cause hypotension and decreased pulmonary arterial pressure.

Generic Name: FENTANYL TRANSDERMAL SYSTEM
Trade Name: Duragesic
Dosage Form: Transdermal system, 25, 50, 75, 100 µg/h
Uses: Indicated for the management of chronic pain in patients requiring opioid analgesia.
Adult Dosage (Transdermal): Systems are replaced every 72 hours. One must first convert the patient from the oral or parenteral opioid to the transdermal system equivalent (10 mg IM or 60 mg oral dose of morphine every 4 hours is approximately equivalent to fentanyl transdermal, 100 µg/h). After 3 days at this dose (initial evaluation of maximum analgesic effect cannot be made before 24 hours of wearing), it may be increased and then maintained for 6 days, after which the dose may be increased further (90 mg/24 h increase of oral morphine is approximately equivalent to 25 µg/h increase in transdermal fentanyl). Discontinuation—after removal it takes $\geq$ 17 hours for fentanyl concentrations to decrease by 50%. Therefore, new analgesics should be titrated based on the patient's report of pain during this washout period.

Generic Name: KETOROLAC TROMETHAMINE
Trade Name: Toradol
Dosage Form: Injection: 15 mg, 30 mg, 60 mg
Uses: Parenterally administered nonsteroidal anti-inflammatory agent with analgesic, anti-inflammatory, and antipyretic activity. Indicated for the short-term management of pain.
Adult Dosage (Parenteral): Loading dose of 30–60 mg IM followed by 15–30 mg every 6 hours. The recommended total daily dose for the first day is 150 mg and 120 mg/d thereafter. The lower end of the recommended dosage range is for patients under 50 kg, greater than 65 years of age, and/or with reduced renal function.
Pediatric Dosage (Parenteral): Safety and efficacy are not established in children.
Contraindications: Hypersensitivity to ketorolac; in patients with complete or partial syndrome of nasal polyps, angioedema, and bronchospastic reactivity to aspirin or other NSAIDs.
Precautions: Patient should be closely monitored for signs and symptoms of GI bleeding. Use with caution in patients with

impaired renal function (BUN and serum creatinine should be monitored), impaired hepatic function or a history of liver disease (monitor LFTs), and elderly patients. Not recommended for use during labor and delivery. Inhibits platelet aggregation and may prolong bleeding time; therefore, patients with coagulation disorders should be closely monitored (effect disappears 24–48 hours after discontinuance of therapy).

Adverse Reactions: Bronchospasm, nausea, GI ulceration, GI bleeding, GI perforation, hepatic injury, nephrotoxicity, fluid retention, headache, drowsiness, sweating, injection pain.

Drug Interactions: None reported (few studied). Based on other NSAIDs, lithium and methotrexate serum concentrations may become elevated with concurrent use.

Generic Name: MEPERIDINE HCl
Trade Name: Demerol
Dosage Forms: Tablets, 50 mg, 100 mg; injection (IM/IV), 25 mg, 50 mg, 75 mg, 100 mg; elixir, 10 mg/mL
Uses: Narcotic analgesic for moderate to severe pain; 80–100 mg of meperidine is approximately equal in analgesic potency to 10 mg of morphine sulfate. Oral doses are about one-half as effective as parenteral doses. Duration of analgesia, 2–4 hours.
Adult Dosage (Oral): 50–150 mg q. 3–4h, prn.
Adult Dosage (Parenteral): 50–150 mg IM q. 3–4h, prn; or slow IV 50–100 mg diluted and titrated.
Pediatric Dosage (Oral): 6 mg/kg/d, divided q. 4h, prn (up to 100 mg/dose).
Pediatric Dosage (Parenteral): Same as oral dosage.
Contraindications: See morphine. Administration of MAO inhibitors within last 14 days. Hypersensitivity to meperidine.
Precautions: See also morphine. Use IV route cautiously since it can cause significant respiratory depression. Avoid subcutaneous injections since they can cause pain and tissue necrosis. Metabolite (normeperidine) has excitatory properties that may precipitate seizures in those with convulsive disorders, renal dysfunction, or receiving high doses.
Adverse Reactions: See morphine.
Drug Interactions: See morphine. With anticonvulsants, decrease in seizure threshold; increase in anticonvulsant dosage may be required. Use with MAO inhibitors can precipitate severe or fatal reactions (hypertensive crisis, vascular collapse).

Generic Name: MORPHINE SULFATE
Trade Name: Morphine
Dosage Forms: Injection (IM/IV/subcutaneous), 2 mg, 4 mg, 6 mg, 8 mg, 10 mg, and 15 mg/mL; tablets, 10 mg, 15 mg, 30 mg; oral solution, 2 mg and 4 mg/mL; oral drops, 20 mg/mL
Uses: Narcotic analgesic for severe pain. Duration of action, 4–5 hours.
Adult Dosage (Oral): Same as parenteral dosage. Use oral solution or drops for best absorption and effects.
Adult Dosage (Parenteral): 5–20 mg IM or subcutaneously q. 4h, prn. For IV administration, 1–10 mg diluted and slowly injected; may repeat small doses q. 5–10 min, cautiously.
Pediatric Dosage (Parenteral): 100–200 μg/kg subcutaneously q. 4h, prn (maximum of 15 mg/dose).
Contraindications: Hypersensitivity to morphine. Bronchial asthma or severe respiratory depression.
Precautions: Addicting. Dose must be decreased by one-half when other CNS depressants are used. IV doses can cause significant hypotension and respiratory depression. May interfere with evaluation of neurologic function or diagnosis of acute abdomen. Vagolytic action may increase ventricular rate (caution in paroxysmal supraventricular tachycardia). Use cautiously in elderly or debilitated patients, those with respiratory disorders, myocardial infarction (decreases systemic vascular resistance), ulcerative colitis, acute abdomen, myxedema, hepatic or renal impairment (if severe), convulsive disorders, prostatic hypertrophy, and head trauma with intracranial lesions or increased intracranial pressure. Use cautiously prior to biliary surgery or during labor (fetal effects). Slows reflexes so ability to perform hazardous tasks may be impaired.

Adverse Reactions: Primarily respiratory, circulatory, and CNS depression. Also euphoria, dysphoria, hallucinations, oliguria, urinary retention, sweating, gastric upset, constipation, and biliary tract spasm (morphine more than meperidine). Also causes histamine release with urticaria, flushing, and wheal formation at IV site. IV doses can cause flushing, tachycardia, bradycardia, hypotension, syncope, shock, significant respiratory depression, and cardiac arrest.

Drug Interactions: Physically incompatible with all barbiturates, benzodiazepines, aminophylline, sodium bicarbonate, and hydrocortisone. Additive CNS depression with other narcotics, sedative-hypnotics, tricyclic antidepressants, alcohol, and antianxiety agents. With anticholinergics and tricyclic antidepressants, additive anticholinergic effects.

Generic Name: PENTAZOCINE
Trade Names: Talwin, Talwin Nx
Dosage Forms: Injection (IM/IV/subcutaneous), 30 mg/mL; tablets (Talwin NX), 50 mg (with 0.5 mg naloxone)
Uses: Non-narcotic analgesic for relief of moderate to severe pain. Onset of analgesia, 15–30 min; duration, 2–3 hours (IM/subcutaneous), 1 hour (IV), and over 3 hours (oral).
Adult Dosage (Oral): 50–100 mg q. 3–4h, prn (up to 600 mg/d).
Adult Dosage (Parenteral): 30–60 mg IM or 30 mg IV, q. 3–4h, prn (up to 360 mg/d).
Contraindications: Hypersensitivity to pentazocine. Not recommended for children under 12 years old.
Precautions: See morphine. Addicting. Pentazocine is a mild narcotic antagonist that may reduce the effectiveness of a previously administered narcotic and may precipitate opiate withdrawal. Causes slowing of reflexes so it can impair ability to perform hazardous tasks. Use cautiously in those with acute myocardial infarction (may increase systemic and arterial pressures). Avoid subcutaneous injections.
Adverse Reactions: Sedation, sweating, dizziness, nausea, euphoria, alterations in mood, dream disturbances, hallucinations are most frequent. Occasional anticholinergic effects, allergic reactions, visual disturbances. After parenteral use, diaphoresis, ulceration and sclerosis of skin and underlying tissues, seizures, respiratory depression, apnea.
Drug Interactions: See morphine.

Generic Name: PROPOXYPHENE
Trade Name: Darvon
Dosage Forms: Tablets, 50 mg, 100 mg with acetaminophen (Darvocet-N, Darvocet-N 100); capsules, 32 mg, 65 mg (plain), 32 mg and 65 mg with aspirin/caffeine (Darvon Compound-32 and Darvon Compound-65)

Uses: Non-narcotic analgesic for relief of mild to moderate pain. Onset of action, 15–60 min; duration of analgesia, 4–6 hours.
Adult Dosage (Oral): 65 mg q. 4–6h, prn, or 100 mg (Darvocet-N 100) q. 4–6h, prn.
Contraindications: Not recommended in children. Hypersensitivity to propoxyphene, pregnancy, suicidal or addiction-prone patients.
Precautions: Addicting. Can slow reflexes and impair ability to perform hazardous tasks.
Adverse Reactions: Dizziness, sedation, light-headedness, nausea, and vomiting are most frequent. Constipation, euphoria, dysphoria, paradoxical excitement, insomnia, minor visual disturbances, and rashes also occur. Chronic ingestion of over 800 mg/d may cause toxic psychosis and convulsions. Acute overdoses cause CNS and respiratory depression, coma, convulsions, pulmonary edema, hypotension, arrhythmias. Toxic serum levels over 2 mg/dL alone or 1 mg/dL when combined with other CNS depressants can be fatal (lethal doses may be 0.5 g or more). Naloxone is used to treat respiratory depression. Hemodialysis is of little value in treatment of overdose.
Drug Interactions: Other CNS depressants, tricyclic antidepressants, alcohol, and muscle relaxants potentiate CNS depression.

SEDATIVE-HYPNOTICS

BARBITURATES

Uses: Sedative-hypnotic. Also used for management of status epilepticus and other acute convulsive episodes, for preoperative sedation, induction of light anesthesia, and prior to otolaryngologic procedures (facilitation of tracheostomy or intubation). Recently, high doses of short-acting barbiturates have been used during cerebral resuscitation as adjuncts to other measures for control of intracranial hypertension.
Dosage Forms: Various preparations are available for parenteral, oral, or rectal use. They may be rapid-acting (duration of minutes, as thiopental sodium IV) short- to intermediate-acting (duration of 5–8 hours, as pentobarbital, secobarbital), or long-acting (duration of 6–10 hours, as phenobarbital).
Contraindications: Hypersensitivity to barbiturates; porphyria; respiratory disease in which dyspnea or obstruction is present.
Precautions: Administer IV doses slowly (less than 50 mg/min); respiratory depression, apnea, laryngospasm, and hypotension can occur with rapid IV infusion rates. Use cautiously during pregnancy, in infants, children, the elderly, and the debilitated, and in those with severe cardiac disease. Severe hepatic or renal impairment can cause drug accumulation. Psychic and/or physical dependence with tolerance may develop. Drug-induced drowsiness can slow reflexes and impair ability to perform hazardous tasks.
Adverse Reactions: Habit-forming, residual sedation ("hangover"), lethargy, paradoxic excitement or hyperactivity in children, hypersensitivity reactions, skin eruptions, serum sickness, and CNS depression. IV use, especially, causes thrombophlebitis, severe respiratory depression, apnea, hypotension, coughing, hiccoughing, laryngospasm, bronchospasm, nausea, and vomiting. Blood levels of 1.5–3.5 mg/dL for short- and intermediate-acting barbiturates and 8–12 mg/dL for long-acting compounds are potentially lethal. Toxic symptoms usually appear at ten times the hypnotic dose and include hypothermia, fever, sluggish or absent reflexes, respiratory depression, hypotension, circulatory collapse, pulmonary edema, miosis, or (in severe cases) mydriasis, oliguria, and coma.
Drug Interactions: With alcohol, tranquilizers, and other CNS depressants, additive CNS and respiratory depression. With coumarin anticoagulants, decreased prothrombin time. Barbiturates stimulate hepatic microsomal enzymes, resulting in increased metabolism of many drugs metabolized in the liver (eg, digitoxin, phenytoin, corticosteroids).

Generic Name: AMOBARBITAL (Barbiturate-derivative)
Trade Names: Amytal, Amytal Sodium
Dosage Forms: Injection (IM/IV), 65 mg–1 g; tablets, 15 mg, 30 mg, 50 mg, 100 mg; oral elixir, 44 mg/5 mL
Uses: Sedative-hypnotic used primarily as anticonvulsant for status epilepticus and acute agitation in psychotic and hysterical states; used in narcoanalysis.
Adult Dosage (Oral): See secobarbital.
Adult Dosage (Parenteral): 130–260 mg IM or slow IV (range, 65–500 mg slow IV). IV administration rate should not exceed 100 mg/min.
Precautions: See barbiturates. Toxic serum levels are about 5 mg/dL.
Adverse Reactions: See barbiturates.
Drug Interactions: See barbiturates.

Generic Name: CHLORAL HYDRATE
Trade Names: Noctec, Chloral Hydrate
Dosage Forms: Capsules, 250 mg, 500 mg; oral syrup, 250 mg/5 mL, 500 mg/5 mL; rectal suppositories, 300 mg, 600 mg, 1000 mg
Uses: Sedative-hypnotic used for nocturnal or preoperative sedation and prior to electroencephalographic (EEG) evaluation. Preferred sedative for anxiety or apprehension in infants, children, and the elderly since it usually produces less paradoxical excitement than do the barbiturates.
Adult Dosage (Oral or Rectal): For sedation, 250 mg tid; for hypnosis, 500–1000 mg; prior to EEG examination, 500–2000 mg.
Pediatric Dosage (Oral or Rectal): For sedation, 15–40 mg/kg/d, divided q. 8h; for hypnosis, 50 mg/kg as a single dose (maximum, 1 g); prior to EEG examination, 20–25 mg/kg as a single dose.
Contraindications: Hypersensitivity to chloral hydrate, marked hepatic or renal impairment, gastritis or esophagitis, severe cardiac disease.
Precautions: Gastric irritant so take doses with meals or with a full glass of fluid. Can cause excitement or delirium in patients experiencing pain. Use cautiously in renal or hepatic impairment, porphyria, or severe cardiac disease (large doses). May be habit-forming; can cause withdrawal symptoms. Drug-induced slowing of reflexes and decreased mental alertness can impair ability to perform hazardous tasks.

Adverse Reactions: Gastric irritation, nausea, vomiting, and diarrhea. CNS depressant effects of drowsiness, dizziness, ataxia, and disorientation. Paradoxical excitement or delirium may occur, as well as rashes and leukopenia. Toxic doses cause gastric necrosis, parenchymatous renal injury, hepatic damage, muscle flaccidity, and profound CNS depression. See also barbiturates.

Drug Interactions: Additive CNS depression with other CNS depressants. Potentiates hypoprothrombinemic effect of oral anticoagulants. Use of IV furosemide within 24 hours of chloral hydrate (especially with post–myocardial infarction patients) may cause a hypermetabolic state characterized by hypertension, sweating, flushing, hot flashes, and variable blood pressure.

Generic Name: ETHCHLORVYNOL
Trade Name: Placidyl
Dosage Forms: Capsules, 100 mg, 200 mg, 500 mg, 750 mg
Uses: Sedative-hypnotic.
Adult Dosage (Oral): 500–750 mg at bedtime for 1 week only (maximum dose, 1 g).
Contraindications: Hypersensitivity to ethchlorvynol; porphyria.
Precautions: See barbiturates. Toxic levels are about 4 mg/dL.
Adverse Reactions: See barbiturates. Also, prolonged coma (days) with fluctuating levels of consciousness may occur with overdoses. Paradoxical excitement and seizures, hypothermia, and pancytopenia may occur. Lethal doses are not well defined. Chronic exposure may produce ataxia, incoordination, tremors, muscle weakness, peripheral neuropathy, slurred speech, and confusion.
Drug Interactions: See barbiturates.

Generic Name: FLURAZEPAM
Trade Name: Dalmane
Dosage Forms: Capsules, 15 mg and 30 mg
Uses: Benzodiazepine derivative (long-acting) for insomnia.
Adult Dosage (Oral): 15–30 mg at bedtime.
Contraindications: Hypersensitivity to flurazepam; pregnancy.
Precautions: Avoid use during pregnancy (possibly teratogenic). Use reduced dosages in elderly or debilitated patients and those with renal or hepatic impairment. Use cautiously in states of mental depression or chronic pulmonary insufficiency. May be habit-forming. May precipitate barbiturate-like withdrawal symptoms if abruptly discontinued after prolonged therapy. Caution patients that additive CNS depression may occur if alcoholic beverages are consumed the day following a dose of flurazepam and for several days after the medication is discontinued.
Adverse Reactions: Drowsiness, dizziness, headache, confusion, disorientation, ataxia, falling, and slurred speech. Also gastric upset, dry mouth, blurred vision, palpitations, shortness of breath, hypotension, genitourinary tract complaints, paradoxical hyperexcitability, pruritus, and rashes.
Drug Interactions: Additive CNS depression with other CNS depressants and tranquilizers.

Generic Name: GLUTETHIMIDE
Trade Name: Doriden
Dosage Forms: Tablets, 0.25 g, 0.5 g; capsules, 0.5 g
Uses: Sedative-hypnotic.
Adult Dosage (Oral): 0.25–0.5 g at bedtime prn.
Contraindications: Hypersensitivity to glutethimide; porphyria.

Precautions: See barbiturates. Hemodialysis or peritoneal dialysis is of little value in overdose treatment. Toxic serum levels usually 1–3 mg/dL or more.
Adverse Reactions: See barbiturates. Lethal adult dose probably 5–20 g. Stupor or coma may alternate with alert, hyperactive behavior (owing to enterohepatic recirculation). Convulsions may occur.
Drug Interactions: See barbiturates.

Generic Name: MIDAZOLAM
Trade Name: Versed
Dosage Form: Injection, 1 mg/mL and 5 mg/mL vials; 5 mg/mL in 2 mL Tel-E-Ject syringe
Uses: Short-acting benzodiazepine that is 3–4 times more potent than diazepam. Indicated for perioperative sedation and to impair memory of perioperative events and for conscious sedation prior to short diagnostic or endoscopic procedures alone or with a narcotic; for induction of general anesthesia before administration of other anesthetic agents; to supplement nitrous oxide and oxygen for surgical procedures.
Adult Dosage (Parenteral): Preoperative sedation/memory impairment of perioperative events—0.07 to 0.08 mg/kg IM 1 hour prior to surgery. Endoscopic/cardiovascular procedures/conscious sedation—initial dose of 1 to 2.5 mg IV over ≥ 2 minutes (30% reduction in patients > 60 years old and when a narcotic is used concurrently); additional doses may be repeated at 2-minute intervals until desired response is achieved (usually a total dose of > 5 mg is not needed). Induction and maintenance of general anesthesia—initially 0.3 mg/kg over 20 to 30 seconds; after 2 minutes additional dosages of 25% of the initial dose (≤ 0.6 mg/kg is usually required) until desired effect; maintenance of anesthesia with incremental doses of 25% of the induction dose; patients > 55 years require a 30% reduction in initial and subsequent doses.
Pediatric Dosage (Parenteral): Induction of anesthesia—0.15 mg/kg/dose initially followed by 0.05 mg/kg/dose every 2 minutes $\times$ 1 to 3 doses as required. Sedation for procedures or preanesthesia—0.08 mg/kg/dose IM $\times$ 1 or 0.3 mg/kg/dose rectal $\times$ 1 (dilute dose in 5 mL normal saline). Sedation during mechanical ventilation—load 0.2 mg/kg IV $\times$ 1 followed by maintenance therapy beginning at 2 μg/kg/min every 30 minutes until light sleep is induced.
Contraindications: Hypersensitivity to benzodiazepines, acute narrow angle glaucoma.
Precautions: Serious cardiorespiratory adverse events (respiratory depression, respiratory arrest, or cardiac arrest) have occurred in patients receiving midazolam. IV should be administered slowly to minimize the risk of these events. Pregnancy category D—use only if potential benefit justifies the possible risk to the fetus. Midazolam does not protect against the increased intracranial pressure or circulatory effects noted following administration of succinylcholine or pancuronium or associated with endotracheal intubation under light general anesthesia. Delayed metabolism in hepatic, renal, and congestive heart failure.
Adverse Reactions: CNS—headache, euphoria, confusion, amnesia, slurred speech, ataxia, oversedation, stupor, coma, emergence delirium, agitation; CV—hypotension, tachycardia; DERM—rash, hives, pruritus, hypersensitivity; RESP—depression, apnea, bronchospasm; MISC—tenderness at injection site,

hiccoughs, elevated intraocular pressure, blurred vision, diplopia, salivation, nausea, vomiting, phlebitis.
Drug Interactions: Potentiates other CNS depressants.

Generic Name: PENTOBARBITAL (Barbiturate-derivative)
Trade Name: Nembutal
Dosage Forms: Injection (IM/IV), 50 mg/mL; capsules, 30 mg, 50 mg, 100 mg; oral elixir, 18.5 mg/5 mL; suppositories, 30 mg to 200 mg
Uses: Sedative-hypnotic for insomnia, preoperative sedation, control of acute convulsive seizures. Also used in adjunctive therapy of intracranial hypertension.
Adult Dosage (Oral): For hypnosis, 100–200 mg at bedtime; for preoperative sedation, 100–150 mg 1 to 1½ hours before surgery.
Adult Dosage (Rectal): Same as oral dosage.
Adult Dosage (Parenteral): For hypnosis, 100–200 mg IM; for preoperative sedation, 150–200 mg IM 1 to 1½ hours before surgery. For acute convulsion, 150–200 mg slowly IV (average initial dose, 100 mg/70 kg); can follow with additional fractional IV doses, up to a total of 200–500 mg. (Wait at least 1 min between each dose to determine its effect.) As adjunct in management of intracranial hypertension (investigational use), 3–5 mg/kg slowly IV (diluted, over 30–60 min), followed by continuous IV infusion of 2 mg/kg/h.
Pediatric Dosage (Oral): For preoperative sedation in a child over 8 years, 3 mg/kg/dose (maximum, 100 mg) given 1½ hours before surgery.
Pediatric Dosage (Rectal): For preoperative sedation in a child 6 months to 8 years, 4 mg/kg/dose (maximum, 120 mg) given 1½ hours before surgery.
Pediatric Dosage (Parenteral): For acute convulsions, 2–6 mg/kg IM or slowly IV; as adjunct in management of intracranial hypertension (investigational use), same as adult dosage.
Contraindications: See barbiturates.
Precautions: See barbiturates.
Adverse Reactions: See barbiturates.
Drug Interactions: See barbiturates.

Generic Name: PHENOBARBITAL
Trade Names: Luminal, Phenobarbital
Dosage Forms: Injection (IM/IV), 65 mg/mL to 325 mg/mL in vials and ampules; tablets, 8 mg to 100 mg; capsules, 16 mg; oral elixir, 4 mg/mL; rectal suppositories, 8 mg to 120 mg
Uses: Barbiturate sedative-hypnotic given parenterally as anticonvulsant for acute seizures and as a sedative for acute agitation and anxiety; orally, given as anticonvulsant for seizure prophylaxis and as a sedative-hypnotic; rectally, used as a sedative-hypnotic.
Adult Dosage (Oral or Parenteral): For sedation, 30–120 mg/d, PO or IM in divided doses, q. 8–12h; for hypnosis, 100–320 mg PO or IM at bedtime (short-term use only).
Pediatric Dosage (Oral or Rectal): For sedation, 6 mg/kg/d in divided doses, q. 8h.
Contraindications: See barbiturates.
Precautions: See barbiturates.
Adverse Reactions: See barbiturates.
Drug Interactions: See barbiturates.

Generic Name: SECOBARBITAL (Barbiturate-derivative)
Trade Name: Seconal
Dosage Forms: Tablets, 50 mg, 100 mg; capsules, 30 mg, 50 mg, 100 mg; injection (IM/IV), 50 mg/mL; suppositories, 30–200 mg; elixir 22 mg/5 mL
Uses: Sedative-hypnotic. See barbiturates.
Adult Dosage (Oral): For hypnosis, 100–200 mg at bedtime; for preoperative sedation, 100–150 mg 1 to 1½ hours before surgery.
Adult Dosage (Parenteral): For hypnosis, 100 mg at bedtime; for acute convulsions, 5–6 mg/kg IM or slow IV, repeated q. 3–4h as needed; for basal hypnosis for anesthesia or otolaryngologic procedures, 50–100 mg slowly IV (up to 250 mg).
Pediatric Dosage (Oral or Rectal): See pentobarbital.
Pediatric Dosage (Parenteral): For acute convulsions, 3–5 mg/kg IM or slow IV, repeated q. 3–4h, prn.
Contraindications: Obstetric deliveries. (See also barbiturates.)
Precautions: See barbiturates.
Adverse Reactions: See barbiturates.
Drug Interactions: See barbiturates.

Generic Name: TEMAZEPAM
Trade Name: Restoril
Dosage Forms: Capsules, 15 mg and 30 mg
Uses: Benzodiazepine derivative (intermediate to short-acting) for insomnia.
Adult Dosage (Oral): 15–30 mg at bedtime.
Contraindications: Pregnancy.
Precautions: Avoid use during pregnancy (may be teratogenic). Use cautiously in elderly or debilitated patients (give reduced dosages), in renal or hepatic impairment, or in states of mental depression. Nocturnal sleep disturbances may be experienced during first or second night after discontinuance of the medication. May be habit-forming. Abrupt discontinuance after prolonged use may precipitate barbiturate-like withdrawal symptoms.
Adverse Reactions: Drowsiness, dizziness, lethargy, weakness, ataxia, anorexia, diarrhea. Rarely, palpitations, nystagmus, paradoxical excitement, or hyperactivity.
Drug Interactions: Additive CNS depression with other CNS depressants and tranquilizers.

Generic Name: THIOPENTAL IV (Barbiturate-derivative)
Trade Name: Pentothal
Dosage Forms: Injection (IV only), 500 mg/20 mL
Uses: Anesthesia for brief procedures, induction anesthesia, anticonvulsant. Also used for narcoanalysis in psychiatric disorders.
Adult Dosage (Parenteral): Dosage must be titrated to response.
Contraindications: Absence of suitable veins for IV administration. Hypersensitivity to barbiturates. Latent or manifest porphyria.
Precautions: Extravasation or intra-arterial injection should be avoided. Test dose of 25–75 mg recommended. Use with caution in advanced cardiac disease, increased intracranial pressure, asthma, myasthenia gravis, and pregnancy.
Adverse Reactions: Repeated doses lead to prolonged anesthesia owing to drug accumulation in fatty tissues. IV reactions as for reactions to IV administration of barbiturates.

Generic Name: TRIAZOLAM
Trade Name: Halcion
Dosage Forms: Tablets, 0.25 mg, 0.50 mg

Uses: Sedative-hypnotic (short-acting benzodiazepine derivative) for short-term management of insomnia.
Adult Dosage (Oral): 0.25–0.50 mg at bedtime as needed.
Contraindications: Hypersensitivity to benzodiazepines, pregnancy.
Precautions: Reduce dosage by 50% for elderly or debilitated patients. See also flurazepam and temazepam.
Adverse Reactions: See flurazepam and temazepam.
Drug Interactions: See flurazepam and temazepam.

SKELETAL MUSCLE RELAXANTS

Generic Name: ATRACURIUM
Trade Name: Tracrium
Dosage Form: Injection, 10 mg/mL in 5 and 10 mL vials (refrigerate)
Uses: Nondepolarizing neuromuscular blocker. Indicated as an adjunct to anesthesia, to induce skeletal muscle relaxation, to facilitate the management of patients undergoing mechanical ventilation, to facilitate tracheal intubation. Renal and hepatic mechanisms as well as plasma cholinesterase are not involved in the metabolism of atracurium. The drug undergoes (1) Hofmann degradation, a pH- and temperature-dependent process in which the drug molecule spontaneously breaks down, and (2) hydrolysis by nonspecific plasma esterases.
Adult Dosage (Parenteral): Should be administered only by or under the supervision of clinicians experienced in the use of this agent. For intubation—0.4 to 0.5 mg/kg IV. Subsequent doses for relaxation must be individualized. Generally, an IV infusion consisting of 250 mg of atracurium in 250 mL of a suitable diluent to run at a rate of 5 to 10 μg/kg/min is used.
Pediatric Dosage (Parenteral): ≥2 years old—same as adult. 1 month to 2 years—0.3 to 0.4 mg/kg followed by a maintenance dose of 0.3 to 0.4 mg/kg every 20 to 45 minutes as required to maintain neuromuscular blockade. The manufacturer does not recommend continuous infusion of the drug in children <2 years of age.
Contraindications: Hypersensitivity to the drug product.
Precautions: Use with caution in patients with pre-existing pulmonary or renal dysfunction (avoid prolonged infusion). Laudanosine, a metabolite of atracurium, exogenously administered in large quantities has been shown to cause CNS excitation and even seizure. Significant blood levels of laudanosine do exist in patients with renal failure who receive atracurium infusions for several days. Release of histamine may occur infrequently with rapid bolus injection of an intubating dose of atracurium. Therefore, administer slowly and cautiously, especially in patients where histamine release may prove hazardous (ie, significant cardiovascular disease and asthma). Conditions of slower circulation time (eg, old age, heart disease) may delay onset. Atracurium has no effect on pain threshold or consciousness. Electrolyte imbalance may alter neuromuscular blockade. Respiratory acidosis, metabolic alkalosis, and hypothermia may result in prolonged neuromuscular blockade. Markedly prolonged neuromuscular blockade can occur in patients with myasthenia gravis. Neuromuscular function should be monitored via peripheral nerve simulators. Inadequate airway protection and risk of aspiration exist. Reversal of neuromuscular blockade—(1) atropine, 7 to 9 μg/kg plus edrophonium, 0.5 to 1 mg/kg, or (2) glycopyrrolate, 7.5 μg/kg, or atropine, 15 μg/kg, plus neostigmine, 40 to 70 μg/kg.
Adverse Reactions: Generally well tolerated except for occasional prolonged neuromuscular blockade and adverse reactions suggestive of histamine release (ie, cutaneous flushing, hypotension, and rarely bronchospasm).
Drug Interactions: See pancuronium.

Generic Name: CARISOPRODOL
Trade Name: Soma
Dosage Forms: Tablets, 350 mg (also with codeine, 16 mg, phenacetin, caffeine)
Uses: Skeletal muscle relaxant used as adjunctive therapy for acute muscle spasms associated with trauma, tension, or inflammation. Ineffective for spasticity caused by neurologic disorders or drug-induced extrapyramidal reactions.
Adult Dosage (Oral): 350 mg tid and at bedtime.
Pediatric Dosage (Oral): For a child 5 years or older, 25 mg/kg/d divided qid.
Contraindications: Acute intermittent porphyria; hypersensitivity to carisoprodol or related compounds, such as meprobamate.
Precautions: Causes mental impairment and reflex slowing. Renal or hepatic impairment. Mild withdrawal symptoms after large doses (100 mg/kg/d).
Adverse Reactions: See methocarbamol. Idiosyncratic reactions after first to fourth dose have occurred; these include CNS derangement, diplopia, temporary vision loss, ataxia, stammering, transient quadriplegia, extreme weakness, confusion, and disorientation.
Drug Interactions: Additive CNS depression with alcohol, tranquilizers, sedative-hypnotics.

Generic Name: CYCLOBENZAPRINE
Trade Name: Flexeril
Dosage Forms: Tablets, 10 mg
Uses: Skeletal muscle relaxant used as adjunctive therapy for painful muscle spasms caused by trauma, tension, or inflammation.
Adult Dosage (Oral): 10 mg tid (range, 20–60 mg/d in divided doses for not more than 2 or 3 weeks).
Contraindications: Hypersensitivity to cyclobenzaprine, hyperthyroidism, MAO inhibitor therapy, severe cardiovascular conditions.
Precautions: Closely related to tricyclic antidepressants so use cautiously in patients with cardiac disease (congestive heart failure, arrhythmias, and acute recovery phase of myocardial infarction). Do not use concurrently or within 14 days of therapy with MAO inhibitors. Use with caution in the elderly and in patients with glaucoma, urinary retention, or other conditions aggravated by anticholinergic effects. Abrupt termination of prolonged therapy may cause a withdrawal syndrome. Caution patients that drug-induced drowsiness can impair ability to perform hazardous tasks.
Adverse Reactions: Frequently, drowsiness, dizziness, lethargy, nervousness, confusion. Anticholinergic effects include dry mouth, blurred vision, urinary retention, tachycardia. Also, gas-

tric upset, unpleasant taste in mouth, rashes, urticaria, facial edema, muscle twitching, weakness, CNS derangements, hypotension, syncope, palpitations, and arrhythmias.

Drug Interactions: With MAO inhibitors, hypertensive crisis and convulsions. Additive CNS depression with other CNS depressants. Additive anticholinergic effects with other anticholinergic agents. Decreased antihypertensive effect with clonidine and guanethidine.

Generic Name: DANTROLENE
Trade Name: Dantrium
Dosage Forms: Capsules, 25, 50, 100 mg; injection, 20 mg/vial
Uses: Skeletal muscle relaxant that does not alter contraction in cardiac or smooth muscle. Indicated for the treatment of malignant hyperthermia (IV), possibly neuroleptic malignant syndrome (IV), chronic spasticity (oral), and prophylaxis of malignant hyperthermia (IV/PO).
Adult Dosage (Parenteral): Malignant hyperthermia—1–2 mg/kg IV via rapid infusion (may be given repeatedly to a total of 10 mg/kg if needed) followed by 2–5 mg/kg IV every 4 hours with continuous monitoring for the first 24 hours after the initial event; then oral administration of 1–2 mg/kg four times daily may be necessary for 1–3 days to prevent recurrence. In patients susceptible to malignant hyperthermia, prophylactic dantrolene can be administered—2.5 mg/kg IV 90 minutes before surgery.
Adult Dosage (Oral): Spasticity—initially 25 mg PO daily, then gradually increase by 25 mg every 4–7 days to a maximum daily dose of 400 mg given in 4 divided doses. Prophylaxis of malignant hyperthermia—1 to 2 mg/kg PO in 4 divided doses for 1 to 2 days prior to surgery, with last dose given approximately 3 to 4 hours before scheduled surgery.
Pediatric Dosage (Parenteral): Dosage is the same as for adults for the treatment of malignant hyperthermia.
Pediatric Dosage (Oral): Chronic spasticity—initially 0.5 mg/kg/dose PO twice daily; then increase frequency to tid-qid at 4- to 7-day intervals; then increase dose by 0.5 mg/kg up to a maximum of 100 mg/24 hours.
Contraindications: Active hepatic disease; when spasticity is utilized to sustain upright posture and balance in locomotion or to obtain or maintain increased function.
Precautions: Fatal and nonfatal liver disorders (greater likelihood in females > 35 years of age) of an idiosyncratic or hypersensitivity type may occur; therefore, baseline liver function studies should be performed prior to the initiation of therapy and at appropriate intervals throughout therapy; therapy should be discontinued if such studies reveal abnormal values unless the benefit far outweighs the risk. Long-term safety and efficacy have not been established. IV use in malignant hyperthermia should not be a substitute for (but rather an adjunct to) known supportive measures such as discontinuing suspected triggering agents, addressing increased oxygen requirements, managing metabolic acidosis, instituting cooling when needed, attending to urinary output, and monitoring electrolyte imbalance. Use with caution in patients with impaired pulmonary and cardiac function. Photosensitization may occur; therefore, patients should be cautioned to take protective measures (ie, sunscreens and protective clothing) against exposure to UV light or sunlight until tolerance is determined. Precautions to prevent extravasation into surrounding tissue when using the IV route (due to the increased pH of the solution) should be instituted. Avoid alcohol and other CNS depressants.
Adverse Reactions: Most frequently reported (and generally transient) include drowsiness, dizziness, weakness, general malaise, fatigue, and diarrhea. Others include GI—hepatitis, constipation, GI bleeding, anorexia, dysphagia, gastric irritation, abdominal cramps; CNS—speech disturbances, seizures, headache, lightheadedness, visual disturbances, diplopia, taste disturbances, insomnia, mental depression and confusion, increased nervousness; CV—tachycardia, erratic blood pressure, phlebitis; GU—increased urinary frequency, hematuria, crystalluria, urinary incontinence, dysuria, urinary retention; DERM—abnormal hair growth, acne-like rash, pruritus, urticaria, eczematoid eruption, sweats, musculoskeletal myalgia, backache; other—fever, chills, feeling of suffocation, excessive tearing, pleural effusion with pericarditis.
Drug Interactions: With warfarin and clofibrate, results in reduced plasma protein binding of dantrolene. With tolbutamide, results in increased plasma protein binding of dantrolene. With estrogens, may be associated with an increased risk for hepatotoxicity in women. With nondepolarizing skeletal muscle relaxants, may have an additive muscle relaxant effect.

Generic Name: DIAZEPAM
Trade Name: Valium
Dosage Forms: Injection (IM/IV), 5 mg/mL; tablets, 2 mg, 5 mg, 10 mg; capsules, 15 mg (sustained-release)
Uses: Benzodiazepine derivative used as skeletal muscle relaxant for adjunctive treatment of acute, painful muscle spasm, including tetany and that caused by trauma, inflammation, or upper motor neuron disorders. Also given for short-term relief of anxiety and management of acute alcohol withdrawal. See also anticonvulsants.
Adult Dosage (Oral): For acute muscle spasm or anxiety, 2–10 mg bid to qid, depending on severity. For acute alcohol withdrawal symptoms, 5–10 mg q. 1–4h as needed during first 24 hours, then decrease dose as tolerated.
Adult Dosage (Parenteral): For acute muscle spasms, 5–10 mg slowly IV; can be repeated in 3–4 hours. For tetany, 5–20 mg slowly IV q. 2–8h as needed.
Pediatric Dosage (Oral): For muscle spasms or adjunctive anticonvulsant therapy in a child over 6 months, 1–2.5 mg tid to qid initially, then increased gradually as needed.
Pediatric Dosage (Parenteral): (IV bolus doses should be given over at least 3 min.) For tetany in a child 1 month to 5 years, 1–2 mg slowly IV, repeated in 3–4 hours as needed; for a child over 5 years, 5–10 mg slowly IV, repeated q. 3–4h as needed.
Contraindications: Hypersensitivity to benzodiazepines. Newborns up to 1 month old, shock, coma, psychosis, acute alcohol withdrawal seizures if vital signs are depressed. Relative contraindications for prolonged use: acute narrow angle and open angle glaucoma.
Precautions: IV doses should be given slowly undiluted and into the injection port closest to the infusion site; flush IV line after administration of dose. Avoid extravasation or intra-arterial administration. Monitor blood pressure and respiration closely since cumulative dose increases. IV administration can cause severe hypotension. IM doses are slowly and erratically absorbed so they are not recommended for acute seizure control. Use with

caution in depressed or suicidal patients. Reduce doses and give cautiously to elderly or debilitated patients, those with hepatic impairment, and infants and children. Higher doses may be required in excessive smokers. May be habit-forming and cause barbiturate-like withdrawal symptoms.

Adverse Reactions: For oral use: drowsiness, ataxia, fatigue, vertigo, dizziness, paradoxical hyperexcitability, hallucinations, nightmares (especially in the elderly), rash, hepatic abnormalities, and jaundice. In addition from parenteral use: tissue necrosis, thrombophlebitis, hypotension, respiratory depression, premature ventricular contractions, laryngospasm, and cardiovascular collapse.

Drug Interactions: Do not mix injection with any other medications or aqueous solutions. Additive CNS depression with other CNS depressants. Cimetidine may impair hepatic metabolism of diazepam so excessive sedation may occur.

Generic Name: METHOCARBAMOL
Trade Name: Robaxin
Dosage Forms: Tablets, 500 mg, 750 mg; injection (IM/IV), 100 mg/mL
Uses: Skeletal muscle relaxant used as adjunctive therapy for acute, painful musculoskeletal conditions and tetanus. Ineffective for spasticity caused by neurologic disorders or drug-induced extrapyramidal reactions.
Adult Dosage (Oral): 1.5 g qid for initial 48–72 hours, then 750 mg–1 g qid (up to 4.5 g/d).
Adult Dosage (Parenteral): 100–300 mg/d IM or IV for up to 3 days. May repeat after 48 hours; for tetany, 100–300 mg IV q. 6h until nasogastric tube can be inserted.
Pediatric Dosage (Parenteral): For tetany, 15 mg/kg or more, slow IV q. 6h (rate under 3 mL/min).
Contraindications: Hypersensitivity to methocarbamol. Renal disease (contraindication with injectable form only).
Precautions: Can dilute IV bolus doses with D_5W or NS. IV bolus rate should not exceed 300 mg/min (3 mL/min undiluted). Avoid extravasation since tissue sloughing can occur. Drug will not mix with blood if aspirated into same syringe. Propylene glycol diluent in injectable form may be nephrotoxic. IV administration causes convulsions; use cautiously in those with epileptic disorders, renal impairment, and metabolic acidosis.
Adverse Reactions: Oral administration may produce sedation, dizziness, lethargy, gastric upset, and allergic reactions. Parenteral administration may produce nausea, vomiting, syncope, hypotension, bradycardia, metallic taste, blurred vision, facial flushing, respiratory depression, thrombophlebitis, anaphylaxis, and convulsions.
Drug Interactions: See carisoprodol.

Generic Name: PANCURONIUM
Trade Name: Pavulon
Dosage Form: Injection, 1 mg/mL in 10 mL vials; 2 mg/mL in 2 and 5 mL ampules (refrigerate)
Uses: Nondepolarizing neuromuscular blocker approximately ⅓ less potent than vecuronium. Indicated as an adjunct to anesthesia, to induce skeletal muscle relaxation; to facilitate the management of patients undergoing mechanical ventilation; to facilitate tracheal intubation.
Adult Dosage (Parenteral): Should be administered only by or under the supervision of clinicians experienced in the use of this agent. For intubation—0.07 to 0.08 mg/kg IV. Subsequent doses for relaxation must be individualized. Generally, subsequent doses are given every 40 to 60 minutes at 25% to 50% of the original dose.
Pediatric Dosage (Parenteral): Newborn (≤1 month)—initially 0.03 mg/kg/dose repeat ×2 at intervals of 5 to 10 minutes as needed, then maintain at 0.03 to 0.09 mg/kg/dose every 0.5 to 4 hours as needed (titrate dose to achieve a dosage interval of 3 to 4 hours). Infant (>1 month)—0.06 to 0.1 mg/kg/dose initially, then maintain at 0.02 to 0.1 mg/kg/dose every 40 to 60 minutes as needed.
Contraindications: Hypersensitivity to the drug product.
Precautions: Use with caution in patients with pre-existing pulmonary, renal, or hepatic disease. Conditions of slower circulation time (eg, old age, heart disease) may delay onset. Pancuronium has no effect on pain threshold or consciousness. Electrolyte imbalance may alter neuromuscular blockade. Respiratory acidosis, metabolic alkalosis, and hypothermia may result in prolonged neuromuscular blockade. Markedly prolonged neuromuscular blockade can occur in patients with myasthenia gravis. Pancuronium administration can precipitate tachycardia as a result of the drug's vagolytic properties. Neuromuscular function should be monitored via peripheral nerve stimulators. Inadequate airway protection and risk of aspiration exist. Reversal of neuromuscular blockade—(1) atropine, 7 to 9 μg/kg, plus edrophonium, 0.5 to 1 mg/kg; or (2) glycopyrrolate, 7.5 μg/kg, or atropine, 15 μg/kg, plus neostigmine, 40 to 70 μg/kg.
Adverse Reactions: Prolonged neuromuscular blockade, tachycardia, salivation, transient rash, hypersensitivity reactions (anaphylactoid).
Drug Interactions: With antibiotics (aminoglycosides, polymyxin B, bacitracin, tetracycline, colistin, clindamycin, lincomycin), may prolong the action of neuromuscular blockers (penicillins and cephalosporins have no effect). With magnesium salts in pre-eclampsia or lithium in psychiatric patients, can result in an increased sensitivity to neuromuscular blockers and prolonged paralysis. With lidocaine, quinidine, and procainamide, may increase sensitivity to neuromuscular blockers. Theophyllines and azathioprine may reverse the blocking effects of neuromuscular blockers. Diuretics may alter neuromuscular blockade via their effect on electrolyte balance.

Generic Name: VECURONIUM
Trade Name: Norcuron
Dosage Forms: Injection, 10 mg powder for injection in 5 and 10 mL vials
Uses: Nondepolarizing neuromuscular blocker. Indicated as an adjunct to anesthesia, to induce skeletal muscle relaxation, to facilitate the management of patients undergoing mechanical ventilation, to facilitate tracheal intubation.
Adult Dosage (Parenteral): Should be administered only by or under the supervision of clinicians experienced in the use of this agent. For intubation—0.08 to 0.1 mg/kg IV. Subsequent doses for relaxation must be individualized. Generally, an IV infusion consisting of 100 mg of vecuronium in 250 mL of a suitable diluent to run at a rate of 1 to 2 μg/kg/min is used.
Pediatric Dosage (Parenteral): (<7 weeks old)—not recommended. (7 weeks to 1 year old)—initially, 0.08 to 0.1 mg/kg/

dose, then maintain at 0.01 to 0.015 mg/kg/dose every 30 to 60 minutes as needed. (>1 year old)—initially, 0.08 to 0.1 mg/kg/dose, then maintain at 0.01 to 0.015 mg/kg/dose every 25 to 40 minutes as needed.

Contraindications: Hypersensitivity to the drug product.

Precautions: Use with caution in patients with pre-existing pulmonary, renal, or hepatic disease. Conditions of slower circulation time (eg, old age, heart disease) may delay onset. Vecuronium has no effect on pain threshold or consciousness. Electrolyte imbalance may alter neuromuscular blockade. Respiratory acidosis, metabolic alkalosis, and hypothermia may result in prolonged neuromuscular blockade. Markedly prolonged neuromuscular blockade can occur in patients with myasthenia gravis. Neuromuscular function should be monitored via peripheral nerve stimulators. Inadequate airway protection and risk of aspiration exist. Reversal of neuromuscular blockade—(1) atropine, 7 to 9 µg/kg, plus edrophonium, 0.5 to 1 mg/kg; or (2) glycopyrrolate, 7.5 µg/kg, or atropine, 15 µg/kg, plus neostigmine, 40 to 70 µg/kg.

Adverse Reactions: Generally well tolerated except for occasional prolonged neuromuscular blockade.

Drug Interactions: See pancuronium.

PLASMA VOLUME EXPANDERS

Generic Name: ALBUMIN (Human)
Trade Names: Normal Serum Albumin, Albutein, others
Dosage Forms: Injection (IV), 250 mg/mL (25%) in 50 mL; 50 mg/mL (5%) in 250 mL, 500 mL
Uses: Plasma volume expander. Also given for hypoproteinemia and as an adjunct to exchange transfusions in the treatment of hyperbilirubinemia and erythroblastosis fetalis.
Adult Dosage (Parenteral): For hypovolemic shock, usual dose is 25 g (100 mL of 25% solution) IV rapidly. May be repeated in 15–30 min (up to 125 g/d, maximum). As plasma volume returns to normal, IV infusion should be slowed to 1 mL/min (or 2–4 mL/min of 5% solution) or less to prevent circulatory overload. For burns, give sufficient amount to raise plasma oncotic pressure to 20 mmHg or total serum protein concentration to 5.2 g/dL.
Pediatric Dosage (Parenteral): Use 5% solution only; can dilute 25% solution (1:4) with NS. All doses given are for 5% concentration: For hypovolemic shock, 10–20 mL/kg/dose slow IV; can repeat in 15–30 min; for burns, 10 mL/kg/dose slow IV with electrolyte solutions; for hyperbilirubinemia, 20 mL/kg slow IV, given 1 to 2 hours before exchange transfusion.
Contraindications:Ცardiac failure, severe anemia.
Precautions: All commercial preparations contain 130–160 mEq sodium per L. Rapid infusion rates (over 1 mL/min for 25% or 4 mL/min for 5% solutions) may cause circulatory overload in patients whose plasma volume has almost returned to normal. Administration of albumin to dehydrated patients may be ineffective unless additional IV fluids are given. Use cautiously in congestive heart failure, pulmonary edema, and those with low cardiac reserve or no albumin deficiency. The rapid rise in blood pressure induced by albumin may reveal bleeding points not apparent at lower pressures in patients with traumatic injuries or those undergoing surgery.
Adverse Reactions: See plasma protein fraction. However, since albumin is more highly purified than plasma protein fraction, it may be less likely to cause adverse allergic reactions and hypotension.

Generic Name: DEXTRAN 40, 70, 75
Trade Names: Rheomacrodex, Dextran 40, Dextran 70, Gentran-40, Gentran-75, Macrodex
Dosage Forms: Injection (IV), Dextran 40 (10%) in 500 mL NS or D_5W; Dextran 70 (6%) in 500 mL/NS or D_5W; Dextran 75 (6%) in 500 mL NS, D_5W, or 10% invert sugar
Uses: Plasma volume expander. Dextran 70 and 75 are high-molecular-weight polymers; Dextran 40 is a low-molecular-weight polymer.
Adult Dosage (Parenteral): For administration of Dextran 40, 10–20 mL/kg slow IV (not to exceed 20 mL/kg/d); if therapy continued for more than 24 hours, total daily dose should not exceed 10 mL/kg/d. For administration of Dextran 70 or 75, 500 to 1000 mL slow IV at 20–40 mL/min initially; reduce to 4 mL/min as plasma volume approaches normal; total dose should not exceed 20 mL/kg/d during first 24 hours and 10 mL/kg/d thereafter.
Pediatric Dosage (Parenteral): Same as adult dosage.
Contraindications: Hypersensitivity to dextrans. Severe congestive heart failure, renal failure, hypervolemic states, bleeding disorders.
Precautions: As for hetastarch. Antigenic potential greater with high-molecular-weight dextrans than with the low-molecular-weight preparations; observe patient closely during the first few minutes of administration. Avoid prolonged therapy over 5 days.
Adverse Reactions: Hypersensitivity reactions include rash, urticaria, pruritus, nasal congestion, dyspnea, chest tightness, and mild hypotension. Angioedema, bronchospasm, and anaphylaxis have occurred, as well as nausea, vomiting, fever, arthralgia, osmotic nephrosis (renal tubular vacuolization), and acute hypotension.

Generic Name: HETASTARCH (Hydroxyethyl starch)
Trade Names: Volex, Hespan
Dosage Forms: Injection (IV), 6% hetastarch in 500 mL normal saline
Uses: Plasma volume expander.
Adult Dosage (Parenteral): 500–1000 mL by IV infusion (up to 20 mL/kg/d or 1500 mL/d). For acute hemorrhagic shock, may be administered at 20 mL/kg/h; for burns and septic shock, administered at less than 20 mL/kg/h.
Contraindications: Severe bleeding disorders; severe congestive cardiac and renal failure with oliguria or anuria.
Precautions: Can cause circulatory overload so central venous pressure should be monitored. Large doses may prolong prothrombin and bleeding times (antiplatelet effect), decrease hematocrit, and dilute plasma proteins. Use cautiously in very young patients, the elderly, and those with congestive heart failure, pulmonary edema, thrombocytopenia, renal or hepatic impairment. Reduce dose by 25%–50% in severe renal impairment.
Adverse Reactions: Minimal antigenic properties, but allergic reactions have been reported, including vomiting, mild fever, chills, itching, parotid gland enlargement, headaches, urticaria, peripheral and periorbital edema, and wheezing.

Generic Name: PLASMA PROTEIN FRACTION (Human)
Trade Name: Plasmanate
Dosage Forms: Injection (IV) (5%), 250 mL, 500 mL
Uses: Plasma volume expander.
Adult Dosage (Parenteral): For hypovolemic shock, 250–500 mL IV infusion at 10 mL/min or less; as plasma volume approaches normal, rate should be slowed to 5–8 mL/min. For hypoproteinemia, 1000–1500 mL/d IV.
Pediatric Dosage (Parenteral): For hypovolemic shock, 5–7 mL/kg infused IV at rate of 10 mL/min or less.
Contraindications: Cardiopulmonary bypass procedures. Severe anemia (possible contraindication).
Precautions: Does not provide coagulation factors. IV rates over 10 mL/min may cause vascular overload with pulmonary edema and cardiac failure. Commercial preparations contain 130–160 mEq sodium per L; must be used cautiously in patients with hepatic, renal, or cardiac failure. See also albumin.
Adverse Reactions: Infrequent, but include flushing, nausea, vomiting, chills, fever, headache, back pain, hypersalivation, erythema, and urticaria.

THYROID/ANTITHYROID AGENTS

Generic Name: LEVOTHYROXINE
Trade Name: Synthroid
Dosage Forms: Tablets, 25 μg, 50 μg, 100 μg, 150 μg, 200 μg, 300 μg; injection (IV), 500 μg vial
Uses: Thyroid preparation for treatment of hypothyroidism or absent thyroid function and cretinism. Given parenterally for treatment of myxedema coma or stupor.
Adult Dosage (Oral): 25–50 μg/d initially as a single dose, increased by 25–50 μg at 2- to 3-week intervals until desired response is obtained (usual maintenance dose, 100–200 μg/d).
Adult Dosage (Parenteral): For myxedema coma without heart disease, 200–500 μg IV to start, repeated in 1–2 days with 100–300 μg; for maintenance, 50–100 μg/d IV until oral doses tolerated. When converting from the oral to IV route, ½ the oral dose should be given.
Pediatric Dosage (Oral): For a child 11 to 20 years, 3 μg/kg/d; for 6 to 10 years, 4 μg/kg/d; for 1 to 5 years, 6 μg/kg/d; for infant to 1 year, 9 μg/kg/d. Doses can be increased every 2 to 5 weeks to desired response (up to 400 μg/d).
Contraindications: Acute myocardial infarction, uncorrected adrenal insufficiency, thyrotoxicosis.
Precautions: Caution required in patients with cardiovascular disease or acute myocardial infarction. The status of other metabolic diseases, including diabetes, adrenal insufficiency, hyperadrenalism, and hypopituitarism, may be affected by changes in thyroid status (may unmask symptoms).
Adverse Reactions: Headache, nervousness, tremor, palpitations, tachycardia, angina, cardiac arrhythmias, diarrhea, abdominal cramps, heat intolerance, diaphoresis, and weight loss may occur. All are dose related and may be avoided by slow dosage increases.
Drug Interactions: With oral anticoagulants, potentiation of hypoprothombinemic effect. With insulin and oral hypoglycemics, decreased hypoglycemic effect. With tricyclic antidepressants, potentiation of antidepressant effects. With phenytoin, possible increase in thyroxine blood level.

Generic Name: PROPYLTHIOURACIL
Trade Name: Propylthiouracil, PTU
Dosage Form: Tablet, 50 mg
Uses: Treatment of hyperthyroidism and thyroid storm (antithyroid).
Adult Dosage (Oral): 100 mg q. 8h initially and continued for 6–8 weeks until patient is euthyroid. Then, dosage is reduced by one third every 4–6 weeks to maintenance levels of 100–150 mg/d. Occasionally, resistant patients may require initial doses of 600–1200 mg/d, divided q. 4–8h.
Pediatric Dosage (Oral): For a child 6–10 years old, 50–150 mg/d until euthyroid, then 50 mg bid. For a child over 10 years, 150–300 mg/d until euthyroid, then 50 mg bid. For a newborn, 5–10 mg/kg/d.
Contraindications: Last few weeks of pregnancy/lactation; hypersensitivity to PTU.
Precautions: Use cautiously in pregnancy and those on anticoagulant therapy. Possible cross-allergenicity with methimazole (low incidence). Potentially serious agranulocytosis can develop; monitor patient carefully during first few months; have patient report any signs and symptoms of fever, sore throat, chills, skin eruptions, rash, or general malaise.
Adverse Reactions: Rashes, urticaria (dose-related). Occasional gastrointestinal disturbances, drowsiness, headache, dizziness, paresthesias, myalgia, arthralgia, hypoprothrombinemia, salivary gland and lymph node enlargement, loss of taste, visual disturbances, and edema may occur. Mild leukopenia (white blood cell count under 4000/mm³) occurs in about 10% of patients treated and is usually not an indication for discontinuation of the drug. However, severe leukopenia, thrombocytopenia, and agranulocytosis require discontinuance. Also drug fever, lupus-like syndrome, and hepatitis have been reported.
Drug Interactions: May potentiate action of oral anticoagulants.

ERGOT ALKALOIDS, OXYTOCICS, ESTROGENS

Generic Name: CONJUGATED ESTROGENS
Trade Name: Premarin
Dosage Forms: Tablets, 0.3 mg, 0.625 mg, 1.25 mg, 2.5 mg; injection (IV), 25 mg
Uses: Estrogen replacement therapy in menopause, dysfunctional uterine bleeding, prostatic carcinoma, estrogen deficiency, osteoporosis. Parenterally, used for emergency treatment of dysfunctional uterine bleeding.
Adult Dosage (Oral): In menopause, 0.3–1.25 mg/d or cyclicly.
Adult Dosage (Parenteral): For emergency uterine bleeding, 25 mg slow IV stat, then 25 mg q. 6–12h prn (given slowly to prevent flushing).

Contraindications: Known or suspected breast cancer if estrogen-dependent neoplasms suspected. Pregnancy. History of thrombophlebitic disorders or active thrombophlebitis. Undiagnosed abnormal vaginal bleeding.

Precautions: With prolonged therapy, use cautiously in renal or hepatic disease and metastatic bone cancer associated with hypercalcemia. Possible increased risk of gallbladder disease or malignant neoplasms. Hypertension, fluid retention, and thromboembolism are all exacerbated.

Adverse Reactions: Nausea, vomiting, abdominal cramps, breakthrough bleeding, amenorrhea, breast enlargement, migraine headaches, cholestatic jaundice, edema, dermatologic changes, mental depression, steepening of corneal curvature, intolerance to contact lenses.

Drug Interactions: With oral anticoagulants, decreased anticoagulant effect. With tricyclic antidepressants, increased antidepressant side-effects.

Generic Name: ERGOTAMINE TARTRATE
Trade Names: Ergomar, Gynergen, Ergostat
Dosage Forms: Tablets (sublingual), 2 mg; tablets (oral), 1 mg; injection (subcutaneous/IM), 0.5 mg/mL; inhalation, 9 mg/mL; also available as Cafergot tablets containing 1 mg ergotamine plus 100 mg caffeine, and Cafergot rectal suppositories containing 2 mg ergotamine plus 100 mg caffeine
Uses: Ergot alkaloid for treatment of migraine (vascular) headaches.
Adult Dosage (Oral): 2–3 mg initially (or 1–2 mg sublingually), then 1–2 mg q. ½–1h to a maximum of 6 mg/d or 10 mg/wk. For inhalation therapy, one inhalation stat, then q. 5 min prn (up to 6/d). Cafergot tablets are given as follows: 2 tablets at start of attack, then 1 tablet q. 30 min prn (maximum of 6 tablets/attack or 10 tablets/wk). For Cafergot suppositories, 1 suppository is given stat; may be repeated once (maximum of 2 suppositories/attack or 4 suppositories/wk).
Adult Dosage (Parenteral): 0.25–0.5 mg IM or subcutaneously to start; repeated once in 2 hours (up to 1 mg/wk).
Contraindications: Pregnancy, occlusive vascular disease, coronary heart disease, hypertension, hepatic or renal impairment, sepsis, severe pruritus, cellulitis. Hypersensitivity to ergot alkaloids.
Precautions: Overdosing or prolonged administration may lead to ergotism and eventual gangrene.
Adverse Reactions: Nausea, vomiting, diarrhea, muscle weakness and pain in extremities, tingling in fingers and toes, localized edema, itching, occasional headaches. Also precordial distress, tachycardia, bradycardia, gangrene (rare).

Generic Name: METHYLERGONOVINE MALEATE
Trade Name: Methergine
Dosage Forms: Tablets, 0.2 mg; injection (IM/IV) 0.2 mg/mL
Generic Name: ERGONOVINE MALEATE
Trade Name: Ergotrate
Dosage Forms: Tablets, 0.2 mg; injection (IM/IV), 0.2 mg/mL
Uses: Used postpartum after placental delivery to produce firm uterine contractions and decrease uterine bleeding.
Adult Dosage (Oral): 0.2 mg bid to qid for 2 days, usually.

Adult Dosage (Parenteral): 0.2 mg IM; can be repeated in 2–4 hours if bleeding is severe.
Contraindications: See ergotamine; toxemia.
Precautions: See ergotamine. Avoid IV administration (can induce hypertensive cerebral vascular accident); if used, administer doses slowly over at least 1 min and monitor blood pressure continuously.
Adverse Reactions: Nausea, vomiting, dizziness, headache, tinnitus, transient hypertension, diaphoresis, temporary chest pain, palpitations, dyspnea.

Generic Name: METHYSERGIDE MALEATE
Trade Name: Sansert
Dosage Form: Tablets, 2 mg
Uses: Serotonin antagonist for prevention and reduction in frequency of vascular headaches (severe and/or uncontrollable ones that necessitate prophylaxis).
Adult Dosage (Oral): 4–8 mg/d with meals (divided doses).
Contraindications: See ergotamine. Also pulmonary disease, collagen or fibrotic disease, valvular heart disease.
Precautions: With long-term uninterrupted treatment, retroperitoneal and pleuropulmonary fibrosis, fibrotic thickening of cardiac valves and murmurs may occur. Continuous administration should not exceed 6 months, with 3–4 weeks of no drug every 6 months.
Adverse Reactions: Cold, numb extremities; leg cramps; girdle and flank pain; urinary obstruction; nausea; vomiting; diarrhea; CNS changes; edema; and flushing.

Generic Name: OXYTOCIN
Trade Names: Pitocin, Syntocinon
Dosage Forms: Injection (IM/IV), 5 U (5000 milliunits)/0.5 mL, 10 U (10,000 milliunits)/1 mL
Uses: Oxytocic agent to induce or stimulate labor. Also used postpartum to prevent or control hemorrhage and to induce abortion.
Adult Dosage (Parenteral): Dilute 10 U (1 mL) in 1000 mL D_5W or NS (concentration, 10 milliunits/mL); administer with controlled infusion device. For labor induction, begin with 1–2 milliunits/min. Gradually increase by 1–2 milliunits/min at 15- to 30-min intervals until contraction pattern similar to normal labor occurs (maximum dose should not exceed 40 milliunits/min). For prevention of postpartum hemorrhage, 10–40 milliunits/min (up to 100 milliunits/min may be needed). To induce abortion, 20–40 milliunits/min (up to 100 milliunits/min may be necessary).
Contraindications: Any contraindication to induction of labor.
Precautions: Hyperstimulation of uterus during labor may lead to uterine tetany (discontinue oxytocin stat). Concurrent administration of vasopressors may cause severe hypertension and cerebral hemorrhage. Avoid IM route since effects may be unpredictable and difficult to control.
Adverse Reactions: Severe water intoxication with convulsions and coma may occur with IV rates exceeding 20 milliunits/min or 24-hour infusions. Hypertensive episodes, subarachnoid hemorrhage, nausea, vomiting, rupture of uterus, anaphylactic reactions, neonatal jaundice, and fetal arrhythmias may occur.
Drug Interaction: Vasopressors (such as vasoconstrictors in anesthetics used for caudal block) may produce severe hypertension.

HEMATINICS

Generic Name: FERROUS SULFATE
Trade Name: Ledermark F20
Dosage Forms: Tablets, 325 mg (containing 65 mg elemental iron, but other strengths available); elixir, 300 mg/5 mL (other strengths available)
Uses: Treatment of iron-deficient anemia.
Adult Dosage (Oral): Usual therapeutic dose, 2–3 mg/kg/d of elemental iron (or 10–15 mg/kg/d of ferrous sulfate) in divided doses, tid (approximately 325 mg tid).
Pediatric Dosage (Oral): (Ferrous sulfate = 20% elemental iron.) For iron deficiency in a child or infant over 2 months, 4–6 mg/kg/d of elemental iron (20–30 mg/kg/d of ferrous sulfate) in divided doses tid. For prophylaxis, 1 mg/kg/d elemental iron (5 mg/kg/d ferrous sulfate) in divided doses tid.
Contraindications: Hemochromatosis, hemosiderosis, hemolytic anemias, peptic ulcer, regional enteritis, ulcerative colitis.
Precautions: Gastric upset can be minimized by taking doses with a small amount of food or milk. Liquid iron preparations may stain teeth or gum membranes in infants. Therapeutic effects after both oral or parenteral iron administration are slow to appear; rises in hemoglobin and hematocrit values may take 3 weeks to appear. Use cautiously in liver or gastrointestinal inflammatory disease. Avoid prolonged therapy (over 6 months) unless clinically indicated; since there is no excretory mechanism for iron, iron overload and hemosiderosis may occur. Avoid use in infants under 8 weeks of age since iron interferes with further vitamin E absorption in these already vitamin E–deficient infants, resulting in hemolytic anemia.
Adverse Reactions: Gastric irritation, black tarry stools, constipation, diarrhea, stained teeth (with liquid forms). Severe, acute poisoning occurs frequently in children; lethal dose for a child 2 to 5 years is 1–2 g elemental iron, but 300–400 mg can be potentially lethal. Toxic symptoms occur in stages: vomiting, gastrointestinal irritation, diarrhea (bloody or tarry), drowsiness, pallor, cyanosis, lassitude, shock, fever, metabolic acidosis, hepatic impairment or necrosis, bleeding, circulatory collapse, convulsions, and death. Treat overdoses with deferoxamine.
Drug Interactions: Vitamin C increases iron absorption. Food and antacids decrease absorption. Tetracycline chelated by iron so tetracycline absorption decreased. Allopurinol increases hepatic concentration of iron.

Generic Name: IRON DEXTRAN
Trade Name: Imferon
Dosage Forms: Injection (IM), 50 mg elemental iron/mL (contains 0.5% phenol); injection (IV), 50 mg elemental iron/mL (without phenol)
Uses: Hematinic for parenteral therapy of iron deficiency anemia when oral administration of iron is not feasible (eg, malabsorption syndrome, gastrointestinal disease, intolerance).
Adult Dosage (Parenteral): Calculated dose is based on hemoglobin deficit. For iron deficiency anemia, total iron requirement needed to replenish iron stores is:

$$\text{Total iron (mg)} = 0.3 \times \text{patient's weight (lb)} \times \left(100 - \frac{100 \times \text{Hgb}}{14.8}\right)$$

where Hgb = patient's observed hemoglobin in g/dL.

For iron replacement secondary to blood loss:

$$\text{Iron deficit (mg)} = \text{weight (kg)} \times 70 \text{ mL/kg} \times \left(0.45 - \frac{\text{Hct}}{100}\right)$$

where Hct = patient's observed hematocrit
Blood volume = 70 mL/kg
(*Note:* This formula does not allow for repletion of iron stores.)

Pediatric Dosage (Parenteral): Use same calculations for adult. For IM doses, do not exceed 0.1 mL (5 mg)/kg/dose.
Contraindications: Hypersensitivity to iron dextran, any anemia other than that caused by iron deficiency.
Precautions: *Do not administer subcutaneously.* To minimize staining of skin, use separate needles to withdraw drug from container and to inject it; use "Z-tract" technique; give doses deeply into upper outer quadrant of buttock, using 2- or 3-in, 19 or 20 gauge needles. Do not give the preparation containing phenol IV. The total calculated dose can be diluted in 250–1000 mL NS; give a 25-mg test dose (0.5 mL) slowly IV over 5 min; if no adverse reaction, administer the remaining solution slowly at 40–60 mL/h. Undiluted IV boluses should be administered no faster than 50 mg/min. Anaphylactic reactions are more frequent with IV route. Use cautiously in those with asthma, history of significant allergies, and renal or hepatic impairment. IV administration may exacerbate or reactivate joint pain or swelling in those with rheumatoid arthritis (use IM route only). Do not give iron dextran injections concurrently with oral iron preparations. See also ferrous sulfate.
Adverse Reactions: IV administration or rapid IV rates can cause anaphylaxis, shock, phlebitis, pain, peripheral vascular flushing, venospasm, arthralgia, myalgia, and fever. IM use can cause pain, inflammation, sterile abscesses, and skin staining. Rare sarcomas have been reported in animals after subcutaneous injections. Other reactions include dyspnea, sweating, fever, chills, backache, urticaria, rashes, nausea, vomiting, headache, paresthesias, syncope, faintness, hypotension, lymphadenopathy, metallic taste, malaise, and seizures.
Drug Interactions: See ferrous sulfate.

MISCELLANEOUS AGENTS FOR OVERDOSE TREATMENT

Generic Name: ACETYLCYSTEINE
Trade Name: Mucomyst
Dosage Forms: Solution, 10% and 20%
Uses: Used investigationally as an antidote for acute acetaminophen overdosage. More effective if given within 24 hours of the acetaminophen ingestion.
Adult Dosage (Oral): Dilute doses of 20% solution with 3 parts cola, citrus juice, or water to achieve a 5% (isotonic) solution. Initially, a loading dose of 140 mg/kg, followed by 70 mg/kg in 4 hours and q. 4h thereafter over a period of 68 hours (eg, 17 maintenance doses). If any of the doses are vomited within 1 hour of administration, repeat the dose. Can also administer doses by duodenal intubation.
Pediatric Dosage (Oral): Same as adult dosage.

Contraindications: Hypersensitivity to acetylcysteine.
Precautions: 20% solutions should be made isotonic (diluted to 5%) to minimize vomiting. Do not administer with activated charcoal since it will inactivate acetylcysteine. Supportive therapy should include gastric emptying by lavage or induction of emesis with syrup of ipecac. Draw blood sample for acetaminophen level stat and again in 4 hours; if 4-hour level has decreased to 120 μg/mL or less with no clinical or laboratory evidence of toxicity, acetylcysteine therapy may be discontinued.
Adverse Reactions: Oral doses are usually well tolerated with the exception of nausea and vomiting.

Generic Name: ACTIVATED CHARCOAL
Trade Names: Activated Charcoal, Actidose
Dosage Forms: Bulk powder; commercial suspension, 50 mg/240 mL
Uses: General-purpose antidote for immediate treatment of ingested poisons, including many drugs and noncorrosive chemicals.
Adult Dosage: Five to 10 times by weight the amount of ingested toxin. Usually 30 g in enough water to make a thick slurry, given orally or via a nasogastric tube (up to 100 g may be necessary).
Pediatric Dosage (Oral): Same as adult dosage.
Contraindications: All ingested corrosives, alkalis, mineral acids, cyanide, ethanol, methanol, organic solvents, iron salts; acetaminophen overdose when acetylcysteine has also been given.
Precautions: *Do not give simultaneously with ipecac syrup since the charcoal will absorb the syrup, rendering it ineffective.* Effectiveness of charcoal may be enhanced if given after induction of emesis. Palatability may be improved if charcoal is mixed in juice or if a small amount of chocolate syrup is added to slurry. (Do not use milk, ice cream, or sherbet for this purpose because they decrease the adsorptive capacity of the charcoal.) May make endoscopy difficult.
Adverse Reactions: None.

Generic Name: AMYL NITRITE
Trade Name: Amyl Nitrite
Dosage Form: Vaporoles for inhalation (0.3 mL)
Uses: For inhalation. Used in preliminary treatment of cyanide and thiocyanate poisoning. Also used as antianginal agent.
Adult and Pediatric Dosage: One vaporole administered by inhalation for 15–30 s of every minute while sodium nitrite solution is being prepared for IV administration. Hold under patient's nose or over Ambu-bag intake valve.

Generic Name: DEFEROXAMINE
Trade Name: Desferal
Dosage Forms: Injection (IM/IV), 500 mg
Uses: Iron-chelating agent for treatment of iron intoxication.
Adult Dosage (Parenteral): Usually, 1 g IM or IV, then 500 mg IM or slow IV q. 4h for two doses. Depending on clinical response, subsequent doses of 500 mg may be given q. 4–12h. (Maximum dose, 6 g/d.)
Pediatric Dosage (Parenteral): 20 mg/kg IM or slow IV, then 10 mg/kg q. 4h for two doses (or q. 4–12h if needed). Maximum dose is 6 g/d.
Contraindications: Severe renal disease or anuria.
Precautions: Gastric aspiration should be done first, then a lavage with 5% sodium bicarbonate to form insoluble iron carbonates. Deferoxamine will turn urine red. IM administration is preferred unless patient is in shock. Slow IV infusion not to exceed 15 mg/kg/h.
Adverse Reactions: Too rapid IV infusion causes histamine release with erythema, urticaria, hypotension, and shock. Also pain and induration at injection site.

Generic Name: FLUMAZENIL
Trade Name: Mazicon
Dosage Form: Injection, 0.1 mg/mL in 5 mL and 10 mL vials
Uses: Imidazobenzodiazepine derivative that antagonizes the actions of benzodiazepines on the central nervous system. Indicated for the complete or partial reversal of the sedative effects of benzodiazepines in cases where general anesthesia has been induced and/or maintained with a benzodiazepine; where sedation has been produced with a benzodiazepine for diagnostic and therapeutic procedures; and for the management of benzodiazepine overdose.
Adult Dosage (Parenteral): For the reversal of conscious sedation or general anesthesia—recommended initial dose is 0.2 mg administered IV over 15 seconds; if desired level of consciousness is not obtained after waiting an additional 45 seconds, then another 0.2-mg dose can be administered and repeated at 60-second intervals (up to a maximum of 4 additional times) to a maximum total dose of 1 mg; in the event of resedation, repeat doses may be administered at 20-min intervals as needed (no more than 3 mg in 1 hour or 1 mg at any one time). Benzodiazepine overdose—initial dose of 0.2 mg over 30 seconds; if desired level of consciousness is not obtained after waiting an additional 30 seconds, then a dose of 0.3 mg can be administered over 30 seconds; further dosages of 0.5 mg can be administered over 30 seconds at 1-minute intervals up to a cumulative dose of 3 mg.
Pediatric Dosage (Parenteral): Safety and efficacy are not established.
Contraindications: Hypersensitivity to flumazenil or benzodiazepines; patient receiving benzodiazepine for control of a potentially life-threatening condition (eg, status epilepticus); patient who is showing signs of serious cyclic antidepressant overdose.
Precautions: In overdose, flumazenil is an adjunct to but not a substitute for proper management of airway, assisted breathing, circulatory access, and adequate clinical evaluation. Reversal of benzodiazepine effects may be associated with the onset of seizures, especially in patients on benzodiazepines for long-term sedation or in overdose cases where the patient is showing signs of serious cyclic antidepressant overdose. May produce convulsions in patients physically dependent on benzodiazepines by precipitation of withdrawal. Use with caution in head injury, psychiatric illness, respiratory disease, alcohol dependence. Dosage adjustment following initial bolus may be required in hepatic disease. Patients who have received flumazenil should be monitored for resedation, respiratory depression, or other residual effects.
Adverse Reactions: Most common include dizziness, injection site pain, increased sweating, headache, and abnormal or blurred vision. Others include seizures, cutaneous vasodilation, nausea and vomiting, agitation, and confusion.

Drug Interactions: No clinically significant reactions have been reported to date.

Generic Name: IPECAC SYRUP
Trade Name: Ipecac Syrup
Dosage Forms: Oral syrup, 30 mL and other sizes
Uses: To induce vomiting in the early management of acute oral drug overdosage and in certain cases of oral poisoning with other toxic substances.
Adult Dosage (Oral): 15 mL with 200–300 mL water to facilitate emetic action; dose can be repeated after 20–30 min if necessary.
Pediatric Dosage (Oral): (Doses should be given with a smaller amount of water.) For a child over 1 year old, 15 mL; for a child 1 year old or younger, 5–10 mL.
Contraindications: Ingestion of caustic or corrosive poisons, strong acids or alkalis, volatile oils, convulsant poisons, and liquid hydrocarbons of low volatility; ingestion of antiemetics more than 1 hour before; simultaneous use of activated charcoal; patients who are unconscious, semicomatose, severely inebriated, convulsing, in shock, or who have lost the gag reflex.
Precautions: Do not confuse syrup of ipecac with ipecac *fluidextract*, which is 14 times more concentrated and toxic. Use cautiously in digitalis overdoses since vomiting potentiates vagal activity and atrioventricular block. Emesis may precipitate seizures in those who have ingested convulsive poisons (eg, strychnine). Ipecac may be cardiotoxic if systemically absorbed instead of vomited; remove from stomach with lavage or activated charcoal if no emesis occurs after second dose.
Adverse Reactions: Usually none with doses of 30 mL or less. Absorption of larger doses can cause gastric upset, cardiotoxicity, and cardiovascular collapse.

Generic Name: LACTULOSE
Trade Names: Chronulac, Cephulac
Dosage Form: Oral syrup, 10 g/15 mL
Uses: Laxative. Also used for prevention and adjunctive treatment of portal-systemic encephalopathy, including hepatic coma and precoma.
Adult Dosage (Oral): For hepatic encephalopathy, 30–45 mL (20–30 g) tid or qid. Dose adjusted q. 1–2 days prn to provide two or three soft stools daily. For acute portal-systemic encephalopathy, 30–45 mL q. 1–2h until laxative effect. As a laxative, 15–30 mL/d (up to 60 mL/d). (*Note:* May also be given as a retention enema of 300 mL lactulose and 700 mL water to be retained 1 hour.)
Contraindications: Low galactose diets (syrup contains galactose).
Precautions: Diabetics (syrup contains sugars).
Adverse Reactions: Flatulence, cramps, nausea, diarrhea.

Generic Name: METHYLENE BLUE INJECTION
Trade Name: Methylene Blue
Dosage Form: Injection (IV), 10 mg/mL (1%)
Uses: Given parenterally to reverse acute methemoglobinemia induced by both organic and inorganic nitrates and nitrites. *Not* recommended for methemoglobinemia caused by cyanide or carbon monoxide poisoning.
Adult Dosage (Parenteral): 1–2 mg/kg/dose (0.1–0.2 mL/kg/dose) slowly IV over several minutes; can be repeated in 1 to 2 hours if necessary to reduce methemoglobin serum levels to less than 40%.
Pediatric Dosage (Parenteral): Same as adult dosage.
Contraindications: Hypersensitivity to methylene blue; intraspinal, intrathecal, IM, or subcutaneous injection.
Precautions: Administer oxygen concurrently. Avoid exceeding recommended dosage or rapidly infusing doses since both can cause additional methemoglobinemia. Usually ineffective in patients with glucose-6-phosphate dehydrogenase deficiency since they lack the necessary methemoglobin-reductase enzymes.
Adverse Reactions: Large IV doses or rapid infusion rates can cause nausea, vomiting, dizziness, mental confusion, abdominal and chest pain, sweating, hypertension, grayish-blue cyanosis, and methemoglobinemia.

Generic Name: NALOXONE HCl
Trade Name: Narcan
Dosage Forms: Injection (IM/IV/subcutaneous), 0.4 mg/mL, 0.02 mg/mL (neonatal)
Uses: Narcotic antagonist. Treatment of narcotic-induced respiratory depression. Also effective in respiratory depression due to pentazocine, propoxyphene, butorphanol, nalbuphine, diphenoxylate, and possibly diazepam. Since its duration of action is short (1 to 4 hours), frequent injections are often needed to maintain adequate respiratory response. Consequently, continuous IV infusions of naloxone have been used to treat prolonged respiratory depression.
Adult Dosage (Parenteral): 0.005–0.025 mg/kg IV (usual dose, 0.4 mg); can be repeated q. 2–3 min as needed. Investigationally, IV loading dose of 3.7 µg/kg followed by constant infusion of 3.7 µg/kg/h has been used (average dose 2 mg/500 mL NS at 0.8 mg/h).
Pediatric Dosage (Parenteral): 0.01 mg/kg IV, IM, or subcutaneously. May be repeated in 2–3 min (until 0.1 mg/kg has been used). Can be injected into umbilical vein in newborns.
Precautions: Ineffective in respiratory depression not due to narcotics (eg, barbiturates, cocaine). If no improvement seen after 2–3 hours, another etiology must be suspected.
Adverse Reactions: In absence of narcotic, naloxone has no activity of its own. Rarely, nausea, vomiting, hypertension, tachycardia, pulmonary edema, and ventricular arrhythmias have been reported in patients with coronary artery disease.

Generic Name: PHYSOSTIGMINE
Trade Name: Antilirium
Dosage Forms: Injection (IV), 1 mg/mL
Uses: Cholinesterase inhibitor for treatment of anticholinergic overdoses.
Adult Dosage (Parenteral): Initially, 2 mg slow IV over 2 min. May be repeated with 1–2 mg until positive response or cholinergic signs develop.
Pediatric Dosage (Parenteral): Initially, 0.5 mg slow IV over 2 min. May be repeated with 0.5 mg IV q. 5 min until positive response or cholinergic signs develop (maximum, 2 mg).
Contraindications: Asthma, chronic airway obstruction gangrene, diabetes, cardiovascular disease, mechanical obstruction of intestinal or genitourinary tracts, concomitant use of depolarizing skeletal muscle relaxants (eg, succinylcholine).
Precautions: Avoid rapid IV infusion rates. Atropine injection should always be available to reverse excess cholinergic effects.

Use cautiously in bronchial disease, epilepsy, parkinsonism, and bradycardia. Facilities and equipment for mechanical ventilation and bronchial aspiration should be readily available. Reduce dosage if nausea, vomiting, or sweating is excessive.

Adverse Reactions: Primarily those of exaggerated cholinergic stimulation: nausea, vomiting, epigastric pain, miosis, sweating, salivation, lacrimation, dyspnea, bronchospasm, CNS stimulation, muscle twitching, weakness, seizures, bradycardia, palpitations, respiratory paralysis, and pulmonary edema. Rapid IV rates cause bradycardia, hypersalivation, respiratory problems, cholinergic crisis with paralysis, coma, and seizures (antidote: IV atropine in a dose of 50% of injected amount of physostigmine to control muscarinic effects and IV pralidoxime for respiratory paralysis and skeletal muscle effects).

Generic Name: SODIUM NITRITE
Trade Name: Sodium Nitrite (contained in Cyanide Antidote Package)
Dosage Forms: Injection (IV), 300 mg/10 mL (3%), 2 vials/package
Uses: Treatment of cyanide and thiocyanate poisoning.
Adult Dosage (Parenteral): To be given *before* the sodium thiosulfate solution: 10 mL (300 mg 3% solution) slow IV push over 2–4 min. Then, leaving needle in place, the sodium thiosulfate infusion is begun immediately.
Pediatric Dosage (Parenteral): 0.2 mL/kg (or 6–8 mg/kg) slow IV push over 2–4 min. Maximum dose, 10 mL.

Generic Name: SODIUM POLYSTYRENE SULFONATE
Trade Name: Kayexalate
Dosage Form: Powder, for oral or rectal use; suspension (in 33% sorbitol), 1.25 g/5 mL
Uses: Ion exchange resin for treatment of hyperkalemia; exchanges approximately 1 mEq potassium/g resin.
Adult Dosage: Prepare a mixture with equal parts resin and sorbitol solution and enough water to make a fluid suspension. For oral use, 15–40 g/d to qid. For rectal use, 30–50 g as needed (up to 1–2 hours initially, then q. 6h, prn). Retain enema for 30–60 min.
Pediatric Dosage: Give 1 g/kg/dose (as a suspension with water and sorbitol) orally or rectally. Retain rectal suspension for 30–45 min; tape buttocks together if necessary.
Precautions: Mixture for administration should be a fluid suspension, *not* a paste. Slow effect (hours). Should not be used alone in emergency situations. Is not selective for potassium; also binds calcium and magnesium. Caution in patients who cannot tolerate sodium load.
Adverse Reactions: Anorexia, nausea, vomiting, gastric irritation, and fecal impaction when given orally. Latter avoided by rectal use and addition of sorbitol to solutions.

Generic Name: SODIUM THIOSULFATE
Trade Name: Sodium Thiosulfate (contained in Cyanide Antidote Package)
Dosage Forms: Injection (IV), 12.5 g/50 mL (25%), 2 vials/package
Uses: Treatment of cyanide and thiocyanate poisoning.
Adult Dosage (Parenteral): To be given immediately *after* the sodium nitrite solution through the same needle left in patient's arm: 12.5 g (50 mL of 25% solution) slow IV push over 10 min. If symptoms recur, regimen may be repeated with half doses of sodium nitrite and sodium thiosulfate.
Pediatric Dosage (Parenteral): Give 30–40 mL (or 1 mL/kg) slow IV push over 10 min using same needle left in patient's arm.

BIBLIOGRAPHY

Benitiz WE, Tatro DS. *The Pediatric Drug Handbook*. 2nd ed. Chicago, Ill: Mosby Year-Book; 1988.

Cada DJ, Covington TR, Hussar DA, et al, eds. *Drug Facts and Comparisons*. New York, NY: JB Lippincott Co; 1992.

Drug Information for the Health Care Professional. 10th ed. Rockville, Md: US Pharmacopeial Convention; 1990.

Eisenberg MS, Copass MK, eds. *Manual of Emergency Medical Therapeutics*. Philadelphia, Pa: WB Saunders Co; 1978.

Emergency Cardiac Care Committee and Subcommittees, American Heart Association. Guidelines for cardiopulmonary resuscitation and emergency cardiac care, III: adult advanced cardiac life support. *JAMA*. 1992;268:2199–2241.

Geffner ES, ed. *The Hospital Pharmacy Compendium of Drug Therapy*. New York, NY: Biomedical Information Corporation; 1981, 1984.

Hansten PD. *Drug Interactions*. 4th ed. Philadelphia, Pa: Lea & Febiger; 1979.

Heinemann CJ. *Emergency Drug Reference*. Kettering, Ohio: Kettering Medical Center; 1981.

Hendeles L, Weinberger M. Guidelines for rapid attainment of therapeutic serum theophylline concentrations. *Am J Hosp Pharm*. 1982;39:249.

Katcher BS, Young LY, Koda-Kimble MA, eds. *Applied Therapeutics: The Clinical Use of Drugs*. 3rd ed. Spokane, Wash: Applied Therapeutics, Inc; 1984.

Knoben JE, Anderson PO, Watanabe AS. *Handbook of Clinical Drug Data*. 4th ed. Hamilton, Ill: Drug Intelligence Publications, Inc; 1978.

Levin RH, Pagliaro LA, eds. *Problems in Pediatric Drug Therapy*. Hamilton, Ill: Drug Intelligence Publications, Inc; 1979.

Marder VJ, Sherry S. Thrombolytic therapy: current status. Part I. *N Engl J Med*. 1988;318:1512–1520.

Marder VJ, Sherry S. Thrombolytic therapy: current status. Part II. *N Engl J Med*. 1988;318:1585–1595.

McEvoy GK. *Drug Information 89*. Bethesda, Md: American Society of Hospital Pharmacists; 1989.

McEvoy GK, McQuarrie GM, eds. *Drug Information 86: The American Hospital Formulary Service*. Bethesda, Md: American Society of Hospital Pharmacists; 1986.

Medical Letter on Drugs and Therapeutics. Handbook of Antimicrobial Therapy, rev ed. New Rochelle, NY: The Medical Letter, Inc; 1986.

Newhaus KL, Werner F, et al. Improved thrombolysis with a modified dose regimen of r-tPA. *J Am Coll Cardiol*. 1989; 14:1566.

Ornato JP, Gonzalez ER, eds. *Drug Therapy in Emergency Medicine*. New York, NY: Churchill Livingstone; 1990.

Phillips RE, Feeney MK. *The Cardiac Rhythms: A Systematic Approach to Interpretation*. Philadelphia, Pa: WB Saunders Co; 1973.

Product Information: Cardizem™ injectable, diltiazem. Kansas City, Mo: Marion Merrell Dow Inc; 1991.

Product Information: Ethmozine™, moricizine. Wilmington, Del: DuPont; 1990.

Product Information: Mazicon™, flumazenil. Nutley, NJ: Roche; 1991.

Product Information. Ticlid™, ticlopidine. Palo Alto, CA: Syntex; 1991.

Shirkey HC, ed. *Pediatric Therapy*. 5th ed. St Louis, Mo: CV Mosby Co; 1975.

Zagola ZP. *The Critical Care Drug Handbook*. St. Louis, Mo: Mosby Year-Book; 1991.

Zipes DP. Management of cardiac arrhythmias: pharmacological, electrical, and surgical techniques. In: Braunwald E, ed. *Heart Disease: A Textbook of Cardiovascular Medicine*. Philadelphia, Pa: WB Saunders Co; 1988:621–657.

APPENDIX 87-A: LIST OF PHARMACOLOGIC/THERAPEUTIC DRUGS AND AGENTS FOR EMERGENCY FACILITIES

Antibiotics
  Erythromycin
  Gentamicin Sulfate
  Oxacillin Sodium
  Penicillins
    Ampicillin
    Benzathine Penicillin
    Penicillin G Potassium
    Penicillin G Procaine
Antihistamine Drugs
  Diphenhydramine
    (Benadryl®)
Autonomic Drugs
  Parasympatholytic (Cholinergic
    Blocking) Agents
    Atropine Sulfate
  Parasympathomimetic
    (Cholinergic) Agents
    Edrophonium Chloride
      (Tensilon®)
    Neostigmine Methylsulfate
    Physostigmine
  Sympathomimetic (Adrenergic) Agents
    Dopamine
    Epinephrine HCl
    Isoproterenol HCl
    Norepinephrine Bitartrate
Blood Formation and Coagulation
  Anticoagulant Reversing Agents
    Aqueous Vitamin K
    Protamine Sulfate
  Anticoagulants
    Heparin Sodium
Cardiovascular Drugs
  Cardiac Drugs
    Bretylium HCl
    Calcium Chloride
    Digoxin
    Lidocaine
    Procainamide HCl
    Propranolol
    Sodium Bicarbonate
    Verapamil HCl
  Hypotensive Agents
    Diazoxide (Hyperstat®)
    Sodium Nitroprusside
      (Nipride®)
    Trimethaphan (Arfonad®)
  Vasodilating Agents
    Amyl Nitrite
    Nitroglycerin
Central Nervous System Drugs
  Analgesics and Antipyretics
    Acetaminophen
    Aspirin
    Codeine
    Meperidine HCl
      (Demerol®)
    Morphine Sulfate
  Anticonvulsants
    Diazepam (Valium®)
    Phenobarbital
    Phenytoin (Dilantin®)
  Narcotic Antagonists
    Naloxone (Narcan®)
  Psychotherapeutic Agents
    Chlorpromazine
      (Thorazine®)
    Diazepam
    Haloperidol
Diagnostic Agents
  Blood Contents
    Reagents for estimating
      blood glucose
      (Dextrostix®)
  Myasthenia Gravis
    Edrophonium Chloride
    Neostigmine Methylsulfate

---

*Common trade names have been selectively mentioned for purposes of clarification. This is not to be construed as any form of endorsement.

Stool Contents
    Stool tests for occult blood
      (Hemoccult®)
    Test tapes for urine bilirubin, blood, sugar, ketones,
      pH, urobilinogen, protein (Bili-Labstix®)

Electrolytic, Caloric, and Water Balance
  Diuretics
    Furosemide (Lasix®)
    Mannitol
  Hypoglycemic Agents
    Dextrose 50% in water
  Replacement Solutions
    Dextrose 5% with water
    Ringer's injections, lactated
    Potassium Chloride
    Sodium Chloride

Eye, Ear, Nose, and Throat Preparations
  Local Anesthetics
    Proparacaine
      (Ophthaine®)
    Tetracaine   } either/or
      (Pontacaine®)

Gastrointestinal Drugs
  Adsorbents
    Charcoal, activated
  Cathartics
    Magnesium Salt
  Emetics and Anti-Emetics
    Ipecac Syrup
    Prochlorperazine
      (Compazine®)

Hormones and Synthetic Substitutes
  Adrenals
    Dexamethasone
      (Decadron®)
    Hydrocortisone
      (Solu-Cortef®)
    Methylprednisolone
      (Solu-Medrol®)
  Insulins and Antidiabetic Agents
    Glucagon HCl
    Insulin, regular
  Thyroid
    Levothyroxine Sodium

Local Anesthetics
  Lidocaine HCl

Serums, Toxoids, and Vaccines
  Serums
    Antivenin, Black Widow Spider Bite, Equine Origin
      (geographic-area-specific)
    Antivenin, Snake-Bite, Polyvalent, Equine Origin
      (geographic-area-specific)
    Rabies Immune Globulin, Human
    Tetanus Immune Globulin
  Toxoids
    Diphtheria and Tetanus Toxoids and Pertussis
      Vaccine Adsorbed
    Tetanus and Diphtheria Toxoids Adsorbed, adult
      and pediatric
    Tetanus Toxoid Adsorbed

Spasmolytics
  Inhalation
    Metaproterenol Sulfate
  Parenteral
    Aminophylline
    Terbutaline Sulfate

Vitamins
  Vitamin B Complex
  Thiamine HCl

Unclassified Agents
  Cyanide Antidote Kit

---

*Reprinted from *Annals of Emergency Medicine* with permission, © copyright 1982.

Appendix. Temperature Conversion*

This table permits one to convert from degrees Celsius to degrees Fahrenheit or from degrees Fahrenheit to degrees Celsius. The conversion is accomplished by first locating in a column printed in boldface type the number that is to be converted. If the number to be converted is in degrees Fahrenheit, one may find its equivalent in degrees Celsius by reading to the left. If the number to be converted is in degrees Celsius, one may find its equivalent in degrees Fahrenheit by reading to the right. Degrees Celsius are identical to degrees Centigrade; however, the word Celsius is preferred for international use.

The approved international symbolic abbreviation for degrees Celsius is °C; for degrees Fahrenheit it is °F. Absolute zero on the Celsius scale is -273.15°C; on the Fahrenheit scale it is -459.67°F. The relation beween degrees Fahrenheit and degrees Celsius may be expressed by
$$°C = 5/9(°F - 32) \text{ or}$$
$$°F = 9/5(°C) + 32.$$

To convert			To convert			To convert		
To °C	←°F or °C→	To °F	To °C	←°F or °C→	To °F	To °C	←°F or °C→	To °F
−273.15	**−459.67**	−	−92.78	**−135**	−211	−28.33	**−19**	−2.2
−267.78	**−450**	−	−90	**−130**	−202	−27.78	**−18**	−0.4
−262.22	**−440**	−	−87.22	**−125**	−193	−27.22	**−17**	1.4
−256.67	**−430**	−	−84.44	**−120**	−184	−26.67	**−16**	3.2
−251.11	**−420**	−	−81.67	**−115**	−175	−26.11	**−15**	5
−245.56	**−410**	−	−78.89	**−110**	−166	−25.56	**−14**	6.8
−240	**−400**	−	−76.11	**−105**	−157	−25	**−13**	8.6
−234.44	**−390**	−	−73.33	**−100**	−148	−24.44	**−12**	10.4
−228.89	**−380**	−	−70.56	**−95**	−139	−23.89	**−11**	12.2
−223.33	**−370**	−	−67.78	**−90**	−130	−23.33	**−10**	14
−217.78	**−360**	−	−65	**−85**	−121	−22.78	**−9**	15.8
−212.22	**−350**	−	−62.22	**−80**	−112	−22.22	**−8**	17.6
−206.67	**−340**	−	−59.44	**−75**	−103	−21.67	**−7**	19.4
−201.11	**−330**	−	−56.67	**−70**	−94	−21.11	**−6**	21.2
−195.56	**−320**	−	−53.89	**−65**	−85	−20.56	**−5**	23
−190	**−310**	−	−51.11	**−60**	−76	−20	**−4**	24.8
−184.44	**−300**	−	−48.33	**−55**	−67	−19.44	**−3**	26.6
−178.89	**−290**	−	−45.56	**−50**	−58	−18.89	**−2**	28.4
−173.33	**−280**	−	−42.78	**−45**	−49	−18.33	**−1**	30.2
−167.78	**−270**	−454	−40	**−40**	−40	−17.78	**0**	32
−162.22	**−260**	−436	−39.44	**−39**	−38.2	−17.22	**1**	33.8
−156.67	**−250**	−418	−38.89	**−38**	−36.4	−16.67	**2**	35.6
−151.11	**−240**	−400	−38.33	**−37**	−34.6	−16.11	**3**	37.4
−145.56	**−230**	−382	−37.78	**−36**	−32.8	−15.56	**4**	39.2
−140	**−220**	−364	−37.22	**−35**	−31	−15	**5**	41
−134.44	**−210**	−346	−36.67	**−34**	−29.2	−14.44	**6**	42.8
−131.67	**−205**	−337	−36.11	**−33**	−27.4	−13.89	**7**	44.6
−128.89	**−200**	−328	−35.56	**−32**	−25.6	−13.33	**8**	46.4
−126.11	**−195**	−319	−35	**−31**	−23.8	−12.78	**9**	48.2
−123.33	**−190**	−310	−34.44	**−30**	−22	−12.22	**10**	50
−120.56	**−185**	−301	−33.89	**−29**	−20.2	−11.67	**11**	51.8
−117.78	**−180**	−292	−33.33	**−28**	−18.4	−11.11	**12**	53.6
−115	**−175**	−283	−32.78	**−27**	−16.6	−10.56	**13**	55.4
−112.22	**−170**	−274	−32.22	**−26**	−14.8	−10	**14**	57.2
−109.44	**−165**	−265	−31.67	**−25**	−13	−9.44	**15**	59
−106.67	**−160**	−256	−31.11	**−24**	−11.2	−8.89	**16**	60.8
−103.89	**−155**	−247	−30.56	**−23**	−9.4	−8.33	**17**	62.6
−101.11	**−150**	−238	−30	**−22**	−7.6	−7.78	**18**	64.4
−98.33	**−145**	−229	−29.44	**−21**	−5.8	−7.22	**19**	66.2
−95.56	**−140**	−220	−28.89	**−20**	−4	−6.67	**20**	68

*Condensed with permission from *Handbook of Chemistry and Physics*, 53rd ed, RC Weast, Ed. Copyright CRC Press Inc, Boca Raton, FL.

To convert			To convert			To convert		
To °C	←°F or °C→	To °F	To °C	←°F or °C→	To °F	To °C	←°F or °C→	To °F
−6.11	21	69.8	23.89	75	167	54.44	130	266
−5.56	22	71.6	24.44	76	168.8	55	131	267.8
−5	23	73.4	25	77	170.6	55.56	132	269.6
−4.44	24	75.2	25.56	78	172.4	56.11	133	271.4
−3.89	25	77	26.11	79	174.2	56.67	134	273.2
−3.33	26	78.8	26.67	80	176	57.22	135	275
−2.78	27	80.6	27.22	81	177.8	57.78	136	276.8
−2.22	28	82.4	27.78	82	179.6	58.33	137	278.6
−1.67	29	84.2	28.33	83	181.4	58.89	138	280.4
−1.11	30	86	28.89	84	183.2	59.44	139	282.2
−0.56	31	87.8	29.44	85	185	60	140	284
0	32	89.6	30	86	186.8	60.56	141	285.8
.56	33	91.4	30.56	87	188.6	61.11	142	287.6
1.11	34	93.2	31.11	88	190.4	61.67	143	289.4
1.67	35	95	31.67	89	192.2	62.22	144	291.2
2.22	36	96.8	32.22	90	194	62.78	145	293
2.78	37	98.6	32.78	91	195.8	63.33	146	294.8
3.33	38	100.4	33.33	92	197.6	63.89	147	296.6
3.89	39	102.2	33.89	93	199.4	64.44	148	298.4
4.44	40	104	34.44	94	201.2	65	149	300.2
5	41	105.8	35	95	203	65.56	150	302
5.56	42	107.6	35.56	96	204.8	66.11	151	303.8
6.11	43	109.4	36.11	97	206.6	66.67	152	305.6
6.67	44	111.2	36.67	98	208.4	67.22	153	307.4
7.22	45	113	37.22	99	210.2	67.78	154	309.2
7.78	46	114.8	37.78	100	212	68.33	155	311
8.33	47	116.6	38.33	101	213.8	68.89	156	312.8
8.89	48	118.4	38.89	102	215.6	69.44	157	314.6
9.44	49	120.2	39.44	103	217.4	70	158	316.4
			40	104	219.2	70.56	159	318.2
10	50	122	40.56	105	221	71.11	160	320
10.56	51	123.8	41.11	106	222.8	71.67	161	321.8
11.11	52	125.6	41.67	107	224.6	72.22	162	323.6
11.67	53	127.4	42.22	108	226.4	72.78	163	325.4
12.22	54	129.2	42.78	109	228.2	73.33	164	327.2
12.78	55	131	43.33	110	230	73.89	165	329
13.33	56	132.8	43.89	111	231.8	74.44	166	330.8
13.89	57	134.6	44.44	112	233.6	75	167	332.6
14.44	58	136.4	45	113	235.4	75.56	168	334.4
15	59	138.2	45.56	114	237.2	76.11	169	336.2
15.56	60	140	46.11	115	239	76.67	170	338
16.11	61	141.8	46.67	116	240.8	77.22	171	339.8
16.67	62	143.6	47.22	117	242.6	77.78	172	341.6
17.22	63	145.4	47.78	118	244.4	78.33	173	343.4
17.78	64	147.2	48.33	119	246.2	78.89	174	345.2
18.33	65	149	48.89	120	248	79.44	175	347
18.89	66	150.8	49.44	121	249.8	80	176	348.8
19.44	67	152.6	50	122	251.6	80.56	177	350.6
20	68	154.4	50.56	123	253.4	81.11	178	352.4
20.56	69	156.2	51.11	124	255.2	81.67	179	354.2
21.11	70	158	51.67	125	257	82.22	180	356
21.67	71	159.8	52.22	126	258.8	82.78	181	357.8
22.22	72	161.6	52.78	127	260.6	83.33	182	359.6
22.78	73	163.4	53.33	128	262.4	83.89	183	361.4
23.33	74	165.2	53.89	129	264.2	84.44	184	363.2

To convert			To convert			To convert		
To °C	←°F or °C→	To °F	To °C	←°F or °C→	To °F	To °C	←°F or °C→	To °F
85	**185**	365	115.56	**240**	464	146.11	**295**	563
85.56	**186**	366.8	116.11	**241**	465.8	146.67	**296**	564.8
86.11	**187**	368.6	116.67	**242**	467.6	147.22	**297**	566.6
86.67	**188**	370.4	117.22	**243**	469.4	147.78	**298**	568.4
87.22	**189**	372.2	117.78	**244**	471.2	148.33	**299**	570.2
87.78	**190**	374	118.33	**245**	473	148.89	**300**	572
88.33	**191**	375.8	118.89	**246**	474.8	149.44	**301**	573.8
88.89	**192**	377.6	119.44	**247**	476.6	150	**302**	575.6
89.44	**193**	379.4	120	**248**	478.4	150.56	**303**	577.4
90	**194**	381.2	120.56	**249**	480.2	151.11	**304**	579.2
90.56	**195**	383	121.11	**250**	482	151.67	**305**	581
91.11	**196**	384.8	121.67	**251**	483.8	152.22	**306**	582.8
91.67	**197**	386.6	122.22	**252**	485.6	152.78	**307**	584.6
92.22	**198**	388.4	122.78	**253**	487.4	153.33	**308**	586.4
92.78	**199**	390.2	123.33	**254**	489.2	153.89	**309**	588.2
93.33	**200**	392	123.89	**255**	491	154.44	**310**	590
93.89	**201**	393.8	124.44	**256**	492.8	155	**311**	591.8
94.44	**202**	395.6	125	**257**	494.6	155.56	**312**	593.6
95	**203**	397.4	125.56	**258**	496.4	156.11	**313**	595.4
95.56	**204**	399.2	126.11	**259**	498.2	156.67	**314**	597.2
96.11	**205**	401	126.67	**260**	500	157.22	**315**	599
96.67	**206**	402.8	127.22	**261**	501.8	157.78	**316**	600.8
97.22	**207**	404.6	127.78	**262**	503.6	158.33	**317**	602.6
97.78	**208**	406.4	128.33	**263**	505.4	158.89	**318**	604.4
98.33	**209**	408.2	128.89	**264**	507.2	159.44	**319**	606.2
98.89	**210**	410	129.44	**265**	509	160	**320**	608
99.44	**211**	411.8	130	**266**	510.8	160.56	**321**	609.8
100	**212**	413.6	130.56	**267**	512.6	161.11	**322**	611.6
100.56	**213**	415.4	131.11	**268**	514.4	161.67	**323**	613.4
101.11	**214**	417.2	131.67	**269**	516.2	162.22	**324**	615.2
101.67	**215**	419	132.22	**270**	518	162.78	**325**	617
102.22	**216**	420.8	132.78	**271**	519.8	163.33	**326**	618.8
102.78	**217**	422.6	133.33	**272**	521.6	163.89	**327**	620.6
103.33	**218**	424.4	133.89	**273**	523.4	164.44	**328**	622.4
103.89	**219**	426.2	134.44	**274**	525.2	165	**329**	624.2
104.44	**220**	428	135	**275**	527	165.56	**330**	626
105	**221**	429.8	135.56	**276**	528.8	166.11	**331**	627.8
105.56	**222**	431.6	136.11	**277**	530.6	166.67	**332**	629.6
106.11	**223**	433.4	136.67	**278**	532.4	167.22	**333**	631.4
106.67	**224**	435.2	137.22	**279**	534.2	167.78	**334**	633.2
107.22	**225**	437	137.78	**280**	536	168.33	**335**	635
107.78	**226**	438.8	138.33	**281**	537.8	168.89	**336**	636.8
108.33	**227**	440.6	138.89	**282**	539.6	169.44	**337**	638.6
108.89	**228**	442.4	139.44	**283**	541.4	170	**338**	640.4
109.44	**229**	444.2	140	**284**	543.2	170.56	**339**	642.2
110	**230**	446	140.56	**285**	545	171.11	**340**	644
110.56	**231**	447.8	141.11	**286**	546.8	171.67	**341**	645.8
111.11	**232**	449.6	141.67	**287**	548.6	172.22	**342**	647.6
111.67	**233**	451.4	142.22	**288**	550.4	172.78	**343**	649.4
112.22	**234**	453.2	142.78	**289**	552.2	173.33	**344**	651.2
112.78	**235**	455	143.33	**290**	554	173.89	**345**	653
113.33	**236**	456.8	143.89	**291**	555.8	174.44	**346**	654.8
113.89	**237**	458.6	144.44	**292**	557.6	175	**347**	656.6
114.44	**238**	460.4	145	**293**	559.4	175.56	**348**	658.4
115	**239**	462.2	145.56	**294**	561.2	176.11	**349**	660.2

To convert			To convert			To convert		
To °C	←°F or °C→	To °F	To °C	←°F or °C→	To °F	To °C	←°F or °C→	To °F
176.67	350	662	210	410	770	271.11	520	968
177.22	351	663.8	211.11	412	773.6	272.22	522	971.6
177.78	352	665.6	212.22	414	777.2	273.33	524	975.2
178.33	353	667.4	213.33	416	780.8	274.44	526	978.8
178.89	354	669.2	214.44	418	784.4	275.56	528	982.4
179.44	355	671	215.56	420	788	276.67	530	986
180	356	672.8	216.67	422	791.6	277.78	532	989.6
180.56	357	674.6	217.78	424	795.2	278.89	534	993.2
181.11	358	676.4	218.89	426	798.8	280	536	996.8
181.67	359	678.2	220	428	802.4	281.11	538	1000.4
182.22	360	680	221.11	430	806	282.22	540	1004
182.78	361	681.8	222.22	432	809.6	283.33	542	1007.6
183.33	362	683.6	223.33	434	813.2	284.44	544	1011.2
183.89	363	685.4	224.44	436	816.8	285.56	546	1014.8
184.44	364	687.2	225.56	438	820.4	286.67	548	1018.4
185	365	689	226.67	440	824	287.78	550	1022
185.56	366	690.8	227.78	442	827.6	288.89	552	1025.6
186.11	367	692.6	228.89	444	831.2	290	554	1029.2
186.67	368	694.4	230	446	834.8	291.11	556	1032.8
187.22	369	696.2	231.11	448	838.4	292.22	558	1036.4
187.78	370	698	232.22	450	842	293.33	560	1040
188.33	371	699.8	233.33	452	845.6	294.44	562	1043.6
188.89	372	701.6	234.44	454	849.2	295.56	564	1047.2
189.44	373	703.4	235.56	456	852.8	296.67	566	1050.8
190	374	705.2	236.67	458	856.4	297.78	568	1054.4
190.56	375	707	237.78	460	860	298.89	570	1058
191.11	376	708.8	238.89	462	863.6	300	572	1061.6
191.67	377	710.6	240	464	867.2	301.11	574	1065.2
192.22	378	712.4	241.11	466	870.8	302.22	576	1068.8
192.78	379	714.2	242.22	468	874.4	303.33	578	1072.4
193.33	380	716	243.33	470	878	304.44	580	1076
193.89	381	717.8	244.44	472	881.6	305.56	582	1079.6
194.44	382	719.6	245.56	474	885.2	306.67	584	1083.2
195	383	721.4	246.67	476	888.8	307.78	586	1086.8
195.56	384	723.2	247.78	478	892.4	308.89	588	1090.4
196.11	385	725	248.89	480	896	310	590	1094
196.67	386	726.8	250	482	899.6	311.11	592	1097.6
197.22	387	728.6	251.11	484	903.2	312.22	594	1101.2
197.78	388	730.4	252.22	486	906.8	313.33	596	1104.8
198.33	389	732.2	253.33	488	910.4	314.44	598	1108.4
198.89	390	734	254.44	490	914	315.56	600	1112
199.44	391	735.8	255.56	492	917.6	316.67	602	1115.6
200	392	737.6	256.67	494	921.2	317.78	604	1119.2
200.56	393	739.4	257.78	496	924.8	318.89	606	1122.8
201.11	394	741.2	258.89	498	928.4	320	608	1126.4
201.67	395	743	260	500	932	321.11	610	1130
202.22	396	744.8	261.11	502	935.6	322.22	612	1133.6
202.78	397	746.6	262.22	504	939.2	323.33	614	1137.2
203.33	398	748.4	263.33	506	942.8	324.44	616	1140.8
203.89	399	750.2	264.44	508	946.4	325.56	618	1144.4
204.44	400	752	265.56	510	950	326.67	620	1148
205.56	402	755.6	266.67	512	953.6	327.78	622	1151.6
206.67	404	759.2	267.78	514	957.2	328.89	624	1155.2
207.78	406	762.8	268.89	516	960.8	330	626	1158.8
208.89	408	766.4	270	518	964.4	331.11	628	1162.4

Temperature Conversion

	To convert			To convert			To convert	
To °C	k°F or °Cl	To °F	To °C	k°F or °Cl	To °F	To °C	k°F or °Cl	To °F
332.22	630	1166	393.33	740	1364	454.44	850	1562
333.33	632	1169.6	394.44	742	1367.6	455.56	852	1565.6
334.44	634	1173.2	395.56	744	1371.2	456.67	854	1569.2
335.56	636	1176.8	396.67	746	1374.8	457.78	856	1572.8
336.67	638	1180.4	397.78	748	1378.4	458.89	858	1576.4
337.78	640	1184	398.89	750	1382	460	860	1580
338.89	642	1187.6	400	752	1385.6	461.11	862	1583.6
340	644	1191.2	401.11	754	1389.2	462.22	864	1587.2
341.11	646	1194.8	402.22	756	1392.8	463.33	866	1590.8
342.22	648	1198.4	403.33	758	1396.4	464.44	868	1594.4
343.33	650	1202	404.44	760	1400	465.56	870	1598
344.44	652	1205.6	405.56	762	1403.6	466.67	872	1601.6
345.56	654	1209.2	406.67	764	1407.2	467.78	874	1605.2
346.67	656	1212.8	407.78	766	1410.8	468.89	876	1608.8
347.78	658	1216.4	408.89	768	1414.4	470	878	1612.4
348.89	660	1220	410	770	1418	471.11	880	1616
350	662	1223.6	411.11	772	1421.6	472.22	882	1619.6
351.11	664	1227.2	412.22	774	1425.2	473.33	884	1623.2
352.22	666	1230.8	413.33	776	1428.8	474.44	886	1626.8
353.33	668	1234.4	414.44	778	1432.4	475.56	888	1630.4
354.44	670	1238	415.56	780	1436	476.67	890	1634
355.56	672	1241.6	416.67	782	1439.6	477.78	892	1637.6
356.67	674	1245.2	417.78	784	1443.2	478.89	894	1641.2
357.78	676	1248.8	418.89	786	1446.8	480	896	1644.8
358.89	678	1252.4	420	788	1450.4	481.11	898	1648.4
360	680	1256	421.11	790	1454	482.22	900	1652
361.11	682	1259.6	422.22	792	1457.6	483.33	902	1655.6
362.22	684	1263.2	423.33	794	1461.2	484.44	904	1659.2
363.33	686	1266.8	424.44	796	1464.8	485.56	906	1662.8
364.44	688	1270.4	425.56	798	1468.4	486.67	908	1666.4
365.56	690	1274	426.67	800	1472	487.78	910	1670
366.67	692	1277.6	427.78	802	1475.6	488.89	912	1673.6
367.78	694	1281.2	428.89	804	1479.2	490	914	1677.2
368.89	696	1284.8	430	806	1482.8	491.11	916	1680.8
370	698	1288.4	431.11	808	1486.4	492.22	918	1684.4
371.11	700	1292	432.22	810	1490	493.33	920	1688
372.22	702	1295.6	433.33	812	1493.6	494.44	922	1691.6
373.33	704	1299.2	434.44	814	1497.2	495.56	924	1695.2
374.44	706	1302.8	435.56	816	1500.8	496.67	926	1698.8
375.56	708	1306.4	436.67	818	1504.4	497.78	928	1702.4
376.67	710	1310	437.78	820	1508	498.89	930	1706
377.78	712	1313.6	438.89	822	1511.6	500	932	1709.6
378.89	714	1317.2	440	824	1515.2	501.11	934	1713.2
380	716	1320.8	441.11	826	1518.8	502.22	936	1716.8
381.11	718	1324.4	442.22	828	1522.4	503.33	938	1720.4
382.22	720	1328	443.33	830	1526	504.44	940	1724
383.33	722	1331.6	444.44	832	1529.6	505.56	942	1727.6
384.44	724	1335.2	445.56	834	1533.2	506.67	944	1731.2
385.56	726	1338.8	446.67	836	1536.8	507.78	946	1734.8
386.67	728	1342.4	447.78	838	1540.4	508.89	948	1738.4
387.78	730	1346	448.89	840	1544	510	950	1742
388.89	732	1349.6	450	842	1547.6	511.11	952	1745.6
390	734	1353.2	451.11	844	1551.2	512.22	954	1749.2
391.11	736	1356.8	452.22	846	1554.8	513.33	956	1752.8
392.22	738	1360.4	453.33	848	1558.4	514.44	958	1756.4

To convert			To convert			To convert		
To °C	←°F or °C→	To °F	To °C	←°F or °C→	To °F	To °C	←°F or °C→	To °F
515.56	**960**	1760	576.67	**1070**	1958	637.78	**1180**	2156
516.67	**962**	1763.6	577.78	**1072**	1961.6	638.89	**1182**	2159.6
517.78	**964**	1767.2	578.89	**1074**	1965.2	640	**1184**	2163.2
518.89	**966**	1770.8	580	**1076**	1968.8	641.11	**1186**	2166.8
520	**968**	1774.4	581.11	**1078**	1972.4	642.22	**1188**	2170.4
521.11	**970**	1778	582.22	**1080**	1976	643.33	**1190**	2174
522.22	**972**	1781.6	583.33	**1082**	1979.6	644.44	**1192**	2177.6
523.33	**974**	1785.2	584.44	**1084**	1983.2	645.56	**1194**	2181.2
524.44	**976**	1788.8	585.56	**1086**	1986.8	646.67	**1196**	2184.8
525.56	**978**	1792.4	586.67	**1088**	1990.4	647.78	**1198**	2188.4
526.67	**980**	1796	587.78	**1090**	1994	648.89	**1200**	2192
527.78	**982**	1799.6	588.89	**1092**	1997.6	650	**1202**	2195.6
528.89	**984**	1803.2	590	**1094**	2001.2	651.11	**1204**	2199.2
530	**986**	1806.8	591.11	**1096**	2004.8	652.22	**1206**	2202.8
531.11	**988**	1810.4	592.22	**1098**	2008.4	653.33	**1208**	2206.4
532.22	**990**	1814	593.33	**1100**	2012	654.44	**1210**	2210
533.33	**992**	1817.6	594.44	**1102**	2015.6	655.56	**1212**	2213.6
534.44	**994**	1821.2	595.56	**1104**	2019.2	656.67	**1214**	2217.2
535.56	**996**	1824.8	596.67	**1106**	2022.8	657.78	**1216**	2220.8
536.67	**998**	1828.4	597.78	**1108**	2026.4	658.89	**1218**	2224.4
537.78	**1000**	1832	598.89	**1110**	2030	660	**1220**	2228
538.89	**1002**	1835.6	600	**1112**	2033.6	661.11	**1222**	2231.6
540	**1004**	1839.2	601.11	**1114**	2037.2	662.22	**1224**	2235.2
541.11	**1006**	1842.8	602.22	**1116**	2040.8	663.33	**1226**	2238.8
542.22	**1008**	1846.4	603.33	**1118**	2044.4	664.44	**1228**	2242.4
543.33	**1010**	1850	604.44	**1120**	2048	665.56	**1230**	2246
544.44	**1012**	1853.6	605.56	**1122**	2051.6	666.67	**1232**	2249.6
545.56	**1014**	1857.2	606.67	**1124**	2055.2	667.78	**1234**	2253.2
546.67	**1016**	1860.8	607.78	**1126**	2058.8	668.89	**1236**	2256.8
547.78	**1018**	1864.4	608.89	**1128**	2062.4	670	**1238**	2260.4
548.89	**1020**	1868	610	**1130**	2066	671.11	**1240**	2264
550	**1022**	1871.6	611.11	**1132**	2069.6	672.22	**1242**	2267.6
551.11	**1024**	1875.2	612.22	**1134**	2073.2	673.33	**1244**	2271.2
552.22	**1026**	1878.8	613.33	**1136**	2076.8	674.44	**1246**	2274.8
553.33	**1028**	1882.4	614.44	**1138**	2080.4	675.56	**1248**	2278.4
554.44	**1030**	1886	615.56	**1140**	2084	676.67	**1250**	2282
555.56	**1032**	1889.6	616.67	**1142**	2087.6	677.78	**1252**	2285.6
556.67	**1034**	1893.2	617.78	**1144**	2091.2	678.89	**1254**	2289.2
557.78	**1036**	1896.8	618.89	**1146**	2094.8	680	**1256**	2292.8
558.89	**1038**	1900.4	620	**1148**	2098.4	681.11	**1258**	2296.4
560	**1040**	1904	621.11	**1150**	2102	682.22	**1260**	2300
561.11	**1042**	1907.6	622.22	**1152**	2105.6	683.33	**1262**	2303.6
562.22	**1044**	1911.2	623.33	**1154**	2109.2	684.44	**1264**	2307.2
563.33	**1046**	1914.8	624.44	**1156**	2112.8	685.56	**1266**	2310.8
564.44	**1048**	1918.4	625.56	**1158**	2116.4	686.67	**1268**	2314.4
565.56	**1050**	1922	626.67	**1160**	2120	687.78	**1270**	2318
566.67	**1052**	1925.6	627.78	**1162**	2123.6	688.89	**1272**	2321.6
567.78	**1054**	1929.2	628.89	**1164**	2127.2	690	**1274**	2325.2
568.89	**1056**	1932.8	630	**1166**	2130.8	691.11	**1276**	2328.8
570	**1058**	1936.4	631.11	**1168**	2134.4	692.22	**1278**	2332.4
571.11	**1060**	1940	632.22	**1170**	2138	693.33	**1280**	2336
572.22	**1062**	1943.6	633.33	**1172**	2141.6	694.44	**1282**	2339.6
573.33	**1064**	1947.2	634.44	**1174**	2145.2	695.56	**1284**	2343.2
574.44	**1066**	1950.8	635.56	**1176**	2148.8	696.67	**1286**	2346.8
575.56	**1068**	1954.4	636.67	**1178**	2152.4	697.78	**1288**	2350.4

Temperature Conversion

To convert			To convert			To convert		
To °C	←°F or °C→	To °F	To °C	←°F or °C→	To °F	To °C	←°F or °C→	To °F
698.89	**1290**	2354	760	**1400**	2552	843.33	**1550**	2822
700	**1292**	2357.6	761.11	**1402**	2555.6	848.89	**1560**	2840
701.11	**1294**	2361.2	762.22	**1404**	2559.2	854.44	**1570**	2858
702.22	**1296**	2364.8	763.33	**1406**	2562.8	860	**1580**	2876
703.33	**1298**	2368.4	764.44	**1408**	2566.4	865.56	**1590**	2894
704.44	**1300**	2372	765.56	**1410**	2570	871.11	**1600**	2912
705.56	**1302**	2375.6	766.67	**1412**	2573.6	876.67	**1610**	2930
706.67	**1304**	2379.2	767.78	**1414**	2577.2	882.22	**1620**	2948
707.78	**1306**	2382.8	768.89	**1416**	2580.8	887.78	**1630**	2966
708.89	**1308**	2386.4	770	**1418**	2584.4	893.33	**1640**	2984
710	**1310**	2390	771.11	**1420**	2588	898.89	**1650**	3002
711.11	**1312**	2393.6	772.22	**1422**	2591.6	904.44	**1660**	3020
712.22	**1314**	2397.2	773.33	**1424**	2595.2	910	**1670**	3038
713.33	**1316**	2400.8	774.44	**1426**	2598.8	915.56	**1680**	3056
714.44	**1318**	2404.4	775.56	**1428**	2602.4	921.11	**1690**	3074
715.56	**1320**	2408	776.67	**1430**	2606	926.67	**1700**	3092
716.67	**1322**	2411.6	777.78	**1432**	2609.6	932.22	**1710**	3110
717.78	**1324**	2415.2	778.89	**1434**	2613.2	937.78	**1720**	3128
718.89	**1326**	2418.8	780	**1436**	2616.8	943.33	**1730**	3146
720	**1328**	2422.4	781.11	**1438**	2620.4	948.89	**1740**	3164
721.11	**1330**	2426	782.22	**1440**	2624	954.44	**1750**	3182
722.22	**1332**	2429.6	783.33	**1442**	2627.6	960	**1760**	3200
723.33	**1334**	2433.2	784.44	**1444**	2631.2	965.56	**1770**	3218
724.44	**1336**	2436.8	785.56	**1446**	2634.8	971.11	**1780**	3236
725.56	**1338**	2440.4	786.67	**1448**	2638.4	976.67	**1790**	3254
726.67	**1340**	2444	787.78	**1450**	2642	982.22	**1800**	3272
727.78	**1342**	2447.6	788.89	**1452**	2645.6	987.78	**1810**	3290
728.89	**1344**	2451.2	790	**1454**	2649.2	993.33	**1820**	3308
730	**1346**	2454.8	791.11	**1456**	2652.8	998.89	**1830**	3326
731.11	**1348**	2458.4	792.22	**1458**	2656.4	1004.44	**1840**	3344
732.22	**1350**	2462	793.33	**1460**	2660	1010	**1850**	3362
733.33	**1352**	2465.6	794.44	**1462**	2663.6	1015.56	**1860**	3380
734.44	**1354**	2469.2	795.56	**1464**	2667.2	1021.11	**1870**	3398
735.56	**1356**	2472.8	796.67	**1466**	2670.8	1026.67	**1880**	3416
736.67	**1358**	2476.4	797.78	**1468**	2674.4	1032.22	**1890**	3434
737.78	**1360**	2480	798.89	**1470**	2678	1037.78	**1900**	3452
738.89	**1362**	2483.6	800	**1472**	2681.6	1043.33	**1910**	3470
740	**1364**	2487.2	801.11	**1474**	2685.2	1048.89	**1920**	3488
741.11	**1366**	2490.8	802.22	**1476**	2688.8	1054.44	**1930**	3506
742.22	**1368**	2494.4	803.33	**1478**	2692.4	1060	**1940**	3524
743.33	**1370**	2498	804.44	**1480**	2696	1065.56	**1950**	3542
744.44	**1372**	2501.6	805.56	**1482**	2699.6	1071.11	**1960**	3560
745.56	**1374**	2505.2	806.67	**1484**	2703.2	1076.67	**1970**	3578
746.67	**1376**	2508.8	807.78	**1486**	2706.8	1082.22	**1980**	3596
747.78	**1378**	2512.4	808.89	**1488**	2710.4	1087.78	**1990**	3614
748.89	**1380**	2516	810	**1490**	2714	1093.33	**2000**	3632
750	**1382**	2519.6	811.11	**1492**	2717.6	1098.89	**2010**	3650
751.11	**1384**	2523.2	812.22	**1494**	2721.2	1104.44	**2020**	3668
752.22	**1386**	2526.8	813.33	**1496**	2724.8	1110	**2030**	3686
753.33	**1388**	2530.4	814.44	**1498**	2728.4	1115.56	**2040**	3704
754.44	**1390**	2534	815.56	**1500**	2732	1121.11	**2050**	3722
755.56	**1392**	2537.6	821.11	**1510**	2750	1126.67	**2060**	3740
756.67	**1394**	2541.2	826.67	**1520**	2768	1132.22	**2070**	3758
757.78	**1396**	2544.8	832.22	**1530**	2786	1137.78	**2080**	3776
758.89	**1398**	2548.4	837.78	**1540**	2804	1143.33	**2090**	3794

| \multicolumn{3}{c}{To convert} | \multicolumn{3}{c}{To convert} | \multicolumn{3}{c}{To convert} |
To °C	←°F or °C→	To °F	To °C	←°F or °C→	To °F	To °C	←°F or °C→	To °F
1148.89	2100	3812	1579.44	2875	5207	2343.33	4250	7682
1154.44	2110	3830	1593.33	2900	5252	2357.22	4275	7727
1160	2120	3848	1607.22	2925	5297	2371.11	4300	7772
1165.56	2130	3866	1621.11	2950	5342	2385.00	4325	7817
1171.11	2140	3884	1635	2975	5387	2398.89	4350	7862
1176.67	2150	3902	1648.89	3000	5432	2412.78	4375	7907
1182.22	2160	3920	1662.78	3025	5477	2426.67	4400	7952
1187.78	2170	3938	1676.67	3050	5522	2440.56	4425	7997
1193.33	2180	3956	1690.56	3075	5567	2454.44	4450	8042
1198.89	2190	3974	1704.44	3100	5612	2468.33	4475	8087
1204.44	2200	3992	1718.33	3125	5657	2482.22	4500	8132
1210	2210	4010	1732.22	3150	5702	2496.11	4525	8177
1215.56	2220	4028	1746.11	3175	5747	2510.00	4550	8222
1221.11	2230	4046	1760	3200	5792	2523.89	4575	8267
1226.67	2240	4064	1773.89	3225	5837	2537.78	4600	8312
1232.22	2250	4082	1787.78	3250	5882	2551.67	4625	8357
1237.78	2260	4100	1801.67	3275	5927	2565.56	4650	8402
1243.33	2270	4118	1815.56	3300	5972	2579.44	4675	8447
1248.89	2280	4136	1829.44	3325	6017	2593.33	4700	8492
1254.44	2290	4154	1843.33	3350	6062	2607.22	4725	8537
1260	2300	4172	1857.22	3375	6107	2621.11	4750	8582
1265.56	2310	4190	1871.11	3400	6152	2635.00	4775	8627
1271.11	2320	4208	1885.00	3425	6197	2648.89	4800	8672
1276.67	2330	4226	1898.89	3450	6242	2662.78	4825	8717
1282.22	2340	4244	1912.78	3475	6287	2676.67	4850	8762
1287.78	2350	4262	1926.67	3500	6332	2690.55	4875	8807
1293.33	2360	4280	1940.56	3525	6377	2704.44	4900	8852
1298.89	2370	4298	1954.44	3550	6422	2718.33	4925	8897
1304.44	2380	4316	1968.33	3575	6467	2732.22	4950	8942
1310	2390	4334	1982.22	3600	6512	2746.11	4975	8987
1315.56	2400	4352	1996.11	3625	6557	2760.00	5000	9032
1321.11	2410	4370	2010.00	3650	6602	2787.78	5050	9122
1326.67	2420	4388	2023.89	3675	6647	2815.56	5100	9212
1332.22	2430	4406	2037.78	3700	6692	2843.33	5150	9302
1337.78	2440	4424	2051.67	3725	6737	2871.11	5200	9392
1343.33	2450	4442	2065.56	3750	6782	2898.89	5250	9482
1348.89	2460	4460	2079.44	3775	6827	2926.67	5300	9572
1354.44	2470	4478	2093.33	3800	6872	2954.44	5350	9662
1360	2480	4496	2107.22	3825	6917	2982.22	5400	9752
1365.56	2490	4514	2121.11	3850	6962	3010.00	5450	9842
1371.11	2500	4532	2135.00	3875	7007	3037.78	5500	9932
1385	2525	4577	2148.89	3900	7052	3065.56	5550	10022
1398.89	2550	4622	2162.78	3925	7097	3093.33	5600	10112
1412.78	2575	4667	2176.67	3950	7142	3121.11	5650	10202
1426.67	2600	4712	2190.56	3975	7187	3148.89	5700	10292
1440.56	2625	4757	2204.44	4000	7232	3176.67	5750	10382
1454.44	2650	4802	2218.33	4025	7277	3204.44	5800	10472
1468.33	2675	4847	2232.22	4050	7322	3232.22	5850	10562
1482.22	2700	4892	2246.11	4075	7367	3260.00	5900	10652
1496.11	2725	4937	2260.00	4100	7412	3287.78	5950	10742
1510	2750	4982	2273.89	4125	7457	3315.56	6000	10832
1523.89	2775	5027	2287.78	4150	7502	3593.33	6500	11732
1537.78	2800	5072	2301.67	4175	7547	3871.11	7000	12632
1551.67	2825	5117	2315.56	4200	7592	4148.89	7500	13532
1565.56	2850	5162	2329.44	4225	7637	4426.67	8000	14432

Subject Index

A

AA. *See* Alcoholics Anonymous
AABB. *See* American Association of Blood Banks
Aase syndrome, 365
ABA. *See* American Burn Association
Abdominal aneurysm, 256, 259, 368
Abdominal hemorrhage, PASG for, 5
Abdominal injuries
 adrenal gland hematomas, adrenal insufficiency and, 257
 basic vs. advanced life support skills, 94
 blunt, 1072–1073
 in children, 543
  acute management of, 550–551
  child abuse and, 542, 601
  with multiple trauma, 549, 550
 nasogastric intubation with, 111
 penetrating, 1072
 peritoneal lavage in, 111
  for children, 550–551
 prehospital management, 110–111
  intravenous therapy, 102
  PASG use and, 110–111
 vascular, 1072–1073
 wound suture removal, 144
Abdominal irradiation, hypomagnesemia and, 306
Abdominal malignancies, acanthosis nigricans and, 429
Abdominal pain, 447–448. *See also* Acute abdomen; Gastrointestinal emergencies
 in adrenal gland hemorrhage, 256
 in adrenal insufficiency, 259
 in appendicitis, 463, 464
 in biliary tract disease, 453–454
 in children, 555–557
 common etiologies and misdiagnoses, 447
 in Crohn's disease, 461
 diabetic ketoacidosis and, 235
 differential diagnosis, 342
 in diverticulitis, 463
 in gynecologic emergencies, 1229–1230, 1233
 in hereditary disorders, 368–371
 in infants, 556–557
 in pancreatitis, 455, 456
 in pelvic inflammatory disease, 1233
 in polyarteritis nodosa, 342
 in pregnancy, 1235–1237
 priorities in managing, 448
 in rheumatoid arthritis, 342
 in systemic lupus erythematosus, 342
 in ulcerative colitis, 462
Abdominal surgery, adrenal insufficiency and, 257
Abdominal thrusts. *See* Heimlich maneuver
Abducens nerve. *See* Cranial nerves
Abetalipoproteinemia, 372
Abortion
 saline, sodium excess from, 267
 self-induced, in battering syndrome, 842
 septic, 1230
 spontaneous, 1230
  in battering syndrome, 842
Abrasions, facial, 1328
Abruptio placentae, 1236, 1237–1238
Abscess, dental, 1331–1333
Absence seizures, 949
Abstinence syndrome. *See* Withdrawal syndrome
Abuse, types of, 837. *See also* Battering syndrome; Child abuse; Domestic violence; Elder abuse; Spouse abuse
Abuser, profile of, 846
 in elder abuse, 847
Acanthosis nigricans, 429
Accelerated idioventricular rhythm (AIVR), 970, 1028, 1030, 1031
Acceleration/deceleration injuries, 1319. *See also* Falls; Motor vehicle accidents
Access to care
 issues in, 6–7
 public education about, 11
 telephone access, 7, 9
Accessory nerve. *See* Cranial nerves
Accidental crises, 859
Accidental Death and Disability . . . (National Research Council), 1
Accidents, as disguised suicide attempts, 835
Accountability issues, 20
Accreditation issues, 27, 45, 46
Acetabular fractures, 215–217
 femoral head fractures and, 217
Acetaminophen (Tylenol; Datril; Panadol), 1435
 for ciguatera fish poisoning, 738, 739
 overdose of, 489
  assay methods, 472
Acetazolamide (Diamox), 1429
 for glaucoma, acute, 1289
 for glaucoma, secondary
  with herpetic keratitis, 1265
  with hyphema, 1285–1286
  with uveitis, 1282
 for high-altitude illness, 682, 684
 for hyperkalemic periodic paralysis, 298, 300
  hypokalemia and, 275, 278
 metabolic acidosis risk with, 321–322
Acetone intoxication, 325
 by inhalant, 805, 806
Acetylcholine, hypomagnesemia and, 304
Acetylcysteine (Mucomyst), 1424
 anaphylaxis risk with, 75
 for corneal ulcers, 1277
 for overdose treatment, 1447–1448
Achilles tendinitis, 346
Achromycin. *See* Tetracycline
Acid, defined, 319
"Acid." *See* LSD
Acid contamination, treatment of, 474
Acid diuresis, in toxicologic emergencies, 475–476
Acid ingestion, in children, 554
Acid-base disturbances, 319–331. *See also specific types*
 anion gap decrease, 327
 anion gap elevation, 323–326
  without acidosis, 326–327
 calcium levels and, 281, 313
 calculation methods of, 319–320
 metabolic acidosis, 320–326
 metabolic alkalosis, 327–329
 physiology of, 320
 potassium and, 273, 293
 in renal failure, treatment of, 1224
 respiratory acidosis, 329–330
 respiratory alkalosis, 330–331
 in shock
  correction procedures, 81
  hypovolemic, 71–72

1463

Acid-base disturbances (*contd.*)
    MAST suit use and, 77
    monitoring for, 82
    in toxicologic emergencies, 470, 473–474
Acidemia. *See also* Diabetic ketoacidosis
    in hypovolemic shock, 71
    lactic, in cardiogenic shock, 73
    metabolic
        as MAST suit complication, 77
        shock and, 71
Acidifying agents, metabolic acidosis and, 322
Acidosis
    hyperkalemia and, 273, 279, 298
    hypokalemia and, 276
    hypothermia and, 664
    in hypovolemic shock, 70–72
    ketoacidosis, 323–324
    lactic, 323
        in cardiogenic shock, 74
        metabolic acidosis and, 323
        in septic shock, 72
    as MAST suit complication, 77
    metabolic. *See* Metabolic acidosis
    in neonate, adrenal insufficiency and, 258
    renal failure and, 1221
    respiratory. *See* Respiratory acidosis
Acinetobacter species
    in corneal ulcers, 1275, 1277
    in pneumonia, 383
ACLS procedures. *See* Advanced cardiac life support
Acoustic nerve. *See* Cranial nerves
Acquired immunodeficiency syndrome (AIDS)
    acute epiglottitis and, 1125
    adrenal insufficiency caused by, 257, 258
    autotransfusions and, 132
    Cryptosporidium-caused diarrhea and, 389
    dermatologic lesions with, 443–444
    encephalitis and, 400, 401
    hypercalcemia and, 317
    rape and, 1250–1251
    substance abuse and, 781, 785
    thrush and, 377
    toxoplasmosis in, 400
    tuberculosis and, 257
Acrolein, as fire byproduct, 494
Acromegaly
    carpal tunnel syndrome and, 347
    hypercalcemia and, 282, 317
Acromioclavicular joint, aspiration or injection of, 1374
Acromioclavicular separations, 198
ACTH. *See* Adrenocorticotropic hormone
Actidose. *See* Charcoal, activated
Actinomyces israelii
    in corneal ulcers, 1275
    in pneumonia, 383
Action potentials
    hypercalcemia and, 283
    hypocalcemia and, 285
    potassium-sodium exchange and, 273–274
Activase. *See* Alteplase recombinant or r-tPA
Activated charcoal. *See* Charcoal, activated
Acupressure, for pain relief, 888
Acupuncture, for headache, 923, 924
Acute abdomen. *See also* Abdominal pain; Gastrointestinal emergencies
    adrenal insufficiency vs., 259
    connective tissue disorders and, 342
    in systemic lupus erythematosus, 342–343
Acute Care Foundation, on PASG, 5
Acute mountain sickness (AMS), 680, 681–683
Acute pain, defined, 877
Acute tubular necrosis (ATN), 1218
    burns and, 418
    differential diagnosis, 1222–1223
    hypercalcemia and, 282
    hypokalemia and, 276, 295
    pathogenesis of, 1220
    pathology of, 1219
Acyclovir (Zovirax), 1418
    for herpes simplex
        encephalitis, 398, 401

    gingivostomatitis, 381
    type 2, 442
    for herpes zoster, 442
    for herpetic whitlow, 408
    pregnancy and, 1239
Addiction, defined, 782
Addison's disease. *See also* Adrenal insufficiency
    hypercalcemia and, 282
    hyperkalemia and, 272, 279
    hyponatremia and, 270
Adenocard. *See* Adenosine
Adenoma sebaceum, 365, 369
Adenomatosis, multiple endocrine, 369, 370
Adenosine (Adenocard), 1381
    for PSVT, 1026, 1028
    for regular, wide QRS tachycardia, 1037
    for Wolff-Parkinson-White syndrome, 1042
Adenosine triphosphate (ATP) synthesis, magnesium balance and, 304
Adenoviruses
    as aseptic meningitis cause, 399
    in common colds, 376
    in pharyngitis, 376, 377
    pneumonia and, 383
    polyarthralgias with, 359
    in shellfish, 733
ADH. *See* Antidiuretic hormone
Adhesive capsulitis (frozen shoulder), 346–347
Adjustment disorder with depressed mood, 831
Adolescents
    abdominal pain in, differential diagnosis, 556
    hydrocarbon aspiration by, 584
    peritonsillar abscess in, 1303–1304
    pneumonia in, 383, 384–385
    sexually transmitted diseases in, 556
    sexual abuse of, 605–608
    suicide attempts by, 590, 591
Adrenal adenomas, 276, 282
Adrenal apoplexy (idiopathic hemorrhage infarction), 256
Adrenal cysts, congenital, 258
Adrenal hemorrhage, 256–257, 258
Adrenal insufficiency
    acute (adrenal crisis), in cancer patients, 508
    etiologies of, 255–258
    hypercalcemia and, 317
    hyperkalemia and, 272
    symptoms of, 258–260
    treatment of, 260
Adrenalin. *See* Epinephrine
Adrenaline, in wound anesthetic, 139, 140
Adrenocorticotropic hormone (ACTH)
    adrenal insufficiency and, 258, 259–260
        secondary, 255
    adrenogenital syndrome and, 277
    Cushing's syndrome and, 276
    as drug, anaphylaxis risk with, 75
    hypothermia and, 666
    in response to injury, 69
Adrenogenital syndrome
    hyperkalemia and, 279
    hypokalemia and, 277
Adrenoleukodystrophy, 258, 259
Adrenomyeloneuropathy, 258, 259
Adriamycin. *See* Doxorubicin
Adson's maneuver, in shoulder-hand syndrome, 347
Adult respiratory distress syndrome (ARDS)
    aspiration-induced, 1166
    venous air embolism and, 708
Advanced cardiac life support (ACLS). *See also* Advanced life support (ALS)
    in arrhythmias, 1090–1091
    defibrillation, 1088–1089, 1090–1091
    drug therapy, 1089–1090
    open chest massage vs. external compression, 1091–1092
    procedures, 1088–1091. *See also specific procedures*
    success of, 1092
Advanced life support (ALS). *See also* Advanced cardiac life support (ACLS)
    ambulance equipment for, 15

    basic life support vs., 2
    EMT-P training for, 3–6
    medical control issues, 20–21
    pediatric, drugs used in, 521–525
    skills required for, 94
    in toxicologic emergencies, 469, 470–471
Advent Christian Church, beliefs and practices, 865
Adventists, beliefs and practices, 865
Advisory Council on Trauma Care Systems (DHEW), 27
Adynamic ileus, 460–461
    burns and, 419
Aerolone. *See* Isoproterenol, inhaled
Aeromonas species, 408
Aerosol inhalation abuse, 805, 806
AFE. *See* Amniotic fluid embolism
Affective disorders, 830–831
    battering syndrome and, 842
Affirmations. *See* Autogenic training
Afibrinogenemia, 366, 372
Afterload
    cardiogenic shock and, 74
    defined, 1052
    in shock diagnosis, 67
Aganglionosis, colonic, 558
Age
    adrenal hemorrhage and, 256
    appendicitis and, 463
    chronic obstructive pulmonary disease and, 1130
    croup syndromes and, 1113, 1114
    headache management and, 917
    heat illness and, 655
    hepatitis A and, 403
    herpes zoster and, 442
    interhospital transfer criteria, 10
    lung function changes with, 1154
    meningitis and, 396, 397, 398
    mononucleosis and, 401
    occult bacteremia and, 530
    pemphigus vulgaris and, 437
    shock risk and, 72
    temporal arteritis and, 917
    urinary tract infections and, 391
Agitation
    drug-induced, 474
    in thyroid storm, 250
AIDS. *See* Acquired immunodeficiency syndrome
Air embolism, 708–709, 1170
    as transfusion complication, 133, 134
Air medical transport, 23–26
    COBRA intent and, 7
    communication with, 8
    criteria for using, 25–26
    increasing use of, 27
    safety issues, 26
Airway, surgical, 1110–1111
Airway constriction, in anaphylaxis, 75
Airway control, 94–99, 1103–1111
    assessment as part of, 1103
    basic vs. advanced life support skills, 94
    for children, 513–515, 517
        with burns, 553
        with corrosive exposure, 554
        in multisystem trauma, 544–545
        unconscious, 591
    in CPR, 1084–1085
    for infants, 1088
    cricothyrotomy for, 99, 1110–1111
    devices for, 95–99
        bag-valve-mask (BVM), 95, 514, 515, 1104
        endotracheal tube, 96–97
        esophageal airway (EOA), 98–99, 1104
        esophageal-tracheal combitube (ETC), 99, 1104
        nasopharyngeal airways, 95–96, 1103–1104
        nasotracheal tube, 98
        oropharyngeal airway, 95–96, 1104
        partial artificial airways, 1103–1104
        for pediatric patients, 95, 97, 514, 517
        pharyngeal-tracheal lumen airway, 99
    in head injuries, 891, 892–893
    in maxillofacial injuries, 1320, 1321
    oxygen supplementation, 1103

partial artificial airways, 1103–1104
in respiratory failure, 1157
in toxicologic emergencies, 469, 470
sedative overdose, 802
Airway damage
with burns, 419, 420
Airway obstruction
in children, 563–570
with fever, 566–570
pathophysiology and, 573–574
with sudden onset, 564–566
chronic, 564
CPR and, 1984–1985
in infants, 1088
in relapsing polychondritis, 340
AIVR. *See* Accelerated idioventricular rhythm
Alaska
air medical transport in, 25
EMS service area, 22
Albinism, 365
Albumin, human (Normal Serum Albumin; Albutein), 1444
Albumin solutions, for shock, 80, 126–127
Albuminemia, anion gap decrease in, 327
Albutein. *See* Albumin, human
Albuterol (Salbutamol)
for anaphylaxis, 86
for hyperkalemia, 300
for hyperkalemic periodic paralysis, 298, 300
inhaled
for asthma, 1132
for obstructive airway disease, 1132, 1133
pediatric dosage, 578
pharmacokinetics of, 1133
Alcohol consumption. *See also* Alcoholism
addiction and withdrawal, 818–819
drowning accidents and, 689–690
epileptic seizures and, 948
extent of, 782
high altitude and, 684
hypothermia and, 662, 666, 671, 672
intoxication and overdose, 817–818
motor vehicle accidents and, 1319
sedatives and, 800
situational syncope and, 961
socioeconomic impact of, 782
as withdrawal treatment, 820
Alcohol metabolism, 816–817
Alcohol sensitivity, in Asians, 372
Alcohol solvents, listed, 756
Alcohol tolerance, 817
Alcohol withdrawal, 818–822
acute confusion with, 954
alcoholic hallucinosis in, 821
delirium tremens in, 306, 819, 821–822
diagnosis of, 820, 821, 822–823
differential diagnosis, 819–820
hypomagnesemia and, 306, 307
mild syndromes, 820–821
opioid withdrawal vs., 798
seizures in, 822, 948–949
treatment of, 820–822
Alcoholic ketoacidosis, 323
Alcoholics Anonymous (AA), referrals to, 823
Alcoholism, 815–825. *See also* Ethanol intoxication; Substance abuse; Toxicologic emergencies
battering syndrome and, 842
detox units, "clearing" patient for, 823–825, 828
diagnosis of, 817, 822–823
screening tests, 827–828
disease concept of, 815–816
emergency departments and, 815, 817–818
crisis counseling, 823
patient behaviors, 818
patient relations, 822–823
hepatitis and, 458
history taking and, 818, 827–828
hypomagnesemia and, 286, 306
morbidity and mortality related to, 815
pancreatitis and, 455
prevalence of, 815

referrals for, 818, 823
"clearing" patient for, 823–825, 828
septic shock risk and, 72
thiamine deficiency with, acute confusion and, 954–955
tolerance and, 817
Aldactone. *See* Spironolactone
Aldehyde solvents, listed, 756
Aldomet. *See* α-Methyldopa
Aldosterone
in acute hemorrhage response, 70
hyperaldosteronism (Conn's syndrome), 276
in injury response, 69
magnesium metabolism and, 286
potassium levels and, 272, 273, 276, 279, 294, 298
Aldosterone antagonist. *See* Spironolactone
Alertness agents, overdose of, 491
Algae, marine, skin reactions from, 741
Aliphatic hydrocarbons
inhalation of, 806
listed, 756
Alkalemia, shock and, 71
Alkali contamination, treatment of, 474
Alkali therapy, for diabetic ketoacidosis, 239
Alkaline diuresis, for toxicologic emergencies, 475
sedative-hypnotic overdose, 804
Alkalosis
congenital, with diarrhea, 328
hypercalcemia and, 313
hypocalcemia and, 281
hypokalemia and, 273, 276, 294
metabolic, 327–329
respiratory, 330–33
at high altitudes, 680
hypocalcemia and, 281
in septic shock, 72
Allergies
anaphylaxis risk with, 75
contact dermatitis and, 432–433
as diarrhea cause, 387
to drugs, skin eruptions, 433–434
to fish or shellfish, 712
to hymenoptera, 643, 644
to local anesthetics, 885
otitis media and, 1309
transfusion reactions, 133, 134
urticaria and, 440
Allopurinol (Zyloprim), 1403
α¹-Antitrypsin deficiency, 366
α-Adrenergic stimulating agents, for PSVT, 1026
α-Blocking agents, for catecholamine crisis, 1067
α-Thalassemia, in Asians, 372
Alprazolam (Xanax), elimination half-life of, 800
ALS. *See* Advanced life support
Alteplase recombinant or r-tPA (Activase), 1400
for acute myocardial infarction, 982
Alternative medicine
for headache prophylaxis, 924
pain management methods, 887–888
spiritual healing methods, 869–870
Altitude-related emergencies, 679–686
decompression sickness (DCS), 706, 707
mountain sickness, 679
acute (AMS), 680, 681–683
chronic (CMS), 685
as headache cause, 918
Aluminum hydroxide phosphate binders, for renal failure, 1224–1225
Aluminum spine boards, costs of, 109
Alupent. *See* Metaproterenol
Alzheimer's disease, 957
Ambulances
communication and, 7, 8, 9
criteria for, 15–16
deployment plans, 16
design criteria developed, 2
in disaster management, 12, 35
diversion policies and, 18
as EMS system components, 15–16
mutual aid issues, 11
record keeping issues, 11–12
Amcill. *See* Ampicillin

Amebiasis, aseptic meningitis and, 399
American Academy of Orthopedic Surgeons, EMT training by, 3
American Academy of Pediatrics (AAP)
on foreign body removal, 515, 516
on child abuse evaluation, 603
on sexual abuse evaluation, 607
on steroids for meningitis, 538
American Association of Blood Banks (AABB)
on autotransfusions, 132
on crystalloid solutions, 126
standards by, 117, 122–124
American Association of Poison Control Centers, ED classification by, 48
American Burn Association (ABA)
burn center criteria by, 47
EMS systems and, 19
American College of Emergency Physicians
disaster defined by, 31
on medical control, 21
American College of Surgeons
on burn center criteria, 47
on interhospital transfer, 10
quality criteria and, 55
on staffing requirements, 21
on tetanus prophylaxis, 155
trauma care standards by, 94
trauma centers and, 18, 49
triage decision scheme, 16, 17
American Heart Association
ACLS standards by, 1088, 1089
ALS standards by, 94
on foreign body removal in children, 515, 516
American Hospital Association
ED classification by, 46
on rural vs. urban facilities, 23
American Medical Association (AMA)
critical care area classification by, 46–49
facilities categorized by, 18, 45–46
quality criteria by, 54, 62
American Red Cross, blood donor guidelines, 118–119, 120
American Society for Testing and Materials (ASTM), EMS standards role, 27
American Trauma Society, founding of, 2
Amicar. *See* ε-Aminocaproic acid
Amikacin (Amikin), 1409
for corneal ulcers, 1278
eye drop preparation, 1268
Amiloride (Midamor), 1430
Amino acid replacement, for renal failure, 1225
ε-Aminocaproic acid (Amicar), 1400
Aminoglycoside antibiotics, 1409–1411
in appendicitis, 465
for colon injury, 465
for necrotizing fasciitis or myositis, 410
for open fractures, 172
for prostatitis, 395
for sepsis, 406
for septic arthritis, 357, 412
for septic shock, 85
for skin infections, marine-associated, 408
for urinary tract infection
with bacteremia, 392
prostatitis, 395
for vertebral column injuries, 187–188
Aminophylline (Aminophyllin), 1425–1426
for anaphylaxis, 86
for asthma
in children, 581
in pregnancy, 1239
calculating dosage of, 482
for congestive heart failure, 1055, 1056
for obstructive airway disease, 1134
for pulmonary edema, 1099
Aminopyrine, anaphylaxis risk with, 75
Amiodarone (Cordarone), 1381–1382
Amitriptyline (Elavil; Endep), 1406. *See also* Antidepressants
for headache, 924
hyponatremia and, 271
overdose of, 484

Ammonia inhalation, 769, 770
  from fires, 494
Ammonium chloride, for acid diuresis, 475
Amniotic fluid embolism (AFE), 1171
Amobarbital (Amytal; Amylobarbitone), 1438.
    See also Barbiturates
  elimination half-life of, 800
  pharmacology of, 801
Amoxapine (Asendin), 486
  overdose of, 473, 486
Amoxicillin (Amoxil; Larotid; Polymox), 1413
  for febrile children under two, 532
  for gonococcal pharyngitis, 378
  for gonorrhea, 1250
  for Lyme disease, 357, 409
  for otitis media, 381, 1309
  for pneumonia, 386
    in children, 586
  for sinusitis, 379
  for urinary tract infections, 393
Amoxicillin-clavulanic acid (Augmentin), 1413–1414
  for animal bites, 158
  for otitis media, 381
  for pneumonia, 386
  for septic arthritis, 411–412
  for sinusitis, 379, 1303
  for urinary tract infections, 393
Amoxil. See Amoxicillin
Amphetamine, 786–787, 789–791
  complications of, 78–90, 784, 790–791
  crystal ("ice"), 790
  history of, 789–790
  hypothermia and, 671
  overdose
    clinical signs, 472, 473, 474
    respiratory alkalosis and, 330
    treatment of, 475–476, 791–793
  pharmacology of, 790
  in pregnancy, effects on neonate, 810
  screening tests for, 786
  as sympathomimetic, 787
Amphojel, for renal failure, 1224
Amphotericin B (Fungizone), 1418–1419
  as diabetes insipidus cause, 268
  as hypokalemia cause, 275
Ampicillin (Polycillin; Amcill), 1414
  for cellulitis, 432
  for cholangitis and sepsis, 454–455
  for corneal ulcers, 1275, 1278
  for gonococcal pharyngitis, 378
  for gonorrhea, 1250
  for infectious mononucleosis, 402
  for meningitis, purulent, 398, 953
    in infants under 3 months, 535
  for otitis media, 381, 1309
  for pelvic inflammatory disease, 1234
  for pneumonia, 386
    in children, 586
  for septic arthritis, 411
  for sinusitis, 379, 1303
  for urinary tract infections, 392, 393
Ampicillin/sulbactam, for animal bites, 158
Amputations, replantation of
  penis, 1208, 1209
  upper extremities, 212
Amrinone lactate (Inocor), 1382
  for congestive heart failure, 1055, 1056
  for shock, 84
Amyl nitrite, 1448
  for hydrogen sulfide poisoning, 756
Amylase-creatinine clearance ratio, in diabetic ketoacidosis, 235
Amylobarbitone. See Amobarbital
Amyloidosis, carpal tunnel syndrome and, 347
Amytal. See Amobarbital
Anaerobic bacteria
  in bite wounds, 155, 156
  OHP as bacteriocidal for, 704
  otitis media, 1309
  in peritonsillar abscess, 569
  in pneumonia, 383
  in retropharyngeal abscess, 569
  in septic arthritis, 410
  in sinusitis, 1302
Anaerobic infections, HBO therapy for, 705
Anaerobic metabolism, indicators of, 71
Anal fissure, 466
Anal reflex loss, in cauda equina syndrome, 193
Analeptic overdose, respiratory alkalosis and, 330
Analgesia; Analgesics, 1435–1438. See also Narcotic analgesics; specific drugs
  for cardiogenic shock, 85
  for dislocations, 173
  emergency room use of, 880–881
  endogenous, 879
  for herpes zoster, 442
  for ocular pain
    corneal abrasion or foreign body, 1270
    herpetic keratitis, 1265
    hyphema, 1284
    uveitis, 1281
  for pancreatitis, 456
  side effects of, 880
  simple, listed, 880
  for sinusitis, 379
  thoracic injuries and, 101
  for vertebral column injuries, 187, 193
  in wound management, 139
Anaphylactoid reactions, 75
Anaphylaxis; Anaphylactic shock
  in children, airway obstruction with, 565
  defined, 75
  in drug reaction, 433
  hymenoptera allergy and, 643, 644
  pathophysiology of, 75
  as transfusion complication, 133, 134
  treatment of, 86–87
Ancef. See Cefazolin
Adrenoleukodystrophy, 259
Anemia
  hemolytic, burns and, 418
  in hereditary disorders, 364, 365
  in lead poisoning, 494
  pernicious, adrenal insufficiency and, 255
  renal failure and, 1226
Anencephaly, 258
Anesthesia
  general
    anaphylaxis risk with, 75
    in wound management, 139
  local, 884–885
    anaphylaxis risk with, 75
    for emergency department, 1453
    reactions to, 884–885
    in wound management, 139–140
  overdose of, clinical signs, 473
  regional blocks, 885
  thyroid storm after, 249
  topical, 885–886
    for endotracheal intubation, 1106
    for oral ulcerations, 1336
  in wound management, 139–140
Anesthesia bag, for ventilation assistance, 99
Anesthetic agents, inhalant abuse with, 805
Aneurysm
  abdominal, 256, 259, 368
  cerebral, subarachnoid hemorrhage and, 939, 940
  as diabetes insipidus cause, 267
"Angel dust." See PCP
Anger, in grieving process, 860
Angiitis, allergic, vasculitis with, 341
Angina
  abdominal, differential diagnosis, 368
  medications for, 1391–1397
  pulmonary artery pressure monitoring with, 83
Angiodysplasia, colonic, 558
Angioedema, in anaphylaxis, 75
Angiography
  in acute myocardial infarction, 982
  in cardiovascular accident, 943
  in cerebral aneurysm, 918
  in headache evaluation, 921
  in intestinal obstruction, 461
  in pulmonary embolism, 1146–1147
  renal
    in blunt trauma, 1197
    in penetrating trauma, 1199
  for upper GI bleeding, 450
Angiokeratoma, in hereditary disorder, 365
Angioneurotic edema, hereditary, 369, 370
Angiotensin, physiology and, 272, 273
Angiotensin II, in response to injury, 69
Angiotensin-converting enzyme inhibitors, hyperkalemia risk with, 298
Anglicans, beliefs and practices, 866
Angulation-rotation fractures, 164
Aniline dye intoxication, 473, 757
Animal bite wounds, 155–156, 157–158, 627–632
  cat bites, 629, 631–632
  dog bites, 627–631
  rabies precautions, 629
Animals, exposure to. See also Animal bite wounds
  acute watery diarrhea and, 389
  occupational disorders, 1162
  pneumonia and, 385
  sepsis and, 406
  skin infections from, 409
  as urticaria cause, 440
Anion gap
  decrease in, 327
  elevation of without acidosis, 326–327
  metabolic acidosis and, 321–326
Anistreplase or APSAC (Eminase), 1400–1401
  for acute myocardial infarction, 982
Ankles
  arthrocentesis of, 355
  fractures of, 226–228
  sprains of, 230–231
  in vertebral column injury, 185
Ankylosing spondylitis
  anterior cord syndrome with, 185
  ocular involvement in, 338, 339
Anointing, as nonmedical healing method, 870
Anorectal abscesses, 407, 408, 466
Anorexia
  in adrenal insufficiency, 259
  in hypercalcemia, 283
  in hypomagnesemia, 286, 304
Anoscopy
  for lower GI bleeding, 451
  in rape examination, 1249
Ansaid. See Flurbiprofen
Anserine bursa, aspiration or injection of, 1374
Anspor. See Cephradine
Antacids
  calcium-containing, hypercalcemia and, 282, 315, 318
  as diarrhea cause, 387
  for hypomagnesemia, 287
Anterior cerebral artery syndrome, 937
Anterior cord syndrome, 184–185
  in cervical spine, 909, 910
Anterior lesions, in ischemic CVA, 937
Anterior-posterior (AP) compression injury, 213, 215
Anthracyclines, toxic reactions to, cardiac, 509
Anthrax, 409
Anti-inflammatory drugs, 1403–1405. See also Corticosteroids; Nonsteroidal anti-inflammatory agents
Antianginal agents, 1391–1397, 1448
Antiarrhythmics, 1381–1391. See also Antidysrhythmic drugs
Antiasthmatic agents, 1424–1428
Antibiotics. See also specific antibiotics; specific conditions
  aminoglycoside, 1409–1411
  anaphylaxis risk with, 75
  cephalosporin, 1411–1413
  as diarrhea cause, 387
  E. coli infection and, 390
  for emergency departments, listed, 1452
  for febrile infants under 3 months, 535
  in fracture management, 168, 172

as gastroenteritis cause, 387, 388
hypothermia and, 671
for marine organism wounds, 731, 732
miscellaneous types of, 1418–1424
for ocular infections, 1275, 1277, 1278
  eye drop preparations, 1268, 1269
oxygen under high pressure (OHP) as, 704
penicillin and penicillin derivatives, 1413–1416
in pregnancy, 1239
renal failure and, 1218–1219, 1225
for respiratory distress, in children, 579
for sepsis, 406–407
in septic shock treatment, 85
sulfonamides, 1417
tetracyclines, 1417–1418
in trauma management, 553
in wound management, 138, 154, 155, 156, 157-158
Antibody screening, 122, 123
Anticholinergics
  behavioral disorders induced by, 474
  for diverticulitis, 463
  for insecticide poisoning, 478
  for obstructive airway disease, 1134
  overdose of
    clinical signs, 472
    physostigmine for, 479–480
    as unconsciousness cause, 591
Anticoagulants, 1400–1403
  adrenal hemorrhage and, 256–257
  for air embolism, 1170
  in cardiogenic shock treatment, 85
  for emergency department, 1452
  hypomagnesemia and, 306
  for pulmonary embolism, 1148
  renal failure and, 1225
  reversing agents, 1452
Anticollagenase, for corneal ulcers, 1277
Anticonvulsants, 1398–1399. *See also* Convulsions; *specific drugs*
  for head injury, 898
  for meningitis, in children under two, 539
  overdose with, 489–491
  for seizures
    intravenous, 946–947
    oral, 949
Antidepressants, 1406–1408
  bicyclic, 487
  for depression, 832
  for headache, 924
  tetracyclic, 486–487
  tricyclic. *See* Tricyclic antidepressants
  as unconsciousness cause, 591
Antidigoxin F(ab) fragments, 492–493
Antidiuretic hormone (ADH)
  in acute hemorrhage response, 70
  in cancer patients, hyponatremia and, 507–508
  hyponatremia and, 270, 271, 272
  hypothermia and, 666
  myxedema coma and, 252
  sodium levels and, 266
Antidumping statute, 42–43
Antidysrhythmic drugs
  in advanced cardiac life support, 1089–1090
  for atrial premature complex, 1001–1002
  multifocal atrial tachycardia and, 1022
  for premature ventricular complexes, 1002–1003, 1005
  for PSVT, 1028
Antiemetics, 1406–1408
  cannabis, 808–809
  for pancreatitis, 456
Antifibrinolytics, 1400–1403
Antifreeze intoxication, 324–325
Antigout agents, 1403–1405
Antihistamines, 1408–1409
  for anaphylaxis, 86
  behavioral disorders induced by, 474
  for emergency department, 1452
  for hymenoptera stings, 644
  for otitis media, 381

overdose of, 491
for scombroid fish poisoning, 739
for urticaria, 441
Antihypertensives, 1391–1397
Antihypoglycemics/hypoglycemics, 1432–1433
Antilirium. *See* Physostigmine
Antimalarial retinopathy, 339
Antimetabolites, as diarrhea cause, 387
Antinausea agents, for headache, 922
Antineoplastic drugs. *See* Chemotherapy
Antipruritics, 1408–1409
Antishock garment. *See* MAST suit
Antivenin treatments
  for black widow spiders, 493, 641
  for emergency department, 1453
  for jellyfish, 721
  for scorpions, 493, 643
  for snakes, 493, 638–639
Antiviral agents
  for herpetic keratitis, 1264
  for uveitis, 1282
Antrenyl. *See* Oxyphenonium
Anturane. *See* Sulfinpyrazone
Aortic aneurysm, as hereditary disorder, 367
Aortic dissection
  acute, 1066, 1081–1082
  in Marfan's syndrome, 371
  syncope and, 960
Aortic injury, 1072, 1081–1082, 1187. *See also* Aortic dissection; Vascular emergencies
Aortic insufficiency, pulmonary edema and, 1097
Aortic outflow obstruction, syncope and, 959–960, 963
Aortic stenosis, syncope and, 959
Aortography
  in blunt chest injury, 1072, 1187
  in renal trauma, 1197, 1199
AP (anterior-posterior) pelvic injuries, 213, 215
APC. *See* Atrial premature complex
Aphthous ulcers, 1336
Apocrine sweat glands, abscess formation in, 431
Appendicitis, 463–465
  in pediatric patients, 464, 555–556
Appetite suppression, amphetamines for, 790
Appropriateness (efficacy) of care, as quality issue, 54, 62
APSAC. *See* Anistreplase or APSAC
AquaMephyton. *See* Phytonadione
Arachnodactyly, 367, 368
Aramine, for PSVT, 1026
Arbovirus, polyarthralgias with, 359
ARDS. *See* Adult respiratory distress syndrome
Arena viruses, as sepsis cause, 406
Arfonad. *See* Trimethaphan camphor sulfonate
Arginine vasopressin (AVP), in response to injury, 69
Arm shock, 72, 73
Armenians
  beliefs and practices, 865
  familial Mediterranean fever in, 369, 370
Arms. *See also* Extremities; Upper extremity injuries
  dysmorphology of, in hereditary disorders, 364, 365
  fractures of
    cast application to, 171
    in children, 165
    humeral shaft, 201–202
    proximal humerus, 201
    subclavian steal syndrome in, 961
Aromatic hydrocarbons, listed, 756
Arrhythmias. *See* Dysrhythmias
Arsenic poisoning, 473, 474, 494. *See also* Metal poisoning
Arsine, as systemic toxin, 774–775
Arsine toxicity, 757
Arterial air embolism, 708–709
Arterial blood gases. *See* Blood gas measurements
Arterial blood pressure. *See also* Pulmonary artery wedge pressure monitoring
  acute myocardial infarction and, 989
  dysrhythmia and, 997–998
  vasopressors and, 84
Arterial trauma. *See* Vascular emergencies

Arterial-central venous oxygen difference, monitoring for shock, 82–83
Arteriography
  in acute aortic dissection, 1082
  in hemoptysis evaluation, 1168
  for lower GI bleeding, 451
  in vascular injury, 1070
    abdominal, 1073
    to extremities, 1073
    intra-arterial injection of foreign substances, 1075
    to neck, 1074
    thoracic, 1071, 1072
Arteriolar dilating agents, in acute myocardial infarction, 993
Arteriovenous fistula, acute, 1070–1071
Arteritis, temporal, 337–338
Arthralgia
  in adrenal insufficiency, 259
  differential diagnosis, 359
  in erythema nodosum, 336
  in hypercalcemia, 283
  in Wegener's granulomatosis, 340
Arthritis
  acute monoarticular, 335, 351–359
    diagnosis of, 353–356
    etiologies of, 351, 356–358
    history taking and, 351–352
    physical examination in, 352–353
  crystal, 357–358
  in elbow, 204
  gonococcal. *See* Gonococcal arthritis
  infectious
    cutaneous lesions in, 336–337
    fever in, 335
  ocular emergencies in, 338
  polyarticular, 358–359
  psoriatic, monoarticular arthritis with, 358
  recurrent, in Lyme disease, 357
  rheumatoid. *See* Rheumatoid arthritis
  septic, 204, 410–412
    diagnosis, of, 351, 352, 356–357, 411
    differential diagnosis, 411
    drug abuse and, 785
    in elbow, 204
    as human bite complication, 156
    pathogenesis of, 411
    treatment of, 411–412
  traumatic, 358
Arthrocentesis
  of knee, 224, 354–355
  in septic arthritis, 411
  techniques, 353–355, 1373–1375
Arthropod-borne viruses, encephalitis and, 400
Arthroscopy, in knee evaluation, 223, 224
AS cells, for transfusions, 117
Ascaris species, biliary obstruction and, 455
Ascites, 459
  acute liver failure and, 458
  in systemic lupus erythematosus, 342
  treatment of, 459
Asendin. *See* Amoxapine
Ashkenazi Jews, hereditary disorders of, 365, 366, 368
Ashman phenomenon, 1008, 1009
Aspergillus species
  in otitis externa, 1310, 1311
  pneumonia and, 383
  sinusitis and, 378, 1302
Asphalt burns, 424
Asphyxia, traumatic, 1188–1189
Asphyxiants. *See also* Inhalation injury
  chemical, 764–769
  physical, 763–764
Aspiration injuries, 1165–1167
  management of, 1166
  pediatric, 515–516, 583–584
    hydrocarbons, 584
    with multiple trauma, 543
    sudden UAO and, 564–565
Aspiration of meconium, 1166–1167

Aspiration pneumonia
  diagnosis of, 385
  prevention of, 1166
  treatment of, 387
Aspirin, 1435
  in acute myocardial infarction treatment, 982–983
  anaphylaxis risk with, 75
  chronic salicylism and, 488
  for gout/pseudogout, 358
  for hypercalcemia, 313
  ingestion of, hyphema and, 1285
  for Lyme disease, 357
  for pain relief, 881
    side effects of, 880
  for polyarticular arthritis, 359
  salicylate emergencies. *See* Salicylates
  serum sickness and, 433
  as urticaria cause, 440
Assault and battery
  domestic violence, 843
  elder abuse, 847
Assay tests, in toxicologic emergencies, 471, 472
Assembly of God, beliefs and practices, 868
Assessment. *See* Evaluation; Quality issues
Association for Air Medical Services, 26
  accreditation and, 27
  guidelines by, 25–26
Asterixis, as hyponatremia sign, 271
Asthma. *See also* Obstructive airway disease
  adrenal insufficiency and, 259
  anaphylaxis risk with, 75
  asphyxia with, 1134–1135
  in children, 580–582
  defined, 1129
  dehydration risk with, 267
  high altitude and, 685
  management guidelines, 1136–1138
  pathogenesis of, 1130
  in pregnancy, 1239
  risk factors for, 1130
  statistics about, 1129–1130
  treatment of
    antibiotics, 1135
    anticholinergics, 1134
    calcium channel blockers, 1136
    magnesium, 308, 1135
    mechanical ventilation, 1134–1135
    methylxanthines, 1134
    oxygen, 1132
    steroids, 1135–1136
    sympathomimetics, 1133
Asystole
  advanced cardiac life support for, 1091
  in hyperkalemia, 280
Atabrine. *See* Quinacrine
Atarax. *See* Hydroxyzine
Ataxia
  as hyponatremia sign, 271
  as toxin ingestion sign, 474
Ataxia telangiectasia, 364, 365, 368
Atenolol (Tenormin), 1391
  for alcohol withdrawal, 820
  for headache prophylaxis, 922, 924
  for ventricular premature complexes, 1005
Athetoid movements, in hypomagnesemia, 304
Athlete's foot (tinea pedis), 436
Ativan. *See* Lorazepam
Atlantic Portuguese man-of-war, 718
Atlanto-occipital dislocations, 188
Atlantoaxial joint destruction, in rheumatoid arthritis, 343
Atlas-dens interval, dislocations and, 188–189
ATN. *See* Acute tubular necrosis
Atopic dermatitis, 429–430
ATP synthesis, magnesium balance and, 304
Atracurium (Tracrium), 1441
Atrial fibrillation, 1009, 1018, 1022–1023
Atrial flutter, 1016, 1018, 1023–1024
Atrial premature complex (APC), 999–1002
  aberration vs. ectopy, 1007–1008, 1009
Atrial standstill (sudden sinus), 1010–1012

Atrioventricular (AV) block, 1013–1017
  treatment for, 984–985, 1013
Atropine, 1382
  in acute myocardial infarction treatment, 984, 985
  behavioral disorders and, 474
  for carbamate toxicity, 757
  for ciguatera fish poisoning, 738
  in CPR
    advanced cardiac life support, 1089, 1090, 1091
    of pediatric patients, 523
  for dysrhythmias
    atrioventricular (AV) block, 1013
    sudden sinus (atrial standstill), 1011
  in endotracheal intubation, 1106
  hypothermia and, 671
  for obstructive airway disease, 1134
  for organophosphate toxicity, 478, 757, 776
  for uveitis, 1281
Atrovent. *See* Ipratropium bromide
Audiologic tests, 1307
Augmentin. *See* Amoxicillin-clavulanic acid
Aura
  with migraine, 916
  with seizure-related syncope, 961
Autogenic training, for pain management, 887
Autoimmune deficiency syndrome. *See* Acquired immunodeficiency syndrome
Autoimmune disorders
  adrenal insufficiency and, 255
  aphthous ulcers and, 1336
  chronic lymphocytic (Hashimoto's) thyroiditis, myxedema coma and, 251
  pemphigus vulgaris, 437
Autonomic drugs, for EDs, listed, 1452
Autonomic dysfunction
  hyperreflexia (dysreflexia), 912–913
  orthostatic syncope and, 961
Autosuggestion, as nonmedical healing method, 870
Autotransfusions, 81, 116, 132–133
AVP. *See* Arginine vasopressin
Avulsion injury, 164, 165
  to face, 1328
  to teeth, 1333–1335
Awareness, defined, 927–928
Axillary hair, in hypocalcemia, 285
Axillary sweating, dehydration sign, 268
Azapropazone (Rheumox), for pain relief, 881
Azathioprine
  aseptic meningitis and, 344
  in systemic lupus erythematosus, pancreatitis and, 342
Azo dye intoxication, 473
Azotemia
  differential diagnosis, 1221–1223
  hematologic disorders with, 1226
  magnesium therapy and, 307
  renal failure and, 1219
AZT. *See* Zidovudine

B

Bacillus anthracis, 409
  in pneumonia, 383
Bacillus cereus
  in food poisoning, 390
  in gastroenteritis, 388
Bacillus fragilis, in septic shock, 85
Bacitracin eye drop preparation, 1268
  for corneal ulcers, 1277, 1278
Back injuries. *See* Cervical spine injuries; Spinal injuries
Back pain
  in adrenal insufficiency, 259
  in cauda equina syndrome, 193
  chronic, in adrenal insufficiency, 159
  in systemic lupus erythematosus, 344
Back wounds, suture removal from, 144
Bacteremia
  differential diagnosis, 406
  Gram-negative, septic shock and, 72

  occult (OB), in febrile children under two, 529–533
  urinary tract infection and, 392
Bacterial infections
  acute confusion with, 953
  acute sepsis in, differential diagnosis, 406
  adrenal insufficiency and, 256
  in appendicitis, 463, 465
  aspiration-induced, 1165
  in biliary tract disease, 453
  bivalve mollusk poisoning and, 731–733
  in children under two, fever in, 529–533
  dermatologic, 430–432
    toxic epidermal necrolysis and, 440
  encephalitis, 400, 401
  epididymitis, 1212
  gastroenteritis, 387–389
  hemoptysis caused by, 1167
  marine organisms and, 731, 742
  meningitis, 535–536
    in infants and children, 533–539, 590
  occupational sources of, 1162
  ocular
    antibiotics for, 1275, 1276, 1277–1278
    corneal ulcers, 1273–1276
    diagnostic tests, 1270–1273
  of oropharynx, 382
  otitis externa, 379–380, 1310, 1311
  otitis media, 380–381, 1309–1310
  peritonsillar abscess and, 569
  pharyngitis, 376
  pneumonia, 383, 384
    in children, 585–586
  prostatitis, 395–396
  purulent, 396–390
  in scombroid fish poisoning, 739
  sinusitis, 378–379, 1302–1303
  substance abuse and, 785
  tracheitis (membranous croup), 569, 1113, 1116–1117
  tracheobronchitis, airway control in children and, 514
  of urinary tract, 391–396
  as urticaria cause, 440
Bacteriuria, in febrile infants, 535
Bacteroides
  in dog bites, 155
  in human bites, 156
  in oropharyngeal infections, 382, 383
Bactrim. *See* Trimethoprim-sulfamethoxazole
"Bag of bones" technique, for intercondylar fractures of distal humerus, 203
Bag-valve-mask (BVM) unit, 95, 514, 515, 1104
  for children, 514, 515, 517, 518, 519
Baha'i, beliefs and practices, 865
Baker's cyst, 346
Balance's sign, 110
Balanitis circinata, in Reiter's syndrome, 358
Balloon tamponade, for upper GI bleeding, 450
Baptists, beliefs and practices, 865
Barbiturates, 1438–1441. *See also* Sedative-hypnotics
  in abstinence syndrome diagnosis, 798
  abstinence syndromes, 804, 805
  for cannabis overdose, 809
  for head injury, 898
  for headache, 922, 923
  hyponatremia and, 271
  hypothermia and, 662
  listed, 800
  near-drowning and, 694, 698
  overdose of, 802–804
    clinical signs, 472, 473, 803
  for pain relief, 882, 883
  pharmacology of, 800–801
  as sedative withdrawal treatment, 805
  serum sickness and, 433
Barium enema
  in irritable bowel syndrome, 463
  in ulcerative colitis, 462
Barium poisoning
  hyperkalemia and, 279
  hypokalemia and, 276, 295

Barium swallow, for esophageal obstruction, 452
Barracuda, attacks by, 714
Barton's fracture, 205
Bartter's syndrome
  hypokalemia and, 275, 294, 296
  treatment of, 278
Basaljel, for renal failure, 1224
Base, defined, 319
Baseball or mallet finger, 207
Basic EMT training, 3
Basic life support (BLS)
  advanced life support vs., 2
  in trauma stabilization, 5
  ambulance equipment for, 15
  CPR procedures, 1083–1088
  for infants and children, 519, 1088
  skills required for, 94
Basilar artery syndrome, 938
Bassen-Kornzweig disease, 372
Bats, exposure to
  pneumonia and, 385
  rabies and, 629
Battering syndrome, 841–842. See also Domestic violence
  defined, 837, 841
  misconceptions about, 842–843
  profile of abused woman, 845
  profile of abuser, 846
  psychologic aspects of, 846
Battery ingestion, 559
Battle's sign, 110
Beclomethasone (Vanceril; Beclovent), 1426
  for asthma in pregnancy, 1239
Bee stings, 75, 643–644
Behavioral disorders. See also Confusion; Psychiatric disorders; specific disorders
  alcohol-induced, 817, 818
  classification of, 47
  drug- or toxin-induced, 474
Behavioral emergencies, ED classification for, 47
Behçet's syndrome, 341
  aseptic meningitis and, 399
  erythema nodosum and, 336–337
  neurologic involvement in, 343
  ocular involvement in, 338–339
  thrombophlebitis in, 341
Bell's palsy, in Lyme disease, 357
Benadryl. See Diphenhydramine
Bends. See Decompression sickness
Benemid. See Probenecid
Bennett's fracture, 208
Benorylate (Benoral), for pain relief, 881
Benoxinate HCl, pharmacologic classification, 885
Bentyl. See Dicyclomine
Benzedrine. See Phenylisopropylamine
Benzene, as systemic toxin, 774
Benzocaine. See Ethylaminobenzoate
Benzodiazepines. See also Sedative-hypnotics
  abstinence syndromes, 804
  extent of use, 800
  for headache, 922
  listed, 800
  overdose of, 472, 491–492, 802–804
  for PCP overdose, 808
  pharmacokinetics and, 484
  pharmacology of, 801
Benzphetamine, as sympathomimetic, 787
Bereavement, uncomplicated, 831
Bernard-Soulier syndrome, 366
β-Adrenergic blocking agents. See also Propranolol
  in acute myocardial infarction treatment, 983, 993
  for alcohol withdrawal, 820
  for asthma, in pregnancy, 1239
  confusion caused by, 474
  for dysrhythmias
    atrial fibrillation, 1022
    atrial flutter, 1024
    premature ventricular complexes, 1005
    PSVT, 1026, 1028
    sudden sinus (atrial standstill), 1011
    Wolff-Parkinson-White syndrome, 1042
  for headache prophylaxis, 924
  for hyperkalemia, 299, 300
  for hyperkalemic periodic paralysis, 298
  for hypertensive emergencies, 1063–1064, 1066, 1067
  hypokalemia risk with, 295
  for obstructive airway disease, 1133
  for thyroid storm, 251
β-Adrenergic stimulating agents, for sudden sinus (atrial standstill), 1011
Betagan. See Levobunolol
Betaxolol (Betoptic)
  for acute glaucoma, 1289
  for hyphema, 1286
Bhopal, India, 747, 751–752
Bicarbonate. See Sodium bicarbonate
Bicarbonate levels, 328
Bicipital tendon, aspiration or injection of, 1374
Bicycle accidents, children in, 541, 542
Bicyclic antidepressants, 487
Bigeminy, rule of, 1008, 1009
Bilateral adrenal venography, adrenal insufficiency and, 257
Biliary tract disease, 453–455
Bilious vomiting, in infants, 557–558
Bilirubin, in pulmonary embolism, 1145
Binding agents, for hypercalcemia, 315–316
Bing v. Theunig, 61
Biofeedback, for headache prophylaxis, 924
Bipolar disorders, 830
  alcoholism and, 824
Birds, exposure to, pneumonia and, 385
Bird's nest filter, for pulmonary embolism, 1148–1149
Birth control pills
  adrenal insufficiency and, 258
  gallstones and, 556
"Biscuit." See Methadone
Bisexual patients, mononucleosis syndrome and, 402
Bismuth subsalicylate, for diarrhea, 389–390
Bite wounds, 155–156, 157–158
  cat, 155, 156, 157, 631–632
  dog, 155, 156, 157, 627–631
  human, 156, 157–158, 632–634
  hymenoptera, 643–644
  rabies precautions, 629
  scorpion, 493, 642–643
  snake, 634–640
    anaphylaxis risk with, 75
    antivenin treatments for, 493, 638–639
    identifying the snake, 650–651
  spider, 493, 640–642
Bitolterol, inhaled, for obstructive airway disease, 1133
Bivalve mollusks, poisoning by, 391, 731–734, 735
Black widow spiders, 640–641
  antivenin for, 493, 641
Bladder drainage, filliform and follower for, 1214, 1215
Bladder injuries, 1202–1205
  iatrogenic, 1202
  management of, 1205
  ruptures, 1202, 1204, 1205
Bladder outlet obstruction, in prostatitis, 395
Blastomyces dermatitidis, in pneumonia, 383
Blastomycosis, adrenal insufficiency and, 258
Bleeding. See also Hemostasis; Vascular emergencies
  from dental extraction, 1335–1336
  epistaxis, 1304–1306
  in hereditary disorders, 364, 365–368
  intraocular
    in glaucoma, 1289
    in hyphema, 1282–1286
  in liver failure, 458
  lower gastrointestinal, 450–451
  in maxillofacial injuries, 1320, 1321
  rectal, hemorrhoids, 465–466
  upper gastrointestinal, 448–450
    early management, 448
    esophageal varices and, 452–453
  vaginal, abnormal, 1230–1231
Bleomycin, toxic pulmonary reactions to, 508
Blindness
  hyphema and, 1282
  sudden
    in systemic lupus erythematosus, 338
    in temporal arteritis, 337, 338
Blocadren. See Timolol
Blood alcohol levels, 816–817
Blood banks
  compatibility testing by, 122–124
  origins of, 116
  regulations and practices, 117–119
Blood culture, indications for. See specific infections
Blood donors, regulations for, 117, 118
Blood filters, 130–131
Blood gas measurements
  in obstructive airway disease, 1131, 1132
  in pediatric respiratory disorders, 576
  in pulmonary embolism, 1145
Blood pressure. See also Hypertension; Hypertensive emergencies; Hypotension
  acute myocardial infarction and, 989, 991–992
  in anaphylaxis, 75
  cervical cord injuries and, 912–913
  dysrhythmia and, 997–998
  interpreting, 66–67
  intracerebral hemorrhage and, 941
  measuring, in shock states, 66
  monitoring, in shock treatment, 81–82
  normal values, 66
  in shock, 66–67
    cardiogenic, 72, 73, 74–75
    monitoring methods, 81–82
    septic, 72
  spinal injuries and, 104
Blood transfusions, 115–125. See also Autotransfusions
  anaphylaxis risk with, 75
  blood substitutes, 80, 81, 127–128
  compatibility testing for, 122–124, 129–130
  complications of, 133–134
  component therapy
    compatibility testing for, 122–124
    functional classifications, 124–125
    preparation standards, 119
    preservative methods, 117
    types of, 119–122
  criteria for ordering, 124
  devices used in, 130–132
  history of, 115–117
  hyperkalemia and, 279
  hypocalcemia and, 284
  hypomagnesemia and, 286, 306
  preservative methods, 116–117
  for shock, 78–79, 80–81, 128–130
    whole blood vs. components, 128–129
  for upper GI bleeding, 448
Blood typing, 122–123
  cross-matching and, 130
  origins of, 116
  universal donors and, 129–130
Blood urea nitrogen (BUN)
  in hypernatremia, 267, 269
  in renal failure, 1221
Blood vessel sutures, 141, 142
Blood volume, in shock, 67–68, 69, 70. See also Fluid replacement
Blood warmers, 131–132
Bloom's syndrome, 364, 372
BLS. See Basic life support
Blundell, James, 116
Blunt trauma
  to abdomen, 1072–1073
  asphyxia from, 1188–1189
  cardiac tamponade with, 203
  to chest, 1181
    myocardial contusion, 1186–1187
  to children, 541
    child abuse, 601
  to diaphragm, 1188
  to extremities, 1073–1074

Blunt trauma (*contd.*)
  to heart, 1081
  to kidneys, 1195–1198
  to larynx, 1313–1317
  to penis, 1208
  to scrotum or testicle, 1209, 1210
  to thorax, 1071–1072
  tracheobronchial, 1188
  vascular, 1070
Boari flap, for ureteral repair, 1202, 1203
Bobcats, rabies and, 629
Body lice, 437
Body position. *See* Position
Body temperature
  conversion chart, 1455–1462
  heat stress and, 653
Boerhaave's syndrome, 452
Bombings. *See* Disaster linkages
Bone, metastatic disease in, 504–505
Bone cancer, presentation of, 504–505
Bone marrow toxicity, from chemotherapy, 509
Bone scan
  in child abuse cases, 604
  in stress fracture, 226
  in vertebral column injury, 187
  in vertebral osteomyelitis, 193
Bordetella pertussis, pharyngitis and, 377
Borrelia burgdorferi, 409
Bowel ischemia or infarction, adrenal insufficiency vs., 259
Bowel obstruction, 459–461
"Boxer's fracture," 208
Boyd, Dr. David, on EMS support, 2
Brachial plexus injury, 198
Brachial splint, coaptation, for humeral shaft fracture, 201
Bracing, for tennis elbow, 204
Bradycardia. *See also* Bradydysrhythmias; Dysrhythmias
  cardiac-pacing systems for. *See* Pacing therapy
  in hyperkalemia, 280
  in hypermagnesemia, 308
  in myxedema coma, 252
  in shock, cardiogenic, 74
Bradydysrhythmias, 1008–1017. *See also* Bradycardia; Dysrhythmias
  atrioventricular (AV) block, 1013–1017
  sudden sinus (atrial standstill), 1010–1012
Bradykinin
  anaphylaxis and, 75
  hypovolemic shock and, 71
Brain, anatomy of, structurally caused coma and, 929–930
Brain abscess
  as acute confusional state cause, 955
  encephalitis and, 400–401
Brain biopsy, in encephalitis, 401
Brain injuries. *See* Head injuries
Brain scan, in encephalitis, 400
Brain stem, consciousness and, 927, 928
Brain tumors
  as acute confusional state cause, 955
  as headache cause, 919
  hyponatremia and, 271
  oncologic emergencies, 502–503
Branhamella catarrhalis, in sinusitis, 1302
Breach, as legal concept, 41
Breast cancer
  acanthosis nigricans and, 429
  adrenal crisis risk with, 508
  adrenal insufficiency and, 257
  chest wall syndrome vs., 348
  as diabetes insipidus cause, 267
  hypercalcemia and, 282, 315, 317
Breathing assistance. *See also* Respiration; Ventilation
  in acute epiglottitis, 1119
  basic vs. advanced life support skills, 94
  for children, 515–519, 544–545, 575
    unconscious, 591
  CPR procedure, 1085
    for infants, 1088

  devices for, 99–100
  in head injuries, 891, 893
  in intracerebral hemorrhage, 942
  for multifocal atrial tachycardia (MAT), 1022
  with multisystem injuries, 99–101, 544–545
  for noncardiogenic pulmonary edema, 1101
  for obstructive airway disease, 1134–1135
  for respiratory failure, 1157
Brethine. *See* Terbutaline
Bretylium tosylate (Bretylol), 1382
  in CPR
    advanced cardiac life support, 1089–1090
    of pediatric patients, 523
    preventive use of, 984
  for ventricular fibrillation, 984
  for ventricular tachycardia, 1030
Brevibloc. *See* Esmolol
Brevital. *See* Methohexital
Bricanyl. *See* Terbutaline
Bristle worms, spine or puncture injuries by, 723–724
Bromides
  anion gap and, 327
  for pain relief, 884
Bronchiolitis, in pediatric patients, 582–583
Bronchitis, chronic. *See also* Obstructive airway disease
  defined, 1129
  occupational sources of, 1163
Bronchoconstriction, in anaphylaxis, 75
Bronchodilators, 1424–1428
  for anaphylaxis, 86
  inhaled
    for asthma, 581, 1132
    for children, 578
  for multifocal atrial tachycardia (MAT), 1022
  for scombroid fish poisoning, 739
Bronchoscopy
  fiberoptic, in hemoptysis evaluation, 1168
  for foreign body, 559
Bronchospastic airway disease, high altitude and, 685
Bronkosol; Bronkometer. *See* Isoetharine
Broselow Resuscitation Tape, children and, 521, 544
Brown recluse spider bites, 641–642
Brown-Séquard syndrome, 184, 909, 910
Brucella species, in septic arthritis, 410
Brucellosis, diagnosis of, 385
Brudzinski's signs, in meningitis
  aseptic, 399
  purulent, 397
Brufen. *See* Ibuprofen
Buddhists, beliefs and practices, 865–866
Buddy taping
  for hand injuries, 209, 210, 211
  for toe injuries, 230
Budget considerations. *See* Financial issues
Build-a-board immobilization device, 109
Bulbocavernosus reflex, loss of, in cauda equina syndrome, 193
Bumetanide (Bumex), 1430
  for congestive heart failure, 1055
  for pulmonary edema, 1099
BUMP screening test for alcoholism, 822, 827
BUN. *See* Blood urea nitrogen
Bupivacaine (Marcaine)
  clinical characteristics and dosage, 884
  pharmacologic classification of, 885
Buprenorphine, for opioid withdrawal, 798–799
Bureau of Health Manpower (Health Resources Administration), EMS grants by, 2
Bureau of Medical Services, data collection guidelines, 11
Burn centers
  categorization of, 19
  transfer of patient to, 427
    checklist, 426
    criteria for, 10, 47–48, 553
Burn shock, 418
Burnett's syndrome. *See* Milk-alkali syndrome
Burning eyes, in Sjögren's disease, 338
Burns, 417–427
  adrenal gland hemorrhage and, 256

  categorization of facilities for, 19
  as cause of death, 419, 420
  in children, 553, 554
  electrical
    as major injuries, 424
    myoglobinuria and, 427
    to upper extremities, 212
  evaluation of, 419–424
    American Burn Association categories, 423–424
    depth indicators, 423
    surface area by age, 554
  first aid measures, 419
  hyperkalemia and, 279, 298
  inhalation injuries, 419, 420
  mafenide acetate for, metabolic acidosis and, 322
  as MAST suit contraindication, 77
  pathophysiology of, 417–419
  prehospital care, 419
  shock following, 418
  succinylcholine for, hyperkalemia risk with, 298
  toxin exposure with, 494
  transfer to burn center for, 427, 553
    checklist, 426
    criteria for, 10, 47–48
  transport and, 419
  trauma associated with, 419, 423
  treatment of
    drug administration, 423, 424
    fluid therapy, 421–423
    in infants and children, 553
    with inhalation injury, 420
    wound management, 424–426
  upper extremity injuries, 212
Burow's solution
  for contact dermatitis, 433
  for fungal infections, 436, 437
  for herpes zoster, 442
Bursae, aspiration and injection of, 1373–1375
Bursitis
  in elbow, 204
  onset of, 352
  septic, 204, 412
  in shoulder, 201
Burst fractures
  of cervical spine, 192–193, 907, 908
  of thoracolumbar spine, 179, 193
Buspirone (Buspar), 1406
"But for" standard, 41
Butabarbital (Butisol), elimination half-life of, 800. *See also* Barbiturates
Butalbital (Fiorinal). *See* Barbiturates
Butazolidin. *See* Phenylbutazone
Butisol. *See* Butabarbital
Butorphanol (Stadol), 1435–1436
Butterfly rash, 336
Buttocks, abscesses on, 407
Butyrophenones, sedative withdrawal and, 804
BVM ventilation. *See* Bag-valve-mask unit

C

Cacao, as sympathomimetic, 787
Café au lait spots, 368, 369, 371
Caffeine, as sympathomimetic, 787
Caffeine overdose, 473, 474, 491
CAGE screening test for alcoholism, 822
Calan. *See* Verapamil
Calcaneocuboid joint injuries, 229
Calcaneus fractures, 228–229, 230
Calciferol. *See* Vitamin D
Calcitonin, for hypercalcemia, 283, 316
Calcitriol. *See* 1,25-Hydroxycalciferol
Calcium administration. *See also specific calcium compounds*
  for ciguatera fish poisoning, 738–739
  hypothermia and, 671
Calcium carbonate antacids, hypercalcemia and, 282
Calcium channel blockers
  for atrial fibrillation, 1022
  for headache prophylaxis, 923, 924
  for obstructive airway disease, 1136

for PSVT, 1026
for Raynaud's phenomenon, 341
Calcium chloride, 1382–1383
  in CPR
    for electromechanical dissociation, 1091
    of pediatric patients, 523, 524
  for hyperkalemia, 281, 299
  for hypermagnesemia, 288, 308
  for hypocalcemia, 285
Calcium gluceptate, for hypocalcemia, 285
Calcium gluconate, 1383
  for chemical burns, 754
  for ciguatera fish poisoning, 738, 739
  for hyperkalemia, 280, 281, 299
  for hypocalcemia, 285
Calcium lactate, for hypocalcemia, 285
Calcium levels, 281. *See also* Hypercalcemia; Hypocalcemia
  adrenal insufficiency and, 259
  in hypercalcemic crisis, 312–313
  interpreting, 311–313
  physiology and, 281, 313
Calf pain, in Baker's cyst, 346
California encephalitis, 400
Caloric testing. *See* Oculovestibular reflex
Campylobacter jejuni
  in food poisoning, 390
  in gastroenteritis, 387, 388
    dysenteric, 390
    treatment and, 389, 390
Cancer. *See also* Neoplastic disorders; Oncologic emergencies; *specific types*
  ED personnel and, 501–502
  hypercalcemia and, 311, 313, 316
  psychosocial factors in, 501–502
Candida infections
  AIDS and, 444
  cutaneous
    adrenal insufficiency and, 258
    hives with, 440
  in diabetic patients, 433
  esophageal, in systemic lupus erythematosus, 342
  esophageal obstruction and, 452
  in intertriginous areas, 437
  otitis externa and, 380, 1310, 1311
  sinusitis and, 1302
  thrush, 377
"Canker sores," 381
Cannabis. *See also* Marijuana
  ingestion of, 808
  intoxication or overdose of, 809
  pharmacologic uses of, 808–809
Capillaries
  increased permeability of, in anaphylaxis, 75
  microthrombi development in, in shock, 71
Capoten. *See* Captopril
Capsulitis, adhesive, 346–347
Captopril (Capoten), 1391–1392
  for congestive heart failure, 1055
Carafate. *See* Sucralfate
Carbamate toxicity
  decontamination procedures, 474
  treatment of, 478, 757
Carbamazepine (Tegretol)
  for alcohol withdrawal, 821
  hyponatremia and, 271
  overdose of, 490
    clinical signs, 472, 473, 490
  for seizures, 949
Carbenicillin (Geopen; Geocillin; Pyopen), 1414
  anion gap elevation and, 327
  for corneal ulcers, 1275, 1278
  eye drop preparation, 1268
  hypokalemia and, 275, 294
  renal failure and, 1225
  in septic shock treatment, 85
Carbocaine. *See* Mepivacaine
Carbohydrate utilization, diabetic ketoacidosis and, 238–239
Carbon dioxide
  asphyxiation injury by, 764

in respiratory acidosis, 329
in respiratory alkalosis, 330
Carbon dioxide dissociation curve, 1154
Carbon dioxide narcosis, in myxedema coma, 252
Carbon monoxide (CO) poisoning, 756, 1159–1161
  asphyxiation injury, 764–767
  diagnosis of, 766, 1161
  differential diagnosis, 477
  HBO therapy for, 704–705, 1161
  as headache cause, 917–918
  mechanism of, 1160
  signs and symptoms of, 472, 474, 477–478, 765, 766, 1160
  smoke inhalation and, 772–773
  smoking and, 765, 1160
  sources of, 1160
  treatment of, 766–767, 1161
    HBO therapy in, 704–705, 756, 767, 1161
Carbon tetrachloride
  inhalant abuse with, 805, 806
  as systemic toxin, 774
Carbonic anhydrase inhibitors, metabolic acidosis risk with, 321–322
Carbuncles, 431
Carcinoma. *See also specific types*
  hypercalcemia and, 281–282
  vertebral osteomyelitis vs., 194
Carcinomatosis
  aseptic meningitis and, 399
  terminal metastatic, adrenal insufficiency and, 257
Cardiac arrest
  in acute myocardial infarction
    CCU transfer routine and, 994
    treatment for, 984
  causes of, 1083
  in children, 513, 514
  hyperkalemia-induced, treatment of, 300
  in hypermagnesemia, 308
  medications for, 1381–1391
Cardiac defibrillation. *See* Defibrillation
Cardiac disorders. *See also specific disorders*
  cannabis use and, 809
  chemotherapy and, 509
  hereditary, 365
  high altitude and, 685
  hypocalcemia and, 281
  hypokalemia and, 295–296
  hypomagnesemia and, 304–305, 306–307
  magnesium therapy for, 307–308
  in systemic lupus erythematosus, 340–341
Cardiac emergencies, 1078–1081
  advanced cardiac life support (ACLS) for, 1088–1091
  asystole, 1091
  basic vs. EMT-P training and, 4
  blunt trauma, 1081, 1186–1187
  ED classification for, 48
  electromechanical dissociation, 1091
  EMS research on, 2
  general principles, 1077
  myocardial contusion, 1081, 1183, 1186–1187
  myocardial rupture, 1081
  open chest massage vs. CPR in, 1091–1092
  penetrating wounds, 1078–1079, 1185–1186
    cardiac tamponade and, 1185
    management algorithm for, 1186
    thoracotomy procedure, 1078–1079
  pericardial tamponade, 1080–1081
  stabilization indications, 5
  ventricular fibrillation, 1090
  ventricular tachycardia, 1090–1091
Cardiac failure, in cardiogenic shock, 75
Cardiac function. *See also* Cardiac output
  dysrhythmia and, 997–998
  hypothermia and, 664, 665
  interrelated parameters in, 1052
  monitoring
    Swan-Ganz catheterization for, 1347–1349
    in toxicologic emergencies, 470
  shock and, 71

Cardiac glycosides, for shock, 84
Cardiac ischemia, acute, 1066
Cardiac life support, advanced (ACLS), 1088–1091
Cardiac massage
  external chest compression vs., 1091–1092
  for ventricular tachycardia, 1030
Cardiac output, 66, 985, 989
  acute myocardial infarction and, 992–993
  blood pressure and, 67
  in cardiogenic shock, 74
  dysrhythmia and, 997–998
  high altitude and, 681
  inotropic agents and, 84
  monitoring, Swan-Ganz catheterization for, 1347–1349
  in septic shock, 72
  stroke and, 66
  syncope and, 959, 960, 963
Cardiac rhythm, influences on, 67. *See also* Dysrhythmias
Cardiac tamponade
  in cancer patient, 504
  as cardiogenic shock cause, 74, 103
  circulation control with, 103
  in penetrating trauma, 1185
Cardiac trauma. *See* Cardiac emergencies
Cardiac-pacing systems. *See* Pacing therapy
Cardiogenic shock, 72–75
  clinical features, 73, 74–75
  etiologies, 74
  as MAST suit contraindication, 77
  monitoring with, 83
  treatment of, 84–85
Cardiomegaly, adrenal insufficiency and, 259
Cardiomyopathy
  as cardiogenic shock cause, 74
  hypertrophic, syncope and, 959, 963
Cardiopulmonary bypass, autotransfusions and, 132
Cardiopulmonary monitoring
  components of, 78
  in near-drowning, 695
Cardiopulmonary resuscitation (CPR), 1083–1092
  advanced life support procedures, 1088–1091
    arrhythmias, 1090–1091
    defibrillation, 1088–1089
    drug therapy, 1089–1090
  basic life support procedures, 1083–1088
    airway, 1084–1085
    breathing, 1085
    chest compression, 1086–1088
    unresponsiveness determination, 1083–1084
  checking patient during, 1087–1088
  chest compression hemodynamics, 1085–1087
  esophageal perforation and, 452
  experimental techniques, 1087
  in near-drowning, 694–695, 698
  of pediatric patients, 513–527
    airway, 513–515
    breathing, 515–519
    circulation, 519–521
    defibrillation, 525
    drug overdose and, 526
    drugs used in, 521–525
    hypoglycemia and, 526
    hypothermia and, 525–526
    hypovolemia and, 526
    infants, 1088
    neonates, 526–527
    pediatric vs. adult, 527
  postresuscitation dysrhythmias, 1091
  success of, 1092
  in toxicologic emergencies, 469
Cardiotoxicity, hyperkalemia-induced, 299
Cardiovascular disorders. *See also specific disorders*
  adrenal insufficiency and, 258–259
  aortic outflow obstruction, syncope with, 959–960
  as CVA risk factor, 341
  emergency department drugs, listed, 1452
  high altitude and, 685
  hypermagnesemia and, 308

Cardiovascular disorders (contd.)
  hypokalemia and, 277
  hypomagnesemia and, 304–305, 306–307
  syncope and, 959–960, 961–962, 963
Cardiovascular function
  amphetamine and, 791
  cardiogenic shock and, 75
  cocaine and, 789
  head injury and, 896
  high altitude and, 681
  hypercalcemia and, 312
  hyperkalemia and, 299
  hypothermia and, 664
  infection and, 72
  near-drowning and, 693
  sedative overdose and, 803
  sympathomimetics and, 787
Cardioversion. See Electrical cardioversion
Cardizem. See Diltiazem
Carisoprodol (Soma), 1441
Carotid artery syndrome, in ischemic CVA, 937
Carotid sinus massage
  for PSVT, 1026
  for regular, wide QRS tachycardia, 1037
  for Wolff-Parkinson-White syndrome, 1042
Carotid sinus syncope, 963. See also Cardiovascular disorders, syncope and
Carotidynia, 916
Carpal injuries, 206
  dislocations, 206
Carpal spasm, in hypocalcemia, 284, 285
Carpal tunnel syndrome, 347
Carpometacarpal (thumb) joint, aspiration or injection of, 1374, 1375
Carpopedal spasm, in hypomagnesemia, 286
Carrel, Alexis, 116
Cartilage-hair hypoplasia, 372
Case review, ALS medical control through, 21
Casts
  for fractures, 169–171
  for upper extremity injuries, 196–197, 198
Cat bites, 155, 156, 157, 629, 631–632
Catapres. See Clonidine
Cataracts, hypocalcemia and, 281, 285
Catecholamines
  in acute hemorrhage response, 70
  in advanced cardiac life support, 1089
    for asystole, 1091
  respiratory alkalosis and, 330
  shock and, 67, 68, 70
Categorization. See also Classification
  of emergency departments (EDs), 45
  of EMS facilities, 18
  horizontal vs. vertical, 18
  as regionalization method, 49–50
Catfishes, spine or puncture wounds by, 726
Catgut sutures, 142
Cathartics, indications for, 475
Catheterization
  for renal obstruction, 1223
  Swan-Ganz, procedure, 1347–1349
  for urinary retention, 1214, 1215
Catheters
  indwelling, septic shock risk and, 72
  for shock treatments, 76
Catholics. See Roman Catholics
Cattle, skin infections from, 409
Cauda equina injuries, steroids and, 104
Cauda equina syndrome, 193
Causalgia, 347
Caustic ingestion
  airway obstruction with, 566
  as esophageal emergency, 451
Cavernous sinus thrombosis, 1296
CCS (command and control system), 8
CCU. See Coronary care unit
CDC. See Centers for Disease Control
Cecal volvulus, 460, 461
  adrenal insufficiency vs., 259
Cefaclor (Ceclor), 1413
  for pneumonia in children, 586
  for urinary tract infections, 393

Cefadroxil (Duricef; Ultracef), 1413
Cefadyl. See Cephapirin
Cefamandole (Mandol), 1412
Cefazolin (Ancef; Kefzol), 1412
  for corneal ulcers, 1277, 1278
  eye drop preparation, 1268
Cefixime (Suprax), 1413
  for otitis media, 381
Cefizox. See Ceftizoxime
Cefobid. See Cefoperazone
Cefonicid (Monocid), 1412
Cefoperazone (Cefobid), 1412
  for marine organism injuries, 731, 732
  for puncture wounds, 154
  for septic arthritis, 357, 411, 412
Cefotaxime (Claforan), 1412
  for ascites, 459
  for marine organism injuries, 731, 732
  for meningitis, 398
    in infants under 3 months, 535
  oxacillin plus, in septic shock treatment, 85
  for sepsis, in infants under 3 months, 535
  for septic gonococcal arthritis, 411
  for urethritis in men, 395
Cefotetan, for cholecystitis, 454
Cefoxitin (Mefoxin), 1412
  for colon injury, 465
  for corneal ulcers, 1278
  for pelvic inflammatory disease, 1234
Ceftazidime (Fortaz; Tazidime), 1412
  for marine organism injuries, 731, 732
  for septic arthritis, 412
Ceftin. See Cefuroxime-axetil
Ceftizoxime (Cefizox), 1412
  for gonococcal dermatitis, 430
  for septic gonococcal arthritis, 411
Ceftriaxone (Rocephin), 1412
  for animal bites, 158
  for gonococcal dermatitis, 430
  for gonococcal pharyngitis, 378
  for gonorrhea or chlamydia, 1233, 1250
  for meningitis or sepsis, in infants under 3 months, 535
  for pneumonia, in children, 586
  for septic arthritis
    in children, 412
    gonococcal, 411
  for urethritis, 395
Cefuroxime (Zinacef), 1412
  for septic arthritis, 357
Cefuroxime-axetil (Ceftin), 1413
  for otitis media, 381
  for pneumonia, 386
  for septic arthritis, 411
  for urethritis in men, 395
Celiac artery stenosis, in hereditary disorder, 371
Cellular anoxia, shock and, 65
Cellular metabolism, shock and, 67
  hypovolemic, 70–71
  septic, 72
Cellular perfusion, shock and, 71
Cellular phones, in RTSS systems, 9
Cellulitis, 431–432
  in cutaneous abscesses, 408
  in elbow, 204
  ocular, 1296, 1297
  as puncture wound complication, in feet, 154
Celsius temperature, conversion chart, 1455–1462
Centers for Disease Control (CDC)
  Clostridium botulinum and, 391
  on gonorrhea treatment, 1233, 1250
  injury control program, 3
  malarial treatment and, 407
  on septic arthritis treatment, 411
  on urethritis treatment, 395
Central arterial pressure monitoring, in shock treatment, 81–82
Central cord syndrome, 184
  in cervical spine, 909–910
Central nervous system
  consciousness and, 927–928

emergency department drugs for, listed, 1452
sympathomimetics and, 787. See also specific drugs
Central nervous system depression
  in diabetic ketoacidosis, 237, 238
  hypothermia and, 662, 666
  in near-drowning, 694
Central nervous system infections, 396–403
  aseptic meningitis, 399–400
  encephalitis and brain abscess, 400–401
  infectious mononucleosis syndrome, 401–403
  purulent meningitis, 396–399
Central nervous system injuries
  assessing
    levels of consciousness, 105
    motor function, 106
    pupillary responses, 107
    sensory function and reflexes, 106
    vital signs, 105–106
  in near-drowning, 697–698
  prehospital care, 107–109
    assessment, 104–107
    history taking, 107
    inspection, 107
  transfer criteria, 10
  types of, 104
Central neurologic lesions
  dehydration risk with, 267
  hypothermia and, 662
  spongy degeneration, 372
Central venous line, placement of, confirming, 103
Central venous pressure monitoring
  cannulation procedures for, 1339–1346
  for near-drowning, 698
  for shock, 82
Central venous-arterial oxygen consumption, monitoring for shock, 82–83
Centrax. See Prazepam
Cephalexin (Keflex), 1413
  for cutaneous abscesses, 408
  for dog bites, 157
  for urinary tract infections, 393
Cephalopods
  envenomation by, 730–731
  food poisoning by, 735
Cephaloridine
  for corneal ulcers, 1278
  eye drop preparation, 1268
Cephalosporins, 1411–1413
  anaphylaxis risk with, 75
  for corneal ulcers, 1275, 1278
  for cutaneous abscesses, 408
  for gonococcal dermatitis, 430
  for meningitis, purulent, 398
  for pneumonias, 386
  for sepsis, 406–407
  for septic arthritis, 357
    in children, 412
    gonococcal, 411
  for sinusitis, 1303
  for skin infections, marine-associated, 409
  for urinary tract infections, 392
  for vertebral column injuries, 187–188
  in wound management, 157, 158
    cat bites, 156
    human bites, 156
Cephalothin (Keflin), 1412
  for corneal ulcers, 1278
  for open fractures, 168
  plus aminoglycoside, for septic shock, 85
Cephapirin (Cefadyl), 1413
Cephazolin, in wound management, 157
Cephradine (Anspor; Velosef), 1413
  for urinary tract infections, 393
Cephulac. See Lactulose
Cerebellar hemorrhage, 942–943
Cerebral aneurysm
  as headache cause, 918
  hyponatremia and, 271
  subarachnoid hemorrhage and, 939, 940
Cerebral artery syndromes, in ischemic CVA, 937–938
Cerebral cortex, awareness and, 927–928

Cerebral decompression sickness, 706
Cerebral edema
  in children, unconsciousness with, 590
  as dehydration treatment risk, 270
  diabetic ketoacidosis and, 241
  HBO therapy for, 709
  high-altitude (HACE), 681, 684–685
  as MAST suit contraindication, 77
  near-drowning and, 697–698
Cerebral hemorrhage, shoulder-hand syndrome and, 347
Cerebral herniation, in infants and children, 592
Cerebral ischemia, in anaphylaxis, 75
Cerebral thrombosis, high altitude and, 685
Cerebrospinal fluid (CSF)
  in aseptic meningitis, 399, 400
  in encephalitis, 400
  leaking, in head injury, 898–899, 901
  in purulent meningitis, 396, 397
    in children under two, 537, 538
Cerebrovascular accident (CVA; Stroke), 935–943.
    See also specific types
  as acute confusional state cause, 955
  anatomy and, 936
  anticoagulation therapy for, 943
  classification of, 934
  diagnostic imaging in, 943
  differential diagnosis, 343
  evaluation of, 936
  as headache cause, 920
  hemorrhagic syndromes, 934, 939–943
  ischemic syndromes, 934, 937–939
  neurologic deficit patterns with, 936–937
  risk factors for, 934, 935
  transient ischemic attack (TIA), 943, 961, 962
Cerebrovascular emergencies
  alcohol withdrawal vs., 819
  in sympathomimetic overdose, 792
Cervical collar, for rheumatoid arthritis, 343
Cervical fusion, for rheumatoid arthritis, 343
Cervical Immobilizer Device, 108, 109
Cervical pain, as headache cause, 917
Cervical spine
  anatomy of, 903–904
  osteoarthritis of, as headache cause, 917
  rheumatoid arthritis and, 343
Cervical spine injuries, 903–913. See also Vertebral column injuries
  airway control with, 95
    nasotracheal tube for, 98
  assessing, prehospital, 104
  basic vs. advanced life support skills and, 94
  in children, 542, 543
  clinical signs of, 911
  compression-type, 906–907
  diagnosis of, 180
  differential diagnosis, 911
  dislocations, 188–190, 905, 906
    stable vs. unstable, 908
  etiologies of, 904, 905
  extension-type, 177, 907
  flexion-rotation-type, 906
  flexion-type, 905–910
  fracture-dislocations, 176, 188, 189, 907, 908
  fractures, 190–192, 905–908
    stable vs. unstable, 908
  management of, 188, 190, 192, 193
    prehospital, 107, 108–109
  pathophysiology of, 904–910
  radiological evaluation of, 911–912
  spinal cord injuries with, 903, 905, 907, 909–910
    anatomical structure and, 908
    diagnosis of, 913
    special problems with, 912–913
  sprains, as headache cause, 917
  statistics on, 903
  subluxations, 189
  treatment of, 913
  upper extremity injuries and, 198
  vertical compression fractures, 177–179
Cervical traction, manual methods, 108
Cervicitis, herpetic, 442

Cervix, culdocentesis at, 1231, 1354
Chance fractures. See Seat-belt fractures
Chancre, 439
Chaplain, as spiritual support source, 864
Charcoal, activated (Actidose), 1448
  in toxicologic emergencies, 475. See also specific toxic substances
Charcot's triad, 454
Cheek, lacerations, 152
Chelating agents, for hypercalcemia, 315–316
Chelation, for cyanide poisoning, 478
Chemical burns. See also Chemical injury; Hazardous materials; Toxicologic emergencies
  of esophagus, 451
  first aid measures, 419
  hospital care, 753–754
  materials causing, 753, 754
  prehospital care, 419
  tar and asphalt, 424
Chemical injury. See also Chemical burns; Hazardous materials; Toxicologic emergencies
  aseptic meningitis and, 399
  clinical signs, 472, 473. See also Toxicologic emergencies
  by combustion products, 477, 494, 747, 757, 761, 772–773
  contact dermatitis, 432–433
  by corrosives, in children, 553–554
  to eyes, 754, 1320
    as priority, 1262
  occupation-related, 761–776, 1162. See also Occupational injuries
  pharyngitis and, 377
  skin and ocular decontamination, 474
  systemic toxins, 755–758
  by toxic gases. See Inhalation injury
Chemical pneumonitis, 385
Chemical spot tests, for drugs, 786
Chemical Transportation Emergency Center (CHEMTREC), 752
Chemosis, in anaphylaxis, 75
Chemotherapy
  complications of, toxic reactions, 508–509
  as gastroenteritis cause, 388
  hypercalcemia and, 317
  toxic reactions to, 508–509
Chernobyl nuclear accident, 747
Chest compression, in CPR
  hemodynamics of, 1086–1087
  of infants, 1088
  practical issues, 1087–1088
Chest deformity, in hereditary disorders, 364, 365, 367
Chest injuries, 1181–1191. See also Cardiac emergencies; specific types or locations of injuries
  aortic emergencies, 1081–1082, 1187
  asphyxia with, 1188–1189
  associated injuries, 1181–1182
  blunt trauma, 1071–1072, 1181, 1186–1187, 1188
  chest wall trauma, 1182–1183
  in children, 543
    with multiple trauma, 545–546, 548, 549
  diaphragmatic, 1188, 1189
  epidemiology of, 1181–1182
  initial assessment of, 1182
  mediastinal trauma, 1185–1188
  penetrating trauma, 1071, 1181, 1185–1186, 1188
  prehospital management, 110
  pulmonary trauma, 1183–1185
  transfer criteria, 10
  treatment procedures, 1189–1191
  types of, 1182
  wound management. See Chest wounds
Chest pain
  in acute aortic dissection, 1066
  in acute myocardial infarction, management of, 985
  in anaphylaxis, 75
  in cardiogenic shock, 75
  in chest wall syndromes, 348
  in myocardial contusion, 1081
  in pneumonia, 384

  in scleroderma, 340, 342
  in systemic lupus erythematosus, 340, 341
Chest percussion, for multifocal atrial tachycardia (MAT), 1022
Chest radiography
  in connective tissue disease, 339, 340
  in head injury, 897
  in obstructive airway disease, 1132
  in pleural effusion, 1169
  in pulmonary edema, 1098
  in pulmonary embolism, 1145
  in respiratory disorder evaluation, pediatric, 576
Chest wall motion, respiratory alkalosis and, 330
Chest wall syndrome, 347–348
Chest wall trauma, 1182–1183
Chest wounds. See also Chest injuries
  open, ventilation with, 99, 101
  penetrating, 1071
    esophageal rupture and, 452
  suture removal from, 144
Cheyne-Stokes respiration, in multisystem trauma, 106
CHF. See Congestive heart failure
Chickenpox. See Varicella
Chilblains, 672
Child abuse, 597–608
  blunt trauma, 601
  bruising and, 598
  burns, 48, 598–599
  consent issues, 42
  documentation of, 602, 604–605, 608
  domestic violence and, 841, 844, 845
  evaluating wounds for, 137
  extraskeletal trauma, 600–601
  fractures, 599–600, 603–604
  frequency of, 597
  head injuries, 542, 600–601, 604
  history taking and, 601, 602, 605
  homicide detection, 601
  indicators of, 597–598
  intentional poisoning, 601, 603
  laboratory evaluation of, 603
  legal issues, 597, 601, 602–603
    documentation and, 604–605
  minor trauma and, 552
  Munchausen's syndrome by proxy, 601–602, 603
  physical examination and, 602
  radiographic imaging of, 603–604
  risk factors for, 597
  scrotum injuries, 560
  sexual, 605–608
  shaken baby syndrome, 589, 600–601
  skin trauma and, 598–599
  subdural hematoma with, 589
  tibia fractures, 226
  as trauma source, 542
Children, grieving process in, 860–861. See also Minors; Pediatric patients
"China White" (fentanyl analogue), 799
Chinese restaurant syndrome, 391
Chlamydia pneumoniae
  in pharyngitis, 376
  in pneumonia, 383, 585, 586
Chlamydia psittaci, in pneumonia, 383
Chlamydia trachomatis
  child sexual abuse and, 1253
  in dysenteric gastroenteritis, 390
  in pelvic inflammatory disease, 1233
  in pneumonia, 383
  in urinary tract infections, 391, 392
  urethritis in men, 394, 395
Chlamydial infections
  perihepatitis, 556
  pneumonia, 383
  rape and, 1250
Chlor-Trimeton. See Chlorpheniramine maleate
Chloral betaine, for pain relief, 884
Chloral hydrate (Noctec; Chloral Hydrate), 1438–1439. See also Sedative-hypnotics
  elimination half-life of, 800
  intoxication or overdose, 325, 492
    clinical signs, 472, 473, 803

Chloral hydrate (contd.)
　for pain relief, 884
　pharmacology of, 802
Chloramphenicol (Chloromycetin), 1419
　for cellulitis, 432
　for corneal ulcers, 1275, 1278
　for encephalitis with brain abscess, 401
　in eye drops or ointment, 1269
　for meningitis
　　in infants under 3 months, 535
　　purulent, 398, 953
　for meningococcemia, 430
　for oropharyngeal infections, 383
　for Rocky Mountain spotted fever, 407, 438
　for sepsis, in infants under 3 months, 535
　for septic arthritis, 412
　in septic shock treatment, 85
　for skin infections, marine-associated, 408
Chlorazepate (Tranxene), overdose of, 491–492
Chlordiazepoxide (Librium), 1406
　for alcohol withdrawal, 820
　elimination half-life of, 800
　overdose of, 491–492
Chlorine inhalation, 769–770
Chloroform, as systemic toxin, 774
Chloroform intoxication, 325
Chloromycetin. See Chloramphenicol
2-Chloroprocaine (Nesacaine), clinical characteristics and dosage, 884
Chloroquine, retinopathy from, 339
Chlorpheniramine maleate (Chlor-Trimeton), for urticaria, 441
Chlorpromazine (Thorazine), 1406–1407
　for acute confusion, psychiatric, 956
　for chemical restraint, of alcohol-intoxicated patient, 818
　for headache, 922
Chlorpropamide
　anaphylaxis risk with, 75
　hyponatremia and, 271
Chlorquine, for malaria, 407
Chlortetracycline, in eye ointment, 1269
Chlorthalidone
　hyperosmolar hyperglycemic nonketotic coma and, 243–244
　as hypokalemia cause, 294
Chlorthiazide, for congestive heart failure, 1055, 1056
Cholangitis
　diagnosis of, 454
　HIV and, 455
　treatment of, 454–455
Cholecystitis
　acalculous, 453
　　HIV and, 455
　acute, 453
　　diagnosis of, 454
　　in pregnancy, 1235–1236
　adrenal insufficiency vs., 259
　in hereditary disorders, 369, 370
Cholecystotomy, for pancreatic disease, 456
Choledyl; Choledyl SA. See Oxtriphylline
Cholelithiasis
　in hereditary disorders, 369
　in pregnancy, 1235
Cholera
　acute watery diarrhea in, 389
　enterotoxin in, 387
　travel and, 389, 732
　treatment of, 389
　Vibrio epidemics, shellfish and, 732
Cholesterol embolism, 1171
Cholestyramine, metabolic acidosis risk with, 322
Choline magnesium trisalicylate (Trilisate), for pain relief, 881
Cholinergic agents
　as diarrhea cause, 387
　as unconsciousness cause, 591
Cholinergic urticaria, 441
Cholinesterase inhibitors, for PSVT, 1026
Chondritis, bilateral auticular, in relapsing polychondritis, 340
Chondrocalcinosis, 356

Chondrodysplasia, metaphyseal, ethnic groups and, 372
Chopart's joint injuries, 229
Christian Church, beliefs and practices, 866
Christian Scientists, beliefs and practices, 865, 866
Christmas disease, 366
"Christmas tree" eruption, in pityriasis rosea, 438
Chromatography, in drug and toxin screening, 471
Chromosomal disorders. See Hereditary disorders
Chronic mountain sickness (CMS), 685
Chronic obstructive pulmonary disease (COPD). See also Obstructive airway disease
　defined, 1129
　headache and, 917
　management guidelines, 1136–1138
　pathogenesis of, 1130
Chronic pain, defined, 877–878
Chronulac. See Lactulose
Church of the Brethren, beliefs and practices, 866–867
Church of Christ, beliefs and practices, 866
Church of God, beliefs and practices, 866
Church of Jesus Christ of Latter-Day Saints (Mormons), beliefs and practices, 866
Chvostek's sign
　in hypocalcemia, 284–285
　in hypomagnesemia, 286–287
Ciguatera fish poisoning, 391, 712, 736–739
Cilastin, for marine organism injuries, 731
Ciliary injection, in uveitis, 1278
Cimetidine (Tagamet), 1433
　for burn patients, 423
　for scombroid fish poisoning, 739
　for upper GI bleeding, 449
Ciprofloxacin (Cipro), 1419
　for dysenteric gastroenteritis, 390
　for gonococcal pharyngitis, 378
　for gonorrhea, 1250
　for marine organism injuries, 731
　for prostatitis, 395–396
　for urethritis in men, 395
　for urinary tract infections, 393
Circulation, controlling
　in acute myocardial infarction, 985, 989–992
　basic vs. advanced life support skills, 94
　with head injuries, 891, 893
　with multisystem injuries, 101–103, 545
　in pediatric patients, 519–521, 545, 591
　in prehospital setting, 101–103
Circulatory system. See also Blood pressure
　high altitude and, 680
　normal function of, 65–66
　in shock, 65, 68
　　cardiogenic, 72–73
　　hypovolemic, 71
　　septic, 72, 73
　　staging of, 101
Circumorbital hemorrhage, assessing for, 110
Cirrhosis
　acute sepsis and, 406
　anion gap decrease in, 327
　esophageal varices and, 452
Citanest. See Prilocaine
Citrate, hypomagnesemia and, 306
Citrobacter species, in pneumonia, 383
Civil defense operations, in disaster linkages, 12
Civil law, 39–40. See also Legal issues
CK levels. See Creatine kinase levels
Claforan. See Cefotaxime
Clams, poisoning by, 391, 731–735
Classification. See also Categorization
　of behavioral disorders, 47
　of emergency departments (EDs), 45–47
　　for behavioral emergencies, 47
　　horizontal, 45–46
　　vertical, 46–47
Clavicle
　absence of, 365
　acromioclavicular separations, 198
　dislocations, 198–199
　fractures, 198
　sternoclavicular dislocations, 198–199

Clavulanate, for animal bites, 158
Clay ingestion, as hypokalemia cause, 294
Clay shoveler's fracture, 906, 908
Cleaning agents
　inhalant abuse with, 805, 806
　as systemic toxins, 774
Clearance, of drugs, 483
Clearinghouse. See National Clearinghouse (National Association of State Emergency Medical Services Directors)
Clenched fist injury, 156, 211
Cleocin. See Clindamycin
Click-murmur syndrome. See Mitral valve prolapse
Clindamycin (Cleocin), 1420
　in appendicitis, 465
　for cholangitis and sepsis, 454–455
　for colon injury, 465
　for corneal ulcers, 1275, 1278
　for cutaneous abscesses, 408
　for human bites, 157
　for necrotizing fasciitis or myositis, 410
　for oropharyngeal infections, 383
　for pelvic inflammatory disease, 1234
　for pneumonias, 387
　in septic shock treatment, 85
Clinoril. See Sulindac
Clonazepam (Clonopin)
　elimination half-life of, 800
　overdose of, 491–492
Clonidine (Catapres; Combi-pres), 1392
　for hypertensive emergencies, 1063
　　catecholamine crisis, 1067
　for opioid withdrawal, 798, 799
　overdose of, clinical signs, 472, 473
　in renal failure treatment, 1225
　withdrawal from, hypertension and, 1066
Clonopin. See Clonazepam
Clorazepate (Tranxene), elimination half-life of, 800
Closed fractures, 161
　reduction of, 168–169
Clostridium botulinum
　bivalve mollusks and, 732
　in food poisoning, 391
　in gastroenteritis, 388
Clostridium difficile
　as cytotoxin, 387
　in gastroenteritis, 387, 388
　dysenteric, 390
Clostridium perfringens
　emphysematous cholecystitis and, 454
　in food poisoning, 390
　in gastroenteritis, 388
　in necrotizing fasciitis or myositis, 410
Clostridium species
　in gastroenteritis, 387, 388
　in necrotizing fasciitis or myositis, 410
　OHP as bacteriocidal for, 704
Clotrimazole (Lotrimin), for fungal infections
　of intertriginous areas, 437
　of skin, 436
　thrush, 378
Cloxacillin (Tegopen), 1414–1415
　for impetigo, 431
　for septic bursitis, 412
Cluster headache, 916, 922–923
CMS (chronic mountain sickness), 685
Coagulopathy
　in cancer patients, 510
　hereditary, 366
　as transfusion reaction, 133, 134
Coaptation brachial splint, for humeral shaft fracture, 201
Coast Guard
　communication with, 8
　in disaster linkages, 12
Cobalt EDTA, for cyanide poisoning, 755
COBRA. See Consolidated Omnibus Budget Reconciliation Act of 1980
Cocaine, 786, 787–789
　abstinence syndrome, 789
　clinical use of, 788, 885. See also Cocaine anesthesia

for pain relief, 885
topical, for uveitis, 1281
complications of, 784, 785, 788–789
crack or free-base, 787, 788
complications of, 789
ingestion by children, 566
extent of abuse, 782, 788
heroin abuse signs vs., 796
history of, 787–788
overdose of
clinical signs, 472, 473, 474, 788–789
respiratory alkalosis and, 330
treatment of, 791–793
pharmacology of, 788, 885
in pregnancy, effects on neonate, 810
screening tests for, 786
as sympathomimetic, 787
Cocaine anesthesia, 788
anaphylaxis risk with, 75
in wound management, 139
Coccidioides immitis, in pneumonia, 383, 384
Coccidioidomycosis
adrenal insufficiency and, 258
diagnosis of, 385
Codeine, 1436
anaphylaxis risk with, 75
for pain relief, 882
Codman, Dr. E. A., quality management and, 55, 58
Coelenterate stings, 717–718, 720
Cola nuts, as sympathomimetic, 787
Colchicine, 1403–1404
for gout, 357
Cold applications, for pain relief, 888
Cold caloric stimulation. *See* Oculovestibular reflex
Cold injury. *See also* Hypothermia
chilblains, 672
frostbite, 672–673
frostnip, 672
Cold medications, overdose of, 491
"Cold shake." *See* Percocet; Percodan
"Cold shock," 72
Cold urticaria, 440, 441
Colds, common, 375–376
Colic, infant, 556–557
Colistin
for corneal ulcers, 1278
in eye drops, 1269
Colitis
antibiotic-associated, 387, 388
pseudomembranous
cytotoxins and, 387
treatment of, 390
ulcerative, 462–463
treatment of, 463
upper GI bleeding with, 449
Collagen disorders. *See* Connective tissue disease
Colles' fractures, 205–206
Colloid solutions
crystalloids vs., 127
for shock, 79, 80, 126–127
Coloboma of the iris, 365
Colon
injuries to, 465
obstruction of, 460–461
Colon cancer
familial polyposis and, 369, 370
obstruction and, 460
Colonic aganglionosis, 558
Colonic angiodysplasia, 558
Colonoscopy
for lower GI bleeding, 451
in small bowel obstruction, 460
in ulcerative colitis, 462
Colorado tick fever, 400
skin infections in, 409
Colposcopy, in rape examination, 1249
Coma, 927–934. *See also* Unconscious patients
in adrenal insufficiency, 259
anatomy of consciousness and, 927–928
assessing for. *See* Levels of consciousness
causes of, 928–931

metabolic lesions, 930
psychogenic, 930–931
structural lesions, 929–930
defined, 927
differential diagnosis, 344
hyperosmolar hyperglycemic nonketotic (HHNK), 242–245
in hypomagnesemia, 304
in infants and children, 589–592
etiologies of, 589–591
management of, 591–592
with multiple trauma, 546, 547
management of patient in, 933–934
myxedema, 251–252
in shock
cardiogenic, 75
hypovolemic, 68, 70
in systemic lupus erythematosus, 343–344
in thyroid storm, 250
in toxicologic emergencies, 472, 473
Combi-pres. *See* Clonidine
Combustion byproducts, 477, 494, 747, 757
in occupational injuries, 761–762
Command and control system (CCS), 8
Comminuted fractures, 161, 163
of cervical spine, 191–192
of wrist, 206
Commission on Life Sciences (NRC), 2–3
Common cold, 375–376
Common law, 39
Communication
emotional/spiritual support through, 871–872
neurolinguistic programming (NLP) and, 872–875
right-brain techniques, 872, 874–875
Communications
in disaster management, 15, 33
EMS system components, 7–9
on-line medical control through, 20
Community, EMS policies and, 7
Compartment syndrome
as elbow injury complication, 202
in forearm, 205
HBO therapy for, 709
as MAST suit complication, 77
in multisystem trauma, 111
as tibia fracture complication, 225
tibial stress fracture vs., 226
Compazine. *See* Prochlorperazine
Competency, refusal of consent and, 42
Compliance, respiratory failure and, 1152
Component therapy
preparation standards, 119
preservative methods, 117
types of, 119–122
Compression fractures, 164, 165
in forearm, 205
of vertebral column, 175, 177–179, 180, 193
calcaneus fractures and, 228, 230
cervical spine, 906–907
differential diagnosis, 186–187
treatment of, 193
Computed tomography (CT scanning)
in adrenal insufficiency, 255, 256, 257
in brain abscess, 400–401
in cerebral aneurysm, 918
in cerebrovascular accident, 943
cerebellar hemorrhage, 942
intracerebral hemorrhage, 941, 942
ischemic, 939
subarachnoid hemorrhage, 940–941
in cervical spine injuries, 911
in child abuse cases, 604
in coma assessment, 930
in head injury, 897
in headache evaluation, 921
in intestinal obstruction, 461
in multiple trauma, in children, 549, 550
in neck injury, vascular, 1074
of pelvic injuries, 214
in renal trauma, 1197
of vertebral column injuries, 186

Computerized Stored Ambulatory Record (COSTAR), 58
Concussion. *See also* Head injuries
acute confusion with, 954
postconcussion headache, 919–920
Condyle fractures, 202–203
Cone shells, spine or puncture injuries by, 722
Conflict theory, of domestic violence, 843
Confusion, 951–957
acute confusional states, 951–953
etiologies of, 953–955
organic vs. psychiatric, 951–952
in adrenal insufficiency, 259
assessment of patient in, 928–929, 955
defined, 927
delirium, 953
in dementia, 956–957
diagnostic problems, 951, 955
drug-induced, 474
in hypercalcemia, 311, 312
psychiatric, 955–957
acute confusion vs., 951–952
in shock, 68
in thyroid storm, 250
toxin-induced, 474
Congenital disorders
alkalosis with diarrhea, 328
cerebral aneurysm, 918
diabetes insipidus, 268
DiGeorge's syndrome, hypocalcemia and, 284
glaucoma, 1289
idiopathic adrenal hypoplasia, 258
intermittent hydronephrosis and, 1211
mercury poisoning (Minamata disease), 494
stridor and, 570
Congestive heart failure (CHF), 1051–1057
acute myocardial infarction and, 993
definition of, 1051
diagnosis of, 1053–1054
drug abuse and, 785
dysrhythmia and, 997
evaluation of, Swan-Ganz catheter in, 1052–1053
functional classes of, 1051–1052
hypokalemia and, 294, 295
hypomagnesemia and, 306–307
hyponatremia and, 270
pathophysiology of, 1052–1053
pulmonary artery pressure monitoring with, 83
septic shock and, 72
symptoms of, 1052
treatment of, 1054–1056
Conjunctival vessels, telangiectasia of, 368
Conjunctivitis. *See also* Ocular emergencies, infections
in acute glaucoma, 1288
culture media for, 1271
obtaining culture specimens in, 1272
Connective tissue disease, 335–348. *See also specific diseases*
cardiac involvement in, 340–341
cutaneous lesions in, 336–337
fever in, 335
gastrointestinal involvement in, 341–343
neurologic involvement in, 343–344
ocular emergencies in, 337–339
pulmonary problems in, 339–340
soft tissue rheumatism, 344–348
Baker's cyst, 346
bursitis, 344–345, 412
shoulder syndromes, 346–348
tendinitis, 345–346
vascular disease with, 341
Conn's syndrome (hyperaldosteronism), 276
Consciousness impairment. *See* Coma; Levels of consciousness; Unconscious patients
Consent, 41–42
refusal of, 42
toxicologic screening and, 786
Consolidated Omnibus Budget Reconciliation Act of 1980 (COBRA), 7
antidumping statute, 42–43
quality management and, 58

Constipation
  in children, 558
    chronic, "overflow" diarrhea and, 558
  in hypercalcemia, 283
  in irritable bowel syndrome, 463
Consultation. See Referrals
Consumer participation
  in EMS policy and planning, 7
  in quality management, 61–62
Consumer Products Safety Commission (CPSC), formation of, 748
Contact dermatitis, 432–433
Continuous positive airway pressure (CPAP)
  for high-altitude pulmonary edema, 684
  for near-drowning, 691, 695–697
Contraceptives, oral. See Birth control pills
Contractility
  cardiac function and, 1052
  in shock diagnosis, 66–67
Contrast media
  anaphylaxis risk with, 75
  renal failure and, 1219
Convulsions
  in children
    febrile, 595–596
    unconsciousness and, 590–591
  in hypomagnesemia, 304
  magnesium for, 307. See also Anticonvulsants
  in systemic lupus erythematosus, 344
Convulsive status epilepticus, defined, 945, 946–947.
    See also Status epilepticus
Cook County Hospital
  first blood bank at, 116
  helicopter transport to, 23
Cooling blanket, for thyroid storm, 250, 251
Coombs test
  in blood cross-matching, 123, 124
  transfusion reaction and, 134
COPD. See Chronic obstructive pulmonary disease; Obstructive airway disease
Coping mechanisms
  communicating, therapeutic metaphors for, 874–875
  in grief response, 859–860
Coproporphyria, hereditary, 370
Coquille vacuum immobilizer, 109
Corals, 720–721
  hydroid, 717–718
Cordarone. See Amiodarone
Corgard. See Nadolol
Corneal blood staining, 1285
Corneal disorders
  abrasions or foreign bodies, 1266–1270
  herpetic keratitis, 1264, 1265–1266
  ulcers (bacterial keratitis), 1273–1276
    antibiotics for, 1275, 1276, 1277–1278
Corneal edema, in acute glaucoma, 1288–1289
Corneal injuries, 1327
Corneal reflex, in unconscious infants or children, 592
Coronary artery disease. See also specific types
  acute myocardial infarction risk with, 965
  high altitude and, 685
  pulmonary edema and, 1097
  in systemic lupus erythematosus, 340–341
Coronary care unit (CCU), transfer to, 994
  in pulmonary edema, 1099
Coronaviruses
  in common colds, 375–376
  in pharyngitis, 376
Corpus callosum, agenesis of, 372
Correction fluid inhalation, 805
Corrosive exposure, in children, 553–554
Corticosteroids, 1428–1429
  for acute epiglottitis, 1123
  in acute myocardial infarction treatment, 982
  for adrenal insufficiency, 259, 260
  adrenal insufficiency (secondary) and, 255–256
    in neonates, 258
  for asthma in pregnancy, 1239
  for carpal tunnel syndrome, 347
  for connective tissue disease
    esophageal candidiasis and, 342
    ocular problems of, 338, 339

for contact dermatitis, 433
for Crohn's disease, 462
for croup, 568
for drug eruptions, 434
for erythema multiforme, 435
for eye disorders, principles of, 1280
for gout/pseudogout, 358
for head injury, 897
for herpes zoster, 442
for hymenoptera stings, 644
for hypercalcemia, 283, 316
  hyperosmolar hyperglycemic nonketotic coma and, 243–244
  hypothermia and, 671
for infectious mononucleosis, 402
for intracranial pressure elevation, 502
for laryngotracheitis (viral croup), 1116
for Lyme disease, 357
for meningitis, in children under two, 538
for myxedema coma, 252
for obstructive airway disease, 1135–1136
  ocular herpes and, 1265
for otitis externa, 380
for respiratory distress, in children, 578–579
for scleritis, 338
for shock
  anaphylactic, 87
  contraindications, 85
spinal cord injuries and, 104
for systemic lupus erythematosus, 344
  ocular lesions of, 338
  pancreatitis from, 342
  as psychosis cause, 344
for temporal arteritis, 338, 917
for thyroid storm, 250, 251
topical
  for otitis externa, 1311
  for sinusitis, 1303
  for uveitis, 1280
for ulcerative colitis, 463
ulcers and, 342
vertebral column injuries and, 187
Cortisporin, for otitis externa, 1311
Corynebacterium diphtheriae, 569–570
  in pharyngitis, 376, 377, 378
Corynebacterium hemolyticum, in pharyngitis, 376
Corynebacterium minutissimum, in erythrasma, 430
Cosmetic repair, antibiotics with, 158
Cost considerations. See Financial issues
COSTAR (Computerized Stored Ambulatory Record), 58
Costochondral cartilage calcification, adrenal insufficiency and, 258
Costochondritis, 348
"Cotton fever," drug abuse and, 786
Cotton sutures, 142
Cough
  in anaphylaxis, 75
  in croup syndromes, 1113, 1114, 1116. See also Croup
  hemoptysis, 1167–1168
  in Wegener's granulomatosis, 340
Cough syncope, 961, 963
Coumadin. See Warfarin sodium
Coumarin compounds, adrenal hemorrhage and, 256–257
Counterimmunoelectrophoresis (CIE)
  in febrile infants under 3 months, 535
  in meningitis diagnosis, 399
Cow's milk, sodium excess in infant from, 267
Cow's milk allergy, in TAR syndrome, 368
Coxiella burnetii (Q fever), pneumonia and, 383, 385
Coxsackieviruses
  oral lesions from, 381
  in pharyngitis, 376, 377
  skin eruptions with, 443
Coyotes, rabies and, 629
CPAP. See Continuous positive airway pressure
CPD-A, for blood storage, 116–117
CPSC. See Consumer Products Safety Commission
Crabs, poisoning by, 735
Crack cocaine. See Cocaine

Cranial nerves, 106. See also specific nerves
  in head injury, 896
  in multisystem trauma, 106
  in unresponsive patients, 931–933
    infants or children, 591–592
Craniopharyngioma, 502
Creatine kinase (CK) levels, acute myocardial infarction and, 970
Creatine levels, renal failure and, 1221
Crescent sign, in Baker's cyst, 346
Cricoarytenoid synovitis, in rheumatoid arthritis, 339
Cricothyrotomy (cricothyroidotomy)
  in acute epiglottitis, 1121–1122
  complications of, 99
  laryngeal trauma and, 1317, 1321
  needle, 1110
    procedure, 1364–1365
  prehospital use of, 99
  surgical, 1110–1111
  for tracheobronchial foreign body, 1308
Criminal activities, sanctions for, 60
Crisis
  definition of, 858–859
  developmental vs. accidental, 859
  dynamics of, 859
  emotional needs in, 858–862
    of grieving family, 860–861
    of grieving patient, 859–860
    of staff, 861–862
  spiritual needs in, 862–865
    nonmedical healing and, 869–870
    religious beliefs and, 865–869
    support techniques, 870–872
Crisis counseling. See also Emotional support; Referrals
  advantages of, 858–859
  for alcoholics, 823
  for rape victim, 1255
  referral as part of, 859
Critical patients
  cardiopulmonary monitoring of, 78
  interhospital transport of, 9–10
  staple closure of wounds in, 149
Critique, in disaster management, 36, 37. See also Evaluation
Crohn's disease, 461–462
  anorectal abscess and, 466
  upper GI bleeding with, 449
Cross-matching blood, 122, 123–124, 129–130
Cross-tolerance, defined, 782
Croup, 1113–1117
  laryngotracheitis (LT), 567–569, 1113–1116
    airway control method and, 514
    epiglottitis vs., 1114
  spasmodic (SC), 565, 1116
Croup score, 568, 1115
Crush injuries
  antibiotics for, 158
  fractures, 163
  HBO therapy for, 709
  to head, 900
  hyperkalemia and, 279, 298
  renal trauma in, 1195, 1223
Crustaceans, poisoning by, 735
Cryoprecipitated AHF, in component therapy, 120
Crypt abscesses, in ulcerative colitis, 462
Cryptococcosis, adrenal insufficiency and, 258
Cryptococcus neoformans, in pneumonia, 383, 384
Cryptosporidium
  acalculous cholecystitis and, 455
  in acute watery diarrhea, 389, 390
  in gastroenteritis, 387, 388
  immunocompromised patients and, 389
Crystal arthritis, 355–356, 357–358
Crystal methamphetamine ("ice"). See Amphetamine
Crystalloid solutions
  colloids vs., 127
  for shock, 79, 80, 126
CSF. See Cerebrospinal fluid
CT scanning. See Computed tomography
Culdocentesis

procedure, 1231, 1354
  in vaginal bleeding evaluation, 1230–1231
Culture
  communication about pain and, 879
  domestic violence and, 843–844
Currant jelly stool, in ileocolic intussusception, 557
Cushing's disease; Cushing's syndrome, 276
  congenital idiopathic adrenal hypoplasia and, 258
  hypokalemia and, 276
Cutaneous lesions
  abscesses, 407–408, 431
  acanthosis nigricans, 429
  AIDS and, 444
  atopic dermatitis, 429–430
  in child abuse, 598–599. *See also* Child abuse
  in connective tissue disease, 336–337
    dermatomyositis, 336
    erythema nodosa, 336–337
    systemic lupus erythematosus, 336
    vasculitis, 337
  drug reactions, 433–434
  in hereditary disorders, 364, 365, 368, 369, 371
  herpetic whitlow, 408
  occupational infections, 408–409
  in scabies, 438–439
  in syphilis, 439–440
Cutaneous oximetry, in obstructive airway disease, 1132
Cutaneous stimulation, for pain management, 888
Cuttlefishes, poisoning by, 735
CVA. *See* Cerebrovascular accident
Cyanide kit, 478, 755, 768
  in hydrogen sulfide poisoning, 756
Cyanide poisoning, 755, 767–768
  clinical signs, 472
  from combustion products, 494, 773
  treatment of, 478, 755
Cyanosis
  in cardiogenic shock, 75
  of distal extremities, in Raynaud's phenomenon, 341
  in toxicologic emergencies, 473
Cyclobenzaprine (Flexeril), 1441–1442
Cyclogyl. *See* Cyclopentolate
Cyclopentolate (Mydrilate; Cyclogyl), for uveitis, 1281
Cycloplegics, 1281
  for corneal ulcers, 1277
  for herpetic keratitis, 1265
  for uveitis, 1280–1281
Cyclosporine, hyperkalemia risk with, 298
Cyclostome poisoning, 712, 736
Cyclothymic disorder, 830
Cyproheptadine (Periactin), 1408
  for headache prophylaxis, 922, 924
Cystic fibrosis, sinusitis, 379
Cystic medial necrosis, as hereditary disorder, 367
Cysticercosis, brain infection and, 400
Cystitis, 391, 392
Cystogram, filling, in multisystem trauma, 112
Cystostomy, suprapubic
  tube for, 1215
  for urethral injury, 1206, 1207, 1208
Cystourethroscopy, in urinary retention, 1214
Cytomegalovirus
  acalculous cholecystitis and, 455
  as aseptic meningitis cause, 399
  in mononucleosis, 401, 402
  pharyngitis and, 377
  pneumonia and, 383, 384
Cytomegalovirus infection, disseminated, hypercalcemia and, 317
Cytotec. *See* Misoprostol
Cytotoxins
  in acute watery diarrhea, 389
  in gastroenteritis, 387, 390

D

Dalmane. *See* Flurazepam
Damages, as legal concept, 41

DAN (Divers Alert Network), hyperbaric chamber referral by, 707, 709
Dantrolene (Dantrium), 1442
Daranide. *See* Dichlorphenamide
Daraprim. *See* Pyrimethamine
Darkfield examination, in syphilis, 439
Darling v. Charleston Community Memorial Hospital, 61
Darvon. *See* Propoxyphene
Dashboard injuries
  hip dislocations, 217
  patellar fractures, 222–223
Data collection. *See* Record keeping
Database
  National Practitioner Data Bank, 55–56, 58, 59, 60
  of physician quality reviews, 55–56, 58, 59, 60
Datril. *See* Acetaminophen
Daunorubicin, cardiac reaction to, 509
DCS. *See* Decompression sickness
Death of patient
  emotional support needs
    of family, 860–861
    of staff, 861–862
  from shock, 70
  spiritual needs of survivors, 864
Death rate. *See* Mortality
Debridement, 140–141. *See also specific types of wounds*
  for burns, 425
  of fracture wounds, 168, 172
Decadron. *See* Dexamethasone
Deceleration injuries, 1319. *See also* Falls; Motor vehicle accidents
Decompression sickness (DCS), 705–707
  altitude, 706, 707
  nitrogen gas and, 764
  treatment of, 707
Decongestants
  for otitis media, 381, 1309
  for sinusitis, 379, 1303
Decontamination procedures
  hazardous materials, 752–753
  occupational toxicologic emergencies, 762–763
  radiation, 618–619, 758–759
Decorticate vs. decerebrate posture, 895
Deep palmar space infections, 211
Deep venous thrombosis (DVT). *See also* Pulmonary embolism; Thromboembolism; Thrombosis
  diagnosis of, 1147–1148
  differential diagnosis, 1144–1145
  high altitude and, 685
  pulmonary embolism and, 1147–1148
  treatment of, 1141
Defecation syncope, 961, 963
Defenses, as legal concept, 41
Deferoxamine (Desferal), 1448
Defibrillation
  in advanced cardiac life support, 1088–1089, 1090, 1091
  blind, indications for, 1083
  EMT-D training in, 6
  methods, 984
  procedure, 1361
Degreasing agents, as systemic toxins, 774
Dehydration
  ADH secretion and, 266
  anion gap elevation in, 327
  clinical signs of, 268
  diagnosis of, 268–269
  diarrhea-caused, in infants and children, 558–559
  etiologies of, 267–268
  as head injury treatment, 897
  heat illness and, 653, 655
  heat syncope and, 655
  hypokalemia test result and, 277–278
  in neonates, adrenal insufficiency and, 258
  pharyngitis and, 377
  polyuric, in hypercalcemia, 311
  prehospital interventions, 270
  treatment of, 269–270
Delirium, 953. *See also* Confusion; Delirium tremens
  in adrenal insufficiency, 259

drug-induced, 474
  in hypercalcemia, 311
Delirium tremens, 821–822
  diagnosis of, 819, 955
  hypomagnesemia vs., 306
  prototypical patient with, 927
Delivery
  amniotic fluid embolism during, 1171
  meconium aspiration in, 1166–1167
  postpartum hemorrhage, 1238
Delta hepatitis, 403, 404, 405, 457
Deltasone. *See* Prednisone
Deltoid function, in vertebral column injury, 183
Demeclocycline
  as diabetes insipidus cause, 268
  in hyponatremia treatment, 272
Dementia, 956–957
Demerol. *See* Meperidine hydrochloride
Deming, Dr. W. Edwards, continuous quality improvement model by, 57
Denial, in grieving process, 859–860
Dengue fever, 406
Dens fractures, 190
  dislocation and, 189
Dental emergencies, 1331–1337
  fractured or avulsed teeth, 1333–1335
  in maxillofacial injury, 1322
  mucosal lacerations, 1336–1337
  odontogenic infection, 1331–1333
  postextraction bleeding, 1335–1336
  temporomandibular joint dislocation, 1335
Dental malocclusion, in mandibular fracture, 1328
Dental pain, differential diagnosis, 1333
Dentoalveolar trauma, 1333–1335
Denture sores or ulcers, 1336, 1337
Denys, John Baptiste, 115
Department of Defense, in National Disaster Medical System, 37
Department of Energy, radiation accident assistance by, 758
Department of Health, Education, and Welfare (DHEW)
  Advisory Council on Trauma Care Systems, 27
  consumer participation support by, 7
  Division of Emergency Services, 3
  EMS projects funded by, 2
  EMT-P training role, 4
  in National Disaster Medical System, 37
Department of Labor, EMT-P training role, 4
Department of Transportation (DOT). *See also* National Highway Traffic Safety Administration
  Basic EMT curriculum by, 3
  EMS systems and, 1–2, 27
  EMT-I level and, 6
  EMT-P training role, 4
  hazardous materials and, 748, 749
  ID codes for immediate evacuation, 751–752
  helicopter transport and, 26
  rural EMS programs and, 23
Dependence, physical vs. psychological, defined, 782
Depilatory ingestion, hypokalemia and, 276
Deployment plans, 16
Depo-Medrol. *See* Methylprednisolone
Depolarization/repolarization, action potential and, 273–274
Depression, 829–835
  atypical, 830
  in battering syndrome, 842
  causes of, 830
  differential diagnosis, 831
  drug-induced, 474
  headache with, 920
  levels and types of, 830–831
  referrals for, 831
    to inpatient care, 831–832
    to outpatient psychotherapy, 831, 832
  sedative-hypnotic abuse and, 800
  suicide risk and, 831, 834
Depressive episodes, 830
DeQuervain's tenosynovitis, 346
  "sprains" vs., 207

Dermatitis
  atopic, 429–430
  contact, 432–433
  marine-associated, 741–742
Dermatographia, urticaria and, 440–441
Dermatologic emergencies. See Burns; Chemical burns; Skin disorders; Skin infections
Dermatomyositis, cutaneous lesions in, 336
Desferal. See Deferoxamine
Designation
  of emergency departments (EDs), 45, 50
  of hospitals, as regionalization method, 49, 50
Designer drugs, 799–800
Desoxycorticosterone acetate, for adrenal insufficiency, 260
Desyrel. See Trazodone
DET (diethyltryptamine), 806–807
Detoxification units, "clearing" alcoholic patient for, 823–825, 828
Developmental crises, 859
Dexamethasone (Decadron), 1428–1429
  adrenal insufficiency and, 260
    secondary, 256
  for high-altitude illness, 682
  for purulent meningitis, 398
    in children under two, 538, 539
  for viral croup, 568
Dexon (polyglycolic acid) sutures, 142
Dextran solutions, 1444
  anaphylaxis risk with, 80
  for frostbite, 673
  for shock, 80, 127
Dextrose, as medication, 1432
DHEW. See Department of Health, Education, and Welfare
Diabetes insipidus
  central, 267–268, 270
  dehydration risk with, 267, 268
  diagnosis of, 269
  nephrogenic, 268, 270
  psychogenic polydipsia vs., 269
  treatment of, 270
Diabetes mellitus
  adrenal insufficiency and, 255
  carpal tunnel syndrome and, 347
  as CVA risk factor, 935
  emergencies associated with, 233–245
    diabetic ketoacidosis (DKA), 233–242
    hyperosmolar hyperglycemic nonketotic coma (HHNK), 242–245
  foot ulcers with, 231
  gallstones and, 455
  hyperkalemia and, 279, 300
  otitis externa and, 380, 1310, 1311
  skin disorders with, 433
  thrush and, 377
  vertebral osteomyelitis and, 193
Diabetic ketoacidosis (DKA), 233–242, 323–324
  acute confusion with, 953
  in children, unconsciousness with, 590
  complications of, 237, 238–239, 241
  diagnosis of, 234–236
  education of patient with, 241–242
  hypokalemia and, 276, 294, 297
  hypomagnesemia and, 286, 306
  pathogenesis of, 233–234, 235
  thyroid storm and, 249
  treatment of, 236–242, 323
    metabolic acidosis risk with, 322, 323–324
Diagnostic agents, for emergency departments, 1452–1453
Diagnostic and Statistical Manual of Mental Disorders (DSM III), 830
Dialysis
  hemodialysis vs. peritoneal, 1227
  for hypercalcemic crisis, 315
  for hyperkalemia, 280–281, 299, 300
  for hypermagnesemia, 308
  for renal failure, 1226–1227
  septic arthritis and, 357
  in toxicologic emergencies, 476
Diamox. See Acetazolamide

Diaphoresis. See also Sweating
  hypokalemia and, 276
  hyponatremia and, 270
  in shock, 68, 70
Diaphragm spasms, intractable hiccups, 454
Diaphragmatic injuries, 1188, 1189
Diarrhea
  acute watery, 389–390
  in anaphylaxis, 75
  chronic, in adrenal insufficiency, 259
  congenital alkalosis with, 328
  in Crohn's disease, 461, 462
  dehydration risk with, 267
  in dysenteric gastroenteritis, 390
  in food poisoning, 390, 391
  in gastroenteritis, 387–389
  hypokalemia and, 275, 294
  hypomagnesemia and, 286, 304, 305
  hyponatremia and, 270
  in irritable bowel syndrome, 463
  metabolic acidosis and, 321
  in neonate, adrenal insufficiency and, 258
  in pediatric patients, 558
    "overflow," 558
  in thyroid storm, 250
  traveler's, 387, 389
  treatment of, 389–390
  in ulcerative colitis, 462
Diastrophic dysplasia, 372
Diazepam (Valium), 1398, 1442–1443
  for acute confusion, psychiatric, 956
  in acute myocardial infarction treatment, 984, 985
  for alcohol-intoxicated patient, 818
  for alcohol withdrawal, 821
  for cannabis overdose, 809
  for cardiogenic shock, 85
  for ciguatera fish poisoning, 738
  elimination half-life of, 800
  for epistaxis, 1306
  for LSD-induced "bad trips," 810
  overdose of, 491–492
  for status epilepticus, 946, 947
    in children, 594
Diazoxide (Hyperstat), 1392
  hyperosmolar hyperglycemic nonketotic coma and, 244
  for hypertensive emergencies, 1062, 1063
  eclampsia, 1066
DIC. See Disseminated intravascular coagulation
Dichloromethane. See Methylene dichloride
Dichlorphenamide (Daranide; Oratrol), for acute glaucoma, 1289
Diclofenac (Voltaren), for pain relief, 881
Dicloxacillin (Dynapen; Veracillin), 1415
  for cutaneous abscesses, 408
  for dog bites, 157
  for human bites, 156, 157
  for impetigo, 431
  for septic bursitis, 412
  for sinusitis, 1303
  for staphylococcal scalded skin syndrome, 431
Dicyclomine (Bentyl), for irritable bowel syndrome, 463
Diet
  headache and, 925
  hyperkalemic periodic paralysis and, 298
  hypokalemia and, 293, 294
  metabolic alkalosis and, 328
  renal failure and, 1225
Diet medication, behavioral disorders and, 474
Diethyltryptamine (DET), 806–807
Diffuse interstitial disease
  in rheumatoid arthritis, 339
  in systemic lupus erythematosus, 339–340
DiFlucan. See Fluconazole
Diflunisal (Dolobid), 1404
  for pain relief, 881
DiGeorge's syndrome, hypocalcemia and, 284
Digital necrosis, in cholesterol embolism, 1171
Digitalis. See also Digoxin
  for atrial flutter, 1034
  hypercalcemia and, 283, 314–315

  hyperkalemia and, 298
  hypokalemia and, 277, 295, 297, 314–315
  hypomagnesemia and, 286, 306–307
  hypothermia and, 671
  nonparoxysmal junctional tachycardia and, 1028
  overdose of, hyperkalemia and, 279
  for PSVT, 1026
  for pulmonary edema, 1099
  renal failure and, 1225
  serum sickness and, 433
  for shock, 84
  for thyroid storm, 250
  ventricular tachycardia and, 1034
Digitalization (triphalangeal thumb), in Holt-Oram syndrome, 363
Digoxin (Lanoxin), 1383. See also Digitalis
  for atrial fibrillation, 1022
  calcium gluconate and, 285
  for congestive heart failure, 1055, 1056
  ectopic atrial tachycardia (EAT) and, 1019
  overdose of
    clinical signs, 473, 492
    treatment of, 477, 492–493
  pharmacokinetics and, 484
  for PSVT, 1028
  for pulmonary edema, 1099
  shock diagnosis and, 66–67
  Wolff-Parkinson-White syndrome and, 1042
Dihydroergotamine, for headache, 922
Diiodohydroxyquin, for dysenteric gastroenteritis, 390
Dilantin. See Phenytoin
Dilaudid. See Hydromorphone
Diltiazem (Cardizem), 1383–1384, 1392
  for atrial fibrillation, 1022
  for atrial flutter, 1024
Dimethoxyamphetamine;
  Dimethoxymethylamphetamine (DOM/STP), 807
  as sympathomimetic, 787
Dimethyltryptamine (DMT), 806
Dinitrobenzene intoxication, 473
Dinitrophenol intoxication, 757
Dinoflagellates
  red tides and, 734
  shellfish poisoning and, 733–734
Diphenhydramine (Benadryl), 1408–1409
  in acute myocardial infarction treatment, 982
  for anaphylaxis, 86, 433
  for drug eruption, 434
  for urticaria, 441
Diphenoxylate
  for diarrhea, 389
  as opioid, 793
Diphenoxylate-atropine (Lomotil)
  overdose of, 472
    in children, 795
  pharmacology of, 795
Diphenylhydantoin. See Phenytoin
Diphosphonate, for hypercalcemia in cancer patients, 316
Diphtheria, 569–570
  pharyngitis and, 378
Diphtheria antitoxin, anaphylaxis risk with, 75
Diphtheroids, in cat bites, 156
Dipivefrin (Propine), for acute glaucoma, 1289
Diplopia, in temporal arteritis, 337
Dipropyltryptamine (DPT), 807
Direct-current cardioversion. See Electrical cardioversion
Disaster, defined, 31
Disaster management, 12, 15, 16, 31–37
  communications in, 8, 33
  hospital care issues, 36
  medical direction in, 32–33
  medical evaluation of, 36–37
  mutual aid issues, 11, 32
  National Disaster Medical System (NDMS), 37
  personnel issues, 33–34
  phases for, 32
  planning issues, 31–32
  prehospital care component, 35
  public participation in, 36

Subject Index 1479

public safety agencies and, 12, 33, 34
training issues, 34
transportation issues, 25, 35–36
triage issues, 34–35
Disciples of Christ, beliefs and practices, 866
Disciplinary measures, National Practitioner Data
　　Bank and, 56
Dislocations, 173–174
　in cervical spine, 188–190, 905, 906
　　stable vs. unstable, 908
　in feet and toes, 230
　hip, 173, 217
　　acetabular fractures and, 215, 216
　　femoral head fractures and, 217–218
　knee, 172, 223, 224
　　anatomy and, 221–222
　temporomandibular joint, 1328, 1335
　upper extremity, 195, 198–199
　　carpal, 206–207
　　elbow, 202, 204
　　shoulder, 199–200
　　sternoclavicular, 198–199
　vertebral column, 188–190
Disopyramide (Norpace), 1384
　for dysrhythmias
　　atrial premature complex, 1002
　　PSVT, 1026, 1028
　　ventricular premature complexes, 1005
　　ventricular tachycardia, 1030, 1034
　for Wolff-Parkinson-White syndrome, 1042
Disorientation. See Confusion
Dispatch
　in communications systems, 7, 8
　staffing issues, 22
Disseminated intravascular coagulation (DIC)
　in cancer patients, 510
　in hypovolemic shock, 71
　in septic shock, 72
　as transfusion reaction, 133, 134
Dissociation, acid-base balance and, 319
Distraction, for pain management, 887
Diuresis. See also Diuretics
　dehydration risk with, 267
　forced
　　for sedative-hypnotic overdose, 804
　　in toxicologic emergencies, 475–476
　hyperkalemia and, 279
　hypocalcemia and, 284
　hypokalemia and, 275–276, 293, 294, 296, 297
　hypomagnesemia and, 286
　as hypothermia response, 666
　metabolic alkalosis and, 327, 328
　self-abuse of, 296
Diuretics, 1429–1432. See also Diuresis; specific kinds
　acute gouty arthritis and, 352
　in acute myocardial infarction treatment, 993
　anaphylaxis risk with, 75
　for ascites, 459
　for congestive heart failure, 1055, 1056
　for hypercalcemic crisis, 315
　for hyperkalemia, 281, 299, 300
　hyperosmolar hyperglycemic nonketotic coma and,
　　243–244
　for hypertensive emergencies, 1064
　hypokalemia and, 275–276
　hyponatremia and, 270
　for pulmonary edema, 1099
　for respiratory distress in children, 579
　urine testing and, 266
Divers; Diving injuries
　arterial air embolism, 708–709
　cervical spine fracture, 192
　dangerous marine organisms and. See Marine
　　organisms
　decompression sickness (DCS) in, 705–707
　hypothermia, 662
　nitrogen and, 764
Divers Alert Network (DAN), hyperbaric chamber
　　referral by, 707, 709, 1161
Diverticulitis, 460, 463
Diving Accident Network. See Divers Alert Network
Division of Emergency Services (DHEW), 3

Division of Injury Control (CDC), research support
　　by, 3
Dizziness, postural, in adrenal insufficiency, 258
DKA (diabetic ketoacidosis), 233–242
DMT (dimethyltryptamine), 806
Dobutamine (Dobutrex), 1384
　in acute myocardial infarction treatment, 984, 992
　for congestive heart failure, 1055, 1056
　for shock, 84
　　septic, 85
Documentation. See Record keeping
Dog bites, 155, 156, 157, 627–631
　complications of, 628
　epidemiology of, 627–628
　rabies precautions, 629
　treatment of, 628–631
Dogfish sharks, spine or puncture wounds by, 724
Dogger Bank itch (sea moss dermatitis), 741
Dolichocephaly, 368
"Dolies" or "Dollies". See Methadone
Doll's eyes reflex. See Oculocephalic maneuver
Dolobid. See Diflunisal
Dolophine. See Methadone
Dolphin fish, poisoning by, 712
DOM. See Dimethoxyamphetamine;
　　Dimethoxymethylamphetamine
Domestic violence (DV), 837–854. See also Child
　　abuse; Elder abuse
　approaches to treatment of, 844
　assailant in, 841, 842, 846
　barriers to identification of, 839–841
　battering syndrome, 841–842
　child abuse and, 841, 844, 845
　documentation of, 843, 853
　emergency department management of, 848–852
　　assessment, 848
　　intervention process, 852–854
　　issues in, 839–841
　extent of, 837–838
　family characteristics and, 844–845
　follow-up care, 853
　health problems with, 841
　history taking and, 839, 840, 841, 848
　　assessment and treatment report, 849–851
　　in battering syndrome, 842
　　questioning techniques, 848, 851–852
　legal issues, 843
　management of victims of, 848–852
　misconceptions about, 842–843
　patient reactions to, 840
　profiles of victims of, 845–846
　psychologic aspects of, 846
　as public health problem, 837
　recommendations for care, 853
　referrals for, 852, 853–854
　suicide attempts and, 841
　terminology, 837
　theories of, 843–844
　types of abuse, 837
Donabedian quality assessment framework, 54–55
Done salicylate nomogram, 488–489
Donnatal, for diverticulitis, 463
Dopamine (Intropin), 1384–1385
　in acute myocardial infarction treatment, 984, 992
　for ciguatera fish poisoning, 738
　for congestive heart failure, 1055, 1056
　for drug reaction, 433
　hypothermia and, 671
　for shock, 84
　　anaphylactic, 87
　　septic, 85
Doppler echocardiogram, in congestive heart failure,
　　1054
Doppler ultrasonography, in deep venous thrombosis,
　　1147
Doriden. See Glutethimide
Dorsal intercalary segment instability (carpal
　　dislocation), 206
DOT. See Department of Transportation
Doxepin (Sinequan), overdose of, 485. See also
　　Antidepressants
Doxorubicin (Adriamycin), cardiac reactions to, 509

Doxycycline (Vibramycin; Vibratabs), 1417
　for corneal ulcers, 1278
　for gonorrhea, 1250
　for gonorrhea or chlamydia, 1233
　for pelvic inflammatory disease, 1234
　for pneumonias, 386
　for septic gonococcal arthritis, 412
　for urethritis in men, 395
　for urinary tract infections, 393
DPT (dipropyltryptamine), 807
Dressings
　for burns, 425
　for eye, 1268, 1270
　for upper extremities, 195, 196–197
　Velpeau stockinette, 200
　in wound management, 156–157
Droperidol, as general anesthesia, 887
Drowning and near-drowning, 689–698
　ambulatory and follow-up care, 698
　definitions, 689
　diagnosis of, 694
　epidemiology and etiology, 689–690
　monitoring requirements in, 698
　multiple injuries with, 694, 695
　pathology of, 690
　pathophysiology of, 690–694
　treatment in, 694–698
　　guidelines for, 696
　　prehospital, 694–695
Drug abuse. See also Alcoholism; Substance abuse
　abstinence syndrome. See Withdrawal syndrome
　as acute confusional state cause, 954
　defined, 782
　factitious headache and, 920
　hepatitis and, 403, 404
　intra-arterial injection of foreign substances, 1075
　intravenous
　　complications of, 784–786
　　vertebral osteomyelitis and, 193
　mononucleosis syndrome and, 402
　overdose and. See Drug overdose
　renal failure and, 1219
　as seizure cause, 948
　sepsis risk with, 406
　septic arthritis and, 352
　septic shock risk and, 72
　sternoclavicular joint monoarthritis and, 351
　types of drugs, 782. See also specific types
　　designer drugs, 799–800
　　hallucinogens, 806–807
　　inhalants, 805–806
　　opioids, 793–799
　　sedative-hypnotics, 800–805
　　sympathomimetics, 786–793
　withdrawal syndrome. See Withdrawal syndrome
Drug overdose. See also specific drugs; Toxicologic
　　emergencies
　alertness agents, 491
　anticonvulsants, 489–491
　antidepressants, 485–487
　catecholamine-induced hypertension from, 1066
　in children or adolescents
　　resuscitation and, 525–526
　　unconsciousness with, 591
　common toxidromes, 591
　medications for, 1447–1450
　methanol and ethylene glycol, 487–488
　over-the-counter medications, 491
　pharmacokinetics and, 480–484
　salicylates, 488–489
　theophylline, 484
Drug reactions. See also specific drugs
　as acute confusional state cause, 954
　antivenin and, 493
　aseptic meningitis and, 399
　to local anesthetics, 884–885
　orthostatic syncope, 961
　phenothiazine dystonia, in children, 565–566
Drug screens, in toxicologic emergencies, 471–474
Drug withdrawal. See Withdrawal syndrome
Drugs, therapeutic, 1377–1450. See also specific
　　drugs; specific types

Drugs, therapeutic (contd.)
  as acute confusional state cause, 954
  anaphylaxis risk with, 75
  anti-inflammatories, 1403–1405, 1428–1429
  antianginal agents, 1391–1397
  antiarrhythmics, 1381–1391
  antiasthmatic agents, 1424–1428
  antibiotics
    aminoglycoside, 1409–1411
    cephalosporin, 1411–1413
    miscellaneous types of, 1418–1424
    penicillin and penicillin derivatives, 1413–1416
    sulfonamides, 1417
    tetracyclines, 1417–1418
  anticoagulants, 1400–1403
  anticonvulsants, 1398–1399
  antidepressants, 1406–1408
  antiemetics, 1406–1408
  antifibrinolytics, 1400–1403
  antigout agents, 1403–1405
  antihistamines/antipruritics, 1408–1409
  antihypertensives, 1391–1397
  bronchodilators, 1424–1428
  for cardiac arrest, 1381–1391
  catecholamine-induced hypertension and, 1066, 1067
  clearance of, 483
  for connective tissue disease, complications of, 342, 343
  corticosteroids, 1428–1429
  in CPR
    advanced cardiac life support, 1089–1090
    of pediatric patients, 521–525
  as diabetes insipidus cause, 268
  diuretics, 1429–1432
  dosage control, for pediatric patients, 521
  elimination of, 482–483
  for emergency departments, listed, 1452–1453
  ergot alkaloids, 1446
  estrogens, 1445–1446
  gastric acid inhibitors, 1433–1434
  as gastroenteritis cause, 387
  as headache cause, 918
  heat illness and, 655
  hematinics, 1447
  hypercalcemia and, 315, 317
  hyperkalemia and, 298
  hyperosmolar hyperglycemic nonketotic coma and, 243–244
  hypoglycemics/antihypoglycemics, 1432–1433
  hypokalemia and, 275–276, 294
  hyponatremia and, 271
  hypothermia and, 662
  illicit, defined, 782
  narcotic and non-narcotic analgesics, 1435–1438
  for overdose treatment, 1447–1450
  oxytocics, 1446
  pharmacokinetics and, 480–484
  plasma volume expanders, 1444–1445
  pregnancy and, 1240
  renal failure and, 1218–1219, 1225–1226
  for respiratory distress, in pediatric patients, 578–579
  sedative-hypnotics, 1438–1441
  shock diagnosis and, 66–67
  skeletal muscle relaxants, 1441–1444
  sulfonamides, 1417
  systemic lupus erythematosus complications, 342, 343
  thyroid/antithyroid agents, 1445
  as toxic epidermal necrolysis cause, 440
  tranquilizers, 1406–1408
  as urticaria cause, 440
  vascular access routes for, 520–521
  vasopressors, 1381–1391
Drugs in Pregnancy and Lactation (Briggs, Freeman, and Yaffe), 1240
Dry mouth, in shock, 70
DSM III (Diagnostic and Statistical Manual of Mental Disorders), 830
Duchenne muscular dystrophy, myotonic dystrophy vs., 369
"Dumping," 7, 42–43
Dunlops' traction, for supracondylar fracture, 202
Duodenal hypomotility, in scleroderma, 342
Duodenal ulcers
  hereditary, 370
  upper GI bleeding with, 449
Durable power of attorney, 42
Duragesic. See Fentanyl transdermal system
Duranest. See Etidocaine
Duricef. See Cefadroxil
Duty, as legal concept, 40, 41
DV. See Domestic violence
DVT. See Deep venous thrombosis
Dye compounds, intoxication by, 473
Dynapen. See Dicloxacillin
Dyrenium. See Triamterene
Dysautonomia, familial (Riley-Day syndrome), 372
Dysenteric gastroenteritis, 390
Dysentery
  bacterial agents in, 387
  etiologies of, 387
  protozoans in, 387
Dysmorphology, in hereditary disease, 361, 363–365
Dysphagia
  esophageal obstruction and, 452
  in systemic lupus erythematosus, 342
Dyspnea, 1095–1096
  in anaphylaxis, 75
  causes of, 1095, 1096
  in congestive heart failure, 1052, 1054
  diagnosis with, 1095–1096
  dysrhythmia and, 997
  in obstructive airway disease, 1129–1138
  paroxysmal nocturnal, 1096
  pulmonary edema and, 1096–1101
  in pulmonary embolism, 1143
  respiratory alkalosis and, 330
  in scleroderma, 340
  in shock, 70
    cardiogenic, 75
  in systemic lupus erythematosus, 339
  in Wegener's granulomatosis, 340
Dysreflexia, autonomic, 912–913
Dysrhythmias, 997–1049
  accelerated idioventricular rhythm, 970, 1028, 1030, 1031
  in acute myocardial infarction
    diagnosis and, 970
    management of, 983–985
  advanced cardiac life support and, 1090–1091
  Ashman phenomenon in, 1008, 1009
  bradydysrhythmias, 1008–1017
    atrioventricular (AV) block, 1013–1017
    sudden sinus (atrial standstill), 1010–1012
  cardiac conduction system and, 998
  cardiac-pacing systems for, 1042–1049
    temporary placement of, 1351–1352
  as cardiogenic shock cause, 74, 85
  diagnosis of, 997, 999
  ectopic beats, 999–1005
    aberration vs., 1007–1008, 1009
    atrial premature complex (APC), 999–1002
    premature ventricular complexes (PVCs), 1002–1005
  hemodynamic consequences of, 997–998
  at high altitude, 681
  in hypomagnesemia, 304, 306–307
  hypothermia and, 664, 671
  magnesium administration for, 307
  parasystole, 1005–1007
  postresuscitation, 1091
  rule of bigeminy and, 1008, 1009
  symptoms attributable to, 997, 998
  syncope and, 959, 960, 962, 963
  tachydysrhythmias, 1018–1037, 1038, 1039
    regular, wide QRS tachycardias, 1034, 1037, 1038, 1039
    supraventricular, 1018–1028, 1029
    ventricular, 1028, 1030–1034
  in toxicologic emergencies, 472–473
  Wolff-Parkinson-White syndrome, 1037, 1040–1042

Dysthymic disorder (depressive neurosis), 830
Dystonia, torsion, 372
Dysuria
  in infections, 391, 392
  in prostatitis, 395
  in urethritis, 394

E

E.E.S. See Erythromycin
Ear medications, for emergency department, 1453
Ear wicks, for otitis externa, 1311
Ears
  burns on, as major injuries, 424
  foreign bodies in, 1307, 1308
  injury repair, 1326–1327
  lacerations of, 153
    wound dressings for, 157
  otitis, 379–381
    externa (swimmer's ear), 379–380, 1310–1311
    media, 380–381, 1309–1310
  in Raynaud's phenomenon, 341
  tympanic membrane perforations, 1306–1307
Eastern equine encephalitis, 400
Eastern Orthodox Church, beliefs and practices, 866
EAT. See Ectopic atrial tachycardia
Eating disorders. See also Anorexia
  hypokalemia and, 294, 296
  in neonate, adrenal insufficiency and, 258
ECGs. See Electrocardiograms
ECG telemetry, 8
Echocardiography, in congestive heart failure, 1054
Echovirus
  in shellfish, 733
  skin eruptions with, 443
Eclampsia, 1066. See also Pre-eclampsia
Economic issues. See Financial issues
"Ecstasy." See Methylenedioxymethamphetamine
Ectopic atrial tachycardia (EAT), 1018, 1019, 1020
Ectopic beats, 999–1005
  aberration vs., 1007–1008, 1009
  atrial premature complex (APC), 999–1002
  premature ventricular complexes (PVCs), 1002–1005
Ectopic pregnancy, 1231–1233
  culdocentesis in, 1230–1231
  diagnosis of, 1229, 1232
  etiologies of, 1232
  pelvic inflammatory disease vs., 1233, 1234
  treatment of, 1232–1233
  vaginal bleeding in, 1230
Eczematous drug eruptions, 434
Edecrin. See Ethacrynic acid
Edema
  in acute mountain sickness (AMS), 681
  high-altitude cerebral (HACE), 681, 684–685
  high-altitude pulmonary (HAPE), 681, 683–684
  as hypokalemia cause, 294
  as hyponatremia cause, 270
Edetic acid, for hypercalcemia, 283
Edrophonium (Tensilon), 1385
  for PSVT, 1026, 1028
  for regular, wide QRS tachycardia, 1037
  for Wolff-Parkinson-White syndrome, 1042
EDs. See Emergency departments
Education, as EMS system component, 11
E.E.S. See Erythromycin
Efficacy (appropriateness), as quality issue, 54, 62
"Eggshell" fractures, of distal phalanx, 207
Ehlers-Danlos disorders, 367
EIA. See Enzyme-linked immunoassay
Eikenella corrodens, in human bite wounds, 156, 632–633
Elasmobranch poisoning, 712, 736
Elavil. See Amitriptyline; Antidepressants
Elbow, 202–204
  arthrocentesis of, 353–354
  aspiration or injection of, 1374, 1375
  dislocations, 202, 204
  fractures, 202–203
  infections, 204
  osteomyelitis in, 204

septic arthritis in, 204
septic bursitis in, 204, 412
subluxation of radial head, 204
tendinitis (tennis elbow), 204
Elbow tendinitis (tennis elbow), 345, 346
Elder abuse, 846–847. *See also* Domestic violence
  burn center referral and, 48
  defined, 837
  extent of, 838
  legal issues, 847
  patterns of, 847
Elderly patients
  acute confusion in, drugs as cause of, 954
  Alzheimer's disease in, 957
  bursitis in, 345
  carbon monoxide poisoning and, 765
  compliance (ventilation) and, 1152
  dehydration risk in, 267
  dementia diagnosis in, 956–957
  diabetic ketoacidosis in
    mortality with, 233
    myocardial infarction and, 235
  epistaxis in, 1305
  gastrointestinal bleeding in, 450
  heat illness and, 655
  herpes zoster in, 442
  hip fractures in, 218, 219, 220
  hyperosmolar hyperglycemic nonketotic coma and, 243, 245
  hypothermia in, 661, 662
    chilblains, 672
  immobility of, hypercalcemia and, 282
  intestinal obstruction in, 460, 461
  leg lacerations in, complications caused by, 154
  meningitis in, etiology of, 396
  monoarticular arthritis in, 351
  myxedema coma and, 252
  otitis externa in, 380
  pharmacokinetic problems in, 483, 484
  rape and, 1253–1254
  rectal prolapse in, 466
  septic arthritis in, 410
  septic shock in, clinical features, 72
  subdural hematoma in, as headache cause, 918
  syncope in, 959, 960, 961–962
  thoracolumbar fractures in, Stryker frame for, 188
  urinary tract infections in, 391
Electrical burns, myoglobinuria and, 427
Electrical cardioversion
  for acute myocardial infarction, 984
  in advanced cardiac life support, 1088–1089
  for atrial fibrillation, 1022
  for atrial flutter, 1024
  for congestive heart failure, 1056
  procedure, 1361
  for PSVT, 1026, 1028
  for ventricular fibrillation, 1034, 1036, 1090
  for ventricular tachycardia, 1030, 1032, 1090–1091
Electrocardiograms (ECGs)
  in acute myocardial infarction, 967–970, 971–982, 986–988
  in aortic outflow obstruction, 959
  of cardiac-pacing systems, 1043, 1044–1045, 1048
  in dysrhythmias, 999–1041
    accelerated idioventricular rhythm (AIVR), 1028, 1030, 1031
    atrial fibrillation, 1009, 1022
    atrial flutter, 1023–1024
    atrioventricular (AV) block, 1013, 1014–1017
    ectopic atrial tachycardia (EAT), 1019, 1020
    ectopic beats, 999–1005, 1008, 1009
    multifocal atrial tachycardia (MAT), 1019, 1021
    nonparoxysmal junctional tachycardia, 1028, 1029
    parasystole, 1005, 1006
    paroxysmal supraventricular tachycardia (PSVT), 1024–1026, 1027
    regular, wide QRS tachycardia, 1034, 1037, 1038, 1039
    sinus slowing, 1010
    sudden sinus (atrial standstill), 1011, 1012
    ventricular fibrillation, 1004, 1034, 1036

ventricular tachycardia, 1004, 1030, 1032–1034
Wolff-Parkinson-White syndrome, 974, 977, 1037, 1040–1042
electrolyte disorders and, 265
in hypercalcemia, 281, 283, 313
in hyperkalemia, 280, 299
in hypocalcemia, 285
in hypokalemia, 277, 278, 295
in hypomagnesemia, 287
hypothermia and, 664, 665
in metabolic alkalosis, 328
in pulmonary embolism, 1145
in syncope, 962, 963
in toxicologic emergencies, 470
Electrocauterization
  for lower GI bleeding, 451
  of wounds, 141
Electroencephalography, in encephalitis, 400
Electrolyte abnormalities, 265–288
  emergency department agents for, 1453
  hydration physiology and, 265–266
  hypercalcemia, 281–284, 311–318
  hyperkalemia, 279–281, 297–300
  hypermagnesemia, 287–288, 308
  hypernatremia, 266–270
  hypocalcemia, 284–285
  hypokalemia, 275–278, 293–297
  hypomagnesemia, 286–287, 304–307
  hyponatremia, 270–272
  in near-drowning, 692–693
  potassium physiology and, 272–275
  in renal failure, 1224–1225
  respiratory problems with, 1155
  sodium physiology and, 266–267
  in toxicologic emergencies, 470
Electrolyte solutions, 292. *See also* Fluid replacement
  for acute watery diarrhea, 389
  for diabetic ketoacidosis, 237–239
  in fluid resuscitation, 126
  for gastroenteritis, 389–390
  for HHNK, 244–245
  for hypercalcemia, 314–315
  for hyperkalemia, 280, 299–300
  for hypokalemia, 278
  for shock, 76
  for thyroid storm, 250
Electromechanical dissociation, advanced cardiac life support for, 1091
Electrophysiological testing, in syncope, 962–963
Elimination, of drugs, 482–483
Ellis-van Creveld syndrome, 372
Embolectomy, for pulmonary embolism, 1148
Emboli. *See also specific types*
  air embolism, 1170
  amniotic fluid embolism, 1171
  cholesterol embolism, 1171
  drug abuse and, 785
  fat embolism, 1170–1171
Embolization, for lower GI bleeding, 451
Emergency Care and Transportation of the Sick and Injured (American Academy of Orthopedic Surgeons), 3
Emergency departments (EDs), 45–50
  acute epiglottitis and, 1119–1120
  acute myocardial infarction and, 982–985, 989–992
  alcoholics and, 815, 817–818, 822–823
  cancer patients and, 501–502
  categorization of, 45
  classification of, 45–47
    for behavioral emergencies, 47
    horizontal, 45–46
    vertical, 46–47
  crisis intervention role of, 835, 852
  domestic violence management in, 839–841, 848–854
    intervention process, 852–854
    questioning techniques, 848, 851–852
  drugs for use in, listed, 1452–1453
  emotional support role, 858–859
    in grief experiences, 859–861
    for staff, 861–862
  headache patients and, 915, 920, 921

holistic health care model for, 857–858
infectious diseases and, 375
liability issues in, 61
number of visits to, 45, 46
OB/GYN emergencies and, 1229
ocular emergencies and, 1259, 1261, 1295
pain management role, 888–889
pain perception and, 879
radiation injury preparedness for, 623–624, 758
rape victims and, 1241–1242, 1245–1246
  elderly, 1254
  evaluation form for, 1256, 1257
  social service referral, 1255
regionalization and, 49
spiritual support role of, 863–865
toxicologic screening in, 786
vascular emergency teamwork by, 1075
Emergency Medical Services (EMS), 1–27
  clinical conditions requiring, 2
  components of, 2, 3–12, 15–20
    access to care, 6–7
    communications, 7–9
    consumer participation, 7
    disaster linkages, 12, 15, 16, 31–37
    evaluation, 19–20
    facilities, 16, 18–19
    mutual aid, 11, 32
    patient transfer, 9–10
    public education, 11
    public safety agencies, 11
    record keeping, 11–12, 13–14
    staffpower and training, 3–6
    transportation, 15–16, 17
  funding for, 1–2, 23, 27
  geographical divisions for, 2
  historical overview, 1–3
  medical control issues, 20–21
  principles of, 3
  in rural areas, 22–23
  staffing issues, 21–22, 27
Emergency Medical Services Act of 1973, 1, 2, 8, 46, 93–94
Emergency Medical Technician-Intermediate National Standard Curriculum, 6
Emergency Medical Technician-Paramedic National Training Course, 4
Emergency medical technicians (EMTs)
  basic EMTs, 3
  CPR successes and, 1092
  destination criteria for, 46
  EMT-I level, 6, 22
  EMT-D level, 6, 22
  EMT-P level, 3–6, 22, 27
  first responders, 6
  registry of, 2
  standards of care and, 94
  training programs for, 2, 3, 4, 6, 94
Emergency procedures. *See* Procedures; *specific types*
Emergentologists, quality issues for, 53–62. *See also* Physicians
Emetics, therapeutic use of, 474–475. *See also* Vomiting
  for ciguatera fish poisoning, 738
  for sedative overdose, 803
Eminase. *See* Anistreplase or APSAC
EMIT. *See* Enzyme-linked immunoassay
Emotional assessment, of abused woman, 848
Emotional lability
  alcohol-induced, 818
  in thyroid storm, 250
Emotional support
  communication and, 871–875
  for disaster EMS personnel, 34
  in grief experiences, 859–861
  in holistic model, 857–858
  patients' needs for, 858–859
  for rape victim, 1241, 1242, 1245
    elderly, 1253–1254
    by first responder, 1244, 1245
  staff's needs for, in death of patient, 861–862
  therapeutic use of self in, 871

Emphysema
  chronic, 1129. See also Obstructive airway disease
    compliance and, 1152
EMS coordinators, 19
EMS. See Emergency Medical Services
EMT-I training, 6, 22
EMT-D training, 6, 22
EMT-P training, 3–6, 22, 27
E-Mycin. See Erythromycin
Enalapril (Vasotec), 1392
  for congestive heart failure, 1055
Enalaprilat (Vasotec IV), 1392
Encephalitis, 400–401
  acute liver failure and, 458
  aseptic meningitis and, 399
  as diabetes insipidus cause, 267
  hyponatremia and, 271
  treatment of, 401
  viral, in infants and children, 590
Encephalopathy
  acute liver failure and, 459
  Addisonian, 259
  differential diagnosis, 259, 343
  hypertensive, 1065
  in polyarteritis nodosa, 343
End-result system, 55
Endep. See Amitriptyline
Endocarditis, infective, drug abuse and, 785
Endocrine disorders
  adrenal insufficiency and, 258, 260
  hypercalcemia and, 282
  multiple endocrine adenomatosis syndromes, 369, 370, 371
  in renal failure, 1226
  thyroid storm, 249–251
Endocrine system
  hypothermia and, 664, 666
  response to injury, 69
Endogenous agents, shock diagnosis and, 66–67
Endogenous pain control mechanism, 879
Endophthalmitis. See Ocular emergencies, infections
Endorphins, in pain theory, 879
Endoscopic sclerotherapy, for esophageal varices, 449, 453
Endoscopy
  for chemical burns of esophagus, 451
  for lower GI bleeding, 451
  for upper GI bleeding, 449–450
Endotracheal intubation, 1104–1110
  in acute epiglottitis, 1119, 1120, 1121–1122
  of children, 514–515, 1106
    indications and guidelines, 579
    with multiple trauma, 544
    techniques, 517–519
    tubes for, 1108
  complications of, 97
  confirmation of, 97
  devices for, 96–97
  equipment for, 1107–1108
  esophageal airways and, 1104–1105
  indications for, 1104–1105
  of infants, techniques, 517–519
  in laryngeal trauma, 1316
  pharyngitis and, 377
  prehospital
    for cardiac tamponade, 103
    confirmation of, 97
    controversy about, 6
    devices for, 96–97
  preparing patient for, 1105–1106
  rapid sequence, 942, 1106–1107
  techniques, 1108–1110, 1366–1369
    for pediatric patients, 517–519
Endotracheal tube (ET), 96–97, 1107–1108
  esophageal obturator airway vs., 99, 1104
Enemas, for acute liver failure, 458
Enophthalmos, assessing for, 110
Entamoeba histolytica, in gastroenteritis, 387, 388
  dysenteric, 390
Enteritis, radiation, 508

Enterobacter species
  in corneal ulcers, 1274, 1275, 1277
  in nosocomial sinusitis, 1302–1303
  in pneumonia, 383
  in urinary tract infections, 391
Enterococci
  in corneal ulcers, 1277
  in urinary tract infections, 391
Enterotoxins
  in acute watery diarrhea, 389, 390
  in dysenteric gastroenteritis, 390
  in food poisoning, 390
  in gastroenteritis, 387, 388
  pathophysiology of, 387
Enteroviruses
  in shellfish, 733
  skin eruptions with, 443
Entonox, as general anesthesia, 886
Environmental Protection Agency (EPA), 747
Environmental stress. See Cold injury; Heat illnesses
Enzyme levels. See Serum enzyme levels; *specific enzymes*
Enzyme-linked immunoassay (EIA or EMIT), in drug screening, 786
EOA. See Esophageal obturator airway
EPA (Environmental Protection Agency), 747
Ephedrine
  as sympathomimetic, 787
  for uveitis, 1281
Epicondyle, lateral, aspiration or injection of, 1374
Epicondyle fractures, 203
Epicondylitis, lateral. See Elbow tendinitis
Epicondylitis, medial, 346
Epidemiology, drowning and, 689–690
Epidermal necrolysis, toxic, 440
Epididymitis, acute, 1212
Epidural anesthesia, 885
Epidural hematoma, 899
  in children, unconsciousness with, 589
Epiglottitis, acute, 1117–1125
  in adults, 1123–1125
  in AIDS patients, 1125
  airway and, 514, 515, 566–567
  in children, 1117–1123
    clinical signs, 1117–1118
    infection associated with, 1118–1119
  croup vs., 1114
  differential diagnosis, 1114, 1120, 1125
  etiologies of, 1117, 1123–1124
  pathology of, 1117
  treatment of, 567, 1119–1123, 1124–1125
Epilepsy. See also Status epilepticus
  defined, 945
  etiology of, 593
  idiopathic vs. symptomatic, 946
  myoclonus, 372
  symptomatic, defined, 945
Epinephrine (Adrenalin; Epinephrine; Sus-Phrine), 1385
  for anaphylaxis, 86, 87, 433
  for asthma, 1132, 1133
  for COPD, 1133
  in CPR
    advanced cardiac life support, 1089, 1090, 1091
    of pediatric patients, 522–523
  for hymenoptera stings, 644
  hypothermia and, 671
  for obstructive airway disease, 1133
  racemic, 1116
    for spasmodic croup, 565
    for viral croup (laryngotracheitis), 568, 1115–1116
  in response to injury, 69
  for scombroid fish poisoning, 739
  self-administration kits, 87
  for uveitis, 1281
  in wound anesthetic, 139, 140
Epiphora, in uveitis, 1278
Episcleritis, in rheumatoid arthritis, 338
Episcopalians, beliefs and practices, 866

Epistaxis, 1304–1306
  maxillofacial injuries and, 110
Epstein-Barr virus
  aseptic meningitis and, 399
  in mononucleosis syndrome, 401–403
  pharyngitis and, 377
Equine encephalitis, 400
Ergot alkaloids, 1446
Ergotamine tartrate (Ergomar; Ergostat; Gynergen), 1446
  for headache, 923
Erysipelas, 432
Erysipelothrix rhusiopathiae, 408
Erythema marginatum rheumaticum, 336
Erythema migrans, 336
  in Lyme disease, 357
Erythema multiforme, 434–435
  oral lesions with, 382
Erythema nodosum, 336–337
Erythrasma, 430
Erythrocyte hemolysis, burns and, 418
Erythrocyte sedimentation rate (ESR), in temporal arteritis, 917
Erythromycin (E.E.S.; Ilosone; E-Mycin), 1420
  anaphylaxis risk with, 75
  for corneal ulcers, 1275
  for cutaneous abscesses, 408
  for dysenteric gastroenteritis, 390
  for erythrasma, 430
  for gastroenteritis, 390
  for gonorrhea, 1250
  for human bites, 157
  for impetigo, 431
  for otitis media, 1309
  for pharyngitis, 378
  for pneumonia, 386
    in children, 586
  for prostatitis, 395
  for scarlet fever, 432
  for septic gonococcal arthritis, 412
  for sinusitis, 1303
  for skin infections, marine-associated, 408
  for urethritis in men, 395
  for urinary tract infections, 393
Erythromycin-sulfamethoxazole (Pediazole), for pneumonia in
children, 586
Erythropoietic protoporphyria, 366
Escharatomy, for burns, indications for, 427
Escherichia coli
  in acute sepsis, 406
  in acute watery diarrhea, 389
  in corneal ulcers, 1274, 1275, 1277
  as enterotoxin, 387
  in gastroenteritis, 387, 388
    dysenteric, 390
  in pneumonia, 383, 386–387
  in prostatitis, 395
  in urinary tract infections, 391
  as vertebral osteomyelitis cause, 194
Esmolol (Brevibloc), 1385–1386
  for atrial fibrillation, 1022
  for PSVT, 1026
Esophageal dysfunction
  in scleroderma, 341–342
  in systemic lupus erythematosus, 342
Esophageal emergencies, 451–452
  chemical burns, 451
  obstruction, 452
    in cancer patients, 505
  penetrating trauma, 1188
  peptic esophagitis, 452
  rupture, 452
  varices, 449, 452–453
Esophageal gastric tube airway, 6, 98
Esophageal obturator airway (EOA), 98–99, 1104
  complications of, 98–99
  endotracheal tube vs., 99
  prehospital use of, 6, 98
Esophageal reflux, 452

Esophageal varices, upper GI bleeding with, 449
Esophageal-tracheal combitube (ETC), 99, 1104
Esophagitis
　peptic, 452
　in systemic lupus erythematosus, 342
Esophagoscopy
　in corrosive ingestion, 554
　for esophagitis diagnosis, 452
　for foreign body, 559
Esophagus
　foreign body in, 1308–1309
　surgery on, adrenal insufficiency and, 257
ESR. *See* Erythrocyte sedimentation rate
Essex-Lopresti injury, 203
Estriol excretion, maternal, congenital adrenal insufficiency and, 258
Estrogen, conjugated (Premarin), 1445–1446
Estrogen therapy, hypercalcemic crisis and, 315
ET. *See* Endotracheal tube
ETC. *See* Esophageal-tracheal combitube
Ethacrynic acid (Edecrin), 1430
　for congestive heart failure, 1055
　for hypercalcemic crisis, 315
　hypokalemia and, 275–276
Ethambutol, for marine-associated skin infections, 409
Ethane, asphyxiation injury by, 764
Ethanol, in over-the-counter drugs, overdose and, 491
Ethanol intoxication, 325, 492. *See also* Alcohol withdrawal; Alcoholism
　assay methods, 472
　behavioral disorders and, 474, 492
　clinical signs, 472, 473, 492
　as diabetes insipidus cause, 268
　hypomagesemia and, 286, 306
　treatment of, 476
Ethchlorvynol (Placidyl), 1439. *See also* Sedative-hypnotics
　abstinence syndrome, 804
　elimination half-life of, 800
　overdose of, 492
　　clinical signs, 472, 492, 803
　　intoxication, 325
　　treatment of, 477, 804
　for pain relief, 882
　pharmacology of, 802
Ethinamate (Valmid), for pain relief, 882
Ethmozine. *See* Moricizine
Ethosuximide, for seizures, 949
Ethyl cellosolve poisoning, 774
Ethyl ether intoxication, 325
Ethylaminobenzoate (Benzocaine)
　intoxication by, 473
　pharmacologic classification, 885
Ethylene dibromide, as systemic toxin, 774
Ethylene glycol intoxication, 324, 487
　assay method, 472
　clinical signs of, 473–474
　treatment of, 476, 487–488, 757
Etidocaine (Duranest), clinical characteristics and dosage, 884
Eucatropine (Euphalmine), for uveitis, 1281
Evaluation. *See also* Quality issues
　ALS medical control through, 20–21
　consumer role in, 61–62
　in disaster management, 36–37
　as EMS system component, 19–20
　record keeping for, 11–12
Evisceration, as MAST suit contraindication, 77
Exanthemic eruptions
　drug reactions, 433–434
　viral, 443
Excision of wounds, 140, 151
Excretory urography
　in blunt trauma, 1196
　in flank pain diagnosis, 1211
　in penetrating trauma, 1198–1199
　in ureteral injury, 1200
　in urethral injury, 1206
Exercise
　excessive

　　adrenal insufficiency and, 259
　　hypokalemia and, 295
　　hyperkalemic periodic paralysis and, 298
Exercise testing, in syncope, 962
Existential concerns of patient, 863
Exogenous agents, shock diagnosis and, 66–67
Exophthalmos, assessing for, 110
Expert witnesses, on duty, 40
Express consent, 41–42
Extension block splint, for hand, 209–210
Extension injuries
　to cervical spine, 907
　to vertebral column, 177
Extensor carpi radialis brevis/longus tendonitis, "sprains" vs., 207
Extensor carpi ulnaris subluxation, "sprain" vs., 207
Extensor tendon lacerations, in wrist and hand, 212
External jugular vein, IV placement in, 102
Extracellular fluid
　in hypovolemic shock, 67–68, 70
　in metabolic alkalosis, 327
Extraocular movements
　in head injury, 895–896
　in unresponsive patients, 932–933
Extremities. *See also* Fractures; *specific extremities*
　blunt injury to, 1073–1074
　dysmorphology of, 363
　erythema multiforme on, 434
　fungal infections on, 435, 436
　penetrating injury to, 1073
　in Raynaud's phenomenon, 341
　upper, 195–212
　vascular emergencies in, 1073–1074
　wound management on
　　splinting, 157
　　suture material, 143
　　suture removal, 144
　　suture technique, 143
Extrication back splint, cost of, 109
Eye drop preparations, 1268, 1269
　for corneal abrasion or foreign body, 1267, 1268, 1270
Eye medications, for emergency department, 1453
Eye movements. *See* Extraocular movements
Eye ointments, 1269
　for corneal abrasion or foreign body, 1268
Eye-opening response, 928
　assessing, 929, 931
　on Glasgow Coma Scale, 929
　in head injury, 894
Eyebrows
　decrease of hair in, 285
　lacerations on, 151
　soft tissue injury of, 1327
Eyelashes, decrease of hair in, 285
Eyelids
　lacerations on, 151–152, 1327
　obtaining culture specimens from, 1272
　retraction and eversion of, 1263
Eyes. *See also* Ocular emergencies
　anatomy of, 1260, 1291–1294
　blood in anterior chamber of (hyphema), 1282–1286
　burn injuries to, as major injuries, 424
　chemical injury to, 754, 1320
　　as priority, 1262
　　treatment of, 1327
　dysmorphology in, in hereditary disorders, 364, 365
　foreign bodies in, 1327
　　corneal abrasions and, 1266–1270
　　removal of, 1263–1264, 1266–1267
　headache cause in, 917
　in maxillofacial injury, 1322
　physical examination of
　　globe exposure for, 1263–1264
　　lid eversion for, 1263–1264
　　lid retraction for, 1263
　in Sjögren's disease, 338
　toxic contamination of, 474
　trauma to, 1327
　　history taking in, 1261–1262

　　orbital floor fractures, 1329–1330
　　treatment of, 1327
　　visual acuity testing in, 1262
　in unresponsive patient evaluation, 931–933

F

Fabry's disease, 364, 365, 370
Face. *See also terms beginning with* Facial
　erysipelas on, 432
　impetigo on, 431
　oral-facial infections, 381–383
　vascular lesions on, 368
Facet joints, dislocation of, 190, 905
Facial injuries. *See also* Maxillofacial injuries; *specific organs*
　abrasion/avulsion, 1328
　airway control with, cricothyrotomy for, 99
　burns, as major injuries, 424
　fractures, 1328–1330
　lacerations, 150–154
　to lips, 1326
　to mouth and tongue, 1326
　wound management
　　debridement, 140
　　dressings, 157
　　suturing, 143, 144
　　topical anesthesia, 140
Facial nerves, 1323
　assessing for trauma, 1322, 1323. *See also* Cranial nerves
Facial pain, 916
　in carotidynia, 916, 920
Facilities
　categorization of, 18
　for disaster managemenet, 36
　as EMS system component, 16, 18–19
　rural vs. urban, 22–23
Faciogenital dysplasia, 364
Factor VIII deficiency (Hemophilia A), 367
Factor IX deficiency (Hemophilia B; Christmas disease), 367
Factor XI deficiency, 366, 372
Factor XIII deficiency, 366
Fahrenheit temperature, conversion chart, 1455–1462
Failure to thrive, adrenal insufficiency and, 258
Fainting. *See* Syncope
Falls
　cervical spine injuries from, 904, 905
　by children, 552
　as cause of death, 541
　great vessel injuries in, 1187
　renal injuries in, 1195
　subdural hematomas from, 899–900
　urethral injuries in, 1206
　vertebral column injuries from, 175, 179
Families, violence in. *See* Child abuse; Domestic violence
Famotidine (Pepcid), 1433
Fanconi's pancytopenia, 364, 365, 366, 368
Fangs, injuries by. *See* Snake bites
Farrington method of immobilization, 108–109
Fascia
　necrotizing infections of, 409–410
　suture material for, 142, 143
　suture technique for, 143
Fasciculations, in hypomagnesemia, 304
Fasciitis, necrotizing, 409–410
Fasciotomy, for frostbite, 673
Fasting
　adrenal insufficiency and, 259
　metabolic alkalosis and, 328
Fat embolism, 1170–1171
Fat excision, 140, 141
Fat pad sign, in elbow radiograph, 202
FATAL DTs screening test for alcoholism, 822, 827
FCC. *See* Federal Communications Commission
FDA. *See* Food and Drug Administration

Fecal impaction in children, "overflow" diarrhea and, 558
Fecal incontinence, in systemic lupus erythematosus, 344
Fecal-oral transmission, of hepatitis A virus, 403
Feces
    occult blood in, in intestinal obstruction, 461
    as wound contamination source, 138
Federal Communications Commission (FCC), EMS communications and, 8
Federal Emergency Management Agency (FEMA)
    in National Disaster Medical System, 37
    on response levels, 31
Feet
    burns on, as major injuries, 424
    dislocations in, 230
    dysmorphology of, in hereditary disorders, 363
    erythema multiforme on, 434
    fractures of, 228–230
        stress-type, 167
    hand-foot-mouth disease, 381–382
    lacerations of, 154–155
    skin abscess in, diabetic ketoacidosis and, 234
    soil-borne infections of, 409
    suture material for, 143
    suture technique for, 143
    ulcers of, 231
    in vertebral column injury, 185
Feldene. See Piroxicam
Felon, 210
FEMA. See Federal Emergency Management Agency
Females
    abuse victim profile, 845
    appendicitis in, 463, 464
    battering of. See Battering syndrome; Domestic violence
    erythema nodosa in, 336
    gynecologic emergencies in, 1229–1234
    herpes simplex 2 infections in, 442
    hydration and, 265
    obstetric emergencies in, 1234–1240
    pseudotumor cerebri in, 919
    urinary tract infections in, 391, 392, 393
Femoral epiphysis, fracture and, in children, 221
Femoral head fractures, 217–218
Femoral neck fractures, 218, 219
    treatment prognosis, 219
Femur
    acute osteomyelitis in, 358
    dislocations of, 173, 174
    fractures of, 162, 217–221
        blood loss risk with, 168
        classifications, 222
        emergency interventions, 222
        knee injuries and, 224
        open, 172, 222
        splinting, 168
Fenbufen (Lederfen), for pain relief, 881
Fenclofenac (Flenac), for pain relief, 881
Fenoprofen (Nalfon), for pain relief, 881
Fenoterol, inhaled, for obstructive airway disease, 1133
Fentanyl (Sublimaze), 1436
    designer drugs from, 799
    for facial lacerations in children, 139
    as opioid, 793
Fentanyl transdermal system (Duragesic), 1436
Feprazone (Methrazone), for pain relief, 881
Ferno-KED immobilization device, 109
Ferrous sulfate (Ledermark F20), 1447
FEV. See Forced expiratory volume
Fever. See also Hyperthermia
    in cancer patients, 505–506
    dehydration risk with, 267
    as headache cause, 917
    in measles, 442
    in neonate, adrenal insufficiency and, 258
    occult bacteremia (OB) with, in children under two, 529–533
    in pediatric patients
        convulsions with, 595–596

    in occult bacteremia, 529–533
    respiratory distress and, 578
    stridor with, 566–570
    under 3 months old, 533–535
    under 2 years old, 529–539
    in pharyngitis, 378
    in polyarteritis nodosa, 342
    polyarticular arthritis with, 358
    in pulmonary embolism, 1144–1145
    rheumatic
        cutaneous lesions of, 336
        polyarticular arthritis with, 358
    in rheumatoid arthritis, 358–359
    in rheumatologic emergencies, 335
    Rocky Mountain spotted, 438
    in roseola infantum, 438
    seizures with, 950
    in septic arthritis, 356
    in systemic lupus erythematosus, 339, 340
    in thyroid storm, 249, 250
    in toxic shock syndrome, 432
    as transfusion reaction, 133, 134
    as vertebral osteomyelitis sign, 194
    in Wegener's granulomatosis, 340
FFP. See Fresh-frozen plasma
Fibrillation
    atrial, 1009, 1018, 1022–1023
    EMT-Ds and, 6
    ventricular, 984, 1004, 1034, 1036
        advanced cardiac life support, 1090
        in cardiac arrest, 1083
        magnesium therapy for, 307
Fibrinogen scan, in deep venous thrombosis, 1147
Fibrinolytic therapy, for pulmonary embolism, 1148
Fibula, fractures of, 226
Fight or flight response, in shock, 70
"Fighter's fracture," 208
Fighting
    dental trauma in, 1333
    renal injuries in, 1195
Filliform and follower, for bladder drainage, 1214, 1215
Filters, for transfusion products, 130–131
Financial issues
    accreditation and, 27
    federal funding sources, 1–2, 27
    in rural vs. urban areas, 22, 23
    staffing and, 22
    state funding variations, 23
    transport of indigent patients, 7
    trauma center designation and, 18
Fingernails, pigmentation of, adrenal insufficiency and, 258
Fingers. See also Hand
    in carpal tunnel syndrome, 347
    dislocations of, 174
    dysmorphology of, in hereditary disorders, 363
    fractures of, 164, 207–208
    immobilization methods, 207, 208, 209, 210
    infections in, 210–211
    "sprains" of, 210
    "trigger" (tendinitis), 346
    upper extremity injuries and, 195, 198
    in vertebral column injury, 184
Finkelstein's test, for DeQuervain's tenosynovitis, 346
Finnish patients, hereditary disorders in, 372
Fiorinal (butalbital), for headache, 923
Fire ant bites or stings, 643–644
Fire department personnel
    collaborating with, 7, 11
    communication with, 8
    as dispatch personnel, 22
    as first responders, 6, 22
Fire injuries. See Burns; Chemical burns; Inhalation injury
Firefighters, chemical injury risk to, 761–762
First responders, 6, 11, 16, 22
Fish poisoning, 391, 711–712, 736–741
    skin infections, 742
Fitz-Hugh-Curtis syndrome, 556, 1233
Flagyl. See Metronidazole

Flail chest, 99, 101, 1182–1183
Flank pain, 1210–1211
    in adrenal gland hemorrhage, 256
Flare
    in glaucoma, 1289
    in uveitis, 1278
Flecainide (Tambocor), for atrial premature complex, 1002
Flenac. See Fenclofenac
Flexeril. See Cyclobenzaprine
Flexion contractures, in adrenal insufficiency, 259
Flexion injuries, to cervical spine, 905–906
Flexion-rotation injuries, to cervical spine, 906
Flexor carpi radialis
    tendinitis, 207
    in vertebral column injury, 184
Flexor digitorum function, in vertebral column injury, 184
Flexor tendon lacerations, in wrist or hand, 212
Flexor tenosynovitis, 211
Florinef. See Fludrocortisone; 9-α-Fluorohydrocortisone
Flosint. See Indoprofen
Fluconazole (DiFlucan), 1420–1421
    for thrush, 378
Fludrocortisone; 9-α-Fluorohydrocortisone (Florinef), 1429
    for adrenal insufficiency, 260
    for hyperkalemia, 281
Flufenamic acid (Meralen), for pain relief, 881
Fluid deficit
    hypernatremia and, 266–270
    hypokalemia and, 294
Fluid excess, hyponatremia and, 270–272
Fluid management. See also Fluid replacement
    emergency department agents for, 1453
    hydration physiology and, 265–266
    pelvic fractures and, 215
    in renal failure, 1223–1224
    for shock, 71, 76
    venous access guidelines, 76
Fluid replacement. See also Blood transfusions; Dehydration; Fluid management
    for acute watery diarrhea, 389
    for adrenal insufficiency, 260
    in appendicitis, 465
    blood components in, 125
    for burns, 420–423
    for cardiac tamponade, 103
    for children
        maintenance requirements, 550
        with multiple trauma, 550
    for ciguatera fish poisoning, 738
    dehydration treatment, 269–270
    diabetes insipidus treatments, 270
    for diabetic ketoacidosis, 236–237
    for dysenteric gastroenteritis, 390
    equipment used for, 130–132
    in field vs. hospital, 5
    for gastroenteritis, 389
    for HHNK, 244–245
    for hypercalcemia, 283, 314, 315
    for hyponatremia, with hypovolemia, 272
    for hypothermia, 671
    for intestinal obstruction, 460, 461
    metabolic acidosis risk with, 322
    for near-drowning, 697
    oral, indications for, 269
    for pancreatitis, 456
    in pediatric patients, 521
        with diarrhea, 558
        intraosseous access for, 520–521
        with respiratory distress, 578
        umbilical access for, 521
        vascular access for, 520
    physiology and, 265–266
    plasma volume expanders for, 1444–1445
    in renal failure, 1223–1224
    Ringer's lactate in, 126
    for shock, 78–81, 84
        anaphylaxis, 86

monitoring with, 81, 82
  physiologic considerations, 79–80
  types of fluids, 78–79, 126–130
 sodium excess treatment, 270
 for thyroid storm, 250
 for toxic epidermal necrolysis, 440
Fluid status, 265–266. *See also* Fluid management; Fluid replacement
Flumazenil (Mazicon), 1448–1449
 for benzodiazepine overdose, 802, 804
Fluorescent treponemal antibody absorption (FTA-ABS) test, 440
Fluorescent-linked immunoassay (FPIA), in drug screening, 786
Fluoroacetate overdose, 472, 473
Fluorocarbon inhalation, 805, 806
9-α-Fluorohydrocortisone. *See* Fludrocortisone
Fluoroscopy, foreign body removal with, 139
Fluosol DA (blood substitute), 81, 128
Fluoxetine, for headache, 924
Flurazepam (Dalmane), 1439
 elimination half-life of, 800
 overdose of, 491–492
 for pain relief, 884
Flurbiprofen (Ansaid), for pain relief, 881
Focal brain disease, confusion as sign of, 955
Focal neurologic signs, in head injury, 895
Focal seizures, 949
 syncope and, 961
Folic acid, for renal failure, 1226
Folliculitis, 431
Follow-up care. *See specific conditions*
Fontanelles, dehydration sign in, 268
Food
 airway obstruction by, in children, 564
 esophageal obstruction by, 452
Food allergies
 anaphylaxis risk with, 75
 to fish or shellfish, 712
 urticaria and, 440
Food and Drug Administration (FDA), blood and component regulations, 116, 117–119
Food poisoning
 gastroenteritis, 390–391
 by marine organisms, 711–712
  fish, 735–741
  shellfish, 390, 391, 731–735
Foot. *See* Feet
Foot-drop, as tibia fracture complication, 224
Football accidents. *See also* Sports injuries
 cervical spine fracture, 192
 renal injuries, 1195
Forced expiratory volume (FEV), respiratory failure and, 1151, 1152
Forced vital capacity (FVC)
 in obstructive airway disease, 1132
 respiratory failure and, 1151, 1152
Forearm injuries, 204–205
 compartment syndrome, 205
 fractures, 204–205
Foreign bodies
 in airway, 559, 564–565, 1308
 in ear, 1307, 1308
 in esophagus, 1308–1309
 in eye, 1327
  corneal abrasions and, 1266–1270
  removal of, 1263–1264, 1266–1267
 in maxillofacial injuries, 1320
 in nose, 1307–1308
 in pediatric patients, 559, 1307–1309
  aspiration of, 515–516, 583–584
  sudden UAO and, 564–565
 in rectum or colon, 465
 wound evaluation for, 139
Foreign substances, intra-arterial injection of, 1075
Forensic specimens
 for child abuse cases, 607
 for rape cases, 1241, 1243–1244, 1251–1252
Formaldehyde inhalation, 769, 774
Fortaz. *See* Ceftazidime
Forum for Quality and Effectiveness in Health Care, 58

Foursquare Church, beliefs and practices, 868
Foxes, rabies and, 629
FPIA. *See* Fluorescent-linked immunoassay
Fracture-dislocations
 of cervical spine, 176, 188, 189, 907, 908
 of foot, 229
 of hip, 217
 of thumb metacarpal, 208
 of vertebral column, 175–176
Fractures, 161–168. *See also* Skeletal injuries; *specific locations*
 basic vs. advanced life support skills, 94
 in cancer patients, 504
 in children, 161, 164, 165, 166
  child abuse, 599–600
  physeal fracture types, 166
 closed, reduction of, 168–169
 closed vs. open, 161
 comminuted, 161
 compression, 164, 165
 crush, 163
 description of, 161
 facial, prehospital care, 110
 fat embolism with, 1170, 1171
 HBO therapy for, 709
 mandibular, 1328
 in multisystem trauma, prehospital care, 111
 oblique, 162
 open, 161
  blood loss risk with, 168
  classification of, 166–168
  treatment of, 172
 open vs. closed, 161
 pathological, 166
 principles of, 161–168
 spiral, 163, 164
 splinting of, in shock response, 76
 stress, 166, 167
  of feet, 167
  of hip, 219
  tibial, 226
 tapping, 161, 163
 tensions, 163–164
 torus, 164, 165
 traction, 163, 164
 transverse, 161, 162, 163
 treatment of, 168–173
  immobilization, 169–172, 173
  manipulation or reduction, 168–169
  splinting, 168, 171–172
Francisella tularensis, 409
 in pneumonia, 383
Frank-Starling mechanism. *See* Preload
FRC. *See* Functional residual capacity
Free water excretion, sodium levels and, 266
Freon, inhalation abuse with, 806
Fresh-frozen plasma
 as colloid solution, 127
 in component therapy, 120, 121
 whole blood vs., 129
Friends (Quakers), beliefs and practices, 868–869
Froimson strap, for tennis elbow, 204
Frostbite, 672–673
Frostnip, 672, 673
Frozen shoulder, 346–347
FTA-ABS test, 440
Fugu poisoning (tetrodotoxism), 740–741
Functional bracing, for humeral shaft fracture, 201–202
Functional residual capacity (FRC), respiratory failure and, 1151, 1152
Funding. *See* Financial issues
Fundoscopic examination, of comatose patient, 931
Fungizone. *See* Amphotericin
Fungus infections
 aseptic meningitis and, 399
 in eye, diagnostic tests, 1272
 occupational sources of, 1162
 pneumonia, 383, 384
 sinusitis, 378, 1302
 of skin, 435–437. *See also specific infections*
 soil-borne, 409

 thrush, 377, 378
 tinea capitis, 435
 tinea corporis, 435–436
 tinea pedis (athlete's foot), 436
Funnel breast, in hereditary disorders, 365
Furosemide (Lasix), 1430
 in acute myocardial infarction treatment, 993
 for congestive heart failure, 1055, 1056
 for hypercalcemia, 283, 314, 315
 for hyperkalemia, 281
 hyperosmolar hyperglycemic nonketotic coma and, 243–244
 for hypertensive emergencies, 1064
 hypokalemia and, 275–276
 hypomagnesemia and, 307
 for hyponatremia, 272
 pharmacokinetics of, 483
 for pulmonary edema, 1099
Furuncles, 431
FVC. *See* Forced vital capacity

G

G-suit. *See* MAST suit
Galeazzi fracture, 205
Gallbladder disease, 453–455
 in pregnancy, 1235–1236
 shoulder-hand syndrome and, 347
Gallstones, 454
 in adolescent girls, 556
 in hereditary disorders, 369, 370
Game fish, injuries by, 729
"Gamekeeper's" thumb, 209
Gamma globulin, anaphylaxis risk with, 75
Gangrene, 409–410
 hyperkalemia and, 279
Gantrisin. *See* Sulfisoxazole
Garamycin. *See* Gentamicin
Gardner-Wells tongs, 188, 913
Gas chromatography, in drug abuse testing, 786
Gas exchange, respiratory failure and, 1152–1153
"Gas gangrene," 410
Gas inhalation. *See* Inhalant abuse; Inhalation injury
Gas-liquid chromatography (GLC), in drug and toxin screening, 471
Gasoline
 inhalation of, 474, 805, 806
 skin or ocular decontamination, 474
Gastric acid inhibitors, 1433–1434
Gastric contents
 analyzing, 471
 inducing emesis of, 474–475
 removing. *See* Gastric lavage
Gastric dilatation
 burns and, 419
 in pediatric trauma, 543
Gastric lavage
 in toxicologic emergencies, 475
  sedative-hypnotic overdose, 803–804
 for upper GI bleeding, 449
Gastric mucosa ulceration, in hypovolemic shock, 71
Gastric outlet obstruction, in cancer patients, 505
Gastric ulcer, endoscopic treatment of, 449
Gastric varices, upper GI bleeding with, 449
Gastrin, hypercalcemia and, 281
Gastrinomas, in multiple endocrine adenomatosis syndromes, 369, 371
Gastritis
 burns and, 419
 in systemic lupus erythematosus, 342
 upper GI bleeding with, 449
Gastrocnemius muscle, rupture of head of, Baker's cyst vs., 346
Gastroenteritis
 acute, 387–389
 in children, 556
 dysenteric, 390
 etiologies of, 387
 fish or shellfish ingestion and, 732, 733
 as radiation complication, 508
 treatment of, 389–390
Gastroesophageal tears, upper GI bleeding with, 449

Gastrointestinal disorders. *See also* Gastrointestinal
        infections
    adrenal insufficiency and, 259
    bleeding, in hereditary disorders, 365
    chemotherapy reactions, 509
    in connective tissue disease, 341–343
    hypercalcemia and, 311, 312
    hypokalemia and, 293, 294
    hypomagnesemia and, 304, 305, 306
    hyponatremia and, 270
    hypothermia and, 666
Gastrointestinal emergencies, 447–466. *See also*
        Gastrointestinal disorders; Gastrointestinal
        infections
    abdominal pain, 447–448
    anal fissure, 466
    anorectal disease, 466
    appendicitis, 463–465
    ascites, 459
    biliary tract disease, 453–455
    in cancer patients, 505
    colon injuries, 465
    Crohn's disease, 461–462
    diverticulitis, 463
    emergency department drugs for, listed, 1453
    esophageal, 451–452
    foreign bodies, 559
    head injury with, 896
    hemorrhoids, 465–466
    hiccups, 454
    irritable bowel syndrome, 463
    liver disease, 456–459
    lower gastrointestinal bleeding, 450–451
        in infants and children, 558
    noninfectious inflammatory bowel disease, 461–463
    pancreatic disease, 455–456
    in pediatric patients, 555–559
    proctitis, 466
    rectal herpes, 466
    rectal injuries, 465
    rectal prolapse, 466
    small bowel and colon disorders, 459–461
    splenic rupture and infarct, 459
    ulcerative colitis, 462–463
    upper gastrointestinal bleeding, 448–450
        in children, 558
        esophageal varices and, 452–453
Gastrointestinal fistulas, hypokalemia and, 294
Gastrointestinal function, hypothermia and, 666
Gastrointestinal infections, 387–391
    acute gastroenteritis, 387–389
    acute watery diarrhea, 389–390
    ascites and, 459
    dysenteric gastroenteritis, 390
    food poisoning, 390–391
    septic shock risk and, 72
Gastrointestinal malignancies
    obstruction and, 505
    thrombophlebitis and, 510
Gate Control Theory of pain, 878–879
Gaucher's disease, 365, 366, 368, 372
General anesthesia, 886–887
    in wound management, 139
General Electric, quality improvement role, 61
General systems theory of domestic violence, 844
Genetics, 361–373. *See also* Hereditary disorders
    basic principles, 361–363
    clinical, 363–365
Genital herpes, 441, 442
Genitourinary injuries
    to bladder, 1202–1205
    to kidneys, 1195–1199
    in multisystem trauma, 111–112, 896
    to penis, 1208–1209
    prehospital care, 111–112
    to scrotum and testicle, 1209, 1210
    to ureters, 1200–1202
    to urethra, 1205–1208
Genitourinary obstructions
    in cancer patients, 505
    flank pain with, 1210–1211

Gentamicin (Garamycin), 1409–1410
    for cholangitis and sepsis, 454–455
    for corneal ulcers, 1275, 1277, 1278
    in eye drops, 1268, 1269
    in eye ointment, 1269
    hypokalemia and, 275
    hypomagnesemia and, 286
    for marine organism injuries, 731, 732
    for meningitis, purulent, 953
    for meningitis or sepsis, in infants under 3 months,
        535
    for open fractures, 172
    for pelvic inflammatory disease, 1234
    for vertebral column injuries, 187–188
Gentamicin-tobramycin, for septic shock, 85
Gentian violet, for thrush, 378, 437
Gentran-40; Gentran-75. *See* Dextran solutions
Geocillin. *See* Carbenicillin
Geopen. *See* Carbenicillin
German measles, 443
Giardia lamblia
    in acute watery diarrhea, 389
    in gastroenteritis, 387, 388
    travel and, 389
    treatment of, 390
Giemsa stain, in eye infection, 1272
Gilles de la Tourette syndrome, 372
Gingivitis, acute necrotizing ulcerative, 382
Gingivostomatitis, in herpes infection, 381
Glanzmann's thrombasthenia, 366
Glasgow Coma Scale, 591, 592
Glaucoma, 1286–1289
    acute, 1288–1289
    chronic, presentation of, 1289
    classifications of, 1287–1288
    congenital, 1289
    defined, 1286
    differential diagnosis, 1288
    as headache cause, 917
    intraocular pressure readings, 1297
    open- vs. closed-angle, 1288
    pathogenesis of, 1286–1287
    primary, types of, 1287
    secondary
        in herpetic keratitis, 1265
        hyphema and, 1282, 1283, 1285, 1286
        types of, 1287–1288
        in uveitis, 1281–1282
GLC. *See* Gas-liquid chromatography
Glenohumeral joint
    aspiration or injection of, 1374, 1375
    dislocations, 199–200
Glomerulonephritis
    differential diagnosis, 1222
    rapidly progressing (RPGN), 1218
    treatment of, 1223
Glossopharyngeal nerve. *See* Cranial nerves
Glucagon, as medication, 1432
Glucocorticoids
    for asthma, in pregnancy, 1239
    for hypercalcemia, 316
    for pemphigus vulgaris, 437
    for thyroid storm, 250
Glucose administration
    in CPR, of pediatric patients, 523, 524
    for diarrhea, 389–390
    for hyperkalemia, 299
    for hypothermia, 671
    for thyroid storm, 250, 251
    in toxicologic emergencies, prehospital care, 469
Glucose levels. *See also* Hyperglycemia;
        Hypoglycemia
    diabetic ketoacidosis and, 236
    in hypernatremia, 267, 269
    hypokalemia and, 296
Glucose-insulin infusion, for hyperkalemia, 280, 281,
    299, 300
Glue sniffing, 805, 806
Glutethimide (Doriden), 1439. *See also*
        Sedative-hypnotics
    abstinence syndrome, 804

    combined with codeine, 801
    elimination half-life of, 800
    overdose of, 472, 492, 803
    for pain relief, 882
    pharmacology of, 801–802
Glycerol (Glycerin), 1430–1431
    for acute glaucoma, 1289
    hypokalemia and, 275–276
    for secondary glaucoma with uveitis, 1282
Glycol ethers, poisoning by, 774
Glycol solvents, listed, 756
Glycosuria, in hypothermia, 666
GM^1, for spinal injuries, 104
God, perceptions of, 864
Goltz's syndrome, 364
Gonococcal arthritis
    age and sex and, 351
    cutaneous lesions of, 336
    presentation of, 359
    septic, 357, 410, 411
Gonococcal dermatitis, 430
Gonococcal eye infection, culture media for, 1270
Gonococcal otitis externa, 1310
Gonococcal pharyngitis, treatment of, 378
Gonococcal proctitis, 466
Gonococcal tenosynovitis, 346
Gonococcal urethritis, 394, 395
Gonorrhea
    pelvic inflammatory disease and, 1233
    rape and, 1250
Gonorrheal epididymitis, 1212
Good Samaritan laws, 41
Goodpasture's syndrome, 1218
Gottron's patches, 336
Gout, 357–358
    age and sex and, 351
    Baker's cyst in, 346
    carpal tunnel syndrome and, 347
    differential diagnosis, 351
    hyperkalemia and, 279
    medications for, 1403–1405
    onset of, 351–352
    polyarticular arthritis with, 359
Government agencies. *See also* specific agencies
    in disaster linkages, 12, 33–34
    in hazardous materials response, 751
    in National Disaster Medical System, 37
    rural EMS services and, 23
Governor's Highway Safety Act (1966), 1, 8
Grace Brethren, beliefs and practices, 866–867
Gram stain
    in aseptic meningitis, 399
    in bacterial meningitis, 397
    in eye infections, 1272, 1273
        corneal ulcers, 1276
    in monoarticular arthritis, 355
    in pneumonia diagnosis, 385
    in septic arthritis, 356
Gram-negative organisms
    in bite wounds, 155, 156
    in corneal ulcers, 1274, 1275
    in encephalitis and brain abscess, 400
    in meningitis, 396
    in otitis media, 1309
    in pneumonia, 383, 384
    in prostatitis, 395
    in septic arthritis, 410, 411
    in urinary tract infections, 391
        prostatitis, 395
    in vertebral osteomyelitis, 193
Grand mal (tonic-clonic) seizures, 945, 948. *See also*
    Seizures
Granulocytopenia
    acute sepsis and, 406
    in cancer patients, 505–506
Granulomas, as diabetes insipidus cause, 267
Granulomatous disease
    adrenal insufficiency and, 257–258
    chronic (CGD), oxygen as drug and, 704
    colitis, in Hermansky-Pudlak syndrome, 365, 366
    cutaneous lesions with, 337

hypercalcemia and, 317
  temporal arteritis with, 337
  Wegener's granulomatosis, 337
Graves' disease, adrenal insufficiency and, 251
Gray platelet syndrome, 366
Grease gun injuries, 155
  to upper extremities, 212
Great vessel trauma, 1187–1188
  acute aortic dissection in, 1081–1082
  general principles, 1077
Greater trochanter, fractures of, 220–221
Greater trochanteric bursa, aspiration or injection of, 1374
Greek Orthodox Church, beliefs and practices, 865, 867
Greene body splint, cost of, 109
Greenfield filter, for pulmonary embolism, 1148
Greenstick fracture, in forearm, 205
Grief
  coping process and, 859–860
  uncomplicated bereavement, 831
Griseofulvin, for fungal infections of scalp or nails, 436
Grouper
  attacks by, 714–715
  poisoning by, 712
Growth hormone, in response to injury, 69
Grunting, in children, 575
Guanabenz (Wytensin), 1392–1393
Guanethidine, for Raynaud's phenomenon, 341
Guided imagery techniques, 874, 875
  for pain management, 887
Guidelines for Development and Operation of Burn Centers (ABA), 47
Guillain-Barré syndrome
  adrenal insufficiency and, 259
  hyponatremia and, 271
Gums
  abscess in, 1331–1333
  pemphigus vulgaris lesions on, 437
  ulcerations of, 1336–1337
    acute necrotizing ulcerative gingivitis, 382
Gunshot wounds. *See also* Penetrating injuries
  acute arteriovenous fistula, 1070
  to bladder, 1202
  to chest, 1181
    intra-abdominal wounds with, 1181–1182
  in children, 541
  evaluating for closure, 139
  to head, 899
  to heart, 1078–1079, 1185–1186
  to kidney, 1199
  to neck, 1074
  penetrating fractures, 163
  to rectum and colon, 465
  to spinal cord, steroids and, 104
  to ureters, 1201
  vascular, 1070
Gustilo-Anderson fracture classification, 166–167
"Gutter" splint, ulnar, 209
Gynecologic emergencies, 1229–1234
  abnormal vaginal bleeding, 1230–1231
  ectopic pregnancy, 1231–1233
  history taking in, 1229
  pelvic inflammatory disease (PID), 1233–1234
  pelvic pain, 1229–1230
Gynecologic procedure, culdocentesis, 1231, 1354
Gynecologic surgery, ureteral injury in, 1200
Gynergen. *See* Ergotamine tartrate

H

H2 receptor antagonist, for anaphylaxis, 86
HACE (high-altitude cerebral edema), 681, 684–685
Hagfish poisoning, 712, 736
Hair, as wound contamination source, 138
Hair follicles, infection of, 431
Halcion. *See* Triazolam
Haldol. *See* Haloperidol
Half-life of drugs, 482, 483
HALFD regimen, for shock, 82

Hallucinations
  in alcohol withdrawal, 821
  auditory, in psychiatric confusion, 955
  drug-induced, 474
  in hypomagnesemia, 304
Hallucinogenic drugs, 806–810
  screening tests for, 786
  sympathomimetics, 787, 799
  types of, 806–807. *See also specific types*
Hallucinosis, alcoholic, 821
Halo traction, 188, 191, 192
Halogen gases, as fire byproduct, 494
Halogenated hydrocarbons, listed, 756
Haloperidol (Haldol), 1407
  for acute confusion, psychiatric, 956
  for alcohol withdrawal, 821
  overdose of, 472, 474
  for PCP intoxication, 808
  reactions to, 474
  sedative withdrawal and, 804
  for systemic lupus erythematosus, 344
Haloprogin (Halotex), for fungal infections of skin, 436
HALT screening test for alcoholism, 822, 827
Hamartoma, in hereditary disorders, 365, 369, 371
Hand-foot-mouth disease, 381–382
Hand-Schüller-Christian disease, as diabetes insipidus cause, 267
Hands, 207–211. *See also* Extremities; Upper extremity injuries
  assessing, 207
    motor function, in vertebral column injury, 184
  burns on, as major injuries, 424
  clenched fist injury to, 156
  dislocations in, 208–209
  dressing and splinting wounds on, 157
  dysmorphology of, in hereditary disorders, 363, 364, 365
  erythema multiforme on, 434
  fractures, 207–208
  immobilization methods, 207, 208, 209, 210
  infections in, 210–211
    clenched fist injury, 156, 211
    cutaneous abscesses, 407, 408
    deep palmar space, 211
    paronychia, 210
    web space abscess, 210–211
  ligamentous injuries, 208–209
  in Raynaud's phenomenon, 341
  shoulder-hand syndrome, 347
  soft tissue injuries, 207
  soft tissue rheumatism in, 347
  suture material for, 143
  suture technique for, 143
  volar plate injuries, 209–210
Hanging cast, for humeral shaft fracture, 201
Hangman's fracture, 191, 907, 908
HAPE (high-altitude pulmonary edema), 681, 683–684
Harvard Community Health Plan, quality control system, 58
Hashimoto's (autoimmune) thyroiditis, 251, 255
Hashish, 808. *See also* Marijuana
HAV. *See* Hepatitis A virus
Hazardous materials, 747–759. *See also* Radiation emergencies; Toxicologic emergencies
  accident prevention with, 751
  decontamination procedures, 752–753
  defined, 747
  evacuation requirements, 751–752
  hospital care guidelines, 753–758
    for dermal injury, 753–754
    for pulmonary injury, 754–755
    for systemic toxins, 755–758
  regulations on, 748–750
  response system for, 750–752
    levels of response, 751
Hazardous materials response (HAZMAT) units, 750–751
Hazardous Materials Transportation Control Act of 1970, 748

HBV. *See* Hepatitis B virus
HCA. *See* Hospital Corporation of America
HCFA. *See* Health Care Financing Administration
HCQIA. *See* Health Care Quality Improvement Act of 1986
Head injuries, 891–901. *See also* Central nervous system injuries; Scalp wounds
  assessing, prehospital, 104–107
  basic vs. advanced life support skills, 94
  causes of, 891
  cervical spine injuries and, 911
  in children, 542, 543–544
    acute management of, 550
    child abuse and, 542, 600–601
    CT scans of, 549
    minor, 552
    unconsciousness with, 589–590
  complications of, 901
  laboratory studies, 896–897
  management of, prehospital, 107–108
  MAST suit use and, 77
  maxillofacial injuries and, 1321
  in multisystem trauma, 896
  neurologic examination in, 894–896
  open, prehospital management, 107
  outcome prediction with, 900–901
  pathophysiology of, 893–894
  patient transport with, 187
  penetrating, 107
  prehospital care, 104–107, 891–892
  purulent meningitis with, 398
  radiologic tests with, 897
  sequelae to, 104
  treatment of, 897–898, 900
  types of, 104
    closed injuries, 899–900
    penetrating or projectile, 899
    scalp and skull, 898–899
    with unconsciousness, 589–590
  wound management, local anesthesia in, 140
Head lice, 437
Head-tilt methods, for CPR, 1084, 1085
Headache, 915–925
  in acute mountain sickness (AMS), 681
  in brain abscess, 400
  in cerebrovascular accident, 940, 941
  cluster, 916
  emergency room problems, 915, 920, 921
  in encephalitis, 400
  etiologies of
    primary (vascular and tension) disorders, 915–916
    secondary (systemic) disorders, 916–921
  evaluation of, 921–922
    warning factors, 921
  facial pain vs., 920
  factitious, 920
  in hypertensive encephalopathy, 1065
  as hyponatremia sign, 271
  in intracerebral hemorrhage, 941
  intracranial pressure and, 502
  in Lyme disease, 357
  in meningitis
    aseptic, 399
    purulent, 397
  migraine. *See* Migraine
  patient education on, 924–925
  in pregnancy, 923
    pre-eclampsia, 1238
  prophylactic therapy for, 923–924
  psychogenic, 920–921
  rebound, 922, 923
  referrals for, 921
  in rheumatoid arthritis, 343
  in subarachnoid hemorrhage, 940, 941
  in temporal arteritis, 338
  treatments for, 922–924
Healing, nonmedical methods of, 869–870
Health Care Financing Administration (HCFA)
  in PRO review process, 58–59, 60
  quality criteria and, 54, 58

Health Care Quality Improvement Act (HCQIA) of 1986, 54
  implications of, 56–57
  National Practitioner Data Bank and, 56
  physician vs. hospital liability and, 61
  PROs and, 58
Health care workers. *See also* Personnel; Staffpower and training
  communication techniques for, 871–872
    neurolinguistic programming (NLP), 872–875
    right-brain communication, 872, 874–875
  emotional support for
    in death of patient, 861–862
    in disaster, 34
  hepatitis B in, 785
  therapeutic use of self by, 871
Health departments, as first responders, 22
Health maintenance organizations (HMOs), quality review systems in, 58
Health Resources Administration, EMS grants by, 2
Health Services Mental Health Administration, EMS grants by, 2
Hearing test, 1307
Heart injuries and disorders. *See* Cardiac emergencies
Heart failure. *See* Congestive heart failure
Heart rate
  bradydysrhythmias, 1008–1017
  cardiac function and, 1052
  in shock diagnosis, 67
  sudden sinus (atrial standstill), 1010–1012
Heart size, adrenal insufficiency and, 259
Heartburn, 452
Heat applications
  for otitis externa, 1311
  for pain relief, 888
  for sinusitis, 1303
Heat illnesses. *See also* Hyperthermia
  dehydration and, 267
  heat cramps, 655–656
  heat edema, 655
  heat exhaustion, 656
  heat stroke, 656–659
    as cause of death, 653
    complications of, 659
    diagnosis of, 656–657
    hypokalemia and, 276
    pathophysiology of, 656
    treatment of, 657–659
  heat syncope, 655
  hyponatremia and, 270
  physiology and, 654
  predicting, 653–654
  risk factors for, 655
Heat injuries, pharyngitis and, 377
Heat loss, types of, 661. *See also* Cold injury; Hypothermia
Heat/cold stimulation, for pain relief, 888
Heavy metal poisoning. *See* Metal poisoning
Heimlich maneuver
  in children, 515–516
  in CPR procedure, 1085
  for near-drowning, 695
  for tracheobronchial foreign body, 1308
Heimlich valve, in tension pneumothorax intervention, 100
Helicopter EMS systems, 23–26
  database system for, 12, 13–14
  interhospital transport by, 9
Helminths, intestinal
  biliary tract disease vs., 455
  gastroenteritis and, 387
Hemangiomas, in hereditary disorders, 364, 365
Hemangiopericytoma, hypokalemia and, 277
Hematinic agents, 1447
Hematocrit, dropping
  in adrenal hemorrhage, 256
  in shock, 70
Hematologic disorders, renal failure and, 1226
Hematologic emergencies, in cancer patients, 509–510
Hematologic response
  to high altitude, 680–681
  to hypothermia, 666
  in near-drowning, 693
Hematoma, Baker's cyst vs., 346
Hematuria
  in bladder injuries, 1202
  renal calculi and, 1210
  renal failure and, 1222, 1223
  in renal injuries, 1195–1196
  in ureteral injuries, 1200
  urinary retention and, 1214
Hemiplegia, in systemic lupus erythematosus, 344
Hemisuccinate, for adrenal insufficiency, 260
Hemochromatosis, idiopathic, 366
Hemocytometer, in urine examination, 392
Hemodialysis
  for hypercalcemic crisis, 315
  for hyperkalemia, 280–281, 299, 300
  for hypermagnesemia, 308
  for renal failure, 1226–1227
  for sedative-hypnotic overdose, 804
  in toxicologic emergencies, 476, 488, 757
Hemodynamics
  in acute myocardial infarction management, 991–992
  cardiogenic shock mortality and, 74
  dysrhythmia and, 997–998
  factors supporting, 66–67
  sedative overdose and, 803
Hemoglobin, stroma-free
  as blood substitute, 81
  for shock, 80
Hemolysis, burns and, 418
Hemolytic anemia, burns and, 418
Hemolytic streptococci, from dog bites, 155
Hemoperfusion, for drug overdose, 476–477, 486
Hemophilia, 366
  mononucleosis syndrome and, 402
Hemophilus influenzae
  in bacterial tracheitis, 569, 1116, 1117
  in cellulitis in children, 432
  in epiglottitis (supraglottitis), 566–567, 1117, 1118, 1122, 1123
  in eye infection, culture media for, 1270
  in febrile children under two, 530, 531, 532
  in meningitis, 396, 398, 399
  in occult bacteremia (OB), in children under two, 530, 531, 532
  in otitis media, 380, 381, 1309
  in pharyngitis, 376
  in pneumonia, 383, 384, 386
    in children, 585, 586
  in septic arthritis, 357, 410, 412
  in sinusitis, 378, 379, 1302, 1303
Hemopneumothorax, 102
Hemoptysis, 1167–1169
  evaluation of, 1167–1168
  management of, 1168–1169
  nontraumatic causes of, 1167
Hemorrhage
  acute
    blood component therapy and, 125
    hypovolemic shock with, 70
  adrenal insufficiency an, 256–257
  in cancer patients, 509–510
  of closed wound, 141
  controlling
    MAST suit in, 77
    PASG in, 5
    in shock response, 76
  gastrointestinal, in pediatric patients, 558–559
Hemorrhagic CVAs. *See* Cerebrovascular accident
Hemorrhagic fevers, as sepsis cause, 406
Hemorrhagic shock. *See* Hypovolemic shock
Hemorrhoids, 465–466
Hemostasis
  with multisystem injuries, 101–102
  in wound management, 141
Hemotherapy. *See* Blood transfusions
Hemothorax, 1184
  emergency autotranfusion from, 132, 133
Hemotympanum, assessing for, 107, 110

Heparin sodium (Heparin), 1401
  adrenal hemorrhage and, 256–257
  for air embolism, 1170
  for frostbite, 673
  hyperkalemia and, 279
  for pulmonary embolism, 1148
Hepatic encephalopathy, 459
Hepatic failure, acute, 458–459
Hepatic insufficiency, respiratory alkalosis and, 330
Hepatitis, 457–458
  diagnosis of, 403–404, 457–458
  etiologies of, 457
  rape and, 1250
  shellfish ingestion and, 733
  treatment of, 458
  viral, 403–405, 457, 458
    aseptic meningitis and, 399
Hepatitis A virus, 403, 404, 405, 457
  diagnosis of, 404
  prevention of, 404
  shellfish and, 733
Hepatitis B virus, 403, 404, 405, 457
  diagnosis of, 404
  drug abuse and, 785
  in health care workers, 785
  polyarthralgias with, 359
  prevention of, 404
  shellfish and, 733
Hepatitis C virus, 403
  diagnosis of, 404
Hepatitis E virus, 403
  diagnosis of, 404
"Herald patch," in pityriasis rosea, 438
Hereditary disorders, 361–373
  adrenal insufficiency, 258
  basic genetics and, 361–363, 371, 373
  clinical genetics and, 363–373
  diagnosis of, 361
  epistaxis in, 1304
  hypoparathyroidism, hypocalcemia and, 284
  pseudohyperkalemia, 279
  pseudohypoparathyroidism, hypocalcemia and, 284
  recessive, ethnic groups and, 372, 373
  as urticaria cause, 440
Hermansky-Pudlak syndrome, 365, 366
Hernia
  inguinal, in infants, 557, 559
  inguinoscrotal, in infants, 559
  intestinal obstruction and, 460
  in infants, 557
Heroin
  abstinence syndromes, 798–799
  complications of, 786, 796–797
  extent of abuse, 782
  as opioid, 793
  overdose of
    clinical signs, 472, 796–797
    differential diagnosis, 797
    treatment of, 796, 797–798
  pharmacology of, 794
Herpangina, 381
Herpes simplex
  AIDS and, 444
  as aseptic meningitis cause, 399
  as cause of death, 442
  encephalitis and, 400
  esophageal obstruction and, 452
  felon vs., 210
  herpetic whitlow, 408
  oral lesions in, 381, 1336
  in pharyngitis, 376, 377
  in pregnancy, 1239
  rectal, 466
  skin lesions in, 441–442
  in urethritis in men, 394
Herpes simplex encephalitis
  diagnosis of, 400
  meningitis vs., treatment and, 398
  treatment of, 401
Herpes zoster, 442
  AIDS and, 444

chest wall syndrome vs., 348
  of oral cavity, 1336
Herpesvirus, in dysenteric gastroenteritis, 390
Herpetic ocular disease, 1264–1266
Herpetic whitlow, 408
Hetastarch; Hydroxyethyl starch (Volex; Hespan; HES), 1444–1445
  in fluid resuscitation, 127
  for shock, 80
Hexachlorophene, in burn cleansing, 424
Hexane inhalation, 806
HHNK. See Hyperosmolar hyperglycemic nonketotic coma
Hiccups, 454
Hidradenitis suppurativa, 431
High altitude
  chronic mountain sickness (CMS) at, 685
  maladaptation syndromes, 681–686
    acute mountain sickness (AMS), 680, 681–683
    high-altitude cerebral edema (HACE), 681, 684–685
    high-altitude pulmonary edema (HAPE), 681, 683–684, 1101
  periodic breathing in sleep at, 684
  physiologic effects of, 680–681
  physiology and, 679–681
  retinal hemorrhage and, 684–685
  underlying medical conditions and, 685
High-pressure liquid chromatography (HPLC), in drug and toxin screening, 471
Highway safety, EMS legislation, 1–2
Hindus, beliefs and practices, 865, 867
Hip
  acetabular fractures, 215–217
  arthrocentesis of, 354
  aspiration or injection of, 1374, 1375
  dislocations, 173, 217
    acetabular fractures and, 215, 216
    femoral head fractures and, 217–218
  fractures
    in children, 221
    classification of, 218–219
    femoral head, 217–218
    femoral neck, 218, 219
    femoral shaft, 219, 220
    intertrochanteric, 218, 219–220
    intracapsular, 218
    statistics on, 218
    subtrochanteric, 220
    trochanteric, 220–221
  multisystem injuries and, 218–219
Hirschprung's disease, 283
Histamine
  anaphylaxis and, 75
  hypovolemic shock and, 71
Histamine receptor antagonists, for upper GI bleeding, 449
Histoplasma capsulatum, in pneumonia, 383, 384
Histoplasmosis
  adrenal insufficiency and, 258
  diagnosis of, 385
History taking
  in acute monoarticular arthritis, 351–352
  adrenal insufficiency and, 255, 256, 260
  alcohol and, 816–817, 818, 822, 827–828
  in biliary tract disease, 453
  for cancer patients, 501–502
  in cerebrovascular accident, 936, 940
  child abuse and, 601, 602, 605
  confusional states and, 951–952
  in congestive heart failure, 1054
  domestic violence and, 839, 840, 841, 848
    assessment and treatment report, 849–851
    in battering syndrome, 842
    questioning techniques, 848, 851–852
    emotional/spiritual support with, 870–872
  encephalitis and, 401
  in epistaxis, 1305
  with head injuries, 892
  head and neck injuries, in multisystem trauma, 107
  in headache, 921

  in hemoptysis evaluation, 1167
  in hereditary disease, 361
  hypokalemia diagnosis and, 296
  in infectious disease, 375, 385
  in maxillofacial injury, 1322
  in multisystem trauma, head and neck injuries, 107
  for OB/GYN patients, 1229
  in obstructive airway disease, 1130–1131
  on pain, 879
  in pneumonia, 385
  in rape case, 1246, 1247
  in seizures, 946, 948, 950
  sexual abuse and, 605–606
  spiritual needs and, 864
  in status epilepticus, 946
  for stridor in infant, 570
  in subarachnoid hemorrhage, 940
  in substance abuse emergencies, 786
  in syncope, 962
  in toxicologic emergencies, 469–470, 471
    occupational, 762, 763
  in upper extremity evaluation, 195
  in upper GI bleeding, 449
  in wound evaluation, 137, 138
HIV. See Human immunodeficiency virus
Hives. See Urticaria
HMOs. See Health maintenance organizations
"Hog." See PCP
Holistic health care model, 857–858
Holt-Oram syndrome, 363, 364, 365
Homatropine, for uveitis, 1281, 1282
Homicide
  in child abuse cases, 601, 603
  domestic violence factors, 838
Homocystinuria, 364, 365
Homosexual patients
  dysenteric gastroenteritis in, 390
  gonococcal proctitis in, 466
  mononucleosis syndrome and, 402
Honeybee stings, 643–644
Horizontal categorization of EMS facilities, 18
Horizontal classification of emergency departments, 45–46
Hormones and substitutes, for emergency department, 1453
Horner's syndrome, with cluster headache, 916
Hornet stings, 643–644
  anaphylaxis risk and, 75
Hospital Corporation of America (HCA), quality management system, 57–58
Hospital-to-ambulance communications, 7–8
Hospital-to-hospital communication, 8
Hospital-to-hospital transfer, 9–10
Hospitals. See also Burn centers; Trauma centers
  air transport services by, 23–24
  categorization of, 45
    as regionalization method, 49–50
  in disaster management, 12, 33, 34, 36
  emergency departments (EDs), 45–50
    categorization of, 45, 49–50
    classification of, 45–49
    designation, 45, 50
    number of visits to, 45, 46
    regionalization and, 49
  as EMS system component, 16, 18–19
    categorization of, 18
  interhospital transport, 9–10
    antidumping statute, 42–43
    indigence issues, 7, 42
  liability of physicians vs., 61
  pediatric care and, 551
  quality of care in, 53–62
  radiation emergency preparedness in, 618–619, 758–759
  record keeping guidelines, 8, 11–12, 13–14
  regionalization of care in, 49
Hot weather. See Heat illnesses
HPLC. See High-pressure liquid chromatography
Human bites, 156, 157–158, 632–634
Human epidermal cells, for burns, 426
Human immunodeficiency virus (HIV)

  AIDS and, 444
  biliary tract disease and, 455
  management of, 402–403
  pneumonia and, 384
  mononucleosis and, 402
  testing for
    with aseptic meningitis, 399
    in rape case, 1250–1251
    with urethritis, 395
  thrush and, 377, 378
Humerus
  acute osteomyelitis in, 358
  fractures of, 201–202, 203
Humidity, heat stress and, 654
Hybridomas, monoclonal antibodies and, 492, 493
Hydantoins, hypothermia and, 671
Hydralazine
  for congestive heart failure, 1055, 1056
  for hypertensive emergencies, 1062–1063
    eclampsia, 1066
  in renal failure treatment, 1225
Hydration, 265–266. See also Fluid management; Fluid replacement
Hydrocarbon aspiration, in children, 584
Hydrocarbon solvents, 756–757
  inhalation abuse with, 805, 806
  listed, 756
  skin or ocular decontamination, 474
  as systemic toxins, 774
Hydroceles, in children, 559–560
Hydrochlorothiazide (HydroDIURIL), 1431
  for hyperkalemia, 281
  as hypokalemia cause, 294
Hydrocortisone (Solu-Cortef), 1429
  for adrenal insufficiency, 260
  for myxedema coma, 252
  for thyroid storm, 250, 251
Hydrocortisone suppositories, for hemorrhoids, 466
HydroDIURIL. See Hydrochlorothiazide
Hydrofluoric acid injury, 754
Hydrogen chloride, as fire byproduct, 494
Hydrogen cyanide, as fire byproduct, 494. See also Cyanide poisoning
Hydrogen ion concentration, 319–320
  pH calculation vs., 320
Hydrogen sulfide poisoning, 755–756, 768–769, 1161
Hydroids, stings by, 717–718
Hydromorphone (Dilaudid)
  for cardiogenic shock, 85
  as opioid, 793
  for pain relief, 882
Hydronephrosis, intermittent, 1211
Hydrosalpinx, 1233, 1234
Hydroxyamphetamine (Paredrine), for uveitis, 1281
Hydroxyapatite synovitis, chronic (Milwaukee shoulder), 351
1,25-Hydroxycalciferol (Calcitriol), for hypocalcemia, 285
Hydroxychloroquine, retinopathy from, 339
Hydroxycobalamin, for cyanide poisoning, 755
Hydroxyethyl starch. See Hetastarch
Hydroxyzine (Atarax; Vistaril), 1409
  for drug eruption, 434
  for urticaria, 441
Hymenoptera bites or stings, 643–644
  anaphylaxis risk and, 75, 87
  prevention program and, 644
Hyoscine (Scopolamine)
  behavioral disorders and, 474
  for uveitis, 1281
Hyperaldosteronism (Conn's syndrome), 276
Hyperalimentation
  hypomagnesia and, 286, 306
  of infants, metabolic acidosis risk with, 322
Hyperbaric oxygenation (HBO) therapy, 701–710
  for air embolism, 708, 709, 1170
  for anaerobic infections, 705
  for carbon monoxide poisoning, 704–705, 756, 767
  complications of, 704
  for cyanide poisoning, 755

Hyperbaric oxygenation (HBO) therapy (contd.)
  for decompression sickness, 705–707
  increased used of, 701
  monoplace facilities, 701, 702
  multiplace facilities, 701–702, 703
  pathophysiology and, 702–704
  portable chamber for, for high-altitude illness, 682–683
  principles of, 702–704
  referral sources, 707, 709, 1161
Hypercalcemia, 281–284, 311–318
  acute confusion with, 953
  in adrenal insufficiency, 259, 260
  anion gap and, 327
  in cancer patients, 506–507
  clinical signs of, 283
  as diabetes insipidus cause, 268
  diagnosis of, 283, 318
    hypercalcemic crisis, 311–313
  etiologies of, 281–283, 313, 317–318
  metabolic alkalosis and, 328
  renal failure and, 1224
  treatment of, 283–284, 314–317
Hypercapnia
  chronic, metabolic alkalosis and, 328
  in respiratory failure, 1155, 1156
Hypercarbia, as headache cause, 917
Hypercube Queuing Model, for deployment, 16
Hypergastrinemia, in hereditary disorder, 370
Hyperglycemia
  acute confusion with, 953
  dehydration treatment and, 270
  in diabetic ketoacidosis, 233–234, 235–236
  in HHNK, 242, 243, 244, 245
  hyperkalemia and, 298
  hyponatremia and, 272
Hyperkalemia, 279–281, 297–300
  in adrenal insufficiency, 259, 260
    in neonate, 258
  as cause of death, 297
  clinical signs of, 280, 299
  diagnosis of, 280, 297–298
  etiologies of, 279, 297–298
  in neonate, adrenal insufficiency and, 258
  nursing care for, 281
  physiology/pathophysiology and, 272–275
  as potassium chloride risk, 296–297
  prehospital care, 281
  renal failure and, 1221, 1225
  treatment of, 280–281, 299–300
Hyperlipemia, hyponatremia and, 272
Hyperlipidemia, as CVA risk factor, 935
Hypermagnesemia, 287–288, 308
  clinical signs of, 287, 308
  diagnosis of, 287
  etiologies of, 287, 308
  treatment of, 287–288, 308
Hypernatremia
  acute confusion with, 953
  anion gap and, 327
  clinical signs of, 268
  diagnosis of, 268–269
  etiologies of, 267–268
  fluid deficit and, 266–270
  in infants and children, unconsciousness with, 590
  pathophysiology of, 266–267
  treatment of, 269–270
Hyperosmolar diuresis, hyperkalemia and, 279
Hyperosmolar hyperglycemic nonketotic coma (HHNK), 242–245
Hyperosmolarity (hypertonicity)
  diagnosis of, 268–269
  hypernatremia and, 267
Hyperosmotic agents
  for acute glaucoma, 1289
  for secondary glaucoma, with uveitis, 1282
Hyperparathyroidism
  in hereditary disorder, 370
  hypercalcemia and, 282, 317–318
  hyperkalemia and, 279
Hyperpepsinogen disorders, hereditary, 369, 370

Hyperphosphatemia, in renal failure, 1224–1225
Hyperpigmentation, adrenal insufficiency and, 258
Hyperproteinemia
  in cancer patient, hypercalcemia and, 313
  hyponatremia and, 272
Hyperpyrexia, acute confusion with, 954
Hyperreflexia
  autonomic, 912–913
  in hypomagnesemia, 287
  in toxicologic emergencies, 472
Hyperreninemia, hypokalemia and, 277
Hyperstat. See Diazoxide
Hypersuggestion, communication and, 873–874
Hypertension. See also Hypertensive emergencies
  burns and, 419
  as CVA risk factor, 935
  esophageal varices and, 452–453
  as headache cause, 917
  medications for, 1391–1397
  ocular. See Glaucoma
  portal, in hereditary disorders, 366
  pregnancy-induced, 1238–1239. See also Pre-eclampsia
    high altitude and, 685
  in renal failure, treatment of, 1225
  in sympathomimetic overdose, 792
Hypertensive emergencies, 1059–1067. See also Hypertension
  accelerated and malignant hypertension, 1064–1065
    defined, 1059, 1064, 1065
    hypokalemia and, 277
    in systemic lupus erythematosus, 341
  acute aortic dissection, 1066
  acute left ventricular failure (acute cardiac ischemia), 1066
  acute myocardial infarction and, 993–994
  catecholamine-induced hypertension, 1066–1067
  defined, 1059
  diagnosis of, 1060
  eclampsia, 1066, 1238
  etiologies of, 1059–1060
  hypertensive encephalopathy, 1065
  intracranial hemorrhage, 1065–1066
  listed, 1059
  pathophysiology of, 1060
  prehospital care, 1064
  terminology, 1059
  treatment of, 1059, 1060–1064
Hypertensive urgency, defined, 1059
Hyperthermia, 653–659. See also Fever; Heat illnesses
  as cardiogenic shock cause, 74
  cervical cord injuries and, 912
  differential diagnosis, 657
  risk factors for, 655
  in toxicologic emergencies, 473
Hyperthyroidism
  heat illness and, 655
  hypercalcemia and, 282
  hypomagnesemia and, 286
  medication for, 1445
  thyroid storm, 249–251
Hypertonia in children, as dehydration sign, 268
Hypertonic albumin-containing fluid demand (HALFD) regimen, in shock treatment, 82
Hypertonic solutions
  hyperkalemia and, 279
  for shock, 80, 92
Hypertonicity, in toxicologic emergencies, 472
Hyperventilation
  alveolar, in hypovolemic shock, 71
  as head injury treatment, 897
  in hypovolemic shock, 71
  in metabolic acidosis, 320–321
  respiratory alkalosis caused by, 330
  underwater swimming and, 690
Hyphema, 1282–1286, 1327
Hypnosis
  legal issues, 873
  as nonmedical healing method, 870, 873–874
  for pain management, 887
Hypoadrenalism. See Adrenal insufficiency
Hypoaldosteronism, hyperkalemia and, 279, 298, 300

Hypocalcemia, 284–285
  clinical signs of, 284–285
  etiologies of, 284
  treatment of, 285
Hypocalcemic tetany, 281
  in children, 566
Hypocapnia
  chronic, anion gap elevation in, 327
  hypovolemic shock and, 71
  metabolic acidosis and, 322
Hypoglossal nerve. See Cranial nerves
Hypoglycemia
  acute confusion with, 953
  in adrenal insufficiency, 259, 260
  alcohol-induced, 824–825
  in children, unconsciousness with, 590
  in infants
    resuscitation and, 526
    unconsciousness with, 590
  as insulin therapy complication, 241
  in myxedema coma, 252
  in neonates, adrenal insufficiency and, 258
Hypoglycemics/antihypoglycemics, 1432–1433
Hypogonadism, adrenal insufficiency and, 255
Hypokalemia, 275–278, 293–297
  clinical signs of, 277, 295–296
  as diabetes insipidus cause, 268
  diagnosis of, 277–278, 296
  etiologies of, 275–277, 293–295
  metabolic alkalosis and, 327, 328
  physiology/pathophysiology and, 272–275
  treatment of, 278, 296–297
    in hypercalcemic crisis, 314–315
Hypomagnesemia, 286–287, 304–307
  clinical signs of, 286–287, 304–305
  diagnosis of, 287
  etiologies of, 286, 305–307
  hypocalcemia and, 284
  hypokalemia and, 294, 297
  treatment of, 287, 307
    in hypercalcemic crisis, 314, 315
Hyponatremia, 270–272
  acute confusion with, 953
  in adrenal insufficiency, 259, 260
  in cancer patients, 507
  in children, unconsciousness with, 590
  diabetic ketoacidosis vs., 235–236
  diagnosis of, 271–272
  hyperkalemia and, 299
  in infants and children, unconsciousness with, 590
  in neonates, adrenal insufficiency and, 258
  treatment of, 272
Hypoparathyroidism
  adrenal insufficiency and, 255
  idiopathic, hypocalcemia and, 284
  metabolic alkalosis and, 328
Hypoperfusion, in shock, 65
Hypopituitarism
  adrenal insufficiency and, 258
  hyperkalemia and, 279
  hyponatremia and, 270
Hypoplastic anemia, hereditary, 365
Hyporeninemic hypoaldosteronism, hyperkalemia and, 279, 298, 300
Hypotension. See also Shock
  in acute myocardial infarction, 992–993
  in adrenal insufficiency, 258–259
  in anaphylaxis, 75
    treatment of, 86–87
  in hypermagnesemia, 308
  interpreting, for shock, 66–67
  in myxedema coma, 252
  orthostatic
    cervical cord injuries and, 912
    as hypovolemia, 70
  postural, heat syncope, 655
  in shock, 68, 74
    cardiogenic, 74–75
    septic, 72
  in thyroid storm, 250
  in toxic shock syndrome, 432
  in toxicologic emergencies, 472

treatment of, MAST suit in, 76–78
upper GI bleeding with, 448
Hypothalamus, lesions in, dehydration risk with, 267
Hypothermia, 661–673, 668–671
  accidental
    acute, 661–662
    gradual (urban or domestic), 661, 662
    subacute, 661, 662
  accidental, 661–662
  acute confusion with, 953–954
  blood gases in, 663–664
  as burn treatment risk, 423, 672
  as cardiogenic shock cause, 74
  cervical cord injuries and, 912
  drowning accidents and, 690, 694
  evaluation of, 667–668
  localized cold injuries, 672–673
  in myxedema coma, 252
  neonatal, 661–662
  in pediatric patients
    acute, 661
    CPR and, 525–526
    resuscitation and, 525–526
  physiologic changes with, 662–667
  prehospital care, 667
  risk factors for, 662
  symptoms of, 663
  in toxicologic emergencies, 473
  treatment of, 672
    cessation indications, 672
    medications for, 671–672
    protocol for, 667
    rewarming methods, 668–671
Hypothyroidism
  adrenal insufficiency and, 260
  hypercalcemia and, 317
  hyponatremia and, 271, 272
  medication for, 1445
  myxedema coma, 251–252
Hypotonia, in hypercalcemia, 311, 312
Hypoventilation, in myxedema coma, 252
Hypovolemia
  ADH secretion and, 266
  in children, 543–544
    resuscitation and, 526
  as dehydration sign, 268
  in hypercalcemic crisis, 314, 315
  hypernatremia and, 270–271
  in hyperosmolar hyperglycemic nonketotic coma, 243
  metabolic alkalosis and, 327
  orthostatic syncope and, 961
  treatment of, metabolic acidosis risk with, 322
Hypovolemic shock, 67–72
  blood component therapy for, 125
  burns and, 418
  as cause of death, 125
  cellular metabolism in, 70–71
  in children, 544
  clinical features of, 68
  extracellular fluid in, 67–68, 70
  in infants, with diarrhea, 558
  in multisystem injuries, prehospital care, 101–103
  resuscitation fluids for, 125–130
  staging of, 101
  upper GI bleeding with, 448
  vasoactive substances and, 71
Hypoxemia
  acute myocardial infarction and, 994
  in near-drowning, 690–691
  respiratory alkalosis and, 330
  in shock, 70, 71
Hypoxia
  acute confusion with, 953
  hypobaric, in altitude illness, 679–680
  in near-drowning, 691
  in respiratory failure, 1155–1156
  in shock, 65
  in systemic lupus erythematosus, 340
  tissue
    pathophysiology of, 331
    respiratory alkalosis and, 330

I

Iatrogenic disorders. *See also* Nosocomial infections
  antimalarial retinopathy, 339
  epistaxis and, 1306
  hypermagnesemia, in toxemia of pregnancy, 308
Iatrogenic injuries
  to bladder, 1202
  to ureters, 1200, 1201
  to urethra, 1205, 1207
Ibuprofen (Motrin), 1404
  as aseptic meningitis cause, 344
  for pain relief, 881
"Ice." *See* Amphetamine
Ice, as burn treatment, precautions, 423
Ichthyosarcotoxism, 736–739
Ichthyosis, adrenal insufficiency and, 258
ICP. *See* Intracranial pressure
ICS (incident command system), 15
ICU. *See* Intensive care unit
Idiopathic infantile hypercalcemia, 283, 317
Idoxuridine (Stoxil), for herpetic keratitis, 1264
Ig preparations, in hepatitis prevention, 404, 405
Ileocolic intussusception, 556, 557
Iletin. *See* Insulin therapy
Ileus
  acute adynamic, burns and, 419
  adynamic, 460–461
  in myxedema coma, 252
  paralytic, 459–460
Illicit drugs, defined, 782
Illinois, hospital liability law in, 61
Ilosone. *See* Erythromycin
Imferon. *See* Iron dextran
Imipenem, for marine organism injuries, 731, 732
Imipenem-cilastatin (Primaxin), 1421
Imipramine (Tofranil)
  for headache, 924
  overdose of, 485
Immobilization. *See also* Casts; *specific injuries*
  hypercalcemia and, 282, 311, 315, 317
  in wound management, 157
Immunities, statutory, 41
  hospital vs. physician responsibility and, 61
Immunoassay
  in drug abuse emergencies, 786
  in toxicologic emergencies, 471
Immunocompromised patients
  acute monoarticular arthritis in, 352, 357, 358
  acute watery diarrhea and, 389
  anorectal abscesses in, 466
  Cryptosporidium and, 389
  encephalitis in, 400
  headache management for, 919
  herpes simplex and, 381
  herpes zoster in, 442
  marine organism injuries and, 731
  meningitis in, 396, 398
  otitis media in, 381
  pneumonia in, 384
  seizures in, 948
  septic arthritis in, 352, 357
  shock risk in, 72
  sinusitis in, 378
  thrush in, 377
Immunosuppressive agents, HHNK and, 244
Impedance plethysmography (IPG), in deep venous thrombosis, 1147–1148
Impetigo, 431
Impingement syndrome (subacromial bursitis), 201
Implied consent, 41–42
Impotence, in cauda equina syndrome, 193
Incest. *See* Sexual abuse
Incident command system (ICS), 15
Inderal. *See* Propranolol
Indigent patients, transfer issues, 7
Indomethacin (Indocin), 1404
  as aseptic meningitis cause, 344
  for ciguatera fish poisoning, 738
  for gout/pseudogout, 357–358
  for hypercalcemia, 283, 316

for hypokalemia, with Bartter's syndrome, 278, 294
  for pain relief, 881
Indoprofen (Flosint), for pain relief, 881
Industrial accidents. *See* Occupational injuries
Industrial exposure, pharyngitis and, 377
Indwelling catheters, septic shock risk and, 72
Infants. *See also* Neonates; Pediatric patients; Premature infants
  abdominal pain in, 556–557
  abuse of. *See* Child abuse
  acute watery diarrhea in, 389
  airway obstruction in, 563
  burns and, 553, 554
  colic in, 556–557
  congenital glaucoma in, 1289
  constipation in, 558
  CPR of, 1088
    drugs in, 521, 522
    hypoglycemia and, 526
    hypothermia and, 525–526
  croup in, 1113–1116
    acute epiglottitis, 1118
  dehydration risk in, 267
  dehydration signs in, 268
  diarrhea in, 558
  fever in, 529–539
    evaluation of, under 3 months, 533–535
    occult bacteremia (OB), 529–533
    stridor with, 566
  foreign body aspiration by, 583–584
  hepatitis B prevention in, 404–405
  hereditary disorders in, 372
  hernias and hydroceles in, 559–560
  idiopathic hypercalcemia in, 283, 317
  ileocolic intussusception in, 556, 557
  impetigo on, 431
  meningitis in, 397, 398
  metabolic emergencies in, 590–591
  neurologic emergencies in, 589–596
  ocular trauma in (hyphema), 1285
  oliguria in, documenting, 268
  pneumonia in, 585–586
  renal thrombosis in, 1211
  respiratory emergencies in. *See* Respiratory emergencies; *specific conditions*
  roseola infantum in, 438
  scrotum problems in, 559
  septic arthritis in, 411
  shaken baby syndrome in, 589, 600–601
  sodium excess in, from cow's milk, 267
  spasmodic croup (SC) in, 565
  stridor in, causes of, 570
  thrush in, 436–437
  unconscious
    etiologies and, 589–591
    management of, 591–592
  vomiting in, 557–558
Infection. *See also* Infectious diseases; Sepsis; *specific diseases*
  as diabetic ketoacidosis risk, 238
  from dog bites, 155
  in hands, 210–211
  as presenting complaint, 375
  septic shock and, 72
  in systemic lupus erythematosus, 335
  thyroid storm and, 249
  as transfusion complication, 133, 134
  of wounds
    antibiotic prophylaxis and, 157–158
    evaluating for, 138
Infectious diseases, 375–412
  as IV drug use risk, 784–785
  as acute confusional state cause, 953
  in cancer patients, 505–506
  of central nervous system, 396–403
    aseptic meningitis, 399–400
    encephalitis and brain abscess, 400–401
    infectious mononucleosis syndrome, 401–403
    purulent meningitis, 393–399
  drug abuse and, 785
  emergency departments and, 375
  esophageal obstruction and, 452

Infectious diseases (contd.)
  gastrointestinal, 387–391
    acute gastroenteritis, 387–389
    acute watery diarrhea, 389–390
    dysenteric gastroenteritis, 390
    food poisoning, 390–391
  as headache cause, 919
  history taking and, 375
  marine-associated, 408–409, 742
  oral-facial, 381–383
  oxygen under high pressure (OHP) for, 704
  in pediatric patients, fever evaluation, 529–559
  of respiratory tract, 375–387
    common cold, 375–376
    otitis, 379–381
    pharyngitis, 376–378
    pneumonia, 382–387
    sinusitis, 378–379
  sepsis as presentation of, 406–407
  of skin and soft tissue, 407–412
    cutaneous abscesses, 407–408
    herpetic whitlow, 408
    necrotizing fasciitis and myositis, 409–410
    occupational skin infections, 408–409
    septic arthritis, 410–412
    septic bursitis, 412
  upper GI bleeding with, 449
  of urinary tract, 391–396
    diagnosis of, 391–392
    differential diagnosis, 392
    in females, 391
    in males, 391, 394–396
    pathophysiology, 391
    treatment of, 392–394
Inferior vena cava (IVC) intraluminal devices, for pulmonary embolism, 1141, 1148–1149
Inflammatory bowel disease
  acute monoarticular arthritis with, 358
  noninfectious, 461–463
    Crohn's disease, 461–462
    diverticulitis, 463
    ulcerative colitis, 462–463
  ocular emergencies in, 338
  polyarticular arthritis with, 359
Inflammatory cells, in uveitis, 1278, 1279
Inflatable splints, 168
Influenza viruses
  in common colds, 376
  in pharyngitis, 376
  pneumonia and, 383
Information, as EMS system component, 11
Infundibular obstruction, 1210–1211
Inguinal abscesses, 407
Inguinal hernia, in infants, 557, 559
Inguinoscrotal hernia, in infants, 559
Inhalant abuse, 805–806
Inhalation injury, 1159–1167. See also Carbon monoxide poisoning; Hazardous materials; specific materials
  with burns, 419, 420
  as major injuries, 424
  by combustion byproducts, 477, 494, 747, 772–773, 1163–1165
    management of, 772–773, 1163–1165
    methemoglobinemia and, 757
    types of materials, 772
  from fires, 494
    pharyngitis and, 377
  in infants and children, airway obstruction from, 566
  management of, 772–773
  metal fume fever, 1161–1162
  occupational sources of, 1162, 1175–1180
  pathophysiology of, 1159
  by toxic gases, 763–773
    chemical asphyxiants, 764–769
    irritant gases, 769–772
    physical asphyxiants, 763–764
Inhalation therapy, in obstructive airway disease, 1132, 1133, 1134. See also Oxygen administration

Inhaled bronchodilators
  for asthma, 581, 1132
  for children, 578
Injury in America, 3
Injury prevention, in EMS planning, 7
Innovar, as general anesthesia, 887
Inocor. See Amrinone lactate
Inotropic agents, for shock, 76, 84
Insect stings, anaphylaxis risk and, 75, 87, 643, 644
Insecticide exposure. See Pesticide exposure
Institute of Medicine (National Academy of Sciences), EMS research role, 3
Instrumentation, septic shock risk and, 72
Insulin
  hypothermia and, 666, 671
  renal failure and, 1225, 1226
  serum sickness and, 433
Insulin deficiency, hyperkalemia and, 298
Insulin therapy, 1432–1433
  adrenal insufficiency and, 259
  anaphylaxis risk with, 75
  complications of, 241
  for diabetic ketoacidosis, 239–241
    hypomagnesemia risk with, 306
  HHNK treatment and, 245
  for hyperkalemia, 280, 300
  hypokalemia risk with, 276, 295, 297
Intensive care unit (ICU), transfer to
  in acute epiglottitis, 1123
  in pulmonary edema, 1099
Interaction theory of domestic violence, 844
Intercondylar fractures, of distal humerus, 203
Intercostal nerve block, 885
Intermittent pain, defined, 878
Intermittent positive-pressure breathing (IPPB), for pulmonary edema, 1099
Internal carotid artery syndrome, 937
Internal jugular vein cannulation, 1343–1346
  in multisystem trauma, 102–103
Interphalangeal joints
  aspiration or injection of, 1374, 1375
  dislocation of, 230
Interstitial edema, as fluid replacement complication, 79
Interstitial fluid, 265
Interstitial pulmonary fibrosis
  in connective tissue disorders, 339, 340
  in rheumatoid arthritis, 339
  in scleroderma, 340
  in systemic lupus erythematosus, 340
Intertriginous lesions, fungal, 437
Intertrochanteric fractures, 218, 219–220
Intestinal hemorrhage, in systemic lupus erythematosus, 342–343
Intestinal obstruction, 459–461
  in pregnancy, 1236
Intestinal perforation, in systemic lupus erythematosus, 342–343
Intra-aortic balloon counterpulsation, 85
  cardiogenic shock prognosis and, 74
Intra-arterial pressure monitoring, in shock treatment, 81–82
Intracapsular fractures of hip, 218
Intracerebral hemorrhage, 941–942
Intracranial emergencies, in infants and children, 589–590
  child abuse, 600–601
Intracranial hemorrhage
  acute confusion with, 954
  as hypertensive emergency, 1065–1066
  prehospital management, 107, 108
Intracranial pressure (ICP)
  cancer and, 502–503
  intracerebral hemorrhage and, 941–942
  meningitis and, in children under two, 537
  monitoring, 898
  near-drowning and, 697–698
  unconsciousness and, in infants or children, 592, 593
Intraocular pressure elevation. See Glaucoma
Intraosseous access, in pediatric patients, 520–521

Intraparenchymal hematoma, 900
Intravenous drug abuse. See also Drug abuse
  complications of, 784–786
  vertebral osteomyelitis and, 193
Intravenous fluid therapy. See also Fluid replacement
  as hypomagnesemia cause, 305
  prehospital
    for cardiac tamponade, 103
    controversy about, 5
    in multisystem trauma, 102–103
Intravenous polygram, in multisystem trauma, 112
Intropin. See Dopamine
Intubation. See also Endotracheal intubation; Nasogastric intubation; Oral intubation
  in chest trauma, 1189
  for laryngotracheitis (viral croup), 1116
  nasotracheal, 98, 1110
    for esophageal burns, 451
  prehospital, controversy about, 6
  retrograde, 1111
Iodides, anaphylaxis risk with, 75
Iodine, for thyroid storm, 250–251
Ipecac syrup, 1449
  indications for, 475
  for sedative-hypnotic overdose, 804
IPG. See Impedance plethysmography
IPPB. See Intermittent positive-pressure breathing
Ipratropium bromide (Atrovent), 1426
  for obstructive airway disease, 1134
Ipsilateral tube thoracostomy, for penetrating chest injury, 1071
Iridocyclitis, in acute glaucoma, 1288
Iridodonesis, 365, 368
Iris, in hereditary disorders, 365
Iritis, in seronegative spondyloarthropathies, 338
Iron, parenteral, anaphylaxis risk with, 75
Iron dextran (Imferon), 1447
Irrigation of wounds, 140
  with fractures, 168
Irritability
  in children, as dehydration sign, 268
  in hypocalcemia, 284
  in metabolic alkalosis, 328
Irritable bowel syndrome, 463
Irritant gases, listed, 769. See also Inhalation injury
Ischemia, myocardial, in hypovolemic shock, 71
Ischemic CVAs. See Cerebrovascular accident
Islam, beliefs and practices, 868
Islet cell cancer, hereditary, 371
Isocyanates, as fire byproduct, 494
Isoetharine, inhaled (Bronkosol; Bronkometer), 1426
  for obstructive airway disease, 1133
  pediatric dosage, 578
  pharmacokinetics of, 1133
Isometheptate (Midrin), for headache, 923
Isoniazid
  overdose of, 490–491
    clinical signs, 472, 474, 491
  scombroid fish poisoning and, 740
Isopropanol intoxication, 325, 492
Isoproterenol (Isuprel), 1386
  in acute myocardial infarction treatment, 984, 985
  for congestive heart failure, 1055
  for dysrhythmias
    atrioventricular (AV) block, 1013
    sudden sinus (atrial standstill), 1011
  hypothermia and, 671
  shock and, 66–67, 84
Isoproterenol, inhaled (Isuprel Mistometer; Norisodrine; Aerolone), 1426–1427
  for obstructive airway disease, 1133
  pharmacokinetics of, 1133
  for respiratory distress in children, 578–579
Isoptin. See Verapamil
Isosorbide dinitrate
  in acute myocardial infarction treatment, 993
  for congestive heart failure, 1055, 1056
Isotretinoin therapy, hypercalcemic crisis and, 315
Isuprel. See Isoproterenol
Isuprel Mistometer. See Isoproterenol, inhaled
Itching. See Pruritus

IV therapy. *See* Fluid replacement; Intravenous fluid therapy
IVC intraluminal devices, for pulmonary embolism, 1141, 1148–1149

J

Jaundice, 456–457
  biliary tract disease and, 453, 454
  clinical signs of, 457
  in thyroid storm, 250
Jaw claudication, in temporal arteritis, 337
JCAHO. *See* Joint Commission on Accreditation of Healthcare Organizations
Jefferson's fracture, 179, 188, 190, 906–907, 908
Jehovah's Witnesses, beliefs and practices, 865, 867
Jellyfish stings, 717, 718–720
  anaphylaxis risk with, 75
Jews
  beliefs and practices, 865, 867
  hereditary disorders in, 365, 366, 368, 369, 370, 372
Johnson, President Lyndon, highway safety and, 1
Johnson, Robert Wood, EMS grants by, 2
Joint Commission on Accreditation of Healthcare Organizations (JCAHO)
  levels of care and, 46
  quality assurance and, 54, 55
    continuous quality improvement model, 57
    multicenter practice parameter studies, 58
    standards development, 62
Joint disorders. *See also* Arthritis; *specific disorders*
  cricoarytenoid synovitis, 339
  differential diagnosis, 351, 356–359
  structural, Baker's cyst with, 346
Joints
  assessing
    aspiration/injection techniques, 353–355, 1373–1375
    fluid analysis, 355–356
    in upper extremity injuries, 195
  dislocations of, 173–174
  infection in, onset of, 351
  subluxations of, 173
Judaism. *See* Jews
Judge-made law, 39
Jugular veins, IV placement in, 102–103, 1343–1346
Jugular venous distention, in cardiogenic shock, 75
Juxtaglomerular cell tumor, hypokalemia and, 277
Juxtaglomerular hyperplasia, 275
Juxtaglomerular hypoplasia, hyperkalemia and, 279

K

K-Lor. *See* Potassium chloride
Kabikinase. *See* Streptokinase
Kanamycin (Kantrex), 1410
Kaolin, for diarrhea, 389
Kaposi's sarcoma (KS), 444
Kaufman's syndrome, 372
Kayexalate. *See* Sodium polystyrene sulfonate
KCL. *See* Potassium chloride
KED immobilization device, 109
Keflex. *See* Cephalexin
Keflin. *See* Cephalothin
Kefzol. *See* Cefazolin
Kehr's sign, 110
Keratic precipitates (KPs), in uveitis, 1279
Keratitis
  bacterial (corneal ulcers), 1273–1276
  herpetic, 1264, 1265–1266
Keratodermia blenorrhagica, in Reiter's syndrome, 358
Keratolytic agents, for fungal infections of skin, 436
Kernig's sign, in meningitis
  aseptic, 399
  purulent, 397
Ketamine, as general anesthetic, 887
  contraindications, 887
  for facial repair in children, 1325

Ketoacidosis, 323–324. *See also* Diabetic ketoacidosis
Ketoconazole (Nizoral), 1421
  for thrush, 378
Ketone loss, hypokalemia and, 275
Ketone solvents, listed, 756
Ketoprofen (Orudis), for pain relief, 881
Ketorolac tromethamine (Toradol), 1436–1437
Khat, as sympathomimetic, 787
Kidneys. *See also* terms beginning with "Renal"
  assessing, in multisystem trauma, 112
  functions of, 1217
  high altitude and, 680
  hypothermia and, 666
  near-drowning and, 693
  rupture of, 1211
  surgery on, adrenal insufficiency and, 257
  trauma to, 1195–1199
  ultrasound examination of, 549–550
Killer whales, 713–714
Kirschner wire fixation, for thumb metacarpal fracture, 208
Klebsiella pneumoniae
  in corneal ulcers, 1274, 1275, 1277
  in nosocomial sinusitis, 1302–1303
  in pneumonia, 383, 384, 386–387
Klebsiella species
  in sinusitis, 1302
  in urinary tract infections, 391
Klippel-Trenaunay-Weber syndrome, 364
Klorvess. *See* Potassium chloride
Klotrix. *See* Potassium chloride
Knee, 221–225
  anatomical considerations, 221–222
  arthrocentesis of, 354–355
  aspiration or injection of, 1373, 1374, 1375
  assessing, in vertebral column injury, 185
  Baker's cyst in, 346
  dislocations of, 173, 223, 224
    anatomy and, 221–222
    vascular emergencies with, 1073
  fractures of, 221
  ligamentous injuries of, 223–224
  Lyme arthritis in, 357
  meniscal tear repair, 224
  monoarticular arthritis in, 351, 352–353
  septic bursitis in, 412
Kocher maneuver, for shoulder dislocation, 199
Koplik's spots, 443
KPs. *See* Keratic precipitates
KS. *See* Kaposi's sarcoma
Kyphosis, congenital, vertebral column injuries vs., 186

L

Labeling requirements, for hazardous materials, 748–750
Labetalol (Normodyne; Trandate), 1394
  for hypertensive emergencies, 1061–1062, 1063
    acute aortic dissection, 1066
    catecholamine crisis, 1067
    eclampsia, 1066
Labor
  preterm
    as abdominal pain cause, 1236–1237
    in trauma, 1238
    thyroid storm and, 249
Laboratory error, hyperkalemia and, 297–298
Lacerations. *See also specific sites*; Wound management
  in children, 552–553
    suturing guidelines, 552–553
  dog bites, 629–630
  dressings for, 156–157
  by marine organisms, 712–715
    treatment of, 715–716
  myocardial, 1078–1079
  of penis, 1208, 1209
  renal, 1196, 1199. *See also* Renal injuries
  of scrotum or testicle, 1209

staple closure of, 149
suturing of. *See* Suturing
tape closure of, 148–149
topical anesthesia for, 885–886
types of, 149–155
in upper extremities, tendon, 212
Lactate levels
  myxedema coma and, 252
  shock prognosis and, 71
Lactate therapy, diabetic ketoacidosis and, 239
Lactic acidemia, in cardiogenic shock, 73
Lactic acidosis, 323. *See also* Metabolic acidosis
  in cardiogenic shock, 74
  etiologies of, 323
  hyperventilation and, 321
  ketoacidosis vs., 323
  in septic shock, 72
Lactic dehydrogenase (LDH) levels
  acute myocardial infarction and, 970
  in pulmonary embolism, 1145
Lactulose (Chronulac; Cephulac), 1449
Lacunar CVA, 938
Laerdal Mask, 95
Lagomorphs (rabbits and hares), rabies and, 629
Laminectomy, vertebral osteomyelitis and, 193
Lampreys, poisoning by, 712, 736
Landsteiner, Karl, blood typing and, 116
Lanoxin. *See* Digoxin
Laparoscopy
  in ectopic pregnancy, 1233
  in pelvic inflammatory disease, 1233
  in vaginal bleeding, 1231
Laparotomy
  in intestinal obstruction, 461
  in shock treatment, 1069
Large bowel obstruction, 460–461
Larotid. *See* Amoxicillin
Laryngeal edema, in anaphylaxis, 75
Laryngeal fracture, cricothyrotomy for, 99
Laryngeal obstruction, in oropharyngeal infection, 382
Laryngeal trauma, 1313–1317
  anatomy and, 1313–1314
  associated injuries, 1314–1315
  clinical signs of, 1315–1316
  etiologies of, 1313
  management of, 1316–1317
Laryngomalacia, as stridor cause, 570
Laryngoscope, in nasotracheal intubation, 98
Laryngospasm in children
  hypocalcemic tetany, 566
  phenothiazine dystonia, 565–566
Laryngotracheitis (LT), 567–569, 1113–1116
  acute epiglottitis vs., 1114, 1120
  airway control method and, 514
  clinical signs, 1114
  diagnosis of, 1115
  treatment of, 1115–1116
Laser treatment, of lower GI bleeding, 451
Lasix. *See* Furosemide
Lassa fever, 406
Lateral condyle fractures, in children, 203
Latex fixation test, in febrile infants under 3 months, 535
Laws. *See also* Legal issues
  hazardous materials regulations, 748–750
  purpose and types of, 39
Laxative abuse
  hypokalemia and, 275, 294, 296
  hypomagnesemia and, 286, 306
Laying on of hands, as nonmedical healing method, 870
LDH. *See* Lactic dehydrogenase levels
Lead poisoning, 473, 474, 493–494. *See also* Metal poisoning
Leading, as communication skill, 873
Lederfen. *See* Fenbufen
Ledermark F20. *See* Ferrous sulfate
Left ventricular failure, acute, 1066
Leg pain
  in Baker's cyst, 346
  in cauda equina syndrome, 193

Legal issues, 39–44
  ALS medical control, 20, 21
  blood collection and tranfusion, 117–119
  breach, 41
  causation, 41
  in child abuse, 597, 602–603
    documentation and, 604–605, 611–616
  consent, 41–42
  consent refusal, 42
  damages, 41
  defenses, 41
  in disaster planning, 32
  domestic violence, 843
  duty, 40
  elder abuse, 847
  facial injuries, 1322, 1325
  forensic specimens, in sexual abuse cases, 607
  hazardous materials, 748–750
  hospital vs. physician responsibility, 61
  hypnosis, 873
  liability, 61
    in ALS medical control, 21
    immunities and, 41
    physician vs. hospital, 61
  National Practitioner Data Bank and, 56
  negligence, 40
  ocular trauma, 1262
  organ transplantation, 43
  rape, 1241, 1243–1244, 1246, 1247
    definitions, 1242, 1243
  sexual abuse, 607, 608
  social engineering and, 40
  suicidal patient, 831–832, 833
  tort law, 39–40
  transfer of patients, 42–43
  tympanic membrane perforation, 1307
  types of laws, 39
Legionella pneumophila, in pneumonia, 383, 384, 385
Legionnaire's disease
  diagnosis of, 385
  renal failure and, 1219
  treatment of, 387
Legs
  erythema nodosum on, 435
  fractures of, 162, 163
    blood loss risk with, 168
    cast application to, 169–170, 171
    open, 172
  lacerations of, 154–155
Lembcke, Dr. Paul, quality studies by, 55
Lens dislocation, in hereditary disorders, 364, 365
Leopard syndrome, 364, 365
Leptospirosis, aseptic meningitis and, 399
Lesser trochanter fractures, 220–221
Lethargy
  as dehydration sign, 268
  in Lyme disease, 357
Leukemia
  acute, hypokalemia and, 276, 294
  hyperkalemia and, 279
Leukocyte count. *See* White blood count
Leukocytoclastic vasculitis, 337
Leukocytosis
  in diabetic ketoacidosis, 235
  hypothermia and, 666
  pseudohyperkalemia and, 279
  in septic arthritis, 356
Levarterenol. *See* Norepinephrine or Levarterenol
Levels of care
  behavioral emergencies and, 47
  for burn patients, 19
  cardiac emergencies and, 48
  JCAHO-recognized, 46
  pediatric/perinatal emergencies and, 48
  toxicologic emergencies and, 48
  trauma and, 49
  in trauma centers, 18
Levels of consciousness, assessing, 105
  in acute confusional states, 952
  AVPU grid, 928
  diagnostic role of, 589
  Glasgow Coma Scale, 591, 592, 894, 928–929

in head injury, 894
in multisystem trauma, 105
in near-drowning, 694
Levels of response, to hazardous materials, 751
Levobunolol HCl (Betagan)
  for acute glaucoma, 1289
  for hyphema, 1286
Levophed. *See* Norepinephrine or Levarterenol
Levorphanol (Levo-Dromoran), for pain relief, 883
Levothyroxine (Synthroid), 1445
Liability issues
  in ALS medical control, 21
  immunities, 41
  physician vs. hospital, 61
Librium. *See* Chlordiazepoxide
Lice, 437
Licensure, National Practitioner Data Bank and, 56
Licorice
  adrenal insufficiency and, 259
  hypokalemia and, 277, 294, 295
Lidocaine (Xylocaine), 1386–1387
  in acute myocardial infarction treatment, 983–984
  in advanced cardiac life support, 1089
  anaphylaxis risk with, 75
  for antidepressant overdose, 485
  clinical characteristics and dosage, 884
  for congestive heart failure, 1056
  in CPR, of pediatric patients, 523
  for dysrhythmias
    PSVT, 1026, 1028
    ventricular premature complexes, 1005
    ventricular tachycardia, 1030, 1034
  in endotracheal intubation, 1106
  for gout, 358
  pharmacologic classification of, 885
  for regular, wide QRS tachycardia, 1037
  for status epilepticus, 947
  toxic reactions to, 139
  for Wolff-Parkinson-White syndrome, 1042
  as wound anesthetic, 139, 140
  in maxillofacial injuries, 1325
LIFE STAR helicopter, 24
LIFE STAR registry, 12, 13–14
Lifeguards, as first responders, 6
Ligamentous injuries
  to ankles, 230–231
  chronic, 226, 231
  to hands, 208–209
  to knee, 223–224
  to wrist, 207
Ligature of wounds, 141. *See also* Suturing
Limited pain, defined, 878
Lipoprotein lipase deficiency, familial, 370
Lips
  injury repair, 1326
  lacerations, 153
  pemphigus vulgaris lesions on, 437
Liquid protein diets, as hypomagnesemia cause, 305, 306
Lisfranc's joint injuries, 229
Lisinopril, for congestive heart failure, 1055
LISS. *See* Low ionic strength solutions
Listeria monocytogenes, in meningitis, 396, 398
Lithium
  anion gap and, 327
  as diabetes insipidus cause, 268
  hypercalcemia, 315, 318
  in hyponatremia treatment, 272
  movement disorders with, 474
  overdose of, clinical signs, 473, 474
  pharmacokinetics and, 484

jaundice, 456–457
respiratory alkalosis and, 330
Liver flukes, biliary obstruction and, 455
Livestock, rabies and, 629
Lobster poisoning, 735
Local anesthesia, 884–885
  agents used for, 884, 885, 1453
  anaphylaxis risk with, 75
  reactions to, 884–885
  in wound management, 139–140
    maxillofacial, 1325
Locked-in syndrome, coma vs., 928
Lofgren's syndrome, 336
  polyarticular arthritis with, 359
Loma Linda Hospital, helicopter transport at, 23
Lomotil. *See* Diphenoxylate-atropine
Loniten. *See* Minoxidil
Loperamide hydrochloride, for diarrhea, 389
Lopressor. *See* Metoprolol
Lorazepam (Ativan)
  for acute confusion, psychiatric, 956
  elimination half-life of, 800
  for meningitis in children under two, 539
  overdose of, 491–492
  for status epilepticus, 946–947
  in children, 594
Lotrimin. *See* Clotrimazole
Low back pain, chronic, in adrenal insufficiency, 259
Low blood pressure. *See* Hypotension
Low ionic strength solutions (LISS), in cross-matching, 123, 124
Lower extremity injuries, 221–231
  anatomy and, 221–222
  ankle fractures, 226–228
  ankle sprains, 230–231
    ligamentous instability and, 226
  dislocations, patellar, 223, 224
  fibula fractures, 226
  foot fractures or dislocations, 228–230
  foot ulcers, diabetic, 231
  fracture classification, 222–223
  knee dislocations, 223–224
  ligamentous, 223–224
  proximal tibia fractures, 224–225
  tibia fractures, 225–226
Lower gastrointestinal bleeding, 450–451
Lower respiratory tract disorders, in children, 573–587
  anatomy/physiology and, 573–574
  clinical evaluation of, 575–576
  etiologies of, 574–575, 576
  laboratory studies, 576–577
  management of, 577–579
Lower, Richard, 115
Loxapine (Loxitane), 486
  overdose of, 486
Loxoscelism (brown recluse spider bite), 641–642
LSD, 806, 809–810
Ludiomil. *See* Maprotiline; Tetracyclic maprotiline
Lugol's solution, for thyroid storm, 250
Lumbar puncture
  in cerebrovascular accident, 941
  contraindications, 397
  in delirium tremens, 955
  as headache cause, 919
  in headache evaluation, 921, 941
  in intracerebral hemorrhage, 942
  in meningitis diagnosis, 397
  of children under two, 536, 537–538
  neurologic indications for, 344
Lumbar spine injuries
  cauda equina syndrome and, 193
  fractures, 192–193
    compression, calcaneus fractures and, 228, 230
    treatment of, 188
  gastrointestinal tract and, 187
  neurologic assessment with, 182
Lumbosacral corset, for thoracolumbar spine fracture, 193
Luminal. *See* Phenobarbital
Luminal defect, in vascular injury, 1070
Lund and Browder burn evaluation method, 421, 422
Lung abscesses, hyponatremia and, 271

Lung cancer
  acanthosis nigricans and, 429
  adrenal insufficiency and, 257
  chest wall syndrome vs., 348
  hypercalcemia and, 282, 317
  hyponatremia and, 271
  SVC obstruction and, 510, 511
Lung function
  gas exchange and, 1152–1153
  near-drowning and, 690–692
  obstructive airway disease and, 1132
  perfusion and, 1153
  ventilation, 1151
  ventilation control, 1154–1156
  ventilation distribution and, 1151–1152
  ventilation/perfusion (V/Q) ratio, 1153–1154
Lung scan, in pulmonary embolism, 1145–1146
Lung volume, respiratory failure and, 1151, 1152
Lupus. See Systemic lupus erythematosus
Lusitrophy, cardiac function and, 1052
Lutherans, beliefs and practices, 867
Lye ingestion
  airway obstruction with, 566
  esophageal burns with, 451
Lyme disease, 409
  arthritis of, 357
  aseptic meningitis, 399
  complications of, 357, 409
  encephalitis and, 400, 401
  skin lesions in, 336, 357, 409
Lymphadenopathy, in infectious mononucleosis, 401
Lymphocytic choriomeningitis, aseptic meningitis and, 399
Lymphoma
  adrenal insufficiency and, 257
  hypercalcemia and, 317
  hyperkalemia and, 279
  hyponatremia and, 271
Lysosomal enzymes, in hypovolemic shock, 71

M

Ma huang (ephedrine), as sympathomimetic, 787
Maalox, for hypomagnesemia, 287
Macrodantin. See Nitrofurantoin
Macrodex. See Dextran solutions
"Madura foot," 409
Mafenide acetate (Sulfamylon)
  for burns, 424, 425
  metabolic acidosis and, 322–323
Mafucci's syndrome, 364
Magill forceps
  in endotracheal intubation, 96
  for foreign body removal, 515
  in nasotracheal intubation, 98
Magnesium administration
  for alcohol withdrawal, 821
  for hypercalcemic crisis, 315
  hypothermia and, 671
  for obstructive airway disease, 308, 1135
Magnesium levels, 285–286, 303–304
  diabetic ketoacidosis and, 239
  hypermagnesemia and, 287–288, 308
  hypomagnesemia and, 286–287, 304–307
  physiology and, 285–286
Magnesium sulfate, 1398
  in advanced cardiac life support, 1090
  for asthma, 308
  for cardiac disorders, 307–308
  for eclampsia, 1066
  for hypomagnesemia, 287, 307
  for magnesium-deficiency seizures, 307
  in myocardial infarction, 1090
  for pre-eclampsia, 1239
  in torsades de pointes, 1090
Magnetic resonance imaging (MRI)
  in brain abscess, 401
  in cardiovascular accident, 943
  in child abuse cases, 604
  in coma assessment, 930
  in headache evaluation, 921
  in knee evaluation, 224

Mahi-mahi, scombrotoxism and, 739
Malabsorption syndromes
  hypocalcemia and, 284
  hypomagnesemia and, 286, 306
  in scleroderma, 342
Malaise
  in hypercalcemia, 283
  in Lyme disease, 357
Malaria
  brain infection and, 400
  sepsis and, 407
Maldistribution, as hypokalemia cause, 293, 294–295
Males
  abuse victim profile, 845–846
  acute intrascrotal pain, 1211–1213
  appendicitis in, 463, 464
  epididymitis in, 1212
  genitourinary injuries in. See Genitourinary injuries
  herpes simplex 2 infections in, 442
  high-altitude pulmonary edema and, 683
  hydration and, 265
  orchitis in, 1212
  prostatitis in, 391
  rape of, 1252
  testicular torsion in, 1212–1213
Malignancies. See also Cancer; Neoplastic disorders; Oncologic emergencies; specific types
  cutaneous lesions in, 337
    acanthosis nigricans, 429
  hypercalcemia and, 313, 316, 317
  hyponatremia and, 271
Mallet or baseball finger, 207
Mallory-Weiss syndrome, 449, 452
Malnutrition, as hypokalemia cause, 294
Malpractice. See also Legal issues; Quality issues
  National Practitioner Data Bank and, 56
  paramedic, responsibility for, 21
  physician vs. hospital responsibility, 61
Malrotation, as vomiting cause in infants, 557–558
Mammalian bites. See Bite wounds
Man-of-war, stings by, 718
Mandelamine. See Methenamine mandelate
Mandible fractures, assessing for, 110
Mandibular fractures, 1322, 1328
Mandol. See Cefamandole
Mania, acute
  confusion in, 955
  in systemic lupus erythematosus, 343
Manic depressive illness. See Bipolar disorders
Manipulation of fractures, 168–169
Mannitol (Mannitol; Osmitrol), 1431
  for ciguatera fish poisoning, 738
  for glaucoma, acute, 1289
  for glaucoma, secondary
    with hyphema, 1286
    with uveitis, 1282
  for head injury, 897
  hyperkalemia and, 279, 280
  hypokalemia and, 275–276
Maprotiline (Ludiomil), 486
  overdose of, 486–487
Marcaine. See Bupivacaine
Marfan's syndrome, 364, 365, 367, 368, 371
Marijuana, 807, 808–809
  extent of use, 782, 808
  paraquat poisoning from, 809
  in pregnancy, effects on neonate, 810
  screening tests for, 786
Marine organisms, 711–742
  Atlantic Portuguese man-of-war, 718
  barracuda, 714
  bivalve mollusks, 731–734, 735
  bristle worms, 723–724
  catfishes, 726
  coelenterates, 717–718, 720
  cone shells, 722
  food poisoning by, 711–712, 731–741. See also specific organisms
    bacterial infections, 731–733
    dinoflagellate intoxication, 733, 734
    ichthyosarcotoxism, 736–739

    neurotropic shellfish poisoning, 735
    paralytic shellfish poisoning (PSP), 734–735
    scrombrotoxism, 739–740
    tetrodotoxism, 740–741
    venerupin shellfish poisoning, 734
    viral infections, 733
  grouper, 714–715
  historical perspective on, 712
  hydroids, 717–718
  injuries by, 711. See also specific organisms
    antibiotic therapy for, 731, 732
    beaks, 730–731
    fangs, 729–730
    lacerations, 712–716
    spine or puncture (invertebrates), 722–724
    spine or puncture (vertebrates), 724–729
    stings, 716–721
  jellyfish, 717, 718–720
  killer whales, 713–714
  marlin, 729
  moray eels, 714
  nematocysts, 717–721
  octopuses, 730–731
  ratfishes, 725–726
  sailfish, 729
  scorpionfishes, 727–728
  sea anemones and sea corals, 720–721
  sea urchins, 722–723
  sea wasps, 719
  sharks, 712–713, 715
    dogfish, 724
  skin infections and, 408–409, 742
  skin reactions caused by, 741
  sponges, 716
  starfish; sea stars, 723
  stingrays, 724–725
  stonefish, 727–728
  surgeonfishes, 728–729
  swordfish, 729
  toadfishes, 728
  venerupin shellfish, 734
  weevers, 726–727
  zebrafish, 727–728
Marlin, injuries by, 729
Maryland, regional trauma system in, 50
Masculinization, in adrenogenital syndrome
  hyperkalemia and, 279
  hypokalemia and, 277
Mass casualty incidents (MCIs), 31. See also Disaster management
  levels of, 32
  medical direction and, 33
  mutual aid issues, 32
  triage issues, 34–35
Mass spectrometry, in drug abuse testing, 786
Massage, for pain relief, 888
MAST suit (military antishock trousers)
  for children, 521, 547
  complications of, 77, 1069
  direct pressure vs., 1069
  indications for, 1069
  in shock treatment, 76–78
MAT. See Multifocal (chaotic) atrial tachycardia
Matching, as communication skill, 873
Mattress sutures
  horizontal, 148
  vertical, 145, 147
Maxillary fractures, 1328–1329
Maxillary space infections, 382–383
Maxillofacial injuries, 1319–1330. See also Dental emergencies
  anatomy and, 1320, 1321, 1323, 1324
  evaluation of, 1321–1323
  fractures and dislocations, 1328–1330, 1335
  prehospital management, 110, 1320
  to soft tissues, 1320, 1325–1328
  wound management, 1325–1326
    anesthesia infiltration, 1325
    cleansing and debriding, 1325–1326
    closure considerations, 1326
    delayed closure, 1325
    dressings, 1326

Maxillofacial injuries (*contd.*)
    follow-up care, 1326
    topical anesthesia, 140, 1325
Mazicon. *See* Flumazenil
MCIs. *See* Mass casualty incidents
McKusick-type dysplasia, 372
McSwain dart, in tension pneumothorax, 100
MDA. *See* Methylenedioxyamphetamine
MDEA. *See* Methylenedioxyethamphetamine
MDI inhaler systems, for asthma, 1132
MDMA. *See* Methylenedioxymethamphetamine
MDTP (meperidine analogue), 799–800
Measles, 442–443
    as aseptic meningitis cause, 399
    German (rubella), 443
    pneumonia and, 383
Mebendazole (Vermox), 1421
Meckel's diverticulum, 558, 559
Meclofenamate sodium (Meclomen), for pain relief, 881
Meconium aspiration, 1166–1167
Media communications, in disaster plan, 15
Medial condyle fractures, 203
Mediastinal trauma, 1185–1188. *See also specific types*
    cardiac tamponade, 1185
    great vessel injury, 1187
    intrathoracic esophageal injury, 1188
    myocardial contusion, 1186–1187
    penetrating cardiac injury, 1185–1186
    tracheobronchial injury, 1188
Medical antishock trousers. *See* MAST suit
Medical control
    as EMS system component, 8
    on-line vs. off-line, 20
    in prehospital care, 20–21
    in rural vs. urban areas, 23
MedicAlert tag, for hymenoptera allergies, 644
Medicare and Medicaid Patient and Program Protection Act of 1987, 60
Medicare/Medicaid
    antidumping statutes and, 43
    false claims penalties, 60
    organ transplantation and, 43
    quality improvement and, 54, 61–62
        National Practitioner Data Bank use, 56
        PRO role in, 58
        sanctions, 60
Medications. *See* Drugs
Meditation, for pain management, 887
    techniques, 874, 875
Mediterranean fever, familial, 369, 370
Mefenamic acid (Ponstel), for pain relief, 881
Melanotic stools, differential diagnosis, 449
Melena, upper GI bleeding with, 449
Membranous croup (bacterial tracheitis), 569, 1113, 1116–1117
Memory impairment, in systemic lupus erythematosus, 343
Men. *See* Males
Meningismus
    in Lyme disease, 357
    in subarachnoid hemorrhage, 940
Meningitis
    alcohol withdrawal vs., 819
    aseptic, 399–400, 536
        diagnosis of, 399
        encephalitis and, 400
        in systemic lupus erythematosus, 344
        treatment of, 399–400
    bacterial. *See* Meningitis, purulent
    as cause of death, 397
    in children under two, 535–539
    as diabetes insipidus cause, 267
    granulomatous, 536
    as headache cause, 919
    hyponatremia and, 271
    in infants under 3 months, 533–535
    purulent, 396–399
        acute confusion with, 953
        diagnosis of, 397
        differential diagnosis, 397
        etiologies of, 396
        in infants and children, 533–539, 590
        pathogenesis of, 396–397
        prevention of, 398–399
        treatment of, 397–398
    as seizure cause, 947
    in systemic lupus erythematosus, 344
    viral, 535, 536
Meningococcemia, 430
    adrenal insufficiency and, 256
    diagnosis of, 406, 430
Meningococcus, in eye infection, culture media for, 1270
Meningoencephalitis
    in Behet's syndrome, 343
    differential diagnosis, 343
Meniscal tears
    Baker's cyst with, 346
    in knee, arthroscopic repair of, 224
Mennonites, beliefs and practices, 867
Menstruation
    canker sores and, 381
    gonococcal arthritis and, 352
Mental disturbances, in systemic lupus erythematosus, 343–344
Mental dysfunction, differential diagnosis, 344
Mental retardation, Bartter's syndrome and, 275
Mental status
    in confusional state, organic vs. psychiatric, 952
    dehydration signs, 268
    in encephalitis, 400
    in hypercalcemia, 283, 311, 312
    in hypernatremia, 268
    in hypocalcemia, 284
    in hypokalemia, 295
    in hypomagnesemia, 287, 304, 305
    in hyponatremia, 271, 272
    in meningitis, purulent, 397
    in metabolic alkalosis, 328
    in shock
        cardiogenic, 74, 75
        hypovolemic, 68
        septic, 72
Meperidine hydrochloride (Demerol), 1437
    for acute confusion, psychiatric, 956
    for acute myocardial infarction, 985
    designer analogues of, 799–800
    for epistaxis, 1306
    for facial wound repair, in children, 1325
    for headache, 922
    as opioid, 793
    overdose of, clinical signs, 472
    for pain relief, 881, 883
    for pancreatitis, 456
    pharmacology of, 794
    seizures induced by, 793–794
    in wound management, 139
Meperidine-promethazine-chlorpromazine, in facial repair in children, 1325
Mephentermine, as sympathomimetic, 787
Mephyton. *See* Phytonadione
Mepivacaine (Carbocaine)
    clinical characteristics and dosage, 884
    pharmacologic classification, 885
Meprobamate. *See also* Sedative-hypnotics
    abstinence syndrome, 804
    anaphylaxis risk with, 75
    elimination half-life of, 800
    overdose of, clinical signs, 472, 803
    pharmacology of, 802
Meralen. *See* Flufenamic acid
Mercury poisoning, 474, 494. *See also* Metal poisoning
    behavioral disorders and, 474
Mescaline, 807, 809
Mesenteric ischemia, diagnosis of, 461
Mesenteric vasculitis
    in rheumatoid arthritis, 342
    in systemic lupus erythematosus, 342–343
Metabolic acidemia
    as MAST suit complication, 77
    shock and, 71
Metabolic acidosis, 320–326
    alcohol withdrawal and, 825
    in cardiac arrest, 1090
    compensatory response in, 320–321
    diagnosis of, 321
    etiologies of
        with increased anion gap, 323–326
        with normal anion gap, 321–322
    hyperkalemia and, 279, 298
    in hyperosmolar hyperglycemic nonketotic coma, 244
    hypokalemia and, 276
    hypothermia and, 664
    in hypovolemic shock, 70–71
    as MAST suit complication, 77
    in toxicologic emergencies, 473–474
    treatment of, 326
Metabolic alkalemia, shock and, 71
Metabolic alkalosis, 327–329
Metabolic disturbances. *See also* Acid-base disturbances; Electrolyte abnormalities; *specific types*
    as acute confusional state cause, 953
    in cancer patients, 506–508
    as coma cause, 930
        in children, 590–591
    hereditary, 369, 370
    in hypokalemia, 295, 296
    in renal failure, treatment of, 1225–1226
    syncope and, 961
Metabolism. *See also* Cellular metabolism
    hyperactive, in thyroid storm, 249
    sodium, 266
Metacarpal fractures, 208
Metacarpophalangeal joints
    aspiration or injection of, 1374, 1375
    clenched fist injury and, 211
    trauma to, 209
Metaclopramide, for headache, 922
Metal poisoning, 493–494
    behavioral disorders and, 474
    food poisoning vs., 390
    metal fume fever, 1161–1162
    movement disorders and, 474
    occupational, 1162
    treatment of, 476
Metaphoric (right-brain) communication, 874–875
Metaphyseal chondrodysplasia, ethnic groups and, 372
Metaproterenol (Metaprel; Alupent), 1427
    inhaled
        for asthma, 1132
        for obstructive airway disease, 1132, 1133
        pediatric dosage, 578
        pharmacokinetics of, 1133
    for obstructive airway disease, 1133
Metaraminol, for shock, 84
Metastatic disease
    chest wall syndrome vs., 348
    hypercalcemia and, 282
    indomethacin and, 283
Metatarsal head osteomyelitis, diabetic foot ulcers and, 231
Metatarsal injuries, fractures and dislocations, 230
Metatarsophalangeal joint
    aspiration or injection of, 1374
    pain in, differential diagnosis, 351
Methadone (Dolophine)
    abstinence syndromes, 798, 799
    adrenal insufficiency and, 258
    as opioid, 793
    for opioid detoxification, 798
    for pain relief, 881, 883
    pharmacology of, 794
Methamphetamine use. *See* Amphetamine
Methane, asphyxiation injury by, 764
Methanol intoxication, 324, 487
    assay method, 472
    clinical signs of, 473–474
    treatment of, 476, 487–488
Methaqualone (Quaalude). *See also* Sedative-hypnotics
    elimination half-life of, 800

overdose of, clinical signs, 472, 803
pharmacology of, 801
Methazolamide (Neptazane)
for acute glaucoma, 1289
for secondary glaucoma, with hyphema, 1285–1286
Methdilazine (Tacaryl), for ciguatera fish poisoning, 738
Methemoglobinemia, 473, 757
nitrite inhalation and, 806
in nitrogen dioxide exposure, 771
treatment of, 479
Methenamine mandelate (Mandelamine), 1422
Methergine. *See* Methylergonovine maleate
Methicillin (Staphcillin), 1415
for corneal ulcers, 1275, 1278
renal failure and, 1218–1219
for staphylococcal scalded skin syndrome, 431
Methimazole, for thyroid storm, 250, 251
Methocarbamol (Robaxin), 1443
Methodists, beliefs and practices, 867–868
Methohexital (Brevital), as general anesthesia, 887
Methotrexate
in ectopic pregnancy, 1233
pulmonary reactions to, 508
Methoxamine (Vasoxyl), 1387
for PSVT, 1026
Methrazone. *See* Feprazone
Methyl alcohol poisoning, 757, 774
Methyl bromide, as systemic toxin, 774
Methyl cellosolve poisoning, 774
Methyl n-butyl ketone, as systemic toxin, 774
α-Methyldopa, 1394
for hypertension, in renal failure, 1225
Methylene blue, 1449
for nitro compound toxicity, 479, 757
Methylene chloride, carbon monoxide poisoning and, 478
Methylene dichloride (dichloromethane), carbon monoxide poisoning and, 765
Methylenedioxyamphetamine (MDA), 787, 799
Methylenedioxyethamphetamine (MDEA), 787
Methylenedioxymethamphetamine (MDMA), 787, 799
Methylergonovine maleate (Methergine), 1446
Methylphenidate (Ritalin)
abuse of, 793
as sympathomimetic, 787
Methylprednisolone (Solu-Medrol; Depo-Medrol)
for asthma, in children, 581
for gout, 358
for obstructive airway disease, 1135–1136
asthma in children, 581
for spinal cord injuries, 104, 913
Methylxanthines, for obstructive airway disease, 1134
Methysergide maleate (Sansert), 1446
for headache prophylaxis, 922, 924
Metolazone (Zaroxolyn), 1431
for congestive heart failure, 1055
Metoprolol (Lopressor), 1394
for acute myocardial infarction, 983
confusion caused by, 474
for dysrhythmias
atrial fibrillation, 1022
premature ventricular complexes, 1005
PSVT, 1026
overdose of, clinical signs, 472
Metric temperature, conversion chart, 1455–1462
Metronidazole (Flagyl), 1422
for cholangitis and sepsis, 454–455
for dysenteric gastroenteritis, 390
for *Giardia* enteritis, 390
for oropharyngeal infections, 383
for pelvic inflammatory disease, 1234
for *Trichomonas* urethritis, 395
Mexilitine (Mexitil), for ventricular premature complexes, 1005
Mezlocillin sodium (Mezlin), 1415
for cholangitis and sepsis, 454–455
Mianserin (Norval), 486, 487
overdose of, 487
Miconazole (MicaTin), for fungal infections

of intertriginous areas, 437
of skin, 436
Microcoleus lyngbyaceus (seaweed), as dermatitis cause, 741
Microthrombi, in shock response, 71
Micturition syncope, 961, 963
Midamor. *See* Amiloride
Midazolam (Versed), 1439–1440
in acute myocardial infarction treatment, 984
elimination half-life of, 800
in endotracheal intubation, 1106
as sedative, for sexual abuse examination, 606
Middle cerebral artery syndrome, 937
Middle Eastern patients, familial Mediterranean fever in, 369, 370
Midrin. *See* Isometheptate
Migraine
in children, 916
cyproheptadine for, 922, 924
cocaine and, 789
etiology of, 915–916
types of, 916
Military antishock trousers. *See* MAST suit
Military trauma
fluid resuscitation in, 126
multisystem injury care and, 93
wound age factors, 137–138
Milk allergy, in TAR syndrome, 368
Milk intake, hypercalcemia and, 282
Milk of Magnesia, for hypomagnesemia, 287
Milk-alkali syndrome (Burnett's syndrome), hypercalcemia and, 282, 313, 317
Miller blade, for endotracheal intubation, 96
of children, 544
Miltown. *See* Meprobamate
Milwaukee shoulder (chronic hydroxyapatite synovitis), 351
Minamata disease, 494
Mineralocorticoid activity, hypokalemia and, 293, 294. *See also specific conditions*
Mineralocorticoids, for hyperkalemic periodic paralysis, 298, 300
Mining injuries, methane asphyxiation, 764
Minnesota tube, in balloon tamponade, 450
Minocycline, in meningitis prevention, 398
Minors, consent issues, 41–42
Minoxidil (Loniten), 1394–1395
for congestive heart failure, 1055
in renal failure treatment, 1225
Miotics, for acute glaucoma, 1289
Mirroring, as therapeutic tool, 872, 873
Misoprostol (Cytotec), 1433–1434
Mist treatment, for laryngotracheitis, 1115
Mithramycin, for hypercalcemia, 283, 316
Mitomycin-C, toxic reactions to, pulmonary, 508
Mitral insufficiency, pulmonary edema and, 1097, 1098
Mitral valve prolapse, premature ventricular complexes and, 1003, 1005
Mobile relay system (MRS), 8, 9
Mobilization. *See* Ambulation
Moist air treatment, for laryngotracheitis, 1115
Molar pregnancy, vaginal bleeding in, 1230
Mollaret's syndrome, aseptic meningitis and, 399
Molluscum contagiosum, AIDS and, 444
Mollusks, poisoning by, 391, 731–735
Monitoring. *See also specific types of injuries*
cardiopulmonary, of critically ill patient, 78
in communications systems, 8
in shock treatment, 76, 81–83
with MAST suit use, 77
for septic shock, 85
Monoarticular arthritis. *See* Arthritis, acute monoarticular
Monocid. *See* Cefonicid
Monofilament sutures, 142
Mononucleosis, 401–403
polyarthralgias with, 359
splenic rupture and, 459
Monosodium glutamate intoxication, 391
Monteggia fracture, 205
Moravians, beliefs and practices, 868

Moraxella catarrhalis
in otitis media, 380, 381
in pneumonia, 383
in sinusitis, 378
in tracheitis, 1116
Moraxella lacunata, in corneal ulcers, 1274
Moray eels, 714
Moricizine (Ethmozine), 1387
Mormons, beliefs and practices, 866
Morning glory seeds, 806
Morphine sulfate (Morphine), 1437
for acute myocardial infarction, 985
anaphylaxis risk with, 75
for cardiogenic shock, 85
for congestive heart failure, 1055–1056
for pain relief, 880–881, 882
side effects of, 881
for pulmonary edema, 1098–1099
sustained-release (MS-Contin), overdose of, 797
Morphology, clinical genetics and, 361, 363–365
Morquio's syndrome, 372
Mortality
diabetic ketoacidosis and, 233
ground vs. air transport and, 24–25
hip fractures and, 218, 219–220
in hyperosmolar hyperglycemic nonketotic coma, 242
military injuries and, 93
myxedema coma and, 252
rural vs. urban areas and, 22
thyroid storm and, 249, 251
trauma as cause of, 93
trauma centers and, 19
Morton's salt substitute, for hypokalemia, 278
Motor function, assessing
in head injury, 894–895, 896
in multisystem trauma, 106
in unconscious infants or children, 591
in vertebral column trauma, 183, 184
Motor response, scoring, 929
Motor vehicle accidents
air transport indications, 25
blunt trauma to heart in, 1081
burns from, 419
cervical spine injuries in, 904, 905
Colles' fractures and, 205
dashboard injuries
hip dislocations, 217
patellar fractures, 222–223
dentoalveolar trauma in, 1333
foreign body emergencies in, 1308, 1309
heart and great vessel injuries in, 1077, 1187–1188
hip fractures from, 218–219, 224
interhospital transfer criteria, 10
knee injuries and, 223
laryngeal trauma in, 1313
maxillofacial injuries and, 1319
mortality from
in children, 541
in rural vs. urban areas, 22
myocardial contusions from, 1081
pediatric injuries in, 541, 542
renal injuries in, 1195
sedative-hypnotic abuse and, 800
tibia fractures from, 226
urethral injuries in, 1205
vertebral column injuries from, 175, 191
Motorcycle accidents
hip dislocations from, 217
tibia fractures from, 226
vertebral column injuries from, 175, 179–180
Motrin. *See* Ibuprofen
Mountain sickness, 679
acute (AMS), 680, 681–683
chronic (CMS), 685
as headache cause, 918
Mouth
infections in, 381–383, 1336–1337
thrush, 377, 378, 436–437
injury repair, 1326
lacerations, 153, 1336, 1337
pemphigus vulgaris in, 437, 1336

Movement disorders, in toxicologic emergencies, 474
Moxalactam (Moxam), 1413
Moynihan, Dr. Daniel, EMS projects and, 2
MPPP (meperidine analogue), 799–800
MRS (mobile relay system), 8, 9
MS-Contin. *See* Morphine sulfate, sustained-release
Mucocutaneous lesions, in syphilis, 439
Mucolipidosis type IV, 372
Mucomyst. *See* Acetylcysteine
Mucor, sinusitis and, 378, 1302
Mucous membranes
    dryness of, as dehydration sign, 268
    fungal infections of, 377, 378, 436–437
    pemphigus vulgaris lesions on, 437
    suture material and technique for, 143
Mucopolysaccharidosis type IVA (Morquio's syndrome), 372
Multicenter practice parameter studies, 58
Multifilament sutures, 142
Multifocal (chaotic) atrial tachycardia (MAT), 1018, 1019, 1021–1022
Multiple myeloma
    carpal tunnel syndrome and, 347
    chest wall syndrome vs., 348
    hypercalcemia and, 282, 313, 317, 318
    hyponatremia and, 272
Multisystem injuries, 93–112
    approaches to
        abdominal injuries, 110–111
        airway control, 95–99, 544–545
        basic vs. advanced skills and, 94
        breathing assistance, 99–101, 544–545
        central nervous system, 104–109
        chest injuries, 110
        for children, 544–552
        circulation control, 101–103, 545
        genitourinary system, 111–112
        maxillofacial area, 110
        monitoring, 545
        pelvis and extremities, 111
        rectum, 111–112
        tetanus immunization, 112
    in battering syndrome, 841, 845, 848
    in children, 541–552
        management guidelines, 544–552
        patterns of injury, 541–542
        physiology and, 542–544
    in drowning or near-drowning, 694, 695
    field management priorities, 94
    head injury with, 896
    hip fractures and, 218–219, 220
    hyperkalemia risk with, 298
    hypokalemia risk with, 295
    laryngeal trauma with, 1314–1315
    pelvic fractures with, 215
    prehospital interventions, 93–112
    primary survey of, 94, 95–103
        in children, 545–547
    radiographic evaluation of, in children, 548–550
    record keeping with, 112
    rectal or colon injuries with, 465
    secondary survey of, 94, 103–112
        in children, 547–548
    succinylcholine for, hyperkalemia risk with, 298
    transport for, 94
    upper extremity injuries with, 195
    vertebral column injuries and, 180, 187
Mumps
    aseptic meningitis and, 399
    orchitis and, 1212
Munchausen's syndrome by proxy, 601–602
Muscle
    necrotizing infections of, 409–410
    suture material for, 142, 143
    suture removal from, 144
    suture technique for, 143
Muscle contraction
    potassium and, 273–274
    in respiration, 1155
Muscle contraction headaches. *See* Tension headaches
Muscle cramping

    heat cramps, 655–656
    hypocalcemia and, 285
Muscle relaxants, 1441–1444
    for dislocations, 173
    in endotracheal intubation, 1107
Muscle spasms, in rheumatoid arthritis, 343
Muscle strain, Baker's cyst vs., 346
Muscle weakness. *See* Weakness
Muscular dystrophy, Duchenne, myotonic dystrophy vs., 369, 370
Musculoskeletal emergencies, 161–174
    in children, 543
    head injury with, 896
Musculoskeletal pain, treatment of, 880
Mushroom poisoning, 391
Muslims, beliefs and practices, 868
Mussels, poisoning by, 391, 731–734
Mutual aid, in EMS systems, 7, 8, 11
    in disaster planning, 32
Myalgia, in adrenal insufficiency, 259
Mycetoma, 409
Mycifradin. *See* Neomycin
Mycobacterial infections
    in eye, diagnostic studies, 1270, 1272
    pneumonia, 383, 384
Mycobacterium avium-intracellulare, in pneumonia, 383
Mycobacterium kansasii, in pneumonia, 383
Mycobacterium marinum
    dermatitis caused by, 742
    skin infections from, 408–409
Mycobacterium tuberculosis
    in eye, culture media for, 1270
    in pneumonia, 383
Mycoplasmal infections
    otitis media and, 380, 1309
    pharyngitis, 376
    pneumonia, 383, 384–385, 386
        in children, 585, 586
Mycostatin. *See* Nystatin
Mydriacyl. *See* Tropicamide
Mydriasis, in shock
    cardiogenic, 75
    hypovolemic, 70
Mydriatics, 1281
    for uveitis, 1280–1281
Mydrilate. *See* Cyclopentolate
Myelitis, transverse, in systemic lupus erythematosus, 344
Myelography, in vertebral column injuries, 186, 193
Myeloma, anion gap and, 327
Myeloma, multiple
    carpal tunnel syndrome and, 347
    chest wall syndrome vs., 348
    hypercalcemia and, 282, 313, 317, 318
    hyponatremia and, 272
Mylanta II, for hypomagnesemia, 287
Myocardial contusion, 1081, 1186–1187
    as cardiogenic shock cause, 74
    sternal fracture and, 1183
Myocardial depressant factor
    cardiogenic shock and, 74
    hypovolemic shock and, 71
Myocardial infarction
    acute, 965–995
        cardiac output and, 992–993
        cardiogenic shock from, 72–75
        ECGs in, 967–970, 971–982, 986–988
        hypertension management, 993–994
        hypokalemia risk with, 296
        hypotension management, 992–993
        immediate interventions, 966, 982
        management of, 982–985, 989–992
        myocardial ischemia effects, 966
        pathogenesis of, 965–966
        physical examination in, 967–982
        prehospital care, 983
        preshock syndrome with, 73–74
        pulmonary edema and, 1097
        symptoms of, 967
        transfer to CCU for, 994

    acute aortic dissection vs., 1082
    in anaphylaxis, 75
    cocaine and, 789, 792
    congestive heart failure and, 993
    diabetic ketoacidosis and, 235
    HHNK and, 244
    pulmonary artery pressure monitoring with, 83
    shoulder-hand syndrome and, 347
    syncope and, 960, 963
    treatment for, adrenal hemorrhage risk with, 256
Myocardial ischemia
    in anaphylaxis, 75
    ECGs in, 969, 971, 973
    effects of, 966
    in hypovolemic shock, 71
    symptoms of, 966
Myocardial rupture, 1081
Myocarditis
    as cardiogenic shock cause, 74
    in systemic lupus erythematosus, 340
Myoclonus
    as hyponatremia sign, 271
    in toxicologic emergencies, 472
Myoclonus epilepsy, 372
Myoglobinuria
    burns and, 418, 427
    electrical burns and, 427
Myositis, 409–410
Myotonic dystrophy, 369, 370
Myringotomy, for otitis media, 381
Myxedema, carpal tunnel syndrome and, 347
Myxedema coma, 251–252

N

Nadolol (Corgard), 1395
    for headache prophylaxis, 922, 924
    for ventricular premature complexes, 1005
Nafcillin (Unipen; Nafcil), 1415
    for cellulitis, 431
    for corneal ulcers, 1275, 1278
    hypokalemia risk with, 294
    for meningitis, purulent, 398
    for oropharyngeal infections, 383
    for sepsis, 406
    for septic arthritis, 357, 412
    for sinusitis, 1303
Nagel, Dr. Eugene, advanced EMT training by, 4
Nail bed, herpetic whitlow of, 408
Nail-bed injuries, 154, 207
Nails
    fungal infections of, 436
    lacerations through, 154
Nalfon. *See* Fenoprofen
Naloxone HCl (Narcan), 1449
    in CPR, of pediatric patients, 523
    for hypothermia, 671
    for pain relief, 881
    for shock, 85, 86
        mechanism of, 87
    in toxicologic emergencies, 479
        meperidine overdose, 794–795
        narcotic overdose, 472
        opioid overdose, 472, 796
        prehospital care, 469
        propoxyphene overdose, 795
        TMF overdose, 799
    in wound management, 139
Naltrexone, for opioid withdrawal, 798, 799
Naphtha inhalation, 806
Naproxen (Naprosyn), 1404–1405
    as aseptic meningitis cause, 344
    for pain relief, 881
Narcan. *See* Naloxone HCl
Narcolepsy, amphetamines for, 790
Narcosis, in hypermagnesemia, 308
Narcotic analgesics, 1436, 1437
    anaphylaxis risk with, 75
    for pain relief, 880–881, 883
    in wound management, 139
Narcotic antagonists, for pain relief, 881

Narcotic-opiate toxicologic syndrome, 472
Narcotics
 in burn treatment, precautions, 423
 for headache, 922
 hyponatremia and, 271
 overdose of
  in children or adolescents, 590
  clinical signs, 472
  naloxone for, 479
 as urticaria cause, 440
NAS. *See* National Academy of Sciences
Nasal disorders. *See* Nose
Nasal intubation. *See* Nasotracheal intubation
Nasal trumpets. *See* Nasopharyngeal airways
Nasogastric intubation
 with abdominal injuries, 111
 for burn patients, 423
 for Crohn's disease, 462
 for lower GI bleeding, 451
 for pancreatitis, 456
 in toxicologic emergencies, 475
 for upper GI bleeding, 449
Nasogastric suction, metabolic alkalosis and, 327
Nasopharyngeal airways, 95–96, 1103–1104
 for children, 517
Nasopharyngeal culture, in otitis media, 1309
Nasotracheal intubation, 98, 1110
 in acute epiglottitis, 1122
 for esophageal burns, 451
 laryngeal trauma and, 1317
 in maxillofacial trauma, 1321
Nasotracheal suctioning, procedure, 1362–1363
National Academy of Sciences (NAS), 1
 EMS research role, 1, 2–3
National Association of EMS Physicians, on PASG, 5
National Association of State Emergency Medical
  Services Directors clearinghouse, 3, 27
 on funding sources, 23
 on number of ambulances, 15–16
 on number and type of EMTs, 4, 6
National Center for Health Services Research, EMS
  grants by, 2
National Clearinghouse. *See* National Association of
  State Emergency Medical Services Directors
  clearinghouse
National Disaster Medical System (NDMS), 37
National EMS Pilots Association, 26
National Fire Protection Association (NFPA),
  hazardous materials placard system, 749
National Flight Nurses Association, 26
National Flight Paramedics Association, 26
National Guard, in disaster linkages, 12
National Highway Traffic Safety Administration, 1–2.
  See also Department of Transportation
 EMS grants by, 2
 helicopter transport and, 26
National Institute for Occupational Safety and Health
  (NIOSH), formation of, 748
National Institutes of Health (NIH)
 on FFP indications, 121
 quality management role, 62
National Leadership Commission on Health Care,
  standards and, 62
National Practitioner Data Bank, 55–56, 58, 59, 60
National Registry of Emergency Medical Technicians
 certification by, 3, 4, 6
 formation of, 2
National Research Council (NRC), 1
 Commission on Life Sciences, 2–3
 EMS research by, 1, 2–3
National Traffic Safety Agency. *See* National
  Highway Traffic Safety Administration
National Training Course, 4
Native American religions, beliefs and practices, 868
Natural disasters. *See* Disaster management
Natural gas, asphyxiation injury by, 764
Nausea. *See also* Nausea and vomiting
 drug-related, atropine for, 985
 with headache, treatments for, 922
Nausea and vomiting
 in acute glaucoma, 1288

 in adrenal insufficiency, 259
 in anaphylaxis, 75
 in brain abscess, 400
 in cancer patients, chemotherapy reactions, 509
 in Crohn's disease, 461–462
 dehydration risk with, 267
 in encephalitis, 400
 in food poisoning, 390
 in gastroenteritis, 387
 in hypercalcemia, 283
 in hypomagnesemia, 286, 304
 as hyponatremia sign, 271
 in meningitis, purulent, 397
 in septic shock, 72
Nazarenes, beliefs and practices, 868
NDMS (National Disaster Medical System), 37
Near-drowning. *See* Drowning and near-drowning
Nebcin. *See* Tobramycin
Nebulization therapy
 MDI with spacer vs., 1132
 for asthma, 578, 581, 1132
 for laryngotracheitis (viral croup), 1115
Neck injuries
 blunt injuries to, 1074–1075
 in children, airway obstruction and, 566
 laryngeal trauma, 1313–1317
 patient transport with, 187
 penetrating injuries to, 1074
 prehospital care, 104–109
 types of, 104
 vascular, 1074–1075
Neck pain
 in cardiogenic shock, 75
 in stroke, 920
Necrobiosis lipoidica diabeticorum, 433
Needle cricothyroidotomy. *See* Cricothyrotomy
  (cricothyroidotomy)
Needle pericardiocentesis. *See* Pericardiocentesis
Needle thoracostomy. *See* Thoracostomy
Negligence, 40, 61. *See also* Legal issues
Neisseria catarrhalis, in otitis media, 1309
Neisseria gonorrhoeae. *See also* Terms beginning with
  Gonococcal
 in corneal ulcers, 1274, 1275
 in gastroenteritis, 388, 390
 in pelvic inflammatory disease, 1233
 in pharyngitis, 376, 378
 in prostatitis, 395
 in septic arthritis, 410, 411
 urethritis in men and, 394, 395
Neisseria meningitidis
 in acute sepsis, 406
 in febrile children under two, 530
 in meningitis, 396, 398
 OHP as bacteriocidal for, 704
 in pharyngitis, 376
 in pneumonia, 383
 in septic arthritis, 410
Nematocysts, stings by, 717–721
Nembutal. *See* Pentobarbital
Neo-Synephrine. *See* Phenylephrine; Phenylephrine
  hydrochloride
Neomycin (Mycifradin; Neomycin), 1410
 eye drop preparation, 1268
 for corneal ulcers, 1277, 1278
Neomycin-lactulose, for acute liver failure, 458
Neonates. *See also* Infants; Premature infants
 adrenal insufficiency etiologies in, 258
 CPR of
  at delivery in ED, 526–527
  drugs in, 521, 522
  endotracheal intubation, 518
  equipment list for, 526
  hypothermia and, 525–526
  umbilical access, 521
 drug abuse in pregnancy and, 810
 heat illness and, 655
 hepatitis B prevention in, 404–405
 hydration and, 265–266
 hypomagnesemia in, 305
 hypothermia in, 661–662

 meconium aspiration by, 1166–1167
 meningitis in, 396, 537
 pharmacokinetic problems in, 483, 484
 pneumonia in, 585
 testicular torsion in, 1213
 vomiting in, 557–558
Neonatology, specialized transport in, 9
Neoplasms. *See* Cancer; Malignancies; *specific types*
Neoplastic disorders
 adrenal insufficiency and, 257
 hereditary, 369, 370–371
Nephritis, acute interstitial, 1223
Nephrocalcinosis, hypercalcemia and, 281, 282
Nephrogenic diabetes insipidus, 268, 270
Nephrolithiasis
 adrenal insufficiency vs., 259
 hypercalcemia and, 281
Nephropathy, hypokalemia and, 293, 294. *See also*
  terms beginning with Renal
Nephrosis, congenital (Finnish), 372
Nephrostomy, percutaneous, in renal obstruction,
  1222, 1223
Nephrotic syndrome, anion gap decrease in, 327
Neptazane. *See* Methazolamide
Nerve conduction, potassium and, 273–274
Nervine toxicity, anion gap and, 327
Nesacaine. *See* 2-Chloroprocaine
Netilmicin (Netromycin), 1410–1411
Neuralgia
 facial pain with, 920
 occipital, 920
 postherpetic, 442
 trigeminal, as facial pain cause, 920
Neurofibromatosis (Von Recklinghausen's disease),
  369, 371
Neuroleptics, for acute psychiatric confusion, 956. *See
  also specific drugs*
Neurolinguistic programming (NLP), 872–875
Neurologic assessment. *See* Neurologic examination
Neurologic disorders
 adrenal insufficiency and, 259
 in cancer patients, 502–504
 in connective tissue disease, 343–344
 hypermagnesemia and, 308
 hypomagnesemia and, 304, 305
 hyponatremia and, 271
 spongy degeneration of central nervous system, 372
Neurologic emergencies, pediatric, 589–596
 etiologies of, 589–591
 febrile convulsions, 595–596
 management of, 591–592
 status epilepticus, 592–595
Neurologic examination
 in acute confusional state, 952
 of comatose patient, 931–933
  Glasgow Coma Scale, 591, 592
  infants and children, 591–592
 for compartment syndrome, of forearm, 205
 in head injury, 892, 894–896
 hypocalcemia signs, 284–285
 in maxillofacial injury, 1322
 prehospital, in multisystem trauma, 104–107
 in shock response, 76
 in syncope, 962
 in systemic lupus erythematosus, importance of,
  344
 in toxicologic emergencies, 470
 in upper extremity injuries, 195
 in vertebral column injury, 181–182
  repeating, 188
 in wrist injury, 205
Neurologic impairment
 in acute liver failure, 458
 in carpal tunnel syndrome, 347
 in cerebrovascular accident, 936–937
 cocaine and, 789
 focal
  in brain abscess, 400
  encephalitis and, 400
  in head injury, 895
  meningitis and, 397

Neurologic impairment (contd.)
  in food poisoning, 391
  in head injury, 894–896
  in hyperosmolar hyperglycemic nonketotic coma, 243
  in hypokalemia, 295
  in hypothermia, 662, 666
  in infectious mononucleosis, 401
  in intracerebral hemorrhage, 941
  in Lyme disease, 357
  in migraine headache, 916
  in PCP intoxication, 808
  in shock, cardiogenic, 75
  in shoulder-hand syndrome, 347
  in systemic lupus erythematosus, 343–344
  in toxicologic emergencies, 472–473
  in vertebral column injuries, 175, 183–185
    assessing for, 180, 181–183
    Stryker frame for, 188
Neuromuscular blocking agents, in endotracheal intubation, 1106, 1107
Neuromuscular impairment
  differential diagnosis, 344, 345
  in hyperkalemia, 299
  in hypokalemia, 277, 295
  hypomagnesemia and, 304, 305
  in soft tissue rheumatism, 344–348
  succinylcholine for, hyperkalemia risk with, 298
Neuropathy, peripheral, differential diagnosis, 343
Neurosis, depressive (dysthymic disorder), 830
Neurotoxins
  as gastroenteritis cause, 387–388
  in shellfish poisoning, 734–735
Neurovascular examination, in upper extremity injury, 195
Neurovascular syndromes
  in hemorrhagic CVA, 939–943
  in ischemic CVA, 937–939
Nevus flammeus, 365
New York State
  antidumping regulations, 43
  hospital liability law in, 61
NFPA. See National Fire Protection Association
Nickel carbonyl toxicity, 757
Nicotine, as sympathomimetic, 787
Niemann-Pick disease, 372
Nifedipine (Procardia), 1395
  for congestive heart failure, 1055
  for headache prophylaxis, 924
  for high-altitude pulmonary edema, 684
  for hypertensive emergencies, 1061, 1063
    catecholamine crisis, 1067
    eclampsia, 1066
  for intra-arterial foreign substance, 1075
  for pulmonary edema, 1099
Night blindness, in hereditary disorders, 372
Night-stick fracture, 205
NIH. See National Institutes of Health
Nikolsky's sign, 437
Nilstat. See Nystatin
Nimodipine (Nimotop), 1395
911 service, 9
NIOSH. See National Institute for Occupational Safety and Health
Nipride. See Sodium nitroprusside
Nitrate intoxication, 473, 757
Nitrite intoxication, 473, 757
  by inhalation, 805, 806
Nitro compound intoxication, 473, 757
  clinical signs, 473, 479
  methylene blue for, 479
Nitro-Bid; Nitro-Dur. See Nitroglycerin
Nitroaniline intoxication, 473
Nitrobenzene intoxication, 473, 757
Nitrofurantoin (Macrodantin), 1422
  renal failure and, 1225
  for urinary tract infections, 393, 394
Nitrogen dioxide inhalation, 770–771
  from fires, 494
Nitrogen gas, asphyxiation injury by, 764
Nitroglycerin (Nitrostat; Nitrol; Nitro-Bid; Transderm-Nitro; Nitro-Dur), 1395–1396
  in acute myocardial infarction treatment, 982, 983, 985, 993
  for congestive heart failure, 1055, 1056
  for hypertensive emergencies, 1061, 1063
  for pulmonary edema, 1099
Nitrol. See Nitroglycerin
Nitronox, for self-administered anesthesia, 886, 889
Nitrophenol intoxication, 473
2-Nitropropane, as systemic toxin, 774
Nitroprusside. See Sodium nitroprusside
Nitroprusside test
  in diabetic ketoacidosis, 235, 236
  in HHNK coma, 244
Nitrosoureas, pulmonary reactions to, 508
Nitrostat. See Nitroglycerin
Nitrous oxide
  abuse of, 805
  as general anesthesia, 886
  in wound management, 139
Nixon, President Richard, EMS Act of 1973 and, 2
Nizoral. See Ketoconazole
NLP (neurolinguistic programming), 872–875
Nocardia asteroides
  in eye infection, culture media for, 1270
  in pneumonia, 383
Noctec. See Chloral hydrate
Nondepolarizing muscle relaxants, in endotracheal intubation, 1106, 1107
Nonparoxysmal junctional tachycardia (NPJT), 1018, 1028, 1029
Nonsteroidal anti-inflammatory agents (NSAIDs), 1403–1405
  anaphylaxis risk with, 75
  for frostbite, 673
  for gout, 357
  for headache, 923
  hyperkalemia risk with, 298
  listed, 881
  meningitis as complication of, 344
  for pain relief, 880
    dosages, 881
  for polyarticular arthritis, 359
  renal failure and, 1225–1226
  septic arthritis and, 357
  side effects of, 880
  for systemic lupus erythematosus, 340
Nonverbal communication, 873
Noonan's syndrome, 364, 365
Norcuron. See Vecuronium
Norepinephrine or Levarterenol (Levophed), 1387–1388
  in acute myocardial infarction treatment, 984, 992
  for drug reaction, 433
  hypothermia and, 671
  in response to injury, 69
  for shock, 84
    diagnosis and, 66–67
    hypovolemic, 68, 70
  spinal injuries and, 104
Norfloxacin (Noroxin), 1422–1423
  for urethritis in men, 395
  for urinary tract infections, 393
Norfloxan, for dysenteric gastroenteritis, 390
Norisodrine. See Isoproterenol, inhaled
Normodyne. See Labetalol
Normovolemia, hyponatremia with, 271
Noroxin. See Norfloxacin
Norpace. See Disopyramide
Norval. See Mianserin
Norwalk virus
  in food poisoning, 390–391, 733
  in gastroenteritis, 388
Norzimelidine, 487
Nose
  foreign bodies in, 1307–1308
  in Raynaud's phenomenon, 341
  trauma to, 1327–1328
    lacerations, 152–153, 157
    wound dressings for, 157
Nose medications, for emergency department, 1453
Nosebleeds, 1304–1306
  maxillofacial injuries and, 110

Nosocomial infections. See also Iatrogenic disorders
  pneumonia, 383
  purulent meningitis, treatment of, 398
  sinusitis, 1302–1303
Novocain. See Procaine hydrochloride
NPJT. See Nonparoxysmal junctional tachycardia
NRC. See National Research Council
NSAIDs. See Nonsteroidal anti-inflammatory agents
Nuchal rigidity
  in aseptic meningitis, 399
  in purulent meningitis, 397
Nuclear scans. See Radionuclide scans
Numorphan. See Oxymorphone
Nurses, on-line medical control by, 20
Nutrition
  emergency department agents for, 1453
  magnesium requirements, 303
  renal failure and, 1225
Nutritional deficit
  as hypokalemia cause, 294
  as hypomagnesemia cause, 305
Nylon sutures, 142
Nystagmus
  hereditary, 370
  as toxin ingestion sign, 474
Nystatin (Mycostatin; Nilstat), 1423
  for thrush, 378, 437

O

O_2PBDs. See Oxygen powered breathing devices
OB. See Occult bacteremia
Obesity
  heat illness and, 655
  interventions for, hypomagnesemia from, 306
OBRA. See Omnibus Budget Reconciliation Act of 1990
Obstetric emergencies, 1234–1240
  history taking in, 1229
Obstipation, in hypercalcemia, 283
Obstructive airway disease, 1129–1138. See also Asthma
  COPD, headache and, 917
  definitions, 1129
  diagnosis of, 1130–1132
  differential diagnosis, 1131
  management algorithms for, 1136, 1137
  pathogenesis of, 1130
  treatment of, 1132–1136
    antibiotics, 1135
    anticholinergics, 1134
    calcium channel blockers, 1136
    disposition and, 1136–1138
    magnesium, 1135
    mechanical ventilation, 1134–1135
    methylxanthines, 1134
    oxygen, 1132
    steroids, 1135–1136
    sympathomimetics, 1133
Obtundation. See Coma
Occipital neuralgia, 920
Occult bacteremia (OB), in febrile children under two, 529–533
  evaluating for, 530–532
  frequency of, 529
  management of, 532–533
Occupational disorders. See also Hazardous materials; specific disorders
  adrenal insufficiency, 256
  arterial air embolism, in divers, 708–709
  asthma, 1130
  carpal tunnel syndrome, 347
  decompression sickness (DCS), 705–707
  hepatitis B, in health care workers, 785
  hypothermia, in divers, 662
  marine organisms and, 711
  metal poisoning, 493–494, 1161–1162
  pharyngitis, 377
  radiation accidents, 617–624, 758–759
  sea moss dermatitis (Dogger Bank itch), 741
  skin infections, 408–409

sponge fisherman's disease, 716
statistics on, 761, 762
Occupational injuries. *See also* Occupational toxicologic emergencies
to penis, 1208
sedative-hypnotic abuse and, 800
statistics on, 761, 762
Occupational Safety and Health Administration (OSHA)
on asphyxiants, 764
formation of, 747
hazardous materials regulations, 748, 750
Occupational toxicologic emergencies. *See also* Chemical injury
decontamination procedures, 762–763
history taking in, 762, 763
management principles, 762–763
systemic toxins, 773–776
toxic gas inhalation, 763–773, 1162, 1175–1180
chemical asphyxiants, 764–769
from fires, 772–773
irritant gases, 769–772
physical asphyxiants, 763–764
toxins listed by occupation, 1175–1180
Octopuses, 730–731
Ocular emergencies, 1259–1289. *See also* Eyes; *Terms beginning with* Eye
in connective tissue disease, 337–339
Behçet's syndrome, 338–339
rheumatoid arthritis, 338
seronegative spondyloarthropathies, 338
Sjögren's disease, 338
systemic lupus erythematosus, 338
temporal arteritis, 337–338
corneal abrasions or foreign bodies, 1266–1270
emergency department and, 1259, 1261, 1295
herpetic ocular disease, 1264–1266
history taking in, 1261–1262
hyphema, 1282–1286
infections, 1296–1297
antibiotics for, 1275, 1276, 1277–1278
cavernous sinus thrombosis, 1296
cellulitis, 1296
corneal ulcers (bacterial keratitis), 1273–1276, 1277–1278
diagnostic tests, 1270–1273
endophthalmitis, treatment of, 1297
terminology, 1295–1296
trauma
corneal abrasions or foreign bodies, 1266–1270
diagnostic studies, 1284
differential diagnosis, 1284
hyphema, 1282–1286
physical examination in, 1262–1264
post-traumatic preseptal cellulitis, 1297
visual acuity testing in, 1262, 1263, 1284
uveitis, 1276, 1277–1282
Oculocephalic maneuver (doll's eyes)
in head injury, 895, 896
in unresponsiveness assessment, 933
psychogenic, 931
Oculomotor nerve. *See* Cranial nerves
Oculomotor ophthalmoplegia, in temporal arteritis, 337
Oculovestibular reflex, 933
in head injury, 895, 896
in infants and children, 592
in psychogenic unresponsiveness, 931
Odontoid (dens) fractures, 190, 907, 908
Odontoid process destruction, in rheumatoid arthritis, 343
Odynophagia, esophageal obstruction and, 452
Office of Technology Assessment, on quality indicators, 53, 54
Ohio Hope II bag, 99–100
OHP. *See* Oxygen under high pressure
Olecranon bursa, aspiration or injection of, 1374
Olecranon bursitis, septic, 204, 412
Olecranon fractures, 203
Olfactory nerve. *See* Cranial nerves
Oliguria
defined, 1218

in dehydration, 268
in renal failure, 1218, 1221
Omeprazole (Prilosec), 1434
Omnibus Budget Reconciliation Acts, 7
on PROs, 58
quality assurance and, 58
Oncologic emergencies, 501–511
adrenal crisis, 506
cardiopulmonary, 510–511
chemotherapy complications, 508–509
hematologic, 509–510
infectious, 505–506
metabolic, 506–508
neurologic, 502–504
pathologic fractures, 504–505
platelet transfusion for, 122
psychosocial factors, 501–502
radiation therapy complications, 508
surgical, 504–505
Ondansetron (Zofran), 1407
"Open book" pelvic injury, 213
Open fractures, 161
blood loss risk with, 168
classification of, 166–168
treatment of, 172
Ophthalmologic disease, as headache cause, 917
Opiates. *See also* Opioids; *specific drugs*
defined, 793
hypothermia and, 662
for pain relief, 880–881, 882
as unconsciousness cause, 591
Opioids, 793–799. *See also specific drugs*
abstinence syndromes, 798–799
defined, 793
extent of abuse, 793
intoxication and overdose of, 795–798
for pain relief, 880–881, 882
pharmacology of, 793, 794–795
in pregnancy, effects on neonate, 810
referral requirements, 799
screening tests for, 786
Optic nerve. *See* Cranial nerves
Oral contraceptives. *See* Birth control pills
Oral intubation
for children, 515
prehospital, controversy about, 6
problems in, 1109–1110
rapid sequence, 942, 1106–1107
techniques, 1108–1109
Oral lesions, herpetic, 381, 1336
Oral mucosa, lacerations of, 1336–1337
Oral secretions, as wound contamination source, 138
Oral-facial infections, 381–383
herpes simplex type 1, 441–442, 1336
measles, 443
syphilis, 439
thrush, 377, 378, 436–437
"Orange book," 3
Oratrol. *See* Dichlorphenamide
Orbital cellulitis, 1296
Orbital floor fractures, 1329–1330
Orchitis, acute, 1212
Ordinances, 39
Organ donation; Organ transplants
air medical transport for, 25
approaching family about, 861
legal issues, 43
Organic solvent toxicity, 474, 756–757
Organometallic compound toxicity, 757
Organophosphate toxicity, 757
diagnosis of, 775–776
hypothermia and, 662
treatment of, 474, 478–479, 757, 776
Ornithinemia with gyrate atrophy of the retina, 372
Oropharyngeal airways, 95–96
children and, 516–517, 544–545
Oropharyngeal infections, 382–383
aspiration pneumonia and, 385
odontogenic, 1331–1333
Oropharyngeal trauma, retropharyngeal abscess and, 569
Orotracheal intubation. *See* Oral intubation

Orthostatic hypotension, as hypovolemia, 70
Orthostatic syncope, 961, 963
Orudis. *See* Ketoprofen
OSHA. *See* Occupational Safety and Health Administration
Osler-Weber-Rendu syndrome, 364, 365, 368
Osmitrol. *See* Mannitol
Osmolar gap, ethylene glycol/methanol intoxication and, 325
Osteoarthritis
Baker's cyst in, 346
central cord syndrome and, 184
Osteogenesis imperfecta, 364
Osteomalacia, hypocalcemia and, 284
Osteomyelitis
as acute monoarticular arthritis cause, 358
drug abuse and, 785
in elbow, 204
foot ulcers and, 231
as human bite complication, 156
as puncture wound complication, in feet, 154
vertebral, 193–194
Osteoporosis
Colles' fractures and, 205
pathological fractures with, 166
in shoulder-hand syndrome, 347
Otitis, 379–381
externa (swimmer's ear), 379–380, 1310, 1311
media, 380–381, 1309–1310
Oto-palatal-digital syndrome, 364
Otolaryngologic emergencies, 1299–1311
acute sinusitis, 1299–1303
epistaxis, 1304–1306
foreign bodies, 1307–1309
peritonsillary abscess (quinsy), 1303–1304
tympanic membrane perforations, 1306–1307
Otorrhea
assessing for, 110
in head injury, 898, 901
Outcomes management, 54, 55, 62
Outrigger, on palmar plaster splint, 209
Ova and parasites, stool examination for, 390
Ovarian masses, in pregnancy, 1236. *See also* Pelvic inflammatory disease; Pelvic pain
Over-the-counter drugs, overdose of, 491
Overflow incontinence, in cauda equina syndrome, 193
Overhead skeletal traction, for supracondylar fracture, 202
Oxacillin (Prostaphlin), 1415–1416
for corneal ulcers, 1275, 1277, 1278
for cutaneous abscesses, 408
eye drop preparation, 1268
for meningitis, purulent, 953
for oropharyngeal infections, 383
for sepsis, 406
for septic arthritis, 412
for septic shock, 85
for sinusitis, 1303
Oxazepam (Serax)
for alcohol withdrawal, 820, 821
elimination half-life of, 800
overdose of, 491–492
Oxtriphylline (Choledyl; Choledyl SA), 1427
Oxycodone, as opioid, 793. *See also* Percocet; Percodan
Oxygen administration
in acute myocardial infarction treatment, 993, 994
for asthma, 1132
for carbon monoxide poisoning, 1161
for congestive heart failure, 1054
for COPD, 1132
in endotracheal intubation, 1106, 1107
for headache, 922–923
for high-altitude illness, 682
humidified, for laryngotracheitis, 1115
for hypothermia, 671
for methemoglobinemia, 479
methods of
compared, 1132
transcutaneous oxygen monitor, 83
for multifocal atrial tachycardia (MAT), 1022

Oxygen administration (contd.)
    for near-drowning, 695–696, 698
    in obstructive airway disease, 1132
    oxygen under high pressure (OHP), in hyperbaric medicine, 702–704
    to pediatric patients
        in CPR, 516, 519, 522
        in respiratory emergencies, 577
    for pulmonary edema
        cardiogenic, 1098, 1099
        noncardiogenic, 1101
    for shock, 76
    in toxicologic emergencies, 477–478
    prehospital care, 469
Oxygen consumption monitoring, for shock, 82–83
Oxygen powered breathing devices (O^2PBDs), contraindicated for children, 516, 519
Oxygen-hemoglobin dissociation curve, 1152, 1153
Oxymetazoline, for sinusitis, 1303
Oxymorphone (Numorphan), as opioid, 793
Oxyphenbutazone (Tandearil), 1405
Oxyphenonium (Antrenyl), for uveitis, 1281
Oxytocin (Pitocin; Syntocinon), 1446
    for postpartum hemorrhage, 1238
Oysters, poisoning by, 391, 731–734
Ozone inhalation, 771

P

Pacemaker. See Pacing therapy
Pacing, as communication skill, 873
Pacing artifacts, 1042, 1043
Pacing catheter, 1351
Pacing therapy, 1042–1049
    in acute myocardial infarction treatment, 985
    components of, 1042
    dual-chamber system, 1047–1049
    for dysrhythmias
        atrioventricular (AV) block, 1013
        recurrent supraventricular bradydysrhythmias, 1011
    system malfunctions, 1043, 1045, 1046–1047
    temporary transvenous pacemaker placement, 1351–1352
Paget's disease, hypercalcemia and, 282
Pain. See also Headache; specific pain locations
    acute vs. chronic, 877–878
    assessment of, 879
    classifications of, 877–878
    communication about, 879
    defined, 877
    emergency room treatment of, 879–880
    management of. See Pain management
    prolonged, defined, 878
    situational factors and, 879
    superficial vs. deep, 877
    theories of, 878–879
        endorphins and, 879
        Gate Control Theory, 878–879
Pain management, 880–889
    in acute myocardial infarction, 985
    alternative modalities for, 887–888
    for chronic pain, 878
    disassociation in, 874
    emergency practitioner's role in, 888–889
    endorphins in, 879
    future directions in, 889
    Gate Control Theory and, 878–879
    general anesthesia for, 886–887
    for headache patients, 922–924
    local anesthesia for, 884–885
    patient control for, 889
    pharmacology of, 880–884
    regional blocks for, 885
    topical anesthesia for, 885–886
    undertreatment problems, 879–880
Pain sensation
    hypothermia and, 666
    physiology of, 877
    time distortion and, 874
Paint gun injuries, 155
Paint remover intoxication, 478
    carbon monoxide and, 765

Paint thinner intoxication, 324, 325
    by inhalant abuse, 805, 806
Palmar plaster splint, 209
Palms, erythema multiforme on, 434
Palpitation, dysrhythmia and, 997
2-PAM. See Pralidoxime
Panadol. See Acetaminophen
Pancreas, hypothermia and, 666
Pancreatic adenomas, hypercalcemia and, 282
Pancreatic cancer
    in hereditary disorders, 370, 371
    hyponatremia and, 271
Pancreatic disease, 455–456
Pancreatic enzyme supplements, anaphylaxis risk with, 75
Pancreatic fistula, metabolic acidosis and, 321
Pancreatitis, 455–456
    acute
        hypocalcemia and, 284
        hypomagnesemia and, 286, 306
        in systemic lupus erythematosus, 342
    adrenal insufficiency vs., 259
    clinical signs of, 455
    diabetic ketoacidosis vs., 235
    diagnosis of, 455–456
    etiologies of, 455
    hereditary, 369, 370
    hypercalcemia and, 281
    hypocalcemia and, 284
    hyponatremia and, 270
    hypothermia and, 666
    treatment of, 456
Pancuronium (Pavulon), 1443
Pancytopenia, Fanconi's, 364, 365, 366, 368
Panniculitis, 336
Papaver somniferum, drugs derived from, 793
Papaverine (Pavabid; Papaverine), 1396
    for intra-arterial foreign substance, 1075
    for pain relief, 882
Papillary muscle rupture, as cardiogenic shock cause, 74
Papilledema
    in brain abscess, 400
    meningitis and, 397
        in children under two, 536, 537
    in pseudotumor cerebri, 919
    in unresponsive patient, 931
Papoose board, in wound management, 139
Papulovesicular lesions, 336
Paracentesis
    for ascites, 459
    indications for, 342
Paracoccidioidomycosis, adrenal insufficiency and, 258
Parainfluenza
    pharyngitis and, 376
    pneumonia and, 383
Parainfluenza viruses, in common colds, 376
Paraldehyde, 1398–1399
    for alcohol withdrawal, 820
    intoxication by, 324
    for pain relief, 884
    for status epilepticus, 947
Paralysis
    ascending, in hyperkalemia, 299
    in cervical spine fracture, 192
    in food poisoning, 391, 734–735
    in hyperkalemia, 299
    in hypermagnesemia, 308
    hypokalemia and, 295
    in incomplete spinal cord injury, 184–185
    periodic
        hyperkalemia and, 279, 298, 300
        hypokalemia and, 276, 294
        treatment of, 278, 300
    in systemic lupus erythematosus, 344
Paralytic ileus, 459–460
Paralytic shellfish poisoning (PSP), 391, 734–735
Paramedics. See also Emergency medical technicians
    accreditation of training for, 27
    CPR successes and, 1092
    as dispatch personnel, 22
    EMT-P training, 3–6

Paranoia, drug-induced, 474
Paraquat poisoning, 809
Parasites
    encephalitis and, 400
    lice, 437
    scabies, 438–439
    stool examination for, 390
Parasympathetic nervous system
    cardiogenic shock and, 74
    in response to injury, 69
Parasympathetic stimulating agents, for PSVT, 1026
Parasympatholytics, 1281
Parasystole, 1005–1007
Parathormone, calcium levels and, 281, 313
    in hyperkalemia, 282
Parathyroid gland, congenital absence of, hypocalcemia and, 284
Parathyroid hormone, magnesium reabsorption and, 304
Parathyroid tumors, hypocalcemia and, 284
    adenoma, 282
    carcinoma, 317–318
Parathyroidectomy, hypocalcemia and, 284
Paredrine. See Hydroxyamphetamine
Paregoric
    for diarrhea, 389
    as opioid, 793
Parenteral fluids. See Hyperalimentation
Paresthesias
    in carpal tunnel syndrome, 347
    in hypocalcemia, 284
    in rheumatoid arthritis, 343
    in shellfish poisoning, 391
    in shoulder-hand syndrome, 347
    in systemic lupus erythematosus, 344
Parkinsonism, MPTP-induced, 799–800
Paronychia, 210
Paroxysmal supraventricular tachycardia (PSVT), 1018, 1024–1028
    Wolff-Parkinson-White syndrome and, 1028, 1037, 1042
Parvovirus, polyarthralgias with, 359
PASG. See Pneumatic anti-shock garment
Pasteurella multocida
    from cat bites, 156, 157, 631, 632
    from dog bites, 155, 630, 632
Pasteurella tularensis, in eye infection, 1271
Patella, fractures of, 222–223
Pathologic fractures, 166
    in cancer patients, 504–505
Patient education
    on diabetic ketoacidosis, 241–242
    on headache, 924–925
Patients
    alcoholic, relations with, 818, 822–823
    communication with, techniques for, 870–875
    death of
        emotional responses to, 860–862
        spiritual responses to, 864
    emotional needs of, 858–860
    evaluation of care by, 62
    holistic model for care of, 857–858
    spiritual needs of, 862–865
    transfer of. See Transfer of patients
Pauciarticular arthritis, differential diagnosis, 351
Pavabid. See Papaverine
Pavulon. See Pancuronium
Payment for care, access and, 6–7
PCBs (polychlorinated biphenyls), 747
PCP (pentachlorophenol) toxicity, 757–758
PCP (phencyclidine) abuse, 807–808
    psychosis and, 808
    screening tests for, 786
Peak expiratory rate (PEFR), in obstructive airway disease, 1132
Peau d'orange
    in hereditary disorder, 368–369
    in inguinal hernia, 559
Pectin, for diarrhea, 389
Pectus excavatum, in hereditary disorders, 364, 365, 367
Pedal spasm

in hypocalcemia, 284
in hypomagnesemia, 286
Pedestrian injuries, to children, 541–542
Pediatric emergencies, ED classification for, 48
Pediatric patients
   abdominal injuries in, 543
      acute management of, 550–551
      child abuse and, 542
      with multiple trauma, 549, 550
   abdominal pain in, 555–557
   abuse of. *See* Child abuse
   acid ingestion by, 554
   acute gastroenteritis in, 387, 388
   acute monoarticular arthritis in, 357, 358
   acute polyarticular arthritis in, 258
   air transport criteria, 26
   airway control devices for, 514, 517
      bag-mask units, 95
      endotracheal tubes, 97
   airway obstruction in, 563–570
      with fever, 566–570
      with sudden onset, 564–566
   anal fissure in, 466
   anaphylaxis in, 565
   ankle fractures in, 227, 228
   ankle sprains in, 230–231
   appendicitis in, 464, 555–556
   arthritis in, septic, 410, 412
   asthma in, 580–582, 1132
   bleeding in, gastrointestinal, 558–559
   bronchiolitis in, 582–583
   burns in, 553, 554
      burn center referral for, 47–48, 553
      child abuse and, 598–599
      evaluation of, 421, 422
      hypertension with, 419
   caustic ingestion by, 566
   chest injuries in, 543
      with multiple trauma, 545–546, 548, 549
   child abuse in. *See* Child abuse
   clavicle fractures in, 198
   common colds in, 375–376
   constipation in, 558
   corrosive ingestion by, 553–554
   coughing in, croup syndromes, 1113, 1114
   CPR of, 513–527
      airway for, 513–515
      breathing assistance, 515–519
      circulation assistance, 519–521
      defibrillation, 525
      drug overdose and, 526
      drugs in, 521–525
      fluid replacement in, 521
      hypoglycemia and, 526
      hypothermia and, 525–526
      hypovolemia and, 526
   croup in, 1113–1117
      bacterial tracheitis (membranous croup), 1113, 1116–1117
      epiglottitis vs., 1114
      laryngotracheitis (LT), 567–569, 1113–1116
      spasmodic, 565, 1113, 1116
      viral, 567–569
   cyanide poisoning in, treatment for, 478
   death of, child abuse homicides, 601
   dehydration in, 268, 270
   diarrhea in, 387, 388, 558
   diphtheria in, 569–570
   dog bites and, 628
   drowning accidents and, 689, 694
   drug overdose in, 491
   dystonic reaction in, 565–566
   ear infections in, 380, 381, 1309–1310
   endotracheal intubation of, 1106
      techniques, 517–519
      tubes for, 1108
   epididymo-orchitis in, 560
   epiglottitis in, 566–567, 1114, 1117–1123
      croup vs., 1114
   erythema nodosa in, 336
   facial infections in, 381
   facial trauma in, analgesia or anesthesia for, 1325
   febrile
      occult bacteremia (OB) in, 529–533
      seizures in, 950
      stridor in, 566–570
      under 2 years old, 529–539
   fluid maintenance requirements in, 550
   foreign body emergencies, 559
      airway obstruction, 564–565, 1308
      aspiration, 515–516, 583–584, 1308
      in ear, 1307, 1308
      in esophagus, 1308–1309
      with multiple trauma, 543
      in nose, 1307–1308
   fractures in
      of ankle, 227, 228
      child abuse, 599–600
      classification of, 161, 164, 165, 166, 167
      of clavicle, 198
      of forearm, 204–205
      of hip, 221
      of tibia, 226
      upper extremity, 198, 202, 203, 204–205, 206
   gastrointestinal bleeding in, 558–559
   gastrointestinal infections in, 387, 388, 389, 390
      acute gastroenteritis, 387, 388
      acute watery diarrhea, 389, 390
      dysenteric gastroenteritis, 390
      presentation and differential diagnosis, 556
   groin and scrotum problems in, 559–560
   head injuries in, 542, 543–544
      acute management of, 550
      child abuse and, 542
      CT scans of, 549
   heat illness and, 655
   hepatitis vaccine for, 458
   hereditary disorders in, 372
      ethnic groups and, 372
      spongy degeneration of central nervous system, 372
      Tay-Sachs disease, 372
   herpetic mouth lesions in, 1336
   high-altitude pulmonary edema and, 683
   hip fractures in, 221
   hydrocarbon aspiration by, 584
   hydroceles in, 559–560
   hypocalcemic tetany in, 566
   hypothermia in, physiology and, 661
   immobilization of, hypercalcemia and, 282
   inhalation injury in, airway obstruction with, 566
   knee dislocations in, 223
   lead poisoning in, 494
   maxillofacial wounds in, anesthetic for, 1325
   measles in, 442–443
   meningitis in, 533–539
      clinical signs of, 536
      diagnosis of, 536–538
      etiologies of, 536
      pathogenesis of, 536
      prevention of, 398–399
      treatment of, 398, 538–539
      unconsciousness with, 590
   meningococcemia in, 430
   metabolic emergencies in, 590–591
   migraine in, 916
      cyproheptadine for, 922, 924
   neck trauma in, 566
   neurologic emergencies in, 589–596
      etiologies of, 589–591
      febrile convulsions, 595–596
      management of, 591–592
      status epilepticus, 592–595
   ocular disorders in, herpetic keratitis, 1265
   ocular trauma in
      hyphema treatment, 1285
      restraint use with, 1284
   oral-facial infections in, 381, 1336
   otitis in, 380, 381, 1309–1310
   patellar dislocations in, 223
   pediculosis capitis (head lice) in, 437
   periodic paralysis in, hyperkalemia and, 279
   peritonsillar abscess in, 569
   pharyngitis in, 377, 378
   pityriasis rosea in, 437–438
   pneumonia in, 383, 585–586
   pneumothorax in, spontaneous, 586–587
   rectal prolapse in, 466
   respiratory emergencies in. *See* Respiratory emergencies; *specific conditions*
   retropharyngeal abscess in, 569
   rheumatoid arthritis in, 358–359
   rubella (German measles) in, 443
   salicylate intoxication or overdose in, 325, 488
   seizures in
      absence, 949
      febrile, 950
   septic arthritis in, 410, 412
   sexual abuse of, 605–608, 1253
   sinusitis in, 379, 1300, 1301, 1302, 1303
   skin disorders in
      atopic dermatitis, 429
      pediculosis, 437
      pityriasis rosea, 437–438
      roseola infantum, 438
   skin infections in
      cellulitis, 432
      fungal, 435
      impetigo, 431
      meningococcemia, 430
      scarlet fever, 432
      staphylococcal scalded skin syndrome, 431
   spasmodic croup (SC) in, 565
   supraglottitis in. *See* Pediatric patients, epiglottitis in
   surgical emergencies in, 541–560
   testicular torsion in, 1213
   thermal injury in, from hot liquid, 566
   toxin ingestion by, 566, 590, 591. *See also* Toxicologic emergencies; *specific substances*
   tracheitis in, 569
   trauma in. *See also* Child abuse; *specific types of trauma*
      as cause of death, 541
      management of, 544–552
      minor, 552–553
      multisystem, 541–552
      patterns of injury, 541–542
      prevention of, 552
      transfer criteria and guidelines, 551–552
      upper airway obstruction (UAO) with, 563–570
   unconscious
      etiologies and, 589–591
      management of, 591–592
   upper extremity injuries in
      clavicle fractures, 198
      forearm fractures, 204–205
      fractures, 198, 202, 203, 204–205
      lateral condyle fractures, 203
      medial condyle and epicondyle fractures, 203
      radial head subluxations, 204
      supracondyle fractures, 202
      wrist fractures, 206
   varicella in, 443
   vertebral column injuries in
      differential diagnosis, 186, 187
      dislocations, 188, 189
   vomiting in, 557–558
   wound management in
      human bites, 156
      maxillofacial injuries, 1325
      premedication, 139
      TAC anesthesia for, 885–886
      tape closure problems, 148
      tetanus prophylaxis, 155
Pediatric trauma centers, 551–552
Pediatric Trauma Score, transfer and, 551, 552
Pediazole. *See* Erythromycin-sulfamethoxazole
Pediculosis, 437
PEEP. *See* Positive end expiratory pressure
Peer review
   clinical consensus panels, 61
   continuous quality improvement models, 57–58
   for quality assurance, 55, 56
Peer review organizations (PROs), 58–61
PEFR. *See* Peak expiratory rate
Pelvic fractures, 213–215
   assessing for, in multisystem trauma, 111
   classification of, 213

Pelvic fractures (contd.)
  multisystem injuries and, 215
  PASG as hemorrhage prevention in, 5
  radiographic assessment of, 213–214
  urethral injury with, 1206
  vascular emergencies with, 1072–1073
Pelvic hemorrhage, PASG for, 5
Pelvic inflammatory disease (PID), 1233–1234
  in young adolescents, 556
Pelvic injuries
  fractures
    blood loss risk with, 168
    management of, 215
  in multisystem trauma, assessing, 111
  transfer criteria, 10
Pelvic pain, as gynecologic emergency, 1229–1230.
    See also Abdominal pain
Pemphigus vulgaris, 382, 437
Pen-Vee K. *See* Penicillin V
Penetrating injuries
  to abdomen, 1072
  to bladder, 1202
  cardiac tamponade with, prehospital interventions, 103
  to chest, 1181
    intra-abdominal injuries with, 1181–1182
    in children, 541
  to diaphragm, 1188
  to esophagus, 452, 1188
  to extremities, 1073
  fractures, 163
  to head, 899
    prehospital interventions, 107
  to heart, 1078–1079, 1185–1186
    cardiac tamponade and, 1185
    management algorithm for, 1186
    pericardial tamponade in, 1080–1081
    thoracotomy procedure, 1078–1079
  to kidneys, 1198–1199
  to penis, 1208, 1209
  to scrotum or testicle, 1209
  to thorax, 1071
  tracheobronchial, 1188
  to urethra, 1205, 1206, 1207
  vascular, 1070
  to vertebral column, 175
Penicillin V (V-Cillin K; Pen-Vee K), 1416. *See also* Penicillin
Penicillin, 1416
  anaphylaxis risk with, 75
  for bacterial meningitis, 953
  for cellulitis, 431, 432
  for cutaneous abscesses, 408
  for gingivitis, 382
  for gonorrhea, 1250
  for impetigo, 431
  for Lyme disease, 357, 409
  for oropharyngeal infections, 382–383
  for otitis media, 381, 1309
  for peritonsillar abscess, 1304
  for pharyngitis, 377, 378
  for pneumonia, 386
  potassium, hyperkalemia and, 279
  procaine, for pneumonia, 386
  for prostatitis, 395
  for scarlet fever, 432
  for septic arthritis, 411, 412
  for septic bursitis, 412
  serum sickness and, 433
  for sinusitis, 379
  for skin infections, marine-associated, 408
  sodium, hypokalemia and, 294
  for toxic shock syndrome, 407
  as urticaria cause, 440
  for Vincent's infection, 1337
  in wound management, 158
    human bites, 156, 157
Penicillin derivatives, 1413–1416
Penicillin G (Pentids; Penicillin G), 1416. *See also* Penicillin
  for cat bites, 156
  for corneal ulcers, 1275, 1277, 1278
  for encephalitis with brain abscess, 401
  for erysipelas, 432
  eye drop preparation, 1268
  for gonorrhea, 1250
  for meningitis, purulent, 398
  for meningococcemia, 430
  for necrotizing fasciitis or myositis, 410
  for pneumonias, 386, 387
  for sepsis, 406
  for syphilis, 440
Penicillin-streptomycin, for open fractures, 168
Penis
  injuries to, 1208–1209
  scaling rash on, in Reiter's syndrome, 358
Pentachlorophenol (PCP) toxicity, 757–758
  acid diuresis and, 476
Pentamidine, for *Pneumocystis carinii* pneumonia, 387
Pentazocine (Talwin), 1437
  as opioid-like, 793
  pharmacology of, 795
Pentecostals, beliefs and practices, 868
Pentids. *See* Penicillin G
Pentobarbital (Nembutal; Pentobarbitone), 1440. *See also* Barbiturates
  elimination half-life of, 800
  pharmacology of, 801
  in sedative withdrawal treatment, 805
Pentothal. *See* Thiopental
Pepcid. *See* Famotidine
Pepsinogen disorders, hereditary, 369, 370
Peptic esophagitis, 452
Peptic ulcer disease
  hereditary, 369, 370
  hypercalcemia and, 281
  shoulder-hand syndrome and, 347
  treatment of, 449
    hypercalcemia risk with, 282
  upper GI bleeding with, 449
Peptostreptococcus, in oropharyngeal infections, 382
Perceptual disorders, drug-induced, 474
Percocet; Percodan
  as opioid, 793
  pharmacology of, 795
Percutaneous nephrostomy, in renal obstruction, 1222, 1223
Percutaneous pinning
  for Colles' fracture, 206
  for femoral neck fracture, 218
  for supracondylar fracture, 202
Percutaneous transtracheal ventilation, in acute epiglottitis, 1121–1122
Perfluorocarbon (PFC), as blood substitute, 128
Perfusion, respiratory failure and, 1153
Periactin. *See* Cyproheptadine
Perianal pain or numbness, in cauda equina syndrome, 193
Periarteritis, vasculitis with, 341
Periarteritis nodosa, pulmonary symptoms and, 340
Periarticular problems
  in acute monoarticular arthritis, 352
  onset of, 352
Pericardial involvement, in systemic lupus erythematosus, 340
Pericardial tamponade, 1080–1081
Pericardiocentesis, 1080–1081, 1190
  for cardiac tamponade, 103
  for electromechanical dissociation, 1091
  procedure, 1358–1360
  risks with, 103
Pericarditis, in systemic lupus erythematosus, 340
Perihepatitis, in adolescent girls, 556
Perinatal emergencies, ED classification for, 48
Perineal abscesses, 407, 408
Perinephric abscess, 1211
Perineum, burns on, as major injuries, 424
Periosteum, suture material for, 142
Peripharyngeal abscesses, 382–383
Peripheral vascular disease, necrotizing fasciitis or myositis and, 409–410
Peripheral vascular resistance
  blood pressure and, 67
  in cardiogenic shock, 74
  in septic shock, 72
Peripheral vasodilation, in anaphylaxis, 75
Peritoneal dialysis
  for hypercalcemic crisis, 315
  for hyperkalemia, 280–281, 299, 300
  for hypermagnesemia, 308
  for renal failure, 1227
  in toxicologic emergencies, 476
Peritoneal involvement, in systemic lupus erythematosus, 342
Peritoneal lavage
  for children, with multiple trauma, 550–551
  indications for, 111
  patient transfer and, 111
  procedure, 111, 1356–1357
Peritonitis
  adrenal insufficiency vs., 259
  ascites and, 459
  in pelvic inflammatory disease, 1233
Peritonsillar abscess (quinsy), 569, 1303–1304
Peritovenous shunt, for ascites, 459
Pernicious anemia
  adrenal insufficiency and, 255
  treatment of, hypokalemia risk with, 276
Persistent pain, defined, 878
Personnel. *See also* Health care workers; Staffpower and training
  in disaster management, 32, 33–34
  identification methods, 15
  psychological help for, 34
  EMS coordinators, 19
Perspiration, dehydration risk with, 267
Pesticide exposure
  atropine for, 478
  decontamination procedures, 474
  ingestion, hypokalemia and, 276
  organophosphate inhalation, 775–776
Peutz-Jeghers syndrome, 369, 370
Peyote, 807
PFC. *See* Perfluorocarbon
PGE inhibitors, for hypercalcemia, 316. *See also* Aspirin; Indomethacin
pH calculations, 210
Phalanges
  hand, fractures of, 207–208
  interphalangeal joints
    aspiration or injection of, 1374, 1375
    dislocation of, 230
  toe, fractures and dislocations of, 230
Pharyngeal swelling, in retropharyngeal abscess, 382–383
  in children, 569
Pharyngeal-tracheal lumen airway, 99
  prehospital use of, 6
Pharyngitis, 376–378
Phenazopyridine (Pyridium), 1423
  intoxication by, 473
Phencyclidine (PCP)
  overdose, clinical signs, 472, 473, 474
  screening tests for, 786
  as sympathomimetic, 787
Phenergan. *See* Promethazine
Phenformin ingestion, lactic acidosis and, 473
Phenmetrazine (Preludin), as sympathomimetic, 787
Phenobarbital (Luminal; Phenobarbital), 1399, 1440
  for alcohol withdrawal, 820
  elimination half-life of, 800
  for meningitis, in children under two, 539
  for neonates, pharmacokinetics and, 483
  overdose of, 490
    assay methods, 472
    treatment of, 475, 477
  for pain relief, 882, 883
  for sedative withdrawal, 805
  for seizures, 949
  for status epilepticus, 946, 947
    in children, 594
Phenol toxicity, 757–758
Phenols, listed, 756

Phenothiazines
  behavioral disorders and, 474
  dystonia from, in children, 565–566
  hypothermia and, 662, 671
  for LSD-induced "bad trips," 810
  movement disorders and, 474
  overdose of
    clinical signs, 472, 473, 474
    treatment of, 477
  for PCP intoxication, 808
  sedative withdrawal and, 804
  as unconsciousness cause, 591
Phenoxybenzamine, for frostbite, 673
Phentolamine, for catecholamine crisis, 1067
Phenylbutazone (Butazolidin), 1405
  for pain relief, 881
  serum sickness and, 433
Phenylephrine; Phenylephrine hydrochloride (Neo-Synephrine)
  for PSVT, 1026
  spinal injuries and, 104
  as sympathomimetic, 787
  for uveitis, 1281
Phenylisopropylamine (Benzedrine), 790, 791
  as sympathomimetic, 787
Phenylpropanolamine (PPA)
  behavioral disorders and, 474
  as sympathomimetic, 787
Phenytoin (Dilantin), 1388, 1399
  behavioral disorders and, 474
  calculating dosage of, 482
  for ciguatera fish poisoning, 738
  for dysrhythmias
    ventricular premature complexes, 1005
    ventricular tachycardia, 1034
  elimination of, 482
  for head injury, 898, 901
  HHNK and, 244
  movement disorders and, 474
  for neonates, pharmacokinetics and, 483
  overdose of, 489–490
    assay methods, 472
    clinical signs, 472, 474, 489
  as overdose treatment, 485
  sedative withdrawal and, 804–805
  for seizures, 947, 949
  serum sickness and, 433
  for status epilepticus, 946, 947
    in children, 594, 595
  in subarachnoid hemorrhage, 941
Pheochromocytoma
  adrenal insufficiency and, 257
  in hereditary disorders, 370
  hypercalcemia and, 282, 317
  respiratory alkalosis and, 330
Pheochromocytoma crisis, 1066
Philadelphia collar, 108, 109
Phillips blade, for endotracheal intubation, 96
Phlebitis. See Thrombophlebitis
Phlebotomy
  potassium level error and, 277, 297
  for pulmonary edema, 1099
Phosgene inhalation, 769, 770
Phosphate binders, in renal failure treatment, 1226
Phosphate depletion
  diabetic ketoacidosis and, 237–239
  hypercalcemia and, 317
Phosphate therapy
  for diabetic ketoacidosis, 239
  for hypercalcemia, 283, 316
Phosphine inhalation, 772
Photographic documentation
  of child abuse, 604
  of facial injuries, 1322
  of rape, 1244, 1245, 1248, 1249
  of sexual abuse, 607
Photophobia
  in meningitis, purulent, 397
  in seronegative spondyloarthropathies, 338
  in Sjögren's disease, 338
  in subarachnoid hemorrhage, 940
Photosensitivity, as drug reaction, 434

Physeal fractures in children, 166, 203
Physical dependence, defined, 782
Physical examination
  in acute monoarticular arthritis, 352–353
  in acute myocardial infarction, 967–982
  in biliary tract disease, 453–454
  child abuse and, 602
  in children
    with appendicitis, 555
    with multiple trauma, 547–548
  in congestive heart failure, 1054
  in epistaxis, 1305–1306
  in glaucoma, 1288–1289
  in head injury, 896
  in headache, 921
  in heart and great vessel trauma, 1077
  in hemoptysis evaluation, 1167–1168
  in hereditary disease, 361, 363–365
  in maxillofacial injury, 1322
  in obstructive airway disease, 1131
  for pain, 879
  in pleural effusion, 1169
  of rape victim, 1245, 1246–1249
    equipment for, 1244
  in sexual abuse, 605, 606–607
  for spouse abuse, 848
  in toxicologic emergencies, 470, 471
  upper extremity injuries, 195
  in upper GI bleeding, 449
  vertebral column injuries, 181
Physicians
  National Practitioner Data Bank, 55–56
  prehospital medical control role, 20, 21
  quality assurance and, 55–56, 60–61
    consumer review, 62
    criminal and civil sanctions, 60
    HCFA/PRO review process, 58–60
    hospital liability and, 61
Physostigmine (Antilirium), 1449–1450
  for anticholinergic drug overdose, 479–480
  for antidepressant overdose, 485
Phytonadione (AquaMephyton; Mephyton; Vitamin K₁), 1401–1402
Piano playing, as DeQuervain's tenosynovitis cause, 346
PID. See Pelvic inflammatory disease
Pigmentation disorders, adrenal insufficiency and, 258
Pilocarpine, for acute glaucoma, 1289
Pilonidal abscesses, 407
Piperacillin (Pipracil), 1416
Pipkin femoral head fracture classification, 217, 218
Pipracil. See Piperacillin
Piroxicam (Feldene), for pain relief, 881
Pitocin. See Oxytocin
Pituitary adenoma, hypercalcemia and, 282
Pituitary extract, anaphylaxis risk with, 75
Pituitary gland disorders. See also Hypopituitarism
Pityriasis rosea, 437–438
Placebos, for pain relief, 881–882
Placenta previa, 1237
Placental abruption, 1236, 1237–1238
Placidyl. See Ethchlorvynol
Plafond fractures, 226
Plague
  diagnosis of, 385
  sepsis and, 406
Planning, in disaster management, 31–32
  personnel issues, 33–34
Plantaris muscle, ruptured, Baker's cyst vs., 346
Plasma
  for acute liver failure, 458
  in component therapy, 120, 121
  for shock, 80
  for upper GI bleeding, 448, 453
  whole blood vs., 128–129
Plasma expanders, for shock, 80, 127
Plasma osmolality
  diabetic ketoacidosis and, 237
  hyperosmolar hyperglycemic nonketotic coma and, 242, 244
Plasma protein fraction, for shock, 127
Plasma refill rates, in hypovolemic shock, 70

Plasma substitutes, for shock, 80
Plasma volume, 265
Plasma volume expanders, 1444–1445
Plasmapheresis, for thyroid storm, 251
Plasmin inhibitor deficiency, 366
Plasmodium falciparum, 406, 407
Plaster of Paris casting, 168–171
Platelet abnormalities
  in cancer patients
    as bleeding cause, 510
    chemotherapy and, 509
  hereditary, 365, 366
  in hypothermia, 666
  in renal failure, 1226
Platelet cyclo-oxygenase deficiency, 366
Platelet transfusions, 120, 121–122
  anaphylaxis risk with, 75
Plethysmography, impedance (IPG), in deep vein thrombosis, 1147–1148
Pleural disease
  in rheumatoid arthritis, 339
  in systemic lupus erythematosus, 339
Pleural effusion, 1169–1170
Pleuritic chest pain, in scleroderma, 340
Plywood spine boards, costs of, 109
Pneumatic anti-shock garment (PASG). See also MAST suit
  in abdominal injuries, 110–111
  controversies about, 5, 111
Pneumatic sleeve, for transfusion delivery, 131
Pneumococcus species, in bacterial tracheitis, 569
Pneumoconiosis, occupational, 1164
Pneumocystis carinii pneumonia, 383, 384
  diagnosis and treatment of, 387
  drug abuse and, 785
Pneumonia, acute, 382–387
  alcohol withdrawal vs., 819
  as cause of death, 383
  diagnosis of, 384–386
  differential diagnosis, 386
  hyponatremia and, 271
  pathogenesis of, 384
  in pediatric patients, 383, 585–586
  treatment of, 386–387
Pneumonitis
  chemical, hydrocarbon aspiration and, 584
  radiation, 508
  in systemic lupus erythematosus, 340
  in Wegener's granulomatosis, 340
Pneumothorax, 1183
  drug abuse and, 786
  hemopneumothorax, 102
  IV management with, 102
  open, 101, 1184
  spontaneous
    in children, 586–587
    in scleroderma, 340
    in tuberous sclerosis, 365
  tension, 1183–1184
    indications of, 100
    as MAST suit contraindication, 77
    prehospital care and, 100–101, 110
    ventilation with, 99, 100–101
Point-of-entry protocols, 20
Poison ivy/oak/sumac, 432, 433
Poisoning. See Toxicologic emergencies
Police personnel
  collaborating with, 7
  communication with, 8
  as first responders, 6
Poliomyelitis
  aseptic meningitis and, 399
  pharyngitis and, 377
Poliovirus, in shellfish, 733
Poloxamer 188, for puncture wounds, 154
Polyarteritis nodosa, 337
  gastrointestinal involvement in, 342
  neurologic involvement in, 343
Polyarticular arthritis, 358–359
Polychlorinated biphenyls (PCBs), 747
Polychondritis, relapsing, pulmonary involvement in, 340

Polycillin. *See* Ampicillin
Polycythemia vera, carpal tunnel syndrome and, 347
Polydipsia
  in hypercalcemia, 283
  in hypokalemia, 296
  psychogenic
    diabetes insipidus vs., 269
    hyponatremia and, 271
Polyester sutures, 142
Polyglactin 910 (Vicryl) sutures, 142
Polyglycolic acid (Dexin) sutures, 142
Polymer fume fever, 1162–1163
Polymox. *See* Amoxicillin
Polymyalgia rheumatica
  carpal tunnel syndrome and, 347
  temporal arteritis and, 337
Polymyxin B-neomycin-gramicin, eye drops and ointment, 1269
Polypeptides, hypovolemic shock and, 71
Polyposis, familial, 369, 370
Polypropylene sutures, 142
Polyradiculoneuropathy, in adrenal insufficiency, 259
Polyuria
  in hypercalcemia, 283, 311, 312
  in hypokalemia, 296
Ponstel. *See* Mefenamic acid
Pontocaine. *See* Tetracaine
Popliteal fossa, Baker's cyst in, 346
Porphyrias
  acute intermittent, hyponatremia and, 271
  as hereditary, 369, 370
Portal hypertension, in hereditary disorders, 366
Portal venous obstruction, prehepatic, in children, 558
Portuguese man-of-war, 718
Position. *See also specific procedures*
  for cervical cord injuries, 912, 913
  in head injury treatment, 897
  in pulmonary edema, 1098
  in respiratory emergencies, of children, 577–578
  in shock treatment, 78
Positive end expiratory pressure (PEEP)
  central venous pressure monitoring and, 82
  for near-drowning, 691, 695–697
  pulmonary artery pressure monitoring and, 83
  for pulmonary edema, noncardiogenic, 1101
Post-term pregnancy, adrenal insufficiency and, 258
Post-traumatic stress, rape trauma syndrome, 1254–1255
Postauricular ecchymosis (Battle's sign), 110
Posterior cerebral artery syndrome, 937
Posterior cord syndrome, 185
Posterior lesions, in ischemic CVA, 937
Postictal states
  in children, 590–591
  confusion in, 954
Postoperative complications
  adrenal insufficiency, 257
  hyponatremia, 271
  small bowel obstruction, 459, 460
  thyroid storm, 249
Postpartum hemorrhage, 1238
Postural drainage, for multifocal atrial tachycardia (MAT), 1022
Posture, in head injury, 895
Potassium administration. *See also* Potassium chloride
  for diabetic ketoacidosis, 237
  for hypercalcemic crisis, 315
  hyperkalemia and, 279, 298
  for hypokalemia, 278, 296–297
  hypothermia and, 671
Potassium chloride (KCL; Klorvess; K-Lor; Slow-K; Klotrix), 1388. *See also* Potassium administration
  in alkaline diuresis, 475
  for ectopic atrial tachycardia (EAT), 1019
  for hypercalcemic crisis, 315
  for hypokalemia, 278, 296–297
  for metabolic alkalosis, 328
Potassium exchange resins, for hyperkalemia, 299
Potassium iodide, for soil-borne skin infections, 409
Potassium levels. *See also* Hyperkalemia; Hypokalemia
  adrenal insufficiency and, 259
  diet and, 294
  in hyperkalemia, 280, 297
  HHNK coma and, 242, 244
  in hypokalemia, 296, 297
  physiology and, 272–275
  renal failure and, 1225
Povidine-iodine solution, for wound irrigation, 140
Power of attorney, durable, 42
PPOs. *See* Preferred Provider Organizations
Pralidoxime, for organophosphate toxicity, 478, 757, 776
Prayer, nonmedical healing through, 874, 875
Prazepam (Centrax), elimination half-life of, 800
Prazosin
  for congestive heart failure, 1055, 1056
  in renal failure treatment, 1225
Pre-eclampsia, 1238–1239. *See also* Hypertension, pregnancy-induced
  defined, 1238
  neonatal adrenal insufficiency and, 258
  thyroid storm and, 249
  treatment for, hypermagnesemia from, 308
Pre-hospital and Disaster Medicine
  on fluid resuscitation in field, 5
  on PASG, 5
Prednisolone, topical, for uveitis, 1282
Prednisone (Deltasone), 1429
  adrenal insufficiency and, 260
  for contact dermatitis, 433
  for drug eruptions, 434
  for headache, 923
  for hypercalcemia, 283
  for infectious mononucleosis, 402
  for toxic epidermal necrolysis, 440
Preferred Provider Organizations (PPOs), quality review systems in, 58
Pregnancy. *See also* Delivery; Ectopic pregnancy; Labor
  abdominal pain in, 1235–1237
  abuse during, 838, 845
  age and, consent issues, 42
  anatomic changes in, 1235
  carbon monoxide exposure and, 478
  carpal tunnel syndrome and, 347
  confirmation of, 1234
  consent issues, 42
  diagnostic procedures and, 1235
  genital herpes in, 1239
  headache in, 923
  high altitude and, 685
  history taking about, 1229
  hypertension in, 1238–1239. *See also* Pregnancy, toxemia of
  as MAST suit contraindication, 77
  medical conditions in, 1239–1240
  mercury exposure and, 494
  phenytoin overdose and, 489
  post-term, neonatal adrenal insufficiency and, 258
  rape and, 1252
  toxemia (pre-eclampsia) of. *See also* Pregnancy, hypertension in
    eclampsia and, 1066
    iatrogenic hypermagnesemia and, 308
    neonatal adrenal insufficiency and, 258
    thyroid storm and, 249
  trauma in, 1238
  urinary tract infections in, 393
  vaginal bleeding in, 1230, 1237–1238
Prehospital interventions. *See also* Prehospital services
  acute epiglottitis, 1119
  acute myocardial infarction, 983
  in bacterial tracheitis, 1117
  burns, 419
  carbon monoxide poisoning, 766
  cardiogenic shock, 74
  congestive heart failure, 1054, 1055
  cyanide poisoning, 478, 755, 768
  dehydration, 270
  head injuries, 891–892
  heat stroke, 657
  hyperkalemia, 281
  hypernatremia, 270
  hypertensive emergencies, 1064
  hypocalcemia, 285
  hypokalemia, 278
  hyponatremia, 272
  hypothermia, 667
  laryngotracheitis, 1115
  maxillofacial injuries, 110, 1320
  multisystem injuries, 93–112. *See also specific types of injuries*
    airway control, 95–99
    breathing assistance, 99–101
    chest area, 110
    circulation control, 101–103
    rectum, 112
    tetanus immunization with, 112
    upper extremity injuries with, 195
  near-drowning, 694–695
  pulmonary edema, 1098
  rape cases, 1244–1245
  status epilepticus, 947
  toxicologic emergencies, 469
  upper extremity injuries, 195
  vertebral column injuries, 187
Prehospital services, 1–27. *See also* Prehospital interventions
  ALS vs. BLS controversies, 5–6
  categorization of facilities for, 18
  communications and, 8
  data collection guidelines, 11
  for evaluation, 20
  in disaster management, 35
  EMS Act of 1973 and, 93–94
  medical control issues, 20–21
  radioactive materials and, 758
  staffing issues, 21–22
  standards of care, 94
Preload
  in cardiogenic shock, 74
  defined, 1052
  in shock diagnosis, 66
Preludin. *See* Phenmetrazine
Premarin. *See* Estrogen, conjugated
Premature infants
  endotracheal intubation of, 518
  pharmacokinetic problems in, 483, 484
Premature ventricular complexes (PVCs), 1002–1005
Premedication, in wound management, 139
Prepatellar bursitis, septic, 412
Presbyterians, beliefs and practices, 868
Preshock syndrome, 73–74
Pressors. *See* Vasopressor agents
Pressure, for pain relief, 888
Pressure dressing, indications for, 141
Pressure (paint and grease) gun injuries, 155
Presyncope, dysrhythmia and, 997
Preterm labor
  as abdominal pain cause, 1236–1237
  in trauma, 1238
Prickly heat, 655
Prilocaine (Citanest)
  clinical characteristics and dosage, 884
  pharmacologic classification of, 885
Prilosec. *See* Omeprazole
Primary survey, multisystem injuries, 94, 95–103
Primaxin. *See* Imipenem-cilastatin
Primidone, for seizures, 949
Primidone overdose, 490
Probenecid (Benemid), 1405
  for gonorrhea, 1250
Procainamide (Pronestyl; Procan; Procan SR), 1388–1389
  in acute myocardial infarction treatment, 984
  in advanced cardiac life support, 1089, 1090
  for dysrhythmias
    atrial fibrillation, 1022
    atrial flutter, 1024
    atrial premature complex, 1002
    PSVT, 1026, 1028
    ventricular premature complexes, 1005
    ventricular tachycardia, 1030, 1034
  hypothermia and, 671

pharmacokinetics and, 484
for Wolff-Parkinson-White syndrome, 1042
Procaine hydrochloride (Novocain)
  anaphylaxis risk with, 75
  clinical characteristics and dosage, 884
  pharmacologic classification of, 885
  as wound anesthetic, 139–140
Procan; Procan-SR. See Procainamide
Procarbazine, pulmonary reactions to, 508
Procardia. See Nifedipine
Procedures
  aspiration and injection of joints, bursae, and tendons, 1373–1375
  closed thoracostomy, 1370–1372
  culdocentesis, 1231, 1354
  defibrillation and electrical cardioversion, 1361
  endotracheal intubation, 1366–1369
  internal jugular vein cannulation, 1343–1346
  nasotracheal suctioning, 1362–1363
  needle cricothyroid puncture, 1364–1365
  pericardiocentesis, 1358–1360
  peritoneal lavage, 1356–1357
  subclavian vein cannulation, 1339–1342
  Swan-Ganz catheterization, 1347–1349
  temporary transvenous pacemaker placement, 1351–1352
Prochlorperazine (Compazine), 1407–1408
  for headache, 922
  for pancreatitis, 456
Proctitis, 466
Proctosigmoidoscopy, in rectal or colon injuries, 465
Progesterone, respiratory alkalosis in pregnancy and, 330
Projectile injuries
  to cervical spine, 904, 905
  to head, 899
Prolonged pain, defined, 878
Promethazine (Phenergan), 1408
Pronestyl. See Procainamide
Propafenone (Rythmol), 1389
Propine. See Dipivefrin
Propoxyphene (Darvon), 1437–1438
  as opioid, 793
  overdose of, clinical signs, 472
  pharmacology of, 795
Propranolol (Inderal), 1389–1390
  in advanced cardiac life support, 1090
  for atrial flutter, 1024
  confusion caused by, 474
  for dysrhythmias
    atrial fibrillation, 1022
    atrial premature complex, 1002
    premature ventricular complexes, 1005
    PSVT, 1026
    ventricular tachycardia, 1034
  for headache prophylaxis, 922, 924
  HHNK coma and, 244
  overdose of, clinical signs, 472, 473
  in renal failure treatment, 1225
  for thyroid storm, 250, 251
Propylthiouracil (PTU), 1445
  for thyroid storm, 250, 251
PROs. See Peer review organizations
Prostaglandin E
  Bartter's syndrome and, 275
  hypercalcemia and, 282
Prostaglandin F2$_\alpha$, for postpartum hemorrhage, 1238
Prostaphlin. See Oxacillin
Prostate gland, in multisystem trauma, 112
Prostatic cancer
  chest wall syndrome vs., 348
  hyponatremia and, 271
Prostatitis
  acute bacterial, 395–396
  urinary tract infections and, 392
Protamine, anaphylaxis risk with, 75
Protective clothing, for hazardous materials response, 750
Protein deficit, as hypomagnesemia cause, 305
Proteus species
  in corneal ulcers, 1274, 1275, 1277

in otitis externa, 380, 1310, 1311
in urinary tract infections, 391
Protocols
  in disaster management, 35
  for prehospital services, 20
Protoporphyria, erythropoietic, 366
Protozoa, bivalve mollusk poisoning and, 733–734
Proventil. See Albuterol (Salbutamol)
Pruritus
  in atopic dermatitis, 429
  of burn wound, 425
  in diabetics, 433
  in drug reaction, 434
  in otitis externa, 1310–1311
Pseudoaneurysms, surgery required for, 1071
Pseudoephedrine, as sympathomimetic, 787
Pseudogout
  age and, 351
  diagnosis of, 356
  hyperkalemia and, 279
  onset of, 351
  polyarticular arthritis with, 359
Pseudohyperkalemia, 279
Pseudohyponatremia, 271
Pseudohypoparathyroidism, 284
Pseudomembranous colitis
  cytotoxins and, 387
  treatment of, 390
Pseudomonas aeruginosa
  in corneal ulcers, 1274, 1275, 1277
  in nosocomial sinusitis, 1302
  in otitis externa, 380, 1310, 1311
  in pneumonia, 383
  as puncture wound complication, 154
  in septic arthritis, 410
  in urinary tract infections, 391
Pseudotumor cerebri, as headache cause, 919
Pseudoxanthoma elasticum (PXE), 367, 368–369, 371
Psilocybin, 807, 809
Psittacosis, 385, 386
Psoriasis, arthritis and, 358, 359
PSP. See Paralytic shellfish poisoning
PSVT. See Paroxysmal supraventricular tachycardia
Psychiatric disorders
  alcoholism and, 824
  confusion in, 951, 955–957
    treatment of, 956
  self-induced, 842
Psychiatric emergencies. See also Depression; Psychiatric disorders; Psychosis; Schizophrenia
  amphetamine and, 790–791, 793
  cocaine and, 789, 793
  ED classification for, 47
  LSD and, 810
  PCP and, 808
  in sexual abuse cases, 606
Psychiatric hospitalization, for suicidal patients, 831–832, 833, 834
Psychiatric patients, abused women as, 838
Psychic healing, 870
Psychogenic headache, 920–921
Psychogenic unresponsiveness, 930–931
Psychologic abuse, 846
  in battering syndrome, 841
  of elders, 847
Psychological dependence, defined, 782
Psychological interventions. See Emotional support
Psychological stress, as syncope cause, 960–961
Psychomotor seizures, acute confusion after, 954
Psychopathology theory of domestic violence, 844
Psychosis
  acute, in adrenal insufficiency, 259
  drug-induced, 474
  headache with, 920
  in systemic lupus erythematosus, 343, 344
  in thyroid storm, 250
Psychosocial component of spirituality, 863
Psychosocial intervention, in child abuse cases, 602–603. See also Social workers
Psychosomatic complaints, in battering syndrome, 841
Psychospiritual support, 863, 870–872
Psychotherapy, referral to

for depressed patients, 831, 832
for pain management, 887
for suicidal patients, 834, 835
Psyllium hydrophilic mucilloid, for diarrhea, 389
Psylocibin, 806
Ptosis, in temporal arteritis, 337, 338
PTU. See Propylthiouracil
Ptychodiscus breve poisoning, 735
Pubic hair abnormalities
  in adrenal insufficiency, 259
  in hypocalcemia, 285
Public education
  for disasters, 36
  as EMS system component, 11
Public Law 96-499, 7
Public Law 101-590, 27
Public opinion, quality issues and, 53
Public safety agencies
  in deployment plans, 16
  in disaster linkages, 12, 33, 34
  as EMS system component, 7, 8, 11
  as first responders, 6
Pufferfish poisoning (tetrodotoxism), 740–741
Pulmonary angiography, in pulmonary embolism, 1146–1147
Pulmonary artery wedge pressure monitoring
  in acute myocardial infarction, 992
  in pulmonary edema, 83
  for shock, 83
  Swan-Ganz catheterization for, 1347–1349
Pulmonary circulation, high altitude and, 680
Pulmonary complications
  of acute myocardial infarction, 993
  of chemotherapy, 508–509
  "shock lung" physiology, 79
Pulmonary disorders. See also Obstructive airway disease
  in connective tissue disease, 339–340
  high altitude and, 685
  hyponatremia and, 271
  magnesium therapy for, 307–308
  physiology and. See Lung function
  pneumonia, 383–387
  respiratory alkalosis and, 330
  situational syncope and, 961
Pulmonary edema
  cardiogenic, 1096–1100
    diagnosis of, 1098–1098
    differential diagnosis, 1098
    etiologies of, 1096–1097
    pathology and pathophysiology, 1097
    treatment of, 1098–1100
  high-altitude (HAPE), 681, 683–684, 1101
  noncardiogenic, 1100–1101
    in acute epiglottitis, 1118, 1122
    diagnosis of, 1101
    differential diagnosis, 1101
    etiologies of, 1100
    medications and, 1100
    pathology and pathophysiology, 1100
    treatment of, 1101
  prehospital care, 1098
  pulmonary artery pressure monitoring with, 83
  in toxicologic emergencies, 472
Pulmonary embolectomy, indications for, 1148
Pulmonary embolism, 1141–1149
  as cardiogenic shock cause, 74
  clinical signs of, 1143–1145
  deep venous thrombosis and, 1147–1148
  diagnostic problems, 1141
  diagnostic studies, 1145–1148
  differential diagnosis, 1144–1145
  epidemiology of, 1142
  high altitude and, 685
  historical view of, 1141
  pathophysiology of, 1142–1143
  risk factors for, 960, 1142
  syncope with, 960, 963
  thyroid storm and, 249
  treatment of, 1148–1149
Pulmonary fibrosis, in Hermansky-Pudlak syndrome, 365, 366

Pulmonary function. *See* Lung function
Pulmonary function tests, in obstructive airway disease, 1132
Pulmonary hemorrhage, in systemic lupus erythematosus, 340
Pulmonary hypertension, pulmonary artery pressure monitoring with, 83
Pulmonary neoplasms, shoulder-hand syndrome and, 347
Pulmonary status monitoring, with MAST suit, 77
Pulmonary toxicity, chemotherapy and, 508–509
Pulmonary trauma, 1183–1185
    contusion, 1184–1185
    hazardous materials and, 754–755
    hemothorax, 1184
    pneumothorax, 1183
        open, 1184
    treatment procedures, 1189–1190
Pulmonary venous pressure, acute myocardial infarction and, 991–992
Pulse oximetry, in pediatric respiratory disorder, 576
Pulse pressure
    in multisystem trauma, 105
    in shock, 66
        hypovolemic, 68, 70
    stroke volume and, 66
Puncture wounds
    dog bites, 630
    in feet, 154
    tetanus prophylaxis for, 155
Punitive damages, 41
Pupillary responses
    in head injury, 895
    in multisystem trauma, 107
    in unresponsive patient, 931–932
PVCs. *See* Premature ventricular complexes
PXE. *See* Pseudoxanthoma elasticum
Pyarthrosis, diabetic foot ulcers and, 231
Pyelonephritis, 391, 392, 1210–1211
Pyloric stenosis, 557
Pyoderma, 430–432
Pyopen. *See* Carbenicillin
Pyridium. *See* Phenazopyridine
Pyrimethamine (Daraprim), 1423
    for malaria, 407
    for toxoplasmosis, 402

Q

Q fever, 383, 385, 386
Quaalude. *See* Methaqualone
Quadriplegia
    in anterior cord syndrome, 184–185
    in hyperkalemia, 299
    in rheumatoid arthritis, 343
    in systemic lupus erythematosus, 344
Quakers, beliefs and practices, 868–869
Quality issues, 53–62. *See also* Evaluation
    AMA/JCAHO criteria, 54, 57
    assessment criteria, 53–54, 58
    COBRA and, 58
    consumer control, 61–62
    continuous improvement models, 57–58
    Donabedian assessment framework, 54–55
    efficacy vs. quality of care, 54
    enforcement and sanctions, 56, 58, 59–50
    Health Care Quality Improvement Act, 54, 56–57
    levels of severity, 59
    multicenter practice parameter studies, 58
    National Practitioner Data Bank, 55–56, 58, 59, 60
    outcomes management, 54, 55, 62
    peer review, 55, 56
    peer review organizations (PROs), 58–61
    procedural, 55
    public opinion and, 53
    standards development, 62
    structural, 54–55
    technical vs. interpersonal, 55
Quality of life, quality of care and, 62
Quibron-T. *See* Theophylline
Quinacrine (Atabrine), 1423
    for *Giardia* enteritis, 390

Quinaglute. *See* Quinidine gluconate
Quinalbarbitone. *See* Secobarbital
Quinidine sulfate (Quinidine), 1390. *See also* Quinidine gluconate; Quinine sulfate
    for dysrhythmias
        atrial fibrillation, 1022
        atrial flutter, 1024
        atrial premature complex, 1002
        PSVT, 1026
        ventricular premature complexes, 1005
        ventricular tachycardia, 1030, 1034
    hypothermia and, 671
    for Wolff-Parkinson-White syndrome, 1042
Quinidine gluconate (Quinaglute), for malaria, 407
Quinine dihydrochloride, for malaria, 407
Quinine sulfate, for malaria, 407
Quinolone antibiotics
    for dysenteric gastroenteritis, 390
    for prostatitis, 395
Quinsy (peritonsillar abscess), 569, 1303–1304

R

Rabbits and hares, rabies and, 629
Rabies precautions, dog bites and, 629
Rabies treatment, anaphylaxis risk with, 75
Rabies virus, encephalitis and, 400
Raccoons, rabies and, 629
Racemic epinephrine. *See* Epinephrine
Radial fractures, 204–205
    in children, 165, 166, 206
    distal, 205–206
    "greenstick" or compression, 205
Radial head fractures, 203
Radial head subluxations, 204
Radial nerve injury, humeral shaft fracture and, 201
Radial slab splints, 171–172
Radial styloid fractures, carpal dislocations and, 206
Radial ulnar joint, radial head fractures and, 203
Radiation emergencies, 617–624, 758–759
    assistance sources in, 758–759
    decontamination procedures, 618–619, 758–759
    ED preparedness for, 623–624, 758
    exposure criteria, 618
    internal contamination, 622–623
    localized injuries, 619–620
    physics and pathophysiology of, 617–618
    prevention of, 622
    total-body injuries, 620–622
        acute radiation syndrome, 620–621
Radiation Emergency Assistance Center/Training Site (REAC/TS), 758–759
Radiation enteritis, 508
Radiation pneumonitis, 508
Radiation therapy
    complications of, as emergencies, 508
    for hyperthyroidism, thyroid storm and, 249
    for intracranial pressure elevation, 502
Radio communications, 8, 9
Radio-telephone switch station (RTSS), 8–9
Radiocarpal (wrist) joint, aspiration or injection of, 1374, 1375
Radiography. *See also* specific types of injuries
    in acute epiglottitis, 1120
    in appendicitis, 464, 556
    in cervical spine injuries, 911–912
    in connective tissue disease, 339, 340
    in Crohn's disease, 462
    in croup, 1114
    in dislocation evaluation, 173, 174
    for esophageal burns, 451
    in febrile infants under 3 months, 535
    in foreign body aspiration, 1308
    in fracture evaluation, 162, 163, 168
    in head injury, 897
    in headache evaluation, 921
    in large bowel obstruction, 460
    in laryngeal trauma, 1316
    in maxillofacial injury, 1322–1323
    in monoarticular arthritis, 356
    in multiple trauma, in children, 548–549
    in obstructive airway disease, 1132

    of pelvis, 213–214
    in pneumonia, 384, 385
    in pulmonary embolism, 1145
    in respiratory disorder evaluation, pediatric, 576
    in septic arthritis, 411
    of shoulder syndromes, 346
    in sinusitis, 379, 1301
    of upper extremity injuries, 195, 198
    of vertebral column injuries, 185–187
    in wound evaluation, 139
        clenched fist injury, 156
        pressure gun injuries, 155
        puncture wounds, 154
Radiohumeral joint, aspiration or injection of, 1374, 1375
Radioiodine-linked immunoassay (RIA), in drug screening, 786
Radionuclide scans
    in biliary tract disease, 454
    in hemoptysis, 1168
    for lower GI bleeding, 451
    in multiple trauma, in children, 549
    in pulmonary embolism, 1145–1146
    renal
        in blunt trauma, 1195–1197
        in penetrating trauma, 1199
    in stress fracture diagnosis, 226
Radius. *See* Extremities; *terms beginning with* Radial; Upper extremity injuries
Range of motion testing, in upper extremities, 195
Ranitidine (Zantac), 1434
    for anaphylaxis, 86
    for upper GI bleeding, 449
Ranson's signs, 456
Rape, 1241–1247. *See also* Sexual abuse
    in battering syndrome, 838, 845
    definitions of, 1242, 1243
    elderly victims of, 1253–1254
    emergency department issues, 1241–1242, 1245–1246
        evaluation form, 1256, 1257
        social service referral, 1255
    follow-up care, 1246, 1251, 1255
    history taking, 1246, 1247
    HIV testing and, 1250–1251
    legal issues, 1241, 1242, 1243–1244, 1246, 1247
        special forensic studies, 1251–1252
    of males, 1252
    myths about, 1242–1243, 1252
    physical examination, 1244, 1246–1249
    pregnancy and, 1252
    prehospital care, 1244–1245
    statistics about, 1242
    STDs and, 1250
Rape kit, 607, 1244
    components of, 1244
Rape trauma syndrome (RTS), 1254–1255
Rape-crisis workers, role of, 1255
Rapid sequence intubation techniques, 942, 1106–1107
Rapidly progressing glomerulonephritis (RPGN), renal failure and, 1218
Rashes. *See also* Cutaneous lesions
    in connective tissue disease, 336
    in Lyme disease, 336, 357, 409
    in measles, 443
    in meningitis, in children under two, 536
    poison ivy/oak/sumac, 432, 433
    in Rocky Mountain spotted fever, 438
    in rubella, 443
    in sepsis diagnosis, 406
    in systemic lupus erythematosus, 336
    in toxic shock syndrome, 432
    urticaria, 440–441
    viral exanthems, 443
Ratfishes
    food poisoning by, 712
    spine or puncture wounds by, 725–726
"Rave" dance parties, MDMA and, 799
Raynaud's phenomenon, 341
    connective tissue disorders and, 341
Rays, poisoning by, 712, 736

"Reasonable conduct" concept, 40
Rebound tenderness, in polyarteritis nodosa, 342
Recombinant tissue type plaminogen activator. *See* Alteplase recombinant or r-tPA
Record keeping
  ALS medical control through, 20–21
  in child abuse cases, 602, 603, 604–605
    Suspected Abuse Form, 611–616
  consent issues and, 42
  in disasters, 36, 37
  in domestic violence cases, 843, 853
  of EMS communications, 8
  as EMS system component, 8, 11–12, 13–14
  in maxillofacial injuries, 1320
  in multisystem trauma, 112
  in ocular trauma, hyphema, 1284, 1285
  on patient transfers, 43
  in rape cases, 1241, 1243–1244
  in sexual abuse cases, 607, 608
    Suspected Abuse Form, 611–616
  in vertebral column injury, 181
Rectal biopsy
  in Crohn's disease, 462
  in ulcerative colitis, 462–463
Rectal bleeding, 450–451
  hemorrhoids, 465–466
Rectal examination
  in children
    for appendicitis, 555
    with multiple trauma, 548
  in rape cases. *See* Rape, physical examination
Rectal injuries, 465
  in multisystem trauma, 112
  in children, 548
  prehospital care, 112
Rectum
  anorectal abscess, 407, 408, 466
  herpes simplex in, 466
  prolapse of, 466
Red blood cells
  anaphylaxis risk with, 75
  in component therapy, 121, 119, 120
Red Cross, in disaster linkages, 12
Red eyes, in seronegative spondyloarthropathies, 338
Red tides, shellfish poisoning and, 734, 735
Reeves Sleeve, 109
Referrals
  for alcoholics, 818, 823
    "clearing" patient for, 823–825, 828
  for depression, 831
  for domestic violence, 846, 853–854
  for headache, 921
  in maxillofacial injury, 1323–1325
  for ocular disorders, 1282
    glaucoma, 1288, 1289
  for ocular trauma, 1285
  for otitis media, 1310
  for peritonsillar abscess, 1303
  for sinusitis, 1303
  for tympanic membrane perforation, 1307
Reflex disorders. *See also* Neurologic disorders
  hypothermia and, 666
  in multisystem trauma, 106–107
  reflex sympathetic dystrophy, 347
  in toxicologic emergencies, 472
  in vertebral column injury, 181–182
Reflux, esophageal, 452
Refraction errors, as headache cause, 917
Refrigerant, inhalation abuse with, 806
Refusal of consent, 42
Regional blocks, for pain relief, 885
  in maxillofacial injury, 1325
Regional Medical Program, EMS grants by, 2
Regionalization of hospital care, 49
  categorization vs. designation, 49–50
  trauma center successes, 19
Regulations, 39
  for quality management, 54, 56, 58–60, 61
Reiter's syndrome
  acute monoarticular arthritis with, 358
  ocular involvement in, 338, 339
  polyarticular arthritis with, 359

Relapsing fever, skin infections in, 409
Relaxation exercises
  for headache prophylaxis, 924
  in nonmedical healing, 874–875
  for pain management, 887
Religion. *See also* Spiritual needs
  beliefs and practices, listed, 865–869
  extrinsic vs. intrinsic orientation, 863
  health care issues, 865
    autotransfusions, 132
  resources for patient care, 864–865
  spiritual healing methods, 869–870
  as spiritual support source, 862
Religiosity
  as spiritual need, 863
  types of, 863, 864
Renal artery occlusion, acute, 1211
Renal artery stenosis, hypokalemia and, 277
Renal calculi, 1210, 1211
  hypercalcemia and, 281, 311
  urinary tract infections and, 392
Renal carcinoma; Renal cell carcinoma
  chest wall syndrome vs., 348
  in hereditary disorders, 370
  hypercalcemia and, 282, 317
Renal colic, adrenal hemorrhage, vs., 256
Renal cysts, 1211
Renal disorders
  flank pain and, 1210
  hereditary, 372
Renal failure, 1217–1227
  acute, hypocalcemia and, 284
  acute confusion with, 953
  burns and, 418
  chronic
    as diabetes insipidus cause, 268
    hyperkalemia and, 298, 300
    hypomagnesemia and, 286
    pulmonary edema and, 1097
  diagnosis of, 1217–1218, 1221
  differential diagnosis, 1221–1223
  etiologies of, 1217–1219
  hypercalcemia and, 282, 317
  hyperkalemia and, 279, 298
  hypermagnesemia and, 308
  hypocalcemia and, 284
  hypokalemia and, 293, 294, 295, 296
  hypovolemic shock and, 71
  metabolic acidosis and, 322
  mortality with, 1221
  pathogenesis of, 1219–1221
  pathology of, 1219
  presentations of, 1217
  prognosis of, 1227
  septic shock and, 72
  as transfusion reaction, 133, 134
  treatment of, 1223–1227
Renal function, 1217
  high altitude and, 680
  near-drowning and, 693
Renal function tests, diabetic ketoacidosis and, 236
Renal injuries, 1195–1199
  associated injuries with, 1195
  blunt trauma, 1073, 1195–1198
  burns, 427
  clinical signs, 1195–1196, 1198
  diagnostic studies, 1196–1197, 1198–1199
  management of, 1197–1198, 1199
  penetrating, 1198–1199
Renal obstruction. *See also* Renal calculi
  differential diagnosis, 1222
  pathology of, 1219
  renal failure and, 1219, 1220–1221
  treatment of, 1223
Renal physiology
  ADH and, 266
  magnesium and, 303–304
  in neonates, pharmacokinetics and, 483
Renal salt-wasting. *See also* Renal wasting
  hypokalemia and, 293
  hyponatremia and, 270
Renal scan

in blunt trauma, 1195–1197
  in penetrating trauma, 1199
Renal shutdown, in shock, 71
Renal stones. *See* Renal calculi
Renal transplants
  hypercalcemia and, 282, 317
  hyperkalemia and, 298
Renal tubular acidosis
  causes of, 322
  hypokalemia and, 275, 293, 294
  hypomagnesemia and, 286
  metabolic acidosis and, 322
Renal tubule damage, with burns, 427
Renal vein thrombosis, acute, 1211
Renal wasting, hypomagnesemia and, 286. *See also* Renal salt-wasting
Rendu-Osler-Weber disease, epistaxis in, 1304
Renin-angiotensin, physiology and, 272, 273
Reoviruses, in shellfish, 733
Replantation of upper extremities, 212
Repolarization, action potential and, 274
Reproductive system, hypothermia and, 667
Reserpine (Serpasil), 1396–1397
  hypothermia and, 662, 673
  for Raynaud's phenomenon, 341
Resident physicians, on-line medical control by, 20
Residual volume (RV), respiratory failure and, 1151, 1152
Resource theory of domestic violence, 844
Resources for Optimal Care of the Injured Patient (American College of Surgeons), 18
Respiration. *See also* Respiratory system
  assessing, in multisystem trauma, 105–106
  physiology of, 1151–1155
    gas exchange, 1152–1153
    musculature role, 1155
    perfusion, 1153
    ventilation, 1151
    ventilation control, 1154–1155
    ventilation distribution, 1151–1152
    ventilation/perfusion (V/Q) ratio, 1153–1154
Respiratory acidosis, 329–330
  in hypovolemic shock, 71–72
  as MAST suit complication, 77
  in myxedema coma, 252
  pathophysiology of, 329–330
Respiratory alkalosis, 330–331
  chronic, metabolic acidosis and, 322
  clinical signs of, 331
  etiologies of, 330–331
  at high altitudes, 680
  hypocalcemia and, 281
  hypokalemia and, 276
  in septic shock, 72
  treatment of, 331
Respiratory arrest, as acute epiglottitis risk, 1119
Respiratory burns, 420
Respiratory depression
  in hypermagnesemia, 308
  in metabolic alkalosis, 328
Respiratory distress syndrome, adult (ARDS)
  hypovolemic shock and, 71
  pulmonary artery pressure monitoring with, 83
  septic shock and, 72
  venous air embolism and, 708
Respiratory emergencies. *See also* Chest injuries; Pulmonary trauma; *specific conditions*
  air embolism, 1170
  amniotic fluid embolism, 1171
  aspiration, 1165–1167
  cholesterol embolism, 1171
  fat embolism, 1170–1171
  hemoptysis, 1167–1169
  inhalation exposure, 1159–1167
    occupational, 1161–1163, 1164
  pediatric, 573–587
    anatomy/physiology and, 573
    clinical evaluation of, 574–576
    etiologies of, 574–575, 576
    laboratory studies, 576–577
    management of, 577–579
    pathophysiology and, 573–574

Respiratory emergencies (contd.)
  pleural effusion, 1169–1170
  tracheobronchial injury, 1188
  traumatic asphyxia, 1188–1189
Respiratory failure, 1151–1157
  in children
    as cardiac arrest cause, 513, 514
    signs of, 575–576
  classification of, 1151
  criteria for, 1155
  etiologies of, 1155–1156
  hypercapnic, 1156
  hypoxic, 1155–1156
  management of, 1156–1157
  physiology and, 1151–1155
    gas exchange, 1152–1153
    perfusion, 1153
    ventilation, 1151
    ventilation distribution, 1151–1152
    ventilation/perfusion ratio, 1153–1154
  ventilation control, 1154–1155
Respiratory irritants, exposure to, 754–755
Respiratory paralysis, hypokalemia and, 295
Respiratory problems. *See also* Pulmonary disorders; *specific disorders; specific symptoms*
  as cardiac arrest cause, in children, 513, 514
  cocaine and, 789
  head injury with, 896
  high altitude and, 680
  hypothermia and, 663–664
  occupational sources of, 1162–1163, 1175–1180
  urticaria and, 440
Respiratory rate
  in pediatric patients, 575
  in septic shock, 72
Respiratory syncytial virus (RSV)
  in children, 582–583
  in common colds, 376
  pneumonia and, 383
Respiratory therapists, asthma among, 1130
Respiratory tract infections, 375–387. *See also* Obstructive airway disease
  bacterial tracheitis, 569
  bronchiolitis, in children, 582–583
  common cold, 375–376
  diphtheria, 569–570
  laryngotracheitis (croup), 514, 567–569
  otitis, 379–381
  pharyngitis, 376–378
  pneumonia, 382–387
    in children, 383, 585–586
  sinusitis, 378–379
Response times, 22
Resting membrane potential, potassium physiology and, 273, 274–275
Restoril. *See* Temazepam
Restraint, of alcohol-intoxicated patient, 818
Resuscitation, shock treatment with, 76
Resuscitation fluids, 125–130. *See also* Electrolyte solutions; Fluid replacement
Resuscitator devices, 99–100
Retinal disease, in systemic lupus erythematosus, 338
Retinal hemorrhage, high-altitude, 684–685
Retinopathy, antimalarial, 339
Retrograde intubation, 1111
Retrograde urethrography, 1207
  in flank pain diagnosis, 1211
  indications for, 1206, 1207
  in urinary retention, 1214
Retrograde urography
  in blunt trauma, 1197
  in flank pain diagnosis, 1211
  in penetrating trauma, 1199
Retroperitoneal disease, hyponatremia and, 270
Retroperitoneal hematoma, vascular injury and, 1072
Retroperitoneal hemorrhage, adrenal insufficiency vs., 259
Retropharyngeal abscesses, 382–383
  in children, 569
Retrosigmoid injuries, pelvic fractures and, 215
Retrosternal burning, in systemic lupus erythematosus, 342

Revised Trauma Score, pediatric transfer and, 551, 552
Reye's syndrome
  liver failure in, 458, 459
  unconsciousness with, 590
Reynolds' pentad, 454
Rh factor
  blood compatibility and, 130
  historical background, 116
Rhabdomyolysis
  in drug overdoses, 472, 789, 793
    acid diuresis and, 476
  hypercalcemia and, 282
  hyperkalemia and, 279
  hypokalemia and, 295
Rheomacrodex. *See* Dextran solutions
Rheumatic fever
  cutaneous lesions of, 336
  pharyngitis and, 377–378
  polyarticular arthritis with, 358
Rheumatism, soft tissue
  Baker's cyst, 346
  bursitis, 344–345, 412
  carpal tunnel syndrome, 347
  chest wall syndrome, 347–348
  shoulder syndromes, 346–347
  shoulder-hand syndrome, 347
  tendinitis, 345–346
Rheumatoid arthritis
  carpal tunnel syndrome and, 347
  cutaneous lesions in, 337
  gastrointestinal involvement in, 342, 343
  neurologic involvement in, 343
  ocular emergencies in, 338
  polyarticular arthritis with, 358–359
  pulmonary involvement in, 339
  septic joints with, 357
  shoulder-hand syndrome and, 347
  tendinitis in, 346
  "trigger finger" in, 346
  vascular involvement in, 341
Rheumatologic emergencies, 335–348. *See also* Connective tissue disease; *specific diseases*
Rheumox. *See* Azapropazone
Rhinorrhea
  in anaphylaxis, 75
  assessing for, 110
  in head injury, 898, 901
Rhinoviruses
  in common colds, 375
  in pharyngitis, 376, 377
  pneumonia and, 383
Rhus plants, contact dermatitis from, 432–433
RIA. *See* Radioiodine-linked immunoassay
Rib fractures, 1182
  intravenous management with, 102
  prehospital management, 110
  thoracolumbar fractures and, 193
Rib tip syndrome (slipping rib), 348
Rickettsia rickettsii
  in Rocky Mountain spotted fever, 438
  sepsis from, 406, 407
Rickettsial infections
  encephalitis, 400, 401
  pneumonia, 383
  Rocky Mountain spotted fever, 438
  sepsis with, 406, 407
Rifampin (Rifadin; Rimactane), 1423
  adrenal insufficiency and, 258
  for marine-associated skin infections, 409
  in meningitis prevention, 398–399
Right-brain communication, 872
  therapeutic metaphors for, 874–875
Riley-Day syndrome, 372
Rimactane. *See* Rifampin
Ringer's lactate; Ringer's solution. *See* Electrolyte solutions; Fluid replacement
Ritalin. *See* Methylphenidate
Ritual, in nonmedical healing, 870
Robaxin. *See* Methocarbamol
Robert Jones dressing (splint), 172, 173
Robertshaw Mask, 95

Robertson-Kihara syndrome, hypokalemia and, 277
Rocephin. *See* Ceftriaxone
Rockfish. *See* Scorpionfishes
Rocky Mountain spotted fever, 438
  acute sepsis and, 406, 407
  as cause of death, 438
  encephalitis and, 400
  skin infections in, 409
Rocky Mountain states, encephalitis in, 400
Rodenticide poisoning, 473
Rodents, rabies and, 629
Roentgenography. *See* Radiography; *specific types of injuries*
Roman Catholics, beliefs and practices, 865, 869
Root injury, to spinal cord, 184
Roseola infantum, 438
Rotary subluxation of the scaphoid, 206
Rotator cuff injuries, 200, 346
Rotaviruses
  in acute watery diarrhea, 389
  in gastroenteritis, 388
  in infants and children, 558
Routing, in communications systems, 8
RPGN. *See* Rapidly progressing glomerulonephritis
RSV. *See* Respiratory syncytial virus
r-TPA. *See* Alteplase recombinant
RTS (rape trauma syndrome), 1254–1255
RTSS. *See* Radio-telephone switch station
Rubella, 443
  pharyngitis and, 376
  polyarthralgias with, 359
Rubeola, pharyngitis and, 376
Rule of bigeminy, 1008
Rule of nines, in burn evaluation, 421
  for infants, 553
Rule of palms, in burn evaluation, 421
Rural EMS services, 22–23
  air transport in, 25
Russian Orthodox Church, beliefs and practices, 869
RV. *See* Residual volume
Rythmol. *See* Propafenone

S

Sacroplexus injuries, pelvic fractures and, 215
Saegesser's sign, 110
Safety issues, in helicopter transport, 26
SAH. *See* Subarachnoid hemorrhage
Sailfish, injuries by, 729
St. Anthony's Hospital (Denver), helicopter transport at, 23–24
St. Louis encephalitis, 400
Salbutamol. *See* Albuterol
Salicylates
  anaphylaxis risk with, 75
  chronic salicylism, 488
  overdose of, 325–326, 488–489
    assay methods, 472
    clinical signs, 472, 473–474, 488
    treatment of, 475, 476, 477
  pharmacokinetics and, 483
  renal failure and, 1225
Saline solution. *See also* Fluid replacement
  for hypercalcemia, 283, 314, 315
  for shock, 76, 80
  for wound irrigation, 140
Salmonella species
  in febrile children under two, 530
  in food poisoning, 390
  in gastroenteritis, 387, 388, 389, 390
Salmonella typhi, in acute sepsis, 406
Salpingectomy, in ectopic pregnancy, 1233
Salpingotomy, in ectopic pregnancy, 1233
Salt craving, in adrenal insufficiency, 259
Salt intake, heat cramps and, 656
Salt substitutes, for hypokalemia, 296
Salt tablets
  caution about, 656
  excessive ingestion of, 267
Salter-Harris fracture classification, 166, 167
  lateral condyle fractures, 203
Salvation Army, beliefs and practices, 869

San Francisco General Hospital, trauma care successes, 19
San Joaquin Valley, coccidioidomycosis and, 385
Sanctions. *See* Quality issues
Sandbag immobilization device, 108, 109
    for vertebral column fracture, 168
"Sandpaper" skin, in scarlet fever, 432
Sarcoidosis
    aseptic meningitis and, 399
    as diabetes insipidus cause, 267
    hypercalcemia and, 282, 318
    polyarticular arthritis with, 359
Saxitoxin, in shellfish poisoning, 734–735
SC. *See* Spasmodic croup
Scabies, 438–439
Scallops, poisoning by, 391, 731–734
Scalp, fungal infections of, 435, 436
Scalp wounds, 898. *See also* Head injuries
    debridement and, 140
    hemostatis techniques, 141
    lacerations, 149–150, 898
        dressings for, 157
    prehospital interventions, 107
    suture material for, 143
    suture removal from, 144
    suture technique for, 143
Scaphoid, rotary subluxation of, 206
Scaphoid fractures, 206
Scapholunate dissociation, 206
Scapula fractures, 199
Scarlet fever, 432
Scheuermann's disease, vertebral column injuries vs., 186
Schizophrenia
    alcohol withdrawal vs., 819
    alcoholism and, 824
    confusion in, 955
    toxic psychosis vs., 474
Schloendorff v. Society of New York Hospitals, 61
SCIWORA (spinal cord injury without radiographic abnormality) syndrome, 543
Scleritis, in rheumatoid arthritis, 338
Scleroderma
    gastrointestinal involvement in, 341–342
    pulmonary involvement in, 340
Sclerotherapy, endoscopic, for esophageal varices, 449, 453
Scoliosis
    congenital, vertebral column injuries vs., 186
    hereditary
        thorax deformities in, 365
        in Von Recklinghausen's disease, 369, 371
Scomboid fish poisoning, 391
Scombrotoxism, 739–740
Scoop stretcher, cost of, 109
Scopolamine, *See* Hyoscine
Scorpion bites, 642–643
    antivenin for, 493, 643
Scorpionfishes, spine or puncture wounds by, 727–728
Scrotum
    acute conditions of
        in infants and children, 559
        intrascrotal pain, 1211–1213
    injuries to, 1209
SDP. *See* Single-donor plasma
Sea anemones and sea corals, 720–721
Sea bather's eruption, 741
Sea moss dermatitis (Dogger Bank itch), 741
Sea nettles, 719
Sea snakes, 729–730
Sea stars, spine or puncture injuries by, 723
Sea urchins, spine or puncture injuries by, 722–723
Sea wasps, 718, 719
Seafood, skin infections from, 408
SEALEASY Mask, 95
Seat belt injuries
    to cervical spine, 904–905
    to larynx, 1313
    to rectum or colon, 465
Seat belt sign, 110
Seat-belt fractures, 164, 177, 192
Seaweed, marine, 741

Secobarbital (Seconal; Quinalbarbitone), 1440. *See also* Barbiturates
    elimination half-life of, 800
    pharmacology of, 801
Secondary survey, multisystem injuries, 94, 103–112
Sedation
    for endotracheal intubation, 1106
    for epistaxis, 1306
    in hyphema treatment, 1284
    for sexual abuse examination, 606
Sedative-hypnotics, 800–805, 1438–1441
    abstinence syndromes, 804–805
        opioid abstinence vs., 798
    alcohol use and, 800
    for alcohol withdrawal, 821
    battering syndrome and, 842
    for headache, 922
    high altitude caution, 684
    history of, 800
    intoxication signs, 802
    listed, 800
    overdose of, 492, 802–804
        clinical signs, 472, 473, 803
        treatment of, 802–804
    for pain relief, 882, 883, 884
    pharmacology of, 800–802
    renal failure and, 1226
    as unconsciousness cause, 591
Seizures, 945–950
    absence, 949
    acute confusion after, 954
    in alcohol withdrawal, 822, 948–949
    approaches to patient with, 945
    in brain abscess, 400
    in children
        as dehydration sign, 268
        with fever, 595–596
    cocaine-related, 792–793
    convulsive status epilepticus, 945, 946–947. *See also* Status epilepticus
    defined, 945
    etiologies of, 945, 946. *See also specific types of seizures*
    febrile, 950
    focal, 949
    generalized tonic-clonic (grand mal), 945, 948
    in head injury, 901
        anticonvulsants for, 898
    in hyperosmolar hyperglycemic nonketotic coma, 243
    in hyponatremia, 271, 272
    idiopathic, defined, 945
    magnesium deficiency and, 286, 307
    morbidity with, 945–946
    normeperidine-induced, 794–795
    partial, 949
    in polyarteritis nodosa, 343
    in subarachnoid hemorrhage, 941
    symptomatic, defined, 945
    syncope and, 961, 962, 963
    in systemic lupus erythematosus, 343
    terminology, 945
    in toxicologic emergencies, 472, 473
Self-mutilation, adrenal insufficiency and, 259
Sellick's maneuver, in endotracheal intubation, 96
Sengstaken-Blakemore tube, in balloon tamponade, 450
Sensory enhancement, in adrenal insufficiency, 259
Sensory function, assessing
    in multisystem trauma, 106
    in vertebral column trauma, 182–183
Sensory impairment
    in carpal tunnel syndrome, 347
    in hypothermia, 666
    in systemic lupus erythematosus, 344
Sensory radiculopathy, in Lyme disease, 357
Sepsis
    acute, 406–407
    adrenal gland hemorrhage and, 256
    adrenal insufficiency and, 256
    community-acquired, 406–407
    differential diagnosis, 406

electrolyte disorders as, 265
in shock response, 71
testing for, in febrile infants under 3 months, 534–535
Septic abortion, signs of, 1230
Septic arthritis, 204, 410–412
    diagnosis of, 351, 352, 356–357, 411
    differential diagnosis, 411
    drug abuse and, 785
    in elbow, 204
    as human bite complication, 156
    pathogenesis of, 411
    treatment of, 411–412
Septic bursitis, 412
Septic shock, 72
    in adrenal insufficiency, 260
    monitoring with, 83
    as transfusion reaction, 134
    treatment of, 85, 86
Septra. *See* Trimethoprim-sulfamethoxazole
Serax. *See* Oxazepam
Serositis, in systemic lupus erythematosus, 342
Serotonergic agents, for headache, 924
Serotonin, hypovolemic shock and, 71
Serpasil. *See* Reserpine
Serratia marcescens
    in corneal ulcers, 1274, 1275
    in pneumonia, 383
    in urinary tract infections, 391
Serum, for emergency department, 1453
Serum albumin. *See* Albumin, human
Serum amylase level, in diabetic ketoacidosis, 235
Serum creatinine, renal failure and, 1221
Serum enzyme levels. *See also specific enzymes*
    in acute myocardial infarction, 970, 982
    in pulmonary embolism, 1145
Serum glutamic oxaloacetate transaminase (SGOT), in pulmonary embolism, 1145
Serum lactate dehydrogenase. *See* Lactic dehydrogenase levels
Serum osmolarity
    in hypernatremia, 267, 268–269
    in hyponatremia, 271, 272
Serum sickness
    as antivenin reaction, 493
    as drug reaction, 433
Seventh Day Adventists, beliefs and practices, 865
Severed parts, replantation of, 212
Sex-linked disorders, adrenal insufficiency and, 258
Sexual abuse, 605–608, 1253
    conditions confused with, 607
    defined, 1243, 1253
    documentation of, 608
    evaluation of, 605–608
    legal issues in, 607, 608
    STD as sign of, 1250, 1253
    treatment of, 608
Sexual activity, urinary tract infections and, 394
Sexual assault. *See also* Rape
    definitions of, 1243
    legal issues in, 1243–1244
Sexual molestation, defined, 1243
Sexually transmitted diseases. *See also specific diseases*
    consent issues, 42
    gonococcal proctitis, 466
    hepatitis A, 403
    hepatitis B, 403, 458
    herpes simplex type 2, 441, 442
    pediculosis, 437
    pelvic inflammatory disease and, 1233
    rape and, 1249, 1250
    rectal herpes, 466
    scabies, 439
    sexual abuse and, 608, 1250
    syphilis, 439–440
    urethritis in men, 394–395
SFH. *See* Stroma-free hemoglobin
SGOT. *See* Serum glutamic oxaloacetate transaminase
Shaken baby syndrome, 589, 600–601

Sharks
    dogfish, spine or puncture wounds by, 724
    food poisoning and, 712, 736
    lacerations by, 712–713, 715
Shearing fractures of vertebral column, 179–180
Sheehan's syndrome, as diabetes insipidus cause, 267
Shellfish poisoning, 390, 391
    bivalve mollusks, 731–734
    paralytic, 391, 734–735
    skin infections, 408
    venerupin, 734
Shigella species
    in food poisoning, 390
    in gastroenteritis, 387, 388
        dysenteric, 390
        treatment and, 389, 390
    in infants and children, 558
Shin splints, tibial stress fractures vs., 226
Shingles (herpes zoster), 442
Shivering, 662
Shock, 65–87
    in adrenal insufficiency, 258–259, 260
    anaphylactic, 75
    blood pressure in, 66–67
    burn, 418
    in cardiac tamponade, 103
    cardiogenic, 72–75
        clinical features, 73, 74–75
        as MAST suit contraindication, 77
        treatment of, 84–85
    in children, 544
    dropping, 256
    emotional, hypersuggestibility and, 874
    etiologies of, 68, 76
    hypovolemic. *See* Hypovolemic shock
    IV management and, site choice for large-bore IV line, 102
    maxillofacial injuries and, 1320, 1321
    monitoring for, 81–83
        in first response, 76
    physiologic effects of, 65–67
    pneumatic anti-shock garment (PASG), controversy about, 5
    resuscitation fluids for, 125–130
    septic, 72
        as transfusion reaction, 134
        treatment of, 85, 86
    spinal, 104
    staging of, 101
    as thyroid storm result, 250
    treatment of, 75–81, 84–87
        first response, 76
        fluid replacement, 78–81, 84
        inotropic and vasopressor agents, 84
        MAST suit in, 76–78
        Trendelenburg position, 78
        vasodilators, 85
    in vascular emergencies, 1069
"Shock lung," physiology of, 79
Shortness of breath. *See* Dyspnea
Shoulder arthritis, shoulder-hand syndrome and, 347
Shoulder injuries, 199–201
    acromioclavicular separations, 198
    adhesive capsulitis (frozen shoulder), 346–347
    bursitis, 201, 344–345
    dislocations, 173, 199–200
    of rotator cuff, 200, 346
    tendinitis, 201, 345–346
Shoulder joint
    arthrocentesis of, 353, 354
    aspiration or injection of, 1374, 1375
Shoulder syndromes, 346–348
    shoulder-hand syndrome (Sudec's atrophy), 347
Shoulder tendinitis, 345–346
Shrimp, poisoning by, 735
Shunt, V/Q ratio and, 1154
Sickle cell disease/sickle cell trait
    abdominal pain in, 369, 370
    burns and, 424
    as diabetes insipidus cause, 268
    high altitude and, 685
    hyphema and, 1286, 1287

hyponatremia and, 271, 272
inhalant abuse and, 805
splenic thrombosis and, 459
SIDS. *See* Sudden infant death syndrome
Sigmoid diverticulitis, obstruction and, 460
Sigmoid volvulus, 460, 461
Sigmoidoscopy
    in Crohn's disease, 462
    in ulcerative colitis, 462
Silk sutures, 142
Silvadene. *See* Silver sulfadiazine
Silver nitrate solution
    for burns, 424, 425
    for erythema multiforme, 435
Silver sulfadiazine (Silvadene), for burns, 424, 425
Simmonds' syndrome, as diabetes insipidus cause, 267
Sinequan. *See* Doxepin
Single-donor plasma (SDP), in component therapy, 120, 121
Sinus arrest (sudden sinus or atrial standstill), 1010–1012
Sinus tachycardia, 1018–1019
Sinusitis
    acute, 378–379, 1299–1303
    anatomy and, 1299–1300
    clinical signs of, 1300–1301
    complications of, 1301, 1302
    diagnosis of, 1301–1302
    differential diagnosis, 1302
    etiologies of, 1300, 1301
    as headache cause, 917
    orbital cellulitis and, 1296
    pathophysiology of, 1300
    treatment of, 1302–1303
Siphonophores, stings by, 718
Sipple's syndrome, hypercalcemia and, 282
Situational syncope, 961, 963
Sjögren's disease, ocular problems in, 338
Skates and rays, poisoning by, 712, 736
Skeletal injuries. *See also* Fractures
    basic vs. advanced life support skills, 94
    in children, 543
Skeletal muscle relaxants. *See* Muscle relaxants
Skiing accidents. *See also* Sports injuries
    "ski pole" thumb, 209
    tibia fractures, 226
Skin
    burn injuries to. *See* Burns
    child abuse indicators, 598–599. *See also* Child abuse
    dehydration signs in, 268
    in hereditary disorders, 364, 365, 368, 369
    hypothermia and, 663
    prickly heat on, 655
    in shock
        cardiogenic, 73, 75
        hypovolemic, 70
        septic, 72
    toxic contamination of, 474
Skin disorders
    acanthosis nigricans, 429
    adrenal insufficiency and, 258
    of AIDS, 443–444
    atopic dermatitis, 429–430
    contact dermatitis, 432–433
    in diabetes mellitus, 433
    drug eruptions, 433–434
    erythema multiforme, 434–435
    erythema nodosum, 435
    heat illness and, 655
    hypothermia and, 662
    marine-associated, 741
    pediculosis, 437
    pemphigus vulgaris, 437
    pityriasis rosea, 437–438
    roseola infantum, 438
    scabies, 438–439
    sponge fisherman's disease, 716
    in syphilis, 439–440
    toxic epidermal necrolysis, 440
    urticaria, 440–441

Skin infections. *See also specific infections*
    AIDS and, 444
    animal-associated, 409
    bacterial, 430–432
    cellulitis, 431–432
    cutaneous abscesses, 407–408, 431
    erythrasma, 430
    fungal, 435–437
    herpes zoster (shingles), 442
    herpetic whitlow, 408
    impetigo, 431
    marine-associated, 408–409, 742
    measles, 442–443
    occupational, 408–409
    pyoderma, 430–432
    Rocky Mountain spotted fever, 438
    rubella, 443
    scarlet fever, 432
    soil-associated, 409
    staphylococcal scalded skin syndrome, 431
    tick-borne, 409
    toxic shock syndrome (TSS), 432
    varicella (chickenpox), 443
    viral, 441–443
Skin substitutes, as burn dressings, 425–426
Skin wounds. *See* Wound management; *specific sites*
Skull fractures, 898–899
    assessing for, 107, 110, 898
    complications of, 901
    epidural hematomas and, 899
    pediatric, 589
Skull radiography, in head injury, 897
Skunk bites, rabies precautions, 629
Sleep aids, overdose of, 491
Sleep apnea
    as daytime headache cause, 917
    at high altitudes, 684
Slice fracture, of thoracic spine, 192
Slice fracture-dislocation, of vertebral column, 164, 176
Slings, for upper extremity injuries
    clavicle fractures, 198
    wounds, 157
Slipping rib (rib tip syndrome), 348
Slo-Phyllin. *See* Theophylline
Slow virus, encephalitis and, 400
Slow-K. *See* Potassium chloride
Small bowel obstruction, 459–460
Small bowel resection, hypomagnesemia and, 306
Smallpox, polyarthralgias with, 359
Smith's fracture, 205
Smoke inhalation, 494, 1163–1165. *See also* Inhalation injury
    management of, 772–773
    pharyngitis and, 377
    treatment of, 1164–1165
Smoking. *See also* Substance abuse
    carbon monoxide and, 765, 1160
    as CVA risk factor, 935
    hypothermia and, 672
    socioeconomic impact of, 782
Snake bites, 634–640
    anaphylaxis risk with, 75
    antivenin treatments for, 493, 638–639
    clinical signs of, 635–636
    effects of venom, 634–635
    epidemiology of, 634
    management of, 636–640
    sea snakes, 729–730
    taxonomy and physiology and, 634
Snapper, poisoning by, 712
Sneezing, in anaphylaxis, 75
Social theory, domestic violence and, 843–844
Social workers
    child abuse and, 602
    domestic abuse and, 854
    elder abuse and, 847
    opioid abuse and, 799
    rape intervention role, 1255
    sexual abuse and, 605–606, 608
Sodium bicarbonate, 1390–1391
    in advanced cardiac life support, 1090

in alkaline diuresis, 475
for antidepressant toxicity, 485
in CPR
  of pediatric patients, 522, 523
  sodium excess from, 26
for cyanide poisoning, 755
for diabetic ketoacidosis, 239
for hyperkalemia, 280, 281, 299, 300
hypothermia and, 671
Sodium chloride, for metabolic alkalosis, 328
Sodium fluoroacetate overdose, clinical signs, 473
Sodium levels. *See also* Hypernatremia; Hyponatremia
adrenal insufficiency and, 258, 259
diabetic ketoacidosis and, 235–236
HHNK coma and, 242, 244
in hyponatremia, 270, 272
myxedema coma and, 252
physiology and, 266
renal failure and, 1225
Sodium nitrite, 1450
for cyanide poisoning, 768
Sodium nitroprusside (Nipride), 1397
in acute myocardial infarction treatment, 993
for congestive heart failure, 1055
for hypertensive emergencies, 1059, 1060–1061, 1063
  acute aortic dissection, 1066
  catecholamine crisis, 1067
  eclampsia, 1066
  intracranial hemorrhage, 1066
in renal failure treatment, 1225
Sodium polystyrene sulfonate (Kayexalate), 1450
for hyperkalemia, 280, 300, 1225
Sodium thiosulfate, 1450
for cyanide poisoning, 768
Soft tissue infections
necrotizing, 409–410
wisdom teeth and, 1332
Soft tissue injuries
basic vs. advanced life support skills, 94
in children, 552, 553
maxillofacial, 1320, 1325–1328
Soft tissue rheumatism
Baker's cyst, 346
bursitis, 344–345
carpal tunnel syndrome, 347
chest wall syndrome, 347–348
shoulder syndromes, 346–347
shoulder-hand syndrome, 347
tendinitis, 345–346
Soil-borne infections, of skin, 409
Soles, erythema multiforme on, 434
Solu-Cortef. *See* Hydrocortisone
Solu-Medrol. *See* Methylprednisolone
Solvent intoxication, 474, 756–757
behavioral disorders and, 474
carbon monoxide and, 478
by inhalant abuse, 805–806
skin or ocular decontamination, 474
Solvents, listed, 756
Soma. *See* Carisoprodol
Sopor. *See* Methaqualone
Spasmodic croup (SC), 565, 1116
Spasmolytics, for emergency department, 1453
Spectinomycin (Trobicin), 1423–1424
for gonococcal dermatitis, 430
for gonococcal pharyngitis, 378
for gonorrhea, 1250
for septic gonococcal arthritis, 411
Spherocytosis, hereditary, 369, 370
Spicules, sponge stings by, 716
Spider bites, 640–642
anaphylaxis risk with, 75
black widow spiders, 493
Spinal cord compression, in cancer patient, 503–504
Spinal cord injuries
assessing for, 181–183
in cervical spine, 903, 905, 907, 909–910
  anatomical structure and, 908
  classifications of, 909
  diagnosis of, 913
  special problems with, 912–913

HBO therapy for, 709
incomplete, 183–185
prehospital interventions, 104
without radiographic abnormality (SCIWORA syndrome), 543
Spinal fusion, vertebral osteomyelitis and, 193
Spinal immobilization, principles of, 108–109
Spinal injuries. *See also* Central nervous system injuries; Cervical spine injuries; Vertebral column injuries
compression fractures, 164, 165
prehospital approaches, 104, 107–109
slice fracture-dislocation, 164
spinal shock, 104, 105
types of, 104
Spinal root injuries, 184
steroids and, 104
Spinal shock, 104, 105, 182
Spine boards
costs of, 109
using, 187
Spines of invertebrates, injuries by, 724–729
Spines of vertebrates, injuries by, 724–729
Spiral fractures, 163, 164
Spiritual needs. *See also* Religion
assessment of, 864
in crisis situations, 862–865
defined, 863
in holistic model, 857–858
nonmedical healing methods, 869–870
religious resources for, 864–865
spiritual distress diagnosis, 862–863
support techniques, 870–875
Spiritual well-being, defined, 863
Spirituality
defined, 862
spiritual distress and, 862–863
Spirochetes, diseases caused by. *See* Lyme disease; Syphilis
Spironolactone (Aldactone), 1431
hyperkalemia and, 272, 279, 298
for hypokalemia, with periodic paralysis, 278
for metabolic alkalosis, 328
Spleen surgery, adrenal insufficiency and, 257
Splenectomy, acute sepsis and, 406
Splenic rupture and infarct, 459
Splenomegaly, in infectious mononucleosis, 401, 402
Splinting
for carpal tunnel syndrome, 347
for dislocations, 173, 174
extremity wounds, 157
fingers, 207
of fractures, 168, 171–172, 173
upper extremity injuries, 195
  clavicle fractures, 198
for vertebral column injuries, 193
Spondyloarthropathies
ocular emergencies in, 338
polyarticular arthritis with, 359
Spondylolisthesis, traumatic, 191
Sponge fisherman's disease, 716
Sponges, stings by, 716
Sporothrix schenckii, 409
Sports injuries. *See also* Divers; Diving injuries; Football accidents; Skiing accidents; Swimming
carbon monoxide poisoning, 765
to cervical spine, 904, 905
high-altitude-related, 679–686
to knee, 223–224
by marine organisms, 711. *See also* Marine organisms
near-drowning, 689–698
stress fractures, 166, 167
of hip, 219
to teeth, 1333
to vertebral column, 175, 192, 193
Spouse abuse. *See also* Battering syndrome; Domestic violence
defined, 837
by men vs. women, 842
misconceptions about, 842–843

Sprains
ankle, 230–231
  ligamentous instability and, 226
finger, differential diagnosis, 210
wrist, differential diagnosis, 207
Sprue, nontropical, hypomagnesemia and, 306
Sputum examination, in pneumonia diagnosis, 385
Squids, poisoning by, 735
Stab wounds
to bladder, 1202
to chest, 1181
  intra-abdominal wounds with, 1181–1182
in children, 541
to head, 899
to heart, 1078–1079, 1185
  mortality in, 1185–1186
Stabilization
COBRA intent and, 7
training controversy about, 5
transfer requirements, 7
Stadol. *See* Butorphanol
Staffpower and training, 3–6
for disasters, 32, 33, 34
EMS coordinators, 19
one-tiered vs. two-tiered systems, 21–22
prehospital care issues, 21–22
in rural vs. urban areas, 22, 23
Standards of care
defenses and, 41
development of, 62
Standing orders, ALS medical control through, 20
Staphcillin. *See* Methicillin
Staphylococcus albus, in otitis externa, 1310
Staphylococcus aureus
in acute sepsis, 406
in bite wounds, 155, 156, 630, 631, 632
in corneal ulcers, 1274, 1275, 1277
in cutaneous abscesses, 407
in encephalitis and brain abscess, 400
in food poisoning, 390
in gastroenteritis, 388
in monoarticular arthritis, 355, 357
in oropharyngeal infections, 382, 383
in osteomyelitis, 358
in otitis externa, 380, 1310, 1311
in otitis media, 380, 1309
in peritonsillar abscess, 569
in pneumonia, 383, 384
  in children, 585, 586
in retropharyngeal abscess, 569
in septic arthritis, 410, 412
in sinusitis, 378, 1302, 1303
in staphylococcal scalded skin syndrome, 431, 440
in toxic epidermal necrolysis, 440
in toxic shock syndrome, 432
in tracheitis, bacterial, 569, 1116, 1117
as vertebral osteomyelitis cause, 193
Staphylococcus epidermidis, in corneal ulcers, 1274
Staphylococcus saprophyticus, in urinary tract infections, 391
Staphylococcus species, skin infections with, 430–432, 440
Staple closure of lacerations, 149
Stare decisis, 39
Starfish, spine or puncture injuries by, 723
Starling's law
cardiogenic shock and, 74
fluid replacement and, 79
shock diagnosis and, 66
Starvation
as diabetes insipidus cause, 268
hypokalemia and, 275
as hypomagnesemia cause, 305
State laws
antidumping regulations, 42–43
organ transplants and, 43
Status epilepticus, 946–947
in children, 592–595
clinical interventions in, 594
complications of, 593
defined, 945
etiologies of, 593, 947

Status epilepticus (contd.)
  history taking in, 946
  treatment of, 594–595, 946–947
Status inconsistency theory of domestic violence, 844
Statutes, 39
Steatorrhea
  hypocalcemia and, 284
  hypomagnesemia and, 286, 306
Steel sutures, 142
"Steeple sign," in croup, 1114
Steinmann pin, in proximal tibia fracture, 225
Stellate ganglion blockade, for Raynaud's phenomenon, 341
Steri-strips, wound closure with, 148–149
Sternal fracture, 1183
Sternoclavicular joint
  dislocations, 198–199
  monoarthritis of, 351
  sprains or subluxations, 199
Sternotomy, for blunt chest trauma, 1072
Sternum dysmorphology, in hereditary disorders, 364, 365
Steroids. See Corticosteroids
Stevens-Johnson syndrome, 434
Stibine, as systemic toxin, 775
Stifneck cervical collar, 108, 109
Still's disease, arthritis with, 358–359
Stimson technique, for shoulder dislocation, 200
Stinging seaweed dermatitis, 741
Stingrays, spine or puncture wounds by, 724–725
Stings
  by insects, anaphylaxis risk and, 75, 87, 643, 644
  by marine organisms, 716–721, 741
Stockinette dressings. See Dressings; specific injuries
Stomach
  adenocarcinoma of, acanthosis nigricans and, 429
  gastric content analysis, for toxin, 471
  surgery on, adrenal insufficiency and, 257
  ulceration of, in systemic lupus erythematosus, 342
Stonefish, spine or puncture wounds by, 727–728
Stool examination
  in acute watery diarrhea, 390
  in bleeding diagnosis, 450–451
  in gastroenteritis, 388–389
  in hemorrhoids, 465
  in ileocolic intussusception, 557
Stoxil. See Idoxuridine
STP. See Dimethoxyamphetamine; Dimethoxymethylamphetamine
Strabismus, as headache cause, 917
Straddle injury, to urethra, 1206, 1207
Strangulation injury, to penis, 1208, 1209
Strawberry nevus, in hereditary disorders, 365
"Strawberry" tongue, in toxic shock syndrome, 406
Streptase. See Streptokinase
Streptococci
  in acute sepsis, 406
  in cat bites, 156
  cellulitis and, 431, 432
  in common colds, 375
  in corneal ulcers, 1274, 1275, 1277
  in cutaneous abscesses, 407
  in dog bites, 155, 630
  in encephalitis and brain abscess, 400
  in febrile children under two, 530, 531, 532
  in human bites, 156
  human bites, 632, 633
  impetigo and, 431
  in meningitis, 396, 398
  in necrotizing fasciitis or myositis, 410
  in occult bacteremia (OB), in children under two, 530, 531, 532
  in oropharyngeal infections, 382
  in otitis externa, 380, 1310, 1311
  in otitis media, 380, 381, 1309
  in pharyngitis, 376, 377, 378
  in pneumonia, 383, 384, 386
    in children, 585, 586
  polyarticular arthritis and, 358
  scarlet fever and, 432
  in septic arthritis, 410
  in sinusitis, 378, 379, 1302

  skin infections with, 430–432
  in tracheitis, bacterial, 569, 1116
Streptokinase (Kabikinase; Streptase), 1402
  for acute myocardial infarction, 982
Streptomycin, 1411
  anaphylaxis risk with, 75
  for corneal ulcers, 1275
  for open fractures, 168
Stress
  crisis and, 858, 859
  as diarrhea cause, 387, 388
  domestic violence and, 844
  hyponatremia and, 271
  as syncope cause, 960–961
Stress disorder, rape trauma syndrome, 1254–1255
Stress fractures, 166, 167
  of feet, 167
  of hip, 219
  tibial, 226
Stridor
  in anaphylaxis, 75, 565
  approach to child with, 1119
  in croup syndromes, 1113, 1115
  in infants and children
    congenital causes of, 570
    with fever, 566–570
    with sudden onset, 564–566
Stroke. See Cerebrovascular accident
Stroma-free hemoglobin (SFH)
  as blood substitute, 81, 127
  problems with, 128
  for shock, 80, 127–128
Strychnine poisoning
  clinical signs, 472
  treatment of, 475–476
Stryker frame, for thoracolumbar fractures, 188
Stupor, in hypomagnesemia, 304
Stupor-coma, prototypical patient in, 927
Sturge-Weber syndrome, 364, 365
Subacromial bursa, aspiration or injection of, 1374
Subacromial bursitis, 201
Subarachnoid hemorrhage (SAH), 900, 939–941
  acute confusion with, 955
  cerebral aneurysm and, 918
  syncope and, 961
Subclavian steal syndrome, 961
Subclavian vein cannulation, 1339–1342
  in multisystem trauma, 103
Subconjunctival hemorrhage, assessing for, 110
Subcutaneous tissue, suture material for, 142
Subcuticular sutures, 144, 145
Subdural hematoma, 899–900
  acute confusion with, 954
  alcohol withdrawal vs., 819
  in children, unconsciousness with, 589
  chronic, as headache cause, 918–919
Subgaleal hematoma, 899
Sublimaze. See Fentanyl
Subluxations, 173
  in cervical spine, 908
  in rheumatoid arthritis, 343
Submandibular space infections, 382
Substance abuse, 781–810. See also Alcoholism; Drug abuse
  adulterants, substitutes, and diluents, 784
  in battering syndrome, 842
  burn center referral and, 48
  complications of, 783
  defined, 782, 783
  extent of, 781–782
  history taking on, 786
  profile of abuser, 783–784
  reaction to abuser, 783–784
  referral for, 783, 784
  socioeconomic effects of, 781
  terminology of, 783–783
  toxicologic screening for, 786
Substance addiction, defined, 782
Substance dependence, defined, 782
Subtrochanteric fractures of hip, 220
Subungual fibromas, 369
Subungual hematoma, of distal phalanx, 207

Subxiphoid pericardial window, 1190
Succinylcholine
  anaphylaxis risk with, 75
  in endotracheal intubation, 1106–1107
  hyperkalemia risk with, 279, 298
Sucralfate (Carafate), 1434
Sudden infant death syndrome (SIDS), adrenal insufficiency and, 258
Sudec's atrophy, 347
Sugar tong splints, 172, 173
Suicidal patients, 829. See also Suicide attempts
  depression and, 831, 834
  evaluation of, 832–833
  legal issues, 831–832, 833
  referral to inpatient care for, 831–832, 833, 834
  types of, 833–835
Suicide
  by adolescents, 541
  sedative-hypnotic abuse and, 800
Suicide attempts. See also Suicidal patients; Toxicologic emergencies
  arsenic ingestion, 494
  in battering syndrome, 842
  domestic violence and, 841
  emergency department role, 833, 834–835
  mercury ingestion, 494
Sulbactam, in animal bite therapy, 158
Sulfa drugs, pregnancy and, 1239
Sulfacetamide, in eye drops or ointment, 1269
Sulfadiazine
  for malaria, 407
  for toxoplasmosis, 402
Sulfamethoxazole/trimethoprim (SMZ/TMP). See Trimethoprim-sulfamethoxazole
Sulfamylon. See Mafenide acetate
Sulfasalazine
  for Crohn's disease, 462
  for ulcerative colitis, 463
Sulfhemoglobinemia, in toxicologic emergencies, 473
Sulfinpyrazone (Anturane), 1405
Sulfisoxazole (Gantrisin), 1417
  in eye drops or ointment, 1269
  for otitis media, 1309
  for urinary tract infections, 393
Sulfites, anaphylaxis risk with, 75
Sulfocysteinuria, 364
Sulfonamides, 1417
  for corneal ulcers, 1275
  as meningitis prevention, 398
  for otitis media, 381
  overdose of, 473
  renal failure and, 1225
  serum sickness and, 433
Sulfur dioxide inhalation, 771–772
  from fires, 494
Sulfur-containing drugs, intoxication by, 473
Sulindac (Clinoril)
  as aseptic meningitis cause, 344
  for pain relief, 881
Sumatriptan, for headache, 923
Sumycin. See Tetracycline
Superior vena cava (SVC) obstruction, in cancer patients, 510–511
Support persons
  death of patient and, 860–861
  depressed patient and, 832
  for rape victim, 1245
Supracondylar fractures, 202
Supraglottitis
  acute. See Epiglottitis, acute
  thermal, from hot liquid, 566
Supravalvular aortic stenosis, idiopathic hypercalcemia of infancy and, 283
Supraventricular tachydysrhythmias, 1018–1028, 1029
  atrial fibrillation, 1009, 1018, 1022–1023
  atrial flutter, 1016, 1018, 1023–1024
  ectopic atrial tachycardia (EAT), 1018, 1019, 1020
  mechanisms of, 1018
  multifocal (chaotic) atrial tachycardia (MAT), 1018, 1019, 1021–1022
  nonparoxysmal junctional tachycardia (NPJT), 1018, 1028, 1029

paroxysmal supraventricular tachycardia (PSVT), 1018, 1024–1028
sinus tachycardia, 1018–1019
Suprax. *See* Cefixime
Surgeonfishes, spine or puncture wounds by, 728–729
Surgical emergencies. *See also* Postoperative complications
  abdominal pain, in children, 555–557
  adrenal gland hemorrhage and, 256
  brain abscess, 401
  in cancer patients, 504–505
  cholecystitis, 454
  Crohn's disease, 462
  cutaneous abscesses, 407
  esophageal varices, 453
  gout or pseudogout precipitated by, 352
  hemoptysis, 1168–1169
  intestinal obstruction, 460, 461
  intracranial pressure elevation, 502
  lower GI bleeding, 451
  necrotizing fasciitis or myositis, 409–410
  pancreatitis, 456
  pediatric, 541–560. *See also specific conditions*
  revascularization, in cardiogenic shock, 74
  upper GI bleeding, 450
Surgical airways, 1110–1111
Surgical patients, air transport criteria, 25–26
Surital. *See* Thiamylal
Sus-Phrine. *See* Epinephrine
Sutilains ointment, burn debridement with, 425
Suturing, 141–148. *See also specific types of wounds*
  of children, guidelines for, 552–553
  ligature technique, 141
  removal guide, 144
  techniques, 142–148
    horizontal mattress sutures, 148
    running/running locking sutures, 148, 149
    simple sutures, 144–145, 146
    subcuticular sutures, 144, 145
    vertical mattress suture, 145, 147
  types of sutures, 141–142, 143
SVC (superior vena cava) syndrome, 510–511
Swan-Ganz catheterization
  in congestive heart failure evaluation, 1052–1053, 1056–1057
  procedure, 1347–1349
  in shock monitoring, 83
Sweating
  adrenal insufficiency and, 258
  decrease in, as dehydration sign, 268
  heat illness and, 654
  profuse. *See* Diaphoresis
"Swimmer's ear," 379–380, 1310–1311
Swimming
  as dermatitis cause, 742
  drowning accidents and, 689–690
Swine, skin infections from, 409
Swinging accidents, renal trauma in, 1195
Swordfish, injuries by, 729
Sympathectomy
  for frostbite, 673
  for Raynaud's phenomenon, 341
Sympathetic nervous system
  cardiogenic shock and, 74
  in response to injury, 69
  in thyroid storm, 249
Sympathomimetic agents, 1281
  abuse of, 796–793. *See also specific drugs*
  acute hypokalemia and, 474
  in advanced cardiac life support, 1089
  listed, 787
  for obstructive airway disease, 1133
  overdose of, catecholamine-induced hypertension from, 1066
  toxicity signs and symptoms, 787
  for uveitis, 1281
  for Wolff-Parkinson-White syndrome, 1042
Syncope, 959–963
  in adrenal insufficiency, 258
  in anaphylaxis, 75
  cardiovascular, 959–960, 961–962, 963
  defined, 959

diagnostic approach to, 959, 960, 961–962
diagnostic procedures in, 962–963
dysrhythmia and, 997
noncardiovascular, 960–962, 963
unheralded, in subarachnoid hemorrhage, 940
of unknown etiology, 961–962, 963
Synovial fluid aspiration, 353–355, 1373–1375
Synovitis
  chronic hydroxyapatite (Milwaukee shoulder), 351
  cricoarytenoid, in rheumatoid arthritis, 339
  onset of, 351–352
Synthetic substances, inhalation injury by, 1162–1163
Synthroid. *See* Levothyroxine
Syntocinon. *See* Oxytocin
Syphilis, 439–440
  AIDS and, 444
  aseptic meningitis and, 399
  as diabetes insipidus cause, 267
  diagnosis of, 439–440
  encephalitis and, 400, 401
  oral lesions with, 382
  rape and, 1250
  serologic testing for, with urethritis, 395
  treatment of, 440
Systemic lupus erythematosus, 335
  acute monoarticular arthritis with, 358
  adrenal insufficiency and, 258
  aseptic meningitis and, 399
  cardiac involvement in, 340–341
  as cause of death, 340, 342
  cutaneous lesions in, 336, 337
  fever in, 335
  gastrointestinal involvement in, 342–343
  neurologic involvement in, 343, 344
  ocular emergencies in, 338
  polyarticular arthritis with, 359
  pulmonary involvement in, 339–340
  vascular involvement in, 341
Systemic toxins, 773–776
  volatile hydrocarbons, 774
Systems theory, of domestic violence, 844
Systolic murmur, syncope and, 959–960

T

"Ts and blues." *See* Pentazocine
TAC solution, as wound anesthetic, 139, 885–886, 1325
Tacaryl. *See* Methdilazine
Tachycardia. *See also* Dysrhythmias; Tachydysrhythmias
  in acute myocardial infarction, management of, 983–984
  in children, 575
  ectopic atrial (EAT), 1018, 1019, 1020
  magnesium therapy for, 307
  multifocal (chaotic) atrial (MAT), 1018, 1019, 1021–1022
  nonparoxysmal junctional (NPJT), 1018, 1028, 1029
  paroxysmal supraventricular (PSVT), 1018, 1024–1028
  in polyarteritis nodosa, 342
  regular, wide QRS, 1034, 1037, 1038, 1039
  in shock
    cardiogenic, 74
    hypovolemic, 68, 70
  sinus, 1018–1019
  in thyroid storm, 249, 250, 251
  ventricular (VT), 1004, 1030, 1032–1034
    advanced cardiac life support, 1090–1091
Tachydysrhythmias, 1018–1037, 1038, 1039. *See also* Dysrhythmias; Tachycardia
  in adrenal insufficiency, 259
  in alcohol withdrawal, 307
  paroxysmal supraventricular tachycardia (PSVT), 1018, 1024–1028
  regular, wide QRS tachycardias, 1034, 1037, 1038, 1039
  supraventricular, 1018–1028, 1029
    atrial fibrillation, 1009, 1018, 1022–1023
    atrial flutter, 1016, 1018, 1023–1024

ectopic atrial tachycardia (EAT), 1018, 1019, 1020
mechanisms of, 1018
multifocal (chaotic) atrial tachycardia (MAT), 1018, 1019, 1021–1022
nonparoxysmal junctional tachycardia (NPJT), 1018, 1028, 1029
sinus tachycardia, 1018–1019
ventricular, 1028, 1030–1034
  accelerated idioventricular rhythm (AIVR), 1028, 1030, 1031
  ventricular fibrillation (VF), 1004, 1034, 1036
  ventricular tachycardia (VT), 1004, 1030, 1032–1034
Tachypnea
  in children, 575
  dehydration risk with, 267
  in pulmonary embolism, 1144
  in shock
    cardiogenic, 73, 74
    hypovolemic, 68
  in systemic lupus erythematosus, 340
Tagamet. *See* Cimetidine
Talonavicular joint injuries, 229
Talus fractures, 228, 229
Talwin. *See* Pentazocine
Tambocor. *See* Flecainide
Tamoxifen, hypercalcemic crisis and, 315, 317
Tampon use, toxic shock syndrome and, 432
Tandearil. *See* Oxyphenbutazone
Tangential excision, for burns, 425
Tape closure of lacerations, 148–149
Tape recording, of EMS communications, 8
Tapping fractures, 161, 163
Tar burns, 424
TAR syndrome. *See* Thrombocytopenia and absent radius
Tarsometatarsal (Lisfranc's joint) injuries, 229
Tay-Sachs disease, 372
Tazidime. *See* Ceftazidime
TBW (total body water), 265–266
TCSA. *See* Toxic Substances Control Act
Tear gas exposure, 754
Teardrop fracture, of cervical spine, 191–192, 907, 908
Tears, absence of, as dehydration sign, 268
TEC solution, as wound anesthetic, 139
Technetium scan. *See also* Radionuclide scan
  for lower GI bleeding, 451
  in stress fracture diagnosis, 226
Technology, interpersonal skills vs., 55
TEE. *See* Transesophageal echocardiography
Teeth
  fracture or avulsion of, 1333–1335
  infections originating in, 382, 1331–1333
  pain or loose sensation in, in fish poisoning, 391
Tegopen. *See* Cloxacillin
Tegretol. *See* Carbamazepine
Telangiectasias, in hereditary disorders, 364, 365
  of conjunctival vessels, 368
  epistaxis in, 1304
Telecommunications, as EMS system component, 7–9
Telemetry
  in CCS system, 8
  as EMS system component, 8
Telephone access, 7, 8, 9
Temazepam (Restoril), 1440
  elimination half-life of, 800
Temperature
  acid-base disturbances and, 321
  acute confusional state and, 953–954
  environmental, wet bulb globe temperature (WBGT), 653–654
  respiratory distress and, in infants and children, 578
Temperature conversion chart, 1455–1462
Temporal arteritis, 337–338
  as headache cause, 917
Temporomandibular joint (TMJ)
  dislocation of, 1328, 1335
  dysfunction of, as headache cause, 917
Tendinitis, 345–346
  elbow. *See* Tennis elbow

Tendinitis (contd.)
  extensor carpi, 207
  flexor carpi, 207
  onset of, 352
  in shoulder, 201
  "sprains" vs., 207
Tendons
  aspiration and injection of, 1373–1375
  suture material for, 142
Tennis elbow, 204, 345, 346
Tenormin. See Atenolol
Tenosynovitis
  acute pyogenic flexor, 211
  DeQuervain's, 346
  "sprains" vs., 207
  as human bite complication, 156
TENS. See Transcutaneous electrical nerve stimulation (TENS)
Tensilon. See Edrophonium
Tension fractures, 163–164
Tension headaches, etiology of, 915, 916
Tension pneumothorax, 1183–1184
  indications of, 100
  as MAST suit contraindication, 77
  prehospital interventions and, 100–101, 110
  ventilation with, 99, 100–101
Terazosin, in renal failure treatment, 1225
Terbutaline (Bricanyl; Brethine), 1427
  inhaled
    pediatric dosage, 578
    pharmacokinetics of, 1133
  for obstructive airway disease, 1133
Terminal patients, EMS service issues, 27
"Terry-Thomas" sign, 206
Testicular injuries, 1209, 1210
Testicular torsion, 1212–1213
Tetanus prophylaxis
  for children, 553
  indications for
    multisystem trauma, 112
    open fractures, 172
    puncture wounds, 154
    vertebral column injuries, 188
  marine organism attack and, 716
  in soft tissue injuries, 1325
Tetanus toxoid, for emergency department, 1453
Tetanus treatment, anaphylaxis risk with, 75
Tetany
  hypocalcemia and, 281
    in children, 566
  hypomagnesemia and, 286, 304
  metabolic alkalosis, and, 328
Tetracaine (Pontocaine)
  clinical characteristics and dosage, 884
  pharmacologic classification, 885
  in wound anesthetic, 139
Tetracaine-adrenaline-cocaine (TAC) solution, as wound anesthetic, 139, 885–886, 1325
Tetrachlorethylene, as systemic toxin, 774
Tetracyclic antidepressants, 486
  overdose of, 486–487
Tetracyclic maprotiline (Ludiomil) overdose, 473
Tetracycline; Tetracyclines (Achromycin; Sumycin), 1417–1418
  anaphylaxis risk with, 75
  for cat bites, 156
  for corneal ulcers, 1278
  in eye drops, 1269
  for gonorrhea, 1250
  for Lyme disease, 357, 409
  for pneumonias, 386
  pregnancy and, 1239
  for Rocky Mountain spotted fever, 407, 438
  for septic gonococcal arthritis, 412
  for skin infections, marine-associated, 408
  for syphilis, 440
  for "urethral syndrome," 392
  for urethritis in men, 395
  for urinary tract infections, 393
Tetrodotoxism, 740–741
THAM. See Tromethamine
Theo-Dur. See Theophylline

Theolair. See Theophylline
Theophylline (Quibron-T; Slo-Phyllin; Theo-Dur; Theolair; Theophylline), 484, 1427–1428
  for asthma
    in children, 581, 582
    in pregnancy, 1239
  calculating blood levels of, 481–482
  for hymenoptera stings, 644
  for obstructive airway disease, 1134
  overdose of, 484
    assay methods, 472
    clinical signs, 473, 474, 484
    treatment of, 475, 476, 477, 484
  pharmacokinetics and, 484
  for respiratory distress, in children, 578
Therapeutic metaphors, 874–875
Thermal injury. See also Burns
  in children, airway obstruction with, 566
  smoke inhalation and, 773
  in upper extremities, 212
Thermal regulation, cervical cord injuries and, 912
Thermometer, wet bulb globe, 653–654
Thermoregulatory disorders, as acute confusional state cause, 953–954
Thiamine deficiency, as acute confusion cause, 954–955
Thiamylal (Surital), as general anesthesia, 887
Thiazides; Thiazide diuretics
  anaphylaxis risk with, 75
  hypercalcemia and, 282, 283, 313, 315, 318
  hyperosmolar hyperglycemic nonketotic coma and, 243–244
  hypokalemia and, 275–276
  hypomagnesemia and, 307
Thin-layer chromatography (TLC)
  in drug screening, 471, 786
  in toxic screening, 471
Thiopental (Pentothal), 1440
  in acute myocardial infarction treatment, 984
  anesthesia, 886
    anaphylaxis risk with, 75
  in endotracheal intubation, 1106
Thioriadazine hydrochloride, hyponatremia and, 271
Third World patients, biliary tract symptoms in, 455
Thirst
  in diabetic ketoacidosis, 234
  physiology and, 266
  sodium levels and, 266
Thomas cervical collar, 109
Thomas splint, 168
Thoracentesis, in pleural effusion, 1169
Thoracic injuries
  as analgesia contraindication, 101
  blunt, 1071–1072
  penetrating, 1071
  ventilation assistance with, prehospital, 99–101
Thoracic spine injuries
  fractures, 192–193
  gastrointestinal tract and, 187
  neurologic assessment with, 182
  shearing fractures, 179–180
  treatment of, 188
Thoracostomy
  complications of, 1190
  for flail chest, 101
  ipsilateral tube, for penetrating chest injury, 1071
  procedure, 1370–1372
  for tension pneumothorax, methods of, 100
  tube insertion, 1189–1190
Thoracotomy
  for blunt chest trauma, 1072
  for cardiac tamponade, 103, 1081
  emergency procedure, 1190
  indications for, 1190
  open chest massage vs. external compression, 1091–1092
  for penetrating cardiac wound, 1078–1079
  for penetrating chest trauma, 1071
  in shock treatment, 1069
Thorax dysmorphology, in hereditary disorders, 363, 364, 365
Thorazine. See Chlorpromazine

Throat culture, in pharyngitis, 377–378
Throat preparations, for emergency department, 1453
Thrombocytopenia
  in cancer patients, 510
  hereditary, 365, 366
Thrombocytopenia and absent radius (TAR syndrome), 364, 365, 366, 368
Thrombocytosis, pseudohyperkalemia and, 279
Thromboembolic disease, 364, 365
  hereditary, 365
  high altitude and, 685
Thromboembolism. See also Pulmonary embolism
  drug abuse and, 785
  treatment for, adrenal hemorrhage risk with, 256
Thrombolytic agents
  for acute myocardial infarction, 982
  cholesterol embolism and, 1171
Thrombophlebitis
  Baker's cyst vs., 346
  in Beñet's syndrome, 341
  migratory, cancer and, 510
  in systemic lupus erythematosus, 341
Thrombosis. See also Cerebrovascular accident
  acute myocardial infarction and, 982
  in cancer patients, 510
Thrush, 377, 378
Thumb
  aspiration or injection of joint, 1374, 1375
  in carpal tunnel syndrome, 347
  dysmorphology of, in hereditary disorders, 363, 364, 365
  "gamekeeper's" or "ski pole," 209
  infections, 210
  metacarpal fractures, 208
Thurston-Holland sign, 166, 167
Thymus, congenital absence of, hypocalcemia and, 284
Thyroid disorders, 249–252
  adenomas, hypercalcemia and, 282
  adrenal insufficiency and, 255
  carcinoma
    chest wall syndrome vs., 348
    medullary, hypocalcemia and, 284
  hypothyroidism, hyponatremia and, 271
  myxedema coma, 251–252
  thyroid storm, 249–251
Thyroid/antithyroid agents, 1445
Thyroidectomy
  acquired hypoparathyroidism from, hypocalcemia and, 284
  for thyroid storm, 250
Thyroiditis
  autoimmune (Hashimoto's)
    adrenal insufficiency and, 255
    myxedema coma and, 251
  silent thyrotoxic, adrenal insufficiency and, 255
  subacute, pharyngitis and, 377
Thyroxine, for myxedema coma, 252
TIA. See Transient ischemic attack
Tibia
  acute osteomyelitis in, 358
  dislocations of, 173, 174
  fractures of, 162, 163, 225–226
    blood loss risk with, 168
    cast application to, 169–170, 171
    classifications, 222
    complications, 225, 226
    open, 226
    proximal tibia, 224–225
Tibiotalar (ankle) joint, aspiration or injection of, 1374, 1375
Tic douloureux, as facial pain cause, 920
Ticarcillin (Ticar), 1416
  for corneal ulcers, 1275, 1277, 1278
  eye drop preparation, 1268
  renal failure and, 1225
  in septic shock treatment, 85
Tick-borne infections. See also Lyme disease; Rocky Mountain spotted fever
  sepsis and, 406
  skin infections in, 409
Ticlopidine (Ticlid), 1402–1403

Tietze's syndrome, 348
Tigan. *See* Trimethobenzamide
Tilt test, in syncope, 963
Time distortion, pain perception and, 874
Timolol (Blocadren), 1397
Timolol (Timoptic)
　for acute glaucoma, 1289
　for secondary glaucoma, with uveitis, 1282
Tinactin. *See* Tolnaftate
Tinea capitis, 435
Tinea corporis, 435–436
Tinea cruris, 435–436
Tinea pedis (athlete's foot), 436
Tinea unguium, 436
Tissue hypoxia
　pathophysiology of, 331
　respiratory alkalosis and, 330
Tissue perfusion
　impairments in. *See* Shock
　vasopressors and, 84
Tissue plasminogen activator, for pulmonary embolism, 1148
TLC. *See* Thin-layer chromatography
TMA. *See* 3,4,5-Trimethoxyamphetamine
TMF (3-methylfentanyl) overdose, 799
TMJ. *See* Temporomandibular joint
Toadfishes, spine or puncture wounds by, 728
Tobacco consumption, extent of, 782. *See also* Smoking
Tobacco products, hypokalemia and, 277
Tobramycin (Nebcin), 1411
　for corneal ulcers, 1275, 1277, 1278
　eye drop preparation, 1268
　gentimicin and, for septic shock, 85
　for marine organism injuries, 731, 732
　for open fractures, 172
Tocainamide (Tocainide), for ventricular premature complexes, 1005
Toes
　dislocations in, 230
　in Raynaud's phenomenon, 341
Tofranil. *See* Imipramine
Toga viruses, as sepsis cause, 406
Tolbutamide, hyponatremia and, 271
Tolerance, defined, 782
Tolmetin sodium (Tolectin), for pain relief, 881
Tolnaftate (Tinactin), for fungal infections of skin, 436
Toluene
　ingestion of, 473
　inhalation of, 805
　as systemic toxin, 774
Tongue injury repair, 1326
　lacerations, 153
　vascular lesions on, 368
Tonic-clonic (grand mal) seizures, 945, 948
　syncope and, 961
Tonsils, peritonsillar abscess (quinsy), 569, 1303–1304
Tooth fractures or avulsions, 1333–1335
Tooth infections, 382, 1331–1333
Tooth pain, in food poisoning, 391
Topical anesthesia, 885–886
　for endotracheal intubation, 1106
　for oral ulcerations, 1336
　in wound management, 139–140
Toradol. *See* Ketorolac tromethamine
Torsades de pointes, 1034, 1035
　advanced cardiac life support, 1090–1091
　hypokalemia and, 295
　magnesium sulfate for, 1090
Torsion dystonia, 372
Tort law, 39–40
Torus fracture, 154, 165, 205
Total body water (TBW), 265–266
　calculating deficit in, 269
　in hypernatremia, 266, 267
Total systemic arterial resistance (TSR)
　acute myocardial infarction and, 989, 991, 992
　dysrhythmia and, 997–998
Tourette syndrome, 372

Tourniquet use
　in acute myocardial infarction treatment, 993
　for congestive heart failure, 1056
　hypercalcemia and, 283, 313
　indications and precautions, 102, 137
　in pulmonary edema, 1098
　as snake bite contraindication, 637
Toxemia of pregnancy. *See* Pre-eclampsia
Toxic epidermal necrolysis, 440
Toxic gas inhalation. *See* Inhalation injury
Toxic ingestion. *See* Toxicologic emergencies
Toxic megacolon, 461
　in Crohn's disease, 462
Toxic shock syndrome (TSS), 406, 407, 432
Toxic Substances Control Act (TSCA) of 1976, 748
Toxicologic emergencies, 469–494. *See also* Hazardous materials; Inhalation injury; *specific toxic substances*
　chemicals and. *See* Chemical burns; Chemical injury
　chemotherapy and, 508–509
　in children
　　child abuse, 601
　　unconsciousness with, 591
　drug abuse. *See* Substance abuse
　ED classification for, 48
　evaluation of, 469–474
　　drug and toxic screens, 471–474
　food poisoning, 390–391
　　by fish, 391, 736–741
　　by shellfish, 390, 391, 731–735
　hazardous materials, 747–759
　marine organism injuries. *See* Marine organisms
　metabolic acidosis and, 324–326
　occupational, 761–776
　　decontamination procedures, 762–763
　　history taking in, 762, 763
　　management principles, 762–763
　　systemic toxins, 773–776
　　toxic gas inhalation, 763–773
　over-the-counter drug overdose, 491
　pharmacokinetics and, 480–484
　prehospital care, 469
　seaweed ingestion, 741
　shellfish poisoning, 731–735
　skin and ocular decontamination, 474
　substance abuse. *See* Substance abuse
　systemic toxins, 773–776
　treatment of, 474–480
　　absorption prevention, 474–475
　　antibodies in, 492–493
　　enhancement of excretion, 475–477
　　physiologic antagonists, 477–480
Toxicologic screening, 471–474
　for drug abuse, 786
Toxin ingestion
　in food poisoning, 390–391
　as gastroenteritis cause, 387, 388
Toxins
　listed by occupation, 1175–1180
　renal failure and, 1218–1219
Toxoids, for emergency department, 1453
Toxoplasma gondii
　in mononucleosis, 401, 402
　pharyngitis and, 377
Toxoplasmosis
　diagnosis of, 401, 402
　encephalitis and, 400
　pathogenesis of, 401
　treatment of, 402
Tracheal obstruction, by tumor, 511
Tracheitis, bacterial (membranous croup), 569, 1113, 1116–1117
Tracheobronchial foreign bodies, 559, 1308
Tracheobronchial injury, 1188
Tracheobronchitis, bacterial, airway control in children and, 514
Tracheostomy
　contraindications, 1321
　in laryngeal trauma, 1316
　pediatric

acute epiglottitis and, 1119, 1122
caution about, 515
for tracheobronchial foreign body, 1308
Tracrium. *See* Atracurium
Traction
　for cervical spine injuries, 913
　for dislocations, 173, 174
　with fracture splint, 168
　for vertebral column injuries, 188
Traction fractures, 163, 164
Traffic policemen, carbon monoxide toxicity and, 766
Training. *See* Staffpower and training
Trandate. *See* Labetalol
Tranquilizers, 1406–1408. *See also* Sedative-hypnotics
　for alcohol withdrawal, 821
Transcellular shifts
　hyperkalemia and, 279, 298
　hypokalemia and, 276, 293, 294–295, 297
Transcutaneous electrical nerve stimulation (TENS), for pain relief, 888, 889
Transcutaneous oxygen monitor, in shock monitoring, 83
Transderm-Nitro. *See* Nitroglycerin
Transesophageal echocardiography (TEE), of thoracic aortic dissection, 1187
Transfer of patient. *See also* Transport of patient
　air vs. ground transport, 25
　to burn center, 427
　　checklist, 426
　　criteria for, 10, 47–48
　in disaster management, 36
　diversion policy and, 18
　as EMS system component, 9–10
　　criteria for, 10
　for inability to pay, requirements for, 7
　indigence issues, 7, 42–43
　legal issues, 7, 42–43
　　indigent patients, 7
　levels of care criteria and, 46
　peritoneal lavage and, 111
　with vertebral column injury, 187, 188
Transfusions. *See also* Blood transfusions; Fluid replacement
　complications of, 133–134
　equipment for, 130–132
Transient ischemic attack (TIA), 943
　syncope and, 961, 962
Transport of patient. *See also* Prehospital interventions; Transfer of patient
　with acute epiglottitis, 1119
　with burns, 419
　with head injuries, 892
　with vertebral column injury, 187
Transport program
　components of, 10
　hospital categorization in, 19
Transportation
　air services, 23–26
　in disaster management, 15, 35–36
　as EMS system component, 15–16, 17
　of hazardous materials, 747, 748–50
　interhospital transfer equipment, 10
Transtracheal aspiration
　complications of, 386
　indications for, 385
　technique, 385–386
Transtracheal ventilation. *See* Percutaneous transtracheal ventilation
Tranxene. *See* Chlorazepate
Trapezius muscle, cervical spine injury and, 182
Trauma. *See also* Fractures; Multisystem injuries; Wound management; *specific types of trauma*
　as acute confusional state cause, 954
　as acute monoarticular arthritis cause, 358
　adrenal gland hemorrhage and, 256
　air transport indications, 25
　basic vs. EMT-P intervention and, 4–5
　burns with, 419, 423
　　burn center referral criteria, 47
　as cause of death, 93
　　in children, 541

1518 EMERGENCY MEDICINE

Trauma (contd.)
  child abuse indicators, 597–598. See also Child abuse
  deceleration injuries, 1319. See also Falls; Motor vehicle accidents
  as diabetes insipidus cause, 267
  domestic violence indicators, 842, 845, 846
  ED classification for, 49
  EMS research on, 2–3
  endocrine response to, 69
  fat embolism in, 1170, 1171
  field management priorities, 94
  as headache cause, 919
  to heart and great vessels, 1077–1082
  hyperbaric oxygenation (HBO) therapy for, 709
  hyperkalemia and, 298
  hypokalemia and, 276
  interhospital transfer criteria, 10
  by marine organisms, shark, 712–713
  mortality rate from, in rural vs. urban areas, 22
  necrotizing fasciitis or myositis and, 409–410
  occupational. See Occupational injuries
  pediatric. See Pediatric patients, trauma in
  pharyngitis and, 377
  in pregnancy, 1238
  reflex response to, 69
  in rural vs. urban areas, mortality rate from, 22
  sexual abuse, 605–608
  small bowel obstruction and, 459, 460
  stabilization in, controversy about, 5–6
  stabilization vs. transport controversy, 5–6
  thyroid storm and, 249
  vascular. See Vascular emergencies; *specific types*
Trauma Care Systems Planning and Development Act (1990), 27
Trauma centers
  categorization as, 18, 49–50
  designation as, 49, 50
  federal funding for, 27
  hyperbaric centers with, 709
  impact of, 94
  levels of care in, 18
  mortality rate and, 19
  pediatric, transfer to, 551–552
  regionalization and, 49–50
  triage decision scheme for, 17
Trauma registries, evaluation role, 19–20
Trauma Score/Injury Severity Score (TRISS), ground vs. air transport and, 24, 25
Trauma society, founding of, 2
Travelers
  dangerous marine organisms and, 711, 712
  diarrhea in, 387, 389
  high-altitude problems in, 679–686
  sepsis in, 406
Travenol, for wound irrigation, 140
Trazodone (Desyrel), 487
  overdose of, 487
Treatment, refusal of consent for, 42
Treatment protocols, for prehospital services, 20
Tremors
  hereditary, 370
  in hypomagnesemia, 287, 304
"Trench mouth" (Vincent's infection), 1336
Trendelenburg position
  for IV placement, 102
  for air embolism, 1170
  for cervical spine injury, 913
  in shock treatment, 78
Treponema pallidum, 439
  in dysenteric gastroenteritis, 390
  in pharyngitis, 376, 377
Triage
  American College of Surgeons scheme, 16, 17
  beginnings of, 93
  in communications systems, 7, 8
  in disaster management, 12, 15, 34–35
  ED classification and, 46–49
  rape victims and, 1245
Triamterene (Dyrenium), 1431–1432
  hyperkalemia and, 279

Triazolam (Halcion), 1440–1441
  elimination half-life of, 800
  overdose of, 491–492
Triceps function, assessing, in vertebral column injury, 184
Trichloroethane intoxication, 325, 805, 806
Trichloroethylene, as systemic toxin, 774
Trichomonas vaginalis, in urethritis in men, 394, 395
Trichuris species, biliary obstruction and, 455
Tricyclic antidepressants
  behavioral disorders induced by, 474
  for depression, importance of referral with, 832
  overdose of, 485–486
    clinical signs, 472, 473, 474, 485
    treatment of, 477, 485–486, 802
  pharmacokinetics and, 483
  as unconsciousness cause, 591
Tridil. See Nitroglycerin
Trifluorothymidine (trifluridine), for herpetic keratitis, 1264
Trigeminal nerve, 1322, 1323. See also Cranial nerves
Trigeminal neuralgia, as facial pain cause, 920
"Trigger finger," 346
Trilisate. See Choline magnesium trisalicylate
Trimethaphan camphor sulfonate (Arfonad), 1397
  in acute myocardial infarction treatment, 993
  for hypertensive emergencies, 1062, 1063
    acute aortic dissection, 1066
Trimethobenzamide (Tigan), 1408
  as dystonia cause, 565–566
Trimethoprim
  for prostatitis, 395
  for urinary tract infections, 393
Trimethoprim-sulfamethoxazole (Bactrim; Septra), 1417
  for animal bites, 157–158
  for cutaneous abscesses, 408
  for dysenteric gastroenteritis, 390
  for marine organism injuries, 731, 732
  for otitis media, 381, 1309
  for pneumonias, 386, 387
  for prostatitis, 395
  for sinusitis, 379
  for urinary tract infections, 392, 393
3,4,5-Trimethoxyamphetamine (TMA), as sympathomimetic, 787
Trinitrotoluene intoxication, 473
Tripelennamine, pentazocine with, 795
Triphalangeal thumb, in Holt-Oram syndrome, 363
Tris Buffer. See Tromethamine
TRISS. See Trauma Score/Injury Severity Score
Trobicin. See Spectinomycin
Trochanteric fractures, 220–221
Trochlear nerve, See also Cranial nerves
Tromethamine (THAM; Tris Buffer), 1391
Tropicamide (Mydriacyl), for uveitis, 1281
Trousseau's sign
  in hypocalcemia, 285
  in hypomagnesemia, 286–287
Trousseau's syndrome, 510
Trunk, fungal infections on, 435, 436
Trunk wounds
  suture material for, 143
  suture technique for, 143
Trypanosomiasis, brain infection and, 400
TSR. See Total systemic arterial resistance
TSS. See Toxic shock syndrome
Tubal ligation, ectopic pregnancy and, 1229
Tube drainage, hypokalemia and, 294
Tuberculosis
  adrenal insufficiency and, 257–258
  aseptic meningitis and, 399
  as diabetes insipidus cause, 267
  pulmonary, hyponatremia and, 271
Tuberculous epididymitis, 1212
Tuberous sclerosis, 364, 365, 369
Tubo-ovarian abscess, 1233, 1234
Tubocurarine, anaphylaxis risk with, 75
Tularemia, 385, 409
  skin infections in, 409
Turbutaline, inhaled, for asthma, 1132

Turning frame, for thoracolumbar fractures, 188
Tylenol. See Acetaminophen
Tympanic membrane perforations, 1306–1307
Tympanocentesis, for otitis media, 381, 1309
Tympanostomy, otitis media and, 1310
Typewriter correction fluid, inhalation of, 805
Typhoid fever, shellfish ingestion and, 731–732
Typhus, encephalitis and, 400
Tyrosinemia, 366, 372

U

UAO (upper airway obstruction), in children, 563–570
UHF communications, 8, 9
Ulcerative colitis. See Colitis, ulcerative
Ulnar fractures, 204–205
  in children, 165, 206
Ultracef. See Cefadroxil
Ultrasonography
  in appendicitis, 464
  for Baker's cyst diagnosis, 346
  in biliary tract disease, 454
  in deep venous thrombosis, 1147
  in multiple trauma, in children, 549–550
  in pelvic inflammatory disease, 1233
  in pre-eclampsia, 1239
  in renal failure, 1222
  in renal trauma, 1197
  in vaginal bleeding evaluation, 1230
Unconscious patients. See also Coma
  airway control with, 95
    clearing an obstruction, 1085
  alcohol overdose, 817
  assessing, 591–592. See also Levels of consciousness
  in head injury
    motor examination in, 896
    pupillary findings, 895
  management of, 933–934
  in near-drowning, treatment of, 697–698
  in opioid overdose, 796, 797
  pediatric, 589–582
    etiologies, 589–591
    management, 591–592
  in sedative-hypnotic overdose, 802, 803
  in sympathomimetic overdose, 792
Uniform Anatomical Gift Act, 43
Unipen. See Nafcillin
Unitarians, beliefs and practices, 869
United States Air Force, hyperbaric chamber referral by, 707
United States government. See *specific departments*
Universalists, beliefs and practices, 869
Unresponsiveness. See Coma; Unconscious patients
"Unsolved fracture" of femoral neck, 218
Upper airway obstruction (UAO), in children, 563–570
Upper extremity injuries, 195–212. See also Extremities; *specific extremities*
  acromioclavicular separations, 198
  amputations, replantation of, 212
  bursitis, subacromial, 201
  carpal, 206–207
  clavicle fractures, 198
  dislocations, 195, 198–199
    carpal, 206–207
    elbow, 202, 204
    in hands, 209
    shoulder, 199–200
    sternoclavicular, 198–199
  dressings for, 195, 196–197
  to elbow, 202–204
  electrical burns, 212
  to forearm, 204–205
  fractures
    carpal, 206
    clavicle, 198
    elbow, 202–203
    forearm, 204–205
    hand and finger, 207–208
    humeral shaft, 201–202

proximal humerus, 201
wrist, 205–207
grease gun injuries, 212
to hand, 207–211
history taking and, 195
ligamentous
  in hand, 209
  in wrist, 207
multisystem injuries and, 195
physical examination, 195
prehospital interventions, 195
proximal humerus fractures, 201
radial head subluxation, 204
radiographic examination, 195, 198
rotator cuff injuries, 200
scapula fractures, 199
to shoulder, 199–201
sternoclavicular dislocations, 198–199
tendon lacerations, 212
to wrists, 205–207
Upper gastrointestinal bleeding, 448–450
  esophageal varices and, 452–453
Upper gastrointestinal infections, 387–388
Upper respiratory infections. *See* Respiratory tract infections
Urea, intravenous
  for acute glaucoma, 1289
  for secondary glaucoma, with uveitis, 1282
Ureaplasma urealyticum, in urethritis in men, 394, 395
Uremia
  hypocalcemia and, 284
  metabolic acidosis and, 323
Ureteral anastomosis, end-to-end, 1202, 1203
Ureteral colic, 1210, 1211
Ureteral injuries, 1200–1202
  diagnosis of, 1200–1201
  etiologies of, 1200
  iatrogenic, 1200, 1201
  management of, 1201–1202, 1203
  traumatic, 1200
Ureteral obstruction, flank pain with, 1210, 1211
Ureteroenterostomy, metabolic acidosis and, 321
Ureteroneocystostomy, 1201–1202
Urethral culture, in urethritis diagnosis, 394
Urethral injuries, 1205–1208
  to bulbous urethra, 1206–1207
  iatrogenic, 1205, 1207
  to membranous urethra, 1205–1206
  pelvic fractures and, 215
  to pendulous urethra, 1207–1208
Urethral obstruction, urinary retention and, 1213–1214
"Urethral syndrome," in women, 391, 392
Urethritis in men, 394–395
Urethrography, retrograde, 1207
  in flank pain diagnosis, 1211
  indications for, 1206, 1207
  in urinary retention, 1214
Uric acid study, in monoarticular arthritis, 356
Urinary analgesics, intoxication by, 473
Urinary bladder, assessing, in multisystem trauma, 111–112
Urinary disorders, flank pain and, 1210
Urinary frequency, in diabetic ketoacidosis, 234
Urinary obstruction, 1210–1211
Urinary retention
  acute, 1213–1214
    diagnosis of, 1214
    management of, 1214, 1215
    pathogenesis of, 1213–1214
  in prostatitis, 395
  in systemic lupus erythematosus, 344
Urinary system injuries. *See* Genitourinary injuries
Urinary tract disorders, in pregnancy, 1236
Urinary tract infections, 391–396
  diagnosis of, 391–392
  differential diagnosis, 392
  in females, 391
  in males, 391, 394–396
  organisms causing, 391
  pathophysiology of, 391

prostatitis, 391
pyelonephritis, 1210
recurrent, 394
septic shock risk and, 72
treatment of, 392–394
urinary retention and, 1214
Urinary tract obstruction, dehydration risk with, 267
Urination
  difficulty in, in cauda equina syndrome, 193
  syncope during, 961, 963
Urine culture
  in prostatitis, 395
  techniques, 392
  urinary tract infection treatment and, 392, 393–394
Urine examination, in urethritis in men, 394
Urine osmolarity
  in diabetes insipidus diagnosis, 269
  in hyponatremia, 272
Urine output
  in cardiogenic shock, 73
  decrease in, in shock, 70
  monitoring
    with MAST suit, 77
    in shock treatment, 81
Urine potassium, normal, 272
Urine testing
  in diabetic ketoacidosis diagnosis, 234
  diuretics and, 266
  in multiple trauma, in children, 548, 550
  in polyarteritis nodosa, 343
  in toxicologic emergencies, 471
  in urinary tract infections, 392
Urography
  excretory
    in flank pain diagnosis, 1211
    in renal trauma, blunt, 1196
    in renal trauma, penetrating, 1198–1199
    in ureteral injury, 1200
    in urethral injury, 1206
  intravenous, in urinary retention, 1214
  retrograde
    in flank pain diagnosis, 1211
    in renal trauma, blunt, 1197
    in renal trauma, penetrating, 1199
Urokinase, for pulmonary embolism, 1148
Urolithiasis, in pregnancy, 1236
Urticaria, 440–441
  in anaphylaxis, 75
  as transfusion reaction, 134
Uterine cervix, culdocentesis of, 1231, 1354
Uterine dysfunction, vaginal bleeding and, 1231
Uterine hemorrhage, postpartum, 1238
Uveitis, 1276, 1277–1282
  in connective tissue disease, 338–339
  differential diagnosis, 1276
  follow-up care, 1282
  granulomatous vs. nongranulomatous, 1280
  signs and symptoms of, 1276, 1277–1280
  treatment of, 1280–1282

V

V-Cillin K. *See* Penicillin V
V/Q (ventilation/perfusion) ratio, 1153–1154
Vaccines
  Hemophilus influenzae (HIB), supraglottitis and, 567
  hepatitis B, 404, 405, 458
  meningococcal, 398
Vagal stimulation, for PSVT, 1026, 1027
Vaginal bleeding, abnormal, 1230–1231
  in early pregnancy, 1230
  in late pregnancy, 1237–1238
Vaginal infections
  assessing for, in rape examination, 1249
  herpetic vaginitis, 442
  urinary tract infections and, 392
Vaginal injuries, pelvic fractures and, 215
Vagus nerve, *See also* Cranial nerves
Valium. *See* Diazepam
Valmid. *See* ethinamate

Valproic acid
  for headache prophylaxis, 924
  overdose of, 490
    clinical signs, 472, 491
  for seizures, 949
Valsalva's maneuver
  for PSVT, 1026
  for Wolff-Parkinson-White syndrome, 1042
Valvular disease, as cardiogenic shock cause, 74
Vanceril. *See* Beclomethasone
Vancomycin (Vancocin), 1424
  for cutaneous abscesses, 408
  eye drop preparation, 1268
    for corneal ulcers, 1275, 1277, 1278
  for meningitis, staphylococcal, 398
  for pseudomembranous colitis, 30
  for sepsis, 406
  for septic arthritis, 357, 412
  in septic shock treatment, 85
Varicella (chickenpox), 443
  herpes zoster and, 442
  oral lesions with, 382
  pneumonia and, 383
  polyarthralgias with, 359
Varicella zoster
  as aseptic meningitis cause, 399
  pharyngitis and, 377
Varices
  esophageal, 449, 452–453
    as bleeding cause, 449
    treatment of, 450
  gastric
    as bleeding cause, 449
    treatment of, 450
Vascular abnormalities, hereditary, 367, 368
Vascular access, in children, 520
Vascular collapse in neonate, adrenal insufficiency and, 258
Vascular disease
  in connective tissue disorders, 341
  as CVA risk factor, 935
  Raynaud's phenomenon, 341
Vascular emergencies, 1069–1075
  in abdomen, 1072–1073
  emergency department team and, 1075
  in extremities, 1073–1074
  injection of foreign substances, 1075
  in neck, 1074–1075
  pathophysiology of, 1069–1071
  sequelae of, 1075
  in thorax, 1071–1072, 1077, 1187
Vascular headaches
  etiology of, 915–916
  patient education on, 925
Vascular spasm, in Raynaud's phenomenon, 341
Vasculitis
  in connective tissue disease, 337, 341, 342
  cutaneous lesions in, 337
  differential diagnosis, 341
  in drug eruptions, 434
  mesenteric, 342
  neurologic involvement in, 343
  renal failure and, 1218, 1222
  in systemic lupus erythematosus, 341, 342
Vaseline gauze, for open chest wounds, 101
Vasoactive substances, in hypovolemic shock, 71
Vasoconstriction, peripheral, in hypovolemic shock, 71
Vasoconstrictors
  in acute myocardial infarction treatment, 984
  hypothermia and, 671
  spinal injuries and, 104
Vasodepressor syncope, 960–961, 963
Vasodilation, in hypovolemic shock, 71
Vasodilators
  for cardiogenic shock, 74, 84
  for catecholamine crisis, 1067
  for congestive heart failure, 1056
  hypothermia and, 672
  for pulmonary edema, 1099
  for Raynaud's phenomenon, 341

Vasopressor agents, 1381–1391
　for anaphylaxis, 86, 87, 433
　for lower GI bleeding, 451
　for shock, 76, 84
　　anaphylactic shock, 87
　　myxedema coma and, 252
　　septic shock, 85
　for upper GI bleeding, 450
　　esophageal varices, 453
Vasotec. See Enalapril
Vasotec IV. See Enalaprilat
Vasoxyl. See Methoxamine
VDRL test, 439, 440
　rape and, 1250
Vecuronium (Norcuron), 1443–1444
Vegetative state, 928
Velosef. See Cephradine
Velpeau stockinette dressing, 200
Venereal disease, consent issues, 42
Venereal Disease Research Laboratory test. See
　　VDRL test
Venerupin shellfish poisoning, 734
Venipuncture, potassium level error and, 277, 297
Venodilators, in acute myocardial infarction treatment,
　　993
Venogram, for thrombophlebitis diagnosis, 346
Venography, contrast, in deep vein thrombosis, 1148
Venom poisoning, antivenins for, 493
Venous access
　drugs delivered by, 520
　in pediatric patients, 520–521
　for shock treatments, 76
Venous air embolism, 708
Venous pressure monitoring. See Central venous
　　pressure monitoring
Venous trauma. See Vascular emergencies
Ventilation, assisted. See also Breathing assistance
　in cardiopulmonary resuscitation, drug therapy vs.,
　　522
　control of, 1154–1156
　hyponatremia and, 271
　with multisystem injuries, 99–101
　　devices for, 99–100
　in near-drowning, 694–695
　for obstructive airway disease, 1134–1135
　of pediatric patients, 517–519
　respiratory failure and, 1151–1152
　in sedative overdose, 803
Ventilation/perfusion (V/Q) ratio, 1153–1154
　mismatch in, 1154
Ventilators, for infants and children, 519, 579
Ventolin. See Albuterol (Salbutamol)
Ventricular contraction sequence, cardiac function
　　and, 1052
Ventricular ectopic beats, 1002–1005
　aberration vs., 1007–1008, 1009
Ventricular fibrillation, 1004, 1034, 1036
　ACLS procedures, 1088–1089
　advanced cardiac life support, 1090
　bretylium tosylate (Bretylol) for, 984
　in cardiac arrest, 1083
　electrical therapy for, 984
　EMT-Ds and, 6
　magnesium therapy for, 307
Ventricular function, acute myocardial infarction and,
　　989–991
Ventricular pacing systems, permanent-demand,
　　1043–1049
Ventricular septal defects, as cardiogenic shock cause,
　　74
Ventricular tachyarrhythmia, in cardiac arrest, 1083
Ventricular tachycardia, 1004, 1030, 1032–1034
　advanced cardiac life support, 1090–1091
Ventricular tachydysrhythmias, 1028, 1030–1034
　accelerated idioventricular rhythm (AIVR), 1028,
　　1030, 1031
　ventricular fibrillation (VF), 1004, 1034, 1036
　ventricular tachycardia (VT), 1004, 1030,
　　1032–1034
Veracillin. See Dicloxacillin
Verapamil (Calan; Isoptin), 1391, 1397
　for atrial fibrillation, 1022
　for atrial flutter, 1024
　for coelenterate stings, 721
　for headache prophylaxis, 922, 924
　for PSVT, 1026, 1028
　for regular, wide QRS tachycardia, 1037
　for Wolff-Parkinson-White syndrome, 1042
Verbal abuse
　in battering syndrome, 841
　defined, 837
Verbal response
　in head injury, 894
　scoring, 928–929
Vermox. See Mebendazole
Versed. See Midazolam
Vertebral artery syndrome, 937–938
Vertebral column injuries, 175–194. See also Cervical
　　spine injuries; Spinal injuries
　cauda equina syndrome, 193
　diagnosis of, 180–183, 188–194
　　motor function examination, 183, 184
　　neurologic examination, 181–182
　　physical examination, 181
　　roentgenographic, 185–187
　　sensory examination, 182–183
　dislocations, 188–190
　extension injuries, 177
　fracture-dislocations, 164, 175–176, 192–193
　fractures, 190–193
　　burst-type, 179, 192, 193
　　classification of, 175–180
　　compression, 175
　　compression/vertical compression, 175, 177–178,
　　　180
　　diagnosis of, 180–183, 190–192, 193
　　seat-belt-type, 164, 177
　　shearing, 179–180
　　splinting, 168
　　stable types, 193
　incomplete neurologic lesions and, 183–185
　infection diagnosis, 19304
　multisystem injuries with, 180, 187
　osteomyelitis diagnosis, 193–194
　patient transport with, 187
　prehospital cautions, 187
　subluxations, 189
　in rheumatoid arthritis, 343
　treatment of, 187–188, 190, 192, 193
Vertebral destruction, in rheumatoid arthritis, 343
Vertebral osteomyelitis, 193–194
Vertical categorization, of EMS facilities, 18
Vertical classification, of emergency departments
　　(EDs), 46–47
Vertical compression fractures, of vertebral column,
　　177–179, 180
Vertical shear pelvic injury, 213
Veterans Administration, in National Disaster Medical
　　System, 37
VF. See Ventricular fibrillation
Vibramycin. See Doxycycline
Vibratabs. See Doxycycline
Vibration, for pain relief, 888
Vibrio cholerae, in gastroenteritis, 387, 388
Vibrio parahaemolyticus
　in food poisoning, 390
　by fish or shellfish, 731, 732
　in gastroenteritis, 388
　dysenteric, 390
Vibrio species, skin infections from, 408
Vicry (polyglactin 910) sutures, 142
Vidarabine, for herpes simplex encephalitis, 401
Vidarabine (Vira-A Ophthalmic Ointment), for
　　herpetic keratitis, 1264
Villous adenomas, hypokalemia and, 294, 296
Viloxazine, 487
　overdose of, 487
Vincent's infections ("trench mouth"), 1336
Vincristine, toxic reactions to, gastrointestinal, 509
Violent behavior. See also Child abuse; Domestic
　　violence
　alcohol-induced, 818
　drug-induced, 474
　substance abuse and, 783
Vira-A ointment. See Vidarabine
Viral exanthems, 443
Viral infections
　acute watery diarrhea, 389
　in animal exposure, 409
　aseptic meningitis, 399–400
　bivalve mollusk poisoning and, 733
　bronchiolitis, in children, 582–583
　common cold, 375–376
　croup (laryngotracheitis), 567–569, 1113–1116
　dermatologic, 441–443
　encephalitis, 400
　　in infants and children, 590
　exanthems, 443
　in eye, diagnostic tests, 1272
　gastroenteritis, 387, 388
　as headache cause, 917
　hepatitis, 403–405, 457, 458
　　liver disease and, 454
　　pharyngitis and, 377
　herpes simplex, 441–442
　herpes zoster, 442
　laryngotracheitis (croup), airway control method
　　and, 514
　measles, 442–443
　meningitis, 535–536
　mononucleosis, 401–403
　ocular, culture media for, 1272
　oral-facial, 381
　otitis externa, 1310
　otitis media, 380, 1309
　pharyngitis, 376–378
　pneumonia, 383
　　in children, 585
　polyarthralgias with, 359
　rubella, 443
　shellfish ingestion and, 733
　sinusitis, 379
　varicella, 443
Virginia, regional trauma system in, 50
Viroptic. See Trifluorothymidine (trifluridine)
Viscus, perforated, adrenal insufficiency vs., 259
Visiting nurse, elder abuse and, 847
Vistaril. See Hydroxyzine
Visual acuity testing, in ocular trauma, 1262, 1263,
　　1284
Visual field losses, in temporal arteritis, 337
Visual impairment
　in acute glaucoma, 1288
　assessing for, 110
　in connective tissue disease, 337–339
　in hyphema, 1285
　in systemic lupus erythematosus, 338
　in temporal arteritis, 337, 338
　terminology for, 1295–1296
　in uveitis, 1278
Visualization techniques, 874–875
Vital capacity, respiratory failure and, 1151, 1152
Vital signs
　assessing
　　in children, 546, 547
　　in multisystem trauma, 105–106, 546
　monitoring, in near-drowning, 698
　spinal shock and, 182
　temperature conversion chart, 1455–1462
　in vertebral column injury, 182, 188
Vitamin A therapy, hypercalcemia and, 315, 318
Vitamin B_{12} therapy, hypokalemia and, 276, 295
Vitamin D (calciferol)
　calcium levels and, 281
　deficiency of, hypocalcemia and, 284
　excess of
　　hypercalcemia and, 282, 313, 315, 317, 318
　　idiopathic hypercalcemia of infancy and, 283
　for hypocalcemia, 285
Vitamin K_1. See Phytonadione
Vitamin therapy
　for ciguatera fish poisoning, 738, 739
　emergency department stock, 1453
　for renal failure, 1226
Vitiligo, adrenal insufficiency and, 255, 258
Vitreous haze, in uveitis, 1279

Vitreous hemorrhage, hyphema and, 1283
Volar plate injuries, 209–220
Volatile screen, in toxicologic emergencies, 471
Volex. *See* Hetastarch; Hydroxyethyl starch
Volkmann's ischemic contracture or paralysis, as elbow injury complication, 202
Voltaren. *See* Diclofenac
Volume regulation. *See* Fluid management
Volunteer agencies, in National Disaster Medical System, 37
Volunteers
  air transport and, 27
  for rural EMS services, 23
Volvulus
  colon obstruction and, 460
  sigmoid, 460, 461
Vomiting. *See also* Nausea and vomiting
  in anaphylaxis, 75
  in children, 557–558
  dehydration risk with, 267
  in esophageal rupture, 452
  in food poisoning, 390, 391
  heartburn and, 452
  hypokalemia and, 275, 294, 296
  hyponatremia and, 270
  induced. *See* Emetics
  in infants, 557–558
  in intestinal obstruction, 459, 460
  metabolic alkalosis and, 327
  in neonates, 557–558
    adrenal insufficiency and, 258
  self-induced, hypokalemia and, 296
  in thyroid storm, 250
Von Hippel-Lindau disease, 370
Von Recklinghausen's disease. *See* Neurofibromatosis
Von Willebrand disease, 366
VT. *See* Ventricular tachycardia

W

Wakefulness, defined, 927
Waldenström's macroglobulinemia, hypokalemia test result and, 277–278
Warfarin sodium (Coumadin), 1403
  emergency reversal of, 121
  pharmacokinetics and, 484
Wasp stings, 643–644
  anaphylaxis risk and, 75
Water deprivation test, 269
Water retention, hyponatremia with, 270
Waterhouse-Friderichsen syndrome, 256
  meningococcemia and, 430
WBC. *See* White blood count
Weakness
  in food poisoning, 391
  in hypercalcemia, 283, 311, 312
  in hyperkalemia, 299
  hypokalemia and, 295
  in shellfish poisoning, 391
  in shock
    cardiogenic, 75
    hypovolemic, 68
  in systemic lupus erythematosus, 344
Weaver v Ward, 40
Web space abscess, in hand, 210–211
Wedge fracture, of cervical spine, 905, 908
Wedworth-Townsend Paramedic Act (California, 1974), 4
Weevers, spine or puncture wounds by, 726–727

Wegener's granulomatosis, 337
  pulmonary involvement in, 340
Weight loss
  in adrenal insufficiency, 259
  amphetamine abuse for, 790
Weil-Felix test, for Rocky Mountain spotted fever, 438
Weil-Marchesani syndrome, 364
Welding, ozone exposure in, 771
Wermer's syndrome, hypercalcemia and, 282
Wernicke-Korsakoff syndrome
  acute confusion with, 954–955
  alcohol withdrawal vs., 819
Wernicke's syndrome, alcohol-induced hypoglycemia and, 825
Western equine encephalitis, 400
Wet bulb globe temperature (WBGT), 653–654
Whales, killer, 713–714
Wheezing
  in anaphylaxis, 75
  in obstructive airway disease, 1129
White blood cell abnormalities
  chemotherapy and, 509
  in renal failure, 1226
White blood count (WBC)
  in acute epiglottitis, 1122
  in appendicitis, 556
  in hypothermia, 666
  occult bacteremia and, 531
  in respiratory disorder evaluation, pediatric, 576
  vertebral osteomyelitis diagnosis, 193
White cell transfusions, anaphylaxis risk with, 75
Wiggers preparation, 125–126
Wilson's disease, 366
Wisforreger blade, for endotracheal intubation, 96
Wiskott-Aldrich syndrome, 366, 368
Withdrawal syndrome (abstinence syndrome)
  as acute confusional state cause, 954
  alcohol vs. drug withdrawal, 819–820. *See also* Alcohol withdrawal
  amphetamine, 790
  cocaine, 789
  defined, 782
  opioids, 798–799
  sedative-hypnotics, 804–805
  seizures in, 949
Wolff-Parkinson-White syndrome, 974, 977, 1037, 1040–1042
  PSVT treatment and, 1028, 1037, 1042
Women. *See* Females
Wood alcohol intoxication, 324, 325
Work-related disorders. *See* Occupational disorders
World Association for Emergency and Disaster Medicine, on PASG, 5
Wound management, 137–158. *See also* Lacerations; *specific types of wounds*
  anesthesia in, 139–140, 885–886
  antibiotics, 138, 157–158
  bite wounds, 155–156
  causative agent and, 138–139
  closure, assessing for, 137, 138, 139
  debridement, 140–141
    with open fractures, 172
  dislocations, 173–174
  dressings, 156–157
    with open fractures, 172
  evaluation, 137–139
    age of wound, 137–138
    causative agents, 138–139
    contamination and infection, 138
    for foreign bodies, 139

excision, 140, 151
fracture wounds, 166–168, 172
hemostasis, 141
immobilization, 157
inflammation interventions, 158
irrigation, 140–141
  with open fractures, 172
marine organism injuries, 715–716, 721, 731. *See also* Marine organisms; *specific kinds*
pressure (paint and grease) gun injuries, 155
staple closure, 149
suturing, 141–148
  removal guide, 144
  techniques, 142–148
  types of sutures, 141–142, 143
tape closure, 148–149
Wren, Christopher, 115
Wrist
  arthrocentesis of, 354
  aspiration or injection of joint, 1374, 1375
  in carpal tunnel syndrome, 347
  erythema multiforme on, 434
Wrist injuries, 205–207
  carpal, 206–207
  carpal tunnel syndrome, 347
  Colles' fracture, 206
  dislocations, 205–206
    isolated, of distal radial ulnar joint, 207
  fractures, 205–206
  radial head fracture and, 203
  "sprains," 207
Wytensin. *See* Guanabenz

X

Xanax. *See* Alprazolam
Xeroderma pigmentosa, 364
Xeroradiography, in wound evaluation, 139
  puncture wounds, 154
Xerox, quality improvement role, 61, 62
Xiphoidalgia, 348
Xylocaine. *See* Lidocaine

Y

Yellowjacket stings, 643–644
  anaphylaxis risk and, 75
Yellowtail (amberjack) poisoning, 712
Yersinia enterocolitica, in gastroenteritis, 387, 388, 390
Yersinia pestis
  in acute sepsis, 406
  in pneumonia, 383

Z

Zantac. *See* Ranitidine
Zebrafish, spine or puncture wounds by, 727–728
Zidovudine (AZT), 1424
Zimelidine, 487
  overdose of, 487
Zinacef. *See* Cefuroxime
Zofran. *See* Ondansetron
Zomepirac (Zomax), for pain relief, 881
Zovirax. *See* Acyclovir
Zygoma fractures, assessing for, 110
Zygomatic fractures, 1329
Zyloprim. *See* Allopurinol